Eczema, 909
Emerging Infections, 76
Emphysema, 348
End of Life, 26
Epidermal Nevus, 1051
Epidermolysis Bullosa, 1237
Episcleritis, 149
Erythema Ab Igne, 1331
Erythema Annulare Centrifugum, 1371
Erythema Multiforme, 1161
Erythema Nodosum, 1169
Erythema Toxicum Neonatorum, 694
Erythrasma, 759
Erythroderma, 1004
Excoriation Disorder, 941
Eye Trauma, 176

F
Family Planning, 10
Fifth Disease, 802
First Trimester Obstetrical Ultrasound, 484
Flat Warts, 832
Folliculitis, 750
Foreign Body, Ear, 202
Fungal Infections, 850

G
Gallstones, 395
Gangrene, Dry, 1400
Gastric Cancer, 381
Gender-Nonconforming Patients, 119
Genital Warts, 837
Genodermatoses, 1364
Geographic tongue, 246
Gingival Overgrowth, 254
Gingivitis, 250
Glaucoma, 157
Global Health, 51
Goitrous Hypothyroidism, 1479
Gonococcal Urethritis, 1409
Gout, 604
Granuloma Annulare, 1141
Graves Disease and Goiter, 1486

H
Hammer Toe, 1386
Hand, Foot, and Mouth Disease, 806
Hand Eczema, 928
Headache, 1513
Heart Failure, 288
Hemangiomas, Childhood, 700
Hemorrhoids, 424
Hereditary and Congenital Vascular Lesions, 1341
Herpes Simplex, 812
Herpes Zoster, 786
Hidradenitis Suppurativa, 738
Hip Fracture, 624
HIV, 1419
Hoarseness, 234
Hordeolum, 132
Hydronephrosis, 440
Hyperlipidemia, 1455
Hypersensitivity Syndromes, 1161
Hypertension, 284, 295
Hypertensive Retinopathy, 165
Hyphema, 176
Hypopigmentation, 1308

I
Impetigo, 745
Inflammatory Bowel Disease, 415
Ingrown Toenail, 1276
Injection-Drug Use, 1595
Intestinal Worms and Parasites, 56, 1404
Intimate Partner Violence, 102
Iodine Deficiency, 60
Iritis, 153
Iron Deficiency, 60
Ischemic Ulcer, 1390

K
Kaposi Sarcoma, 1419
Keloids, 1359
Keratoacanthoma, 1079
Kidney Stones, 435
Knee Injury, 628
Kwashiorkor, 57

L
Larynx (Hoarseness), 234
Leishmaniasis, 64
Lentigo Maligna, 1084
Leprosy, 69
Lesbian Gay Bisexual Transgender Health Issues, 115
Leukoplakia, 263
Lice, 892
Lichen Planus, 991
Lichen Simplex Chronicus, 941
Liver Disease, 386
Lung Cancer, 366
Lupus: Systemic and Cutaneous, 1183
Lyme Disease, 1425

M
Major Depressive Disorders, 1500
Malaria, 61
Malnutrition, 57
Marasmus, 57
Mastitis, 562
Measles, 797
Melanoma, 1112
  Conjunctival, 135
Melasma, 1303
Mental Health, 1500
Metatarsal Fracture, 621
Methamphetamine, 1580
Micronutrient Deficiencies, 59
Middle East Respiratory Syndrome (MERS), 85
Milia, Newborn, 694
Molluscum Contagiosum, 820
Mongolian Spots, 694
Morphea, 1204
Mycobacterium, 69
Mycosis fungoides, 1124

N
Nail Variants, Normal, 1263
Nasal Polyps, 209
Necrobiosis Lipoidica, 1450
Necrotizing Fasciitis, 776
Neurofibromatosis, 1539
Neuropathic Ulcer, 1393
Nevus Sebaceous, 1051
Nummular Eczema, 936

O
Obesity, 1463
Obstetrical Ultrasound
  First Trimester, 484
  Second Trimester, 488
  Third Trimester, 493
Olecranon Bursitis, 609
Onychomycosis, 1280
Opioid Crisis, 1552
Oropharyngeal Cancer, 267
Osteoarthritis, 585
Osteopenia, 1471
Osteoporosis, 1471
Otitis Externa, 197
Otitis Media, Acute, 188
Otitis Media with Effusion, 188

(*continued on next page*)

TOPIC INDEX

P
Paget Disease of the Breast, 573
Paget Disease of the External Genitalia, 530
Pain, Chronic, 1607
Papilledema, 168
Parasites, Intestinal, 56, 1404
Paronychia, 1287
Pemphigoid Gestationis, 480
Pemphigus, 1226
Peptic Ulcer Disease, 376
Perianal Dermatitis, 712
Pericardial Effusion, 292
Periodontal Disease (Periodontitis), 250
Pharyngitis, 227
Photosensitivity, 1324
Pigmented Nail Disorders, 1269
Pitted Keratolysis, 756
Pityriasis Lichenoides et Varioliformis Acuta, 1239
Pityriasis Rosea, 984
Plantar Warts, 844
Pneumonia, 316
Polycystic Kidneys, 445
Porphyria Cutanea Tarda, 1235
Postinflammatory Hyperpigmentation, 1316
Preauricular Tags, 205
Pregnancy and Birth, 18
Prostate Cancer, 462
Prurigo Nodularis, 941
Pruritic Urticarial Papules and Plaques of Pregnancy, 477
Pseudofolliculitis, 733
Psoriasis, 964
Psoriatic Nails, 1292
Psychocutaneous Disorders, 941
Pterygium, 128
Pulmonary Embolus, 358
Pustular Diseases of Childhood, 708
Pyoderma Gangrenosum, 1147
Pyogenic Granuloma, 1032

R
Radius Fracture, Distal, 616
Reactive Arthritis, 999
Red Eye, 180
Renal Cell Carcinoma, 450
Retinopathy
  Diabetic, 161
  Hypertensive, 165
Rheumatoid Arthritis, 590
Rosacea, 725

S
Sarcoidosis, 1153
Scabies, 898
Scarlet Fever, 223
Scarring Alopecia, 1256
Schizophrenia, 1500
Scleral Pigmentation, 135
Scleritis, 149
Scleroderma, 1204
Sebaceous Hyperplasia, 1021
Seborrheic Dermatitis, 957
Seborrheic Keratosis, 1014
Second Trimester Obstetrical Ultrasound, 488
Self-Inflicted Dermatoses, 941
Severe Acute Respiratory Syndrome (SARS), 85
Sexual Abuse, Child, 96
Sexual Assault, Adult, 108
Shingles, 786
Sinusitis, 212
Skin Cancer, 1064
  Dermoscopy, 1132
Skin Changes
  Normal Childhood, 694
  Pregnancy, 472
Skin Infectious Diseases, 67
Skin Tag, 1010
  Preauricular, 205
Social Justice, 40
Spitz Nevus, 1057
Sports-Related Head Injury, 1517
Squamous Cell Carcinoma, 1103
Steroids, Topical and Intralesional, 681
Stevens-Johnson Syndrome, 1161
Strawberry Tongue, 223
Subdural Hematoma, 1526
Substance Abuse Disorder, 1546
Subungual Hematoma, 1298
Sun Damage, 1064
Syphilis, 1412

T
Terminology, Skin Disorders, 640
Third Trimester Obstetrical Ultrasound, 493
Tinea Capitis, 861
Tinea Corporis, 868
Tinea Cruris, 875
Tinea Pedis, 880
Tinea Versicolor, 887
Tobacco Addiction, 1558
Torus Palatinus, 221
Toxic Epidermal Necrolysis, 1161
Trachoma, 66
Traction Alopecia, 1252
Transgender Patients, 119
Trichomonas Vaginitis, 519
Trichotillomania, 1252
Tuberculosis, 325
Tuberculosis-HIV Coinfection, 71
Typhoid Fever, 54

U
Ultrasound, Obstetrical
  First Trimester, 484
  Second Trimester, 488
  Third Trimester, 493
Urethritis in Men, Gonococcal, 1409
Urinary Sediment, 430
Urticaria, 949
Uveitis, 153

V
Vaginitis, 497
  Atrophic, 501
  Trichomonas, 519
Vascular Lesions, Hereditary and Congenital, 1341
Vascular Malformations, Childhood, 700
Vascular Skin Lesions, Acquired, 1336
Vasculitis, 1174
Vector-Borne Diseases, 61
Venous Insufficiency, 310
Vitamin A Deficiency, 59
Vitiligo, 1308
Vulvar Intraepithelial Neoplasia, 534

W
Warts
  Common, 826
  Flat, 832
  Genital, 837
  Plantar, 844
West Nile Virus, 79
Worms, Intestinal, 1404

X
Xanthomas, 1455
X-Linked Ichthyosis, 1364

Z
Zika, 76
Zoster, 786
Zoster Ophthalmicus, 792

THE COLOR ATLAS AND SYNOPSIS OF FAMILY MEDICINE

NOTICE

THE COLOR ATLAS AND SYNOPSIS OF FAMILY MEDICINE

Third Edition

EDITORS

Richard P. Usatine, MD

Professor of Family and Community Medicine
Professor of Dermatology and Cutaneous Surgery
Program Director, Underserved Family Medicine Dermatology Fellowship
Assistant Director, Medical Humanities Education
University of Texas Health, San Antonio
Founding Director, Skin Clinic, University Health System
San Antonio, Texas

Mindy A. Smith, MD, MS

Clinical Professor, Department of Family Medicine
Michigan State University
East Lansing, Michigan
Honorary Associate, Department of Family Medicine
and Community Health
University of Wisconsin School of Medicine and Public Health
Deputy Editor, *Essential Evidence Plus*
Associate Medical Editor, *FP Essentials*

E.J. Mayeaux, Jr., MD

Professor and Chairman, Department of Family
and Preventive Medicine
Professor of Obstetrics and Gynecology
University of South Carolina School of Medicine
Chairman, Palmetto Health—USC Medical Group
Department of Family Medicine
Columbia, South Carolina

Heidi S. Chumley, MD, MBA

Professor, Behavioral and Clinical Medicine
Executive Dean
American University of the Caribbean School of Medicine
St. Maarten

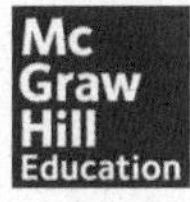

New York Chicago San Francisco Lisbon London Madrid Mexico City
Milan New Delhi San Juan Seoul Singapore Sydney Toronto

The Color Atlas and Synopsis of Family Medicine, Third Edition

2 3 4 5 6 7 8 9 LWI 26 25 24 23

ISBN 978-1-259-86204-5
MHID 1-259-86204-6

This book was set in Minion Pro by Aptara, Inc.
The editors were Amanda Fielding and Harriet Lebowitz.
The production supervisor was Richard Ruzycka.
Project management was provided by Dinesh Pokhriyal, Aptara, Inc.
The cover designers were Thorsten Trotzenberg and W2 Design.
The designer was Alan Barnett.

Library of Congress Cataloging-in-Publication Data

Names: Usatine, Richard, editor. | Smith, Mindy A., editor. | Mayeaux, E.J., Jr., editor. | Chumley, Heidi S., editor.
Title: The color atlas and synopsis of family medicine / editors, Richard P. Usatine, Mindy A. Smith, E.J. Mayeaux, Jr., Heidi S. Chumley.
Other titles: Color atlas of family medicine
Description: Third edition. | New York : McGraw-Hill Education, [2019] | Preceded by The color atlas of family medicine / editors, Richard P. Usatine… et al. 2nd ed. 2013. | Includes bibliographical references and index.
Identifiers: LCCN 2018030686 | ISBN 9781259862045 (adhesive - hard) | ISBN 9781259862052 (E-ISBN)
Subjects: | MESH: Family Practice | Atlases
Classification: LCC R729.5.G4 | NLM WB 17 | DDC 610–dc23 LC record available at https://na01.safelinks.protection.outlook.com/?url=https%3A%2F%2Flccn.loc.gov%2F2018030686&data=01%7C01%7Cleah.carton%40mheducation.com%7Cc929d109621c4f5e88fb08d5dd341422%7Cf919b1efc0c347358fca0928ec39d8d5%7C0&sdata=wklYVzvHWQhQpvXHekc%2FjueJ0ZVaL6awYkv37nLXZ6E%3D&reserved=0

DEDICATION

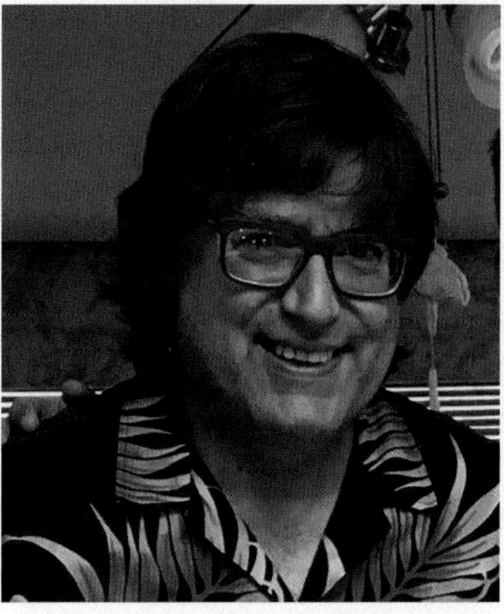

Jeff Meffert, MD

Dr. Meffert started his career as a family physician and then went on to become an exceptional board-certified dermatologist. Jeff and his wife, Paula Lyons, graduated from the University of Texas Health Sciences Center (UTHSCSA) Family Medicine Residency Program more than 30 years ago. He and his wife (still a practicing family physician) volunteered in our student-run free clinics. Jeff has contributed a number of photographs to all of our color atlases and was always helpful when we asked him for an image.

Jeff recently passed away from pancreatic cancer at the age of 60. He was known for his great sense of humor and excellent teaching. He had been happily teaching family physicians dermatology for decades. When he was the program director for the UTHSCSA Dermatology Residency Program he had welcomed our Underserved Family Medicine Dermatology Fellows as learners alongside his dermatology residents. His family has had to deal with too many tragedies, including the death of his oldest son just a few months before his diagnosis of pancreatic cancer. Jeff was a fine photographer and one of the smartest dermatologists. He was also an active editor and writer with an interest in medical ethics. His family, friends, residents, students, patients, and colleagues miss him greatly. We dedicate this book to Jeff as he touched so many lives in a positive way as a great man, a great doctor, and a great teacher.

COVER IMAGES

FRONT COVER

Top left: Dermoscopy of a pigmented basal cell carcinoma that shows leaf-like structures (Figure 177-20B, page 1099; *Richard P. Usatine, MD*).

Top right: Sclerodactyly in a woman with scleroderma showing tight skin over the fingers and some flexion deformities (Figure 190-2, page 1204; *Richard P. Usatine, MD*).

Middle: Distal clavicular fracture (Figure 104-4, page 614; *E.J. Mayeaux, Jr., MD*).

Bottom left: Keratoacanthoma on the nose of a 29-year-old HIV positive man with a central keratin core (Figure 174-5, page 1080; *Richard P. Usatine, MD*).

Bottom middle: Episcleritis showing inflammation of only the conjunctival and episcleral tissue (Figure 19-5, page 151; *Richard P. Usatine, MD*).

Bottom right: Psoriatic plaque (Figure 110-4, page 641; *Richard P. Usatine, MD*).

BACK COVER

Left to right:

Cryotherapy of a pyogenic granuloma using a Cryo Tweezer. The young girl tolerated the cryotherapy well (Figure 167-11, page 1036; *Richard P. Usatine, MD*).

A labial melanotic macule. This is benign (Figure 110-1, page 641; *Richard P. Usatine, MD*).

A weight-bearing dorsoplantar plain radiograph showing a laterally deviated hallux resulting in a bunion (Figure 217-2, page 1382; *Naohiro Shibuya, DPM*).

Bullous fixed drug eruption with a dusky color and an annular pink border on the ankle (Figure 212-21, page 1354; *Richard P. Usatine, MD*).

CONTENTS

Contributors xi
Preface xix
Acknowledgments xxi

PART I
LEARNING WITH IMAGES AND DIGITAL PHOTOGRAPHY

1 An Atlas to Enhance Patient Care, Learning, and Teaching....2

PART II
THE ESSENCE OF FAMILY MEDICINE

2 Doctor–Patient Relationship....6
3 Family Planning 10
4 Pregnancy and Birth.... 18
5 End of Life 26
6 Social Justice 40
7 Global Health 51
8 Zika, Ebola, and Other Emerging Infections 76

PART III
PHYSICAL AND SEXUAL ABUSE AND LGBT HEALTH ISSUES

9 Child Physical Abuse 90
10 Child Sexual Abuse 96
11 Intimate Partner Violence 102
12 Adult Sexual Assault.... 108
13 Lesbian Gay Bisexual Transgender Health Issues 115

PART IV
OPHTHALMOLOGY

14 Pterygium 128
15 Hordeolum and Chalazion 132
16 Scleral and Conjunctival Pigmentation.... 135
17 Corneal Foreign Body and Corneal Abrasion 139
18 Conjunctivitis 144
19 Scleritis and Episcleritis.... 149
20 Uveitis and Iritis 153
21 Glaucoma.... 157
22 Diabetic Retinopathy 161
23 Hypertensive Retinopathy.... 165
24 Papilledema 168
25 Age-Related Macular Degeneration.... 172
26 Eye Trauma—Hyphema.... 176
27 Differential Diagnosis of the Red Eye 180

PART V
EAR, NOSE, AND THROAT

Section A: Ear

28 Otitis Media: Acute Otitis and Otitis Media with Effusion . 188
29 Acute Otitis Externa.... 197
30 Ear: Foreign Body.... 202
31 Chondrodermatitis Nodularis Helicis and Preauricular Tags....205

Section B: Nose and Sinus

32 Nasal Polyps 209
33 Sinusitis 212

Section C: Mouth and Throat

34 Angular Cheilitis.... 218
35 Torus Palatinus 221
36 Scarlet Fever and Strawberry Tongue 223
37 Pharyngitis.... 227
38 The Larynx (Hoarseness).... 234

PART VI
ORAL HEALTH

39 Black Hairy Tongue 242
40 Geographic Tongue 246
41 Gingivitis and Periodontal Disease 250
42 Gingival Overgrowth 254
43 Aphthous Ulcer.... 258
44 Leukoplakia.... 263
45 Oropharyngeal Cancer.... 267
46 Early Childhood Caries.... 271
47 Adult Dental Caries 275

PART VII
THE HEART AND CIRCULATION

Section A: Central

48 Coronary Artery Disease.... 280
49 Hypertension.... 284
50 Heart Failure 288
51 Pericardial Effusion 292
52 Bacterial Endocarditis 297

Section B: Peripheral

53 Clubbing.... 307
54 Venous Insufficiency 310

PART VIII
THE LUNGS

55 Pneumonia.... 316
56 Tuberculosis.... 325

CONTENTS

57 Asthma ... 336
58 Chronic Obstructive Pulmonary Disease ... 348
59 Pulmonary Embolism ... 358
60 Lung Cancer ... 366

PART IX
GASTROINTESTINAL

61 Peptic Ulcer Disease ... 376
62 Gastric Cancer ... 381
63 Liver Disease ... 386
64 Gallstones ... 395
65 Colon Polyps ... 401
66 Colon Cancer ... 407
67 Inflammatory Bowel Disease ... 415
68 Hemorrhoids ... 424

PART X
GENITOURINARY

69 Urinary Sediment ... 430
70 Kidney Stones ... 435
71 Hydronephrosis ... 440
72 Polycystic Kidneys ... 445
73 Renal Cell Carcinoma ... 450
74 Bladder Cancer ... 456
75 Prostate Cancer ... 462

PART XI
WOMEN'S HEALTH

Section A: Pregnancy

76 Skin Findings in Pregnancy ... 472
77 Pruritic Urticarial Papules and Plaques of Pregnancy ... 477
78 Pemphigoid Gestationis ... 480
79 First Trimester Obstetrical Ultrasound ... 484
80 Second Trimester Obstetrical Ultrasound ... 488
81 Third Trimester Obstetrical Ultrasound ... 493

Section B: Vaginitis and Cervicitis

82 Overview of Vaginitis ... 497
83 Atrophic Vaginitis ... 501
84 Bacterial Vaginosis ... 508
85 *Candida* Vulvovaginitis ... 513
86 *Trichomonas* Vaginitis ... 519
87 *Chlamydia* Cervicitis ... 524

Section C: Vulva

88 Paget Disease of the External Genitalia ... 530
89 Vulvar Intraepithelial Neoplasia ... 534

Section D: Colposcopy

90 Colposcopy: Normal and Noncancerous Findings ... 540
91 Colposcopy of Low-Grade Lesions ... 545
92 Colposcopy of High-Grade Lesions ... 550
93 Colposcopy of Cervical Cancer ... 556

Section E: Breast

94 Breast Abscess and Mastitis ... 562
95 Breast Cancer ... 566
96 Paget Disease of the Breast ... 573

PART XII
MUSCULOSKELETAL PROBLEMS

97 Arthritis Overview ... 578
98 Osteoarthritis ... 585
99 Rheumatoid Arthritis ... 590
100 Ankylosing Spondylitis ... 595
101 Back Pain ... 599
102 Gout ... 604
103 Olecranon Bursitis ... 609
104 Clavicular Fracture ... 613
105 Distal Radius Fracture ... 616
106 Metatarsal Fracture ... 621
107 Hip Fracture ... 624
108 Knee Injury ... 628
109 Dupuytren Disease ... 635

PART XIII
DERMATOLOGY

Section A: Foundations of Dermatology

110 Terminology of Skin Disorders ... 640
111 Dermoscopy ... 649
112 Topical and Intralesional Steroids ... 681
113 Biopsy Principles and Techniques ... 688

Section B: Childhood Dermatology

114 Normal Skin Changes ... 694
115 Childhood Hemangiomas ... 700
116 Pustular Diseases of Childhood ... 708
117 Diaper Rash and Perianal Dermatitis ... 712

Section C: Acneiform and Follicular Disorders

118 Acne Vulgaris ... 717
119 Rosacea ... 725
120 Pseudofolliculitis and Acne Keloidalis Nuchae ... 733
121 Hidradenitis Suppurativa ... 738

Section D: Bacterial

122 Impetigo ... 745
123 Folliculitis ... 750
124 Pitted Keratolysis ... 756

125 Erythrasma 759
126 Cellulitis 765
127 Abscess 771
128 Necrotizing Fasciitis 776
Section E: Viral
129 Chickenpox 780
130 Zoster 786
131 Zoster Ophthalmicus 792
132 Measles 797
133 Fifth Disease 802
134 Hand Foot Mouth Syndrome 806
135 Herpes Simplex 812
136 Molluscum Contagiosum 820
137 Common Warts 826
138 Flat Warts 832
139 Genital Warts 837
140 Plantar Warts 844
Section F: Fungal
141 Fungal Overview 850
142 Candidiasis 856
143 Tinea Capitis 861
144 Tinea Corporis 868
145 Tinea Cruris 875
146 Tinea Pedis 880
147 Tinea Versicolor 887
Section G: Infestations
148 Lice 892
149 Scabies 898
150 Cutaneous Larva Migrans 906
Section H: Dermatitis/Allergic
151 Atopic Dermatitis 909
152 Contact Dermatitis 919
153 Hand Eczema 928
154 Nummular Eczema 936
155 Psychocutaneous Disorders 941
156 Urticaria and Angioedema 949
Section I: Papulosquamous Conditions
157 Seborrheic Dermatitis 957
158 Psoriasis 964
159 Pityriasis Rosea 984
160 Lichen Planus 991
161 Reactive Arthritis 999
162 Erythroderma 1004
Section J: Benign Neoplasms
163 Skin Tag 1010
164 Seborrheic Keratosis 1014
165 Sebaceous Hyperplasia 1021
166 Dermatofibroma 1026
167 Pyogenic Granuloma 1032
Section K: Nevi
168 Benign Nevi 1038
169 Congenital Melanocytic Nevi 1046
170 Epidermal Nevus and Nevus Sebaceus 1051
171 Dysplastic Nevus and Spitz Nevus 1057
Section L: Sun Damage and Early Skin Cancer
172 Sun Damage and Skin Cancer Prevention 1064
173 Actinic Keratosis and Bowen Disease 1072
174 Keratoacanthoma 1079
175 Lentigo Maligna 1084
176 Cutaneous Horn 1089
Section M: Skin Cancer
177 Basal Cell Carcinoma 1093
178 Squamous Cell Carcinoma 1103
179 Melanoma 1112
180 Cutaneous T-Cell Lymphoma 1124
181 Advanced Dermoscopy of Skin Cancer 1132
Section N: Infiltrative Immunologic
182 Granuloma Annulare 1141
183 Pyoderma Gangrenosum 1147
184 Sarcoidosis 1153
Section O: Hypersensitivity Syndromes
185 Erythema Multiforme, Stevens-Johnson Syndrome, and Toxic Epidermal Necrolysis 1161
186 Erythema Nodosum 1169
187 Vasculitis 1174
Section P: Connective Tissue Disease
188 Lupus: Systemic and Cutaneous 1183
189 Dermatomyositis 1194
190 Scleroderma and Morphea 1204
Section Q: Bullous Disease
191 Overview of Bullous Diseases 1213
192 Bullous Pemphigoid 1220
193 Pemphigus 1226
194 Other Bullous Diseases 1235
Section R: Hair and Nail Conditions
195 Alopecia Areata 1245
196 Traction Alopecia and Trichotillomania 1252
197 Scarring Alopecia 1256
198 Normal Nail Variants 1263
199 Pigmented Nail Disorders 1269
200 Ingrown Toenail 1276
201 Onychomycosis 1280
202 Paronychia 1287
203 Psoriatic Nails 1292
204 Subungual Hematoma 1298
Section S: Pigmentary and Light-Related Conditions
205 Melasma 1303
206 Vitiligo and Hypopigmentation 1308

CONTENTS

207 Postinflammatory Hyperpigmentation 1316
208 Photosensitivity.................................... 1324
209 Erythema Ab Igne.................................. 1331

Section T: Vascular

210 Acquired Vascular Skin Lesions 1336
211 Hereditary and Congenital Vascular Lesions................ 1341

Section U: Other Skin Disorders

212 Cutaneous Drug Reactions 1346
213 Keloids 1359
214 Genodermatoses.................................... 1364
215 Erythema Annulare Centrifugum 1371

PART XIV

PODIATRY

216 Corn and Callus 1376
217 Bunion Deformity 1381
218 Hammer Toe 1386
219 Ischemic Ulcer 1390
220 Neuropathic Ulcer 1393
221 Charcot Arthropathy 1396
222 Dry Gangrene 1400

PART XV

INFECTIOUS DISEASES

223 Intestinal Worms and Parasites........................ 1404
224 Gonococcal and Chlamydia Urethritis 1409
225 Syphilis.. 1412
226 AIDS and Kaposi Sarcoma 1419
227 Lyme Disease...................................... 1425

PART XVI

ENDOCRINE

228 Diabetes Overview 1432
229 Acanthosis Nigricans 1442
230 Diabetic Dermopathy................................ 1447
231 Necrobiosis Lipoidica................................ 1450
232 Hyperlipidemia and Xanthomas....................... 1455
233 Obesity 1463
234 Osteoporosis and Osteopenia 1471
235 Goitrous Hypothyroidism............................ 1479
236 Graves Disease and Goiter 1486
237 Acromegaly 1493

PART XVII

THE BRAIN AND NERVOUS SYSTEM

238 Mental Health 1500
239 Headache 1513
240 Sports-Related Head Injury........................... 1517
241 Cerebral Vascular Accident........................... 1521
242 Subdural Hematoma 1526
243 Dementia 1531
244 Bell Palsy 1535
245 Neurofibromatosis 1539

PART XVIII

SUBSTANCE ABUSE

246 Substance Abuse Disorder............................ 1546
247 The Opioid Crisis and the War on Drugs 1552
248 Smoking and Tobacco Addiction...................... 1558
249 Alcohol Use Disorder 1571
250 Methamphetamine................................. 1580
251 Cocaine 1587
252 Injection-Drug Use................................. 1595

APPENDIX

A Interpreting Evidence-Based Medicine.................. 1604
B Chronic Pain 1607

Subject Index... 1619

Cathy Abbott, MD
Assistant Professor
Michigan State University
East Lansing, Michigan

Frank Aguirre, MD
Assistant Clinical Professor, Department of Obstetrics and Gynecology
University of South Carolina School of Medicine—Palmetto Health USC Medical Group
Columbia, South Carolina

Kari-Claudia M. Allen, MD, MPH
Assistant Professor
Department of Family and Preventive Medicine
University of South Carolina School of Medicine—Palmetto Health USC Medical Group
Columbia, South Carolina

Anna Allred, MD
Critical Care Anesthesiologist
Greater Houston Anesthesiology
Houston, Texas

Jim Anderst, MD, MSCI
Division of Child Abuse and Neglect
Professor of Pediatrics
Children's Mercy Hospital
UMKC School of Medicine
Kansas City, Missouri

Athena Andreadis, MD
Assistant Professor
Behavioral and Clinical Medicine
American University of the Caribbean School of Medicine
St. Maarten

Nehman Moses Andry, MD
Associate Professor/Clinical
Clerkship Director
University of Texas Health, San Antonio—Joe R. & Teresa Lozano Long School of Medicine
Department of Family & Community Medicine
Sacramento, California

Khaled Z. Aqeel, MD, MBA
Assistant Professor of Family Medicine
Louisiana State University Health Science Center
Shreveport, Louisiana
Medical Director of BAART Norwood
BayMark Health Services
Sacramento, California

Michael J. Babcock, MD
Colorado Springs Dermatology Clinic
Colorado Springs, Colorado

Edward Bae, MD
Resident
Department of Internal Medicine, North Shore Medical Center
Salem, Massachusetts
Department of Dermatology, Roger Williams Medical Center
Providence, Rhode Island

Yoon-Soo Cindy Bae, MD
Clinical Assistant Professor of Dermatology
New York University Medical Center
Associate, Laser & Skin Surgery Center New York
New York, New York

Jeffrey H. Baker, MD
Assistant Professor
Department of Family and Community Medicine
Penn State College of Medicine
Hershey, Pennsylvania

Pavela G. Bambekova, BS
Medical Student
Long School of Medicine
University of Texas Health, San Antonio
San Antonio, Texas

Jonathan C. Banta, MD
Dermatologist
Captain, United States Air Force

Austin Baraki, MD
Internal Medicine
University of Texas Health, San Antonio
San Antonio, Texas

Luke M. Baudoin, MD
Associate Professor of Family Medicine
Louisiana State University Health Center
Shreveport, Louisiana

Elbert M. Belk, MD
Adjunct Assistant Professor
Department of Family and Community Medicine
University of Texas Health, San Antonio
San Antonio, Texas

Ruth E. Berggren, MD
Professor of Medicine, Infectious Diseases
Director
The Center for Medical Humanities & Ethics
University of Texas Health, San Antonio
San Antonio, Texas

Steven N. Bienvenu, MD
Pediatric Medicine
University Health Shreveport
Shreveport, Louisiana

J. Michael Blair, MD
Internal Medicine Resident
Houston, Texas

CONTRIBUTORS

Jacqueline Bucher, MD
Dermatology Resident
University of Texas Health, San Antonio
San Antonio, Texas

Jordan E. Buckley, MD
Dermatology Resident
University of Texas Health Science Center
Houston, Texas

Margaret L. Burks, MD
Clinical Fellow, Diabetes, Endocrinology, & Metabolism
Vanderbilt Eskind Diabetes Clinic
Nashville, Tennessee

Tanya Burrell, MD
Assistant Professor of Pediatrics
Children's Mercy Hospital
UMKC School of Medicine
Kansas City, Missouri

Lina M. Cardona, MD
Family Physician
Graduate, Underserved Family Medicine Dermatology Fellowship
Orlando, Florida

Charles Carter, MD
Associate Professor of Family Medicine
University of South Carolina School of Medicine
Columbia, South Carolina

Gina Chacon, MD
Senior Associate Consultant
Internal Medicine
Mayo Clinic Health System
La Crosse, Wisconsin

Naira Chobanyan, MD, PhD
Doctor of Medical Sciences, Professor
Behavioral and Clinical Medicine
American University of the Caribbean School of Medicine
St. Maarten

Beth Choby, MD
Associate Professor
Department of Medical Education
University of Tennessee College of Medicine
University of Texas Health Sciences Center
Associate Professor
Baptist Family Medicine Residency Program
Memphis, Tennessee

Sigrid M. Collier, MD, MPH
Dermatology Resident
University of Minnesota
Minneapolis, Minnesota

Alissa M. Collins, MD
Laryngology Fellow
University of Texas Health, San Antonio
San Antonio, Texas

Harry Colt, MD
Maine—Dartmouth Family Medicine Residency
Augusta, Maine

Danielle B. Cooper, MD
Associate Professor
Resident Program Director
Department of Obstetrics and Gynecology
Louisiana State University Health
Shreveport, Louisiana

Andrea L. Darby-Stewart, MD
Associate Director, HonorHealth Family Medicine Residency
Clinical Associate Professor, Family and Community Medicine
University of Arizona College of Medicine
Phoenix, Arizona

Tammy J. Davis, MD
Professor of Clinical Family Medicine
Louisiana State University Health—Shreveport, School of Medicine
Shreveport, Louisiana

John E. Delzell, Jr, MD, MSPH
Vice President for Medical Education
Northeast Georgia Health System
Gainesville, Georgia

Francis J. DeMarco, MD
Family Medicine Chief Resident
Louisiana State University Health Science Center
Shreveport, Louisiana

David Ojeda Díaz, DDS
Clinical Assistant Professor of Oral Medicine
Department of Comprehensive Dentistry
University of Texas Health, San Antonio, School of Dentistry
San Antonio, Texas

Lucia Diaz, MD
Assistant Professor of Dermatology and Pediatrics
University of Texas Dell Medical School
Austin, Texas

Laura M. Dominguez, MD
Assistant Professor of Otolaryngology
University of Texas Health, San Antonio
San Antonio, Texas

Kaley K. El-Arab, BS
Medical Student
University of Texas Health, San Antonio
San Antonio, Texas

Bettina Suzanne Fehr, MD
Assistant Professor
Department of Psychiatry
University of Texas Southwestern Medical Center
Dallas, Texas

Cathy M. Feller, MD
Chief Resident
Department of Family Medicine
University of North Carolina School of Medicine
Chapel Hill, North Carolina

Lindsey B. Finklea, MD
Adjunct Assistant Professor
Dermatology and Cutaneous Surgery
University of Texas Health
San Antonio, Texas

Kelli H. Foulkrod, MS, LPC, LPA
Psychotherapist
Organic Mental Health Center, PLLC
Austin, Texas

Robert Christopher Gilson, MD
Medical Student
Long School of Medicine
University of Texas Health, San Antonio
San Antonio, Texas

Bridget Godwin, MD
Assistant Professor of Pediatrics, Perelman School of Medicine—University of Pennsylvania
Attending Physician, Division of Gastroenterology, Hepatology & Nutrition
Children's Hospital of Philadelphia
Philadelphia, Pennsylvania

Radha Raman Murthy Gokula, MD, CMD
Geriatrician & Palliative Medicine Consultant
University of Toledo Medical Center
Assistant Professor
Department of Family Medicine
University of Toledo
Toledo, Ohio

Wanda C. Gonsalves, MD
Professor and Vice Chair
Department of Family and Community Medicine
University of Kentucky
Lexington, Kentucky

M. Joyce Green, MD
Assistant Professor
Department of Family and Community Medicine
Penn State College of Medicine
Hershey, Pennsylvania

Mary Kelly Green, MD
Ophthalmology, Private Practice
Marble Falls, Texas
Clinical Assistant Professor
Department of Ophthalmology
University of Texas Health Science Center
San Antonio, Texas

Sujatha Gubbala, MD
Resident, Department of Family Medicine
Louisiana State University Health—Shreveport
Shreveport, Louisiana

Jeffrey Guy, MD
Professor of Orthopedic Surgery
University of South Carolina School of Medicine
Co-Director of Sports Medicine
Palmetto Health/USC Orthopedic Center
Medical Director—USC Athletic Training Program
Medical Director USC Gamecocks/Athletic Department
Columbia, South Carolina

Alfonso Guzman, Jr, MD
Family Physician
Graduate, Underserved Family Medicine Dermatology Fellowship
San Antonio, Texas

Matthew S. Haldeman, MD
Global Health Fellow, MPH Candidate
Department of Family Medicine
University of South Carolina School of Medicine
Columbia, South Carolina

Jeffrey W. W. Hall, MD
Director Palmetto Health/USC Travel Clinic
Global Health Fellowship Director
Associate Professor of Clinical Family and Preventive Medicine
Department of Family and Preventive Medicine
Columbia, South Carolina

Meredith M. Hancock, MD
Medical/Surgical Dermatologist
Marshfield Clinic Health System
Marshfield, Wisconsin

Jimmy H. Hara, MD
Associate Dean for Graduate Medical Education
Professor, Family Medicine
Charles Drew University of Medicine and Science
Los Angeles, California

J. William Hayden, Jr, MD, EdD
Professor
Behavioral and Clinical Medicine
American University of the Caribbean
St. Maarten

Ronni Hayon, MD
Assistant Professor
Department of Family Medicine and Community Health
University of Wisconsin School of Medicine and Public Health
Madison, Wisconsin

David Henderson, MD
Associate Dean, Student Affairs
Associate Dean, Multicultural and Community Affairs
Associate Professor, Family Medicine
University of Connecticut School of Medicine
Farmington, Connecticut

CONTRIBUTORS

Donald L. Hilton Jr, MD
Adjunct Associate Professor of Neurosurgery
Spine Fellowship Program Director
Department of Neurosurgery
University of Texas Medical School at San Antonio
San Antonio, Texas

Nathan Hitzeman, MD
Faculty, Sutter Health Family Medicine Residency Program
Sacramento, California

Jan Hood, MD
Professor of Clinical Family Medicine
LSU Health Sciences Center—Shreveport
Shreveport, Louisiana

Michaell A. Huber, DDS
Professor & Diplomate American Board of Oral Medicine
Department of Comprehensive Dentistry
University of Texas Health, San Antonio School of Dentistry
San Antonio, Texas

Karen A. Hughes, MD
Clinical Faculty
North Mississippi Medical Center Family Medicine Residency Program
Tupelo, Mississippi

Guy Huynh-Ba, DDS, MS
Professor
Department of Periodontics
The University of Texas Health Science Center at San Antonio (UTHSCSA)
San Antonio, Texas

Carlos Roberto Jaén, MD, PhD
Professor and Chair of Family and Community Medicine
Holly Distinguished Chair, Patient-Centered Medical Home
Long School of Medicine
University of Texas Health, San Antonio
San Antonio, Texas

Sarah J. James, DO
Assistant Professor
University of Wisconsin Department of Family Medicine and Community Health
Madison, Wisconsin

Asif Jawaid, DO
Chief Cardiology Fellow
Broward Health Medical Center
Fort Lauderdale, Florida

Adeliza S. Jimenez, MD
Department of Family Medicine
Partner Physician, Southern California Permanente Medical Group
Downey, California

Anne E. Johnson, MD
Psychiatrist, North Texas Veterans Health Administration
Dallas, Texas

Megha Madhukar Kapoor, MD
Assistant Professor
Department of Radiology
MD Anderson Cancer Center
Houston, Texas

Jonathan B. Karnes, MD
Medical Director, MDFMR Dermatology Services
Maine Dartmouth Family Medicine Residency
Clinical Assistant Professor, Geisel School of Medicine at Dartmouth
Augusta, Maine

Jennifer Tickal Keehbauch, MD
Associate Professor
Department of Family Medicine
Loma Linda School of Medicine
Loma Linda, California

Nancy D. Kellogg, MD
Professor, Pediatrics
Division Chief of Child Abuse
University of Texas Health, San Antonio
San Antonio, Texas

Amor Khachemoune, MD
Mohs Micrographic Surgeon & Dermatopathologist
The Department of Veterans Affairs New York Harbor Healthcare System
Brooklyn, New York

Barbara Kiersz-Mueller, DO
Family Physician
Austin, Texas

Robert L. Kraft, MD
Associate Director, Smoky Hill Family Medicine Residency Program
Assistant Clinical Professor
University of Kansas School of Medicine
Wichita, Kansas

Jennifer Krejci-Manwaring, MD
Adjunct Clinical Professor
University of Texas Health, San Antonio
South Texas Veterans Health Care
Limmer Hair Transplant Center, Medical Director
San Antonio, Texas

Emily Krodel, MD
Assistant Professor of Family and Preventive Medicine
Palmetto Health USC Medical Group
Columbia, South Carolina

Javier La Fontaine, DPM, MS
Professor of Podiatry
Department of Plastic Surgery
UT Southwestern Medical Center
Dallas, Texas

Maria J. LaPlante, MD
Family Physician, former Dermatology Fellow
Valley Health Warren Memorial Multispecialty Clinic
Front Royal, Virginia

Matthew J. Lenhard, MD
Assistant Professor
Department of Obstetrics and Gynecology
University of South Carolina School of Medicine
Columbia, South Carolina

Konstantinos Liopyris, MD
Research Fellow
Memorial Sloan Kettering Cancer Center and Department of Dermatology
University of Athens, A. Sygros Hospital
Athens, Greece

Leo Lopez III, MD
Postdoctoral Fellow
National Clinician Scholars Program
Yale University
New Haven, Connecticut

Juanita Lozano-Pineda, DDS, MPH
Associate Professor, Department of Comprehensive Dentistry
University of Texas Health, San Antonio School of Dentistry
San Antonio, Texas

Phyllis D. MacGilvray, MD
Associate Professor /Clinical and Vice Chair for Medical Student Education
Department of Family & Community Medicine
University of Texas Health, San Antonio
San Antonio, Texas

Ashfaq A. Marghoob, MD
Attending Physician, Dermatology Service
Memorial Sloan Kettering Skin Cancer Center
Hauppauge, New York

Nathan S. Martin, MD
Assistant Professor
Department of Family Medicine and Emergency Medicine
Louisiana State University Health Science Center
Shreveport, Louisiana

Angie Mathai, MD
Associate Clinical Professor
Department of Pediatrics
Division of Internal Medicine—Pediatrics
East Carolina University Brody School of Medicine
Greenville, North Carolina

Melissa M. Mauskar, MD
Assistant Professor
Department of Dermatology
University of Texas Southwestern Medical Center at Dallas
Dallas, Texas

Christopher G. Mazoue, MD
Associate Professor, Department of Orthopedic Surgery
University of South Carolina School of Medicine
Columbia, South Carolina

Maria D. McColgan, MD, MEd
Assistant Professor
Departments of Pediatrics and Emergency Medicine
Director, Child Protection Program
Drexel University College of Medicine
Philadelphia, Pennsylvania

Carolyn Milana, MD
Associate Professor of Clinical Pediatrics
Interim Chair, Department of Pediatrics
Medical Director for Quality, Stony Brook Children's Hospital
Stony Brook, New York

Vineet Mishra, MD
Adjunct Associate Professor of Dermatology
University of California—San Diego
Department of Vascular Surgery, Dermatology, and Mohs Surgery
Scripps Clinic, San Diego

Caitlin Morgan, MD
Resident, Department of Family Medicine
Texas A&M Health Science Center
Bryan, Texas

Tenley E. Murphy, MD
Assistant Professor, Department of Family and Preventive Medicine
University of South Carolina School of Medicine
Columbia, South Carolina

Munima Nasir, MD
Assistant Professor
Department of Family & Community Medicine
Penn State Health Hershey Medical Center
Hershey, Pennsylvania

Cristian Navarrete-Dechent, MD
Department of Dermatology
Facultad de Medicina
Pontificia Universidad Catolica de Chile
Santiago, Chile

Anjeli Nayar, MD
96 MDOS Internal Medicine
Assistant Professor of Medicine, Uniformed Services University of the Health Sciences (USUHS)

Enrique R. Perez-Rodriguez, MD
Internal Medicine
University of Texas Health, San Antonio
Medical Review Officer
Soba Recovery Center—Texas
San Antonio, Texas

Allison Pye, MD
Department of Dermatology, McGovern Medical School
University of Texas Health Science Center at Houston
Houston, Texas

CONTRIBUTORS

Anoop Patel, MD
Urgent Care Medicine
Houston, Texas

Sahand Rahnama-Moghadam, MD, MS
Assistant Professor of Dermatology
Indiana University
Indianapolis, Indiana

Brian Z. Rayala, MD
Associate Professor
Department of Family Medicine
University of North Carolina School of Medicine
Chapel Hill, North Carolina

Suraj G. Reddy, MD
Albuquerque Dermatology Associates, PA
Albuquerque, New Mexico

Alan Remde, MD
Director research and curriculum
St. Luke's University Health Network
Faculty, Family Medicine Residency—Warren
Phillipsburg, New Jersey

Catherine Reppa, MD
Assistant Professor, Department of Ophthalmology and Visual Sciences
Texas Tech Health Science Center
Lubbock, Texas

Karl T. Rew, MD
Associate Professor
Departments of Family Medicine and Urology
University of Michigan Medical School
Ann Arbor, Michigan

Ayelet Rishpon, MD
Department of Dermatology
Tel-Aviv Sourasky Medical Center
Dermatology Service
Memorial Sloan Kettering Cancer Center
New York, New York

Nina Rivera, DO
Cardiology Fellow
Broward Health Medical Center
Fort Lauderdale, Florida

Charles L. Roeth, MD
Cardiologist, Methodist Physicians
San Antonio, Texas

Mark Jason Sanders, MD
Assistant Professor
Division of Community and General Pediatrics
Department of Pediatrics
University of Texas Health Medical School at Houston
Houston, Texas

Khashayar Sarabi, MD
Internal & Integrative Medicine
Irvine, California

Shehnaz Zaman Sarmast, MD
Dermatologist, Skin Specialist
Allen/Addison, Texas

Andrew D. Schechtman, MD
Adjunct Clinical Assistant Professor
Stanford University School of Medicine
Stanford Health Care—O'Connor Hospital Family Medicine
Faculty, Residency Program
San Jose, California

Paige M. Seeker, MD
University of Texas Health, San Antonio
San Antonio, Texas

Adriana Segura, DDS, MS
Professor
Associate Dean for Academic, Faculty and Student Affairs
Department of Comprehensive Department and Department of Pediatrics
School of Dentistry
University of Texas Health, San Antonio
San Antonio, Texas

Jarrett Sell, MD
Associate Professor
Department of Family and Community Medicine
Penn State Health Hershey Medical Center
Hershey, Pennsylvania

Amit Sharma, DO
Department of Family Medicine
Adjunct Clinical Assistant Professor
Lake Erie College of Osteopathic Medicine Arnot Ogden Medical Center
Elmira, New York

Andrew Shedd, MD
Associate Residency Director
Ultrasound Director
Department of Emergency Medicine
JPS Health Network
Fort Worth, Texas

Angela D. Shedd, MD
Faculty Associate Dermatologist
UT Southwestern Monty and Tex Moncrief Medical Center
Fort Worth, Texas

Maureen K. Sheehan, MD, MHA
Associate Professor, Division of Vascular Surgery
University of Texas Health San Antonio
San Antonio, Texas

Danish Sheikh, DO
Cardiology
Broward Health Medical Center
Fort Lauderdale, Florida

Naohiro Shibuya, DPM, MS
Professor
Texas A&M University
College of Medicine
Bryan, Texas

Leslie A. Shimp, PharmD, MS
Professor, College of Pharmacy
University of Michigan
Ann Arbor, Michigan

Valerie Fisher Shiu, MD
Dermatology Resident
University of Texas Health at San Antonio
San Antonio, Texas

C. Blake Simpson, MD
Professor
Department of Otolaryngology-Head and Neck Surgery
University of Texas Health at San Antonio
San Antonio, Texas

Isac P. Simpson, DO
Family Physician
Graduate, Underserved Family Medicine Dermatology Fellowship
Simpson DermCare and Family Medicine
Idaho Falls, Idaho

Stacy L. Speedlin, PhD
Visiting Assistant Professor
University of Texas at San Antonio
San Antonio, Texas

Linda Speer, MD
Professor & Chair
Department of Family Medicine
College of Medicine and Life Sciences
University of Toledo
Toledo, Ohio

Shaun Spielman, MD
Assistant Professor of Clinical Family Medicine
Louisiana State University Health
Shreveport, Louisiana

Julie Scott Taylor, MD, MSc
Chief Academic Officer and Senior Associate Dean, Academic and Student Affairs
Professor, Behavioral and Clinical Medicine
American University of the Caribbean School of Medicine
St. Maarten
Adjunct Professor of Family Medicine
Alpert Medical School of Brown University
Providence, Rhode Island

Theresa Thuy Vo, MD
Family Physician
Graduate, Underserved Family Medicine Dermatology Fellowship
Dallas, Texas

Alexis Rae Tracy, MD
Internal Medicine Resident
University of California San Diego
San Diego, California

Ana Treviño Sauceda, MD
Adjunct Clinical Professor
University of Texas Health, San Antonio
San Antonio, Texas

Anisha R. Turner, MD
Emergency/Family Medicine Resident Physician
Louisiana State University Health
Shreveport, Louisiana

Ernest E. Valdez, DDS
The Orsatti Dental Group
San Antonio, Texas

Cynthia M. Villanueva Ramos, MD
Family Physician, former Dermatology Fellow
Department of Family and Community Medicine
University of Texas Health Science Center at San Antonio—School of Medicine
University Medical Associates
San Antonio, Texas

Holly H. Volz, MD
Assistant Professor of Dermatology and Cutaneous Surgery
University of Texas Health, San Antonio
San Antonio, Texas

Yu Wah, MD
Clinical Assistant Professor
Family and Community Medicine
Graduate, Underserved Family Medicine Dermatology Fellowship
University of Texas Health Science Center at Houston
Houston, Texas

Daniel Wallis, MD
Internal Medicine Resident
Lubbock, Texas

Candice Weiner-Johnson, MD
University Health Hospital and
Louisiana State University Health—Shreveport, School of Medicine
Department of Family Medicine and Emergency Medicine
Shreveport, Louisiana

Mark L. Willenbring, MD
Founder and CEO, ALLTYR
Saint Paul, Minnesota

Brian D. Williams, MD, MPH
Community Preceptor
St. Joseph Hospital
Bruner Family Medicine
Denver, Colorado

James O. Williams, Jr, MD
Assistant Professor, Department of Family and Preventive Medicine
University of South Carolina School of Medicine
Columbia, South Carolina

CONTRIBUTORS

Leah T. Williams, MD
Family Medicine Resident
Louisiana State University Health—Shreveport, School of Medicine
Shreveport, Louisiana

Jennifer L. Wipperman, MD, MPH
Assistant Professor
Family and Community Medicine
University of Kansas School of Medicine—Wichita
Wichita, Kansas

Matthew Witthaus, MD
Academic Family Medicine Fellow
Department of Family and Community Medicine
Saint Louis University School of Medicine
St. Louis, Missouri

Zachary J. Wolner, MD
Memorial Sloan Kettering Cancer Center
Department of Dermatology
New York, New York

Tiffanie C. Wong, DO
Family Physician
Graduate, Underserved Family Medicine Dermatology Fellowship
Tampa, Florida

Jenny Yeh, MD
Dermatology Resident, PGY-4
University of Texas Health, San Antonio
San Antonio, Texas

Oriol Yélamos, MD
Dermatology Department, Hospital Clínic de Barcelona
Universitat de Barcelona
Barcelona, Spain

Jana K. Zaudke, MD, MA
Medical Director
Caritas Clinics
Kansas City, Kansas

PREFACE

Family physicians probably see a wider variety of rashes, eye conditions, foot disorders, lumps and bumps, and undifferentiated problems than any other specialty. Over the past 10 years we have published two comprehensive atlases to aid in diagnosis using visible signs and internal imaging. In this third edition, we have decided that our book and all its electronic forms is more than an atlas—it is a comprehensive guide to all of family medicine. Therefore, the new name for our third edition is ***The Color Atlas and Synopsis of Family Medicine***.

We have assembled more than 2400 outstanding clinical images for the third edition of the most comprehensive atlas and synopsis of family medicine ever produced. Some photographs will amaze you; all will inform you about the various conditions that befall our patients.

We were gratified by the great response to the first two editions. The smartphone, tablet, and web versions were also very well received and are again available for the third edition. Readers sent in a number of suggestions for additions, and we have taken those to heart, with new coverage of fundamental conditions.

New in the third edition are:

- New chapters that expand the scope of the book, including chapters on mental health, the opioid crisis, dementia, sports-related head injury, and LGBT health issues. To expand on our Global Health chapter, we have added a chapter on Zika, Ebola, and other emerging infections.
- A strengthened dermatology area with a new Foundations of Dermatology section that includes a comprehensive dermoscopy chapter, and chapters on dermatology terminology, topical and intralesional steroids, and biopsy principles and techniques. Because dermoscopy (the use of a handheld scope with light and magnification) is revolutionizing the diagnosis or all kinds of skin, nail, and hair conditions, we have incorporated more dermoscopy throughout the dermatology chapters. In this edition, we have added a separate advanced chapter on dermoscopy devoted to the diagnosis of skin cancers. By diagnosing skin cancers early, we can save lives. For providers interested in more procedural medicine, the chapters on intralesional steroids and biopsy techniques will help provide a foundation for these procedures.
- To make the management section more valuable and user-friendly, we have divided management into first-line and second-line therapies whenever possible.

It took many people many years to create all three editions of ***The Color Atlas (and Synopsis) of Family Medicine***. For me it is a life work that started with little notebooks that I kept in my white coat pocket to take notes during my residency. It then took on color and images as I kept a film camera at work and took photographs with my patients' permission of any interesting clinical finding that I might use to teach medical students and residents the art and science of medicine. I was inspired by many great family physicians, including Dr. Jimmy Hara, who had the most amazing 35-mm slide collection of clinical images. His knowledge of medicine is encyclopedic, and I knew that his taking photographs had something to do with that. Also, I realized that these photographs would greatly enhance my teaching of others. As I began to expand my practice to see more dermatology cases, my photograph collection skyrocketed. Digital photography made it more affordable and practical to take and catalogue many new images.

The Color Atlas and Synopsis of Family Medicine is written for family physicians and all healthcare providers involved in primary care. It can also be invaluable to medical students, residents, internists, pediatricians, and dermatologists. It is available electronically for iPad, iPhone, iPod Touch, all Android devices, Kindle, and on the web through Access Medicine. These electronic versions have allowed healthcare providers to access the images and content rapidly at the point-of-care.

> *One doctor wrote, "As a teacher and learner in Family Medicine and Dermatology, this atlas is an invaluable resource. Excellent quality pictures look great on the iPad. My patients appreciate seeing pictures of other people with the same medical conditions as theirs. Concise and evidence-based recommendations are just what we need in the busy setting of primary care. It is one of my most frequently referenced books/apps. A must-have for every teacher, learner, or practitioner of Family Medicine or primary care."*

The third edition of ***The Color Atlas and Synopsis of Family Medicine*** is for anyone who loves to look at clinical photographs for learning, teaching, and practicing medicine. The first chapter begins with an introduction to learning with images and digital photography. The core of the book focuses on medical conditions organized by anatomic and physiologic systems. Both adult and childhood conditions are included, as this book covers healthcare from birth to death. There are special sections devoted to the essence of family medicine, physical/sexual abuse, women's health, and substance abuse.

The collection of clinical images is supported by evidence-based information that will help the healthcare provider diagnose and manage common medical problems. The text is concisely presented with many easy-to-access bullets as a quick point-of-care reference. Each chapter begins with a patient story that ties the photographs to the real-life stories of our patients. The photographic legends are also designed to connect the images to the people and their human conditions. Strength of recommendation ratings are cited throughout so that the science of medicine can be blended with the art of medicine for optimal patient care (see table below).

Because knowledge continues to advance after any book is written, use the online resources presented in many of the chapters to keep up with the newest changes in medicine. Care deeply about your patients and enjoy your practice, as it is a privilege to be a healthcare provider and healer.

Strength of Recommendation (SOR)	Definition
A	Recommendation based on consistent and good-quality patient-oriented evidence.*
B	Recommendation based on inconsistent or limited-quality patient-oriented evidence.*
C	Recommendation based on consensus, usual practice, opinion, disease-oriented evidence, or case series for studies of diagnosis, treatment, prevention, or screening.*

*See Appendix A on pages 1603–1606 for further information.

ACKNOWLEDGMENTS

This book could not have been completed without the contributions of many talented physicians, healthcare professionals, and photographers. We received photographs from people who live and work across the globe. Each photograph is labeled and acknowledges the photographer and contributor. Some photographs were previously published in the Photo Rounds column of the *Journal of Family Practice*. For these we thank Frontline Medical Communications, for generously sharing these photographs with our readers. Being the founding editor of this column in 2005 has given me the opportunity to see a great collection of clinical photographs over many years submitted by authors around the world.

There are some people who contributed so many photographs that it is appropriate to acknowledge them upfront in the book. Paul Comeau was the professional ophthalmology photographer at University of Texas Health Sciences Center at San Antonio (UTHSCSA). His beautiful photographs of the external and internal eye make the ophthalmology section of this book so rich and valuable. The dermatology division at UTHSCSA contributed much of their expertise in photography, writing, and reviewing the extensive dermatology section. During the past 12 years, I was fortunate to work closely with the dermatology faculty and residents and they contributed generously to our book. Dr. Eric Kraus gave us many wonderful photographs, especially for the section on bullous diseases. He also gave us open access to the 35-mm slides collected by the Division of Dermatology. Drs. Robert Gilson and Jeff Meffert also contributed photographs to many chapters. Many dermatology residents wrote chapters and contributed photographs. Dr. Jack Resneck, Sr., from Louisiana, scanned his slides from more than 40 years of practice and gave them to Dr. E.J. Mayeaux, Jr., for use. Dr. Resneck's vast dermatologic experiences add to our atlas.

The UTHSCSA Head and Neck Department contributed many photographs for this book. We especially thank Drs. Frank Miller, Randy Otto, and Blake Simpson for their contributions. UTHSCSA pediatrics faculty contributed to our chapters on child abuse and otitis media. We are fortunate to have Dr. Nancy Kellogg contribute her photographs and expertise in caring for abused children to the book. Dr. Dan Stulberg, a Professor of Family Medicine in New Mexico, with a passion for photography and dermatology, contributed many photographs throughout our book.

We thank our learners, many of whom coauthored chapters with us. Medical students, residents, and fellows from the Underserved Family Medicine Dermatology fellowship and junior faculty members coauthored chapters and contributed photographs with great enthusiasm to the creation of this work. It was a pleasure to mentor these young writers and experience with them the rewards of authorship.

We thank Dr. Kelly Green for reviewing and improving the ophthalmology section. She not only went over each chapter word by word, but she also made sure that our photographs were properly described and labeled. Dr. Green was a former student of mine, and I am proud to see the wonderful ophthalmologist that she has become.

Of course, we would have no book without the talented writing and editing of my coeditors, Drs. Mindy A. Smith, E.J. Mayeaux, and Heidi Chumley. They each bring years of clinical and educational experience to the writing of this work. Dr. Mayeaux contributed many of his own photographs, especially in women's healthcare, where he is an international expert. I value their friendship along with what they contributed to this new edition.

Most of all we need to thank our patients, who generously gave their permission for their photographs to be taken and published in this book. Although some photos are not recognizable, we have many photos of the full face that are very recognizable and were generously given to us by our patients with full written permission to be published as is. For photographs that were taken decades ago in which written consents were no longer available, we have used bars across the eyes to make the photos less recognizable—verbal consent was always obtained for these images.

The last section of this book is dedicated to understanding substance abuse (chemical dependency) and its treatment. This could not have been done without the generous contributions of the dedicated staff and the women residents at Alpha Home, a nonprofit alcohol and drug treatment program in San Antonio. The medical students and faculty (including Dr. Usatine every Monday evening) from University of Texas Health, San Antonio, spend two to three evenings a week providing free healthcare to these women who are bravely facing their addictions and fighting to stay sober one day at a time. Their pictures taken at the Usatine Wellness Center have been generously added to our book with their permission.

I (Richard Usatine) thank my family for giving me the support to see this book through. It has taken much time from my family life, and my family has supported me through the long nights and weekends it takes to write and edit a book while continuing to practice and teach medicine. I am fortunate to have a loving wife, two wonderful children, and one very cute grandson who add meaning to my life and allowed me to work hard on the creation of this new work.

Dr. Mindy Smith adds, "I thank my partner, Ted, and daughter, Jenny, for their support and willingness to listen and advise when I struggle with phrasing and wording in my writing and editing. I also thank my brother, Fred, who does the lion's share of looking after our beloved parents, now in their 90s, so that I can continue to do my work in the place that I love. And last to the friends who sustain me—Diane, Matt, Virginia, Leslie S, Jim, Marg, and Sally."

Dr. E.J. Mayeaux adds, "I would like to think my co-editors for the camaraderie and teamwork. I would like to especially thank Dr. Richard Usatine for his vision and leadership in creating the Color Atlas family of books. Thanks for inviting us all along for the ride."

Dr. Heidi Chumley adds, "I would like to thank my husband and co-author, Dr. John Delzell, and my children for their incredible support during a very challenging time. I would also like to thank my American University of the Caribbean family for the privilege to lead such an amazing university."

Finally, we all thank James Shanahan, Harriet Lebowitz, and Amanda Fielding from McGraw-Hill.

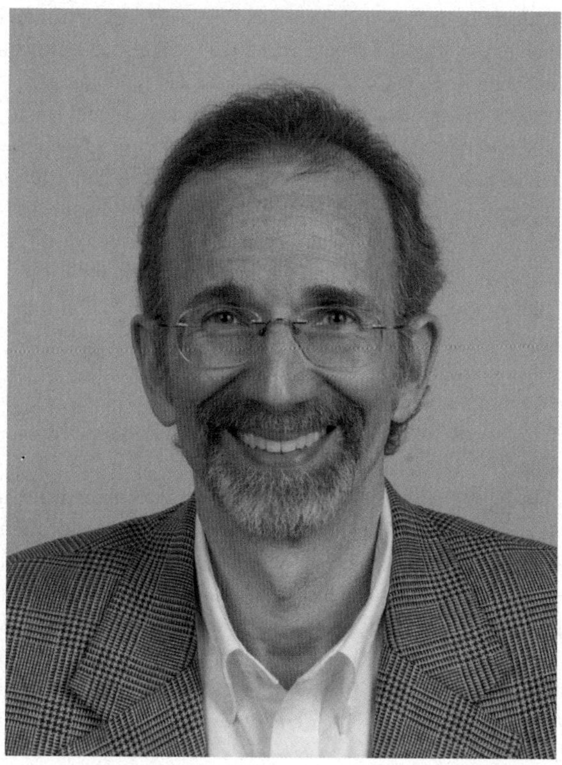

Richard P. Usatine, MD, has devoted his career to teaching health care providers at all levels and providing compassionate health care to underserved and vulnerable populations. He is a Professor of Family Medicine and Dermatology and Cutaneous Surgery at University of Texas Health, San Antonio. He received his MD from Columbia College of Physicians and Surgeons and completed his family medicine residency at UCLA. He is a principal author of 10 books and the lead author of 8 books including *Dermatological and Cosmetic Procedures in Office Practice, Cutaneous Cryosurgery* and all three editions of the *Color Atlas of Family Medicine.* He has published over 120 journal articles and has won numerous teaching and humanitarian awards. In 2000, Dr. Usatine was the national recipient of the Humanism in Medicine Award by the Association of American Medical Colleges.

Dr. Usatine founded the University Health System Skin Clinic in 2006. He is the program director of the only Underserved Dermatology Family Medicine Fellowship Program in the United States. He is also involved in teaching family medicine, internal medicine and dermatology residents at the University of Texas Health, San Antonio. He is the Founding Director of a program that includes 6 student-run free clinics and two medical student electives associated with these clinics. Dr. Usatine has been an active member of his university's global health program and has been the faculty leader for one global health trip yearly since 2009. His work in dermatology and global health has helped to inform those sections of this book.

Dr. Usatine has been the national chair of the yearly Skin Course put on by the American Academy of Family Physicians since 2006. He began teaching dermoscopy to primary care providers in 2009 and now teaches dermoscopy to international audiences. He co-developed a free interactive app for smart phones and tablets called "Dermoscopy: Two Step Algorithm." He is the first family physician to be elected to the board of the International Dermoscopy Society. Dr. Usatine has also developed over 80 dermatology instructional videos and the Interactive Dermatology Atlas website. His clinical photography has been used in many books, monographs, journal articles and educational websites (including VisualDx and the American Cancer Society). He is the associate editor of the Journal of Family Practice and the author of Photo Rounds Friday on the journal website. Dr. Usatine is the family medicine editor for VisualDx.

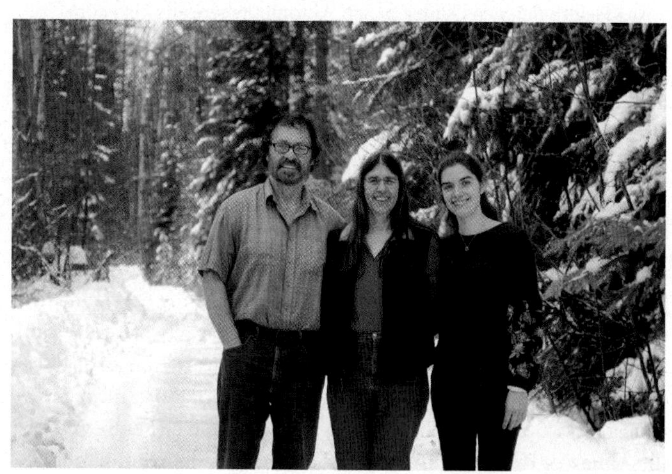

Mindy Ann Smith, MD, MS, is a Clinical Professor in the Department of Family Medicine, College of Human Medicine at Michigan State University and an Honorary Associate in the Department of Family Medicine and Community Health at the University of Wisconsin School of Medicine and Public Health where she provides mentorship for faculty members. She is an Associate Medical Editor for AAFP *FP Essentials* and Deputy Editor for *Essential Evidence Plus.* Her work has resulted in 57 papers published in peer-review journals, hundreds of published book chapters and 12 books. She reviews study documents for the Environmental Protection Agency on behalf of Citizens for a Clean Columbia, is an executive committee member for the Kootenay Library Federation, and chairs the Patient Advisory Committee for the Kootenay-Boundary Collaborative Services Committee, which works to transform the local delivery of primary care in that region of British Columbia, Canada. She is shown here with her partner Ted and daughter Jenny at her BC home.

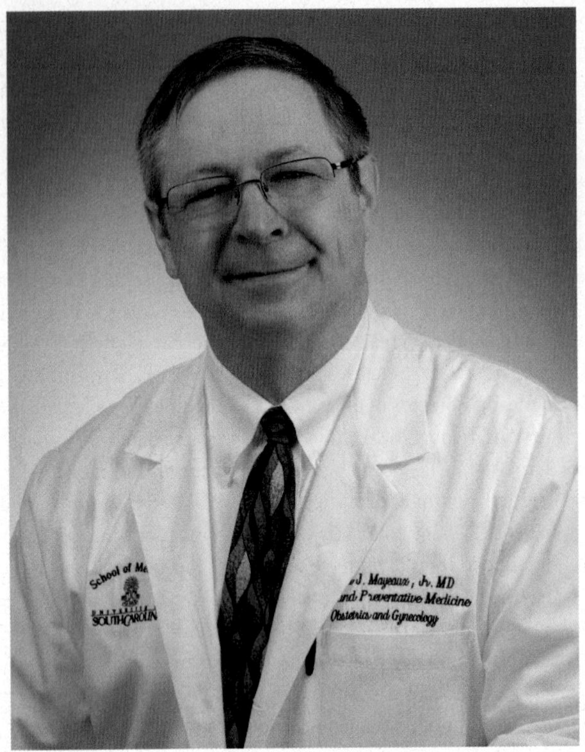

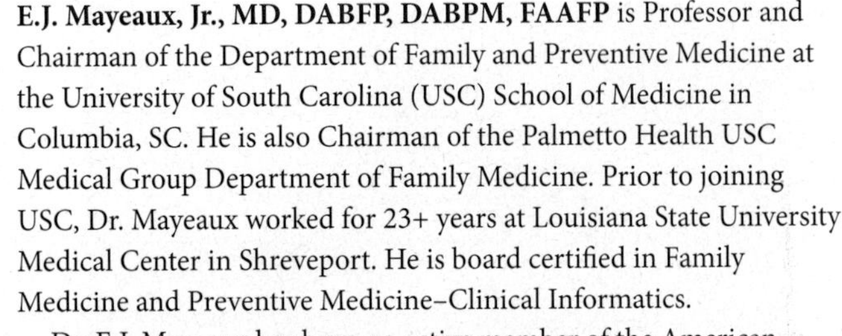

E.J. Mayeaux, Jr., MD, DABFP, DABPM, FAAFP is Professor and Chairman of the Department of Family and Preventive Medicine at the University of South Carolina (USC) School of Medicine in Columbia, SC. He is also Chairman of the Palmetto Health USC Medical Group Department of Family Medicine. Prior to joining USC, Dr. Mayeaux worked for 23+ years at Louisiana State University Medical Center in Shreveport. He is board certified in Family Medicine and Preventive Medicine–Clinical Informatics.

Dr. E.J. Mayeaux has been an active member of the American Society for Colposcopy and Cervical Pathology (ASCCP) and the International Federation for Colposcopy and Pathology of the Cervix (IFCPC) since 1996. He was President of ASCCP in 2014. He has served on the executive board of the IFCPC since 2014. He is the lead editor of *Modern Colposcopy*, 3rd edition, the flagship publication on colposcopy from the ASCCP.

Dr. Mayeaux is a well-respected educator who regularly is invited to teach worldwide. He has published and edited 9 books including the *Color Atlas of Family Medicine* and the *Essential Guide to Primary Care Procedures*, both of which are available in multiple languages. Dr. Mayeaux's clinical expertise includes women's health topics such as cervical disease, HPV disease, HPV vaccination, skin diseases and patient literacy as it relates to clinical medicine. He has dedicated the majority of his professional life to the study and practice of women's health.

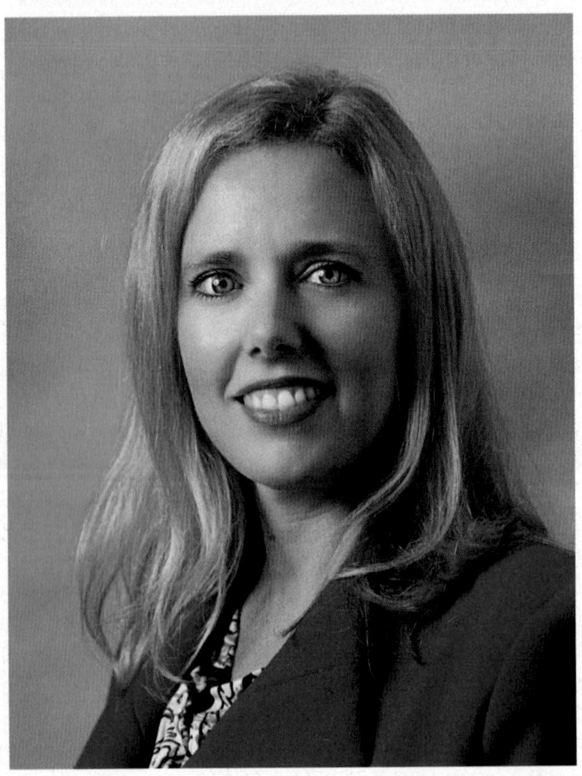

Heidi Chumley, MD, MBA is Executive Dean at American University of the Caribbean School of Medicine (AUC), an international medical school with campuses on island Sint Maarten and in the United Kingdom. Prior to joining AUC, she worked for eight years at the University of Kansas School of Medicine, serving as Senior Associate Dean for Medical Education and Vice Chancellor for Education Resources and Interprofessional Education.

Dr. Chumley earned her medical degree from the University of Texas Health Science Center in San Antonio, where she also completed her residency in family medicine and a fellowship in academic leadership. She earned an executive MBA, with emphasis on Latin America and the Caribbean, at University of Miami. From 1999 to 2013, she practiced full-scope family medicine in Academic Health Centers in Texas and Kansas.

Dr. Chumley's career has focused on changing medical education by increasing access for those from educationally disadvantaged settings, and creating curriculum and culture conducive to promoting social accountability and community engagement. She led the development of the first national clerkship curriculum for the Society of Teachers of Family Medicine (STFM), for which she and her team won an STFM Presidential Award. She has authored numerous articles in medical education, served as an editor on five textbooks, and currently sits on the Annals of Family Medicine Board of Directors. In her current role, she is most proud of the high percentage of AUC graduates who choose family medicine and work in underserved areas.

PART I

LEARNING WITH IMAGES AND DIGITAL PHOTOGRAPHY

Strength of Recommendation (SOR)	Definition
A	Recommendation based on consistent and good-quality patient-oriented evidence.*
B	Recommendation based on inconsistent or limited-quality patient-oriented evidence.*
C	Recommendation based on consensus, usual practice, opinion, disease-oriented evidence, or case series for studies of diagnosis, treatment, prevention, or screening.*

*See Appendix A on pages 1603–1606 for further information.

1 AN ATLAS TO ENHANCE PATIENT CARE, LEARNING, AND TEACHING

Richard P. Usatine, MD

People only see what they are prepared to see.
—Ralph Waldo Emerson

Whether you are viewing **Figure 1-1** in a book, in an aquarium, or in the sea, you immediately recognize the image as a fish. Those of you who are more schooled in the classification of fish might recognize that this is an angelfish, with the tail resembling the head of the angel and the posterior fins representing the wings. If you are truly prepared to see this fish in all its splendor, you would see the blue circle above its eye as the crown of the queen angelfish.

Making a diagnosis in medicine often involves the kind of pattern recognition needed to identify a queen angelfish. This is much the same as recognizing a beautiful bird or the painting of a favorite artist. If you are prepared to look for the clues that lead to the identification (diagnosis), you will see what needs to be seen. How can we be best prepared to see these clues? One method is to see printed and electronic images of patients who have the diagnoses before you encounter your patient with this diagnosis. The memory of a powerful visual image can become hardwired into your brain for ready recall.

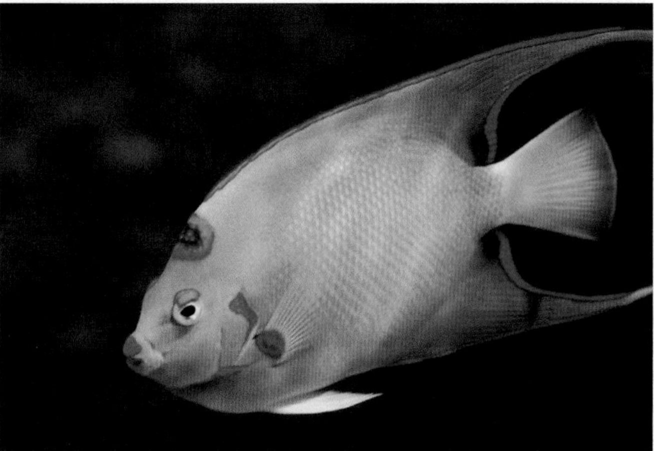

FIGURE 1-1 Queen angelfish (*Holacanthus ciliaris*). (*Reproduced with permission from Sam Thekkethil. http://www.flickr.com/photos/natureloving.*)

In medicine it also helps to know where and how to look to find the clues you may need when the diagnosis cannot be made at a single glance. For example, a patient with inverse psoriasis may present with a rash under the breast that has been repeatedly and unsuccessfully treated with antifungal agents for candidiasis or tinea (**Figures 1-2** and **1-3**). The prepared clinician knows that *not* all erythematous plaques under the breast are fungal and looks for clues such as nail changes (**Figures 1-2** and **1-4**) or scaling erythematous plaques around the elbows, knees, or umbilicus (**Figure 1-3**). Knowing where to look and what to look for is how an experienced clinician makes the diagnosis of psoriasis.

USING OUR SENSES

As physicians we collect clinical data through sight, sound, touch, and smell. Although physicians in the past used taste to collect data, such as tasting the sweet urine of a patient with diabetes, this sense is rarely, if ever, used in modern medicine. We listen to heart sounds, lung sounds, bruits, and percussion notes to collect information for diagnoses. We touch our patients to feel lumps, bumps, thrills, and masses. We occasionally use smell for diagnosis. Unfortunately, the smells of disease are rarely pleasant. Even the fruity odors of *Pseudomonas* are not like the sweet fruits of a farmers' market. Of course, we also use the patient's history, laboratory data, and more advanced imaging techniques to diagnose and manage patients' illnesses.

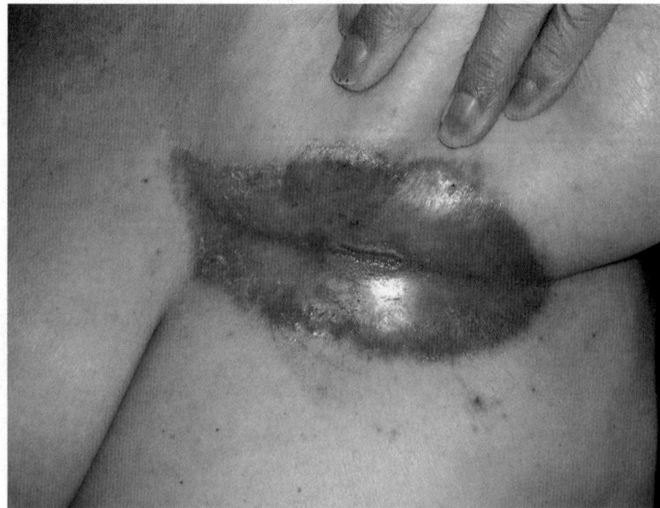

FIGURE 1-2 Inverse psoriasis under the breast that might appear to be a fungal infection to the untrained eye. Note the splinter hemorrhages in the nail of the third digit that provide a clue that the patient has psoriasis. (*Reproduced with permission from Richard P. Usatine, MD.*)

THIS THIRD EDITION DELIVERS MORE IMAGES AND INFORMATION

It was our belief in the value of visual imagery that led to the development of the first edition of *The Color Atlas of Family Medicine*. We delivered more than 1500 images to doctors around the world, first as a large color textbook and then as an interactive electronic application for easy use on the iPhone, iPad, and all Android devices. Our images were so valuable for learning and practicing medicine that they were requested for use and then incorporated into other primary care and specialty textbooks, websites, continuing medical education (CME) presentations, and test-preparation services. Now it is our pleasure to bring you our third edition of *The Color Atlas of Family Medicine* with more than 2XXX clinical images. It became clear in the second edition that this resource was so much more than a "color atlas" that we have expanded the name now to *The Color Atlas and Synopsis of Family Medicine.*

We also have added many new chapters on such important topics as Zika, Ebola, and other emerging infections; LGBT health issues; dermatology terminology; dermoscopy, including dermoscopy of skin cancer; topical and intralesional steroids; biopsy principles and techniques; sun damage and skin cancer prevention; disorders of hyperpigmentation; mental health; sports-related head injury; dementia; and the opioid epidemic. Although these topics were covered to some extent in the first edition, we decided to create these new chapters so that the text and images would become an updated comprehensive resource for the full range of family medicine. Electronic applications for our third edition will be available in all major platforms at the same time that the new book is released.

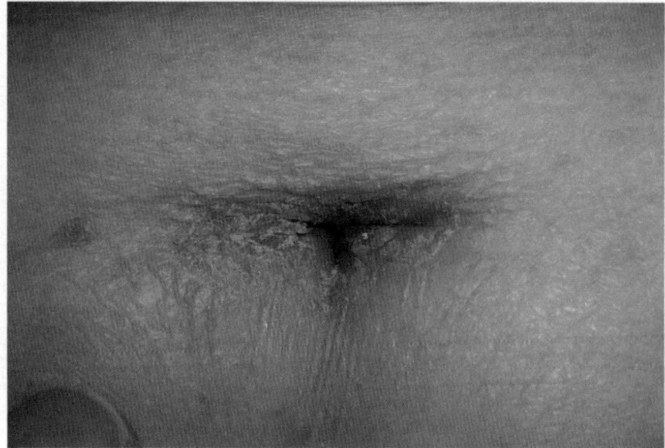

FIGURE 1-3 The patient in **Figure 1-2** with inverse psoriasis had a typical psoriatic plaque in the umbilicus. This was the only other area involved besides the breasts and the nails but easily could have been missed without the knowledge of where to look for the clues needed to make the diagnosis. (*Reproduced with permission from Richard P. Usatine, MD.*)

EXPANDING OUR INTERNAL IMAGE BANKS

The larger our saved image bank in our brain, the better clinicians and diagnosticians we can become. The expert clinician has a large image bank stored in memory to call on for rapid pattern recognition. Our image banks begin to develop in medical school when we view pictures in lectures and textbooks. We then begin to develop our own clinical image bank through our clinical experiences. Our references are printed color atlases and those color atlases available on the Internet and electronically.

Studying and learning the patterns from any atlas can enhance your expertise by enlarging the image bank stored in your memory. An atlas takes the clinical experiences of clinicians over decades and gives it to you as a single reference. We offer you an updated, modern, comprehensive color atlas of family medicine, with all organ systems including oral health, dermatology, podiatry, and the eye.

USING IMAGES TO MAKE A DIAGNOSIS

We all see visible clinical findings on patients that we do not recognize. When this happens, open this book and look for a close match. Use the list inside the front cover, the Table of Contents, or the index to direct you to the section with the highest yield photos. If you find a direct image match, you may have found the diagnosis. Read the text and see if the history and physical examination match your patient. Perform or order tests to confirm the diagnosis, if needed.

If you cannot find the image in our book, try the Internet and the Google search engine. Try a Google image search and follow the leads. Of course this is easiest to do if you have a good differential diagnosis and want to confirm your impression. If you don't have a diagnosis in

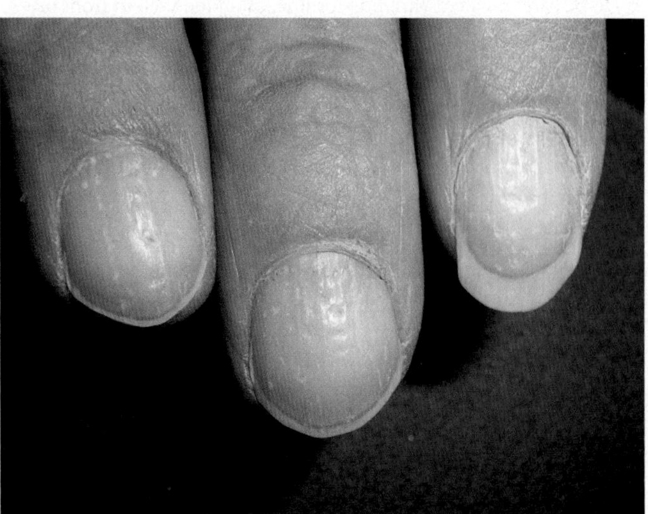

FIGURE 1-4 When the diagnosis of psoriasis is being considered, look at the nails for pitting or other nail changes such as splinter hemorrhages, onycholysis, or oil spots. This is a good example of nail pitting in a patient with psoriasis. (*Reproduced with permission from Richard P. Usatine, MD.*)

TABLE 1-1 Free Clinical Image Collections on the Internet

DermIS	www.dermis.net	Derm Information Systems from Germany
Dermnet	www.dermnet.com	From Thomas Habif, MD
Interactive Derm Atlas	www.dermatlas.net	From Richard P. Usatine, MD
ENT	www.entusa.com	From an ENT physician
Eye	www.eyerounds.org	From University of Iowa
Images of all types	https://commons.wikimedia.org	Wikimedia Commons
Infectious Diseases	https://phil.cdc.gov	CDC Public Health Image Library
Radiology	https://medpix.nlm.nih.gov/home	MedPix
Skinsight	https://www.skinsight.com	Logical Images

mind, you may try putting in descriptive words and look for an image that matches what you are seeing. If the Google image search does not work, try a Web search and look at the links for other clues.

Finally, there are dedicated atlases on the Internet for organ systems that can help you find the needed image. Most of these atlases have their own search engines, which can help direct you to the right diagnosis.

Table 1-1 lists some of the best resources currently available online.

USING IMAGES TO BUILD TRUST IN THE PATIENT–PHYSICIAN RELATIONSHIP

If you are seeing a patient with a mysterious illness that remains undiagnosed and you figure out the diagnosis, you can often bridge the issues of mistrust and anxiety by showing the patient a picture of another person with the diagnosis. Use our atlas for that purpose and supplement it with the Internet. This is especially important for a patient who has gone undiagnosed or misdiagnosed for some time. "Seeing is believing" for many patients. Ask first if they would want to see some pictures of other persons with a similar condition; most will be very interested. The patient can see the similarities between their condition and the other images and feel reassured that your diagnosis is correct. Write down the name of the diagnosis for your patient to take home, as many will want to research their diagnosis on the Internet.

Do be careful when searching for images on the Web in front of patients. Sometimes what pops up is not "pretty" (or, for that matter, G or PG rated). I turn the screen away from the patients before initiating the search and then censor what I will show them.

If you teach, model this behavior in front of your students. Show them how reference books and the Internet at the point of care can help with the care of patients.

TAKING YOUR OWN PHOTOGRAPHS

Images taken by you with your own camera of your own patients complete with their own stories are more likely to be retained and retrievable in your memory because they have a context and a story to go with them. We encourage you to use a digital camera (within a smartphone or a stand-alone camera) and take your own clinical photos. Of course, always ask permission before taking any photograph of a patient. Explain how the photographs can be used to teach other doctors and to create a record of the patient's condition at this point in time. If the photograph will be identifiable, ask for written consent; for patients younger than age 18 years, ask the parent to sign. Store the photos in a manner that avoids any Health Insurance Portability and Accountability Act (HIPAA) privacy violations, such as on a secure server or on your own computer with password protection and data encryption. These photographs can directly benefit the patient when, for example, following nevi for changes. Also, take photos of a lesion or rash before performing a biopsy. Those images may be very useful if you need to refer the patient to a surgical oncologist or Mohs surgeon for additional surgery. While these images may be entered into some electronic health records (EHRs), they can also be sent via secure messaging or protected email.

Digital photography is a wonderful method for practicing, teaching, and learning medicine. You can show patients pictures of conditions on parts of their bodies that they could not see without multiple mirrors and some unusual body contortions. You can also use the zoom view feature on the smartphone or camera to view or show a segment of the image in greater detail. Children generally love to have their photos taken and will be delighted to see themselves on the screen of your smartphone or camera.

Smartphone and digital photography makes the recording of photographic images essentially free, easier to do, and easier to maintain. Digital photography also gives you immediate feedback. Not only does this give you immediate gratification to see your image displayed instantaneously on the smartphone or camera, but also it alerts you to poor-quality photographs that can then be retaken while the patient is still in the office. This speeds up the learning curve of the photographer in a way that could not happen with film photography. Pay close attention to focus and lighting, as poorly focused and lit photographs are not very helpful.

OUR GOALS

Many of the images in this atlas are from my collected works over the past 33 years of my practice in family medicine and dermatology. My patients have generously allowed me to photograph them so that their photographs could help the physicians and patients of the future. To these photos, we have added images that represent decades of experiences by other family physicians and specialists. Family physicians who have submitted their images to Photo Rounds in the *Journal of Family Practice* are also sharing their photos with you.

It is our goal to provide you with a wide range of images of common and uncommon conditions, as well as the knowledge you need to make the diagnosis and manage the patient. We want to help you be the best diagnostician you can be. We can all aspire to be a clinician like Sir William Osler and have the detective acumen of Sherlock Holmes. The images collected for this work can move you in that direction by helping you to be prepared to see what you need to see.

PART II

THE ESSENCE OF FAMILY MEDICINE

Strength of Recommendation (SOR)	Definition
A	Recommendation based on consistent and good-quality patient-oriented evidence.*
B	Recommendation based on inconsistent or limited-quality patient-oriented evidence.*
C	Recommendation based on consensus, usual practice, opinion, disease-oriented evidence, or case series for studies of diagnosis, treatment, prevention, or screening.*

*See Appendix A on pages 1603–1606 for further information.

2 DOCTOR–PATIENT RELATIONSHIP

Mindy A. Smith, MD, MS

PATIENT STORY

Patient stories, particularly if we listen attentively and nonjudgmentally, provide us with a window into their lives and experiences. These stories help us to know our patients in powerful ways, and that knowledge about the patient, as someone special, provides the context, meaning, and clues about their symptoms and illnesses that can lead to healing. At our best, we serve as witness to their struggles and triumphs, supporter of their efforts to change and grow, and guide through the medical maze of diagnostic and therapeutic options. Sometimes, their stories become our own stories—those patients whom we will never forget because their stories have changed our lives and the way we practice medicine (**Figure 2-1**).

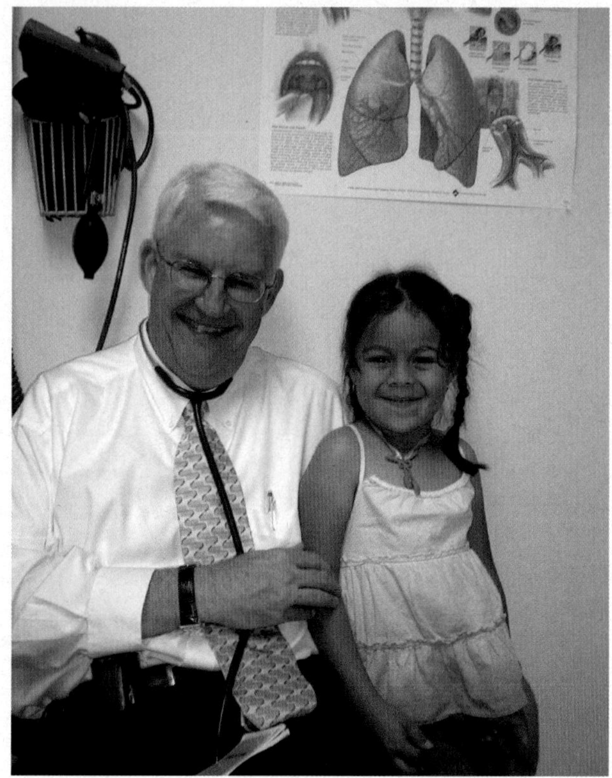

FIGURE 2-1 Dr. Jim Legler caring for a young girl in a free clinic within a transitional housing village for homeless families. He is a family physician who volunteers every week to care for the 40 families working their way out of homelessness. He had been caring for Kimberly and her family for many months at the time this photograph was taken. Dr. Legler serves as a role model for students interested in primary care of the underserved. He is known for his kindness and compassion to all his patients.

WHAT PATIENTS WANT FROM THEIR PHYSICIAN

As part of the future of family medicine (FFM) initiative, 1031 telephone interviews of the general public were conducted in 2002.[1] Most patients strongly agreed that they wanted to take an active role in their healthcare (82% and 91%, patients with family physicians and patients with general internists, respectively), they wanted their physicians to treat a wide variety of medical problems but refer to a specialist when necessary (88% and 84%), and they wanted a physician who looks at the whole person—emotional, psychological, and physical (73% and 74%). In addition, of 39 possible attributes of physicians, most patients viewed the following as the most important attributes/services that drive overall satisfaction with their physician:

- Does not judge; understands and supports.
- Always honest, direct.
- Acts as partner in maintaining health.
- Treats both serious and nonserious conditions.
- Attends to emotional and physical health.
- Listens to me.
- Encourages healthier lifestyle.
- Tries to get to know me.
- Can help with any problem.
- Someone I can stay with as I get older.

WHAT PHYSICIANS WANT FROM AND FOR PATIENTS

Although the types and intensity of relationships with patients differ, our positive and negative experiences with patients shape us as clinicians, influence us in our personal relationships, and shape the character of our practices. Arthur Kleinman, in his prologue to *Patients and Doctors: Life-Changing Stories from Primary Care*, wrote, "We all seem to want (or demand) experiences that matter, but maybe what is foremost is that we want experiences in which *we* matter." There is perhaps no greater satisfaction than the belief that what we do and who we are matters to those we care for in both our personal and professional lives.[2] A positive relationship with a patient is one of mutual growth. This concept of doctor–patient reciprocity is not new and can be found in the writings of Erasmus, more than 500 years ago, arising from a classical conception of friendship.[3]

As clinicians, we want patients to be healthier and improved in some meaningful way after our encounter with them. Meaningful elements common to healing practices across cultures include:[4]

- Providing a meaningful explanation for the sickness.
- Expressing care and concern.
- Offering the possibility of mastery and control over the illness or its symptoms.

The 300 family physicians who were interviewed as part of the FFM initiative stated that the following things completely captured the essence of what they found most satisfying about being a family physician:[1]

- The deep relationships developed with patients over the years (54%).
- The variety—no day is ever the same (54%).
- Offers me a strong sense of purpose because I can make a real difference in people's lives (48%).
- Don't spend their days taking care of illness, but take care of the whole patient (**Figure 2-2**) (46%).

LEARNING FROM PATIENTS

To learn from patients, clinicians must do the following:

- Move outside of their worldview and accept the patient's point of view and belief system.
- Let go of stereotypes, biases, and dogma.
- Use active empathic listening, see the patient in context, and adopt reflective and reflexive practices.[5]
- Emphasize patient dignity and control within a supportive team, which may include family, friends, aides, and community resources.
- Graciously accept differences of opinion or patient refusal without abandoning the patient.
- Look at each patient encounter as a cross-cultural event.[4] Western medical training acculturates clinicians into a world seen in large part as one of problems and solutions; this is often at odds with patients' need to find meaning in the illness episode, be heard and acknowledged, and learn to live a quality life with chronic illness.

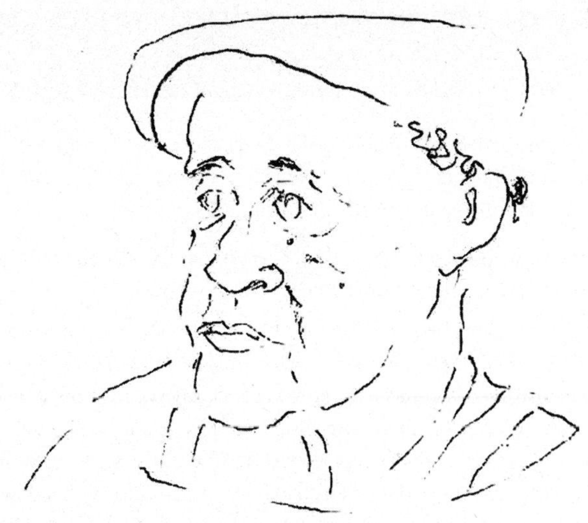

FIGURE 2-2 Dr. Alan Blum is a family physician who has been doing sketches of his patients for decades now. When he presents his drawings of his patients, he reads his poetic stories that go with the drawings. Some of his drawings have been published in *JAMA*. Here is the poem that goes with this man's story:

"Gov'ment gave me a chance
to get a hearin' aid for free.
But when I went to th' doctor,
he say,
'Well, cap'n,
there gonna be a lot o' things
you don't want to hear!'"

BENEFITS OF A GOOD DOCTOR–PATIENT RELATIONSHIP

Beyond the benefit of enhancing the medical experience for both clinicians and patients, data that support developing a good doctor–patient relationship include the following:

- Patients who are satisfied with their physicians are three times more likely to follow a prescribed medical regimen.[6]
- Patients with diabetes cared for by physicians with high empathy scores (based on the physician's self-administered Jefferson Scale of Empathy) were significantly more likely to have good control based on hemoglobin A_{1C} than were patients of physicians with low empathy scores (56% and 40%, respectively).[7] In another study, patients with diabetes whose physicians had high empathy scores had lower combined rates of hyperosmolar state, diabetic ketoacidosis, and coma compared with patients of physicians with moderate and low empathy scores (4.0 vs. 7.1 and 6.5 per 1000 patients, respectively).[8]
- Patients who reported an established relationship with a primary care provider (PCP) were less likely to currently smoke than those who lacked a PCP relationship (26.5% and 62.3%, respectively).[9]
- There is a direct link between patient satisfaction and the amount of information that physicians provide.[10]
- There is also a strong positive correlation between patient satisfaction, recall, and understanding and physician's partnership building (e.g., enlisting patient input).[10]
- Provision of health information to patients influences patient decision-making in important ways.

ESSENTIALS OF GOOD DOCTOR–PATIENT RELATIONSHIP

Although the doctor–patient relationship may be viewed as a contract for providing services, Candib argues that this view does not fit well with developing a healing relationship that must be based on "unconditional positive regard," beneficence, caring, and a moral basis of conduct.[11] Furthermore, contracts fail to deal with the unpredictable and fail to acknowledge the power inequality between physicians and patients. To counter this power imbalance, Candib emphasizes the need for clinicians to use that power to empower the patient.

Caring is an essential feature of a good doctor–patient relationship. Caring, as connectedness with a patient, evolves from the relationship. Within the context of this relationship, the clinician makes the patient feel known, pays attention to the meaning that a symptom or illness has in the patient's life, expresses real feeling (separate from reflecting back the patient's feelings), and practices devotion (e.g., a willingness at times to do something extra for the patient).[12] In a survey of 485 patients attending a routine healthcare visit, physician-prompted patient expressions of concern, physician understanding of the patient's healthcare preferences and values, and a patient–physician interaction outside of the exam room were associated with patient ratings of positive physician relational communication.[13] To provide caring to patients, however, clinicians must take care of themselves.

Effective patient communication is also important in relationship building and results in improved health outcomes,[14,15] decreased costs,[16] and increased patient satisfaction.[17,18] Authors of a systematic review found that verbal behaviors of primary care physicians related to improved patient satisfaction were empathy, encouragement, patient-centeredness, and time spent on history taking and health education.[19] Verbal behaviors related to adherence to medication were humor/tension release and patient-centeredness, while one-way conversation flow hindered adherence.[19] Interestingly, in this age of technology to enhance patient communication, one study found that use of partnership-building language and supportive talk was low with electronic communication compared to in-person communication.[20]

SKILLS FOR BUILDING GOOD DOCTOR–PATIENT RELATIONSHIPS

- One strategy for improving communication with patients is using the patient-centered interview.[21] This technique focuses on eliciting the patient's agenda in order to address their concerns more promptly.
- Incorporating the BATHE (Background, Affect, Trouble and Handling of their current situation, and Empathy) method into the standard patient interview was found to increase 8 of 11 measures of patient satisfaction.[22] The clinician begins with an open-ended question about the patient's concerns, asks about how the patient feels in relation to the issues revealed, asks the patient what troubles them most (area of greatest concern), assesses the patient's coping skills to assist patients in generating their own solutions to problems, and validates their experience (expresses empathy).
- Motivational interviewing (MI) is another technique that can enhance the doctor–patient relationship through strengthening a person's own motivation and commitment to change.[23] This process includes understanding patient's values, careful listening, encouraging patient choice, and resisting the urge to fix things for the patient; the technique focuses on enhancing patient self-efficacy. Although evidence is limited, MI may have positive effects on chronic disease treatment adherence,[24] diabetes care,[25] health habits,[26] and uptake of health screening.[27]
- Patients who are informed and involved in decision-making are more adherent to medical recommendations and carry out more health-related behavior change such as exercise, smoking cessation, and dietary modification.[28] To engage successfully in shared decision-making, patients need both information and power to participate in the choice.[29] In one study, of patients' perceptions of shared decision-making, coming to a mutually agreed-upon decision appeared to be more important than the process of getting to that decision.[30]
- Physician communication skills can be improved with training.[31] Similarly, patients can be trained to increase active participation with their health providers without increasing visit length, although data do not show a relationship between patient communication training and improved health outcomes.[32]

REFERENCES

1. American Academy of Family Physicians. *Future of Family Medicine Project.* http://www.aafp.org/about/initiatives/future-family-medicine.html. Accessed June 2017.
2. Kleinman A. Prologue. In: Borkan J, Reis S, Steinmetz D, Medalie JH, eds. *Patients and Doctors: Life-Changing Stories from Primary Care.* Madison, WI: University of Wisconsin Press; 1999:ix.
3. Albury WR, Weisz GM. The medical ethics of Erasmus and the physician-patient relationship. *Med Humanit.* 2001;27(1):35-41.
4. Brody H. Family and community—reflections. In: Borkan J, Reis S, Steinmetz D, Medalie JH, eds. *Patients and Doctors: Life-Changing Stories from Primary Care.* Madison, WI: University of Wisconsin Press; 1999:67-72.
5. Medalie JH. Learning from patients—reflections. In: Borkan J, Reis S, Steinmetz D, Medalie JH, eds. *Patients and Doctors: Life-Changing Stories from Primary Care.* Madison, WI: University of Wisconsin Press; 1999:50.
6. Rosenberg EE, Lussier MT, Beaudoin C. Lessons for clinicians from physician-patient communication literature. *Arch Fam Med.* 1997;6:279-283.
7. Hojat M, Louis DZ, Markham FW, et al. Physicians' empathy and clinical outcomes for diabetic patients. *Acad Med.* 2011;86(3): 359-364.
8. Del Canale S, Louis DZ, Maio V, et al. The relationship between physician empathy and disease complications: an empirical study of primary care physicians and their diabetic patients in Parma, Italy. *Acad Med.* 2012;87(9):1243-1249.
9. DePew Z, Gossman W, Morrow LE. Association of primary care physician relationship and insurance status with reduced rates of tobacco smoking. *Chest.* 2010;138(5):1278-1279.
10. Hall JA, Roter KL, Katz NR. Meta-analysis of correlates of provider behavior in medical encounters. *Med Care.* 1988;26:657-675.
11. Candib LM. *Medicine and the Family—A Feminist Perspective.* New York: Basic Books; 1995:119-145.
12. Candib LM. *Medicine and the Family—A Feminist Perspective.* New York, NY: Basic Books; 1995:206-239.
13. Shay LA, Dumenci L, Siminoff LA, et al. Factors associated with patient reports of positive physician relational communication. *Patient Educ Couns.* 2012;89(1):96-101.
14. Stewart MA. Effective physician-patient communication and health outcomes: a review. *CMAJ.* 1995;152(9):1423-1433.
15. Kaplan SH, Greenfield S, Ware JE. Assessing the effects of physician-patient interactions on the outcomes of chronic disease. *Med Care.* 1989;27(3 Suppl):S110-S127.
16. Epstein RM, Franks P, Shields CG, et al. Patient-centered communication and diagnostic testing. *Ann Fam Med.* 2005;3(5):415-421.
17. Little P, Everitt H, Williamson I, et al. Observational study of effect of patient centredness and positive approach on outcomes of general practice consultations. *BMJ.* 2001;323(7318):908-911.
18. Bertakis KD, Roter D, Putnam SM. The relationship of physician medical interview style to patient satisfaction. *J Fam Pract.* 1991;32:175-181.
19. Beck RS, Daughtridge R, Sloane PD. Physician-patient communication in the primary care office: a systematic review. *J Am Board Fam Pract.* 2002;15(1):25-38.
20. Alpert JM, Dyer KE, Lafata JE. Patient-centered communication in digital medical encounters. *Patient Educ Couns.* 2017;100(10): 1852-1858.
21. Brown J, Stewart M, McCracken E, et al. The patient-centered clinical method. 2. Definition and application. *Fam Pract.* 1986; 3:75-79.
22. Leiblum SR, Schnall E, Seehuus M, DeMaria A. To BATHE or not to BATHE: patient satisfaction with visits to their family physician. *Fam Med.* 2008;40(6):407-411.
23. Miller WR, Rollnick S. *Motivational Interviewing: Helping People Change* (Third Edition). New York: Guilford, 2013.
24. Schaefer MR, Kavookjian J. The impact of motivational interviewing on adherence and symptom severity in adolescents and young adults with chronic illness: a systematic review. *Patient Educ Couns.* 2017;100(12):2190-2199.
25. Thepwongsa I, Muthukumar R, Kessomboon P. Motivational interviewing by general practitioners for Type 2 diabetes patients: a systematic review. *Fam Pract.* 2017;34(4):373-383.
26. Lee WW, Choi KC, Yum RW, et al. Effectiveness of motivational interviewing on lifestyle modification and health outcomes of clients at risk or diagnosed with cardiovascular diseases: A systematic review. *Int J Nurs Stud.* 2016;53:331-341.
27. Miller SJ, Foran-Tuller K, Ledergerber J, Jandorf L. Motivational interviewing to improve health screening uptake: a systematic review. *Patient Educ Couns.* 2017;100(2):190-198.
28. DiMatteo R. Health behaviors and care decisions: an overview of professional-patient communication. In: Gochman DS, ed. *Handbook of Health Behavior Research II: Provider Determinants.* New York: Plenum Press, 1997:5-22.
29. Joseph-Williams N, Elwyn G, Edwards A. Knowledge is not power for patients: a systematic review and thematic synthesis of patient-reported barriers and facilitators to shared decision making. *Patient Educ Couns.* 2014;94(3):291-309.
30. Shay LA, Lafata JE. Understanding patient perceptions of shared decision making. *Patient Educ Couns.* 2014;96(3): 295-301.
31. Berkhof M, Van Rijssen HJ, Schellart AJM, et al. Effective training strategies for teaching communication skills to physicians: an overview of systematic reviews. *Patient Educ Couns.* 2011;84(2): 152-162.
32. D'Agostino TA, Atkinson TM, Latella LE, et al. Promoting patient participation in healthcare interactions through communication skills training: a systematic review. *Patient Educ Couns.* 2017;100(7): 1247-1257.

3 FAMILY PLANNING

E.J. Mayeaux, Jr., MD

PATIENT STORY

Your patient is a 25-year-old married woman who wants to postpone having children for another 2 years while she finishes graduate school. She and her husband are currently using condoms, but would like to change to something different. She is in good health and does not smoke. You take this opportunity to discuss with her all the methods available to prevent pregnancy. First, you determine what she knows about the methods and if she has any preferences. She tells you that she is specifically interested in either the *hormonal vaginal ring* (NuvaRing) (**Figure 3-1**) or an *intrauterine device* that releases a hormone (**Figure 3-2**). You participate in shared decision-making as she comes up with the method that best fits her lifestyle and health issues.

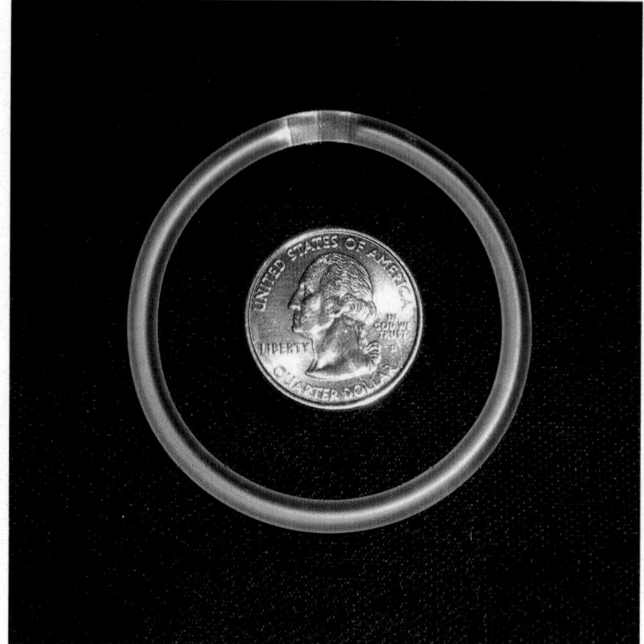

FIGURE 3-1 NuvaRing is a combined hormonal intravaginal contraceptive ring. The flexible material of the ring allows for easy insertion and removal. Note the size in comparison to a quarter. (*Reproduced with permission from Richard P. Usatine, MD.*)

INTRODUCTION

Contraception, like most other medical interventions, requires informed decision-making for best outcomes. Each birth control method has its inherent risks and benefits. Each method has its barriers to use, such as compliance, cost, and social stigmas. By educating patients appropriately and letting them know beforehand of potential side effects, we can greatly increase adherence and satisfaction.

An unintended pregnancy may be either unwanted (occurred when no children or no more children were desired) or mistimed. Unintended pregnancy most often results from nonuse, inconsistent use, or incorrect use of effective contraceptive methods. Unintended pregnancy is associated with an increased risk of adverse outcomes for the mother and baby. For instance, a woman may not be in optimal health for childbearing or have missed the opportunity for preconception or early prenatal care such as taking folic acid, quitting tobacco use, and abstaining from alcohol and drugs.[1] Good communication and shared decision-making between providers and patients may minimize these risks.

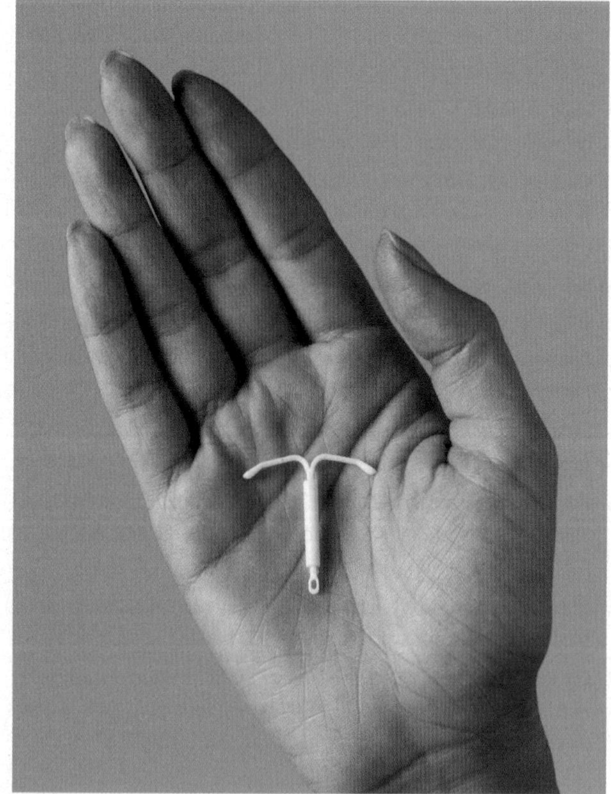
FIGURE 3-2 Mirena (levonorgestrel-releasing intrauterine system) provides effective contraception for at least 5 years. (*Reproduced with permission from Bayer HealthCare Pharmaceuticals Inc.*)

EPIDEMIOLOGY

- In 2011, 45% of pregnancies were unintended, which is a decline from 51% in 2008. During this period, the rate of unintended pregnancies decreased 18% from 54 to 45 unintended pregnancies per 1000 women for ages 15–44 years.[2] Approximately half of these occurred in women using reversible contraception.[3]
- Large declines (44%) also occurred among teenagers ages 15–17 years. However, unintended pregnancy rates per 1000 women were highest among women ages 18–24 years, had incomes <100% of the federal poverty level, had not graduated from high school, or who were cohabiting women and had never been married. Among teenagers 15–19 years of age, 3 of every 4 pregnancies were unintended.[2]

TABLE 3-1 Contraceptive Methods, Effectiveness, and Reversibility

Effectiveness	Pregnancy Rate	Reversibility	Method
Highly	<1 pregnancy/100 women/year	Permanent Reversible	Female and male sterilization Intrauterine devices Contraceptive implants
Moderate	6–12 pregnancies/100 women/year	Reversible	Combined hormonal contraceptives Injectable progestin
Less	>17 pregnancies/100 women/year	Reversible	Barrier methods Fertility awareness–based methods Lactational amenorrhea method Coitus interruptus Spermicides

- The most commonly used contraceptive methods in the United States are oral contraceptive pills (OCPs), male condoms, and female sterilization.[4]
- Long-acting reversible forms of contraception are increasingly popular. Encouraging these methods may help lower the unintended pregnancy rate. Gaps or discontinuation of use of short-acting methods leads to unintended pregnancy.[5]
- Newer contraceptives often have improved side-effect profiles or have more convenient delivery systems that may not require daily patient adherence. Having a wide range of contraceptive options helps patients find a method that will work best for them.
- This chapter focuses on contraceptive methods available in the United States and the considerations one must address when counseling patients on their choice of method.

CONSIDERATIONS

- No contraception method is perfect. Each individual or couple must balance the advantages and disadvantages of each method and decide which offers the best choice. Providers should help the patient make the appropriate decision based on many factors that are unrelated to their medical history or to the side-effect profile of the method, such as the likelihood of compliance and access to follow up. Contraceptive methods can be broken down into four groups based on how effective they are in pregnancy prevention and reversibility (**Table 3-1**).
- Some important considerations in choosing a contraceptive method are its efficacy (**Figure 3-3**), potential side effects, failure rates, and noncontraceptive benefits. See **Table 3-2**.
- Smoking increases the risks of the most dangerous side effects of estrogen-containing contraceptives. This is an important issue in helping a patient choose the safest and the best method. Encouraging smoking cessation is always a good intervention, but one might avoid prescribing an estrogen-containing contraceptive until the patient can truly quit smoking.
- Avoid estrogen-containing contraceptives in women with hypertension or migraine with aura. In both cases, the theoretical or proven risk of stroke outweighs the advantages.

HIGHLY EFFECTIVE METHODS

- In 2017, four intrauterine devices (IUDs) were available in the United States: the copper-containing IUD (Cu-IUD) and three levonorgestrel-releasing IUDs. Fewer than 1 woman in 100 becomes

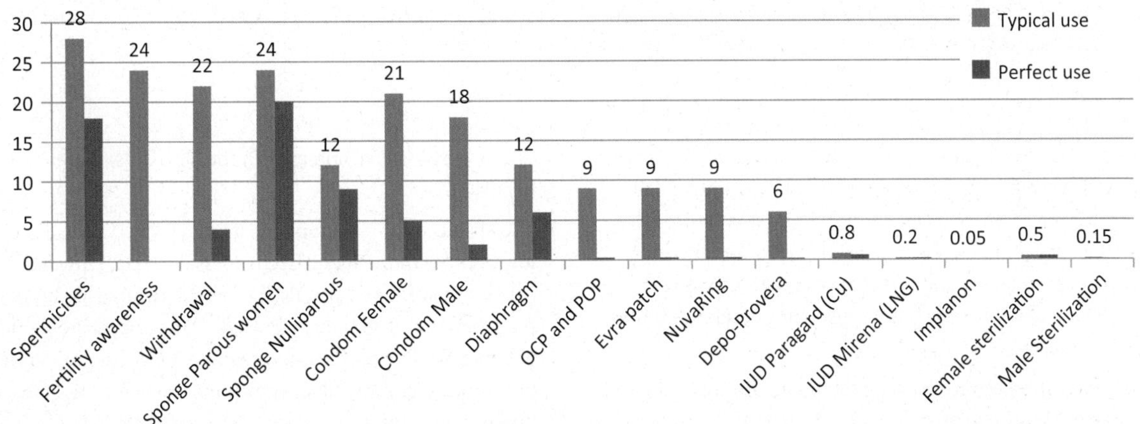

FIGURE 3-3 Women experiencing a pregnancy during 1 year of use. U.S. Selected Practice Recommendations for Contraceptive Use, 2013. (Data from Division of Reproductive Health, National Center for Chronic Disease Prevention and Health Promotion, Centers for Disease Control and Prevention (CDC): U.S. Selected Practice Recommendations for Contraceptive Use, 2013: adapted from the World Health Organization selected practice recommendations for contraceptive use, 2nd edition, *MMWR Recomm Rep.* 2013;62(RR-05):1-60)

TABLE 3-2 Contraceptive Options Available in the United States in 2012

Method	Unintended Pregnancies with 1 Year of Use (%)		Noncontraceptive Benefits	Use with Breastfeeding
	Typical Use	Theoretical		
None	85	85	—	—
Spermicide	29	18	None	Yes
Withdrawal	27	4	None	Yes
Periodic abstinence (fertility awareness)	25	3–5	None	Yes
Diaphragm with spermicide	16	6	None	Yes
Female condom	21	5	Prevents STDs	Yes
Male condom	15	2	Prevents STDs	Yes
OCPs—combined and progestin-only	8	0.3	Regulation of menstrual cycle and dysmenorrhea, possible decrease in ovarian and endometrial cancer risk, decrease acne	No
Contraceptive patch	8	0.3	Same as OCPs	No
Vaginal ring	8	0.3	Same as OCPs	No
Depo-Provera	3	0.3	Same as OCPs	Yes
Copper-containing IUD	0.8	0.6	None	Yes
Levonorgestrel IUD	0.2	0.2	Regulation of menstrual cycles and dysmenorrhea	Yes
Female sterilization	0.5	0.5	None	Yes
Male sterilization	0.15	0.10	None	Yes
Etonogestrel implant	0.05	0.05	Same as OCPs	Safety conditional

OCP, oral contraceptive pill; IUD, intrauterine device; STD, sexually transmitted disease.
Data from Trussell J. Contraceptive efficacy. In Hatcher RA, Trussell J, Nelson AL, et al., eds. *Contraceptive Technology*, 20th rev ed. New York: Ardent Media; 2011:827-1010; Herndon EJ, Zieman M. New contraceptive options. *Am Fam Physician*. 2004;69:853–860; Herndon EJ, Zieman M. *Improving Access to Quality Care in Family Planning: Medical Eligibility Criteria for Contraceptive Use*, 2nd ed. Geneva, Switzerland: Reproductive Health and Research, World Health Organization, 2000. Available at: http://whqlibdoc.who.int/publications/2004/9241562668.pdf (accessed July 4, 2006); Speroff L, Fritz MA. *Clinical Gynecologic Endocrinology and Infertility*, 7th ed. Philadelphia: Lippincott Williams & Wilkins, 2005.

pregnant in the first year of using IUDs with typical use.[6] IUDs are long-acting and reversible, and they can be used by women of all ages and by parous and nulliparous women. IUDs do not protect against sexually transmitted diseases (STDs); concomitant consistent and correct use of latex condoms reduces the risk for STDs. IUDs can be inserted at any time if it is reasonably certain that the woman is not pregnant.

- There are three levonorgestrel-releasing IUDs containing a total of either 13.5 mg or 52 mg levonorgestrel. The Mirena IUD releases levonorgestrel and provides effective contraception for at least 5 years (see **Figure 3-2**). Copper-containing IUDs are another long-term option lasting up to 10 years; however, they may be associated with dysmenorrhea and irregular vaginal bleeding some of the time. Twenty percent of women have amenorrhea after 1 year of use with Mirena, and as with the Cu-IUDs, there is a risk of expulsion.
- The absolute risk of ectopic pregnancy with IUD use is extremely low because of the high effectiveness of IUDs. However, if a woman becomes pregnant during IUD use, the relative likelihood of ectopic pregnancy is greatly increased.[7] Paracervical block might reduce patient pain during IUD insertion. Misoprostol for cervical dilatation is not recommended for routine use before IUD insertion, but it might be helpful in women with a recent failed insertion.[1] Prophylactic antibiotics are generally not recommended for any IUD insertion. Current IUDs are not associated with pelvic inflammatory disease (PID) or tubal infertility. The IUD expulsion rate is 3% to 5% in adult women and 5% to 22% in adolescents, and prior expulsion is not a contraindication to another IUD placement.[8]

- The etonogestrel implant (Nexplanon) is a *single rod implant* for subdermal use (**Figure 3-4**). It is long-acting (up to 3 years), reversible, and can be used by women of all ages, including adolescents. It must be removed or replaced by the end of the third year. The implant is 4 cm in length with a diameter of 2 mm and contains 68 mg of the synthetic progestin etonogestrel (ENG). It does not contain estrogen or latex and is radiopaque. The contraceptive effect of the ENG implant involves suppression of ovulation, increased viscosity of the cervical mucus, and alterations in the endometrium. In the first year of use, it had the lowest failure rate of any form of contraception, including tubal ligation.[6] The effectiveness of Nexplanon in women who weigh more than 130% of their ideal body weight has not been studied. Problems with Nexplanon are similar to those with other progestin-only contraceptives (acne and gaining weight).
- Laparoscopic, abdominal, and hysteroscopic female sterilization are available in the United States. Because these methods are intended to be irreversible, all women should be appropriately counseled about the permanency of these methods and the availability of highly effective, long-acting, reversible methods of contraception. Hysteroscopic tubal occlusion (Essure) is a newer outpatient sterilization technique (**Figures 3-5** to **3-7**). The device is a flexible microcoil designed to promote tissue growth in the fallopian tubes. It does not require any incisions and can be performed without general anesthesia, typically in less than 30 minutes. There is a 3-month waiting period after the device is placed when an alternative birth control must be used. At the 3-month follow-up visit, a hysterosalpingogram is performed to document that the tubes have been blocked.

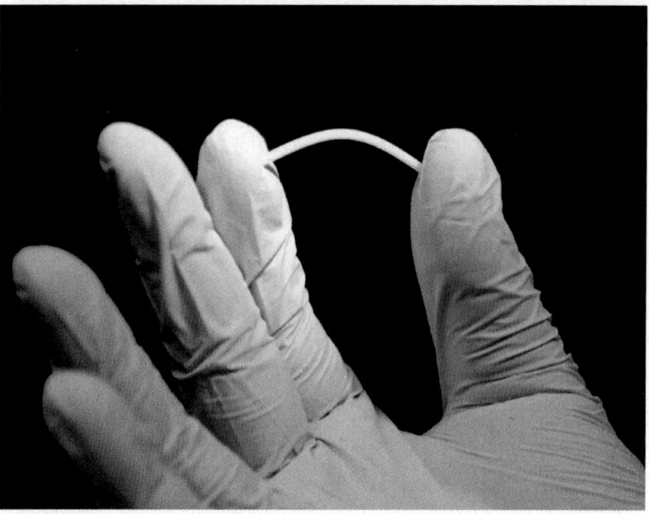

FIGURE 3-4 Nexplanon implantable subcutaneous contraceptive system. The insertion device is a sharp trocar, and the implant is made of a soft Silastic tube. *(Reproduced with permission from E .J. Mayeaux Jr., MD.)*

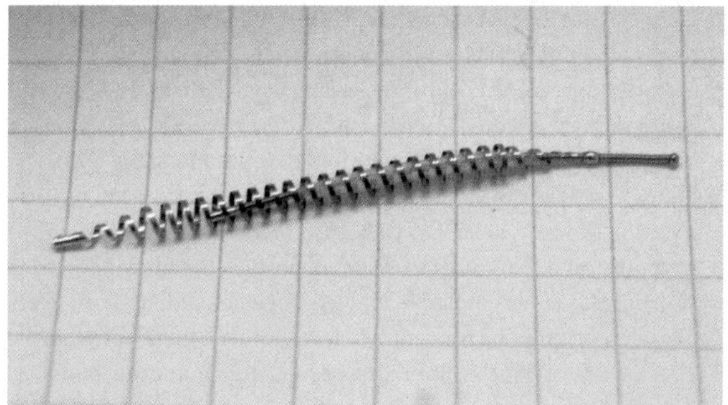

FIGURE 3-5 Essure tubal occlusion device for permanent sterilization. It is placed within the fallopian tubes using a vaginal approach and a hysteroscope. *(Reproduced with permission from Jay Berman, MD.)*

MODERATELY EFFECTIVE METHODS

- Combined hormonal contraceptives (CHCs) contain both estrogen and a progestin. Examples include various formulations of combined oral contraceptive (COC), a transdermal contraceptive patch, and a vaginal contraceptive ring. Approximately 9 of 100 women become pregnant in the first year of use of CHCs with typical use.[6] These methods are reversible and can be used by women of all ages. CHCs are generally used for 21–24 consecutive days, followed by 4–7 hormone-free days. The Centers for Disease Control and Prevention (CDC) recommends providing a year to 13 months of CHCs since this has been shown to increase continuation of the method.[9]
- The *combination contraceptive patch* releases 150 mcg of norelgestromin and 20 mcg ethinyl estradiol daily and has the same mechanism of action as OCPs (**Figure 3-8**). It is applied weekly for 3 weeks, followed by a patch-free week during which menses occur. Recommended application sites include the upper arm, buttocks, and torso (excluding the back and breasts). It has similar efficacy to OCPs but may be less effective in women weighing more than 90 kg (198 lb). In the rare instance of patch detachment, it must be replaced. The progesterone in the patch may decrease the severity of acne.
- In addition to the traditional 20 to 35 mcg ethinyl estradiol (EE) OCPs, 30 and 20 mcg EE in combination with the new progestogen *drospirenone* (Yasmin, YAZ, others) are available. Drospirenone has some antimineralocorticoid activity and has been shown to decrease the water retention, negative affect, and appetite changes

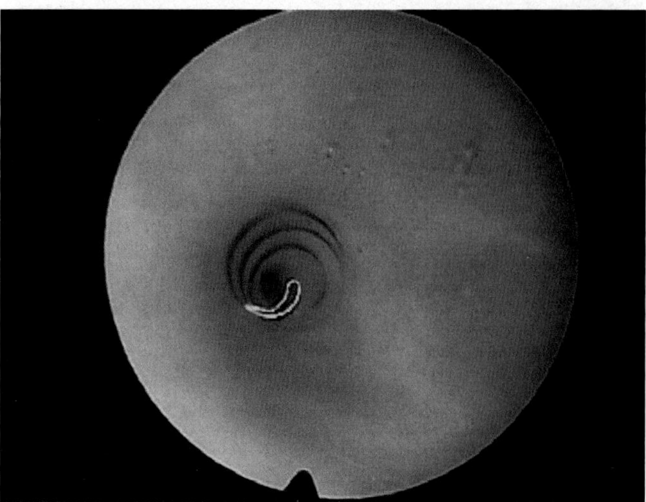

FIGURE 3-6 Hysteroscopic view showing the coiled Essure device within a fallopian tube immediately after it was implanted. *(Reproduced with permission from Jay Berman, MD.)*

that are commonly associated with menstrual cycle changes.[5] Serum potassium levels should be monitored when women are at a risk for hyperkalemia. The progesterone in these pills often helps in decreasing the severity of acne. Beyaz, Safyral, and Rajani are similar but also have the addition of folate. If a patient becomes pregnant while taking these pills, her folate levels would be adequate to prevent neural tube defects.

- *Extended OCP* regimens with 84 days of levonorgestrel-EE pills and 7 days of nonhormonal pills are available. They have similar advantages to other OCPs except that the patient has only four periods a year. Another extended OCP regimen combining levonorgestrel and ethinyl estradiol has been released in which there are no nonhormonal pills at all (Lybrel).
- The *hormonal vaginal ring* (NuvaRing) releases 120 mcg etonogestrel and 15 mcg ethinyl estradiol daily and does not require daily attention (see **Figure 3-1**). It is placed in the vagina for 3 weeks at a time (with 1 week off). Withdrawal bleeding occurs during the ring-free week. The vaginal ring is associated with a lower incidence of breakthrough bleeding than standard OCPs.
- Progestin-only injectable contraceptives (DMPA, 150 mg intramuscularly or 104 mg subcutaneously) are approved for use in the United States. DMPA can be used by women of all ages and is reversible, although return to fertility may be delayed with extended use. Weight gain and bleeding irregularities are known issues with this method.[1] The is a newer form given every 3 months, but given subcutaneously (SQ) instead of intramuscularly (IM). The SQ version provides 30% less hormone, 104 versus 150 mg per injection. It works at least as well as IM preparation does as a contraceptive, and also works as well as Lupron Depot for endometriosis pain with fewer hot flashes and less bone loss. If long-term use is considered, it may be prudent to select another contraceptive, discuss the risk of possible bone loss, or consider monitoring bone density in women using either version of Depo-Provera for more than 2 years. These medications can increase the incidence of acne and weight gain in some women as a result of the androgenic effects of the progesterone.

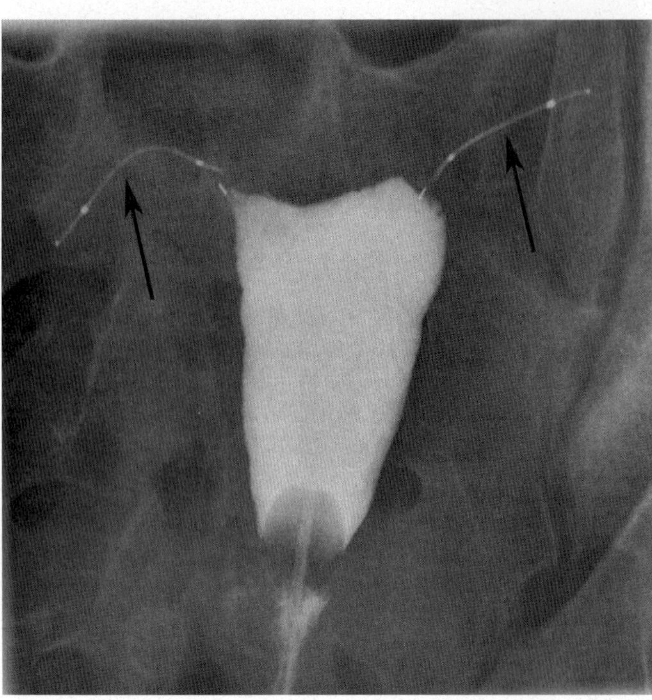

FIGURE 3-7 Hysterosalpingogram (HSG) with bilateral Essure devices within the fallopian tubes (*arrows*). Contrast material distends the uterine cavity but does not enter the cornua, fallopian tubes, or peritoneal cavity, indicating successful occlusion. The black/gray bubble in the white-appearing uterus is the HSG catheter balloon. (*Reproduced with permission from E.J. Mayeaux Jr., MD.*)

LESS EFFECTIVE METHODS

- There are many less effective methods that may be used singly or in combination with other contraceptive methods. Condoms, sponge, withdrawal, and spermicides must be used correctly every time with every sexual encounter. Fertility awareness–based methods (**Table 3-3**) require abstinence from sexual activity or the use of condoms on fertile days.[10] The newest methods such as the Standard Days Method and the Two Day Method may be more effective due to ease of use.[1,11]

STARTING AND SWITCHING METHODS

- Once a desired method is chosen, recommended examinations and tests should be done prior to or with initiation of specific contraceptive method (**Table 3-4**). Performing nonrecommended testing is discouraged, because unnecessary testing may be a barrier to obtaining or using effective contraception.
- Routine pregnancy testing for every woman starting contraception is not necessary.[1] For many patients, a detailed history provides an

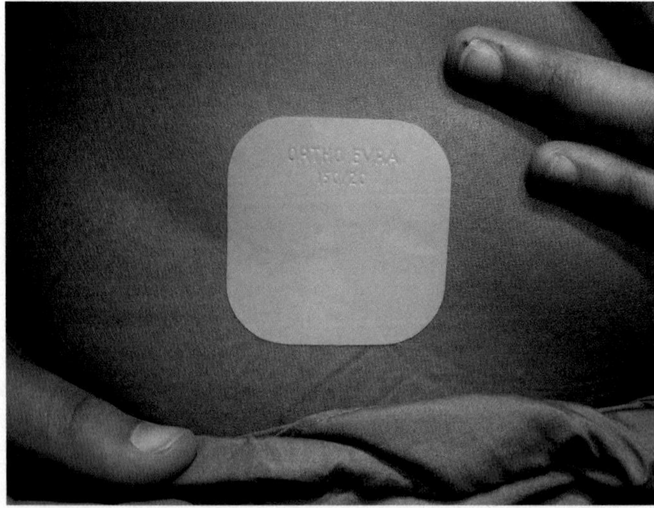

FIGURE 3-8 The Ortho Evra combined hormonal contraceptive patch. The patch is changed weekly for 3 weeks, then left off for 1 week per cycle. (*Reproduced with permission from E.J. Mayeaux, Jr., MD.*)

TABLE 3-3 Natural Family Planning Methods

Method	Description
Basal body temperature charting	Helps identify the menstrual luteal phase by identifying the postovulatory increase in basal body temperature. All other days are of the menstrual cycle are considered fertile
Calendar calculation	Predicts the fertile period by menstrual dating against a standard menstrual cycle
Standard Days Method	A simplified calendar method that assumes a cycle length of 26 to 32 days and sets a 12-day fertile period from days 8 through 19
Cervical mucus monitoring	Identifies the beginning and end of the fertile period by detecting changes in the cervical secretions
Lactational amenorrhea	Uses typical suppression of ovulation during breastfeeding as a method. The effectiveness is limited to 6 months postpartum
Symptothermal method	Based on cervical mucus monitoring; calendar calculations and/or basal body temperature charting monitoring to increase accuracy of identification of the fertile period
Two Day Method	Uses cervical secretions to indicate fertility. The woman checks for cervical secretions at least twice a day. If she notices secretions of any type, color, or consistency either "today" or "yesterday," she considers herself fertile

Data from Smoley BA, Robinson CM. Natural family planning. *Am Fam Physician.* 2012;86(10):924-928 and Germano E, Jennings V. New approaches to fertility awareness-based methods: incorporating the Standard Days and TwoDay Methods into practice. *J Midwifery Womens Health.* 2006;51(6):471-477.

accurate assessment of pregnancy risk in a woman starting a contraceptive method. When history leaves the clinician uncertain of pregnancy status, there are several recommendations from the CDC for establishing reasonable certainty on a negative pregnancy status. These criteria are highly accurate with a negative predictive value of 99% to 100% in ruling out pregnancy among nonpregnant women (**Table 3-5**).[1] If a woman meets at least one of these criteria, the healthcare provider can be reasonably certain that she is not pregnant. A urine pregnancy test may also be done based on clinical judgment of need and bearing in mind the limitations of the accuracy of pregnancy testing. If a woman has had unprotected sexual intercourse within the last 5 days, consider offering emergency contraception (either a Cu-IUD or emergency contraceptive pills) if pregnancy is not desired. Similar considerations must be made when starting or switching contraceptive methods (**Table 3-6**).

PATIENT EDUCATION

For some contraceptive methods to be effective, the patient must be willing to use them consistently and correctly. Other methods do not require any action on the part of the patient. Patients will need to understand the benefits and risks of the method they choose and how to be best assured that the method is working for them. If patients are aware of the possible side effects, they can address any such effect with their physician if an adverse effect occurs.

FOLLOW-UP

Monitor for side effects, level of usage, and tolerability. The contraceptive choice should be periodically reexamined, as the patient may want to switch to a different method of contraception as needs and circumstances change. Assess any changes in health status, including medications, which would change the appropriateness of the contraceptive method. Consider performing an examination to check for the presence of the IUD strings in IUD users.

PATIENT RESOURCES

- Managing Contraception website has a choices section that is good for patients, **http://managingcontraception.com/.**
- CDC website, **https://www.cdc.gov/reproductivehealth/contraception/index.htm.**
- ACOG website, **https://www.acog.org/Patients.**
- Georgetown University Institute for Reproductive Health—Standard Days Method, the TwoDay Method, and the Lactational Amenorrhea Methods, **http://www.irh.org**
- NURX—a website and mobile app that provides easy HIPAA-compliant access to birth control in a number of states in the United States. It involves remote physician review in the patient's state and provides direct delivery to the home, **https://app.nurx.com/**

PROVIDER RESOURCES

- Contraceptive Technology Table of Contraceptive Efficacy, **http://www.contraceptivetechnology.org/table.html.**
- American Family Physician. "New Contraceptive Options," **http://www.aafp.org/afp/20040215/853.html.**
- World Health Organization. *Medical Eligibility Criteria for Contraceptive Use*, **http://www.who.int/reproductivehealth/publications/family_planning/clinical/en/.**

TABLE 3-4 Recommended Examinations and Tests Prior to Initiation of Specific Contraceptive Methods

Examination or Test	Contraceptive Method and Class							
Examination	**LNG and Cu-IUD**	**Implant**	**Injectable**	**CHC**	**POP**	**Condom**	**Diaphragm or Cervical Cap**	**Spermicide**
Blood pressure	C	C	C	A	C	C	C	C
Weight (BMI)	—*	—*	—*	—*	—*	C	C	C
Clinical breast exam	C	C	C	C	C	C	C	C
Bimanual exam and cervical inspection	A	C	C	C	C	C	**	C
Laboratory Test								
Glucose	C	C	C	C	C	C	C	C
Lipids	C	C	C	C	C	C	C	C
Liver enzymes	C	C	C	C	C	C	C	C
Hemoglobin	C	C	C	C	C	C	C	C
Thrombogenic mutations	C	C	C	C	C	C	C	C
Cervical Ca screening	C	C	C	C	C	C	C	C
STD screening	<24 years†	C	C	C	C	C	C	C
HIV screening	C	C	C	C	C	C	C	C

Class A: essential and mandatory in all circumstances for safe and effective use of the contraceptive method.
Class B: contributes substantially to safe and effective use, but implementation may be considered within the public health and/or service context; risk of not performing an examination or test should be balanced against the benefits of making the contraceptive method available.
Class C: does not contribute substantially to safe and effective use of the contraceptive method.
CHC = Combined hormonal contraceptives, IUD = intrauterine device, LNG = levonorgestrel, POP = progestin-only pill; STD = sexually transmitted disease.
*Weight (BMI) measurement is not needed to determine medical eligibility for any method, but measuring weight or BMI at baseline might be helpful for monitoring any changes perceived to be associated with their contraceptive method.
**A bimanual examination (not cervical inspection) is needed for diaphragm fitting.
†Most women do not require additional STD screening at the time of IUD insertion if they have already been screened according to CDC's *STD Treatment Guidelines* (http://www.cdc.gov/std/treatment). If a woman has not been screened according to guidelines, screening can be performed at the time of IUD insertion and insertion should not be delayed. Women with purulent cervicitis or current chlamydial infection or gonorrhea should not undergo IUD insertion.
Data from U.S. Selected Practice Recommendations for Contraceptive Use, 2013: adapted from the World Health Organization. Selected practice recommendations for contraceptive use, 2nd edition. *MMWR Recomm Rep.* 2013; 62(RR-05):1-60.

TABLE 3-5 How to Be Reasonably Certain That a Woman Is Not Pregnant

In a woman who can give a reliable history with no symptoms or signs of pregnancy and any one of the following criteria:

- Is ≤7 days after the start of normal regular menses
- Has not had sexual intercourse since the start of last normal menses
- Has been correctly and consistently using a reliable method of contraception
- Is ≤7 days after spontaneous or induced abortion
- Is within 4 weeks postpartum
- Is fully or nearly fully breastfeeding (≥85% of feedings are breastfeeds), amenorrheic, and <6 months postpartum

TABLE 3-6 When to Start Using Specific Contraceptive Methods and When to Use Backup Contraceptive Methods

Contraceptive Method	When to Start*	Additional Contraception (i.e., Backup) Needed
Copper-containing IUD	Anytime	Not needed
Levonorgestrel-releasing IUD	Anytime	If >7 days after menses started, use backup method or abstain for 7 days.
Implant	Anytime	If >5 days after menses started, use backup method or abstain for 7 days.
Injectable	Anytime	If >7 days after menses started, use backup method or abstain for 7 days.
Combined hormonal contraceptive	Anytime	If >5 days after menses started, use backup method or abstain for 7 days.
Progestin-only pill	Anytime	If >5 days after menses started, use backup method or abstain for 2 days.

*If the provider is reasonably certain the woman is not pregnant.
Data from U.S. Selected Practice Recommendations for Contraceptive Use, 2013: adapted from the World Health Organization selected practice recommendations for contraceptive use, 2nd edition. *MMWR Recomm Rep.* 2013; 62(RR-05):1-60.

REFERENCES

1. Curtis KM, Jatlaoui TC, Tepper NK, et al. U.S. Selected Practice Recommendations for Contraceptive Use, 2016. *MMWR Recomm Rep.* 2016;65(4):1-66.
2. Finer LB, Zolna MR. Declines in unintended pregnancy in the United States, 2008–2011. *N Engl J Med.* 2016;374(9):843-852.
3. Kost K, Singh S, Vaughan B, et al. Estimates of contraceptive failure from the 2002 National Survey of Family Growth. *Contraception.* 2008;77:10.
4. Piccinino LJ, Mosher WD. Trends in contraceptive use in the United States: 1982–1995. *Fam Plann Perspect.* 1998;30:4-10, 46.
5. Raine TR, Foster-Rosales A, Upadhyay UD, et al. One-year contraceptive continuation and pregnancy in adolescent girls and women initiating hormonal contraceptives. *Obstet Gynecol.* 2011; 117(2 Pt 1):363-371.
6. Trussell J. Contraceptive failure in the United States. *Contraception.* 2011;83(5);397-404.
7. Herndon EJ, Zieman M. New contraceptive options. *Am Fam Physician.* 2004;69:853-860.
8. Marnach ML, Long ME, Casey PM. Current issues in contraception. *Mayo Clin Proc.* 2013;88(3):295-299.
9. Steenland MW, Rodriguez MI, Marchbanks PA, Curtis KM. How does the number of oral contraceptive pill packs dispensed or prescribed affect continuation and other measures of consistent and correct use? A systematic review. *Contraception.* 2013;87:605-610.
10. Smoley BA, Robinson CM. Natural family planning. *Am Fam Physician.* 2012;86(10):924-928.
11. Germano E, Jennings V. New approaches to fertility awareness-based methods: incorporating the Standard Days and TwoDay Methods into practice. *J Midwifery Womens Health.* 2006;51(6): 471-477.

4 PREGNANCY AND BIRTH

Beth Choby, MD
Mindy A. Smith, MD, MS
Leslie A. Shimp, PharmD, MS

PATIENT STORY

As a longtime pregnancy care provider, I found it difficult to choose a single story as representative of pregnancy and birth. Most of the stories are meaningful because of the context of the relationship with the woman and the family—a few are tragic and yet filled with grace and the amazing strength displayed by even the very young. Some are truly epic tales, and all are learning opportunities. Pregnancy experiences are filled with consternation at the myriad of changes, discomforts, and worries. They are filled with laughter as women's bodies alter in amazing ways; we waddle, unconsciously rest plates on our bellies, and lose sight of our feet (**Figure 4-1**). Our partners and/or supportive others alternate between reassurance and befuddlement. And then a child appears, miraculously from a space that seems far too small to accommodate, and (regardless of the outcome) a new journey begins.

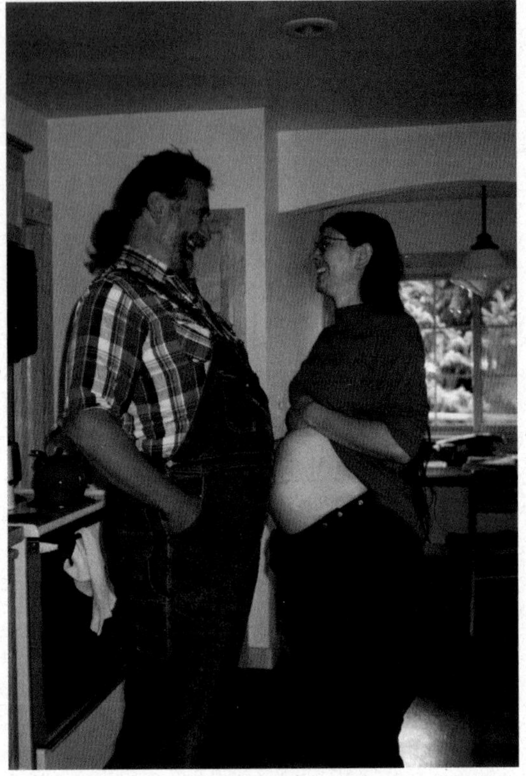

FIGURE 4-1 Dr. Mindy A. Smith and her husband, Gary, touching bellies during Mindy's pregnancy with Jenny.

EPIDEMIOLOGY

- Planned pregnancy—Approximately 85% of sexually active women not using a contraceptive method will become pregnant over the course of a year.
- Unplanned pregnancy—The unintended pregnancy rate in the United States is around 50 pregnancies annually per 1000 women.[1] A single act of intercourse at a random time in the menstrual cycle carries a 4% to 6% risk of pregnancy; risk increases to around 30% if intercourse occurs from 5 days prior to and within 24 hours after ovulation.[2,3]
    - Unintended pregnancy (defined as a mistimed pregnancy or one not desired at the time of conception) can result from lack of use of a contraceptive or contraceptive failure.
    - Unintended pregnancy occurs among women of all ages, socioeconomic status, and marital status. Although unintended pregnancies are often associated with teens, 41% of pregnancies among women 35 to 39 years of age and 51% of those among women older than 40 years are unintended.[4]
    - Some unintended pregnancies end in abortion. A total of 664,435 legally induced abortions occurred in the United States in 2013 (12.5 per 1000 women aged 15 to 44 years; 200 abortions per 1000 live births).[5] During 2004 to 2013, the percentage of abortions in adolescents ages 15–19 years decreased by 31%; rates in other age groups also decreased, with the exception of women over age 40 years, where rates remained stable.[5]
    - Of all abortions for which gestational age was reported, 66% were performed at ≤8 weeks' gestation.[5]
- While maternal mortality has declined dramatically compared to the 1900s, recent data show an increase in the pregnancy-related

mortality ratio (17.8 deaths per 100,000 live births in 2009 compared to 7.2 deaths in 1987).[6] The maternal mortality rate in 2013–2014 in 27 states and the District of Columbia rose significantly from 20.6 maternal deaths per 100,000 live births (2008–2009) to 25.4 in 2013–2014; the rate for mothers over 40 years of age was 269.9—18 times the 14.7 rate in 25- to 29-year-olds.[7] Reasons for this increase are unclear. Use of statewide computerized data linkage, changes in the way death is coded in ICD-10, and the addition of a pregnancy checkbox to the 2003 standard U.S. death certificate may be factors.

 - Traditional causes of pregnancy-related mortality (i.e., hemorrhage, sepsis, hypertensive disorders of pregnancy) have declined, with the emergence of cardiovascular and other medical conditions becoming more important contributors to U.S. maternal mortality. From 2006 to 2009, cardiovascular conditions accounted for over one third of all pregnancy-related deaths. When combined with other medical conditions, they accounted for half of total pregnancy-related deaths.[6]
 - Major racial disparities continue to exist. Maternal mortality (2013–2014) in non-Hispanic black women was 56.3 per 100,000 live births compared with 20.3 per 100,000 live births in non-Hispanic whites and 15.1 per 100,000 live births in Hispanics.[7] African-American women have 2.7 times the risk of pregnancy-related death compared with whites.

- Care delivery by family physicians (**Figure 4-2**)—Nineteen percent of family physicians perform deliveries as a regular part of their practice.[8]
- Care outcomes by family physicians—Several studies compare outcomes between family physicians and obstetricians, primarily for comparable patients at low maternal risk (although proportions of high-risk patients are frequently similar across disciplines). One retrospective population-based Canadian cohort study found a similar risk of perinatal mortality and adverse maternal outcomes in vaginal or cesarean deliveries done by family physicians and obstetricians.[9] Another study comparing cesarean delivery outcomes between rural family physicians and obstetricians found no increased risk to patients when the surgery was performed by family physicians.[10] A 2013 Cochrane review found that most childbirth outcomes did not differ by healthcare provider, including perineal trauma, labor induction/augmentation, cesarean delivery, postpartum hemorrhage, length of stay, Apgar scores, neonatal intensive care admission, or breastfeeding initiation.[11]

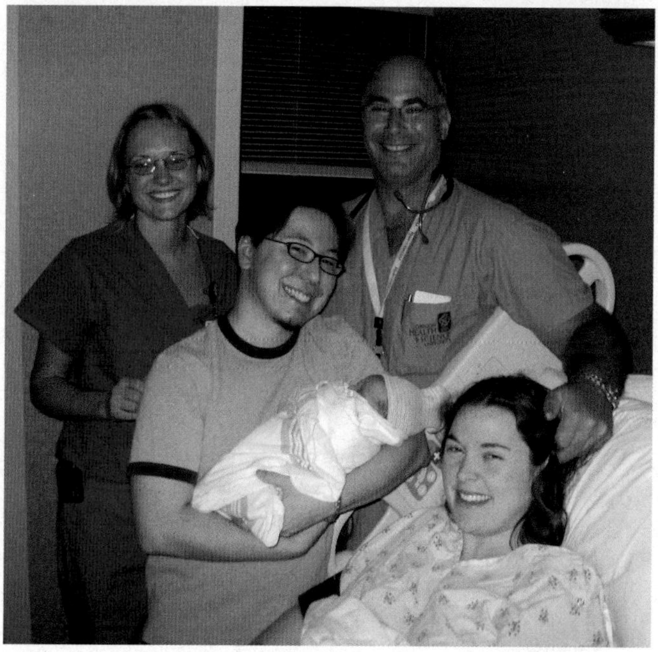

FIGURE 4-2 Family physicians Drs. Scott Fields and Katherine Schlessman have just delivered Jennifer Kam's baby. Dr. Fields has known Jennifer (daughter of Dr. John Saultz—Oregon's Chair of Family Medicine) since she was 6 years old. This is a happy event for all.

ETIOLOGY AND PATHOPHYSIOLOGY

- The most fertile period for women is the several days prior to ovulation and ends 24 hours after ovulation.[12] The ovum can be fertilized for only 12 to 24 hours after ovulation.
- Sperm usually remain viable for 3 days after intercourse.
- Once the egg is fertilized, it is transported to the uterine cavity in approximately 2 to 3 days. Implantation occurs approximately 6 to 7 days after fertilization following cell division that forms a blastocyst.[12]
- Pregnancy is defined by the National Institutes of Health, the American College of Obstetricians and Gynecologists, and the

Food and Drug Administration as implantation of the blastocyst in the endometrium.[13]

- The precise cause of labor is unknown, but the physiologic changes prior to labor onset include decreased placental progesterone secretion and stimulation of prostaglandin production (E_2 and $F_{2\alpha}$) from the decidua, uterine endometrium, and fetal membranes.
- Labor is defined as progressive dilation of the cervix with uterine contractions. Bloody show (blood-tinged mucus from the vagina), indicating extrusion of the mucus plug, often predicts labor onset.

DIAGNOSIS

A detailed menstrual history should be obtained with the goal of accurately determining the first day of the most recent menstrual cycle. This date is traditionally used to calculate the estimated date of delivery (EDD) by using Naegele's rule (EDD = [first day of last menstrual period minus 3 months] plus 7 days). The rule is most useful in women who have regular 28-day cycles followed by an abrupt cessation of menses.

CLINICAL FEATURES

- Common early symptoms include amenorrhea, nausea, fatigue, and breast tenderness.
- Signs of pregnancy include the following:
  - Alterations in the skin (e.g., a hyperpigmented streak appearing below the umbilicus [linea nigra] and a reddish hyperpigmentation over the bridge of the nose and cheeks [chloasma]) (**Figure 4-3**).
  - Alterations in the vulva, vagina, and cervix (i.e., bluish discoloration [Chadwick sign] caused by vascular engorgement of the pelvic organs and softening of the cervix [Hegar sign]).

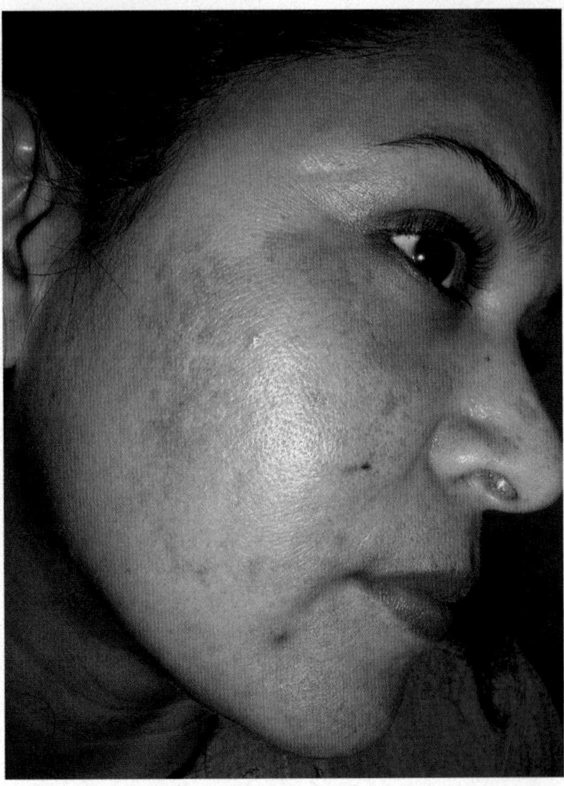

FIGURE 4-3 Chloasma (melasma) in a young woman after having children. This hyperpigmentation over the cheeks and nose is sometimes called the mask of pregnancy. (*Reproduced with permission from Richard P. Usatine, MD.*)

LABORATORY

- Pregnancy tests are an accurate marker for pregnancy. Urine (qualitative) or serum (quantitative) are tested for β-human chorionic gonadotropin (HCG).
  - Urine tests are generally positive around the time of the first missed period. β-HCG concentrations in the range of 5 to 50 mIU/mL are detectable in qualitative urine samples.
  - Home pregnancy test kits detect β-HCG in the urine. β-HCG is detectable within 1 to 2 weeks after fertilization, but a pregnancy cannot be detected prior to implantation. The highest sensitivity (97%) of home pregnancy tests is at 1 week after the first day of the missed period.
  - Serum pregnancy tests detect β-HCG at levels as low as 2 to 4 mIU/mL and mean levels closely correspond with gestational age during the first trimester. In healthy gestations, β-HCG levels double every 1.4 to 2 days, increasing exponentially until the fetus is 8 to 10 weeks old. Levels then decline somewhat and remain steady throughout the pregnancy. A minimum increase of 66% is expected every 48 hours. An appropriate rise in β-HCG levels on two quantitative (serum) pregnancy tests drawn 48 hours apart is reassuring for normal pregnancy development.

IMAGING

- Transvaginal ultrasound may be used to confirm and date a pregnancy. Sonographic landmarks such as the gestational sac and fetal pole correlate highly with β-HCG levels.
    - The gestational sac is generally seen when the pregnancy is 4.5 to 5 weeks along and the β-HCG level is greater than 1000 mIU/mL.
    - The double decidual sign is a thick, hyperechoic (white) ring that surrounds the gestational sac. The yolk sac is the early nourishment for the embryo, seen at 6 weeks when β-HCG levels are greater than 2500 mIU/mL.
    - The fetal pole is seen at 7 weeks' gestation with β-HCG levels more than 5000 mIU/mL.
    - Ultrasound measurements of the gestational sac and the crown to rump length (**Figure 4-4**) of the fetus are a very accurate means of establishing the EDD. First trimester transvaginal ultrasound confirms gestational age within ±5–7 days.

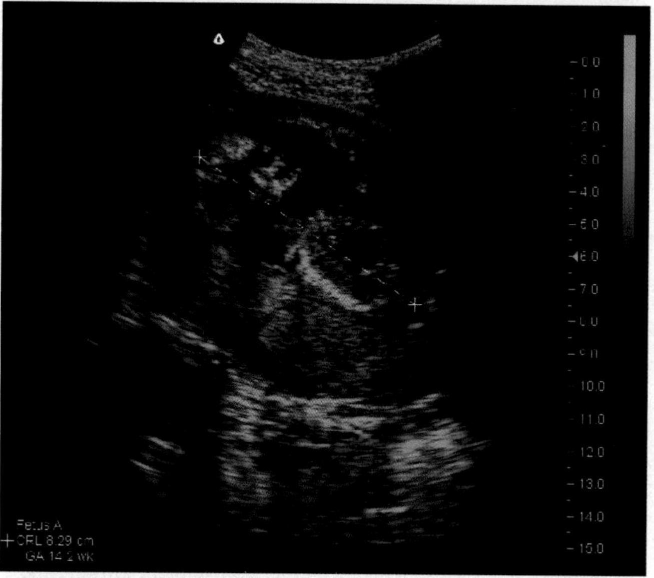

FIGURE 4-4 First trimester ultrasound showing crown to rump length. *(Reproduced with permission from Richard P. Usatine, MD.)*

DIFFERENTIAL DIAGNOSIS

The differential diagnosis of pregnancy includes several gynecologic and nongynecologic conditions. Conditions presenting with an enlarged uterus or abdominal mass include the following:

- Uterine leiomyomas—benign tumors arising from uterine smooth muscle cells. Although most women with symptomatic leiomyomas are in the age range of 30 to 40 years, tumors are occasionally found in adolescents. Myomas occur as single or multiple tumors and range in size from microscopic to large masses. A 20-cm myoma often mimics pregnancy with increased abdominal girth and fullness, but can be distinguished on ultrasound.
- Large adnexal masses and tuboovarian abscesses (TOAs)—The bimanual examination often distinguishes between an adnexal mass and an enlarged uterus. TOA is associated with cervical motion tenderness and abdominal pain. Both conditions can be further evaluated by transvaginal ultrasonography.

Conditions that can present with amenorrhea include the following:

- Hyperthyroidism (see Chapter 236, Graves Disease and Goiter)—Reproductive symptoms can include hypomenorrhea, irregular menses, infertility, and decreased libido. Graves disease is the most common cause among younger patients and common symptoms are nervousness, fatigue, heat intolerance, and tachycardia. Hyperthyroidism is confirmed by a subnormal or undetectable level of thyroid-stimulating hormone (TSH) and elevated level of thyroxine (T_4).
- Sheehan syndrome is a form of acquired hypopituitarism; pituitary apoplexy (sudden neurologic impairment resulting from cerebrovascular disorder) can occur in the postpartum period and may result in severe hypoglycemia and hypotension. Acute symptoms include severe headache and bilateral visual changes; long-term symptoms depend on which hormones are deficient (i.e., TSH, follicle-stimulating hormone [FSH], and luteinizing hormone [LH]; prolactin; adrenocorticotropin hormone [ACTH]; and growth hormone [GH]) and the extent of the hormone deficiency. Diagnosis is

made when low levels of trophic hormones are seen in conjunction with low levels of target hormones.

- Premature menopause—Menopause, defined as permanent amenorrhea in a previously cycling woman, is considered premature when it occurs before the age of 40 years; approximately 10% of women are menopausal by the age of 46 years. Vasomotor symptoms (e.g., hot flashes) and menstrual irregularity usually precede cessation of menses, the latter by approximately 4 years. An FSH level greater than 40 mIU/mL helps to confirm, but may drop again if ovulatory cycles return.

Conditions that can present with symptoms of pregnancy include the following:

- Ectopic pregnancy is an important diagnosis to exclude in women with a positive pregnancy test, abdominal pain, or vaginal bleeding. Transvaginal ultrasound in combination with serial β-HCG measurements is useful to delineate between intrauterine and ectopic gestation. Heterotopic pregnancies (i.e., concomitant intrauterine and ectopic pregnancies) are seen in 1 in 30,000 gestations.
- Pseudopregnancy is a psychiatric condition in which a woman thinks she is pregnant when she is not. She may have symptoms and behaviors consistent with a diagnosis of pregnancy, including weight gain, abdominal pain, and sensations of fetal movement. Confirmatory lab work is negative, although the woman often cannot be convinced of these results.

MANAGEMENT

- Decision-making—Many women and their partners find themselves facing an unplanned pregnancy. Options include continuing the pregnancy and caring for the infant, continuing the pregnancy and placing the infant with an adoptive family, or ending the pregnancy via medical or surgical abortion. Couples need support and information to assist them with this decision.
- Methods to prevent or terminate an unwanted pregnancy include the following:
    - Emergency contraceptives (ECs)—These oral methods can be used after unprotected intercourse or contraceptive failure to prevent pregnancy. These agents are not abortifacients and prevent pregnancy by preventing or delaying ovulation. They do not disrupt an already established pregnancy and are considered to have little to no influence on postovulation events.[14] There are no evidence-based medical contraindications to their use.
        - The levonorgestrel product Plan B One-Step reduces the likelihood of pregnancy by 95% if taken within 24 hours, 85% within 24–48 hours, and 58% if taken within 49–72 hours of unprotected intercourse.[15] Clinical trials demonstrate reasonable efficacy rates up to 120 hours postcoitus. Side effects include heavier menstrual bleeding (31%) and nausea (14–23%). The standard dosing regimen is one 1.5-mg tablet as soon as possible within 72 hours of unprotected intercourse. Levonorgestrel single dose (Plan B One-step; Take action; Next Choice one dose; My way; After pill; After a EContra EZ) has been available as a nonprescription product without age restrictions since 2013. It is less effective in women with a body mass index (BMI) over 25 and ineffective for women with a BMI over 30 kg/m^2 (failure rate of 5.8%).[15] The mechanism of action is delay/inhibition of ovulation. It does not affect an existing pregnancy and will not harm a fetus.
        - Ulipristal acetate (ella) is a selective progesterone receptor modulator that is also FDA approved as an emergency contraceptive for use for up to 5 days after unprotected intercourse or contraceptive failure. It is given as a single 30-mg dose; ella is only available by prescription. The most common side effects include mild to moderate headache, nausea, dysmenorrhea, and abdominal pain. The mechanism of action is prevention/delay of the LH surge and follicular rupture with delay of ovulation in 79% of cases. Ella is more effective than levonorgestrel 72 to 120 hours after unprotected intercourse.[16] Ella may make progestin-based contraceptives less effective, so a barrier method of birth control (e.g., condom) should be used in addition to hormonal contraceptives for the remainder of that same menstrual cycle.
        - Use of oral contraceptives containing ethinyl estradiol, plus either levonorgestrel or norgestrel, is the least effective method with the most side effects. It is not considered first-line EC and should be offered as the last option if other methods are unavailable.
    - Medical abortion (i.e., use of medications to induce an abortion)—Medical abortions account for 20.8% of the abortions performed in the United States.[17] Medical abortion is an option for women who wish to terminate a pregnancy up to 70 days' gestation (calculated from the first day of the last menstrual period). The efficacy of the various regimens ranges from 88% to 99%. Regimens including 200 mg of oral mifepristone followed by 800 mcg of misoprostol vaginally from 6 to 8 hours to 72 hours afterwards been shown to be most effective with fewer side effects and lower cost. SOR Ⓐ Side effects of medical abortion using mifepristone and misoprostol include nausea (20% to 52%), thermoregulatory dysfunction (i.e., warmth, fever, chills, hot flashes; 9% to 56%), dizziness (12% to 37%), headache (10% to 37%), vomiting (5% to 30%), and diarrhea (1% to 27%).[18]
    - Surgical (aspiration) abortion—This method can be performed in the office up to 13 weeks' gestation and has a low rate of major complications. A Cochrane review found no data showing that any one procedure (manual or electrical vacuum aspiration or dilation and curettage) is superior.[19]
- Pregnancy care—Despite the widespread use of prenatal care, evidence of its effectiveness is limited. Prenatal care offered by family physicians likely benefits both maternal and infant health by encouraging long-term health maintenance within a continuity relationship and increasing the likelihood that those infants receive timely care. Routine visits provide opportunities for screening, management of complications, anticipatory guidance, and educational activities.
    - First trimester care includes a detailed history to identify medical, health habit, and prior pregnancy problems requiring management (e.g., use of safer medications for pregnancy, smoking cessation, prior gestational diabetes).

An initial pelvic examination is appropriate to detect anatomic defects of the reproductive tract and to screen for gonorrhea and chlamydia.

Screening laboratory tests include blood type (D [Rh] factor), hepatitis B surface antigen, Venereal Disease Research Laboratory (VDRL) (syphilis), urine culture, and human immunodeficiency virus (HIV) for high-risk women. SOR Ⓐ

Blood pressure and weight are monitored.

Folic acid–fortified multivitamin supplements once daily are recommended. SOR Ⓐ Authors of a Cochrane review found that use of multivitamin supplements provided consistent protection against neural tube defects, although no clear benefit for other birth defects (e.g., congenital cardiovascular defects, cleft lip, or miscarriage) was demonstrated.[20] Folic acid (400 to 800 mcg/day) ideally should be started in the preconception period and continued during pregnancy.

Iron supplementation of at least 30 mg of elemental iron is recommended orally daily (may start in the second trimester). SOR Ⓒ Although demonstrated to increase hemoglobin levels in maternal blood in both the antenatal and postnatal periods, there is limited information related to clinical maternal and infant outcomes.[21]

Common chronic medical conditions that may require treatment modification or more intense monitoring include asthma (e.g., lowest dose of steroids and stress-dose coverage in labor), hypertension (e.g., safer medication such as α-methyldopa and discontinuation of diuretics [metabolic abnormalities] and angiotensin-converting enzyme inhibitors [adverse fetal effects]), thyroid disease (e.g., increased thyroid hormone dose is usually needed), and seizure disorders (e.g., anticonvulsant teratogen risk; 50% have worsening seizures).

- Second trimester care includes continued monitoring, support, and education. Women should be queried about new symptoms and fears, including direct questions about intimate partner violence (present in up to 20% of pregnant women).

Routine measurement of maternal weight, blood pressure, fundal height, and fetal heart tones are conducted. SOR Ⓒ

Second trimester screening includes counseling regarding maternal serum tests. The quadruple test combines serum markers of maternal serum α-fetoprotein, estriol, β-HCG, and inhibin A, and detects 86% of infants with Down syndrome (trisomy 21), with a false positive rate of 8.2%. Cell free fetal DNA (cffDNA; Materni T21) screening is an option for women older than age 35 years or with increased risk for aneuploidy. It can be performed any time after 9–10 weeks' gestation.[22] CffDNA is not recommended in low-risk pregnancies. Women with abnormal screening should undergo diagnostic ultrasound and be offered amniocentesis. One-hour Glucola (gestational diabetes) and an antibody screen for Rh-negative women are obtained around gestational age of 24–28 weeks.

Ultrasound at 18 to 20 weeks' gestation is standard of care in many regions; however, current evidence fails to associate routine ultrasound screening in pregnancy with improved fetal outcomes.[23]

Counseling to encourage a healthful diet and moderate exercise.

- Third trimester care includes preparation for birth and newborn care, monitoring, and support.

Evidence-based recommendations include repeat screening for hepatitis B, syphilis, gonorrhea, and chlamydia in high-risk populations (i.e., women younger than age 25 years with two or more sexual contacts, women who are sex workers, and women with prior history of syphilis or gonorrhea) and universal screening for group B streptococcus (GBS) at 35 to 37 weeks' gestation.

Breastfeeding for 6 months should be encouraged and birth preferences discussed (**Figure 4-5**).

Childbirth classes are often recommended, but evidence supporting their benefit is lacking.

- Labor and birthing:

Labor—Labor is defined as regular uterine contractions and progressive cervical dilation. Effacement, the process of thinning of the cervix, occurs before and during labor. Traditionally, labor is classified by three stages:

a. First stage is divided into latent (1 to 24+ hours), characterized by milder and less frequent contractions, and active, where the cervix dilates from 4 cm to complete (10 cm), characterized by stronger, regular contractions lasting 60 seconds or more. Research suggests that active labor may begin once 6 cm cervical dilation is reached. Recommendations for duration of first stage labor have been lengthened, permitting a slower rate of cervical change prior to arrest of descent being diagnosed.[24]
b. Second stage begins with complete cervical dilation and ends with the birth of the baby—averaging 20 minutes in multiparas and 50 minutes in primiparas.
c. Third stage is from the delivery of the baby to delivery of the placenta (up to 30 minutes is considered normal).

Birthing requires flexibility and patience. Traditional labor interventions such as withholding food and drink, giving enemas, and perineal shaving have no evidence to support their routine use. Many options are available to increase comfort and ease the process of labor and birth. For example:

a. Ambulation and frequent position changes (e.g., side, upright) during labor.
b. The presence of a supportive labor companion (e.g., partner, doula).
c. Pain control options include supportive others, physical contact, massage, warm showers, inhaled nitrous oxide, opioid pain control, and regional analgesia (e.g., blocks and epidurals). Authors of a Cochrane review of 38 studies involving 9658 women found epidural anesthesia, compared most often to opioid use during labor, provided better pain relief but an increased risk of instrumental delivery.[25] In a second Cochrane review of 15,752 women, there was no difference in duration of the second stage of labor, risk for instrumented (vacuum or forceps) delivery, cesarean delivery, or infant Apgar scores in women receiving "early" vs. "late epidurals" (<4–5 cm cervical dilation vs. >4–5 cm dilation, respectively).[26]

There is no evidence to support routine electronic fetal monitoring, episiotomy, or supine birth positions.[27]

Women who are culture positive for GBS should receive antibiotic prophylaxis when in labor (e.g., intravenous penicillin G [PCN G] in nonallergic women).

PATIENT EDUCATION

- Pregnancy detection with home pregnancy test kits—The first morning urine is the best specimen for testing. The most accurate results are obtained by waiting at least 1 week after the date of the expected period to test. Common reasons for a false-negative test include testing too early (i.e., on or before the first day of a missed period), using a waxed cup for urine collection, soap residue in the container used to collect urine, or testing refrigerated urine.
- Pregnancy prevention—Use of contraceptives dramatically reduces the likelihood of unplanned pregnancy (only 9% of women per year using oral contraceptives become pregnant, and of women whose partners are using a condom only 18% become pregnant).[28] Many pregnancies occur when a woman discontinues a contraceptive method and does not begin use of another method prior to intercourse; women should be encouraged to have a backup method they can use if the chosen method proves unsatisfactory (see Chapter 3, Family Planning) and should be educated about the availability of emergency contraception.
- Abortion choices—Since the FDA approval of mifepristone for elective first trimester termination, medical abortion is increasingly common. In 2013, approximately 20% of abortions were performed using combinations of mifepristone and/or misoprostol.[5]
- Pregnancy planning begins with preconception care, ideally occurring 3 to 6 months prior to conception, to discuss health promotion, risk assessment, and medical intervention.
- Environmental exposures that adversely affect the fetus should be minimized (e.g., pesticides, paint thinner/strippers, fertilizers, and heavy metals). Women who work in hospital settings should avoid exposure to ionizing radiation, chemotherapeutic agents, and misoprostol.
- Intake of 400 mcg/day of folic acid prior to and during the early part of pregnancy reduces the risk of neural tube defects. SOR Ⓐ
- Certain heritable genetic diseases can be diagnosed in individuals prior to becoming pregnant (e.g., sickle cell disease, cystic fibrosis).
- Optimal treatment of chronic medical conditions (e.g., diabetes, epilepsy, hypertension) may reduce fetal loss and adverse effects. Switching to the least teratogenic medication options available to effectively treat the condition is critical.
- Smoking cessation and alcohol avoidance should be encouraged.
- Immunizations (e.g., rubella, varicella) can be provided.
- Patients should be encouraged to discuss their delivery preferences and their practitioner's practice style with respect to the routine use of technology.

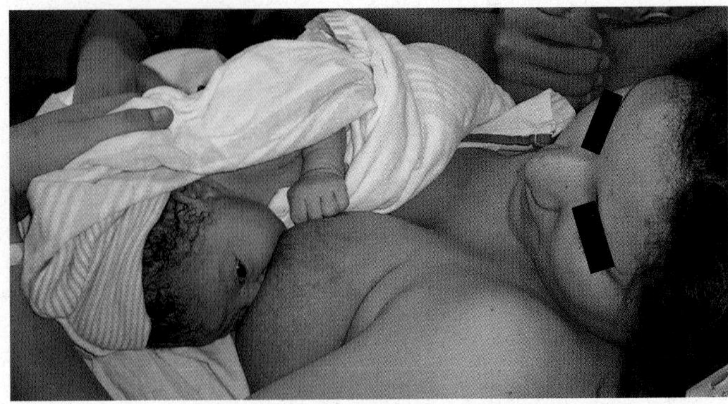

FIGURE 4-5 We are privileged to observe this newborn baby breastfeeding for the first time immediately after the delivery performed by Dr. Richard P. Usatine. (*Reproduced with permission from Richard P. Usatine, MD.*)

PATIENT RESOURCES

- **https://womenshealth.gov/pregnancy/**
- **https://ec.princeton.edu/questions/dose.html**

PROVIDER RESOURCES

- **https://www.nlm.nih.gov/medlineplus/pregnancy.html**
- **https://www.cdc.gov/pregnancy/**
- **https://www.cdc.gov/ncbddd/pregnancy_gateway/index.html**

REFERENCES

1. Finer LB, Zolna MR. Unintended pregnancy in the United States: incidence and disparities. *Contraception.* 2011;84:478-485.
2. Wilcox AJ, Dunson DB, Weinberg CR, et al. Likelihood of conception with a single act of intercourse: providing benchmark rates for assessment of post-coital contraceptives. *Contraception.* 2001;63:211-215.
3. Glasier A, Cameron ST, Blithe D, et al. Can we identify women at risk of pregnancy despite using emergency contraception? Data from randomized trials of ulipristal acetate and levonorgestrel. *Contraception.* 2011;84:363-367.
4. Seibert C, Barbouche E, Fagan J, et al. Prescribing oral contraceptives for women older than 35 years of age. *Ann Intern Med.* 2003;138:54-64.
5. Jatlaoui TC, Ewing A, Mandel MG, et al. Abortion surveillance—United States 2013. *MMWR Surveill Summ.* 2016;65(12):1-44.
6. Creanga AA, Berg CJ, Ko JY, et al. Maternal mortality and morbidity in the United States: where are we now? *J Women's Health.* 2014;23(1):3-9.
7. MacDorman MF, Declercq E, Thoma ME. Trends in maternal mortality by sociodemographic characteristics and cause of death in 27 states and the District of Columbia. *Obstet Gynecol.* 2017;129(5):811-818.
8. American Academy of Family Physicians. *Facts About Family Medicine. 2015.* Leawood, KS: American Academy of Family Physicians, 2015.
9. Aubrey-Bassler K, Cullen RM, Simms A, et al. Outcomes of deliveries by family physicians or obstetricians: a population-based cohort study using an instrumental variable. *CMAJ.* 2015;187(15): 1125-1130.
10. Homan FF, Olson AL, Johnson DJ. A comparison of cesarean delivery outcomes for rural family physicians and obstetricians. *J Am Board Fam Med.* 2013;26(4):366-372.
11. Sandall J, Soltani H, Gates S, et al. Midwife-led continuity models versus other models of care for childbearing women. *Cochrane Database Syst Rev.* 2013;(8):CD004667.
12. Hatcher RA, Namnoun AB. The menstrual cycle. In: Hatcher RA, Trussell J, Stewart FH, et al, eds. *Contraceptive Technology*, 20th ed. New York: Ardent Media; 2012:69-76.
13. Stewart FH, Trussell J, Van Look PFA. Emergency contraception. In: Hatcher RA, Trussell J, Stewart FH, et al, eds. *Contraceptive Technology*, 18th ed. New York: Ardent Media; 2004:279-303.
14. Batur P, Kransdorf LN, Casey PM. Emergency contraception. *Mayo Clinical Proc.* 2016;91(6):802-807.
15. Rome ES, Issac V. Sometimes you do get a second chance. Emergency contraception for adolescents. *Pediatr Clin N Am.* 2017;64:371-380.
16. Mazza D. Ulipristal acetate: an update for Australian GPs. *Royal Coll Aust GP.* 2017;46(5):301-304.
17. Pazol K, Creanga AA, Jamieson DJ. Abortion surveillance—United States, 2012. *MMWR.* 2015;64(SS10):1-40.
18. ACOG practice bulletin. Clinical management guidelines of obstetrician-gynecologists. Number 67, October 2005. Medical management of abortion. *Obstet Gynecol.* 2005;106(4):871-882.
19. Kulier R, Cheng L Fekih A, et al. Surgical methods for first trimester termination of pregnancy. *Cochrane Database Syst Rev.* 2009;(3):CD002900.
20. De-Regil LM, Pena-Rosas JP, Fernandez-Gaziola AC, et al. Effects and safety of periconceptional supplementation for preventing birth defects. *Cochrane Database Syst Rev.* 2015;14(12):CD007950.
21. Pena-Rosas JP, De-Regil LM, Garcia-Casal MN, et al. Daily oral iron supplementation during pregnancy. *Cochrane Database Syst Rev.* 2015;7:CD004736.
22. Dashe J. Aneuploidy screening in pregnancy. *Obstet Gynecol.* 2016;128(1):181-194.
23. Ewigman BG, Crane JP, Frigoletto FD, et al. Effect of prenatal ultrasound screening on perinatal outcome. RADIUS Study Group. *N Engl J Med.* 1993;329:821-827.
24. Spong C, Berghella V, Wenstrom KD, et al. Preventing the first cesarean delivery: summary of a joint Eunice Kennedy Shriver National Institute of Child Health and Human Development, Society for Maternal-Fetal Medicine and American College of Obstetricians and Gynecologists Workshop. *Obstet Gynecol.* 2012;120(5):1181-1193.
25. Anim-Somuah M, Smyth RMD, Jones L. Epidural versus non-epidural or no analgesia in labour. Cochrane Database Syst Rev. 2011;(12):CD000331.
26. Sng BL, Leong WL, Zeng Y, et al. Early versus late initiation of epidural analgesia for labour. *Cochrane Database Syst Rev.* 2014;(10):CD007238.
27. Berghella V, Baxter JK, Chauhan SP. Evidence-based labor and delivery management. *Am J Obstet Gynecol.* 2008;199(5): 445-454.
28. Planned Parenthood. *All About Birth Control Methods.* https://www.plannedparenthood.org/learn/birth-control. Accessed May 2017.

5 END OF LIFE

Radha Raman Murthy Gokula, MD, CMD
Mindy A. Smith, MD, MS

PATIENT STORY

A 72-year-old woman is being cared for at home at the end of life. She is dying from metastatic breast cancer. She is a social worker and planned meticulously for her end of life, including choosing home hospice, designating her medical power of attorney, and completing her last will and testament. The home hospice nurse visits daily and helps with many aspects of comfort care during her remaining days. In between visits, her family helps her stay clean and comfortable as she is now bedbound. They bring her water to sip, and soft food and medications as needed. Her doctor in conjunction with the hospice program has provided liquid morphine and a liquid benzodiazepine that helps tremendously with her pain and anxiety. The family members are able to administer these medications according to the schedule provided by the hospice nurse. The metastatic cancer has spread to many bones and leg muscles, and in the last weeks the morphine and benzodiazepine have truly contributed to her comfort. The hospice program has provided a music thanatologist to play the harp for her now that it is clear that her death is imminent **(Figure 5-1)**. In the last hours of her life, the family plays her favorite music as she peacefully passes away with her two sons on either side of the bed, each holding a hand.

Music thanatology uses harp and voice at the bedside to provide live music that attempts to respond to the patient's physiologic needs. Authors of a before-and-after study of 65 patients found that patients had decreased levels of agitation and wakefulness, and breathing was slower and deeper after the music vigil.[1] In another paper, family members reported benefits for both themselves and their loved one, with perceived improvement in the patient's breathing, relaxation, pain, and ability to sleep.[2]

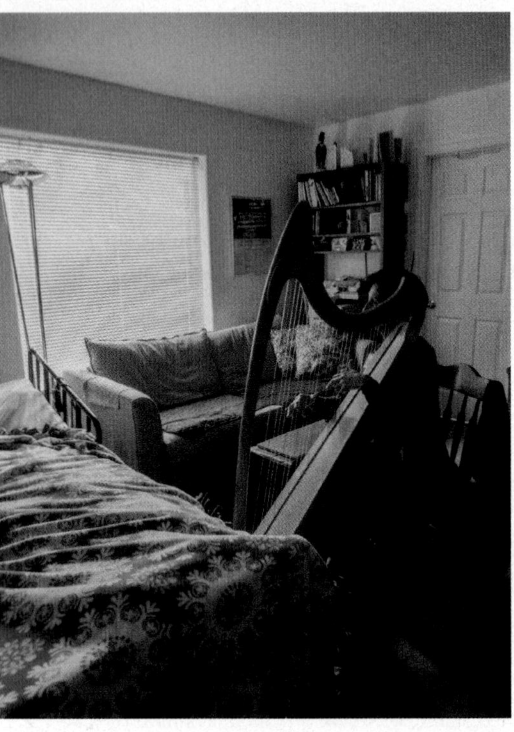

FIGURE 5-1 Music thanatologist playing the harp at the bedside of a dying woman on home hospice. Her family members are also listening as the woman both plays the harp and sings to comfort the patient. *(Reproduced with permission from Richard P. Usatine, MD.)*

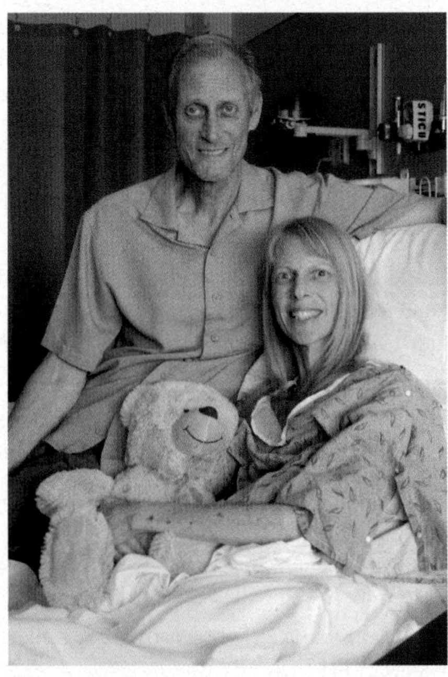

FIGURE 5-2 This 53-year-old woman is on the palliative care service at the hospital. She has been battling B cell lymphoma. Her husband is very supportive. She told her provider, "I don't know when I'm going to be able to go home, and I'm scared of having to come back. . . . But I have faith. Things will work out as they should." *(Reproduced with permission from Bryant Huang.)*

INTRODUCTION

End-of-life care is care delivered to patients of all ages who have a very short life expectancy **(Figure 5-2)**. This care is focused on meeting the patient's emotional and physical needs for symptom relief and general comfort care and offering patient and family support. Patients at the end of life are fragile and require complex care and, therefore, are at higher risk of compromised safety, medical complications, and medical errors. Addressing these issues requires different approaches—patient and family preferences and quality of life are key factors in the balance between safety and quality of life. Early referral to palliative care, along with concurrent treatment, is vital to optimizing outcomes.

The five basic principles of palliative care are:[3]

1. Respect the goals, preferences, and choices of the person.
2. Look after their medical, emotional, social, and spiritual needs.
3. Support the needs of family members.

TABLE 5-1 Elements of Palliative Care and Domains of End-of-Life Quality of Care

Palliative Care Elements	Quality of Care Domains
• Improve family and caregiver relationship	• Physical and emotional symptom management
• Symptom management	• Support of function, autonomy, personal dignity, and self-respect
• Education and prognostication to align with treatment goals	• Advanced care planning
• Supportive care	• Aggressive symptom control near death
• Assistance with advance directives	• Patient and family satisfaction
• Care coordination with other specialists	• Patient's assessment of overall quality of life and well-being
• Referrals with interprofessional team members	• Family burden—emotional and financial
• Provider continuity	• Survival time
• Bereavement services	• Provider continuity and skill
• Shared decision-making	• Bereavement services

Information from Lynn J. Measuring quality of care at the end of life: a statement of principles. *J Am Geriatr Soc.* 1997;45:526-527; Virdun C, Luckett T, Davidson PM, Phillips J. Dying in the hospital setting: a systematic review of quantitative studies identifying the elements of end-of-life care that patients and their families rank as being most important. *Palliat Med.* 2015;29(9):774-796.

4. Help patients and their families access needed healthcare providers and appropriate care settings.
5. Provide excellence in care at the end of life.

Elements of palliative care and the quality-of-care domains for end of life are shown in **Table 5-1**.

EPIDEMIOLOGY

- In 2015, life expectancy at birth was 78.8 years for the total U.S. population.[4] For males, life expectancy changed from 76.5 years in 2014 to 76.3 years in 2015. For females, life expectancy decreased 0.1 year from 81.3 years in 2014 to 81.2 years in 2015.
- In 2013 the proportion of persons over 80 years of age was 13.7% and was projected to reach 20.9% in 2050.[5]
- According to National Health Center statistics, there were approximately 2.63 million deaths in the United States in 2015.[4] The 10 leading causes of death (heart disease, cancer, chronic lower respiratory diseases, unintentional injuries, stroke, Alzheimer disease, diabetes, influenza and pneumonia, kidney disease, and suicide) remained the same as in 2014. These 10 leading causes accounted for 74.2% of all deaths in the United States in 2015.[6]
- The 2015 U.S. infant mortality rate was 589.5 infant deaths per 100,000 live births.
- The age breakdown for causes of death in 2014 are as follows:[7]
  - For children ages 1 to 9 years, leading causes of death were accidents (31.5%), other, cancer, congenital malformations, homicide, heart disease, and influenza and pneumonia.
  - Among patients ages 10 to 24 years, leading causes of death were external causes (i.e., accidents, homicide, and suicide), followed by cancer and heart disease. As age increases, there is a trend toward chronic conditions being responsible for deaths.
  - The major causes of death in the population ages 25 to 44 years were accidents, other, cancer, heart disease, suicide, homicide, and chronic liver disease.
  - For those ages 45 to 64 years, leading causes of death were cancer, heart disease, other, accidents, liver disease, and chronic respiratory diseases.
  - The common causes of death in persons older than age 65 years are heart disease, other, cancer, chronic lower respiratory disease, stroke, and Alzheimer disease.
- About one-third of all deaths in the United States in 2000 and 2010 were inpatient hospital deaths.[8] Average length of stay for patients who died was 7.9 days compared to 4.8 days for all patients in 2010.

According to data from the National Hospice and Palliative Care Organization, 44.6% of all deaths in the United States were under the care of a hospice program, with an estimated 1.65 million patients receiving hospice care.[9]

- Although whites have traditionally used hospice services more than blacks, authors of a study of Medicare beneficiaries in North and South Carolina who died in 2008 found a racial disparity in hospice use in only 30% of their 128 counties; in these counties, the mean proportion of whites vs. blacks enrolled in hospice was 41.3% vs. 28.7%.[10] Counties with a racial disparity had more hospital beds and specialists, suggesting that blacks may be more likely to use acute care services at end of life.

ETIOLOGY AND PATHOPHYSIOLOGY

Although the causes of death are multifactorial, the following are the major modifiable contributors:

- Tobacco use—Of all adults in the United States in 2015, 15.1% smoke cigarettes; more adult men smoke than adult women (16.7%

vs. 13.6%, respectively) and the highest smoking rates are among adults ages 25 to 44 years (17.7%) and American Indians/Alaska Natives (21.9%).[11] It is estimated that nearly 1 of every 5 deaths each year in the United States is attributable to smoking.[12] Smoking increases the risk of developing emphysema (10- to 13-fold), heart and cardiovascular disease (2- to 4-fold), and many cancers (1.4- to 3-fold).[11]

- Poor diet—Diets that are high in fat (>40% of calories consumed) are associated with increased risk of breast, colon, endometrial, and prostate cancer. Diet is important in controlling diabetes, heart disease, obesity, and chronic renal disease.
- Physical inactivity—Those who exercise regularly live longer and are healthier; exercise reduces the risk of cardiovascular disease and hypertension and improves function in those with depression, osteoarthritis, and fibromyalgia. Unfortunately, as of 2016, only 51.7% of U.S. adults met Physical Activity Guidelines for aerobic activity and only 21.7% met guidelines for both aerobic activity and muscle strengthening.[12a]
- Alcohol consumption—The past-year prevalence of consuming alcohol among adults in the United States, reported in 2009–2011, was 70.5%. Past-month excessive drinking was reported by 35.4% of men and 23.7% of women, and 4.5% of men and 2.5% of women reported alcohol dependence over the past year.[13] Excess alcohol drinking includes binge drinking (4 or more drinks for women and 5 or more drinks for men on a single occasion), heavy drinking (8 or more drinks for women and 15 or more drinks for men per week), drinking while pregnant, or drinking when under age 21 years.[14] Excess consumption (>3 drinks per day) is associated with mood disorders (10% to 40%), cirrhosis (15% to 20%), and neuropathy (5% to 15%); it increases the risk of pancreatitis (3-fold) as well as cancers of the breast (1.4-fold), esophagus (3-fold), and rectum (1.5-fold).[14] In addition, based on data from 2009, an estimated 30.2 million people (12%) ages 12 years or older reported driving under the influence of alcohol at least once in the past year.[15]
- Injury—In 2014, 199,752 people died because of injury, accounting for 7.6% of all deaths.[7] The majority of injury-related deaths are unintentional. Falls are the leading mechanism of injury-related death for elderly people, whereas for adults 35 to 53 years of age, poisoning is the leading mechanism of injury-related death.[16] Motor vehicles in traffic are the leading mechanism of injury-related death for all other age groups, except for children younger than age 2 years.[16] Many of these deaths are preventable.
- Sexual behaviors—Sexually transmitted infections (STIs) are among the most common infectious diseases and affect approximately 20 million people in the United States each year. Sexually transmitted diseases (STDs) are associated with increased risk of HIV/AIDS; in 2014, there were approximately 1.1 million persons living with HIV in the United States.[17] Causes of death from AIDS include infections (especially pulmonary and central nervous system), cancer (especially Kaposi sarcoma and non-Hodgkin lymphoma), cardiomyopathy, and nephropathy.
- Illicit use of drugs—Drug addiction remains a major problem in the United States. The Centers for Disease Control and Prevention report a 2015 prevalence rate of 10.1% for illicit drug use in the past month for those age 12 years and over.[18] According to data from the National Institute on Drug Abuse Monitoring the Future Survey 2016 of 45,473 eighth to 12th grade students, past-month marijuana use was reported by 22.5% of high school seniors, although lifetime use of most illicit drugs (e.g., ecstasy 2.7%, cocaine 2.3%), in addition to cigarettes (10.5% past month) and alcohol (33.2% past month), continues to fall. Misuse of prescription drugs in the past year among 12th graders included amphetamines (6.7%) and opioids other than heroin (4.8%).[19] Cocaine is associated with death from respiratory depression, cardiac arrhythmias, and convulsions; methamphetamine use is associated with life-threatening hypertension, cardiac arrhythmia, subarachnoid and intracerebral hemorrhage, ischemic stroke, convulsions, and coma.
- Microbial agents—Microbial agents remain a major cause of death and disability with continued discovery of new agents and increasing drug resistance. Although it is difficult to ascertain whether an infectious agent caused death or was incidental to death, an expert panel of investigators in New Mexico, based on autopsy data, found that 85% (106 of 125) of the deaths (late 1994 to mid-1996) were identified as infectious-disease related.[20]
- Toxic agents—Toxic agents include poisons and environmental toxins. In the United States in 2015, there were 52,404 poisoning deaths; the vast majority (84%) were unintentional and 10% were suicides.[21] The highest percentage of drug-poisoning deaths involved heroin (a 3-fold increase from 2010); opioid pain medications were involved in 24%. In a 10-year cross-sectional study of drug-related deaths in Wisconsin, 3410 (71%) were unintentional and 1053 (22%) were suicides.[22] The most common drugs identified were opioid analgesics, cocaine, antidepressants, benzodiazepines, and methadone.

DIAGNOSIS

In 2014, apart from cancer, chronic diseases such as cardiovascular disease, chronic respiratory infections, stroke, diabetes mellitus, Alzheimer disease, and nephrotic syndromes were in the top 10 conditions causing death in the United States.[23] Early diagnosis, prognostication, and referral to hospice or palliative care for end-stage disease will help improve quality of life and reduce healthcare costs by avoiding unnecessary hospitalizations and use of treatments that do not work.

Approximately 70% of all deaths are preceded by a disease/condition such that it is reasonable to plan for dying soon. In 2015, the Institute of Medicine published "Dying in America; Improving Quality and Honoring Individual Preferences near End of Life." This document provides guidelines for person-centered, family-oriented palliative and hospice care for patients with chronic illnesses and includes triggers for hospice referral based on patient performance status, clinical signs and types of malignancy.[23] These diseases/conditions include:

- Cancer that is widespread, aggressive, or metastatic and for patients who no longer seek chemotherapy. Other clues include a decline in performance status (Karnofsky score ≤50% where a person needs considerable assistance and medical care, or ECOG performance status ≥3 where a person is confined to bed or wheelchair more than 50% of waking time and capable of only limited self-care) and/

or malignant ascites, multiple brain metastases, malignant bowel obstruction, malignant pleural or pericardial effusions, serum albumin ≤2.5 mg/dL, or meningeal carcinomatosus.[24]

- Dementia with an inability to ambulate, bathe, or dress without assistance; associated urinary or fecal incontinence; inability to meaningfully communicate; or associated with life-threatening infections (e.g., septicemia), multiple stage 3 or 4 skin ulcers, inability to maintain sufficient fluid and calorie intake, or failure to thrive (including a temporal decline in functional status) and 10% weight loss or albumin <2.5 g/dL.
- Patients confined to bed or who require assistance with all basic activities of daily living.
- Patients with a body mass index less than 22 and/or those who refuse or do not respond to enteral or parenteral nutritional support.
- Heart disease that is poorly responsive to optimal medical treatment, New York Heart Association (NYHA) class IV, or congestive heart failure with poor ejection fraction (≤20%) (**Figure 5-3**). Based on data from multiple studies including SUPPORT, Framingham, and IMPROVEMENT, 1-year mortality estimates are as follows: NYHA Class II (mild symptoms), 5% to 10%; Class III (moderate symptoms), 10% to 15%; Class IV (severe symptoms), 30% to 40%. Independent predictors of poor prognosis in patients with heart failure include recent cardiac hospitalization, renal insufficiency (creatinine ≥1.4 mg/dL), systolic blood pressure less than 100 mm Hg and/or pulse greater than 100 beats/min, treatment-resistant ventricular dysrhythmias, treatment resistant-anemia, hyponatremia, cachexia, reduced functional capacity, and comorbidities (e.g., diabetes).[25] Other indicators of poor prognosis include persistent angina despite maximal treatment and ejection fraction less than 20%.
- HIV/AIDS with CD4 count less than 25 or persistent viral load greater than 100,000 copies/mL plus at least one of the following: wasting (loss of 33% of lean body mass); major AIDS-defining refractory infection (e.g., *Cryptosporidium* infection) or malignancy (e.g., central nervous system or systemic lymphoma); progressive multifocal leukoencephalopathy; renal failure; Palliative Performance Status (PPS) less than 50%; advanced AIDS dementia complex; or significant functional decline in the activities of daily living.
- Neurologic disease (e.g., Parkinson disease, amyotrophic lateral sclerosis, multiple sclerosis, muscular dystrophy, and myasthenia gravis) that is associated with rapid progression and/or critical nutritional state, life-threatening infections in the preceding 12 months, stage 3 or 4 skin ulcers, critically impaired breathing capacity and declined ventilator support, or life-threatening complications (e.g., recurrent aspiration, sepsis).
- Pulmonary disease, including disabling dyspnea at rest or with minimal exertion, increased emergency department visits and/or hospitalizations, hypoxemia on room air (oxygen saturation <88%), hypercapnia (PCO_2 >50 mmHg), cor pulmonale, unintentional progressive weight loss, or resting tachycardia greater than 100 beats/min.
- End-stage renal disease with progressive decline in those not seeking dialysis (or not a candidate), with a calculated creatinine clearance less than 10 (<15 for patients with diabetes) or serum creatinine greater than 8 mg/dL (>6 mg/dL for patients with diabetes).

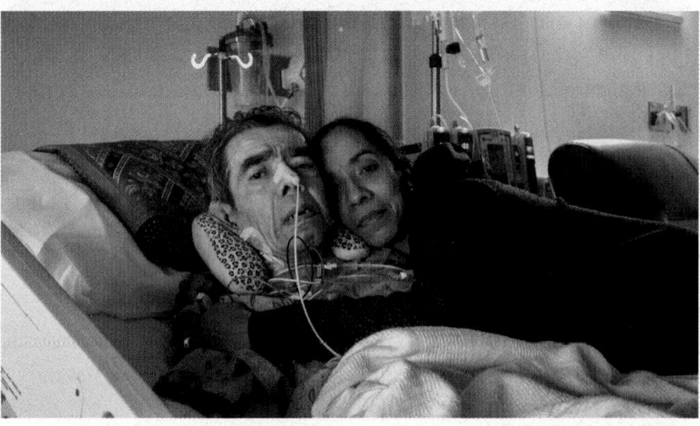

FIGURE 5-3 A 78-year-old man with severe aortic stenosis clings to life while he awaits transfer to home hospice. He is shown here with his daughter and says, "They called the priest to administer the last rites several days ago, but I said no. I'm not leaving my daughter. She's my youngest. I love everything about her. And I have 14 cats waiting for me back home. One day at a time." (*Reproduced with permission from Bryant Huang.*)

- End-stage liver disease with prothrombin time/international normalized ratio (INR) >5 sec/1.5, serum albumin <2.5 g/dL, progressive decline in those with refractory ascites, spontaneous bacterial peritonitis, hepatorenal syndrome, hepatic encephalopathy, or recurrent variceal bleeding despite treatment.
- Stroke associated with coma in the acute phase; coma with abnormal brainstem response, absent verbal response, absent withdrawal response to pain, or serum creatinine greater than 1.5 mg/dL at day 3; dysphagia and insufficient intake of fluids and calories; poor functional status; poststroke dementia; Palliative Performance Scale (PPS) ≤40% with ≥10% weight loss in 6 months or ≥7.5% weight loss in 3 months; serum albumin <2.5 g/dL.
- Nonspecific terminal illness characterized by a rapid decline, disease progression, or progressive weight loss; dysphasia with aspiration; increase in emergency department visits and/or hospitalizations; worsening pressure ulcers despite optimum care; or a decline in systolic blood pressure below 90 mm Hg.

Unfortunately, physicians are often reluctant to make this determination, resulting in palliative and hospice care not being offered until very late during the illness. In addition, physicians often believe that they must be able to predict a life expectancy of less than 6 months with certainty to institute hospice care.

The National Hospice and Palliative Care Organization has evidence-based guidelines available for its members on determining prognosis for many noncancer conditions. Fast-facts are evidence-based guidelines for disease conditions like heart failure and chronic obstructive pulmonary disease (COPD) that are published by the palliative care network of Wisconsin to serve as eligibility for hospice in chronic disease states (www.mypcnow.org/fast-facts). Another resource that includes a prognosis calculator is www.eprognosis.org, maintained by University of California, San Francisco Geriatrics and Palliative Medicine Department.

Two validated instruments that may help clinicians estimate prognosis are the PPS and the Karnofsky Performance Scale (KPS).

- The PPS, version 2 (http://www.palliative.org/NewPC/professionals/tools/pps.html), rates information on ambulation, activity and evidence of disease, self-care, intake, and consciousness level. In a retrospective cohort study, the PPS was found to be a strong predictor of survival when applied at admission to patients in palliative care.[26] In this study, median survival time at PPS of 10% was 1 day, survival with PPS of 20% was 2 days, at PPS of 30% survival was 9 days, while at PPS of 60% median survival was 40 days. In a more recent study of PPS rating and survival among outpatients with advanced cancer, median survival for patients with PPS ratings of 70, 60, and 50 were approximately 6, 3, and 2 months, respectively, but only 24% of survival estimates were accurate.[27] The authors suggest that the PPS score be used for care discussions.
- The KPS (http://www.hospicepatients.org/karnofsky.html) is often used to follow the course of illness and is based on performance status ranging from normal (100%) to dead (0%).

CLINICAL FEATURES

Common physical symptoms reported by dying patients:[28]

- Fatigue and weakness (90%).
- Constipation (87%).
- Dyspnea (80% to 90% of those with lung cancer, COPD, or heart disease).
- Nausea (up to 70%).
- Pain (36% to 90%).
- Insomnia.
- Other GI symptoms, including dry mouth, anorexia, vomiting, diarrhea, and dysphagia.
- Fecal and urinary incontinence.
- Dizziness.
- Swelling and numbness of the extremities.

Common mental and psychological symptoms reported by dying patients:[28]

- Depression (75% symptomatic; <25% with major depression) and feelings of hopelessness, anxiety, and/or irritability.
- Confusion and delirium (up to 85% at the end stage).

PATIENT SAFETY AT END OF LIFE

Patient safety is part of optimal healthcare and, at the end of life, needs to be addressed systematically. The Agency for Healthcare Research and Quality provides guidance for practitioners and healthcare systems in their evidence report/technical assessment document "Making Health Care Safer II."[29] This report covers topics such as adverse drug events, infection control, surgical issues, hospitalized elders with respect to falls and delirium, and creating a safety culture. Although safety practices can improve care, some can be problematic at the end of life. Examples include wearing mask and gloves for contact isolation that can prevent intimacy and balancing multiple medications to treat symptoms with their untoward effects such as delirium, falls, and constipation. Even documentation of advance directives can be considered a safety concern if these have been incorrectly recorded, were inadequately discussed, or are no longer consistent with patient preferences.[30]

An author of a literature review identified many areas for consideration in balancing patient needs at end of life and patient safety.[30] Some of these issues are:

- High-alert medications (opioids): priority of treating pain vs. medication errors and adverse events.
- Delirium: a natural consequence of dying and side effect of symptom-control medications vs. a consequence of overly aggressive symptom management.
- Falls: patient goals for freedom of movement vs. fall prevention to prevent fracture.
- Pressure ulcers: comfort of current position vs. need to reposition, which can cause pain.

MANAGEMENT

Management often begins with communicating bad news to patients and families about likely or imminent death. This task can be extremely difficult. In cases where the patient is not deemed legally competent, make sure that the legal decision maker is present. In addition, if the patient is a non-English speaker, consider obtaining a skilled medical interpreter rather than relying on a family member. Providers may find the following P-SPIKES approach useful:[31]

- Preparation—Review information to be presented and practice.
- Setting—Arrange time and place, ensure privacy, and include important support persons.
- Perception of patient—Inquire about the patient's and the family's understanding of the illness.
- Information needs—Find out about what the patient and family need to be told and in how much detail.
- Knowledge of the condition—Provide bad news sensitively and slowly, warning them that bad news is imminent and checking to see whether there is understanding.
- Empathy and exploration—Acknowledge the feelings expressed, give the patient and family time to react, and remind them that you are not abandoning them.
- Summary/strategic planning—Discuss next steps or schedule follow-ups to do this if more time is needed.

Another approach to delivering bad news in the hospital setting is ABCDE, which follows an Ask-Tell-Ask approach in communication.[32] The steps are: advance preparation, building a therapeutic environment/relationship, communicating well, dealing with patient/family reactions, and encouraging and validating emotions.

Roles for the primary care provider include consultation, providing anticipatory guidance, providing support and comfort, and assisting with identifying and managing symptoms (including pain control) in alignment with the patient's goals (**Figure 5-4**). This can include physical, psychosocial, and spiritual aspects of care.

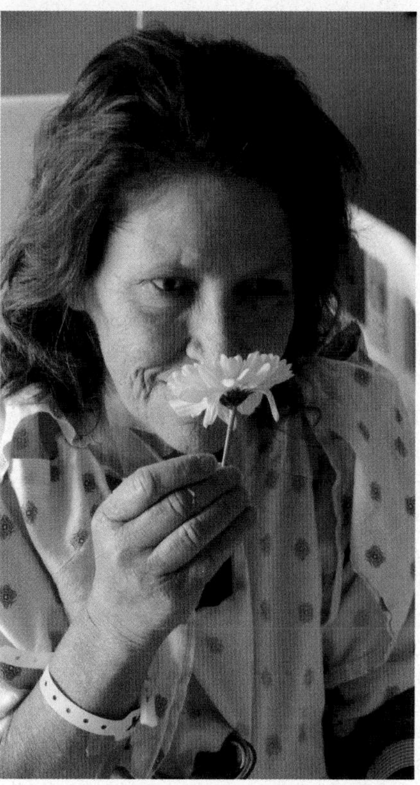

FIGURE 5-4 This 57-year-old woman is currently receiving palliative care in the hospital. She has chronic kidney disease and end-stage liver disease. Her provider is keeping her company to prevent her from being alone on her wedding anniversary. She holds a simple yellow flower, her favorite color. She notes that "Death is not something to be feared. Death is part of life, and life is a beautiful journey." *(Reproduced with permission from Bryant Huang.)*

In assisting dying patients and their families/caregivers with making decisions about their care, clinicians should be prepared to discuss the following:

- Realistic treatment options for cure or palliation of the primary disease process.
- Advance directives and withholding of life-sustaining treatment.
- Cultural beliefs and preferences (e.g., truth-telling vs. protecting the patient, religious beliefs).
- Preferences for place of care for those dying, involvement of others, and symptom management.

Many factors are important in providing optimal care to the dying. In a study of factors considered important to seriously ill patients, recently bereaved family members, and physicians involved in end-of-life care, investigators found the following:[33]

- There was a general agreement on the items relating to having preferences in writing, symptom control, being kept clean, experiencing physical touch, good communication and knowing what to expect, getting one's affairs in order and achieving a sense of completion, and maintaining dignity and a sense of humor.
- Patients reported wanting to remain mentally aware, not be a burden, and noted the importance of prayer and being at peace with God. They were not as concerned about dying at home.
- Family members reported wanting to use all the treatment options and to help patients avoid pain, shortness of breath, and suffering.

COMMUNICATION IN PRIMARY CARE AT END OF LIFE

Effective provider–patient communication at end of life can improve outcomes for patients and families, enhance clinician satisfaction, and lower healthcare costs. However, there are many barriers to effective communication.[34] For clinicians, barriers include lack of professional training on prognostication or end-of-life care, low confidence in initiating these conversations, and personal distress, especially in cases where the clinician knows the patient well. System barriers include lack of care coordination across specialties, poor documentation and lack of institutional commitment to communication with clinicians. Cultural and patient factors also influence communication and asking about expectations and past experiences helps set the stage for more effective communication.

During communication, it is critical for the clinical team to display empathy; this can be enhanced by using an evidence-based approach known as NURSE: **n**aming, **u**nderstanding, **r**espect, **s**upporting, and **e**xploring. Phrases that one should consider to ease the discussion are:[35]

- Initiating conversation: "I am sorry to have to tell you this." "I know this is not good news." "I wish I had better news."
- Eliciting patient preferences: "Would you rather I speak with you about this or your daughter?" "Some people want to be very involved in medical decision making and some people want their doctor to just give them a recommendation—how do you feel about that?"
- To facilitate empathy: "I can see how upsetting this is." "Is it okay if I hold your hand?"

One should avoid phrases like, "There is nothing more we can do for you," "I know what this must be like," and "I understand what you are going through."

ADVANCE DIRECTIVES

Advance directives and advance care planning (ACP) continue to be poorly utilized. Clinicians should consider outpatient and inpatient opportunities to introduce these concepts with the goals of empowering the patient and understanding the patient's preferences if they are too sick to speak for themselves.

ACP is an important part of patient-centered care to ensure that the patient's preferences, needs and values guide clinical decisions. Resources to help healthcare providers can be obtained during workshops at national meetings of the American Academy of Family Physicians, the American Academy of Hospice and Palliative Medicine, or the American Geriatrics Society. Following protocols such as SPIKES and ABCDE helps providers systematically discuss goals of care.

Recently Medicare has created codes to pay for ACP. The three opportunities in primary care in which you can readily introduce ACP discussions are: (1) during a routine visit with no recent health changes, (2) after recent illness or hospitalization, and (3) in follow-up after exacerbation of health conditions.[36]

To assist in ACP, possible scenarios can be discussed, such as recovery from an acute event (specifying acceptable interventions) and persistent vegetative state (preferences for life-sustaining interventions).

- The National POLST (physician orders for life-sustaining treatment) Paradigm Task Force is a program designed to improve the quality of end-of-life care based on effective communication of patient wishes, documentation of medical orders, and a commitment by healthcare professionals to honor these wishes. Information can be found at **http://closure.org** and includes web-based resources for patients and health providers. In addition, advance directives can be stored at sites like POL-ST; this feature can be particularly helpful for homeless patients.[37]
- Advance directive documents are of two broad types: instructional directives and proxy designations.
    - Instructional directives, such as living wills, describe decisions about care and healthcare. These can be general or specific. Only 26% of 7946 U.S. adults who participated in the 2009 or 2010 HealthStyles Survey reported completing advance directives; many non-completers reported lack of knowledge about the document.[38] Specific forms do not have to be used, and oral directives may be enforceable.[39]
    - Proxy designations—Appointing an individual or individuals to make medical decisions (i.e., durable power of attorney for healthcare).

Legal aspects—The United States Supreme Court ruled that patients have a right to decide about refusing or terminating medical interventions. Many states have their own statutory forms for living wills.

- The American College of Physicians and the American Society of Internal Medicine End-of-Life Care Consensus Panel note that life-sustaining treatment may be withheld for patients unable to speak for themselves if it is believed to be the patient's wish, the surrogate decision maker states that it is the patient's wish, and/or it is in the patient's best interests to do so.[39]
- The prescription of high-dose opioids to relieve pain in terminally ill patients that result in death will not lead to criminal prosecution, provided it was the physician's intent to relieve suffering.[39]

HOSPICE CARE AND SERVICES

Hospice care refers to care when curative interventions have been judged to be no longer beneficial. This type of care can be delivered in many settings, including home, hospital, and special residential facilities. More than 1.6 million Americans received hospice care in 2014, and more than 85% of hospice patients used the Medicare Hospice Benefit (MHB).[40]

- The types of hospice services include physician and nursing care, home health aides, pastoral care, counseling, respite care, and bereavement programs.
- Hospice eligibility general guidelines include fulfilling the criteria for end-stage disease as outlined above and documenting both the patient's and family's decision on palliative care rather than curative care. In addition, documentation of significant functional decline is important using validated instruments like FAST (Functional Assessment Staging), PPS, BADLs (Basic Activities of Daily Living), and/or NYHA Class IV heart disease. Other criteria include weight loss of 7.5% or 10% in the preceding 3 to 6 months, respectively, or serum albumin <2.5 g/dL.

Physicians should be aware of the MHB covered under Medicare Part A (physician services are billed under Medicare Part B).[41] In the

United States, the MHB pays for 80% of all hospice care including medical, nursing, counseling, and bereavement services to terminally ill patients and their families. Medicare beneficiaries who choose hospice care receive noncurative medical and support services for their terminal illness. Home care may be provided along with inpatient care if needed and a variety of other services that are not covered by Medicare. Eligibility criteria are:

- Patient eligible for Medicare Part A or Medicaid.
- Patient is terminally ill, that is, patient's physician and the medical director of hospice certify that the patient is terminally ill and has a life expectancy of 6 months or less if the disease runs its normal course. If the medical director is the patient's physician, only one signature is required.
- Patient chooses hospice care and signs a Medicare hospice benefits form. This process is reversible, and patients may at a future time elect to return to Medicare Part A.
- Hospice care is provided by a Medicare-certified hospice program.
- Under Medicare, do not resuscitate (DNR) status cannot be used as a requirement for admission.

Length of benefits:

- Entitled to receive hospice care as long as he or she meets the eligibility criteria.
- Hospice benefit consists of two 90-day benefit periods, followed by an unlimited number of 60-day benefit periods.
- Benefit periods may be used consecutively or at intervals.
- Patient needs to be certified terminally ill at the beginning of each period.
- No lifetime limit to hospice care for Medicare beneficiaries.
- If patient experiences remission of the disease and is discharged from hospice, the patient can be eligible for hospice care in the future without any regard to the previous use of hospice services.
- The same rules apply for Medicaid patients.

Services covered include physician, nurse, dietician, medical social services, medical supplies and equipment, outpatient drugs for symptom management and pain relief, and home care (e.g., aids, physical, occupational, and speech therapy). Other included services are as follows:

- Short-term general inpatient care for problems that cannot be managed at home—most commonly intractable pain or delirium.
- Short-term respite care—up to 5 days to permit family caregivers to take a break (can incur a 5% copayment).
- Counseling in home for patient and family.
- Bereavement, pastoral, and spiritual support for patient and family.
- Payment of consulting physician fees at 100% of Medicare allowance.
- Physician, nurse, social worker, and counselor on-call availability 24 hours a day, 7 days a week.

Services not covered include active treatment of terminal illness (except for symptom management and pain control of the terminal illness), care provided by a physician or facility that has not contracted with the patient's hospice agency, and continuous nursing assistant or nursing home room-and-board charges.

Medicare's first hospice demonstration project, 35 years ago, carried out both curative and hospice services at end of life to reduce barriers to hospice and palliative care and help patients and families receive care that was aligned with their preferences. Novel approaches are under development to help deliver more intensive services at end of life and reduce numbers of long-stay patients. These services may include palliative chemotherapy, radiation, and intravenous (IV) therapies.[40]

PALLIATIVE CARE

Palliative care is care focused on preventing, relieving, reducing, or soothing symptoms of disease without effecting a cure. As such, it is not restricted to patients who are dying, but can be used along with a curative therapy.

Many hospitals have inpatient palliative care services to assist patients, families, and primary care providers in delivering this type of care. It is vital that primary care providers be trained and prepared to recognize a patient's palliative care needs, provide prognostication and ACP, and, when appropriate, make timely referrals to this type of service.

General approach to palliative care focuses on four broad domains: managing physical symptoms, managing psychological symptoms, addressing social needs. and understanding spiritual needs. Exploring physical and psychological causes along with symptom evaluation will give clues to underlying causes and aid in effective treatment to enhance quality of life.

- Needs assessment—Clinicians should focus on the four domains and try to understand the degree of difficulty and how much the identified problem interferes with the patient's life.
- Setting goals and continuous reassessment—Goals for care include improving symptoms, delaying disability, finding peace, and providing for the loved ones. Plan times to review these goals as the course of the illness changes or progresses.
- Pain management—There is no reason that patients need to suffer, particularly at the end of life. Barriers to managing pain successfully include limited ability of providers to assess pain severity, fear of sanction/prosecution, and lack of knowledge (including awareness of guidelines).
    - Assessment of pain—Important aspects include periodicity (e.g., continuous), location, intensity, modifying factors, effects of treatments, and impact on the patient. Tools such as Wong Baker FACES (www.wongbakerfaces.org) and the Pain Assessment in Advanced Dementia (PAINAD; https://www.mdcalc.com/pain-assessment-advanced-dementia-scale-painad) scale are helpful to assess pain severity.
    - Intervention—This includes nonpharmacologic treatment (e.g., massage, positioning, transcutaneous electrical nerve stimulation [TENS], physical therapy), pain medications, and other palliative procedures (e.g., nerve blocks, radiotherapy, acupuncture).
    - Pain medications may be approached in a stepwise fashion from nonopioids (e.g., acetaminophen [4 g/day], ibuprofen [1600 mg/day]), to mild opioids (e.g., codeine [30 mg every 4 hours] or hydrocodone [5 mg every 4 hours]), to stronger opioids (e.g., morphine 2.5 to 10 mg every 4 hours).[42] Doses should be titrated

as needed. Side effects (e.g., constipation, nausea, and drowsiness) should be anticipated and prevented (e.g., laxatives and antiemetic) or treated. Patients may become tolerant to these side effects after approximately 1 week.
  - Specific pain syndromes may require additional consideration. These include:
    - Continuous pain, which requires round-the-clock dosing, rescue medication, and regular assessment and readjustment. If rescue medication is needed, increase the daily opioid dose the next day by the total dose of rescue medication. For longer duration of action, transdermal fentanyl may be considered (100 mcg/h is equianalgesic to morphine 4 mg/h and has a duration of 48 to 72 hours).
    - Neuropathic pain (arising from disordered, ectopic nerve signals), which is typically shock-like or burning. Medications to consider in addition to opioids are gabapentin (100 to 300 mg daily or up to 3 times daily), 5% lidocaine patch (3 patches daily for a maximum of 12 hours), tramadol (50 to 100 mg 1 to 3 times daily), and tricyclic antidepressants (10 to 25 mg at bedtime titrated to 75 to 150 mg).
  - Adjunctive analgesic medications are those that potentiate opioid effects. These include the above treatments for neuropathic pain, glucocorticoids (e.g., dexamethasone once daily), clonidine, and baclofen.
  - Adjuvant therapies like neural blockade, radiation therapy, physical and occupational therapy, lymphedema therapy, massage, acupuncture, relaxation therapy, and cognitive behavioral therapy (CBT) can also be helpful for pain management.[43]
  - Legal concerns to opioid prescribing—Physicians may be unwilling or uncomfortable with providing high-dose opioids out of fear that they would be hastening the patient's death. However, the assumption that opioids appropriately titrated to control pain hasten death is not supported by medical evidence. In addition, as noted above, the physician's intent to relieve suffering, despite the risk of death, is ethical and unlikely to result in prosecution.

Control of common symptoms:[44]

- Constipation—Due to medications, inactivity, poor nutritional/hydration, limited fiber intake, confusion, intestinal obstruction, and comorbidities such as diabetes mellitus, hypothyroidism, and hypercalcemia. The treatment goal is one bowel movement every 1 to 2 days. Constipation prophylaxis should be started for all patients taking regular opiate regimens. Options include increasing fiber, stool softeners (e.g., sodium docusate [Colace] 300 to 600 mg/day orally), stimulant laxatives (e.g., prune juice ½ to 1 glass/day, senna [Senokot] 2 to 4 tablets/day, bisacodyl 5 to 15 mg/day orally or per rectum), and osmotic laxatives (e.g., lactulose 15 to 30 mL every 4 to 8 hours, polyethylene glycol [Miralax] 1 tablespoon in 4 to 8 oz of fluid daily, magnesium hydroxide [milk of magnesia] 15 to 60 mL/day).
- Dyspnea—Occurs in 90% of patients with COPD, 70% of patients with lung cancer, and 65% with heart failure.[45] When possible, treat reversible causes (e.g., infection, hypoxia). Options include opioids (e.g., codeine 30 mg every 4 hours, morphine 5 to 10 mg every 4 hours) and anxiolytics (e.g., lorazepam 0.5 to 2 mg oral/sublingual/IV, diazepam 5 to 10 mg oral/IV). A parenteral infusion or long-acting opiate can also be tried, with bolus dosing for breakthrough pain; nebulized opiates are ineffective for dyspnea.[46] For patients with a history of respiratory disease, consider bronchodilators and/or glucocorticoids. Oxygen is commonly prescribed, although data do not support its effectiveness in improving the sensation of breathlessness.[46] The inexpensive and simple practice of blowing ambient air on the patient's face may help relieve dyspnea.
- For those with excessive secretions, hyoscyamine (Levsin; 0.125 to 0.5 sublingual or subcutaneously every 4 hours), atropine 1% ophthalmic drops (1 or 2 drops every 6 hours), glycopyrrolate (Robinul; 1 mg oral or 0.2 to 0.4 mg subcutaneously every 4 hours), or scopolamine 1.5 mg transdermal (1 or 2 patches every 72 hours) may be considered.
- Fatigue—Seen in 80% of patients.[46] May be due to disease factors (e.g., heart failure, tumor necrosis factor), cachexia, dehydration, anemia, hypothyroidism, and medications. Options include decreasing activity, increasing exercise as tolerated, changing medications, or prescribing glucocorticoids (e.g., methylprednisolone or dexamethasone once daily). Modafinil, an analeptic drug, may also be considered (initial dose: 200 mg).
- Nausea and vomiting—Mediated through multiple brain receptor pathways. First-line medications include haloperidol (0.5 to 2 mg orally or IV every 4 to 8 hours), chlorpromazine (12.5 to 25 mg IV or 25 to 50 mg orally every 6 to 8 hours), metoclopramide (Reglan; 5 to 20 mg orally or IV every 6 hours), and prochlorperazine (5 to 10 mg orally or IV every 6 to 8 hours), which target dopaminergic pathways. Anticholinergic medications such as transdermal scopolamine can be used as second-line agents. Synthetic cannabinoids (e.g., dronabinol [Marinol; 5 to 10 mg orally, rectally or sublingually every 6 to 8 hours]) and medical marijuana (if approved for medical use) can also be considered as second-line agents for nausea control.[44]
- Anorexia/cachexia—Defined by loss of muscle mass, metabolic derangements, increased resting energy expenditure, fatigue and loss of performance and experienced in most end-stage chronic diseases. Effects of treatments used are short lived, and there is no survival benefit. A multidrug regimen (medroxyprogesterone, eicosapentaenoic acid, L-carnitine, thalidomide), diet, exercise, and nutritional program was shown to improve lean body mass and fatigue in patients with advanced cancers.[47] Family distress is common due to lack of knowledge about the limited benefit of nutrition and hydration in the last weeks of life.
- Spiritual distress—The FICA tool (Faith or Beliefs, Importance or Influence, Community, Address issues; https://www.hpsm.org/documents/End_of_Life_Summit_FICA_References.pdf) can be used to elicit a spiritual history to improve well-being and mental health. Addressing spiritual distress may improve quality of life and increase hospice use at end of life. Four spiritual themes that dominate in 80% of patients with cancer are coping mechanisms to help endure illness, impact of spiritual and religious beliefs in life, connectedness with a higher power, and community relationships.[48]
- Depression—Present in 60% of patients.[45] Because many of the somatic symptoms used to diagnose depression in healthy individuals are present in patients who are dying, psychological criteria become more important in making treatment decisions. Options include counseling, exercise, and medications (e.g., selective

serotonin reuptake inhibitors); low doses should be used initially (e.g., fluoxetine 10 mg/day) and increased as needed. Psychostimulants (e.g., dextroamphetamine or methylphenidate 2.5 to 5 mg twice daily) may be considered if rapid onset of action is needed when the prognosis is <6 months; these may be used in conjunction with traditional antidepressants.

- Anxiety—Often due to the uncertain course of illness along with fear of uncontrolled symptoms and death. Multifactorial interventions such as environmental modifications and CBT can help along with provider support and medications. Benzodiazepines provide short-term benefit, and selective serotonin receptor inhibitors can be used for long-term management.
- Delirium—Due to metabolic abnormalities (liver failure, electrolyte disturbance, vitamin B_{12} deficiency), infection, brain tumors, medications, and multiple other causes. Options include treating reversible causes and medications including neuroleptics (e.g., haloperidol 0.5 to 5 mg orally/subcutaneous/IM/IV every 1 to 4 hours, risperidone 1 to 3 mg every 12 hours) and anesthetics (propofol 0.3 to 2 mg/h continuous infusion). Anxiolytics may exacerbate delirium and must be used cautiously (e.g., lorazepam 0.5 to 2 mg oral/IM/IV).
- Fever—Treatment depends on care goals and life expectancy. Treated with antipyretic medications (nonsteroidal anti-inflammatory drugs, acetaminophen, or corticosteroids) if causing discomfort.

ADDRESSING SOCIAL NEEDS

Considerations include economic burden and caregivers.

- The U.S. health insurance system is neither universal nor comprehensive, and many patients and their families find themselves under tremendous financial strain.
- In a study of Medicare fee-for-service beneficiaries, aged 70 years or older, who died in 2005–2010, investigators examined end-of-life costs for 1702 individuals.[49] Patients were stratified into four cohorts: those with high probability of dementia, those with heart disease, those with cancer, and those with other causes of death.
  - The mean adjusted total healthcare spending in the last 5 years was $287,038 among those with dementia and $183,001 among individuals in the other three groups.
  - Average out-of-pocket and informal care costs were also higher for the dementia group ($61,522 and $83,022, respectively) compared to the other groups ($34,068 and $38,272, respectively). This out-of-pocket spending represented 32% of wealth measured 5 years before death for the dementia group vs. 11% for non-dementia decedents.
- The proportion of out-of-pocket spending was greater for blacks (84%), those with less than high school education (48%), and unmarried/widowed women (58%).
- Families/caregivers often need outside help, such as providing personal care for the patient (such as bathing), psychological or spiritual counseling, respite care, or making arrangements for the body after death.
- Primary care providers can facilitate encounters with family and friends by offering their presence and suggestions about easing the visits (e.g., reading to the patient, sharing music, or creating a videotape, audiotape, or scrapbook).
- Hospice and social workers can offer great assistance to patients and families in addressing these needs.

Understanding spiritual needs:

- Approximately 70% of dying patients become more religious or spiritual at the end of life.
- As noted by Steinhauser and colleagues, patients noted the importance of prayer and being at peace with God.[33]
- Physicians should ask about and support patient and family expressions of spirituality and consider encouraging pastoral care, as desired.

PATIENT AND FAMILY EDUCATION

It is very important to involve patients and their families in discussion at an early stage, as most want to know their diagnosis and prognosis. Nurses can play a key role education regarding ACP, symptom management, improved self-care, and therapeutic choices. Overall, there is strong association between therapeutic communication and patient satisfaction as well as quality of care.[50] Patients and families can be encouraged to begin ACP at home; a good starting point can be found at The Conversation Project (http://theconversationproject.org).

The Carer Support Needs Assessment Tool (CSNAT; http://csnat.org/) is an evidence-based tool used to assess caregiver support needs in 14 domains. Although very detailed, the tool can be used for both research and clinical practice.[51]

- The role of the primary care physician should be discussed, particularly if other providers are involved in the care of the patient. Possible roles include consultation about care needs, anticipatory guidance on prognosis and expected symptoms, provision of support and comfort, and assistance with managing symptoms.
  - Assessment of the family includes their understanding of diagnosis and prognosis and identifying the primary caregiver, decision maker, and support systems in the family with consideration of cultural and ethnic backgrounds. It is important to listen to build trust.
  - Frequent family meetings may help the patient and family feel supported and improve patient satisfaction and quality of life/death. Topics to discuss include prognosis and disease trajectory and treatment options that align with the patient's care goals.
- Families often suffer emotionally, spiritually, and financially as they care for the patient. Family members can experience a sense of hopelessness, anger, guilt, and powerlessness when they cannot relieve the suffering of their terminally ill family member.
- Families who need to provide care for a terminally ill patient should be made aware of community resources and the provisions in the Family and Medical Leave Act.[52]
- It is not unusual to see hidden family conflicts resurface in the face of a terminal illness, and any emotional tension that exists between the caregivers and patient can impede care. Physicians should be sensitive to the conflicts and cultural influences and closely observe

how patients and their families are communicating so that they can better support them, allowing them to express their emotions and concerns and referring them to appropriate counselors or support groups when needed.[53,54]

- Children should not be excluded from this process, and the physician, with permission, can help in determining what children already know about the illness and in providing accurate information about the diagnosis, prognosis, and treatment expectations for the dying family member. Also advise caregivers to try to maintain the children's daily schedule and routines of the family as much as possible, monitor for problems at school, encourage questions, and plan activities (e.g., reading a story) when visiting ill family members. It may be helpful to inform teachers and counselors at school about the family situation and request that the teachers let the parent know if the child is having any difficulty or talks about worries.
- Consider counseling for the child if the child requests help or displays symptoms of depression or anxiety that interfere with school, home, or peers; risk-taking behavior; or significant discord with others.

RECOGNIZING DYING AT END OF LIFE

Recognizing dying can be complex. Dying is associated with reduction in performance status, fluctuating level of conscious, social withdrawal, weakness and fatigue, and reduced oral intake.

Patient and family education should focus on the following:

- Social withdrawal—Initial withdrawal is from the surroundings, then worldly interests decline, and finally withdrawal from family, ultimately leading to loss of communication.
- Decreasing nutritional requirements—There is a decreased need for fluids and solids; fluids are usually preferred and should follow what the patient wants rather than force-feeding.
- Disorientation—There is increased confusion with time, place, and person. Usually patients talk about seeing people who have already died or state that their death is nearing. Redirecting the patient is necessary only if asked for or if the patient is distressed.
- Decreased senses—Hearing and vision decrease. Using soft lights helps to decrease visual hallucinations. Speak softly and gently, as patients hear even at the end of life. Hearing is the last of the five senses to be lost.
- Restlessness—Also called "terminal restlessness" and is caused by the change in the body's metabolism. Reassurance is important, and appropriate symptom management with medications may be helpful.
- Sleep—There is increased time spent in sleep that may be due to changes in the body's metabolism or natural to the underlying disease process. Spending time at the bedside can help capture the time when the patient is most alert.
- Incontinence is often not a problem until death is very near. Absorbent pads can be placed under the patient for greater comfort and cleanliness, or a urinary catheter may be used for comfort care. The amount of urine will decrease and becomes darker at the end of life.

Physical changes to be expected include the following:

- Skin color changes including flushing, bluish hue to the skin, and cold sensation of the skin. Skin may have a jaundiced look when the patient is approaching death. The arms and legs of the body may become cool to the touch. The hands and feet become purplish. The knees, ankles, and elbows are blotchy. These symptoms are a result of decreased circulation.
- Blood pressure decreases; the pulse may increase or decrease.
- Body temperature can fluctuate; fever is common.
- Increased perspiration along with clamminess.
- Respirations may increase, decrease, or become irregular; there may be periods of cessation of breathing (apnea).
- Congestion can present as a rattling sound in the lungs and/or upper throat. This occurs because the patient is too weak to clear the throat or cough. The congestion can be affected by positioning, may be very loud, and sometimes comes and goes. Elevating the head of the bed and swabbing the mouth with oral swabs may be helpful.
- The patient may enter a coma before death and not respond to verbal or tactile stimuli.

END-OF-LIFE CARE IN NURSING HOMES

There are challenges to providing end-of-life care for patients in nursing homes. Authors of a study of family member perceptions of care in this setting reported problems with poor communication, lack of effective pain management, gaps with hospice collaboration, unmet expectations and information needs, and resident care issues.[55]

- Shift changes can result in suboptimal care and late communication with families.
- Primary care clinicians may be late in responding to requests for better pain management after families observed the patient's moaning and grimacing.
- Inadequate staffing may result in families having to provide direct care such as hydrating the patients or asking for a medication refill.
- Care concerns raised by families often included hydration/nutrition, falls, bedsores, and medical equipment failure.

Primary care providers can ameliorate some of these concerns through shared advance directives, anticipatory medication prescribing, care coordination and anticipatory guidance, and involving families and care team members in identifying and meeting the dying patient's needs.

FOLLOW-UP

Withdrawal of life-sustaining treatment:

- Evidence-based criteria for guiding physicians through this process are lacking; however, general consensus exists based on ethical and clinical principles in the care of these patients.[56,57]
  - Withdrawal of life-sustaining treatment can be considered when curative care is not possible and supportive or other treatment is no longer desired and does not provide patient comfort.

- Withholding life-sustaining treatment is morally, ethically, and legally equivalent to withdrawing life support. Any treatment given to the patient can be withdrawn or withheld. In conducting these discussions with patients and their families, consider a patient's information-sharing preferences (e.g., a preference for limited information), minimum acceptable quality of life and functional status, whether the patient can understand the consequences of life-sustaining treatment, whether procedures offered conflict with the patient's values, and the patient's need for advice and guidance.[58]
- Treat withdrawal of life-sustaining treatment as equivalent to a medical procedure and fulfill all formalities (e.g., informed consent) prior to the procedure.
- If withdrawal of one life-sustaining treatment is indicated, consider withdrawing all existing treatments for the patient; this does not include withdrawing comfort care.

- A consensus should be reached with the healthcare team and family that is in the best interest of the patient. The following steps should be taken for withdrawal of life support:[57]
  - Informed consent.
  - Appropriate setting and monitoring.
  - Sedation and analgesia.
  - Having a plan for withdrawal (information about the protocol can be found in fast facts at https://www.capc.org).
  - Pastoral, nursing, and emotional support.
  - Documentation.
  - Interventions to improve care during withdrawal of life-sustaining treatment that can be considered are consultation with an ethics committee, palliative care team, family conferences, and a standardized order form for withdrawing life-sustaining therapies.[59]

Grief and bereavement follow-up:

- Manifestations of grief consist of both psychological symptoms (e.g., sadness, anxiety, emotional lability, apathy, impaired concentration) and physical symptoms (anorexia, change in weight, trouble initiating or maintaining sleep, fatigue, headache). In the first month following a death, it is important to reassure surviving family members and friends that these manifestations of grief are normal and to offer support, suggestions for symptom management, and coping resources.
- Subsequent follow-up visits should be used to assess the progress of mourning and to identify depression; if the latter is identified, consider counseling and pharmacotherapy.
- Usually, the primary physician is notified of the death and may be required to make the pronouncement (based on lack of vital signs and lack of response to noxious stimulus) and complete the death certificate (noting cause of death and contributing medical conditions).
- Following the death of the patient, personal expressions of condolence from the primary care provider(s) and staff should be encouraged and range from cards to attending visitation and the funeral; based on personal experience, the latter can assist with grieving and closure for the physician.

PATIENT RESOURCES

- Caring Connections—**https://www.caringinfo.org.**
- Get Palliative Care—**www.getpalliativecare.org.**
- Caregivers Action Network— **http://caregiveraction.org/.**
- National Hospice and Palliative Care Organization—**https://www.nhpco.org.**

Online State Specific Living Will Forms—**https://www.doyourownwill.com/free-living-wills.html.**

PROVIDER RESOURCES

- American Academy of Hospice and Palliative Medicine—**http://www.aahpm.org/.**
- National Hospice and Palliative Care Organization—**https://www.nhpco.org.**
- American Pain Society—**https://www.ampainsoc.org.**
- American Society for Bioethics and Humanities—**http://www.asbh.org.**
- American Society of Law, Medicine and Ethics—**http://www.aslme.org.**
- End-of-Life Care Consensus Panel—American College of Physicians–American Society of Internal Medicine—**https://www.acponline.org/clinical-information/ethics-and-professionalism.**
- The EPEC Project (Education resource online)—**http://bioethics.northwestern.edu/programs/epec/.**
- Palliative Care Matters—**http://www.pallcare.info.**

SUGGESTED READINGS

- Baugher R, Calija M. *A Guide to the Bereaved Survivor*. Newcastle, WA; 1998. [ISBN:0-9635975-0-7.]
- Brown LK, Brown M. *When Dinosaurs Die: A Guide to Understanding Death*. Little, Brown & Company; 1996. [ISBN:0-316-11955-5.]
- Callanan M, Kely P. *Final Gifts: Understanding the Special Awareness, Needs and Communications of the Dying*. Bantam Books; 1992. [ISBN: 0-553-37876-7.]
- Gawande A. *Being Mortal*. Picador; 2017. [ISBN: 9781250076229]
- Hanson W. *The Next Place*. Waldman House Press; 1997. [ISBN: 0-931674-32-8.]
- Heegaard M. *When Someone Special Dies: Children Can Learn to Cope with Grief*. Woodland Press; 1988. [ISBN:0-9620502-0-2.]
- Lattanzi-Licht M, Mahoney JJ, Miller GW. *The National Hospice Organization Guide to Hospice Care: The Hospice Choice: In Pursuit of A Peaceful Death*. Simon & Schuster; 1998. [ISBN:0-684-82269-5.]
- Ray MC. *I Am Here to Help: A Hospice Workers Guide to Communicating with Dying People and Their Loved Ones*. Hospice Handouts, McRay Company; 1992. [ISBN:0-963611-0-1.]
- Traisman ES. *Fire in My Heart, Ice in My Veins: A Journal for Teenagers Experiencing a Loss*. Centering Corporation; 1992. [ISBN:1-56123-056-1.]

REFERENCES

1. Freeman L, Caserta M, Lund D, et al. Music thanatology: prescriptive harp music as palliative care for the dying patient. *Am J Hosp Palliat Care*. 2006;23(2):100-104.
2. Ganzini L, Rakoski A, Cohn S, Mularski RA. Family members' views on the benefits of harp music vigils for terminally-ill or dying loved ones. *Palliat Support Care*. 2015;13(1):41-44.
3. Von Gunten CF. Interventions to manage symptoms at the end of life. *J Palliat Med*. 2005;8 (Suppl 1):S88-S94.
4. National Center for Health Statistics. *Deaths and Mortality*. https://www.cdc.gov/nchs/fastats/deaths.htm. Accessed October 2017.
5. Ortman JM, Velkoff VA, Hogan H. An aging nation: the older population in the United States. *Current Population Reports*. May 2014, https://www.census.gov/prod/2014pubs/p25-1140.pdf. Accessed October 2017.
6. Murphy SL, Xu J, Kochanek KD. Deaths: preliminary data for 2014. *National Vital Statistics Reports*; Vol. 65 No. 4. Hyattsville, MD: National Center for Health Statistics.
7. Heron M. *Deaths: Leading causes for 2014. National Vital Statistics Reports*; Vol. 65 No. 5. Hyattsville, MD: National Center for Health Statistics. June 30, 2016.
8. National Center for Health Statistics. *Trends in Inpatient Hospital Deaths: National Hospital Discharge Survey, 2000–2010*. https://www.cdc.gov/nchs/products/databriefs/db118.htm. Accessed October 2017.
9. National Hospice and Palliative Care Organization. *Hospice Facts and Figures*. https://www.nhpco.org/press-room/press-releases/hospice-facts-figures. Accessed October 2017.
10. Johnson KS, Kuchibhatla M, Payne R, Tulsky JA. Race and residence: intercounty variation in black-white differences in hospice use. *J Pain Symptom Manage*. 2013;46(5):681-690.
11. Centers for Disease Control and Prevention. Cigarette smoking among adults—United States, 2005–2015. *Morb Mortal Wkly Rep*. 2016;65(44):1205-1211.
12. U.S. Department of Health and Human Services. The Health Consequences of Smoking—50 Years of Progress: A Report of the Surgeon General. Atlanta: U.S. Department of Health and Human Services, Centers for Disease Control and Prevention, National Center for Chronic Disease Prevention and Health Promotion, Office on Smoking and Health, 2014.

12a. National Center for Health Statistics. *Fastfacts: Exercise and Physical Activity*, https://www.cdc.gov/nchs/fastats/exercise.htm. Accessed October 2017.

13. Esser MB, Hedden SL, Kanny D, et al. Prevalence of alcohol dependence among US adult drinkers, 2009–2011. https://www.cdc.gov/pcd/issues/2014/14_0329.htm. Accessed October 2017.
14. Centers for Disease Control and Prevention. *Fact Sheets—Alcohol Use and Your Health*. https://www.cdc.gov/alcohol/fact-sheets/alcohol-use.htm. Accessed October 2017.
15. National Institute on Drug Abuse. *InfoFacts: Nationwide Trends*. http://www.drugabuse.gov/publications/infofacts/nationwide-trends. Accessed March 2012.
16. United States Department of Health and Human Services. *Injury in the United States: 2007 Chartbook*. http://www.cdc.gov/nchs/data/misc/injury2007.pdf. Accessed October 2017.
17. Centers for Disease Control and Prevention. *HIV Basics*. https://www.cdc.gov/hiv/basics/statistics.html. Accessed October 2017.
18. Centers for Disease Control and Prevention. *Illegal Drug Use*. https://www.cdc.gov/nchs/fastats/drug-use-illegal.htm. Accessed October 2017.
19. National Institute on Drug Abuse. *Monitoring the Future Survey 2016 Results*. https://www.drugabuse.gov/related-topics/trends-statistics/infographics/monitoring-future-2016-survey-results. Accessed October 2017.
20. Wolfe MI, Nolte KB, Yoon SS. *Fatal Infectious Disease Surveillance in a Medical Examiner Database. Emerg Infect Dis*. 2004;10(1): 48-53.
21. Centers for Disease Control and Prevention. *NCHS Data on Drug-Poisoning Deaths*. https://www.cdc.gov/nchs/data/fact-sheets/factsheet_drug_poisoning.htm. Accessed October 2017.
22. Nordstrom DL, Yokoi-Shelton ML, Zosel A. Using multiple cause-of-death data to improve surveillance of drug-related mortality. *J Public Health Manag Pract*. 2013;19(5):402-411.
23. Institute of Medicine (IOM). *Dying in America: Improving Quality and Honoring Individual Preferences near the End of Life*. Washington, DC: The National Academies Press; 2015.
24. EPEC™-O: Education in Palliative and End-of-Life Care – Oncology (Original Curriculum). https://www.cancer.gov/resources-for/hp/education/epeco/self-study. Accessed October 2017.
25. Reisfield GM, Wilson GR. *Prognostication in Heart Failure. Fast Facts and Concepts #143*. https://www.mypcnow.org/blank-fj2d4. Accessed October 2017.
26. Lau F, Downing GM, Lesperance M, et al. Use of Palliative Performance Scale in end-of-life prognostication. *J Palliative Med*. 2006;9(5):1066-1075.
27. Myers J, Kim A, Flanagan J, Selby D. Palliative Performance Scale and survival among outpatients with advanced cancer. *Support Care Cancer*. 2015;23(4):913-918.
28. Emanuel EJ. Palliative and end-of-life care. In: Kasper DL, Fauci AS, Hauser SL, et al, eds. *Harrison's Principles of Internal Medicine*, 19th ed. New York: McGraw-Hill; 2016:Chapter 10.
29. Shekelle PG, Wachter RM, Pronovost PJ, et al. *Making Health Care Safer II: An Updated Critical Analysis of the Evidence for Patient Safety Practices*. Comparative Effectiveness Review No. 211. (Prepared by the Southern California-RAND Evidence-based Practice Center under Contract No. 290-2007-10062-I.) AHRQ Publication No. 13-E001-EF. Rockville, MD: Agency for Healthcare Research and Quality; March 2013. www.ahrq.gov/research/findings/evidence-based-reports/ptsafetyuptp.html. Accessed October 2017.
30. Dy SM. Patient safety and end-of-life care: common issues, perspectives, and strategies for improving care. *Am J Hosp Palliat Care*. 2016;33(8):791-796.
31. Buckman R. *How to Break Bad News: A Guide for Health Care Professionals*. Baltimore, MD: Johns Hopkins University Press; 1992.

32. Rabow MW, McPhee, SJ. Beyond breaking bad news: how to help patients who suffer. *West J Med.* 1999;171:260-263.
33. Steinhauser KE, Christakis NA, Clipp EC, et al. Factors considered important at the end of life by patients, family physicians, and other care providers. *JAMA.* 2000;284(19):1476-1482.
34. Lakin JR, Block SD, Billings JA, et al. Improving communication about serious illness in primary care. *JAMA Intern Med.* 2016;176(9):1380-1387.
35. Minichiello TA, Ling D, Ucci DK. Breaking bad news: a practical approach for the hospitalist. *J Hosp Med.* 2007;2:415-421.
36. Lakin JR, Block SD, Struck BD, et al. Advance care planning in the outpatient geriatric medicine setting. *Prim Care.* 2017;44(3): 511-518.
37. Hubbell SA. Advance care planning with individuals experiencing homelessness: literature review and recommendations for public health practice. *Public Health Nurs.* 2017;34(5):472-478.
38. Rao JK, Anderson LA, Lin FC, Laux JP. Completion of advance directives among U.S. consumers. *Am J Prev Med.* 2014;46(1): 65-70.
39. Meisel A, Snyder L, Quill T; American College of Physicians—American Society of Internal Medicine End-of-Life Care Consensus Panel. Seven legal barriers to end-of-life care: myths, realities and grains of truth. *JAMA.* 2000;284(19):2495-2501.
40. Harrison KL, Connor SR. First Medicare demonstration of concurrent provision of curative and hospice services for end-of-life care. *Am J Public Health.* 2016;106(8):1405-1408.
41. Turner R. *Fast Facts and Concepts No. 82 and 83. Medicare Hospice Benefit Part 1.* January 2003. End-of-Life Physician Education Resource Center. https://www.mypcnow.org/blank-jvz8r. Accessed October 2017.
42. World Health Organization. *Pain Ladder.* www.who.int/entity/cancer/palliative/painladder/en/. Accessed October 1, 2017.
43. Kogan M, Cheng S, Rao S, et al. Integrative medicine for geriatric and palliative care. *Med Clin N Am.* 2017;101:1005-1029.
44. Albert RH. End-of-life care: managing common symptoms. *Am Fam Physician.* 2017;95(6):356-361.
45. Singer AE, Meeker D. Symptom trends in the last year of life from 1998 to 2010: a cohort study. *Ann Intern Med.* 2015;162(3): 175-178.
46. Clemens KE, Quednau I, Klaschik E. Use of oxygen and opioids in the palliation of dyspnoea in hypoxic and non-hypoxic palliative care patients: a prospective study. *Support Care Cancer.* 2009;17:367-377.
47. Mantovani G. Randomized phase III clinical trial of five different arms of treatment in 332 patients with cancer cachexia. *Eur Rev Med Pharmacol Sci.* 2010;14(4):292-301.
48. Alcorn SR, Balboni MJ, Prigerson HG, et al. "If God wanted me yesterday, I wouldn't be here today": religious and spiritual themes in patients' experiences of advanced cancer. *J Palliat Med.* 2010;3(5):581-588.
49. Kelley AS, McGarry K, Gorges R, Skinner JS. The burden of health care costs in the last 5 years of life. *Ann Intern Med.* 2015;163(10):729-736.
50. Ke LS, Huang X, O'Connor M, Lee S. Nurses' views regarding implementing advance care planning for older people: a systematic review and synthesis of qualitative studies. *J Clin Nurs.* 2015;24:2057-2073.
51. Ewing G, Grande G; National Association for Hospice at Home. Development of a Carer Support Needs Assessment Tool (CSNAT) for end-of-life care practice at home: a qualitative study. *Palliat Med.* 2013;27(3):244-256.
52. Department of Labor, Wage and Hour Division. *Family and Medical Leave Act.* http://www.dol.gov/whd/fmla/. Accessed October 2017.
53. Larson DG, Tobin DR. End of life conversations: evolving practice and theory. *JAMA.* 2000;284:1573-1578.
54. Della Santina C, Bernstein RH. Whole patient assessment, goal planning, and inflection points: their role in achieving quality end-of life care. *Clin Geriatr Med.* 2004;20:595-620.
55. Oliver DP, Washington K, Kruse LR, et al. Hospice family members' perceptions of and experiences with end-of-life care in the nursing home. *J Am Med Dir Assoc.* 2014;15:744-750.
56. Jonsen AR, Seigler M, Winslade WJ. *Clinical Ethics: A Practical Approach to Ethical Decisions in Clinical Medicine,* 4th ed. New York: McGraw-Hill; 1998.
57. Gordon DR. Principles and practice of withdrawing life-sustaining treatments. *Crit Care Clin.* 2004;20:435-451.
58. Billings JA, Krakauer EL. On patient autonomy and physician responsibility in end-of-life care. *Arch Intern Med.* 2011;171(9): 849-853.
59. Curtis JR. Interventions to improve care during withdrawal of life-sustaining treatments. *J Palliat Med.* 2005;8(Suppl 1):S116-S131.

6 SOCIAL JUSTICE

Mindy A. Smith, MD, MS
Richard P. Usatine, MD

Of all the forms of inequality, injustice in health care is the most shocking and inhumane.
—Martin Luther King, Jr.

The first question which the priest and the Levite asked was "If I stop to help this man, what will happen to me?" But . . . the Good Samaritan reversed the question: "If I do not stop to help this man, what will happen to him?"
—Martin Luther King, Jr.

PATIENT STORIES

For this third edition of the *Color Atlas*, we decided to focus on what we consider some of the most pressing social justice issues that face our country—issues that also influence healthcare and over which health providers have some influence. Most of us carry the stories of patients who were victims of racism, bullying, and hatred that sometimes escalated to direct violence or, more insidiously, undermined confidence, health, and self-esteem. All of us are aware of health disparities. What we may not realize is that data confirm that an individual's health is more strongly linked to their zip code than their genetic code; it is estimated that social and economic factors contribute 40% to health outcomes compared to 30% for health behaviors, 20% for clinical care, and 10% for the physical environment.[1] In fact, a Medline search using the terms racism and health yielded 970 articles linking the two in the last 5 years.

The U.S. Office of Disease Prevention and Health Promotion has set goals for 2020 to achieve health equity, eliminate disparities, and improve the health of all groups.[2] To set our sights on this goal, we, as health providers and educators, need to act by speaking out against social injustice, participating in anti-hate groups, reaching out to our communities and beyond, and creating safe and welcoming spaces in our clinical offices. Our most vulnerable patients should expect nothing less.

RACISM

- According to the Southern Poverty Law Center (SPLC), there were 917 active hate groups in the United States in 2016.[3] In addition, since this past presidential election, there has been a dramatic rise in hate violence and incidents of harassment and intimidation. The SPLC fights racial and social injustice through exposing and monitoring hate groups, creating materials to teach tolerance in our schools, and using the courts and other forms of advocacy to fight on behalf of victims of bigotry and discrimination.
- Authors of a meta-analysis of 293 predominantly U.S. studies published between 1983 and 2013 found that racism was associated with poorer mental, physical, and general health.[4] These negative effects were not moderated by age, sex, birthplace or education.
- Among black American women, perceived racism was most strongly associated with adverse birth outcomes.[5]
- That racism is still a systemic problem, negatively influencing health and healthcare, was described in a 2014 article by Feagin and Bennefield.[6] They noted the following:
    - Whites are dominant in heading medical associations, hospital systems, and public health institutions. As of 2014, the National Institutes of Health (NIH) director and six deputy directors were white, as were 23 of 27 directors of NIH agencies, and 83% of senior investigators.
    - Access continues to be a critical issue. For example, black women cared for by white physicians are not as well educated as white women about preventive care, are not screened as effectively, and are not referred as often to state-of-the-art treatment. African Americans, Latinos, Native Americans, and Asian Americans receive a poorer quality of healthcare, including diagnostic testing and treatments such as innovative cancer treatments, cardiac catheterization, and kidney transplants.
    - Both implicit bias (negative attitudes and associations with persons of color) and white-racial framing (racial stereotypes and prejudices; racist ideologies, images, and narratives) are prevalent and contribute to provision of inequitable healthcare, likely affecting morbidity and mortality rates for populations of color.
    - Solutions may include creation of a well-run nationalized health system, anti-poverty campaigns, counter-framing through publicly voicing experiences of institutional racism by people of color, and teaching about commonplace racist framing to medical providers.
- Dr. Jennifer Edgoose, MD, MPH, is an associate professor, family physician, and educator who began her career working at a federally qualified health center in South Tacoma, WA. She joined the faculty at the University of Wisconsin School of Medicine and Public Health, Department of Family Medicine and Community Health in 2010. Her clinical focus is on vulnerable populations and bridging differences. She is founder and chair of the department's Diversity, Equity and Inclusion Committee and serves on the health-equity team for Family Medicine for America's Health, striving to develop a national agenda and resources to promote family medicine's move toward social accountability and health equity. She is ethnically Korean but considers herself a "yellow person" who grew up as a daughter of immigrants in rural America.
    - Dr. Edgoose and her colleagues have been developing materials for health professionals and educators to combat racism in healthcare. This effort was prompted by the admission of a 100% white class to her residency program in 2014 and the recognition that more needed to be done to address diversity, inclusion, and disparity. As she began exploring the depth of local disparities, she realized that she didn't want to teach about disparities but about "inequities" and not just about race but about racism.
    - When asked to describe episodes of racism that she has experienced personally or professionally, she described rushing to attend a precipitous delivery only to have the most junior nursing assistant in the room cry out "thank goodness, the Nepalese interpreter has arrived!" She also described racism toward her patients with sickle

cell disease. In one instance, an entire floor of nurses accused a patient of pretending to lose her opiate prescriptions on discharge. When Dr. Edgoose insisted they look where they might store such items, a nurse found the prescription in her own nursing station. Dr. Edgoose states, "We must constantly strive to reflect on these everyday episodes that should eat at our souls, as these have enormous consequences for chronically maligned groups of people."

- Unable to find materials for addressing racism in medicine, Dr. Edgoose looked elsewhere and found many resources including those shown in Provider Resources at the end of this chapter. A toolkit that she developed along with national colleagues contains examples of resources and activities that many educators are using to teach these topics. Intended as a facilitator's guide, sections of the toolkit focus on how to address these topics. The toolkit can be downloaded from the Society of Teachers of Family Medicine at: https://resourcelibrary.stfm.org/viewdocument/toolkit-for-teaching-about-racism-i.
- When asked about what clinicians can do to become involved in advocacy against racism, she replied: "The first step is to confront racial privilege intentionally on a personal level. The next critical step is to advocate for diversification of leadership in the organizations to which we belong. Studies in the business sector show that the best way to diversify an organization is not to provide diversity training but rather to specifically assure diversity in the people at the top. Invariably, I have found keeping issues of health equity, let alone diversity and inclusion, on the table is an ongoing problem unless there is diversity of voice and opinion in decision-making bodies."

- **What You Can Do:** In working with our patients from diverse backgrounds, we can strive toward greater health equity by spending time listening to their health concerns, particularly their background stories and context, provide thoughtful explanations and education using the teach-back method to ensure understanding, incorporate interpreters and language-appropriate materials when needed, and engage in shared decision-making, cautioning ourselves to present all options fairly.

UNIVERSAL HEALTHCARE AND IMPROVED ACCESS TO CARE

- In 2015, in the United States, about 29 million people (9.1%) were without health insurance for the entire year, a drop from 10.4% or 33 million in 2014.[7] At the time of this writing, however, about 22 million more could lose insurance if proposed legislation is adopted. The consequences for those who are uninsured can be dire.
  - In 2002, the Institute of Medicine concluded that those who were uninsured had poorer health and that gaining insurance could decrease their all-cause mortality.[8]
  - Lack of insurance is associated with lower use of preventive services and reduces the likelihood of detection and treatment for common problems such as hypertension, diabetes, and depression.[9]
  - In a systematic review of evidence from studies on the relationship between insurance coverage and all-cause mortality, survival appears to be decreased among the uninsured.[9] These authors concluded in a second paper that single-payer reform was the best way to increase insurance coverage, improve benefits, and reduce costs.[10]
- Lack of insurance disproportionately affects Hispanics (16.2% are uninsured), followed by blacks (11.1%), Asians (7.5%), and non-Hispanic whites (6.7%)[7] (**Figures 6-1** and **6-2**).

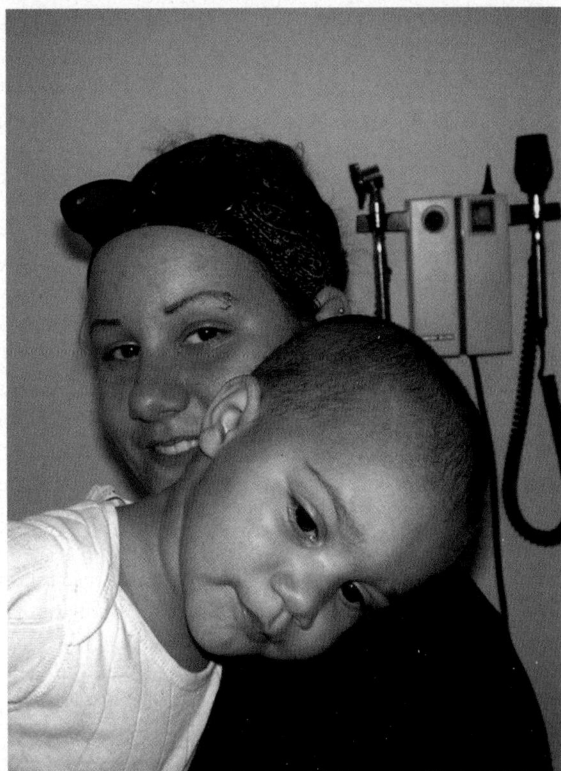

FIGURE 6-1 This mother and child are being cared for in the University of California at Los Angeles (UCLA)/Salvation Army free clinic run by medical students for homeless families in a transitional housing village. The boy had a bacterial infection on his leg and required antibiotics. The computer system in a pharmacy rejected his name and number, but, fortunately, the family doctor advocated for this child and the medicine was obtained. (*Reproduced with permission from Richard P. Usatine, MD.*)

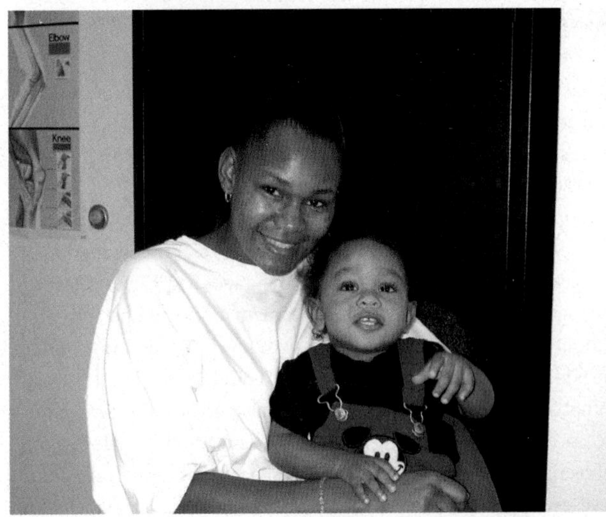

FIGURE 6-2 This 18-year-old mother has had type I diabetes since age 13 years. As a single mom she qualified for one of the living units within the Salvation Army transitional housing village. The week before this photo was taken, she presented to the student-run free clinic with diabetic ketoacidosis secondary to running out of her insulin. She knew that she needed her insulin but the pharmacy would not fill it because her insurance appeared to have lapsed in the computer system. After many calls to many pharmacies with no luck, her needed insulin was obtained from another free clinic in town. She survived without hospitalization and was feeling much better at the time of this photograph. (*Reproduced with permission from Richard P. Usatine, MD.*)

- In 2007, 62% of personal bankruptcies were caused by medical bills, a rise of almost 50% since 2001.[11] Importantly, of those bankruptcies, three quarters of the individuals were insured at the time of their illness.
- The Affordable Care Act resulted in considerable progress in reducing uninsured rates (absolute rate reduction of 6.9% from 2010 to 2015), reducing debt and improving perceived health status.[12]
- Physicians for a National Health Plan (PNHP), a nonprofit research and education organization of 20,000 physicians, medical students, and health professionals, advocates for a universal, comprehensive single-payer national health program. PNHP is not a new organization. Founded in 1987, this organization provides the latest news on this issue, speakers, slides, and many other single-payer resources. In 2016, a 39-member working group created "Beyond the Affordable Care Act: A Physicians' Proposal for Single-Payer Health Care Reform."[13] This proposal outlines the general structure of a single-payer system for the United States, including coverage and eligibility; physician and outpatient care payment; global budgeting of hospitals; health planning and capital investments; coverage for medications, devices, and supplies; the establishment of a national long-term care program; cost containment; and single-payer financing.
    - Sen. Bernie Sanders has introduced single-payer legislation in the U.S. Senate. The Medicare For All Act (S.1804), filed September 13, 2017, would cover all U.S. residents for medically necessary services, including primary and preventive care, with copays for some drugs but no copay for medical services.
    - **What You Can Do:** Become informed about the policy and political issues that affect our patients' access to health insurance and healthcare. Regardless of your political party, look at the proposals for health policy changes and consider how they will affect your patients. Advocate to your representatives and professional organizations for improved access to health insurance and healthcare.
- Provision of healthcare for all also requires improved access to both primary care and specialty services. In addition to lack of insurance, other barriers to care include cost, specialist availability, limited patient knowledge about healthcare, fear of discrimination, and fear of deportation.
    - Access to mental health services is particularly difficult in many areas of the United States. In a study based on National Health Interview Survey data, unmet need for mental healthcare increased from 4.3 million in 1997 to 7.2 million in 2010.[14] The likelihood of unmet need was higher among children (ages 2 to 17 years); working-age adults (ages 18–64 years); women; uninsured persons (about 5-fold higher); and persons with low incomes, those in fair or poor health, and those with chronic conditions.
    - **What You Can Do:** Primary care clinicians can help improve these access barriers by providing services based on a sliding-scale fees, volunteering in free clinics, partnering with paraprofessionals and mid-level providers to expand appointment slots and hours, and increasing use of videoconferencing and telemedicine for specialist consultation.
- Approximately 56.7 million Americans live with disabilities and these patients are more likely to experience difficulties or delays in accessing healthcare.[15] Barriers include inaccessible medical diagnostic equipment such as examination tables, weight scales, and imaging technologies; noninclusive health or wellness programs designed for people without disabilities; transportation problems; inaccurate or inadequate knowledge or stigmatizing attitudes of clinicians about

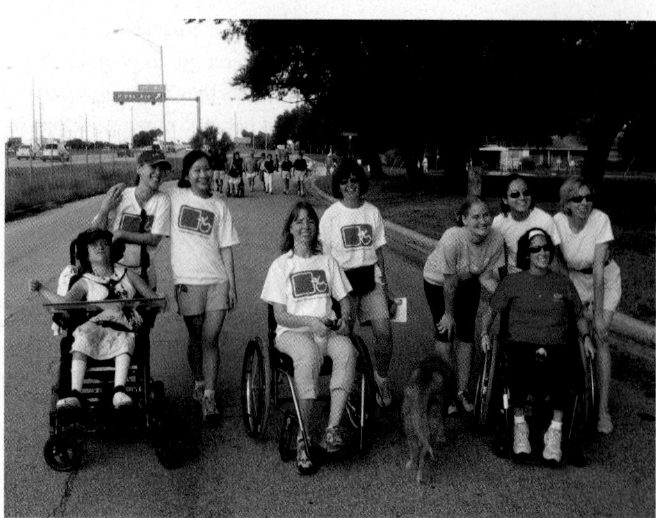

FIGURE 6-3 Dr. Woodard, a disability educator and advocate, her daughter Anika, and dog Nikki are part of a team of University of South Florida (USF) medical students, faculty, and family who participated in a "wheel-a-thon" to raise money for Tampa's first fully accessible playground. Teaching medical students the therapeutic value of sports and recreation for people with disabilities is an important aspect of the USF curriculum.

disabling conditions; and communication barriers, such as failure to accommodate deaf patients who require sign-language interpreters.[15] Dr. Laurie Woodard, shown in Figure 6-3, created and implemented a curriculum for training healthcare students about the capabilities and needs of individuals with disabilities. The curriculum includes a panel discussion, home visits, a service-learning project and sensitivity training.

- **What You Can Do:** Clinicians can improve care for their patients with disabilities through acquiring additional equipment, providing home visits, educating ourselves and our staff on disabling conditions, and identifying local resources such as transportation and interpretive services or resources available from the American Foundation for the Blind, National Federation of the Blind, National Association of the Deaf, or The Arc of the United States.

SUPPORTING MIGRANT AND IMMIGRANT HEALTH

- There is a pervasive fear that migrants and immigrants cause a drain on the healthcare system. In fact, the immigrant population starts off being healthier than their native-born counterparts. This may be due to many factors including selection (healthier individuals being more likely to successfully emigrate), bias in reporting due to underuse of medical care, or healthier risk profiles (e.g., less obesity) from their countries of origin.
  - In the 2007 National Survey of Children's Health, immigrant children in each racial/ethnic group had a lower prevalence of depression and behavioral problems; asthma; attention deficit disorder or attention-deficit/hyperactivity disorder; developmental delay; learning disability; speech, hearing, and sleep problems; school absence; and one or more chronic conditions than native-born children.[16]
  - In another population-based retrospective cohort from Canada, there was a lower adjusted risk of cardiovascular events or mortality among immigrants (adjusted hazard ratio [HR] 0.76, 95% confidence interval [CI] 0.74–0.78) after accounting for baseline differences; this benefit persisted beyond 10 years from immigration.[17] However, this healthy-immigrant advantage was not found among more recent refugees, immigrants with no previous education, and those who were unmarried.
- For some immigrants, health status declines over time in residence in the United States. In one study, having spent more than 10 cumulative years in the United States had borderline significance in predicting health decline ($p = .052$).[18] Having health insurance appears to attenuate worsening health.[19]
  - In six industrialized nations, including the United States, immigrant women from sub-Saharan Africa, Latin America, and the Caribbean were at higher risk of pre-eclampsia (OR: 1.72 and 1.63, respectively) and eclampsia (OR: 2.12 and 1.55, respectively), after adjustment for parity, maternal age, and destination country.[20] Stress may be one factor increasing risk; in another study, there were significant associations between lifetime stress and preterm birth in immigrant mothers compared with U.S.-born mothers.[21]
  - Despite expansion of health insurance coverage by the Affordable Care Act, an estimated 11.2 million undocumented immigrants in the United States remain uncovered.[12] Among uninsured immigrants, there is a stronger negative association between length of stay and health compared to immigrants with health insurance. Uninsured immigrants are also almost two times less likely than insured immigrants to have received preventive screenings, such as a Pap smear or prostate exam.[19]
- Dr. Kate Lemler Hughey is a clinical lecturer, family physician, and educator in the Department of Family Medicine at the University of Michigan (UM). She became interested in the challenges faced by immigrants after living and working outside the United States for 1 year. In 2016, she completed a fellowship in community medicine and health disparities through the UM Department of Family Medicine. The focus of her clinical practice is to provide culturally aware and language-concordant primary care for patients who identify as Latinx or Hispanic. Her scholarly work includes community-based participatory research on risk for unintended pregnancy and barriers to contraception use in this demographic. She is a member of the UM Asylum Collaborative and provides medical exams, legal affidavits, and expert witness services for local immigrants and refugees seeking asylum status. At the UM Medical School, she is core faculty for the Global Health and Disparities Path of Excellence, a longitudinal, co-curricular track for students interested in global and domestic health disparities, including migrant/immigrant health. Outside the university, she is active with community and grassroots organizations to promote immigrant rights.
  - U.S. Immigration and Customs Enforcement activity and deportations increased in 2017, particularly in places like Washtenaw County, MI, which is within 100 miles of an international border. Dr. Hughey believes that this directly affects patients and their physical and mental health. Many patients are afraid to come to their visits, and their blood pressure and diabetes are unmonitored or uncontrolled. Several pregnant women will not come to prenatal visits for fear of apprehension outside their homes. Families seek assistance navigating emergency documents that describe custody plans for their citizen children in the event of parent deportation—these children cry and worry at school, unable to focus because of fear that their parents will be gone at the end of the day. The parents experience symptoms of depression and anxiety and must balance seeking needed healthcare with the risk of leaving their own homes. Families often must choose between the wage earnings of a primary income earner and the risk of this person being detained or deported on their way to work. These situations affect mental health, nutrition, neighborhood safety, chronic medical conditions, and many other factors that influence a person's or family's overall health.
  - Dr. Hughey writes, "As I got to know my patients, I heard most describe leaving situations of violence, poverty, war, or political oppression on their journey to the U.S. Now, in my community, these same patients contribute economically and culturally in vital ways. Quality healthcare for all of us living in this country makes us all healthier and safer." She notes that many medical professional organizations have resources available to help in the care of immigrants and migrants (listed later in this chapter). Most states have an immigrant rights organization that can be found through a simple Internet search.
  - **What You Can Do:** Like any group, immigrants to the United States are a diverse group of people with different life experiences, resources, goals, and legal statuses. Remembering to

simply ask patients about their experiences without making assumptions is useful to better understand an individual's situation.

- Those who fear deportation may be reluctant to volunteer their documentation status, so it is important to provide assurance that this information is confidential and not recorded in the medical chart or elsewhere. Some providers prefer a general policy where documentation status is not elicited at any point during a visit. This should not limit discussion regarding symptoms or routine care that may be affected by immigration status or processes, but can help patients feel that they can share this information in a safe environment.
- Make available a list of local immigrant resources in commonly spoken languages to be given to patients who affirm they would like this information. Language-appropriate care is crucial to the care of any person who does not speak the dominant language. Trained healthcare interpreters (rather than family members, community members, or bilingual staff members) help to ensure that communication is clear and effective; these services may be available by phone or in person.
- Seek out community leaders for assistance in making your practice more supportive of this population. Possible contacts include leaders of local houses of worship, local immigrant rights centers, or leaders of community coalitions or neighborhood committees.
- Social media is a useful way to hear about events related to immigration—consider attending a meeting and introducing yourself to its organizers. Let these community leaders tell you about their needs and listen carefully to their concerns and suggestions for how you can help. Share what you learn with your own organization, advocating for awareness and policy change.
- Local officials also have regular meetings and publicize current events and proposals on the Internet or via mailing lists. Consider attending a county commissioners' meeting, for example, or contacting your local representatives with questions or thoughts about immigration health and policy.
- Become involved in your state-level professional organization. For example, the Michigan Academy of Family Physicians hosts an annual advocacy day with representatives in the state's capital.

ENVIRONMENTAL PROTECTION AND SOCIAL JUSTICE

- There are many threats to our health and the health of our planet. These include air pollution, climate change, lack of clean drinking water, deforestation, overpopulation, and use of toxic pesticides.
- Research has established the following connections with respect to air pollution and climate change and individual health:
    - Exposure to fine-particle outdoor air pollution is a leading risk factor for mortality, especially dangerous for the young and old and those with cardiovascular or lung disease, especially asthma.[22] Air pollution contributes to both development of cardiovascular disease and the triggering of cardiac events.[23] In an analysis of public health burden of air pollution in Sydney, Australia, investigators estimated that reducing fine-particle air pollution by 10% over 10 years would result in about 650 fewer premature deaths and about 700 fewer respiratory and cardiovascular hospital visits.[24]
    - Adverse health aspects related to climate change include heat-related disorders and consequences of warmer temperatures including heat stress; decreased air quality and reduced crop yields; infections including vector-borne and waterborne diseases; and mental health disorders, such as posttraumatic stress disorder and depression associated with natural disasters.[25] We have recently witnessed unprecedented loss of life from extensive wildfires, floods, and hurricanes linked to climate change.
- The Environmental Protection Agency (EPA) currently attempts to protect us from six air pollutants—carbon monoxide, lead, nitrogen oxides, ground-level ozone, particle pollution, and sulfur oxides. Further information about these can be found on the websites of both the EPA and the Centers for Disease Control and Prevention (CDC) (the websites are listed later). The CDC also provides air quality resources for health providers, including current air quality information and tool kits for assisting patients with asthma and heart disease about risks associated with air pollution.
    - The burning of fossil fuels (coal, oil, natural gas, and gasoline) is one of the major contributors to air pollution. Climate change is attributed to increased emissions of carbon dioxide (CO_2), a greenhouse gas.
    - **What You Can Do:** Use and promote energy-efficient vehicles or electric cars and alternative energy sources for our homes and offices. With respect to climate change, in addition to donating money to disaster funds and participating as volunteers in affected communities, clinicians can take steps to prepare for emergencies. The CDC provides information on emergency preparedness and response for the public and health providers, including information on outbreaks, training, and tools (https://www.emergency.cdc.gov).
- Most data on health effects of water pollution come from countries outside the United States; for example, in China, water pollution was negatively associated with mental health and self-reported physical health.[26] Sources of water pollution in this country include improper disposal of municipal and industrial effluents, indiscriminate applications of agrochemicals, and agricultural runoff. In addition, and more insidious, are sources of contamination in urban areas that find their way into groundwater and wastewater systems; these include hormones, antibiotics, endocrine disruptors, human and veterinary pharmaceuticals, X-ray contrast media, disinfection by-products, algal toxins, and taste-and-odor compounds.[27] Potential health effects from these chemicals include carcinogenesis (plasticizers), thyroid disease (perifluorinated compounds), lower reproductive function (UV filters), and liver disease (algal toxins).
    - The Centers for Disease Control and Prevention Healthy Places Site (https://www.cdc.gov/healthyplaces/healthtopics/water.htm) lists suggestions for a low-impact development approach to conserve natural systems and hydrologic functions of any site by capturing, cleansing, and reusing water from precipitation events (e.g., creating greenroofs, porous paving systems); integrating reuse of wastes and water in a way that protects public health while preserving the integrity of ecological and biological

systems; protecting and incorporating natural aquatic systems (e.g., wetlands and streams); preserving natural open spaces and minimizing land disturbance; and protecting watersheds and water resources through greenfield development practices.

- The water crisis in Flint, Michigan, is one example of both adverse health effects of contaminated water and the crucial role played by a local pediatrician, Dr. Mona Hanna-Attisha. Briefly, in 2014, the city of Flint, as a temporary cost-cutting measure while awaiting a new pipeline, changed its drinking water source from the Detroit Water and Sewage Department (sourced from the Detroit River and Lake Huron) to the Flint River—a watershed with a history of bacterial contamination and many sources of pollution including industrial complexes, landfills, and farms laden with pesticides and fertilizer. The corrosiveness of the water allowed lead from aging water pipes to leach into the drinking water system. In February 2016, the EPA notified the Michigan Department of Environmental Quality (MEDQ) about dangerously elevated lead levels in the water at the home of a Flint resident.[28]
    - Dr. Hanna-Attisha was greatly concerned about the situation of lead exposure, a potent neurotoxin, and its effects on Flint's pregnant women and children. In the face of false reassurances by the MEDQ and the Flint mayor, she and her colleagues undertook a retrospective study of all children younger than 5 years of age who had a blood lead level processed through the Hurley Medical Center's laboratory 9 months before and 9 months after the water source change.[29] They found the percentage of elevated blood levels increased from 2.4% to 4.9%; in those living in high water-lead-level areas, children's elevated blood lead level percentages increased from 4% to 10.6%. Following release of her findings and those of the Virginia Tech research team studying Flint's water in September 2015, the Michigan Department of Health and Human Services began testing drinking water, and the following month, the city switched back to Detroit water.[28]
    - Years later, the residents of Flint are still dealing with the consequences of the toxic exposures that occurred from drinking tap water in their homes and schools. In March 2017, a federal judge approved a $97 million settlement, in which the state of Michigan agrees to replace lead or galvanized steel water lines in the City of Flint.
- One of the authors, Dr. Mindy Smith, secured funding through EPA for a technical adviser to assist her local community in providing input and understanding results of a remedial investigation and feasibility study and is actively participating in document review and public outreach for a Superfund site. As secretary and board member of Citizens for a Clean Columbia (**Figure 6-4**), she writes biannual newsletters, participates in local cleanup efforts, (**Figure 6-5**), serves as liaison to other environmental groups, and attends local community events to educate the public about study results and potential health effects of river, soil, beach, and sediment contaminants. She also worked with a passionate local resident, Jamie Paparich, who has been deeply committed to documenting and understanding community health problems, to develop an Internet-based health survey of current and past residents; this effort led to an epidemiologic survey confirming a cluster of ulcerative colitis cases in the community.
- **What You Can Do:** Health providers can make significant inroads in protecting their patients and communities by being aware of potential water contaminants, watching for illness clusters, and

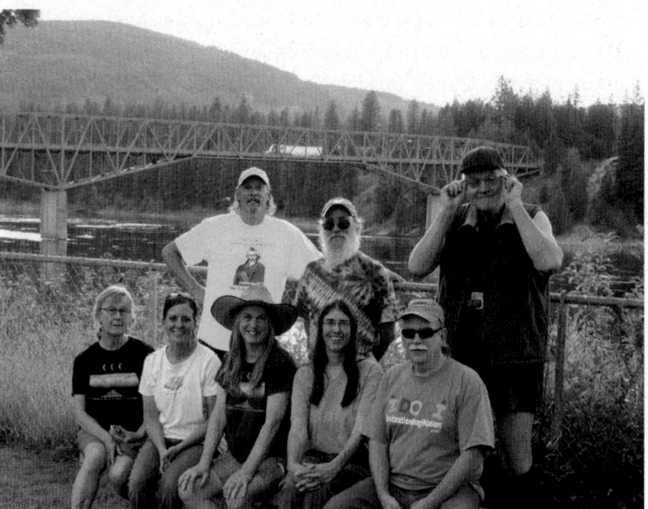

FIGURE 6-4 Board members and technical adviser of Citizens for a Clean Columbia (CCC), a nonprofit, volunteer organization focused on advocating for the health of the Upper Columbia River and Lake Roosevelt (www.cleancolumbia.org).

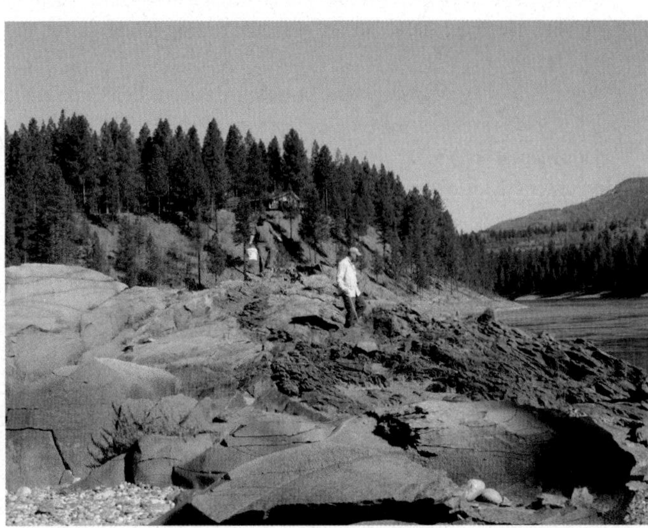

FIGURE 6-5 Columbia River shoreline cleanup event with members of CCC.

reporting to health departments and the EPA when appropriate. We can also lobby for restriction of chemicals with high water-pollution potential and ecotoxicologic risk; development of wastewater and drinking water treatment technologies to remove organic chemicals; additional research into health and ecological risks of organic chemicals, chemical transport, and natural attenuation processes; and ecologically friendly alternatives.[27]

- Pesticides are chemicals intended to kill unwanted insects, plants, molds, and rodents. Exposure to pesticides can occur through unintentional exposure via agricultural work or presence in the immediate area during and right after application of pesticides, through chemical residue on food or plants (e.g., grass), or through intentional exposures during suicide attempts. Routes of exposure are dermal, inhalation, oral, and eyes. The World Health Organization estimated that 1 million serious unintentional poisonings and as many as 25 million minor poisonings occur each year worldwide, with an addition 2 million people hospitalized for suicide attempts with pesticides.[30] Organophosphate and carbamate insecticides, strychnine rodenticides, and paraquat herbicides are among the more toxic pesticides. Based on data from the National Institute for Occupational Safety and Health, the highest rates of pesticide poisoning in the United States (>3.89/100,000) occurred in the states of Washington, Idaho, Wyoming, Nebraska, and New Mexico.[31]
    - U.S. poison centers received 130,136 calls about pesticides from 2006 to 2010, with an average of 20,116 cases (17.8%) treated in healthcare facilities annually; this included an annual average of 7385 emergency room visits (2006 to 2008) and 1419 annual hospitalizations (2005 to 2009).[32] The annual cost associated with pesticide exposures was estimated at nearly $200 million USD, excluding costs from lost work time, hospital physician fees, and pesticide-induced cancers.
    - Acute effects of pesticide exposure depend on route of exposure and allergic response. Adverse effects include dermatitis, cough and wheezing, gastrointestinal symptoms (nausea, vomiting), and headache. In one study, acute respiratory effects were reported in 48% of the 4974 cases of acute pyrethrin/pyrethroid-related illness; these pesticides are used most commonly in and around homes.[33] Exposures were most often from spills/splashes, improper storage, and failure to evacuate during pesticide application.
    - In addition to death from acute poisoning, serious health effects of pesticides include neurologic disorders, depression,[34] neurodevelopmental and behavioral disorders such as attention-deficit/hyperactivity disorder, diabetes,[35] lymphocytic leukemia, and brain tumors.[36] In one study, for each 1.0 mcg/L of pesticide in groundwater, tested from residential wells, the risk of Parkinson disease increased by 3% (adjusted odds ratio [AOR] 1.03; 95% confidence interval, 1.02–1.04).[37]
- **What You Can Do:** Recognize and be prepared to treat acute pesticide poisoning. Some pesticides, such as organophosphates and carbamates, can be diagnosed by specific laboratory tests (e.g., depressed red blood cell cholinesterase levels) and have available antidotal therapy. In addition, educate patients about risks of pesticide exposure, lobby for comprehensive pesticide labeling and marketing practices that incorporate health considerations, and support bans on cosmetic use of pesticides.

CARING FOR PERSONS EXPERIENCING HOMELESSNESS

- According to the 2017 Annual Homeless Point in Time Assessment, 553,742 persons were homeless on a single night in January 2017; 35% were in unsheltered locations.[38]
- Homelessness among families with children decreased 5.4% nationwide after 2016, while local communities report the number of persons experiencing long-term chronic homelessness and the number of veterans increased.[38] The number of unaccompanied homeless youth and children in 2017 was estimated to be 40,799.[38]
- Even before the massive fires of 2017, the City and County of Los Angeles reported a nearly 26% increase in overall homelessness since 2016, primarily among persons found in unsheltered locations.[38] In many of the high-cost cities of our country, the severe shortage of affordable housing is leading to increased homelessness.[38]
- With all the hurricanes and fires in 2017, many families are finding themselves homeless for the first times in their lives. While this may be temporary for many families, this is putting additional pressure on affordable housing for those living in poverty.
- Persons experiencing homelessness are three to six times more likely to become ill, four times more likely to be hospitalized, and three to four times more likely to die at a younger age compared to non-homeless persons.[39] Disability and mental illness contribute to chronic homelessness.
- First-time homelessness is independently associated with alcohol-use disorders (AOR = 1.34), drug-use disorders (AOR = 2.51), and poverty (AOR = 1.34).[40]
- Compared to the general population, incidence of tuberculosis (TB) is nearly 10-fold higher among homeless persons, and these individuals are less likely to complete treatment.[41]
- Annual death rates among the homeless vary based on reporting source; for example, in Georgia, rates ranged from 40 deaths annually based on medical examiner reports to 191 deaths based on information provided by shelters.[42]
- In a study of deaths of 128 homeless persons in Fulton County, Georgia, almost all were men (98%) with an average age of 46 years.[43] The estimated crude death rate, based on a homeless population of 10,000 to 15,000, was 281 to 426 per 100,000 for persons reported to the medical examiner.
    - More than half (55%) died or were found dead outdoors. Of the persons who died indoors, 29 (23%) were found in vacant buildings and 3 died at shelters.
    - Cause of death, based on the medical history, investigation scene information, circumstances of death, and autopsy and toxicologic studies (when performed) was classified as natural (71), accidental (40), homicide (10), or suicide (4). Natural deaths included alcohol related (42), hypertension or heart disease (13), and lung disease (4). Nearly half of unintentional deaths from injuries were due to alcohol (18 of 54 deaths) or fire.
- Persons experiencing homelessness are often extremely poor and socially isolated; the latter is considered a significant contributor to being homeless. Many medical conditions are caused by or

exacerbated by the adverse living conditions and lack of healthcare experienced by the homeless. These include:
  - Psychiatric illnesses and substance abuse disorders.
  - Physical health problems, including injuries from trauma, respiratory disease (e.g., TB), scabies and pediculosis infestations, and chronic illnesses such as diabetes.
- Dr. Richard Usatine is a professor of Family and Community Medicine. He has worked with individuals and families experiencing homelessness for 34 years. Their stories and lives have touched his heart and soul in profound ways. He writes, "The homeless in America are at the bottom of our society in dire poverty and lacking a stable living environment. Losing a job and a home and suffering with mental illness and addictions make the homeless one of the most vulnerable populations in our wealthy country. Caring for them with compassion brings joy to the heart."
  - In 1984, Dr. Usatine began to provide healthcare to homeless people at the Venice Family Clinic, a free clinic in Venice, California. Along with Mary Smith, a seasoned nurse practitioner who had years of experience working with the homeless, he delivered healthcare to the homeless of Los Angeles both in the free clinic and in the surrounding shelters. Dr. Usatine was also the medical director of a nurse-practitioner–run full-time free clinic in the largest homeless shelter on skid row of Los Angeles. Working with Aaron Strehlow, NP, PhD, they made care accessible to the approximately 1000 homeless persons staying in that shelter daily.
  - He first established two student-run clinics for homeless families and individuals with the medical students of UCLA. He states that the "passion and motivation of the students to serve this vulnerable population has been a tremendous inspiration to him throughout his career." After moving to San Antonio, Texas, Dr. Usatine worked with medical students, his colleagues, and the Center for Medical Humanities and Ethics to establish six more student-run free clinics, including one for homeless families and another for women in a residential drug and alcohol treatment home (**Figures 6-6** and **6-7**).
- **What You Can Do:** Join with medical learners to create clinics for persons experiencing homelessness and seek opportunities to bring services to homeless shelters. Advocate for affordable housing in your community. Today, more than ever, there is a shortage of housing units that people with low income can afford. As the gap between income and housing costs grows, more people face homelessness.
  - Work and partner with the best organizations in your community that serve persons experiencing homelessness. One model that stands out is the Haven for Hope Transformational Campus in San Antonio, Texas. They work with 140 partner organizations to provide more than 300 comprehensive services. The services offered include short-term residential housing on campus, primary care, substance abuse and mental health treatment, dental care, vision care, employment services, education services, life-skills training, legal services, childcare, housing assistance and an on-site animal kennel. This approach gives people the best chance of success by addressing root causes of homelessness while providing the wrap-around services needed to break the cycle of homelessness.
- The Haven for Hope approach is based on the philosophy that the individual is at the center of all services. Providers recognize and understand the role trauma plays in the lives of those served, and they work with clients to help them recover from conditions associated with mental health, substance abuse, and trauma. Dr. Usatine

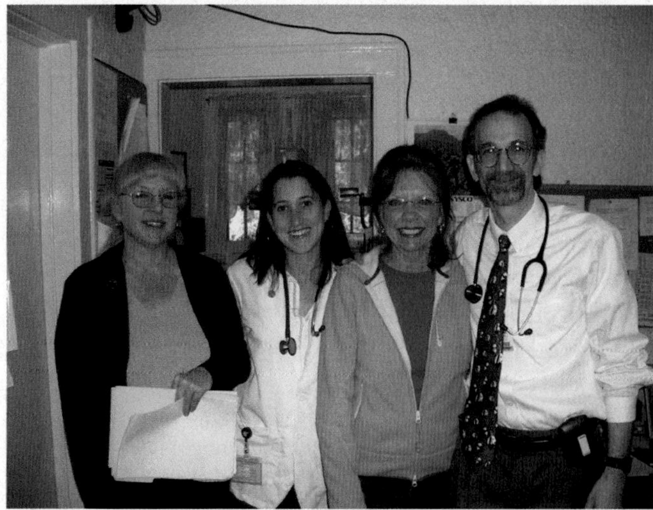

FIGURE 6-6 To help women recovering from substance abuse, the students and faculty of University of Texas Health Sciences Center San Antonio partnered with Alpha Home to open a free clinic on site. Alpha Home is a residential treatment unit with a 40-year track record of helping women become clean and sober. Prior to the opening of this clinic within the home in which the women reside, most of these uninsured women would go to the crowded university emergency department for healthcare. Many went without healthcare for fear that a 36-hour wait would drive them back to drugs and alcohol. The photograph shows (from left to right) Melanie Lane, the head counselor; Amy Cantor, the student founder; Julie Wisdom-Wild, the CEO; and Richard P. Usatine, the faculty founder and advisor.

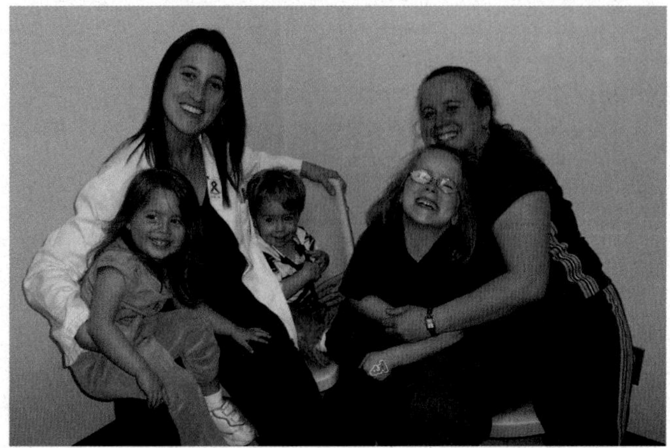

FIGURE 6-7 Amy Cantor as a fourth-year medical student in the Humanism Fellowship caring for a family at the second student-run clinic established in San Antonio. The mom and her four children have been reunited at the San Antonio Metropolitan Ministries Transitional Living and Learning Center. We saw this family almost weekly in our clinic and helped them make the transition from homelessness to independence. (*Reproduced with permission from Richard P. Usatine, MD.*)

and the students from UT Health San Antonio partner with Haven for Hope to make a difference in the lives of the families and individuals receiving help on this campus.

- Dr. Usatine states that this is one of the most rewarding aspects of his work and encourages other family physicians and healthcare providers to find community partners like Haven for Hope. When these partners don't exist, advocate for developing programs like this in your own community. Those interested in replicating this transformational village in their communities are welcome to tour the facility and learn from the experience of creating this collaborative and comprehensive program for persons experiencing homelessness.
- Listen to your patients' stories to increase your compassion for their suffering and appreciation for their courage under adversity. Listen without judgment, and the listening will help your patients heal their wounds. Do this with students in attendance so their compassion will grow from example.
- Create courses in your medical schools and healthcare schools so students can receive credit and recognition for their work with vulnerable populations. Dr. Usatine created two courses in the medical school, "Homelessness and Addiction" for first- and second-year medical students and "Humanism in Medicine" for senior students. More than 120 students participate each year in monthly seminars and volunteer work in the student-run free clinics. Community partners are involved in facilitating the seminars and some, like the philanthropist Mr. Bill Greehey, have become important financial supporters of the program. Dr. Usatine encourages other faculty members to create free clinics with connected courses and work with community partners and philanthropists. This approach leads to success in delivering healthcare services and immunizing students against the loss of compassion and increased cynicism that can develop in medical education. The philosophy of "The Center for Medical Humanities Ethics" espoused by Dr. Usatine is "preparing tomorrow's healers to act with compassion and justice."
- Comments from the participating students are:
  - I used to think of homelessness as a self-induced scenario, but through my work in the clinics and through this course, I have learned about the many reasons that homelessness occurs, most of which are external.
  - It is our calling to care for these people with full compassion and no sense of judgment, because we do not know what led them to their situation.
  - Persons experiencing homelessness are desperately in need of basic care, and good health is so important to their reentry into the working world. These basic steps of caring for people and preventing progression of illness help to prevent disastrous declines in health that they likely couldn't recover from without resources. These are the obvious reminders that healthcare is not a given in our society. Some people desperately need it and we can be there for them. Further, it strengthens our connection with these communities and breaks down any judgmental barriers.
  - I have learned that everyone has a life story that you should take the time to listen to and appreciate.
  - Homeless families can get so much hope from having someone who cares about them and actually takes the time to show that they care.
  - I never realized how many families and children are homeless. It was definitely eye opening. Also, I've learned that these patients have many serious medical problems because they have not had consistent medical care.

PROVIDER RESOURCES

Racism

- Southern Poverty Law Center, **https://www.splcenter.org.**
- Camara Jones Allegories on Race and Racism, **https://www.youtube.com/watch?v=GNhcY6fTyBM**
- Dorothy Roberts "The Problem with Raced-Based Medicine," **https://www.ted.com/talks/dorothy_roberts_the_problem_with_race_based_medicine.**

Access to Healthcare

- American Academy of Family Physicians, **http://www.aafp.org/online/en/home/policy.html.**
- Kaiser Family Foundation, **http://www.kff.org/uninsured/index.cfm.**
- American Foundation for the Blind, **https://www.afb.org/default.aspx.**
- National Association for the Deaf, **https://www.nad.org/.**

Immigrants and Migrants

- American Academy of Pediatrics, AAP Statement on Protecting Immigrant children, **https://www.aap.org/en-us/about-the-aap/aap-press-room/Pages/AAPStatementonProtectingImmigrantChildren.aspx.**
- Centers for Disease Control and Prevention, **https://www.cdc.gov/immigrantrefugeehealth/about-refugees.html.**
- World Health Organization. Overcoming migrants' barriers to health, **http://www.who.int/bulletin/volumes/86/8/08-020808.pdf.**

Environment

- National Center for Environmental Health, **https://www.cdc.gov/nceh/.**
- Healthy Places, **https://www.cdc.gov/healthyplaces/healthtopics/water.htm.**
- Environmental Protection Agency. Environmental Matter, **https://www.epa.gov/environmental-topics.**
- Centers for Disease Control and Prevention. Air Quality Resources for Professionals, **https://www.cdc.gov/air/resources.htm** and Air Pollutants, **https://www.cdc.gov/air/pollutants.htm.**

Homelessness

- National Alliance to End Homelessness, **http://www.naeh.org.**
- Student-run Free Clinics in San Antonio, **http://www.studentrunclinics.org.**
- The Society of Student-run Free Clinics, **http://www.studentrunfreeclinics.org.**
- Haven for Hope, **http://www.havenforhope.org.**

REFERENCES

1. County Health Rankings & Road Maps. *County Health Rankings Model.* http://www.countyhealthrankings.org/resources/county-health-rankings-model. Accessed July 2017.
2. Office of Disease Prevention and Health Promotion. *Disparities.* https://www.healthypeople.gov/2020/about/foundation-health-measures/Disparities. Accessed July 2017.
3. Southern Poverty Law Center, www.splcenter.org. Accessed August 2017.
4. Paradies Y, Ben J, Denson N, et al. Racism as a determinant of health: a systematic review and meta-analysis. *PLoS One.* 2015;10(9):e0138511.
5. Black LL, Johnson R, VanHoose L. The relationship between perceived racism/discrimination and health and black American women: a review of the literature from 2003-2013. *J Racial Ethn Health Disparities.* 2015;2(1):11-20.
6. Feagin J, Bennefield Z. Systemic racism and U.S. health care. *Soc Sci Med.* 2014;103:7-14.
7. Barnett JC, Vornovitsky M. *U.S. Census Bureau, Health Insurance Coverage in the United States: 2015.* Report No. P60-257. Washington, DC: U.S. Government Printing Office; 2015. https://www.census.gov/library/publications/2016/demo/p60-257.html. Accessed August 2017.
8. Institute of Medicine; Committee on the Consequences of Uninsurance. *Care Without Coverage: Too Little, Too Late.* Washington, DC: National Academies Press; 2002.
9. Woolhandler S, Himmelstein DU. The relationship of health insurance and mortality: is lack of insurance deadly? *Ann Intern Med.* 2017;167(6):424-431.
10. Woolhandler S, Himmelstein DU. Single-payer reform: the only way to fulfill the president's pledge of more coverage, better benefits, and lower costs. *Ann Intern Med.* 2017;166(8):587-588.
11. Himmelstein DU, Thorne D, Warren E, Woolhandler S. Medical bankruptcy in the United States, 2007: results of a national study. *Am J Med.* 2009;122(8):741-746.
12. Obama B. United States health care reform: progress to date and next steps. *JAMA.* 2016;316(5):525-532.
13. Physicians for a National Health Program. *Beyond the Affordable Care Act: A Physicians' Proposal for Single-Payer Health Care Reform.* http://www.pnhp.org/nhi. Accessed August 2017.
14. Roll JM, Kennedy J, Tran M, Howell D. Disparities in unmet need for mental health services in the United States, 1997-2010. *Psychiatr Serv.* 2013;64(1):80-82.
15. Peacock G, Iezzoni L, Harkin TR. Health care for Americans with disabilities—25 years after the ADA. *N Engl J Med.* 2015;373(10):892-893.
16. Singh GK, Yu SM, Kogan MD. Health, chronic conditions, and behavioral risk disparities among U.S. immigrant children and adolescents. *Public Health Rep.* 2013;128(6):463-479.
17. Okrainec K, Bell CM, Hollands S, Booth GL. Risk of cardiovascular events and mortality among a population-based cohort of immigrants and long-term residents with diabetes: are all immigrants healthier and if so, for how long? *Am Heart J.* 2015;170(1):123-132.
18. Brown HS, Wilson KJ, Angel JL. Mexican immigrant health: health insurance coverage implications. *J Health Care Poor Underserved.* 2015;26(3):990-1004.
19. Lee S, O'Neill A, Park J, et al. Health insurance moderates the association between immigrant length of stay and health status. *J Immigr Minor Health.* 2012;14(2):345-349.
20. Urquia ML, Glazier RH, Gagnon AJ, et al. Disparities in pre-eclampsia and eclampsia among immigrant women giving birth in six industrialised countries. *BJOG.* 2014;121(12):1492-1500.
21. Tsai HJ, Surkan PJ, Yu SM, et al. Differential effects of stress and African ancestry on preterm birth and related traits among U.S. born and immigrant Black mothers. *Medicine.* 2017;Feb;96(5):e5899.
22. Guillerm N, Cesari G. Fighting ambient air pollution and its impact on health: from human rights to the right to a clean environment. *Int J Tuberc Lung Dis.* 2015;19(8):887-897.
23. Franklin BA, Brook R, Arden Pope C 3rd. Air pollution and cardiovascular disease. *Curr Probl Cardiol.* 2015;40(5):207-238.
24. Broome RA, Fann N, Cristina TJ, et al. The health benefits of reducing air pollution in Sydney, Australia. *Environ Res.* 2015;143(Pt A):19-25.
25. Patz JA, Frumkin H, Holloway T, et al. Climate change: challenges and opportunities for global health. *JAMA.* 2014;312(15):1565-1580.
26. Wang Q, Yang Z. Industrial water pollution, water environment treatment, and health risks in China. *Environ Pollut.* 2016;218:358-365.
27. Pal A, He Y, Jekel M, et al. Emerging contaminants of public health significance as water quality indicator compounds in the urban water cycle. *Environ Int.* 2014 Oct;71:46-62.
28. CNN Library. *Flint Water Crisis Fast Facts.* http://www.cnn.com/2016/03/04/us/flint-water-crisis-fast-facts/index.html. Accessed November 2017.
29. Hanna-Attisha M, LaChance J, Sadler RC, Champney Schnepp A. Elevated blood lead levels in children associated with the Flint drinking water crisis: a spatial analysis of risk and public health response. *Am J Pub Health.* 2016;106(2):283-290.
30. Jeyaratnam J. Acute pesticide poisoning: a major global health problem. *World Health Stat Q.* 1990;43(3):139-144.
31. National Institute for Occupational Safety and Health. *Pesticide Illness & Injury Surveillance.* https://www.cdc.gov/niosh/topics/pesticides/. Accessed November 2017.
32. Langley RL, Mort SA. Human exposures to pesticides in the United States. *J Agromed.* 2012;17(3):300-315.
33. Hudson NL, Kasner EJ, Beckman J, et al. Characteristics and magnitude of acute pesticide-related illnesses and injuries associated with pyrethrin and pyrethroid exposures—11 states, 2000–2008. *Am J Ind Med.* 2014;57(1):15-30.
34. Beard JD, Hoppin JA, Richards M, et al. Pesticide exposure and self-reported incident depression among wives in the Agricultural Health Study. *Environ Res.* 2013;126:31-42.
35. Evangelou E, Ntritsos G, Chondrogiorgi M, et al. Exposure to pesticides and diabetes: a systematic review and meta-analysis. *Environ Int.* 2016;91:60-68.

36. Roberts JR, Karr CJ; Council on Environmental Health. Pesticide exposure in children. *Pediatrics.* 2012;130(6):e1765-1788.

37. James KA, Hall DA. Groundwater pesticide levels and the association with Parkinson disease. *Int J Toxicol.* 2015;34(3):266-273.

38. U.S. Department of Housing and Urban Development. *Homelessness Declines in Most Communities of the U.S. with Increases Reported in High-Cost Areas.* [Press release.] https://www.hud.gov/press/press_releases_media_advisories/2017/HUDNo_17-109. Accessed December 2017.

39. Maness DL, Khan M. Care of the homeless: an overview. *Am Fam Physician.* 2014;89(8):634-640.

40. Thompson RG Jr, Wall MM, Greenstein E, et al. Substance-use disorders and poverty as prospective predictors of first-time homelessness in the United States. *Am J Public Health.* 2013; 103(Suppl 2):S282-288.

41. Bamrah S, Yelk Woodruff RS, Powell K, et al. Tuberculosis among the homeless, United States, 1994–2010. *Int J Tuberc Lung Dis.* 2013;17(11):1414-1419.

42. Centers for Disease Control and Prevention. Enumerating deaths among homeless persons: comparison of medical examiner data and shelter-based reports—Fulton County, Georgia, 1991. *MMWR Morb Mortal Wkly Rep.* 1993;42(37): 719, 725-726.

43. Hanzlick R, Parrish RG. Deaths among the homeless in Fulton County, GA, 1989-90. *Public Health Rep.* 1993;108(4): 488-491.

7 GLOBAL HEALTH

Ruth E. Berggren, MD
Tiffanie C. Wong, DO
Richard P. Usatine, MD

COMMUNITY STORY

Common River is a U.S.-based nongovernmental organization (NGO) implementing a community development program in Aleta Wondo, Ethiopia. This NGO is founded on the principle of positive deviance, in which local best practices are identified and replicated to maximize agricultural production (organically grown coffee is produced in this region), as well as to improve the nutritional status, health, and education of orphaned and vulnerable children. Since 2009, a group from the University of Texas School of Medicine has traveled annually to Aleta Wondo to provide school health screening and free healthcare, including treatment of endemic helminth infections, trachoma, and skin diseases, while collaborating with and supporting the local government-sponsored health clinic (**Figures 7-1A** and **B**). In **Figure 7-1C**, the schoolchildren of Common River are looking at the new group of American medical students that have just arrived in Africa. In the coming week, these children will receive oral albendazole to treat intestinal parasites and have complete physical exams to detect and treat other common conditions, such as head lice, tinea capitis, trachoma, and foot infections. Note that many of the children are barefoot. In **Figure 7-1D**, a group of women has just completed their women's literacy class for the day. Improving women's literacy can improve the health of the entire community.

WHAT IS GLOBAL HEALTH?

For years, the term *international health* has described health work in resource-limited settings with an emphasis on tropical diseases, communicable diseases, and illness caused by poor nutrition and inadequate access to water, sanitation, and maternal care.[1] More recently, *global health* is commonly used to emphasize mutual sharing of experience and knowledge, in a bilateral exchange between industrialized nations and resource-limited countries, and the emphasis is expanding to include noncommunicable diseases and chronic illness.[2] One definition of global health, proposed by the Consortium of Universities for Global Health Executive Board, is "an area for study, research, and practice that places a priority on improving health and achieving equity in health for all people worldwide."[1] This chapter focuses on a few conditions commonly encountered in developing nations, emphasizing communicable diseases and malnutrition.

Ethical dilemmas abound when professionals from resource-rich settings leave their familiar environment and apply their practices in a severely resource limited setting. Consider, for example, breastfeeding guidelines in the setting of maternal-to-child HIV prevention. National protocols differ depending on resource availability. In some settings, telling an HIV-positive mother not to breastfeed (because breast milk can transmit HIV) may sentence her infant to near-certain death from diarrhea. If a program overturns local teaching about exclusive

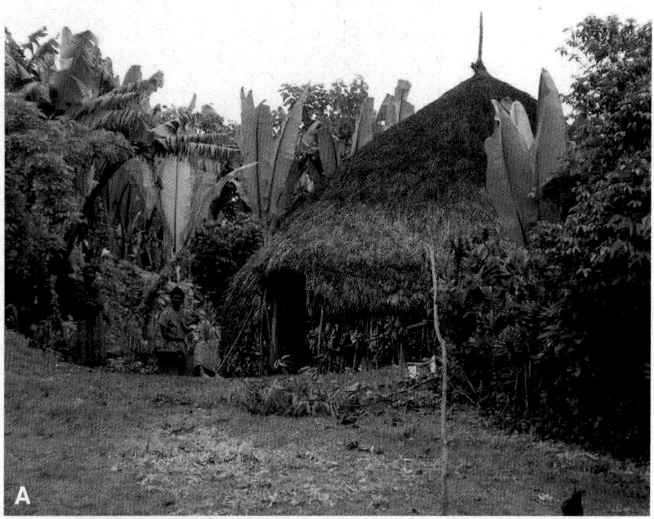

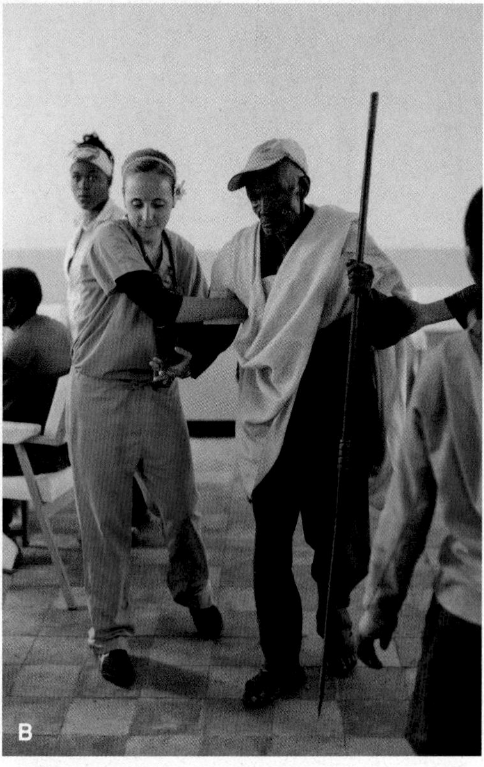

FIGURE 7-1 **A.** Many people still live in extreme poverty with no running water and electricity. This is a typical dwelling in rural Ethiopia. This one is inhabited by a grandmother, her grandchild, and a cow. The photograph was taken after a home visit to provide IM ceftriaxone to the child after her release from the local hospital where she was treated for a neck abscess and cellulitis. The medical team was staying at Common River and originated from the University of Texas. (*Reproduced with permission from Richard P. Usatine, MD.*) **B.** A University of Texas medical student helps an elderly man to a chair where he will be seen by the medical team working in Aleta Wondo. One of the local nursing students is observing the clinical activity. (*Reproduced with permission from Lester Rosebrock.*) (*continued*)

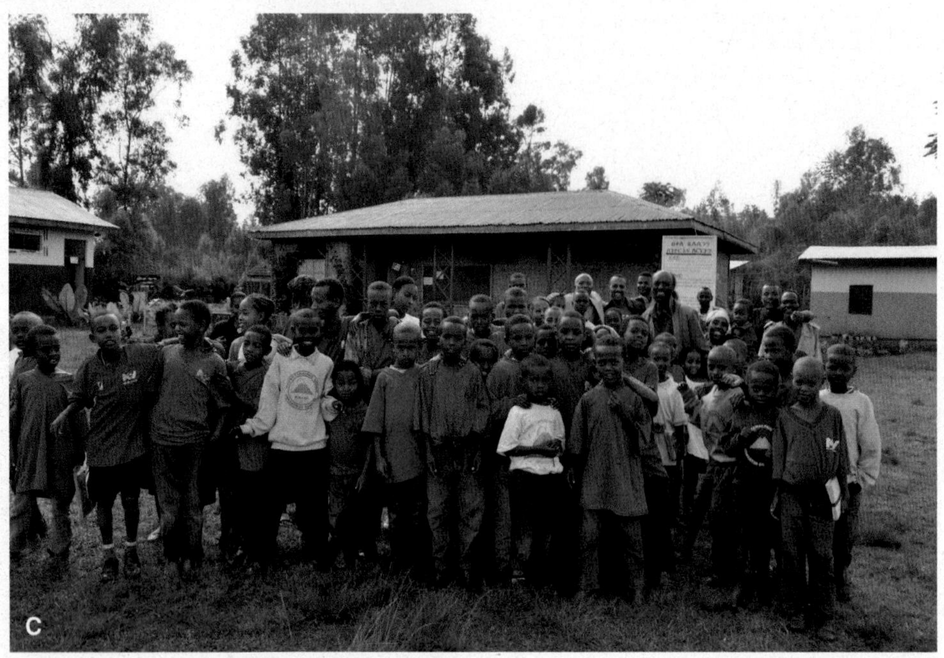

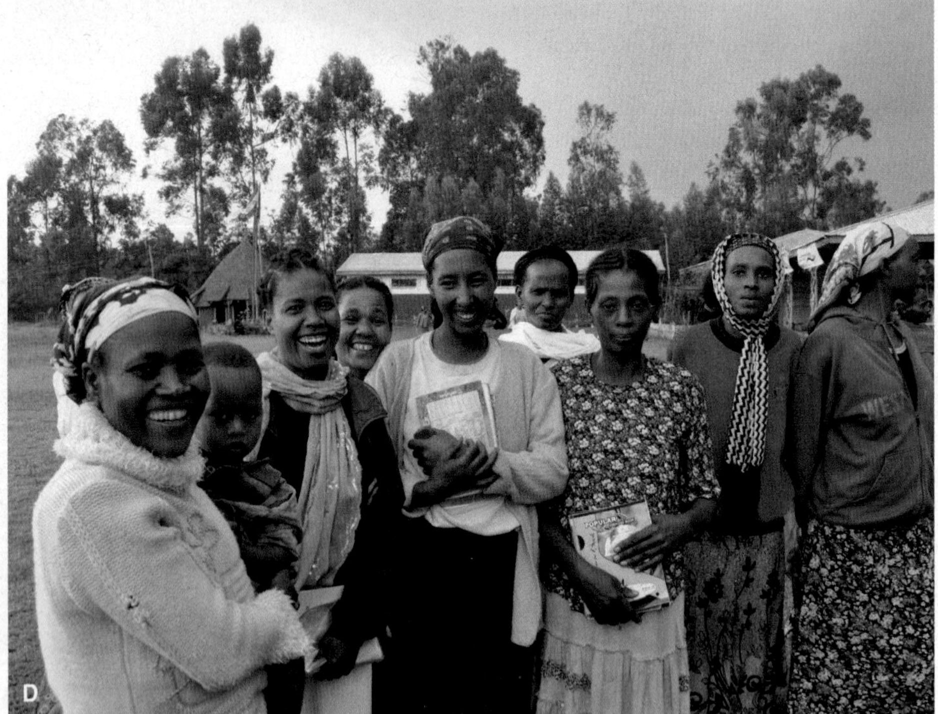

FIGURE 7-1 (*Continued*) **C.** The schoolchildren of Common River in rural Ethiopia greet the new group of American medical students that have just arrived in Africa. **D.** Smiling women who have just completed their women's literacy class for the day. Improving women's literacy is a great way to raise the health status of the community. (*Reproduced with permission from Richard P. Usatine, MD.*)

breastfeeding, it must ensure a safe and sustainable alternative form of infant feeding. Imposing the standards of industrialized nations in a community that cannot afford to continue to provide these standards can undo years of program development. Care must be taken not to undermine the trust a community has placed in local health providers, as this can ultimately increase morbidity rather than relieve suffering. Working with local health providers is essential so that a short trip can result in extended benefits to the community (**Figure 7-2**).

This chapter briefly introduces some of the relevant subject areas with which global health providers should familiarize themselves when preparing for international work. Statistics that aid in understanding the state of a nation's health relative to other countries are the mortality rate of children younger than age of 5 years old and adult life expectancy. Least-developed countries report that as many as 127 of 1000 children die before age 5 years (Chad), compared to 3 to 4 per 1000 in developed countries (Japan, Canada),[3] and adult life expectancy ranges from 50 or 52 years at birth (Chad, Swaziland) to 83 or 85 years (Japan, Hong Kong).[4] Another important parameter by which to compare the health status of countries is that of maternal mortality, defined as the number of maternal deaths per 100,000 live births. These figures, together with basic epidemiology of disease, provide important insights into public health priorities for populations.

What statistics do not provide, however, is the level of importance ascribed to a particular health issue by a community. It is necessary to acknowledge and address the needs expressed by communities themselves, in order of their own priorities, so as to achieve sustained improvements in health outcomes. All health improvements ultimately rely on long-term behavioral changes, whether dietary, pill taking, physical activity, or hygiene related. Group behavioral change requires buy-in from the population with approbation and influence of local leadership.

A useful method of creating a positive impact is to make use of ongoing peer-to-peer adult education techniques through the introduction of community health clubs. This can be effective for empowering resource-limited communities to develop their priorities, and to advocate for their community health and development needs.[5] It is best to learn about and collaborate with the local and governmental community health activities before launching any intervention, be it clinical, infrastructural, or preventive.

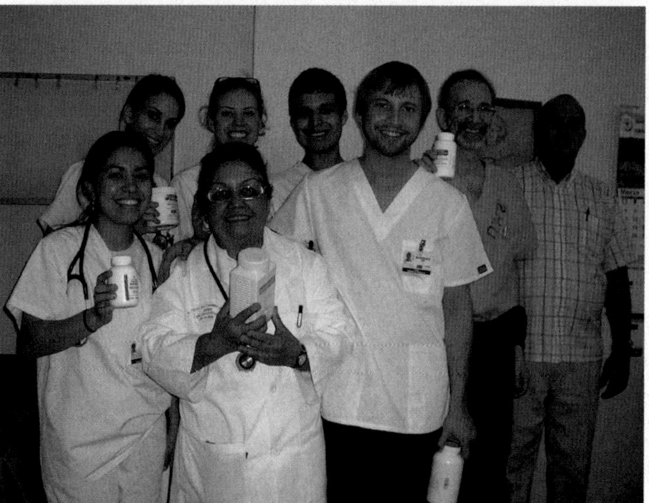

FIGURE 7-2 The physician in the front of this picture is pleased to receive medications that are unavailable to her hospital in rural Panama. Before shipping or bringing medications abroad, it is essential to learn what practicing physicians need. Bringing redundant or nearly expired meds or short-term supplies of expensive brand medications causes more harm than good. Donated medications should be locally relevant generics that are not expired. The WHO list of essential medications may be helpful in planning (http://www.who.int/medicines/publications/essentialmedicines/en/index.html). *(Reproduced with permission from Richard P. Usatine, MD.)*

WATER AND SANITATION

Many diseases in resource-poor settings are traceable to deficits in clean water supply and storage, lack of soap for bathing, and lack of functioning infrastructure to manage human waste (garbage collection, latrines) (**Figure 7-3**). Some of the most important ones include typhoid fever, cholera, and intestinal parasites.

Lack of governmental and public health infrastructure in the developing world leads to large populations living without clean running water. The World Health Organization (WHO) and UNICEF estimate that 844 million persons are without access to basic drinking water services, 2.5 billion people (37% of the world's population) are without access to basic sanitation services, and 892 million people worldwide still practice open defecation.[6]

Water and sanitation deficiencies are responsible for most of the global burden of diarrheal disease. The most common diarrheal disease of returning travelers is caused by enterotoxigenic *Escherichia coli*. All over the world, young and malnourished children die of preventable diarrhea caused by rotavirus, *E. coli*, *Salmonella*, *Shigella*, and *Campylobacter*.

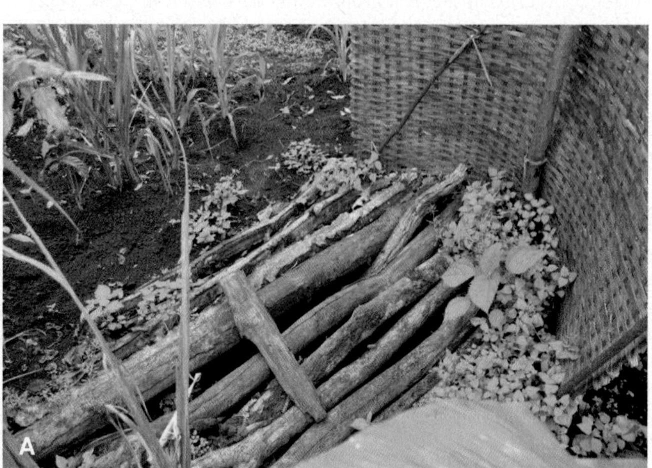

FIGURE 7-3 **A.** A covered pit latrine serving the needs of an Ethiopian family. The latrine is located on the edge of the garden near their home and presents a fall hazard for young children. *(Reproduced with permission from Richard P. Usatine, MD.)* *(continued)*

Diseases that are particularly deadly as a result of lack of access to clean water include typhoid fever and cholera. Intestinal parasites, while usually not deadly, do lead to chronic problems with malnutrition and anemia, which themselves contribute to cyclical poverty and disease because they lead to impaired learning, reduced productivity, and vulnerability to other infectious diseases.

TYPHOID FEVER

Typhoid fever, also known as enteric fever, is an acute systemic illness caused by the invasive bacterial pathogen *Salmonella typhi*. *Salmonella* is ingested in contaminated water or food, invades the mucosal surface of the small intestine, and causes bacteremia, with seeding of the liver, spleen, and lymph nodes.

EPIDEMIOLOGY

Typhoid fever is mainly found in countries with poor sanitary conditions. Because most such countries do not routinely confirm the diagnosis with blood cultures, the disease is highly underreported. Outbreaks of typhoid are often seen in the rainy season, and in areas where human fecal material washes into sources of drinking water. Shallow water tables and improperly placed latrines are environmental risk factors for typhoid. Globally there are 16 to 33 million cases annually, with up to a half a million deaths every year.[7]

CLINICAL PRESENTATION

Patients develop an acute systemic illness with prolonged fever, malaise, and abdominal pain after ingesting contaminated food or water. This truly nonspecific syndrome may include headache, mild cough, and constipation, with nausea and vomiting. Diarrhea may be present, but it is not the rule. After a 10- to 20-day incubation period, there is a stepwise progression of fever over a period of 3 weeks, and the patient may display a transient rash described as rose spots (2- to 4-mm pink macules on the torso, which fade on pressure). Temperature pulse dissociation with relative bradycardia despite high fever may be noted in fewer than 25% of patients. In the second week, the patient becomes more toxic and may develop hepatosplenomegaly. Untreated, typhoid can progress to include delirium, neurologic complications, and intestinal perforation caused by a proliferation of *Salmonella* in the Peyer patches (lymphoid tissue) of the intestinal mucosa. Although the mortality rate for untreated typhoid is 20%, early antibiotic therapy can decrease mortality. Approximately 1% to 4% of those who recover from acute typhoid fever become carriers of the disease who continue to shed *Salmonella* in their stool despite not being ill.[7]

DIAGNOSIS

Culture of blood, stool, rectal swab, or bone marrow.[8]

DIFFERENTIAL DIAGNOSIS[9]

- Malaria (often clinically indistinguishable from typhoid; empiric therapy for both malaria and typhoid may be warranted if diagnostic testing is unavailable).
- Enteroinvasive *E. coli*
- *Campylobacter*
- Paratyphoid fever (*Salmonella para typhi*, other less virulent Salmonellae)

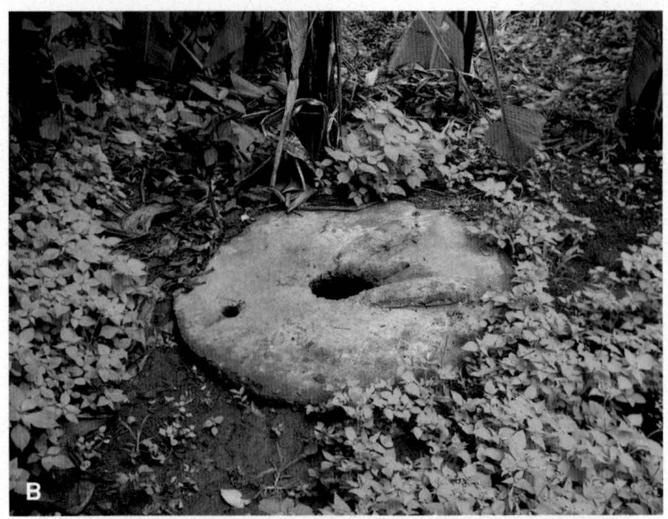

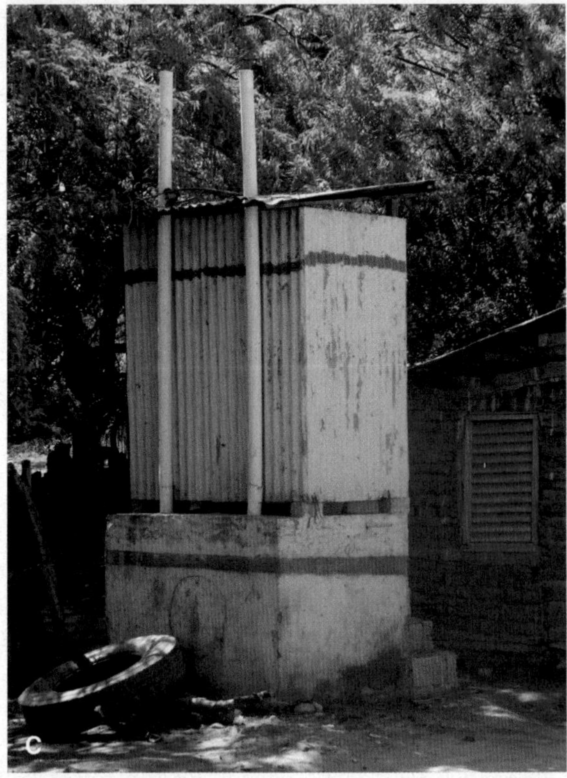

FIGURE 7-3 (*Continued*) **B.** An Ethiopian pit latrine, which offers no mitigation for flies and is situated in proximity to the water table below. Heavy rains will lead to contamination of the water supply with fecal pathogens. (*Reproduced with permission from Richard P. Usatine, MD.*) **C.** An elevated, ventilated improved pit latrine can protect the water table and reduce flies. Air circulates down the squat hole, into the pit and up through the pipe. To ensure unhindered flow of air, the top of the vent pipe must be 0.5 meter above the top of the shelter. The latrine interior is kept dark so the main light source in the pit comes from the vent pipe. Flies are attracted to the light, but the pipe has a fly-proof screen at the top, so they cannot escape and eventually die.[9] Many countries consider the ventilated improved pit latrine to be the minimum standard for improved sanitation. (*Reproduced with permission from Jason Rosenfeld, MPH.*)

- Dengue fever (mosquito-borne arbovirus infection spread by *Aedes aegypti*)
- Rickettsial diseases (typhus, spotted fever, Q fever)
- Brucellosis
- Leptospirosis
- Heat stroke

MANAGEMENT

Prompt diagnosis and initiation of antibiotic therapy is essential and lifesaving. Oral rehydration therapy should be initiated first, followed by IV fluids if vomiting cannot be controlled and for patients with altered mental status or hypovolemic shock. Antibiotic resistance patterns differ with geographic location.

For Africa and resource-limited settings in the Americas, the first choice is chloramphenicol 1 g PO daily for 10 to 14 days, or ciprofloxacin. Historically, trimethoprim-sulfamethoxazole 960 mg PO twice daily for 10 to 14 days has been used,[8] but there has been increasing drug resistance to sulfa in these areas. In Asia, where multidrug resistant *S. typhi* strains are well described, ciprofloxacin (500 to 750 mg twice daily), ceftriaxone (60 mg/kg IV daily), or azithromycin (500 mg daily) may be used for 7 to 14 days.[8,10,11] Azithromycin should only be used in mild disease. Some guidelines advocate the use of dexamethasone, 3 mg/kg IV, followed by 1 mg/kg every 6 hours for 2 days in the setting of shock or altered mental status.[8] See vaccine information at the end of this chapter.

CHOLERA

Cholera is an acute, diarrheal disease caused by *Vibrio cholerae*. It is usually transmitted by contaminated water or food and is associated with pandemics in countries that lack public health infrastructure and resources for sanitation. Although the infection is often mild or asymptomatic, in 5% to 10% of patients it can be severe and life-threatening.[12]

EPIDEMIOLOGY

V. cholerae reservoirs occur in brackish and salt water, as well as estuaries. Although the organism occurs in association with copepods and zooplankton, its largest reservoir is in humans. Cholera pandemics have been reported in south Asia, Africa, and Latin America. Characteristically, cholera outbreaks occur in countries that have suffered destruction of public health infrastructure (collapse of water supplies, sanitation, and garbage collection systems). The 2010 outbreak in post-earthquake Haiti has been traced to UN peacekeeping soldiers, whose waste contaminated a major Haitian river used for bathing, irrigation, and drinking water. In just 10 months, 300,000 cases were reported, of whom 4500 died, and the outbreak has continued to wax and wane with the rainy seasons for years.[13] A large infective dose is necessary for infection, and although only approximately 10% of those infected fall ill, the infection can be fatal for young children, the elderly, and malnourished individuals.

PATHOPHYSIOLOGY

V. cholerae is a motile, gram-negative rod. After ingestion via contaminated water or food, it must survive the acid environment of the stomach before colonizing the mucosal surface of the small intestine. The organism is noninvasive and not associated with bloody diarrhea. Rather, it makes a potent toxin causing massive secretion of electrolyte-rich fluid into the gut lumen. Human-to-human contact spread virtually never occurs. Transmission through contaminated food or water is the rule.[14]

Clinical presentation ranges from mild watery diarrhea to acute, fulminant watery diarrhea that looks like rice water. After an incubation period of 18 to 40 hours, patients may lose up to 30 L of fluid daily, with resulting metabolic acidosis and electrolyte disturbances. Severe dehydration can lead to death in a matter of hours. Vomiting, when present, starts after the onset of diarrhea. Profoundly dehydrated patients present with decreased skin turgor, sunken eyes, and lethargy. Children, but not adults, may have mild fever. Cramping caused by loss of calcium and potassium is common.[14]

DIFFERENTIAL DIAGNOSIS AND LABORATORY TESTS

Early presentation may resemble enterotoxigenic *E. coli*; however, the syndrome is quickly distinguishable because of the extreme volume of "rice water" secretory diarrhea that is the result of cholera toxin. *V. cholerae* may be confirmed by stool culture, polymerase chain reaction (PCR) for toxin genes, or dark-field microscopy with specific antisera, which will immobilize the *V. cholerae*.[15] In areas with limited or no laboratories available, there is a Crystal VC dipstick rapid test which can provide early warnings that an outbreak of cholera is occurring. However, as the sensitivity and specificity of the test is not optimal, it is still recommended to be confirmed by culture based methods.[16] The Centers for Disease Control and Prevention (CDC) states that confirmation of cholera by stool specimen culture or rectal swab remains the gold standard. For transport, Cary Blair medium is used, and for identification, thiosulfate-citrate-bile-salts (TCBS) agar is recommended.[16]

MANAGEMENT

Water, sanitation, and hygiene education is essential, as is education about recognizing the symptoms and immediately seeking medical attention while initiating oral rehydration. Optimally, rehydration should commence with reconstitution of WHO-distributed oral rehydration salts (ORS), which is available in all but the most remote areas of the world. Hydration is the mainstay of therapy, and replacement of fluids should be calibrated to match losses. ORS should be prepared with previously boiled water and consumed within 24 hours of reconstitution. IV or intraosseous hydration with Ringer lactate solution should be initiated if the patient is vomiting or in danger of hypovolemic shock. The volume needed to rehydrate a cholera patient is often underestimated; for this reason, collection and measurement of the watery stool in a bucket placed under the cholera cot is recommended.

Antibiotics are recommended for severe cases of cholera; options include[17]:

1. Tetracyclines
2. Doxycycline 300 mg orally as single dose (contraindicated in pregnancy) has been shown to be equivalent to tetracycline treatment. Single dosing offers ease of administration.
3. Ofloxacin, Trimethoprim-sulfamethoxazole (TMP-SMX), and ciprofloxacin are effective.

4. Azithromycin 1 g orally as single dose (more effective than either erythromycin or ciprofloxacin; appropriate first-line therapy for children and in pregnancy)
5. Erythromycin 250 mg PO daily for 3 days is appropriate and effective for children and pregnant women.

It has been shown that zinc supplementation can significantly reduce the duration (8 fewer hours of diarrheal illness) and severity of diarrhea (10% less diarrheal stool volume) in children suffering from cholera. As a result the CDC now recommends to immediately start supplementation with 10 to 20 mg of zinc daily when available for pediatric cholera.[18]

PREVENTION OF DISEASES SECONDARY TO CONTAMINATED WATER

Drinking purified or treated water, good hand-washing practices, and avoidance of contaminated food are essential. Travelers should be reminded not to brush their teeth with tap water and to avoid having potentially contaminated ice added to their beverages. Carbonated beverages are safe, as the carbonation process is bactericidal. Community education about hand washing and treatment of water is essential. In communities lacking running water (**Figure 7-4**), home storage of drinking water should be in containers with protective lids. Local guidelines regarding addition of chlorine to home stored water containers should be followed.

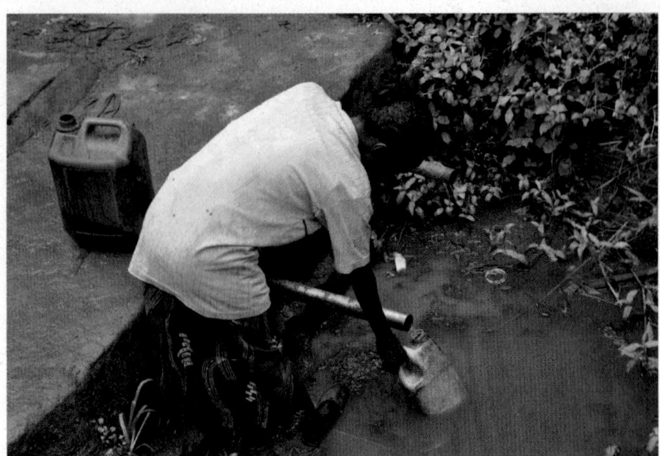

FIGURE 7-4 In this Ethiopian community without running water, water is collected in Jerry cans. Thousands of women carry these heavy, filled cans for miles after filling them up from this single pipe. The local town has provided one single pipe as the water source for the community. Although there is muddy water below, the water coming from the pipe appears clear, although it is likely to harbor bacteria and parasites. *(Reproduced with permission from Richard P. Usatine, MD.)*

INTESTINAL PARASITES

EPIDEMIOLOGY AND GEOGRAPHIC DISTRIBUTION

One-third of the world's population is infected with intestinal parasites, and although many parasitic infections are asymptomatic, some have serious health consequences. Especially affected are pregnant women and children, for whom hookworm-associated anemia results in maternal mortality, low-birth-weight babies, growth stunting, and impaired learning. The CDC recommends predeparture albendazole treatment as a single 600-mg dose (200 mg for children 12–23 months) and ivermectin two doses of 200 μg/kg orally once a day for 2 days prior to departure to the United States for all Middle Eastern, Asian, North African, Latin American, and Caribbean refugees. All African refugees who did not originate from counties where loa loa infection is endemic follow the same predeparture regimen with the addition of Praziquantel 40mg/kg divided into two doses. For those African refugees who originate where loa loa is endemic, they do not receive presumptive ivermectin for strongyloidiasis and treatment is deferred until arrival in the United States. This deferment of treatment is due to known rare cases of encephalopathy, a reaction due to loa loa microfilarial load.[19]

CLINICAL PRESENTATION

Abdominal pain, cramps, bloating, anorexia, anemia, fatigue, growth stunting of children, hepatomegaly (schistosomiasis).

DIAGNOSIS

Stool for ova and parasite studies (**Figure 7-5**). Note that these will not reliably detect *Strongyloides* or schistosomiasis; serologic testing is available for the latter. Eosinophilia is an important diagnostic clue for the presence of parasites; the finding of persistent eosinophilia warrants a careful diagnostic evaluation for parasitic infection.

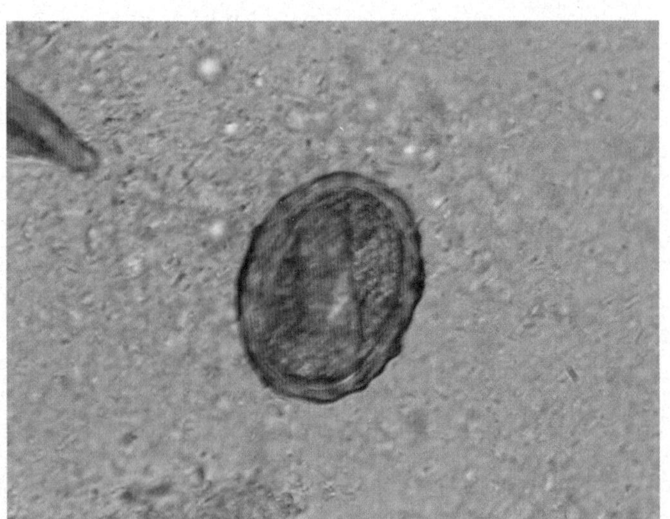

FIGURE 7-5 *Ascaris* egg found in the stool of a child with intestinal parasites. In most developing countries *Ascaris* is treated empirically with albendazole; stool studies are not always available or may not be cost effective. *(Reproduced with permission from Richard P. Usatine, MD.)*

TREATMENT

▶ Adults

Albendazole 400 mg orally as single dose will eradicate hookworm and *Ascaris*, but not *Trichuris* in most people.[20] Eradication of *Trichuris trichiura* requires three daily doses of albendazole or adding ivermectin to mebendazole.[21]

▶ Children 12 months to 2 years

Albendazole 200 mg orally as a single dose.[22] *S. stercoralis* requires 7 days of albendazole at 400 mg twice daily. For schistosomiasis, praziquantel is effective against all species of schistosomes. Give two doses of 20 mg/kg PO 4 to 6 hours apart (3 doses 4 hours apart for *Schistosoma japonicum*).[23]

PREVENTION

Preventative measures include proper management of human waste, hand washing after defecation and before cooking, and wearing shoes (prevents hookworm and *Strongyloides*). WHO guidelines recommend mass treatment of school children in endemic areas with single-dose albendazole therapy once every 6 months.

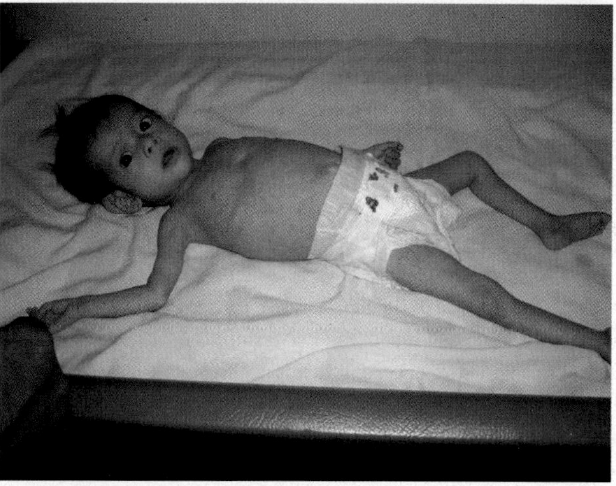

FIGURE 7-6 This 12-month-old Bolivian child with marasmus presented to medical attention with pneumonia. She has severe growth stunting and atrophied limbs, and she looks miserable. Her presentation highlights the association between malnutrition and infection. (*Reproduced with permission from Carolina Clark.*)

MALNUTRITION

Types of malnutrition include:

- Kwashiorkor
- Marasmus
- Micronutrient deficiencies

A global shift is underway, from diseases of undernutrition to overnutrition in tandem with industrialization and advances in transportation and technology. In spite of this global shift, about a quarter of the world's preschool children demonstrate growth stunting caused by nutritional deficiencies. In resource-poor countries, adult obesity and childhood undernutrition may coexist within the same families. The causes of this seeming paradox include many factors associated with poverty: the vulnerability of preschool children to infection when sanitation is inadequate, lack of nutrition education, decreased physical activity with increasing availability of technology and transportation, and mass marketing of inexpensive, calorie-rich foods.

Two classic presentations of malnutrition in children are important to recognize because they signal a patient who is immunocompromised and vulnerable not only to infection but also to preventable developmental delay. The accompanying photographs show an emaciated child with marasmus (severe, nonedematous malnutrition caused by calorie deprivation; **Figure 7-6**), and a puffy child with kwashiorkor (severe, edematous protein energy malnutrition; **Figure 7-7**). Marasmic kwashiorkor is another descriptor, illustrating the high level of overlap in the etiology and presentation of these extreme forms of malnutrition.[24] Whenever possible, one should avoid hospitalizing these children for nutritional rehabilitation, as hospitalization will expose them to many infectious pathogens that could be lethal during their vulnerable period of "nutritional AIDS."[25]

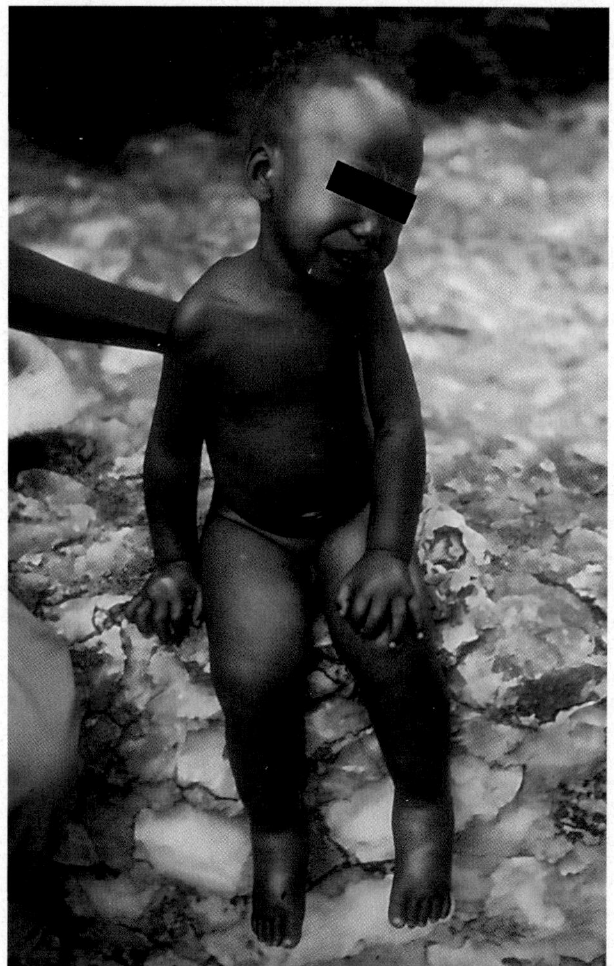

FIGURE 7-7 This 2-year-old child presented with classic signs and symptoms of kwashiorkor, a severe form of protein-energy malnutrition. The word *kwashiorkor*, from a Ghanaian language, refers to the sickness a child develops when it is weaned from breastfeeding. In countries with limited protein sources, newly weaned children are especially vulnerable to this disease. They present with depigmentation, red discoloration of the hair, distended abdomens, and peripheral edema. (*Reproduced with permission from Ruth Berggren, MD.*)

DIAGNOSIS

Growth chart monitoring is important for earliest detection of weight loss, growth stunting, or failure to gain height and weight over time.

In most resource-poor countries, growth monitoring is implemented by trained community health workers, who refer mothers for nutrition and education programs upon detecting faltering growth in children younger than the age of 5 years. Children often fail to gain weight normally after an episode of infectious diarrhea or malaria; this should be followed by a period of rapid catchup growth. If a child becomes reinfected before catchup growth is complete, the child will fall further behind on the growth curve.

Depending on the relative protein content of the diet, patients develop marasmus (calorie deprivation), characterized by emaciation and listlessness (see **Figure 7-6**), or kwashiorkor, "the disease of weaning"—protein-energy malnutrition. Kwashiorkor is characterized by red discoloration of the hair (**Figure 7-8**), which is also brittle, puffy eyes, bloated bellies, and pitting edema of the extremities (see **Figure 7-7**). These children feel miserable and are lethargic and uninterested in food. The differential diagnosis of kwashiorkor includes nephrotic syndrome, renal failure, or right-side congestive heart failure.

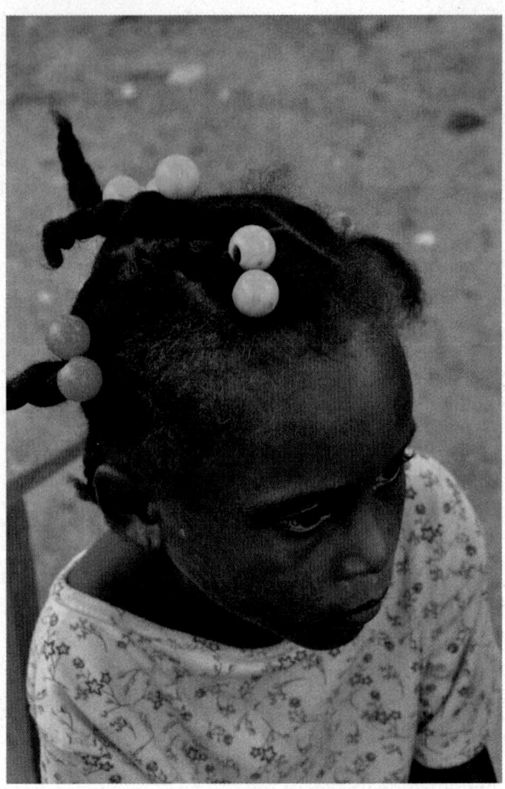

FIGURE 7-8 Child with kwashiorkor, protein-calorie malnutrition and red hair. The red hair is a result of the kwashiorkor. *(Reproduced with permission from Richard P. Usatine, MD.)*

PATHOPHYSIOLOGY

Childhood malnutrition, and especially kwashiorkor, may begin when a breastfeeding mother weans her child from the breast. Deprived of protective maternal antibodies and protein source, weaning infants begin sampling their contaminated environments and ingesting pathogens. Production of cytokines such as tumor necrosis factor (TNF)-α during infectious episodes suppresses appetite and impedes nutritional recovery.[25]

Micronutrient deficiencies coexist,[24] and deficiencies of vitamin A and zinc, in particular, predispose children to increased morbidity from subsequent infections. When parents are unable to replace protein requirements of weaning infants, children eat whatever locally available calorie sources (grains, cereals, bread, fruit) they can find. The poor in many developing countries lack protein sources, and toddlers are frequently not prioritized when meat, milk, or eggs become available.

As a result of severe protein deficiency, hypoalbuminemia and decreased intravascular oncotic pressure lead to edema, and the classic puffy appearance of the child with kwashiorkor. For years it was believed that children with kwashiorkor are disproportionately deprived of protein, whereas children with marasmus are deprived of both protein and carbohydrate calories proportionally; it now appears there is a great deal of overlap between these two presentations of severe malnutrition.[24]

MANAGEMENT

The endless cycle of infection leading to poor appetite and weight loss leading to malnutrition and further risk of infection[25] can be difficult to break unless mothers of malnourished children are taught to introduce calorie-dense weaning food supplements and snacks. Many countries have locally produced ready-to-use therapeutic foods (RUTF),[24] offering products like Plumpy'nut, or Haiti's Nourimanba, made from peanut butter, milk powder, vegetable oil, sugar, and a vitamin mix.[26]

These therapeutic foods are a useful adjunct to breaking the cycle of infection, anorexia, weight loss, and malnutrition, but they are not a substitute for educating mothers about how to rehabilitate their malnourished child using locally available and affordable foods. Nonmeat protein substitutes, such as red beans, and locally available green leafy vegetables are easier for mothers to obtain than meat, cow's milk, or expensive imported food supplements.

MICRONUTRIENT DEFICIENCIES

VITAMIN A DEFICIENCY

In contrast to marasmus and kwashiorkor, growth stunting is a more subtle syndrome affecting 200 million children who are younger than the age of 5 years. A variety of micronutrient deficiencies are believed to contribute to stunting syndrome and to accompany developmental delays, reduced cognitive function, impaired immunity, and future risk of obesity and hypertension.[27] There are four micronutrient deficiencies of global importance, each with associated clinical syndromes that should be recognized. All can be associated with growth stunting in children, who may present with abnormally short stature but relatively normal weight for height.

Vitamin A is a critical regulator of immune function, which is required for maintaining the integrity of mucosal surfaces. Vitamin A supplementation in countries with malnutrition reduces blindness (from xerophthalmia) as well as the morbidity of infectious diseases (especially measles, diarrhea, and respiratory infections). **Figure 7-9** shows a photograph of blindness caused by vitamin A deficiency. In 2009, the WHO estimated that clinical vitamin A deficiency (night blindness) and biochemical vitamin A deficiency (serum retinol concentration <0.70 μmol/L) affected 5.2 and 190 million preschool-age children, respectively.[28] About 250,000 to 500,000 children develop blindness caused by vitamin A deficiency every year, and half of these die within 12 months of losing sight.[29]

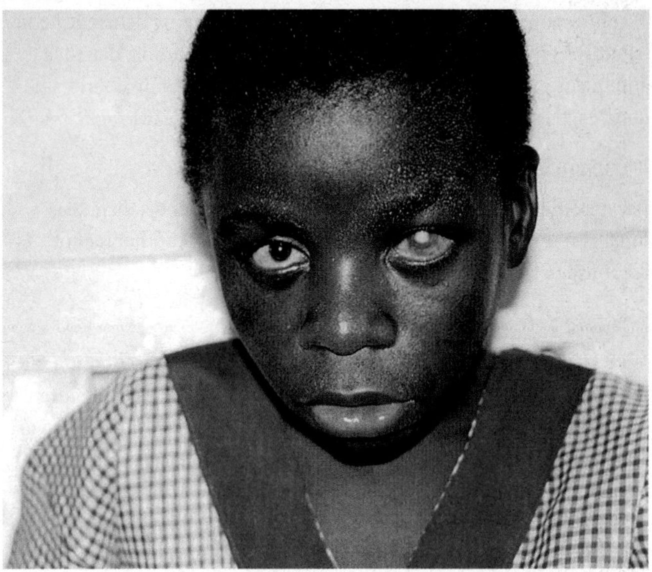

FIGURE 7-9 Child with severe xerophthalmia of the left eye secondary to vitamin A deficiency.[32] *(Used with permission from SIGHT AND LIFE, www.sightandlife.org.)*

▶ Clinical presentation

The earliest presentation of vitamin A deficiency is poor night vision, which may progress to night blindness, xerophthalmia, ulceration, and scarring of the cornea, followed ultimately by blindness. Vitamin A deficiency is also associated with anemia and is particularly dangerous in patients with measles, for whom mortality rates are high.

▶ Management

A meta-analysis of 43 trials involving 216,000 children younger than the age of 5 years who were given vitamin A supplements revealed striking reductions in mortality and morbidity. Seventeen of these trials reported a 24% reduction in mortality, and 7 trials reported a 28% reduction in mortality associated with diarrhea. Vitamin A reduced diarrhea and measles incidence. Vitamin A significantly reduces morbidity, mortality, and eye disease. Vitamin A supplements are recommended to all children who are at risk in low- and middle-income countries.[30] Most countries implement WHO guidelines for vitamin A supplementation synchronized with childhood vaccine schedules.

ZINC DEFICIENCY

Zinc plays a central role in cellular growth, differentiation, and metabolism. It is necessary for physical growth and GI and immune function. Many zinc studies show improved growth of children and decreased infections when supplements are given to vulnerable populations. Studies suggest that the global prevalence of zinc deficiency approaches 31%, especially in Africa, the eastern Mediterranean, and South Asia.[31]

▶ Clinical presentation

The most common presentation of zinc deficiency is nonspecific and may include growth stunting, delayed sexual maturation, dermatitis, and defective immunity. Zinc deficiency is associated with decreased macrophage chemotaxis, decreased neutrophil activity, and decreased

T-cell responses.[25] It is widely acknowledged that zinc deficiency contributes significantly to child mortality from pneumonia, diarrhea, and malaria. A rare but characteristic presentation of profound zinc deficiency is acrodermatitis enteropathica (**Figure 7-10**).

▶ Diagnosis

Because there is no good biomarker for zinc deficiency, diagnosis must rest on clinical suspicion and documentation of therapeutic response to supplementation.

▶ Management

WHO guidelines for diarrhea recommend use of low-concentration ORS together with routine zinc supplementation for 10 to 14 days. Children older than age 6 months should get 20 mg daily; infants younger than age 6 months should get 10 mg daily.[33] Zinc supplementation decreases the duration and volume of diarrheal stools by 25% and 30%, respectively. More importantly, 14 days of zinc supplementation for a diarrheal episode reduces the incidence of diarrhea and pneumonia in the subsequent 2 to 3 months, reduces hospital admissions for diarrhea, and brings approximately a 50% reduction in noninjury deaths in the year following the treatment.[34] Unfortunately, zinc supplementation benefits are still not widely known by healthcare workers in developing countries.[35]

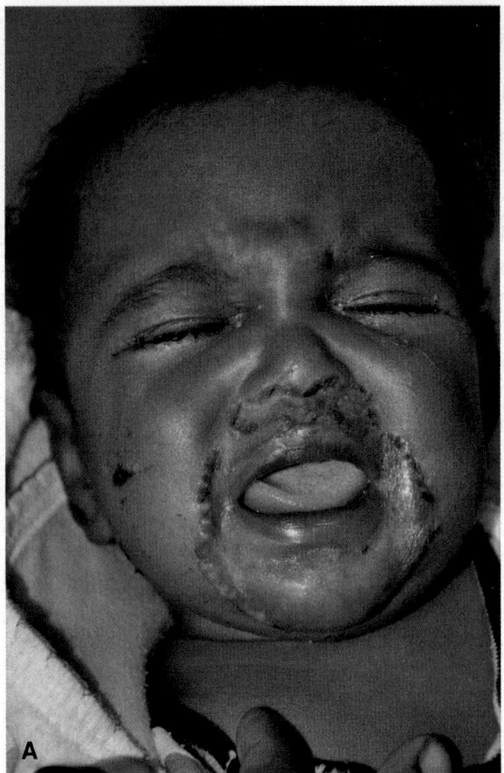

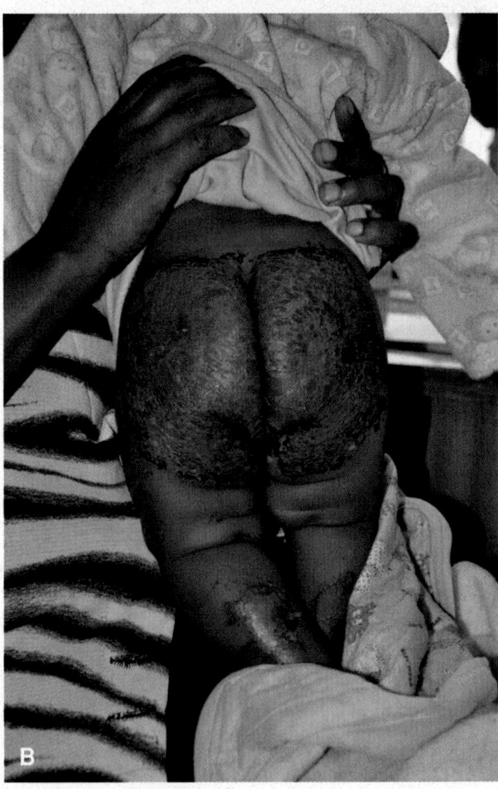

FIGURE 7-10 Acrodermatitis enteropathica caused by a zinc deficiency. Zinc supplementation is a standard recommendation from WHO in treatment of childhood diarrhea. Even children who do not have skin findings of zinc deficiency benefit with reduced duration of diarrhea and reduced mortality from all infectious causes in the ensuing months after receiving supplementation. Note the typical lesions around the **(A)** mouth and **(B)** buttocks. (*Reproduced with permission from Richard P. Usatine, MD.*)

IRON

Iron deficiency is the most common micronutrient deficiency in the world, and 2 billion people (nearly one-third of the global population) are anemic. In resource-limited countries, iron-deficiency anemia is either caused or aggravated by malaria, intestinal parasites such as hookworm, and other chronic infections such as HIV, tuberculosis, or schistosomiasis. Iron deficiency causes enormous morbidity and contributes 20% of global maternal mortality. Because the consequences include impaired cognition and physical development, increased risk of illness in children and reduced work productivity, iron deficiency is a real barrier to economic development in resource-poor countries.[36] As with zinc and vitamin A, iron deficiency can be detrimental to host immunity, causing decreased neutrophil chemotaxis.[25]

▶ Interventions

The WHO has developed a three-pronged strategy for addressing global iron deficiency: increasing iron uptake through dietary diversification and supplementation, improvement of nutritional status, and controlling infections, especially worms. In countries with significant iron-deficiency anemia, malaria, and helminth infections, these interventions can restore individual health as well as raise national productivity levels, thereby interrupting the cycle of poverty and disease.[36]

IODINE

Insufficient dietary iodine can significantly lower the IQ of whole populations and is the leading preventable cause of brain damage. Although iodine deficiency is easily solved through food fortification costing 2 cents per person annually, a prevalence of 60% to 90% iodine deficiency among school-age children is observed in multiple African, Asian, and eastern Mediterranean countries. There is tremendous variance of iodine deficiency within individual countries, and deficiency is not linked to poor or disadvantaged districts.[37] Iodine deficiency occurs where the soil has low iodine content because of past glaciation or repeated leaching effects of precipitation. Food crops grown in iodine-deficient soil provide inadequate dietary iodine.[38]

▶ Clinical presentation

Because iodine is required for thyroid hormone synthesis, iodine deficiency results in hypothyroidism and goiter (**Figure 7-11**). Congenital iodine deficiency results in a form of profound cognitive impairment known as *cretinism*. Other consequences include stillbirths, deaf-mutism, subclinical hyper- or hypothyroidism, impaired mental function, and retarded physical development.[38]

▶ Interventions

Iodine may be supplied in tablets or liquid form and taken daily; in adults, 150 μg/day is sufficient for thyroid function, and an adult multivitamin typically contains 150 μg of iodine per tablet, but this is impractical. Population-based interventions should include iodization of salt, and in some developing countries, eradication of iodine deficiency has been accomplished by adding iodine drops to well water.

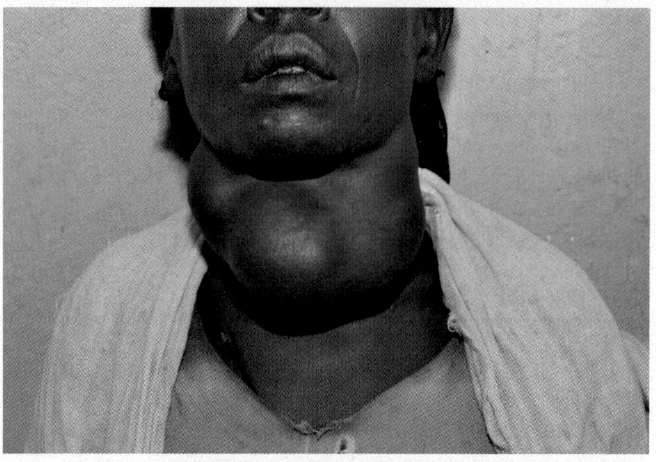

FIGURE 7-11 Massive goiter caused by iodine deficiency. This woman is from a country in Africa where iodine is not routinely supplemented in the diet and goiter is endemic. (*Reproduced with permission from Richard P. Usatine, MD.*)

VECTOR-BORNE DISEASES

MALARIA

Malaria is a protozoan infection spread by the *Anopheles* mosquito vector in endemic areas. Of the four species of malaria (*Plasmodium falciparum*, *Plasmodium ovale*, *Plasmodium malariae*, and *Plasmodium vivax*), *P. falciparum* is the most important to address, because if unrecognized and untreated, it can be rapidly fatal. Only *P. falciparum* exhibits high levels of parasitemia in blood, and it is the only type of malaria that causes sequestration of parasitized erythrocytes in microvasculature. This unique feature of *P. falciparum* is responsible for the severe end-organ damage, including renal failure, acute respiratory distress syndrome, and coma, that is seen with untreated disease.[39]

▶ Epidemiology and geographic distribution

There are more than 200 million cases of malaria in the world every year; in 2016 there were an estimated 216 million cases worldwide.[40] According to the WHO, in 2015 there were an estimated 429,000 deaths from malaria, with 90% of these deaths occurring in Africa.[41] Most of the deaths caused by malaria occur in children younger than age 5 years. *P. falciparum*, *P. vivax*, *P. malariae*, and *P. ovale* are globally distributed in the tropics. *P. vivax* is more common in Asia, South America, Oceania, and India. *P. ovale* is found mainly in West Africa, and *P. malariae* is much less common than *P. vivax* or *P. falciparum*.

The risk for malaria varies greatly within a given country, and depends on altitude (higher altitudes have lower risk), season (greatest risk in rainy season), and urbanization (rural areas have greater risk than urban areas). Thus, travelers should be aware of these differences and plan for prophylaxis accordingly.

The CDC publication, *Health Information for International Travel*, is available online at http://www.cdc.gov/travel/ and should be consulted for updates about regional patterns of malaria risk, as well as drug resistance and guidelines, which are subject to frequent changes.[42]

▶ Clinical presentation

After a 1- to 3-week incubation period following the bite of an infected female mosquito, patients develop a nonspecific syndrome of high fever, headache, myalgia, and shaking chills. This syndrome is frequently accompanied by nausea, vomiting, and back pain, and occasional diarrhea. Splenomegaly and anemia (related to hemolysis) are common in all 4 types of malaria.

As untreated *P. falciparum* progresses, there is a risk of cerebral malaria, which is caused by parasitized erythrocytes sequestered in the capillaries of the brain, with secondary metabolic consequences. Cerebral malaria is characterized by severe headache and altered consciousness. These patients may also develop acute respiratory distress syndrome (ARDS), hypoglycemia, acidosis, and shock in the setting of hyperparasitemia. Untreated patients with cerebral malaria ultimately progress to coma, respiratory failure, and death.[43]

▶ Differential diagnosis

The initial presentation of malaria is so nonspecific that it mimics influenza (without the respiratory symptoms), enteric fever (see section on typhoid), dengue fever, rickettsial infections, brucellosis, and leishmaniasis. If hemolysis has been extensive, the patient may present with jaundice, and viral hepatitis or leptospirosis may also be on the differential diagnosis.[39]

▶ Laboratory diagnosis

Malaria is usually diagnosed by light microscopy of peripheral blood smears prepared with a Giemsa, Field, or modified Wright stain (**Figures 7-12** and **7-13**). A thick-and-thin smear should be obtained whenever possible in every febrile patient in whom malaria is suspected, especially from febrile travelers returning from malaria endemic areas. Thin smears allow relative quantification and speciation of parasites when the parasitemia is high; thick smears are useful to rule in malaria, especially when parasitemia is low. Because a single negative smear does not rule out malaria, the test must be repeated on at least 3 occasions at 12- to 24-hour intervals. If all 3 sets are negative, the diagnosis of malaria is essentially ruled out.[44] Patients with high levels of parasitemia (>5%) have a worse prognosis, and should be considered for inpatient care.

Other diagnostic modalities include the fluorochrome acridine orange stain for fluorescence microscopy and PCR. PCR is more sensitive and specific than microscopy, can confirm species, and also detect drug resistance mutations. However the limitation of PCR is that it can only be performed in reference laboratories, and so the results are not often available quickly enough for routine diagnosis.[44] Rapid antigen assays using fingerstick blood samples on cards impregnated with specific antibodies are alternative methods for laboratory diagnosis of malaria. In the United States, the U.S. Food and Drug Administration has approved the BinaxNOW Malaria test, which, although costly, is convenient for rapid field use. Unfortunately, this and other immunochromatographic strip assays are not able to determine parasite load.[42]

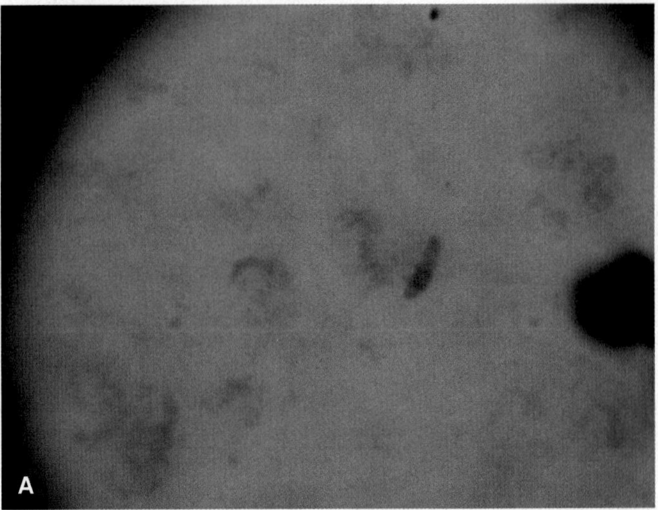

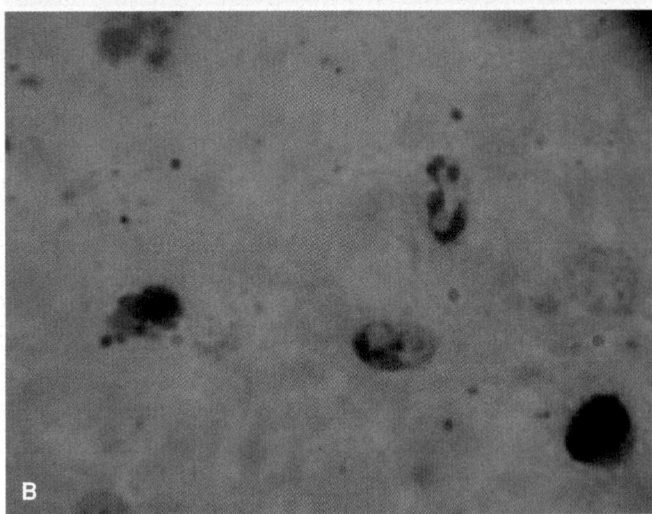

FIGURE 7-12 **A.** *Plasmodium falciparum* with a banana-shaped gametocyte. Of all the species of malaria, *P. falciparum* is the most likely to cause severe morbidity and mortality. **B.** *Plasmodium falciparum* with chromatin in rings. (*Reproduced with permission from Richard P. Usatine, MD.*)

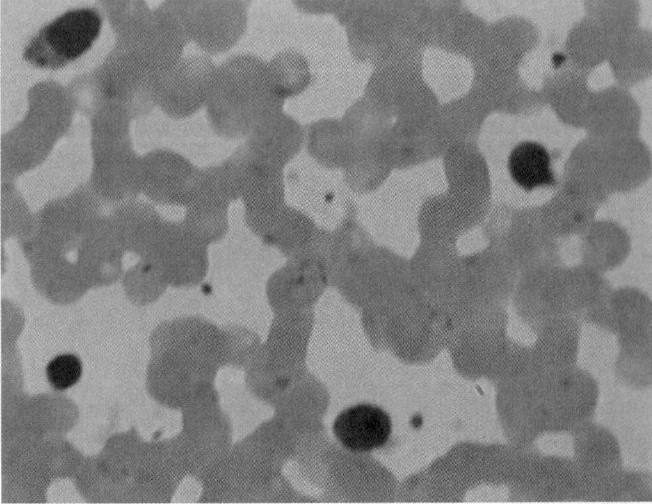

FIGURE 7-13 Blood smear for malaria diagnosis showing *Plasmodium vivax*. Rapid field tests are now available but still more expensive than microscopy. (*Reproduced with permission from Richard P. Usatine, MD.*)

▶ Treatment

Many cases of malaria can be treated effectively with oral medication, and parenteral therapy is reserved for severe disease or for patients who are vomiting. Before prescribing therapy, determine which species is most likely involved based on microscopy or rapid diagnostic test; consider the geographic area and local drug resistance patterns.

The determination of the infecting *Plasmodium* species is of the upmost importance prior to treatment. For instance, *P. falciparum* and *P. knowlesi* can cause rapidly progressive severe illness or death. Other species such as *P. vivas* and *P. ovale* require treatment for the hypnozoite forms that have the potential to remain dormant in the liver and can cause a relapsing infection. In terms of *P. falciparum* and *P. vivax* species, they have significantly different drug resistance patterns in differing geographic regions which need to be reviewed prior to treatment.[44]

After the patient has been given the first dose of medication, the patient should be observed for an hour. Vomiting can be managed with metoclopramide, 10 mg orally, and if the vomiting occurs within 30 minutes, the full initial dose can be repeated. The WHO recommends artemisinin-based combination treatments (ACTs) as first-line for uncomplicated *P. falciparum*. The WHO currently recommends five different ACTs for use against *P. falciparum* malaria and the choice of agent should be based on therapeutic efficacy studies against local strains of *P. falciparum* malaria.[45] Artemisinin based combination therapies include artemether plus lumefantrine, artesunate plus amodiaquine, artesunate plus mefloquine, dihydroartemisinin plus piperaquine, and artesunate plus sulfadoxine-pyrimethamine.[46] Artemisinin and derivatives should not be given as monotherapy.

For U.S.-returning travelers:

- Quinine + doxycycline: quinine 10 mg/kg 3 times daily for 7 days and doxycycline twice daily for 7 days

  or

- Atovaquone-proguanil: atovaquone 20 mg/kg per day, proguanil 8 mg/kg per day for 3 days.

Treatment of severe P. falciparum

All cases of severe malaria should be managed as medical emergencies. Give IV or IM artesunate, artemether, or quinine dihydrochloride (not available in the United States).

In the United States, give quinidine gluconate, 10 mg base/kg (up to 600 mg) in 0.9% saline by rate-controlled IV infusion over 1 to 2 hours, followed by a maintenance dose of 0.02 mg base/kg per minute with electrocardiogram (ECG) monitoring until patient can take oral drugs. Quinine and quinidine must never be given by IV bolus because of the potential for fatal hypotension.

Patients with cerebral malaria should undergo lumbar puncture to rule out bacterial meningitis (**Figure 7-14**) and their blood glucose should be checked every 4 hours because of the significant risk of hypoglycemia in severe malaria. Careful hemodynamic monitoring and management of seizures (with intravenous benzodiazepines) are essential. As there are many considerations to keep in mind in regards to malaria, there is a 24-hour CDC malaria hotline which provides advice to clinicians on the diagnosis and treatment that can be reached toll free at 855-856-4713.[44]

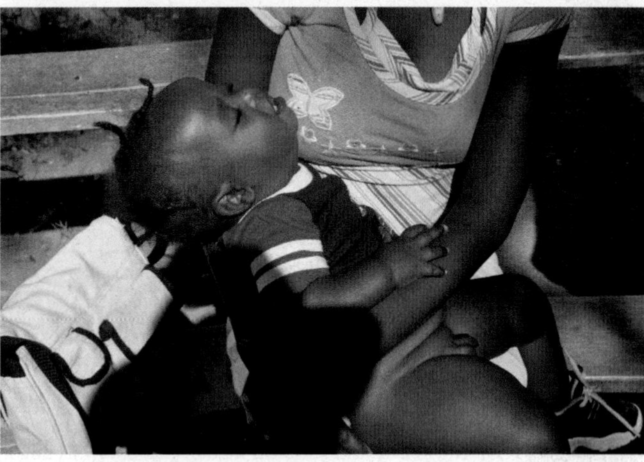

FIGURE 7-14 Meningitis in a child with a very rigid neck. Cerebral malaria should be in the differential diagnosis for this child. Most bacterial meningitis in children can now be prevented by vaccines that are frequently still not available in developing countries. (*Reproduced with permission from Richard P. Usatine, MD.*)

▶ Prevention

Prevention measures are a public health priority and should include mosquito control, elimination of standing water in households and gardens, insect repellant containing at least 10% to 50% diethyltoluamide (DEET; 30% DEET provides 6 to 8 hours of protection), and permethrin-impregnated bed nets. Since 2010, prevention and control measures have reduced malaria mortality by 29% among all age groups and by 35% among children under 5.[41]

Prevention for travelers

Choice of chemoprophylaxis depends on drug resistance patterns for *P. falciparum* in the country being visited. Generally, prophylaxis should start 1 week before arrival and should continue through 4 weeks after leaving the endemic area. In the case of atovaquone-proguanil, prophylaxis may start the day before arrival and end 7 days after departure. Drugs commonly used in prophylaxis include atovaquone-proguanil (Malarone, which is expensive in the United States), mefloquine (may cause central nervous system side effects), and doxycycline (causes photosensitivity). Chloroquine can be used only in a few areas; chloroquine-susceptible malaria is restricted to the Caribbean, Central America, and parts of the Middle East.

RESOURCES

- Centers for Disease Control and Prevention. *Malaria*—**http://www.cdc.gov/malaria.**
- Centers for Disease Control and Prevention. *Malaria hotline*—855-856-4713 (toll free, M-F 9 a.m.–5 p.m. EST). Hotline provides healthcare providers with assistance with diagnosis or management of suspected cases of malaria. For emergency consultation after hours, call 770-488-7100 and request to speak with a CDC Malaria Branch clinician.
- World Health Organization. **http://www.who.int/malaria/en/.**

LEISHMANIASIS

Leishmaniasis is a vector-borne disease transmitted by the sandfly. It can be divided into two major forms: a cutaneous form, which is the most common, and the visceral form. There is also a more rare mucocutaneous form that can cause significant facial disfigurement around the nose and mouth.

Synonyms

Kala-azar is another name for visceral leishmaniasis.

Epidemiology

- New World (the Western Hemisphere) leishmaniasis is found in Mexico, Central America, and South America. Old World (the Eastern Hemisphere) leishmaniasis is found in India, Africa, the Middle East, southern Europe, and parts of Asia.
- Most leishmaniasis diagnosed in the United States occurs in travelers returning from endemic tourist destinations in Latin America, such as Costa Rica as well as military personnel who served in endemic areas, such as Iraq or Afghanistan.
- Some cutaneous leishmaniasis cases acquired in the United States have been reported in Texas and Oklahoma.[47]

Etiology and pathophysiology

- Leishmaniasis is caused by more than 20 species of the protozoan genus *Leishmania*.
- Leishmaniasis is transmitted to people through the bite of the sandfly.
- The intracellular amastigotes of *Leishmania* replicate within macrophages.
- The disease can also be transmitted like any bloodborne infection, but human-to-human transmission is rare.

Risk factors

- Living in and traveling to endemic countries.
- Rural areas have a higher prevalence of disease in the endemic countries.
- Not protecting the skin from sandfly bites during the time from dusk to dawn.
- Blood transfusions, needle sharing in injection-drug users, needlestick injuries, and congenital transmission also are all reported risk factors for visceral leishmaniasis.[48]

Diagnosis

Clinical features

- Six weeks after a sandfly bite, the cutaneous form may be localized to a single ulcer or nodule (**Figure 7-15**) or may be disseminated widely (**Figure 7-16**).

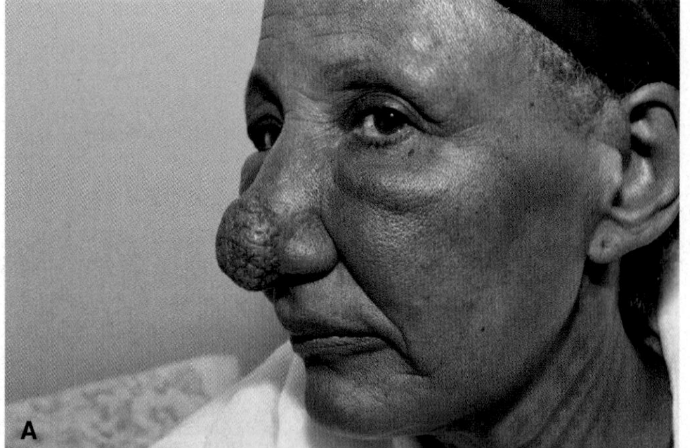

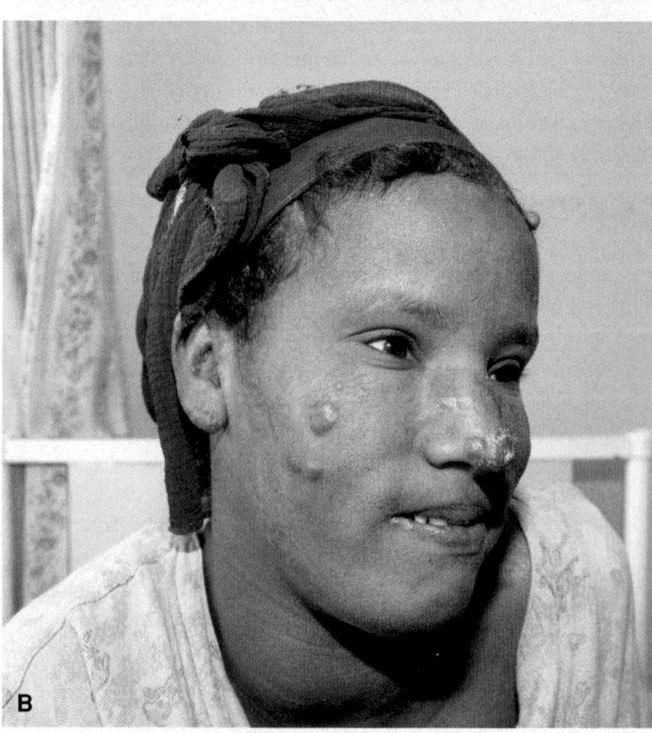

FIGURE 7-15 Examples of leishmaniasis on the face. Lesions emerge in the site of the sandfly bite; the nose is commonly affected, as seen in the women in figures A and B from Africa. (*Reproduced with permission from Richard P. Usatine, MD.*)

- After a 2- to 6-month incubation period, the visceral form can involve the liver, spleen, and bone marrow and causes systemic illness. The patient may present with fever, anemia, night sweats, weight loss, and an enlarged abdomen because of hepatosplenomegaly.[49]
- Mucocutaneous leishmaniasis affects the nose and mouth and may affect the nasal septum and palate (**Figure 7-17**). This form may occur months to years after what appears to be healing of cutaneous leishmaniasis.

Distribution

- A cutaneous form of leishmaniasis has a predilection for the nose and face (see **Figure 7-15**).
- Cutaneous leishmaniasis is also commonly seen on the extremities. Note that the sandfly would generally have more access to bite the face and extremities where clothing is less likely to be a protective barrier.
- Disseminated cutaneous leishmaniasis can be seen from the head to the toes (see **Figure 7-16**).

Laboratory testing

- Cutaneous leishmaniasis may be diagnosed by clinical appearance and a biopsy or a scraping of the ulcer. A Giemsa stain will demonstrate parasites in the skin smears taken from the edge of an active ulcer.[49] In some centers, PCR is available and is considered the method of choice.[50]
- Visceral leishmaniasis is diagnosed from a blood sample or a bone marrow biopsy. Several serologic agglutination tests (direct agglutination test [DAT] or fluorescent allergosorbent test [FAST]) are highly sensitive for detection of leishmania antibodies. Culture of a bone marrow aspirate or PCR improves diagnostic yield.[49]

▶ Differential diagnosis

- The differential diagnosis of cutaneous leishmaniasis includes leprosy, sarcoidosis, pyoderma gangrenosum, primary syphilis, and venous stasis ulcers.
- The differential diagnosis of visceral leishmaniasis includes malaria, typhoid fever, and lymphoma.

▶ Management

Nonpharmacologic

- Wound care for ulcers.

Medications

- The main drugs used to treat leishmaniasis include sodium stibogluconate (available from the CDC) and meglumine antimonate.[51,52] Other medications used include miltefosine (the only oral drug for leishmaniasis), fluconazole, and liposomal amphotericin b (this is the only drug with FDA approval for visceral leishmaniasis in the United States).[51,52] Amphotericin b is the standard of care in India because of antimonial resistance.[50]

Surgery

- Plastic surgery may be used to treat the disfigurement of mucocutaneous or cutaneous leishmaniasis.

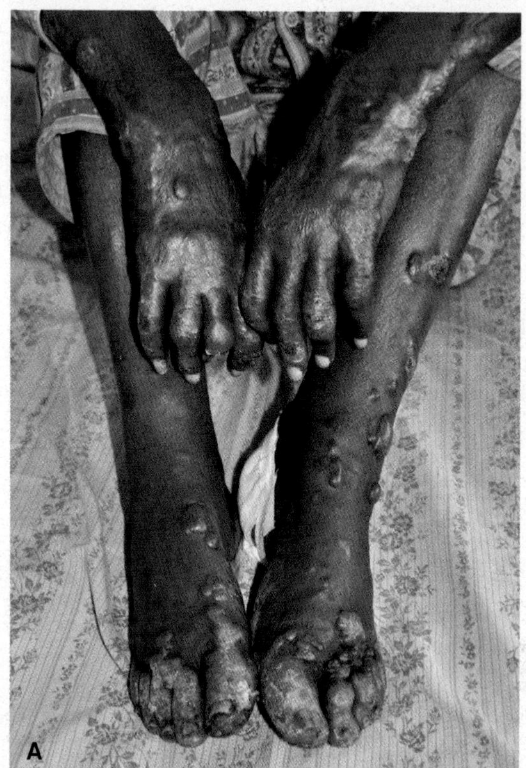

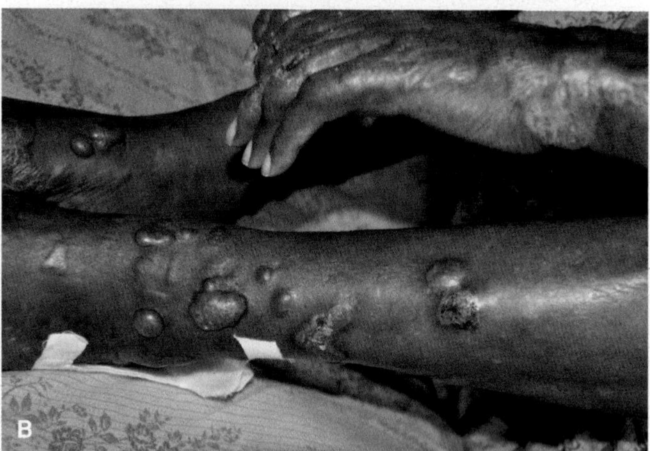

FIGURE 7-16 Diffuse leishmaniasis in an African man with involvement from the face to the toes. The multiple nodules look like lepromatous leprosy, but by skin snip testing, the diagnosis of leishmaniasis was confirmed. Figures **A** and **B** show different views of the same patient. *(Reproduced with permission from Richard P. Usatine, MD.)*

PREVENTION OF VECTOR-BORNE DISEASES

Prevention is a public health priority that must include vector (mosquito and sandfly) control, elimination of standing water in households and gardens, insect repellant containing 20% to 30% DEET, and permethrin-coated bed nets. Sandflies and *Anopheles* mosquitoes bite from dusk to dawn, but the *Aedes aegypti* vector of dengue fever bites any time during the day, making daytime use of mosquito repellant especially important in dengue-endemic areas.

PROGNOSIS

- Cutaneous leishmaniasis does resolve spontaneously in some cases; in other cases it may persist and resist treatments. The prognosis is related to the severity of the case and the community of the host. Even in those cases that resolve, scarring is frequent.
- Visceral leishmaniasis is fatal if not diagnosed and treated.

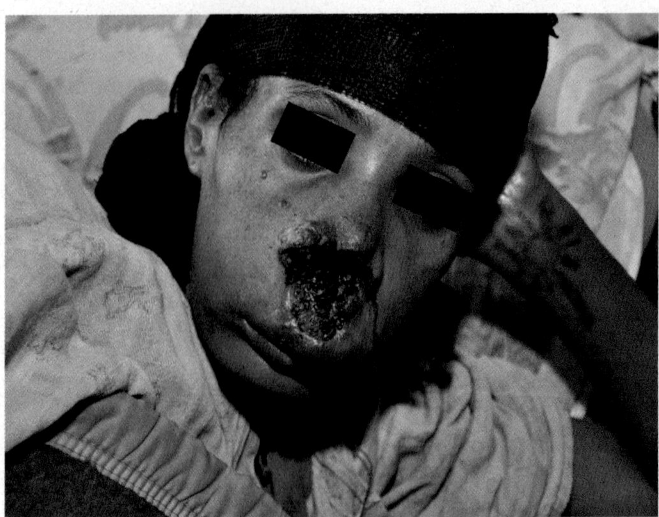

FIGURE 7-17 Severe mucocutaneous leishmaniasis causing destruction of the nose. (*Reproduced with permission from Richard P. Usatine, MD.*)

RESOURCES

- PubMed Health. *Leishmaniasis*—**http://www.ncbi.nlm.nih.gov/pubmedhealth/PMH0002362/.**
- Centers for Disease Control and Prevention. *Parasites–Leishmaniasis*—**http://www.cdc.gov/parasites/leishmaniasis/.**

EYES—TRACHOMA

EPIDEMIOLOGY AND GEOGRAPHIC DISTRIBUTION

Chlamydia trachomatis is the leading infectious cause of blindness, accounting for 1.4% of the world's blindness. Globally, trachoma is responsible for the blindness or impairment of about 1.9 million people.[53] Blindness from trachoma is irreversible. Trachoma is associated with poor sanitation, inadequate water supply, and lack of personal hygiene. It is transmitted from person to person via unwashed fingers, flies that have been in close contact with discharge from the eyes or nose of an infected person, and close family contact (sharing of face towels and bedclothes). Trachoma is endemic in Africa (especially in the driest regions), Central and South America, Asia, and the Middle East. As part of a resolution by the WHO, 10 countries have reported achieving major elimination goals to eradicate trachoma as of July 1, 2017. In addition, the countries of Mexico, Morocco, and Oman have been validated by the WHO as having eliminated trachoma as a public health problem.[53]

CLINICAL PRESENTATION

Patients experience inflammation of the eye with watery discharge, itching, burning, and blurry vision. Examination of the tarsal conjunctiva reveals follicles (round swellings that are paler than the surrounding conjunctiva, at least 0.5 mm in diameter). With progression, intense trachomatous inflammation develops, producing inflammatory thickening of the tarsal conjunctiva, which appears red and thickened with numerous follicles (**Figure 7-18**).

Eventually, trachoma causes scarring, with white lines or bands in the tarsal conjunctiva as well as trichiasis, in which eyelashes turn inward and begin to rub against the cornea, and entropion, or inward

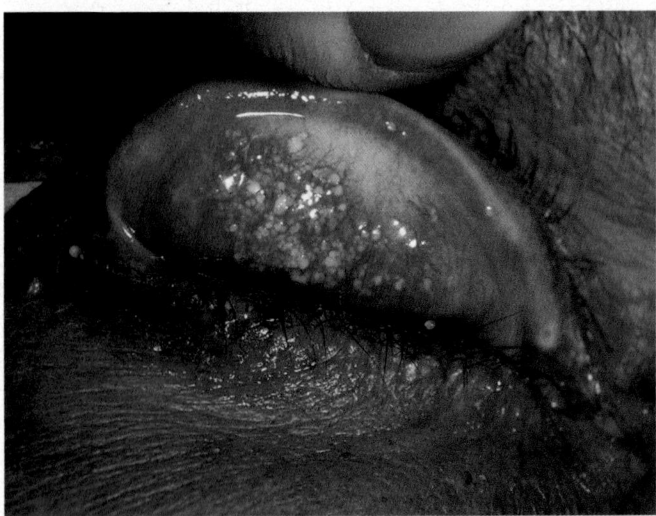

FIGURE 7-18 Trachoma causing prominent follicles on the upper eyelid in a person infected with *C. trachomatis*. Note how flipping the eyelid is needed to see the follicles under the upper eyelid. (*Reproduced with permission from Richard P. Usatine, MD.*)

turning of the eyelid itself. With time, this chronic rubbing causes corneal opacity and blindness (**Figure 7-19**).

DIAGNOSIS

Although laboratory diagnostic testing is available for staining *C. trachomatis* in scrapings from the tarsal plate, most settings where trachoma is endemic do not offer this resource, and visual inspection of the everted upper eyelid must suffice. Each eye should be examined for trichiasis and corneal opacities. The upper eyelid is everted by asking the patient to look down, holding eyelashes between thumb and finger, and everting the lid using a cotton-tipped applicator. The everted lid is then checked for follicles, inflammation, and scarring. The differential diagnosis of trachoma includes allergic conjunctivitis (which can also produce follicles of the tarsal plate), and bacterial or viral conjunctivitis.

MANAGEMENT

- Azithromycin, 1 g single oral dose for adults and 20 mg/kg for children in a single dose.
- In pregnancy: erythromycin 500 mg twice daily for 7 days.
- Less effective: topical erythromycin and tetracycline.[11]
- In some settings, surgery is available to correct entropion and trichiasis.

RISK FACTORS

- Poor hygiene
- Poor sanitation
- Crowded households
- Lack of availability of clean water
- Increased household fly density

PREVENTION

Preventive measures include community hygiene education, use of soap and water for washing hands and faces, and control of flies through use of ventilated improved pit (VIP) latrines. The WHO has developed the acronym "SAFE" for the global elimination of trachoma:

S Surgery for entropion and trichiasis

A Antibiotics for infectious trachoma

F Facial cleanliness to reduce transmission

E Environmental improvements such as control of disease-spreading flies and access to clean water[54]

SKIN

INFECTIOUS SKIN DISEASES

Many of the skin diseases encountered in resource-limited countries are secondary to crowded living conditions and lack of clean water and soap. Scabies mites and human lice are endemic in many populations that are unable to wash frequently. If clean water is scarce, it is more likely to be used for drinking and cooking than bathing. In developed countries, we take clean running water (hot and cold), soap, and shampoo for granted. In developing countries, even if water

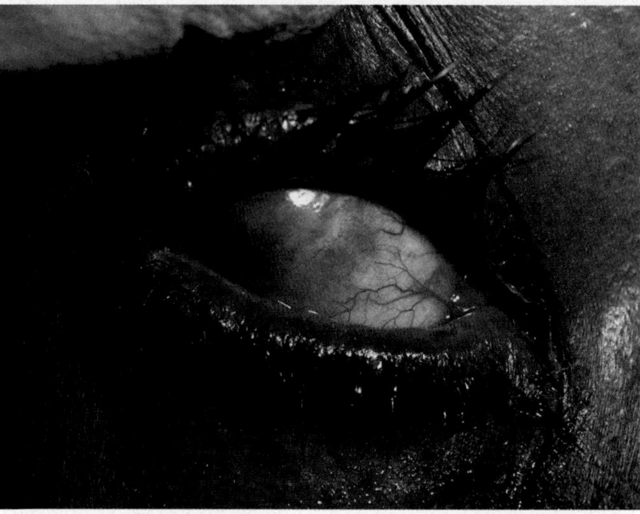

FIGURE 7-19 Blindness caused by untreated trachoma. Although this is one of the most common causes of blindness worldwide, trachoma is easily treatable with a single dose of oral azithromycin. Prevention is achieved through better access to water and soap, together with education about the three "Fs": flies, fingers, facial hygiene. (*Reproduced with permission from Richard P. Usatine, MD.*)

is available, it may not be accessible as warm running water for showers or baths.

When an intervention as simple as mass distribution of free soap for personal hygiene draws enormous crowds to a mobile clinic, the vastness of inequality in access to basic health measures around the world becomes painfully obvious. So although people recognize the importance of access to soap and clean water, the absence of this luxury results in skin infections and infestations that are highly prevalent and spread from person-to-person (**Figure 7-20**).

We can divide the skin diseases into infestations and bacterial, viral, and fungal infections. All of these skin infections are covered in the dermatology section of this book. Here we highlight some cases seen in developing countries.

Scabies (see Chapter 149, Scabies) is caused by a human mite that burrows under the skin causing itching and leading to scratching. The itching and scratching may keep the person awake at night and may lead to bacterial superinfections (**Figure 7-21**). Scabies is spread by direct skin contact (**Figures 7-22** and **7-23**), shared bedding and clothing, and occasionally by fomites. Transmission rates increase substantially in resource-poor conditions that are prone to overcrowding. Scabies can occur in any setting but over the past century has become less prevalent in temperate regions and is more common in tropical, humid regions.[55] The diagnosis of scabies is clinical: common characteristics are pruritus (worse at night), rash (erythematous papules often with signs of excoriations), and linear burrows (often found about the wrists or webs of the fingers). Scabies is part of the WHO list of neglected tropical diseases, estimated to affect more than 130 million people globally at any one time. The effect of scabies extends beyond simple pruritus and insomnia; it has become a major underlying cause of high rates of bacterial skin infections.[56] Mass drug administration programs are currently being attempted to use ivermectin to control scabies in endemic communities around the world.[57]

Human lice (see Chapter 148, Lice) exist as three separate species that are known as head lice, body lice, and pubic lice. Schoolchildren are particularly at risk for head lice, and in areas with limited head washing, the majority of kids may be infested. Body lice live on clothing and feed on the blood of their host. Body lice are more prevalent on adults who bathe rarely and wear the same unwashed clothing day after day. Pubic lice are transmitted through sexual contact and are not known to be more prevalent in developing countries. Water and hygiene issues do predispose to increased head and body lice in developing countries.

Bacterial infections of the skin (see Chapter 122, Impetigo) are ubiquitous throughout the world. Impetigo is a superficial bacterial infection that presents with honey crusts (**Figure 7-24**) or bullae. Good hygiene can prevent impetigo, and therefore it is not surprising that many cases of impetigo will be seen in countries that lack access to soap and clean water. Impetigo is often secondary to other skin diseases such as scabies or fungal infections that create breaks in the skin barrier function. Cases of secondarily infected scabies and tinea are seen commonly in developing countries and without treatment can lead to fatal complications such as sepsis.

Viral infections of the skin (see Chapters 129, Chickenpox; 130, Zoster; 131, Zoster Ophthalmicus; 132, Measles; 133, Fifth Disease; 134, Hand, Foot, and Mouth Disease; 135, Herpes Simplex; 136, Molluscum Contagiosum; 137, Common Warts; 138, Flat Warts; 139,

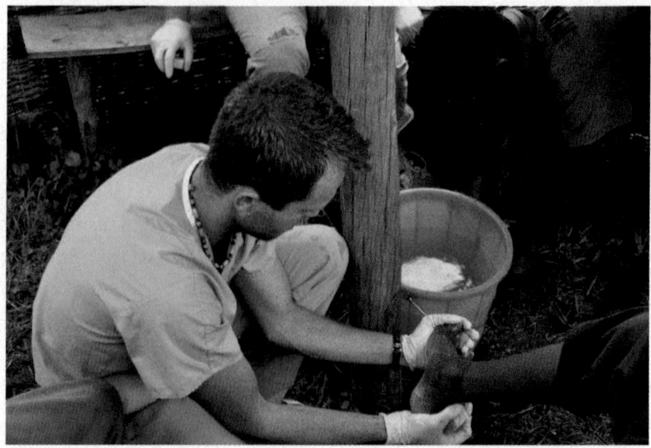

FIGURE 7-20 An American medical student is washing the feet of Ethiopian schoolchildren to treat skin infections and to educate them on preventive hygiene measures. (*Reproduced with permission from Richard P. Usatine, MD.*)

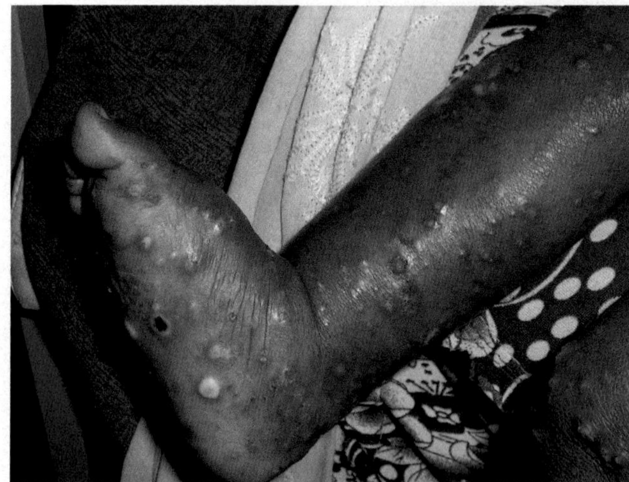

FIGURE 7-21 Badly superinfected scabies with pustules and crusting sores on this young child's leg. (*Reproduced with permission from Richard P. Usatine, MD.*)

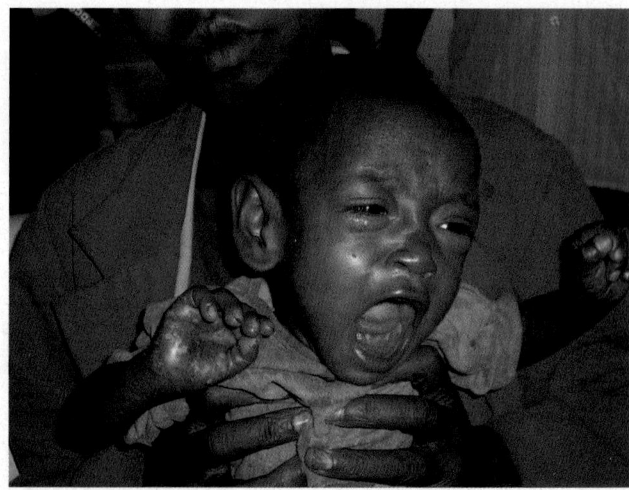

FIGURE 7-22 A malnourished baby with marasmus is infested with scabies seen on the hands and arms. Lack of adequate nutrition also is a risk factor for many infections and diseases. The scabies infestation is a marker for scarcity of clean water; the consequences of both may be contributing to the child's irritability and poor feeding. (*Reproduced with permission from Richard P. Usatine, MD.*)

Genital Warts; and 140, Plantar Warts) include herpes simplex, varicella zoster, molluscum contagiosum, and human papilloma virus infections. These infections are seen commonly in HIV-infected persons who are not receiving optimal antiretroviral therapy. In countries with a high prevalence of HIV-infected persons, a severe case of molluscum, warts, or shingles in a young person should prompt a clinician to consider HIV testing, if possible. Molluscum infections and warts are so ubiquitous throughout the world that it is important to realize that healthy people with healthy immune systems can get these infections, too. Viral exanthems caused by such diseases as varicella and measles may be more prevalent in countries where vaccinations are less available.

Fungal infections of the skin (see Chapters 141, Fungal Overview; 142, Candidiasis; 143, Tinea Capitis; 144, Tinea Corporis; 145, Tinea Cruris; 146, Tinea Pedis; and 147, Tinea Versicolor) can occur from the head down to the toes. Heat, humidity, and lack of bathing are predisposing factors to fungal skin infections. Therefore tropical developing countries provide good environments for tinea capitis (**Figure 7-25**), tinea corporis, and tinea pedis.

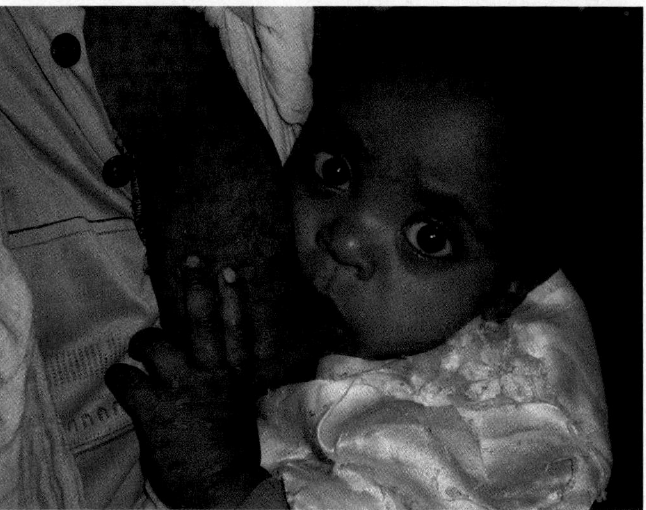

FIGURE 7-23 Scabies infestation covering the mother's breast and her baby's hand. With poor access to healthcare, this infestation would likely remain untreated, and could lead to bacterial superinfection and impetigo on the baby's skin. (*Reproduced with permission from Richard P. Usatine, MD.*)

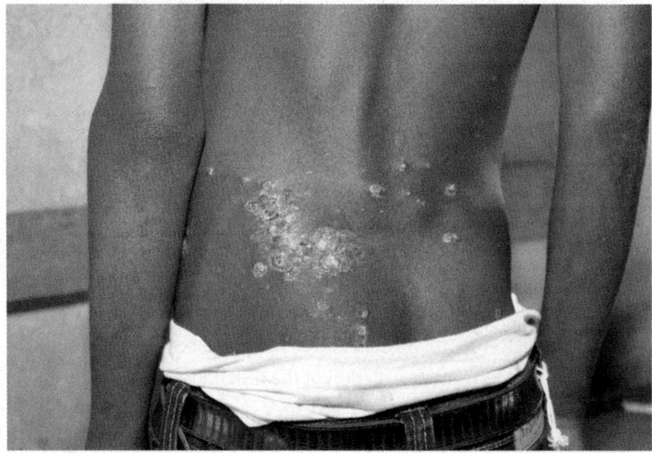

FIGURE 7-24 Impetigo caused by a bacterial infection on the buttocks of this child in Haiti. Impetigo is more prevalent when there is inadequate hygiene and lack of access to healthcare. (*Reproduced with permission from Richard P. Usatine, MD.*)

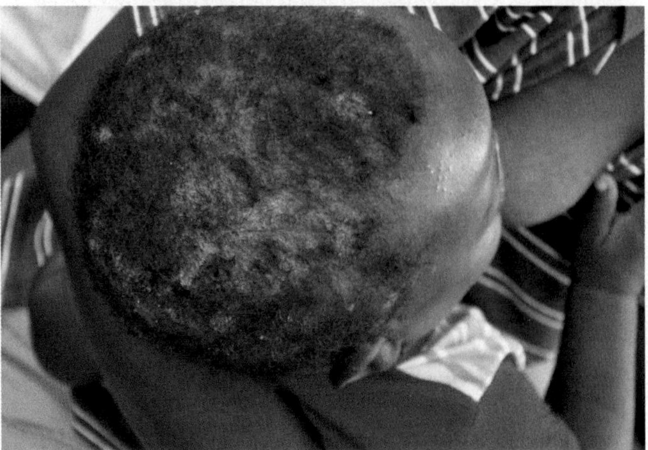

FIGURE 7-25 Tinea capitis in this young boy living in a developing country. Many children live with untreated tinea capitis in developing countries because of limited hygiene resources and poor access to healthcare. (*Reproduced with permission from Richard P. Usatine, MD.*)

MYCOBACTERIUM (LEPROSY AND TUBERCULOSIS-HIV COINFECTION)

LEPROSY

▶ Patient story

A young boy presents with significant changes to his face (**Figure 7-26**). The boy and his father are from rural Africa, and it is obvious to the physician that the boy has lepromatous leprosy. The father is also examined, and he has more subtle signs of leprosy present (several patches of hypopigmented anesthetic skin). A slit-skin exam is performed on the ear lobe of the boy, and many acid-fast bacilli, characteristic of *Mycobacterium leprae*, are found. The boy is started on the WHO-standard multidrug therapy using rifampin, clofazimine, and dapsone. The father is also examined and treated.

▶ Introduction

Leprosy (Hansen disease) is caused by *M. leprae* and is still endemic in many parts of the developing world where there is poverty and poor access to clean water. At one time, persons with leprosy were called "lepers" and isolated to leper colonies because the disease was disfiguring and the communities were afraid that it was highly contagious. Current science and epidemiology tell us that leprosy is transmitted via droplets from the nose and mouth during close and frequent contact over a period of years, and not by casual contact. Thus doctors working with patients who have leprosy are at no real risk of becoming infected. Issues related to stigma and discrimination still do exist.

▶ Epidemiology

- There were 216,108 new cases reported in the world by 145 countries in 2016.[58]
- The United States reported 178 new cases in 2015.[59]
- Since 1990, more than 14 million leprosy patients have been cured, about 4 million from 2000 to 2010.[60]

▶ Etiology and pathophysiology

- The clinical manifestations of leprosy depend on the immunologic reaction to the infection. The two opposite ends of the spectrum consist of:
  - Lepromatous leprosy, in which there is a strong antibody response and a poor cell-mediated community resulting in larger amounts of *M. leprae* in the tissues (see **Figure 7-26**).
  - Tuberculoid leprosy, in which there is a strong cell-mediated immunity and a poor antibody response resulting in less *M. leprae* in the tissues. This tends to present with hypopigmented anesthetic patches (**Figure 7-27**).
- There is also borderline leprosy, in which there is a mixed cell-mediated immunity and antibody response showing features of both lepromatous leprosy and tuberculoid leprosy.
- Treatment regimens differ depending on whether the patient has paucibacillary (fewer organisms) or multibacillary leprosy. Lepromatous leprosy and borderline lepromatous leprosy are most likely to be multibacillary.

▶ Risk factors

- Poverty and living in an endemic area
- Inadequate access to clean water and poor hygiene
- Living in the household of an infected person
- Eating or handling armadillos, as these animals are natural hosts for *M. leprae*

▶ Diagnosis

Clinical features

- Facial features include leonine facies, madarosis (loss of eyebrows as seen in **Figure 7-26**), elongated and dysmorphic earlobes, and saddle-nose deformities from destruction of the nasal cartilage and bone.
- Visible skin changes include nodules in lepromatous leprosy, hypopigmented patches in tuberculoid (see **Figure 7-27**) and borderline leprosy, and annular saucer-like lesions in borderline leprosy.
- Nerve involvement can cause a clawhand (flexion contractures of the fingers as seen in **Figure 7-28**), wristdrop, footdrop, Bell palsy, hammertoes, and sensory neuropathy leading to neurotropic ulcers and traumatic blisters.
- Eye involvement can cause corneal anesthesia, keratitis, episcleritis, lagophthalmos (the inability to close the eyelid completely), and blindness.
- Advanced untreated leprosy can lead to shortening and/or loss of fingers as a result of bone resorption in hands that have become anesthetic and not protected from repeated trauma (**Figure 7-29**).

Distribution

The nodules of lepromatous leprosy are mostly seen on the face and ears but can be seen in other areas. Hypopigmented patches can be seen anywhere on the body, including the face.

Laboratory testing

- In obvious cases of leprosy, the slit-skin exam done on the ear lobe for bacillary index is the most important test to determine if the patient has multibacillary or paucibacillary leprosy.

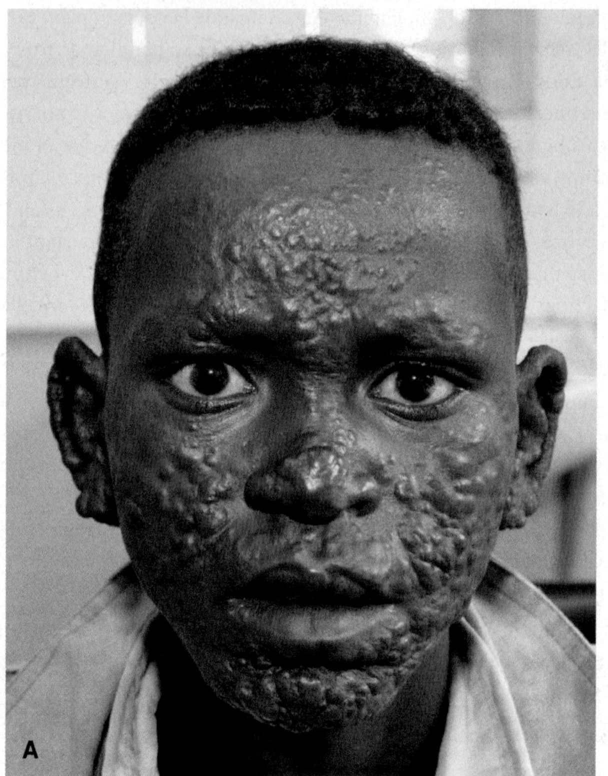

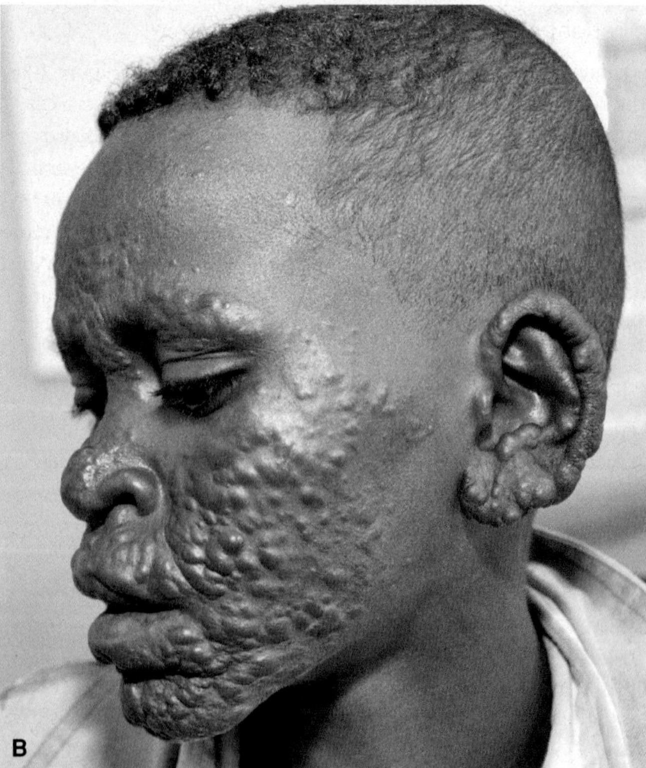

FIGURE 7-26 Lepromatous leprosy with leonine facies in a young boy. **A.** Note the loss of eyebrows, called madarosis. **B.** Also note the prominent ear involvement. (*Reproduced with permission from Richard P. Usatine, MD.*)

- In cases that are suspicious for leprosy (especially outside of endemic areas), a skin punch biopsy of a suspicious lesion is useful for finding *M. leprae* in the tissues.

▶ Differential diagnosis

Superficial mycoses, vitiligo, and cutaneous filariasis all cause changes in pigmentation similar to leprosy. Infiltrated lesions that resemble leprosy include those of leishmaniasis, psoriasis, and sarcoidosis.[52]

▶ Management

Early diagnosis and multidrug therapy are essential to reducing the disease burden of leprosy worldwide. The WHO has supplied multidrug therapy free of cost to leprosy patients in all endemic countries.[61]

- Leprosy is curable, and treatment in an early stage can prevent disability.
- Multidrug therapy is a combination of rifampin, dapsone, and clofazimine for multibacillary leprosy patients, and rifampin and dapsone for paucibacillary patients.
- Duration of multidrug therapy is 12 to 24 months for multibacillary and 6 months for paucibacillary patients.[62]
- Treatment with a single antileprosy drug will always result in development of drug resistance to that drug and is therefore an unethical practice.
- Strategies to increase early access to care and provide easy-to-obtain free multidrug treatment are essential to eliminating leprosy in the world. Research on a preventive vaccine continues in tandem with *Mycobacterium tuberculosis* vaccine research.[63]
- Comprehensive treatment of advanced cases with neuropathy should include foot and hand care to prevent further damage to these insensitive limbs.[62]
- Surgical management for some leprosy-associated problems, such as tendon transfer to correct the clawhand, may be available in some centers.[64]

TUBERCULOSIS AND HIV

▶ Epidemiology

Tuberculosis (TB) is a very common HIV-associated infection and causes at least 37% of HIV-associated deaths worldwide.[65] In 2016 alone, the WHO estimated there were 1 million HIV-associated new cases of TB, the majority of who live in sub-Saharan Africa (**Figure 7-30**). Globally, about one-third of HIV-infected people are coinfected with TB (at least 11 million people) (**Figure 7-31**) and 54% of these individuals did not have access to care.[65]

▶ Pathogenesis

TB is transmitted by aerosolized respiratory droplet nuclei (see Chapter 56, Tuberculosis). Weakened cell-mediated immunity in HIV-infected individuals allows more rapid disease progression and causes higher mortality rates from TB. At the same time, untreated TB infection accelerates immunologic decline in HIV infection. Because these two diseases preferentially afflict populations with reduced access to medications and supportive care, the emergence of multidrug-resistant TB has become an increasing threat.

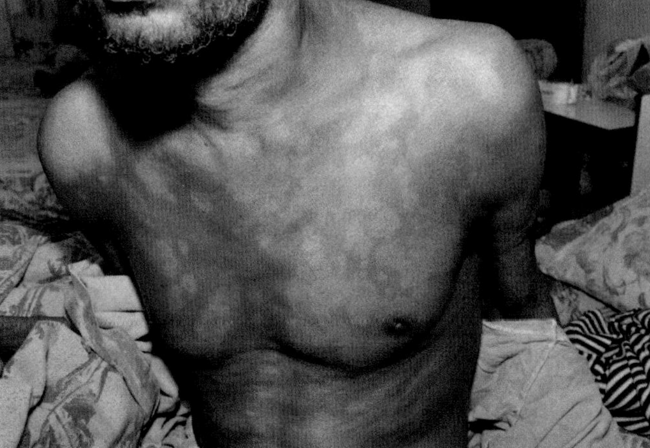

FIGURE 7-27 Multibacillary leprosy with hypopigmented patches. These patches are commonly numb due to cutaneous nerve damage from mycobacterial infection. *(Reproduced with permission from Richard P. Usatine, MD.)*

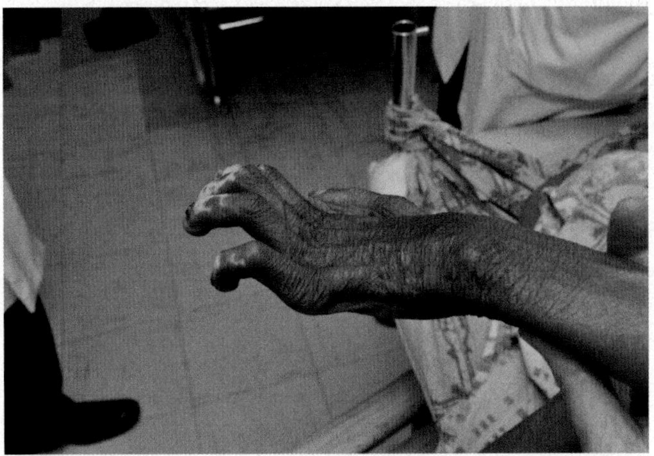

FIGURE 7-28 Clawhand caused by the neurologic damage of leprosy. This condition may be amenable to surgical intervention involving tendon transfer. *(Reproduced with permission from Richard P. Usatine, MD.)*

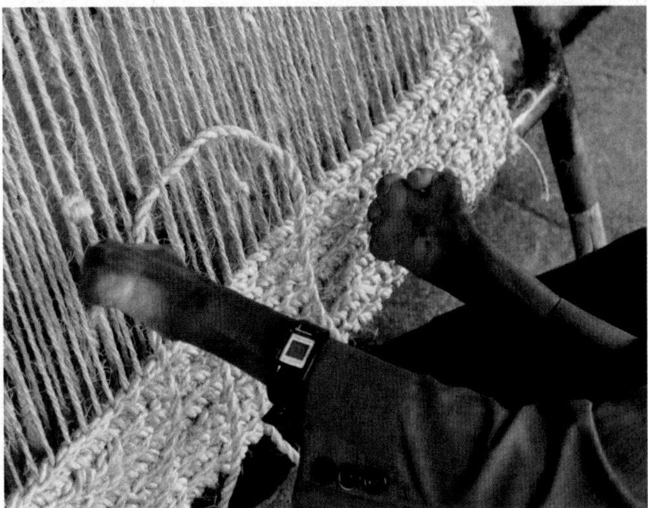

FIGURE 7-29 Leprosy has caused this older man to lose his fingers, but he continues to lead a productive life weaving rugs for sale at a leprosy hospital. *(Reproduced with permission from Richard P. Usatine, MD.)*

▶ Clinical presentation

The clinical presentation of TB in an HIV-infected person with a relatively preserved immune system (CD4+ T-cell count greater than 350 cells/μL) is identical to that seen in HIV-negative patients. With increasing immunodeficiency, however, TB often presents atypically. Chest radiographs may not demonstrate classic findings of upper lobe fibronodular or cavitary disease, and extrapulmonary presentations (lymphadenitis, pleuritis, pericarditis, meningitis) are seen. Tuberculous lymphadenitis and cutaneous TB (designated scrofula when it affects the neck) are illustrated in **Figures 7-32, 7-33** and **7-34**.

▶ Diagnosis

HIV screening should be performed in all patients diagnosed with TB, and HIV-infected patients should be screened annually for *M. tuberculosis* with purified protein derivative (PPD) skin testing, chest x-ray, and/or blood test for interferon-γ release assay (IGRA) depending on availability. Patients with low CD4 cell counts (below 200 cells/μL) commonly have poorly reactive skin tests for TB, and thus need a careful history of exposures, review of symptoms, and monitoring of the chest x-ray for evidence of active disease, with repeat TB screening when the CD4 cell count rises above 200 cells/μL.

▶ Management

Latent TB infection

HIV-positive patients with latent tuberculosis infection (LTBI) should have a chest x-ray and three sputum smears for acid-fast bacilli to rule out active disease. Once active TB is ruled out, isoniazid prophylaxis should be initiated regardless of age for any HIV-positive person with the following characteristics: (a) a positive diagnostic test for LTBI, or (b) a negative LTBI test but with evidence of old or poorly healed fibrotic lesions on chest x-ray, or (c) negative LTBI diagnostic test, but the person is in close contact with a person with infectious pulmonary TB.

Duration of LTBI prophylaxis: Isoniazid 300 mg daily or twice weekly for 9 months given with vitamin B_6 (pyridoxine, 25 mg daily). An alternative regimen of 12 doses of once-weekly isoniazid-rifapentine has recently been validated. Pyridoxine prevents isoniazid-associated peripheral neuropathy.[66]

Active M. tuberculosis *disease*

Any HIV-positive patient with cough and pulmonary infiltrates should be placed in respiratory isolation until TB is ruled out by three separately obtained sputum smears (Ziehl-Neelsen) with cultures sent for acid-fast bacilli. This rule applies even when the chest radiograph does not demonstrate cavitary or upper lobe infiltrates. Smear-negative, culture-positive *M. tuberculosis* is not uncommon.

Treatment regimens for HIV-TB coinfected patients are largely identical to those of TB mono-infected patients. It is important not to start antiretroviral therapy (ART) and TB therapy simultaneously, to avoid confusion about drug allergies and side effects. In addition, there is a risk of immune reconstitution syndrome (IRIS [immune reconstitution inflammatory reaction]: inflammatory response that worsens manifestations of any opportunistic infection) when ART is started too soon after initiating TB medication.

Guidelines for ART in TB coinfection are specific. If the CD4 cell count is less than 50, ART should start within 2 weeks of TB therapy. If the CD4 count is greater than 50, ART should start within 8 weeks

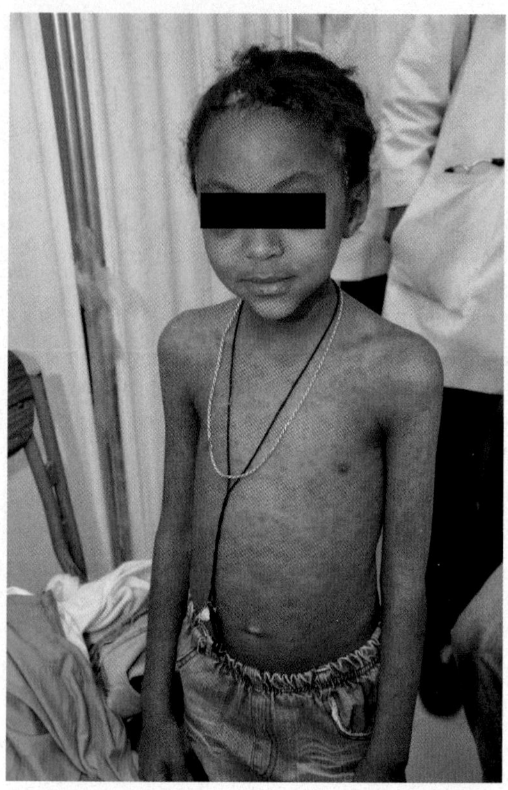

FIGURE 7-30 Young girl who acquired HIV at birth and now has papular pruritic eruption. One in three children born to HIV-infected mothers may be infected; mother-to-child transmission is preventable with simple and affordable antiviral regimens. Fortunately this girl had no signs or symptoms of tuberculosis. (*Reproduced with permission from Richard P. Usatine, MD.*)

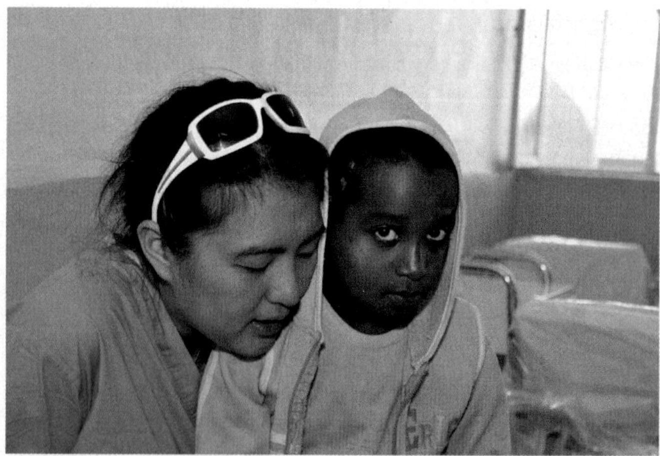

FIGURE 7-31 Young Ethiopian girl with HIV since birth who has neck swelling secondary to tuberculosis. She also has tinea capitis. HIV is a highly stigmatizing disease in most cultures, and clinicians can play an important role in mitigating community stigma by modeling compassionate care. (*Reproduced with permission from Richard P. Usatine, MD.*)

of TB therapy. If IRIS does occur, both ART and TB treatment should be continued while managing the IRIS.[67]

Directly observed therapy (DOT) for TB is strongly recommended for HIV-TB coinfected patients.

PROVIDER AND PATIENT RESOURCES

- Traveler's Health from the Centers for Disease Control and Prevention is a comprehensive site that includes information on more than 200 international destinations, travel vaccinations, diseases related to travel, illness and injury abroad, finding travel health specialists, insect protection, safe food and water, and a survival guide—**http://wwwnc.cdc.gov/travel/.**
- The Yellow Book 2018 is available online as a reference for those who advise international travelers about health risks—**http://wwwnc.cdc.gov/travel/page/yellowbook-home.htm.**
- Detailed vaccine information for travel can be obtained at the CDC website on vaccinations. This includes information on yellow fever vaccine, typhoid vaccine and routine vaccines—**http://wwwnc.cdc.gov/travel/page/vaccinations.htm.**
- Vaccine information can be looked up by specific destination on the traveler's health website—**http://wwwnc.cdc.gov/travel/.**
- U.S. Department of State International Travel Site, including country-specific information, travel alerts, and travel warnings—**http://travel.state.gov/travel/travel_1744.html.**

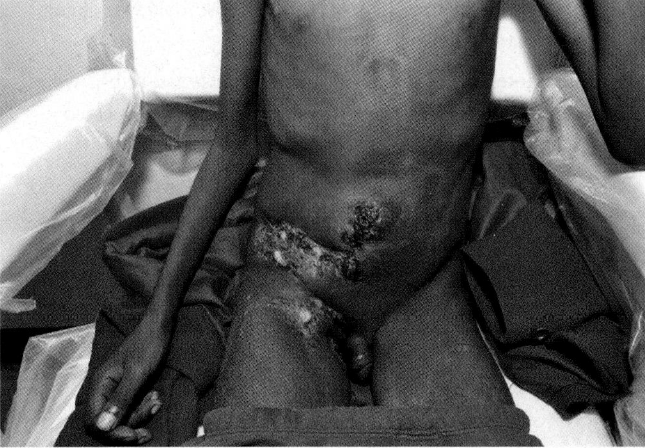

FIGURE 7-32 Scrofula in the inguinal area caused by *M. tuberculosis*. The patient appears systemically ill with weight loss. (*Reproduced with permission from Richard P. Usatine, MD.*)

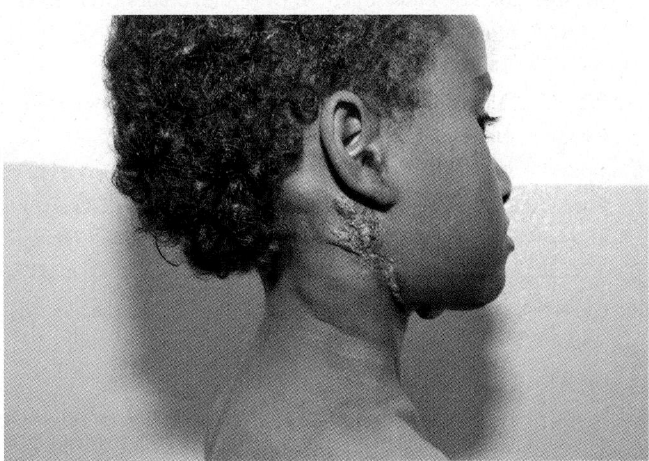

FIGURE 7-33 Scrofula of the neck caused by *M. tuberculosis* in a child. Chronic drainage and fistulous tract formation are commonly associated with this entity, and therapy is the same as for pulmonary tuberculosis. (*Reproduced with permission from Richard P. Usatine, MD.*)

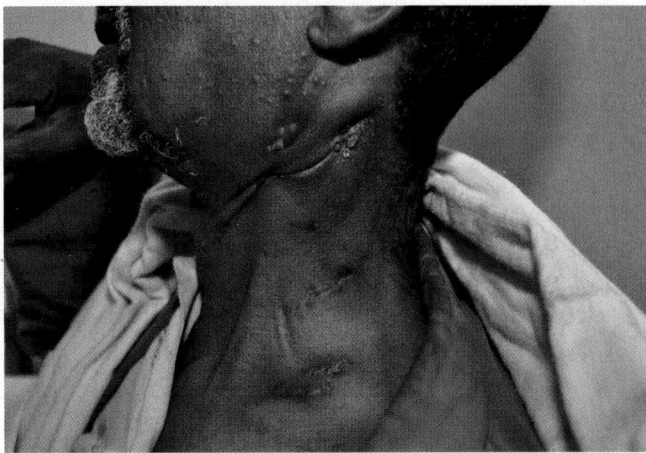

FIGURE 7-34 Scrofula of the neck caused by *M. tuberculosis* in an adult who did not complete his tuberculosis treatment. The long duration of therapy leads to challenges for adherence, and drug-resistant tuberculosis commonly results. (*Reproduced with permission from Richard P. Usatine, MD.*)

CONCLUSION

Medical students and health professionals are increasingly drawn to global health for reasons ranging from the desire for enhanced cultural understanding, to the mission to work for global health equity, to alleviate suffering, or to broaden medical experience beyond their geographic boundaries. Whatever one's personal motivation, such experiences should never be undertaken without disciplined preparation. Medical professionals should learn in advance of their travels about the culture, language, and expressed needs and priorities of the local government and health providers and their service populations. In addition, they need to learn about the diagnoses and locally appropriate management of prevalent diseases in the population they plan to serve. Equally important, they should take appropriate preventive measures (vaccines, malaria prophylaxis) to protect their own health. Lack of personal and professional preparation can easily turn the tide from net benefit to major burdens for host country organizations. Ultimately, well-prepared medical educators and clinicians, wherever they may come from, are uniquely positioned to share knowledge that saves lives and leads to a more equitable world.

REFERENCES

1. Kaplan JP, Bond TC, Merson MH, et al. Towards a common definition of global health. *Lancet* 2009;373:1993-1995.
2. Brown TM, Cueto M, Fee E. The World Health Organization and the transition from "international" to "global" public health. *Am J Public Health* 2006;96:62-72.

3. The World Bank. *Indicators of Health.* https://data.worldbank.org/indicator. Accessed January 2018.
4. Central Intelligence Agency. *The World Factbook.* https://www.cia.gov/library/publications/the-world-factbook/. Accessed January 2018.
5. Waterkeyn J, Carincross S. Creating demand for sanitation and hygiene through community health clubs: a cost-effective intervention in two districts in Zimbabwe. *Soc Sci Med* 2005;61(9):1958-1970.
6. UNICEF and WHO. *Progress on Drinking Water and Sanitation 2017 Update.* https://www.unicef.org/publications/files/Progress_on_Drinking_Water_Sanitation_and_Hygiene_2017.pdf. Accessed January 2018.
7. Epstein J, Hoffman S. Typhoid fever. In: Guerrant RL, Walker DH, Weller PF, eds. *Tropical Infectious Diseases; Principles, Pathogens & Practice.* 2nd ed. Philadelphia, PA: Elsevier; 2006:220-240.
8. Araujo-Jorge T, Callan M, Chappuis F, et al. Multisystem diseases and infections. In: Eddleston M, Davidson R, Brent A, Wilkinson R, eds. *Oxford Handbook of Tropical Medicine.* 3rd ed. New York, NY: Oxford University Press; 2008:665-739.
9. World Health Organization. *VIP and ROEC Latrines.* www.who.int/water_sanitation_health/hygiene/emergencies/fs3_5.pdf. Accessed January 2018.
10. Boggild AK, Van Voorhis WC, Liles WC. Travel-acquired illnesses associated with fever. In: Jong E, Sanford E, eds. *Travel and Tropical Medicine Manual.* 4th ed. Philadelphia, PA: Saunders Elsevier; 2008.
11. Gilbert D, Moellering R, Eliopoulos G, Chambers H, Saag M. *The Sanford Guide to Antimicrobial Therapy.* 41st ed. Sperryville, VA: Antimicrobial Therapy; 2011.
12. Centers for Disease Control and Prevention. *Cholera General Information.* http://www.cdc.gov/cholera/general/index.html. Accessed January 2018.
13. Cravioto A, Lanata CF, Lantagne DS, Nair GB. *Final Report of the Independent Panel of Experts on the Cholera Outbreak in Haiti 2011.* http://www.un.org/News/dh/infocus/haiti/UN-cholera-report-final.pdf. Accessed September 2012.
14. Levine MM, Gotuzzo E, Sow SO. Cholera infections. In: Guerrant RL, Walker DH, Weller PF, eds. *Tropical Infectious Diseases; Principles, Pathogens & Practice.* 2nd ed. Philadelphia, PA: Elsevier; 2006:273-282.
15. Penny ME. Diarrhoeal diseases. In: Eddleston M, Davidson R, Brent A, Wilkinson R, eds. *Oxford Handbook of Tropical Medicine.* 3rd ed. New York, NY: Oxford University Press; 2008:213-267.
16. Centers for Disease Control and Prevention. *Cholera Diagnosis and Detection.* http://www.cdc.gov/cholera/diagnosis.html. Accessed January 2018.
17. Centers for Disease Control and Prevention. *Recommendations for the Use of Antibiotics for the Treatment of Cholera.* http://www.cdc.gov/cholera/treatment/antibiotic-treatment.html. Accessed January 2018.
18. Centers for Disease Control and Prevention. *Cholera—Zinc Treatment.* https://www.cdc.gov/cholera/treatment/zinc-treatment.html. Accessed January 2018.
19. Centers for Disease Control and Prevention. *Guidelines for Overseas Presumptive Treatment for Strongyloidiasis, Schistosomiasis, and Soil Transmitted Helminth Infections.* http://www.cdc.gov/immigrantrefugeehealth/guidelines/overseas/intestinal-parasites-overseas.html. Accessed January 2018.
20. Keiser J, Utzinger J. Efficacy of current drugs against soil-transmitted helminth infections: systematic review and meta-analysis. *JAMA.* 2008;299(16):1937-1948.
21. Knopp S, Mohammed K, Speich B, et al. Mebendazole administered alone or in combination with ivermectin against *Trichuris trichiura*: a randomized controlled trial. *Clin Infect Dis.* 2010;51(12):1420-1428.
22. World Health Organization. *Model Formulary for Children, 2010.* http://www.who.int/selection_medicines/list/WMFc_2010.pdf. Accessed January 2018.
23. Mendelson M. Gastroenterology. In: Eddleston M, Davidson R, Brent A, Wilkinson R, eds. *Oxford Handbook of Tropical Medicine.* 3rd ed. New York, NY: Oxford University Press; 2008:269-327.
24. Alderman H, Shekar M. Nutrition, food security and health. In: Kliegman RM, Behrman RE, Jenson HB, et al, eds. *Nelson Textbook of Pediatrics.* 19th ed. St. Louis, MO: Saunders; 2011.
25. Kosek M, Black R, Keusch G. Nutrition and micronutrients in tropical infectious diseases. In: Guerrant RL, Walker DH, Weller PF, eds. *Tropical Infectious Diseases; Principles, Pathogens & Practice.* 2nd ed. Philadelphia, PA: Elsevier; 2006:36-52.
26. Diop el HI, Dossou NI, Ndour MM, et al. Comparison of the efficacy of a solid ready-to-use food and a liquid, milk-based diet for the rehabilitation of severely malnourished children: a randomized trial. *Am J Clin Nutr.* 2003;78:302-307.
27. Branca F, Ferrari M. Impact of micronutrient deficiencies on growth: the stunting syndrome. *Ann Nutr Metab.* 2002;46 Suppl 1:8-17.
28. World Health Organization. *Global Prevalence of Vitamin A Deficiency in Populations at Risk 1995-2005.* In: WHO Global Database on Vitamin A Deficiency. http://whqlibdoc.who.int/publications/2009/9789241598019_eng.pdf. Accessed January 2018.
29. World Health Organization. *Micronutrient Deficiencies: Vitamin A Deficiency.* http://www.who.int/nutrition/topics/vad/en/index.html. Accessed January 2018.
30. Mayo-Wilson E, Imdad A, Herzer K, et al. Vitamin A supplements for preventing mortality, illness, and blindness in children aged under 5: systematic review and meta-analysis. *BMJ.* 2011;343:d5094.
31. Brown K, Wuehler S, Peerson J. The importance of zinc in human nutrition and estimation of the global prevalence of zinc deficiency. *Food Nutr Bull.* 2001;22:113-169.
32. Burgess A. Mother and child undernutrition—vitamin A deficiency. *So Sudan Med J.* 2008;1:13. http://www.southsudanmedicaljournal.com/assets/images/Articles/feb08/image2.jpg. Accessed September 2012.
33. World Health Organization. *Implementing the New Recommendations of the Clinical Management of Diarrhea. Guidelines for Policy Makers and Programme Managers.* Geneva, Switzerland: World Health Organization; 2006. http://whqlibdoc.who.int/publications/2006/9241594217_eng.pdf. Accessed January 2018.

34. Baqui AH, Black RE, Shams EA, et al. Effect of zinc supplementation started during diarrhoea on morbidity and mortality in Bangladeshi children: community randomised trial. *BMJ.* 2002; 325:1059.

35. Brown K, Wuehler S, Peerson J. The importance of zinc in human nutrition and estimation of the global prevalence of zinc deficiency. *Food Nutr Bull.* 2001. http://archive.unu.edu/unupress/food/fnb22-2.pdf. Accessed September 2012.

36. World Health Organization. *Micronutrient Deficiencies. Iron Deficiency Anaemia.* http://www.who.int/nutrition/topics/ida/en/index.html. Accessed January 2018.

37. Horton S, Miloff A. Iodine status and availability of iodized salt: an across-country analysis. *Food Nutr Bull.* 2010;31: 214-220.

38. World Health Organization. *Iodine Status Worldwide.* http://whqlibdoc.who.int.publications/2004/9241592001.pdf. Accessed January 2018.

39. Day N. Malaria. In: Eddleston M, Davidson R, Brent A, Wilkinson R, eds. *Oxford Handbook of Tropical Medicine.* 3rd ed. New York, NY: Oxford University Press; 2008:31-65.

40. Centers for Disease Control. *Malaria.* https://www.cdc.gov/malaria/. Accessed January 2018.

41. World Health Organization. *10 Facts on Malaria.* http://www.who.int/features/factfiles/malaria/en/index.html. Accessed January 2018.

42. Ashley E, White N. Malaria diagnosis and treatment. In: Jong E, Sanford E, eds. *Travel and Tropical Medicine Manual.* 4th ed. Philadelphia, PA: Saunders Elsevier; 2008:303-321.

43. Hoffman S, Campbell C, White N. Malaria. In: Guerrant RL, Walker DH, Weller PF, eds. *Tropical Infectious Diseases; Principles, Pathogens & Practice.* 2nd ed. Philadelphia, PA: Elsevier; 2006:1024-1062.

44. Centers for Disease Control. *Treatment of Malaria (Guidelines for Clinicians).* July 2013. http://www.cdc.gov/malaria/resources/pdf/clinicalguidance.pdf. Accessed January 2018.

45. World Health Organization. *Guidelines for the treatment of malaria.* 3rd ed. April 2015. http://www.who.int/malaria/publications/atoz/9789241549127/en/. Accessed January 30, 2018.

46. World Health Organization. *Q&A for artemisinin resistance.* March 2018. http://www.who.int/malaria/media/artemisinin_resistance_qa/en/. Accessed April 10, 2018.

47. Centers for Disease Control and Prevention. *Parasites—Leishmaniasis.* http://www.cdc.gov/parasites/leishmaniasis/. Accessed January 2018.

48. Singh S. New developments in diagnosis of leishmaniasis. *Indian J Med Res.* 2006;123:311-330.

49. Ryan T. Dermatology. In: Eddleston M, Davidson R, Brent A, Wilkinson R, eds. *Oxford Handbook of Tropical Medicine.* 3rd ed. New York, NY: Oxford University Press; 2008:566.

50. Schwartz E. Leishmaniasis. In: Jong E, Sanford E, eds. *Travel and Tropical Medicine Manual.* 4th ed. Philadelphia, PA: Saunders Elsevier; 2008:532-542.

51. Pub Med Health. *Leishmaniasis.* http://www.ncbi.nlm.nih.gov/pubmedhealth/PMH0002362/. Accessed September 15, 2012.

52. Pearson R, Weller P, Guerrant R. Chemotherapy of parasitic diseases. In: Guerrant RL, Walker DH, Weller PF, eds. *Tropical Infectious Diseases; Principles, Pathogens & Practice.* 2nd ed. Philadelphia, PA: Elsevier; 2006:142-168.

53. World Health Organization. *WHO Guidelines for the treatment of Chlamydia trachomatis.* http://www.who.int/reproductivehealth/publications/rtis/chlamydia-treatment-guidelines/en/. Accessed January 2018.

54. Yorston D. Ophthalmology. In: Eddleston M, Davidson R, Brent A, Wilkinson R, eds. *Oxford Handbook of Tropical Medicine.* 3rd ed. New York, NY: Oxford University Press; 2008:523.

55. Karimkhani C, Colombara DV, Drucker AM, et al. The global burden of scabies: a cross-sectional analysis from the Global Burden of Disease Study 2015. *Lancet Infect Dis.* 2017;17(12):1247-1254.

56. Currie BJ. Scabies and global control of neglected tropical diseases. *N Engl J Med.* 2015;373(24):2371-2372.

57. Thomas J, Peterson GM, Walton SF, et al. Scabies: an ancient global disease with a need for new therapies. *BMC Infect Dis.* 2015;15;250.

58. World Health Organization. *Leprosy; Fact Sheet No.101.* http://www.who.int/mediacentre/factsheets/fs101/en/index.html. Accessed January 2018.

59. Health Resources & Services Administration. *Hansen's Disease Data & Statistics.* https://www.hrsa.gov/hansens-disease/data-and-statistics.html. Accessed January 2018.

60. Global Leprosy Situation, 2012. *Wkly Epidemiol Rec.* 2012;87(34):317-328.

61. World Health Organization. *Leprosy Elimination. WHO Multidrug Therapy.* http://www.who.int/lep/mdt/en/index.html. Accessed January 2018.

62. Meyers W. Leprosy. In: Guerrant, RL, Walker DH, Weller PF, eds. *Tropical Infectious Diseases; Principles, Pathogens & Practice.* 2nd ed. Philadelphia, PA: Elsevier; 2006:436.

63. Gormus BJ, Meyers WM. Under-explored experimental topics related to integral mycobacterial vaccines for leprosy. *Expert Rev Vaccines.* 2003;2(6):791-804.

64. Sapienza A, Green S. Correction of the claw hand. *Hand Clin.* 2012;28(1):53-66.

65. World Health Organization. *TB/HIV FACTS 2011-2012.* http://www.who.int/tb/areas-of-work/tb-hiv/tbhiv_factsheet_2016.pdf. Accessed January 2018.

66. Johnson J, Ellner J. Tuberculosis and atypical mycobacterial infections. In: Guerrant RL, Walker DH, Weller PF, eds. *Tropical Infectious Diseases; Principles, Pathogens & Practice.* 2nd ed. Philadelphia, PA: Elsevier; 2006:411.

67. National Institutes of Health Clinical Guidelines Portal. *Considerations for Antiretroviral Use in Patients with Coinfections; Mycobacterium Tuberculosis Disease with HIV Coinfection.* http://www.aidsinfo.nih.gov/guidelines/html/1/adult-and-adolescent-treatment-guidelines/27/. Accessed January 2018.

8 ZIKA, EBOLA, AND OTHER EMERGING INFECTIONS

Jeffrey W. W. Hall, MD
Matthew S. Haldeman, MD

PATIENT STORY

A 35-year-old graduate student at the local university returned from visiting his family in Liberia over the summer. He has been back in the United States for a week, and three days ago he began having fevers up to 40°C (104°F). He has had shaking chills, significant body aches, and a faint papular rash noted on his torso. Initial laboratory studies include a single negative malaria smear and a negative malaria rapid diagnostic test. A CBC reveals WBC count of 5000 with a left shift noted, and his platelet count is low at 120,000. Upon further history, the student reported a tick bite while visiting his family in the rural parts of the country. He reports no known contact with ill people or participation in any funerals or burial rituals in the country. He is admitted to the hospital for supportive management. Because of his history of recent travel to western Africa, the Centers for Disease Control and Prevention (CDC) is notified, and serologies for Ebola, dengue, chikungunya, and African tick-bite fever are sent. In addition to careful fluid and electrolyte management, he is empirically started on doxycycline for the possibility of rickettsial diseases while awaiting the results of the serologic tests. After 24 hours, his fever improves, and he is monitored for vascular leakage and hypotension, but recovers well. IgM for dengue ultimately returns positive.

INTRODUCTION

Travel has dramatically increased over the past 50 years, both in number of travelers and in distances traveled. Diseases once isolated to restricted geographic areas now must often be included in the differential diagnosis and management of people throughout the world. Failure to diagnose certain critical illnesses not only can lead to worsened clinical outcomes, but also may pose a significant public health threat. Diagnosing emerging infections can be difficult because many of them have nonspecific findings in early stages, and definitive testing often requires reference laboratory testing that may take days to weeks for results. Clinicians need to be aware of current disease outbreaks in their areas, and they need to obtain relevant travel history, including the patient's travel destinations, activities while traveling, insect bites, water exposure, prophylaxis used, and the timing of symptoms relevant to travel.

ZIKA

SYNONYMS: None

▶ Epidemiology

Zika virus was originally described in monkeys in the Zika Forest of Uganda in 1947, with the first human case described in 1952.[1] The first Zika outbreak outside of Africa and Asia was described in Yap Island in Micronesia in 2007.[2] Subsequently, the largest known outbreak of Zika virus was identified in Brazil in 2015, and the causal link between Zika infection in pregnancy and serious fetal anomalies such as microcephaly was identified.[3] The first locally acquired case of Zika in the United States was diagnosed on July 7, 2016.[4] A list of countries and regions with active Zika transmission is maintained by the CDC.[5]

ETIOLOGY/PATHOPHYSIOLOGY

Zika disease is caused by a flavivirus that is primarily transmitted through the bites of *Aedes aegypti* and *Aedes albopictus* mosquitoes.[6] Less common means of transmission include sexual transmission, vertical transmission from a mother to child, blood transfusion, or through laboratory/healthcare-related exposures. Although clinical illness in adults is often mild, infection during pregnancy can be devastating, because Zika virus appears to be neurotoxic to developing fetal neural progenitor cells. An estimated 10% of infants will be affected to some degree, with approximately 15% of infants having Zika-associated birth defects if infected during the first trimester.[7] Zika-associated birth defects include a range of neurologic defects in the infant, including a fetal brain disruption sequence resulting in clinical microcephaly.[8]

RISK FACTORS

The two greatest risk factors for Zika infection are exposure to *Aedes aegypti* mosquitoes and living in and traveling to countries with active Zika transmission. Regions with active Zika infection at the time of this writing include Central/South America, the Caribbean, Papua New Guinea, and some Pacific Islands (**Figure 8-1**).[9] *Aedes* mosquitoes are well adapted to urban living with their ability to breed in both human-made and natural containers. They bite both indoors and outdoors, and they feed primarily during the daytime, but can bite at night.[10]

Sexual transmission of Zika has also been described. Viable Zika virus persists in semen longer than in blood or other fluids. Interim recommendations are that men wait to conceive for at least 6 months after Zika symptom onset or last Zika exposure.[11]

DIAGNOSIS

▶ Clinical features

Clinical symptoms for Zika infection are generally mild and nonspecific, including fever, joint pain, and conjunctivitis. A generalized maculopapular rash is frequently seen.[12] Headache and myalgia are also reported. Guillain-Barré syndrome has been occasionally associated with Zika Infection. Fetal abnormalities due to exposure in utero include microcephaly, and long-term sequelae are being investigated (**Figure 8-2**).

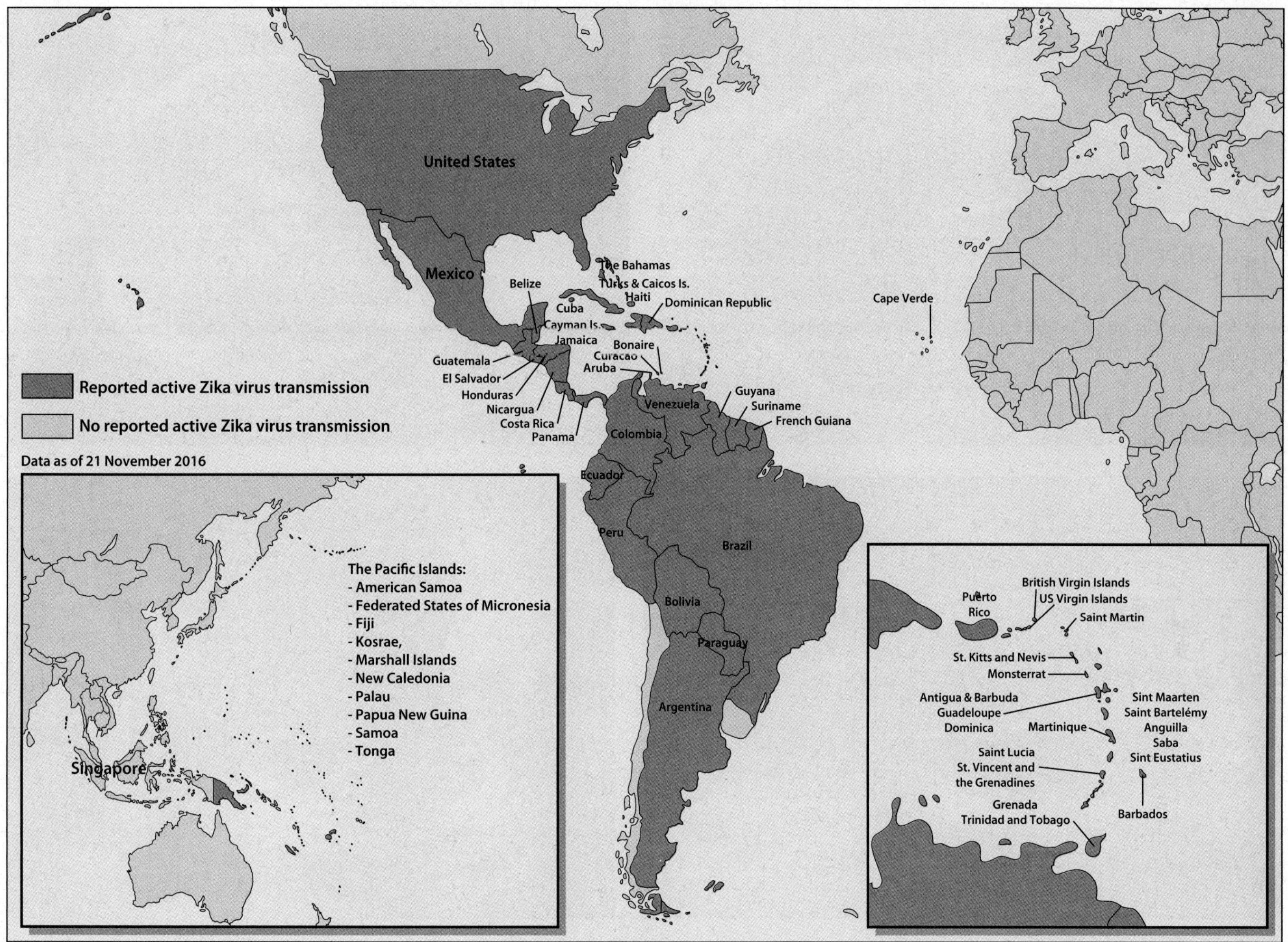

FIGURE 8-1 Shading indicates countries and territories where mosquito-borne transmission of Zika virus has been reported. It does not necessarily indicate that mosquito-borne transmission is occurring throughout the entire country or territory. *(Reproduced with permission from Centers for Disease Control and Prevention (CDC).)*

▶ Laboratory testing

Zika viral RNA often is detectable for up to 2 weeks after exposure, but may be present for up to 12 weeks. The absence of viremia does not exclude a recent infection, so a negative RNA test should be confirmed with Zika IgM antibody. Zika IgM antibodies typically develop by day 4 to 7 of illness.

Testing algorithms for asymptomatic people, including pregnant women, is a rapidly evolving science. RNA nucleic acid testing (NAT) is recommended to be done on both urine and serum specimens for up to 2 weeks following exposure/start of symptoms or up to 12 weeks if IgM is positive. In nonpregnant women, testing should be performed on blood and urine specimens during the first 2 weeks after symptom onset for suspected cases. The URL for the CDC-recommended algorithm is listed in Provider Resources. Because symptoms of Zika significantly overlap with those of chikungunya and dengue infections, consider testing samples for anti-dengue and anti-chikungunya antibodies as well.[13]

▶ Imaging

The CDC recommends that all infants born to mothers with recent Zika virus infection have postnatal neuroimaging and also be tested for Zika virus, as this may correlate with future developmental abnormalities.[7] During pregnancy, serial fetal ultrasounds every 3 to 4 weeks are recommended in pregnant women with presumed or confirmed Zika or unspecified flavivirus infection.

DIFFERENTIAL DIAGNOSIS

- Other flavivirus infection
  - Dengue
  - Chikungunya
  - West Nile virus
- Other nonspecific causes of fever in the tropics
  - Malaria
  - Bacterial infection
  - Alternate viral infection: influenza, mononucleosis, etc.
  - Rickettsial diseases
- Other causes of congenital fetal malformations
  - Cytomegalovirus (CMV)
  - Toxoplasmosis
  - Congenital syphilis

MANAGEMENT

- The treatment of Zika is generally supportive, including analgesics and antipyretics. Aspirin should be avoided. SOR Ⓒ

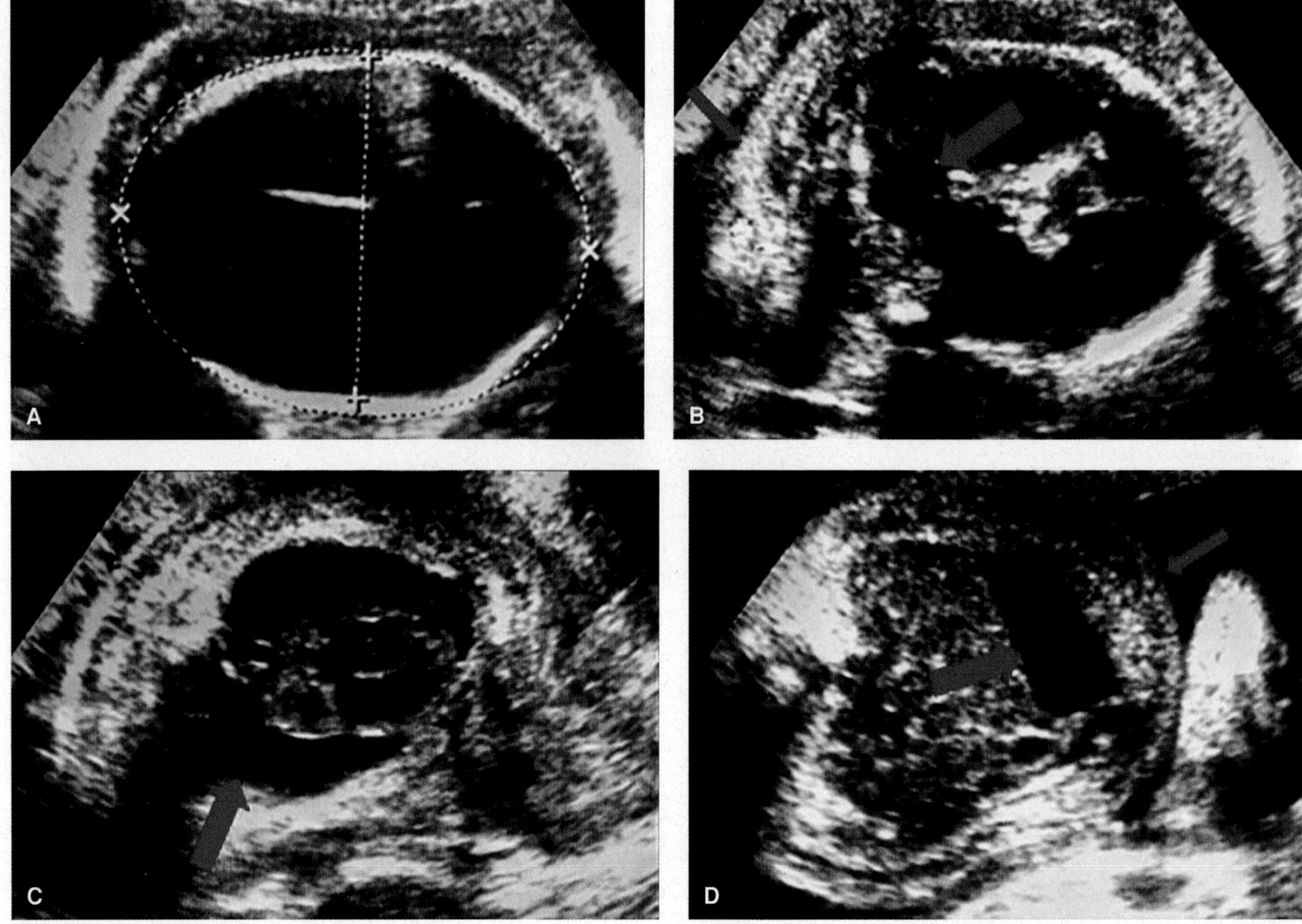

FIGURE 8-2 Axial ultrasound views of the fetus at the 30th gestational week showing (**A**) cranium with severe microcephaly (215 mm) and hydranencephaly; (**B**) posterior fossa with destruction of the cerebellar vermis *(wide arrow)* and nuchal edema *(thin arrow)*; (**C**) thorax with bilateral pleural effusions *(arrow)*; and (**D**) abdomen with ascites *(wide arrow)* and subcutaneous edema *(thin arrow)*. (*Reproduced with permission from Wikipedia Commons/Sarno M, Sacramento G, Khouri R, et al. https://commons.wikimedia.org/wiki/File:Zika-Virus-Infection-and-Stillbirths-A-Case-of-Hydrops-Fetalis-Hydranencephaly-and-Fetal-Demise-pntd.0004517.g001.jpg.*)

- Patients with Zika infection are advised to practice mosquito prevention strategies for 2 weeks following exposure or symptom resolution to decrease the risk of spread. SOR Ⓒ
- Male patients are advised to avoid attempts at conceiving with their partner for 6 months following symptoms or exposure. SOR Ⓒ

PREVENTION

Avoiding exposure is the best prevention. Patients can be advised to avoid travel to endemic areas, especially if pregnant. If travel is unavoidable, or if patients live in endemic areas, they should employ mosquito prevention strategies: wear long-sleeved shirt/long pants, use a permethrin-treated bed net, apply insect repellant, and treat clothes with permethrin. Condoms may reduce the risk of sexual transmission. Vaccine trials are ongoing.

PROGNOSIS

Zika infection in adults or children is typically a mild disease with a good prognosis. Outpatient management is typical, and hospitalization is rarely necessary. If infection occurs during pregnancy, the incidence of serious congenital malformations, including microcephaly, is estimated to be approximately 10%, and is up to 15% of infants when exposure takes place during the first trimester.[7]

PATIENT RESOURCES

- CDC website on Zika. **https://www.cdc.gov/zika/about/index.html.**

PROVIDER RESOURCES

- CDC Web tool for Zika Virus testing. **https://www.cdc.gov/zika/hc-providers/index.html.**
- Tiered algorithm for arbovirus detection for suspected cases of chikungunya, dengue, or Zika. **https://www.cdc.gov/zika/pdfs/denvchikvzikv-testing-algorithm.pdf.**
- Testing and interpretation recommendations for a pregnant woman with possible exposure to Zika virus—United States (including U.S. territories). **https://www.cdc.gov/zika/pdfs/testing_algorithm.pdf.**
- *New England Journal of Medicine. Zika Virus.* **http://www.nejm.org/page/zika-virus.**

WEST NILE VIRUS

▶ Epidemiology

West Nile virus (WNV) is the most common vector-borne viral disease in the United States, causing more than 40,000 total reported cases and 2000 deaths between 1999 and 2015.[14,15] It was first discovered in 1937 in Uganda, and currently has a worldwide range including Africa, the Middle East, southern Europe, western Russia, southwestern Asia, and Australia. The wide geographic range stems from the virus's ability to infect many species of birds and mosquitoes. It was first identified in the Americas in New York City in 1999, and has since become endemic in all 48 states of the continental United States and all Canadian provinces.[16]

ETIOLOGY/PATHOPHYSIOLOGY

West Nile virus is a flavivirus that is spread to humans from the bite of an infected *Culex* mosquito (**Figure 8-3**). An estimated 25% of people infected will develop clinical symptoms known as West Nile fever. Roughly 1 in 200 infected people will develop neuroinvasive disease including meningitis, encephalitis, or acute flaccid paralysis.

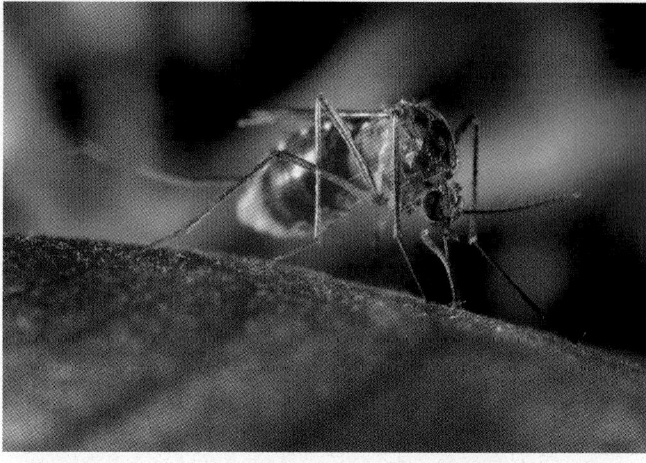

FIGURE 8-3 Close-up photograph of *Culex quinquefasciatus*, one of the many *Culex* mosquito species that transmits West Nile virus to humans through its bite. (*Reproduced with permission from Centers for Disease Control and Prevention (CDC)/James Gathany.*)

RISK FACTORS

The risk factors are travel or living in an endemic area during the *Culex* mosquito season. Endemic regions include all of Africa, the Middle East, southern Europe/Russia, India, parts of SE Asia and Australia, North America including all of the United States and Mexico, and more recently parts of South America.[17] More than 90% of infections in North America occur during the summer months from July to September. Any age can be infected, although people over the age of 65 have a 16-fold increase in risk in developing neuroinvasive disease compared to those ages 16–24.

DIAGNOSIS

▶ Clinical features

West Nile fever can range from a mild infection resolving after several days to an incapacitating illness persisting for months. The incubation period is around 2 to 14 days. Symptoms include sudden onset of headache, weakness, myalgias, and low-grade fever. A nonspecific rash often develops at the time of defervescence. The rash is described as a morbilliform, maculopapular, nonpruritic rash over the torso and extremities. There is no strong age predilection for this manifestation of WNV.

West Nile neuroinvasive disease has several clinical syndromes in addition to those of West Nile fever. West Nile meningitis includes meningeal signs, photophobia, or phonophobia. Nausea and vomiting are often more pronounced. West Nile encephalitis includes a depressed or altered level of consciousness or personality change lasting more than 24 hours. Symptoms can include parkinsonian symptoms, including a coarse tremor, as well as delirium, coma, and death. Acute flaccid paralysis is an acute onset of limb weakness progressing rapidly over 48 hours. Such paralysis is usually asymmetric, hyporeflexic, and without loss of sensation. Of those with acute paralysis, 80% also have meningitis or encephalitis.

▶ Laboratory testing

Total leukocyte counts are usually normal or slightly elevated. Cerebrospinal fluid (CSF) studies often show normal glucose, mildly elevated protein levels, and mild pleocytosis with a lymphocytic predominance. WNV-specific IgM antibody in serum can make the diagnosis. Convalescent testing may be required if initial testing is negative at the time of clinical presentation. Neuroinvasive disease is diagnosed with WNV IgM in cerebrospinal fluid. WNV viral polymerase chain reaction (PCR) testing is highly specific, but generally less sensitive because of the transient and low levels of viremia.

▶ Imaging

Neuroimaging studies are usually normal. Occasionally focal lesions or leptomeningeal enhancement is noted.

DIFFERENTIAL DIAGNOSIS

- Bacterial meningitis
- Other causes of viral meningitis
- Other viral encephalitides, including:
  - Varicella encephalitis
  - Herpes encephalitis
  - St. Louis encephalitis
  - Japanese encephalitis
  - Enteroviral encephalitis
  - Eastern equine encephalitis, Western equine encephalitis

MANAGEMENT

- Management is supportive

PREVENTION

- Mosquito control and avoiding mosquito bites in areas of active transmission

PROGNOSIS

Most patients with uncomplicated West Nile fever will ultimately make a full recovery, although patients with neuroinvasive disease have approximately a 10% fatality rate.[16] Those patients with West Nile encephalitis often have persistent weakness or neurocognitive deficits lasting up to a year or longer. One third of patients with acute flaccid paralysis will recover to full strength, one third will have some improvement, and one third will have little to no improvement.[16]

FOLLOW-UP

- West Nile virus is a nationally notifiable disease.

PATIENT RESOURCES

- West Nile Virus Advocacy. **http://www.westnilevirusadvocacy.org**

PROVIDER RESOURCES

- CDC website on WNV. **https://www.cdc.gov/westnile/index.html.**

DENGUE

SYNONYMS: Breakbone fever, dengue hemorrhagic fever

▶ Epidemiology

Dengue is endemic in more than 100 countries globally, and it is the most common arboviral disease in the world. The World Health Organization reported 3 million suspected or confirmed cases of Dengue in 2015.[18] Most cases in the United States are travel related, but local transmission has occurred in Florida, Texas, and Hawaii.

ETIOLOGY/PATHOPHYSIOLOGY

Dengue virus is caused by four different flavivirus serotypes that are transmitted person to person by *Aedes aegypti* and *Aedes albopictus* mosquitoes. The incubation period is short, usually only 4 to 7 days.[19] Patients are classified as having either dengue fever or severe dengue. The hallmark of severe dengue is systemic vascular permeability. This results in edema, fluid accumulation, and hemoconcentration and often progresses to end-organ hypoperfusion and shock. Hemorrhagic manifestations, including thrombocytopenia, a decrease in fibrinogen level, and an increase in the activated partial-thromboplastin time,[20] are also frequently seen in severe cases. The mechanisms behind hemorrhagic manifestations are incompletely understood.

RISK FACTORS

Living in and traveling to endemic countries or areas is the major risk factor for acquiring dengue fever (**Figure 8-4**). *Aedes* mosquitoes are well adapted to urban living, bite both indoors and outdoors, with biting activity greatest during the daytime.[10] Patients previously infected with a different serovar of the dengue virus are at greater risk of progression to severe dengue.

DIAGNOSIS

▶ Clinical features

Dengue fever often presents as an abrupt onset of a nonspecific febrile illness within a week after travel to an endemic area. Dengue fever can be completely asymptomatic, cause a mild nonspecific febrile illness, or cause "classic dengue fever" (with or without progression to severe dengue), which consists of three phases (**Figure 8-5**):

- Febrile phase (days 0 to 4–7)
  - Fever, retro-orbital headache, severe myalgias and arthralgias, nausea, vomiting, changes in taste, possible lymphadenopathy, and generalized rash. When seen, the rash is referred to as "generalized erythroderma with islands of sparing" (see **Figure 8-6**). Petechiae may be seen at sites of compression.
- Critical phase (lasts 2 days after febrile phase)
  - Defervescence occurs, other symptoms may persist
  - This period involves the greatest risk of progression to severe dengue—closely monitor urine output, hematocrit, and physical exam for signs of capillary leak and edema.
- Progression either to severe dengue or to convalescence/recovery

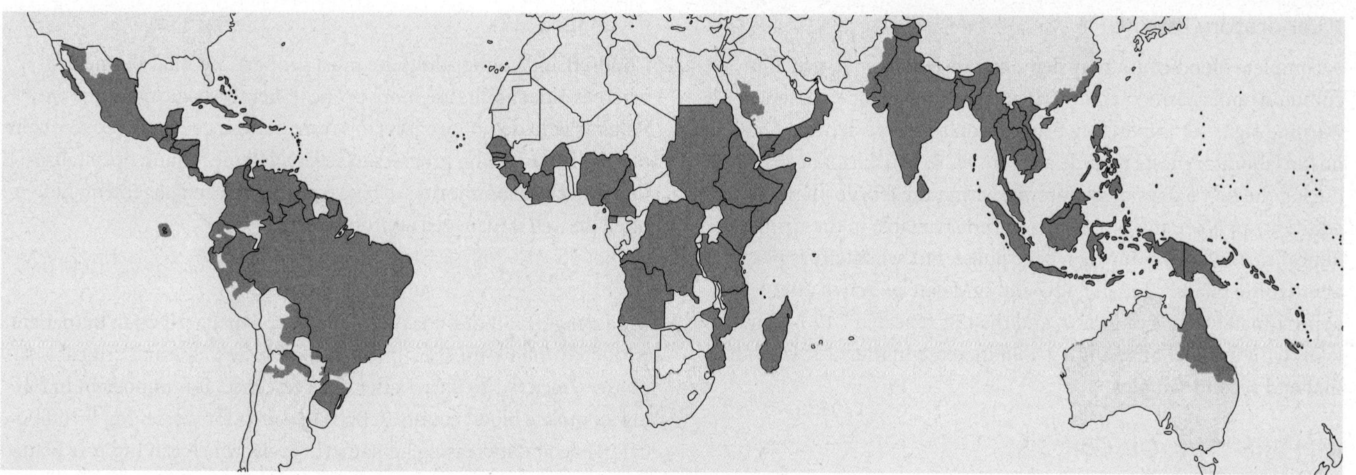

FIGURE 8-4 Distribution map showing regions with risk of dengue transmission. (*Reproduced with permission from Centers for Disease Control and Prevention (CDC). http://www.cdc.gov/dengue/epidemiology/index.Html.*)

A presumptive diagnosis is made with an appropriate exposure history, fever, and two of the following:[21]

- Nausea/vomiting
- Rash
- Myalgias, arthralgias, headache
- Positive tourniquet test
  - The tourniquet test is a simple test for signs of microvascular fragility in a patient with potential dengue fever. To perform, a blood pressure cuff is inflated over the upper arm to midway between systolic and diastolic pressures, and this is held for 5 minutes. Afterwards, it is deflated and the skin is examined for 1–2 minutes for signs of new petechiae. The test is considered positive if there are >10–20 new petechiae present over an area of skin that is 2.5 cm (1 in.) square
- Leukopenia
- Any warning sign.

Warning signs for impending progression to severe dengue include:

- Abdominal pain/tenderness
- Persistent vomiting
- Clinical fluid accumulation
- Mucosal bleed
- Lethargy, restlessness
- Liver enlargement >2 cm
- Increase in hematocrit (Hct) concurrent with rapid decrease in platelet count

Criteria for severe dengue include

- Severe plasma leakage leading to shock or fluid accumulation with respiratory distress
- Severe bleeding

  Severe organ involvement including aspartate transaminase (AST) or alanine transaminase (ALT) >1000, impaired consciousness, or other end-organ dysfunction.

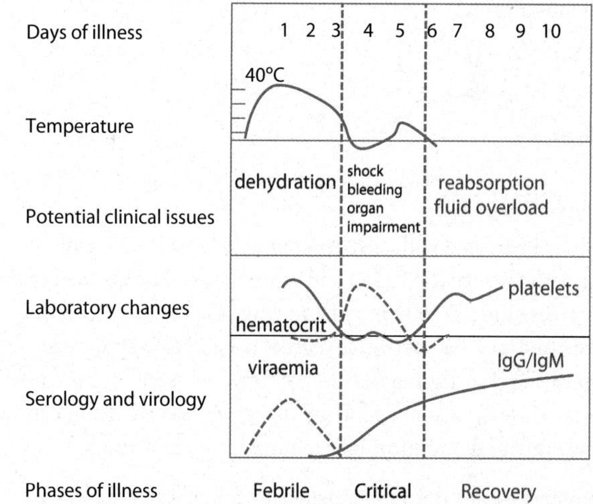

FIGURE 8-5 Course of dengue fever. (*Reproduced with permission from Wikimedia Commons/Graham Beards. https://commons.wikimedia.org/wiki/File:Course_of_Dengue_illness.png.*)

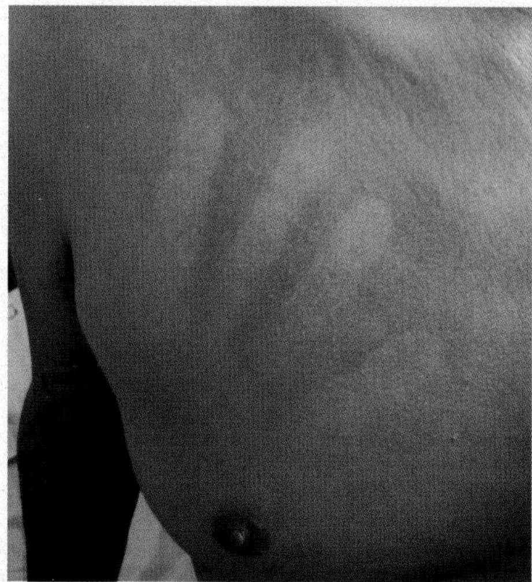

FIGURE 8-6 Rash in dengue fever, showing generalized erythroderma. Handprint demonstrates blanching. Classically, patients will have scattered small areas of normal skin color, termed *islands of sparing*. (*Reproduced with permission from Wikipedia Commons/Ranjan Premaratna. https://commons.wikimedia.org/wiki/File:Early_Dengue_Fever_Rash_2014.jpg.*)

▶ Laboratory testing

A complete blood count may demonstrate leukopenia, which is common, and a rising hematocrit and thrombocytopenia, which are warning signs for impending progression to severe dengue. Diagnostic laboratory tests include a serum PCR, which can be drawn during the first 5 days of symptoms, within the febrile phase. In addition, an NS-1 antigen detection (not available in the United States) can be drawn during febrile phase, but sensitivity is poor after febrile phase.[22] Finally, IgG and IgM can be drawn after approximately day 4 of illness, and the test repeated 7 to 14 days later, with the goal of seeing a 4-fold increase in titers between the first and second samples.

DIFFERENTIAL DIAGNOSIS

- Malaria
- Other viral hemorrhagic fevers
- Sepsis with disseminated intravascular coagulation
- Chikungunya
- Yellow fever
- Rickettsial diseases
- Influenza

MANAGEMENT

Fever may be treated with acetaminophen. Nonsteroidal anti-inflammatory drugs (NSAIDs) and aspirin should be avoided as they may increase the risk of hemorrhage. Have the patient use insect repellant and/or a bed net while febrile to avoid infecting other mosquitoes and spreading the disease. Have the patient drink plenty of fluids, if tolerated, and get plenty of rest. For severe dengue, more intensive inpatient monitoring is required, which includes:[23]

- Monitoring urine output, hematocrit, and vital signs closely
- Giving judicious fluids (oral if tolerated, and/or IV normal saline or Ringer's Lactate) if hypotensive, hematocrit rises, or urine output falls. Avoid large-volume IV fluid administration given high risk of fluid overload
- Use of colloids (such as albumin, if available) for persistent hypotension after two or three boluses of isotonic saline
- Transfusion of packed red blood cells (PRBCs) or whole blood can be indicated for clinically significant bleeding, a rapid drop in hematocrit, or poor urine output despite IV fluid administration.

Corticosteroids have not demonstrated benefit SOR Ⓒ and platelet transfusions do not decrease the risk of severe bleeding SOR Ⓒ. In addition, use of half-normal saline can worsen ascites and pleural effusions SOR Ⓒ, and IV fluids are not needed if oral intake is adequate SOR Ⓒ.[23]

PREVENTION

Mosquito control and avoidance strategies are the most important methods of prevention. This includes wearing long-sleeved shirt/long pants, use of a permethrin-treated bed net, frequent applications of insect repellant, and spraying clothes with permethrin. A tetravalent vaccine has been developed and is licensed for use in 14 countries as of February 2017.[24]

PROGNOSIS

Children and young adults are most prone to vascular permeability, whereas older adults are more prone to hemorrhagic manifestions.[20] Patients who do not progress to severe dengue generally recover completely. Patients who progress to severe dengue require hospitalization and close monitoring, often requiring ICU management, but often do well if managed appropriately.

FOLLOW-UP

Mild dengue without warning signs can be managed as an outpatient with daily follow-up visits through the febrile phase and critical phase, which is 1 to 2 days after defervescence. It is important to follow complete blood counts (CBCs) to watch for worsening thrombocytopenia and increasing hematocrit levels, which can indicate hemoconcentration, along with any other clinical signs of intravascular volume depletion. Patients with warning signs or coexisting conditions should be observed inpatient. Patients meeting criteria for severe dengue will require inpatient treatment.

PATIENT RESOURCES

- Centers for Disease Control and Prevention. *Dengue.* **https://www.cdc.gov/dengue/.**

PROVIDER RESOURCES

- Centers for Disease Control and Prevention. *Dengue.* **https://www.cdc.gov/dengue/index.html.**
- WHO fact sheet. *Dengue and Severe Dengue.* **http://www.who.int/mediacentre/factsheets/fs117/en/.**

CHIKUNGUNYA

EPIDEMIOLOGY

The virus was identified in modern-day Tanzania during an epidemic in 1952. Subsequent outbreaks were noted in Asia during the 1950s and 1960s.[25] Urban outbreaks have subsequently occurred in India, Italy, France, and the Americas.

ETIOLOGY/PATHOPHYSIOLOGY

Chikungunya is an alphavirus that is spread by infected *Aedes aegypti* and *Aedes albopictus* mosquitoes (same as for Zika and dengue). More than 85% of chikungunya infections are clinically symptomatic.

RISK FACTORS

Living in and traveling to endemic countries or areas is the major risk factor (**Figure 8-7**). *Aedes* mosquitoes are well adapted to urban living and bite both indoors and outdoors, with biting activity greatest during the daytime. Chikungunya outbreaks are often intense but are more limited in duration than those of dengue or West Nile virus.

DIAGNOSIS

▶ Clinical features

Chikungunya fever has an abrupt onset with a brief incubation period averaging 3 days. Fever lasts approximately 1 week. Myalgias

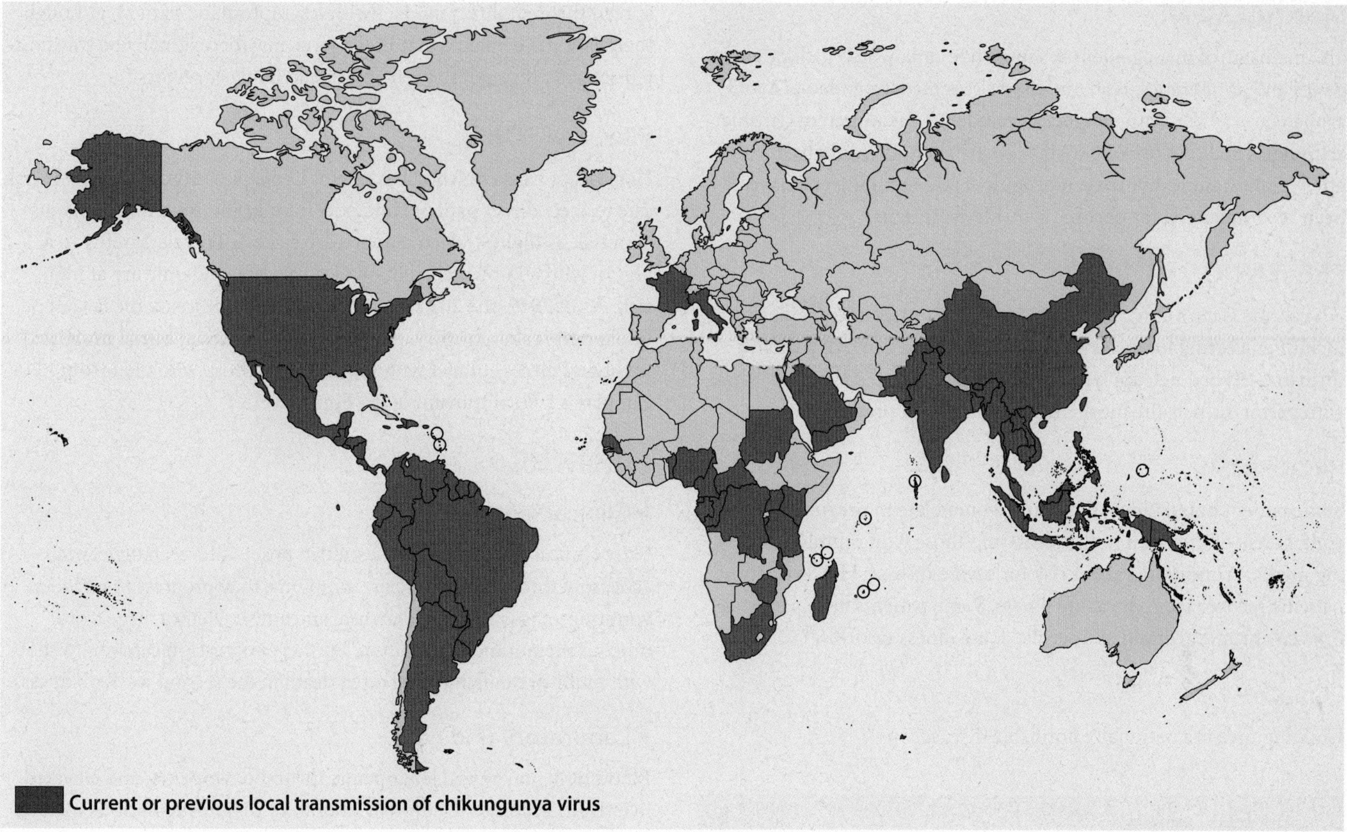

Current or previous local transmission of chikungunya virus

FIGURE 8-7 Map showing distribution of Chikungunya. (*Reproduced with permission from Centers for Disease Control and Prevention (CDC). https://www.cdc.gov/chikungunya/geo/index.html.*)

and severe, symmetric joint pains, most commonly in the bilateral hands and feet, are present in more than 90% of patients. A maculopapular rash on the trunk can occur in 20% to 80% of patients. The rash has been known to involve the face, arms, legs, palms, and soles (**Figure 8-8**). Severe chikungunya fever generally is limited to older patients with comorbid conditions, or very young children. These patients can rarely progress to encephalitis, myocarditis, multi-organ failure and death. Up to 50% of patients can have an arthritis that persists long-term after the acute illness resolves, which mimics rheumatoid arthritis.

▶ Laboratory findings

Routine laboratory testing in acute chikungunya often reveals lymphopenia, thrombocytopenia, and elevated aminotransferase levels. Diagnostic testing for chikungunya includes viral PCR, which is typically positive during the first week after onset of symptoms.[26] Also, viral IgM, if obtained, is typically positive by day 5 of illness. If this initial acute-phase serology is negative, a second convalescent-phase sample should also be obtained for more definitive diagnosis.[26]

DIFFERENTIAL DIAGNOSIS

- Malaria
- Dengue and other arboviral infections
- Rickettsial infections
- Zika
- Influenza.

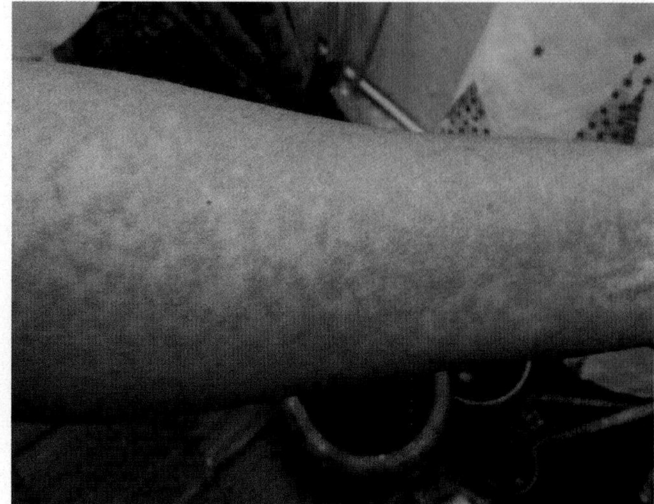

FIGURE 8-8 Maculopapular rash of Chikungunya. (*Reproduced with permission from Wikipedia Commons/EEIM. https://commons.wikimedia.org/wiki/File:Chikungu%C3%B1a_2_en_Col.JPG*)

MANAGEMENT

The mainstay of management is supportive care, which includes analgesics and antipyretics, rest, oral fluids. It is recommended to avoid aspirin or NSAIDs until dengue is excluded.[27] Treatment of chronic arthralgias includes use of NSAIDs, corticosteroids, and physiotherapy.[26] Chloroquine, hydroxychloroquine, and methotrexate have been recommended for chronic arthritis symptoms.

PREVENTION

No vaccine is currently available. Mosquito control and avoidance, including wearing long-sleeved shirt/long pants, using of a permethrin-treated bed net, applying insect repellant, and spraying clothes with permethrin, is the most effective method of prevention.

PROGNOSIS

Some patient populations, including women late in pregnancy (which confers risk of infection to the fetus) and those with multiple underlying medical conditions, are at risk for severe disease. However, most patients recover from the acute illness. Some patients have persistent or even chronic arthralgias after the acute illness resolves.[26]

FOLLOW-UP

Chikungunya is a nationally notifiable disease.

PATIENT RESOURCES

- Centers for Disease Control and Prevention. *Chikungunya Virus.* **http://www.cdc.gov/chikungunya.**

PROVIDER RESOURCES

- Centers for Disease Control and Prevention. *Chikungunya Virus: Information for Health Care Professionals.* **https://www.cdc.gov/chikungunya/hc/index.html.**
- World Health Organization. *Media Centre: Chikungunya Fact Sheet.* **http://www.who.int/mediacentre/factsheets/fs327/en/.**

EBOLA

▶ Epidemiology

Ebola virus disease (EVD) was first identified in 1976 near the Ebola River in what is now the Democratic Republic of Congo.[28] Ebola virus disease outbreaks had been in smaller villages until 2014, when the disease hit urban centers in Liberia, Sierra Leone, and Guinea to cause nearly 30,000 cases and 12,000 deaths. The 2014 outbreak also spread to Nigeria (one traveler), the United States, Mali, and Senegal.

ETIOLOGY/PATHOPHYSIOLOGY

Ebola virus disease, caused by a virus in the family Filoviridae, is a zoonotic disease that is introduced to human populations through contact with infected bats, primates, or other rainforest animals. Ebola spreads human to human through direct contact with bodily fluids and contaminated materials. The incubation period from exposure to onset of symptoms is 2 to 21 days. Nearly all infections are spread through direct contact with a symptomatic patient, although there is some evidence that Ebola virus may occasionally be transmitted sexually through the semen of male Ebola survivors.[29]

RISK FACTORS

Healthcare workers who take care of Ebola patients are at notable risk due to their direct patient contact. Viremia, and therefore transmission risk, is highest when patients are sickest. Travelers going to a region with a known current or recent Ebola epidemic are at high risk. As of 2017, the 2014 West Africa Ebola outbreak, the largest Ebola outbreak in history, is subsiding. Traditional burial practices involving direct contact with the bodies of those who died from Ebola can play a role in transmission (**Figure 8-9**).

DIAGNOSIS

▶ Clinical features

Early clinical features include a sudden onset of fever, fatigue, headache, sore throat, and myalgias. Symptoms may progress to include vomiting, epigastric pain, diarrhea, and a rash. Hemorrhage from mucous membranes is common. Further progression can lead to shock with multi-organ failure and often death in the second week of illness.

▶ Laboratory findings

Blood tests may reveal leukopenia, thrombocytopenia, and elevated liver transaminases. Definitive laboratory diagnostic options include viral PCR, which is the current standard method of diagnosis, as well as rapid antigen testing ("ReEBOV," which is slightly less sensitive/specific than PCR) and serology testing.[30]

DIFFERENTIAL DIAGNOSIS

- Malaria
- Dengue
- Chikungunya
- Typhoid
- Meningitis
- Other viral hemorrhagic fevers
- Yellow fever.

MANAGEMENT

Stringent contact precautions in full personal protective equipment are critical to protect healthcare workers. Aggressive supportive care including hemodynamic monitoring and fluid and electrolyte replacement may improve survival.[31]

PREVENTION

All bodily fluids, including those sent for laboratory confirmation, must be handled as though potentially highly infectious. Multiple candidate vaccines are in development, with rVSV-ZEBOV currently performing well both in safety and immunogenicity trials.[32]

PROGNOSIS

Mortality of Ebola Virus disease in West Africa ranges from 37% to 74%.[31] Mortality of those patients treated in the United States and Europe with critical care facilities was 18.5%.

FOLLOW-UP

Male patients who survive Ebola should have their semen tested by PCR for virus at 3 months after onset of disease. If positive, they should be tested every month until semen tests negative twice.

PATIENT RESOURCES

- Centers for Disease Control and Prevention. *Ebola (Ebola Virus Disease).* **https://www.cdc.gov/vhf/ebola/index.html.**
- World Health Organization. *Media Centre: Ebola Virus Disease Fact Sheet.* **http://www.who.int/mediacentre/factsheets/fs103/en/.**

PROVIDER RESOURCES

- Centers for Disease Control and Prevention. *Ebola (Ebola Virus Disease): U.S. Healthcare Workers and Settings.* **https://www.cdc.gov/vhf/ebola/healthcare-us/index.html.**
- World Health Organization. *Ebola Virus Disease.* **http://www.who.int/ebola/en/.**

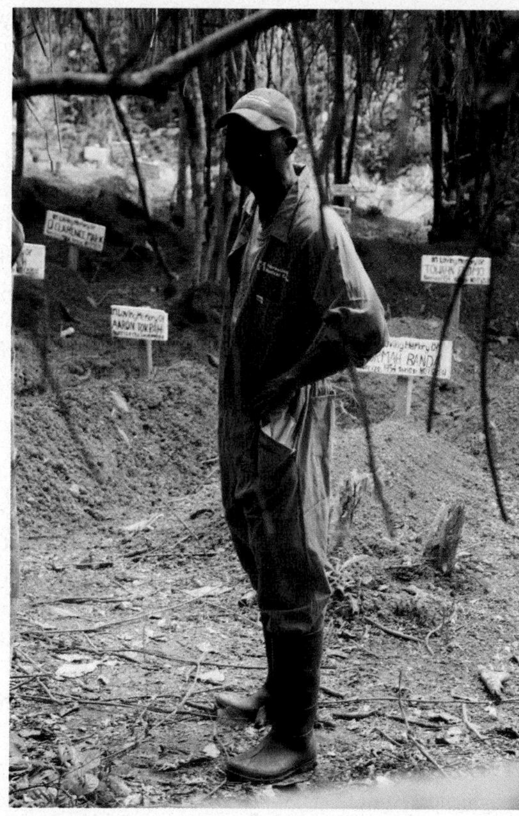

FIGURE 8-9 Burial worker standing near graves of recent Ebola victims in Suakoko, Liberia, in 2014. (*Reproduced with permission from Wikipedia Commons/Brien Vorhees. https://commons.wikimedia.org/wiki/File:Ebola_treatment_unit_visit_141122-A-QE750-081.jpg,*)

MIDDLE EAST RESPIRATORY SYNDROME (MERS) AND SEVERE ACUTE RESPIRATORY SYNDROME (SARS)

EPIDEMIOLOGY

MERS was first reported in September 2012 in Saudi Arabia. Subsequent cases, mostly in early 2014, were noted throughout the Middle East, specifically the United Arab Emirates (UAE), Qatar, Jordan, Oman, Kuwait, Yemen, Lebanon, and Iran. Currently, almost all cases originate from the Arabian Peninsula.[33]

The first reported cases of SARS were noted in November 2002, with the epidemic ending July 2003. SARS initially emerged from Guangdong, China, but rapidly spread throughout China and then worldwide to 29 countries, with more than 8000 cases and nearly 744 deaths. No new cases have been reported worldwide since 2004.[34]

ETIOLOGY/PATHOPHYSIOLOGY

Both viruses are RNA viruses and belong to the family Coronaviridae. Pathophysiology of both viruses is poorly understood, but both seem to have a predilection for the lower respiratory tract.[33] Concerning MERS transmission, the virus has been detected both in bats and dromedary camels (**Figure 8-10**), but there is uncertainty as to which acts as a reservoir for the virus. Human-to-human transmission is possible among close contacts and in the healthcare setting, but sustained community transmission has not been seen. Median incubation period is 5 days, but can range from 2 to 14 days.[33,35]

Concerning SARS, a precursor virus has been found in *Rhinolophus* bats, but the virus likely adapted and jumped to humans from civet cats and other small mammals sold in markets, which serve as reservoirs. Human-to-human transmission occurs primarily via the

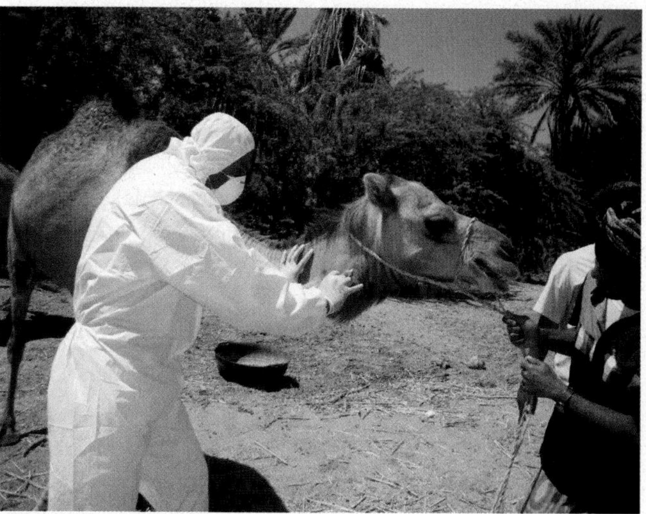

FIGURE 8-10 Veterinarian extracting blood sample from a camel's neck for evaluation during investigation into first reported MERS-CoV case in Haramout, Yemen. (*Reproduced with permission from Centers for Disease Control and Prevention (CDC)/Awadh Mohammed Ba Saleh.*)

respiratory route, but it can also be spread via the fecal-oral route.[34] Incubation period is 2 to 7 days.[36]

RISK FACTORS

Risk factors for MERS include travelers to the Arabian Peninsula, especially if they have close contact with sick individuals or exposure to healthcare settings. Per the World Health Organization (WHO), groups at high risk for severe MERS include patients with diabetes, kidney failure, chronic lung disease, or immunocompromised state.[33] As of 2017, the risk is minimal given the absence of cases since 2004. If recurrent outbreak does occur, travel to afflicted areas would confer high risk.

DIAGNOSIS

▶ Clinical features

Symptoms of MERS include a mild, nonspecific illness or even the patient being completely asymptomatic. This may quickly progress to severe acute respiratory failure with multi-organ dysfunction, and sometimes rapidly leads to fatality.[33] MERS progresses more quickly to respiratory failure than does SARS.[37]

SARS, like MERS, may be asymptomatic or a mild, nonspecific illness. Symptomatic patients present initially with fever, myalgias, sore throat, rhinorrhea and chills/rigors, but they then often rapidly progress to cough and dyspnea. Subsequently, rapid progression to acute respiratory failure may occur.[34,38] Extrapulmonary symptoms, such as diarrhea and headache, may also be present.[37]

▶ Laboratory testing

For MERS, real-time reverse transcriptase (RT)-PCR, performed on multiple lower respiratory tract specimens (includes expectorated sputum, bronchoalveolar lavage aspirate, endotracheal aspirate) is ideal. RT-PCR may also be performed on upper respiratory, stool, and serum specimens.[33]

For SARS, real-time RT-PCR should be performed on at least two samples from at least two sites, obtained as early in the disease process as possible. Paired acute-phase and convalescent-phase serologic samples should also be obtained for enzyme-linked immunosorbent assay (ELISA) testing, with the latter obtained at least 28 days after onset of illness. A "positive" serology is one where the convalescent-phase sample has either turned positive, or the titer has had at least a 4-fold increase. Most patients have detectable antibodies within 2 weeks of symptom onset.[39] Other laboratory findings may include a CBC that shows lymphopenia and/or thrombocytopenia and elevated liver function tests.[33]

DIFFERENTIAL DIAGNOSIS

- Pneumonia, bacterial or viral (see Chapter 55, "Pneumonia")
- Influenza
- Legionella
- Acute pulmonary edema, cardiogenic and non-cardiogenic (see Chapter 50, "Heart Failure")
- Viral upper respiratory tract infection (URI) with exacerbation of underlying chronic pulmonary disease

MANAGEMENT

Management includes supportive care, which may include critical care with mechanical ventilation. No specific antiviral therapy is currently recommended.[33] SOR Ⓒ Data from in vitro trials, animal studies, and case reports demonstrate possible efficacy of the use of convalescent plasma, interferon (IFN)-β/ribavirin combination therapy, and lopinavir for the treatment of MERS, but these therapies are investigational at this time.[40] Standard, contact, and airborne precautions are recommended.

PREVENTION

No vaccine is currently available for either MERS or SARS. Travelers to the Arabian Peninsula (MERS) or to a region with an outbreak of SARS should engage in frequent handwashing, avoid contact with sick individuals, and avoid touching the eyes, nose, and mouth. High-risk groups (per WHO, as discussed earlier) are advised to avoid the following: contact with camels, drinking raw camel milk or urine, or eating undercooked meat, particularly camel meat.[33]

PROGNOSIS

MERS has a high mortality rate, with ~40% of confirmed cases becoming fatal. Patients with comorbidities are at higher risk of mortality.[33] SARS has a lower case-fatality rate than does MERS.[37] In the 2002–2003 epidemic, there were 744 fatalities in 8096 cases.[34]

PATIENT RESOURCES

- Centers for Disease Control and Prevention. *Middle East Respiratory Syndrome (MERS).* **https://www.cdc.gov/coronavirus/mers/about/index.html.**
- Centers for Disease Control and Prevention. *Severe Acute Respiratory Syndrome (SARS).* **https://www.cdc.gov/sars/about/index.html.**

PROVIDER RESOURCES

- Centers for Disease Control and Prevention. *Middle East Respiratory Syndrome (MERS): Information for Healthcare Professionals.* **https://www.cdc.gov/coronavirus/mers/hcp.html.**
- CDC website for SARS for Healthcare Professionals. **https://www.cdc.gov/sars/who/clinicians.html.**

REFERENCES

1. Centers for Disease Control and Prevention. *Zika History.* https://www.cdc.gov/zika/about/overview.html. Accessed February 2017.
2. Duffy MR, Chen TH, et al. Zika virus outbreak on Yap Island, Federated States of Micronesia. *N Engl J Med.* 2009;360: 2536-2543.
3. Rasmussen SA, Jamieson DJ, et al. Zika virus and birth defects—reviewing the evidence for causality. *N Engl J Med.* 2016;374: 1981-1987.

4. Chen L, Hafeez F, Curry CL, Elgart G. Cutaneous eruption in a U.S. woman with locally acquired Zika virus infection. *N Engl J Med.* 2017;376:400-401.
5. Centers for Disease Control and Prevention. *All Countries & Territories with Active Zika Virus Transmission.* https://www.cdc.gov/zika/geo/active-countries.html. Accessed February 2017.
6. Centers for Disease Control and Prevention. *Transmission and Risks.* https://www.cdc.gov/zika/transmission/index.html. Accessed February 2017.
7. Reynolds MR, Jones AM, Petersen EE, et al. Vital Signs: Update on Zika virus–associated birth defects and evaluation of all U.S. infants with congenital Zika virus exposure—U.S. Zika Pregnancy Registry, 2016. *MMWR Morb Mortal Wkly Rep.* 2017;66:366-373.
8. Russell K, Oliver SE, Lewis L, et al. Update: interim guidance for the evaluation and management of infants with possible congenital Zika virus infection—United States, August 2016. *MMWR Morb Mortal Wkly Rep.* 2016; 65:870-878.
9. Centers for Disease Control and Prevention. *All Countries and Territories with Active Zika Virus Transmission.* https://www.cdc.gov/zika/geo/active-countries.html. Accessed March 2017.
10. White GB, Faust C: Medical acarology and entomology. In: Farrar J, Hotez PJ, Junghanss T, et al, eds. *Manson's Tropical Diseases.* 23rd ed. Philadelphia, PA: Elsevier Saunders, 2014:1263.
11. Peterson EE, Meany-Delman D, et al. Update: interim guidance for preconception counseling and prevention of sexual transmission of Zika virus for persons with possible Zika virus exposure—United States, September 2016. *MMWR Morb Mortal Wkly Rep.* 65:1077-1081
12. Centers for Disease Control and Prevention. *Clinical Evaluation & Disease.* https://www.cdc.gov/zika/hc-providers/preparing-for-zika/clinicalevaluationdisease.html. Accessed February 2017.
13. Oduyebo T, Igbinosa I, Petersen EE, et al. Update: interim guidance for health care providers caring for pregnant women with possible Zika virus exposure—United States, July 2016. *MMWR Morb Mortal Wkly Rep.* 2016; 65:739-744.
14. Centers for Disease Control and Prevention. Final Cumulative Maps and Data for 1999–2015, https://www.cdc.gov/westnile/statsmaps/cummapsdata.html. Accessed February 2017.
15. Lindsey NP, Lehman JA, Staples JE, Fischer M. West Nile virus and other nationally notifiable arboviral diseases—United States, 2014. *MMWR Morb Mortal Wkly Rep.* 2015;64(34):929-934.
16. Petersen LR, Brault AC, Nasci RS. West Nile virus: review of the literature. *JAMA.* 2013;310(3):308-315.
17. Young PR, Ng LF, Hall RA, et al. Arbovirus infections. In: Farrar J, Hotez PJ, Junghanss T, et al, eds. *Manson's Tropical Diseases,* 23rd ed. Philadelphia, PA: Elsevier Saunders; 2014:152-153.
18. World Health Organization. *Dengue Control/Epidemiology.* http://www.who.int/denguecontrol/epidemiology/en/. Accessed February 2017.
19. Centers for Disease Control and Prevention. *Dengue/Epidemiology.* https://www.cdc.gov/dengue/epidemiology/index.html. Accessed February 2017.
20. Simmons CP, Farrar JJ, Vinh Chau N, Wills B. Dengue. *N Engl J Med.* 2012; 366:1423-1432.
21. World Health Organization. *Dengue: Guidelines for Diagnosis, Treatment, Prevention, and Control, New Edition.* Geneva, Switzerland: World Health Organization; 2009.
22. Tomashek KM, Sharp TM, Margolis HS. Dengue. In: Brunette GW, ed. CDC *Health Information for International Travel 2016.* New York, NY: Oxford University Press; 2016:171-177.
23. Centers for Disease Control and Prevention. *Dengue Case Management.* https://www.cdc.gov/dengue/resources/dengue-clinician-guide_508.pdf. Accessed February 2017.
24. Sanofi Pasteur. Dengue Vaccine Registered in 14 Countries. http://dengue.info/. Accessed February 2017.
25. Weaver SC, Lecuit M. Chikungunya virus and the global spread of a mosquito-borne disease. *N Engl J Med.* 2015; 372: 1231-1239
26. Staples JE, Hills SL, Powers AM. Chikungunya. In: Brunette GW, ed. CDC *Health Information for International Travel 2016.* New York, NY: Oxford University Press; 2016:161-163.
27. Huntington MK, Allison J, Nair D. Emerging vector-borne diseases. *Am Fam Physician.* 2016; 94:551-557.
28. World Health Organization. *Ebola Virus Disease.* http://www.who.int/mediacentre/factsheets/fs103/en/. Accessed February 2017.
29. Christie A, Davies-Wayne G, Cordier-Lasalle T, et al. Possible sexual transmission of Ebola virus—Liberia, 2015. *MMWR.* 64(17);479-481.
30. World Health Organization. *First Antigen Rapid Test for Ebola through Emergency Assessment and Eligible for Procurement.* http://www.who.int/medicines/ebola-treatment/1st_antigen_RT_Ebola/en/. Accessed March 2017.
31. Uyeki TM, Mehta AK, Davey RT, et al. Clinical management of Ebola virus disease in the United States and Europe. *N Engl J Med.* 2016; 374:636-646
32. World Health Organization. Final Trial Results Confirm Ebola Vaccine Provides High Protection against Disease. http://www.who.int/mediacentre/news/releases/2016/ebola-vaccine-results/en/. Accessed March 2017.
33. Watson JT, Gerber SI. Middle East Respiratory Syndrome (MERS). In: Brunette GW, ed. CDC *Health Information for International Travel 2016.* New York, NY: Oxford University Press; 2016:161-163.
34. McNamara PS, Rogier Van Doorn H. Respiratory viruses and atypical bacteria. In: Farrar J, Hotez PJ, Junghanss T, et al, eds. *Manson's Tropical Diseases.* 23rd ed. Philadelphia, PA: Elsevier Saunders; 2014:218.
35. Hui DS. Epidemic and emerging coronaviruses (severe acute respiratory syndrome and Middle East respiratory syndrome). *Clin Chest Med.* 2017;38(1):71-86.
36. Donnelly CA, Ghani AC, Leung GM, et al. Epidemiological determinants of spread of causal agent of severe acute respiratory syndrome in Hong Kong. *Lancet.* 2003;361(9371):1761.

37. Hui DS, Memish ZA, Zumla A. Severe acute respiratory syndrome vs. the Middle East Respiratory Syndrome. *Curr Opin Pulm Med.* 2014;20(3):233-241.
38. Centers for Disease Control and Prevention. *Severe Acute Respiratory Syndrome (SARS), Clinical Guidance on the Identification and Evaluation of Possible SARS-CoV Disease among Persons Presenting with Community-Acquired Illness (version 2).* https://www.cdc.gov/sars/clinical/guidance.html. Accessed March 2017.
39. Centers for Disease Control and Prevention. *Severe Acute Respiratory Syndrome (SARS), III. Diagnostic Assays, Supplement F: Laboratory Guidance.* https://www.cdc.gov/sars/guidance/f-lab/assays.html. Accessed March 2017.
40. Mo Y, Fisher D. A review of treatment modalities for Middle East Respiratory Syndrome. *J Antimicrob Chemother.* 2016;71(12):3340-3350.

PART III

PHYSICAL AND SEXUAL ABUSE AND LGBT HEALTH ISSUES

Strength of Recommendation (SOR)	Definition
A	Recommendation based on consistent and good-quality patient-oriented evidence.*
B	Recommendation based on inconsistent or limited-quality patient-oriented evidence.*
C	Recommendation based on consensus, usual practice, opinion, disease-oriented evidence, or case series for studies of diagnosis, treatment, prevention, or screening.*

*See Appendix A on pages 1603–1606 for further information.

9 CHILD PHYSICAL ABUSE

Tanya Burrell, MD
Jim Anderst, MD, MSCI

PATIENT STORIES

CASE 1

A 1-month-old child was seen in the emergency room for bruising. Physical examination revealed bruises to the buttocks, chest, and eye. The parents reported that the child received the buttock bruise (**Figure 9-1**) after being dropped by the father, that the chest bruise was from the child's seat belt, and the eye bruise was from accidentally hitting the child with an elbow while cosleeping. The social worker was consulted in the emergency room, and found no concerning "red flags" in the family. The emergency room physician felt the findings were because of inexperienced parents. The child was sent home with the parents, and the emergency room later reported the case to Child Protective Services (CPS) in hopes of providing the family with support services. A child abuse pediatrician (CAP) was consulted by CPS to review the case the next day. The CAP requested that the child be brought back to the hospital emergently for further evaluation. A skeletal survey, including oblique views of the ribs, at that time showed a healing fracture of the eighth posterior rib (**Figure 9-2**). A head CT and liver function tests were performed to screen for occult trauma, and laboratory tests were done to evaluate for a bleeding diathesis. All results were negative. Law enforcement was contacted and coinvestigated with CPS. The child was placed in the home of a relative. Two weeks later, a repeat skeletal survey showed new bone formation over the right femur, indicating a healing fracture.

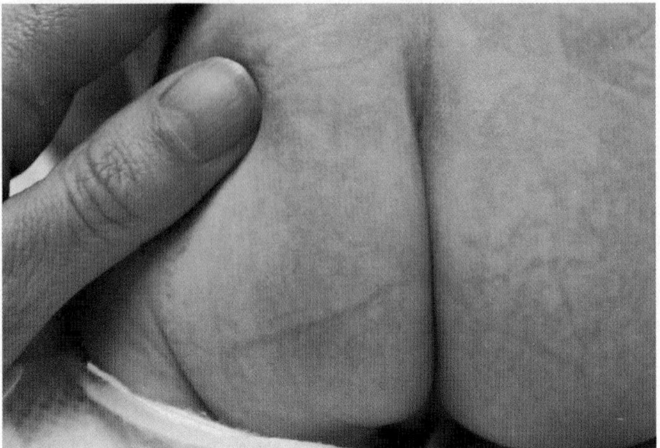

FIGURE 9-1 Bruising to the left buttock noted in a 1-month-old child. Any bruising on an immobile child is highly concerning for child physical abuse. Bleeding disorders must be considered in the differential diagnosis. (*Reproduced with permission from James Anderst, MD, MS.*)

CASE 2

A 15-month-old child is brought to the emergency department by the police after a relative called 911. The child and his mother attended a family gathering where concerned relatives viewed the mother's story that the child "falls a lot" with suspicion. On examination there were many signs of physical abuse (**Figures 9-3** to **9-5**). His face was covered with bruises, especially around the right eye and cheek (see **Figure 9-3**). His axilla showed signs of being gouged with fingernails (see **Figure 9-4**). In the emergency department, the child was evaluated by a forensic nurse examiner trained in child-abuse photo documentation. The child was admitted to the hospital and the police, hospital social workers, and CPS were notified. Although an initial skeletal survey did not show any fractures, a repeat skeletal survey and oblique views of the ribs were done 2 weeks later showing eight healing rib fractures. Repeat skeletal surveys are recommended in children younger than 4 years of age who are confirmed or suspected victims of abuse (see **Figure 9-5**). The child was then referred to a CAP, who assessed mechanisms of injuries, reexamined the child, and interpreted the initial and follow-up skeletal surveys.

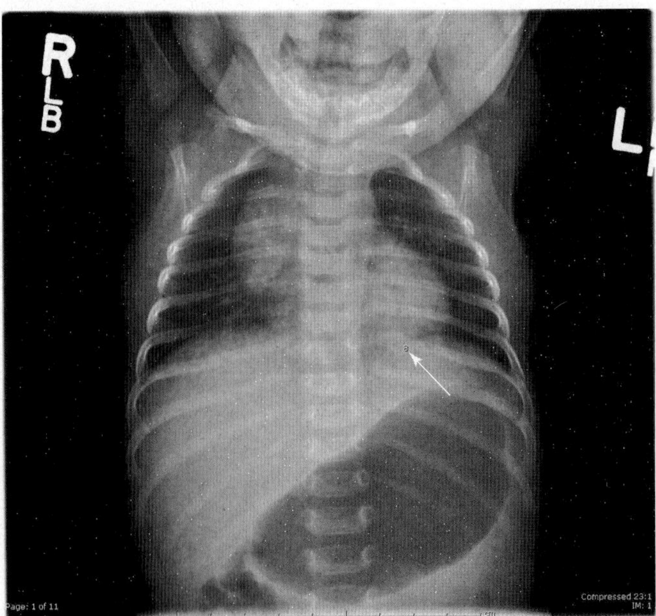

FIGURE 9-2 Healing eighth posterior rib fracture in the same child from Figure 9-1. A skeletal survey is indicated in any child younger than 2 years of age where suspicions of physical abuse exist. (*Reproduced with permission from James Anderst, MD, MS.*)

INTRODUCTION

The appropriate identification of child physical abuse is critical. Misdiagnoses in either direction (missed abuse or inappropriate diagnosis of abuse) are extremely harmful to the child and family. A careful evaluation of each case, coupled with an application of the existing scientific data on child physical abuse, may result in improved outcomes for the child and family.

EPIDEMIOLOGY

- Child maltreatment occurs in 9.4 per 1000 children, with highest rate of victimization in the birth to 1 year age group (24.4 per 1000).
- The Department of Health and Human Services compilation of State CPS Child Maltreatment 2014 had 3.6 million CPS referrals filed in 2014, with 702,000 confirmed child victims.[1] Of these:
  - Seventy-five percent were neglected.
  - Seventeen percent were physically abused.
  - Eight percent were sexually abused.
  - Six percent were psychologically abused.
- The majority (78.1%) of perpetrators were a parent of the victim.
- Medical personnel made only 9.2% of the referrals to CPS.

RISK FACTORS

Caregiver factors associated with child abuse include the following:[2]

- Inappropriate parental expectations of the child.
- Low self-esteem
- Poor impulse control
- Substance abuse
- Young maternal or paternal age
- Depression or other mental illness
- Caregiver abused as a child.

Factors specific to the child that are associated with abuse:[2]

- Prematurity
- Disabilities
- Chronic illness
- Unplanned pregnancy
- Unwanted child
- Emotional/behavioral difficulties of the child.

Environmental factors associated with abuse:

- Family or intimate partner violence
- Poverty
- Social isolation
- Nonbiologically related male in the home
- Unemployment
- Single parent.

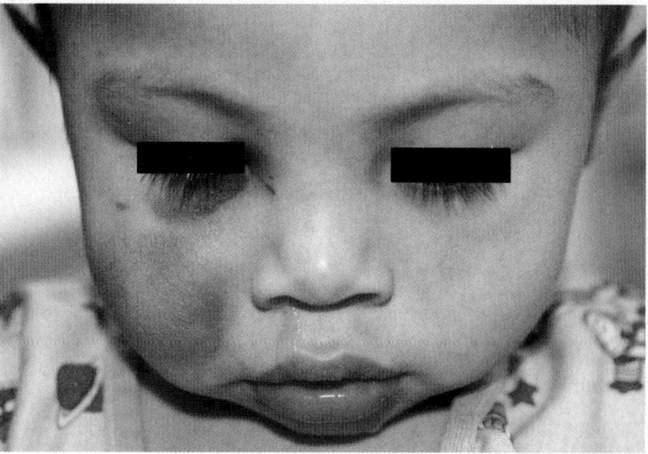

FIGURE 9-3 A 15-month-old boy who has been physically abused by his mother's boyfriend for several weeks. There is bruising under both eyes, with the greatest degree of bruising seen under the right eye and on the right cheek. The boy is in the emergency department after concerned relatives called the police. (*Reproduced with permission from James Anderst, MD, MS.*)

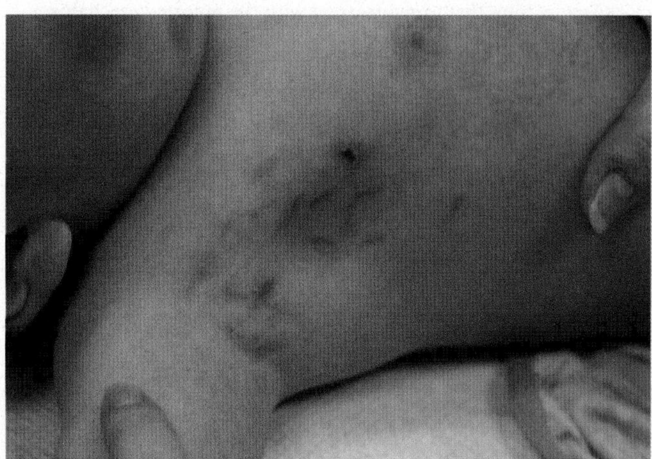

FIGURE 9-4 Same 15-month-old boy from **Figure 9-3** with multiple fingernail gouges in his right axilla. Some are fresh and one appears to be older and somewhat crusted. Injuries in different stages of healing may indicate chronicity of abuse. (*Reproduced with permission from James Anderst, MD, MS.*)

DIAGNOSIS

CONCERNING HISTORY[2]

- History inconsistent with child's developmental stage
- Injuries inconsistent with history given
- History changes over time
- History differs among witnesses
- Delay in seeking medical care (must consider family's access to care and availability of transportation)
- Sibling blamed
- Magical injury—no one knows how it happened.

CLINICAL FEATURES

- Bruising:[3,4]
  - In children who are not independently mobile
  - In mobile children:
    - Seen away from bony prominences
    - Facial bruising to the cheeks or mouth
    - To the ears, buttocks, neck abdomen, and back of the legs
  - In the shape of an imprint of an object or hand, or a ligature (object used to tie or bind tightly)
  - Multiple bruises in clusters
- Burns:[5]
  - Inconsistent with history (**Figure 9-6**)
  - Stocking/glove distribution
  - Well-demarcated edges
  - Symmetrical burns
- Fractures:[6,7]
  - Rib fractures
  - Fractures in immobile children that are not attributable to birth injury
  - Multiple fractures and/or multiple fractures of different ages
  - Fractures in the absence of a history of trauma
  - Any fracture that is inconsistent with the reported mechanism.
- Intracranial injury:
  - Highly variable clinical presentation; however, presence of apnea, retinal hemorrhages, and/or rib fractures is more strongly associated with inflicted (versus noninflicted) intracranial injury[8,9]
  - Mild abusive head injury may present with isolated vomiting or fussiness[10]
- Oral lesions—Torn frenula (**Figure 9-7**), palatal petechiae, contusions, or lacerations (typically from a bottle, finger, or other object forced into the child's mouth)[10,11]
- Failure to thrive and signs of malnutrition as a result of intentional withholding of food and/or liquids.

LABORATORY STUDIES AND IMAGING

- Concerning bruising that is not obviously abusive—Prothrombin time/partial thromboplastin time (PT/PTT), complete blood count (CBC), von Willebrand testing, factor 8 and factor 9 levels.[12] Testing best done in collaboration with a CAP or pediatric hematologist.

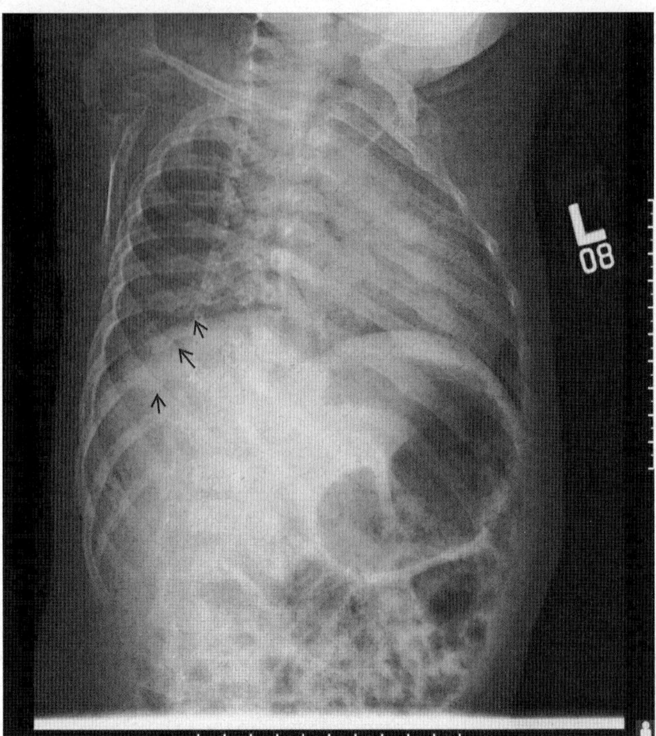

FIGURE 9-5 Same boy from **Figure 9-3** with oblique X-ray showing healing rib fractures with callus in eight different locations as marked by the *arrows*. The degree of callus formation shows that these rib fractures are not new. Oblique radiographs should be requested in addition to a "skeletal survey" because lateral rib fractures are best seen with this view. (*Reproduced with permission from James Anderst, MD, MS.*)

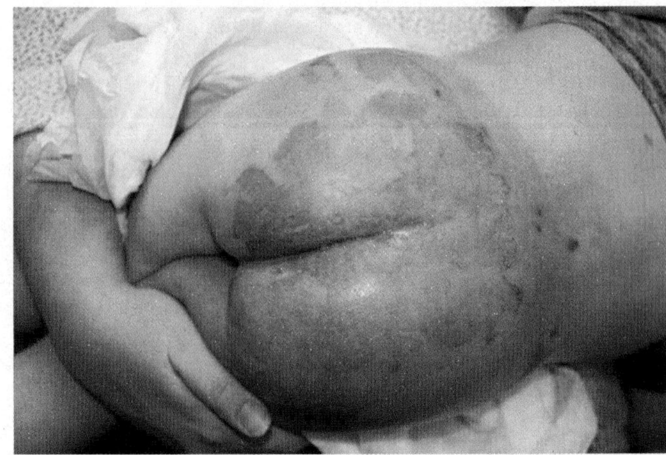

FIGURE 9-6 Toddler with second degree burns to the buttocks. The caregiver reported that the child fell into a bathtub of hot water, sustaining the burns. Scene investigation showed that there was no bathtub in the home where the burn occurred. The caregiver eventually admitted to dipping the child into a sink full of extremely hot water. (*Reproduced with permission from James Anderst, MD, MS.*)

- Detection of occult abdominal trauma—Liver function tests (LFTs), amylase, lipase, urinalysis; CT of abdomen recommended if laboratory results are elevated or urinalysis positive for blood.[13]
- Detection of occult fractures—Skeletal survey (including oblique views of the ribs) in children younger than 2 years of age or nonverbal children; consider radionuclide bone scan to look for acute fractures, or a follow-up skeletal survey 2 weeks after initial presentation.[14]
- Detection of occult intracranial injury—CT/MR of head in all young children, even if there are no clinical signs of intracranial injury; ophthalmology examination for retinal hemorrhages if intracranial hemorrhage is present.[15,16]

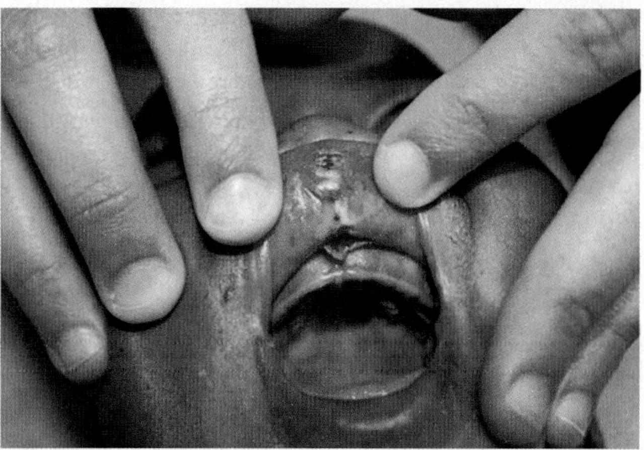

FIGURE 9-7 Torn frenulum in an immobile infant resulting from a caregiver violently jamming a bottle into the infant's mouth. The child presented with a chief complaint of excessive crying. A thorough physical exam identified the torn frenulum. (*Reproduced with permission from James Anderst, MD, MS.*)

DIFFERENTIAL DIAGNOSIS

- Bruises and other skin findings:
  - Accidental bruises—Any bruising in an infant or precruiser is very concerning for abuse.[3,4] Accidental bruising is much more common in cruising or walking children. Any inflicted bruising or skin markings (including those from spanking or other punishment) lasting more than 24 hours constitutes abuse.[17] Ear bruising is very specific for abuse (**Figure 9-8**).[3,4,18] It is not possible to accurately date bruises.[19] Accidental bruising is typically located on the shins, lower arms, under chin, forehead, hips, elbows, and bony prominences. Looplike bruising is suspicious for blows with a cord or a looped belt (**Figure 9-9**)
  - Bruising with tracking of blood (subgaleal hematoma) can be seen with severe injuries to the head from violent hair pulling (**Figure 9-10**)
  - Bleeding disorders—Familial history, abnormal coagulation laboratory test results, vitamin K deficiency
  - Other rare diseases associated with bruising—Ehlers-Danlos, Henoch-Schönlein purpura, phytophotodermatitis (skin reaction to psoralens, most commonly found in limes), osteogenesis imperfecta (brittle bones)
  - Skin discoloration—Common examples are allergic shiners (dark, puffy lower eyelids) and Mongolian spots (macular blue-gray pigmentation usually on the sacral area of normal infants, usually present at birth or appear within the first weeks of life) (see Chapter 114, Normal Skin Changes)
- Burns:
  - Accidental burns (splash marks more often seen)
  - Bullous impetigo, cellulitis, scalded skin syndrome, diaper rash
  - Chemical burn caused by senna-containing laxatives
  - Drug reaction
- Fractures from other diseases occurring in infants and young children:
  - Osteogenesis imperfecta—A congenital disorder with bone fragility; patients may have repeated fractures after mild trauma that heal readily. Other features seen in some cases include blue sclera, easy bruising, and deafness
  - Rickets—Usually from vitamin D deficiency; consider in exclusively breastfed infants, dark-skinned children, children with little sun exposure. The metaphyses show widening and cupping with irregular calcification as a result of poor calcification of osteoid

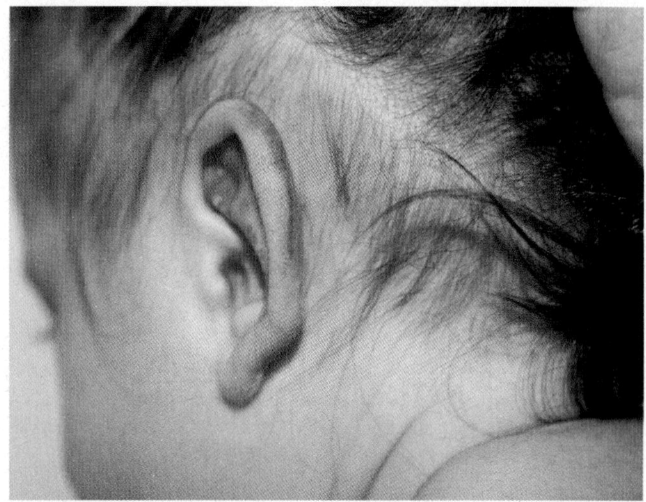

FIGURE 9-8 Bruising of the ear in a young boy from a violent slap to the head by a caregiver. Ear bruising is rarely accidental. (*Reproduced with permission from James Anderst, MD, MS.*)

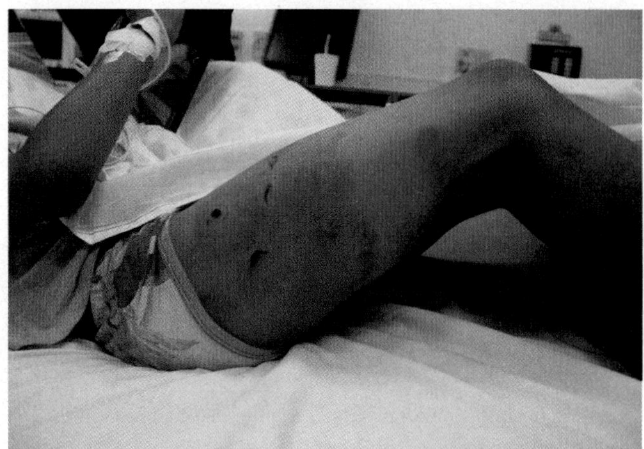

FIGURE 9-9 Patterned loop marks to a young girl. Loop-shaped bruises are often caused by electrical cords (or other similar objects). Blows with flexible objects produce patterns that tend to conform to the curved surfaces of the body, whereas inflexible objects may produce a discontinuous pattern over curved surfaces. (*Reproduced with permission from James Anderst, MD, MS.*)

- Failure to thrive from other causes including improper mixing of formula, breastfeeding difficulty, organic diseases such as cystic fibrosis, HIV, metabolic disorders, celiac disease, and renal disease[20]
- Intracranial bleeding—Other causes include accidental injury, infection, coagulation disorders, birth injury, and rare metabolic conditions (glutaric aciduria)
- Cultural practices—Coining (**Figure 9-11**), cupping, moxibustion (cultural practice of burning herbs on skin).

MANAGEMENT

- Emergent care first; treat injuries, burns, failure to thrive accordingly
- Careful examination of the skin and oral cavity, palpation for bony tenderness or callus formation, signs of abdominal trauma or neurologic abnormalities
- Document the history provided by caregivers and physical findings accurately, including pictures
- Consider consultation with a CAP or a family physician with additional training or expertise. Child abuse pediatrics is a subspecialty of pediatrics requiring an additional 3 years of fellowship training required for eligibility for board certification
- In cases where the injury was truly caused by an accidental mechanism, the role of neglect must be considered
- Mandated reporting:
    - All 50 states require that all professionals who work with children report suspected child abuse and neglect
    - Reporter of abuse is granted legal immunity
    - Once the case is reported, further collaboration with CPS or law enforcement is usually necessary to ensure appropriate outcomes.[21]

PATIENT EDUCATION

- Prevention programs:[22]
    - Home visitation programs have been shown to reduce child abuse and child mortality
    - Nursery-based prevention of abusive head trauma
    - Specific models of primary care may reduce abuse
    - Population-based prevention
    - Parent–child interactive therapy (PCIT) reduces repeat abuse.[23,24]

FOLLOW-UP

- If there is suspicion of fractures, obtain repeat skeletal X-ray in 2 weeks to look for evidence of healing fractures
- Siblings of abused children should be interviewed and examined for findings concerning for abuse
- Counseling for child and family as appropriate
- Frequent follow-up with primary care provider to evaluate for signs of abuse and neglect
- Report to CPS.

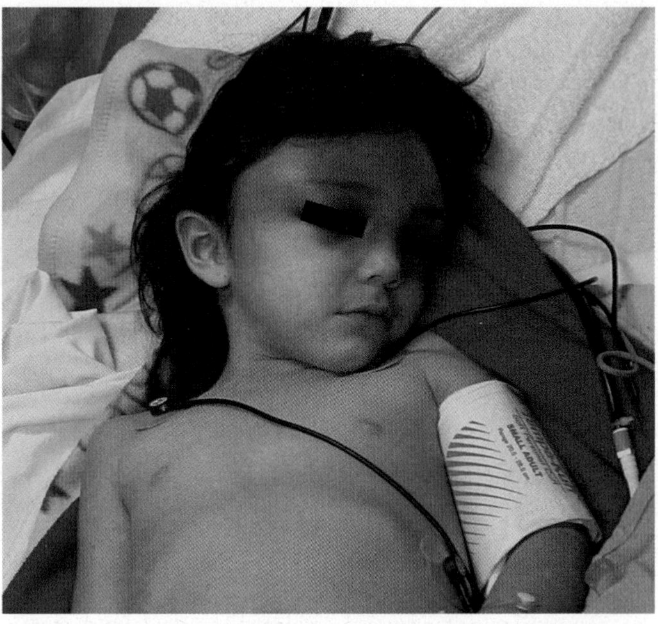

FIGURE 9-10 Young girl with severe subgaleal hematoma with extensive blood tracking into the upper face after being lifted off the ground by her hair. Blood tracking after significant injury is most commonly seen on the face, although some injuries to the genitals may also track into the perineum. (*Reproduced with permission from James Anderst, MD, MS.*)

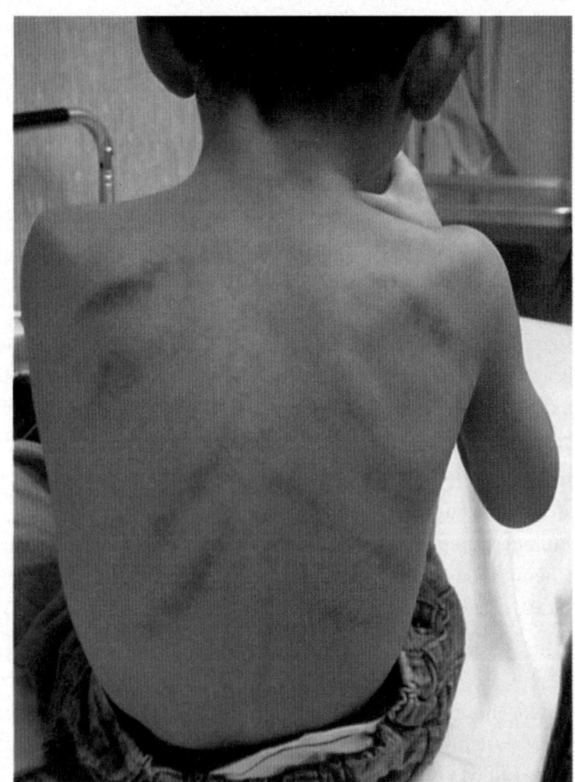

FIGURE 9-11 Young boy with the marks of coining on his back. A coin was rubbed across his back, leaving ecchymoses over bony prominences, with the intent to help the child heal from an acute illness. This cultural practice is more common among Asian immigrants to this country and mimics child abuse. (*Reproduced with permission from Maria McColgan, MD.*)

PATIENT RESOURCES

- Child Help—**http://childhelp.org.**
- Prevent Child Abuse America—**http://www.preventchildabuse.org.**

PROVIDER RESOURCES

- Child Protector phone app to aid in the medical/forensic evaluation of physical abuse—**http://www.childrensmercy.org/childprotector/.**
- American Academy of Pediatrics Clinical Report. *The Evaluation of Suspected Child Physical Abuse*—**http://pediatrics.aappublications.org/content/early/2015/04/21/peds.2015-0356.**
- The American Professional Society on the Abuse of Children—**www.apsac.org.**
- Child Abuse Evaluation & Treatment for Medical Providers—**http://www.childabusemd.com/index.shtml.**

REFERENCES

1. U.S. Department of Health & Human Services, Administration for Children and Families, Administration on Children, Youth and Families, Children's Bureau. (2016). *Child maltreatment 2014.* http://www.acf.hhs.gov/programs/cb/research-data-technology/statistics-research/child-maltreatment. Accessed December 2016.
2. Christian CW; American Academy of Pediatrics, Committee on Child Abuse and Neglect. The evaluation of suspected child physical abuse. *Pediatrics.* 2015;135(5):e1337-e1354.
3. Maguire S, Mann MK, Sibert J, Kemp A. Are there patterns of bruising in childhood which are diagnostic or suggestive of abuse? A systematic review. *Arch Dis Child.* 2005;90:182-186.
4. Kemp AM, Dunstan F, Nuttall D, et al. Patterns of bruising in preschool children—a longitudinal study. *Arch Dis Child.* 2015;100(5):426-431.
5. Maguire S, Moynihan S, Mann M, et al. A systematic review of the features that indicate intentional scalds in children. *Burns.* 2008;34(8):1072-1081.
6. Maguire S. Which injuries may indicate child abuse? *Arch Dis Child Educ Pract Ed.* 2010;95:170-177.
7. Flaherty EG, Perez-Rossello JM, Levine MA, et al. Evaluating children with fractures for child physical abuse. *Pediatrics.* 2014;133(2):e477-e489.
8. Maguire S, Pickerd N, Farewell D, et al. Which clinical features distinguish inflicted from non-inflicted brain injury? A systematic review. *Arch Dis Child.* 2009;94:860-867.
9. Maguire S, Kemp AM, Lumb R, Farewell D. Estimating the probability of abusive head trauma: a pooled analysis. *Pediatrics.* 2011;128(3):e550-e564.
10. Sheets LK, Leach ME, Koszewski IJ, et al. Sentinel injuries in infants evaluated for child physical abuse. *Pediatrics.* 2013;131:701-707.
11. Jenny C, Hymel KP, Ritzen A, et al. Analysis of missed cases of abusive head trauma. *JAMA.* 1999;282(7):621-626.
12. Anderst J, Carpenter S, Abshire T, and the Section on Hematology/Oncology and Committee on Child Abuse and Neglect. Evaluation for bleeding disorders in suspected child abuse. *Pediatrics.* 2013;131(4):e1314-e1322.
13. Lindberg D, Makoroff K, Harper N, et al. Utility of hepatic transaminases to recognize abuse in children. *Pediatrics.* 2009;124(2):509-516.
14. American Academy of Pediatrics Section on Radiology. Diagnostic imaging of child abuse. *Pediatrics.* 2009;123(5):1430-1435.
15. Rubin DM, Christian CW, Bilaniuk L, et al. Occult head injury in high risk abused children. *Pediatrics.* 2003;111(6):1382-1386.
16. Greiner MV, Berger RP, Thackeray JD, Lindberg DM. Dedicated retinal examination in children evaluated for physical abuse without radiographically identified traumatic brain injury. *J Pediatr.* 2013;163(2):527-531.
17. American Academy of Pediatrics, Committee on Child Abuse and Neglect. When inflicted skin injuries constitute child abuse. *Pediatrics.* 2002;110(3):644-645.
18. Pierce MC, Kaczor K, Aldrige A, et al. Bruising characteristics discriminating physical child abuse from accidental trauma. *Pediatrics.* 2010;125(1):67-74.
19. Maguire S, Mann MK, Sibert J, Kemp A. Can you age bruises accurately in children? A systematic review. *Arch Dis Child.* 2005;90:187-189.
20. Block RW, Krebs NF. Failure to thrive as a manifestation of child neglect. *Pediatrics.* 2005;116(5):1234-1237.
21. Anderst J, Kellogg N, Jung I. Is the diagnosis of physical abuse changed when Child Protective Services consults a Child Abuse Pediatrics subspecialty group as a second opinion? *Child Abuse Negl.* 2009;33(8):481-489.
22. Flaherty EG, Stirling J, Committee on Child Abuse and Neglect. The pediatrician's role in child maltreatment prevention. *Pediatrics.* 2010; 126(4):833-841.
23. Timmer SG, Urquiza AJ, Zebell NM, McGrath JM. Parent-child interaction therapy: application to maltreating parent-child dyads. *Child Abuse Negl.* 2005;29(7):825-842.
24. Hakman M, Chaffin M, Funderburk B, Silovosky J. Change trajectories for parent-child interaction sequences during parent-child interaction therapy for child physical abuse. *Child Abuse Neglect.* 2009;33:461-470.

10 CHILD SEXUAL ABUSE

Nancy D. Kellogg, MD
Maria D. McColgan, MD, MEd

PATIENT STORY

A 12-year-old girl is being seen for chronic abdominal pain by her family physician. The physician asks the mother to step out of the room and does a complete history including the HEADSS (home life, education level, activities, drug use, sexual activity, suicide ideation/attempts) questions. The girl tearfully reports that her stepfather has been touching her in her private areas when her mother is not home. On examination with a female nurse chaperone in the room, the physician finds that the girl's hymen initially appears normal (**Figure 10-1**). However, when the girl is more carefully examined with a cotton-tip applicator, a healed posterior hymenal transection is seen (**Figure 10-2**). When the girl is asked whether any other types of sexual abuse occurred with her stepfather, she admits to repeated penile penetration. Although rare, sometimes the examination reveals more than what the child is willing to disclose about the abuse. Partial disclosures of abuse are common in children. In addition, the findings of sexual abuse tend to be subtle and are easily missed if a careful examination and special techniques are not used. Attempts are made to reassure the girl that this should never happen and that this is not her fault. Her mother is brought back into the room, and after a sensitive discussion, the police are called and Child Protective Services (CPS) notified.

HEADSS is an acronym that provides a framework for interviewing adolescents and children about health risks. The questions start from easiest and least sensitive to more sensitive questions that need to be asked:

H—home

E—education

A—activities

D—depression and drugs

S—sex and sexual abuse

S—suicide

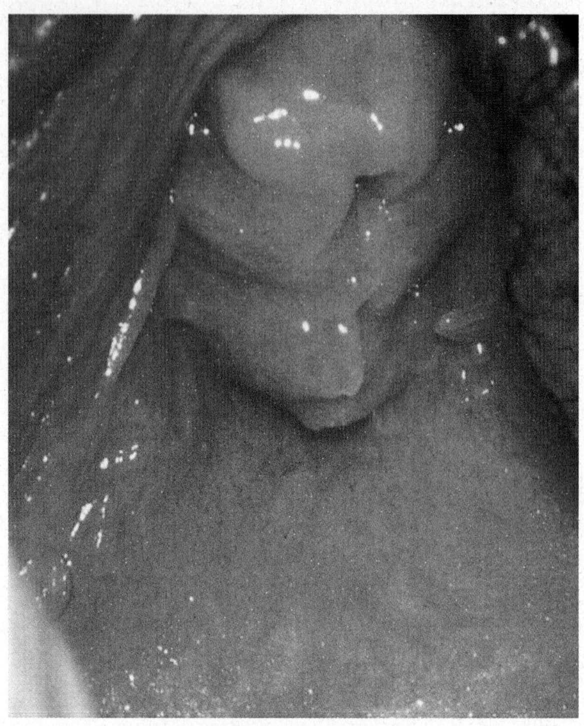

FIGURE 10-1 Typical appearance of the hymen and perihymenal tissues in a 12-year-old girl. Once females have entered puberty, the hymen becomes redundant with overlapping folds and is more difficult to examine for subtle signs of acute or healed injury. (*Reproduced with permission from Nancy D. Kellogg, MD.*)

EPIDEMIOLOGY

- The U.S. Department of Health and Human Services compilation of CPS data in FY 2014 indicates there were 702,000 children confirmed as victims of abuse.[1] Of these, 8.3% were victims of sexual abuse. Not included in these numbers are several thousand additional victims who are sexually assaulted by nonfamily members; these cases are reported to law enforcement but not CPS.
- By age 17, 26.6% of girls and 5.1% of boys will experience sexual abuse and/or assault.[2]
- Up to 50% of abusive sexual acts involve penetration of the vagina, anus, or oral cavity, or oral–genital contact.[3] In general, penetrative types of abuse are associated with poorer medical and mental health outcomes.

ETIOLOGY AND PATHOPHYSIOLOGY

Child sexual abuse occurs when a child is involved in sexual activities that he or she cannot comprehend, for which the child is developmentally unprepared and cannot or does not give consent, and/or that violate laws. All states have laws that require physicians to report a suspicion of abuse to child protection or law enforcement agencies.

Most sexual abuse involves an adult perpetrator the child knows and is expected to trust who uses deception and position of authority to gain the child's acquiescence and accommodation to the abuse;[4] it is not unusual for the abuse to progress from less to more severe and intrusive sexual acts, and for the child to wait months or years to disclose the abuse.

DIAGNOSIS

CLINICAL FEATURES

- Child victims of sexual abuse may have behavior changes, depression, increased sexual behaviors, somatic complaints (e.g., headaches or abdominal pain, constipation, enuresis/encopresis, genital/anal pain), or may be asymptomatic.
- Child may present to a medical provider for the following reasons:
  - Child has disclosed abuse (most common); it is rare for the abuse to be witnessed. Referrals to specialized programs with clinicians trained in the assessment of child sexual abuse is recommended, and these programs are generally accessible in most areas of the United States.
  - Caregiver suspects abuse and presents to the clinician because of behavioral or physical symptoms.
  - Child is brought for routine care and sexual abuse is suspected based on clinical findings (e.g., acute or healed genital injuries, vaginal discharge in a prepubertal child, lesions suggestive of human papillomavirus [HPV] or herpes simplex virus [HSV]).
- Recent studies show that fewer than 5% of child sexual abuse victims have physical examination findings indicative of penetrative trauma because the type of sexual act either does not result in tissue damage or because when tissue damage occurs, most injuries heal quickly and completely.[5–7] In a study of 36 pregnant adolescents, only two had evidence of penetrative trauma.[8] The medical diagnosis relies predominantly on the child's history, and clinicians should remember that "normal" does not mean "nothing happened."
- Tips for doing the physical examination:
  - The anogenital inspection should utilize an optimal direct light source, magnification, and appropriate examination positions and techniques.
  - Recommended examination positions include supine frogleg or lithotomy, supine knee-chest and prone knee-chest. Prepubertal children can be placed in supine knee-chest position for inspection of perianal tissues. Prone knee-chest position is particularly important to confirm any posterior (between the 4 and 8 o'clock positions of the hymen in supine) defects of the hymen that are seen in supine position.
  - Various examination techniques include labial separation and traction (gently pulling the labia outward and inferiorly), gluteal lifting in prone knee-chest, and using a cotton-tipped applicator for separating tissues.

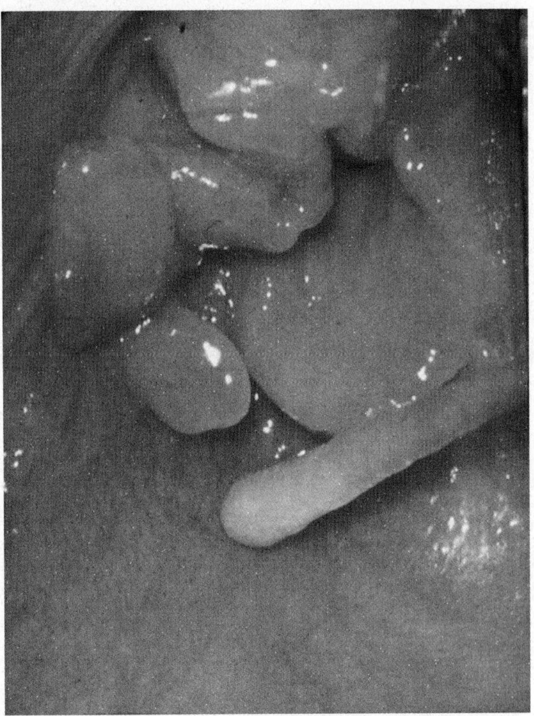

FIGURE 10-2 Hymenal cleft visible when the girl in **Figure 10-1** is more carefully examined using a saline moistened cotton-tip applicator to gently separate and demonstrate the edges of the hymen. This injury was caused by sexual abuse and may have been missed without the more careful examination. (*Reproduced with permission from Nancy D. Kellogg, MD.*)

- In some cases, it may help to have an assistant gently squirt a small amount of nonbacteriostatic saline onto the hymen as the examiner uses gentle labial traction; this procedure is used to free folded hymenal edges.
  - A speculum examination and use of a cotton-tipped applicator to separate hymenal edges are traumatic procedures for prepubertal females and should not be used.
  - Most findings of anal trauma can be visualized by gently spreading the anal folds.
- Physical findings concerning for abuse include:[9]
  - Abrasions, lacerations, or bruising of the hymen, perihymenal structures, vagina, or perianal tissues[10] (**Figures 10-3, 10-4, and 10-5**).
  - Healed hymenal transection between 4 and 8 o'clock that extends to the base of the hymen[9] (see **Figure 10-2**).

LABORATORY TESTS AND IMAGING

- Forensic evidence collection if sexual assault occurred less than 72 to 96 hours (protocols vary from region to region) prior to clinical presentation (consider referring to an emergency department or rape crisis center skilled in performing forensic evidence collection on children).
- Approximately 5% of sexually abused children and adolescents acquire a sexually transmitted infection (STI) from the abuse[9] (**Figure 10-6**).
- Consider STI testing in all postpubescent patients and in prepubescent children with a history of genital contact with any orifice.
- Chlamydia and gonorrhea nucleic acid amplification tests (NAATs) can be used in prepubertal (urine) and postpubertal (urine, vaginal, anal) patients; culture or NAAT is recommended for *Trichomonas* testing.[10]
- HIV, hepatitis B (if unimmunized), rapid plasma reagin (RPR) (for syphilis; positive RPR results should be confirmed with treponemal-specific test).
- Culture (or PCR) for HSV1 and HSV2 if ulcers or vesicles are present (see **Figure 10-6**).
- Condylomata acuminata is a clinical diagnosis, and biopsy is required only if lesions are atypical or resistant to treatment (molluscum contagiosum is a mimic and not sexually transmitted in children). HPV vaccination of patients 9 years and older should be initiated, or provided if incomplete.[10]
- Pregnancy testing in postpubescent children; consider prophylaxis (e.g., Plan B) if the event occurred less than 96 hours prior to evaluation.
- Consider follow-up examinations 2 to 3 weeks after an acute assault to complete testing for STIs with prolonged incubation periods, assess resolution of injuries, and ensure emotional recovery.

DIFFERENTIAL DIAGNOSIS

In females, the following may be confused with abuse:

- Straddle injury (or other accidental trauma)—This occurs when a child falls onto an object. Bruising or lacerations to the labia majora, labia minora, or posterior fourchette may be seen.

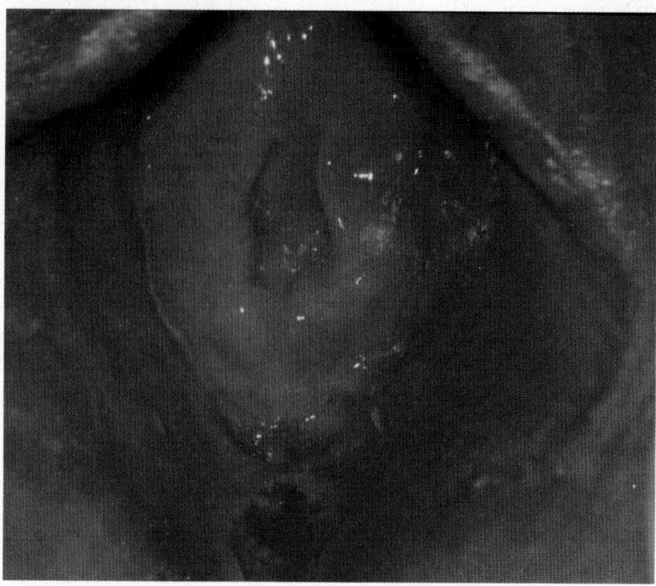

FIGURE 10-3 A 10-year-old girl with an acute tear of the posterior vestibule after recent sexual assault by a stranger. The posterior vestibule is the most common location for acute penetrative trauma in females. (*Used with permission from Nancy D. Kellogg, MD.*)

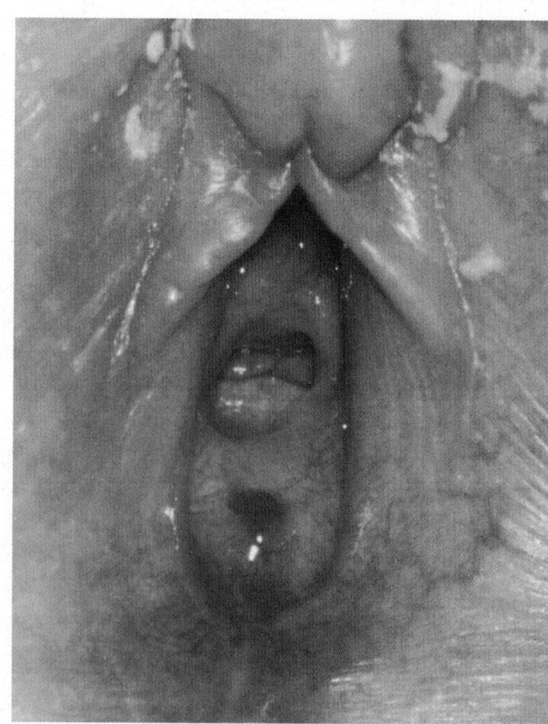

FIGURE 10-4 Acute hymenal hematoma in a prepubertal girl from penile penetration/contact. One reason why the considerable majority of examinations are normal may be that contact is more common than complete penetration and injuries resulting from penile contact are uncommon or are minor injuries that heal quickly and completely within days. (*Reproduced with permission from Nancy D. Kellogg, MD.*)

Although rare, accidental penetrating injury involving perihymenal tissues occurs, but rarely.

- Anatomic variants of normal, including shallow hymenal notches, anterior hymenal clefts, midline vestibule white lines, perineal defects, and narrow hymenal rims.
- Vulvovaginitis (e.g., nonspecific vaginal flora, shigella, streptococcus, poor hygiene, candidiasis)—Complaints include vaginal irritation or itching and vaginal discharge; wet prep and/or culture may be helpful.
- Lichen sclerosus et atrophicus is a cutaneous disease not caused by sexual abuse. It may present with bleeding, bruising, and/or vulvar itching, and the examination shows subepidermal hemorrhages and/or atrophic changes with areas of hypopigmentation over the vulva, perineum, and/or anus, an "hourglass" configuration (**Figure 10-7**).
- Anogenital irritation or bleeding—Causes may be infectious (pinworms, candidiasis, group B streptococcal infection), irritative (overgrowth of normal flora, sensitivity to laundry detergent or fabric softeners, sequelae of pubic hair shaving), or anatomic (urethral prolapse, dehiscence of a labial adhesion) (**Figure 10-8**).
- Normal physiologic leukorrhea—Scant, whitish tenacious discharge in pubertal females. Wet mount is normal.

In males, the following may be confused with abuse:

- Accidental trauma (e.g., penis caught in zipper)—History should support pattern of injury. Most intentionally inflicted injuries of male genitals are physical, not sexual, abuse.
- Phimosis—Unretractable foreskin. Irritation and redness occurs as a result of trapped debris.

Additional findings that may be confused with abuse:

- Anal fissure(s), which is a superficial excoriation or tear that extends from the anal verge into the anal canal, may or may not cause pain or bleeding during bowel movements. Sometimes, but not always, associated with diarrhea or constipation.
- Perianal venous pooling is sometimes mistaken for bruising.

MANAGEMENT

- Children may present with nonspecific behavioral and physical symptoms (but no disclosure of abuse) that include chronic stomachaches or headaches, school difficulties, mood changes, and sleeping difficulties. These children should be questioned in a careful and nonleading manner about the possibility of sexual abuse. For example, the clinician may state: "I treat other children who have problems like you do with school and headaches. Some of these children have told me about things that have happened to their body or feelings that made them sad, scared, or confused. Has anything like that ever happened to you?"
- Take a history from the child if necessary to make a medical diagnosis and to determine appropriate testing, treatment, and the need to report suspected abuse to child protection or law enforcement. The clinician may opt not to take a history if the child was or will be interviewed elsewhere; in this case, information necessary to

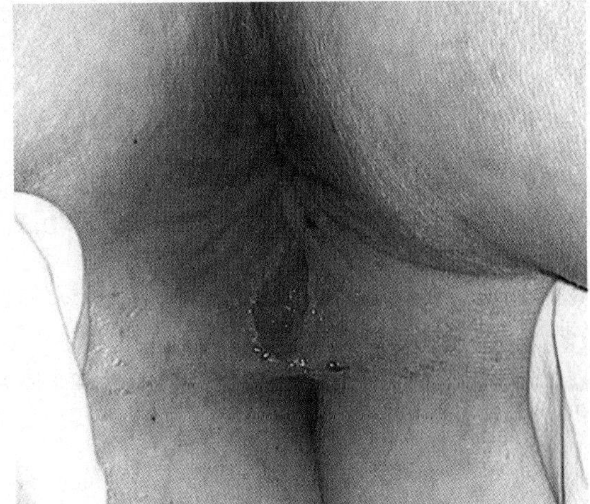

FIGURE 10-5 Acute rectal laceration in a young boy who was sexually abused by a relative. More than 95% of anal examinations in children with a history of anal penetration are normal or nonspecific. (*Reproduced with permission from Nancy D. Kellogg, MD.*)

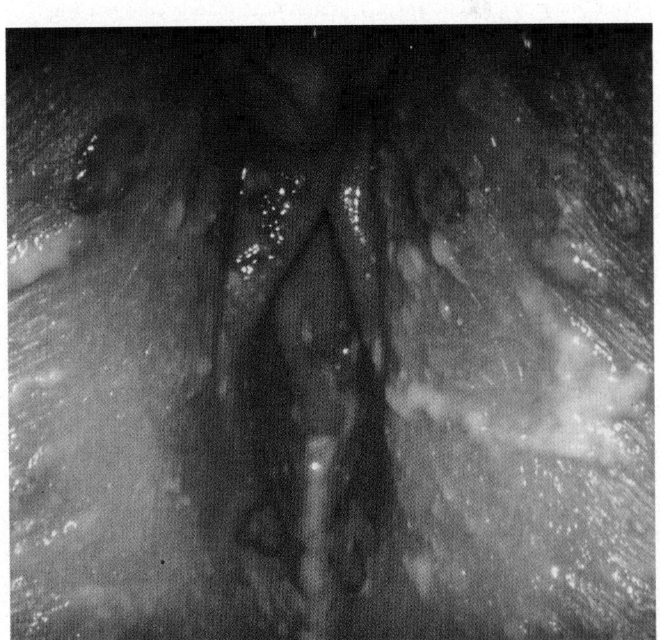

FIGURE 10-6 Herpes simplex virus (HSV) type 1 infection on the vulva of a prepubertal girl caused by sexual abuse. HSV type 1 of the genitals from sexual contact is increasing in prevalence relative to HSV type 2 infections of the genitals. (*Reproduced with permission from Nancy D. Kellogg, MD.*)

determine what type of medical assessment and testing should be obtained from other sources.
  - Ensure that the parent is not in the room for the history. A parent or other support person may be present for the physical examination, if the child wishes.
  - Use open-ended questions, such as "What happened?" or "Tell me more" as opposed to suggestive questions such as "Did Daddy touch your private parts?"
  - Take careful notes and document with quotations whenever possible.
- Clinicians should utilize community resources with expertise in the evaluation of sexual abuse or assault. If none are available, the clinician should:
  - Conduct a full physical examination including genitalia. Elicit cooperation from the child by explaining all procedures and earning his or her trust.
  - Consider STI and pregnancy prophylaxis for postpubertal patients who are evaluated within 96 hours of the assault.
  - Withhold STI treatment in asymptomatic prepubescent children until STI tests are confirmed positive, as the incidence of STI in asymptomatic prepubertal children is relatively low.
  - Consult with an infectious disease specialist regarding HIV prophylaxis. If HIV prevalence is high in local regions, assailant risk factors are unknown or high for HIV, and if the child is evaluated within 72 hours of a high-risk exposure, then HIV prophylaxis may be appropriate.
  - Examine closely for signs of physical and emotional abuse and neglect.

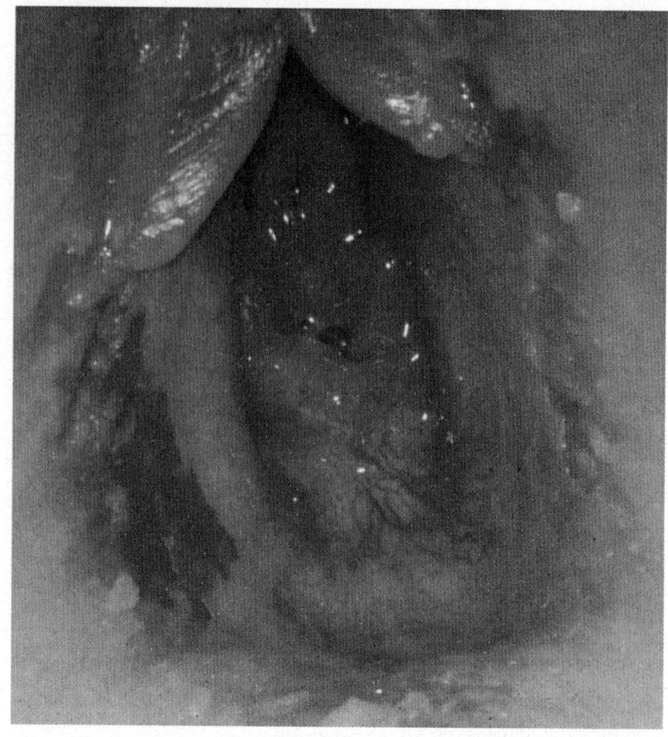

FIGURE 10-7 Lichen sclerosus et atrophicus in a young girl. This is a cutaneous disease, but commonly confused with sexual abuse because of the subepidermal hemorrhages. (*Reproduced with permission from Nancy D. Kellogg, MD.*)

FOLLOW-UP

- Laws vary by state; however, all states have mandated reporting laws (see Child Welfare Information Gateway, http://www.childwelfare.gov).
- All victims of sexual abuse and their families should be referred to local counseling agencies and to a Children's Advocacy Center, or other child abuse agency if available in the community.

PATIENT EDUCATION

At well-child visits, provider should discuss touches that make children sad, scared, or confused, or that give them an "uh-oh" feeling inside, and encourage parents to reinforce these themes at home.

PATIENT RESOURCES

- Child Help—**http://childhelp.org.**
- National Child Abuse Hotline, **1-800-422-4453.**
- Prevent Child Abuse America—**http://www.preventchildabuse.org.**
- National Center for Missing and Exploited Children—**http://www.missingkids.com.**

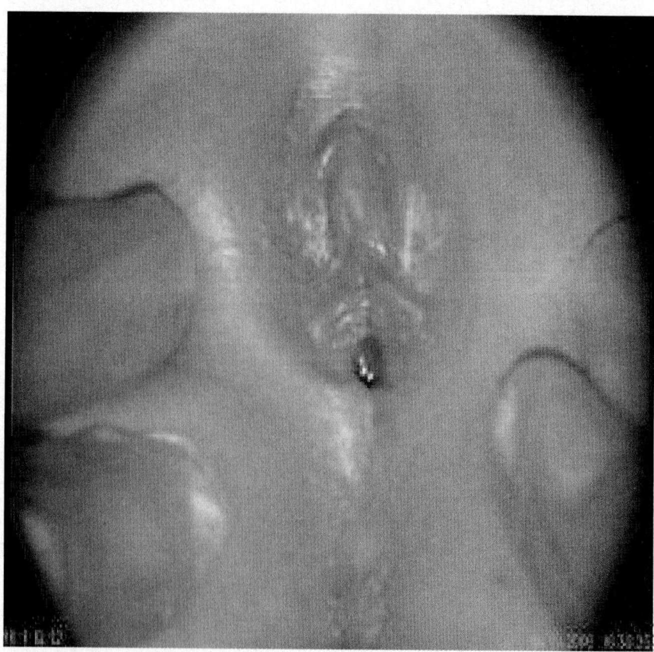

FIGURE 10-8 Labial adhesion can be confused with scarring secondary to child sexual abuse. This acquired condition is common in prepubertal girls and thought to be related to hygiene, irritation, and possibly trauma. (*Reproduced with permission from Maria D. McColgan, MD.*)

PROVIDER RESOURCES

- The American Academy of Pediatrics Guidelines for the Evaluation of Sexual Abuse of Children—**http://pediatrics.aappublications.org/content/103/1/186.full.**

REFERENCES

1. U.S. Department of Health and Human Services. Administration of Children, Youth and Families. *Child Maltreatment: 2008.* Washington, DC: Government Printing Office; 2010.
2. Finkelhor D, Shattock A, Turner HA, Hamby SL. The lifetime prevalence of child sexual abuse and sexual assault assessed in late adolescence. *J Adolesc Health.* 2014;55(3):329-333.
3. Finkelhor D. Current information on the scope and nature of child sexual abuse. *Future Child.* 1994;4(2):31-53.
4. Summit R. Child sexual abuse accommodation syndrome. *Child Abuse Negl.* 1983;7(2):177-193.
5. Berenson AB, Chacko MR, Weimann CM, et al. A case-control study of anatomic changes resulting from sexual abuse. *Am J Obstet Gynecol.* 2000;182(4):820-831.
6. Heger A, Ticson L, Velasquez O, et al. Children referred for possible sexual abuse: medical findings in 2384 children. *Child Abuse Negl.* 2002;26(6-7):645-659.
7. Adams JA, Harper K, Knudson S, Revilla J. Examination findings in legally confirmed child sexual abuse: it's normal to be normal. *Pediatrics.* 1994;94(3):310-317.
8. Kellogg ND, Menard SW, Santos A. Genital anatomy in pregnant adolescents: "normal" does not mean "nothing happened." *Pediatrics.* 2004;113(1):e67-e69.
9. Adams JA, Kellogg ND, Farst KJ, et al. Updated guidelines for the medical assessment and care of children who may have been sexually abused. *J Pediatr Adolesc Gynecol.* 2015;29(2):81-87.
10. Sena AC, Hsu KK, Kellogg N, et al. Sexual assault and sexually transmitted infections in adults, adolescents and children. *Clin Infect Dis.* 2015;61 Suppl 8:S856-864.

11 INTIMATE PARTNER VIOLENCE

Mindy A. Smith, MD, MS

PATIENT STORY

A woman who fled her abusive boyfriend is observed sitting at a table with other women in a residential chemical dependency treatment program. Her bruised face could not be missed (**Figure 11-1**). The program physician asked to speak with her and learned that her boyfriend beat her when she told him that she was voluntarily entering this program. The boyfriend was also an addict and had been physically abusive to her before. The violence escalated when she said that she needed help to stop the alcohol and drugs. She left him and did not believe that he would follow her. The program management assured her that they would not let him on the premises and would do all they could to keep her safe while she was recovering. **Figure 11-2** was taken 2 months later, when her face was healing along with her mind and spirit. She completed the 90-day program and is currently working and actively following a 12-step program.

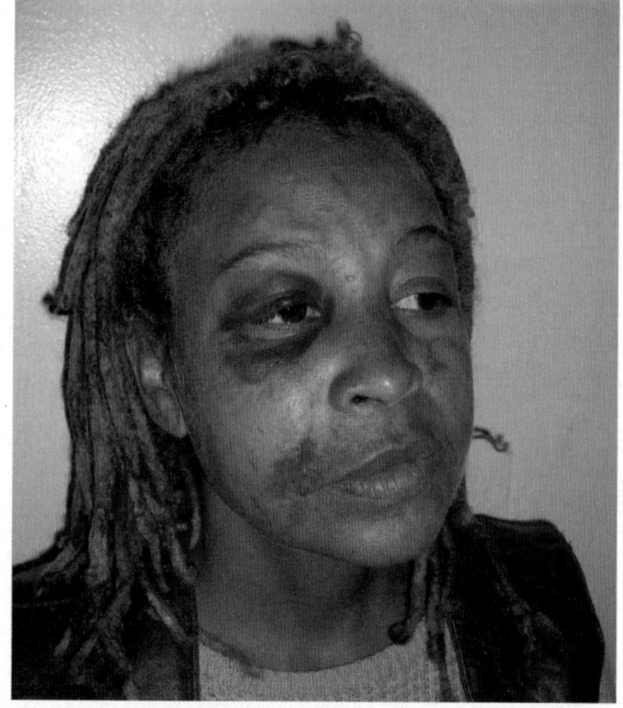

FIGURE 11-1 Bruising caused by intimate partner violence in a woman who fled her abusive boyfriend. *(Reproduced with permission from Richard P. Usatine, MD.)*

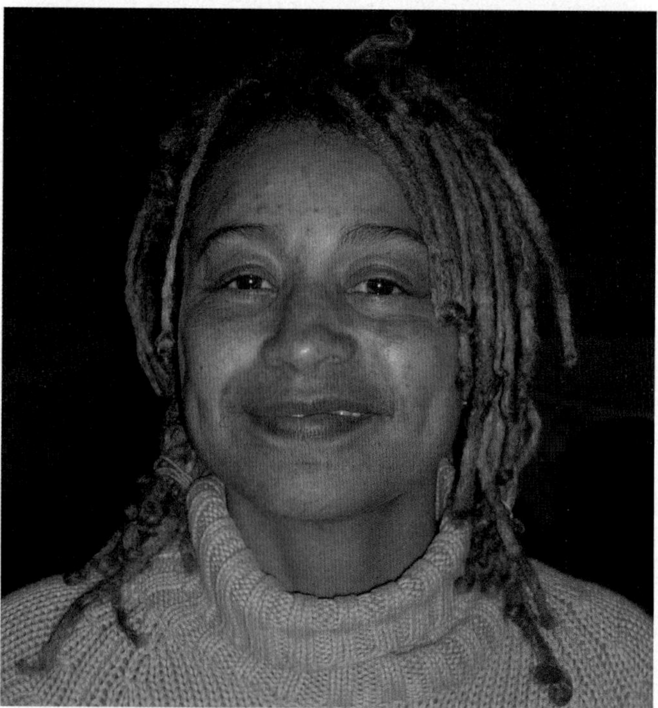

FIGURE 11-2 Photograph of the woman in **Figure 11-1** taken 2 months later. Her facial and psychological wounds are healing. *(Reproduced with permission from Richard P. Usatine, MD.)*

INTRODUCTION

Intimate partner violence (IPV) is defined as an intimate partner's physical, emotional (stalking or psychological aggression), or sexual abuse.[1] Physical violence is the intentional use of physical force with the potential for causing death, disability, injury, or harm. Physical violence includes scratching; pushing; biting; punching; use of a weapon; and use of restraints or one's body, size, or strength against another person.[1] Physical violence also includes coercing another person to commit these acts. Common to all IPV forms is a pattern of coercion and control.

EPIDEMIOLOGY

IPV affects about 36% of women and 29% of men in the United States during their lifetimes.[2]

- An estimated 10 to 12 million men and women in the United States experience physical violence by a current or former intimate partner; more than 1 in 5 women (22.3%) and nearly 1 in 7 men (14.0%) experience severe lifetime physical violence by an intimate partner.[3,4]
- Physical violence by an intimate partner can result in direct injury including death (1095 women and 241 men in 2010; Bureau of Justice, 2011), adverse psychological and social consequences, and impaired endocrine and immune systems through chronic stress and other mechanisms.[5] IPV victimization also increases the odds of having a substance use disorder, particularly alcohol and cannabis, for both men and women.[6]
- Lifetime stalking by an intimate partner was reported by 9.2% of women and 2.5% of men in the 2011 National Intimate Partner and Sexual Violence Survey (NIPSVS).[2]

- Nearly 1 in 6 women are battered by a partner during pregnancy.[7] These pregnant women are more likely to experience poor weight gain, infection, and hypertensive disorders of pregnancy and are at higher risk for preterm delivery and delivery of a low-birth-weight infant.
- According to the National Violence Against Women Survey, more than 200,000 women age 18 years and older were raped by intimate partners in the 12 months preceding the survey.[8] Sexual violence is discussed in Chapter 12.
- In a national caregiver survey of more than 4500 children, 17.3% of the children had witnessed an assault between parental partners in their lifetime and 6.1% had witnessed an assault in the past year.[1,9] Children may become injured themselves. One study found that children of abused mothers were 57 times more likely to have been harmed because of IPV between their parents, compared to children of nonabused mothers.[10]
- Clinicians identify only a small number of victims (<10%).[1] Only about 20% of IPV rapes or sexual assaults, 25% of physical assaults, and 50% of cases of stalking directed toward women are reported; fewer events against men are reported.[5]

RISK FACTORS

Risk factors for IPV include the following[11]:

- Individual factors—Prior history of physical or psychological abuse (strong risk factor), social isolation, witnessing or experiencing violence as a child, being young, less educated, unemployed, heavy user of alcohol or illicit drugs, mental health problems (e.g., depression, borderline or antisocial personality traits), and engaging in aggressive or delinquent behavior as a youth.
- Relationship factors—Relationship factors include couples with income, educational, or job status disparities or in which there is dominance and control of the relationship by one partner over the other, economic stress, and marital conflict or instability.
- Community factors—Community factors include poverty and associated factors or weak community sanctions against IPV (e.g., police unwilling to intervene).

DIAGNOSIS

Ask patients directly or through questionnaires about violence at routine visits or when presenting with clues (as below). SOR C Data are lacking, however, that identification produces positive outcomes.[12] It is important to use patient-centered approaches.

- Questions that may be asked include general questions about how things are going at home or more specific questions about experiences of nonviolent (e.g., insulting, threatening) or violent (e.g., grabbing, punching, beating, forced sex) abusive acts.
- Five screening instruments are highly accurate—Hurt, Insult, Threaten, Scream (HITS); Ongoing Violence Assessment Tool; Slapped, Threatened, Throw; Humiliation, Afraid, Rape, Kick; and the Woman Abuse Screening Tool (WAST).[13] In a study of screening tools, women preferred self-completed approaches (versus face-to-face), although no differences in prevalence were found for method or screening instrument.[14] In a predominantly Hispanic population, investigators found the Spanish version of the four-question instrument HITS to be moderately reliable with good validity compared with WAST for Spanish-speaking patients[15]; HITS has also been validated with male victims.[16]

CLINICAL FEATURES

Clues on patient history include the following:

- Chronic pain syndromes (e.g., headache, backache, stomachache, or pelvic pain).
- Depression.
- Drug and alcohol abuse.
- Frequent late of missed appointments or late entry into prenatal care.
- Somatic symptoms such as menstrual or sexual health problems, headaches, dizziness, palpitations, shortness of breath, generalized fatigue, and insomnia.[17]

Clues on physical examination:

- Physical injury—Most physical injuries are minor (e.g., contusions, lacerations, abrasions) but include broken bones, traumatic brain injury, and knife wounds (see **Figures 11-1** to **11-3**).
  - Ocular injuries can include soft-tissue injuries, corneal abrasions, orbital fractures, lens dislocation, retinal detachment, visual field loss, double vision, and blindness (see **Figure 11-1**).
  - Trauma to the mouth and lips may be accompanied by fractures, broken teeth, tongue lacerations, and altered taste and smell.
  - Injuries suspicious for abuse are those only in areas covered by clothing, injuries in different stages of healing, and injuries that show a defensive wound pattern, particularly on the hands or arms.
  - Upper torso injury carries a high risk of injury to cervical spine, large vessels of the neck, and chest and lungs.
- Depression or symptoms of posttraumatic stress disorder (e.g., emotional detachment, sleep disturbances, flashbacks, replaying assault in mind).
- Evidence of forced sexual assault.
- Presence of sexually transmitted infections.

MANAGEMENT

- Initial evaluation, following identification of abuse, is to assess for immediate danger to the patient and any children (e.g., Do you feel it is safe to go home tonight? Where is your partner?). If danger is perceived, assist the patient in finding a safe place to go (**Figures 11-4** and **11-5**).
- Document all findings and include photographs (with date), if possible (**Figure 11-6**).
- Develop a safety plan. This should include:
  - A safe physical location that is not known to the abuser,
  - Transportation to that location, and
  - A list of items to take or a packed suitcase—clothes, keys, cash, valuable documents, telephone numbers, prescriptions, something meaningful for each child.
- Address the needs of any children.

- Listen to the patient empathically and nonjudgmentally, express concern for health and future safety, affirm a commitment to helping, and provide education and information on community resources.
- Data on effective intervention programs are scarce.
  - Intensive advocacy (more than 12 hours) may improve short-term quality of life and reduce physical abuse at 1–2 years postintervention for women recruited from domestic violence shelters or refuges.[18] Brief advocacy may provide small short-term mental health benefits and reduce abuse,[19] particularly among pregnant women and for less severe abuse.
  - Women residents in a domestic violence shelter showed improvement in psychological distress symptoms and less health care utilization following a social support intervention.[20]
  - A randomized controlled trial (RCT) of a psychobehavioral intervention for pregnant women reduced recurrent episodes of IPV victimization (odds ratio [OR] 0.48, 95% confidence interval [CI], 0.29, 0.80); number needed to treat = 17). Women who reported minor episodes of IPV were less likely to experience further episodes during pregnancy, and women with either minor or major IPV episodes were less likely to experience further IPV postpartum.[21] Early childhood visitation may also be helpful in reducing IPV.[22]
  - Use of computerized self-paced IPV prevention modules reduced physical and sexual IPV victimization and severe injury at 12-month follow-up in an RCT of women in New York City community corrections.[23]
  - Community-provided trauma-focused cognitive behavioral therapy (CBT) was effective in reducing stress symptoms and anxiety in an RCT of 7- to 14-year-old children exposed to IPV.[24]
  - In a Cochrane review of CBT for abusive men, only four small trials could be combined and no significant effect was found for reduced risk of violence (relative risk [RR], 0.86; 95% CI, 0.54, 1.38); the authors concluded that there were too few trials to determine effectiveness.[25]

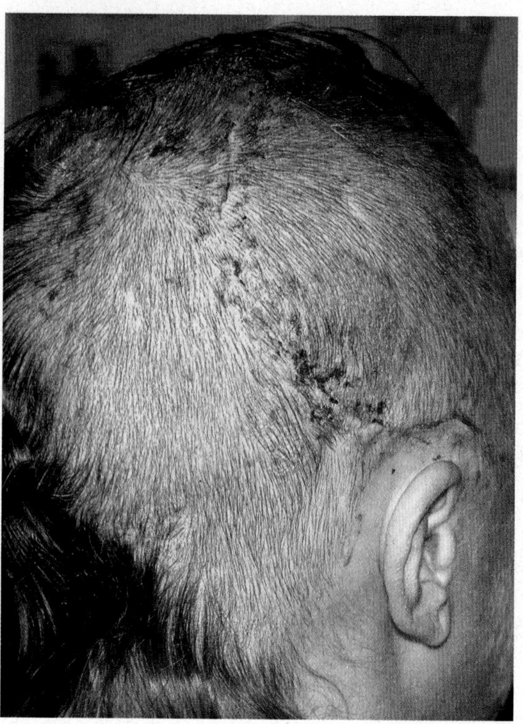

FIGURE 11-3 A woman with a large craniotomy wound that was needed to evacuate her intracranial bleeding secondary to being beaten over the head with a board by her fiancé. *(Reproduced with permission from Richard P. Usatine, MD.)*

SCREENING AND PREVENTION

- The U.S. Preventive Services Task Force (USPSTF) recommends that clinicians screen women of childbearing age for IPV and provide intervention services or referral to those who screen positive.[26] SOR Ⓑ Evidence was insufficient to assess the balance of benefits and harms of screening elderly or vulnerable adults. The USPSTF found evidence that IPV can be accurately identified using available screening instruments, that advocacy interventions can mitigate the adverse health outcomes of IPV, and that screening causes minimal harm. However, rates of identification from screening interventions are low relative to expected rates, and it is unclear whether there are improved outcomes for women screened for IPV in healthcare settings.[12]
- In one RCT, computer screening increased detection and opportunities to discuss IPV in a busy family medicine practice.[27]

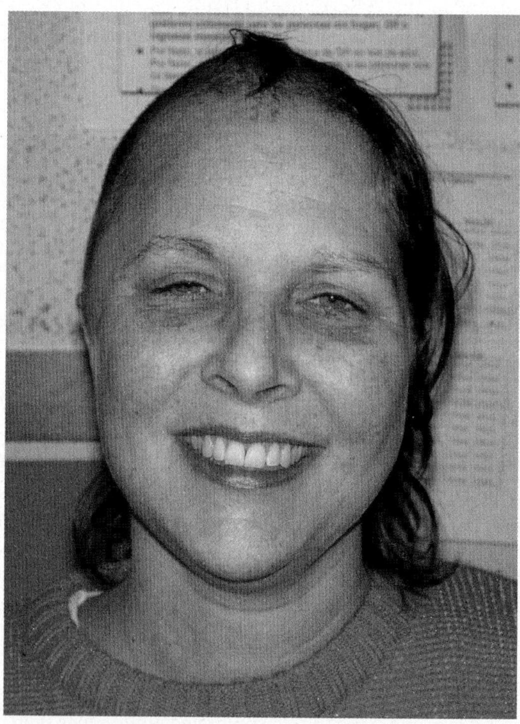

FIGURE 11-4 Frontal view of the woman in **Figure 11-3** at a homeless shelter. She was putting her life back together again with the help of the shelter and the providers at the clinic. *(Reproduced with permission from Richard P. Usatine, MD.)*

PROGNOSIS

- Many individuals (or people) are not ready to leave an abusive relationship for a variety of reasons. In one study, duration of abuse was less than 1 year to 5 median years, and in 3% to 5% of instances, IPV persisted for longer than 20 years.[28]
- Women who are abused have a higher risk of posttraumatic stress disorder, depression (1 in 6 abused women will attempt suicide), insomnia, nightmares, and alcohol (16-fold risk of alcohol use) and drug abuse (9-fold risk over nonabused patient).[1]
- IPV for women also decreases the odds of completing substance abuse treatment.[29]
- In one study, women reporting IPV in the year prior to pregnancy were at increased risk for high blood pressure or edema (adjusted OR 1.37 to 1.40), vaginal bleeding (adjusted OR 1.54 to 1.66), severe nausea, vomiting, or dehydration (adjusted OR 1.48 to 1.63), and kidney infection or urinary tract infection (adjusted OR 1.43 to 1.55), in addition to preterm delivery (adjusted OR 1.37), low-birth-weight infant (adjusted OR 1.17), and an infant requiring intensive care unit care (adjusted OR 1.31 to 1.33) compared with those not reporting IPV.[30]
- In another study, infants of mothers exposed to IPV were more likely to experience low birth weight, neonatal hospitalization, and postneonatal hospitalization.[31]
- In one primary care cross-sectional study, children of parents reporting both IPV and parental psychological distress (n = 88; 0.5%) were more likely to fail at least one developmental milestone.[32]

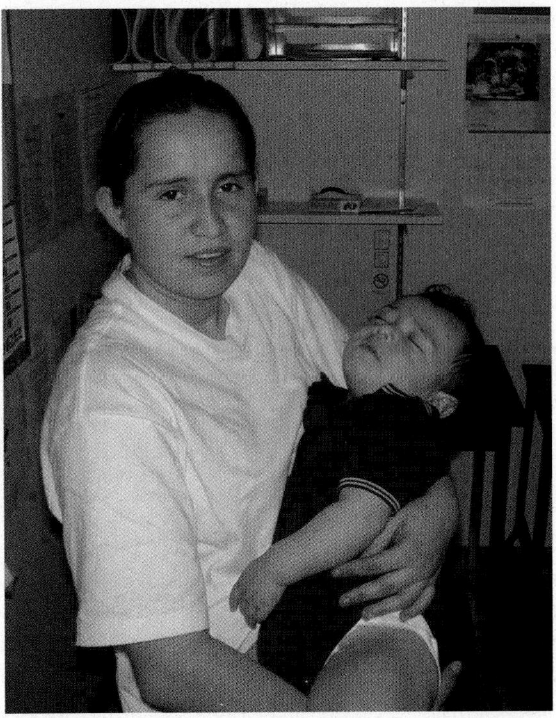

FIGURE 11-5 A young, Hispanic mom with her baby at a clinic in a homeless shelter. She had fled her abusive husband with her child. (*Reproduced with permission from Richard P. Usatine, MD.*)

FOLLOW-UP

- Plan for the next visit and provide ongoing support, as it often takes time for individuals (or people) to leave an abusive relationship.
- Monitor for depression, insomnia, nightmares, and alcohol and drug abuse.
- If pregnant, monitor for miscarriage, preterm delivery, and low birth weight.
- Children exposed to IPV also should be monitored because they are at risk of behavioral problems including aggression, anxiety/depression, and inattention/hyperactivity, especially if parental mental health disorders or substance abuse are also present.[33,34]

PATIENT EDUCATION

- Assist patients in recognizing the cycle of abuse, that is, violence followed by remorse/apology, tension-building period (patient may experience fear, isolation, forced dependency, intermittent reward), followed by another episode of violence.
- Provide victim education and information on community resources (see Patient Resources below).
- Acknowledge that leaving may take time.
- Recovery from abuse may include shame and guilt, but often leads to an improved sense of self and self-worth.

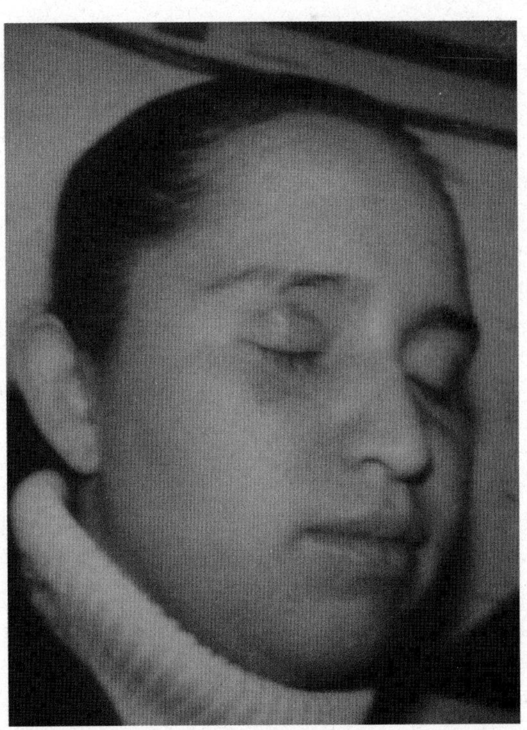

FIGURE 11-6 A copy of a photograph, which the woman had in her purse, showing her black eyes after being beaten by her husband the month before. Out of fear for her life and the well-being of her child, she left her husband. (*Reproduced with permission from Richard P. Usatine, MD.*)

- In a follow-up study of women exiting a shelter, women who were employed, who reported higher quality of life, and who had people in their networks who provided practical help and/or were available to talk about personal matters were less likely to be re-victimized.[35]

PATIENT RESOURCES

- National Domestic Violence Hotline connects individuals to help in their area by using a nationwide database that includes detailed information about domestic violence shelters, other emergency shelters, legal advocacy and assistance programs, and social service programs. Help is more than 170 languages, 24 hours a day, 7 days a week—**www.ndvh.org.**

  Hotline: 800-779-SAFE (7233)

  TTY: 800-787-3224 available for the deaf, deaf-blind, and hard of hearing.
- National Coalition Against Domestic Violence is a membership organization that includes service programs, reading lists, advocacy, educational materials, and coordinates a national collaborative effort to assist battered women in removing the physical scars of abuse—**www.ncadv.org.**
- Centers for Disease Control and Prevention—**https://www.cdc.gov/ViolencePrevention/intimatepartnerviolence/index.html.**

PROVIDER RESOURCES

- CDC—**http://www.cdc.gov/ViolencePrevention/intimatepartnerviolence/index.html.**
- Futures without Violence—**http://www.futureswithoutviolence.org.**
- Institute on Domestic Violence in the African American Community—**http://www.idvaac.org.**

REFERENCES

1. Centers for Disease Control. *Intimate Partner Violence: Definitions.* https://www.cdc.gov/violenceprevention/intimatepartnerviolence/definitions.html. Accessed January 2017.
2. Black MC, Basile KC, Breiding MJ, et al. *National Intimate Partner and Sexual Violence Survey: 2010 Summary Report.* Atlanta, GA: National Center for Injury Prevention and Control, Centers for Disease Control and Prevention; 2011.
3. Breiding MJ, Basile KC, Smith SG, et al. *Intimate Partner Violence Surveillance: Uniform Definitions and Recommended Data Elements, Version 2.0.* Atlanta (GA): National Center for Injury Prevention and Control, Centers for Disease Control and Prevention; 2015.
4. Sumner SA, Mercy JA, Dahlberg LL, et al. Violence in the United States: status, challenges, and opportunities. *JAMA.* 2015;314(5):478-488.
5. Centers for Disease Control. *Intimate Partner Violence: Consequences.* https://www.cdc.gov/violenceprevention/intimatepartnerviolence/consequences.html. Accessed January 2017.
6. Afifi TO, Henriksen CA, Asmundson GJ, Sareen J. Victimization and perpetration of intimate partner violence and substance use disorders in a nationally representative sample. *J Nerv Ment Dis.* 2012;200(8):684-691.
7. Agency for Healthcare Research and Quality. https://*www.ahrq.gov/professionals/prevention-chronic-care/healthier-pregnancy/preventive/partnerviolence.html.* Accessed January 2017.
8. Centers for Disease Control. *CDC Injury Fact Book.* https://stacks.cdc.gov/view/cdc/11438/. Accessed January 2017.
9. MacMillan HL, Wathen CN. Children's exposure to intimate partner violence. *Child Adolesc Psychiatr Clin N Am.* 2014;23(2):295-308.
10. Parkinson GW, Adams RC, Emerling FG. Maternal domestic violence screening in an office-based pediatric practice. *Pediatrics.* 2001;108(3):E43.
11. Centers for Disease Control. *Intimate Partner Violence: Risk and Protective Factors.* https://www.cdc.gov/violenceprevention/intimatepartnerviolence/riskprotectivefactors.html. Accessed January 2017.
12. O'Doherty LJ, Taft A, Hegarty K, et al. Screening women for intimate partner violence in healthcare settings: abridged Cochrane systematic review and meta-analysis. *BMJ.* 2014;348:g2913.
13. Nelson HD, Bougatsos C, Blazina I. Screening women for intimate partner violence: a systematic review to update the U.S. Preventive Services Task Force recommendation. *Ann Intern Med.* 2012;156(11):796-808.
14. MacMillan HL, Wathen CN, Jamieson E, et al. Approaches to screening for intimate partner violence in health care settings: a randomized trial. *JAMA.* 2006;296(5):530-536.
15. Chen PH, Rovi S, Vega M, et al. Screening for domestic violence in a predominantly Hispanic clinical setting. *Fam Pract.* 2005;22(6):617-623.
16. Shakil A, Donald S, Sinacore JM, Krepcho M. Validation of the HITS domestic violence screening tool with males. *Fam Med.* 2005;37(3):193-198.
17. Eberhard-Gran M, Schei B, Eskild A. Somatic symptoms and diseases are more common in women exposed to violence. *J Gen Intern Med.* 2007;22:1668-1673.
18. Rivas C, Ramsay J, Sadowski L, et al. Advocacy interventions to reduce or eliminate violence and promote the physical and psychosocial well-being of women who experience intimate partner abuse. *Cochrane Database Syst Rev.* 2015;(12):CD005043.
19. Hegarty K, O'Doherty L, Taft A, et al. Screening and counselling in the primary care setting for women who have experienced intimate partner violence (WEAVE): a cluster randomised controlled trial. *Lancet.* 2013;382(9888):249-258.
20. Contantino R, Kim Y, Crane PA. Effects of a social support intervention on health outcomes in residents of a domestic violence shelter: a pilot study. *Issues Ment Health Nurs.* 2005;26(6):575-590.
21. Kiely M, El-Mohandes AA, El-Khorazaty MN, et al. An integrated intervention to reduce intimate partner violence in pregnancy: a randomized controlled trial. *Obstet Gynecol.* 2010;115(2 Pt 1):273-283.
22. Bair-Merritt MH, Jennings JM, Chen R, et al. Reducing maternal intimate partner violence after the birth of a child: a randomized controlled trial of the Hawaii Healthy Start Home Visitation Program. *Arch Pediatr Adolesc Med.* 2010;164(1):16-23.

23. Gilbert L, Goddard-Eckrich D, Hunt T, et al. Efficacy of a computerized intervention on HIV and intimate partner violence among substance-using women in community corrections: a randomized controlled trial. *Am J Public Health.* 2016;106(7):1278-1286.
24. Cohen JA, Mannarino AP, Iyengar S. Community treatment of posttraumatic stress disorder for children exposed to intimate partner violence: a randomized controlled trial. *Arch Pediatr Adolesc Med.* 2011;165(1):16-21.
25. Smedslund G, Dalsbø TK, Steiro AK, et al. Cognitive behavioural therapy for men who physically abuse their female partner. *Cochrane Database Syst Rev.* 2007;(3):CD006048.
26. Moyer VA; U.S. Preventive Services Task Force. Screening for intimate partner violence and abuse of elderly and vulnerable adults: U.S. Preventive Services Task Force recommendation statement. *Ann Intern Med.* 2013;158(6):478-486.
27. Ahmad F, Hogg-Johnson S, Stewart DE, et al. Computer-assisted screening for intimate partner violence and control: a randomized trial. *Ann Intern Med.* 2009;151(2):93-102.
28. Thompson RS, Bonomi AE, Anderson M, et al. Intimate partner violence: prevalence, types, and chronicity in adult women. *Am J Prev Med.* 2006;30(6):447-457.
29. Lipsky S, Krupski A, Roy-Bryne P, et al. Effect of co-occurring disorders and intimate partner violence on substance abuse treatment outcomes. *J Subst Abuse Treat.* 2010;38(3): 231-244.
30. Silverman JG, Decker MR, Reed E, Raj A. Intimate partner violence victimization prior to and during pregnancy among women residing in 26 U.S. states: associations with maternal and neonatal health. *Am J Obstet Gynecol.* 2006;195(1):140-148.
31. Pavey AR, Gorman GH, Kuehn D, et al. Intimate partner violence increases adverse outcomes at birth and in early infancy. *J Pediatr.* 2014;165(5):1034-1039.
32. Gilbert AL, Bauer NS, Carroll AE, Downs SM. Child exposure to parental violence and psychological distress associated with delayed milestones. *Pediatrics.* 2013;132(6):e1577-1583
33. Whitaker RC, Orzol SM, Kahn RS. Maternal mental health, substance use, and domestic violence in the year after delivery and subsequent behavior problems in children at age 3 years. *Arch Gen Psychiatry.* 2006;63(5):551-560.
34. McFarlane J, Maddoux J, Cesario S, et al. Effect of abuse during pregnancy on maternal and child safety and functioning for 24 months after delivery. *Obstet Gynecol.* 2014;123(4): 839-847.
35. Bybee D, Sullivan CM. Predicting re-victimization of battered women 3 years after exiting a shelter program. *Am J Community Psychol.* 2005;36(1-2):85-96.

12 ADULT SEXUAL ASSAULT

Mindy A. Smith, MD, MS

PATIENT STORIES

CASE 1

A 19-year-old college woman presents to the office after being raped 3 weeks ago. She went out on a date and was forced to have sex against her will. She states that she had been a virgin and that he made her bleed by penetrating her vagina with his penis. She tried to stop him, but was afraid to fight too hard because he was a strong man and was drunk. She is in tears as she tells her story. She waited so long to come in for help because she did not know where to turn. She took emergency contraception (EC) immediately, and a home pregnancy test taken last night was negative. She wants to be checked for any sexually transmitted infections (STIs). Upon examination, there is a tear of her hymen at the 5-o'clock position that has healed (**Figure 12-1**). There are no signs of infection, and sexually transmitted infection (STI) screening is performed. She is afraid to prosecute but would like to be referred to a rape-counseling program.

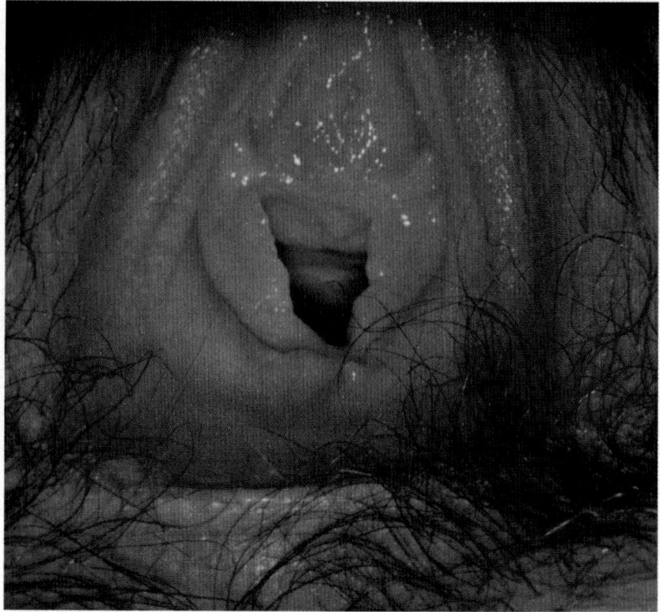

FIGURE 12-1 External genitalia of a 19-year-old college girl showing the tear of her hymen at approximately the 5-o'clock position. This was the result of date rape 3 weeks before the photograph was taken. *(Reproduced with permission from Nancy D. Kellogg, MD.)*

CASE 2

A 47-year-old woman is seen in follow-up for depression. She admits to being raped in a parking lot several months prior but did not report it to the police. She is continuing to have intrusive nightmares and flashbacks of the event. She is having difficulty concentrating at work and does not feel comfortable in social situations.

INTRODUCTION

Sexual violence is a sexual act that is committed or attempted by another person without freely given consent of the victim or against someone who is unable to consent or refuse.[1] It may involve actual or threatened physical force, use of guns or other weapons, coercion, intimidation, or pressure. Sexual violence includes unwanted penetration (completed or attempted with or without alcohol/drug facilitation) defined as physical insertion, however slight, of the penis into the vulva; contact between the mouth and the penis, vulva, or anus; or physical insertion of a hand, finger, or other object into the anal or genital opening of another person. Sexual violence also includes unwanted sexual contact (intentional touching either directly or through clothing of the genitals, anus, groin, breast, inner thigh, or buttocks against a victim's will or when a victim is unable to consent) and noncontact unwanted sexual experiences, such as voyeurism, intentional exposure to exhibitionism, undesired exposure to pornography, verbal or behavioral sexual harassment, threats of sexual violence, or taking nude photographs of a sexual nature of another person without his or her consent or knowledge or of a person unable to consent or refuse.

EPIDEMIOLOGY

- Based on the National Intimate Partner and Sexual Violence Survey (NISVS; 2010) of more than 16,000 adults, nearly 1 in 5 women

(18.3%) and 1 in 71 men (1.4%) in the United States has been raped.[2] More than half of the women were raped by an intimate partner (see Chapter 11, Intimate Partner Violence) and 40.8% were raped by an acquaintance. Among men, more than half were raped by an acquaintance and 15.1% by a stranger.[2]
  - Unwanted sexual contact was reported in the NISVS by 27.2% of women and 11.7% of men.[2]
  - Lifetime stalking victimization was reported by 1 in 6 women (16.2%) and 1 in 19 men (5.2%) in the NISVS.[2]
- In an interview survey of 15,162 women and men aged 16–74 years living in Britain, completed non volitional sex was reported by 9.8% (95% CI 9.0–10.5) of women and 1.4% (1.1–1.7) of men.[3]
- Most victims of sexual assault are young:
  - In the NISVS, most women (79.6%) experienced their first completed rape before age 25 years and 42.2% before the age of 18 years.[2] More than one-quarter of male victims of completed rape (27.8%) experienced their first rape before they were 11 years of age.
  - Similar findings were reported in another national survey where 60.4% of female and 69.2% of male victims were first raped before age 18 years.[4] A quarter of females were first raped before age 12 years.
  - In the British survey, median age at most recent occurrence of completed non-volitional sex was 18 years for women and 16 years for men.[3]
- In surveys of college students, annually 10% of women described a rape, 17% reported an attempted rape, 26% reported unwanted sexual coercion, and 63% experienced unwanted sexual contact.[5]
- Women in substance abuse treatment are a particularly high-risk group for having experienced violence. In one study, 89% reported a history of interpersonal violence and 70% reported a history of sexual assault.[6]
- Men are most often the perpetrators of sexual violence,[2] even among male victims.
  - In a community sample of 423 young single men interested in dating women who completed baseline and 1-year follow-up interviews, one quarter reported having made a woman engage in some type of sexual activity during the past year when they knew she was unwilling or unable to consent.[7] These men were more likely to objectify women and report pressure from friends to have sex by any means.
- According to the FBI Uniform Crime Reports, there were an estimated 79,770 rapes reported to law enforcement in 2013, or 25.2 per 100,000 women, a decrease of 6.3% from 2012 and 10.6% lower than 2009.[8] Most women, however, do not report being raped to the police:
  - As in the cases presented in this chapter, most cases of sexual assault go unreported (only about 1 in 5 women report their rape to police).[9] Reasons for failing to report include fear of reprisal, shame, fear of the justice system, and failure to define the act as rape. Furthermore, according to victim accounts in the NISVS, only 37% of the rapes reported to police resulted in the rapist being criminally prosecuted, and of those prosecuted, less than half (46.2%) were convicted of a crime.[2]

ETIOLOGY AND PATHOPHYSIOLOGY

- Two types of factors are believed to contribute to sexual violence—*vulnerability factors* that increase the likelihood that a person will suffer harm and *risk factors* that increase the likelihood that a person will cause harm. Neither vulnerability nor risk factors are direct causes of sexual violence.[4]

RISK FACTORS

Vulnerability factors for sexual assault, in addition to young age and female sex, include[10–12]:

- Prior history of sexual violence.
- Being disabled (physical, psychiatric illness, or cognitive impairment).
- Pregnancy.
- Poverty, homelessness.
- Having many sexual partners or being involved in sex work.
- Consuming alcohol or illicit drugs.

Risk factors for perpetration include[10,13]:

- Alcohol and drug use.
- Childhood history of physical or sexual abuse and/or witnessed family violence as a child.
- Coercive sexual fantasies.
- Preference for impersonal sex.
- Hostility toward women.
- Association with sexually aggressive and delinquent peers.
- Family environment characterized by physical violence and few resources.
- Poverty and lack of employment opportunities.
- Societal norms that support sexual violence, male superiority, and sexual entitlement.
- Weak laws and policies related to gender equity.

DIAGNOSIS

It is recommended that patients be asked directly about violence during routine visits, when seen in the emergency department, or when presenting with substance abuse, depression, and/or physical clues (as listed below) to identify those who are suffering from the aftermath of sexual or physical violence.

CLINICAL FEATURES

- Based on a retrospective case series in England of 83 rape cases in women, most had bruises and scratches to the extremities, 27% had genital/anal injuries, 20% sustained injuries to the chest/breasts, and 18% had injuries to the face; only 15 (18%) had no injury.[14]
- Women who are raped are significantly more likely than nonraped women to experience genital injuries and STIs, and have significantly greater difficulties with aspects of reproductive/sexual functioning, including dyspareunia, endometriosis, menstrual irregularities, and chronic pelvic pain.[15]

- Many women suffer psychological trauma following sexual assault such as posttraumatic stress disorder (PTSD) symptoms[1]:
    - Immediate psychological consequences include confusion, anxiety, withdrawal, fear, guilt, intrusive recollections, emotional detachment, and flashbacks.
    - Some victims may attempt suicide after being raped (**Figure 12-2**).

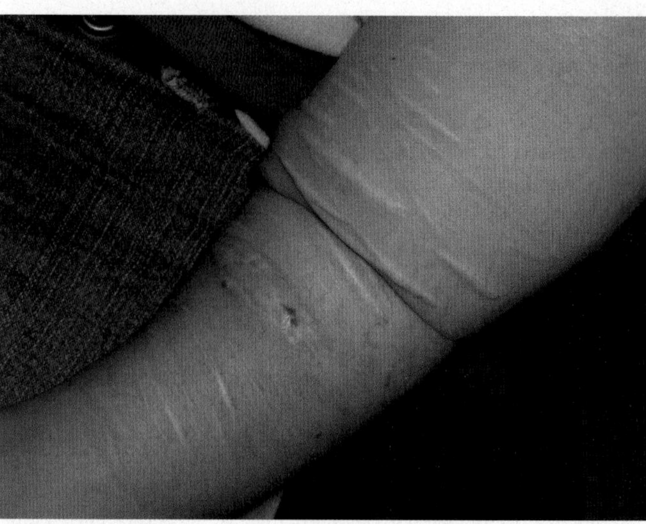

FIGURE 12-2 The damaged arm of a 26-year-old woman who was raped 5 years prior to this photograph. After being raped, she became suicidal and began cutting her arm repeatedly. The additional malformation of the arm is secondary to osteomyelitis from previous intravenous drug use. (*Reproduced with permission from Richard P. Usatine, MD.*)

MANAGEMENT

NONPHARMACOLOGIC

Following a sexual assault, many people (or individuals) report that they thought they were going to be killed. The survivor may be terrified and unable to provide a complete history of the assault. It is important to provide support and reassurance of immediate safety, and to obtain informed consent for examination, procedures, and contact of others. With permission, the clinician should contact a rape crisis worker and the police, although the survivor decides whether or not to file criminal charges; in general, notification of law enforcement is not required if the patient is an adult age 18 years or older and is not disabled, mentally ill, or elderly. In these cases, reporting is done only if the patient gives his or her consent. Injury caused by any weapon or incidents involving life-threatening assault, however, must be reported to the law enforcement agency (per statute) irrespective of reporting the sexual assault.[16]

- A guideline is available from the U.S. Department of Justice for sexual assault medical forensic examinations.[16] Steps in the evaluation are reviewed briefly below. A medical forensic evaluation is appropriate if the assault occurred within 72 hours up to 5 to 7 days of presentation.[16] A Standard Sexual Assault Forensic Evidence (SAFE) Kit should be used for gathering forensic evidence. Consider obtaining evidence even if a patient does not appear interested initially in reporting the assault.
- The patient should be assessed for safety and immediate mental health needs. The history includes details of the assault (e.g., date, time, location, descriptors of assailant[s]), type of bodily and sexual contact (orifice[s] penetrated, objects used), and sexual activity or bathing/washing since the assault.[11,16] Laws in all 50 states strictly limit the evidentiary use of a survivor's previous sexual history, including evidence of previously acquired STIs, as part of an effort to undermine the credibility of the survivor's testimony.[17]
- Treat traumatic injuries—Physical examination should include observations of emotional state and descriptions of clothing and stains. Gently, and with permission, examine for lacerations, abrasions, ecchymoses, and bites. A body chart may be useful for documenting the size, type, color, and location of any injuries. A genital examination should be conducted by an experienced clinician in a way that minimizes further trauma to the survivor; examination is directed by history.
- Test and treat for STI—A guideline for managing STI following sexual assault is available through the Centers for Disease Control and Prevention (CDC).[17]
    - Trichomoniasis, bacterial vaginosis (BV), gonorrhea, and chlamydial infection are the most frequently diagnosed infections

following sexual assault. As the prevalence of these infections is high among sexually active women, their presence after an assault does not necessarily signify acquisition during the assault.

- Nucleic acid amplification tests (NAATs) are recommended for *Neisseria gonorrhoeae* and *Chlamydia trachomatis* at the sites of completed or attempted penetration.[17]
- Wet mount or point-of-care testing of a vaginal swab specimen for *Trichomonas vaginalis* infection. The wet mount also should be examined for evidence of BV and candidiasis, especially if vaginal discharge, malodor, or itching is present.
- Collect a serum sample for immediate evaluation for HIV, hepatitis B, and syphilis, and obtain serum or urine for a pregnancy test in reproductive-aged women. Obtain toxicology and/or alcohol test if a patient has altered mental status, reports blackouts, or is concerned that he/she may have been drugged.[16]

MEDICATIONS

The following prophylactic regimen is suggested as preventive therapy:

- Hepatitis B vaccination, with hepatitis B immune globulin if the assailant is known to be hepatitis B surface antigen positive, is administered to sexual assault victims at the time of the initial examination if they have not been previously vaccinated. Follow-up doses of vaccine should be administered 1 to 2 and 4 to 6 months after the first dose.
- Human papilloma virus (HPV) vaccination in 2 doses, with the second dose given 6–12 months after the initial dose, is recommended for females and males through ages 9 to 26 years. The newest vaccine is 9-valent, thereby protecting persons against 9 HPV types. For persons 9 through 14 years of age, this HPV vaccine can be given using a 2-dose or 3-dose schedule. For the 2-dose schedule, the second shot should be given 6–12 months after the first shot. For persons 15 through 26 years of age, the nine 9-valent vaccine is given using a 3-dose schedule; the second shot should be given 2 months after the first shot, and the third shot should be given 6 months after the first shot.
- Regardless of gender, an empiric antimicrobial regimen for *Chlamydia*, gonorrhea, and *Trichomonas* is ceftriaxone 250 mg IM in a single dose **plus** azithromycin 1 g orally (single dose) **plus** metronidazole 2 g orally (single dose) **or** tinidazole 2 g orally in a single dose. Clinicians should counsel patients about the possible benefits and toxicities associated with these treatment regimens, such as gastrointestinal (GI) side effects. If alcohol has been consumed by the victim, metronidazole or tinidazole can be taken at home rather than observed to avoid drug–alcohol interaction.
- HIV seroconversion has occurred in persons whose only known risk factor was sexual assault or sexual abuse, but the risk is probably low (in consensual sex, the risk for HIV transmission from vaginal intercourse is 0.1% to 0.2%, for receptive anal intercourse the risk is 0.5% to 3%, and for oral sex the risk is substantially lower).[17]
- The healthcare provider should assess available information concerning HIV-risk behaviors of the assailant(s) (e.g., a man who has sex with other men and/or injected drug or crack cocaine use), local epidemiology of HIV/AIDS, and exposure characteristics of the assault. Specific circumstances of an assault that might increase risk for HIV transmission are trauma, including bleeding, with vaginal, anal, or oral penetration; exposure of mucous membranes to ejaculate; viral load in ejaculate (e.g., multiple assailants); the presence of an STI or genital lesions in the assailant or survivor; involvement of multiple assailants; and local epidemiology of HIV.
- If HIV postexposure prophylaxis (PEP) is offered, the following information should be discussed with the patient: (a) the possible benefit and known toxicities of antiretrovirals; (b) the close follow-up that will be necessary; (c) the benefit of adherence to recommended dosing; and (d) the necessity of early initiation to optimize potential benefits (as soon as possible after and up to 72 hours after the assault). Providers should emphasize that PEP appears to be well tolerated and that severe adverse effects are rare.
- Specialist consultation on PEP regimens is recommended. If the victim and clinician decide that PEP is warranted, provide enough medication to last until the next return visit and reevaluate the victim 3 to 7 days after initial assessment and assess tolerance of medications.[17] If assistance with PEP-related decisions is needed, call the National Clinician's Post Exposure Prophylaxis Hotline (PEP Line) (telephone: 888–448–4911).
- If PEP is started, perform a complete blood count (CBC) and serum chemistry at baseline (initiation of PEP should not be delayed pending results).
- Collect samples for legal evidence. Most emergency departments have rape or sexual assault kits containing instructions for gathering material to support legal charges; all samples must be carefully labeled and kept under supervision. Details of these procedures may be found elsewhere.[16]
- Reproductive-age female survivors should be evaluated for pregnancy, if appropriate, and offered EC if desired. Providers might also consider antiemetic medications, particularly if an EC containing estrogen is provided.
- Consider tetanus prophylaxis if skin wounds occurred and the patient is not up-to-date on tetanus immunization.
- Arrange for safety.
- Provide written information about the visit and any instructions given to the patient.

REFERRAL

- If the victim is amenable, refer for advocacy or counseling. In one randomized clinical trial (RCT) of Congolese sexual-violence survivors, group psychotherapy reduced PTSD symptoms and combined depression and anxiety symptoms and improved functioning compared to individual support.[18]
- If you are not the primary healthcare provider, arrange for follow-up medical care.

PREVENTION

- Authors of a systematic review of data from health and law enforcement surveillance systems identified the most effective violence prevention strategies for all types of interpersonal violence as parent and family-focused programs, early childhood education, school-based programs, therapeutic or counseling interventions, and public policy.[19]

- Although dating violence prevention–intervention programs have not been uniformly successful, women should be counseled about strategies for avoiding future victimization (e.g., recognition of dangerous situations, limiting use of alcohol, safety with friends). One program, Safe Dates, was shown in an RCT to be effective in preventing or interrupting sexual violence perpetration.[20] In another RCT of 893 first-year college women, resistance training consisting of four 3-hour units providing education and skills in risk assessment, overcoming emotional barriers in acknowledging danger, and verbal and physical self-defense strategies reduced the incidence of completed rape by nearly half (5.2% vs. 9.8% in the control group).[21]
- Life skills and educational programs can also encourage men to take greater responsibility for their actions and have greater respect for others. Although not many programs have been formally evaluated, there are reports of reduced violence against women in communities in Cambodia, the Gambia, South Africa, Uganda, and the United Republic of Tanzania attributed to these programs.[10] Other prevention efforts include media campaigns, written materials, victim risk-reduction techniques (e.g., self-defense, awareness), men's activism groups (e.g., Men Can Stop Rape), school-based programs, and legal and policy responses (e.g., encourage reporting, broadening the definition of rape and sexual assault).[10,22] In designing programs, information provided in documents prepared for the CDC may be useful.[22]

Health providers can also become involved in prevention activities at multiple levels:

- The United States Preventive Services Task Force recommends screening women of childbearing age for intimate partner violence and providing or referring women who screen positive to intervention services (see Chapter 11, Intimate Partner Violence.[23] SOR B
- Strengthening individual knowledge and skills through skill-building programs in high schools or training bystanders to safely interrupt sexist and harassing behavior.
- Promoting community education by sponsoring activities such as plays that reinforce positive cultural norms and portray responsible sexual behavior or developing awards to recognize responsible media coverage.
- Educating other community leaders and providers, such as little league coaches, prison guards, nursing home providers.
- Fostering coalitions and networks to promote community understanding and strategies to prevent sexual violence.
- Changing organizational practices such as implementation and enforcement of sexual harassment policies in schools and workplaces; implementing environmental safety measures such as adequate lighting and emergency call boxes.
- Influencing policies and legislation such as offering comprehensive sex education programs in middle and high schools, including violence prevention.

PROGNOSIS

- More than 32,000 pregnancies result yearly from rape (approximately 5% of rapes result in pregnancy).[10]
- In one follow-up study of post-partum women with a history of abuse, there was a greater risk for murder for 8 months after delivery, depression at 4, 8, 16, and 20 months after delivery, and PTSD for 24 months among the 24 women reporting abuse, including sexual abuse, during pregnancy compared to the 22 women reporting abuse only outside of pregnancy.[24] Children living with mothers who were abused during pregnancy had more problems with depression and anxiety.
- Chronic psychological consequences—In a meta-analysis of 17 case-control and 20 cohort studies (N = 3,162,318 participants), there was an association between sexual abuse and a lifetime diagnosis of anxiety disorder (odds ratio [OR], 3.09; 95% confidence interval [CI], 2.43 to 3.94), depression (OR, 2.66; 95% CI, 2.14 to 3.30), eating disorders (OR, 2.72; 95% CI, 2.04 to 3.63), PTSD (OR, 2.34; 95% CI, 1.59 to 3.43), sleep disorders (OR, 16.17; 95% CI, 2.06 to 126.76), and suicide attempts (OR, 4.14; 95% CI, 2.98 to 5.76).[25]
- Chronic somatic consequences—Authors of a meta-analysis of 23 studies found associations between sexual abuse and lifetime diagnosis of functional GI disorders (OR, 2.43; 95% CI, 1.36 to 4.31), nonspecific chronic pain (OR, 2.20; 95% CI, 1.54 to 3.15), psychogenic seizures (OR, 2.96; 95% CI, 1.12 to 4.69), and chronic pelvic pain (OR, 2.73; 95% CI, 1.73 to 4.30).[26] Significant associations with rape included lifetime diagnosis of fibromyalgia (OR, 3.35; 95% CI, 1.51 to 7.46), chronic pelvic pain (OR, 3.27; 95% CI, 1.02 to 10.53), and functional GI disorders (OR, 4.01; 95% CI, 1.88 to 8.57).
- Sexual revictimization occurs in about half of women who have experienced an act of sexual abuse.[27] Among these women, odds of PTSD were 4.3 to 8.2 times higher than non-victimized women compared to 2.4 to 3.5 times higher for single-episode victims.[27]

FOLLOW-UP

Follow-up visits provide an opportunity to (a) provide support and advocacy; (b) evaluate for resolution and healing of injury and current symptoms; (c) detect new infections acquired during or after the assault; (d) complete hepatitis B immunization, if indicated; (e) complete counseling and treatment for other STIs; and (f) monitor side effects and adherence to PEP, if prescribed.[16]

- Initial follow-up should be within 1 to 2 weeks following the assault.
- Provide ongoing support—Survivors of sexual abuse report strained relationships with family, friends, and intimate partners, including less emotional support and less frequent contact with friends and relatives.[10] In addition, only about half of victims keep this appointment, so outreach efforts may be needed.
- Review results of tests and discuss the plan for redraw of Venereal Disease Research Laboratory (VDRL) 3 months after exposure and HIV in 6 weeks and 3 and 6 months (if initial test results were negative).
- Long-term support, monitoring, and treatment:
  - For women suffering from PTSD, medications that may be useful include selective serotonin reuptake inhibitors and risperdal.[28] Cognitive-Processing Therapy and Prolonged Exposure have been the most useful therapies for treating PTSD, depression, and anxiety in female rape victims.[29] However, more than one-third of women retain the diagnosis of PTSD or drop out of treatment.[29]

PATIENT EDUCATION

- Recovery from sexual assault is a slow process. In one study, one-third of survivors reported recovery within 1 year but one-quarter thought that they had not recovered after 4 to 6 years.[30]
- Counseling, and sometimes medication, is available to help control symptoms and treat depression and PTSD, and patients should be encouraged to report and seek help for continuing difficulties.

PATIENT RESOURCES

- National Sexual Violence Resource Center serves as a comprehensive collection and distribution center for information, statistics, and resources related to sexual violence—**http://www.nsvrc.org.**
- Centers for Disease Control and Prevention. *Sexual Violence*—**http://www.cdc.gov/ViolencePrevention/sexualviolence/index.html.**
- National Domestic Violence Hotline (**http://www.thehotline.org/**), 1-800-799-SAFE; National Sexual Assault Hotline (**https://www.rainn.org/**), 1-800-656-HOPE.

PROVIDER RESOURCES

- A National Protocol for Sexual Assault Medical Forensic Examinations: Adults/Adolescents, 2nd ed—**https://www.ncjrs.gov/pdffiles1/ovw/241903.pdf.**
- United States Department of Justice—Office on Violence Against Women, offers links to resources—**http://www.ovw.usdoj.gov/sexassault.htm.**
- Assistance with PEP decisions can be obtained by calling the National Clinician's Post-Exposure Prophylaxis Hotline (PEP Line), 1-888-448-4911.
- National Sexual Violence Resource Center serves as a comprehensive collection and distribution center for information, statistics, and resources related to sexual violence—**http://www.nsvrc.org.**
- The American College of Obstetricians and Gynecologists provides publications about violence against women, intimate partner violence, sexual violence, adolescent dating violence, and patient education materials in both English and Spanish—**http://www.acog.org.**
- A directory of sexual assault centers in the United States can be obtained from the following URL— **https://www.nsvrc.org/find-help.**

REFERENCES

1. Centers for Disease Control and Prevention. *Sexual Violence: Definitions.* https://www.cdc.gov/violenceprevention/sexualviolence/definitions.html. Accessed April 2018.
2. Black MC, Basile KC, Breiding MJ, et al. *The National Intimate Partner and Sexual Violence Survey (NISVS): 2010 Summary Report.* Atlanta, GA: National Center for Injury Prevention and Control, Centers for Disease Control and Prevention; 2011. https://www.cdc.gov/violenceprevention/pdf/NISVS_Report2010-a.pdf. Accessed April 2018.
3. Macdowall W, Gibson LJ, Tanton C, et al. Lifetime prevalence, associated factors, and circumstances of non-volitional sex in women and men in Britain: findings from the third National Survey of Sexual Attitudes and Lifestyles (Natsal-3). *Lancet.* 2013;382(9907):1845-1855.
4. Basile KC, Chen J, Lynberg MC, Saltzman LE. Prevalence and characteristics of sexual violence victimization. *Violence Vict.* 2007;22(4):437-448.
5. Koss MP. Detecting the scope of rape: a review of prevalence research methods. *J Interpers Violence.* 1993;8:198-222.
6. Lincoln AK, Liebschutz JM, Chernoff M, et al. Brief screening for co-occurring disorders among women entering substance abuse treatment. *Subst Abuse Treat Prev Policy.* 2006;1:26.
7. Jacques-Tiura AJ, Abbey A, Wegner R, et al. Friends matter: protective and harmful aspects of male friendships associated with past-year sexual aggression in a community sample of young men. *Am J Public Health.* 2015;105(5):1001-1007.
8. Federal Bureau of Investigation. *Crime in the United States 2013: Rape.* Washington, DC: U.S. Department of Justice; 2013. https://ucr.fbi.gov/crime-in-the-u.s/2013/crime-in-the-u.s.-2013/violent-crime/rape. Accessed March 2017.
9. National Institute of Justice. *Extent, Nature, and Consequences of Rape Victimization: Findings from the National Violence Against Women Survey (2006).* https://www.ncjrs.gov/pdffiles1/nij/210346.pdf. Accessed March 2012.
10. World Health Organization. *World Report on Violence and Health, Sexual Violence.* Chapter 6. http://www.who.int/violence_injury_prevention/violence/global_campaign/en/chap6.pdf. Accessed March 2017.
11. Williams A. Managing adult sexual assault. *Aust Fam Physician.* 2004;33(10):825-828.
12. Basile KC, Breiding MJ, Smith SG. Disability and risk of recent sexual violence in the United States. *Am J Public Health.* 2016;106(5):928-933.
13. Centers for Disease Control and Prevention. *Sexual Violence. Risk and Protective Factors.* https://www.cdc.gov/violenceprevention/sexualviolence/riskprotectivefactors.html. Accessed April 2018.
14. Bower L, Dalton ME. Female victims of rape and their genital injuries. *BJOG.* 1997;104:617-620.
15. Weaver TL. Impact of rape on female sexuality: review of selected literature. *Clin Obstet Gynecol.* 2009;52(4):702-711.
16. A National Protocol for Sexual Assault Medical Forensic Examinations: Adults/Adolescents, 2nd ed. https://www.ncjrs.gov/pdffiles1/ovw/241903.pdf. Accessed April 2018.
17. Centers for Disease Control and Prevention. *2015 Sexually Transmitted Diseases Treatment Guidelines. Sexual Assault and Abuse and STDs.* https://www.cdc.gov/std/tg2015/sexual-assault.htm. Accessed March 2017.
18. Bass JK, Annan J, McIvor Murray S, et al. Controlled trial of psychotherapy for Congolese survivors of sexual violence. *N Engl J Med.* 2013;368(23):2182-2191.

19. Sumner SA, Mercy JA, Dahlberg LL, et al. Violence in the United States: status, challenges, and opportunities. *JAMA*. 2015;314(5):478-488.
20. Foshee V, Bauman KE, Ennett ST, et al. Assessing the long-term effects of the Safe Dates program and a booster in preventing and reducing adolescent dating violence victimization and perpetration. *Am J Public Health*. 2004;94:619-624.
21. Senn CY, Eliasziw M, Barata PC, et al. Efficacy of a sexual assault resistance program for university women. *N Engl J Med*. 2015;372(24):2326-2335.
22. Centers for Disease Control and Prevention. *Sexual Violence: Prevention Strategies*. https://www.cdc.gov/violenceprevention/sexualviolence/prevention.html. Accessed April 2018.
23. Moyer VA; U.S. Preventive Services Task Force. Screening for intimate partner violence and abuse of elderly and vulnerable adults: U.S. Preventive Services Task Force recommendation statement. *Ann Intern Med*. 2013;158(6):478-486.
24. McFarlane J, Maddoux J, Cesario S, et al. Effect of abuse during pregnancy on maternal and child safety and functioning for 24 months after delivery. *Obstet Gynecol*. 2014;123(4):839-847.
25. Chen LP, Murad MH, Paras ML, et al. Sexual abuse and lifetime diagnosis of psychiatric disorders: systematic review and meta-analysis. *Mayo Clin Proc*. 2010;85(7):618-629.
26. Paras ML, Murad MH, Chen LP, et al. Sexual abuse and lifetime diagnosis of somatic disorders: a systematic review and meta-analysis. *JAMA*. 2009;302(5):550-561.
27. Walsh K, Danielson CK, McCauley JL, et al. National prevalence of posttraumatic stress disorder among sexually revictimized adolescent, college, and adult household-residing women. *Arch Gen Psychiatry*. 2012;69(9):935-942.
28. Padala PR, Madison J, Monnahan M, et al. Risperidone monotherapy for post-traumatic stress disorder related to sexual assault and domestic abuse in women. *Int Clin Psychopharmacol*. 2006;21(5):275-280.
29. Vickerman KA, Margolin G. Rape treatment outcome research: empirical findings and state of the literature. *Clin Psychol Rev*. 2009;29:431-448.
30. Burgess AW, Holmstrom LL. Adaptive strategies and recovery from rape. *Am J Psychiatry*. 1979;136:1278-1282.

13 LESBIAN GAY BISEXUAL TRANSGENDER HEALTH ISSUES

Ronni Hayon, MD
Jarrett Sell, MD
Matthew Witthaus, MD

CARE FOR SEXUAL-MINORITY PATIENTS

PATIENT STORY

Ana is a 35-year-old woman who presents for a routine physical. In the past, you have discussed her social history and learned that she is divorced, has one child from that relationship, and has had a healthy relationship with her current live-in boyfriend for about 5 years. In reviewing her social history today, you inquire about relationships and she shares that she and her boyfriend have an open relationship and that she has had one new male partner and two new female partners in the past 3 months. She identifies as bisexual and polyamorous. She is "fluid bonded" (does not use barrier methods) with her primary partner, but uses barriers with her other partners. You offer STI screening today and together plan for regular screening in the future.

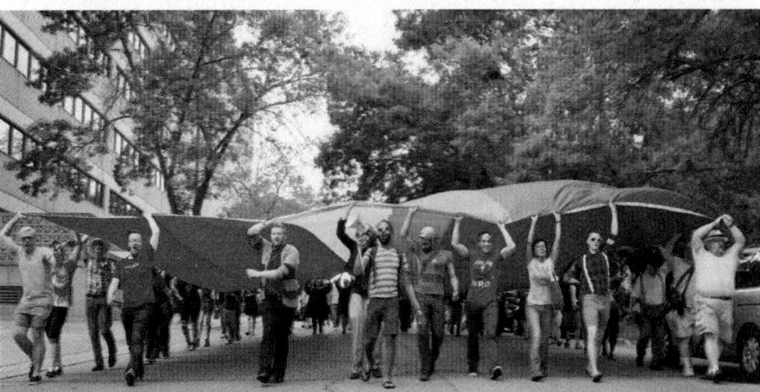

FIGURE 13-1 Marchers at a marriage equality rally in Madison, Wisconsin, holding a rainbow flag, sometimes referred to as the gay pride flag or LGBT pride flag. The rainbow flag is a symbol of lesbian, gay, bisexual, transgender and queer pride, and of LGBTQ social movements. (*Reproduced with permission of Dutcher Photography LLC.*)

INTRODUCTION

The term "sexual minority" is an umbrella term that encompasses people whose sexual orientation, practices or identity differ from that of the larger surrounding society (**Figures 13-1** and **13-2**). Most commonly, it is used to refer to people who identify as lesbian, gay, bisexual, or queer.[1] **Table 13-1** lists descriptions of sexual minority populations.

- Population-based surveys show prevalence rates of sexual-minority adults in the United States ranging from 2.2% to 4.0%, depending on which survey is used.[2] Depending on how these questions are asked, and how safe respondents feel about answering these sensitive questions, surveys may not be an accurate reflection of prevalence and may underestimate rates of same-sex attraction and sexual behaviors.
- Based on 2013 National Health Interview Survey (NHIS) data, the Centers for Disease Control and Prevention (CDC) reported that among adults in the United States, 1.6% identified as gay or lesbian, 0.7% identified as bisexual, and 1.1% identified as "something else," declined to answer, or stated "I don't know."[3] NHIS data also showed significant differences in health status, healthcare service utilization, health-related behaviors, and healthcare access when comparing sexual minority people to those who identify as straight.

Cultural competency is an important aspect of providing care to sexual-minority patients. General tips for providing sensitive care include using open-ended questions with neutral language when taking social histories, avoiding assumptions about sexual behaviors, posting nondiscrimination statements that include sexual orientation, and displaying posters and reading materials that are inclusive of and friendly to sexual-minority patients.

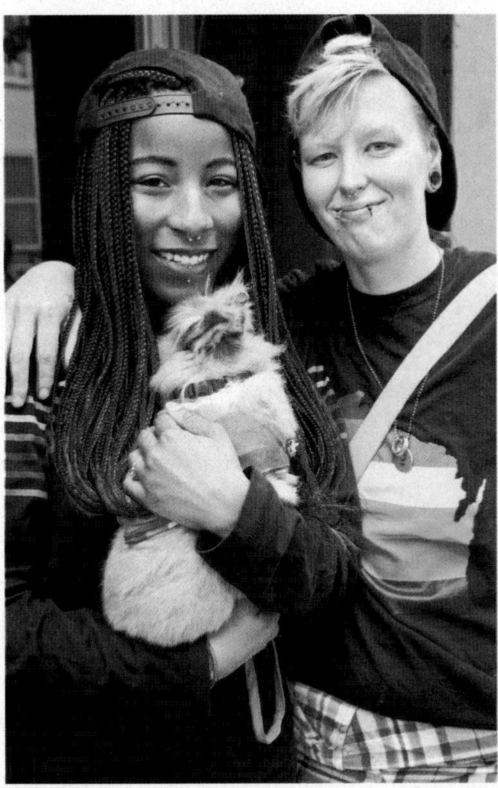

FIGURE 13-2 Two young people at a marriage equality rally in Madison, Wisconsin. (*Reproduced with permission of Dutcher Photography LLC.*)

TABLE 13-1 Sexual Minority Identities/Behaviors

Asexuality	Sexual orientation characterized by little to no sexual attraction to others. Distinct from celibacy, which is a choice rather than a sexual orientation. Also distinct from sexual interest/arousal disorders, defined in DSM-5, which, by definition, cause significant distress. Like heterosexual or other sexual-minority people, asexual individuals have emotional needs that can be met through a rich variety of relationships, friendships, and partnerships.[36,68,69]
Bisexuality	Sexual or romantic attraction, or sexual activity, with members of both sexes.
Nonmonogamy	Umbrella term that describes a relationship in which two people are not sexually exclusive. Includes many types of relationships that vary in structure, degree of sexual openness, and emotional attachment.[70]
Open relationship	Consensual nonmonogamous relationship that centers around a primary couple who agree to sexual contact with others (e.g., long-term dyad who has sexual contact with a 3rd partner), while maintaining the primary relationship as a priority. Partners outside the primary dyad are considered secondary.[70]
Pansexuality	Sexual orientation characterized by enduring physical, romantic, and/or emotional attractions to people of all genders and sexes. This includes, but is not limited to, gender-expansive people.[67]
Polyamory	Also somewhat of an umbrella term. Relationship-oriented approach to nonmonogamy where multiple consensual relationships are practiced with a focus on consent, ethical behavior, and agreement.[71]
Queer	Traditionally, a pejorative term used against people who were LGBTQ or perceived to be so. Recently, the term has been reclaimed by the LGBTQ community. "Queer" can be used as an umbrella term for LGBTQ to describe a sexual orientation that breaks binary thinking and recognizes sexual orientation and gender as potentially fluid, and as a simple label to describe a complex and varied set of sexual behaviors and desires. *Given its history as a slur, unless given express permission, clinicians should not use this term to describe or refer to their patients.*[66]
Swinging	Sex-oriented approach to nonmonogamy. A couple may seek sexual partners outside the primary relationship, but the focus is on sexual exploration rather than emotional attachments/intimacy with multiple partners.[71]

DSM, Diagnostic and Statistical Manual of Mental Disorders; LGBT, lesbian, gay, bisexual, transgender, queer.

MEDICAL ISSUES

SEXUAL HEALTH

- Obtain a complete sexual history (behavior, orientation, identity, function, and contentment—see **Table 13-2**).
  - Keep in mind that behavior may not always correlate with identity (e.g., a male who identifies as heterosexual but has sexual contact with other men).
- Sexually transmitted infections (STIs)
  - Epidemiology
    - Men who have sex with men (MSM) experience disproportionately higher rates of STIs than straight men.
    - Human immunodeficiency virus (HIV) disproportionately affects MSM and transgender women (woman who was assigned male gender at birth).
    - In 2014, most (67%) of new HIV infections were in MSM and over half of the people living with HIV were MSM.[4]

TABLE 13-2 Aspects of Sexual History for Sexual Minority Patients

Behavior	Gender of partners Number of current and lifetime partners Type of relationships (e.g., monogamous, open relationship, casual) Safer sex practices (e.g., condoms, vaccinations, pre-exposure prophylaxis) Transactional sex (sex in exchange for money, food, drugs or shelter)
Orientation and identity	Sexual orientation is the inclination to develop romantic and sexual feelings for or relationships with the same or different gender Sexual identity is how individuals describe their sexuality (e.g., lesbian, gay, bisexual, straight)
Function and contentment	Sexual desire and drive Sexual functioning (e.g., pleasure, arousal, orgasm, erectile dysfunction, vaginal atrophy)
Safety	Past or current sexual abuse or IPV
STI history	Personal and partner history of STI

IPV, intimate partner violence; STI, sexually transmitted infection.
Information from Daskalakis DC, Radix A, Mayer G. Sexual health. In: Makadon HJ, Mayer KH, Potter J, Goldhammer H, eds. *Fenway Guide to Lesbian, Gay, Bisexual & Transgender Health*, 2nd ed. Chelsea, MI: Sheridan Books; 2015:289-324.

TABLE 13-3 Sexually Transmitted Disease Screening Recommendations

HIV	One lifetime screen for all persons ages 13–64 years Screen all who seek evaluation and treatment for STIs Retest at least annually for those at increased risk of acquiring HIV*
Syphilis	At least annually for sexually-active MSM and people participating in transactional sex Screen every 3-6 months for MSM who have multiple or anonymous partners Screen at least once for persons in adult correctional facilities
Chlamydia and gonorrhea	Annual screening for all sexually active women <25 years Annual screening for women >25 years with risk factors** Annual screening for people who are HIV+ Screen every 3–6 months in MSM with risk factors*** Urine NAAT if insertive intercourse in preceding year Rectal NAAT if receptive anal intercourse in preceding year Pharyngeal NAAT for GC only if receptive oral sex in preceding year
Hepatitis B	Screen MSM once with serum antigen and vaccinate if uninfected and no documentation of past vaccination
Hepatitis C	Annually for HIV positive MSM Annually for all injection drug users One lifetime screening for all persons born between 1945 and 1965

*Includes: MSM who themselves or their sex partners have had more than one sex partner since their most recent HIV test, injection drug users and their sex partners, persons participating in transactional sex, sex partners of HIV-infected persons.
**New or multiple sex partners, sex partner with an STI, inconsistent condom use if not in mutually monogamous relationship, previous or concurrent STI, transactional sex.
***Sex with multiple or anonymous partners, sex in relation to illicit drug use, partners participating in these activities.
GC, *Neisseria gonorrhoeae*; HIV, human immunodeficiency virus; MSM, men who have sex with men; NAAT, nucleic acid amplification test; STI, sexually transmitted infection.
Information from: Moyer VA. Screening for HIV: U.S. Preventive Services Task Force Recommendation Statement. *Ann Intern Med.* 2013;159(1):51-60; Centers for Disease Control and Prevention. Revised recommendations for HIV testing of adults, adolescents, and pregnant women in health-care settings. *MMWR.* 2006;55(No. RR-14):1-17; U.S. Preventive Services Task Force. Screening for syphilis infection: Recommendation Statement. *Ann Fam Med.* 2004;2(4):362-365. doi:10.1370/afm.215; Workowski KA, Bolan GA. Sexually transmitted diseases treatment guidelines, 2015. *MMWR Recomm Rep.* 2015;64(No. RR-3):1-137; LeFevre ML. Screening for chlamydia and gonorrhea: U.S. Preventive Services Task Force Recommendation Statement. *Ann Intern Med.* 2014;161(12): 902-910; Garg S, Taylor LE, Grasso C, Mayer KH. Prevalent and incident hepatitis C virus infection among HIV-infected men who have sex with men engaged in primary care in a Boston community health center. *Clin Infect Dis.* 2013;56(10):1480-1487; Moyer VA. Screening for hepatitis C virus in adults: U.S. Preventive Services Task Force Recommendation Statement. *Ann Intern Med.* 2013;159(5):349-358.

        - In a 2013 meta-analysis, 19% of transgender women worldwide were HIV positive.[5]
        - Syphilis also disproportionately affects MSM. The CDC estimated in 2015 that 60% of primary and secondary cases of syphilis occurred in MSM.[6]
        - MSM who are HIV positive are thought to be at increased risk for sexually acquired hepatitis C.[7]
    - Screening recommendations are displayed in **Table 13-3**.
    - Education and counseling for risk reduction
        - Educate on relative risk of different sexual practices allowing patients to determine the level of risk they are willing to accept.
        - Activities with highest to lowest risk: receptive anal intercourse, insertive anal intercourse, distantly followed by receptive and insertive oral sex.[8]
        - Insertive sex toys shared between partners can transmit HIV, hepatitis A, and hepatitis B. Reduce risk by not sharing toys, cleaning with bleach, and using them with condoms.[9]
        - Barrier use, such as latex condoms, decreases the risk of HIV and STI transmission.[8,9]
        - Avoid even brief unprotected anal penetration, as HIV is present in pre-ejaculate.[10]

PREVENTIVE CARE

- Immunizations
    - All routine immunizations per CDC guidelines.
    - Special considerations for MSM: Hep A, Hep B vaccines recommended.[11]
- Cancer Screening
    - Mammogram and Pap smear: per U.S. Preventive Services Task Force (USPSTF) guidelines. Same screening recommendations as for straight women.[12,13]
        - Lesbian and bisexual women are 10 times less likely to receive cervical cancer screening than straight women, even though they are just as likely to develop cervical cancer.[13]

- Anal cancer screening with anal Pap smear: Although some experts recommend yearly screening,[14] there are insufficient data to support routine screening with anal Pap smears, even among high-risk groups (MSM, HIV-positive or immunosuppressed patients).[15]
  - If anal Pap is performed, abnormal results should be followed with high-resolution anoscopy, which is not available in all settings.[16]
- Weight Management
  - Lesbian and bisexual women are more likely to be overweight and obese than straight women.[17]
  - Gay and bisexual men are more likely to have body dissatisfaction and eating disorders than straight men.[18,19]

SUBSTANCE USE

- Tobacco
  - Twenty-seven percent of gay and lesbian adults and 29% of bisexual adults reported being current smokers compared to 19% of straight adults in the 2013 NHIS.[3]
- Alcohol
  - Thirty-five percent of gay and lesbian adults and 41% of bisexual adults reported having five or more drinks in one day at least once in the past year compared to 26% of straight adults in the NHIS.[3]
- Drug Use
  - Stimulants (methamphetamine and cocaine), erectile dysfunction drugs (PDE5 inhibitors), and alkyl nitrites ("poppers") are associated with high-risk sexual behavior and higher rates of HIV among MSM.[20–23]

PSYCHOSOCIAL ISSUES

COMING OUT

- "Coming out" is a lifelong process in which LGBTQ people disclose their sexual orientation or identity to others.
  - Positive consequences may include finding support through family, the LGBTQ community, and/or positive romantic relationships that help validate one's true sense of self (**Figure 13-3**).[24]
  - Negative consequences may include discrimination, rejection, and violence.
- Healthcare providers can help by normalizing the romantic and sexual attraction of the patient.[25]

MENTAL HEALTH

- Primary care providers should routinely screen sexual-minority patients for mental health disorders, bullying and victimization.[26,27] See Patient Resources below for a list of resources for behavioral health.
- Minority stress model: explains how stigma, prejudice, and discrimination create a hostile and stressful social environment that causes mental health problems for LGBTQ individuals.[28]
  - Stressors are unique, chronic and socially based (e.g., experience of prejudice events, expectations of rejection, hiding and concealing, internalized homophobia, and ameliorative coping processes).[28]
  - Minority stress has been shown to increase the odds of experiencing a physical health problem.[29]

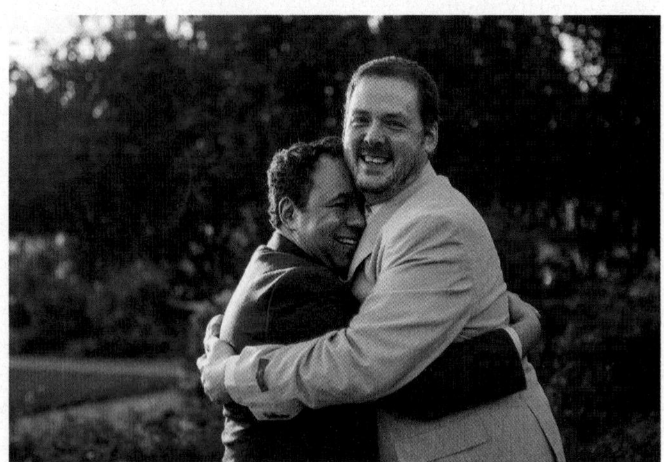

FIGURE 13-3 Daniel and Seth embracing on their wedding day. *(Reproduced with permission of Dutcher Photography LLC.)*

- Gay and bisexual males in high school have been shown to have significantly higher odds of suicidal ideation and suicide attempts than straight males.[30]
- LGB individuals who report recent discrimination or who report not discussing discrimination have higher rates of mood, anxiety, and substance use disorders and higher odds of mental health disorders, respectively.[31]
- LGB young adults who experienced higher levels of family rejection were more likely to report a suicide attempt, high levels of depression, and more likely to use illegal drugs than peers who experience no or low levels of family rejection.[32]

HOMELESSNESS

- In a 2012 Williams Institute survey of Homeless Youth Organizations, 39% of all of their clients identified as LGB and 26% of clients utilizing housing programs identified as LGB (making this an overrepresented group).[33]

FAMILY PLANNING (see Patient Resources below)

- Adoption and Foster Parenting
  - Same-sex couples are four times more likely to be raising an adopted child and six times more likely to be raising a foster child than their different-sex counterparts.[34]
  - Adopting children can take 12–36 months to match the adoptive parent(s) and child.[35]
  - Public adoptions are approximately $2000, whereas private adoptions range from $20,000 to $35,000.[35]
- Assisted Reproduction
  - Options include donor insemination, in vitro fertilization (IVF), surrogacy.
  - Insurance coverage and costs are variable.

CARE OF TRANSGENDER AND GENDER-NONCONFORMING PATIENTS

PATIENT STORY

Gavin is a 25-year-old patient who was assigned female at birth but has been living for many years in accordance with his male gender identity. He presents to discuss starting gender-affirming therapy with testosterone. Gavin is employed at the state university and has a long-term non-transgender male partner. He wonders if his benefits, which are administered by the state, will cover gender-related care. He has never had a Pap smear, and expresses significant fear and worry about this sort of exam. He asks if having a Pap smear is a requirement for starting hormones. He also mentions that he and his partner would like to have children someday, but they are not ready to be parents right now, and he very much wants to start hormones as soon as possible.

INTRODUCTION

The terms "transgender," "gender nonconforming," "trans," and "gender-expansive" are umbrella terms that broadly encompass anyone whose identity or behavior falls outside of stereotypical gender norms (**Figure 13-4**). More narrowly defined, it refers to an individual whose gender identity (internal sense of being male, female, or something else) does not match their assigned birth sex. Some

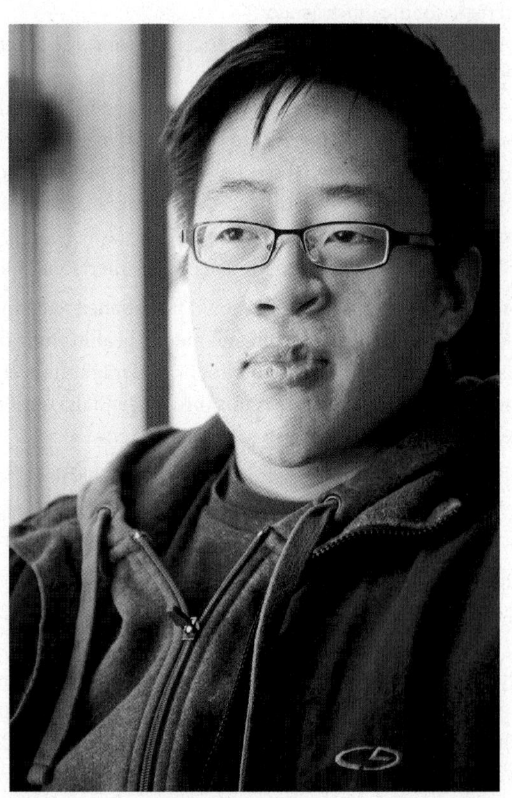

FIGURE 13-4 Ray M, a trans-identified person and roller derby enthusiast. (*Reproduced with permission of Dutcher Photography LLC.*)

transgender people will choose to pursue gender-affirming therapies such as hormonal medications and/or surgeries, but not all transgender individuals desire these interventions.

As with sexual-minority populations, cultural competency is an important aspect of providing care to gender-nonconforming patients. General tips for providing sensitive care include using open-ended questions with neutral language when taking social histories, asking which name and pronouns to use, avoiding unnecessary questioning about gender, avoiding assumptions about gender identity or plans for transition, having gender-neutral bathrooms available to patients, and posting nondiscrimination statements that include gender identity and expression.

DIAGNOSIS OF GENDER DYSPHORIA

- The definition of Gender Dysphoria in children, adolescents and adults is found in the *Diagnostic and Statistical Manual of Mental Disorders* (DSM-5).[36] Diagnosing gender dysphoria requires associated clinically significant distress or impairment in social, occupational, or other important areas of functioning.
    - To diagnose Gender Dysphoria in adolescents and adults, two of the following criteria must also be met[36]:
        - A marked incongruence between one's experienced/expressed gender and primary and/or secondary sex characteristics (or in young adolescents, the anticipated secondary sex characteristics).
        - A strong desire to be rid of one's primary and/or secondary sex characteristics because of a marked incongruence with one's experienced/expressed gender (or in young adolescents, a desire to prevent the development of the anticipated secondary sex characteristics).
        - A strong desire for the primary and/or secondary sex characteristics of the other gender.
        - A strong desire to be of the other gender (or some alternative gender different from one's assigned gender).
        - A strong desire to be treated as the other gender (or some alternative gender different from one's assigned gender).
        - A strong conviction that one has the typical feelings and reactions of the other gender (or some alternative gender different from one's assigned gender).
    - DSM-5 should be consulted for diagnostic criteria for children.
- A complete history and physical should be obtained with an emphasis on sexual development and mental health, while fully assessing any chronic medical conditions that might impact care.
    - Consider delaying sensitive exams (breast, genitals) until rapport is established.
- Health disparities: Recent data from the Behavioral Risk Factors Surveillance System show that gender-minority people are more likely to report depression, be overweight, be unemployed, have lower income, be uninsured, and have unmet medical needs due to cost.[37]

LABORATORY TESTING

- For individuals interested in starting gender-affirming hormone therapy, consider baseline labs that may be affected by hormones (complete blood count [CBC], complete metabolic panel [CMP], lipids).[38] SOR Ⓒ
- Consider bone density testing, coagulation testing, or cardiovascular risk stratification if patient is at risk.[38] SOR Ⓒ

DIFFERENTIAL DIAGNOSIS

- Gender nonconformity (behavior and appearance that does not conform to social gender expectations while maintaining a gender identity that is congruent with birth sex).
- Body dysmorphic disorder (distress due to a perceived issue with one's appearance).
- Mood disorders (see Chapter 238, Mental Health).
- A systematic review demonstrated a co-occurrence of gender dysphoria and autism spectrum disorder.[39]

MANAGEMENT

- Individuals who identify as transgender or gender nonconforming may opt to not pursue medical or surgical treatment options for a variety of reasons. Care should be individualized with the goal of maximizing overall health and psychological well-being.[40]
- Discuss family planning before initiating treatment. SOR Ⓒ
    - The Ethics Committee of the American Society for Reproductive Medicine concluded that denial of access to fertility services for transgender individuals is not justified.[41]

▶ Nonpharmacologic treatment

- Phytoestrogens and other herbals have not been adequately studied in cross-sex hormone therapy, but may be options explored by patients.
- Mental health providers with gender experience can assist with diagnosis and exploration of management options.

▶ Medications

- To begin gender-affirming hormone therapy, The World Professional Association for Transgender Health (WPATH) Standards of Care recommend that an individual demonstrate the following[40]:
    - Persistent, well-documented gender dysphoria.
    - Capacity to make a fully informed decision and consent for treatment.
    - Demonstrable knowledge of what hormones can and cannot do.
    - Reasonably controlled medical and/or mental health conditions.
    - A letter of support from a qualified mental health professional to the prescribing clinician is recommended, but not required.

Feminizing treatment

- Goals of feminizing hormones should be individualized and may include breast growth, fat/muscle redistribution, and reduction in gender dysphoria.
- A combination of estrogen and an anti-androgen is typically used for feminizing hormone therapy in the following dose ranges:
    - Oral estradiol 2–6 mg/d divided twice daily.
    - Transdermal estradiol patches 0.1–0.4 mg weekly or biweekly.
    - Estradiol valerate 5–20 mg intramuscularly (IM) every 2 weeks.
    - Spironolactone 100–400 mg/d orally (cyproterone acetate is used in Europe).
    - Finasteride 2.5–5 mg/day.
- Ask about nonprescription treatment. A cross-sectional study showed that one in four trans women self-prescribe gender-affirming hormones before being evaluated at a gender clinic.[42]

- Monitoring
  - Recommendations from the Endocrine Society include checking testosterone, estradiol, CBC, CMP, and lipids every 3 months in the first year of treatment and then 1–2 times annually. Prolactin can also be monitored periodically for those on estrogen.[38] SOR C
  - Monitoring recommendations from the University of California at San Francisco (UCSF) Center of Excellence for Transgender Health highlight more conservative monitoring strategies and the limited evidence available to guide testing frequency.[43]
  - Goal serum estradiol is typically 100–200 pg/mL and goal total testosterone is <55 ng/dL.
- Estradiol can be given transdermally, orally or sublingually. The bioavailability of sublingual estradiol is greater than oral and bypasses the liver, which is thought to reduce thromboembolic risk.[44]
  - Topical or injectable estrogen is considered less thrombogenic than oral and safer for use at older ages (35–45 years).[45] SOR C
  - Ethinyl estradiol should be avoided due to higher risk of thromboembolic disease and cardiovascular disease.[45] SOR B
- The addition of progestins has not been shown to improve breast growth, although patients often anecdotally report achieving a more natural breast shape with its use.[46] Potential adverse effects include depression, weight gain, and dyslipidemia.
- A prospective cohort study of 53 trans women followed for 12 months on cyproterone acetate and estradiol found the following significant effects[47]:
  - Three of 53 had transient elevation of liver enzymes.
  - Increased breast tenderness, hot flashes, emotional lability.
  - Decreased libido.
  - Increased fasting insulin, total body fat mass, and prolactin.
  - Decreased waist-hip ratio, lean mass, total cholesterol, and low-density lipids.

Masculinizing treatment

- Goals of masculinizing hormones using testosterone should be individualized and may include facial and body hair growth, clitoral enlargement, fat/muscle redistribution, and reduction in gender dysphoria.
- Monitoring:
  - Recommendations from the Endocrine Society include checking testosterone, CMP, CBC, and lipids every 3 months and then every 6–12 months while on treatment.[38] SOR C
  - Monitoring recommendations from the UCSF Center of Excellence for Transgender Health highlight more conservative monitoring strategies and the limited evidence available to guide testing frequency.[43]
  - Goal serum total testosterone is typically 300–750 ng/dL.
- Testosterone is typically prescribed as testosterone cypionate 50–200 mg IM every 2 weeks OR 25–100 mg IM once weekly OR as varying doses of transdermal testosterone (patches, gel, or cream). Note that this is a painful injection and requires frequent visits for ongoing therapy. Subcutaneous testosterone is not FDA approved but may be an effective alternative to intramuscular injections.[48,49]
- A prospective cohort study of 53 trans men followed for 12 months on injectable testosterone undecanoate every 3 months found the following significant effects[47]:
  - Increased sexual desire, voice instability, and clitoral pain.
  - Increased acne, facial/body hair, and androgenic alopecia.
  - Increased waist-hip ratio, muscle mass, triglycerides, total cholesterol, and low-density lipids.
  - Decreased total body fat mass and high-density lipids.
  - Two of 53 had erythrocytosis.
  - Two of 53 had liver enzyme elevation.

▶ Surgical management

- WPATH recommends one referral/letter of support for breast/chest surgery and two referrals for genital surgery from qualified health professionals.[40]
- Common surgical techniques for male-to-female gender confirmation in trans women consist of facial feminization surgery, voice surgery, breast augmentation, orchiectomy, and vaginoplasty.
- Common surgical techniques for female-to-male gender confirmation in trans men include bilateral subcutaneous mastectomy (with chest reconstruction) and phalloplasty procedures.
- A retrospective cohort study showed that 62.4% of trans women reported a decrease in sexual desire and 71% of trans men reported an increase in sexual desire after gender-confirmation surgery.[50]

PREVENTION

▶ Cancer

- Transgender individuals should continue to be screened in accordance with cancer screening recommendations for the general population based on organs that remain present, such as a prostate in transgender women or a cervix in transgender men.[38] SOR C
- An increase in breast cancer risk in transgender individuals was not seen with gender-affirming hormone therapy in a U.S. Veterans Health Administration cohort study[51] nor a Dutch cohort[52] when compared to the general population.
  - Offer screening mammography every 2 years to transgender women who have been on gender-affirming hormones for 5–10 years and who are ≥50 years.[43]
- No patients developed hormone-related cancers in a single-center cross-sectional study of 100 patients after gender confirmation surgery and, on average, 10 years of gender-affirming hormones.[53]

▶ Cardiovascular and thromboembolic risk

- The incidence of cardiovascular mortality has been found to be 123 per 100,000 person-years in male to female (MTF) people (95% CI: 73–173) and 15 per 100,000 person-years in female to male (FTM) people (95% CI: 1–68).[45]
- A retrospective cohort study of 816 FTM patients showed a 20-fold higher risk of thromboembolic disease.[54]
- Several cohort studies of FTM on testosterone up to a median duration of 18.5 years have not shown an increase in cardiovascular morbidity or mortality.[45]
- Several studies in older non-transgender men have shown an increased risk of cardiovascular disease with use of testosterone,[55–57] but it is not clear if this applies to trans men; studies in this population are often smaller and with younger participants.

▶ Bone health

- One quarter of trans women had osteoporosis in a single-center cross-sectional study of 100 patients after gender-confirmation surgery and, on average, 10 years of gender-affirming hormones.[53]

▶ Human immunodeficiency virus (HIV) prevention

- Recommend a single lifetime HIV screening test in accordance with USPSTF/AAFP/AAP recommendations for all patients, with more frequent testing based on risk. SOR Ⓐ
- Consider pre-exposure prophylaxis for at-risk transgender women who have a high risk of HIV.[58] SOR Ⓒ
    - Authors of a systematic review found a prevalence of HIV infection of 19.1% in transgender women worldwide.[5]
    - In 2008 in the United States, authors of a systematic review found that 27.7% of MTF people tested positive for HIV, with 56.3% of African-American MTF individuals being HIV-infected.[59]

▶ Mental health

- In an observational study in Chicago and Boston, young transgender women (ages 16–29 years) had a 41.5% prevalence of one or more mental health or substance dependence diagnoses.[60]
- A cohort study of 73 socially transitioned transgender prepubescent children did not show higher rates of depression and only minimally higher rates of anxiety compared with a matched control group—demonstrating the importance of social and community support.[61]
- Gay–straight alliances, which are school-based organizations for LGBTQ youth, have been shown in a meta-analysis to significantly lower rates of youth's self-reports of homophobic victimization, fear for safety, and hearing homophobic remarks (**Figure 13-5**).[62]

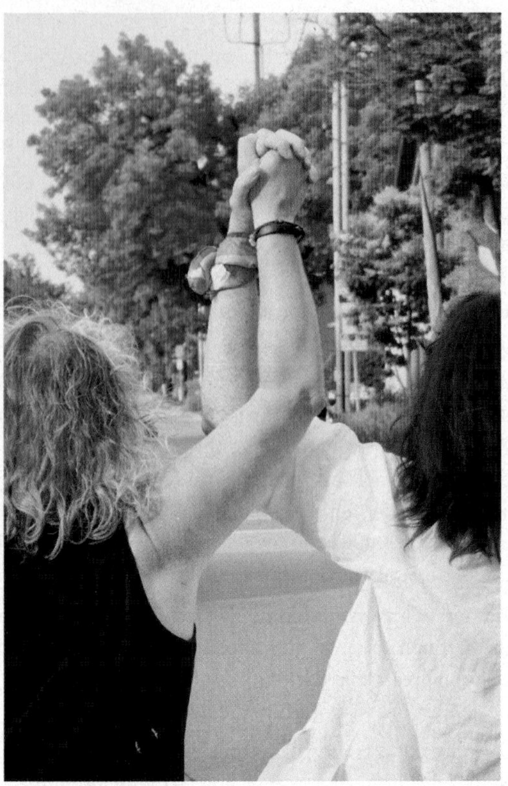

FIGURE 13-5 Two people marching hand in hand at a marriage equality rally in Madison, Wisconsin. (*Reproduced with permission of Dutcher Photography LLC.*)

PROGNOSIS

- The number of children with gender dysphoria that persists into adulthood has been reported as 2.2% to 30% for natal males and 12% to 50% in natal females.[36,63]
- A retrospective cohort study of 127 adolescents with gender dysphoria showed that the intensity of early gender dysphoria was predictive of persistence, and that natal girls were more likely to have gender dysphoria persist into adolescence.[64]
- A systematic review of the effects of hormone therapy found three uncontrolled prospective cohort studies that identified improvements in psychological functioning and quality of life a year after initiation of hormone therapy.[65]
- A cohort study of 966 MTF individuals with 18.5 years of median follow-up showed that total mortality was 51% higher than in the general population. This increased mortality was due to suicide, acquired immunodeficiency syndrome, cardiovascular disease, and drug abuse. No increase was observed in total cancer mortality, but lung and hematologic cancer mortality rates were elevated.[48]

FOLLOW-UP

- See patients starting gender-affirming hormone therapy every 3 months for the first year and then every 6–12 months for monitoring of laboratory testing, physical changes, and a current understanding of medical and mental health.

PATIENT RESOURCES

- AdoptUSKids: **adoptuskids.org**.
- CDC: Lesbian, Gay, Bisexual, and Transgender Health: **www.cdc.gov/lgbthealth**.
- Family Equality Council (FEC): **www.familyequality.org**.
- Fenway Health's Violence Recovery Program: **http://fenwayhealth.org/care/behavioral-health/violence-recovery/** (provides counseling, support groups, advocacy and referral services to LGBTQ victims).
- GLBT National Help Center/Hotline: **https://www.glbthotline.org**.
- Human Rights Campaign (HRC): **www.hrc.org**.
- Lambda Legal: **www.lambdalegal.org**.
- National Alliance on Mental Illness: LGBTQ Information and Resources webpage. **https://www.nami.org/Find-Support/LGBTQ**.
- National LGBT Health Education Center, a program of the Fenway Institute: **www.lgbthealtheducation.org**.
- Parents, Families, and Friends of LGBT People (PFLAG): **www.pflag.org**.
- Path2Parenthood: **www.path2parenthood.org/start-your-journey**.
- The Trevor Project: **www.thetrevorproject.org** (provides crisis intervention and suicide prevention to LGBTQ young people ages 13–24 years)
- Transline, a national online transgender medical consultation service: **http://project-health.org/transline/**.

PROVIDER RESOURCES

- American Psychological Association: Guidelines for psychological practice with lesbian, gay, and bisexual clients: **http://www.apa.org/pi/lgbt/resources/guidelines.aspx**.
- Endocrine Treatment of Transsexual Persons: An Endocrine Society Clinical Practice Guideline, 2009. **https://academic.oup.com/jcem/article/94/9/3132/2596324.**
- Center Link: Database of LGBT community centers across the United States and the world. **www.lgbtcenters.org**.
- Center of Excellence for Transgender Health, University of California, San Francisco (UCSF): **http://transhealth.ucsf.edu.**
- LGBT Health and Human Services Toolkit: A toolkit to help professionals recognize and measure risky health behaviors among LGBT individuals and assess their level of social support, social isolation, self-esteem, access to healthcare, and general attitudes and knowledge. Includes scoring guides. **http://lgbttobacco.org/files/AI_Eval_Indicator_Toolkit.pdf**.
- The World Professional Association for Transgender Health (WPATH) *Standards of Care,* 7th ed. **https://www.wpath.org/.**

REFERENCES

1. Mayer KH, Bradford JB, Makadon HJ, et al. Sexual and gender minority health: what we know and what needs to be done. *Am J Public Health*. 2008;98(6):989-995.
2. Gates GJ. *LGBT Demographics: Comparisons among Population-Based Surveys Executive Summary*. NHIS; 2014. https://williaminstitute.law.ucla.edu/wp-content/uploads/lgbt-demogs-sep-2014.pdf. Accessed August 2017.
3. Ward BW, Dahlhamer JM, Galinsky AM, Joestl SS. Sexual orientation and health among U.S. adults: national health interview survey, 2013. *Natl Health Stat Report*. 2014;(77):1-10. http://www.ncbi.nlm.nih.gov/pubmed/25025690. Accessed January 2015.
4. Hess K, Dailey A, Johnson AS, et al. Diagnoses of HIV infection in the United States and dependent areas, 2015. *HIV Surveill Rep*. 2015;3(27). http://www.cdc.gov/hiv/library/reports/hiv-surveillance.html. Accessed August 2017.
5. Baral SD, Poteat T, Strömdahl S, et al. Worldwide burden of HIV in transgender women: a systematic review and meta-analysis. *Lancet Infect Dis*. 2013;13(3):214-222.
6. Centers for Disease Control. Sexually transmitted disease surveillance 2015. *Cent Dis Control Prev*. 2015:1-156.
7. Garg S, Taylor LE, Grasso C, Mayer KH. Prevalent and incident hepatitis C virus infection among HIV-infected men who have sex with men engaged in primary care in a Boston community health center. *Clin Infect Dis*. 2013;56(10):1480-1487.
8. Varghese B, Maher JE, Peterman TA, et al. Reducing the risk of sexual HIV transmission: quantifying the per-act risk for HIV on the basis of choice of partner, sex act, and condom use. *Sex Transm Dis*. 2002;29(1):38-43.
9. Workowski KA, Bolan GA, Centers for Disease Control and Prevention. Sexually transmitted diseases treatment guidelines, 2015. *MMWR Recomm Reports* 2015;64(RR-03):1-137. http://www.ncbi.nlm.nih.gov/pubmed/26042815. Accessed August 2017.
10. Pudney J, Oneta M, Mayer K, et al. Pre-ejaculatory fluid as potential vector for sexual transmission of HIV-1. *Lancet*. 1992; 340(8833):1470.
11. Centers for Disease Control and Prevention. *Recommended Immunization Schedule for Adults Aged 19 Years or Older by Medical Conditions and Other Indications, United States, 2018.* https://www.cdc.gov/vaccines/schedules/hcp/imz/adult-conditions.html. Accessed March 2018.
12. Screening for breast cancer: U.S. Preventive Services Task Force recommendation statement. *Ann Intern Med*. 2009;151(10):716-726.
13. Peitzmeier SM. *Promoting Cervical Cancer Screening Among Lesbians and Bisexual Women*; 2013. http://fenwayhealth.org/documents/the-fenway-institute/policy-briefs/PolicyFocus_cervicalcancer_web.pdf. Accessed August 2017.
14. Panel on Antiretroviral Guidelines for Adults and Adolescents. *Guidelines for the Use of Antiretroviral Agents in HIV-1-Infected Adults and Adolescents*; 2016. http://aidsinfo.nih.gov/contentfiles/lvguidelines/AdultandAdolescentGL.pdf. Accessed September 9, 2017.
15. Liszewski W, Ananth AT, Ploch LE, Rogers NE. Anal Pap smears and anal cancer: what dermatologists should know. *J Am Acad Dermatol*. 2014;71(5):985-992.
16. Dandapani SV, Eaton M, Thomas CR, Pagnini PG. HIV-positive anal cancer: an update for the clinician. *J Gastrointest Oncol*. 2010; 1(1):34-44.

17. Boehmer U, Bowen DJ, Bauer GR. Overweight and obesity in sexual-minority women: evidence from population-based data. *Am J Public Health.* 2007;97(6):1134-1140.
18. French SA, Story M, Remafedi G, et al. Sexual orientation and prevalence of body dissatisfaction and eating disordered behaviors: a population-based study of adolescents. *Int J Eat Disord.* 1996;19(2):119-126.
19. Siever MD. Sexual orientation and gender as factors in socioculturally acquired vulnerability to body dissatisfaction and eating disorders. *J Consult Clin Psychol.* 1994;62(2):252-260.
20. Koblin BA, Husnik MJ, Colfax G, et al. Risk factors for HIV infection among men who have sex with men. *AIDS.* 2006;20(5):731-739.
21. Lea T, Mao L, Bath N, et al. Injecting drug use among gay and bisexual men in Sydney: prevalence and associations with sexual risk practices and HIV and hepatitis C infection. *AIDS Behav.* 2013;17(4):1344-1351.
22. Rajasingham R, Mimiaga MJ, White JM, et al. A systematic review of behavioral and treatment outcome studies among HIV-infected men who have sex with men who abuse crystal methamphetamine. *AIDS Patient Care STDs.* 2012;26(1):36-52.
23. Plankey MW, Ostrow DG, Stall R, et al. The relationship between methamphetamine and popper use and risk of HIV seroconversion in the multicenter AIDS cohort study. *J Acquir Immune Defic Syndr.* 2007;45(1):85-92.
24. Meyer I, Dean L. Stigma and sexual orientation: understanding prejudice against lesbians, gay men, and bisexuals. In: Herek GM, ed. *Stigma and Sexual Orientation: Understanding Prejudice Against Lesbians, Gay Men, and Bisexuals.* SAGE Publications; 1998:160-186.
25. Greenfield J. Coming out: the process of forming a positive identity. In: Makadon HJ, Mayer KH, Potter J, Goldhammer H, eds. *The Fenway Guide to Lesbian, Gay, Bisexual and Transgender Health.* 2nd ed. American College of Physicians; 2015:49-77. https://books.google.com/books?id=tFUkQG_hfMYC&pg=PT61&lpg=PT61&dq=Coming+Out:+The+Process+of+Forming+a+Positive+Identity&source=bl&ots=XoQvm33gJd&sig=i-oCRnbgv-IdSukybrJ9uZusHhQ&hl=en&sa=X&ved=0ahUKEwi0w_jV3frVAhXly4MKHaaUAckQ6AEIKDAA#v=onepage&q=Coming%25. Accessed August 2017.
26. McNamara MC, Ng H. Best practices in LGBT care: a guide for primary care physicians. *Cleve Clin J Med.* 2016;83(7):531 541.
27. Society for Adolescent Health and Medicine. Recommendations for promoting the health and well-being of lesbian, gay, bisexual, and transgender adolescents: a position paper of the Society for Adolescent Health and Medicine. *J Adolesc Health.* 2013;52(4):506-510.
28. Meyer IH. Prejudice, social stress, and mental health in lesbian, gay, and bisexual populations: conceptual issues and research evidence. *Psychol Bull.* 2003;129(5):674-697.
29. Frost DM, Lehavot K, Meyer IH. Minority stress and physical health among sexual minority individuals. *J Behav Med.* 2015;38:1-8.
30. Remafedi G, French S, Story M, et al. The relationship between suicide risk and sexual orientation: results of a population-based study. *Am J Public Health.* 1998;88(1):57-60.
31. McLaughlin KA, Hatzenbuehler ML, Keyes KM. Responses to discrimination and psychiatric disorders among black, Hispanic, female, and lesbian, gay, and bisexual individuals. *Am J Public Health.* 2010;100(8):1477-1484.
32. Ryan C, Huebner D, Diaz RM, Sanchez J. Family rejection as a predictor of negative health outcomes in white and Latino lesbian, gay, and bisexual young adults. *Pediatrics.* 2009;123(1):346-352.
33. Durso LE, Gates GJ. *Serving Our Youth: Findings from a National Survey of Services Providers Working with Lesbian, Gay, Bisexual and Transgender Youth Who Are Homeless or At Risk of Becoming Homeless.* Los Angeles; 2012. https://williamsinstitute.law.ucla.edu/wp-content/uploads/Durso-Gates-LGBT-Homeless-Youth-Survey-July-2012.pdf. Accessed August 2017.
34. Gates GJ. *LGBT Parenting in the United States.* Los Angeles; 2013. http://williamsinstitute.law.ucla.edu/wp-content/uploads/LGBT-Parenting.pdf. Accessed August 2017.
35. Center NLHE. *Pathways to Parenthood for LGBT People*; 2013. https://www.lgbthealtheducation.org/wp-content/uploads/Pathways-to-Parenthood-for-LGBT-People.pdf. Accessed August 2017.
36. American Psychiatric Association. *Diagnostic and Statistical Manual of Mental Disorders, 5th Edition (DSM-5).* American Psychiatric Association; 2016.
37. Streed CG, McCarthy EP, Haas JS. Association between gender minority status and self-reported physical and mental health in the United States. *JAMA Intern Med.* 2017;63(6):985-997.
38. Hembree WC, Cohen-Kettenis P, Delemarre-Van De Waal HA, et al. Endocrine treatment of transsexual persons: an endocrine society clinical practice guideline. *J Clin Endocrinol Metab.* 2009; 94(9):3132-3154.
39. Glidden D, Bouman WP, Jones BA, Arcelus J. Gender dysphoria and autism spectrum disorder: a systematic review of the literature. *Sex Med Rev.* 2016;4(1):3-14.
40. Coleman E, Bockting W, Botzer M, et al. Standards of care for the health of transsexual, transgender, and gender-nonconforming people, version 7. *Int J Transgenderism.* 2012;13(4):165-232.
41. Ethics Committee of the American Society for Reproductive Medicine. Access to fertility services by transgender persons: an Ethics Committee opinion. *Fertil Steril.* 2015;104(5):1111-1115.
42. Mepham N, Bouman WP, Arcelus J, et al. People with gender dysphoria who self-prescribe cross-sex hormones: prevalence, sources, and side effects knowledge. *J Sex Med.* 2014;11(12): 2995-3001.
43. Deutsch MB. *Guidelines for the Primary and Gender Affirming Care of Transgender and Gender Nonconforming People: Overview of Feminizing Hormone Therapy.* http://transhealth.ucsf.edu/trans?page=guidelines-feminizing-therapy. Accessed August 2017.
44. Price TM, Blauer KL, Hansen M, et al. Single-dose pharmacokinetics of sublingual versus oral administration of micronized 17 beta-estradiol. *Obstet Gynecol.* 1997;89(3):340-345.
45. Gooren LJ, Wierckx K, Giltay EJ. Cardiovascular disease in transsexual persons treated with cross-sex hormones: reversal of the traditional sex difference in cardiovascular disease pattern. *Eur J Endocrinol.* 2014;170(6):809-819.

46. Meyer WJ, Webb A, Stuart CA, et al. Physical and hormonal evaluation of transsexual patients: a longitudinal study. *Arch Sex Behav*. 1986;15(2):121-138.

47. Wierckx K, Van Caenegem E, Schreiner T, et al. Cross-sex hormone therapy in trans persons is safe and effective at short-time follow-up: results from the European network for the investigation of gender incongruence. *J Sex Med*. 2014;11(8):1999-2011.

48. Asscheman H, Giltay EJ, Megens JAJ, et al. A long-term follow-up study of mortality in transsexuals receiving treatment with cross-sex hormones. *Eur J Endocrinol*. 2011;164(4):635-642.

49. Spratt DI, Stewart I, Savage C, et al. Subcutaneous injection of testosterone is an effective and preferred alternative to intramuscular injection: demonstration in female-to-male transgender patients. *J Clin Endocrinol Metab*. 2017;102(7):2349-2355.

50. Wierckx K, Elaut E, Van Hoorde B, et al. Sexual desire in trans persons: associations with sex reassignment treatment. *J Sex Med*. 2014;11(1):107-118.

51. Brown GR, Jones KT. Incidence of breast cancer in a cohort of 5,135 transgender veterans. *Breast Cancer Res Treat*. 2015;149(1):191-198.

52. Gooren LJ, van Trotsenburg MAA, Giltay EJ, van Diest PJ. Breast cancer development in transsexual subjects receiving cross-sex hormone treatment. *J Sex Med*. 2013;10(12):3129-3134.

53. Wierckx K, Mueller S, Weyers S, et al. Long-term evaluation of cross-sex hormone treatment in transsexual persons. *J Sex Med*. 2012;9(10):2641-2651.

54. van Kesteren PJ, Asscheman H, Megens JA, Gooren LJ. Mortality and morbidity in transsexual subjects treated with cross-sex hormones. *Clin Endocrinol (Oxf)*. 1997;47(3):337-342.

55. Basaria S, Coviello AD, Travison TG, et al. Adverse events associated with testosterone administration. *N Engl J Med*. 2010;363(2):109-122.

56. Finkle WD, Greenland S, Ridgeway GK, et al. Increased risk of non-fatal myocardial infarction following testosterone therapy prescription in men. *PLoS One*. 2014;9(1):e85805.

57. Vigen R. Association of testosterone therapy with mortality, myocardial infarction, and stroke in men with low testosterone levels. *JAMA*. 2013;310(17):1820-1836.

58. Centers for Disease Control and Prevention. *Preexposure Prophylaxis for the Prevention of HIV Infection in the United States—2017 Clinical Practice Guideline*. https://www.cdc.gov/hiv/pdf/risk/prep/cdc-hiv-prep-guidelines-2017.pdf. Accessed April 2018.

59. Herbst JH, Jacobs ED, Finlayson TJ, et al. Estimating HIV prevalence and risk behaviors of transgender persons in the United States: a systematic review. *AIDS Behav*. 2008;12(1):1-17.

60. Reisner SL, Biello KB, White Hughto JM, et al. Psychiatric diagnoses and comorbidities in a diverse, multicity cohort of young transgender women: baseline findings from Project Lifeskills. *JAMA Pediatr*. 2016;2115(5):481-486.

61. Olson KR, Durwood L, DeMeules M, McLaughlin KA. Mental health of transgender children who are supported in their identities. *Pediatrics*. 2016;137(3):1-8.

62. Marx RA, Kettrey HH. Gay-straight alliances are associated with lower levels of school-based victimization of LGBTQ+ youth: a systematic review and meta-analysis. *J Youth Adolesc*. 2016;45(7):1269-1282.

63. Wallien MSC, Cohen-Kettenis PT. Psychosexual outcome of gender-dysphoric children. *J Am Acad Child Adolesc Psychiatry*. 2008;47(12):1413-1423.

64. Steensma TD, McGuire JK, Kreukels BPC, et al. Factors associated with desistence and persistence of childhood gender dysphoria: a quantitative follow-up study. *J Am Acad Child Adolesc Psychiatry*. 2013;52(6):582-590.

65. White Hughto JM, Reisner SL. A systematic review of the effects of hormone therapy on psychological functioning and quality of life in transgender individuals. *Transgender Health*. 2016;1(1):21-31.

66. Somerville, SB. *Queer | Keywords for American Cultural Studies*. http://keywords.nyupress.org/american-cultural-studies/essay/queer/. Accessed September 2017.

67. GLAAD. *What Is Pansexuality? 4 Pan Celebs Explain in Their Own Words*. https://www.glaad.org/tags/pansexual. Accessed April 2018.

68. The Asexual Visibility and Education Network. *About Asexuality*. http://www.asexuality.org/?q=overview.html. Accessed September 2017.

69. Prause N, Graham CA. Asexuality: classification and characterization. *Arch Sex Behav*. 2007;36:341-356.

70. Sheff E. Seven forms of non-monogamy: exploring the wide world of extra-dyadic sexual relationships. *Psychol Today*. 2014. https://www.psychologytoday.com/blog/the-polyamorists-next-door/201407/seven-forms-non-monogamy. Accessed September 2017.

71. Johnson AL. Counseling the Polyamorous Client: Implications for Competent Practice. 2013. https://www.researchgate.net/publication/316439079_Counseling_the_Polyamorous_Client_Implications_for_Competent_Practice. Accessed April 2018.

PART IV

OPHTHALMOLOGY

Strength of Recommendation (SOR)	Definition
A	Recommendation based on consistent and good-quality patient-oriented evidence.*
B	Recommendation based on consistent and good-quality patient-oriented evidence.*
C	Recommendation based on consensus, usual practice, opinion, disease-oriented evidence, or case series for studies of diagnosis, treatment, prevention, or screening.*

*See Appendix A on pages 1603–1606 for further information.

14 PTERYGIUM

Heidi S. Chumley, MD, MBA
Athena Andreadis, MD

PATIENT STORY

A 50-year-old man has spent most of his adult life working outdoors in southern Texas near the Mexico border. He denies any problems with his vision, but wonders what is growing on his eye and if it should be removed (**Figure 14-1**). His eyes are often dry and irritated. He is diagnosed with a pterygium and instructed that it does not need to be removed unless it interferes with his vision in the future. Liquid tears are suggested for his dry and irritated eyes. He is also instructed to wear wraparound sunglasses to avoid UV exposure and irritation from wind and dust.

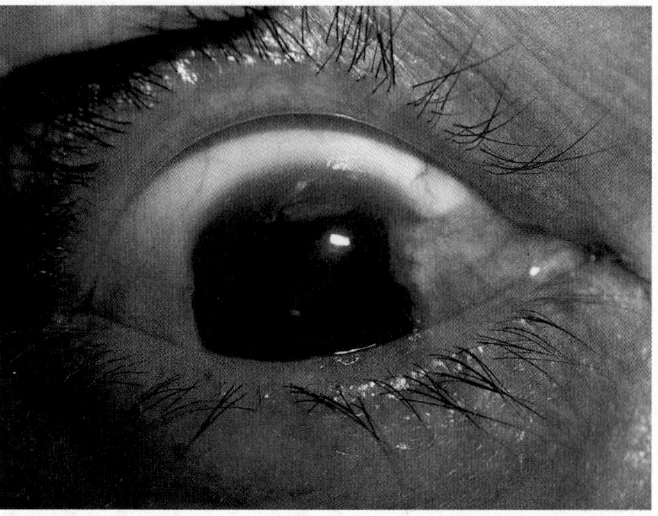

FIGURE 14-1 A nasal pterygium. (*Reproduced with permission from Richard P. Usatine, MD.*)

INTRODUCTION

A pterygium is a generally benign growth of fibroblastic tissue on the eye of an adult with chronic UV exposure. Pterygia can be unilateral or bilateral, are usually located on the nasal side, and extend to the cornea. Pterygia often require no treatment, but can be removed surgically if they interfere with vision. Patients with dry eyes are prone to the development and progression of pterygia.

EPIDEMIOLOGY

- Pterygium most often develops between the ages of 20 and 50 years.
- The frequency of pterygium increases with sun exposure and age. In a population-based study (Indonesia), it was found that the prevalence ranged from 3% (in 21- to 29-year-olds) to 18% (older than 50 years of age).[1] In rural China, the prevalence was 3.76% and also increased with age.[2]
- In one study carried out in Australia, it was found that sun exposure is consistently the greatest risk factor, contributing 43% of the risk.[3]

ETIOLOGY AND PATHOPHYSIOLOGY

- A pterygium is a proliferation of fibrovascular tissue on the surface of the eye, which extends onto the cornea.
- The etiology of pterygium is incompletely understood; however, chronic UV exposure is accepted as a causative agent. Chronic inflammation and oxidative stress may also play a role in pathogenesis.
- Pterygia have features seen in malignant tissues, such as normal tissue invasion and high recurrence rate.[4] Pterygia can be associated with premalignant lesions.[4]

RISK FACTORS

Risk factors are related to chronic UV exposure:

- Living in low-latitude, low-precipitation area.[2]
- Male gender.[2]

DIAGNOSIS

CLINICAL FEATURES

- Redness, itching, and/or irritation of the involved eyes (some are symptom free).
- Visual blurring if the pterygium grows over the visual axis. Even if not obscuring the visual axis, the pterygium can cause poor vision by leading to irregular and high astigmatism.
- Pterygia are diagnosed clinically by their distinctive appearance (**Figures 14-1** to **14-4**).

TYPICAL DISTRIBUTION

Unilateral or bilateral.

- Nasal or nasal and temporal.
- Consider another diagnosis with a unilateral temporal distribution.

BIOPSY

Not indicated; however, excised pterygia are sent for histologic examination because of their association with premalignant lesions.[4]

DIFFERENTIAL DIAGNOSIS

- Pinguecula is a yellowish patch or nodule on the conjunctiva and does not extend onto the cornea (**Figure 14-5**).
- Conjunctivitis is conjunctival infection with discomfort and eye discharge (see Chapter 18, Conjunctivitis).
- Squamous cell carcinoma of the conjunctiva is rare. Consider carcinoma when a unilateral growth is noted on the temporal side. Also consider malignancy if there are grossly aberrant-appearing blood vessels on the surface of the eye. Patients with abnormal immune systems (e.g. cancer, HIV) are at particular risk for ocular surface malignancy.

MANAGEMENT

NONPHARMACOLOGIC

Avoid sun exposure and use UV filtering sunglasses when sun exposure is unavoidable.

MEDICATIONS

Nonprescription artificial tears and/or topical lubricating drops to soothe the inflammation. Ophthalmologists will occasionally prescribe a short course of topical corticosteroid anti-inflammatory drops when symptoms of the pterygia are more intense.

SURGICAL

- Pterygia are usually treated when they interfere with vision or when they cause significant irritation or pain (**Figure 14-3**). The standard therapy is surgical removal.
- Pterygia have a high rate of recurrence. Conjunctival autografting and an antifibrotic treatment (e.g., mitomycin-C) can be used intraoperatively to lower recurrence.[5]

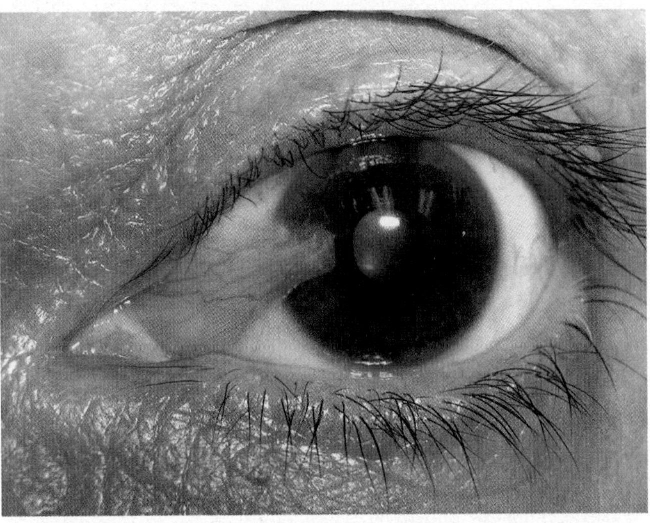

FIGURE 14-2 Pterygium that has grown onto the cornea but not covered the visual axis. This fibrovascular tissue has the shape of a bird's wing (literal definition of pterygium). The small vessels are prominent in this view. *(Reproduced with permission from Richard P. Usatine, MD.)*

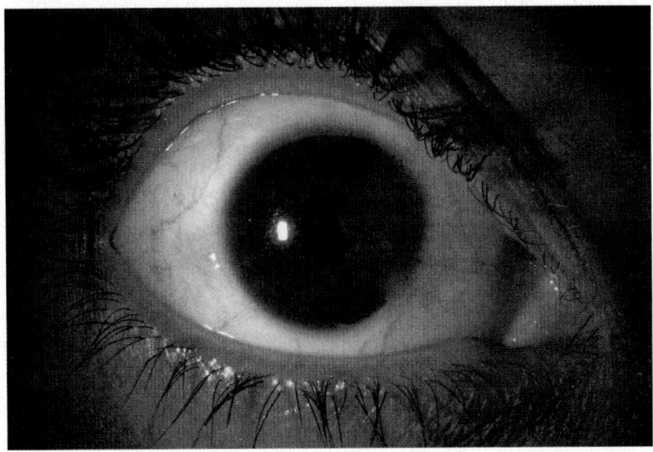

FIGURE 14-3 A pterygium that has grown over the visual axis and is interfering with this person's vision. The patient plans to undergo surgery. *(Reproduced with permission from Paul D. Comeau.)*

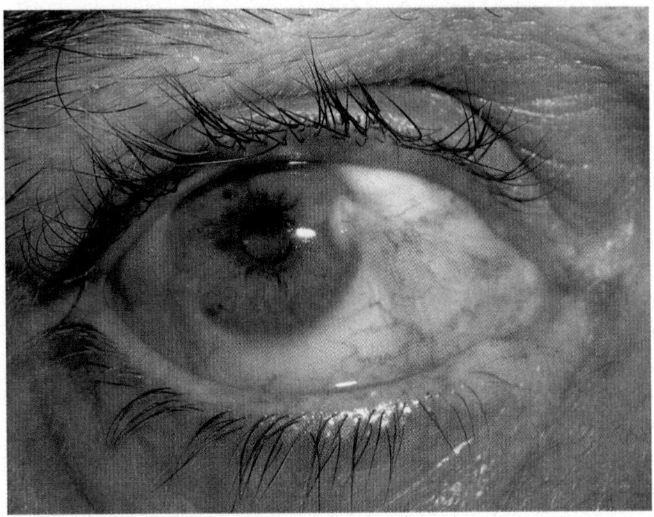

FIGURE 14-4 Bilateral pterygia growing over the cornea. *(Reproduced with permission from Richard P. Usatine, MD.)*

ASSOCIATED RISKS

- Pterygia affect astigmatism[6,7] and are associated with increased rates of macular degeneration; however, it is unclear whether treatment reduces this risk.
- Eyes with a pterygium or previous pterygium surgery (but not pinguecula) have a higher risk of incident late age-related maculopathy (ARM) (odds ratio [OR] 3.3, 95% confidence interval [CI], 1.1 to 10.3) and early ARM (OR 1.8, 95% CI, 1.1 to 2.9).[8]

PREVENTION

All persons (including school-aged children) should use sunglasses with 100% UV protection to protect the eyes from UV damage **(Figure 14-6)**. Sunglasses should fit close to the eye to block scattered or reflected light in addition to direct light.[9]

PROGNOSIS

Most pterygia do not require surgical treatment. Pterygia that interfere with vision and are removed have a high chance of recurrence.

FOLLOW-UP

No specific follow-up is needed; however, consider monitoring vision during annual examinations because of the increased risk of age-related macular degeneration.

PATIENT EDUCATION

Wraparound sunglasses are helpful to avoid UV exposure and irritation from wind and dust. Liquid tears are suggested for dry and irritated eyes.

PATIENT RESOURCES

- MedlinePlus: Pterigium—**https://medlineplus.gov/ency/article/001011.htm.**

PROVIDER RESOURCES

- Fisher JP. *Pterygium*—**http://emedicine.medscape.com/article/1192527.**

REFERENCES

1. Gazzard G, Saw SM, Farook M, et al. Pterygium in Indonesia: prevalence, severity and risk factors. *Br J Ophthalmol.* 2002;86(12):1341-1346.
2. Liang QF, Xu L, Jin XY, et al. Epidemiology of pterygium in aged rural population of Beijing, China. *Chin Med J (Engl).* 2010;123(13):1699-1701.
3. McCarty CA, Fu CL, Taylor HR. Epidemiology of pterygium in Victoria, Australia. *Br J Ophthalmol.* 2000;84(3):289-292.

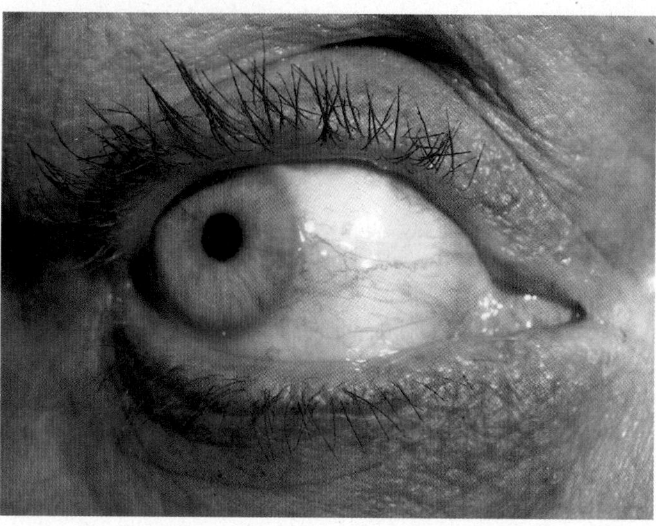

FIGURE 14-5 Pinguecula nodule on conjunctiva that does not extend to the cornea. Note the yellow color. *(Reproduced with permission from Richard P. Usatine, MD.)*

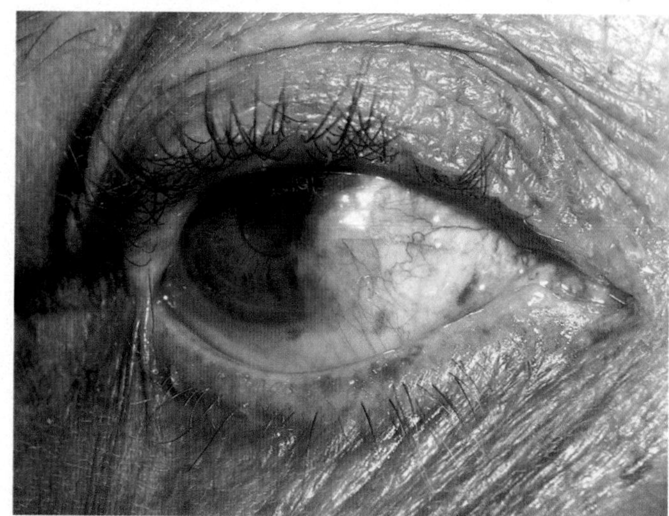

FIGURE 14-6 Nasal pterygium growing over the visual axis in a man living close to the equator. The patient did not use sunglasses. The melanosis within the pterygium is benign. *(Reproduced with permission from Richard P. Usatine, MD.)*

4. Chui J, Coroneo MT, Tat LT, et al. Ophthalmic pterygium: a stem cell disorder with premalignant features. *Am J Pathol.* 2011;178(2): 817-827.
5. Detorakis ET, Spandidos DA. Pathogenetic mechanisms and treatment options for ophthalmic pterygium: trends and perspectives. *Int J Mol Med.* 2009;23(4):439-447.
6. Ashaye AO. Refractive astigmatism and size of pterygium. *Afr J Med Med Sci.* 2002;31(2):163-165.
7. Kampitak K. The effect of pterygium on corneal astigmatism. *J Med Assoc Thai.* 2003;86(1):16-23.
8. Pham TQ, Wang JJ, Rochtchina E, Mitchell P. Pterygium/pinguecula and the five-year incidence of age-related maculopathy. *Am J Ophthalmol.* 2005;139(3):536-537.
9. Wang SQ, Balaqula Y, Osterwalder U. Photoprotection: a review of the current and future technologies. *Dermatol Ther.* 2010;23(1): 31-47.

15 HORDEOLUM AND CHALAZION

Heidi S. Chumley, MD, MBA

PATIENT STORY

A 35-year-old woman presented with a tender nodule on the upper eyelid along with crusting and erythema to both eyelids (**Figure 15-1**). The upper eyelid had a large external hordeolum. When the lower eyelid was inverted an internal hordeolum was also present. The physician recommended that she apply warm moist compresses to her eyelids four times a day. Her hordeola resolved within 7 days.

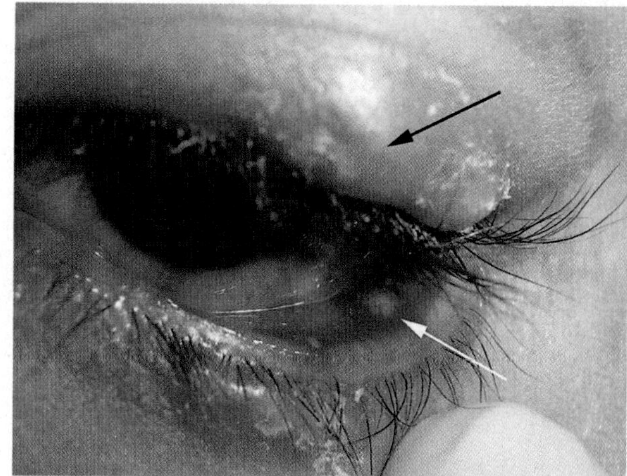

FIGURE 15-1 External hordeolum (*black arrow*) and an internal hordeolum (*white arrow*). (*Reproduced with permission from Richard P. Usatine, MD.*)

INTRODUCTION

A hordeolum is an acute painful infection of the glands of the eyelid, usually caused by bacteria. Hordeola can be located on the internal or external eyelid. Internal hordeola that do not completely resolve become cysts called chalazia. External hordeola are commonly known as styes.

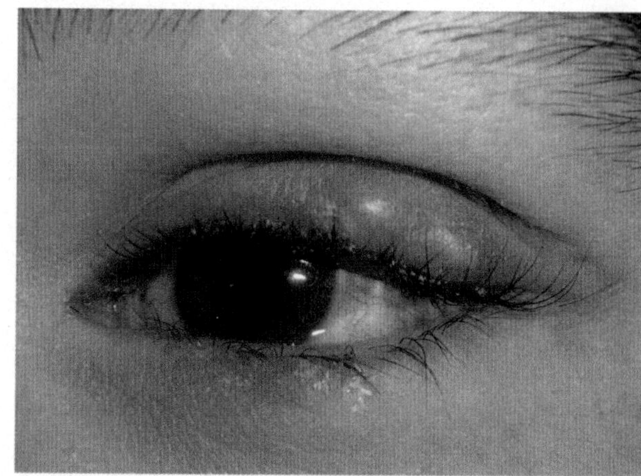

FIGURE 15-2 External hordeolum on upper lid with surrounding erythema. (*Reproduced with permission from Richard P. Usatine, MD.*)

SYNONYMS

Stye (external hordeolum).

EPIDEMIOLOGY

- Unclear incidence or prevalence in the United States, but often stated to be more common in school-aged children and adults 30 to 50 years old.
- In one study in school-aged children in Brazil, the prevalence of chalazion was found to be 0.2% and that of hordeolum was 0.3%.[1]

ETIOLOGY AND PATHOPHYSIOLOGY

HORDEOLUM (ACUTELY TENDER NODULE IN THE EYE)

- Infection in the meibomian gland (internal hordeolum), often resolves into a chalazion (**Figure 15-1**).
- Infection in the Zeiss or Moll glands (external hordeolum) (**Figures 15-2** and **15-3**).
- *Staphylococcus aureus* is the causative agent in most cases.

CHALAZION

- Meibomian gland becomes blocked, often in a patient with blepharitis.
- Blocked meibomian gland's duct releases gland contents into the soft tissue of eyelid.

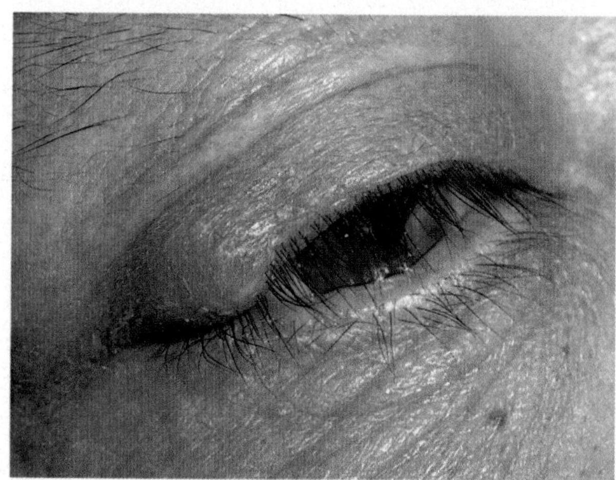

FIGURE 15-3 External hordeolum with visible purulence and the normal contour of the eyelid is disrupted. (*Reproduced with permission from Richard P. Usatine, MD.*)

- Gland contents cause a lipogranulomatous reaction (**Figure 15-4**).
- Reaction can cause acute tenderness and erythema, which then resolves into a chronic nodule (**Figure 15-5**).
- *Demodex* mites have been associated with chalazia.[2]

RISK FACTORS

- Hordeolum: *Staphylococcus aureus* blepharitis, previous hordeolum
- Chalazion: seborrheic blepharitis and rosacea

DIAGNOSIS

Hordeolum and chalazion are clinical diagnoses.

Hordeolum:

- Tenderness and erythema localized to a point on the eyelid (see **Figures 15-1** to **15-3**).
- Conjunctival injection may be present.
- Fever, preauricular nodes, and vision changes should be absent.
- Laboratory tests are generally not indicated.
- Chalazion is a nontender nodule on the eyelid.

DIFFERENTIAL DIAGNOSIS

Eyelid masses:

- Hidrocystoma—benign cystic lesion that grows on the edge of the eyelids and is filled with clear fluid (**Figure 15-6**).
- Xanthelasma—yellowish plaques, generally near medial canthus (see Chapter 232, Hyperlipidemia).
- Molluscum contagiosum—waxy nodules with central umbilication; generally multiple (see Chapter 136, Molluscum Contagiosum).
- Sebaceous cell carcinoma—rare cancer seen in middle-aged and elderly patients; difficult to distinguish from recurrent chalazion or unilateral chronic blepharitis without biopsy.
- Basal cell carcinoma—pearly nodule, often with telangiectasias or central ulceration; more common on lower medial eyelid (see Chapter 177, Basal Cell Carcinoma).
- Herpes zoster ophthalmicus—vesicular lesions on an erythematous base (see Chapter 131, Zoster Ophthalmicus).

MANAGEMENT

Hordeolum (internal):

- No studies of non-surgical interventions (compresses, lid scrubs, antibiotics, steroids) met criteria for inclusion in a Cochrane study. No evidence for or against non-surgical interventions for acute internal hordeolum.[3] SOR Ⓐ
- Treat as described below for external hordeolum.

Hordeolum (external):

- Warm soaks, three to four times a day for 15 minutes, will elicit drainage in most cases. SOR Ⓒ

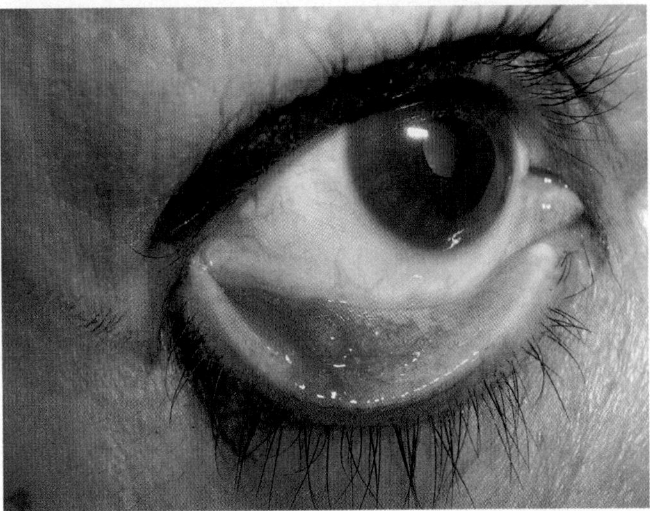

FIGURE 15-4 Chalazion viewed from internal eyelid showing the yellow lipogranulomatous material. (*Reproduced with permission from Richard P. Usatine, MD.*)

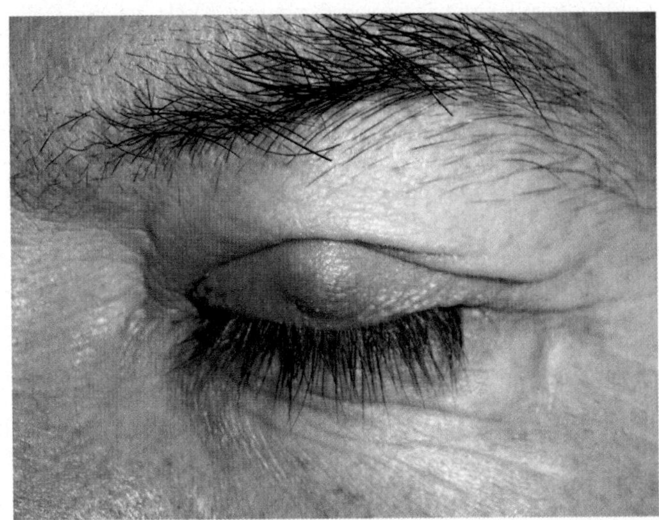

FIGURE 15-5 Chalazion present for 4 months with minimal symptoms but cosmetically unappealing. (*Reproduced with permission from Richard P. Usatine, MD.*)

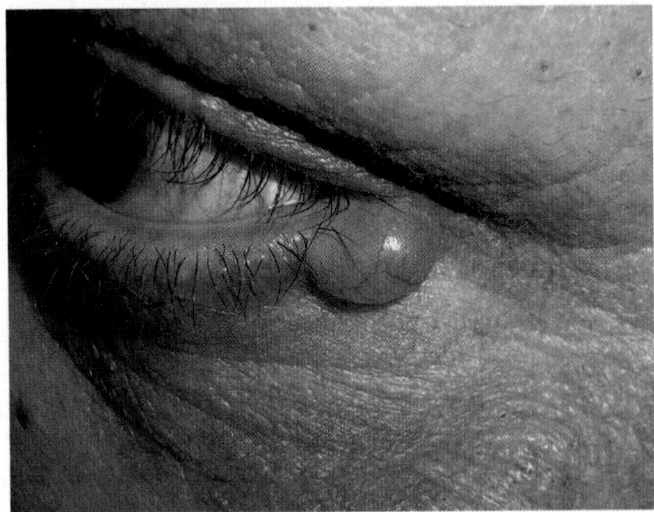

FIGURE 15-6 Hidrocystoma showing telangiectasias. The cyst was easily resected and the fluid was clear. (*Reproduced with permission from Richard P. Usatine, MD.*)

- Topical antibiotics (e.g., bacitracin ophthalmic ointment) may be beneficial for recurrent or spontaneously draining hordeolum. SOR C
- Cases that do not respond to warm soaks or that are extremely painful and swollen may be incised and drained with a small incision using a #11 blade. Make the incision on either the internal or external eyelid depending on where the hordeolum is pointing. A chalazion clamp can be used to protect the globe from damage. SOR C
- Antibiotics do not provide benefit after incision and drainage.[4] SOR B
- Systemic antibiotics are usually not needed unless patient has preseptal cellulitis. SOR C

Chalazion:

- First-line: Treat conservatively with lid hygiene and warm compresses applied 2-3 times daily. In one study, 46% responded. Treatment may require weeks to months.[5] SOR C
- Second-line: Injection with steroid (e.g., 0.3 mL triamcinolone acetonide) or incision and curettage. SOR B
  - A meta-analysis of 288 patients in trials comparing triamcinolone injection with incision and curettage found resolution rates of 72.5% and 86.7%, respectively.[6] SOR B
  - One comparative study of 30 patients found triamcinolone injection to be more comfortable for the patient while providing a comparable response to incision and curettage.[7] SOR B

The chalazion is usually drained from the internal eyelid using a chalazion clamp to protect the globe. After anesthetizing the area, a #11 blade is carefully used to open the chalazion. A chalazion curette helps to scoop out the lipogranulomatous material. No suturing is needed.

REFERRAL

Refer to an ophthalmologist if the hordeolum or chalazion is interfering with vision and not responding to therapy. If a surgical intervention is needed and you lack experience doing such a procedure, refer to a colleague with experience.

PREVENTION

Eyelid hygiene, keeping the area around the eyelid clean, may prevent hordeola.

PROGNOSIS

Chalazia can persist for years if untreated. Some patients are prone to recurrence of hordeola and chalazia.

FOLLOW-UP

A hordeolum with significant purulence and swelling should be reevaluated in 2 to 3 days or referred to an ophthalmologist. Warm compresses are slow to work for a chalazion, so follow-up should be no sooner than 1 month if nonsurgical treatment is prescribed.

PATIENT EDUCATION

Hordeolum commonly responds to warm soaks and topical antibiotics. It often recurs and can develop into a chronic chalazion, which may need to be treated with surgical removal or a steroid injection.

PATIENT RESOURCES

- The American Academy of Ophthalmology—**http://www.geteyesmart.org/eyesmart/diseases/chalazion-stye.cfm.**
- The American Academy of Family Physicians has a patient handout in English or Spanish on stye—**http://familydoctor.org/familydoctor/en/diseases-conditions/sty.html.**

PROVIDER RESOURCES

- Hordeolum and Stye in Emergency Medicine—**http://emedicine.medscape.com/article/798940.**
- Chalazion—**http://emedicine.medscape.com/article/1212709.**
- Chalazion Injection Demonstration—**http://www.youtube.com/watch?v=yYCCkDZwKgg.**
- Chalazion incision and curettage—**https://www.youtube.com/watch?v=4W0dO3b-M7U.**

REFERENCES

1. Garcia CA, Pinheiro FI, Montenegro DA, et al. Prevalence of biomicroscopic findings in the anterior segment and ocular adnexa among schoolchildren in Natal, Brazil. *Arq Bras Oftalmol São Paulo.* 2005;68(2):167-170.
2. Schear MJ, Milman T, Steiner T, et al. The association of *Demodex* with chalazia: a histopathologic study of the eyelid. *Int Ophthalmol.* 2014;34(5):1049-1053.
3. Lindsley K, Nichols JJ, Dickersin K. Non-surgical interventions for acute internal hordeolum. *Cochrane Database Syst Rev.* 2017;(1):CD007742.
4. Hirunwiwatkul P, Wachirasereechai K. Effectiveness of combined antibiotic ophthalmic solution in the treatment of hordeolum after incision and curettage: a randomized, placebo-controlled trial: a pilot study. *J Med Assoc Thai.* 2005;88(5):647-650.
5. Goawalla A, Lee V. A prospective randomized treatment study comparing three treatment options for chalazia: triamcinolone acetonide injections, incision and curettage and treatment with hot compresses. *Clin Exp Ophthalmol.* 2007;35(8):706-712.
6. Aycinena AR, Achiron A, Paul M, Burgansky-Eliash Z. Incision and curettage versus steroid injection for the treatment of chalazia: a meta-analysis. *Ophthal Plast Reconstr Surg.* 2016;32(3):220-224.
7. Biuk D, Matić S, Barać J, et al. Chalazion management—surgical treatment versus triamcinolon application. *Coll Antropol.* 2013;37 Suppl 1:247-250.

16 SCLERAL AND CONJUNCTIVAL PIGMENTATION

Heidi S. Chumley, MD, MBA

PATIENT STORY

A 40-year-old white man came to see his physician about a brown spot in his eye (**Figure 16-1**). He noticed this spot many years ago, but became concerned after recently reading information on the Internet about ocular melanoma. He thinks the spot has changed in size. He denies any eye discomfort or visual changes. He was referred for a biopsy, and the pathology showed a benign nevus that did not require further treatment.

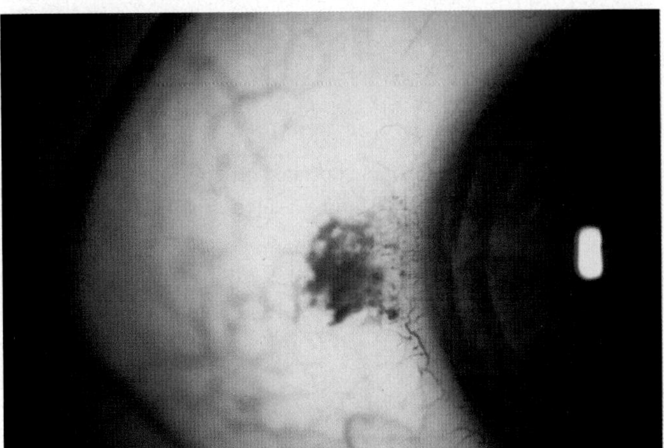

FIGURE 16-1 Scleral nevus. Unilateral localized distinct area of dark pigmentation on sclera. (*Reproduced with permission from Paul D. Comeau.*)

INTRODUCTION

Scleral and conjunctival pigmentation is common and usually benign. Nevi can be observed and referred if they change in size. Primary acquired melanosis (PAM) must be biopsied because PAM with atypia has malignant potential, whereas PAM without atypia does not. Conjunctival melanoma is rare, but deadly.

EPIDEMIOLOGY

There is little information on the prevalence of ocular pigmentation other than complexion-associated melanosis (physiologic or racial melanosis).

- In a study of pigmented lesions referred for biopsy, investigators reported that 52% were nevi, 21% were PAM, and 25% were melanoma.[1]
- Scleral and conjunctival nevi (see **Figures 16-1** and **16-2**) are the most common cause of ocular pigmentation in light-skinned races. The pigmentation is generally noticeable by young adulthood and is more common in whites.[2]
- Complexion-associated melanosis (**Figure 16-3**) is seen in 90% of black patients.[3] It can be congenital and often presents early in life.
- PAM (**Figure 16-4**) is generally noted in middle-aged to older adults[4,5] and is also more common in whites.
- Conjunctival melanoma (**Figures 16-5** to **16-7**) is rare; the incidence of conjunctival melanoma in Denmark was 0.5/1,000,000/year.[6]

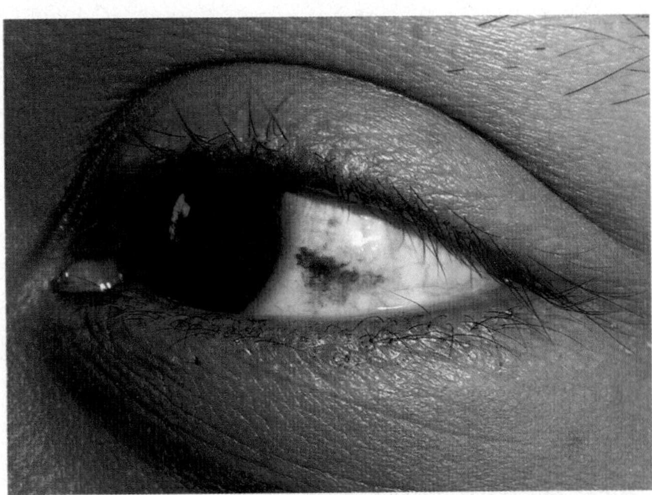

FIGURE 16-2 Conjunctival nevus. Unilateral localized distinct area of pigmentation on the conjunctiva of a 17-year-old Hispanic female. (*Reproduced with permission from Richard P. Usatine, MD.*)

ETIOLOGY AND PATHOPHYSIOLOGY

The etiology of scleral or conjunctival nevi is not well understood. Complexion-associated melanosis is genetically determined. Conjunctival melanoma is associated with BRAF mutations,[6] appears to be related to mucosal and cutaneous melanomas,[6] and can arise from PAM with severe atypia, nevi, or de novo.[7,8]

RISK FACTORS

- In non-Hispanic whites, the incidence of conjunctival melanoma increases as latitude decreases.[9]
- Fair-skinned individuals are at higher risk for conjunctival melanoma.

DIAGNOSIS

Definitive diagnosis of pigmented ocular lesions is by biopsy.

CLINICAL FEATURES

- Benign nevi and complexion-associated melanosis are stable over time, whereas PAM and melanoma change.
- Melanoma, compared to PAM, was more common in older patients (61 vs 54 years); and had intralesional cysts (7% vs 0%), feeder vessels (48% vs 10%), intrinsic vessels (33% vs 4%), or hemorrhage (3% vs <1%).[10]

TYPICAL DISTRIBUTION

- Complexion-associated melanosis is typically bilateral and symmetrical.
- Nevi, PAM, and melanoma are typically unilateral; however, one study found that 13% of PAM cases were bilateral.[8]

LABORATORY TESTING

- None indicated, other than biopsy.

IMAGING

- Diagnosis is made by biopsy; however, ultrasound biomicroscopy and anterior segment optical coherence tomography aid in diagnosis.[11]

BIOPSY

- Eighty-seven percent of biopsy-proven nevi do not change over time.[4]
- Features seen more commonly in malignancy: ulceration, hemorrhage, change in color, and formation of new vessels around the lesion.
- Pathologic factors of conjunctival melanoma with a higher mortality rate include increased tumor thickness, location on the palpebral, caruncular or forniceal conjunctiva, increased mitotic activity, lymphocytic invasion, and association with PAM.[12]

DIFFERENTIAL DIAGNOSIS

Pigmented areas on the sclera or conjunctiva include the following:

- Benign nevi—Unilateral and stable over time (see **Figures 16-1** and **16-2**).
- Complexion associated melanosis (physiologic or racial melanosis)—Bilateral and symmetric, most common circumlimbally, and relatively consistent throughout patient's life (see **Figure 16-3**).
- PAM—Typically unilateral, often multifocal indistinct areas of dark pigmentation, and can progress to malignancy over time (see **Figure 16-4**). This term is used clinically when the histology is not known.
- Secondary acquired melanosis—Seen with hormonal changes or after trauma to the conjunctiva with irradiation, chemical irritation, or chronic inflammation.

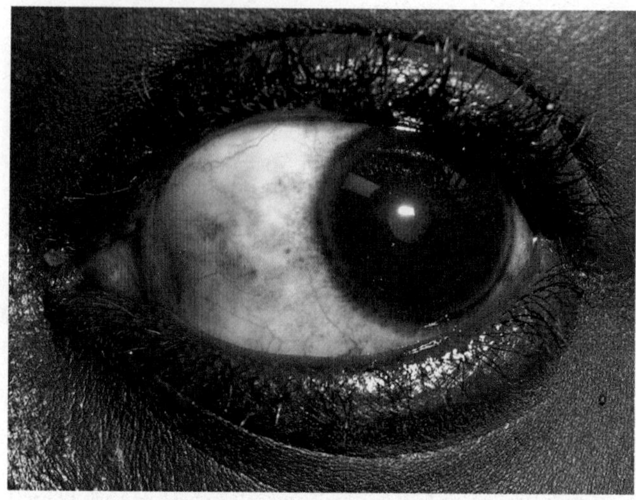

FIGURE 16-3 Complexion-associated (physiologic or racial) melanosis. Flat conjunctival pigmentation present bilaterally starting at the limbus and most prominent in the interpalpebral zone is likely to be racial melanosis in a darkly pigmented patient. (*Reproduced with permission from Richard P. Usatine, MD.*)

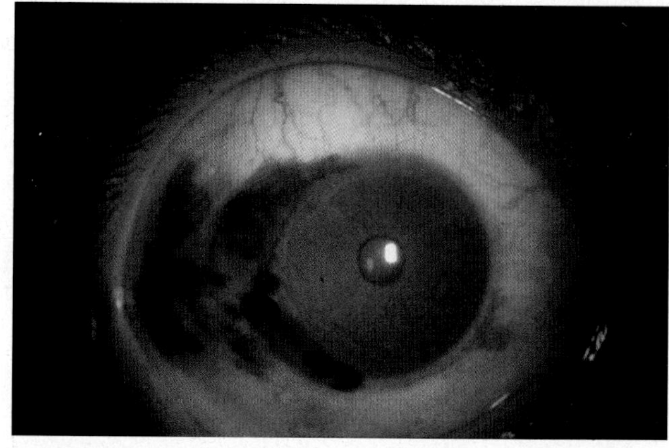

FIGURE 16-4 Primary acquired melanosis (PAM). Multiple unilateral indistinct areas of dark pigmentation. (*Reproduced with permission from Paul D. Comeau.*)

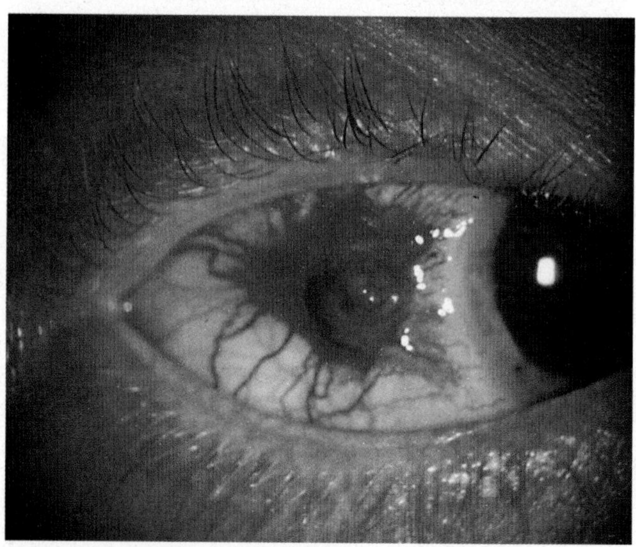

FIGURE 16-5 Conjunctival melanoma. Unilateral, nodular lesion with irregular contours and colors, and surrounded by hyperemic vessels. (*Reproduced with permission from Paul D. Comeau.*)

- Conjunctival melanoma—Unilateral, nodular, with variegated color and size changes (see **Figures 16-5** to **16-7**).
- Alkaptonuria—Rare disease accompanied by dark urine and arthritis.
- Nevus of Ota (also known as oculodermal melanocytosis)—Blue-gray scleral pigment involving the periorbital skin as well (**Figure 16-8**). It is more common in the Asian population but can be seen in any population. It can also be bilateral. Most importantly, these persons should be followed by an ophthalmologist because they are at higher risk for glaucoma and possibly melanoma.

MANAGEMENT

- Complexion-associated melanosis and nevi can be monitored for changes without a biopsy.
- Refer any changing pigmented lesion in the eye to a specialist who can perform a biopsy.
- Biopsy-proven PAM without atypia does not require excision, but must be monitored for stability. SOR Ⓒ
- PAM with atypia is generally removed with large margins because of its potential for conversion into melanoma.[4] SOR Ⓒ
- The primary treatment for conjunctival melanoma is surgical removal. Cryotherapy, radiotherapy, and chemotherapy may be used as adjunct therapy.[11] SOR Ⓒ

PREVENTION

To decrease risk of conjunctival melanoma, use sunglasses that protect the eye from UV radiation. SOR Ⓒ

PROGNOSIS

In one study, PAM without atypia or with mild atypia did not progress into melanoma. Thirteen percent of PAM cases with severe atypia did progress. The risk of melanoma increases as PAM covers more of the iris circumference (see **Figure 16-4**).[7] In one study, conjunctival melanoma arose from PAM, nevi, and de novo. Melanoma arising de novo had a worse prognosis. Other bad factors were fornix location and nodular tumor.[8]

FOLLOW-UP

Follow-up is based on the type of lesion. Nevi and complexion-associated melanosis that have not changed can be monitored without biopsy. PAM requires close follow-up because of its potential conversion to melanoma. Patients with nevus of Ota should be monitored for glaucoma and melanoma.

PATIENT EDUCATION

Most pigmentation in the eye is benign and does not change over time. Discuss the importance of reporting any changing pigmented lesion, even in the eye.

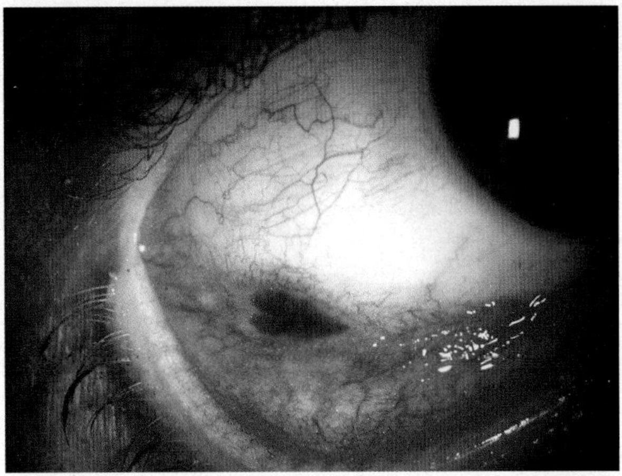

FIGURE 16-6 Early photo of conjunctival melanoma with irregular borders and variations in color. (*Reproduced with permission from Paul D. Comeau.*)

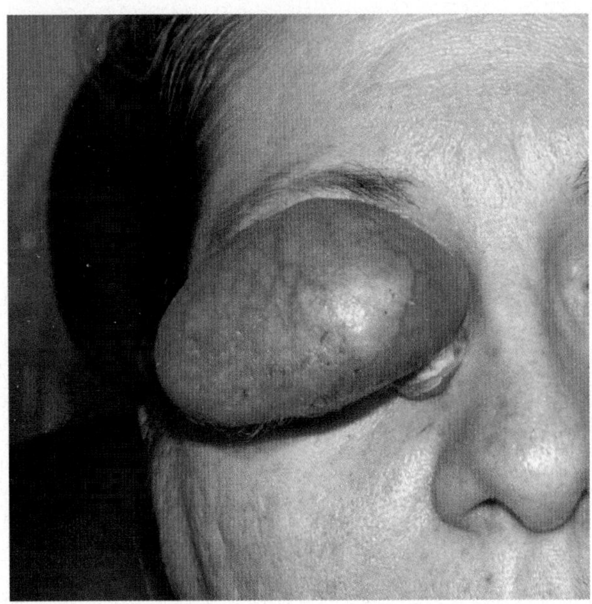

FIGURE 16-7 Conjunctival melanoma, 1 year after the previous photo, in a patient who initially declined treatment. (*Reproduced with permission from Paul D. Comeau.*)

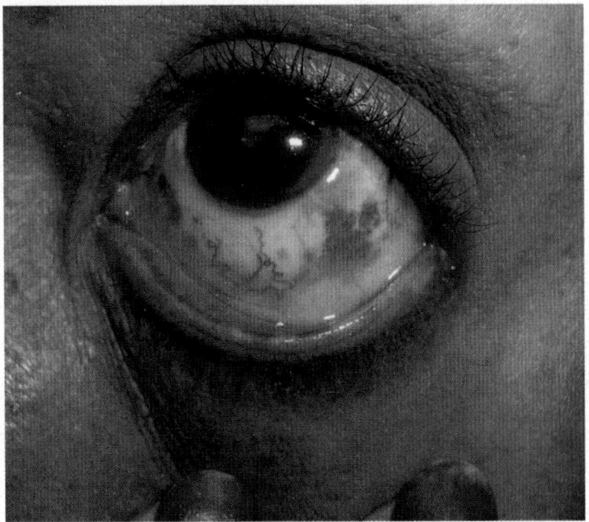

FIGURE 16-8 Nevus of Ota (also known as oculodermal melanocytosis). Unilateral blue-gray ocular pigmentation with periorbital hyperpigmentation. (*Reproduced with permission from Richard P. Usatine, MD.*)

PATIENT RESOURCES

- American Academy of Ophthalmology (**http://www.aao.org**). Information on nevi and ocular melanoma. *What Is a Nevus?*—**http://www.geteyesmart.org/eyesmart/diseases/nevus.cfm.**
- Ocular Melanoma Foundation. *About Ocular Melanoma*—**http://www.ocularmelanoma.org/disease.htm.**

PROVIDER RESOURCES

- *Conjunctival Melanoma*—**http://emedicine.medscape.com/article/1191840.**

REFERENCES

1. Shields CL, Demirci H, Karatza E, Shields JA. Clinical survey of 1643 melanocytic and nonmelanocytic conjunctival tumors. *Ophthalmology.* 2004;111(9):1747-1754.
2. Shields CL, Fasiudden A, Mashayekhi A, Shields JA. Conjunctival nevi: clinical features and natural course in 410 consecutive patients. *Arch Ophthalmol.* 2004;122(2):167-175.
3. Singh AD, Campos OE, Rhatigan RM, et al. Conjunctival melanoma in the black population [review]. *Surv Ophthalmol.* 1998;43(2):127-133.
4. Folberg R, Mclean IW, Zimmerman LE. Conjunctival melanosis and melanoma. *Ophthalmology.* 1984;91(6):673-678.
5. Seregard S, af Trampe E, Månsson-Brahme E, et al. Prevalence of primary acquired melanosis and nevi of the conjunctiva and uvea in the dysplastic nevus syndrome. A case-control study. *Ophthalmology.* 1995;102(10):1524-1529.
6. Larsen AC. Conjunctival malignant melanoma in Denmark: epidemiology, treatment and prognosis with special emphasis on tumorigenesis and genetic profile. *Acta Ophthalmol.* 2016 (94) Thesis 1:1-27.
7. Shields CL, Markowitz JS, Belinsky I, et al. Conjunctival melanoma: outcomes based on tumor origin in 382 consecutive cases. *Ophthalmology.* 2011;118(2):389-395.
8. Shields JA, Shields CL, Mashayekhi A, et al. Primary acquired melanosis of conjunctiva: risks for progression to melanoma in 311 eyes. *Ophthalmology.* 2008;115(3):511-519.
9. Yu GP, Hu DN, McCormick SA. Latitude and incidence of ocular melanoma. *Photochem Photobiol.* 2006;82(6):1621-1626.
10. Shields CL, Alset AE, Boal NS, et al. Conjunctival tumors in 5002 cases. Comparative analysis of benign versus malignant counterparts. The 2016 James D. Allen Lecture. *Am J Ophthalmol.* 2017; 173:106-133.
11. Vora GK, Demirci H, Marr B, Mruthyunjaya P. Advances in the management of conjunctival melanoma. *Surv Ophthalmol.* 2017; 62(1):26-42.
12. Shields CL, Shields JA, Gunduz K, et al. Conjunctival melanoma: Risk factors for recurrence, exenteration, metastasis, and death in 150 consecutive patients [comment]. *Arch Ophthalmol.* 2000; 118(11):1497-1507.

17 CORNEAL FOREIGN BODY AND CORNEAL ABRASION

J. William Hayden, Jr, MD, EdD
Heidi S. Chumley, MD, MBA

PATIENT STORY

A 28-year-old man felt something fly into his eye while he was using a table saw without wearing protective eye gear. He presented with pain, tearing, photophobia, and thought that something was still in his eye. On examination with a slit lamp, the physician noted that he had a wood chip that had penetrated the cornea (**Figures 17-1** and **17-2**). He was referred to an ophthalmologist who successfully removed the foreign body. He was treated with a short course of topical nonsteroidal anti-inflammatory drugs (NSAIDs) for pain relief and had complete healing.

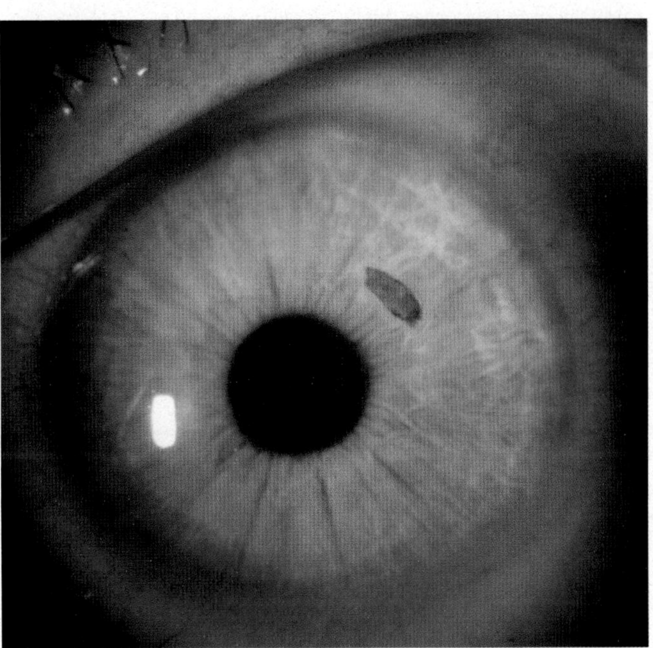

FIGURE 17-1 Wood chip is visible in the cornea on close inspection of the eye. (*Reproduced with permission from Paul D. Comeau.*)

INTRODUCTION

Corneal abrasions are often caused by eye trauma, retained foreign bodies, chemical splash, or improper contact lens use. Such abrasions can cause an inflammatory response. Eyes that have had prior corneal abrasions or eyes that have an underlying corneal epithelial abnormality may experience spontaneous defects that are referred to as recurrent erosions.[1] Corneal abrasions are detected using fluorescein and a UV light. A corneal foreign body can be seen during a careful physical examination with a good light source or slit lamp. Nonpenetrating foreign bodies can be removed by an experienced physician in the office using topical anesthesia. Refer all penetrating foreign bodies to an ophthalmologist.

SYNONYMS

Corneal abrasion is sometimes referred to as a corneal epithelial defect, a broader term that refers to all corneal defects, whether traumatic, spontaneous, acquired, or genetic.

EPIDEMIOLOGY

- Corneal abrasions with or without foreign bodies are common; however, the prevalence or incidence of corneal abrasions in the general population is unknown.
- Corneal abrasions accounted for 85% of closed-eye injuries in adults presenting to an emergency department.[2]
- In professional sports, such as major league baseball, 33% of all eye injuries are corneal abrasions. In professional basketball, corneal abrasions account for 12% of eye injuries, while 1 in 10 college basketball players sustains an eye injury, usually corneal abrasion, each year.[3,4]

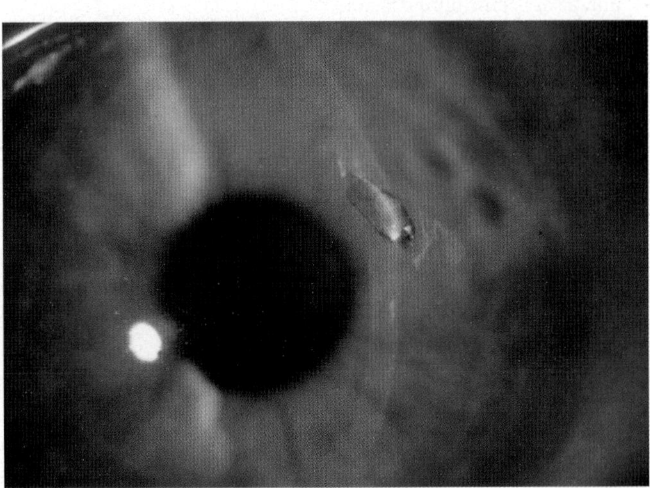

FIGURE 17-2 Slit-lamp examination reveals this wood chip has penetrated the cornea. (*Reproduced with permission from Paul D. Comeau.*)

- Incidence of corneal abrasion for patients undergoing general anesthesia is as high as 44% due to surface trauma from surgical drapes, anesthetic masks, or exposure.[4]

ETIOLOGY AND PATHOPHYSIOLOGY

- The cornea overlies the iris and provides barrier protection, filters UV light, and refracts light onto the retina.
- Abrasions in the cornea can be caused by:
  - Direct injury from a foreign body
  - Extended contact lens wear
  - Eye makeup applications
  - Thermal/chemical burns (e.g., ear drops mistaken for eyedrops)
  - UV keratitis from arc welding or tanning beds
  - "Snow blindness" from bright sun exposure without sun glasses while skiing
  - Eyelid margin injuries
  - Iatrogenic—inadvertent injury by healthcare workers
- The inflammatory reaction causes the symptoms and can persist for several days after the foreign object is out.

RISK FACTORS

- Those with occupations such as metal workers, woodworkers, miners, and landscapers have an increased risk of corneal injuries from foreign bodies.[5]
- Participating in sports such as wrestling, hockey, lacrosse, or racquetball raises the risk of corneal abrasions from ocular trauma.[5]
- Ventilated neonates (as a result of mask pressure on the orbit) or sedated patients (as a result of disruption of the blink reflex, and subsequent corneal exposure) are at increased risk for corneal abrasions.[5]
- Unconscious patients in intensive care who have lost their corneal reflexes are at increased risk.
- Contact lenses, especially soft extended wear, increase the risk of developing an infected abrasion and resultant corneal ulcer, referred to as infectious keratitis. Improper lens cleaning and storage are contributing factors.[1]

DIAGNOSIS

CLINICAL FEATURES

History and physical:

- History of ocular trauma or eye rubbing (although corneal abrasions can occur with no trauma history, as in recurrent corneal erosion syndrome).
- History of contact lens wear.
- History of ocular or perioral herpes virus infection.
- Symptoms of pain, eye redness, photophobia, and a foreign-body sensation.
- If the source of eye discomfort is unclear, a detailed history should include recent engagement in sports activities, UV light exposure, use of eye makeup, contact lens use, and occupation.
- Initial physical examination should exclude open globe penetrating injury as well as hyphema (blood in the anterior chamber of the eye). Both conditions require immediate consultation with an ophthalmologist.[1]
- If penetrating injury is possible, perform the Seidel test. (Apply a moistened fluorescein strip to the site of injury. Using a slit lamp and cobalt blue light, look for streaming aqueous fluid appearing as a dark stream within a pool of bright green dye.)[6]
- Check for foreign body with direct visualization or a slit lamp (**Figure 17-3**).
- Under cobalt-blue filtered light and fluorescein application, corneal abrasion appears as a bright green area indicating disruption in the corneal epithelium (**Figure 17-4**).

LABORATORY TESTING

- Culture if an infection is suspected. Corneal abrasion resulting from contaminated materials, such as farm instruments or vegetable matter, is the most common cause of bacterial and fungal ulcers.[4]

IMAGING

- If physical examination is equivocal, imaging may be useful to determine if a foreign body has perforated the cornea. An object that has fully perforated the cornea has passed through the cornea and will be located in the anterior segment or posterior segment of the eye, making it difficult to see without imaging technology.
- CT or spiral CT (1-mm axial and coronal cuts) can detect nonmetallic and metallic foreign bodies.
- If you suspect a metallic foreign body, the initial study can be an orbital radiograph. Avoid MRI if the history suggests a possible metal foreign body.
- B-scan ultrasound and ultrasound biomicroscopy can also visualize intraocular foreign bodies and may be useful in some cases.
- In vivo confocal microscopy (IVCM) is an emerging noninvasive imaging and diagnostic tool that can be helpful in the diagnosis of hidden corneal foreign bodies, permitting visualization of the entire corneal thickness.[7]

DIFFERENTIAL DIAGNOSIS

- Uveitis or iritis—Usually unilateral 360-degree perilimbal injection, eye pain, photophobia, and vision loss (see Chapter 20, Uveitis and Iritis).
- Bacterial and fungal keratitis or corneal ulcerations—Diffuse erythema with ciliary injection often with miosis; eye discharge; pain, photophobia, and vision loss depending on the location of ulceration (**Figures 17-5** and **17-6**). There is often a history of trauma, herpes simplex virus (HSV), or contact lens wear. Patients should see an ophthalmologist urgently.
- Conjunctivitis—Conjunctival injection; eye discharge; gritty or uncomfortable feeling; no vision loss, history of respiratory infection, or contacts with others who have red eyes (see Chapter 18, Conjunctivitis).

- Acute-angle closure glaucoma—Cloudy cornea and scleral injection; eye pain with ipsilateral headache; severe vision loss, acutely elevated intraocular pressure (see Chapter 21, Glaucoma).
- With traumatic injuries, always consider intraocular foreign body.

MANAGEMENT

NONPHARMACOLOGIC

- Confirm diagnosis with fluorescein and a UV light (for abrasion) if no foreign body is readily visible (see **Figure 17-4**).
- For chemical splash injuries, measure pH in inferior fornix. If pH is <6.5 or >7.5, initiate irrigation with normal saline or Ringer lactate solution using a Morgan irrigation lens. Pretreat with a topical eye anesthetic. Goal is a neutral pH after 20–30 minutes irrigation depending on the irritant substance.[1]
- Carefully inspect for a foreign body. Evert both upper and lower eyelids for full visualization. Slit-lamp visualization and the Seidel test may be needed to determine corneal penetration (see **Figure 17-2**).
- Remove (or refer for removal) nonpenetrating foreign bodies. Apply a topical anesthetic, such as proparacaine or tetracaine. Remove with irrigation, a foreign-body spud, a wet-tipped cotton applicator, or a fine-gauge needle.
- Remove contact lenses until cornea is healed.[8] SOR Ⓒ
- Avoid patching in corneal abrasions smaller than 10 mm; it does not help.[9] SOR Ⓐ Patching is also contraindicated for use in patients with corneal abrasions caused by contact lenses.[1]
- Rust rings created by foreign bodies containing iron should be treated as corneal abrasions. Rust rings will usually resorb gradually after 2 to 3 days. Persistent rust rings may be debrided with an electric burr by trained clinicians. Routine removal of rust rings at the time of foreign body removal is not recommended because of potential damage to Bowman membrane with resultant scarring.[1]

MEDICATIONS

- Prescribe ophthalmic NSAIDs (diclofenac, ketorolac tromethamine 0.5%) for pain if needed.[10] SOR Ⓐ
- Consider topical antibiotics. SOR Ⓒ Chloramphenicol ointment reduced the risk of recurrent ulcer in a prospective, nonplacebo, controlled trial.[11] Although chloramphenicol is rarely used in the United States, other ophthalmic antibiotics, such as erythromycin ointment, are used for corneal abrasions. SOR Ⓒ
- Abrasions secondary to contact lenses may become infected corneal ulcers, especially by *Pseudomonas* and amoebic species. For this reason, antibiotic coverage for gram-negative organisms is recommended (gentamicin, tobramycin, ciprofloxacin).[4]
- Although routine tetanus prophylaxis is unnecessary, consider tetanus prophylaxis for tetanus-prone "dirty" eye injuries produced by organic matter or dirt as per Centers for Disease Control and Prevention guidelines.[2] SOR Ⓒ
- For large abrasions, topical cycloplegics and mydriatics may be considered for pain and photophobia, although some literature reviews question their effectiveness.[3] SOR Ⓑ

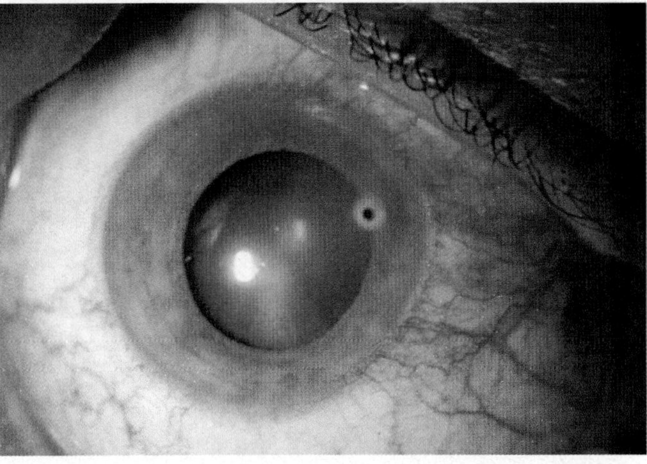

FIGURE 17-3 Metallic foreign body with rust ring within the corneal stroma and conjunctival injection. (*Reproduced with permission from Paul D. Comeau.*)

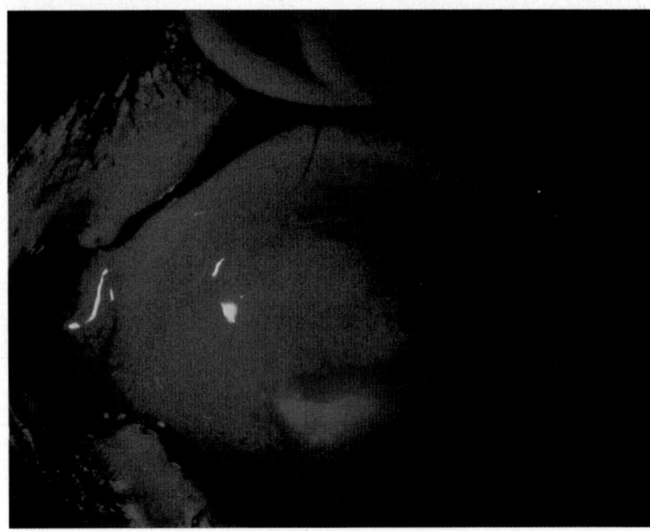

FIGURE 17-4 Fluorescein stains green, indicating corneal abrasion. (*Reproduced with permission from Paul D. Comeau.*)

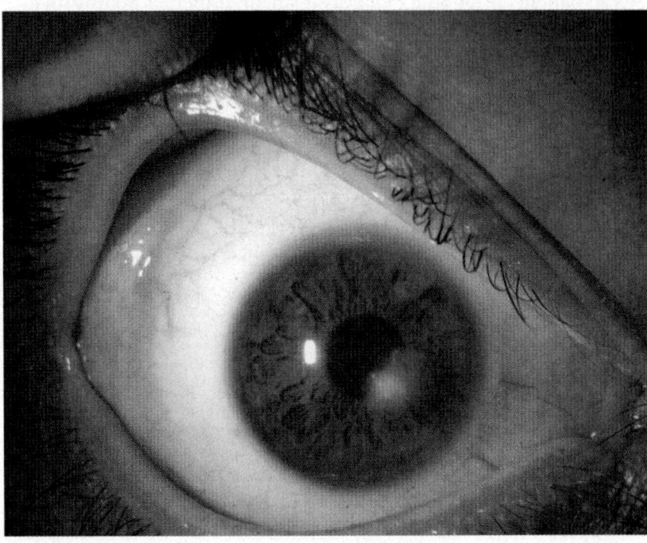

FIGURE 17-5 Small corneal ulcer in the visual axis. (*Reproduced with permission from Paul D. Comeau.*)

- Medications to avoid[1,4,12]:
  - Topical steroids
  - Repeated use of topical anesthetic drops
  - Neomycin due to high incidence of sensitivity reactions.

REFERRAL

- Immediate referral is indicated in the following cases[3]:
  - Open globe injury
  - Hyphema
  - Scleral or corneal laceration
  - Diffuse subconjunctival hemorrhage
  - Abnormal shaped pupil
  - Corneal infiltrate, white spot, or opacity suggestive of ulceration
  - Foreign body that cannot be removed
  - Hypopyon (pus in the anterior chamber)[4]
- Refer penetrating foreign bodies to an experienced eye surgeon.

PREVENTION

Eye protection should be worn for high-risk occupations such as auto mechanics, metalworking, welding, or mining, as well as recreational activities and contact sports.

For unconscious patients or those with neuropathies such as Bell palsy that prevent voluntary eyelid closure, tape the eyelid(s) closed.

Contact lens wearers should follow manufacturers' recommendations for use, cleansing, and replacement.

PROGNOSIS

Prognosis is generally good. Development of infection or a rust ring worsens prognosis due to risk for corneal ulcers, as essentially all corneal ulcers begin as an abrasion.[4]

FOLLOW-UP

See all patients in 24 hours for reassessment. If there is no improvement, look for an initially overlooked foreign body or a full-thickness injury. Refer to an ophthalmologist if patient is not improving.

Urgent referral to an ophthalmologist is indicated in the following cases[4]:

- A larger epithelial defect
- Purulent discharge
- A drop in vision more than one to two lines on a Snellen chart
- A child or infant with persistent discharge or unwillingness to open eyes
- Corneal abrasions that remain unhealed after 3 to 4 days.

PATIENT EDUCATION

- Advise patients in specific professions (e.g., woodworking, metalworking) and those who play sports, such as racquetball or hockey, to wear eye protection for primary prevention.

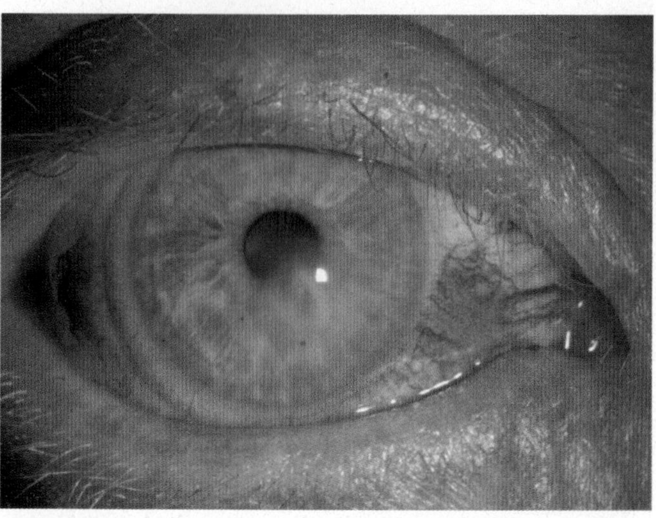

FIGURE 17-6 Larger corneal ulcer partially obscuring the visual axis. *(Reproduced with permission from Paul D. Comeau.)*

- Advise patients with corneal abrasions that healing usually occurs within 2 to 3 days, and they should report persistent pain, redness, and photophobia.
- Patients should be advised not to sleep in contact lenses, even if labeled "extended wear."

PATIENT RESOURCES

- FamilyDoctor.org. Patient handout on *Corneal Abrasions*—**http://familydoctor.org/familydoctor/en/prevention-wellness/staying-healthy/first-aid/corneal-abrasions.html.**

PROVIDER RESOURCES

- Cao C. *Corneal Foreign Body Removal*—**http://emedicine.medscape.com/article/82717.**

REFERENCES

1. Jacobs DS. *Corneal Abrasions and Corneal Foreign Bodies: Management.* UpToDate Website. https://www.uptodate.com/contents/corneal-abrasions-and-corneal-foreign-bodies-management. Accessed April 2018.
2. Oum BS, Lee JS, Han YS. Clinical features of ocular trauma in emergency department. *Korean J Ophthalmol.* 2004;18(1):70-78.
3. Bashour M, Hampton R, et al. *Corneal Foreign Body.* Medscape Website. http://emedicine.medscape.com/article/1195581-overview. Accessed April 2017.
4. Verma A, Dahl A, et al. *Corneal Abrasion.* Medscape Website. http://emedicine.medscape.com/article/1195402-overview. Accessed April 2017.
5. Wilson SA, Last A. Management of corneal abrasions. *Am Fam Physician.* 2004;1(70):123-128.
6. Pokhrel PK, Loftus SA. *Ocular Emergencies.* American Family Physician Website. http://www.aafp.org /afp/2007/0915/p829.html. Accessed April 2017.
7. Xu Z, Yu X, Li Z, Wang L. The role of in vivo confocal microscopy in the diagnosis of hidden corneal foreign bodies. *J Int Med Res.* 2014;42(1):145-152.
8. Weissman BA. *Care of the Contact Lens Patient: Reference Guide for Clinicians.* St Louis, MO: American Optometric Association; 2000.
9. Turner A, Rabiu M. Patching for corneal abrasion. *Cochrane Database Syst Rev.* 2006 Apr 19;(2):CD004764.
10. Weaver CS, Terrell KM. Evidence-based emergency medicine. Update: do ophthalmic nonsteroidal anti-inflammatory drugs reduce the pain associated with simple corneal abrasion without delaying healing [review]? *Ann Emerg Med.* 2003;41(1):134-140.
11. Upadhyaya MP, Karmacharyaa PC, Kairalaa S, et al. The Bhaktapur eye study: ocular trauma and antibiotic prophylaxis for the prevention of corneal ulceration in Nepal. *Br J Ophthalmol.* 2001; 85:388-392.
12. Messman A, Hooker EA, et al. *Ocular Injuries: New Strategies in Emergency Department Management.* Evidence-based Emergency Medicine Website. http://www.ebmedicine.net/topics.php?paction=showTopic&topic_id=469. Accessed April 2017.

18 CONJUNCTIVITIS

Heidi S. Chumley, MD, MBA
Richard P. Usatine, MD

PATIENT STORY

A 35-year-old woman presents with 2 days of redness and tearing in her eyes (**Figure 18-1**). She has some thin matter in eyes, but neither eye has been glued shut when she awakens. She does not have any trouble seeing once she blinks to clear any accumulated debris. Both eyes are uncomfortable and itchy, but she is not having any severe pain. She does not wear contact lenses and has not had this problem previously. The patient was diagnosed with viral conjunctivitis and scored −1 on the clinical scoring system (see "Diagnosis" below). She was instructed about eye hygiene and recovered in 3 days.

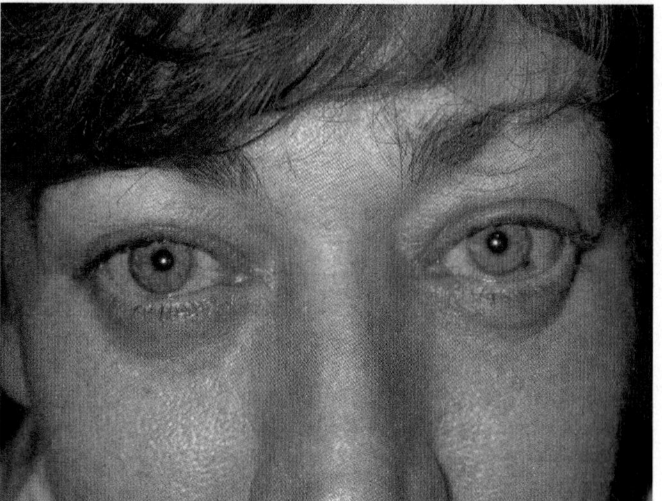

FIGURE 18-1 Viral conjunctivitis demonstrating bilateral conjunctival injection with little discharge. The patient has an incidental left eye conjunctival nevus. (*Reproduced with permission from Richard P. Usatine, MD.*)

INTRODUCTION

Conjunctivitis, inflammation of the membrane lining the eyelids and globe, presents with injected pink or red eye(s), eye discharge ranging from mild to purulent, eye discomfort or gritty sensation, and no vision loss. Conjunctivitis is most commonly infectious (viral or bacterial) or allergic, but can be caused by irritants. Diagnosis is clinical, based on differences in symptoms and signs.

SYNONYMS

Pink eye.

EPIDEMIOLOGY

- Infectious conjunctivitis is common and often occurs in outbreaks, making the prevalence difficult to estimate.
- In the United States:
  - The estimated annual incidence rate for conjunctivitis is 22,000 per 1 million people per year[1]
  - Viral conjunctivitis is more common than bacterial conjunctivitis
  - Allergic conjunctivitis had a point prevalence of 6.4% and a lifetime prevalence of 40% in a large population study in the United States from 1988 to 1994[2]
  - The direct healthcare costs related to conjunctivitis are estimated to be $800 million per year.[1]
- Worldwide, *Chlamydia trachomatis* is a common cause of conjunctivitis in adults and newborns. In 2016, almost 2 million people worldwide lost their eyesight to chlamydial eye infections.[3] Blindness due to chlamydial infection is rare in the United States because of neonatal prophylactic treatment programs.

ETIOLOGY AND PATHOPHYSIOLOGY

Conjunctivitis is predominately infectious (bacterial or viral) or allergic, and the most common etiologies vary by age and geographic location.

- Neonatal conjunctivitis is often caused by *C. trachomatis* and *Neisseria gonorrhoeae.*[4]
- Children younger than 6 years are more likely to have a bacterial than viral conjunctivitis (**Figure 18-2**). In the United States, the most common bacterial causes are *Haemophilus* species and *Streptococcus pneumoniae* accounting for almost 90% of cases in children.[5]
- Children age 6 years or older are more likely to have viral or allergic causes for conjunctivitis.[5] Adenovirus is the most common viral cause.

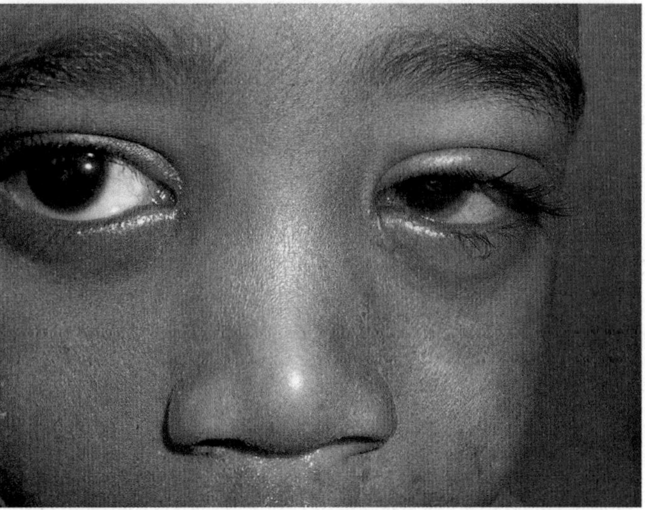

FIGURE 18-2 Unilateral conjunctivitis in a 4-year-old child. The child's age and purulent discharge are consistent with a bacterial etiology. (*Reproduced with permission from Richard P. Usatine, MD.*)

DIAGNOSIS

- To distinguish conjunctivitis from other causes of a red eye, ask about pain and check for vision loss. Patients with a red eye and intense pain or vision loss that does not clear with blinking are unlikely to have conjunctivitis and should undergo further evaluation.
- Always ask about contact lens use, as this can be a risk factor for all types of conjunctivitis, including bacterial conjunctivitis (**Figure 18-3**).
- Typical clinical features of any type of conjunctivitis may include eye discharge, gritty or uncomfortable feeling, one or both pink eyes, and no vision loss. The infection usually starts in one eye, and progresses to involve the other eye days later.
- Bacterial conjunctivitis (see **Figures 18-2** to **18-4**) has a more purulent discharge than viral or allergic conjunctivitis.
- A clinical scoring system has been developed to distinguish bacterial from other causes of conjunctivitis in healthy adults who did not wear contact lenses. A score of +5 to −3 is determined as follows:
    - Two glued eyes (+5); one glued eye (+2); history of conjunctivitis (−2); eye itching (−1).
    - A score of +5, +4, or +3 is useful in ruling in bacterial conjunctivitis with specificities of 100%, 94%, and 92%, respectively.
    - Scores of −1, −2, or −3 are useful in ruling out bacterial conjunctivitis with sensitivities of 98%, 98%, and 100%, respectively.[6]

Allergic conjunctivitis is typically bilateral and accompanied by eye itching. Giant papillary conjunctivitis is a type of allergic reaction, most commonly to soft contact lenses (**Figure 18-5**).

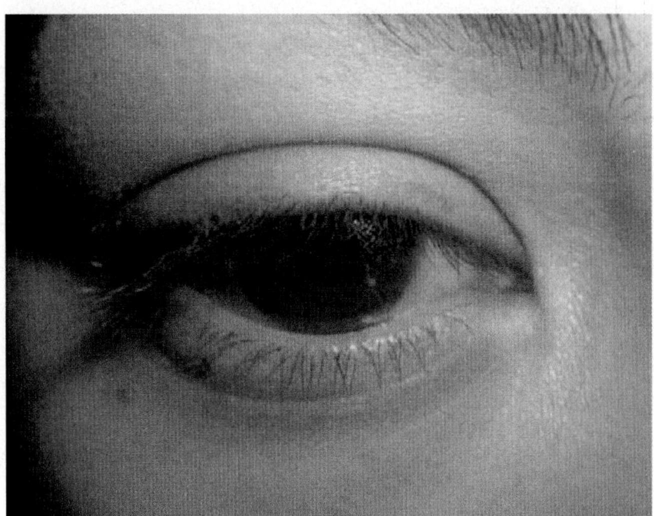

FIGURE 18-3 Bacterial conjunctivitis with a small amount of discharge. The patient was unable to clean her contacts while being evacuated from a hurricane-threatened Houston and the conjunctivitis was bilateral. (*Reproduced with permission from Richard P. Usatine, MD.*)

LABORATORY TESTING

- An in-office rapid test for adenoviral conjunctivitis (RPS AdenoPlus) has a sensitivity of 90% and a specificity of 96% compared to viral cell culture with confirmatory immunofluorescence staining.[7]

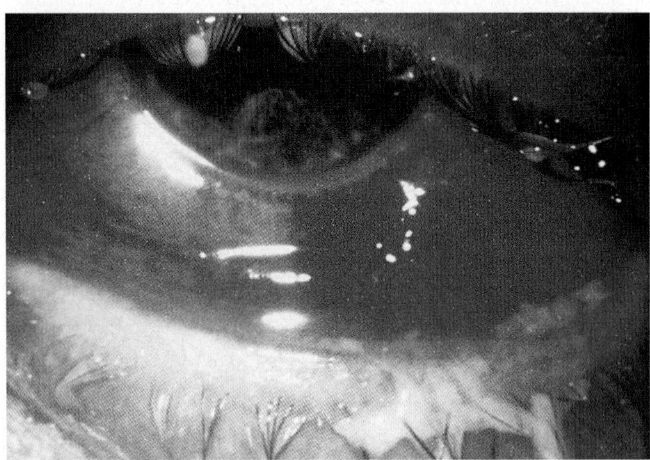

FIGURE 18-4 Gonococcus conjunctivitis has a copious discharge. This severe case resulted in partial blindness. (*Reproduced with permission from Centers for Disease Control and Prevention [CDC].*)

DIFFERENTIAL DIAGNOSIS

- Episcleritis—Segmental or diffuse inflammation of episclera (pink color), mild or no discomfort but can be tender to palpation, and no vision disturbance (see also Chapter 19, Scleritis and Episcleritis).
- Scleritis—Segmental or diffuse inflammation of sclera (dark red, purple, or blue color), severe boring eye pain often radiating to head and neck, and photophobia and vision loss (see also Chapter 19, Scleritis and Episcleritis).
- Uveitis or iritis—360-degree perilimbal injection, eye pain, photophobia, and vision loss. Frequently treated initially as conjunctivitis without resolution (see also Chapter 20, Uveitis and Iritis).
- Keratitis or corneal ulcerations—Diffuse conjunctival injection, often with miosis (constriction of pupil), eye discharge, pain, photophobia, and vision loss depending on the location of ulceration. Herpes keratitis is a diagnosis that should not be missed (**Figures 18-6** and **18-7**). The use of fluorescein and a UV light can help identify dendritic ulcers or other corneal damage and prompt an emergent referral to an ophthalmologist (**Figure 18-7**). Contact lens wearers should urgently see an ophthalmologist for keratitis.
- Acute-angle closure glaucoma—Cloudy cornea and scleral injection, eye pain with ipsilateral headache, elevated intraocular pressure, and severe vision loss (see also Chapter 21, Glaucoma).
- A foreign body in the eye can cause conjunctival injection and lead to a bacterial superinfection. If the foreign body is not easily dislodged with conservative measures, or appears to be superinfected with ulceration or leukocyte infiltrate, prompt referral to an ophthalmologist is required (**Figure 18-8**).

Trachoma is an eye infection caused by *C. trachomatis* that is rare in the United States but common in the rural areas of some developing countries. It is a leading cause of blindness in the developing world. Poverty and poor hygiene are major risk factors. Once the eye is infected, follicles can be seen on the upper tarsal conjunctiva upon eyelid eversion (**Figure 18-9**). Superior tarsal conjunctival scarring leads to entropion, which causes corneal scarring and ultimately blindness (**Figure 18-10**).

Vernal conjunctivitis is a severe recurrent form of allergic conjunctivitis that is more common in the summer (not the spring). The term *vernal* refers to the springtime, and therefore it is now referred to as "warm weather conjunctivitis" rather than "spring catarrh." Giant papillae that look like a cobblestone pattern may be seen in this condition. It occurs primarily in young boys, and typically ceases to recur seasonally with age.

MANAGEMENT

Hand hygiene can control the spread of infectious conjunctivitis.

Most acute conjunctival infections are viral and resolve without treatment. Following are the categories of patients who have a high probability of bacterial conjunctivitis and who are treated with topical antibiotics:

- Children younger than age 6 years.[5]

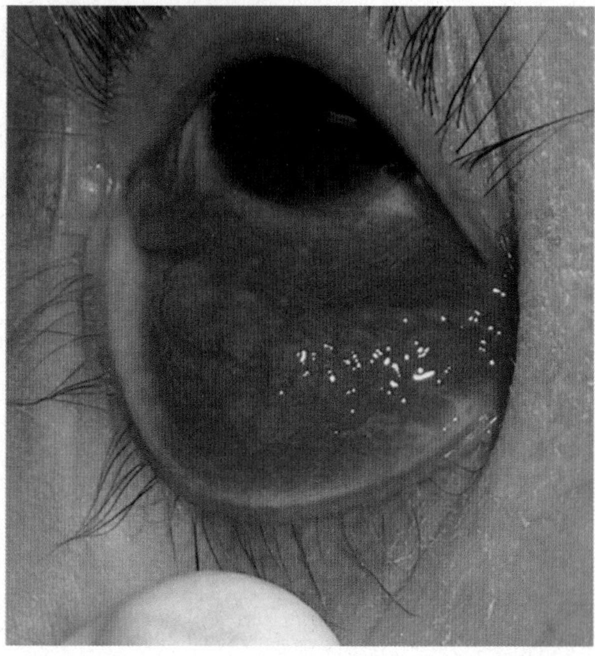

FIGURE 18-5 Giant papillary conjunctivitis in a contact lens wearer. *(Reproduced with permission from Mike Johnson, MD.)*

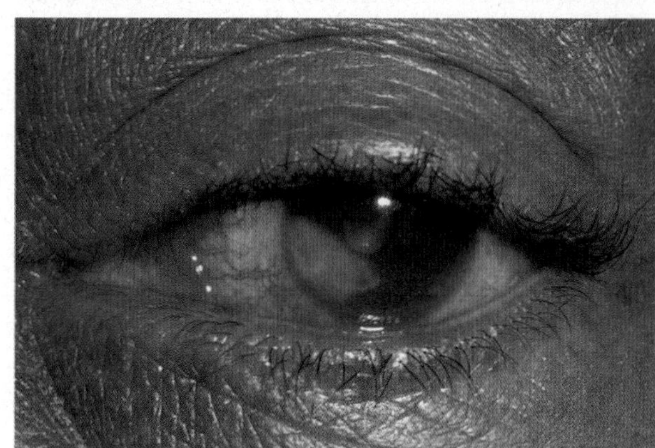

FIGURE 18-6 Herpetic keratitis in a 56-year-old woman staying in a shelter after Hurricane Katrina. *(Reproduced with permission from Richard P. Usatine, MD.)*

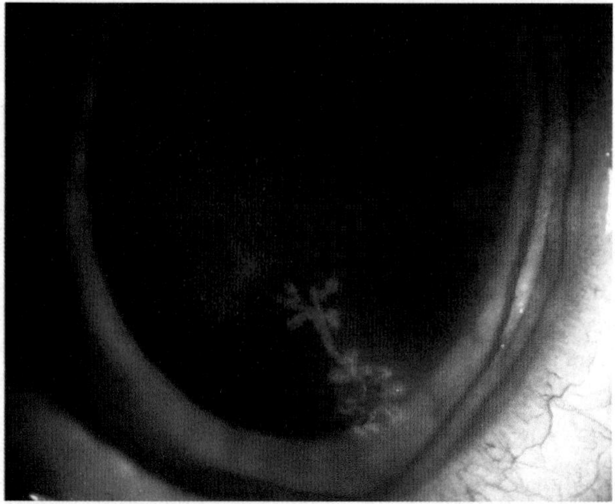

FIGURE 18-7 Slit-lamp view of a dendritic ulcer with fluorescein uptake from herpetic keratitis. *(Reproduced with permission from Paul D. Comeau.)*

- Azithromycin 1.5% ophthalmic solution twice daily for 3 days resulted in a clinical and microbiologic cure in 47.1% (day 3) and 89.2% (day 7) of children. This dosing regimen provides equivalent efficacy to 4 times a day dosing of tobramycin.[8]
- Children age 6 or older or adults who score +3 or above on the clinical scoring system for bacterial conjunctivitis.
  - Antibiotics from the following drug classes have been shown to be effective in randomized, controlled trials: aminoglycosides, fluoroquinolones, macrolides, and sulfonamides.[9]
  - Azithromycin 1% ophthalmic solution 1 drop twice a day for 2 days, then 1 drop once a day for 3 days is a convenient dosing schedule.[9]
- Delayed antibiotic prescription decreased antibiotic use by nearly 50% and provided similar symptom control compared to immediate antibiotics.[10]

Allergic conjunctivitis can be treated with antihistamines, mast-cell stabilizers, nonsteroidal anti-inflammatory agents, corticosteroids, and immunomodulatory agents.[9]

REFERRAL

- Refer patients who have vision loss, copious purulent discharge (this could represent gonococcal disease, which must be cultured, and which can cause vision loss), severe pain, lack of response to therapy, or a history of herpes simplex or zoster eye disease to an ophthalmologist.
- Any patient who may need ocular steroid should be seen by an ophthalmologist. There is a severe risk for complications with the use of ocular steroids.

PREVENTION

Good hygiene practices with washing of the hands and face with soap and water.

FOLLOW-UP/RETURN TO SCHOOL

Routine follow-up is generally not needed if symptoms resolve in 3 to 5 days.

State health departments have no consensus on when children with conjunctivitis can return to school. A literature-based review suggests the best strategy is excluding children from school until they are asymptomatic.[11]

PATIENT EDUCATION

- Most adults and children older than age 6 years have a nonbacterial cause of conjunctivitis.
- Remove contact lenses until conjunctivitis has resolved.
- Avoid touching the face or rubbing the eyes and wash hands immediately afterwards.
- Do not share face towels, eye makeup, or contact lens cases.
- Inform your physician immediately if you experience eye pain or vision loss.

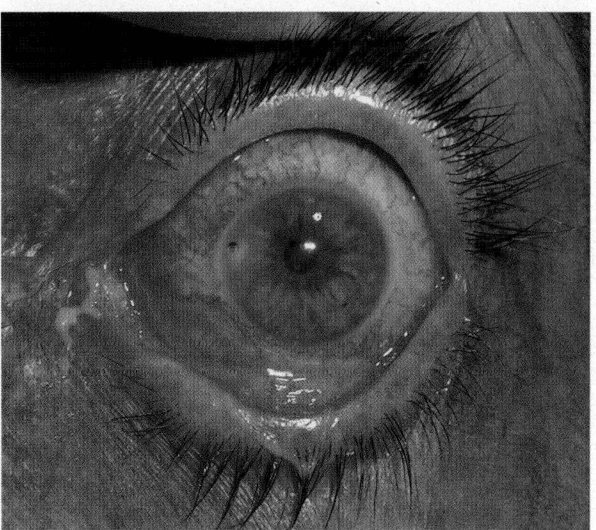

FIGURE 18-8 Conjunctivitis caused by a foreign body in the eye of a machinist. The ground metal speck is seen on the cornea, and the corneal infiltrate, along with a purulent discharge, indicate a bacterial superinfection. (*Reproduced with permission from Richard P. Usatine, MD.*)

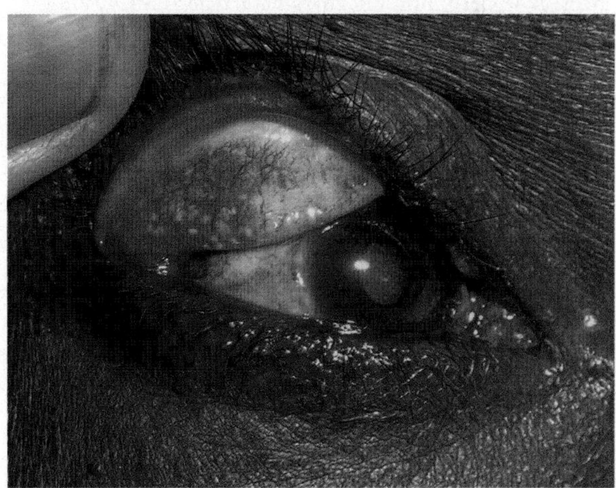

FIGURE 18-9 Trachoma showing many white follicles on the underside of the upper eyelid. (*Reproduced with permission from Richard P. Usatine, MD.*)

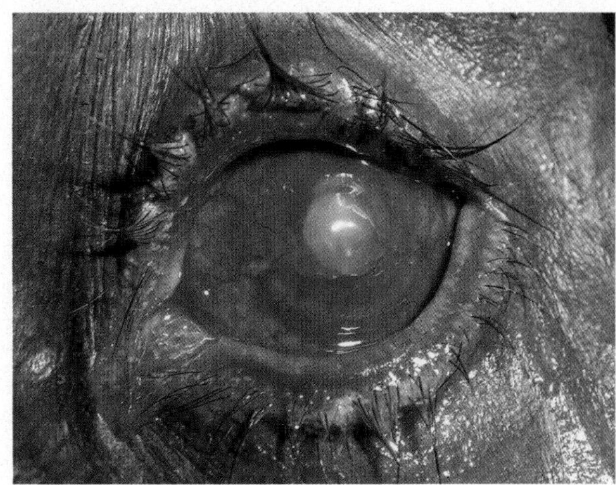

FIGURE 18-10 Advanced trachoma with blindness as a consequence of cornea opacities. Note the deep conjunctival injection and purulent discharge from the *C. trachomatis* infection. (*Reproduced with permission from Richard P. Usatine, MD.*)

PATIENT RESOURCES

- PubMed Health. *Conjunctivitis (Pink Eye)*—**http://www.ncbi.nlm.nih.gov/pubmedhealth/PMH0002005/.**
- American Academy of Ophthalmology. *Conjunctivitis: What Is Pink Eye?*—**http://www.geteyesmart.org/eyesmart/diseases/conjunctivitis.cfm.**
- Centers for Disease Control and Prevention has patient information in English and Spanish at **http://www.cdc.gov.**
- Centers for Disease Control and Prevention. *Conjunctivitis (Pink Eye)*—**http://www.cdc.gov/conjunctivitis/index.html.**
- The Livestrong foundation has auditory patient information on YouTube. *Conjunctivitis Health Byte*—**http://www.youtube.com/watch?v=O8LkDfbLCaY**; and *A Healthy Byte: Pink Eye*—**http://www.youtube.com/watch?v=Hp28hS7XYCo&feature=relmfu.**

PROVIDER RESOURCES

- A comprehensive review article on conjunctivitis—**https://www.ncbi.nlm.nih.gov/pmc/articles/PMC4049531/**

REFERENCES

1. Schneider JE, Scheibling CM, Degall D, et al. Epidemiology and economic burden of conjunctivitis: a managed care perspective. *J Manage Care Med.* 2014;17(1):78-83.
2. Singh K, Axelrod S, Bielory L. The epidemiology of ocular and nasal allergy in the United States, 1988–1994. *J Allergy Clin Immunol.* 2010;126(4):778-783.
3. Satpathy G, Behera HS, Ahmed NH. Chlamydial eye infections: current perspectives. *Indian J Ophthalmol.* 2017;65(2):97-102.
4. Centers for Disease Control and Prevention. *Conjunctivitis (Pink-Eye) in Newborns.* https://www.cdc.gov/conjunctivitis/newborns.html. Accessed October 2017.
5. Meltzer JA, Kunkov D, Crain EF. Identifying children at low risk for bacterial conjunctivitis. *Arch Pediatr Adolesc Med.* 2010;164:263-267.
6. Rietveld RP. Predicting bacterial cause in infectious conjunctivitis: cohort study on informativeness of combinations of signs and symptoms. *BMJ.* 2004;329:206-210.
7. Sambursky R, Trattler W, Tauber S, et al. Sensitivity and specificity of the AdenoPlus test for diagnosing adenoviral conjunctivitis. *JAMA Ophthalmol.* 2013;131(1):17-21.
8. Bremond-Gignac D, Nezzar H, Bianchi PE, et al. Efficacy and safety of azithromycin 1.5% eye drops in paediatric population with purulent bacterial conjunctivitis. *Br J Ophthalmol.* 2014;98(6):739-745.
9. Azari AA, Barney NP. Conjunctivitis. A systematic review of diagnosis and treatment. *JAMA.* 2013;310(16):1721-1729.
10. Everitt HA, Little PS, Smith PW. A randomized controlled trial of management strategies for acute infective conjunctivitis in general practice. *BMJ.* 2006;333(7563):321.
11. Ohnsman CM. Exclusion of students with conjunctivitis from school: policies of state departments of health. *J Pediatr Ophthalmol Strabismus.* 2007;44(2):101-105.

19 SCLERITIS AND EPISCLERITIS

Heidi S. Chumley, MD, MBA
Mary Kelly Green, MD

PATIENT STORY

A 45-year-old woman presents with 1 day of increasing eye pain, eye redness, and blurred vision. On examination, there is scleral injection and exquisite globe tenderness to palpation (**Figure 19-1**). Her review of systems is positive for morning stiffness and swelling in both of her hands. The patient was urgently referred to an ophthalmologist who diagnosed her with scleritis. Her visual acuity was reduced minimally. A slit lamp exam revealed injected sclera with a bluish hue in the affected eye and rare anterior chamber cells. The posterior segment was normal.

The ophthalmologist prescribed an oral nonsteroidal anti-inflammatory drug (NSAID), specifically indomethacin, as it effectively crosses the blood-brain barrier and gets good levels in the eye.

Her rheumatoid factor was positive, so she was also referred to a rheumatologist.

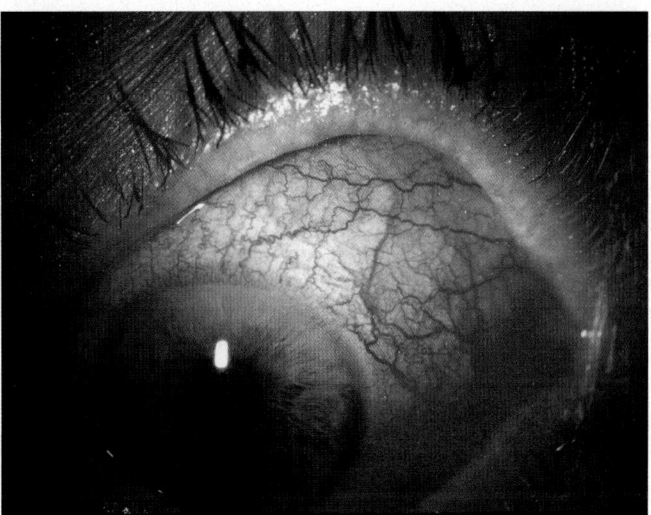

FIGURE 19-1 Scleritis in a patient with eye pain and exquisite globe tenderness. Untreated, this can result in loss of vision. (*Reproduced with permission from Paul D. Comeau.*)

INTRODUCTION

Episcleritis and scleritis are inflammations of the deeper layers of the eye, the vascular episclera, and the avascular sclera. Episcleritis presents with segmental eye redness, discomfort but not severe pain, and no vision loss. Scleritis can have overlying episcleritis, but also has a violaceous hue, is usually painful, and may cause vision loss. Scleritis typically has an associated underlying condition (autoimmune or infectious) that should be identified and treated. Scleritis is treated with oral NSAIDs, systemic glucocorticoids, or immunosuppressive medications. Patients with scleritis are often referred to an ophthalmologist, as vision loss is common.

EPIDEMIOLOGY

Scleritis:

- In a community-based population study[1]:
  - Incidence: 4.1 cases/100,000 person years
  - More common in women than men (6.4 vs. 2.3/100,000 person years)
  - Median age at diagnosis: 56 years; 50% of cases diagnosed between ages 42 and 60
- In tertiary referral centers[2]:
  - 35.8% of patients with scleritis had an associated systemic illness, most commonly (24.8%) a connective tissue or vasculitic disease
  - Scleritis was diagnosed before the systemic disease in 38.7% of patients

Episcleritis:

- In a community-based population study[1]:
  - Incidence: 21.7 cases/100,000 person years
  - More common in women than men (26.0 vs. 17.7/100,000 person years)
  - Median age at diagnosis: 45; 50% of cases diagnosed between ages 32 and 54
- In tertiary referral centers[2]:
  - 27.1% of patients with episcleritis had an associated systemic illness, most commonly (15.3%) a connective tissue or vasculitic disease
- Nodular or recurrent episcleritis is more likely to be associated with an underlying systemic condition than is an isolated episode of simple episcleritis.

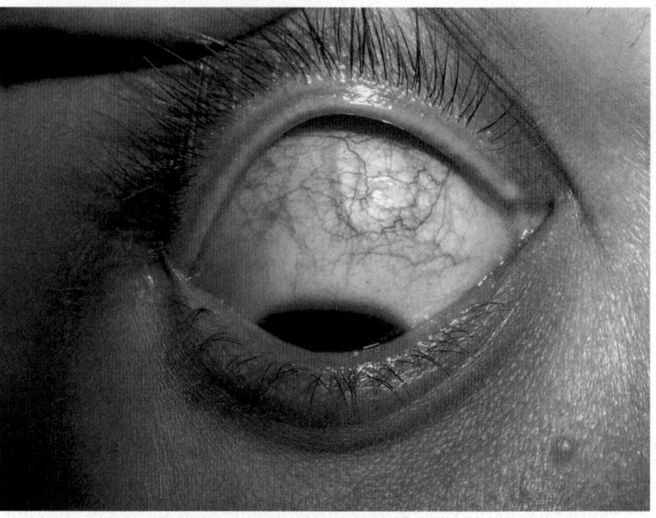

FIGURE 19-2 Scleritis in a young woman with rheumatoid arthritis. Note the violaceous deep vessel engorgement. (*Reproduced with permission from Richard P. Usatine, MD.*)

ETIOLOGY AND PATHOPHYSIOLOGY

- Scleritis and episcleritis are inflammatory conditions causing congestion of the deeper 2 of the 3 vascular layers (conjunctival, episcleral, and scleral plexuses) overlying the avascular sclera.
- Scleritis often occurs with episcleritis; episcleritis does not involve the sclera and does not progress to scleritis.
- Scleritis disrupts vascular architecture and may cause vision loss; episcleritis does not.
- Causes of scleritis:
  - Systemic autoimmune diseases such as rheumatoid arthritis (**Figure 19-2**), Wegener granulomatosis (**Figure 19-3**), seronegative spondyloarthropathies, relapsing polychondritis, polyarteritis nodosa, and systemic lupus erythematosus (SLE)
  - Infections (*Pseudomonas*, tuberculosis, syphilis, herpes zoster)
  - Less common causes include Behçet syndrome, gout, and sarcoidosis
  - Idiopathic
- Causes of episcleritis:
  - Most often idiopathic
  - May be associated with any of the conditions listed above, especially if the presentation is nodular or recurrent

DIAGNOSIS

CLINICAL FEATURES

Scleritis:

- Segmental or diffuse inflammation of sclera (violaceous, purple, blue, or dark red color), with overlying episcleral and conjunctival inflammation (**Figures 19-1** to **19-3**).
- Severe, boring eye pain often radiating to head and neck that worsens with eye movement. However, 20% of patients may not have pain, including those with the necrotizing type (scleromalacia perforans) and those taking immunosuppressive agents prior to the onset of scleritis.[3]
- Photophobia and vision loss.

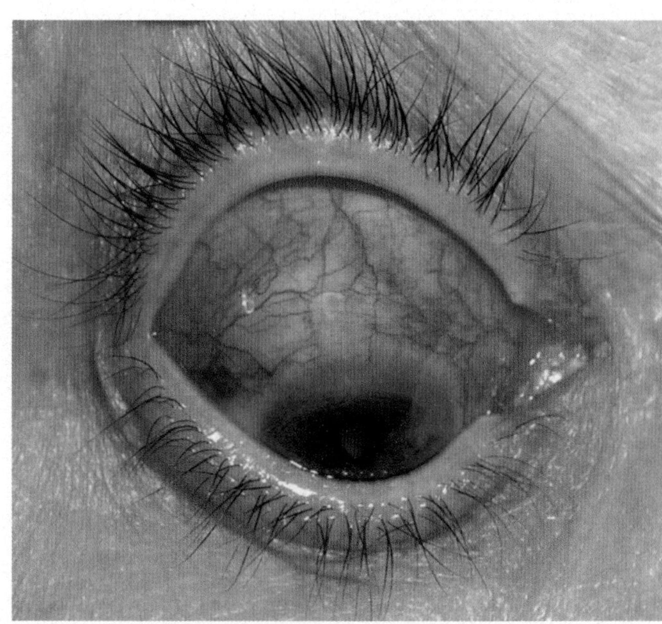

FIGURE 19-3 Scleritis in a patient with Wegener granulomatosis. Deep vessels are affected, giving the eye a purplish or blue hue. (*Reproduced with permission from Everett Allen, MD.*)

Episcleritis:

- Segmental or diffuse inflammation of episclera (pink color) and overlying conjunctival vessel injection (**Figures 19-4** and **19-5**).
- Mild if any discomfort but can be tender to palpation.
- No vision disturbance.
- Scleritis and episcleritis are often distinguished by history and physical examination features; however, when scleritis has extensive overlying episcleritis, the diagnosis becomes more difficult. Scleritis must be differentiated from episcleritis because scleritis requires treatment and an evaluation for underlying medical conditions.
- Ten percent phenylephrine blanches inflamed episcleral and conjunctival vessels, but not scleral vessels; in scleritis, this can reveal a focus of scleral engorgement covered by episcleral injection.
- Scleritis and episcleritis, as opposed to iritis with overlying episcleral injection, often have areas of focal tenderness to palpation. These can be elicited with a sterile cotton swab after applying a topical anesthetic.

Typical distribution:

- Scleritis can be posterior (posterior to the medial and lateral rectus muscles) or anterior:
    - Posterior scleritis can produce serous retinal detachments and subretinal exudates and is often associated with uveitis (inflammation of the iris, ciliary body, or choroid)
    - Anterior scleritis can be diffuse, nodular, necrotizing with inflammation or necrotizing without inflammation[3]
- Scleritis is bilateral in 50% of patients.[3]
- Episcleritis is often segmental, but can be diffuse, and is typically benign.

LABORATORY TESTING

In scleritis, if an associated systemic disease has not been previously diagnosed, consider ordering these tests: complete blood count, metabolic panel, urinalysis, antineutrophil cytoplasmic antibody, antinuclear antibody, rheumatoid factor, anticyclic citrullinated peptide antibodies, rapid plasma reagin, and Lyme antibody in Lyme endemic regions.

IMAGING

- In scleritis, if an associated systemic disease has not been previously diagnosed, consider the following: chest radiographs, sinus CT, or sacroiliac joint radiographs.
- To diagnose posterior scleritis, ophthalmic ultrasound or orbital CT can demonstrate scleral thickening.

BIOPSY

An ophthalmologist may rarely perform a biopsy when it is important to distinguish among scleritis caused by rheumatic diseases, infections, or sarcoidosis.

- Rheumatic—Zonal necrotizing granulomatous scleral inflammation with loss of anterior scleral tissue.
- Infectious—Necrotizing scleritis with microabscesses.
- Sarcoid—Sarcoidal granulomatous inflammation can be identified in cases of sarcoidosis.

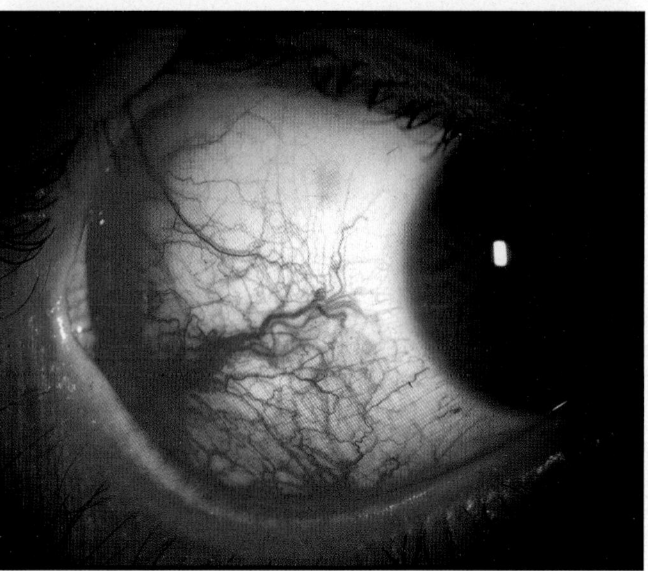

FIGURE 19-4 Episcleritis showing inflammation of the conjunctival and episcleral tissue with associated vascular engorgement. A sector of this eye is involved, and that is typical. Vessels were blanched with 2.5% phenylephrine, which helped distinguish this from scleritis. *(Reproduced with permission from Paul D. Comeau.)*

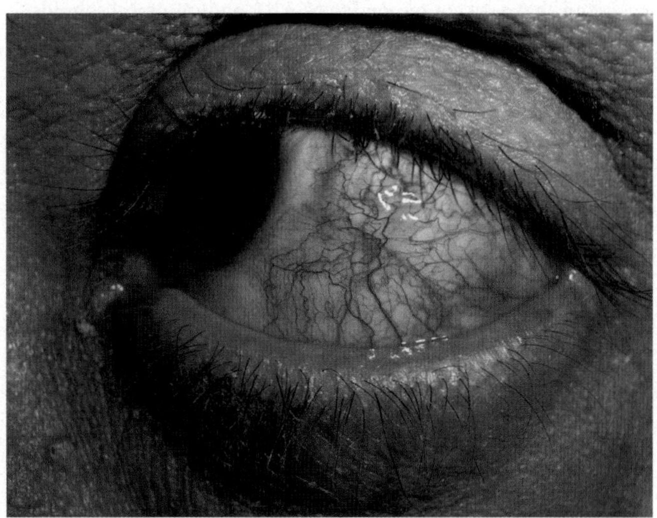

FIGURE 19-5 Episcleritis showing inflammation of only the conjunctival and episcleral tissue. Note the absence of violaceous color that is seen in scleritis. *(Reproduced with permission from Richard P. Usatine, MD.)*

DIFFERENTIAL DIAGNOSIS

Causes of red eye, other than scleritis and episcleritis:

- Uveitis or iritis—360 degrees limbal injection, eye pain, photophobia, and vision loss (see Chapter 20, Uveitis and Iritis).
- Keratitis or corneal ulcerations—Diffuse erythema with limbal injection often with pupillary constriction; eye discharge; pain, photophobia, and vision loss depending on location of ulceration.
- Conjunctivitis—Conjunctival injection, eye discharge, gritty or uncomfortable feeling, no vision loss (see Chapter 18, Conjunctivitis).
- Acute-angle closure glaucoma—Cloudy cornea and scleral injection; eye pain with ipsilateral headache; severe vision loss (see Chapter 21, Glaucoma).

MANAGEMENT

For patients presenting with scleritis who do not have a previously diagnosed associated systemic condition, a search for an underlying cause is indicated, particularly if the scleritis is recurrent.

- Evaluate for signs and symptoms of rheumatoid arthritis, Wegener granulomatosis (respiratory or renal symptoms), polyarteritis nodosa (ocular involvement may precede systemic disease by years), relapsing polychondritis (vasculitis around ear or nose cartilage or trachea), and seronegative spondyloarthropathies (inflammatory back pain, arthritis, and inflammatory bowel symptoms).
- Evaluate for signs, symptoms, and risk factors for infection including eye trauma, recent ocular surgery, recurrent herpes simplex or varicella zoster, or risk factors for tuberculosis.
- Evaluate for signs and symptoms of gout and sarcoidosis.

MEDICATIONS

- Scleritis is initially treated with systemic NSAIDs and/or topical steroids; however, in one study only 47% of patients responded to 2 drops of 1% prednisolone every 2 hours for up to 2 weeks.[4] SOR B
- Scleritis that does not respond to NSAIDs and/or topical steroids may need systemic steroids, subconjunctival steroids, or immune modulators. SOR C
- Episcleritis often resolves spontaneously. Eye redness and irritation improve by 50% in less than a week. Treatment with topical NSAIDs was no better than artificial tears on measures of redness and comfort.[5] SOR B

REFERRAL

- If you suspect scleritis, refer the patient to an ophthalmologist immediately. This is especially important if there is any visual loss or eye pain.
- If episcleritis is not resolved, refer to an ophthalmologist.

PROGNOSIS

- Simple episcleritis improves in 7 to 10 days. Episcleritis that is nodular or associated with an underlying disease may take 2 to 3 weeks to resolve.
- Patients who smoke may take longer to recover from episcleritis or scleritis. One retrospective trial demonstrated that patients who smoked and had episcleritis or scleritis were 5.4 times more likely to have a delayed response of more than 4 weeks to any medication (95% confidence interval [CI] = 1.9 to 15.5).[6]
- Vision loss occurs in 15% of patients with scleritis; risk factors for vision loss include necrotizing scleritis (odds ratio [OR] 6.63), infectious cause (OR 4.44), ocular hypertension (OR 3.19), and posterior scleritis (OR 2.33).[2]

FOLLOW-UP

- Advise patients with episcleritis to return for any increases in eye pain, changes in vision, or no improvement in 1 week.
- Advise patients with scleritis to pursue follow-up testing for underlying systemic illnesses. If none is found, consider retesting, as the diagnosis of scleritis precedes the diagnosis of an associated illness in almost 40% of patients.[2]

PATIENT EDUCATION

- Reassure patients with episcleritis of its generally benign nature and that oral NSAIDs may be used for discomfort.
- Advise patients with scleritis of its association with systemic illnesses and the need for further work-up.

PATIENT RESOURCES

- Episcleritis and Scleritis—**https://patient.info/health/episcleritis-and-scleritis-leaflet.**

PROVIDER RESOURCES

- Episcleritis and Scleritis—**http://www.patient.co.uk/doctor/Scleritis-and-Episcleritis.htm.**

REFERENCES

1. Homayounfar G, Nardone N, Borkar DS, et al. Incidence of scleritis and episcleritis: results from the Pacific Ocular Inflammation Study. *Am J Ophthalmol.* 2013;156(4):752-758.
2. De la Maza MS, Molina N, Gonzalez-Gonzalez LA, et al. Clinical characteristics of a large cohort of patients with scleritis and episcleritis. *Ophthalmology.* 2012;119(1):43-50.
3. Galor A, Thorne JE. Scleritis and peripheral ulcerative keratitis. *Rheum Dis Clin North Am.* 2007;33(4):835-854.
4. McMullen M, Kovarik G, Hodge WG. Use of topical steroid therapy in the management of nonnecrotizing anterior scleritis. *Can J Ophthalmol.* 1999;34(4):217-221.
5. Williams CP, Browning AC, Sleep TJ, et al. A randomised, double-blind trial of topical ketorolac vs artificial tears for the treatment of episcleritis. *Eye (Lond).* 2005;19(7):739-742.
6. Boonman ZF, de Keizer RJ, Watson PG. Smoking delays the response to treatment in episcleritis and scleritis. *Eye (Lond).* 2005;19(9):945-955.

20 UVEITIS AND IRITIS

Heidi S. Chumley, MD, MBA

PATIENT STORY

A 28-year-old man presented with sudden onset of a right red eye, severe eye pain, tearing, photophobia, and decreased vision. He denied eye trauma. His review of systems was positive for lower back pain and stiffness over the past year. On examination, he had a ciliary flush (**Figure 20-1**) and decreased vision. He was referred to an ophthalmologist who confirmed the diagnosis of acute anterior uveitis. He was found to be HLA-B27 positive with characteristics of ankylosing spondylitis. His uveitis was treated with topical steroids.

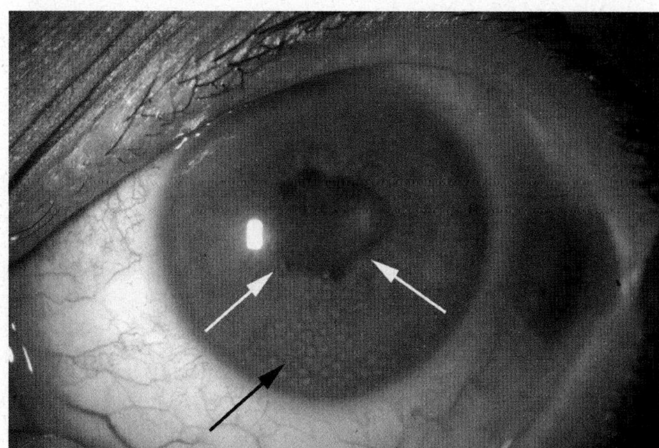

FIGURE 20-1 Acute anterior uveitis with corneal endothelial white cell aggregates (*black arrow*) and posterior synechiae formation (iris adhesions to the lens, *white arrows*). (*Reproduced with permission from Paul D. Comeau.*)

INTRODUCTION

Uveitis is inflammation of any component of the uveal tract: iris (anterior), ciliary body (intermediate), or choroid (posterior). Most uveitis is anterior and is also called iritis. Uveitis is caused by trauma, inflammation, or infection and the most common etiologies vary by location in the uveal tract. Patients present with vision changes and, if uveitis is anterior, eye pain, redness, tearing, and photophobia. All patients with uveitis should be referred to an ophthalmologist.

SYNONYMS

Anterior uveitis includes iritis and iridocyclitis. *Iritis* is when the inflammation is limited to the iris. If the ciliary body is involved too, then it is called *iridocyclitis*. Posterior uveitis includes choroiditis and chorioretinitis.

EPIDEMIOLOGY

- In a large population study in Hawaii, the annual incidence of uveitis was 24.9 per 100,000 person years and the prevalence was 58 per 100,000 population.[1]
- Occurs at any age, but most commonly between 25 and 64 years, and nearly equivalent between men and women.[1]
- 73% of uveitis cases are anterior (also called iritis); 6% are intermediate; 21% are posterior or panuveitis.[1]
- In children, juvenile rheumatoid arthritis is the most common associated systemic disease, present in over 50% of cases associated with a systemic disease and 20% of all uveitis cases in children.[2]
- In the United States, noninfectious uveitis accounts for 10% of legal blindness.[3]

ETIOLOGY AND PATHOPHYSIOLOGY

- Uveitis can be caused by trauma, infections, inflammation, or, rarely, neoplasms. Most likely causes differ by location.[4]

- Iritis—Trauma is common (**Figure 20-2**). In nontraumatic cases, causes include idiopathic (50%); seronegative spondyloarthropathies, that is, ankylosing spondylitis, reactive arthritis, psoriatic arthritis, inflammatory bowel disease (20%); and juvenile idiopathic arthritis (10%). Infections are less common and include herpes, syphilis, and tuberculosis.[4]
- Intermediate—Most are idiopathic[4] (**Figure 20-3**).
- Posterior—Toxoplasmosis is the most common, followed by idiopathic.[4]
- Panuveitis (affecting all layers)—Idiopathic (22% to 45%) and sarcoidosis (14% to 28%).[4] Unilateral panuveitis is often endophthalmitis (endogenous or related to trauma or surgery). Bilateral panuveitis can be caused by sarcoidosis or syphilis.

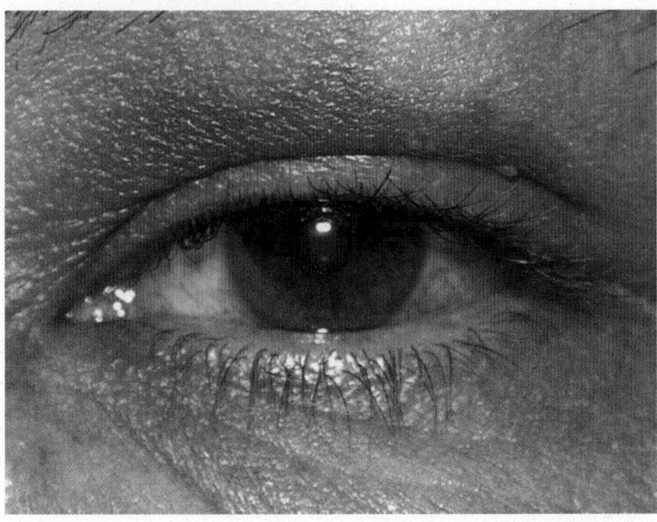

FIGURE 20-2 A young man with traumatic iritis (anterior uveitis) after being hit in the eye with a baseball. He has photophobia and eye pain. (*Reproduced with permission from Richard P. Usatine, MD.*)

RISK FACTORS

Patients with Behçet disease and ankylosing spondylitis have uveitis more commonly than the general population (relative risk of 4 to 20) because of human leukocyte antigen (HLA) associations.[5]

DIAGNOSIS

CLINICAL FEATURES

Anterior acute uveitis presents with:

- Usually unilateral eye pain, redness, tearing, photophobia, and decreased vision.
- 360-Degree perilimbal injection, which is most intense at the limbus (see **Figures 20-1, 20-2,** and **20-4**).
- History of eye trauma, an associated systemic disease, or risk factors for infection.
- Severe anterior uveitis may cause a hypopyon from layering of leukocytes and fibrous debris in the anterior chamber (**Figure 20-4**). Behçet syndrome and HLA-B27 disease are the only two common noninfectious causes of hypopyon.

Intermediate and posterior uveitis:

- Presents with altered vision or floaters.
- Often there is no pain, redness, tearing, or photophobia.

Sarcoid uveitis presents with:

- Panuveitis (anterior, intermediate, and posterior).
- Gradual and usually a bilateral onset.
- Few vision complaints unless cataracts or glaucoma develops.
- Characteristic findings on slit-lamp examination (i.e., mutton-fat keratic precipitates, posterior iris synechiae).[6]

Typical distribution:

- Anterior uveitis is typically unilateral and sarcoid uveitis is typically bilateral.

LABORATORY AND RADIOGRAPHIC TESTING

- Consider laboratory testing if the cause of uveitis is not readily apparent: complete blood count, basic metabolic panel, urinalysis, and erythrocyte sedimentation rate.[7]
- Consider HLA-B27 for patients with recurrent anterior uveitis.[7]

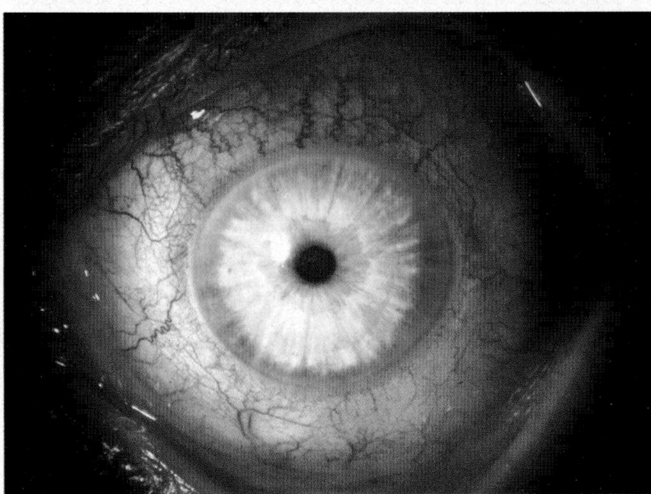

FIGURE 20-3 Idiopathic intermediate uveitis. The ciliary flush is perilimbal injection from dilation of blood vessels adjacent to the cornea, extending 3 mm into the sclera. Perilimbal injection may appear as a violet hue around the limbus with blurring of individual vessels. (*Reproduced with permission from Paul D. Comeau.*)

- Serology for syphilis and a chest radiograph to identify sarcoidosis or tuberculosis may also be indicated when other tests are normal.[7]

DIFFERENTIAL DIAGNOSIS

Causes of red eye, other than uveitis:

- Scleritis—Segmental or diffuse inflammation of sclera (dark red, purple, or blue color); severe, boring eye pain often radiating to head and neck; and photophobia and vision loss (see Chapter 19, Scleritis and Episcleritis).
- Episcleritis—Segmental or diffuse inflammation of episclera (pink color), mild or no discomfort but can be tender to palpation, and no vision disturbance (see Chapter 19, Scleritis and Episcleritis).
- Keratitis or corneal ulcerations—Diffuse erythema with ciliary injection often with constricted pupil; eye discharge; and pain, photophobia, and vision loss depending on the location of ulceration. Frequently associated with trauma, a history of herpes simplex virus (HSV) infection, or contact lens wear. Needs urgent evaluation by an ophthalmologist. There will be staining of the cornea with fluorescein.
- Conjunctivitis—Conjunctival injection, eye discharge, gritty or uncomfortable feeling, and no vision loss (see Chapter 18, Conjunctivitis). Recent history of red eye contacts or URI symptoms.
- Acute-angle closure glaucoma—Cloudy cornea and scleral injection, eye pain with ipsilateral headache, and severe vision loss (see Chapter 21, Glaucoma). May be a family history of same.

MANAGEMENT

Refer patients for any red eye along with loss of vision to an ophthalmologist. Patients with uveitis warrant additional examinations by the ophthalmologist.

- Traumatic uveitis—Dilated funduscopy for other ocular trauma, measurement of intraocular pressure, gonioscopy to evaluate for angle recession and risk for future glaucoma, and treatment may include steroid and/or cycloplegics for comfort.
- Nontraumatic uveitis—Slit-lamp examination and laboratory tests to assist with diagnosis of underlying cause; treatment is based on underlying cause but is usually topical steroid drops with or without cycloplegia.
- Therapeutic dilation is used to break the posterior synechiae that can occur (**Figure 20-5**).

PROGNOSIS

Uveitis causes vision loss, cataract, and often glaucoma if treatment is delayed or not provided. 5-year risk in non-infectious intermediate, posterior, or panuveitis[8]:

- 66% for any ocular complication, compared to 24% in controls.
- 35% for cataract, compared to 13% in controls.
- 29% for visual disturbance, compared to 9% in controls.
- 20% for glaucoma, compared to 9% in controls.
- 5% for blindness/low vision, compared to 0.5% in controls.

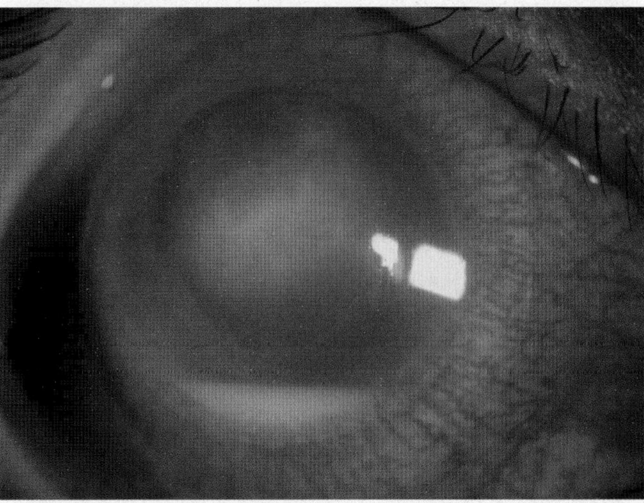

FIGURE 20-4 Hypopyon with severe anterior uveitis, showing layering of leukocytes and fibrinous debris in the anterior chamber. May be sterile or infectious. An intense ciliary flush is seen. Most commonly seen in HLA-B27-positive patients with uveitis. Hypopyon may also be a presenting sign of malignancy (retinoblastoma and lymphoma). (*Reproduced with permission from Paul D. Comeau.*)

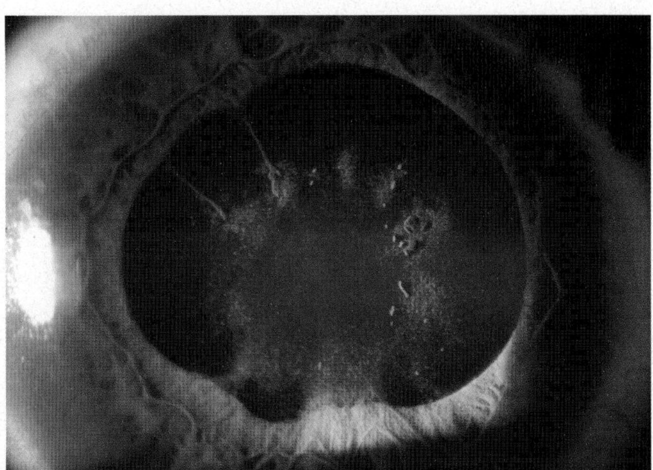

FIGURE 20-5 This patient with uveitis had posterior synechiae that are attachments of the iris to the anterior capsule of the lens. Therapeutic dilation broke the synechiae, but left residual pigment on the anterior capsule. (*Reproduced with permission from Paul D. Comeau.*)

HLA-B27 disease is the most common etiology for anterior uveitis, and is associated with recurrent, bilateral anterior uveitis.

FOLLOW-UP

Appropriate follow-up is based on the underlying cause.

PATIENT EDUCATION

- See a physician immediately for a red eye with loss of vision.
- A series of tests may be performed to determine the cause of the uveitis; however, the underlying cause is often elusive.

PATIENT RESOURCES

- **http://www.ncbi.nlm.nih.gov/pubmedhealth/PMH0002000/.**

PROVIDER RESOURCES

- **http://emedicine.medscape.com/article/1209123-overview#a1.**

REFERENCES

1. Acharya NR, Than VM, Esterberg E, et al. Incidence and prevalence of uveitis: results from the Pacific Ocular Inflammation Study. *JAMA Ophthal.* 2013;131(11):1406-1412.
2. BenEzra D, Cohen E, Maftzir G. Uveitis in children and adolescents. *Br J Ophthal.* 2005;89(4):444-448.
3. Gritz DC, Wong IG. Incidence and prevalence of uveitis in northern California; the Northern California Epidemiology of Uveitis Study. *Ophthalmology.* 2004;111(3):491-500.
4. Brazis PW, Stewart M, Lee AG. The uveo-meningeal syndromes. *Neurologist.* 2004;10(4):171-184.
5. Capsi RR. A look at autoimmunity and inflammation in the eye. *J Clin Invest.* 2010;120(9):3073-3083.
6. Pasadhika S, Rosenbaum JT. Ocular sarcoidosis. *Clin Chest Med.* 2015;36(4):669-683.
7. Harman LE, Margo CE, Roetzheim RG. Uveitis: the collaborative diagnostic evaluation. *Am Fam Physician.* 2014;15(90):711-716.
8. Dick AD, Tundia N, Sorg R, et al. Risk of ocular complications in patients with noninfectious intermediate uveitis, posterior uveitis, or panuveitis. *Ophthalmology.* 2016;123(3):655-662.

21 GLAUCOMA

Heidi S. Chumley, MD, MBA

PATIENT STORY

A 50-year-old black man was noted to have a large cup-to-disc ratio during a funduscopic examination by his primary care provider (**Figure 20-1**). The patient reported no visual complaints. Further evaluation revealed elevated intraocular pressure and early visual field defects. He was started on medication to lower his intraocular pressure. He remained asymptomatic, and his visual field defects did not progress for the next several years.

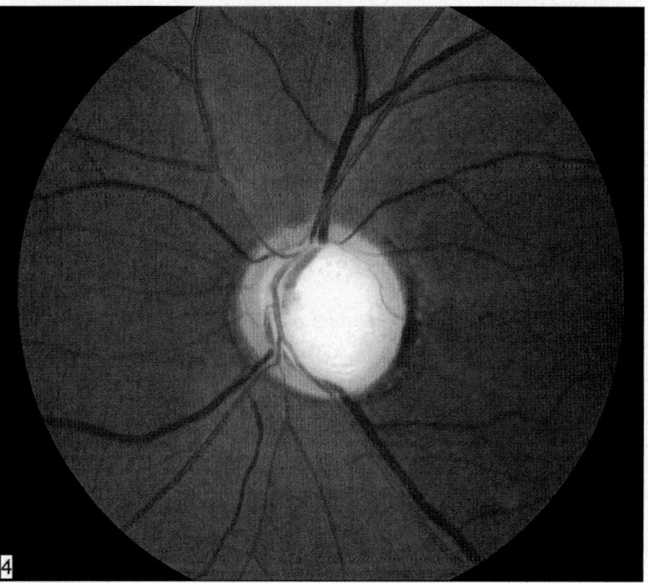

FIGURE 21-1 A 50-year-old man with glaucoma has an increased optic cup-to-disc ratio of 0.8. Median cup-to-disc ratio is 0.2 to 0.3, but varies considerably among individuals. (*Reproduced with permission from Paul D. Comeau.*)

INTRODUCTION

Glaucoma is a leading cause of blindness in the United States and globally. Open-angle glaucoma is an acquired loss of retinal ganglion cells characterized by either normal or increased intraocular pressure (IOP), a large cup-to-disc ratio, and visual field defects. Open-angle glaucoma is treated by reducing IOP, most commonly with eye drops. Angle-closure glaucoma, which is much less common, is an acute increase in IOP from a mechanical obstruction that must be treated emergently to preserve vision.

EPIDEMIOLOGY

- In 2013, an estimated 65 million people worldwide had glaucoma.[1]
- The prevalence of glaucoma in the global population between ages 40 and 80 is 3.54%; Africa has the highest prevalence of open-angle glaucoma (4.2%); Asia has the highest prevalence of angle-closure glaucoma.[1]
- The incidence of primary open-angle glaucoma was 8.3 per 100,000 population in people older than 40 years in a Minnesota population study.[2]
- According to a population-based study, a family history of glaucoma increased the risk of having glaucoma (odds ratio [OR] = 3.08).[3]

ETIOLOGY AND PATHOPHYSIOLOGY

- Glaucoma pathophysiology is incompletely understood, but the level of IOP correlates with the acquired loss of retinal ganglion cells and resulting irreversible vision loss.[4]
- The ciliary body secretes aqueous humor, which drains through the trabecular meshwork and/or the uveoscleral outflow pathway; the balance between secretion and outflow determines IOP.[4]
    - In open-angle glaucoma, resistance in the trabecular meshwork impedes outflow
    - In angle-closure glaucoma, the drainage pathways is obstructed

- High systemic blood pressure affects ocular circulation and is associated with glaucoma progression.[5]
- IOP can cause mechanical stress on the posterior structures of the eye, with consequent damage to optic nerve fibers.[4]
- Optic nerve atrophy is seen as optic disc cupping and irreversible visual field loss. Compare **Figures 21-1** and **21-2** to see the difference between abnormal (**Figure 21-1**) and normal (**Figure 21-2**) optic disc cupping.

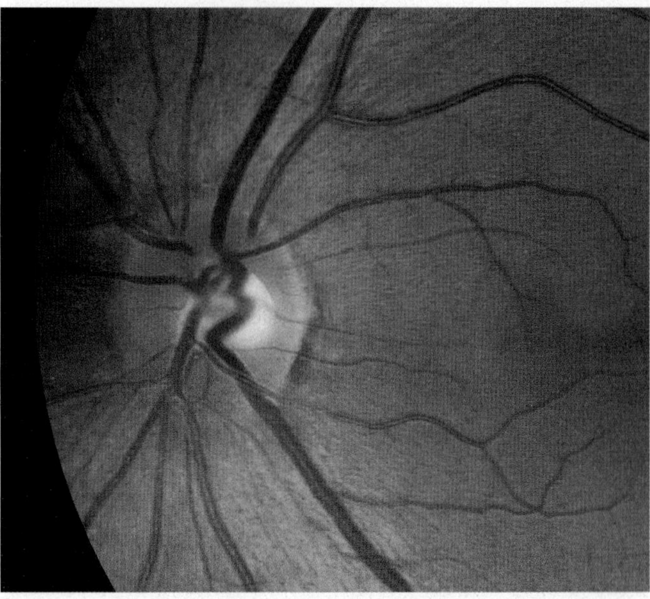

FIGURE 21-2 Normal eye with a normal cup-to-disc ratio of 0.4. A cup-to-disc ratio of more than 0.5 requires further evaluation. (*Reproduced with permission from Paul D. Comeau.*)

RISK FACTORS

Open-angle risk factors include:

- Nonmodifiable: age older than 50 years, first-degree family history, and African ancestry.[4]
- Modifiable: high IOP, high or low BP, use of systemic or topical steroids, and maybe diabetes mellitus.[4]
- Several genes are associated with glaucoma, including the MYOC gene, which encodes myocilin. This gene is found in approximately 5% of adults with open-angle glaucoma; 90% of MYOC gene carriers develop glaucoma.[4]

Acute closed-angle glaucoma is more common in persons of Asian descent.[1]

DIAGNOSIS

CLINICAL FEATURES

- Open-angle glaucoma:
  - History—Usually asymptomatic, occasionally "tunnel vision."
  - Positive family history
  - Physical examination
    - Elevated IOP; however, IOP was below 21 mm Hg in 76% of patients diagnosed with primary open angle glaucoma in a large population-based study.[6]
    - Optic cupping asymmetry; cup-to-disc ratio asymmetry of ≥0.20 has a 22.7% sensitivity, 97.7% specificity, 7% positive predictive value, and +9.9 likelihood ratio for disc plus field defined glaucoma.[7]
    - Loss of peripheral vision by automated perimetry (typically bilateral, but may be asymmetric).
- Acute closed-angle glaucoma:
  - History—Painful red eye (unilateral), vision loss, headache, nausea, halos around lights, and vomiting (**Figure 21-3**).
  - Physical examination—Shallow anterior chamber, optic cupping and elevated IOP, injection of the conjunctiva, and cloudy cornea (**Figure 21-3**).
- Typical distribution
  - Open-angle glaucoma is typically bilateral
  - Closed-angle glaucoma is typically unilateral. However, there is risk for the other eye to undergo the same process, as the

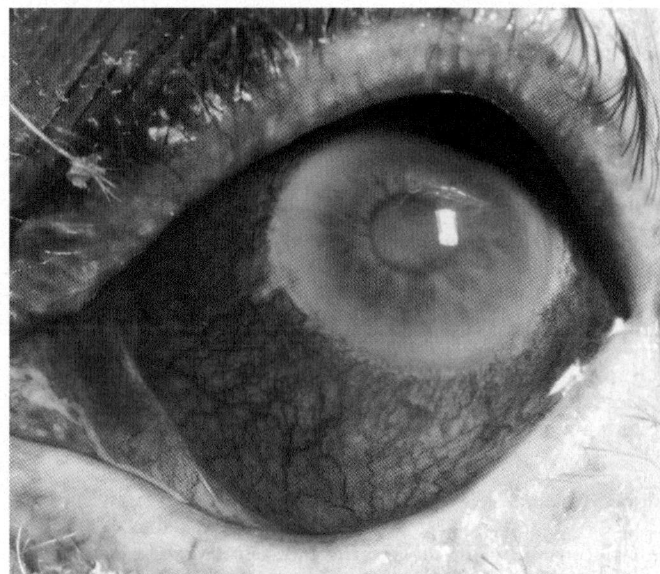

FIGURE 21-3 Acute closed-angle glaucoma with a painful red eye, vision loss, headache, nausea, and vomiting. This is a phacomorphic (i.e., lens induced) secondary acute angle closure. The mature cataract increased in anteroposterior (AP) diameter, thus moving the lens-iris diaphragm forward and closing off the angle as well as the pupil, resulting in high intraocular pressure, injected conjunctiva, and a cloudy cornea. (*Reproduced with permission from Gilberto Aquirre.*)

abnormal anatomically narrow angle is usually present in the other eye, too

DIFFERENTIAL DIAGNOSIS

Glaucoma is the most common cause of optic disc cupping and is sometimes accompanied by elevated IOP.

- Optic disc cupping without elevated IOP can be caused by[8]:
  - Physiologic cupping (**Figure 21-2**)
  - Congenital optic-disc anomalies (i.e., coloboma or tilted discs)
  - Ischemic (i.e., compression by tumors), traumatic (closed-head injury), or hereditary optic neuropathies
- Glaucomatous optic disc cupping compared to other causes has[8]:
  - Larger cup-to-disc ratios (compare **Figure 21-1** to **Figure 21-2**)
  - Vertical (as opposed to horizontal) elongation of the cup
  - Disc hemorrhages

MANAGEMENT

- Treat with topical agents to decrease IOP by 20% to 40%, which has been demonstrated to decrease glaucoma progression.[9] SOR Ⓐ Many medications are available including[4]:
  - Nonspecific β-blockers (e.g., timolol 0.5%, once or twice a day).
  - Prostaglandin analogs (e.g., latanoprost 0.005%, once a day).
  - Carbonic anhydrase inhibitors (e.g., dorzolamide 2%, 2 to 3 times a day).
  - α-Agonists (e.g., brimonidine 1.0%, 2 to 3 times a day).
- Selective laser trabeculoplasty has shown promise as an initial therapy in open-angle glaucoma; an ongoing multicenter randomized controlled trial is comparing this procedure to medical therapy.[10]

REFERRAL

- Emergently refer patients with suspected angle-closure glaucoma to an ophthalmologist (see **Figure 21-3**).
- Evaluate (or refer for evaluation) patients with abnormal optic nerve cupping (cup-to-disc ratio of greater than 0.5; difference in cup-to-disc ratio of 0.2 or greater between eyes; asymmetric cup), or increased IOP measured by tonometry, or visual field deficits.
- Document the location and extent of visual field deficits with automated perimetry.
- Refer patients with shallow anterior chambers, severe far-sightedness (hyperopia), or previous history of acute angle-closure glaucoma to an ophthalmologist.
- Refer for surgical evaluation if you are unable to medically reduce the IOP.

PREVENTION

- Screening—According to the U.S. Preventive Services Task Force (https://www.ahrq.gov/professionals/clinicians-providers/guidelines-recommendations/guide/section2b.html#Glaucoma), there is insufficient evidence to recommend for or against population screening for open-angle glaucoma. However, African Americans have been underrepresented in trials. Previously screening has been recommended for African Americans older than age 40 years, whites older than age 65 years, and patients with a family history of glaucoma.[4] SOR Ⓒ

PROGNOSIS

Most patients with open-angle glaucoma, provided they are treated, will not lose vision.

Angle-closure glaucoma must be treated emergently to prevent vision loss.

FOLLOW-UP

Patients with glaucoma should have regular measurements of their IOP and visual fields to follow treatment efficacy.

PATIENT EDUCATION

Advise patients that glaucoma is a progressive disease requiring continued therapy to prevent vision loss.

PATIENT RESOURCES

- Glaucoma research foundation website has information on treatment, research progress, personal stories, and practical tips at **www.glaucoma.org.**
- **http://www.ncbi.nlm.nih.gov/pubmedhealth/PMH0002587/.**

PROVIDER RESOURCES

- Acute angle-closure glaucoma—**http://emedicine.medscape.com/article/798811.**
- Primary open-angle glaucoma—**http://emedicine.medscape.com/article/1206147.**

REFERENCES

1. Tram YC, Li X, Wong TY, et al. Global prevalence of glaucoma and projections of glaucoma burden through 2040: a systematic review and meta-analysis. *Ophthalmology*. 2014;121(11):2081-2090.
2. Erie JC, Hodge DO, Gray DT. The incidence of primary angle-closure glaucoma in Olmsted County, Minnesota. *Arch Ophthalmol.* 1997;115(2):177-181.
3. Leske MC, Warheit-Roberts L, Wu SY. Open-angle glaucoma and ocular hypertension: the Long Island Glaucoma Case-control Study. *Ophthalmic Epidemiol.* 1996;3(2):85-96.
4. Weinreb RN, Aung T, Medeiros FA. The pathophysiology and treatment of glaucoma: a review. *JAMA*. 2014;311(18):1901-1911.

5. Jürgens C, Grossjohann R, Tost FH. Relationship of systemic blood pressure with ocular perfusion pressure and intraocular pressure of glaucoma patients in telemedical home monitoring. *Med Sci Monit.* 2012;18(11):MT85-89.

6. Chan MPY, Broadway DC, Khawaja AP, et al. Glaucoma and intraocular pressure in EPIC-Norfolk Eye Study: cross sectional study. *BMJ.* 2017;358:j3889.

7. Qiu M, Boland MV, Ramulu PY. Cup-to-disc ratio asymmetry in U.S. adults: prevalence and association with glaucoma in the 2005–2008 National Health and Nutrition Examination Survey. *Ophthalmology.* 2017;124(8):1229-1236.

8. Piette SD, Sergott RC. Pathological optic-disc cupping. *Curr Opin Ophthalmol.* 2006;17(1):1-6.

9. Heijl A, Leske MC, Bengtsson B, et al. Reduction of intraocular pressure and glaucoma progression: results from the Early Manifest Glaucoma Trial. *Arch Ophthalmol.* 2002;120(10): 1268-1279.

10. Lamoureux EL, Mcintosh R, Constantinou M, et al. Comparing the effectiveness of selective laser trabeculoplasty with topical medication as initial treatment (the Glaucoma Initial Treatment Study): study protocol for a randomised controlled trial. *Trials.* 2015;16:406.

22 DIABETIC RETINOPATHY

Heidi S. Chumley, MD, MBA
Mary Kelly Green, MD

PATIENT STORY

A 38-year-old man saw a physician for the first time in 10 years after noticing visual loss in his left eye. His history revealed many risk factors for and symptoms of diabetes mellitus (DM). On an undilated funduscopic examination, his physician was able to see some hemorrhages and hard exudates. A fingerstick in the office showed a blood glucose level of 420 mg/dL. He was treated for DM and referred to an ophthalmologist to be evaluated for diabetic retinopathy (**Figure 22-1**).

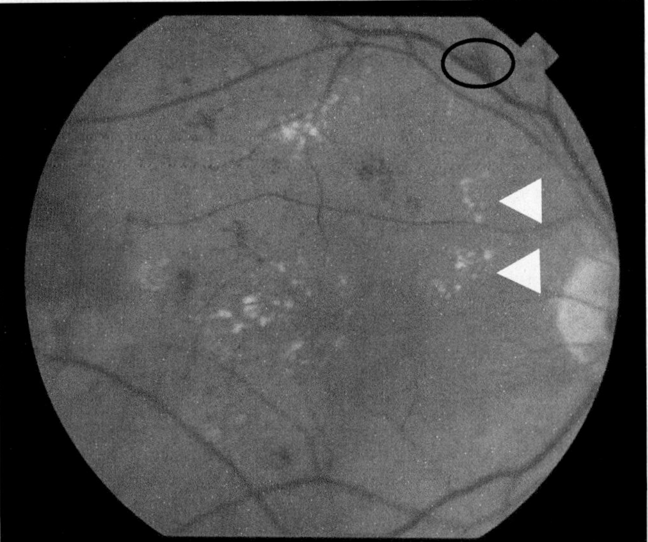

FIGURE 22-1 Dilated funduscopic photograph demonstrating microaneurysms (small red swellings attached to vessels), which are often the first change in diabetic retinopathy. Also present are flame hemorrhages (*black oval*) and hard exudates (*yellow*). Some of the hard exudates are demonstrated with *white arrowheads*. This case is an example of diabetic nonproliferative retinopathy. (*Reproduced with permission from Paul D. Comeau.*)

INTRODUCTION

Diabetic retinopathy (DR) is a leading cause of blindness in the United States. Nonproliferative DR is characterized by microaneurysms, macular edema, cotton-wool spots, superficial (flame) or deep (dot-blot) hemorrhages, and exudates. Proliferative DR also has neovascularization of the retina, optic nerve head, or iris. Because patients may be asymptomatic until vision loss occurs, screening is indicated in all diabetic patients. Excellent glycemic control lowers a patient's risk of developing DR.

EPIDEMIOLOGY

- In developed nations, DR is a common cause of blindness, accounting for 14.4% of blindness in working-age adults.[1]
- In prevalence studies from 33 countries, diabetic retinopathy was present in 27.9% of all patients with known diabetes and 10.5% of patients with newly diagnosed diabetes; prevalence is higher in developing countries.[2]
- In a community-based study, 29% of adults older than age 40 years with DM had DR. Prevalence in black patients was higher than in white patients (38.8% vs. 26.4%).[3]
- Nine years after diabetes diagnosis, 28% of diabetes type 2 patients and 24% diabetes type 1 patients developed diabetic retinopathy.[4]

ETIOLOGY AND PATHOPHYSIOLOGY

- Hyperglycemia results in microvascular complications including retinopathy.
- Metabolic and signaling abnormalities found in diabetes and inflammation, in the presence of hyperglycemia, play key roles in the development of DR.[5]
- In nonproliferative retinopathy, microaneurysms weaken vessel walls. Vessels then leak fluid, lipids, and blood resulting in macular edema, exudates, and hemorrhages (**Figures 22-1** and **22-2**).

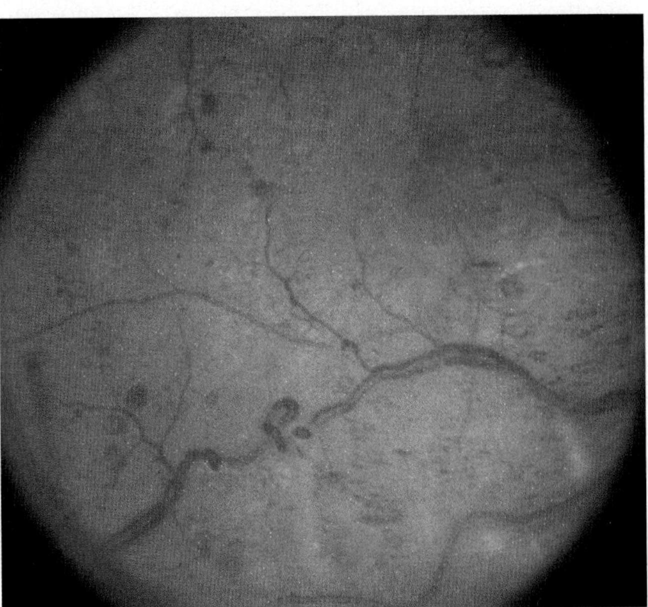

FIGURE 22-2 Very severe nonproliferative diabetic retinopathy with multiple deep dot-blot hemorrhages, venous beading, and looping. This patient may benefit from panretinal photocoagulation. (*Reproduced with permission from Paul D. Comeau.*)

- Cotton-wool spots result when small vessel occlusion causes focal ischemia to the superficial nerve fiber layer of the retina.
- In proliferative retinopathy, new blood vessels form in response to ischemia (**Figure 22-3**).

RISK FACTORS

- Poor glycemic control (higher $HgbA_{1c}$), longer duration of diabetes, and use of insulin therapy.[6]
- Hypertension.[6]
- Studies report inconsistent associations with obesity, hyperlipidemia, gender, or smoking.[6]
- Myopia is protective.[6]

DIAGNOSIS

Definitive diagnosis is made by an eye specialist who may use any of the following:

- Dilated funduscopic examination or review of high-quality retinal photographs; ophthalmologist-read fundus photographs accurately detect diabetic retinopathy and are particularly useful in rural or underserved areas.[7]
- Fluorescein angiography.
- Optical coherence tomography, which measures retinal thickness and provides information on macular edema.

CLINICAL FEATURES

- Central vision loss as a result of macular edema or macular ischemia.
- Nonproliferative retinopathy—Microaneurysms are seen initially (mild), followed by macular edema, cotton-wool spots, superficial (flame) or deep (dot-blot) hemorrhages, and exudates (**Figure 22-1** shows moderate, and **Figure 22-2** shows severe).
- Proliferative retinopathy—Neovascularization, that is, growth of new blood vessels on the optic disc (**Figure 22-3**), retina, or iris.

DIFFERENTIAL DIAGNOSIS

Retinopathy is also seen with other systemic illnesses and infections including:

- Hypertensive retinopathy—arterial narrowing or atrioventricular nicking in addition to cotton-wool spots (see Chapter 23, Hypertensive Retinopathy).
- HIV retinopathy—Cotton-wool spots and infections such as *Cytomegalovirus*.

MANAGEMENT

Control diabetes and vascular risk factors:

- Glycemic control lowers the risk of retinopathy. Reducing $HgbA_{1c}$ from 9% to 7% reduces the risk to develop DR by 76% and slows DR progression by 54%.[8] SOR Ⓐ

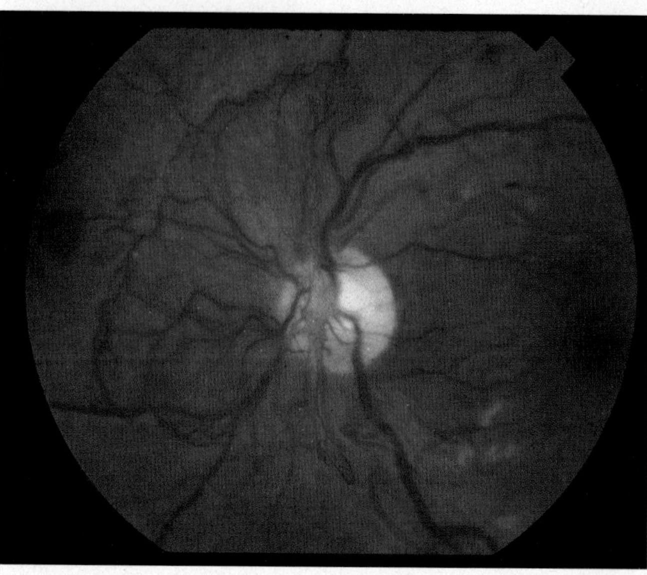

FIGURE 22-3 Proliferative diabetic retinopathy showing newly developed, porous, friable blood vessels. New vessels can be seen on the optic disc and peripheral retina. Panretinal photocoagulation may help prevent vitreous hemorrhage, retinal detachment, and neovascular glaucoma. *(Reproduced with permission from Paul D. Comeau.)*

- Intensive blood pressure control lowers risk and progression of DR (estimated RR 0.78; 95% CI 0.63 to 0.97).[9] SOR A
- Treatment with angiotensin-converting enzyme inhibitors (ACEIs) or angiotensin receptor blockers (ARBs) in type 1 DM or an ARB in type 2 DM has been shown to reduce retinopathy progression independent of blood pressure control.[10] SOR B
- Fenofibrate slows progression of DR and decreases the need for invasive treatment in patients with type 2 diabetes.[11] SOR B
- Patients with high lipids have more hard exudates and a higher risk of vision loss, but it is unclear if lipid control changes outcomes. SOR C

REFERRAL

Work with an ophthalmologist to prevent vision loss:

- Complications of DR are vitreous hemorrhage (**Figure 22-4**), retinal detachment, and neovascular glaucoma. Each of these complications can result in devastating vision loss.
- Ophthalmologists will determine when retinal photocoagulation is indicated (**Figure 22-5**). Photocoagulation reduces the risk of severe visual loss by more than 50%.[12] SOR A
- Intravenous ranibizumab was noted to produce similar outcomes to panretinal photocoagulation in a randomized, controlled trial in patients with proliferative diabetic retinopathy.[13]

FIGURE 22-4 This vitreous hemorrhage occurred when friable neovascular membranes broke spontaneously. The patient described a "shower of red dots" obscuring the vision and then loss of vision in that eye. (*Reproduced with permission from Paul D. Comeau.*)

PREVENTION

Prevent DR by preventing development of type 2 DM or tightly controlling type 1 or type 2 DM.

Screen patients with DM for DR based on national recommendations[10]:

- Type 1 DM—Adults and children older than age 10 years: screen for retinopathy 5 years after diagnosis and at regular intervals as recommended by an eye specialist.
- Type 2 DM—Screen for retinopathy at diagnosis and then annually.

Patients can be referred to an eye specialist, or screened using telemedicine or retinal photographs taken during outreach screenings or in primary care offices.[7,10]

Patients without DR and with well-controlled diabetes may be screened every 2 years instead of annually.[10,14]

FOLLOW-UP

Once DR is diagnosed, frequency of examination is set by the ophthalmologist.

PATIENT EDUCATION

Preventing retinopathy by controlling diabetes and hypertension leads to better vision outcomes than any available treatment.[8,9]

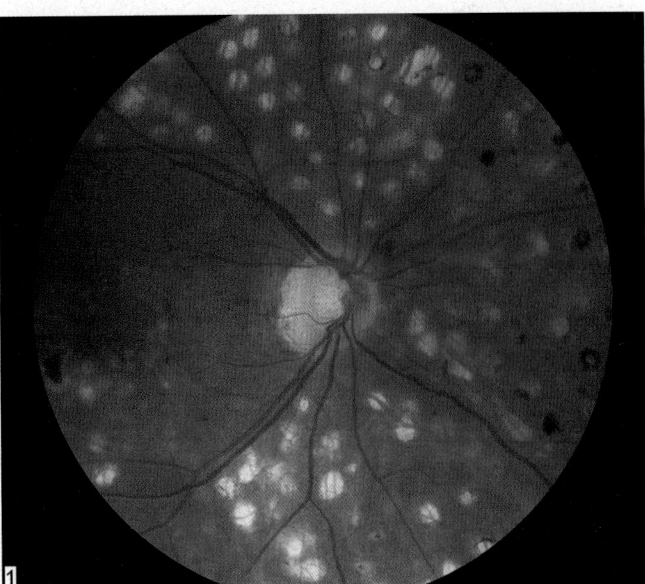

FIGURE 22-5 Panretinal photocoagulation is the application of laser burns to the peripheral retina. The ischemic peripheral retina is treated with thousands of laser spots to presumably eliminate vasogenic factors responsible for the development of neovascular vessels. Laser spots cause scarring of the retina and choroid. The scars may be hypotrophic (*white spots*) or hypertrophic (*black spots*). (*Reproduced with permission from Paul D. Comeau.*)

PATIENT RESOURCES

- National Eye Institute—**http://www.nei.nih.gov/health/diabetic/.**

PROVIDER RESOURCES

- **http://emedicine.medscape.com/article/1225122.**

REFERENCES

1. Liew G, Michaelides M, Bunce C. A comparison of the causes of blindness certifications in England and Wales in working age adults (16–64 years), 1999–2000 with 2009–2010. *BMJ Open.* 2014;12:4(2):e004015.
2. Ruta LM, Magliano DJ, Lemesurier R, et al. Prevalence of diabetic retinopathy in type 2 diabetes in developing and developed countries. *Diabet Med.* 2013;30(4):387-398.
3. Zhang X, Saaddine JB, Chou CF, et al. Prevalence of diabetic retinopathy in the United States, 2005–2008. *JAMA.* 2010;304(6):649-656.
4. Martín-Merino E, Fortuny J, Rivero-Ferrer E, García-Rodríguez LA. Incidence of retinal complications in a cohort of newly diagnosed diabetic patients. *PLoS One.* 2014;9(6):e100283.
5. Arboleda-Velasquez JF, Valdez C, Marko CK, D'Amore PA. From pathobiology to the targeting of pericytes for the treatment of diabetic retinopathy. *Curr Diab Rep.* 2015;15(2):573.
6. Wat N, Wong RL, Wong IY. Associations between diabetic retinopathy and systemic risk factors. *Hong Kong Med J.* 2016;22(6):589-599.
7. Raman R, Bhojwani DN, Sharma T. How accurate is the diagnosis of diabetic retinopathy on telescreening? The Indian scenario. *Rural Remote Health.* 2014;14(4):2809.
8. Aiello LP; DCCT/EDIC Research Group. Diabetic retinopathy and other ocular findings in the diabetes control and complications trial/epidemiology of diabetes interventions and complications study. *Diabetes Care.* 2014;37(1):17-23.
9. Do DV, Wang X, Vedula SS, et al. Blood pressure control for diabetic retinopathy. *Cochrane Database Syst Rev.* 2015;1:CD006127.
10. American Diabetes Association. Standards of medical care in diabetes—2017. *Diabetes Care.* 2017;40(Suppl 1):S91-S93.
11. Sharma N, Ooi JL, Ong J, Newman D. The use of fenofibrate in the management of patients with diabetic retinopathy: an evidence-based review. *Aust Fam Physician.* 2015;44(6):367-370.
12. Evans JR, Michelessi M, Virgili G. Laser photocoagulation for proliferative diabetic retinopathy. *Cochrane Database Syst Rev.* 2014;(11):CD011234.
13. Gross JG, Glassman AR, Jampol LM, et al. Panretinal photocoagulation vs intravitreous ranibizumab for proliferative diabetic retinopathy: a randomized clinical trial. *JAMA.* 2015;314(20):2137-2146.
14. Echouffo-Tcheugui JB, Ali MK, Roglic G, et al. Screening intervals for diabetic retinopathy and incidence of visual loss: a systematic review. *Diabet Med.* 2013;30(11):1272-1292.

23 HYPERTENSIVE RETINOPATHY

Heidi S. Chumley, MD, MBA
Mary Kelly Green, MD

PATIENT STORY

A 37-year-old man comes in for a physical examination and is noted to have a blood pressure of 198/142 mm Hg. He has no symptoms at the time. The physician performs a dilated funduscopic examination and notes optic disc edema, cotton wool spots, flame hemorrhages, dot-blot hemorrhages, arteriovenous nicking, and exudates (**Figure 23-1**). Fortunately, the remainder of the neurologic exam and the ECG are normal. The patient is sent to the emergency department to be evaluated further and treated for a hypertensive emergency.

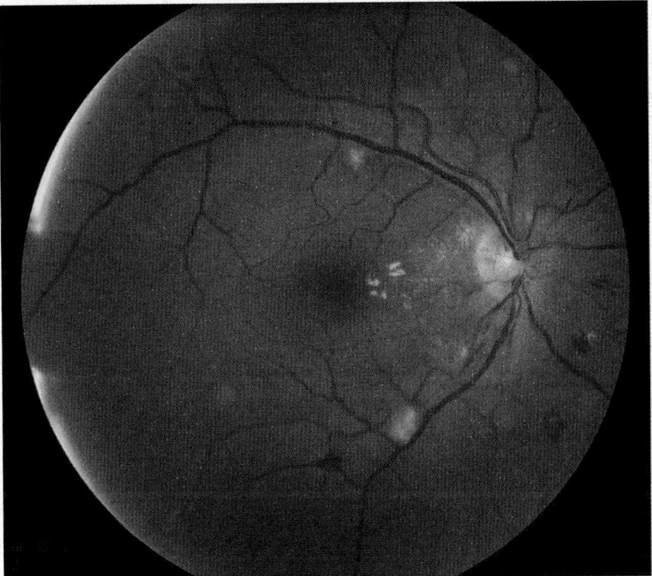

FIGURE 23-1 Hypertensive retinopathy with optic disc edema, cotton wool spots, flame hemorrhages, dot-blot hemorrhages, arteriovenous nicking, and exudates. (*Reproduced with permission from EyeRounds.org and The University of Iowa.*)

INTRODUCTION

Hypertensive retinopathy (HR) develops from elevated blood pressure. HR is diagnosed clinically by the presence of classic retinal findings seen on funduscopic examination or digital retinal photographs in a patient with hypertension. HR can result in vision loss. Treatment is control of blood pressure.

EPIDEMIOLOGY

- Prevalence of 7.7% (black) versus 4.1% (white) in a population study of men and women between 49 and 73 years of age without diabetes.[1]
- Patients with moderate HR are 2 to 3 times more likely to have a stroke than those without HR at the same level of blood pressure control independent of other risk factors.[2]

ETIOLOGY AND PATHOPHYSIOLOGY

High blood pressure results in these retinal findings[3]:

- Retinal vessels become narrow and straighten at diastolic blood pressure (DBP) of 90 to 110 mm Hg.
- Arteriovenous "nicking" (white oval in **Figure 23-1**) occurs when the arteriolar wall enlarges from arteriosclerosis, compressing the vein. Patients with hypertension are at risk for central and branch retinal vein occlusions, which can result in significant vision loss.
- Microaneurysms and flame hemorrhages (**Figures 23-1** and **23-2**) result from the increased intravascular pressure. Cotton-wool spots (*dashed arrow* in **Figure 23-2**) represent ischemia of the nerve fiber layer. Hard exudates indicate vascular leakage (*white arrowheads* in Chapter 22, **Figure 22-1**).

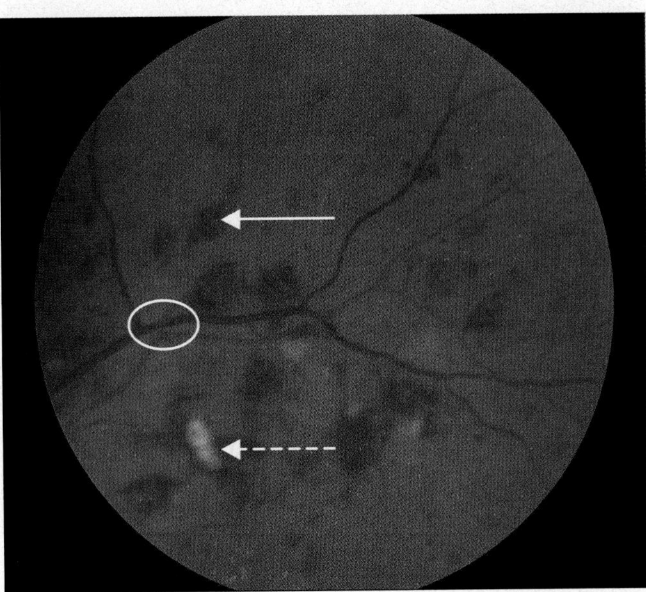

FIGURE 23-2 More advanced hypertensive retinopathy with flame hemorrhages (*white arrow*), arteriovenous nicking (*white oval*), and cotton-wool spots (*dashed arrow*). (*Reproduced with permission from Paul D. Comeau.*)

- DBP 110 to 115 mm Hg causes leakage of plasma proteins and blood products resulting in retinal hemorrhages and hard exudates (**Figures 23-1** to **23-4**).
- Optic nerve swelling occurs at DBP of 130 to 140 mm Hg (**Figure 23-3**).

DIAGNOSIS

The diagnosis is made clinically from typical retinal findings in a patient with hypertension. These findings can be seen using funduscopic examination or by viewing retinal digital images. Retinal digital images have a higher interobserver reliability than funduscopic examination.[4]

CLINICAL FEATURES

In order of increasing severity:

- Mild arteriolar narrowing.
- Severe arteriolar narrowing plus arteriovenous nicking.
- Retinal hemorrhages, microaneurysms, hard exudation, cotton-wool spots.
- Swelling of the optic nerve head and macular star, also called accelerated or malignant HR.

TYPICAL DISTRIBUTION

- Bilateral and symmetrical.

LABORATORY TESTING

- Laboratory tests are not needed to make the diagnosis.
- Recommended tests for patients with hypertension include urinalysis, blood glucose, hematocrit, serum potassium, creatinine, calcium, and a fasting lipid profile.
- 12-Lead ECG is also recommended.

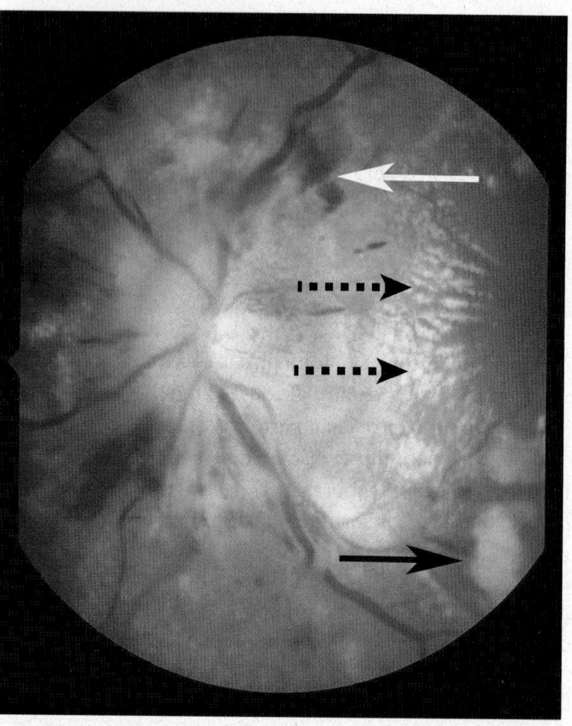

FIGURE 23-3 Malignant hypertensive retinopathy with optic nerve head edema (papilledema), flame hemorrhages (*white arrow*), cotton-wool spots (*black arrow*), and macular edema with exudates (*dashed arrows*). The patient was admitted to the hospital to treat malignant hypertension aggressively. (*Reproduced with permission from Paul D. Comeau.*)

DIFFERENTIAL DIAGNOSIS

Retinal vessel narrowing, atrioventricular nicking, microaneurysms, retinal hemorrhages, hard exudates, and cotton-wool spots are also seen in other conditions that impair blood flow, including:

- Diabetic retinopathy (see Chapter 22, Diabetic Retinopathy).
- Radiation retinopathy.
- Venous or carotid artery occlusive disease.
- Systemic illnesses such as collagen vascular disease.
- Hematologic diseases such as anemia and leukemia.
- Systemic infectious diseases such as HIV.

Optic nerve swelling and a macular star (blurring of the macula in a starlike pattern) also occur in:

- Neuroretinitis.
- Diabetic papillopathy.
- Radiation optic retinopathy.
- Optic neuritis.
- Intracranial disease.

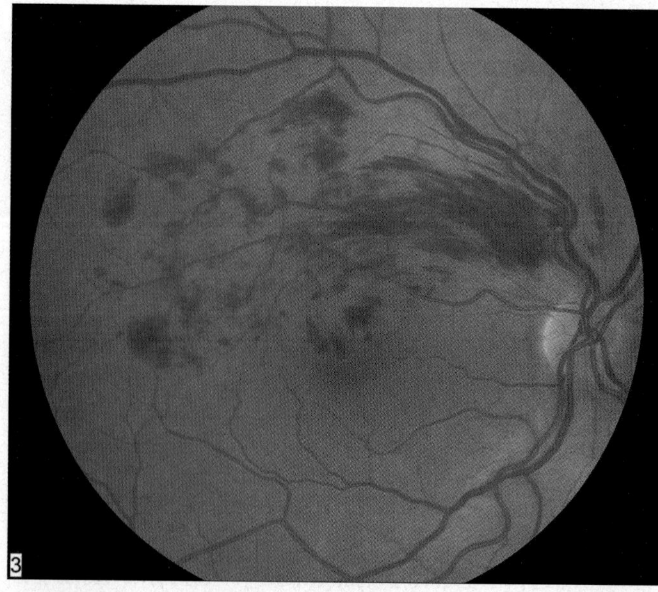

FIGURE 23-4 Branch retinal vein occlusion of a major retinal vein associated with hypertension. The patient noted new onset of blurred vision and visual field constriction. Flame hemorrhages are seen along the course of the obstructed vein. (*Reproduced with permission from Paul D. Comeau.*)

MANAGEMENT

Patients with funduscopic findings of HR should have their blood pressure measured and treated to the goals listed below to reduce the risk of heart and cerebrovascular disease.[5] SOR Ⓐ

- In patients ≥60 years of age, lower blood pressure to <150/90 mm Hg. SOR Ⓐ
- In patients between ages 30 and 59 years, lower diastolic blood pressure to <90 mm Hg (SOR Ⓐ), and systolic blood pressure to <140 mm Hg.
- In patients between ages 18 and 29 years, lower diastolic blood pressure to <90 mm Hg. SOR Ⓒ
- In patients over the age of 18 with diabetes mellitus or chronic kidney disease, lower blood pressure to <140/90 mm Hg. SOR Ⓒ
- Nonpharmacologic:
    - Assist patients in smoking cessation. This will result in the greatest benefit in morbidity and mortality.
    - Reduce weight or maintain normal body mass index (BMI).
    - Eat a diet rich in fruits and vegetables and low in saturated fats.
    - Reduce sodium to less than 6 g of sodium chloride per day.
    - Engage in regular physical activity for 30 minutes most days of the week.
    - Limit alcohol to 2 drinks per day in men and 1 drink per day in women.
- Medications:
    - In the non-black population, initiate therapy with a thiazide diuretic, calcium channel blocker, angiotensin-converting enzyme inhibitor, or angiotensin receptor blocker (ARB).[5] SOR Ⓑ
    - In the black population, initiate therapy with a thiazide diuretic or a calcium channel blocker.[5] SOR Ⓑ
    - If goal BP is not reached in 1 month, increase the dose or add a second medication.[5] SOR Ⓒ
    - Evaluate and manage other risk factors for cardiovascular disease, including high cholesterol and diabetes.

REFERRAL

Patients experiencing acute visual disturbances should be referred for evaluation of hemorrhage or optic nerve edema (see **Figures 23-3** and **23-4**).

PREVENTION

- Maintain normal blood pressure through a healthy lifestyle and medications when needed.
- Patients with hypertension alone do not require routine funduscopic examination, unless they also have diabetes mellitus.[6] SOR Ⓐ

PROGNOSIS

- Prognosis is associated with severity of hypertension retinopathy. Visual loss is uncommon; however, hypertensive retinopathy is associated with cerebrovascular and cardiovascular morbidity and mortality.
- In persons with well-controlled hypertension, mild and moderate retinopathy were related to an increased risk of cerebral infarction (mild retinopathy: hazard ratio, 1.96 [95% confidence interval, 1.09–3.55]; and moderate retinopathy: hazard ratio, 2.98 [95% confidence interval, 1.01–8.83]).[2]
- Hypertensive retinopathy is associated with more severe coronary artery disease in women.[7]

FOLLOW-UP

Once diagnosed with hypertension, patients should be seen every month until blood pressure is controlled and then every 3 to 6 months.[4] SOR Ⓒ

PATIENT EDUCATION

- HR does not require treatment other than lowering blood pressure unless acute vision changes occur.
- Control of blood pressure typically reverses HR findings, except for optic nerve edema, which may result in permanent vision loss.
- Control of blood pressure also reduces the risk of heart attack and stroke.

PATIENT RESOURCES

- **http://www.ncbi.nlm.nih.gov/pubmedhealth/PMH0001994/.**

PROVIDER RESOURCES

- **http://emedicine.medscape.com/article/1201779.**
- Guidelines to manage hypertension in adults at **https://jamanetwork.com/journals/jama/fullarticle/1791497.**

REFERENCES

1. Wong TY, Klein R, Duncan BB, et al. Racial differences in the prevalence of hypertensive retinopathy. *Hypertension*. 2003;41(5):1086-1091.
2. Ong YT, Wong TY, Klein R, et al. Hypertensive retinopathy and risk of stroke. *Hypertension*. 2013;62(4):706-711.
3. Luo BP, Brown GC. Update on the ocular manifestations of systemic arterial hypertension. *Curr Opin Ophthalmol*. 2004;15(3):203-210.
4. Castro AF, Silva-Turnes JC, Gonzalez F. Evaluation of retinal digital images by a general practitioner. *Telemed J E Health*. 2007;13(3):287-292.
5. James PA, Oparil S, Carter BL, et al. 2014 evidence-based guideline for the management of high blood pressure in adults: report from the panel members appointed to the Eighth Joint National Committee (JNC 8). *JAMA*. 2014;5;311(5):507-520.
6. van den Born BJ, Hulsman CA, Hoekstra JB, et al. Value of routine funduscopy in patients with hypertension: systematic review. *BMJ*. 2005;331(7508):73.
7. Gopinath B, Chiha J, Plant AJ, et al. Associations between retinal microvascular structure and the severity and extent of coronary artery disease. *Atherosclerosis*. 2014;236(1):25-30.

24 PAPILLEDEMA

Heidi S. Chumley, MD, MBA

PATIENT STORY

A 29-year-old obese woman presented with chronic headaches that were worse in the morning or while lying down. She denied nausea or other neurologic symptoms. She had no other medical problems and took no medications. On examination, she had a visual acuity of 20/20 in both eyes, bilateral papilledema (**Figure 24-1**), no spontaneous venous pulsations (SVPs), and no other neurologic signs. She had a brain MRI showing no mass or hydrocephalus, and elevated intracranial pressure measured by lumbar puncture. She was diagnosed with idiopathic intracranial hypertension and was followed closely for any changes in her vision. She was started on acetazolamide and assisted with a weight-loss program. Her symptoms resolved over the course of 18 months.

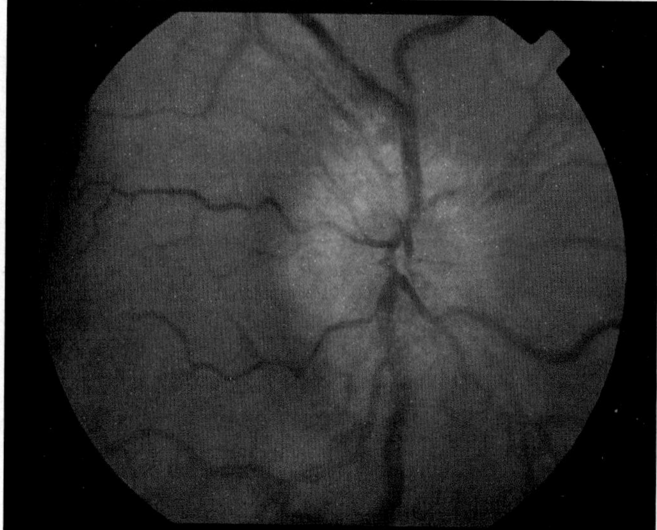

FIGURE 24-1 Papilledema from increased intracranial pressure. The optic disc is elevated and hyperemic with engorged retinal veins. The entire optic disc margin is blurred. Optic neuropathies can also have blurring of the entire disc margin, but often, only part of the disc is blurred. (*Reproduced with permission from Paul D. Comeau.*)

INTRODUCTION

The term *papilledema* refers specifically to optic disc swelling related to increased intracranial pressure. When no localizing neurological signs or space-occupying lesion is present, idiopathic intracranial hypertension (IIH) is a likely cause in patients younger than age 45 years, especially obese women. Patients with IIH usually present with daily pulsatile headache with nausea and often have transient visual disturbances and/or pulsatile tinnitus. Patients often report a "whooshing" sound that they hear. Bilateral papilledema and visual field defects on a perimetry test are found in almost all patients. Elevated opening pressure on lumbar puncture is required for the diagnosis.

SYNONYMS

For IIH: *Pseudotumor cerebri* or *benign intracranial hypertension.*

EPIDEMIOLOGY

IIH occurs in:

- 0.9 per 100,000 people and 3.5 per 100,000 women in the United States.[1]
- 19 per 100,000 obese women ages 20 to 44 years.[1]
- Prevalence may be increasing with increasing obesity.[1]
- Mean age of diagnosis is approximately 30 years.[1]

ETIOLOGY AND PATHOPHYSIOLOGY

The optic disc swells because of elevated intracranial pressure from any cause. In IIH, the cerebral spinal fluid pressure is increased. The cause of this increase in unknown, but a current hypothesis implicates arterial flow in the transverse sinus due to a combination of increased arterial flow and low-grade stenosis.[2]

RISK FACTORS

IIH:

- Obesity and female gender (post-pubertal).[1]
- Hypervitaminosis A.[1]

DIAGNOSIS

Patients with papilledema should undergo imaging, preferably MRI, followed by lumbar puncture. MRI will reveal many causes of increased intracranial pressure.

IIH is a diagnosis of exclusion in patients with symptoms of increased intracranial pressure (headache, transient visual disturbances). IIH was overdiagnosed in 40% of cases in one study, primarily due to inaccurate ophthalmologic examination of obese young women.[3]

Each of the following must be present for diagnosis[4]:

- Papilledema, typically bilateral; in the unusual absence of papilledema, the diagnosis can be made with a VI nerve palsy.
- Normal neurological examination except for cranial nerve abnormalities, most commonly VI nerve palsy.
- Normal brain parenchyma; no hydrocephalus, mass, or structural lesion; and no abnormal meningeal enhancement on MRI with and without gadolinium (contrast-enhanced CT may be used).
- Normal cerebrospinal fluid (CSF) composition.
- Elevated lumbar puncture opening pressure ≥250 mm CSF in adults.

The diagnosis may be made in the absence of papilledema and VI nerve palsy if specific radiographic findings are present.

CLINICAL FEATURES

Papilledema:

- Appears as blurring of the optic disc, but may be challenging to see in an undilated eye with an office ophthalmoscope.
- Spontaneous venous pulsations are retinal vein pulsations at the optic disc, which are seen in >90% of patients with normal intracranial pressure, but are absent when the CSF pressure is above 190 mm Hg.[5]

IIH:

- More than 90% of patients with IIH are obese women of childbearing age. Look for a different diagnosis in children, men, and older patients.[1]
- Common symptoms include chronic daily headache, pulsatile tinnitus, transient visual changes, and papilledema.[2] Acute onset is unusual and should prompt exploration of other causes.
- Difficulty in thinking or concentrating is frequently reported. New studies indicate cognitive impairment, particularly in learning and memory.[6]
- SVPs are typically absent in IIH patients. As the CSF pressure may be transiently normal in IIH, the presence of SVPs does not preclude IIH, but indicates that the CSF pressure is normal at that moment.[5]

TYPICAL DISTRIBUTION

Papilledema is symmetric and bilateral in the overwhelming majority of cases (see **Figures 24-1** and **24-2**). Highly asymmetric optic disc swelling was noted in 3.6% of patients with IIH.[7]

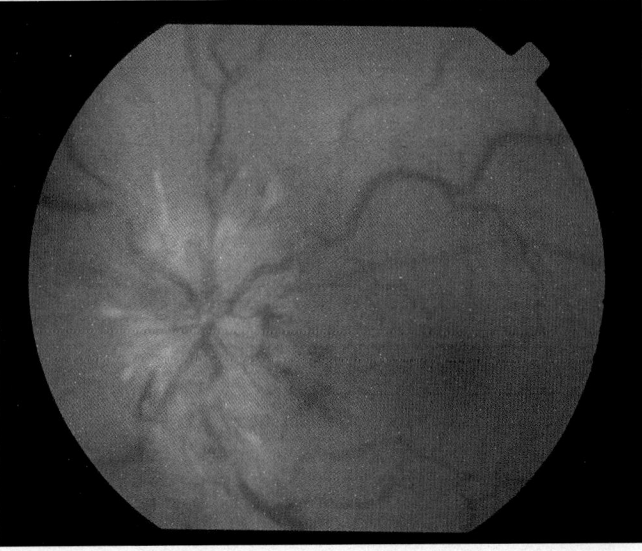

FIGURE 24-2 Severe acute papilledema with papillary flame hemorrhages and cotton-wool spots that obscure the disc vessels. The blurred edges of the optic disc appear as a starburst. (*Reproduced with permission from Paul D. Comeau.*)

LABORATORY TESTING

Cerebral spinal fluid is typically sent for cell count and culture.

IMAGING

- Traditionally, imaging was used to rule out intracranial mass or venous sinus obstruction.
  - MRI with and without gadolinium in obese women of childbearing years
  - MRI with and without gadolinium and magnetic resonance venography in atypical patients to rule out cavernous venous sinus thrombosis, a rare diagnosis that can mimic IIH
- Several methods of noninvasive monitoring of intracranial pressure, such as optic nerve sheath diameter and pupillometry, show promise as tools that may mitigate the need for recurrent lumbar punctures to monitor pressures.[8]

DIFFERENTIAL DIAGNOSIS

Papilledema:

- Pseudopapilledema or optic disc drusen, an optic nerve anomaly that elevates the optic disc surface and blurs the disc margins, which can be caused by calcifications in the optic nerve head.
- Optic neuropathies, swelling of all or parts of one or both discs, which can be caused by ischemia or demyelination (as in multiple sclerosis) and may be seen in 1% to 2% of patients with diabetes mellitus type 1 or 2.[9]

Elevated intracranial pressure can also be caused by obstructing lesions, medical conditions, or medications[2]:

- Mass lesions, hydrocephalus, venous sinus or jugular venous thrombosis, and meningeal infections.
- Addison disease, hypoparathyroidism, chronic obstructive pulmonary disease (COPD), sleep apnea, renal failure, pulmonary hypertension, and severe anemia.
- Antibiotics in the tetracycline family, vitamin A, anabolic steroids, lithium, and corticosteroid withdrawal.

MANAGEMENT

Papilledema:

- Refer for urgent imaging to determine the underlying cause of the elevated intracranial pressure and assess the need for interventions to preserve vision.

IIH:

- In many cases, IIH is self-limiting, presents without visual symptoms, and will resolve over several years without loss of vision.

In patients with IIH with mild visual loss:

- Place on a low-sodium diet.[10] SOR Ⓐ
- Start acetazolamide 500 mg twice a day (1 g/day) and titrate to highest tolerable dose up to 4 g/day.[10] SOR Ⓐ

Patients with significant or worsening visual disturbances:

- Refer to an ophthalmologist to guide therapy.
- Treatment may be required to lower the intracranial pressure to prevent optic nerve damage and irreversible loss of vision.
- Surgical options, including transverse sinus stenting, are used in some cases.[11]

PREVENTION

Maintenance of ideal body weight may prevent IIH.

PROGNOSIS

Although approximately two-thirds of patients with IIH present with visual impairment, the majority of patients improve.

Patients who are male, have higher grade papilledema, and present with visual loss at baseline are more likely to fail treatment.[12]

FOLLOW-UP

Patients should be followed every 3 to 6 months by a physician who can adequately view the entire optic disc and document visual acuity and visual field deficits. They should be seen immediately for any visual changes.

PATIENT EDUCATION

Advise patients with new papilledema of the need for an evaluation for dangerous causes of increased intracranial pressure, such as intracranial masses or underlying medical illnesses. Also advise patients that IIH often resolves spontaneously over several years, but they should report any visual changes immediately.

PATIENT RESOURCES

- The Intracranial Hypertension Research Foundation has information for patients at **www.ihrfoundation.org.**

PROVIDER RESOURCES

- The Intracranial Hypertension Research Foundation has information for medical professionals including ongoing research studies and information on patient registries at **www.ihrfoundation.org.**

REFERENCES

1. Chen J, Wall M. Epidemiology and risk factors for idiopathic intracranial hypertension. *Int Ophthalmol Clin.* 2014;54(1):1-11.
2. Wall M. Update on idiopathic intracranial hypertension. *Neurol Clin.* 2017;35(1):45-57.
3. Fisayo A, Bruce BB, Newman NY, Biousse V. Overdiagnosis of idiopathic intracranial hypertension. *Neurology.* 2016;86(4):341-350.

4. Friedman DL, Liu GT, Digre KB. Revised diagnostic criteria for the pseudotumor cerebri syndrome in adults and children. *Neurology*. 2013;81(13):1159-1165.
5. Jacks AS, Miller NR. Spontaneous retinal venous pulsation: aetiology and significance. *J Neurol Neurosurg Psychiatry*. 2003; 74(1):7-9.
6. Kharkar S, Hernandez R, Batra S, et al. Cognitive impairment in patients with pseudotumor cerebri syndrome. *Behav Neurol*. 2011;24(2):143-148.
7. Bidot S, Bruce BB, Saindane AM, et al. Asymmetric papilledema in idiopathic intracranial hypertension. *J Neuroophthalmol*. 2015;35(1):31-36.
8. Khan MN, Shallwani H, Khan MU, Shamim MS. Noninvasive monitoring intracranial pressure—A review of available modalities. *Surg Neurol Int*. 2017;8:51.
9. Bayraktar Z, Alacali N, Bayraktar S. Diabetic papillopathy in type II diabetic patients. *Retina*. 2002;22(6):752-758.
10. NORDIC Idiopathic Intracranial Hypertension Study Group Writing Committee, Wall M, McDermott MP, Kieburtz KD, et al. Effect of acetazolamide on visual function in patients with idiopathic intracranial hypertension and mild visual loss: the idiopathic intracranial hypertension treatment trial. *JAMA*. 2014; 311(16):1641-1651.
11. Dinkin MJ, Patsalides A. Venous sinus stenting for idiopathic intracranial hypertension: where are we now? *Neurol Clin*. 2017; 35(1):59-81.
12. Wall M, Falardeau J, Fletcher WA, et al; NORDIC Idiopathic Intracranial Hypertension Study Group. Risk factors for poor visual outcome in patients with idiopathic intracranial hypertension. *Neurology*. 2015;85(9):799-805.

25 AGE-RELATED MACULAR DEGENERATION

Heidi S. Chumley, MD, MBA

PATIENT STORY

A 78-year-old white woman presents with loss of central vision that has gradually worsened over the past 6 months. Fully independent before, she can no longer drive and has difficulty with activities of daily living. Her peripheral vision remains normal. Funduscopic examination reveals macular depigmentation and drusen (yellowish-colored subretinal deposits on the macula) (**Figure 25-1**). She is diagnosed with dry, age-related macular degeneration. After her physician discusses the available information about antioxidants and therapeutic options, she decides to start antioxidants and see an ophthalmologist to discuss laser, surgical, or medical treatments.

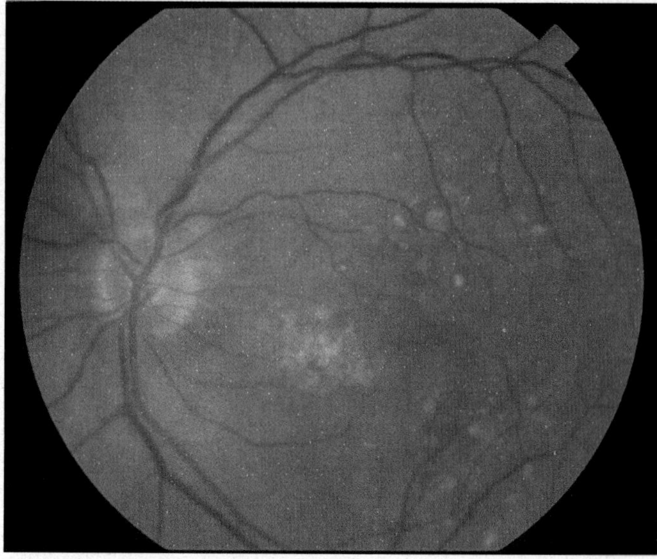

FIGURE 25-1 Intermediate, dry, age-related macular degeneration with macular depigmentation and drusen (yellowish-colored subretinal deposits on the macula). This patient has central vision distortion. *(Reproduced with permission from Paul D. Comeau.)*

INTRODUCTION

Age-related macular degeneration (AMD) causes central vision loss in elderly patients. The pathophysiology of AMD is incompletely understood, but involves chronic changes in the retina and retinal pigment epithelium mediated by environmental and genetic factors. AMD is diagnosed by ophthalmoscopic detection of drusen. Healthy lifestyle decreases the risk of development and progression of AMD. Refer patients to an ophthalmologist to evaluate for intravitreal injections, laser photocoagulation or photodynamic therapy, or surgery.

EPIDEMIOLOGY

AMD is the leading cause of irreversible vision loss in the industrialized world.

- Globally, AMD is estimated to affect 196 million persons by 2020 and 228 million persons by 2040.[1]
- Prevalence is higher in Europeans (12.3%) than in Asians (7.4%) or Africans (7.5%).[1]
- Annual incidence of late AMD in American whites is 3.5 per 1000 persons ≥50 years of age and approximately quadruples per decade in age.[2]
- Smoking increases risk in women (relative risk [RR] 2.5 for current smokers; 2.0 for former smokers).[3]
- AMD aggregates in families, but the specific genetic and familial risk factors are not clear.[3]

ETIOLOGY AND PATHOPHYSIOLOGY

AMD affects central but not peripheral vision. Environment and genetic attributes increase risk of these pathologic changes with aging.[4]

- Oxidative stress from the buildup of free oxygen radicals causes retinal pigment epithelial (RPE) injury.

- RPE injury evokes a chronic inflammatory response. The complement system is involved, and specific polymorphisms of complement genes are associated with advanced disease and progression.[4]
- RPE injury/inflammation forms an abnormal extracellular matrix (ECM), which alters diffusion of nutrients to the retina and RPE.
- The abnormal ECM and diffusion leads to retinal atrophy and new vessel growth.

RISK FACTORS

- For late AMD, strong risk factors are age, current cigarette smoking, previous cataract surgery (replaced lens provides less eye protection from sunlight), and family history of AMD.
- Moderate risk factors include higher body mass index, history of cardiovascular disease, hypertension, and high plasma fibrinogen.
- Weak or inconsistent risk factors include gender, ethnicity, diabetes, iris color, history of cerebrovascular disease, total cholesterol, high-density lipoprotein, and triglyceride levels.[5]

DIAGNOSIS

Diagnosis is clinical and made by ophthalmoscopy. AMD can be dry (early, intermediate, or late) or wet (always considered late).

- Early dry—May have no vision change; drusen present (**Figure 25-2**).
- Intermediate dry—Distortion in the center of vision; multiple medium-size drusen (see **Figure 25-1**).
- Advanced dry—(Nonexudative) Significant central vision loss from breakdown of support tissues around the macula.
- Advanced wet—(Exudative) Gradual or sudden significant loss of vision; new onset of distortion in vision (straight lines appear wavy); abnormal blood vessels grow under the macula and can cause hemorrhage (**Figure 25-3**). Late changes include subretinal scarring and retinal atrophy (**Figure 25-4**).

CLINICAL FEATURES

- Symptoms that occur before vision loss include metamorphopsia (distorted vision) and central scotoma (impaired vision at the point of fixation).[6]
- Vision loss is central. Peripheral and night vision are generally not affected.
- Drusen (yellowish-colored subretinal deposits on the macula) is the classic physical examination finding. The following classification scheme has been proposed[7]:
  - Early AMD: medium drusen (63 to 125 μm), without AMD-related pigmentary abnormalities
  - Intermediate AMD: large drusen (≥125 μm) or medium drusen with pigmentary abnormalities
  - Late AMD: geography atrophy or neovascular changes

TYPICAL DISTRIBUTION

- Bilateral, although usually one eye is affected before the other.

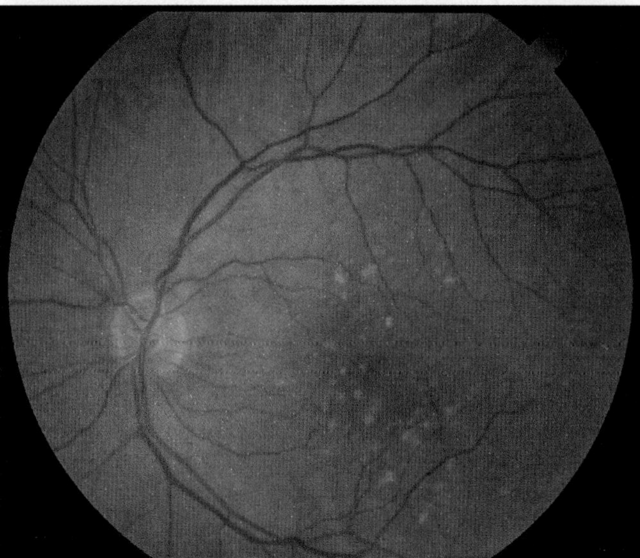

FIGURE 25-2 Early, dry, age-related macular degeneration demonstrating drusen, yellowish-colored subretinal deposits on the macula. Patients may have no visual complaints at this stage. *(Reproduced with permission from Paul D. Comeau.)*

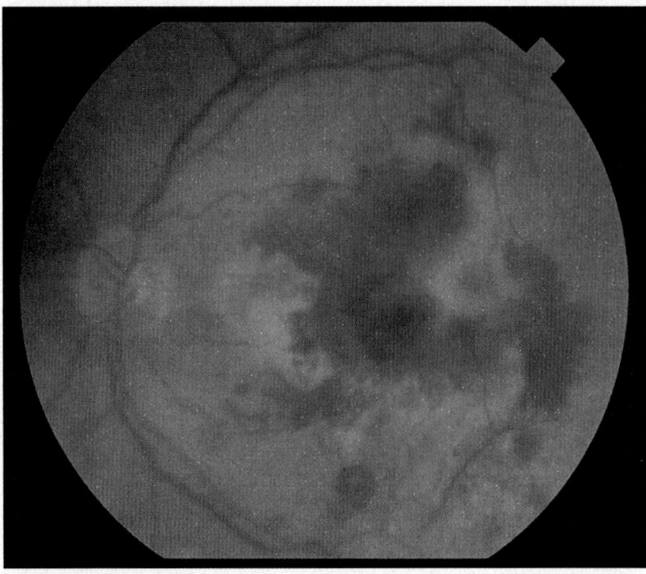

FIGURE 25-3 Late, wet, age-related macular degeneration (exudative) with subretinal hemorrhages. Patients usually have significant central vision loss. *(Reproduced with permission from Paul D. Comeau.)*

ANCILLARY TESTING

Amsler grid may be used to detect changes in central vision. Optical coherence tomography (OCT) and fluorescein angiography are most commonly used to assess for leakage from abnormal blood vessels. If leakage is present, this indicates that anti-vascular endothelial growth factor (VEGF) treatment may help.

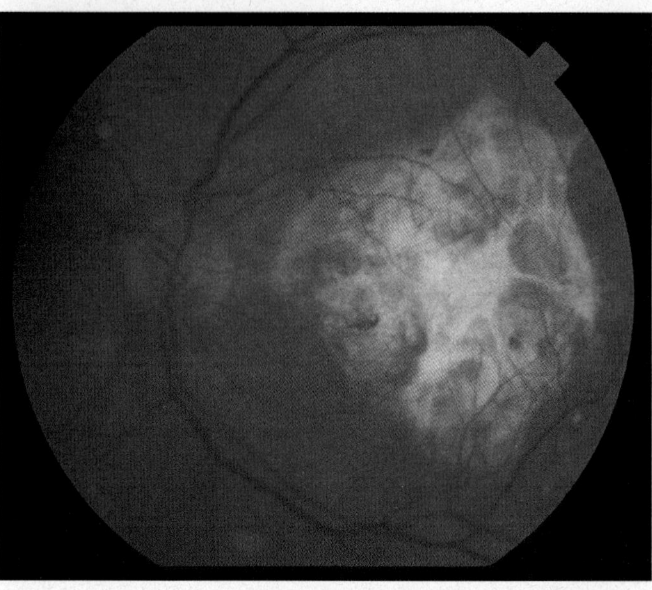

FIGURE 25-4 Late, wet, age-related macular degeneration (exudative) with subretinal scarring. Patients usually have significant central vision loss resulting from destruction of tissue around the macula. *(Reproduced with permission from Paul D. Comeau.)*

DIFFERENTIAL DIAGNOSIS

Vision loss in the elderly can also be caused by any of the following[8]:

- Glaucoma (open-angle)—Often asymptomatic until late in the disease, but then has visual field defects instead of central vision loss; funduscopic examination may reveal a large cup-to-disc ratio (see Chapter 21, Glaucoma).
- Diabetic retinopathy—May have central vision loss with macular edema; funduscopic examination demonstrates microaneurysms, cotton-wool spots, hemorrhages, and exudates (see Chapter 22, Diabetic Retinopathy).
- Cataracts—Blurred vision or glare; lens opacities seen when examining the red reflex.

Drusen can also be seen with:

- Pigmented nevi and choroidal malignant melanoma.
- Retinal detachment.
- Glomerulonephritis, particularly membranoproliferative glomerulonephritis type II.

MANAGEMENT

Refer to ophthalmologist to evaluate for treatments such as intravitreal injections, laser photocoagulation or photodynamic therapy, or surgery.[9]

- Nonpharmacologic:
  - Healthy lifestyle that includes diet, exercise, and no smoking.
- Medications:
  - Intraocular injections of several different anti-VEGFs (i.e., pegaptanib and ranibizumab) reduce the risk of visual acuity loss in patients with advanced neovascular AMD. SOR Ⓐ
- Complementary/alternative therapy:
  - Consider antioxidants (vitamin C, 500 mg; vitamin E, 400 IU; and beta-carotene, 15 mg) plus 80 mg zinc per day to decrease the risk of worsening vision loss in patients with intermediate to advanced AMD.[9] SOR Ⓑ
  - Avoid beta-carotene for smokers or people who have smoked in the last 10 years.

REFERRAL

- Most patients are treated by an ophthalmologist, and treatment may include intravitreal injections, laser photocoagulation or photodynamic therapy, or surgery.
- Urgently refer a patient with a history of dry AMD and acute changes in vision (distortion of lines, objects) to an ophthalmologist for evaluation and treatment.

PREVENTION

- Healthy diet—People with healthy diets, compared with non-healthy diets, were 46% less likely to develop AMD.[10]
- Physical activity—Active people, compared to inactive people, were 54% less likely to develop AMD.[10]
- Healthy behaviors—People with a healthy diet who exercised and did not smoke, compared with people without these healthy behaviors, were 71% less likely to develop AMD.[10]
- Regular intake of age-related eye disease study (AREDS) formula (vitamins A, C, and E, and zinc) may reduce the risk of AMD.[11]

PROGNOSIS

- The risk of progression to late AMD increases with increasing age and severity of drusen and reaches nearly 50% within 10 years in the oldest patients with large drusen at baseline.[12]
- Women and current smokers are at a higher risk of progression to late AMD.[12]
- 50% of patients with intermediate AMD progressed to late AMD within 5 years.[7]

FOLLOW-UP

Patients with ARM and AMD should have regular follow-up with an ophthalmologist.

PATIENT EDUCATION

- AMD can cause a loss of vision leading to an inability to read and drive, thereby affecting many activities of daily living.
- A healthy lifestyle may prevent development or progression of AMD.
- Treatment options are available that decrease the risk of vision loss.
- Most patients with AMD need to see an ophthalmologist regularly in addition to their primary care physician.

PATIENT RESOURCES

- The National Eye Institute has information for patients—**https://nei.nih.gov/health/maculardegen/.**

PROVIDER RESOURCES

- A tool for calculating the risk of advanced AMD is available at: **http://caseyamdcalc.ohsu.edu.**
- Exudative AMD—**https://emedicine.medscape.com/article/1226030-overview.**
- Nonexudative AMD—**https://emedicine.medscape.com/article/1223154-overview.**

REFERENCES

1. Wong WL, Su X, Li X. Global prevalence of age related macular degeneration and disease burden projection for 2020 and 2040: a systematic review and meta-analysis. *Lancet Glob Health.* 2014;2(2):e106-116.
2. Rudnicka AR, Kapetanakis VV, Jarrar Z, et al. Incidence of late-stage age-related macular degeneration in American whites: systematic review and meta-analysis. *Am J Ophthalmol.* 2015;160(1):85-93.
3. Seddon JM, Chen CA. The epidemiology of age-related macular degeneration. *Int Ophthalmol Clin.* 2004;44(4):17-39.
4. Gemenetzi M, Lotery AJ. The role of epigenetics in age-related macular degeneration. *Eye.* 2014;28(12):1407-1417.
5. Chakravarthy U, Wong TY, Fletcher A, et al. Clinical risk factors for age-related macular degeneration: a systematic review and meta-analysis. *BMC Ophthalmol.* 2010;10:31.
6. Kokotas H, Grigoriadou M, Petersen MB. Age-related macular degeneration: genetic and clinical findings. *Clin Chem Lab Med.* 2011;49(4):601-616.
7. Ferris FL 3rd, Wilkinson CP, Bird A, et al. Clinical classification of age-related macular degeneration. *Ophthalmology.* 2013;120(4):844-851.
8. Pelletier AL, Rojas-Roldan L, Coffin J. Vision loss in older adults. *Am Fam Physician.* 2016;94(3):219-226.
9. Yonekawa Y, Kim IK. Clinical characteristics and current treatment of age-related macular degeneration. *Cold Spring Harb Perspect Med.* 2015;5(1):a017178.
10. Mares JA, Voland RP, Sondel SA, et al. Healthy lifestyles related to subsequent prevalence of age-related macular degeneration. *Arch Ophthalmol.* 2011;129(4):470-480.
11. Wong IY, Koo SC, Chan CW. Prevention of age-related macular degeneration. *Int Ophthalmol.* 2011;31(1):73-82.
12. Chew EY, Clemons TE, Agrón E, et al. Ten-year follow-up of age-related macular degeneration in the age-related eye disease study: AREDS report no. 36. *JAMA Ophthalmol.* 2014;132(3):272-277.

26 EYE TRAUMA—HYPHEMA

Heidi S. Chumley, MD, MBA

PATIENT STORY

A 22-year-old man was hit in the eye with a baseball and presented to the emergency department with eye pain and redness and decreased visual acuity. There was a collection of blood in his anterior chamber (**Figure 26-1**) and he was diagnosed with a hyphema. He was given an eye shield for protection, advised to take acetaminophen for pain, and counseled not to engage in sporting activities until his hyphema resolved. He saw his physician daily for the next 2 days, during which his vision improved. His hyphema resolved in 5 days.

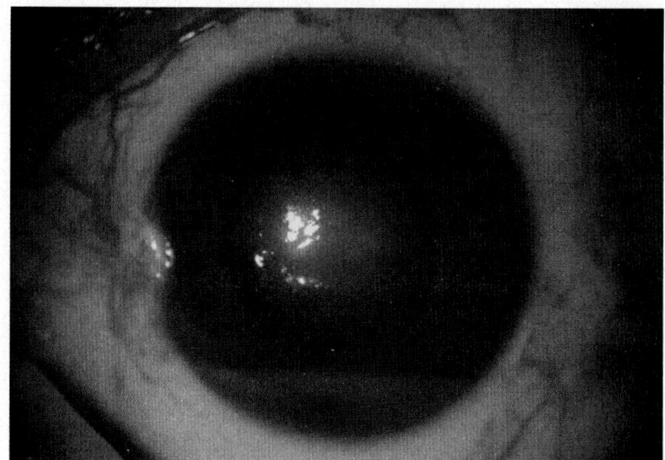

FIGURE 26-1 Layering of red blood cells in the anterior chamber following blunt trauma. This grade 1 hyphema has blood filling in less than one-third of the anterior chamber. *(Reproduced with permission from Paul D. Comeau.)*

INTRODUCTION

Hyphema, blood in the anterior chamber, can be seen following eye trauma or as a result of clotting disturbances, vascular abnormalities, or mass effects from neoplasms. Traumatic hyphema occurs more often in boys and men, often related to work or sports. Hyphema typically resolves in 5 to 7 days, but some cases are complicated by rebleeding.

EPIDEMIOLOGY

- Eye injuries are common among children, with a rate of 14.31 per 1000 children. Over 60% of injuries occur in males. The most common diagnosis is contusion/abrasion.[1]
- Traumatic hyphema is more common in males (20.2 per 100,000) than females (4.1 per 100,000).[2]
- Sixty percent of hyphemas result from sports injuries.[3] Sports with higher risk for eye injuries include paintball, baseball/softball, basketball, soccer, fishing, ice hockey, racquet sports, fencing, lacrosse, and boxing.

ETIOLOGY AND PATHOPHYSIOLOGY

- A hyphema is a collection of blood, mostly erythrocytes, that layer within the anterior chamber.
- Trauma is the most common cause, often resulting from a direct blow from a projectile object such as a ball, air pellet or BB, rock, or fist.
- Direct force to the eye (blunt trauma) forces the globe inward, distorting the normal architecture.
- Intraocular pressure rises instantaneously, causing the lens/iris/ciliary body to move posteriorly, thus disrupting the vascularization with resultant bleeding.
- Intraocular pressure continues to rise, and bleeding stops when this pressure is high enough to compress the bleeding vessels.
- A fibrin-platelet clot forms and stabilizes in 4 to 7 days; this is eventually broken down by the fibrinolytic system and cleared through the trabecular meshwork.

DIAGNOSIS

The diagnosis of hyphema is clinical, depending on the classic appearance of blood layering in the anterior chamber.

CLINICAL FEATURES

History and physical:

- Layered blood in the anterior chamber.
- History of eye trauma or risk factor for nontraumatic hyphema.
- Increased intraocular pressure (32%).
- Decreased vision.
- Hyphemas are classified according to the amount of blood in the anterior chamber[4]:
  - Grade 1: Less than one-third of the anterior chamber (see **Figure 26-1**); 58% of all hyphemas
  - Grade 2: One-third to one-half of the anterior chamber; 20% of all hyphemas
  - Grade 3: One-half filled to almost completely filled anterior chamber; 14% of all hyphemas
  - Grade 4: Completely filled anterior chamber; 8% of all hyphemas
- Eye trauma without hyphema (**Figures 26-2 and 26-3**) can lead to subconjunctival hemorrhage, anterior uveitis, and/or distortion of the normal architecture, including globe rupture.

LABORATORY TESTING

- Consider laboratory tests to evaluate for bleeding disorders: bleeding time, electrophoresis for sickle cell trait, platelet count, prothrombin and partial thromboplastin time, and liver tests.

IMAGING

- Consider CT imaging if a mechanism of injury suggests an associated orbital fracture or concern for orbital or intraocular foreign body.

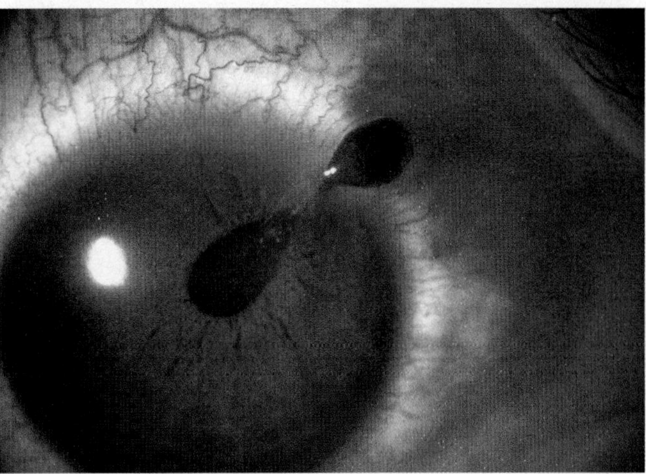

FIGURE 26-2 This young patient was hit in the eye with the corner of a laminated name card. The sharp edge perforated the cornea and pulled a portion of the iris out of the wound. Note the abnormal configuration of the pupil (dyscoria). No hyphema noted. This patient required emergent surgical repair. (*Reproduced with permission from Lo MW, Chalfin S. Retrobulbar anesthesia for repair of ruptured globes, Am J Ophthalmol. 1997;123(6):833-835. Photo contributor: Paul D. Comeau.*)

DIFFERENTIAL DIAGNOSIS

Hyphema is an unmistakable physical examination finding that can be caused by any of the following:

- Trauma—History of trauma, including nonaccidental trauma (i.e., child abuse).
- Blood clotting disturbances—Personal or family history of bleeding disorder, little or no trauma, and black race (increased incidence of sickle trait and disease).
- Medication-induced anticoagulation—Chronic use of aspirin or warfarin and little or no trauma.
- Neovascularization—Diabetes with diabetic retinopathy, history of other ocular disease (central retinal vein occlusion), or history of prior eye surgery (cataract); without trauma, often painless, sudden, blurry vision.
- Melanoma or retinoblastoma—Variety of presentations depending on the size and location; hyphema occurs when mass effect sheers the lens/iris/ciliary body causing bleeding.

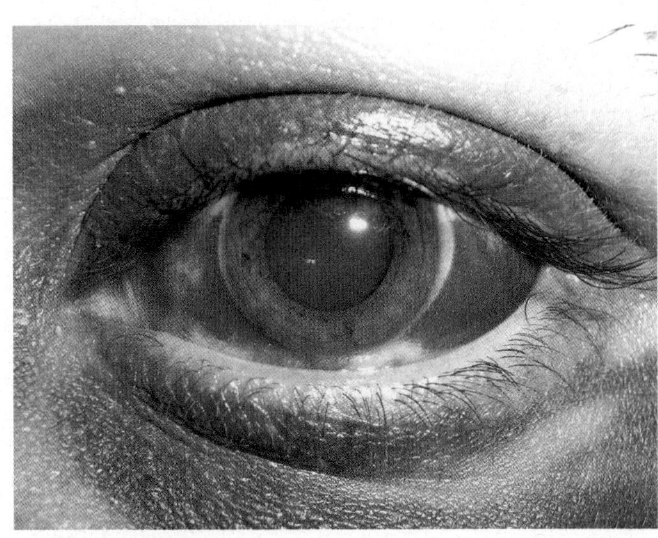

FIGURE 26-3 Subconjunctival hemorrhage and eyelid ecchymosis following accidental trauma. There was no hyphema present. (*Reproduced with permission from Richard P. Usatine, MD.*)

- Abnormal vasculature, that is, juvenile xanthogranuloma—Red to yellow papules and nodules in the eyes, skin, and viscera, most often present by 1 year of age.

MANAGEMENT

- Most hyphemas resolve in 5 to 7 days; management strategies protect the eye and decrease complications, including rebleeding.
- Evaluate or refer for evaluation for elevated intraocular pressure and other associated injuries. Urgent referral if concern for globe rupture.

A recent Cochrane review evaluated these interventions: antifibrinolytic agents, corticosteroids, cycloplegics, miotics, aspirin, conjugated estrogens, eye patching, head elevation, and bed rest.

- No interventions had a significant effect on visual acuity.
- Aminocaproic acid (antifibrinolytic) use resulted in a slower resolution of the primary hyphema.
- Antifibrinolytics: aminocaproic acid and tranexamic acid reduced the rate of secondary hemorrhage.[5]

NONPHARMACOLOGIC

- Eye patching, head elevation, and bed rest do not independently affect visual acuity.[5] However, experts recommend patching and shielding the injured eye and allowing the patient to remain ambulatory as part of a comprehensive treatment plan.[4] SOR Ⓒ

MEDICATIONS

- Although controversy remains about the best treatment, each of the following has been demonstrated to lower the risk of rebleeding in randomized controlled trials:
  - Oral antifibrinolytic agents (aminocaproic acid 50 mg/kg every 4 hours for 5 days, not to exceed 30 g/day, or tranexamic acid 75 mg/kg per day divided into 3 doses).[6] SOR Ⓒ
  - Topical aminocaproic acid (30% in a gel vehicle 4 times a day) is as effective as oral.[6] SOR Ⓒ
  - Avoid aspirin and nonsteroidal anti-inflammatory drugs (NSAIDs), which have been associated with higher rates of rebleeding.
  - Use acetaminophen, if needed, for pain.

REFERRAL OR HOSPITALIZATION

- Signs of a violated globe, such as a perforation of the cornea, conjunctiva, or sclera; distorted ocular architecture; or exposed and/or distorted uveal tissue such as the iris (causing a peaked pupil), require immediate surgical evaluation and repair (see **Figure 26-2**).
- Surgical intervention has been recommended for patients with persistent total hyphema or prolonged elevated intraocular pressure.
- Outpatient management is acceptable for adults and children if patient is likely to be able to follow the treatment plan.[6,7] SOR Ⓑ

PREVENTION

Ninety percent of sports-related eye injuries can be prevented with appropriate eyewear.[8]

Mandates for protective eyewear reduced severe eye injuries by nearly 70% in high school field hockey.[9]

PROGNOSIS

The percentage of patients who regain 20/40 vision varies by severity of the hyphema: grade I, 80%; grade III, 60%; grade IV, 35%.[4]

FOLLOW-UP

Patients should be monitored daily for the first 5 or more days by a provider familiar with caring for hyphemas. Patient with a hyphema should be followed subsequently for signs of angle recession and high intraocular pressure, which predisposes the patient to traumatic glaucoma, an insidious cause of blindness in patients with a history of trauma.

PATIENT EDUCATION

- Complications include rebleeding, decreased visual acuity, posterior or peripheral anterior synechiae, corneal bloodstaining, glaucoma, and optic atrophy. Patients may need surgical or medical management for glaucoma.
- Patients who are more likely to rebleed include black patients (irrespective of sickle cell/trait status),[10,11] patients with a grade 3 or 4 hyphema, and patients with high initial intraocular pressure.
- Warn patients that they may have angle recession from traumatic causes of the hyphema. This will predispose the patient to a lifetime risk of traumatic glaucoma, which can cause blindness without any symptoms. These patients need to be monitored regularly by an ophthalmologist for increased pressure and glaucomatous nerve changes.

PATIENT RESOURCES

- The National Eye Institute has information for parents, teachers, and coaches at **https://nei.nih.gov/sports/**

PROVIDER RESOURCES

- The National Eye Institute has a variety of handouts suitable for displaying or giving to patients at **https://nei.nih.gov/healthyeyestoolkit/d_resources**

REFERENCES

1. Armstrong GW, Kim JG, Linakis JG, et al. Pediatric eye injuries presenting to United States emergency departments: 2001–2007. *Graefes Arch Clin Exp Ophthalmol.* 2013:251(3):629-636.
2. Kennedy RH, Brubaker RF. Traumatic hyphema in a defined population. *Am J Ophthalmol.* 1988;106(2):123.
3. Schein OD, Hibberd PL, Shingleton BJ, et al. The spectrum and burden of ocular injury. *Ophthalmology.* 1988;95(3):300-305.
4. Nash DL. Hyphema. Medscape. *https://emedicine.medscape.com/article/1190165-overview.* Accessed October 2017.

5. Gharaibeh A, Savage HI, Scherer RW, et al. Medical interventions for traumatic hyphema. *Cochrane Database Syst Rev.* 2013;(12): CD005431.

6. Walton W, Von HS, Grigorian R, Zarbin M. Management of traumatic hyphema. *Surv Ophthalmol.* 2002;47(4):297-334.

7. Rocha KM, Martins EN, Melo LA Jr, Moraes NS. Outpatient management of traumatic hyphema in children: prospective evaluation. *J AAPOS.* 2004;8(4):357-361.

8. Harrison A, Telander DG. Eye injuries in the youth athlete: a case-based approach. *Sports Med.* 2002;l31(1):33-40.

9. Kriz PK, Zurakowski D, Almquist JL, et al. Eye protection and risk of eye injuries in high school field hockey. *Pediatrics.* 2015; 136(3):521-527.

10. Lai JC, Fekrat S, Barron Y, Goldberg MF. Traumatic hyphema in children: risk factors for complications. *Arch Ophthalmol.* 2001; 119(1):64-70.

11. Spoor TC, Kwitko GM, O'Grady JM, Ramocki JM. Traumatic hyphema in an urban population. *Am J Ophthalmol.* 1990;109(1): 23-27.

27 DIFFERENTIAL DIAGNOSIS OF THE RED EYE

Heidi S. Chumley, MD, MBA
Richard P. Usatine, MD

PATIENT STORY

A 41-year-old man wakes up with eyes that are reddened bilaterally (**Figure 27-1**). He has some burning and itching in the eyes, but no pain. He describes minimal crusting on his eyelashes. Examination shows no loss of vision, no foreign bodies, and pupils that are equal, round, and reactive to light. He is diagnosed with viral conjunctivitis, which does not require antibiotic treatment. He is advised about methods to prevent spreading conjunctivitis to others and is asked to notify the physician immediately if he experiences eye pain or loss of vision. He recovers spontaneously without complications after a few days.

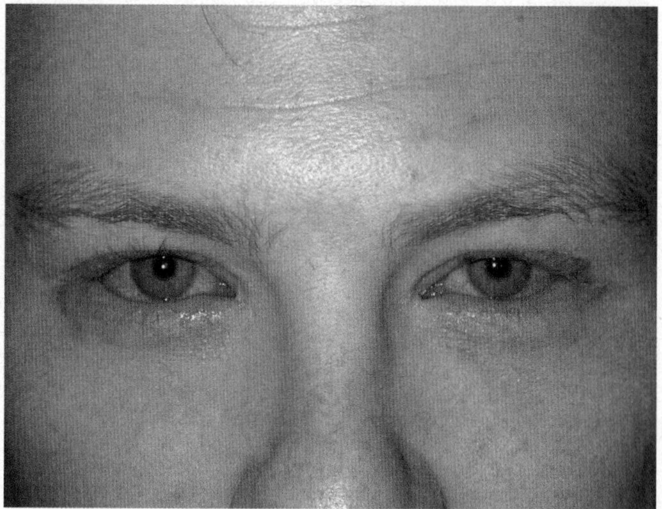

FIGURE 27-1 Bilateral viral conjunctivitis in a 41-year-old man. *(Reproduced with permission from Richard P. Usatine, MD.)*

INTRODUCTION

A red eye signifies ocular inflammation. The differential diagnosis includes both benign and sight-threatening conditions. The pattern of redness; presence/absence of eye pain or photophobia, vision loss, or eye discharge; involvement of cornea; and visual acuity are helpful in differentiating among causes (see **Table 27-1**). Although most red eyes seen in the primary care setting are a result of viral conjunctivitis, several causes of red eye require urgent referral.

EPIDEMIOLOGY

- An acute red eye or eyes is a common presentation in ambulatory and emergency departments.
- Conjunctivitis is the most common cause of a nontraumatic red eye in primary care.

ETIOLOGY AND PATHOPHYSIOLOGY

Red eye is caused by any of the following:

- Infectious or noninfectious inflammation of any layer of the eye (conjunctivitis, episcleritis, scleritis, uveitis, keratitis).
- Eyelid pathology (blepharitis, entropion, i.e., inward turning of the eyelid, or other eyelid malposition).
- Acute glaucoma (usually angle closure).
- Trauma.
- Subconjunctival hemorrhage.

TABLE 27-1 Clinical Features in the Diagnosis of Red Eye

	Conjunctivitis	Episcleritis	Scleritis	Uveitis	Keratitis	Closed-Angle Glaucoma	Subconjunctival Hemorrhage	Ocular Rosacea
Redness	Diffuse	Segmental; pink	Segmental or diffuse; dark red, purple, or blue	360-Degree perilimbal (worse at limbus)	Diffuse, ciliary injection	Diffuse, scleral	Blotchy, outside vessels	Diffuse
Eye pain	No	Mild, may be tender to touch	Severe, boring	Sometimes	Usually	Yes	No, unless caused by trauma	No
Vision loss	No	No	Sometimes	Sometimes	Maybe, depending on location	Yes	No	In severe cases
Discharge	Usually	No	No	No	Maybe	No	No	No
Photophobia*	No	No	Yes	Yes, if anterior	Yes	Yes	No	Sometimes
Pupil	Normal	Normal	Normal	Constricted	Normal to constricted	Mild dilation, less responsive	Normal; unless affected by trauma	Normal
Cornea	Clear	Clear	Clear	Clear to hazy	Hazy	Usually hazy	Clear	Clear or neovascularization, cloudy
Associated diseases	URI, allergy, exposure	Occasional systemic disease	Systemic disease	Systemic disease, idiopathic	Contact lenses, HSV or varicella, rosacea	Causes headaches, nausea, vomiting, GI symptoms	HTN, trauma, Valsalva, cough, blood thinners	Acne rosacea (can exist without also), blepharitis

HSV, herpes simplex virus; HTN, hypertension; URI, upper respiratory infection.
*For identifying serious causes of red eye, the presence of photophobia elicited with a penlight in a general practice had a positive predictive value of 60% and a negative predictive value of 90%.[5]

DIFFERENTIAL DIAGNOSIS

An acute red eye can be caused by any of the following:

- Conjunctivitis—Conjunctival injection, eye discharge, gritty or uncomfortable feeling, and no vision loss (**Figures 27-1** to **27-4**) (see also Chapter 18, Conjunctivitis).
- Episcleritis—Segmental or diffuse inflammation of episclera (pink color), mild or no discomfort, but can be tender to palpation, and no vision disturbance (**Figure 27-5**) (see also Chapter 19, Scleritis and Episcleritis).
- Scleritis—Segmental or diffuse inflammation of sclera (dark red, purple, or blue color), severe boring eye pain often radiating to head and neck, and photophobia and vision loss (**Figure 27-6**) (see also Chapter 19, Scleritis and Episcleritis).
- Keratitis or corneal ulcerations—Diffuse erythema with ciliary injection often with pupillary constriction; eye discharge; and pain, photophobia, vision loss depending on the location of ulceration (**Figure 27-7**). Often associated with the use of contact lenses.
- Subconjunctival hemorrhage (**Figure 27-8**)—Bright red subconjunctival blood; usually not painful; can present after significant coughing/sneezing, after trauma, or in the setting of dry eyes with minor trauma from rubbing with a finger. Not vision-threatening.
- Ocular rosacea—Eye findings present in more than 50% of people with facial rosacea. Can present as blepharitis, conjunctivitis, or episcleritis or cause corneal ulcerations and neovascularization (**Figures 27-9** and **27-10**).
- Uveitis or iritis—A 360-degree injection, which is most intense at the limbus, eye pain, photophobia, and vision loss (**Figure 27-11**) (see also Chapter 20, Uveitis and Iritis).
- Trauma causing globe injury, or hemorrhage into the anterior chamber called hyphema (**Figures 27-12** and **27-13**) (see Chapter 26, Eye Trauma—Hyphema).
- Pterygium—Fibrovascular tissue on the surface of the eye extending onto the cornea (**Figure 27-14**) (see also Chapter 14, Pterygium).
- Hypopyon is a term for visible white cells (pus) layered out in the anterior chamber. It may be caused by inflammation of the iris or an eye infection. The inflammation and/or infection also causes the conjunctiva and sclera to become red (**Figure 27-15**).
- Acute-angle closure glaucoma—Cloudy cornea and scleral injection, shallow anterior chamber (check other eye if difficult to assess chamber depth in the red eye), eye pain with ipsilateral headache, and severe vision loss (see also Chapter 21, Glaucoma).
- Eyelid pathology—Blepharitis (inflammation of the eyelid) (**Figure 27-16**). Entropion is a turning inward of the eyelid and can cause irritation to the conjunctiva and cornea.

The Edinburgh Red Eye Diagnostic Algorithm demonstrated a diagnostic accuracy of 72% in primary care.[1]

CLINICAL FEATURES

Primary care providers need to distinguish more serious from less serious causes of red eye. The following clinical features increased the likelihood of a serious eye condition.[2]

- Anisocoria of >1 mm, with smaller pupil in red eye [LR +6.5]

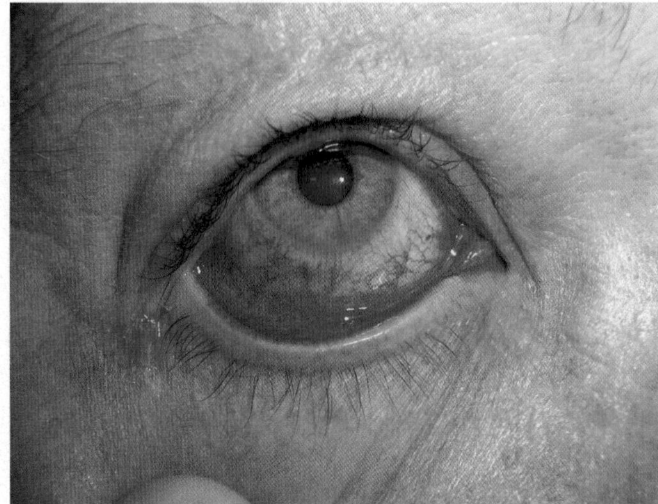

FIGURE 27-2 Bacterial conjunctivitis in a contact lens user. *(Reproduced with permission from Richard P. Usatine, MD.)*

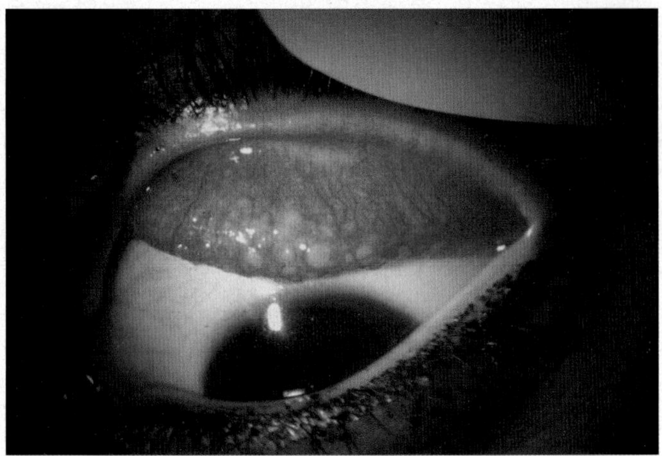

FIGURE 27-3 Giant papillary conjunctivitis secondary to contact lens use. *(Reproduced with permission from Paul D. Comeau.)*

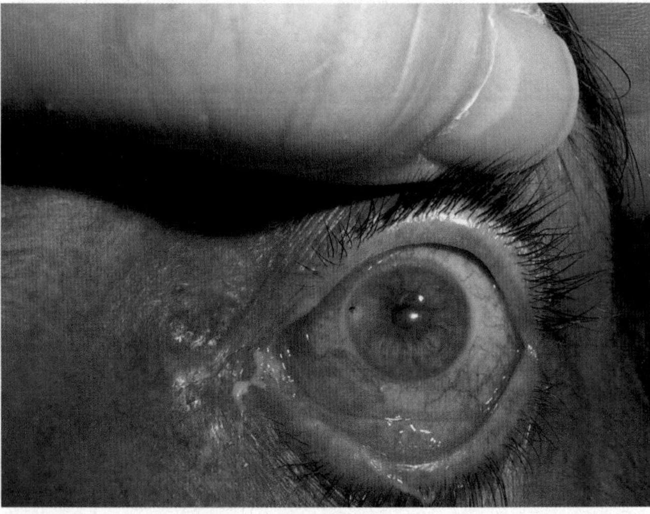

FIGURE 27-4 Conjunctival irritation caused by a fleck of metal (at 9-o'clock position) that was embedded in the eye of a man who was grinding steel. *(Reproduced with permission from Richard P. Usatine, MD.)*

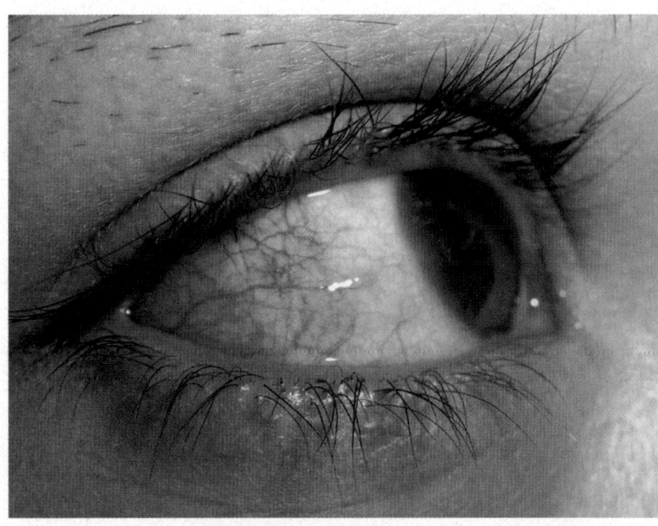

FIGURE 27-5 Episcleritis showing a sector of erythema. (*Reproduced with permission from Richard P. Usatine, MD.*)

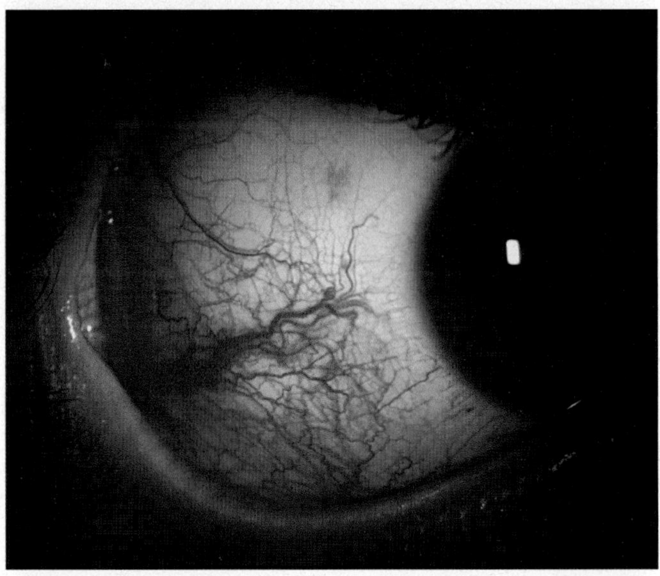

FIGURE 27-6 Scleritis with deeper, darker vessels than the episcleritis. (*Reproduced with permission from Paul D. Comeau.*)

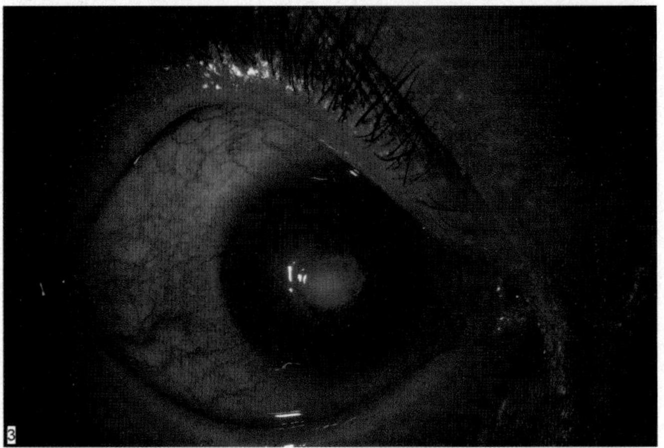

FIGURE 27-7 Diffuse ciliary injection and cloudy cornea demonstrating keratitis with corneal ulcer formation and a leukocyte infiltrate. (*Reproduced with permission from Paul D. Comeau.*)

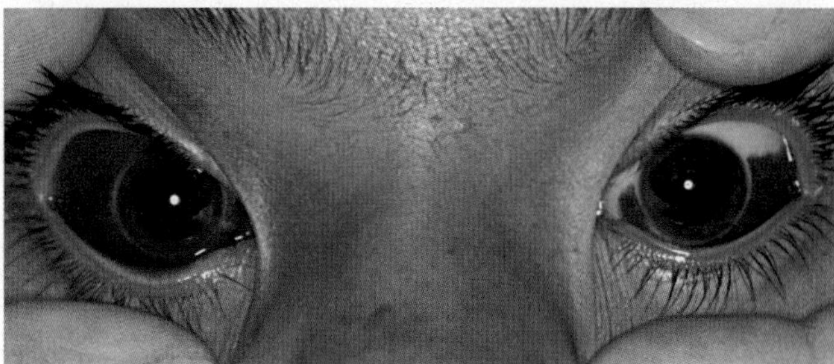

FIGURE 27-8 Subconjunctival hemorrhage secondary to trauma. (*Reproduced with permission from Paul D. Comeau.*)

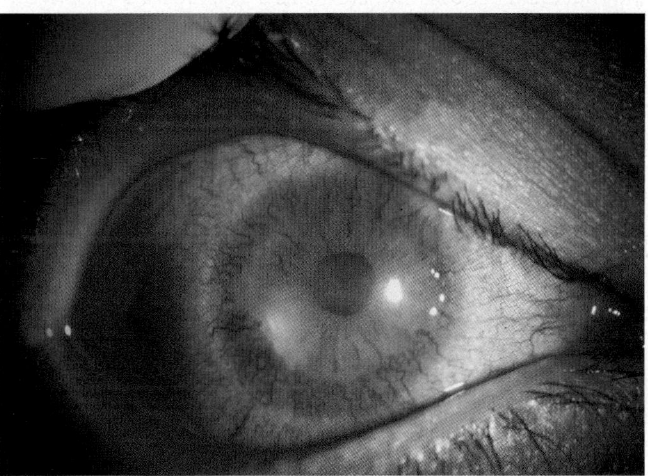

FIGURE 27-9 Ocular rosacea with new vessels growing onto the cornea. Many patients with rosacea have some ocular findings including blepharitis (inflammation of the eyelid), conjunctivitis (most common), episcleritis (rare), keratitis, or corneal ulceration/neovascularization. (*Reproduced with permission from Paul D. Comeau.*)

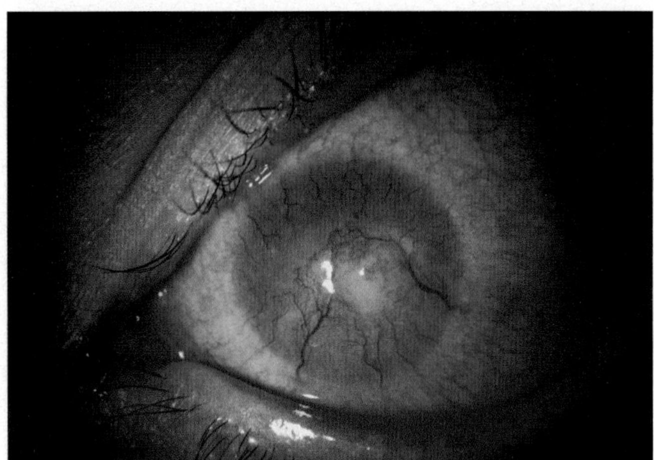

FIGURE 27-10 Severe ocular rosacea with blood vessels growing over the cornea leading to blindness. (*Reproduced with permission from Paul D. Comeau.*)

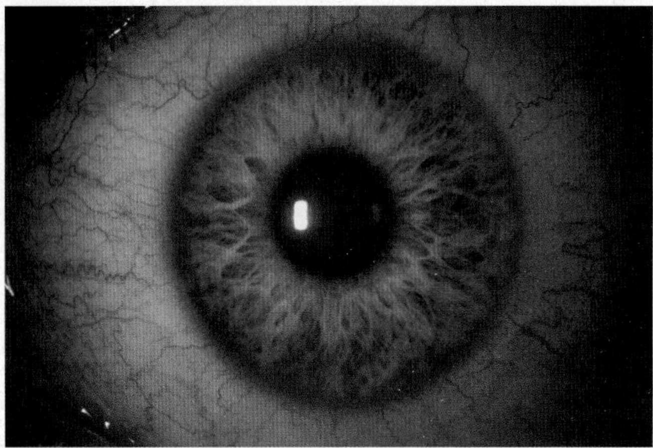

FIGURE 27-11 Iritis (anterior uveitis) with a limbal flush, red to purple perilimbal ring. For contrast, note the perilimbal area is not involved in conjunctivitis, as best seen in **Figure 25-2**. This patient has eye pain and vision loss, which are also absent in conjunctivitis. (*Reproduced with permission from Paul D. Comeau.*)

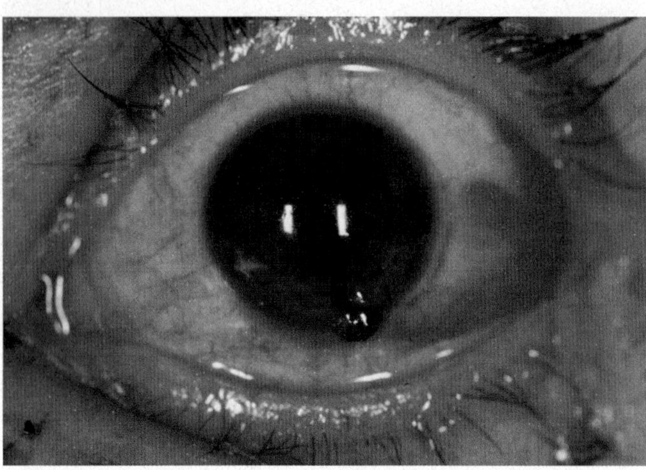

FIGURE 27-12 Trauma to the eye resulting in an open globe injury with extrusion of some of the iris through the cornea and an abnormal pupil. There is conjunctival injection and hemorrhage causing this red eye. (*Reproduced with permission from Paul D. Comeau.*)

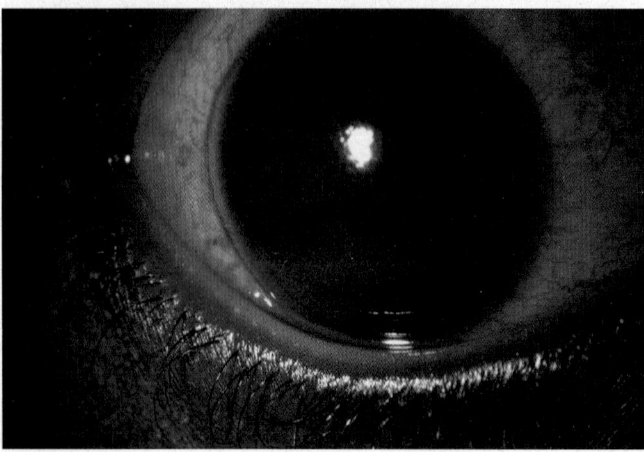

FIGURE 27-13 Hyphema with red cells in the anterior chamber and an inferior blood clot. (*Reproduced with permission from Paul D. Comeau.*)

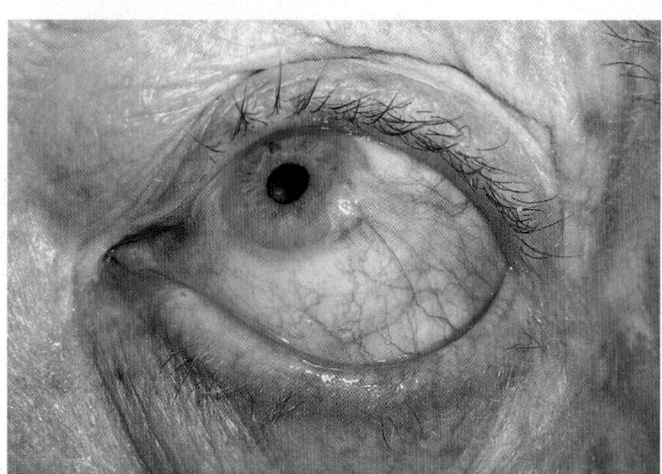

FIGURE 27-14 Pterygium often become irritated and injected. (*Reproduced with permission from Richard P. Usatine, MD.*)

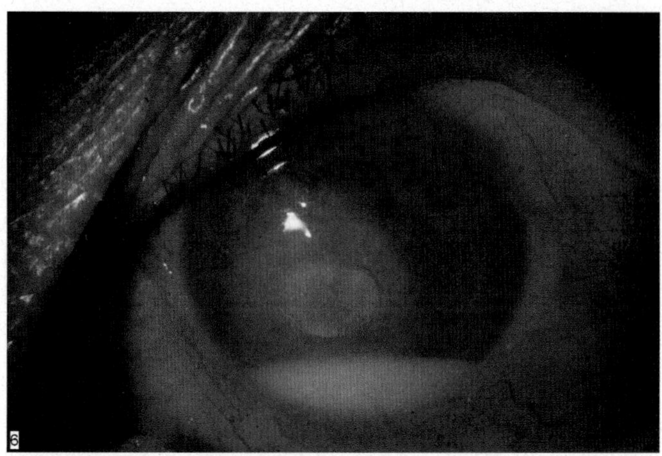

FIGURE 27-15 Hypopyon with white cells layered in the anterior chamber. (*Reproduced with permission from Paul D. Comeau.*)

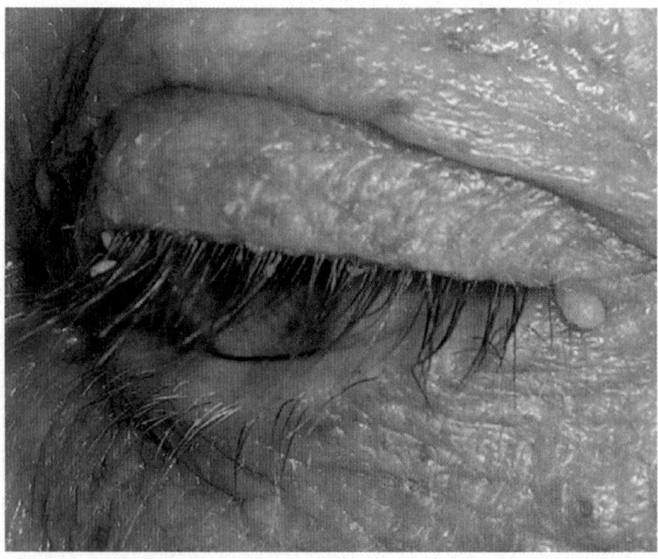

FIGURE 27-16 Blepharitis showing erythema of the eyelids and flaking in the eyelashes. Note the scale that has accumulated in the eyelashes. (*Reproduced with permission from Richard P. Usatine, MD.*)

- Photophobia when light directed at red eye [LR +8.3]
- Photophobia in red eye when light directed at normal eye [LR +28.8]
- Pain in the red eye on convergence [LR +21.4]

MANAGEMENT

Treatment for specific causes is discussed in the corresponding chapters.

Refer patients with any of the following to an ophthalmologist[3,4]: SOR Ⓒ

- Visual loss.
- Moderate or severe pain.
- Severe, purulent discharge.
- Corneal involvement.
- Conjunctival scarring.
- Lack of response to therapy.
- Topical steroid therapy.
- Recurrent episodes.
- Open globe or perforation.
- History of herpes simplex virus (HSV) eye disease.
- History of contact lens wear.

PROGNOSIS

Prognosis depends on underlying cause (see corresponding chapters).

FOLLOW-UP

Timing of follow-up and need for further testing is determined by the underlying cause (see corresponding chapters).

PATIENT EDUCATION

Advise patients to notify their physician immediately for eye pain (other than gritty discomfort) and/or loss of vision.

PATIENT RESOURCES

- FamilyDoctor.org. An algorithm to help patients determine when to seek care: *Eye Problems*—**https://familydoctor.org/symptom/eye-problems/.**

PROVIDER RESOURCES

- The Edinburgh Red Eye Algorithm to assist with diagnosis—**http://www.nhslothian.scot.nhs.uk/Services/A-Z/Ophthalmology/GPs/Documents/Red%20Eye%20A%20and%20E%20sheet%20008.pdf.**

REFERENCES

1. Timlin H, Butler L, Wright M. The accuracy of the Edinburgh Red Eye Diagnostic Algorithm. *Eye.* 2015;29(5):619-624.
2. Narayana S, McGee S. Bedside diagnosis of the red eye: a systematic review. *Am J Med.* 2015;128(11):1220-1224.
3. American Academy of Ophthalmology Cornea/External Disease Panel, Preferred Practice Patterns Committee. *Conjunctivitis.* San Francisco, CA: American Academy of Ophthalmology; 2003:25.
4. Cronau H, Kankanala RR, Mauger T. Diagnosis and management of red eye in primary care. *Am Fam Physician.* 2010;81(2):137-144.
5. Yaphe J, Pandher K. The predictive value of the penlight test for photophobia for serious eye pathology in general practice. *Fam Pract.* 2003;20(4):425-427.

PART V

EAR, NOSE, AND THROAT

Strength of Recommendation (SOR)	Definition
A	Recommendation based on consistent and good-quality patient-oriented evidence.*
B	Recommendation based on inconsistent or limited-quality patient-oriented evidence.*
C	Recommendation based on consensus, usual practice, opinion, disease-oriented evidence, or case series for studies of diagnosis, treatment, prevention, or screening.*

*See Appendix A on pages 1603–1606 for further information.

SECTION A EAR

28 OTITIS MEDIA: ACUTE OTITIS AND OTITIS MEDIA WITH EFFUSION

Brian Z. Rayala, MD

PATIENT STORY

A 15-month-old boy is brought by both parents to his family physician with a 2-day history of fever, irritability, and frequent tugging of his left ear. This was preceded by a 1-week history of nasal congestion, cough, and rhinorrhea. On otoscopy, his left tympanic membrane (TM) appears erythematous, cloudy, bulging, and exudative (**Figure 28-1**). His left TM fails to move on pneumatic otoscopy. The physician diagnoses acute otitis media and decides with the parents to prescribe a 10-day course of amoxicillin; the child recovers uneventfully.

In follow-up 2 months later, the child appears healthy and is meeting all his developmental milestones. On otoscopic examination, air–fluid levels are seen in the right ear (**Figure 28-2**). The physician explains the diagnosis of otitis media with effusion to the parents and arranges follow-up. Three months later, the effusion is completely resolved.

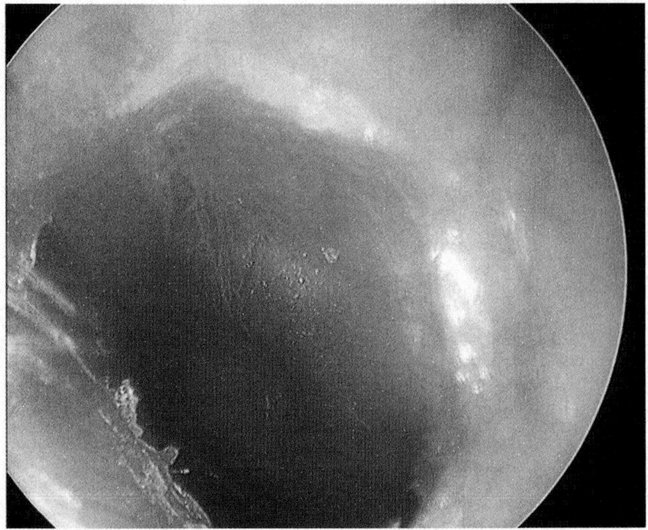

FIGURE 28-1 Acute otitis media in the left ear of a 15-month-old patient with marked erythema and bulging of the tympanic membrane. The malleus and light reflex are not visible. (*Reproduced with permission from William Clark, MD.*)

INTRODUCTION

Acute otitis media (AOM) is the most common diagnosis for acute office visits for children.[1] AOM is characterized by middle-ear effusion in a patient with signs and symptoms of acute illness (e.g., fever, irritability, otalgia). Otitis media with effusion (OME) is a disorder characterized by fluid in the middle ear in a patient without signs and symptoms of acute ear infection; it is also very common in childhood.

SYNONYMS

AOM: acute suppurative, purulent, or bacterial otitis media.[2]

OME: glue ear; secretory, nonsuppurative, serous, or mucoid otitis media.[2]

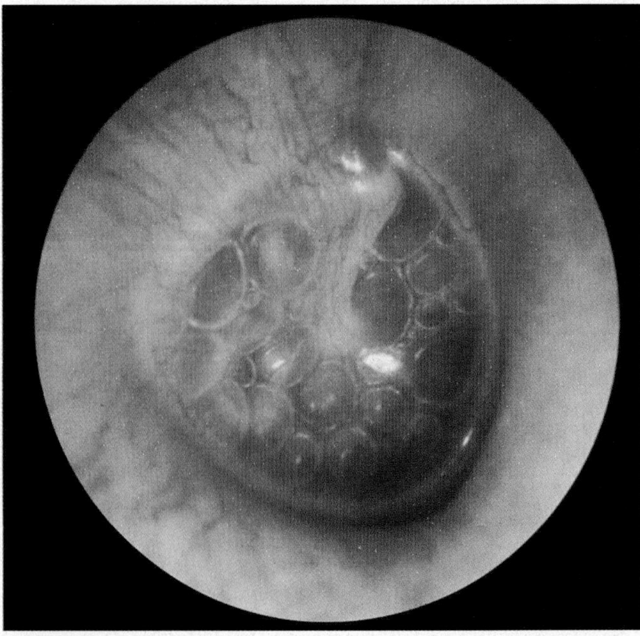

FIGURE 28-2 Otitis media with effusion (OME) in the right ear. Note multiple air–fluid levels in this slightly retracted, translucent, nonerythematous tympanic membrane. (*Reproduced with permission from Frank Miller, MD.*)

EPIDEMIOLOGY

- AOM accounted for $5 billion of the total national health expenditure in 2000; more than 40% was incurred for children between 1 and 3 years of age.[1]
- It is estimated that 60% to 80% of children in the United States develop AOM by 1 year of age and that 80% to 90% develop AOM by 2 to 3 years of age.[3,4]

- The highest incidence occurs between 6 and 24 months of age.[3,4]
- AOM is the most common reason for outpatient antibiotic treatment in the United States.[5] A national survey in 1992 revealed that 30% of all antibiotics prescribed for children younger than age 18 years was for treatment of AOM.[6]
- In the United Kingdom, 87% of AOM cases receive antibiotics.[7]
- OME is diagnosed in 2.2 million children yearly in the United States.[8]
- Approximately 90% of children (80% of individual ears) have OME at some time before school age, most often between ages 6 months and 4 years.[8]
- The combined direct and indirect health care costs of OME amount to $4 billion annually.

ETIOLOGY AND PATHOPHYSIOLOGY

AOM is often preceded by upper respiratory symptoms such as cough and rhinorrhea.

- Pathogenesis of AOM includes[9]:
    - Eustachian tube dysfunction (usually a result of an upper respiratory infection) and subsequent tube obstruction
    - Increased negative pressure in the middle ear
    - Accumulation of middle-ear fluid
    - Microbial growth
    - Suppuration (that leads to clinical signs of AOM)
- Most common pathogens in the United States and United Kingdom are[10,11]:
    - Strains of *Streptococcus pneumoniae* not in the heptavalent pneumococcal vaccine (PCV7) (after introduction of PCV7 vaccine in 2000)
    - Nonencapsulated (nontypable) *Haemophilus influenzae* (NTHi)
    - *Moraxella catarrhalis*
    - *Staphylococcus aureus*
- Viruses account for 16% of cases. Respiratory syncytial viruses, rhinoviruses, influenza viruses, and adenoviruses have been the most common isolated viruses.[12]

OME most commonly follows AOM; it may also occur spontaneously.

- Fluid limits sound conduction through the ossicles and results in decreased hearing.
- Reasons for the persistence of fluid in otitis media remain unclear, although potential etiologies include allergies, biofilm, and physiologic features.
- "Glue ear" refers to extremely viscous mucoid material within the middle ear and is a distinct subtype of OME.

RISK FACTORS

- The most important risk factors for AOM include young age and attendance at daycare centers.
- Other risk factors include[13]:
    - White race.
    - Male gender.

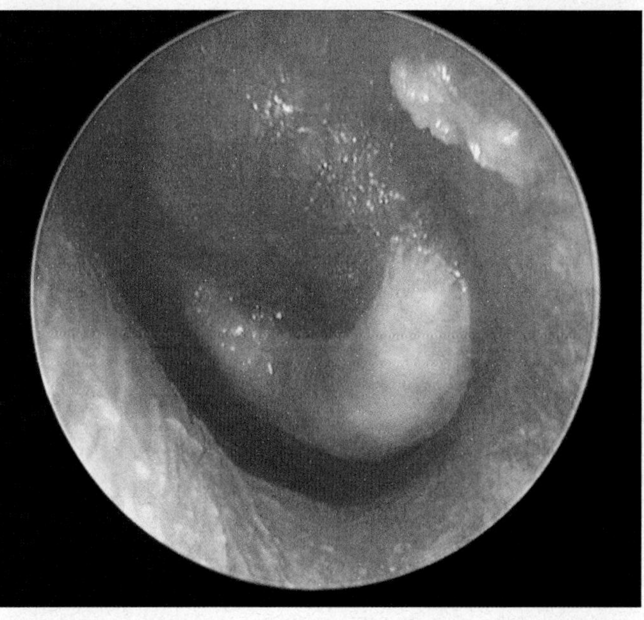

FIGURE 28-3 Acute otitis media, stage of suppuration. Note presence of purulent exudate behind the tympanic membrane (TM), the outward bulging of the TM, prominence of the posterosuperior portion of the drum, and generalized TM edema. The *white area* is tympanosclerosis from a previous infection. (*Reproduced with permission from William Clark, MD.*)

   - History of enlarged adenoids, tonsillitis, or asthma.
   - Multiple previous episodes.
   - Bottle feeding.
   - History of ear infections in parents or siblings.
   - Use of a soother or pacifier.
- Secondhand smoke is a risk factor when parents smoke at home.
- Risk factors for OME include age 6 years or younger, large number of siblings, low socioeconomic group, frequent upper respiratory tract infection, tobacco exposure, daycare attendance, and bottle feeding.[14]

DIAGNOSIS

CLINICAL FEATURES OF AOM

- 2013 American Academy of Pediatrics (AAP) clinical practice guidelines has refined the diagnosis of AOM as[15]:
   - Moderate to severe bulging of the TM (**Figure 28-3**), *or* new-onset otorrhea in the absence of acute otitis externa. SOR B
   - Mild bulging of the TM (**Figure 28-1**) *and* recent onset (<48 hours) of otalgia (i.e., holding, tugging, rubbing of ear in nonverbal child) or intense TM erythema (**Figures 28-4** and **28-5**). SOR C
   - Diagnosis of AOM should not be made in the absence of middle ear effusion (MEE) on pneumatic otoscopy or tympanometry. SOR B
      - MEE presents as limited or absent TM mobility on pneumatic otoscopy, i.e., the TM does not move during air insufflation, often accompanied by retraction of the TM during the initial stages of the disease (**Figure 28-4**).

CLINICAL FEATURES OF OME

- The most common symptom, present in more than half of patients, is mild hearing loss. This is usually identified when parents express concern regarding their child's behavior, performance at school, or language development.
- Absence of signs and symptoms of acute illness assists in differentiating OME from AOM.
- Common otoscopic findings include:
   - Air–fluid levels or bubbles (**Figure 28-2**).
   - Cloudy TM (**Figure 28-3**) in contrast to the normal TM (**Figure 28-6**).
   - Redness of the TM may be present in approximately 5% of ears with OME.
- Clinicians should use pneumatic otoscopy to document presence of MEE when diagnosing OME. Pneumatic otoscopy should be performed to determine the presence of MEE in a child presenting with otalgia, hearing loss, or both. SOR A
   - Impaired mobility of the TM is the hallmark of MEE.
   - According to a meta-analysis, impaired mobility on pneumatic otoscopy has a pooled sensitivity of 94% and specificity of 80%, and positive likelihood ratio of 4.7 and negative likelihood ratio of 0.075.[16]
- When the clinical diagnosis remains uncertain after performing or attempting pneumatic otoscopy in children suspected to have OME, the clinician should perform tympanometry to establish the presence or absence MEE.[8] SOR B

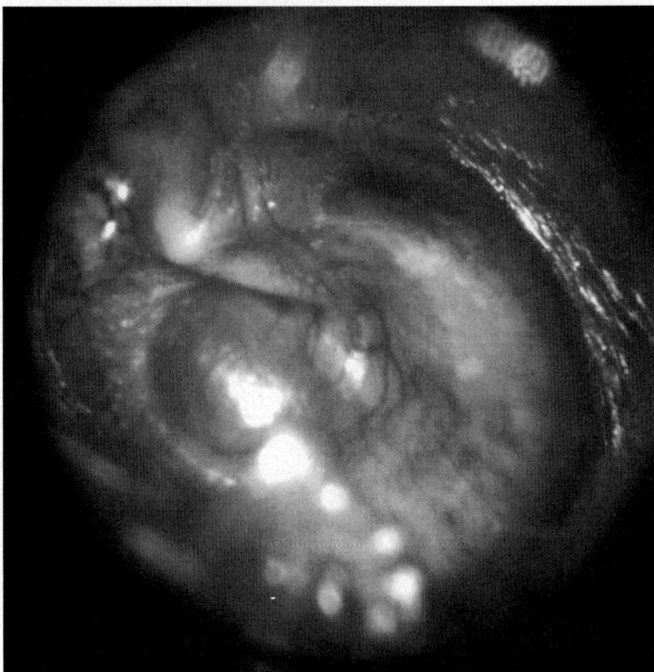

FIGURE 28-4 Otitis media with effusion in the left ear showing retraction of the tympanic membrane and straightening of the handle of the malleus as the retraction pulls the bone upward. (*Reproduced with permission from Glen Medellin, MD.*)

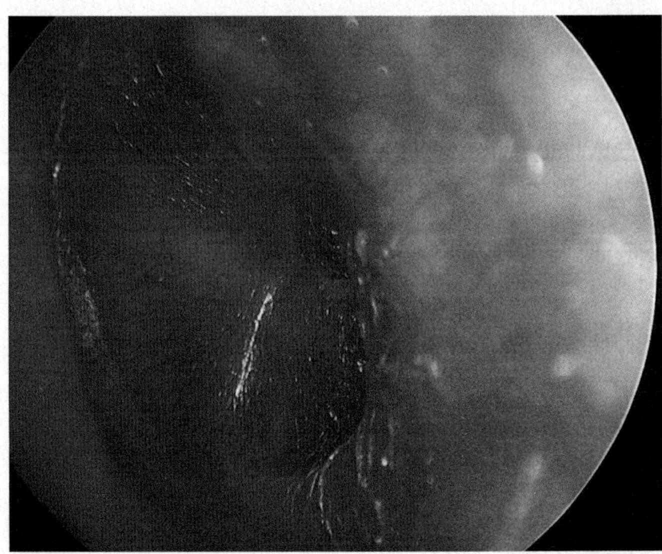

FIGURE 28-5 Early acute otitis media at the stage of eustachian tube obstruction. Note the slight retraction of the tympanic membrane, the more horizontal position of the malleus, and the prominence of the lateral process. (*Reproduced with permission from William Clark, MD.*)

LABORATORY TESTS AND IMAGING

- Because AOM and OME are clinical diagnoses, diagnostic testing has a limited role. When clinical presentation and physical examination (including otoscopy) do not establish the diagnosis, the following can be used as adjunctive techniques:
  - Tympanometry—This procedure records compliance of the TM by measuring reflected sound. AOM and OME will plot as a reduced or flat waveform. This technique requires patient cooperation but provides more objective data.
  - Acoustic reflectometry—This procedure, like tympanometry, measures sound reflectivity from the middle ear. With this test, the clinician can distinguish air- or fluid-filled space without requiring an airtight seal of the ear canal.
  - Middle ear aspiration—For patients with AOM, aspiration may be warranted if the patient is toxic, immunocompromised, or has failed prior courses of antibiotics.

DIFFERENTIAL DIAGNOSIS

The key differentiating feature between AOM and OME is the absence of signs and symptoms of acute illness in OME (e.g., fever, irritability, otalgia). Otoscopic findings may be similar. Other clinical entities that may be confused with AOM and OME include:

- Otitis externa—Otitis externa presents with otalgia, otorrhea, and mild hearing loss, all of which can be present in AOM. Tragal pain on physical exam and signs of external canal inflammation on otoscopic exam differentiate it from AOM. Careful ear irrigation if tolerated may be helpful to visualize the TM to differentiate otitis externa from AOM (see Chapter 29, Acute Otitis Externa).
- Otitic barotrauma—This often presents with severe otalgia. Key historical features include recent air travel, scuba diving, or ear trauma, preceded by an upper respiratory infection.
- Cholesteatoma—Unlike AOM, this is a clinically silent disease in its initial stages. Presence of white keratin debris in the middle ear cavity (on otoscopy) is diagnostic (**Figures 28-7** and **28-8**).
- Foreign body—A foreign body may present with otalgia. Otoscopy reveals presence of foreign body (see Chapter 30, Ear: Foreign Body).
- Bullous myringitis—Bullous myringitis is often associated with viral or mycoplasma infection as well as usual AOM pathogens; in approximately one-third of patients, there is a component of sensorineural hearing loss. Otoscopy shows serous-filled bullae on the surface of the TM (**Figure 28-9**). Patients present with severe otalgia.
- Chronic suppurative otitis media (CSOM)—Otoscopy shows TM perforation and otorrhea; history reveals a chronically draining ear and recurrent middle-ear infections with or without hearing loss.
- Referred otalgia—This is rare in children and in cases of bilateral otalgia. Should be considered in cases of otalgia that do not fit clinical features of AOM. Referred pain usually from other head and neck structures (e.g., teeth, jaw, cervical spine, lymph and salivary glands, nose and sinuses, tonsils, tongue, pharynx, meninges).
- Mastoiditis—Mastoiditis may be differentiated from simple AOM by presence of increasing pain and tenderness over the mastoid bone in a patient with AOM who has not been treated with antibiotics, or

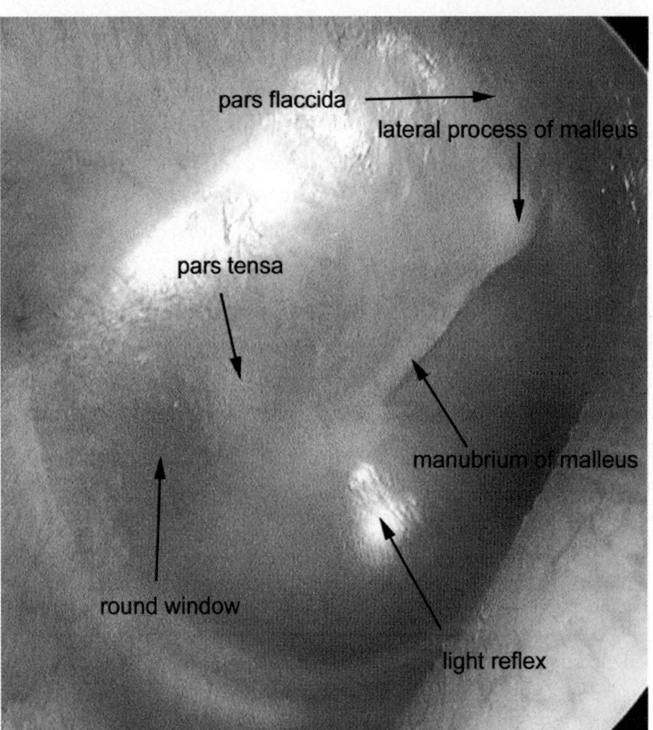

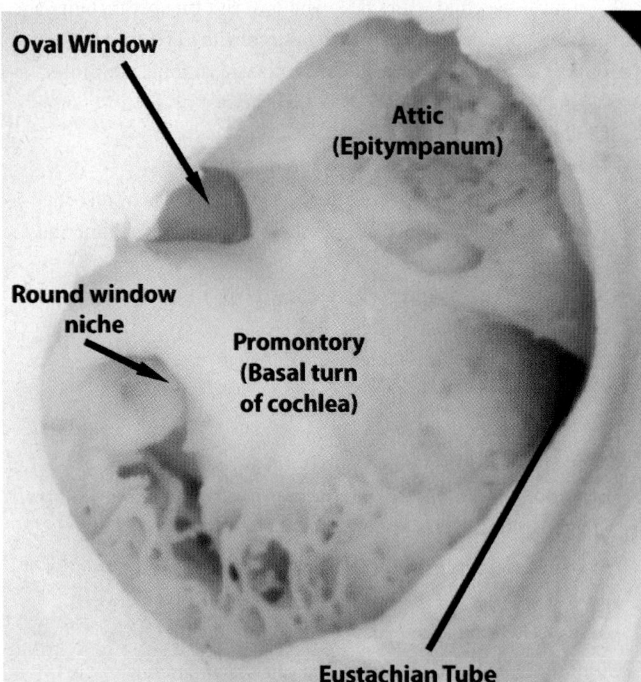

FIGURE 28-6 Normal right tympanic membrane with comparison using normal bony landmarks of the inner ear. The ossicles were removed in this dissection. (*Reproduced with permission from William Clark, MD.*)

recurrence of mastoid pain and tenderness in patients treated with antibiotics. Recurrence or persistence of fever, as well as progressive otorrhea, are other historical clues. The mastoid swelling may cause the pinna to protrude further than normal (**Figure 28-10**).

- Traumatic perforation of the TM (**Figure 28-11**)—A hole in the TM is seen without purulent drainage.

MANAGEMENT

FIRST LINE

NONPHARMACOLOGIC

Antibiotics are not necessary to treat uncomplicated AOM in an otherwise healthy child.[17,18] SOR Ⓐ

Management of OME primarily consists of watchful waiting. Most cases resolve spontaneously within 3 months; only 5% to 10% last 1 year or longer. Treatment depends on duration and associated conditions. The following options should be considered:

- Document the laterality, duration of effusion, and presence and severity of associated symptoms at each assessment of the child with OME. SOR Ⓒ
- Distinguish the child with OME who is at risk for speech, language, or learning problems from other children with OME and more promptly evaluate hearing, speech, language, and need for intervention in children at risk. SOR Ⓒ Risk factors for developmental difficulties include:
  - Permanent hearing loss independent of OME
  - Suspected or diagnosed speech and language delay or disorder
  - Autism spectrum disorder and other pervasive developmental disorders
  - Syndromes (e.g., Down) or craniofacial disorders that include cognitive, speech, and language delays
  - Blindness or uncorrectable visual impairment
  - Cleft palate with or without associated syndrome
  - Developmental delay
- Manage the child with OME who is not at risk with expectant observation for 3 months from the date of effusion onset (if known) or diagnosis (if onset is unknown). SOR Ⓐ
- Hearing test is recommended when OME persists for 3 months or longer or at any time if language delay, learning problems, or significant hearing loss is suspected in a child with OME. SOR Ⓒ
- Autoinflation with nasal balloon, in one systematic review, provided short-term benefits, although 12% of children ages 3 to 10 years were unable to use it. The balloon is held outside the nose and can be purchased from Otovent. A 2013 Cochrane review concluded that autoinflation, given its low cost and safety, should be considered while waiting for the natural resolution of OME, but further research is needed to better inform duration of treatment and long-term outcomes.[19] SOR Ⓐ

MEDICATIONS

- Monotherapy with either oral acetaminophen (paracetamol) or ibuprofen appears effective in reduction of otalgia within the first 48 hours in children with AOM, but there is insufficient evidence of

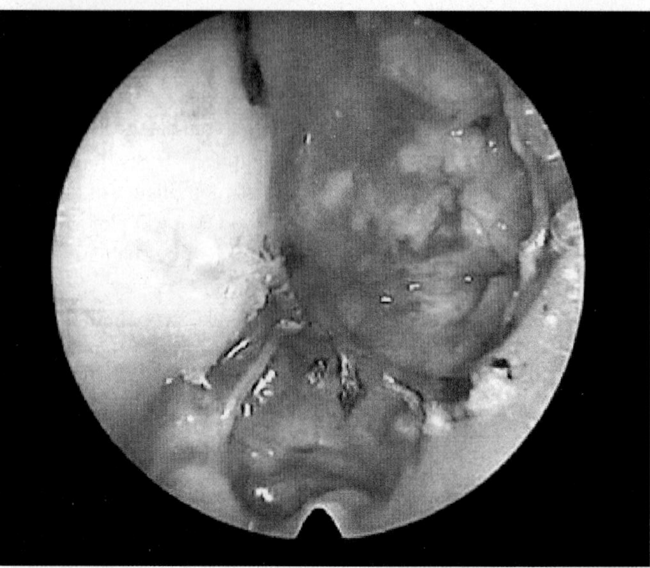

FIGURE 28-7 Cholesteatoma. (*Reproduced with permission from Vladimir Zlinsky, MD, in Roy F. Sullivan, PhD. Audiology Forum: Video Otoscopy, www.rcsullivan.com.*)

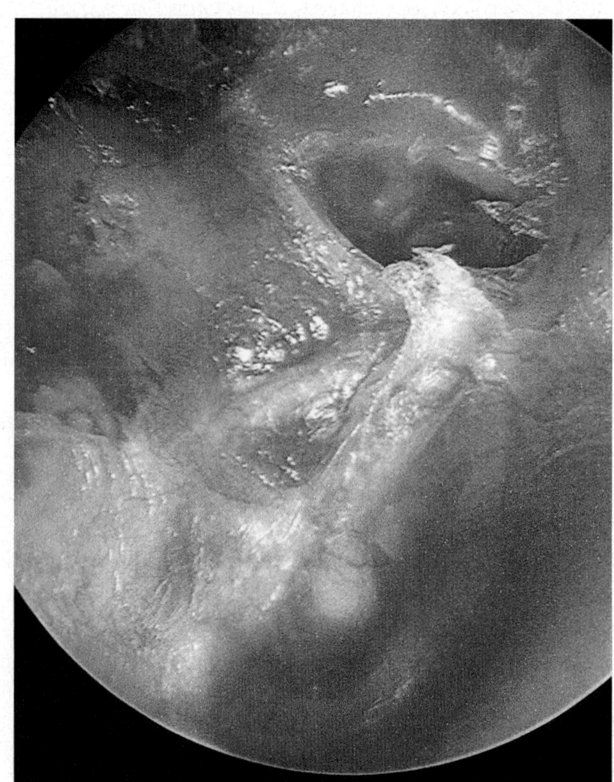

FIGURE 28-8 Primary acquired cholesteatoma with debris removed from the attic retraction pocket. (*Reproduced with permission from William Clark, MD.*)

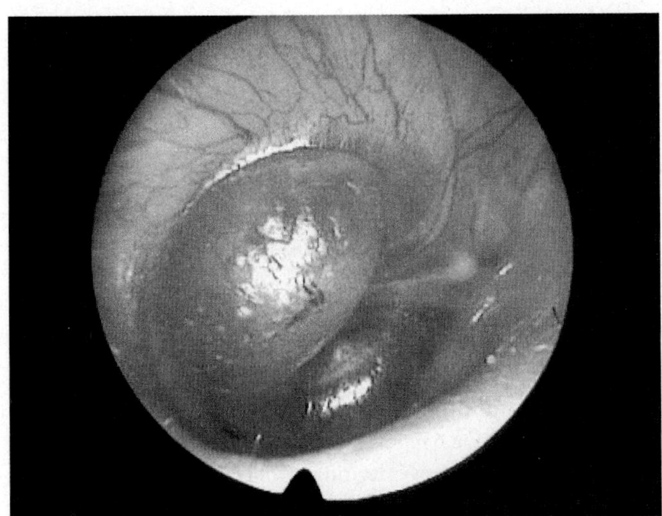

FIGURE 28-9 Bullous myringitis can be differentiated from otitis media with effusion by identifying a serous-filled bulla on the surface of the tympanic membrane. (*Reproduced with permission from Vladimir Zlinsky, MD, in Roy F. Sullivan, PhD. Audiology Forum: Video Otoscopy, www.rcsullivan.com.*)

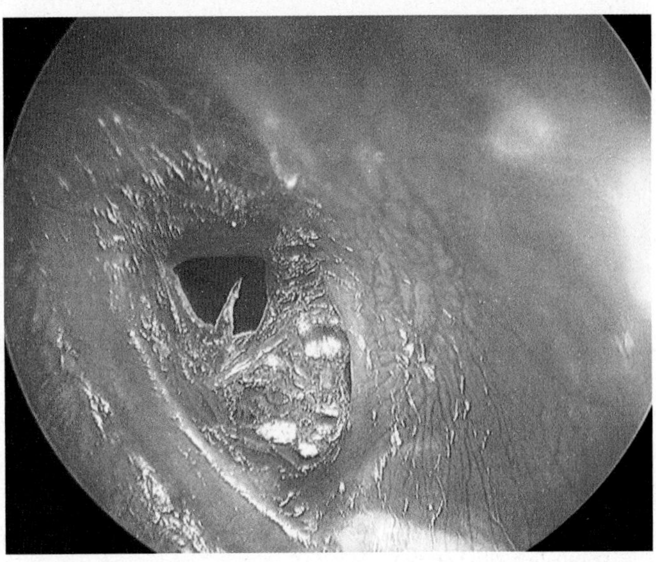

FIGURE 28-11 Traumatic perforation of the left tympanic membrane. (*Reproduced with permission from William Clark, MD.*)

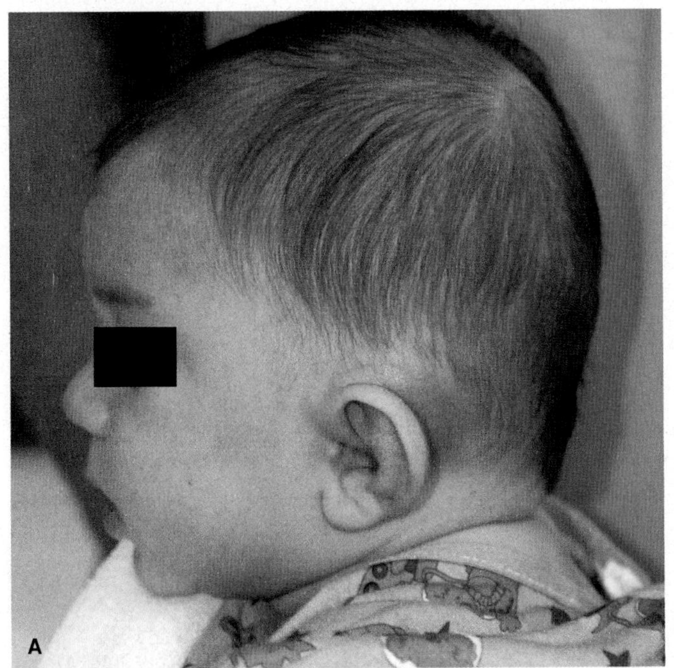

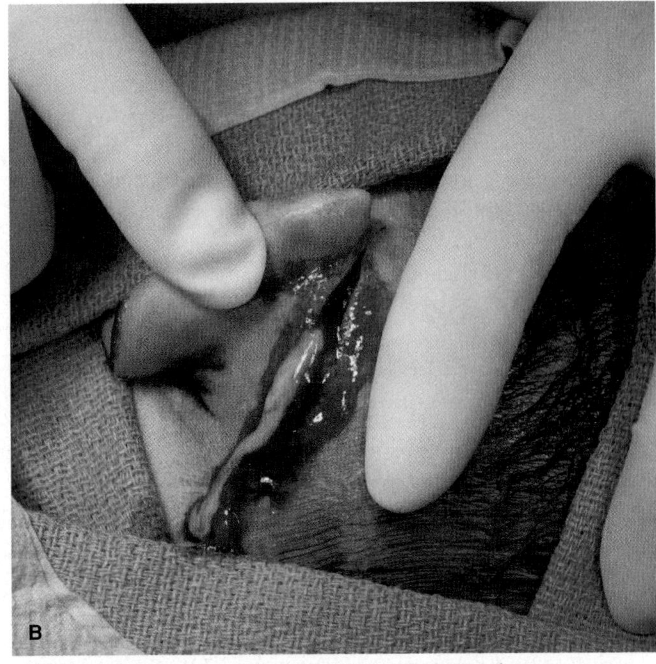

FIGURE 28-10 **A.** Mastoiditis in a young boy with recurrent otitis media. Note the erythema and swelling behind the ear. The ear is sticking out more than the other side. **B.** Surgical drainage was performed under general anesthesia. (*Reproduced with permission from William Clark, MD.*)

the superiority of one medication over the other. Furthermore, there is insufficient evidence that combined therapy is superior to monotherapy.[20] SOR Ⓐ

SECOND LINE

MEDICATIONS

- Antibiotics seem to be most beneficial in children younger than 2 years of age with bilateral AOM (number needed to treat [NNT] 4), or in children with both AOM and otorrhea (NNT 3). Among healthy children with mild disease in developed nations, expectant management is a reasonable approach. SOR Ⓐ
- Antibiotics may reduce symptoms of AOM but increase the risk of adverse effects. SOR Ⓐ
    - Antibiotics appear to reduce pain at 2 to 3 days (NNT 20) and at 4 to 7 days (NNT 16), but increase risk of adverse effects such as diarrhea, vomiting, and rash (number needed to harm [NNH] 14) compared with placebo.[13]
    - In comparison to placebo, antibiotics modestly decrease TM perforations (NNT 33) and development of contralateral AOM (NNT 11).[18] Antibiotics do not, however, decrease abnormal tympanometry findings at 3 months or decrease late AOM recurrences.
    - In high-income settings, immediate antibiotic treatment (i.e., given at initial consultation) does not appear to be therapeutically better than expectant management for pain reduction at 3 to 7 days or at 11 to 14 days, tympanometric abnormalities at 4 weeks, tympanic perforations, and AOM recurrences. More importantly, no serious complications occurred in children managed expectantly and in those treated with immediate antibiotics.
    - Antibiotics effective in treating AOM include amoxicillin, amoxicillin/clavulanic acid, ampicillin, penicillin, erythromycin, azithromycin, trimethoprim-sulfamethoxazole, and cephalosporins. Although data are limited, amoxicillin may be more effective than macrolide antibiotics and cephalosporins and is a good initial choice, given that its low cost and variety of flavors and formulations make it appealing to children and parents.
    - Once- or twice-daily amoxicillin, alone or in combination with clavulanate, appears comparable with three times daily dosing in children with AOM.[21]
    - Except for ceftriaxone and azithromycin, short courses of antibiotics (less than 7 days) have higher 1-month treatment failure (NNH 33) compared to longer courses (7 days or longer). However, this needs to be balanced against higher gastrointestinal adverse events associated with longer treatment courses.[22]
    - If watchful waiting is chosen as the initial approach for a healthy child with AOM, no antibiotic prescription compared to delayed prescription (i.e., handing a prescription with instructions to delay initiation unless the child worsens) appears to result in the lowest rate of antibiotic usage and has similar parental satisfaction and clinical outcomes.[23]
- Authors of a 2006 Cochrane review found limited evidence for efficacy of analgesic ear drops 30 minutes after application in children 3 years and older with AOM.[24] SOR Ⓐ
- Antihistamines and decongestants should not be used for OME.[8] SOR Ⓐ
- Antimicrobials and corticosteroids (systemic or intranasal) are not recommended for OME. SOR Ⓐ

COMPLEMENTARY AND ALTERNATIVE THERAPY

- There is conflicting evidence that zinc supplementation reduces the occurrence of AOM in healthy children younger than 5 years living in developing countries.[25] SOR Ⓑ

REFERRAL

- Refer to specialist (otolaryngologist, audiologist, or speech-language pathologist) if: SOR Ⓒ
    - Persistent fluid for 4 or more months with persistent hearing loss.
    - Associated speech delay.
    - Structural abnormalities of TM or middle ear.
- Tympanostomy tubes for children with recurrent AOM (3 or more episodes of AOM in 6 months, or 4 or more AOM episodes in 1 year) modestly improves hearing in the first 6 months after insertion, but efficacy drops beyond 9 months and is comparable to the natural history of the disease in children not receiving tympanostomy tubes. Because long-term effectiveness is uncertain, clinicians should consider possible adverse effects (e.g., tympanosclerosis in one third of children; **Figures 28-12** and **28-13**) before surgery is undertaken.[26] SOR Ⓐ
- Prompt insertion of tympanostomy tubes in healthy children under 3 years of age with persistent MEE does not improve cognitive development, language acquisition, or speech development up to 9 to 11 years of age compared with waiting 6 to 9 months for the effusion to resolve before placing the tubes.[27] Moreover, delayed insertion of tubes helps children avoid getting tubes altogether.[27] SOR Ⓐ
- When a child under 4 years becomes a surgical candidate, tympanostomy tube insertion is the preferred initial procedure. For children 4 years and older, tympanostomy tubes, adenoidectomy, or both should be considered. SOR Ⓑ

PREVENTION

- The currently licensed PCV7 administered during infancy has modest beneficial effects for the prevention of AOM in low-risk infants. However, in high-risk infants, PCV7 given in early infancy and in older children with prior AOM does not decrease the incidence of AOM. Rigorous systematic reviews of newer trials of recently licensed, multivalent pneumococcal vaccines for the prevention of AOM are still unavailable.[28] SOR Ⓐ
- Influenza vaccination in infants and children under the age of 6 years modestly decreases the incidence of AOM and the use of antibiotics, but there are limited data on safety.[29] SOR Ⓐ

PROGNOSIS

- Without antibiotics, AOM resolves within 24 hours in approximately 60% of children and within 3 days in approximately 80% of children. Rate of suppurative complications if antibiotics are withheld is 0.13%.[30]
- Most cases of OME resolve spontaneously within 3 months; only 5% to 10% last 1 year or longer. However, effusion will recur in 30% to 40% of patients.

FOLLOW-UP

- If a patient with AOM fails to respond to the initial management option within 48 to 72 hours, the clinician should reassess the patient to confirm AOM and exclude other causes of illness. If AOM is confirmed in a patient initially managed with observation, the clinician should begin antibiotics. If the patient was initially managed with antibiotics, the clinician should change antibiotics. SOR B
- Potentially serious complications of AOM, such as mastoiditis or facial nerve involvement, require urgent referral.
- There is no consensus in the medical community regarding timing of posttreatment follow-up of AOM or who should be receiving follow-up. There is some evidence that parents can be reliable predictors in the resolution or persistence of AOM.[31]
- Low-risk children with persistent OME should be reexamined at 3- to 6-month intervals until MEE has resolved or when significant hearing loss or structural abnormalities of the TM or middle ear cavity are diagnosed or suspected. SOR C

PATIENT EDUCATION

- Patient education should focus on identification, prevention, and control of risk factors (see above).
- Parents should be made aware of the high rates of spontaneous resolution of AOM and potential adverse effects of antibiotics.
- Patients should be informed that the natural history of OME is spontaneous resolution.
  - Periodic follow-up to monitor resolution of MEE is important.
  - If MEE is persistent and signs and symptoms of hearing loss, language difficulties, and learning problems arise, additional treatment may be considered.

PATIENT RESOURCES

AOM

- **http://www.nlm.nih.gov/medlineplus/ency/article/000638.htm.**
- **https://www.nidcd.nih.gov/health/ear-infections-children.**
- **https://familydoctor.org/condition/ear-infection.**
- **http://kidshealth.org/en/kids/ear-infection.html.**
- **http://www.nhs.uk/conditions/Otitis-media/Pages/Introduction.aspx.**

OME

- **https://familydoctor.org/condition/otitis-media-with-effusion.**
- **https://medlineplus.gov/ency/article/007010.htm.**

PROVIDER RESOURCES

AOM

- The diagnosis and management of acute otitis media. *Pediatrics.* 2013;131(3):e964-e999.
- **www.gpnotebook.co.uk (otitis media).**
- **http://www.gpnotebook.co.uk/simplepage.cfm?ID=1928234161.**

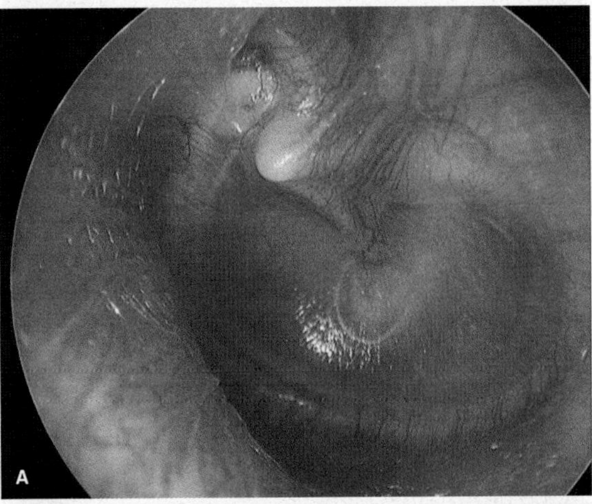

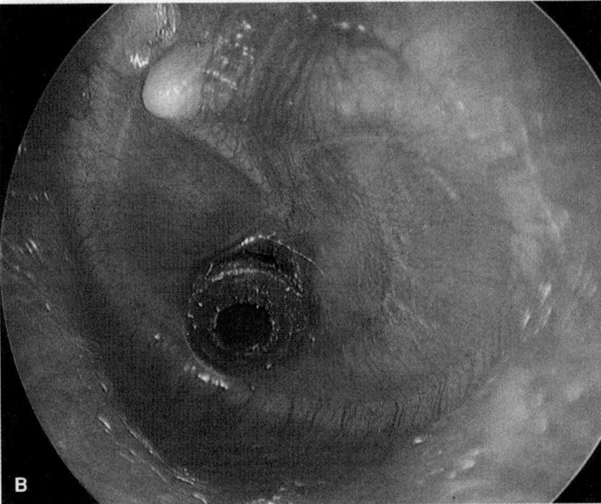

FIGURE 28-12 A. Left tympanic membrane™ of a 9-year-old girl with recurrent acute otitis media and chronic TM retractions prior to polyethylene (PE) tube placement. The circular area near the center of the TM is caused by the TM being retracted against the promontory of the medial wall of the middle ear. B. A fluoroplastic PE tube is placed in the anterior-inferior quadrant of the TM of a 9-year-old girl with recurrent acute otitis media. It is black because it is impregnated with silver oxide to retard the growth of bacterial microfilms. (*Reproduced with permission from William Clark, MD.*)

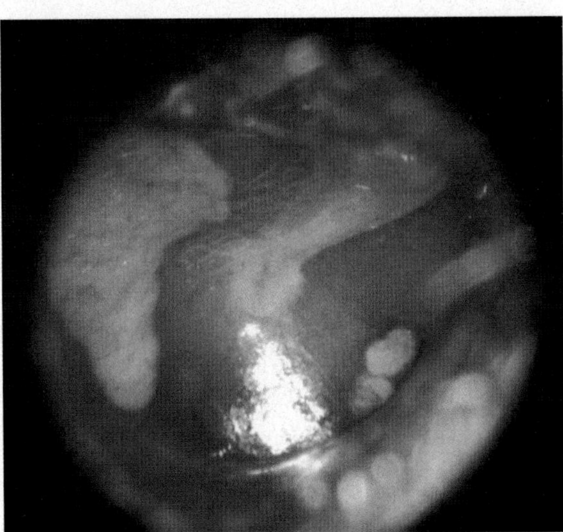

FIGURE 28-13 Tympanosclerosis as the result of previous recurrent episodes of otitis media and polyethylene (PE) tube placement. (*Reproduced with permission from Glen Medellin, MD.*)

OME

- Clinical Practice Guideline: Otitis Media with Effusion (Update). *Otolaryngol Head Neck Surg.* 2016;154(1 Suppl):S1-S41.

REFERENCES

1. Bondy J, Berman S, Glazner J, Lezotte D. Direct expenditures related to otitis media diagnoses: extrapolations from a pediatric Medicaid cohort. *Pediatrics.* 2000;105(6):E72.
2. RAND Corporation. *Quality of Care for Children and Adolescents: A Review of Selected Clinical Conditions and Quality Indicators.* http://www.rand.org/pubs/monograph_reports/MR1283.html. Accessed March 2017.
3. Teele DW, Klein JO, Rosner BA. Epidemiology of otitis media during the first seven years of life in children in greater Boston: a prospective, cohort study. *J Infect Dis.* 1989;160(1):83-94.
4. Paradise JL, Rockette HE, Colborn DK, et al. Otitis media in 2253 Pittsburgh-area infants: prevalence and risk factors during the first two years of life. *Pediatrics.* 1997;99(3):318-333.
5. Del Mar C, Glasziou P, Hayem M. Are antibiotics indicated as initial treatment for children with acute otitis media? A meta-analysis. *BMJ.* 1997;314:1526-1529.
6. Nyquist AC, Gonzales R, Steiner JF, Sande MA. Antibiotic prescribing for children with colds, upper respiratory tract infections, and bronchitis. *JAMA.* 1998;279:875.
7. Venekamp RP, Damoiseaux RA, Schilder AG. Acute otitis media in children. *Am Fam Physician.* 2017;95(2):109-110.
8. Rosenfeld RM, Shin JJ, Schwartz SR, et al. Clinical practice guideline: otitis media with effusion (update). *Otolaryngol Head Neck Surg.* 2016;154(1 Suppl):S1-S41.
9. Rovers MM, Schilder AG, Zielhuis GA, Rosenfeld RM. Otitis media. *Lancet.* 2004;363:465.
10. Casey JR, Adlowitz DG, Pichichero ME. New patterns in the otopathogens causing acute otitis media six to eight years after introduction of pneumococcal conjugate vaccine. *Pediatr Infect Dis J.* 2010;29(4):304-309.
11. McEllistrem MC. Acute otitis media due to penicillin-nonsusceptible *Streptococcus pneumoniae* before and after the introduction of the pneumococcal conjugate vaccine. *Clin Infect Dis.* 2005; 40(12):1738-1744.
12. Ruuskanen O, Arola M, Heikkinen T, Ziegler T. Viruses in acute otitis media: increasing evidence for clinical significance. *Pediatr Infect Dis J.* 1991;10:425-427.
13. Froom J, Culpepper L, Jacobs M, et al. Antimicrobials for acute otitis media? A review from the International Primary Care Network. *BMJ.* 1997;315:98-102.
14. Williamson I. Otitis media with effusion in children. *Clin Evid.* 2011;01:502-531.
15. Lieberthal AS, Carroll AE, Chonmaitree T, et al. The diagnosis and management of acute otitis media. *Pediatrics.* 2013;131(3):e964-e999.
16. Takata GS, Chan LS, Morphew T, et al. Evidence assessment of the accuracy of methods of diagnosing middle ear effusion in children with otitis media with effusion. *Pediatrics.* 2003;112: 1379-1387.
17. Gamboa S, Park MK, Wanserski G, Lo V. Clinical inquiries. Should you use antibiotics to treat acute otitis media in children? *J Fam Pract.* 2009;58(11):602-604.
18. Venekamp RP, Sanders SL, Glasziou PP, et al. Antibiotics for acute otitis media in children. *Cochrane Database Syst Rev.* 2015;(6): CD000219.
19. Perera R, Glasziou PP, Heneghan CJ, et al. Autoinflation for hearing loss associated with otitis media with effusion. *Cochrane Database Syst Rev.* 2013;(5):CD006285.
20. Sjoukes A, Venekamp RP, van de Pol AC, et al. Paracetamol (acetaminophen) or non-steroidal anti-inflammatory drugs, alone or combined, for pain relief in acute otitis media in children. *Cochrane Database Syst Rev.* 2016;(12):CD011534.
21. Thanaviratananich S, Laopaiboon M, Vatanasapt P. Once or twice daily versus three times daily amoxicillin with or without clavulanate for the treatment of acute otitis media. *Cochrane Database Syst Rev.* 2013;(12):CD004975.
22. Kozyrskyj A, Klassen TP, Moffatt M, Harvey K. Short-course antibiotics for acute otitis media. *Cochrane Database Syst Rev.* 2010;(9): CD001095.
23. Spurling GK, Del Mar CB, Dooley L, et al. Delayed antibiotics for respiratory infections. *Cochrane Database Syst Rev.* 2013;(4):CD004417.
24. Foxlee R, Johansson A, Wejfalk J, et al. Topical analgesia for acute otitis media. *Cochrane Database Syst Rev.* 2006;(3):CD005657.
25. Gulani A, Sachdev HS. Zinc supplements for preventing otitis media. *Cochrane Database Syst Rev.* 2014;(6):CD006639.
26. Lau L, Mick P, Nunez DA. Grommets (ventilation tubes) for hearing loss associated with otitis media with effusion in children. *Cochrane Database Syst Rev.* 2018;(4):CD004741.
27. Paradise JL, Feldman HM, Campbell TF, et al. Tympanostomy tubes and developmental outcomes at 9 to 11 years of age. *N Engl J Med.* 2007;356:300-302.
28. Fortanier AC, Venekamp RP, Boonacker CW, et al. Pneumococcal conjugate vaccines for preventing otitis media. *Cochrane Database Syst Rev.* 2014;(4):CD001480.
29. Norhayati MN, Ho JJ, Azman MY. Influenza vaccines for preventing acute otitis media in infants and children. *Cochrane Database Syst Rev.* 2015;(3):CD010089.
30. Rosenfeld RM. Natural history of untreated otitis media. *Laryngoscope.* 2003;113:1645-1657.
31. Hathaway TJ, Katz HP, Dershewitz RA, Marx TJ. Acute otitis media: who needs posttreatment follow-up? *Pediatrics.* 1994;94(2 Pt 1): 143-147.

29 ACUTE OTITIS EXTERNA

Brian Z. Rayala, MD

PATIENT STORY

A 40-year-old woman with type 2 diabetes presents to her family physician with a 2-day history of bilateral otalgia, otorrhea, and hearing loss. Symptoms started in the right ear and then rapidly spread to the left ear. She had a low-grade fever and was systemically ill. The external ear was swollen with honey-crusts (**Figures 29-1** and **29-2**). The external auditory canal (EAC) was narrowed and contained purulent discharge (**Figure 29-3**). Ear, nose, and throat (ENT) was consulted, and she was admitted to the hospital for the presumptive diagnosis of malignant otitis externa. The MRI showed some destruction of the temporal bone. She was started on IV ciprofloxacin, and the ear culture grew out *Pseudomonas aeruginosa* sensitive to ciprofloxacin. The patient responded well to treatment and went home on oral ciprofloxacin 5 days later.

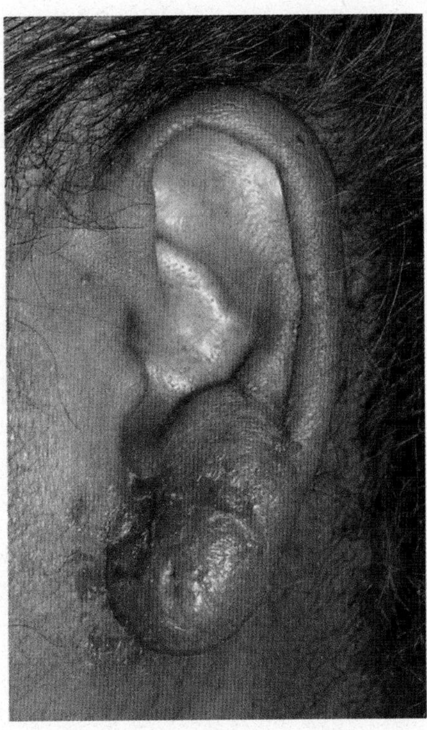

FIGURE 29-1 Malignant/necrotizing otitis externa in a 40-year-old woman with diabetes. Note the swelling and honey-crusts of the pinna. The external auditory canal and temporal bone were involved. *(Reproduced with permission from E.J. Mayeaux, MD.)*

INTRODUCTION

Acute otitis externa (AOE) is among the most common clinical conditions presenting as acute ear pain in the primary care setting. AOE is defined as acute inflammation, often with infection, of the EAC.[1]

SYNONYMS

Swimmer's ear.

EPIDEMIOLOGY

- Incidence of AOE is not known precisely; its lifetime incidence was estimated at 10% in one study.[2]
- Occurs more in adults than in children.

ETIOLOGY AND PATHOPHYSIOLOGY

- Common pathogens, which are part of normal EAC flora, include aerobic organisms predominantly (*P. aeruginosa* and *Staphylococcus aureus*) and, to a lesser extent, anaerobes (*Bacteroides* and *Peptostreptococcus*). Up to a third of infections are polymicrobial. A small proportion (<10%) of AOE is caused by fungal pathogens (e.g., *Aspergillus* and *Candida* species). Fungal AOE is associated with prior antibiotic use and seen frequently in humid environments (i.e., tropical and subtropical settings).[1]
- Pathogenesis of AOE includes the following:
  - Trauma, the usual inciting event, leads to breach in the integrity of EAC skin
  - Skin inflammation and edema ensue, which, in turn, leads to pruritus and obstruction of adnexal structures (e.g., cerumen glands, sebaceous glands, and hair follicles)

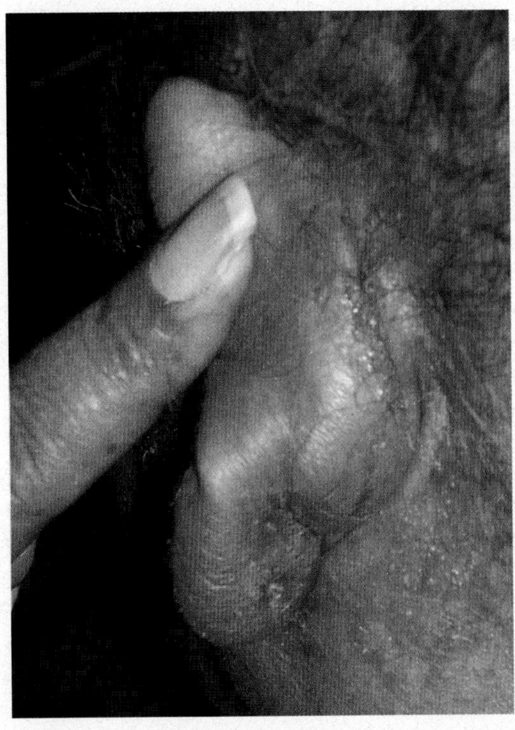

FIGURE 29-2 Another view of the malignant/necrotizing otitis externa. *(Reproduced with permission from E.J. Mayeaux, MD.)*

- Pruritus leads to scratching, which results in further skin injury
- Consequently, the milieu of the EAC is altered (i.e., change in quality and quantity of cerumen, increase in pH of EAC, and dysfunctional epithelial migration)
- Finally, the EAC becomes a warm, alkaline, and moist environment—ideal for growth of different pathogens

RISK FACTORS[3]

- Environmental factors:
  - Moisture—Macerates skin of EAC, elevates pH, and removes protective cerumen layer (from swimming, perspiration, high humidity)
  - Trauma—Leads to injury of EAC skin (from cotton buds, finger-nails, hearing aids, ear plugs, paper clips, match sticks, mechanical removal of cerumen)
  - High environmental temperatures
- Host factors:
  - Anatomical—Wax and debris accumulate and lead to moisture retention (e.g., a narrow or hairy ear canal)
  - Cerumen—Absence or overproduction of cerumen (leads to loss of the protective layer and moisture retention, respectively)
  - Chronic dermatologic disease (e.g., atopic dermatitis, psoriasis, seborrheic dermatitis)
  - Immunocompromise (e.g., chemotherapy, HIV, AIDS)

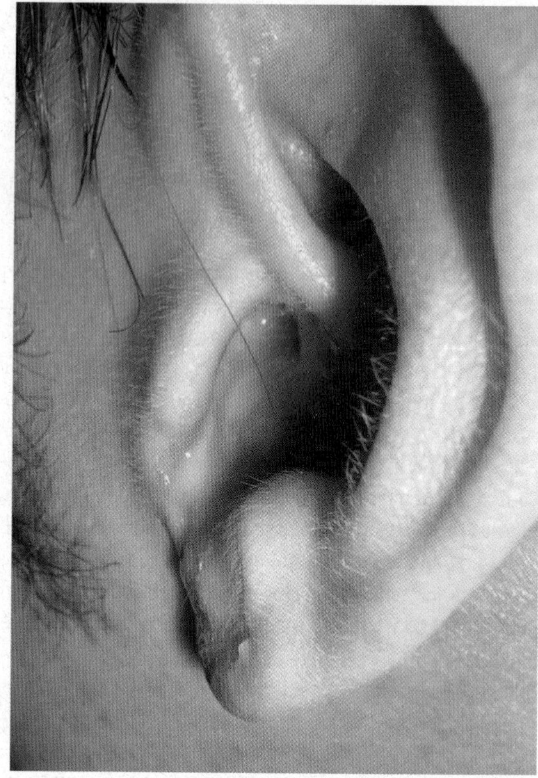

FIGURE 29-3 Chronic suppurative otitis media with purulent discharge chronically draining from the ear of this 25-year-old man. This image could be seen in acute otitis media with perforation of the tympanic membrane or in a purulent otitis externa. *(Reproduced with permission from Richard P. Usatine, MD.)*

DIAGNOSIS

CLINICAL FEATURES

- AOE can either be localized, like a furuncle, or generalized (**Figure 29-4**). The latter is known as "diffuse AOE," or simply AOE. Seborrheic dermatitis of the external ear and EAC can be diffuse or generalized (see **Figure 29-4**).
- Forms of (diffuse) OE:
  - Acute (<6 weeks; **Figures 29-5** and **29-6**).
  - Chronic (>3 months)—May cause hearing loss and stenosis of the EAC (**Figure 29-7**).
  - Necrotizing or malignant form—Defined by destruction of the temporal bone, usually in patients with diabetes or who are otherwise immunocompromised; often life-threatening (see **Figure 29-1**).
- Elements of diagnosis of diffuse AOE include[4]:
  - Rapid onset (within 48 hours) in the past 3 weeks, AND
  - Symptoms of EAC inflammation, including otalgia, itching, or fullness, with or without loss of hearing or jaw pain, AND
  - Signs of EAC inflammation, including tenderness of tragus or pinna, with or without otorrhea (see **Figure 29-3**), regional lymphadenitis, tympanic membrane (TM) erythema, or cellulitis of pinna and adjacent skin.
- Establishing the integrity of the TM (through direct visualization) and the absence of middle-ear effusion (through pneumatic otoscopy) is crucial in differentiating AOE from other diagnoses (e.g., suppurative otitis media, cholesteatoma).

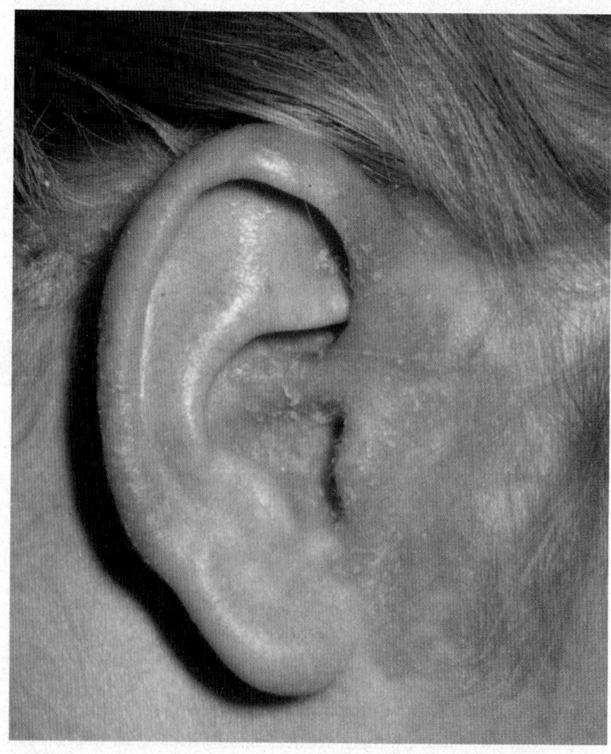

FIGURE 29-4 Seborrheic dermatitis causing erythema and greasy scale of the external ear and ear canal. The seborrheic dermatitis itself causes breaks in the skin, and the coexisting pruritus may lead the patient to damage their own ear canal. All this can become secondarily infected. *(Reproduced with permission from Eric Kraus, MD.)*

LABORATORY AND IMAGING

- Because AOE is mostly a clinical diagnosis, diagnostic testing has a limited role. When a patient fails to respond to empiric treatment, obtaining a culture of aural discharge may help guide proper choice of treatment (antibacterial vs. antifungal agents).
- If necrotizing or malignant AOE is suspected, CT or MRI of the ear/skull base is warranted.

DIFFERENTIAL DIAGNOSIS

- Chronic suppurative otitis media—Otoscopy shows TM perforation; history reveals a chronically draining ear and recurrent middle-ear infections with or without hearing loss (see **Figure 29-3**).
- Seborrheic dermatitis involving the external ear and EAC can lead to inflammation and breaks in the skin (see **Figure 29-4**). The coexisting pruritus may lead the patient to damage their own ear canal. This can all become secondarily infected and become an infected AOE.
- Acute otitis media with perforated TM—Presents with purulent drainage from the canal in the setting of ear pain and clinical signs or symptoms of acute illness such as fever. If the TM is visible, it will be red with a perforation; see Chapter 28, Otitis Media: Acute Otitis and Otitis Media with Effusion.
- Foreign body in the EAC—Otoscopy, with or without aural toilet, confirms presence of foreign body (that incites an inflammatory response, leading to otalgia and otorrhea); see Chapter 30, Ear: Foreign Body.
- Otomycosis—Pruritus is generally more prominent and EAC inflammation (otalgia and otorrhea) is less pronounced; fungal organisms have a characteristic appearance in the EAC.
- Contact dermatitis—Usually caused by ototopical agents (e.g., neomycin, benzocaine, propylene glycol); seen in patients with poor response to empiric AOE treatment; prominent clinical features include pruritus, erythema of conchal bowl, crusting, and excoriations.

FIGURE 29-5 Acute otitis externa showing purulent discharge and narrowing of the ear canal. (*Reproduced with permission from Roy F. Sullivan, PhD. Audiology Forum: Video Otoscopy, www.rcsullivan.com.*)

MANAGEMENT

FIRST LINE

MEDICATIONS

- The management of AOE should include an assessment of pain. The clinician should recommend analgesic treatment based on the severity of pain.[4] SOR B
- Treat uncomplicated AOE using topical treatments instead of systemic therapies. Additional oral antibiotics are not required.[3] SOR B
- There is very limited evidence to support the use of steroid-only drops.[3] SOR B
- Meta-analyses of topical treatments show comparable efficacy of various therapies, hence choice of topical therapy may be dictated by other factors including ototoxicity, contact sensitivity, availability, cost, dosing schedule, and possibility of developing antibiotic resistance.[3] SOR B
  - Evidence from one trial of low quality found no difference in clinical efficacy between quinolone and nonquinolone drops. Quinolones are more expensive than nonquinolones[3] SOR B

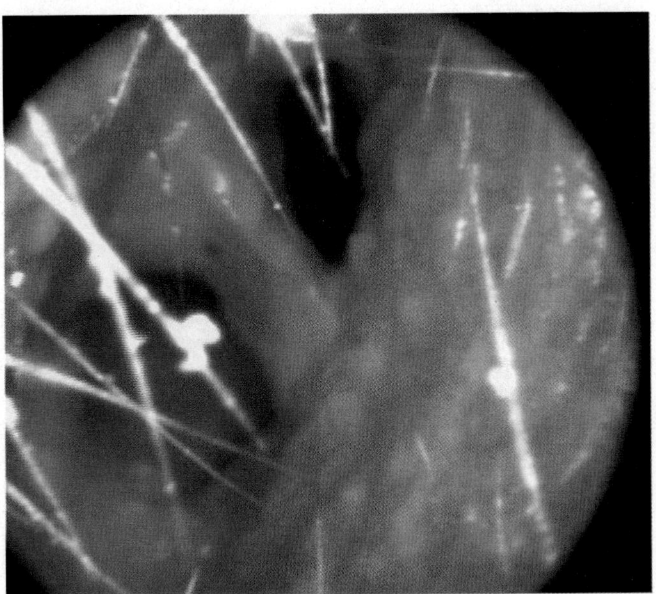

FIGURE 29-6 Acute otitis externa in an older man who wears a hearing aid. Note the viscous purulent discharge and narrowing of the ear canal. (*Reproduced with permission from Roy F. Sullivan, PhD. Audiology Forum: Video Otoscopy, www.rcsullivan.com.*)

- There is some evidence indicating that patients treated with topical preparations containing antibiotics and steroids benefit from reduced swelling, redness, otorrhea, and use of pain medications compared to preparations without steroids. There is a suggestion that high-potency steroids may be more effective than low-potency steroids (in terms of severe pain, inflammation, and swelling)[3] SOR B
- Current options for topical preparations for AOE include:
  - Ciprofloxacin/dexamethasone otic—note that this has a high-potency steroid and a quinolone
  - Ciprofloxacin/hydrocortisone otic—note that this has a low-potency steroid
  - Ofloxacin otic—another quinolone but without the steroid
  - Neomycin/polymyxin B/hydrocortisone otic—avoid this if there is a perforated tympanic membrane because of the aminoglycoside neomycin
  - Avoid the use of aminoglycosides containing ophthalmic solutions for the ear
  - Acetic acid otic—within the first week, acetic acid appears comparable to antibiotic/steroid ear drops. But beyond 1 week, acetic acid appears inferior to antibiotic/steroid solution[3] SOR B

- The standard advice of using topical treatment for 7 to 10 days may lead to incomplete treatment for some and overtreatment for others. Better advice is to use ear drops for at least 1 week and extend treatment for a few days beyond complete resolution of symptoms, but no more than 2 weeks total.[3] SOR B

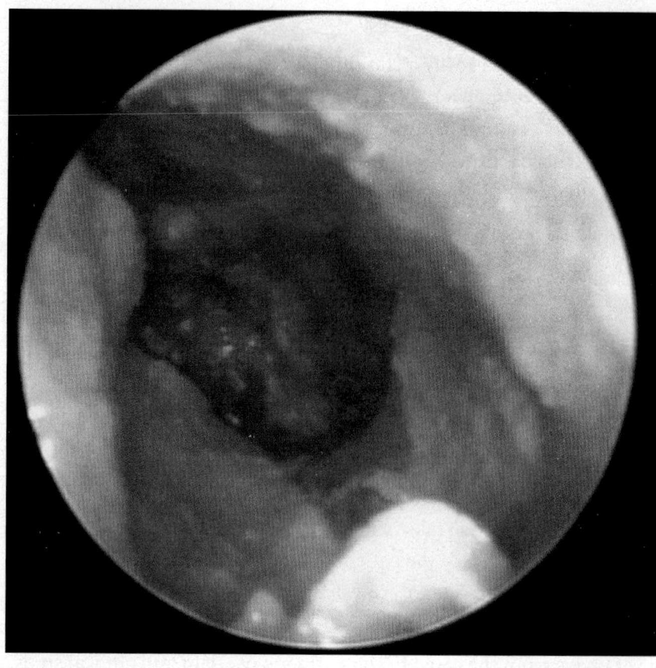

FIGURE 29-7 Chronic otitis externa in an older woman who wears a hearing aid. The ear canal is not narrowed but is coated with a purulent discharge. (*Reproduced with permission from Roy F. Sullivan, PhD. Audiology Forum: Video Otoscopy, www.rcsullivan.com.*)

SECOND LINE

NONPHARMACOLOGIC

- The effectiveness of ear cleaning is unknown.[3] SOR B
- The effectiveness of specialist aural toilet (use of operating microscope to mechanically remove material from external canal) for treating OE is unknown.[1] SOR C

MEDICATIONS

- Evidence from one low-quality trial suggests a glycerin-ichthammol medicated wick may provide better pain relief in early severe AOE than a triamcinolone/gramicidin/neomycin/nystatin medicated wick.[3] SOR B
- Evidence to support use of topical antifungal agents (with or without steroids) in AOE is lacking.[3] SOR B

PREVENTION

- There is insufficient evidence to recommend preventive interventions for AOE, including topical acetic acid, topical corticosteroids, and water exclusion.[3] SOR B

PROGNOSIS

- AOE often resolves within 6 weeks but can recur.
- Symptoms typically resolve after 6 days of treatment with antibiotic/steroid drops.

FOLLOW-UP

- Lack of clinical response after 48 to 72 hours of therapy warrants reevaluation to confirm the diagnosis of AOE and to rule out other causes.[4] SOR Ⓑ
- Treatment failure should be considered if a patient remains symptomatic beyond 2 weeks of therapy. The clinician should explore alternative treatment options.[3] SOR Ⓑ

PATIENT EDUCATION

- To avoid recurrent infections[5]:
  - Recommend that patients not use cotton swabs inserted into the ear canal
  - Minimize use of soap to clean the ears since formation of an alkali residue in the EAC may neutralize the normal acidic pH of the ear canal
  - Advise against swimming in polluted waters
  - Adequately empty residual water from the ear canal after bathing and swimming. This can be done by turning the head and/or holding a facial tissue on the outside of the ear to act as a wick.
- Consider ear drops for swimmers who get frequent AOE. A combination of a 2:1 ratio of 70% isopropyl alcohol and acetic acid may be used after each episode of swimming to assist in drying and acidifying the ear canal.[5] SOR Ⓒ
- Do not use earplugs while swimming because they may irritate or injure the ear canal, leading to AOE.[5]

PATIENT RESOURCES

- **https://familydoctor.org/condition/otitis-externa-swimmers-ear.**

PROVIDER RESOURCES

- Rosenfeld RM, Schwartz SR, Cannon CR, et al. Clinical practice guideline: acute otitis externa. *Otolaryngol Head Neck Surg.* 2014;150(1 Suppl):S1-S24.
- **http://emedicine.medscape.com/article/994550-overview.**
- **http://emedicine.medscape.com/article/994550-treatment.**

REFERENCES

1. Schaefer P, Baugh RF. Acute otitis externa: an update. *Am Fam Physician.* 2012;86(11):1055-1061.
2. Raza SA, Denholm SW, Wong JC. An audit of the management of otitis externa in an ENT casualty clinic. *J Laryngol Otol.* 1995;109:130-133.
3. Kaushik V, Malik T, Saeed SR. Interventions for acute otitis externa. *Cochrane Database Syst Rev.* 2010;(1):CD004740.
4. Rosenfeld RM, Schwartz SR, Cannon CR, et al. Clinical practice guideline: acute otitis externa. *Otolaryngol Head Neck Surg.* 2014;150(1 Suppl):S1-S24.
5. Waitzman AA. *Otitis Externa Treatment & Management.* Updated July 2016. http://emedicine.medscape.com/article/994550-treatment#d10. Accessed April 2017.

30 EAR: FOREIGN BODY

Brian Z. Rayala, MD

PATIENT STORY

A 3-year-old girl is brought by her parents to an urgent care facility after a day of crying, irritability, scant otorrhea, and frequent pulling of her right ear. Otoscopy reveals an erythematous, swollen external auditory canal (EAC) where a bead is wedged (**Figure 30-1**). The patient is referred to an otolaryngologist and the bead is removed using an operating microscope for visualization.

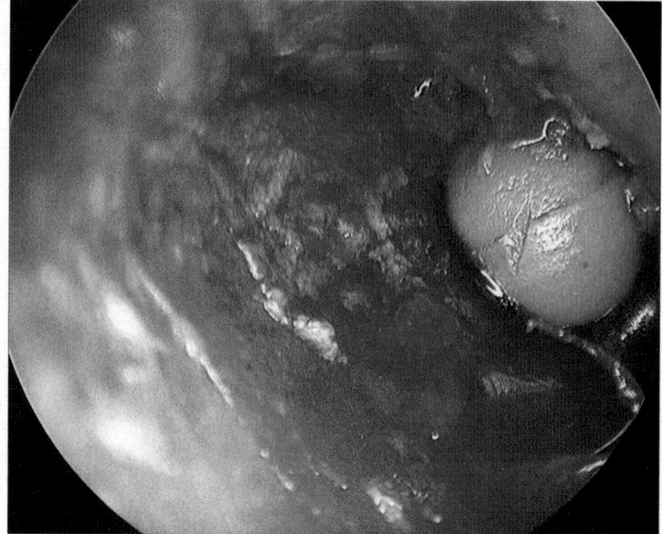

FIGURE 30-1 Foreign body (bead) in the ear canal of a 3-year-old girl with reactive tissue around it. *(Reproduced with permission from William Clark, MD.)*

INTRODUCTION

- Children with ear foreign bodies (FBs) usually present with otalgia, otorrhea, or decreased hearing. At times, symptoms may be non-specific, such as irritability and crying. Other times, the presentation is asymptomatic.

EPIDEMIOLOGY

- Ear FBs are commonly seen in children ages 1 to 6 years.[1–3]
- Equal male-to-female ratio in the pediatric population.[4]

ETIOLOGY AND PATHOPHYSIOLOGY

- Most common FBs in children include[5]:
  - Inanimate objects such as beads (see **Figure 30-1**), cotton tips, paper, toy parts, crayons (**Figure 30-2**), eraser tips, food, or organic matter, including sand (**Figure 30-3**), sticks, and stones.
  - Insects (**Figure 30-4**).
- Pathogenesis includes some of the key elements of otitis externa (see Chapter 29, Acute Otitis Externa):
  - Initial breakdown of the skin-cerumen barrier (caused by presence of FB)
  - Skin inflammation and edema leading to subsequent obstruction of adnexal structures (e.g., cerumen glands, sebaceous glands, and hair follicles)
  - FB reaction leading to further skin injury
  - In the case of alkaline battery electrochemical reaction, severe alkaline burns can occur

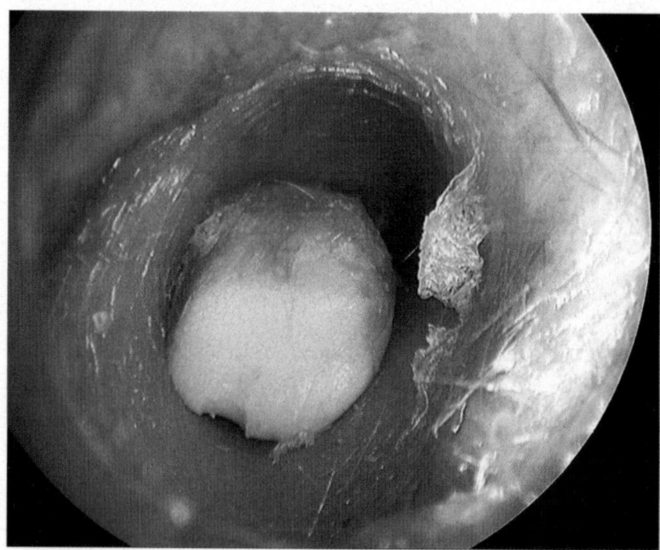

FIGURE 30-2 Piece of a crayon in the ear canal of a 4-year-old boy. *(Reproduced with permission from William Clark, MD.)*

RISK FACTORS

- Children with attention-deficit/hyperactivity disorder (ADHD) may be more likely to self-insert FBs, and ADHD should be considered in children with ear FBs who are older than age 5 years.[6]

DIAGNOSIS

CLINICAL FEATURES

- Key historical features include:
  - Otalgia
  - Otorrhea or otorrhagia
  - Mild hearing loss
  - Irritability, crying
  - History suspicious for FB insertion or witnessed FB insertion
- Some children may be asymptomatic.
- Hallmark of diagnosis includes visualization of FB on otoscopy (see **Figures 30-1** through **30-4**).
- Otoscopy may reveal signs of EAC inflammation (e.g., edema, erythema, aural discharge) (see **Figure 30-1**).

LABORATORY AND IMAGING

- Aural FB is a clinical diagnosis. Laboratory and imaging studies have very limited use.

DIFFERENTIAL DIAGNOSIS

- Otitis externa—Presents with otalgia, otorrhea, and mild hearing loss, all of which can be present in ear FB. Absence of FB on otoscopic exam is the key differentiating factor (see Chapter 29, Acute Otitis Externa).
- Acute otitis media (with or without perforated tympanic membrane [TM])—Otoscopy shows absence of FB and presence of middle-ear inflammation and effusion (i.e., bulging, erythematous, cloudy, immobile TM). Patients present with clinical signs or symptoms of acute illness like fever (see Chapter 28, Otitis Media: Acute Otitis and Otitis Media with Effusion).
- Chronic suppurative otitis media—Otoscopy shows absence of FB and presence of TM perforation; history reveals a chronically draining ear and recurrent middle-ear infections with or without hearing loss.

MANAGEMENT

PROCEDURES

- Adequate immobilization of the child (sedation if necessary) and proper instrumentation allow the uncomplicated removal of many ear FBs in the pediatric population.[7] SOR C
  - The use of general anesthesia is preferred in very young children and in children of any age with ear FBs whose contour, composition, or location predispose to traumatic removal in the ambulatory setting[7] SOR C
- Ear FBs can be removed by irrigation, suction, or instrumentation. The type of procedure depends on the type of FB being removed.
  - Small inorganic objects can be removed from the EAC by irrigation. Contraindication to irrigation includes:
    - Perforated TM
    - Vegetable matter—Irrigation causes swelling of the vegetable matter which leads to further obstruction
    - Alkaline (button) battery—Irrigation enhances leakage and potential for liquefaction necrosis and severe alkaline burns

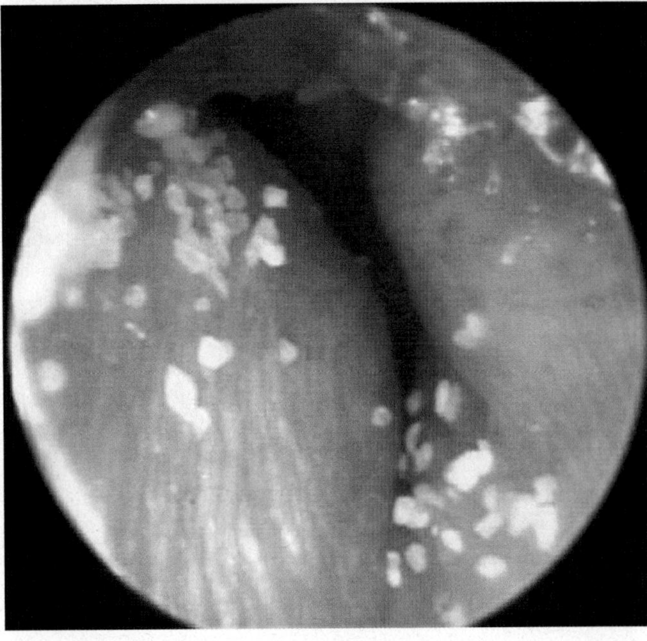

FIGURE 30-3 Beach sand granules with exostosis in the ear of a cold water surfer. The exostoses are common in cold water swimmers and surfers. (*Reproduced with permission from Roy F. Sullivan, PhD. Audiology Forum: Video Otoscopy, www.rcsullivan.com.*)

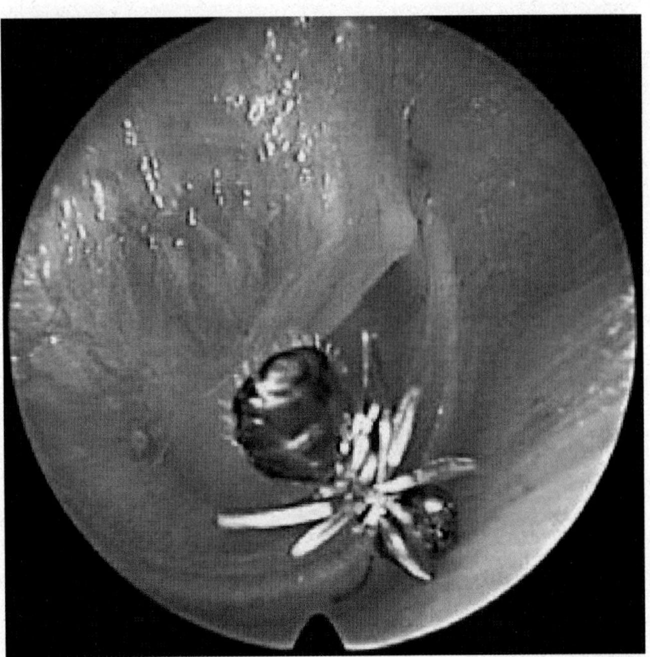

FIGURE 30-4 Ant in the ear canal. (*Reproduced with permission from Vladimir Zlinsky, MD in Roy F. Sullivan, PhD. Audiology Forum: Video Otoscopy, www.rcsullivan.com.*)

- Objects with protruding surfaces or irregular edges may be removed with alligator forceps under direct visualization
- Objects that are round or breakable can be removed using a wire loop, a curette, or a right-angle hook that is slowly advanced beyond the object and carefully withdrawn
- Cyanoacrylate adhesive (e.g., "superglue") has been used to remove tightly wedged, smooth, round FBs
- Live insects should be killed before removing them (by irrigation or forceps). Instilling alcohol or mineral oil into the auditory canal can kill them

REFERRAL

Referral to otolaryngology should be considered if:

- More than one attempt has been carried out without success.[8]
- More than one instrument is needed for removal.[7]
- Patients have firm, rounded FBs (see **Figure 30-1**).[9]
- Patients have FBs with smooth, nongraspable surfaces (see **Figure 30-1**).[10]

PREVENTION

- Efforts should focus on preventing small children from having access to tiny objects (e.g., beads, small toys).

PROGNOSIS

- Several retrospective studies from urban emergency departments showed that emergency physicians successfully removed most FBs (53% to 80%) with minimal complications and no need for operative removal.[7–10]

FOLLOW-UP

- Follow-up is very important, especially in cases where EAC inflammation or infection is likely (e.g., numerous attempts, use of numerous instruments, protracted exposure to the FB).

PATIENT EDUCATION

- Parents should be informed that successful removal depends a great deal on the length of time the FB has remained in the EAC.

PATIENT RESOURCES

- **http://www.emedicinehealth.com/foreign_body_ear/article_em.htm.**
- **http://www.webmd.com/pain-management/tc/objects-in-the-ear-topic-overview.**

PROVIDER RESOURCES

- **http://www.entusa.com/external_ear_canal.htm.**
- **https://medlineplus.gov/ency/article/000052.htm.**
- **http://emedicine.medscape.com/article/763712-overview.**

REFERENCES

1. Balbani AP, Sanchez TG, Butugan O, et al. Ear and nose foreign body removal in children. *Int J Pediatr Otorhinolaryngol.* 1998; 46:37-42.
2. Mishra A, Shukla GK, Bhatia N. Aural foreign bodies. *Indian J Pediatr.* 2000;67:267-269.
3. Ansley JF, Cunningham MJ. Treatment of aural foreign bodies in children. *Pediatrics.* 1998;101:638-641.
4. Baker MD. Foreign bodies of the ears and nose in childhood. *Pediatr Emerg Care.* 1987;3:67-70.
5. Ryan C, Ghosh A, Wilson-Boyd B, et al. Presentation and management of aural foreign bodies in two Australian emergency departments. *Emerg Med Australas.* 2006;18:372-378.
6. Perera H, Fernando SM, Yasawardena AD, et al. Prevalence of attention deficit hyperactivity disorder (ADHD) in children presenting with self-inserted nasal and aural foreign bodies. *Int J Pediatr Otorhinolaryngol.* 2009;73(10):1362-1364.
7. Ansley JF, Cunningham MJ. Response to O'Donovan. Glue ear and foreign body. *Pediatrics.* 1999;103(4):857.
8. Marin JR, Trainor JL. Foreign body removal from the external auditory canal in a pediatric emergency department. *Pediatr Emerg Care.* 2006;22:630-634.
9. Thompson SK, Wein RO, Dutcher PO. External auditory canal foreign body removal: management practices and outcomes. *Laryngoscope.* 2003;113:1912-1915.
10. DiMuzio J Jr, Deschler DG. Emergency department management of foreign bodies of the external ear canal in children. *Otol Neurotol.* 2002;23:473-475.

31 CHONDRODERMATITIS NODULARIS HELICIS AND PREAURICULAR TAGS

Linda Speer, MD

PATIENT STORY

A 44-year-old white man presents with a painful nodule on his right ear for 1 year (**Figure 31-1**). He has a long history of occupational sun exposure but no skin cancers. He states that it is too painful to sleep on his right side because of the ear nodule. He tried to remove it once with nail clippers but it bled too much. The patient is told that this is likely a benign condition called chondrodermatitis nodularis helicis. A shave biopsy/removal is performed for diagnostic and therapeutic purposes. It is explained to the patient that this could be a skin cancer because of his sun exposure history. The biopsy confirms chondrodermatitis nodularis helicis, and he is counseled to use sun protection.

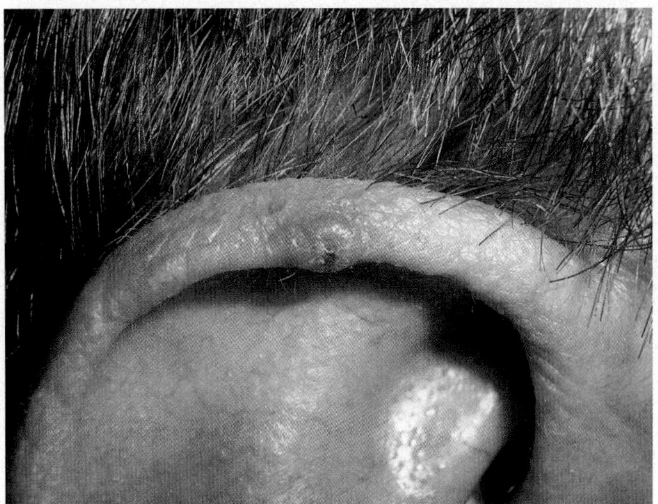

FIGURE 31-1 Chondrodermatitis nodularis helicis on the right ear of a 44-year-old man. (*Reproduced with permission from Richard P. Usatine, MD.*)

INTRODUCTION

Chondrodermatitis nodularis helicis is a benign neoplasm of the ear cartilage commonly believed to be related to excessive pressure, for example, during sleep, and sun exposure. The result is a localized overgrowth of cartilage, and subsequent skin changes. Preauricular tags are malformations of the external ear.

SYNONYMS

Chondrodermatitis nodularis chronica helicis.

EPIDEMIOLOGY

CHONDRODERMATITIS NODULARIS

- The incidence of chondrodermatitis nodularis has not been determined.
- Occurs most commonly in men older than 40 years of age, but older women can also be affected.

PREAURICULAR TAGS

- Occur in approximately 1 of 10,000 to 12,500 births without predilection for gender or race.
- Ear malformations may occur in isolation or as part of a constellation of abnormalities, often involving the renal system. Children have a 5-fold risk of hearing impairment (8 of 10,000 vs. 1.5 of 10,000).[1]
- Several chromosomal abnormalities include preauricular tags as one of the phenotypic expressions.
- The Goldenhar syndrome includes preauricular skin tags, bilateral limbal dermoids of the eye, and eyelid colobomas.

ETIOLOGY AND PATHOPHYSIOLOGY

CHONDRODERMATITIS NODULARIS HELICIS

- In rare cases, especially when occurring at younger ages, the lesion may be related to an underlying disease associated with microvascular injury, such as vasculitis or other necrobiotic collagen disease.[2]

PREAURICULAR TAGS

- Arise from remnants of supernumerary brachial hillocks.[3]
- Early stage embryology involves the formation of several slitlike structures on the side of the head, the branchial clefts. The three hillocks between the first four clefts eventually form the structure of the outer ear. Preauricular tags are generally minor malformations arising from remnants of supernumerary branchial hillocks.[4]

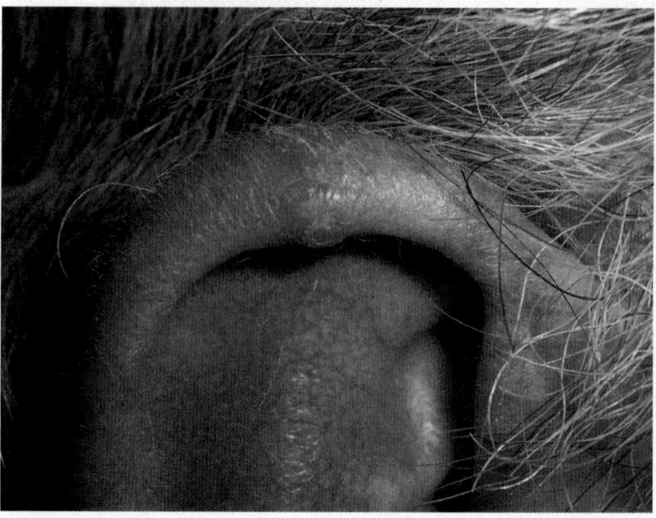

FIGURE 31-2 Chondrodermatitis nodularis on the helix of the right ear in a 62-year-old man. Note the pearly appearance, which may be seen with a basal cell carcinoma. (*Reproduced with permission from Richard P. Usatine, MD.*)

DIAGNOSIS

CLINICAL FEATURES OF CHONDRODERMATITIS

- Firm, painful nodule 3–20 mm in size (**Figures 31-1** to **31-4**).
- The helix is most often affected especially in men (**Figures 31-1** and **31-2**). The antihelix is affected more often in women (**Figures 31-3** and **31-4**).
- Overlying skin normal in color or erythematous; a central ulcer may be present.

CLINICAL FEATURES OF PREAURICULAR TAGS

- Fleshy knob in front of the ear (**Figures 31-5** and **31-6**).
- Present from the time of birth.
- Generally asymptomatic.

TYPICAL DISTRIBUTION

- Chondrodermatitis is located at the helix or antihelix of the ear. The right ear is more often affected than the left.
- Preauricular tags may be unilateral or bilateral, more often present on the left.

BIOPSY

- Often required for chondrodermatitis nodularis to rule out malignancy, especially when occurring in individuals with actinic damage and/or history of other skin cancers.
- Not indicated for preauricular tag.

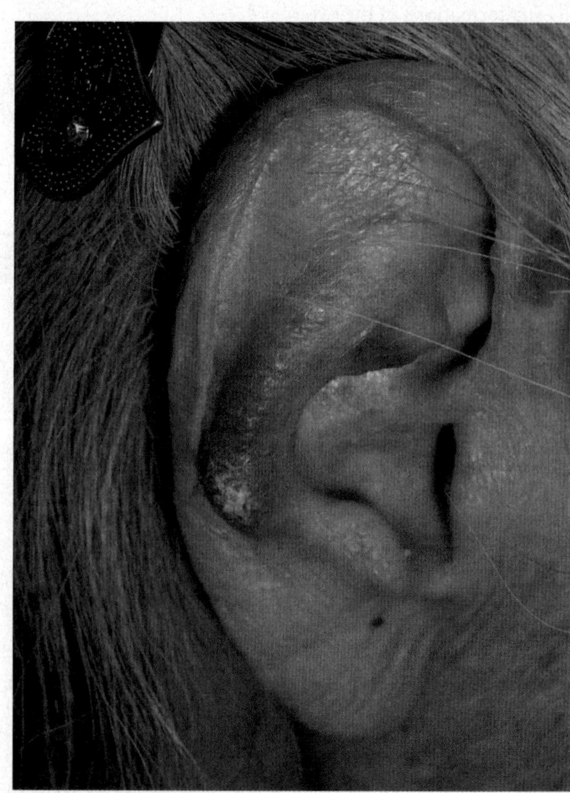

FIGURE 31-3 Chondrodermatitis nodularis on the antihelix of the right ear of an 86-year-old woman. Note the erythema and scale. A shave biopsy was performed to make sure this was not a squamous cell carcinoma. (*Reproduced with permission from Richard P. Usatine, MD.*)

DIFFERENTIAL DIAGNOSIS

- Chondrodermatitis nodularis helicis may be confused with skin cancer, especially squamous cell carcinoma (SCC; see Chapter 178, Squamous Cell Carcinoma). In SCC, the overlying skin is often ulcerated and the tumor has poorly defined margins.
- The key issue in diagnosis of preauricular tags is whether the ear tags are an isolated anomaly or part of a syndrome involving vital

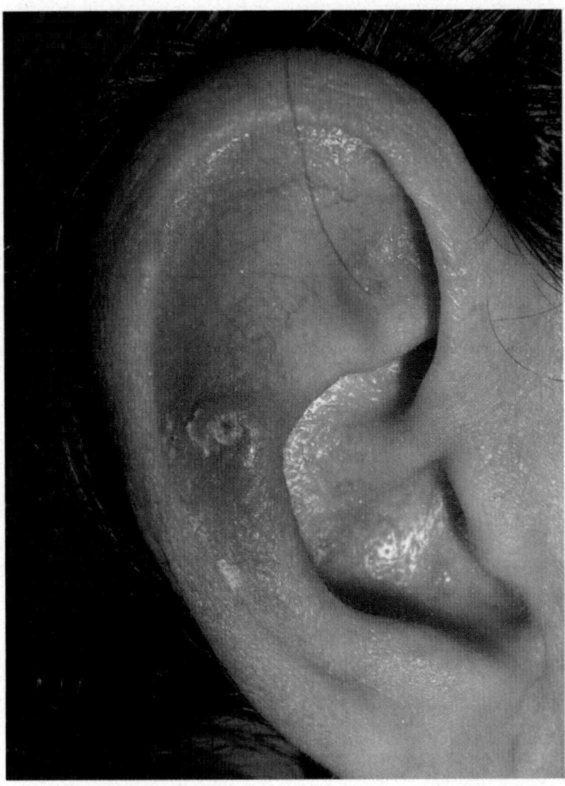

FIGURE 31-4 Chondrodermatitis nodularis on the antihelix of the right ear of a 52-year-old woman. Note the pearly nodule with central scale. A shave biopsy was performed to rule out basal cell carcinoma and squamous cell carcinoma. (*Reproduced with permission from Richard P. Usatine, MD.*)

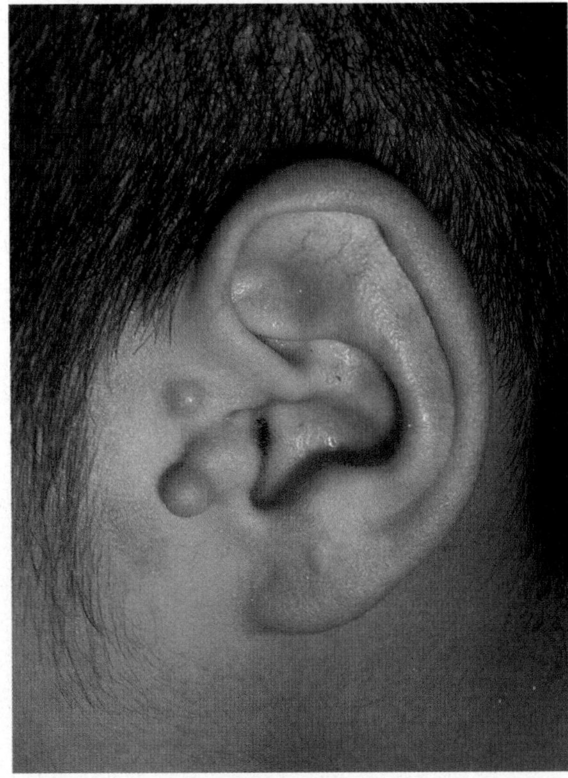

FIGURE 31-5 Preauricular tags in a young boy. (*Reproduced with permission from Richard P. Usatine, MD.*)

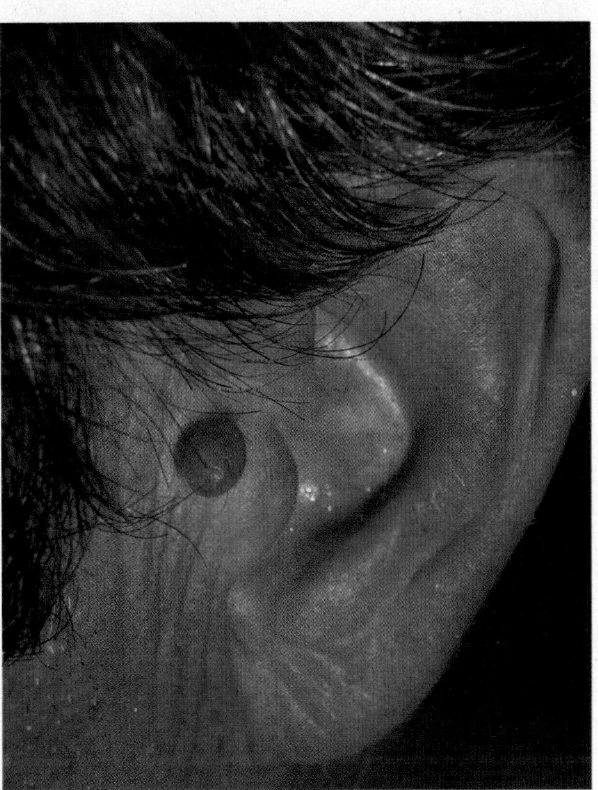

FIGURE 31-6 Preauricular tag present since birth in a 59-year-old man. The patient has never had any renal abnormalities or related medical problems. He wants it removed for cosmetic purposes. (*Reproduced with permission from Richard P. Usatine, MD.*)

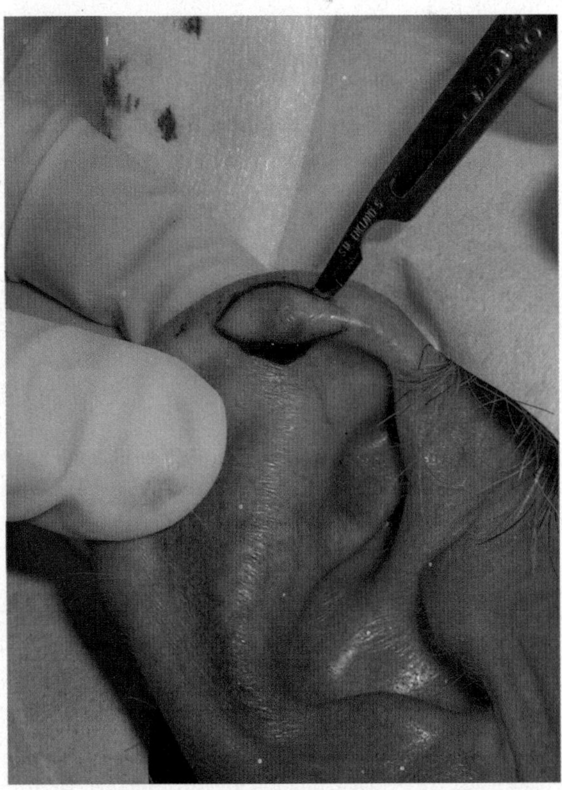

FIGURE 31-7 Elliptical excision of chondrodermatitis nodularis helicis. (*Reproduced with permission from Richard P. Usatine, MD.*)

organs, especially the kidneys. There is no consensus about whether children with ear tags who otherwise appear to be healthy should be evaluated with renal ultrasound.[4,5]

MANAGEMENT

Chondrodermatitis nodularis is treated with the following:

NONPHARMACOLOGICAL

- A pressure-relieving prosthesis or donut-shaped pillow can be used.[6,7] SOR C This can also be created by cutting a hole from the center of a bath sponge. The sponge can then be held in place with a headband if needed. A special prefabricated pillow is available from http://www.cnhpillow.com/.

PROCEDURES

- Shave biopsy can be used to make the diagnosis and may relieve symptoms temporarily. SOR C
- Cryotherapy, intralesional steroids, or curettage and electrodesiccation can be performed after the result from the shave biopsy is known and there is no malignancy. SOR C
- Photodynamic therapy (combines a photosensitizer with a specific type of light to kill nearby cells) has been reported to decrease pain in case reports.[8] SOR C
- A small elliptical excision of the nodule with removal of inflamed cartilage provides excellent results (**Figure 31-7**).[9,10] SOR C

Preauricular tags can be left alone or surgically excised for cosmetic reasons. SOR C

FOLLOW-UP FOR CHONDRODERMATITIS NODULARIS

- Recurrences are common and may require further treatment.

PATIENT EDUCATION

- Chondrodermatitis nodularis is a benign lesion that tends to recur; therapeutic options can be discussed.
- There is a low risk of urinary tract abnormalities in children who have apparently isolated preauricular tags and an increased risk of hearing impairment.

PATIENT RESOURCES

- A special prefabricated pillow is available that helps relieve pressure on the ear. For more information, contact: CNH Pillow, PO Box 1247, Abilene, TX 79604; phone (800) 255-7487; **http://www.cnhpillow.com/.**
- Preauricular tags—**http://nlm.nih.gov/medlineplus/ency/article/003304.htm.**

PROVIDER RESOURCES

- To learn how to perform an easy elliptical excision of chondrodermatitis nodularis helicis refer to the text and DVD: Usatine R, Pfenninger J, Stulberg D, Small R. *Dermatologic and Cosmetic Procedures in Office Practice*. Text and DVD. Philadelphia, PA: Elsevier; 2012.
- Marks VJ, Papa CA. **http://emedicine.medscape.com/article/1119141-overview.**
- Preauricular tags—**http://emedicine.medscape.com/article/845288-overview.**

REFERENCES

1. Roth DA, Hildesheimer M, Bardenstein S, et al. Preauricular skin tags and ear pits are associated with permanent hearing impairment in newborns. *Pediatrics.* 2008;122(4):e844-e890.
2. Magro CM, Frambach GE, Crowson AN. Chondrodermatitis nodularis helices as a marker of internal disease associated with microvascular injury. *J Cutan Pathol.* 2005;32:329-333.
3. Ostrower ST. Preauricular cysts, pits, and fissures. Updated Feb 7, 2017. http://emedicine.medscape.com/article/845288-overview. Accessed March 2017.
4. Deshpande SA, Watson H. Renal ultrasound not required in babies with isolated minor ear abnormalities. *Arch Dis Child Fetal Neonatal Ed.* 2006;91:F29-F30.
5. Kohelet D, Arbel E. A prospective search for urinary tract abnormalities in infants with isolated preauricular tags. *Pediatrics.* 2000;105:E61.
6. Sanu A, Koppana R, Snow DG. Management of chondrodermatitis nodularis chronica helicis using a "donut pillow". *J Laryngol Otol.* 2007;121(11):1096-1098.
7. Moncrieff M, Sassoon EM. Effective treatment of chondrodermatitis nodularis chronica helicis using a conservative approach. *Br J Dermatol.* 2004;150:892-894.
8. Pellegrino M, Taddeucci P, Mei S, et al. Chondrodermatitis nodularis chronics helicis and photodynamic therapy: a new therapeutic option? *Dermatol Ther.* 2011;24(1):144-147.
9. Rex J, Ribera M, Bielsa I, et al. Narrow elliptical skin excision and cartilage shaving for treatment of chondrodermatitis nodularis. *Dermatol Surg.* 2006;32:400-404.
10. Hudson-Peacock MJ, Cox NH, Lawrence CM. The long-term results of cartilage removal alone for the treatment of chondrodermatitis nodularis. *Br J Dermatol.* 1999;141:703-705.

SECTION B NOSE AND SINUS

32 NASAL POLYPS

Linda Speer, MD

PATIENT STORY

A 35-year-old man complains of unilateral nasal obstruction for the past several months of gradual onset. On examination of the nose, a nasal polyp is found (**Figure 32-1**).

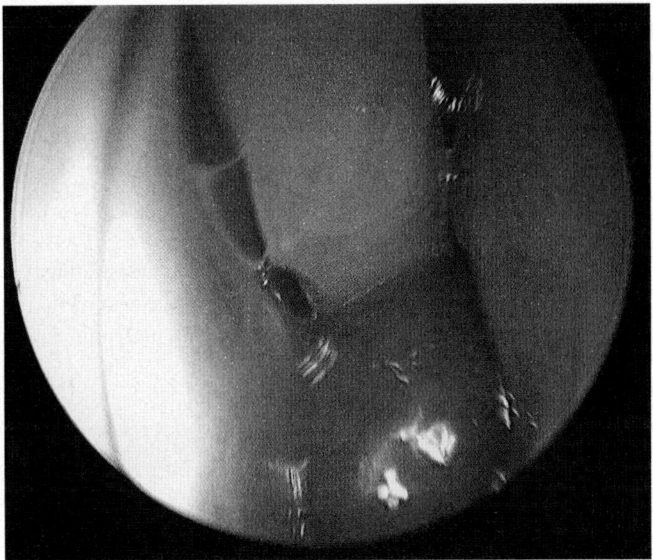

FIGURE 32-1 Nasal polyp in left middle meatus with normal surrounding mucosa. (*Reproduced with permission from William Clark, MD.*)

INTRODUCTION

Nasal polyps are benign lesions arising from the mucosa of the nasal passages, including the paranasal sinuses. They are most commonly semitransparent.

EPIDEMIOLOGY[1]

- Prevalence of 1% to 4% of adults; 0.1% of children of all races and classes.
- The male-to-female ratio in adults is approximately 2-4:1.
- Peak age of onset is 20 to 40 years; rare in children younger than 10 years.
- Associated with the following conditions:
  - Nonallergic and allergic rhinitis and rhinosinusitis
  - Asthma—In 20% to 50% of patients with polyps
  - Cystic fibrosis
  - Aspirin intolerance—In 8% to 26% of patients with polyps
  - Alcohol intolerance—In 50% of patients with polyps

ETIOLOGY AND PATHOPHYSIOLOGY

- The precise cause of nasal polyp formation is unknown.
- Infectious agents causing desquamation of the mucous membrane may play a triggering role.
- Activated epithelial cells appear to be the major source of mediators that induce an influx of inflammatory cells, including eosinophils prominently; these in turn lead to proliferation and activation of fibroblasts.[2] Cytokines and growth factors play a role in maintaining the mucosal inflammation associated with polyps.
- Food allergies are strongly associated with nasal polyps.

DIAGNOSIS

CLINICAL FEATURES

- The appearance is usually smooth and rounded (**Figure 32-1**).

- Moist and translucent (**Figure 32-2**).
- Variable size.
- Color ranging from nearly none to deep erythema.

TYPICAL DISTRIBUTION

- The middle meatus (origin from the ethmoid sinus) is the most common location. Nasal polyps are frequently bilateral.

LABORATORY AND IMAGING

- Consider allergy testing.
- In children with multiple polyps, order sweat test to rule out cystic fibrosis.
- CT of the nose and paranasal sinuses may be indicated to evaluate extent of lesion(s) (**Figure 32-3**).

BIOPSY

- Not usually indicated. Histology typically shows pseudostratified ciliary epithelium, edematous stroma, epithelial basement membrane, and proinflammatory cells with eosinophils present in 80% to 90% of cases.

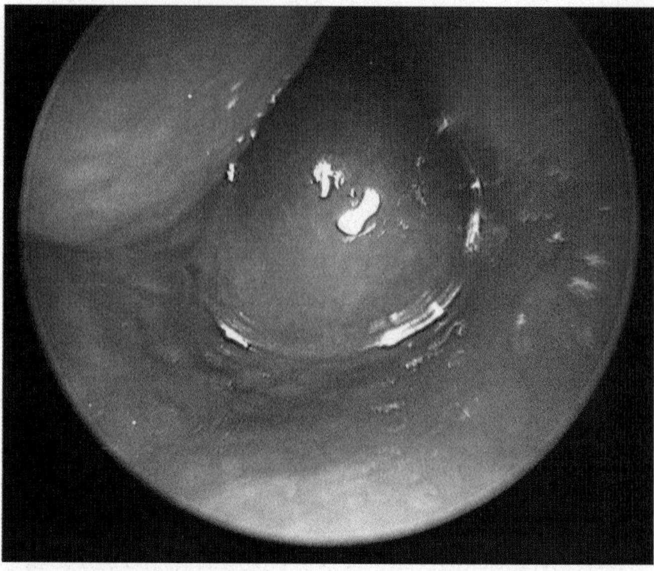

FIGURE 32-2 Nasal polyp in right nasal cavity in a patient with inflamed mucosa from allergic rhinitis. (*Reproduced with permission from William Clark, MD.*)

DIFFERENTIAL DIAGNOSIS

Many relatively rare conditions can cause an intranasal mass including (in adults):

- Papilloma—About 1% of nasal tumors, affecting about 1 in 100,000 adults per year. Locally invasive, these tend to recur especially if excision is not complete. Papillomas are of unknown etiology but are associated with chronic sinusitis, air pollution, and viral infections. They are irregular and friable in appearance and bleed easily.[3]
- Meningoencephalocele—Grayish gelatinous appearance.[4]
- Nasopharyngeal carcinoma—Firm, often ulcerated.
- Pyogenic granuloma—Relatively common benign vascular neoplasm of skin and mucous membranes (see Chapter 167, Pyogenic Granuloma).[5]
- Chordoma—Locally invasive neoplasms with gelatinous appearance that arise from notochordal (embryonic) remnants. Occurs in all age groups (mean age: 48 years).[6]
- Glioblastoma—Rare manifestation of the most common kind of brain tumor in adults.

Conditions that may mimic nasal polyp in children include:

- Rhabdomyosarcoma—Malignant tumor of childhood originating from striated muscle.
- Dermoid tumor—Inclusion cysts of ectodermal epithelial elements, usually manifest before 20 years of age. May grow slowly.
- Hemangioma—Congenital, abnormal proliferation of blood vessels that may occur in any vascularized tissue (see Chapter 115, Childhood Hemangiomas).
- Neuroblastoma—Unusual presentation of relatively common malignancy of childhood.
- Meningoencephalocele—Grayish gelatinous appearance.

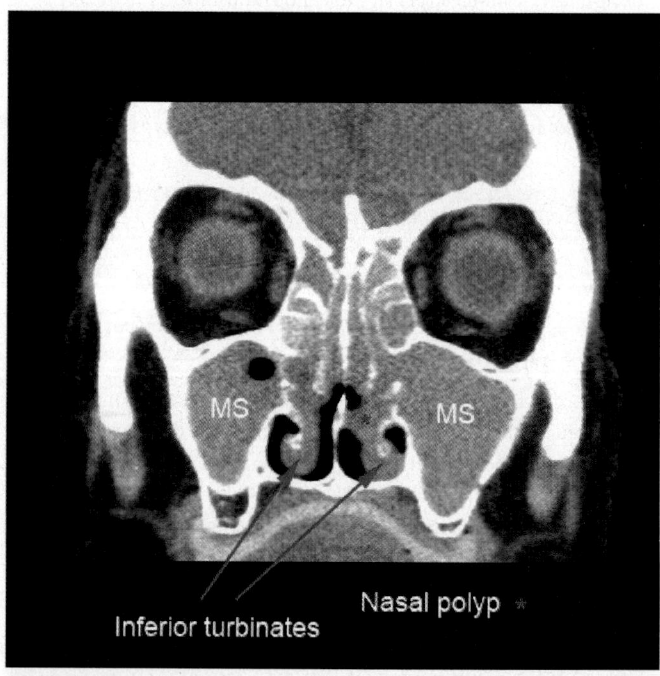

FIGURE 32-3 CT scan showing polyps (*asterisk*) and bilateral opacified maxillary sinuses (*MS*). Note that the nasal polyp appears to be coming from the left maxillary sinus and is above the inferior turbinate. (*Reproduced with permission from Richard P. Usatine, MD.*)

- Angiofibroma—Locally invasive neoplasm that appears as a firm grayish mass. Bleeds easily. Occurs in young males ages 7 to 19 years. Undetermined etiology.[7]
- Pyogenic granuloma (see Chapter 167, Pyogenic Granuloma).[5]

MANAGEMENT

MEDICATIONS

- Evidence is lacking to demonstrate superiority of surgical versus medical approaches to treatment.[8]
- Medical treatment consists of intranasal corticosteroids.[9] SOR Ⓐ
- An initial short course (2 to 4 weeks) of oral steroids may be considered in severe cases.[10,11] SOR Ⓐ
- Steroid treatment reduces polyp size, but does not generally resolve them. Corticosteroid treatment is also useful preoperatively to reduce polyp size.
- Oral doxycycline 100 mg daily for 20 days was shown to decrease polyp size, providing benefit for 12 weeks in one randomized controlled trial.[12] SOR Ⓑ
- Topical nasal decongestants may provide some symptom relief, but do not reduce polyp size.[13] SOR Ⓑ
- Montelukast reduces symptoms when used as an adjunct to oral and inhaled steroid therapy in patients with bilateral nasal polyposis.[14] SOR Ⓑ

PROCEDURES

- Surgical excision is often required to relieve symptoms.
- Consider immunotherapy for patients with allergies.

PROGNOSIS

- Lesions are benign and tend to recur. They do not evolve into more serious conditions over time if left untreated.[15]

FOLLOW-UP

- Periodic reevaluation is recommended because recurrence rates are high.[16]

PATIENT EDUCATION

- Patients should be informed about the benign nature of nasal polyps and their tendency to recur.

PATIENT RESOURCES

- **http://www.mayoclinic.org/diseases-conditions/nasal-polyps/home/ovc-20267294.**
- **http://www.nlm.nih.gov/medlineplus/ency/article/001641.htm.**

PROVIDER RESOURCES

- **http://emedicine.medscape.com/article/994274-overview.**
- **http://emedicine.medscape.com/article/861353-overview.**

REFERENCES

1. McClay JE. *Nasal Polyps.* http://emedicine.medscape.com/article/994274-overview. Accessed March 2017.
2. Pawliczak R, Lewandowska-Polak A, Kowalski ML. Pathogenesis of nasal polyps: an update. *Curr Allergy Asthma Rep.* 2005;5:463-471.
3. Sadeghi N. *Sinonasal Papillomas.* http://emedicine.medscape.com/article/862677-overview. Accessed March 2017.
4. Kumar KK, Ganapathy K, Sumathi V, et al. Adult meningoencephalocele presenting as a nasal polyp. *J Clin Neurosci.* 2005;12:594-596.
5. Hoving EW. Nasal encephaloceles. *Childs Nerv Syst.* 2000;16:702-706.
6. Palmer CA. *Chordoma.* http://emedicine.medscape.com/article/250902-overview. Accessed March 2017.
7. Tewfik TL. *Juvenile Nasopharyngeal Angiofibroma.* http://emedicine.medscape.com/article/872580. Accessed March 2017.
8. Rimmer J, Fikkens W, Chong LY, Hopkins C. Surgical versus medical interventions for chronic rhinosinusitis with nasal polyps. *Cochrane Database Syst Rev.* 2014;(12):CD006991.
9. Joe SA, Thambi R, Huang J. A systematic review of the use of intranasal steroids in the treatment of chronic rhinosinusitis. *Otolaryngol Head Neck Surg.* 2008;139(3):340-347.
10. Martinez-Devesa P, Patiar S. Oral steroids for nasal polyps. *Cochrane Database Syst Rev.* 2011;6(7):CD005232.
11. Vaidyanathan S, Barnes M, Williamson P, et al. Treatment of chronic rhinosinusitis with nasal polyposis with oral steroids followed by topical steroids: a randomized trial. *Ann Intern Med.* 2011;154(5):293-302.
12. Van Zele T, Gevaert P, Holtappels G, et al. Oral steroids and doxycycline: two different approaches to treat nasal polyps. *J Allergy Clin Immunol.* 2010;125(5):1069-1076.e4.
13. Johansson L, Oberg D, Melem I, Bende M. Do topical nasal decongestants affect polyps? *Acta Otolaryngol.* 2006:126:288-290.
14. Stewart RA, Ram B, Hamilton G, et al. Montelukast as an adjunct to oral and inhaled steroid therapy in chronic nasal polyposis. *Otolaryngol Head Neck Surg.* 2008;139(5):682-687.
15. Oscarsson M, Johansson I, Bende M. What happens with untreated nasal polyps over time? A 13-year prospective study. *Ann Otol Rhinol Laryngol.* 2016;125(9):710-715.
16. Vento SI, Ertama LO, Hytonen ML, et al. Nasal polyposis: clinical course during 20 years. *Ann Allergy Asthma Immunol.* 2000;85:209-214.

33 SINUSITIS

Mindy A. Smith, MD, MS

PATIENT STORY

A 55-year-old woman reports sinus pressure for the past 2 weeks along with headache, rhinorrhea, postnasal drip, and cough that followed a cold 3 weeks ago. She has chronic allergic rhinitis, but now the pressure on the right side of her face has become intense and her right upper molars are painful. The nasal discharge has become discolored and she feels feverish. She is diagnosed clinically with right maxillary sinusitis and elects antibiotic treatment with amoxicillin. Two weeks later when her symptoms have persisted, a CT is ordered and she is found to have air-fluid levels in both maxillary sinuses and loculated fluid on the right side (**Figures 33-1** and **33-2**). The antibiotic is changed to amoxicillin/clavulanate and she is given information about nasal saline irrigation for symptom relief. If the symptoms don't improve, the clinician plans to send her to ear, nose, and throat (ENT) for further evaluation.

FIGURE 33-1 Bilateral maxillary sinusitis on axial CT. Note that fluid levels are greater on the right. (*Reproduced with permission from Chris McMains, MD.*)

INTRODUCTION

Rhinosinusitis is symptomatic inflammation of the paranasal sinuses, nasal cavity, and their epithelial lining.[1] Mucosal edema blocks mucous drainage, creating a culture medium for viruses and bacteria. Rhinosinusitis is classified by duration as acute (<4 weeks), subacute (4 to 12 weeks), or chronic (>12 weeks).

EPIDEMIOLOGY

- Rhinosinusitis is common in the United States, with an age-adjusted prevalence of 11.7% of the adult population in 2015.[2] The prevalence is increased in women and in individuals living in the southern United States.
- Only 10% of adults with symptoms of sinusitis actually have bacterial infection; in contrast 60% of children with sinusitis have a bacterial cause.[3] Of adult patients with acute viral sinusitis accompanying an upper respiratory tract infection (URI), only 0.5% to 2.5% develop superimposed acute bacterial sinusitis.[4]
- The prevalence of chronic rhinosinusitis in patients referred for evaluation of potential chronic rhinosinusitis, based on symptoms, ranges from 65% to 80%.[1]
- Children average 6 to 8 colds per year. In one study of 112 children with URIs, 8% developed sinusitis.[5]

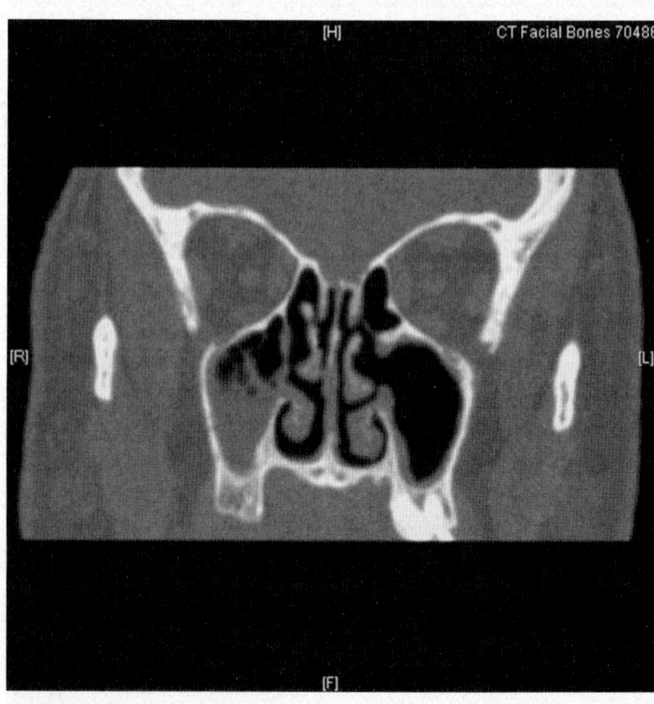

FIGURE 33-2 Maxillary sinusitis on coronal CT of same patient. (*Reproduced with permission from Chris McMains, MD.*)

ETIOLOGY AND PATHOPHYSIOLOGY

- Sinus cavities are lined with mucus-secreting respiratory epithelium. The mucus is transported by ciliary action through the sinus ostia (openings) to the nasal cavity. Under normal conditions, the paranasal sinuses are sterile cavities and there is no mucus retention.

- Bacterial sinusitis occurs when ostia become obstructed or ciliary action is impaired, causing mucus accumulation and secondary bacterial overgrowth.
- The causes of sinusitis include[6]:
  - Infection—Most commonly viral (e.g., rhinovirus, parainfluenza, and influenza) followed by bacterial infection (e.g., *Streptococcus pneumoniae, Haemophilus influenzae, Moraxella catarrhalis,* and *Staphylococcus aureus*).[4] In immunocompromised patients, fulminant fungal sinusitis may occur (e.g., rhinocerebral mucormycosis—**Figure 33-3**). Biofilms may play a role in recalcitrant disease.[7]
  - Noninfectious obstruction—Allergic, polyposis, barotrauma (e.g., deep-sea diving, airplane travel), chemical irritants, tumors (e.g., squamous cell carcinoma, granulomatous disease, inverting papilloma), and conditions that alter mucus composition (e.g., cystic fibrosis).

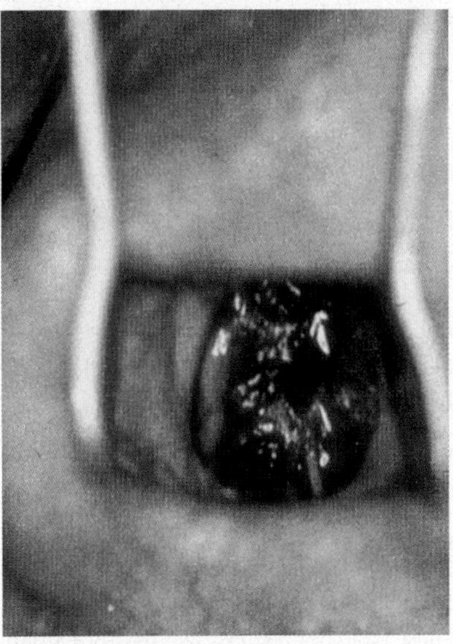

FIGURE 33-3 Mucormycosis sinusitis in a patient with diabetes showing the classic black nasal discharge. (*Reproduced with permission from Randal A. Otto, MD.*)

DIAGNOSIS

The diagnosis is based on the clinical picture with typical symptoms listed below. Symptoms arising from viral infection generally peak by day 5 or before.

- Acute bacterial rhinosinusitis is diagnosed when symptoms are present for 10 days or longer or when symptoms worsen after initial stability or improvement ("double worsening" or "double sickening"); it can also be presumed in patients with unusually severe presentations or extrasinus manifestations of infection.[1]
- Similar diagnostic criteria are used for children—persistent illness with any quality of nasal discharge or daytime cough or both lasting more than 10 days without improvement OR worsening course OR severe onset (i.e., concurrent fever [≥39°C/102.2°F] and purulent nasal discharge for at least 3 consecutive days).[8]
- Chronic rhinosinusitis is diagnosed after 12 or more weeks based on two or more of: mucopurulent drainage (anterior, posterior, or both), nasal obstruction (congestion), facial pain-pressure-fullness, or decreased sense of smell AND inflammation documented by purulent mucus or edema in the middle meatus or anterior ethmoid region, polyps in nasal cavity or the middle meatus, and/or radiographic imaging showing inflammation of the paranasal sinuses.[1]

CLINICAL FEATURES

- Most cases are seen in conjunction with viral upper respiratory infections and represent sinus inflammation rather than infection.[4]
- The American Academy of Otolaryngology guideline recommends a diagnosis of acute rhinosinusitis with up to 4 weeks of purulent nasal drainage accompanied by nasal obstruction; facial pain, pressure, or fullness; or both.[1] Other guidelines do not require presence of purulent nasal drainage for diagnosis.[4] The Infectious Disease Society of America recommends a diagnosis of acute sinusitis with up to 4 weeks of at least 2 major symptoms (the above or hyposmia or anosmia) or one major symptom and at least two minor symptoms (i.e., headache; ear pain, pressure, or fullness; halitosis; dental pain; cough; and fatigue).[9]
- Localizing symptoms include facial pain or pressure over the involved sinus when bending over or supine (i.e., forehead in frontal sinusitis, cheek with maxillary sinusitis, between the eyes with ethmoid sinusitis, and neck and top of the head with sphenoid

sinusitis) and maxillary tooth pain, most commonly the upper molars; the latter is seen more often with bacterial sinusitis.

- In a study of patients with chronic rhinosinusitis, diagnosis based on symptoms was problematic, and only dysosmia (impairment in the sense of smell) and the presence of polyps could distinguish between normal and abnormal radiographs.[10]

TYPICAL DISTRIBUTION

- Most sinus infections involve the maxillary sinus followed in frequency by the ethmoid (anterior), frontal, and sphenoid sinuses; however, most cases involve more than one sinus.[5]
- Children are more likely to have inflammation in the posterior ethmoid and sphenoid sinuses.[11]

LABORATORY AND IMAGING

- Routine culture of nasal or nasopharyngeal secretions is not recommended, as these have not been shown to differentiate between bacterial and viral rhinosinusitis. Culture may be considered for patients with immune compromise who have persistent symptoms despite initial antibiotic treatment.[4]
- If culture is needed because of suspected bacterial resistance or persistence of infection, one meta-analysis found endoscopically directed middle meatal cultures to be reasonably sensitive (80.9%), specific (90.5%), and accurate (87.0%; 95% confidence interval, 81.3% to 92.8%) compared with maxillary sinus taps.[12]
- Radiography should not be obtained for patients meeting diagnostic criteria for acute rhinosinusitis, unless a complication or alternate diagnosis is suspected.[1] If performed in cases of clinical uncertainty or for complications (e.g., orbital, intracranial, or soft-tissue involvement), the American College of Radiology (ACR) recommends computed tomography (CT) without contrast or magnetic resonance imaging (MRI) without and with contrast.[13] (**Figures 33-4** and **33-5**) There are considerable limitations to the sensitivity of plain films, especially in diagnosing ethmoid and sphenoid disease.
- For children, ACR recommends CT of the paranasal sinuses without contrast or magnetic resonance imaging if there are orbital or intracranial complications.[14]
- Nasal endoscopy, identifying purulent material within the drainage area of the sinuses, may be useful in diagnosing acute sinusitis.[12] In one case series of patients with suspected chronic rhinosinusitis, the addition of endoscopy to symptom criteria had similar sensitivity (88.7% vs. 84.1%) but significantly improved specificity (66% vs. 12.3%) using CT as the gold standard.[15]
- For chronic rhinosinusitis, inflammation is documented objectively using anterior rhinoscopy, nasal endoscopy, or CT.

REFER OR HOSPITALIZE

- Potentially life-threatening complications include subperiosteal orbital abscess, meningitis, epidural or cerebral abscess, and cavernous sinus thrombosis (**Figures 33-6** and **33-7**).
- The risk of frontal sinusitis includes eroding through the frontal bone forward and causing a Pott's puffy tumor, spreading into the brain and cavernous sinuses (**Figure 33-5**).
- Orbital abscess is highly dangerous and can be the result of spread from the frontal or ethmoid sinuses (**Figure 33-6**).

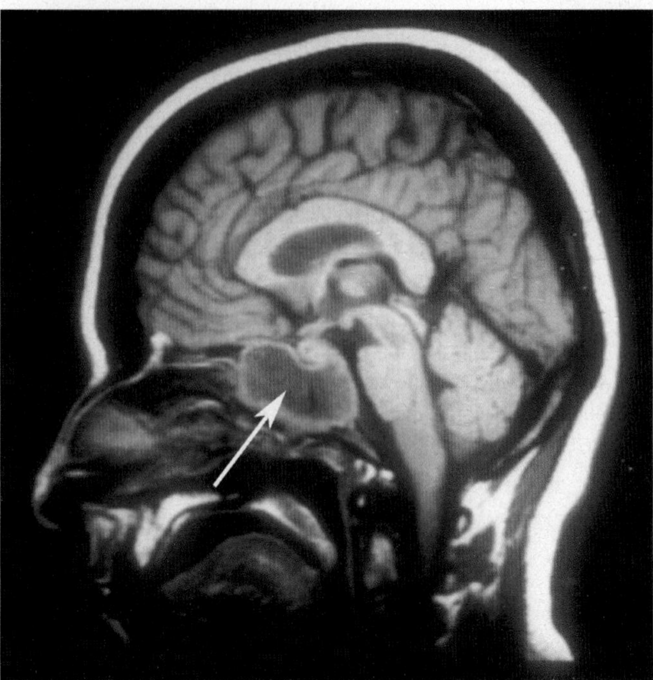

FIGURE 33-4 Mucopyocele in the sphenoid sinus (*arrow*) as a complication of bacterial sinusitis. (*Reproduced with permission from Randal A. Otto, MD.*)

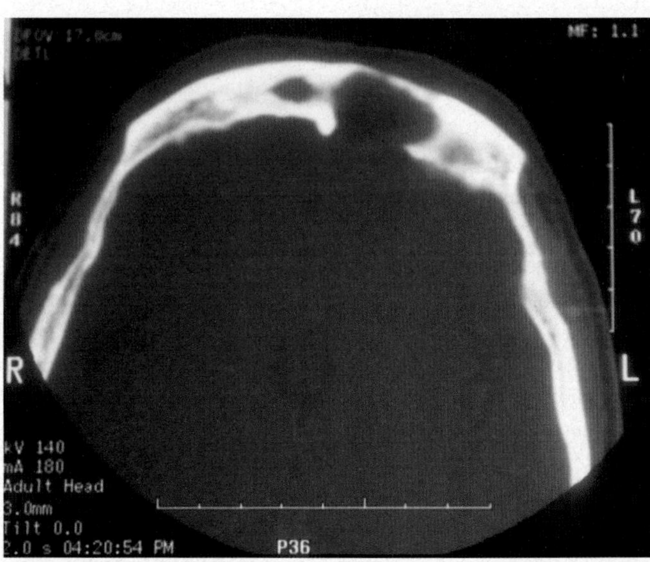

FIGURE 33-5 Frontal sinusitis eroded through the frontal bone inward toward the brain threatening such complications as a brain abscess and cavernous sinus thrombosis. Seen on CT scan. (*Reproduced with permission from Randal A. Otto, MD.*)

- In immunocompromised patients, fulminant fungal sinusitis may cause orbital swelling, cellulitis, proptosis, ptosis, impairment of extraocular motion, nasopharyngeal ulceration, epistaxis, and bony erosion. Nasal mucosa may appear black (**Figure 33-3**), blanched white, or erythematous.
- Hospitalized patients may be critically ill with "fever of unknown origin" and without localizing symptoms. Infections in these patients are often polymicrobial including *Pseudomonas aeruginosa, Klebsiella pneumoniae,* and *Enterobacter.*[16]

DIFFERENTIAL DIAGNOSIS

- Upper respiratory tract infections—These are common infections, primarily viral (most commonly rhinovirus), that cause 2 to 4 infections per year in adults and 6 to 8 infections per year in children. Infections are self-limited (lasting approximately 7 to 10 days) and typical symptoms include rhinorrhea, nasal congestion, sore throat, and cough. URI often precedes acute sinusitis.
- Allergic rhinitis—Sneezing, itching, watery rhinorrhea.
- Tumor (usually squamous cell carcinoma)—Rare; unilateral epistaxis or discharge and obstruction, recurrent sinusitis, sinus pain.

Other causes of facial pain include:

- Migraine headache or cluster headache—Moderate to severe head pain that is usually deep seated, persistent, and pulsatile. There is a history of multiple occurrences, and head pain may be associated with nausea, vomiting, photophobia, and scotomata. Attacks last 4 to 72 hours.
- Trigeminal neuralgia—Painful condition characterized by excruciating, paroxysmal, shocklike pain lasting seconds to minutes along the distribution of the trigeminal nerve (ophthalmic, maxillary, and/or mandibular branches). Pain may be triggered by face washing, air draft, or chewing.
- Dental pain—Tooth pain may be secondary to caries or gingivitis. When caries extend into the tooth pulp, the tooth becomes sensitive to percussion and hot and cold food and beverages. If pulp necrosis occurs, pain becomes severe, sharp, throbbing, and often worse when supine. Abscess formation results in pain, swelling, and erythema of the gum and surrounding tissue, and possibly purulent drainage.
- Temporal arteritis—Unilateral pounding headache that may be associated with visual changes and systemic symptoms (e.g., fever, weight loss, muscle aches). Onset is usually older adults (older than age 50 years), and laboratory testing reveals an elevated erythrocyte sedimentation rate (>50).

MANAGEMENT

Duration of illness assists in decision making, as most patients improve without specific treatment. A period of watchful waiting for up to 7 days is consistent with guidelines[1]; up to 3 days is recommended for children.[8] Treatment of symptoms, including pain, is important.

FIRST LINE

NONPHARMACOLOGIC

- Nasal saline irrigation for acute upper respiratory tract infection in adults is generally not helpful, although data are limited[17]; one large

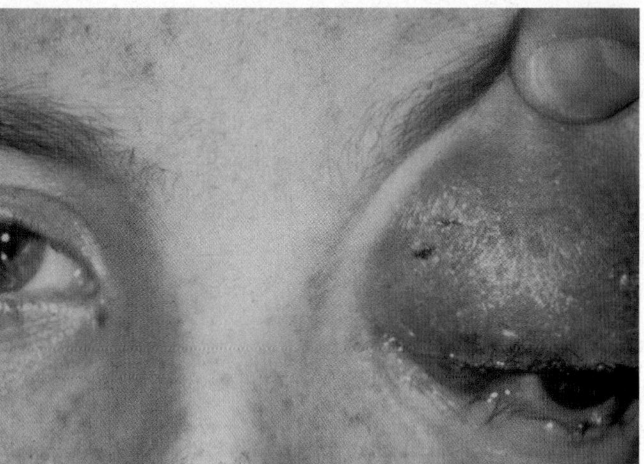

FIGURE 33-6 Right orbital abscess with proptosis as a complication of frontal sinusitis eroding through the superior orbital bones. (*Reproduced with permission from Randal A. Otto, MD.*)

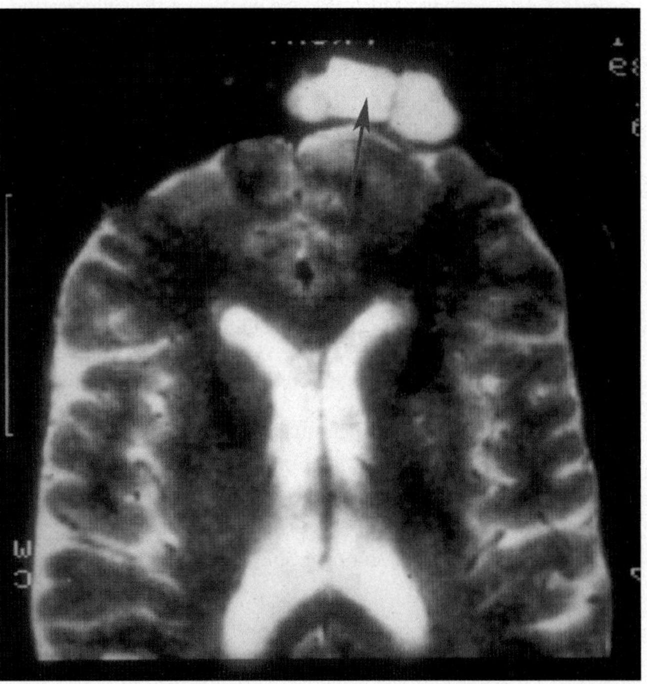

FIGURE 33-7 Mucopyocele (*red arrow*) in the right frontal sinus seen on MRI scan as a complication of frontal sinusitis. (*Reproduced with permission from Randal A. Otto, MD.*)

trial in children found benefit in reducing nasal secretions and nasal breathing. SOR B In adults with chronic sinusitis, nasal saline irrigation alone may provide symptom relief.[18] SOR B High-volume saline irrigation in addition to topical steroids is considered first-line therapy for symptoms in chronic rhinosinusitis.[19]

MEDICATIONS

- Analgesics (acetaminophen or nonsteroidal antiinflammatory drugs alone or in combination with an opioid) should be used for pain.[1]
- Oral and topical (nasal) decongestants are NOT recommended for adults or children based on lack of randomized controlled trials (RCTs) demonstrating effectiveness.[1,20] Topical agents can cause rebound nasal congestion after discontinuation. Antihistamines may be helpful in patients with sinusitis and allergic rhinitis.[4]
- Topical corticosteroids appear to be of benefit in improvement and resolution of symptoms for acute sinusitis.[21] SOR B Oral steroids do not appear to be of benefit for acute disease.[22] For patients with chronic rhinosinusitis and nasal polyps, consider a short course of systemic corticosteroids (1–3 weeks), a short course of doxycycline (3 weeks), or a leukotriene antagonist.[19]
- Patients with uncomplicated acute bacterial rhinosinusitis may be offered watchful waiting with symptomatic treatment (if there is assurance of follow-up) or antibiotics.[1] Patients who fail to improve after 7 days or who have severe symptoms may be offered oral antibiotics. SOR A
    - Adults—Amoxicillin (500 to 1000 mg orally three times daily or 875 mg orally twice daily) for 5–10 days or amoxicillin/clavulanate (500 mg of amoxicillin and 125 mg of clavulanate orally three times daily or 875 mg of amoxicillin and 125 mg of clavulanate orally twice daily) for 5–10 days; the higher doses are recommended for patients at high risk of having an amoxicillin-resistant organism, from regions with high endemic rates (>10%) of invasive *S. pneumoniae*, those with severe infection, age >65 years, recent hospitalization, antibiotic use within the past month, or those who are immunocompromised.[1] For patients allergic to penicillin, use doxycycline.[4]
    - Children—Amoxicillin (45 to 90 mg/kg divided twice daily).[8] For children with moderate to severe illness or those younger than 2 years, attending childcare, or who have recently been treated with an antimicrobial, consider high-dose amoxicillin-clavulanate (80–90 mg/kg per day of the amoxicillin component with 6.4 mg/kg per day of clavulanate in 2 divided doses with a maximum of 2 g per dose).[8]
- In a Cochrane review of 10 high-quality trials evaluating antibiotic treatment for acute rhinosinusitis, antibiotics shortened time to cure in only five per 100 at any time point between 7 and 14 days and caused adverse effects in 27% (vs. 15% with placebo).[23] Comparisons between classes of antibiotics showed no significant differences.[1]
- The modest benefit of antibiotics for improving rates of clinical cure or improvement at 7 to 12 days (number needed to treat = 7–18) must be weighed against the risks of harm (primarily gastrointestinal, but also skin rash, vaginal discharge, headache, dizziness, and fatigue [number needed to harm = 8–12]).[4]

COMPLEMENTARY AND ALTERNATIVE MEDICINE

- With respect to alternative therapy, there is limited evidence that Sinupret and bromelain may be effective adjunctive treatments in acute rhinosinusitis.[24] SOR B

SECOND LINE

PROCEDURES

- Surgery and intravenous antibiotics are primarily used for complications, including abscess and cases with orbital involvement.[6]
- Patients with fungal sinusitis are treated with aggressive debridement and adjunctive antifungals (e.g., amphotericin).[6]
- Based on three RCTs, endoscopic sinus surgery is not superior to medical treatment; in one study there was a lower relapse rate (2.4% vs. 5.6% without surgery).[25] SOR B Patients should be selected based on the severity of disease (frequency of antibiotics/oral steroid use), comorbidities (asthma, cystic fibrosis, aspirin sensitivity, etc.), and overall clinical picture (presence of polyps or fungal disease).
- Cochrane authors found lack of supporting evidence for use of endoscopic balloon sinus ostial dilation vs. conventional surgical modalities in the management of patients with chronic rhinosinusitis who failed medical treatment.[26]

PREVENTION

- Smoking increases the risk for sinusitis; patients should be counseled about cessation.[1]

PROGNOSIS

- Cure or improvement rate for acute sinusitis within 2 weeks is high in both the placebo group (73%–85%) and the antibiotic group (77%–88%).[4]
- For patients with chronic sinusitis, a retrospective study of medical treatment reported treatment success in about half of patients (N = 74); 26 patients had partial resolution, and 45 patients underwent surgery. Facial pressure/pain, mucosal inflammation, and higher endoscopic severity grade predicted treatment failure.[27]

FOLLOW-UP

- For those adults who fail treatment after 7 days of antibiotic therapy,[1] a nonbacterial cause or resistant organism should be considered. Patients initially treated with amoxicillin without clavulanate can be treated with high-dose amoxicillin plus clavulanate, doxycycline, a respiratory fluoroquinolone (levofloxacin or moxifloxacin), or the combination of clindamycin plus a third-generation oral cephalosporin (cefixime or cefpodoxime).[1]
- For children who fail initial treatment with amoxicillin, use amoxicillin-clavulanate; for those who fail the latter, use clindamycin and cefixime OR linezolid and cefixime OR levofloxacin based on community resistance patterns.[8] SOR C

PATIENT EDUCATION

- Nasal congestion, purulent rhinitis, and facial pain following a cold may indicate a sinus infection. Symptoms due to a cold usually abate within 1 week.
- Patients can consider nasal saline irrigation and topical nasal steroids.
- Patients should be encouraged to see their primary care provider if symptoms persist or worsen after 10 days, suggesting bacterial infection that may benefit from antibiotic treatment.

PATIENT RESOURCES

- **https://www.cdc.gov/antibiotic-use/community/for-patients/common-illnesses/sinus-infection.html.**
- **https://familydoctor.org/?s=sinusitis.**

PROVIDER RESOURCES

- Wald ER, Applegate KE, Bordley C, et al. Clinical practice guideline for the diagnosis and management of acute bacterial sinusitis in children aged 1 to 18 years. *Pediatrics.* 2013;132(1):e262-280.
- Rosenfeld RM, Piccirillo JF, Chandrasehar SS, et al. Clinical practice guideline (update): adult sinusitis. *Otolaryngol Head Neck Surg.* 2015;152(2 Suppl):S1-S39.

REFERENCES

1. Rosenfeld RM, Piccirillo JF, Chandrasehar SS, et al. Clinical practice guideline (update): adult sinusitis. *Otolaryngol Head Neck Surg.* 2015;152(2 Suppl):S1-S39.
2. Centers for Disease Control and Prevention. *Summary Health Statistics: National Health Interview Survey, 2015.* https://ftp.cdc.gov/pub/Health_Statistics/NCHS/NHIS/SHS/2015_SHS_Table_A-2.pdf. Accessed January 2017.
3. Centers for Disease Control and Prevention. *Sinus Infection.* https://www.cdc.gov/antibiotic-use/community/for-patients/common-illnesses/sinus-infection.html. Accessed April 2018.
4. Rosenfeld RM. Clinical Practice. Acute sinusitis in adults. *N Engl J Med.* 2016;375(10):962-970.
5. Revai K, Dobbs LA, Nair S, et al. Incidence of acute otitis media and sinusitis complicating upper respiratory tract infection: the effect of age. *Pediatrics.* 2007;119(6):e1408-e1412.
6. Rubin MA, Gonzales R, Sande MA. Infections of the upper respiratory tract. In: Kasper DL, Braunwald E, Fauci AS, et al, eds. *Harrison's Principles of Internal Medicine.* New York, NY: McGraw-Hill; 2005:185-188.
7. Ramakrishnan Y, Shields RC, Elbadawey MR, Wilson JA. Biofilms in chronic rhinosinusitis: what is new and where next? *J Laryngol Otol.* 2015;129(8):744-751.
8. Wald ER, Applegate KE, Bordley C, et al. Clinical practice guideline for the diagnosis and management of acute bacterial sinusitis in children aged 1 to 18 years. *Pediatrics.* 2013;132(1):e262-280.
9. Chow AW, Benninger MS, Brook I, et al. IDSA clinical practice guideline for acute bacterial rhinosinusitis in children and adults. *Clin Infect Dis.* 2012;54(8):e72-e112.
10. Bhattacharyya N. Clinical and symptom criteria for the accurate diagnosis of chronic rhinosinusitis. *Laryngoscope.* 2006;116 (7 Pt 2 Suppl 110):1-22.
11. Gordts F, Clement PA, Destryker A, et al. Prevalence of sinusitis signs on MRI in a non-ENT pediatric population. *Rhinology.* 1997;35:154-157.
12. Benninger MS, Payne SC, Ferguson BJ, et al. Endoscopically directed middle meatal cultures versus maxillary sinus taps in acute bacterial maxillary rhinosinusitis: a meta-analysis. *Otolaryngol Head Neck Surg.* 2006;134(1):3-9.
13. American College of Radiology ACR Appropriateness Criteria: Sinonasal Disease. https://acsearch.acr.org/docs/69502/Narrative/. Accessed January 2017.
14. American College of Radiology ACR Appropriateness Criteria: Sinusitis—Child. https://acsearch.acr.org/docs/69442/Narrative/. Accessed January 2017.
15. Bhattacharyya N, Lee LN. Evaluating the diagnosis of chronic rhinosinusitis based on clinical guidelines and endoscopy. *Otolaryngol Head Neck Surg.* 2010;143(1):147-151.
16. van Zanten ARH, Dixon JM, Nipshagen MD, et al. Hospital-acquired sinusitis is a common cause of fever of unknown origin in orotracheally intubated critically ill patients. *Crit Care.* 2005; 9(5):R583-R590.
17. King D, Mitchell B, Williams CP, Spurling GKP. Saline nasal irrigation for acute upper respiratory tract infections. *Cochrane Database Syst Rev.* 2015;(3):CD006821.
18. Chong LY, Head K, Hopkins C, et al. Saline irrigation for chronic rhinosinusitis. *Cochrane Database Syst Rev.* 2016;(2):CD0011995.
19. Rudmik L, Soler ZM. Medical therapies for adult chronic sinusitis. *JAMA.* 2015;334(9):926-939.
20. Shaikh N, Wald ER. Decongestants, antihistamines and nasal irrigation for acute sinusitis in children. *Cochrane Database Syst Rev.* 2014;(4):CD007909.
21. Zalmanovici Trestioreanu A, Yaphe J. Intranasal steroids for acute sinusitis. *Cochrane Database Syst Rev.* 2013;(4):CD005149.
22. Venekamp RP, Bonten MJ, Rovers MM, et al. Systemic corticosteroid monotherapy for clinically diagnosed acute rhinosinusitis: a randomized controlled trial. *CMAJ.* 2012;184(14):E751-757.
23. Lemiengre MB, van Driel ML, Merenstein D, et al. Antibiotics for clinically diagnosed acute rhinosinusitis in adults. *Cochrane Database Syst Rev.* 2012;(4):CD006089.
24. Guo R, Canter PH, Ernst E. Herbal medicines for the treatment of rhinosinusitis: a systematic review. *Otolaryngol Head Neck Surg.* 2006;135(4):496-506.
25. Khalil HS, Nunez DA. Functional endoscopic sinus surgery for chronic rhinosinusitis. *Cochrane Database Syst Rev.* 2006;3: CD004458.
26. Ahmed J, Pal S, Hopkins C, Jayaraj S. Functional endoscopic balloon dilation of sinus ostia for chronic rhinosinusitis. *Cochrane Database Syst Rev.* 2011;(2):CD008515.
27. Lal D, Scianna JM, Stankiewicz JA. Efficacy of targeted medical therapy in chronic rhinosinusitis, and predictors of failure. *Am J Rhinol Allergy.* 2009;23:396-400.

SECTION C MOUTH AND THROAT

34 ANGULAR CHEILITIS

Linda Speer, MD
Richard P. Usatine, MD

PATIENT STORY

A middle-aged woman presents to your office with soreness at the corners of her mouth for 4 months (**Figure 34-1**). On examination, she has cracking and fissures at the right corner of her mouth. She is diagnosed with angular cheilitis and treated with nonprescription nystatin ointment twice daily. Within 2 weeks she is fully healed.

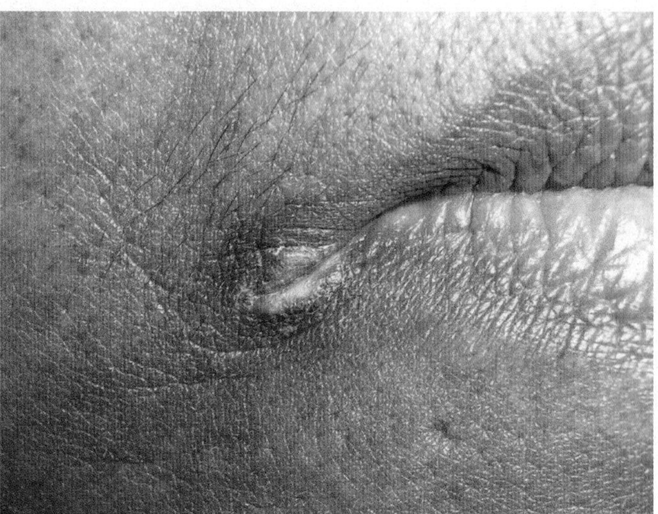

FIGURE 34-1 Angular cheilitis (perlèche). Note dry, erythematous, and fissured appearance. (*Reproduced with permission from Richard P. Usatine, MD.*)

INTRODUCTION

Angular cheilitis is an inflammatory lesion of the commissure or corner of the lip characterized by scaling and fissuring.

SYNONYM

Perlèche, angular cheilosis, commissural cheilitis, angular stomatitis.

EPIDEMIOLOGY

- Most common in the elderly, people with inflammatory bowel disease, and people with Down syndrome.[1–3] In one study of institutionalized elderly patients in Scotland, angular cheilitis was present in 25% of patients.[4]

ETIOLOGY AND PATHOPHYSIOLOGY

- Maceration is the usual predisposing factor. Microorganisms, most often *Candida albicans*, can then invade the macerated area (**Figure 34-2**).[5]
- It may also occur in infants and children related to drooling, thumb sucking, and lip licking (**Figure 34-3**).
- Lip licking can cause a contact dermatitis to the saliva along with perlèche (**Figure 34-4**). Perlèche is derived from the French word *lecher*, meaning "to lick."
- Historically associated with vitamin B deficiency, which is rare in developed countries.

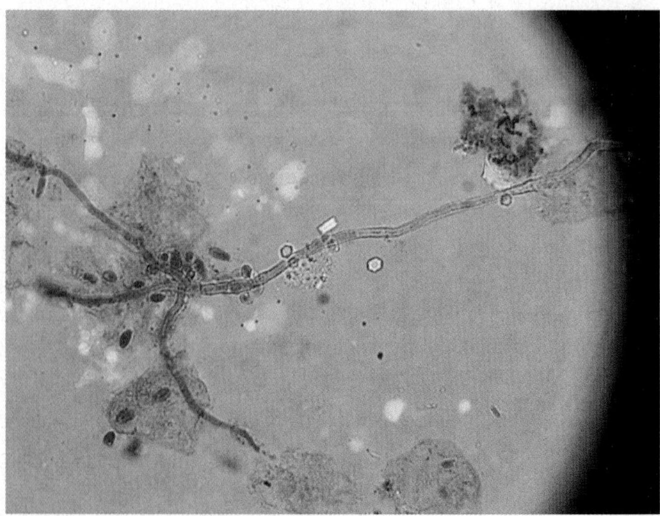

FIGURE 34-2 *Candida albicans* seen under the microscope after gently scraping a case of angular cheilitis and using KOH on the slide. (*Reproduced with permission from Richard P. Usatine, MD.*)

RISK FACTORS

- Maceration that can be related to poor dentition, deep facial wrinkles, orthodontic treatment, or poorly fitting dentures in the elderly (**Figure 34-5**).

- Other risk factors include incorrect use of dental floss causing trauma, or diseases that enlarge the lips such as orofacial granulomatosis.
- Atopic dermatitis (**Figure 34-6**).
- HIV or other types of immunodeficiency may lead to a more severe case of angular cheilitis with overgrowth of *Candida* (**Figure 34-7**).
- Use of isotretinoin, which dries the lips and predisposes to angular cheilitis.

DIAGNOSIS

CLINICAL FEATURES

- Erythema and fissuring at the corners of the mouth, without exudates or ulceration (see **Figures 34-3** to **34-7**).

TYPICAL DISTRIBUTION

- Corners of the mouth (oral commissures or angles of the mouth), hence the names commissural cheilitis and angular cheilitis.

LABORATORY

- A light scraping of the corner of the mouth can be placed on a slide with KOH to look for *Candida* (see **Figure 34-2**).

BIOPSY

- Not usually indicated.

DIFFERENTIAL DIAGNOSIS

- Impetigo—Yellowish crusts or exudates are characteristic of impetigo but not angular cheilitis (see Chapter 122, Impetigo).
- Herpes simplex (cold sores)—Initial blisters, followed by shallow ulcers, are characteristic of herpes simplex, but not angular cheilitis (see Chapter 135, Herpes Simplex).

MANAGEMENT

NONPHARMACOLOGIC

- Attempt to relieve precipitating causes such as poorly fitting dentures.
- Counsel patients to stop licking their lips if this is part of the cause (see **Figure 34-4**).
- Recommend protective petrolatum or lip balm as needed.
- Counsel patients to stop using tobacco, either chewing or smoking.

MEDICATIONS

- Recommend topical antifungal creams or ointments, such as clotrimazole, to be applied twice daily.[6] SOR Ⓑ
- Low-potency topical corticosteroid, such as 1% hydrocortisone cream twice daily, may be added to treat the inflammatory component. SOR Ⓑ
- Nystatin lozenges work well, but their use is limited because of their unpleasant taste.[6] SOR Ⓒ If thrush is also present, prescribe clotrimazole troches for treatment of both conditions.

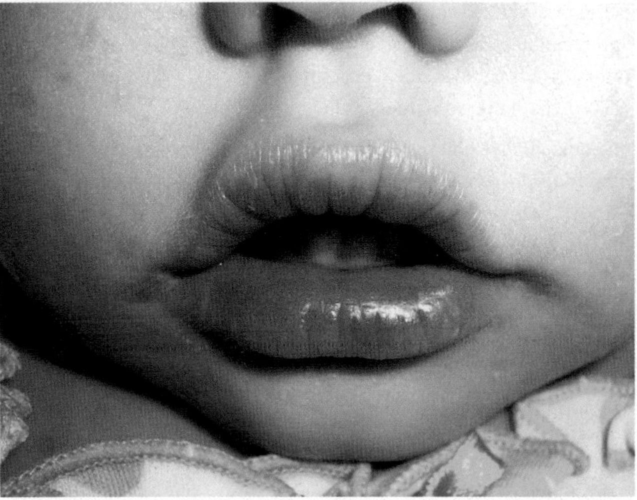

FIGURE 34-3 Angular cheilitis in a 1-year-old girl with widespread atopic dermatitis on her extremities. (*Reproduced with permission from Richard P. Usatine, MD.*)

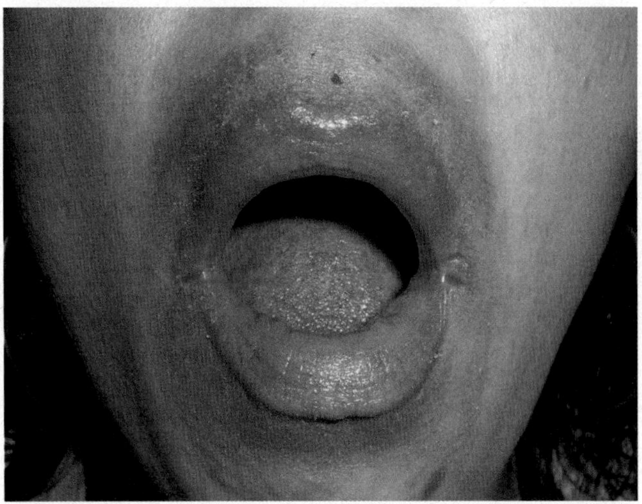

FIGURE 34-4 Perlèche in a woman with contact dermatitis related to lip licking. (*Reproduced with permission from Richard P. Usatine, MD.*)

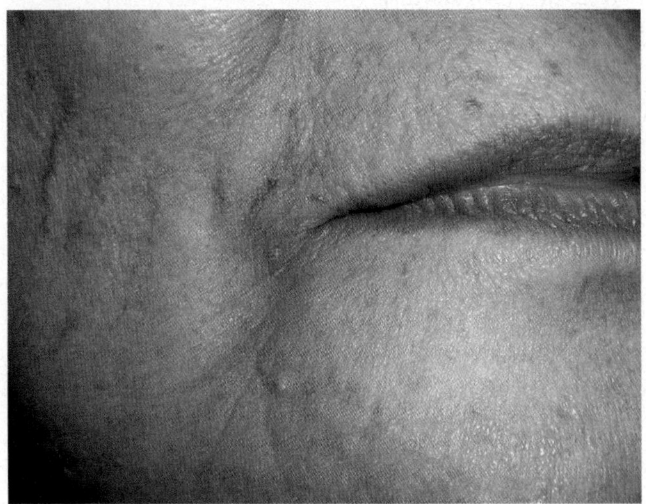

FIGURE 34-5 Angular cheilitis in an elderly woman. Note the wrinkles line extending downward from the corner of her mouth indicating some change in her facial anatomy that can predispose to this condition. The perlèche started while she was waiting for her dentures to be repaired. (*Reproduced with permission from Richard P. Usatine, MD.*)

- One randomized controlled study showed that medicated chewing gum can decrease the risk of angular cheilitis in older occupants of nursing homes. Consider recommending xylitol-containing gum to elderly patients with angular cheilitis.[7] SOR B
- Ozonized olive oil applied topically twice daily was associated with lesion improvement or resolution in one small observational study.[8] SOR C

PREVENTION

Attempt to identify predisposing factors and correct if possible, such as:

- Edentulousness.
- Poorly fitting dentures.
- Drooling.
- Lip licking (see **Figure 34-4**).
- Atopic dermatitis (see **Figures 34-3** and **34-6**).

Protective lip balm may be helpful to prevent recurrences if the patient is not allergic to chemicals within the product. Plain petrolatum is often the safest product for dry lips.

PATIENT EDUCATION

- Encourage patients to identify and correct predisposing factors (as above). Protective lip balm may be helpful.

PATIENT AND PROVIDER RESOURCES

- **http://www.stevedds.com (search Angular Cheilitis).**
- **http://www.ncemi.org/cse/cse0409.htm.**

REFERENCES

1. Al-Maweri SA, Tarakii B, Al-Sufvani GA, et al. Lip and oral lesions in children with Down syndrome. A controlled study. *J Clin Exp Dent*. 2015;7(2):e284-e288.
2. Pereira MS, Munerato MC. Oral manifestations of inflammatory bowel diseases: two case reports. *Clin Med Res*. 2016;14(1):46-52.
3. Skrzsat A, Olczak-Kovalszyk D, Turska-Szybka A. Crohn's disease should be considered in children with inflammatory oral lesions. *Acta Paediatr*. 2017;106(2):199-203.
4. Samaranayake LP, Wilkieson CA, Lamey PJ, MacFarlane TW. Oral disease in the elderly in long-term hospital care. *Oral Dis*. 1995;1(3): 147-151.
5. Sharon V, Fazel N. Oral candidiasis and angular cheilitis. *Dermatol Ther*. 2010;23(3):230-242.
6. Skinner N, Junker JA, Flake D, Hoffman R. Clinical inquiries. What is angular cheilitis and how is it treated? *J Fam Pract*. 2005;54(5):470-471.
7. Simons D, Brailsford SR, Kidd EA, Beighton D. The effect of medicated chewing gums on oral health in frail older people: a 1-year clinical trial. *J Am Geriatr Soc*. 2002;50(8):1348-1353.
8. Kumar T, Arora N, Puri G, et al. Efficacy of ozonized olive oil in the management of oral lesions and conditions: a clinical trial. *Contemp Clin Dent*. 2016;7(1):51-54.

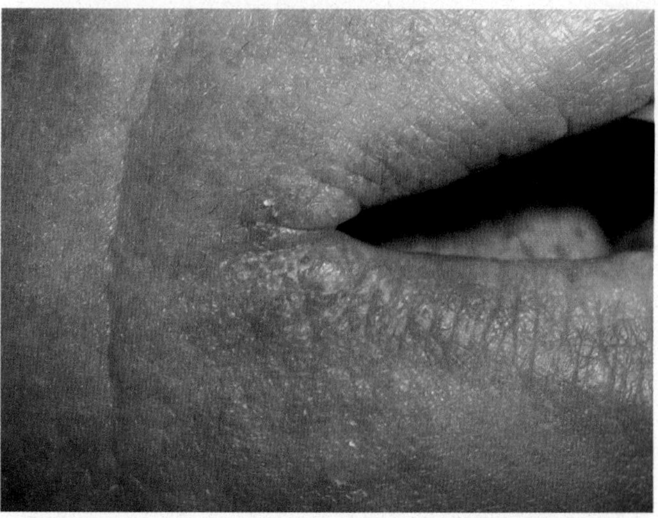

FIGURE 34-6 Angular cheilitis in a woman with atopic dermatitis. (*Reproduced with permission from Richard P. Usatine, MD.*)

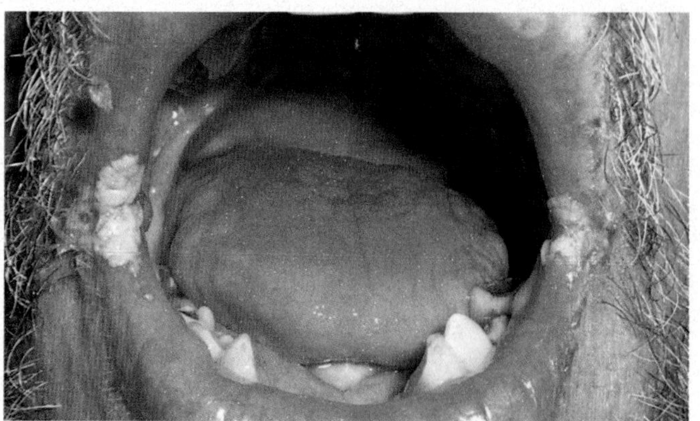

FIGURE 34-7 Severe angular cheilitis in an HIV-positive man with thrush. Note the obvious white *Candida* growth on both corners of his mouth. (*Reproduced with permission from Richard P. Usatine, MD.*)

35 TORUS PALATINUS

Linda Speer, MD
Mindy A. Smith, MD, MS

PATIENT STORY

An elderly woman is in the office for a physical examination. While looking in her mouth, you see a torus at the midline on the hard palate (**Figure 35-1**). She states that she has had this for her whole adult life and it does not bother her. You explain to her that it is a torus palatinus and that nothing needs to be done. She is pleased to know the name of this lump and even happier to know that it is not harmful.

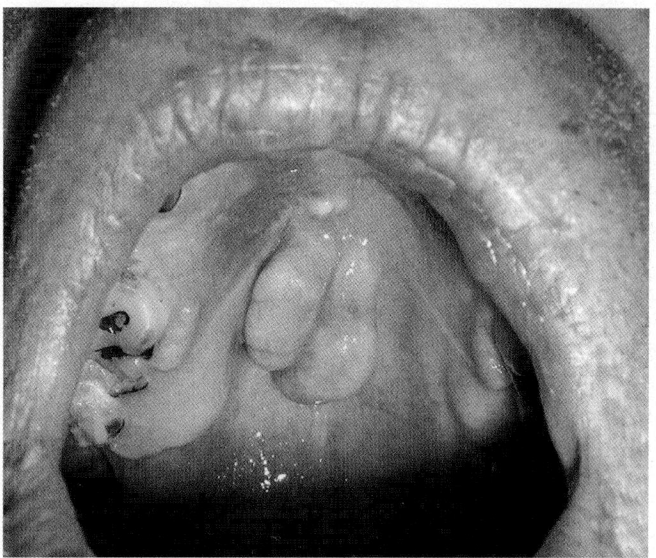

FIGURE 35-1 Torus palatinus in a 67-year-old man. The patient was asymptomatic and this was an incidental finding. (*Reproduced with permission from Richard P. Usatine, MD.*)

INTRODUCTION

Torus palatinus is a benign bony exostosis (bony growth) occurring in the midline of the hard palate. Torus mandibularis often presents as multiple benign bony exostoses on the floor of the mouth. Two less common tori are the torus maxillaris, located near the upper premolars and torus auditivus, usually located on the floor of the external acoustic meatus.[1]

EPIDEMIOLOGY

- Most common bony maxillofacial exostosis, unclear origin.
- Usually in adults older than 30 years of age.
- Prevalence of torus palatinus ranges from 9.5% to 26.9%; among ethnic groups, the range is wider (0.9% in Vietnamese to 33.8% among African Americans).[2] Prevalence of torus mandibularis is about 6%.[1]
- More common in women than men for torus palatinus; the reverse is true for torus mandibularis.[1]
- Some populations seem to be more predisposed (e.g., Middle Eastern).[3]
- An autosomal dominant inheritance is postulated for the oral tori.[1]

DIAGNOSIS

CLINICAL FEATURES

- Hard lump protruding from the hard palate into the mouth covered with normal mucous membrane (**Figure 35-2**).
- Small size (<2 mm) appear most frequent (70% to 91%).[2]
- Shapes include flat, nodular, lobular, or spindle-shaped; nodular appear most common.[2]

TYPICAL DISTRIBUTION

- Midline hard palate.

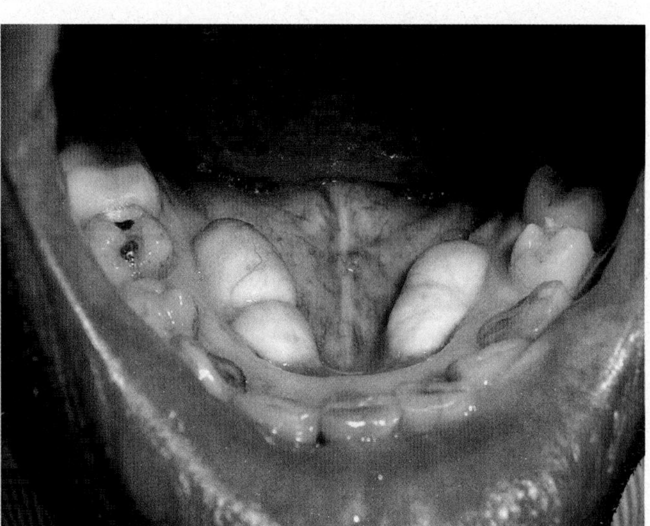

FIGURE 35-2 Torus mandibularis seen under the tongue caused by bony exostoses. Note these are bilateral and appear similar to a torus palatinus. Although this patient had multiple untreated dental problems, the tori were asymptomatic and this was an incidental finding. (*Reproduced with permission from Richard P. Usatine, MD.*)

DIFFERENTIAL DIAGNOSIS

- Torus mandibularis is also a bony exostosis but is found under the tongue. These appear similar to a torus palatinus but are usually bilateral (80%) rather than midline (see **Figure 35-2**).
- Squamous cell carcinoma is not as hard and the mucous membranes are usually ulcerated. Mucous membranes are normal in appearance with torus palatinus unless traumatized.
- Adenoid cystic carcinoma is a rare tumor that can start in a minor salivary gland over the hard palate. Note that this tumor will not be midline as found in the torus palatinus. If a suspected torus is not midline, a biopsy is needed to rule out this potentially fatal carcinoma (**Figure 35-3**).

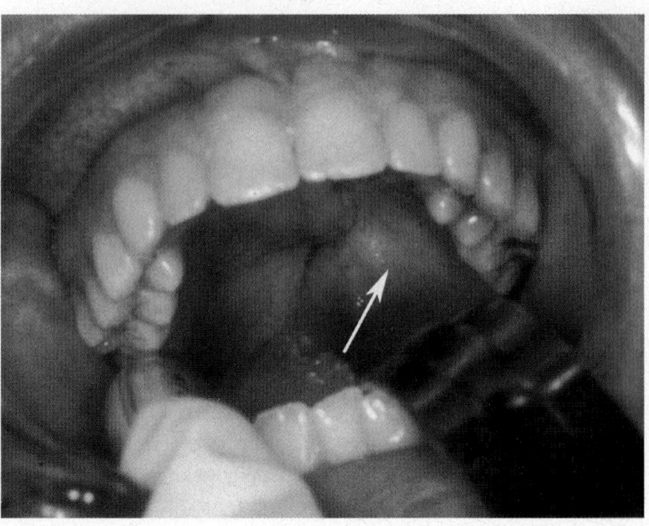

FIGURE 35-3 Adenoid cystic carcinoma in a 22-year-old woman. The arrow points to this unilateral tumor that should not be confused with a torus palatinus. (*Reproduced with permission from Randal A. Otto, MD.*)

MANAGEMENT

- Excision can be considered if the lesion interferes with function, such as the fit of dentures. This is performed as an outpatient procedure.[4,5]
- Sometimes removed because of disturbances of phonation, traumatic inflammation or ulcer, aesthetic reasons, or as source of autogenous cortical bone for grafts in periodontal surgery.[2]

PROGNOSIS

- Very slow growing; can stop growth spontaneously.[2]
- Surgical complications include perforation of nasal cavities, palatine nerve damage, bone necrosis, hemorrhage, and fracture of palatine bone.[2]

PATIENT EDUCATION

- Patients should be informed about the benign nature of the lesion and that removal can be considered, if bothersome.

PATIENT RESOURCES

- **http://fpnotebook.com/Dental/Palate/TrsPltns.htm.**

REFERENCES

1. Loukas M, Hulsberg P, Tubbs RS, et al. The tori of the mouth and ear: a review. *Clin Anat.* 2013;26:953-960.
2. García-García AS, Martínez-González JM, Gómez-Font R, et al. Current status of the torus palatinus and torus mandibularis. *Med Oral Patol Oral Cir Bucal.* 2010;15(2):e353-e360.
3. Yildiz E, Deniz M, Ceyhan O. Prevalence of torus palatinus in Turkish school children. *Surg Radiol Anat.* 2005;27:368-371.
4. Al-Quran FA, Al-Dwairi ZN. Torus palatinus and torus mandibularis in edentulous patients. *J Contemp Dent Pract.* 2006;7:112-119.
5. Cagirankaya LB, Dansu O, Hatipoglu MG. Is torus palatinus a feature of a well-developed maxilla? *Clin Anat.* 2004;17:623-625.

36 SCARLET FEVER AND STRAWBERRY TONGUE

Mark Jason Sanders, MD
Linda Speer, MD

PATIENT STORY

A 7-year-old boy is brought to the family physician's office with a rough red rash on his trunk (**Figures 36-1** and **36-2**) along with fever and a sore throat. The sandpaper rash and signs consistent with strep pharyngitis lead the physician to diagnose scarlet fever. The physician explains the diagnosis to the mother, and oral Pen VK is prescribed. The boy feels markedly better by the next day, and the mother continues to give the penicillin for the full 10 days as directed to prevent rheumatic fever.

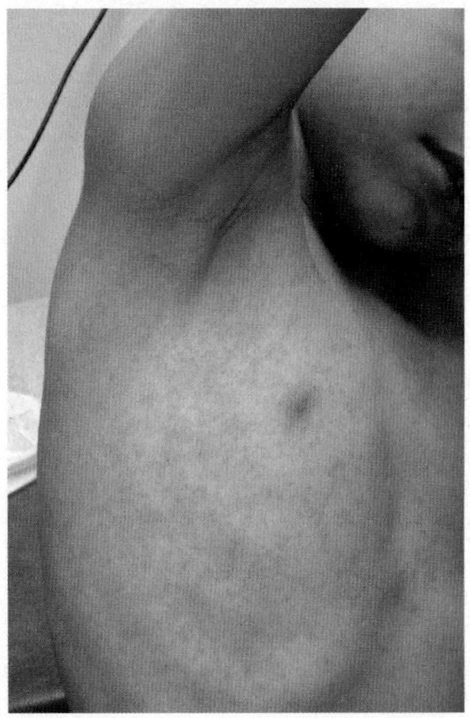

FIGURE 36-1 Sandpaper rash on the trunk and in the axilla of a 7-year-old boy with scarlet fever. *(Reproduced with permission from Richard P. Usatine, MD.)*

INTRODUCTION

Scarlet fever is an illness caused by toxin-producing group A β-hemolytic streptococci. Most commonly, scarlet fever evolves from an exudative pharyngitis.

Strawberry tongue may be observed in patients with scarlet fever, and usually develops within the first 2 to 3 days of illness. A white or yellowish coating usually precedes the classic red tongue with white papillae (**Figure 36-3**).

EPIDEMIOLOGY

- Scarlet fever is predominately seen in school-age children with no gender predilection.
- Majority related to strep pharyngitis, with 1 in 10 developing scarlet fever (**Figures 36-1**, **36-2**, and **36-4**).
- Prevalent in late fall to early spring.
- Strawberry tongue (see **Figure 36-4**) is most commonly seen in children in association with scarlet fever or Kawasaki disease.
- Can be present with other group A *Streptococcus* (strep) infections.
- In cases of strep, a white membrane through which the papillae are seen can initially cover the tongue, followed by desquamation of the membrane (with the appearance as in **Figure 36-4**).

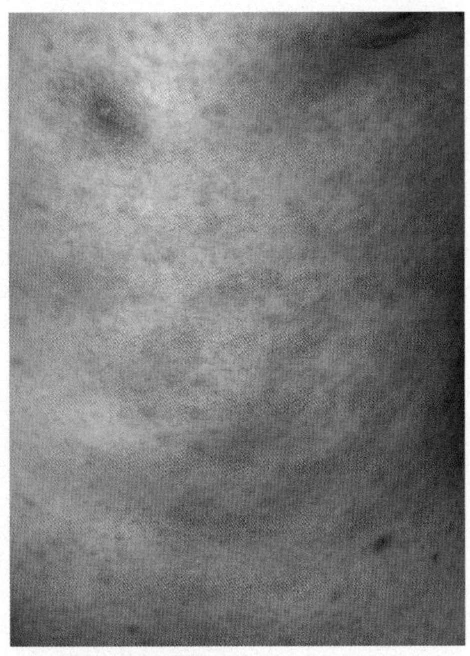

FIGURE 36-2 Scarlatiniform rash comprising small papules and erythema on the trunk of a febrile child with strep pharyngitis. *(Reproduced with permission from Richard P. Usatine, MD.)*

ETIOLOGY AND PATHOPHYSIOLOGY

- Transmission of *Streptococcus* occurs via respiratory secretions.
- Virulent *Streptococcus pyogenes* (group A streptococcus or GAS) incubate more than 2 to 7 days. M protein serotypes of GAS are typically more invasive with greater potential for progression to rheumatic fever or acute glomerulonephritis if untreated.[1]
- Fever and rash are related to pyrogenic A–C and erythrogenic exotoxins produced by GAS.[2]

- Infection may originate from other sites such as skin (e.g., cellulitis), and then seed blood (bacteremia) or organ systems (e.g., pneumonia).
- Strawberry tongue results from a general inflammatory response during the early course of the disease.

DIAGNOSIS

CLINICAL FEATURES

- Headache, sore throat, cervical lymphadenopathy, abdominal pain, nausea and vomiting, decreased oral intake, malaise, and fever may precede rash. Cough is usually not present.
- Oropharyngeal findings include:
  - Strawberry tongue—Erythematous and sometimes edematous tongue with prominent papillae (see **Figure 36-4**).
- May be covered by a white membrane/coating through which the papillae can be seen.
- Not typically painful.
- Forchheimer spots—Palatal and uvular petechiae and erythematous macules.
- Initial sandpaper rash, associated with blanching erythema and occasional pruritus, erupts in 1 to 2 days (see **Figures 36-1** to **36-3**).[2]
- Pastia lines are pink or red lines seen in the body folds (especially elbows and axilla) during scarlet fever. Linear hyperpigmentation may persist after the rash fades (see **Figure 36-1**).
- Desquamation of the skin (especially of the hands and feet) ensues in 3 to 4 days as rash fades and can persist for 2 to 4 weeks.[1]

TYPICAL DISTRIBUTION

- Progresses centrally (torso) to peripherally (extremities) and can be prominent on the face, chest, palms, fingers, and toes.[1]

LABORATORY TESTS AND IMAGING

- Throat swab for rapid strep testing (screening) and/or culture (confirmation) is usually performed.
- Complete blood count (CBC), if indicated, to look for:
  - Elevation of white blood cell count with left shift
  - Elevated platelet count—Seen with Kawasaki disease (after 1 week)
- Antistreptolysin-*O* titer is obtained to confirm prior infection or support suspected poststreptococcal complication, such as rheumatic fever.[3]
- Acute phase reactants (C-reactive protein [CRP] and erythrocyte sedimentation rate [ESR]) may be elevated and may be useful in monitoring nonsuppurative complications such as rheumatic fever.[4]
- If Kawasaki disease is suspected, two-dimensional echocardiography or angiography is obtained to detect coronary artery abnormalities. The initial echocardiogram should be performed as soon as the diagnosis is suspected to establish a baseline for longitudinal follow-up of coronary artery morphology, left ventricular and left valvular function, and the evolution and resolution of pericardial effusion when present.[4] SOR Ⓒ

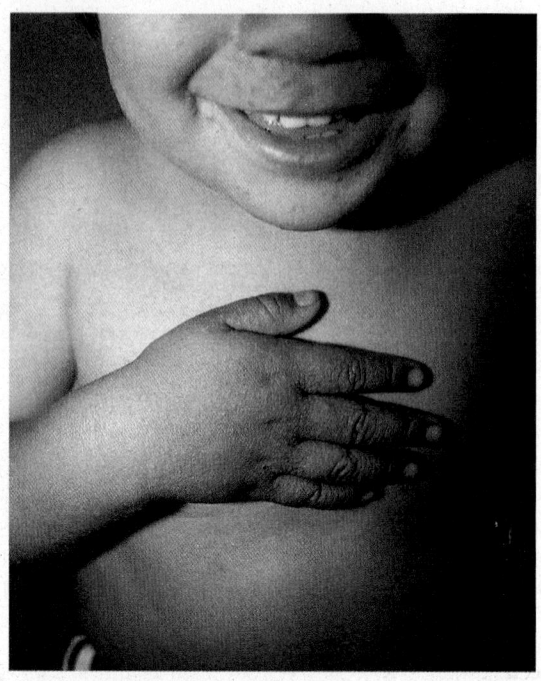

FIGURE 36-3 Sandpaper rash (scarlatiniform) seen prominently on the hand of a child recovering from strep pharyngitis. (*Reproduced with permission from Richard P. Usatine, MD.*)

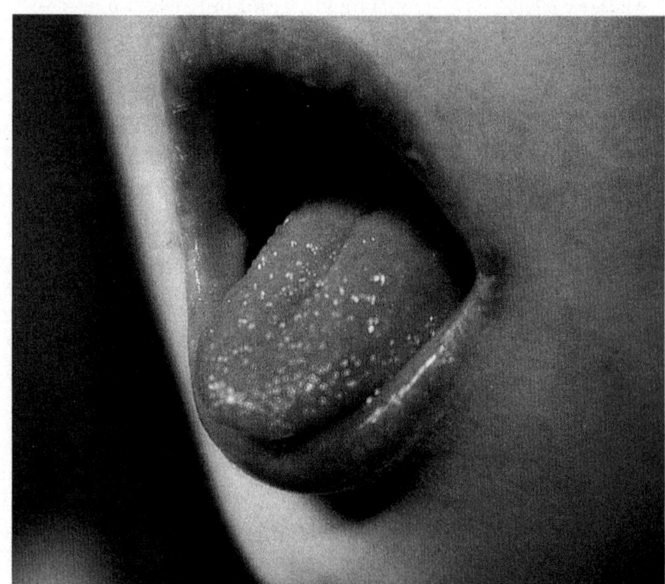

FIGURE 36-4 Strawberry tongue in a child with scarlet fever caused by strep pharyngitis; note marked erythema and prominent papillae. (*Reproduced with permission from Richard P. Usatine, MD.*)

DIFFERENTIAL DIAGNOSIS

The rash of scarlet fever may be confused with the following:

- Allergic/contact dermatitis—Often localized to areas of contact; prominent pruritus and skin vesicles often in linear streaks (see Chapter 151, Atopic Dermatitis and Chapter 152, Contact Dermatitis).
- Viral exanthem—Many viral exanthems have prodromal phases with fever followed by skin rashes that can be macular or maculopapular including measles (see Chapter 132, Measles), rubella (tender retroauricular, cervical, and occipital lymphadenopathy, and rash starts on face and spreads and fades quickly), and roseola (rash occurs at the end of a period of 3 to 5 days of high fever). Lack of sandpaper feel and oral findings help distinguish.
- Staphylococcal scalded skin syndrome—Rash may also follow a prodrome of malaise and fever but is macular, brightly erythematous, and initially involves the face, neck axilla, and groin. Skin is markedly tender and large areas of the epidermis peel away.
- Erythema toxicum—Rash of newborns; often blotchy, evanescent, macular erythema that can include pale yellow or white wheals or papules on an erythematous base (see Chapter 114, Normal Skin Changes).

The differential diagnosis for strawberry tongue includes:

- Kawasaki disease (**Figure 36-5**) is an acute childhood systemic vasculitis with predilection for the coronary arteries, of unknown etiology but presumed caused by a pathogen that triggers an exaggerated autoimmune response.[5] Fever persists at least 5 days, and there must be the presence of at least four principal features including the following[4]:
    - Changes in extremities—Acute: Erythema of palms, soles; edema of hands and feet. Subacute: Periungual peeling of fingers and toes in weeks 2 and 3
    - Polymorphous exanthem
    - Bilateral bulbar conjunctival injection without exudate
    - Changes in lips and oral cavity—Erythema, lips cracking, strawberry tongue, diffuse injection of oral and pharyngeal mucosae
    - Cervical lymphadenopathy (>1.5 cm diameter), usually unilateral
- Viral stomatitis with eruptive lingual papillitis—Lack of other features for scarlet fever or Kawasaki disease will assist in differentiating.
- Red-colored food dyes—History is helpful; edema and prominent papillae will be absent.

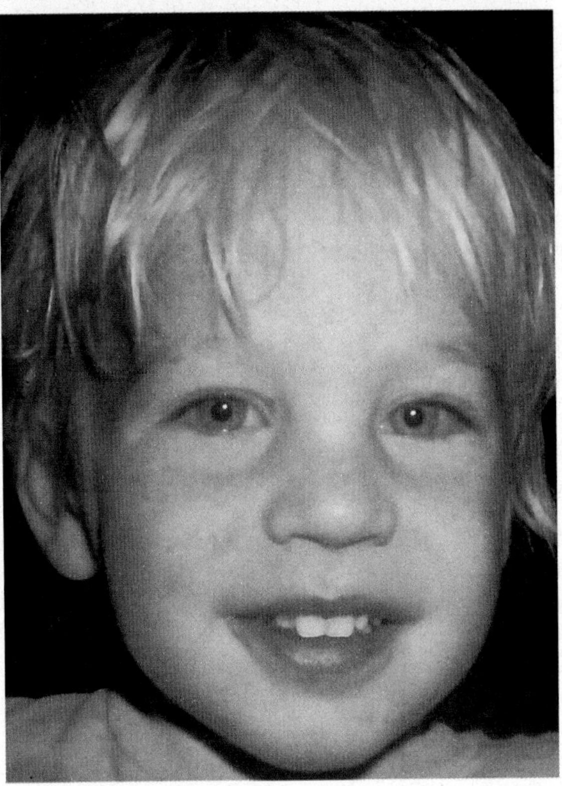

FIGURE 36-5 Child recovering from Kawasaki disease. Note the conjunctival injection that still remains. (*Reproduced with permission from Greg Thompson, MD.*)

MANAGEMENT

NONPHARMACOLOGIC

- Supportive care with oral fluids and age-appropriate symptomatic measures, such as salt-water gargles, and an antipyretic as needed are recommended.

MEDICATIONS

- For scarlet fever and strawberry tongue caused by group A *Streptococcus*:
    - Oral penicillin (penicillin VK 500 mg divided twice daily or 250 mg divided 4 times daily for 10 days for adults or 25 to

50 mg/kg per day divided 4 times daily for 10 days for children) or macrolide (erythromycin base 500 mg 4 times daily for 10 days for adults or erythromycin estolate 20 mg/kg per day or succinate 40 mg/kg per day divided twice daily for 10 days for children) in penicillin-allergic patients for 10 days.[6] SOR Ⓐ
    - Cephalosporins are an efficacious alternative (e.g., cefuroxime axetil 250 mg twice daily for 10 days for adults or 20 mg/kg per day divided twice daily for 10 days for children); cephalosporins were better than penicillin in a meta-analysis.[7] SOR Ⓐ
    - Symptoms typically resolve in 4 to 7 days
- For strawberry tongue caused by Kawasaki disease:
    - Intravenous gamma globulin (IVIG), 2 g/kg in a single infusion, within 7 to 10 days of onset for Kawasaki disease to reduce subsequent coronary artery abnormalities.[4] SOR Ⓐ Additional IVIG infusion may be considered if defervescence is not achieved in the first 1 to 2 days.[8]
    - In the acute phase, aspirin is also administered at 80 to 100 mg/kg per day in 4 doses with IVIG followed by low-dose aspirin (3 to 5 mg/kg per day) until the patient shows no evidence of coronary changes by 6 to 8 weeks after the onset of illness.[4] SOR Ⓒ

REFERRAL OR HOSPITALIZATION

- Hospitalization should be considered if a patient is dehydrated or exhibits cardiorespiratory instability. It should also be considered for cases of complicated scarlet fever, streptococcal toxic shock, staphylococcal scalded skin, rheumatic fever, acute glomerulonephritis, or Kawasaki disease (when suspected).
- Cardiology, infectious disease, or nephrology consultation may be indicated in the most severe cases.

PREVENTION

- In a randomized clinical trial of 222 kindergarten children, administration of *Streptococcus salivarius* K12 (a probiotic strain strongly antagonistic to the growth of *Streptococcus pyogenes*) reduced the incidence of streptococcal pharyngotonsillitis and otitis media but not scarlet fever compared to the control group during the 6-month trial and at 3-months follow-up.[9] It is available in a number of different over-the-counter brands.

PROGNOSIS

Scarlet fever usually follows a benign course. Rarely it is complicated by septic shock and multi-organ failure, suppurative complications such as peritonsillar abscess, or nonsuppurative complications such as rheumatic fever or poststreptococcal glomerulonephritis

FOLLOW-UP

- Routine follow-up is not required unless illness is protracted or a complication is suspected.
- For patients with uncomplicated Kawasaki disease, echocardiographic evaluation should be performed at the time of diagnosis, at 2 weeks, and at 6 to 8 weeks after onset of the disease.[4] SOR Ⓒ

Recent studies show that repeat echocardiography performed 1 year after the onset of the illness is unlikely to reveal coronary artery enlargement in patients whose echocardiographic findings were normal at 4 to 8 weeks.[4]

PATIENT EDUCATION

- Contact physician for fever recurrence, atypical or persistent rash, and new symptoms or potential complications (meningitis, sinusitis, otitis media, oropharyngeal abscess, pneumonia, acute glomerulonephritis, or rheumatic fever).
- Completion of a prescribed antibiotic course is encouraged to decrease the incidence of recurrence and potential complications.[3]

PATIENT RESOURCES

- CDC patient information—**https://www.cdc.gov/features/scarletfever/index.html.**

PROVIDER RESOURCES

- CDC for clinicians—**https://www.cdc.gov/groupastrep/diseases-hcp/scarlet-fever.html.**

REFERENCES

1. Cunningham MW. Pathogenesis of group A streptococcal infections. *Clin Microbiol Rev.* 2000;13(3):470-511.
2. Cherry JD. Contemporary infectious exanthems. *Clin Infect Dis.* 1993;16(2):199-205.
3. Hahn RG, Knox LM, Forman TA. Evaluation of poststreptococcal illness. *Am Fam Physician.* 2005;71(10):1949-1954.
4. Newburger JW, Takahashi M, Gerber MA, et al. Diagnosis, treatment, and long-term management of Kawasaki disease: a statement for health professionals from the Committee on Rheumatic Fever, Endocarditis and Kawasaki Disease, Council on Cardiovascular Disease in the Young, American Heart Association. *Circulation.* 2004;110(17):2747-2771.
5. Saguil A, Fargo M. Diagnosis and management of Kawasaki disease. *Am Fam Physician.* 2015;91(6):365-371.
6. Gilbert DN, Moellering RC, Eliopoulos GM, et al. *The Sanford Guide to Antimicrobial Therapy 2010.* 40th ed. Sperryville, VA: Antimicrobial Therapy, Inc.; 2010.
7. Casey JR, Pichichero ME. Meta-analysis of cephalosporin versus penicillin treatment of group A streptococcal tonsillopharyngitis in children. *Pediatrics.* 2004;113(4):866-882.
8. Freeman AF, Shulman ST. Kawasaki disease: summary of the American Heart Association guidelines. *Am Fam Physician.* 2006;74(7):1141-1148.
9. Di Pierro F, Colombo M, Giuliani MG, et al. Effect of administration of *Streptococcus salivarius* K12 on the occurrence of streptococcal pharyngo-tonsillitis, scarlet fever and acute otitis media in 3 years old children. *Eur Rev Med Pharmacol Sci.* 2016;20(21):4601-4606.

37 PHARYNGITIS

Brian D. Williams, MD, MPH
Richard P. Usatine, MD
Mindy A. Smith, MD, MS

PATIENT STORY

A 27-year-old woman complains of 2 days of sore throat, fever, and chills. She is unable to swallow anything other than liquids because of severe odynophagia. She denies any congestion or cough. On examination, she has bilateral tonsillar erythema and exudate (**Figure 37-1**). Her anterior cervical lymph nodes are tender. Based on the presence of fever, absence of cough, tender lymphadenopathy, and tonsillar exudate, you believe that she has a high probability of group A β-hemolytic *Streptococcus* (GABHS) pharyngitis. A rapid antigen detection test confirms the diagnosis, and you prescribe antibiotics.

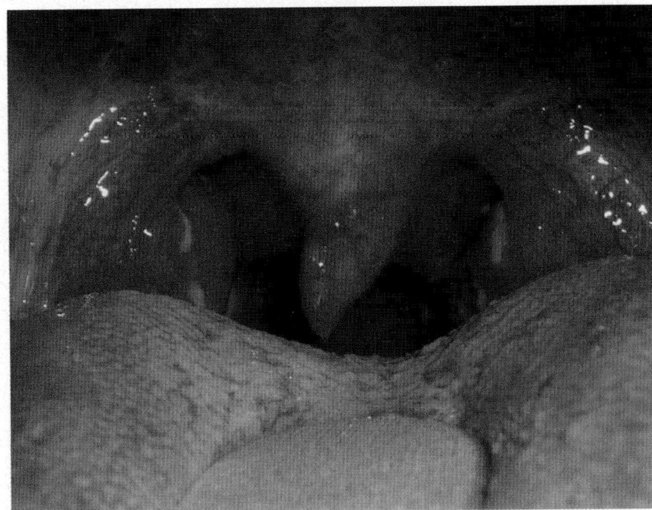

FIGURE 37-1 Strep pharyngitis showing tonsillar exudate and erythema. (*Reproduced with permission from Richard P. Usatine, MD.*)

INTRODUCTION

Pharyngitis is inflammation of the pharyngeal tissues and is usually associated with pain. The complaint of "sore throat" is a common one in the primary care office and can be accompanied by other symptoms and signs including throat scratchiness, fever, headache, malaise, rash, joint and muscle pains, and swollen lymph nodes.

EPIDEMIOLOGY

- Pharyngitis accounts for 1% of primary care visits.[1]
- Viral infections account for an estimated 60% to 90% of cases of pharyngitis.
- In patients ages 16–20 years, 1 in 13 presenting with sore throat have mononucleosis.[2]
- Bacterial infections are responsible for between 5% and 30% of pharyngitis cases, depending on the age of the population (higher rates among children ages 4–7 years) and season (highest in winter).
- The GABHS accounts for 5% to 15% of pharyngitis in adults and 20% to 30% in children.[3] Up to 38% of cases of tonsillitis are because of GABHS.
- Acute rheumatic fever is currently rare in the United States.
- Up to 14% of deep neck infections result from pharyngitis.[4]

ETIOLOGY AND PATHOPHYSIOLOGY

- Some viruses, such as adenovirus, cause inflammation of the pharyngeal mucosa by direct invasion of the mucosa or secondary to suprapharyngeal secretions.[5] Other viruses, such as rhinovirus, cause pain through stimulation of pain nerve endings by mediators, such as bradykinin.
- The GABHS releases exotoxins and proteases. Erythrogenic exotoxins are responsible for the development of the scarlatiniform exanthem (**Figure 37-2**).[6] Secondary antibody formation because of

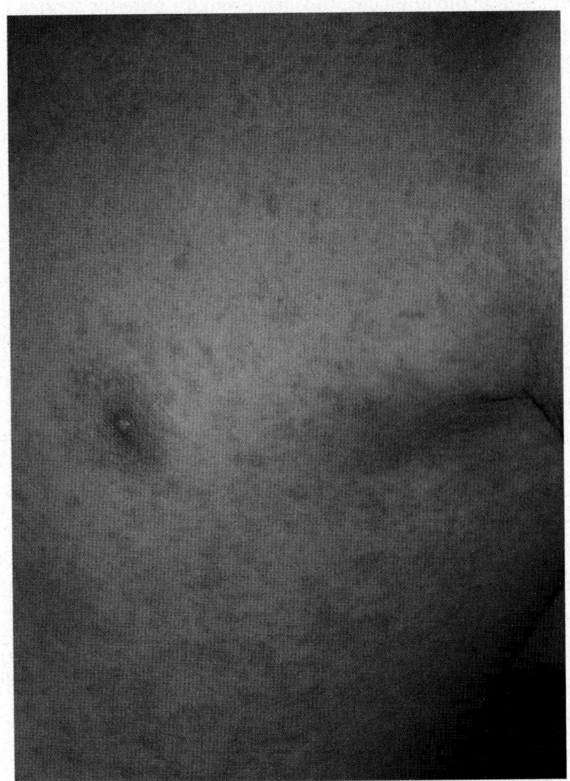

FIGURE 37-2 Scarlatiniform rash in scarlet fever. This 7-year-old boy has a typical sandpaper rash with his strep throat and fever. The erythema is particularly concentrated in the axillary area. (*Reproduced with permission from Richard P. Usatine, MD.*)

cross-reactivity with the M protein (a virulence factor located peripherally on the cell wall) may result in rheumatic fever and valvular heart disease.[6] Antigen–antibody complexes may lead to acute poststreptococcal glomerulonephritis.

- Untreated GABHS pharyngitis can result in suppurative complications including bacteremia, otitis media, meningitis, mastoiditis, cervical lymphadenitis, endocarditis, pneumonia, or peritonsillar abscess formation (**Figure 37-3**). Nonsuppurative complications include rheumatic fever and poststreptococcal glomerulonephritis.

RISK FACTORS

- GABHS: children aged 5 to 15 years, exposure to GABHS, presentation in winter or early spring.
- Immune deficiency.
- Chronic irritation (e.g., allergies, cigarette smoking).

DIAGNOSIS

CLINICAL FEATURES

- Rhinorrhea, cough, oral ulcers, and/or hoarseness are more consistent with a viral etiology.[3] Rigors, cough, and epidemic make influenza more likely. Posterior cervical, inguinal or axillary adenopathy; palatine petechiae; and splenomegaly make mononucleosis more likely,[2] as does fatigue.
- Rapid-onset odynophagia, tonsillar exudates, anterior cervical lymphadenopathy, and fever are consistent with streptococcal pharyngitis.
- Not all tonsillar exudates are caused by streptococcal pharyngitis. Mononucleosis and other viral pharyngitis can cause tonsillar exudates (**Figures 37-4** and **37-5**). The positive predictive value for tonsillar exudate in strep throat is only 31%; that is, 69% of patients with tonsillar exudate will have a non-streptococcal cause.
- Para- and supratonsillar edema with medial and/or anterior displacement of the involved tonsil and uvular displacement to the contralateral side suggest peritonsillar abscess (see **Figure 37-3**). Trismus and anterior cervical lymphadenopathy with severe tenderness to palpation are additional findings.
- Palatal petechiae can be seen in all types of pharyngitis (**Figure 37-6**).
- A sandpaper rash is suggestive of scarlet fever (see **Figure 37-2**, and Chapter 36, Scarlet Fever and Strawberry Tongue).
- Lymphoid hyperplasia can cause a cobblestone pattern on the posterior pharynx or palate from viral infections, gastroesophageal reflux disease (GERD), or allergies (**Figure 37-7**). Although it usually is more suggestive of a viral infection or allergic rhinitis, lymphoid hyperplasia can be seen in strep pharyngitis (**Figure 37-8**).
- The following criteria are helpful in the diagnosis of GABHS pharyngitis[7]:
    - Fever or temperature of 38°C (100.4°F) (1 point)
    - Absence of cough (1 point)
    - Tender anterior cervical lymph nodes (1 point)
    - Tonsillar swelling or exudates (1 point)

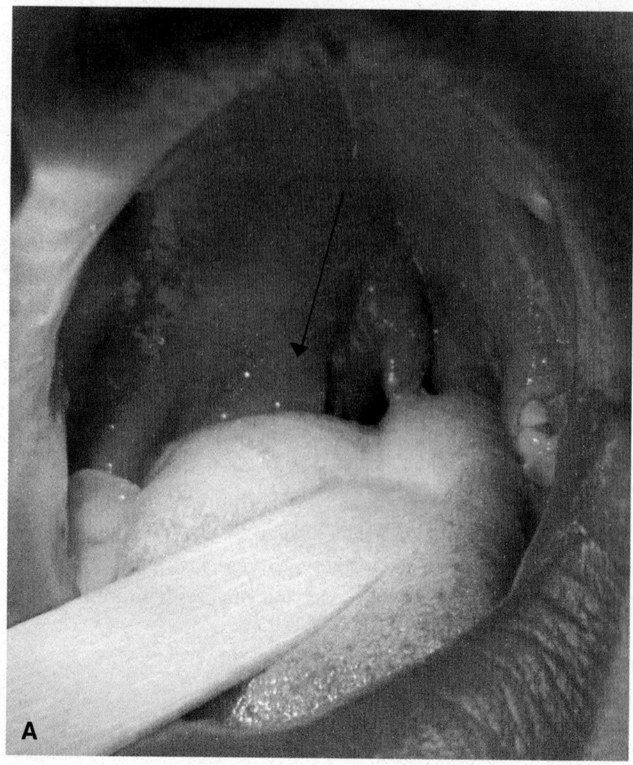

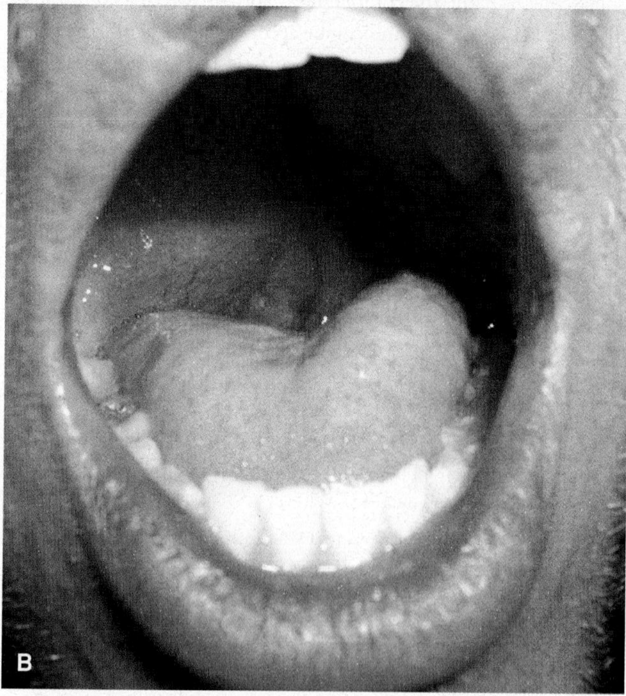

FIGURE 37-3 A. Peritonsillar abscess on the right showing uvular deviation away from the side with the abscess. (*Reproduced with permission from James Heilman, MD.*) B. Peritonsillar abscess with swelling and anatomic distortion of the right tonsillar region. (*Reproduced with permission from Charlie Goldberg, MD, and The Regents of the University of California.*)

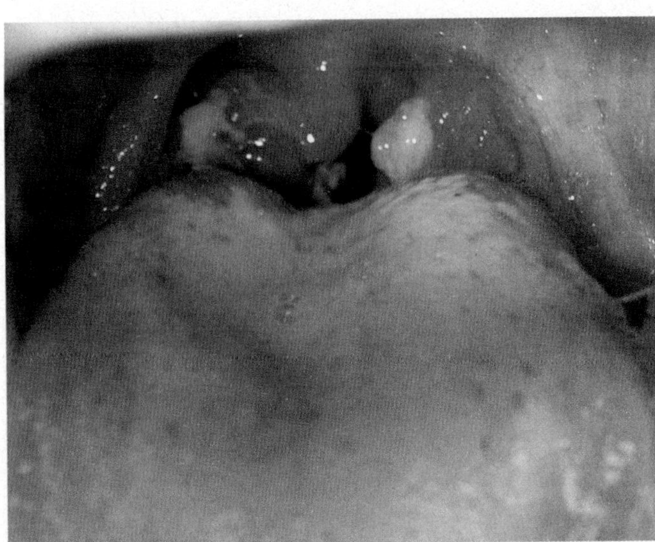

FIGURE 37-4 Mononucleosis in a young adult with considerable tonsillar exudate. (*Reproduced with permission from Richard P. Usatine, MD.*)

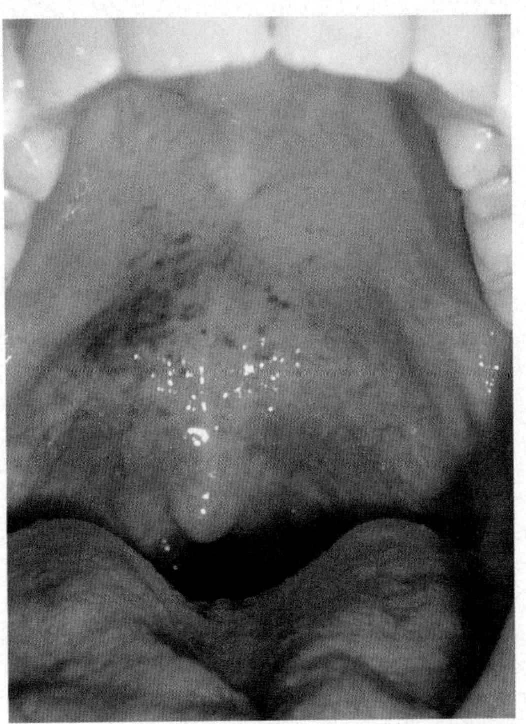

FIGURE 37-6 Viral pharyngitis with visible palatal petechiae. Palatal petechiae can be seen in all types of pharyngitis. (*Reproduced with permission from Richard P. Usatine, MD.*)

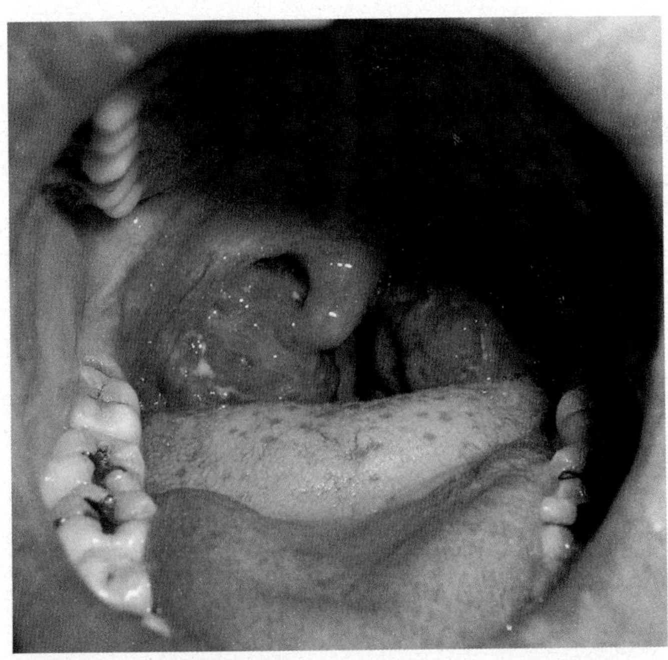

FIGURE 37-5 Viral pharyngitis in a young adult showing enlarged cryptic tonsils with some erythema and exudate. (*Reproduced with permission from Richard P. Usatine, MD.*)

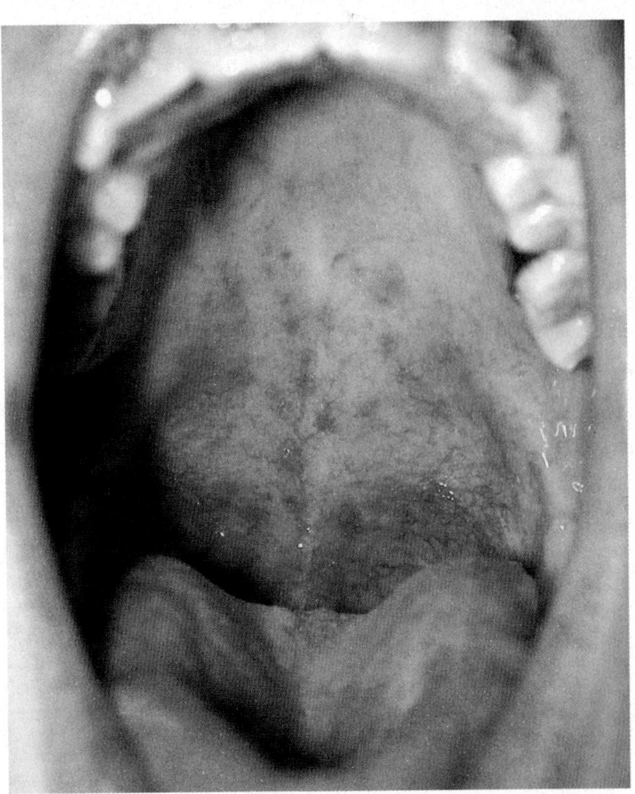

FIGURE 37-7 Viral pharyngitis with prominent vascular injection of the soft palate and lymphoid hyperplasia. (*Reproduced with permission from Richard P. Usatine, MD.*)

- Age:
  - <5 years (1 point)
  - 5 to 15 years (0 points)
  - >15 years (−1 point)

The probability of GABHS is approximately 12% with <2 points, 29% with 2 or 3 points, and approximately 55% with 4 to 5 points.[7]

LABORATORY TESTS AND IMAGING

- Rapid antigen detection testing (RADT) can be used to diagnose GABHS. Authors of a Cochrane review found a sensitivity of 85.6% and specificity of 95.4% in children.[8] The authors concluded, based on these results, that of 100 children with strep throat, 86 would be correctly detected with the rapid test while 14 would be missed and not receive antibiotic treatment. Conversely, among 100 children with non-streptococcal sore throat, 95 would be correctly classified with the rapid test while 5 would be misdiagnosed as having strep throat.
- The Infectious Disease Society of America (IDSA) recommends RADT for all patients with pharyngitis except for children under age 3 years or when sore throat is accompanied by overt viral features as above.[9] The Centers for Disease Control and Prevention/American College of Physicians also support testing using RADT or culture in adult patients with symptoms suggestive of group A streptococcal pharyngitis.[10]
- The gold standard for the diagnosis of streptococcal infection is a positive throat culture. However, GABHS is part of the normal oropharyngeal flora in many patients, and the definitive diagnosis of acute streptococcal pharyngitis must include both the clinical signs of acute infection and a positive throat culture.
  - Throat culture is recommended by IDSA for children and adolescents with a negative RADT. However, a throat culture is not considered necessary for adults with a negative RADT, because of the low likelihood that it will change management.[9]
  - The IDSA does not recommend routine follow-up posttreatment throat culture or RADT.[9]
- False-positive tests for streptococcal infection can occur when the patient is colonized with GABHS but is not the cause of the acute disease.
- False-negative tests for streptococcal infection can occur from poor sampling technique.
- A positive mono spot (likelihood ratio in the first week of illness: 5.7) and/or greater than 40% atypical lymphocytes on the peripheral smear (likelihood ratio: 39) indicate mononucleosis.[11]
- Viral cultures obtained from vesicles can be obtained in Coxsackievirus and herpes infections, but the diagnosis is usually based on clinical suspicion and findings.
- Ultrasonography can assist in the diagnosis and localization of peritonsillar abscess, and computed tomography scan should be obtained if further extension into the deeper neck is suspected.[12]

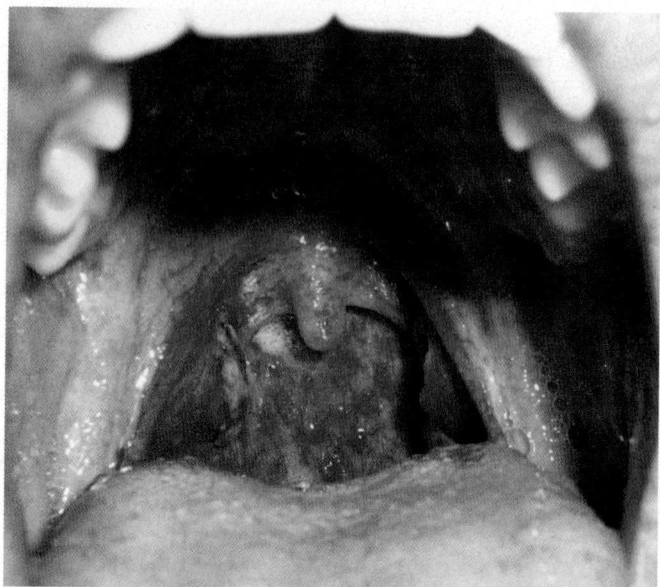

FIGURE 37-8 Strep pharyngitis with dark necrotic area on right tonsil and prominent lymphoid hyperplasia in a cobblestone pattern on the posterior pharynx. (*Reproduced with permission from Richard P. Usatine, MD.*)

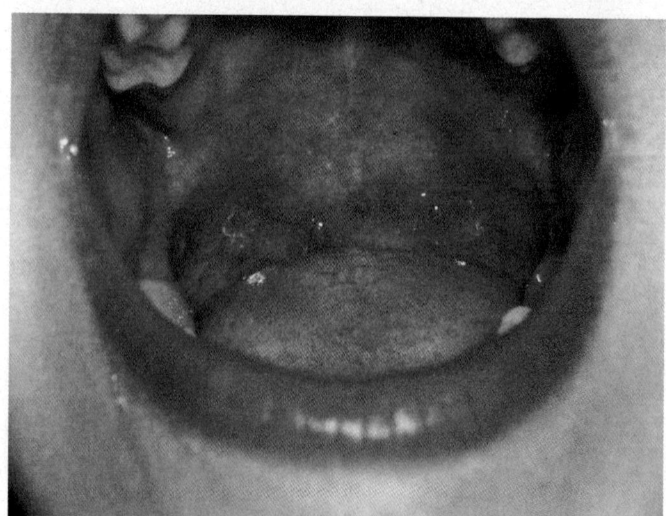

FIGURE 37-9 Herpangina in a child caused by Coxsackievirus A16. (*Reproduced with permission from Emily Scott, MD.*)

DIFFERENTIAL DIAGNOSIS

- Infectious mononucleosis—Nausea, anorexia without vomiting, uvular edema, generalized symmetric lymphadenopathy, and lethargy particularly in teenagers and young adults, is more suggestive of acute mononucleosis (Epstein-Barr virus [EBV]) although the pharyngeal examination has a similar appearance to GABHS (see **Figure 37-4**). Hepatosplenomegaly is indicative of EBV in this group.

- Herpangina/Coxsackievirus infection—Oropharyngeal vesicles and ulcers indicate herpangina, which is caused by Coxsackievirus A16 in most cases (**Figure 37-9**).
- Oral *Candida*—Whitish plaques of the oropharyngeal mucosa indicate oral *Candida*/thrush, which is mainly found in infants but can be found in adults with immunosuppression (see Chapter 142, Candidiasis).
- Sexually transmitted infections—Primary human immunodeficiency virus, gonococcal, and syphilitic pharyngitis can all present with the symptom of sore throat. Although uncommon, these diagnoses should be considered in high-risk populations.
- Primary herpes gingivostomatitis causes oral ulcers and pain in the mouth. The wide distribution of ulcers with the first case of herpes simplex virus (HSV)-1 distinguishes this infection from other types of pharyngitis (see Chapter 135, Herpes Simplex).
- Cytomegalovirus (CMV)—Primary CMV infection in the immunocompetent host is usually asymptomatic. In the immunocompromised host, CMV may present with a mononucleosis-like syndrome clinically indistinguishable from EBV infection.
- Deep neck infections—Asymmetry of the neck, neck masses, and any displacement of the peripharyngeal wall should raise suspicion. Associated shortness of breath may be a warning sign of impending airway obstruction. Other complications include aspiration, thrombosis, mediastinitis, and septic shock.
- Epiglottitis—Rapid-onset fever, malaise, sore throat, and drooling in the absence of coughing characterize acute epiglottitis, especially when presenting in children. Progression of the disease can lead to life-threatening airway obstruction. Fortunately, this is a rare condition because of the preventive effect of the *Haemophilus influenzae* type b (HIB) vaccine.
- Supraglottitis—Similar symptoms to epiglottitis, although seen in adults. Sore throat and painful swallowing are the most common presenting symptoms, seen in more than 90% of cases. Muffled voice and drooling, dyspnea, stridor, and cough are reported in less than 50% of cases. No definite organism is identified in most cases. Unlike epiglottitis in children, HIB is responsible for less than 20% of adult cases but still accounts for the majority of positive cultures. Mortality rates have been reported up to 20%. Currently more common than epiglottitis, because of HIB vaccine.
- Diphtheria—A rare condition in the United States today, as most patients have been immunized. However, it needs to be considered, especially in unvaccinated and immigrant populations. Pharyngeal diphtheria presents with sore throat, low-grade fever, and malaise. The pharynx is erythematous with a grayish pseudomembrane that cannot be scraped off. Complications include myocarditis resulting in acute and severe congestive heart failure (CHF), endocarditis, and neuropathies.
- Other bacterial causes—Non–group A *Streptococcus, Fusobacterium necrophorum, Mycoplasma pneumoniae, Chlamydophila pneumoniae*, and *Arcanobacterium haemolyticum* have all been isolated as bacterial causes of pharyngitis; not as clinically significant, but all generally respond to treatments prescribed for strep pharyngitis.

MANAGEMENT

FIRST LINE

NONPHARMACOLOGIC

- Hydration with plenty of liquids (children and adults).
- Salt-water gargles (children and adults).
- Lozenges for comfort (adults only).
- Age-appropriate dosing of acetaminophen (e.g., 1 g every 6 hours for adults) and ibuprofen may be used for symptomatic relief of fever and pain. Doses can be alternated as needed.

MEDICATIONS

- Antibiotic use—Use a clinical prediction rule (given above [see "Clinical Features"]) and/or RADT or culture for determining need to treat for GABHS[9–11]: SOR Ⓐ Antibiotics for GABHS shorten symptom duration by about 1 day and prevent suppurative (otitis media, sinusitis, and peritonsillar abscess) and nonsuppurative (rheumatic fever) complications. Conversely, antibiotics have a 20% rate of adverse effects compared with 5% for placebo.[11]
    - Low probability (patients with predominantly viral symptoms, adults scoring 0 points on the modified Center score, negative RADT in an adult, negative throat culture): Treat symptomatically without antibiotics.
    - Intermediate probability (test and treatment based on result of RADT or culture): Patients with 1 to 3 points (probability of GABHS is approximately 18%) should undergo a rapid antigen test and be treated with antibiotics if positive.[11]
    - High probability (patients with 4 to 5 points on the modified Center score, all those with positive RADT or culture) should be considered for antibiotic treatment.
- For suspected or proven GABHS, penicillin V 500 mg orally 2 times daily for 10 days continues to be the treatment of choice for adolescents and adults.[9] Oral cephalexin (20 mg/kg/dose twice daily [max = 500 mg/dose]), cefadroxil (30 mg/kg once daily [max = 1 g]), clindamycin (7 mg/kg/dose 3 times daily [max = 300 mg/dose]), azithromycin (12 mg/kg once daily [max = 500 mg/dose]), OR clarithromycin (7.5 mg/kg/dose twice daily [max = 250 mg/dose]) can be used in penicillin-allergic patients. Penicillin G 1.2 million U IM single dose may be used for adults (<27 kg: 600,000 U) if unable to tolerate oral medication. For children: Pen VK 250 mg twice or 3 times daily OR amoxicillin 50 mg/kg once daily for 10 days. In some cases amoxicillin 25 mg/kg per day in divided doses every 12 hours is preferred because of palatability.
- Needle aspiration or incision and drainage AND combination Penicillin G (600 mg IV every 6 hours for 24 to 48 hours) with metronidazole (15 mg/kg IV more than 1 hour followed by 7.5 mg/kg IV more than 1 hour every 6 to 8 hours) is recommended for peritonsillar abscess, based primarily on case series.[13]

SECOND LINE

- Steroids (e.g., dexamethasone single 10-mg injection) can be used in severe tonsillitis in patients without immunocompromise. SOR Ⓒ Authors of a Cochrane review of eight trials of pharyngitis found a reduction of 6 hours to onset of pain relief with corticosteroids and mean time to complete resolution of pain by 14 hours.[14] Number needed to treat was <4 to prevent one person continuing to experience pain at 24 hours. The IDSA does not recommend use of corticosteroids as adjunctive treatment.[9] There are insufficient data to determine efficacy of steroids for patients with mononucleosis.[15]

- In extreme cases of pharyngitis, 1 teaspoon of viscous lidocaine 2% in a half glass of water gargled 20 to 30 minutes before meals helps the odynophagia. This is typically only recommended in rare cases because of risk of aspiration, potential toxicity of lidocaine, and the risk for oral mucosal burns—consider hospitalization if symptoms are this severe.

REFERRAL

- If signs of airway impairment are present, the patient should be immediately transported to an emergency department. Intubation can be extremely difficult and risky.
- Refer patients with peritonsillar abscess to ear, nose, and throat (ENT). Incision and drainage is the treatment of choice in addition to using systemic antibiotics.
- Consider ENT referral for tonsillectomy in proven recurrent GABHS cases, or under certain other conditions (e.g., antibiotic allergies/intolerances) with recurrence.[16]

PROGNOSIS

- Sore throat, regardless of the cause, is typically self-limiting. Typical symptoms last 3 to 4 days.
- Longer-term complications are rare, but antibiotic treatment to prevent these sequelae remains justification for treatment. Antibiotics shorten the duration of illness by approximately 1 day and can reduce the risk of rheumatic fever by approximately two-thirds in communities where this complication is common.[11] However, GI symptoms such as mild diarrhea are common side effects of antibiotic therapy.

FOLLOW-UP

Follow up if clinically deteriorating, especially if swallowing or breathing becomes more difficult or severe headache develops.

PATIENT EDUCATION

- The treatment for most cases of non-GABHS pharyngitis is education. Explain to patients the difference between a viral and a bacterial infection to help them understand why antibiotics were prescribed or not prescribed. Antibiotic treatment for a patient with an obvious viral infection is inappropriate, despite patient requests. Studies demonstrate that spending time with the patient to explain the disease process is associated with greater patient satisfaction than prescribing an antibiotic.[17,18]
- Rest, liquids, and analgesics should be encouraged.
- Patients receiving antibiotics should be reminded to complete the entire course, even if symptoms improve. Common antibiotic side effects, such as rash, nausea, and diarrhea, should be reviewed.
- Patients with mononucleosis and splenomegaly should be warned to avoid contact sports because of the risk of splenic rupture.

PATIENT RESOURCES

- **https://familydoctor.org/condition/sore-throat/.**
- **www.nlm.nih.gov/medlineplus/ency/article/000639.htm.**
- Mononucleosis information for patients—**https://medlineplus.gov/infectiousmononucleosis.html.**

PROVIDER RESOURCES

- Free clinical calculator online: Modified Centor Score for Strep Pharyngitis—**http://www.mdcalc.com/modified-centor-score-for-strep-pharyngitis.**

REFERENCES

1. U.S. Department of Health and Human Services. Ambulatory Medical Care Utilization Estimates for 2007. *Vital Health and Statistics*, Series 13, Number 169, April 2011. https://www.cdc.gov/nchs/data/series/sr_13/sr13_169.pdf. Accessed April 2018.
2. Ebell MH, Call M, Shinholser J, Gardner J. Does this patient have infectious mononucleosis?: The rational clinical examination systematic review. *JAMA*. 2016;315(14):1502-1509.
3. Shulman ST, Bisno AL, Clegg HW, et al. Clinical practice guideline for the diagnosis and management of group A streptococcal pharyngitis: 2012 update by the Infectious Diseases Society of America. *Clin Infect Dis*. 2012;55(10):1279-1282.
4. Bottin R, Marioni G, Rinaldi R, et al. Deep neck infection: a present-day complication. A retrospective review of 83 cases (1998–2001). *Eur Arch Otorhinolaryngol.* 2003;260(10):576-579.
5. Aung K, Ojha A, Lo C. *Viral Pharyngitis*. Updated July 2017. http://www.emedicine.medscape.com/article/225362. Accessed October 2017.
6. Carrillo-Marquez MA. *Bacterial Pharyngitis*. Updated March 2016. http://emedicine.medscape.com/article/225243. Accessed October 2017.
7. Ebell MH. Diagnosis of streptococcal pharyngitis. *Am Fam Physician*. 2014;89(12):976-977.
8. Cohen JF, Bertille N, Cohen R, Chalumeau M. Rapid antigen detection test for group A streptococcus in children with pharyngitis. *Cochrane Database Syst Rev*. 2016;(7):CD010502.
9. Shulman ST, Bisno AL, Clegg HW, et al. Clinical practice guideline for the diagnosis and management of group A streptococcal pharyngitis: 2012 update by the Infectious Diseases Society of America. *Clin Infect Dis*. 2012;55(10):e86-e102.
10. Harris AM, Hicks LA, Qaseem A, High Value Care Task Force of the American College of Physicians and for the Centers for Disease Control and Prevention. Appropriate antibiotic use for acute respiratory tract infection in adults: advice for high-value care from the American College of Physicians and the Centers for Disease Control and Prevention. *Ann Intern Med*. 2016;164:425-434.
11. Ebell MH. Sore throat. In: Sloane PD, Slatt LM, Ebell MH, et al, eds. *Essentials of Family Medicine*. Baltimore, MD: Lippincott Williams & Wilkins; 2012:207-216.

12. Maroldi R, Farina D, Ravanelli M, et al. Emergency imaging assessment of deep neck space infections. *Semin Ultrasound CT MR*. 2012;33(5):432-442.

13. Powell J, Wilson JA. An evidence-based review of peritonsillar abscess. *Clin Otolaryngol*. 2012;37(2):136-145.

14. Hayward G, Thompson MJ, Perera R, et al. Corticosteroids as standalone or add-on treatment for sore throat. *Cochrane Database Syst Rev*. 2012;(10):CD008268.

15. Rezk E, Nofal YH, Hamzeh A, et al. Steroids for symptom control in infectious mononucleosis. *Cochrane Database Syst Rev*. 2015;(11):CD004402.

16. Baugh RF, Archer SM, Mitchell RB, et al. Clinical practice guideline: tonsillectomy in children. *Otolaryngol Head Neck Surg*. 2011;144(1 Suppl):S1-S30.

17. Hamm RM, Hicks RJ, Bemben DA. Antibiotics and respiratory infections: are patients more satisfied when expectations are met? *J Fam Pract*. 1996;43(1):56-62.

18. Ong S, Nakase J, Moran GJ, et al. Antibiotic use for emergency department patients with upper respiratory infections: prescribing practices, patient expectations, and patient satisfaction. *Ann Emerg Med*. 2007;50(3):213-220.

38 THE LARYNX (HOARSENESS)

Alissa M. Collins, MD
C. Blake Simpson, MD
Laura M. Dominguez, MD

PATIENT STORY

A 67-year-old man with a 40-pack-year history of smoking presents with worsening hoarseness that began approximately 6 weeks ago. He complains of globus sensation and difficulty swallowing solid foods. He denies odynophagia, otalgia, hemoptysis, and hematemesis. There is no associated cough, and he has not had any constitutional symptoms such as fevers, chills, or recent weight loss.

Hoarseness in a middle-aged man with the above symptoms is very common, and the differential diagnosis is long (all the diseases below are possibilities in this case scenario). The patient's smoking history and duration of symptoms should raise concern for a possible laryngeal malignancy. However, more common diagnoses such as laryngopharyngeal reflux (LPR) and benign vocal fold (cord) lesions should be considered as well.

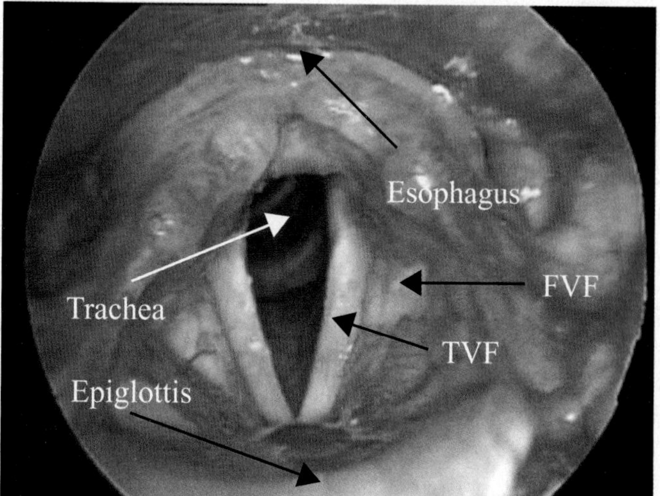

FIGURE 38-1 Normal larynx (true and false vocal folds). *FVF*, False vocal fold; *TVF*, true vocal fold (cord). (*Reproduced with permission from C. Blake Simpson, MD.*)

INTRODUCTION

The evaluation of hoarseness typically involves first ruling out the most serious pathologies, such as laryngeal squamous cell carcinoma (SCC) in adults or recurrent respiratory papillomatosis (RRP) in children, and then proceeding with a more focused and subtle evaluation to uncover any of the many benign pathologies that affect the larynx. Treatment of these benign pathologies must take into account the patient's lifestyle and voice needs. It also often incorporates education on vocal hygiene, which involves increasing hydration, decreasing mucus and vocal abuse, and reducing acid reflux if a factor.

SYNONYMS AND DEFINITIONS

- Hoarseness, dysphonia, vocal strain, breathiness, raspiness.
- Vocal cords, true vocal cords, true vocal folds, glottis (**Figure 38-1**).
- False vocal folds, false vocal cords (mucosal folds in the supraglottis, just superior to the true vocal folds and separated from the true folds by the ventricle).
- Flexible fiberoptic laryngoscopy, nasopharyngeal scope (NP scope), transnasal fiberoptic laryngoscopy.
- Stroboscopy, videolaryngostroboscopy (VLS), strobe exam.

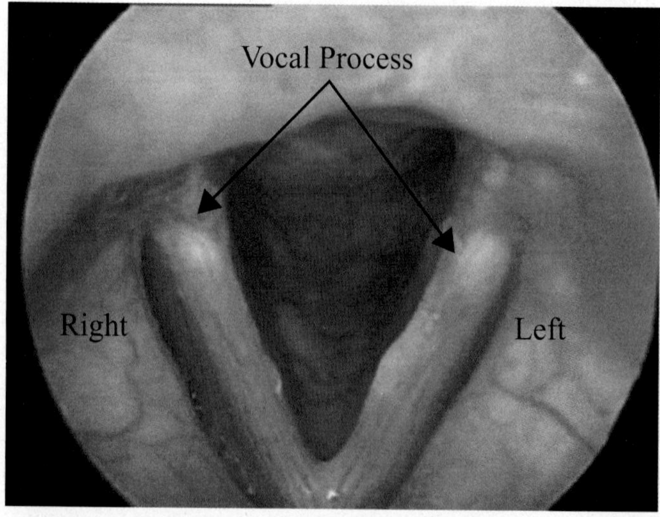

FIGURE 38-2 Laryngitis—diffuse erythema and inflammation, irregular vocal fold edges. (*Reproduced with permission from C. Blake Simpson, MD.*)

EPIDEMIOLOGY

- The most common cause of hoarseness in adults and children overall is viral infection causing laryngitis (**Figure 38-2**).

- LPR disease may be present in up to 50% of patients presenting with voice and laryngeal disorders.[1] It is less commonly the sole cause of hoarseness (**Figures 38-3** and **38-4**).
- Hoarseness can be a symptom of laryngeal cancer. It is estimated there were 13,000 new diagnoses of laryngeal cancer in the United States in 2017. The average age at diagnosis is 65 with a strong male predominance.[2] SCC accounts for 95% of laryngeal cancer[1] (**Figure 38-5**).
- RRP represents the most common benign neoplasm of the larynx among children and should be considered in children with chronic hoarseness. A known risk factor for juvenile onset is the triad of a firstborn child (75%), teenage mother, and vaginal delivery. The incidence of RRP in the United States is 4.3 per 100,000 children and 1.8 per 100,000 adults.[3] There is a known association between cervical human papillomavirus (HPV) infection in the mother and juvenile-onset RRP, but the precise mode of transmission is unclear. The risk of a child contracting RRP after delivery from an actively infected mother with genital HPV ranges from 0.25% to 3%.[4] Because cesarean section does not prevent RRP in all cases, routine prophylactic cesarean section in mothers with active condyloma acuminata is currently *not* recommended. There is no published research regarding the impact the HPV vaccine has had on the incidence of RRP (**Figures 38-6** and **38-7**).

ETIOLOGY AND PATHOPHYSIOLOGY

- Laryngitis is a nonspecific term to describe inflammation of the larynx from any cause. Most commonly this is due to a viral upper respiratory infection. Compare the anatomy of the normal larynx (see **Figure 38-1**) with that of acute laryngitis (see **Figure 38-2**), with the primary differences being in the diffuse erythema and edema of the vocal folds and the often transient irregularities of the vocal fold medial edge as compared to the straight medial edge of the normal vocal fold. Laryngeal symptoms result from dry throat, mucous stasis, and recurrent trauma from coughing and throat clearing.
- LPR must be differentiated from gastroesophageal reflux disease (GERD), in which acid reflux is more likely to cause heartburn, indigestion, and regurgitation and does not necessarily reach the larynx or upper aerodigestive tract. LPR is more likely to present with frequent throat clearing, dry cough, hoarseness, and globus sensation, and does not include heartburn in more than 60% of patients. The larynx is highly sensitive to even small amounts of acid or pepsin. Thus, patients who do not have severe enough reflux to cause esophagitis, with its associated symptoms of GERD, may still develop symptomatic laryngeal mucosal injury, with its associated symptoms of LPR.[1,5–7]
- SCC has a multifactorial etiology, but 90% of patients have a history of heavy tobacco and/or alcohol use. These risk factors have a synergistic effect. Other independent risk factors include a history of RRP, employment as a painter or metalworker, exposure to diesel or gasoline fumes, and exposure to therapeutic doses of radiation.
- Most cases of RRP are caused by HPV-6 and HPV-11.[8] Onset is predominantly in young children, although an adult-onset variant exists. Its course is unpredictable and highly variable. Tracheal and bronchopulmonary spread can occur. Bronchopulmonary spread is

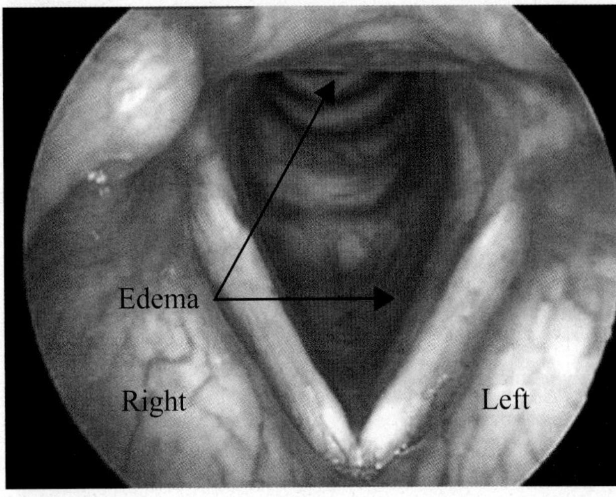

FIGURE 38-3 Laryngopharyngeal reflux (LPR). Postcricoid region edema (normal is less full and nearly concave) and edema just inferior to the true vocal fold edge (infraglottic edema) indicative of chronic inflammation from reflux, often called "pseudosulcus." Other findings of LPR not seen in this image include thick mucus and mucosal erythema. (*Reproduced with permission from C. Blake Simpson, MD.*)

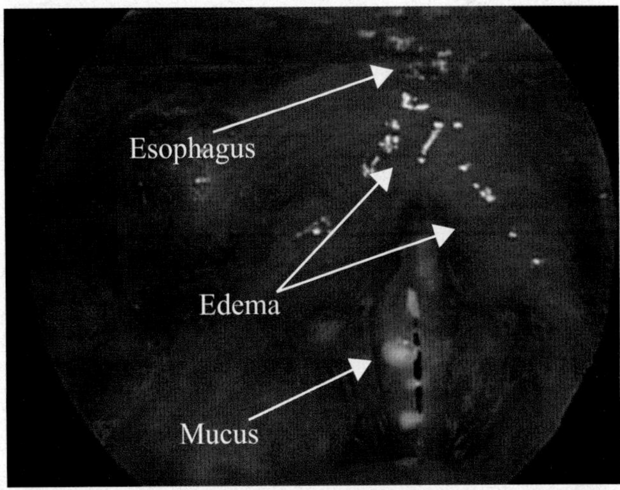

FIGURE 38-4 Laryngopharyngeal reflux during phonation with diffuse erythema, inflammation, and thick mucus. (*Reproduced with permission from C. Blake Simpson, MD.*)

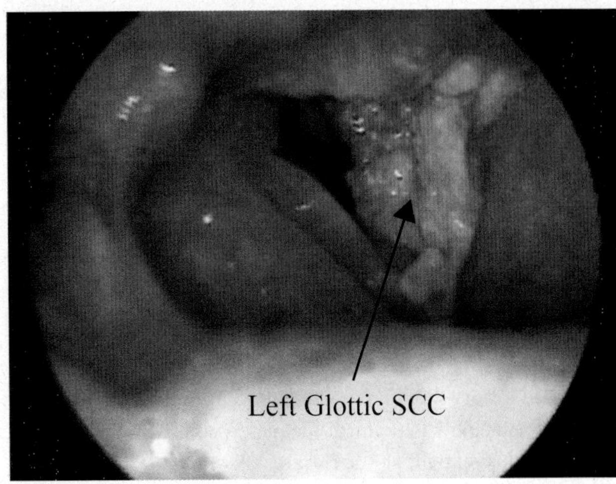

FIGURE 38-5 Squamous cell carcinoma (SCC), advanced stage with left true vocal cord paralysis. (*Reproduced with permission from C. Blake Simpson, MD.*)

uniformly fatal as a consequence of the lack of surgical options. Malignant transformation to SCC is rare.

- Vocal cord nodules are benign lesions arising from mechanical trauma (vocal abuse or misuse) and are often described as a "callus" of the vocal folds (**Figure 38-8**). They are a common cause of dysphonia in singers, teachers, and other professional voice users. Vocal cord polyps or cysts can arise from vocal abuse, a blocked mucous gland, vocal fold hemorrhage, a background of polypoid corditis (see below), or idiopathic etiologies (**Figures 38-9** and **38-10**). Vocal cord granulomas are associated with LPR, chronic cough, frequent throat clearing, and/or intubation trauma and rarely require surgery.[9]
- Causes of vocal cord paresis or paralysis are myriad[1,10]:
  - Iatrogenic surgical injury (anterior spine fusion, carotid endarterectomy, thyroidectomy) is most common (25%)
  - Nonlaryngeal malignancy (mediastinal, bronchopulmonary, and skull base) (24%)
  - No identifiable cause (idiopathic), often assumed to be viral (20%)
  - Nonsurgical trauma (penetrating/blunt injury and intubation injury) (10%)
  - Neurologic causes (stroke, central nervous system [CNS] tumors, multiple sclerosis [MS], and amyotrophic lateral sclerosis [ALS]) (8%).
  - Inflammatory/infectious disease (2% to 5%).
- Presbyphonia is a diagnosis of exclusion denoting vocal changes from aging of the larynx (gradually weakening voice, poor vocal projection, and vocal "roughness"). Hoarseness in patients older than 60 years of age is most commonly a result of benign vocal fold lesions, followed by malignancy and vocal fold paralysis. Once a thorough evaluation has been done to rule out organic causes, presbyphonia is the cause of hoarseness in approximately 10% of elderly patients; it is characterized by atrophied vocal folds.[11]

DIAGNOSIS

CLINICAL FEATURES

- Key historical and physical examination findings can help differentiate benign pathology from potentially more serious problems:
  - Otalgia (ear pain)—Often a source of referred pain from primary laryngeal and pharyngeal carcinomas; it is not typically seen with benign pathologies.
  - Dysphagia and odynophagia (pain when swallowing)—Nonspecific complaints, but potentially worrisome for obstructing lesions or reactive pharyngeal edema.
  - Stridor or dyspnea—"Noisy breathing" with respiratory distress should be evaluated urgently to rule out impending airway obstruction. Less-severe dyspnea may be noted by patients with vocal cord paralysis caused by air escape during speech; a detailed history should reveal that it occurs only during speech or from the inability to perform adequate Valsalva maneuver as a result of loss of tight glottic closure.
  - Globus pharyngeus—The persistent or intermittent nonpainful sensation of a lump or foreign body in the throat. This is commonly associated with LPR.

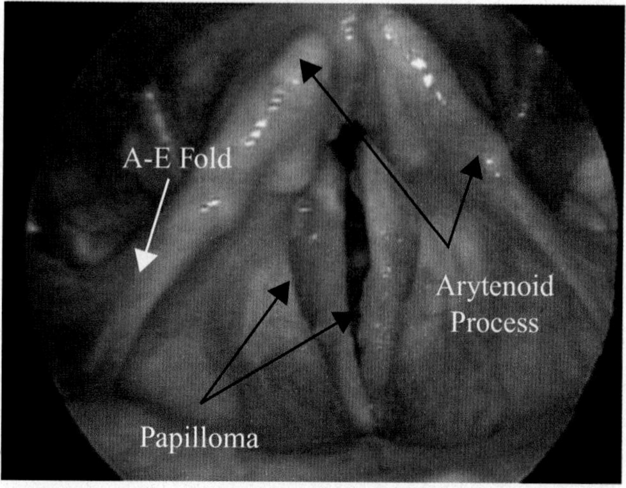

FIGURE 38-6 Adult recurrent respiratory papillomatosis. Aryepiglottic fold (*A-E fold*). (*Reproduced with permission from C. Blake Simpson, MD.*)

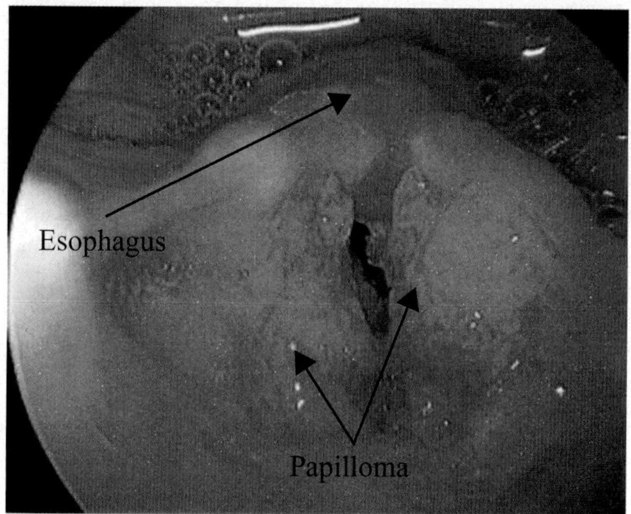

FIGURE 38-7 Recurrent respiratory papillomatosis in a 3-year-old child. The papillomas are nearly obstructing the airway and have required debridement. (*Reproduced with permission from C. Blake Simpson, MD.*)

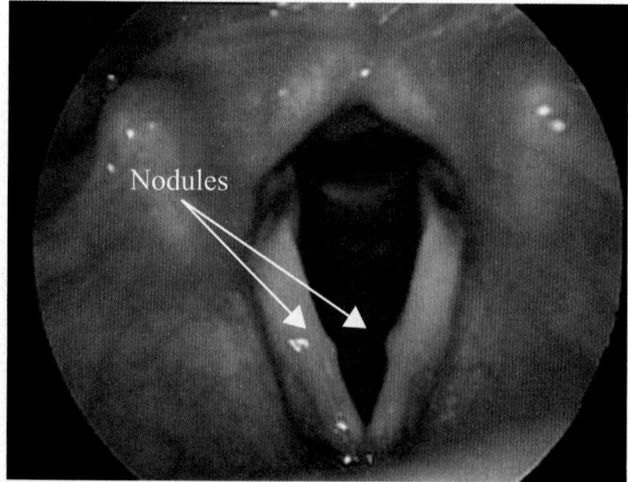

FIGURE 38-8 Vocal cord nodules. (*Reproduced with permission from C. Blake Simpson, MD.*)

- Neck mass—Associated unilateral or bilateral lymphadenopathy, typically painless, is suspicious for a laryngeal neoplasm until proven otherwise.
- Timing—Onset, duration, and frequency of symptoms are important.

- Red flags for laryngeal carcinoma include a history of smoking and/or alcohol abuse, dysphonia, neck mass, weight loss or severe dysphagia, presence of stridor (often initially noted with sleep or when lying flat), and otalgia.
- LPR symptoms include hoarseness, throat clearing, "postnasal drip," chronic cough, dysphagia, globus pharyngeus, and sore throat. "Heartburn" is *not* a requisite symptom!
- Hallmark of diagnosis is direct visualization of the larynx, often performed by an otolaryngologist with a flexible laryngoscopic exam. Stroboscopy is added to the evaluation when visualization of the mucosal vibration or "wave" of the vocal folds is necessary. Assessment of the mucosal wave aids in determining the depth of a lesion within the vocal fold and the severity of its effect on the voice.

LABORATORY AND IMAGING

- Laboratory studies are not usually helpful, except in the rare case that a previously undiagnosed rheumatologic disease presents with vocal complaints as the initial symptom.
- Plain films of the chest are useful to rule out bronchopulmonary or mediastinal masses as a cause of vocal cord paralysis, but are generally not helpful for primary laryngeal lesions.
- A CT of the neck and chest with contrast is useful in ruling out pathology along the length of the recurrent laryngeal nerve in cases of unexplained vocal cord paralysis and in cases suspicious for carcinoma, especially if there is associated cervical lymphadenopathy. A chest X-ray is sometimes used to replace the chest CT.
- An MRI with and without gadolinium offers the best imaging for suspected primary CNS or skull base lesions; this is typically added to the work-up for vocal cord paralysis when evidence of high vagal injury such as weakness in palate elevation is present.
- Referral to a gastroenterologist for *dual-channel* 24-hour pH probe monitoring (*while on antireflux medications*) is a useful diagnostic tool for patients with suspected LPR.

BIOPSY

- Biopsy is typically reserved for lesions suspicious for carcinoma and is performed by an otolaryngologist in either the clinic or operating room under direct visualization.

DIFFERENTIAL DIAGNOSIS

- Laryngitis (see **Figure 38-2**).
- Laryngopharyngeal reflux (see **Figures 38-3** and **38-4**).
- SCC (see **Figure 38-5**).
- Laryngeal papillomatosis (see **Figures 38-6** and **38-7**).
- Vocal cord nodule (see **Figure 38-8**).
- Vocal cord polyp (see **Figure 38-9**).
- Vocal cord cyst (see **Figure 38-10**).

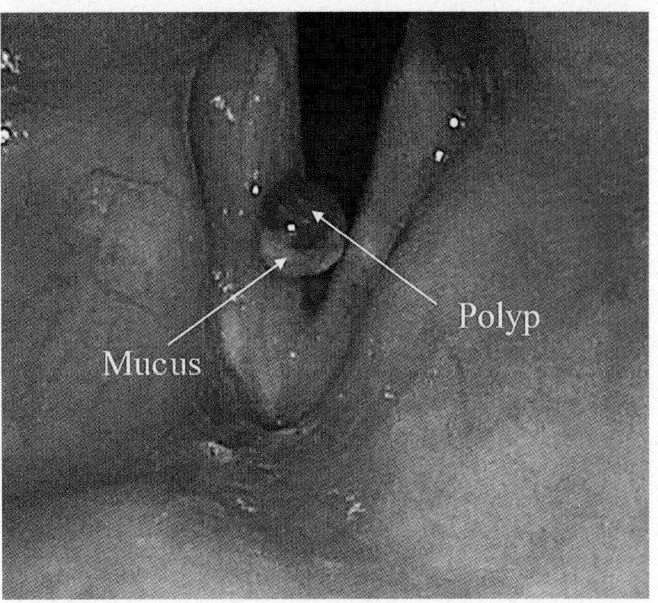

FIGURE 38-9 Right vocal cord polyp with thick mucus collecting around it. (*Reproduced with permission from Alissa Collins, MD.*)

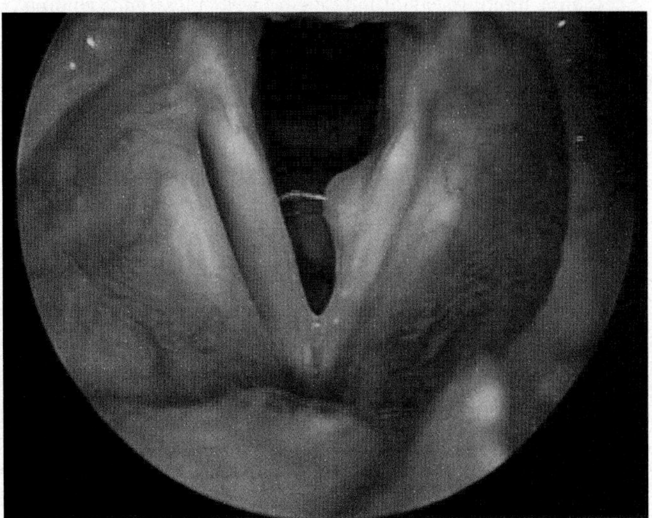

FIGURE 38-10 Left vocal cord cyst. (*Reproduced with permission from Laura Dominguez, MD.*)

- Vocal cord paresis or paralysis.
- Presbyphonia.
- Neurologic disorders (MS, Parkinson disease, ALS, and essential tremor).
- Systemic diseases (granulomatosis with polyangiitis [GPA], sarcoidosis, rheumatoid arthritis).

MANAGEMENT

- Laryngitis—Empiric treatment is aimed at alleviating symptoms such as cough and thinning nasal/pharyngeal secretions. Hydration is critical for healing (increased water intake, steam showers, humidifiers, and saunas may help). Throat clearing should be discouraged and voice rest encouraged. Talking should be conserved, not prohibited. Inform patients that whispering causes even more vocal strain than normal speech. Guaifenesin can be helpful for thinning upper airway secretions. Antibiotics are rarely indicated, as most cases are viral. There is a lack of evidence to support the routine use of steroids in the treatment of adults with acute laryngitis.[12]
- Vocal cord nodules, polyps, and cysts—Initial management involves voice therapy accompanied by medical treatment of dehydration, allergies, sinonasal secretions (postnasal drip), and LPR. Refractory disease may require surgical excision.
- Laryngeal papillomatosis—Most patients have a recalcitrant course that requires periodic surgical debridement by an otolaryngologist to prevent airway obstruction. In severe cases, a tracheostomy may be indicated. Periods of spontaneous remission may occur. Adjuvant therapies include intralesional injection with cidofovir or bevacizumab, indole-3-carbinol, mumps vaccine, celecoxib, and control of LPR/GERD.[13] It is hoped the administration of the newest HPV vaccines (4- and 9-valent) will decrease the incidence of RRP over time. Some practitioners administer the vaccine in a nonprophylactic manner to patients with existing RRP, although there is no strong evidence currently to support a treatment effect of the vaccine.[3,4,14]
- LPR—Mainstay treatment involves patient education to modify diet and behavior (avoidance of acidic or greasy foods, tobacco cessation, limiting alcohol and caffeine, weight loss, and avoiding meals shortly before lying down). Medical therapy consists of *twice* daily proton pump inhibitors (PPIs) 30 to 60 minutes before meals, which can often be weaned after several months of therapy. Some patients benefit from adding an H_2-blocker, such as ranitidine 300 mg, at bedtime.
- SCC—Multidisciplinary management is best. Depending on the staging and extent of disease, patients often receive one or more modalities of treatment including surgery, radiation, and chemotherapy.
- Vocal cord paresis or paralysis—Treatment is targeted at the underlying disorder. Some patients may be candidates for surgical intervention to reposition the paralyzed cord medially with an implant. With a mobile vocal fold on the contralateral side, the airway is rarely compromised by medialization of the paralyzed vocal fold. These procedures restore voice quality and often alleviate chronic aspiration problems.
- Neurologic diseases—Laryngeal complaints can be associated with MS, myasthenia gravis, Parkinson disease, ALS, and essential tremor. In addition to managing the underlying disorder, a trial of voice therapy is sometimes useful. Botulinum toxin injection into the vocal folds has been used successfully to treat vocal tremor.[15]
- Systemic diseases—Diseases such as GPA, sarcoidosis, relapsing polychondritis, and rheumatoid arthritis rarely may involve the larynx. Voice and swallowing problems in these patients should be evaluated by an otolaryngologist for possible therapies to improve the voice and to rule out associated airway stenosis.
- Presbyphonia—This is a diagnosis of exclusion. Once organic etiologies have been ruled out, a trial of voice therapy is recommended before considering surgical options, such as vocal fold injection augmentation to plump the atrophied vocal fold.

FOLLOW-UP

- Urgent referral to an otolaryngologist for flexible laryngoscopic examination of the larynx is advisable when the history and physical are suspicious for carcinoma.
- When symptoms worsen or fail to resolve, referral to an otolaryngologist (or laryngologist) is indicated.
- Patients suspected of having LPR should be seen approximately 6 to 8 weeks after initiating empiric therapy with a PPI and lifestyle measures. An otolaryngology and/or gastroenterology consultation is indicated when symptoms do not improve after optimized behavioral and medical management or for patients who require long-term PPI therapy (longer than 12 months). Some of these patients, particularly those with chronic cough or long-standing requirement for PPIs, may require transnasal esophagoscopy (performed in the otolaryngologist's office) or esophagogastroduodenoscopy (performed by a gastroenterologist in the endoscopy suite). Recent evidence has pointed to chronic cough as an independent indicator of esophageal adenocarcinoma, and Barrett esophagus should be ruled out in any patient requiring long-term PPI use.[16]

PATIENT EDUCATION

- In cases of nonmalignant pathology, vocal hygiene and other lifestyle measures often play an important role in treatment. Efforts should focus on increasing hydration, decreasing caffeine intake, tobacco cessation, and prevention of excessive alcohol use.
- Vocal cord nodules, polyps, and cysts typically occur in professional voice users (clergy, auctioneers, teachers, singers, etc.). Speech therapists can be integral in preventing and healing lesions by teaching patients how to avoid vocal misuse.
- Benign laryngeal pathology may be improved, but not necessarily resolved, by controlling both gastroesophageal and LPR disease. Patients should be educated about GERD/LPR risk factors:
    - Spicy, acidic, or greasy foods
    - Tobacco and alcohol abuse
    - Caffeinated beverages (especially carbonated sodas)
    - Citric juices, tomato sauces, chocolate, mints
    - Obesity
    - Eating meals within 2 to 3 hours of lying down

PATIENT RESOURCES

- **http://www.entnet.org/healthinfo/index.cfm.**
- **http://www.entusa.com.**

PROVIDER RESOURCES

- **http://www.entnet.org/content/clinical-practice-guideline-hoarseness-dysphonia.**
- **http://www.ucdvoice.org/gallery.html.**
- **https://www.voicedoctor.net.**

REFERENCES

1. Ossoff R, Shapshay S, Woodson G, Netterville J. *The Larynx.* Philadelphia, PA: Lippincott Williams & Wilkins; 2003.
2. National Cancer Institute. *SEER Cancer Stat Facts: Laryngeal Cancer.* http://seer.cancer.gov/statfacts/html/laryn.html. Accessed January 2018.
3. Derkay CS. Recurrent respiratory papillomatosis. *Laryngoscope.* 2001;111:57-69.
4. Gallagher TQ, Derkay CS. Recurrent respiratory papillomatosis: update 2008. *Curr Opin Otolaryngol Head Neck Surg.* 2008;16: 536-542.
5. Simpson CB. Patient of the month program: breathy dysphonia. *American Academy of Otolaryngol Head Neck Surg.* 2002;31(7):19-28.
6. Koufmann JA, Amin MA, Panetti M. Prevalence of reflux in 113 consecutive patients with laryngeal and voice disorders. *Otolaryngol Head Neck Surg.* 2000;123:385-388.
7. Koufman JA, Aviv JE, Casiano RR, Shaw GY. Laryngopharyngeal reflux: position statement of the committee on speech, voice, and swallowing disorders of the American Academy of Otolaryngology—Head and Neck Surgery. *Otolaryngol Head Neck Surg.* 2002;127:32-38.
8. Donne AJ, Hampson L, Homer JJ, Hampson IN. The role of HPV type in recurrent respiratory papillomatosis. *Int J Pediatr Otorhinolaryngol.* 2010;74(1):7-14.
9. Karkos PD, George M, Van Der Veen J, et al. Vocal process granulomas: a systematic review of treatment. *Ann Otol Rhinol Laryngol.* 2014;123(5):314-320.
10. Benninger MS, Gillen JB, Altman JS. Changing etiology of vocal fold immobility. *Laryngoscope.* 1998;108:1346-1349.
11. Kendall K. Presbyphonia: a review. *Curr Opin Otolaryngol Head Neck Surg.* 2007;15:137-140.
12. Schwartz SR, Cohen SM, Dailey SH, et al. Clinical practice guideline: hoarseness (dysphonia). *Otolaryngol Head Neck Surg.* 2009;141(3Suppl 2):S1-S31.
13. Carifi M, Napolitano D, Morandi M, Dall'Olio D. Recurrent respiratory papillomatosis: current and future perspectives. *Ther Clin Risk Manag.* 2015;11:731-738.
14. Tjon Pian Gi RE, San Giorgi MR, Pawlita M, et al. Immunological response to quadrivalent HPV vaccine in treatment of recurrent respiratory papillomatosis. *Eur Arch Otorhinolaryngol.* 2016; 273:3231-3236.
15. Gurey LE, Sinclair CF, Blitzer A. A new paradigm for the management of essential vocal tremor with botulinum toxin. *Laryngoscope.* 2013;123:2497-2501.
16. Reavis KM, Morris CD, Gopal DV, et al. Laryngopharyngeal reflux symptoms better predict the presence of esophageal adenocarcinoma than typical gastroesophageal reflux symptoms. *Ann Surg.* 2004;239(6):849-858.

PART VI

ORAL HEALTH

Strength of Recommendation (SOR)	Definition
A	Recommendation based on consistent and good-quality patient-oriented evidence.*
B	Recommendation based on inconsistent or limited-quality patient-oriented evidence.*
C	Recommendation based on consensus, usual practice, opinion, disease-oriented evidence, or case series for studies of diagnosis, treatment, prevention, or screening.*

*See Appendix A on pages 1603–1606 for further information.

39 BLACK HAIRY TONGUE

Richard P. Usatine, MD
Wanda C. Gonsalves, MD
David Ojeda Díaz, DDS

PATIENT STORY

A 60-year-old man who smokes presents to the physician's office smelling of alcohol. He complains of a black discoloration of his tongue and a gagging sensation on occasion. He admits to smoking 1 to 2 packs per day along with drinking at least 6 to 8 beers per day. The patient brushes his teeth infrequently and has not seen a dentist for a long time. On physical exam, his teeth are stained and his tongue is brown, coated with a hairlike appearance toward the posterior two-thirds (**Figure 39-1**). Diagnoses include black hairy tongue (BHT), poor oral hygiene, and tobacco and alcohol addiction.

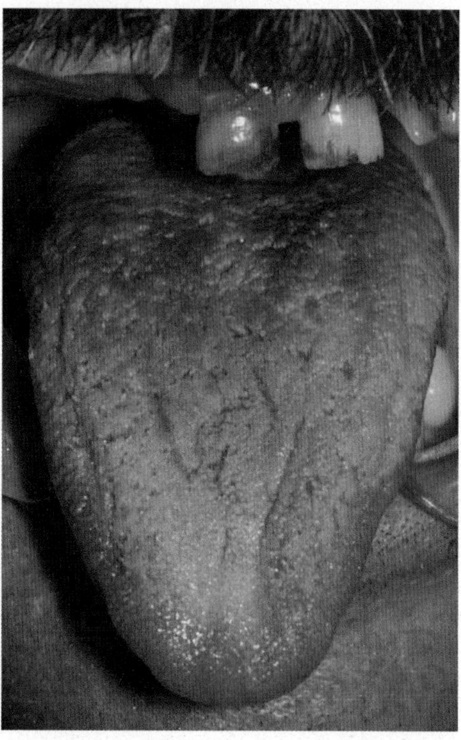

FIGURE 39-1 Black hairy tongue showing elongated filiform papillae with brown discoloration in a man who is a heavy smoker and drinker. Note the tobacco-stained teeth. (*Reproduced with permission from Brad Neville, DDS.*)

INTRODUCTION

BHT is a benign disorder characterized by the reactive hypertrophy of the filiform papillae of the tongue, which results in the clinical elongation of the papillae,[1] providing the hairlike appearance of the dorsum of the tongue.[2]

SYNONYMS

Hyperkeratosis of the tongue, lingua villosa nigra.

EPIDEMIOLOGY

The prevalence of BHT varies depending on the risk factors in the population being studied. However, several studies have consistently reported a higher prevalence in males compared with females.[1] Increasing age also showed a positive correlation with a prevalence nearly 40% in patients over 60 years old.[3]

- It can be as high as 57% in persons incarcerated or addicted to drugs.[4]
- The prevalence in Minnesota schoolchildren was 0.06%.[5]
- In Turkish dental patients, the highest prevalence was 54% in heavy smokers.[3]

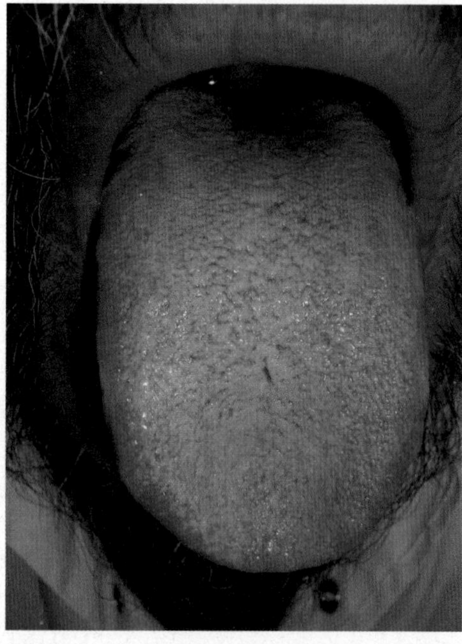

FIGURE 39-2 Drug-induced black hairy tongue with yellowish-brown elongated filiform papillae in a patient taking a broad-spectrum antibiotic. (*Reproduced with permission from Richard P. Usatine, MD.*)

ETIOLOGY AND PATHOPHYSIOLOGY

- BHT (**Figure 39-1**) is a disorder characterized by the hypertrophy of filiform papillae and its defective desquamation that leads to an accumulation of keratinized layers.[1,4,6]

- These papillae, which are normally about 1 mm in length, may become as long as 12 mm.
  - The elongated filiform papillae can then collect debris, bacteria, fungus, or other foreign materials which cause the characteristic black coloration.[1]
- In an extensive literature review of reported cases of drug-induced BHT, 82% of the cases were caused by antibiotics (**Figure 39-2**).[2]
- Medication-induced xerostomia (dry mouth), tobacco, and radiation therapy can lead to BHT.[2]

RISK FACTORS[2]

- Tobacco (smoking and chewing).
- Alcoholism and drug abuse (especially drugs that are smoked).
- Poor oral hygiene.
- Medication-induced xerostomia (dry mouth).
- Oxidizing mouthwashes (containing peroxide).
- Radiotherapy of the head and neck region.
- Excessive drinking of black tea or coffee.

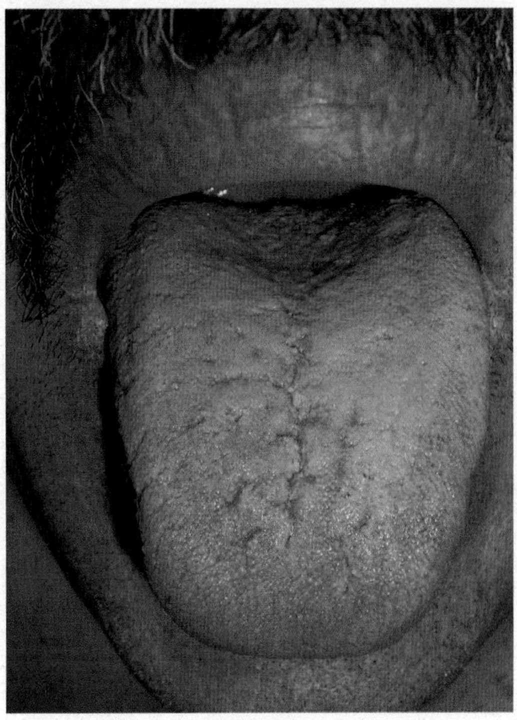

FIGURE 39-3 Black hairy tongue that also is furrowed in a heavy smoker. Note this man also has angular cheilitis, poor dentition, and halitosis. (*Reproduced with permission from Richard P. Usatine, MD.*)

DIAGNOSIS

CLINICAL FEATURES

- Patients may be asymptomatic. However, the accumulation of debris in the elongated papillae may cause taste alterations, nausea, gagging, halitosis, and pain or burning of the tongue.[2] Also depending on the severity of the clinical appearance, BHT could have an emotional and psychological impact on the patient.

The diagnosis is made by visual inspection:

- BHT may exhibit a thick coating of black, brown, or yellow discoloration, depending on foods ingested, tobacco use, and amount of coffee or tea consumed (**Figure 39-3**).

TYPICAL DISTRIBUTION

The lesion is restricted to the dorsum of the tongue, anterior to the circumvallate papillae, rarely involving the tip or sides of the tongue.

LABORATORY TESTS

Consider performing a KOH preparation or *Candida* culture to rule out associated candidiasis.

DIFFERENTIAL DIAGNOSIS

- Black tongue can occur with the ingestion of bismuth subsalicylate or minocycline. Although the tongue has a black coating, the papillae are not elongated. Without the hypertrophy of papillae, this is not a BHT (**Figure 39-4**).
- Chemotherapy-induced pigmentations—Could appear as diffused brown patches on the tongue.[7] The lack of the hairy appearance and a good medical history would rule out BHT.

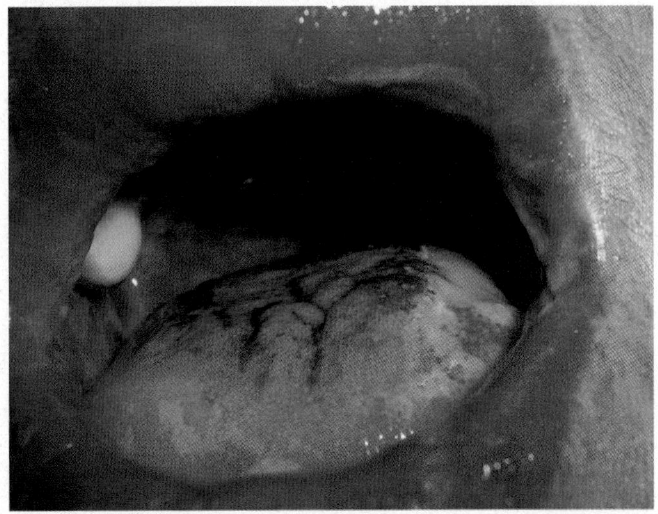

FIGURE 39-4 Black tongue without elongated papillae in a woman with untreated pemphigus vulgaris. Note the palatal erosions along with the black color of the tongue. The black color was gone in 2 days after prednisone was initiated and the patient was able to eat again. (*Reproduced with permission from Richard P. Usatine, MD.*)

- Oral hairy leukoplakia—Appears as faint white vertical keratotic streaks typically on the lateral side of the tongue (**Figure 39-5**). Do not confuse BHT with oral hairy leukoplakia, an Epstein-Barr virus–related condition typically affecting the lateral tongue bilaterally in immunocompromised patients, especially those with HIV infection.
- Oral candidiasis—White plaques typically found on the buccal mucosa, tongue, and palate; when removed, has an erythematous base. The white color should make this easy to distinguish from BHT (see Chapter 142, Candidiasis).

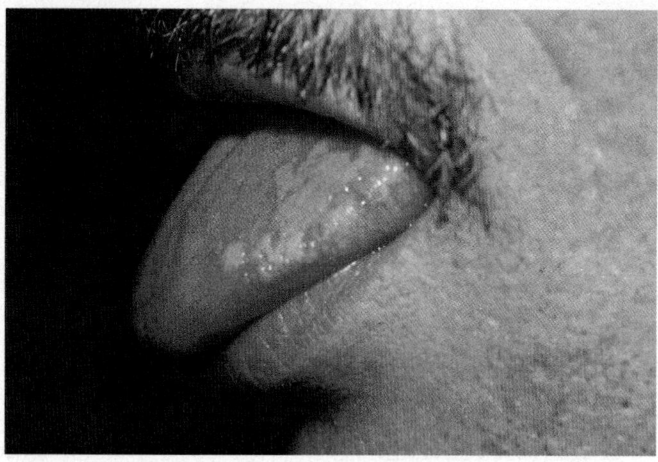

FIGURE 39-5 Oral hairy leukoplakia caused by Epstein-Barr virus on the tongue of a man with AIDS. (*Reproduced with permission from Richard P. Usatine, MD.*)

MANAGEMENT

NONPHARMACOLOGIC

- Avoidance of predisposing risk factors (e.g., tobacco, alcohol, and antibiotics). SOR C
- Stop the offending medication in drug-induced BHT whenever possible.[2] SOR B
- Regular tongue brushing using a soft toothbrush or tongue scraper. SOR C

MEDICATIONS

- Dilute Dakin's solution (sodium hypochlorite 0.5%) 1:4 with water to make a 0.125% solution. Then brush the tongue using this solution with a spare toothbrush twice a day. When improved this can be reduced to once a day. SOR C
- If candidiasis is present, an oral antifungal is indicated. If there is no liver disease, the preferred regimen for oral candidiasis is fluconazole 100–200 mg daily for 14 days. An alternative is clotrimazole troches 5 times a day for 14 days. Nystatin is less effective. Fluconazole-treated HIV patients with oropharyngeal candidiasis were more likely to remain disease-free than were those treated with other antifungal agents.[6] SOR A

REFERRAL

Patients with poor oral hygiene should be referred to a dentist. All patients should be encouraged to see a dentist at least twice yearly.

PREVENTION

Good oral hygiene and avoidance of risk factors.

PROGNOSIS

BHT is generally a self-limited disorder, so the prognosis should be excellent with good oral hygiene and treatment.

PATIENT EDUCATION

Tell patients to brush their teeth and tongue twice a day or to use a tongue scraper. Address addictions and offer help to quit. Suggest that patients eat firm foods, like fresh apples, that will help to clean the tongue.

PATIENT RESOURCES

- American Academy of Oral Medicine. *Hairy Tongue.* Patient, patient condition information—**http://www.aaom.com/index.php?option=com_content&view=article&id=133:hairy-tongue&catid=22:patient-condition-information&Itemid=120.**

PROVIDER RESOURCES

- Medscape. *Hairy tongue*—**http://emedicine.medscape.com/article/1075886-overview#showall.**

REFERENCES

1. Gurvits GE, Tan A. Black hairy tongue syndrome. *World J Gastroenterol.* 2014;20:10845-10850.
2. Thompson DF, Kessler TL. Drug-induced black hairy tongue. *Pharmacotherapy.* 2010;30(6):585-593.
3. Sarti GM, Haddy RI, Schaffer D, Kihm J. Black hairy tongue. *Am Fam Physician.* 1990;41:1751-1755.
4. Harada Y, Gaafar H. Black hairy tongue. A scanning electron microscopic study. *J Laryngol Otol.* 1977;91:91-96.
5. Redman RS. Prevalence of geographic tongue, fissured tongue, median rhomboid glossitis, and hairy tongue among 3,611 Minnesota schoolchildren. *Oral Surg Oral Med Oral Pathol.* 1970;30:390-395.
6. Albougy HA, Naidoo S. A systematic review of the management of oral candidiasis associated with HIV/AIDS. *SADJ.* 2002;57(11):457-466.
7. Alawi F. Pigmented lesions of the oral cavity: an update. *Dent Clin North Am.* 2013;57(4):699-710.

40 GEOGRAPHIC TONGUE

Ernest E. Valdez, DDS
Richard P. Usatine, MD
Wanda C. Gonsalves, MD
David Ojeda Díaz, DDS

PATIENT STORY

A 23-year-old male medical student presents to the physician's office complaining of his tongue's "strange appearance." He denies pain or discomfort and is unsure how long the lesions have been present. The lesions seem to change areas of distribution on the tongue. The examination reveals large, well-delineated, shiny and smooth, erythematous spots on the surface of the tongue (**Figure 40-1**). The diagnosis is geographic tongue (benign migratory glossitis). The physician explains that it is benign and that no treatment is needed unless symptoms develop.

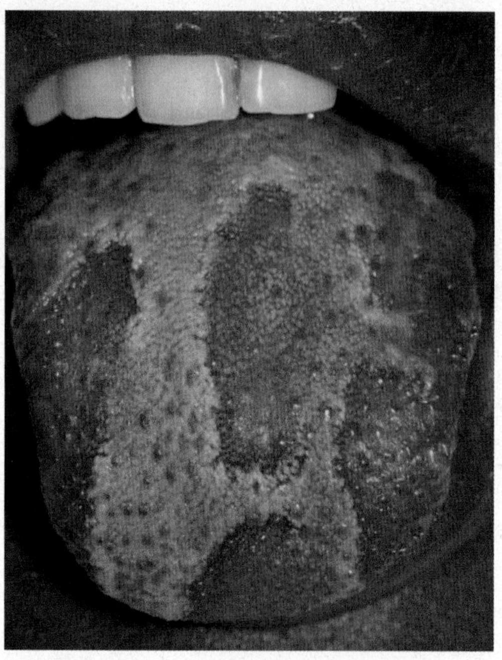

FIGURE 40-1 Geographic tongue (benign migratory glossitis). Note the pink continents among the white oceans. *(Reproduced with permission from Gonsalves WC, Chi AC, Neville BW: Common oral lesions: Part I. Superficial mucosal lesions, Am Fam Physician. 2007; 75(4):501-507.)*

INTRODUCTION

Geographic tongue is a chronic, benign, usually asymptomatic, inflammatory disorder of the mucosa of the dorsum and lateral borders of the tongue. Geographic tongue is characterized by circinate, irregularly shaped erythematous patches bordered by a white keratotic band. The central erythematous patch represents loss of filiform papillae of tongue epithelium. Geographic tongue presents with a migratory pattern.

SYNONYMS

Benign migratory glossitis, geographic stomatitis.

EPIDEMIOLOGY

- Multiple studies have shown a prevalence ranging from 1% to 12.7% in the general population.[1]
- Predilection for the second and third decades of life.[1]
- No gender bias.[1]
- Some studies have shown an increased frequency in patients with anxiety or increased stress, allergies, pustular psoriasis, type 1 diabetes, fissured tongue, or hormonal disturbances.[2]

ETIOLOGY AND PATHOPHYSIOLOGY

- Geographic tongue is a common oral inflammatory condition of unknown etiology.
- Studies shows that geographic tongue is the oral lesion most commonly associated with psoriasis based on the histologic appearance and the presence of a common genetic marker.[2,3]

DIAGNOSIS

CLINICAL FEATURES

- The diagnosis is made by visual inspection and history of the lesion. The lesions are suggestive of a geographic map (hence geographic tongue) with pink continents surrounded by whiter oceans (see **Figure 40-1**).
- Geographic tongue consists of large, well-delineated, shiny, and smooth, erythematous patches surrounded by a white halo (**Figure 40-2**).
- Tongue lesions exhibit central erythema because of atrophy of the filiform papillae and are usually surrounded by slightly elevated, curving, white-to-yellow elevated borders (**Figures 40-1** and **40-2**).
- The condition typically waxes and wanes over time so the lesions appear to be migrating (hence migratory glossitis).
- Lesions may last days, months, or years. The lesions do not scar.
- Most patients are asymptomatic, but some patients may complain of pain or burning, especially when eating spicy foods.
- Suspect systemic intraoral manifestations of psoriasis or reactive arthritis if the patient has psoriatic skin lesions or has conjunctivitis, urethritis, arthritis, and skin involvement suggestive of reactive arthritis (see Chapter 161, Reactive Arthritis).

TYPICAL DISTRIBUTION

- The lesions are typically found on the anterior two-thirds of the dorsal tongue mucosa.
- Ectopic signs of geographic tongue can occur less frequently on the ventral aspect of the tongue, the buccal and labial mucosa, and rarely on the palate. In these instances, it is called migratory stomatitis.[4]

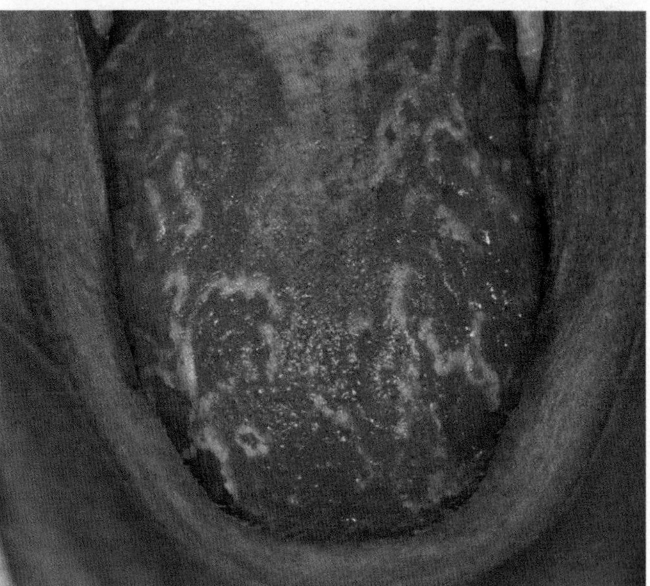

FIGURE 40-2 Geographic tongue lesions in a 71-year-old woman. Note the white halos around the pink areas of atrophy of filiform papillae. (*Reproduced with permission from Michael Huber, DMD.*)

DIFFERENTIAL DIAGNOSIS

- Erythroplakia or leukoplakia—May be suspected when lesions affect the soft palate (see Chapter 44, Leukoplakia).
- Lichen planus—Reticular forms are characterized by interlacing white lines commonly found on the buccal mucosa, or erosive forms, characterized by atrophic erythematous areas with central ulceration and surrounding radiating striae (see Chapter 160, Lichen Planus) (**Figure 40-3**).
- Psoriasis—Intraoral lesions have been described as red or white plaques associated with the activity of cutaneous lesions (see Chapter 158, Psoriasis) (**Figure 40-4**).
- Reactive arthritis—A condition characterized by the triad of "urethritis, arthritis, and conjunctivitis"; may have rare intraoral lesions described as painless ulcerative papules on the buccal mucosa and palate (see Chapter 161, Reactive Arthritis).
- Fissured tongue—An inherited condition in which the tongue has fissures that are asymptomatic. Although it has been called a *scrotal tongue* in the past, the term *fissured tongue* is preferred by patients (**Figure 40-5**).

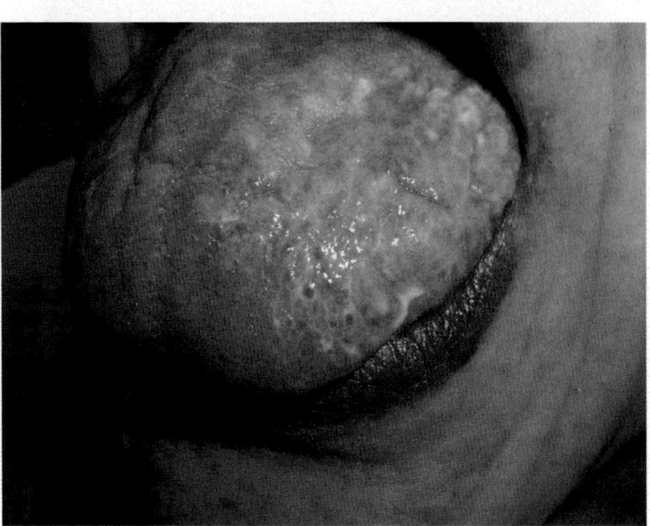

FIGURE 40-3 Lichen planus of the tongue. There are white striae; the surface is smooth in the affected area because of the loss of papillae. (*Reproduced with permission from Richard P. Usatine, MD.*)

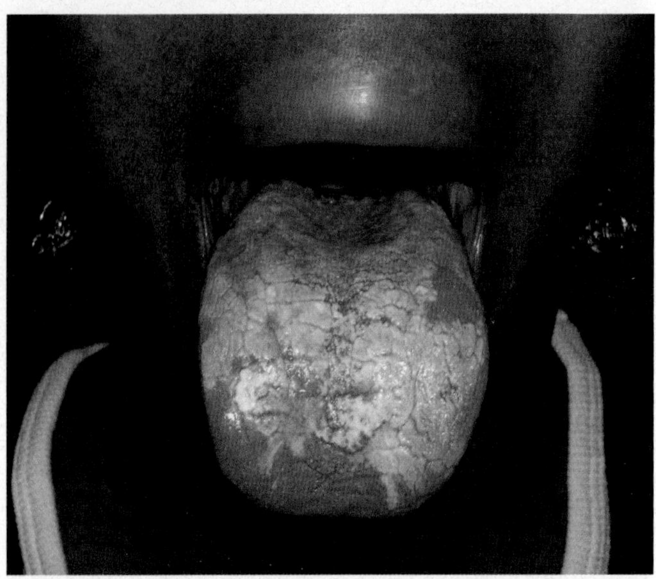

FIGURE 40-4 White plaques on the tongue of a black woman with severe cutaneous plaque psoriasis. A histologic specimen would appear similar to geographic tongue. (*Reproduced with permission from E.J. Mayeaux, Jr., MD.*)

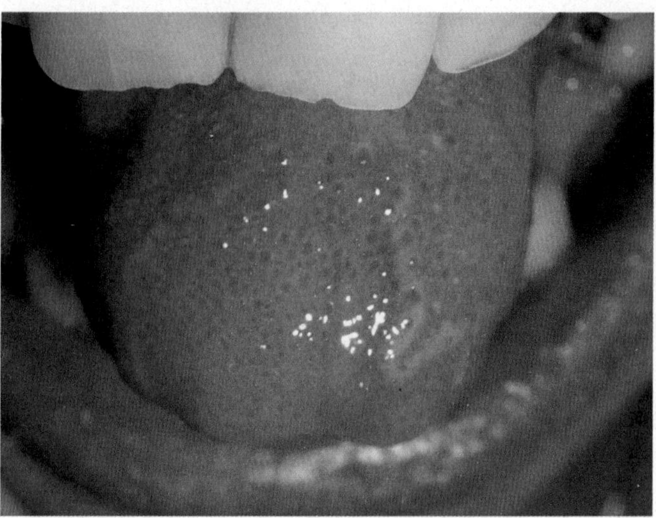

FIGURE 40-6 A mild asymptomatic case of geographic tongue. Note the atrophic filiform papillae and the subtle white halo. (*Reproduced with permission from Richard P. Usatine, MD.*)

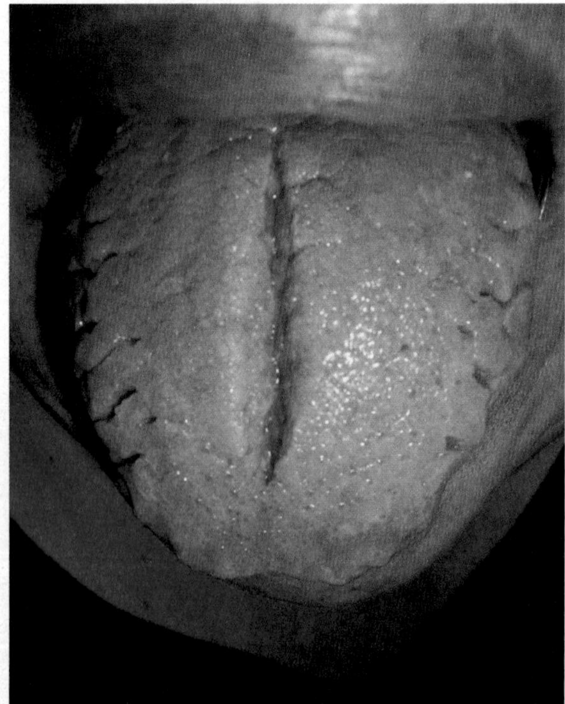

FIGURE 40-5 Fissured tongue present since birth. Although this has also been called a *scrotal tongue*, the preferred terminology is now *fissured tongue*, for obvious reasons. (*Reproduced with permission from Richard P. Usatine, MD.*)

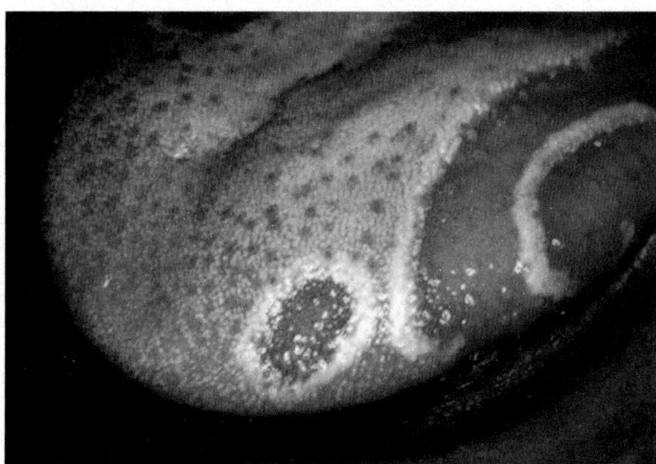

FIGURE 40-7 Geographic tongue with more severe symptomatology, including pain and a burning sensation when eating spicy foods. The contrast between the normal tongue tissue and the pink atrophic papillae is striking. (*Reproduced with permission from Ellen Eisenberg, DMD.*)

MANAGEMENT

Most individuals are asymptomatic and do not require treatment (**Figure 40-6**).

- For symptomatic cases, several treatments have been proposed but not proven effective with good clinical trials[5,6]:
    - Topical steroids such as triamcinolone dental paste (Oralone or Kenalog in Orabase) SOR Ⓒ
    - Supplements such as zinc, vitamin B_{12}, niacin, and riboflavin SOR Ⓒ
    - Antihistamine mouth rinses (e.g., diphenhydramine elixir 12.5 mg per 5 mL diluted in a 1:4 ratio with water) SOR Ⓒ
    - Topical anesthetic rinses[5,6] SOR Ⓒ

Geographic tongue can rarely present as persistent and painful (**Figure 40-7**). In one case report, 0.1% tacrolimus ointment was applied twice daily for 2 weeks with significant improvement of symptoms.[7] SOR Ⓒ

No treatment has been proven to be uniformly effective.[8]

FOLLOW-UP

Tell the patient to contact you if the symptoms continue past 10 days (of consistent treatment) and to go to the emergency department immediately if:

- The tongue swells significantly;
- The patient has trouble breathing; or
- The patient has trouble talking or chewing/swallowing.

PATIENT EDUCATION

Patients should be reassured of the condition's benign nature. Tell patients with geographic tongue to avoid irritating spicy foods and liquids.

PATIENT RESOURCES

- American Academy of Oral Medicine. *Geographic Tongue*—**http://www.aaom.com/index.php?option=com_content&view=article&id=131:geographic-tongue&catid=22:patient-condition-information&Itemid=120.**

PROVIDER RESOURCES

- Medscape. *Geographic Tongue*—**http://emedicine.medscape.com/article/1078465.**
- Mayo Clinic. *Geographic Tongue*—**http://www.mayoclinic.org/diseases-conditions/geographic-tongue/home/ovc-20319483.**

REFERENCES

1. Scariot R, Dias TB, Olandoski M, et al. Host and clinical aspects in patients with benign migratory glossitis. *Arch Oral Biol.* 2017;73:259-268.
2. Alikhani M, Khalighninejad N, Ghalaiani P, et al. Immunologic and psychologic parameters associated with geographic tongue. *Oral Surg Oral Med Oral Pathol Oral Radiol.* 2014;118:68-71.
3. Espelid M, Bang G, Johannessen AC, et al. Geographic stomatitis: report of 6 cases. *J Oral Pathol Med.* 1991;20:425-428.
4. Flores IL, Santos-Silva AR, Coletta RD, et al. Widespread red oral lesions. *J Am Dent Assoc.* 2013;144(11):1257-1260.
5. Abe M, Sogabe Y, Syuto T, et al. Successful treatment with cyclosporin administration for persistent benign migratory glossitis. *J Dermatol.* 2007;34:340-343.
6. Reamy BV, Derby R, Bunt CW. Common tongue conditions in primary care. *Am Fam Physician.* 2010;81:627-634.
7. Ishibashi M, Tojo G, Watanabe M, et al. Geographic tongue treated with topical tacrolimus. *J Dermatol Case Rep.* 2010;4:57-59.
8. Gonsalves W, Chi A, Neville B. Common oral lesions: part 1. Superficial mucosal lesions. *Am Fam Physician.* 2007;75:501-507.

41 GINGIVITIS AND PERIODONTAL DISEASE

Richard P. Usatine, MD
Wanda C. Gonsalves, MD
Guy Huynh-Ba, DDS, MS

PATIENT STORY

A 35-year-old woman presents to clinic for a routine physical examination. She says that for the last 6 months her gums bleed when she brushes her teeth. She reports smoking 1 pack of cigarettes per day. The oral examination finds generalized plaque and red swollen interdental papilla (**Figure 41-1**). The physician explains to her that she has gingivitis and that she should brush twice daily and use floss daily. The physician tells her that smoking is terrible for her health in all ways, including her oral health. The physician offers her help to quit smoking and refers her to a dentist for a cleaning and full dental examination.

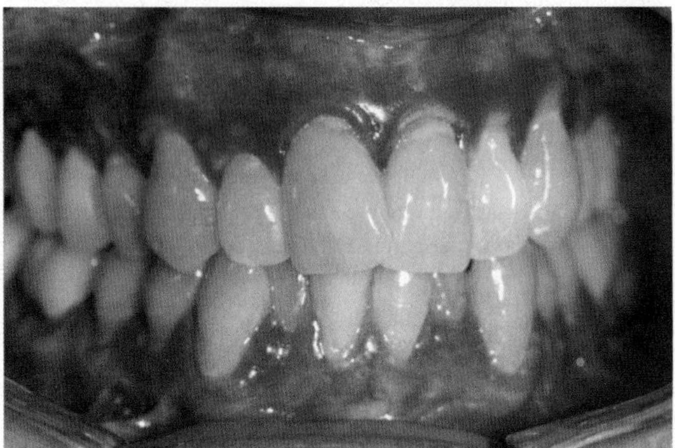

FIGURE 41-1 Chronic gingivitis in which the interdental papillae are edematous and blunted. There is some loss of gingival tissue. The gums bleed with brushing. (*Reproduced with permission from Gerald Ferretti, DMD.*)

INTRODUCTION

Gingivitis is the inflammation of the gingiva (gums). Gingivitis alone does not affect the underlying supporting structures of the teeth and is reversible (see **Figure 41-1**).

Periodontitis (periodontal disease) is a chronic inflammatory disease, which includes gingivitis along with loss of connective tissue and bone support for the teeth. It damages alveolar bone (the bone of the jaw in which the roots of the teeth are connected) and the periodontal ligaments that hold the roots in place. It is a major cause of tooth loss in adults (**Figures 41-2** to **41-4**).

EPIDEMIOLOGY

- Gingivitis and periodontal diseases are the most common oral diseases in adults.
- It is estimated that 45.9% of adults 30 years of age or older in the United States have periodontal disease. In that overall population, 8.9% have a severe form.[1]
- The prevalence and severity of periodontitis is increased in Hispanic, non-Hispanic black, Asian, low–socioeconomic status, and smoker populations. The prevalence increases with age, reaching 70% for the age group >65 years, and men are more frequently affected than women (see **Figure 41-4**).
- Periodontal disease has been shown in studies to be associated with atherosclerotic cardiovascular diseases, hospital-acquired pneumonia, and chronic kidney disease.[2]
- Periodontal disease has also been associated with adverse pregnancy outcomes including preterm birth, low birth weight, and pre-eclampsia.[3,4]

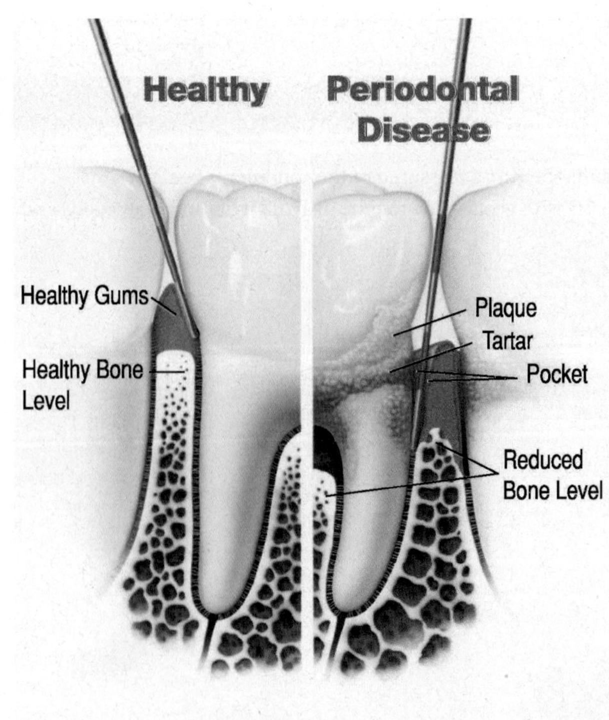

FIGURE 41-2 Healthy periodontal anatomy versus periodontal disease. (*Reproduced with permission from the American Academy of Periodontology; http://www.perio.org/consumer/2a.html.*)

ETIOLOGY AND PATHOPHYSIOLOGY

- Periodontal diseases are caused by bacteria in dental plaque that create an inflammatory response in gingival tissues (gingivitis) or in the soft tissue and bone supporting the teeth (periodontitis).
- The normal healthy gingival attachments form the gingival cuff around the tooth to help protect the underlying bone and teeth from the bacteria of the mouth.
- Gingivitis is caused by a reversible inflammatory process that occurs as the result of prolonged exposure of the gingival tissues to plaque and tartar (see **Figure 41-2**).
- Gingivitis may be classified by appearance (e.g., ulcerative, hemorrhagic), etiology (e.g., drugs, hormones), duration (e.g., acute, chronic), or by quality (e.g., mild, moderate, or severe).
- A severe form, acute necrotizing ulcerative gingivitis (ANUG) (**Figure 41-5**), also known as Vincent disease or trench mouth, is associated with α-hemolytic streptococci, anaerobic fusiform bacteria, and non-treponemal oral spirochetes. The term *trench mouth* was coined in World War I when ANUG was common among soldiers in the trenches. Predisposing factors now include HIV, malnutrition, and stress.[5]
- The most common form of gingivitis is chronic gingivitis induced by plaque (see **Figure 41-1**). This type of gingivitis occurs in half of the population 4 years of age or older. The inflammation worsens as mineralized plaque forms calculus (tartar) at and below the gum line (sulcus). The plaque that covers calculus causes destruction of bone (an irreversible condition), which may result in tooth mobility and ultimately in tooth loss.
- Gingivitis may persist for months or years without progressing to periodontitis. This suggests that host susceptibility plays an important role in the development of periodontal disease.[6]

RISK FACTORS

Risk factors that contribute to the development of periodontal disease include poor oral hygiene, smoking, diabetes, obesity, increased alcohol consumption, environmental factors (e.g., crowded teeth and mouth breathing), and comorbid conditions, such as a weakened immune status (e.g., HIV, steroids), low educational attainment, and low income.[1,6–10]

DIAGNOSIS

CLINICAL FEATURES

- Simple or marginal gingivitis first cause swelling of the interdental papillae and later affect the gingiva and dental interface (see **Figures 41-1** to **41-4**).
- Mild gingivitis is painless and may bleed when brushing or eating hard foods.
- ANUG (see **Figure 41-5**) is painful, ulcerative, and edematous and produces halitosis and bleeding gingival tissue. Patients with ANUG may have systemic symptoms such as myalgias and fever.

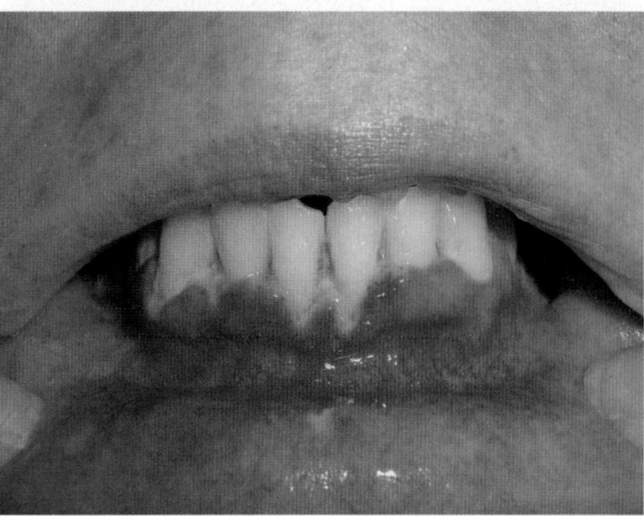

FIGURE 41-3 Severe periodontal disease in a woman who smokes and is addicted to cocaine. Note the blunting of the interdental papillae and the dramatic loss of gingival tissue. (*Reproduced with permission from Richard P. Usatine, MD.*)

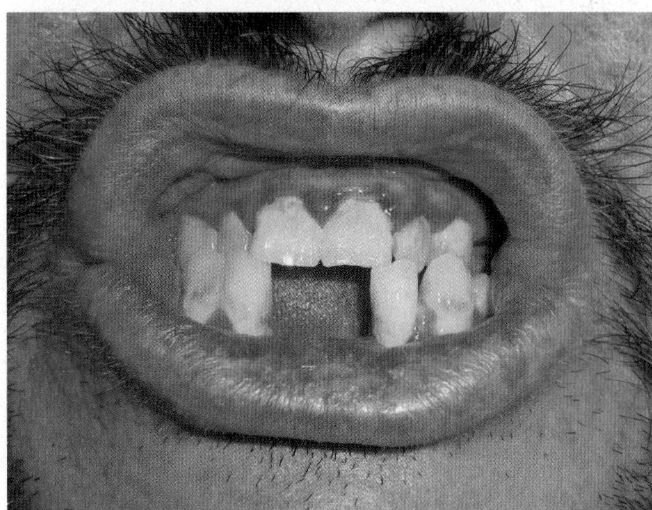

FIGURE 41-4 Severe periodontal disease in a man addicted to tobacco and alcohol. Note the edematous and blunted interdental papilla. This homeless man has already lost two teeth secondary to his severe periodontal disease. (*Reproduced with permission from Richard P. Usatine, MD.*)

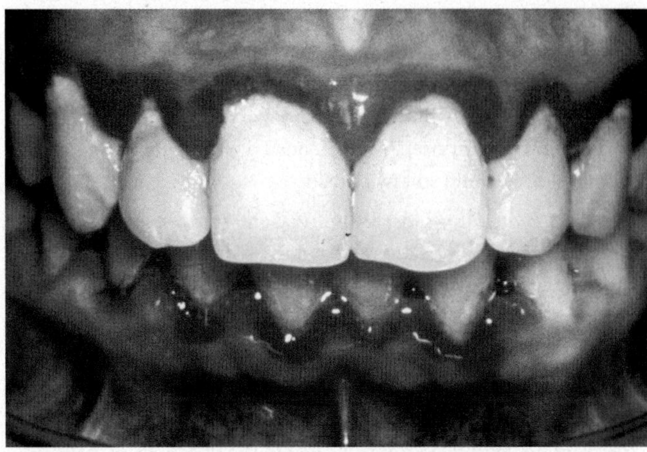

FIGURE 41-5 Acute necrotizing ulcerative gingivitis (ANUG) with intense erythema and ulcerations around the teeth. This is an acute infectious process. (*Reproduced with permission from Gerald Ferretti, DMD.*)

TYPICAL DISTRIBUTION

Gingivitis begins at the gingival and dental margins and may extend toward the alveolar ridge.

LABORATORY STUDIES AND IMAGING

Radiographs of the mouth are used to evaluate for bone loss in periodontal disease.

DIFFERENTIAL DIAGNOSIS

- Gingivitis can be from poor dental hygiene only or secondary to conditions that affect the immune system such as diabetes, Addison disease, HIV, and pregnancy.
- Gingival hyperplasia is an overgrowth of the gingiva with various etiologies, including medications such as calcium channel blockers, phenytoin, and cyclosporine. This can occur with or without coexisting gingivitis (see Chapter 42, Gingival Overgrowth).

MANAGEMENT

- Recommend smoking cessation for all patients who smoke.[8] SOR Ⓐ Offer help to support the patients' smoking cessation efforts with behavioral counseling and pharmacologic methods (see Chapter 248, Smoking and Tobacco Addiction). SOR Ⓐ
- Recommend alcohol cessation for patients with alcoholism and refer to Alcoholics Anonymous (AA) or another resource. For patients in whom alcohol use is heavy but addiction has not been diagnosed, at least recommend a decrease in alcohol use (see Chapter 249, Alcohol Use Disorder).[10] SOR Ⓑ
- Dental experts recommend tooth brushing twice a day and flossing daily.[11,12] SOR Ⓒ However, a Cochrane systematic review failed to show a benefit for daily flossing on plaque and clinical parameters of gingivitis.[13] SOR Ⓐ
- Studies suggest that electric toothbrushes may have an additional benefit over manual brushing, but given the current limitations of the existing literature, the effect size of such an advantage remains to be determined. Toothbrushing, with a manual or powered toothbrush, remains the primary mean to reduce plaque and gingivitis. SOR Ⓒ
- Systematic reviews indicate that there is strong evidence supporting the efficacy of chlorhexidine as an antiplaque, antigingivitis mouthrinse.[14] SOR Ⓐ Mouthwashes should not be used as a replacement for tooth brushing. Chlorhexidine oropharyngeal 0.12% is available as a generic mouthrinse. Recommended dosing is 15 mL to swish (for 30 seconds) and spit twice daily.
- The treatments with chlorhexidine (gel and spray) achieved a significant reduction in plaque and gingival bleeding in children with special needs. The parents/caregivers preferred the administration of chlorhexidine in spray form.[15] SOR Ⓑ
- In patients with ANUG, treatment involves antibiotics, nonsteroidal anti-inflammatory drugs (NSAIDs), and topical 2% viscous lidocaine for pain relief. Oral rinses with saline, hydrogen peroxide 3% solution, or chlorhexidine 0.12% may be of benefit. SOR Ⓒ
- Antibiotics recommended for ANUG include metronidazole, penicillin VK, erythromycin, doxycycline, and clindamycin. SOR Ⓒ
- Everyone should receive ongoing care from a dental professional for prevention and treatment of periodontal disease.

PREVENTION

- No smoking or tobacco use at all.
- Avoid alcohol and drug abuse.
- Good oral hygiene with tooth brushing and flossing.
- Dental visits at least twice yearly even during pregnancy.

PATIENT EDUCATION

- There is no safe level of smoking. Quitting is crucial to good health.
- Drink alcohol in moderation or not at all.
- Practice good oral hygiene to remove plaque (i.e., brush twice a day and use floss daily).
- Consider use of chlorhexidine-containing mouthrinse.
- Consult a dentist for regular check-ups, especially when the condition does not improve after using good oral hygiene.
- Pregnancy is not a contraindication for dental visits and cleaning.

FOLLOW-UP

Follow up patients with ANUG closely. All patients need regular dental care and follow-up with their dentist.

PATIENT RESOURCES

- American Academy of Periodontology—*Gum Disease Information* **https://www.perio.org/consumer/gum-disease.htm.**
- The European Federation of Periodontology—*What Is Periodontitis?* **https://www.efp.org/patients/what-is-periodontitis.html.**

PROVIDER RESOURCES

- Stephen JM. *Gingivitis*—**http://emedicine.medscape.com/article/763801.**

REFERENCES

1. Eke PI, Dye BA, Wei L, et al. Update on prevalence of periodontitis in adults in the United States: NHANES 2009 to 2012. *J Periodontol.* 2015;86:611-622.
2. Linden GJ, Lyons A, Scannapieco FA. Periodontal systemic associations: review of the evidence. *J Periodontol.* 2013 Apr; 84(4 Suppl):S8-S19.
3. Corbella S, Taschieri S, Del Fabbro M, et al. Adverse pregnancy outcomes and periodontitis: a systematic review and meta-analysis exploring potential association. *Quintessence Int.* 2016;47(3):193-204.
4. Ide M, Papapanou PN. Epidemiology of association between maternal periodontal disease and adverse pregnancy outcomes—systematic review. *J Periodontol.* 2013;84(4 Suppl):S181-S194.

5. Herrera D, Alonso B, de Arriba L, et al. Acute periodontal lesions. *Periodontol 2000.* 2014;65(1):149-177.
6. Kornman KS. Mapping the pathogenesis of periodontitis: a new look. *J Periodontol.* 2008;79(8 Suppl):1560-1568.
7. Casanova L, Hughes FJ, Preshaw PM. Diabetes and periodontal disease: a two-way relationship. *Br Dent J.* 2014;217(8):433-437.
8. Hanioka T, Ojima M, Tanaka K, et al. Causal assessment of smoking and tooth loss: a systematic review of observational studies. *BMC Public Health.* 2011;11:221.
9. Boillot A, El Halabi B, Batty GD, et al. Education as a predictor of chronic periodontitis: a systematic review with meta-analysis population-based studies. *PLoS One.* 2011;6(7):e21508.
10. Wang J, Lv J, Wang W, Jiang X. Alcohol consumption and risk of periodontitis: a meta-analysis. *J Clin Periodontol.* 2016;43(7): 572-583.
11. Chapple IL, Van der Weijden F, Doerfer C, et al. Primary prevention of periodontitis: managing gingivitis. *J Clin Periodontol.* 2015 Apr;42 Suppl 16:S71-S76.
12. Van der Weijden FA, Slot DE. Efficacy of homecare regimens for mechanical plaque removal in managing gingivitis: a meta review. *J Clin Periodontol.* 2015;42 Suppl 16:S77-S91.
13. Berchier CE, Slot DE, Haps S, Van der Weijden GA. The efficacy of dental floss in addition to a toothbrush on plaque and parameters of gingival inflammation: a systematic review. *Int J Dent Hyg.* 2008;6:265-279.
14. Gunsolley JC. Clinical efficacy of antimicrobial mouthrinses. *J Dent.* 2010;38 Suppl 1:S6-S10.
15. Chibinski AC, Pochapski MT, Farago PV, et al. Clinical evaluation of chlorhexidine for the control of dental biofilm in children with special needs. *Community Dent Health.* 2011;28:222-226.

42 GINGIVAL OVERGROWTH

Richard P. Usatine, MD
Wanda C. Gonsalves, MD
Guy Huynh-Ba, DDS, MS

PATIENT STORY

A 31-year-old woman with a history of seizure disorder notices increasing gum enlargement (**Figure 42-1**). She is unemployed and does not have dental insurance. She has not been to a dentist in at least 10 years. She brushes her teeth only once a day and does not floss at all. She has been on phenytoin (Dilantin) since early childhood, and this does prevent her seizures. You talk to her about dental hygiene and refer her to a low-cost dental clinic that cares for persons with limited resources.

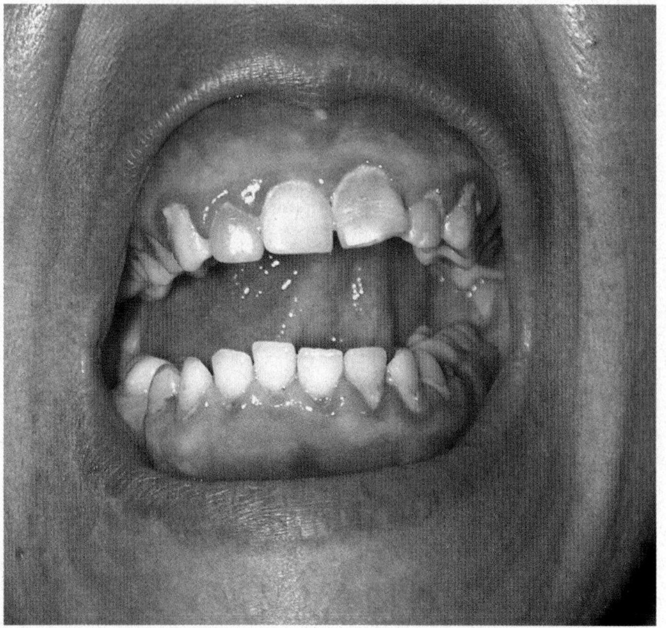

FIGURE 42-1 Gingival overgrowth secondary to phenytoin (Dilantin) in a woman with epilepsy. (*Reproduced with permission from Richard P. Usatine, MD.*)

INTRODUCTION

Gingival overgrowth (hyperplasia) can be hereditary or induced as a side effect of systemic drugs, such as phenytoin, cyclosporine, or calcium channel blockers. Besides the cosmetic effect, it can make good oral hygiene more difficult to maintain.

SYNONYMS

Gingival hyperplasia, drug-induced gingival overgrowth (DIGO), hereditary gingival fibromatosis.

EPIDEMIOLOGY

- The prevalence of phenytoin-induced gingival hyperplasia is estimated at 15% to 50% in patients taking the medication[1,2] (**Figures 42-1** and **42-2**).
- In patients receiving cyclosporine for more than 3 months, the incidence of gingival overgrowth (GO) can approach 70%[3] (**Figure 42-3**).
- The incidence of gingival hyperplasia has been reported as 10% to 20% in patients treated with calcium channel blockers in the general population.[2]

ETIOLOGY AND PATHOPHYSIOLOGY

- Although the etiology of GO is not entirely known, risk factors known to contribute to GO include the following: nonspecific chronic inflammation associated with poor hygiene, hormonal changes (pregnancy), medications (calcium channel blockers, phenytoin, and cyclosporine), and systemic diseases (leukemia, sarcoidosis, and Crohn disease).
    - Studies suggest that phenytoin, cyclosporine, and nifedipine interact with epithelial keratinocytes, fibroblasts, and collagen to lead to an overgrowth of gingival tissue in susceptible individuals.[2]
    - More than 15 drugs have been shown to cause GO.

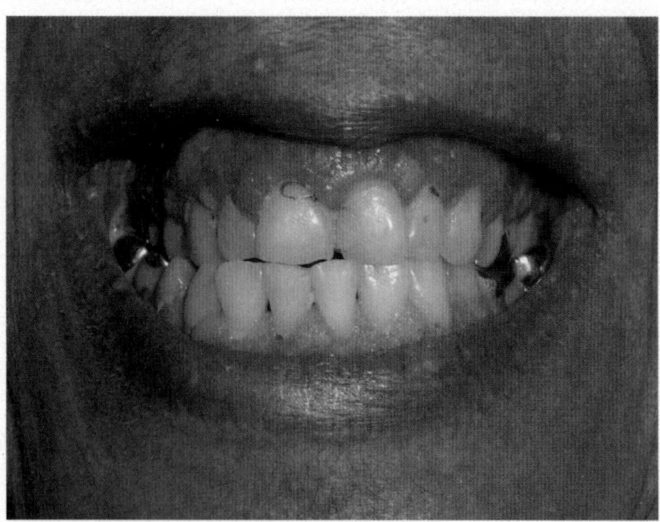

FIGURE 42-2 Multiple tiny hamartomas on the gums from Cowden disease with gingival overgrowth secondary to phenytoin. (*Reproduced with permission from Richard P. Usatine, MD.*)

   ◦ The most common nonreversible DIGO is caused by phenytoin (see **Figures 42-1** and **42-2**).
- Histopathologically, tissue enlargement is the result of proliferation of fibroblasts, collagen, and chronic inflammatory cells.

RISK FACTORS

- Prolonged use of phenytoin, cyclosporine, or calcium-channel blockers (especially nifedipine).
- Pregnancy.
- Systemic diseases (leukemia, sarcoidosis, and Crohn disease).
- Poor oral hygiene and the presence of periodontal disease.

DIAGNOSIS

SIGNS AND SYMPTOMS

- The diagnosis is made by visual inspection and by obtaining a thorough history (see **Figures 42-1** to **42-3**).
- The gingiva appears edematous and bulky with loss of its stippling. It may be soft or firm.
- Inflamed gingiva that are red and friable. They may bleed easily with minor trauma from eating, brushing the teeth or flossing.

TYPICAL DISTRIBUTION

Lobular gingival enlargement occurs first at the interdental papillae and anterior facial gingiva approximately 2 to 3 months after starting the drug and increases in maximum severity in 12 to 18 months (see **Figure 42-3**).

LABORATORY TESTS

Consider checking a complete blood count (CBC) with differential count to investigate for leukemia if there is not an obvious etiology.

IMAGING

The periodontist or oral medicine specialist may order bitewing radiographs and periapical films to evaluate for the presence of periodontal disease.

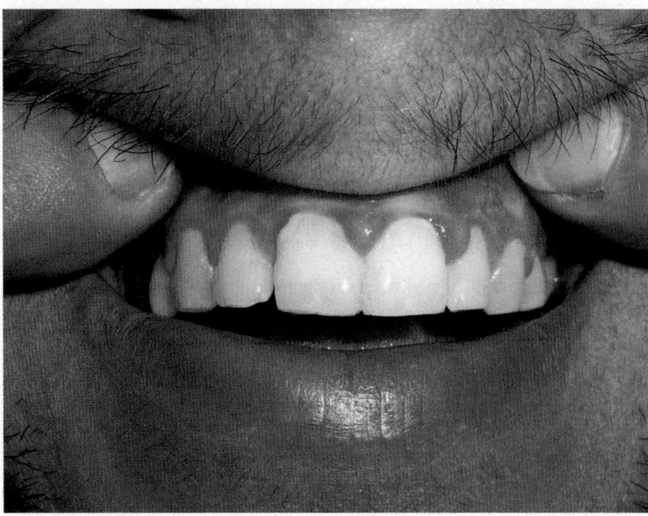

FIGURE 42-3 Gingival overgrowth secondary to cyclosporine use for 1 year to treat severe plaque psoriasis. Note the blunted and thickened interdental papillae. (*Reproduced with permission from Richard P. Usatine, MD.*)

DIFFERENTIAL DIAGNOSIS

- Generalized gingivitis—Gums around the teeth become inflamed. This condition often occurs with poor oral hygiene (see Chapter 41, Gingivitis and Periodontal Disease).
- Pregnancy gingivitis—Inflamed gums. More than half of pregnant women will develop gingivitis during pregnancy because of hormonal changes.
- Pyogenic granuloma—A small red bump that may bleed and grow to approximately half an inch. These are most often found on the skin but can occur in the mouth secondary to trauma or pregnancy. When they occur in pregnancy, they are sometimes called a pregnancy tumor. In reality, these are not pyogenic or granulomatous but are a type of lobular capillary hemangioma (see Chapter 167, Pyogenic Granuloma) (**Figure 42-4**).

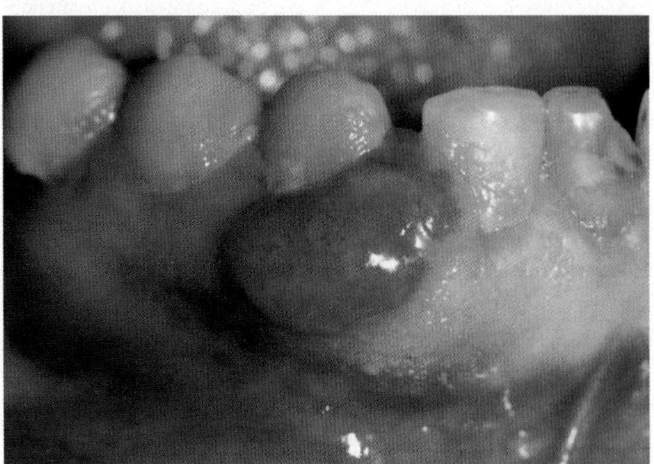

FIGURE 42-4 Pyogenic granuloma growing rapidly on the gums after minor trauma. (*Reproduced with permission from Gonsalves WC, Chi AC, Neville BW. Common oral lesions: part II. Masses and neoplasia, Am Fam Physician. 2007;75(4):509-512.*)

- Leukemia—Leukemic cells may infiltrate the oral soft tissues, producing a diffuse, boggy, nontender swelling of the gingiva that may ulcerate or bleed.

MANAGEMENT

NONPHARMACOLOGIC

- Consider referral for nonsurgical periodontal treatment including motivation and oral hygiene instruction and cleanings at least every 3 months to control plaque.[4] SOR B
- The use of a powered toothbrush, together with oral hygiene instruction, reduces GO for pediatric transplantation patients on cyclosporine. In one study, the sonic toothbrushing and oral hygiene instruction group had less severe GO after 12 months than did the control group.[5] SOR B
- If possible, stop drugs that induce gingival hyperplasia as discontinuing the medications may reverse the condition in most cases (except phenytoin).
- If drugs cannot be stopped, try reducing the dose, if possible, as gingival hyperplasia can be dose dependent.

MEDICATIONS

- Tacrolimus is an alternative to cyclosporine to prevent transplant rejection; it causes less GO. In one study on the prevalence of gingival growth after renal transplantation, GO occurred in 29% of patients treated with tacrolimus and in 60% of patients treated with cyclosporine.[6] SOR B In another study, switching patients from cyclosporine to tacrolimus reduced GO in the first month after the change was made.[7] SOR B
- Case reports have reported regression of overgrowth with both oral metronidazole and azithromycin. In one randomized controlled trial (RCT), patients with GO were randomized to receive either 1 course of 5 days of azithromycin or 7 days of metronidazole. The extent of GO was measured at 0, 2, 4, 6, 12, and 24 weeks, and azithromycin was found to be more effective than metronidazole.[3] SOR B
- Azithromycin with an oral hygiene program resulted in a reduction in cyclosporine-induced GO, whereas oral hygiene alone improved oral symptoms (pain, halitosis, and gum bleeding) but did not decrease cyclosporine-induced GO.[8] Patients were randomized into two groups, both receiving oral hygiene instructions, with the treatment group receiving 3 days of azithromycin 500 mg daily. They were evaluated after 15 and 30 days, and only the azithromycin group had a reduction in GO.[8] SOR B
- Chlorhexidine 12% (Peridex) once before going to bed or Biotene mouthwash after meals is recommended for patients who are known to be at risk for gingivitis.[2] SOR C Warn patients that chlorhexidine 12% will taste bad and can stain the teeth. This staining can be removed with a dental cleaning. This information should help improve adherence to the use of this mouthwash.

REFERRAL

- For patients who do not respond to the above measures, refer to a dental health professional for possible gingivectomy. This can be done with a scalpel or a laser.

PREVENTION

Ensure healthy periodontal tissue prior to starting calcium channel blockers or phenytoin, or before any organ transplantation in which cyclosporine will be prescribed.

Folic acid supplementation, 0.5 mg per day, is associated with prevention of GO in children taking phenytoin monotherapy. Of patients in the folic acid arm, 21% developed GO, as compared with 88% receiving placebo.[1] SOR B

PATIENT EDUCATION

Advise patients to practice good oral hygiene (i.e., brush at least twice a day and floss at least once a day) and have regular follow-up with their dental health professional to monitor for worsening periodontal disease.

FOLLOW-UP

- Patients should be monitored by a periodontist or an oral medicine specialist as long as the patients are taking medicines that induce gingival hyperplasia.

PATIENT RESOURCES

- The American Academy of Oral Medicine (AAOM), *Gingival Enlargement*—**http://www.aaom.com/index.php%3Foption=com_content&view=article&id=132:gingival-enlargement&catid=22:patient-condition-information&Itemid=120.**

PROVIDER RESOURCES

- Mejia L. *Drug-Induced Gingival Hyperplasia*—**https://emedicine.medscape.com/article/1076264-overview.**
- American Academy of Periodontology (AAP). *Informational Paper: Drug-Associated Gingival Enlargement*—**http://www.joponline.org/doi/pdf/10.1902/jop.2004.75.10.1424.**

REFERENCES

1. Arya R, Gulati S, Kabra M, et al. Folic acid supplementation prevents phenytoin-induced gingival overgrowth in children. *Neurology*. 2011;76:1338-1343.
2. Mejia L. *Drug-Induced Gingival Hyperplasia*. http://emedicine.medscape.com/article/1076264. Accessed January 2012.

3. Chand DH, Quattrocchi J, Poe SA, et al. Trial of metronidazole vs. azithromycin for treatment of cyclosporine-induced gingival overgrowth. *Pediatr Transplant.* 2004;8:60-64.

4. Pejcic A, Djordjevic V, Kojovic D, et al. Effect of periodontal treatment in renal transplant recipients. *Med Princ Pract.* 2014;23(2):149-153.

5. Smith JM, Wong CS, Salamonik EB, et al. Sonic tooth brushing reduces gingival overgrowth in renal transplant recipients. *Pediatr Nephrol.* 2006;21:1753-1759.

6. Cota LO, Aquino DR, Franco GC, et al. Gingival overgrowth in subjects under immunosuppressive regimens based on cyclosporine, tacrolimus, or sirolimus. *J Clin Periodontol.* 2010;37:894-902.

7. Parraga-Linares L, Almendros-Marques N, Berini-Aytes L, Gay-Escoda C. Effectiveness of substituting cyclosporin A with tacrolimus in reducing gingival overgrowth in renal transplant patients. *Med Oral Patol Oral Cir Bucal.* 2009;14:e429-e433.

8. Ramalho VL, Ramalho HJ, Cipullo JP, et al. Comparison of azithromycin and oral hygiene program in the treatment of cyclosporine-induced gingival hyperplasia. *Ren Fail.* 2007;29:265-270.

43 APHTHOUS ULCER

Richard P. Usatine, MD
Wanda C. Gonsalves, MD
David Ojeda Díaz, DDS

PATIENT STORY

A 58-year-old man presents with a 1-year history of painful sores in his mouth (**Figures 43-1** to **43-4**). He has lost 20 pounds over the past year because it hurts to eat. The ulcers come and go, but are found on his tongue, buccal mucosa, and inner lips. Prior to the onset of these lesions, the patient had been in good health and was not on any medications. The physician recognized his condition as recurrent aphthous ulcers. No underlying systemic diseases were found on work-up. The patient was started on oral prednisone and given dexamethasone oral elixir to swish and swallow. Within 1 week the patient was able to eat and drink liquids comfortably and began regaining his lost weight. Long-term management of his problem required the use of other medications so as to successfully taper him off prednisone without recurrences.

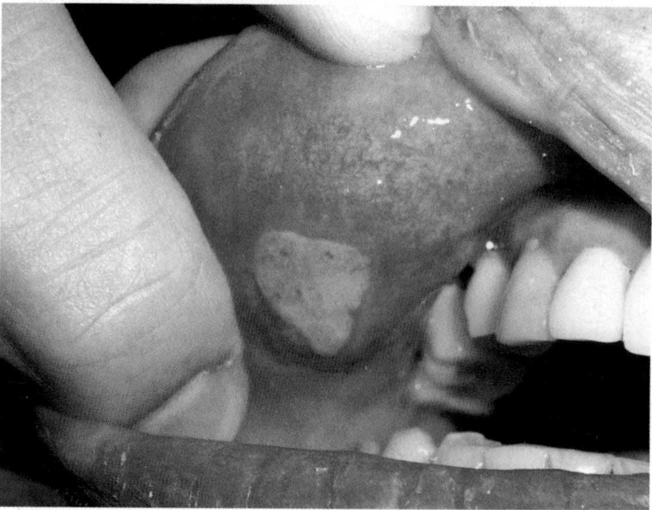

FIGURE 43-1 Major aphthous ulcer on the buccal mucosa of a 58-year-old man who has been suffering with recurrent aphthous stomatitis for the past year. (*Reproduced with permission from Richard P. Usatine, MD.*)

INTRODUCTION

Aphthous ulcers are the most frequent form of ulcerations in the oral cavity. They can present as a single or multiple ulcerations, and with an occasional or recurrent pattern. They vary in size, but typically present as a round and shallow ulceration with a well-defined erythematous halo. Aphthous ulcers are painful and may interfere with oral function such as eating and speaking. Oral trauma, stress, and systemic diseases can contribute to the occurrence of these ulcers, but no precise etiology is apparent. The disabling character of this condition makes the patient seek medical evaluation. The medical management of recurrent aphthous stomatitis (RAS) can be frustrating and sometime requires aggressive treatment aimed at pain relief and prevention.

SYNONYMS

Canker sores, recurrent aphthous ulcer (RAU), aphthous stomatitis, RAS.

EPIDEMIOLOGY

- Approximately 20% of the general population is affected by RAS,[1] but the incidence rate varies from 5% to 60% according to the population studied.[2]
- In children, prevalence of RAS can be as high as 39% and is influenced by the presence of RAS in one or both parents.[1] A study showed that children with a RAS-positive parent have a 90% chance of developing RAS.[3]
- RAS is more common in people younger than age 40 years, with a peak between ages of 10 and 19 years,[1] in women, in whites, in nonsmokers, and in people with high levels of stress and high socioeconomic status.[4]

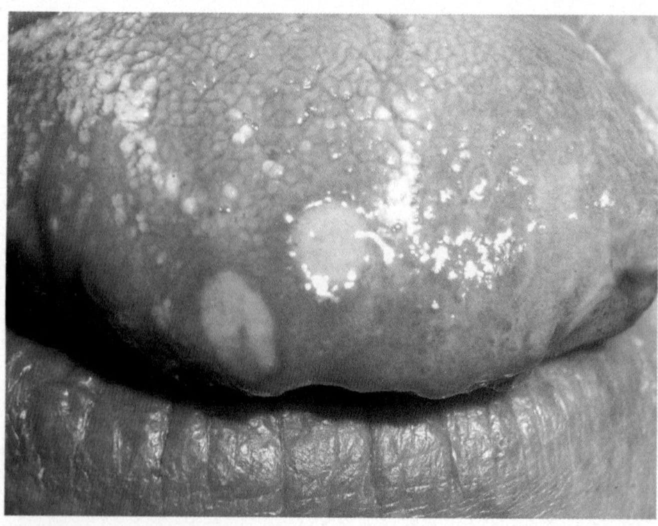

FIGURE 43-2 Two aphthous ulcers on the tongue of a 58-year-old man with recurrent aphthous stomatitis. (*Reproduced with permission from Richard P. Usatine, MD.*)

ETIOLOGY AND PATHOPHYSIOLOGY

- The precise etiology and pathogenesis of this condition remains unclear, although a variety of host and environmental factors have been implicated.
- The immunopathogenesis likely involves a cell-mediated immune response mechanism, which includes T cells and tumor necrosis factor-α (TNF-α) activation by other leukocytes such as macrophages and mast cells. This inflammatory process might be initiated by the effect of TNF-α on endothelial cells stimulating the neutrophils.[2]
- From the cellular perspective, lymphocytes infiltrate the epithelium developing intraepithelial edema, which triggers an inflammatory response characterized by localized vasculitis and keratinocyte vacuolization, resulting in a papule formation. The papule then ulcerates and is infiltrated by neutrophils, lymphocytes, and plasma cells initiating the healing process and regeneration of the epithelium.[2]
- A positive family history is seen in about one-third of RAS patients. A genetic predisposition is suggested by an increased frequency of HLA types A2, A11, B12, and DR2.[4]

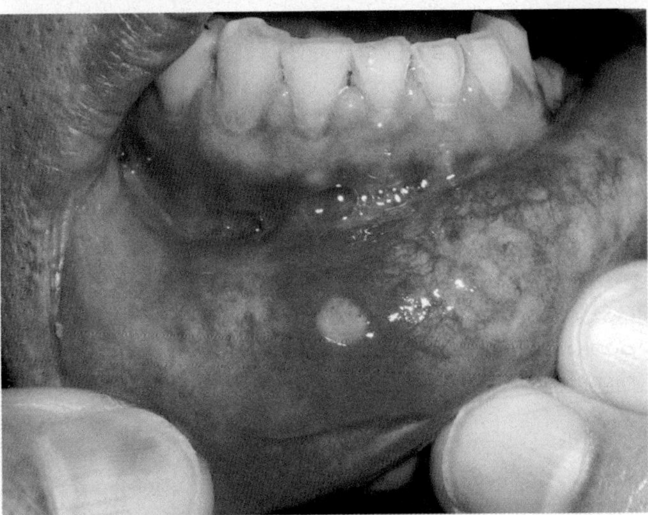

FIGURE 43-3 Minor aphthous ulcer occurring simultaneously with major aphthous ulcers on the buccal mucosa and tongue of a 58-year-old man with recurrent aphthous ulcers. (*Reproduced with permission from Richard P. Usatine, MD.*)

RISK FACTORS

- Oral trauma.
- Stress and anxiety.
- Systemic diseases (celiac disease, Crohn disease, Behçet syndrome, HIV, reactive arthritis, cyclic neutropenia).
- Medications (nonsteroidal anti-inflammatory drugs [NSAIDs], β-blockers, angiotensin-converting enzyme inhibitors [ACEIs]).
- Nutritional and vitamin deficiencies (zinc, iron, B_{12}, folate).
- Food and chemical sensitivities.
- Psychological stress.

DIAGNOSIS

CLINICAL FEATURES

History:

- Symptoms may begin with a prodromal burning sensation that lasts 2 to 48 hours before the ulcer appears,[1] and the pain is exacerbated by moving the area affected by the ulcer.
- Eating often hurts, especially foods and drinks with a high acid content.
- Ask about family history.
- Ask about recurrences and onset in relation to the use of medications.
- Ask about GI symptoms, genital ulcers, HIV risk factors, and joint pain.

Physical:

- The ulcers are rounded, center covered with yellowish-gray pseudomembrane surrounded by a well-defined erythematous halo. These could be solitary or multiple (**Figure 43-5**).

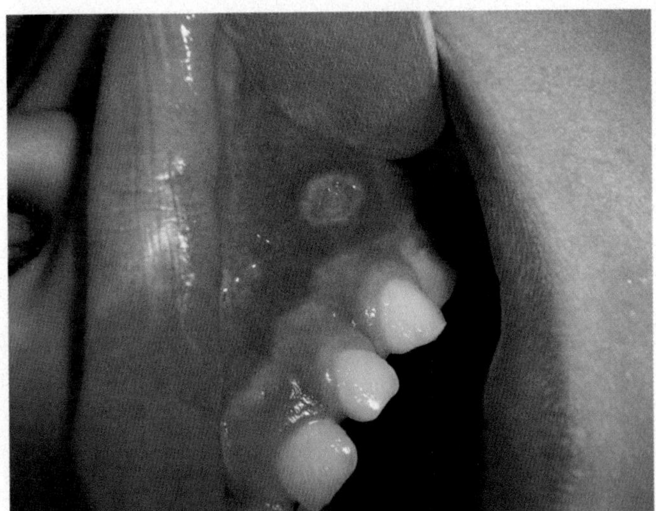

FIGURE 43-4 Aphthous ulcer located on unkeratinized (movable) mucosa in a 5-year-old girl. It is slightly raised, round, with a white-yellow necrotic center and surrounding erythema. (*Reproduced with permission from Richard P. Usatine, MD.*)

- Three clinical variations are described based on the size of the ulcers: Minor (4 to 9 mm) the most common form, usually heals in 7 to 10 days without scarring formation. Major (>1 cm) usually heals in 15 to 20 days and may result in scarring. Herpetiform (<3 mm) is usually multiple and manifests as a cluster. This term is used to describe the clinical appearance of the ulcers and does not suggest the presence of herpes simplex virus (HSV) (see **Figure 43-5**).

TYPICAL DISTRIBUTION

RAS usually involves non-keratinizing mucosa (e.g., labial mucosa, buccal mucosa, ventral tongue). Aphthous ulcers spare the attached gingiva and the hard palate (non-movable mucosa).

LABORATORY TESTS

Consider complete blood count (CBC), ferritin, B_{12}, folate, erythrocyte sedimentation rate (ESR), viral culture, KOH, skin biopsy, and HIV testing, if indicated. In case of RAS in patients older than 40 years, consider pertinent testing to rule out celiac disease, Crohn disease, Behçet syndrome, reactive arthritis, and cyclic neutropenia.

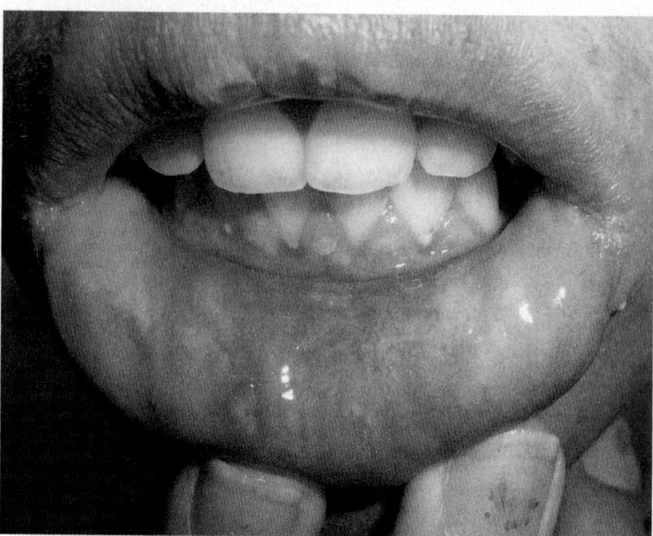

FIGURE 43-5 Behçet syndrome characterized by recurrent oral and genital ulcers in a 17-year-old girl. *(Reproduced with permission from Richard P. Usatine, MD.)*

DIFFERENTIAL DIAGNOSIS

- Primary oral herpes simplex virus (primary gingivostomatitis)—Begins as vesicular lesions, which quickly ulcerate on all mucosal lesions in the mouth. It is accompanied by systemic manifestations such as fever, malaise, anorexia, and sore throat. The ulcers are located on movable and non-movable oral mucosa (includes attached gingiva and hard palate). Lesions may also appear on keratinized surfaces such as the lip (see Chapter 135, Herpes Simplex).
- Herpangina causes multiple ulcers in the mouth, especially on the soft palate and the anterior fauces. It is caused by Coxsackievirus A16 in most cases. The distribution of the ulcers is different than in aphthous ulcers.
- Oral cancer—Ulcerative lesion that will not resolve by 2 weeks (see Chapter 45, Oropharyngeal Cancer).
- Erythema multiforme (EM)—Mucocutaneous lesion preceded by infection with HSV, *Mycoplasma pneumoniae*, or exposure to certain drugs or medications. Oral lesions begin as patches and evolve into large shallow erosions and ulcerations with irregular borders. Common sites include the lip, tongue, buccal mucosa, floor of the mouth, and soft palate. The presence of targetoid skin lesions should help differentiate EM from RAS (see Chapter 185, Erythema Multiforme, Stevens-Johnson Syndrome, and Toxic Epidermal Necrolysis).
- Erosive lichen planus—Erythematous ulcerative lesion with surrounding striae (see Chapter 160, Lichen Planus).
- Behçet syndrome—A condition with multiple ulcerative lesions that resemble aphthae involving the soft palate and oropharynx, infrequent sites for routine aphthae. Common cutaneous lesions include the genital and ocular mucosa (**Figure 43-6**).
- Hand, foot, and mouth disease presents as mucocutaneous lesions involving the hand, foot, and mouth caused by enterovirus. Any area of mucosa may be involved. Lesions resolve within 1 week (see Chapter 134, Hand Foot Mouth Syndrome).

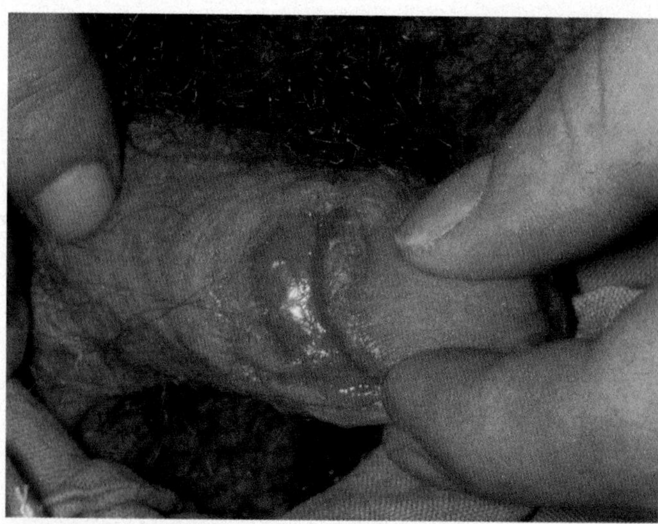

FIGURE 43-6 Ulcer on the penis in a patient with Behçet syndrome. *(Reproduced with permission from Richard P. Usatine, MD.)*

MANAGEMENT

FIRST LINE

Most isolated aphthae require no treatment or only periodic topical therapy. For the following topical medications, patients should be instructed to dab the area of ulcer dry, apply the gel, paste, or cream, and then avoid eating or drinking for at least 30 minutes:

- Topical corticosteroids, such as fluocinonide gel or dexamethasone elixir, can promote healing and lessen the severity of RAS.[5] SOR Ⓒ
- Amlexanox 5% paste (Aphthasol) reduces ulcer size, pain duration, and healing time.[6] It is nonprescription and the paste is applied directly to ulcers four times a day until ulcers heal.[6] SOR Ⓑ
- Lidocaine 1% cream applied to aphthous ulcers was found to reduce pain intensity compared to the placebo cream.[7] SOR Ⓑ Lidocaine also can be prescribed in 2% jelly.

SECOND LINE

In severe RAS cases, systemic therapy with oral steroids, montelukast, colchicine, pentoxifylline, dapsone, clofazimine, or thalidomide may need to be considered:

- Both prednisone and montelukast were effective in reducing the number of aphthous ulcers and improving pain relief and ulcer healing when compared with placebo in a randomized controlled trial (RCT).[8] Prednisone was more effective than montelukast in pain cessation ($P < 0.0001$) and in accelerating ulcer healing ($P < 0.0001$). Montelukast may be useful in cases of RAS where pharmacologic therapy for long periods is needed and prednisone is to be avoided.[8] In this study, prednisone was given 25 mg daily for 15 days, 12.5 mg daily for 15 days, 6.25 mg daily for 15 days, and then 6.25 mg on alternate days for 15 days. Montelukast 10 mg daily was given every evening and then on alternate days for the second month.[8] SOR Ⓑ
- In one RCT, 5 mg per day prednisolone was compared with 0.5 mg per day colchicine in the treatment of RAS. Both colchicine and prednisolone treatments significantly reduced RAS. No significant differences in size and number of lesions, recurrence and severity of pain, and duration of pain-free period were seen between the two treatment groups. Colchicine (52.9%) had significantly more side effects than prednisolone (11.8%), so the prednisolone seems to be a better alternative in reducing the signs and symptoms of RAS in the short term.[9] SOR Ⓑ However, long-term prednisolone and/or prednisone has many adverse effects to be avoided.
- Clofazimine 100 mg daily for 30 days and then 100 mg every other day has been studied in a partially blinded RCT for the prevention of RAS. A greater percentage of individuals in the clofazimine group had no further aphthous episodes (17% to 44%) compared with the other groups (<6%).[10] Clofazimine has many risks and should only be prescribed by clinicians familiar with this medication.
- A multicenter cohort analysis of thalidomide for severe RAS found that low-dose maintenance regimens of thalidomide appear to be effective.[11] However, adverse events were reported by 84% (77 of 92) of patients. If thalidomide is to be considered, refer the patient to a specialist with experience using this toxic drug.[11] SOR Ⓑ Thalidomide is associated with severe birth defects and can only be obtained in the United States through a special program.
- One small study compared the clinical response of multiple systemic drugs (dapsone, thalidomide, colchicine, and pentoxifylline) in 21 patients with RAS.[12] All the patients were given a 2-week course of prednisone for symptom relief before any of the other systemic medications were started. Dapsone (100 mg/day) given for 1 to 6 months (mean 4.2 months) showed excellent-to-moderate improvement in symptoms in 89% of patients. However, moderate-to-severe side effects were reported in 66% of the patients, requiring the discontinuation of the medication. Anemia, hemolysis, and jaundice were found in 33% of patients. The same study investigated pentoxifylline (400 mg three times daily) in a different group of patients with RAS.[12] Forty percent reported moderate improvement (shorter healing time, less severe lesions, and lower recurrence rate), 20% reported complete remission, and 20% reported no benefit. Few side effects were reported for pentoxifylline. Although pentoxifylline was the least effective of all the medications tested, it is by far the safest of the four medications.

COMPLEMENTARY AND ALTERNATIVE THERAPY

Vitamin C was shown to reduce the frequency of minor RAS and the severity of pain by 50% in a small group of teens. They were given 2000 mg/m^2 per day of ascorbate.[13]

REFERRAL

Refer patients with a persistent or atypical oral ulcer that does not heal after 2–3 weeks of treatment to an oral medicine specialist (especially in patients with oral cancer risk factors such as tobacco and alcohol use). SOR Ⓒ

Consider referring children with periodic fever with aphthous stomatitis, pharyngitis, and adenitis (PFAPA) syndrome for tonsillectomy or adenotonsillectomy. A meta-analysis found little evidence to support surgery, but the authors concluded that surgery is an option when symptoms markedly interfere with the child's quality of life and medical treatment has failed.[14] SOR Ⓒ

PREVENTION

Oral vitamin B_{12} was studied in an RCT of primary care patients. A sublingual dose of 1000 mcg of vitamin B_{12} was used by patients in the intervention group for 6 months. During the last month of treatment more participants in the intervention group reached a status of "no aphthous ulcers" (74.1% vs. 32.0%; $P < 0.01$). The treatment worked regardless of the serum vitamin B_{12} level.[15] SOR Ⓑ

PATIENT EDUCATION

Recurrent lesions that do not respond to treatment and severe cases should be seen by their oral health provider or primary care physician to look for an underlying cause. Foods that are spicy or acidic worsen pain and should be avoided.

PATIENT RESOURCES

- American Academy of Oral Medicine. *Canker Sores*—**http://www.aaom.com/index.php?option=com_content&view=article&id=82:canker-sores&catid=22:patient-condition-information&Itemid=120.**

PROVIDER RESOURCES

- Medscape. *Aphthous Stomatitis*—**https://emedicine.medscape.com/article/1075570.**

REFERENCES

1. Akintoye SO, Greenberg MS. Recurrent aphthous stomatitis. *Dent Clin North Am.* 2014; 58(2):281-297.
2. Ricky C, Alison B, Roy R III. Recurrent aphthous stomatitis. *Clin Dermatol.* 2016;34:475-481.
3. Miller MF, Garfunkel AA, Ram CA, Ship II. The inheritance of recurrent aphthous stomatitis. Observations and susceptibility. *Oral Surg Oral Med Oral Pathol.* 1980;49(5):409-412.
4. Messadi DV, Younai F. Aphthous ulcers. *Dermatol Ther.* 2010;23: 281-290.
5. Casiglia JM. Recurrent aphthous stomatitis: etiology, diagnosis, and treatment. *Gen Dent.* 2002;50:157-166.
6. Bailey J, McCarthy C, Smith RF. Clinical inquiry. What is the most effective way to treat recurrent canker sores? *J Fam Pract.* 2011;60:621-632.
7. Descroix V, Coudert AE, Vige A, et al. Efficacy of topical 1% lidocaine in the symptomatic treatment of pain associated with oral mucosal trauma or minor oral aphthous ulcer: a randomized, double-blind, placebo-controlled, parallel-group, single-dose study. *J Orofac Pain.* 2011;25:327-332.
8. Femiano F, Buonaiuto C, Gombos F, et al. Pilot study on recurrent aphthous stomatitis (RAS): a randomized placebo-controlled trial for the comparative therapeutic effects of systemic prednisone and systemic montelukast in subjects unresponsive to topical therapy. *Oral Surg Oral Med Oral Pathol Oral Radiol Endod.* 2010;109:402-407.
9. Pakfetrat A, Mansourian A, Momen-Heravi F, et al. Comparison of colchicine versus prednisolone in recurrent aphthous stomatitis: a double-blind randomized clinical trial. *Clin Invest Med.* 2010;33: E189-E195.
10. de Abreu MA, Hirata CH, Pimentel DR, Weckx LL. Treatment of recurrent aphthous stomatitis with clofazimine. *Oral Surg Oral Med Oral Pathol Oral Radiol Endod.* 2009;108:714-721.
11. Hello M, Barbarot S, Bastuji-Garin S, et al. Use of thalidomide for severe recurrent aphthous stomatitis: a multicenter cohort analysis. *Medicine (Baltimore).* 2010;89:176-182.
12. Mimura MA, Hirota SK, Sugaya NN, et al. Systemic treatment in severe cases of recurrent aphthous stomatitis: an open trial. *Clinics (Sao Paulo).* 2009;64(3):193-198.
13. Yasui K, Kurata T, Yashiro M, et al. The effect of ascorbate on minor recurrent aphthous stomatitis. *Acta Paediatr.* 2010;99:442-445.
14. Garavello W, Pignataro L, Gaini L, et al. Tonsillectomy in children with periodic fever with aphthous stomatitis, pharyngitis, and adenitis syndrome. *J Pediatr.* 2011;159:138-142.
15. Volkov I, Rudoy I, Freud T, et al. Effectiveness of vitamin B_{12} in treating recurrent aphthous stomatitis: a randomized, double-blind, placebo-controlled trial. *J Am Board Fam Med.* 2009;22:9-16.

44 LEUKOPLAKIA

Michaell A. Huber, DDS
Wanda C. Gonsalves, MD

PATIENT STORY

A 57-year-old female smoker presents at the physician's clinic with a 7-month history of a nonpainful white patch below her tongue. She admits to drinking 2 to 3 beers in the evening and smoking 1 pack of cigarettes per day. Your examination reveals a painless white, thick lesion with fissuring below the tongue (**Figure 44-1**). A biopsy shows this to be premalignant and the patient is told that she must stop smoking and drinking. She is also referred to an oral surgeon for further evaluation of her dysplasia.

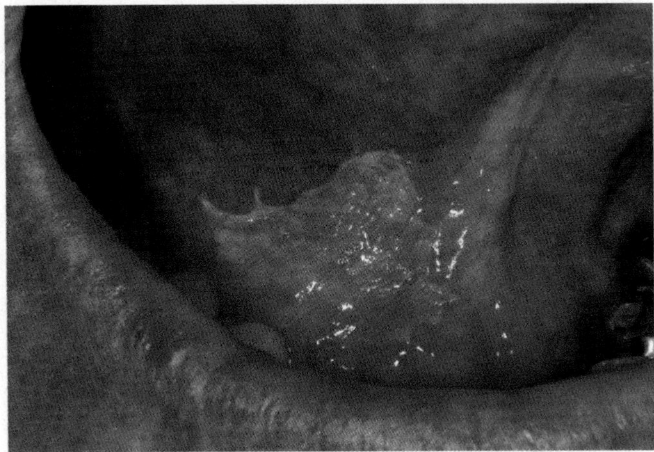

FIGURE 44-1 Homogenous leukoplakia on the lateral tongue presenting with a uniform surface plaque and surface cracks in a patient with a long smoking history. A 4-mm punch biopsy was performed and showed moderate dysplasia. (*Reproduced with permission from Michaell Huber, DDS.*)

INTRODUCTION

The World Health Organization defines leukoplakia as a clinical term used to recognize "white plaques of questionable risk having excluded (other) known diseases or disorders that carry no increased risk for cancer."[1,2] For all types of leukoplakia (see "Clinical Features" below) the risk of malignant transformation is approximately 1%, with a much higher risk associated with leukoplakias manifesting a red and/or highly variable (e.g., nodular or verrucous) surface texture component.

The term *erythroplakia* is reserved for a purely red lesion, which is described as a "fiery red patch that cannot be characterized clinically or pathologically as any other definable disease."[1,2] It may be flat or slightly depressed and exhibits a smooth or granular surface texture. The majority of erythroplakias will undergo malignant transformation.

SYNONYMS

Homogenous leukoplakia; nonhomogenous leukoplakia; speckled leukoplakia; nodular leukoplakia; verrucous leukoplakia; proliferative verrucous leukoplakia; erythroleukoplakia; erythroplakia; erythroplasia.

EPIDEMIOLOGY

- Leukoplakia occurs in 0.5% to 2.0% of adults and is most frequently seen in middle-age and older men.[1]
- Erythroplakia occurs in approximately 0.02% to 0.83% of adults and is most commonly observed in middle-age and elderly persons, with no gender distinction.[1]

ETIOLOGY AND PATHOPHYSIOLOGY

- Both leukoplakia and erythroplakia likely represent clinical changes associated with the underlying multistep progression of alterations at the molecular level underlying the development of dysplasia and subsequent carcinoma.

- For all types of leukoplakia, the risk of malignant transformation is approximately 1%, with a much higher risk associated with nonhomogenous leukoplakias or leukoplakias manifesting a red component.[1]
- For erythroplakia, the risk of malignant transformation is extremely high, with approximately 90% of cases demonstrating either dysplasia or carcinoma at the time of biopsy.[3]

RISK FACTORS

- Smoking, alcohol, and areca nut exposure are the most prominent risk factors for leukoplakia and erythroplakia, and create a synergistic effect when combined.[4]
- Human papillomavirus (HPV) is a recognized risk factor for oropharyngeal cancer, but its association with leukoplakia and erythroplakia is undetermined.[4]
- Up to 27% of leukoplakias are idiopathic.[5]

DIAGNOSIS

- Both leukoplakia and erythroplakia are clinical working diagnoses of exclusion, to be applied when other conditions have been excluded.

CLINICAL FEATURES

- Leukoplakia may be characterized as either homogenous or nonhomogenous.[1,2]
- Homogenous leukoplakia (**Figure 44-1**) presents uniformly as a thin surface plaque with possible shallow surface cracks.[2]
- Nonhomogenous leukoplakia (**Figures 44-2** and **44-3**) may be further characterized as speckled (white predominant with interspersed red component); nodular (small polypoid outcrops, may be red or white); or verrucous (corrugated or folded surface appearance).[2] Proliferative verrucous leukoplakia (PVL) is a variant form of nonhomogenous leukoplakia characterized by multifocal involvement and relentless progression to carcinoma (70%–100%).[4] PVL more commonly affects women and is not associated with tobacco exposure.
- Erythroplakia (**Figure 44-4**) presents as a distinct flat or slightly depressed red lesion with a smooth or granular surface texture.[1,2]

TYPICAL DISTRIBUTION

- Both leukoplakia and erythroplakia may occur on any oropharyngeal mucosal site.[4,5]
- Lesions affecting the floor of the mouth, ventral/lateral tongue, and possibly the soft palatal complex, are associated with a increased risk for malignant transformation.[4–6]
- Idiopathic leukoplakias demonstrate a significantly higher risk of malignant transformation compared to risk-associated variants.[5]

LABORATORY

A biopsy is required to determine the histologic characterization of the lesion. Usually a 4-mm punch biopsy is a good start, but be wary of a false negative as a consequence of sampling error. If the lesion appears suspicious, refer to an ear, nose, and throat (ENT) surgeon, oral and maxillofacial surgeon, or oral medicine specialist, even with a negative result.

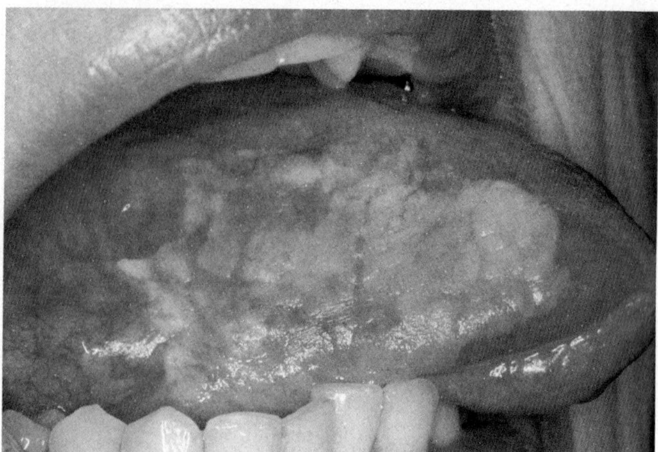

FIGURE 44-2 Nonhomogenous leukoplakia of the right ventral tongue in a 54-year-old white woman. Although she is a nonsmoker, she did have moderate alcohol exposure. Previous biopsy 6 years ago revealed hyperkeratosis. New biopsy indicated moderate to severe dysplasia. Patient was managed with total excision of the leukoplakia and an AlloDerm graft. (*Reproduced with permission from Michaell Huber, DDS.*)

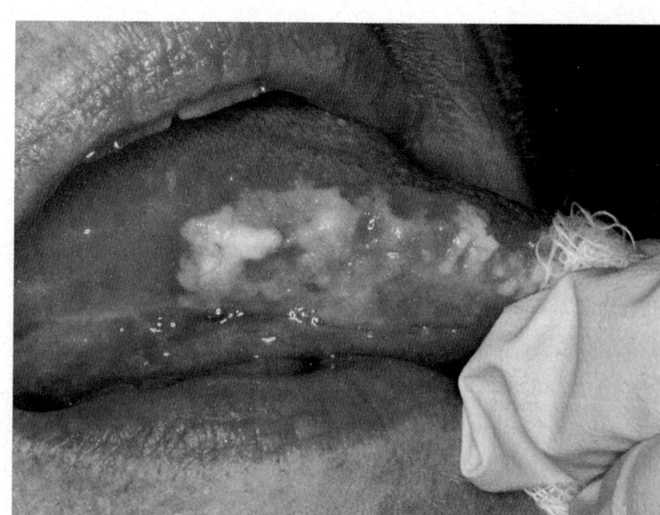

FIGURE 44-3 Leukoplakia (nonhomogenous) with moderate dysplasia on the lateral border of the tongue of a 65-year-old woman with a long history of smoking. She presented with discomfort and a noticeable white plaque on her tongue; a biopsy proved this to be moderate dysplasia. This was the third white dysplastic lesion she had developed in this area. A new excision will be performed and close follow-up is needed. Even though she quit smoking a few years ago, the damage done has led to a relentless dysplastic process. (*Reproduced with permission from Ellen Eisenberg, DMD.*)

DIFFERENTIAL DIAGNOSIS[1,2]

- Aspirin/chemical burn—Determined by history.
- Candidosis—Typically symmetrical and wipes off.
- Discoid lupus—Concurrent cutaneous lesions, circumscribed mucosal lesion with central erythema, radiating white lines, histopathology.
- Oral hairy leukoplakia—Characteristic clinical presentation (bilateral tongue), histopathologic evidence of Epstein-Barr virus (EBV).
- Lichen planus—Presence of striations, symmetrical presentation.
- Lichenoid lesion—Presence of striations, temporal association with trigger agent (e.g., new drug, dental material, home care product).
- Linea alba—Parallel to line of occlusion, often bilateral.
- Morsicatio—Habitual chewing or biting habit of the oral mucosa, often bilateral (**Figure 44-5**).
- Nicotine stomatitis—Smoking habit, characteristic appearance (**Figure 44-6**).
- Snuff patch—Characteristic folded, corrugated appearance at site of tobacco placement.
- White sponge nevus—Familial history, symmetrical pattern, and other mucosal sites often involved.

MANAGEMENT

MEDICATIONS

- There are no pharmacologic regimens to manage either leukoplakia or erythroplakia.

SURGERY

- All leukoplakias and erythroplakias should be excised and biopsied to determine the presence of epithelial dysplasia, carcinoma in situ, or squamous cell carcinoma.[1,4,6,7] SOR Ⓒ
- Watchful waiting is not recommended without a baseline histologic diagnosis.

REFERRAL

- Refer as appropriate to an oral and maxillofacial surgeon, an oral medicine expert, or an ENT surgeon.

PREVENTION AND SCREENING

- Risk reduction measures are to be encouraged.
- Ensure that a thorough and disciplined soft-tissue examination is accomplished on a routine basis.

PROGNOSIS

- Highly variable for leukoplakia; it may ultimately regress and disappear, persist, or progress to eventual carcinoma. Leukoplakia may recur after excision.[7–9]
- Erythroplakia almost always progresses to cancer.[1,3]

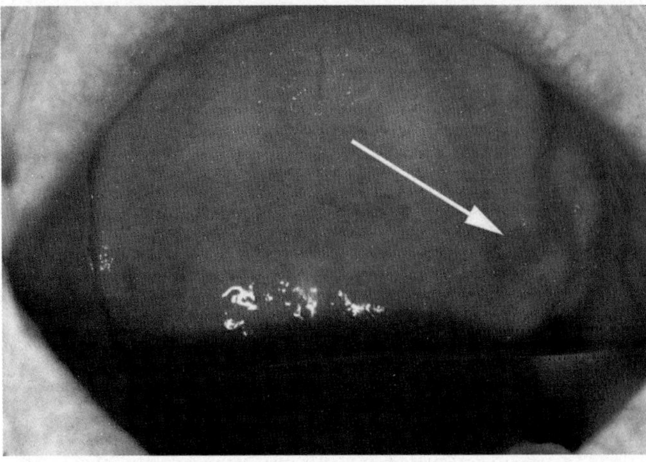

FIGURE 44-4 Erythroplakia with red patch (*arrow*) on the upper alveolar ridge of an edentulous person. (*Reproduced with permission from Gerald Ferritti, DMD.*)

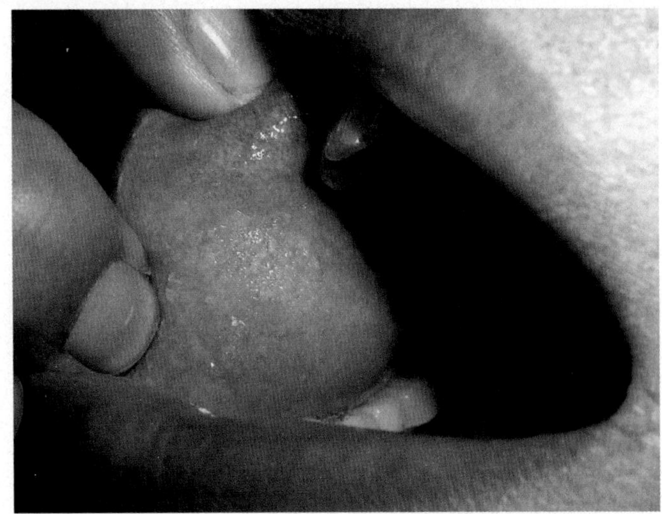

FIGURE 44-5 Morsicatio—leukoplakia caused by habitual chewing and biting of the oral mucosa. This young man only reluctantly acknowledged this habit upon further questioning of his bilateral leukoplakia. (*Reproduced with permission from Richard P. Usatine, MD.*)

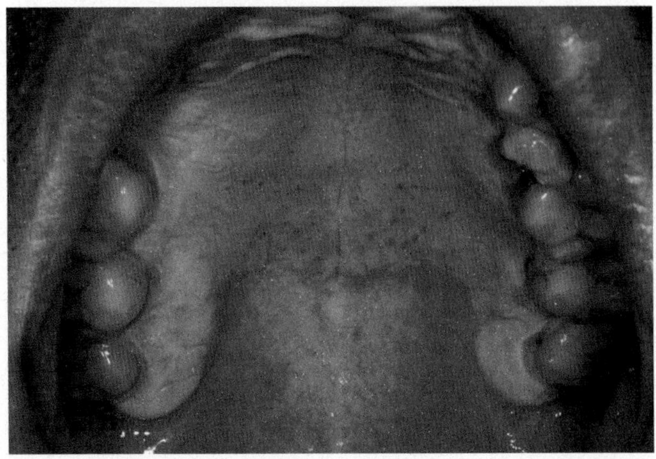

FIGURE 44-6 Nicotine stomatitis is observed in smoker. Note the hyperkeratosis affecting the hard palate and the erythematous minor salivary duct orifices. (*Reproduced with permission from Michaell Huber, DDS.*)

FOLLOW-UP

- Routine monitoring (e.g., every 3 to 6 months) for recurrence or change should be done.[6–8] SOR C
- Risk factor elimination is essential and may reduce the risk of recurrence.[1,7,10]

PATIENT EDUCATION

- Counsel patients who use tobacco (e.g., smoke or smokeless tobacco) to quit. Ask if they are ready to quit at each visit, and sign a contract with them that specifies the date and time they will quit. Provide tools (see "Patient Resources" below) they can use to quit (see Chapter 248, Smoking and Tobacco Addiction).

PATIENT RESOURCES

- American Lung Association. *How to Quit Smoking*—**http://www.lung.org/stop-smoking/i-want-to-quit/how-to-quit-smoking.html.**
- QuitSmokingSupport.com. **http://www.quitsmokingsupport.com.**
- Centers for Disease Control and Prevention. *Quit Smoking*—**http://www.cdc.gov/tobacco/quit_smoking/index.htm.**

PROVIDER RESOURCES

- Tobacco Use and Dependence Guideline Panel. *Treating Tobacco Use and Dependence: 2008 Update.* Rockville, MD: US Department of Health and Human Services; 2008. **http://www.ncbi.nlm.nih.gov/books/NBK63952/.**
- National Cancer Institute. *Cigarette Smoking: Health Risks and How to Quit (PDQ®)—Health Professional Version*—**https://www.cancer.gov/about-cancer/causes-prevention/risk/tobacco/quit-smoking-hp-pdq.**

REFERENCES

1. van der Waal I. Potentially malignant disorders of the oral and oropharyngeal mucosa; terminology, classification and present concepts of management. *Oral Oncol.* 2009;45:317-323.
2. Warnakulasuriya S, Johnson NW, van der Waal I. Nomenclature and classification of potentially malignant disorders of the oral mucosa. *J Oral Pathol Med.* 2007;36:575-580.
3. Huber MA, Tantiwongkosi B. Oral and oropharyngeal cancer. *Med Clin North Am.* 2014;98(6):1299-1321.
4. Villa A, Woo SB. Leukoplakia—a diagnostic and management algorithm. *J Oral Maxillofac Surg.* 2017;75(4):723-734.
5. Napier SS, Speight PM. Natural history of potentially malignant oral lesions and conditions: an overview of the literature. *J Oral Pathol Med.* 2008;37:1-10.
6. Reibel J. Prognosis of oral pre-malignant lesions: significance of clinical, histopathological, and molecular biological characteristics. *Crit Rev Oral Biol Med.* 2003;14:47-62.
7. Lodi G, Porter S. Management of potentially malignant disorders: evidence and critique. *J Oral Pathol Med.* 2008;37:63-69.
8. Holmstrup P, Vedtofte P, Reibel J, Stoltze K. Oral premalignant lesions: is a biopsy reliable? *J Oral Pathol Med.* 2007;36:262-266.
9. Holmstrup P, Vedtofte P, Reibel J, Stoltze K. Long-term treatment outcome of oral premalignant lesions. *Oral Oncol.* 2006;44:461-474.
10. Vladimirov BS, Schiodt M. The effect of quitting smoking on the risk of unfavorable events after surgical treatment of oral potentially malignant lesions. *Int J Oral Maxillofac Surg* 2009;38:1188-1193.

45 OROPHARYNGEAL CANCER

Michaell A. Huber, DDS
Wanda C. Gonsalves, MD

PATIENT STORY

A 66-year-old man presents to the physician's office with a nonhealing painful lesion on the roof of his mouth (**Figure 45-1**). The lesion has increased in size recently and he is worried because his dad died from oral cancer. Your patient has smoked since he was 11 years old by getting cigarettes from his dad. He admits to being a heavy drinker. A biopsy shows squamous cell carcinoma, and the patient is referred to a head and neck surgeon.

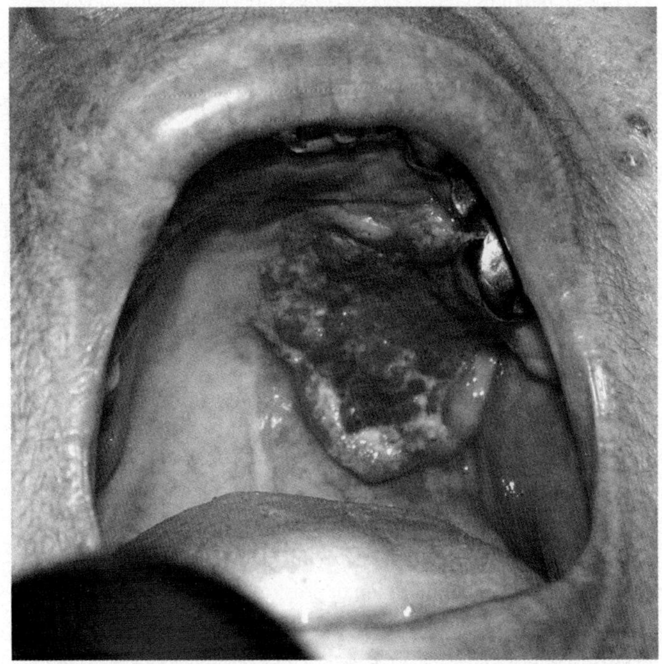

FIGURE 45-1 Squamous cell carcinoma of the palate of a 66-year-old man who smokes and drinks. (*Reproduced with permission from Frank Miller, MD.*)

INTRODUCTION

In spite of the relative ease for the healthcare provider to accomplish a visual and tactile examination of the oropharyngeal cavity, fully two-thirds of oropharyngeal cancers (OPCs) will present with advanced disease at the time of diagnosis.[1] Ninety percent of OPCs are of the squamous cell type. Concern has been raised that practitioners are missing early disease by not accomplishing a thorough soft-tissue examination on a routine basis.[2] However, the fact that more than 35% of patients do not see a dentist on a routine basis likely contributes to the diagnostic delay.[3] The 5-year survival rate for patients diagnosed from 2006 to 2012 is 68% for whites and 47% for blacks.[4]

SYNONYMS

Oral cancer; oral squamous cell carcinoma; mouth cancer; site specific (e.g., gingival cancer, tongue cancer, lip cancer).

EPIDEMIOLOGY

- In the United States, an estimated 48,000 OPC cases occur annually, accounting for approximately 4.1% of malignancies among men and 1.6% of malignancies among women.[1]
- The median age at diagnosis is 62 years, and more than 73% of cases occur after the age of 55 years.[4]
- Incidence rates vary from a low of 4.0 per 100,000 Hispanic women to a high of 17.4 per 100,000 white men.[4]
- Up to 35% of OPC patients will develop a new primary tumor within 5 years.[5]

ETIOLOGY AND PATHOPHYSIOLOGY

- Typical OPC develops from a complex multistep progression marked by a series of mutations at the molecular level, followed by phenotypic changes and subsequent clinically observable changes affecting the squamous epithelium.[6]

RISK FACTORS

- Tobacco use is the major risk factor for OPC and is implicated in approximately 75% of cases.[7]
- Alcohol use is a major risk factor, and the combined use of tobacco and alcohol increases the risk of OPC far more than either alone.[7]
- Human papillomavirus (HPV) (especially HPV 16) is a newly recognized major risk factor for carcinomas affecting the lingual and palatine tonsils.[8]
- Other risk factors include betel quid chewing, low intake of fruits and vegetables, immunosuppression, and maté drinking.[9]
- Excess sun exposure is the major risk factor for cancer of the lip.[7]

DIAGNOSIS

- A scalpel biopsy is required to establish the diagnosis.[5,10]

CLINICAL FEATURES

- OPC may affect any area of the oropharyngeal cavity.
- Early OPC often presents as a leukoplakia or erythroplakia (see **Figure 45-1**). High-risk sites are the floor of the mouth and ventrolateral tongue (**Figure 45-2**).
- Features of more advanced disease include induration, persistent ulceration, tissue proliferation or erosion, pain or paresthesia, loss of function, and lymphadenopathy (**Figures 45-3** to **45-5**).[10]
- HPV-associated carcinomas are often less visible and share signs and symptoms (e.g., sore throat, hoarseness, earaches, enlarged lymph nodes) of tonsillitis and pharyngitis. More advanced symptoms include dysphagia, hemoptysis, and weight loss.[9,10]
- Lip cancer typically presents as a relapsing or persistent chronic scab, plaque, crust, or ulceration (**Figure 45-6**). Antecedent actinic cheilosis is commonly observed.
- Nonsquamous type cancers (e.g., salivary gland tumors, melanoma, sarcomas) often present as a submucosal nodular swelling or mass (**Figures 45-7** and **45-8**).

TYPICAL DISTRIBUTION

- OPCs occur most commonly (in order of frequency) on the tongue, floor of mouth, and lower lip vermilion. The lymphoepithelial tissues of the Waldeyer ring (lateral tongue extending to the lateral soft palate and tonsillar area) has the greatest risk of developing an HPV-associated OPC.[8]

LABORATORY

- A scalpel biopsy is required to establish the diagnosis. An excisional biopsy is preferred to better ensure all suspicious tissue is available for histologic assessment. Confirmed cases are staged using the TNM (tumor, nodes, metastases) scheme.[9]

DIFFERENTIAL DIAGNOSIS

- OPC is capricious and may initially mimic any number of benign conditions such as aphthae, chronic ulcerative conditions, pharyngitis, and tonsillitis.

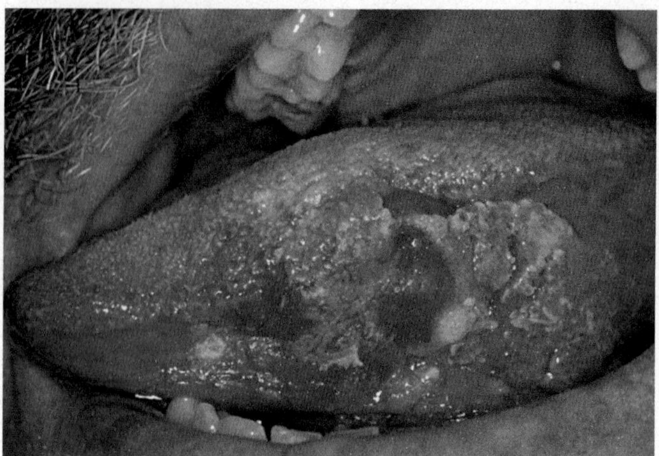

FIGURE 45-2 Squamous cell carcinoma on the lateral side of the tongue. This is a broad erythroleukoplakic plaque with surface ulcerations. *(Reproduced with permission from Ellen Eisenberg, DMD.)*

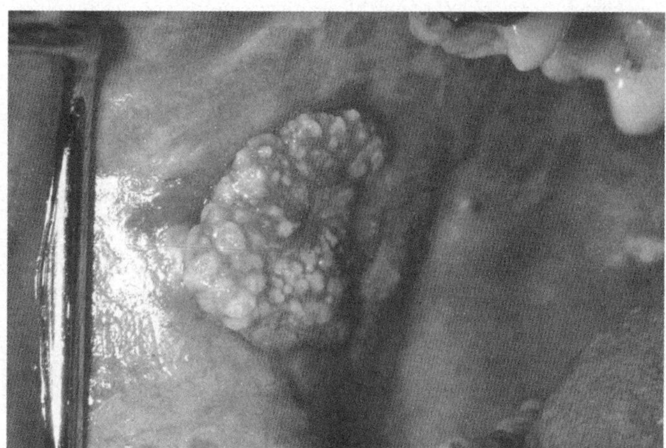

FIGURE 45-3 Squamous cell carcinoma arising on the buccal mucosa. *(Reproduced with permission from Gerald Ferritti, DDS.)*

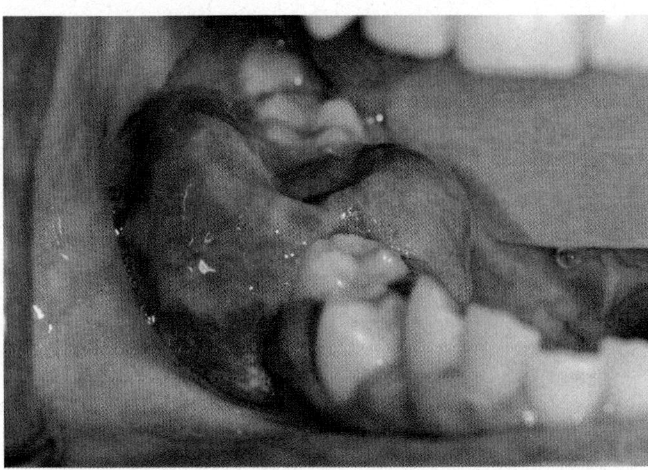

FIGURE 45-4 Exophytic cancer of the mouth. (*Reproduced with permission from Gerald Ferritti, DDS.*)

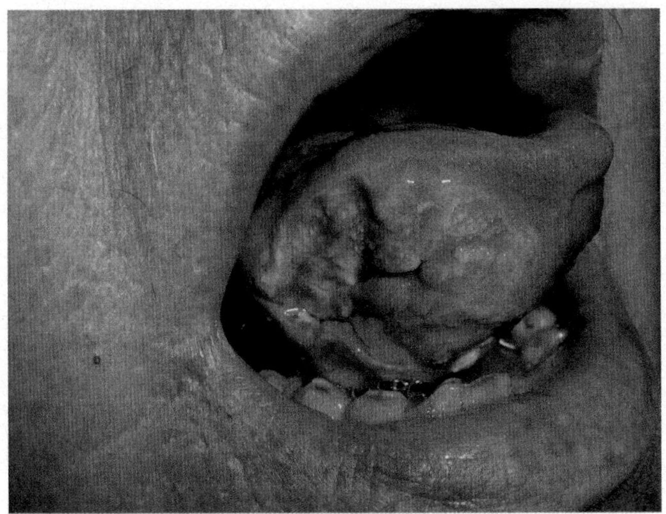

FIGURE 45-5 Squamous cell carcinoma manifesting chronic ulceration with induration on the right side of the tongue in a woman with a long history of smoking and alcohol abuse. (*Reproduced with permission from Richard P. Usatine, MD.*)

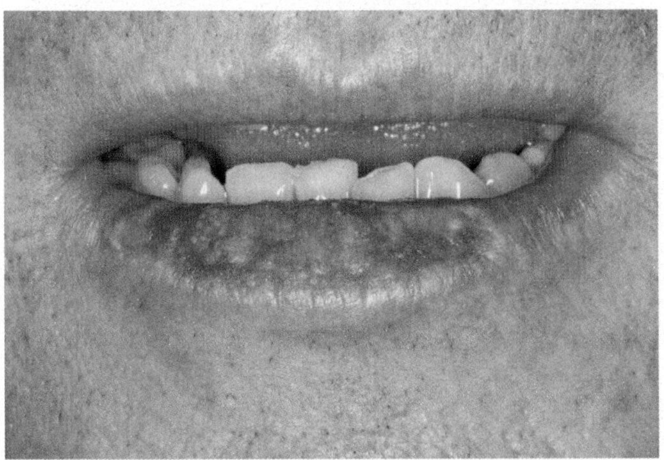

FIGURE 45-6 Squamous cell carcinoma of the lower lip in a 51-year-old man, managed with vermilionectomy. (*Reproduced with permission from Michaell Huber, DDS.*)

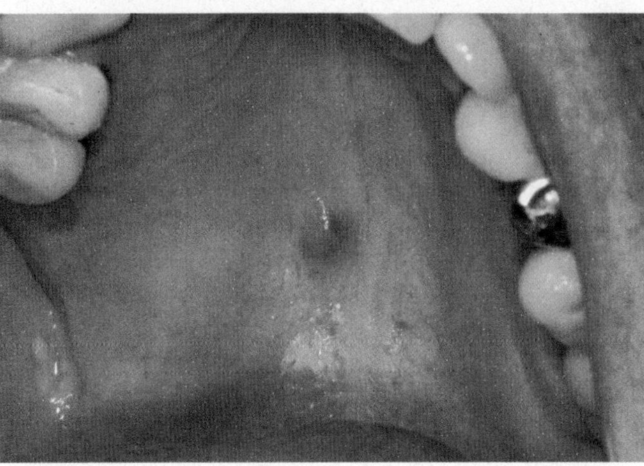

FIGURE 45-7 A 58-year-old man with well-defined soft bluish diascopy-positive nodule of unknown duration. Although a benign vascular lesion was the biopsy-proven diagnosis, a minor salivary gland tumor or Kaposi sarcoma were considered as possible diagnoses. (*Reproduced with permission from Michaell Huber, DDS.*)

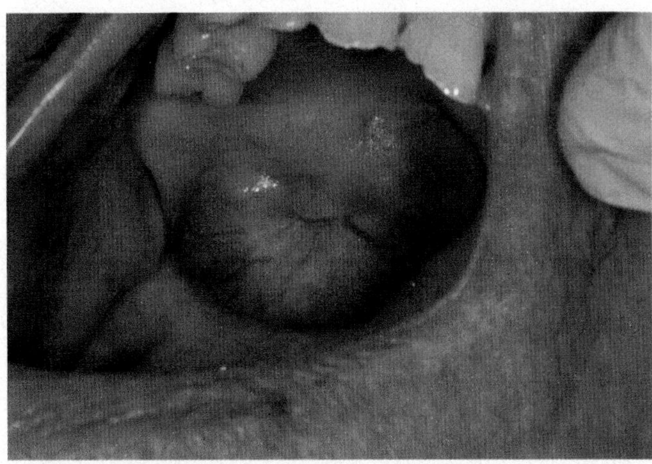

FIGURE 45-8 An 80-year-old Hispanic woman with a 25-year history of palatal mass, which she stated only recently started getting bigger. A low-grade adenocarcinoma of the palate was confirmed with biopsy. (*Reproduced with permission from Michaell Huber, DDS.*)

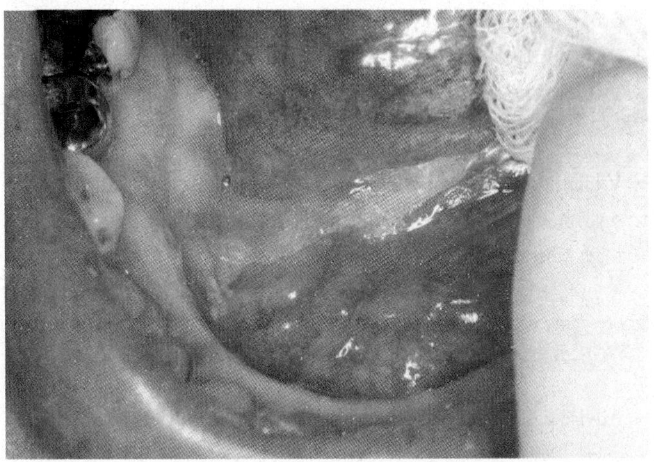

FIGURE 45-9 A 64-year-old woman with faint leukoplakia and a history of a hot coffee burn. Upon 2-week follow-up, the leukoplakia was still present and an excisional biopsy revealed carcinoma in situ completely excised. She was recommended for close monitoring. (*Reproduced with permission from Michaell Huber, DDS.*)

- Any lesion deemed suspicious or equivocal at discovery should be referred to an expert (oral and maxillofacial surgeon, an oral medicine expert, or an ear, nose, and throat [ENT] surgeon) for further assessment or immediate biopsy.
- Findings deemed innocuous should be reevaluated within 2 weeks for resolution and referred to an expert for further assessment or undergo biopsy if still present (**Figure 45-9**).

MANAGEMENT

- Confirmed OPC is best managed by the oncology team whose members deliver all indicated therapeutic antitumor modalities and provide appropriate adjunctive services such as dental care and nutritional, psychological, and social support. TNM staging is useful for treatment planning and prognostication.
- The principal therapeutic modalities are surgery, radiotherapy, and chemotherapy.[11,12]
- The use of one treatment over another depends on the size, location, and stage of the primary tumor, the patient's ability to tolerate treatment, and the patient's desires.[11,12]
- Surgical excision is the preferred modality for most well-defined and accessible solid tumors; however, it has its limitations for inaccessible or more advanced tumors demonstrating lymph node involvement and/or metastasis.[11,12]
- Radiotherapy may be either an effective alternative to surgery or a valuable adjunct to surgery and/or chemotherapy in the locoregional treatment of malignant head and neck tumors.[11,12]
- Protocols using concomitant chemoradiotherapy improve both locoregional control and survival.[12]

PROGNOSIS

- Early OPCs (stage I and stage II) of the lip and oral cavity are highly curable, with 5-year survival rates exceeding 90%.[11]
- Later stage OPCs (stage III and stage IV) have a more guarded prognosis with 5-year survival rates ranging from 25% to 63%.[1]

FOLLOW-UP

- Vigilant posttherapy follow-up is required (every 6 months).
- Posttherapy OPC patients are at risk for developing a second primary tumor, 3% to 7% per year.[12]

PATIENT EDUCATION

- Advise patients to discontinue smoking and/or drinking alcohol.

PATIENT RESOURCES

- The Oral Cancer Foundation—**http://www.oralcancerfoundation.org.**
- National Cancer Institute. *Oral Cavity and Oropharyngeal Cancer Prevention (PDQ®)—Patient Version*—**https://www.cancer.gov/types/head-and-neck/patient/oral-prevention-pdq.**

PROVIDER RESOURCES

- The Oral Cancer Foundation—**http://www.oralcancerfoundation.org.**
- National Cancer Institute. *Lip and Oral Cavity Cancer Treatment (PDQ®)—Health Professional Version*—**https://www.cancer.gov/types/head-and-neck/hp/lip-mouth-treatment-pdq.**
- National Cancer Institute. *Oropharyngeal Cancer Treatment (PDQ®)—Health Professional Version*—**https://www.cancer.gov/types/head-and-neck/hp/oropharyngeal-treatment-pdq.**
- Medscape Reference. *Cancers of the Oral Mucosa*—**http://emedicine.medscape.com/article/1075729-overview.**

REFERENCES

1. Siegel RL, Miller KD, Jemal A. Cancer Statistics, 2016. *Cancer J Clin*. 2016;66:7-30.
2. Mignogna MD, Fedele S, Lo Russo L, et al. Oral and pharyngeal cancer: lack of prevention and early detection by health care providers. *Eur J Cancer Prev*. 2001;10(4):381-383.
3. Pleis JR, Ward BW, Lucas JW. Summary health statistics for U.S. adults: National Health Interview Survey, 2009. National Center for Health Statistics. *Vital Health Stat 10*. 2010;(249):1-207.
4. National Cancer Institute, Surveillance Epidemiology and End Results. *SEER Stat Fact Sheets: Oral Cavity and Pharynx*. http://seer.cancer.gov/statfacts/html/oralcav.html. Accessed December 2016.
5. Lingen MW, Kalmar JR, Karrison T, Speight PM. Critical evaluation of diagnostic aids for the detection of oral cancer. *Oral Oncol*. 2008;44(1):10-22.
6. Malik UU, Zarina S, Pennington SR. Oral squamous cell carcinoma: key clinical questions, biomarker discovery, and the role of proteomics. *Arch Oral Biol*. 2016;63:53-65.
7. National Cancer Institute. *Oral Cavity and Oropharyngeal Cancer Prevention (PDQ)—Health Professional Version*. https://www.cancer.gov/types/head-and-neck/hp/oral-prevention-pdq. Accessed December 2016.
8. Cleveland JL, Junger ML, Saraiya M, et al. The connection between human papillomavirus and oropharyngeal squamous cell carcinomas in the United States. *J Am Dent Assoc*. 2011;142:915-924.
9. Huber MA, Tantiwongkosi B. Oral and oropharyngeal cancer. *Med Clin North Am*. 2014;98(6):1299-321.
10. Rethman MP, Carpenter W, Cohen EEW, et al. Evidence-based clinical recommendations regarding screening for oral squamous cell carcinomas. *J Am Dent Assoc*. 2010;141:509-520.
11. National Cancer Institute. *Lip and Oral Cavity Cancer Treatment (PDQ)—Health Professional Version*. https://www.cancer.gov/types/head-and-neck/hp/lip-mouth-treatment-pdq. Accessed December 2016.
12. National Cancer Institute. *Oropharyngeal Cancer Treatment (PDQ)—Health Professional Version*. https://www.cancer.gov/types/head-and-neck/hp/oropharyngeal-treatment-pdq. Accessed December 2016.

46 EARLY CHILDHOOD CARIES

Adriana Segura, DDS, MS
Wanda C. Gonsalves, MD

PATIENT STORY

A mother brings her 18-month-old son to the physician's clinic for his well-child examination. He is almost weaned from his bottle, but still drinks from a bottle to go to sleep. During the day, he uses a sippy cup to drink everything—from milk to soda. His mother has started giving him apple juice in the bottle instead of milk because he tends to get constipated. On performing an oral examination, the physician notices that several of his teeth have "white spots" (**Figure 46-1**). The physician discusses dental hygiene and treats him with topical fluoride gel.

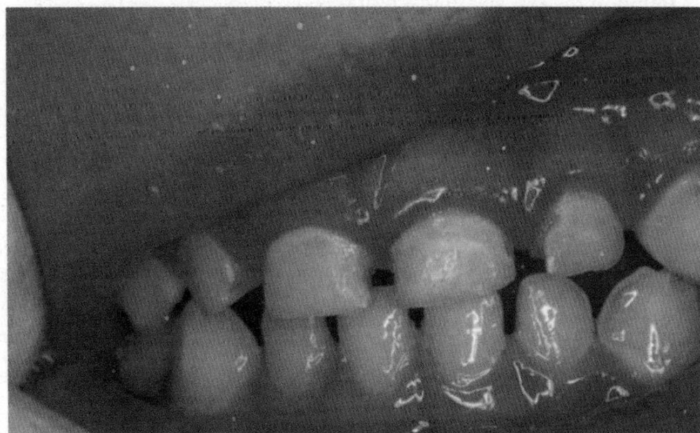

FIGURE 46-1 Demineralization at gingival margins characterized by whitish discolorations. (*Reproduced with permission from Gerald Ferretti, DMD.*)

INTRODUCTION

Dental caries continues to be the most prevalent chronic disease problem facing infants and children. The American Academy of Pediatric Dentistry, American Academy of Pediatrics, and American Dental Association recommend that a child's first visit to a dentist should occur 6 months after the eruption of the first tooth or at 1 year of age. Providing a dental home by age 1 year allows the health provider to complete a risk assessment, provide an introduction to dentistry, and provide anticipatory guidance. It is important to be able to recognize disease and to provide prevention strategies early on to the parents/caregivers.

SYNONYMS

Nursing bottle caries, baby bottles caries.

EPIDEMIOLOGY

- Early childhood caries (ECC; tooth decay) is the single most common chronic childhood disease. It is 5 times more common than asthma and 7 times more common than hay fever among children 5 to 7 years of age.[1]
- Approximately 37% of children ages 2–8 years had experienced dental caries in primary teeth in 2011–2012.[2]
- Disparities in oral health exist. In 2011, 27% of Hispanic children had dental caries in permanent teeth compared to 18% of non-Hispanic children.[2]
- ECC is defined as "the presence of one or more decayed (noncavitated or cavitated lesions), missing (as a consequence of caries), or filled tooth surfaces in any primary tooth in a child 71 months of age or younger" (**Figures 46-2** to **46-4**).[3]
- Consequences of ECC include poor self-esteem, diminished physical development, decreased ability to learn, higher risk of new caries, and added cost.[3]

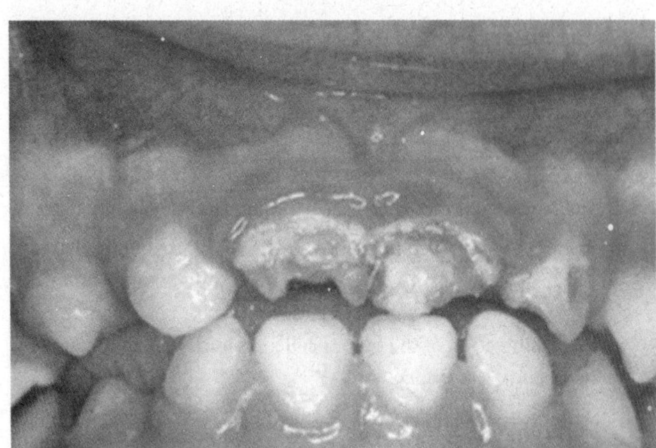

FIGURE 46-2 Central maxillary incisors with severe tooth decay, and bilateral maxillary lateral incisors with demineralized area near gingival line (yellow-brownish discolorations). The upper incisors are often the first teeth involved in nursing-bottle caries. (*Reproduced with permission from Gerald Ferretti, DMD.*)

ETIOLOGY AND PATHOPHYSIOLOGY

- Dental caries is a multifactorial, infectious, communicable disease caused by the demineralization of tooth enamel (see **Figure 46-1**) in the presence of a sugar substrate and acid-forming cariogenic bacteria, *Streptococcus mutans* (also known as *mutans streptococci*), which is considered to be the primary strain causing decay that are found in the soft gelatinous biofilm.
- Caries can develop at any time after tooth eruption. Early teeth are principally susceptible to caries caused by the transmission of *S. mutans* from the mouth of the caregiver or sibling(s) to the mouth of the infant or toddler. This type of tooth decay is called baby bottle tooth decay, nursing bottle caries, or ECC.

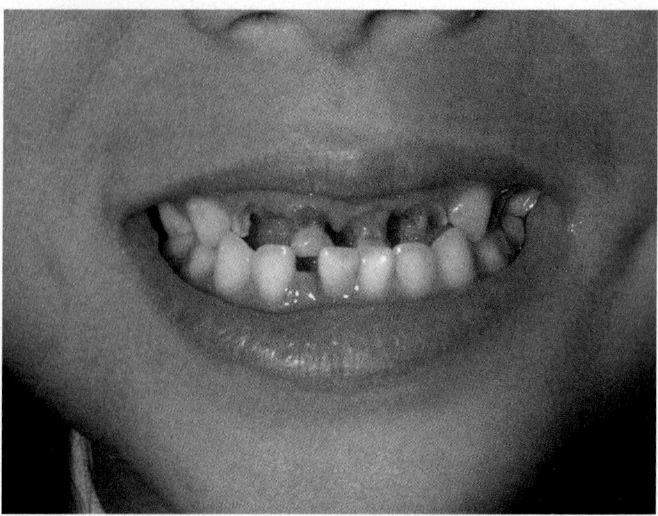

FIGURE 46-3 Severe ECC in a 4-year-old with severe decay of all four maxillary incisors. (*Reproduced with permission from Richard P. Usatine, MD.*)

RISK FACTORS

Risk factors for caries development include:

- Frequent consumption of liquids containing sugar.
- Repetitive use of a "sippy cup" containing sugars (juice, milk, formula, soda).
- Consumption of sticky foods.
- Human breast milk is uniquely superior in providing the best possible nutrition to infants and, by itself, has been shown to be noncariogenic.[4]
- Nighttime bottle feeding and caregiver with caries.
- Drinking unfluoridated community water or bottled water, which usually lacks fluoride.
- Low socioeconomic status.
- Taking medications that contain sugar or cause dryness.
- Lack of good oral hygiene practices.
- Subnormal saliva and function.

DIAGNOSIS

CLINICAL FEATURES

- Demineralized areas develop on the tooth surfaces, between teeth, and on pits and fissures. These areas are painless and appear clinically as opaque or brown spots (see **Figure 46-1**). White-spot lesions are the first indication the demineralization has started.
- Infection that is allowed to progress forms a cavity that can spread to and through the dentin (the component of the tooth located below the enamel) and to the pulp (composed of nerves and blood vessels; an infection of the pulp is called pulpitis) causing pain, necrosis, and, perhaps, an abscess.

TYPICAL DISTRIBUTION

Demineralized (white or brown spots) and carious lesions generally occur at the margins of the gingiva at upper incisors, and later first and second molars in pits and grooves of occlusal surfaces. Lower incisors are rarely affected.

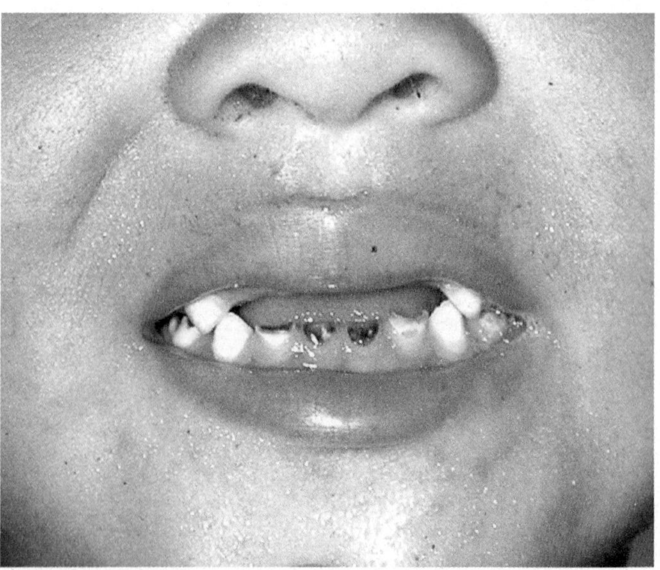

FIGURE 46-4 Severe ECC in a 3-year-old with multiple areas of cavitary lesions involving the mandibular incisors and missing maxillary incisors secondary to decay. (*Reproduced with permission from Richard P. Usatine, MD.*)

TABLE 46-1 Supplemental Fluoride Dosage Schedule

	Concentration of Fluoride in Water		
Age	<0.3 ppm F	0.3 to 0.6 ppm F	>0.6 ppm F
Birth to 6 months	0	0	0
6 months to 3 years	0.25 mg	0	0
3 to 6 years	0.50 mg	0.25 mg	0
6 to at least 16 years	1.00 mg	0.50 mg	0

Reproduced with permission from The Guideline on Fluoride Therapy (2008 revision) is Copyright © 2007–2008 by the American Academy of Pediatric Dentistry and is reproduced with their permission. http://www.aapd.org/media/Policies_Guidelines/G_fluoridetherapy.pdf

LABORATORY AND IMAGING

Demineralized lesions may not be seen on radiographs, but advanced carious lesions between and on the occlusal surfaces are detected by X-ray.

MANAGEMENT

- Counsel patients about the importance of good oral hygiene practices and perform a caries risk assessment during well-child examination visits.[5,6] SOR Ⓑ
- Refer to the dental health professional for the application of pit and fissure sealants.[5,6] SOR Ⓑ
- Before prescribing supplemental fluoride, the primary care provider must determine the fluoride concentration in the child's primary source of drinking water. If fluoridated water is not available in the community, natural sources of fluoride are well water exposed to fluorite minerals and certain fruits and vegetables grown in soil irrigated with fluoridated water.[7] SOR Ⓑ
- Fluoride supplementation is not recommended for use by persons who live in communities whose water is optimally fluoridated (0.7 to 1.2 parts per million [ppm] or >0.6 mg/L). See **Table 46-1** for fluoride supplementation.[7] SOR Ⓐ
- Advise the caregiver to take the child to a dentist by age 1 year.[6] SOR Ⓒ
- Application of fluoride varnishes twice per year in moderate to high-risk children has been shown to prevent caries in demineralized enamel.[8] SOR Ⓐ

FOLLOW-UP

Ensure that any child whose teeth have "white spots" or visible caries is taken to a dentist for evaluation and treatment so the teeth can be saved from decay or repaired.

PATIENT EDUCATION[6]

- Give the child's caregiver anticipatory guidance that is appropriate to the child's age and dental development. Before the teeth erupt, the caregiver should use a washcloth or cotton gauze to clean a baby's mouth and to transition the child to tooth brushing. SOR Ⓒ
- A "smear" of fluoridated toothpaste (approximately 0.1 mg fluoride) should be considered for children younger than 3 years of age (**Figure 46-5**).[6] SOR Ⓑ

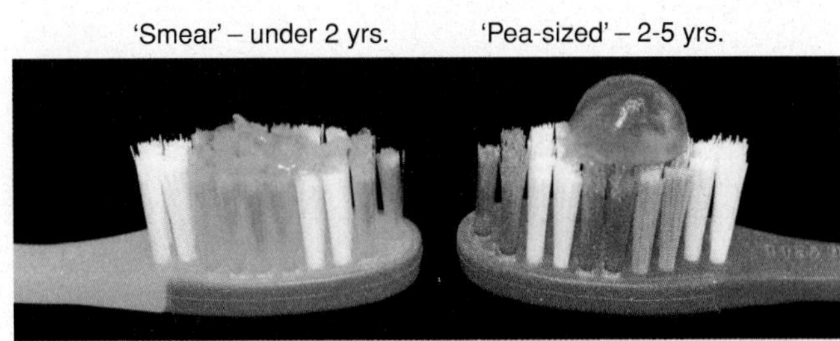

FIGURE 46-5 Comparison of a "smear" (*left*) with a "pea-sized" (*right*) amount of toothpaste. (*Reproduced with permission from Richard P. Usatine, MD.*)

- A "pea size" amount of toothpaste (approximately 0.2 mg fluoride) is appropriate for children 3 through 6 years of age.[6] SOR B
- The caregiver should brush the child's teeth until the child is capable of doing an adequate job (usually around age 7 years).
- Educate caregivers about the benefits of fluoride and fluorosis, and the possible side effects of using too much fluoride (see **Table 46-1**).
- Advise caregivers to teach the child to drink from a "sippy cup" as soon as possible and to avoid giving the child milk, juice, or soda in either a bottle or sippy cup when putting the child to bed.

Breastfeeding by itself is noncariogenic but, when supplemented with other carbohydrates, can place the child at risk for caries.[4,9]

The American Academy of Pediatric Dentistry (AAPD) promotes breastfeeding for infants but recommends cessation of ad libitum breastfeeding as the first primary tooth begins to erupt and other dietary carbohydrates are introduced.[9] SOR C

PATIENT RESOURCES

- Douglass JM, Douglass AB, Silk HJ. Your baby's teeth. *Am Fam Physician.* 2004;70:2121. **http://www.aafp.org/afp/2004/1201/p2121.html.**
- **http://www.mychildrensteeth.org/education/.**
- **http://www.mouthhealthy.org/en/babies-and-kids.**
- **https://www.healthychildren.org/English/healthy-living/oral-health/Pages/Brush-Book-Bed.aspx.**

PROVIDER RESOURCES

- American Academy of Pediatric Dentistry—**http://www.aapd.org.**
- Smiles for Life: A National Oral Health Curriculum—**http://www.smilesforlifeoralhealth.org.**
- American Academy of Pediatrics (AAP). *Bright Futures Oral Health Risk Assessment Tool*—**https://www.aap.org/en-us/Documents/oralhealth_RiskAssessmentTool.pdf.**

REFERENCES

1. U.S. Department of Health and Human Services. *Oral Health in America: A Report of the Surgeon General—Executive Summary.* Rockville, MD: U.S. Department of Health and Human Services, National Institute of Dental and Craniofacial Research, National Institutes of Health, 2000. http://www.nidr.nih.gov/sgr/execsumm.htm. Accessed April 2012.
2. Dye BA, Thornton-Evans G, Li X, Iafolla TJ. *Dental Caries and Sealant Prevalence in Children and Adolescents in the United States, 2011–2012.* NCHS Data Brief, No 191. Hyattsville, MD: National Center for Health Statistics; 2015.
3. American Academy of Pediatric Dentistry, Council on Clinical Affairs. *Policy on Early Child Caries (ECC: Classifications, Consequences, and Prevention Strategies (Revised 2016).* http://www.aapd.org/media/policies_guidelines/p_eccclassifications.pdf. Accessed February 2017.
4. Iida H, Auinger P, Billings RJ, Weitzman M. Association between infant breastfeeding and early childhood caries in the United States. *Pediatrics.* 2007;120;944-952.
5. American Academy of Pediatrics, Section on Oral Health. Maintaining and improving the oral health of young children. Policy statement. *Pediatrics* 2014;134:1224-1229.
6. American Academy of Pediatric Dentistry, Clinical Affairs Committee. *Guideline on Caries-risk Assessment and Management for Infants, Children, and Adolescents (Revised 2014).* http://www.aapd.org/media/Policies_Guidelines/P_ECCClassifications1.pdf. Accessed February 2017.
7. American Academy of Pediatric Dentistry, Council on Clinical Affairs. *Guideline on Fluoride Therapy. (Revised 2014).* http://www.aapd.org/media/Policies_Guidelines/G_FluorideTherapy1.pdf. Accessed February 2017.
8. Adair SM. Evidence base use of fluoride in contemporary pediatric dental medicine. *Pediatr Dent.* 2006;28(2):133-142, discussion 192-198.
9. American Academy of Pediatric Dentistry, Council on Clinical Affairs. *Policy on Dietary Recommendation for Infants, Children and Adolescents (Revised 2012).* http://www.aapd.org/media/Policies_Guidelines/P_DietaryRec1.pdf. Accessed February 2017.

47 ADULT DENTAL CARIES

Juanita Lozano-Pineda, DDS, MPH
Wanda C. Gonsalves, MD

PATIENT STORY

A 41-year-old man experiencing homelessness presents to a clinic on "skid row" with a toothache (**Figure 47-1**). He has a history of alcoholism and smoking. Many of his teeth are loose and a number of his teeth have fallen out in the past year. He acknowledges that he does not floss or brush his teeth regularly. He has been sober for 60 days now and wants help to get his teeth fixed. He states that no one will hire him with his teeth as they are. He also has pain in a molar and wants something for the pain until he can see a dentist. On oral examination, you see missing teeth, generalized plaque, and teeth with multiple brown caries.

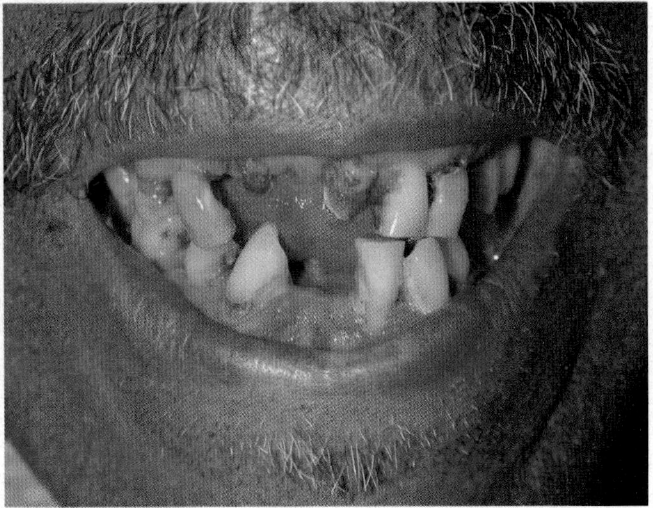

FIGURE 47-1 Severe caries in a man experiencing homelessness. *(Reproduced with permission from Richard P. Usatine, MD.)*

INTRODUCTION

Dental caries is a multifactorial disease that is primarily caused by an interaction between bacteria and fermentable carbohydrates producing acid that has potential to demineralize the tooth surface over time. Host factors, such as the plaque (biofilm) adherence, quality and quantity of saliva, immune system response, use of fluoride, and a diet that is caries-promoting, play a role in the formation of incipient demineralized lesions that progress to dental caries. Caries risk is impacted by factors that may be behavioral, biologic, environmental, lifestyle-related, and physical. Age, diabetes, ethnic origin, gingival recession, smoking, and socioeconomic status are frequently associated with high caries prevalence.[1]

SYNONYMS

Dental decay, dental cavities, cavitated lesions.

EPIDEMIOLOGY

- Many adults (e.g., 27.3% of those 20 to 34 years of age, 27% of those 35 to 49 years of age, and 25.5% of those 50 to 64 years of age) have untreated dental caries (**Figure 47-2**).[2]
- Approximately one in five of the older adults in the United States (e.g., 18.5% of those 65 to 74 years of age, and 19.4% of those 75 years of age and over) continue to have untreated dental caries.[2]
- Black and Hispanic adults, younger adults, and those with lower incomes and less education have more untreated decay.[3]
- Adults over 65 are predisposed to a higher prevalence of root caries than younger populations due to an increase in exposed root surfaces from gingival recession (**Figure 47-3**). This prevalence is difficult to estimate due to existing tooth loss that confounds the data.[4]
- An association between tobacco use and caries among adults is not conclusive; however, tobacco use is associated with increased caries development during adolescence.[5]

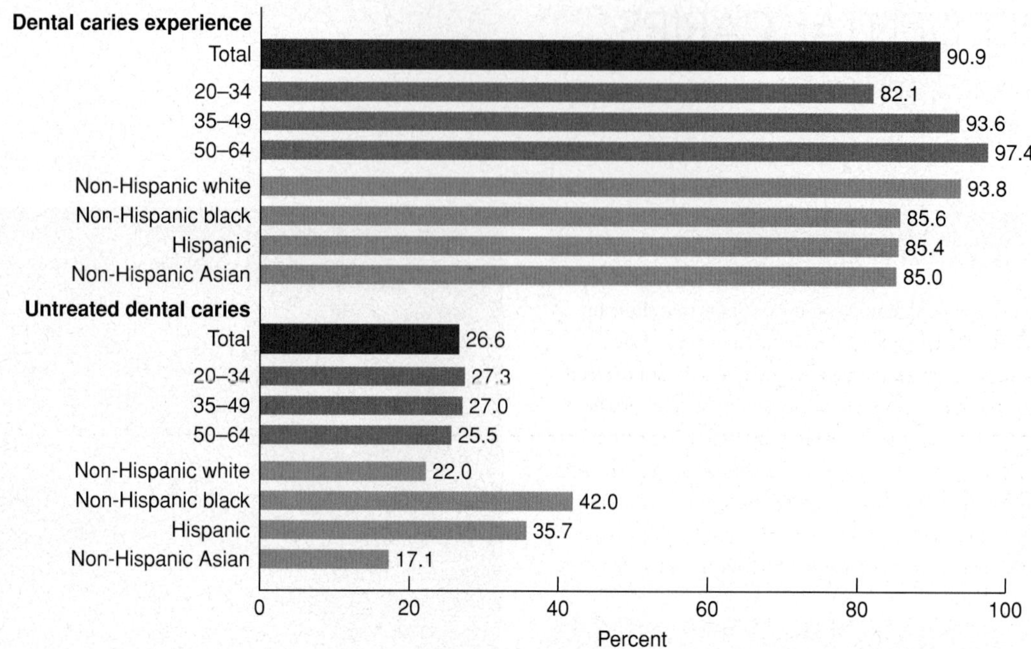

FIGURE 47-2 Dental caries in the United States. (*Data from CDC/NCHS, National Health and Nutrition Examination Survey, 2011–2012. https://www.cdc.gov/nchs/products/databriefs/db197.htm*

ETIOLOGY AND PATHOPHYSIOLOGY

- Dental caries result from the activity of dental bacterial plaque, a complex biofilm containing microorganisms that demineralize and proteolyze tooth enamel and dentin through their action on the fermentation of sucrose and other sugars. The main organism is *Streptococcus mutans.*
- A caries-promoting diet that is high in sugar or acid increases the demineralization process. A cariostatic diet that contains calcium helps buffer the acidity and increase remineralization of the tooth's enamel surface.
- Low saliva flow and low pH also increase demineralization; the lack of saliva to buffer the acidity from plaque and diet increases caries risk.
- Dental caries progression or reversal depends on the balance between demineralization and remineralization. If caries is untreated and progresses, it eventually destroys enough tooth structure that either the unsupported tooth fractures, or the caries reaches the tooth's pulp (nerve tissue) and leads to infection that can progress through the pulp to the tooth's root apex and surrounding bone.
- Plaque also impacts the gingival tissues; if it is not removed regularly, it may calcify with the minerals in the saliva and form calculus (tartar).

RISK FACTORS

The risk factors for adult caries include[6,7]:

- Increased acidic environment that may be a result of:
  - A diet that is high in fermentable carbohydrates and/or acid
  - High quantity of bacteria/poor oral hygiene
  - Physical and medical disabilities that often prevent proper oral hygiene
  - Acid reflux
  - Bulimia
- Low saliva flow and dry mouth:
  - Medications that decrease saliva flow (tricyclic antidepressants, antihistamines, steroids, diuretics) and subsequently also decrease the saliva's pH
  - Illicit drugs such as methamphetamine and cocaine that dry the mouth
  - Radiation to the head and neck that may damage salivary glands
  - Sjögren syndrome affects saliva glands and decreases flow rate
- The presence of existing restorations or oral appliances.
- Inadequate fluoride exposure does not allow for the benefits of remineralization.
- Gingival recession exposing root surfaces (see **Figure 47-3**) that demineralize at a higher pH.
- Existing restorations or appliances that may lead to accumulation of bacteria, if not cleansed daily.
- Low socioeconomic status with limited or no access to medical or dental care.

DIAGNOSIS

Caries can be diagnosed clinically through visual examination of the teeth, where lesions range from a white spot (incipient) to a large cavitated lesion. Radiographically, the carious lesion appears radiolucent (as a consequence of demineralization or cavitation) within a radiopaque, calcified tooth structure.

CLINICAL FEATURES

- Dental caries initially present as a painless white spot (demineralization of enamel) and if contributing risk factors are not modified, it progresses to a brownish discoloration, with eventual cavitation into the dentin. Pain is usually not felt until the caries progresses into the dentin and/or approximates the pulp. It presents only when stimulated with cold or sweets, and rarely with heat, subsiding shortly after stimulus removal. Once the caries infects the nerve, it leads to pulpal necrosis. The patient may present with pain that is spontaneous, triggered with heat and lingers, is more severe, and may be accompanied with soft-tissue swelling.

TYPICAL DISTRIBUTION

Any enamel, exposed dentin, or cementum surface, including occlusal, interproximal, and root surfaces.

LABORATORY AND IMAGING

An X-ray will show the extent of the cavity, but not all demineralized areas.

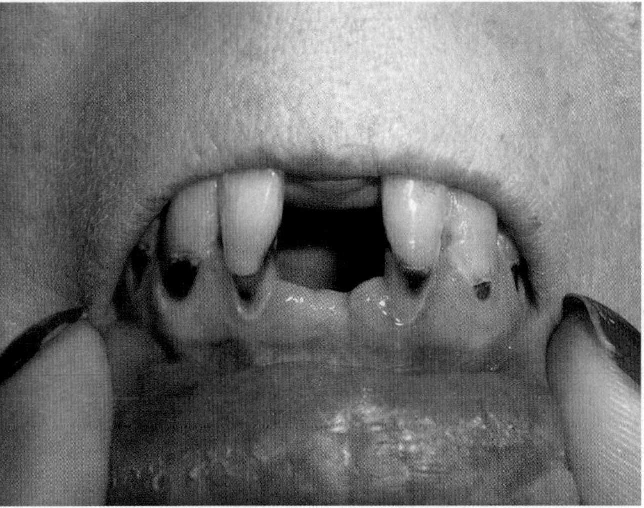

FIGURE 47-3 Root caries in a woman with a history of substance abuse. Note the severe gingival recession that has exposed the darkened roots. She has lost all of her upper teeth and is beginning to lose her lower teeth. Some gingival recession is part of normal aging, but this is severe due to her substance abuse and neglect of her dental health. *(Reproduced with permission from Richard P. Usatine, MD.)*

DIFFERENTIAL DIAGNOSIS

- Fluorosis—Mild fluorosis may present as white spot lesions with an appearance that is similar to the "white-spot" incipient carious lesions.
- Dark staining in the tooth's deep pits and fissures that may be a result of tobacco use or tartar buildup.
- Trauma—Usually involves maxillary incisors; common in sports, accidents, violence, and epilepsy.
- Tooth erosion—Results from consumption of carbonated beverages and fruit drinks, repeated vomiting associated with eating disorders, gastroesophageal reflux, and alcoholism.
- Tooth attrition—Wearing down of teeth because of tooth grinding (bruxism) or an abrasive diet.
- Tooth abrasion—Caused by brushing with a hard toothbrush and using abrasive toothpaste.
- Bulimia can cause destruction of the teeth because of the gastric acids (**Figure 47-4**).

MANAGEMENT

- Demineralized lesions ("white spots") and caries—Topical fluorides such as varnishes (5% NaF; 23,000 parts per million [ppm] F^-) that are applied by dental health providers or the primary care physician twice a year have been shown to decrease dental caries by 21%.[7]
- Fluoride mouth rinses (0.2% NaF, 900 ppm F^-) are effective in controlling caries when used daily.[7]
- Refer to a dental health professional for sealant placement of deep pits and fissures.[8]
- Refer patients with "white spots" and dental caries to a dental professional for treatment and/or restoration.
- Patients with xerostomia may be treated with saliva substitutes such as Oralbalance in the Biotene product range.

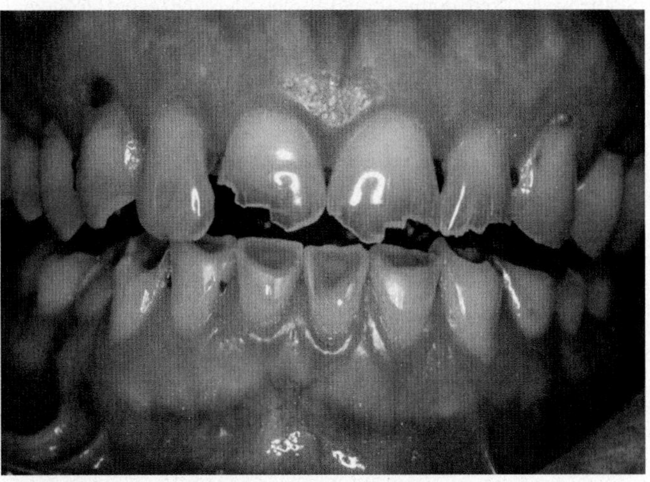

FIGURE 47-4 Destruction of the teeth in woman with bulimia. The gastric acids have dissolved the enamel. *(Reproduced with permission from Richard P. Usatine, MD.)*

PREVENTION AND SCREENING

Most oral disease, including cavities, is preventable. Proper oral hygiene (daily brushing and flossing), daily exposure to fluoride (systemic or topical), along with a healthy diet that is not high in sugar, can prevent the formation and/or progression of dental caries. Visual screening can detect caries at the early stages.

PROGNOSIS

The prognosis for lesions that are detected during their early stages or prior to approximating the tooth's nerve is very good. Removal of the carious portion of the tooth and placement of a filling will restore the tooth to function and prevent further progression of the cavity.

FOLLOW-UP

Remind adult patients who have incipient "white-spot" caries or active caries to go to a dentist for treatment. Patients with large caries should be referred for immediate treatment.

PATIENT EDUCATION

- Advise patients to maintain good oral hygiene by brushing their teeth twice daily with a small-headed, soft to medium hardness brush using a toothpaste that contains fluoride. Electric toothbrushes may be useful for those with poor manual dexterity. Counsel patients to floss once daily to remove plaque and food particles from between the teeth.
- Suggest that patients use antiplaque mouthwashes containing chlorhexidine to inhibit *S. mutans*, but caution patients that such mouthwashes may increase dental staining. This can be minimized with thorough brushing and flossing before using the mouthrinse.[9]
- Patients with xerostomia (dry mouth) should be advised to practice good oral hygiene, to increase water intake, and to avoid acidic and sugary foods. Chewing sugar-free gum will induce salivation.
- Patients with xerostomia should also be advised to avoid alcohol-containing mouth rinses, as alcohol also dries the mouth.
- Advise patients that plaque formation may be reduced by chewing sugar-free gum and eating raw fruits and vegetables, which reduces bacteria through mechanical cleansing of the tooth surfaces.
- Patients who use asthma inhalers should be advised to rinse their mouth out with water after inhaler use to decrease the amount of residue that is left in the oral cavity. Many inhalers contain lactose, a fermentable sugar.
- Eating calcium-containing foods, such as milk and cheese, helps buffer the acidic environment and helps with remineralization.
- Advise patients to visit a dental professional at least once a year for a cleaning and examination.

PATIENT RESOURCES

- American Dental Association. *Mouth Healthy*—**http://www.mouthhealthy.org/en.**
- CDC Dental caries—**https://www.cdc.gov/healthywater/hygiene/disease/dental_caries.html.**

PROVIDER RESOURCES

- Smiles for Life: A National Oral Health Curriculum—**http://www.smilesforlifeoralhealth.org.**
- Centers for Disease Control and Prevention. *Working to Improve Oral Health for All Americans At A Glance 2016*—**https://www.cdc.gov/chronicdisease/resources/publications/aag/oral-health.htm.**
- World Health Organization. *Oral Health*—**http://www.who.int/oral_health/en/.**

REFERENCES

1. Ritter AV, Preisser JS, Chung Y, et al; X-ACT Collaborative Research Group. Risk indicators for the presence and extent of root caries among caries-active adults enrolled in the Xylitol for Adult Caries Trial (X-ACT). *Clin Oral Investig.* 2012;16(6):1647-1657.
2. Dye BA, Thornton-Evans G, Li X, Iafolla TJ. *Dental caries and tooth loss in adults in the United States, 2011–2012.* NCHS data brief, no 197. Hyattsville, MD: National Center for Health Statistics; 2015.
3. National Institute of Dental and Craniofacial Research. *Dental Caries (Tooth Decay) in Adults (Age 20 to 64).* http://www.nidcr.nih.gov/DataStatistics/FindDataByTopic/DentalCaries/DentalCariesAdults20to64.htm. Accessed November 2017.
4. Hayes M, De Mata C, Cole M, et al. Risk indicators associated with root caries in independently living older adults. *J. Dentistry.* 2016; 51:8-14.
5. Holmén A, Strömberg U, Magnusson K, Twetman S. Tobacco use and caries risk among adolescents—a longitudinal study in Sweden. *BMC Oral Health.* 2013;13:31.
6. Stookey G.K. The effect of saliva on dental caries. *J Am Dent Assoc.* 2008;139(suppl):S11-S17.
7. Cappelli DP, Mobley CC. *Prevention in Clinical Oral Health Care.* St. Louis, MO: Elsevier; 2008.
8. National Institutes of Health, Consensus Development Conference Statement, March 26–28, 2001. *Diagnosis and Management of Dental Caries Throughout Life.* http://consensus.nih.gov/2001/2001DentalCaries115html.htm. Accessed November 2017.
9. Chlorhexidine Gluconate 0.12% Antigingivitis Oral Rinse. *Product Monograph Pr Peridex® Oral Rinse.* http://solutions.3mcanada.ca/3MContentRetrievalAPI/BlobServlet?lmd=1326817103000&locale=en_CA&assetType=MMM_Image&assetId=1319218897052&blobAttribute=ImageFile. Accessed November 2017.

PART VII

THE HEART AND CIRCULATION

Strength of Recommendation (SOR)	Definition
A	Recommendation based on consistent and good-quality patient-oriented evidence.*
B	Recommendation based on inconsistent or limited-quality patient-oriented evidence.*
C	Recommendation based on consensus, usual practice, opinion, disease-oriented evidence, or case series for studies of diagnosis, treatment, prevention, or screening.*

*See Appendix A on pages 1603–1606 for further information.

SECTION A CENTRAL

48 CORONARY ARTERY DISEASE

John E. Delzell, Jr, MD, MSPH
Heidi S. Chumley, MD, MBA

PATIENT STORY

A 45-year-old man began having chest pressure with exertion that was relieved with rest. He did not have diabetes, high blood pressure, or high cholesterol and had never had a myocardial infarction. His examination and resting ECG were normal. On the basis of the testing modalities available, he was scheduled for exercise stress testing. After a positive test, he underwent coronary angiography that demonstrated a significant stenosis in the left coronary artery (**Figure 48-1**). He underwent a stenting procedure and was placed on aspirin and cholesterol-lowering medication.

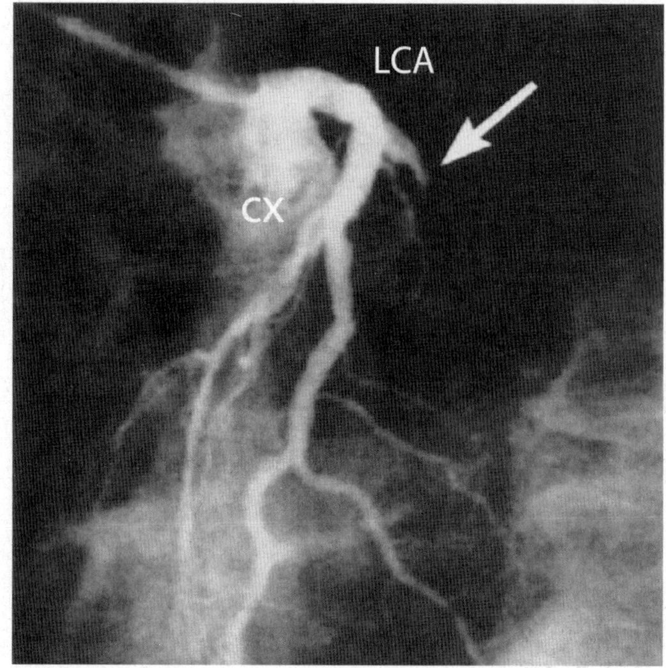

FIGURE 48-1 Coronary arteriogram demonstrating severe stenosis (*white arrow*) in the left coronary artery (*LCA*). Note that the circumflex artery (*CX*) is patent.

INTRODUCTION

In the United States, a person dies of coronary heart disease every 39 seconds. Coronary heart disease is a manifestation of atherosclerotic disease and has many modifiable risk factors. Patients with and without coronary heart disease should be advised to stop smoking, maintain normal blood pressure and cholesterol levels, exercise, achieve or maintain a normal weight, and control diabetes mellitus if present.

EPIDEMIOLOGY

- Coronary heart disease (CHD) is the leading cause of death in the United States, responsible for approximately 600,000 deaths in 2014.[1] The mortality rate has steadily declined for the past 30 years.
- Each year, 790,000 myocardial infarctions occur (first and recurrent) with a 14% mortality rate.[1]
- Approximately 92.1 million U.S. adults have cardiovascular disease.[1]
- In 2012, the prevalence of CHD among U.S. adults older than 18 years of age was higher in men than in women (12.1% vs. 9.7%) and higher in people with a less-than-high-school-diploma education (13.6% vs. 10.4% for college graduates).[2]
- In 2014, prevalence of heart disease was similar among white (10.9%), black (10.8%), and Hispanic (7.8%) persons.[2]

ETIOLOGY AND PATHOPHYSIOLOGY

- CHD is one of several manifestations of atherosclerotic disease, which begins with endothelium dysfunction.[3]

- Endothelium, when normal, balances vasoconstrictors and vasodilators, impedes platelet aggregation, and controls fibrin production.
- Dysfunctional endothelium encourages macrophage adhesion, plaque growth, and vasoconstriction by recruiting inflammatory cells into the vessel walls, the initiating step of atherosclerosis.
- The vessel wall lesions develop a cap of smooth muscle cells and collagen to become fibroadenomas.
- The vessels with these lesions undergo enlargement, allowing progression of the plaque without compromising the lumen.
- Two-thirds of acute coronary events are from plaque disruption and thrombus formation, instead of progressive narrowing of the coronary artery lumen.[2]
- Plaques most likely to rupture (high-risk plaques) have a large core of lipids, many macrophages, decreased vascular smooth muscle cells, and a thin fibrous cap.
- After plaque rupture, the exposed lipid core triggers a superimposed thrombus that occludes the vessel.
- Increased thrombosis is triggered by known cardiac risk factors including elevated low-density lipoprotein (LDL) cholesterol, cigarette smoking, and hyperglycemia.
- The other one-third of acute coronary events occurs at the site of very stenotic lesions (**Figure 48-2**).[3]

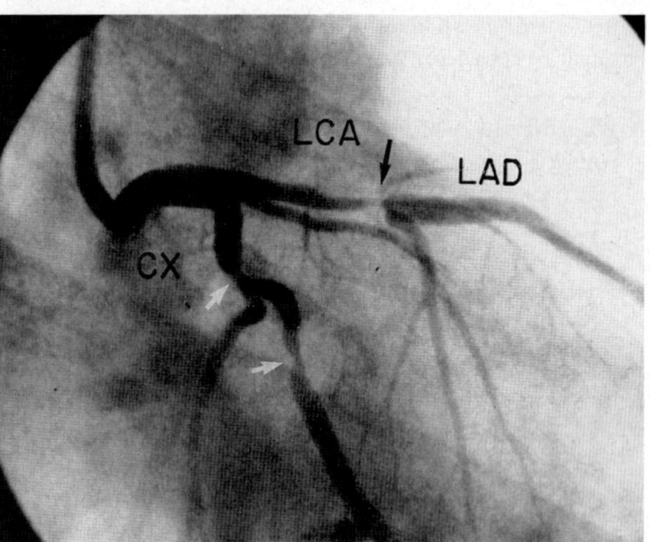

FIGURE 48-2 Coronary angiogram of a left coronary artery (*LCA*) with a tight stenosis in the proximal left anterior descending (*LAD*) artery (*black arrow*). The circumflex artery (*CX*) has two moderately severe stenoses (*white arrows*).

RISK FACTORS

- Family history of premature paternal or sibling myocardial infarction increases risk of heart disease by 50%.[1]
- Tobacco use and secondhand smoke exposure increase the risk of CHD and smoking cessation decreases the risk.[1]
- High total cholesterol, high LDL, and/or low high-density lipoprotein (HDL) are independent risk factors.
- Physical inactivity has a relative risk of CHD of 1.5 to 2.4.[1]
- Overweight or obesity increases risk of heart disease by 20% (men and women) and 46% (men)/64% (women), respectively.[1]
- Diabetes mellitus increases risk of heart disease (hazard ratio 2.5).[1]
- Eighty percent of deaths from CVD can be prevented by healthier lifestyles including tobacco cessation, physical activity, control of blood pressure, and maintaining a healthy weight.[1]

DIAGNOSIS

CLINICAL FEATURES

- Typical angina is chest pain or pressure, brought on by exertion or stress, and relieved with rest or nitroglycerin.
- Atypical angina has two of the three features of typical angina; however, women with coronary artery disease report more neck, throat, or jaw pain.[4]
- Noncardiac chest pain has zero to one of the three features of typical angina.

LABORATORY TESTING

- Risk factor assessment—Lipid profile and fasting blood glucose.

- Acute coronary syndrome—Cardiac-specific troponin is preferred; should be measured at presentation and again 3–6 hours after onset of symptoms.
- When troponin cutoff is 0.1 g/L, sensitivity is 93%, specificity is 91%, positive likelihood ratio (LR+) is 10.33, and negative likelihood ratio (LR−) is 0.08.

COMMON NONINVASIVE TESTING[5]

- Exercise treadmill testing—Sensitivity 52% and specificity 71%, LR+ 1.79, LR+ 0.68.
- Stress echocardiogram—Sensitivity 85% and specificity 77%, LR+ 3.70, LR− 0.19.
- Stress thallium—Sensitivity 87% and specificity 64%, LR+ 2.42, LR− 0.20.

Newer methods being tested include CT and MRI[6]:

- CT for coronary calcium has minimal benefit but only in those with intermediate cardiovascular risk (10%–20% 10-year CV risk)[6,7]
- Coronary CT angiography is not recommended for assessment of asymptomatic patients.[6,7]
- MRI is not recommended for assessment of asymptomatic patients.[6,7]

DIFFERENTIAL DIAGNOSIS

Chest pain can be caused by several conditions including:

- Cardiac—Pericarditis—slower onset of pain, pain aggravated by movement or inspiration, characteristic ECG changes. Aortic dissection—acute onset with tearing type chest or upper back pain, shortness of breath, widening on mediastinum on chest X-ray
- Respiratory—Pneumothorax—acute onset with shortness of breath and characteristic radiographic findings; pneumonia—often accompanied by fever, cough, shortness of breath/hypoxia, and/or radiographic findings; pulmonary embolism—acute onset of shortness of breath, positive ventilation-perfusion scan, or spiral CT.
- GI—Gastroesophageal reflux—related to eating, responds to H_2 blockers or proton pump inhibitor (PPI).
- Musculoskeletal—Costochondritis—chest muscles tender to palpation.

MANAGEMENT

NONPHARMACOLOGIC

- Advise patients with coronary artery disease to stop smoking.[8] SOR A
- Recommend 30 minutes of physical activity 5 to 7 days per week.[1,8] SOR B
- Advise patients in weight management with a goal body mass index (BMI) of 18.5 to 24.9.[8] SOR B

MEDICATIONS

Managing risk factors:

- Lower LDL cholesterol with statin therapy (hydroxymethylglutaryl coenzyme A [HMG-CoA] reductase inhibitors) to decrease all-cause mortality (relative risk [RR] 0.90), cardiovascular mortality (RR 0.80), fatal and nonfatal myocardial infarction (MI) (RR 0.82 and 0.74).[8] SOR A
- Lower blood pressure to 140/90 or 130/80 mm Hg (with diabetes or chronic renal disease); treat patients who are post-MI with a β-blocker, thiazide diuretic, or aldosterone antagonist.[8,9] SOR A
- Prescribe aspirin (75–162 mg) for all patients with coronary artery disease.[8] SOR A
- Prescribe a P2Y12 receptor antagonist such as clopidogrel in combination with aspirin after acute coronary syndrome (ACS) or stent placement.[8] SOR A
- Prescribe a β-antagonist—Several trials demonstrate mortality decreases of 25% to 40% with various β-blockers used in the acute MI or post-MI period.[8]

Treat symptoms:

- Nitroglycerin sublingual or spray for immediate relief of angina.[10,11] SOR B
- Long-acting nitrates or calcium antagonists if β-blockers are contraindicated, do not control symptoms, or have unacceptable side effects.[10,11] SOR B

REFERRAL OR HOSPITALIZATION

- Refer patients with positive noninvasive testing to be evaluated for cardiac catheterization.
- Consult with cardiologists and cardiothoracic surgeons to determine optimal management.
- Patients with greater than 50% stenosis of left main, proximal stenosis of three major arteries, or significant stenosis of the proximal left anterior descending and one other major artery are treated with coronary bypass surgery.[12] SOR A
- Percutaneous coronary intervention (PCI) typically involves balloon dilation plus stent placement. Drug-eluting stents decrease the risk of restenosis.[12]

PREVENTION

Prevention of CHD is accomplished by risk factor control. In a study of older men that examined the risk factors of smoking, high LDL, high blood pressure, and no aspirin use, the number needed to treat (NNT) to prevent one cardiovascular outcome were: 22, 8, 6, and 5 when 1, 2, 3, and 4 risk factors were controlled, respectively.[10]

FOLLOW-UP

Follow-up frequency is based on the extent of illness and symptoms and may include primary care and subspecialty care. Patients should have ongoing evaluation of risk factors and symptoms every 4 to 12 months. Patients who have new or changing ischemic symptoms should undergo stress testing to evaluate for their risk of further cardiac events.[10] SOR C

PATIENT EDUCATION

Advise patients in the importance of lifestyle modification and medications in the long-term management of CHD.

PATIENT RESOURCES

- PubMed Health. *Coronary Heart Disease*—**http://www.ncbi.nlm.nih.gov/pubmedhealth/PMH0004449/.**
- The American Heart Association has information about the warning signs of heart attacks and living a healthy lifestyle at **http://www.americanheart.org.**

PROVIDER RESOURCES

- Boudi FB. *Coronary Artery Atherosclerosis*—**https://reference.medscape.com/refarticle-srch/153647-overview.**
- Online calculator for pre- and posttest probability of coronary artery disease based on history and physical—**http://www.soapnote.org/cardiovascular/chest-pain-evaluation/.**
- The National Heart, Lung, and Blood Institute—**https://www.nhlbi.nih.gov/health-topics/coronary-heart-disease.**

REFERENCES

1. Benjamin EJ, Blaha MJ, Chiuve SE, et al. On behalf of the American Heart Association Statistics Committee and Stroke Statistics Subcommittee. Heart Disease and Stroke Statistics—2017 Update: A Report From the American Heart Association. *Circulation.* 2017;135:0.
2. Blackwell DL, Lucas JW, Clarke TC. Summary health statistics for U.S. adults: National Health Interview Survey, 2012. National Center for Health Statistics. *Vital Health Stat.* 2014;10(260).
3. Viles-Gonzalez JF, Fuster V, Badimon JJ. Atherothrombosis: a widespread disease with unpredictable and life-threatening consequences. *Eur Heart J.* 2004;25(14):1197-1207.
4. Philpott S, Boynton PM, Feder G, Hemingway H. Gender differences in descriptions of angina symptoms and health problems immediately prior to angiography: the ACRE study. Appropriateness of Coronary Revascularisation study. *Soc Sci Med.* 2001; 52(10):1565-1575.
5. Pryor DB, Shaw L, McCants CB, et al. Value of the history and physical in identifying patients at increased risk for coronary artery disease. *Ann Intern Med.* 1993;118(2):81-90.
6. Budoff MJ, Achenbach S, Blumenthal RS, et al. Assessment of Coronary Artery Disease by Cardiac Computed Tomography: A Scientific Statement From the American Heart Association Committee on Cardiovascular Imaging and Intervention, Council on Cardiovascular Radiology and Intervention, and Committee on Cardiac Imaging, Council on Clinical Cardiology. *Circulation.* 2006;114:1761-1791.
7. Greenland P, Alpert JS, Beller GA. 2010 ACCF/AHA Guideline for Assessment of Cardiovascular Risk in Asymptomatic Adults: A Report of the American College of Cardiology Foundation/American Heart Association Task Force on Practice Guidelines. *Circulation.* 2010;122:e584-e636.
8. Smith SC, Benjamin EJ, Bonow RO, et al. AHA/ACCF Secondary Prevention and Risk Reduction Therapy for Patients With Coronary and Other Atherosclerotic Vascular Disease: 2011 Update. *Circulation.* 2011;124:2458-2473.
9. *The Seventh Report of the Joint National Committee on Prevention, Detection, Evaluation and Treatment of High Blood Pressure (JNC 7).* http://www.nhlbi.nih.gov/guidelines/hypertension/index.htm. Accessed September 2012.
10. Gibbons RJ, Chatterjee K, Daley J. ACC/AHA/ACP–ASIM Guidelines for the Management of Patients With Chronic Stable Angina: Executive Summary and Recommendations: A Report of the American College of Cardiology/American Heart Association Task Force on Practice Guidelines (Committee on Management of Patients With Chronic Stable Angina). *Circulation.* 1999;99:2829-2848.
11. Gibbons RJ, Abrams J, Chatterjee K, et al. ACC/AHA 2002 guideline update for the management of patients with chronic stable angina: a report of the American College of Cardiology/American Heart Association Task Force on Practice Guidelines (Committee to Update the 1999 Guidelines for the Management of Patients with Chronic Stable Angina). *JACC.* 2007;50(23): 2264-2274.
12. Anderson JL, Adams CD, Antman EM, et al. 2011 ACCF/AHA Focused Update Incorporated Into the ACC/AHA 2007 Guidelines for the Management of Patients With Unstable Angina/Non–ST-Elevation Myocardial Infarction. *JACC.* 2011; 57(19): e215-367.

49 HYPERTENSION

John E. Delzell, Jr, MD, MSPH
Heidi S. Chumley, MD, MBA

PATIENT STORY

A 40 year-old man presents to his family doctor after getting his blood pressure checked at a local health fair. His blood pressure was measured as 180/100 mm Hg. He has no symptoms or complaints. His blood pressure today was 178/98 mm Hg. Based on these two readings, he is diagnosed with stage 2 hypertension. He has a significant family history of essential hypertension. His examination is normal other than an enlarged and laterally displaced point of maximal impulse on cardiac examination. His body mass index is normal. His physician orders a urinalysis, complete blood count (CBC), fasting lipid profile, and a chemistry panel that includes serum glucose, potassium, creatinine, and calcium. An ECG shows left ventricular hypertrophy (**Figure 49-1**). He is counseled regarding lifestyle changes, started on two medications, and asked to follow-up within a couple of weeks.

INTRODUCTION

Hypertension (HTN) is a major risk factor for both myocardial infarction and stroke. Primary HTN constitutes 90% of HTN cases. Initial treatment includes lifestyle modifications and medications. Most patients require at least two medications to achieve control. Patients who cannot be controlled on three medications should undergo a work-up for secondary causes.

EPIDEMIOLOGY

- 29% of U.S. adults older than age 18 years have HTN.[1]
- Blood pressure is controlled in approximately 50% of adults with HTN.[1]
- Blood pressure control is lowest among those without health insurance (29%), Mexican Americans (37%), and younger adults ages 18 to 39 years (31%).[1,2]
- In the United States, HTN contributes to 1 of every 7 deaths and to half of the cardiovascular disease-related deaths.[2]
- Cost of HTN to the U.S. healthcare system is estimated to be \$93.5 billion per year.[2]

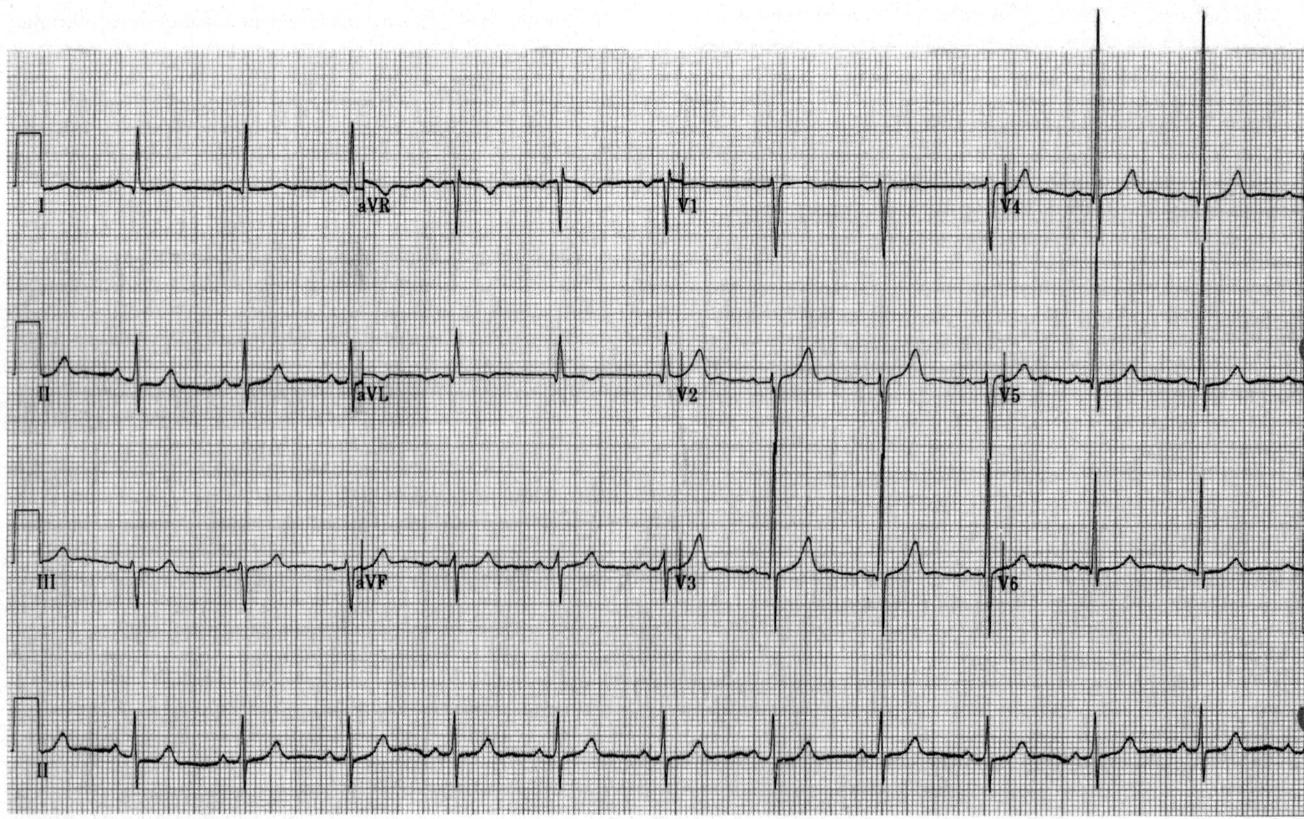

FIGURE 49-1 EKG showing left ventricular hypertrophy in this 58-year-old man with current blood pressure of 178/98. Note how S V_1 + R V_5 > 35 mm. Also his ECG shows left axis deviation and nonspecific ST changes in the high lateral leads (I and aVL). *(Reproduced with permission from Gary Ferenchick, MD.)*

ETIOLOGY AND PATHOPHYSIOLOGY

- Primary HTN (>90% of patients)—A specific cause is unknown, but environmental factors (salt intake, excess alcohol intake, obesity) and genetics both play a role.
- Secondary HTN (5% to 10% of patients)—Causes include medications, kidney disease, renal artery stenosis (**Figure 47-2**), thyroid disease, hyperaldosteronism, and sleep apnea. Rare causes include coarctation of the aorta, Cushing syndrome and pheochromocytoma.

RISK FACTORS

- Family history.
- Genetic predisposition.
- Obesity.
- High sodium chloride intake.
- Medications, including oral contraceptives, NSAIDs, decongestants, and some antidepressants.
- Substances, including caffeine, licorice, amphetamines, cocaine, tobacco.

DIAGNOSIS

Average of two or more seated blood pressure readings on two or more office visits. Diagnosis can be made based on systolic (SBP) or diastolic (DBP) blood pressures.[3]

- Prehypertension—SBP 120 to 139 mm Hg or DBP 80 to 89 mm Hg.
- Stage 1 HTN—SBP 140 to 159 mm Hg or DBP 90 to 99 mm Hg.
- Stage 2 HTN—SBP equal to or greater than 160 mm Hg or DBP equal to or greater than 100 mm Hg.
- In 2017, the ACC/AHA released new hypertension diagnostic criteria.[4] The new criteria lowers the threshold for the diagnosis of hypertension to systolic BP 130 or diastolic BP 80. Some national organizations including the AAFP[5] have decided not to endorse these new guidelines but instead continue to endorse the most recent guideline from the JNC 8.[6]

CLINICAL FEATURES

- Often asymptomatic.
- When blood pressure is high, patients may have headaches or vision changes. Even higher pressures may lead to confusion, chest pain/myocardial ischemia, pulmonary edema, stroke or hematuria.
- Hypertensive retinopathy may be present (**Figure 49-3** and Chapter 23, Hypertensive Retinopathy).
- An S4 can be an early finding on physical examination.
- Long standing HTN may lead to left ventricular hypertrophy which may be identified as an enlarged laterally displaced point of maximal impulse, abnormal ECG (**Figure 47-1**), or abnormal chest radiograph.
- Abdominal bruits may be present with renal artery stenosis.

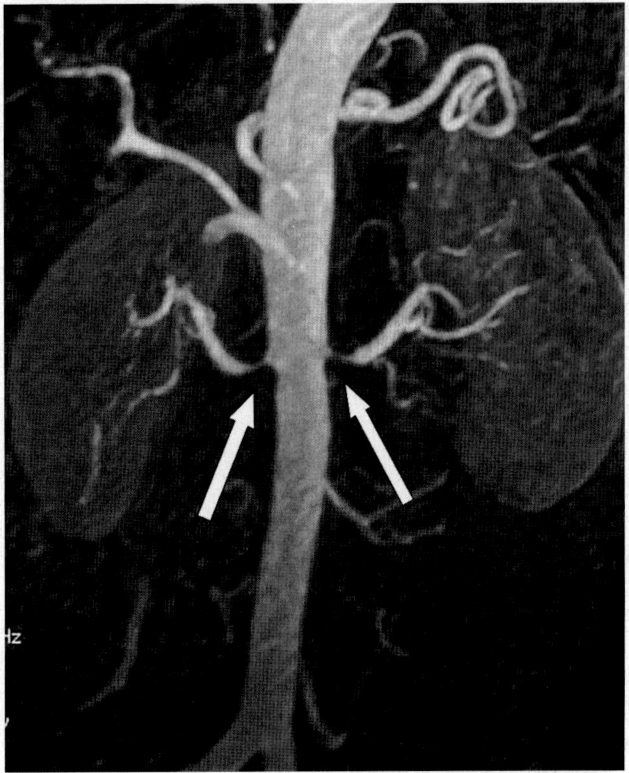

FIGURE 49-2 Angiogram revealing bilateral renal artery stenosis (*arrows*), one of the more common causes of secondary hypertension, most often a result of atherosclerotic disease in older patients. (*Reproduced with permission from Fuster V, Walsh R, Harrington RA: Hurst the Heart, 13th ed. New York, NY: McGraw-Hill Education; 2011.*)

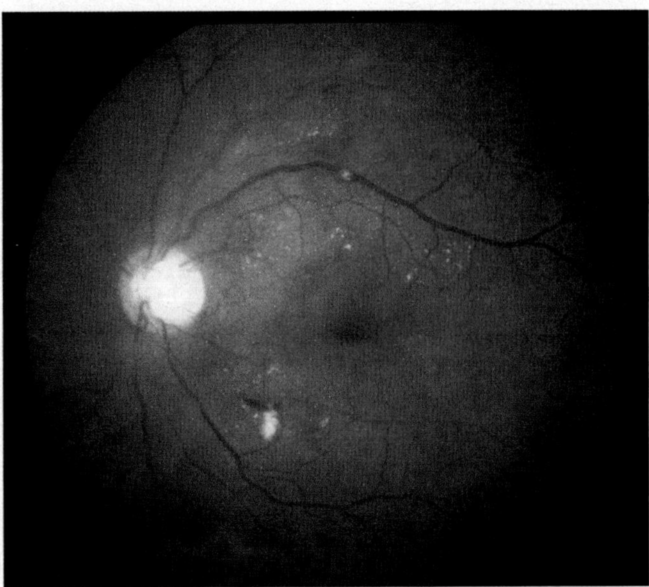

FIGURE 49-3 Hypertensive and diabetic retinopathy with dot-blot hemorrhages, a flame hemorrhage, and hard exudates. The arterioles are attenuated from the hypertension. (*Reproduced with permission from Carrie Cooke.*)

LABORATORY TESTING

- Before initiating therapy for presumed primary HTN perform the following tests: urinalysis, CBC, fasting lipid profile, and chemistry panel, including fasting blood glucose, potassium, creatinine, and calcium.
- Consider testing for thyroid disorders with a thyroid-stimulating hormone (TSH) if signs or symptoms of hyperthyroidism are present.
- For patients with abnormal screening tests, signs indicating a secondary cause, or inadequate control on three medications:
  - Serum aldosterone and plasma renin activity in patients with hypokalemia.
  - 24-hour urine protein and creatinine for suspected renal disease.
  - A 24-hour urine free cortisol or a dexamethasone suppression test for suspected Cushing syndrome.
  - Plasma and urine catecholamines or metanephrines for suspected pheochromocytoma.
  - Parathyroid hormone level for suspected hyperparathyroidism.
- ECG on all patients with HTN.
- Chest radiograph is not necessary for patients diagnosed with primary HTN; however, if obtained, cardiomegaly may be present. If coarctation of the aorta is expected, rib notching may be present.
- Echocardiogram may demonstrate left ventricular hypertrophy.
- Renal artery stenosis can be seen on magnetic resonance angiography or by angiography (**Figure 49-2**).
- Renal ultrasound may demonstrate small or absent kidney.

DIFFERENTIAL DIAGNOSIS

- Falsely elevated blood pressure readings can be a result of improper cuff size (too small with a large arm diameter) or method (patient not seated, arm in incorrect position, etc.).
- Acute elevations in blood pressure may be caused by substances (e.g., tobacco, caffeine, cocaine).
- White coat HTN is defined as blood pressure that is consistently over 140/90 mm Hg in the presence of a healthcare provider with an ambulatory monitoring average of less than 135/85 mm Hg.

MANAGEMENT

NONPHARMACOLOGIC

- Weight reduction if overweight or obese.
- DASH (dietary approaches to stop hypertension) diet, rich in fruits and vegetables, aimed at reducing sodium intake and eating a variety of foods rich in nutrients that help lower blood pressure, such as potassium, calcium, and magnesium.
- Low-fat diet.
- Low dietary sodium chloride.
- Regular aerobic exercise.
- Moderate alcohol intake: no more than two drinks per day for men and one per day for women.
- Smoking cessation for cardiovascular risk reduction (see Chapter 248, Smoking and Tobacco Addiction).

MEDICATIONS

- Start a thiazide-type diuretic in most patients. An angiotensin converting enzyme inhibitor (ACEI) may be the initial choice in white males.[3,6]
- Patients with Stage 2 HTN should be started on two medications upon diagnosis.
- Consider starting two medications when blood pressure is 20/10 mm Hg higher than goal. Goal is 140/90 mm Hg or 130/80 mm Hg in patients with diabetes or chronic kidney disease.
- Add an ACEI, angiotensin receptor blocker (ARB), β-blocker (BB), or calcium channel blocker (CCB) if control is not achieved with initial agent.
- Specific medications have compelling indications in these situations:
  - Heart failure—Diuretic, BB, ACEI, ARB, aldosterone antagonist (AA).
  - Post myocardial infarction—BB, ACEI, AA.
  - Diabetes—Diuretic, BB, ACEI, ARB, CCB.
  - Chronic kidney disease—ACEI, ARB.
  - Recurrent stroke prevention—Diuretic, ACEI.

REFERRAL OR HOSPITALIZATION

- Refer patients in whom adequate blood pressure control is not obtained.
- Women with HTN who are planning a pregnancy or who become pregnant should be referred to a provider with experience managing chronic HTN during pregnancy.

PREVENTION

Healthy lifestyle for all persons, including weight reduction (if overweight or obese), use of DASH diet, initiation and maintenance of adequate physical activity, and moderate alcohol intake.

PROGNOSIS

- Risk of cardiovascular disease increases as blood pressure increases.
- Between 115/75 and 185/115 mm Hg, every increase of 20 mm Hg systolic BP or 10 mm Hg diastolic BP doubles the risk of cardiovascular disease for adults ages 40 to 70 years.[7]

FOLLOW-UP

- Schedule visits monthly until blood pressure goal is obtained.
- Consider more frequent visits for patients with stage 2 HTN or significant comorbid conditions.
- Patients with controlled HTN should be seen every 3 to 6 months.

PATIENT EDUCATION

- HTN is a chronic disease requiring lifelong lifestyle modifications and one or more daily medications for most patients.
- Adequate control of HTN reduces the risk for heart attack and stroke.

PATIENT RESOURCE

- The National Heart Lung and Blood Institute. *What Is High Blood Pressure?*—**http://www.nhlbi.nih.gov/health/health-topics/high-blood-pressure.**

PROVIDER RESOURCES

- The Seventh Report of the Joint National Committee on Prevention, Detection, Evaluation, and Treatment of High Blood Pressure (JNC 7)— **https://www.nhlbi.nih.gov/files/docs/guidelines/express.pdf.**
- The Eighth Report of the Joint National Committee on Prevention, Detection, Evaluation, and Treatment of High Blood Pressure (JNC 8)—**https://jamanetwork.com/journals/jama/fullarticle/1791497.**

REFERENCES

1. Egan BM, Zhao Y, Axon RN. US trends in prevalence, awareness, treatment and control of hypertension, 1988–2008. *JAMA* 2010; 303(2):2043-2050.
2. Centers for Disease Control and Prevention. Vital signs: prevalence, treatment, and control of hypertension—United States, 1999–2002 and 2005–2008. *MMWR Morb Mortal Wkly Rep.* 2011; 60:103-108.
3. Chobanian AV1, Bakris GL, Black HR, et al. National Heart, Lung, and Blood Institute Joint National Committee on Prevention, Detection, Evaluation, and Treatment of High Blood Pressure; National High Blood Pressure Education Program Coordinating Committee. The Seventh Report of the Joint National Committee on Prevention, Detection, Evaluation, and Treatment of High Blood Pressure: the JNC 7 report. *JAMA*. 2003;289 (19):2560-2572.
4. Whelton PK, Carey RM, Aronow WS, et al. 2017 ACC/AHA guideline for the prevention, detection, evaluation, and management of high blood pressure in adults. *J Am College Cardiol.* doi:10.1016/j.jacc.2017.11.006.
5. AAFP. *AAFP Decides to Not Endorse AHA/ACC Hypertension Guideline.* https://www.aafp.org/news/health-of-the-public/20171212notendorseaha-accgdlne.html. Accessed January 2018.
6. James PA, Oparil S, Carter BL. 2014 Evidence-Based Guideline for the Management of High Blood Pressure in Adults: report from the panel members appointed to the Eighth Joint National Committee (JNC 8). *JAMA*. 2014;311(5):507-520.
7. Lewington S, Clarke R, Qizilbash N, et al. Age-specific relevance of usual blood pressure to vascular mortality: a metaanalysis of individual data for one million adults in 61 prospective studies. *Lancet.* 2002;360:1903-1913.

50 HEART FAILURE

Heidi S. Chumley, MD, MBA
Nina Rivera, DO
John E. Delzell, Jr, MD, MSPH

PATIENT STORY

A 60-year-old man presents to the emergency department with exertional shortness of breath increasing in severity over the past several days, along with paroxysmal nocturnal dyspnea and orthopnea. He does not have a history of heart failure or previous myocardial infarction. On examination, it was found that he had a third heart sound and an elevated jugular venous pressure. His chest radiograph showed cardiomegaly (**Figure 50-1**) and his B-type natriuretic peptide (BNP) was elevated at 600 pg/mL. He was diagnosed with heart failure, evaluated for underlying causes including coronary artery disease, and treated initially with an angiotensin-converting enzyme inhibitor (ACEI) and a loop diuretic. Later, he will be started on a β-blocker and an aldosterone receptor antagonist.

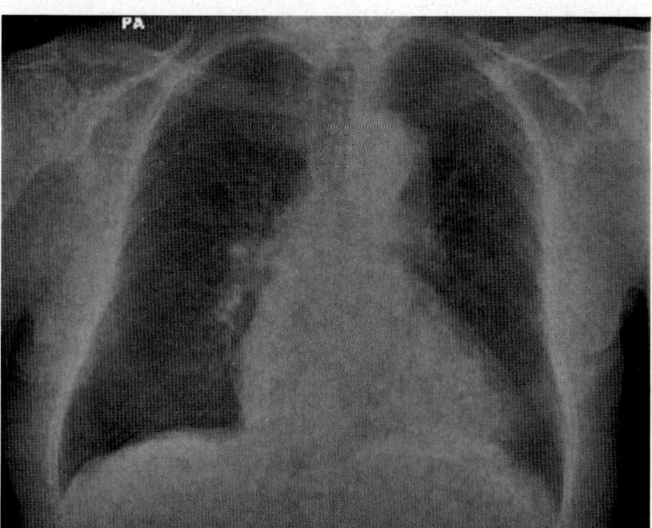

FIGURE 50-1 Cardiomegaly demonstrated in a posteroanterior (PA) view. The widest part of the heart is greater than 50% of the diameter of the chest. (*Reproduced with permission from Heidi Chumley, MD.*)

INTRODUCTION

Heart failure (HF) is common and increases with age. HF is a clinical syndrome that has multiple etiologies, all of which lead to a decrease in heart pumping capacity. There are two main types of heart failure: heart failure with reduced ejection fraction (HFrEF), also referred to as systolic HF, and heart failure with preserved ejection fraction (HFpEF) or diastolic HF.[1] ACEIs and β-blockers with or without aldosterone antagonists and angiotensin II blockers are the main pharmacologic therapies.

SYNONYMS

Congestive heart failure (CHF), systolic or diastolic dysfunction.

EPIDEMIOLOGY

- The prevalence of HF in the community increases with age: 0.7% (45 to 54 years); 1.3% (55 to 64 years); 1.5% (65 to 74 years); and 8.4% (75 years or older).[2]
- In the United States, the prevalence of HF is more than 5.8 million and the annual incidence is approximately 550,000.[3]
- There are race-related differences in the risk of HF, with the prevalence among black men and women about twice that of whites.[4]
- More than 40% of patients in the community with HF have an ejection fraction greater than 50%.[5]
- At age 40 years, the lifetime risk for HF is 21.0% (95% confidence interval [CI] 18.7% to 23.2%) for men and 20.3% (95% CI 18.2% to 22.5%) for women.[5]
- Survival rate is 50% at 5 years after diagnosis.[1]

ETIOLOGY AND PATHOPHYSIOLOGY

- The most common cause of heart failure is ischemia, but heart pumping capacity can decline from several causes (i.e., myocardial infarction or ischemia, hypertension, valvular dysfunction, cardiomyopathy, or infections such as endocarditis or myocarditis).
- Cardiac dysfunction activates the adrenergic and renin-angiotensin-aldosterone systems.
- These systems provide short-term compensation, but chronic activation leads to myocardial remodeling and eventually worsening of cardiac function.
- Norepinephrine, angiotensin II, aldosterone, and tissue necrosis factor each contributes to disease progression.
- Angiotensin II directly causes cell death through necrosis and apoptosis, as well as cardiac hypertrophy.

CLASSIFICATIONS

- Two types of classifications: Stages of HF and New York Heart Association functional classifications[1]:

American College of Cardiology/American Heart Association	
Stage A	At risk but no structural disease or symptoms
Stage B	Structural disease but no symptoms
Stage C	Structural disease with current or previous symptoms
Stage D	Refractory disease
New York Heart Association	
I	Ordinary activity does not cause any symptoms
II	No symptoms at rest but symptoms with ordinary activity
III	No symptoms at rest but symptoms with less than ordinary activity
IV	Symptoms at rest

DIAGNOSIS

Many history, examination, radiographic, ECG, and laboratory features are helpful in making the diagnosis of HF for patients presenting with dyspnea in the emergency department.[6]

CLINICAL FEATURES

- History and physical
  - History of HF (LR + [likelihood ratio] = 5.8), myocardial infarction (LR+ = 3.1).[6]
  - Symptoms of paroxysmal nocturnal dyspnea (LR+ = 2.6), orthopnea (LR+ = 2.2), edema (LR+ = 2.1).[6]
  - Examination finding of third heart sound (LR+ = 11), hepatojugular reflex (LR+ = 6.4), jugular venous distention (LR+ = 5.1), rales or crackles (LR+ = 2.8), lower extremity edema (LR+ = 2.3).[6]

LABORATORY AND ANCILLARY TESTING

- Laboratory value of BNP ≥250 (LR+ = 4.6); BNP <100 decreases likelihood of HF.[6]
- BNP cutoff points may be different in patients with renal insufficiency, obesity, or advanced age.
- ECG finding of atrial fibrillation (LR+ = 3.8), T-wave changes (LR+ = 3.0), any abnormality (LR+ = 2.2). A normal ECG lowers likelihood (LR− = 0.640).[6]

IMAGING

- Radiographic finding of pulmonary venous congestion (**Figure 50-2**) (LR+ = 12.0), interstitial edema (LR+ = 12.0), alveolar edema (LR+ = 6.0), cardiomegaly (**Figures 50-1** to **50-3**) (LR+ = 3.3).[6]

DIFFERENTIAL DIAGNOSIS

Gradually increasing shortness of breath can also be caused by:

- Chronic obstructive pulmonary disease may have dyspnea with exertion but does not have orthopnea; chest radiograph shows a normal-size heart, hyperinflated lungs, and flattened diaphragm; pulmonary function tests may be abnormal.
- Deconditioning has a normal chest radiograph.
- Metabolic acidosis from any cause can be differentiated with an arterial blood gas.
- Anxiety has episodic shortness of breath, not associated with exertion, and a normal chest radiograph.
- Neuromuscular weakness may have abnormal pulmonary function tests and a normal chest radiograph.
- Pneumonia may have fever and an infiltrate on chest radiograph.

MANAGEMENT

NONPHARMACOLOGIC

- Telemonitoring of patients with known HF for arrhythmias reduced all-cause mortality (relative risk [RR] 0.66). Telemonitoring and structure telephone support reduced HF related hospitalization (RR 0.79 and 0.77, respectively).[7]
- Exercise rehabilitation increases quality of life and decreases hospital admissions in patients with left ventricular systolic dysfunction.[8]
- Modest salt restriction is reasonable for most patients with HF but there is insufficient evidence to determine if this has an effect on mortality in patients with HF.[1,9]

MEDICATIONS

Individually, ACE-Is, β-blockers, and aldosterone antagonists (AAs) lower mortality and should be considered for all patients without contraindications. Detailed treatment recommendations can be found in the 2013 ACCF/AHA Guidelines for the Management of Heart Failure.[1]

- Prescribe an ACE-I. SOR Ⓐ ACE-Is lower overall mortality rates by 23% and decrease hospitalization. Use in all patients with HFrEF unless there is a contraindication.[1,10]

- Prescribe a β-blocker. SOR Ⓐ Use one of the three beta blockers (bisoprolol, carvedilol, and sustained release metoprolol) that have been shown to reduce mortality. β-Blockers (BBs) reduce mortality by 32%.[11] Begin at a small dose and double the dose every 2 to 4 weeks until the target dose is reached or the patient cannot tolerate the increased dose. One study demonstrating a decrease in mortality had a large percentage of patients in the control and intervention groups already on an ACEI, indicating that the two together may decrease mortality more than an ACEI alone.[1,10] SOR Ⓑ
- Prescribe an AA for patients with HFrEF and an EF <35%. Use when the creatinine is less than 2.5 mg/dL (men) and 2.0 mg/dL in women; monitor renal function and potassium.[10] SOR Ⓐ AAs lowered mortality by 30% and should be used in patients who are already taking ACE-I and BB.[1] SOR Ⓑ
- Consider an angiotensin II receptor blocker (ARB) for patients who cannot tolerate an ACEI. Combining the use of an ACEI with an ARB is not recommended.[1] SOR Ⓒ
- Combination of hydralazine and isosorbide dinitrate in addition to ACE-I, BB, and AA reduces mortality in African American patients with NYHA class III or IV.[1] SOR Ⓐ
- Loop diuretics (e.g., furosemide or bumetanide) should be used in patients with evidence of fluid retention. Combine with ACEI, β-blocker, AA as above.[1] Associated with worse outcomes, including higher mortality when used alone.[11]
- Calcium channel blockers are not recommended in HF.[1] SOR Ⓐ
- Digoxin reduces hospitalizations and improves clinical symptoms, but does not lower mortality. Consider adding digoxin when patients have symptoms despite adequate therapy with ACEI, β-blockers, and AA.[1,11] SOR Ⓑ

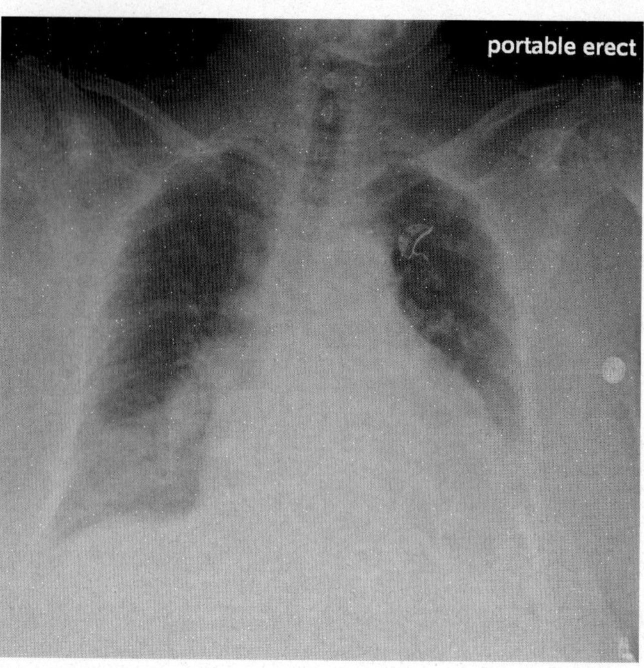

FIGURE 50-2 Cardiomegaly with pulmonary venous congestion and bilateral pleural effusions. (*Reproduced with permission from Heidi Chumley, MD.*)

REFERRAL OR HOSPITALIZATION

- Refer for evaluation for cardiac resynchronization therapy in patients with left ventricular ejection fraction (LVEF) less than 35% and QRS greater than 150 milliseconds.[1] A recent meta-analysis demonstrated that cardiac resynchronization therapy decreased all-cause mortality and hospitalizations for HF in patients with New York Heart Association (NYHA) class II. Number needed to treat (NNT) = 12 to prevent 1 hospitalization.[12]
- Refer for evaluation for implantable cardiac defibrillator (ICD) placement in patients with NYHA class II-IV and LVEF less than 35%. SOR Ⓒ ICDs have been shown to reduce mortality up to 30% and may offer greater risk reduction than antiarrhythmic medical therapy for some patients.[1]

PROGNOSIS

Absolute mortality is high in patients with HF.

- Patients with preserved ejection fraction (>50%) have a mortality rate of 121 per 1000 patient years. Patients with reduced ejection fraction (<40%) have a mortality rate of 141 per 1000 patient years.[13]
- Five-year mortality rate after hospitalization for HF is 42.3%.[1]

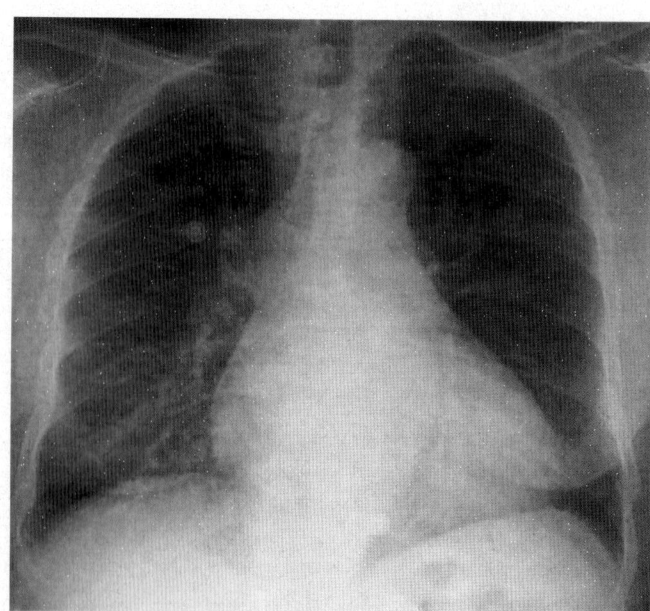

FIGURE 50-3 Cardiomegaly with increased pulmonary vasculature and Kerley B lines (2- to 3-cm horizontal lines in the lower lung fields). (*Reproduced with permission from Heidi Chumley, MD.*)

FOLLOW-UP

Close follow-up in many forms, including telemedicine and structured telephone visits, can reduce hospitalizations and mortality.[7]

PATIENT EDUCATION

Fluid and sodium restriction are still recommended by the ACCF/AHA guidelines, but a recent Cochrane review found no evidence of mortality improvements.[9]

PATIENT RESOURCES

- **http://www.ncbi.nlm.nih.gov/pubmedhealth/PMH0001211/.**
- The National Heart, Lung, and Blood Institute has patient information on HF at **http://www.nhlbi.nih.gov/health/health-topics/topics/hf/.**

PROVIDER RESOURCES

- Yancy et al.[1] 2013 Guideline for the management of heart failure—**http://circ.ahajournals.org/content/128/16/1810.**
- Yancy et al. 2017 Focused update of 2013 Guideline for the management of heart failure—**http://www.onlinejacc.org/content/70/6/776?_ga=2.162007100.1680271014.1514559843-204072263.1514559843.**

REFERENCES

1. Yancy CW, Jessup M, Bozkurt B, et al. 2013 ACCF/AHA Guideline for the Management of Heart Failure: a report of the American College of Cardiology Foundation/American Heart Association Task Force on Practice Guidelines. *Circulation.* 2013;128(16):e240-e327.
2. Redfield MM, Jacobsen SJ, Burnett JC Jr, et al. Burden of systolic and diastolic ventricular dysfunction in the community: appreciating the scope of the heart failure epidemic [see comment]. *JAMA.* 2003;289(2):194-202.
3. Roger VL. Epidemiology of heart failure. *Circ Res.* 2013;113(6):646-659.
4. Go AS, Mozaffarian D, Roger VL, et al. Heart disease and stroke statistics—2013 update: a report from the American Heart Association. *Circulation.* 2013;127:e6-e245.
5. Lloyd-Jones DM, Larson MG, Leip EP, et al. Lifetime risk for developing congestive heart failure: The Framingham Heart Study [see comment]. *Circulation.* 2002;106(24):3068-3072.
6. Wang CS, FitzGerald JM, Schulzer M, et al. Does this dyspneic patient in the emergency department have congestive heart failure [review]? *JAMA.* 2005;294(15):1944-1956.
7. Inglis SC, Clark RA, McAlister FA, et al. Which components of heart failure programmes are effective? A systematic review and meta-analysis of the outcomes of structured telephone support or telemonitoring as the primary component of chronic heart failure management in 8323 patients: Abridged Cochrane review. *Eur J Heart Fail.* 2011;139(9):1028-1040.
8. Mant J, Al-Mohammad A, Swain S, Laramée P; Guideline Development Group. Management of chronic heart failure in adults: synopsis of the national institute for health and clinical excellence guideline. *Ann Intern Med.* 2011;155(4):252-259.
9. Adler AJ, et al. Reduced dietary salt for the prevention of cardiovascular disease. *Cochrane Database Syst Rev.* 2014;(12):CD009217.
10. Mielniczuk L, Stevenson LW. Angiotensin-converting enzyme inhibitors and angiotensin II type I receptor blockers in the management of congestive heart failure patients: what have we learned from recent clinical trials [review]? *Curr Opin Cardiol.* 2005;20(4):250-255.
11. Yan AT, Yan RT, Liu PP. Narrative review: pharmacotherapy for chronic heart failure: evidence from recent clinical trials [review]. *Ann Intern Med.* 2005;142(2):132-145. [Summary for patients in *Ann Intern Med.* 2005;142(2):I53.]
12. Adabag S, Roukoz H, Anand IS, Moss AJ. Cardiac resynchronization therapy in patients with minimal heart failure: a systematic review and meta-analysis. *J Am Coll Cardiol.* 2011;58(9):935-941.
13. Meta-analysis Global Group in Chronic Heart Failure. The survival of patients with heart failure with preserved or reduced left ventricular ejection fraction: an individual patient data meta-analysis. *Eur Heart J.* 2012;33(14):1750-1757.

51 PERICARDIAL EFFUSION

Asif Jawaid, DO
John E. Delzell, Jr, MD, MSPH
Heidi S. Chumley, MD, MBA

PATIENT STORY

A 30-year-old woman presented to her family physician with increasing shortness of breath over the past 2 weeks. Two weeks ago she developed a flulike illness and felt like she never recovered. She denied chest pain or edema, did not take any medications, and had not had any recent trauma or surgery. She had a normal examination. Her chest radiograph showed a classic globular heart as demonstrated in **Figure 51-1**. She had nonspecific ST changes on her ECG. An echocardiogram confirmed pericardial effusion (**Figure 51-2**). The underlying etiology was not elucidated, but she recovered spontaneously over the next several months.

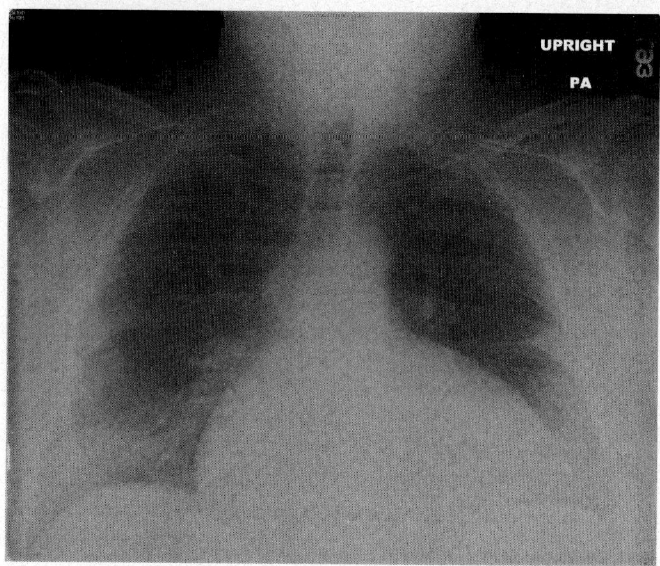

FIGURE 51-1 Globular cardiac silhouette or classic "water-bottle heart" seen with a pericardial effusion can be difficult to distinguish from cardiomegaly on plain radiographs. *(Reproduced with permission from Heidi Chumley, MD.)*

INTRODUCTION

Pericardial effusion is an abnormal amount of fluid that may accumulate in the pericardial space. The pericardial space normally contains 15–50 mL of fluid, which serves as lubrication between the visceral and parietal layers of the pericardium. The speed at which a pericardial effusion develops has a great impact on a patient's symptoms. Pericardial effusions are commonly found in the general population, and the incidence increases with age. They can be caused by cardiac disease or surgery, connective tissue disorders, neoplasms, infections, renal disease, hypothyroidism, or medications; however, a cause is identified only 50% of the time. The definitive diagnosis is made by echocardiography.

EPIDEMIOLOGY

- Six-and-a-half percent of adults (<1% ages 20 to 30 years; 15% older than 80 years of age) had echocardiogram findings consistent with pericardial effusion in a population-based study of 5652 adults and adult family members of participants in the Framingham Heart Study.[1]
- Few large studies have characterized the population prevalence of pericardial effusion; however, the available data consistently show that pericardial effusion is more prevalent than is clinically evident.
- Seventy-seven percent of patients after cardiac surgery for valves or bypass have pericardial effusions, which rarely (<1%) require treatment (**Figure 51-3**).[2]
- Forty percent of healthy pregnant women have small, asymptomatic pericardial effusions in the third trimester.[3]

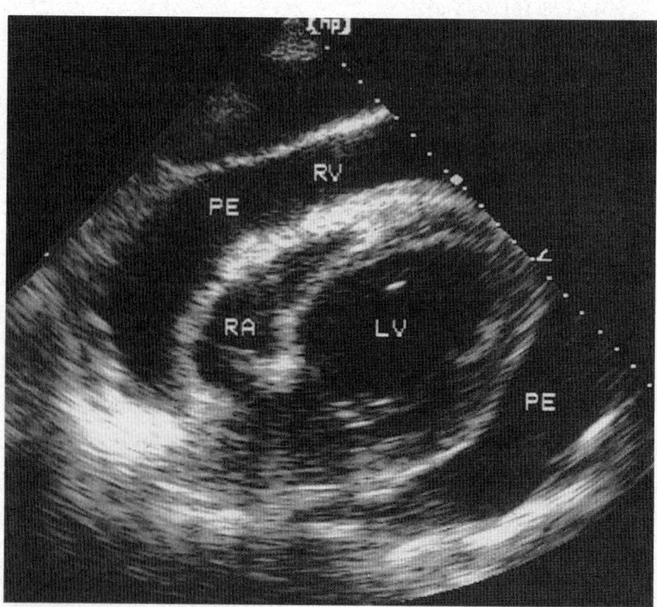

FIGURE 51-2 Echocardiogram showing right ventricular (*RV*) compression from a pericardial effusion (*PE*). *LV*, left ventricle; *RA*, right atrium. *(Reproduced with permission from Heidi Chumley, MD.)*

ETIOLOGY AND PATHOPHYSIOLOGY

Pericardial effusion, acute or chronic, occurs when there is increased production or decreased drainage of pericardial fluid allowing accumulation in the pericardial space. The underlying etiology is clinically apparent approximately 25% of the time and can be determined with testing in another 25% of cases, leaving 50% of cases idiopathic.[4] Most idiopathic cases have small effusions. Moderate to large pericardial effusions have an identifiable cause in 90%.[5]

The normal pericardium can stretch to accommodate a small amount of fluid without a significant change in intrapericardial pressure, although once this pericardial reserve volume is surpassed, the pressure-volume curve becomes steep. Rapid accumulation of pericardial fluid may cause elevated intrapericardial pressures with as little as 80 mL of fluid, while slowly progressing effusions can grow to 2 L without symptoms.

RISK FACTORS

Underlying causes include:

- Congestive heart failure from other cardiac diseases, such as rheumatic heart disease, cor pulmonale, or cardiomyopathy.[6]
- After cardiac surgery or myocardial infarction.[2]
- Connective tissue disorders (scleroderma, lupus erythematosus, rheumatoid arthritis).[6,7]
- Neoplasms: benign (atrial myxoma); primary malignant (mesothelioma); secondary malignant (i.e., lung or breast cancer).[6]
- Chronic renal disease (uremia or hemodialysis) or other causes of hypoalbuminemia.[8]
- Infections: acute (enterovirus, adenovirus, influenza virus, *Streptococcus* pneumonia, *Coxiella burnetii*—responsible for Q fever) or chronic (tuberculosis, fungus, parasites).[4]
- Medications (procainamide, hydralazine) or after radiation.[6]
- Severe hypothyroidism with myxedema.[6]

DIAGNOSIS

Clinical features, chest radiograph, and electrocardiogram suggest pericardial effusion, which is confirmed by echocardiogram. The underlying etiology is identifiable in approximately 50% of cases.[7]

CLINICAL FEATURES

Signs and symptoms occur when the volume of fluid is large enough to affect hemodynamics. Rapid accumulation of pericardial fluid may cause elevated intrapericardial pressures with as little as 80 mL of fluid. Chronic pericardial effusion allows stretching over time and may require up to 2 L to cause significant symptoms[6]:

- Hypotension, increased jugular venous pressure, and soft heart sounds form the classic **Beck's triad** of acute cardiac tamponade, but all three are present only in approximately 30% of cases.[6]
- Common symptoms include anorexia (90%), dyspnea (78%), cough (47%), and chest pain (27%).[6]
- Common physical examination findings include pulsus paradoxus (77% with acute tamponade, 30% with chronic effusions), sinus tachycardia (50%), jugular venous distention (45%), hepatomegaly, and peripheral edema (35%).[6]

LABORATORY AND ANCILLARY TESTING

- Electrocardiogram is abnormal in 90%. Findings include low QRS voltage and nonspecific ST-T changes (59% to 63%) and electrical alternans (0% to 10%).[6]
- When the diagnosis remains unclear, pericardial fluid can be sent for cell count and differential, protein, lactate dehydrogenase, glucose, Gram stain, bacterial cultures, fungal cultures, mycobacterial acid-fast stain and culture, and tumor cytology.
- Measure rheumatoid factor, antinuclear antibody, and complement levels when collagen vascular disease is suspected.[6] Check HIV status in at-risk patients.

When there is no obvious cause, ordering this set of specific tests determined the underlying etiology more often than seen in historic controls (27.3% vs. 3.9%; $p < 0.001$).[9]

- Aerobic and anaerobic blood cultures.
- Throat swab cultures for influenza, adenovirus, and enterovirus.
- Serologic tests for *Cytomegalovirus*, influenza, *C. burnetii*, *Mycoplasma* pneumonia, and *Toxoplasma*.
- Blood tests for antinuclear antibody (ANA) and thyroid-stimulating hormone (TSH).

IMAGING

- Chest radiograph shows a globular enlarged cardiac silhouette (see **Figure 51-1**) (sensitivity 78%, specificity 34% with moderate or severe effusions) and pericardial fat stripe (**Figure 51-3**) (sensitivity 22%, specificity 92%).[6]
- Echocardiography is the preferred imaging test. Echo can be used to quantify volume of pericardial effusion (correlation to amount of fluid withdrawn 0.7).[10] Echo-free, as opposed to echogenic, fluid is associated with a lower risk of constrictive pericarditis or recurrent pleural effusion.[11]
- CT scanning, typically done for another purpose, can demonstrate the presence of a pericardial effusion, **but does not quantify volume as well as echocardiography** (correlation to amount of fluid withdrawn 0.4).[10]

DIFFERENTIAL DIAGNOSIS

- Congestive heart failure has many similar signs and symptoms (dyspnea, jugular venous distention, hepatomegaly, and edema) but may have pulmonary rales, which are unusual in pericardial effusions. A lateral radiograph in a patient with congestive heart failure (without pleural effusion) should have a normal thin pericardium (**Figure 51-4**).
- Pleural effusions may also present with dyspnea, but have different physical examination and radiographic findings.
- Acute pericarditis (without pericardial effusion) can present with chest pain and nonspecific ECG changes also seen with pericardial effusion. In contrast, acute pericarditis often has elevated inflammatory markers and a normal chest radiograph.[12]

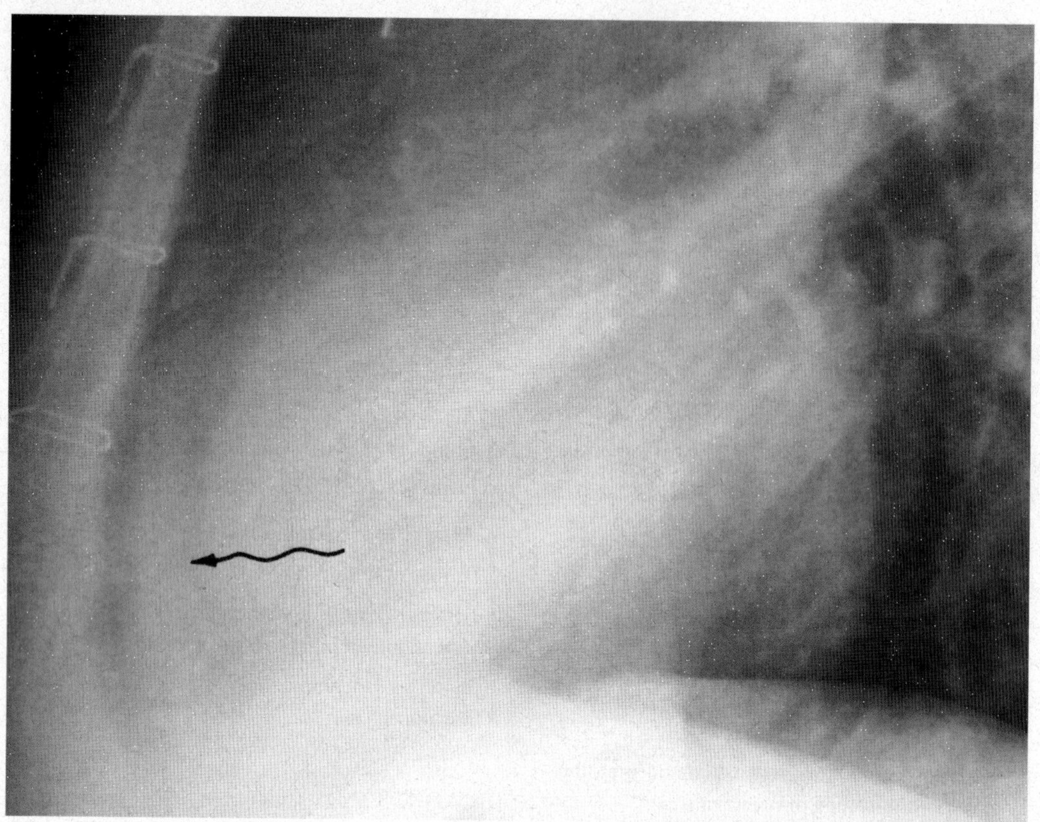

FIGURE 51-3 Moderate pericardial effusion is seen as a wide pericardium (*arrow*). (*Reproduced with permission from Heidi Chumley, MD.*)

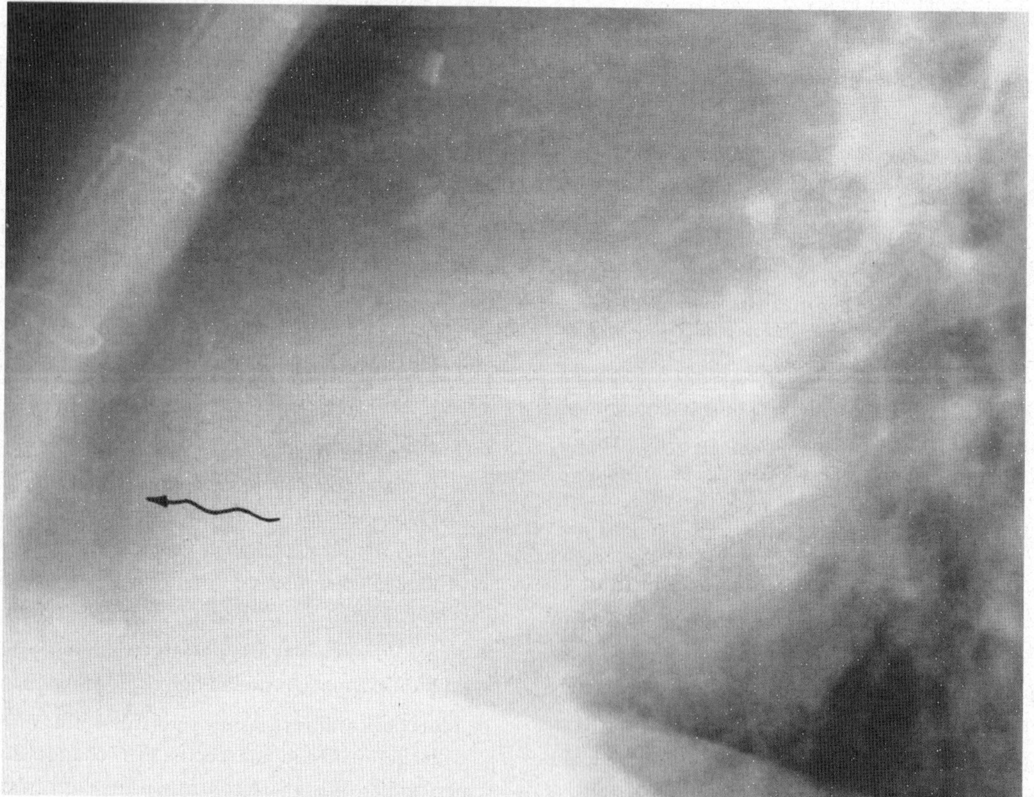

FIGURE 51-4 The lateral view demonstrates the normal thin pericardium (*arrow*), which should be less than 2 mm. (*Reproduced with permission from Heidi Chumley, MD.*)

MANAGEMENT

Most acute idiopathic or viral pericarditis occurrences are self-limited and respond to treatment with a nonsteroidal anti-inflammatory drug (NSAID).[7] Colchicine or prednisone may be administered for severe inflammatory pericardial effusions or when NSAID treatment has failed. Colchicine is preferred over steroids (unless specifically indicated), as the latter is associated with an increased incidence of recurrent pericarditis.[13]

Pharmacotherapy for pericardial effusion includes use of the following agents, depending on the etiology:

- **NSAIDs** (e.g., indomethacin, ibuprofen, naproxen, diclofenac, ketoprofen, aspirin)
- **Corticosteroids** (e.g., prednisone, methylprednisolone, prednisolone)
- **Anti-inflammatory agents** (e.g., colchicine)
- **Antibiotics** (e.g., vancomycin, ceftriaxone, ciprofloxacin, isoniazid, rifampin, pyrazinamide, ethambutol)
- **Antineoplastic therapy** (e.g., systemic chemotherapy, radiation)
- **Sclerosing agents** (e.g., tetracycline, doxycycline, cisplatin, 5-fluorouracil)
- Treat any identified underlying cause.
- When the diagnosis is unclear and the patient is hemodynamically stable, NSAIDs may be beneficial, especially if inflammatory markers are elevated.

Pericardiocentesis:

- Required when there is hemodynamic compromise. Also useful when the pericardial effusion is large or suspected to be secondary to a bacterial infection or neoplastic process.
- Pericardiocentesis should be performed under local anesthesia as follows: Elevate the patient to a 45-degree angle. Insert a needle in the angle between the left costal arch and the xiphoid process, directed 15-degrees posterior, and angled toward the head or either shoulder. Complications are reduced when this procedure is guided by echocardiography. Fluid often reaccumulates. An indwelling catheter can be placed for up to 72 hours without increasing the risk of infection, until a more permanent procedure can be performed to decrease the likelihood of reaccumulation.
- Sclerosing therapy reduces the recurrence of symptoms from reaccumulation or the need for a repeat procedure for 30 days in more than 70% of patients. A caustic substance such as bleomycin or tetracycline is instilled into the pericardial space and held there for up to 4 hours.
- Other options to reduce recurrence include balloon pericardiotomy performed in a cardiac catheterization laboratory, radiation therapy, and surgery (i.e., pericardial window).

PROGNOSIS

Prognosis depends on the underlying cause.

In a study of older adults undergoing echocardiography for reasons other than a pericardial effusion, patients with an incidental small pericardial effusion had a higher 1-year mortality (26%) than did patients without an effusion (11%).[14]

FOLLOW-UP

Follow-up is based on the underlying cause. Pericardial effusions often disappear when the underlying illness resolves, and reappear when the underlying illness does not resolve (metastatic cancer).

PATIENT EDUCATION

- The underlying cause of a pericardial effusion is identified only 50% of the time; however, specific tests should be done to find treatable causes.
- In patients without an obvious underlying illness, infections (such as the flu, Q fever, or tuberculosis) and cancer are the two most commonly identified causes of pericardial effusions.

PATIENT RESOURCES

- MedlinePlus—**https://medlineplus.gov/pericardialdisorders.html.**
- Mayo Clinic Health Information—**https://www.mayoclinic.org/diseases-conditions/pericardial-effusion/diagnosis-treatment/drc-20353724.**

PROVIDER RESOURCES

- **https://emedicine.medscape.com/article/157325-overview.**
- **https://emedicine.medscape.com/article/80602-overview.**

REFERENCES

1. Savage DD, Garrison RJ, Brand F, et al. Prevalence and correlates of posterior extra echocardiographic spaces in a free-living population based sample (the Framingham study). *Am J Cardiol.* 1983;51(7):1207-1212.
2. Ikaheimo MJ, Huikuri HV, Airaksinen KE, et al. Pericardial effusion after cardiac surgery: incidence, relation to the type of surgery, antithrombotic therapy, and early coronary bypass graft patency. *Am Heart J.* 1988;116(1 Pt 1):97-102.
3. Ristic AD, Seferovic PM, Ljubic A, et al. Pericardial disease in pregnancy. *Herz.* 2003;28(3):209-215.
4. Levy PY, Corey R, Berger P, et al. Etiologic diagnosis of 204 pericardial effusions. *Medicine (Baltimore).* 2003;82(6):385-391.
5. Imazio M, Spodick DH, Brucato A, et al. Controversial issues in the management of pericardial diseases. *Circulation.* 2010;121(7):916-928.
6. Karam N, Patel P, deFilippi C. Diagnosis and management of chronic pericardial effusions. *Am J Med Sci.* 2002;322(2):79-87.
7. Adler Y, Charron P, Imazio M, et al. 2015 ESC guidelines for the diagnosis and management of pericardial diseases. *Eur Heart.* 2015;J36:2921-2964.
8. Stolz L, Valenzuela J, Situ-LaCasse E, et al. Clinical and historical features of emergency department patients with pericardial effusions. *World J Emerg Med.* 2017;8(1):29-33.

9. Levy PY, Moatti JP, Gauduchon V, et al. Comparison of intuitive versus systematic strategies for aetiological diagnosis of pericardial effusion. *Scand J Infect Dis.* 2005;37(3):216-220.
10. Liebowitz D, Perlman G, Planer D, et al. Quantification of pericardial effusions by echocardiography and computed tomography. *Am J Cardiol.* 2011;107(2):331-335.
11. Kim SH, Song JM, Jung IH, et al. Initial echocardiographic characteristics of pericardial effusion determine the pericardial complications. *Int J Cardiol.* 2009;136(2):151-155.
12. Imazio M, Gaita F, LeWinter M. Evaluation and treatment of pericarditis: a systematic review. *JAMA* 2015;314:1498-1506.
13. Izadi A, Bozorgi A, HajHossein Talasaz A, et al. Efficacy of colchicine versus placebo for the treatment of pericardial effusion after open-heart surgery: a randomized, placebo-controlled trial. *Am Heart J.* 2015;170(6):1195-1201.
14. Mitiku TY, Heidenreich PA. A small pericardial effusion is a marker of increased mortality. *Am Heart J.* 2011;161(1): 152-157.

52 BACTERIAL ENDOCARDITIS

Danish Sheikh, DO
John E. Delzell, Jr, MD, MSPH

PATIENT STORY

A 25-year-old man presented to the office because he had been feeling tired and feverish for several weeks. He admitted to injecting heroin regularly in the last 2 months. On examination, he was febrile and had a heart murmur of which he was previously unaware. His fingernails showed splinter hemorrhages (**Figure 52-1**). His funduscopic examination revealed Roth spots (**Figures 52-2** and **52-3**). An echocardiogram demonstrated vegetation on the tricuspid valve. He was hospitalized and treated empirically for bacterial endocarditis. After his blood cultures returned *Staphylococcus aureus*, his regimen was adjusted based on sensitivities and continued for 6 weeks.

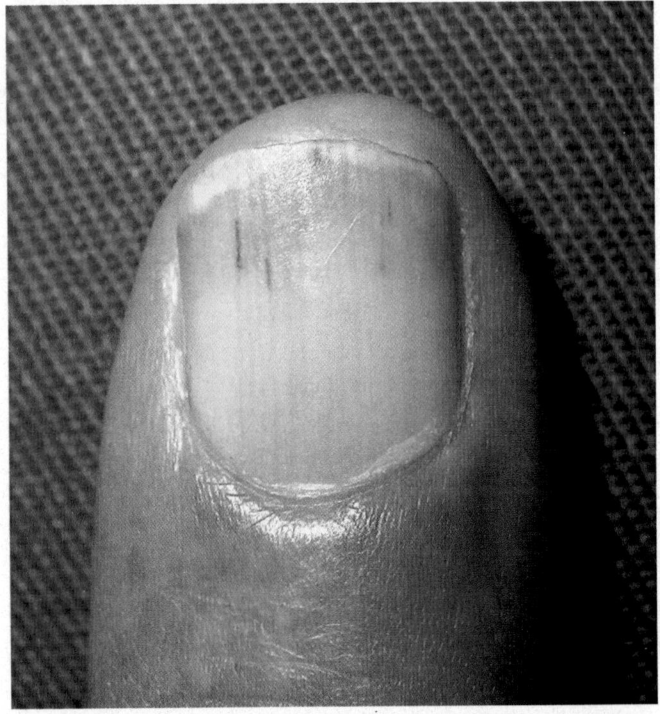

FIGURE 52-1 Splinter hemorrhages appearing as red linear streaks under the nail plate and within the nail bed. Although endocarditis can cause this, splinter hemorrhages are more commonly seen in psoriasis and trauma. *(Reproduced with permission from Richard P. Usatine, MD.)*

INTRODUCTION

Bacterial endocarditis is a serious infection seen most commonly in patients with prosthetic valves; injection drug users; patients with HIV, especially those who use intravenous (IV) drugs; and patients who are immunosuppressed. Diagnosis is made using the Duke Criteria. Treatment is IV antibiotics or surgical valve replacement. Mortality, even with treatment, is 26% to 37%.

EPIDEMIOLOGY

- 3 to 7.0 cases per 100,000 patient years.[1]
  - Historically more common in men; however, the incidence in women is increasing. Men 8.6 to 12.7 and women 1.4 to 6.7 cases per 100,000 person years, respectively[1]
  - Average age has increased from 46.5 years (1980–1984) to 70 years (2001–2006)[1]
  - Incidence in IV drug users is 3 per 1000 person years or 1% to 5% per year[2]
  - Incidence in HIV-positive IV drug users is 13.8 per 1000 person years[2]
  - Incidence of vegetations forming on intracardiac devices has increased from 13.8% (1998) to 18.9%[3]
- Morbidity and mortality is increasing. It is ranked the 3rd or 4th most common cause of life-threatening infection.[1]
- Seen in immunosuppressed patients with central venous catheters or hemodialysis patients.
  - Fifty percent healthcare-associated, 43% community-acquired, and 7.5% nosocomial[4]
  - Mortality ranges from 16% to 37%[5]
- Patients with endocarditis who require surgery is increasing, now about 50%[1]

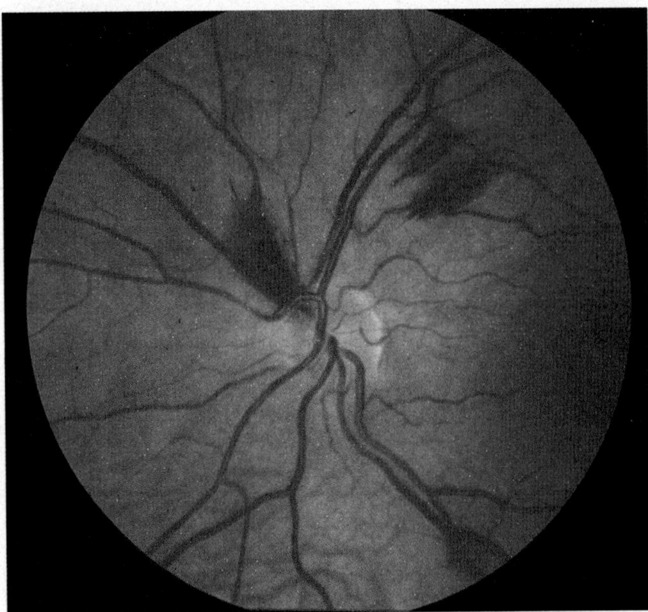

FIGURE 52-2 Roth spots that are retinal hemorrhages with white centers seen in bacterial endocarditis. These can also be seen in leukemia and diabetes. *(Reproduced with permission from Paul D. Comeau.)*

- Prosthetic valve endocarditis makes up 10% to 15% of endocarditis cases.[6]
  - Incidence of 0.1% to 2.3% person year[6]
  - Can occur early (2 months after surgery) or late

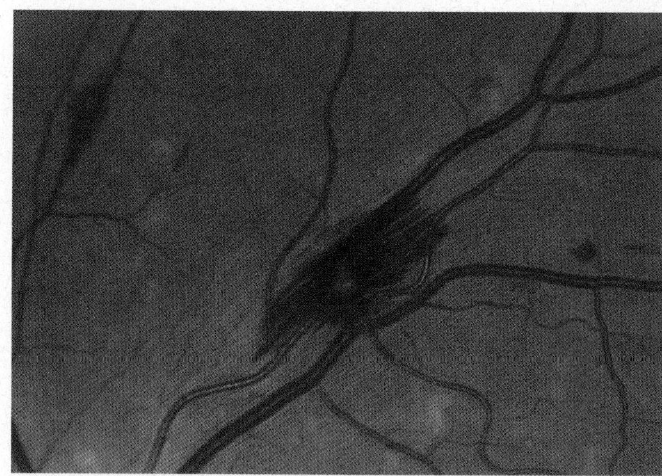

FIGURE 52-3 Close-up of a Roth spot, which is actually a cotton-wool spot surrounded by hemorrhage. The cotton wool comes from ischemic bursting of axons, and the hemorrhage comes from ischemic bursting of an arteriole. (*Reproduced with permission from Paul D. Comeau.*)

ETIOLOGY AND PATHOPHYSIOLOGY

- Endothelium is injured by mechanical or inflammatory processes.
- Microbes adhere to compromised endothelium during transient bacteremia.
- Common organisms include *S. aureus* (IV drug users, nosocomial infections, prosthetic valve patients), *Streptococcus gallolyticus* (previously known as *S. bovis*, seen in elderly patients), enterococci (nosocomial infections), and *Staphylococcus epidermidis* (early infection in prosthetic valve patients).
- Blood contacts subendothelial factors, which promotes coagulation.
- Pathogens bind and activate monocyte, cytokine, and tissue factor production, enlarging the vegetations on the heart valves.
- The vegetations enlarge and damage the heart valves (**Figure 52-4**). This process can lead to death if not treated adequately in time.
- Septic emboli can occur, most commonly to the brain, spleen, or kidney.[6]

RISK FACTORS

- Prosthetic heart valve.
- Injection drug use.
- HIV infection.
- Immunodeficiency.

DIAGNOSIS

I. Modified Duke Criteria[1]
   A. The Modified Duke criteria use a combination of history, physical examination, laboratory, and echocardiogram findings, and have a sensitivity of approximately 80% across several studies.
   B. Definition of Infective Endocarditis
      i. Definite Endocarditis
         1. Pathological Criteria
            a. Microorganisms demonstrated by culture/histological review of vegetation specimen
            b. Abscess formation
         2. 2 Major Criteria; 1 Major criterion and 3 minor criteria; OR 5 minor criteria
      ii. Possible Endocarditis
         1. 1 Major criterion and 1 minor criterion; OR 3 minor criteria
      iii. No Endocarditis
         1. Definite alternative diagnosis explaining signs and symptoms
         2. Resolution of endocarditis with <4 days of antibiotic therapy

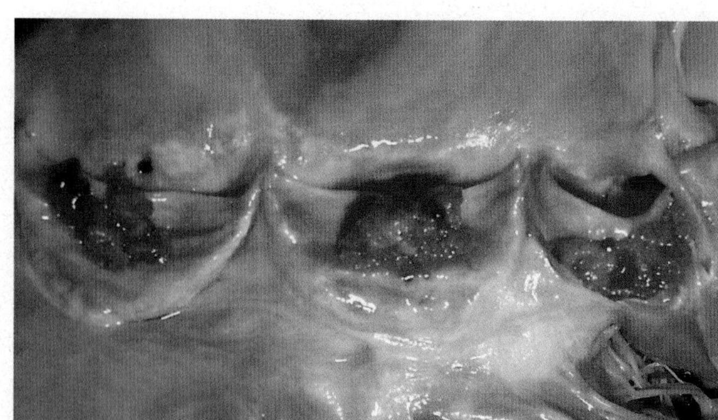

FIGURE 52-4 Pathology specimen of a patient who died of bacterial endocarditis. Bacterial growth can be seen on the three cusps of this heart valve. (*Reproduced with permission from Larry Fowler, MD.*)

3. No pathological or histological evidence of infection in patients treated with <4 days of antibiotics
4. Does not meet criteria for definite or possible endocarditis

C. Major Criteria
   i. Positive blood cultures
      1. Three sets of blood cultures from different venipunctures sites with the first and last culture being no different than one hour apart
      2. Minimum of two blood cultures showing infection required to designate "Positive Blood cultures"
      3. A single culture positive for *Coxiella burnetii* or anti–phase 1 IgG antibody titer ≥1:800 is sufficient to designate as "positive"
      4. Organisms
         a. *Staphylococcus aureus*—most common in United States
         b. *Streptococci viridans*
         c. *Streptococcus gallolyticus (bovis)*
         d. HACEK group (*Haemophilus, Actinobacillus, Cardiobacterium, Eikenella, Kingella*)
         e. Community-acquired enterococci
      5. Microorganisms present on recurrent blood cultures drawn at least 12 hours apart.
   ii. Endocardial involvement as evidenced by:
      1. Echocardiogram evidence of vegetation, abscess, or new partial dehiscence of a prosthetic valve.
      2. New valvular regurgitation.
   iii. Echocardiogram findings consistent with infected vegetation (NOTE: This was previously a minor criterion). Echocardiogram should be performed on any patient with suspected endocarditis.

D. Minor Criteria
   i. Predisposition (e.g., heart condition such as a congenital or acquired valvular defect, injection drug use, prior history of endocarditis).
   ii. Temperature >38°C (100.4°F).
   iii. Clinical signs: arterial emboli, septic pulmonary infarcts, mycotic aneurysms, intracranial hemorrhages, Janeway lesions (**Figures 52-5** and **52-6**).
   iv. Glomerulonephritis, Osler nodes, Roth spots, or positive rheumatoid factor (see **Figures 52-2**, **52-3**, and **52-6**).
   v. Positive blood culture not meeting major criteria.

CLINICAL FEATURES

- Fever—Seen in 85% to 99% of patients, typically low-grade, approximately 39°C (102.2°F).
- New or changing heart murmur—Seen in 20% to 80% of patients.
- Septic emboli—Seen in up to 60%, largely dependent on the size (>10 mm) and mobility of the vegetation.
- Intracranial hemorrhages—Seen in 30% to 40% of patients, bleeding from septic emboli or cerebral mycotic aneurysms.
- Mycotic aneurysms—Aneurysms resulting from infectious process in the arterial wall, most commonly in the thoracic aorta, also found in the cerebral arteries.
- Janeway lesions—Very rare, flat, painless, red to bluish-red spots on the palms and soles (**Figures 52-5** and **52-6**).

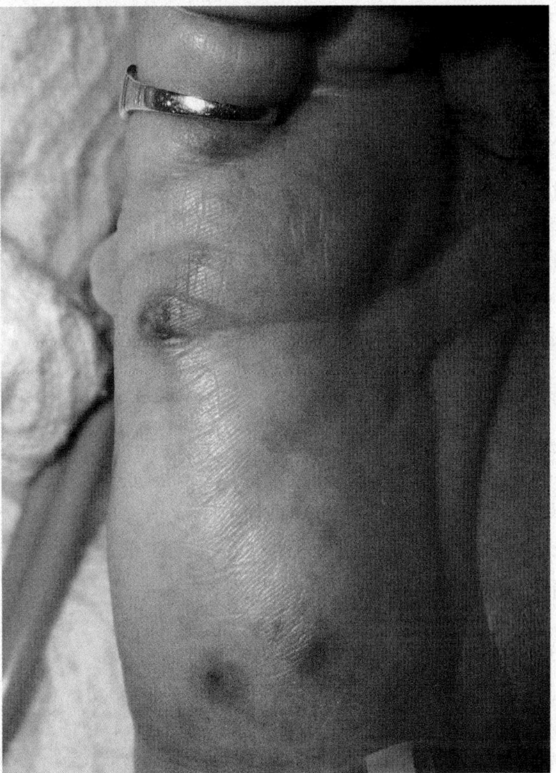

FIGURE 52-5 Janeway lesions on the palm of a woman hospitalized with acute bacterial endocarditis. These were not painful. (*Reproduced with permission from David A. Kasper DO, MBA.*)

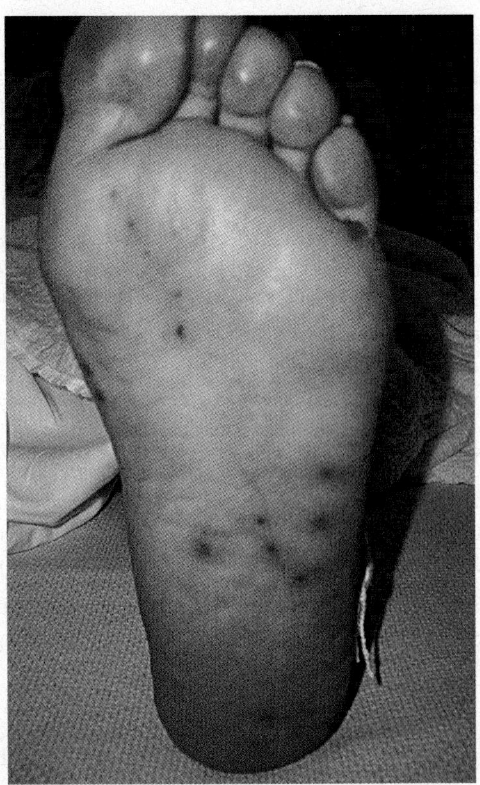

FIGURE 52-6 Osler node causing pain within pulp of the big toe in the same woman hospitalized with acute bacterial endocarditis. (Osler nodes are painful—remember "O" for Ouch and Osler.) Note the multiple painless flat Janeway lesions over the sole of the foot. (*Reproduced with permission from David A. Kasper DO, MBA.*)

- Splinter hemorrhages—Red, linear streaks in the nail beds of the fingers or toes (**Figure 52-1**).
- Glomerulonephritis—Immune mediated; can result in hematuria and renal insufficiency, occurs in approximately 15% of patients with endocarditis.
- Osler nodes—Tender, subcutaneous nodules in the pulp of the digits (**Figure 52-6**).
- Roth spots—Retinal hemorrhages from microemboli, seen in approximately 5% of endocarditis (**Figures 52-2** and **52-3**).
- Positive rheumatoid factor—Seen in up to 50% of patients.

TYPICAL DISTRIBUTION

- Native endocarditis: Mitral valve is most common location (prior rheumatic fever or mitral valve prolapse), followed by aortic (prior rheumatic fever, calcific aortic stenosis of bicuspid valve).
- Prosthetic valve endocarditis: Site of any prosthetic valve.
- In IV drug users: Tricuspid valve, followed by aortic.[2]

LABORATORY AND ANCILLARY TESTING

In addition to blood cultures, consider a complete blood count for anemia and leukocytosis, erythrocyte sedimentation rate (ESR) (elevated in approximately 90%), and urinalysis for proteinuria or microscopic hematuria (seen in approximately 50%).

- Positive blood culture—First two sets of cultures are positive in 90%.[6]

IMAGING

- Abnormal echocardiogram in 85%.[7]
- If transthoracic echocardiogram is normal and endocarditis is still suspected, order a transesophageal echocardiogram (TEE).[6] SOR Ⓒ
  - TEE should be ordered in all patients with history of prosthetic valves, when there is concern of abscess formation, and when poor cardiac windows are expected (obese, history of chronic obstructive pulmonary disease [COPD], previous thoracic surgery)[1]
  - If initial TEE is negative for endocarditis but there is a high suspicion, repeat TEE in 3–5 days to look for changes[1]
  - Repeat TEE if there are clinical signs of complication of the disease
  - Transthoracic echocardiogram may be done after completion of antibiotic therapy to establish a new baseline[1]
  - Vegetation >10 mm have a higher risk of embolization
- Cardiac MRI and CT scans are currently being studied as imaging modalities to diagnose endocarditis, but no clear guidelines and recommendations have yet been established.
- 3D TEE may be useful in detecting vegetations and their effect on the surrounding structures, but resolution is not high enough for routine use.[1]

DIFFERENTIAL DIAGNOSIS

Fever without a clear cause may be seen with:

- Connective tissue disorders—Typically with other signs depending on the disorder, negative blood cultures, normal echocardiogram.
- Fever of unknown origin—Negative blood cultures or positive cultures with atypical organisms, normal echocardiogram in noncardiac causes.
- Intra-abdominal infections—Fever and positive blood cultures, normal echocardiogram.
- Echocardiogram findings similar to bacterial endocarditis may be seen with:
  - Noninfective vegetations—No fever and negative blood cultures
  - Cardiac tumors—Embolic complications, right or left heart failure, often located off valves in cardiac chambers, negative blood cultures
  - Cusp prolapse—No fever and negative blood cultures
  - Myxomatous changes—Extra connective tissue in the valve leaflets
  - Lambl excrescences—Stranding from wear and tear on the valve, most commonly aortic, no fever, and negative blood cultures

MANAGEMENT

- Draw blood cultures (three sets) and admit suspected cases to the hospital for IV antibiotics. SOR Ⓒ
- Consider infectious disease consultation. SOR Ⓒ

MEDICATIONS

- Start antibiotics empirically SOR Ⓒ for specific regimens (**Table 52-1**).
  - Do not use gentamicin for right-sided *Staphylococcus*-related native valve endocarditis[1,8]
  - Do not use gentamicin to treat methicillin-sensitive *Staphylococcus aureus* (MSSA) or methicillin-resistant *Staphylococcus aureus* (MRSA)
  - Clindamycin is not recommended for treatment of infective endocarditis due to high rate of recurrence
  - Patients with vancomycin-resistant *Staphylococcus* should be managed by an infectious disease consultant
- Alter antibiotics based on culture results.[1] SOR Ⓐ
- Anticoagulation and aspirin are not indicated for infective endocarditis and are contraindicated with cerebral complications or aneurysms.

SURGICAL CONSULTATION

- Surgical excision of infected tissue has a 10% to 16% mortality rate in the immediate postop period.[9,10]
- Consider surgical consultation when:
  - Congestive heart failure is severe with mitral or aortic regurgitation
  - Fever and/or bacteremia persist for 5–7 days despite adequate antibiotic therapy, abscesses or perivalvular involvement occurs, fungal organisms are identified, or heart block occurs[1]
  - Embolic events recur on adequate antibiotic therapy or the risk of embolic events is high because of vegetations larger than 10 mm. SOR Ⓒ
  - Consider postponing surgery in cases with large ischemic stroke or hemorrhagic stroke.

TABLE 52-1 Medications

Native Valve Endocarditis[1]		
Organisms	**Drug**	**Dose**
S. viridans and S. gallolyticus (bovis)		
Highly penicillin susceptible	**Duration: 4 weeks**	
	Aqueous crystalline penicillin G sodium	12–18 million U/24 h IV either continuously or in 4 or 6 equally divided doses
		OR
	Ceftriaxone sodium	2 g/24 h IV/IM in 1 dose
		OR
	Vancomycin hydrochloride (If unable to tolerate penicillin or ceftriaxone)	30 mg/kg per 24 h IV in 2 equally divided doses
	Duration: 2 weeks	
	Aqueous crystalline penicillin G sodium	12–18 million U/24 h IV either continuously or in 6 equally divided doses
		OR
	Ceftriaxone sodium	2 g/24 h IV or IM in 1 dose
		PLUS
	Gentamicin sulfate	3 mg/kg per 24 h IV or IM in 1 dose
Relatively penicillin resistant	**Duration: 4 weeks**	
	Aqueous crystalline penicillin G sodium	24 million U/24 h IV either continuously or in 4–6 equally divided doses
		OR
	Vancomycin hydrochloride (If not able to tolerate penicillin or ceftriaxone)	30 mg/kg per 24 h IV in 2 equally divided doses
	Duration: 2 weeks	
	Gentamicin sulfate	3 mg/kg per 24 h IV or IM in 1 dose
Staphylococci		
Oxacillin susceptible	**Duration: 6 weeks**	
	Nafcillin or oxacillin	12 g/24 h IV in 4–6 equally divided doses
		OR
	Cefazolin (if penicillin allergic)	6 g/24 h IV in 3 equally divided doses
Oxacillin resistant	**Duration: 6 weeks**	
	Vancomycin	30 mg/kg per 24 h IV in 2 equally divided doses (keep trough between 10 and 15 mcg/mL)
		OR
	Daptomycin	≥8 mg/kg/dose (dose adjustment per infectious disease consultant)

(continued)

TABLE 52-1 Medications (*Continued*)

Native Valve Endocarditis[1]		
Organisms	**Drug**	**Dose**
Enterococcus		
Penicillin susceptible		**Duration: 4–6 weeks**
	Ampicillin sodium	2 g IV every 4 h
		OR
	Aqueous penicillin G sodium	18–30 million U/24 h IV either continuously or in 6 equally divided doses
		PLUS
	Gentamicin sulfate	3 mg/kg ideal body weight in 2–3 equally divided doses
		Duration: 6 weeks
	Double β-lactam ampicillin	2 g IV every 4 h
		PLUS
	Ceftriaxone	2 g IV every 12 h
Aminoglycoside resistant		**Duration: 6 weeks**
	Double β-lactam ampicillin	2 g IV every 4 h
		PLUS
	Ceftriaxone	2 g IV every 12 h
Penicillin resistant in patients not able to tolerate β-lactams		**Duration: 6 weeks**
	Vancomycin	30 mg/kg per 24 h IV in 2 equally divided doses
		PLUS
	Gentamicin	3 mg/kg per 24 h IV or IM in 3 equally divided doses
Resistant to penicillin, aminoglycoside, and vancomycin		**Duration: >6 weeks**
	Linezolid	600 mg IV or orally every 12 h
		OR
	Daptomycin	10–12 mg/kg per dose
HACEK Organisms (*Haemophilus* species, *Aggregatibacter* species, *Cardiobacterium hominis*, *Eikenella corrodens*, and *Kingella* species)		
		Duration: 4 weeks
	Ceftriaxone sodium	2 g/24 h IV or IM in 1 dose
		OR
	Ampicillin sodium	2 g IV every 4 h
		OR
	Ciprofloxacin	1000 mg/24 h orally or 800 mg/24 h IV in 2 equally divided doses

TABLE 52-1 Medications (*Continued*)

Prosthetic Valve/Material Endocarditis[1]		
	Drug	Dose
S. viridans and S. gallolyticus (bovis)		
Penicillin susceptible	**Duration 6 weeks**	
	Aqueous crystalline penicillin G sodium	24 million U/24 h IV either continuously or in 4–6 equally divided doses
		OR
	Ceftriaxone sodium	2 g/24 h IV or IM in 1 dose
		Plus or minus 2 weeks duration of:
	Gentamicin sulfate	3 mg/kg per 24 h IV or IM in 1 dose
		OR
	Vancomycin hydrochloride (if not able to tolerate penicillin or ceftriaxone)	30 mg/kg per 24 h IV in 2 equally divided doses
Relatively or fully penicillin resistant	**Duration: 6 weeks**	
	Aqueous crystalline penicillin G sodium	24 million U/24 h IV either continuously or in 4–6 equally divided doses
		OR
	Ceftriaxone sodium	2 g/24 h IV or IM in 1 dose
		PLUS
	Gentamicin sulfate	3 mg/kg per 24 h IV or IM in 1 dose
		OR
	Vancomycin hydrochloride (if not able to tolerate penicillin or ceftriaxone)	30 mg/kg per 24 h IV in 2 equally divided doses
Staphylococci		
Oxacillin susceptible	**Duration: ≥6 weeks**	
	Nafcillin or oxacillin	12 g/24 h IV in 6 equally divided doses
		PLUS
	Rifampin	900 mg per 24 h IV or orally in 3 equally divided doses
		PLUS
	Gentamicin (for 2 weeks)	3 mg/kg per 24 h IV or IM in 2 or 3 equally divided doses
Oxacillin resistant	**Duration: ≥6 weeks**	
	Vancomycin	30 mg/kg 24 h in 2 equally divided doses (keep trough between 10 and 15 mcg/mL)
		PLUS
	Rifampin	900 mg/24 h IV/PO in 3 equally divided doses
		PLUS
	Gentamicin (for 2 weeks)	3 mg/kg per 24 h IV/IM in 2 or 3 equally divided doses

(*continued*)

TABLE 52-1 Medications (*Continued*)

Prosthetic Valve/Material Endocarditis[1]		
	Drug	**Dose**
Enterococcus		
Penicillin susceptible	**Duration: 4–6 weeks**	
	Ampicillin sodium	2 g IV every 4 h
		OR
	Aqueous penicillin G sodium	18–30 million U/24 h IV either continuously or in 6 equally divided doses
		PLUS
	Gentamicin sulfate	3 mg/kg ideal body weight in 2–3 equally divided doses
	Duration: 6 weeks	
	Ampicillin	2 g IV every 4 h
		PLUS
	Ceftriaxone	2 g IV every 12 h
Penicillin susceptible, gentamicin resistant	**Duration: 6 weeks**	
	Ampicillin	2 g IV every 4 h
		PLUS
	Ceftriaxone	2 g IV every 12 h
Penicillin resistant in patients not able to tolerate β-lactams	**Duration: 6 weeks**	
	Vancomycin	30 mg/kg per 24 h IV in 2 equally divided doses
		PLUS
	Gentamicin	3 mg/kg per 24 h IV or IM in 3 equally divided doses
Penicillin resistant, aminoglycosides and vancomycin	**Duration: >6 weeks**	
	Linezolid	600 mg IV or orally every 12 h
		OR
	Daptomycin	10–12 mg/kg per dose
HACEK Organisms (*Haemophilus* species, *Aggregatibacter* species, *Cardiobacterium hominis*, *Eikenella corrodens*, and *Kingella* species)		
	Duration: 4 weeks	
	Ceftriaxone sodium	2 g/24 h IV or IM in 1 dose
		OR
	Ampicillin sodium	2 g IV every 4 h
		OR
	Ciprofloxacin	1000 mg/24 h orally or 800 mg/24 h IV in 2 equally divided doses

PREVENTION

- Prophylactic antibiotics are ***recommended*** for high-risk patients before certain procedures[11]: SOR B
  - Patients with prosthetic cardiac valves
  - Patients with previous bacterial endocarditis
  - Cardiac transplant recipients with cardiac valvuloplasty
  - Patients with these congenital heart defects: unrepaired cyanotic congenital defects, heart defects repaired with prosthetic material within the last 6 months, congenital heart defects with a residual defect at or adjacent to the site of a prosthetic device
- Prophylactic antibiotics are only for patients undergoing one of the following:
  - Any dental procedure that involves manipulation of gingival tissue or the periapical region of teeth or perforation of the oral mucosa SOR C
  - Respiratory procedures involving incision or biopsy of the respiratory mucosa such as a tonsillectomy or adenoidectomy SOR C
  - Procedures on infected skin or musculoskeletal tissue
- Prophylactic antibiotics are ***not recommended*** for patients with mitral valve prolapse.
- Endocarditis prophylaxis is ***not recommended*** for patients undergoing gastrointestinal or genitourinary procedures. SOR B
- Antibiotic regimens:
  - Prescribe a one-dose regimen taken 30 minutes to 1 hour before the procedure[11]:
  - Amoxicillin 2.0 g orally for adults, 50 mg/kg for children
  - If unable to take oral medications:
    - Adults—Ampicillin 2.0 g IM or IV *or* cefazolin/ceftriaxone 1 g IM or IV
    - Children—Ampicillin 50 mg/kg 30 minutes before the procedure; *or* cefazolin or ceftriaxone 50 mg/kg IM or IV
  - Penicillin allergic:
    - Adults—Clindamycin 600 mg PO, IM, or IV; *or* azithromycin or clarithromycin 500 mg orally
    - Children—Clindamycin 20 mg/kg orally, IM, or IV; *or* azithromycin/clarithromycin 15 mg/kg orally
  - If allergy to penicillin is *not* anaphylaxis, angioedema, or urticaria, may also use cephalexin 2.0 g PO for adults, 50 mg/kg PO for children; *or* cefazolin or ceftriaxone 1 g IM or IV for adults, 50 mg/kg for children.

PROGNOSIS

Bacterial endocarditis requires early detection and aggressive antibiotic therapy to decrease mortality.

- Thirty-day mortality is 16% to 25%.[5]
- Ninety-day mortality is 14.5%.[5]
- Greater than 6-month mortality is 20% to 37%.[5]
- Myocardial infarction (MI) occurs in about 5.5%; stroke and central nervous system (CNS) infection occur in about 13.3%.

FOLLOW-UP

- Most patients with bacterial endocarditis will require 4 to 6 weeks of IV antibiotics.
- Depending on the antibiotics, some patients will need to have medication levels monitored.
- Repeat blood cultures to ensure response to therapy.
- An echocardiogram at the end of treatment provides baseline imaging, as patients with endocarditis are at risk for recurrence.[1] SOR C
- Patients with history of IV drug abuse should be established in a rehab program.[1] SOR C
- Patients should follow up with a dental evaluation.[1] SOR C
- Patients should be educated on signs and symptoms of recurrence and complications that can occur from endocarditis.[1] SOR C

PATIENT EDUCATION

- Bacterial endocarditis is a serious disease with a significant mortality rate.
- Finish all antibiotics and keep follow-up appointments to ensure adequate treatment.
- Mortality remains elevated even 6 months after an episode.
- Recurrence is common, especially if risk factors remain (i.e., immunosuppression or IV drug use).

PATIENT RESOURCES

- The American Heart Association has information about who is at risk for bacterial endocarditis and a printable wallet card for at-risk patients, available in English or Spanish—**http://www.heart.org/HEARTORG/Conditions/CongenitalHeartDefects/TheImpactofCongenitalHeartDefects/Infective-Endocarditis_UCM_307108_Article.jsp.**

PROVIDER RESOURCES

- The 2007 American Heart Association guidelines on endocarditis prophylaxis—**http://circ.ahajournals.org/content/116/15/1736.full.pdf.**
- 2015 Guidelines on Infective Endocarditis: Diagnosis, Antimicrobial Therapy, and Management of Complications—**http://circ.ahajournals.org/content/early/2015/09/15/CIR.0000000000000296.**
- MdCalc has an interactive website with the modified Duke criteria for infective endocarditis—**https://www.mdcalc.com/duke-criteria-infective-endocarditis.**

REFERENCES

1. Baddour LM, Wilson WR, Bayer AS, et al. Infective endocarditis in adults: diagnosis, antimicrobial therapy, and management of complications. *Circulation.* 2015;132:1435-1486.

2. Wilson LE, Thomas DL, Astemborski J, et al. Prospective study of infective endocarditis among injection drug users. *J Infect Dis.* 2002;185(12):1761-1766.
3. Bor DH, Woolhandler S, Nardin R, et al. Infective endocarditis in the U.S., 1998–2009: a nationwide study. *PLoS One.* 2013;8(3): e60033.
4. de Sa DD, Tleyjeh IM, Anavekar NS, et al. Epidemiological trends of infective endocarditis: a population-based study in Olmsted County, Minnesota. *Mayo Clin Proc.* 2010;85(5): 422-426.
5. Nomura A, Omata F, Furukawa K. Risk factors of mid-term mortality of patients with infective endocarditis. *Eur J Clin Microbiol Infect Dis.* 2010;29(11):1355-1360.
6. Prendergast BD. The changing face of infective endocarditis. *Heart.* 2006;92(7):879-885.
7. Habib G. Management of infective endocarditis. *Heart.* 2006; 92(1):124-130.
8. Falagas ME, Matthaiou DK, Bliziotis IA. The role of aminoglycosides in combination with a beta-lactam for the treatment of bacterial endocarditis: a meta-analysis of comparative trials. *J Antimicrob Chemother.* 2006;57(4):639-647
9. Fayad G, Leroy G, Devos P, et al. Characteristics and prognosis of patients requiring valve surgery during active infective endocarditis. *J Heart Valve Dis.* 2011;20(2):223-228.
10. Mokhles MM, Ciampichetti I, Head SJ, et al. Survival of surgically treated infective endocarditis: a comparison with the general Dutch population. *Ann Thorac Surg.* 2011;91(5):1407-1412.
11. Wilson W, Taubert KA, Gewitz M, et al. Prevention of infective endocarditis: a guideline from the American Heart Association. *Circulation.* 2007;116:1736-1754.

SECTION B PERIPHERAL

53 CLUBBING

Heidi S. Chumley, MD, MBA
John E. Delzell, Jr, MD, MSPH

PATIENT STORY

A 31-year-old man with congenital heart disease has had these clubbed fingers since his childhood (**Figures 53-1** and **53-2**). A close view of the fingers shows a widened club-like distal phalanx. He has learned to live with the limitations from his congenital heart disease and his fingers do not bother him at all.

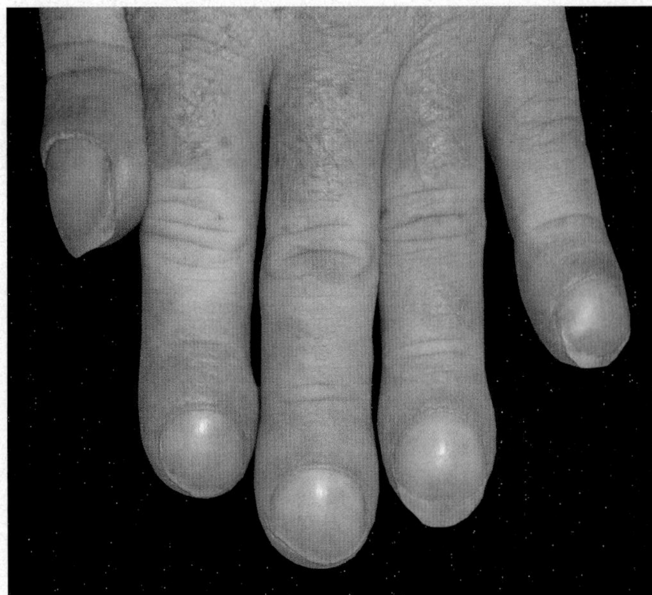

FIGURE 53-1 Clubbing of all the fingers in a 31-year-old man with congenital heart disease. Note the thickening around the proximal nail folds. (*Reproduced with permission from Richard P. Usatine, MD.*)

INTRODUCTION

Clubbing is a physical examination finding first described by Hippocrates in 400 BC. Clubbing can be primary (pachydermoperiostosis or hypertrophic osteoarthropathy) or secondary (pulmonary, cardiac, or GI disease or HIV). Diagnosis is clinical, based on nail fold angles and phalangeal depth ratios. The treatment is to correct the underlying cause, after which clubbing may resolve.

SYNONYMS

Hippocratic nails or fingers, drumstick fingers.

EPIDEMIOLOGY

Prevalence in the general population is unknown:

- One percent of adult patients admitted to a general medicine or service.[1]
- Thirty-eight percent and 15% of patients with Crohn disease and ulcerative colitis, respectively.[2]
- Thirty-three percent and 11% of patients with lung cancer and chronic obstructive pulmonary disease (COPD), respectively.[3]
- Forty percent of patients admitted to a general medicine service with clubbing had a serious medical condition.[1]

ETIOLOGY AND PATHOPHYSIOLOGY

- The etiology of clubbing is poorly understood.
- Increased connective tissue growth and angiogenesis in the nail bed result in the remodeling of the finger into a club shape.

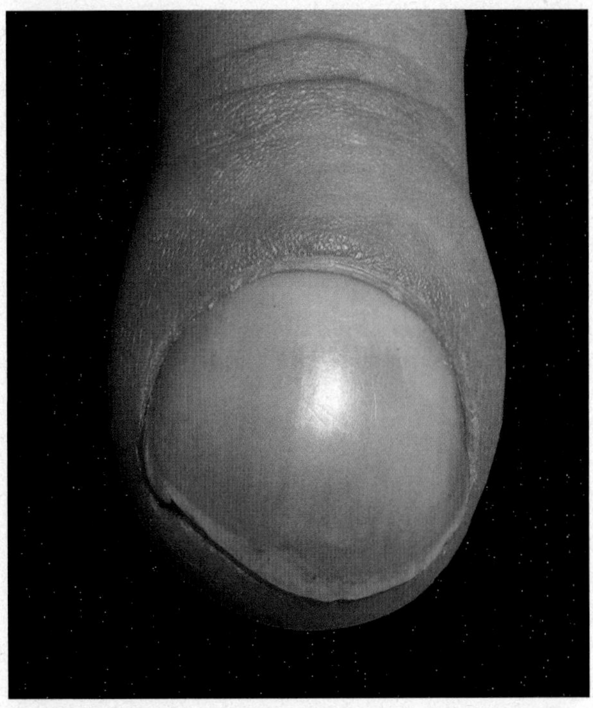

FIGURE 53-2 Close-up view of a clubbed finger. (*Reproduced with permission from Richard P. Usatine, MD.*)

- Cytokine release, specifically megakaryocyte release of platelet-activated growth factor and aggregated platelet release of vascular endothelial growth factor, plays a key role.[4]

RISK FACTORS

- Family history.
- History of a disease associated with clubbing such as bronchogenic carcinoma, lymphoma, tuberculosis, cyanotic heart disease, primary biliary cirrhosis, cirrhosis, inflammatory bowel disease or HIV.[5]

DIAGNOSIS

CLINICAL FEATURES

- History of present illness: Gradual onset of painless enlargement at the ends of the fingers and toes.
  - Family history suggests primary hypertrophic osteoarthropathy/familial clubbing.
  - Social history to identify exposure to asbestos, coal mine dust, and pigeons; tobacco use as risk factor for lung cancer; HIV and tuberculosis risk factors.
- Review of systems: Constitutional, pulmonary, cardiac, GI, and musculoskeletal symptoms for clues to an underlying disease.[5]

PHYSICAL EXAMINATION

- Abnormal nail fold angles[6] (**Figure 53-3**).
  - Profile angle (*ABC*) ≥180 degrees.
  - Hyponychial (*ABD*) ≥192 degrees.
  - Phalangeal depth ratio (*BE:GF*) ≥1[6] (**Figure 53-3**).
- Schamroth sign, obliteration of the diamond shape normally created when dorsal surfaces of 2 corresponding fingers are opposed (**Figure 53-4**). LR+ (likelihood ratio) 7.60 to 8.40 and LR– 0.14 to 0.25.[7]

TYPICAL DISTRIBUTION

- Bilateral; involves all fingers and often toes.
- Rarely unilateral or involving only one or some digits (consider neurologic or traumatic insult to extremity).

LABORATORY TESTING

Laboratory testing is useful to evaluate for secondary causes. Consider:

- HIV testing if risk factors present.
- Complete blood count (CBC) and blood cultures if systemic symptoms (fever, night sweats, weight loss) are present.
- Thyroid-stimulating hormone (TSH)/thyroxine (T_4) if exophthalmos or pretibial myxedema is present.
- Liver function tests (LFTs), hepatitis serologies for right upper quadrant (RUQ) tenderness or jaundice.

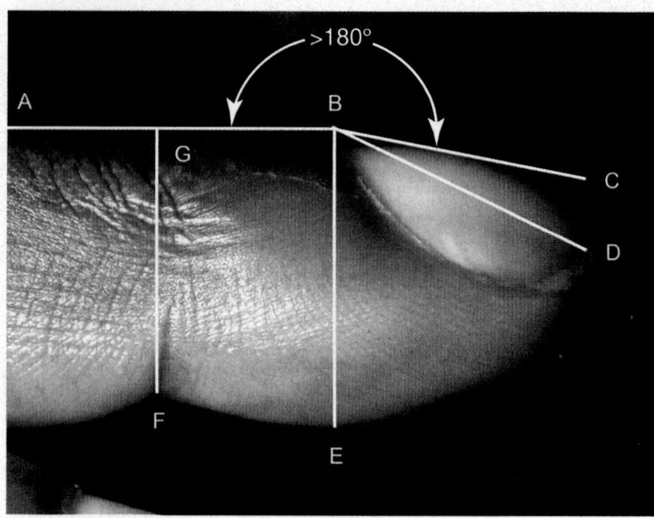

FIGURE 53-3 Clubbing of fingers in a 55-year-old man with chronic obstructive pulmonary disease. Abnormal profile angle (*ABC*) and hyponychial angle (*ABD*); distal phalangeal depth (*BE*) greater than interphalangeal depth (*GF*). (*Reproduced with permission from Richard P. Usatine, MD.*)

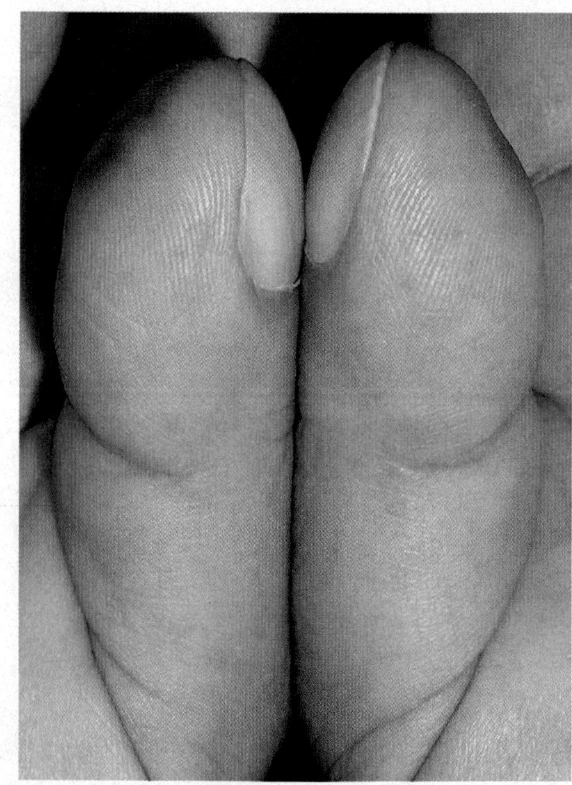

FIGURE 53-4 Schamroth sign. Loss of the normal diamond shape formed when right and left thumbs are opposed in a person with clubbing of the fingers. (*Reproduced with permission from Richard P. Usatine, MD.*)

IMAGING

- Screening chest radiograph if an underlying cause is not identified.
- Plain radiograph of the hand can distinguish clubbed from non-clubbed by measuring nail bed greater than or equal to 3 mm.[8]
- Ultrasound measurement of the soft tissue depth under the nail and the ratio of distal phalangeal depth to interphalangeal depth may also be useful to identify clubbing.[9]

DIFFERENTIAL DIAGNOSIS

PRIMARY CLUBBING

- Hypertrophic osteoarthropathy (HOA)—Clubbing, periostosis, and arthritis or arthralgias.
  - Primary HOA, also known as pachydermoperiostosis, is an autosomal dominant disorder.
  - Secondary HOA is often associated with pulmonary neoplasms.
- Familial clubbing, now thought to be an incomplete form of primary HOA.

SECONDARY CLUBBING

Secondary clubbing can be caused by many conditions, including[5]:

- Pulmonary—Idiopathic pulmonary fibrosis, malignancy, asbestosis, COPD, and cystic fibrosis.
- Cardiac—Congenital heart disease, endocarditis, atrioventricular malformations, or fistulas.
- GI—Inflammatory bowel disease, cirrhosis, and celiac disease.
- HIV infection—Clubbing was found in 36% of patients with HIV in one study.[10]

MANAGEMENT

- Clubbing improves with the management of the underlying disease.
- Evaluate patients without an obvious associated disease with a chest radiograph to screen for lung cancer.[5] SOR Ⓒ
- Evaluate patients with COPD and a phalangeal depth ratio greater than 1 for lung cancer.[3] (LR 3.9) SOR Ⓑ

PROGNOSIS

Prognosis depends on the underlying process. Clubbing usually completely reverses after successful treatment of the underlying process.

FOLLOW-UP

Follow-up is dependent on the underlying disease process.

PATIENT EDUCATION

Clubbing may be secondary to many different types of disease, some very serious.

PATIENT RESOURCES

- MedlinePlus—**http://www.nlm.nih.gov/medlineplus/ency/article/003282.htm.**

PROVIDER RESOURCES

- Chan[5] provides an algorithm useful in identifying the underlying cause of clubbing. **https://www.racgp.org.au/afp/2015/march/evaluation-of-digital-clubbing/**.

REFERENCES

1. Vandemergel X, Renneboog B. Prevalence, aetiologies and significance of clubbing in a department of general internal medicine. *Eur J Intern Med.* 2008;19:325-329.
2. Kitis G, Thompson H, Allan RN. Finger clubbing in inflammatory bowel disease: its prevalence and pathogenesis. *Br Med J.* 1979; 2(6194):825-828.
3. Baughman RP, Gunther KL, Buchsbaum JA, Lower EE. Prevalence of digital clubbing in bronchogenic carcinoma by a new digital index. *Clin Exp Rheumatol.* 1998;16(1):21-26.
4. Dubrey S, Pal S, Singh S, Karagiannis G. Digital clubbing: forms, associations and pathophysiology. *Br J Hosp Med (Lond).* 2016;77(7):403-408.
5. Chan CW. Evaluation of digital clubbing. *Aust Fam Phys.* 2015;44(3):113-116.
6. Myers KA, Farquhar DR. The rational clinical examination. Does this patient have clubbing [comment]? *JAMA.* 2001;286(3): 341-347.
7. Pallares-Sanmartin A, Leiro-Fernandez V, Cebreiro TL, et al. Validity and reliability of the Schamroth sign for the diagnosis of clubbing. *JAMA.* 2010;304(2):159-161.
8. Moreira AL, Porto NS, Moreira JS, et al. Clubbed fingers: radiological evaluation of the nail bed thickness. *Clin Anat.* 2008;21(4):314-318.
9. Roy HS, Wang Z, Ran H, et al. Diagnosis of digital clubbing by high-frequency ultrasound imaging. *Int J Dermatol.* 2013;52(1): 1-5.
10. Dever LL, Matta JS. Digital clubbing in HIV-infected patients: an observational study. *AIDS Patient Care STDS.* 2009;23(1):19-22.

54 VENOUS INSUFFICIENCY

Maureen K. Sheehan, MD, MHA

PATIENT STORY

A 45-year-old woman presents to her physician's office with complaints of heaviness and fatigue in her legs (**Figure 54-1**). She does not experience the symptoms in the morning, but they become more noticeable as the day progresses and with prolonged standing. When she stands for many hours, she develops swelling in both of her legs. The symptoms are concentrated over her medial calf, where she has prominent tortuous veins. She first noted the veins approximately 20 years ago when she was pregnant. Initially, they did not cause her any discomfort but have progressively enlarged now and over the past 10 years have become increasingly painful. She recalls that her mother had similar veins in her legs.

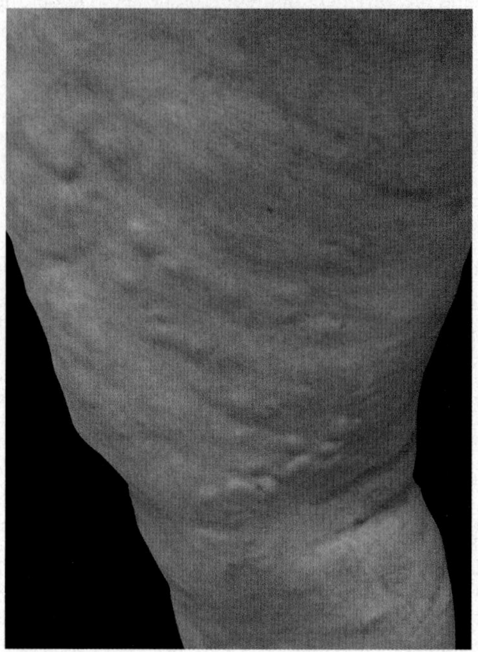

FIGURE 54-1 Uncomplicated varicose veins of thigh. (*Reproduced with permission from Maureen K. Sheehan, MD.*)

INTRODUCTION

Venous insufficiency, or improperly functioning valves in the venous system, can lead to a variety of symptoms, including, but not limited to, heaviness and/or swelling in the legs with prolonged standing, leg fatigue or aching, bleeding from leg varices, skin changes, and ulcerations. The prevalence is higher in industrialized nations and ranges from 15% to 30% of the U.S. population.

SYNONYMS

Varicose veins, venous stasis.

EPIDEMIOLOGY

- Varies by definition and region, but generally venous insufficiency affects 27% of the population.[1]
- Prevalence estimates vary by some reports, indicating a prevalence of 10.4% to 23% in men and 29.5% to 39% in women.[2,3]
- More frequent in women as compared to men.
- Symptomatic in more than two-thirds of those affected.
- Varicose veins are notable only in half of patients with venous insufficiency.[4]

ETIOLOGY AND PATHOPHYSIOLOGY

- Most frequently it is a result of valvular dysfunction.
- Valvular dysfunction may be primary or secondary (result of trauma, deep venous thrombosis [DVT], or May-Thurner syndrome).
- It may affect deep system (i.e., femoral veins), superficial system (i.e., saphenous vein), or both.
- The superficial system is involved in 88% of cases either alone or in conjunction with the deep system.
- Dysfunction leads to loss of compartmentalization of veins, leading to distention and increased pressure (**Figures 54-1** and **54-2**).

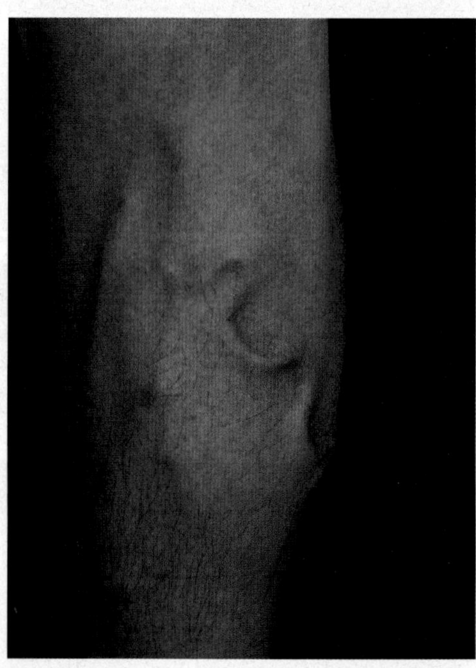

FIGURE 54-2 Varicose veins of posterior calf *without* hemosiderin deposition, lipodermatosclerosis, or ulceration. (*Reproduced with permission from Maureen K. Sheehan, MD.*)

- Increased pressure in veins is transmitted to microvasculature leading to basement membrane thickening, increased capillary elongation, and visual skin changes (**Figures 54-3** and **54-4**).

RISK FACTORS

- Family history.
- DVT.
- Female gender.
- Estrogen increase (hormone replacement, pregnancy, oral contraceptive pills).
- Age.
- Obesity.
- Prolonged standing.

DIAGNOSIS

SYMPTOMS

- Heaviness, fatigue, and edema; not present immediately in the morning; gets worse with prolonged standing or walking; relieved with elevation.

TYPICAL DISTRIBUTION

- Varicose veins can be present anywhere on the leg depending on affected segments or tributaries; ulcers from venous disease tend to be near the medial malleoli (**Figure 54-5**).

TESTS

- Duplex scanning to assess valve closure; normal valve closure is <0.5 to 1.0 seconds depending on vein.

DIFFERENTIAL DIAGNOSIS

- Arterial ulcers—Tend to be at toes, shin, and pressure points (heels or sides of feet).
- Diabetic ulcers—Occur at ambulatory pressure points, mostly at first metatarsal head.
- Malignancy (basal cell or squamous cell carcinoma).
- Chronic infectious diseases (osteomyelitis, leprosy).
- Vasculitides—Irregular border, black necrosis, erythema, or bluish or purplish discoloration of adjacent tissue.

MANAGEMENT

- Graduated compression hose for superficial or deep system insufficiency: SOR C
  - 15 to 20 mm Hg—Minor reflux and minimal symptoms.
  - 20 to 30 mm Hg—Moderate to severe reflux and symptoms; moderate edema; postsurgical.
  - 30 to 40 mm Hg—Severe reflux and symptoms; severe edema.

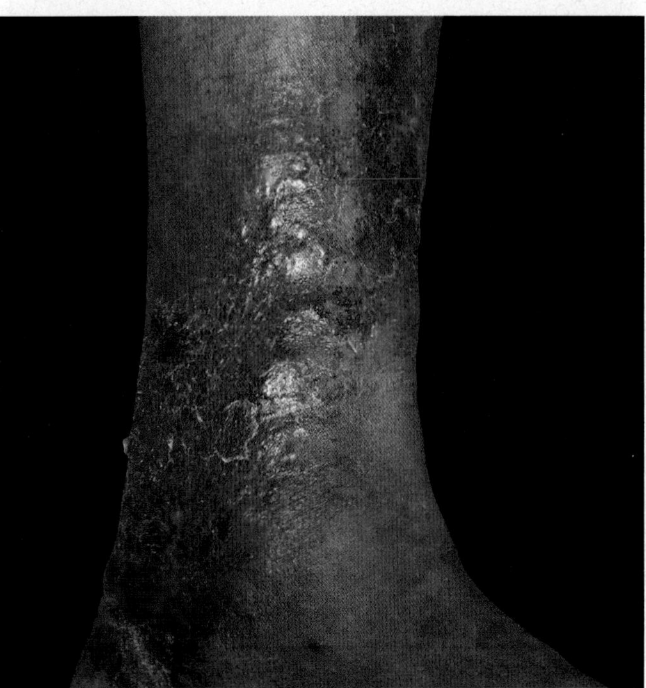

FIGURE 54-3 Lipodermatosclerosis with hemosiderin deposition. *(Reproduced with permission from Maureen K. Sheehan, MD.)*

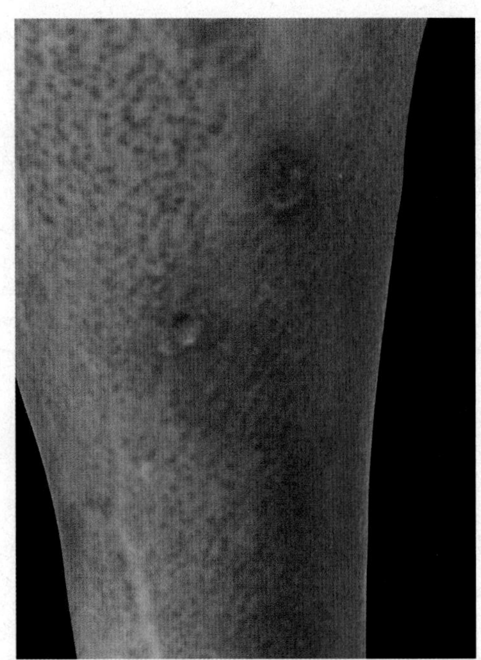

FIGURE 54-4 Healed ulcers with hemosiderin deposition. *(Reproduced with permission from Maureen K. Sheehan, MD.)*

- Compression bandage for open ulcer.[5] SOR Ⓑ
- Compression hose treat symptoms, not underlying pathophysiology. Effective only when being worn.
- If superficial system is involved, surgical intervention is available through endovenous ablation, nonthermal ablation (i.e. glue, foam), or with stripping and ligation.[6]
- If only deep system involvement, then compression hose is the mainstay of therapy. SOR Ⓒ
- When superficial and deep systems are affected, treatment of superficial system leads to improvement of deep system reflux in one-third of patients.
- A study randomizing patients to stripping and ligation versus compression therapy demonstrated an improved quality of life in the surgical arm.[7] SOR Ⓐ
- Endovenous therapy uses radiofrequency or laser energy to ablate vein. Because the vein is usually accessed with a needle under ultrasound guidance, an incision is avoided in most instances. Tumescence is needed for analgesia and effectiveness.
- Foamed sclerotherapy has been shown to be less effective than endovenous ablation in some studies.[8]
- Mechanochemical ablation has been shown to be less painful than radiofrequency ablation, but long-term effectiveness not known.[9]
- Cyanoacrylate adhesive has been shown to be as safe and effective as other thermal and nonthermal ablative methods at 3-year follow-up.[10]
- Decreased postoperative pain and analgesic use in patients undergoing endovenous ablation compared to those undergoing stripping and ligation.[11] SOR Ⓐ
- Adjunctive phlebectomies or sclerotherapy for branch varicosities may be necessary with either operative approach.

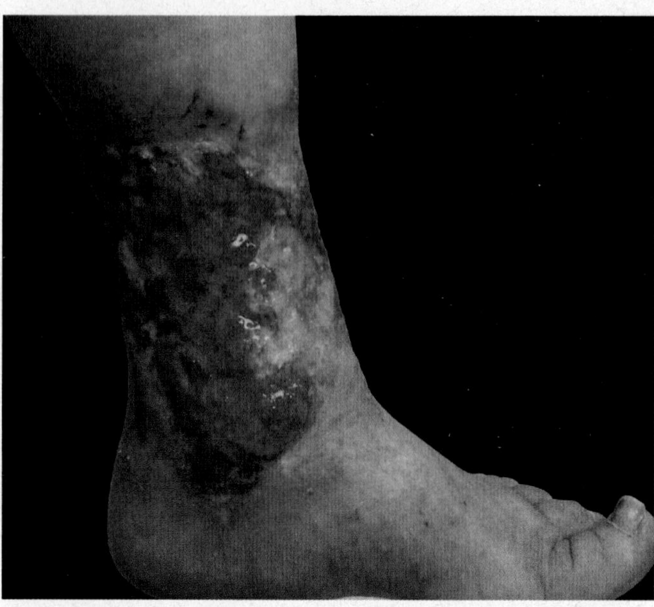

FIGURE 54-5 Venous stasis ulcer in the typical location around the medial malleolus. (*Reproduced with permission from Maureen K. Sheehan, MD.*)

PREVENTION

Patients at risk for developing venous insufficiency (genetics, occupations with prolonged standing, etc.) may benefit from compression hose use.

PROGNOSIS

Majority of patients with venous insufficiency live a full and complete life without significant sequelae. Those with only superficial involvement tend to have greater relief with treatment than those with superficial and deep or only deep system involvement. Most patients obtain relief from interventions such as compression hose or surgery.

FOLLOW-UP

- It depends on the treatment and severity of disease.
- Unna boots for ulceration need to be changed at least weekly.
- Compression hose needs to be replaced every 6 months.
- Following surgical intervention, follow-up depends on intervention. Stripping and ligation require wound checks, whereas endovenous ablations require ultrasound monitoring.

PATIENT EDUCATION

Venous insufficiency is not merely a cosmetic concern. Long-standing disease can give rise to skin changes (see **Figures 54-3** and **54-4**) and ulcers (see **Figure 54-5**). Compliance with compression hose is necessary. Compression hose only treats symptoms, not the underlying disease process. Even after surgical intervention, new varicose veins may appear, as the process is chronic.

PATIENT RESOURCES

- MedlinePlus. *Venous Insufficiency*—**http://www.nlm.nih.gov/medlineplus/ency/article/000203.htm.**
- MedlinePlus. *Varicose Veins*—**https://medlineplus.gov/varicoseveins.html.**
- MedlinePlus. *Stasis Dermatitis and Ulcers*—**https://medlineplus.gov/ency/article/000834.htm.**

PROVIDER RESOURCES

- Medscape. *Venous Insufficiency*—**https://emedicine.medscape.com/article/1085412-overview.**
- American College of Phlebology—**http://www.phlebology.org.**

REFERENCES

1. White JV, Ryjewski C. Chronic venous insufficiency. *Perspect Vasc Surg Endovasc Ther.* 2005;17:319-327.
2. Beebe-Dimmer JL, Pfeifer JR, Engle JS, Schottenfeld D. The epidemiology of chronic venous insufficiency and varicose veins. *Ann Epidemiol.* 2005;15:175-184.
3. Mundy L, Merlin TL, Fitridge RA, Hiller JE. Systematic review of endovenous laser treatment for varicose veins. *Br J Surg.* 2005;92:1189-1194.
4. Reichenberg J, Davis M. Venous ulcers. *Semin Cutan Med Surg.* 2005;24:216-226.
5. Cullum N, Nelson EA, Fletcher AW, Sheldon TA. Compression for venous leg ulcers. *Cochrane Database Syst Rev.* 2000;(3):CD000265.
6. Puggioni A, Lurie F, Kistner RL, et al. How often is deep venous reflux eliminated after saphenous vein ablation? *J Vasc Surg.* 2003;38:517-541.
7. Michaels JA, Brazier JE, Campbell WB, et al. Randomized clinical trial comparing surgery with conservative treatment for uncomplicated varicose veins. *Br J Surg.* 2006;93:175-181.
8. Bootun R, Lane TR, Dharamarajah B, et al. Intra-procedural pain score in a randomized controlled trial comparing mechanochemical ablation to radiofrequency ablation: the Multicentre Venfit versus Clarivein for varicose veins trial. *Phlebology.* 2016;31(1):61-65.
9. van der Velden SK, Biemans AA, De Maeseneer MG, et al. Five-year results of a randomized clinical trial of conventional surgery, endovenous laser ablation and ultrasound-guided foam sclerotherapy in patients with great saphenous varicose veins. *Br J Surg.* 2015;102(10):1184-1194.
10. Almeida JI, Javier JJ, Mackay EG, et al. Thirty-six-month follow-up of first-in-human use of cyanoacrylate adhesive for treatment of saphenous vein incompetence. *J Vasc Surg Venous Lymphat Disord.* 2017;5(5):658-666.
11. Rautio T, Ohinmaa A, Perala J, et al. Endovenous obliteration versus conventional stripping operation in the treatment of primary varicose veins: a randomized controlled trial with the comparison of the costs. *J Vasc Surg.* 2002;35:958-965.

PART VIII

THE LUNGS

Strength of Recommendation (SOR)	Definition
A	Recommendation based on consistent and good-quality patient-oriented evidence.*
B	Recommendation based on inconsistent or limited-quality patient-oriented evidence.*
C	Recommendation based on consensus, usual practice, opinion, disease-oriented evidence, or case series for studies of diagnosis, treatment, prevention, or screening.*

*See Appendix A on pages 1603–1606 for further information.

55 PNEUMONIA

Mindy A. Smith, MD, MS

PATIENT STORY

Max is a 65-year-old man who presents with a "terrible cough" and fever of several days' duration. He has just returned from a business trip and is feeling quite run down. His cough is productive, with rusty-colored sputum. He is otherwise healthy and is a nonsmoker. His chest x-ray is similar to the one shown in **Figure 55-1**. He is diagnosed with probable bacterial pneumonia and is placed on antibiotics. You note that he has never had vaccinations against influenza or pneumococcus, and you offer these to him at a follow-up visit when he is well.

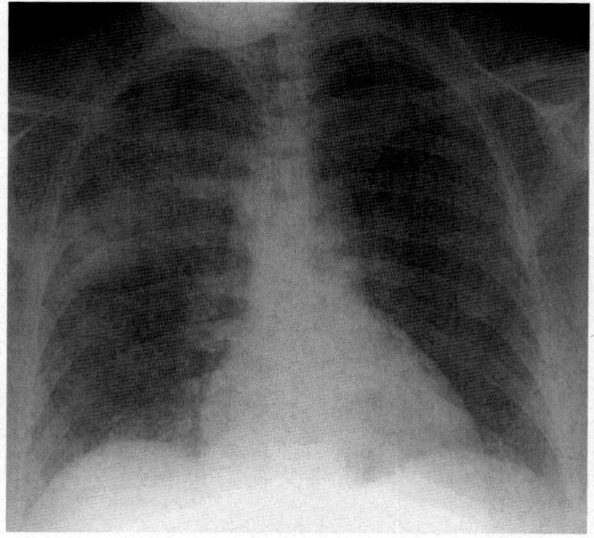

FIGURE 55-1 Chest x-ray (CXR) showing right upper lobe consolidation. *(Reproduced with permission from Miller WT: Diagnostic Thoracic Imaging. New York, NY: McGraw-Hill Education; 2006.)*

INTRODUCTION

Pneumonia refers to an infection in the lower respiratory tract (distal airways, alveoli, and interstitium of the lung). Community-acquired pneumonia (CAP) has traditionally referred to pneumonia occurring outside of the hospital setting. More recently, a subgroup of CAP has been identified that is associated with healthcare risk factors (e.g., prior hospitalization, dialysis, nursing home residence, immunocompromised state); this form of pneumonia has been classified as healthcare-associated pneumonia (HCAP), although definitions of HCAP vary. While severity and excess mortality are associated with HCAP, as well as a slight increase in multidrug-resistant (MDR) pathogens, most studies do not support either a causal relationship between MDR and excess mortality or demonstrate benefit from broad-spectrum antibiotic coverage.[1] It is likely that excess mortality is a result of underlying patient-related factors (e.g., older age, comorbidities, higher initial severity).[1,2] This chapter primarily addresses CAP.

EPIDEMIOLOGY

- Three to 4 million adults per year in the United States are diagnosed with CAP (8 to 15 per 1000 persons/year).[3,4]
- Annual incidence rate of CAP requiring hospitalization for adults: 24.8 cases (95% confidence interval [CI], 23.5 to 26.1) per 10,000 adults. The incidence rate among adults 65 to 79 years of age was 63.0 cases per 10,000 adults and for those 80 years of age or older was 164.3 cases per 10,000 adults.[5]
- Annual incidence rate of CAP requiring hospitalization for children: 15.7 cases (95% CI, 14.9 to 16.5) per 10,000 children. The highest rate was among children younger than age 2 years (62.2 cases per 10,000 children).[6]
- Of the 10% to 20% of patients with CAP admitted to the hospital,[3,4] 10% to 20% are admitted to the intensive care unit (ICU).[7]
- Increased incidence in men and in blacks versus whites.[3]
- CAP is the most frequent cause of death caused by infectious disease in the United States and the eighth leading cause of death

overall (2014).[7,8] Influenza and pneumonia were responsible for 55,227 deaths or 2.1% of the total deaths in 2014.[8]

- Economic burden associated with CAP is estimated at more than $12 billion annually in the United States.[7]

ETIOLOGY AND PATHOPHYSIOLOGY

- In a study of children hospitalized with CAP (N = 254), the cause of the disease (identified in 85% of cases) was most often viral (62%, with 30% having evidence of both viral and bacterial pathogens).[9] The most common pathogens were *Streptococcus pneumoniae* (37%), respiratory syncytial virus (RSV, 29%), and rhinovirus (24%). Dual bacterial infections were found in 19 patients; only 1 patient of 125 tested had a positive blood culture. Similar findings were reported in a study of hospitalized children in three U.S. hospitals; the cause of disease was detected in 81% with one or more viruses detected in 1472 (66%), bacteria in 175 (8%), and both bacterial and viral pathogens in 155 (7%).[6] RSV was the most common viral pathogen, followed by rhinovirus, and *Staphylococcus aureus (27% of whom 77% had methicillin-resistant S. aureus) was the most common bacterial pathogen followed by Streptococcus pyogenes (20%), viridans streptococcus (17%), Chlamydia pneumoniae (15%), and Haemophilus influenzae (11%).*
- In a study of adults hospitalized with CAP in five hospitals in Chicago and Nashville, a pathogen was detected in 853 (38%).[5] Viral pathogens were most common (N = 530 [23%]) followed by bacteria in 247 (11%), bacterial and viral pathogens in 59 (3%), and a fungal or mycobacterial pathogen in 17 (1%). The most common viral pathogens were human rhinovirus (9%) and influenza virus (6%), and the most common bacterial pathogen was *S. pneumoniae* (5%).
- Most common route of infection is microaspiration of oropharyngeal secretions colonized by pathogens. In this setting, *S. pneumoniae* and *H. influenzae* are the most common pathogens.
- Pneumonia secondary to gross aspiration occurs postoperatively or in those with central nervous system disorders; anaerobes and Gram-negative bacilli are common pathogens.
- Hematogenous spread, most often from the urinary tract, results in *Escherichia coli* pneumonia, and hematogenous spread from intravenous catheters or in the setting of endocarditis may cause *S. aureus* pneumonia.
- *Mycobacterium tuberculosis* (TB), fungi, *Legionella*, and many respiratory viruses are spread by aerosolization. Reported incidence rates of atypical pathogens vary greatly; for example, *Legionella* species were identified in patients with CAP in 1.3% (defined as positive urine antigen),[10] 1.4% (defined as 4-fold rise in antibody titer or a single titer of ≥400),[11] and 18.9% (defined as 4-fold rise in antibody titer of 128),[12] with coinfection with another pathogen in approximately 10%.
- Etiology is unknown in up to 70% of cases of CAP.

RISK FACTORS[3,4,13]

- Age older than 70 years (relative risk [RR], 1.5 vs. 60- to 69-year-olds).
- Smoking more than 20 cigarettes/day (odds ratio [OR], 2.77; 95% confidence interval [CI], 1.14 to 6.7).
- Alcohol consumption (RR, 9).
- Asthma (RR, 4.2), chronic bronchitis (OR, 2.22; 95% CI, 1.13 to 4.37), and other chronic lung diseases or pulmonary edema.
- Previous respiratory infection (OR, 2.73; 95% CI, 1.75 to 4.26).
- Uremia.
- Immunosuppression (RR, 1.9).
- Malnutrition.
- Acid-suppressing drugs (proton pump inhibitors and histamine-2 receptor antagonist; OR, 1.27; 95% CI, 1.11 to 1.46 and OR, 1.22; 95% CI, 1.09 to 1.36, respectively).[14]

DIAGNOSIS

The history can provide clues to the likely pathogen[3]:

- Alcoholism—Consider *S. pneumoniae, Klebsiella, S. aureus*, and anaerobes.
- Chronic obstructive pulmonary disease—Consider *S. pneumoniae, H. influenzae*, and *Moraxella.*
- Uncontrolled diabetes mellitus—Consider *S. pneumoniae* and *S. aureus.*
- Sickle-cell disease—Consider *S. pneumoniae.*
- HIV with low CD4 count—Consider *S. pneumoniae, Pneumocystis jiroveci, H. influenzae, Cryptococcus*, and TB.

CLINICAL FEATURES

- Constellation of symptoms includes cough, fever, chills, pleuritic chest pain, and sputum production. Patients may also complain of fatigue, myalgia, and headache.[4] Patients with viral or atypical pathogens (e.g., *Mycoplasma, Chlamydia*) often present with fever, nonproductive cough, and constitutional symptoms developing over several days; patients with *Legionella* pathogens may present initially with GI symptoms.[4]
- Signs include increased respiratory rate, dullness to percussion, bronchial breathing, egophony, crackles, wheezes, and pleural-friction rub. Lung findings in atypical pneumonia may be more diffuse.
- In a diagnostic study conducted in primary care centers in 12 European countries, the optimal combination of factors for prediction of pneumonia included absence of runny nose and presence of breathlessness, crackles and diminished breath sounds on auscultation, tachycardia, and fever, with a receiver operating characteristic (ROC) curve area of 0.70 (0.65 to 0.75).[15]

LABORATORY STUDIES

- Sputum Gram stain may be helpful in determining etiology in hospitalized patients. Pretreatment Gram stain and culture of expectorated sputum should be performed only if a good-quality specimen is obtained; indications are the same as for blood cultures listed below.[16] An adequate specimen has more than 25 white blood cells (WBCs) and fewer than 10 epithelial cells per high-powered field. For intubated patients with severe CAP, an endotracheal aspirate sample should be obtained.[16]

- Testing of induced sputum has established merit primarily for detection of TB and *P. jiroveci.* SOR Ⓐ Special stains are needed for detecting TB, *P. jiroveci*, and fungi.
- Blood cultures are not recommended routinely for nontoxic, fully immunized children with CAP managed in the outpatient setting.[17] SOR Ⓑ Blood cultures should be obtained in children who fail to demonstrate clinical improvement and in those who have progressive symptoms or clinical deterioration after initiation of antibiotics.[17] SOR Ⓑ
- Blood cultures are recommended for children requiring hospitalization for presumed bacterial CAP that is moderate to severe, particularly those with complicated pneumonia.[17] SOR Ⓒ
- Routine diagnostic tests to identify an etiologic agent are optional for adult outpatients with CAP.[16] SOR Ⓒ Blood cultures should be considered in ambulatory patients with a temperature higher than 38.5°C (101.3°F) or lower than 36°C (96.8°F) and in those who are homeless or abusing alcohol.[3] SOR Ⓒ
- Blood cultures (two sets prior to administration of antibiotics) are suggested for hospitalized patients who meet clinical indications (i.e., cavitary infiltrates, leukopenia, active alcohol abuse, chronic severe liver disease, asplenia, positive pneumococcal urinary antigen, or pleural effusion) or are admitted to the ICU.[16] SOR Ⓐ Blood cultures are positive in 6% to 20% of hospitalized patients.[3] Investigators in a Canadian study found that blood cultures had limited usefulness in the routine management of patients admitted to the hospital with uncomplicated CAP; only 1.97% (15 of 760 patients) had a change of therapy directed by blood culture results.[18]
- Sensitive and specific tests for the rapid diagnosis of influenza virus and other respiratory viruses should be used in the evaluation of children with CAP.[17] A positive influenza test may decrease both the need for additional diagnostic studies and antibiotic use, while guiding appropriate use of antiviral agents in both outpatient and inpatient settings.[17] SOR Ⓐ Serology (4-fold rise in immunoglobulin [Ig] M titer) may also be useful in diagnosing *Mycoplasma pneumoniae, Chlamydia pneumoniae, Legionella pneumoniae, Legionella pneumophila,* and other viral pneumonia.[16] SOR Ⓒ
- Urinary antigens may be useful in diagnosing Legionnaire's disease (*L. pneumophila*) and *S. pneumoniae* and are recommended in patients with severe CAP.[16] SOR Ⓑ Urinary antigen detection tests are not recommended for the diagnosis of pneumococcal pneumonia in children, as false-positive tests are common.[17]
- Procalcitonin, a peptide precursor of calcitonin used as a biomarker of bacterial infection and sepsis, has been used in the emergency department setting to distinguish between pneumonia (increased level) and an exacerbation of asthma.[19] In one study, use of guidelines including measurement of procalcitonin versus standard guidelines in patients with lower respiratory infection reduced exposure to antibiotics (mean duration: 5.7 vs. 8.7 days).[20] However, in the 12-country study cited earlier, the addition of C-reactive protein to the constellation of signs and symptoms improved diagnostic accuracy, but not addition of procalcitonin.[15]
- Pulse oximetry should be performed in patients with pneumonia and suspected hypoxemia. The presence of hypoxemia should guide decisions regarding site of care and further diagnostic testing. SOR Ⓑ

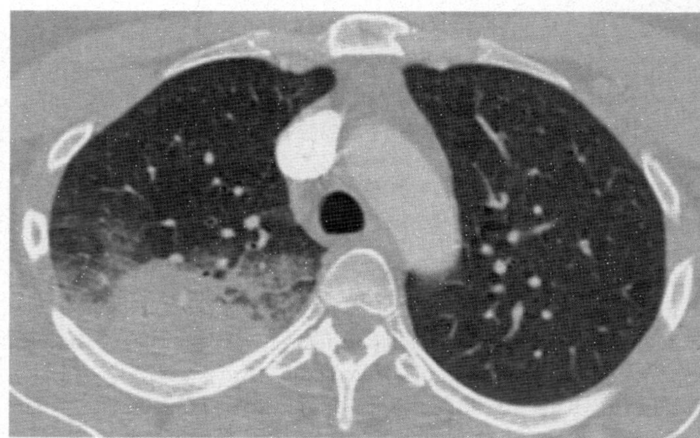

FIGURE 55-2 CT scan of the patient in **Figure 55-1** demonstrating a confluent region of lung consolidation with ground-glass opacification on the margins of the consolidated lung commonly seen in bacterial pneumonia. (*Reproduced with permission from Miller WT: Diagnostic Thoracic Imaging. New York, NY: McGraw-Hill Education; 2006.*)

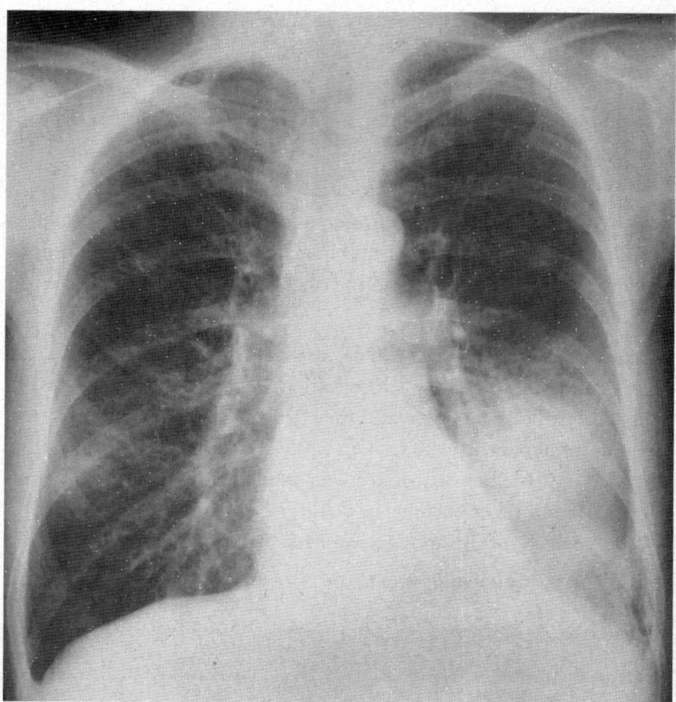

FIGURE 55-3 Posteroanterior CXR consolidation in the left lower lobe occupying all 3 basilar segments. There is blunting of the left costophrenic angle indicating a parapneumonic effusion. (*Reproduced with permission from Miller WT: Diagnostic Thoracic Imaging. New York, NY: McGraw-Hill Education; 2006.*)

IMAGING

Routine chest X-ray (CXR) is not necessary for the confirmation of suspected CAP in children who are well enough to be treated in the outpatient setting (after evaluation in the office, clinic, or emergency department setting).[17] SOR Ⓐ CXR, posteroanterior and lateral, should be obtained in patients with suspected or documented hypoxemia, significant respiratory distress, those who failed initial antibiotic therapy, and hospitalized patients. SOR Ⓑ

The diagnosis of pneumonia in adults based on clinical history and examination is only 47% to 69% sensitive and 58% to 75% specific; thus CXR is considered a standard part of evaluation.[3,16] The presence of new infiltrate in conjunction with clinical features is diagnostic. If the initial CXR is negative in a patient with clinical features of pneumonia, the CXR should be repeated in 24 to 48 hours, or a chest CT should be considered. SOR Ⓒ Ultrasound appears useful for diagnosis of CAP and evaluation of pleural effusion.[20,21] In one study, the combination of auscultation and lung ultrasound increased the positive likelihood ratio (LR) for CAP to 42.9 (95% CI, 10.8–170.0) and decreased the negative LR to 0.04 (95% CI, 0.02–0.09).[21] Point-of-care ultrasound was also useful in children for diagnosing pneumonia by visualizing lung consolidation with sonographic air bronchograms (overall sensitivity 86%, specificity of 89%, positive LR of 7.8 and negative LR of 0.2).[22]

There are four general patterns of pneumonia seen on CXR[3]:

- Lobar—Consolidation involves the entire lobe (**Figures 55-1** to **55-5**). A cavity with an air–fluid level is sometimes seen within the area of consolidation representing abscess formation (**Figure 55-5**).
- Bronchopneumonia—Patchy involvement of one or several lobes that may be extensive (**Figures 55-6** and **55-7**), usually in the dependent lower and posterior lungs (see **Figure 55-3**).
- Interstitial pneumonia—Inflammatory process involves the interstitium; usually patchy and diffuse (**Figure 55-8**). A nodular interstitial pattern is seen in patients with histoplasmosis (**Figure 55-9**), miliary TB, pneumoconiosis, and sarcoidosis.
- Miliary pneumonia—Numerous discrete lesions from hematogenous spread (see Chapter 56, Tuberculosis).

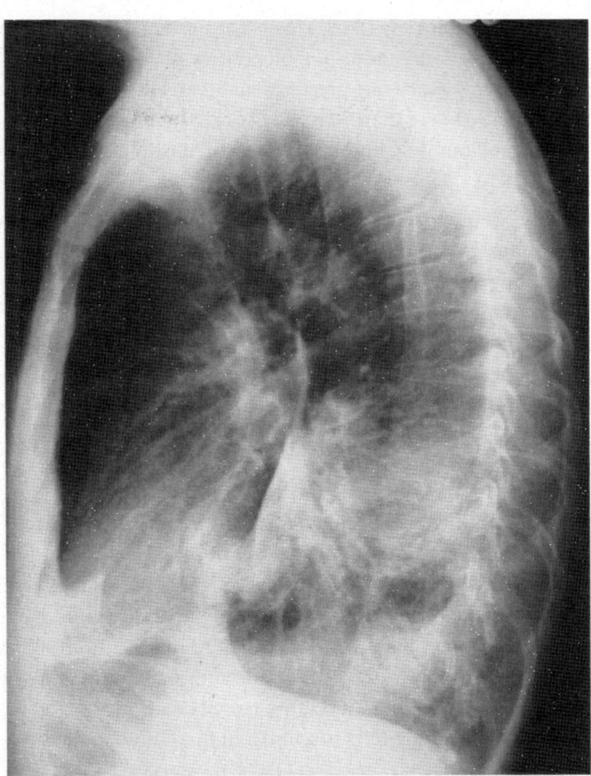

FIGURE 55-4 Lateral CXR of the patient in **Figure 55-3** showing posterior displacement of the major fissure indicating some atelectasis of the left lower lobe. (*Reproduced with permission from Miller WT: Diagnostic Thoracic Imaging. New York, NY: McGraw-Hill Education; 2006.*)

DIFFERENTIAL DIAGNOSIS

- Upper respiratory illnesses, including bronchitis, can cause cough, fever, chills, and sputum production with a negative CXR.
- Pulmonary embolus should be considered in patients with pleuritic chest pain or hypoxia and a negative CXR (see Chapter 59, Pulmonary Embolism).
- Asthma can cause cough, wheezing, dyspnea, and hypoxia, with the CXR negative unless mucous plugging causes collapse of airways (see Chapter 57, Asthma).

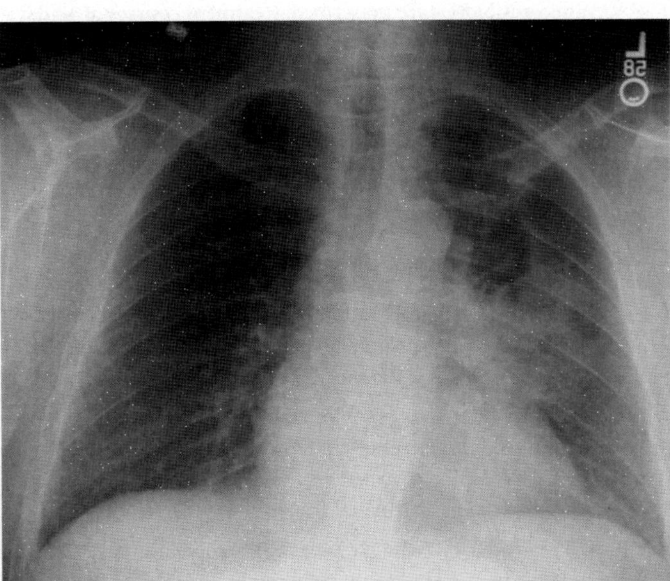

FIGURE 55-5 CXR showing a consolidation in the left upper lobe; note oval lucency that represents cavitation within the infiltrate. This patient had *Klebsiella* pneumonia. (*Reproduced with permission from Miller WT: Diagnostic Thoracic Imaging. New York, NY: McGraw-Hill Education; 2006.*)

MANAGEMENT

Initial determination of severity of illness is used to identify patients with CAP who may be candidates for outpatient treatment.[16]

- Respiratory rate more than 30 breaths/min without underlying disease is single best predictor.

- British Thoracic Society (BTS) rule—The presence of one or more of the following four: confusion; blood urea nitrogen greater than 7 mmol/L; respiratory rate greater than 30 breaths/min; systolic blood pressure lower than 90 mm Hg or diastolic blood pressure lower than 60 mm Hg. If none are present, mortality rate is 2.4%; 1 present, 8%; 2 present, 23%; 3 present, 33%; and all 4 present, 80%.
- A number of other severity scores are available (e.g., CURB-65 criteria [confusion, uremia, respiratory rate, low blood pressure, age 65 years or greater] and prognostic models such as the Pneumonia Severity Index [PSI]).[4,16]
- Assessment of oxygen consumption/hypoxia.

FIRST LINE

NONPHARMACOLOGIC

- The Infectious Diseases Society of America/American Thoracic Society recommend a cautious trial of noninvasive ventilation for patients with hypoxemia or respiratory distress unless they require immediate intubation because of severe hypoxemia (arterial oxygen pressure/fraction of inspired oxygen [PaO_2/FiO_2] ratio <150) and bilateral alveolar infiltrates.[16] Cochrane authors found that use of noninvasive ventilation reduced the risk of death in the ICU in addition to shortening ICU stay and length of intubation.[23]
- One small randomized controlled trial (RCT) (N = 40) found continuous positive airway pressure (CPAP) delivered by helmet improved oxygenation more quickly than oxygen therapy alone (median: 1.5 vs. 48 hours, respectively) in patients with CAP and moderate hypoxemic acute respiratory failure.[24]

MEDICATIONS

Antimicrobial therapy is not routinely required for preschool-age children with CAP because of the high proportion with viral disease.[16] SOR Ⓐ When antibiotics are prescribed, treatment courses of 10 days are recommended. SOR Ⓒ

- Amoxicillin is first-line therapy for previously healthy, appropriately immunized infants and preschool-age children with mild to moderate CAP suspected to be of bacterial origin.[17] SOR Ⓑ Authors of a Cochrane review supported use of amoxicillin (or co-trimoxazole) as first-line therapy.[25]
- Amoxicillin is also recommended for previously healthy, appropriately immunized school-age children and adolescents with mild to moderate CAP with consideration of atypical pathogens.[17] SOR Ⓑ If atypical pathogens are suspected clinically, macrolide antibiotics should be prescribed and diagnostic testing performed.
- Influenza antiviral therapy should be administered as soon as possible (within 48 hours) to children with moderate to severe CAP consistent with influenza virus infection during widespread local circulation of influenza viruses.[17] SOR Ⓑ
- For children with CAP who are inpatients, ampicillin or penicillin G should be administered to the fully immunized infant or school-age child when local epidemiologic data document lack of substantial high-level penicillin resistance for invasive *S. pneumoniae*.[17,25] Empiric therapy with a third-generation parenteral cephalosporin (ceftriaxone or cefotaxime) should be prescribed for hospitalized

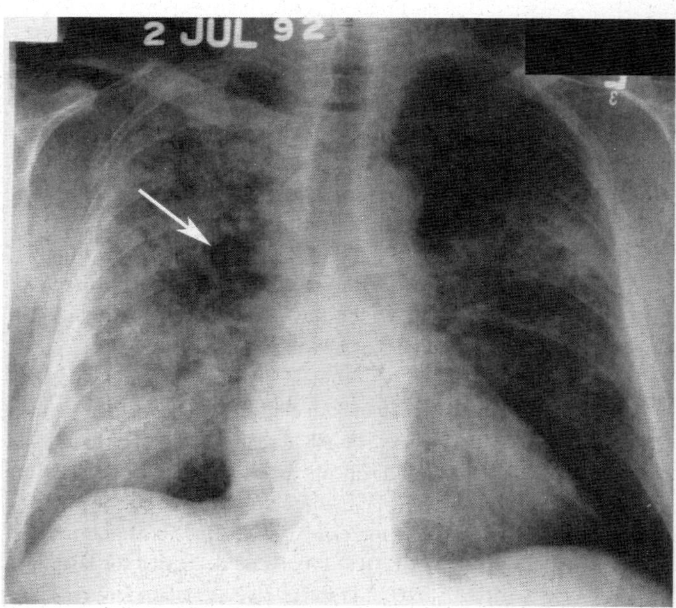

FIGURE 55-6 This patient has bilateral pulmonary infiltrates worsening despite antibiotics characteristic of severe bronchopneumonia. Note air bronchograms (*arrows*) on the right side. He was diagnosed with *Legionella* pneumonia. (*Reproduced with permission from Miller WT: Diagnostic Thoracic Imaging. New York, NY: McGraw-Hill Education; 2006.*)

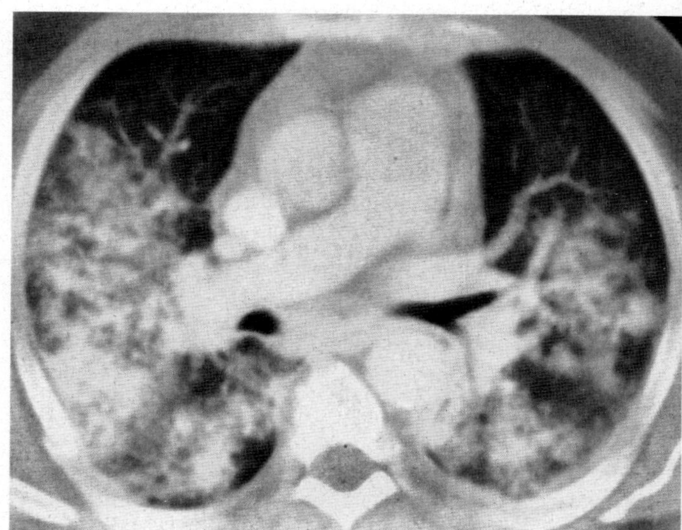

FIGURE 55-7 CT scan of the patient in **Figure 55-6** at the level of the main pulmonary arteries showing extensive pulmonary consolidation in both lungs caused by *Legionella pneumonia*. (*Reproduced with permission from Miller WT: Diagnostic Thoracic Imaging. New York, NY: McGraw-Hill Education; 2006.*)

infants and children who are not fully immunized, in regions where local epidemiology of invasive pneumococcal strains documents high-level penicillin resistance, or for infants and children with life-threatening infection.[17] SOR Ⓑ

- For children who are inpatients, empiric combination therapy with a macrolide (oral or parenteral) in addition to a β-lactam antibiotic should be prescribed when *M. pneumoniae* and *C. pneumoniae* are significant considerations; diagnostic testing should be performed.[17] SOR Ⓑ For children hospitalized with severe and very severe CAP, penicillin/ampicillin plus gentamicin is superior to chloramphenicol.[25]
- Vancomycin or clindamycin (based on local susceptibility data) should be provided in addition to β-lactam therapy for hospitalized children if clinical, laboratory, or imaging characteristics are consistent with infection caused by *S. aureus*.[17] SOR Ⓒ

Empiric antibiotic treatment for **adults** with CAP includes[16]:

- Outpatient, uncomplicated (previously healthy, no risk factors for drug-resistant *S. pneumoniae* [DRSP] infection)—Macrolide (erythromycin, azithromycin, or clarithromycin) SOR Ⓐ or doxycycline. SOR Ⓒ Authors of a Cochrane review did not find sufficient evidence to determine antibiotic choice for the treatment of CAP in ambulatory patients.[26]
- Outpatient with comorbidities (e.g., cardiac disease, diabetes mellitus) or risk factors for DRSP—Respiratory fluoroquinolone (i.e., levofloxacin [750 mg], moxifloxacin, and gemifloxacin) or β-lactam **plus** macrolide. SOR Ⓐ In regions with high rate (>25%) of macrolide-resistant *S. pneumoniae*, consider use of an alternate agent.
- Hospitalized patient (non-ICU)—Respiratory fluoroquinolone **or** β-lactam (preferred agents include cefotaxime, ceftriaxone, and ampicillin; ertapenem for selected patients) **plus** macrolide combination. SOR Ⓐ Doxycycline can be considered as an alternative to the macrolide.
  - Treatment should be started in the emergency room for patients admitted from there. Initiation of antibiotics within 4 to 8 hours of hospital arrival is associated with relative reductions of 5% to 43% in mortality, based on observational studies.[27]
  - In a cluster-randomized crossover trial with antibiotic treatment strategies for non-ICU hospitalized patients with CAP, beta-lactam monotherapy was noninferior to beta-lactam–macrolide combination or fluoroquinolone monotherapy with respect to 90-day mortality.[28] However, in an RCT of patients admitted in Switzerland with moderately severe CAP, although mortality, ICU admission, complications, length of stay (LOS), and 90-day pneumonia recurrence did not differ between those on β-lactam alone vs. β-lactam and macrolide combination, 30-day readmissions were higher in the monotherapy arm (7.9% vs 3.1%).[29] Clinical stability was delayed in those infected with atypical pathogens and PSI IV pneumonia with monotherapy.
  - A Cochrane review, however, did not find benefit in survival or clinical efficacy using empirical atypical coverage in hospitalized patients with CAP.[30]
- If the etiology of CAP is identified on the basis of reliable microbiologic methods, antimicrobial therapy should be directed at that pathogen.

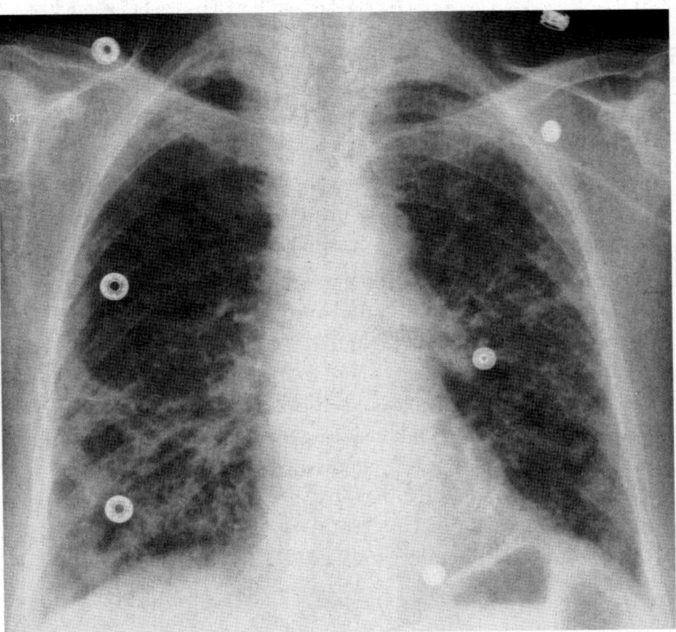

FIGURE 55-8 CXR showing basilar predominant interstitial lung disease in this 70-year-old woman; given her age, idiopathic pulmonary fibrosis is the most likely diagnosis. (*Reproduced with permission from Miller WT: Diagnostic Thoracic Imaging. New York, NY: McGraw-Hill Education; 2006.*)

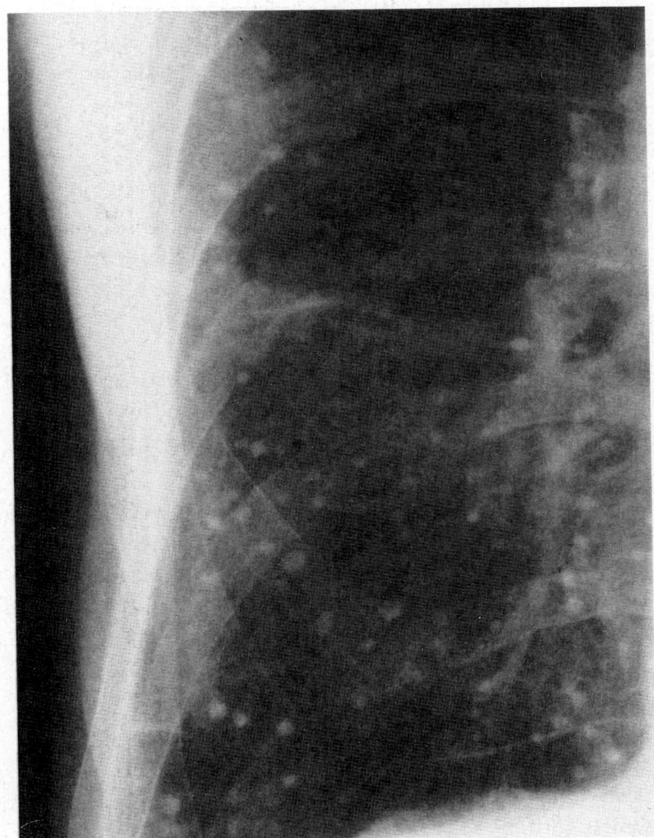

FIGURE 55-9 Nodular interstitial pattern with many calcified granulomas in a patient with histoplasmosis. (*Reproduced with permission from Schwartz DT, Reisdorff EJ. Emergency Radiology. New York, NY: McGraw-Hil Education; 2000.*)

- Early treatment (within 48 hours of the onset of symptoms) with oseltamivir or zanamivir is recommended for influenza A.[16]
- Duration of therapy—A minimum of 5 days. SOR A The patient should be afebrile for 48 to 72 hours and have no more than one CAP-associated sign of instability (e.g., temperature >37.8°C [100°F], tachycardia, respiratory rate >24 breaths/min, hypotension, oxygen saturation <90%, unable to maintain oral intake, altered mental status) before discontinuing antibiotics.[16]
- Corticosteroid treatment in adults with CAP is associated with a decreased risk of acute respiratory distress syndrome (RR 0.21–0.24) and may reduce hospital LOS and time to clinical stability[31,32]; among hospitalized patients, there was reduced need for mechanical ventilation and possibly reduced all-cause mortality but increased frequency of hyperglycemia requiring treatment.[30,32] Among children hospitalized with CAP, adjunctive steroids reduced hospital LOS, but only in conjunction with concomitant β-agonist therapy (i.e., likely only children with acute wheezing benefit).[33] Steroid use without β-agonist therapy increased LOS and readmission.

SECOND LINE

NONPHARMACOLOGIC

- Based on limited data, chest physiotherapy cannot be recommended as part of routine care for adults with pneumonia.[34] Positive expiratory pressure (versus no physiotherapy) and osteopathic manipulative treatment (OMT, versus placebo therapy) appear to slightly reduce the duration of hospital stay (by 2.02 and 1.4 days, respectively). OMT may also reduce duration of antibiotic use by 1 to 2 days.[35]

MEDICATIONS

- In children with CAP who are outpatients, amoxicillin-clavulanate and cefpodoxime may be alternative second-line drugs.[25]

HOSPITALIZATION

- Children and infants who have moderate to severe CAP, as defined by several factors including respiratory distress and hypoxemia, should be hospitalized for management, including skilled pediatric nursing care.[17] SOR A
- Infants younger than 3 to 6 months of age with suspected bacterial CAP, children and infants with suspected or documented CAP caused by a pathogen with increased virulence (e.g., community-acquired methicillin-resistant *S. aureus* [MRSA]), and children and infants for whom there is concern about careful observation at home or who are unable to comply with therapy or follow-up are likely to benefit from hospitalization.[17] SOR C
- For adults, severity-of-illness scores can be used to identify patients with CAP who may be candidates for outpatient treatment. SOR A Consider hospitalization if the patient has severe CAP (CURB-65 ≥2 or BTS score >0); or has hypoxia, worsening symptoms, or preexisting conditions that compromise safety of home care; or for patients who fail to improve in more than 72 hours.[3,16]

PREVENTION

- Vaccination—Children should be immunized with vaccines for bacterial pathogens including *S. pneumoniae*, *H. influenzae* type b, and pertussis to prevent CAP.[17] SOR A Pneumococcal polysaccharide vaccine is recommended for persons 65 years of age and older, and for those with selected high-risk concurrent diseases.[16] SOR B All infants 6 months of age or older, children, adolescents, persons 50 years of age or older, others at risk for influenza complications, and healthcare workers should be immunized annually with vaccines for influenza virus to prevent CAP.[16,17] SOR A Vaccination status should be assessed at the time of hospital admission for all patients and appropriate vaccines offered at discharge.[16] SOR C
- Smoking cessation assistance should be offered to patients who smoke (see Chapter 248, Smoking and Tobacco Addiction).
- To prevent spread of respiratory pathogens, respiratory hygiene measures should be practiced.[16] These include the coughing into the elbow and use of hand hygiene and masks or tissues for patients with cough, particularly in outpatient settings and emergency departments.
- Authors of a Cochrane review of six RCTs found that zinc supplementation in children (aged 2 to 59 months) was associated with reduced risk of pneumonia.[36]

PROGNOSIS

- Patients on adequate therapy for CAP should demonstrate clinical (and laboratory) signs of improvement within 48 to 72 hours.[17]
- Overall mortality rate from pneumonia in the United States is 15.9 deaths per 100,000.[37]
- Outpatient mortality rate is 1%. The mortality rate for those who require admission to the hospital averages 12%, and the mortality rate for patients with severe CAP in the ICU setting approaches 40%.[3] In a multihospital study in Canada, 9% (N = 89) of patients died in-hospital, 10% died at 30 days, and 247 (26%) died by 1 year. In-hospital mortality was higher among patients with admission hypoglycemia.[38]
- Using a large database, guideline concordant therapy for CAP (65% of cases) was associated with decreased in-hospital mortality (OR, 0.70; 95% CI, 0.63 to 0.77), sepsis (OR, 0.83; 95% CI, 0.72 to 0.96), renal failure (OR, 0.79; 95% CI, 0.67 to 0.94), and reduced hospital LOS and duration of parenteral therapy (0.6 days for both).[39]

FOLLOW-UP

- Assess need and provide pneumococcal and influenza vaccination at hospital discharge or follow-up.
- Monitor improvement and treat comorbid illness (which may worsen).
- In children, repeat CXRs (inpatient or outpatient) are not routinely required if recovery from an episode of CAP is uneventful.[17] SOR B

Follow-up chest radiographs should be obtained in patients with complicated pneumonia with worsening respiratory distress or clinical instability, or in those with persistent fever that is not responding to therapy over 48 to 72 hours. SOR Ⓒ Repeat CXR at 4 to 6 weeks after the diagnosis of CAP should be obtained in patients with recurrent pneumonia involving the same lobe and in patients with lobar collapse at initial CXR with suspicion of an anatomic anomaly, chest mass, or foreign-body aspiration.[17] SOR Ⓑ

- In adults, repeat CXRs until clear if the patient is older than 40 years or smokes, as 2% of such patients may have underlying cancer.[3]

PATIENT EDUCATION

- Patients who smoke should be offered cessation assistance.
- Improvement is expected in healthy outpatients younger than age 65 years in 48 to 72 hours with their returning to work or school in approximately 4 to 5 days and complete improvement within 2 weeks.
- In hospitalized patients, clinical stability is expected in 3 to 7 days; mortality is 12% with 70% developing a complication such as respiratory failure, congestive heart failure, shock, dysrhythmia, myocardial infarction, GI bleeding, or renal insufficiency.[3]

PATIENT RESOURCES

- MedlinePlus. *Pneumonia*—**https://medlineplus.gov/pneumonia.html.**
- Centers for Disease Control and Prevention. *Pneumonia*—**https://www.cdc.gov/nchs/fastats/pneumonia.htm.**

PROVIDER RESOURCES

- Lee JS, Giesler DL, Gellad WF, Fine MJ. Antibiotic therapy for adults hospitalized with community-acquired pneumonia: a systematic review. *JAMA*. 2016;315(6):593-602.
- Infectious Diseases Society of America. The management of community-acquired pneumonia in infants and children older than 3 months of age: clinical practice guidelines by the Pediatric Infectious Diseases Society and the Infectious Diseases Society of America. **http://www.idsociety.org/Guidelines/Patient_Care/IDSA_Practice_Guidelines/Infections_By_Organ_System-81567/Lower/Upper_Respiratory/Community-Acquired_Pneumonia_(CAP)_in_Infants_and_Children/.**
- American Thoracic Society. *Infectious Diseases Society of America/American Thoracic Society Consensus Guidelines on the Management of Community-Acquired Pneumonia in Adults*—**https://www.thoracic.org/statements/resources/mtpi/idsaats-cap.pdf.**

REFERENCES

1. Ewig S, Welte T, Torres A. Is healthcare-associated pneumonia a distinct entity needing specific therapy? *Curr Opin Infect Dis.* 2012;25(2):166-175.
2. Chalmers JD, Taylor JK, Singanayagam A, et al. Epidemiology, antibiotic therapy, and clinical outcomes in health care-associated pneumonia: a UK cohort study. *Clin Infect Dis.* 2011;55(2):107-113.
3. Marrie TJ, Campbell GD, Walker DH, Low DE. Pneumonia. In: Kasper DL, Braunwald E, Fauci AS, et al, eds. *Harrison's Principles of Internal Medicine*, 16th ed. New York, NY: McGraw-Hill; 2005:1528-1541.
4. Butt S, Swiatlo E. Treatment of community-acquired pneumonia in an ambulatory setting. *Am J Med.* 2011;124(4);297-300.
5. Jain S, Self WH, Wunderink RG, et al. Community-acquired pneumonia requiring hospitalization among U.S. adults. *N Engl J Med.* 2015;373:415-427.
6. Jain S, Williams DJ, Arnold SR, et al. Community-acquired pneumonia requiring hospitalization among U.S. children. *N Engl J Med.* 2015;372:835-845.
7. File TM. Case studies of lower respiratory tract infections: community-acquired pneumonia. *Am J Med.* 2010;123(4 Suppl):S4-S15.
8. Centers for Disease Control and Prevention. *Deaths: Final Data for 2014.* https://www.cdc.gov/nchs/data/nvsr/nvsr65/nvsr65_04.pdf. Accessed January 2017.
9. Juvén T, Mertsola J, Waris M, et al. Etiology of community-acquired pneumonia in 254 hospitalized children. *Pediatr Infect Dis J.* 2000;19(4):293-298.
10. Micek ST, Kollef KE, Reichley RM, et al. Health care-associated pneumonia and community-acquired pneumonia: a single-center experience. *Antimicrob Agents Chemother.* 2007;51(10):3568-3573.
11. Marrie TJ, Raoult D, La Scola B. *Legionella*-like and other amoebal pathogens as agents of community-acquired pneumonia. *Emerg Infect Dis.* 2001;7(6):1026-1029.
12. Benson RF, Drozanski WJ, Rowbatham TJ, et al. Serologic evidence of infection with 9 *Legionella*-like amoebal pathogens in pneumonia patients. Proceedings of the 95th ASM General Meeting; May 21-25, 1995; Washington, DC. [Abstract C-200, p. 35.]
13. Almirall J, Bolibar I, Balanzo X, Gonzalez CA. Risk factors for community-acquired pneumonia in adults: a population-based case control study. *Eur Respir J.* 1999;13(2):349-355.
14. Eom CS, Jeon CY, Lim JW, et al. Use of acid-suppressive drugs and risk of pneumonia: a systematic review and meta-analysis. *CMAJ.* 2011;183(3):310-319.
15. van Vugt SF, Broekhuizen BD, Lammens C, et al. Use of serum C reactive protein and procalcitonin concentrations in addition to symptoms and signs to predict pneumonia in patients presenting to primary care with acute cough: diagnostic study. *BMJ.* 2013;346:f2450.
16. Mandell LA, Wunderink RG, Anzueto A, et al. Infectious Diseases Society of America/American Thoracic Society consensus guidelines on the management of community-acquired pneumonia in adults. *Clin Infect Dis.* 2007;44 Suppl 2:S27-S72.
17. Bradley JS, Byington CL, Shah SS, et al. The management of community-acquired pneumonia in infants and children older than 3 months of age: clinical practice guidelines by the Pediatric Infectious Diseases Society and the Infectious Diseases Society of America. *Clin Infect Dis.* 2011;55(7):e25-e76.

18. Campbell SG, Marrie TJ, Anstey R, et al. The contribution of blood cultures to the clinical management of adult patients admitted to the hospital with community-acquired pneumonia: a prospective observational study. *Chest.* 2003;123(4):1142-1150.
19. Badfadhel M, Clark TW, Reid C, et al. Procalcitonin and C-reactive protein in hospitalized adult patients with community-acquired pneumonia or exacerbation of asthma or COPD. *Chest.* 2011;139 (6):1410-1418.
20. Schuetz P, Christ-Crain M, Thomann R, et al. Effect of procalcitonin-based guidelines vs standard guidelines on antibiotic use in lower respiratory tract infections: the ProHOSP randomized controlled trial. *JAMA.* 2009;302(10):1059-1066.
21. Reissig A, Copetti R, Mathis G, et al. Lung ultrasound in the diagnosis and follow-up of community-acquired pneumonia: a prospective, multicenter, diagnostic accuracy study. *Chest.* 2012; 142(4):965-972.
22. Shah VP, Tunik MG, Tsung JW. Prospective evaluation of point-of-care ultrasonography for the diagnosis of pneumonia in children and young adults. *JAMA Pediatr.* 2013;167(2):119-125.
23. Zhang Y, Fang C, Dong BR, Wu T, Deng JL. Oxygen therapy for pneumonia in adults. *Cochrane Database Syst Rev.* 2012;(3): CD006607.
24. Cosentini R, Brambilla AM, Aliberti S, et al. Helmet continuous positive airway pressure vs oxygen therapy to improve oxygenation in community-acquired pneumonia: a randomized, controlled trial. *Chest.* 2010;138(1):114-120.
25. Lodha R, Kabra SK, Pandey RM. Antibiotics for community-acquired pneumonia in children. *Cochrane Database Syst Rev.* 2013;(6):CD004874.
26. Pakhale S, Mulpuru S, Verheij TJM, et al. Antibiotics for community acquired pneumonia in adult outpatients. *Cochrane Database Syst Rev.* 2014;(10):CD002109.
27. Lee JS, Giesler DL, Gellad WF, Fine MJ. Antibiotic therapy for adults hospitalized with community-acquired pneumonia: a systematic review. *JAMA.* 2016;315(6):593-602.
28. Postma DF, van Werkhoven CH, van Elden LJ, et al; CAP-START Study Group. Antibiotic treatment strategies for community-acquired pneumonia in adults. *N Engl J Med.* 2015;372(14):1312-1323.
29. Garin N, Genné D, Carballo S, et al. β-Lactam monotherapy vs β-lactam-macrolide combination treatment in moderately severe community-acquired pneumonia: a randomized noninferiority trial. *JAMA Intern Med.* 2014;174(12):1894-1901.
30. Robenshtok E, Shefet D, Gafter-Gvili A, et al. Empiric antibiotic coverage of atypical pathogens for community-acquired pneumonia in hospitalized adults. *Cochrane Database Syst Rev.* 2012;(9): CD004418.
31. Wan YD, Sun TW, Liu ZQ, et al. Efficacy and safety of corticosteroids for community-acquired pneumonia: a systematic review and meta-analysis. *Chest.* 2016;149(1):209-219.
32. Siemieniuk RA, Meade MO, Alonso-Coello P, et al. Corticosteroid therapy for patients hospitalized with community-acquired pneumonia: a systematic review and meta-analysis. *Ann Intern Med.* 2015;163(7):519-528.
33. Weiss AK, Hall M, Lee GE, et al. Adjunct corticosteroids in children hospitalized with community-acquired pneumonia. *Pediatrics.* 2011;127(2):e255-e263.
34. Reynolds JH, McDonald G, Alton H, Gordon SB. Pneumonia in the immunocompetent patient. *Br J Radiol.* 2010;83(996):998-1009.
35. Yang M, Yan Y, Yin X, et al. Chest physiotherapy for pneumonia in adults. *Cochrane Database Syst Rev.* 2010;(2):CD006338.
36. Lassi ZS, Moin A, Bhutta ZA. Zinc supplementation for the prevention of pneumonia in children aged 2 months to 59 months. *Cochrane Database Syst Rev.* 2016;(12):CD005978.
37. Centers for Disease Control and Prevention. *Pneumonia.* https://www.cdc.gov/nchs/fastats/pneumonia.htm. Accessed January 2017.
38. Gamble JM, Eurich DT, Marrie TJ, Majumdar SR. Admission hypoglycemia and increased mortality in patients hospitalized with pneumonia. *Am J Med.* 2010;123(6):556.e11-e16.
39. McCabe C, Kirchner C, Zhang H, et al. Guideline-concordant therapy and reduced mortality and length of stay in adults with community-acquired pneumonia: playing by the rules. *Arch Intern Med.* 2009;169(16):1525-1551.

56 TUBERCULOSIS

Mindy A. Smith, MD, MS

PATIENT STORY

A 20-year-old man presents to the emergency department with a persistent cough for 3 weeks, low-grade fever, and night sweats. His chest X-ray shows mediastinal and right hilar lymphadenopathy and right upper lobe consolidation concerning for primary tuberculosis (**Figure 56-1**). Upon review of the radiograph, the emergency room staff admits the patient to a single room with negative pressure. The patient is placed in respiratory isolation, sputum is sent for acid-fast bacillus (AFB) stain and cultures, and the results show acid-fast bacilli consistent with *Mycobacterium* spp. (**Figure 56-2**). While culture results are pending, the patient is started on four antituberculosis drugs. Fortunately, the sputum culture result shows *pansusceptible Mycobacterium tuberculosis*, and his treatment continues with directly observed therapy through the local city health department.

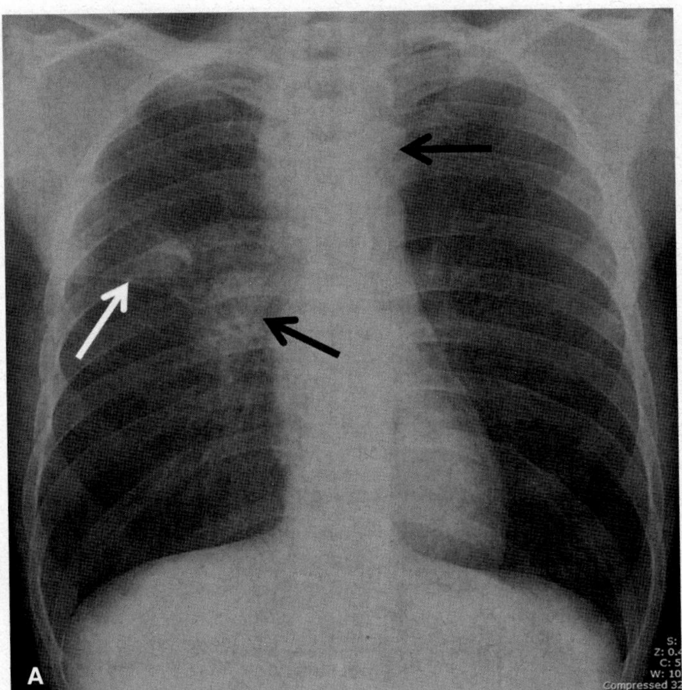

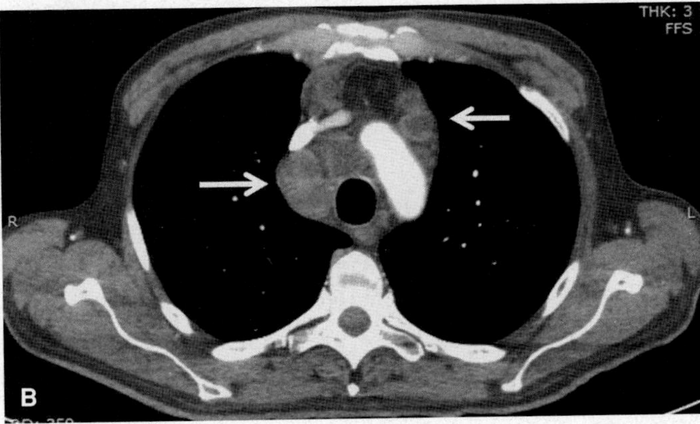

FIGURE 56-1 Typical presentation of a primary pulmonary tuberculosis infection in a 20-year-old man. **A.** Frontal chest radiograph shows mediastinal and right hilar lymphadenopathy (*black arrows*) and right upper lobe consolidation (*white arrow*). **B.** Contrast-enhanced CT demonstrates low-density enlarged mediastinal lymph nodes with rim peripheral enhancement consistent with necrotizing lymphadenopathy (*arrows*). (*Reproduced with permission from Carlos Santiago Restrepo, MD.*)

INTRODUCTION

Tuberculosis (TB) is a bacterial infection caused by *M. tuberculosis*, an obligate intracellular pathogen that is aerobic, acid fast, and non-encapsulated. TB primarily involves the lungs, although other organs are involved in one-third of cases. Improvements in diagnostics, drugs, vaccines, and understanding of biomarkers of disease activity are expected to change future management of this devastating world-wide disease.

EPIDEMIOLOGY

- Among individuals who were HIV-negative, all-form TB incidence worldwide in 2013 was 7.1 million (6.9 million to 7.3 million), prevalence was 11.2 million (10.8 million to 11.6 million), and number of TB-related deaths was 1.3 million (1.2 million to 1.4 million).[1]
- A total of 9557 TB cases (3.0 per 100,000 persons) were reported in the United States in 2015; the incidence has been relatively stable since 2013.[2] The highest incidence rates were recorded in California, Georgia, New York, and Texas.
- The multidrug-resistant (MDR) TB rate in the United States was 1.2% (88 cases) in 2010, a rate that remains relatively stable in the United States.[1] MDR TB rates are highest in India, China, the Russian Federation, South Africa, and Bangladesh.[3] Global incidence of MDR TB in children was estimated at 3.2%[4]; isoniazid-resistant TB in children was estimated at 12.1% in 2010, with the highest proportion reported in the European region at 26.1%.[5]
- Based on 2015 data, 66.4% of reported U.S. cases of *M. tuberculosis* occurred in foreign-born individuals (case rate 13 times higher than U.S.-born individuals).[2]
- There were 493 reported deaths from TB in the United States in 2014 (a 11% decrease from 2013).[2]

- Prophylactic treatment of those with latent TB (infection without active disease—diagnosed by tuberculin skin test [TST] conversion from negative to positive or by an interferon-γ release assay [IGRA] performed on blood) can reduce the risk of active TB by 90% or more.[6] SOR Ⓐ

ETIOLOGY AND PATHOPHYSIOLOGY[6]

- Infection is transmitted by aerosolized respiratory droplet nuclei.
- Approximately 10% of those infected develop active TB, usually within 1 to 2 years of exposure; risk factors for the development of active TB are listed below.
- There are three host responses to infection—immediate nonspecific macrophage and likely neutrophil ingestion of those bacilli reaching the alveoli, later tissue-damaging response (delayed-type hypersensitivity reaction), and specific macrophage activating and potentially neutrophil-related response. The latter, if effective, walls off infection into granulomas. Recent evidence suggests that mycobacteria themselves may promote granuloma formation and these granulomas are dynamic, blurring distinctions between latent and active TB.[3]
- The disease process usually localizes to the middle and upper lung zones accompanied by hilar and paratracheal lymphadenopathy (as the tubercle bacilli spread from lung to lymphatic vessels). The primary focus usually heals spontaneously and may disappear entirely or, if encapsulated by fibroblasts and collagen fibers, be visible as a calcified lung nodule (Ghon complex) (**Figure 56-3**).

RISK FACTORS

Risk factors for infection or progression to active TB include[2,3,6]:

- Minority and foreign-born populations (subject to overcrowding and malnutrition).
- HIV (relative risk [RR] for progression to active TB 100) and other immunocompromised states (e.g., cancer, treatment with tumor necrosis factor antagonists) (RR [progression to active TB] 10). Because of the high susceptibility of HIV-infected patients, 12% of worldwide TB cases are HIV-associated, with sub-Saharan Africa accounting for 4 of every 5 of these cases.[3]
- Chronic diseases such as diabetes mellitus (RR 3) or chronic renal failure/hemodialysis (RR [infection and progression to active TB] 10 to 25 for renal failure).
- Malignancy.
- Genetic susceptibility.
- Bariatric surgery or jejunoileal bypass recipients (RR [progression to active TB] 30 to 60) recipients.
- Injection drug users (RR [progression to active TB] 10 to 30).
- Smoking (RR 2 for progression and infection).
- Personnel who work or live in high-risk settings (e.g., prisons, long-term care facilities, and hospitals).
- Adult women (ratio 2:1 adult man).
- Older age (both infection and progression).
- Children younger than 4 years of age who are exposed to high-risk individuals.

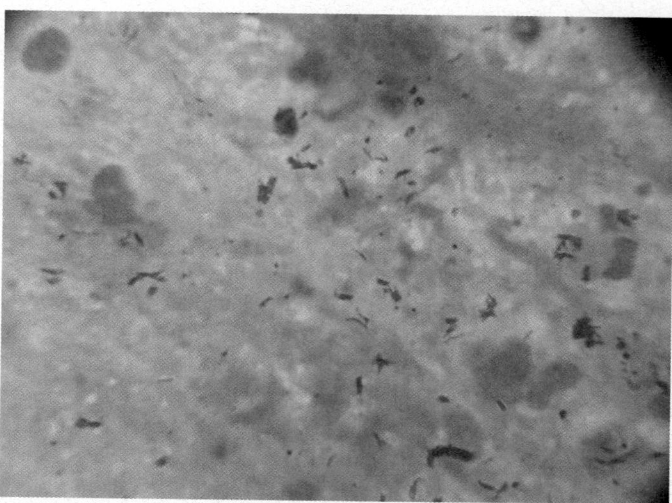

FIGURE 56-2 The acid-fast bacilli of *Mycobacterium tuberculosis* seen with acid-fast staining at 100 power with oil immersion microscopy. *(Reproduced with permission from Richard P. Usatine, MD.)*

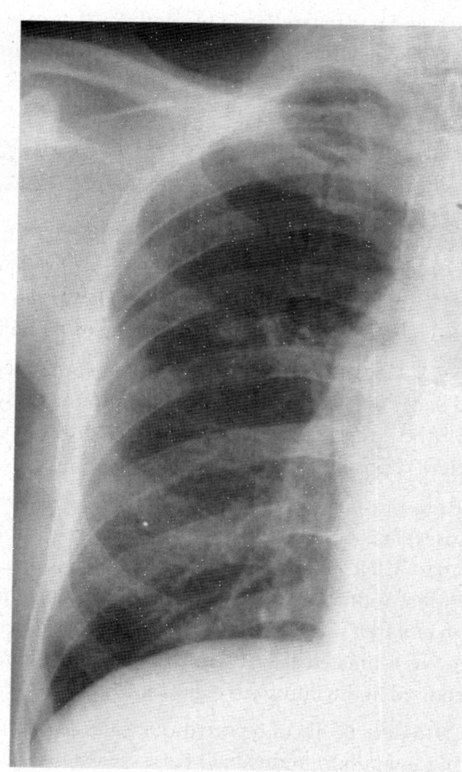

FIGURE 56-3 Primary tuberculosis may coalesce into a small granuloma in the upper lobe, referred to as a Ghon complex. *(Reproduced with permission from Miller WT: Diagnostic Thoracic Imaging. New York, NY: McGraw-Hill Education; 2006.)*

- Recent infection (<1 year) (RR [progression to active TB] 12.9 vs. old infection).
- Fibrotic lung lesions (spontaneously healed) (RR [progression to active TB] 2 to 20).
- Silicosis (RR [infection] 3 and RR [progression to active TB] 30).
- Malnutrition (RR [progression to active TB] 2).
- In a study of hospital personnel, only the percentage of low-income persons within the employee's residential postal zone was independently associated with conversion (odds ratio [OR] 1.39, 95% confidence interval [CI], 1.09 to 1.78).[7]

DIAGNOSIS

The diagnosis of active TB requires a high index of suspicion. Targeted testing for latent TB using an IGRA is recommended for individuals 5 years and older who are (1) are likely to be infected with *M. tuberculosis*, (2) have a low or intermediate risk of disease progression, (3) for whom it has been decided that testing for latent TB is warranted, and (4) either have a history of bacille Calmette-Guérin (BCG) vaccination or are unlikely to return to have their TST read; a TST is an acceptable alternative.[8] Those at risk of infection include household contacts or recent exposure to an infected person, mycobacteriology laboratory personnel, immigrants from high-burden countries (>20/100,000 persons), and residents or employees of high-risk congregate settings. If positive, a second confirmatory test with either an IGRA or TST is suggested. In general, unless mandated by law or through a credentialing body, testing for latent TB infection in individuals who are low risk for infection or progression is not recommended.[8] These tests are described below.

Manifestations of active TB can be classified as pulmonary or extrapulmonary. TB can affect any organ system.

CLINICAL FEATURES

The disease may be asymptomatic (1 in 4 culture-confirmed cases from active case finding in Asia).[3]

Pulmonary TB:

- Early nonspecific signs and symptoms: fever, night sweats, fatigue, anorexia, weight loss.
- Later nonproductive cough (lasting 2 to 3 weeks) or cough with purulent sputum.
- Patients with extensive disease may develop dyspnea or acute respiratory distress syndrome.
- Physical examination findings are also nonspecific with crackles or rhonchi.

Extrapulmonary TB, caused by hematogenous spread, occurs in the following order of frequency[6]:

- Lymph nodes: painless swelling of cervical and supraclavicular nodes (scrofula) (**Figure 56-4**).
- Pleura: pleural effusion with exudates.
- Genitourinary tract: may cause urethral stricture, kidney damage, or infertility (in women, affects the fallopian tubes and endometrium).
- Bones and joints: pain in the spine (Pott disease, **Figure 56-5**), hips, or knees.

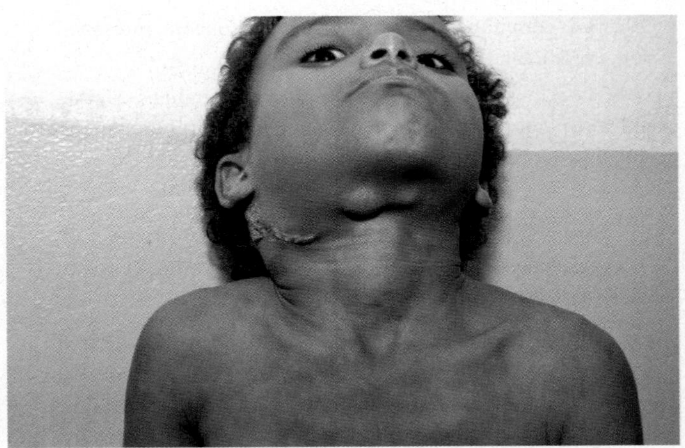

FIGURE 56-4 Young boy in Africa with scrofuloderma and large cervical and submandibular lymphadenopathy from tuberculosis. (*Reproduced with permission from Richard P. Usatine, MD.*)

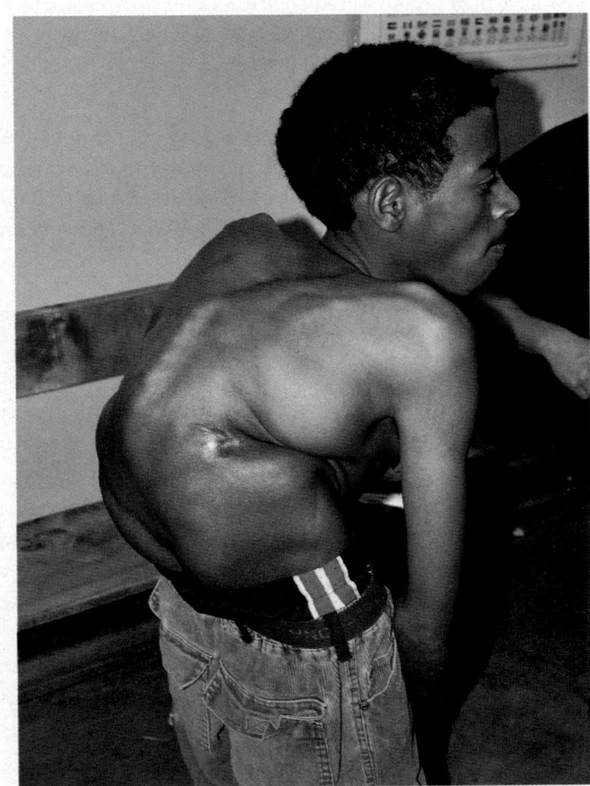

FIGURE 56-5 Pott disease from tuberculosis infection of the spine resulting in a severe kyphoscoliosis. Note the skin ulceration on the right and the severe deformity caused by this disease. (*Reproduced with permission from Richard P. Usatine, MD.*)

- Other less common sites are meninges, peritoneum, intestines, skin, eye, ear, and pericardium.
- TB of the skin (scrofuloderma) shows as skin ulcerations (**Figures 56-4** and **56-6**) in the inguinal or cervical region along with lymphadenopathy.

SKIN TESTING AND RAPID TESTING

Positive results on either a TST or IGRA in the absence of active TB establish a diagnosis of latent TB infection.

- TST with purified protein derivative (PPD) is not useful in diagnosing active TB but is used to detect latent infection in exposed or high-risk individuals. A positive test is 10 mm induration at the inoculation site or 5 mm induration in a patient who is immunocompromised, evaluated in 48 to 72 hours after test placement.
- Two commercially produced IGRAs are licensed for use in the United States and in many other countries: QuantiFERON-TB Gold (QFT-G, Cellestis Limited, Carnegie, Victoria, Australia) and TSPOT.TB (Oxford Immunotec, Inc., Oxford, England) as an aid for diagnosing *M. tuberculosis* infection.[3]
- IGRAs detect the release of interferon-g in fresh heparinized whole blood from sensitized persons when it is incubated with mixtures of synthetic peptides using antigens present in *M. tuberculosis*. Advantages include no need for a return visit and greater specificity than skin testing. Disadvantages include cost, availability, and lack of supporting data that these tests improve patient outcomes.
- IGRAs have high negative predictive values for progression to active TB, similar to those for a TST (99.7% and 99.4%, respectively) and higher positive predictive values than TST (2.7% vs. 1.5%, respectively).[9]
- Slightly higher sensitivity and specificity have been demonstrated for IGRAs compared to TST in children younger than 5 years, and these tests can be used as supporting tools to detect latent TB infection in this group.[10] However, the ATA/IDSA/CDC guidelines recommend TST as the preferred test.[8]

LABORATORY AND ANCILLARY TESTING

- Nonspecific findings include mild anemia and leukocytosis.
- Urinalysis may show "sterile" pyuria and hematuria with urinary tract involvement.
- Acid-fast bacilli may be seen on acid-fast staining from sputum or pleural or peritoneal fluid (**Figure 56-2**). The ATS/IDSA/CDC guidelines recommend AFB smear microscopy for all patients suspected of having pulmonary TB (traditionally on 3 specimens obtained 8–12 hours apart).[8] AFB may also be seen upon staining tissue from fine-needle aspiration or biopsy of lymph nodes or other tissues as above. Sputum processing with bleach or sodium hydroxide and centrifugation and use of fluorescent microscopy is associated with increased sensitivity of smear microscopy.[3]
- Definitive diagnosis is based on culture of sputum (3 sets of samples collected 8 to 24 hours apart), urine (3 morning specimens—positive in 90% with urinary tract infection), or from tissue or bone biopsy using automated liquid culture systems. *M. tuberculosis* is slow growing and may take 4 to 8 weeks to identify. One culture isolate from each mycobacterial culture-positive patient should be submitted to a regional genotyping laboratory for genotyping.[8]
- The ATS/IDSA/CDC guidelines recommend that a nucleic acid amplification test (NAAT) be performed on the initial specimen from patients with suspected pulmonary or extrapulmonary TB. TB is unlikely in patients with a positive AFB smear but negative NAAT, although a negative NAAT cannot be used to rule out TB when AFB smears are negative.[8] Once identified, testing for drug sensitivity should be performed.
- Obtaining baseline liver enzymes is recommended for patients older than age 35 years, or for those with a history of liver disease, HIV infection, pregnancy (or within 3 months postdelivery), concomitant hepatotoxic therapy, or regular alcohol use.
- Testing vision, including color vision, is suggested prior to initiating and throughout treatment with ethambutol (EMB), which can cause irreversible cumulative toxicity to the optic nerve.
- Biomarkers of disease activity on T cells are an area of active investigation[11]; however, a simple, inexpensive point-of-care test is still not available.

IMAGING

- Chest X-ray (CXR) is the diagnostic test of choice and classically shows upper lobe infiltrates with cavitation and/or lymphadenopathy (**Figures 56-1** and **56-7**).
- Other patterns of TB seen on CXR include a solitary nodule (Ghon complex) (**Figure 56-3**) and diffuse infiltrates that may represent bronchogenic spread (**Figure 56-8**).
- CXR in children and young adults often shows an infiltrate with hilar and paratracheal lymphadenopathy (**Figures 56-1** and **56-9**).
- In disseminated (miliary) TB, innumerable tiny nodules are seen throughout both lungs on CXR and CT (**Figure 56-10**).
- Reactivation TB may show large cavities in both upper lobes associated with bronchiectasis and fibronodular opacities (**Figure 56-11**).
- X-ray, CT, or MRI of bone may show destructive lesions. Spinal MRI has a sensitivity of approximately 100% and specificity of 88% for detecting tuberculous lesions before deformity develops.[12]

BIOPSY

Histology reveals granulomas with caseating necrosis.

DIFFERENTIAL DIAGNOSIS

Because any pattern on CXR may be seen with active TB, the differential diagnosis includes:

- Bacterial or viral pneumonia—Sputum or blood culture may reveal the infecting organism, and the patient will usually respond to antibacterial drugs and/or time.
- Fungal respiratory infections—These patients usually have a history of travel to or living in an area where histoplasmosis or coccidioidomycosis is endemic.
- Acute histoplasmosis is usually asymptomatic or causes only mild symptoms, and CXR typically shows hilar adenopathy with or

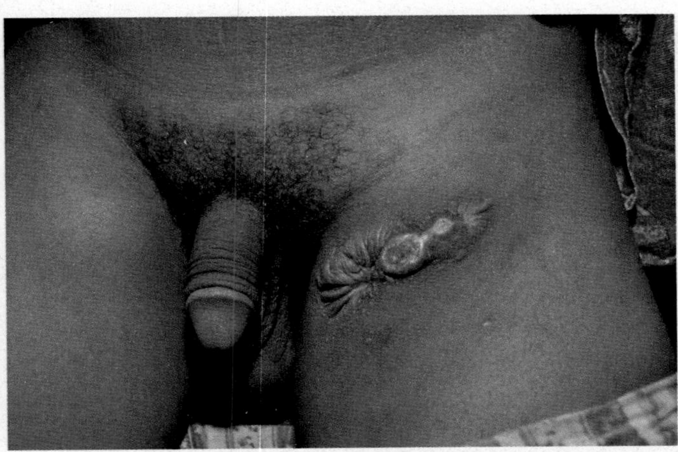

FIGURE 56-6 Young adult man in Africa with scrofuloderma showing an ulcerated lesion on one side and inguinal adenopathy on the other side. *(Reproduced with permission from Richard P. Usatine, MD.)*

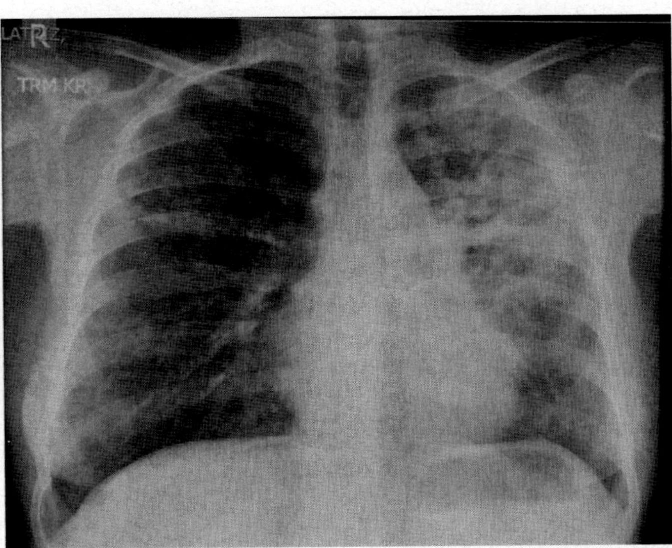

FIGURE 56-8 A 23-year-old woman with pulmonary tuberculosis. There is increased density of the lung parenchyma in the upper left lobe with a heterogeneous pattern showing areas of consolidation, fibrosis, and bullae. Other sections of the lung show a micronodular pattern. There is a retraction of the mediastinum toward the left. This whole pattern is consistent with pulmonary tuberculosis. *(Reproduced with permission from Richard P. Usatine, MD.)*

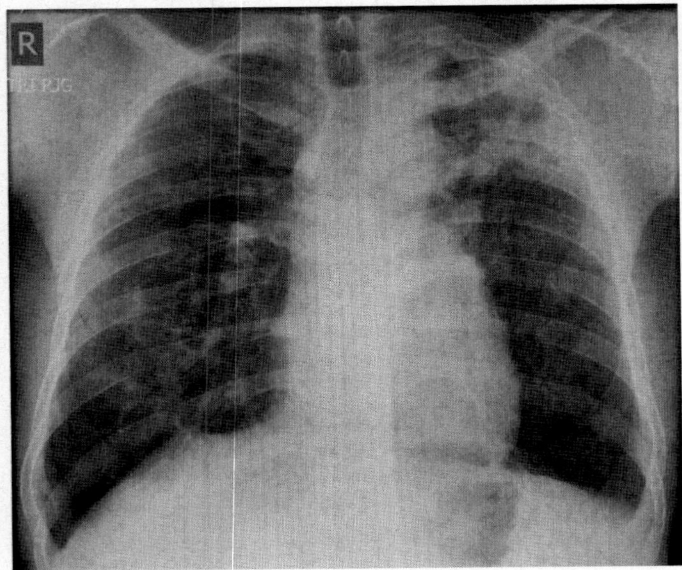

FIGURE 56-7 A 36-year-old man with pulmonary tuberculosis. There is an opacity in the left pulmonary apex associated with a cavity consistent with fibrosis and scarring changes of pulmonary tuberculosis. Also, there is an infiltrate in the right lung. *(Reproduced with permission from Richard P. Usatine, MD [upper block only].)*

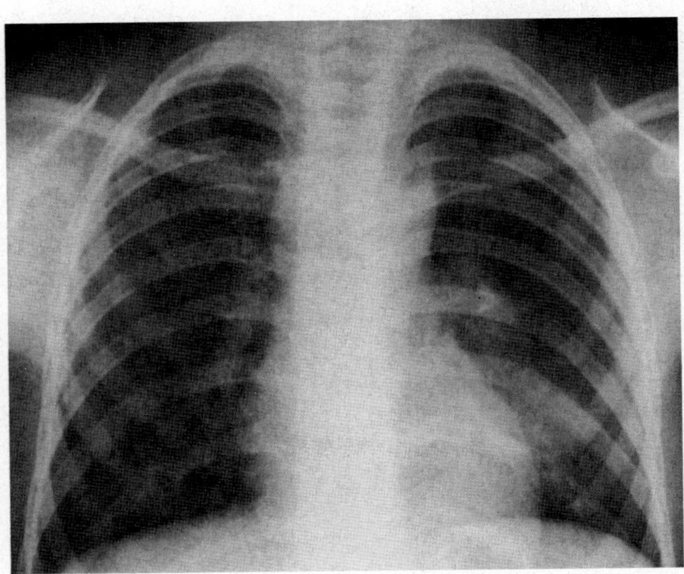

FIGURE 56-9 Primary tuberculosis in a child; note the left lower lobe infiltrate and the left hilar lymphadenopathy and right paratracheal adenopathy. *(Reproduced with permission from Schwartz DT and ReisdorffEJ. Emergency Radiology. New York, NY: McGraw-Hill Education; 2000.)*

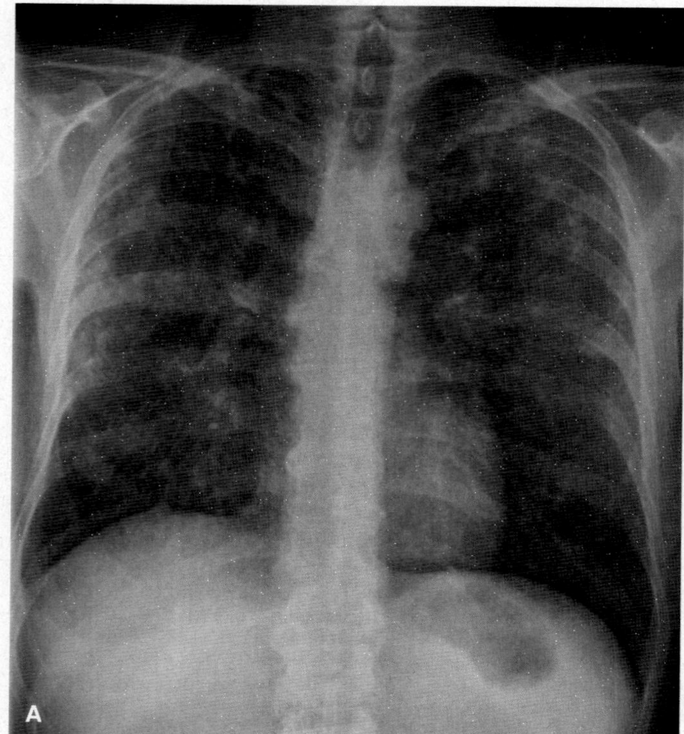

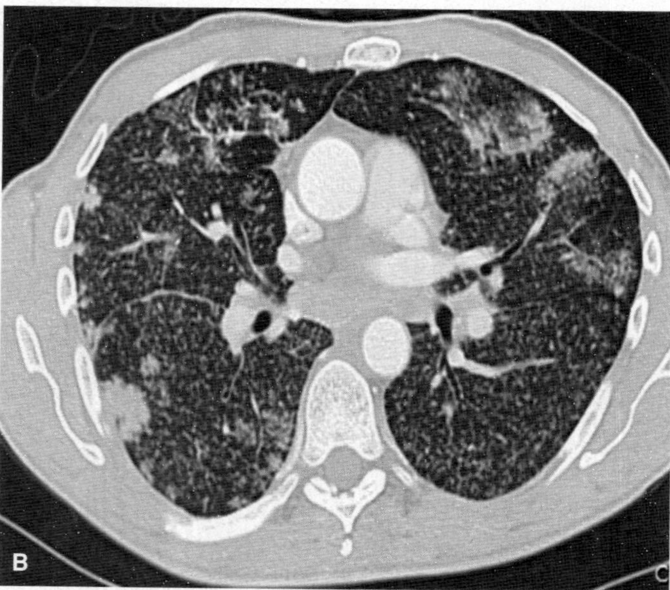

FIGURE 56-10 Disseminated (miliary) tuberculosis with tiny innumerable nodules throughout both lungs. **A.** Chest X-ray. **B.** CT scan. (*Reproduced with permission from Carlos Santiago Restrepo, MD.*)

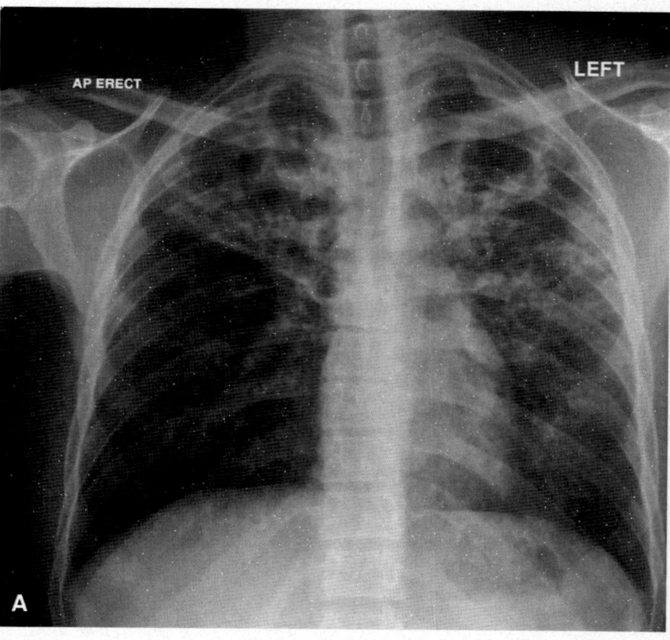

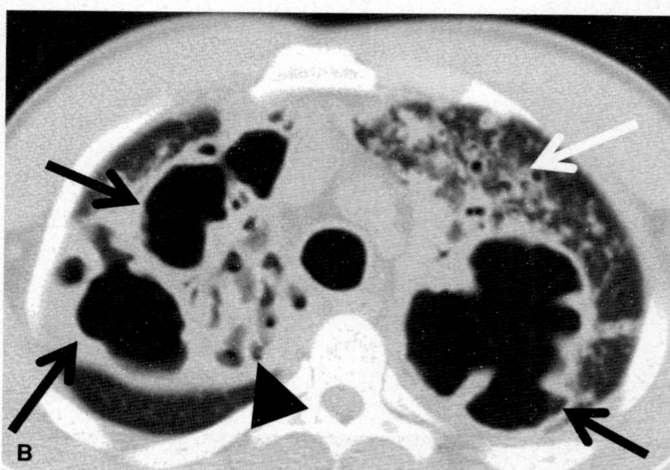

FIGURE 56-11 Reactivation tuberculosis with cavitary lesions in the upper lobes of a 35-year-old man. **A.** Frontal chest radiograph depicts large cavitary lesions in both upper lobes associated with bronchiectasis and fibronodular opacities. **B.** Noncontrast chest CT confirms the presence of irregular cavities in both upper lobes (*black arrows*), nodules (*white arrow*), and bronchiectasis (*black arrowhead*). (*Reproduced with permission from Carlos Santiago Restrepo, MD.*)

without pneumonitis (**Figure 56-12**); patients with chronic pulmonary histoplasmosis have gradually increasing cough, weight loss, and night sweats, and CXR shows uni- or bilateral fibronodular, apical infiltrates; positive serology or culture, immunodiffusion test, or lung biopsy can be diagnostic.

- Coccidiomycosis has similar clinical features to TB, and CXR may show infiltrate, hilar adenopathy, and pleural effusion; serologic tests are useful in the diagnosis.
- Sarcoidosis—No TB contacts, dyspnea and cough, hilar adenopathy on CXR, skin lesions help to differentiate along with serum angiotensin-converting enzyme level or biopsy. Pathology shows noncaseating granulomata (see Chapter 184, Sarcoidosis).

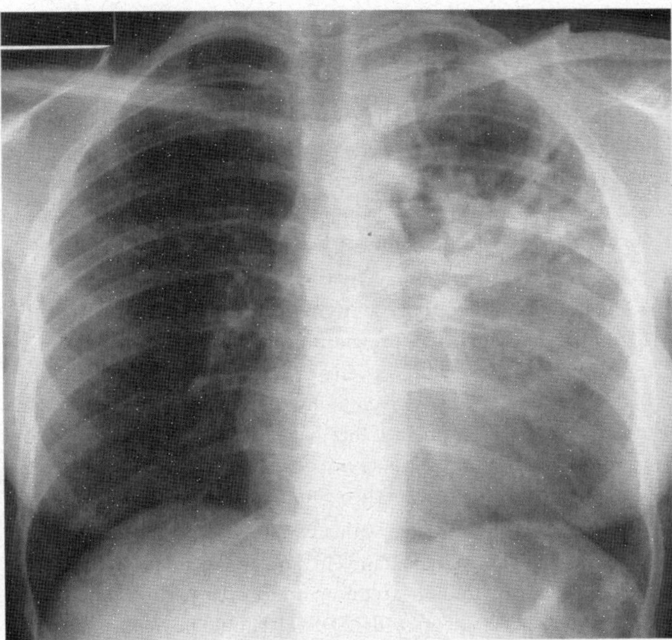

FIGURE 56-12 Histoplasmosis in a 33-year-old man with a 6-month history of fatigue. Chest X-ray shows a 4-cm mass overlying the right hilum and a lumpy contour of the left hilum that indicates lymphadenopathy. Histoplasmosis was diagnosed on bronchoscopy. (*Reproduced with permission from Miller WT: Diagnostic Thoracic Imaging. New York, NY: McGraw-Hill Education; 2006.*)

MANAGEMENT

Patients may be managed by their primary care provider, by public health departments, or jointly, but in all cases the health department is ultimately responsible for ensuring availability of appropriate diagnostic and treatment services and for monitoring results of therapy.

FIRST LINE

MEDICATIONS

Treatment of TB is focused on curing the individual patient and minimizing transmission. Factors favoring delayed or no treatment include patient and clinical factors (increased concern for adverse effects, no TB exposure, stable with atypical features for TB, or alternate diagnosis considered), testing features (imaging not consistent with TB, AFB-smear positive or negative AND rapid molecular test negative), and low transmission risk.[13]

For adult patients with *active TB,* 4 drugs are used for TB with unknown organisms or suspected drug resistance. Review the patient's current medications to avoid drug interactions. Clinically significant drug-drug interactions with rifampin, for example, include lowered concentrations of many antiviral and anti-infective agents as well as cardiovascular, hypoglycemic, hypolipidemic, psychotropic drugs and warfarin.[13] The following regimen is recommended by the ATS/CDC/IDSA guidelines (which can be accessed through the CDC at https://www.cdc.gov/tb/)[13]: SOR Ⓑ

- Two-month initial treatment phase with isoniazid (INH, 5 mg/kg daily [typically 300 mg] or 15 mg/kg once, twice or thrice weekly [typically 900 mg]), rifampin (RIF, 10 mg/kg daily, twice or thrice weekly [typically 600 mg]), pyrazinamide (PZA, dosed by weight category from 1000 to 2000 mg daily, or twice weekly from 2000 to 4000 mg, or thrice weekly from 1500 to 3000 mg); and EMB (dosed by weight category from 800 to 1600 mg daily, or 2000 to 4000 mg twice weekly, or 1200 to 2400 mg thrice weekly). For patients with reduced renal function, PZA is recommended at 25 to 35 mg/kg/dose thrice weekly and EMB at 20 to 25 mg/kg/dose thrice weekly. For pregnant women, the decision to include PZA is made on a case-by-case basis, although its inclusion is recommended by the World Health Organization.
- If treatment is initiated after drug susceptibility test results demonstrate that the patient's isolate is susceptible to both INH and RIF, EMB is not necessary.[13]

- Daily dosing is the preferred regimen, but 5-days-a-week drug administration by directly observed therapy (DOT) is an acceptable alternative.
- Four-month continuation phase with INH and rifampin; treatment is extended to 7 months for patients with cavitary pulmonary TB who remain sputum-positive after initial treatment or if pregnant and PZA is not used. Breastfeeding is encouraged for women who are deemed noninfectious and are being treated with first-line agents.
- To prevent INH-related neuropathy, pyridoxine at 25–50 mg/day is given, especially to those at higher risk for neuropathy (e.g., alcoholic, malnourished, pregnant or lactating women, HIV-infection, and those with diabetes or chronic renal disease).[13] SOR Ⓐ Pyridoxine is also given to infants, children, and adolescents undergoing INH treatment if they have nutritional deficiencies, symptomatic HIV infection, or are breastfeeding. In patients with peripheral neuropathy, experts recommend a dose of 100 mg/day.
- Drug-resistant TB is treated with a variety of injectable drugs including streptomycin, kanamycin, and amikacin, or oral drugs, including fluoroquinolones, ethionamide, cycloserine, and *p*-aminosalicylic acid.[6] Patients with MDR TB should be managed in consultation with an expert in the disease.
- For children, a 4-drug regimen (INH [10–15 mg/kg daily or 20–30 mg/kg twice weekly], RIF [10–20 mg/kg daily or twice weekly], PZA [30–40 mg/kg daily or 50 mg/kg twice weekly], and EMB [15–25 mg/kg daily or 50 mg/kg twice weekly]) for 2 months followed by INH and RIF for 4 months is the preferred regimen with suspected or confirmed pulmonary TB.[13]
- Details for treatment in special situations such as patients with HIV infection and patients with extrapulmonary TB are provided in the ATS/CDC/IDSA guidelines.[13] In HIV-infected adults with newly diagnosed TB, early antiretroviral therapy improves survival if the patient's CD4+ T-cell count is less than 0.050 × 109 cells/L; early treatment, however, increases TB-associated immune reconstitution inflammatory syndrome twofold.[14] For adult patients with *latent TB*, treatment should be initiated after the possibility of active TB has been excluded.[15]
- Persons with high priority for treatment of latent TB include those who have either a positive IGRA result *or* a reaction to the TST of 5 mm or larger *and* who have HIV infection, recent contact with a TB case, radiographic changes consistent with old TB, an organ transplant, or immunosuppression. Patients are also high priority if they have a positive IGRA result *or* a TST of 10 mm or larger *and* are recent (<5 years) immigrants, injection drug users, residents and employees of high-risk congregate settings, mycobacteriology laboratory personnel, children under age 4 years, or children or adolescents exposed to adults in high-risk categories. The following options are preferred:
    - INH 5 mg/kg for adults and 10–15 mg/kg for children daily (maximum 300 mg) or 15 mg/kg for adults and 20–30 mg/kg for children twice weekly via DOT for 9 months. SOR Ⓐ
- In an open-label, randomized noninferiority trial comparing 3 months of once-weekly DOT with rifapentine plus INH with 9 months of self-administered daily INH (300 mg) in subjects at high risk for TB, rates of TB were comparable (7 of 3986 subjects in the combination-therapy group [cumulative rate, 0.19%] and in 15 of 3745 subjects in the INH-only group [cumulative rate, 0.43%]) and completion rates were higher.[16] Three additional RCTs (Brazil, South Africa, and International) have shown that this combination regimen administered weekly for 12 weeks as DOT is as effective for preventing TB as other regimens and is more likely to be completed than the U.S. standard regimen of 9 months of INH daily without DOT.[15]
- Refusal of treatment for latent TB in another study at 32 clinics was 17.1% (95% CI, 14.5% to 20.0%) and 52.7% (95% CI, 48.5% to 56.8%) failed to complete the recommended course.[17]

SECOND LINE

NONPHARMACOLOGIC

- There are insufficient data to support use of free food or nutritional supplements on improving treatment outcome or quality of life in individuals with TB in the United States.[18] Although plasma levels of zinc, vitamin D, vitamin E, and selenium improve with supplementation, there is no evidence of clinical benefit.

MEDICATION

- Second-line regimens for active TB include 3 times weekly INH, RIF, PZA, and EMB for 24 weeks (use with caution in patients with HIV or cavitary disease) and daily INH, RIF, PZA, and EMB for 14 doses followed by twice-weekly doses for 12 doses.[13]
- Second-line drugs for active TB include cycloserine, ethionamide, streptomycin, amikacin/kanamycin, capreomycin, *para*-amino salicylic acid, levofloxacin, and moxifloxacin.
- For latent TB, 6-month therapy with INH (5 mg/kg daily [maximum 300 mg] or 15 mg/kg twice weekly [maximum 900 mg] via DOT) may be considered for adults who are not HIV-infected and have no fibrotic lesions on CXR.[15] SOR Ⓑ The standard treatment regimen is preferred for HIV-infected people taking antiretroviral therapy (ART) and children 2 to 11 years of age. Pyridoxine supplementation is provided as noted above.
- A 4-month regimen of RIF (10 mg/kg daily [maximum 600 mg] for adults) can be considered for persons who cannot tolerate INH or who have been exposed to INH-resistant TB.[15] It should not be used to treat HIV-infected persons taking some combinations of ART. For children, the American Academy of Pediatrics recommends 6 months of daily therapy at 10–20 mg/kg of RIF.[15]
- Rifapentine (dosed by weight with 900 mg maximum; a rifamycin derivative) plus INH (15 mg/kg; 900 mg maximum) for 3 months via DOT once weekly can be used for adults and children over age 12 years.[15] SOR Ⓑ Authors of a meta-analysis found that therapies containing rifamycins for 3 months or more were potentially more efficacious at preventing active TB than INH alone.[19]
- Adjuvant corticosteroid treatment in patients with active TB did not reduce all-cause mortality, although there may be some short-term clinical benefit.[20]

PREVENTION

- There is no currently available vaccine with adequate effectiveness for the prevention of TB,[3] although approximately 10 vaccines are in the clinical trial phase.[21] BCG vaccine, first released in 1921, can prevent up to 50% of TB cases.[22]

- BCG vaccine also has a protective effect against meningitis and disseminated TB in children, although it does not appear to prevent primary infection or reactivation of latent pulmonary infection, the principal source of bacillary spread in many communities.
- In clinical trials in Guinea-Bissau, vaccination at birth of low-birth-weight infants decreased mortality, whereas revaccination of children with BCG appeared to increase mortality, resulting in early discontinuation of the trial.[23,24] A recent trial of a new vaccine in previously BCG-vaccinated infants was not effective in preventing TB incidence or conversion compared to controls.[25] The CDC recommends that BCG vaccine be considered only for very select persons who meet specific criteria and in consultation with a TB expert.[26]
- In an RCT, the use of primary INH prophylaxis did not improve tuberculosis disease-free survival among HIV-infected children or tuberculosis infection-free survival among HIV-uninfected children immunized with BCG vaccine.[27]
- In an evidence report on primary care screening for latent TB, authors were unable to identify any trials evaluating benefit of screening vs. no screening.[28] TST and IGRAs were moderately sensitive and highly specific within countries with low TB burden. In the single large treatment trial of patients with latent TB and fibrotic pulmonary lesions, 6 months of daily INH versus placebo reduced the absolute risk of active TB at 5 years from 1.4% to 0.5% but increased the absolute risk for hepatotoxicity from 0.1% to 0.5%. The U.S. Preventive Services Task Force recommends screening for latent tuberculosis infection (LTBI) in populations at increased risk. SOR Ⓑ
- For prevention of progression to active TB, the CDC recommends that the following groups receive treatment for latent TB (as discussed above):
  - People with HIV infection
  - People with recent (in the last 2 years) TB infection
  - Infants, young children, and the elderly
  - People who inject illegal drugs
  - People with immunosuppressing comorbidities
  - People inadequately treated for TB in the past
- CDC consensus-based recommendations to prevent TB spread include administrative measures such as education, training, risk assessment, and testing exposed workers; environmental controls such as use of exhaust hoods and controlling air flow; and respiratory-protective equipment.[29]

PROGNOSIS

- Without treatment, approximately one-third of individuals with active TB will die within 1 year and half within 5 years. Of those who survive 5 years, 60% will have undergone spontaneous remission and the remainder will continue to be infectious.[30]

FOLLOW-UP SOR Ⓒ

- Patients are considered contagious until they have been on adequate chemotherapy for a minimum of 2 weeks, have 3 negative AFB sputum cultures (collected in 8- to 24-hour intervals with 1 early morning specimen), and show clinical improvement.[31]
- Monitor clinical recovery including weight, medication adverse effects (e.g., vision if on EMB), and compliance with treatment monthly; risk factors for noncompliance include lack of motivation, lack of perceived vulnerability, and poverty. The ATS/CDC/IDSA guidelines also recommend monthly testing of liver function in patients at high risk of hepatotoxicity (e.g., alcohol use, prior liver injury) and creatinine and/or platelet count if there are baseline abnormalities.[13]
- Monitor response to treatment—Monthly sputum cultures should be obtained until culture negative (80% expected by 2 months). If culture positive at 3 or more months, consider drug resistance or treatment failure and institute additional evaluation and treatment. For those with extrapulmonary TB, monitor clinically.[6,13]
- CXR is not used for monitoring treatment, as clearing lags behind clinical improvement. A CXR should be completed at the end of treatment for later comparison if reactivation is suspected.[6]
- Monitor drug toxicity[6,13]:
  - GI side effects and pruritus are common and can generally be managed without suspending treatment. Symptoms may be minimized by taking medication at bedtime or use of antacids or proton pump inhibitors.
  - Hepatitis is the most common serious adverse event (symptoms include dark urine and decreased appetite); elevation of liver enzymes up to 3 times normal occurs in 20% and is of no clinical importance. Treatment (INH, PZA, or RIF) should be discontinued for elevations of 5 times or more or with symptoms and drugs reintroduced one at a time after liver function has normalized.
  - Hypersensitivity reactions usually require discontinuing treatment. The presence of skin itching without mucous membrane involvement or systemic signs can be managed with an antihistamine. Suspect thrombocytopenia from RIF with a petechial rash.
  - Hyperuricemia and arthralgias may occur with PZA and can be managed with aspirin; the drug should be discontinued if the patient develops gouty arthritis.
  - Autoimmune thrombocytopenia may be caused by RIF and requires discontinuing the drug.
  - Optic neuritis may occur with EMB, and the drug should be discontinued. Visual acuity and color vision testing monthly if EMB is used for more than 2 months or in doses greater than 15 to 20 mg/kg.[13] If vision does not improve with discontinuation of EMB, consider discontinuing INH, which can also rarely cause optic neuritis.

PATIENT EDUCATION

- Identifying and testing household and other intimate contacts and maintaining follow-up are extremely important for preventing spread, insuring cure, and monitoring for drug toxicity (as below). The potential severity of TB should be emphasized.
- If available, patients should consider receiving treatment through a short course program composed of five distinct elements: political commitment; microscopy services; drug supplies; surveillance and monitoring systems and use of highly efficacious regimens; and DOT.[32] Although data are conflicting about the benefits of such programs, they may be better equipped to provide the intense

services needed, especially in resource-poor communities. DOT is recommended for the 3-month combination RIF and INH treatment.

- TB is not spread through direct contact, sharing food, or kissing. The best prevention of progression and spread is to take the prescribed medications regularly for the recommended duration and to avoid unnecessary contact with people from outside the household (e.g., avoid work, daycare facilities, or schools) for the first 2 weeks of treatment and until the patient has three negative AFB sputum cultures and feels better.
- Authors of a Cochrane review found that patient education and counseling interventions may improve completion of treatment for patients with latent TB.[33]

PATIENT RESOURCES

- Centers for Disease Control and Prevention. *Tuberculosis (TB)*—**http://www.cdc.gov/tb/.**
- MedlinePlus. *Tuberculosis*—**http://www.nlm.nih.gov/medlineplus/tuberculosis.html.**

PROVIDER RESOURCES

- Centers for Disease Control and Prevention. *Tuberculosis (TB)*—**http://www.cdc.gov/tb/.**
- Lewinsohn DM, Leonard MK, LoBue PA, et al. Official American Thoracic Society (ATS)/Infectious Diseases Society of America (IDSA)/Centers for Disease Control and Prevention Practice Guidelines: Diagnosis of tuberculosis in adults and children. *Clin Infect Dis*. 2014;64(2):111-115. **https://www.cdc.gov/tb/publications/guidelines/testing.htm.**
- Nahid P, Dorman SE, Alipanah N, et al. Official American Thoracic Society/Centers for Disease Control and Prevention/Infectious Diseases Society of America Clinical Practice Guidelines: Treatment of drug-susceptible tuberculosis. *Clin Infect Diseases*. 2016;63(7):e147-e195. **https://www.cdc.gov/tb/publications/guidelines/treatment.htm.**
- Occupational Safety & Health Administration. *Tuberculosis*—**http://www.osha.gov/SLTC/tuberculosis/index.html.**

REFERENCES

1. Murray CJ, Ortblad KF, Guinovart C, et al. Global, regional, and national incidence and mortality for HIV, tuberculosis, and malaria during 1990-2013: a systematic analysis for the Global Burden of Disease Study 2013. *Lancet*. 2014;384(9947):1005-1070.
2. Centers for Disease Control and Prevention. *Trends in Tuberculosis, 2015 (Fact Sheet)*. http://www.cdc.gov/tb/publications/factsheets/statistics/tbtrends.htm. Accessed January 2017.
3. Lawn SD, Zumla AI. Tuberculosis. *Lancet*. 2011;378(9785):57-72.
4. Jenkins HE, Tolman AW, Yuen CM, et al. Incidence of multidrug-resistant tuberculosis disease in children: systematic review and global estimates. *Lancet*. 2014;383(9928):1572-1579.
5. Yuen CM, Jenkins HE, Rodriguez CA, et al. Global and regional burden of isoniazid-resistant tuberculosis. *Pediatrics*. 2015;136(1):e50-e59.
6. Escalante P. In the clinic. Tuberculosis. *Ann Intern Med*. 2009;150(11):ITC61-614.
7. Bailey TC, Fraser VJ, Spitznagel EL, Dunagan WC. Risk factors for a positive tuberculin skin test among employees of an urban, Midwestern teaching hospital. *Ann Intern Med*. 1995;122(8):580-585.
8. Lewinsohn DM, Leonard MK, LoBue PA, et al. Official American Thoracic Society (ATS)/Infectious Diseases Society of America (IDSA)/Centers for Disease Control and Prevention Practice Guidelines: Diagnosis of tuberculosis in adults and children. *Clin Infect Dis*. 2017;64(2):111-115.
9. Diel R, Loddenkemper R, Nienhaus A. Predictive value of interferon-γ release assays and tuberculin skin testing for progression from latent TB infection to disease state: a meta-analysis. *Chest*. 2012;142(1):63-75.
10. Ge L, Ma JC, Han M, et al. Interferon-γ release assay for the diagnosis of latent *Mycobacterium tuberculosis* infection in children younger than 5 years: a meta-analysis. *Clin Pediatr (Phila)*. 2014;53(13):1255-1263.
11. Adekambi T, Ibegbu CC, Cagle S, et al. Biomarkers on patient T cells diagnose active tuberculosis and monitor treatment response. *J Clin Invest*. 2015;125(5):1827-1838.
12. Jain AK. Tuberculosis of the spine: a fresh look at an old disease. *J Bone Joint Surg Br*. 2010;92(7):905-913.
13. Nahid P, Dorman SE, Alipanah N, et al. Official American Thoracic Society/Centers for Disease Control and Prevention/ Infectious Diseases Society of America Clinical Practice Guidelines: Treatment of drug-susceptible tuberculosis. *Clin Infect Dis*. 2016; 63(7):e147-e195.
14. Uthman OA, Okwundu C, Gbenga K, et al. Optimal timing of antiretroviral therapy initiation for HIV-infected adults with newly diagnosed pulmonary tuberculosis: a systematic review and meta-analysis. *Ann Intern Med*. 2015;163(1):32-39.
15. Centers for Disease Control and Prevention. *Treatment Regimens for Latent TB Infection*. https://www.cdc.gov/tb/topic/treatment/ltbi.htm. Accessed February 2017.
16. Sterling TR, Villarino ME, Borisov AS, et al. Three months of rifapentine and isoniazid for latent tuberculosis infection. *N Engl J Med*. 2011;365(23):2155-2166.
17. Horsburgh CR Jr, Goldberg S, Bethel J, et al. Latent TB infection treatment acceptance and completion in the United States and Canada. *Chest*. 2010;137(2):401-409.
18. Grobler L, Nagpal S, Sudarsanam TD, Sinclair D. Nutritional supplements for people being treated for active tuberculosis. *Cochrane Database Syst Rev*. 2016;(6):CD006086.
19. Stagg HR, Zenner D, Harris RJ, et al. Treatment of latent tuberculosis infection: a network meta-analysis. *Ann Intern Med*. 2014; 161(6):419-428.
20. Critchley JA, Orton LC, Pearson F. Adjunctive steroid therapy for managing pulmonary tuberculosis. *Cochrane Database Syst Rev*. 2014;(11):CD011370.

21. Kaufmann SH, Hussey G, Lambert PH. New vaccines for tuberculosis. *Lancet.* 2010;375(9731):2110-2119.
22. Colditz GA, Brewer TF, Berkley CS, et al. Efficacy of BCG vaccine in the prevention of tuberculosis. Meta-analysis of the published literature. *JAMA.* 1994;271(9):698-702.
23. Aaby P, Roth A, Ravn H, et al. Randomized trial of BCG vaccination at birth to low-birth-weight children: beneficial nonspecific effects in the neonatal period? *J Infect Dis.* 2011;204(2):245-252.
24. Roth AE, Benn CS, Ravn H, et al. Effect of revaccination with BCG in early childhood on mortality: randomised trial in Guinea-Bissau. *BMJ.* 2010;340:c671.
25. Tameris MD, Hatherill M, Landry BS, et al. Safety and efficacy of MVA85A, a new tuberculosis vaccine, in infants previously vaccinated with BCG: a randomised, placebo-controlled phase 2b trial. *Lancet.* 2013;381(9871):1021-1028.
26. Centers for Disease Control and Prevention. Fact Sheets. *BCG Vaccine.* https://www.cdc.gov/tb/publications/factsheets/prevention/bcg.htm. Accessed February 2017.
27. Madhi SA, Nachman S, Violari A, et al. Primary isoniazid prophylaxis against tuberculosis in HIV-exposed children. *N Engl J Med.* 2011;365(1):21-31.
28. Kahwati LC, Feltner C, Halpern M, et al. Primary care screening and treatment for latent tuberculosis infection in adults: evidence report and systematic review for the US Preventive Services Task Force. *JAMA.* 2016;316(9):970-983.
29. Centers for Disease Control and Prevention. *Infection Control in Health-Care Settings.* https://www.cdc.gov/tb/topic/infectioncontrol/default.htm. Accessed January 2017.
30. Raviglione MC, O'Brien RJ. Tuberculosis. In: Kasper DL, Braunwald E, Fauci AS, et al., eds. *Harrison's Principles of Internal Medicine*, 16th ed. New York, NY: McGraw-Hill; 2005:953-966.
31. Centers for Disease Control and Prevention. *Menu of Suggested Provision For State Tuberculosis Prevention and Control Laws.* https://www.cdc.gov/tb/programs/laws/menu/isolation.htm. Accessed February 2017.
32. Davies PD. The role of DOTS in tuberculosis treatment and control. *Am J Respir Med.* 2003;2(3):203-209.
33. M'Imunya JM, Kredo T, Volmink J. Patient education and counselling for promoting adherence to treatment for tuberculosis. *Cochrane Database Syst Rev.* 2012;(5):CD006591.

57 ASTHMA

Mindy A. Smith, MD, MS

PATIENT STORY

A 32-year-old Hispanic woman presents to your office with a chronic cough for 3 months. She states the cough is dry and started with a cold 3 months ago. She denies fever, chills, and night sweats. She has never been diagnosed with asthma or lung disease in the past. She has had persistent dry coughs that linger on after getting colds in the past. She is not sure what wheezing is but she has noticed a tight feeling in her chest at night with some whistling sound. On physical examination, her lungs are clear and she is moving air well. She is 5 feet tall and weighs 220 pounds, giving her a body mass index (BMI) of 43. Her peak expiratory flow (PEF) in the office is at 80% of predicted. Even though she is not wheezing, her history and physical exam are highly suspicious for asthma. You prescribe a short-acting β_2-agonist rescue inhaler with spacer and order pulmonary function tests (PFTs). You have your nurse provide asthma education (including proper use of an inhaler) and suggestions for weight loss.

The patient returns 1 week later and the cough is much improved. You review her PFTs (**Figure 57-1**) and note that she has reversible bronchospasm especially in the small airways ($FEF_{25\%-75\%}$ shows a 70% improvement with inhaled albuterol). **Table 57-1** lists the meaning of typical abbreviations used with PFTs. Her lung volumes (**Figure 57-1B**) show hyperinflation with a high residual volume and normal diffusing capacity. The whole picture is consistent with asthma. An asthma action plan is created and a referral to a nutritionist is offered to help the patient with her obesity.

TABLE 57-1 Pulmonary Function Tests: Key to Abbreviations

DLCO	Diffusing capacity of lung (using carbon monoxide measuring)
DL/VA	Diffusing capacity divided by alveolar volume
ERV (L)	Expiratory reserve volume
$FEF_{25\%}$ (L/s)	Forced expiratory flow rate when 25% of the FVC has been exhaled (slope of FVC curve at 25% exhaled)
$FEF_{25-75\%}$ (L/s)	Forced expiratory flow between 25% and 75% of capacity—same as maximal mid expiratory flow (MMFR)
$FEF_{50\%}$ (L/s)	Forced expiratory flow rate when 50% of the FVC has been exhaled
$FEF_{75\%}$ (L/s)	Forced expiratory flow rate when 75% of the FVC has been exhaled
FEF_{max} (L/s)	Forced expiratory flow maximum
FEV_1 (L)	Forced vital capacity at 1 second
FEV_1/FVC %	FEV_1 divided by FVC
$FIF_{50\%}$ (L/s)	Forced inspiratory flow at 50% capacity
FITC (L)	Forced inspiratory vital capacity
FVC (L)	Forced vital capacity
IC (L)	Inspiratory capacity
Raw	Airway resistance
RV (L)	Residual volume
RV/TLC	Residual volume divided by total lung capacity
SVC (L)	Slow vital capacity
TGV (L)	Thoracic gas volume
TLC (L)	Total lung capacity
VA (L)	Alveolar volume

INTRODUCTION

Asthma is a chronic inflammatory airway disorder with variable airflow obstruction and bronchial hyperresponsiveness that is at least partially reversible, spontaneously or with treatment (e.g., β_2-agonist treatment). Patients with asthma have recurrent episodes of wheezing, breathlessness, chest tightness, and cough (particularly at night or in the early morning).

EPIDEMIOLOGY

- Estimated prevalence of asthma in noninstitutionalized adults older than age 18 years in the United States (2014) is approximately 7.4% (17.7 million cases).[1] There are 6.3 million children (8.6%) who currently have asthma. Prevalence is highest among African-American children (10.3%).[2]
- The number of deaths from asthma in 2014 was 3651 (1.1/100,000 population).[1]
- Asthma was recorded on the medial record in 6.5% of visits to office-based physicians (2013).[1]
- Asthma was the first-listed diagnosis for 493,000 hospital discharges in 2010 with an average length of stay of 3.6 days.[1]
- Estimated yearly costs associated with asthma in the United States are approximately $56 billion with direct costs of about $3259 per person and indirect costs of about $2.2 billion.[3]

	Pre-Bronch			Post-Bronch		
	Pred	Actual	%Pred	Actual	%Pred	%Chng
— SPIROMETRY —						
FVC (L)	3.14	3.27	104	3.69	117	+12
FEV_1 (L)	2.64	2.16	81	2.68	101	+24
FEV_1/FVC (%)	85	66	77	73	85	+9
$FEF_{25-75\%}$ (L/s)	3.14	1.44	45	2.47	78	+70
FEF_{Max} (L/s)	6.14	4.83	78	6.73	109	+39
$FEF_{25\%}$ (L/s)	5.06	2.88	56	4.70	92	+62
$FEF_{50\%}$ (L/s)	4.36	1.72	39	2.82	64	+64
$FEF_{75\%}$ (L/s)	1.79	0.69	38	1.28	71	+86
FIVC (L)		3.24		3.75		+15
$FIF_{50\%}$ (L/s)	4.18	5.09	121	5.45	130	+6

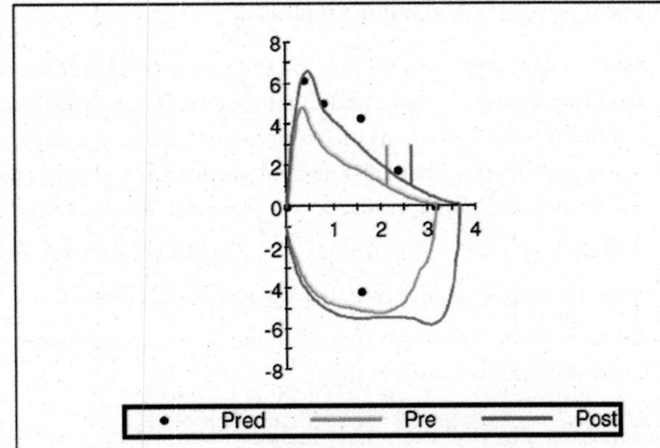

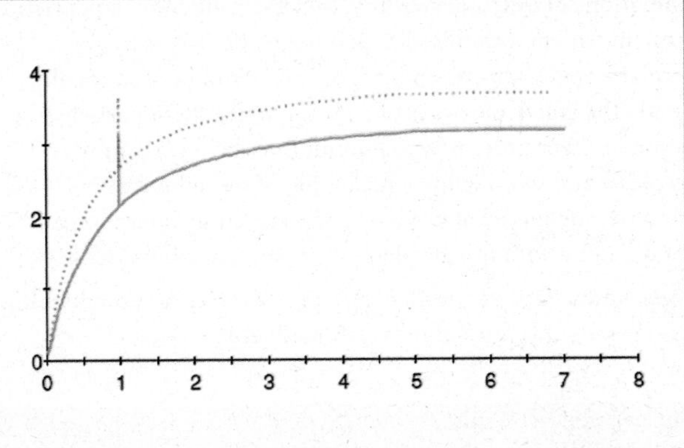

	Pre-Bronch			Post-Bronch		
	Pred	Actual	%Pred	Actual	%Pred	%Chng
— LUNG VOLUMES —						
SVC (L)	3.14	3.17	101			
TLC (Pleth) (L)	4.30	5.12	119			
RV (Pleth) (L)	1.23	1.95	158			
RV/TLC (Pleth) (%)	29	38	131			
TGV (L)	2.32	3.33	143			
Raw (cmH_2O/L/s)	1.86	3.71	199			
ERV (L)	1.16	1.38	118			
IC (L)	1.98	1.79	90			
— DIFFUSION —						
DLCOunc (mL/min/mm H_2)	17.53	27.25	155			
DLCOcor (mL/min/mm H_2)	17.53					
VA (L)	4.30	5.11	118			
DL/VA (mL/min/mm Hg)	4.08	5.33	130			

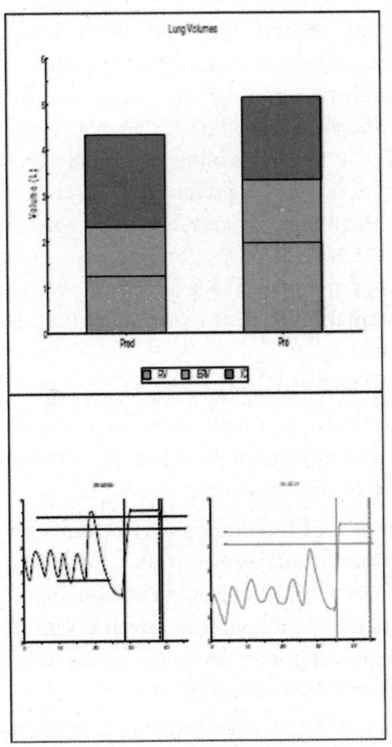

B

FIGURE 57-1 Pulmonary function tests in a woman with suspected asthma. **A.** Spirometry before and after bronchodilation with flow volumes loops and graph of forced vital capacity. The FEV_1 is normal, but the FEV_1/FVC ratio and $FEF_{25-75\%}$ are reduced. Following administration of bronchodilators, there is a good response especially in the small airways as represented by $FEF_{25-75\%}$. **B.** Lung volumes are all increased (especially the residual volume), indicating overinflation and air trapping. The diffusing capacity is normal. Conclusions: Minimal airway obstruction, overinflation, and a response to bronchodilators are consistent with a diagnosis of asthma. The patient has minimal obstructive airways disease of the asthmatic type. *%Chng*, percent change; *%Pred*, percent predicted; *Pre-Bronch*, prebronchodilation; *Pred*, predicted; *Post-Bronch*, postbronchodilation. See **Table 57-1** for additional abbreviation explanations. (*Reproduced with permission from Richard P. Usatine, MD.*)

ETIOLOGY AND PATHOPHYSIOLOGY

- Although the precise cause is unknown, early exposure to airborne allergens (e.g., house-dust mite, cockroach antigens) and childhood respiratory infections (e.g., respiratory syncytial virus, parainfluenza) are associated with asthma development.
- In addition to environmental factors, asthma has an inherited component, although the genetics involved remain complex.[4] There are a number of asthma-risk genetic loci that have been identified.[5] A nested case-control study found that genetic variation in the ATPAF1 gene predisposed children of different racial backgrounds to asthma.[6]
- The pulmonary obstruction characterizing asthma results from combinations of mucosal swelling, mucus production, constriction of bronchiolar smooth muscles, and neutrophils (the last is particularly important in smokers or those with occupational asthma). The smaller airways of children make them particularly susceptible. Over time, airway smooth muscle hypertrophy and hyperplasia and remodeling (thickening of the subbasement membrane, subepithelial fibrosis, and vascular proliferation and dilation), along with mucus plugging, complicate the disease.
- Allergen-induced acute bronchospasm involves immunoglobulin-E (IgE)-dependent release of mast cell mediators.

RISK FACTORS

- Based on a cohort study, early life (first 5 years) risk factors for diagnosed asthma at age 10 years include[7]:
  - Family history of asthma (maternal [odds ratio (OR), 2.26; 95% confidence interval (CI), 1.24 to 3.73]; paternal [OR, 2.30; 95% CI, 1.17 to 4.52]; sibling [OR, 2.00; 95% CI, 1.16 to 3.43]).
  - Recurrent chest infections at 1 year of age (OR, 2.67; 95% CI, 1.12 to 6.40) and 2 years of age (OR, 4.11; 95% CI, 2.06 to 8.18).
  - Atopy at 4 years of age (OR, 7.22; 95% CI, 4.13 to 12.62).
  - Parental smoking at 1 year of age (OR, 1.99; 95% CI, 1.15 to 3.45).
  - Male gender (OR, 1.72; 95% CI, 1.01 to 2.95).
- Authors of a systematic review and meta-analysis found pre- or postnatal passive smoke exposure was associated with at least a 20% increased risk of incident wheezing.[8]
- Recent use of acetaminophen has also been associated with asthma symptoms in adolescents (OR, 1.43; 95% CI, 1.33 to 1.53 and OR, 2.51; 95% CI, 2.33 to 2.70 for at least once a year and at least once a month use vs. no use, respectively).[9] One possible mechanism is through acetaminophen reducing the immune response and prolonging rhinovirus infection.[10]
- Other modifiable risk factors include adult and childhood obesity,[11,12] rapid increase in BMI in the first 2 years of life (hazard ratio 1.3 [95% CI, 1.1–1.5]),[13] and tobacco smoking. In one study, consumption of salty snacks (OR 4.8; 95% CI, 1.50 to 15.8) was strongly associated with the presence of asthma symptoms, especially in children with television/video-game viewing of more than 2 hours per day.[14]

DIAGNOSIS

The diagnosis of asthma is made on clinical suspicion (presence of symptoms of recurrent and partially reversible airflow obstruction and airway hyperresponsiveness) and confirmed with spirometry.[4] Alternative diagnoses should be excluded.

CLINICAL FEATURES

Asthma's most common symptoms are recurrent wheezing, difficulty breathing, chest tightness, and cough. An absence of wheezing or normal physical exam does not exclude asthma.[4] In fact, up to 25% of patients with asthma have normal physical exams even though abnormalities are seen on pulmonary function testing.[15] As part of the diagnosis of asthma, ask about the following[4]:

- Pattern of symptoms and precipitating factors. Symptoms often occur or worsen at night and during exercise, viral infection, exposure to inhalant allergens or irritants (e.g., tobacco smoke, wood smoke, airborne chemicals), changes in weather, strong emotional expression (laughing hard or crying), menstrual cycle, and stress.[4]
- Family history of asthma, allergy, or atopy in close relatives.
- Social history (e.g., daycare, workplace, social support).
- History of exacerbations (e.g., frequency, duration, treatment) and impact on patient and family.

Findings on physical exam may include[4]:

- Upper respiratory tract—Increased nasal secretion, mucosal swelling, and/or nasal polyp.
- Lungs—Decreased intensity of breath sounds is the most common (33% to 65% of patients).[15] Additional findings may include wheezing, prolonged phase of forced exhalation, use of accessory respiratory muscles, appearance of hunched shoulders, and chest deformity. During a severe exacerbation of asthma, minimal airflow may result in no audible wheezing.
- Skin—Atopic dermatitis and/or eczema (see Chapters 151, Atopic Dermatitis; 153, Hand Eczema; and 154, Nummular Eczema). There is a strong association between asthma, allergic rhinoconjunctivitis, and eczema (**Figure 57-2**), although the "atopic or allergic triad," with the coexistence of all three conditions at one time (**Figure 57-3**), is not very common. Children with asthma are also more likely to develop pityriasis alba, a chronic skin disorder characterized by patches of lighter skin mainly on the face (**Figure 57-4**). In a U.S. study of children with physician-confirmed atopic dermatitis (N = 2270), 38% reported symptoms of asthma and allergic rhinitis on a survey[16]; similarly, in a population study in Taiwan using the National Insurance register, of the 66,446 individuals diagnosed with atopic dermatitis, approximately 50% had a concomitant diagnosis of allergic rhinitis and/or asthma.[17] Data support a sequence of atopic manifestations beginning typically with atopic dermatitis in infancy followed by allergic rhinitis and/or asthma in later stages.[18]

Findings in patients with status asthmaticus (prolonged/severe asthma attack that is not responsive to standard treatment) may include[15]:

- Tachycardia (heart rate >120 beats/min) and tachypnea (respiratory rate >30 breaths/min).

- Use of accessory respiratory muscles.
- Pulsus paradoxus (inspiratory decrease in systolic blood pressure >10 mm Hg).
- Mental status changes (due to hypoxia and hypercapnia).
- Paradoxical abdominal and diaphragmatic movement on inspiration.

LABORATORY TESTING

The National Asthma Education and Prevention Program (NAEPP) recommends spirometry for all patients older than 4 years of age to determine airway obstruction that is at least partially reversible (**Figures 57-1, 57-5,** and **57-6**).[3] SOR Ⓑ

- Assess severity—Severity is defined as the intrinsic intensity of the disease process.[4] The NAEPP divides severity into four groups: intermittent, persistent-mild, persistent-moderate, and persistent-severe (**Table 57-2**).
- Initially, severity can be assessed in the office, urgent, or emergency care setting with predicted forced expiratory volume in 1 second (FEV_1) or PEF; a value of less than 40% indicates a severe exacerbation. A value of equal to or greater than 70% predicted FEV_1 or PEF is a goal for discharge from the emergency care setting.
- Once asthma control is achieved, severity can be assessed by the step of care required for control (see Medications).

Additional tests that may be useful include[4]:

- Pulmonary function testing if a diagnosis of chronic obstructive pulmonary disease (COPD), restrictive lung disease, or vocal cord dysfunction is considered.
- Bronchoprovocation (using methacholine, histamine, cold air, or exercise challenge) if spirometry is normal or near-normal and asthma is still suspected; a negative test is helpful in ruling out asthma.
- Pulse oximetry or arterial blood gas if hypoxia is suspected (e.g., cyanosis, rapid respiratory rate).
- In the emergency room setting, B-type natriuretic peptide can help distinguish between heart failure and pulmonary disease.[15]

IMAGING

A chest X-ray (CXR) is not useful for asthma diagnosis but is helpful for excluding other diseases (e.g., pneumonia) or identifying comorbidity (e.g., heart failure). The main finding on CXR is hyperinflation (occurring in approximately 45% of patients with asthma).[15] Hyperinflation is manifested by the following:

- Increased anteroposterior (AP) diameter.
- Increased retrosternal air space (**Figure 57-7**).
- Infracardiac air.
- Low-set flattened diaphragms (best assessed in lateral chest).
- Vertical heart.

Atelectasis is another finding seen during acute severe episodes (**Figure 57-8**).

Similarly, for patients with severe asthma, the European Respiratory Society/American Thoracic Society (ERS/ATS) guidelines recommend high-resolution computed tomography only when the presentation is atypical.[19]

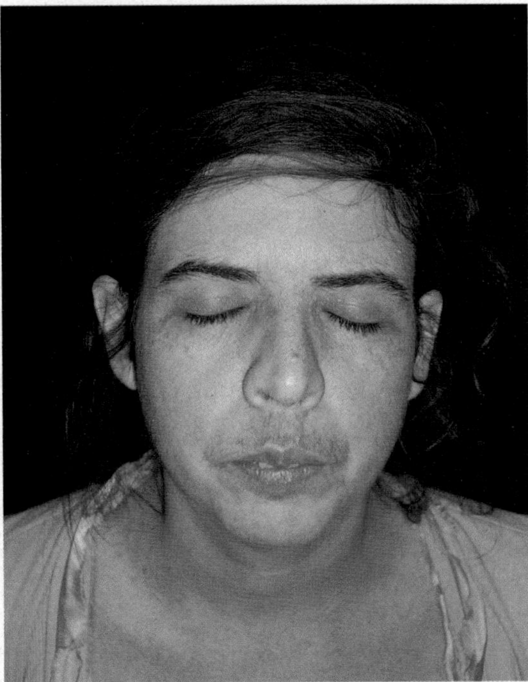

FIGURE 57-2 Patient with severe asthma, atopic dermatitis, and allergic rhinitis—atopic triad. *(Reproduced with permission from Richard P. Usatine, MD.)*

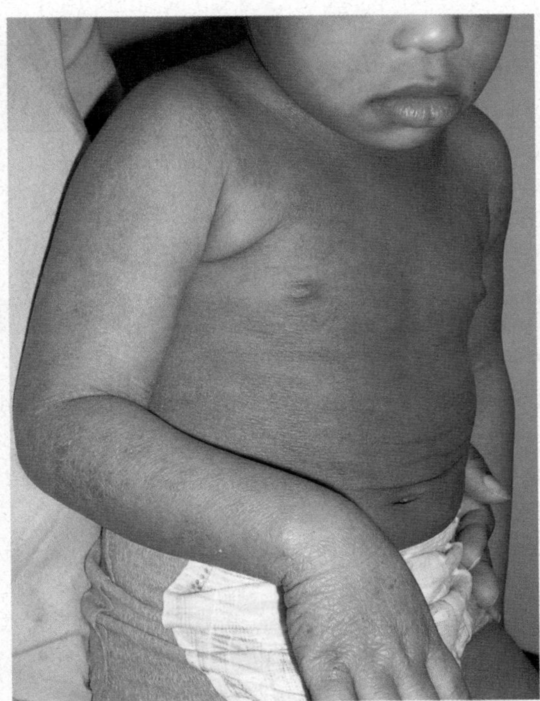

FIGURE 57-3 Two-year-old child with the "atopic triad" showing skin manifestations of atopic dermatitis. *(Reproduced with permission from Richard P. Usatine, MD.)*

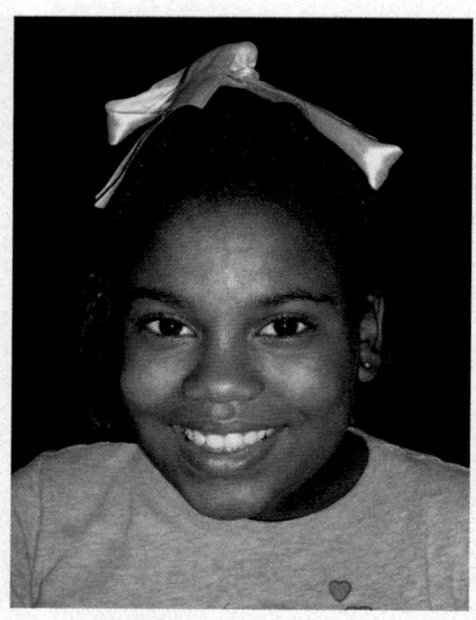

FIGURE 57-4 Ten-year-old girl with pityriasis alba, atopic dermatitis, and asthma under control. (*Reproduced with permission from Richard P. Usatine, MD.*)

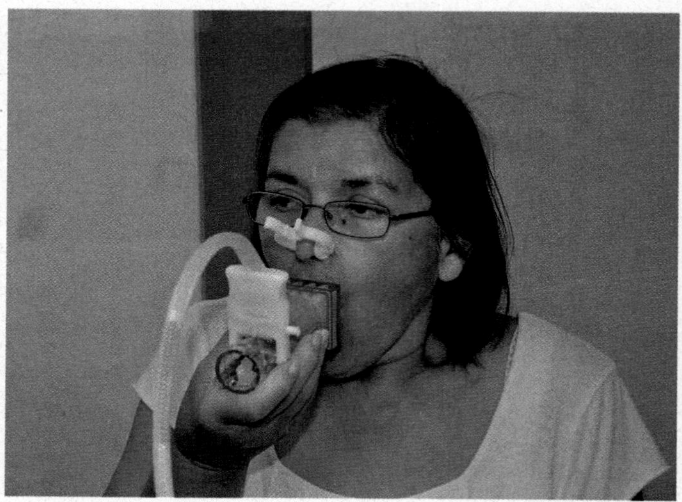

FIGURE 57-6 Patient having pulmonary function tests. (*Reproduced with permission from Richard P. Usatine, MD.*)

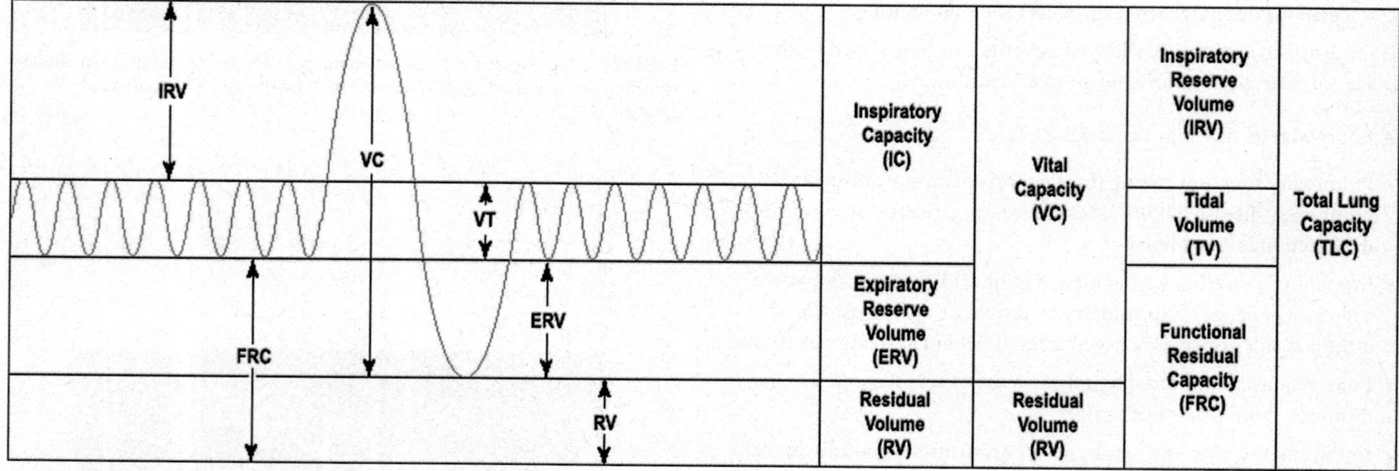

FIGURE 57-5 Graph of lung volumes showing the relationship of tidal volume to vital capacity and other important lung volumes. (*Reproduced with permission from Wikimedia Commons and Vihsadas at http://commons.wikimedia.org/wiki/File:LungVolume.jpg*)

TABLE 57-2 Classification of Asthma Severity

	Intermittent	Mild Persistent	Moderate Persistent	Severe Persistent
Symptoms	≤2 days/week	More than 2 days per week	Daily	Throughout the day
Nighttime Awakenings	≤2 times/month	3–4 times per month	Greater than once per week but not nightly	Nightly
Inhaler Use for Symptom Control (Rescue Use)	≤2 days/week	>2 days per week, but not daily	Daily	Several times per day
Interference with Normal Activity	None	Minor limitation	Some limitation	Extremely limited
Lung Function	FEV_1 >80% predicted and normal between exacerbations	FEV_1 >80% predicted	FEV_1 >60%–80% predicted	FEV_1 less than 60% predicted

Source: National Asthma Education and Prevention Program. *Guidelines for the Diagnosis and Management of Asthma*—http://www. nhlbi.nih.gov/guidelines/asthma/asthsumm.pdf.

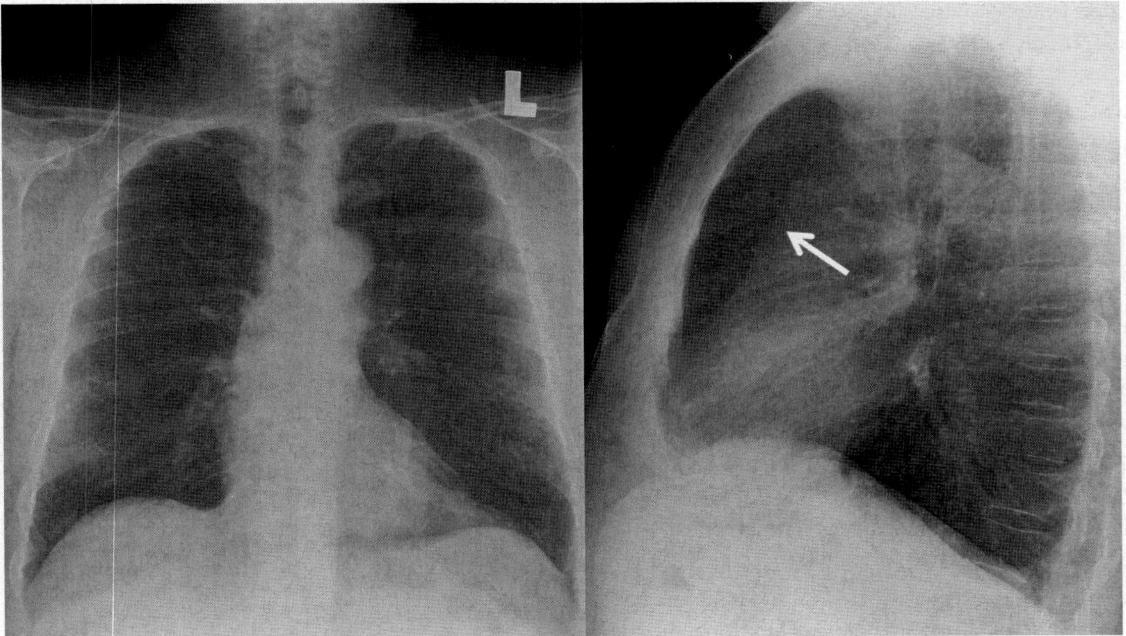

FIGURE 57-7 Acute asthma exacerbation with increased lung volumes on chest X-ray. The lateral projection reveals enlargement of the retrosternal clear space (*arrow*). (*Reproduced with permission from Carlos Santiago Restrepo, MD.*)

DIFFERENTIAL DIAGNOSIS

The differential diagnosis of an infant or child with wheezing includes[4]:

- Upper airway disease (e.g., allergic rhinitis, sinusitis)—Exam or imaging helps differentiate.
- Airway obstruction (foreign body, vascular rings, vocal cord dysfunction, tracheal stenosis, enlarged lymph node or tumor, infection, cystic fibrosis, heart disease)—Imaging helps differentiate.
- Other causes, such as recurrent cough or reflux. Cough-variant asthma (only cough) occurs especially in young children.

The differential diagnosis of an adult with episodic wheezing, chest tightness, cough, and difficulty breathing includes:

- COPD—Usually begins after age 40 years with dyspnea (persistent or progressive or worse with exercise), chronic cough (even if intermittent or nonproductive) and/or sputum production, and/or a history of COPD risk factors, including a family history of COPD (see Chapter 58, Chronic Obstructive Pulmonary Disease).
- Chronic bronchitis—A clinical diagnosis defined as the presence of cough and sputum production of at least 3 months in two consecutive years[20]; although often seen in patients with COPD, chronic bronchitis can occur in patients with normal spirometry.
- Pneumonia—Symptoms include fever, chills, and pleuritic chest pain; physical findings include dullness to percussion, bronchial breathing, egophony (E to A change), and crackles with area of infiltrate/pneumonia usually confirmed on CXR (see Chapter 55, Pneumonia).
- Tuberculosis—Any age; symptoms of chronic cough. CXR shows infiltrate; positive culture confirms (see Chapter 56, Tuberculosis).

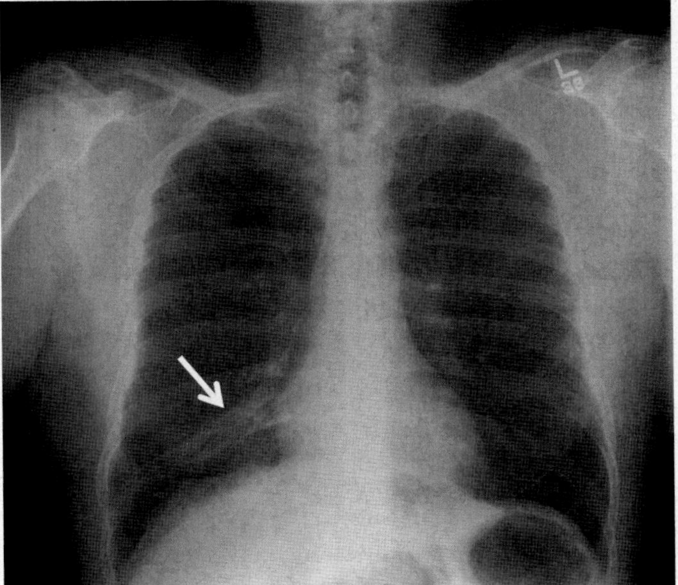

FIGURE 57-8 Acute asthma exacerbation in a 28-year-old man. Frontal chest radiograph demonstrates increased lung volumes and ill-defined opacity in the right infrahilar region consistent with middle lobe segmental atelectasis (*arrow*). (*Reproduced with permission from Carlos Santiago Restrepo, MD.*)

- Congestive heart failure—Nonspecific basilar crackles, CXR shows cardiomegaly, echocardiogram confirms (see Chapter 50, Heart Failure).
- Cough due to drugs (e.g., angiotensin-converting enzyme inhibitor) or vocal cord dysfunction—Identified on medication history or PFT.
- Asthma may occur in conjunction with these conditions.

MANAGEMENT

NAEPP outlines four components of care: assessment and monitoring, provision of education, control of environmental factors and comorbid conditions, and use of medications.[4] The goals of asthma therapy are twofold[4]:

- Reduce impairment—Prevent chronic symptoms, require infrequent (twice weekly or less) use of rescue inhaler, maintain near-normal pulmonary function, maintain normal activity levels, meet patient and family expectations and satisfaction with care.
- Reduce risk—Prevent recurrent exacerbations and minimize need for emergency or hospital care, prevent loss of lung function (for children, prevent reduced lung growth), and provide optimal pharmacotherapy while minimizing side effects and adverse effects.

FIRST LINE

NONPHARMACOLOGIC

- Exercise should be encouraged. In a randomized controlled trial (RCT) of aerobic exercise in patients with persistent asthma, the group randomized to exercise showed significant improvements in physical limitations, frequency of symptoms, health-related quality of life, number of asthma-symptom–free days, and anxiety and depression levels over the control group (education and breathing exercises only).[21]
- Advise smokers with asthma to stop smoking (see Chapter 248, Smoking and Tobacco Addiction) and parents and partners of patients to stop or avoid smoking near persons with asthma. For patients exposed to secondhand smoke in the home, use of high-efficiency particulate-arresting (HEPA) air cleaners was shown in one RCT to decrease unscheduled asthma visits for children ages 6 to 12 years; there was no difference between groups in parent-reported symptoms.[22]
- Provide patient education. SOR Ⓐ Pediatric asthma education was shown in a metaanalysis to reduce mean number of hospitalizations and emergency department (ED) visits and the odds of an ED visit for asthma.[23] Reduction in hospital and ED visits and missed work/school also has been shown for self-management education with written asthma action plans and physician review.[15] In one RCT, peer-led asthma education compared to adult-led education was associated with more positive attitudes at 6 months and higher quality of life at 6 and 9 months.[24]
- Consider interventions to control home environmental triggers; comprehensive individual programs may reduce symptom days.[15] SOR Ⓑ
    - Many people who have asthma are allergic to dust mites **(Figure 57-9)**. Two relatively easy interventions to decrease dust mite exposure are to encase pillows and mattresses in special

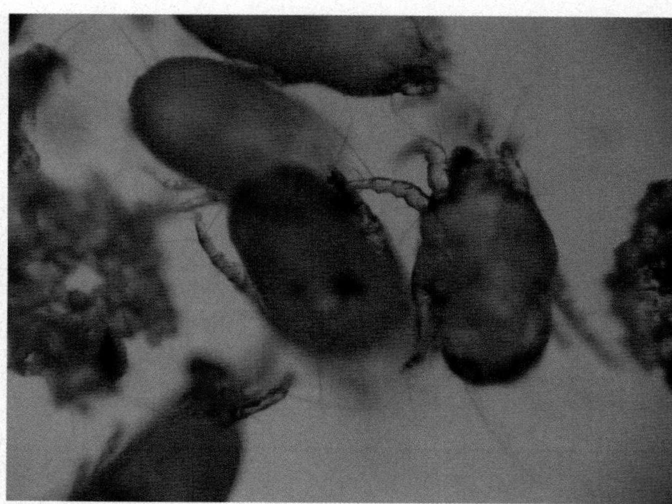

FIGURE 57-9 Dust mites under the microscope. Dust mites are a common allergen for patients who suffer from asthma and allergic rhinitis. Environmental control to minimize dust mite exposure can help control asthma for some individuals. *(Reproduced with permission from Richard P. Usatine, MD.)*

dust-mite–proof covers and wash bed sheets and blankets each week in hot water.[4]
  - Other suggestions for reducing environmental triggers can be found in the NAEPP reference[4] at http://www.nhlbi.nih.gov/guidelines/asthma/asthsumm.pdf.

MEDICATIONS

To determine appropriate medication management, assess severity based on symptoms, medication usage, and lung function (**Figure 57-1**). In addition, assess risk based on number of exacerbations requiring systemic steroids. For children, severity is assessed through symptoms, nighttime awakenings, interference with normal activity, and lung function—the latter if the child is older than 4 years of age. Risk is assessed by exacerbations requiring systemic steroids and treatment-related adverse effects.[4] A chart for children is available in the NAEPP reference to facilitate these assessments and includes treatment protocols.[4]

For youths age 12 years and up and adults, persistent asthma can then be divided into mild, moderate, or severe; these categories are matched to steps of medications described below. The ERS/ATS guideline also suggests that treatment for severe asthma in adults be guided by clinical criteria and sputum eosinophil counts performed in centers experienced in using this technique rather than by clinical criteria alone.[19]

Children are categorized as controlled, not-well controlled, or very poorly controlled with steps of care suggested as well. Treatment for asthma can be stepped up or down the stages as clinically indicated. The NAEPP six steps of care with respect to asthma medications are[4]:

- **Step 1:** For all patients of all ages with intermittent asthma, an inhaled short-acting β_2-agonist (SABA) is recommended. SOR Ⓐ Metered-dose inhalers with spacers are at least as effective (with fewer side effects) as nebulized treatment for most patients.
- **Step 2:** Low-dose inhaled corticosteroids (ICSs) are the preferred long-term control therapy for all ages with persistent asthma. SOR Ⓐ Cochrane authors reported that regular use of ICS at low or medium daily doses, however, is associated with a reduction in linear growth velocity (mean 0.48 cm/year) and a 0.61-cm change from baseline in height during a one1-year treatment period in children with mild to moderate persistent asthma.[25] Growth suppression appears to be maximal during the first year of therapy.
  - In an RCT of preschool-age children with recurrent wheezing (N = 278), intermittent budesonide inhalation suspension (1 mg twice daily for 7 days, starting early during a predefined respiratory tract illness) was as effective as a daily low-dose regimen (0.5 mg nightly) in preventing acute exacerbations (about 1 fewer per patient-year) while reducing mean exposure to budesonide.[26] In addition, authors of a Cochrane review found two trials showing that in children and adults with mild persistent asthma, intermittent ICS at the time of exacerbation reduced the subsequent need for oral corticosteroids by half.[27]
- **Step 3:** Combination low-dose ICSs and long-acting β_2-agonist (LABA) or medium-dose ICSs are equally preferred options in patients older than 4 years of age.[4] SOR Ⓑ Authors of a Cochrane review found that combination ICS-LABA in children was similar to ICS alone with respect to exacerbations but improved lung function and linear growth, the latter compared to higher dose ICS.[28] There was a tend towards increased risk of hospitalization with use of LABA. In adolescents and adults with sub-optimal control on low- dose ICS alone, combination LABA/ICS was more effective in reducing the risk of exacerbations than a higher dose of ICS.[29]
  - For patients age 4 years and younger, low-dose ICSs and LABA are suggested initially by NAEPP, followed by increasing the ICS dose if persistent low lung function and more than 2 days per week of impairment.[4]
  - One trial of step-up therapy for children with not-well-controlled persistent asthma on ICSs found that although combination ICS-LABA was most likely to result in a best response, some children had a best response to doubling ICSs or combination ICSs-LTRA.[30]
- **Step 4:** Combination medium-dose ICS and LABA.
- **Step 5:** Combination high-dose ICS and LABA.
- **Step 6:** Combination high-dose ICS and LABA plus oral corticosteroid.

In patients with severe allergic asthma, the ERS/ATS recommends a trial of omalizumab, a monoclonal antibody that binds to immunoglobulin E, for both adults and children.[19] The NAEPP suggests consideration of omalizumab in patients older than 11 years who have allergies or for adults who require step 5 or 6 care (severe asthma).[4] In an RCT with inner-city children, adolescents, and young adults (N = 419) with persistent asthma, omalizumab reduced symptom days and the proportion of subjects who had 1 or more exacerbations (30.3% vs. 48.8% on placebo).[31]

SECOND LINE

NONPHARMACOLOGIC

- Breathing exercises for asthma may reduce symptoms but data are limited by poor study methodology.[32]
- Dietary changes may also be useful. In a cross-sectional study, greater adherence to a Mediterranean-type diet was associated with a lower prevalence of asthma symptoms.[33]

MEDICATIONS

- **Step 2:** Alternatives to ICSs include cromolyn inhaler, leukotriene receptor antagonist (LTRA), nedocromil, or theophylline. LTRAs are less effective than ICSs but better than placebo.[4] SOR Ⓐ Authors of a systematic review and meta-analysis found LTRA's as monotherapy improved asthma control vs. placebo (RR for exacerbation 0.60 [95% CI, 0.44 to 0.81]).[34] Their role as add-on to ICS was less clear.
- **Step 3:** Alternatives to ICS and LABA or medium-dose ICSs are low-dose ICS plus LTRA (less effective than ICS and LABA), theophylline, or zileuton.[4] Authors of a Cochrane review did not find benefit of the addition of LTRAs to ICS on need for rescue oral corticosteroids or hospital admission compared to the same or an increased dose of ICS in children and adolescents with mild to moderate asthma.[35] Theophylline requires monitoring serum concentration levels. Zileuton is less desirable because of limited supporting data and the need to monitor liver function.
- **Step 4:** Alternatives to medium-dose ICS and LABA are combination medium-dose ICS plus LTRA, theophylline, or zileuton (see above).[4]

Other drug options:

- Long-acting muscarinic antagonists (LAMAs): In patients with severe asthma, tiotropium add-on appears to reduce exacerbations over LABA/ICS alone; no differences were noted in quality of life.[36] For patients taking ICSs without LABA, the addition of LAMA reduces the likelihood of exacerbations but additional benefits remain unknown.[37]
- To assist with smoking cessation, consider nicotine-replacement therapy (bupropion [150 mg, twice daily], varenicline [1 mg twice daily], nortriptyline [75 to 100 mg daily], or nicotine replacement [gum, inhaler, spray, patch]) and supportive counseling and follow-up; using these interventions improves rates of smoking cessation from 50% to up to twofold (see Chapter 248, Smoking and Tobacco Addiction).[38–40] SOR Ⓐ
- In patients with persistent asthma attributed to allergies, consider allergy immunotherapy.[4] SOR Ⓑ One metaanalysis concluded that specific immunotherapy for patients with positive skin tests resulted in a reduction in need for increased medications (number needed to treat = 5) and another study in patients with high IgE found immunotherapy reduced exacerbations.[41]

For patients with a mild *exacerbation* of asthma (dyspnea with activity, PEF ³70% predicted or personal best), SABAs, and sometimes oral corticosteroids, are used for home management of patients following their action plan. NAEPP does not recommend doubling the dose of ICSs for home management versus oral steroids for exacerbations.[4] Authors of a Cochrane review concluded that a short course of oral steroids was effective in reducing relapses, hospitalizations, and use of SABA without an apparent increase in side effects.[42] For children, a single day or 2-day regimen of dexamethasone [0.6 mg/kg (max 16 mg) orally once daily for 1–2 days] single or 2-dose regimens of dexamethasone is an alternative to a 5-day course of prednisone.[43] For adults, a simple course of prednisone 40 mg per day for 5 days works well in clinical practice.

- Moderate exacerbation (dyspnea interferes with usual activity, PEF 40% to 69% predicted or personal best) usually requires an office or ED visit; SABA and oral corticosteroids (typically 40 mg prednisone for adults and 1 to 2 mg/kg per day of prednisolone liquid in children in two divided doses) are recommended for 3 to 10 days (5 days will usually be sufficient). SOR Ⓐ SABA can be administered every 20 minutes as needed and the addition of inhaled ipratropium bromide may reduce the need for hospitalization (0.68 to 0.75).[5] SOR Ⓐ Symptoms usually abate in 1 to 2 days.
- Severe exacerbation (dyspnea at rest, PEF <40% predicted or personal best) usually requires an ED visit, and hospitalization is likely—combination SABA-anticholinergic nebulized treatment hourly or continuously as needed, oral corticosteroids, adjunctive treatment as needed (see below). Symptoms last for longer than 3 days after treatment begins.
- Life-threatening exacerbation (too dyspneic to speak, diaphoresis, PEF <25% predicted or personal best) requires an ED visit and/or hospitalization; consider intensive care unit, SABA-anticholinergic, intravenous corticosteroids, and adjunctive therapies.
- Oxygen therapy—Use to correct hypoxia in patients with moderate to life-threatening exacerbations; maintain O_2 saturation above 90%.[4,5] SOR Ⓒ
- Consider intravenous magnesium sulfate or heliox-driven albuterol nebulization if severe exacerbation and unresponsive to treatment after initial assessments.
- Monitor response to treatment with serial assessments of FEV_1 or PEF. Pulse oximetry may be useful in children for assessing initial severity—a result of less than 92% to 94% after 1 hour is an indication for hospitalization.[4] For adults, pulse oximetry may be useful for severe episodes or when unable to perform lung function testing; repeat assessments for hypoxia are useful for predicting need for hospitalization, as are signs and symptoms at 1 hour posttreatment.
- Patients with severe or life-threatening exacerbation unresponsive to initial treatments may require intubation and mechanical ventilation. Drowsiness may be a symptom of impending respiratory failure.
- The following should not be used as they have no supporting evidence and may delay effective treatment: drinking large volumes of liquids; breathing warm, moist air; using nonprescription products, such as antihistamines or cold remedies; and pursed-lip and other forms of breathing.[4] In addition, the NAEPP does not recommend use of methylxanthines, antibiotics (except as needed for comorbid conditions), aggressive hydration, chest physical therapy, mucolytics, or sedation in the ED or hospital setting.[4]

REFERRAL

- Consider referral to an asthma specialist if signs and symptoms are atypical, if there are problems in assessing other diagnoses, or if additional specialized testing is needed.
- Referral or consultation should also be considered if there are difficulties achieving or maintaining control of asthma, if the patient required more than two bursts of oral systemic corticosteroids in 1 year or has an exacerbation requiring hospitalization, or if immunotherapy or omalizumab is considered.[4]
- Consultation with an asthma specialist should be conducted for patients with persistent asthma requiring step 4 care or higher and considered if a patient requires step 3 care.[4]

PREVENTION AND SCREENING

- Smoking cessation and avoidance of secondhand smoke while limiting occupational exposures and exposure to indoor air pollution may be preventive.
- Influenza and pneumococcal vaccination are recommended.[4] SOR Ⓑ
- Despite limited data, vitamins A, D, and E; zinc; fruits and vegetables; and a Mediterranean diet may be useful for the prevention of asthma.[44] In addition, raw cow's milk consumption appears protective (adjusted OR, 0.59; 95% CI, 0.46 to 0.74).[45]

PROGNOSIS

- More than half of children with asthma will no longer have symptoms by age 6 years.[5]
- In a meta-analysis, maternal asthma was associated with an increased risk of low birth weight (relative risk [RR], 1.46; 95% CI 1.22 to 1.75),

small for gestational age (RR, 1.22; 95% CI 1.14 to 1.31), preterm delivery (RR, 1.41; 95% CI 1.22 to 1.61), and preeclampsia (RR, 1.54; 95% CI 1.32 to 1.81).[46] The RR of preterm delivery and preterm labor became nonsignificant with active asthma management. Pregnancy does not appear to increase asthma severity, provided women continue to use their prescribed medications.[47]

- Among children, factors predictive of an asthma exacerbation include bronchiolitis or pneumonia during infancy, maternal eczema, paternal history of hay fever, asthma symptoms lasting 3 or more months/year, more than four scheduled physician visits for asthma in the previous year, and use of certain medications (SABAs, anti-inflammatory medications, and one or more courses of oral steroids) in the prior year.[48]
- For patients with an asthma exacerbation, the following factors place a patient at higher risk of asthma-related death; these patients should be advised to seek medical care early during an exacerbation[4]:
  - Previous severe exacerbation (e.g., intubation or intensive care unit admission for asthma)
  - Two or more hospitalizations or more than three ED visits in the past year
  - Use of more than two canisters of SABA per month
  - Difficulty perceiving airway obstruction or the severity of worsening asthma
  - Low socioeconomic status or inner-city resident

FOLLOW-UP

Many patients have asthma that is not well controlled. In a cross-sectional study of 29 pediatric practices (N = 2429), 46% reported uncontrolled asthma (defined as a Childhood Asthma Control Test [C-ACT] or the Asthma Control Test [ACT] less than or equal to 19).[49]

The NAEP 2007 guidelines recommend the following:[4]

- At each visit ask about frequency and intensity of symptoms and functional limitations currently or recently experienced (impairment). Severity can be measured by the step of care required to maintain control.[4] SOR Ⓒ
- In addition, at each visit, assess the likelihood of either asthma exacerbations, progressive decline in lung function (or lung growth for children), or risk of medication adverse effects. A patient self-assessment sheet rating asthma control (e.g., symptoms, PEF) and medication use is available in the NAEPP reference.[4] Provision of a visually standardized, interpreted peak-flow graph to assist in understanding when to add medication or contact a healthcare provider may reduce need for oral steroids and urgent care visits.[50]
- For patients on medications, monitor treatment effectiveness ("Have you noticed a difference, for example, less breathlessness?") and side effects. Observe inhaler technique at least once to ensure optimal delivery.
- For smokers, encourage cessation.
- Document exacerbations/hospitalizations—This may indicate a need for additional treatment.
- Monitor for comorbidities (e.g., heart disease, chronic lung disease) and maximize control of those conditions.

PATIENT EDUCATION

- Smoking cessation should be strongly and repeatedly encouraged. Exercise should also be encouraged along with weight loss, if obese, or maintenance of a healthy weight.
- The NAEPP suggests that key educational messages include basic facts about asthma, the role of medications (i.e., rescue/short-term vs. control/long-term), and patient skills (e.g., correct inhaler technique, self-monitoring).
- Creation of an asthma action plan can be helpful in promoting self-management and greater understanding of warning signs of worsening asthma. An example of an action plan can be found in the NAEPP document.[4] Asthma action plans usually use three zones, similar to traffic lights, with green zone representing good control (i.e., few symptoms, PEF 80% to 100%), yellow zone representing worsening or not-well-controlled asthma (i.e., mild to moderate symptoms, PEF 50% to 80%), and red zone representing an alert or warning (i.e., severe symptoms, PEF <50%), with advice to seek emergency care if not better after 15 minutes of rescue medication use and unable to reach their healthcare provider. Each zone contains instructions for management that the primary care provider can modify.

PATIENT RESOURCES

For general information, these sites are helpful:

- Centers for Disease Control and Prevention. *Asthma's Impact on the Nation*—**https://www.cdc.gov/asthma/impacts_nation/asthmafactsheet.pdf.**
- American Lung Association. *Asthma*—**http://www.lung.org/lung-health-and-diseases/lung-disease-lookup/asthma/.**
- MedlinePlus. *Asthma*—**http://www.nlm.nih.gov/medlineplus/asthma.html.**
- US Department of Health and Human Services. *Managing Asthma. A guide for schools.* **https://www.nhlbi.nih.gov/files/docs/resources/lung/NACI_ManagingAsthma-508%20FINAL.pdf.**

PROVIDER RESOURCES

- National Asthma Education and Prevention Program. *Guidelines for the Diagnosis and Management of Asthma*—**http://www.nhlbi.nih.gov/guidelines/asthma/asthsumm.pdf.**
- Centers for Disease Control and Prevention. *FastStats: Asthma*—**http://www.cdc.gov/nchs/fastats/asthma.htm.**

REFERENCES

1. Centers for Disease Control and Prevention. *Asthma FastStats.* http://www.cdc.gov/nchs/fastats/asthma.htm. Accessed February 2017.
2. Centers for Disease Control and Prevention. *Asthma Data, Statistics and Surveillance.* https://www.cdc.gov/asthma/asthmadata.htm. Accessed May 2018.
3. Asthma and Allergy Foundation of America. *Cost of Asthma on Society.* http://www.aafa.org/page/cost-of-asthma-on-society.aspx. Accessed February 2017.

4. *National Asthma Education and Prevention Program Expert Panel Report 3 (2007)*. http://www.nhlbi.nih.gov/guidelines/asthma/asthsumm.pdf. Accessed February 2012.
5. Myers RA, Himes BE, Gignoux CR, et al. Further replication studies of the EVE Consortium meta-analysis identifies 2 asthma risk loci in European Americans. *J Allergy Clin Immunol.* 2012; 130(6):1294-301.
6. Schauberger EM, Ewart SL, Arshad SH, et al. Identification of ATPAF1 as a novel candidate gene for asthma in children. *J Allergy Clin Immunol.* 2011;128(4):753-760.
7. Arshad SH, Kurukulaaratchy RJ, Fenn M, Matthews S. Early life risk factors for current wheeze, asthma, and bronchial hyperresponsiveness at 10 years of age. *Chest.* 2005;127(2):502-508.
8. Burke H, Leonardi-Bee J, Hashim A, et al. Prenatal and passive smoke exposure and incidence of asthma and wheeze: systematic review and meta-analysis. *Pediatrics.* 2012;129(4):735-744.
9. Beasley RW, Clayton TO, Crane J, et al. Acetaminophen use and risk of asthma, rhinoconjunctivitis, and eczema in adolescents: International Study of Asthma and Allergies in Childhood Phase Three. *Am J Respir Crit Care Med.* 2011;183(2):171-178.
10. Holgate ST. The acetaminophen enigma in asthma. *Am J Respir Crit Care Med.* 2011;183(2):147-151.
11. Bhatt NA, Lazarus A. Obesity-related asthma in adults. *Postgrad Med.* 2016;128(6):563-566.
12. Papoutsakis C, Priftis KN, Drakouli M, et al. Childhood overweight/obesity and asthma: is there a link? A systematic review of recent epidemiologic evidence. *J Acad Nutr Diet.* 2013;113(1):77-105.
13. Rzehak P, Wijga AH, Keil T, et al. Body mass index trajectory classes and incident asthma in childhood: results from 8 European Birth Cohorts—a Global Allergy and Asthma European Network initiative. *J Allergy Clin Immunol.* 2013;131(6):1528-1536.
14. Arvaniti F, Priftis KN, Papadimitriou A, et al. Salty-snack eating, television or video-game viewing, and asthma symptoms among 10- to 12-year-old children: the PANACEA study. *J Am Diet Assoc.* 2011;111(2):251-257.
15. Roett MA, Gillespie C. Asthma. In: Sloane PD, Slatt LM, Ebell MH, Smith MA, Power D, Viera AJ, et al., eds. *Essentials of Family Medicine.* Philadelphia, PA: Lippincott Williams & Wilkins; 2011:607-623.
16. Kapoor R, Menon C, Hoffstad O, et al. The prevalence of atopic triad in children with physician-confirmed atopic dermatitis. *J Am Acad Dermatol.* 2008;58(1):66-73.
17. Hwang CY, Chen YJ, Lin MW, et al. Prevalence of atopic dermatitis, allergic rhinitis and asthma in Taiwan: a national study 2000-2007. *Acta Derm Venereol.* 2010;90(6):589-594.
18. Spergel JM. From atopic dermatitis to asthma. *Ann Allergy Asthma Immunol.* 2010;105(2):99-106.
19. *International ERS/ATS Guidelines on Definition, Evaluation and Treatment of Severe Asthma.* Available at https://www.guideline.gov/summaries/summary/48457/international-ersats-guidelines-on-definition-evaluation-and-treatment-of-severe-asthma. Accessed February 2017.
20. Global Initiative for Chronic Obstructive Lung Disease (GOLD). *Global Strategy for the Diagnosis, Management and Prevention of COPD.* 2011. http://www.goldcopd.org. Accessed January 2012.
21. Mendes FA, Goncalves RC, Nunes MP, et al. Effects of aerobic training on psychosocial morbidity and symptoms in patients with asthma: a randomized clinical trial. *Chest.* 2010;138(2):331-337.
22. Lanphear BP, Hornung RW, Khoury J, et al. Effects of HEPA air cleaners on unscheduled asthma visits and asthma symptoms for children exposed to secondhand tobacco smoke. *Pediatrics.* 2011; 127(1):93-101.
23. Coffman JM, Cabana MD, Halpin HA, Yelin EH. Effects of asthma education on children's use of acute care services: a meta-analysis. *Pediatrics.* 2008;121(3):575-586.
24. Rhee H, Belyea MJ, Hunt JF, Brasch J. Effects of a peer-led asthma self-management program for adolescents. *Arch Pediatr Adolesc Med.* 2011;165(6):513-519.
25. Zhang L, Prietsch SOM, Ducharme FM. Inhaled corticosteroids in children with persistent asthma: effects on growth. *Cochrane Database Syst Rev.* 2014;(7):CD009471.
26. Zeiger RS, Mauger D, Bacharier LB, et al. Daily or intermittent budesonide in preschool children with recurrent wheezing. *N Engl J Med.* 2011;365(21):1990-2001.
27. Chong J, Haran C, Chauhan BF, Asher I. Intermittent inhaled corticosteroid therapy versus placebo for persistent asthma in children and adults. *Cochrane Database Syst Rev.* 2015;(7):CD011032.
28. Chauhan BF, Chartrand C, Ni Chroinin M, Milan SJ, Ducharme FM, et al. Addition of long-acting beta$_2$-agonists to inhaled corticosteroids for chronic asthma in children. *Cochrane Database Syst Rev.* 2015;(11):CD007949.
29. Ducharme FM, Ni Chroinin M, Greenstone I, Lasserson TJ. Addition of long-acting beta$_2$-agonists to inhaled steroids versus higher dose inhaled steroids in adults and children with persistent asthma. *Cochrane Database Syst Rev.* 2010;(4):CD005733.
30. Lemanske RF Jr, Mauger DT, Sorkness CA, et al. Step-up therapy for children with uncontrolled asthma receiving inhaled corticosteroids. *N Engl J Med.* 2010;362(11):975-985.
31. Busse WW, Morgan WJ, Gergen PJ, et al. Randomized trial of omalizumab (anti-IgE) for asthma in inner-city children. *N Engl J Med.* 2011;364(11):1005-1015.
32. Freitas DA, Holloway EA, Bruno SS, Chaves GSS,Fregonezi GAF, Mendonça KMPP, et al. Breathing exercises for adults with asthma. *Cochrane Database of Systematic Reviews.* 2013, Issue;(10. Art. No.:):CD001277.
33. Arvaniti F, Priftis KN, Papadimitriou A, et al. Adherence to the Mediterranean type of diet is associated with lower prevalence of asthma symptoms, among 10–12 year old children: the PANACEA study. *Pediatr Allergy Immunol.* 2011;22(3):283-289.
34. Miligkos M, Bannuru RR, Alkofide H, et al. Leukotriene-receptor antagonists versus placebo in the treatment of asthma in adults and adolescents: a systematic review and meta-analysis. *Ann Intern Med.* 2015;163(10):756-767.
35. Chauhan BF, Ben Salah R, Ducharme FM. Addition of anti-leukotriene agents to inhaled corticosteroids in children with persistent asthma. *Cochrane Database Syst Rev.* 2013;(10): CD009585.
36. Kew KM, Dahri K. Long-acting muscarinic antagonists (LAMA) added to combination long-acting beta$_2$-agonists and inhaled

corticosteroids (LABA/ICS) versus LABA/ICS for adults with asthma. *Cochrane Database Syst Rev*. 2016;(1):CD011721.

37. Anderson DE, Kew KM, Boyter AC. Long-acting muscarinic antagonists (LAMA) added to inhaled corticosteroids (ICS) versus the same dose of ICS alone for adults with asthma. *Cochrane Database Syst Rev*. 2015;(8):CD011397.
38. Hughes JR, Stead LF, Hartmann-Boyce J, Cahill K, et al. Antidepressants for smoking cessation. *Cochrane Database Syst Rev*. 2014;(1):CD000031.
39. Stead LF, Perera R, Bullen C, et al. Nicotine replacement therapy for smoking cessation. *Cochrane Database Syst Rev*. 2012;(11): CD000146.
40. Stead LF, Bergson G, Preciado N, et al. Physician advice for smoking cessation. *Cochrane Database Syst Rev*. 2013;(5):CD000165.
41. Lin SY, Erekosima N, Kim JM, et al. Sublingual immunotherapy for the treatment of allergic rhinoconjunctivitis and asthma: a systematic review. *JAMA*. 2013;309(12):1278-1288.
42. Rowe BH, Spooner CH, Ducharme FM, et al. Corticosteroids for preventing relapse following acute exacerbations of asthma. *Cochrane Database Syst Rev*. 2007;(3):CD000195.
43. Keeney GE, Gray MP, Morrison AK, et al. Dexamethasone for acute asthma exacerbations in children: a meta-analysis. *Pediatrics*. 2014;133(3):493-499.
44. Nurmatov U, Devereux G, Sheikh A. Nutrients and foods for the primary prevention of asthma and allergy: systematic review and meta-analysis. *J Allergy Clin Immunol*. 2011;127(3):724-733. e1-e30.
45. Loss G, Apprich S, Waser M, et al. The protective effect of farm milk consumption on childhood asthma and atopy: the GABRIELA study. *J Allergy Clin Immunol*. 2011;128(4):766-773.e4.
46. Murphy VE, Namazy JA, Powell H, et al. A meta-analysis of adverse perinatal outcomes in women with asthma. *BJOG*. 2011;118(11):1314-1323.
47. Belanger K, Hellenbrand ME, Holford TR, Bracken M. Effect of pregnancy on maternal asthma symptoms and medication use. *Obstet Gynecol*. 2010;115(3):579-567.
48. Forno E, Fuhlbrigge A, Soto-Quiros ME, et al. Risk factors and predictive clinical scores for asthma exacerbations in childhood. *Chest*. 2010;138(5):1156-1165.
49. Liu AH, Gilsenan AW, Stanford RH, et al. Status of asthma control in pediatric primary care: results from the pediatric Asthma Control Characteristics and Prevalence Survey Study (ACCESS). *J Pediatr*. 2010;157(2):276-281.
50. Janson SL, McGrath KW, Covington JK, et al. Objective airway monitoring improves asthma control in the cold and flu season: a cluster randomized trial. *Chest*. 2010;138(5):1148-1157.

58 CHRONIC OBSTRUCTIVE PULMONARY DISEASE

Mindy A. Smith, MD, MS

PATIENT STORY

A 74-year-old woman and longtime smoker presents with fatigue and shortness of breath. She has not seen a physician for many years and says she has been basically healthy. On physical examination, she is found to be pale and mildly cachectic, and her lips are cyanotic. Her breath sounds are distant, although crackles can be heard in both lung bases. Her heart sounds are best heard in the epigastrium; a third heart sound is present. She has mild peripheral edema. Her resting pulse oximetry is 74%. Her chest X-ray (CXR) shows emphysema (**Figure 58-1**), and her echocardiogram confirms heart failure.

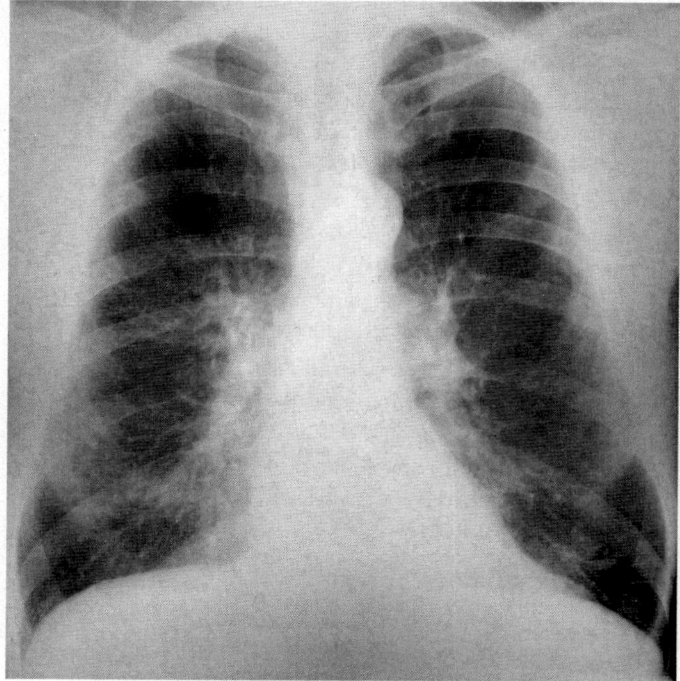

FIGURE 58-1 Emphysema with mild hyperinflation and increased interstitial markings. *(Reproduced with permission from Miller WT: Diagnostic Thoracic Imaging. New York, NY: McGraw-Hill Education; 2006.)*

INTRODUCTION

Chronic obstructive pulmonary disease (COPD) is defined as a disease state characterized by persistent airflow limitation that is usually progressive and associated with an enhanced chronic inflammatory response of the lung and airways to noxious particles or gases.[1] COPD is preventable and treatable. Some patients have significant extrapulmonary effects (particularly cardiac) that may contribute to disease severity. Worldwide, tobacco smoke is the primary cause of COPD (**Figure 58-2**).

SYNONYMS

Emphysema (technically refers to destruction of the alveoli).

EPIDEMIOLOGY

- Estimated prevalence of COPD in adults older than age 18 years in the United States (2014) is about 15.7 million cases, or 6.4% of the population.[2] Prevalence rate varies greatly between states, from <4% in Hawaii, Colorado, and Utah to >9% in Alabama, Tennessee, Kentucky, and West Virginia.[3]
- Third leading cause of death in the United States (2014).[2] Mortality rates have declined for men from 1999 to 2014 (57 per 100,000 to 44.3 per 100,000) and remained fairly stable for women (35.3 per 100,000 to 35.6 per 100,000).[3]
- In a study in Latin America, prevalence rates ranged from 7.8% to 19.7% of the population[4]; a prevalence of between 3% and 11% has been reported in never-smokers.[1] This high rate among never-smokers is most likely related to indoor cooking with open wood fires.
- In a Swedish study of COPD (birth cohorts from 1919 to 1950), the 10-year cumulative incidence rate of COPD was 13.5% using Global Initiative for Chronic Obstructive Lung Disease (GOLD) criteria (**Table 58-1**) based on 1109 patients with baseline

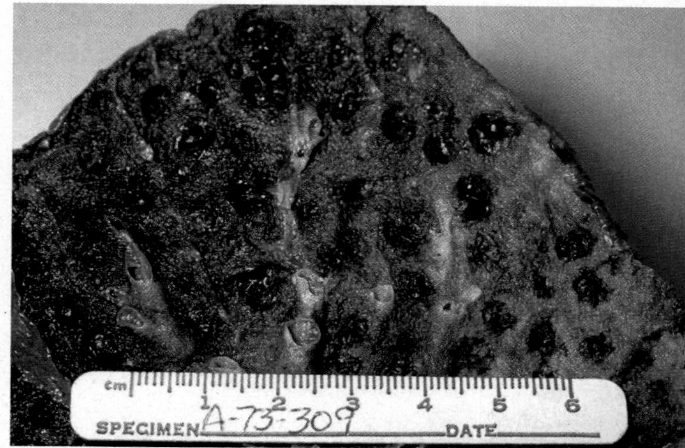

FIGURE 58-2 Gross pathology of lung showing centrilobular emphysema caused by tobacco smoking. Close-up of cut surface shows multiple cavities lined by heavy black carbon deposits. *(Reproduced with permission from Centers for Disease Control and Prevention [CDC] and Dr. Edwin P. Ewing, Jr.)*

TABLE 58-1 COPD Severity—GOLD Grade

Grade	FEV_1/FVC	FEV_1
Mild COPD (GOLD 1)	<0.7	≥80% predicted
Moderate COPD (GOLD 2)	<0.7	<80% but ≥50% predicted
Severe COPD (GOLD 3)	<0.7	<50% but ≥30% predicted
Very severe COPD (GOLD 4)	<0.7	<30% predicted or FEV_1 <50% with respiratory failure or right-sided heart failure

Abbreviations: FEV_1, forced expiratory volume in 1 second; *FVC*, forced vital capacity.

respiratory symptoms (76.6% of the original symptomatic cohort and 16.7% of the total cohort).[5]

- Estimated direct costs associated with COPD in the United States are more than $29 billion with additional indirect costs of $20.4 billion.[1]

ETIOLOGY AND PATHOPHYSIOLOGY

- Mediated by chronic inflammatory responses to environmental factors, especially cigarette smoke, that result in recruitment of inflammatory cells in terminal airspaces and release of elastolytic proteinases that damage the extracellular lung matrix and cause ineffective repair of elastin and other matrix components.
- Oxidative stress may be an important amplifying mechanism in COPD development and exacerbations.[1] In addition, there appears to be an imbalance between proteases and antiproteases in the lungs of patients with COPD.
- The inflammatory process leads to obstruction and later fibrosis of small airways and the destruction of lung parenchyma. Circulating inflammatory mediators may contribute to muscle wasting and cachexia and worsen comorbidities such as heart failure and diabetes.[1]
- Gas exchange abnormalities result in hypoxemia and hypercapnia.
- Pulmonary hypertension may occur as a result of hypoxic vasoconstriction of small pulmonary arteries.
- Genetic mutations (e.g., α_1-antitrypsin deficiency [1% to 2% of cases; affects 1 in 2000 to 5000 individuals]) are present in some patients. Suspect a genetic mutation when emphysema is found in a patient age 45 to 50 years or younger, a positive family history of COPD, primarily basilar disease, or a minimal smoking history.[6] Single-nucleotide polymorphisms at three loci—TNS1, GSTCD, and HTR4—are associated with COPD, as is genetic variation in the transcription factor SOX5.[7,8]
- Acute exacerbations of COPD are most commonly triggered by upper respiratory tract infections; other precipitating causes include air pollution, although a specific trigger cannot be identified in about one third of severe exacerbations.[1]

RISK FACTORS

- Smoking (direct and passive)—COPD relative risk (RR) for ever smoking is 2.89 (95% CI, 2.63 to 3.17) and RR for current smoking is 3.51 (95% CI, 3.08 to 3.99).[9]
- Airway hypersensitivity (15% of the population attributable risk).[1]
- Occupational exposures (e.g., gold and coal mining, cotton textile dust).[1,2,6] The estimated fraction of COPD attributed to work exposures is 19.2% overall and 31.1% among never smokers.[1]
- Indoor air pollution from burning wood and other biomass fuels, particularly with open fires, poorly functioning stoves, and poorly ventilated dwellings.[1]
- Reduced maximal attained lung function (e.g., preterm vs. full-term infants).[1]
- Infections (e.g., early childhood infection, chronic bronchitis, HIV, tuberculosis).[1]
- Poverty.
- Parental history of COPD (odds ratio [OR] 1.73).[10]
- α_1-Antitrypsin deficiency (genetic disorder).
- In a study of 2138 patients with COPD, nearly one third (31%) reported a total of 1452 COPD exacerbations requiring hospital admission over 3 years.[11] The most important risk factor was a prior history of COPD exacerbation requiring hospital admission; other risk factors were more severe airflow limitation, poorer health status, older age, radiologic evidence of emphysema, and higher WBC count.

DIAGNOSIS

A diagnosis of COPD should be considered in a patient older than age 40 years with dyspnea (persistent or progressive or worse with exercise), chronic cough (even if intermittent or nonproductive) and/or sputum production, and/or a history of COPD risk factors including a family history of COPD.[1]

CLINICAL FEATURES

- COPD's three most common symptoms are cough, sputum production, and exertional dyspnea. In one study of newly diagnosed patients, most presented with cough (85%) and exertional dyspnea (70%); almost half (45%) reported increased sputum production.[12] Most patients were classified in GOLD stage 0 to 1 (42%) or 2 (46%) (see **Table 58-1**).
- Patients may also report chest tightness, often following exertion; fatigue, weight loss, and anorexia are symptoms later in the disease.
- Several validated questionnaires are available to assess symptoms in patients with COPD; GOLD recommends either the Modified

British Medical Research Council (MMRC) questionnaire (https://www.mdcalc.com/mmrc-modified-medical-research-council-dyspnea-scale) or the 8-question COPD Assessment Test (CAT; http://catestonline.org) or the COPD Control Questionnaire (CCQ; http://www.ccq.nl).[1]

- Assessment of exacerbations is important for management decisions. Ask about number of previous episodes/hospitalizations, comorbidities, previous treatment, and use of mechanical ventilation.[1]
- Physical findings may include:
  - Tobacco odor and nicotine staining of fingernails.
  - Increased expiratory phase or expiratory wheezing.
  - Signs of hyperinflation—Barrel chest, poor diaphragmatic excursion.
  - Use of accessory muscles of respiration—Intercostals, sternocleidomastoid, and scalene muscles.
  - Late in illness—Cyanosis of the lips and nail beds, wasting, and *cor pulmonale* (right-sided heart failure—signs include increased jugular-venous distention, right ventricular heave, third heart sound, ascites, and peripheral edema).

LABORATORY TESTING

Postbronchodilator spirometry secures the diagnosis and provides the severity classification[1,13]: SOR Ⓑ

- At risk—Chronic cough and sputum production with normal spirometry.

Additional tests that may be useful in management are sputum culture (in acute exacerbations to assist in confirming pneumonia), complete blood count (to identify anemia or polycythemia), and pulse oximetry or blood gases (confirms hypoxia when peripheral oxygen saturation is <92% or respiratory failure [PCO_2 >45]).[1]

- A serum level of α_1-antitrypsin should be measured if you suspect a genetic mutation (young age at presentation [≤45 years], lower lobe emphysema, family history, minimal smoking history).
- Exercise (walking) tests to assess disability or response to rehabilitation.[1]

IMAGING

A CXR is not useful for diagnosis but is helpful for excluding other diseases or identifying comorbidity (e.g., heart failure). Findings on CXR include[3]:

Hyperinflation manifested by the following (**Figures 58-1** to **58-3**):

- Increased anteroposterior (AP) diameter.
- Increased retrosternal air space.
- Infracardiac air.
- Low-set flattened diaphragms (best assessed in lateral chest).
- Vertical heart.
- Bullae are difficult to recognize in CXR but are easily seen on CT (**Figures 58-4** to **58-8**).
- Paucity of vascular markings in periphery (see **Figure 58-2**).
- Pulmonary hypertension (CXR shows enlarged central pulmonary arteries).
- α_1-Antitrypsin deficiency leads to early COPD even in nonsmokers. See **Figure 58-9** for advanced pulmonary emphysema in a 30-year-old woman with α_1-antitrypsin deficiency. The CXR shows increased lung volumes, flattening of the diaphragms, and a vertical heart. A CT may show extensive panlobular emphysema of the mid and lower lung zones (**Figure 58-10**). The vascular markings are prominent in the upper lobes, demonstrating "cephalization" of flow.

A chest CT scan is the current definitive test for emphysema, but the findings do not influence treatment.[6] Cystic and bullous lesions are better delineated with CT scan (see **Figures 58-4, 58-5**, and **58-7**), and collapsing airways with inspiration and expiration can also be demonstrated with CT. Chest CT is recommended if surgery is contemplated.[1]

Echocardiography is suggested if features of cor pulmonale are present.

DIFFERENTIAL DIAGNOSIS

The differential diagnosis of an individual with persistent productive cough and dyspnea includes:

- Asthma—Begins before age 40 years in most (often in childhood), usually episodic and characterized by increased responsiveness to stimuli (e.g., allergens, occupational exposures). This condition is reversible with bronchodilators (see Chapter 57, Asthma).
- Chronic bronchitis—A clinical diagnosis defined as the presence of cough and sputum production of at least 3 months in 2 consecutive years[1]; although often seen in patients with COPD and associated with development and/or acceleration of fixed airflow limitation, chronic bronchitis can occur in patients with normal spirometry.
- Pneumonia—Symptoms include fever, chills, and pleuritic chest pain; physical findings include dullness to percussion, bronchial breathing, egophony (E to A change), and crackles with area of infiltrate/pneumonia usually confirmed on CXR (see Chapter 55, Pneumonia).
- Tuberculosis—Any age; symptoms of chronic cough. CXR shows infiltrate; positive culture confirms (see Chapter 56, Tuberculosis).
- Congestive heart failure—Nonspecific basilar crackles; CXR shows cardiomegaly; echocardiogram confirms (see Chapter 50, Heart Failure).
- Lung cancer—Symptoms may occur with central or endobronchial growth of the tumor (e.g., cough, hemoptysis, wheeze, stridor, dyspnea), collapse of airways from tumor obstruction (e.g., post-obstructive pneumonitis), involvement of the pleura or chest wall (e.g., pleuritic chest pain), or from regional spread of the tumor (e.g., dysphagia, hoarseness from recurrent laryngeal nerve paralysis). Findings on CXR or chest CT may be focal or unilateral and tissue confirms diagnosis (see Chapter 60, Lung Cancer).

Any of these processes/illnesses may occur in conjunction with emphysema.

MANAGEMENT

Management of COPD is based on symptoms, risk or history of exacerbations, and severity/predicted survival. GOLD places patients into four categories as shown in **Table 58-2**. The updated 2016 GOLD report includes an appendix on Asthma COPD Overlap Syndrome.[1]

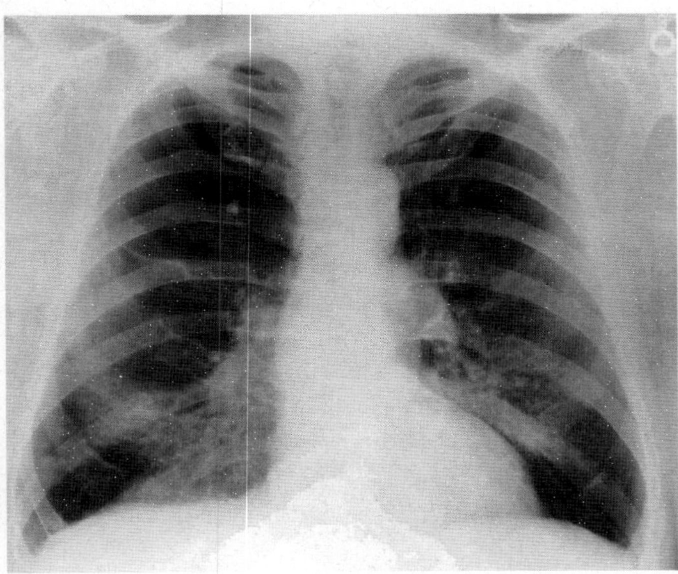

FIGURE 58-3 Posteroanterior (PA) radiograph showing flattened hemidiaphragms and decreased vascular markings from hyperinflation as a result of air trapping in a patient with COPD. (*Reproduced with permission from Miller WT: Diagnostic Thoracic Imaging. New York, NY: McGraw-Hill Education; 2006.*)

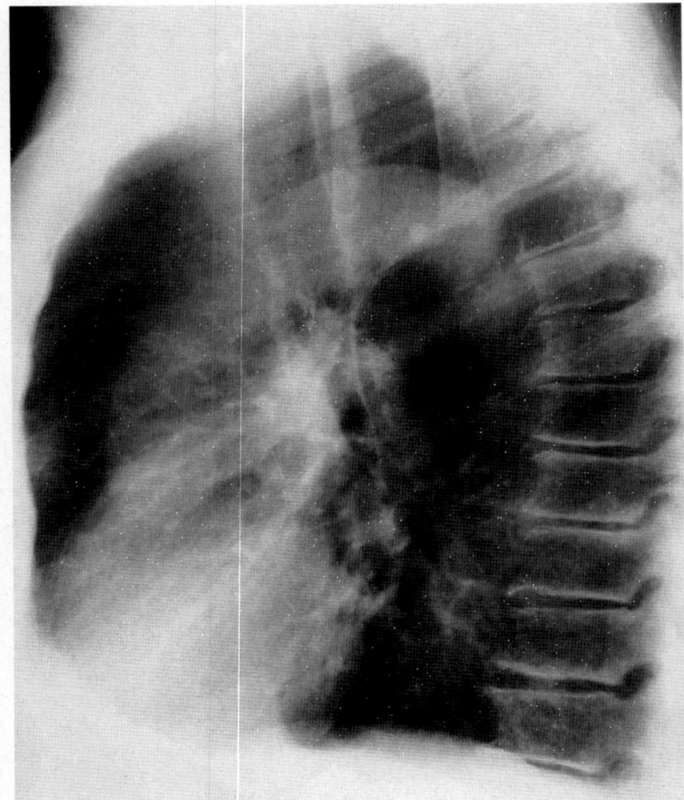

FIGURE 58-4 Lateral view in the patient in **Figure 58-3** showing increased anteroposterior (AP) diameter from hyperinflation as a result of air trapping in a patient with COPD. (*Reproduced with permission from Miller WT: Diagnostic Thoracic Imaging. New York, NY: McGraw-Hill Education; 2006.*)

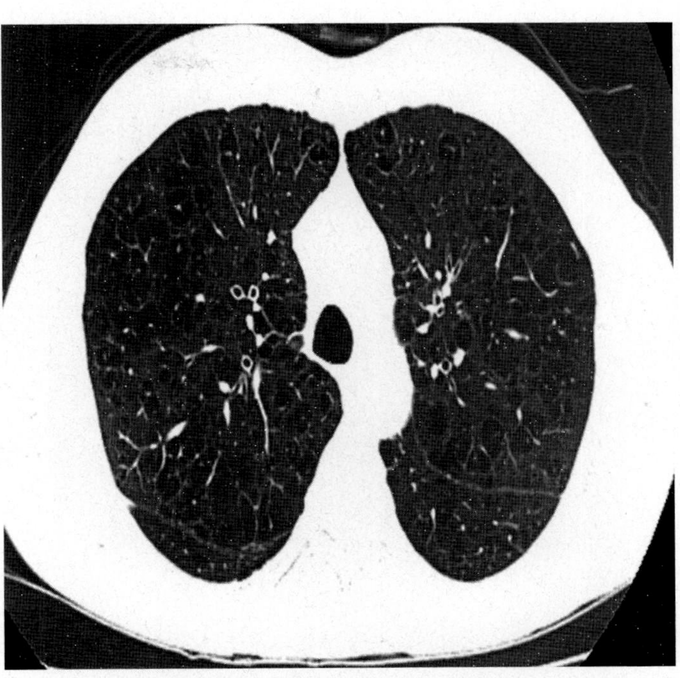

FIGURE 58-5 Centrilobular emphysema seen on high-resolution CT of the chest. Diffuse emphysematous changes throughout both lungs are seen as darker round areas of cystlike lesions. (*Reproduced with permission from Carlos S. Restrepo, MD.*)

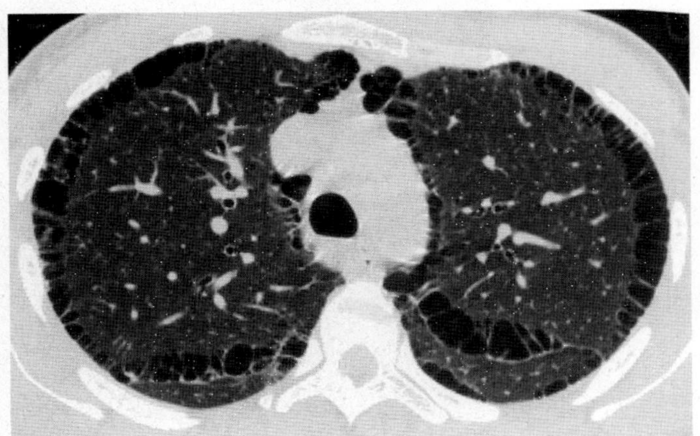

FIGURE 58-6 CT at the level of the aortic arch showing a pattern of cysts in the subpleural lung with an upper-lung zone predominance characteristic of mild paraseptal emphysema. (*Reproduced with permission from Miller WT: Diagnostic Thoracic Imaging. New York, NY: McGraw-Hill Education; 2006.*)

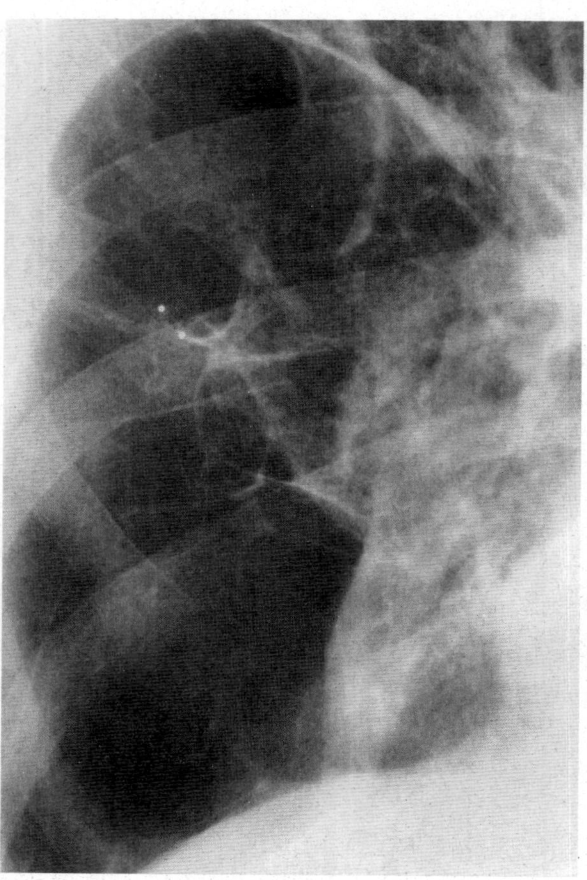

FIGURE 58-7 Close-up of CXR showing multiple large bullae in a patient with COPD. (*Reproduced with permission from Miller WT: Diagnostic Thoracic Imaging. New York, NY: McGraw-Hill Education; 2006.*)

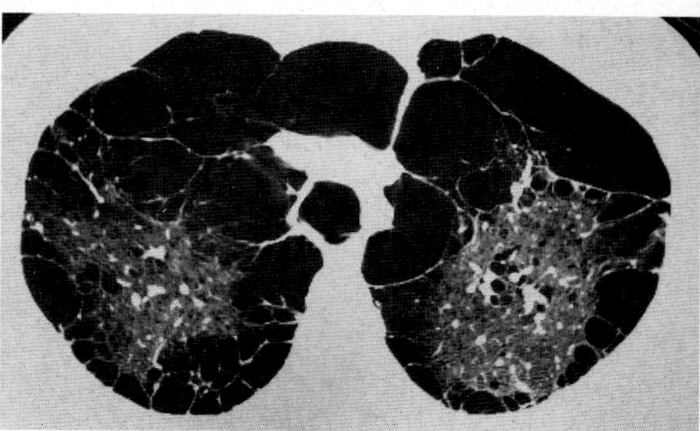

FIGURE 58-8 CT scan of the patient in **Figure 58-6** (at the level of the pulmonary veins) showing multiple large peripheral bullae; the patient was diagnosed with severe paraseptal emphysema. (*Reproduced with permission from Miller WT: Diagnostic Thoracic Imaging. New York, NY: McGraw-Hill Education; 2006.*)

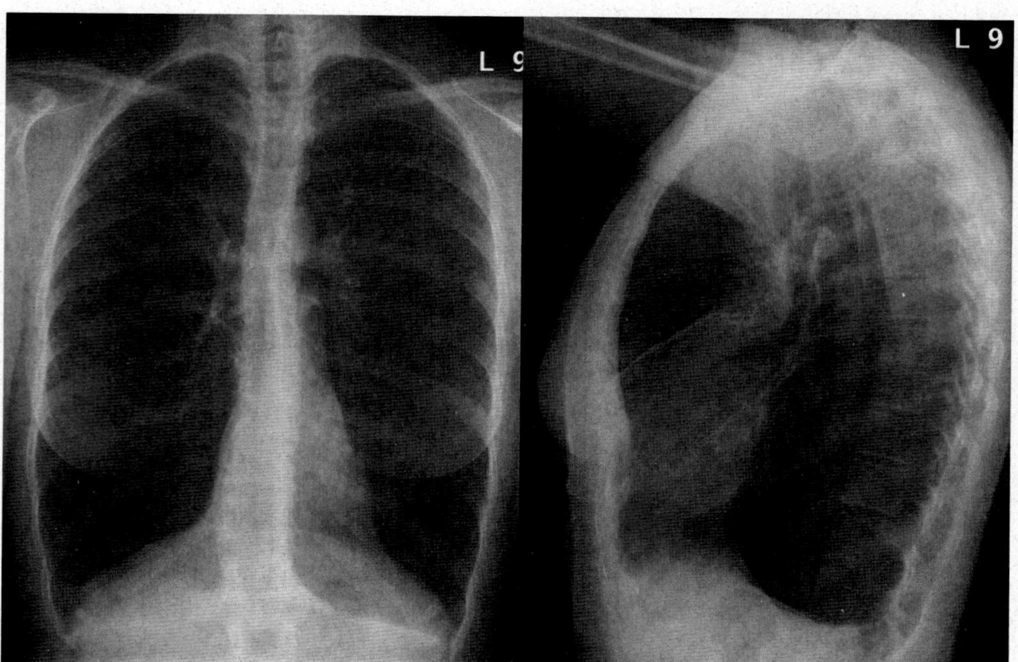

FIGURE 58-9 Advanced pulmonary emphysema in a 30-year-old woman with α_1-antitrypsin deficiency. The CXR shows increased lung volumes, flattening of the diaphragms, and a vertical heart. (*Reproduced with permission from Carlos S. Restrepo, MD.*)

TABLE 58-2 Recommended Management of COPD based on GOLD grade and exacerbation history

Patient Group	Description	Nonpharmacological Treatment	Medications (First Choice)
A	Few symptoms (CAT score <10) and 0–1 exacerbations per year, and/or mild impairment (GOLD 1 or 2)*	Smoking cessation, physical activity, vaccinations	Short-acting bronchodilator (anticholinergic OR beta$_2$-agonist as needed)
B	More symptoms (CAT score ≥10) and 0–1 exacerbations per year; and/or mild impairment (GOLD 1 or 2).*	Smoking cessation, physical activity, vaccinations, pulmonary rehabilitation	Long-acting bronchodilator (anticholinergic OR beta$_2$-agonist)
C	Few symptoms (CAT score <10) and ≥2 exacerbations per year, and/or severe impairment (GOLD 3 or 4).*	Smoking cessation, physical activity, vaccinations, pulmonary rehabilitation	Inhaled corticosteroid AND Long-acting bronchodilator OR combination long-acting beta-agonist and anticholinergic
D	More symptoms (CAT score ≥10) and ≥2 exacerbations per year, and/or severe impairment (GOLD 3 or 4).*	Smoking cessation, physical activity, vaccinations, pulmonary rehabilitation	As for C PLUS oxygen (15–20 hours daily) as appropriate

*See laboratory testing.
Abbreviations: CAT = COPD Assessment Test; GOLD = Global Initiative for Chronic Obstructive Lung Disease.

FIRST LINE

NONPHARMACOLOGIC

Nonpharmacologic therapies that should be considered for all patients are[1]:

- Smoking cessation (pharmacotherapy and nicotine replacement increase abstinence rates). SOR Ⓐ
- Influenza and pneumococcal vaccination, which are most effective in the elderly. SOR Ⓑ Also consider vaccination against herpes zoster, as patients with COPD are at increased risk (adjusted hazard ratio [HR] 1.68, 95% CI, 1.45 to 1.95), especially if using inhaled steroids (adjusted HR 2.09, 95% CI, 1.38 to 3.16) or oral steroids (adjusted HR 3.00, 95% CI, 2.40 to 3.75).[14]
- Patient education (multidisciplinary and self-management training) improves patient outcomes and reduces costs and hospitalizations.[1,15] SOR Ⓐ
- Pulmonary rehabilitation programs decrease hospitalization at 6 to 12 months, increase quality of life, and improve dyspnea and exercise capacity.[1,6] SOR Ⓐ Pulmonary rehabilitation may increase survival and improve recovery following hospitalization.[1] SOR Ⓑ
- There are no clear benefits of continuous positive pressure ventilation in patients with COPD unless they have coexisting sleep apnea, in which case there is an associated improvement in survival and decrease in risk of hospitalization.[1]

For patients with an *acute exacerbation* of COPD (defined as an increase in symptoms and change in the amount and character of the sputum and anticipated to occur about 1 to 3 times a year in patients with moderate or severe COPD), the following assessments and nonpharmacologic interventions are recommended[1]:

- Assess severity SOR Ⓒ—Physical signs of a more severe exacerbation include use of accessory muscles of respiration, paradoxical chest wall movements, worsening (or new onset) cyanosis, new

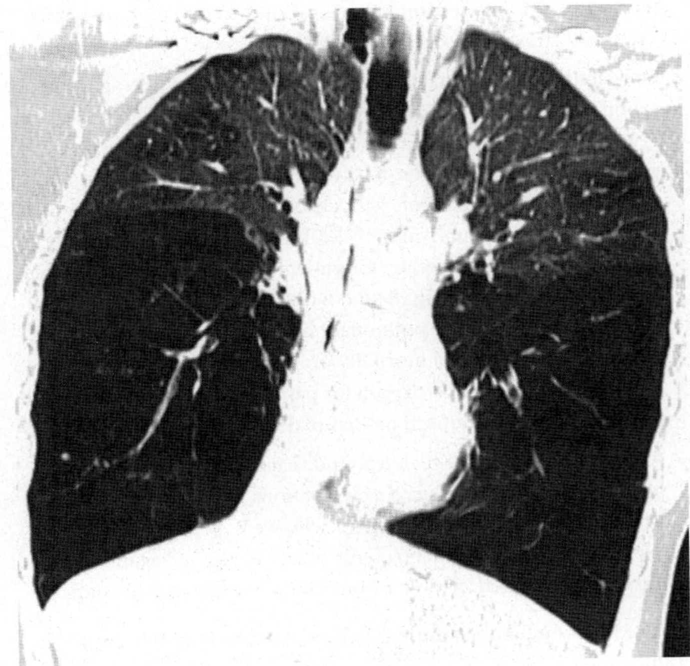

FIGURE 58-10 CT of the chest in the same 30-year-old woman with α_1-antitrypsin deficiency. Coronal reformation of the CT demonstrates extensive panlobular emphysema of the mid and lower lung zones, which is a typical distribution of this condition. The vascular markings are more prominent in the upper lobes, showing "cephalization" of flow. (*Reproduced with permission from Carlos S. Restrepo, MD.*)

peripheral edema, hemodynamic instability, or worsening mental status. Consider pulse oximetry.

- Consider CXR for those with moderate to severe symptoms and focal lung findings to exclude other diagnoses.
- Consider an ECG if suspecting cardiac complication or comorbidity.
- Consider a complete blood count (to identify anemia, polycythemia, or leukocytosis) and a theophylline level if on theophylline at admission. Consider sputum or blood cultures if clinically appropriate (e.g., purulent sputum, fever).
- Consider blood gas for those with moderate to severe symptoms, advanced COPD, history of hypercarbia, or mental status changes.
- Hospitalize—Based on clinical judgment; recommended in those with marked increase in symptom intensity or onset of new physical signs (e.g., cyanosis); frequent exacerbations; older age; the presence of respiratory acidosis, hypercarbia, hypoxemia; severe underlying COPD or serious comorbidities (e.g., heart failure); failure to respond to outpatient treatment; or poor home support.[1] SOR C

MEDICATIONS

For patients with *stable COPD*, only smoking cessation and oxygen therapy for those with hypoxia at rest have been clearly shown to improve outcome.[1] SOR A

- To assist with smoking cessation, consider antidepressant therapy (bupropion [150 mg, twice daily], varenicline [1 mg twice daily], nortriptyline [75 to 100 mg daily]), or nicotine replacement (gum, inhaler, spray, patch) and supportive counseling and follow-up; using these interventions improves rates of smoking cessation by up to twofold (see Chapter 248, Smoking and Tobacco Addiction).[1,16,17] SOR A Combining pharmacotherapy with behavioral support increases smoking cessation success compared to a minimal intervention or usual care.[18]
- Oxygen therapy is initiated for patients who have a resting O_2 saturation <89% (PaO_2 ≤55 mm Hg [7.3 kPa], confirmed twice over a 3-week period, or <89% in a patient with pulmonary hypertension, right-sided heart failure, or polycythemia); chronic administration (<15 hours/day) in patients with chronic respiratory failure is associated with greater survival.[1] SOR B The British Thoracic Society recommends oxygen therapy for patients with stable COPD with a resting PaO_2 ≤60 mm Hg (8 kPa) with evidence of peripheral edema, polycythemia or pulmonary hypertension.[19] A recent trial, however, failed to find a mortality or hospitalization benefit of long-term supplemental oxygen for patients with stable COPD and resting or exercise-induced moderate desaturation.[20]
- Authors of a Cochrane review found that use of continuous prophylactic antibiotics reduced exacerbations in patients with COPD who were frequent exacerbators or who were on supplemental oxygen. Benefits to individual patients must be weighed against potential harms to society created by antibiotic overuse and resistance.[21]

The following are recommended for symptomatic relief (see **Table 58-2**):

- Short-acting inhaled bronchodilators—β-agonists (e.g., albuterol) or anticholinergic agents (e.g., ipratropium bromide)—intermittent use; SOR A these agents are comparable in efficacy, and the choice of agent should be based on side effects, cost, and patient preference.[1]
- Inhaled long-acting bronchodilator (β-agonists or anticholinergic)—Regular treatment is more effective, but more costly.[1] SOR A β-Agonists may cause tachycardia and tremor, and anticholinergics can cause dry mouth, blurred vision, and urinary outlet obstruction. Salmeterol reduces the risk of hospitalization but has no effect on mortality or the rate of lung function decline.
- Combination long-acting β-agonists with inhaled anticholinergic agents can provide incremental benefit for symptoms.[1,22] SOR B They may also be used in combination with inhaled corticosteroids to improve health status and reduce exacerbations in patients with moderate SOR B to severe COPD SOR A.[1] In a recent randomized controlled trial (RCT), combination long acting β-agonist plus anticholinergic (indacaterol-glycopyrronium) was more effective than salmeterol-fluticasone in preventing COPD exacerbations in patients with a history of exacerbation during the previous year.[23]
- Inhaled long-acting anticholinergic (tiotropium, glycopyrronium)—Both have a duration of action of 24 hours and reduce exacerbations and improve symptoms.[1] SOR A Adverse effects include dry mouth[1]; mortality was increased with use of tiotropium mist inhaler (2.4% vs. 1.6% on placebo; number needed to harm over 1 year = 124)[24]; the Respimat inhaler appears safe.
- Inhaled glucocorticoids—Regular use is associated with improved quality of life and a small decrease in the frequency of exacerbations (approximately half-a-day per month), but an increase in oral candidiasis, easy bruising, and bone loss (the last shown for long-term triamcinolone acetonide).[1] SOR A These agents are recommended for patients with moderate to severe COPD or for frequent exacerbations. In patients at low risk of exacerbation, steroids can be withdrawn safely provided patients continue use of long-acting bronchodilators.[25] Parenteral steroids do not benefit patients with stable COPD. In a Cochrane review comparing inhaled glucocorticoids with long-acting β-agonists, the authors concluded that effects were comparable on most outcomes, including reduced frequency of exacerbation, with β-agonists conferring a small additional benefit in lung function while inhaled corticosteroid therapy showed a small advantage in health-related quality of life but increased the risk of pneumonia.[26]

For patients with *an acute exacerbation* of COPD, the three classes of medications commonly used are bronchodilators, corticosteroids, and antibiotics.

- Inhaled bronchodilators—Both β-agonists and anticholinergics can be used alone or in combination; metered-dose inhalers with proper patient instruction perform as well as nebulized treatments and are less expensive; nebulizers can be considered for sicker patients.[1] SOR A
- Glucocorticoid—Use oral (prednisone 40 mg/day for 5 days) or intravenous glucocorticoids if the patient is unable to tolerate oral medication. Steroids decrease recovery time, hospital length of stay, and relapse rates.[1] SOR A
- Antibiotics—Treating COPD with antibiotics is controversial. Authors of a Cochrane review concluded that antibiotics were helpful for patients admitted to the ICU with severe exacerbations but did not significantly affect mortality or length of stay for other hospitalized patients or for outpatients.[27] GOLD recommends the use of antibiotics for 5 to 10 days for patients with increased dyspnea,

sputum volume, and sputum purulence, and for patients who require mechanical ventilation.[1] SOR Ⓑ Antibiotics can be considered for those with two of these three symptoms, provided that one is increased sputum purulence, but should primarily be used for patients with clinical evidence of bacterial infection who are moderately or severely ill.[1] SOR Ⓒ

- The choice of antibiotic does not appear to influence outcome and should be based on local bacterial resistance and severity of disease. For exacerbations of lesser severity, use narrow-spectrum antibiotics such as amoxicillin with or without clavulanic acid, doxycycline, or a macrolide.[1] For exacerbations of greater severity or with frequent exacerbations, cultures can help direct antibiotic choice. SOR Ⓒ
- Oxygen therapy—Use to maintain O_2 saturation at 88% to 92%.[1] SOR Ⓒ
- Noninvasive mechanical ventilation (NIV) decreases mortality and the need for intubation, and reduces hospital length of stay.[1] SOR Ⓐ However, patients may find it difficult to tolerate. It should be considered for patients with severe dyspnea (e.g., use of accessory muscles) and/or respiratory acidosis (pH <7.35 and/or $PaCO_2$ >6.0 kPa, 45 mm Hg).[1]
- Mechanical ventilation support should be considered for patients with the above indications who are unable to tolerate NIV and for those with respiratory pauses with loss of consciousness, diminished consciousness, massive aspiration or inability to remove respiratory secretions, severe hemodynamic instability unresponsive to fluids or vasoactive drugs, heart rate less than 50 beats per minute with loss of alertness, severe ventricular arrhythmias, and respiratory or cardiac arrest.[1] SOR Ⓒ

COMPLEMENTARY AND ALTERNATIVE THERAPY

- There is supporting evidence for immunostimulant therapy (reduced hospital days), cineole (a constituent of eucalyptus oil on reducing severity and duration of exacerbations and improved lung function, dyspnea, and quality of life), and ginseng (on lung function and quality of life) in patients with COPD.[28–30] SOR Ⓑ
- Cochrane authors concluded that tai chi improved walking distance over usual care but data were inconclusive with respect to other outcomes.[31] SOR Ⓑ
- Acupuncture may improve 6-minute walk distance during exercise for patients with COPD.[32]

REFERRAL

Reasons to consider referral include diagnostic uncertainty; severe disease, including onset of cor pulmonale; assessment for oxygen, corticosteroid, or pulmonary rehabilitation therapy; surgical assessment (bullous lung disease, severe disease); rapid decline in FEV_1; early onset or family history of COPD; frequent infections; and hemoptysis. There are treatments available for α_1-antitrypsin deficiency, and these patients should be referred to a pulmonologist for evaluation and treatment.

SECOND LINE

MEDICATIONS

- Theophylline—Mildly effective for symptoms SOR Ⓐ and reduction in exacerbations SOR Ⓑ, but associated with nausea and risk of toxicity with high blood levels.[1]
- Mucolytic agents (e.g., guaifenesin, carbocysteine, potassium iodide)—Produce a small decrease in the frequency of exacerbations (0.5 fewer exacerbations/year) and in disability days.[33] SOR Ⓐ GOLD does not recommend these medications for routine use.[1]
- Phosphodiesterase-4 inhibitor (roflumilast) can be considered for patients with moderate to severe COPD who are already on an inhaled bronchodilator. It is prescribed as a 500-mcg oral daily dose. Authors of a Cochrane review found benefit over placebo in improving lung function and reducing likelihood of exacerbations, but little impact on quality of life.[34] Side effects include nausea, diarrhea, weight loss, and headache. The role of these agents in COPD management is unclear.

SURGERY

Two surgical therapies with the best supporting evidence may be considered for patients with severe disease despite optimal medical therapy:

- Lung volume reduction surgery (LVRS)—A procedure in which parts of the lung are removed to reduce hyperinflation. Patients with upper lobe predominant disease and low postrehabilitation exercise capacity appear to gain the most symptom benefit and improved survival (54% vs. 39.7%).[1] SOR Ⓐ However, in one RCT, there was a high risk of death within the first 30 days following surgery, resulting in a significantly higher mortality rate at 3 years; at 5 years, survival was similar to medical therapy and quality of life was possibly superior.[35] This procedure can also be performed bronchoscopically.
- Lung transplantation—GOLD lists recommended criteria of a BODE (body mass, obstruction, dyspnea, exercise) index (see Prognosis) of 7–10 with at least one of the following: history of exacerbation with acute hypercapnia; pulmonary hypertension, cor pulmonale, or both despite oxygen therapy; and FEV_1 <20% predicted with either diffusing capacity of the lung for carbon monoxide <20% predicted or homogenous distribution of emphysema.[1] SOR Ⓒ Lung transplantation has potential for improving quality of life and exercise capacity, but complications are many and include postoperative mortality, bronchiolitis obliterans, and opportunistic infections. Of course it is major surgery with very high costs and significant risks.

PREVENTION AND SCREENING

- The best prevention for COPD is to not smoke or to quit smoking. Limiting occupational exposures and exposure to indoor air pollution is also preventive.
- GOLD recommends active case finding but not general population screening.[1] The U.S. Preventive Services Task Force also recommends against screening asymptomatic adults for COPD using spirometry.[36]

PROGNOSIS

- In a longitudinal study of 227 patients with COPD in Japan, 5-year survival was 73%; level of dyspnea but not FEV_1 was correlated with survival rates.[37]
- Severity classification (see "Laboratory Testing" above) can be used in predicting risk of exacerbations (1.1 to 1.3 for severe and 1.2 to 2.0 for very severe), hospitalizations per year (0.11 to 0.2 for moderate,

0.25 to 0.3 for severe, and 0.4 to 0.54 for very severe), or 3-year mortality (11% for moderate, 15% for severe, 24% for very severe).[1]

- The BODE index is a composite measure using body mass, obstruction (FEV_1, % predicted), dyspnea (MMRC score), and exercise (6-minute walking distance) to predict mortality. The risk of death from respiratory causes increases by more than 60% for each 1-point increase in BODE score.[38] An online calculator is available at http://reference.medscape.com/calculator/bode-index-copd.
- In-hospital mortality of patients admitted for hypercapnic exacerbation with acidosis is approximately 10%, and mortality at 1-year postdischarge for those requiring mechanical ventilation is 40%.[1] Hospitalization for COPD increases risk of death, which has been reported as 23% at 1-year and 79% at 9-year follow-up.[39,40]

FOLLOW-UP

Patients should be followed regularly for disease progression or development of complications.

- At each visit ask about symptoms, activity, and sleep. For smokers, encourage cessation. Symptom questionnaires can be used (every 2 to 3 months using CAT suggested by GOLD) for monitoring.
- For patients on medications, monitor treatment effectiveness ("Have you noticed a difference, for example less breathlessness?") and side effects. Observe inhaler technique at least once to ensure optimal delivery.
- Document exacerbations/hospitalizations; this may indicate a need for additional treatment.
- Monitor for comorbidities (e.g., heart disease, hypertension, osteoporosis, anxiety/depression, lung cancer, infections, metabolic syndrome, and diabetes) and maximize control of those conditions. The GOLD reference provides information on management of these conditions in patients with COPD.[1]
- Additional concerns for patients with severe COPD include need for long-term oxygen and need for specialist referral, including social services; biyearly evaluation should be considered. Hospice referral may also be appropriate.
- Unfortunately, comprehensive management programs for patients with severe COPD do not appear beneficial.[41,42]

PATIENT EDUCATION

Smoking cessation should be strongly and repeatedly encouraged. Progressive exercise should also be encouraged. Activities that brace the arms and allow use of accessory muscles of respiration are better tolerated—these include pushing a cart, walker, or wheelchair, and use of a treadmill.

PATIENT RESOURCES

For general information, these sites are helpful:

- American Lung Association—**http://www.lung.org/lung-health-and-diseases/lung-disease-lookup/copd/.**
- *Journal of the American Medical Association*, Chronic Obstructive Pulmonary Disease, Patient Page with good diagram—**http://jamanetwork.com/journals/jama/fullarticle/182970.**
- MedlinePlus—**https://medlineplus.gov/copd.html.**
- The Family of COPD Support Programs, COPD Support, Inc. This website provides information and links to support groups—**http://www.copd-support.com.**

PROVIDER RESOURCES

- Evidence-based guidelines are available on GOLD (GOLD) at—**http://www.goldcopd.org.**

REFERENCES

1. Global Initiative for Chronic Obstructive Lung Disease (GOLD). *Global Strategy for the Diagnosis, Management and Prevention of Chronic Obstructive Pulmonary Disease (Updated 2016)*. Accessed April 2017. Available from goldcopd.org/.
2. Centers for Disease Control and Prevention. *Chronic Obstructive Pulmonary Disease.* https://www.cdc.gov/copd/index.html. Accessed January 2017.
3. Centers for Disease Control and Prevention. *Chronic Obstructive Pulmonary Disease (COPD). Data and Statistics.* http://www.cdc.gov/copd/data.html. Accessed January 2017.
4. Menezes AM, Perez-Padilla R, Jardim JR, et al. Chronic obstructive lung disease in five Latin American cities (the PLATINO study): a prevalence study. *Lancet.* 2005;366:1875-1881.
5. Lindberg A, Jonsson AC, Ronmark E, et al. Ten-year cumulative incidence of COPD and risk factors for incident disease in asymptomatic cohort. *Chest.* 2005;127:1544-1552.
6. Reilly JJ, Silverman EK, Shapiro SD. Chronic obstructive pulmonary disease. In: Kasper DL, Braunwald E, Fauci AS, et al., eds. *Harrison's Principles of Internal Medicine*, 16th ed. New York, NY: McGraw-Hill; 2005:1547-1554.
7. Soler Artigas M, Wain LV, Repapi E, et al. Effect of five genetic variants associated with lung function on the risk of chronic obstructive lung disease, and their joint effects on lung function. *Am J Respir Crit Care Med.* 2011;184(7):786-795.
8. Hersh CP, Silverman EK, Gascon J, et al. SOX5 is a candidate gene for chronic obstructive pulmonary disease susceptibility and is necessary for lung development. *Am J Respir Crit Care Med.* 2011; 183(11):1482-1489.
9. Forey BA, Thornton AJ, Lee PN. Systematic review with meta-analysis of the epidemiological evidence relating smoking to COPD, chronic bronchitis and emphysema. *BMC Pulm Med.* 2011;11:36.
10. Hersh CP, Hokanson JE, Lynch DA, et al. Family history is a risk factor for COPD. *Chest.* 2011;140(2):343-350.
11. Müllerova H, Maselli DJ, Locantore N, et al. Hospitalized exacerbations of COPD: risk factors and outcomes in the ECLIPSE cohort. *Chest.* 2015;147(4):999-1007.

12. Kornmann O, Beeh KM, Beier J, et al. Global Initiative for Obstructive Lung Disease. Newly diagnosed chronic obstructive pulmonary disease. Clinical features and distribution of the novel stages of the Global Initiative for Obstructive Lung Disease. *Respiration.* 2003;70:67-75.

13. Qaseem A, Wilt TJ, Weinberger SE, et al. Diagnosis and management of stable chronic obstructive pulmonary disease: a clinical practice guideline update from the American College of Physicians, American College of Chest Physicians, American Thoracic Society, and European Respiratory Society. *Ann Intern Med.* 2011;155(3):179-191.

14. Yang YW, Chen YH, Wang KH, et al. Risk of herpes zoster among patients with chronic obstructive pulmonary disease: a population-based study. *CMAJ.* 2011;183:E275-E280.

15. Gadoury MA, Schwartzman K, Rouleau M, et al. Chronic Obstructive Pulmonary Disease axis of the Respiratory Health Network, Fonds de la recherche en sante du Quebec (FRSQ). Self-management reduces both short- and long-term hospitalisation in COPD. *Eur Respir J.* 2005;26(5):853-857.

16. Hughes JR, Stead LF, Hartmann-Boyce J, et al. Antidepressants for smoking cessation. *Cochrane Database Syst Rev.* 2014;(1):CD000031.

17. Stead LF, Perera R, Bullen C, et al. Nicotine replacement therapy for smoking cessation. *Cochrane Database Syst Rev.* 2012;(11):CD000146.

18. Stead LF, Koilpillai P, Fanshawe TR, Lancaster T. Combined pharmacotherapy and behavioural interventions for smoking cessation. *Cochrane Database Syst Rev.* 2016;(3):CD008286.

19. Hardinge M, Annandale J, Bourne S, et al. British Thoracic Society guidelines for home oxygen use in adults. *Thorax.* 2015;70 Suppl 1:i1-i43.

20. Long-Term Oxygen Treatment Trial Research Group. A randomized trial of long-term oxygen for COPD with moderate desaturation. *N Engl J Med.* 2016;375(17):1617-1627.

21. Herath SC, Poole P. Prophylactic antibiotic therapy for chronic obstructive pulmonary disease (COPD). *Cochrane Database Syst Rev.* 2013;(11):CD009764.

22. Oba Y, Sarva ST, Dias S. Efficacy and safety of long-acting β-agonist/long acting muscarinic antagonist combinations in COPD: a network meta-analysis. *Thorax.* 2016;71(1):15-25.

23. Wedzicha JA, Banerji D, Chapman KR, et al. Indacaterol-glycopyrronium versus salmeterol-fluticasone for COPD. *N Engl J Med.* 2016;374(23):2222-2234.

24. Singh S, Loke YK, Enright PL, Furberg CD. Mortality associated with tiotropium mist inhaler in patients with chronic obstructive pulmonary disease: systematic review and meta-analysis of randomised controlled trials. *BMJ.* 2011;342:d3215.

25. Magnussen H, Disse B, Rodriguez-Roisin R, et al. Withdrawal of inhaled glucocorticoids and exacerbations of COPD. *N Engl J Med.* 2014 2;371(14):1285-1294.

26. Spencer S, Evans DJ, Karner C, Cates CJ. Inhaled corticosteroids versus long-acting beta(2)-agonists for chronic obstructive pulmonary disease. *Cochrane Database Syst Rev.* 2011;(12):CD007033.

27. Vollenweider DJ, Jarrett H, Steurer-Stey CA, et al. Antibiotics for exacerbations of chronic obstructive pulmonary disease. *Cochrane Database Syst Rev.* 2012;(12):CD010257.

28. Collet JP, Shapiro P, Ernst P, et al. Effects of an immunostimulating agent on acute exacerbations and hospitalizations in patients with chronic obstructive pulmonary disease. The PARI-IS Study Steering Committee and Research Group. Prevention of Acute Respiratory Infection by an Immunostimulant. *Am J Respir Crit Care Med.* 1997;158:1719-1724.

29. Worth H, Schacher C, Dethlefsen U. Concomitant therapy with Cineole (Eucalyptole) reduces exacerbations in COPD: a placebo-controlled double-blind trial. *Respir Res.* 2009;10:69.

30. An X, Zhang AL, Yang AW, et al. Oral ginseng formulae for stable chronic obstructive pulmonary disease: a systematic review. *Respir Med.* 2011;105:165-176.

31. Ngai SPC, Jones AYM, Tam WWS. Tai Chi for chronic obstructive pulmonary disease (COPD). *Cochrane Database Syst Rev.* 2016;(6):CD009953.

32. Suzuki M, Muro S, Ando Y, et al. A randomized, placebo-controlled trial of acupuncture in patients with chronic obstructive pulmonary disease (COPD): the COPD-acupuncture trial (CAT). *Arch Intern Med.* 2012;172(11):878-886.

33. Poole P, Chong J, Cates CJ. Mucolytic agents for chronic bronchitis or chronic obstructive pulmonary disease. *Cochrane Database Syst Rev.* 2015;(7):CD001287.

34. Chong J, Leung B, Poole P. Phosphodiesterase-4 inhibitors for chronic obstructive pulmonary disease. *Cochrane Database Syst Rev.* 2013;(11):CD002309.

35. Kaplan RM, Sun Q, Naunheim KS, Ries AL. Long-term follow-up of high-risk patients in the National Emphysema Treatment Trial. *Ann Thorac Surg.* 2014;98(5):1782-1789.

36. United States Preventive Services Task Force. *Screening for Chronic Obstructive Pulmonary Disease Using Spirometry.* https://www.uspreventiveservicestaskforce.org/Page/Document/Update-SummaryFinal/chronic-obstructive-pulmonary-disease-screening?ds=1&s=copd. Accessed January 2017.

37. Nishimura K, Izumi T, Tsukino M, Oga T. Dyspnea is a better predictor of 5-year survival than airway obstruction in patients with COPD. *Chest.* 2002;121:1434-1440.

38. Celli BR, Cote CG, Martin JM, et al. The body-mass index, airflow obstruction, dyspnea, and exercise capacity index in chronic obstructive pulmonary disease. *N Engl J Med.* 2004;350(10):1005-1012.

39. Groenewegen KH, Schols AM, Wouters EF. Mortality and mortality-related factors after hospitalization for acute exacerbation of COPD. *Chest.* 2003;124:459-467.

40. Gudmundsson G, Ulrik CS, Gislason T, et al. Long-term survival in patients hospitalized for chronic obstructive pulmonary disease: a prospective observational study in the Nordic countries. *Int J Chron Obstruct Pulmon Dis.* 2012;7:571-576.

41. Fan VS, Gaziano JM, Lew R, et al. A comprehensive care management program to prevent chronic obstructive pulmonary disease hospitalizations: a randomized, controlled trial. *Ann Intern Med.* 2012;158(10):673-83.

42. Kruis AL, Boland MR, Assendelft WJ, et al. Effectiveness of integrated disease management for primary care chronic obstructive pulmonary disease patients: results of cluster randomised trial. *BMJ.* 2014 Sep 10;349:g5392.

59 PULMONARY EMBOLISM

Munima Nasir, MD
M. Joyce Green, MD
Mindy A. Smith, MD, MS

PATIENT STORY

A 52-year-old woman developed acute shortness of breath 3 weeks after a hysterectomy. She denied leg pain or swelling. She has no chronic medical problems and takes no medications. Her pulse is 105 beats/min, respiratory rate is 20 breaths/min, and the rest of her examination is unremarkable. She had an elevated hemidiaphragm on chest X-ray (CXR). These findings placed her at moderate risk for pulmonary embolism (PE) based on the Geneva score. Chest CT demonstrated a moderate-sized PE like the one shown in **Figure 59-1**. She was treated with anticoagulation without complications.

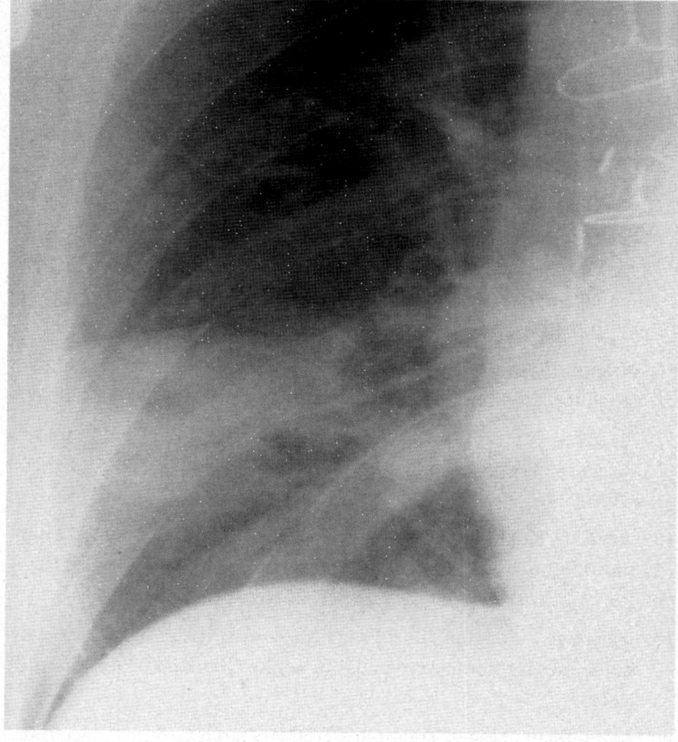

FIGURE 59-1 CXR showing a wedge-shaped pulmonary infarction with the base on the pleural surface and the apex at the tip of a pulmonary artery catheter; the catheter caused the occlusion of a peripheral artery. (*Reproduced with permission from Miller WT: Diagnostic Thoracic Imaging. New York, NY: McGraw-Hill Education; 2006.*)

INTRODUCTION

PE is a thromboembolic occlusion (total or partial) of one or more pulmonary arteries, usually arising from venous thromboembolism (VTE).

SYNONYMS

PE is also known as pulmonary thromboembolism and VTE as deep venous thrombosis (DVT).

EPIDEMIOLOGY

- In a report based on national surveillance data from 2007 to 2009, the estimated mean annual incidence of hospitalization with VTE in adults in the United States was 547,596. PE is diagnosed in an estimated mean 277,549 annual hospitalizations.[1]
- In one population-based retrospective medical record review from Olmstead County, Minnesota, the average annual incidence of in-hospital VTE was 960.5 per 10,000 person years, more than 100 times greater than that among community residents.[2] PE accounted for most of the age-related increase among hospital cases.
- Authors of one meta-analysis concluded that nearly 1 in every 4 to 5 patients presenting with an exacerbation of chronic obstructive pulmonary disease has a PE; presenting signs and symptoms did not distinguish patients with and without PE.[3]
- In a meta-analysis of randomized controlled trials (RCTs) of patients on VTE prophylaxis, the pooled rates of symptomatic DVT were 0.63% (95% confidence interval [CI], 0.47% to 0.78%) following knee arthroplasty and 0.26% (95% CI, 0.14% to 0.37%) following hip arthroplasty. The pooled rates for PE were 0.27% (95% CI, 0.16% to 0.38%) following knee arthroplasty and 0.14% (95% CI, 0.07% to 0.21%) following hip arthroplasty.[4]

- Authors of a meta-analysis of 12 studies concluded that PEs were noted as incidental findings in 2.6% (95% CI 1.9, 3.4) of chest CT studies.[5]

ETIOLOGY AND PATHOPHYSIOLOGY

- PE is most commonly caused by embolization of a thrombus from a proximal leg or pelvic vein that enters the pulmonary artery circulation and obstructs a vessel. PE may also be caused by an upper-extremity thrombus (**Figure 59-1**); fat embolus; hair, talc, or cotton embolus from IV drug use; or amniotic fluid embolus.[6]
- PE results from vascular endothelial injury, which promotes platelet adhesion, blood flow stasis, and/or hypercoagulation, causing more coagulants to accumulate than usual and resulting in obstruction. Although most PEs are asymptomatic and do not alter physiology, PE can cause:
  - Increased pulmonary, vascular, and airway resistance
  - Impaired gas exchange
  - Alveolar hyperventilation
  - Decreased pulmonary compliance
  - Right ventricular (RV) dysfunction
  - Only approximately 10% of emboli cause pulmonary infarction; most PEs are multiple and involve the lower lobes[7]

RISK FACTORS

Factors associated with increased risk of VTE based on a cohort study are[8]:

- Pregnancy or postpartum (adjusted odds ratio [OR] 8.3)
- Recent sepsis (adjusted OR 4)
- Malignancy (adjusted OR 2.3)
- History of VTE (adjusted OR 2.1)
- Central venous access (adjusted OR 1.8)
- Other risk factors for PE include hormonal treatment (i.e., combined estrogen/progestogen oral contraceptives [OCs] or menopausal hormone therapy), use of antipsychotics, obesity, smoking, chronic obstructive pulmonary disease, immobility, bed rest for more than 3 days, and clotting disorders.

Several risk-scoring systems are available:

- Through a prospective open cohort study, a risk prediction model or algorithm using many of the above factors, the QThrombosis, was developed and validated. This model quantifies absolute risk of thrombosis at 1 and 5 years among patients who do not have a history of venous thrombosis; a family history of thrombosis; and are not pregnant, taking anticoagulants, or have symptoms suggestive of a thrombosis.[9] An online calculator can be found at QThrombosis risk calculator (http://www.qthrombosis.org/index.php).
- The Rogers risk score can be used to predict risk of postoperative VTE after general and vascular surgery.[10] This scoring system of 15 variables including patient, laboratory and operative characteristics was based on a cohort study with independent derivation and validation cohorts. This system helps identify patients at risk for postoperative VTE and to institute appropriate perioperative prophylactic measures.

DIAGNOSIS

A history and physical examination should be completed to assess risk factors and determine whether the patient is clinically stable and to determine the clinical probability of PE.

CLINICAL FEATURES

- Dyspnea—The most common symptom; tachycardia is the most common sign. Sudden onset of dyspnea is the best single predictor (positive likelihood ratio [LR+] 2.7).
- Chest pain—May be caused by a small, peripheral PE with pulmonary infarction.
- Other signs—Include fever, neck vein distention, and accentuated pulmonic component of the second heart sound.
- Massive PE—May present with shock, syncope, and cyanosis.

When the clinical presentation raises the suspicion of PE, it should prompt further objective testing. Diagnosis begins with initial risk stratification based on the presence of persistent hypotension to identify patients with high risk of early mortality.

- Emergency CT angiography or bedside transthoracic echocardiography is recommended for patients with suspected high-risk PE with sustained hypotension.[11]
- For patients without high suspicion of PE, the use of prediction rules allows classification of patients with suspected PE into distinct categories of clinical or pretest probability that correspond to an increasing prevalence of confirmed PE.[11,12]
- Validated diagnostic clinical decision rules include the following; online calculators are available for each:
  - Wells clinical decision rule
  - Revised Geneva score
  - Pisa model, which appears more accurate than Wells or Geneva models
  - Pulmonary Embolism Rule-Out Criteria (PERC)
- The American College of Physicians (ACP) recommends that clinicians use validated clinical prediction rules to estimate pretest probability in patients in whom acute PE is being considered.[12]

LABORATORY STUDIES AND ECG

- The combination of clinical decision rules and sensitive plasma D-dimer is used to rule out a PE (sensitive but not specific).[13,14] SOR B The ACP recommends obtaining a high-sensitivity D-dimer measurement as the initial diagnostic test in patients who have an intermediate pretest probability of PE or in patients with low pretest probability of PE who do not meet all Pulmonary Embolism Rule-Out Criteria.[12] ACP recommends that clinicians NOT obtain D-dimer measurements or imaging studies in patients with a low pretest probability of PE and who meet all PERC criteria (https://www.mdcalc.com/perc-rule-pulmonary-embolism) or in patients with a high pretest probability of PE.[12]
  - Several D-dimer assays are available. The quantitative enzyme-linked immunosorbent assay (ELISA) has a diagnostic

sensitivity of 95% or better and can therefore be used to exclude PE in patients with either a low or a moderate pretest probability.[11,15,16]

 - Clinicians should use age-adjusted D-dimer thresholds in patients older than 50 years to determine whether imaging is warranted.[12] Clinicians should not obtain any imaging studies in patients with a D-dimer level below the age-adjusted cutoff.

- An ECG may be indicated to search for alternative diagnoses. The most frequent, sensitive, and specific ECG finding for PE is T-wave inversion in leads V1 to V4, which is indicative of RV strain. Other findings include tachycardia, new-onset atrial fibrillation or flutter, S in lead I, Q and inverted T in lead III, and a QRS axis greater than 90 degrees.
- Arterial blood gas is obtained if clinically indicated. A platelet count should be obtained prior to initiation of fondaparinux.[17]

IMAGING

- The American College of Radiology (ACR) recommends chest X-ray for patients with acute chest pain and intermediate probability with a negative D-dimer or low pretest probability.[18] CXR is often nonspecific; dyspnea with a near-normal CXR should suggest PE. Findings that may be seen on CXR include:
  - Triad of basal infiltrate, blunted costophrenic angle, and elevated hemidiaphragm.
  - Infiltrates similar to pneumonia (**Figure 59-2**) that may be diagnosed using CT (**Figure 59-3**).
  - A peripheral wedge-shaped density (see **Figure 59-1**).
  - Decreased vascular markings (**Figure 59-4**).
- ACR recommends CT angiography (CTA) of the chest with intravenous (IV) contrast, CT chest with IV contrast or CXR for patients with acute chest pain and intermediate probability with a positive D-dimer or high pretest probability.
  - CTA (spiral or helical) is considered the imaging method of choice by the European Society of Cardiology (**Figure 59-5**).[11] ACP recommends that clinicians obtain imaging with CT pulmonary angiography (CTPA) in patients with high pretest probability of PE.[12]
- ACP also recommend that clinicians should reserve ventilation-perfusion scans for patients who have a contraindication to CTPA or if CTPA is not available.[12] A V/Q scan is considered the initial test for patients with high probability of PE who have renal insufficiency or dye allergy. A high-probability scan for PE (positive predictive value of 90%) has 2 or more segmental perfusion defects with normal ventilation.
- For pregnant women with suspected PE, the American Thoracic Society/Society of Thoracic Radiology recommend CXR as the initial study followed by lung scintigraphy (V/Q scan) if the CXR is normal, and CTPA if the V/Q scan is nondiagnostic.[19]
- If the CTPA or lung scan is nondiagnostic, a leg ultrasound with compression is usually performed. If positive for a DVT, proceed with treatment as below. If normal or nondiagnostic, other testing such as a pulmonary angiogram is suggested.
- Pulmonary angiography is generally reserved for patients with nondiagnostic CTPA, lung scans, or leg ultrasound, and for patients

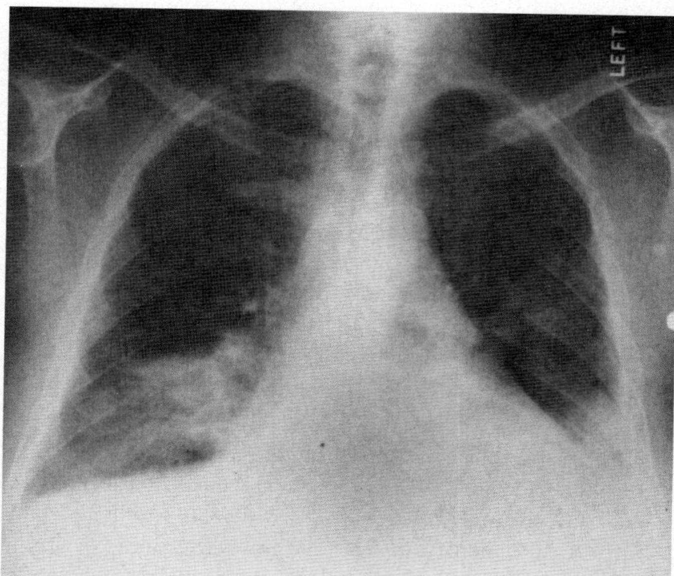

FIGURE 59-2 CXR showing bilateral pulmonary infiltrates thought to represent pneumonia. (*Reproduced with permission from Miller WT: Diagnostic Thoracic Imaging. New York, NY: McGraw-Hill Education; 2006.*)

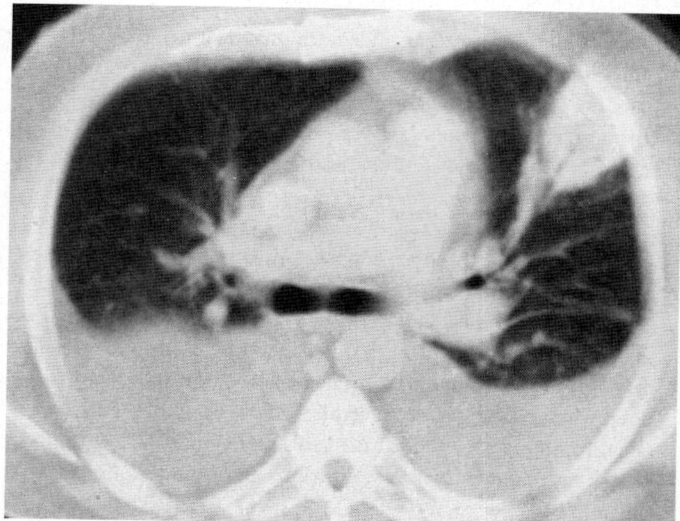

FIGURE 59-3 CT scan from the patient in **Figure 59-2** demonstrates several large, wedge-shaped pulmonary opacities with air bronchograms characteristic of pulmonary infarcts. (*Reproduced with permission from Miller WT: Diagnostic Thoracic Imaging. New York, NY: McGraw-Hill Education; 2006.*)

who will undergo embolectomy or catheter-directed thrombolysis. ACR also recommends pulmonary angiography in circumstances where a specific diagnosis (i.e., PE) is considered necessary for proper patient management and before placement of an inferior vena cava (IVC) filter.[19] An intraluminal filling defect may be seen along with truncated arteries associated with regions of diminished perfusion (**Figure 59-6**).

DIFFERENTIAL DIAGNOSIS

The differential diagnosis of a symptomatic PE includes:

- Pneumonia—Symptoms include chills, fever, and pleuritic chest pain. Physical findings include dullness to percussion and crackles with area of infiltrate usually confirmed on CXR (see Chapter 55, Pneumonia).
- Congestive heart failure—History of previous heart failure or myocardial infarction; symptoms of paroxysmal nocturnal dyspnea, orthopnea, or the presence of bilateral lower extremity edema, third heart sound, hepatojugular reflex, and jugular venous distention. CXR may show pulmonary venous congestion, interstitial or alveolar edema, and cardiomegaly (see Chapter 50, Heart Failure).
- Pneumothorax—History of previous pneumothorax or chronic obstructive pulmonary disease, or current rib fracture; physical findings include absence of breath sounds, and CXR may show free air, an elevated hemidiaphragm, or a shift of the mediastinum to the contralateral side with a tension pneumothorax.

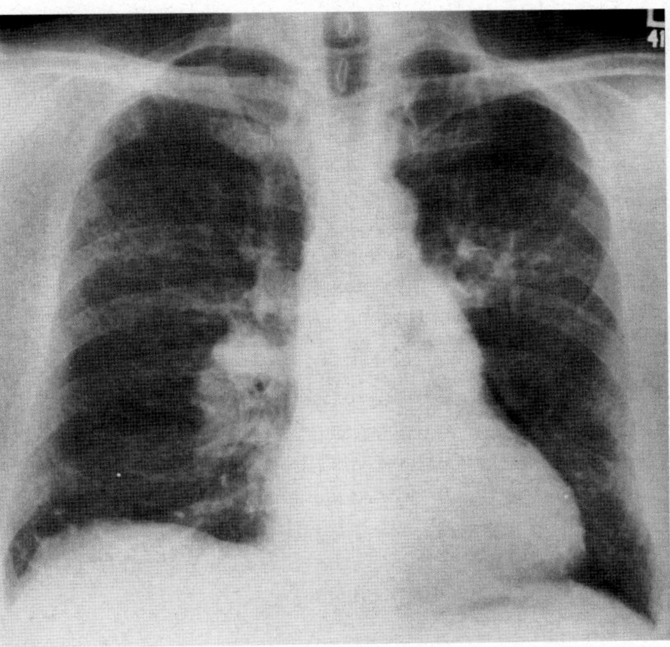

FIGURE 59-4 Pulmonary embolism: Westermark sign, an avascular zone because of obstructed vessel from a blood clot. In this patient, both lung apices and the mid to lower thorax have decreased vascular markings. Note the fusiform enlargement of both hila and the prominent pulmonary artery mediastinal shadow characteristic of pulmonary hypertension. (*Reproduced with permission from Miller WT: Diagnostic Thoracic Imaging. New York, NY: McGraw-Hill Education; 2006.*)

MANAGEMENT

FIRST LINE

MEDICATION

▶ Initial treatment of stable patients with suspected or diagnosed PE

- Treatment of asymptomatic PE (found incidentally) and that of symptomatic PE are similar.[20] SOR Ⓑ
- In patients without cancer, initial treatment of acute PE is with a novel oral anticoagulant (NOAC) for the first 3 months.[21–24] SOR Ⓐ NOACs not requiring initial parental anticoagulation include:
  - Rivaroxaban (Xarelto): 15 mg twice daily for 3 weeks (followed by 20 mg once-daily dosing; avoid if creatinine clearance <30 mL/min).
  - Apixaban (Eliquis): 10 mg orally twice daily for 7 days, then 5 mg twice daily.
- Alternatively, NOAC therapy can be started after 5–10 days of parenteral anticoagulant.[20] These include:
  - Dabigatran (Pradaxa): 150 mg twice daily (avoid if creatinine clearance <30 mL/min).
  - Edoxaban (Savaysa): 60 mg once daily (30 mg once daily if creatinine clearance is 15–50 mL/min, if body weight ≤60 kg, or with concomitant use of certain p-glycoprotein inhibitors).

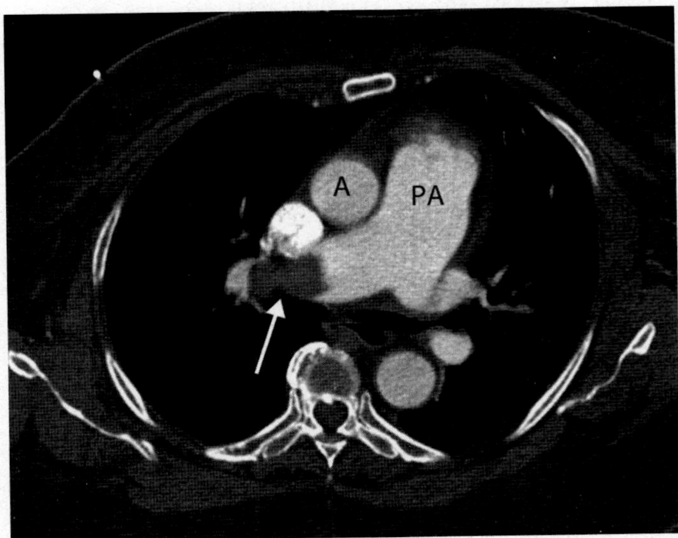

FIGURE 59-5 Acute pulmonary embolism with likely pulmonary arterial hypertension. There is an intraluminal filling defect, consistent with an acute pulmonary embolism (*white arrow*). The pulmonary arterial trunk (*PA*) is larger than the adjacent ascending aorta (*A*), suggesting pulmonary arterial hypertension, likely due to the large PE. (*Reproduced with permission from Elsayes KM, Oldham SAA. Introduction to Diagnostic Radiology. New York, NY; McGraw-Hill Education; 2014.*)

▶ Treatment of patients with high-risk PE, shock, or hypotension

- IV unfractionated heparin (UFH) is the drug of choice for treating patients with high-risk PE with shock or hypotension.[20] SOR Ⓐ
- Based on the updated CHEST guideline, thrombolytic therapy is recommended if shock is present, unless an absolute contraindication exists.[20] SOR Ⓑ Suggestions are to consider thrombolytic therapy if PE is associated with hypotension and without high bleeding risk,[20] or in intermediate- to high-risk patients if clinical signs of hemodynamic decompensation occur.[20,25–28] SOR Ⓑ

▶ Anticoagulation for patients with acute PE and cancer[20]

- The drug of choice for patients with acute PE with cancer is low-molecular-weight heparin (LMWH) which, is considered superior to vitamin K antagonist (VKA) therapy. SOR Ⓑ
- If patient has active cancer, recommendations are for extended anticoagulant therapy (beyond the first 3–6 months) provided the patient is not at high risk of bleeding. SOR Ⓐ

▶ Long-term anticoagulation[20]

- In patients with acute PE without cancer, recommendations are to use NOACs such as dabigatran, rivaroxaban, apixaban, or edoxaban over VKA as long-term therapy due to decreased side effects, particularly intracranial bleeding. SOR Ⓑ
- The duration of anticoagulant therapy varies based on risk factor assessment. If transient risk factors exist (surgical or nonsurgical), then recommendations are to anticoagulate for 3 months. SOR Ⓐ
- If unprovoked or idiopathic PE occurs, then oral anticoagulation is recommended for at least 3 months. SOR Ⓐ If a second unprovoked PE occurs, recommendations are >3 months (indefinite duration) on oral anticoagulants for patients at low risk of bleeding and at least 3 months for patients at high risk of bleeding.
- In patients with cancer, extended anticoagulation (beyond the first 3–6 months) should be considered for an indefinite period or until the cancer is cured. SOR Ⓒ

SECOND LINE

NONPHARMACOLOGIC

- In patients with acute DVT, compression stockings are not routinely recommended to prevent post-thrombotic syndrome, but are recommended for use in high-risk patients (e.g., older age, obesity, smoker, varicose veins at baseline, thrombophilia).[11,13,29–31] SOR Ⓑ

MEDICATION[20]

- If therapy other than NOAC is desired, recommended alternatives include parenteral anticoagulants to be given in parallel with a VKA. SOR Ⓐ
  - Options for parental anticoagulation include subcutaneous LMWH, which is suggested over IV UFH or subcutaneous UFH. SOR Ⓑ
  - Start VKA early (same day as parenteral anticoagulation) over delayed start. SOR Ⓐ

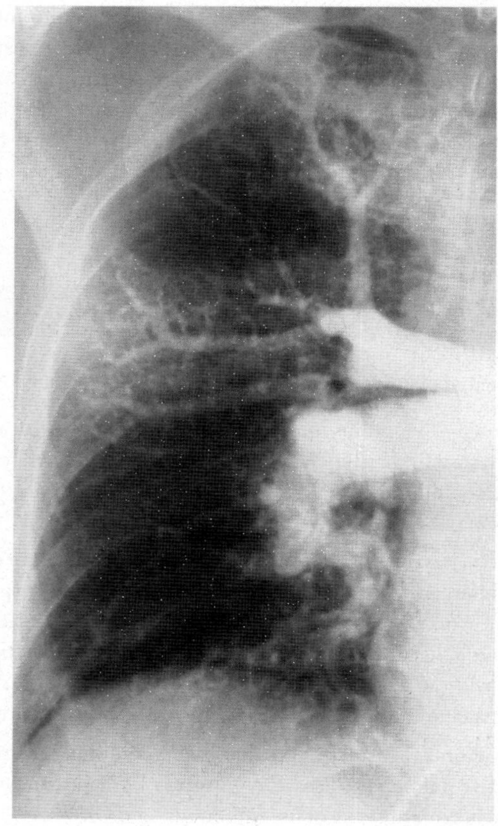

FIGURE 59-6 Pulmonary angiogram in the patient in **Figure 59-4** showing abruptly truncated pulmonary arteries associated with regions of diminished perfusion typical of chronic pulmonary emboli. (*Reproduced with permission from Miller WT: Diagnostic Thoracic Imaging. New York, NY: McGraw-Hill Education; 2006.*)

- Initial warfarin dose ranges from 2 to 10 mg. One option is to start with an initial warfarin dose of 10 mg once daily for 2 days; subsequent dosing should be based on international normalized ratio (INR). SOR Ⓑ The recommended target INR is 2.5 (INR range 2–3). SOR Ⓐ
- When treating with parenteral anticoagulation, recommendations are to treat for at least 5 days on parental therapy AND until INR ≥2 for at least 24 hours. SOR Ⓐ

- For patients with cancer, if LMWH is not used, recommendations are to use VKA therapy for long-term anticoagulation over NOACs such as dabigatran or rivaroxaban.[20]

SURGERY AND PROCEDURES

▶ Vena cava filters

- In patients with acute PE who are treated with anticoagulants, the CHEST guideline recommends against the use of an IVC filter.[20]
- A vena cava filter may be considered if anticoagulant therapy is contraindicated (SOR Ⓐ) or if there is recurrence of PE despite adequate anticoagulation.[4,32,33] SOR Ⓒ

▶ Other procedures

- Invasive procedures, such as catheter-based thrombus removal, are not recommended for most patients. However, based on the CHEST guideline, catheter-based thrombus removal is recommended in patients with acute PE with clinical signs of shock, hypotension, high bleeding risk, or failed thrombolysis.[20,34–37] SOR Ⓒ
- Highly compromised patients who are unable to receive thrombolytic therapy or whose critical status does not allow sufficient time to infuse thrombolytic therapy may be treated with pulmonary embolectomy.[17] SOR Ⓒ
- Surgery may also be considered in submassive acute PE with clinical evidence of poor prognosis (e.g., new hemodynamic instability, worsening respiratory failure, severe right ventricular dysfunction, or major myocardial necrosis)[37] or with intermediate- to high-risk PE if anticipated bleeding risk with thrombolysis is high.[20] SOR Ⓒ

REFERRAL OR HOSPITALIZATION

- Consider consultation with a coagulation specialist for patients with recurrent VTE, if alternative anticoagulants are being considered, if there is an increased risk of bleeding, and for pregnant women.
- Patients with cardiovascular or respiratory compromise should be admitted to the intensive care unit. Patients with symptomatic PE are usually hospitalized because of decreased cardiopulmonary reserve.[17] One open-label trial with 344 patients found no significant differences between inpatient and outpatient treatment, with only 1 patient dying in each group.[38] However, 2 outpatients had major bleeding in the first 14 days and 3 by 90 days, versus no patients in the inpatient group.

PREVENTION

- ACP recommends assessing thromboembolism and bleeding risk in medical patients (including patients with stroke) prior to starting prophylaxis against VTE.[39] The use of the IMPROVE combined risk calculator or the QThrombosis risk calculator is helpful.
- Following major orthopedic surgery (total hip replacement, knee replacement, or hip fracture surgery), American College of Chest Physicians (ACCP) recommends antithrombotic prophylaxis for minimum of 10–14 days.[40] SOR Ⓑ They also recommend dual prophylaxis with antithrombotic agent plus intermittent pneumatic compression device (IPCD) during hospital stay. SOR Ⓒ
- For abdominal and abdominal-pelvic surgery, the ACCP recommends thromboprophylaxis as well.[41] The Rogers and Caprini score will help determine the type of prophylaxis to be used.
- For long-distance travelers (e.g., flights >8 hours), avoidance of constrictive clothing around the lower extremities or waist, maintenance of adequate hydration, and frequent calf muscle contraction are recommended.[17] SOR Ⓒ In high-risk individuals, consider use of graduated compression stockings providing 15 to 30 mm Hg of pressure at the ankle or a single prophylactic dose of LMWH, injected prior to departure.[17] SOR Ⓒ

PROGNOSIS

- In a large multicenter study of 1880 patients with acute PE, mortality rate directly attributed to PE was 1% (95% CI, 0% to 1.6%).[42] Mortality from hemorrhage was 0.2% and the all-cause 30-day mortality rate was 5.4% (95% CI, 4.4% to 6.6%). Delay in initiating anticoagulation appeared to be a mortality factor, as only 3 of 20 patients with fatal PE had systemic anticoagulation initiated before diagnostic confirmation; another 3 of these 20 received a fibrinolytic agent. These figures were much improved over a 3-country registry of 2110 patients with acute PE from 1999 where the 3-month mortality rate was 15.3%.[43]
- In one study of 42 patients with acute PE, adverse events occurred in 7.4% at 30 days. Factors associated with those events included altered mental state (OR 6.8; 95% CI, 2.0 to 23.3), shock on admission (OR 2.8; 95% CI, 1.1 to 7.5), and cancer (OR 2.9; 95% CI, 1.2 to 6.9).[44]
- Pulmonary hypertension develops in approximately 5% of patients following PE.[45]

FOLLOW-UP

- Patients on warfarin should be monitored using a standard protocol. Patients on LMWH do not require routine monitoring except for pregnant women, in whom monitoring with anti-Xa levels is recommended.[17] SOR Ⓒ
- PE is slow to resolve; based on 4 imaging studies, the percentage of patients with residual pulmonary thrombi was 87% at 8 days after diagnosis, 68% after 6 weeks, 65% after 3 months, 57% after 6 months, and 52% after 11 months.[46]

PATIENT EDUCATION

- Patients taking warfarin should be instructed about the importance of remaining on oral anticoagulation for at least 3 months and use of compression stockings to decrease the likelihood of recurrence. Patients should also be counseled about the signs and symptoms of bleeding, to ask about potential drug interactions before starting a new medication, and about the importance of laboratory monitoring.

- Use of an anticoagulation service or home self-monitoring[47] may be considered to improve adherence and reduce complications.
- Avoidance of periods of prolonged immobilization is suggested.

PATIENT RESOURCES

- National Heart, Lung, and Blood Institute. *What Is Pulmonary Embolism?*—**http://www.nhlbi.nih.gov/health-topics/pulmonary-embolism.**

PROVIDER RESOURCES

- MedlinePlus. *Pulmonary Embolism*—**https://medlineplus.gov/pulmonaryembolism.html.**
- American Thoracic Society. *Evaluation of Suspected Pulmonary Embolism in Pregnancy*—**https://www.thoracic.org/statements/resources/pvd/evaluation-of-suspected-pulmonary-embolism-in-pregnancy.pdf.**

REFERENCES

1. Centers for Disease Control and Prevention. Venous thromboembolism in adult hospitalizations—United States, 2007–2009. *MMWR Morb Mortal Wkly Rep.* 2012;61(22):401-404.
2. Heit JA, Melton LJ, Lohse CM, et al. Incidence of venous thromboembolism in hospitalized patients vs. community residence. *Mayo Clinic Proc.* 2001;76(11):1102-1110.
3. Rizkallah J, Man SF, Sin DD. Prevalence of pulmonary embolism in acute exacerbations of COPD: a systematic review and meta-analysis. *Chest.* 2009;135(3):786-793.
4. Januel JM, Chen G, Ruffieux C, et al. Symptomatic in-hospital deep vein thrombosis and pulmonary embolism following hip and knee arthroplasty among patients receiving recommended prophylaxis: a systematic review. *JAMA.* 2012;307(3):294-303.
5. Dentali F, Ageno W, Becattini C, et al. Prevalence and clinical history of incidental, asymptomatic pulmonary embolism: a meta-analysis. *Thromb Res.* 2010;125(6):518-522.
6. Silverstein MD, Heit JA, Mohr DN, et al. Trends in the incidence of deep vein thrombosis and pulmonary embolism. A 25-year population-based study. *Arch Intern Med.* 1998;158:585-593.
7. Moser KM. Venous thromboembolism. *Am Rev Respir Dis.* 1990; 141:235-249.
8. Bahl V, Hu HM, Henke PK, et al. A validation study of a retrospective venous embolism risk scoring method. *Ann Surg.* 2010; 251(2):344-350.
9. Hippisley-Cox J, Coupland C. Development and validation of risk prediction algorithm (QThrombosis) to estimate future risk of venous thromboembolism: prospective cohort study. *BMJ.* 2011; 343;4656.
10. Rogers SO Jr, Kilaru RK, Hosokawa P, et al. Multivariable predictors of postoperative venous thrombolic events after general and vascular surgery: results in the Patient Safety in Surgery study. *J Am Coll Surg.* 2007; 204(6):1211-1121.
11. Konstantinides SV, Torbicki A, Agnelli G, et al. 2014 ESC guidelines on the diagnosis and management of acute pulmonary embolism. *Eur Heart J.* 2014:35(43):3033-3069, 3069a-3069k.
12. Raja AS, Greenberg JO, Qaseem A, et al. Evaluation of patients with suspected acute pulmonary embolism: best practice advice from the Clinical Guidelines Committee of the American College of Physicians. *Ann Intern Med.* 2015;163(9):701-711.
13. American College of Emergency Physicians Clinical Policies Committee; Clinical Policies Committee Subcommittee on Suspected Pulmonary Embolism. Clinical policy: critical issues in the evaluation and management of adult patients presenting with suspected pulmonary embolism. *Ann Emerg Med.* 2003;41(2): 257-270.
14. Lucassen W, Geersing GJ, Erkens PM, et al. Clinical decision rules for excluding pulmonary embolism: a meta-analysis. *Ann Intern Med.* 2011;155(7):448-460.
15. Di Nisio M, Squizzato A, Rutjes AW, et al. Diagnostic accuracy of D-dimer test for exclusion of venous thromboembolism: a systematic review. *J Thromb Haemost.* 2007;5(2):296-304.
16. Perrier A, Roy PM, Aujesky D, et al. Diagnosing pulmonary embolism in outpatients with clinical assessment, D-dimer measurement, venous ultrasound, and helical computed tomography: a multicenter management study. *Am J Med.* 2004;116(5):291-299.
17. Ansell J, Hirsh J, Hylek E, et al. Pharmacology and management of the vitamin K antagonists: American College of Chest Physicians Evidence-Based Clinical Practice Guidelines (8th Edition). *Chest.* 2008;133(6 Suppl):160S-198S.
18. American College of Radiology. ACR Appropriateness Criteria.® *Suspected Pulmonary Embolism.* Available at https://acsearch.acr.org/docs/69404/Narrative/. Accessed April 2017.
19. Leung AN, Bull TM, Jaeschke R, et al. An official American Thoracic Society/Society of Thoracic Radiology clinical practice guideline: evaluation of suspected pulmonary embolism in pregnancy. *Am J Respir Crit Care Med.* 2011;184(10):1200-1208.
20. Kearon C, Akl EA, Ornelas J, et al. Antithrombotic therapy for VTE disease. CHEST guideline and expert panel report. *Chest.* 2016;149(2):315-352.
21. Castellucci LA, Cameron C, Le Gal G, et al. Clinical and safety outcomes associated with treatment of acute venous thromboembolism: a systematic review and meta-analysis. *JAMA.* 2014; 312(11):1122-1135.
22. Gomez-Outes A, Terleira-Fernandez AI, Lecumberri R, et al. Direct oral anticoagulants in the treatment of acute venous thromboembolism: a systematic review and meta-analysis. *Thromb Res.* 2014;134(4):774-782.
23. van der Hulle T, Kooiman J, den Exter PL, et al. Effectiveness and safety of novel oral anticoagulants as compared with vitamin K antagonists in the treatment of acute symptomatic venous thromboembolism: a systematic review and meta-analysis. *J Thromb Haemost.* 2014;12(3):320-328.

24. Chai-Adisaksopha C, Crowther M, Isayama T, Lim W. The impact of bleeding complications in patients receiving target-specific oral anticoagulants: a systematic review and meta-analysis. *Blood.* 2014;124(15):2450-2458.

25. Kline JA, Nordenholz KE, Courtney DM, et al. Treatment of submassive pulmonary embolism with tenecteplase or placebo: cardiopulmonary outcomes at 3 months: multicenter double-blind, placebo-controlled randomized trial. *J Thromb Haemost.* 2014; 12(4):459-468.

26. Sharifi M, Bay C, Skrocki L, et al. Moderate pulmonary embolism treated with thrombolysis (from the "MOPETT" Trial). *Am J Cardiol.* 2013;111(2):273-277.

27. Meyer G, Vicaut E, Danays T, et al. Fibrinolysis for patients with intermediate-risk pulmonary embolism. *N Engl J Med.* 2014;370 (15):1402-1411.

28. Wang TF, Squizzato A, Dentali F, Ageno W. The role of thrombolytic therapy in pulmonary embolism. *Blood.* 2015;125(14): 2191-2199.

29. Kahn SR, Comerota AJ, Cushman M, et al. The postthrombotic syndrome: evidence-based prevention, diagnosis, and treatment strategies: a scientific statement from the American Heart Association. *Circulation.* 2014;130(18):1636-1661.

30. Prandoni P, Lensing AW, Prins MH, et al. Below-knee elastic compression stockings to prevent the post-thrombotic syndrome: a randomized, controlled trial. *Ann Intern Med.* 2004;141(4):249-256.

31. Kahn SR, Shapiro S, Wells PS, et al. Compression stockings to prevent post-thrombotic syndrome: a randomised placebo controlled trial. *Lancet.* 2014;383(9920):880-888.

32. Avgerinos ED, Chaer RA. Catheter-directed interventions for acute pulmonary embolism. *J Vasc Surg.* 2015;61(2):559-565.

33. Jaff MR, McMurtry MS, Archer SL, et al. Management of massive and submassive pulmonary embolism, iliofemoral deep vein thrombosis, and chronic thromboembolic pulmonary hypertension: a scientific statement from the American Heart Association. *Circulation.* 2011;123(16):1788-1830.

34. Kuo WT, Gould MK, Louie JD, et al. Catheter-directed therapy for the treatment of massive pulmonary embolism: systematic review and meta-analysis of modern techniques. *J Vasc Interv Radiol.* 2009;20(11):1431-1440.

35. Kucher N, Boekstegers P, Muller OJ, et al. Randomized, controlled trial of ultrasound-assisted catheter-directed thrombolysis for acute intermediate-risk pulmonary embolism. *Circulation.* 2014; 129(4): 479-486.

36. Kuo WT, Banerjee A, Kim PS, et al. Pulmonary Embolism Response to Fragmentation, Embolectomy, and Catheter Thrombolysis (PERFECT): initial results from a prospective multicenter registry. *Chest.* 2015;148(3):667-673.

37. Fukuda I, Taniguchi S, Fukui K, et al. Improved outcome of surgical pulmonary embolectomy by aggressive intervention for critically ill patients. *Ann Thorac Surg.* 2011;91(3):728-732.

38. Aujesky D, Roy PM, Verschuren F, et al. Outpatient versus inpatient treatment for patients with acute pulmonary embolism: an international, open-label, randomised, non-inferiority trial. *Lancet.* 2011;378(9785):41-48.

39. Kahn SR, Lim W, Dunn AS, et al; American College of Chest Physicians. Prevention of VTE in nonsurgical patients: Antithrombotic Therapy and Prevention of Thrombosis, 9th ed: American College of Chest Physicians Evidence-Based Clinical Practice Guidelines. *Chest.* 2012;141(2 Suppl):e195S-226.

40. Falck-Ytter Y, Francis CW, Johanson NA, et al. Prevention of VTE in orthopedic surgery patients: Antithrombotic Therapy and Prevention of Thrombosis, 9th ed: American College of Chest Physicians Evidence-Based Clinical Practice Guidelines. *Chest.* 2012; 141(2 Suppl):e278S-325S.

41. Gould MK, Garcia DA, Wren SM, et al. Prevention of VTE in nonorthopedic surgical patients: Antithrombotic Therapy and Prevention of Thrombosis, 9th ed: American College of Chest Physicians Evidence-Based Clinical Practice Guidelines. *Chest.* 2012;141(2 Suppl):e227S-77S.

42. Pollack CV, Schreiber D, Goldhaber SZ, et al. Clinical characteristics, management, and outcomes of patients diagnosed with acute pulmonary embolism in the emergency department: initial report of EMPEROR (Multicenter Emergency Medicine Pulmonary Embolism in the Real World Registry). *J Am Coll Cardiol.* 2011; 59(6):700-706.

43. Goldhaber SZ, Visani L, De Rosa M. Acute pulmonary embolism: clinical outcomes in the International Cooperative Pulmonary Embolism Registry (ICOPER). *Lancet.* 1999;353:1386-1389.

44. Sanchez O, Trinquart L, Caille V, et al. Prognostic factors for pulmonary embolism: the prep study, a prospective multicenter cohort study. *Am J Respir Crit Care Med.* 2010;181(2): 168-173.

45. Kearon C. Natural history of venous thromboembolism. *Circulation.* 2003;107:I22-I30.

46. Nijkeuter M, Hovens MM, Davidson BL, Huisman MV. Resolution of thromboemboli in patients with acute pulmonary embolism: a systematic review. *Chest.* 2006;129:192-197.

47. Menéndez-Jándula B, Souto JC, Oliver A, et al. Comparing self-management of oral anticoagulant therapy with clinic management. *Ann Intern Med.* 2005;142(1):1-10.

60 LUNG CANCER

Mindy A. Smith, MD, MS

PATIENT STORY

A 60-year-old woman presents with a solid, nontender, movable mass on her upper chest that's been present for 6 months. It began as a dime-size mass and has been growing more rapidly over the past month (**Figure 60-1A**). She has lost 10 pounds over the last year without dieting. She has smoked 1 pack of cigarettes daily since age 18 years and gets short of breath easily. Her "smoker's cough" has gotten worse in the last few months and occasionally she coughs up some blood-tinged sputum. Her family physician excised the mass in the office and sent it to pathology (**Figure 60-1B**). When the result demonstrated squamous cell carcinoma of the lung, a chest X-ray (CXR) was ordered (**Figure 60-2A**). The radiologist suggested a CT to confirm the diagnosis (**Figure 60-2B**). The patient chose to have no treatment and passed away in 10 months of her lung cancer.

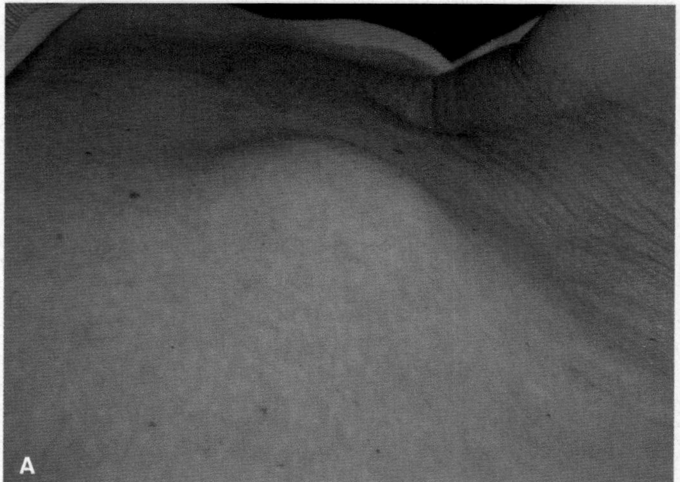

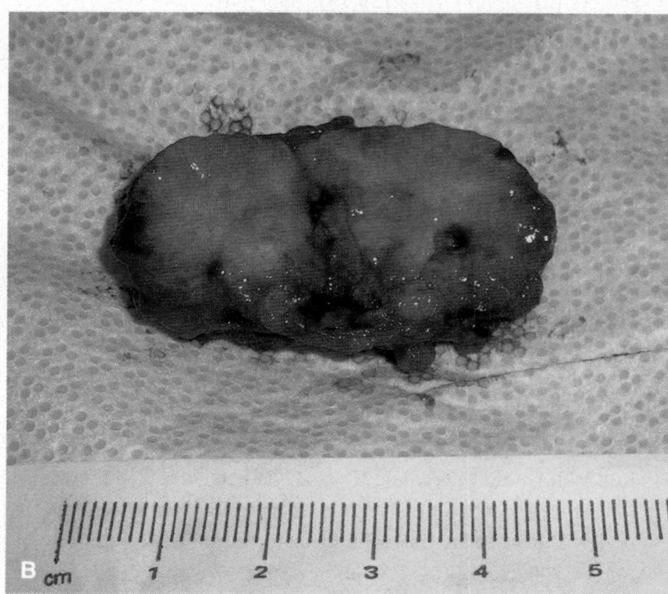

FIGURE 60-1 **A.** Growing chest nodule in a 60-year-old woman who smoked tobacco her whole adult life. The pathology demonstrated metastatic squamous cell carcinoma from the lung. **B.** The resected nodule was surgically removed by the family physician in the office. *(Reproduced with permission from Leonard Chow, MD, and Ross Lawler, MD.)*

INTRODUCTION

Lung cancer is a malignant neoplasm of the lung arising from respiratory epithelium (bronchi, bronchioles/alveoli), most commonly adenocarcinoma or squamous cell carcinoma.

EPIDEMIOLOGY

- In 2013, lung cancer was diagnosed in 212,584 people in the United States (111,907 men and 100,677 women) and there were 156,176 deaths from the disease.[1]
- Black men have the highest age-adjusted incidence rates (87.3/100,000) followed by white men (68.1/100,000), and then white women (51.8/100,000) and black women (50.0/100,000); Hispanic men (36.6/100,000) and women (24.8/100,000) have the lowest incidence rates.[2]
- Risk increases with age; at age 60 years, 1.96% of men will develop lung cancer in 10 years and 5.01% in 20 years.[1] Among women at age 60 years, 1.5% will develop lung cancer in 10 years and 3.89% in 20 years. Median age at diagnosis is 70 years.[1]
- Estimates for 2016: lung cancer was the leading cause of cancer deaths, accounting for 13.3% of all cancer diagnoses and 26.5% of all cancer deaths.[2]

ETIOLOGY AND PATHOPHYSIOLOGY

- Lung cancer begins in the lungs, spreading to regional lymph nodes and regional structures (e.g., trachea, esophagus). Extrathoracic metastases are common (found at autopsy in 50% to 95%), and sites include brain, bone, and liver.[3]

- Likely caused by a multistep process involving both carcinogens and tumor promoters; a number of genetic mutations (e.g., epidermal growth factor receptor [EGFR] mutations) are present in lung cancer cells, including activation of dominant oncogenes and inactivation of tumor-suppressor oncogenes.[3]
- There are two main groupings of lung cancer: non–small cell lung cancer (NSCLC; most common) and small cell lung cancer (SCLC). The four major cell types responsible for 88% of cases[3] are:
  - Adenocarcinoma (including bronchoalveolar)—32% of cases
  - Squamous or epidermoid carcinoma—29% of cases
  - Small cell (or oat cell) carcinoma—18% of cases
  - Large cell (or large cell anaplastic)—9% of cases
- Adenocarcinoma, squamous carcinoma, and large cell are classified together under NSCLC because of similar diagnostic, staging, and treatment approaches.
- Adenocarcinoma and squamous carcinoma have defined premalignant precursor lesions with lung tissue morphology ranging from hyperplasia to dysplasia and carcinoma in situ.

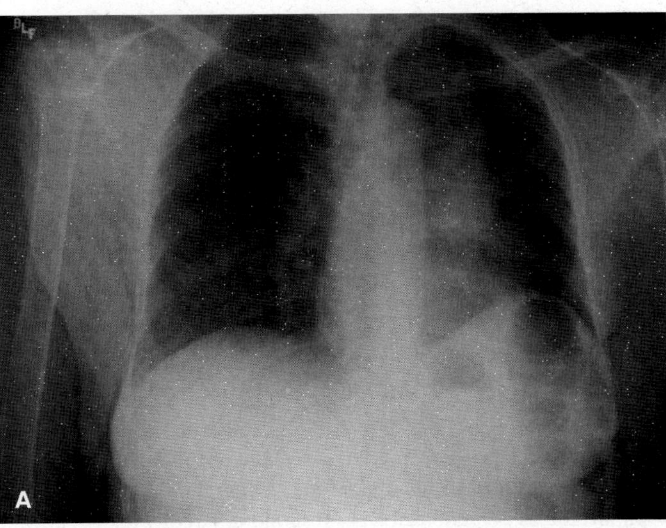

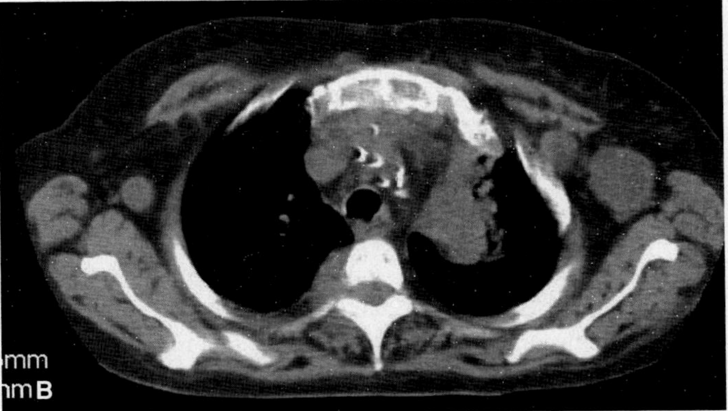

FIGURE 60-2 **A.** Chest X-ray showing squamous cell carcinoma of the lung. **B.** CT scan demonstrating the architecture of the squamous cell carcinoma of the lung. (*Reproduced with permission from David A. Kasper, DO, MBA.*)

RISK FACTORS

- Smoking is the major risk factor; smoking is linked to 80% to 90% of lung cancers, and each year passive smoking results in death due to lung cancer of about 7300 people who never smoked.[4] In 2015, 15.1% of adults in the United States were smokers; rates were higher in men than women (16.7% vs. 13.6%) and highest among non-Hispanic American Indians/Alaska Natives (21.9%).[5] In the 2015 Youth Risk Behavior Survey, daily smoking was reported by 2.3% of high school students, and 10.8% reported smoking cigarettes on 1 or more of the 30 days preceding the survey[6] (Chapter 248, Smoking and Tobacco Addiction).
- Occupations and exposures that increase risk of lung cancer include asbestos mining and processing, pesticide manufacturing (arsenic), and metallurgy (chromium).[4] Home exposure to asbestos or radon and diesel exhaust also increase risk.[4]
- Radiation therapy to the chest.[4]
- Family or personal history of lung cancer.
- Beta-carotene supplementation in current smokers (small increased risk).
- Hormone therapy (women). In the Women's Health Initiative, although incidence of lung cancer was not significantly increased, death from lung cancer (primarily NSCLC) was increased (73 vs. 40 deaths; 0.11% vs. 0.06%).[7]

DIAGNOSIS

Signs and symptoms depend on location, tumor size and type, and the presence of local or distant spread.

- Five percent to 15% of patients are asymptomatic—The cancer is found on chest imaging performed for another reason.[3]

- Systemic symptoms (e.g., anorexia, cachexia, weight loss [seen in 30% of patients]) may be seen, but the cause is unknown.

The diagnosis of lung cancer requires tissue confirmation through the safest and least-invasive procedure.[8] Procedures include sputum cytology, bronchoscopy, lymph node biopsy, operative specimen, fine needle aspiration (e.g., endobronchial ultrasound-guided transbronchial approach for mediastinal or hilar lymph nodes or CT-guided transthoracic approach for peripheral tumors), biopsy under CT guidance, or cell block from pleural effusion.[3,8] The specific procedures recommended depend on tumor location and success with the initial procedure.[8]

- Immunohistochemistry (e.g., thyroid transcription factor 1 for adenocarcinoma or P63 for squamous carcinoma) is used to help differentiate between cell types when morphologic criteria used in resections are not apparent.[9,10] Differentiation is important, as different cell types respond differently to treatment.
- In a meta-analysis of 14 studies, technetium-99m methoxy isobutyl isonitrile (Tc-MIBI) single photon emission CT appears useful in detecting malignant lung lesions, with an area under the receiver-operating characteristic curves of 0.906.[11]

CLINICAL FEATURES

- The most common symptoms at diagnosis are worsening cough or chest pain.[4] Symptoms may occur in the following situations[3]:
  - Central or endobronchial growth of the tumor may produce cough, hemoptysis, wheezing, stridor, and dyspnea.
  - Collapse of airways from tumor obstruction may cause post-obstructive pneumonitis.
  - Involvement of the pleura or chest wall may cause pleuritic chest pain, dyspnea on a restrictive basis, or lung abscess from tumor cavitation.
  - Regional spread of the tumor may cause tracheal obstruction; dysphagia from esophageal spread; hoarseness from recurrent laryngeal nerve paralysis; dyspnea and elevated hemidiaphragm from phrenic nerve paralysis; and Horner syndrome (enophthalmos, ptosis, miosis, ipsilateral loss of sweating from sympathetic nerve paralysis).
  - Spread to lymph nodes may be detected as firm masses in the supraclavicular area, axilla, or groin.
  - Extrathoracic metastases are common (found at autopsy in 50% to 95%) and may cause neurologic symptoms with brain metastases; pain and fracture with bone metastases; cytopenias or leukoerythroblastosis from bone marrow involvement; and liver dysfunction from metastases to the liver.
  - Paraneoplastic syndromes are common in SCLC and include endocrine syndromes (seen in 12%), such as hypercalcemia and hypophosphatemia from elevated parathyroid hormone or parathyroid-hormone related peptide; hyponatremia from secretion of antidiuretic hormone; electrolyte disturbances as seen with secretion of adrenocorticotropic hormone; and Lambert-Eaton myasthenic syndrome (primarily proximal muscle weakness, abnormal gait, fatigue, autonomic dysfunction, paresthesias). The most common paraneoplastic syndromes in SCLC are the syndrome of inappropriate antidiuresis (15% to 40% of patients with SCLC) and Cushing syndrome (2% to 5% of patients with SCLC).[8]
  - Skeletal and connective tissue syndromes including clubbing (seen in 30%, especially with NSCLC) and hypertrophic pulmonary osteoarthropathy with pain and swelling from periostitis (1% to 10%, especially with adenocarcinoma).
  - Skin nodules from lung cancer metastases may not be painful but are a poor prognostic sign (**Figures 60-1** and **60-2**).

LABORATORY TESTING

- Molecular testing for mutational profiles is standard for NSCLC with the rapid development of targeted therapies. Specifically, identification of activating EGFR mutations is the best predictor for response to EGFR-tyrosine kinase inhibitors.[14] In one multicenter study in Spain, EGFR mutations were found in 16.6% (350 of 2105) of patients and were more frequent in women (69.7%), in never smokers (66.6%), and in those with adenocarcinomas (80.9%).[15]

IMAGING

- For an incidental lung nodule >1 cm, the American College of Radiology (ACR) recommends transthoracic needle biopsy, whole-body fluorine-18-2-fluoro-2-deoxy-D-glucose-positron emission tomography (FDG-PET), or computed tomography (CT) of the chest without contrast.[16] If the nodule is <1 cm and suspicion of malignancy is low, chest CT without contrast or watchful waiting with follow-up CT is appropriate. When suspicion of malignancy is moderate to high, chest CT without contrast is recommended.
- For peripheral nodules, radial endobronchial ultrasound can be useful in confirming in real time the best location for bronchoscopic sampling and increase diagnostic yield.[8] If a tumor is associated with mediastinal adenopathy, endoscopic/bronchoscopic mediastinal biopsy is recommended.
- CXR may be useful as baseline if not already performed, and a chest CT scan should be performed; these tests may show a nodule (**Figures 60-3** and **60-4**) or diffuse lung abnormalities often confused with pneumonia (**Figures 60-5** to **60-7**).

TYPICAL DISTRIBUTION[3]

- Squamous cell carcinoma and SCLC tend to present as central masses with endobronchial growth.
- Other NSCLCs tend to present as peripheral masses, frequently with pleural involvement.

BIOPSY: HISTOLOGY[3]

- SCLCs have scant cytoplasm, hyperchromatic nuclei with fine chromatin pattern, nucleoli that are indistinct, and diffuse sheets of cells.
- NSCLCs have abundant cytoplasm, pleomorphic nuclei with coarse chromatin pattern, prominent nucleoli, and glandular or squamous architecture.

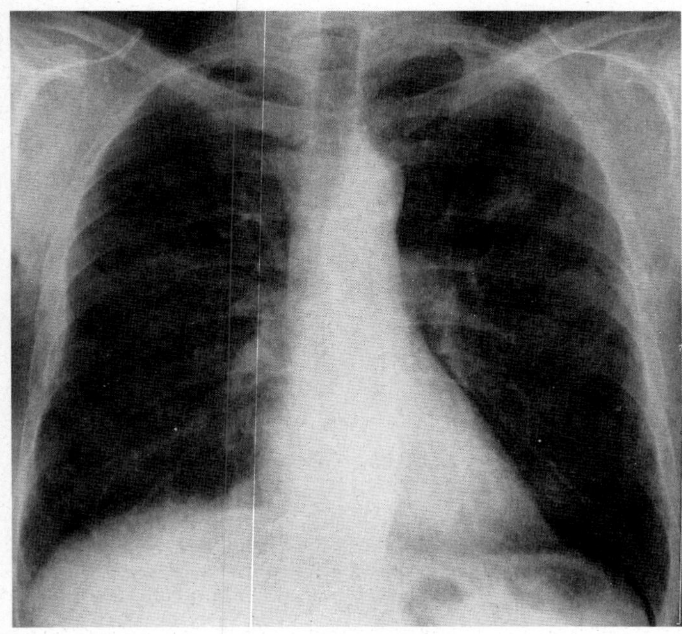

FIGURE 60-3 Chest X-ray demonstrating a 2.5-cm irregular nodule in the left upper lobe. A CT scan was ordered which is shown in Figure 60-4. (*Reproduced with permission from Miller WT: Diagnostic Thoracic Imaging. New York, NY: McGraw-Hill Education; 2006.*)

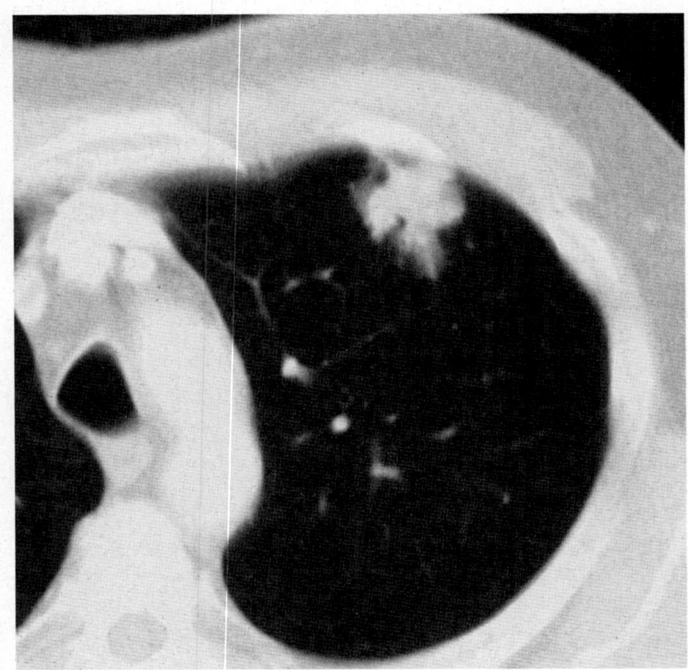

FIGURE 60-4 CT scan of the patient in Figure 60-3 shows a spiculated mass confirmed at surgery to be an adenocarcinoma. (*Reproduced with permission from Miller WT: Diagnostic Thoracic Imaging. New York, NY: McGraw-Hill Education; 2006.*)

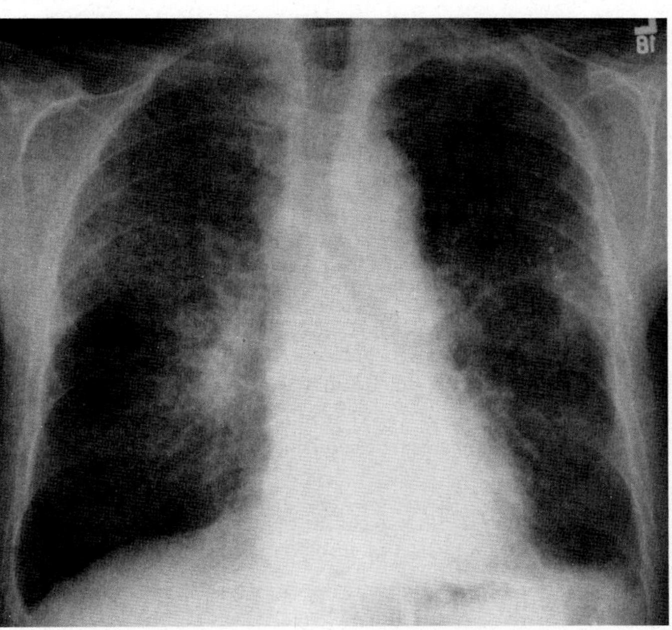

FIGURE 60-5 Diffuse lung abnormality seen on chest X-ray best characterized as ground-glass opacity, slightly worse in the right upper lobe. Open biopsy demonstrated bronchoalveolar carcinoma. (*Reproduced with permission from Miller WT: Diagnostic Thoracic Imaging. New York, NY: McGraw-Hill Education; 2006.*)

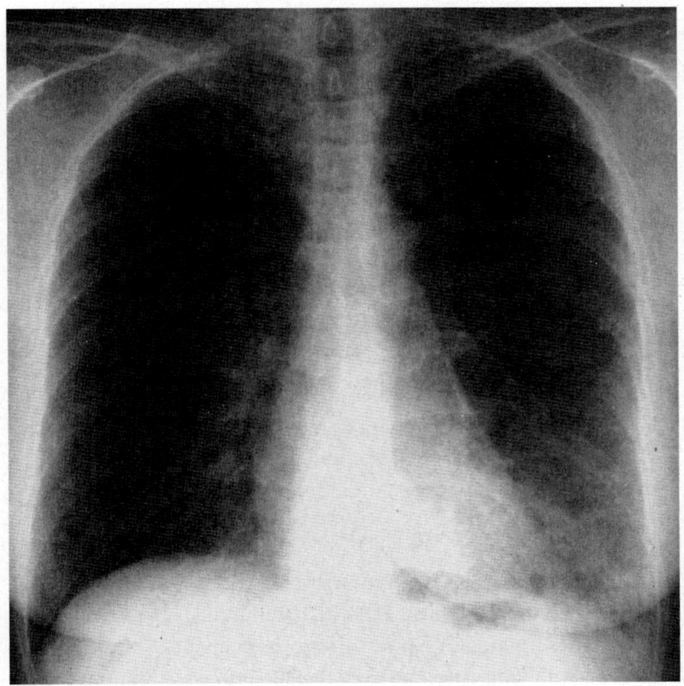

FIGURE 60-6 Chest X-ray showing local area of consolidation in the left lower lobe. Worsening consolidation for the subsequent 2 months despite antibiotic treatment led to a surgical biopsy, which confirmed bronchoalveolar carcinoma. (*Reproduced with permission from Miller WT: Diagnostic Thoracic Imaging. New York, NY: McGraw-Hill Education; 2006.*)

DIFFERENTIAL DIAGNOSIS

The differential diagnosis of an individual with lung findings (e.g., productive cough and dyspnea) includes:

- Chronic obstructive pulmonary disease—Most common symptoms are cough, sputum production, and exertional dyspnea. Although hemoptysis may occur, imaging (chest CT is most definitive) will not show a tumor. There is an increased risk of lung cancer in these patients (Chapter 58, Chronic Obstructive Pulmonary Disease).
- Pneumonia—Symptoms include fever, chills, and pleuritic chest pain; physical findings include dullness to percussion, bronchial breathing, egophony (E to A change), and crackles with area of infiltrate (pneumonia usually confirmed on CXR; see Chapter 55, Pneumonia).

Both these processes may occur in conjunction with lung cancer.

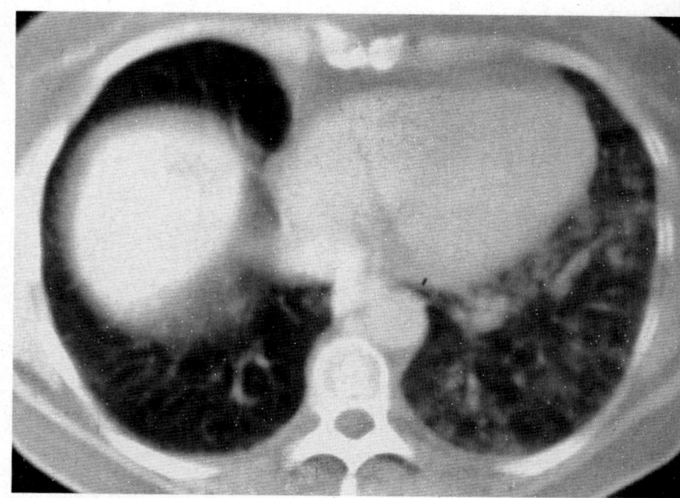

FIGURE 60-7 CT at the level of the bases in the patient in **Figure 60-6** showing areas of ground-glass opacification in the left lower lobe and lingula. (*Reproduced with permission from Miller WT: Diagnostic Thoracic Imaging. New York, NY: McGraw-Hill Education; 2006.*)

MANAGEMENT

Treatment is based on staging and cell type; both anatomic (e.g., physical location of tumor) and physiologic (e.g., patient's ability to withstand treatment) factors are considered. All patients should undergo the following[3,9]: SOR Ⓒ

- Complete history and physical.
- Laboratory tests—Complete blood count with differential and platelets, electrolytes, glucose, calcium, phosphorus, and renal and liver function tests.

For staging purposes for NSCLC the ACR recommends the following imaging[17]:

- CT chest scan with contrast, if there are no strong contraindications, and an FDG-PET from skull base to midthigh. Although this approach spares more patients from stage-inappropriate surgery, the strategy appears to incorrectly upstage disease in some patients and, in one randomized controlled trial (RCT), did not affect overall mortality.[18]
- If a patient has neurologic symptoms or an adenocarcinoma larger than 3 cm or mediastinal adenopathy, MRIs of the head without and with contrast are recommended.[17]
- In addition, for patients with non–small cell tumors who may be candidates for curative surgery or radiotherapy, obtain pulmonary function tests, coagulation tests, and possibly cardiopulmonary exercise testing.[3]

For staging of patients with SCLC, ACR recommends[17]:

- CT chest and abdomen with contrast and MRIs of the head without and with contrast. Perform FDG-PET from skull base to midthigh, if a diagnostic chest CT has not already been obtained. Staging for patients with lung cancer is based on the TNM classification system, where T describes the size of the tumor, N describes any regional lymph node involvement, and M notes the presence or absence of distant metastases (**Box 60-1**).[19] At diagnosis, approximately 16% have localized disease, 22% have regional disease (spread to regional lymph nodes), and 57% have distant metastases.[2]

BOX 60-1 TNM Staging of Lung Cancer

- Stage 0—Carcinoma in situ (Tis N0 M0)
- Stage IA—Tumor size 2 centimeters (cm) or smaller (1a) or tumor size >2 cm but <3 cm (1b) (T1a,b N0 M0)
- Stage IB—Tumor size >3 cm but <5 cm (2a) and has any of the following: involves the main bronchus (>2 cm distal to the carina), invades visceral pleura, or associated with atelectasis or obstructive pneumonitis extending to the hilar region (T2a N0 M0)
- Stage IIA—Tumor size >5 cm but <7 cm (2b) (T2b N0 M0, T1a,b N1 M0, T2a N1 M0)
- Stage IIB—Tumor size >5 cm but <7 cm (2b) or tumor size >7 cm or directly invades the chest wall, diaphragm, phrenic nerve, mediastinal pleura, parietal pericardium; or tumor in the main bronchus <2 cm distal to the carina but without carina involvement; or associated atelectasis or obstructive pneumonitis of the entire lung or separate tumor nodule(s) in the same lobe as the primary (T3) (T2b N1 M0, T3 N0 M0)
- Stage IIIA—Any size tumor including a tumor that invades the mediastinum, heart, great vessels, trachea, recurrent laryngeal nerve, esophagus, vertebral body, carina or separate tumor in a different ipsilateral lobe to that of the primary (T4) (T1a,b or T2a,b N2 M0, T3 N1or 2 M0, T4 N0 or 1 M0)
- Stage IIIB—T4 N2 M0, any T N3 M0
- Stage IV—Tumor has spread to distant sites (any T any N M1)

T, tumor (size and extent); N, regional lymph nodes (N0, no regional lymph node metastasis; N1, metastasis in ipsilateral peribronchial and/or ipsilateral hilar lymph nodes and intrapulmonary nodes, including involvement by direct extension; N2, metastasis in ipsilateral mediastinal and/or subcarinal lymph node[s]; N3, metastasis in contralateral mediastinal, contralateral hilar, ipsilateral or contralateral scalene, or supraclavicular lymph node[s]); M, metastases (M0, no distant metastasis; M1, distant metastasis).

FIRST LINE

NONPHARMACOLOGIC

Supportive care for the patient and family and palliative care of the patient should be provided by a multidisciplinary team and include adequate pain relief.

- Early palliative care was shown in one trial to improve quality of life and mood and increase median survival (11.6 months vs. 8.9 months) for patients with metastatic NSCLC compared to those receiving standard care.[20]
- Smoking cessation—Continued smoking is associated with a significantly increased risk of all-cause mortality and recurrence in early stage NSCLC and of all-cause mortality, development of a second primary tumor, and recurrence in all but stage IV SCLC.[21] Using life-table modeling, these investigators estimated that 5-year survival in 65-year-old patients with early-stage NSCLC who quit smoking would increase from 33% (for those who continued to smoke) to 70%, and for those with limited-stage SCLC, from 29% (continued smokers) to 63% (quitters) (Chapter 248, Smoking and Tobacco Addiction).

MEDICATIONS

- Pain medication should be provided as needed (Chapter 5, End of Life). Opioids, such as codeine or morphine, may reduce cough.
- Adjuvant chemotherapy in patients with NSCLC, with or without postoperative radiotherapy, increases 5-year survival by approximately 4%.[9,22]
- Preoperative chemotherapy in patients with NSCLC increases survival by approximately 6% (absolute benefit) at 5 years.[23] Advantages of preoperative chemotherapy include early start on potential micrometastases and higher adherence to therapy.[9]
- Maintenance therapy with either cytotoxic agents or tyrosine kinase inhibitor agents (or switch therapy) can be considered as it appears to increase overall survival for patients with nonprogressive NSCLC.[24] In patients with advanced EGFR mutation–positive NSCLC, erlotinib, gefitinib, and afatinib all demonstrated prolonged progression-free survival compared to cytotoxic chemotherapy.[25]
- Management of patients with SCLC includes combination platinum-based chemotherapy, surgery (in selected cases of limited stage of disease), and radiation therapy.[26,27] SOR Ⓐ Authors of a Cochrane review, however, found that platinum-based chemotherapy regimens did not offer a significant benefit in survival or overall tumor response compared with non–platinum-based regimens, and poor survival was seen in both groups.[28] Targeted therapies have not proved beneficial for patients with SCLC.[26]

SURGERY AND RADIATION

Management of patients with NSCLC includes the following:

- Localized stages I and II—Pulmonary resection and appropriate nodal dissection. SOR Ⓐ Evidence is conflicting about whether video-assisted thoracoscopic surgery offers advantages over standard lobectomy; either technique can be used.[9,29]
- In patients undergoing resection, intraoperative systematic mediastinal lymph node sampling or dissection is recommended for accurate staging.[29] Although data are limited, a Cochrane review concluded that resection combined with complete mediastinal lymph node dissection is associated with a modest survival improvement

compared with resection combined with systematic sampling of mediastinal nodes in patients with stages I to IIIA NSCLC.[30]

- For patients with stage I disease who are not surgical candidates, external-beam radiotherapy is recommended; stereotactic body radiation therapy or percutaneous ablation can be considered as a treatment option.[29] SOR B
- Stage IIIB—Concurrent chemo/radiation therapy.[31]
- Stage IV—Options include radiation therapy to symptomatic local sites, chemotherapy or molecular targeted agents, chest tube for malignant effusion, and consideration of resection of primary or isolated brain or adrenal metastases.[3,29] A Cochrane review concluded that chemotherapy improves overall survival in patients with advanced NSCLC (absolute improvement in survival of 9% at 12 months [20% to 29%] or absolute increase in median survival of 1.5 months [from 4.5 months to 6 months]).[32]
- Curative radiotherapy should be considered for patients with good performance status and inoperable stages I to III disease.[29]

Management of patients with very limited (stage I) SCLC is surgical resection and adjuvant combined cisplatin-based chemotherapy, possibly with prophylactic cranial irradiation.[26]

- Other patients with limited-stage SCLC (stages II to III) should be offered thoracic irradiation concurrently with the first or second cycle of chemotherapy or following completion of chemotherapy if there has been at least a good partial response within the thorax.[3,26] Prophylactic cranial irradiation should be considered if nonprogressive after induction treatment.[26]
- For patients with extensive disease (stage IV), limited data support prolonged survival (added 63 to 84 days) using chemotherapy.[33] Supportive care plus palliative thoracic irradiation should be considered following chemotherapy (combination etoposide and cisplatin for non-Asian patients and irinotecan and cisplatin for Asian patients).[26]
- For patients who are not candidates for chemotherapy, palliative radiotherapy should be considered to improve thoracic symptoms.[26,34] Other targeted therapies, based on molecular testing of tumor mutational profiles (e.g., erlotinib for mutant EGFR) should be considered.

SECOND LINE

NONPHARMACOLOGIC

- Authors of a Cochrane review found that nursing interventions to manage breathlessness reduced symptoms and improved performance status, and structured nursing programs delayed clinical deterioration.[35]

MEDICATION

- Authors of a meta-analysis found a higher overall (hazard ratio [HR] 0.92, 95% CI 0.86–0.98) and progression-free survival (HR 0.75, 95% CI 0.66–0.85) in patients receiving combination antiangiogenic agents with chemotherapy versus chemotherapy alone. They propose that these be considered first-line agents.[36]
- Medications that are useful for symptom management are reviewed in the 2013 American College of Chest Physicians guideline and include anticonvulsants or tricyclic antidepressants for neuropathic pain, corticosteroids or macrolides for cough associated with radiation therapy, and bisphosphonates for painful bone metastastases.[37]

COMPLEMENTARY AND ALTERNATIVE THERAPY

- In a small RCT of patients with NSCLC on chemotherapy, nutritional intervention with 2.2 g of fish oil per day provided a benefit on maintenance of weight and muscle mass over standard care.[38] Fish oil also increased the response to chemotherapy in those with advanced NSCLC and may provide a survival benefit (trend).[39]

PREVENTION

- Avoid smoking/smoking exposure or quit, if already smoking (Chapter 248, Smoking and Tobacco Addiction). Avoid workplace and home exposures (listed in risk factors).
- Daily aspirin appears to protect against lung adenocarcinoma.[40]
- The U.S. Preventive Services Task recommends annual screening for lung cancer with low-dose CT in adults ages 55 to 80 years who have a 30 pack-year smoking history and currently smoke or have quit within the past 15 years. Screening should be discontinued once a person has not smoked for 15 years or develops a health problem that substantially limits life expectancy or the ability or willingness to have curative lung surgery.[41] SOR B
- The National Lung Screening Trial (N = 53,454 patients at high risk for lung cancer) reported lower mortality from lung cancer after three annual screenings for patients randomized to low-dose CT versus single-view posteroanterior chest radiography (247 deaths from lung cancer per 100,000 person-years and 309 deaths per 100,000 person-years, respectively).[42] There was also reduced all-cause mortality in this group by 6.7%. The risk of false positives with low-dose CT, however, is high (33% after two screenings),[43] and there is potential for radiation-induced cancer.

PROGNOSIS

- Perioperative mortality from a large database of over 18,000 lung cancer resections performed at 111 participating centers was 2.2% and composite morbidity and mortality occurred in 8.6%.[44] Predictive factors of mortality included pneumonectomy, bilobectomy, performance status, induction chemoradiation, steroids, age, and renal dysfunction, among other factors.
- Adverse prognostic factors for NSCLC include presence of pulmonary symptoms, large tumor size (>3 cm), nonsquamous histology, metastases to multiple lymph nodes within a TNM-defined nodal station, and vascular invasion.[12]
- The overall 5-year relative survival from lung cancer (SEER data 2001–2007) was 17.7%.[2]
- Five-year survival decreases by stage at diagnosis ranging from 55.2% for localized disease to 4.3% for those with distant metastases.[2]
- For SCLC, median survival for patients with limited-stage disease is approximately 16 to 24 months (14% survive to 5 years).[13]
- Following lung cancer resection, there is a 1% to 2% risk per patient per year that a second lung cancer will occur.[3] For patients with SCLC, second primary tumors are reported in 2% to 10% of patients per year.[26]

FOLLOW-UP

Surveillance for the recognition of a recurrence of the original lung cancer and/or the development of a metachronous tumor should be coordinated through a multidisciplinary team approach.

- This team should develop a lifelong surveillance plan appropriate for the individual circumstances of each patient immediately following initial curative-intent therapy.[3] SOR C
- The Program in Evidence-Based Care 2014 guideline recommends the following for curatively treated patients:[45]
  - Clinical evaluations to include medical history, physical examination, and chest imaging every 3 months in the first 2 years, every 6 months in year 3, and annually thereafter.
  - Work-up for recurrence if constitutional symptoms (e.g., dysphagia, sweats, weight loss), pain, neurologic symptoms (e.g., headache), or respiratory symptoms occur.
  - Management of symptoms to improve quality of life.

PATIENT EDUCATION

- Smoking cessation, never initiating smoking, and avoidance of occupational and environmental exposure to carcinogenic substances are recommended to reduce the risk of recurrence or a second primary in curatively treated patients. In patients with metastatic disease, although smoking cessation has little effect on overall prognosis, it may improve respiratory symptoms.
- Information about local hospice services and support groups should be provided. The Lung Cancer Alliance website, listed in "Patient Resources" below, can be used to find support groups.

PATIENT RESOURCES

- National Cancer Institute. *Lung Cancer*—**http://www.cancer.gov/cancertopics/types/lung.**
- Mayo Clinic. *Lung Cancer*—**www.mayoclinic.com/health/lung-cancer/DS00038.**
- American Lung Association—**www.lung.org.**
- Lung Cancer Alliance. Support groups for patients and families can be found at the following website—**http://www.lungcancer-alliance.org/get-help-and-support/coping-with-lung-cancer/support-groups.html.**

PROVIDER RESOURCES

- MedlinePlus. *Lung Cancer*—**www.nlm.nih.gov/medlineplus/lungcancer.html.**
- National Cancer Institute. *Lung Cancer*—**https://www.cancer.gov/types/lung/hp.**

REFERENCES

1. Centers for Disease Control and Prevention. *Lung Cancer Statistics.* http://www.cdc.gov/cancer/lung/statistics/index.htm. Accessed February 2017.
2. National Cancer Institute. *Cancer Stat Facts: Lung and Bronchus Cancer.* http://seer.cancer.gov/statfacts/html/lungb.html. Accessed February 2017.
3. Minna JD. Neoplasms of the lung. In: Kasper DL, Braunwald E, Fauci AS, et al., eds. *Harrison's Principles of Internal Medicine*, 16th ed. New York, NY: McGraw-Hill; 2005:506-516.
4. Centers for Disease Control and Prevention. *What are the Risk Factors for Lung Cancer.* https://www.cdc.gov/cancer/lung/basic_info/risk_factors.htm. Accessed February 2017.
5. Centers for Disease Control and Prevention. *Fast Facts and Fact Sheets.* https://www.cdc.gov/tobacco/data_statistics/fact_sheets/index.htm. Accessed February 2017.
6. Centers for Disease Control and Prevention. *Youth Risk Behavior Surveillance—2015.* https://www.cdc.gov/healthyyouth/data/yrbs/pdf/2015/ss6506_updated.pdf. Accessed February 2017.
7. Chlebowski RT, Schwartz AG, Wakelee H, et al. Oestrogen plus progestin and lung cancer in postmenopausal women (Women's Health Initiative trial): a post-hoc analysis of a randomised controlled trial. *Lancet.* 2009;374(9697):1243-1251.
8. National Guideline Clearinghouse (NGC). *Guideline Summary: Establishing the Diagnosis of Lung Cancer: Diagnosis and Management of Lung Cancer, 3rd ed: American College of Chest Physicians Evidence-Based Clinical Practice Guidelines.* In: National Guideline Clearinghouse (NGC). Rockville, MD: Agency for Healthcare Research and Quality (AHRQ); 2013 May 01. Accessed February 2017. Available: http://www.chestnet.org/Guidelines-and-Resources/CHEST-Guideline-Topic-Areas/Thoracic-Oncology.
9. Goldstraw P, Ball D, Jett JR, et al. Non-small-cell lung cancer. *Lancet.* 2011;378(9804):1727-1740.
10. National Guideline Clearinghouse (NGC). Guideline Summary: Diagnostic Surgical Pathology in Lung Cancer: Diagnosis and Management of Lung Cancer, 3rd ed: American College of Chest Physicians Evidence-Based Clinical Practice Guidelines. In: National Guideline Clearinghouse (NGC) [website]. Rockville, MD: Agency for Healthcare Research and Quality (AHRQ); 2013 May 01. Accessed February 2017. Available: https://www.guideline.gov.
11. Zhang S, Liu Y. Diagnostic performances of ^{99m}Tc-methoxy isobutyl isonitrile scan in predicting the malignancy of lung lesions: a meta-analysis. *Medicine (Baltimore).* 2016;95(18):e3571.
12. National Cancer Institute. *Non-Small Cell Lung Cancer Treatment (PDQ)—Health Professional Version.* https://www.cancer.gov/types/lung/hp/non-small-cell-lung-treatment-pdq. Accessed February 2017.
13. National Cancer Institute. *Small Cell Lung Cancer Treatment (PDQ)—Health Professional Version.* https://www.cancer.gov/types/lung/hp/small-cell-lung-treatment-pdq. Accessed February 2017.
14. Dacic S. Molecular diagnostics of lung carcinomas. *Arch Pathol Lab Med.* 2011;135(5):622-629.
15. Rosell R, Moran T, Queralt C, et al. Screening for epidermal growth factor receptor mutations in lung cancer. *N Engl J Med.* 2009;361(10):958-967.
16. American College of Radiology Appropriateness Criteria. *Radiographically Detected Solitary Pulmonary Nodule* (2012). https://acsearch.acr.org/docs/69455/Narrative/. Accessed February 2017.

17. American College of Radiology Appropriateness Criteria. Non-invasive Clinical Staging of Bronchogenic Carcinoma (2013). https://acsearch.acr.org/docs/69456/Narrative/. Accessed February 2017.
18. Fischer B, Lassen U, Mortensen J, et al. Preoperative staging of lung cancer with combined PET-CT. *N Engl J Med.* 2009;361(1):32-39.
19. Goldstraw P, Crowley J, Chansky K, et al. The IASLC Lung Cancer Staging Project: proposals for the revision of the TNM stage groupings in the forthcoming (seventh) edition of the TNM Classification of malignant tumours. *J Thorac Oncol.* 2007;2(8):706-714.
20. Temel JS, Greer JA, Muzikansky A, et al. Early palliative care for patients with metastatic non-small-cell lung cancer. *N Engl J Med.* 2010;363(8):733-742.
21. Parsons A, Daley A, Begh R, Aveyard P. Influence of smoking cessation after diagnosis of early stage lung cancer on prognosis: systematic review of observational studies with meta-analysis. *BMJ.* 2010;340:b5569.
22. Burdett S, Pignon JP, Tierney J, et al., for the Non-Small Cell Lung Cancer Collaborative Group. Adjuvant chemotherapy for resected early-stage non-small cell lung cancer. *Cochrane Database Syst Rev.* 2015;(3):CD011430.
23. Burdett S, Stewart L, Rydzewska L. Chemotherapy and surgery versus surgery alone in non-small cell lung cancer. *Cochrane Database Syst Rev.* 2007;(3):CD006157.
24. Zhang X, Zhang J, Xu J, et al. Maintenance therapy with continuous or switch strategy in advanced non-small cell lung cancer: a systematic review and meta-analysis. *Chest.* 2011;140(1):117-126.
25. Greenhalgh J, Dwan K, Boland A, et al. First-line treatment of advanced epidermal growth factor receptor (EGFR) mutation positive non-squamous non-small cell lung cancer. *Cochrane Database Syst Rev.* 2016;(5):CD010383.
26. van Meerbeeck JP, Fennell DA, DeRuysscher DKM. Small-cell lung cancer. *Lancet.* 2011;378(9804):1741-1755.
27. Kong FM, Lally BE, Chang JY, et al. ACR Appropriateness Criteria radiation therapy for small-cell lung cancer. *Am J Clin Oncol.* 2013;36(2):206-213.
28. Amarasena IU, Chatterjee S, Walters JAE, et al. Platinum versus non-platinum chemotherapy regimens for small cell lung cancer. *Cochrane Database Syst Rev.* 2015;(8):CD006849.
29. Carr LL, Finigan JH, Kern JA. Evaluation and treatment of patients with non-small cell lung cancer. *Med Clin North Am.* 2011;95(6):1041-1054.
30. Manser R, Wright G, Hart D, et al. Surgery for local and locally advanced non-small cell lung cancer. *Cochrane Database Syst Rev.* 2005;(1):CD004699.
31. Gewanter RM, Movsas B, Rosenzweig KE, et al. *Expert Panel on Radiation Oncology—Lung. ACR Appropriateness Criteria Non-surgical Treatment for Non-Small-Cell Lung Cancer: Good Performance Status/Definitive Intent.* Reston, VA: American College of Radiology; 2014. https://www.guideline.gov/summaries/summary/48303. Accessed February 2017.
32. Non-Small Cell Lung Cancer Collaborative Group. Chemotherapy and supportive care versus supportive care alone for advanced non-small cell lung cancer. *Cochrane Database Syst Rev.* 2010;(5):CD007309.
33. Pelayo Alvarez M, Westeel V, Cortés-Jofré M, Bonfill Cosp X. Chemotherapy versus best supportive care for extensive small cell lung cancer. *Cochrane Database Syst Rev.* 2013;(11):CD001990.
34. Stevens R, MacBeth F, Toy E, et al. Palliative radiotherapy regimens for non-small cell lung cancer. *Cochrane Database Syst Rev.* 2015;(1):CD002143.
35. Rueda JR, Solà I, Pascual A, Subirana Casacuberta M. Non-invasive interventions for improving well-being and quality of life in patients with lung cancer. *Cochrane Database Syst Rev.* 2011;(9):CD004282.
36. Zhang L, Cao F, Wang Y, et al. Antiangiogenic agents combined with chemotherapy in the first-line treatment of advanced non-small-cell lung cancer: overall and histology subgroup-specific meta-analysis. *Oncol Res Treat.* 2014;37(12):710-718.
37. *Symptom Management in Patients with Lung Cancer: Diagnosis and Management of Lung Cancer, 3rd ed: American College of Chest Physicians Evidence-Based Clinical Practice Guidelines.* 2013. https://www.guideline.gov/summaries/summary/46179/symptom-management-in-patients-with-lung-cancer-diagnosis-and-management-of-lung-cancer-3rd-ed-american-college-of-chest-physicians-evidencebased-clinical-practice-guidelines?q=Lung+Cancer. Accessed February 2017.
38. Murphy RA, Mourtzakis M, Chu QS, et al. Nutritional intervention with fish oil provides a benefit over standard of care for weight and skeletal muscle mass in patients with nonsmall cell lung cancer receiving chemotherapy. *Cancer.* 2011;117(8):1775-1782.
39. Murthy RA, Mourizakis M, Chu QS, et al. Supplementation with fish oil increases first-line chemotherapy efficacy in patients with advanced nonsmall cell lung cancer. *Cancer.* 2011;117(16):3774-3780.
40. Rothwell PM, Fowkes FG, Belch JF, et al. Effect of daily aspirin on long-term risk of death due to cancer: analysis of individual patient data from randomised trials. *Lancet.* 2011;377(9759):31-41.
41. United States Preventive Services Task Force. *Lung Cancer: Screening.* https://www.uspreventiveservicestaskforce.org/Page/Document/UpdateSummaryFinal/lung-cancer-screening?ds=1&s=Lung%20Cancer. Accessed February 2017.
42. National Lung Screening Trial Research Team, Aberle DR, Adams AM, Bery CD, et al. Reduced lung-cancer mortality with low-dose computed tomographic screening. *N Engl J Med.* 2011;365(5):395-409.
43. Croswell JM, Baker SG, Marcus PM, et al. Cumulative incidence of false-positive test results in lung cancer screening: a randomized trial. *Ann Intern Med.* 2010;152(8):505-512.
44. Kozower BD, Sheng S, O'Brien SM, et al. STS database risk models: predictors of mortality and major morbidity for lung cancer resection. *Ann Thorac Surg.* 2010;90(3):875-881.
45. Follow-up and surveillance of curatively treated lung cancer patients. 2014 Consensus Developed by Program in Evidence-based Care (PEBC). https://www.guideline.gov/summaries/summary/48566/followup-and-surveillance-of-curatively-treated-lung-cancer-patients?q=Lung+Cancer. Accessed February 2017.

PART IX

GASTROINTESTINAL

Strength of Recommendation (SOR)	Definition
A	Recommendation based on consistent and good-quality patient-oriented evidence.*
B	Recommendation based on inconsistent or limited-quality patient-oriented evidence.*
C	Recommendation based on consensus, usual practice, opinion, disease-oriented evidence, or case series for studies of diagnosis, treatment, prevention, or screening.*

*See Appendix A on pages 1603–1606 for further information.

61 PEPTIC ULCER DISEASE

Mindy A. Smith, MD, MS

PATIENT STORY

A 41-year-old man presents with a 4-month history of epigastric pain. The pain is dull, achy, and intermittent; there is no radiation of the pain and it has not changed in character since it began. Coffee intake seems to exacerbate the symptoms, whereas eating or drinking milk helps. Infrequently, he is awakened at night by the pain. He reports no weight loss, vomiting, melena, or hematochezia. On examination, there is mild epigastric tenderness with no rebound or guarding. The remainder of the examination is unremarkable. A stool antigen test is positive for *Helicobacter pylori*, and the patient is treated for peptic ulcer disease with eradication therapy.

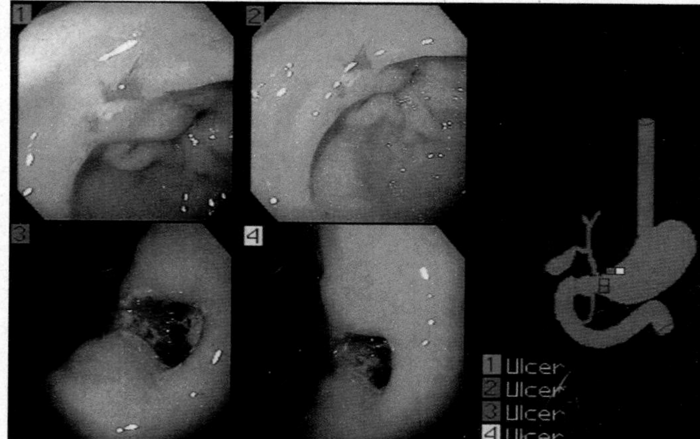

FIGURE 61-1 Endoscopic pictures of a gastric ulcer. Plates 1 and 2 show erosions. Note that the bleeding is from biopsy. Plates 3 and 4 show a large crater with evidence of recent bleeding. Both are consistent with severe ulcer disease. (*Reproduced with permission from Michael Harper, MD.*)

INTRODUCTION

Peptic ulcer disease (PUD) is a disease of the gastrointestinal (GI) tract characterized by a break in the mucosal lining of the stomach or duodenum due to pepsin and gastric acid secretion. This damage is greater than 5 mm in size and with a depth reaching the submucosal layer.[1]

EPIDEMIOLOGY

- PUD is a common disorder affecting approximately 4.5 million people annually in the United States. It encompasses both gastric and duodenal ulcers (**Figures 61-1** and **61-2**).[2]
- One-year point prevalence is 1.8%, and the lifetime prevalence is 10% in the United States.[2]
- Prevalence is similar in both sexes, with increased incidence with age.[1] Duodenal ulcers most commonly occur in patients between the ages of 30 and 55 years, whereas gastric ulcers are more common in patients between the ages of 55 and 70 years.[2]
- PUD incidence in *H. pylori*–infected individuals is approximately 1% per year (6- to 10-fold higher than uninfected subjects).[1]
- Physician office visits and hospitalizations for PUD have decreased in the past few decades.[1]
- The incidence of peptic ulcers is declining, possibly as a result of the increasing use of proton pump inhibitors and eradication of *H. pylori* infection.

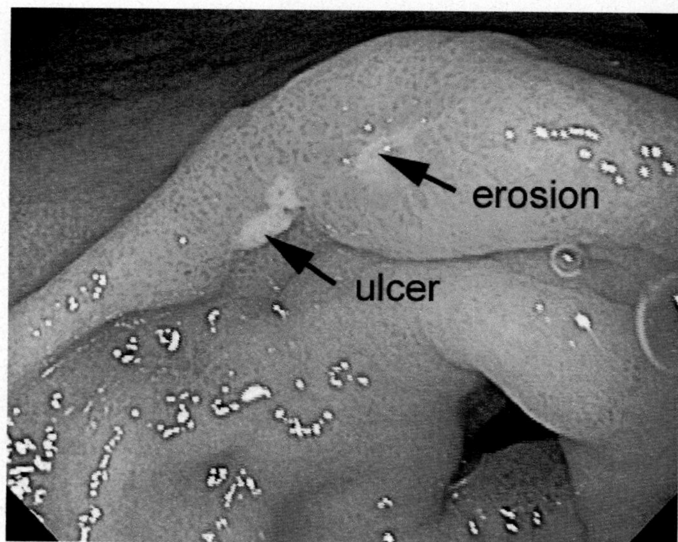

FIGURE 61-2 Endoscopic view of a pyloric ulcer and an erosion of the mucosa. The ulcer and erosion are benign peptic ulcer disease and not malignant. (*Reproduced with permission from Marvin Derezin, MD.*)

ETIOLOGY AND PATHOPHYSIOLOGY

- Causes of PUD include:
  - Nonsteroidal anti-inflammatory drugs (NSAIDs), chronic *H. pylori* infection, and acid hypersecretory states such as Zollinger-Ellison syndrome.[2]

- Uncommon causes include *Cytomegalovirus* (especially in transplantation recipients), systemic mastocytosis, Crohn disease, lymphoma, and medications (e.g., alendronate).[2]
- Up to 10% of ulcers are idiopathic.[2]

- Infection with *H. pylori*, a short, spiral-shaped, microaerophilic Gram-negative bacillus, is the leading cause of PUD. It is associated with up to 70% to 80% of duodenal ulcers.[2]
- *H. pylori* colonize the deep layers of the gel that coats the mucosa and disrupt its protective properties, causing release of certain enzymes and toxins. These make the underlying tissues more vulnerable to damage by digestive juices and thus cause injury to the stomach (**Figures 61-1** to **61-3**) and duodenal cells.[1]
- NSAIDs are the second most common cause of PUD and account for many *H. pylori*–negative cases.
- NSAIDs and aspirin inhibit mucosal cyclooxygenase activity, reducing the level of mucosal prostaglandin and causing defects in the protective mucous layer.
- There is a 10% to 20% prevalence of gastric ulcers and a 2% to 5% prevalence of duodenal ulcers in long-term NSAID users.[2] The annual risk of a life-threatening ulcer-related complication is 1% to 4% in long-term NSAID users, with older patients having the highest risk.[3]

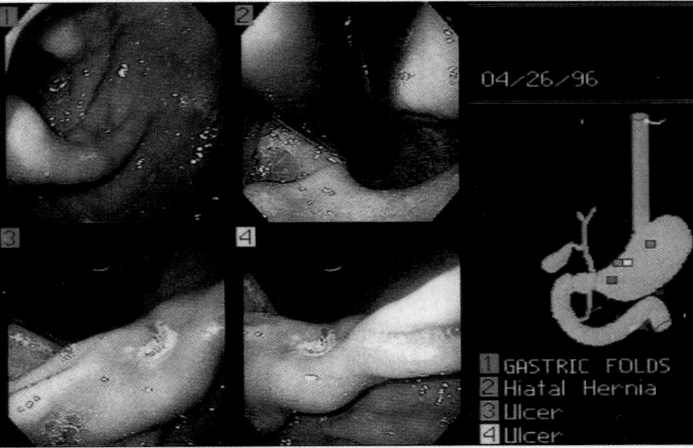

FIGURE 61-3 Stomach ulcer in a patient with a hiatal hernia. (*Reproduced with permission from Michael Harper, MD.*)

RISK FACTORS

- Severe physiologic stress—Burns, central nervous system trauma, surgery, and severe medical illness increase the risk for secondary (stress) ulceration.[4]
- Smoking—Evidence that tobacco use is a risk factor for duodenal ulcers is not conclusive, with several studies producing contradictory findings. However, smoking in the setting of *H. pylori* infection may increase the risk of relapse of PUD.[5]
- Alcohol use—Ethanol is known to cause gastric mucosal irritation and nonspecific gastritis. Evidence that consumption of alcohol is a risk factor for duodenal ulcer is inconclusive.[5]
- Medications—Corticosteroids alone do not increase the risk for PUD; however, they can potentiate ulcer risk in patients who use NSAIDs concurrently.[4]

DIAGNOSIS

CLINICAL FEATURES

- Epigastric pain (dyspepsia), the hallmark of PUD, is present in 80% to 90% of patients; however, this symptom is not sensitive or specific enough to serve as a reliable diagnostic criterion for PUD. Pain is typically described as gnawing or burning, occurring 1 to 3 hours after meals and relieved by food or antacids. It can occur at night, and sometimes radiates to the back.[2] Only 20% to 25% of patients with suggestive symptoms have ulcer disease at endoscopy.[4]
- Other dyspeptic symptoms including belching, bloating, and distention are common but also not specific features of PUD, as they are commonly encountered in many other conditions.

- Additional symptoms include fatty food intolerance, heartburn, and chest discomfort.
- Nausea and anorexia may occur with gastric ulcers.
- Significant vomiting and weight loss are unusual with uncomplicated ulcer disease and suggest gastric outlet obstruction or gastric malignancy.[2]
- Twenty percent of patients with ulcer complications such as bleeding and nearly 61% of patients with NSAID-related ulcer complications have no antecedent symptoms.
- Rare and nonspecific physical findings include:
  - Epigastric tenderness
  - Heme-positive stool
  - Hematemesis or melena in cases of GI bleeding

TYPICAL DISTRIBUTION

- Duodenal ulcers occur most often in the first portion of the duodenum (>95%), with approximately 90% of ulcers located within 3 cm of the pylorus.[1]
- Benign gastric ulcers are located most commonly in the antrum (60%) and at the junction of the antrum and body on the lesser curvature (25%) (see **Figure 61-3**).[1]

LABORATORY STUDIES

- In most patients with uncomplicated PUD, routine laboratory tests are not helpful.[4]
- All patients with PUD or a history of PUD should be tested for *H. pylori*.[6] Patients under age 60 years who have no alarm symptoms (listed below) can be considered for noninvasive testing with either a fecal antigen test or urea breath tests to detect active disease.[6] Point-of-care urea breath tests are available.
- Obtaining a serum gastrin may be useful in patients with recurrent, refractory, or complicated PUD and in patients with a family history of PUD to screen for Zollinger-Ellison syndrome.[1]

IMAGING

- Upper endoscopy is the procedure of choice for the diagnosis of duodenal and gastric ulcers (see **Figures 61-1** to **61-3**).[2]
- Endoscopy provides better diagnostic accuracy than barium radiography and affords the ability to biopsy for the presence of malignancy and *H. pylori* infection. Endoscopy is usually reserved for the following situations:
  - Patients with alarm symptoms (e.g., bleeding, dysphagia, severe pain, abdominal mass, recurrent vomiting, weight loss) or age older than 59 years. It should be noted, however, that alarm features have poor diagnostic accuracy for malignancy.[7]
  - Patients who fail initial therapy.
  - Patients whose symptoms recur after appropriate therapy.
- Duodenal ulcers are virtually never malignant and do not require biopsy.[2]
- Gastric ulcers should be biopsied because 3% to 5% of benign-appearing gastric ulcers prove to be malignant.[2]
- Upper GI (UGI) series has limited accuracy in distinguishing benign from malignant gastric ulcers; therefore, all patients diagnosed this way should be reevaluated with endoscopy after 8 to 12 weeks of therapy.

DIFFERENTIAL DIAGNOSIS

Disease processes that may present with "ulcer-like" symptoms include:

- Nonulcer or functional dyspepsia (FD)—The most common diagnosis among patients seen for upper abdominal discomfort; it is a diagnosis of exclusion. Dyspepsia has been reported to occur in up to 30% of the U.S. population.
- Gastroesophageal reflux—Classic symptoms are heartburn (i.e., substernal pain that may be associated with acid regurgitation or a sour taste) aggravated by bending forward or lying down, especially after a large meal. Endoscopy is considered if symptoms fail to respond to treatment (e.g., histamine-2-receptor agonist, proton pump inhibitor [PPI]) or red flag signs and symptoms occur.
- Gastric cancer—Most patients do not become symptomatic until late in the disease; symptoms include upper abdominal pain, postprandial fullness, anorexia and mild nausea, vomiting (especially with pyloric tumors), weight loss, and a palpable mass. Endoscopic biopsy is used to make this diagnosis (see Chapter 62, Gastric Cancer).
- Biliary colic is characterized by discrete, intermittent episodes of pain that should not be confused with other causes of dyspepsia.
- Gastroduodenal Crohn disease—Symptoms include epigastric pain, nausea, and vomiting. On endoscopy, patients often have *H. pylori*–negative gastritis and may develop gastric outlet obstruction. Extraintestinal manifestations include erythema nodosum, peripheral arthritis, conjunctivitis, uveitis, and episcleritis. Endoscopy shows an inflammatory process with skip lesions, fistulas, aphthous ulcerations, and rectal sparing. Small bowel involvement is seen on imaging with longitudinal and transverse ulceration (cobblestoning) in addition to segmental colitis and frequent stricture (see Chapter 67, Inflammatory Bowel Disease).

MANAGEMENT

- The approach to patients with dyspepsia includes performing endoscopy for patients with red flag symptoms or who are older than age 59 years. For patients who have an ulcer identified on endoscopy, eradication of *H. pylori* is attempted (as below) and a PPI is continued for 4 to 8 weeks. For those without an ulcer on endoscopy, treatment with a PPI or H_2 blocker is provided.[3]
- For patients without red flag findings, testing and treating for *H. pylori*; counseling to avoid smoking, alcohol, and NSAIDs; and appropriate use of antisecretory therapy for 4 weeks will be successful in most patients.[3]

MEDICATIONS

- The goals of treatment of active *H. pylori*–associated ulcers are to relieve dyspeptic symptoms, to promote ulcer healing, and to eradicate *H. pylori* infection. Eradication of *H. pylori* is better than ulcer-healing drug therapy for duodenal ulcer healing (persistent ulcer in 12.4% vs. 18.7%) and, compared to no treatment, prevents both duodenal (12.9% vs. 64.4%) and gastric ulcer recurrence (16.3% vs. 52.4%).[8] Trial data quality, however, is low.
- Traditional triple therapy with PPI, clarithromycin, and amoxicillin for 14 days is reserved for patients with no previous history of macrolide exposure who reside in areas where clarithromycin resistance among *H. pylori* isolates is known to be low.[6]
- Four-drug combinations, given for 10–14 days, currently provide the best results and consist of two general combinations: (a) a PPI, amoxicillin, clarithromycin, metronidazole/tinidazole given either sequentially or concomitantly, or (b) a PPI, a bismuth, tetracycline HCl, and metronidazole/tinidazole.[6] SOR Ⓐ Sequential therapy consists of a PPI and amoxicillin for 5–7 days followed by a PPI, clarithromycin, and a nitroimidazole for 5–7 days (quality of evidence for this treatment is low).
- Treat NSAID-induced ulcers with cessation of NSAIDs, if possible, and an appropriate course of standard ulcer therapy with a H_2-receptor antagonist or a PPI. If NSAIDs are continued, prescribe a PPI. SOR Ⓐ
- *H. pylori*–negative ulcers that are not caused by NSAIDs can be treated with appropriate antisecretory therapy, either H_2-receptor antagonist or PPI. SOR Ⓐ
- For patients with bleeding peptic ulcers, high-dose PPIs do not reduce rates of rebleeding, surgical intervention, or mortality after endoscopic treatment compared with non–high-dose PPIs.[9] In addition, for endoscopically treated high-risk bleeding ulcers, intermittent-dose PPIs were comparable to bolus PPI followed by infusion for 72 hours with respect to rebleeding within 7 days.[10]
- For patients who experience blood loss from severe acute UGI bleeding, a restrictive policy for transfusion (hemoglobin <7 g/dL) was associated with better survival (95% vs. 91%), less rebleeding, and fewer complications.[11]

SURGERY

- For perforated ulcers, laparoscopic repair and open repair appear comparable with respect to operative duration and complications, but hospital length of stay and postoperative pain are less with laparoscopy.[12]

PREVENTION

- In a large randomized controlled trial of PUD prevention in 2426 patients taking low-dose acetylsalicylic acid who were at risk for ulcer development (e.g., prior ulcer, GI symptoms and erosions, age older than 65 years), esomeprazole 40 mg or 20 mg reduced the rate of endoscopically confirmed peptic ulcer development (1.5% and 1.1%, respectively) versus placebo (7.4%).[13]
- Authors of a meta-analysis found the use of prophylactic H_2 blockers to prevent stress ulcers was not necessary in patients receiving enteral nutrition and that such therapy was associated with pneumonia and higher risk of hospital mortality.[14] In another meta-analysis, PPIs were similar to H_2-receptor antagonists in terms of stress-related UGI bleeding prophylaxis, pneumonia, and mortality among patients admitted to intensive care units,[15] although authors of a more recent meta-analysis found small differences in clinically important UGI bleeding in favor of PPIs but not other differences.[16]

PROGNOSIS

- Mortality rate is approximately 1 per 100,000 cases.[4]
- When the underlying cause is addressed, the prognosis is excellent.
- With the eradication of *H. pylori* infection, ulcer recurrence rate has decreased from 60%–90% to approximately 10%–20%.[4]
- The incidence of perforation is approximately 0.3% per patient year, and the incidence of obstruction is approximately 0.1% per patient year.[4]

FOLLOW-UP

- Endoscopy is required to document healing of gastric ulcers and to rule out gastric cancer; this is performed 6 to 8 weeks after the initial diagnosis.
- Confirmation of *H. pylori* eradication is recommended using a urea breath test, fecal antigen test, or biopsy-based testing whenever *H. pylori* infection is identified and treated.[6] Testing is performed at least 4 weeks after the completion of antibiotic therapy and after PPI therapy has been withheld for 1–2 weeks.
- Confirmation of healing with endoscopy is required in all patients with ulcer complicated by bleeding, perforation, or obstruction.
- For patients without initial endoscopy who have persistent symptoms following initial treatment, the PPI or H_2 blocker can be continued for another 4 to 8 weeks.[3] If there is inadequate response to therapy, endoscopy and evaluation for hypersecretory states should be considered.
- Osteoporosis is associated with PUD, especially among patients treated with PPI; osteoporosis developed after 1 year.[17]

PATIENT EDUCATION

- Patients with PUD should be encouraged to eat balanced meals at regular intervals, avoid heavy alcohol use, and avoid smoking (which has been shown to retard the rate of ulcer healing and increase the frequency of recurrences); stress reduction counseling might be helpful in individual cases.

PATIENT RESOURCES

- National Digestive Diseases Information Clearing House—**https://www.niddk.nih.gov/health-information/digestive-diseases/peptic-ulcers-stomach-ulcers.**
- MedlinePlus. Peptic Ulcer-**https://medlineplus.gov/pepticulcer.html.**

PROVIDER RESOURCES

- **http://emedicine.medscape.com/article/181753-overview.**

REFERENCES

1. Del Valle J. Peptic ulcer disease and related disorders. In: Kasper DL, Braunwald E, Fauci AS, et al, eds. *Harrison's Principles of Internal Medicine*, 16th ed. New York, NY: McGraw-Hill; 2005: 1746-1762.
2. McPhee SJ, Papadakis MA, Tierney LW Jr. *Current Medical Diagnosis and Treatment*. New York, NY: McGraw-Hill; 2007.
3. Ramakrishnan K, Salinas RC. Peptic ulcer disease. *Am Fam Physician*. 2007;76(7):1005-1012.
4. Anand BS. *Peptic Ulcer Disease*. http://emedicine.medscape.com/article/181753-overview. Updated January 2017. Accessed February 2017.
5. Aldoori WH, Giovannucci EL, Stampfer MJ, et al. A prospective study of alcohol, smoking, caffeine, and the risk of duodenal ulcer in men. *Epidemiology*. 1997;8(4):420-424.
6. Chey WD, Leontiadis GI, Howden CW, Moss SF. American College of Gastroenterology clinical guideline: treatment of *Helicobacter pylori* infection. *Am J Gastroenterol*. 2017;112:212-238.
7. Khademi H, Radmard A-R, Malekzadeh F, et al. Diagnostic accuracy of age and alarm symptoms for upper GI malignancy in patients with dyspepsia in a GI clinic: a 7-year cross-sectional study. *PLoS One*. 2012;7(6):e39173.
8. Ford AC, Gurusamy KS, Delaney B, et al. Eradication therapy for peptic ulcer disease in *Helicobacter pylori* positive patients. *Cochrane Database Syst Rev*. 2016;(4):CD003840.
9. Wang CH, Ma MH, Chou HC, et al. High-dose vs non-high-dose proton pump inhibitors after endoscopic treatment in patients with bleeding peptic ulcer: a systematic review and meta-analysis of randomized controlled trials. *Arch Intern Med*. 2010;170(9): 751-758.
10. Sachar H, Vaidya K, Laine L. Intermittent vs continuous proton pump inhibitor therapy for high-risk bleeding ulcers: a systematic review and meta-analysis. *JAMA Intern Med*. 2014;174(11):1755-1762.
11. Villanueva C, Colomo A, Bosch A, et al. Transfusion strategies for acute upper gastrointestinal bleeding. *N Engl J Med*. 2013;368(1): 11-21.
12. Ge B, Wu M, Chen Q, et al. A prospective randomized controlled trial of laparoscopic repair versus open repair for perforated peptic ulcers. *Surgery*. 2016;159(2):451-458.
13. Scheiman JM, Devereaux PJ, Herlitz J, et al. Prevention of peptic ulcers with esomeprazole in patients at risk of ulcer development treated with low-dose acetylsalicylic acid: a randomised, controlled trial (OBERON). *Heart*. 2011;97(10):797-802.
14. Marik PE, Vasu T, Hirani A, Pachinburavan M. Stress ulcer prophylaxis in the new millennium: a systematic review and meta-analysis. *Crit Care Med*. 2010;38(11):2222-2228.
15. Lin PC, Chang CH, Hsu PI, et al. The efficacy and safety of proton pump inhibitors vs histamine-2 receptor antagonists for stress ulcer bleeding prophylaxis among critical care patients: a meta-analysis. *Crit Care Med*. 2010;38(4):1197-1205.
16. Alhazzani W, Alenezi F, Jaeschke RZ, et al. Proton pump inhibitors versus histamine 2 receptor antagonists for stress ulcer prophylaxis in critically ill patients: a systematic review and meta-analysis. *Crit Care Med*. 2013;41(3):693-705.
17. Wu CH, Tung YC, Chai CY, et al. Increased risk of osteoporosis in patients with peptic ulcer disease: a nationwide population-based study. *Medicine (Baltimore)*. 2016;95(16):e3309.

62 GASTRIC CANCER

Mindy A. Smith, MD, MS

PATIENT STORY

A 72-year-old Japanese immigrant was brought in by his family with complaints of difficulty eating, vague abdominal pain, and weight loss. Endoscopy and biopsy confirmed gastric adenocarcinoma (**Figure 62-1**). Liver metastases were found on abdominal CT. The family and the patient chose only comfort measures, and the patient died 6 months later.

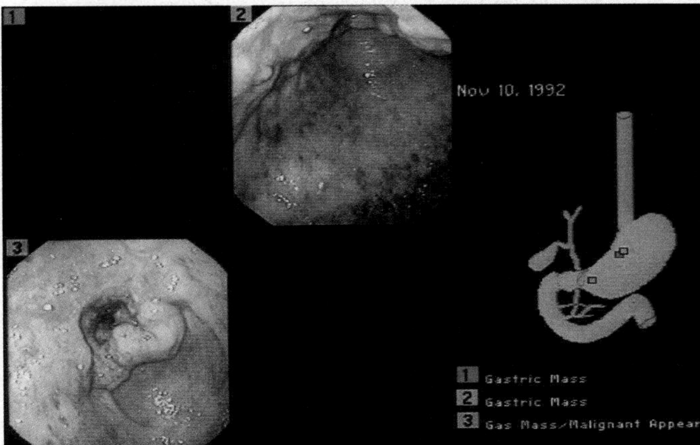

FIGURE 62-1 Endoscopy showing a raised and irregular mass in the antrum of the stomach deforming the pylorus. It fills the distal one-half of the antrum. The lesion was hard when probed with biopsy forceps. Biopsy indicated adenocarcinoma. (*Reproduced with permission from Michael Harper, MD.*)

INTRODUCTION

Gastric cancer, also known as stomach cancer, is a malignant neoplasm of the stomach, usually adenocarcinoma.

EPIDEMIOLOGY

- Based on Surveillance Epidemiology and End Results (SEER) data (2009–2013), an estimated 26,370 people will be diagnosed with gastric cancer, and 10,730 will die of this cancer in 2016.[1] The male-to-female ratio is about 2:1.[2] The median age at diagnosis is 70 years (typical range 60–84 years)[2] and median age at death from gastric cancer is 73 years.[1]
- Gastric cancer occurs in 7.4 per 100,000 men and women annually. In 2013, an estimated 79,843 people in the United States had gastric cancer, with a lifetime risk of 0.9%.[1]
- Highest rates of gastric cancer occur in eastern Asia, eastern Europe, and South America.[2]

ETIOLOGY AND PATHOPHYSIOLOGY

- Over 90% percent of gastric cancers are adenocarcinomas with the remainder lymphomas, carcinoid tumors, and GI stromal tumors.[3]
- Exogenous and endogenous factors (see "Risk Factors" below) contribute to the development of gastric cancer.[2]
    - Genetic factors—Oncogenic pathways identified in most gastric cancers are the proliferation/stem cell, nuclear factor-κB, and Wnt/β-catenin; interactions between them appear to influence disease behavior and patient survival.[4] There are several autosomal dominant genetic syndromes associated with gastric cancer—hereditary diffuse gastric cancer caused by a germline mutation in the *CDH1* gene; Lynch syndrome, which involves defective DNA mismatch repair; juvenile polyposis syndrome; and Peutz-Jeghers syndrome.[2,5]
    - Gastric tumors are classified for staging using the T (tumor) N (nodal involvement) M (metastases) system. Two important prognostic factors are depth of invasion through the gastric wall (less than T2 [tumor invades muscularis propria]) and presence or absence of regional lymph node involvement (N0). Changes made to the classification system in the seventh edition of the

American Joint Commission's *Cancer Staging Manual* for gastric cancer demonstrate better survival discrimination.[6]
- Gastric cancer spreads in multiple ways[3]:
  - Local extension through the gastric wall to the perigastric tissues, omenta, pancreas, colon, or liver.
  - Lymphatic drainage through numerous pathways leads to multiple nodal group involvement (e.g., intra-abdominal, supraclavicular) or seeding of peritoneal surfaces with metastatic nodules occurring on the ovary, periumbilical region, or peritoneal cul-de-sac.
  - Hematogenous spread is also common with liver metastases.

RISK FACTORS

- Modifiable risk factors—*Helicobacter pylori* infection (relative risk [RR] 2.56; 95% confidence interval [CI] 1.99 to 3.29 in low-risk settings), cigarette smoking (RR 1.53; 95% CI 1.42 to 1.65), alcohol use (RR 1.20; 95% CI 1.01 to 1.44 for heavy drinkers), dietary salt (RR 1.08 for each gram consumed), and low vegetable consumption.[2]
- Atrophic gastritis (including postsurgical vagotomized patients) and pernicious anemia (RR 6.8; 95% CI 2.6 to 18.1) are conditions that favor the growth of nitrate-converting bacteria.[2] In addition, intestinal-type cells that develop metaplasia and possibly atypia can replace the gastric mucosa in these patients. Genetic polymorphisms (e.g., interleukin-1B-511, interleukin-1RN, and tumor necrosis factor-α) also appear to play a role. Familial adenomatous polyposis and hereditary nonpolyposis colorectal cancer are also risk factors.[5]
- Additional risk factors—Low socioeconomic class, lower educational level, exposure to certain pesticides (e.g., those who work in the citrus fruit industry in fields treated with 2,4-dichlorophenoxyacetic acid [2,4-D], chlordane, propargite, and trifluralin[7]), radiation exposure, and blood type A.

DIAGNOSIS

CLINICAL FEATURES[3]

- Asymptomatic, if superficial and/or early.
- Upper abdominal pain that ranges from vague to severe.
- Postprandial fullness.
- Anorexia and mild nausea.
- Nausea and vomiting occur with pyloric tumors.
- Late symptoms include weight loss and a palpable mass (regional extension).
- Late complications include peritoneal and pleural effusions and obstruction of the gastric outlet.
- Physical signs are also late features and include[8]:
  - Palpable enlarged stomach with succussion splash (splashing sound on shaking, indicative of the presence of fluid and air in a body cavity).
  - Enlarged liver.
  - Rarely, enlarged, firm to hard, lymph nodes (i.e., left supraclavicular [Virchow]), periumbilical region (Sister Mary Joseph node), and peritoneal cul-de-sac (Blumer shelf; palpable on vaginal or rectal examination).

TYPICAL DISTRIBUTION

- Based on SEER data from 1988 to 2001, gastric tumors occur most often in the cardia (25.5%) and gastric antrum (20.7%), followed by the lesser curvature (9.9%), body (7.4%) and greater curvature (4.3%), and fundus (4.1%). Overlapping lesions were reported in 9.8%, and no specific information was available in 15.2%.[9]

IMAGING, ENDOSCOPY, AND SPECIAL TESTS

- Diagnosis can be made on endoscopy (**Figures 62-1** and **62-2**) with biopsy of suspicious lesions.[5]
- Urgent referral for endoscopy (within 2 weeks) is recommended for patients with dyspepsia who also have alarm symptoms (GI bleeding, dysphagia, progressive unexplained weight loss, persistent vomiting, unexplained iron-deficiency anemia, epigastric mass or lymphadenopathy, family history of gastric cancer [onset <50 years]), or whose dyspepsia is persistent and they are older than age 55 years.[2] SOR Ⓒ Use of alarm features, however, only has a pooled positive likelihood ratio of 2.74 (95% CI 1.47 to 5.24).[10]
- Double-contrast radiography is an alternative to endoscopy, especially for patients with dysphagia, and can detect large primary tumors, but distinguishing benign from malignant disease is difficult.[3]
- Although endoscopy is not necessary when radiography demonstrates a benign-appearing ulcer with evidence of complete healing at 6 weeks, some authors recommend routine endoscopy, biopsy, and brush cytology when any gastric ulcer is identified.[3]
- Some gastric polyps (adenomas, hyperplastic) have malignant potential and should be removed.[11]
- Work-up includes[5]: SOR Ⓒ
  - Chest, abdominal, and pelvic CT with oral and IV radiocontrast
  - Endoscopic ultrasound if no evidence of metastatic disease
  - Positron emission tomography/CT if no evidence of metastatic disease and if clinically indicated
  - Biopsy of metastatic disease as clinically indicated
  - HER2-neu testing if metastatic adenocarcinoma is documented or suspected
  - Nutritional assessment

LABORATORY STUDIES

- A hemoglobin or hematocrit can identify anemia, present in approximately one third of patients.
- Comprehensive chemistry profile can assist in assessing the patient's clinical state and any liver involvement.[5]
- Circulating microRNA R-21 obtained from serum or plasma appears to be a potential biomarker for detection of gastric cancer, with an area under the receiver-operating characteristic curve of 0.91.[12]
- Exhaled breath sampling for analysis of volatile organic compounds is another potential tool for gastric cancer diagnosis with an area under the receiver-operating characteristic curve of 0.98.[13]

DIFFERENTIAL DIAGNOSIS

- Peptic ulcer—Typical symptoms include epigastric pain (described as a gnawing or burning), occurring 1 to 3 hours after meals and relieved by food or antacids. Patients may also have nausea and vomiting, bloating, abdominal distention, and anorexia. Endoscopy confirms diagnosis (see Chapter 61, Peptic Ulcer Disease).

- Nonulcer dyspepsia—Includes gastroesophageal reflux disease and functional dyspepsia. Classic symptoms of gastroesophageal reflux disease are heartburn (i.e., substernal pain that may be associated with acid regurgitation or a sour taste) aggravated by bending forward or lying down, especially after a large meal; individual symptoms, however, do not help to distinguish these patients from those with peptic ulcer disease. Endoscopy is considered if symptoms fail to respond to treatment (e.g., histamine-2 receptor agonist, proton pump inhibitor) or red flag signs/symptoms occur (e.g., bleeding, dysphagia, severe pain, weight loss).
- Chronic gastritis—Includes autoimmune (body-predominant) and *H. pylori*–related (antral-predominant) types; mucosal inflammation (primarily lymphocytes) may progress to atrophy and metaplasia. Abdominal pain and dyspepsia are common symptoms, and patients may have pernicious anemia.
- Esophagitis—May be mechanical or infectious (primarily viral and fungal). Symptoms include heartburn (retrosternal wave-like pain that may radiate to the neck or jaw) and painful swallowing (odynophagia); regurgitation of sour or bitter-tasting material may occur with obstruction. Barium swallow or esophagoscopy can be used to establish the diagnosis.
- Esophageal cancer—Relatively uncommon malignancy of two cell types: squamous cell cancers (largely related to smoking, excessive alcohol consumption, and other agents causing mucosal trauma) and adenocarcinomas (usually arising in the distal esophagus related to reflux disease). Symptoms include progressive dysphagia and weight loss; the diagnosis is confirmed on esophagoscopy and biopsy.

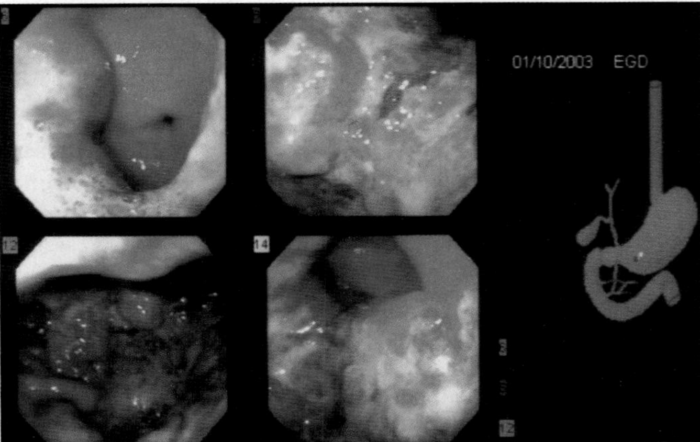

FIGURE 62-2 Endoscopy showing a deep ulcer with yellow-brown exudate in center of mass, consistent with cancer. Pathology confirmed a high-grade, diffuse, large B-cell lymphoma of the stomach. (*Reproduced with permission from Michael Harper, MD.*)

MANAGEMENT

- Patients may be best managed by an experienced multidisciplinary team. In general, tumors with local invasion or distant metastases are not amenable to curative treatment, and curative treatment is based, in part, on whether patients are medically able to tolerate surgery.[2,5] Expert consensus from the National Comprehensive Cancer Network (NCCN) Practice Guidelines for treatment is[5]:
  - For early cancers (in situ or T1a or b) and medically fit, endoscopic surveillance or surgery is recommended.
  - For T2 and higher in patients who are medically fit with tumors that are potentially resectable, surgery with or without perioperative chemotherapy or perioperative chemoradiation is recommended.
  - For those with locoregional disease that is surgically unresectable, concurrent fluoropyrimidine or taxane-based chemoradiation or chemotherapy is recommended, or palliative care if the patient is not a surgical candidate.

PHARMACOLOGIC

- Chemotherapy using 5-fluorouracil (5-FU) and doxorubicin with or without cisplatin or mitomycin C is somewhat helpful (partial response in 30% to 50%).[2] The European Organization for Research and Treatment of Cancer (EORTC)—Gastrointestinal Cancer Group notes improved outcomes for resectable gastric cancer using a strategy of perioperative (pre- and postoperative) chemotherapy or postoperative chemoradiotherapy.[14] SOR Ⓐ For patients with

T2N0 resected tumors with no residual, the NCCN recommends fluoropyrimidine (fluorouracil or capecitabine) followed by fluoropyrimidine-based chemoradiation, and then fluoropyrimidine for selected patients with T2N0 lesions or T3 or T4 lesions.[7]

- In a meta-analysis, three-drug regimens containing 5-FU, an anthracycline, and cisplatin administered as adjunct therapy appeared to have the best survival rates,[15] and another meta-analysis confirmed that postoperative adjuvant chemotherapy based on 5-FU regimens was associated with reduced risk of death in gastric cancer in patients with resectable cancer compared with surgery alone (hazard ratio [HR] 0.82; 95% CI 0.76 to 0.90) with an absolute 5-year survival benefit of 5.7%.[16] SOR Ⓐ
- EORTC—Gastrointestinal Cancer Group found that no chemotherapy combination was an accepted gold standard and that in the treatment of unresectable, locally advanced, or metastatic gastric or gastroesophageal junction adenocarcinoma, response rates were poor.[14]
- About 20% of patients with gastric cancer have tumors with amplification of HER2. Use of targeted treatment with Herceptin (trastuzumab) plus chemotherapy (cisplatin with capecitabine or 5-FU) increases survival by several months compared to chemotherapy alone[17]; this is now accepted therapy.[2]

REFERRAL FOR SURGERY OR PROCEDURES

- Complete resection including adjacent lymph nodes is recommended for T1 tumors and surgery following neoadjuvant therapy for T2 or higher lesions.[2,7] For resectable gastric adenocarcinoma, EORTC-Gastrointestinal Cancer Group recommends free-margin surgery with at least D1 resection (perigastric lymph nodes) combined with removal of a minimum of 15 lymph nodes.[14]
- In a meta-analysis of six trials comparing D1 with D2 (extended lymph node dissection—hepatic, left gastric, celiac, and splenic arteries, as well as those in the splenic hilum) gastrectomy for patients with resectable gastric cancer, postoperative morbidity and 30-day mortality rate were higher in the D2 group; 5-year survival was similar.[18] Authors of a recent review article noted that most high-volume centers perform a modified (spleen-sparing) D2 dissection.[2]
- In a meta-analysis, laparoscopy-assisted distal gastrectomy compared to conventional distal gastrectomy was associated with lower morbidity, less pain, faster bowel function recovery, and shorter hospital stay; anastomotic and wound complications and mortality rates were similar.[19]
- The use of chemoradiation is less well supported by data.[2] Radiation is useful for palliation for pain.

PREVENTION

- Aspirin use reduces the risk of GI cancers (20-year cancer death HR 0.65; 95% CI 0.54, 0.78); the latent period before an effect on death was seen for gastric cancer was more than 5 years.[20]
- Adherence to a relative Mediterranean diet is associated with a reduced risk of gastric cancer (HR 0.67; 95% CI 0.47, 0.94).[21]
- Limited data are available regarding prevention of gastric cancer, but in a population of poorly nourished Chinese subjects, combined supplementation with beta-carotene, α-tocopherol, and selenium reduced the incidence of and mortality rate from gastric cancer and the overall mortality rate from cancer by 13% to 21%.[22]
- Consuming more fruits and vegetables: In a Swedish study, intake of 2–5 servings of fruit and vegetables daily decreased gastric cancer risk compared to consuming <1 serving daily (hazard ratio 0.56, 95% CI 0.34 to 0.93).[23] In a meta-analysis, consumption of large amounts of allium vegetables (onions, garlic, shallots, leeks, chives) was associated with a reduced risk of gastric cancer (odds ratio [OR] 0.54; 95% CI 0.43 to 0.65).[24]
- Despite limited data, a meta-analysis of six studies conducted primarily in Asia found a reduced gastric cancer risk (0.6% absolute risk reduction) with eradication of *H. pylori* infection.[25] Eradication of *H. pylori* following resection of early gastric cancer reducing the risk of developing metachronous gastric carcinoma.[2]
- Screening for gastric cancer in Japan has led to a greater number of cases of gastric cancer being detected in an early stage.

PROGNOSIS

- Surgical morbidity (e.g., anastomotic leaks, infection) occurs in approximately 25% of patients, and operative mortality is approximately 3%.[26]
- Overall 5-year relative survival based on SEER 2006–2012 data was 30.4%.[9] Five-year relative survival for all stages by race and gender was 27.4% for white men; 32.1% for white women; 25.6% for black men; and 34.4% for black women.[27]
- Five-year relative survival for localized disease is 66.9%, for spread to regional nodes is 30.9%, and for metastatic disease is 5%.[9]
- Median survival for grade of tumor decreases from well-differentiated tumors (22.6 months) to undifferentiated (7.6 months).[9]

FOLLOW-UP

- Recurrences occur in the first 8 years.
- The NCCN guideline recommends clinical evaluation every 3–6 months for the first 2 years and every 6–12 months for the next 3 years, then annually; laboratory testing and imaging are performed if clinically indicated.[7] Patients following gastrectomy should be monitored for nutritional deficiency (e.g., vitamin B_{12} and iron). Patients with recurrence may benefit from additional surgery or chemotherapy if they are medically fit.[2]
- Isolated liver metastasis identified on CT, however, may be resectable.
- Tumor markers have been used with some success to detect subclinical recurrences but are not yet in routine use.[28]

PATIENT EDUCATION

- Surgery with perioperative chemotherapy is potentially curative; operative mortality is approximately 3%.[20]
- Early postoperative complications include anastomotic failure, bleeding, ileus, cholecystitis, pancreatitis, pulmonary infections, and thromboembolism. Further surgery may be required for anastomotic leaks.[8]

- Late mechanical and physiologic complications include dumping syndrome, vitamin B_{12} deficiency, reflux esophagitis, and bone disorders, especially osteoporosis.
- Postgastrectomy patients often are immunologically deficient.

PATIENT RESOURCES

- National Cancer Institute—**http://www.cancer.gov/cancertopics/types/stomach/.**
- MedlinePlus—**http://www.nlm.nih.gov/medlineplus/stomachcancer.html.**

PROVIDER RESOURCES

- National Cancer Institute—**https://www.cancer.gov/types/stomach/hp.**

REFERENCES

1. National Cancer Institute. http://seer.cancer.gov/statfacts/html/stomach.html. Accessed March 2017.
2. Thrumurthy SG, Chaudry MA, Hochhauser D, Mughal M. The diagnosis and management of gastric cancer. *BMJ*. 2013; 347;f6367.
3. Mayer R. Gastrointestinal tract cancer. In: Kasper DL, Braunwald E, Fauci AS, et al, eds. *Harrison's Principles of Internal Medicine*, 16th ed. New York, NY: McGraw-Hill; 2005:523-533.
4. Ooi CH, Ivanova T, Wu J, et al. Oncogenic pathway combinations predict clinical prognosis in gastric cancer. *PLoS Genet*. 2009; 5(10):e1000676.
5. National Comprehensive Cancer Network Practice Guidelines in Oncology. *Gastric Cancer*. Version 3.2016. https://www.nccn.org/professionals/physician_gls/f_guidelines.asp. Accessed March 2017.
6. McGhan LJ, Pockai BA, Gray RJ, et al. Validation of the updated 7th edition AJCC TNM staging criteria for gastric adenocarcinoma. *J Gastrointest Surg*. 2012;16(1):53-61, discussion 61.
7. Mills PK, Yang RC. Agricultural exposures and gastric cancer risk in Hispanic farm workers in California. *Environ Res*. 2007;104(2):282-289.
8. Cabebe EC. *Gastric Cancer Clinical Presentation*. http://emedicine.medscape.com/article/278744-clinical. Updated January 2017. Accessed March 2017.
9. Key C, Meisner ALW. *Cancers of the Esophagus, Stomach, and Small Intestine*. http://seer.cancer.gov/publications/survival/surv_esoph_stomach.pdf. Accessed March 2017.
10. Vakil N, Moayyedi P, Fennerty MB, Talley NJ. Limited value of alarm features in the diagnosis of upper gastrointestinal malignancy: systematic review and meta-analysis. *Gastroenterology*. 2006;131:390-401.
11. Goddard AF, Badreldin R, Pritchard DM, et al. The management of gastric polyps. *Gut*. 2010;59(9):1270-1276.
12. Zhu X, Lv M, Wang H, Guan W. Identification of circulating micro RNAs as novel potential biomarkers for gastric cancer detection: a systematic review and meta-analysis. *Dig Dis Sci*. 2014;59(5):911-919.
13. Kumar S, Huang J, Abbassi-Ghadi N, et al. Mass spectrometric analysis of exhaled breath for the identification of volatile organic compound biomarkers in esophageal and gastric adenocarcinoma. *Ann Surg*. 2015;262(6):981-990.
14. Van Cutsem E, Van de Velde C, Roth A, et al. Expert opinion on management of gastric and gastro-oesophageal junction adenocarcinoma on behalf of the European Organisation for Research and Treatment of Cancer (EORTC)—gastrointestinal cancer group. *Eur J Cancer*. 2008;44(2):182-194.
15. Wagner AD, Grothe W, Haerting J, et al. Chemotherapy in advanced gastric cancer: a systematic review and meta-analysis based on aggregate data. *J Clin Oncol*. 2006;24(18):2903-2909.
16. GASTRIC (Global Advanced/Adjuvant Stomach Tumor Research International Collaboration) Group, Paoletti X, Oba K, Burzykowski T, et al. Benefit of adjuvant chemotherapy for resectable gastric cancer: a meta-analysis. *JAMA*. 2010;303(17):1729-1737.
17. Bang YJ, Van Cutsem E, Feyereislova A, et al. Trastuzumab in combination with chemotherapy versus chemotherapy alone for treatment of HER2-positive advanced gastric or gastro-oesophageal junction cancer (ToGA): a phase 3, open-label, randomised controlled trial. *Lancet*. 2010;376:687-697.
18. Memon MA, Subramanya MS, Khan S, et al. Meta-analysis of D1 versus D2 gastrectomy for gastric adenocarcinoma. *Ann Surg*. 2011;253(5):900-911.
19. Hosono S, Arimoto Y, Ohtani H, Kanamiya Y. Meta-analysis of short-term outcomes after laparoscopy-assisted distal gastrectomy. *World J Gastroenterol*. 2006;12(47):7676-7683.
20. Rothwell PM, Fowkes FG, Belch JF, et al. Effect of daily aspirin on long-term risk of death due to cancer: analysis of individual patient data from randomised trials. *Lancet*. 2011;377(9759):31-41.
21. Buckland G, Agudo A, Luján L, et al. Adherence to a Mediterranean diet and risk of gastric adenocarcinoma within the European Prospective Investigation into Cancer and Nutrition (EPIC) cohort study. *Am J Clin Nutr*. 2010;91(2):381-390.
22. Huang HY, Caballero B, Chang S, et al. The efficacy and safety of multivitamin and mineral supplement use to prevent cancer and chronic disease in adults: a systematic review for a National Institutes of Health state-of-the-science conference. *Ann Intern Med*. 2006;145(5):372-385.57(1):69-74.
23. Larsson SC, Bergkvist L, Wolk A. Fruit and vegetable consumption and incidence of gastric cancer: a prospective study. *Cancer Epidemiol Biomarkers Prev*. 2006;15:1998-2001.
24. Zhou Y, Zhuang W, Hu W, et al. Consumption of large amounts of Allium vegetables reduces risk for gastric cancer in a meta-analysis. *Gastroenterology*. 2011;141(1):80-89.
25. Fuccio L, Zagari RM, Eusebi LH, et al. Meta-analysis: can *Helicobacter pylori* eradication treatment reduce the risk for gastric cancer? *Ann Intern Med*. 2009;151(2):121-128.
26. Zilberstein B, Abbud Ferreira J, Cecconello I. Management of postoperative complications in gastric cancer. *Minerva Gastroenterol Dietol*. 2011;57(1):69-74
27. National Cancer Institute. *Surveillance, Epidemiology and End Results Program*. https://seer.cancer.gov/csr/1975_2013/results_single/sect_24_table.08.pdf. Accessed March 2017.
28. Fareed KR, Kaye P, Soomro IN, et al. Biomarkers of response to therapy in oesophago-gastric cancer. *Gut*. 2009;58(1):127-143.

63 LIVER DISEASE

Mindy A. Smith, MD, MS
Angie Mathai, MD

PATIENT STORY

A 64-year-old woman presents with complaints of itchy skin and fatigue. She is noted on physical examination to have scleral icterus and jaundice (**Figure 63-1**). Laboratory testing revealed elevated liver enzymes, particularly the serum alkaline phosphatase and γ-glutamyltranspeptidase, and positive antinuclear and anti-mitochondrial antibodies. A liver biopsy confirmed primary biliary cirrhosis. Two months later, she vomited up some blood and on endoscopy was found to have esophageal varices from her portal hypertension (**Figure 63-2**).

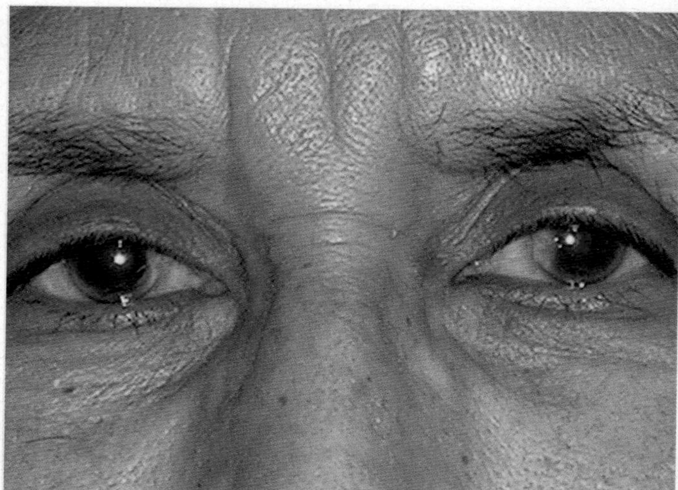

FIGURE 63-1 Scleral icterus in a 64-year-old Hispanic woman with primary biliary cirrhosis. (*Reproduced with permission from Javid Ghandehari, MD.*)

INTRODUCTION

Liver disease can be caused by any number of metabolic, toxic, microbial, circulatory, or neoplastic insults resulting in direct liver injury or from obstruction of bile flow or both. Liver injury falls anywhere on the spectrum from transient abnormalities in biomarkers to life-threatening multiorgan failure. Cirrhosis refers to the development of liver fibrosis with resulting architectural distortion and the formation of regenerative nodules.

SYNONYMS

The following terms refer to various types of liver diseases: hepatic failure, hepatic dysfunction, alcoholic hepatitis, viral hepatitis, cirrhosis, hepatocellular disease, cholestatic disease, liver fibrosis.

EPIDEMIOLOGY

Common causes of liver disease include:

- Nonalcoholic fatty liver disease (NAFLD)—Present in about 30% of adults in the United States; now the most common cause of liver disease worldwide.[1] NAFLD is believed responsible for 90% of cases of elevated liver enzymes without an identifiable cause (e.g., viral hepatitis, alcohol, genetic, medications).[2]
- Alcohol, excessive use—Approximately 5% of the population are at risk; this includes women who drink more than two drinks per day and men who drink more than three drinks per day.[3]
- Drug-induced liver disease[4]:
  - Drugs causing hepatitis include phenytoin, captopril, enalapril, isoniazid, amitriptyline, and ibuprofen.
  - Drugs causing cholestasis include oral contraceptives, erythromycin, and nitrofurantoin.
  - Drugs causing hepatitis and cholestasis include azathioprine, carbamazepine, statins, nifedipine, verapamil, amoxicillin/clavulanic acid, and trimethoprim-sulfamethoxazole.

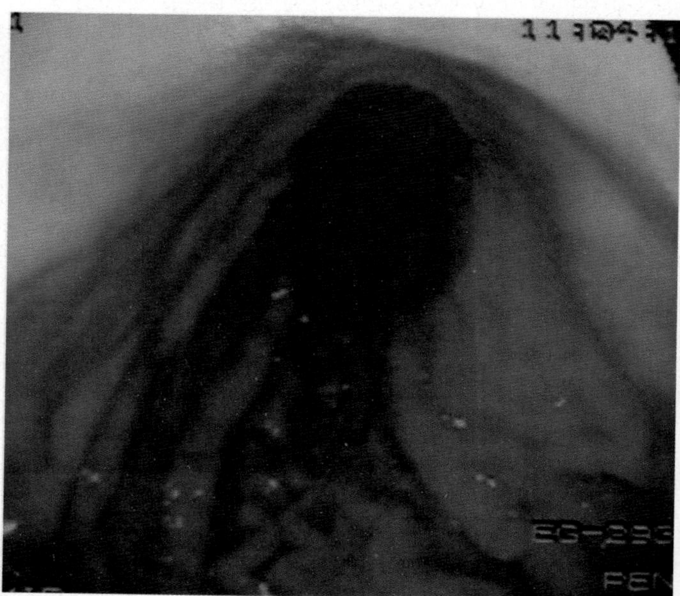

FIGURE 63-2 Esophageal varices in the patient in **Figure 63-1** secondary to her cirrhosis and portal hypertension. (*Reproduced with permission from Javid Ghandehari, MD.*)

- Infectious disease—Viral hepatitis, infectious mononucleosis, *Cytomegalovirus*, and coxsackievirus are most common. Viral hepatitis infections include:
  - Hepatitis A—Anti–hepatitis A virus prevalence in the U.S. population is 35%, a stable frequency of infection over the past decade, representing both natural and vaccine-induced immunity; there are no chronic infections.[5] Universal infant vaccination has occurred since 2006. Incidence rates continue to decline with 1239 cases reported in 2014 (0.4 per 100,000).[6]
  - Hepatitis B—Five percent to 10% of volunteer blood donors in the United States have evidence of prior infection, with 1% to 10% of those infected progressing to chronic hepatitis B virus (HBV) infection.[5] An estimated 2.2 million people have chronic hepatitis B.[7] In 2014 there were 19,200 reported cases.
    - Transfusion risk of acquiring HBV infection is 1 in 230,000.[5] Perinatal transmission correlates with the presence of HBe antigen (Ag) and high-level viral replication; 90% of HBeAg-positive mothers transmit HBV infection to their infants compared to 10% to 15% of anti-HBe–positive mothers.[5]
    - Three phases of chronic HBV infection have been identified: immune-tolerant phase (almost exclusively in children with perinatally acquired infection in whom HBV is nonpathogenic), immune-active phase (host response to HBV with liver inflammation), and inactive phase (seroconvert to antibody to HBeAg).
  - Hepatitis C—In the United States, 1.6% of the general population have had hepatitis C virus (HCV); prevalence of HCV in the 1945–1965 birth cohort is 3.2% (representing three quarters of those infected).[5] About 85% of patients develop chronic infection and up to 50% with chronic infection develop cirrhosis.[5] In 2014, there were approximately 30,500 cases of acute hepatitis C reported in the United States, and 2.7–3.9 million people had chronic hepatitis C.
    - Transfusion-associated hepatitis C is very rare at about 1 in 2.3 million.[8]

Less common disorders include:

- Genetic inheritance—Wilson disease (defective copper transport with copper toxicity; autosomal recessive with 1 per 40,000 affected), hemochromatosis (disorder of iron storage; autosomal recessive—among individuals of northern European heritage, 1 in 10 individuals is a heterozygous carrier and 0.3% to 0.5% have the disease), α_1-antitrypsin deficiency (autosomal recessive with 1% to 2% of patients with chronic obstructive pulmonary disease affected).
- Autoimmune liver disease—Eleven percent to 23% of patients with chronic liver disease and accounts for approximately 6% of liver transplantations in the United States.[9]
- Primary biliary cirrhosis (approximately 5 per 100,000 persons worldwide)—A disease of unknown etiology characterized by inflammatory destruction of the small bile ducts and gradual liver cirrhosis (**Figures 63-1** and **63-2**).

ETIOLOGY AND PATHOPHYSIOLOGY

To understand liver disease, the anatomy and key functions are briefly described here.

- The hepatic artery (20%) and the portal vein (80%) provide the vascular supply of the liver.[3] The liver is organized functionally into acini, which are divided into three zones[3]:
  - Zone 1—The portal areas where blood enters from both sources
  - Zone 2—The hepatocytes and sinusoids where blood flows
  - Zone 3—The terminal hepatic veins
- Hepatocytes, the predominant cells in the liver, perform several vital functions, including the synthesis of essential serum proteins (e.g., albumin, coagulation factors); production of bile and its carriers (e.g., bile acids, cholesterol); regulation of nutrients (e.g., glucose, lipids, amino acids); and metabolism and conjugation of lipophilic compounds (e.g., bilirubin, various drugs) for excretion into the bile or urine.[3]
- There are two basic patterns of liver disease and one mixed pattern[3]:
  - Hepatocellular—Features of this type are direct liver injury, inflammation, and necrosis. Examples are alcoholic and viral hepatitis.
  - Cholestatic (obstructive)—Involves inhibition of bile flow. Examples are gallstone disease, malignancy, primary biliary cirrhosis, and some drug-induced disease.
  - Both patterns—Evidence of direct damage and obstruction. Examples are cholestatic form of viral hepatitis and some drug-induced diseases.
- Cirrhosis occurs following irreversible hepatic injury with hepatocyte necrosis resulting in fibrosis and distortion of the vascular bed. This, in turn, can cause portal hypertension.
- The spectrum of NAFLD ranges from hepatic steatosis (fat deposition in liver cells) to nonalcoholic steatohepatitis (NASH) and cirrhosis.[2] In NAFLD, steatosis occurs when free fatty acids, released in the setting of insulin resistance, are taken up by the liver; the same process can occur in alcoholism. The presence of these fatty acids leads to inflammation from other insults to the liver including oxidative stress, upregulation of inflammatory mediators, and dysregulated apoptosis, producing NASH, fibrosis, and sometimes cirrhosis (occurs in approximately 20% of patients with NASH).[2]

RISK FACTORS

- Risk factors for liver disease include[3]:
  - Alcohol and intravenous drug use.
  - Drugs (e.g., oral contraceptives).
  - Personal and sexual habits.
  - Travel to underdeveloped countries.
  - Exposure to contaminant in food (e.g., shellfish) or individuals with liver disease (includes needle stick injuries).
  - Family history.
  - Remote or recent blood transfusion.
- Risk factors for progressive NAFLD and the more advanced form NASH are central obesity, hypertension, dyslipidemia, type 2 diabetes mellitus, and metabolic syndrome.[1]

DIAGNOSIS

The goals of diagnosis are to determine the etiology and severity of the liver disease, and, where appropriate, the stage of the disease, including whether it is acute or chronic, early or late during the disease, and whether there is cirrhosis present and to what degree.

CLINICAL FEATURES

- Patients with NAFLD are usually asymptomatic.
- Constitutional symptoms in patients with liver disease include fatigue (most common; especially following activity), weakness, anorexia, and nausea.
- Skin alterations[3]:
  - Jaundice (hallmark of obstructive pattern and reliable marker of severity)—Best seen in the sclera or below the tongue; the latter is particularly useful in dark-skinned individuals. Not detected until serum bilirubin levels reach 2.5 mg/dL (43 μmol/L). Early, jaundice may manifest as dark (tea colored) urine and later with light-colored stools. Jaundice without dark urine is usually from indirect hyperbilirubinemia, as seen in patients with hemolytic anemia or Gilbert syndrome.
  - Palmar erythema—Can be seen in both acute and chronic disease but also seen in normal individuals and during pregnancy (**Figure 63-3**).
  - Spider angiomas (superficial, tortuous arterioles that flow outward from the center)—Also seen in both acute and chronic disease, in normal individuals, and during pregnancy (**Figure 63-4**).
  - Excoriations—Pruritus is prominent in acute obstructive disease and in chronic cholestatic diseases such as primary biliary cirrhosis.
  - Palpable purpura—Seen with HCV and chronic HBV.
- Abdominal distention/bloating—Secondary to ascites (accumulation of excess fluid within the peritoneal cavity) (**Figure 63-5**).
  - Ascites may be detected on examination by shifting dullness on percussion (ascitic fluid will flow to the most dependent portions of the abdomen and the air-filled intestines will float on top of this fluid. The fluid–air interface is detected with the patient supine and then turned onto the side where the "line" shifts upward) (**Figures 63-6** and **63-7**).
- Pain in the right upper quadrant (caused by stretching or irritation of the Glisson capsule surrounding the liver) with tenderness on examination in the liver area. Severe pain is most typical of gallbladder disease, liver abscess, and severe veno-occlusive disease. Pain and fever in a patient with ascites should suggest the diagnosis of spontaneous bacterial peritonitis (SBP).
- Hepatomegaly and splenomegaly (congestive splenomegaly from portal hypertension)—Seen in patients with cirrhosis, venoocclusive disease, malignancy, and alcoholic hepatitis.[3]
- Features of hyperestrogenemia in men including gynecomastia (**Figure 63-8**) and testicular atrophy.
- Physical signs of specific liver disease include:
  - Kayser-Fleischer rings—Brown copper pigment deposits around the periphery of the cornea seen in Wilson disease (**Figure 63-9**).
  - Excessive skin pigmentation (slate gray hue/bronzing), diabetes mellitus, polyarticular arthropathy, congestive heart failure, and hypogonadism (hemochromatosis).
  - Cachexia, wasting, and firm hepatomegaly (primary hepatocellular carcinoma or metastatic liver disease).
- Features of patients with advanced disease include muscle wasting, ascites, edema, dilated abdominal veins (e.g., caput medusa—collateral veins seen radiating from the umbilicus),

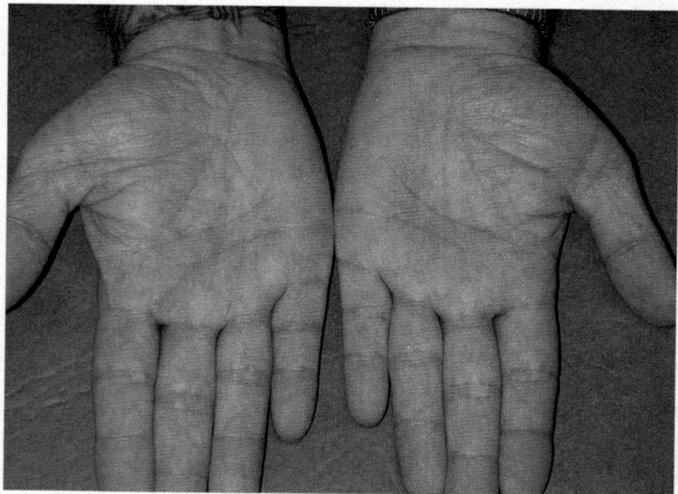

FIGURE 63-3 Palmar erythema in a man with cirrhosis secondary to alcoholism. (*Reproduced with permission from Richard P. Usatine, MD.*)

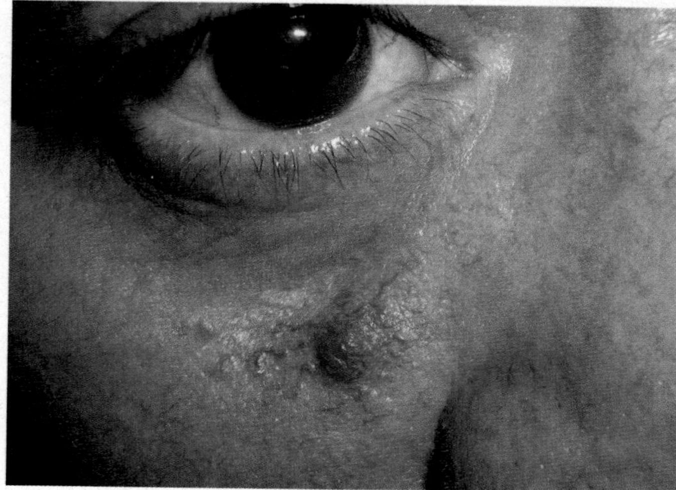

FIGURE 63-4 Spider angioma on the face of a woman with cirrhosis secondary to chronic hepatitis C. (*Reproduced with permission from Richard P. Usatine, MD.*)

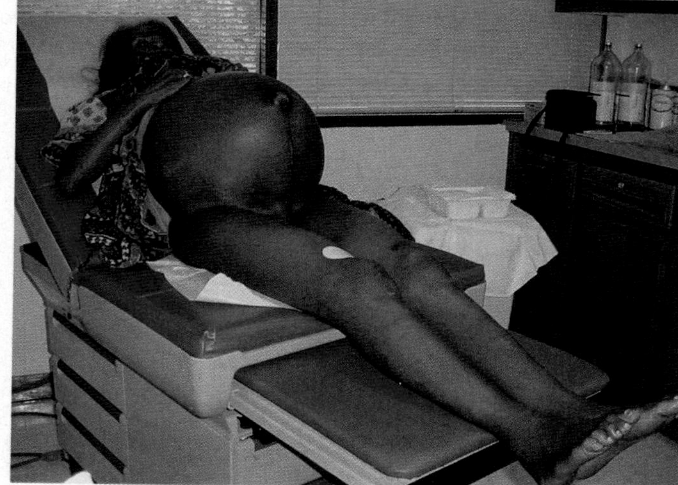

FIGURE 63-5 Tense ascites in a woman with cirrhosis from her alcoholism. An umbilical hernia is also seen from the increased intra-abdominal pressure. (*Reproduced with permission from Richard P. Usatine, MD.*)

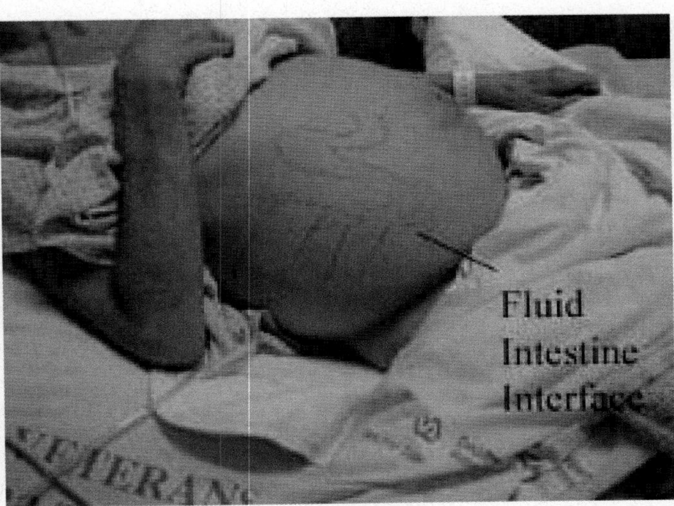

FIGURE 63-6 Patient with ascites and jaundice; lines drawn demonstrate the position of the fluid dullness to percussion (*solid stripes*), intestines (*tubular structure*), and the fluid intestine interface (*dotted line*). (*Reproduced with permission from Charlie Goldberg, MD, copyright University of California, San Diego.*)

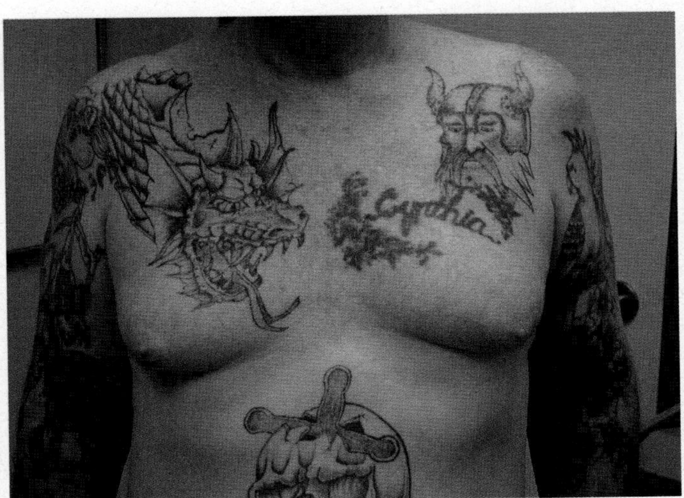

FIGURE 63-8 Gynecomastia in a man with cirrhosis secondary to alcoholism. (*Reproduced with permission from Richard P. Usatine, MD.*)

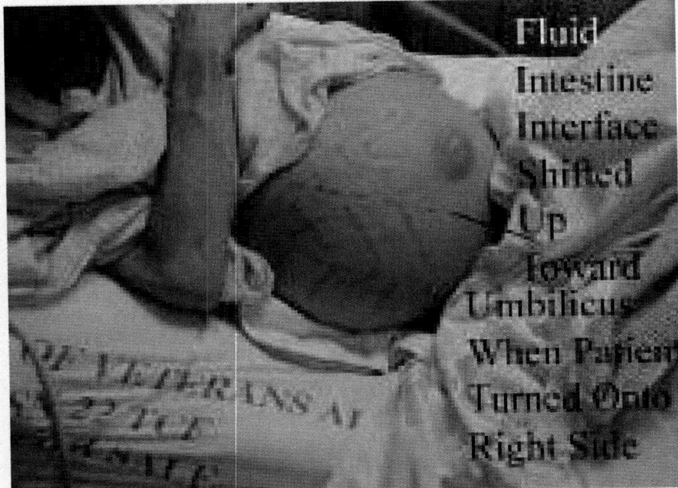

FIGURE 63-7 When patient is turned to the right side, the fluid intestine interface is shifted upward as shown; this is the sign called *shifting dullness*. (*Reproduced with permission from Charlie Goldberg, MD, copyright University of California, San Diego.*)

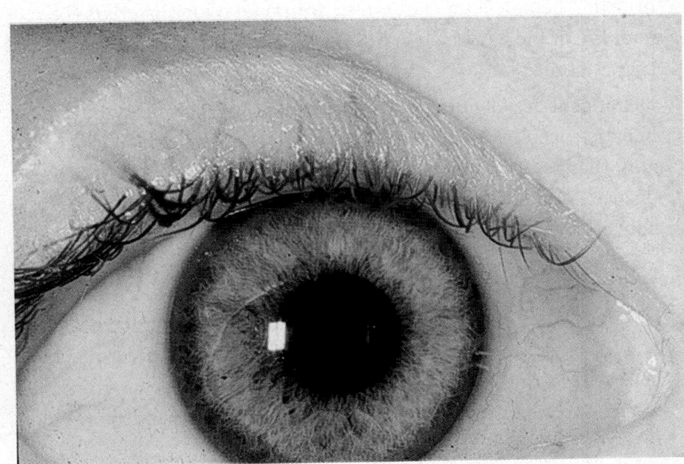

FIGURE 63-9 Kayser-Fleischer ring around the cornea in a patient with Wilson disease. (*Reproduced with permission from Marc Solioz, University of Berne.*)

TABLE 63-1 Patterns of Liver Disease with Usual Laboratory Features, Differential Diagnosis, and Key Components of Diagnostic Work-up

Liver Pattern	AST	ALT	AlkP	GGT	TB	Differential Dx	Diagnostic Work-up
Acute—Hepatocellular	↑	↑↑	Usually normal	↑	Usually normal	Hepatitis A/B/C	Hepatitis panel
						Autoimmune hepatitis	Antinuclear Ab Smooth muscle Ab
						Mononucleosis	Monospot
						Wilson disease	Ceruloplasmin screen Urinary copper
						Tylenol overdose	Tylenol level
						Alcoholic hepatitis	Ammonia level History of alcohol use
						Drug ingestion	Toxicology screen History of drug use
Acute—Cholestatic	Often normal	↑	↑↑	↑↑	↑	Gallstones	Ultrasound
						Mass, hepatic or biliary	MRI MRCP
						Fatty infiltration	Ultrasound
						Biliary duct dilatation	Ultrasound
						Primary biliary cirrhosis	Antimitochondrial Ab
						Primary sclerosing cholangitis	ERCP with biopsies
Chronic—Hepatocellular	↑	↑↑	Usually normal	Usually normal	May be ↑	Hepatitis B/C	Hepatitis panel
						Hemochromatosis	Iron saturation and ferritin
						Wilson disease	Ceruloplasmin screen Urinary copper
						α_1-Antitrypsin deficiency	α_1-Antitrypsin serum level
Chronic—Cholestatic	Usually normal	↑	↑↑	↑↑	↑	Primary sclerosing cholangitis	Antimitochondrial Ab pANCA Ultrasound MRCP ERCP

Abbreviations: Ab, antibody; AST, aspartate aminotransferase; AlkP, alkaline phosphatase; ALT, alanine aminotransferase; dx, diagnosis; ERCP, endoscopic retrograde cholangiopancreatography; GGT, γ-glutamyl transferase; MRCP, magnetic resonance cholangiopancreatography; pANCA, peripheral antinuclear cytoplasmic antibody; TB, total bilirubin.

bruising, hepatic fetor (i.e., sweet, ammonia odor), asterixis (i.e., flapping of the hands when extended), and mental confusion, stupor, or coma.[3]

- Hepatic failure, defined as the occurrence of signs and symptoms of hepatic encephalopathy, may begin with sleep disturbance, personality changes, irritability, and mental slowness.[3] Mental confusion, disorientation, or coma may occur later along with physical signs as above.

LABORATORY TESTING

- Initial evaluation with bilirubin, albumin, alanine aminotransferase (ALT), aspartate aminotransferase (AST), γ-glutamyl transpeptidase (GGT), and alkaline phosphatase (AlkP).[3] **Table 63-1** provides the diagnostic interpretation of the patterns of liver biochemical markers.
    - In acute disease (duration <6 months) with a hepatocellular pattern (see **Table 63-1**), consider infections, ingestions, or Wilson disease.
    - In acute disease with a cholestatic pattern (see **Table 63-1**), consider obstructing gallstones or masses, primary biliary cirrhosis, and cholangitis.
    - In chronic disease (duration >6 months) with hepatocellular pattern (see **Table 63-1**) or mixed pattern (↑ALT, ↑AlkP), consider hemochromatosis, Wilson disease, and α_1-antitrypsin deficiency. Because many of the acute processes can also cause a chronic picture, consider work-up for hepatitis B or C (hepatitis B surface antigen [HBsAg] and anti-HCV), autoimmune hepatitis, alcoholic disease, chronic drug ingestion, or structural abnormalities. Anti-HCV supports and HCV RNA testing establishes the diagnosis of chronic hepatitis C.[5]
    - In chronic disease with cholestatic pattern, consider primary sclerosing cholangitis (see **Table 63-1**).
    - In patients with NAFLD, elevations in ALT and AST are usually no more than 4 times the upper limit of normal; ALT usually predominates.[2] Offer testing for liver fibrosis with enhanced fibrosis liver test (score 10.5 or above is indicative) or with the

NAFLD fibrosis score—the latter calculated using age, body mass index, presence or absence of hyperglycemia, platelet count, albumin level, and ratio of AST to ALT.[1]

- Bilirubin, albumin, and prothrombin time along with the presence or absence of ascites and hepatic encephalopathy are part of the Child-Pugh classification of cirrhosis that has been used to estimate the likelihood of survival and complications of cirrhosis; it is also used to determine candidacy for liver transplantation.[10] Another scoring system, the model for end-stage liver disease (MELD), which uses the international normalized ratio, serum bilirubin, and serum creatinine, is a reliable measure of mortality risk in patients with end-stage liver disease, regardless or cause, and is also used to prioritize liver transplantations (http://www.mayoclinic.org/gi-rst/mayomodel5.html).[11] Modification of MELD adding serum sodium and following the change in MELD score have been proposed to improve predictive accuracy, but it is not clear that these are superior to MELD.[12]

- Suspected SBP can be confirmed following paracentesis of the ascitic fluid showing a polymorphonuclear leukocyte count greater than 250 cells/mm.[5]
- It may be possible to predict significant fibrosis and inflammation among patients with chronic hepatitis B using noninvasive markers, thereby limiting the number of biopsies needed. Serum microRNA profiles may serve as noninvasive biomarkers for HBV infection.[13] The aspartate aminotransferase-to-platelet ratio index (APRI) is a marker that can identify hepatitis C–related fibrosis with a moderate degree of accuracy. This information may limit biopsies in patients with chronic hepatitis C.[14]

IMAGING

Ultrasound is best for detection of NAFLD. It is most accurate when there is greater than 30% steatosis; use of liver elasticity can help distinguish severe from mild fibrosis.[2] MRI reliably detects lesser degrees of steatosis (down to 3%). NAFLD can usually be diagnosed by history, serologies, and abdominal imaging, although biopsy may be needed to judge severity.

BIOPSY

Liver biopsy is the gold standard for diagnosing those with acute disease where the etiology is unclear or for those with chronic disease (e.g., chronic hepatitis B, hepatitis C) to assist in disease staging and prognosis.

MANAGEMENT

Management decisions are based on the etiology, acuity, and severity of the disease.

- NAFLD/NASH—Diet and exercise have been shown to decrease liver enzymes, although it is not known if there is histologic improvement as well.[2] In one study of overweight and obese adolescents, hepatic steatosis was associated with a greater intake of fat and fried foods.[15] Other treatments for obesity, such as medication or bariatric surgery, may also be useful (see Chapter 233, Obesity). Treatment of other risk factors, such as hypertension and hyperlipidemia, should be undertaken. Authors of a Cochrane review found only low-quality trials showing no benefit of antioxidants, bile acids, or thiazolidinediones compared to no intervention for people with NAFLD.[16] For patients with NASH, consider treatment with 800 IU vitamin E or 30 mg pioglitazone daily; however, it is not clear whether these treatments will improve patient-oriented outcomes.[1]
- Alcoholic cirrhosis—Discontinue alcohol and provide supportive therapy; prednisone (40 mg/d) is used for patients with severe alcoholic hepatitis, defined as a MELD >20.[17] Alcoholic hepatitis is treated with either glucocorticoids or pentoxifylline.[17] However, in a recent RCT of 1103 patients with alcoholic hepatitis, neither prednisolone nor pentoxifylline improved survival.[18]
- Drug-induced disease—Withdrawal of agent. Routine screening of asymptomatic patients on statins is no longer recommended. Withdrawal of statins usually results in resolution of elevated transaminases within 2 months. The same statin could be continued at a lower dose or another statin could be started.[19]
- Viral hepatitis—Hepatitis A and acute hepatitis B are treated supportively; virtually all patients recover without specific treatment.
    - Chronic hepatitis B (CHB) is treated based on the presence or absence of compensated or decompensated cirrhosis, HBeAg status, HBV DNA, and ALT elevation with one of 7 U.S. Food and Drug Administration (FDA)-approved drugs including injectable or pegylated interferon alpha, lamivudine, adefovir, dipivoxil, entecavir, telbivudine, or tenofovir.[20] A comparison of these different agents with respect to sustained virologic response and side effects can be found in this reference.[21]
        - The American Association for the Study of Liver Diseases (AASLD) recommends pegylated interferon, entecavir, or tenofovir as preferred initial therapy for adults with immune-active CHB.[21] They recommend against antiviral therapy in adults with immune-tolerant CHB and suggest monitoring ALT every 6 months for potential transition to immune-active or -inactive CHB. National Institute for Health and Care Excellence (NICE) guidelines are also available.[22]
        - For patients with decompensated cirrhosis, lamivudine and telbivudine significantly decrease mortality and disease severity.[23]
        - All persons with chronic hepatitis B who are not immune to hepatitis A should receive 2 doses of hepatitis A vaccine 6 to 18 months apart.
        - Newborns of HBV-infected mothers should receive hepatitis B immunoglobulin and hepatitis B vaccine at delivery and complete the recommended vaccination series.[24] SOR Ⓐ
    - Hepatitis C is currently treated with pegylated interferon and ribavirin; these drugs are combined with protease inhibitors telaprevir and boceprevir in adult patients with HCV genotype 1.[25] NICE guidelines are also available for chronic hepatitis C.[26]
        - There has been an explosion of new medications for hepatitis C. FDA-approved medications for treatment of hepatitis C can be found at http://www.hepatitisc.uw.edu/page/treatment/drugs. These second-generation direct-acting antivirals (DAAs) can be used to treat hepatitis C without interferon.[25] While there are still significant side effects, the courses are shorter and side effects are generally better tolerated. The sustained viral response rates are generally better than older treatments, but costs run around $100,000 for a typical 12-week course. DAAs cure HCV infection in more than 95% of patients which reduces need for liver transplantation and improves quality of life; however, safety issues include the potential recurrence of aggressive hepatocellular

carcinoma and flares of HBV in patients with overt or occult HBV infection.[27] The Infectious Disease Society of America and AASLD are good sources for the newest treatment guidelines.
    - Patients with hepatitis C should be vaccinated against hepatitis A and hepatitis B if they are seronegative for these other forms of hepatitis. SOR Ⓑ
- Wilson disease is treated with a copper-chelating agent, D-penicillamine or trientine, and zinc acetate.[28]
- Hemochromatosis is treated with weekly or twice-weekly phlebotomy; maintenance phlebotomy is typically achieved with 1 unit of blood removed every 2–3 months.[28]
- Primary biliary cirrhosis is managed with ursodiol (13 to 15 mg/kg per day) single dose, most effective if initiated early; antihistamines, naltrexone, or rifampin for pruritus; and eventual liver transplantation.[28] SOR Ⓐ
- Autoimmune hepatitis is treated with glucocorticoid therapy (20–60 mg prednisone) with or without azathioprine (50 mg/day).[28] Oral budesonide, in combination with azathioprine, induces and maintains remission in patients with noncirrhotic autoimmune hepatitis, with a low rate of steroid-specific side effects.[29]

Management of the complications of cirrhosis includes:

- Control ascites with salt restriction (2 g per day of NaCl), fluid restriction if hyponatremic (1000 mL per day), and gentle diuresis to avoid electrolyte disturbance (spironolactone 100 to 200 mg per day) with or without furosemide (40 to 80 mg per day).[30] SOR Ⓐ Recent treatment guidelines are available from the Japanese Society of Gastroenterology.[31]
- SBP is treated with empiric antibiotic therapy (e.g., intravenous cefotaxime 2 g every 8 hours). SOR Ⓐ
- Portal hypertension may be managed with shunting.

PREVENTION AND SCREENING

- Maintaining normal weight and treating obstructive sleep apnea and diabetes may help prevent NAFLD.
- Screen for alcohol abuse using structured questionnaires (e.g., CAGE [cutting, annoyance, guilt, eye-opener], Alcohol Use Disorders Identification Test [AUDIT]). Encourage abstinence and consider naltrexone or acamprosate in combination with counseling.[23]
- Risk for hepatitis A can be minimized by avoidance of susceptible foods in high-risk countries.
- For hepatitis B, Centers for Disease Control and Prevention (CDC) recommendations include avoidance of high-risk behavior and blood contact, vaccination of risk groups, postexposure prophylaxis with anti–hepatitis B immunoglobulin, and cleaning of wound after exposure to infectious blood.
- Screen for HBV infection in pregnant women at their first prenatal visit SOR Ⓐ and in persons at high risk for infection such as those engaging in unprotected sex with multiple partners and living with someone who has chronic hepatitis B. SOR Ⓑ[32]
- Hepatitis C risk can be decreased by avoidance of intravenous drug use, tattooing, and unprotected sexual intercourse. Authors of a meta-analysis of screening for hepatitis C found that point-of-care tests for blood are highly accurate. Screen persons at high risk for HCV infection such as exposed healthcare workers and intravenous illicit drug users, and offer one-time screening for HCV infection to adults born between 1945 and 1965.[26]
- Patients with chronic liver disease should be vaccinated with hepatitis A and hepatitis B vaccines.
- Screen patients with mild elevations of liver enzymes (above normal but less than 5 times the upper limit of normal) for hepatitis B and hepatitis C.[33]

PROGNOSIS

- Thirty percent of patients with NAFLD show histologic progression of fibrosis over 5 years, and approximately 3% eventually develop cirrhosis.[2] Of those with NASH, 15% to 20% may develop cirrhosis. Leading causes of death appear to be cardiovascular disease, cancer (including hepatocellular carcinoma), and liver-related disease. Recurrence of hepatocellular carcinoma is higher in patients with NASH.[2]
- Patients presenting with a high clinical suspicion of alcoholic hepatitis should have their risk for poor outcome stratified using the MDF. Continued alcohol use is associated with disease progression.[34]
- Most cases of hepatitis B are self-limiting. If the HBsAg test remains positive 6 months after the disease onset, the patient is likely to have become a hepatitis B carrier. The carrier status is confirmed by a positive HBsAg test at 12 months.[7]
- Hepatitis C becomes chronic more often than hepatitis B; this occurs in approximately 50% to 90% of patients. The average time from primary infection to liver disease to cirrhosis is 21 years. Twenty percent to 30% develop cirrhosis as early as 5 to 7.5 years after contracting the disease. Standard treatment is more effective for genotypes 2 and 3 than for genotypes 1 and 4.[20] HCV is a leading cause of hepatocellular carcinoma, affecting 15,000 persons annually; treatment resulting in a sustained virologic response at any stage is associated with reduced risk.[35] In observational studies, HCV is also associated with increased cardiovascular mortality (odds ratio [OR] 1.65) and cerebrovascular events (OR 1.3).[36]
- Approximately 50% of patients with autoimmune hepatitis will die within 5 years without treatment. Steroids can induce remission with survival rates similar to the general population.[9] The majority of patients with autoimmune hepatitis achieves complete remission within 3 months but requires long-term or permanent immunosuppressive therapy; such therapy is usually well tolerated. Ten-year survival in well-managed patients is 80% to 98%.[28]
- In the absence of cirrhosis and diabetes, phlebotomy prevents further tissue damage and guarantees a normal life expectancy in patients with hemochromatosis.[28]
- Primary sclerosing cholangitis is a progressive process with a probability of transplant-free survival of 18 years in asymptomatic patients and of 8.5 years in symptomatic patients.[37]
- Cirrhosis can be reversible if the cause is removed; this is especially true for chronic hepatitis C.[30] Mortality is high in patients with decompensation and in those who develop complications such as portal hypertension and bleeding esophageal varices; these patients should be considered for liver transplantation.

FOLLOW-UP

- Hepatitis B virus carriers with high risk for hepatocellular carcinoma (HCC) (e.g., men older than 45 years of age, those with cirrhosis, and individuals with a family history of HCC), should be screened periodically with both a-fetoprotein and ultrasonography.[20] SOR Ⓐ Detailed recommendations for follow-up for patients with chronic hepatitis B and C can be found in the NICE guidelines.[22,26]
- Patients who survive an episode of SBP should receive long-term prophylaxis with daily norfloxacin or trimethoprim-sulfamethoxazole.[30] SOR Ⓐ

PATIENT EDUCATION

- Patients with liver disease should be counseled about avoidance of alcohol and medications that may cause liver injury. They should avoid aspirin use (coagulation impaired) and use acetaminophen at lower doses (2 g per day).
- For those with infectious causes of liver disease, prevention of the spread of disease should be emphasized, including limiting alcohol, safe-sex practices, and avoiding needle sharing. Screening for sexual contacts and household members should be offered along with vaccination for hepatitis B, if nonimmune and noninfected. SOR Ⓐ

PATIENT RESOURCES

- MedlinePlus has a wealth of information for patients with kinds of liver diseases—**http://www.nlm.nih.gov/medlineplus/.**

PROVIDER RESOURCES

- Kwo PY, Cohen SM, Lim JK. ACG Clinical Guideline: Evaluation of abnormal liver chemistries. *Am J Gastroenterol.* 2017;112(1):18-35.
- O'Shea RS, Dasarathy S, McCullough AJ; Practice Guideline Committee of the American Association for the Study of Liver. Alcoholic liver disease. *Hepatology.* 2010;51(1):307-328.

REFERENCES

1. Rinella ME. Nonalcoholic fatty liver disease: a systematic review. *JAMA.* 2015;313(22):2263-2273.
2. Lewis JR, Mohanty SR. Nonalcoholic fatty liver disease: a review and update. *Dig Dis Sci.* 2010;55(3):560-578.
3. Ghany M, Hoofnagle JH. Approach to the patient with liver disease. In: Kasper DL, Fauci AS, Hauser SL, et al, eds. *Harrison's Principles of Internal Medicine*, 19th ed. McGraw-Hill; 2014.
4. Dientag JL, Isselbacher KJ. Toxic and drug-induced hepatitis. In: Kasper DL, Braunwald E, Fauci AS, et al. *Harrison's Principles of Internal Medicine*, 16th ed. New York, NY: McGraw-Hill; 2005: 1840.
5. Dienstag JL. Acute viral hepatitis. In: Kasper DL, Fauci AS, Hauser SL, et al, eds. *Harrison's Principles of Internal Medicine*, 16th ed. New York, NY: McGraw-Hill; 2014.
6. Centers for Disease Control and Prevention. *Surveillance for Viral Hepatitis—United States, 2014*. http://www.cdc.gov/hepatitis/Statistics/index.htm. Accessed April 2017.
7. Centers for Disease Control and Prevention. *Hepatitis B FAQs for Health Professionals.* https://www.cdc.gov/hepatitis/hbv/hbvfaq.htm#overview. Accessed May 2018.
8. Centers for Disease Control and Prevention. *Viral Hepatitis: Hepatitis C FAQs for the Public.* https://www.cdc.gov/hepatitis/hcv/cfaq.htm. Accessed April 2017.
9. Wolf DC, Raghuraman UV. *Autoimmune Hepatitis.* http://emedicine.medscape.com/article/172356-overview#a6. Accessed April 2017.
10. Kamath PS, Wiesner RH, McDiarmid SV, et al. A model to predict survival in patients with end-stage liver disease. *Hepatology.* 2001;33(2):464-470.
11. Asrani SK, Kim WR. Model for end-stage liver disease: end of the first decade. *Clin Liver Dis.* 2011;15(4):685-698.
12. Kim HJ, Lee HW. Important predictor of mortality in patients with end-stage liver disease. *Clin Mol Hepatol.* 2013;19(2):105-115.
13. Li LM, Hu ZB, Zhou ZX, Chen X. Serum microRNA profiles serve as novel biomarkers for HBV infection and diagnosis of HBV-positive hepatocarcinoma. *Cancer Res.* 2010;70(23):798-807.
14. Lin ZH, Xin YN, Dong QJ, Wang Q. Performance of the aspartate aminotransferase-to-platelet ratio index for the staging of hepatitis C-related fibrosis: an updated meta-analysis. *Hepatology.* 2011; 53(3):726-736.
15. Mollard RC, Sénéchal M, MacIntosh AC, et al. Dietary determinants of hepatic steatosis and visceral adiposity in overweight and obese youth at risk of type 2 diabetes. *Am J Clin Nutr.* 2014;99(4): 804-812.
16. Lombardi R, Onali S, Thorburn D, et al. Pharmacological interventions for non-alcohol related fatty liver disease (NAFLD): an attempted network meta-analysis. *Cochrane Database Syst Rev.* 2017;(3):CD011640.
17. Mailliard ME, Sorrell NF. Alcoholic liver disease. In: Kasper DL, Fauci AS, Hauser SL, et al, eds. *Harrison's Principles of Internal Medicine*, 19th ed. New York, NY: McGraw-Hill; 2014.
18. Thursz MR, Richardson P, Allison M, et al. Prednisolone or pentoxifylline for alcoholic hepatitis. *N Engl J Med.* 2015;372(17): 1619-1628.
19. Gillett RC Jr, Norrell A. Considerations for safe use of statins: liver enzyme abnormalities and muscle toxicity. *Am Fam Physician.* 2011;83(6):711-716.
20. Dienstag JL. Chronic hepatitis. In: Kasper DL, Fauci AS, Hauser SL, et al, eds. *Harrison's Principles of Internal Medicine*, 19th ed. New York, NY: McGraw-Hill; 2014.
21. AASLD Guidelines for Treatment of Chronic Hepatitis B. https://www.aasld.org/sites/default/files/guideline_documents/hep28156.pdf. Accessed May 2018.
22. National Guideline Clearinghouse (NGC). Guideline Summary: *Hepatitis B (Chronic). Diagnosis and Management of Chronic Hepatitis B in children, Young People and Adults.* In: National Guideline Clearinghouse (NGC) [website]. Rockville, MD: Agency for Healthcare Research and Quality (AHRQ); June 2013. Accessed April 2017. https://www.guideline.gov.

23. Huang Y, Wu H, Wu S, et al. A meta-analysis of nucleos(t)ide analogues in patients with decompensated cirrhosis due to hepatitis B. *Dig Dis Sci*. 2013;58(3):815-823.

24. Centers for Disease Control and Prevention. *Viral Hepatitis. Perinatal Transmission*. https://www.cdc.gov/hepatitis/hbv/perinatalxmtn.htm. Accessed April 2017.

25. Zhu GQ, Zou ZL, Zheng JN, et al. Systematic review and network meta-analysis of randomized controlled trials: comparative effectiveness and safety of direct-acting antiviral agents for treatment-naive hepatitis C genotype 1. *Medicine (Baltimore)*. 2016;95(9): e3004.

26. National Guideline Clearinghouse (NGC). *Guideline Summary: Management of Hepatitis C. A National Clinical Guideline*. In: National Guideline Clearinghouse (NGC) [website]. Rockville, MD: Agency for Healthcare Research and Quality (AHRQ); July 2013. Accessed April 2017. https://www.guideline.gov.

27. Salmon D, Mondelli MU, Maticic M, Arends JE; ESCMID Study Group for Viral Hepatitis. The benefits of hepatitis C virus cure: Every rose has thorns. *J Viral Hepat*. 2018;25(4):320-328.

28. Bacon BR. Genetic, metabolic, and infiltrative diseases affecting the liver. In: Kasper DL, Fauci AS, Hauser SL, et al, eds. *Harrison's Principles of Internal Medicine*, 19th ed. New York, NY: McGraw-Hill; 2014.

29. Manns MP, Woynarowski M, Kreisel W, Lurie Y. Budesonide induces remission more effectively than prednisone in a controlled trial of patients with autoimmune hepatitis. *Gastroenterology*. 2010;139(4):1198-1206.

30. Bacon BR. Cirrhosis and its complications. In: Kasper DL, Fauci AS, Hauser SL, et al, eds. *Harrison's Principles of Internal Medicine*, 19th ed. New York, NY: McGraw-Hill; 2014.

31. Fukui H, Saito H, Ueno Y, et al. Evidence-based clinical practice guidelines for liver cirrhosis 2015. *J Gastroenterol*. 2016;51(7):629-650.

32. U.S. Preventive Services Task Force. Available at https://www.uspreventiveservicestaskforce.org/BrowseRec/Search?s=hepatitis+B. Accessed April 2017.

33. Senadhi V. A paradigm shift in the outpatient approach to liver function tests. *South Med J*. 2011;104(7):521-525.

34. O'Shea RS, Dasarathy S, McCullough AJ; Practice Guideline Committee of the American Association for the Study of Liver. Alcoholic liver disease. *Hepatology*. 2010;51(1):307-328.

35. Morgan RL, Baack B, Smith BD, et al. Eradication of hepatitis C virus infection and the development of hepatocellular carcinoma: a meta-analysis of observational studies. *Ann Intern Med*. 2013;158(5 Pt 1):329-337.

36. Petta S, Maida M, Macaluso FS, et al. Hepatitis C virus infection is associated with increased cardiovascular mortality: a meta-analysis of observational studies. *Gastroenterology*. 2016;150(1):145-155.

37. Parés A. Primary sclerosing cholangitis: diagnosis, prognosis and treatment. *Gastroenterol Hepatol*. 2011;34(1):41-52.

64 GALLSTONES

Mindy A. Smith, MD, MS

PATIENT STORY

A 44-year-old woman reports frequent episodes of severe pain in the mid and upper right side of her abdomen that usually occurs shortly after her evening meal and sometimes at night. She is obese, but otherwise healthy. The pain lasts for several hours and is steady and often causes vomiting. On physical examination, she complains of slight tenderness in the right upper quadrant (RUQ). An ultrasound confirms the presence of gallstones (**Figure 64-1**).

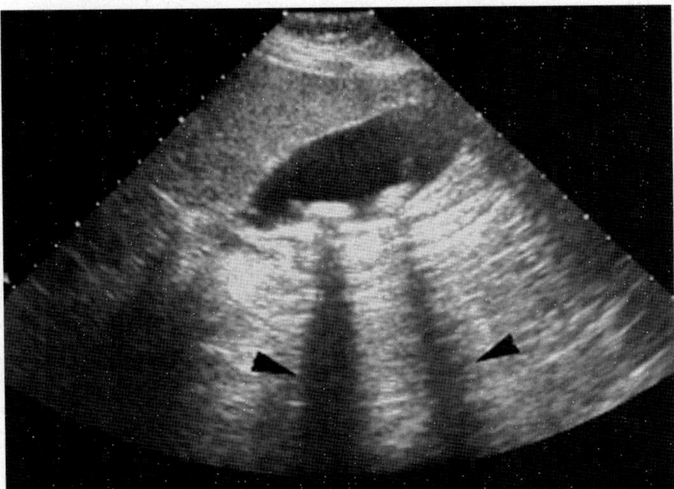

FIGURE 64-1 Ultrasound showing two echogenic gallstones in the gallbladder. Note the absence of echoes posterior to the gallstone, called "shadowing" (*arrowheads*). (*Reproduced with permission from Brunicardi F, Andersen D, Billiar T, et al: Schwartz's Principles of Surgery, 9th ed. New York, NY: McGraw-Hill Education; 2010.*)

INTRODUCTION

Gallstones are concretions (inorganic masses), usually composed of cholesterol, that form in the gallbladder or bile duct. They are formed by concretion (joining together of adjacent parts and hardening) or accretion (growth by addition or adherence of parts normally separated) of normal and/or abnormal bile constituents.

EPIDEMIOLOGY

- Based on autopsy data, 20% of women and 8% of men have gallstones. Similar figures for gallstone prevalence of 16.6% in women 7.9% in men were reported in the third National Health and Nutrition Examination Survey.[1] Prevalence is highest among Mexican Americans (26.7% of women and 8.9% of men) and lowest among African Americans (13.9% of women and 5.3% of men).
- In a Swedish incidence study of 621 randomly selected individuals ages 35 to 85 years, 42 (8.3%) of the 503 subjects available at 5 years developed gallstones; this yielded an incidence for newly developed gallstones of 1.39 per 100 person years.[2]
- Among pregnant women, 5% to 12% have gallstones and 20% to 30% have gallbladder sludge (thick mucous material containing cholesterol crystals and mucin thread or mucous gels). Gallbladder sludge is a possible precursor form of gallstone disease.[1]
- Gallstones form in about 10%–20% of persons with rapid weight reduction through very-low-calorie dieting.[1] In a follow-up study of patients undergoing bariatric surgery, 32.5% of 117 patients undergoing gastric bypass and 25.5% of 51 patients undergoing sleeve gastrectomy developed gallstones.[3]
- Patients with asymptomatic gallstones have a 2% to 4% risk per year of developing symptoms during the first 5 years following diagnosis, and a 1% to 2% risk per year of developing symptoms thereafter.[1] The incidence of gallstone complications is 0.1% to 0.3% and is preceded by warning signs.[1]
- Gallstone disease is responsible for approximately 10,000 deaths per year in the United States. Most (7000) of these deaths are attributable to acute gallstone complications (e.g., cholecystitis, pancreatitis, cholangitis).[4]

- Although gallbladder cancers most often occur in the setting of stones (91% of 34 patients with gallbladder cancer in one study),[5] gallbladder cancer is rare. An incidence rate of 0.28% for incidental gallbladder carcinoma was reported in a Swiss database study of a population of more than 30,000 patients undergoing laparoscopic cholecystectomy.[6]
- Gallbladder polyps are often detected incidentally; prevalence ranges from 4.3% to 6.9%.[7] Malignant transformation appears to be rare and is associated with polyp characteristics (>1.5 cm, solitary, sessile, or symptomatic) and patient characteristics (age over 50 years, diabetes).[7]

ETIOLOGY AND PATHOPHYSIOLOGY

- There are two types of gallstones: cholesterol stones (90% in Western industrialized countries) and pigment stones (primarily calcium bilirubinate).
- The solute components of bile include bile acids, lecithin and other phospholipids, and unesterified cholesterol.[1] Cholesterol gallstones form when there is excess cholesterol or an abnormal ratio of cholesterol to bile acids and lecithin.
- Excess biliary cholesterol can occur from an increase in secretion of cholesterol caused by obesity, high-cholesterol diet, clofibrate therapy, or a genetic predisposition to increased hydroxymethylglutaryl-coenzyme A reductase.
- The excess cholesterol becomes supersaturated and can precipitate out of solution in a process called *nucleation*, forming solid cholesterol monohydrate crystals that can become trapped in gallbladder mucus, producing sludge, and/or grow and aggregate to form cholesterol gallstones. In most individuals with supersaturated bile, the time that bile remains in the gallbladder is less than the time required for crystals to nucleate.[1]
- Gallbladder hypomotility is a predisposing and possibly necessary factor in stone formation because of the failure to completely empty supersaturated or crystal-containing bile.[1] Situations associated with hypomotility include pregnancy, prolonged parenteral nutrition, surgery, burns, and use of oral contraceptives or estrogen therapy.
- The presence of gallbladder sludge (a thick, mucous material composed of lecithin-cholesterol liquid crystals, cholesterol monohydrate crystals, calcium bilirubinate, and mucin gels) implies a disruption of the normal balance between gallbladder mucin secretion and elimination and that nucleation of biliary solutes has occurred. Although sludge can disappear completely or reappear, in one study, 14% of 96 patients with sludge developed gallstones.[1]
- Pigmented stones occur when increasing amounts of unconjugated bilirubin in bile precipitate to form stones. Bilirubin, a yellow pigment derived from the breakdown of heme, is actively secreted into bile by liver cells. In situations of high heme turnover, such as chronic hemolytic states (e.g., sickle cell anemia), calcium bilirubinate can crystallize from solution and form stones.
- Chronic gallstones may cause progressive fibrosis of the gallbladder wall and loss of function.
- Gallbladder polyps appear to be associated with fat metabolism.

RISK FACTORS

- Genetic mutations can result in reduction of bile acids and lecithin that predispose some patients to stone formation. In one study, a single-nucleotide polymorphism of the gene encoding the hepatic cholesterol transporter ABCG5/G8 was found in 21% of patients with gallstones compared to only 9% of the general population.[1] A high prevalence of gallstones is found in first-degree relatives of patients with gallstones and among Native Americans, Chilean Indians, and Chilean Hispanics.[1]
- In a case-control study, the prevalence of gallstones was 28.6% in first-degree relatives of subjects with gallstones versus 12.4% in first-degree relatives of subjects without gallstones (relative risk [RR] 1.80, 95% confidence interval [CI] 1.29 to 2.63).[4]
- Other risk factors for gallstones include rapid weight loss (10% to 20% of these patients form stones),[1] increasing age, liver or ileal disease, and cystic fibrosis.

DIAGNOSIS

CLINICAL FEATURES

- Symptoms of gallstones are caused from inflammation or obstruction as stones migrate into the cystic or common bile duct (CBD).
  - Biliary colic is a steady, severe pain or ache, usually of sudden onset, located in the epigastrium or RUQ. Pain episodes last between 30 minutes and 5 hours and may radiate to the interscapular area, right scapula, or right shoulder.
  - Gallstone-related pain may be precipitated by a fatty meal, a regular meal, or a large meal followed by a prolonged fast.
  - Pain is recurrent and often nocturnal.
- RUQ tenderness may be elicited on physical examination.
- Nausea and vomiting are common.
- Accompanying fever and chills suggests a complication of gallstones. Complications are more common in patients with a calcified gallbladder or in those who have had a previous episode of acute cholecystitis.[1]

LABORATORY STUDIES

- No laboratory testing is usually indicated as the results are usually normal. However, an elevated γ-glutamyl transpeptidase (GGT), elevated bilirubin, and/or alkaline phosphatase suggests a CBD stone. In a study of patients with acute calculous gallbladder disease, investigators found a 1-in-3 chance of CBD stones when the γ-glutamyl transpeptidase level was above 90 U/L and a 1-in-30 chance when the level was less than 90 U/L.[8]

IMAGING

- Ultrasound (US) is the diagnostic test of choice and is 95% accurate for stones as small as 1.5 mm in diameter (see **Figure 64-1**).[1] Shadowing, a discrete acoustic shadow caused by the absorption and reflection of sound by the stone that changes with patient positioning, is an important diagnostic feature that is shown in **Figures 64-1** and **64-2**.

- In one study, high-resolution US was more accurate than endoscopic US or CT in differentiating benign disease from malignancy in cases with gallbladder polypoid lesions.[9]
- In patients with obesity undergoing laparoscopic Roux-en-Y gastric bypass, however, laparoscopic US may be useful, particularly for identifying gallbladder polyps.[10]
- Gallstones may be seen on plain film, but only calcified stones are seen (**Figures 64-3** and **64-4**). This includes only 10% to 15% of cholesterol stones and about half of pigmented stones.[1] Stones may be single or multiple, and the gallbladder wall may be calcified (referred to as a porcelain gallbladder, **Figure 64-5**), indicating severe chronic cholecystitis or adenocarcinoma.
- CT is less sensitive and more expensive than ultrasound for the detection of gallstones (**Figures 64-6** and **64-7**). However, CT can detect both radiopaque stones and radiolucent stones.
- Endoscopic retrograde cholangiopancreatography (ERCP) can be used for imaging bile ducts. Stones in bile appear as filling defects in the opacified ducts. ERCP is usually performed in conjunction with endoscopic retrograde sphincterotomy and gallstone extraction.
- Intraductal US was useful in 95 patients highly suspected of choledocholithiasis but with negative ERCP; bile duct stones were identified in 31 patients.[11]
- The National Institute for Health and Care Excellence recommends magnetic resonance (MR) CP if US fails to detect bile duct stones when the bile duct is dilated and/or liver enzymes are elevated or endoscopic US if MRCP fails to make a diagnosis.[12]

DIFFERENTIAL DIAGNOSIS

Severe epigastric and RUQ pain can be seen in the following conditions:

- Acute cholecystitis—Pain may radiate to the back, and fever is usually present. Physical examination can reveal RUQ rigidity and guarding with a positive Murphy sign (RUQ pain worsening with deep inspiration while the examiner maintains steady pressure below the right costal margin). White blood count, serum amylase, aspartate transaminase, and alanine transaminase may all be elevated.
- Pancreatitis—Pain is in the midepigastrium and left upper quadrant, but may radiate to the RUQ. Abdominal distention and diminished bowel sounds may be present. Elevations in lipase and amylase are found and pancreatic pseudocysts or abscess may be present on ultrasound.
- Peptic ulcer disease—Pain may be described as burning and is usually epigastric and often relieved by antacids. Onset is 1 to 3 hours after meals or following nonsteroidal anti-inflammatory drug usage. Stool hemoccult testing may be positive. An ulcer may be visualized on upper GI barium swallow or endoscopy (Chapter 61, Peptic Ulcer Disease).
- Hepatitis—Other symptoms and signs include malaise, anorexia, pruritus, tender liver, and low-grade fever. Jaundice may be present and urine may be dark (i.e., bilirubinuria). Aspartate transaminase and alanine transaminase are elevated (Chapter 63, Liver Disease).

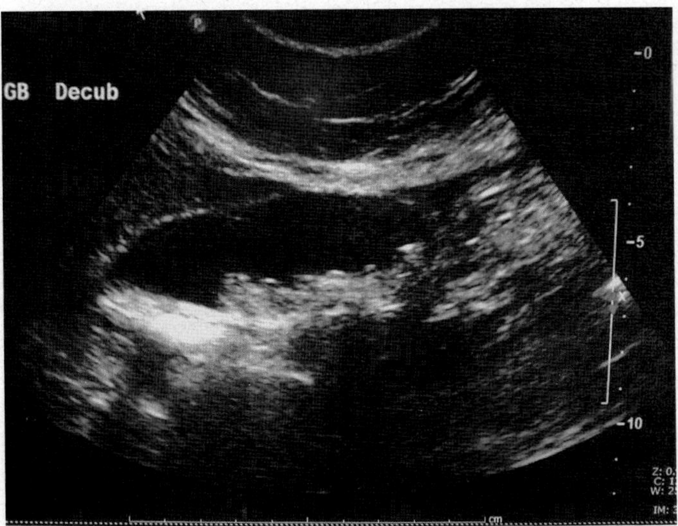

FIGURE 64-2 Gallstones visible in the gallbladder of a 43-year-old woman with right upper quadrant pain and a positive Murphy sign. *(Reproduced with permission from Jeff Russell, MD.)*

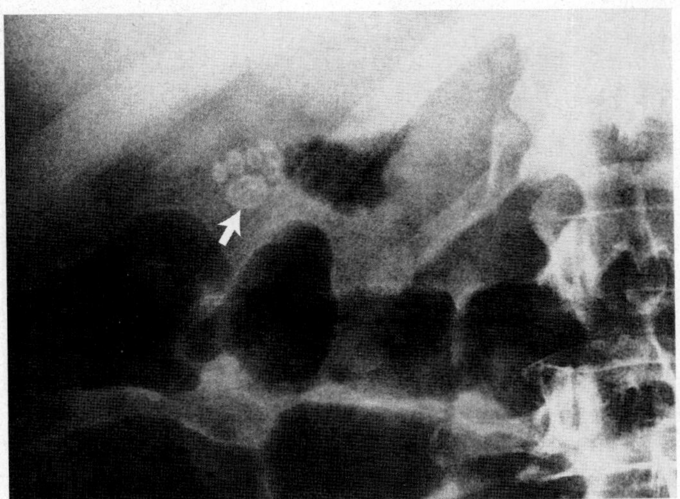

FIGURE 64-3 Plain film showing multiple gallstones (*white arrow*). *(Reproduced with permission from Schwartz DT, Reisdorff EJ. Emergency Radiology. New York, NY: McGraw-Hill Education; 2000.)*

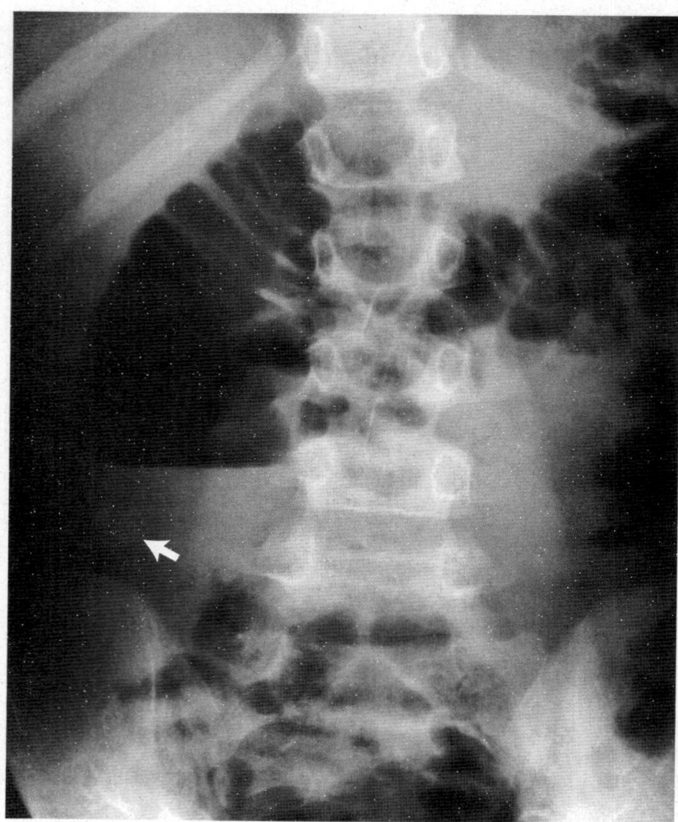

FIGURE 64-4 Gallstone ileus in an elderly patient with diabetes; note dilated loops of small bowel and an ectopic gallstone (*arrow*). (*Reproduced with permission from Schwartz DT, Reisdorff EJ. Emergency Radiology. New York, NY: McGraw-Hill Education; 2000.*)

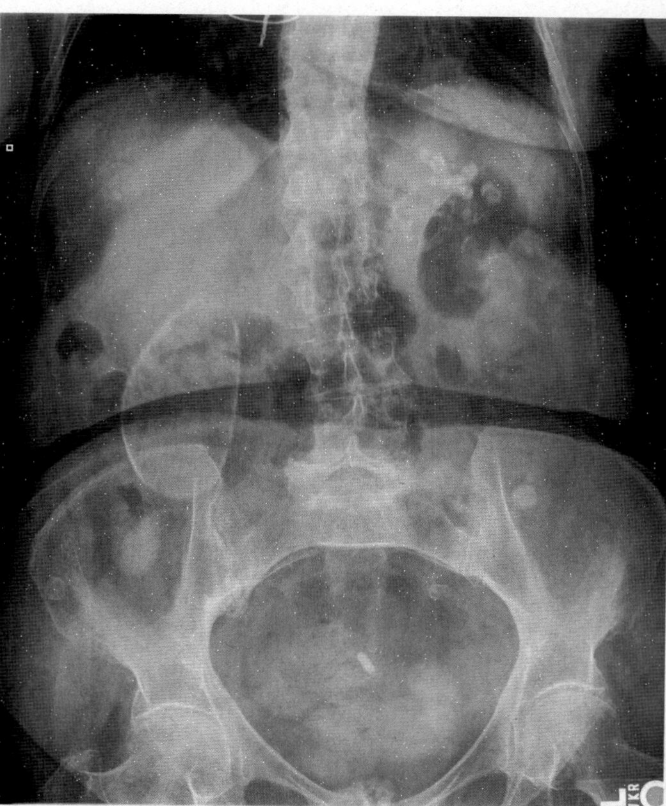

FIGURE 64-5 Porcelain gallbladder is a term used to describe calcification of the gallbladder wall. In this case it is due to severe chronic cholecystitis and not adenocarcinoma. (*Reproduced with permission from Vimalachandran P, Paknikar J. Recurrent right upper quadrant abdominal pain. J Fam Pract. 2016;65(10):723-724. Frontline Medical Communications. Inc.*)

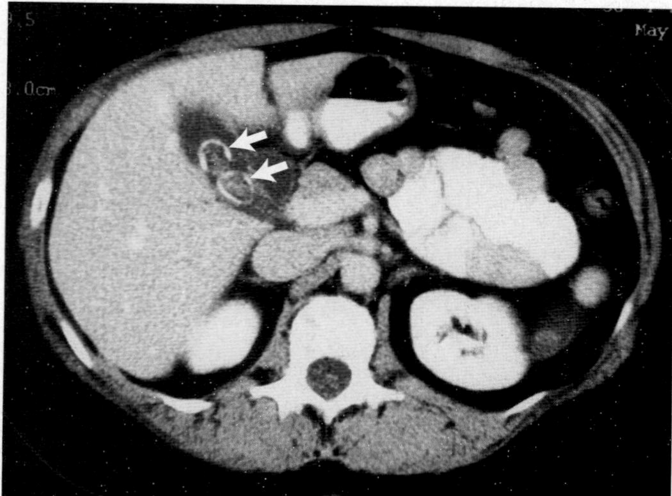

FIGURE 64-6 CT scan showing two large gallstones that have a rim of calcification (*large arrows*). (*Reproduced with permission from Schwartz DT, Reisdorff EJ. Emergency Radiology. New York, NY: McGraw-Hill Education; 2000.*)

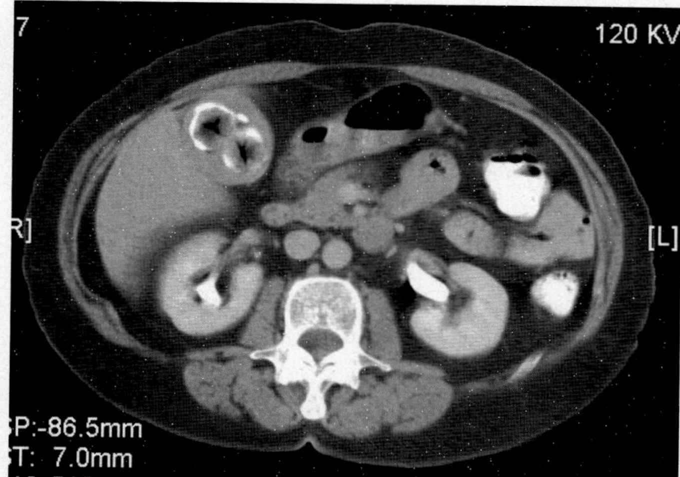

FIGURE 64-7 Radiographic Mercedes-Benz sign seen on a CT cut through the gallbladder (the gallstones produce a black pattern that resembles a Mercedes-Benz logo in the center). (*Reproduced with permission from Mike Freckleton, MD.*)

MANAGEMENT

FIRST LINE

- Silent gallstones may be managed expectantly; prophylactic cholecystectomy is unwarranted based on the few who develop symptoms over time and the very low rate of complications (annually 0.1% to 0.3%).[1] There are no randomized controlled trials comparing cholecystectomy to watchful waiting for silent gallstones.[13] SOR C
- Cholecystectomy should be offered to patients with symptomatic gallstones, a prior complication of gallstones, or the presence of an underlying condition (e.g., calcified gallbladder) that predisposes the patient to increased risk of complications.[1,12]
- Laparoscopic cholecystectomy is the surgical treatment of choice because of the low rate of complications (4%) and mortality (<0.1%), shortened hospital stay, and reduced cost.[1] Conversion to an open laparotomy is infrequent (5%).[1]
- A Cochrane review found no differences in mortality or complications among open, small-incision, and laparoscopic cholecystectomy, but quicker recovery favors minimally invasive procedures; small-incision cholecystectomies appear to have shorter operative time and lower cost.[14] Authors of a systematic review reported a high procedure failure rate with single-incision laparoscopic cholecystectomy over the conventional procedure.[15]
- Early laparoscopic cholecystectomy (<7 days from symptom onset) during acute cholecystitis has comparable outcomes to delayed cholecystectomy and may shorten hospital stay.[16]
- For patients with gallbladder and CBD stones, intraoperative endoscopic sphincterotomy during laparoscopic cholecystectomy appears as safe and effective as preoperative endoscopic sphincterotomy followed by laparoscopic cholecystectomy and is associated with significantly shorter hospital stay.[17] Endoscopic papillary balloon dilation in addition to endoscopic sphincterotomy may reduce the rate of recurrent stones.[18]

SECOND LINE

- Medical therapy with ursodeoxycholic acid may be considered for patients with functioning gallbladders and small stones (<10 mm).[1] Approximately 50% of these patients will have complete dissolution of stones in 6 to 24 months, but recurrences are common (see "Prognosis" below).[1]

PREVENTION

- Medical therapy can be used to prevent gallstone formation in patients with expected rapid weight loss caused by very-low-calorie diets or bariatric surgery. In one study, ursodeoxycholic acid at a dose of 500 mg daily for 6 months reduced the incidence of gallstones over placebo (3% vs. 22%, respectively, at 12 months) and cholecystectomy (4.7% vs. 12%, respectively).[19]

PROGNOSIS

- Abdominal pain resembling biliary colic may persist in up to 30% of patients despite cholecystectomy (called postcholecystectomy syndrome).[20] In one follow-up survey of 573/1300 patients following cholecystectomy (44% response rate), preoperative pain resolved in 90% but postoperative pain was reported in 25%; in 10% of these patients the postoperative pain was the same quality and location as the preoperative pain, and in 17% a new abdominal pain developed, most often in the periumbilical area.[21] In a study of 100 consecutive patients, 13% had persistent pain following laparoscopic cholecystectomy.[22]
- In the follow-up survey noted above, nonpain symptoms all decreased in prevalence following cholecystectomy, including indigestion (14%), fatty food intolerance (19%), and heartburn (13%). Diarrhea, however, was present in similar percentages pre- and postoperatively (19% and 21%, respectively).[21]
- Following medical therapy, recurrences are common (30% to 50% at 3- to 5-year follow-up).[1]

FOLLOW-UP

- Approximately 5% to 10% of patients develop chronic diarrhea, attributed to increased bile salts reaching the colon, following cholecystectomy. Diarrhea is usually mild and can be managed with nonprescription antidiarrheal agents (e.g., loperamide).
- Postcholecystectomy pain may be related to recurrent stones, choledocholithiasis, biliary dyskinesia, inflammatory scarring or strictures involving the sphincter of Oddi or the CBD, and dilation of cystic duct remnants; ultrasound or MRCP may be useful in identification of the cause, and some may be amenable to surgical management.[23,24]

PATIENT EDUCATION

- Patients with asymptomatic gallstones may be managed expectantly—The rates of developing symptoms and complications should be reviewed. They should be encouraged to report symptoms of biliary colic and acute cholecystitis or pancreatitis (described above).
- Laparoscopic cholecystectomy appears to be very successful for symptom resolution, although chronic diarrhea may occur and abdominal pain may persist or new pain develop in approximately one-quarter of patients.[20]

PATIENT RESOURCES

- National Digestive Diseases Information Clearinghouse Gallstones (NDDIC). *Gallstones*—**https://www.niddk.nih.gov/health-information/digestive-diseases/gallstones.**
- American Academy of Family Physicians (AAFP)—**https://familydoctor.org/condition/gallstones/.**

PROVIDER RESOURCES

- Abraham S, Rivero HG, Erlikh I, et al. Surgical and nonsurgical management of gallstones—**http://www.aafp.org/afp/2014/0515/p795.html.**
- Heuman DM. Cholelithiasis—**http://emedicine.medscape.com/article/175667-overview.**
- National Institute of Diabetes and Digestive and Kidney Diseases. Gallstone—https://www.niddk.nih.gov/health-information/digestive-diseases/gallstones.

REFERENCES

1. Greenberger NJ, Paumgartner G. Diseases of the gallbladder and bile ducts. In: Kasper DL, Fauci AS, Hauser SL, et al, eds. *Harrison's Principles of Internal Medicine*, 19th ed. New York, NY: McGraw-Hill; 2014.
2. Halldestam I, Kullman E, Borch K. Incidence of and potential risk factors for gallstone disease in a general population sample. *Br J Surg.* 2009;96(11):1315-1322.
3. Coupaye M, Calabrese D, Sami O, et al. Evaluation of incidence of cholelithiasis after bariatric surgery in subjects treated or not treated with ursodeoxycholic acid. *Surg Obes Relat Dis.* 2016;13(4):681-685.
4. Attili AF, De Santis A, Attili F, et al. Prevalence of gallstone disease in first-degree relatives of patients with cholelithiasis. *World J Gastroenterol.* 2005;11(41):6508-6511.
5. Ishak G, Ribeiro FS, Costa DS, et al. Gallbladder cancer: 10 years of experience at an Amazon reference hospital. *Rev Col Bras Cir.* 2011;38(2):100-104.
6. Glauser PM, Strub D, Käser SA, et al. Incidence, management, and outcome of incidental gallbladder carcinoma: analysis of the database of the Swiss association of laparoscopic and thoracoscopic surgery. *Surg Endosc.* 2010;24(9):2281-2286.
7. Andrén-Sandberg A. Diagnosis and management of gallbladder polyps. *N Am J Med Sci.* 2012;4(5):203-211.
8. Peng WK, Sheikh Z, Paterson-Brown S, Nixon SJ. Role of liver function tests in predicting common bile duct stones in acute calculous cholecystitis. *Br J Surg.* 2005;92(10):1241-1247.
9. Jang JY, Kim SW, Lee SE, et al. Differential diagnostic and staging accuracies of high resolution ultrasonography, endoscopic ultrasonography, and multidetector computed tomography for gallbladder polypoid lesions and gallbladder cancer. *Ann Surg.* 2009;250(6):943-949.
10. Kothari SN, Obinwanne KM, Baker MT, et al. A prospective, blinded comparison of laparoscopic ultrasound with transabdominal ultrasound for the detection of gallbladder pathology in morbidly obese patients. *J Am Coll Surg.* 2013;216(6):1057-1062.
11. Kim DC, Moon JH, Choi HJ, et al. Usefulness of intraductal ultrasonography in icteric patients with highly suspected choledocholithiasis showing normal endoscopic retrograde cholangiopancreatography. *Dig Dis Sci.* 2014;59(8):1902-1908.
12. National Institute for Health and Care Excellence. *Gallstone Disease Overview.* http://pathways.nice.org.uk/pathways/gallstone-disease. Accessed March 2017.
13. Gurusamy KS, Samraj K. Cholecystectomy for patients with silent gallstones. *Cochrane Database Syst Rev.* 2007;(1):CD006430.
14. Keus F, Gooszen HG, van Laarhoven CJHM. Open, small-incision, or laparoscopic cholecystectomy for patients with symptomatic cholecystolithiasis. An overview of Cochrane Hepato-Biliary Group reviews. *Cochrane Database Syst Rev.* 2010;(1):CD008318.
15. Trastulli S, Cirocchi R, Desiderio J, et al. Systematic review and meta-analysis of randomized clinical trials comparing single-incision versus conventional laparoscopic cholecystectomy. *Br J Surg.* 2013;100(2):191-208.
16. Gurusamy KS, Davidson C. Gluud C, et al. Early versus delayed laparoscopic cholecystectomy for acute cholecystitis. *Cochrane Database Syst Rev.* 2013;(6):CD005440.
17. Gurusamy K, Sahay SJ, Burroughs AK, Davidson BR. Systematic review and meta-analysis of intraoperative versus preoperative endoscopic sphincterotomy in patients with gallbladder and suspected common bile duct stones. *Br J Surg.* 2011;98(7):908-916.
18. Mu H, Gao J, Kong Q, et al. Prognostic factors and postoperative recurrence of calculus following small-incision sphincterotomy with papillary balloon dilation for the treatment of intractable choledocholithiasis: a 72-month follow-up study. *Dig Dis Sci.* 2015;60(7):2144-2149.
19. Miller K, Hell E, Lang B, Lengauer E. Gallstone formation prophylaxis after gastric restrictive procedures for weight loss: a randomized double-blind placebo-controlled trial. *Ann Surg.* 2003;238(5):697-702.
20. Gui GP, Cheruvu CV, West N, et al. Is cholecystectomy effective treatment for symptomatic gallstones? Clinical outcomes after long-term follow-up. *Ann R Coll Surg Engl.* 1998;80:25-32.
21. Lublin M, Crawford DL, Hiatt JR, Phillips EH. Symptoms before and after laparoscopic cholecystectomy for gallstones. *Am Surg.* 2004;70(10):863-866.
22. Luman W, Adams WH, Nixon SN, et al. Incidence of persistent symptoms after laparoscopic cholecystectomy: a prospective study. *Gut.* 1996;39(6):863-866.
23. Perera E, Bhatt S, Dogra VS. Cystic duct remnant syndrome. *J Clin Imaging Sci.* 2011;1:2.
24. Girometti R, Brondani G, Cereser L, et al. Post-cholecystectomy syndrome: spectrum of biliary findings at magnetic resonance cholangiopancreatography. *Br J Radiol.* 2010;83(988):351-361.

65 COLON POLYPS

Mindy A. Smith, MD, MS
Cathy Abbott, MD

PATIENT STORY

A 62-year-old woman presents to her physician for routine annual examination. She has no known family history of colon disease and is asymptomatic. Stool cards and flexible sigmoidoscopy were recommended and on flexible sigmoidoscopy a 2.4-cm polyp was noted at 35 cm. A colonoscopy was performed and additional polyps were identified in the descending colon and cecum (**Figure 65-1**).

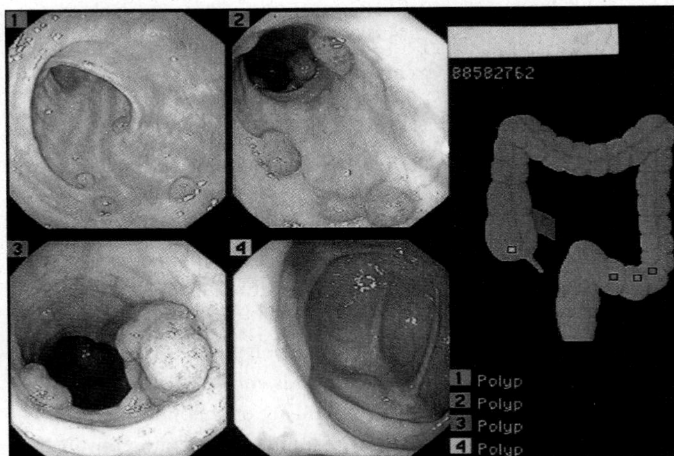

FIGURE 65-1 Colon polyps seen on colonoscopy. (*Reproduced with permission from Michael Harper, MD.*)

INTRODUCTION

Colon polyps are growths that arise from the epithelial cells lining the colon.

EPIDEMIOLOGY

- More than 30% of middle-aged and elderly patients are found to have adenomatous polyps on screening and based on autopsy surveys; fewer than 1% will become malignant.[1] The lifetime risk of colon cancer is 4.4%.[2]
- In the first round of screening in the Bowel Cancer Screening Programme in England, of over 1 million subjects aged 60–69 years, 2.5% of men and 1.5% of women had an abnormal test. About 40% underwent subsequent colonoscopy revealing higher risk adenomas (n = 6543) and cancer (n = 1772) in 43% and 11.6% of men and 29% and 7.8% of women investigated.[3]
- Patients with an adenomatous polyp have a 30% to 50% risk for developing another adenoma and are at higher risk for colon cancer.[1] This risk is greatest in the first 4 years after diagnosis of the first polyp, and greater if a villous adenoma or more than 3 polyps were found.
- Familial adenomatous polyposis of the colon is a rare autosomal dominant disorder associated with a deletion in the long arm of chromosome 5. Thousands of adenomatous polyps appear in the large colon, generally by age 25 years, and colorectal cancer develops in almost all these patients by age 40 years.[1] Other hereditary polyposis syndromes include Gardner syndrome, Turcot syndrome, Peutz-Jeghers syndrome, and MYH-associated polyposis, familial juvenile polyposis.[1]

ETIOLOGY AND PATHOPHYSIOLOGY

- There are several types of colon polyps, including:
  - Hyperplastic polyps—These contain increased numbers of glandular cells with decreased cytoplasmic mucus and an absence of nuclear hyperchromatism, stratification, or atypia. They are thought to be benign, with the exception of those associated with hyperplastic polyposis syndrome (a familial disorder with multiple [>30] hyperplastic polyps proximal to the sigmoid colon

with 2 or more >10 mm).[4] The percentage of polyps reported to be in this category ranges from 12% to 90%.[4,5]
  - Adenomatous polyps—These may be tubular, villous (papillary), or tubulovillous; villous polyps are most likely to become malignant.[1] In a case series of 582 patients who had a polyp removed, 81% were adenomatous, including 65.0% that were tubular, 25.8% tubulovillous, 7.2% villous adenomas, and 0.5% mixed adenomatous hyperplastic polyps; 12 (1.4%) were invasive carcinomas.[5]
    - Adenomatous polyps may be pedunculated or sessile; cancers more frequently develop in sessile polyps.[1]
    - Adenomatous polyps that are >1 cm, contain a substantial (>25%) villous component, or have high-grade dysplasia are at higher risk of malignancy.[4]
  - Villous adenomas can cause hypersecretory syndromes characterized by hypokalemia and profuse mucous discharge; these more frequently harbor carcinoma in situ or invasive carcinoma than other adenomas.[4]
  - Nonneoplastic hamartoma (juvenile polyp)—These are benign cystic polyps with mucus-filled glands, most commonly found in male children, ages 2 to 5 years, and are often found as singular lesions, but additional polyps are found on panendoscopy in 40% to 50% of children. Juvenile polyps in adolescence may be associated with hereditary syndromes that carry malignant potential.[6]
  - Inflammatory polyps are found in patients with inflammatory bowel disease (see Chapter 67, Inflammatory Bowel Disease).
- A series of genetic/molecular changes have been found that are thought to represent a multistep process from normal colon mucosa to malignant tumor.[1] These include:
  - Point mutations in the K-*ras* protooncogene leading to gene activation, hypomethylation of DNA leading to gene activation, deletion of DNA at the site of a tumor-suppressor gene, allelic loss at the site of a tumor-suppressor gene on chromosome 18q and at chromosome 17p, associated with mutations in the *p53* tumor-suppressor gene.[1]
  - This results in an altered proliferative pattern and polyp formation.
  - Mutational activation of an oncogene, coupled with loss of tumor-suppressor genes, leads to malignant transformation.
  - Serrated polyps, which have in the past been characterized as hyperplastic polyps, are now known to have epigenetic alterations that may develop into colon cancers by another pathway—the CpG-island-methylation-phenotype pathway.[7]
  - Patients with familial polyposis inherit a germline alteration that leads into the above pathway.
- Insulin resistance, with increased concentrations of insulin-like growth factor type I, may also stimulate proliferation of the intestinal mucosa.[1]

RISK FACTORS

- Older age—99% of cases occur in people older than age 40 years and 85% in those older than age 60 years.[8]
- Family history—Present in 10% to 20% of cases.[8]
- Diet appears to be associated with colon polyps and colon cancer. Animal fats in red meat may alter anaerobes in the gut microflora, increasing conversion of normal bile acids to carcinogens. Also, increased cholesterol is associated with an enhanced risk of development of adenomas.[1]
- Inflammatory bowel disease, primarily ulcerative colitis (8%–30% after 25 years).[1]
- There may be an association between *Helicobacter* exposure and colonic polyps.[9]
- Excess body weight increases the risk for colon adenoma (relative risk [RR] 1.19; 95% confidence interval [CI] 1.13–1.26).[10]
- Moderate and heavy alcohol consumption increases risk of colorectal serrated polyp (RR 1.19 and 1.6, respectively).[11]

DIAGNOSIS

CLINICAL FEATURES

- Usually asymptomatic.
- Patients may experience overt or occult rectal bleeding.
- Change in bowel habits—Diarrhea or constipation can occur, often with decreased stool caliber.
- Secretory villous adenomas can occasionally manifest as a syndrome of severe diarrhea with massive fluid and electrolyte loss.[4]

TYPICAL DISTRIBUTION

- Colon cancers are more commonly seen in the left (about 2/3 to 3/4) vs. right colon.[3]
- Juvenile polyps are usually found in the rectosigmoid region.

LABORATORY TESTING

- Occult blood in the stool is found in less than 5% of patients with polyps.[1] Of the 2% to 4% of asymptomatic patients who have heme-positive stool on screening, 20% to 30% will have polyps.[1]
- For patients with a family history of familial adenomatous polyposis, DNA testing may be performed from peripheral blood mononuclear cells to detect the adenomatous polyposis coli *(APC)* gene mutation; this can lead to a definitive diagnosis before the development of polyps.[1] SOR Ⓒ A positive test finding only indicates susceptibility, not the actual presence of a polyp.[4]

IMAGING AND ENDOSCOPIC FEATURES

- Polyps may be identified on barium enema (**Figures 65-2** and **65-3**), flexible sigmoidoscopy, or colonoscopy (including virtual computer tomography colonoscopy) (**Figures 65-1** and **65-4**).
- A polyp is defined as grossly visible protrusion from the mucosal surface, although adenomas can also be flat or even depressed.[12]
- Colonoscopy must be subsequently performed to identify additional lesions and remove all lesions.
- Narrow-band imaging colonoscopy can be useful for distinguishing between benign and malignant polyps.[13]
- Synchronous lesions occur in one third of cases (**Figure 65-1**).

BIOPSY

- Polyps upon removal are sent for histology to determine type and whether dysplasia or carcinoma in situ is present (**Figure 65-5**).

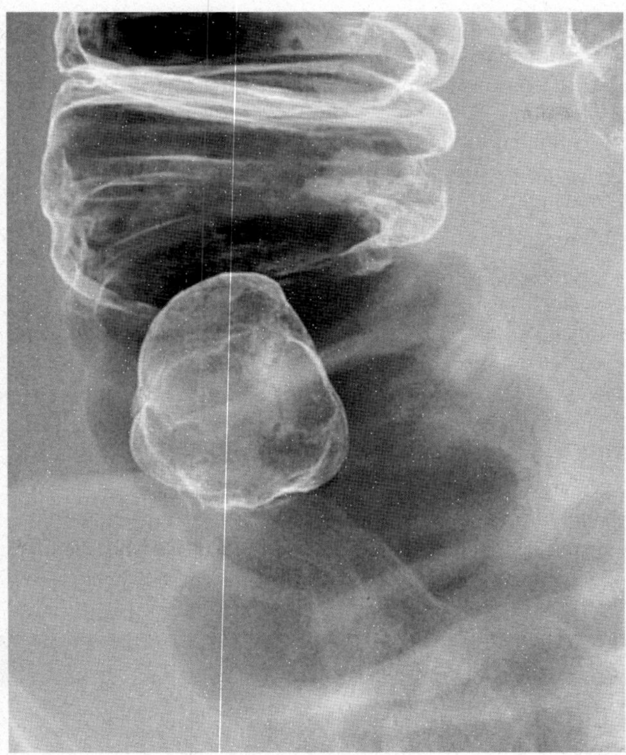

FIGURE 65-2 A 69-year-old woman with a family history of colon cancer presented for screening. Her hemoccult test was positive. Her double-contrast barium enema (air contrast) demonstrated a large colonic polyp, which was found on surgery to be highly dysplastic. (*Reproduced with permission from E.J. Mayeaux, Jr., MD.*)

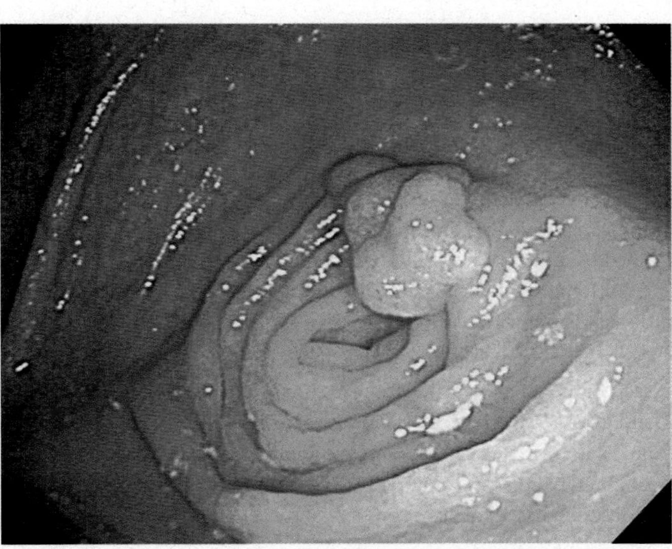

FIGURE 65-4 Polyp in the cecum seen on colonoscopy. (*Reproduced with permission from Marvin Derezin, MD.*)

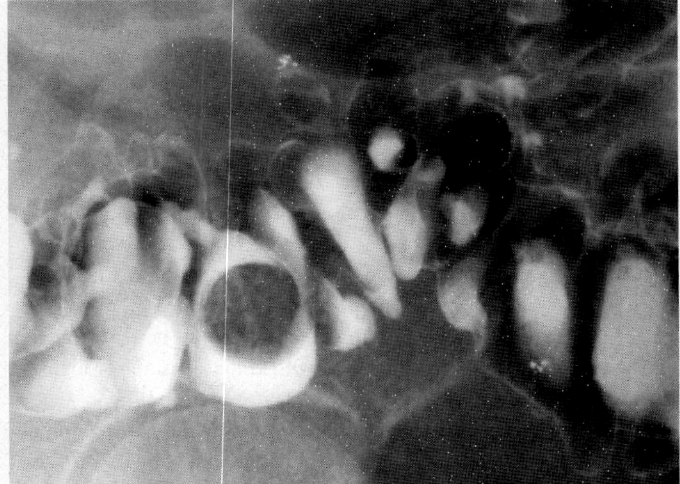

FIGURE 65-3 While getting a barium enema for other reasons, this patient was found to have a large colonic polyp. Biopsy of the polyp demonstrated early-stage colon cancer, which was treated by surgical resection. (*Reproduced with permission from E.J. Mayeaux, Jr., MD.*)

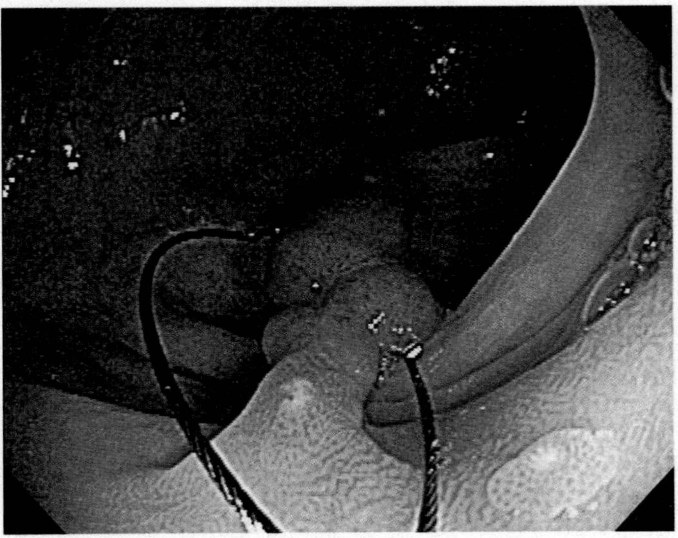

FIGURE 65-5 Polypectomy being performed through the colonoscope. (*Reproduced with permission from Marvin Derezin, MD.*)

DIFFERENTIAL DIAGNOSIS

Other causes of rectal bleeding include:

- Infectious agents—*Salmonella, Shigella*, certain *Campylobacter* species, enteroinvasive *Escherichia coli, Clostridium difficile*, and *Entamoeba histolytica* can cause bloody, watery diarrhea and are identified by culture. Bacterial toxins may be identified with *C. difficile*. Additional symptoms include fever and abdominal pain, and the disease is often self-limited.
- Hemorrhoids and fissures—Bleeding is usually bright red blood and seen in the toilet or with wiping after bowel movements. Hemorrhoids can sometimes be visible as a protruding mass often associated with pruritus, and fissures are identified as a cut or tear occurring in the anus (see Chapter 68, Hemorrhoids). Hemorrhoidal pain is described as a dull ache, but may be severe if thrombosed.
- Diverticula—Bleeding is usually abrupt in onset, painless, and may be massive but often stops spontaneously. These may be seen on endoscopy or on radiographic study.
- Vascular colonic ectasias—Bleeding tends to be chronic, resulting in anemia. Bleeding source may be identified during colonoscopy but a radionuclide scan or angiography may be needed.
- Colon cancer—Other symptoms include abdominal cramping, tenesmus (i.e., urgency with a feeling of incomplete evacuation), narrow-caliber stool, occasional obstruction, and, rarely, perforation. Imaging studies often can distinguish and biopsy confirms malignancy (see Chapter 66, Colon Cancer).
- Inflammatory bowel disease—This includes ulcerative colitis and Crohn disease; symptoms include diarrhea, tenesmus, passage of mucus, and cramping abdominal pain (see Chapter 67: Inflammatory Bowel Disease). Extraintestinal manifestations are more common in Crohn disease and include skin involvement (e.g., erythema nodosum), rheumatologic symptoms (e.g., peripheral arthritis, symmetric sacroiliitis), and ocular problems (e.g., uveitis, iritis). Diagnosis may be made on endoscopy.

MANAGEMENT

- Removal of a polyp may be completed during sigmoidoscopy or colonoscopy (**Figure 65-5**).
- Authors of a systematic review of large colorectal polyps found that endoscopic treatment was successful in 90.3% (95% CI 88.2% to 92.5%); perforation occurred in 1.5% (96/6595 polyps). The remainder underwent surgical removal.[14]

PREVENTION

- Primary prevention of colon cancer should be encouraged (see Chapter 66, Colon Cancer).
  - Dietary alterations may be useful:
    - Decreasing animal fats, as diets high in animal fats are thought to be a major risk factor based on epidemiologic studies. However, in the Women's Health Initiative study, a low-fat dietary intervention did not reduce the risk of colorectal cancer in postmenopausal women during 8.1 years of follow-up.[15]
    - Increasing water consumption to 8 glasses per day may be helpful.
    - Diets high in flavonols (fruits, vegetables, and tea) are associated with decreased risk of colon polyps, possibly by reducing serum interleukin (IL)-6, which is associated with inflammation and carcinogenesis.[16]
  - Calcium supplements (1200 mg per day) have been shown to reduce the development of adenomatous polyps.[17] SOR Ⓐ
  - Low-dose aspirin (81 mg per day) was found to decrease recurrent adenomas, including those containing advanced neoplasms.[18,19] SOR Ⓑ In patients with familial adenomatous polyposis, once-daily treatment with 25 mg rofecoxib significantly decreased the number and size of rectal polyps in one randomized trial.[20]
  - Smoking cessation.[21]
  - Increasing physical activity reduces the risk of advanced polyps and neoplasia, possibly by decreasing insulin resistance.[22]

PROGNOSIS

- Polyp recurrence rate after endoscopic mucosal resection was 13.1% based on a meta-analysis of 30 studies with 3404 patients.[23] Piecemeal resection was associated with a higher recurrence rate than en bloc resection; recurrence was not influenced by use of argon plasma coagulation.
- Patients with a polyp with tubulovillous features or with more than 3 polyps larger than 10 mm are at increased risk for further aggressive lesions on follow-up colonoscopy, and untreated patients with polyps larger than 10 mm are at increased risk for colon cancer both at the site of the polyp and at other sites.[24] Serrated polyps also confer higher risk of subsequent malignancy.[25]

FOLLOW-UP

- Secondary prevention of colon cancer should be maximized through screening and removal of additional or recurrent polyps or colon cancer in these patients (see Chapter 66, Colon Cancer). Although there is debate regarding the frequency of screening, the American Cancer Society, the U.S. Multi-Society Task Force on Colorectal Cancer, and the American College of Radiology updated guideline recommends repeat colonoscopy at the following intervals[26]:
  - Every 5 to 10 years for those with 1 to 2 small tubular adenomas with low-grade dysplasia after initial polypectomy.
  - Every 3 years for patients with 3 to 10 adenomas or 1 adenoma larger than 1 cm or any adenoma with villous features or high-grade dysplasia.
  - Less than every 3 years for patients with more than 10 adenomas.
  - At 2 to 6 months to verify complete removal in patients with sessile adenomas that are removed piecemeal.
- Although screening options that enable detection of both adenomatous polyps and colon cancer include flexible sigmoidoscopy, colonoscopy, double-contrast barium enema, and CT colonography

(use of dyes or other visual enhancements during colonoscopy), authors of a Cochrane review found that chromoscopic colonoscopy enhances the detection of polyps in the colon and rectum.[27] This form of colonoscopy can be used to identify flat polyps, increasing the sensitivity of colonoscopy, and may allow for detection of high-risk polyps without the need for biopsy.

PATIENT EDUCATION

- Attention to lifestyle factors can contribute to decreasing the risk of colon polyps.
- Patients should be encouraged to undergo screening for colon cancer starting at age 50 years and continuing until age 75 years.[28] SOR Ⓐ Recommended screening test options are fecal occult blood testing (guaiac-based fecal occult blood test, fecal immunochemical test [FIT], or multitargeted stool DNA test; annually or every 1 or 3 years for the DNA test), flexible sigmoidoscopy (with or without FIT every 5 years), CT colonography every 5 years, or colonoscopy every 10 years.
- Patients diagnosed with polyps should be encouraged to engage in continued surveillance for polyps and colon cancer. Those at increased risk for a subsequent advanced neoplasia (see above) should have a follow-up colonoscopy at 3 or fewer years.[26] SOR Ⓑ For other patients, follow-up is recommended at 5 to 10 years.[26] SOR Ⓒ

PATIENT RESOURCES

- **https://www.niddk.nih.gov/health-information/digestive-diseases/colon-polyps.**
- **http://www.mayoclinic.org/diseases-conditions/colon-polyps/basics/definition/con-20031957.**

PROVIDER RESOURCES

- **http://emedicine.medscape.com/article/172674-overview.**

REFERENCES

1. Mayer R. Lower gastrointestinal cancers. In: Kasper DL, Fauci AS, Hauser SL, et al, eds. *Harrison's Principles of Internal Medicine*, 19th ed. New York, NY: McGraw-Hill; 2014.
2. National Cancer Institute. *Cancer Stat Facts: Colorectal Cancer.* http://seer.cancer.gov/statfacts/html/colorect.html. Accessed March 2017.
3. Logan RF, Patnick J, Nickerson C, et al; English Bowel Cancer Screening Evaluation Committee. Outcomes of the Bowel Cancer Screening Programme (BCSP) in England after the first 1 million tests. *Gut.* 2012;61(10):1439-1446.
4. Enders GH. *Colonic Polyps.* http://emedicine.medscape.com/article/172674-overview. Accessed March 2017.
5. Khan A, Shrier I, Gordon PH. The changed histologic paradigm of colorectal polyps. *Surg Endosc.* 2002;16(3):436-440.
6. Barnard J. Gastrointestinal polyps and polyp syndromes in adolescents. *Adolesc Med Clin.* 2004;15(1):119-129.
7. Noffsinger AE. Serrated polyps and colorectal cancer: new pathway to malignancy. *Annu Rev Pathol.* 2009;4:343-364.
8. Ballinger AB, Anggiansah C. Colorectal cancer. *BMJ.* 2007;335:715-718, 1059.
9. Abbass K, Gul W, Beck G, et al. Association of *Helicobacter pylori* infection with the development of colorectal polyps and colorectal cancer. *South Med J.* 2011;104(7):473-476.
10. Ben Q, An W, Jiang Y, et al. Body mass index increases risk for colorectal adenomas based on meta-analysis. *Gastroenterology.* 2012;142(4):762-772.
11. Wang YM, Zhou QY, Zhu JZ, et al. Systematic review with meta-analysis: alcohol consumption and risk of colorectal serrated polyp. *Dig Dis Sci.* 2015;60(7):1889-1902.
12. Anderson JC. Risk factors and diagnosis of flat adenomas of the colon. *Expert Rev Gastroenterol Hepatol.* 2011;5(1):25-32.
13. McGill SK, Evangelou E, Ioannidis JP, et al. Narrow band imaging to differentiate neoplastic and non-neoplastic colorectal polyps in real time: a meta-analysis of diagnostic operating characteristics. *Gut.* 2013;62(12):1704-1713.
14. Hassan C, Repici A, Sharma P, et al. Efficacy and safety of endoscopic resection of large colorectal polyps: a systematic review and meta-analysis. *Gut.* 2016;65(5):806-820.
15. Beresford SA, Johnson KC, Ritenbaugh C, et al. Low-fat dietary pattern and risk of colorectal cancer: the Women's Health Initiative Randomized Controlled Dietary Modification Trial. *JAMA.* 2006;295(6):643-654.
16. Bobe G, Albert PS, Sansbury LB, et al. Interleukin-6 as a potential indicator for prevention of high risk adenoma recurrence by dietary flavonols in the polyp prevention trial. *Cancer Prev Res (Phila).* 2010;3(6):764-775.
17. Weingarten MAMA, Zalmanovici Trestioreanu A, Yaphe J. Dietary calcium supplementation for preventing colorectal cancer and adenomatous polyps. *Cochrane Database Syst Rev.* 2008;(1):CD003548
18. Baron JA, Cole BF, Sandler RS, et al. A randomized trial of aspirin to prevent colorectal adenomas. *N Engl J Med.* 2003;348(10):891-899.
19. Ishikawa H, Mutoh M, Suzuki S, et al. The preventive effects of low-dose enteric-coated aspirin tablets on the development of colorectal tumours in Asian patients: a randomised trial. *Gut.* 2014;63(11):1755-1759.
20. Higuchi T, Iwama T, Yoshinaga K, et al. A randomized, double-blind, placebo-controlled trial of the effects of rofecoxib, a selective cyclooxygenase-2 inhibitor, on rectal polyps in familial adenomatous polyposis patients. *Clin Cancer Res.* 2003;9(13):4756-4760.
21. Botteri E, Iodice S, Raimondi S. Cigarette smoking and adenomatous polyps: a meta-analysis. *Gastroenterology.* 2008;134:388-395.
22. Wolin KY, Yan Y, Colditz GA. Physical activity and risk of colon adenoma: a meta-analysis. *Br J Cancer.* 2011;104(5):882-885.
23. Ortiz AM, Bhargavi P, Zuckerman MJ, Othman MO. Endoscopic mucosal resection recurrence rate for colorectal lesions. *South Med J.* 2014;107(10):615-621.

24. Hassan C, Pickhardt PJ, Kim DH, et al. Systematic review: distribution of advanced neoplasia according to polyp size at screening colonoscopy. *Aliment Pharmacol Ther*. 2010;31(2):210-217.

25. Holme Ø, Bretthauer M, Eide TJ, et al. Long-term risk of colorectal cancer in individuals with serrated polyps. *Gut*. 2015;64(6): 929-936.

26. Levin B, Lieberman DA, McFarland B, et al. Screening and surveillance for the early detection of colorectal cancer and adenomatous polyps, 2008: a joint guideline from the American Cancer Society, the US Multi-Society Task Force on Colorectal Cancer, and the American College of Radiology. *Gastroenterology*. 2008; 134:1570-1595.

27. Brown SR, Baraza W, Din S, Riley S. Chromoscopy versus conventional endoscopy for the detection of polyps in the colon and rectum. *Cochrane Database Syst Rev*. 2016;(4):CD006439.

28. United States Preventive Services Task Force. *Colorectal Cancer: Screening*. https://www.uspreventiveservicestaskforce.org/Page/Document/UpdateSummaryFinal/colorectal-cancer-screening2?ds=1&s=colon%20cancer Accessed March 2017.

66 COLON CANCER

Mindy A. Smith, MD, MS

PATIENT STORY

A 72-year-old man reports rectal bleeding with bowel movements over the past several months and the stool seems narrower with occasional diarrhea. He has a history of hemorrhoids but now is not experiencing rectal irritation or itching, as with previous episodes. His medical history is significant for controlled hypertension and a remote history of smoking. On digital rectal examination, his stool sample tests positive for blood but anoscopy fails to identify the source of bleeding. On colonoscopy, a mass is seen at 30 cm (**Figure 66-1**). A biopsy was obtained and pathology confirmed adenocarcinoma.

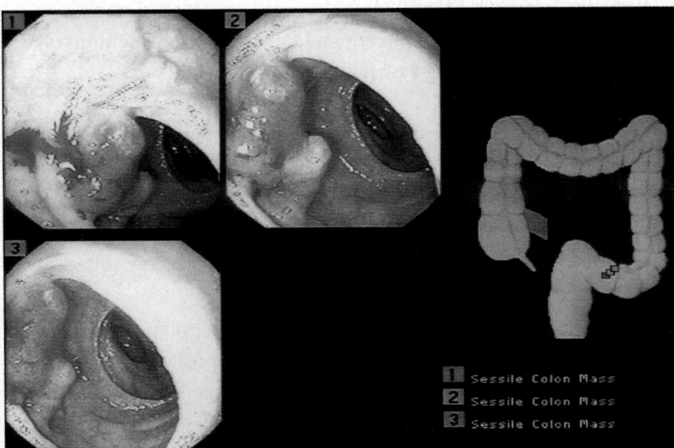

FIGURE 66-1 A sessile colon mass seen at 30 cm. At surgery, this was found to be a Duke stage A adenocarcinoma. *(Reproduced with permission from Michael Harper, MD.)*

INTRODUCTION

Colorectal cancer (CRC) is a malignant neoplasm of the colon, most commonly adenocarcinoma. There has been a slow decline in both the incidence and mortality from colon cancer, although it is the second leading cause of cancer death in the United States.[1]

EPIDEMIOLOGY

- In 2013, 136,119 people in the United States were diagnosed with CRC and there were 51,813 associated deaths.[1]
- Incidence increases with age and is higher in men than women.[1] Of every 100 men who are 60 years old today, 1 to 2 will get colorectal cancer by the age of 70 years. Of every 100 women who are 70 years old today, 1 to 2 will get colorectal cancer by the age of 80 years.[1]
- Colon carcinoma rates are higher in blacks than in whites and lowest among American Indians and Alaska Natives.[1]
- Individuals with a first-degree relative with CRC were at slightly increased risk of developing CRC (hazard ratio [HR], 1.23; 95% confidence interval [CI], 1.07–1.42); risk was higher in those with 2 or more first-degree relatives with CRC (HR, 2.04; 95% CI, 1.44–2.86).[2]

ETIOLOGY AND PATHOPHYSIOLOGY

- Colon cancer appears to be a multipathway disease with tumors usually arising from adenomatous polyps or serrated adenomas; mutational events occur within the polyp, including activation of oncogenes and loss of tumor-suppressor genes.[3]
- The probability of a polyp undergoing malignant transformation increases for the following cases[4]:
  - The polyp is sessile, especially if villous histology or flat.
  - Larger size—Malignant transformation is rare if smaller than 1.5 cm, 2% to 10% if 1.5 to 2.5 cm, and 10% if larger than 2.5 cm.
- Serrated polyps are associated with an increased risk of detection of synchronous advanced neoplasia (odds ratio 2.05; 95% CI, 1.38–3.04).[5]

- Strong associations with CRC risk are found in eight variants of five genes (adenomatous polyposis coli [APC], CHEK2, DNMT3B, MLH1, and MUTYH), moderate associations for two variants in two genes (GSTM1 and TERT), and weak associations for 52 variants in 45 genes.[6] In addition, in a large genome-wide association study, investigators identified polymorphisms close to nucleic acid binding protein 1 (which encodes a DNA-binding protein involved in DNA repair) as being associated with CRC risk.[7]

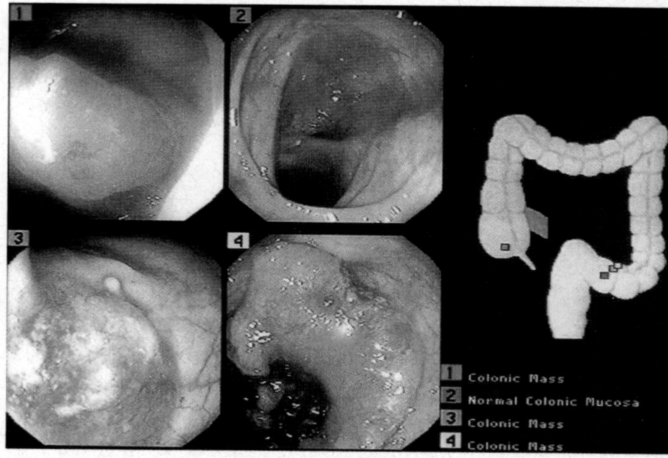

FIGURE 66-2 Plate 2 in this series shows normal cecum. The remaining frames show a large friable mass. Biopsy confirmed adenocarcinoma. The tumor was resected and determined to be Duke stage B adenocarcinoma. Colonoscopy 3 years later was negative. *(Reproduced with permission from Michael Harper, MD.)*

RISK FACTORS[4,8]

- Older age and male sex.
- Ingestion of red and processed meat, eggs, and possibly sugars and cheese.
- Hereditary syndromes—Familial adenomatous polyposis (virtually all develop CRC by age 40 years) and nonpolyposis syndromes (9/10 men and 7/10 women develop CRC by age 70 years).
- Family history of colon cancer in a first-degree relative.
- Inflammatory bowel disease (5% risk after 20 years), gallbladder disease, diabetes, or metabolic syndrome.
- *Helicobacter pylori* infection.
- Prior cancer, especially childhood cancers.
- Smoking.
- Alcohol consumption.
- Following removal of adenomas that are large (20 mm or more) or with high-grade dysplasia (1% by around 4 years).
- Obesity.
- Ionizing radiation.

DIAGNOSIS

The diagnosis of CRC is sometimes made following a positive screening test (i.e., digital rectal examination, fecal occult blood test [FOBT], sigmoidoscopy, colonoscopy, or barium enema). For patients who have symptoms and signs suggestive of CRC, the confirmative diagnostic test most commonly performed is colonoscopy with biopsy. Colonoscopy allows direct visualization of the lesion, examination of the entire large bowel for synchronous and metachronous lesions, and an ability to obtain tissue for histologic diagnosis.

CLINICAL FEATURES

Symptoms vary, primarily based on anatomic location, as follows[4]:

- Right-sided colon tumors more commonly ulcerate, occasionally causing anemia without change in stool or bowel habits.
- Tumors in the transverse and descending colon often impede stool passage, causing abdominal cramping, occasional obstruction, and rarely perforation (**Figure 66-2**).
- Tumors in the rectosigmoid region are associated more often with hematochezia, tenesmus (i.e., urgency with a feeling of incomplete evacuation), narrow caliber stool, and uncommonly, anemia.
- Physical signs, often appearing later in the disease, include weight loss and cachexia; abdominal distention, discomfort or tenderness; abdominal or rectal mass; ascites; and rectal bleeding.

TYPICAL DISTRIBUTION

Colon cancers are more commonly seen in the left (about 2/3 to 3/4) vs. right colon.[9]

LABORATORY TESTING

- Preoperative carcinoembryonic antigen (CEA)—An elevated CEA level can be used to monitor for recurrence. Pretreatment CEA (C-Stage) is an independent predictor of overall mortality (60% increased risk) in patients with colon cancer.[10] CEA may be elevated for reasons other than colon cancer, such as pancreatic or hepatobiliary disease; elevation does not always reflect cancer or disease recurrence.
- Circulating cell-free nucleic acids are under investigation as biomarkers in CRC screening.[11]
- For patients being considered for anti–epidermal growth factor receptor therapy, RAS mutational testing is needed.[12] Mutational analysis should include KRAS and NRAS codons 12; 13 of exon 2; 59 and 61 of exon 3; and 117 and 146 of exon 4.
- BRAF p.V600 mutational analysis should be performed in CRC tissue for prognostic stratification and in deficient MMR tumors with loss of MLH1 to evaluate for Lynch syndrome risk.[12]
- Oncologists also order mismatch repair status testing in patients with CRCs to identify patients at high risk for Lynch syndrome and/or prognostic stratification.[12]

IMAGING, ENDOSCOPY, AND WORK-UP

- Colonoscopy of the entire colon is recommended to identify additional neoplasms or polyps (**Figures 66-1** and **66-2**).
- The American College of Radiology (ACR) notes that imaging for colon cancer is best used to identify advanced T stage and distant metastases.[13] Locoregional nodal staging is less accurate and of marginal clinical utility. Imaging modalities for distant metastases may include MRI (pelvis), CT (chest, abdomen and pelvis), or positron emission tomography (PET) CT scan (whole body), all performed without and with contrast.
- For rectal tumors, ACR recommends transrectal rectum ultrasound (for early-stage tumors) or MRI for locoregional pretreatment staging, or CT if unable to undergo MRI.[13] Multiphase contrast-enhanced MRI or contrast-enhanced CT is used for evaluation of distant metastases.
- At surgery, surgeons perform an examination of the liver, pelvis, hemidiaphragm, and full length of the colon for evidence of tumor spread.[4]

BIOPSY

Colonic adenocarcinomas may be microscopically well-differentiated or poorly differentiated glandular structures. Biopsy is usually performed during colonoscopy.

DIFFERENTIAL DIAGNOSIS

Other causes of abdominal pain in patients in this age group:

- Inflammatory bowel disease, which includes ulcerative colitis and Crohn disease (see Chapter 67, Inflammatory Bowel Disease); symptoms include bloody diarrhea, tenesmus, passage of mucus, and cramping abdominal pain. Extraintestinal manifestations, more common in Crohn disease, include skin involvement (e.g., erythema nodosum), rheumatologic symptoms (e.g., peripheral arthritis, symmetric sacroiliitis), and ocular problems (e.g., uveitis, iritis). Diagnosis may be made with endoscopy.
- Diverticulitis—Patients present with fever, anorexia, lower left-sided abdominal pain, and diarrhea. Abdominal distention and peritonitis may be found on physical examination. Diagnosis is clinical or made using abdominal CT scan.
- Appendicitis—Initial symptoms include periumbilical or epigastric abdominal pain that over time becomes more severe and localized to the right lower quadrant. Additional symptoms include fever, nausea, vomiting, and anorexia.

Other causes of rectal bleeding:

- Infectious agents—*Salmonella, Shigella*, certain *Campylobacter* species, enteroinvasive *Escherichia coli, Clostridium difficile*, and *Entamoeba histolytica* can cause bloody, watery diarrhea and are identified by culture test. Bacterial toxins may be identified with *C. difficile*. Additional symptoms include fever and abdominal pain, and the disease is often self-limited.
- Hemorrhoids (see Chapter 68, Hemorrhoids) and fissures—Bleeding is usually bright red and seen in the toilet or with wiping after bowel movements. Hemorrhoids can sometimes be visible as a protruding mass often associated with pruritus, and fissures are identified as a cut or tear occurring in the anus. Hemorrhoidal pain is described as a dull ache but may be severe if thrombosed.
- Diverticula—Bleeding is usually abrupt in onset, painless, and may be massive, but often stops spontaneously. These may be seen during endoscopy or in radiographic study.
- Vascular colonic ectasias—Bleeding tends to be chronic, resulting in anemia. Bleeding source may be identified during colonoscopy, but a radionuclide scan or angiography may be needed.
- Colon polyp (see Chapter 65, Colon Polyps)—Usually asymptomatic, although abdominal pain, diarrhea, or constipation can occur, often with decreased stool caliber. Imaging studies often can distinguish, and biopsy confirms absence of malignancy.

Other causes of intestinal obstruction include adhesions, peritonitis, inflammatory bowel disease, fecal impaction, strangulated bowels, and ileus.

MANAGEMENT

- Treatment for colon cancer is based on TNM stage with surgery recommended for stages 0 to II, surgery and adjuvant chemotherapy for stage III, and stage IV with multiple options (**Table 66-1**).[14] Similarly, treatment for rectal cancer is based on TNM stage with polypectomy or surgery recommended for stage 0, surgery with or without chemoradiation for stage 1, and surgery with multiple other options for stages II–IV as shown in **Table 66-1**.[15] Management of rectal cancer is somewhat different than for colon cancer because of its higher risk of recurrence and poorer prognosis.

MEDICATIONS

- For colon cancer, many drug combinations are used for adjuvant chemotherapy, most containing a combination of 5-fluorouracil (5-FU), irinotecan and/or oxaliplatin.[14] Chemotherapy is of

TABLE 66-1 Treatment Recommendations for Colon and Rectal Cancer

Stage (TNM)	Dukes	Standard Treatment	Adjuvant Treatment
		Colon Cancer	
O (Tis, N0, M0)		Surgery	None
I (T1 or 2, N0, M0)	A	Surgery	None
IIA-C (T3 or 4a/b, N0, M0)	B	Surgery	None*
IIIA-C (T1-4, N1-2b, M0)	C	Surgery	Chemotherapy
IVA/B and recurrent (Any T, Any N, M1a or 1b)		Surgery	Chemotherapy and targeted therapy
IV with liver metastases		Surgery	Chemotherapy†, ablation
		Rectal Cancer	
0 (Tis, N0, M0)		Polypectomy or surgery	
I (T1 or 2, N0, M0)	A	Surgery	With or without chemoradiation
IIA-C (T3 or 4a/b, N0, M0) IIIA-C (T1-4, N1-2b, M0)	B C	Surgery	Preoperative radiation or pre- or postoperative chemoradiation
IVA/B and recurrent (Any T, Any N, M1a or 1b)		Surgery	Multiple options‡
IV with liver metastases		Surgery	Chemotherapy†, ablation

Abbreviations: is, in situ; N, regional lymph nodes (N1, metastases in 1–3 regional lymph nodes; N1c, tumor deposit(s) in subserosa, mesentery, or nonperitonealized pericolic or perirectal tissues without regional nodal metastasis; N2a, metastases in 4–6 lymph nodes; N2b, metastases in 7 or more regional lymph nodes); M, distant metastasis (M1a, metastases confined to one organ or site; M1b, metastases in more than one organ or peritoneum); T, primary tumor (T1, tumor invades submucosa; T2, tumor invades muscularis propria; T3, tumor invades into pericolorectal tissues; T4a, tumor penetrates to surface of visceral peritoneum; T4b, tumor invades or is adherent to other organs or structures).
*May be helpful for high-risk patients.
†Options include neoadjuvant or adjuvant chemotherapy or intra-arterial therapy.
‡Options include radiation therapy, first-line chemotherapy and targeted therapy, second-line chemotherapy, and palliative therapy.
Data from National Cancer Institute. *Colon Cancer Treatment (PDQ®)-Health Professional Version.* https://www.cancer.gov/types/colorectal/hp/colon-treatment-pdq; *Rectal Cancer Treatment (PDQ®)-Health Professional Version.* https://www.cancer.gov/types/colorectal/hp/rectal-treatment-pdq. Accessed February 2017.

marginal benefit for those with stage III colon cancer, with absolute improvement in overall survival at 3 or 5 years of about 5%.[14] In one trial, a reduction in relapse rate and a modest increase in 3-year disease-free survival were also seen in patients with Duke B and C colon cancer by adding oxaliplatin to 5-FU–leucovorin; however, overall survival is improved for only a subgroup of patients.[16]

- For patients with stage II (Duke B) tumors (**Table 66-1**), authors of a Cochrane review found no difference in overall survival but a significant difference in disease-free survival (relative risk 0.83; 95% CI, 0.75–0.92) with adjuvant chemotherapy.[17] Adjuvant chemotherapy is considered in patients with stage 2 colon cancer and high-risk features for recurrence such as inadequate lymph node sampling, T4 disease, involvement of visceral peritoneum, or a poorly differentiated histology.[14]
- The addition of intraportal chemotherapy administered during radical surgery with adjuvant chemotherapy for treating stage II and III colon cancer improved disease-free and metastatic-free survival at 3 years but not overall survival; neutropenia was higher in the combination arm.[18]
- Differences in survivorship likely complicate treatment decisions. In a cohort study, younger (<50 years) patients at stages I–IV were more likely to receive adjuvant chemotherapy but experienced only minimal gain in adjusted survival compared with their older counterparts who received less treatment.[19] Similarly, in older (>69 years) patients identified from Swedish databases, adjuvant chemotherapy compromised the 5-year overall survival (OS) of older patients with stage II CRC and had no effect on those with stage III CRC.[20]
- For patients with metastatic colon cancer (stage IV), first-line multiagent chemotherapy can be considered, although data are limited on effectiveness.[14]
- For patients with rectal cancer, neoadjuvant (preoperative chemoradiation) therapy is the preferred treatment option for stages II and III disease because of improved resectability and sphincter preservation; complication rates, however, are higher than with surgery alone.[15] There are many drug combinations which are similar to those used for colon cancer.[15]

SURGERY OR OTHER TREATMENTS

- Total resection of the tumor is completed for attempted cure or for symptoms; open surgery or laparoscopic techniques may be used, as CRC outcomes appear comparable.[14,15]
- For superficial lesions, local excision or polypectomy with clear margins is performed. For colon cancers, wide surgical resection and reanastomosis is usually used. For rectal cancers, surgical options include transanal local excision and transanal endoscopic microsurgery for select T1/T2 N0 rectal cancers; total mesorectal excision with autonomic nerve preservation techniques via low-anterior resection; and total mesorectal excision via abdominoperineal resection for patients who are not candidates for sphincter-preservation, with a permanent end-colostomy.
- For patients with metastatic disease (stage IV), treatment options are shown in **Table 66-1**.
- Total colonic resection is performed for patients with familial polyposis and multiple colonic polyps.
- As noted above, preoperative chemoradiation therapy is used for stage II or III rectal tumors. Patients treated with radiation therapy, however, have increased chronic bowel dysfunction, anorectal sphincter dysfunction (if the sphincter was surgically preserved), and sexual dysfunction compared to patients who undergo surgical resection alone.[15] Authors of a Cochrane review of 4 trials of patients with resectable rectal cancer found no evidence of improved survival although treatment may improve local control.[21]

PREVENTION AND SCREENING

- Primary prevention—Increased dietary fiber (conflicting evidence), garlic, milk, and possibly increased ingestion of fruit, vegetables, and fish.[8,22] High levels of physical activity also appear protective.[8] Low-dose aspirin is also associated with a lower risk of colon cancer and death from colon cancer,[23] although authors of a recent meta-analysis found benefit on overall survival from post-CRC diagnosis aspirin use (HR 0.84; 95% CI 0.75–0.94) but not pre-diagnosis aspirin use.[24]
- Individuals who undergo at least one round of screening for colon cancer have a reduced risk of death from bowel cancer. For example, in the Minnesota Colon Cancer Control Study with 46,551 participants, those randomized to annual or biennial screening with fecal occult-blood testing vs. usual care had similar all-cause mortality but a lower risk of CRC mortality (RR with annual screening 0.68; 95% CI 0.56 to 0.82 and RR with biennial screening 0.78; 95%CI 0.65 to 0.93) through 30 years of follow-up.[25] In addition, early polyp removal by colonoscopy with polypectomy is associated with a reduced risk for colorectal cancer in the population setting.[26]
- Recommended screening test options are fecal occult blood testing (guaiac-based fecal occult blood test, fecal immunochemical test [FIT], or multitargeted stool DNA test; annually or every 1 or 3 years for the DNA test), flexible sigmoidoscopy (with or without FIT every 5 years), CT colonography every 5 years, or colonoscopy every 10 years.[27] The U.S. Preventive Services Task Force (USPSTF) recommends screening for colorectal cancer in adults, beginning at age 50 years and continuing until age 75 years.[27] SOR Ⓐ

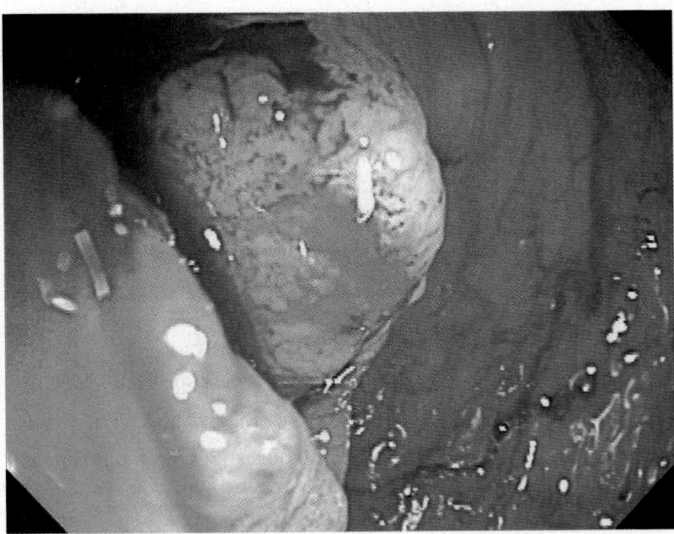

FIGURE 66-3 Adenocarcinoma in the cecum found on colonoscopy. *(Reproduced with permission from Marvin Derezin, MD.)*

Examples of colonoscopy pictures are shown in **Figures 66-1** to **66-3**.

- Double-contrast barium enema—This test offers an alternative means of whole-bowel examination, but is less sensitive than colonoscopy or CT colonography, and there is no direct evidence that it is effective in reducing mortality rates. **Figures 66-4** and **66-5** display classic "apple-core deformities" of the colon from colon cancers.

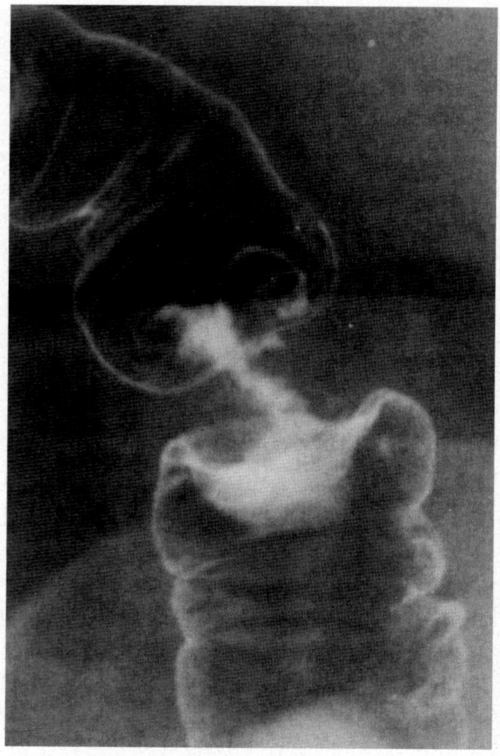

FIGURE 66-4 An "apple core" lesion on barium enema is consistent with colon cancer. The patient is a 72-year-old African-American man who presented with weight loss. A complete blood count demonstrated moderate anemia and his hemoccult cards were positive. *(Reproduced with permission from E.J. Mayeaux, Jr., MD.)*

PROGNOSIS[1,28]

- Localized CRC; 5-year survival: 90.1%.
- Cancer involving regional lymph nodes; 5-year survival: 71.2%.
- Distant metastases (i.e., lung, liver); 5-year survival: 13.5%.
- In addition to node involvement and metastases, poor outcome is associated with[4]:
  - Number of regional lymph nodes involved
  - Tumor penetration or perforation through the bowel wall
  - Histology of poor differentiation
  - Tumor adherence to adjacent organs
  - Venous invasion
  - Bowel obstruction or perforation.
  - Elevated preoperative CEA (i.e., >5 ng/mL)
  - Aneuploidy
  - Specific chromosomal deletion (e.g., allelic loss on chromosome 18q)

FOLLOW-UP

- Staging is based on tumor depth and spread (see **Table 66-1**) and predicts survival as above.[28] Most (80%) of recurrences occur in the first 3 years after resection of the primary tumor.[29]
- Optimal follow-up intervals have not been established. Surveillance recommendations are provided by the National Comprehensive Cancer Network as follows[29]:
  - Stage I disease: Colonoscopy at 1, 3, and then every 5 years if normal. If an advanced adenoma is detected, repeat colonoscopy in 1 year.
  - Stage II/III disease:
    - Office visits and CEA evaluations should be performed every 3–6 months for the first 2 years of follow-up. For those with stage III CRC (and at the discretion of the patient and physician for stage II CRC), continue every 6 months for a total of 5 years.
    - CEA at baseline and every 3–6 months for 2 years, then, for those with stage III CRC (and at the discretion of the patient and physician for stage II CRC), continue every 6 months for a total of 5 years.
    - Colonoscopy should be performed at 1 and 3 years post-resection (or 3–6 months if no baseline colonoscopy), then every 5 years if normal. If an advanced adenoma is detected, repeat colonoscopy in 1 year.
    - Chest, abdominal, and pelvic CT scans are recommended every 6 to 12 months (category 2B for more frequently than annually) for up to 5 years for those with stage III CRC or stage II at high risk of recurrence.
  - For patients with stage IV CRC, after curative intent surgery and adjuvant therapy, obtain CEA every 3–6 months for 2 years, then

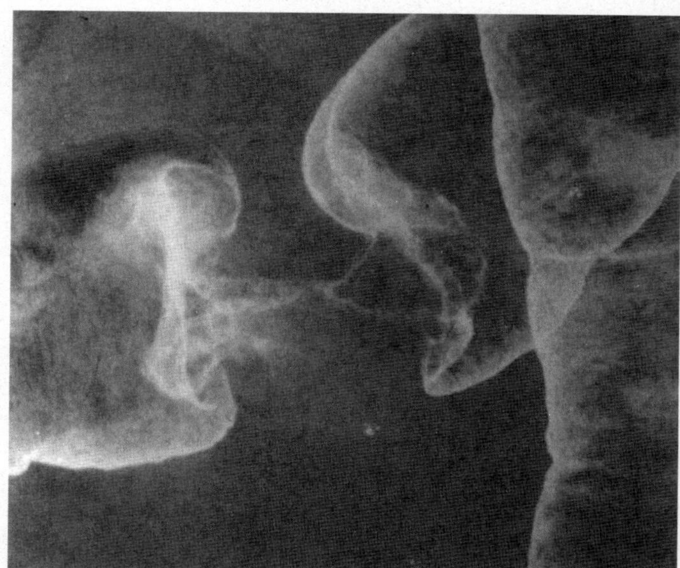

FIGURE 66-5 A barium enema reveals a large "apple core" lesion consistent with colon cancer. The patient is a 66-year-old man who had a barium enema performed as part of the work-up for weight loss and vague abdominal pain. *(Reproduced with permission from E.J. Mayeaux, Jr., MD.)*

every 6 months for a total of 5 years. Perform contrast-enhanced CT scans of the chest, abdomen, and pelvis every 3–6 months for the first 2 years, then every 6–12 months for 5 years.

PATIENT EDUCATION

- Encourage patients to follow a healthy lifestyle including smoking cessation as appropriate, exercise, maintaining a healthy weight, and eating a diet high in fruits, vegetables, and fish. Low-dose aspirin improves disease-specific survival and reduces recurrence; risks should be discussed.
- Most recurrences occur within the first 3 to 4 years, so survival at 5 years is a good indication of cure.[4]
- Surveillance for recurrence should be conducted over the first 5 years following treatment as noted above. In addition to identifying recurrence, a second tumor is found in 3% to 5%, and adenomatous polyps will be found in more than 15% of patients over that period.[4]

PATIENT RESOURCES

- **www.nlm.nih.gov/medlineplus/ency/article/000262.htm.**
- **https://www.cancer.gov/types/colorectal/patient/colon-treatment-pdq.**

PROVIDER RESOURCES

- **https://www.cancer.gov/types/colorectal/hp/colon-treatment-pdq.**
- **http://emedicine.medscape.com/article/277496-overview.**

REFERENCES

1. Centers for Disease Control and Prevention. *Colorectal Cancer Statistics*. https://www.cdc.gov/cancer/colorectal/statistics/index.htm. Accessed February 2017.
2. Schoen RE, Razzak A, Yu KJ, et al. Incidence and mortality of colorectal cancer in individuals with a family history of colorectal cancer. *Gastroenterology*. 2015;149(6):1438-1445.
3. Jass JR. Classification of colorectal cancer based on correlation of clinical, morphological, and molecular features. *Histopathology*. 2007;50:113-130.
4. Mayer R. Gastrointestinal tract cancer. In: Kasper DL, Braunwald E, Fauci AS, et al, eds. *Harrison's Principles of Internal Medicine*, 16th ed. New York, NY: McGraw-Hill; 2005:523-533.
5. Gao Q, Tsoi KK, Hirai HW, et al. Serrated polyps and the risk of synchronous colorectal advanced neoplasia: a systematic review and meta-analysis. *Am J Gastroenterol*. 2015;110(4):501-509.
6. Ma X, Zhang B, Zheng W. Genetic variants associated with colorectal cancer risk: comprehensive research synopsis, meta-analysis, and epidemiological evidence. *Gut*. 2014;63(2):326-336.
7. Peters U, Jiao S, Schumacher FR, et al. Identification of genetic susceptibility loci for colorectal tumors in a genome-wide meta-analysis. *Gastroenterology*. 2013;144(4):799-807.
8. Cancer Research UK. *Bowel Cancer Risk Factors*. http://www.cancerresearchuk.org/health-professional/cancer-statistics/statistics-by-cancer-type/bowel-cancer/risk-factors. Accessed February 2017.
9. Logan RF, Patnick J, Nickerson C, et al. Outcomes of the Bowel Cancer Screening Programme (BCSP) in England after the first 1 million tests. *Gut*. 2012;61(10):1439-1446.
10. Thirunavukarasu P, Sukumar S, Sathaiah M, et al. C-stage in colon cancer: implications of carcinoembryonic antigen biomarker in staging, prognosis, and management. *J Natl Cancer Inst*. 2011; 103(8):689-697.
11. Tóth K, Barták BK, Tulassay Z, Molnár B. Circulating cell-free nucleic acids as biomarkers in colorectal cancer screening and diagnosis. *Expert Rev Mol Diagn*. 2016;16(2):239-252.
12. Zeehnbauer B, Temple-Smolkin R, Monzon FA. Guidelines for colorectal cancer testing: evidence-based practice recommendations. *J Mol Diagn*. 2017;19(2):183-186.
13. ACR Appropriateness Criteria pretreatment staging of colorectal cancer. https://www.acr.org/Clinical-Resources/ACR-Appropriateness-Criteria. Accessed May 2018.
14. National Cancer Institute. *Colon Cancer Treatment (PDQ)-Health Professional Version*. https://www.cancer.gov/types/colorectal/hp/colon-treatment-pdq. Accessed February 2017.
15. National Cancer Institute. *Rectal Cancer Treatment (PDQ)-Health Professional Version*. https://www.cancer.gov/types/colorectal/hp/rectal-treatment-pdq. Accessed February 2017.
16. André T, Boni C, Navarro M, et al. Improved overall survival with oxaliplatin, fluorouracil, and leucovorin as adjuvant treatment in stage II or III colon cancer in the MOSAIC trial. *J Clin Oncol*. 2009;27 (19):3109-3116.
17. Figueredo A, Coombes ME, Mukherjee S. Adjuvant Therapy for Completely Resected Stage II Colon Cancer. *Cochrane Database Syst Rev*. 2008;(3):CD005390.
18. Chang W, Wei Y, Ren L, et al. Randomized controlled trial of intraportal chemotherapy combined with adjuvant chemotherapy (mFOLFOX6) for stage II and III colon cancer. *Ann Surg*. 2016; 263(3):434-439.
19. Kneuertz PJ, Chang GJ, Hu CY, et al. Overtreatment of young adults with colon cancer: more intense treatments with unmatched survival gains. *JAMA Surg*. 2015;150(5):402-409.
20. Yang L, Ma Q, Yu YY, et al. Efficacy of surgery and adjuvant therapy in older patients with colorectal cancer: a STROBE-compliant article. *Medicine (Baltimore)*. 2014;93(28):e266.
21. Resende HM, Jacob LFP, Quinellato LV, et al. Combination chemotherapy versus single-agent chemotherapy during preoperative chemoradiation for resectable rectal cancer. *Cochrane Database Syst Rev*. 2015;(10):CD008531.
22. National Cancer Institute. *Colorectal Cancer Prevention*. https://www.cancer.gov/types/colorectal/hp/colorectal-prevention-pdq. Accessed February 2017.
23. Rothwell PM, Wilson M, Elwin CE, et al. Long-term effect of aspirin on colorectal cancer incidence and mortality: 20-year follow-up of five randomised trials. *Lancet*. 2010;376(9754): 1741-1750.

24. Li P, Wu H, Zhang H, et al. Aspirin use after diagnosis but not prediagnosis improves established colorectal cancer survival: a meta-analysis. *Gut.* 2015;64(9):1419-1425.

25. Shaukat A, Mongin SJ, Geisser MS, et al. Long-term mortality after screening for colorectal cancer. *N Engl J Med.* 2013;369(12):1106-1114

26. Brenner H, Chang-Claude J, Seiler CM, et al. Protection from colorectal cancer after colonoscopy: a population-based, case-control study. *Ann Intern Med.* 2011;154(1):22-30.

27. U.S. Preventive Services Task Force. *Colorectal Cancer: Screening.* https://www.uspreventiveservicestaskforce.org/Page/Document/UpdateSummaryFinal/colorectal-cancer-screening2?ds=1&s=colon%20cancer. Accessed February 2017.

28. National Cancer Institute. *Cancer Stat Facts: Colorectal Cancer.* http://seer.cancer.gov/statfacts/html/colorect.html. Accessed February 2017.

29. National Comprehensive Cancer Network. *Colon Cancer.* November 23, 2016. https://www.nccn.org/professionals/physician_gls/pdf/colon.pdf. Accessed February 2017.

67 INFLAMMATORY BOWEL DISEASE

Mindy A. Smith, MD, MS

PATIENT STORY

A 20-year-old man presents with several days of diarrhea with a small amount of rectal bleeding with each bowel movement. This is his second episode of bloody diarrhea; the first seemed to resolve after several days and occurred several weeks ago. He has cramps that occur with each bowel movement, but feels fine between bouts of diarrhea. He has no travel history outside of the United States. He is of Jewish descent and has a cousin with Crohn disease. Colonoscopy shows mucosal friability with superficial ulceration and exudates confined to the rectosigmoid colon, and he is diagnosed with ulcerative colitis (**Figure 67-1**).

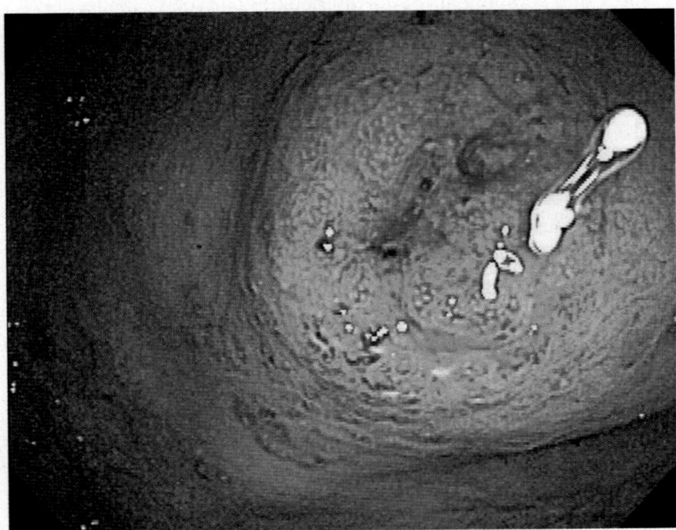

FIGURE 67-1 Ulcerative colitis in the rectosigmoid colon as viewed through the colonoscope. (*Reproduced with permission from Marvin Derezin, MD.*)

INTRODUCTION

Inflammatory bowel disease (IBD) comprises ulcerative colitis (UC) and Crohn disease (CD). The intestinal inflammation in UC is usually confined to the mucosa and affects the rectum with or without parts or the entire colon (pancolitis) in an uninterrupted pattern. In CD, inflammation is often transmural and affects primarily the ileum and colon, often discontinuously. CD, however, can affect the entire GI tract from mouth to anus.

EPIDEMIOLOGY

- Incidence of UC in the West is 8 to 14 per 100,000 people and 6 to 15 per 100,000 people for CD.[1] Prevalence for UC and CD in North America (one of the highest rates in the world) is 37.5 to 248.6 per 100,000 people and 16.7 to 318.5 per 100,000 people, respectively; IBD therefore affects an estimated 1.3 million people in the United States.[2] Rates of IBD are increasing both in the West and in developing countries.[1]
- Age of onset is 30 to 40 years for UC and 20 to 30 years for CD. A bimodal distribution with a second peak at ages 60 to 70 years has been reported but not confirmed.[1] Pediatric patients account for up to 20% of cases.
- Predilection for those of Jewish ancestry (especially Ashkenazi Jews) followed in order by non-Jewish whites and African Americans, Hispanics, and Asians.[1]
- Inheritance (polygenic) plays a role with a concordance of 38% to 58% for CD and 6% to 18% for UC in monozygous twins and a risk of about 10% in first-degree relatives of an incidence IBD case.[2]

ETIOLOGY AND PATHOPHYSIOLOGY

- Unknown etiology—Current theory is that colitis is an inappropriate response to microbial gut flora or a lack of regulation of intestinal immune cells in a genetically susceptible host with failure of the normal suppression of the immune response and tissue repair.[2,3]

- Genetic regions containing nucleotide oligomerization domain 2 (NOD2; encodes an intracellular sensor of peptidoglycan), autophagy genes (regulate clearing of intracellular components like organelles), and components of the interleukin-23–type 17 helper T-cell (Th17) pathway are associated with IBD; the autophagy gene, *ATG16L1*, is associated with CD.[3]
- Multiple bowel pathogens (e.g., *Salmonella, Shigella* species, and *Campylobacter*) may trigger UC. This is supported by a large cohort study where the hazard ratio of developing IBD was 2.4 (95% confidence interval [CI], 1.7 to 3.3) in the group who experienced a bout of infectious gastroenteritis compared with the control group; the excess risk was greatest during the first year after the infective episode.[4] People with IBD also have depletion and reduced diversity of some members of the mucosa-associated bacterial phyla, but it is not known whether this is causal or secondary to inflammation.[3]
- Other abnormalities found in patients with IBD include increased permeability between mucosal epithelial cells, defective regulation of intercellular junctions, infiltration into the lamina propria of innate (e.g., neutrophils) and adaptive (B and T cells) immune cells with increased production of tumor necrosis factor a and increased numbers of CD4+ T cells, mucosal accumulation of cytotoxic, granzyme B-expressing CD19(+) and IgA(+) cells, dysregulation of intestinal CD4+ T-cell subgroups, and the presence of circulating antimicrobial antibodies (e.g., antiflagellin antibodies).[3,5] Many of the therapeutic approaches target these areas.
- Psychological factors (e.g., major life change, daily stressors) are associated with worsening symptoms.
- Patients with long-standing UC are at higher risk of developing colon dysplasia and cancer; this is believed to be a developmental sequence (see "Prognosis" below).

RISK FACTORS

- Smokers are at increased risk for CD and tend to have more severe disease, whereas former smokers and nonsmokers are at greater risk for UC.[1,2]
- Environmental factors appear to be important triggers, especially of CD in children.[1]
- Appendectomy reduces the risk of UC.[1]

DIAGNOSIS

The diagnosis depends on the clinical evaluation, sigmoid appearance, histology, and a negative stool for bacteria, *Clostridium difficile* toxin, and ova and parasites.[2]

CLINICAL FEATURES

- Major symptoms of UC—Diarrhea, rectal bleeding, tenesmus (i.e., urgency with a feeling of incomplete evacuation), passage of mucus, and cramping abdominal pain.
- Symptoms in patients with CD depend on the location of disease; patients become symptomatic when lesions are extensive or distal (e.g., colitis), when systemic inflammatory reaction is present, or when disease is complicated by stricture, abscess, or fistula. Gross blood and mucus in the stool are less frequent, and systemic symptoms, extracolonic features, pain, perineal disease, and obstruction are more common.[2] There is no relationship between symptoms and anatomical damage.[1]
- UC is classified by severity based on the clinical picture and results of endoscopy[6]; treatment is based on disease classification, including extent of disease (see Typical Distribution, below).
  - Mild: Fewer than 4 stools per day, with or without blood, no signs of systemic toxicity, and a normal erythrocyte sedimentation rate (ESR).
  - Moderate: More than 4 stools per day but with minimal signs of toxicity.
  - Severe: More than 6 bloody stools per day, and evidence of toxicity demonstrated by fever, tachycardia, anemia, and elevated ESR.
  - Fulminant: May have more than 10 bowel movements daily, continuous bleeding, toxicity, abdominal tenderness and distention, a blood transfusion requirement, and colonic dilation on abdominal plain films.
- Extraintestinal manifestations are present in 25% to 40% of patients with IBD, but are more common in CD than UC[2,7]:
  - Dermatologic (2% to 34%)—Erythema nodosum (10%) (see Chapter 186, Erythema Nodosum) that correlates with disease activity and pyoderma gangrenosum (nonhealing ulcer surrounded by violaceous borders) in 1% to 12% of patients (see Chapter 183, Pyoderma Gangrenosum).[2]
  - Rheumatologic—Peripheral arthritis (5% to 20%), spondylitis (1% to 26%, but nearly all those positive for human leukocyte antigen B27), and symmetric sacroiliitis (<10%).
  - Ocular—Conjunctivitis, uveitis, iritis, and episcleritis (0.3% to 5%—see Chapter 18, Conjunctivitis, and Chapter 20, Uveitis and Iritis).[7]
  - Hepatobiliary—The most serious complication in this category is primary sclerosing cholangitis; although 75% of patients with this disease have UC, only 5% of those with UC and 2% of patients with CD develop it.[7] Hepatic steatosis (fatty liver) and cholelithiasis can also occur (see Chapter 63, Liver Disease, and Chapter 64, Gallstones).
  - Cardiovascular—Increased risk of deep venous thrombosis, pulmonary embolus, and stroke (because of a hypercoagulable state from thrombocytosis and gut losses of antithrombin III among other factors); endocarditis; myocarditis; and pleuropericarditis (see Chapter 59, Pulmonary Embolism, and Chapter 52, Bacterial Endocarditis).[2]
  - Bone—Osteoporosis and osteomalacia from multiple causes including medications, reduced physical activity, inflammatory-mediated bone resorption, vitamin D deficiency, and calcium and magnesium malabsorption (see Chapter 234, Osteoporosis and Osteopenia). Fracture risk in patients with IBD is 1 per 100 patient years (40% higher than the general population).[7]
  - Renal—Nephrolithiasis, obstructive uropathy, and fistulization of the urinary tract occur in 6% to 23% (see Chapter 70, Kidney Stones).[7]

- Extraintestinal manifestations may occur prior to the diagnosis of IBD. For example, 10% to 30% of patients with IBD-related arthritis develop arthritis prior to IBD diagnosis.[7]
- Severe complications include toxic colitis (15% initially present with catastrophic illness), massive hemorrhage (1% of those with severe attacks), toxic megacolon (i.e., transverse colon diameter >5 to 6 cm) (5% of attacks; may be triggered by electrolyte abnormalities and narcotics), and bowel obstruction (caused by strictures and occurring in 10% of patients).[1]
- On endoscopy in patients with CD, rectal sparing is frequent and cobblestoning of the mucosa is often seen. Small bowel involvement is seen on imaging in addition to segmental colitis and frequent strictures (see **Figure 67-5**).

TYPICAL DISTRIBUTION

- At presentation, about one-third of patients with UC have disease localized to the rectum, another third has disease present in the colorectum distal to the splenic flexure, and the remainder has disease proximal to the splenic flexure; pancolitis is present in one quarter.[1] Adults appear to always have rectal involvement, which is not the case for children. Over time (20 years), half will have pancolitis (see **Figure 67-1**).[8]
- In patients with CD, lesions occur in equal proportions in the ileum, colon, or both; 10% to 15% have upper GI lesions, 20% to 30% present with perianal lesions, and about half eventually develop perianal disease. Fifteen percent to 20% of patients have or have had a fistula.[1]
- The Montreal classification system is most often used for classifying disease extent in adults with both UC and CD[9]:
  - For UC, there are three categories—E1: proctitis (limited to rectum), E2: left sided (limited to colonic mucosa distal to splenic flexure), and E3: extensive (extends proximal to splenic flexure)
  - For CD, there are three major categories:
    - Age of onset—A1: ≤16 years, A2: 17–40 years, A3: >40 years
    - Location—L1: ileal, L2: colonic, L3 ileocolonic, L4 isolated upper GI (L4 can be added to first three categories)
    - Behavior—B1: non-stricturing, B2: stricturing, B3: penetrating (+p if perianal disease)

LABORATORY TESTS

- Acute disease can result in a rise of acute-phase reactants (e.g., C-reactive protein) and elevated ESR (rare in patients with just proctitis). C-reactive protein is elevated in nearly all patients with CD and in approximately half of patients with UC.[10]
- Obtain hemoglobin (to assess for anemia) and platelets (to assess for reactive thrombocytosis).
- Of the biomarkers available to detect IBD, fecal calprotectin and lactoferrin are most commonly used.[10] The former is an indirect measure of neutrophil infiltrate in the bowel mucosa, and the latter is an iron-binding protein secreted by mucosal membranes and found in neutrophil granules and serum. Although the optimal threshold value for calprotectin in detecting IBD is unknown, a study of adult patients suspected of having IBD based on clinical evaluation reported a sensitivity and specificity of the test of 93% and 96%, respectively.[11] Test characteristics for lactoferrin are lower at 80% and 82%. Among children, fecal calprotectin had a pooled sensitivity of 99% and a specificity of 65%.[12]
- Stool should be examined to rule out infectious causes including *C. difficile*; the incidence of *C. difficile* is increasing in patients with UC and is associated with a more severe course in those with IBD.[13]

ENDOSCOPY AND IMAGING

Imaging has become more important for patients with IBD, not only for diagnosis in symptomatic patients but for early detection and treatment of inflammation in asymptomatic patients with CD and for monitoring inflammation and disease complications.[14]

- Colonoscopy with ileoscopy and mucosal biopsy from multiple sites should be performed in the initial evaluation of IBD and for differentiating UC from CD (**Figures 67-1** to **67-5**).[9] SOR Ⓑ It is the best test for detection of colonic inflammation.[6,11]
- Colonoscopy can show pseudopolyps in both active UC (**Figure 67-3**) and inactive UC (**Figure 67-4**). Risks of ileocolonoscopy include perforation, limited small bowel evaluation and inability to stage penetrating disease.[14]
- For children with suspected IBD, upper endoscopy (EGD) is recommended at the time of ileocolonoscopy to evaluate the presence and extent of upper GI tract involvement.[9]
- Capsule endoscopy (CE) is a less invasive technique for evaluating the small intestine in patients with CD and is more sensitive than radiologic and endoscopic procedures for detecting small bowel lesions and mucosal inflammation.[9,14] SOR Ⓑ CE is recommended for patients with suspected CD but negative ileocolonoscopy[9]; CE should not be performed in patients with CD known or suspected to have obstruction. Patency capsule, small-bowel follow-through; CT enterography; OR magnetic resonance (MR) enterography should be performed before CE in patients with known small-bowel CD involvement.[9] The major risk is retention.[14]
- In adult patients with initial presentation of symptomatic CD, the American College of Radiology (ACR) recommends CT of the abdomen and pelvis with IV contrast OR CT enterography.[15] MR enterography may be substituted, but may not be well tolerated; any of these three tests is an acceptable alternative for adults with an acute exacerbation. CT enterography OR MR enterography are equivalent alternatives for diagnosing children or for adult patients with nonacute or indolent initial presentation and mild to moderate abdominal pain or cramping, or for surveillance in stable disease.[15]
- Combination imaging and endoscopic techniques are recommended—it is no longer sufficient to only detect the presence of CD as knowing its subtype, location, and severity helps guide treatment.[15]
- Small intestine contrast ultrasonography may be an alternative to invasive testing (area under receiver operating characteristic curve 0.93) but is not currently recommended by ACR.[16]

DIFFERENTIAL DIAGNOSIS

- Infections of the colon—*Salmonella, Shigella* species, and *Campylobacter* have a similar appearance with bloody diarrhea and

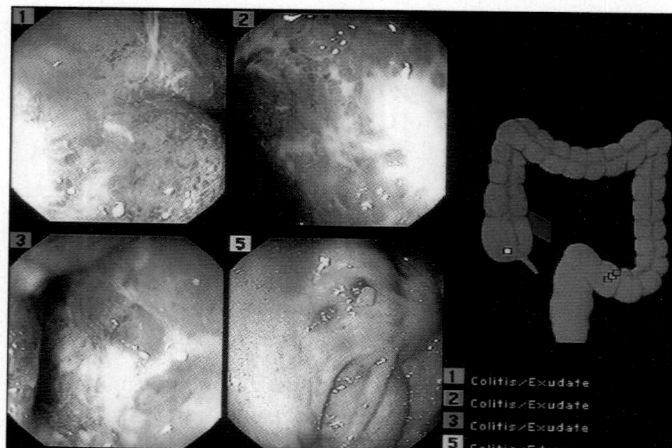

FIGURE 67-2 Endoscopic image showing friability and exudates over superficial ulceration in the sigmoid colon. There is edema in the cecum that, all together, indicates pancolitis. Biopsy confirmed ulcerative colitis. (*Reproduced with permission from Michael Harper, MD.*)

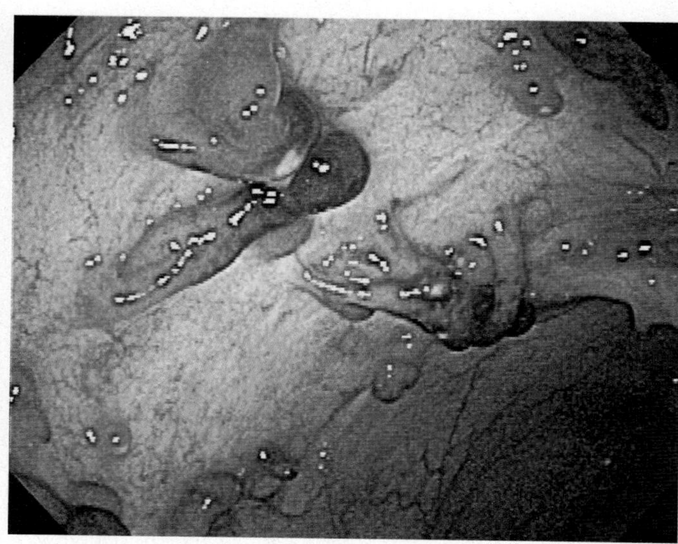

FIGURE 67-4 Pseudopolyps in "inactive" ulcerative colitis viewed through colonoscope. (*Reproduced with permission from Marvin Derezin, MD.*)

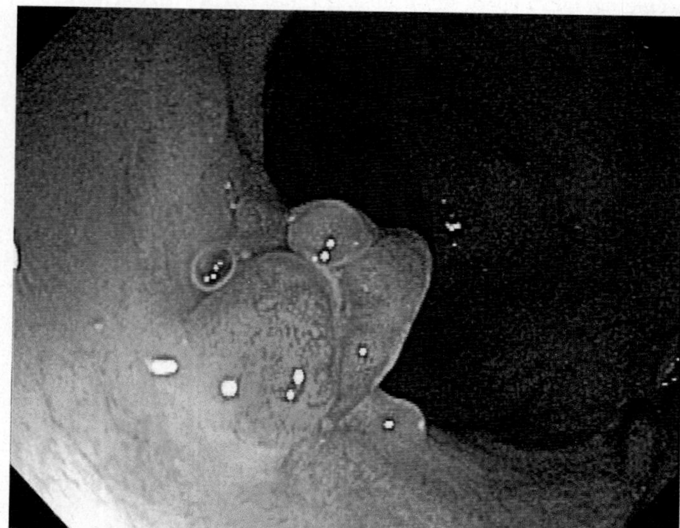

FIGURE 67-3 Pseudopolyps in "active" ulcerative colitis viewed through colonoscope. (*Reproduced with permission from Marvin Derezin, MD.*)

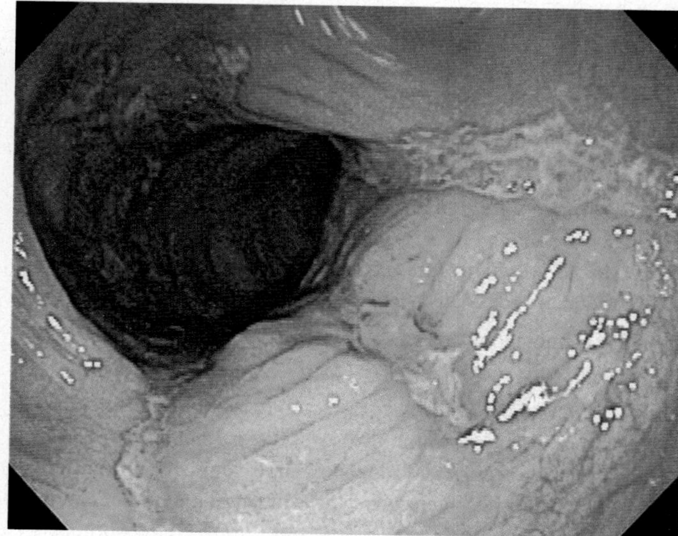

FIGURE 67-5 Crohn colitis with deep longitudinal ulcers and normal-appearing tissue between. The biopsies that showed normal tissue between the ulcers clinched the diagnosis for Crohn disease. Ulcerative colitis is diffuse, whereas CD often skips areas as seen in this patient's colon. (*Reproduced with permission from Marvin Derezin, MD.*)

abdominal pain, but disease is usually self-limited, and stool culture can confirm the presence of these bacteria. *C. difficile* and *Escherichia coli* can also mimic IBD.

- Numerous infectious agents including *Mycobacterium*, *Cytomegalovirus*, and protozoan parasites can mimic UC in immunocompromised patients.
- Ischemic colitis—May present with sudden onset of left lower quadrant pain, urgency to defecate, and bright red blood via rectum. It can be chronic and diffuse and should be considered in elderly patients following abdominal aorta repair or when a patient has a hypercoagulable state. Endoscopic examination often demonstrates normal rectal mucosa with a sharp transition to an area of inflammation in the descending colon or splenic flexure (**Figure 67-6**).
- Colitis associated with nonsteroidal anti-inflammatory drugs (NSAIDs)—Clinical features of diarrhea and pain, but may be complicated by bleeding, stricture, obstruction, and perforation. History is helpful, and symptoms improve with withdrawal of the agent.

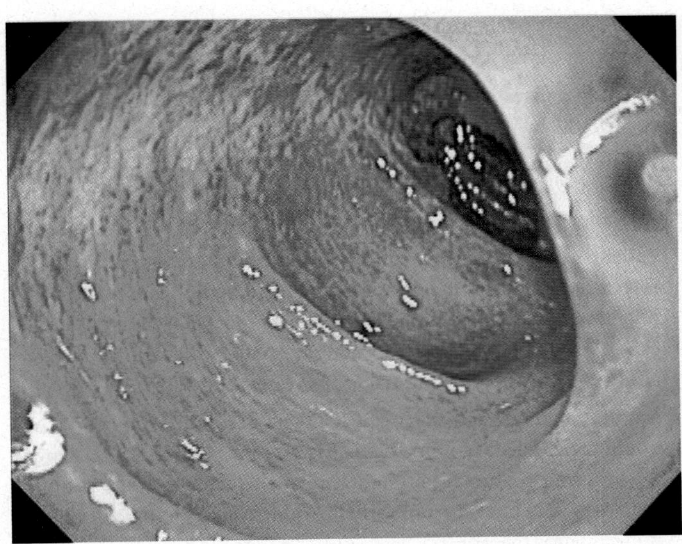

FIGURE 67-6 Ischemic colitis in an elderly patient. (*Reproduced with permission from Marvin Derezin, MD.*)

MANAGEMENT

FIRST LINE

MEDICATION

Treatment of acute disease in patients with UC (treatment algorithms can be found in the reference provided) is based on disease activity as follows[17]:

- Mild to moderate distal disease—Oral aminosalicylates (ASAs), topical mesalamine, or topical steroids.[6] SOR Ⓐ An oral 5-ASA agent can be a prodrug (e.g., sulfasalazine, 4 to 6 g/day), a drug with a pH-dependent coating (e.g., Asacol, 2.4 to 4.8 g/day), or a slow-release agent (Pentasa, 2 to 4 g/day). Mesalamine suppositories (1 g/day) are the best way to induce remission in patients with proctitis.[17] Rectal suppositories or enemas should also be used to improve medication delivery when treating active distal colitis, and a combination of oral and rectal mesalamine is better than monotherapy for stopping rectal bleeding (89% vs. 46% [oral only] or 69% [rectal only]).[6,17] SOR Ⓐ Fifty percent to 75% of patients will show clinical improvement with 2 g/day of 5-ASA, and a similar percentage will maintain remission with doses of 1.5 to 4 g/day.[2]
- Mild to moderate extensive colitis—Oral sulfasalazine (titrated to 4 to 6 g/day) or 5-ASA (up to 4.8 g/day) with or without topical therapy. SOR Ⓐ Oral steroids are generally reserved for patients refractory to combined oral and topical ASA therapy or for those with severe symptoms requiring more prompt improvement.[6] SOR Ⓐ
- Severe colitis—Patients presenting with toxicity should be admitted to the hospital for IV steroids (methylprednisolone, 40 to 60 mg/day, or hydrocortisone, 200 to 300 mg/day).[6,17] SOR Ⓒ Otherwise, treat with oral prednisone, oral ASA drugs, and topical medications with the addition of infliximab, an anti-tumor necrosis factor (TNF) biologic agent (5 mg/kg by intravenous infusion) if refractory to treatment and urgent hospitalization is not necessary.[6] SOR Ⓐ Infliximab is contraindicated in patients with active infection, untreated latent tuberculosis, preexisting demyelinating

disorder or optic neuritis, moderate to severe congestive heart failure, or current or recent malignancies.

- Fulminant disease—Patients should be treated as above with IV glucocorticoid and maintained without oral intake and with use of a decompression tube if small bowel ileus is present.[6] IV cyclosporine (2 to 4 mg/kg per day) or infliximab may be considered for patients who are not improving on maximal medical therapy as above.
- Patients with CD are treated similarly except that there is limited response to mesalamine or cyclosporin and better response to nutritional therapy. A research tool called the CD Activity Index can be used to monitor disease activity (online calculator available at http://www.ibdjohn.com/cdai/. Accessed May 2018).
- Mild to moderate active ileocolic CD—Budesonide (9 mg daily) or prednisone if distal colonic disease is present.[17] Nutrition therapy is the first-line treatment for children. Patients with weight loss or strictures may benefit from early introduction of biologic or immunomodulator therapy.[17]
- Severe CD in any location—Initial treatment with oral or intravenous steroids; anti–tumor necrosis factor therapy is reserved for patients who do not respond to initial therapy. In a single-center cohort study of 614 patients treated with infliximab, only 10.9% were not primary responders by 12 weeks, and sustained benefit was seen in 63% who received long-term treatment (mean follow-up: 55 months).[18] Management also includes nutritional support and treatment of iron deficiency.
- Side effects of biologic therapy include serious infections, induction of autoimmune phenomena, and neurotoxicity.[19] However, in a report of a cohort of 734 patients with IBD treated with infliximab, the most commonly observed systemic side effects were skin eruptions including psoriasiform eruptions in 20%; two patients developed tuberculosis, but none of the 16 patients with positive skin tests who received prophylaxis.[20]

SURGERY

Surgery (total proctocolectomy with ileostomy or continence-preserving operation, i.e., ileal pouch–anal anastomosis [IPAA]) is performed in approximately half of patients with UC within 10 years of disease onset. Indications for surgery in patients with IBD include[2,6]: SOR Ⓒ

- Intractable or fulminant disease.
- Toxic megacolon (UC).
- Massive hemorrhage.
- Colonic obstruction or perforation.
- Extracolonic disease.
- Colon cancer or dysplasia in flat mucosa,[8] SOR Ⓑ or for cancer prophylaxis.
- Stricture, refractory fistula, or abscess (CD).

SECOND LINE

NONPHARMACOLOGIC

- Dietary restriction based on IgG4 titers tested against 16 common food types using enzyme-linked immunosorbent assay (ELISA) improved CD activity and quality of life; the most commonly excluded food items were milk, beef, pork, and eggs.[21]

MEDICATIONS

- For patients with UC who have mild to moderate active proctitis and do not respond to topical mesalamine, adding a topical corticosteroid should be considered. In patients refractory to oral ASAs or topical corticosteroids, mesalamine enemas or suppositories may still be effective.[6] SOR Ⓐ An oral steroid (e.g., prednisone, 40 to 60 mg/day) or infliximab (induction regimen of 5 mg/kg IV at weeks 1, 2, and 6) can be added for patients with mild to moderate local disease who have an inadequate response to initial therapy; the latter is often reserved for patients who do not respond to or tolerate steroids.[6] SOR Ⓒ
- Mild to moderate extensive UC:
  - Immunomodulators (6-mercaptopurine and azathioprine) are effective for patients who do not respond to oral steroids and continue to have moderate disease.[6] SOR Ⓐ
  - Patients who are steroid refractory, intolerant, or steroid-dependent despite adequate doses of a thiopurine can be considered for infliximab induction as above.[6] SOR Ⓐ
  - In a randomized controlled trial (RCT) of infliximab monotherapy, azathioprine monotherapy, or the 2 drugs combined in 239 tumor necrosis factor-α antagonist–naive adults with moderate to severe UC, combination therapy was more likely to result in corticosteroid-free remission at 16 weeks than either monotherapy (39.7% vs. 22.1% with infliximab and 23.7% with azathioprine).[22]
- Severe UC—If patient fails to improve within 3 to 5 days of medical therapy, colectomy SOR Ⓑ or IV cyclosporine SOR Ⓐ should be considered.[6] Antibiotics have no proven efficacy without proven infection, and parenteral nutrition has not been shown to be of benefit as primary therapy for UC.[6] Patients with postsurgical pouchitis can be treated with metronidazole or ciprofloxacin.[2]
- Mild to moderate active ileocolic CD—For patients who do not tolerate steroids or in cases where steroids are ineffective, biologic therapy with infliximab, adalimumab, or certolizumab pegol is appropriate. Methotrexate (25 mg/week) is also effective.[17]
- Thalidomide may be a treatment option for patients with IBD who are refractory to other first- and second-line treatment.[23]

PROCEDURE

- Fecal microbiota transplantation has been tested in patients with UC and appears to improve clinical remission, but there are few RCTs.[24]

COMPLEMENTARY/ALTERNATIVE THERAPY

- *Tripterygium wilfordii* Hook F (TwHF), a traditional Chinese medicine for CD, at high dose (2 mg/kg daily), was more effective in reducing clinical recurrence than low-dose treatment or mesalazine (3 g/d) in one RCT of 137 patients (of 198 initially enrolled) (9.8% vs. 22% and 29%, respectively).[25] Side effects were more common for high-dose TwHF but not withdrawal due to adverse effects.

PROGNOSIS

- In UC (**Figure 67-7**), disease flares and remissions with mucosal healing occur; remission is seen in about half of patients within a year of onset.[1] Those who have complete clinical and endoscopic remission have a significantly decreased risk of colectomy.[1] Disease activity lessens over time with longer periods of remission. In a population study of 1575 patients with UC in Denmark, 13% had no relapse, 74% had 2 or more relapses, and 13% had active disease every year for 5 years after diagnosis.[26]

- The probability of colectomy over 25 years for those with UC is 20% to 30%.[1] Colectomy is not necessarily curative, as pouchitis episodes occur in half of these patients by 5 years postoperatively, and in up to 10% of cases, pouchitis is chronic and often refractory to antibiotic treatment.[1]
- Overall mortality is not increased for patients with UC, unless there is severe disease.[1] Although UC-related mortality from liver disease or colorectal cancer is increased, there is a decreased rate of death from pulmonary cancer and other tobacco-related diseases.[1]
- Recurrence postoperatively is the norm for patients with CD; only 5% have normal endoscopy at 10-years follow-up, and symptoms occur about 2 to 3 years after anatomical lesions are found.[27] Natural progression of the disease with or without surgery is variable with spontaneous and treatment-related remissions, especially of more superficial lesions. Only approximately 10% to 15% of patients have chronic continuous disease.[1]
- Most patients with CD (60% to 80%) require surgery by the time they have had the disease for 20 to 30 years (estimated at 3% to 5% per year) and greater than 10% eventually require fecal diversion, especially in patients with colorectal disease or anal stenosis.[1]
- Factors associated with poor prognosis in IBD are younger age and more extensive disease. Other factors associated with poor prognosis are pouchitis and extraintestinal manifestations at surgery (IPAA) for UC and need for steroids at presentation for CD.[1]
- Mortality rate for CD is slightly increased (standardized mortality ratio = 1.52); most deaths are connected to malnutrition, postoperative complications, and intestinal cancer.
- Both patients with UC and CD are at increased risk for colorectal cancer. The risk increases with duration and extent of disease and decreases following successful treatment.[28] Colorectal cancer is rare within the first 7 years of colitis onset and increases at a rate of approximately 0.5% to 1% per year thereafter, which is likely associated with histologic disease activity.[10] It is not clear if anti-inflammatory medications reduce this risk.
- Patients with cholestasis should be evaluated for primary sclerosing cholangitis and subsequent cholangiocarcinoma.[6]
- Bisphosphonates should be considered to protect against bone mineral loss in patients with IBD, especially if they are on daily steroids.[29]

FOLLOW-UP

- Support and patient education should be provided to address medication side effects, the uncertain nature of the disease, and potential

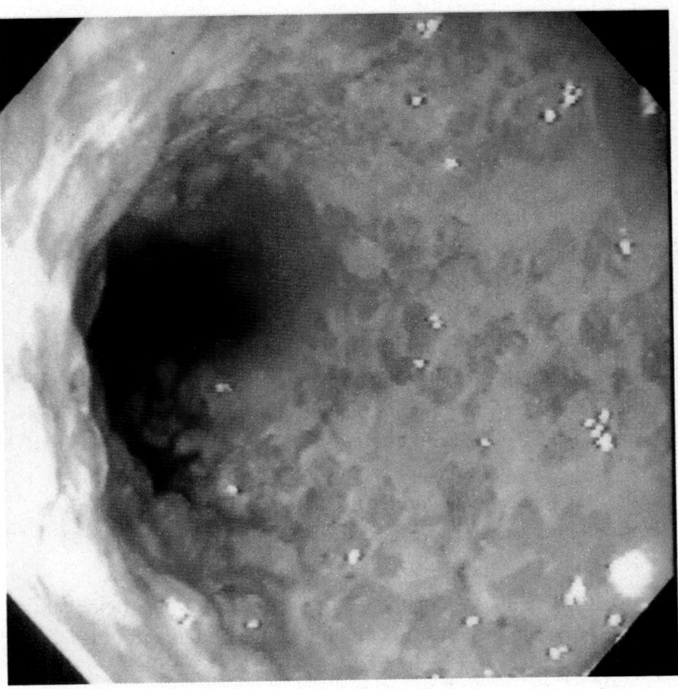

FIGURE 67-7 Ulcerative colitis in a 27-year-old man presenting with rectal bleeding. *(Reproduced with permission from Mark Koch, MD.)*

complications. Discuss medication adherence in patients with apparent inadequate treatment response.

- For maintenance of remission of mild to moderate distal disease—Mesalamine suppositories (proctitis) or enemas (distal colitis) can be dosed as infrequently as every third night.[6] SOR Ⓐ Patients, however, prefer oral therapy.[17] Sulfasalazine, mesalamine compounds, and balsalazide are also effective in maintaining remission; the combination of oral and topical mesalamine is more effective than either one alone.[6] SOR Ⓐ If these fail, thiopurines and infliximab may be effective.[6] SOR Ⓐ
- For maintenance of remission of mild to moderate extensive colitis—Sulfasalazine, olsalazine, mesalamine (2.4 g/day), and balsalazide are effective in reducing relapses; chronic steroid use should be avoided.[6] SOR Ⓐ Infliximab can be used for maintenance of remission in patients who respond to infliximab induction.[6] SOR Ⓐ For patients who relapse despite therapy, azathioprine or 6-mercaptopurine can be used (number needed to treat to prevent 1 recurrence is 5).[17]
- For patients with severe colitis, long-term remission is significantly enhanced with the addition of maintenance 6-mercaptopurine.[6] SOR Ⓑ
- Per the Toronto Consensus Statements for the Management of IBD in Pregnancy, women on 5-ASA, thiopurine, or anti-TNF monotherapy for maintenance should generally continue therapy throughout pregnancy unless very low risk; if low risk for recurrence, consider discontinuing anti-TNF therapy or switching from combination therapy to monotherapy.[30] Systemic corticosteroid or anti-TNF therapy is recommended for mild to moderate disease flares for women on optimized 5-ASA or thiopurine therapy.
- Periodic bone mineral density assessment is recommended for patients on long-term corticosteroid therapy (>3 months).[31] SOR Ⓐ
- Annual ophthalmologic examinations are recommended for patients on long-term corticosteroid therapy.[31] SOR Ⓒ
- Patients with long-standing IBD are at higher risk of developing colon dysplasia and cancer. For patients with pancolitis, the risk is 0.5% to 1% per year after 8 to 10 years of disease.[1] Surveillance colonoscopy with multiple biopsies should be performed every 1 to 2 years beginning after 8 to 10 years of disease.[6] SOR Ⓑ
- It is possible to monitor patients for intestinal ulcerations or thickening using noninvasive techniques (assays for C-reactive protein, fecal calprotectin and lactoferrin; videocapsule and MR imaging) and treat them earlier to prevent disease progression, but it is not known if this is a more effective strategy.[1,14] In addition, biomarkers may be useful for assessing mucosal healing, predicting relapse, and making therapeutic adjustments.[10]

PATIENT EDUCATION

- Patients should be informed about the unpredictable course of IBD and the need for frequent contact with an experienced provider for medical management, support, and surveillance.
- Smoking cessation should be stressed, particularly for patients with CD.[2]

PATIENT RESOURCES

- National Digestive Diseases Information Clearinghouse, *Ulcerative Colitis*—**https://www.niddk.nih.gov/health-information/digestive-diseases/ulcerative-colitis.**
- National Digestive Diseases Information Clearinghouse, *Crohn's Disease*—**https://www.niddk.nih.gov/health-information/digestive-diseases/crohns-disease.**
- Crohn's and Colitis Foundation of America—**http://www.crohnscolitisfoundation.org.**

PROVIDER RESOURCES

- *Ulcerative Colitis.* **http://emedicine.medscape.com/article/183084-overview.**
- *Crohn Disease.* **http://emedicine.medscape.com/article/172940-overview.**
- Burger D, Travis S. Conventional medical management of IBD. *Gastroenterology.* 2011;140(6):1827-1837.

REFERENCES

1. Cosnes J, Gower-Rousseau C, Seksik P, Cortot A. Epidemiology and natural history of inflammatory bowel diseases. *Gastroenterology.* 2011;140(6):1785-1794.
2. Friedman S, Blumberg RS. Inflammatory bowel disease. In: Kasper DL, Fauci AS, Hauser SL, et al, eds. *Harrison's Principles of Internal Medicine*, 19th ed. New York, NY: McGraw-Hill; 2014.
3. Abraham C, Cho J. Inflammatory bowel disease. *N Engl J Med.* 2009;361:2066-2078.
4. Garcia Rodriguez LA, Ruigomez A, Panes J. Acute gastroenteritis is followed by an increased risk of inflammatory bowel disease. *Gastroenterology.* 2006;130(6):1588-1594.
5. Cupi ML, Sarra M, Marafini I, et al. Plasma cells in the mucosa of patients with inflammatory bowel disease produce granzyme B and possess cytotoxic activities. *J Immunol.* 2014;192(12):6083-6091.
6. Kornbluth A, Sachar D; Practice Committee of the American College of Gastroenterology. Ulcerative colitis practice guidelines in adults: American College of Gastroenterology, Practice Parameters Committee. *Am J Gastroenterol.* 2010;105:501-523.
7. Levine JS, Burakoff R. Extraintestinal manifestations of inflammatory bowel disease. *Gastroenterol Hepatol (N Y).* 2011;7(4):235-241.
8. Langholz E, Munkholm P, Davidsen M, et al. Changes in extent of ulcerative colitis: a study on the course and prognostic factors. *Scand J Gastroenterol.* 1996;31:260-266.
9. American Society for Gastrointestinal Endoscopy Standards of Practice Committee, Shergill AK, Lightdale JR, Bruining DH, et al. The role of endoscopy in inflammatory bowel disease. *Gastrointest Endosc.* 2015;81(5):1101-1121.
10. Lewis JD. The utility of biomarkers in the diagnosis and therapy of inflammatory bowel disease. *Gastroenterology.* 2011;140(6):1817-1826.

11. van Rheenen PF, Van de Vijver E, Fidler V. Faecal calprotectin for screening of patients with suspected inflammatory bowel disease: diagnostic meta-analysis. *BMJ.* 2010;341:c3369.

12. Holtman GA, Lisman-van Leeuwen Y, Reitsma JB, Berger MY. Noninvasive tests for inflammatory bowel disease: a meta-analysis. *Pediatrics.* 2016 Jan;137(1).

13. Ananthakrishnan AN, McGinley EL, Binion DG. Excess hospitalization burden associated with *Clostridium difficile* in patients with inflammatory bowel disease. *Gut.* 2008;57:205-210.

14. Fletcher JG, Fider JL, Bruining DH, Huprich JE. New concepts in intestinal imaging for inflammatory bowel disease. *Gastroenterology.* 2011;140(6):1795-1806.

15. ACR Appropriateness Criteria. https://www.acr.org/Clinical-Resources/ACR-Appropriateness-Criteria. Accessed May 2018.

16. Zhu C, Ma X, Xue L, et al. Small intestine contrast ultrasonography for the detection and assessment of Crohn disease: a meta-analysis. *Medicine (Baltimore).* 2016 Aug;95(31):e4235.

17. Burger D, Travis S. Conventional medical management of inflammatory bowel disease. *Gastroenterology.* 2011;140(6): 1827-1837.

18. Schnitzler F, Fidder H, Ferrante M, et al. Long-term outcome of treatment with infliximab in 614 patients with Crohn's disease: results from a single-centre cohort. *Gut.* 2009;58:492-500.

19. Van Assche G, Vermeire S, Rutgeerts P. Safety issues with biological therapies for inflammatory bowel disease. *Curr Opin Gastroenterol.* 2006;22(4):370-376.

20. Fidder H, Schnitzler F, Ferrante M, et al. Long-term safety of infliximab for the treatment of inflammatory bowel disease: a single-centre cohort study. *Gut.* 2009;58(4):501-508.

21. Gunasekeera V, Mendall MA, Chan D, Kumar D. Treatment of Crohn's disease with an IgG4-guided exclusion diet: a randomized controlled trial. *Dig Dis Sci.* 2016;61(4):1148-1157.

22. Panaccione R, Ghosh S, Middleton S, et al. Combination therapy with infliximab and azathioprine is superior to monotherapy with either agent in ulcerative colitis. *Gastroenterology.* 2014;146(2): 392-400.e3.

23. Bramuzzo M, Ventura A, Martelossi S, Lazzerini M. Thalidomide for inflammatory bowel disease: systematic review. *Medicine (Baltimore).* 2016;95(30):e4239.

24. Sun D, Li W, Li S, et al. Fecal microbiota transplantation as a novel therapy for ulcerative colitis: a systematic review and meta-analysis. *Medicine (Baltimore).* 2016;95(23):e3765.

25. Sun J, Shen X, Dong J, et al. *Tripterygium wilfordii* Hook F as maintenance treatment for Crohn's disease. *Am J Med Sci.* 2015; 350(5):345-351.

26. Jess T, Riis L, Vind I, et al. Changes in clinical characteristics, course, and prognosis of inflammatory bowel disease during the last 5 decades: a population-based study from Copenhagen, Denmark. *Inflamm Bowel Dis.* 2007;13:481-489.

27. Olaison G, Smedh K, Sjodahl R. Natural course of Crohn's disease after ileocolic resection: endoscopically visualized ileal ulcers preceding symptoms. *Gut.* 1992;33:331-335.

28. Ullman TA, Itzkowitz SH. Intestinal inflammation and cancer. *Gastroenterology.* 2011;140(6):1807-1816.

29. Yao L, Wang H, Dong W, et al. Efficacy and safety of bisphosphonates in management of low bone density in inflammatory bowel disease: a meta-analysis. *Medicine (Baltimore).* 2017;96(3):e5861.

30. Nguyen GC, Seow CH, Maxwell C, et al. Toronto Consensus Statements for the Management of IBD in Pregnancy. *Gastroenterology.* 2016;150(3):734-757.

31. Lichtenstein GR, Abreu MT, Cohen R, Tremaine W. American Gastroenterological Association Institute medical position statement on corticosteroids, immunomodulators, and infliximab in inflammatory bowel disease. *Gastroenterology.* 2006;130(3):935-939.

68 HEMORRHOIDS

Mindy A. Smith, MD, MS
Jeffrey H. Baker, MD

PATIENT STORY

A 42-year-old woman presents to the office with rectal pressure and occasional bright red blood on the toilet paper when wiping after bowel movements (**Figure 68-1**). She has had difficulty with constipation off and on for many years and had large hemorrhoids during her last pregnancy. Physical examination confirms the diagnosis of external hemorrhoids.

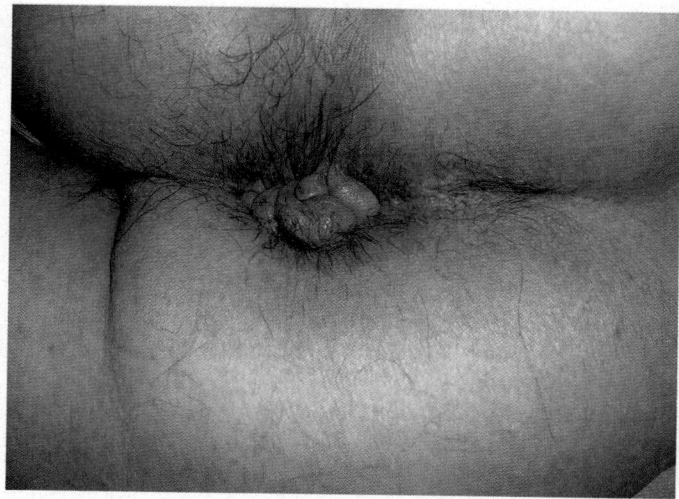

FIGURE 68-1 External hemorrhoid that is symptomatic. The patient had some bleeding with bowel movements. (*Reproduced with permission from Richard P. Usatine, MD.*)

INTRODUCTION

Hemorrhoids are cushions of highly vascular structures found within the submucosa of the anal canal. They become pathologic when swollen or inflamed.

SYNONYMS

Piles.

EPIDEMIOLOGY

- More than 1 million people in Western civilization suffer from hemorrhoids each year.[1]
- Estimated at 5% prevalence in the general population.[2]
- Approximately half of those older than age 50 years have experienced hemorrhoidal symptoms at some time.[2]
- More frequent in whites and in those of higher socioeconomic status.[2]

ETIOLOGY AND PATHOPHYSIOLOGY

- Three hemorrhoidal cushions (comprised of subepithelial connective tissue, elastic tissue, blood vessels, and smooth muscle) surround and support distal anastomoses between the terminal branches of the superior and middle rectal arteries and the superior, middle, and inferior rectal veins.[2] The hemorrhoidal cushions have several functions, including maintaining fecal continence by engorging with blood and closing the anal canal and by protecting the anal sphincter during defecation.
- Hemorrhoidal tissue provides important sensory information, enabling the differentiation between solid, liquid, and gas and subsequent decision to evacuate.[2]
- Abnormal swelling of the anal cushions can occur from several causes (see "Risk Factors" below) resulting in increased pressure, with dilation and engorgement of the arteriovenous plexuses.

Increased pressure can lead to stretching of the suspensory muscles, laxity of connective tissue, and eventual prolapse of rectal tissue through the anal canal.[2] The engorged anal mucosa is easily traumatized, leading to rectal bleeding. Prolapse predisposes to incarceration and strangulation.

- Hemorrhoids are classified with respect to their position relative to the dentate line.
  - Internal hemorrhoids (**Figure 68-2**) develop above the dentate line and are covered by columnar epithelium of anal mucosa. Internal hemorrhoids lack somatic sensory innervation.
  - External hemorrhoids (**Figure 68-1**) arise distal to the dentate line. They are covered by stratified squamous epithelium and receive somatic sensory innervation from the inferior rectal nerve.
- Hemorrhoids are further classified into four stages of disease severity[1,2]:
  - Stage I—Enlargement and bleeding
  - Stage II—Protrusion of hemorrhoids with spontaneous reduction
  - Stage III—Protrusion of hemorrhoids with manual reduction possible
  - Stage IV—Irreducible protrusion of hemorrhoids usually containing both internal and external components with or without acute thrombosis or strangulation

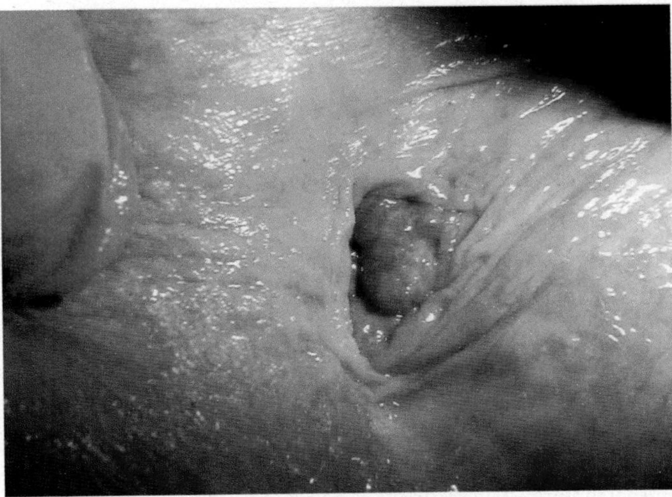

FIGURE 68-2 A large prolapsed internal hemorrhoid. *(Reproduced with permission from Charlie Goldberg, MD, and the Regents of the University of California.)*

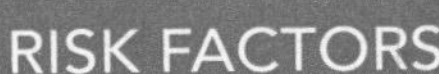

RISK FACTORS

- Family history of hemorrhoids.
- Personal history of constipation, diarrhea, and/or prolonged straining at stool.
- Pregnancy.
- Prolonged sitting or heavy lifting.

DIAGNOSIS

CLINICAL FEATURES

- Bleeding described as bright red blood (a result of the high blood oxygen content within the arteriovenous anastomoses) seen in the toilet or with wiping after bowel movements.
- Protrusion/mass (see **Figure 68-1**).
- Pain described as a dull ache or severe if thrombosed.
- Inability to maintain personal hygiene/staining/soiling due to prolapse.
- Pruritus, also due to prolapse.
- Diagnosis is made on visual inspection and anoscopy, with and without straining:
  - Physical findings of swollen blood vessels protruding from the anus (see **Figure 68-1**).
  - Excoriations may also be seen on the skin surrounding the anus.
  - A thrombosed hemorrhoid will be tender and firm and appear as a circular purplish bulge adjacent to the anal opening (**Figure 68-3**). There may be a black discoloration if there is accompanying necrosis.
  - Internal hemorrhoids may be visualized on anoscopy as swollen purple blood vessels arising above the dentate line.

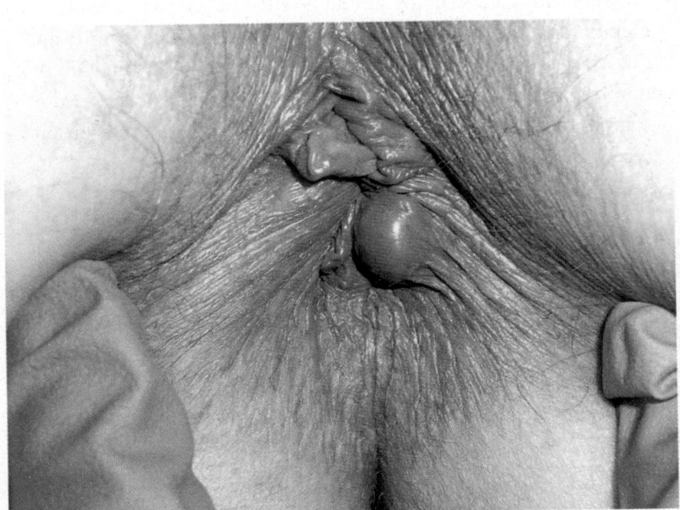

FIGURE 68-3 Thrombosed external hemorrhoid prior to elliptical excision and healing by secondary intention. Note how the hemorrhoid is at the typical 5 o'clock position. *(Reproduced with permission from Yu Wah, MD.)*

- Other physical findings that may accompany hemorrhoids are redundant tissue and skin tags (**Figure 68-4**) from old thrombosed external hemorrhoids.

DIFFERENTIAL DIAGNOSIS

- Rectal prolapse—Full-thickness circumferential protrusion appearing as a bluish, tender perianal mass. More common in women (sixfold higher incidence) and associated with other pelvic-floor disorders (e.g., cystocele, urinary incontinence). It can present as an anal mass with bleeding.[1]
- Condyloma acuminata (see Chapter 139, Genital Warts)—Appear as flesh-colored, exophytic lesions on perianal skin. They may be flat, verrucous, or pedunculated.
- Anal tumors—Tumors in the rectosigmoid region are associated with hematochezia, tenesmus (i.e., urgency with a feeling of incomplete evacuation), and narrow-caliber stool; a firm mass may be found on rectal examination or seen outside the rectum.
- Inflammatory bowel disease (see Chapter 67, Inflammatory Bowel Disease)—Associated diarrhea, rectal bleeding, tenesmus, passage of mucus, and cramping abdominal pain.
- Signs of infection or abscess formation—Tender mass, sometimes feeling fluctuant, with overlying skin erythema (**Figure 68-5**). If cellulitis is also present, skin may have a woody, hard feel. Fistulas may also form and an opening may be seen on the buttock.
- Fissures—A cut or tear occurring in the anus that extends upwards into the anal canal. Common and occurring at all ages; fissures cause pain during bowel movements in addition to bleeding (**Figure 68-4**).

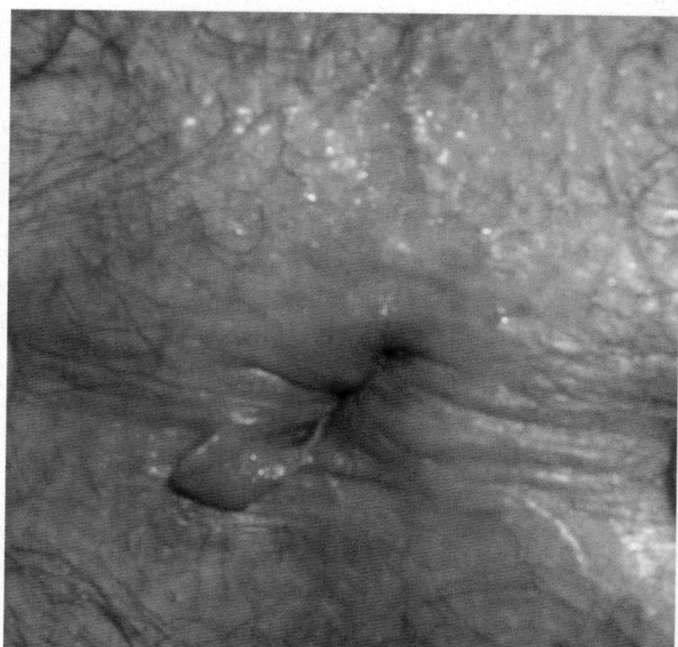

FIGURE 68-4 Rectal fissure with prominent skin tag. (*Reproduced with permission from Charlie Goldberg, MD, copyright University of California, San Diego.*)

MANAGEMENT

NONPHARMACOLOGIC

- Patients with hemorrhoids should be encouraged to increase dietary fiber and/or add a fiber supplement to reduce severity and duration of symptoms. In a Cochrane review of seven small randomized controlled trials (RCTs), fiber supplements decreased symptoms (e.g., pain, itching, and bleeding) by 53% in the group receiving fiber.[3] SOR Ⓐ
- There are no data supporting use of sitz baths.

MEDICATIONS

- Short course of a topical steroid cream or suppositories, twice daily. SOR Ⓒ
- For acute thrombosed external hemorrhoids, a small RCT of 98 patients treated nonsurgically found improved complete pain relief at 7 days with a combination of topical nifedipine 0.3% and lidocaine 1.5% compared with lidocaine alone (86% vs. 50%, respectively).[4] Resolution at 14 days was reported for 92% versus 45.8%, respectively.
- Use stool softener and encourage adequate fluid intake if constipation is a factor. SOR Ⓒ

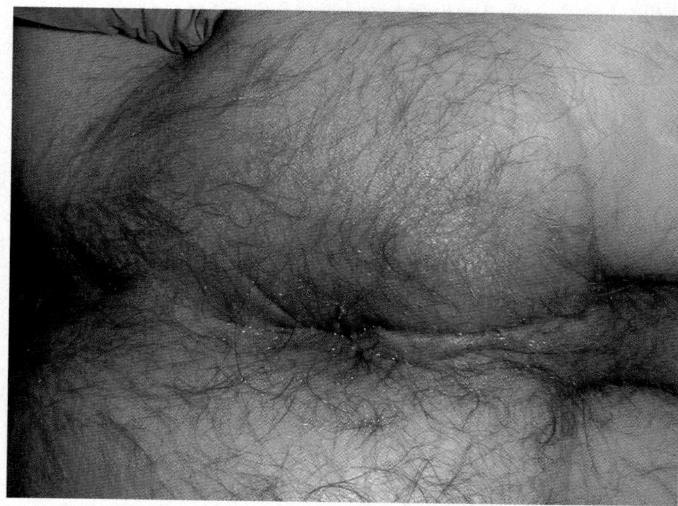

FIGURE 68-5 Perirectal abscess: Note surrounding erythema that extends onto the right buttock. (*Reproduced with permission from Charlie Goldberg, MD, copyright University of California, San Diego.*)

PROCEDURES

- Internal hemorrhoids
  - Data are limited to retrospective studies and case series for most procedures.
  - Stages I to II hemorrhoids can be treated with sclerotherapy (1 to 5 mL of sclerosing agent such as sodium tetradecyl sulfate injected via a 25-gauge needle into the submucosa of the hemorrhoidal complex).[1] Sclerotherapy, however, carries a high risk of postprocedure pain (70%). Urinary retention, abscess formation, and sepsis have also been reported; the author of a review recommends that only two sites be sclerosed at one time to reduce risk.[2] Recurrence rates are as high as 30%.[2]
  - Stages II and III internal hemorrhoids can be treated with rubber band ligation. Two bands are placed around the engorged tissue, producing ischemia and fibrosis of the hemorrhoid.
    - Authors of a meta-analysis of RCTs assessing two or more treatment modalities for symptomatic hemorrhoids found rubber band ligation superior to sclerotherapy for stage I to II hemorrhoids with no difference in complication rate.[5]
    - In a Cochrane review of three methodologically poor trials comparing excisional hemorrhoidectomy with banding for grade III hemorrhoids, results with hemorrhoidectomy were better than banding for resolution of symptoms but were associated with increased postprocedural pain, higher complication rate, and more time off work.[6]
    - Patients on anticoagulants may be better candidates for another procedure with less bleeding risk.[2]
    - Success rates of 50% to 100% are reported, depending on time to follow-up; there is a recurrence rate of 68% at 4 to 5 years.[2]
    - Complications are uncommon (<1%) and include pain, abscess formation, urinary retention, bleeding, band slippage, and sepsis.[2]
    - Use of local anesthetic infiltration in the hemorrhoidal segment may significantly reduce postprocedure pain.[7]
  - Lower stage hemorrhoids can also be treated with infrared photocoagulation (IPC), bipolar electrocautery, laser therapy, or low-voltage direct current (the last works for higher-grade hemorrhoids). IPC is initially successful in 88% to 100% of patients.[2]
- External hemorrhoids
  - Based on retrospective studies, excision is the most effective treatment for thrombosed external hemorrhoids. This procedure is associated with lower recurrence rates (6.5% in one study) and faster symptom resolution.[8] SOR B
  - Acutely thrombosed external hemorrhoids may also be safely excised in the office or emergency department for patients who present within 48 to 72 hours of symptom onset. A local anesthetic containing epinephrine is used, followed by elliptical incision (not extending beyond the anal verge or deeper than the cutaneous layer) and excision of the thrombosed hemorrhoid and overlying skin. Simple incision and clot evacuation is inadequate therapy for complete resolution, although it may relieve pain. A pressure dressing is applied for several hours, after which time the wound is left to heal by secondary intention.
  - Intrasphincteric injection of botulinum toxin provided more effective pain relief at 24 hours than saline injection for patients with thrombosed external hemorrhoids not undergoing surgery.[9]

REFERRAL FOR SURGERY

- Surgeries for hemorrhoids include open and closed excision, harmonic scalpel, LigaSure tissue-sealing device, Doppler-guided transanal hemorrhoidal ligature, and stapled hemorrhoidopexy.[2] The ultimate need for surgical management is uncommon (5% to 10%).[2] The major complication is postoperative pain that can delay work return for 2 to 4 weeks.[2]
- Indications for surgery include:
  - Failure of nonsurgical treatment (persistent bleeding or chronic symptoms).[8]
  - Grades III and IV hemorrhoids with severe symptoms.[8]
  - Combined internal and external hemorrhoids with significant prolapse (grades III and IV).[10]
  - Presence of other anorectal conditions (e.g., anal fissure or fistula) requiring surgery.
  - Patient preference.
- Stage IV hemorrhoids can be treated with traditional excision or surgery using stapling. Authors of a Cochrane review of 12 RCTs comparing conventional hemorrhoidectomy with stapling hemorrhoidopexy in patients with grades I to III hemorrhoids found a lower long-term recurrence rate (9 of 476 [1.9%] vs. 37 of 479 [7.7%], respectively) in patients who had conventional hemorrhoidectomy (number needed to treat = 17).[11] Another meta-analysis of 14 RCTs confirmed higher rates of prolapse recurrence with stapling (odds ratio: 5.5).[12] In an open-label RCT in patients with grades II to IV hemorrhoids, stapling hemorrhoidopexy compared to excision caused less postoperative pain, had a similar complication rate, but was associated with a diminished quality of life score after 24 months.[13]
- Use of perianal local anesthetic infiltration provides significant postoperative pain relief.[14] SOR A
  - Combination acetaminophen and nonsteroidal anti-inflammatory agents or cyclooxygenase (COX)-2–selective inhibitors should be used when possible for pain control, as opioids may be constipating. There are no data supporting any particular drug over another.[11] SOR B
  - Stapled hemorrhoidectomy reduces pain compared with other surgical techniques.[11] SOR A
  - Other medications that can be considered as analgesic adjuncts are laxatives and metronidazole started before surgery.[11] SOR A
- Complications of surgery include transient urinary retention (up to 34%), infection (rare), bleeding (2%), fecal incontinence (if sphincter muscle damage), anal stenosis, and rectal prolapse.

PROGNOSIS

Most hemorrhoids resolve spontaneously or with medical therapy alone. The recurrence rate with nonsurgical therapy is 10% to 50% over a 5-year period and, for surgical treatment, less than 10%.

FOLLOW-UP

- After excision of a thrombosed hemorrhoid, patient instructions should include initial bed rest for several hours, sitz baths 3 times daily, stool softeners, and topical or systemic analgesia. SOR C The patient should return in 48 to 72 hours for a wound check.

- Similar instructions are used for patients postoperatively with respect to bed rest (1 to 2 days), sitz baths, stool softeners, and adequate fluid intake. Pain control is discussed above.

PATIENT EDUCATION

- Patients should be counseled to avoid aggravating factors including constipation and prolonged sitting.
- Advise patients who elect rubber band ligation that complications, based on one follow-up study, include pain (at 1 week, 75% of patients were pain-free and 7% were still experiencing moderate-to-severe pain), rectal bleeding (in 65% on the day after banding, persisting in 24% at 1 week), and relatively low satisfaction (only 59% were satisfied with their experience and would undergo the procedure again).[15]
- Advise patients who elect or are recommended for surgery about potential complications of infection, thrombosis, ulceration, and incontinence.

PATIENT RESOURCES

- **http://www.nlm.nih.gov/medlineplus/hemorrhoids.html.**
- **https://www.niddk.nih.gov/health-information/digestive-diseases/hemorrhoids.**
- **http://www.aafp.org/afp/2011/0715/p215.html.**

PROVIDER RESOURCES

- *Hemorrhoids*—**http://emedicine.medscape.com/article/775407.**

REFERENCES

1. Gerhart SL, Bulkley G. Common diseases of the colon and anorectum and mesenteric vascular insufficiency. In: Kasper DL, Braunwald E, Fauci AS, et al, eds. *Harrison's Principles of Internal Medicine*, 16th ed. New York. NY: McGraw-Hill; 2005:1801-1802.
2. Sneider EB, Maykel JA. Diagnosis and management of symptomatic hemorrhoids. *Surg Clin North Am.* 2010;90(1):17-32.
3. Alonso-Coello P, Guyatt G, Heels-Ansdell D, et al. Laxatives for the treatment of hemorrhoids. *Cochrane Database Syst Rev.* 2005;(4):CD004649.
4. Perrotti P, Antropoli C, Molino D, et al. Conservative treatment of acute thrombosed external hemorrhoids with topical nifedipine. *Dis Colon Rectum.* 2001;44:405-409.
5. MacRae H, McLeod R. Comparison of hemorrhoidal treatments: a meta-analysis. *Can J Surg.* 1997;40(1):14-17.
6. Shanmugam V, Thaha MA, Rabindranath KS, et al. Rubber band ligation versus excisional haemorrhoidectomy for haemorrhoids. *Cochrane Database Syst Rev.* 2005;3:CD005034.
7. Sajid MS, Bhatti MI, Caswell J, et al. Local anaesthetic infiltration for the rubber band ligation of early symptomatic haemorrhoids: a systematic review and meta-analysis. *Updates Surg.* 2015;67(3):3-9.
8. Mounsey AL, Henry SL. Clinical inquiries. Which treatments work best for hemorrhoids? *J Fam Pract.* 2009;58(9):492-493.
9. Patti R, Arcara M, Bonventre S, et al. Randomized clinical trial of botulinum toxin injection for pain relief in patients with thrombosed external haemorrhoids. *Br J Surg.* 2008;95(11):1339-1343.
10. Rivadeneira DE, Steele SR, Tement C; on behalf of the Standards Practice Task Force of the American Society of colon and Rectal Surgeons, et al. Practice parameters for the management of hemorrhoids. *Dis Colon Rectum.* 2011;54:1059-1064.
11. Jayaraman S, Colquhoun PH, Malthaner RA. Stapled versus conventional surgery for hemorrhoids. *Cochrane Database Syst Rev.* 2006;(4):CD005393.
12. Giordano P, Gravante G, Sorge R, et al. Long-term outcomes of stapled hemorrhoidopexy vs conventional hemorrhoidectomy: a meta-analysis of randomized controlled trials. *Arch Surg.* 2009;144(3):266-272.
13. Watson AJ, Hudson J, Wood J; eTHoS Study Group. Comparison of stapled haemorrhoidopexy with traditional excisional surgery for haemorrhoidal disease (eTHoS): a pragmatic, multicenter, randomised controlled trial. *Lancet.* 2016;388(10058):2375-2385.
14. Joshi GP, Neugebauer EA; PROSPECT Collaboration. Evidence-based management of pain after haemorrhoidectomy surgery. *Br J Surg.* 2010;97(8):1155-1168.
15. Watson NF, Liptrott S, Maxwell-Armstrong CA. A prospective audit of early pain and patient satisfaction following out-patient band ligation of haemorrhoids. *Ann R Coll Surg Engl.* 2006;88(3):275-279.

PART X

GENITOURINARY

Strength of Recommendation (SOR)	Definition
A	Recommendation based on consistent and good-quality patient-oriented evidence.*
B	Recommendation based on inconsistent or limited-quality patient-oriented evidence.*
C	Recommendation based on consensus, usual practice, opinion, disease-oriented evidence, or case series for studies of diagnosis, treatment, prevention, or screening.*

*See Appendix A on pages 1603–1606 for further information.

69 URINARY SEDIMENT

Mindy A. Smith, MD, MS
Richard P. Usatine, MD

PATIENT STORY

A 47-year-old woman presents to the office with severe right flank pain that does not radiate. Dipstick urinalysis shows hematuria, and microscopic examination confirms the presence of many red blood cells per high-power field (**Figure 69-1**). There is no pyuria or bacteriuria. The physician gives her some pain medication and sends her to get a non-contrast helical computed tomography (CT). The CT scan shows a stone in the right ureter and some mild hydronephrosis. Fortunately for the patient, she passes the stone when urinating after the imaging study is complete.

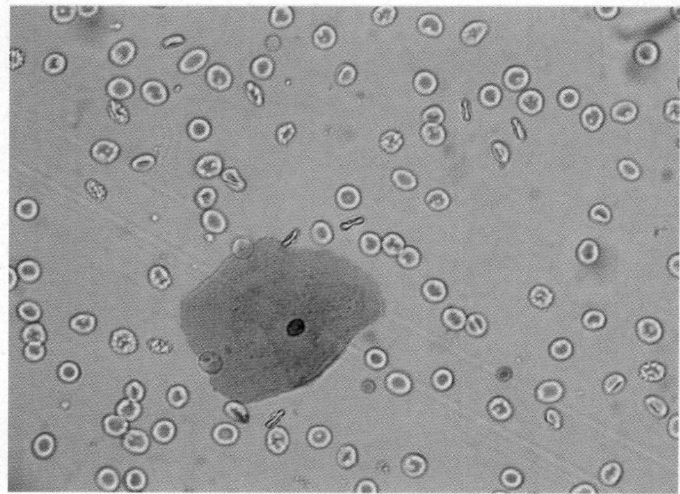

FIGURE 69-1 Red blood cells (RBCs) seen in the urine of a woman passing a kidney stone. Some of the RBCs are crenated and there is one epithelial cell visible. (*Reproduced with permission from Richard P. Usatine, MD.*)

INTRODUCTION

Examination of the urinary sediment is a test frequently done for evaluation of patients with suspected genetic/intrinsic (e.g., systemic lupus nephritis, renal sarcoidosis, sickle cell disease, glomerulonephritis, interstitial nephritis), anatomic (e.g., arteriovenous malformation), obstructive (e.g., kidney or bladder stones, benign prostatic hypertrophy), infectious, metabolic (e.g., coagulopathy), traumatic, or neoplastic disease of the urinary tract. Potential findings of red or white blood cells, casts, bacteria, or neoplastic cells help in directing further evaluation of a patient's problem.

EPIDEMIOLOGY

- A finding of microscopic hematuria (defined by the American Urological Association [AUA] as ≥3 red blood cells [RBCs]/high-power field [HPF]) on a single microscopic urinalysis in an asymptomatic person is common and most often a result of menses, allergy, exercise, viral illness, or mild trauma.[1,2]
- One study of servicemen, conducted for a period of 10 years, found an incidence of 38%.[1]
- In one UK population study, first episode of hematuria resulted in a noncancer or cancer diagnosis within 90 days in 17.5% of women (95% confidence interval [CI], 16.4% to 18.6%) and 18.3% of men (95% CI, 17.4% to 19.3%).[3]
- Persistent (>3 RBCs/HPF over 3 specimens) and significant hematuria (>100 RBCs/HPF or gross hematuria) was associated with significant lesions in 9.1% of more than 1000 patients.[1]
- In a review of hematuria, approximately 5% of patients with significant microscopic hematuria (>3 RBCs/HPF on 2 of 3 properly collected specimens during a 2- to 3-week period)[3] and up to 40% of patients with gross hematuria had a neoplasm.[4]
- Isolated pyuria (>2 to 10 white blood cells per high-power field [WBCs/HPF]) is uncommon, as inflammatory processes in the urinary tract are usually associated with hematuria.[1]

- Glomerulonephritides, although rare, account for about 20% of cases of chronic kidney disease and present with variable amounts of proteinuria and hematuria.[5] Annual incidence for IgA nephropathy is estimated as 2.5 cases per 100,000 adults, 1.2 per 100,000 for membranous glomerulonephritis, 0.6–0.8 per 100,000 for minimal change disease and focal segmental glomerulosclerosis, and 0.2 per 100,000 for membranoproliferative glomerulonephritis.
- In a laboratory study from 88 institutions, 62.5% of urinalysis tests received a manual microscopic evaluation of the urinary sediment, usually triggered by an abnormal urinalysis. New information was obtained 65% of the time because of the manual examination.[6]

ETIOLOGY AND PATHOPHYSIOLOGY

- Hematuria (**Figure 69-1**) has many causes including[1]:
    - Idiopathic (increasing incidence in the young)
    - Stones
    - Neoplasms (increasing incidence with increase in age)
    - Trauma
    - Infection/inflammation including acute cystitis, urethritis, pyelonephritis, and prostatitis
    - Benign prostatic hypertrophy
    - Metabolic abnormalities, including hypercalcemia and hyperuricemia
    - Glomerular diseases such as immunoglobulin (Ig) A nephropathy, hereditary nephritis, and thin basement membrane disease
- Hematuria with dysmorphic RBCs or RBC casts (**Figure 69-2**) and excess protein excretion (>500 mg/dL) indicates glomerulonephritis.
- Gross hematuria suggests a postrenal source in the collecting system.
- Pyuria (**Figure 69-3**) is often the result of urinary tract infection (UTI). Sterile pyuria can be seen with tuberculosis (TB); genitourinary TB is seen in approximately 30% of extrapulmonary TB cases and can be diagnosed using polymerase chain reaction techniques or identifying acid-fast bacilli on urine culture.[7]
    - The presence of bacteria (>10^2 organisms per mL or >10^5 using a midstream urine specimen) suggests infection. A urinalysis with 10 bacteria per HPF is highly suggestive (specificity 99%) of infection (positive likelihood ratio [LR+] 85).[3]
    - Asymptomatic bacteriuria is found in 4% to 15% of pregnant women, usually *Escherichia coli*.
    - The presence of WBC casts (**Figure 69-4**) with bacteria indicates pyelonephritis.
- WBCs and/or WBC casts can be seen in tubulointerstitial processes such as interstitial nephritis, systemic lupus erythematosus, or transplant rejection.
- Urinary casts are formed only in the distal convoluted tubule (DCT) or in the collecting duct (distal nephron).
- Hyaline casts are formed from mucoprotein secreted by the tubular epithelial cells within the nephrons. These translucent casts are the most common type of cast and can be seen in normal persons after vigorous exercise or with dehydration. Low urine flow and concentrated urine from dehydration can contribute to the formation of hyaline casts (**Figure 69-5**).

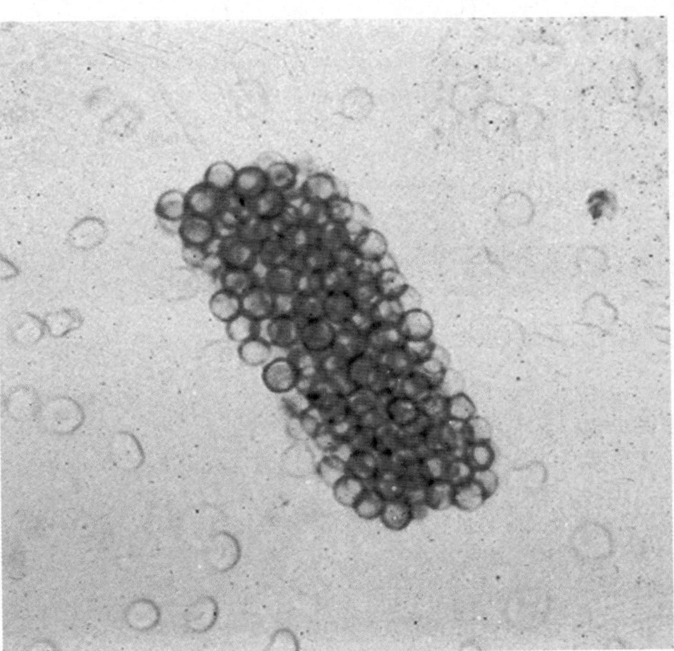

FIGURE 69-2 An RBC cast caused by bleeding into the tubule from the glomerulus. These casts are seen in glomerulonephritis, IgA nephropathy, lupus nephritis, Goodpasture syndrome, and Wegener granulomatosis. RBC casts are always pathologic. *(Reproduced with permission from Agnes B. Fogo, MD, Vanderbilt University.)*

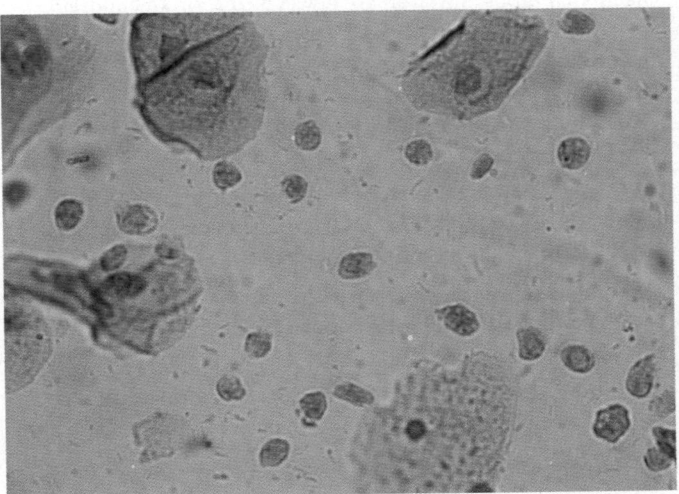

FIGURE 69-3 Pyuria and bacteriuria in a woman with a urinary tract infection (UTI). A simple stain was added to the wet mount of spun urine. Although there are epithelial cells present, the culture demonstrated a true UTI and not merely a contaminated urine. *(Reproduced with permission from Richard P. Usatine, MD.)*

- Granular casts are the second most common type of cast seen (**Figure 69-6**). These casts can result from the breakdown of cellular casts or the inclusion of aggregates of albumin or immunoglobulin light chains. They can be classified as fine or coarse based on the size of the inclusions. There is no diagnostic significance to the classification of fine or coarse.

RISK FACTORS

- Risk factors for cancer in patients with microscopic hematuria include[4]:
  - Smoking
  - Age older than 40 years
  - Medical history of gross hematuria, urologic disease, or pelvic radiation
  - Occupational exposure to chemicals or dyes
  - Analgesic abuse
- Constipation (for UTI in children).
- Family history for glomerulonephritis.

DIAGNOSIS

CLINICAL FEATURES

- Other signs and symptoms of glomerular disease include various degrees of renal failure, edema, oliguria, and hypertension; massive weight gain and edema can occur with nephrotic syndrome.[5]
- Hematuria is often asymptomatic in patients with glomerular disease or metabolic abnormalities. Renal stones can cause pain in the ipsilateral flank and/or abdomen with radiation to the ipsilateral groin, testicle, or vulva or irritative symptoms of frequency, urgency, and dysuria, if located in the bladder.
- Symptoms of UTI include dysuria, nocturia, urgency, frequency, offensive odor of urine, or a combination of these; positive likelihood ratios, however, are low (1.3 to 2.3).[8] In children, pain (abdominal pain [LR+ 6.3; 95% CI, 2.5 to 16.0] or back pain [LR+ 3.6; 95% CI, 2.1 to 6.1]), in addition to dysuria, frequency, or both (LR+ 2.2 to 2.8), and new-onset urinary incontinence (LR+ 4.6; 95% CI, 2.8 to 7.6) increased the likelihood of a UTI.[9]
- In infants, findings of previous UTI (LR+ 2.3 to 2.9), fever higher than 40°C (104°F) (LR+ 3.2 to 3.3), and suprapubic tenderness (LR+ 4.4) were the most useful for identifying UTI.
- Symptoms of pyelonephritis include chills and rigor, fever, nausea and vomiting, and flank pain; positive likelihood ratios are 1.5 to 2.5.
- Family history of renal failure or microscopic hematuria or history of trauma, weight loss, and changes in urine volume may be useful.

LABORATORY TESTING AND IMAGING

The work-up for persistent or significant hematuria, including hematuria in patients taking antiplatelet or anticoagulant therapy, includes the following[1]:

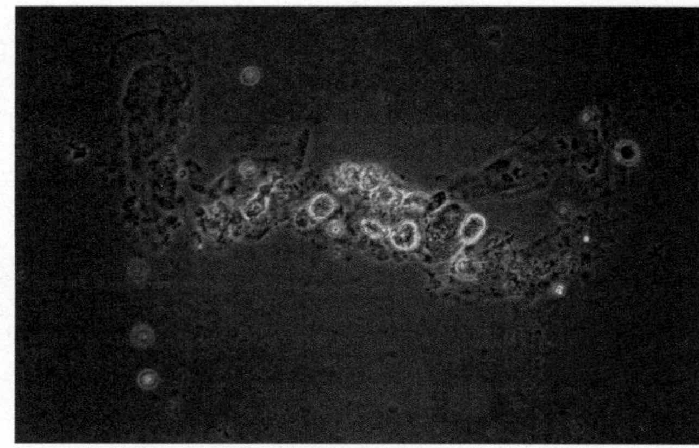

FIGURE 69-4 WBC casts seen in pyelonephritis. These can be differentiated from a clump of WBCs by their cylindrical shape and the presence of a hyaline matrix. (*Reproduced with permission from Agnes B. Fogo, MD, Vanderbilt University.*)

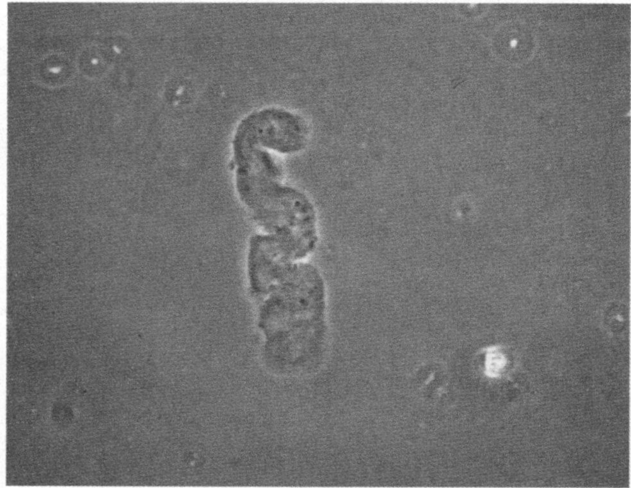

FIGURE 69-5 Hyaline casts are translucent and proteinaceous. These are the most common casts found in the urine and can be seen in normal individuals. Concentrated urine with low flow, usually caused by dehydration, exercise, and/or diuretics, can lead to hyaline cast formation. (*Reproduced with permission from Agnes B. Fogo, MD, Vanderbilt University.*)

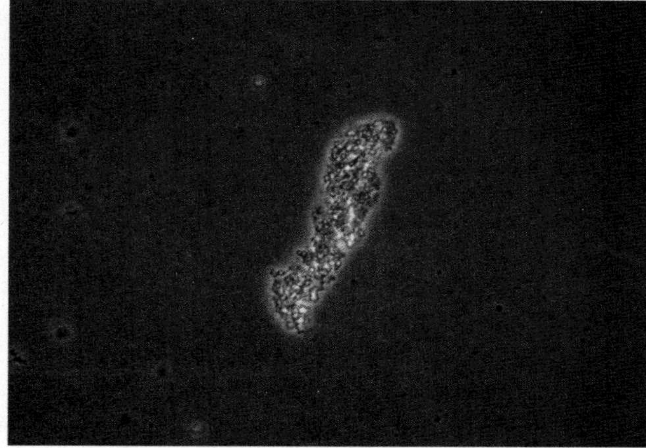

FIGURE 69-6 Coarse granular cast. All granular casts indicate underlying renal disease. These are nonspecific and may be seen in diverse renal conditions. (*Reproduced with permission from Agnes B. Fogo, MD, Vanderbilt University.*)

- Urinary sediment looking for dysmorphic cells or RBC casts (see **Figure 69-2**) and a 24-hour urine sample for proteinuria.
  - If positive, suspect glomerular disease and consider blood cultures, antiglomerular basement membrane antibody, antineutrophil cytoplasmic antibody, phospholipase A2 receptor (membranous glomerulonephritis), complement, cryoglobulins, hepatitis serologies, Venereal Disease Research Laboratory (VDRL), HIV, and antistreptolysin O; a renal biopsy is required for definitive diagnosis of glomerulonephritis.[5]
  - If negative and the sediment contains WBCs (see **Figure 69-3**) or WBC casts (see **Figure 69-4**), suspect infection and obtain a urine culture and susceptibility test if pyelonephritis is suspected; *E. coli* is the most common organism (more than 80%) in uncomplicated cystitis. WBCs seen in conjunction with many epithelial cells, particularly in women, can indicate a contaminated specimen, and a new clean catch urine specimen should be obtained if possible.
  - If negative and no WBCs, obtain a hemoglobin electrophoresis, urine cytology, urinalysis (UA) from family members looking for hematuria or signs of glomerular disease, and a 24-hour urine for calcium and uric acid.
- The AUA recommends obtaining renal function testing, cystoscopy, and CT urography after potential causes of hematuria such as infection, menstruation, and urologic procedures are ruled out and repeat urinalysis confirms microscopic hematuria after treatment of identified causes.[2] If the patient is unable to undergo CT urography, consider magnetic resonance (MR) urogram or retrograde pyelograms in combination with non-contrast CT, MRI, or ultrasound.
- In all adult patients with persistent hematuria not due to vigorous exercise, presence of infection or viral illness, or present or recent menstruation, the American College of Radiology (ACR) recommends obtaining CT urography (CT abdomen and pelvis without and with contrast).[10] In patients with generalized renal parenchymal disease and in children, ultrasound of the kidneys and bladder is recommended.
  - If the above is negative or high risk for cancer, perform cystoscopy.
  - If the above is positive, an open renal biopsy may be indicated.
  - If the above is negative, consider periodic follow-up (6, 12, 24, and 36 months).
- If RBC casts (see **Figure 69-2**) are seen on UA in addition to proteinuria, also consider nephrotic syndrome caused by diabetes or amyloidosis.
- Note that RBC casts are fragile and are best seen in a fresh urine specimen (see **Figure 69-2**).

MANAGEMENT

Treatment will depend on the underlying etiology:

- The American College of Physicians (ACP) recommends urology referral for patients with gross hematuria, even if self-limited, and consider referral for cystoscopy and imaging in adults with microscopically confirmed hematuria in the absence of some demonstrable benign cause.[11]
- Cystitis is treated with appropriate antibiotics based on knowledge of the sensitivities of *E. coli* in your practice location (nitrofurantoin [100 mg twice daily for 5 days], trimethoprim-sulfamethoxazole [1 double-strength tablet twice-daily for 3 days], or fosfomycin [3 g single dose] are first-line agents).[12] Symptoms usually improve within 24 to 36 hours.
- Uncomplicated pyelonephritis is treated with appropriate antibiotics as an outpatient (oral ciprofloxacin [500 mg twice daily]) for 7 days with or without an initial 400-mg intravenous dose when resistance is not known to exceed 10%).[12] The urine should always be cultured in pyelonephritis to help guide therapy. Pregnant women may need hospitalization.
- Glomerulonephritides are treated with supportive measures to prevent progression including maintaining a systolic blood pressure of 120–129 mm Hg, using an angiotensin-converting enzyme inhibitor or angiotensin receptor blocker therapy to control blood pressure and reduce proteinuria, and limiting protein intake to 0.8 g/day.[5] Immunosuppression is considered in patients with IgA nephropathy who are at risk for progressive disease or patients with membranous glomerulonephritis who are progressing. Corticosteroids are used in the treatment of patients with minimal change disease and focal segmental glomerulosclerosis.[5]
- See Chapter 70 (Kidney Stones) for management of patients with kidney stones, Chapter 73 (Renal Cell Carcinoma) for renal cell carcinoma, and Chapter 74 (Bladder Cancer) for bladder cancer.

PREVENTION AND SCREENING

- The U.S. Preventive Services Task Force concluded that there was insufficient evidence to assess the balance of benefits and harms of screening for bladder cancer in asymptomatic adults.[13] The positive predictive value of screening is less than 10% in asymptomatic persons, including higher-risk populations. The ACP recommends against screening urinalysis for cancer detection in asymptomatic adults.[11]

FOLLOW-UP

- The AUA recommends annual microscopic urinalysis for patients with microscopic hematuria and a negative work-up.[2] If persistent microscopic hematuria is documented, consider repeat anatomic evaluation within 3 to 5 years or sooner, if clinically indicated. Repeat urinalysis can be discontinued if negative after 2 years.

PROVIDER RESOURCES

- *Urinalysis*—**http://library.med.utah.edu/WebPath/TUTORIAL/URINE/URINE.html.**
- *Microscopic Hematuria*—**http://www.auanet.org/education/guidelines/asymptomatic-microhematuria.cfm.**

REFERENCES

1. Denker BM, Brenner BM. Azotemia and urinary abnormalities. In: Kasper DL, Braunwald E, Fauci AS, et al, eds. *Harrison's Principles of Internal Medicine*, 16th ed. New York, NY: McGraw-Hill; 2005:250-251.
2. Davis R, Jones JS, Barocas DA, et al. Diagnosis, evaluation and follow-up of asymptomatic microscopic hematuria (AMH) in adults: AUA guideline. *J Urol.* 2012;188(6 Suppl):2473-2481.
3. Jones R, Charlton J, Latinovic R, Gulliford MC. Alarm symptoms and identification of non-cancer diagnoses in primary care: cohort study. *BMJ.* 2009;339:b3094.
4. Margulis V, Sagalowsky AI. Assessment of hematuria. *Med Clin North Am.* 2011;95:153-159.
5. Floege J, Amann K. Primary glomerulonephritides. *Lancet.* 2016; 387:2036-2048.
6. Tworek JA, Wilkinson DS, Walsh MK. The rate of manual microscopic examination of urine sediment: a College of American Pathologists Q-Probes study of 11,243 urinalysis tests from 88 institutions. *Arch Pathol Lab Med.* 2008;132(12): 1868-1873.
7. Goonewardene S, Persad R. Sterile pyuria: a forgotten entity. *Ther Adv Urol.* 2015;7(5):295-298.
8. Bergus GR. Dysuria. In: Sloane PD, Slatt LM, Ebell MH, et al, eds. *Essentials of Family Medicine*, 6th ed. Baltimore, MD: Lippincott Williams & Wilkins; 2012:327-336.
9. Shaikh N, Morone NE, Lopez J, et al. Does this child have a urinary tract infection? *JAMA.* 2007;298(24):2895-2904.
10. American College of Radiology. *ACR Appropriateness Criteria Hematuria.* https://acsearch.acr.org/docs/69490/Narrative/. Accessed April 2017.
11. Nielsen M, Qaseem A; High Value Care Task Force of the American College of Physicians. Hematuria as a marker of occult urinary tract cancer: advice for high-value care from the American College of Physicians. *Ann Intern Med.* 2016;164(7): 488-497.
12. Gupta K, Hooton TM, Naber KG, et al; Infectious Diseases Society of America, European Society for Microbiology and Infectious Diseases. International clinical practice guidelines for the treatment of acute uncomplicated cystitis and pyelonephritis in women: a 2010 update by the Infectious Diseases Society of America and the European Society for Microbiology and Infectious Diseases. *Clin Infect Dis.* 2011;52(5):e103-e120.
13. Moyer VA; U.S. Preventive Services Task Force. Screening for bladder cancer: U.S. Preventive Services Task Force recommendation statement. *Ann Intern Med.* 2011;155(4):246-251.

70 KIDNEY STONES

Karl T. Rew, MD
Mindy A. Smith, MD, MS

PATIENT STORY

A 55-year-old woman presents with severe pain in the right flank. The pain began suddenly after supper and increased dramatically over the next hour. Urinalysis shows blood but no signs of infection. Abdominal X-ray reveals bilateral renal stones (**Figure 70-1**). A noncontrast CT scan confirms multiple bilateral renal stones, with an obstructing right distal ureteral stone and enlargement of the right kidney (**Figure 70-2**). She is subsequently found to have hyperparathyroidism, which is the cause of her multiple stones.

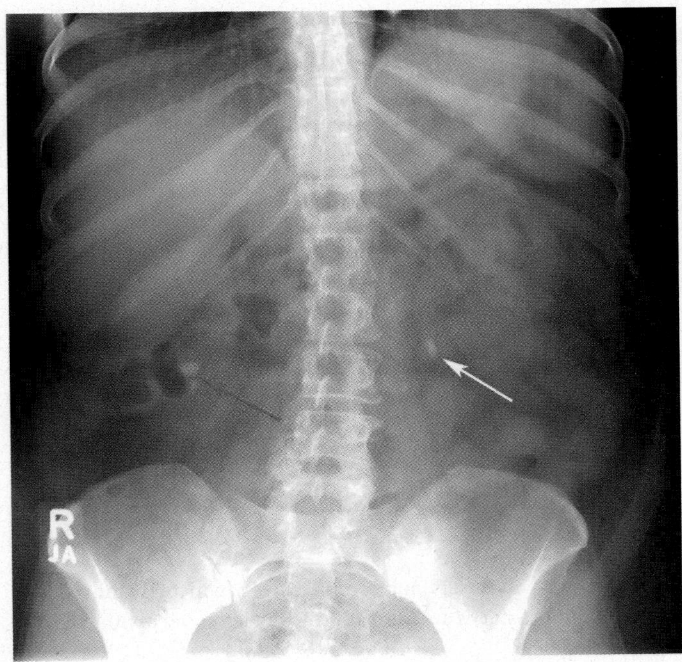

FIGURE 70-1 Plain X-ray of the abdomen in a 55-year-old woman showing several stones in the right kidney (*red arrow*) and a large left ureteral stone (*white arrow*) adjacent to the L2-L3 disc space.

INTRODUCTION

A kidney stone is a solid mass that forms when minerals crystallize and collect in the urinary tract. Kidney stones can cause pain and hematuria and may lead to complications, such as urinary tract obstruction and infection.

SYNONYMS

Kidney stone, nephrolithiasis, renal calculus, renal stone, urinary tract stone, ureterolithiasis, urolithiasis.

EPIDEMIOLOGY

- The prevalence of kidney stones is increasing worldwide across all age, gender, and racial/ethnic groups. This is due to multiple causes, but is clearly associated with increasing rates of obesity and diabetes.[1,2]
- Data from 2007–2010 show that 8.8% of adults in the United States reported having kidney stone disease, including 10.6% of men and 7.1% of women.[2]
- Men between the ages of 40 and 60 years have the highest risk of stones; for women, the risk peaks in their 50s.[3]
- Black (non-Hispanic) and Hispanic Americans have lower rates of kidney stones than white Americans.[2,4]
- Calcium oxalate and calcium phosphate stones are the most common, occurring in 75% to 85% of patients. Struvite (magnesium ammonium phosphate) stones occur in 5% of cases. Uric acid stones occur in 5% to 10% of patients, and cystine stones occur in 1% of cases. Other types of stones are less common.[5]
- Calcium stones are more common in men than in women (ratio 2:1), although this gender gap is narrowing.[1] Struvite stones are more common in women than in men (ratio 3:1).[5]

ETIOLOGY AND PATHOPHYSIOLOGY

- Kidney stones form when there is supersaturation of otherwise soluble materials, usually from increased excretion of these compounds or dehydration. Urine pH is a factor in stone formation because urinary phosphate increases in alkaline urine, whereas uric acid predominates in acidic urine (pH <5.5). Higher urine citrate can decrease stone formation.
- Struvite stones are caused by infection with urea-splitting bacteria, mainly *Proteus*.
- Uric acid stones form in patients with gout or hyperuricemia caused by other causes, including myeloproliferative disorders, chemotherapy, and Lesch-Nyhan syndrome.
- Cystine stones occur in patients with an inherited defect of dibasic amino acid transport.
- Struvite, cystine, and uric acid stones can become quite large, filling the renal pelvis and extending into the calyces to form staghorn calculi (**Figure 70-3**).

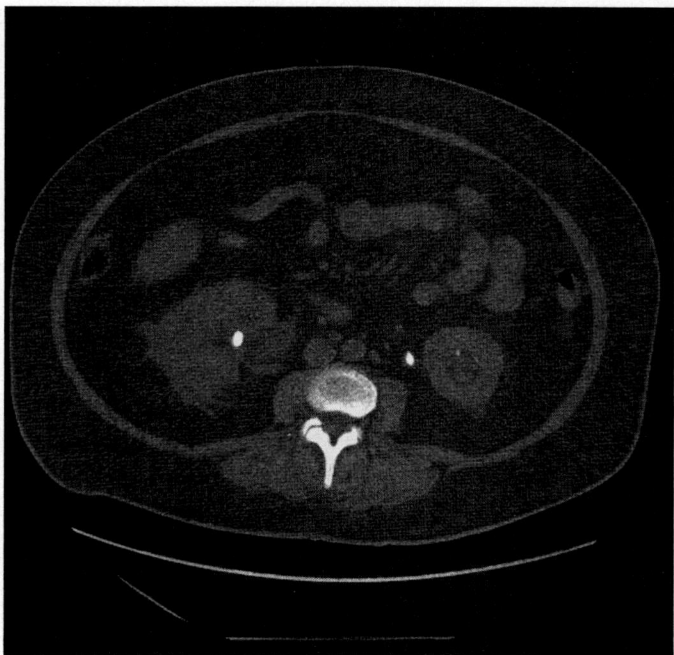

FIGURE 70-2 Noncontrast CT of the abdomen and pelvis of the same woman showing several of the stones seen in **Figure 70-1**, including a nonobstructing stone in the interpolar region of the right kidney. Because the right ureter is obstructed by a distal stone (not visible on this image), the right kidney is enlarged, with collecting system dilation and perinephric stranding. The large left proximal ureteral stone seen in this image is only partially obstructing, causing mild dilation in the left kidney collecting system. Several small stones are visible in the left kidney, and the left kidney is somewhat atrophied from chronic obstruction.

RISK FACTORS

Infections, genetic defects, and certain drugs can increase the risk of stones, but most stones are idiopathic. Risk factors vary with type of stone, as follows:

- Calcium stones are more likely in patients who are obese[6] and in those with diets higher in animal protein, salt, and oxalate-containing foods.
- Although bariatric surgery is effective for treating obesity, kidney stones are common after bariatric surgery and may increase in frequency with malabsorptive procedures.[7]
- Contrary to popular belief, calcium in the diet does not lead to calcium stones; in fact, adequate dietary calcium can prevent calcium stones by trapping oxalate in the GI tract.
- Patients with poor urinary drainage or indwelling catheters are at risk for *Proteus* urinary tract infections and struvite stones.
- Uric acid stones are associated with acidic urine, which is more common in obese patients with metabolic syndrome and insulin resistance, and in patients with chronic diarrhea.

DIAGNOSIS

CLINICAL FEATURES

- Kidney stones are often asymptomatic. Subsequent stone passage into the ureter usually causes pain and hematuria. The pain of renal colic typically begins suddenly in the ipsilateral flank or abdomen and progresses in waves, gradually increasing in intensity over the next 20 to 60 minutes. As the stone moves downward, pain may be felt in the ipsilateral groin, testis, or vulva.
- Obstructing stones cause hydronephrosis, with an associated constant dull flank pain. Stones in the bladder may cause frequency, urgency, dysuria, or recurrent urinary tract infections.

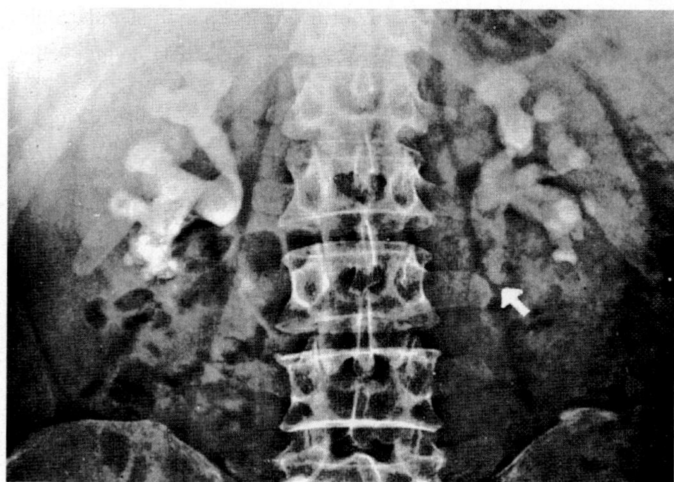

FIGURE 70-3 Bilateral staghorn calculi. (*Reproduced with permission from Doherty GM. Current Surgical Diagnosis and Treatment. New York, NY: McGraw-Hill Education; 2006.*)

LABORATORY

- Urinalysis usually reveals microscopic hematuria and limited pyuria. Gross hematuria is possible.
- Because treatment depends on stone type, stone capture and analysis is recommended. SOR Ⓒ.
- Additional work-up is recommended for adults with recurrent stones and for children with a first stone.[4] This includes a 24-hour urine collection for pH, volume, oxalate, and citrate, with simultaneous serum tests for calcium, uric acid, electrolytes, and creatinine. In patients with elevated serum calcium, parathyroid hormone (PTH) should be measured.

IMAGING

- Plain abdominal X-ray will demonstrate most calcium, struvite, and cystine stones. It is recommended for patients with a prior radiopaque stone (see **Figure 70-1**).
- Noncontrast helical CT (**Figures 70-4** and **70-5**) has largely replaced intravenous urography for patients with a suspected urinary tract stone because it is rapid, exposes patients to less radiation, requires no contrast, and may provide clues to diagnoses outside the urinary system. Although uric acid stones are typically radiolucent (not seen on standard X-rays), they often can be detected with CT.
- Ultrasound can be used to monitor uric acid stones (typically radiolucent), to assess hydronephrosis, or to avoid using X-rays in children and pregnant women.

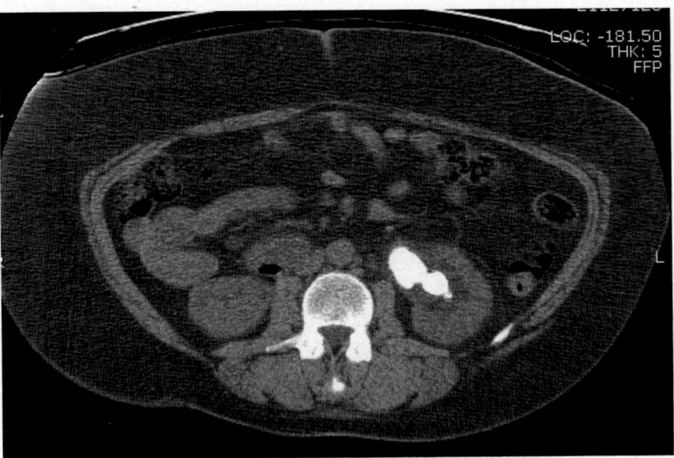

FIGURE 70-4 An unenhanced CT performed on a 49-year-old woman with known renal stones reveals a large left staghorn calculus. The striated appearance of the left renal cortex is seen in obstruction, infection, and ischemia. (*Reproduced with permission from Michael Freckleton, MD.*)

DIFFERENTIAL DIAGNOSIS

Stones within the bladder may mimic urinary tract infection (UTI). Helpful indicators of UTI are a urine dipstick positive for nitrates (positive likelihood ratio [LR+] 26.5) and urinary sediment showing 10 or more bacteria/high-power field (LR+ 85).

Other causes of hematuria include:

- Infection (e.g., UTI, sexually transmitted infection, schistosomiasis).
- Cancer of the bladder (see Chapter 74, Bladder Cancer), ureters, or kidney (see Chapter 73, Renal Cell Carcinoma).
- Renal disease (glomerulonephritis, immunoglobulin [Ig] A nephropathy, lupus nephritis, hemolytic uremic syndrome).
- In men, prostatitis, benign prostatic hypertrophy, or prostate cancer (see Chapter 75, Prostate Cancer); or following trauma.

Other causes of flank and lower pelvic/groin pain include:

- Gynecologic conditions in women (ovarian torsion, cyst, or ectopic pregnancy), which can often be distinguished on ultrasound. Pelvic inflammatory disease can also present with pain and is diagnosed based on clinical examination and culture.
- In men, epididymitis, prostatitis, or testicular torsion may cause pain that can be confused with kidney stones. Testicular tumors rarely cause pain. Physical examination can help differentiate these conditions.
- Cholelithiasis—Biliary colic is usually described as a steady, severe pain or ache, usually of sudden onset, located in the epigastrium or right upper quadrant (RUQ) (see Chapter 64, Gallstones). RUQ

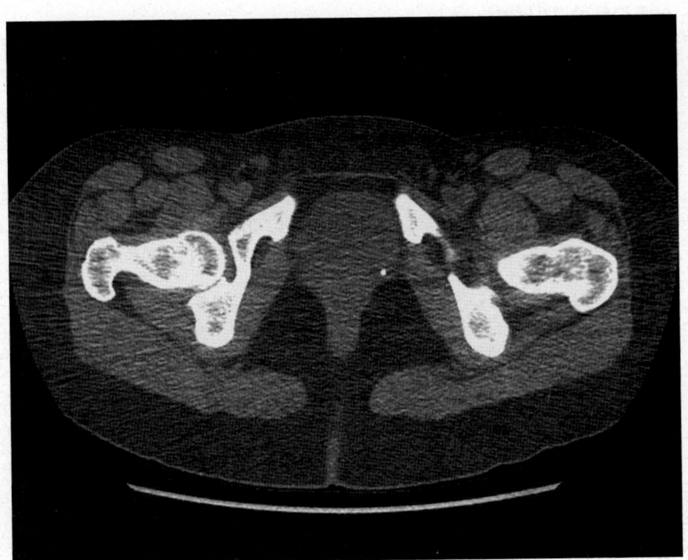

FIGURE 70-5 Noncontrast CT of the abdomen and pelvis in a 33-year-old woman showing a 3-mm obstructing stone in the distal ureter, just proximal to the ureterovesical junction.

tenderness may be elicited on physical examination, and ultrasound usually shows stones in the gallbladder.

- Urologic disorders including ureteropelvic junction obstruction, renal subcapsular hematoma, and renal cell carcinoma (see Chapter 73, Renal Cell Carcinoma). Imaging assists in differentiating these from kidney stones.

Abdominal pain from kidney stones may be confused with:

- Colitis, appendicitis, and diverticulitis—Systemic symptoms such as fever are often seen. Symptoms of colitis include diarrhea, rectal bleeding, tenesmus (i.e., urgency with a feeling of incomplete evacuation), passage of mucus, and cramping abdominal pain (see Chapter 67, Inflammatory Bowel Disease). GI symptoms with kidney stones are limited to nausea and vomiting from stimulation of the celiac plexus.
- Peptic ulcer disease—Epigastric pain is the hallmark, along with dyspeptic symptoms (see Chapter 61, Peptic Ulcer Disease). Stool antigen test can confirm *Helicobacter pylori* infection. Upper endoscopy is the preferred procedure for diagnosing ulcers.
- Abdominal aortic aneurysm—Peak incidence is usually in the sixth and seventh decades. Pain is described as severe and tearing, localized to the front or back of the chest, and associated with diaphoresis. Syncope and weakness may also occur.

MANAGEMENT

NONPHARMACOLOGIC

- Adequate fluid intake is essential—drinking enough water to produce 2.5 liters of urine per day is recommended for most patients.[8,9] SOR Ⓑ
- Stones smaller than 5 mm are likely to pass spontaneously. About three-fourths of distal ureteral stones and about half of proximal ureteral stones will pass spontaneously. The 3-mm distal ureteral stone shown in **Figure 70-3** passed spontaneously.

MEDICATIONS

- Medical expulsive therapy with α-adrenergic blockers (such as tamsulosin) or calcium-channel blockers can increase the chance of stone passage, particularly for larger stones (5–10 mm).[10,11] SOR Ⓑ
- Effective pain control should be provided using nonsteroidal anti-inflammatory drugs (NSAIDs) and narcotics if needed. NSAIDs may need to be avoided in patients with poor renal function or when planning lithotripsy, due to an increased risk of perinephric bleeding.

COMPLEMENTARY AND ALTERNATIVE THERAPY

- Lemon juice is a source of citrate for prevention of calcium stones.[12] For prevention of struvite stones, urine can be acidified with cranberry juice.[8] Other supplements have been suggested as potentially protective against renal stones, but study results are conflicting.

PROCEDURES

- Stones that do not pass spontaneously or with medical expulsive therapy can be treated with lithotripsy or removed via ureteroscopy. Large stones may require percutaneous nephrolithotomy (PCNL) or open surgery.

REFERRAL

- Urgent urologic consultation is recommended for patients with urinary tract stones and urosepsis, anuria, or renal failure. Urologic consultation is recommended for patients with refractory pain and nausea, extremes of age, major comorbidities, or stones larger than 5 mm. SOR Ⓒ

Indications for operative intervention:

- Infection.
- Persistent symptoms of flank pain, nausea, and vomiting.
- Failure to pass a ureteral stone after an appropriate trial of observation (2 to 4 weeks).

PREVENTION

- Foods high in oxalate should be avoided by those who form calcium oxalate stones, including rhubarb, spinach, Swiss chard, beets, apricots, figs, kiwi, many soy products, chocolate, and most nuts and seeds. See Patient Resources: The Oxalate Content of Foods.
- Uric acid stones are prevented with a low-purine diet. High-purine foods to avoid include most fish, shellfish, and meats (especially game meats and organ meats), and protein supplements such as brewer's yeast. Alkalinizing the urine with potassium citrate may be helpful.
- Low-calcium diets should not be used in patients with calcium stones. A low-calcium diet can increase stone formation and lower bone mineral density.

Additional treatments may be warranted based on the type of stone:

- Patients with high urine calcium and recurrent calcium-containing stones can be treated with a thiazide diuretic (reduces recurrence by 50% over 3 years). Hypokalemia should be avoided because low serum potassium reduces urinary citrate.
- Idiopathic stone disease can be treated with fluids and potassium citrate (2 g/day).
- For cystine stones, increasing fluid intake, alkalinizing the urine to a pH ≥7.5, and a diet low in sodium and animal protein are recommended.

PROGNOSIS

- Half of patients with a first calcium-containing stone have a recurrence within 10 years.
- Twenty-five percent of struvite stones recur if there was incomplete removal of the stone.
- Long-term complications are uncommon. The proportion of nephrolithiasis-related end-stage renal disease (ESRD) appears small (3.2%).

FOLLOW-UP

- A follow-up consultation to discuss kidney stone prevention is important for all patients with an initial stone. Patients started on medical therapy should be reevaluated with a 24-hour urine in 3 months. Those with a history of recurrent stones should be seen at least annually.

PATIENT EDUCATION

Maintaining water intake of at least 2 to 3 L/day (to keep urine specific gravity around 1.005) is recommended for most patients as this fluid level has been shown to reduce recurrences by half. Dietary information is available (see "Patient Resources" below).

PATIENT RESOURCES

- National Kidney and Urologic Diseases Information Clearinghouse. *Kidney Stones*—**http://kidney.niddk.nih.gov/health-information/urologic-diseases/kidney-stones/.**
- National Kidney and Urologic Diseases Information Clearinghouse. *Eating, Diet, and Nutrition for Kidney Stones*—**http://kidney.niddk.nih.gov/health-information/urologic-diseases/kidney-stones/eating-diet-nutrition.**
- *The Oxalate Content of Foods*—**https://regepi.bwh.harvard.edu/health/Oxalate/files.**

PROVIDER RESOURCES

- American Urological Association. *Medical Management of Kidney Stones: AUA Guideline*—**https://www.auanet.org/education/guidelines/management-kidney-stones.cfm.**
- European Association of Urology. *Guidelines on Urolithiasis*, update March 2015—**http://uroweb.org/wp-content/uploads/22-Urolithiasis_LR_full.pdf.**

REFERENCES

1. Sorokin I, Mamoulakis C, Miyazawa K, et al. Epidemiology of stone disease across the world. *World J Urol.* 2017;35(9):1301-1320.
2. Scales CD Jr, Smith AC, Hanley JM, Saigal CS; Urologic Diseases in America Project. Prevalence of kidney stones in the United States. *Eur Urol.* 2012;62(1):160-165.
3. Curhan GC. Epidemiology of stone disease. *Urol Clin North Am.* 2007;34(3):287-293.
4. Worcester EM, Coe FL. Calcium kidney stones. *N Engl J Med.* 2010:363:954-963.
5. Asplin JR, Coe FL, Favus MJ. Nephrolithiasis. In: Longo DL, Fauci AS, Kasper DL, et al, eds. *Harrison's Principles of Internal Medicine*, 18th ed. New York, NY: McGraw-Hill; 2012. http://www.accessmedicine.com/content.aspx?aID=9131116. Accessed December 2011.
6. Taylor EN, Stampfer MJ, Curhan GC. Obesity, weight gain, and the risk of kidney stones. *JAMA.* 2005;293(4):455-462.
7. Lieske JC, Mehta RA, Milliner DS, et al. Kidney stones are common after bariatric surgery. *Kidney Int.* 2015;87(4):839-845.
8. Frasetto L, Kohlstadt I. Treatment and prevention of kidney stones: an update. *Am Fam Physician.* 2011;84(11):1234-1242.
9. Pearle MS, Goldfarb DS, Assimos DG, et al; American Urological Association. Medical management of kidney stones: AUA guideline. *J Urol.* 2014;192(2):316-324.
10. Hollingsworth JM, Rogers MA, Kaufman SR, et al. Medical therapy to facilitate urinary stone passage: a metaanalysis. *Lancet.* 2006;368:1171-1179.
11. Wang RC, Smith-Bindman R, Whitaker E, et al. Effect of tamsulosin on stone passage for ureteral stones: a systematic review and meta-analysis. *Ann Emerg Med.* 2017;69(3):353-361.e3.
12. Kang DE, Sur RL, Haleblian GE, et al. Long-term lemonade based dietary manipulation in patients with hypocitraturic nephrolithiasis. *J Urol.* 2007;177(4):1358-1362.

71 HYDRONEPHROSIS

Mindy A. Smith, MD, MS

PATIENT STORY

A 74-year-old man presented with a 2-day history of severe, steady pain radiating down to the lower abdomen and left testicle. He has had urinary frequency, nocturia, hesitancy, and urinary dribbling for several years with slight worsening with time. CT scan revealed left-sided hydronephrosis (**Figure 71-1**). In this patient, an irregular mass was seen at the left ureterovesical junction compressing the bladder. Prostate cancer was found on biopsy.

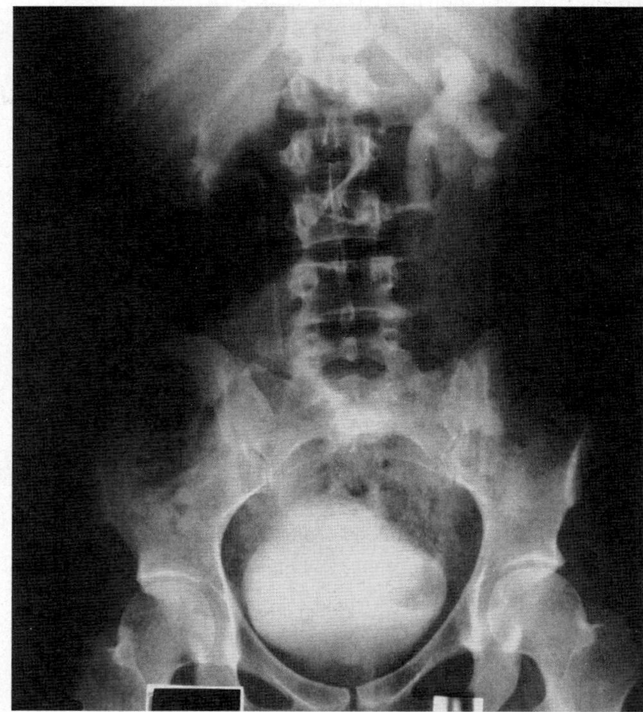

FIGURE 71-1 Intravenous urogram showing left hydronephrosis and hydroureter. (*Reproduced with permission from Schwartz DT, Reisdorff EJ. Emergency Radiology. New York, NY: McGraw-Hill Education; 2000.*)

INTRODUCTION

Hydronephrosis refers to distention of the renal calyces and pelvis of one or both kidneys by urine. Hydronephrosis is not a disease but a physical result of urinary blockage that may occur at the level of the kidney, ureters, bladder, or urethra. The condition may be physiologic (e.g., occurring in up to 80% of pregnant women) or pathologic.

SYNONYMS

- Hydronephrosis with infection is also called pyonephrosis.

EPIDEMIOLOGY

- The most common cause of congenital bilateral hydronephrosis is posterior urethral valves (in males). Other causes include narrowing of the ureteropelvic or ureterovesicular junction.
- Using a large European database for surveillance of congenital malformations (EUROCAT), authors found a prevalence of congenital hydronephrosis of 11.5 cases per 10,000 births; the majority (72%) was in males.[1]
- Ureteropelvic junction obstruction is one of the most common congenital abnormalities of the urinary tract causing hydronephrosis, occurring in approximately 1 in 5000 to 8000 live births.[2]
- Authors of one systematic review reported a mean prevalence of 15% for postnatal primary vesicoureteral reflux (VUR) in children after prenatally detected hydronephrosis.[3] Of the remaining cases, 53% had no postnatal anomalies and 29% had other anomalies (e.g., duplicate collecting systems; **Figure 71-2**).
- Among acquired causes in adults, pelvic tumors, renal calculi, and urethral stricture predominate.[4] If renal colic is present, renal stone is likely present (90% in one study).[5]
- Hydronephrosis is common in pregnancy because of the compression from the enlarging uterus and functional effects of progesterone.

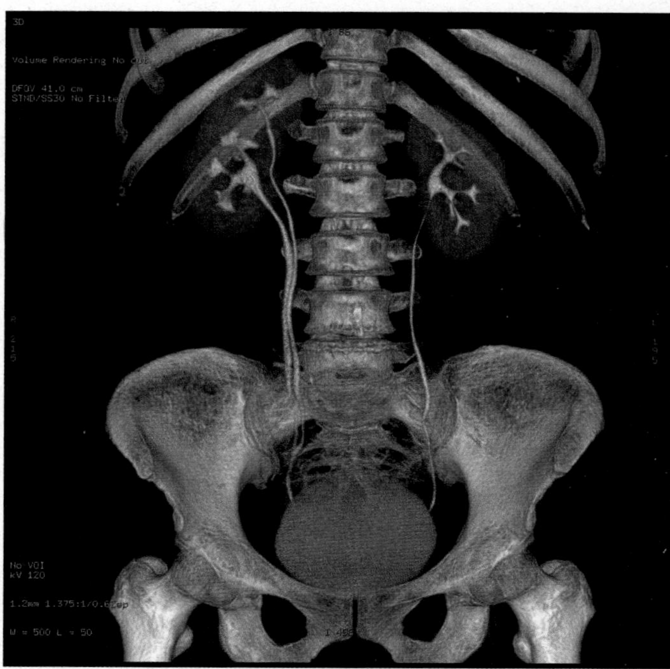

FIGURE 71-2 Duplicate right ureter seen with three-dimensional rendering of a CT urogram. (*Reproduced with permission from Karl T. Rew, MD.*)

ETIOLOGY AND PATHOPHYSIOLOGY

- Bilateral hydronephrosis is caused by a blockage to urine flow occurring at or below the level of the bladder or urethra.
- Unilateral hydronephrosis is caused by a blockage to urine flow occurring above the level of the bladder.
- Multiple causes result in this condition including congenital (e.g., VUR), acquired intrinsic (e.g., calculi, inflammation, and trauma), and acquired extrinsic (e.g., pregnancy or uterine leiomyoma, retroperitoneal fibrosis). Within these groupings, obstruction may be a result of mechanical (e.g., benign prostatic hypertrophy) or functional (e.g., neurogenic bladder) defects.
- Urinary obstruction causes a rise in ureteral pressure leading to declines in glomerular filtration, tubular function (e.g., ability to transport sodium and potassium or adjust urine concentration), and renal blood flow.
- If obstruction persists, tubular atrophy and permanent nephron loss can occur.

DIAGNOSIS

- In children, the diagnosis of hydronephrosis or megaureter is often made by a routine ultrasound.
- A work-up for hydronephrosis in adults is often triggered by the discovery of azotemia (caused by impaired excretory function of sodium, urea, and water). Sudden or new onset of hypertension (because of the increased renin release with unilateral obstruction) may also trigger an investigation. A first step in the evaluation is to perform bladder catheterization. If diuresis occurs, the obstruction is below the bladder neck.

CLINICAL FEATURES

- Pain is the symptom that most commonly leads an adult patient to seek medical attention. This is caused by distention of the collecting system or renal capsule. The pain is often described as severe, steady, and radiating down to the lower abdomen, testicles, or labia. Flank pain with urination is pathognomonic for VUR.
- Disturbed excretory function or difficulty in voiding: Oliguria and anuria are symptoms of complete obstruction, whereas polyuria and nocturia occur with partial obstruction (impaired concentrating ability causes osmotic diuresis).
- Fever or dysuria can occur with associated urinary tract infection (UTI).
- The physical examination may reveal distention of the kidney or bladder. Rectal exam may show an enlarged prostate or rectal/pelvic mass, and pelvic examination may reveal an enlarged uterus or pelvic mass.

LABORATORY TESTING

- Urinalysis may show hematuria, pyuria, proteinuria, or bacteriuria but the sediment is often normal.[3]
- Assess renal function (blood urea nitrogen [BUN], creatinine).
- Urodynamic testing may be indicated for patients with neurogenic bladder or other suspected bladder causes of hydronephrosis.

IMAGING

- Ultrasound imaging has a sensitivity and specificity of 90% for identifying the presence of hydronephrosis if no diuresis occurs following bladder catheterization.[4]
- If a source remains unidentified, an IV urogram (**Figures 71-1** and **71-3**) and/or CT scan (**Figure 71-4**) should be obtained to diagnose intra-abdominal or retroperitoneal causes.
- One study of magnetic resonance (MR) pyelography (vs. ultrasound and urography) reported a sensitivity in detecting stones, strictures, and congenital ureteropelvic junction obstructions of 68.9%, 98.5%, and 100%, respectively, with a specificity of 98%.[6] Accuracy regarding the level of obstruction was high (100%).
- Antegrade urography (percutaneous placement of ureteral catheter) or retrograde urography (cystoscopic placement of ureteral catheter) may be needed in patients with azotemia and poor excretory function or in those at high risk of acute renal failure from IV contrast (i.e., diabetes, multiple myeloma).
- A voiding cystourethrogram is useful in the diagnosis of VUR and bladder neck and urethral obstructions.
- For children identified in the prenatal period with hydronephrosis, the American Urological Association (AUA) recommends a voiding cystourethrogram if there is high-grade hydronephrosis, hydroureter, or an abnormal bladder on ultrasound (late-term prenatal or postnatal), or for children who develop a UTI on observation.[7] SOR Ⓒ Given the unproven value in diagnosing and treating VUR, an observational approach without screening may be taken for children with lesser grades of prenatally detected hydronephrosis (Society for Fetal Urology [SFU] grade 1 or 2).
- This approach of limiting voiding cystourethrogram was evaluated retrospectively with respect to UTI in a population of 87 infants with prenatal hydronephrosis without anatomic abnormalities.[8] Postnatal voiding cystourethrogram was performed in 52 patients (60%) of whom 7 had VUR and none of the 7 had UTI. Six infants developed febrile UTIs—half immediately following catheterization.
- In one study, the Urinary Tract Dilation classification system was found to be reliable in assessing postnatal hydronephrosis and independently predicted the likelihood of surgical intervention; in contrast, the SFU grades were predictive of likelihood of resolution.[9] This system was developed by a consensus panel and consists of six categories based on ultrasonographic findings: (1) anterior-posterior renal pelvic diameter; (2) calyceal dilation; (3) renal parenchymal thickness; (4) renal parenchymal appearance; (5) bladder abnormalities; and (6) ureteral abnormalities stratified by gestational age and time of recognition.[10]

DIFFERENTIAL DIAGNOSIS

Hydronephrosis is usually found during an investigation for symptoms such as flank pain or renal failure. Following are other causes of flank pain:

- Pyelonephritis—Fever, chills, nausea, vomiting, and diarrhea often occurring with or without symptoms of cystitis.

- Cholelithiasis—Pain is more typical in the epigastrium and right upper quadrant (biliary colic) and often nausea and vomiting occurs (see Chapter 64, Gallstones).
- Other urologic disorders include ureteropelvic junction obstruction, renal subcapsular hematoma, and renal cell carcinoma (see Chapter 73, Renal Cell Carcinoma).

Causes of unexplained renal failure in adults:

- Hypoperfusion (prerenal failure).
- Acute tubular necrosis (ATN), interstitial, glomerular, or small vessel disease (intrarenal failure).
- Hypoperfusion and ATN account for most cases of acute renal failure.

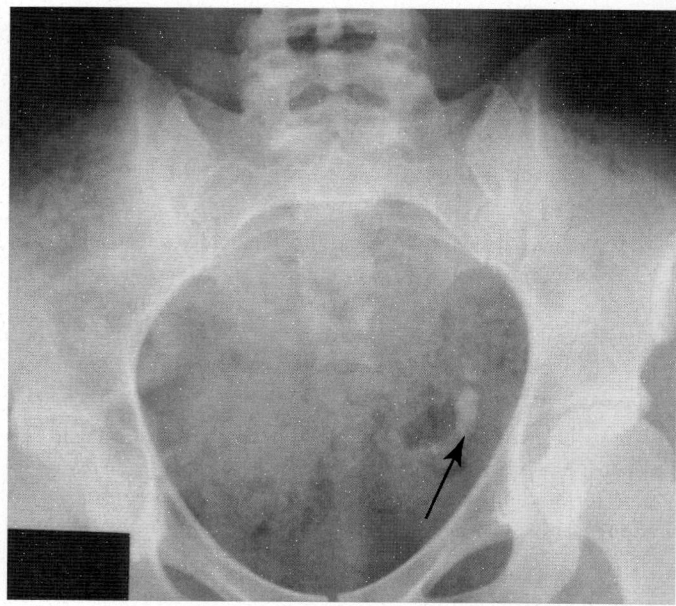

FIGURE 71-3 Large irregular calcification (*arrow*) representing ureterolithiasis in the left side of the pelvis in the patient in **Figure 71-1**. (*Reproduced with permission from Schwartz DT, Reisdorff EJ. Emergency Radiology. New York, NY: McGraw-Hill Education; 2000.*)

MANAGEMENT

NONPHARMACOLOGIC

- Spontaneous resolution or decrease in urinary tract dilation is expected for most cases of neonatal hydronephrosis and primary megaureter diagnosed prenatally.[11,12]
- Functional causes may be treated by frequent voiding or catheterization (intermittent preferred).[13] SOR B

MEDICATIONS

- Children younger than 1 year of age with VUR complicated by a history of febrile UTI or higher grades of VUR (grades III to V) should be placed on prophylactic antibiotics (sulfamethoxazole/trimethoprim or nitrofurantoin).[14] SOR B Authors of a systematic review of 21 articles with 3876 infants found low rates of UTI in children with low-grade hydronephrosis regardless of use of antibiotics (2.2% on prophylaxis vs. 2.8% not receiving prophylaxis), whereas among children with high-grade hydronephrosis, patients receiving prophylactic antibiotics had a significantly lower UTI rate (14.6% vs. 28.9% not receiving prophylaxis), with a number needed to treat to prevent one UTI of 7.[15]
- Adult patients with hydronephrosis, complicated by infection, should be treated with appropriate antibiotics for 3 to 4 weeks. Chronic or recurrent unilateral infections may require nephrectomy. SOR A
- Anticholinergic drugs (e.g., oxybutynin, tolterodine) are recommended for patients with neurogenic bladder.[13] SOR B
- α-Adrenergic blockade in children with neurogenic bladder can also be considered, but studies are lacking.[13] SOR C

PROCEDURES AND SURGERY

- Hydronephrosis with infection is a urologic emergency that can be treated by prompt drainage using retrograde stent insertion or percutaneous nephrostomy.[16] For pregnant women, the former is associated with minimal radiation to the fetus and is the treatment of choice.
- Pyeloplasty is a surgical technique for repairing an obstruction between the ureter and kidney that involves excising the obstructing segment with reanastomosis of the ureter. For children with ureteropelvic junction obstruction, three basic procedures (open

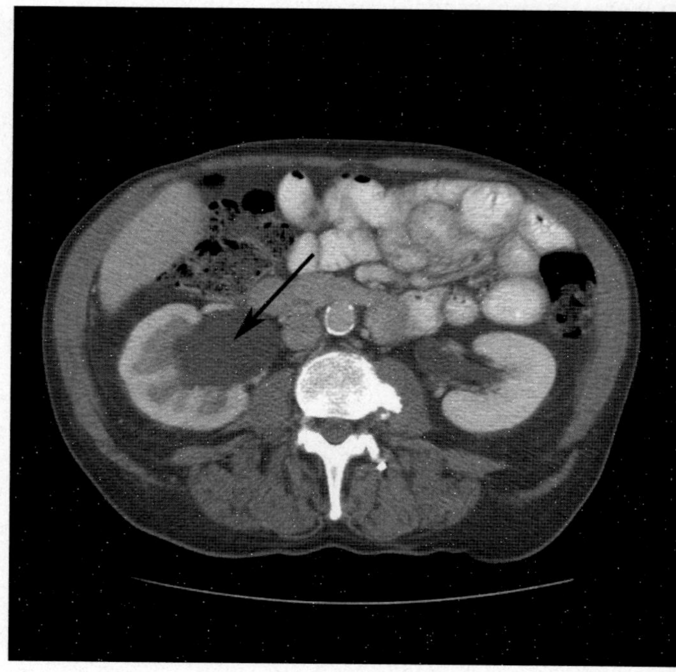

FIGURE 71-4 Right-sided hydronephrosis (*arrow*) seen on CT. (*Reproduced with permission from Karl T. Rew, MD.*)

pyeloplasty [OP], endopyelotomy, and laparoscopic pyeloplasty [LP]) can be used for treatment; early surgery is only needed in approximately 15% to 20% of patients.[17] In one review of largely retrospective data, OP and LP had higher success rates than endopyelotomy (94.1% and 95.9% to 97.2% vs. 62% to 83%, respectively).[18]

- Treatment for VUR includes surgical repair (ureteral reimplantation or ureteroneocystostomy) or endoscopic injection of a bulking agent. Surgical repair is recommended for higher grades of persistent reflux and is based on age, antibiotic failure, and whether reflux is unilateral or bilateral; surgery does not reduce rates of febrile UTI.[19]
- The American College of Radiology (ACR) recommends percutaneous antegrade ureteral stenting or percutaneous nephrostomy for afebrile nonanuric patients with acute hydronephrosis.[20] In a septic patient with acute obstruction, ACR recommends retrograde ureteral stenting followed by stone removal when infection is controlled.[20]
- Patients with renal failure can be treated with dialysis. SOR Ⓐ
- Elective surgery for drainage is performed for persistent pain or progressive loss of renal function. SOR Ⓒ

PREVENTION AND SCREENING

- The prevalence of VUR in siblings of an index case is 27.4% and in offspring 35.7%; severe reflux is identified in approximately 10% of screened patients.[21] Because of the lack of randomized controlled trials of treated versus untreated screened siblings with VUR regarding health outcomes, the best screening strategy is not known. One cost analysis estimated that it would require screening 30 to 430 asymptomatic siblings 1 year of age to prevent 1 febrile UTI at a cost of $56,000 to $820,000 per averted episode.[22]

PROGNOSIS

Prognosis depends on the underlying etiology.

FOLLOW-UP

- Neonates and children with unresolved hydronephrosis or megaureter should be followed periodically with urine cultures, serum creatinine, ultrasonography, and possibly renal scan.[14]
- Prognosis for an adult patient depends on the duration and completeness of the obstruction and associated complications such as infection; complete obstruction for 1 to 2 weeks may be followed by partial return of renal function, but after 8 weeks, recovery is unlikely.[4]
- Postobstructive diuresis can cause loss of sodium, potassium, and magnesium that may require replacement in the setting of hypovolemia, hypotension, or electrolyte imbalance.

PATIENT EDUCATION

- Education regarding VUR should include a discussion of the treatment rationale, treatment approaches, and likely adherence with the care plan.

PATIENT RESOURCES

- National Kidney Foundation (800-622-9010) or **www.kidney.org.**
- National Institutes of Health, MedlinePlus. *Bilateral Hydronephrosis*—**http://www.nlm.nih.gov/medlineplus/ency/article/000474.htm.**

PROVIDER RESOURCES

- Lusaya DG, Lerma EV. *Hydronephrosis and Hydroureter*—**http://emedicine.medscape.com/article/436259-overview.**
- Guideline: Screening of the neonate/infant with prenatal hydronephrosis. In: American Urologic Association Education and Research. *Management and Screening of Primary Vesicoureteral Reflux in Children: AUA Guideline*. Linthicum, MD: American Urologic Association Education and Research; 2010:1-12. **https://www.auanet.org/education/guidelines/vesicoureteral-reflux-a.cfm.**
- Guideline: *ACR Appropriateness Criteria® Treatment of Urinary Tract Obstruction*. [online publication]. **https://acsearch.acr.org/docs/69353/Narrative/.** Accessed May 2018.

REFERENCES

1. van Eerde AM, Meutgeert MH, de Jong TP, Giltay JC. Vesico-ureteral reflux in children with prenatally detected hydronephrosis: a systematic review. *Ultrasound Obstet Gynecol.* 2007;29(4):463-469.
2. Turk TMT, Polcari AJ, Sharma SK, Fulmer BR. *Pyeloplasty*. http://emedicine.medscape.com/article/448299-overview#a0199. Accessed March 2017.
3. Garne E, Loane M, Wellesley D, et al. Congenital hydronephrosis: prenatal diagnosis and epidemiology in Europe. *J Pediatr Urol.* 2009;5(1):47-52.
4. Seifter JL. Urinary tract obstruction. In: Kasper DL, Fauci AS, Hauser SL, et al, eds. *Harrison's Principles of Internal Medicine*, 19th ed. New York, NY: McGraw-Hill; 2014.
5. Pepe P, Motta L, Pennisi M, Aragona F. Functional evaluation of the urinary tract by color-Doppler ultrasonography (CDU) in 100 patients with renal colic. *Eur J Radiol.* 2005;53(1):131-135.
6. Blandino A, Gaeta M, Minutoli F, et al. MR pyelography in 115 patients with a dilated renal collecting system. *Acta Radiol.* 2001; 42(5):532-536.
7. Screening of the neonate/infant with prenatal hydronephrosis. In: American Urological Association Education and Research. *Management and Screening of Primary Vesicoureteral Reflux in Children: AUA Guideline*. Linthicum, MD: American Urological Association Education and Research; 2010:1-12.
8. St Aubin M, Willihnganz-Lawson K, Varda BK, et al. Society for fetal urology recommendations for postnatal evaluation of prenatal hydronephrosis—will fewer voiding cystourethrograms lead to more urinary tract infections? *J Urol.* 2013;190(4 Suppl): 1456-1461.
9. Hodhod A, Capolicchio JP, Jednak R, et al. Evaluation of urinary tract dilation classification system for grading postnatal hydronephrosis. *J Urol.* 2016;195(3):725-730.

10. Nguyen HT, Benson CB, Bromley B, et al. Multidisciplinary consensus on the classification of prenatal and postnatal urinary tract dilation (UTD classification system). *Pediatr Urol.* 2014;10(6):982-998.
11. Shukla AR, Cooper J, Patel RP, et al. Prenatally detected primary megaureter: a role for extended followup. *J Urol.* 2005;173(4): 1353-1356.
12. Upadhyay J, McLorie GA, Bolduc S, et al. Natural history of neonatal reflux associated with prenatal hydronephrosis: long-term results of a prospective study. *J Urol.* 2003;169(5):1837-1841.
13. Management of neurogenic bladder in children. In: Tekgül S, Riedmiller H, Gerharz E, et al. *Guidelines on Paediatric Urology.* Arnhem, The Netherlands: European Association of Urology, European Society for Paediatric Urology; 2009:31-41. https://uroweb.org/wp-content/uploads/22-Paediatric-Urology.pdf. Accessed March 2017.
14. Management of infants less than one year of age with vesicoureteral reflux. In: American Urological Association Education and Research. *Management and Screening of Primary Vesicoureteral Reflux in Children: AUA Guideline.* Linthicum, MD: American Urological Association Education and Research; 2010:1-11. https://www.auanet.org/education/guidelines/vesicoureteral-reflux-a.cfm. Accessed March 2017.
15. Braga LH, Mijovic H, Farrokhyar F, et al. Antibiotic prophylaxis for urinary tract infections in antenatal hydronephrosis. *Pediatrics.* 2013;131(1):e251-261.
16. Ramsey S, Robertson A, Ablett MJ, et al. Evidence-based drainage of infected hydronephrosis secondary to ureteric calculi. *J Endourol.* 2010;24(2):185-189.
17. Madsen MG, Nørregaard R, Frøkiær J, Jørgensen TM. Urinary biomarkers in prenatally diagnosed unilateral hydronephrosis. *J Pediatr Urol.* 2011;7(2):105-112.
18. Gallo F, Schenone M, Giberti C. Ureteropelvic junction obstruction: which is the best treatment today? *J Laparoendosc Adv Surg Tech A.* 2009;19(5):657-662.
19. Estrada CR, Cendron M. *Vesicoureteral Reflux Treatment and Management.* Updated November 21, 2015. http://emedicine.medscape.com/article/439403-treatment#a1128. Accessed March 2017.
20. National Guideline Clearinghouse (NGC). Guideline summary: ACR Appropriateness Criteria radiologic management of urinary tract obstruction. https://www.acr.org/Clinical-Resources/ACR-Appropriateness-Criteria. Accessed May 2018.
21. Skoog SJ, Peters CA, Arant BS Jr, et al. Pediatric Vesicoureteral Reflux Guidelines Panel summary report: clinical practice guidelines for screening siblings of children with vesicoureteral reflux and neonates/infants with prenatal hydronephrosis. *J Urol.* 2010; 184(3):1145-1151.
22. Routh JC, Grant FD, Kokorowski P, et al. Costs and consequences of universal sibling screening for vesicoureteral reflux: decision analysis. *Pediatrics.* 2010;126(5):865-871.

72 POLYCYSTIC KIDNEYS

Mindy A. Smith, MD, MS

PATIENT STORY

A 43-year-old woman with newly diagnosed hypertension reports persistent bilateral flank pain. She has a family history of "kidney problems." On urinalysis, she is noted to have microscopic hematuria. An ultrasound and abdominal computed tomography (CT) scan show bilateral polycystic kidneys (**Figure 72-1**).

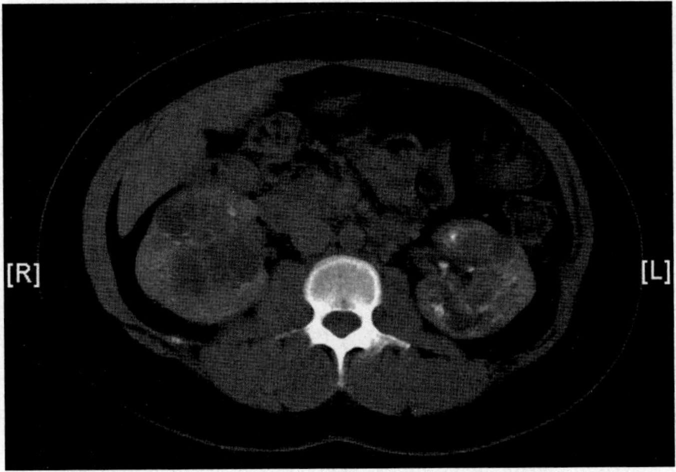

FIGURE 72-1 Polycystic kidneys in a 43-year-old woman with hematuria. (*Reproduced with permission from Michael Freckleton, MD.*)

INTRODUCTION

Polycystic kidney disease (PKD) is a manifestation of a group of inherited disorders resulting in renal cyst development. In the most common form, autosomal-dominant polycystic kidney disease (ADPKD), extensive epithelium-lined cysts develop in the kidney; in some cases, abnormalities also occur in the liver, pancreas, brain, arterial blood vessels, or a combination of these sites.

EPIDEMIOLOGY

- Most common tubular disorder of the kidney, affecting 1 in 339 to 1 in 492 individuals, based on autopsy studies.[1]
- Autosomal dominant in 80% to 85% of cases, rarely as an autosomal recessive trait.[1]
- ADPKD accounts for approximately 4.7% of cases of end-stage renal disease (ESRD).[2]
- Most frequently seen in the third and fourth decades of life, but can be diagnosed at any age.
- Very early-onset ADPKD (under 2 years of age) occurs in only 1% to 2% of affected children.[1]

ETIOLOGY AND PATHOPHYSIOLOGY

- ADPKD results from mutations in either of 2 genes that encode plasma membrane–spanning polycystin 1 (PKD1) and polycystin 2 (PKD2).[3] Polycystins regulate tubular and vascular development in the kidneys and other organs (liver, brain, heart, and pancreas). PKD1 and PKD2 are colocalized in primary cilia and appear to mediate Ca^{2+} signaling as a mechanosensor, essential for maintaining the differentiated state of epithelia lining tubules in the kidney and biliary tract.[4] These mutations result in many abnormalities including increased proliferation and apoptosis and loss of differentiation and polarity.[5]
- Almost universally associated with different forms of cystic kidney disease is activation of the mammalian target of rapamycin (mTOR) pathway, a protein kinase complex that promotes anabolic programs in response to nutrients, growth factors, and cellular energy levels.[1]

- Macrophages infiltrate kidney cysts in patients with ADPKD. Macrophage migration inhibitory factor accumulates in cyst fluid of ADPKD kidneys and likely promotes cystic epithelial cell proliferation by activating mTOR and other pathways.[6]
- Few (1% to 5%) nephrons develop cysts.
- Remaining renal parenchyma shows varying degrees of tubular atrophy, interstitial fibrosis, and nephrosclerosis.
- Cysts are also found in other organs such as liver (**Figure 72-2**), spleen, pancreas, and ovaries. Liver cysts are found in up to 80% of patients with ADPKD.[3] There is also an increased incidence of intracranial aneurysms (5% to 12%).
- Autosomal-recessive PKD (ARPKD) is the neonatal form of PKD that is associated with enlarged kidneys and biliary dysgenesis.[4] The genetic mutation in PKHD1 (polycystic kidney hepatic disease 1) involves a protein, fibrocystin, that is also localized to cilia/basal body and complexes with PKD2. This large, receptor-like protein is thought to be involved in the tubulogenesis and/or maintenance of duct-lumen architecture of epithelium.
- Rare syndromic forms of PKD include defects of the eye, central nervous system, digits, and/or neural tube.[4]
- A variant of PKD is glomerulocystic kidney (GCK), which refers to a kidney with greater than 5% cystic glomeruli.[7] This condition is usually diagnosed in young patients. Although PKD-associated gene mutations have been excluded in many cases, there is a familial form of GCK presenting with cystic kidneys, hyperuricemia, and isosthenuria (concentration similar to plasma).[7]

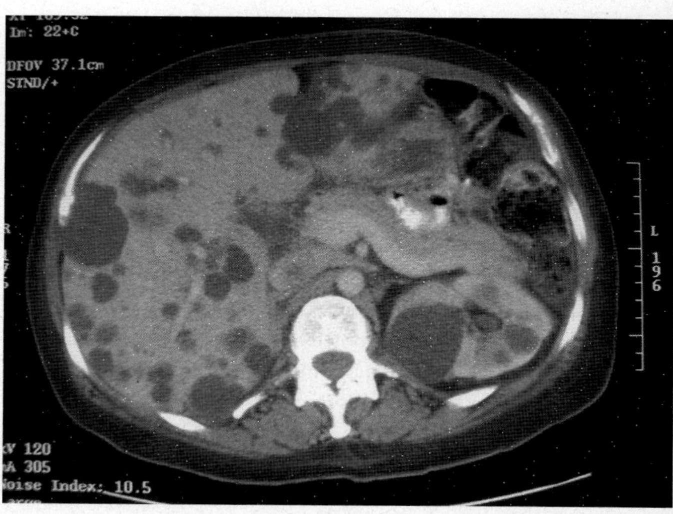

FIGURE 72-2 CT scan showing multiple liver cysts and multiple cysts in both kidneys in a patient with polycystic kidney disease. (*Reproduced with permission from Ves Dimov, MD, Section of Allergy, Asthma and Immunology, Department of Pediatrics, Department of Medicine, University of Chicago, ClinicalCases.org.*)

DIAGNOSIS

Family history is a useful tool for diagnosing early ADPKD.

CLINICAL FEATURES

- Chronic flank pain due to the mass effect of enlarged kidneys.
- Acute pain with infection, kidney stone, obstruction, or hemorrhage into a cyst.
- Enlarged liver can cause dyspnea, early satiety, esophageal reflux, lower extremity edema, and abdominal or low back pain.[2]
- Hypertension is common in adults (75%) and may be present in 10% to 30% of children.
- Kidney stones (calcium oxalate and uric acid) develop in 15% to 20% of affected individuals because of urinary stasis from distortion of the collecting system, low urine pH, and low urinary citrate (see Chapter 70, Kidney Stones).
- Nocturia may also be present from impaired renal concentrating ability.

LABORATORY TESTING

- Gross or microscopic hematuria (60%).[3] Obtain a urinalysis to document hematuria and a complete blood count or hemoglobin to identify anemia.

IMAGING

- Diagnosis often made with ultrasound. More than 80% of patients have cysts present by age 20 years and 100% by age 30 years. In one

REFERENCES

1. Ong AC, Devuyst O, Knebelmann B, et al. Autosomal dominant polycystic kidney disease: the changing face of clinical management. *Lancet*. 2015;385(9981):1993-2002.
2. Srivastava A, Patel N. Autosomal dominant polycystic kidney disease. *Am Fam Physician*. 2014;90(5):303-307.
3. Grantham JJ. Autosomal dominant polycystic kidney disease. *Ann Transplant*. 2009;14(4):86-90.
4. Harris PC, Torres VE. Polycystic kidney disease. *Annu Rev Med*. 2009;60:321-337.
5. Park EY, Woo YM, Park JH. Polycystic kidney disease and therapeutic approaches. *BMB Rep*. 2011;44(6):359-368.
6. Chen L, Zhou X, Fan LX, et al. Macrophage migration inhibitory factor promotes cyst growth in polycystic kidney disease. *J Clin Invest*. 2015;125(6):2399-2412.
7. Lennerz JK, Spence DC, Iskandar SS, et al. Glomerulocystic kidney: one hundred-year perspective. *Arch Pathol Lab Med*. 2010; 134(4):583-605.
8. Nicolau C, Torra R, Bandenas C, et al. Autosomal dominant polycystic kidney disease types 1 and 2: assessment of US sensitivity for diagnosis. *Radiology*. 1999;213(1):273-276.
9. Sweeney WE Jr, Avner ED. Diagnosis and management of childhood polycystic kidney disease. *Pediatr Nephrol*. 2011;26(5):675-692.
10. Barua M, Pei Y. Diagnosis of autosomal-dominant polycystic kidney disease: an integrated approach. *Semin Nephrol*. 2010;30(4): 356-365.
11. Cohen BA, Barash I, Kim DC, et al. Intraobserver and interobserver variability of renal volume measurements in polycystic kidney disease using a semiautomated MR segmentation algorithm. *AJR Am J Roentgenol*. 2012;199(2):387-393.
12. Klahr S, Breyer JA, Beck GJ, et al. Dietary protein restriction, blood pressure control, and the progression of polycystic kidney disease. Modification of Diet in Renal Disease Study Group. *J Am Soc Nephrol*. 1995;6(4):1318.
13. Patch C, Charlton J, Roderick PJ, Gulliford MC. Use of antihypertensive medications and mortality of patients with autosomal dominant polycystic kidney disease: a population-based study. *Am J Kidney Dis*. 2011;57(6):856-862.
14. Schrier R, McFann K, Johnson A, et al. Cardiac and renal effects of standard versus rigorous blood pressure control in autosomal-dominant polycystic kidney disease: results of a seven-year prospective randomized study. *J Am Soc Nephrol*. 2002;13(7):1733-1739.14.
15. Schrier RW, Abebe KZ, Perrone RD, et al. Blood pressure in early autosomal dominant polycystic kidney disease. *N Engl J Med*. 2014;371(24):2255-2266.
16. Zeltner R, Poliak R, Stiasny B, et al. Renal and cardiac effects of antihypertensive treatment with ramipril vs metoprolol in autosomal dominant polycystic kidney disease. *Nephrol Dial Transplant*. 2008;23(2):573-579.
17. He Q, Lin C, Ji S, Chen J. Efficacy and safety of mTOR inhibitor therapy in patients with early-stage autosomal dominant polycystic kidney disease: a meta-analysis of randomized controlled trials. *Am J Med Sci*. 2012;344(6):491-497.
18. Hogan MC, Masyuk TV, Page LJ, et al. Randomized clinical trial of long-acting somatostatin for autosomal dominant polycystic kidney and liver disease. *J Am Soc Nephrol*. 2010;21(6):1052-1061.
19. Hogan MC, Mashu, Bergstralh E, et al. Efficacy of 4 years of octreotide long-acting release therapy in patients with severe polycystic liver disease. *Mayo Clin Proc*. 2015;90(8):1030-1037.
20. Torres VE, Chapman AB, Devuyst O, et al; TEMPO 3:4 Trial Investigators. Tolvaptan in patients with autosomal dominant polycystic kidney disease. *N Engl J Med*. 2012;367(25): 2407-2418.
21. Jacquet A, Pallet N, Kessler M, et al. Outcomes of renal transplantation in patients with autosomal dominant polycystic kidney disease: a nationwide longitudinal study. *Transpl Int*. 2011;24(6): 582-587.
22. Alam A, Perrone RD. Management of ESRD in patients with autosomal dominant polycystic kidney disease. *Adv Chronic Kidney Dis*. 2010;17(2):164-172.
23. Bae KT, Grantham JJ. Imaging for the prognosis of autosomal dominant polycystic kidney disease. *Nat Rev Nephrol*. 2010;6(2): 96-106.
24. Johnston O, O'Kelly P, Donohue J, et al. Favorable graft survival in renal transplant recipients with polycystic kidney disease. *Ren Fail*. 2005;27(3):309-314.
25. Gonçalves S, Guerra J, Santana A, et al. Autosomal-dominant polycystic kidney disease and kidney transplantation: experience of a single center. *Transplant Proc*. 2009;41(3):887-890.
26. Yu TM, Chuang YW, Yu MC, et al. New-onset atrial fibrillation is associated with polycystic kidney disease: a nationwide population-based cohort study. *Medicine (Baltimore)*. 2016;95(4):e2623.
27. Vora N, Perrone R, Bianchi DW. Reproductive issues for adults with autosomal dominant polycystic kidney disease. *Am J Kidney Dis*. 2008;51(2):307-318.

73 RENAL CELL CARCINOMA

Mindy A. Smith, MD, MS

PATIENT STORY

A 56-year-old man with hypertension presents with a 2-week history of left-sided flank pain. Urinalysis shows microscopic hematuria and a CT scan (**Figures 73-1** and **73-2**) demonstrates a solid left renal mass. Work-up for metastatic disease was negative. A biopsy confirmed renal cell carcinoma, and a radical nephrectomy was performed.

FIGURE 73-1 Renal cell carcinoma. CT shows solid mass in the left kidney (*arrow*). (*Reproduced with permission from Michael Freckleton, MD.*)

INTRODUCTION

Renal tumors are a heterogeneous group of kidney neoplasms derived from the various parts of the nephron. Each type of tumor possesses distinct genetic characteristics, histologic features, and, to some extent, clinical phenotypes that range from benign (approximately 20% of small masses) to high-grade malignancy. Ninety percent to 95% of kidney neoplasms are renal cell carcinomas (RCCs).[1]

EPIDEMIOLOGY

- RCC comprises 2% to 3% of all visceral malignant diseases in adults and is the ninth most common cancer.[1] These cancers are more common in men than women (approximately 1.6:1).[2] The incidence in the United States is increasing.
- A similar percentage was reported for children in the Children's Oncology Group study in which 3.7% of 3250 patients enrolled were found to have unilateral RCC (median age, 12.9 years [range, 1.9–22.1 years].[3] The male-to-female ratio was approximately 1:1.
- An estimated 62,700 cases in the United States were diagnosed and approximately 14,240 deaths occurred in 2016 from kidney and renal pelvis cancer (2.4% of all cancer deaths).[4] The age-adjusted incidence rate was 15.6 per 100,000 persons with a median age at diagnosis of 64 years.[4]
- Lifetime risk of kidney and renal pelvis cancer is 1.6% (approximately 1 in 63 people will be diagnosed during their lifetime).[4]
- Approximately 2% to 3% of cases are familial (e.g., von Hippel-Lindau syndrome).[1]
- Metastatic disease at presentation occurs in 10% to 33%; the most common sites of distant metastases (in descending order) are lung (with or without mediastinal or hilar nodes), bone, upper abdomen (including the tumor bed, adrenal gland, contralateral kidney, and liver), brain, and other sites (e.g., skin, spleen, heart, diaphragm, gut, connective tissue, and pancreas).[2,5] In the report of children with RCC, distant metastases were present in 23 cases (19.2%).[3]

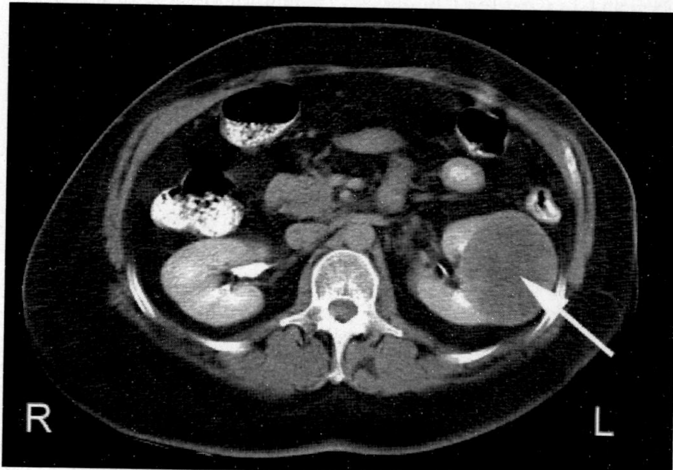

FIGURE 73-2 CT with contrast in the same patient shows the solid hypodense renal cell carcinoma mass (*arrow*) in the left kidney and contrasting normal parenchyma. The contrast is taken up better by the remaining normal kidney tissue and the tumor becomes more visible. (*Reproduced with permission from Michael Freckleton, MD.*)

ETIOLOGY AND PATHOPHYSIOLOGY

The majority of renal tumors fall into the following categories[1]:

- Clear cell carcinoma (from high lipid content) (60% to 80%).
- Papillary carcinoma (5% to 15%), further delineated into type 1 and the more aggressive type 2.
- Chromophobic tumors (3% to 10%) and other rare subtypes, such as medullary, which occurs almost exclusively in patients with sickle cell trait.
- Among children, translocation morphology was the most common followed by papillary and renal medullary carcinoma.[3]
- Renal-cell carcinoma is highly vascular. Tumor cells appear to proliferate primarily through dysregulation of the vascular endothelial growth factor pathway.

RISK FACTORS[1]

- Smoking (relative risk 2 to 3).
- Obesity.
- Hypertension.
- Acquired cystic disease and end-stage renal disease, including dialysis treatment.
- Family history of the disease.

DIAGNOSIS

Most presentations are incidental (identified during other tests) and, consequently, although the incidence has increased, more cancers are diagnosed at early stages.[1] Despite this fact, mortality rates have also increased.

CLINICAL FEATURES

- Hematuria (40%) and flank pain (40%).
- Weight loss and anemia (approximately 33%).
- Flank mass (approximately 25%).
- The classic triad of hematuria, flank pain, and flank mass occurs in 5% to 10% of patients.
- Other reported symptoms include night sweats, bone pain, fatigue, and sudden onset of left varicocele.
- Systemic symptoms may be caused by metastases or paraneoplastic syndromes, such as parathyroid hormone-related protein (causing hypercalcemia and renal stones), renin (causing hypertension), or erythropoietin (causing erythrocytosis).[1]

LABORATORY TESTING

Potentially useful studies: SOR Ⓒ

- Hemoglobin (anemia).
- Liver chemistries (metastatic disease or paraneoplastic syndrome).
- Urinalysis (hematuria—gross or microscopic).
- Urine cytology (neoplastic cells).
- The National Comprehensive Cancer Network (NCCN) also suggests a comprehensive metabolic panel as part of the initial work-up.[6] If a urothelial carcinoma is suspected (e.g., central mass), urine cytology should be considered.
- Two biomarkers, aquaporin 1 (AQP1) and perilipin 2 (PLIN2), detected in urine have area under the receiver operating characteristic curve ranging from 0.99 to 1.00 for differentiating clear cell and papillary RCC from benign tumors and bladder or prostate cancers.[7]

IMAGING

- The work-up for indeterminate renal masses suggested by the American College of Radiology (ACR) includes either CT scan of the abdomen (**Figures 73-1** to **73-3**) (solid renal mass; signs suggestive of renal vein or caval thrombus include filling defects, enlargement of the vessel, and rim enhancement) or abdominal MRI (slightly more sensitive and tends to upgrade cystic lesions; **Figure 73-4**); either scan should be done without and with contrast.[8]
- An ultrasound (US) of the kidney retroperitoneal may help to clarify a mass that is probably a hyperdense cyst (the most common renal mass).
- Authors of a meta-analysis found that MRI with diffusion-weighted MRI had moderate accuracy for determining benign versus malignant renal masses and high-grade versus low-grade clear cell RCCs.[9]
- Angiography can be used to define vascular anatomy before nephron-sparing surgery.[8]

For the purpose of staging an RCC, ACR recommends[8]:

- CT of the abdomen without and with contrast.
- Chest X-ray (CXR; tumor may extend into the hilar lymph nodes); chest CT can be considered for detecting small pulmonary metastases and metastatic mediastinal lymph nodes.
- MRI if patient is unable to undergo CT with contrast.
- Bone scans and brain MRI should be reserved for patients with abnormal blood chemistries, symptoms, or large and locally aggressive or metastatic primary renal cancers.

Staging is based on the TNM staging system. T1 and T2 are based on tumor size (<7 cm are T1, with further subclassification into T1a and T1b using a cut-off of 4 cm). Tumors with extrarenal extension into perinephric/renal sinus fat, renal vein, or inferior vena cava are staged T3 and those with adjacent organ involvement are T4. The classification of tumors as low vs. moderate- to high-risk for disease recurrence is based on pathologic tumor stage.

BIOPSY

A renal biopsy is only needed on occasion based on the appearance and size of the mass; US, CT, or MRI can be used for image guidance.[5]

- Authors of a systematic review of 20 studies of biopsy of clinically localized renal masses suspicious for RCC found high diagnostic accuracy with core biopsy when a diagnostic result was obtained;

however, the nondiagnostic rate was 14.1%, and 90.4% of those undergoing surgery were found to have malignancy.[10] Although most patients with negative biopsies did not undergo surgery, among patients undergoing complete removal, 36.7% with a negative biopsy had malignant disease on surgical pathology (negative predictive value 63.3%). Direct complications were uncommon and primarily included hematoma.

DIFFERENTIAL DIAGNOSIS

The differential diagnosis of a renal mass includes:

- Simple cysts.
- Renal calculi/nephrolithiasis (see Chapter 70, Kidney Stones).
- Benign neoplasms (infrarenal hematoma, adenoma, angiomyolipoma [see **Figure 73-4**], and oncocytoma).
- Inflammatory lesions (focal bacterial nephritis, abscess, pyelonephritis, and renal tuberculosis); patients often present with systemic signs and symptoms of infection such as fever and chills.
- Other primary or metastatic tumors (neoplastic tumors involving the kidney include squamous cell carcinoma of the collecting system, transitional cell carcinomas of the renal pelvis or collecting system, sarcoma, lymphoma, nephroblastoma, and melanoma). These can frequently be differentiated from RCC on CT scan, but biopsy may be necessary.

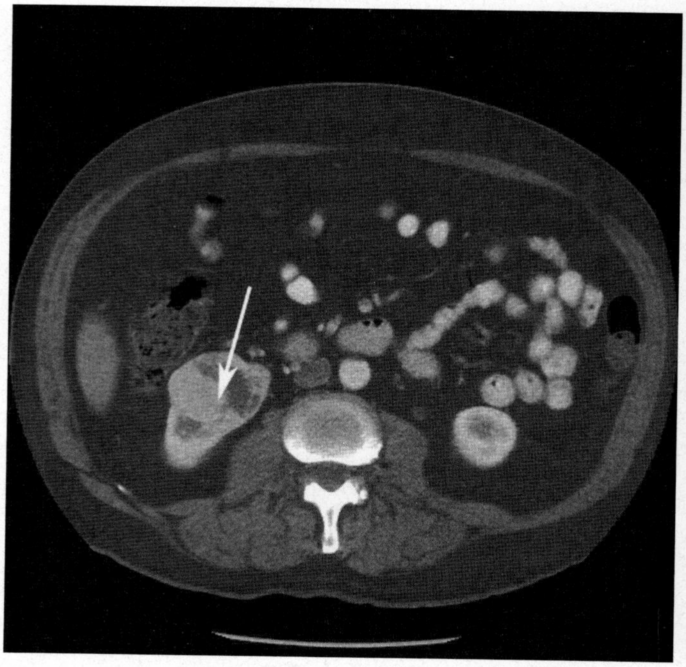

MANAGEMENT

Because an increasing number of tumors are identified early (tumor size <4 cm) and may be slow growing with low risk of early progression, some authors are advocating initial active surveillance.[11] For patients with biopsy-confirmed RCC undergoing active surveillance, ACR recommends annual cross-sectional abdominal scanning (CT or MRI) within 6 months to establish a growth rate.[5] Continued imaging (US, CT, or MRI) is recommended at least annually along with annual CXR to assess for pulmonary metastases. SOR Ⓒ

MEDICATIONS

- The NCCN recommends enrollment in a clinical trial or pazopanib or sunitinib as preferred first-line therapy for stage IV surgically unresectable tumors of predominantly clear cell histology.[6] For non-clear cell histology, a clinical trial or sunitinib are preferred.
- For metastatic RCC, improvement in survival (4 to 5 months), but not cure, has been reported for targeted therapies, primarily those using anti-vascular endothelial growth factor receptor (VEGFR) agents (bevacizumab, sorafenib, sunitinib, pazopanib, tivozanib, or axitinib) or mammalian target of rapamycin (mTOR) inhibitors (temsirolimus or everolimus) usually compared to interferon-α.[12] One placebo-controlled trial reported a small (1 month) benefit on quality of life using pazopanib vs. sunitinib.[13]
- In a recent randomized clinical trial (RCT), progression-free survival was 3.7 months longer with cabozantinib, a tyrosine kinase inhibitor, than with everolimus for patients with RCC that had progressed despite VEGFR-targeted therapy.[14] Similarly, nivolumab, a

FIGURE 73-3 CT in a 70-year-old man demonstrating a heterogeneous solid mass in the midportion to lower pole of the right kidney (*arrow*), consistent with a primary renal cancer. The mass contains low-attenuation, likely necrotic, components and is exophytic. (*Reproduced with permission from Karl T. Rew, MD.*)

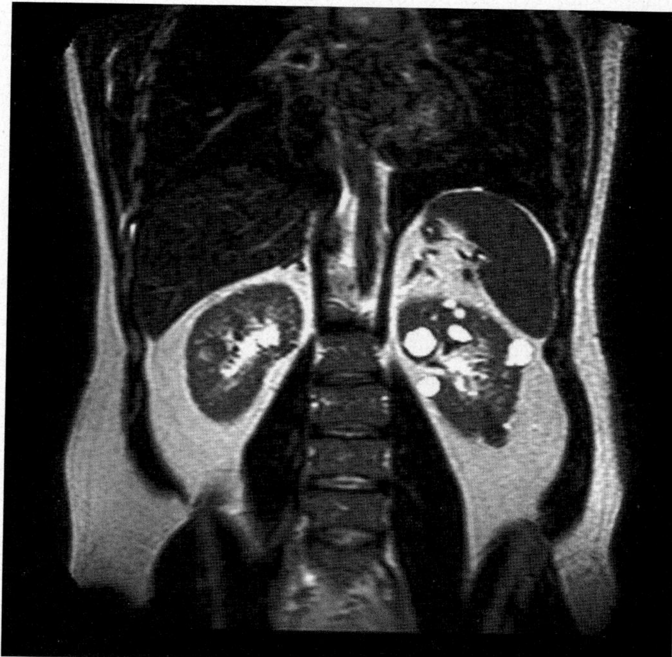

FIGURE 73-4 Patient with tuberous sclerosis. MRI shows multiple angiomyolipomas in the kidneys with several lesions suspicious for renal cancer. (*Reproduced with permission from Karl T. Rew, MD.*)

programmed death 1 checkpoint inhibitor, improved survival by 5.4 months compared to everolimus in previously treated patients with clear-cell RCC.[15]

- For patients with high-grade T1b or greater with completely resected non-metastatic RCC, a large RCT failed to demonstrate improved survival with either adjuvant sunitinib or sorafenib compared to placebo (median disease-free survival was 5.8 years, 6.1 years, and 6.6 years, respectively).[16] There was substantial treatment discontinuation from toxicity and 5 treatment-related deaths.

SURGERY

- For localized disease, partial nephrectomy for small tumors and radical nephrectomy (complete removal of the kidney and Gerota fascia) for large tumors is the gold standard.[1] SOR Ⓑ For T1a tumors, the NCCN recommends either partial (preferred) or radical nephrectomy, active surveillance for selected patients, or thermal ablation for selected patients.[6] For stage T1b, II, and III tumors, partial or radical nephrectomy is recommended.
- Similar to lumpectomy for localized breast cancer, partial nephrectomy for small tumors in the presence of a normal contralateral kidney appears to have similar outcomes to radical nephrectomy, based on observational data. Complications are uncommon and include urinary leak (3% to 5%) and hemorrhage (1%).[1] Advantages include better preservation of renal function, which is associated with fewer hospitalizations and lower risk of cardiac events and mortality.[1]
- In one long-term follow-up study, 5- and 10-year cancer-specific survival for nephron-sparing surgery in these cases was 98.5% and 96.7% for tumors less than 4 cm, respectively, and for imperative indications (solitary kidney) they were 89.6% and 76%, respectively. Chronic renal failure requiring dialysis was reported in 9 patients (11.2%) with a solitary kidney.[17] These procedures can be performed via open, laparoscopic, or robotically assisted laparoscopic procedures; comparison studies are lacking.
- Percutaneous cryoablation or radiofrequency ablation of smaller (≤3.5 cm) renal masses is an alternative treatment[18,19]; outcomes for the 2 methods appear comparable, but the procedures have not been compared in a randomized trial.[20] Limitations of thermoablation include high local recurrence compared to surgery, lack of long-term data, and subsequent fibrosis that may compromise subsequent surgery if needed.
- For patients with larger tumors or local extension, radial nephrectomy offers a 40% to 60% chance of cure.[1] Laparoscopic approaches are frequently used, but data from RCTs comparing these approaches are limited.[21]
- NCCN recommends nephrectomy and surgical metastasectomy for a potentially surgically resectable solitary metastatic site.[6] In cases of a potentially resectable primary with multiple metastatic sites, NCC recommends cytoreductive nephrectomy in selected patients.
- Regional lymphadenectomy is controversial.
- Resection of solitary metastasis should be considered.[6,22] In a systematic review of data on 311 surgically and 73 nonsurgically treated patients with RCC metastatic to pancreas, metastases were single in approximately 60% of both groups. Surgery appeared to improve overall survival at 2 and 5 years (80.6% and 72.6%, respectively, for the surgical group, and 41% and 14%, respectively, in unresected patients).[23]

FOLLOW-UP

There is no standardized follow-up regimen based on evidence. The NCCN recommends a history, physical exam, comprehensive metabolic panel, and other tests every 6 months for 2 years and annually for up to 5 years after diagnosis for patients on active surveillance (stage T1a).[6] In addition, abdominal imaging (CT or MRI) is recommended within 6 months to determine growth rate, then annually, along with CXR or chest CT. Other testing is based on symptoms.

- For patients following nephrectomy (stages I–III): a baseline abdominal scan should be completed within 3–12 months following surgery and, if negative, annually for 3 years after partial nephrectomy and at the physician's discretion after radical nephrectomy. If stage II or III, follow-up with history, physical exam every 3–6 months for 3 years, then annually for 5 years after radical nephrectomy. Laboratory testing is performed every 6 months for 2 years, then annually for 5 years.
- The NCCN recommends follow-up every 6 to 16 weeks for patients with relapse or surgically unresectable stage IV disease, with imaging at the same interval based on physician discretion and patient clinical status.[6]
- The ACR recommends a follow-up CXR and CT or MRI of the abdomen without and with contrast for patients who have been treated for RCC by radical nephrectomy or nephron-sparing surgery.[5] Most recurrences occur within 2 to 3 years after initial resection.[5]
- For patients with T1 tumors, most surveillance protocols recommend a history, physical examination, laboratory tests, and CXR be obtained every 6 to 12 months for 2–3 years and then yearly until year 5.[5,6] Others have suggested no imaging if the tumor is less than 2.5 cm. Most protocols do not recommend surveillance with abdominal CT for patients with T1 tumors.
- For patients with T2 primary tumors, a history, physical examination, laboratory tests, and CXR is recommended annually or every 6 months for 3 years, then annually thereafter till year 5.[5] Protocols vary widely, with some not recommending abdominal CT at all, while others recommend CT at intervals ranging from annually for 3 years to once in year 2 and year 5.
- For patients with T3 or T4 primary tumors, most protocols recommend a history, physical examination, laboratory tests, and CXR be obtained every 6 months for a few years, then annually thereafter.[5] Most also recommend abdominal CT every 3 to 6 months for 3 years after surgery and less frequently (yearly or every other year) thereafter.

PROGNOSIS

- The clinical course is highly variable, and spontaneous remissions have occurred; overall 5-year survival is 73.7% (2006–2012).[4] Five-year survival has improved for all stages since 1992–1995 and was reported as 92.5% for localized cancer and 11.6% for advanced disease in 2006–2012.[4]

- In a meta-analysis of 300 cases, small tumors had an average growth rate of 0.28 cm per year.[24] Although follow-up for most patients was only 2 to 3 years, only 1% of these patients developed metastases.
- In addition to tumor size, prognosis is related to tumor subtype, stage, and nuclear grade; locally aggressive tumors are reported in 5.6% to 8% of patients with RCCs <4 cm.[2]
- Among patients initially treated with partial or radical nephrectomy, local or metastatic recurrences develop in approximately 20% to 50% (20% to 30% of patients with localized tumors).[5,6]
- For papillary RCC, one study found incidental detection, T classification, M classification, vascular invasion, and tumor necrosis extent were independent prognostic factors of disease-specific survival.[25]
- For advanced RCC, a multivariate analysis with 246 patients found performance status 1 versus 0 (hazard ratio [HR] 1.95, $p < 0.0001$), high alkaline phosphatase (HR 1.5, $p = 0.002$), and lung metastasis only (HR 0.73, $p = 0.028$) were overall survival predictors.[26]

PATIENT EDUCATION

Several prognostic algorithms, or nomograms, for RCC survival are available that may be useful in counseling patients about their probable clinical course and facilitating treatment planning; the most widely used is from Memorial Sloan Kettering Cancer Center (www.mskcc.org).[6]

PATIENT RESOURCES

- National Kidney Foundation (800-622-9010) or **http:www.kidney.org.**
- National Institutes of Health, MedlinePlus. *Kidney Cancer*—**http://www.nlm.nih.gov/medlineplus/kidneycancer.html.**

PROVIDER RESOURCES

- National Cancer Institute Surveillance Epidemiology and End Results. *Cancer Stat Facts: Kidney and Renal Pelvis Cancer*—**http://seer.cancer.gov/statfacts/html/kidrp.html.**
- National Kidney Foundation—**https://www.kidney.org/atoz/content/how-can-i-find-clinical-trial.**

REFERENCES

1. Rini BI, Campbell SC, Escudier B. Renal cell carcinoma. *Lancet.* 2009;373:1119-1132.
2. Vikram R, Casalino DD, Remer EM, et al. Expert Panel on Urologic Imaging. ACR Appropriateness Criteria® renal cell carcinoma staging. [online publication]. Reston, VA: American College of Radiology (ACR); 2011. 8 pp. https://www.guideline.gov/summaries/summary/49920/acr-appropriateness-criteria—renal-cell-carcinoma-staging?q=renal+cell+carcinoma. Accessed January 2017.
3. Geller JI, Ehrlich PF, Cost NG, et al. Characterization of adolescent and pediatric renal cell carcinoma: A report from the Children's Oncology Group study AREN03B2. *Cancer.* 2015;121(14):2457-2464.
4. National Cancer Institute. *SEER Stat Fact Sheets: Kidney and Renal Pelvis.* http://seer.cancer.gov/statfacts/html/kidrp.html. Accessed January 2017.
5. Casalino DD, Remer EM, Bishoff JT, et al, Expert Panel on Urologic Imaging. ACR Appropriateness Criteria® post-treatment follow-up of renal cell carcinoma. [online publication]. Reston (VA): American College of Radiology (ACR); 2013. 9 pp. https://www.guideline.gov/summaries/summary/47680/acr-appropriateness-criteria--posttreatment-followup-of-renal-cell-carcinoma?q=renal+cell+carcinoma. Accessed January 2017.
6. Motzer RJ, Jonasch E, Agarwal N, et al. NCCN clinical practice guidelines in oncology: kidney cancer. *J Natl Compr Canc Netw.* 2015;13(2):151-159.
7. Morrissey JJ, Mobley J, Figenshau RS, et al. Urine aquaporin 1 and perilipin 2 differentiate renal carcinomas from other imaged renal masses and bladder and prostate cancer. *Mayo Clin Proc.* 2015;90(1):35-42.
8. Heilbrun ME, Casalino DD, Beland MD, et al. Expert Panel on Urologic Imaging. ACR Appropriateness Criteria indeterminate renal mass [online publication]. Reston, VA: American College of Radiology (ACR); 2014. 11 pp. https://www.guideline.gov/summaries/summary/48291/acr-appropriateness-criteria--indeterminate-renal-mass?q=ACR+Appropriateness+Criteria%C2%AE+Indeterminate+Renal+Masses+. Accessed January 2017.
9. Kang SK, Zhang A, Pandharipande PV, et al. DWI for renal mass characterization: systematic review and meta-analysis of diagnostic test performance. *AJR Am J Roentgenol.* 2015;205(2):317-324.
10. Patel HD, Johnson MH, Pierorazio PM, et al. Diagnostic accuracy and risks of biopsy in the diagnosis of a renal mass suspicious for localized renal cell carcinoma: systematic review of the literature. *J Urol.* 2016;195(5):1340-1347.
11. Jewett MA, Zuniga A. Renal tumor natural history: the rationale and role for active surveillance. *Urol Clin North Am.* 2008;35(4):627-634.
12. Coppin C, Kollmannsberger C, Le L, et al. Targeted therapy for advanced renal cell cancer (RCC): a Cochrane systematic review of published randomised trials. *BMJ (Int Ed).* 2011;108(10):1556-1563.
13. Beaumont JL, Salsman JM, Diaz J, et al. Quality-adjusted time without symptoms or toxicity analysis of pazopanib versus sunitinib in patients with renal cell carcinoma. *Cancer.* 2016;122(7):1108-1115.
14. Choueiri TK, Escudier B, Powles T, et al. Cabozantinib versus everolimus in advanced renal-cell carcinoma. *N Engl J Med.* 2015;373(19):1814-1823.
15. Motzer RJ, Escudier B, McDermott DF, et al. Nivolumab versus everolimus in advanced renal-cell carcinoma. *N Engl J Med.* 2015;373(19):1803-1813.
16. Haas NB, Manola J, Uzzo RG, et al. Adjuvant sunitinib or sorafenib for high-risk, non-metastatic renal-cell carcinoma (ECOG-ACRIN E2805): a double-blind, placebo-controlled, randomised, phase 3 trial. *Lancet.* 2016;387(10032):2008-2016.

17. Roos FC, Pahernik S, Brenner W, Thuroff JW. Imperative and elective indications for nephron-sparing surgery for renal tumors: long-term oncological follow-up. *Aktuelle Urol.* 2010;(Suppl 1): S70-S76.

18. Uppot RN, Harisinghani MG, Gervais DA. Imaging-guided percutaneous renal biopsy: rationale and approach. *AJR Am J Roentgenol.* 2010;194(6):1443-1449.

19. Venkatesan AM, Wood BJ, Gervais DA. Percutaneous ablation in the kidney. *Radiology.* 2011;261(2):375-391.

20. Pirasteh A, Snyder L, Boncher N, et al. Cryoablation vs. radiofrequency ablation for small renal masses. *Acad Radiol.* 2011;18(1): 97-100.

21. Nabi G, Cleves A, Shelley M. Surgical management of localised renal cell carcinoma. *Cochrane Database Syst Rev.* 2010;(3):CD006579. (withdrawn).

22. Karam JA, Rini BI, Varella L, et al. Metastasectomy after targeted therapy in patients with advanced renal cell carcinoma. *J Urol.* 2011;185(2):439-444.

23. Tanis PJ, van der Gaag NA, Busch OR, et al. Systematic review of pancreatic surgery for metastatic renal cell carcinoma. *Br J Surg.* 2009;96(6):579-592.

24. Chawla SN, Crispen PL, Hanlon AL, et al. The natural history of observed enhancing renal masses: meta-analysis and review of the world literature. *J Urol.* 2006;175:425-431.

25. Klatte T, Remzi M, Zigeuner RE, et al. Development and external validation of a nomogram predicting disease specific survival after nephrectomy for papillary renal cell carcinoma. *J Urol.* 2010; 184(1):53-58.

26. Lars PN, Tangen CM, Conlon SJ, et al. Predictors of survival of advanced renal cell carcinoma: long-term results from Southwest Oncology Group Trial S8949. *J Urol.* 2009;181(2):512-516.

74 BLADDER CANCER

Karl T. Rew, MD
Mindy A. Smith, MD, MS

PATIENT STORY

A 68-year-old man, who is a retired painter and in good health, comes to the office at the insistence of his wife. He reports that his urinary stream has become slow, and he has occasional dysuria. He has no major medical problems, although he continues to smoke one pack of cigarettes per day. His urinalysis in the office shows microscopic hematuria. An irregular mass is seen in the bladder on CT scan (**Figure 74-1**). Cystoscopy shows a bladder tumor (**Figure 74-2**). Complete endoscopic resection is performed and confirms transitional cell carcinoma.

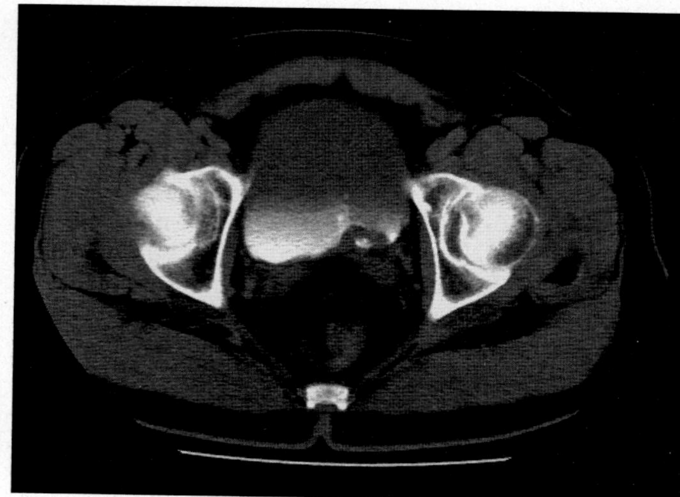

FIGURE 74-1 CT with contrast reveals a bladder cancer in a 68-year-old man with hematuria. (*Reproduced with permission from Michael Freckleton, MD.*)

INTRODUCTION

Bladder cancer is a malignant neoplasm of the bladder, almost exclusively urothelial (transitional cell) carcinoma.

EPIDEMIOLOGY

- In 2013, there were approximately 438,068 men and 149,358 women alive in the United States who had a history of cancer of the urinary bladder.[1]
- An estimated 76,960 new cases (58,950 men and 18,010 women) were diagnosed and approximately 16,390 deaths occurred from bladder cancer in 2016.[1] Mean age at diagnosis is 73 years.
- The age-adjusted incidence rate (based on 2009 to 2013 data) was 20.1 per 100,000 men and women per year with a male-to-female ratio of approximately 4:1. For both men and women, bladder cancer is most prevalent in white non-Hispanics, followed by blacks, Hispanics, Asian/Pacific Islanders, and American Indian/Alaska Natives.[1]

ETIOLOGY AND PATHOPHYSIOLOGY

- More than 95% are transitional cell cancers, and the remainder are nonurothelial neoplasms, including primarily squamous cell, adenocarcinoma, and small cell carcinoma[2,3] (**Figures 74-1** to **74-4**). Rare forms include nonepithelial neoplasms (approximately 1%), including benign tumors, such as hemangiomas or lipomas, and malignant tumors, such as angiosarcomas.[3]
- Transitional cells line almost all of the urinary tract, including the renal pelvis, the ureters and the bladder, and the proximal two thirds of the urethra. Ninety percent of transitional cell tumors develop in the bladder, 8% in the renal pelvis, and 2% in the ureters or urethra.[2]
- At presentation, 75% of tumors are non–muscle invasive, 20% are muscle invasive, and 5% are metastatic.[2]

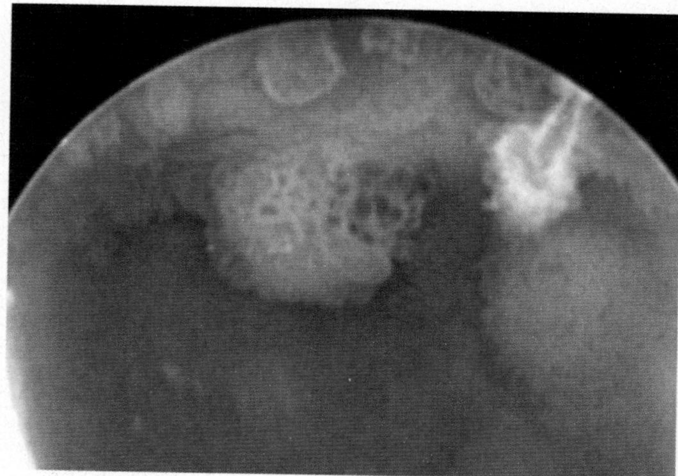

FIGURE 74-2 Cystoscopic view of the transitional cell carcinoma in the man in **Figure 74-1**. (*Reproduced with permission from Carlos Enrique Bermejo, MD.*)

- The most common transitional cell tumor is a low-grade papillary lesion on a central stalk that is friable, tends to bleed, and has a high risk of recurrence but rarely progresses to become muscle invasive. Carcinoma in situ, however, is a high-grade flat tumor considered a precursor of the more lethal muscle-invasive bladder cancer.[2]
- Bladder tumor cells are also graded based on their appearance and behavior into well-differentiated or low-grade (grade 1), moderately well-differentiated or moderate-grade (grade 2), and poorly differentiated or high-grade (grade 3).
- The most common sites of metastasis are lymph nodes, peritoneal organs, and lungs; brain and bone metastases are rare.[4,5] Non–muscle-invasive lesions may remain indolent for years.[2]

RISK FACTORS

- The primary risk factor is smoking (odds ratio increased by 3- to 4-fold; 50% attributable risk). Other risk factors include exposure to pelvic radiation[6]; the drugs cyclophosphamide, phenacetin, and chlornaphazine; and chronic infection, including the parasite *Schistosoma haematobium* and genitourinary tuberculosis.[2,3]
- There is an increased risk in certain occupations, particularly those involving exposure to aromatic amines used in the dye, rubber, and pharmaceutical industries (such as benzidine and beta-naphthylamine). Painters, varnishers, and those exposed to hair dyes have had increased risk in some studies.[3,7,8]
- The impact of diet, including coffee and alcohol, is unclear. Environmental pollution is an area of concern. Arsenic contamination in drinking water increases risk. Secondary smoke exposure appears to increase risk, particularly in women who never smoked.[3,8]
- Risk is doubled in first-degree relatives of patients with bladder cancer, indicating a genetic predisposition.[3,8,9]

DIAGNOSIS

CLINICAL FEATURES

- Hematuria is present in 80% to 90%. When there is microscopic hematuria, approximately 2% have bladder cancer, and with gross hematuria approximately 20% have bladder cancer.[3,4]
- Irritative voiding (i.e., dysuria, frequency, urgency) is the most common symptom.
- Obstructive symptoms may occur if the tumor is located near the urethra or bladder neck.

LABORATORY

- Urine microscopy and culture to rule out bladder infection.[3]
- Urine cytology (high specificity [90% to 95%] but low sensitivity [23% to 60%]), CT urogram of the abdomen and pelvis with and without contrast (see **Figures 74-1, 74-3, and 74-4**), and cystoscopy with biopsy (see **Figure 74-2**) comprise the basic work-up.[2,4] Fluorescence cystoscopy (use of photosensitizer instilled into the

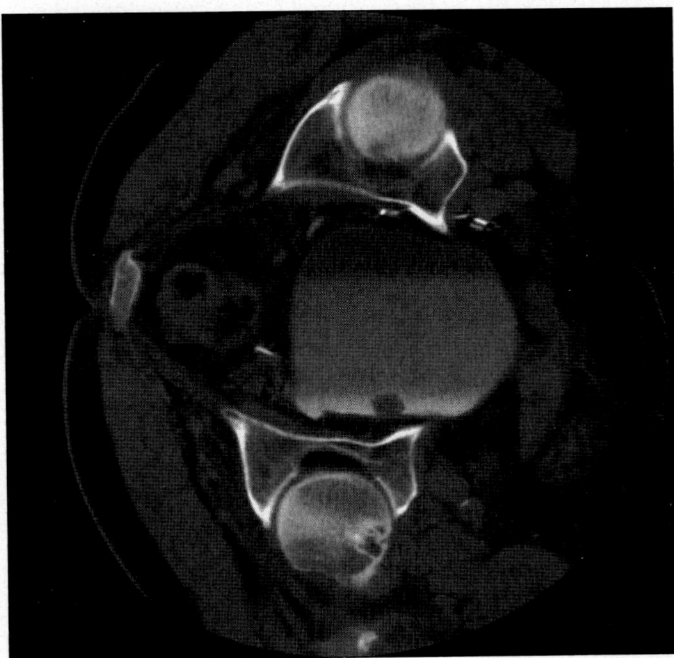

FIGURE 74-3 CT with contrast of a small transitional cell carcinoma of the bladder that was barely visible until the patient was scanned on side. A small bladder diverticulum is visible as well. (*Reproduced with permission from Michael Freckleton, MD.*)

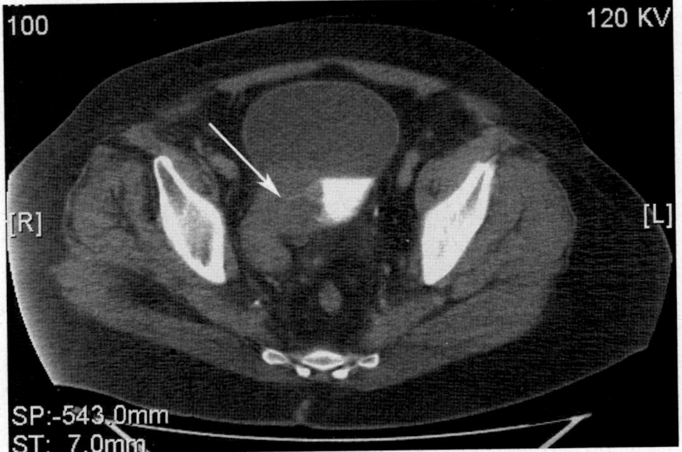

FIGURE 74-4 CT of locally invasive transitional cell carcinoma (*arrow*) of the bladder, extending outside of the bladder in a 71-year-old man. The carcinoma on the patient's right is displacing the contrast toward the left side of the patient's bladder. (*Reproduced with permission from Michael Freckleton, MD.*)

bladder) can enhance detection of flat neoplastic lesions like carcinoma in situ (CIS).[3,4]

- Bladder wash cytology during cystoscopy detects most CIS.[3]
- A complete blood count, blood chemistry tests (including alkaline phosphatase), liver function tests, CT or MRI of the chest or abdomen, and a bone scan may be needed for suspected metastatic disease.[2,3] Bone scanning may be limited to patients with bone pain or elevated levels of serum alkaline phosphatase.[4]
- Tumor markers such as fluorescence in situ hybridization (FISH) analysis and nuclear matrix protein (NMP) 22 identify changes in cells in the urine; they are more sensitive than urine cytology for low-grade tumors and have equivalent sensitivity for high-grade tumors and CIS.[10] As specificity is low, tumor markers should not be used for diagnosis.

IMAGING

- For pretreatment staging of invasive bladder cancer, the American College of Radiology (ACR) recommends a chest X-ray (with chest CT if equivocal), CT urogram of the abdomen and pelvis (without and with contrast), or MRI (especially in cases where patients are unable to undergo contrast injection), and possibly intravenous urography (IVU); contrast-enhanced MRI is preferred over CT for local staging.[4] SOR Ⓒ
- The European Association of Urology (EAU) recommends multidetector-row CT (MDCT) of the chest, abdomen, and pelvis as the optimal form of staging for patients with confirmed muscle-invasive bladder cancer, including MDCT urography for examination of the upper urinary tracts.[5] If MDCT is not available, alternatives are excretory urography and a chest X-ray. SOR Ⓑ

BIOPSY

- Diagnosis is made by cystoscopy, biopsy, and histology.

DIFFERENTIAL DIAGNOSIS

- Among adult patients with microscopic hematuria, most patients have benign pathology, such as urinary tract infection, with only 2% having bladder cancer.[3]
- Among adult patients with gross hematuria, 22% have benign cystitis and 15% to 20% have bladder cancer or another urothelial cancer such as kidney cancer.[3]

MANAGEMENT

FIRST LINE

MEDICATIONS

Neoadjuvant cisplatin-containing combination chemotherapy (administered prior to main treatment) improves overall 5-year survival by 5% to 7% and should be considered in muscle-invasive bladder cancer irrespective of definitive treatment.[5,11] SOR Ⓐ It is not recommended for patients with performance status of 2 or more and impaired renal function or for primary therapy for localized bladder cancer.[5]

- The role of adjuvant chemotherapy (usually administered after surgery) for invasive bladder cancer is under debate. A review and meta-analysis of 13 trials (N = 945) found a 23% relative reduction in the risk of death for chemotherapy compared to control patients (hazard ratio for survival 0.77; 95% CI 0.59, 0.99), and also showed evidence of a disease-free survival benefit for these patients.[12]
- Cisplatin-containing combination chemotherapy is first-line therapy for patients with metastatic disease, and treated patients can achieve a median survival of up to 14 months.[5,13] SOR Ⓐ

SURGICAL

Depends on the extent (depth and grade) or spread of the disease (**Table 74-1**). Recommendations have been provided by the American Urological Association and Society of Urologic Oncology (AUA/SUO, 2016)[13] and the EAU (2016)[5] as summarized below:

- Non–muscle-invasive disease (80% of cases)—Complete endoscopic resection with or without intravesical treatment (bacille Calmette-Guérin [BCG] weekly for 6 weeks or interferon or mitomycin C). SOR Ⓒ Low-grade tumors (Ta tumors) can be treated with resection alone or with a single postoperative dose of intravesical chemotherapy. SOR Ⓑ In a meta-analysis of three trials, tumor recurrence was significantly lower with intravesical BCG, but there was no difference in disease progression or survival.[14] SOR Ⓑ BCG treatment causes urinary frequency (71%), cystitis (67%), hematuria (23%), fever (25%),[15] and, rarely, systemic granulomatous infection requiring antituberculosis treatment.
- For Ta, Tis, or T1 tumors that are initially histologically confirmed as high grade, the AUA recommends repeat resection and additional intravesical therapy (induction course of BCG followed by maintenance therapy).[13] SOR Ⓐ A Cochrane review based on five small trials found that immunotherapy with intravesical BCG following surgery benefits patients with medium/high risk Ta or T1 bladder cancer on delaying tumor recurrence.[15] Additional Cochrane reviews found intravesical BCG more effective than intravesical epirubicin or mitomycin C in reducing tumor recurrence (the latter only for patients at high risk of recurrence)[16,17]; mitomycin C, however, was equivalent to BCG for disease progression and survival. SOR Ⓐ
- Persistent or recurrent non–muscle-invasive disease—Repeat resection with an induction course of BCG; maintenance BCG or mitomycin C is recommended or consideration of intravesical chemotherapy (valrubicin or gemcitabine). SOR Ⓑ For treatment failure of patients with non–muscle-invasive bladder tumors, EAU recommends radical cystectomy for those with high-grade tumors and cystectomy for other patients with T1 tumors.[5] SOR Ⓑ Delay in cystectomy for these patients increases the risk of progression and cancer-specific death.[5]
- Recurrent high-grade T1 tumors or disease that extends to muscle or lymph nodes—Radical cystectomy and pelvic lymphadenectomy with or without systemic chemotherapy.[3,5] SOR Ⓒ In men, radical cystectomy includes removal of the prostate, seminal vesicles, and proximal urethra, resulting in impotence. In women, the uterus, ovaries, and anterior vaginal wall are removed. Most patients

TABLE 74-1 Bladder Cancer Categories, Stage, and 5-Year Survival Rate

Tumor Category	Stage of Tumor*	Description	5-Year Survival
Non–muscle-invasive disease			95.9%
Ta	Stage 0 (N0,M0)	Non–muscle-invasive papillary carcinoma	
Tis	Stage 0 (N0,M0)	Carcinoma in situ	
T1	Stage I (N0,M0)	Tumor invading the lamina propria	
Muscle-invasive disease			70.2%
T2a	Stage II (N0,M0)	Tumor grown into inner half of muscle layer	
T2b	Stage II (N0,M0)	Tumor grown into outer half of muscle layer	
T3†	Stage III (N0,M0)	Tumor through muscle layer into fatty tissue	
T4a	Stage III (N0,M0)	Tumor beyond fatty tissue into nearby organs‡	
T4b	Stage IV (N0,M0)	Tumor beyond into pelvic or abdominal wall‡	
Lymph node			34.5%
N0	Stage IV	No lymph node involvement	
N1	Stage IV	Spread to single lymph node in true pelvis	
N2	Stage IV	Spread to 2 or more lymph nodes in true pelvis	
N3		Spread to nodes along the common iliac artery	
Metastatic disease			5.2%
M0	Stage IV	No distant spread	
M1		Cancer has spread to distant sites*	

*Determined by combining the tumor category with presence or absence and number of lymph nodes involved (N), and presence or absence or distant spread (e.g., distant lymph nodes, bones, lungs, and liver).
†Also divided into *a* (microscopic spread into fatty tissue) and *b* (visible spread on imaging or to the eye).
‡Also divided into *a* (spread to prostate or uterus/vagina) and *b* (spread to pelvic or abdominal wall).
Information based on SEER data. https://seer.cancer.gov/csr/1975_2013/browse_csr.php?sectionSEL=27&pageSEL=sect_27_table.08.html. Accessed March 2017.

receive cutaneous reservoirs (bowel or orthotopic neobladder) drained by intermittent self-catheterization.

- Chemotherapy is not used for nonurothelial cancers, such as squamous cell carcinoma or adenocarcinoma, which are primarily treated with cystectomy.[3]
- Upper urinary tract recurrence—Radical nephroureterectomy. SOR B

SECOND LINE

- In a Cochrane review of three trials comparing radical radiotherapy followed by surgery (salvage cystectomy) versus radical cystectomy, overall survival was better with radical cystectomy.[18] SOR A
- External-beam radiotherapy alone is considered an option for patients unfit for cystectomy or to stop the bleeding from a tumor when local control cannot be achieved by transurethral manipulation because of extensive local tumor growth.[5] SOR C

PREVENTION

Eliminate active and passive smoking.[5] SOR C

PROGNOSIS

- Tumor grade is an important prognostic factor for determining risk of recurrence and progression. Other factors associated with increased risk of progression are large tumor size, the presence of CIS, diffuse disease, infiltration of lymphatic or vascular spaces, and prostatic urethral involvement.[13]
- Performance status, ranging from 0 (fully active) to 4 (completely disabled), and the presence or absence of visceral metastases are independent prognostic factors for survival.
- The EAU working group suggests use of the weighted European Organization for Research and Treatment of Cancer (EORTC) scoring system to estimate recurrence and progression risk.[19] Factors include number, size, category, and grade of tumors; prior recurrence; and concomitant CIS. Scores range from 0 to 17 for recurrence and 0 to 23 for progression. These scores are translated into probabilities for 1-year and 5-year recurrence (15% and 31%, respectively, for a score of 0, and 61% to 78%, respectively, for a score of 10 to 17) and 1-year and 5-year progression (0.2% and 0.8%, respectively, for a score of 0, and 17% to 45%, respectively, for a score of 14 to 23).
- Five-year survival rates for non–muscle-invasive disease are 95.9%; muscle-invasive with localized spread, 70.2%; with lymph node involvement, 34.5%; and with distant metastatic spread of disease, 5.2% (see **Table 74-1**). The 5-year survival rate for all grades and stages combined is 77%.[1]

FOLLOW-UP

- Recurrence rates overall are 50% with a median time of recurrence at 1 year (0.4 to 11 years). Between 5% and 20% will progress to a more advanced stage. Patients should be seen every 3 months for the first year. SOR Ⓒ The ACR and EAU recommend stopping oncologic surveillance after 5 years of normal follow-up, to be replaced by functional surveillance (e.g., renal function).[4,5]

- For patients with high-grade Ta and T1 disease, cystoscopy, urinalysis, and urine cytology are recommended every 3 months for 2 years, then every 6 months for 2 years, then annually. Imaging of the upper tract collecting system is performed every 1 to 2 years.[3,4]
- For patients with muscle-invasive disease, laboratory tests (liver function test, creatinine clearance, electrolyte panel) in addition to a chest X-ray are recommended every 6 to 12 months with imaging of upper urinary tract, abdomen, and pelvis for recurrence every 3 to 6 months for 2 years, and then as clinically indicated.[3]
- For patients undergoing bladder-sparing surgery, urine cytology with or without biopsy is conducted every 3 months for 1 year, then at increasing intervals.[3]
- For patients undergoing cystectomy, urine cytology is conducted every 6 to 12 months, and for those undergoing cystectomy and cutaneous diversion, urethral wash cytology is recommended every 6 to 12 months.[3]
- For patients with cystectomy and continent orthotopic diversion, vitamin B_{12} level should be checked annually.[3,20]
- Bladder tumor markers from voided urine will likely improve detection of recurrence in the future, but data are still insufficient to warrant use of tumor markers instead of cystoscopic follow-up.[4,21]

PATIENT EDUCATION

- The most important primary prevention for muscle-invasive bladder cancer is to eliminate active and passive smoking.
- Tumor recurrence and progression risk can be estimated from clinical and pathologic factors[3]; this information may help in joint decision making for primary treatment and follow-up intervals.

PATIENT RESOURCES

- MedlinePlus. *Bladder Cancer.* **www.nlm.nih.gov/medlineplus/bladdercancer.html.**
- National Cancer Institute. *Bladder Cancer.* **https://www.cancer.gov/types/bladder.**
- Cancer Research UK. *About Bladder Cancer.* **http://cancerhelp.cancerresearchuk.org/type/bladder-cancer/about/.**
- We Are Macmillan. CancerSupport. *Bladder Cancer.* **http://www.macmillan.org.uk/Cancerinformation/Cancertypes/Bladder/Bladdercancer.aspx.**

PROVIDER RESOURCES

- *Cancer State Facts: Bladder Cancer*—**http://seer.cancer.gov/statfacts/html/urinb.html.**
- Bladder Cancer Treatment (PDQ)—Health Professional Version—**https://www.cancer.gov/types/bladder/hp/bladder-treatment-pdq.**

REFERENCES

1. *SEER Cancer Statistics Review 1975–2013.* https://seer.cancer.gov/csr/1975_2013/results_merged/sect_27_urinary_bladder.pdf. Accessed January 2017.
2. Scher HI, Rosenberg JE, Motzer RJ. Bladder and renal cell carcinomas. In: Kasper D, Fauci A, Hauser S, et al, eds. *Harrison's Principles of Internal Medicine*, 19th ed. New York, NY: McGraw-Hill; 2014. http://accessmedicine.mhmedical.com/content.aspx?bookid=1130§ionid=69858213. Accessed February 2017.
3. Sharma S, Ksheersagar P, Sharma P. Diagnosis and treatment of bladder cancer. *Am Fam Physician.* 2009;80(7):717-723.
4. American College of Radiology (ACR), Expert Panel on Urologic Imaging. *ACR Appropriateness Criteria Pretreatment Staging of Invasive Bladder Cancer (2012).* https://acsearch.acr.org/docs/69370/Narrative/. Accessed May 2018.
5. Alfred Witjes J, Lebret T, Compérat EM, et al. Updated 2016 EAU Guidelines on Muscle-invasive and Metastatic Bladder Cancer. *Eur Urol.* 2017;71(3):462-475.
6. Keehn A, Ludmir E, Taylor J, Rabbani F. Incidence of bladder cancer after radiation for prostate cancer as a function of time and radiation modality. *World J Urol.* 2017;35(5):713-720.
7. Rew KT. Causation in genitourinary problems. In: Melhorn JM, Talmage JB, Ackerman WE III, Hyman MH, eds. *AMA Guides to the Evaluation of Disease and Injury Causation.* 2nd ed. Chicago, IL: American Medical Association; 2014.
8. Burger M, Catto JW, Dalbagni G, et al. Epidemiology and risk factors of urothelial bladder cancer. *Eur Urol.* 2013;63(2):234-241. Review. PMID: 22877502
9. Aben KK, Witjes JA, Schoenberg MP, et al. Familial aggregation of urothelial cell carcinoma. *Int J Cancer.* 2002;98(2):274-278.
10. Gutiérrez Baños JL, Rebollo Rodrigo MH, Antolín Juárez FM, Martín García B. NMP 22, BTA stat test and cytology in the diagnosis of bladder cancer: a comparative study. *Urol Int.* 2001;66(4):185-190.
11. Advanced Bladder Cancer Meta-analysis Collaboration. Neoadjuvant chemotherapy for invasive bladder cancer. *Cochrane Database Syst Rev.* 2005;(2):CD005246.
12. Leow JJ, Martin-Doyle W, Rajagopal PS, et al. Adjuvant chemotherapy for invasive bladder cancer: a 2013 updated systematic review and meta-analysis of randomized trials. *Eur Urol.* 2014;66(1):42-54.
13. Chang SS, Boorjian SA, Chou R, et al. Diagnosis and treatment of non-muscle invasive bladder cancer: AUA/SUO guideline. *J Urol.* 2016;196(4):1021-1029.
14. Shelley MD, Wilt TJ, Court J, et al. Intravesical bacillus Calmette-Guerin is superior to mitomycin C in reducing tumour recurrence in high-risk superficial bladder cancer: a meta-analysis of randomized trials. *BJU Int.* 2004;93(4):485-490.
15. Shelley M, Court JB, Kynaston H, et al. Intravesical bacillus Calmette-Guérin in Ta and T1 bladder cancer. *Cochrane Database Syst Rev.* 2000;(4):CD001986.

16. Shang PF, Kwong J, Wang ZP, et al. Intravesical bacillus Calmette-Guérin versus epirubicin for Ta and T1 bladder cancer. *Cochrane Database Syst Rev.* 2011;(5):CD006885.

17. Shelley M, Court JB, Kynaston H, et al. Intravesical bacillus Calmette-Guérin versus mitomycin C for Ta and T1 bladder cancer. *Cochrane Database Syst Rev.* 2003;(3):CD003231.

18. Shelley M, Barber J, Wilt T, Mason M. Surgery versus radiotherapy for muscle invasive bladder cancer. *Cochrane Database Syst Rev.* 2002;(1):CD002079.

19. Babjuk M, Böhle A, Burger M, et al. EAU guidelines on non-muscle-invasive urothelial carcinoma of the bladder: update 2016. *Eur Urol.* 2017;71(3):447-461.

20. Ganesan T, Khadra MH, Wallis J, Neal DE. Vitamin B12 malabsorption following bladder reconstruction or diversion with bowel segments. *ANZ J Surg.* 2002;72(7):479-482.

21. Lokeshwar VB, Habuchi T, Grossman HB, et al. Bladder tumor markers beyond cytology: International consensus panel on bladder tumor markers. *Urology.* 2005;66:35-63.

75 PROSTATE CANCER

Charles Carter, MD
Kari-Claudia M. Allen, MD, MPH

PATIENT STORY

A 55-year-old African-American man in relatively good health comes to the office after having had a prostate-specific antigen (PSA) test performed as part of a workplace health screening. He denies lower urinary tract symptoms, has normal erectile function, and denies weight loss and bone pain. He has no major medical problems, but his father and uncle had prostate cancer. His PSA is 9.3 ng/mL, and he chooses to have a prostate biopsy. Pathology demonstrates prostate cancer with a World Health Organization International Society of Urological Pathology (WHO-ISUP) Grade of 1 (**Figure 75-1**).

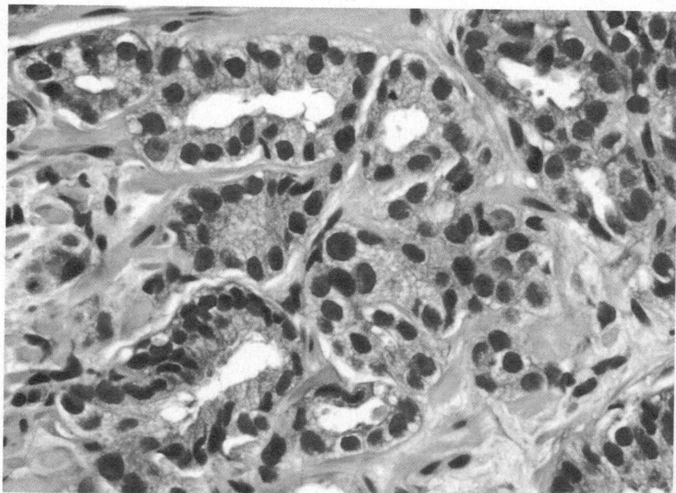

FIGURE 75-1 Microscopic image of biopsy demonstrating glands with enlarged nuclei and prominent nucleoli (hematoxylin and eosin [H&E] staining). The patient was diagnosed with prostate cancer with a Gleason grade of 1. (*Reproduced with permission from E.J. Mayeaux, Jr., MD.*)

INTRODUCTION

Prostate cancer (**Figure 75-2**) is the most common non-dermatologic cancer in men.[1] The advent of PSA testing and resulting widespread use led to an increase in prostate cancer diagnosis. However, this proved controversial because of uncertain benefits and clear harms. Regardless, PSA testing remains a common test in the evaluation of male urogenital complaints. Once prostate cancer has been diagnosed in a patient, multiple factors such as Gleason score, PSA level, stage at diagnosis, and life expectancy are all considered in risk stratification and treatment options.

EPIDEMIOLOGY

- Prostate cancer is the third leading cause of cancer death in American men. In 2017 the estimated incidence of new prostate cancer cases in the United States was 161,360, with 26,730 prostate cancer–related deaths.[1]
- The relative risk of prostate cancer is 74% higher in black males than non-Hispanic white males. While exact mechanisms are uncertain this is thought to be attributable to inherited susceptibility.[1] In 2013, black men had the highest incidence rate of prostate cancer, followed by non-Hispanic white, Hispanic, American Indian/Alaskan Native, and Asian/Pacific Islander men **(Figure 75-3).**
- Mortality risk is also greatest in black males. Although cancer deaths have been steadily decreasing since the early 1990s in men of all races, the death rate remains twice as high in black males as in any other group.[1] Data from 2010–2014 demonstrate a prostate cancer death rate of 42.8 per 100,000 men in black males, compared with 18.7 per 100,000 in white males and 8.8 per 100,000 in Asian males.[2]
- For non-Hispanic white males, the lifetime probability of developing invasive prostate cancer is 12.9%. Incidence increases with age, with the highest probability being in men 70 years of age or older (9.1% or 1 in 11).[1]
- Five-year relative survival rates for prostate cancer are greater than 99% for cancers diagnosed at the local and regional stages. This figure drops to 29% for cancer diagnosed after metastasis.[1]
- Globally, prostate cancer is the second most common cancer in men, with over 1.1 million cases diagnosed in 2012.[3]

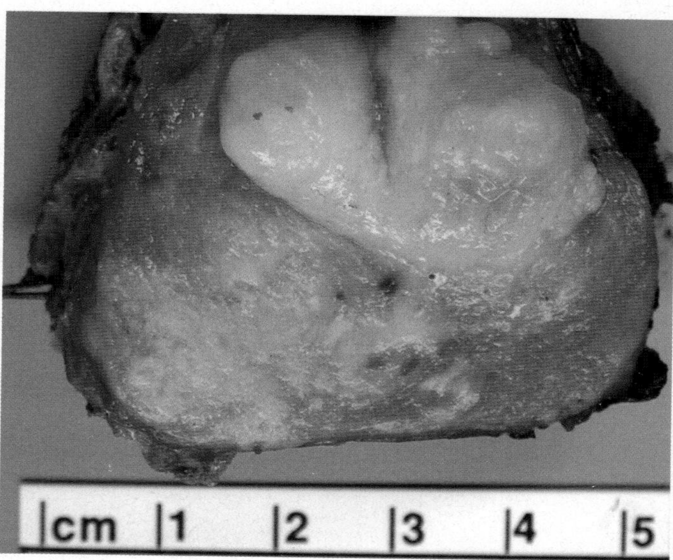

FIGURE 75-2 Photograph showing adenocarcinoma on the left lower side of the specimen and bilateral benign prostatic hypertrophy toward the top. (*Reproduced with permission from E.J. Mayeaux, Jr., MD.*)

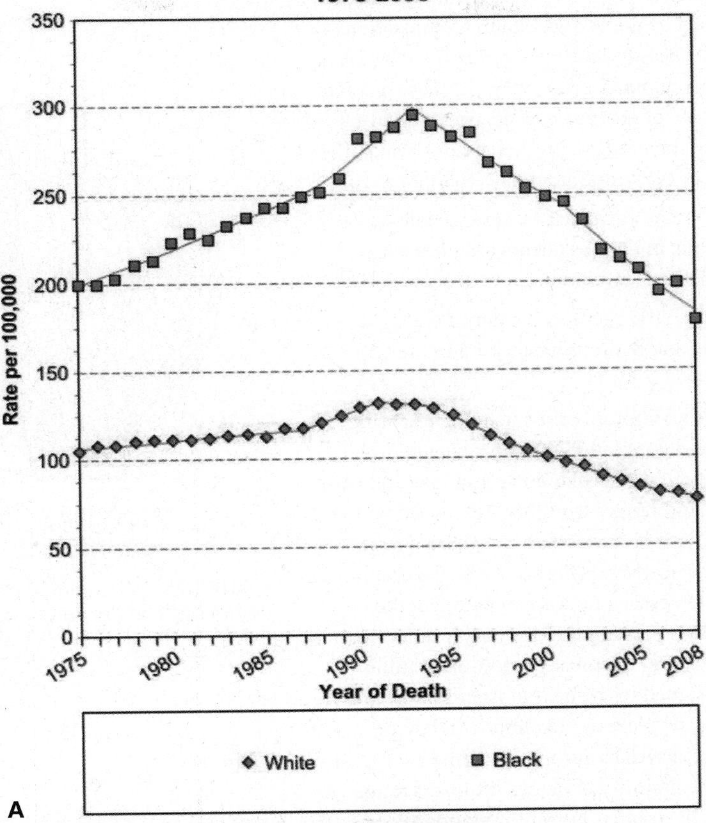

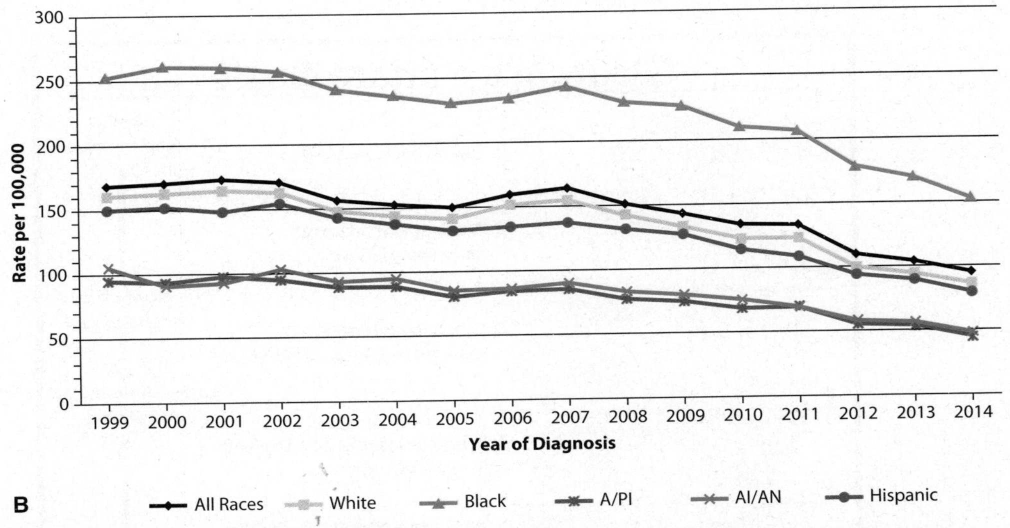

FIGURE 75-3 **A.** Age-adjusted U.S. prostate cancer mortality rates by race and ethnicity in males older than the age of 50 years. Note the higher mortality in blacks. **B.** Incidence rates of prostate cancer in the U.S. from 1999 to 2013 by race and ethnicity in males. Note the higher incidence rate in black males. *(Reproduced with permission from the Centers for Disease Control and Prevention.)*

ETIOLOGY AND PATHOPHYSIOLOGY

- Prostate cancers are a histologically heterogenous group of malignant tumors that are classified by the World Health Organization (WHO) grading system and Gleason scoring. Approximately 95% of prostate cancers are adenocarcinomas, originating from the prostate glands and ducts. The other 5% of prostate cancers originate from transitional epithelial cells in the urethra (urothelial carcinoma), the support tissues (sarcomas), or the lymphoid tissues (lymphoma).[4]
- Although most adenocarcinomas are acinar in type, histologic variants include ductal carcinoma, mucinous adenocarcinoma, signet ring cell carcinoma, and small cell carcinoma.
- Of prostate adenocarcinomas, 70% occur in the peripheral zone, 20% in the transitional zone, and approximately 10% in the central zone (**Figure 75-4**).
- The Gleason score is the most commonly used histologic scoring system for prostate cancer and correlates with tumor aggressiveness. The Gleason score is based on the glandular architectural pattern of prostate cancer cells and ranges from 2 to 10.[5] Based on the growth pattern and differentiation, tumors are categorized from 1 (least aggressive) to 5 (most aggressive) (**Figure 75-5**). To account for the fact that most biopsies reveal a mixture of patterns, the Gleason score is calculated by summing the two most predominant types. The first score is assigned to the most predominant tumor pattern and the second is assigned to the next most common tumor pattern. A higher score indicates a greater likelihood of having non–organ-confined disease, as well as a worse outcome after treatment of localized disease. The majority of detected tumors range from 5 to 10.[5] The newer ISUP Grade is becoming standard and is scored 1–5 based on glandular appearance and Gleason score.[6]
- Patterns of spread include direct extension, hematogenous, and lymphatic.
- Lymphatic spread occurs to the hypogastric, obturator, external iliac, presacral, common iliac, and paraaortic nodes.[7]

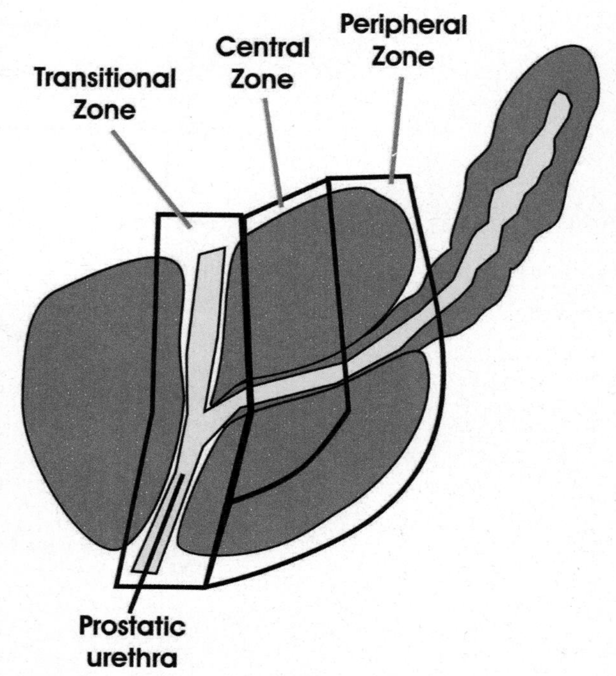

FIGURE 75-4 Diagram of prostate zones. Most prostate adenocarcinomas occur in the peripheral zone. (*Reproduced with permission from E.J. Mayeaux, Jr., MD.*)

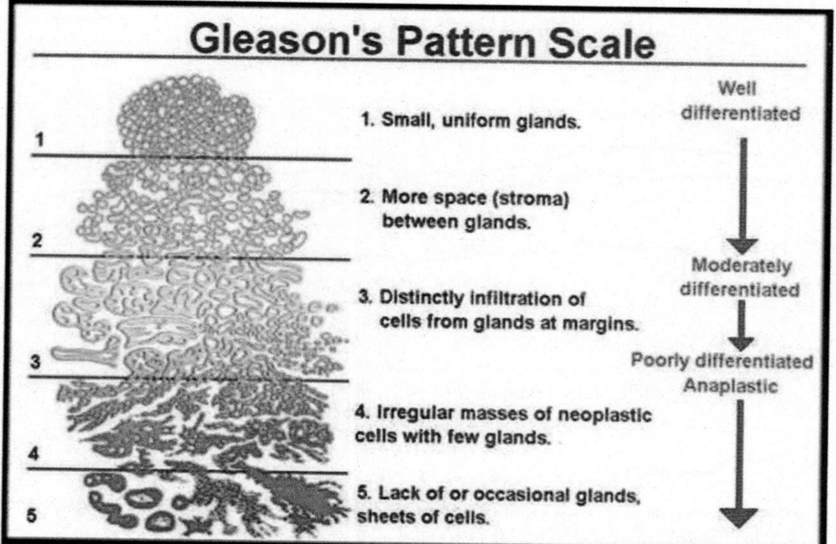

FIGURE 75-5 Gleason scoring of prostate cancer. (*Reproduced with permission from Gleason, DF. Histologic grading and clinical staging of prostatic carcinoma. In Tannenbaum M. Urologic Pathology: The Prostate. Philadelphia, PA: Lea and Febiger; 1977.*)

- 90% of distant metastases are osseous.
- Visceral metastases to lung, liver, and adrenals are less commonly seen without bone involvement.[7]

RISK FACTORS

The following factors increase the risk of developing prostate cancer[1]:

- First-degree relative (father, son, or brother) with prostate cancer
- African ancestry (highest documented rates are in U.S. and Caribbean men of African descent)
- Increasing age
- Inherited genetic conditions, such as BRCA1 or BRCA2, and Lynch syndrome
- Smoking is associated with risk of fatal prostate cancer

DIAGNOSIS

CLINICAL FEATURES

- Most prostate cancers are asymptomatic.
- Prostate cancer can be associated with urinary obstructive symptoms or hematuria, but these are usually a result of other causes.
- Rarely, bone pain can be an initial symptom. This generally represents advanced disease.
- A prostatic nodule on digital rectal examination (DRE) is not always specific for a carcinoma and can underestimate the extent of disease when it does represent a carcinoma. A positive biopsy is as likely to occur in the opposite lobe of the prostate as it is from an abnormal area detected on physical exam.[8]

STAGING

- The most widely used staging of prostate cancer is the American Joint Committee on Cancer (AJCC) TNM system.
- The TNM system is based on the extent of the primary tumor extension (T category); whether the cancer has spread to local lymph nodes (N category); whether the cancer has metastasized to other regions of the body (M category); the PSA level at the time of diagnosis; and the Gleason grade based on biopsy.
- There are two stages: clinical and pathologic.
- Clinical staging is based on the combined results of the DRE, lab tests, prostate biopsy, and imaging.
- Pathologic staging is based on the clinical staging, in addition to the findings of surgical exploration.

LABORATORY TESTING

▶ PSA

- Prostate-specific antigen (PSA) is a glycoprotein produced primarily by the epithelial cells that line the acini and ducts of the prostate gland, urethra, and bulbourethral gland. Because of its concentration within the prostatic tissue, serum PSA levels are normally very low.[9]
- Disruption of the normal prostatic architecture, such as by prostatic disease, inflammation, or trauma, allows greater amounts of PSA to enter the general circulation.[9]
- Several sources will cite data on the sensitivity and specificity of the PSA diagnostic tool. However, there is no cutoff value that determines a "positive" or "negative" test result, as there remains some risk of having prostate cancer even with undetectable PSA levels, due to the operating characteristics of the test.[10]
- In asymptomatic men with PSA levels less than 2.0 ng/mL, the risk of prostate cancer is considered to be very low. Reference levels vary by age range, and the upper limit of normal increases as men get older. It is generally accepted that PSA levels >10.0 ng/mL should be further investigated with biopsy.[11]
- The European Randomized Study of Screening for Prostate Cancer (ERSPC) and the Prostate, Lung, Colorectal, and Ovarian (PCLO) Cancer Screening Trials are two widely accepted studies that addressed PSA-based screening for prostate cancer, and specifically looked at prostate cancer–specific mortality as primary endpoints. The ERSPC study, the largest randomized cohort study of >182,000 men, showed that men screened with PSA testing had a 29% reduction in risk of dying from prostate cancer compared with unscreened men.[12]
- The PCLO, an American study that enrolled approximately 76,000 men, showed no significant difference in the prostate-specific or overall mortality of the screened and unscreened cohorts at 15 years of follow-up.[13,14]
- Since the advent of PSA screening, the incidence of prostate cancer cases diagnosed at advanced stages has declined significantly, and death rates from prostate cancer as reported in the National Cancer Database have declined at the rate of 1% per year since 1990.[15] However, screening asymptomatic men remains controversial, as there are potential benefits for some men but also clear harms, including overdiagnosis and overtreatment as well as no clear mortality benefit. The number needed to screen to prevent 1 prostate cancer death and up to 3 instances of metastasis is 1000. Of those 1000 men screened, approximately 240 will require further evaluation, and 100 will have a positive biopsy. Thus, many "positive" PSA tests are false positives. Furthermore, up to 50% of the men with positive biopsies would have cancer that would not become significant during their lifetime. Finally, many men experience serious harms from treatment including surgical complications, urinary incontinence, and impotence.[16]
- Screening in men with family histories and African-American men is a consideration based on their elevated risk. The USPTSF examined screening in these elevated risk groups but was unable to find sufficient evidence to inform a separate recommendation for these patients (**Table 75-1**).[16]
- For patients considering PSA testing, recommendations encourage clinicians to involve patients in a shared decision discussion focusing on the risks, benefits, limitations, and uncertainties about PSA-based testing. Decision aids may also be helpful. These factors should be weighed in consideration of the patient's personal values and goals relative to the testing, as well as the patient's willingness to pursue further evaluation for abnormal tests. Life expectancy is also a consideration, as men over 70 or those with life expectancy less than 10 years are unlikely to experience the potential benefits.[16]

TABLE 75-1 Recommendations Regarding Prostate Cancer Screening

	American Cancer Society*	American Urological Association†	US Preventive Services Task Force‡
Universal PSA-based screening	No	No	No
Digital rectal exam	Optional addition if using PSA testing	Not recommended for screening	Not recommended for screening
PSA recommendation	For asymptomatic men with a 10-year life expectancy, give the opportunity for screening. High-risk men prior to age 50, average-risk at age 50. Screening uses PSA with or without DRE.	Recommends individualized screening decisions for high-risk men ages 40–54. Shared-decision for men ages 55–69. If testing is performed, it should occur every 2 years. Recommends against screening men under age 40.	Recommends informing men ages 55–69 of the benefits and harms of PSA-based screening and be allowed to make an informed decision. Recommends against screening men 70 and older.
Informed consent	Yes	Yes	Yes
Testing in patients with limited (<10-year) life expectancy	No	No	No
Notes		Recommend against community-based screening (ex: health fairs)	

Abbreviations: DRE, digital rectal examination; PSA, prostate-specific antigen.

*Wolf AM, et al. American Cancer Society guideline for the early detection of prostate cancer: update 2010. *Ca Cancer J Clin.* 2010; 60:70-98.

†AUA Carter HB, et al. *Early Detection of Prostate Cancer: AUA Guideline.* 2013. American Urological Association Education and Research, Inc.

‡US Preventive Services Task Force. Screening for Prostate Cancer: US Preventive Services Task Force Recommendation Statement. *JAMA.* 2018;319(18):1901–1913.

IMAGING

▶ Transrectal ultrasound

- Transrectal ultrasound (TRUS) is also known as prostate sonogram or endorectal ultrasound. It is performed to assess prostate volume and guide prostate biopsy.
- A hypoechoic lesion detected on TRUS has a 30% chance of being carcinoma. After the standard 12-needle biopsy has been performed, additional areas of echogenicity are biopsied. This technique can increase the detection rate by 3.5%.[17]
- TRUS is not recommended as a screening tool.

▶ Bone scan

- Radionuclide imaging is routinely used to evaluate for disseminated disease.
- Likelihood of a positive bone scan is predicted by PSA level >20 and Gleason score of 8 or greater.[18] American Urological Association (AUA) guidelines recommend against bone scan in patients with low-risk tumors.[19]

▶ CT scan and MRI

- CT scans and pelvic MRI are part of evaluating staging, metastasis, and treatment for intermediate-risk tumors and above but are not recommended for low-risk disease evaluation.[19] They may also play a role in active surveillance.

▶ Prostate biopsy

- Performed with local anesthesia and ultrasound guidance using a spring-loaded biopsy needle to obtain 12 prostate biopsy specimens. The patient may experience significant discomfort despite the anesthetic.
- The percentage of positive cores, length, or percentage of cancer per core can provide predictive information.
- Lower GI tract cleansing enemas and prophylactic antibiotics are routinely used.
- Harms including bleeding, prostate and urinary infection, and pain.

DIFFERENTIAL DIAGNOSIS

- Prostatitis—Infection or inflammation of the prostate. This is often associated with perineal or suprapubic pain, dysuria, and urinary frequency, whereas prostate cancer is often asymptomatic.
- Benign prostatic hyperplasia—An enlarged prostate that may cause obstructive lower urinary tract symptoms. There is no relative increase in the risk of developing prostate cancer. Prostate hyperplasia may also elevate the PSA test.
- Prostatic intraepithelial neoplasia (PIN)—High-grade PIN has been noted as a precursor to prostate carcinoma.[20]
- Atypical glands on biopsy—The probability of detecting cancer following an atypical diagnosis is approximately 40%. Often a repeat biopsy is recommended with increased sampling of the atypical site.

MANAGEMENT

- One by-product of PSA testing has been a shift to a more complex and multifactorial management approach due to increased diagnosis of cancers that are not likely to negatively impact the patient. General considerations guiding management include age, and health status, Gleason score, initial serum PSA, estimated tumor volume, tumor stage and risk assessment, life expectancy, and patient values and goals relative to treatment.
- Treatment options through a shared decision model should be explained so that patients can make an informed decision about which treatment best fits their values and goals. SOR Ⓐ
- The AUA has developed a risk assessment strategy for localized tumors.[19] Lower risk tumors have PSA <10 ng/mL, ISUP Grade group 1, T1–T2a stage. In addition, very low-risk tumors also have <34% of biopsy cores positive, no core with >50% cancer, and PSA density <0.15 ng/mL.[19]
- Watchful waiting and active surveillance are the two least invasive management options. Watchful waiting involves the patient forgoing treatment and further surveillance, often because the risk of treatment may outweigh the benefit to the patient, but palliative treatment for symptoms, such as pain or urinary difficulties, can be offered as necessary. In contrast, active surveillance delays treatment but monitors for disease progression over time in patients who are likely to die with the disease rather than from the disease. Treatment is considered if significant disease progression is detected. This involves PSA testing and periodic biopsy.[19] This is the recommended approach for very low-risk individuals SOR Ⓐ and most low-risk individuals.[19] SOR Ⓑ They are also options for men choosing not to undergo immediate therapy at the time of diagnosis.
- For more advanced risk disease there are many treatment options. Radical prostatectomy or radiation plus androgen deprivation therapy are recommended for localized disease in these patients.[19] SOR Ⓐ Radical prostatectomy is performed through either open or robotic-assisted **(Figure 75-6)** techniques. Risks include typical perioperative risks as well as urinary incontinence and erectile dysfunction.

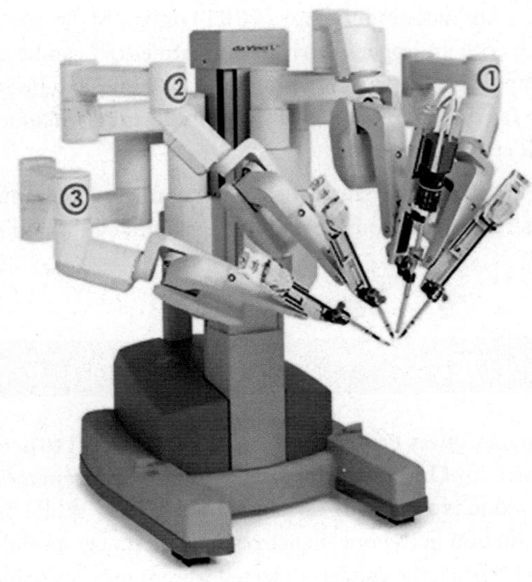

FIGURE 75-6 The DaVinci robot: three working arms and a camera. The robot allows for better visualization of the pelvic anatomy. (*Reproduced with permission from Intuitive Surgical.*)

- External beam radiation therapy (EBRT) or brachytherapy is often combined with androgen deprivation treatment. It can be used without androgen deprivation but guidelines advise there is less evidence for this approach.[19] SOR Ⓑ Side effects can include rectal and bladder symptomatology.
- Local ablation, high-intensity focal ultrasound, cryotherapy, and chemotherapy are options depending on tumor status and patient selection.

PREVENTION

- The Prostate Cancer Prevention Trial (PCPT) sought to determine the prevalence of histologically proven prostate cancer among men randomized to receive daily finasteride or placebo. While there was 24.8% reduction in the prevalence of prostate cancer among men taking finasteride, the cancers detected were significantly higher grade tumors.[21] Therefore, finasteride is not recommended for prostate cancer prevention.[22]
- More recently, the Selenium and Vitamin E Cancer Prevention Trial (SELECT) found that although selenium does not prevent prostate cancer, vitamin E supplementation is associated with a significantly increased risk of prostate cancer.[23]

PROGNOSIS

- The optimal management and outcomes for patients with prostate cancer vary according to a patient's age, overall health status, treatment options, personal preferences, and tumor grade and risk assessment.

PATIENT EDUCATION

- Patients should be provided balanced and objective information about the risks and benefits of screening, post-screening testing, and the various treatment options for prostate cancer. Clinicians should assist patients in finding a course of prevention and treatment that fits their individual needs. For patients diagnosed with prostate cancer, seeking multiple treatment opinions from different specialists is recommended.[19] SOR Ⓑ (See Patient and Provider Resources.)
- Risk assessment calculations can be useful in discussions with patients to help them decide about screening, biopsy, and treatment (Provider Resources).

PATIENT RESOURCES

- United States Preventive Services Task Force—**www.screeningforprostatecancer.org.**
- Men's Health Network—**http://www.menshealthnetwork.org.**
- National Cancer Institute—**https://www.cancer.gov/types/prostate.**
- Links to prostate cancer online prediction tools are listed under Provider Resources below and are useful for patients in their discussions with physicians.

PROVIDER RESOURCES

- American Cancer Society—**https://www.cancer.org/cancer/prostate-cancer/detection-diagnosis-staging.htmL.**
- The Prostate Cancer Prevention Trial Prostate Cancer Risk Calculator (PCPTRC) provides a person's estimated risk of biopsy-detectable prostate cancer and high-grade prostate cancer—**http://deb.uthscsa.edu/URORiskCalc/Pages/uroriskcalc.jsp.**
- National Cancer Institute (NCI). *Prostate Cancer*—**https://www.cancer.gov/types/prostate/hp.**
- National Comprehensive Cancer Network (NCCN)—**http://www.nccn.org/professionals/physician_gls/f_guidelines.asp.**
- Prostate-Specific Antigen-Based Screening for Prostate Cancer: Evidence Report and Systematic Review for the US Preventive Services Task Force—**https://www.uspreventiveservicestaskforce.org/Page/Document/final-evidence-review/prostate-cancer-screening1.**

REFERENCES

1. American Cancer Society. *Cancer Facts & Figures 2017*. Atlanta, GA: American Cancer Society; 2017.
2. National Center for Health Statistics, Centers for Disease Control and Prevention. https://www.cdc.gov/nchs/index.htm. Accessed June 5, 2018.
3. American Cancer Society. *Global Cancer Facts and Figures*, 3rd Edition. https://www.cancer.org/content/dam/cancer-org/research/cancer-facts-and-statistics/global-cancer-facts-and-figures/global-cancer-facts-and-figures-3rd-edition.pdf. Accessed June 5, 2018.
4. Lie AK. Histology of Prostate Cancer. *Oncolex Oncology Encyclopedia*. http://oncolex.org/Prostate-cancer/Background/Histology. Accessed June 4, 2018.
5. Gleason, DF. Histologic grading and clinical staging of prostatic carcinoma. In: Tannenbaum M. *Urologic Pathology: The Prostate*. Philadelphia, PA: Lea and Febiger; 1977:171-197.
6. Epstein JI, Zelefsky MJ, Sjoberg DD, et al. A contemporary prostate cancer grading system: A validated alternative to the Gleason score. *Eur Urol*. 2016;69(3):428-435.
7. Wein A. *Clinical Manual of Urology*. 3rd ed. New York, NY: McGraw-Hill; 2001.
8. McNaughton-Collins M, Ransohoff DF, Barry MJ. Early detection of prostate cancer: serendipity strikes again. *JAMA*. 1997;278:1516-1519.
9. Ramos CG, Carvahal GF, Mager DE, et al. The effect of high grade prostatic intraepithelial neoplasia on serum total and percentage of free prostate specific antigen levels. *J Urol*. 1999;162:1587.
10. Thompson IM, Ankerst DP, Chi C, et al. Operating characteristics of prostate-specific antigen in men with an initial PSA level of 3.0 ng/mL or lower. *JAMA*. 2005;294:66-70.
11. Jacobsen SJ, Bergstralh EJ, Guess HA, et al. Predictive properties of serum prostate-specific antigen testing in a community-based setting. *Arch Intern Med*. 1996;156:2462-2468.

12. Schröder FH, Hugosson J, Roobol MJ, et al. Screening and prostate-cancer mortality in a randomized European study. *N Engl J Med.* 2009;360:1320-1328.

13. Andriole GL, Crawford ED, Grubb RL 3rd, et al. Prostate cancer screening in the randomized Prostate, Lung, Colorectal, and Ovarian Cancer Screening Trial: mortality results after 13 years of follow-up. *J Natl Cancer Inst.* 2012;104:125-132.

14. Pinsky PF, Prorok PC, Yu K, et al. Extended mortality results for prostate cancer screening in the PLCO trial with median follow-up of 15 years. *Cancer.* 123:4,592-599.

15. Mettlin CJ, Murphy GP, Rosenthal DS et al. The National Cancer Data Base report on prostate carcinoma after the peak in incidence rates in the US. The American College of Surgeons Commission on Cancer and the American Cancer Society. *Cancer.* 1998;83:1679.

16. US Preventive Services Task Force. Screening for Prostate Cancer: US Preventive Services Task Force Recommendation Statement. *JAMA.* 2018;319(18): 1901-1913.

17. Gosselaar C, Roobol MJ, Roemeling S, et al. The value of an additional hypoechoic lesion-directed biopsy core for detecting prostate cancer. *BJU Int.* 2008;101:685-690.

18. Merdan S, Womble PR, Miller DC, et al. Toward better use of bone scans among men with early-stage prostate cancer. *Urology.* 2014;84(4):793-798.

19. Sanda MG, Chen RC, Crispino T, et al. Clinically localized prostate cancer: AUA/ASTRO/SUO guideline. 2017 American Urological Association Education and Research, Inc. http://www.auanet.org/guidelines/clinically-localized-prostate-cancer-new-(aua/astro/suo-guideline-2017). Accessed June 5, 2018.

20. Epstein JI, Herawi M. Prostate needle biopsies containing prostatic intraepithelial neoplasia or atypical foci suspicious for carcinoma: implications for patient care. *J Urol.* 2006;175(3 Pt 1):820-834.

21. Crawford ED, Andriole GL, Marberger M, Rittmaster RS. Reduction in the risk of prostate cancer: future directions after the Prostate Cancer Prevention Trial. *Urology.* 2010;75(3):502-509.

22. U.S. Food and Drug Administration. *FDA Drug Safety Communication: 5-alpha Reductase Inhibitors (5-ARIs) May Increase the Risk of a More Serious Form of prostate cancer.* https://www.fda.gov/Drugs/DrugSafety/ucm258314.htm. Accessed June 2017.

23. Klein EA, Thompson IM Jr, Tangen CM, et al. Vitamin E and the risk of prostate cancer: the Selenium and Vitamin E Cancer Prevention Trial (SELECT). *JAMA.* 2011;306(14):1549-1556.

PART XI

WOMEN'S HEALTH

Strength of Recommendation (SOR)	Definition
A	Recommendation based on consistent and good-quality patient-oriented evidence.*
B	Recommendation based on inconsistent or limited-quality patient-oriented evidence.*
C	Recommendation based on consensus, usual practice, opinion, disease-oriented evidence, or case series for studies of diagnosis, treatment, prevention, or screening.*

*See Appendix A on pages 1603–1606 for further information.

SECTION A PREGNANCY

76 SKIN FINDINGS IN PREGNANCY

E.J. Mayeaux, Jr., MD

PATIENT STORY

A 32-year-old G3P2 woman presents with persistent itching in her 31st week of pregnancy. The itching is constant and worse at night. Her pregnancy had been uncomplicated, and she has no past history of medical problems. Many excoriations are noted and there are no blisters (**Figure 76-1**). She has no jaundice or scleral icterus. Her transaminases were greater than 300 and her total bilirubin was elevated at 2.1. Her bile salts were elevated and her hepatitis panel was negative. The ultrasound showed gallstones, but no obstruction was seen. A diagnosis of "intrahepatic cholestasis of pregnancy" was made, and the patient was treated with oral ursodiol (a bile salt binding agent) and topical 1% hydrocortisone cream. The bile salts and transaminases were decreased and the patient's pruritus improved but did not resolve until after delivery.[1]

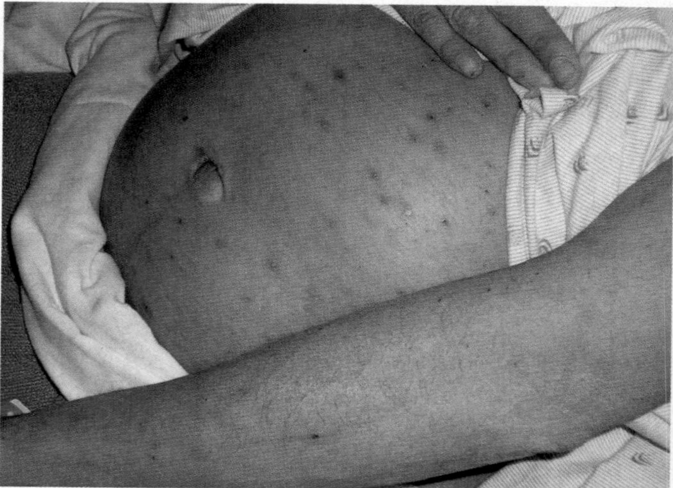

FIGURE 76-1 Pruritus and excoriations in a patient with intrahepatic cholestasis of pregnancy. All the lesions are secondary to patient scratching. (*Reproduced with permission from Richard P. Usatine, MD.*)

INTRODUCTION

Maternal skin and skin structures undergo numerous changes during pregnancy. There are two general categories of pregnancy-associated skin conditions: (a) benign skin conditions associated with normal hormonal changes of pregnancy (striae gravidarum, hyperpigmentation, hair and vascular changes), and (b) pregnancy-specific dermatoses (prurigo of pregnancy, intrahepatic cholestasis of pregnancy, pustular psoriasis of pregnancy).

SYNONYMS

- Striae gravidarum—Stretch marks.
- Atopic eruption of pregnancy, eczema in pregnancy, prurigo of pregnancy, and pruritic folliculitis of pregnancy.
- Spider telangiectasias—Spider nevi or spider angiomas.
- Intrahepatic cholestasis of pregnancy—Pruritus gravidarum.

EPIDEMIOLOGY

- Almost all pregnant women develop some increase in skin pigmentation. This usually occurs in discrete areas, probably because of differences in melanocyte density.
- Striae gravidarum (stretch marks) occur in up to 90% of pregnant women by the third trimester.[2]

- Spider telangiectasias occur in approximately 66% of light-complected and 10% of dark-complected pregnant women, primarily appearing on the face, neck, and arms. The condition is most common during the first and second trimesters.[3] Palmar erythema occurs in approximately two-thirds of light-complected and up to one-third of dark-complected pregnant women.[2]
- Hemorrhoidal, saphenous, and vulvar varicosities occur in approximately 40% of pregnant women.[3]
- Prurigo of pregnancy (now called atopic eruption of pregnancy) occurs with an incidence of approximately 1 in 300 to 1 in 450 pregnancies.[4,5]
- Intrahepatic cholestasis of pregnancy occurs in approximately 1 of 146 to 1293 pregnancies in the United States.[3]

ETIOLOGY AND PATHOPHYSIOLOGY

- The most common skin pigmentary change is darkening of the linea alba (**Figure 76-2**), which is then called the linea nigra.[6] It may span from the pubic symphysis to the umbilicus or all the way to the xiphoid process.
- The skin around the areola may also darken and develop a reticular type pattern. Other anatomic areas that develop hyperpigmentation are the nipples, axillae, vulva, perineum, anus, inner thighs, and neck.[7] Darkening may also occur in nevi during pregnancy.
- As pregnancy progresses, increased eccrine activity may result in hyperhidrosis (increased sweating) and/or miliaria ("prickly heat").[8] Apocrine activity decreases during pregnancy but increases postpartum, so hidradenitis suppurativa improves during pregnancy but may rebound later.[8]
- Hypertrophy of sebaceous glands produces small, brown papules on the areolae (Montgomery tubercles, **Figure 76-3**) in up to half of pregnant women. They usually regress postpartum.[8]
- Stretch marks (striae distensae, striae gravidarum) begin as pink/violaceous linear patches in the sixth to seventh month of gestation and are a common cosmetic concern among pregnant women (**Figure 76-4**). They evolve into hypopigmented linear depressions. They are most common on the abdomen, breasts, and thighs, but may also arise on the lower back, buttocks, and upper arms.[8] The cause of striae is multifactorial and includes physical factors (e.g., actual stretching of the skin) and hormonal factors (e.g., adrenocortical steroids, estrogen, and relaxin). Although striae fade postpartum, they do not completely disappear.
- Spider angiomas, arterial spiders, or spider nevi may develop, especially in white women. They occur mostly on the neck, face, upper chest, arms, and hands.[6] Almost all regress postpartum.
- Palmar erythema may develop and may be limited to the thenar or hypothenar eminence, or may be diffuse and mottled.[8]
- Acrochordons (skin tags) may develop, enlarge, or increase on the face, neck, axillae, chest, groin, and inframammary area during the second half of pregnancy. Some may regress postpartum.[9]
- Keloids, leiomyomas, dermatofibromas, and neurofibromas may enlarge during pregnancy.[9]
- Scalp hair appears thicker during pregnancy as a result of slowing of the normal progression of hairs to the telogen ("resting") stage,

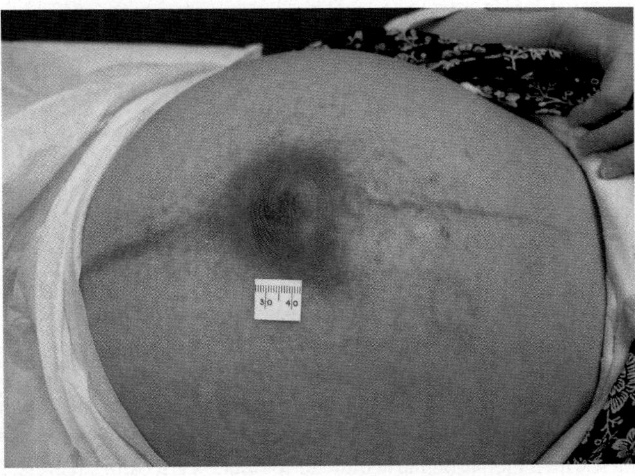

FIGURE 76-2 Darkened linea alba (linea nigra) in a pregnant patient. *(Reproduced with permission from Dan Stulberg, MD.)*

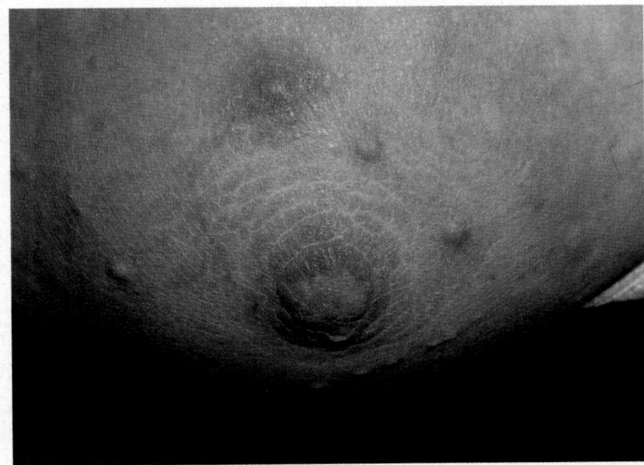

FIGURE 76-3 Montgomery tubercles in a pregnant woman. The brown papules on the areola are caused by hypertrophy of the normal sebaceous glands. *(Reproduced with permission from Richard P. Usatine, MD.)*

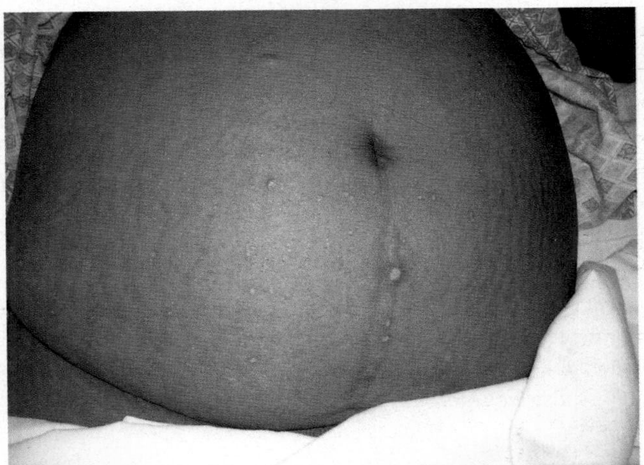

FIGURE 76-4 Atopic eruption of pregnancy. Note the erythematous, excoriated papules on the trunk. This patient's lesions resolved about 2 weeks postpartum. She also demonstrates pink/violaceous linear patches known as striae distensae or striae gravidarum. *(Reproduced with permission from E.J. Mayeaux, Jr., MD.)*

thereby creating a relative increase in anagen hair. Hair loss (telogen effluvium) is common 1 to 5 months postpartum as the percentage of telogen hairs in the scalp normalizes or increases (**Figure 76-5**).[9] Telogen effluvium resolves within 15 months postpartum, but the scalp hair may never return to prepregnancy thickness.[9]

- Hirsutism may occur on the face, arms, legs, back, and suprapubic region.[9] Hirsutism appears to be a result of increased levels of ovarian and placental androgens. Frontoparietal hair loss (androgenic alopecia) may develop late in pregnancy but usually resolves postpartum.
- Saphenous, vulvar, and hemorrhoidal varicosities may increase in number and/or size (see Chapter 68, Hemorrhoids). This may be because of increased blood volume, increased venous pressure, or genetic predisposition. Jacquemier sign refers to venous distention in the vestibule and vagina and is associated with vulvar varicosities, which are particularly difficult to treat.[8] Varicosities regress, at least partially, postpartum.
- Vascular type tumors may develop or enlarge during pregnancy. Pyogenic granulomas (**Figure 76-6**) (granuloma gravidarum, pregnancy tumor, pregnancy epulis) are reddish purple papules that are made up of granulation tissue (see Chapter 167, Pyogenic Granuloma). They usually begin in the first half of pregnancy and then partially regress postpartum. They most commonly appear on the gingiva, but are also common on fingers. Hemangiomas, subcutaneous hemangioendotheliomas, and glomangiomas (glomus tumors) may also occur.
- Atopic eruption of pregnancy is a related group of eczematous problems most common in patients with an atopic background during the second or third trimester, but has been reported in all trimesters. It accounts for over 50 percent of all pregnancy dermatoses.[10] Prurigo of pregnancy presents with erythematous, excoriated papules on the extensor surfaces of the limbs and trunk.[4,5] Lesions are grouped and may appear eczematous. Pruritic folliculitis of pregnancy presents with scattered follicle-based papules and pustules that initially appear on the abdomen but may spread to the trunk and extremities. The eruption usually resolves in the immediate postpartum period, although it can persist for months. This should not be confused with intrahepatic cholestasis of pregnancy, which is most common in the third trimester and has no primary skin lesions (see **Figure 76-4**).
- Intrahepatic cholestasis of pregnancy is usually diagnosed based on clinical history and presentation. Patients demonstrate severe pruritus (with or without jaundice), involvement of the palms and soles, and no primary skin lesions. Laboratory findings consistent with cholestasis confirm the diagnosis. Elevated bilirubin levels may or may not be found.[2] The etiology remains controversial. It usually resolves in the mother postpartum without specific treatment (see **Figure 76-1**) but carries significant potential morbidity for the fetus, including prematurity, meconium-stained amniotic fluid, intrauterine demise, and an increased risk for neonatal respiratory distress syndrome.

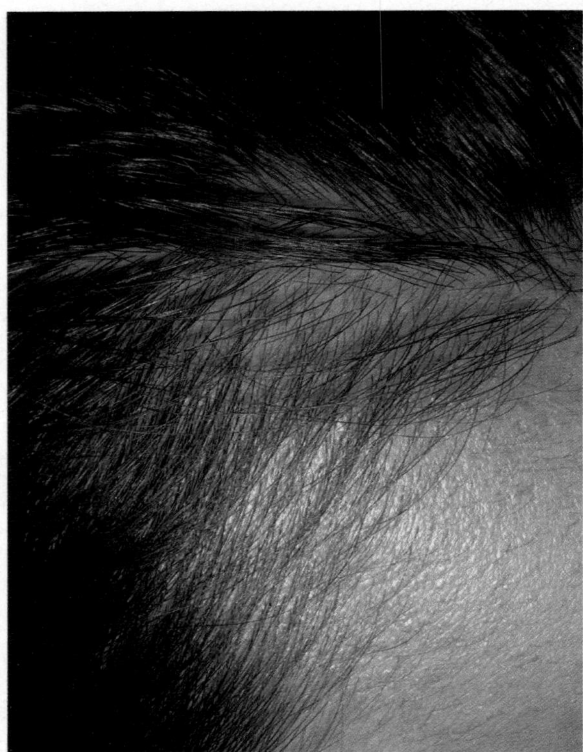

FIGURE 76-5 Telogen effluvium causing a hair loss in a young woman 1 month postpartum. The hair loss was most visible near the temples. There was no scalp inflammation or scarring. A gentle hair pull test produced four hairs in the telogen phase (with a visible bulb). Her hair returned to normal within 1 year of this visit. (*Reproduced with permission from Richard P. Usatine, MD.*)

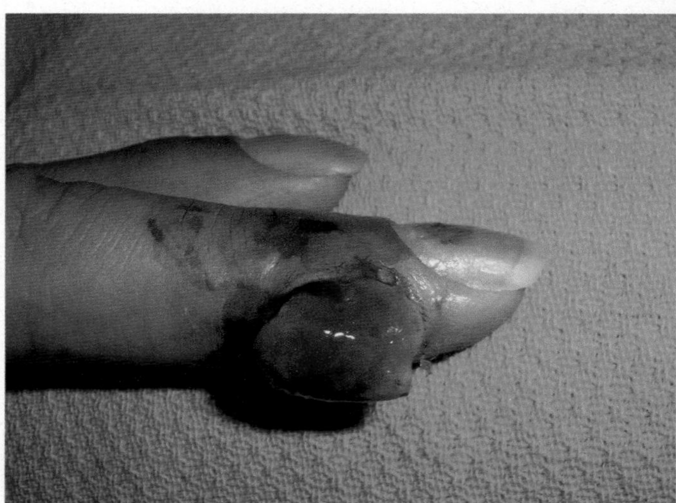

FIGURE 76-6 Pyogenic granuloma in a pregnant woman. (*Reproduced with permission from Richard P. Usatine, MD.*)

RISK FACTORS

Striae gravidarum are more common in women who are younger, nonwhite, have larger babies, and have higher body mass indices.[2] There is a familial predisposition to striae gravidarum, and women with preexisting breast or thigh striae are also more prone to this condition.[11]

Intrahepatic cholestasis of pregnancy is associated with a family history of the condition. It is associated with human leukocyte antigen-A31 and -B8.[3] It often recurs in subsequent pregnancies, and patients have a higher risk of gallstones or a family history of gallstones. It is associated with a higher risk of premature delivery, meconium-stained amniotic fluid, and intrauterine demise.

DIAGNOSIS

- Diagnosis of most conditions is made by identifying characteristic clinical features occurring during pregnancy.
- Laboratory testing for elevated serum bile acid levels and alkaline phosphatase levels is used to confirm the diagnosis of intrahepatic cholestasis of pregnancy.
- Skin biopsy for histopathologic examination and/or direct immunofluorescence staining is necessary if the diagnosis is uncertain or if pemphigoid gestationis or pustular psoriasis of pregnancy is suspected.

MANAGEMENT

FIRST LINE

NONPHARMACOLOGIC

- Changes such as hypertrophy of sebaceous glands, spider angiomas, palmar erythema, and varicosities usually regress postpartum and often require only symptomatic or no therapy. SOR Ⓒ
- Varicosities may be treated with leg elevation, compression with support hose, sleeping on the left side to ease uterine pressure on the great veins, exercise, and avoidance of long periods of standing or sitting SOR Ⓒ (see Chapter 54, Venous Insufficiency).[2]

MEDICATIONS

- The primary treatment for any pruritus in pregnancy is symptomatic. SOR Ⓒ Topical low-potency to mid-potency corticosteroids are safe and can give symptomatic relief of itching.
- Oral antihistamines such as diphenhydramine may be used to relieve itching.[2] SOR Ⓒ See Chapters 77, Pruritic Urticarial Papules and Plaques of Pregnancy, and 78, Pemphigoid Gestationis, for specific treatment of various pruritic diseases in pregnancy.
- Treatment of stretch marks after pregnancy with 0.1% tretinoin was reported to be beneficial but **should not be used** during pregnancy because of the risk of birth defects with any retinoid.[12] SOR Ⓑ
- The pruritus of intrahepatic cholestasis of pregnancy may be treated with oral antihistamines. More severe cases require ursodeoxycholic acid (ursodiol [Actigall]) to relieve pruritus and improve cholestasis while reducing adverse fetal outcomes.[2]

SURGICAL

- Persistent, bothersome pyogenic granulomas can be excised and should be sent to pathology to rule out amelanotic melanoma (see Chapter 167, Pyogenic Granuloma). SOR Ⓒ
- Physical lesions such as skin tags, fibromas, and angiomas may be treated by local surgical or destructive therapies. SOR Ⓒ
- Laser treatment (585-nm and pulsed-dye laser) may be used to treat striae after pregnancy.[2]

SECOND LINE

COMPLEMENTARY AND ALTERNATIVE THERAPY

- Many creams, emollients, and oils containing vitamin E, cocoa butter, aloe vera lotion, and olive oil are used to attempt to prevent striae. However, there is no evidence that these treatments are effective. Limited evidence suggests that *Centella asiatica* extract plus α-tocopherol and collagen-elastin hydrolysates and tocopherol, essential fatty acids, panthenol, hyaluronic acid, elastin, and menthol may be helpful.[13] The safety of using *Centella asiatica* and other components during pregnancy is unclear.[14]

FOLLOW-UP

Conditions should be monitored during pregnancy and the patient regularly reassured. Postpartum, the patient may be followed or treated as needed.

PATIENT EDUCATION

The primary aim of treatment for most skin conditions in pregnancy is to relieve symptoms, as many conditions improve or resolve postpartum. Those conditions that do not resolve can usually be safely treated postpartum when there is no risk to the pregnancy.

PATIENT RESOURCES

- ACOG Education Pamphlet. *Skin Conditions during Pregnancy*—**http://www.acog.org/Patients/FAQs/Skin-Conditions-During-Pregnancy.**
- Netdoctor. *Skin Changes during Pregnancy*—**http://www.netdoctor.co.uk/conditions/pregnancy-and-family/a9135/skin-changes-during-pregnancy/.**
- WebMD. *Skin Problems of Pregnancy*—**http://www.webmd.com/baby/features/skin-problems-of-pregnancy#1.**

PROVIDER RESOURCES

- Dermnet NZ. *Skin Problems in Pregnancy*—**http://www.dermnetnz.org/topics/skin-problems-in-pregnancy.**
- Common skin conditions during pregnancy. *Am Fam Physician.* 2007;75(2):211-218. **http://www.aafp.org/afp/2007/0115/p211.html.**

REFERENCES

1. Orr B, Usatine RP. Pruritus in pregnancy. *J Fam Pract.* 2007;56(11):913-916.
2. Tunzi M, Gray GR. Common skin conditions during pregnancy. *Am Fam Physician.* 2007;75:211-218.

3. Kroumpouzos G, Cohen LM. Dermatoses of pregnancy. *J Am Acad Dermatol.* 2001;45:1-19.
4. Roger D, Vaillant L, Fignon A, et al. Specific pruritic diseases of pregnancy: a prospective study of 3192 pregnant women. *Arch Dermatol.* 1994;130:734-739.
5. Holmes RC, Black MM. The specific dermatoses of pregnancy. *J Am Acad Dermatol.* 1983;8(3):1405-1412.
6. Esteve E, Saudeau L, Pierre F, et al. Physiological cutaneous signs in normal pregnancy: a study of 60 pregnant women. *Ann Dermatol Venereol.* 1994;121:227-231.
7. Muzaffar F, Hussain I, Haroon TS. Physiologic skin changes during pregnancy: a study of 140 cases. *Int J Dermatol.* 1998;37(6):429-431.
8. Martin AG, Leal-Khouri S. Physiologic skin changes associated with pregnancy. *Int J Dermatol.* 1992;31(6):375-378.
9. Winton GB, Lewis CW. Dermatoses of pregnancy. *J Am Acad Dermatol.* 1982;6(6):977-998.
10. Ambros-Rudolph CM, Müllegger RR, Vaughan-Jones SA, et al. The specific dermatoses of pregnancy revisited and reclassified: results of a retrospective two-center study on 505 pregnant patients. *J Am Acad Dermatol.* 2006;54:395-404.
11. Chang AL, Agredano YZ, Kimball AB. Risk factors associated with striae gravidarum. *J Am Acad Dermatol.* 2004;51(6):881-885.
12. Rangel O, Arias I, García E, Lopez-Padilla S. Topical tretinoin 0.1% for pregnancy-related abdominal striae: an open-label, multicenter, prospective study. *Adv Ther.* 2001;18:181-186.
13. Young GL, Jewell D. Creams for preventing stretch marks in pregnancy. *Cochrane Database Syst Rev.* 2000;(2):CD000066.
14. Ernst E. Herbal medicinal products during pregnancy: are they safe? *BJOG.* 2002;109:227-235.

77 PRURITIC URTICARIAL PAPULES AND PLAQUES OF PREGNANCY

E.J. Mayeaux, Jr., MD

PATIENT STORY

A 26-year-old pregnant woman presents at 36 weeks of gestation with a progressive itchy rash. The rash started within the abdominal striae (**Figure 77-1**) and spread to her proximal extremities. This is her first pregnancy and she has never had any rashes like this before. The itching "is maddening." The patient is diagnosed with pruritic urticarial papules and plaques of pregnancy (PUPPP) and treated with topical steroids and oral antihistamines.

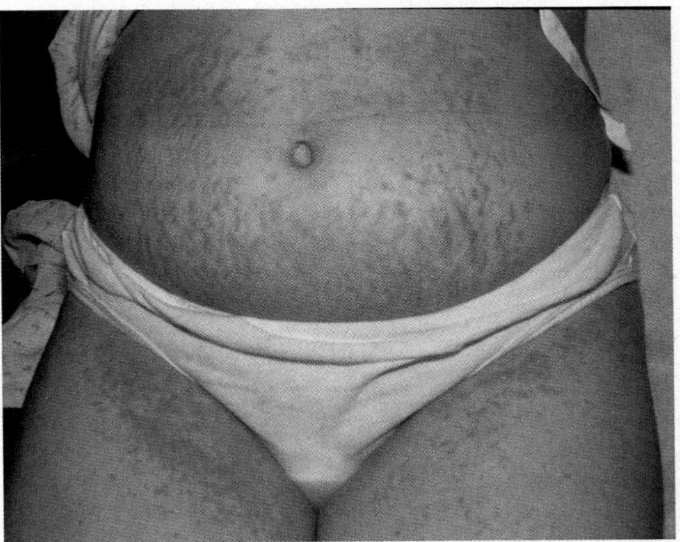

FIGURE 77-1 Pruritic urticarial papules and plaques of pregnancy (PUPPP) presenting as pruritic striae on the abdomen. *(Reproduced with permission from Richard P. Usatine, MD.)*

INTRODUCTION

PUPPP is a dermatosis of pregnancy characterized by a self–limiting pruritic papulovesicular or urticarial eruption on the abdomen, trunk, and limbs. Other than maternal itching, PUPPP poses no increased risk of fetal or maternal morbidity.[1]

SYNONYMS

- Polymorphic eruption of pregnancy.
- Toxic erythema of pregnancy.
- Linear immunoglobulin (Ig) M dermatosis of pregnancy.
- Bourne toxemic rash of pregnancy.
- Nurse's late-onset prurigo.

EPIDEMIOLOGY

- The incidence of PUPPP is 1 in 160 to 1 in 300 pregnancies, making it the most common defined dermatosis of pregnancy.[2]
- Nulliparous patients account for more than 75% of patients with classic PUPPP.[3]
- PUPPP is also more common with multiple gestations, possibly because of increased abdominal distention or higher hormone levels.[4]
- The rate of recurrence with subsequent pregnancies is unknown.

ETIOLOGY AND PATHOPHYSIOLOGY

- The etiology of PUPPP is unknown. PUPPP is more common with excessive stretching of the skin, possibly because of damage to connective tissue, which could result in exposure of antigens that trigger an inflammatory response.[2,5] The disease may also represent an immunologic reaction to circulating fetal antigens.

- Onset of PUPPP is usually late in the third trimester, but it may develop postpartum.[1,3] There are case reports of first- and second-trimester disease.[3] Pruritus may worsen after delivery, but generally resolves by 15 days postpartum. The PUPPP may resolve prior to delivery.

RISK FACTORS

- The disorder is more common with first pregnancies.[6]
- Multiple gestations.[6]
- Familial occurrences have been reported.[4]

DIAGNOSIS

CLINICAL FEATURES

PUPPP is usually diagnosed by its characteristic findings on history and physical examination. PUPPP typically presents with erythematous papules and plaques within striae with periumbilical sparing late in the third trimester (**Figures 77-1** and **77-2**). Extreme pruritus is a hallmark of the disease and is present in all patients.[1]

TYPICAL DISTRIBUTION

Abdominal striae are the most common initial site.[3] The lesions usually spread to the extremities and coalesce to form urticarial plaques (**Figures 77-3** and **77-4**). The face, palms, soles, and periumbilical region are usually spared. White halos often surround the erythematous papules and are target-like, exhibiting three distinct rings of color.[3]

LABORATORY TESTING

There are no related laboratory abnormalities.

BIOPSY

Biopsy is not necessary when the clinical picture is classic. When the diagnosis is uncertain, perform a punch biopsy and consider immunofluorescent studies. IgM or IgA deposits may be found at the dermoepidermal junction or around blood vessels. It is preferable to biopsy a lesion off the abdomen to avoid wound-healing problems on a distended abdomen.

DIFFERENTIAL DIAGNOSIS

- Pemphigoid gestationis can be differentiated from PUPPP by its bullous lesions (see Chapter 78, Pemphigoid Gestationis).
- Erythema multiforme produces target lesions that may affect the palms and soles (see Chapter 185, Erythema Multiforme, Stevens-Johnson Syndrome, and Toxic Epidermal Necrolysis).
- Drug reactions produce various types of erythematous eruptions on the trunk and extremities. History of a new drug exposure helps to distinguish this from PUPPP (see Chapter 212, Cutaneous Drug Reactions).
- Scabies infestations produce severe itching from the mite burrows that are common between the fingers and in areas of skin folds (see Chapter 149, Scabies).

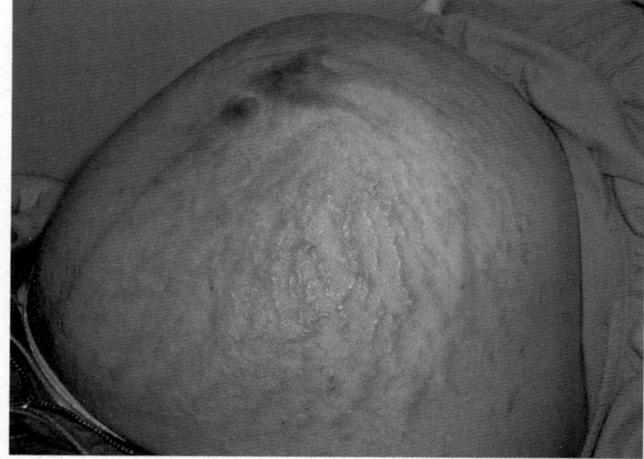

FIGURE 77-2 Pruritic urticarial papules and plaques of pregnancy (PUPPP) occurring in the first pregnancy of a 20-year-old woman during her third trimester. Note how it involves the striae of her abdomen. She also has darkening of her linea alba and umbilicus. (*Reproduced with permission from Rachel Giese, MD.*)

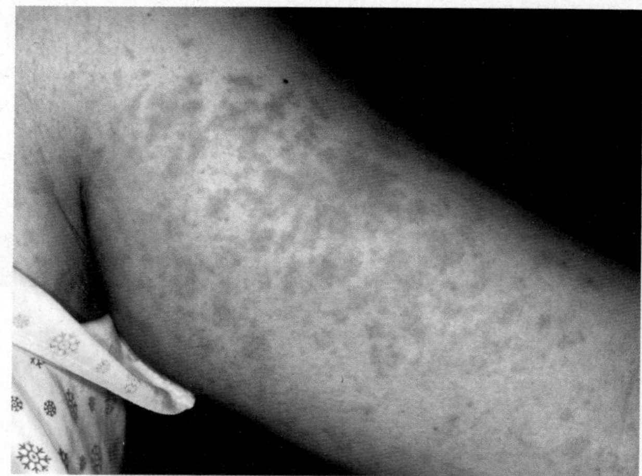

FIGURE 77-3 Pruritic urticarial papules and plaques of pregnancy (PUPPP) on the arm. (*Reproduced with permission from Richard P. Usatine, MD.*)

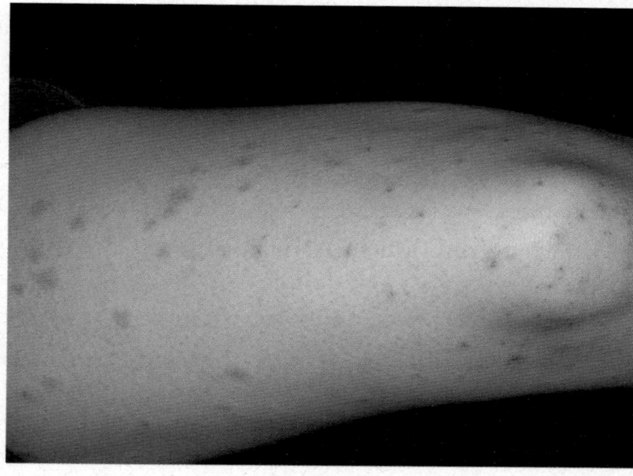

FIGURE 77-4 Pruritic urticarial papules and plaques of pregnancy (PUPPP) on the leg. (*Reproduced with permission from Richard P. Usatine, MD.*)

- Viral exanthems may produce all types of erythematous eruptions that can be pruritic at times. The history of a fever along with upper respiratory symptoms should help to differentiate these eruptions from PUPPP (see Chapters 132, Measles, and 133, Fifth Disease).

MANAGEMENT

FIRST LINE

- Symptom control is the main goal. Aggressive therapy is not recommended because the condition is self-limiting. SOR Ⓒ
- General symptom relief measures such as cool baths, frequent application of emollients, wet soaks, or cool packs applied to the skin provide some symptomatic relief.[7] SOR Ⓒ
- First-line pharmacologic therapy consists of topical steroids and oral antihistamines to alleviate symptoms. SOR Ⓒ
- Start with a mid-potency topical corticosteroid such as 0.1% triamcinolone cream or ointment bid to tid. Pregnancy class B. SOR Ⓒ High-potency, topical, corticosteroids such as fluocinonide may be applied sparingly bid to tid as severity warrants. Pregnancy class B. SOR Ⓒ
- The patient may be given the choice of the steroid vehicle as either a cream or an ointment. In this case both vehicles work, and the one that will work best is the one that the patient will actually use. SOR Ⓒ
- Diphenhydramine 25 to 50 mg PO bid to qid or similar antihistamines may be used for symptomatic relief of pruritus. Pregnancy class B. SOR Ⓒ

SECOND LINE

In severe cases, oral prednisone, 40 to 60 mg daily, may induce a rapid resolution of symptoms.[7] SOR Ⓒ

- Early delivery to relieve symptoms is rarely required.

PROGNOSIS

Apart from itching and related discomfort, the prognosis for the mother is unaffected. It generally lasts 4 to 6 weeks and resolves within 2 weeks postpartum, although the course is variable.[8] Recurrence of the condition in subsequent pregnancies is rare and tends to be less severe than the first episode.[7]

Pruritus may worsen immediately after delivery, but generally resolves by 2 weeks postpartum.

FOLLOW-UP

Routine prenatal and postpartum care should be continued.

PATIENT EDUCATION

- When discussing treatment options, inform the patient that the condition is self-limited, so therapy is based on making the patient comfortable while minimizing the potential risks involved in the use of medications.[6]
- Symptom control with topical steroids and antihistamines is the main goal.

PATIENT RESOURCES

- VeryWell. *PUPPP Is an Itchy Rash during Pregnancy*—**http://dermatology.about.com/cs/pregnancy/a/puppp.htm.**
- DermNet NZ. *Polymorphic Eruption of Pregnancy*—**http://dermnetnz.org/reactions/puppp.html.**
- ACOG Education Pamphlet. *Skin Conditions During Pregnancy*—**http://www.acog.org/Patients/FAQs/Skin-Conditions-During-Pregnancy.**

PROVIDER RESOURCES

- EMedicine. *Polymorphic Eruption of Pregnancy*—**https://emedicine.medscape.com/article/1123725-overview.**
- Medscape Today. *Specific Pregnancy Dermatoses: Pruritic Urticarial Papules and Plaques of Pregnancy*—**http://www.medscape.com/viewarticle/707663_3.**
- Tunzi M, Gray GR. Common skin conditions during pregnancy. *Am Fam Physician*. 2007;75:211-218. **http://www.aafp.org/afp/2007/0115/p211.html.**

REFERENCES

1. Yancey KB, Hall RP, Lawley TJ. Pruritic urticarial papules and plaques of pregnancy. Clinical experience in twenty-five patients. *J Am Acad Dermatol*. 1984;10:473.
2. Vaughan Jones SA, Black MM. Pregnancy dermatoses. *J Am Acad Dermatol*. 1999;40:233.
3. Aronson IK, Bond S, Fiedler VC, et al. Pruritic urticarial papules and plaques of pregnancy: clinical and immunopathologic observations in 57 patients. *J Am Acad Dermatol*. 1998;39:933.
4. Kroumpouzos G, Cohen LM. Specific dermatoses of pregnancy: an evidence-based systematic review. *Am J Obstet Gynecol*. 2003; 188:1083.
5. Beckett MA, Goldberg NS. Pruritic urticarial plaques and papules of pregnancy and skin distention. *Arch Dermatol*. 1991;127:125.
6. Tunzi M, Gray GR. Common skin conditions during pregnancy. *Am Fam Physician*. 2007;75:211-218.
7. Ahmadi S, Powell FC. Pruritic urticarial papules and plaques of pregnancy: current status. *Australas J Dermatol*. 2005; 46:53-60.
8. Roger D, Vaillant L, Fignon A, et al. Specific pruritic diseases of pregnancy. A prospective study of 3192 pregnant women. *Arch Dermatol*. 1994;130:734-739.

78 PEMPHIGOID GESTATIONIS

E.J. Mayeaux, Jr., MD

PATIENT STORY

A 37-year-old pregnant woman presented to the hospital with severe preeclampsia. After all medical methods were tried and failed to control her severe preeclampsia, a joint decision was made to induce labor to save the life of the mother. The pregnancy was too early for the fetus to survive. The following day she began to develop the lesions seen in **Figures 78-1** through **78-4**. A diagnosis of pemphigoid gestationis was made. Her past history includes antiphospholipid syndrome with multiple pregnancy losses but two live children. This was her third episode of pemphigoid gestationis. A photograph of her previous episode is included to see how similar the periumbilical bulla was to her current episode of pemphigoid gestationis (**Figure 78-5**). A new biopsy was not performed given that her previous biopsy was on file and the clinical picture was consistent with a recurrence of this disease. She was treated with oral prednisone and began to improve rapidly.

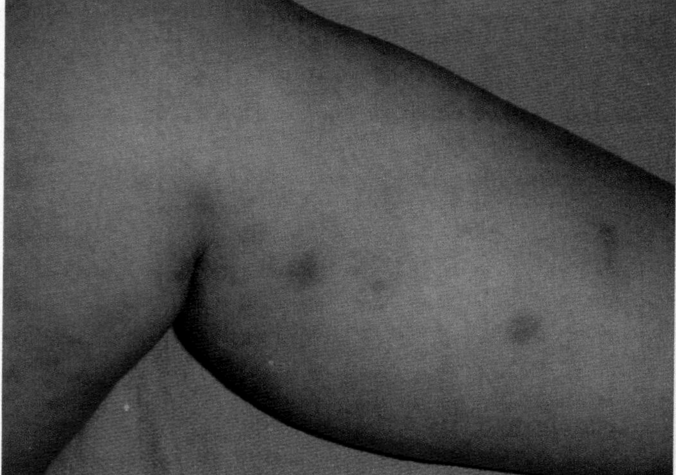

FIGURE 78-1 Pemphigoid gestationis in the pruritic papular stage. The lesions resemble the target lesions of erythema multiforme. (*Reproduced with permission from Richard P. Usatine, MD.*)

INTRODUCTION

Pemphigoid gestationis is a rare autoimmune bullous dermatosis of pregnancy. The disease was originally known as herpes gestationis because of its visual similarities to herpes simplex infection. However, that term has fallen out of favor because pemphigoid gestationis is not associated with active or prior herpes virus infection.

SYNONYMS

Herpes gestationis (confusing, as this condition is not related to the herpes virus).

EPIDEMIOLOGY

- Pemphigoid gestationis is a rare disease that occurs in 1 in 1700 to 1 in 50,000 pregnancies.[1,2]
- Pemphigoid gestationis has an estimated prevalence of 1 case in 50,000 to 60,000 pregnancies in the United States.
- It has been linked to the presence of human leukocyte antigen (HLA)-DR3, HLA-DR4, or both.[3]
- It is rarely associated with molar pregnancies and choriocarcinoma.[3]

ETIOLOGY AND PATHOPHYSIOLOGY

- Pemphigoid gestationis is defined as a bullous or blistering disease that is associated with pregnancy or with trophoblastic tumors.

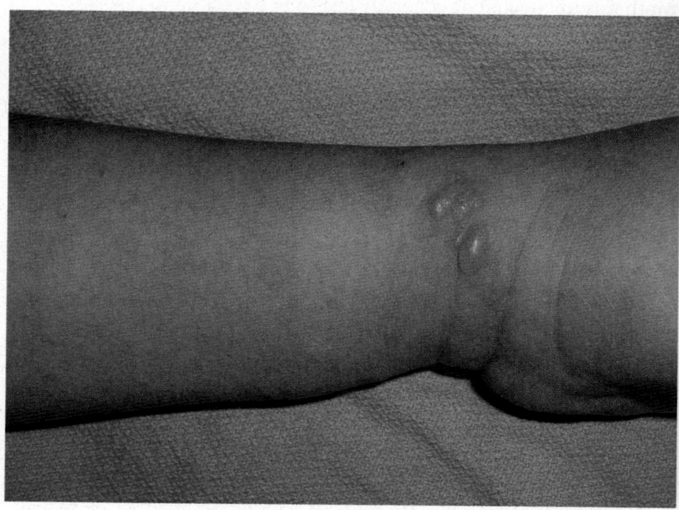

FIGURE 78-2 Pemphigoid gestationis with bullous lesions on the wrist. (*Reproduced with permission from Richard P. Usatine, MD.*)

- The pathophysiology of the disease involves circulating immunoglobulin G1 (IgG1) autoantibodies directed against the bullous pemphigoid antigen (BP180 or collagen XVII), a basement membrane zone transmembrane hemidesmosomal glycoprotein.[4]
- The primary site of autoimmunity sensitization appears to be the placenta, since the autoantibodies bind in the chorionic and amniotic epithelia and in the epidermis.[5]
- When the inflammatory response is activated, the hemidesmosomes are destroyed and the epidermis separates from the dermis.[2]
- It is unknown why some patients form these antibodies.
- Rarely, pemphigoid gestationis persists for years postpartum.[1,2]
- There is no scarring from the lesions.

RISK FACTORS

Pemphigoid gestationis in a prior pregnancy.

DIAGNOSIS

CLINICAL FEATURES: HISTORY AND PHYSICAL

- Pemphigoid gestationis typically erupts during the second or third trimester and, rarely, postpartum and first trimester. Symptoms may abate at the end of pregnancy; however, flares can occur immediately after delivery.
- Pruritus sometimes precedes the rash, and vesicles may develop early.
- The initial manifestations are erythematous urticarial patches and plaques, which typically start around the umbilicus. The lesions progress to tense vesicles (see **Figures 78-1** to **78-5**).

TYPICAL DISTRIBUTION

The rash begins on the trunk around the umbilicus as pruritic papules or plaques and may progress to bullae (see **Figures 78-4** and **78-5**).[1,2] Lesions may occasionally be seen on the palms and soles, and rarely on the face or mucous membranes.

LABORATORY TESTING

Although less commonly used for diagnosis than skin biopsy, measurement of serum levels of anti-BP180 antibodies by an enzyme-linked immunosorbent assay can be used for diagnosis. The levels of circulating anti-BP180 antibodies correlate with the disease severity and may be used to monitor the response to treatment.[6]

BIOPSY

Skin biopsy including the edge of a blistering lesion reveals a subepidermal vesicle with a perivascular lymphocytic and eosinophilic infiltrate.

- Eosinophils may appear at the dermoepidermal junction and inside the vesicle; the degree of eosinophilia correlates with disease severity.
- Basal cell necrosis and papillae edema are usually present.
- A skin biopsy of perilesional skin for indirect immunofluorescent staining shows complement 3 in a homogeneous linear band at the basement membrane. This is pathognomonic for pemphigoid gestationis.

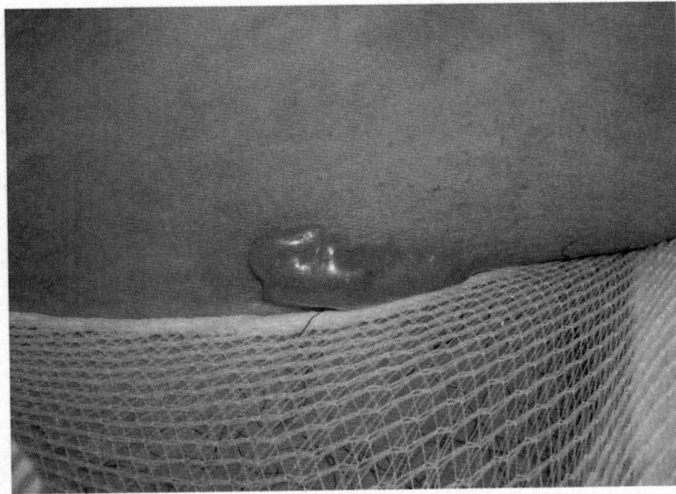

FIGURE 78-3 Pemphigoid gestationis. Close-up of a bullous lesion on the abdomen. *(Reproduced with permission from Richard P. Usatine, MD.)*

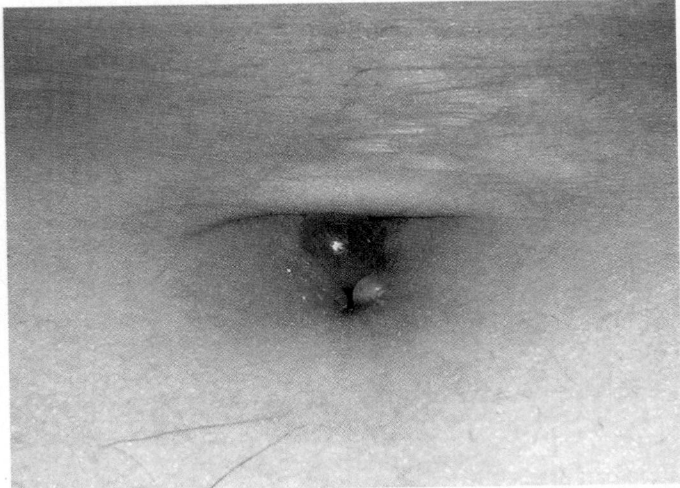

FIGURE 78-4 Pemphigoid gestationis with a bulla in the umbilicus. Lesions typically begin in the periumbilical region. *(Reproduced with permission from Richard P. Usatine, MD.)*

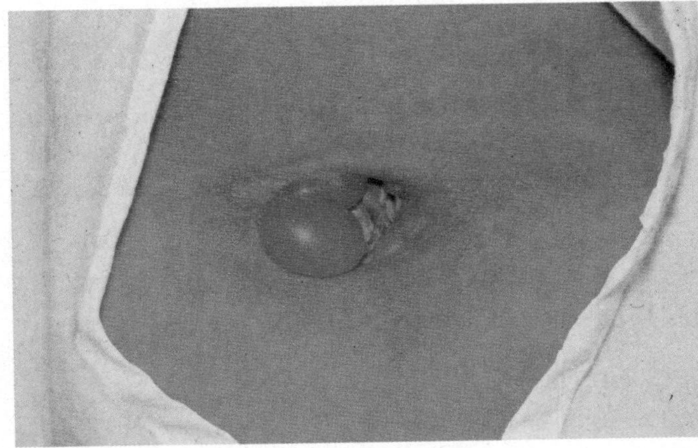

FIGURE 78-5 Close-up of a large bulla in the umbilicus in a previous case of pemphigoid gestationis in the same patient 5 years before. *(Reproduced with permission from Richard P. Usatine, MD.)*

DIFFERENTIAL DIAGNOSIS

- Papular urticarial papules and plaques of pregnancy (PUPPP) may mimic pemphigoid gestationis, especially early in the disease. However, PUPPP usually begin in the striae, whereas pemphigoid gestationis is usually periumbilical. Most importantly, PUPPP does not develop large bullae as does pemphigoid gestations (see Chapter 77, Pruritic Urticarial Papules and Plaques of Pregnancy).
- Dermatitis herpetiformis is a very pruritic, vesicular skin eruption. It is a chronic recurrent symmetric vesicular eruption that is usually associated with gluten-induced enteropathy. Men are more often affected than women (see Chapter 191, Overview of Bullous Disease).
- Erythema multiforme secondary to pregnancy, infection, or drug exposure can mimic pemphigoid gestationis. Biopsy with routine histology can usually distinguish between these disorders (see Chapter 185, Erythema Multiforme, Stevens-Johnson Syndrome, and Toxic Epidermal Necrolysis).
- Contact dermatitis and drug reactions may have a similar appearance and history of exposure to a contact allergen, or medication can help to distinguish between these reactions and pemphigoid gestationis (see Chapters 152, Contact Dermatitis, and 212, Cutaneous Drug Reactions).
- Bullous pemphigoid produces similar lesions, but rarely starts in pregnancy or starts around the umbilicus (see Chapter 192, Bullous Pemphigoid).
- Urticaria may appear similar to early pemphigoid gestationis (see Chapter 156, Urticaria and Angioedema).

MANAGEMENT

FIRST LINE

MEDICATIONS

- High-potency topical steroids (Group 2 and 3) and oral antihistamines should be administered in early or mild cases, but are usually ineffective in more severe or systemic cases. SOR C
- Systemic steroids, such as prednisone (0.5 mg/kg per day), are effective to control most cases.[7] SOR C The dose may be tapered and eventually discontinued in many pregnancies.
- Severe persistent postpartum disease often require higher doses of systemic steroids (prednisone up to 2 mg/kg per day.)

NONPHARMACOLOGIC

Tepid baths, compresses, and emollients may help alleviate pruritus.

SECOND LINE

- Alternative immunosuppressive and anti-inflammatory therapies that have been successfully used in a few patients include azathioprine, intravenous immunoglobulins, cyclosporine, cyclophosphamide, doxycycline and nicotinamide, rituximab, and immunopheresis.[8]

PROGNOSIS

Pemphigoid gestationis typically regresses spontaneously without scarring within weeks to months after delivery. It may recur in subsequent pregnancies or may be precipitated by the use of oral contraceptives.

FOLLOW-UP

- Follow-up of the mother and child are essential because of the following issues:
  - The fetus during a pregnancy in which the mother has pemphigoid gestationis is at risk for growth restriction and prematurity.
  - Mild placental insufficiency may result from an immune response between placental antigens and the disease-related antibodies.[9]
- Cutaneous involvement in infants of affected mothers is rare (5% to 10% have urticarial, vesicular, or bullous lesions) and abates with clearance of the maternal antibodies.[10]
- The mother is at high risk of recurrent pemphigoid gestationis with subsequent pregnancies and at an increased lifetime risk of Graves disease.[2,11]

PATIENT EDUCATION

- Pemphigoid gestationis may abate prior to delivery, but 75% of patients flare postpartum, requiring reinstatement of treatment.
- At least 25% of patients will flare with oral contraceptive pill use.
- Most cases spontaneously resolve in the weeks to months following delivery.
- The disease usually recurs with future pregnancies and often worsens with repeated episodes, but may also skip some pregnancies.[2,9]

PATIENT RESOURCES

- VeryWell. *Pemphigoid Gestationis*—**https://www.verywellfamily.com/pemphigoid-gestationis-1068861.**
- DermNet NZ. *Pemphigoid Gestationis*—**http://www.dermnetnz.org/topics/pemphigoid-gestationis/.**
- Merck Manual (Consumer version). *Pemphigoid Gestationis*—**http://www.merckmanuals.com/home/women-s-health-issues/complications-of-pregnancy/pemphigoid-gestationis/.**

PROVIDER RESOURCES

- eMedicine. *Pemphigoid Gestationis*—**http://emedicine.medscape.com/article/1063499-overview.**
- ARUP. *Pemphigoid Gestationis: Herpes Gestationis*—**https://arupconsult.com/content/pemphigoid-gestationis.**
- Tunzi M, Gray GR. Common skin conditions during pregnancy. *Am Fam Physician*. 2007;75:211-218—**http://www.aafp.org/afp/2007/0115/p211.pdf.**
- Merck Manual (Professional version). *Pemphigoid Gestationis*—**https://www.merckmanuals.com/professional/gynecology-and-obstetrics/abnormalities-of-pregnancy/pemphigoid-gestationis.**

REFERENCES

1. Roger D, Vaillant L, Fignon A, et al. Specific pruritic diseases of pregnancy. A prospective study of 3192 pregnant women. *Arch Dermatol.* 1994;130:734.
2. Shornick JK. Dermatoses of pregnancy. *Semin Cutan Med Surg.* 1998;17:172.
3. Tunzi M, Gray GR. Common skin conditions during pregnancy. *Am Fam Physician*. 2007;75:211-218.
4. Di Zenzo G, Calabresi V, Grosso F, et al. The intracellular and extracellular domains of BP180 antigen comprise novel epitopes targeted by pemphigoid gestationis autoantibodies. *J Invest Dermatol.* 2007;127:864.
5. Sadik CD, Lima AL, Zillikens D. Pemphigoid gestationis: toward a better understanding of the etiopathogenesis. *Clin Dermatol.* 2016; 34:378.
6. Huilaja L, Surcel HM, Bloigu A, Tasanen K. Elevated serum levels of BP180 antibodies in the first trimester of pregnancy precede gestational pemphigoid and remain elevated for a long time after remission of the disease. *Acta Derm Venereol.* 2015;95:843.
7. Jenkins RE, Hern S, Black MM. Clinical features and management of 87 patients with pemphigoid gestationis. *Clin Exp Dermatol.* 1999;24(4):255-259.
8. Henry S. Recognizing presentations of pemphigoid gestationis: a case study. *Case Rep Obstet Gynecol.* 2014;415163. http://dx.doi.org/10.1155/2014/415163.
9. Jenkins RE, Shornick JK, Black BL. Pemphigoid gestationis. *J Eur Acad Dermatol Venereol.* 1993;2:163.
10. Shimanovich I, Brocker EB, Zillikens D. Pemphigoid gestationis: new insights into pathogenesis lead to novel diagnostic tools. *BJOG.* 2002;109:970-976.
11. Jenkins RE, Hern S, Black MM. Clinical features and management of 87 patients with pemphigoid gestationis. *Clin Exp Dermatol.* 1999;24:255.

79 FIRST TRIMESTER OBSTETRICAL ULTRASOUND

Danielle B. Cooper, MD
E.J. Mayeaux, Jr., MD

PATIENT STORY

A 22-year-old woman presents with last menstrual period approximately 2 months ago complains of morning sickness, but is otherwise feeling well. A urine pregnancy test confirms she is pregnant. **Figure 79-1** shows a fetus of 9 weeks estimated gestational age (EGA).

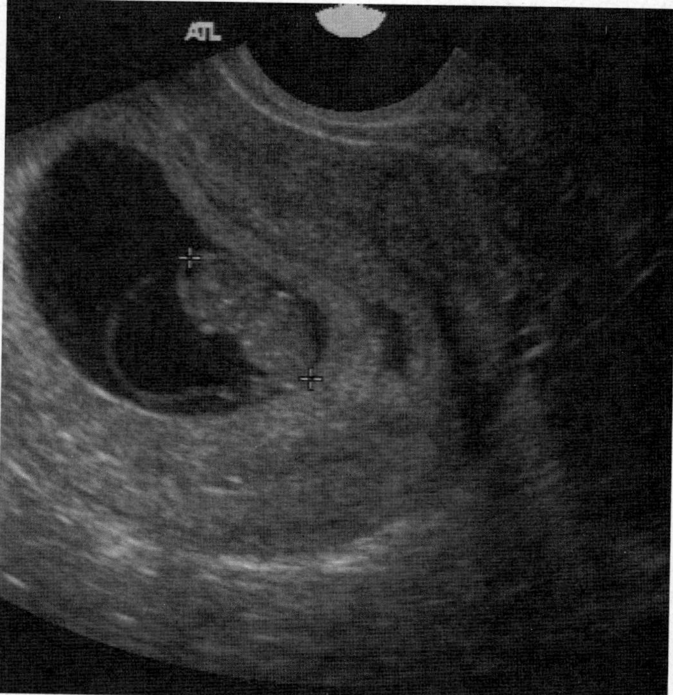

FIGURE 79-1 Ultrasound examination of a fetus of 9 weeks estimated gestational age. The ultrasound was performed with a vaginal probe and the membranes are visible. (*Reproduced with permission from E.J. Mayeaux, Jr., MD.*)

INTRODUCTION

Obstetrical ultrasound has become a vital tool in our ability to properly care for the pregnant patient. Vast technologic improvements have made visualization of the pregnancy even better and improved our diagnostic capabilities, ranging from the normal pregnancy to the extremely early ectopic pregnancy. Ultrasonography (US) allows for a relatively detailed assessment of fetal gestational age, development, number of fetuses, fetal anatomy, placental location, and uterine or ovarian pathology. Most pregnancies in the United States undergo ultrasound imaging for various indications.

SYNONYMS

Dating scan.

EPIDEMIOLOGY

- Women who receive antenatal care have lower maternal and perinatal mortality and better pregnancy outcomes.[1] However, the optimal components of prenatal care have not been rigorously examined in well-designed studies.
- In the United States in 2003, 84.1% of pregnant women obtained prenatal care in the first trimester, and only 3.5% received no care or initiated prenatal care in the third trimester.
- A first trimester ultrasound is performed either transabdominally or transvaginally before 14 weeks.

ETIOLOGY AND PATHOPHYSIOLOGY

- Ultrasound is used to estimate gestational age and to calculate the expected date of delivery (EDD). Ultrasound is especially helpful when menses are irregular, the last menstrual period (LMP) is unknown, or in patients who conceived while using hormonal contraceptives. A Cochrane review noted that with more accurate dating, there was a reduction in intervention for postterm pregnancy.[2] The earlier in pregnancy a scan is performed, the more accurate the age assessment from crown to rump length. The initial age assignment should not be revised on subsequent scans.[3]

- The Routine Antenatal Diagnostic Imaging with Ultrasound (RADIUS) trial was a randomized trial of routine obstetrical ultrasound screening.[4] It included more than 15,000 women in the United States. The trial showed that routine ultrasound screening was associated with a significantly increased detection of fetal anomalies, but no improvement in any perinatal outcome, including mortality, preterm birth, birth weight, and neonatal morbidity.
- First trimester vaginal bleeding is found in 20% to 40% of pregnancies. The differential diagnoses include possible spontaneous abortion, ectopic pregnancy, and gestational trophoblastic disease.
- Ectopic pregnancy causes a significant degree of morbidity and mortality if untreated, often through tubal rupture with potentially life-threatening hemorrhage. Identification of an intrauterine pregnancy effectively excludes the possibility of an ectopic pregnancy in almost all cases, unless conception involved assisted reproductive technology (ART). A heterotopic pregnancy refers to the combination of intrauterine pregnancy and a concurrent ectopic pregnancy. These used to be extremely rare, estimated at 1 in 30,000 pregnancies, but with ART the rate has risen to 1.5 per 1000 pregnancies.[5]
- Threatened, inevitable, incomplete, or complete spontaneous abortion may cause first trimester bleeding. Up to one-third of recognized pregnancies end in early pregnancy loss. Ectopic pregnancy may also be a concern. US may be used to determine if a gestational sac or yolk sac is present in the uterus.
- First trimester transvaginal ultrasound used in conjunction with serum screening is the most sensitive noninvasive technique to detect aneuploidy. When performed in the first trimester, nuchal translucency (**Figure 79-2**) as well as serum pregnancy-associated plasma protein A (PAPP-A) and β-human chorionic gonadotropin (β-hCG) levels are evaluated, which effectively detect 82% to 87% of trisomy 21. Integrated screening would also include a quad screen in the second trimester, which carries a 94% to 96% detection rate.[6]

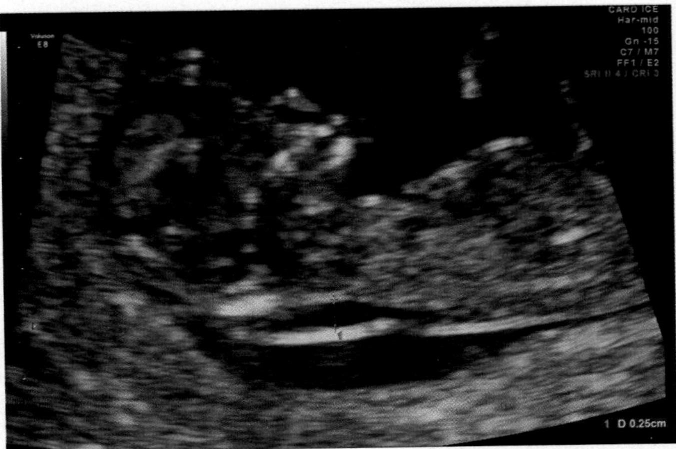

FIGURE 79-2 Ultrasound examination of a fetus of 11 weeks 2 days with nuchal translucency (>2 mm is abnormal at this gestational age). *(Reproduced with permission from E.J. Mayeaux, Jr., MD.)*

DIAGNOSIS

- The goals of a basic first trimester ultrasound examination include[3]:
  - Confirm the presence of an intrauterine (or evaluate suspected extrauterine) pregnancy
  - Assess gestational age
  - Determine fetal viability
  - Evaluate the cause of vaginal bleeding
  - Evaluate pelvic or lower abdominal pain
  - Determine whether a multiple gestation is present
  - Confirm fetal cardiac activity
  - Evaluate maternal pelvic organs for congenital or acquired abnormalities
  - Screen for fetal aneuploidy
  - Evaluate suspected hydatiform mole
- Fetal crown-rump length is used to calculate gestational age and may be performed via the transvaginal or transabdominal route. Because the variation in size from fetus to fetus is minimal in the

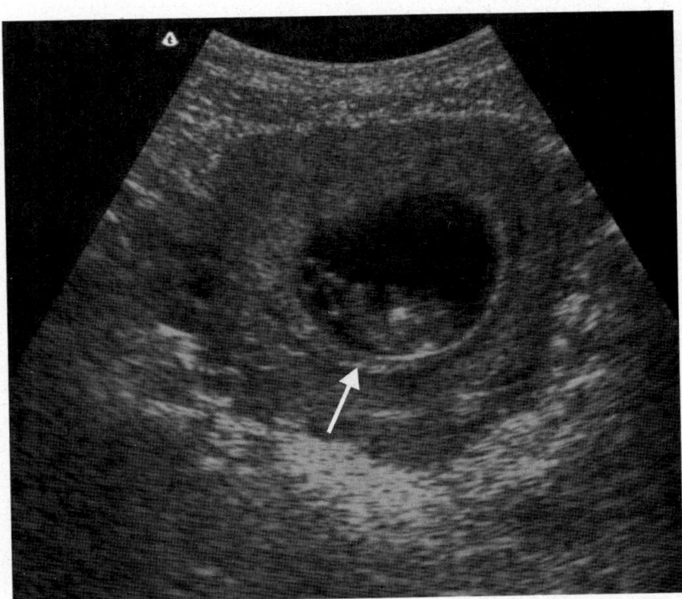

FIGURE 79-3 Ultrasound examination of a 9-week EGA twin with abdominal probe. The *arrow* is pointing to the yolk sac. Only one of the twins is visible. *(Reproduced with permission from E.J. Mayeaux, Jr., MD.)*

first trimester and minimal flexion, this is the optimal time to obtain an estimate of gestational age. Transvaginal US is typically used early for evaluation of the gestational sac, yolk sac, and developing embryo, whereas transabdominal US usually provides better visualization later in the first trimester. In obese patients, transvaginal US in early pregnancy can provide better visualization for more accurate dating.

- During the first 5 weeks of pregnancy, the endometrium has a "trilaminar" appearance and usually does not show distinct evidence of an intrauterine pregnancy. The gestational sac is the first detectable sign on ultrasound. Initial gestational age measurements are based on diameter of the sac. The yolk sac (**Figure 79-3**) is the first anatomic structure to appear within the gestational sac around the fifth week of gestation. A gestational sac diameter of 25 mm or greater with an empty or no fetal pole yolk sac indicates an abnormal gestation.[7] Caution should be used in presumptively diagnosing a gestational sac in the absence of a definitive embryo or yolk sac, as this could be a pseudogestational sac associated with ectopic pregnancy.[7]
- The embryonic disc becomes visible at about a gestational age of 5 to 6 weeks.[8] If the embryo is visible, but too small to measure, detection of cardiac activity establishes a gestational age of approximately 6 weeks. Cardiac motion should be observed when the embryo is 7 mm or greater in length. If cardiac activity is not seen in the embryo <7 mm, then a subsequent scan in 10–14 days will be needed to assess cardiac activity.[7] Direct measurement of the crown-rump length of the embryo provides the most accurate estimate of gestational age once the fetal pole is evident (**Figure 79-4**). The crown-rump length is the mean of three measurements of the longest straight-line length of the embryo from the outer margin of the cephalic pole to the rump. The crown-rump length is a more accurate indicator of gestational age than is the mean gestational sac diameter.
- The biparietal diameter may be used later in the first or early second trimester (**Figure 79-5**). It is highly reproducible and can predict gestational age within 7 days when measured between 14 and 20 weeks of gestation. The biparietal diameter should be measured on a plane of section that intersects both the third ventricle and thalami. The falx cerebri should be visible. The cursors are placed on the outer edge of the proximal skull and the inner edge of the distal skull to take the measurement. The femur length can be assessed by 10 weeks' gestation but is more accurate after 20 weeks' gestation.
- The uterus and adnexal structures should be evaluated. Presence, location, and size of adnexal masses should be documented. The presence, location, and size of leiomyomas should be recorded and followed thought the pregnancy.[7]
- To assess an individual's risk in the first trimester for fetal aneuploidy, a nuchal translucency (see **Figure 79-2**) can be measured with simultaneous serum biochemistry.[6] Fetal nuchal translucency is the sonographic appearance of subcutaneous edema in the fetal neck. It is the maximal thickness of the sonolucent zone (fluid accumulation) between the inner aspect of the fetal skin and the outer aspect of the soft tissue overlying the cervical spines or the occipital bone measured at 10–14 weeks gestation. The fetus must be in the neutral position, with the head in line with the spine. An enlarged nuchal translucency is independently associated with fetal aneuploidy and structural malformations.[6]

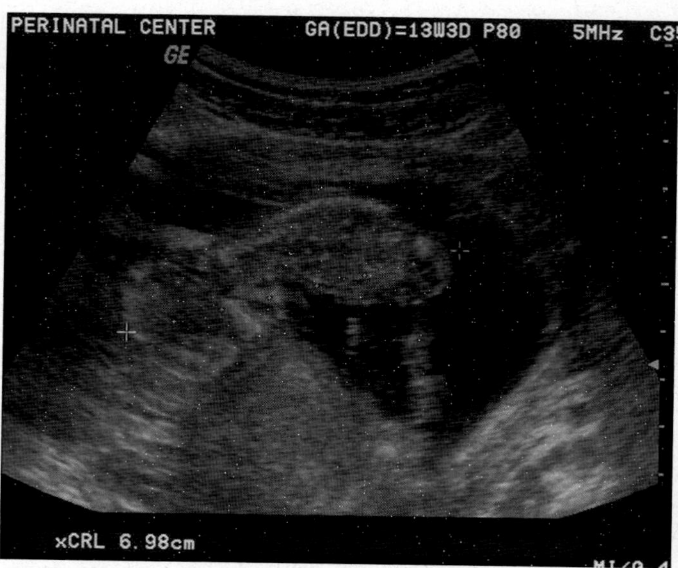

FIGURE 79-4 Ultrasound examination of a 13-week 3-day fetus by dates showing the head and spine with crown-to-rump length measurement of 6.98 cm. This represents an EGA of 13 weeks 3 days by ultrasound estimation (equal to dates). *(Reproduced with permission from E.J. Mayeaux, Jr., MD.)*

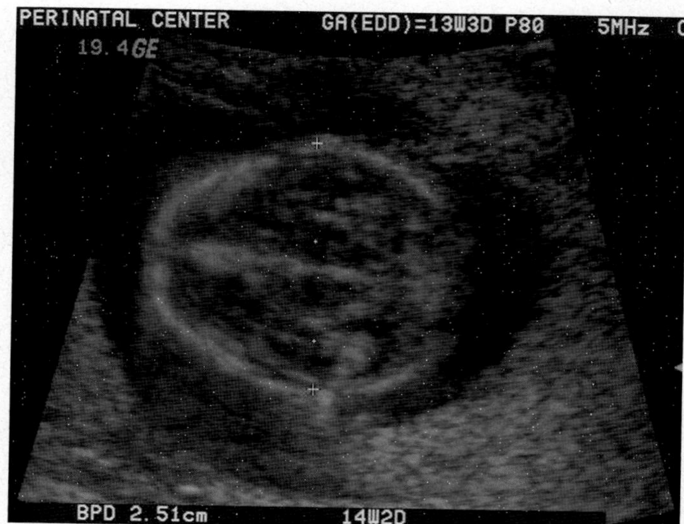

FIGURE 79-5 Ultrasound examination of the same 13-week 3-day fetus showing the biparietal diameter of 2.51 cm producing an EGA of 14 weeks 2 days. A 1-week disparity is within the measurement error of ultrasound at this stage of the pregnancy. *(Reproduced with permission from E.J. Mayeaux, Jr., MD.)*

PATIENT RESOURCES

- Obstetric ultrasound by Dr. Joseph Woo—**http://www.ob-ultrasound.net.**
- ACOG Frequently Asked Questions—**http://www.acog.org/Patients/FAQs/Ultrasound-Exams.**
- RadiologyInfo.org—**http://www.radiologyinfo.org/en/info.cfm?pg=obstetricus.**

PROVIDER RESOURCES

- Obstetric Ultrasound by Dr. Joseph Woo—**http://www.ob-ultrasound.net.**
- Obstetric Ultrasound Examinations—**http://www.aium.org/resources/guidelines/obstetric.pdf.**

REFERENCES

1. Villar J, Bergsjo P. Scientific basis for the content of routine antenatal care. Philosophy, recent studies, and power to eliminate or alleviate adverse maternal outcomes. *Acta Obstet Gynecol Scand.* 1997;76:1.
2. Whitworth M, Bricker L, Neilson J P, Dowsell T. Ultrasound for fetal assessment in early pregnancy. *Cochrane Database Syst Rev.* 2010;(4):CD007058.
3. Doubilet PM. Ultrasound evaluation of the first trimester. *Radiol Clin North Am.* 2014;52(6):1191-1199.
4. Ewigman BG, et al. Effect of prenatal ultrasound screening on perinatal outcome. RADIUS Study Group. *N Engl J Med.* 1993; 329:821.
5. Clayton HB, Schieve LA, Peterson HB, et al. A comparison of heterotopic and intrauterine-only pregnancy outcomes after assisted reproductive technologies in the United States from 1999 to 2002. *Fertil Steril.* 2007;87(2):303.
6. Screening for fetal aneuploidy. ACOG Practice Bulletin No. 163. American College of Obstetricians and Gynecologists. *Obstet Gynecol.* 2016;127:e123-137.
7. American College of Obstetricians and Gynecologists. Ultrasound in pregnancy. ACOG Practice Bulletin No. 175. *Obstet Gynecol.* 2016;128:e241-256.
8. Levi CS, Lyons EA, Lindsay DJ. Early diagnosis of nonviable pregnancy with endovaginal US. *Radiology.* 1988;167:383.

80 SECOND TRIMESTER OBSTETRICAL ULTRASOUND

Danielle B. Cooper, MD
E.J. Mayeaux, Jr., MD

PATIENT STORY

A 23-year-old pregnant gravida 2, para 1 woman is being seen for ultrasound because of her uncertain dates. Her best recollection of her last period gave her an estimated gestational age (EGA) of 19 weeks. Her vital signs are normal and her fundal height is 20 cm. **Figures 80-1** to **80-3** are still images taken from her ultrasound examination demonstrating an EGA of 21 weeks and 6 days by measurement of the baby's biparietal diameter (BPD), head circumference (HC), abdominal circumference (AC), and femur length (FL). All four measurements allow the computer to calculate an estimated fetal weight of 431 g. The pregnancy proceeded without complications, and the patient delivered a healthy boy at $40^{3/7}$ weeks based on the ultrasound-calculated estimated date of delivery. No interventions were needed for postdates because of the ultrasound calculations earlier in the pregnancy.

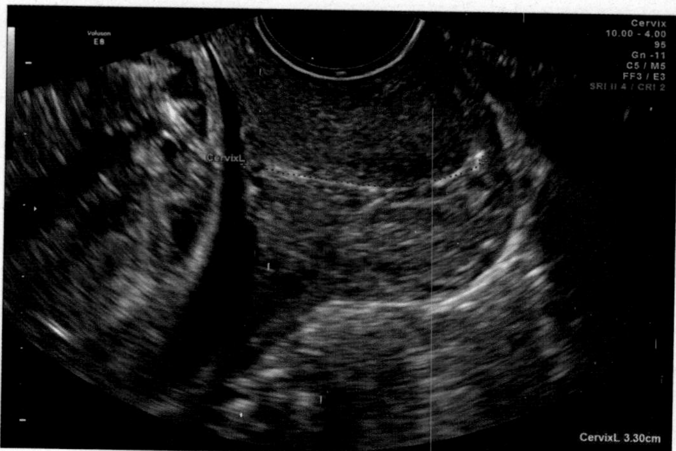

FIGURE 80-1 Transvaginal cervical length of a 24-week uterus. The hyperechoic line identifies the glandular tissue of the cervix and correct positioning to include the entire cervix. Measurement is from the internal os traced out to the external os. The fetal head is visible in this shot but not necessary for the measurement. (*Reproduced with permission from Danielle Cooper, MD.*)

INTRODUCTION

The ideal time to perform an anatomic survey is between 18 and 20 weeks' gestation. The fetus has developed all of its organ systems and is large enough that these can be visualized in detail. Fetal biometry can be obtained to calculate a gestational age and has an accepted error margin of ±7–10 days. If resources are limited or patient costs are an issue, the second trimester ultrasound provides the most bang for the buck.

INDICATIONS FOR ULTRASOUND

- Second and third trimester ultrasound examination can be used to determine fetal number and presentation, and for documentation of fetal cardiac activity, placental location, and amniotic fluid volume.
- Second trimester extends from 14w 0d to 27w 6d and is a good time to perform ultrasound for fetal assessment for gestational age and weight. It is also an integral part of performing diagnostic amniocentesis.
- If only a single ultrasound can be performed on a patient, optimal timing is 18 to 20 weeks. Fetal anatomy is best seen during this interval. If fetal abnormalities are detected, a more detailed examination (level 2 ultrasound) by a specialized sonographer is indicated.
- Ultrasound examination is indicated to establish the number of fetuses and chorionicity when a multiple gestation pregnancy is suspected. Risk factors for a multiple gestation pregnancy include assisted reproductive technology, family history of twins (or higher multiples), and uterine size larger than that expected by menstrual dating. The number of fetuses can be best established by obtaining an image that includes a cross-section of all fetal poles that have distinct cardiac activity within a single frame.

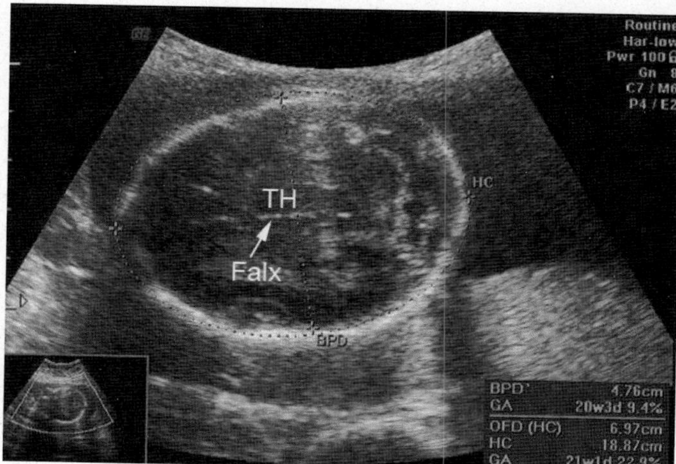

FIGURE 80-2 Ultrasound examination of a 21-week estimated gestational age (EGA) fetus showing measurement of the baby's biparietal diameter (*BPD*) and head circumference (*HC*). Note the presence of the *falx cerebri* and the thalamus (*TH*) to ensure the measurement is at the right anatomic level. (*Reproduced with permission from E.J. Mayeaux, Jr., MD.*)

- Cervical length in second trimester to screen for preterm labor in women at high risk for preterm delivery.

The placental location, appearance, and relationship to the internal cervical os should be recorded.[1]

SYNONYMS

Second trimester anatomy scan, fetal anatomy scan, TIFFA (targeted imaging for fetal anomalies).

PATHOPHYSIOLOGY

- Fetal abnormalities that may be reliably diagnosed by ultrasound include achondroplasia, anencephaly, cleft lip, clubfoot, duodenal atresia, fetal hydrops, gastroschisis, hydrocephalus, omphalocele, transposition of the great vessels, cardiac, pulmonary and renal abnormalities, and spina bifida. If anomalies are suspected, a level 2 ultrasound with a perinatologist is indicated.
- Up to 5% of pregnancies will have placentas that partially or completely cover the internal cervical os at 16 to 18 weeks of gestation. Only 1 in 10 of these will continue to cover the internal os in the late third trimester.[2] Placentas that are clear of the cervix in early pregnancy will not encroach on it later.

INDICATIONS FOR ULTRASOUND IN SECOND TRIMESTER

- Evaluating the possibility of a fetal anomaly is best done by ultrasound examination after 16 weeks of gestation, as earlier examination may be limited by fetal size and development.
- The sensitivity and specificity of the procedure for detecting congenital abnormalities varies depending on the specific defect, the gestational age, the quality of the ultrasound unit, and the skill of the ultrasonographer.
- Ultrasound examination is the main diagnostic modality used to evaluate second and third trimester bleeding. The major placental causes of vaginal bleeding at this time are placenta previa and abruptio placentae. A transvaginal obstetric ultrasound examination can identify placental location and is safe even when placenta previa is present. Preterm labor is another cause of vaginal bleeding, and the cervical length can be measured transvaginally to assess this risk. The normal cervical length can be seen in **Figure 80-1**. The images should be obtained after the mother has emptied her bladder to avoid displacement of the anterior lower uterine segment, thus producing a false-positive test.[3]
- Fetal intrauterine growth–limiting disorders are more likely when the uterine size is less than appropriate for gestational age, a prior pregnancy has been affected by growth restriction, with maternal hypertension, and in multiple gestations. Ultrasound cannot distinguish between a constitutionally small fetus and a pathologically small fetus. Decreased amniotic fluid volume and below-normal interval growth make placental insufficiency more likely.

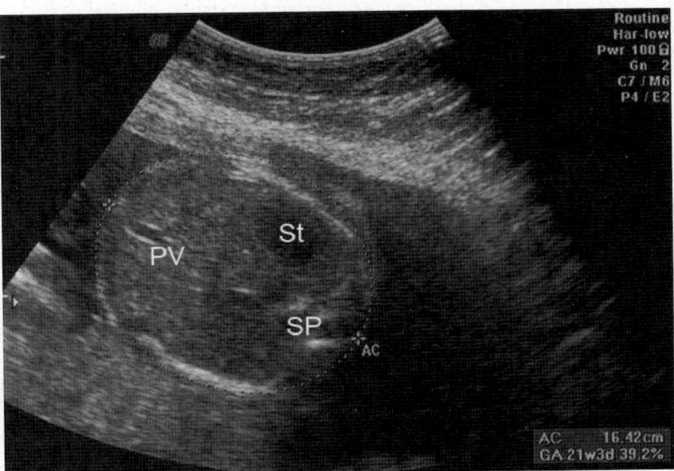

FIGURE 80-3 Ultrasound examination of a 21-week estimated gestational age (EGA) fetus showing measurement of the baby's abdominal circumference (*AC*). Note how the stomach (*St*), spine (*SP*), and portal vein (*PV*) are all visible to ensure that the measurement is at the right anatomic level. (*Reproduced with permission from E.J. Mayeaux, Jr., MD.*)

PERFORMING THE PROCEDURE

- The four standard biometric parameters commonly used to estimate gestational age and/or fetal weight in the second trimester are BPD, HC (see **Figure 80-2**), AC (see **Figure 80-3**), and FL (**Figure 80-4**).[4] They are usually obtained by transabdominal ultrasound examination, and the fetal weight is calculated.
- The BPD (see **Figure 80-2**) is a highly reproducible measurement and can predict gestational age within ±7 days when the ultrasound is performed between 14 and 20 weeks' gestation, although the best time to get an accurate date is in the first trimester. The BPD should be measured on a plane that includes both the third ventricle and the thalamus. The cursors are placed on the outer edge of the proximal skull, and the inner edge of the distal skull and the BPD measured.
- The cephalic index is ratio of the BPD and the occipitofrontal diameter multiplied by 100. It should be used where the BPD may be inaccurate, such as with breech presentations, oligohydramnios, premature rupture of the membranes, and neural tube abnormalities.
- The measurement of fetal HC also accurately estimates gestational age and is especially useful in the setting of growth disorders (see **Figure 80-2**). The accuracy decreases in the second half of pregnancy. The HC should be measured on the same plane that includes the third ventricle, the thalamus, the cavum septum pellucidum anteriorly, and the tentorial hiatus posteriorly. Unlike the BPD measurements, the HC measurement is obtained by placing the cursors on the outer margins of the calvarium bilaterally.
- The AC (see **Figure 80-3**) is the least accurate in predicting gestational age, being accurate within 2 weeks in the second trimester. It is most often used for estimations of fetal weight and interval growth evaluations rather than fetal dating. The AC measurement is a transverse section through the upper abdomen that should demonstrate the following fetal landmarks: fetal stomach, umbilical vein, and portal sinus. The kidneys and cord insertion should not be visible. The measurement should be taken at the level of the largest diameter of the fetal liver where the right and left portal veins join. The four calipers are placed around the abdomen on the skin edge to draw a circular line for AC measurement.
- FL (see **Figure 80-4**) can be measured and is accurate to within 1 week before 20 weeks' gestation. The provider should align the transducer along the long axis of the femoral bone and visualize either the femoral head or the greater trochanter proximally, and the end of the femur or the femoral condyle distally. The provider should ensure that the femur and not another long bone in the arm or leg is being measured. Calipers should be placed at the bone and cartilage junction and measure only ossified bone, not including the femoral head.
- Aside from the fetal biometry for a complete anatomic scan, providers must also visualize fetal brain including ventricles, choroid plexus, the posterior fossa and septum pellucidum. The fetal face including the nasal bone, upper lip and palate, orbits, and mandible should be documented. A four-chamber view of the fetal heart, the left and right outflow tracts, and the diaphragm and lungs should be seen. The fetal abdomen including liver, stomach, kidneys, cord insertion, bladder, umbilical arteries, and genitalia should be seen. The fetal spine, upper limbs including hand opening, and feet should be documented for a complete anatomic survey.[1]
- Many providers will often show expectant parents images of the baby's face (**Figures 80-5** and **80-6**), hands (**Figure 80-7**), and sex (**Figures 80-8** and **80-9**).

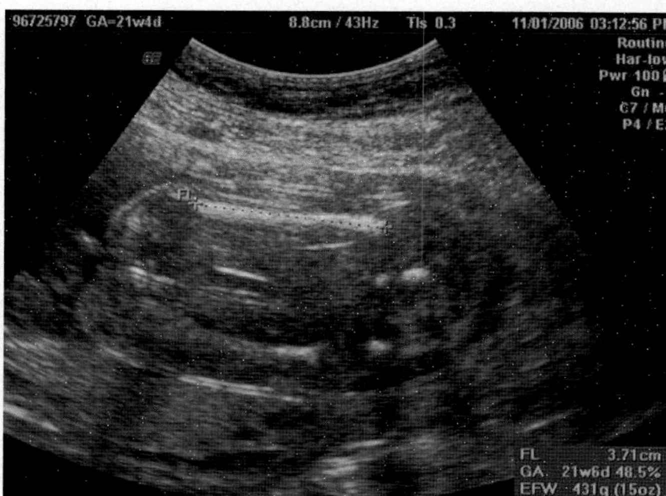

FIGURE 80-4 Ultrasound measurement of the same baby's femur length giving an estimated gestational age (EGA) of 21 weeks and 6 days. Note the buttocks and penis are visible. All four measurements from **Figures 80-1** to **80-3** and this figure allow the computer to calculate an estimated fetal weight (EFW) of 431 grams. (*Reproduced with permission from E.J. Mayeaux, Jr., MD.*)

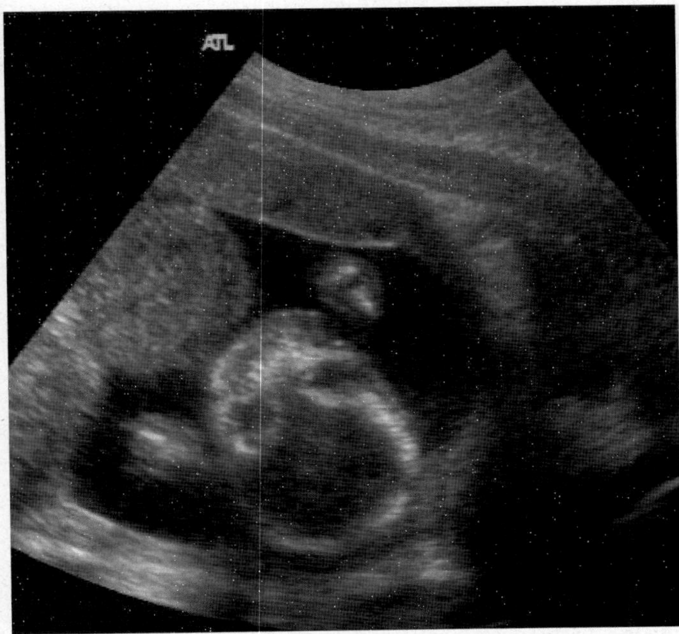

FIGURE 80-5 Ultrasound examination of a 15-week estimated gestational age (EGA) fetus showing the baby's face. (*Reproduced with permission from E.J. Mayeaux, Jr., MD.*)

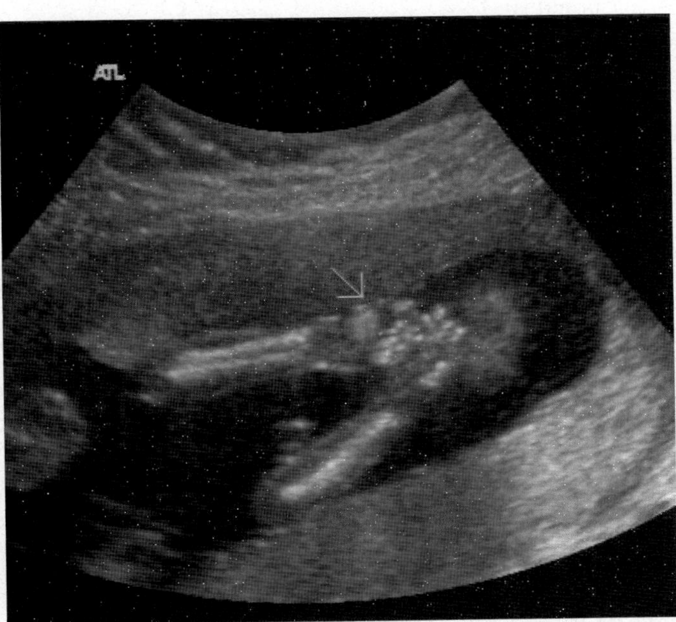

FIGURE 80-7 Ultrasound examination of a 19-week estimated gestational age (EGA) fetus showing the baby's hands and forearms. *Arrow* is pointing at the right hand. (*Reproduced with permission from E.J. Mayeaux, Jr., MD.*)

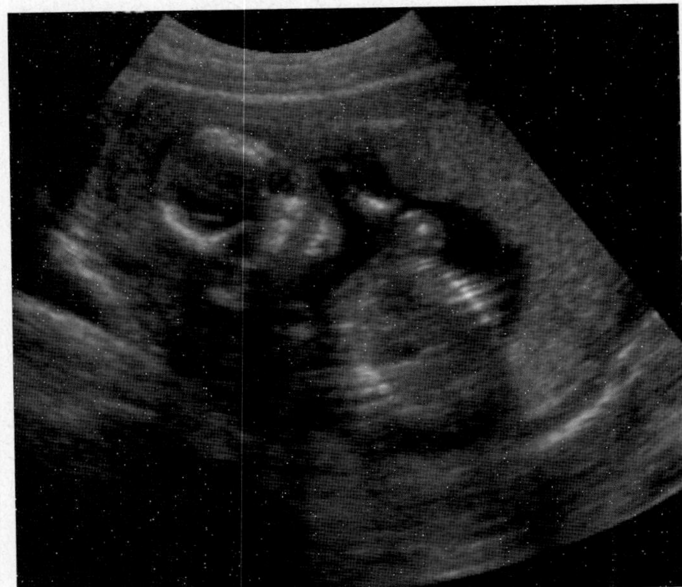

FIGURE 80-6 Ultrasound examination of a 15-week estimated gestational age (EGA) fetus showing another view of the baby's face. (*Reproduced with permission from E.J. Mayeaux, Jr., MD.*)

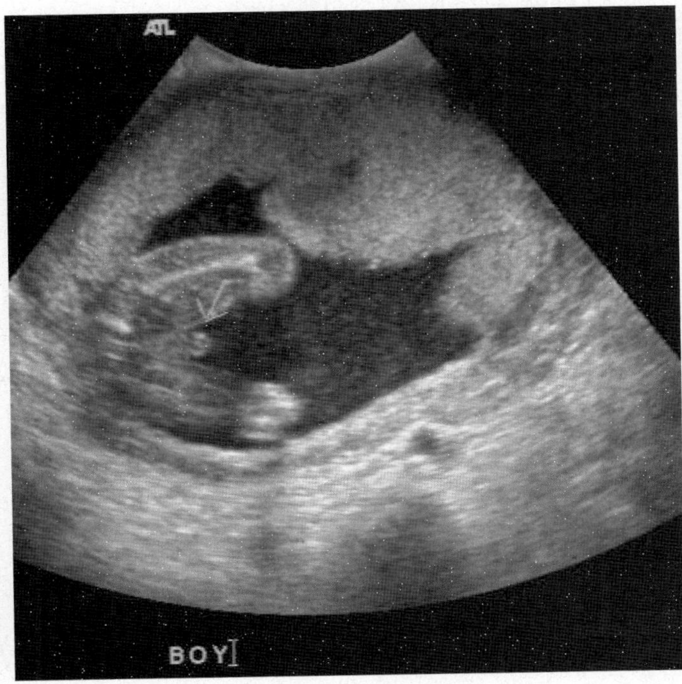

FIGURE 80-8 Ultrasound examination of a 19-week estimated gestational age (EGA) fetus showing the baby is a boy (*arrow*). (*Reproduced with permission from E.J. Mayeaux, Jr., MD.*)

- The placenta and its relationship to the cervix should be examined for signs of placenta previa.

Cervical length or funneling of the cervix should be measured if there is a history of or current evidence of preterm labor or history of incompetent cervix. Cervical length is determined as the distance between the internal and external os. In patients at risk for cervical shortening or incompetence, the operator can apply fundal pressure or scan the patient in the standing position to help identify these women[3] (**Figure 80-10**).

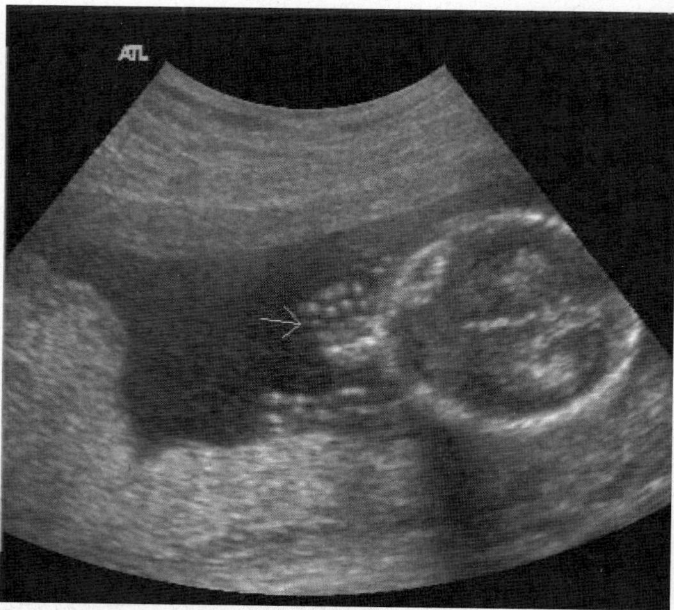

FIGURE 80-9 Ultrasound examination of a 19-week estimated gestational age (EGA) fetus sucking his thumb (*arrow*). The two hemispheres of the brain are visible with the falx cerebri in between. (*Reproduced with permission from E.J. Mayeaux, Jr., MD.*)

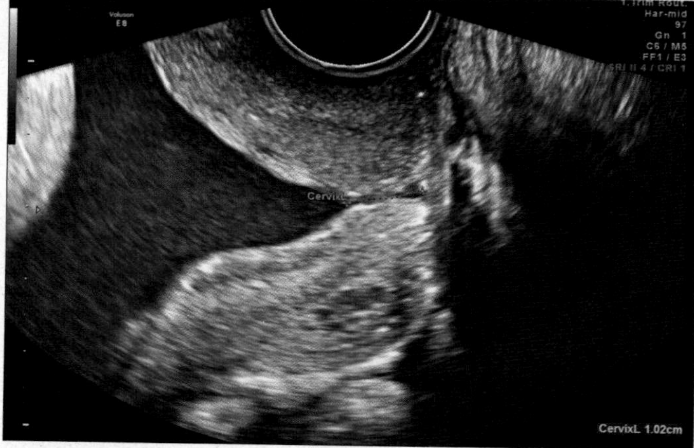

FIGURE 80-10 Transvaginal cervical length (CL) of a 27-week uterus at risk for preterm labor. CL is 1.02 cm. The "V" quality of the lower uterine segment and opening of the internal os significantly increase this patient's risk for preterm labor. (*Reproduced with permission from Danielle Cooper, MD.*)

PATIENT RESOURCES

- ACOG Frequently Asked Questions—**http://www.acog.org/Patients/FAQs/Ultrasound-Exams.**
- March of Dimes pregnancy education center—**http://www.marchofdimes.com/pregnancy/ultrasound-during-pregnancy.aspx.**

PROVIDER RESOURCES

- Obstetric Ultrasound Examinations—**http://www.aium.org/resources/guidelines/obstetric.pdf.**
- Perinatology.com. Level II Ultrasound—**http://www.perinatology.com/ultrasound.htm.**
- Obstetric Ultrasound by Dr. Joseph Woo—**http://www.ob-ultrasound.net.**

REFERENCES

1. American Institute of Ultrasound in Medicine. AIUM practice guideline for the performance of obstetric ultrasound examinations. *J Ultrasound Med.* 2013;32:1083-1101.
2. Townsend RR, Laing FC, Nyberg DA, et al. Technical factors responsible for "placental migration": sonographic assessment. *Radiology.* 1986;160:105.
3. Expert Panel of Women's Imaging. Assessment of the Gravid Cervix. American College of Radiology. Date of origin 1999, last review date 2014. https://acsearch.acr.org/docs/69464/Narrative/ Accessed May 2018.
4. Hadlock FP. Sonographic estimation of fetal age and weight. *Radiol Clin North Am.* 1990;28:39.

81 THIRD TRIMESTER OBSTETRICAL ULTRASOUND

Danielle B. Cooper, MD
E.J. Mayeaux, Jr., MD

PATIENT STORY

A 26-year-old woman gravida 3, para 2-0-0-2 at 30 weeks' gestation with routine prenatal care is concerned because her sister had a fetal demise at 34 weeks and she thinks her baby is moving less. A biophysical profile is performed, and the patient is reassured of normal fetal status (**Figures 81-1** to **81-4**).

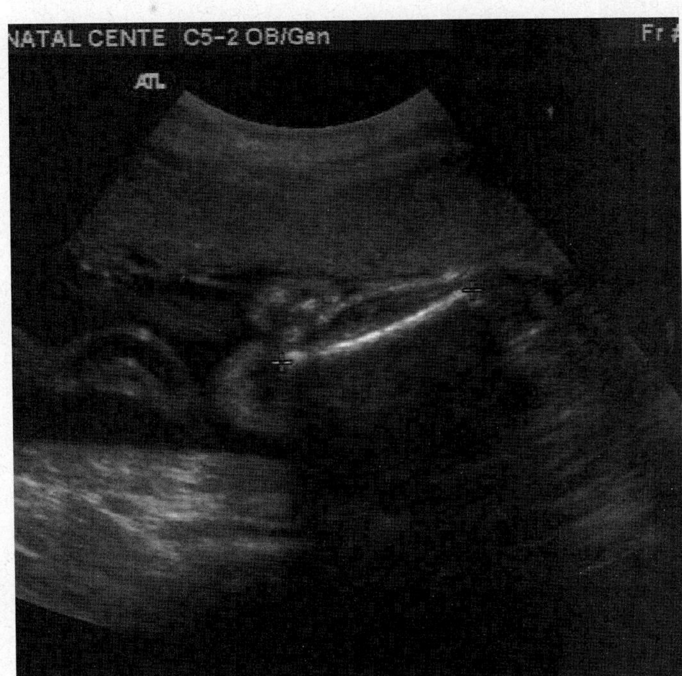

FIGURE 81-1 Ultrasound examination of a 27-week estimated gestational age (EGA) fetus showing measurement of the baby's humerus. *(Reproduced with permission from E.J. Mayeaux, Jr., MD.)*

INTRODUCTION

Ultrasound in the third trimester of pregnancy is most often used to determine fetal number, presentation, and growth issues. This later pregnancy scan is also used to document fetal cardiac activity, placental location, and amniotic fluid volume, as well as provide a method for antenatal fetal assessment.

INDICATIONS FOR USE

- A Cochrane review of 8 studies showed no difference in obstetric, antenatal, or neonatal morbidity between low-risk women undergoing routine late ultrasound examination after 24 weeks and those who did not.[1] In addition, there was no difference in perinatal outcome measures, such as admission to a neonatal intensive care unit, birth weight less than 10th percentile, or perinatal mortality.
- Hydrops fetalis is the accumulation of fluid in 2 or more fetal compartments, usually a result of immune pathologic conditions (**Figure 81-5**). Nonimmune hydrops will also be apparent on ultrasound and may be the result of severe anemias, congenital infections, heart or lung disease, chromosomal abnormalities, or fetal liver disease. Serial ultrasound examinations are useful for following pregnancies at risk for developing hydrops or to determine treatment. The middle cerebral artery peak-systolic velocity (MCA-PSV) is a noninvasive tool to predict fetal anemia.[2] A 2009 systematic review provides compelling evidence that Doppler interrogation of the MCA-PSV performs well as a screening tool for severe fetal anemia of any etiology.[3]
- Ultrasound may also be used to evaluate third trimester bleeding. The major placental causes of vaginal bleeding that must be considered are placenta previa (**Figure 81-6**) and abruptio placentae.
- Ultrasound can safely image maternal abdominal organs during pregnancy. Ovarian cysts, uterine leiomyoma, renal obstruction, and gallbladder or liver disease can be evaluated without using ionizing radiation.

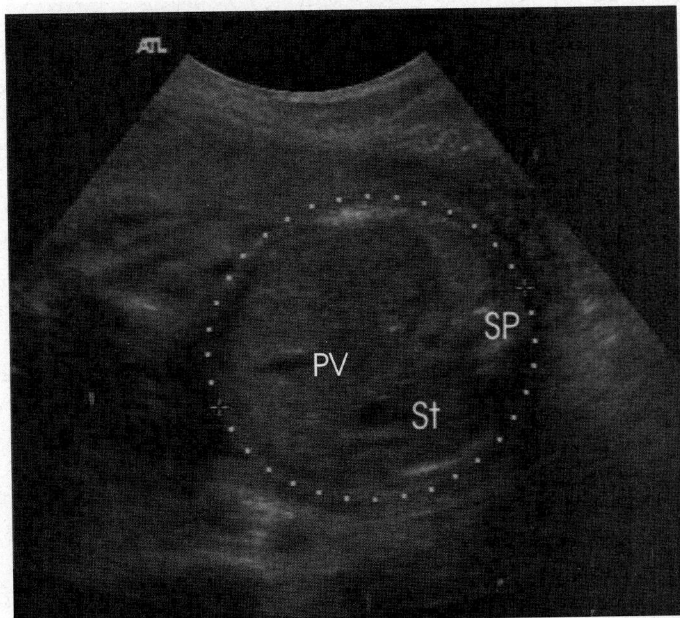

FIGURE 81-2 Ultrasound examination of a 27-week estimated gestational age (EGA) fetus showing the baby's stomach (*St*), abdomen, spine (*SP*), and left portal vein (*PV*). *(Reproduced with permission from E.J. Mayeaux, Jr., MD.)*

Pregnancies complicated by fetal growth restriction and preeclampsia should be evaluated with umbilical artery Doppler sonography. It is recommended for fetal surveillance and monitoring well-being. The values measured are peak-systolic frequency shift (S) and

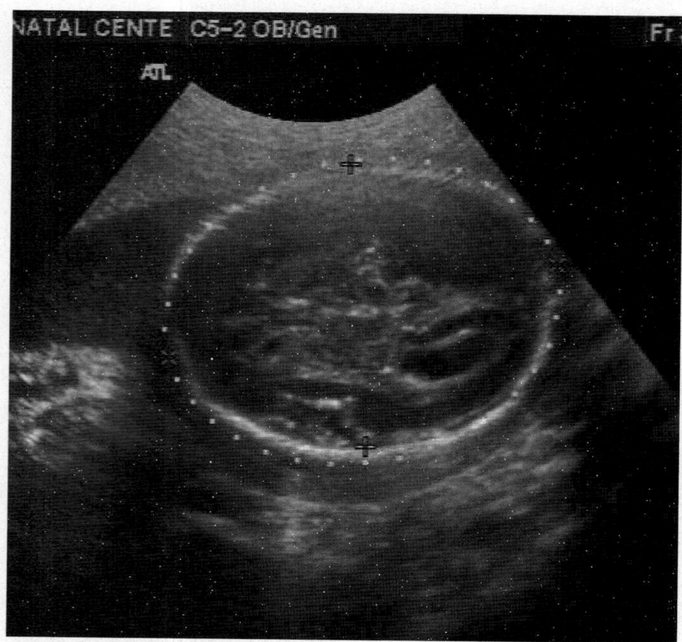

FIGURE 81-3 Ultrasound examination of a 27-week estimated gestational age (EGA) fetus showing measurement of the baby's biparietal diameter (BPD). (*Reproduced with permission from E.J. Mayeaux, Jr., MD.*)

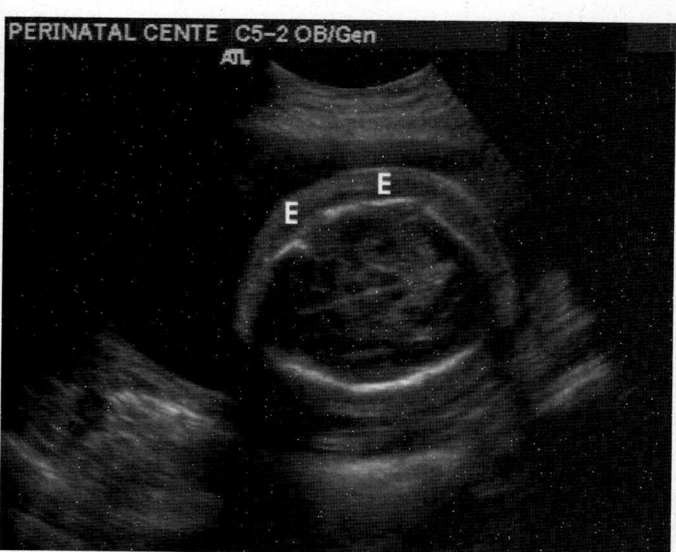

FIGURE 81-5 Ultrasound examination showing scalp edema (*E*) associated with hydrops fetalis. (*Reproduced with permission from E.J. Mayeaux, Jr., MD.*)

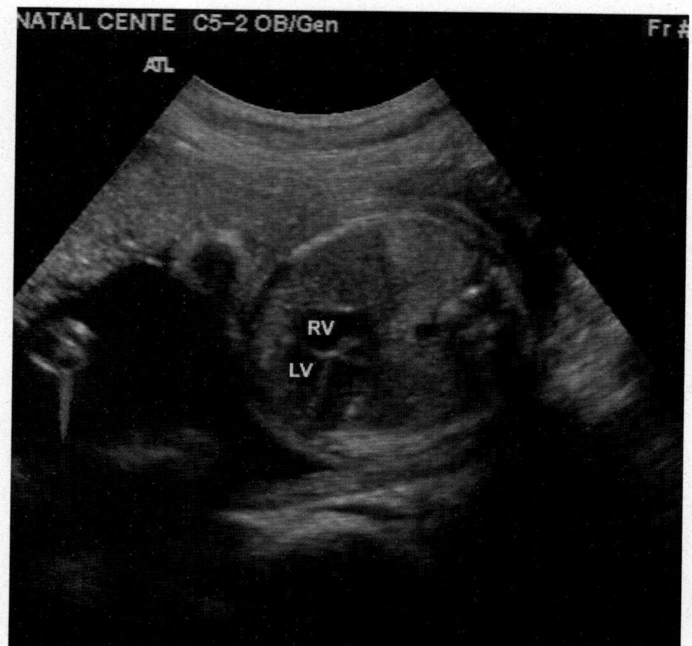

FIGURE 81-4 Ultrasound examination of a 27-week estimated gestational age (EGA) fetus showing all four chambers of the baby's heart. (*Reproduced with permission from E.J. Mayeaux, Jr., MD.*)

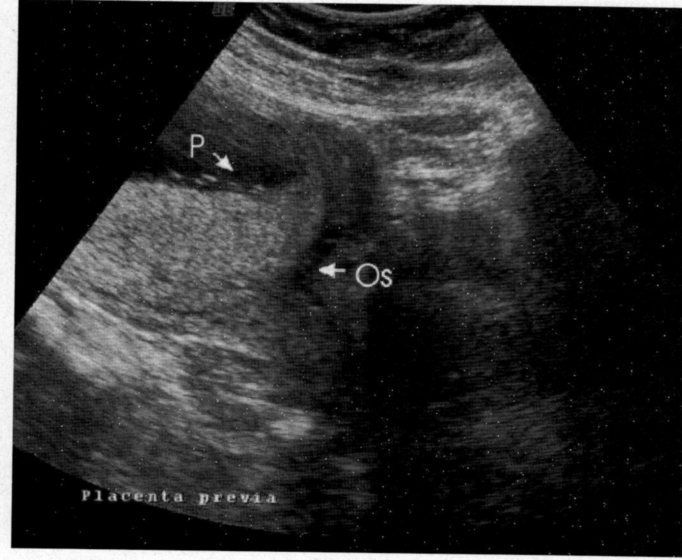

FIGURE 81-6 Ultrasound examination showing the placenta (*P*) covering the cervical os (*Os*) in placenta previa. (*Reproduced with permission from E.J. Mayeaux, Jr., MD.*)

end-diastolic frequency shift (D) of an umbilical artery. This S-to-D ratio gives information about downstream impedance to flow. For example, uteroplacental insufficiency will show rising impedance to fetal placental vascular bed, which shows a decline in end-diastolic velocity and an overall increase in these Doppler indices.[4] Randomized clinical trial and their meta-analyses have shown the effectiveness of ultrasound in decreasing perinatal morbidity.[4,5]

If there is an increased risk for in utero fetal demise or significant risk factors for fetal anemia, then fetal surveillance can be performed with the biophysical profile (BPP). This is the sonographic assessment of four fetal variables: fetal breathing, fetal tone, fetal movement, and the amniotic fluid volume, plus the results of the nonstress testing.[4] Scoring is either a 0 or 2 for each parameter with a total of 10 points possible. Fetal breathing is present if the episode lasts for at least 20 seconds. Flexion and extension seen determines scoring for fetal tone. At least 3 gross body movements must be seen in the 30-minute time period of the BPP to receive 2 points. Amniotic fluid volume is considered normal (2 points) with at least a single 2 × 2 cm pocket seen.[4]

VALUE OF ULTRASOUND IN THIRD TRIMESTER

- Ultrasound-based determination of estimated date of delivery (EDD) has been shown to improve dating and thus reduce intervention for postterm pregnancy. One randomized controlled trial evaluated the effect of routine ultrasound examinations at 18 and 32 weeks of gestation on the accuracy of dating and pregnancy outcome in a low-risk population.[6] They found that ultrasound screening reduced the incidence of induced labor for postterm pregnancy by 70%, and also reduced the incidence of induction for all causes. They also found that the proportion of 5-minute Apgar scores less than 8 and the need for positive pressure ventilation were both lower in the screened group.
- Although ultrasound EDD determination as late as 34 weeks can reduce the number of pregnancies diagnosed as postterm, first trimester ultrasound in a low-risk population is more effective than later ultrasound in decreasing postterm pregnancy.
- Accurate assessment of gestational age is important so as not to inappropriately initiate tocolysis for near-term labor.
- Twin pregnancies are at increased risk of complications, such as fetal heart rate abnormalities and complications as a result of malpresentation. When both twins are found on ultrasound to be vertex (42% of twins), a trial of labor with the goal of a vaginal delivery is appropriate. When one twin is nonvertex (38% of twins), options include cesarean delivery of both twins, or attempted vaginal delivery of one or both twins.[7,8]
- Parents are now paying for 4D ultrasounds (3D images in real time, time being the fourth dimension) so that they can see and get pictures of their developing child. Although the 4D ultrasound is not a standard medical device (**Figure 81-7**), it is being used to better characterize certain anomalies, such as facial clefts, neural tube defects, and skeletal malformations.[9] There are no well-documented harmful effects to the fetus from diagnostic ultrasound examination used appropriately.[10] Nevertheless, examinations should be performed only for valid medical reasons,[10] for the shortest amount of time, and with the lowest level of acoustic energy that allows diagnostic evaluation.[11]

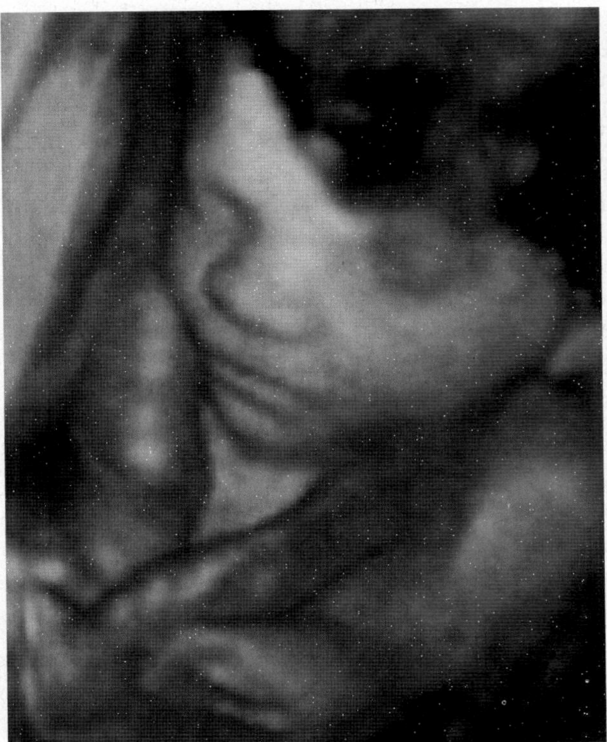

FIGURE 81-7 Three-dimensional (3D) ultrasound showing a 25-week fetus. (*Reproduced with permission from E.J. Mayeaux, Jr., MD.*)

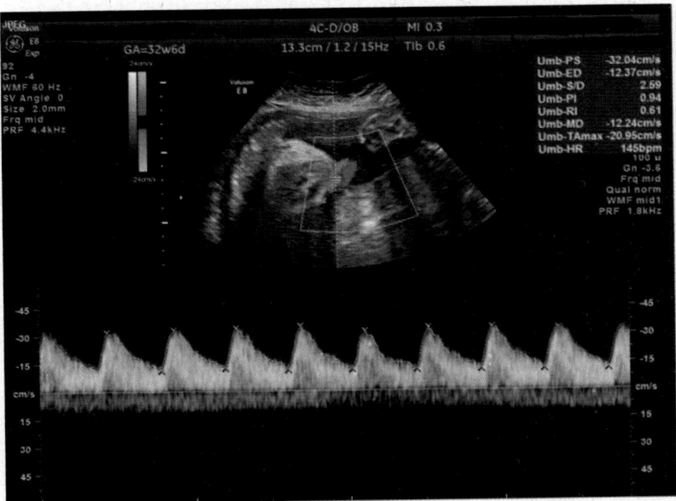

FIGURE 81-8 Umbilical artery Doppler of 32 week 6 day infant with S/D 2.59, which is normal. (*Reproduced with permission from E.J. Mayeaux, Jr., MD.*)

If there is suspicion of unusual fetal growth, restricted or macrosomic, a third trimester growth scan is obtained for evaluation and continued plan of care.

The BPP is a noninvasive, easily performed, accurate means for predicting the presence of significant fetal compromise. Approximately 70% to 90% of late fetal deaths display evidence of fetal compromise prior to demise.[4] Ultrasound detection of these fetal signs can allow appropriate intervention to ideally prevent adverse fetal sequelae.

Umbilical artery (**Figure 81-8**) and middle cerebral artery Doppler measurements should be integrated with other existing modalities of antepartum fetal monitoring to determine their clinical usefulness.[4]

FOLLOW-UP

- Once BPPs are initiated in women requiring fetal surveillance, this test should be repeated on a weekly or twice weekly basis until delivery.

When a patient has placenta previa diagnosed on ultrasound, advise patient to avoid coitus, digital cervical examination, and exercise. Counsel her to seek immediate medical attention if there is any vaginal bleeding or uterine contractions. Advise her that cesarean delivery is the delivery route of choice.[12]

PATIENT RESOURCES

- ACOG Frequently Asked Questions—**http://www.acog.org/Patients/ FAQs/Ultrasound-Exams.**
- March of Dimes pregnancy education center—**http://www.marchofdimes.com/pregnancy/ultrasound-during-pregnancy.aspx.**

PROVIDER RESOURCES

- Obstetric Ultrasound Examinations—**http://www.aium.org/resources/guidelines/obstetric.pdf.**
- OB-GYN ultrasound online—**http://www.fetalsono.com/index.html.**
- Perinatology.com. Level 2 ultrasound—**http://www.perinatology.com/ultrasound.htm.**

REFERENCES

1. Bricker L, Neilson JP. Routine ultrasound in late pregnancy (after 24 weeks' gestation). *Cochrane Database Syst Rev.* 2007;(4): CD001451.
2. Mari G; Collaborative Group for Doppler Assessment of the Blood Velocity in Anemic Fetuses. Noninvasive diagnosis by Doppler ultrasonography of fetal anemia due to maternal red-cell alloimmunization. *N Engl J Med.* 2000;342:9-14.
3. Pretlove SJ, Fox CE, Khan KS, Kilby MD. Noninvasive methods of detecting fetal anemia: a systematic review and meta-analysis. *BJOG.* 2009;116:1558-1567.
4. American College of Obstetricians and Gynecologists. Antepartum fetal surveillance. Practice Bulletin No. 145. *Obstet Gynecol.* 2014;124:182-192.
5. Maulik D, Mundy D, Heitmann E, Maulik D. Evidence based approach to umbilical artery Doppler fetal surveillance in high risk pregnancies: an update. *Clin Obstet Gynecol.* 2010;53(4): 869-878.
6. Eik-Nes SH, Salvesen KA, Okland O, Vatten LJ. Routine ultrasound fetal examination in pregnancy: the "Alesund" randomized controlled trial. *Ultrasound Obstet Gynecol.* 2000;15:473.
7. Chasen ST, Spiro SJ, Kalish RB, Chervenak FA. Changes in fetal presentation in twin pregnancies. *J Matern Fetal Neonatal Med.* 2005;17:45.
8. Dodd JM, Crowther CA. Evidence-based care of women with a multiple pregnancy. *Best Pract Res Clin Obstet Gynaecol.* 2005; 19:131.
9. Goncalves LF, Lee W, Espinoza J, Romero R. Three- and 4-dimensional ultrasound in obstetric practice: does it help? *J Ultrasound Med.* 2005;24:1599-1624.
10. American College of Obstetricians and Gynecologists. Ultrasound in pregnancy. Practice Bulletin No. 175. *Obstet Gynecol.* 2016;128:1459-1460.
11. Reddy UM, Abuhamad A, Saade GR. Fetal imaging. *Semin Perinatol.* 2013;37:289.
12. Bhide A, Prefumo F, Moore J, et al. Placental edge to internal os distance in the late third trimester and mode of delivery in placenta praevia. *BJOG.* 2003;110:860.

SECTION B VAGINITIS AND CERVICITIS

82 OVERVIEW OF VAGINITIS

E.J. Mayeaux, Jr., MD

PATIENT STORY

A 39-year-old woman presented to her physician with a malodorous vaginal discharge. On exam, a thin white discharge was seen covering the introitus (**Figure 82-1**). A speculum exam revealed a thin whitish gray discharge and a distinct fishy odor. The pH of the discharge was 4.6, and 40% of the epithelial cells on her wet prep were clue cells (**Figure 82-2**). She was diagnosed with bacterial vaginosis and treated with oral metronidazole.

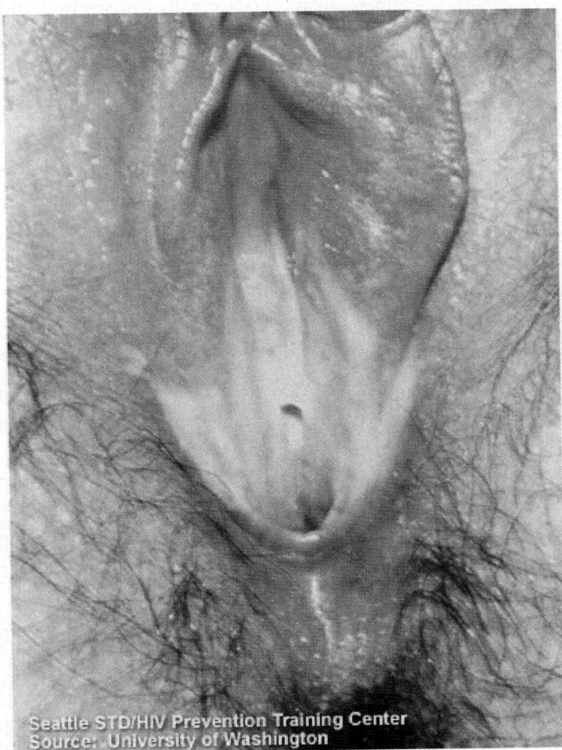

FIGURE 82-1 Thin white discharge from bacterial vaginosis seen covering the introitus prior to speculum exam. (*Reproduced with permission from Seattle STD/HIV Prevention Training Center, University of Washington.*)

INTRODUCTION

Vaginal discharge is a frequent presenting complaint in primary care. The three most common causes are bacterial vaginosis, candidiasis, and trichomoniasis. However, a significant number of patients with vaginal discharge will have some other condition, such as atrophic vaginitis. Providers must refrain from "diagnosing" a vaginitis based solely on the color and consistency of the discharge, as this may lead to misdiagnosis and may miss concomitant infections.[1]

EPIDEMIOLOGY

The reported rates of chlamydia and gonorrhea are highest among females ages 15 to 19 years. Adolescents are at greater risk for sexually transmitted diseases (STDs) because they frequently have unprotected intercourse, are biologically more susceptible to infection, are often engaged in partnerships of limited duration, and face multiple obstacles to utilization of health care.[1] Bacterial vaginosis, *Candida* vulvovaginitis, and trichomoniasis account for over 90% of vaginal infections.[2]

ETIOLOGY AND PATHOPHYSIOLOGY

- The quantity and quality of normal vaginal discharge in healthy women vary. Physiologic leukorrhea refers to generally nonmalodorous, mucous, white or yellowish vaginal discharge in the absence of a pathologic cause. It is not accompanied by signs and symptoms, such as pain, pruritus, burning, erythema, or tissue friability. However, slight malodor and irritative symptoms can be normal for some women at certain times.[3] Physiologic leukorrhea is usually a result of estrogen-induced changes in cervicovaginal secretions.
- Noninfectious causes of vaginitis include irritants (e.g., scented panty liners, spermicides, povidone-iodine, soaps and perfumes,

and some topical drugs) and allergens (e.g., latex condoms, topical antifungal agents, chemical preservatives) that produce hypersensitivity reactions.

- Before starting an examination, determine whether the patient douched recently, because this can lower the yield of diagnostic tests and increase the risk of pelvic inflammatory disease.[4] Patients who have been told not to douche will sometimes start wiping the vagina with soapy washcloths, which also irritates the vagina and cervix and may cause a discharge. Douching is associated with increases in bacterial vaginosis and acquisition of sexually transmitted infections when exposed. However, recent studies indicate that douching with plain water once a week or less did not disturb normal flora.[5,6]
- There are many causes of vaginitis in humans. Infectious causes include bacterial vaginosis (40% to 50% of cases) (see **Figures 82-1** and **82-2**), vulvovaginal candidiasis (20% to 25%), and trichomonas (15% to 20%) (**Figure 82-3**).[7] Less common causes include atrophic vaginitis, foreign body (especially in children), cytolytic or desquamative inflammatory vaginitis, streptococcal vaginitis, ulcerative vaginitis, and idiopathic vulvovaginal ulceration associated with HIV infection.
- Rarer noninfectious causes include chemicals, allergies, hypersensitivity, contact dermatitis, trauma, postpuerperal atrophic vaginitis, erosive lichen planus, collagen vascular disease, Behçet syndrome, and pemphigus syndromes.

FIGURE 82-2 A wet mount of vaginal discharge in saline under high-power light microscopy. Note the presence of vaginal epithelial cells, smaller white blood cells (polymorphonucleocytes), and bacteria. The bacteria are the coccobacilli of *Gardnerella vaginalis* covering the cell membranes of the two vaginal epithelial cells near the lower end of the field. These are clue cells seen in patients with bacterial vaginosis. (*Reproduced with permission from Richard P. Usatine, MD.*)

DIAGNOSIS

CLINICAL FEATURES

- Examine the external genitalia for irritation or discharge (see **Figure 82-2**). Speculum examination is done to determine the amount and character of the discharge (**Figure 82-4**). A chlamydia and gonorrhea test should always be done in sexually active females with a vaginal discharge. Look closely at the cervix for discharge and signs of infection, dysplasia, or cancer (see **Figure 82-3**). Bimanual examination may show evidence of cervical, uterine, or adnexal tenderness. **Table 82-1** shows diagnostic values for examination of vaginitis.
- Vaginal pH testing can be helpful in the diagnosis of vaginitis. The pH can be checked by applying pH paper to the vaginal sidewall. Do not place the pH paper in contact with the cervical mucus, blood, or semen as these may distort the results. A pH above 4.5 is seen with menopausal patients, trichomonas infection, or bacterial vaginosis. Vaginal pH may be altered (usually elevated) by contamination with lubricating gels, semen, douches, amniotic fluid and intravaginal medications.
- Wet preps are obtained by applying a cotton-tipped applicator to the vaginal sidewall and placing the sample into normal saline. A drop of the suspension is then placed on a slide and examined microscopically for the presence and number of white blood cells (WBCs), trichomonads, candidal hyphae, or clue cells (**Figure 82-1**).
- A KOH prep is made by adding a drop of potassium hydroxide (KOH) solution to a drop of saline suspension of the discharge. The KOH lyses epithelial cells in 5 to 15 minutes (faster if the slide is warmed briefly) and allows easier visualization of yeasts. The use of KOH with dimethyl sulfoxide (DMSO) allows for quicker lyses of the epithelial cells and immediate examination of the smear.

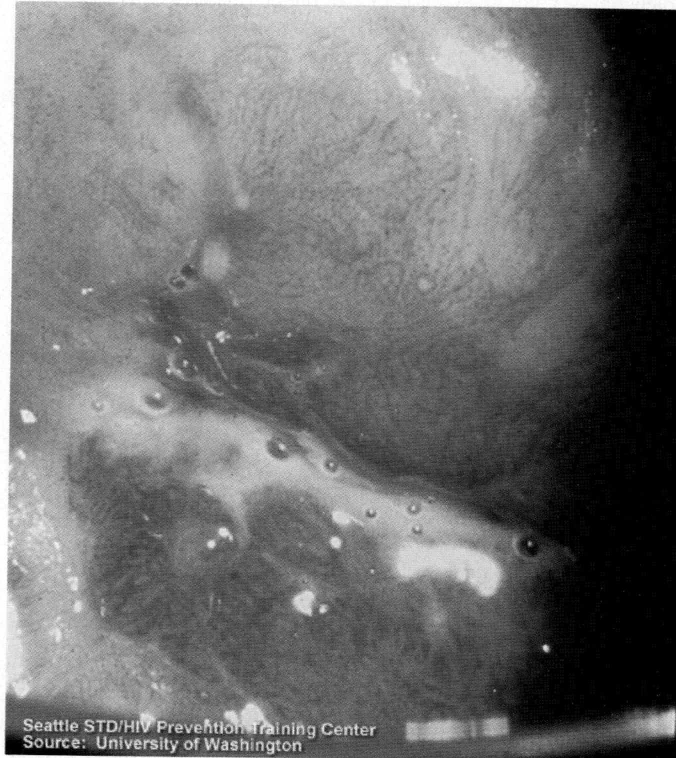

FIGURE 82-3 Colposcopic view of the cervix in a patient infected with *Trichomonas vaginalis*. Note the frothy discharge with visible bubbles and the cervical erythema. (*Reproduced with permission from Seattle STD/HIV Prevention Training Center, University of Washington.*)

TABLE 82-1 Diagnostic Values for Vaginal Infections

Diagnostic Criteria	Normal	Bacterial Vaginosis	*Trichomonas* Vaginitis	*Candida* Vulvovaginitis
Vaginal pH	3.8 to 4.2	>4.5	4.5	<4.5 (usually)
Discharge	White, thin, flocculent	Thin, white, gray	Yellow, green, or gray, frothy	White, curdy, "cottage cheese"
Amine odor "whiff" test	Absent	Fishy	Fishy	Absent
Microscopic	Lactobacilli, epithelial cells	Clue cells, adherent cocci, no white blood cells	Trichomonads, white blood cells >10/hpf	Budding yeast, hyphae, pseudohyphae

Abbreviations: hpf, high-power field.
Reproduced with permission from E.J. Mayeaux, Jr., MD.

- Another diagnostic procedure is the "whiff" test, which is performed by placing a drop of KOH on a slide of the wet prep and smelling for a foul, fishy odor. The odor is indicative of anaerobic overgrowth or infection. The "whiff" test is positive if the fishy amine odor is detected during the exam, and it is then not necessary to add KOH and "whiff" again.

LABORATORY TESTING

- Cultures for *Candida* species or *Trichomonas vaginalis* may be performed. Nucleic acid amplification tests are highly sensitive tests for *Neisseria gonorrhoeae*, *Chlamydia*, and *Chlamydia trachomatis* that can be performed on genital specimens or urine. Urine screening for gonorrhea, chlamydia, or both using nucleic acid amplification tests (NAATs) can be applied successfully in difficult-to-reach adolescents.[8] NAATs are also available for trichomoniasis, *Gardnerella*, *Candida*, and *Mycoplasma genitalium*.

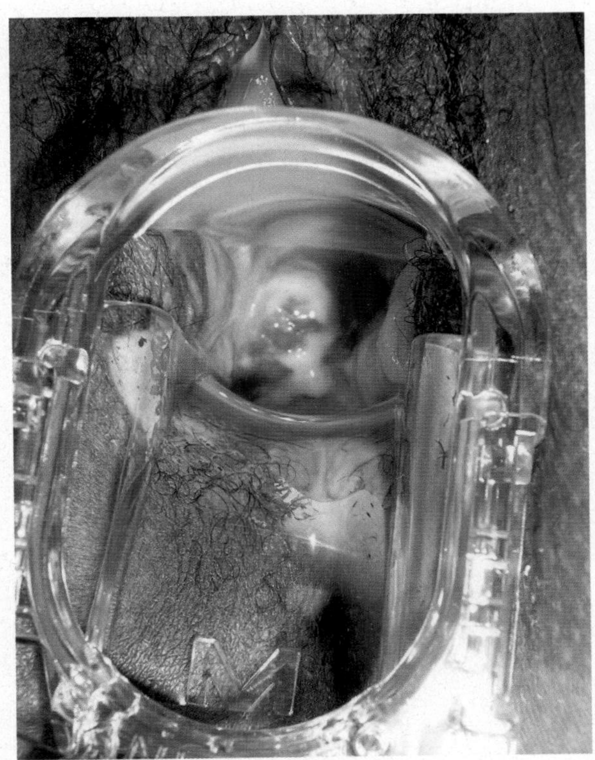

FIGURE 82-4 Speculum exam showing mucopurulent discharge with a friable-appearing cervix. (*Reproduced with permission from Richard P. Usatine, MD.*)

MANAGEMENT

- Management is based on the identification of the causative agent.
- Treatment for physiologic leukorrhea is unnecessary.
- Management of vaginal irritants and allergens involves identifying and eliminating the offending agents. However, irritants and allergens can often be difficult to identify.
- Health food store lactobacilli are the wrong strain and do not adhere well to the vaginal epithelium. Ingestion of live-culture, nonpasteurized yogurt does not significantly change the incidence of candidal vulvovaginitis or bacterial vaginosis.[9]

PATIENT RESOURCES

- Centers for Disease Control and Prevention. *Sexually Transmitted Diseases* page—**http://www.cdc.gov/std/.**
- Planned Parenthood. *Vaginitis.*—**https://www.plannedparenthood.org/learn/health-and-wellness/vaginitis.**
- Illinois Department of Public Health. *Vaginitis*—**www.idph.state.il.us/public/hb/hbvaginitis.htm.**

PROVIDER RESOURCES

- Centers for Disease Control and Prevention. *Sexually Transmitted Diseases Treatment Guidelines, 2010*—**http://www.cdc.gov/std/treatment/2010/STD-Treatment-2010-RR5912.pdf.**
- Centers for Disease Control and Prevention. *Self-Study STD Module—Vaginitis*—**https://www2a.cdc.gov/stdtraining/self-study/vaginitis/.**
- Centers for Disease Control and Prevention. *Vaginitis slides*—**https://www.cdc.gov/std/ready-to-use/vaginitis/vaginitis-slides-2013.pdf.**
- eMedicine—**http://emedicine.medscape.com/article/257141-overview.**
- American Family Physician—**https://www.aafp.org/afp/2018/0301/p321.html.**

REFERENCES

1. Centers for Disease Control and Prevention. *Sexually Transmitted Disease Surveillance 2001*. Atlanta, GA: U.S. Department of Health and Human Services, CDC, 2002.
2. Sobel JD. Vulvovaginitis in healthy women. *Compr Ther.* 1999; 25:335-346.
3. Anderson M, Karasz A, Friedland S. Are vaginal symptoms ever normal? A review of the literature. *MedGenMed.* 2004;6:49.
4. Zhang J, Thomas AG, Leybovich E. Vaginal douching and adverse health effects: a meta-analysis. *Am J Public Health.* 1997;87: 1207-1211.
5. Hassan S, Chatwani A, Brovender H, et al. Douching for perceived vaginal odor with no infectious cause of vaginitis: a randomized controlled trial. *J Low Genit Tract Dis.* 2011;15(2):128-133.
6. Zhang J, Hatch M, Zhang D, et al. Frequency of douching and risk of bacterial vaginosis in African-American women. *Obstet Gynecol.* 2004;104(4):756-760.
7. Sobel JD. Vaginitis. *N Engl J Med.* 1997;337:1896-1903.
8. Monroe KW, Weiss HL, Jones M, Hook EW 3rd. Acceptability of urine screening for *Neisseria gonorrhoeae* and *Chlamydia trachomatis* in adolescents at an urban emergency department. *Sex Transm Dis.* 2003;30:850-853.
9. Pirotta M, Gunn J, Chondros P, et al. Effect of lactobacillus in preventing post-antibiotic vulvovaginal candidiasis: a randomised controlled trial. *BMJ.* 2004;329:548.

83 ATROPHIC VAGINITIS

Frank Aguirre, MD
E.J. Mayeaux, Jr., MD

PATIENT STORY

A 60-year-old woman with vaginal dryness and irritation is seen to follow up on an inflammatory Pap smear. She denies discharge, odor, douching, and sexually transmitted disease (STD) exposure. She does admit to some postcoital bleeding. Her cervix has atrophic changes and an endocervical polyp (**Figure 83-1**). The polyp was removed easily with a ring forceps, and no dysplasia was found on pathology.

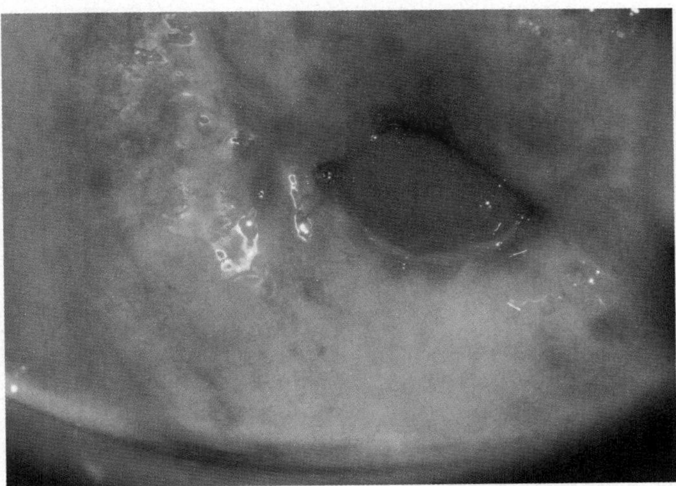

FIGURE 83-1 Colposcopic photograph (scanning objective with 10× eyepiece) demonstrating atrophic vaginitis. Note thinned white epithelium, friable epithelium with bleeding, and a cervical polyp. *(Reproduced with permission from E.J. Mayeaux, Jr., MD.)*

INTRODUCTION

Vaginal atrophy caused by estrogen deficiency is common and usually is asymptomatic. It can, however, be the etiology of such problems as recurrent urinary tract infections, vaginal dryness, dyspareunia, postcoital spotting, or recurrent bacterial vaginosis.

SYNONYMS

Vaginal atrophy, vulvovaginal atrophy, urogenital atrophy, senile vaginitis.

EPIDEMIOLOGY

- The average age of menopause is 51 years in the United States.
- Approximately 5% of women experience menopause after age 55 years (late menopause), and another 5% experience the transition between the ages of 40 and 45 years (early menopause). This means that in the United States, most women will live a significant portion of their lives during menopause. In addition, women who undergo surgical menopause will experience these symptoms at a typically younger age. To a lesser extent, women who undergo ovarian suppression without estrogen supplementation (progestin-only contraceptives) are susceptible to atrophic changes in their lower genital tract.
- Vaginal dryness occurs in approximately 3% of women of reproductive age, 4% to 21% of women in the menopausal transition, and 47% of women 3 years postmenopause.[1] Internationally, 39% of women experience menopause-related vaginal discomfort.[2]

ETIOLOGY AND PATHOPHYSIOLOGY

- Prior to menopause, estrogen stimulates vaginal epithelial cells to produce glycogen, which is then released into the vagina and converted to glucose. This supports vaginal flora that includes *Lactobacillus*, which converts it to lactic acid and decreases the vaginal pH to the 3.5–4.5 typically seen in vaginal secretions.[3] After menopause, circulating estrogen levels dramatically decrease to a level at least one-sixth their premenopausal levels.[4] Changes that occur in the vaginal and cervical epithelium include proliferation of connective tissue, loss of elastin, thinning of the epithelium (**Figure 83-2**), and hyalinization of collagen.

- The age of onset of menopause appears to be predominantly genetic but seems to be lowered by smoking and malnutrition and increased by body mass index (BMI) and increasing parity.[5]
- A long-term decrease in estrogen is generally necessary before symptoms become apparent. Genital symptoms include decreased vaginal lubrication, dryness, burning, dyspareunia, leukorrhea, itching, and yellow malodorous discharge.
- Urinary symptoms, such as frequency, hematuria, urinary tract infection, dysuria, and stress incontinence, are usually late symptoms. Over time, the lack of vaginal lubrication and vaginal elasticity often results in sexual dysfunction.
- Cervical polyps (see **Figure 83-1**) are pedunculated tumors that usually arise from the endocervical canal mucosa and are common in patients with atrophic vaginitis. Many will show squamous metaplasia, and they may develop squamous dysplasia. Polyps are most commonly asymptomatic unless they bleed.
- Menopause is the most common cause of atrophic vaginitis. In premenopausal women, radiation therapy, chemotherapy, immunologic disorders, and bilateral oophorectomy may greatly decrease production of ovarian estrogen and lead to atrophic vaginitis. While lactation can influence vaginal dryness, it is unusual for it to cause the severe symptoms of vaginal atrophy. Anti-estrogen medications such as tamoxifen may also result in atrophic vaginitis. Women who are naturally estrogen deficient prior to menopause, smoke cigarettes, or have not given vaginal birth tend to have more severe symptoms.[4]

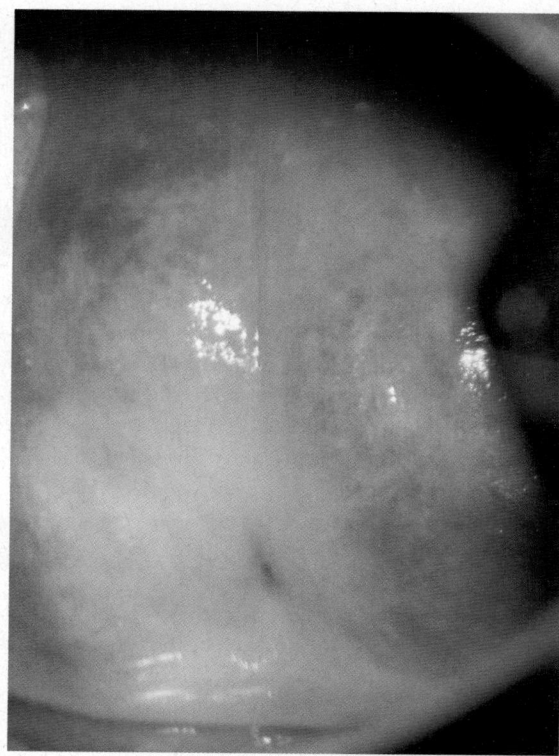

FIGURE 83-2 Colposcopic photograph (scanning objective with 10× eyepiece) demonstrating atrophic cervicovaginitis. Note thin white epithelium, relative dryness, and a barely visible cervical os. *(Reproduced with permission from E.J. Mayeaux, Jr., MD.)*

RISK FACTORS

- Age.
- Family history of early menopause.
- Bilateral oophorectomy.
- Spontaneous premature ovarian failure.
- Antiestrogenic medications effects, such as tamoxifen, danazol, medroxyprogesterone acetate.
- Gonadotropin-releasing hormone agonists (leuprolide, nafarelin, goserelin), or antagonists (ganirelix).
- Prolactin elevation as a result of hypothalamic-pituitary disorders with secondary reduction of estrogen secretion. This includes breastfeeding, although the effect is usually not as severe as in menopause.
- Certain chemotherapeutic agents.
- Pelvic radiation therapy.
- Severe systemic lupus erythematosus or rheumatoid arthritis (because of hypothalamic hypogonadism or primary ovarian insufficiency) combined with glucocorticoid therapy cause combined suppression of ovarian and adrenal activity.

DIAGNOSIS

CLINICAL FEATURES

- Diagnosis is primarily clinical, based on characteristic symptoms and findings. When quantification of atrophy and relative metrics are needed, a vaginal maturation index has been used.[6] Many women with symptoms of vaginal atrophy do not discuss their condition with a healthcare provider because they believe their symptoms are a normal part of the aging process.[7]
- Atrophic vaginal and cervical epithelium appears pale, smooth, relatively dry, and shiny (see **Figure 83-2**). Inflammation with patchy erythema, petechiae, and friability is common in more advanced cases. Elevated pH (greater than 5) of vaginal fluid is common. The external genitalia may demonstrate diminished elasticity, turgor of skin, sparsely distributed pubic hair, dryness of labia, erythema (**Figure 83-3**), and fusion of the labia minora.[8]

LABORATORY TESTING

- Laboratory tests to confirm hypoestrogenic findings are typically not necessary.
- Serum estradiol levels of less than 20 pg/mL support a clinical diagnosis of a low-estrogenic state. However, values are very laboratory dependent and most assays are not sufficiently sensitive or reliable for diagnosis of hypoestrogenic states without clinical signs and symptoms.
- Because of significant perimenopausal variability, there is no isolated serum follicle-stimulating hormone (FSH) level that is diagnostic of menopause. A clinical diagnosis of menopause is only supported with persistent amenorrhea. Evaluations of FSH variations, even for the same patient, do not necessarily remain elevated or increase with time following the "actual" final menstrual event. As a result, FSH levels greater than 40 mIU/mL need to be interpreted cautiously. Serum testing becomes significantly less variable >2 years after menopause.[9,10] The steady-state FSH level for a given patient is markedly influenced by BMI.[11]
- A Papanicolaou smear can confirm the presence of urogenital atrophy. Cytologic examination of smears from the upper one-third of the vagina shows an increased proportion of parabasal cells and a decreased percentage of superficial cells.
- An elevated vaginal pH level (>5), monitored by a pH strip in the vaginal vault, is commonly seen with vaginal atrophy.[4]

IMAGING

- Testing for associated osteoporosis should be considered if not previously performed.

DIFFERENTIAL DIAGNOSIS

- Atrophic vaginitis symptoms can be mimicked or exacerbated by co-infection of candidiasis, trichomoniasis, or bacterial vaginosis. These can be identified by wet prep, pH, and whiff test (see Chapter 84, Bacterial Vaginosis).
- Sexually transmitted diseases, including gonorrhea, trichomonas, and chlamydia, also may coexist with or mimic atrophic vaginitis.

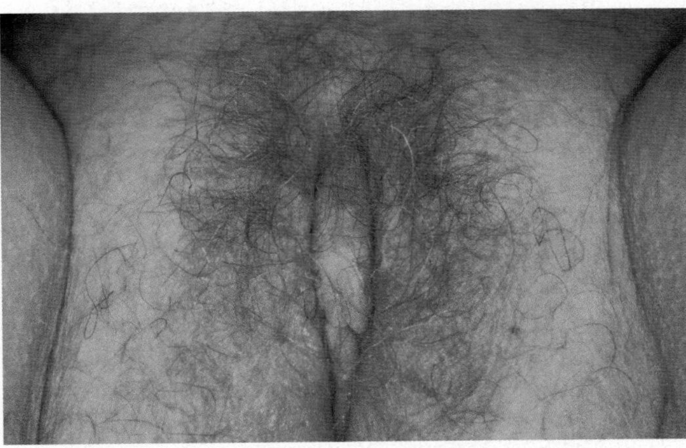

FIGURE 83-3 The vulva of a postmenopausal woman demonstrating thinning of the hair and thinning and erythema of vulvar skin associated with atrophic vulvitis. (*Reproduced with permission from Gordon Davis, MD, Arizona Vulva Clinic, Inc.*)

Cultures or nucleic acid amplification tests can identify these infections. It is important not to assume a diagnosis of solely atrophic vaginitis in the postmenopausal patient who presents with urogenital complaints (see Chapter 82, Overview of Vaginitis).

- Contact dermatitis because of environmental agents (e.g., perfumes, deodorants, soaps, panty liners, perineal pads, spermicides, lubricants, or tight fitting/synthetic clothing) may cause erythema, itching, burning, or pain (see Chapter 152, Contact Dermatitis).
- Vulvovaginal lichen planus, which may produce labial fusion (see Chapter 160, Lichen Planus).
- Lichen sclerosus et atrophicus (LSEA) does produce atrophy of the vulva and can be mistaken for the atrophy of estrogen deficiency. It can be recognized by the hourglass configuration of the atrophy around the vulva and perianal region (**Figure 83-4**) and is usually confirmed with biopsy. LSEA is treated with a high-potency steroid ointment rather than estrogen.

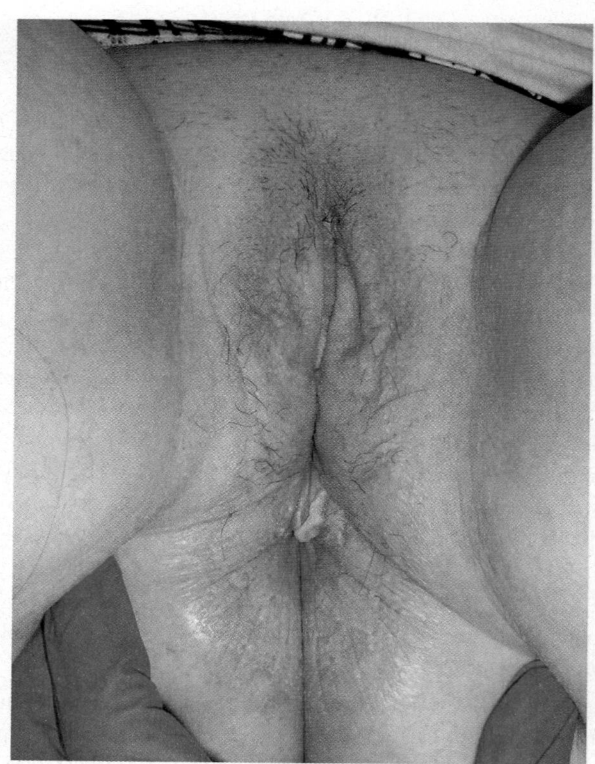

FIGURE 83-4 Lichen sclerosus with atrophy of the vulva in this 53-year-old woman. Lichen sclerosus can be recognized by the hourglass configuration of the atrophy around the vulva and perianal region. (*Reproduced with permission from Richard P. Usatine, MD.*)

MANAGEMENT

FIRST LINE

Per the North American Menopause Society (NAMS) and the American College of Obstetricians and Gynecologists (ACOG), first-line treatment of vaginal dryness and dyspareunia includes nonpharmacologic approaches of vaginal moisturizers and lubricants detailed below.[12,13] Pharmacologic estrogen-based approaches have additional advantages but also may have other systemic risks that may exclude certain patient populations. As a further note, patients who smoke will likely have worsened symptoms, as cigarettes further worsen the degree of estrogen deficiency.[14] SOR Ⓐ

NONPHARMACOLOGIC

- Nonhormonal vaginal treatments have been shown to be helpful for treatment of symptoms of vaginal dryness and dyspareunia. The treatments are divided into local vaginal moisturizers and lubricants. Vaginal lubricants (**Table 83-1**) are intended to be used for short-term lubrication usually related to facilitating sexual activity. In contrast, vaginal moisturizers (**Table 83-2**) are designed to be absorbed into the skin and bind to the vaginal epithelium. The moisturizer components are intended to increase local moisture content and decrease pH so as to address more chronic complaints of vaginal dryness. As a result, moisturizers are applied regularly, and their effects can last 2–4 days. Some patients may choose to use both a regular moisturizer and a lubricant to maintain comfort during intercourse. Sexual activity has been shown to encourage vaginal elasticity and pliability, especially in the presence of a lubricative response to sexual stimulation. Other evaluations comparing relative degrees of effectiveness can be found in review article by Sinha and Ewies.[15] One open-label study indicated that Replens, a bioadhesive vaginal moisturizer, was a safe and effective alternative to estrogen vaginal cream, with both therapies exhibiting statistically significant increases in vaginal moisture, vaginal fluid volume, and vaginal elasticity.[16] SOR Ⓐ
- Vaginal lubricants can be divided into water-based, silicon-based, and oil-based options. The water-based options are popular because

TABLE 83-1 Nonprescription Vaginal Lubricants (Partial List)

Product	Components	Osmolality
Vaginal Lubricants (a Sampling of Water-Based Options)		
Femglide	Water, polyoxyethylene, methylparaben, and sodium carbomer	Hypo-osmotic (32 mOsm/kg)
Pre-Seed	Water, hydroxyethylcellulose (HEC), Pluronic 127, sodium chloride, arabinogalactan, sodium phosphate, carbomer, methylparaben, sodium hydroxide, and potassium phosphate	Iso-osmotic (314 mOsm/kg)
KY-Jelly	Water, chlorhexidine gluconate, hydroxyethyl cellulose, gluconodeltalactone, glycerin, methylparaben, and sodium hydroxide	Moderately hyper-osmotic (2463 mOsm/kg)
Astroglide	Water, glycerin, propylene glycol, polyquaternium 15, methylparaben, and propylparaben	Hyper-osmotic (5848 mOsm/kg)
Vaginal Lubricants (a Few Examples of Silicon-Based Options)		
ID Millennium	Cyclomethicone, dimethicone, and dimethiconol	N/A
Pjur Eros	Cyclopentasiloxane, dimethicone, and dimethiconol	N/A
Pink	Dimethicone, vitamin E, aloe vera, dimethiconol, and cyclomethicone	N/A
Vaginal Lubricants (Common Oil-Based Examples)		
Coconut oil	Can use regular cooking grade coconut oil. Has antifungal properties. Easier clean-up.	Solid at room temperature, liquid at body temperature
Almond oil	Recommend "sweet" almond oil	Avoid for those with almond allergies
Olive oil	Pure olive oil or refined olive oil has improved lubrication over extra virgin oil.	May be harder to clean up, some report "spicy" sensation

TABLE 83-2 Non-prescription Vaginal Moisturizers (Partial List)

Product	Components	Directions for Use
Vaginal Moisturizers		
Bio-adhesive polycarbophil-based gel (Replens)	Purified water, glycerin, mineral oil, polycarbophil, carbopol 974P, hydrogenated palm oil, glyceride, and sorbic acid	One application (2.5 g) three times per week for an initial period of 3 months and then every 3 days or as needed.
Water based Natural ingredients (Emerita)	Purified water, glycerin, pentyleneglycol, hydroxyl ethyl cellulose, sorbitol, xylitol, *Aloe barbadensis* (aloe vera) leaf juice, tocopheryl acetate (vitamin E), retinylpalmitate, *Calendula officinalis* (calendula) flower extract, *Chamomile larecutita* (matricaria) extract, *Panax* ginseng root extract, allantoin, squalane, sodium hydroxyl methylglycinate, disodium EDTA, citric acid	Apply daily or as needed.
Bi-polymer bioadhesive gel (RepHresh)	Purified water USP, glycerin, polycarbophil, carbomer 934P, ethylparaben sodium, methylparaben sodium, propylparaben sodium, sodium hydroxide.	Apply once every 3 days or less frequently, as needed.
Hyaluronic acid based (Hyalo GYN and Hyalo-femme, and Repadina)	Hyaluronic acid derivative (see specific product labels for detailed ingredients)	Apply once every 3 days for 30 days and then apply as needed.

they are easy to clean up and do not stain clothing. Patient preference for the various options can be guided by three issues. The first relates to whether the product has glycerin. For patients with a tendency toward yeast infections, a glycerin-based lubricant should be avoided. The second is that vaginal irritation can be increased with lubricants with higher osmolarity.[17] The third is that one of the listed lubricants (KY-Jelly) contains a microbicide. It is unknown to what degree this might impact the vaginal flora for specific patients. For a partial list of options for water-based vaginal lubricants, see **Table 83-1**.

- Silicone-based lubricants tend to last longer, are not absorbed by the skin, and decrease friction well, but are also more difficult to clean up as they do not dissolve in water. As a result, they require soap for full external cleanup.
- Among the simplest and most accessible options for most patients are the natural oil-based lubricants such as coconut oil, olive oil, or almond oil (see **Table 83-1**). Contact dermatitis can be an issue with any of these oils or other products.
- Water-based and silicone-based vaginal lubricants are compatible with latex condom use. Oil-based lubricants are not and may damage latex-based condoms. Silicon-based lubricants are not compatible with silicon-based sex toys.

SECOND LINE

- Estrogen replacement therapy relieves menopausal symptoms, including atrophic vaginitis.[18] SOR Ⓐ Routes of administration include oral, transdermal, and intravaginal. Risks associated with estrogen use include stroke and venous thromboembolism. For women who still have their uterus, the additional estrogen-increased risk of endometrial hyperplasia or malignancy is usually mitigated with the addition of progestin medications. This addition carries further risks of breast cancer depending on the progestin type. Further risks of coronary heart disease with combined hormonal treatment may also be dependent on progestin type. Progesterone has not been found to increase either the risk of occurrence of breast cancer or the risk of coronary heart disease among the general population and hence is preferred.[19,20] Risks of complications are least for the intravaginal route and then increase for transdermal systemic treatments, and are highest for oral routes. Relief of systemic symptoms is usually minimal with intravaginal estrogen supplementation.
- A Cochrane review found that estrogen creams, pessaries, vaginal tablets, and the estradiol vaginal ring appeared to be equally effective for the symptoms of vaginal atrophy.[18] SOR Ⓐ One trial found significant side effects following conjugated equine estrogen cream administration when compared to tablets, causing uterine bleeding, breast pain, and perineal pain. Another trial found significant endometrial overstimulation following use of the conjugated equine estrogen cream when compared to the estrogen vaginal ring. Women appeared to favor the estradiol-releasing vaginal ring for ease of use, comfort of product, and overall satisfaction.[18] SOR Ⓐ This variation in adverse effects between methods is thought to be primarily due to inevitable variation in absorbed dosages between patients. Applied creams are fundamentally less precise in terms of delivery of estrogen. Good data show that more reliable doses and reduced adverse effects are achieved with either the vaginal tablet or vaginal ring methods of topical estrogen delivery.
- The amount of estrogen and the duration of time required to eliminate symptoms depend on the degree of vaginal atrophy and vary among patients. Progestin therapy should be considered in any woman with an intact uterus to avoid causing endometrial hyperplasia or cancer. When oral estrogen is used at typical doses, atrophic symptoms will persist in 10% to 25% of patients.[21]
- Topical administration of estrogen is an excellent focal treatment for genitourinary symptoms of atrophy. Exposure of other organs can be minimized if low doses of topical vaginal estrogens are used. Studies suggest that absorption rates with vaginal topical therapy either stay the same or decrease with treatment duration because the initially thinned atrophic vaginal mucosa, which is initially a minimal barrier to entry into systemic circulation, may become a greater barrier as it thickens with treatment.[22]
- Vaginal estrogen therapy available in the United States are conjugated estrogens cream (0.625 mg conjugated estrogens/g, 0.5 g of cream intravaginally twice weekly) and estradiol cream (100 mcg estradiol/g of cream, 1 g of cream intravaginally administered daily for 2 weeks, then decreased to 0.3 g of cream 1 to 3 times per week), tablet (10 mcg estradiol/tablet intravaginally daily for 2 weeks then twice weekly), and ring (0.5 mcg estradiol/day, released over 90 days). Estriol, an estrogen analog, is also available in a vaginal cream through compounding pharmacies and more generally in Europe and some other countries. Estriol has relatively lower estrogen agonist strength per gram than estradiol.
- Vaginal estrogen therapy results in some estrogen absorption into the circulation, although to a lesser degree than oral or transdermal estrogen treatment. In one study, systemic absorption was 30% lower in a study of vaginal versus conjugated estrogen therapy.[23] SOR Ⓑ
- Progestin therapy may not be necessary to protect against endometrial hyperplasia in women treated with the low-dose ring or intravaginal tablet when used as approved. The systemic estrogen absorption with use of the vaginal creams is difficult to quantify, so many experts recommend use of an opposing progestin for women treated chronically with vaginal estrogen cream.[24] SOR Ⓒ If progestin therapy is elected, oral micronized progesterone can be used in a continuous manner (100 mg nightly because of sedative effects).

FOLLOW-UP

- Follow-up is needed for all patients placed on estrogen therapy to monitor for estrogen-related side effects and to ensure against overuse. Otherwise, follow-up can be as needed.

PATIENT EDUCATION

- Discuss the risks and benefits of estrogen replacement therapy with patients interested in the use of estrogens. Vaginal moisturizers and lubricants (nonprescription) may safely help prevent vaginal dryness as well as pain during intercourse.

PATIENT RESOURCES

- MedlinePlus. *Atrophic Vaginitis*—**www.nlm.nih.gov/medlineplus/ency/article/000892.htm.**
- Harvard Medical School. *Atrophic Vaginitis*—**http://www.health.harvard.edu/womens-health/vaginal-atrophy-atrophic-vaginitis.**

PROVIDER RESOURCES

- eMedicine. *Vaginitis*—**http://emedicine.medscape.com/article/257141.**
- eMedicine. *Vulvovaginitis*—**http://emedicine.medscape.com/article/797497.**
- Bachmann GA, Nevadunsky NS. Diagnosis and treatment of atrophic vaginitis. *Am Fam Physician.* 2000;61(10):3090-3096.—**http://www.aafp.org/afp/2000/0515/p3090.html.**

REFERENCES

1. Dennerstein L, Dudley EC, Hopper JL, et al. A prospective population-based study of menopausal symptoms. *Obstet Gynecol.* 2000;96:351.
2. Nappi RE, Kokot-Kierepa M. Women's voices in the menopause: results from an international survey on vaginal atrophy. *Maturitas.* 2010;67:233.
3. Stika CS. Atrophic vaginitis. *Dermatol Ther.* 2010;23(5):514-522.
4. Pandit L, Ouslander JG. Postmenopausal vaginal atrophy and atrophic vaginitis. *Am J Med Sci.* 1997;314:228-231.
5. de Bruin JP, Bovenhuis H, van Noord PA, et al. The role of genetic factors in age at natural menopause. *Hum Reprod.* 2001;16:2014-2018.
6. Greendale GA, Zibecchi L, Petersen L, et al. Development and validation of a physical examination scale to assess vaginal atrophy and inflammation. *Climacteric.* 1999;2:197-204.
7. Bachmann GA, Nevadunsky NS. Diagnosis and treatment of atrophic vaginitis. *Am Fam Physician.* 2000;61:3090.
8. Johnston SL, Farrell SA, Bouchard C, et al. The detection and management of vaginal atrophy. *J Obstet Gynaecol Can.* 2004;26:503.
9. Burger HG, Dudley EC, Hopper JL, et al. Prospectively measured levels of serum follicle-stimulating hormone, estradiol, and the dimeric inhibins during the menopausal transition in a population-based cohort of women. *J Clin Endocrinol Metab.* 1999;84:11:4025-4030.
10. Randolph J Jr, Zheng H, Sowers MR, et al. Change in follicle-stimulating hormone and estradiol across the menopausal transition: effect of age at the final menstrual period. *J Clin Endocrinol Metab.* 2011;96(3):746-754.
11. Freeman EW, Sammel MD, Lin H, Gracia CR. Obesity and reproductive hormone levels in the transition to menopause. *Menopause.* 2010;17(4):718-726.
12. Management of symptomatic vulvovaginal atrophy: 2013 position statement of The North American Menopause Society. *Menopause.* 2013;20(9):888-902.
13. ACOG Practice Bulletin No. 141: Management of menopausal symptoms. *Obstet Gynecol.* 2014;123:202-216.
14. Tansavatdi K, McClain B, Herrington DM. The effects of smoking on estradiol metabolism. *Minerva Ginecol.* 2004;56:105.
15. Sinha A, Ewies AA. Non-hormonal topical treatment of vulvovaginal atrophy: an up-to-date overview. *Climacteric.* 2013;16(3):305-312.
16. Nachtigall LE. Comparative study: Replens versus local estrogen in menopausal women. *Fertil Steril.* 1994;61:178.
17. Adriaens E, Remon JP. Mucosal irritation potential of personal lubricants relates to product osmolality as detected by the slug mucosal irritation assay. *Sex Transm Dis.* 2008;35(5):512-516.
18. Lethaby A, Ayeleke RO, Roberts H. Local oestrogen for vaginal atrophy in postmenopausal women. *Cochrane Database Syst Rev.* 2016;(8): CD001500.
19. L'Hermite M. HRT optimization, using transdermal estradiol plus micronized progesterone, a safer HRT. Climacteric. 2013 Aug; 16 Suppl 1:44-53.
20. Asi N, Mohammed K, Haydour Q, et al. Progesterone vs. synthetic progestins and the risk of breast cancer: a systematic review and meta-analysis. *Syst Rev.* 2016;5:121.
21. Smith P, Heimer G, Lindskog M, Ulmsten U. Oestradiol-releasing vaginal ring for treatment of postmenopausal urogenital atrophy. *Maturitas.* 1993;16:145-154.
22. Santen RJ. Vaginal administration of estradiol: effects of dose, preparation and timing on plasma estradiol levels. *Climacteric.* 2015;18(2):121-134.
23. Dorr MB, Nelson AL, Mayer PR, et al. Plasma estrogen concentrations after oral and vaginal estrogen administration in women with atrophic vaginitis. *Fertil Steril.* 2010;94:2365.
24. Bachmann G, Bouchard C, Hoppe D, et al. Efficacy and safety of low-dose regimens of conjugated estrogens cream administered vaginally. *Menopause.* 2009;16:719.

84 BACTERIAL VAGINOSIS

E.J. Mayeaux, Jr., MD
Richard P. Usatine, MD
Tammy J. Davis, MD
Candice Weiner-Johnson, MD

PATIENT STORY

A 31-year-old woman presents with a malodorous vaginal discharge for 3 weeks. There is no associated vaginal itching or pain. She is married and monogamous. She admits to douching about once per month to prevent odor but it is not working this time. On examination, her discharge is visible (**Figure 84-1**). It is thin and off-white. Wet prep examination shows that more than 50% of the epithelial cells are clue cells (**Figure 84-2**). The patient is diagnosed with bacterial vaginosis and treated with oral metronidazole 500 mg bid for 7 days with good results.

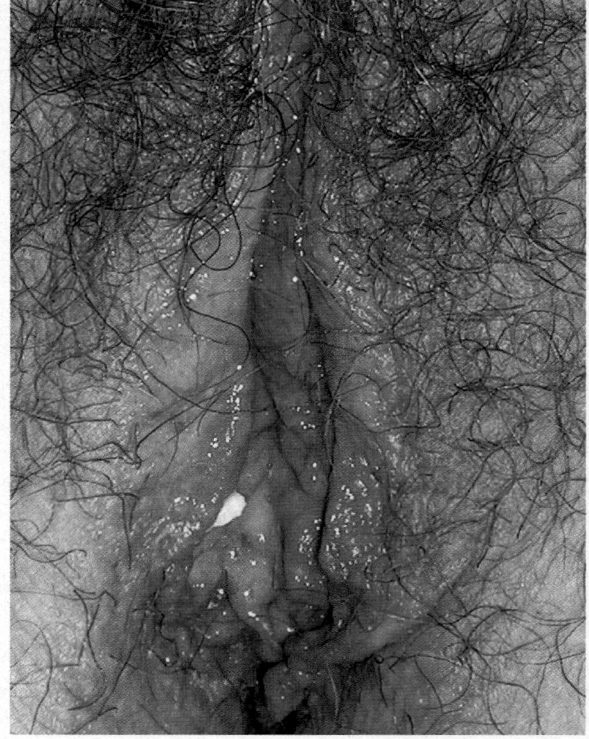

FIGURE 84-1 A 31-year-old woman with homogeneous, thin white malodorous vaginal discharge of bacterial vaginosis. (*Reproduced with permission from Richard P. Usatine, MD.*)

INTRODUCTION

Bacterial vaginosis (BV) is a clinical syndrome resulting from alteration of the vaginal ecosystem. It is called a vaginosis, not a vaginitis, because the tissues themselves are not actually infected, but only have superficial involvement. While it is the most common cause of vaginal discharge, bacterial vaginosis generally does not result in dyspareunia, dysuria, burning, pruritus, or vaginal inflammation on its own. Women with BV are at increased risk for the acquisition of HIV, *Neisseria gonorrhoeae*, *Chlamydia trachomatis*, and herpes simplex virus (HSV)-2, and they have increased risk of complications after gynecologic surgery.[1-4]

BV is associated with adverse pregnancy outcomes, including lower implantation rates,[5] premature rupture of membranes, preterm labor, preterm birth,[6] low birth weight,[3] intra-amniotic infection, late miscarriage,[6] postpartum fever, and postpartum endometritis. However, the only established benefit of BV therapy in pregnant women is the reduction of symptoms and signs of vaginal infection.[1,2]

SYNONYMS

- Vaginal bacteriosis.
- *Corynebacterium* vaginale vaginosis/vaginitis.
- *Gardnerella vaginalis* vaginosis.
- *Haemophilus vaginalis* vaginitis.
- Nonspecific vaginitis.
- Anaerobic vaginosis.

EPIDEMIOLOGY

- BV is estimated to be the most prevalent cause of vaginal discharge or malodor in women presenting for care in the United States, causing 40% to 50% of vaginal discharge cases in women of childbearing age.[6] However, more than 50% of women with BV are asymptomatic.[1,2] BV accounts for more than 10 million outpatient visits per year.[4] The worldwide prevalence is estimated at 29% of women 14–49 years of age and in half of African-American women.[7]

ETIOLOGY AND PATHOPHYSIOLOGY

- Hydrogen peroxide–producing *Lactobacillus* is the most common organism composing normal vaginal flora.[1,2] In BV, normal vaginal lactobacilli are replaced by high concentrations of anaerobic bacteria such as *Mobiluncus*, *Prevotella*, *Gardnerella*, *Bacteroides*, and *Mycoplasma* species.[1,2,4]
- The hydrogen peroxide produced by the *Lactobacillus* may help in inhibiting the growth of atypical flora.
- *Gardnerella* is not a part of the normal vaginal flora, as it is not present in all women or in prepubertal girls.[8] However, it has been present in nearly 100% of women diagnosed with BV.[7] Sexual transmission of *Gardnerella vaginalis* may be responsible for the initiation of BV. *Gardnerella* has the greatest capacity to adhere to epithelial cells and produce a biofilm that creates a scaffolding for normally dormant vaginal anaerobes to compete with *Lactobacillus*. A symbiotic relationship between *G. vaginalis* and ammonia-producing anaerobes leads to a more alkaline pH.[8,9] *Gardnerella* biofilms are capable of withstanding 5 times the concentration of hydrogen peroxide and 8 times the concentration of lactic acid than a planktonic culture.[10]
- The odor of BV is caused by the aromatic amines produced by the altered bacterial flora in the vagina. These aromatic amines include putrescine and cadaverine—aptly named to describe their unpleasant odor.

RISK FACTORS

- Multiple male or female partners.[1,2,11]
- A new sex partner.[1,2]
- Douching.[12]
- Lack of condom use.[1,2]
- Lack of vaginal lactobacilli.[1,2]
- Prior BV infection.[1,2]
- Cigarette smoking.[12,13]
- Lack of use of hormonal contraceptives.[3,14]

DIAGNOSIS

CLINICAL FEATURES

- Symptomatic patients present with an unpleasant, "fishy smelling" discharge that is more noticeable after coitus (the basic pH of seminal fluid is like doing the whiff test with KOH) or during menses.[5] There may be pruritus, but not as often as seen with *Candida* vaginitis. The physical examination should include inspection of the external genitalia for irritation or discharge. Speculum examination is done to determine the amount and character of the discharge. A nucleic acid amplification test for *N. gonorrhoeae*,

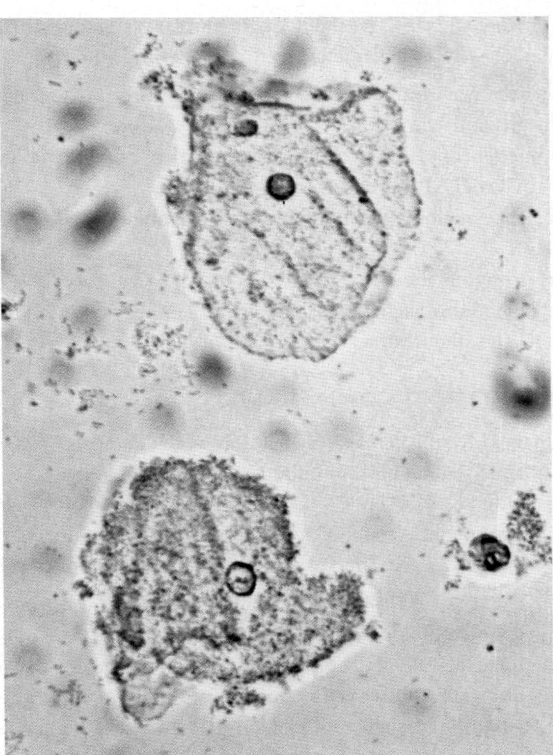

FIGURE 84-2 Clue cell and bacteria seen in bacterial vaginosis. The lower cell is a clue cell covered in bacteria while the upper cell is a normal epithelial cell. Light microscope under high power. (*Reproduced with permission from E.J. Mayeaux, Jr., MD.*)

Chlamydia, and/or *C. trachomatis* (or similar test) should be performed on genital specimens (urethral or cervical) or urine.

- BV is usually clinically diagnosed by finding three of the following four signs and symptoms:
  - Homogeneous, thin, white discharge that smoothly coats the vaginal walls (**Figures 84-3** and **84-4**).
  - Presence of clue cells on microscopic examination (see **Figure 84-2**).
  - pH of vaginal fluid >4.5.
  - A fishy odor of vaginal discharge before or after addition of 10% KOH (i.e., the whiff test).[1,2,15]

LABORATORY TESTING

- Vaginal pH testing can be very helpful in the diagnosis of vaginitis. The normal vaginal pH is usually 3.5 to 4.5. A pH above 4.5 is seen with menopausal patients, *Trichomonas* infection, or BV. A small piece of pH paper is touched to the vaginal discharge during the exam or on the speculum. Do not test a wet-prep sample if saline has been added because the saline alters the pH.
- Wet preps are obtained using a cotton-tipped applicator applied to the vaginal sidewall, placing the sample of discharge into normal saline (not water). Observe for clue cells, number of white blood cells, trichomonads, and candidal hyphae. Clue cells are squamous epithelial cells whose borders are obscured by attached bacteria. More than 20% to 25% of epithelial cells seen in BV should be clue cells (see **Figure 84-2**).
- A proline aminopeptidase test card (Pip Activity Test Card), a DNA probe-based test for high concentrations of *G. vaginalis* (Affirm VP III), and the OSOM BVBLUE test have shown acceptable performance characteristics compared with Gram stain (gold standard).[1,2] However, they are more costly than traditional testing without clear advantages.
- Although a test card is available for the detection of elevated pH and trimethylamine, it has low sensitivity and specificity and is not recommended by the Centers for Disease Control and Prevention (CDC).[1,2]
- Culture of *G. vaginalis* is not recommended as a diagnostic tool because it is not specific.
- Pap tests are not useful for the diagnosis of BV because of their low sensitivity.[1,2]

DIFFERENTIAL DIAGNOSIS

- *Trichomonas* also may have the odor of aromatic amines and, therefore, easily confused with BV at first glance. Look for the strawberry cervix on examination and moving trichomonads on the wet prep (see Chapter 86, *Trichomonas* Vaginitis).
- *Candida* vaginitis tends to present with a cottage-cheese–like discharge and vaginal itching (Chapter 85, *Candida* Vulvovaginitis).
- Gonorrhea and chlamydia should not be missed in patients with vaginal discharge. Consider testing for these sexually transmitted diseases (STDs) based on patients' risk factors and the presence of purulence clinically and white blood cells on the wet prep (see Chapter 87, *Chlamydia* Cervicitis).

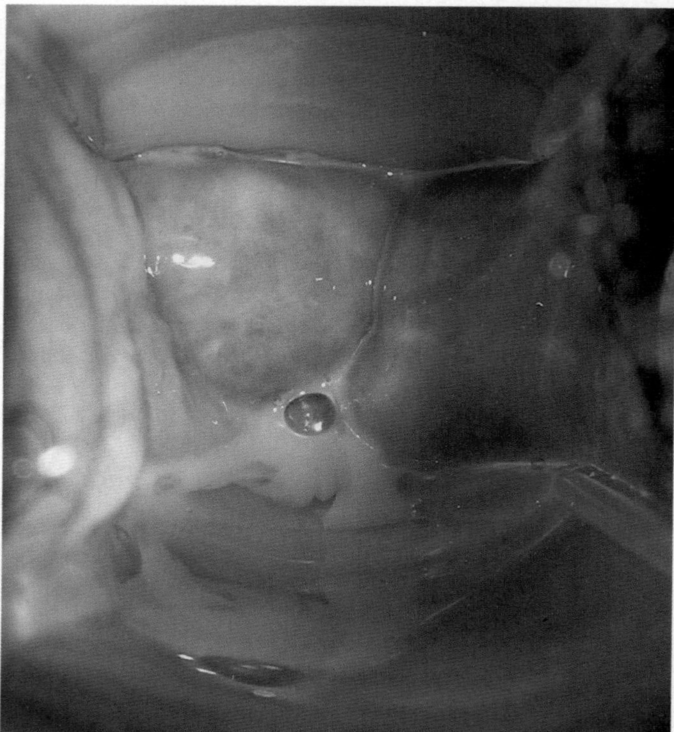

FIGURE 84-3 A homogeneous, off-white creamy malodorous discharge that adheres to the vaginal walls and pools in the vaginal vault in a woman with bacterial vaginosis. *(Reproduced with permission from Richard P. Usatine, MD.)*

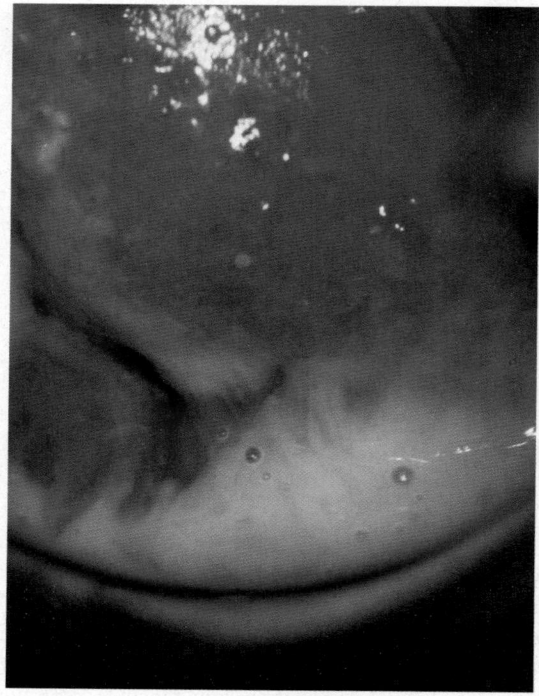

FIGURE 84-4 Close-up view of the cervix showing the white homogeneous discharge of bacterial vaginosis. Note the lack of clumping or "cottage-cheese" appearance usually found with *Candida* infections. *(Reproduced with permission from E.J. Mayeaux, Jr., MD.)*

MANAGEMENT

FIRST LINE

- Treatment is recommended for women with symptoms and women undergoing some gynecologic procedures.[15] SOR A
- Treatment of male sex partners has not been beneficial in preventing the recurrence of BV[2,16] SOR A; however, circumcision of male partners has shown to reduce recurrence.[3]
- Patients should avoid vaginal use of douching and antiseptic materials.[17] SOR C
- The established benefits of therapy for BV in nonpregnant women are to (a) relieve vaginal symptoms and signs of infection and (b) reduce the risk for infectious complications after abortion or hysterectomy.[1,2] SOR A Other potential benefits include a reduction in risk for receiving and transmitting sexually transmitted infections (STIs).[1,2,5,18] SOR B **Table 84-1** shows CDC-recommended treatments.
- Best practice guidelines recommend treatment with metronidazole 500 mg twice daily for 5–7 days.[15] SOR A Metronidazole 2 g single-dose therapy has the lowest efficacy for BV and is no longer a recommended or alternative regimen.[2] Metronidazole should not be taken with alcohol due to a disulfiram-like reaction.[15] Clindamycin cream is oil-based and might weaken latex condoms and diaphragms for 5 days after use. Topical clindamycin preparations should not be used in the second half of pregnancy.[1,2]
- The only established benefit of therapy for BV in pregnant women is to relieve vaginal symptoms and signs of infection.[1,2] SOR A Additional potential benefits of therapy include (a) reducing the risk for infectious complications associated with BV during pregnancy, (b) reducing the risk for other infections (e.g., other STDs or HIV), and (c) treating women with additional preterm labor risk factors before 20 weeks.[15] Multiple studies and meta-analyses have not demonstrated an association between metronidazole use during pregnancy and teratogenic or mutagenic effects in newborns.[1,2,19] SOR A Intravaginal clindamycin cream has been associated with adverse outcomes if used in the latter half of pregnancy.[1,2]

TABLE 84-1 CDC Recommended Regimens SOR A

Metronidazole 500 mg orally twice a day for 7 days
OR
Metronidazole gel 0.75%, 1 full applicator (5 g) intravaginally, once a day for 5 days
OR
Clindamycin cream 2%, 1 full applicator (5 g) intravaginally at bedtime for 7 days
CDC Alternative Regimens SOR A
Tinidazole 2 g orally once daily for 2 days
OR
Tinidazole 1 g orally once daily for 5 days
OR
Clindamycin 300 mg orally twice a day for 7 days
OR
Clindamycin ovules 100 mg intravaginally once at bedtime for 3 days
CDC Recommended Regimens for Pregnant Women SOR A
Metronidazole 500 mg orally twice a day for 7 days
OR
Metronidazole 250 mg orally three times a day for 7 days

Data from Centers for Disease Control and Prevention.[2]

SECOND LINE

- One randomized trial for persistent BV indicated that metronidazole gel 0.75% twice per week for 6 months after completion of a recommended regimen was effective in maintaining a clinical cure for 6 months.[20] SOR B
- Limited data suggest that oral nitroimidazole followed by intravaginal boric acid and suppressive metronidazole gel for those women in remission might be an option in women with recurrent BV.[3,4] SOR B
- Though it was once thought that cleaning sex toys between uses would help decrease transfer of BV between female partners, a small randomized trial demonstrated no reduction in BV persistence.[21]
- It is unnecessary to treat male sexual partners.[2]

COMPLEMENTARY AND ALTERNATIVE THERAPY

- Extended ingestion of live-culture, nonpasteurized yogurt may theoretically increase colonization by lactobacilli and decrease the episodes of BV.[5,22] SOR C However, health food store lactobacilli are the wrong strain and are not well retained by the vagina.
- The efficacy of exogenous lactobacillus recolonization with probiotic lactobacilli vaginal gelatin capsules has been reported in two small trials.[23,24]

PREVENTION

- Avoidance of risk factors is recommended, although asymptomatic BV is common.
- The evidence is insufficient to assess the impact of screening for BV in pregnant women at high risk for preterm delivery.[1,2]

FOLLOW-UP

- Follow-up visits are unnecessary in nonpregnant women if symptoms resolve.[1,2]
- Treatment of BV in asymptomatic pregnant women who are at high risk for preterm delivery might prevent adverse pregnancy outcomes. Therefore, a follow-up evaluation 1 month after completion of treatment should be considered to evaluate whether therapy was effective.[1,2] SOR C
- If symptoms do recur, consider a treatment regimen different from the original regimen to treat recurrent disease.[1,2] SOR C

PATIENT EDUCATION

- Avoid consuming alcohol during treatment with metronidazole and for 24 hours thereafter. Women should be advised to return for additional therapy if symptoms recur because recurrence of BV is up to 40% within 3 months of treatment and the long-term cure rate is low.[5,25,26]

PATIENT RESOURCES

- Centers for Disease Control and Prevention. *Bacterial Vaginosis Fact Sheet*—**http://www.cdc.gov/std/BV/STDFact-Bacterial-Vaginosis.htm.**
- Family Doctor.org from the AAFP—**https://familydoctor.org/condition/bacterial-vaginosis/.**
- MedicineNet.com—**http://www.medicinenet.com/bacterial_vaginosis/article.htm.**

PROVIDER RESOURCES

- Centers for Disease Control and Prevention. *2015 Sexually Transmitted Diseases Treatment Guidelines*—**https://www.cdc.gov/std/tg2015/.**

REFERENCES

1. Centers for Disease Control and Prevention. *Guidelines for Treatment of Sexually Transmitted Diseases*. https://www.cdc.gov/std/tg2015/default.htm. Accessed June 2018.
2. Centers for Disease Control and Prevention. *Guidelines for Treatment of Sexually Transmitted Diseases*. https://www.cdc.gov/std/tg2015/bv.htm. Accessed January 2017.
3. BMC Infectious Diseases. *Making inroads into improving treatment of bacterial vaginosis—striving for long-term cure.* https://bmcinfectdis.biomedcentral.com/articles/10.1186/s12879-015-1027-4. Accessed December 2016.
4. Reichman O, Akins R, Sobel JD. Boric acid addition to suppressive antimicrobial therapy for recurrent bacterial vaginosis. *Sex Transm Dis.* 2009;36:732-734.
5. Mastromarino P, Vitali B, Mosca L. Bacterial vaginosis: a review on clinical trials with probiotics. *New Microbiol.* 2013;36:229-238.
6. Cochrane library. *Antibiotics for Treating Bacterial Vaginosis in Pregnancy.* http://www.cochrane.org/CD000262/PREG_antibiotics-for-treating-bacterial-vaginosis-in-pregnancy. Accessed December 2016.
7. Allsworth JE, Peipert JF. Prevalence of bacterial vaginosis: 2001-2004 National Health and Nutrition Examination Survey data. *Obstet Gynecol.* 2007;109:113.
8. Schwebke J, Muzny C, Josey W. Role of *Gardnerella vaginalis* in the pathogenesis of bacterial vaginosis: a conceptual model. *J Infect Dis.* 2014;210:338-343.
9. Verstraelen H, Swidsinski A. The biofilm in bacterial vaginosis: implications for epidemiology, diagnosis and treatment. *Curr Opin Infect Dis.* 2013;26:86.
10. Muzny C, Schwebke J. Biofilms: an underappreciated mechanism of treatment failure and recurrence in vaginal infections. *Clin Infect Dis.* 2015;61:601-606.
11. Gorgos LM, Marrazzo JM. Sexually transmitted infections among women who have sex with women. *Clin Infect Dis.* 2011;53 Suppl 3:S84-S91.
12. Morris M, Nicoll A, Simms I, et al. Bacterial vaginosis: a public health review. *BJOG.* 2001;108:439.
13. Bradshaw CS, Walker SM, Vodstrcil LA, et al. The influence of behaviors and relationships on the vaginal microbiota of women and their female partners: the WOW Health Study. *J Infect Dis.* 2014;209:1562.
14. Bradshaw CS, Vodstrcil LA, Jocking JS, et al. Recurrence of bacterial vaginosis is significantly associated with posttreatment sexual activities and hormonal contraceptive use. *Clin Infect Dis.* 2013;56:777.
15. National Guideline Clearinghouse (NGC). Guideline summary: UK national guideline for the management of bacterial vaginosis 2012. https://www.bashhguidelines.org/media/1041/bv-2012.pdf. Accessed June 2018.
16. Cochrane library. *Antibiotic treatment for the sexual partners of women with bacterial vaginosis.* http://www.cochrane.org/CD011701/STI_antibiotic-treatment-sexual-partners-women-bacterial-vaginosis Accessed June 18.
17. Martius J, Krohn MA, Hillier SL, et al. Relationships of vaginal lactobacillus species, cervical *Chlamydia trachomatis,* and bacterial vaginosis to preterm birth. *Obstet Gynecol.* 1988;71:89-95.
18. Mitchell C, Marrazzo J. Bacterial vaginosis and the cervicovaginal immune response. *Am J Reprod Immunol.* 2014;6:555-563.
19. Burtin P, Taddio A, Ariburnu O, et al. Safety of metronidazole in pregnancy: a meta-analysis. *Am J Obstet Gynecol.* 1995;172 (2 Pt 1):525-529.
20. Sobel JD, Ferris D, Schwebke J, et al. Suppressive antibacterial therapy with 0.75% metronidazole vaginal gel to prevent recurrent bacterial vaginosis. *Am J Obstet Gynecol.* 2006;194:1283-1289.
21. Marrazzo JM, Thomas KK, Ringwood K. A behavioural intervention to reduce persistence of bacterial vaginosis among women who report sex with women: results of a randomized trial. *Sex Transm Infect.* 2011;87:399.
22. Baylson FA, Nyirjesy P, Weitz MV. Treatment of recurrent bacterial vaginosis with tinidazole. *Obstet Gynecol.* 2004;104(5 Pt 1): 931-932.
23. Anukam KC, Osazuwa E, Osemene GI, et al. Clinical study comparing probiotic *Lactobacillus* GR-1 and RC-14 with metronidazole vaginal gel to treat symptomatic bacterial vaginosis. *Microbes Infect.* 2006;8:2772.
24. Ya W, Reifer C, Miller LE. Efficacy of vaginal probiotic capsules for recurrent bacterial vaginosis: a double-blind, randomized, placebo-controlled study. *Am J Obstet Gynecol.* 2010;203:120.
25. Klebanoff MA, Nansel TR, Brotman RM, et al. Personal hygienic behaviors and bacterial vaginosis. *Sex Transm Dis.* 2010;37:94.
26. Morris M, Nicoll A, Simms I, et al. Bacterial vaginosis: a public health review. *BJOG.* 2001;108:439.

85 *CANDIDA* VULVOVAGINITIS

E.J. Mayeaux, Jr., MD

PATIENT STORY

A 35-year-old woman presents with severe vaginal and vulvar itching. She also complains of a thick white discharge. **Figure 85-1** demonstrates the appearance of her vulva and introitus, and **Figure 85-2** shows her cervix. **Figure 85-3** shows the wet prep with pseudohyphae. Treatment with a nonprescription intravaginal preparation was successful.

INTRODUCTION

Vulvovaginal candidiasis (VVC) is a common fungal infection in women of childbearing age. Pruritus is accompanied by a thick, odorless, white vaginal discharge. VVC is not a sexually transmitted disease. On the basis of clinical presentation, microbiology, host factors, and response to therapy, VVC can be classified as either uncomplicated or complicated.[1] Uncomplicated VVC is characterized by sporadic or infrequent symptoms, mild-to-moderate symptoms, and the patient is nonimmunocompromised. Complicated VVC is characterized by recurrent (four or more episodes in 1 year) or severe VVC, non-*albicans* candidiasis, or the patient has uncontrolled diabetes, debilitation, or immunosuppression.[1]

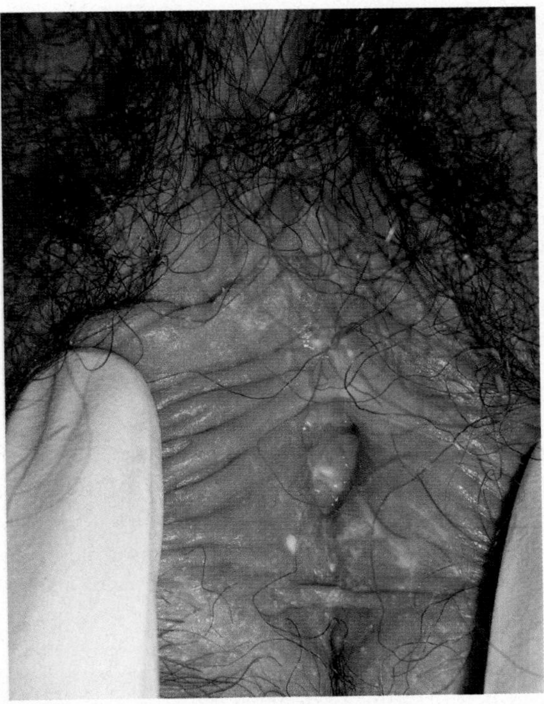

FIGURE 85-1 *Candida* on the vulva and introitus showing whitish patches with erythema. (*Reproduced with permission from Richard P. Usatine, MD.*)

SYNONYMS

Yeast vaginitis, yeast infection, candidiasis, moniliasis.

EPIDEMIOLOGY

- VVC accounts for approximately one third of vaginitis cases.[1]
- *Candida* species are part of the lower genital tract flora in 20% to 50% of healthy asymptomatic women.[2]
- VVC is most common in reproductive-age women and is uncommon in postmenopausal women. Seventy-five percent of all women in the United States will experience at least one episode of VVC. Of these, 40% to 45% will have two or more episodes within their lifetime.[1] In patient surveys, 29%–49% of premenopausal women report having had at least one lifetime episode of VVC, and 55% of female university students report having had at least one healthcare provider–diagnosed episode by age 25 years.[3]
- It is a frequent iatrogenic complication of antibiotic treatment, secondary to altered vaginal flora (**Figure 85-4**).
- Recurrent vulvovaginal candidiasis (RVVC) is defined as four or more episodes of symptomatic VVC in 1 year. Nine percent of women report having had RVVC. In women with an initial infection, the probability of RVVC was 10% by age 25 years, and 25% by age 50 years.[4] Recurrent yeast vaginitis is usually caused by relapse,

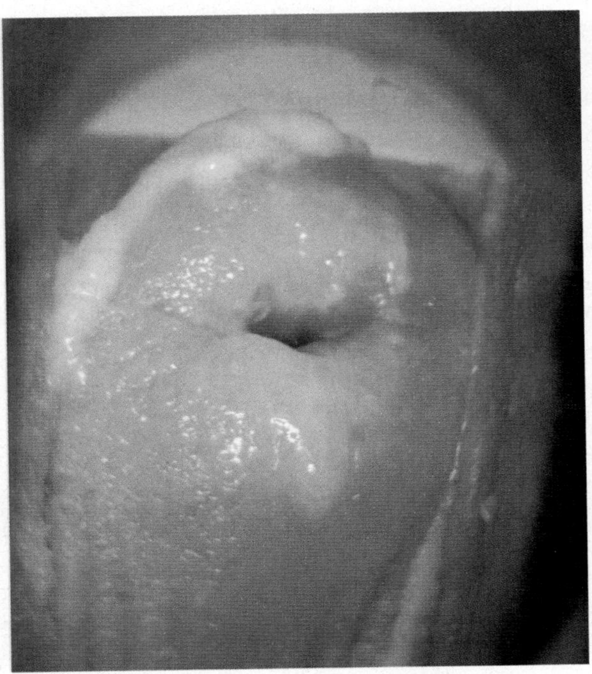

FIGURE 85-2 *Candida* vaginitis visible on the cervix. Note the thick white adherent "cottage-cheese-like" discharge. (*Courtesy E.J. Mayeaux, Jr., MD.*)

and less often by reinfection. Recurrent infection may be caused by *Candida* recolonization of the vagina from the rectum.[5]

ETIOLOGY AND PATHOPHYSIOLOGY

- Most vulvovaginal Candidiasis is caused by *Candida albicans* (**Figure 85-3**).[1,6] *Candida glabrata* now causes a significant percentage of all *Candida* vulvovaginal infections.[7] This organism is more resistant to the nonprescription imidazole creams. It can mutate out of the activity of treatment drugs much faster than *albicans* species.[8]
- VVC is not associated with a reduction in vaginal lactobacilli.[9]
- The disease is suggested by pruritus in the vulvar area, together with erythema of the vagina and vulva (see **Figures 85-1, 85-2,** and **85-4**). The familiar reddening of the vulvar tissues is caused by an ethanol by-product of the *Candida* infection. This ethanol compound also produces pruritic symptoms. A scalloped edge with satellite lesions is characteristic of the erythema on the vulva.
- VVC can occur concomitantly with sexually transmitted diseases (STDs).
- The pathogenesis of recurrent VVC is poorly understood, and most women with these recurrences have no apparent predisposing or underlying conditions.[1]
- The rectum is probably the source of organisms in most patients, since cultures of the gastrointestinal tract and vagina often show identical *Candida* species.[10]

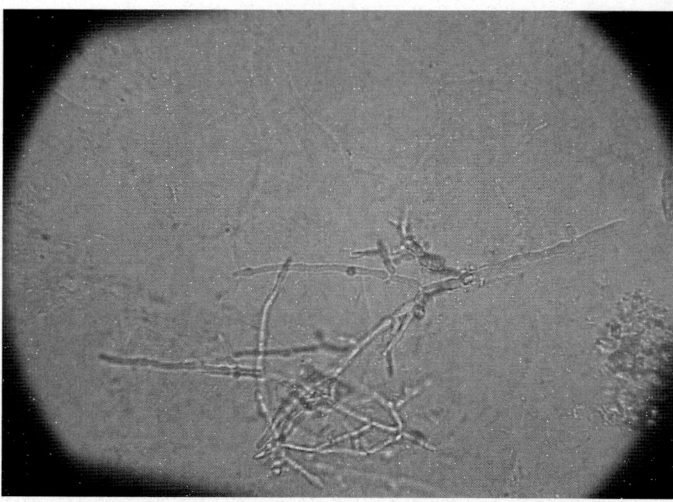

FIGURE 85-3 Wet mount with KOH of *Candida albicans* in a woman with *Candida* vaginitis. Seen under high power demonstrating branching pseudohyphae and budding yeast. (*Reproduced with permission from Richard P. Usatine, MD.*)

RISK FACTORS[11,12]

- Diabetes mellitus.
- Recent antibiotic use (see **Figure 85-4**).
- Increased estrogen levels, including higher-estrogen oral contraceptive use, pregnancy, and estrogen therapy.
- Immunosuppression (**Figure 85-5**).
- Incontinence and adult diapers (see **Figure 85-4**).
- Contraceptive devices (vaginal sponges, diaphragms, and intrauterine devices).
- Genetic susceptibility.
- Behavioral factors—VVC may be linked to orogenital and, less commonly, anogenital sex.
- Spermicides are **not associated** with *Candida* infection.
- There is no high-quality evidence showing a link between VVC and hygienic habits or wearing tight or synthetic clothing.

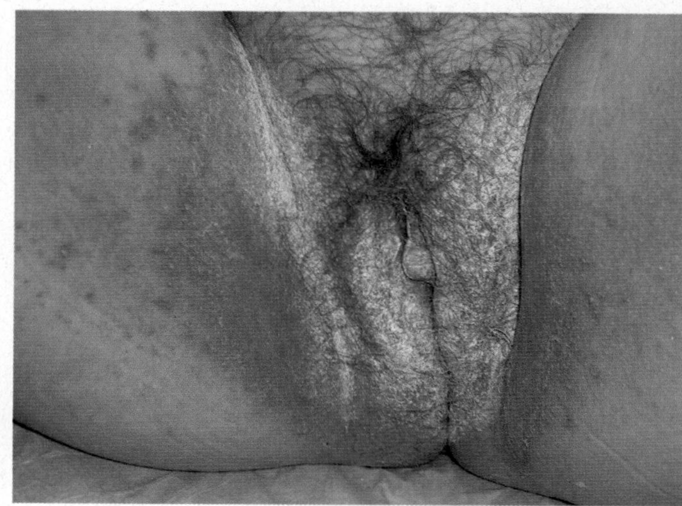

FIGURE 85-4 Red pruritic rash in the vulva and inguinal areas of this 46-year-old woman who suffered a stroke with significant residual hemiparesis. Diagnosis was confirmed with a KOH microscopic examination. The case was particularly severe secondary to her use of an adult diaper for incontinence and a preceding course of antibiotics. (*Reproduced with permission from Richard P. Usatine, MD.*)

DIAGNOSIS

CLINICAL FEATURES

- The diagnosis is usually suspected by characteristic findings (see **Figures 85-1, 85-2,** and **85-4**). Typical symptoms include pruritus, vaginal soreness, dyspareunia, and external dysuria. Typical signs include vulvar edema, fissures, excoriations, or thick, curdy vaginal discharge with no or minimal odor.[1]

LABORATORY TESTING

- Vaginitis solely caused by *Candida* generally has a vaginal pH of less than 4.5.
- The wet prep, KOH smear, or Gram stain may demonstrate yeast and/or pseudohyphae (**Figures 85-3** and **85-6**). Wet preps may also demonstrate white blood cells, trichomonads, candidal hyphae, or clue cells.
- The KOH prep is made by adding a drop of KOH solution to a drop of saline suspension of the discharge. The KOH lyses epithelial cells in 5 to 15 minutes (faster if the slide is warmed) and allows easier visualization of candidal hyphae or yeast.[1] Swartz-Lamkins stain (potassium hydroxide, a surfactant, and blue dye) may facilitate diagnosis by staining the yeast organisms a light blue.[13]
- Nucleic acid amplification testing (NAAT) is also available for *Candida*. The detection of vaginal yeast by this method is most commonly performed in the central laboratory, but some forms may also be feasible for office practice, and all are more sensitive than wet mount. A negative test result, however, was not found to be sensitive enough to rule out yeast and avoid a culture.[1,6] SOR Ⓐ
- Fungal culture with Sabouraud agar, Nickerson medium, or Microstix-*Candida* medium should be considered in patients with symptoms and a negative KOH because *C. glabrata* does not form pseudohyphae or hyphae and is not easily recognized on microscopy. If the wet mount is negative and *Candida* cultures cannot be done, empiric treatment can be considered for symptomatic women with any sign of VVC on examination.[1] SOR Ⓒ Asymptomatic women should not be cultured, as 10% to 20% of women harbor *Candida* spp. and other yeasts in the vagina.[1] SOR Ⓐ
- Vaginal cultures should be obtained from patients with RVVC to confirm the clinical diagnosis and to identify unusual species, including non-*albicans* species, particularly *C. glabrata* (*C. glabrata* does not form pseudohyphae or hyphae and is not easily recognized on microscopy).[1] SOR Ⓑ *C. glabrata* and other non-*albicans* *Candida* species are observed in 10% to 20% of patients with RVVC.[1]
- Given the frequency at which RVVC occurs in the immunocompetent healthy population, the occurrence of RVVC alone should not be considered an indication for HIV testing.[1] SOR Ⓒ

DIFFERENTIAL DIAGNOSIS

- Trichomoniasis can be confused with candidiasis because patients may report itching and a discharge in both diagnoses. Look for the strawberry cervix on examination and moving trichomonads on the wet prep (Chapter 86, *Trichomonas* Vaginitis).
- Bacterial vaginosis can be confused with candidiasis because patients may report a discharge and an odor in both diagnoses. The odor is usually much worse in bacterial vaginosis, and the quality of the discharge can be different. The wet prep should allow for differentiation between these two infections (Chapter 84, Bacterial Vaginosis).
- Gonorrhea and *Chlamydia* should not be missed in patients with vaginal discharge. Consider testing for these STDs based on patients' risk factors and the presence of purulence clinically and white blood cells on the wet prep (Chapter 87, *Chlamydia* Cervicitis).

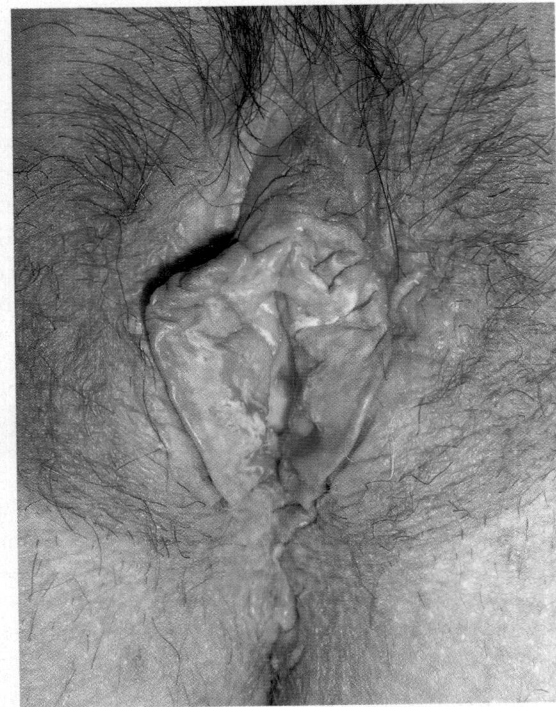

A

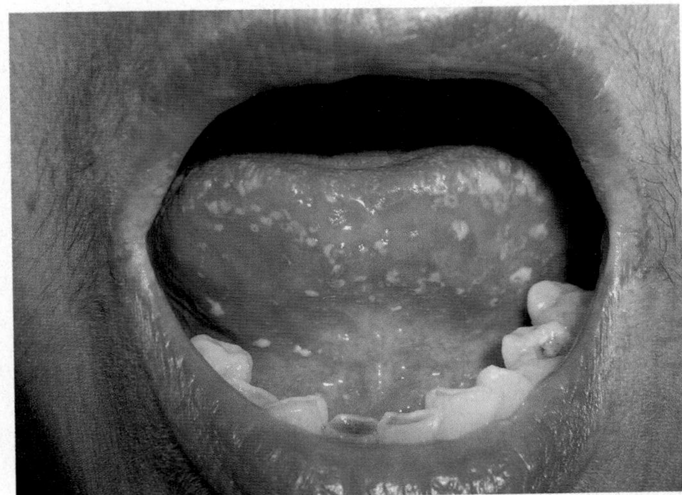

B

FIGURE 85-5 **A.** *Candida* vulvovaginitis in a 52-year-old woman with pemphigus vulgaris on prednisone and mycophenolate to control her immunobullous disease. **B.** The patient also has *Candida* thrush in her mouth secondary to her immunosuppression. (*Reproduced with permission from Richard P. Usatine, MD.*)

- Cytolytic vaginosis, or Döderlein cytolysis, can be confused with candidiasis. Cytolytic vaginosis is produced by a massive desquamation of epithelial cells related to excess lactobacilli in the vagina. The signs and symptoms are similar to *Candida* vaginitis, except no yeast are found on wet prep. The wet prep will show an overgrowth of lactobacilli. The treatment is to discontinue all antifungals and other agents or procedures that alter the vaginal flora.
- Hypersensitivity reactions, allergic or chemical reactions, and contact dermatitis conditions may produce vaginal itching and irritation with a normal vaginal pH.

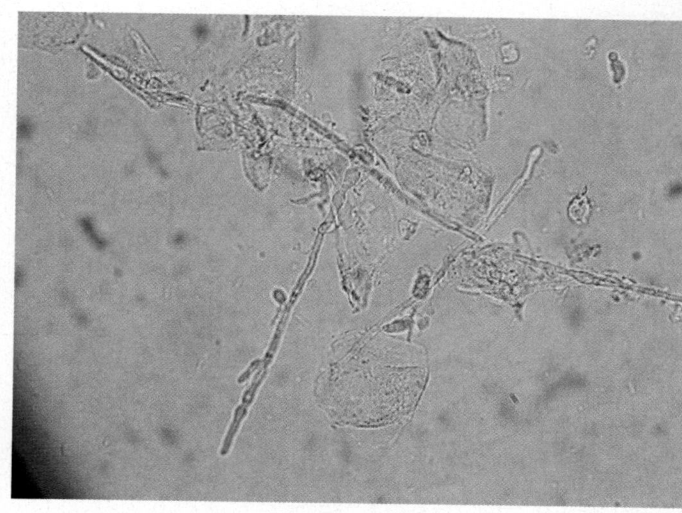

FIGURE 85-6 Wet mount with saline showing *Candida* in a woman with *Candida* vaginitis. Note how the branching pseudohyphae and budding yeast can be seen even though the epithelial cells have not been lysed by KOH. (*Reproduced with permission from Richard P. Usatine, MD.*)

MANAGEMENT

NONPHARMACOLOGIC

- VVC is not usually acquired through sexual intercourse; treatment of sex partners is not recommended but may be considered in women who have recurrent infection. Some male sex partners might have balanitis (Chapter 142, Candidiasis) and might benefit from treatment.[1] SOR Ⓐ
- Any woman whose symptoms persist after using a nonprescription preparation or who has a recurrence of symptoms within 2 months should be evaluated with office-based testing, as they are not necessarily more capable of diagnosing themselves even with prior diagnosed episodes of VVC, and delay in the treatment of other vulvovaginitis etiologies can result in adverse clinical outcomes.[1] SOR Ⓐ

MEDICATIONS

FIRST LINE

- Women with typical symptoms and a positive test result should receive treatment. Short courses of topical formulations effectively treat uncomplicated VVC (**Table 85-1**).[1] SOR Ⓐ Topical azole drugs are more effective than nystatin and result in clinical cure and negative cultures in 80% to 90% of patients who complete therapy. SOR Ⓐ The creams and suppositories in **Table 85-1** are oil-based and might weaken latex condoms and diaphragms.[1]
- The cure rates with single-dose oral fluconazole and all the intravaginal treatments are equal.[14] Fluconazole (Diflucan) 150-mg single dose has become very popular, but may have clinical cure rates of approximately only 70%. SOR Ⓐ Systemic allergic reactions are possible with the oral agents.
- The oral agents ketoconazole and itraconazole also appear to be effective.[1] SOR Ⓑ
- VVC frequently occurs during pregnancy. Only topical azole therapies, applied for 7 days, are recommended for use among pregnant women.[1] SOR Ⓒ
- The optimal treatment of non-*albicans* VVC remains unknown. Options include longer duration of therapy (7 to 14 days) with topical therapy or a 100-mg, 150-mg, or 200-mg oral dose of fluconazole every third day for a total of 3 doses.[1] SOR Ⓒ
- Severe VVC (i.e., extensive vulvar erythema, edema, excoriation, and fissure formation) is associated with lower clinical response

TABLE 85-1 Centers for Disease Control and Prevention Recommended Treatment Regimens

Intravaginal Agents
Clotrimazole 1% cream, 5 g intravaginally for 7 to 14 days
Clotrimazole 2% cream, 5 g intravaginally for 3 days
Clotrimazole 100-mg vaginal suppositories, one intravaginally for 3 days
Miconazole 2% cream, 5 g intravaginally for 7 days
Miconazole 4% cream, 5 g intravaginally daily for 3 days
Miconazole 100-mg vaginal suppository, 1 suppository for 7 days
Miconazole 200-mg vaginal suppository, 1 suppository for 3 days
Miconazole 1200-mg vaginal suppository, 1 suppository for 1 day
Tioconazole 6.5% ointment, 5 g intravaginally in a single application
Terconazole 0.4% cream, 5 g intravaginally for 7 days*
Terconazole 0.8% cream, 5 g intravaginally for 3 days*
Terconazole 80-mg vaginal suppository, 1 suppository for 3 days*
Oral Agent
Fluconazole 150-mg oral tablet, 1 tablet in single dose*

*Prescription only in the United States.
Data from the Centers for Disease Control and Prevention.[1]

rates in patients treated with short courses of topical or oral therapy. Either 7 to 14 days of topical azole or 150 mg of fluconazole in two sequential doses (second dose 72 hours after initial dose) is recommended.[1] SOR C The Infectious Diseases Society of America recommends 10 to 14 days of a topical or oral azole, followed by fluconazole 150 mg once per week for 6 months.[15] SOR C

SECOND LINE

- Nystatin 100,000 units intravaginally daily for 14 days.[1]

COMPLEMENTARY AND ALTERNATIVE THERAPY

- If RVVC occurs, 600 mg of boric acid in a gelatin capsule is recommended, administered vaginally once daily for 2 weeks. This regimen has clinical and mycologic eradication rates of approximately 70%.[1] SOR B
- *Lactobacillus acidophilus* does not adhere well to the vaginal epithelium, and it does not significantly change the incidence of candidal vulvovaginitis.[5,15-17] This should be considered an unproven therapy in the United States.
- There is no evidence from randomized trials that other complementary and alternative (CAM) therapies, such as garlic, tea tree oil, yogurt, or douching, are effective for the treatment or prevention of VVC caused by *C. albicans*.[18,19]

PREVENTION

MAINTENANCE REGIMENS

- Oral fluconazole (i.e., 100-mg, 150-mg, or 200-mg dose) weekly for 6 months is the first line of treatment. If this regimen is not feasible, some specialists recommend topical clotrimazole 200 mg twice a week, clotrimazole (500-mg dose vaginal suppositories once weekly), or other topical treatments used intermittently.[1] SOR C
- Suppressive maintenance antifungal therapies are effective in reducing RVVC.[1] SOR A However, 30% to 50% of women will have recurrent disease after maintenance therapy is discontinued. Routine treatment of sex partners is controversial. *C. albicans* azole resistance is rare in vaginal isolates, and susceptibility testing is usually not warranted for individual treatment guidance.

PROGNOSIS

- Women with underlying debilitating medical conditions (e.g., those with uncontrolled diabetes or those receiving corticosteroid treatments) do not respond as well to short-term therapies. Efforts to correct modifiable conditions should be made, and more prolonged (i.e., 7 to 14 days) conventional antimycotic treatment is necessary.[1] SOR C
- Symptomatic VVC is more frequent in HIV-seropositive women and correlates with severity of immunodeficiency. In addition, among HIV-infected women, systemic azole exposure is associated with the isolation of non–*C. albicans* species from the vagina. According to the available data, therapy for VVC in HIV-infected women should not differ from that for seronegative women.[1] SOR C

FOLLOW-UP

- Patients should be instructed to return for follow-up visits only if symptoms persist or recur within 2 months of onset of initial symptoms.[1]

PATIENT EDUCATION

- Studies show that women who were previously diagnosed with VVC are not necessarily more likely to be able to diagnose themselves.[1] Any woman whose symptoms persist after using a nonprescription preparation, or who has a recurrence of symptoms within 2 months, should be evaluated with office-based testing. Explain that unnecessary or inappropriate use of nonprescription preparations can lead to a delay in the treatment of other vulvovaginitis etiologies, which can result in adverse clinical outcomes.[1]

PATIENT RESOURCES

- FamilyDoctor.org from AAFP. *Yeast Infections*—**https://familydoctor.org/condition/yeast-infections/.**
- MedicineNet. *Yeast Infection (in Women and Men)*—**http://www.medicinenet.com/yeast_vaginitis/article.htm.**
- WebMD. *Vaginal Yeast Infections*—**http://women.webmd.com/tc/vaginal-yeast-infections-topic-overview.**
- Womenshealth.gov. *Vaginal Yeast Infections Fact Sheet*—**https://www.womenshealth.gov/a-z-topics/vaginal-yeast-infections.**
- MedlinePlus. *Yeast Infections*—**http://www.nlm.nih.gov/medlineplus/yeastinfections.html.**
- eMedicine Health. *Candidiasis*—**http://www.emedicinehealth.com/candidiasis_yeast_infection/article_em.htm.**

PROVIDER RESOURCES

- Centers for Disease Control and Prevention. *2015 Sexually Transmitted Diseases Treatment Guidelines*—**https://www.cdc.gov/std/tg2015/default.htm.**
- American Family Physician. Vaginitis: Diagnosis and Treatment. *Am Fam Physician*. 2011; *Am Fam Physician*. 2011;83(7): 807-815.—**http://www.aafp.org/afp/2011/0401/p807.html.**
- eMedicine. *Candidiasis*—**emedicine.medscape.com/article/213853-overview.**
- eMedicine. *Vulvovaginitis*—**http://emedicine.medscape.com/article/2188931-overview.**

REFERENCES

1. Workowski KA, Bolan GA; Centers for Disease Control and Prevention. Sexually transmitted diseases treatment guidelines, 2015. *MMWR Recomm Rep*. 2015;64:1. https://www.cdc.gov/std/tg2015/default.htm. Accessed June 2018.

2. Goldacre MJ, Watt B, Loudon N, et al. Vaginal microbial flora in normal young women. *Br Med J.* 1979;1:1450.
3. Geiger AM, Foxman B, Gillespie BW. The epidemiology of vulvovaginal candidiasis among university students. *Am J Public Health.* 1995;85:1146.
4. Foxman B, Muraglia R, Dietz JP, et al. Prevalence of recurrent vulvovaginal candidiasis in 5 European countries and the United States: results from an internet panel survey. *J Low Genit Tract Dis.* 2013;17:340.
5. Shalev E, Battino S, Weiner E, et al. Ingestion of yogurt containing acidophilus compared with pasteurized yogurt as prophylaxis for recurrent candidal vaginitis and bacterial vaginosis. *Arch Fam Med.* 1996;5:593-596.
6. Cohen DA, Nsuami M, Etame RB, et al. A school-based chlamydia control program using DNA amplification technology. *Pediatrics.* 1998;(1):101.
7. Sobel JD. Vulvovaginal candidosis. *Lancet.* 2007;369:1961.
8. Horowitz BJ, Giaquinta D, Ito S. Evolving pathogens in vulvovaginal candidiasis: implications for patient care. *J Clin Pharmacol.* 1992;32:248.
9. Zhou X, Westman R, Hickey R, et al. Vaginal microbiota of women with frequent vulvovaginal candidiasis. *Infect Immun.* 2009;77:4130.
10. Bertholf ME, Stafford MJ. Colonization of *Candida albicans* in vagina, rectum, and mouth. *J Fam Pract.* 1983;16:919.
11. Foxman B. The epidemiology of vulvovaginal candidiasis: risk factors. *Am J Public Health.* 1990;80:329.
12. Sobel JD. *Candida* vaginitis. *Infect Dis Clin Pract (Baltim Md).* 1994;3:334.
13. Swartz JH, Lamkins BE. A rapid, simple stain for fungi in skin, nail scrapings, and hair. *Arch Dermatol.* 1964;89:89.
14. Sobel JD, Brooker D, Stein GE, et al. Single oral dose fluconazole compared with conventional clotrimazole topical therapy of *Candida* vaginitis. *Am J Obstet Gynecol.* 1995;172:1263-1268.
15. Pappas PG, Kauffman CA, Andes D, et al. Clinical practice guidelines for the management of candidiasis: 2009 update by the Infectious Diseases Society of America. *Clin Infect Dis.* 2009;48:503.
16. Pirotta M, Gunn J, Chondros P, et al. Effect of lactobacillus in preventing post-antibiotic vulvovaginal candidiasis: a randomised controlled trial. *BMJ.* 2004;329:548.
17. Witt A, Kaufmann U, Bitschnau M, et al. Monthly itraconazole versus classic homeopathy for the treatment of recurrent vulvovaginal candidiasis: a randomized trial. *BJOG.* 2009;116:1499.
18. Van Kessel K, Assefi N, Marrazzo J, Eckert L. Common complementary and alternative therapies for yeast vaginitis and bacterial vaginosis: a systematic review. *Obstet Gynecol Surv.* 2003;58(5): 351-358.
19. Boskey ER. Alternative therapies for bacterial vaginosis: a literature review and acceptability survey. *Altern Ther Health Med.* 2005;11(5):38-43.

86 TRICHOMONAS VAGINITIS

E.J. Mayeaux, Jr., MD
Richard P. Usatine, MD

PATIENT STORY

A 17-year-old teen presents with vaginal itching, odor, and discharge for several weeks. She has one partner who is asymptomatic. Speculum examination shows a cervix (**Figure 86-1**) with a copious foamy white discharge with a fishy odor. Wet mount shows trichomonads swimming in saline (**Figures 86-2** and **86-3**). The trichomonads are larger than white blood cells (WBCs) and have visible flagella and movement. She is diagnosed with trichomoniasis and treated with 2 g of metronidazole in a single dose. The patient is tested for other sexually transmitted diseases (STDs) and her partner is treated with the same regimen.

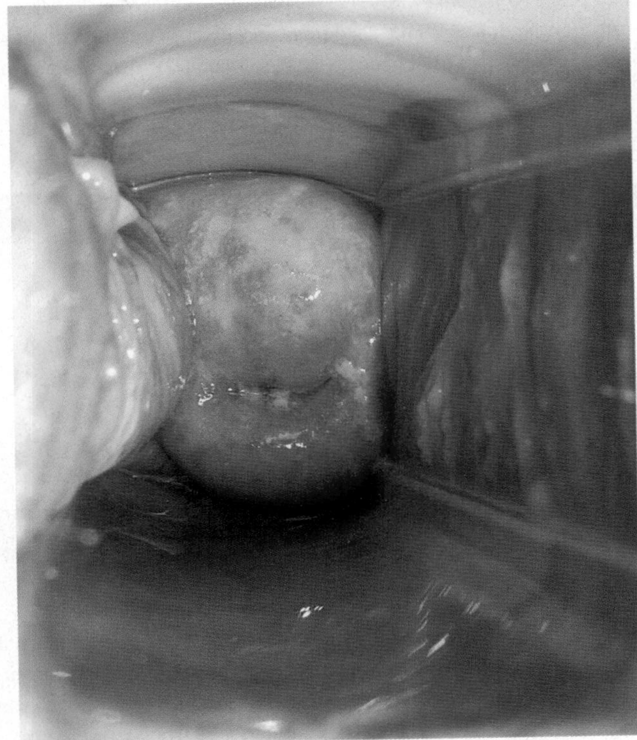

FIGURE 86-1 Speculum examination showing the strawberry cervix pattern seen with *Trichomonas* infections. This strawberry pattern is caused by inflammation and punctate hemorrhages on the cervix. There is a scant white discharge. (*Reproduced with permission from Richard P. Usatine, MD.*)

INTRODUCTION

Trichomonas vaginitis is a local infection caused by the protozoan *Trichomonas vaginalis* that is associated with vaginal discharge and irritation. The patient often has an itch and an odor along with the discharge but may be asymptomatic.

SYNONYMS

Trichomoniasis, trich, tricky monkeys.

EPIDEMIOLOGY

- Trichomoniasis is the most prevalent nonviral sexually transmitted infection in the United States, affecting an estimated 3.7 million persons.[1]
- The worldwide prevalence of trichomoniasis is estimated to be 180 million cases per year; these cases account for 10% to 25% of all vaginal infections.[2]
- Cross-sectional data from the 2003–2004 U.S. National Health and Nutrition Examination Survey (NHANES) shows 3% of female adolescents (aged 14 to 19 years) had laboratory evidence of infection with *T. vaginalis*.[3]

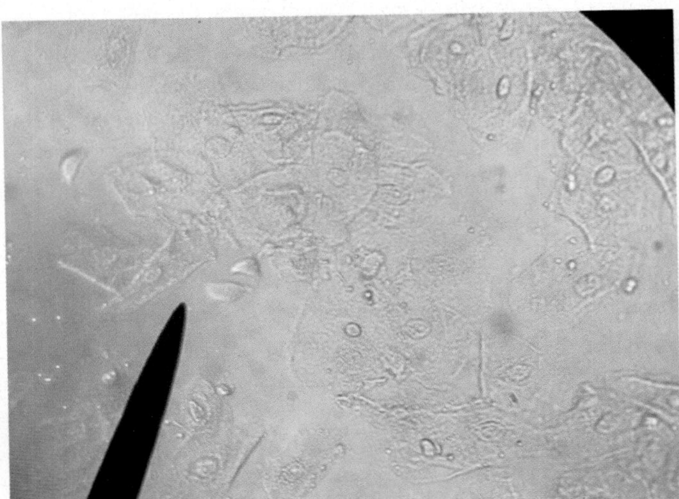

FIGURE 86-2 Wet mount showing *Trichomonas* in saline under low power. There are two visible trichomonads to the right and above the tip of the pointer. The largest cells are vaginal epithelial cells with visible nuclei. (*Reproduced with permission from Richard P. Usatine, MD.*)

ETIOLOGY AND PATHOPHYSIOLOGY

- *Trichomonas* infection is caused by the unicellular protozoan *T. vaginalis*.[4]
- The majority of men (90%) infected with *T. vaginalis* are asymptomatic, but many women (50%) report symptoms.[5]

- The infection is predominantly transmitted via sexual contact. The organism can survive up to 48 hours at 10°C (50°F) outside the body, making transmission from shared undergarments or from infected hot spas possible although extremely unlikely.
- *Trichomonas* infection is associated with low-birth-weight infants, premature rupture of membranes, and preterm delivery in pregnant patients.[6]
- In a person coinfected with HIV, the pathology induced by *T. vaginalis* infection can increase HIV shedding. *Trichomonas* infection may also act to expand the portal of entry for HIV in an HIV-negative person. Studies from Africa have suggested that *T. vaginalis* infection may increase the rate of HIV transmission by approximately twofold.[7]

RISK FACTORS[3]

- New or multiple partners.
- A history of STDs.
- Exchanging sex for payment or drugs.
- Injection drug use.
- Douching.[4]

DIAGNOSIS

CLINICAL FEATURES

- The physical examination should include inspection of the external genitalia for irritation or discharge (**Figures 86-1** and **86-4**). Speculum examination is done to determine the amount and character of the discharge and to look for the characteristic strawberry cervix (**Figure 86-5**). This strawberry pattern is caused by inflammation and punctate hemorrhages on the cervix.
- Typically, women with trichomoniasis have a diffuse, malodorous, yellow-green discharge (see **Figure 86-4**) with vulvar irritation.[4] Vaginal and vulvar itching and irritation are common.
- It should be determined whether the patient douched recently, because this can lower the yield of diagnostic tests. Patients who have been told not to douche will sometimes start wiping the vagina with soapy washcloths to "keep clean" as an alternative. This greatly irritates the vagina and cervix, lowers test sensitivity, and may cause a discharge.

TYPICAL DISTRIBUTION

- In infected women, *Trichomonas vaginalis* may be found in the vagina, urethra, and paraurethral glands. Other sites include the cervix and Bartholin and Skene glands.

LABORATORY TESTING

- Because of the high prevalence of trichomoniasis, testing should be performed in women seeking care for vaginal discharge. Screening should be considered for women with risk factors.[4]
- The use of highly sensitive and specific nucleic acid amplification tests (NAATs) is recommended by the Centers for Disease Control and Prevention (CDC).

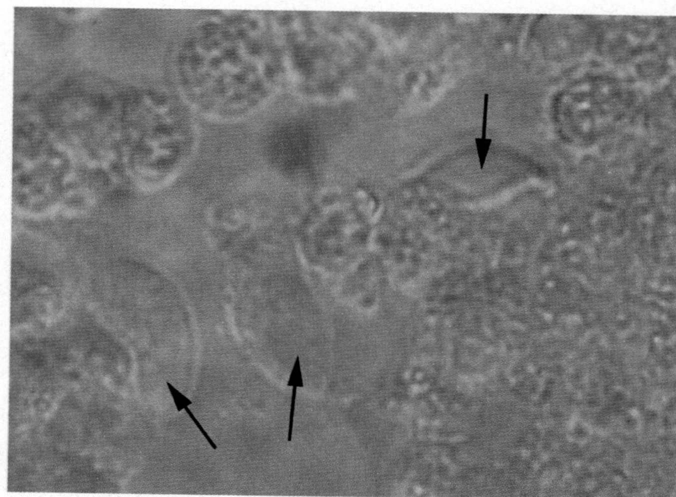

FIGURE 86-3 Wet mount showing *Trichomonas* (*arrows*) in saline under high power. The smaller, more granular cells are white blood cells. (*Reproduced with permission from Richard P. Usatine, MD.*)

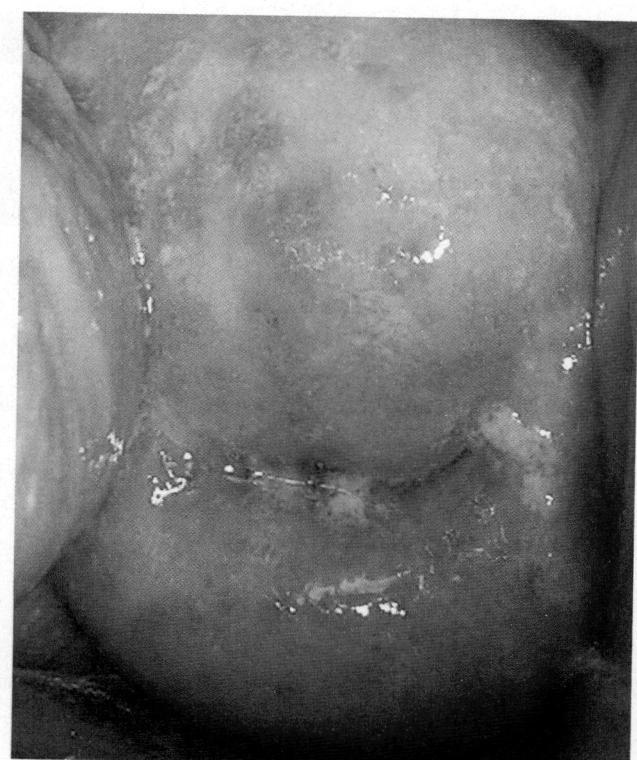

FIGURE 86-4 Close-up of strawberry cervix in a *Trichomonas* infection demonstrating inflammation and punctate hemorrhages. (*Reproduced with permission from E.J. Mayeaux, Jr., MD.*)

- Wet preps are obtained using a cotton-tipped applicator applied to the vaginal sidewall, placing the sample of discharge into normal saline (not water). A drop of the suspension is then placed on a slide, covered with a coverslip, and carefully examined with the low-power and high-dry objective lenses. Under the microscope, observe for motile trichomonads, which are often easy to visualize because of their lashing flagella (see **Figure 86-2**).
- Wet prep has a sensitivity of only approximately 60% to 70% and requires immediate evaluation of wet preparation slide for optimal results.[4] One study found that 20% of samples for wet prep became negative by 10 minutes, 35% samples by 30 minutes, and 78% by 2 hours. They concluded that in order to maximize the sensitivity of this test, all specimens should be examined immediately after they are taken.[8]
- The OSOM Trichomonas Rapid Test and the Affirm VP III are FDA-cleared for trichomoniasis in women. Both tests are performed on vaginal secretions at the point of care and have sensitivity greater than 83% and a specificity greater than 97%. The results of the OSOM Trichomonas Rapid Test are available in approximately 10 minutes, and results of the Affirm VP III are available within 45 minutes. False-positive tests might occur, especially in populations with a low prevalence of disease.[4]
- An FDA-approved polymerase chain reaction (PCR) assay for detection of gonorrhea and chlamydial infection (Amplicor, manufactured by Roche Diagnostic Corp.) has been modified to test for *T. vaginalis* in vaginal or endocervical swabs and in urine from women and men, with sensitivity ranges from 88% to 97% and specificity from 98% to 99%.[9]
- APTIMA *T. vaginalis* Analyte Specific Reagents (ASR; manufactured by Gen-Probe, Inc.) also can detect *T. vaginalis* RNA using the same instrumentation platforms available for the FDA-cleared APTIMA Combo2 assay for diagnosis of gonorrhea and chlamydial infection. Published validation studies found sensitivity ranging from 74% to 98% and specificity from 87% to 98%.[10]
- A vaginal pH above 4.5 is seen with menopausal patients, *Trichomonas* infection, or bacterial vaginosis.[5]
- Culture is a sensitive and highly specific method of diagnosis. In women in whom trichomoniasis is suspected but not confirmed by microscopy, vaginal secretions should be cultured for *T. vaginalis*.[4]
- A nucleic acid amplification test for *Neisseria gonorrhoeae* and/or *Chlamydia trachomatis* should be performed on all patients with *Trichomonas*.
- Although trichomonas may be detected on Pap testing, the sensitivity is low, and Pap testing is not indicated in adolescents unless they are HIV infected.[11]

DIFFERENTIAL DIAGNOSIS

- Bacterial vaginosis and *Trichomonas* may have the odor of aromatic amines, and therefore may easily be confused with each other. Look for clue cells and trichomonads on the wet prep to differentiate between the two (Chapter 84, Bacterial Vaginosis).
- *Candida* vaginitis tends to present with a cottage-cheese-like discharge and vaginal itching (Chapter 85, *Candida* Vulvovaginitis).

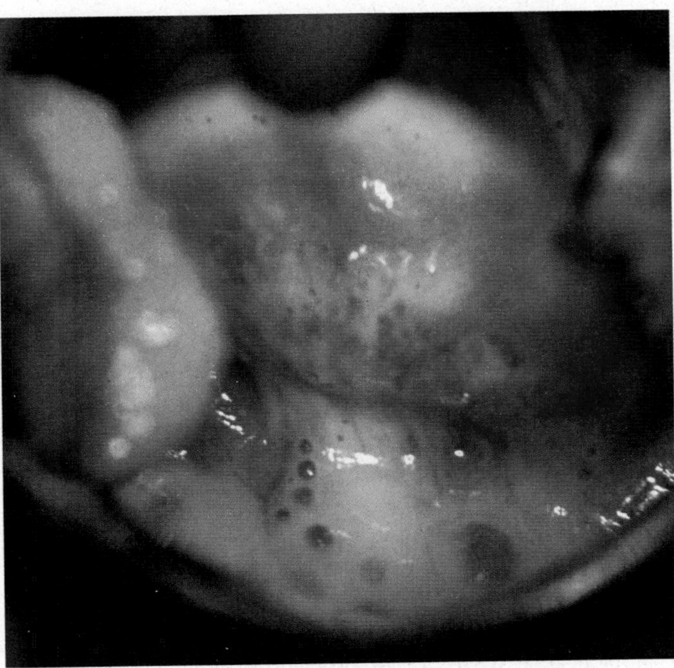

FIGURE 86-5 Speculum examination demonstrating the thick yellow-green discharge that may be seen in *Trichomonas* infection. The discharge can also be frothy white. (*Reproduced with permission from Richard P. Usatine, MD.*)

- Gonorrhea and *Chlamydia* and should not be missed in patients with vaginal discharge. Consider testing for these STDs based on patients' risk factors and the presence of purulence clinically and WBCs on the wet prep (Chapter 87, *Chlamydia* Cervicitis).

MANAGEMENT

FIRST LINE

- **Table 86-1** shows the CDC-recommended treatments for *T. vaginalis* infections. Metronidazole 2 g orally as a single dose or 500 mg bid for 7 days (including pregnant patients) are the best treatments by Cochrane analysis.[12] SOR Ⓐ
- Tinidazole (Tindamax), a second-generation nitroimidazole, is indicated as a one-time dose of 2 g for the treatment of trichomoniasis (including metronidazole-resistant trichomoniasis).[4] SOR Ⓐ It is effective therapy in nonresistant and resistant *T. vaginalis*.[13,14] The contraindications (including ethyl alcohol [EtOH]) to the use of tinidazole are similar to those for metronidazole.
- Alcohol consumption should be eliminated during treatment with nitroimidazoles. To reduce the possibility of a disulfiram-like reaction, abstinence from alcohol use should continue for 24 hours after completion of metronidazole or 72 hours after completion of tinidazole.[4]
- Pregnant women may be treated with 2 g of metronidazole in a single dose. Metronidazole is pregnancy category B. Vaginal trichomoniasis is associated with adverse pregnancy outcomes, particularly premature rupture of membranes, preterm delivery, and low birth weight. Unfortunately, data do not suggest that metronidazole treatment results in a reduction in perinatal morbidity, and treatment may even increase prematurity or low birth weight.[4] Treatment of *T. vaginalis* might relieve symptoms of vaginal discharge in pregnant women and might prevent respiratory or genital infection of the newborn and further sexual transmission. The CDC recommends that clinicians counsel patients regarding the potential risks and benefits of treatment during pregnancy.[4]

SECOND LINE

- Some strains of *T. vaginalis* can have diminished susceptibility to metronidazole. Low-level metronidazole resistance has been identified in 2% to 5% of cases of vaginal trichomoniasis. These infections should respond to tinidazole or higher doses or longer durations of metronidazole. High-level resistance is rare.[15]
- Metronidazole gel is 50% less efficacious for the treatment of trichomoniasis than oral preparations and is not recommended.[4]

PREVENTION

- Patients should be instructed to avoid sex until they and their sex partners are cured (i.e., when therapy has been completed and patient and partner[s] are asymptomatic).[4]
- Spermicidal agents such as nonoxynol-9 reduce the rate of transmission of *Trichomonas*.[16]
- The risk of acquiring infection can be reduced by consistent use of condoms and limiting the number of sexual partners.

TABLE 86-1 Centers for Disease Control and Prevention Recommended Regimens for Pregnant and Nonpregnant Patients SOR Ⓐ

Metronidazole 2 g orally in a single dose
OR
Tinidazole 2 g orally in a single dose
CDC Alternative Regimen SOR Ⓐ
Metronidazole 500 mg orally twice a day for 7 days

Recommendations from Centers for Disease Control and Prevention. Sexually transmitted diseases treatment guidelines, 2015.[2,4]

FOLLOW-UP

- Because of the high rate of reinfection among patients in whom trichomoniasis was diagnosed, rescreening at 3 months following initial infection is recommended.[4]

PATIENT EDUCATION

- *T. vaginalis* infection in pregnant women is associated with two- to threefold increased risk for HIV acquisition, preterm birth, and other adverse pregnancy outcomes.[4]
- The CDC recommends that unless prohibited by law or regulations, medical providers should routinely offer expedited partner therapy (EPT) to heterosexual patients with *Trichomonas* infection when the provider cannot confidently ensure that all of a patient's sex partners from the prior 60 days will be treated.[1] The CDC website contains information on which states allow or prohibit EPT (see Provider Resources below).

PATIENT RESOURCES

- Centers for Disease Control and Prevention information—**https://www.cdc.gov/dpdx/trichomoniasis/index.html.**
- MedlinePlus—**http://www.nlm.nih.gov/medlineplus/ency/article/001331.htm.**
- Centers for Disease Control and Prevention. *Trichomoniasis*—**http://www.cdc.gov/std/trichomonas/default.htm.**
- PubMed Health. *Trichomoniasis*—**http://www.ncbi.nlm.nih.gov/pubmedhealth/PMH0002307/.**
- MedlinePlus. *Trichomoniasis*—**http://www.nlm.nih.gov/medlineplus/trichomoniasis.html.**
- eMedicine Health. *Trichomoniasis*—**http://www.emedicinehealth.com/trichomoniasis/article_em.htm.**

PROVIDER RESOURCES

- Medscape. *Trichomoniasis*—**http://emedicine.medscape.com/article/230617.**
- Trichomoniasis in Emergency Medicine—**http://emedicine.medscape.com/article/787722.**

- Centers for Disease Control and Prevention. *2015 Guidelines for Treatment of Sexually Transmitted Diseases: Trichomoniasis*—**https://www.cdc.gov/std/tg2015/trichomoniasis.htm.**
- Centers for Disease Control and Prevention. *Legal Status of Expedited Partner Therapy (EPT)*—**https://www.cdc.gov/std/ept/legal/default.htm.**

REFERENCES

1. Satterwhite CL, Torrone E, Meites E, et al. Sexually transmitted infections among US women and men: prevalence and incidence estimates, 2008. *Sex Transm Dis.* 2013;40:187-193.
2. Weinstock H, Berman S, Cates W Jr. Sexually transmitted diseases among American youth: incidence and prevalence estimates, 2000. *Perspect Sex Reprod Health.* 2004;36(1):6-10.
3. Forhan SE, Gottlieb SL, Sternberg MR, et al. Prevalence of sexually transmitted infections among female adolescents aged 14 to 19 in the United States. *Pediatrics.* 2009;124:1505.
4. Workowski KA, Bolan GA; Centers for Disease Control and Prevention. Sexually transmitted diseases treatment guidelines, 2015. *MMWR Recomm Rep.* 2015;64(RR-03):1-137.
5. Gjerdngen D, Fontaine P, Bixby M, et al. The impact of regular vaginal pH screening on the diagnosis of bacterial vaginosis in pregnancy. *J Fam Pract.* 2000;49:3-43.
6. Cotch MF, Pastorek JG 2nd, Nugent RP, et al. *Trichomonas vaginalis* associated with low birth weight and preterm delivery: the Vaginal Infections and Prematurity Study Group. *Sex Transm Dis.* 1997;24:353-360.
7. Sorvillo F, Smith L, Kerndt P, Ash L. *Trichomonas vaginalis*, HIV, and African-Americans. *Emerg Infect Dis.* 2001;7(6):927-932.
8. Kingston MA, Bansal D, Carlin EM. "Shelf life" of *Trichomonas vaginalis. Int J STD AIDS.* 2003;14(1):28-29.
9. Van Der PB, Kraft CS, Williams JA. Use of an adaptation of a commercially available PCR assay aimed at diagnosis of chlamydia and gonorrhea to detect *Trichomonas vaginalis* in urogenital specimens. *J Clin Microbiol.* 2006;44:366-373.
10. Nye MB, Schwebke JR, Body BA. Comparison of APTIMA *Trichomonas vaginalis* transcription-mediated amplification to wet mount microscopy, culture, and polymerase chain reaction for diagnosis of trichomoniasis in men and women. *Am J Obstet Gynecol.* 2009;200:188-197.
11. Lobo TT, Feijó G, Carvalho SE, et al. A comparative evaluation of the Papanicolaou test for the diagnosis of trichomoniasis. *Sex Transm Dis.* 2003;30(9):694-699.
12. Epling J. What is the best way to treat trichomoniasis in women? (Cochrane review) *Am Fam Physician.* 2001;64:1241-1243.
13. Mammen-Tobin A, Wilson JD. Management of metronidazole-resistant *Trichomonas vaginalis*—a new approach. *Int J STD AIDS.* 2005;16(7):488-490.
14. Hager WD. Treatment of metronidazole-resistant *Trichomonas vaginalis* with tinidazole: case reports of three patients. *Sex Transm Dis.* 2004;31(6):343-345.
15. Kirkcaldy RD, Augostini P, Asbel LE, et al. Trichomonas vaginalis antimicrobial drug resistance in 6 US cities, STD Surveillance Network, 2009–2010. *Emerg Infect Dis.* 2012;18(6):939-943.
16. d'Oro LC, Parazzini F, Naldi L, La Vecchia C. Barrier methods of contraception, spermicides, and sexually transmitted diseases: a review. *Genitourin Med.* 1994;70:410.

87 *CHLAMYDIA* CERVICITIS

E.J. Mayeaux, Jr., MD
Richard P. Usatine, MD

PATIENT STORY

A 16-year-old girl presents to clinic with a complaint of vaginal discharge. She has only one sexual partner but is unsure if her partner may have had other sexual contacts. On physical examination, there is ectopy and some mucoid discharge (**Figure 87-1**). The cervix bled easily while obtaining discharge and cells for a wet mount and genetic probe test. The wet mount showed many white blood cells (WBCs) but no visible pathogens. The patient was treated with 1 g of azithromycin taken in front of a clinic nurse. She was tested for HIV, syphilis, *Trichomonas*, GC, and *Chlamydia* and given a follow-up appointment in 1 week. The genetic probe test was positive for *Chlamydia* and all the other examinations were negative. This information was given to the patient on her return visit and safe sex was discussed.

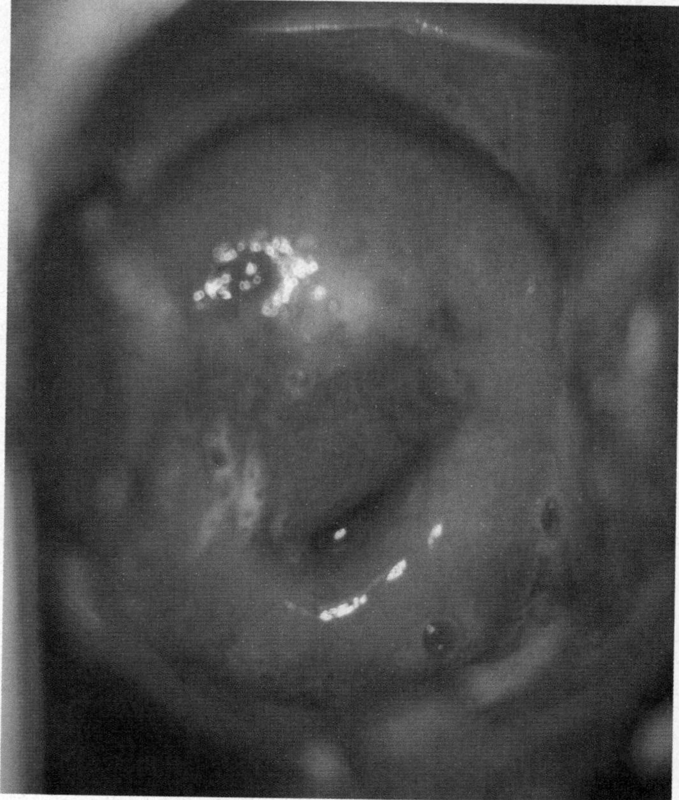

FIGURE 87-1 Chlamydial cervicitis with ectopy, mucoid discharge, and irritation. The cervix is inflamed and friable. (*Reproduced with permission from E.J. Mayeaux, Jr., MD.*)

INTRODUCTION

Chlamydia trachomatis causes genital infections that can result in pelvic inflammatory disease (PID), ectopic pregnancy, and infertility. Asymptomatic infection is common among both men and women, so healthcare providers must rely on screening tests to detect disease. The Centers for Disease Control and Prevention (CDC) recommends annual screening of all sexually active women ages 25 years and younger, and of older women with risk factors, such as having a new sex partner or multiple sex partners.[1]

EPIDEMIOLOGY

- A very common STD, *Chlamydia* is the most frequently reported infectious disease in the United States (excluding human papillomavirus [HPV]).[1] An estimated 1.2 million cases are reported to the CDC annually in the United States.[2]
- The World Health Organization (WHO) estimates there are 140 million cases of *Chlamydia trachomatis* infection worldwide every year.[3]
- The CDC estimates that screening and treatment programs can be conducted at an annual cost of $175 million. Every dollar spent on screening and treatment saves $12 in complications that result from untreated *Chlamydia*.[4]
- *Chlamydia* is common among sexually active adolescents and young adults.[5] As many as 1 in 10 adolescent girls tested for *Chlamydia* is infected. Based on reports to the CDC provided by states that collect age-specific data, teenage girls have the highest rates of chlamydial infection. In these states, 15- to 19-year-old girls represent 46% of infections and 20- to 24-year-old women represent another 33%.[4]
- Cross-sectional data from the 2003–2004 U.S. National Health and Nutrition Examination Survey (NHANES) shows that 4% of female adolescents (ages 14–19 years) had laboratory evidence of infection with *Chlamydia trachomatis*.[6]

ETIOLOGY AND PATHOPHYSIOLOGY

- *C. trachomatis* is a small Gram-negative bacterium with unique biologic properties among living organisms. *Chlamydia* is an obligate intracellular parasite that has a distinct life cycle consisting of two major phases: the small elementary bodies that attach and penetrate into cells, and the metabolically active reticulate bodies that form large inclusions within cells.
- It has a long growth cycle, which explains why extended courses of treatment are often necessary. Immunity to infection is not long-lived, so reinfection or persistent infection is common.
- The infection may be asymptomatic and the onset often indolent. Symptoms of infection when present in women are most commonly abnormal vaginal discharge, vaginal bleeding (including after intercourse), and dysuria. Only 2%–4% of infected men reported any symptoms.[7]
- *Chlamydia* can cause cervicitis, endometritis, PID, infertility, perihepatitis (Fitz-Hugh-Curtis syndrome) urethritis, and epididymitis. It may produce poor neonatal outcomes including premature rupture of membranes, preterm labor, low birth weight, infant death, conjunctivitis, and pediatric pneumonia.[8] Of exposed babies, 50% develop conjunctivitis and 10% to 16% develop pneumonia.[1] Perinatal *Chlamydia* is the leading cause of infectious blindness in the world, which is particularly worrisome because adolescents are at increased risk for infection and have more barriers to healthcare screening.[9]
- *Chlamydia* infections may lead to reactive arthritis, which presents with arthritis, conjunctivitis, and urethritis. Past or ongoing *C. trachomatis* infection may be a risk factor for ovarian cancer.[10,11]
- Up to 40% of women with untreated *Chlamydia* will develop PID. Undiagnosed PID caused by *Chlamydia* is common. Of those with PID, 20% will become infertile; 18% will experience debilitating, chronic pelvic pain; and 9% will have a life-threatening tubal pregnancy. Tubal pregnancy is the leading cause of first-trimester, pregnancy-related deaths in American women.[4]

RISK FACTORS[1,2,12]

- Adolescents and young adults.
- Nonwhite populations.
- Multiple and new sexual partners.
- Poor socioeconomic conditions.
- Single marital status.
- Nonbarrier contraceptive use.
- History of prior STD.

DIAGNOSIS

CLINICAL FEATURES

- The cervix is inflamed, friable, and may bleed easily with manipulation. The cervix may show ectopy (columnar cells on the ectocervix). The discharge is usually mucoid or mucopurulent (**Figures 87-1** to **87-3**).[8]

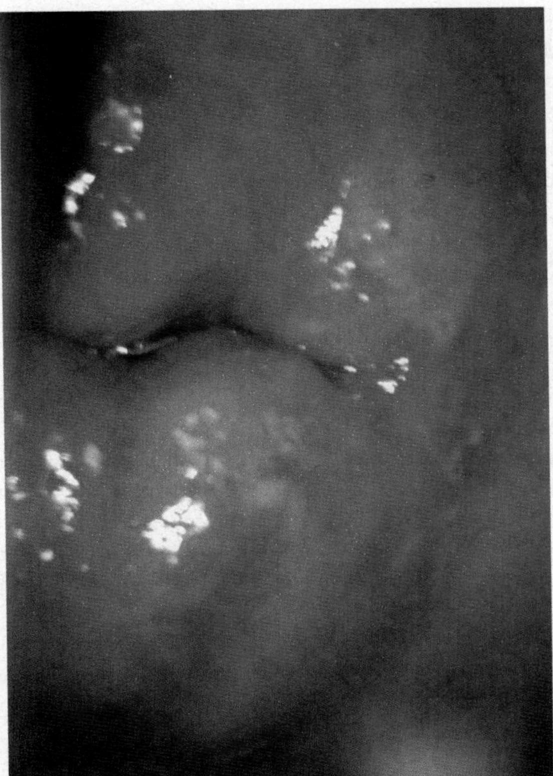

FIGURE 87-2 This patient presented with spotting after intercourse. She has cervicitis with ectopy, friability, and bleeding. NAAT was positive for *Chlamydia*. *(Reproduced with permission from E.J. Mayeaux, Jr., MD.)*

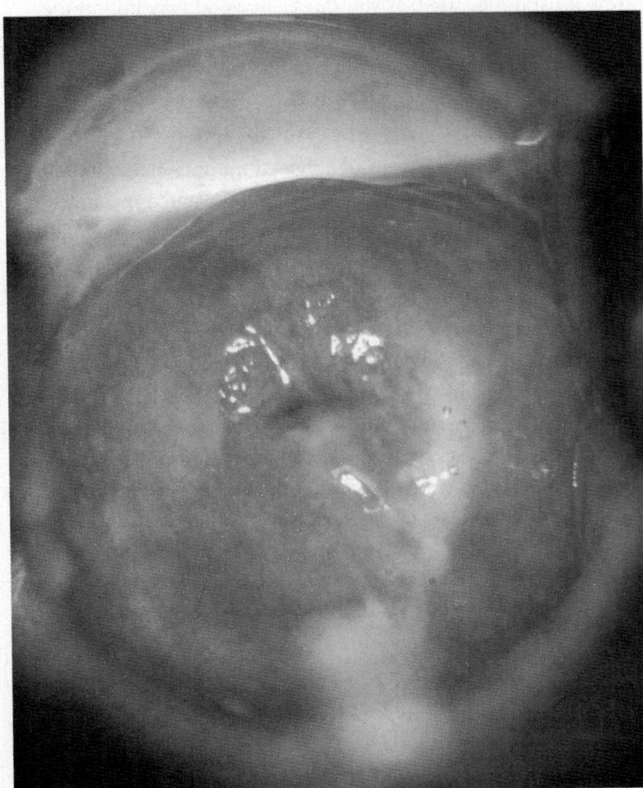

FIGURE 87-3 This patient only complained of a mild discharge. A NAAT test was positive for *Chlamydia*. The rest of her work-up was negative. *(Reproduced with permission from E.J. Mayeaux, Jr., MD.)*

- Persons who have receptive anal intercourse can acquire a rectal infection that presents as anal pain, discharge, or bleeding. Persons who engage in oral sex can acquire a pharyngeal infection that may present as an irritated throat.[8]
- Swab test—A white cotton-tip applicator is placed in the endocervical canal and removed to view. A visible mucopurulent discharge constitutes a positive swab test for *Chlamydia* (**Figure 87-4**). This is not specific for *Chlamydia*, as other genital infections can cause a mucopurulent discharge, and is not recommended for diagnosis.

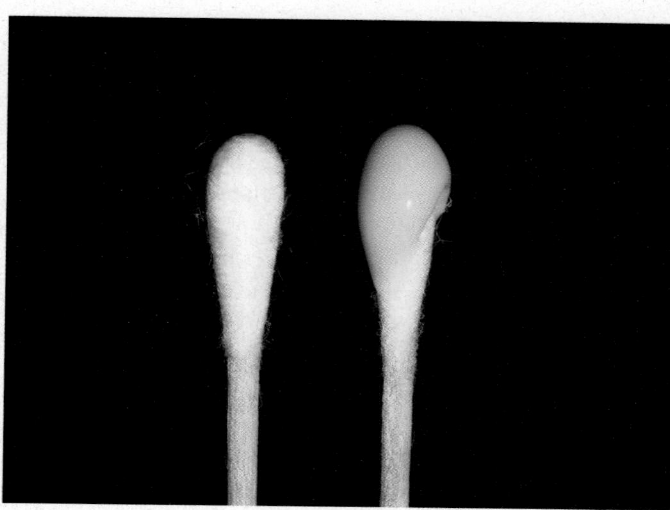

FIGURE 87-4 Mucopurulent discharge on the right swab from a cervix infected with *Chlamydia* (positive swab test). (*Reproduced with permission from Richard P. Usatine, MD.*)

LABORATORY TESTING

- A significant proportion of patients with *Chlamydia* are asymptomatic, providing a reservoir for infection.
- All pregnant women aged <25 years and other women at increased risk for infection (e.g., those who have a new sexual partner, more than one sex partner, a sex partner with concurrent partners, or a sex partner who has a sexually transmitted infection) should be routinely screened for *Chlamydia trachomatis* at the first prenatal visit.[1] Women aged <25 years and those at increased risk for *Chlamydia* also should be retested during the third trimester to prevent maternal postnatal complications and chlamydial infection in the neonate.
- A wet prep is usually negative for other organisms. Only WBCs and normal flora are seen, so the test is not adequate for *Chlamydia*.
- *Chlamydia* cannot be cultured on artificial media because it is an obligate intracellular organism. Tissue culture is required to grow the live organism. When testing for *Chlamydia*, a wood-handled swab must not be used, as substances in wood may inhibit the *Chlamydia* organism. Culture has sensitivity of 70% to 100% and a specificity of almost 100%, which makes it the gold standard.[1]
- The enzyme-linked immunosorbent assay (ELISA) technique (Chlamydiazyme) has a sensitivity of 70% to 100% and a specificity of 97% to 99%.[5] Fluorescein-conjugated monoclonal antibodies test (MicroTrak) has a sensitivity of 70% to 100% and a specificity of 97% to 99%.[5] Because of better sensitivity, nucleic acid amplification techniques (NAATs) testing is preferred.[1]
- *C. trachomatis* can be detected using NAATs on swabs or voided urine specimens. These tests are often used for testing to detect gonorrhea and *Chlamydia*. NAATs have been used successfully in difficult-to-reach adolescents ("street kids") as well as in pediatric emergency departments and school-based settings.[13,14] Screening in school-based settings was associated with significant reduction in *Chlamydia* rates during a 1-year period. Self-collected vaginal swab specimens perform at least as well as with other approved specimens using NAATs.[15] NAATs can be performed on endocervical, urethral, vaginal, pharyngeal, rectal, or urine samples. The accuracy of NAATs on urine samples has been found to be nearly identical to that of samples obtained directly from the cervix.[16]
- Rectal and oropharyngeal *C. trachomatis* infection in persons engaging in anal or oral intercourse can be diagnosed by testing at the site of exposure. Although not FDA-cleared for this use, NAATs have demonstrated improved sensitivity and specificity compared with culture for the detection at rectal sites[17] and at oropharyngeal sites in men.[18] Self-collected rectal swabs are a reasonable alternative to clinician-collected rectal swabs for

C. trachomatis screening by NAAT, especially when clinicians are not available or when self collection is preferred over clinician collection.[1]

- Certain NAATs have been FDA-cleared for use on liquid-based cytology specimens, although test sensitivity using these specimens might be lower.[19]
- Persons who undergo testing for *Chlamydia* should be tested for other STDs as well.[1]

DIFFERENTIAL DIAGNOSIS

- Gonorrhea frequently coexists with *Chlamydia* and should be tested for when a patient is thought to have *Chlamydia*. The discharge of gonorrhea may be more purulent, but this is not always the case.
- Bacterial vaginosis—The aromatic amine odor and clue cells help to distinguish between these infections (Chapter 84, Bacterial Vaginosis).
- Trichomoniasis—Look for the strawberry cervix and *Trichomonas* on the wet prep. There may also be a positive whiff test (see Chapter 86, *Trichomonas* Vaginitis).

MANAGEMENT

NONPHARMACOLOGIC

- Patients diagnosed with *Chlamydia* cervicitis should be tested for other STDs.[1]

MEDICATIONS

FIRST LINE

- **Table 87-1** shows CDC recommended treatments for *Chlamydia*. Azithromycin (Zithromax) 1000 mg one-time dose is easy and may be directly observed in the clinic.[1] SOR Ⓐ It is the first-line therapy for *Chlamydia* during pregnancy.
- Medications for chlamydial infections are best dispensed on site and the first dose directly observed to maximize medication adherence.[1]
- Partners need treatment. The CDC recommends that unless prohibited by law or regulations, medical providers should routinely offer expedited partner therapy (EPT) to heterosexual patients with *Chlamydia* infection when the provider cannot confidently ensure that all of a patient's sex partners from the prior 60 days will be treated.[1] The CDC website contains information on which states allow or prohibit EPT (see Provider Resources below).

SECOND LINE

- Other treatments include doxycycline 100 mg PO bid × 7 days.[1] SOR Ⓐ Avoid dairy products around time of dosing.
- Erythromycin might be less efficacious than either azithromycin or doxycycline, mainly because of the frequent occurrence of GI side effects that can lead to nonadherence.

TABLE 87-1 Centers for Disease Control and Prevention Recommended Regimens SOR Ⓐ

Azithromycin 1 g orally in a single dose
OR
Doxycycline 100 mg orally twice a day for 7 days
CDC Alternative Regimens
Erythromycin base 500 mg orally 4 times a day for 7 days
OR
Erythromycin ethylsuccinate 800 mg orally 4 times a day for 7 days
OR
Ofloxacin 300 mg orally twice a day for 7 days
OR
Levofloxacin 500 mg orally once daily for 7 days
CDC Recommended Regimens in Pregnancy
Azithromycin 1 g orally in a single dose
Alternative Regimens in Pregnancy
Amoxicillin 500 mg orally 3 times a day for 7 days
OR
Erythromycin base 500 mg orally 4 times a day for 7 days
OR
Erythromycin base 250 mg orally 4 times a day for 14 days
OR
Erythromycin ethylsuccinate 800 mg orally 4 times a day for 7 days
OR
Erythromycin ethylsuccinate 400 mg orally 4 times a day for 14 days

Recommendations from the Centers for Disease Control and Prevention. *Sexually Transmitted Diseases Treatment Guidelines, 2015.*[1]

- Ofloxacin (Floxin) 300 mg po bid × 7 days is an alternative that should be taken on an empty stomach.[1] SOR Ⓐ It is contraindicated in children or pregnant and lactating women, but may also cover *Neisseria gonorrhoeae* infection. Levofloxacin 500 mg orally for 7 days is another fluoroquinolone alternative.[1] SOR Ⓐ
- A meta-analysis of 12 randomized clinical trials of azithromycin versus doxycycline for the treatment of genital chlamydial infection demonstrated that the treatments were equally efficacious, with microbial cure rates of 97% and 98%, respectively.[20] SOR Ⓐ
- *C. trachomatis* detected from an oropharyngeal specimen should be treated with azithromycin or doxycycline. The efficacy of other antimicrobial regimens remains unknown.[1]

REFERRAL OR HOSPITALIZATION

- With evidence of complications such as a tuboovarian abscess or severe PID.

PREVENTION

- Individuals who are sexually active should be aware of the risk of STDs and that ways of avoiding infection include mutual monogamy and appropriate barrier protection. Consistent condom and cervical diaphragm use reduces the risk for infection with *Chlamydia*.[1]

PROGNOSIS

- Treatment failures with full primary therapies are quite rare. Reinfection is very common and is related to nontreatment of sexual partners or acquisition from a new partner.

FOLLOW-UP

- Any person who tests positive for *Chlamydia* or gonorrhea, along with women who test positive for *Trichomonas*, should be rescreened 3 months after treatment, regardless of whether they believe that their sex partners were treated.[1] Retesting using NAATs at <3 weeks after completion of therapy is not recommended because of false-positive results resulting from the continued presence of nonviable organisms. Unless prohibited by law or regulations, medical providers should routinely offer expedited partner therapy (EPT) to heterosexual patients with *Chlamydia* infection when the provider cannot confidently ensure that all of a patient's sex partners from the prior 60 days will be treated.[1]
- NAATs test-of-cure to document chlamydial eradication 3–4 weeks after completion of therapy is recommended because severe sequelae can occur in mothers and neonates if the infection persists. If *Chlamydia* is detected during the first trimester, repeat testing for reinfection should also be performed within 3 to 6 months, or in the third trimester.[1]

PATIENT EDUCATION

- To minimize transmission, persons treated for *Chlamydia* should be instructed to abstain from sexual intercourse for 7 days after single-dose therapy or until completion of a 7-day regimen.
- To minimize the risk for reinfection, patients also should be instructed to abstain from sexual intercourse until all of their sex partners are treated.[1]

PATIENT RESOURCES

- eMedicine Health. *Cervicitis*—**http://www.emedicinehealth.com/cervicitis/article_em.htm.**
- eMedicine Health. *Chlamydia*—**http://www.emedicinehealth.com/chlamydia/article_em.htm.**
- CDC patient information—**http://www.cdc.gov/std/Chlamydia/STDFact-Chlamydia.htm.**

PROVIDER RESOURCES

- CDC. *Sexually Transmitted Diseases (STDs) 2015: Diseases Characterized by Urethritis and Cervicitis*—**https://www.cdc.gov/std/tg2015/urethritis-and-cervicitis.htm.**
- *Chlamydial Genitourinary Infections*—**http://emedicine.medscape.com/article/214823-overview.**
- *Cervicitis*—**http://emedicine.medscape.com/article/253402.**
- CDC Expedited Partner Therapy—**https://www.cdc.gov/std/ept/.**

REFERENCES

1. Workowski KA, Bolan GA; Centers for Disease Control and Prevention. Sexually transmitted diseases treatment guidelines, 2015. *MMWR Recomm Rep.* 2015;64(RR-03):1-137.
2. Centers for Disease Control and Prevention. *Sexually Transmitted Disease Surveillance, 2009—Chlamydia.* http://www.cdc.gov/std/stats09/default.htm. Accessed December 2011.
3. World Health Organization. *Chlamydia Trachomatis. Initiative for Vaccine Research.* http://www.who.int/vaccine_research/diseases/soa_std/en/index.html. Accessed December 2011.
4. Centers for Disease Control and Prevention. http://www.cdc.gov/std/Chlamydia/STDFact-Chlamydia.htm. Accessed December 2012.
5. Skolnik NS. Screening for *Chlamydia trachomatis* infection. *Am Fam Physician.* 1995;51:821-826.
6. Forhan SE, Gottlieb SL, Sternberg MR, et al. Prevalence of sexually transmitted infections among female adolescents aged 14 to 19 in the United States. *Pediatrics.* 2009;124:1505.
7. Schillinger JA, Dunne EF, Chapin JB, et al. Prevalence of *Chlamydia trachomatis* infection among men screened in 4 U.S. cities. *Sex Transm Dis.* 2005;32(2):74-77.
8. Mishori R, McClaskey EL, Winkleprins VJ. *Chlamydia trachomatis* infections: screening, diagnosis, and management. *Am Fam Physician.* 2012;86(12):1127-1132.
9. Hu VH, Harding-Esch EM, Burton MJ, et al. Epidemiology and control of trachoma: systematic review. *Trop Med Int Health.* 2010;15(6):673-691.
10. Martius J, Krohn MA, Hillier SL, et al. Relationships of vaginal lactobacillus species, cervical *Chlamydia trachomatis,* and bacterial vaginosis to preterm birth. *Obstet Gynecol.* 1988;71:89-95.
11. Ness RB, Goodman MT, Shen C, Brunham RC. Serologic evidence of past infection with *Chlamydia trachomatis,* in relation to ovarian cancer. *J Infect Dis.* 2003;187:1147-1152.
12. Datta SD, Sternberg M, Johnson RE, et al. Gonorrhea and *Chlamydia* in the United States among persons 14 to 39 years of age, 1999 to 2002. *Ann Intern Med.* 2007;147:89.
13. Monroe KW, Weiss HL, Jones M, Hook EW 3rd. Acceptability of urine screening for *Neisseria gonorrhoeae* and *Chlamydia trachomatis* in adolescents at an urban emergency department. *Sex Transm Dis.* 2003;30:850.

14. Rietmeijer CA, Bull SS, Ortiz CG, et al. Patterns of general health care and STD services use among high-risk youth in Denver participating in community-based urine *Chlamydia* screening. *Sex Transm Dis.* 1998;25:457.

15. Doshi JS, Power J, Allen E. Acceptability of chlamydia screening using self-taken vaginal swabs. *Int J STD AIDS.* 2008;19: 507-509.

16. Cook RL, Hutchison SL, Østergaard L, et al. Systematic review: noninvasive testing for *Chlamydia trachomatis* and *Neisseria gonorrhoeae. Ann Intern Med.* 2005;142(11):914-925.

17. Bachmann LH, Johnson RE, Cheng H, et al. Nucleic acid amplification tests for diagnosis of *Neisseria gonorrhoeae* and *Chlamydia trachomatis* rectal infections. *J Clin Microbiol.* 2010; 48:1827-1832.

18. Bachmann LH, Johnson RE, Cheng H, et al. Nucleic acid amplification tests for diagnosis of *Neisseria gonorrhoeae* oropharyngeal infections. *J Clin Microbiol.* 2009;47:902-907.

19. Chernesky M, Freund GG, Hook E, III, et al. Detection of *Chlamydia trachomatis* and *Neisseria gonorrhoeae* infections in North American women by testing SurePath liquid-based Pap specimens in APTIMA assays. *J Clin Microbiol.* 2007;45:2434-2438.

20. Lau C-Y, Qureshi AK. Azithromycin versus doxycycline for genital chlamydial infections: a meta-analysis of randomized clinical trials. *Sex Transm Dis.* 2002;29:497-502.

SECTION C VULVA

88 PAGET DISEASE OF THE EXTERNAL GENITALIA

E.J. Mayeaux, Jr., MD

PATIENT STORY

A 60-year-old woman presented with vulvar pruritus for 1 year that is now constant. On physical examination, there is one large red lesion surrounded by white epithelium (**Figure 88-1**). A 3-mm punch biopsy was done of the white island within the red lesion using local anesthesia. The pathology showed Paget disease of the vulva. The patient underwent a wide local excision of the involved area and no malignancy was found.

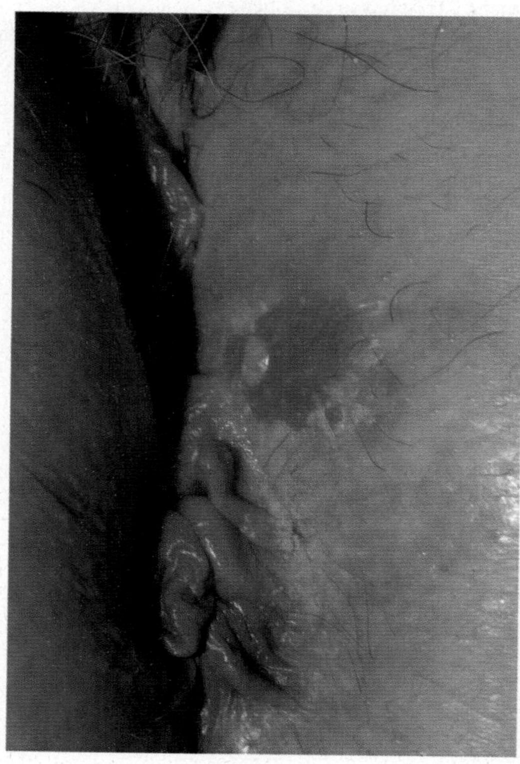

FIGURE 88-1 Paget disease of the vulva. Note the red lesion with the "white island." *(Reproduced with permission from Hope Haefner, MD.)*

INTRODUCTION

Paget disease of the external genitalia is an uncommon primary cutaneous adenocarcinoma of apocrine gland-bearing skin. The most commonly involved site is the vulva, although perineal, perianal, scrotal, and penile skin may also be affected. Less commonly, the axilla, buttocks, thighs, eyelids, and external auditory canal may be found.[1] It is morphologically and histologically identical to Paget disease of the nipple except for the anatomic location.

SYNONYMS

Extramammary Paget disease.

EPIDEMIOLOGY

- The incidence of extramammary Paget disease is approximately is 0.7 per 100,000 persons per year in Europe.[2]
- It accounts for 1–2% of all vulvar malignancies.[2,3]
- The female-to-male ratio is 3 to 4.5 to 1.[4]
- Most patients are white and in their sixth or seventh decade of life.[5]
- Approximately 4% to 25% of patients with genital Paget disease have an underlying neoplasm.[5-7] Associated malignancies include carcinomas of the Bartholin glands, urethra, bladder, vagina, cervix, endometrium, or adnexal apocrine tissue. Only a minority of cases represent a direct extension of an underlying carcinoma.
- Perianal Paget disease (**Figure 88-2**) is associated with underlying colorectal carcinoma in 25% to 35% of cases.

ETIOLOGY AND PATHOPHYSIOLOGY

- Extramammary Paget disease probably arises from apocrine gland tissue, usually as a primary cutaneous adenocarcinoma. The epidermis becomes infiltrated with neoplastic cells showing glandular differentiation. The tumor cells may originate from apocrine gland ducts or from keratinocytic stem cells.

RISK FACTORS

- Extramammary Paget disease should be considered in any patient with chronic dermatitis of the groin, vulva, scrotal, or perianal area. Patients with Paget disease of the external genitalia often present with nonresolving eczematous lesions in the groin, genitalia, perineum, or perianal area.[2,8]

DIAGNOSIS

CLINICAL FEATURES

- Lesions present on the vulva as geographic red macules that often appear excoriated or have an eczematoid appearance (**Figures 88-1** to **88-3**). The lesions are often dotted with small, white patches (islands of tissue). Other lesions may be erythematous, eczematous, or leukoplakic plaques (**Figure 88-4**).[3]
- Pruritus occurs in approximately 70% of patients.[3] Patients may also experience burning, pain, or no symptoms other than the lesion.[7]
- The lesions are well-demarcated and have slightly raised edges.
- Vulvar Paget disease is similar in gross appearance to Paget disease of the breast.

TYPICAL DISTRIBUTION

- It is usually multifocal and may occur anywhere on the vulva, mons, perineum, perianal area, inner thigh, nipple, or bladder. It occurs less often in males (see **Figures 88-3** and **88-4**).

LABORATORY TESTING

- The appearance is similar to superficial melanoma, and sometimes special stains using markers that separate malignant melanocytes from Pagetoid cells may be necessary to identify the correct neoplasm.

IMAGING

- Imaging studies should be used to augment physical and endoscopic examination to assess possible undetected internal malignancy.

BIOPSY

- Biopsy of gross lesions must be performed to determine the diagnosis and the depth and nature of stromal invasion. A punch biopsy should be taken from the center of the lesion and include underlying dermis and connective tissue so the depth of stromal invasion can be determined. If multiple abnormal areas are present, then multiple biopsies should be taken.
- The diagnosis is made by identification of "pagetoid" cells in the epidermis.
    - These cells are round in shape and considerably larger than the surrounding keratinocytes or melanocytes.

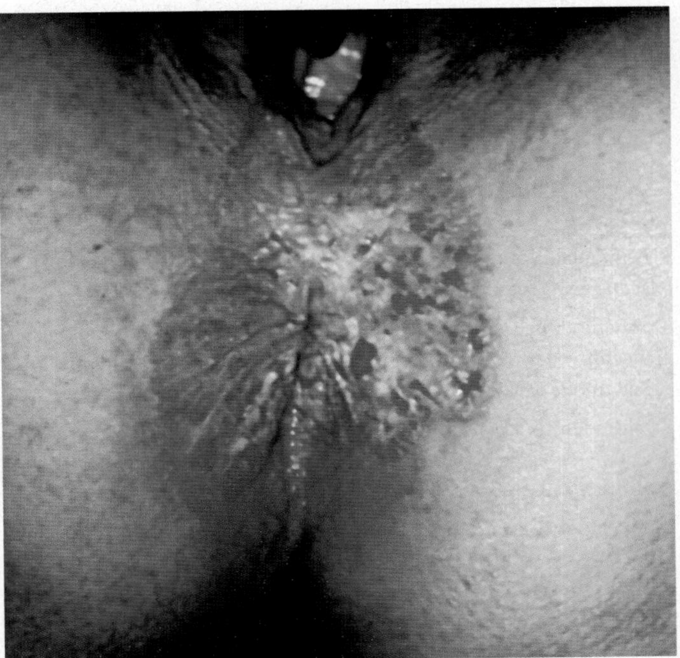

FIGURE 88-2 Perianal Paget disease. Note the appearance is very similar to vulvar Paget disease. *(Reproduced with permission from Richard P. Usatine, MD.)*

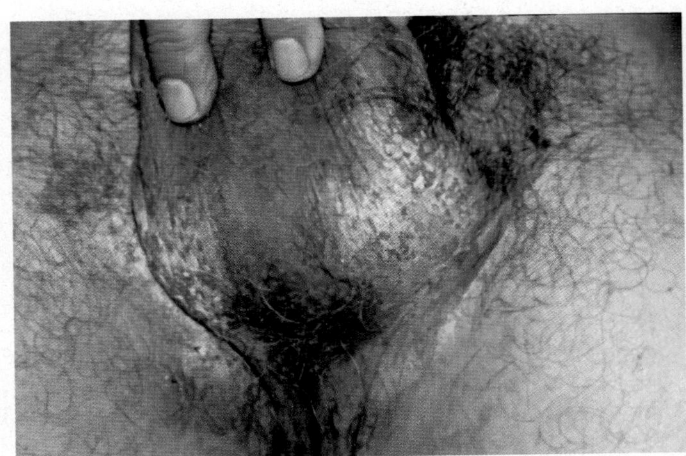

FIGURE 88-3 Paget disease of the scrotum. *(Reproduced with permission from Richard P. Usatine, MD.)*

- The cytoplasm is pink, and the nuclei are large, round, and have prominent nucleoli.
- The pagetoid cells cluster and form small nests in the rete pegs, but single cells spread into the superficial epidermis.

DIFFERENTIAL DIAGNOSIS[3,9]

- Leukoplakia is an elevated white plaque seen before applying of acetic acid (see Chapter 89, Vulvar Intraepithelial Neoplasia).
- Squamous cell carcinoma of the vulva can appear as expanding ulcerative lesions but without the "white islands" (see Chapter 178, Squamous Cell Carcinoma).
- Hidradenitis suppurativa also tends to form in apocrine areas but usually presents as chronic recurring abscesses (see Chapter 121, Hidradenitis Suppurativa).
- Amelanotic melanoma of the vulva can occur, although vulvar melanoma is usually a pigmented lesion with irregular borders. Vulvar melanoma accounts for 5% of primary vulvar neoplasms and occurs predominantly in postmenopausal white women (see Chapter 179, Melanoma).
- Condylomata acuminata (genital condylomas) are common and, when flat or excoriated, may be confused with vulvar Paget disease. More than one third of women have associated cervical intraepithelial neoplasia. Exophytic condylomas are typically verrucous and usually occur in clusters along the vulvar surface (see Chapter 139, Genital Warts).
- Herpes simplex viruses 1 and 2 are associated with ulcerative genital lesions and characteristic systemic symptoms (see Chapter 135, Herpes Simplex).
- Fungal infections commonly affect the vulva and are usually caused by *Candida albicans*. Patients present with vulvar itching and burning. On inspection, the skin surface is red and may demonstrate small satellite lesions. A white "cottage cheese" discharge may also be present. Tinea cruris presents as a reddened area with raised sharp borders that occurs along the inner aspect of the thigh and often extends into the perianal and perineal region (see Chapter 142, Candidiasis).
- Lichen sclerosus is grossly and histologically similar to morphea (circumferential or localized scleroderma), which appears as white sclerotic or atrophic areas (**Figure 88-5**).
- Other dermatoses, including seborrheic or contact dermatitis, psoriasis, lichen planus, and lichen simplex chronicus, can resemble Paget disease when these conditions occur in the vulva or perineum.

MANAGEMENT

FIRST LINE

SURGICAL

- Treatment usually consists either of wide local excision with frozen sections or vulvectomy, if the disease is more extensive.[3,6,7] SOR Ⓑ Local recurrence is common even in the face of negative surgical margins, presumably because the disease tends to be multicentric or from microscopic extension of disease beyond the margins.[6]
- Treatment with Mohs micrographic surgery may have a lower recurrence rate.[9] SOR Ⓑ

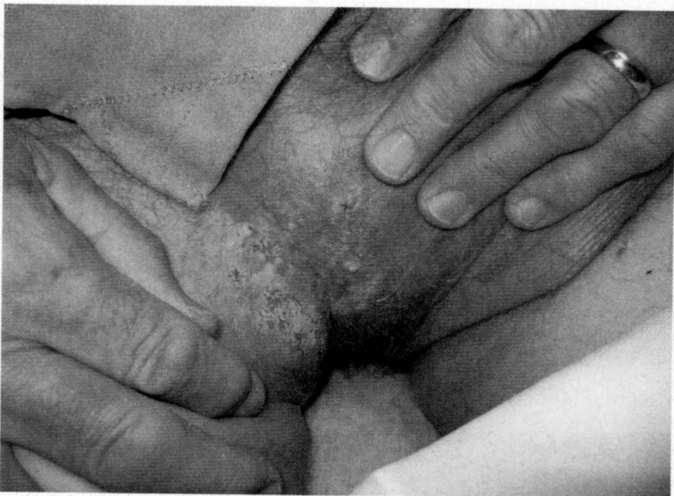

FIGURE 88-4 Paget disease of the scrotum and inguinal area. Note the white plaques with erythema that could be mistaken for *Candida* or tinea. (*Reproduced with permission from Richard P. Usatine, MD.*)

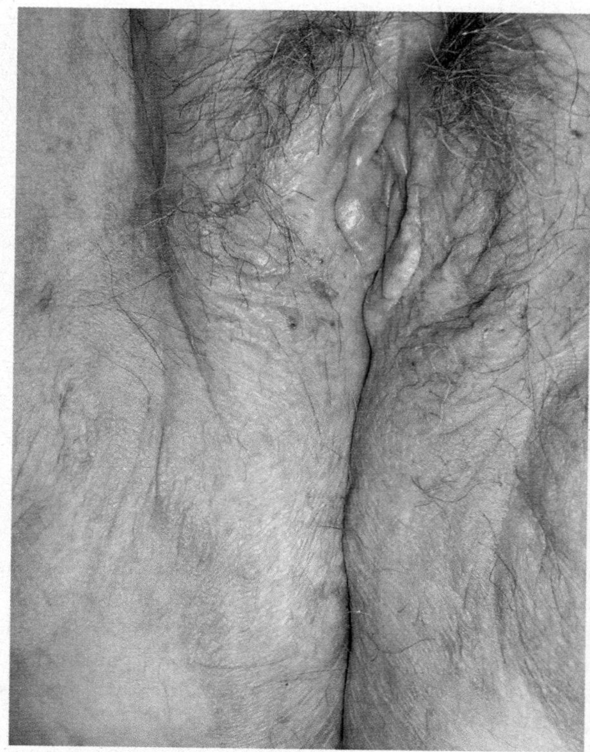

FIGURE 88-5 Lichen sclerosus (et atrophicus) of vulva showing white sclerotic plaques and epidermal atrophy. Note that this is flat and atrophic and lacks the thick white plaques of Paget disease. (*Reproduced with permission from Richard P. Usatine, MD.*)

SECOND LINE

- Topical imiquimod 5% cream applied 3 times weekly for 16 weeks has been shown to induce complete resolution in a patient with perineal disease.[10-12] SOR B However, more studies are needed to define the exact role for this off-label therapy in this disease.
- The role of radiation therapy and chemotherapy (topical and systemic) in the treatment of vulvar Paget disease is not well defined, but may be an option for some patients. SOR C
- Radion therapy is used as a primary treatment option in patients with invasive disease, patients not eligible for surgery, with recurrence after surgery, and as adjuvant postoperative therapy.[2]

PROGNOSIS

- The prognosis for Paget disease of the external genitalia confined to the epidermis is excellent. The rate of invasive malignant conversion is low, and the cutaneous disease may extend over a period of 10 to 15 years without evidence of metastases. The prognosis depends mainly on the early diagnosis with definitive surgical treatment. Full recovery is possible in patients with purely epidermal disease and negative margins after micrographic surgery.
- Perianal disease, male genital disease, dermal invasion, and lymph node metastasis are poor prognostic indicators.[3]
- The recurrence rate of primary tumors after standard surgical excision is 30% to 60%. The rate after excision with Mohs micrographic surgery is 8% to 26%.[9,13]

FOLLOW-UP

- Long-term follow-up is indicated because of the 8% to 60% risk of recurrence (even years after initial therapy) and the increased risk of noncontiguous carcinoma.[9,13]
- The patient's vulva should be inspected annually and biopsy performed with any suggestion of abnormality.
- Screening and surveillance for tumors at other sites (breast, lung, colorectum, gastric, pancreas, and ovary) following national guidelines and U.S. Preventive Services Task Force guidelines should be considered.

PATIENT RESOURCES

- OncoLink. *Paget's Disease of the Vulva*—**https://www.oncolink.org/frequently-asked-questions/cancers/gynecologic/general-concerns/paget-s-disease-of-the-vulva.**
- University of Arkansas for Medical Sciences. *Paget's Disease of the Vulva*—**https://uamshealth.com/medicalservices/womenshealth/gynecologist/vulvar/vulvardisorders/pagetsdisease/.**
- Baylor College of Medicine. *Paget's Disease of the Vulva*—**https://www.bcm.edu/healthcare/care-centers/obstetrics-gynecology/conditions/pagets-disease-vulva.**

PROVIDER RESOURCES

- Medscape. *Extramammary Paget Disease*—**http://emedicine.medscape.com/article/1100397-overview.**
- DermNet NZ. *Extramammary Paget Disease*—**http://dermnetnz.org/site-age-specific/extra-mammary-paget.html.**
- Anton C, da Costa Luiz AV, Carvalho FM, Baracat EC, Carvalho JP. Clinical treatment of vulvar Paget's disease: a case report. **https://www.ncbi.nlm.nih.gov/pmc/articles/PMC3129957/.**
- van der Linden M, Meeuwis KAP, Bulten J, Bosse T, van Poelgeest MIE, de Hullu JA. Paget disease of the vulva. *Critical Reviews in Oncology/Hematology.* 2016;101, 60-74. **http://www.croh-online.com/article/S1040-8428(16)30048-8/abstract.**

REFERENCES

1. Heymann WR. Extramammary Paget's disease. *Clin Dermatol.* 1993;11(1):83-87.
2. van der Linden M, Meeuwis KAP, Bulten J, et al. Paget disease of the vulva. *Crit Rev Oncol Hematol.* 2016;101:60–74.
3. Shepherd V, Davidson EJ, Davies-Humphreys J. Extramammary Paget's disease. *Br J Obstet Gynaecol.* 2005;112:273-279.
4. Chanda JJ. Extramammary Paget's disease: prognosis and relationship to internal malignancy. *J Am Acad Dermatol.* 1985;13(6):1009-1014.
5. Parker LP, Parker JR, Bodurka-Bevers D, et al. Paget's disease of the vulva: pathology, pattern of involvement, and prognosis. *Gynecol Oncol.* 2000;77:183.
6. Fanning J, Lambert HC, Hale TM, et al. Paget's disease of the vulva: prevalence of associated vulvar adenocarcinoma, invasive Paget's disease, and recurrence after surgical excision. *Am J Obstet Gynecol.* 1999;180:24.
7. Bakalianou K, Salakos N, Iavazzo C, et al. Paget's disease of the vulva. A ten-year experience. *Eur J Gynaecol Oncol.* 2008;29(4):368-370.
8. Bagby CM, MacLennan GT. Extramammary Paget's disease of the penis and scrotum. *J Urol.* 2009;182(6):2908-2909.
9. Hendi A, Brodland DG, Zitelli JA. Extramammary Paget's disease: surgical treatment with Mohs micrographic surgery. *J Am Acad Dermatol.* 2004;51:767.
10. Sendagorta E, Herranz P, Feito M, et al. Successful treatment of three cases of primary extramammary Paget's disease of the vulva with Imiquimod—proposal of a therapeutic schedule. *J Eur Acad Dermatol Venereol.* 2010;24(4):490-492.
11. Hatch KD, Davis JR. Complete resolution of Paget disease of the vulva with imiquimod cream. *J Low Genit Tract Dis.* 2008;12(2):90-94.
12. Marchitelli, C, Peremateu MS, Sluga MC, et al. Treatment of primary vulvar Paget disease with 5% imiquimod cream. *J Low Genit Tract Dis.* 2014;18(4):347-350.
13. Coldiron BM, Goldsmith BA, Robinson JK. Surgical treatment of extramammary Paget's disease. A report of six cases and a reexamination of Mohs micrographic surgery compared with conventional surgical excision. *Cancer.* 1991;67(4):933-938.

89 VULVAR INTRAEPITHELIAL NEOPLASIA

E.J. Mayeaux, Jr., MD

PATIENT STORY

A 63-year-old black woman presents with a "knot" on her labia majora (**Figures 89-1** and **89-2**). She is a smoker but is otherwise healthy. The lesion is occasionally pruritic but is generally asymptomatic. She found it approximately 6 months ago, and it has been slowly increasing in size. There is no significant family history of cancer. On physical exam, she is found to have exophytic condyloma acuminata around the introitus and a papule that the patient called a "knot." A 3-mm punch biopsy is performed and demonstrates vulvar intraepithelial neoplasia (VIN) III (high-grade squamous intraepithelial lesion [HSIL]). The patient is referred to gynecologic oncology.

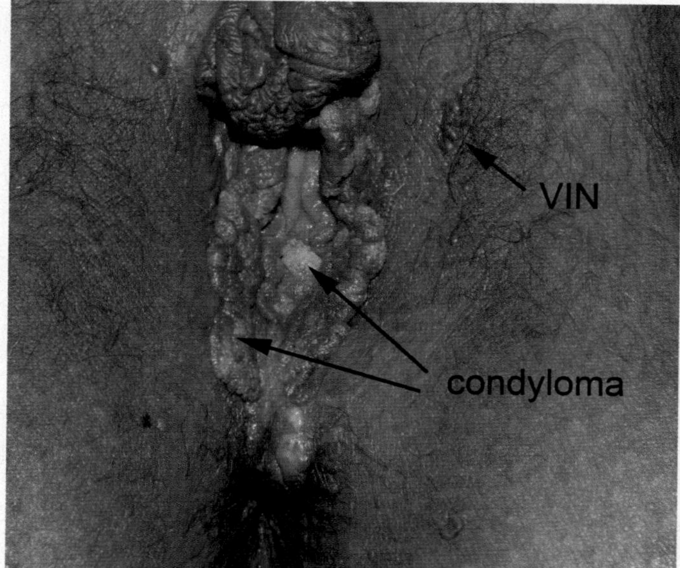

FIGURE 89-1 Patient with multiple exophytic condyloma and vulvar intraepithelial neoplasia III. The large clitoral hood is an incidental finding unrelated to the vulvar intraepithelial neoplasia. *(Reproduced with permission from Hope Haefner, MD.)*

INTRODUCTION

Vulvar intraepithelial neoplasia is a premalignant condition of the vulva. Vulvar dysplasia and cancer are less common than cervical cancer. It is associated with high-risk human papillomavirus (HPV) infection, but not to the same extent as cervical disease.

In the 2004 International Society for the Study of Vulvar Diseases nomenclature, VIN was broken into two main categories[1]:

- VIN usual type—Dysplasia highly associated with high-risk HPV infection. There is no evidence that what was previously called VIN I is a cancer precursor, so the term VIN was restricted to high-grade lesions (formerly termed VIN II and VIN III) in which treatment to prevent progression to cancer is indicated.[2] The term condyloma acuminatum is now used for lesions previously referred to as VIN I.
- VIN differentiated type—Lesions that are not high-risk HPV associated and have a worse prognosis.

In 2012, the Lower Anogenital Squamous Terminology (LAST) project of the American Society for Colposcopy and Cervical Pathology and the College of American Pathology described changes in the terminology in which condyloma acuminatum is referred to as vulvar low-grade squamous intraepithelial lesion (LSIL) and VIN II, III is referred to as vulvar HSIL.[3]

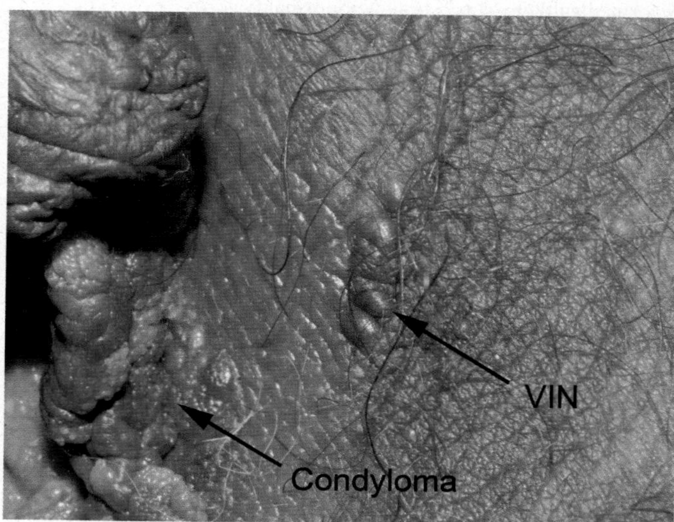

FIGURE 89-2 Close-up of the same patient with vulvar intraepithelial neoplasia III on the labia majora. *(Reproduced with permission from Hope Haefner, MD.)*

EPIDEMIOLOGY

- Vulvar cancer is the fourth most common gynecologic cancer (following cancer of the endometrium, ovary, and cervix) and accounts for 5% of lower female genital tract malignancies.[4] There are approximately 3900 new cases and 870 deaths each year in the United States from this disease.[4]
- Worldwide, vulvar cancer is rare, especially in developing countries. Approximately 27,000 cases are reported annually, making the incidence rate between 1 and 1.5 per 100,000 women.[5]
- Seventy-five percent of VIN cases occur in premenopausal women, with no racial predisposition.

- Although the rate of invasive vulvar carcinoma has remained stable in the past two decades, the incidence of in situ disease (VIN) has more than doubled. This may be the result of improved surveillance and treatment of VIN, or the apparent increase in cases of VIN in younger women.[6]
- VIN usual type is most commonly found in the interlabial grooves, posterior fourchette, and perineum and is often multifocal. Confluent or multifocal lesions exist in up to two-thirds of women with VIN.[7]
- VIN differentiated type comprises less than 5% of VIN and typically occurs in postmenopausal women. It is most commonly unifocal and unicentric and is often associated with lichen sclerosus. Differentiated VIN is probably a precursor of HPV-negative vulvar cancer.[8]

ETIOLOGY AND PATHOPHYSIOLOGY

- VIN is the associated preneoplastic condition that is associated with the loss of epithelial cell maturation and nuclear abnormalities.
- The cervix, vagina, vulva, anus, and lower 3 cm of rectal mucosa are derived from the embryonic cloaca. Most squamous intraepithelial lesions in this area affect multiple anatomic sites.
- HPV 16 is estimated to contribute to approximately 77% of VIN usual lesions.[9]
- The risk of neoplastic progression appears to be lower with VIN than with cervical intraepithelial neoplasia. VIN I has minimal malignant potential, but VIN III often progresses to invasive cancer if left untreated (see "Biopsy" below).[10]

RISK FACTORS[11]

- Risk factors are similar to those for vaginal and cervical dysplasia:
  - High-risk HPV infection
  - Cigarette smoking
  - Altered immune status
  - Lichen sclerosus (VIN differentiated)

DIAGNOSIS

CLINICAL FEATURES

- The vulva is best examined using a good source of white light and magnification from a handheld magnifying lens or a colposcope. The examination should be systematic and incorporate all aspects of the vulvar surface. Vulvar examination may be aided by dilute acetic acid solution, which acts on the vulva much the same way as it does on the cervix and vagina. More acetic acid solution and a longer soaking time are required to achieve the acetowhite effect.
- VIN often appears as raised plaques and papules on the surface of the vulva and perineum (see **Figures 89-1** and **89-2**).
- Approximately one quarter of these lesions are pigmented (usually brown).
- Fifty percent of VINs are white (leukoplakia) or become acetowhite after soaking with dilute acetic acid (**Figure 89-3**).
- Lesions may occasionally be red and ulcerate (**Figure 89-4**). White areas may also indicate malignant changes (**Figures 89-5** and **89-6**).

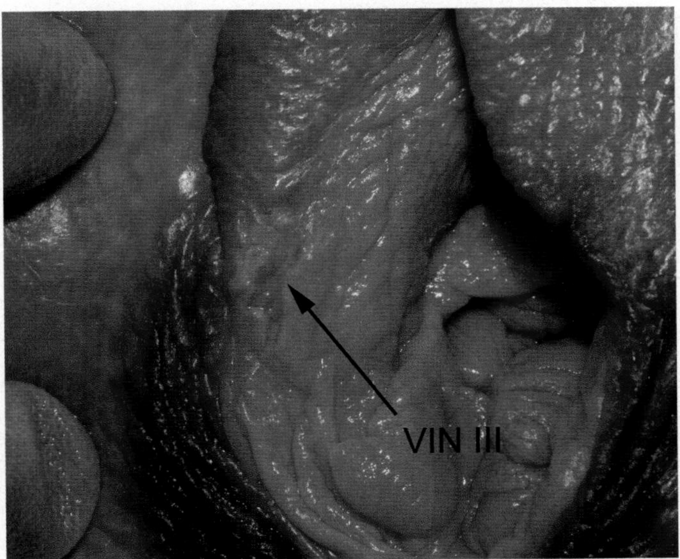

FIGURE 89-3 Diffuse white vulvar intraepithelial neoplasia III with ulceration. (*Reproduced with permission from Hope Haefner, MD.*)

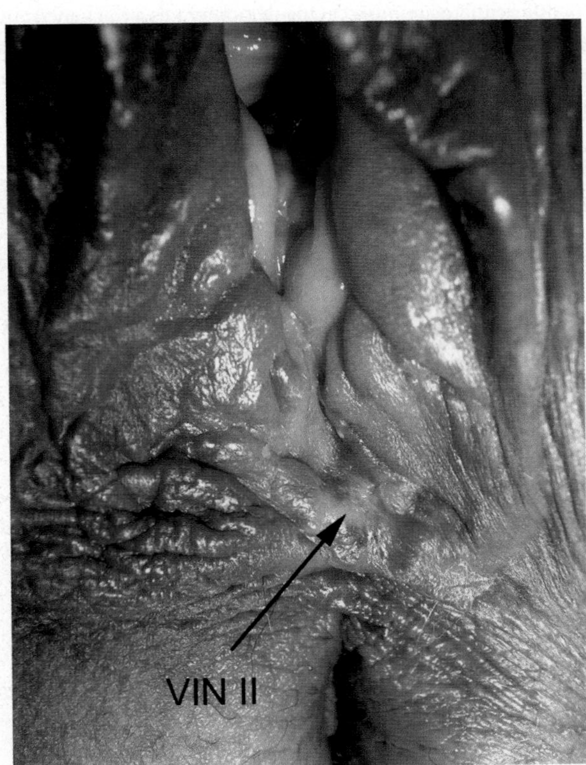

FIGURE 89-4 A small painful ulcer turned out to be vulvar intraepithelial neoplasia II on punch biopsy. A 3-mm punch biopsy was performed on the edge of the ulcer. (*Reproduced with permission from Richard P. Usatine, MD.*)

- VIN can appear warty, so lesions that are diagnosed as condyloma but do not respond to conservative therapy should be biopsied to rule out VIN.
- More than 40% of patients presenting with vulvar dysplasia are without symptoms. Of patients with symptoms, pruritus is the most common.[12]
- Lesions may become confluent, involving the labia majora, minora, and perianal skin.

TYPICAL DISTRIBUTION

- Unlike cervical intraepithelial neoplasia, VIN is usually multifocal and can be located throughout the vulva, anus, and perineum. The interlabial grooves, posterior fourchette, and perineum are the most frequent locations (see **Figures 89-1** to **89-6**).

BIOPSY

- Tissue biopsy is necessary for a definitive diagnosis of abnormal or ambiguous areas. After infiltration with lidocaine and epinephrine, 3-mm punch biopsies are performed in all suspicious areas. Bleeding can be stopped with a chemical hemostatic agent or electrocautery. Small biopsy sites usually do not need to be sutured and will heal well by secondary intention, although pain may be reduced by suturing. Areas of ulceration should be sampled along the edge (see **Figure 89-4**).
- On histology, VIN usual may be graded as condyloma, VIN II (moderate dysplasia), or VIN III (severe dysplasia, carcinoma in situ) based on the depth of epithelial involvement. VIN II and III is now preferentially be reported as HSIL.
- VIN differentiated (simplex) type demonstrates a thickened epithelium with elongated and anastomosing rete ridges. The atypia is confined to the parabasal and basal portion of the rete pegs. The lower cell layers usually stain positively for p53.[13]

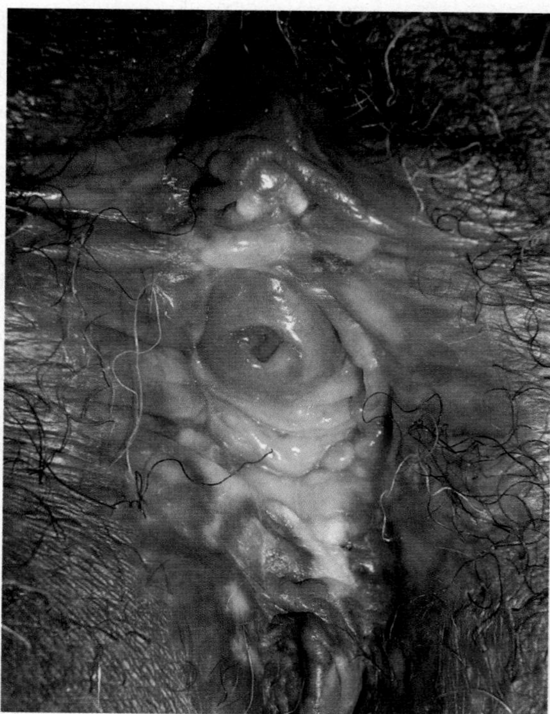

FIGURE 89-5 A 59-year-old woman with long history of condyloma presents with a vaginal irritation. In addition to her cystocele after her hysterectomy, she is found to have *Trichomonas* and evidence of atrophic changes. However, the most concerning areas are the leukoplakia at the 6-, 11-, and 12-o'clock positions. These are most suspicious for vulvar intraepithelial neoplasia. (*Reproduced with permission from Richard P. Usatine, MD.*)

DIFFERENTIAL DIAGNOSIS

- Micropapillae of the inner labia minora have commonly been misinterpreted as being secondary to HPV. Micropapillomatosis is a condition in which the vestibular papillae are atypically prominent. It is a benign normal variant.
- Sebaceous hyperplasia may be found as multiple small yellowish papules from Hart line (junction of the keratinized skin and mucosa) to the junction of the hair-bearing skin. This is a benign condition.
- HPV causes condylomata acuminata (genital condyloma). More than one third of women have associated cervical intraepithelial neoplasia. Exophytic condylomas are typically verrucous and usually occur in clusters. They can be found at any site along the vulvar surface, and diagnosis is usually made by their characteristic appearance (see Chapter 139, Genital Warts).
- Herpes simplex viruses 1 and 2 produce grouped vesicles and ulcers and are associated with genital lesions (see Chapter 135, Herpes Simplex).
- Molluscum contagiosum lesions appear as small papules with central umbilicated cores that contain a cheesy material (see Chapter 136, Molluscum Contagiosum).

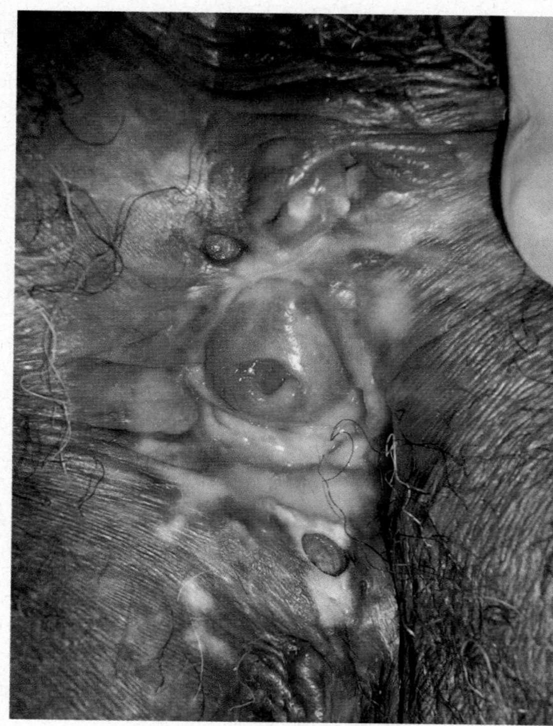

FIGURE 89-6 The woman in **Figure 89-5** after punch biopsies are performed of the most suspicious areas. Both biopsies show moderate epithelial dysplasia, vulvar intraepithelial neoplasia II along with associated human papillomavirus changes. (*Reproduced with permission from Richard P. Usatine, MD.*)

- Secondary syphilis usually appears as a gray, plaque-like lesion (condyloma lata) (see Chapter 225, Syphilis).
- Granuloma inguinale produces small red lesions that appear from 3 weeks to 3 months after inoculation. These evolve into erosive ulcerations resulting in fibrosis and loss of superficial labial structures.
- Fungal infections commonly affect the vulva and are usually caused by *Candida albicans*. Patients present with vulvar itching and burning. On inspection, the skin surface is red and may demonstrate small satellite lesions. A white "cottage cheese" discharge may also be present (see Chapter 85, *Candida* Vulvovaginitis).
- Tinea cruris presents as a reddened area with raised sharp borders that occurs along the inner aspect of the thigh and often extends into the perianal and perineal region (see Chapter 145, Tinea Cruris).
- Lichen sclerosus is grossly and histologically similar to morphea (circumferential or localized scleroderma) and appears as white atrophic patches with erythema and loss of hair. Areas suspicious for VIN should be biopsied (**Figure 89-7**).
- Other dermatoses including psoriasis, lichen planus, and lichen simplex chronicus may present on the vulva and be confused with VIN.
- Nevi are benign melanocytic skin tumors that may occur in any area of the body, including the vulva.

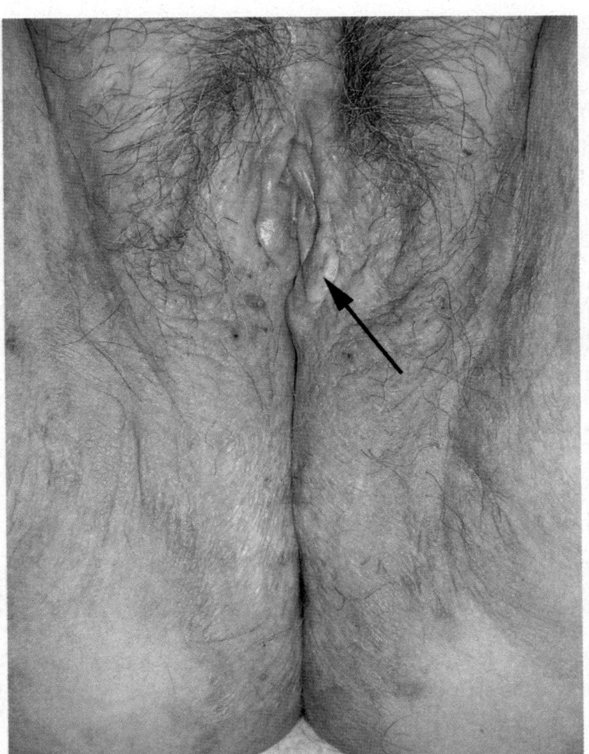

FIGURE 89-7 A 55-year-old woman with lichen sclerosus (et atrophicus). A biopsy was taken at the site indicated by the arrow to confirm the diagnosis and make sure that there was no vulvar intraepithelial neoplasia arising in that area. (*Reproduced with permission from Richard P. Usatine, MD.*)

MANAGEMENT

NONPHARMACOLOGIC

- If the biopsy reveals condyloma, either observation or treatment with topical medications or surgical modalities (see Chapter 139, Genital Warts). Patients with VIN I can be followed by close observation.[14] SOR Ⓐ

MEDICATIONS

- Imiquimod cream is a topical immune response modifier that is FDA-approved for the treatment of anogenital warts, actinic keratosis, and certain basal cell carcinomas.[15] It has been used to treat multifocal VIN II or III in a few small pilot studies. The cream is self-administered 3 times per week for periods of 6 to 34 weeks.[15] SOR Ⓑ
- 5-Fluorouracil (5-FU) cream has been a traditional treatment for VIN that causes a chemical desquamation of the lesion.[16] It may result in significant burning, pain, inflammation, edema, and occasional painful ulcerations. Biopsy to exclude invasive disease is mandatory prior to 5-FU treatment.[16] SOR Ⓑ

SURGICAL

- Wide surgical excision is the primary treatment for VIN II or III. VINs may be treated with ablation on non–hair-bearing epithelium. Colposcopy guided CO_2 laser is most commonly performed, although some providers perform a loop electrosurgical excision procedure.[14] SOR Ⓑ
- Differentiated VINs and any lesions in hair-bearing areas are generally treated with a wide local excision. Resected VIN specimens should be examined for residual disease in the margin.[17] SOR Ⓑ

PREVENTION

- The bivalent vaccine (Cervarix) , the quadrivalent (Gardasil) vaccine, and the 9-valent vaccine (Gardasil) all prevent infection by HPV 16 and 18 and are effective at preventing VIN when given prophylactically. Vaccine efficacy against any VIN lesion (regardless of HPV type) in HPV-naïve patients was 75% (22% to 94%).[18]

PROGNOSIS

- Surgical excision success is dependent on margin status. Most recurrences will occur within 2 years.
- The frequency of recurrence after vulvectomy, partial vulvectomy, local excision, and laser ablation was 19, 18, 22, and 23% respectively.[19]

FOLLOW-UP

- Because of the potential for disease persistence and recurrence, patients should be followed every 6 months for at least a year after treatment.[14]

PATIENT EDUCATION

- The diagnosis of high-grade dysplasia of the lower genital tract confers an increased risk of additional dysplasias and cancers for at least 20 years.[20] Continuing surveillance is necessary.

PATIENT RESOURCES

- Oncolink. *Vulvar Cancer*—**https://www.oncolink.org/frequently-asked-questions/cancers/gynecologic/vulvar-cancer.**
- International Society for the Study of Vulvovaginal Disease. *Vulvar Cancer*—**http://www.issvd.org/document_library/VulvarCancer.pdf.**
- Cancer Research UK. *Vulval Intraepithelial Neoplasia (VIN)*—**http://www.cancerresearchuk.org/about-cancer/vulval-cancer/stages-types-grades/vulval-intraepithelial-neoplasia.**
- Patient.info. *Vulval Intraepithelial Neoplasia*—**https://patient.info/health/vulval-intraepithelial-neoplasia.**

PROVIDER RESOURCES

- Pathology Outlines. Usual type vulvar intraepithelial neoplasia (uVIN)—www.pathologyoutlines.com/topic/vulvaVIN.html.
- eMedicine. *Malignant Vulvar Lesions*—**http://emedicine.medscape.com/article/264898-overview.**
- ACOG. *Management of Vulvar Intraepithelial Neoplasia*—**https://www.acog.org/Resources-And-Publications/Committee-Opinions/Committee-on-Gynecologic-Practice/Management-of-Vulvar-Intraepithelial-Neoplasia.**

REFERENCES

1. Sideri M, Jones RW, Wilkinson EJ, et al. Squamous vulvar intraepithelial neoplasia: 2004 modified terminology, ISSVD Vulvar Oncology Subcommittee. *J Reprod Med.* 2005;50:807.
2. Committee on Gynecologic Practice of American College Obstetricians and Gynecologists. ACOG Committee Opinion No. 509: Management of vulvar intraepithelial neoplasia. *Obstet Gynecol.* 2011;118:1192.
3. Waxman AG, Chelmow D, Darragh TM, et al. Revised terminology for cervical histopathology and its implications for management of high-grade squamous intraepithelial lesions of the cervix. *Obstet Gynecol.* 2012;120(6):1465-1471.
4. Jemal A, Murray T, Ward E, et al. Cancer statistics, 2005. *CA Cancer J Clin.* 2005;55:10-30.
5. Ferlay J, Shin HR, Bray F, et al. Estimates of worldwide burden of cancer in 2008: GLOBOCAN 2008. *Int J Cancer.* 2010;127(12): 2893-2917.
6. Sturgeon SR, Brinton LA, Devesa SS, Kurman RJ. In situ and invasive vulvar cancer incidence trends (1973-87). *Am J Obstet Gynecol.* 1992;166:1482-1485.
7. Friedrich EG Jr, Wilkinson EJ, Fu YS. Carcinoma in situ of the vulva: a continuing challenge. *Am J Obstet Gynecol.* 1980;136:830.
8. Roma AA, Hart WR. Progression of simplex (differentiated) vulvar intraepithelial neoplasia to invasive squamous cell carcinoma: a prospective case study confirming its precursor role in the pathogenesis of vulvar cancer. *Int J Gynecol Pathol.* 2007;26:248.
9. Insinga RP, Liaw KL, Johnson LG, Madeleine MM. A systematic review of the prevalence and attribution of human papillomavirus types among cervical, vaginal, and vulvar precancers and cancers in the United States. *Cancer Epidemiol Biomarkers Prev.* 2008; 17(7):1611-1622.
10. Jones RW, Rowan DM. Vulvar intraepithelial neoplasia III: a clinical study of the outcome in 113 cases with relation to the later development of invasive vulvar carcinoma. *Obstet Gynecol.* 1994; 84:741-745.
11. Modesitt SC, Waters AB, Walton L, et al. Vulvar intraepithelial neoplasia III: occult cancer and the impact of margin status on recurrence. *Obstet Gynecol.* 1998;92:962-966.
12. van Seters M, van Beurden M, de Craen AJ. Is the assumed natural history of vulvar intraepithelial neoplasia III based on enough evidence? A systematic review of 3322 published patients. *Gynecol Oncol.* 2005;97:645.
13. Fox H, Wells M. Recent advances in the pathology of the vulva. *Histopathology.* 2003;42:209.
14. Haefner H, Mayeaux EJ Jr. Vulvar abnormalities. In: Mayeaux EJ Jr, Cox T, eds. *Modern Colposcopy*, 3rd ed. Philadelphia, PA: Lippincott Williams & Wilkins; 2011:432-471.
15. Le T, Menard C, Hicks-Boucher W, et al. Final results of a phase 2 study using continuous 5% imiquimod cream application in the primary treatment of high-grade vulva intraepithelial neoplasia. *Gynecol Oncol.* 2007;106:579-584.
16. Krupp PJ, Bohm JW. 5-fluorouracil topical treatment of in situ vulvar cancer. A preliminary report. *Obstet Gynecol.* 1978;51:702-706.

17. Di Saia PJ, Rich WM. Surgical approach to multifocal carcinoma in situ of the vulva. *Am J Obstet Gynecol.* 1981;140:136-145.
18. The FUTURE I/II Study Group; Dillner J, Kjaer SK, Wheeler CM, et al. Four year efficacy of prophylactic human papillomavirus quadrivalent vaccine against low grade cervical, vulvar, and vaginal intraepithelial neoplasia and anogenital warts: randomised controlled trial. *BMJ.* 2010;340:c3493.
19. van Seters M, van Beurden M, de Craen AJ. Is the assumed natural history of vulvar intraepithelial neoplasia III based on enough evidence? A systematic review of 3322 published patients. *Gynecol Oncol.* 2005;97:645.
20. Soutter WP, Sasieni P, Panoskaltsis T. Long-term risk of invasive cervical cancer after treatment of squamous cervical intraepithelial neoplasia. *Int J Cancer.* 2006;118:2048-2055.

SECTION D COLPOSCOPY

90 COLPOSCOPY: NORMAL AND NONCANCEROUS FINDINGS

E.J. Mayeaux, Jr., MD

PATIENT STORY

A 21-year-old woman presents for her well-woman examination. She has been followed by her provider for many years and has no complaints. She has been sexually active for a little more than 2 years with one mutually monogamous partner. She does not smoke, has never had a sexually transmitted disease (STD), and uses oral contraceptive pills for contraception. On speculum examination, her cervix appears normal (**Figure 90-1**) and a Papanicolaou (Pap) test is performed.

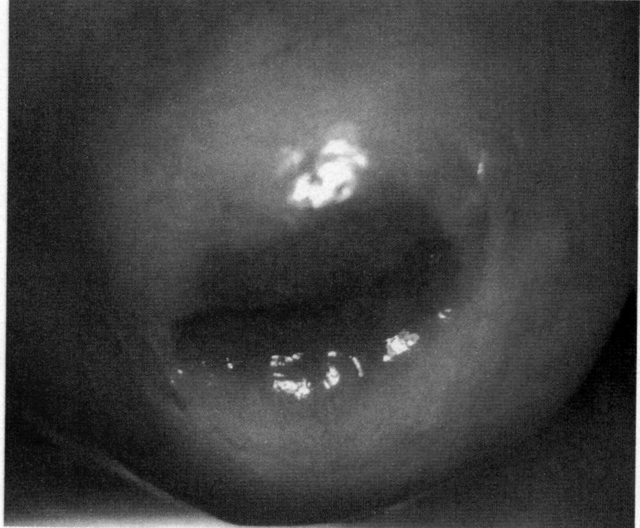

FIGURE 90-1 Normal cervix as seen through a colposcope without the application of vinegar. The red color around the os is produced by columnar cells and the lighter pink on the remainder of the cervix result from normal squamous cells. The presence of visible columnar cells outside the internal os is called ectropion and is a normal finding in young women and women on estrogen-containing contraception. The junction between the two cell types and colors is the squamo-columnar junction. (*Reproduced with permission from E.J. Mayeaux, Jr., MD.*)

INTRODUCTION

The colposcope is an optical instrument using light and magnification that helps distinguish dysplasia and cancer from benign cervical and vaginal findings (**Figure 90-2**). Colposcopy (*colpo:* vagina; *scope:* to look) literally means to look into the vagina. Primary indications for colposcopy include certain abnormal Pap test results or an abnormal appearing cervix. Colposcopically directed biopsies have a higher yield than biopsies done without the benefit of a colposcope, thereby decreasing the risk of false-negative biopsies.

SYNONYMS

- Nabothian cysts are also called mucinous retention cysts or epithelial cysts.
- An ectropion is also known as a persistent juvenile transformation zone or cervical erosion.

EPIDEMIOLOGY

- Colposcopy is the diagnostic test to evaluate patients with an abnormal cervical screening test (cytology and/or human papillomavirus high-risk HPV [HR-HPV] testing) or abnormal-appearing cervix. The Papanicolaou test (Pap smear, Pap test) is a commonly employed screening test for dysplasia and cancer of the vagina and uterine cervix. More than 50 million Pap tests are performed each year in the United States.[1] The Pap test is a cytologic examination of cells taken from the cervical transformation zone (**Figures 90-3** and **90-4**) with or without a HR-HPV test.

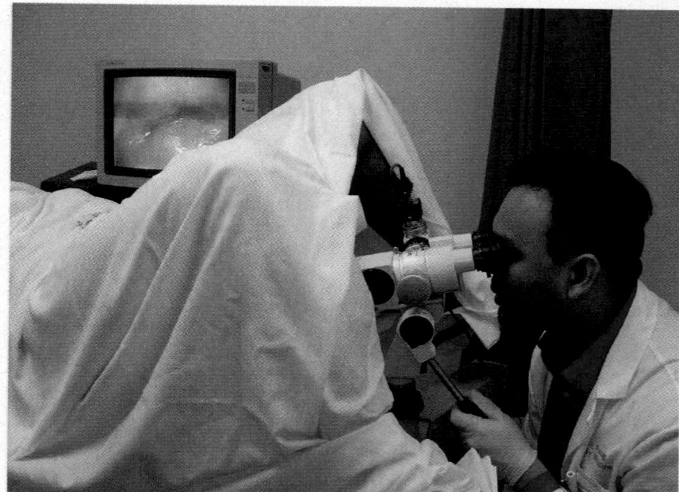

FIGURE 90-2 The family physician is looking at the cervix directly through the colposcope lenses, and the image is also visible on the monitor for learners and/or the patient to see. (*Reproduced with permission from E.J. Mayeaux, Jr., MD.*)

- Nabothian cysts are common and benign and are considered a normal feature of the adult cervix. They may occur singly, or multiple cysts may be found simultaneously (**Figures 90-4** and **90-5**).[2]
- Infections of the lower female genital tract are common and can produce a number of cervical epithelial changes (**Figure 90-6**).
- Cervical epithelial atrophy may occur in hypoestrogenic states and cause the cervix to appear pale and the squamocolumnar junction to retract into the cervical os (**Figure 90-7**).
- Endocervical polyps are the most common benign neoplasms of the uterine cervix (**Figures 90-7** and **90-8**) and are most commonly found incidentally during pelvic examination. They are most common in the fourth to sixth decades of life and usually are asymptomatic, but may cause vaginal discharge or postcoital spotting.[3] Most polyps are benign, with the incidence of malignancy being approximately 1 in 1000.[4] Endocervical polyps must be differentiated from endometrial polyps (**Figure 90-9**), which may look similar. Endometrial polyps are often associated with additional endometrial polyps and sometimes with neoplasia, so they are removed using hysteroscopy or endometrial curettage.

ETIOLOGY AND PATHOPHYSIOLOGY

- Colposcopy entails the use of a field microscope to examine the cervix and vagina. The cervix and vagina are examined under magnification, and all abnormal areas are identified.
- If the cervical colposcopy is satisfactory, the entire transformation zone (TZ) is examined and the extent of all lesions is visualized (see **Figure 90-3**). Directed biopsies of the most abnormal areas are performed to obtain a tissue diagnosis.
- Colposcopy begins after visualization of the cervix prior to application of acetic acid to look for leukoplakia and abnormal vessels. Acetic acid 3% to 5% is applied with a cotton ball held in a ring forceps or with a rectal swab. Scan the cervix with low power (typically 5×) and determine if the entire TZ, including the entire squamocolumnar junction (SCJ), can be seen. The borders of all lesions must be entirely visible (not disappearing into the canal) for the examination to be adequate.
- Most of the normal cervical findings are derived from the physiologic transformation of the exposed columnar epithelium to squamous epithelium (see **Figures 90-1** and **90-3**). Noncancerous findings may include epithelial thinning and whitening as a result of lack of estrogen, and polyp formations. The damage to the cervical epithelium from various infections often produces inflammation, friability, discharge, and bleeding.

DIAGNOSIS

CLINICAL FEATURES

- Normal colposcopic findings include[5]:
  - Original squamous epithelium, which is a featureless, smooth, pink epithelium without gland openings or nabothian cysts (see **Figure 90-4**).
  - Columnar epithelium is a single-cell layer, mucus-producing epithelium that extends between the endometrium and the

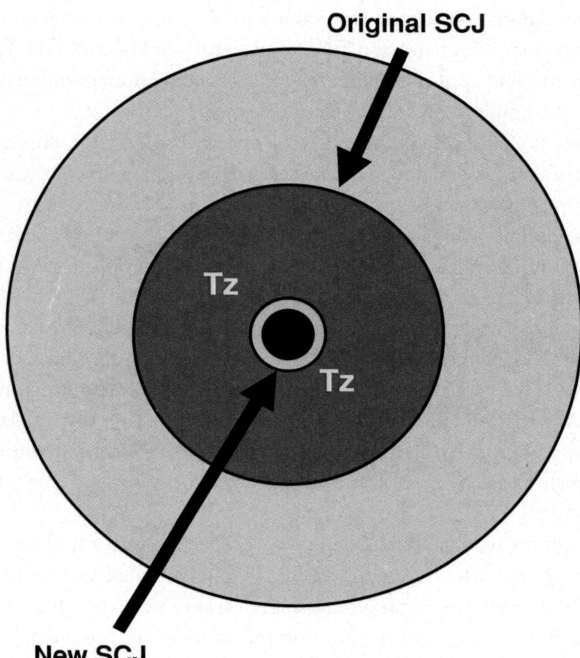

FIGURE 90-3 Schematic demonstration of the development of the transformation zone. The transformation zone extends from the original (prepubertal) squamocolumnar junction to the new (current) squamocolumnar junction. This transformation zone is the area at highest risk for cervical cancer. (*Reproduced with permission from E.J. Mayeaux, Jr., MD.*)

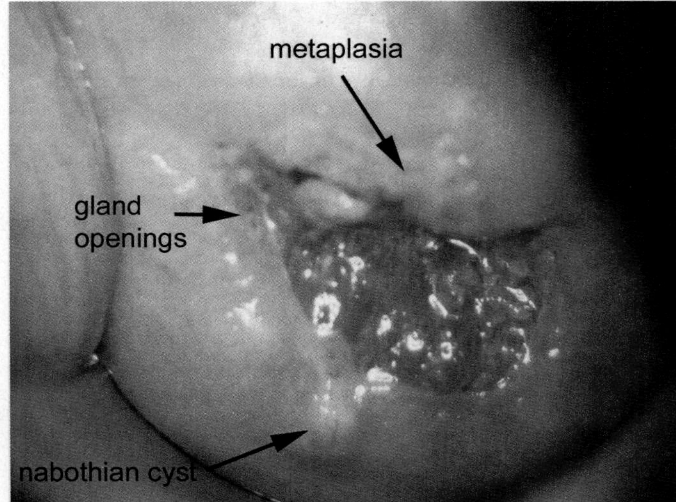

FIGURE 90-4 Normal transformation zone viewed with colposcopy. Note the squamocolumnar junction separating the red columnar epithelium from the pink squamous epithelium. Gland openings, nabothian cysts, and metaplasia are all part of this normal transformation zone. There is a white area of normal metaplasia on the anterior lip and a yellowish nabothian cyst on the posterior lip. (*Reproduced with permission from E.J. Mayeaux, Jr., MD.*)

squamous epithelium. Columnar epithelium appears red and irregular with stromal papillae and clefts (see **Figure 90-4**). With acetic acid application and magnification, columnar epithelium has a grapelike or "sea-anemone" appearance.
  - SCJ is a clinically visible line seen on the ectocervix or within the distal canal, which demarcates endocervical tissue from squamous (or squamous metaplastic) tissue (see **Figure 90-4**).
  - Squamous metaplasia is the physiologic, normal process whereby columnar epithelium transforms into squamous epithelium. At the SCJ, it appears as a "ghostly white" or white-blue film with the application of acetic acid. It is usually sharply demarcated toward the cervical os and has very diffuse borders peripherally (see **Figure 90-4**).
  - TZ is the geographic area between the original squamous epithelium (before puberty) and the current SCJ. It may contain gland openings, nabothian cysts, and islands of columnar epithelium surrounded by metaplastic squamous epithelium (see **Figures 90-3** and **90-4**).
  - In some women, the juvenile type TZ persists into adulthood or is present after trauma or childbirth and is termed an ectropion (**Figure 90-10**). It has a reddish appearance similar to granulation tissue. Ectropion is common in adolescents, pregnant women, and those taking estrogen-containing contraceptives. Although it is usually asymptomatic, vaginal discharge and postcoital bleeding may occur.[6]
- Other nondysplastic colposcopic findings:
  - Nabothian cysts are normal areas of mucus-producing epithelium that are "roofed over" with squamous epithelium (see **Figures 90-4** and **90-5**). They may appear translucent or opaque, whitish to yellow, and can range from a few millimeters to several centimeters in size. They always occur in the cervical TZ. They are usually asymptomatic and do not require any treatment.[2]
  - Cervicitis from an infection may make colposcopic assessment for dysplasia and cervical cancer difficult. Cervicitis appears as friable, inflamed epithelium, often in the presence of a vaginal discharge. *Trichomonas* may cause an inflamed cervix that has a strawberry appearance (see **Figure 90-6** and Chapter 86, *Trichomonas* Vaginitis).
  - Atrophic vaginal or cervical epithelium is frequently white and easily traumatized (see **Figure 90-7** and Chapter 83, Atrophic Vaginitis).
  - Cervical polyps (see **Figures 90-7** and **90-8**) are focal benign hyperplastic protrusions of the endocervical folds. They usually appear as polypoid growths protruding for the cervical os.[3]

BIOPSY

- The colposcope is used to examine the cervix for signs of dysplasia or cancer before performing cervical biopsies (see Chapters 91, Colposcopy of Low-Grade Lesions; 92, Colposcopy of High-Grade Lesions; and 93, Colposcopy of Cervical Cancer, for details of suspicious colposcopic findings).

DIFFERENTIAL DIAGNOSIS

- Friability from infections must be differentiated from dysplastic changes by a history of possible exposure to STDs, presence of discharge, wet prep, and STD testing.

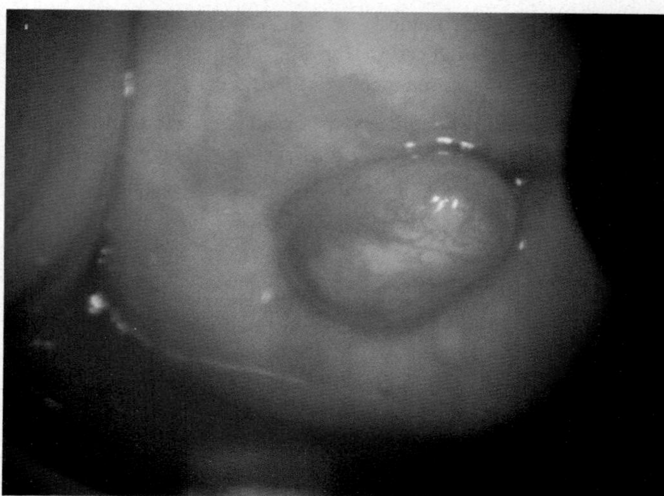

FIGURE 90-5 Colposcopic view of a large polypoid Nabothian cyst. Note the typical yellowish color and dilated vessels. (*Reproduced with permission from E.J. Mayeaux, Jr., MD.*)

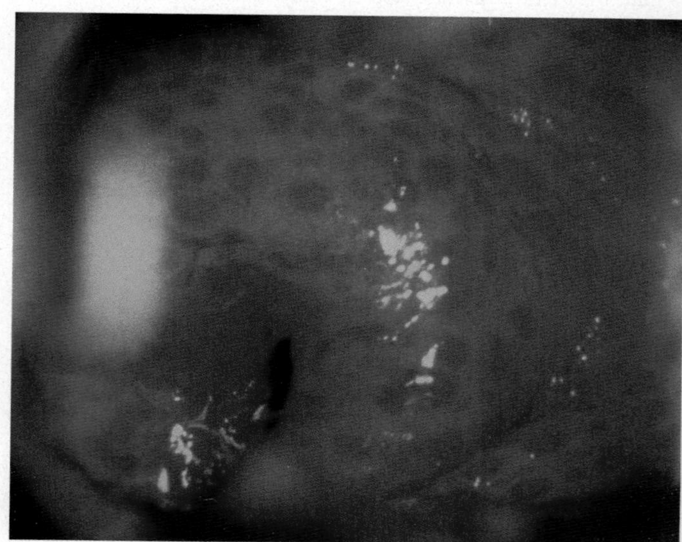

FIGURE 90-6 Colposcopic view of *Trichomonas* infection. Note disruption of the epithelium with petechiae and pinpoint bleeding producing the "strawberry" cervix. (*Reproduced with permission from E.J. Mayeaux, Jr., MD.*)

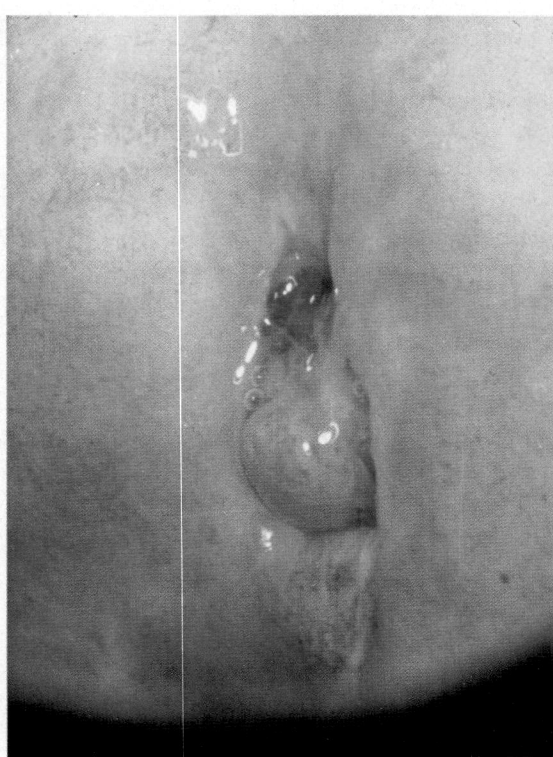

FIGURE 90-7 Colposcopic view of cervical atrophy and a benign endocervical polyp in a postmenopausal woman. Note the pale epithelium and the polyp extending from the cervical os. (*Reproduced with permission from E.J. Mayeaux, Jr., MD.*)

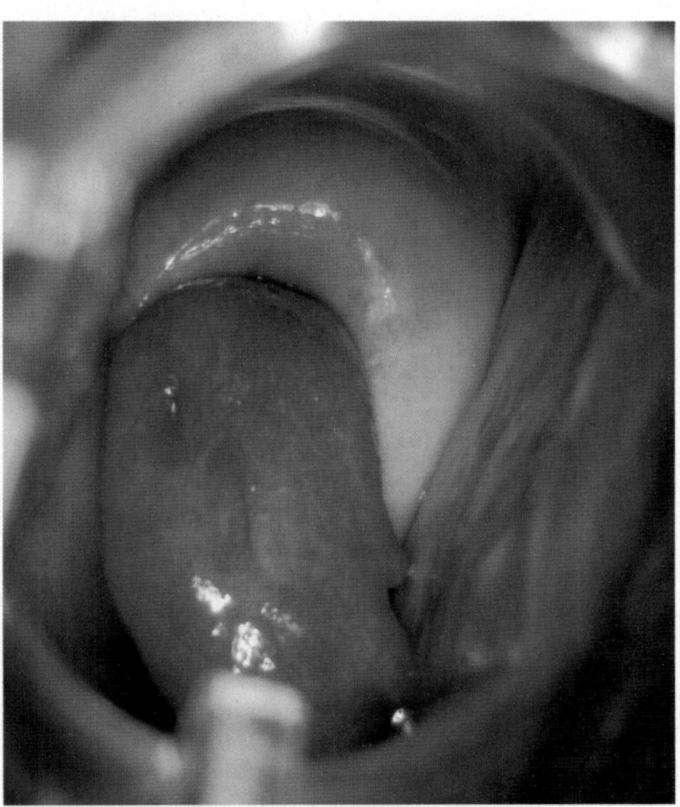

FIGURE 90-9 A large endometrial polyp extending through the os. These polyps are typically removed in conjunction with hysteroscopy or dilatation and curettage because they frequently have a large blood supply and may be associated with additional lesions. (*Reproduced with permission from E.J. Mayeaux, Jr., MD.*)

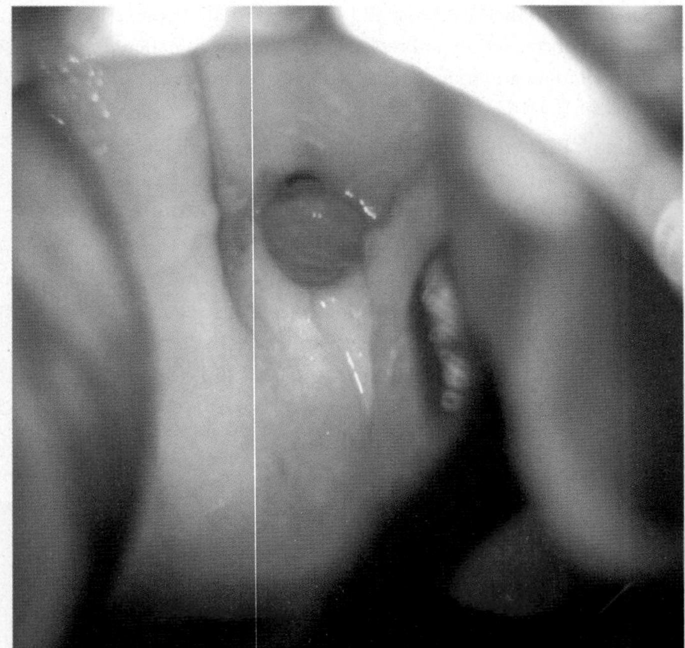

FIGURE 90-8 Colposcopic view of an endocervical polyp. Ring forceps were used to identify the base of the polyp, and after the polyp was found to be arising from the wall of the cervical canal, it was twisted off without complications. (*Reproduced with permission from E.J. Mayeaux, Jr., MD.*)

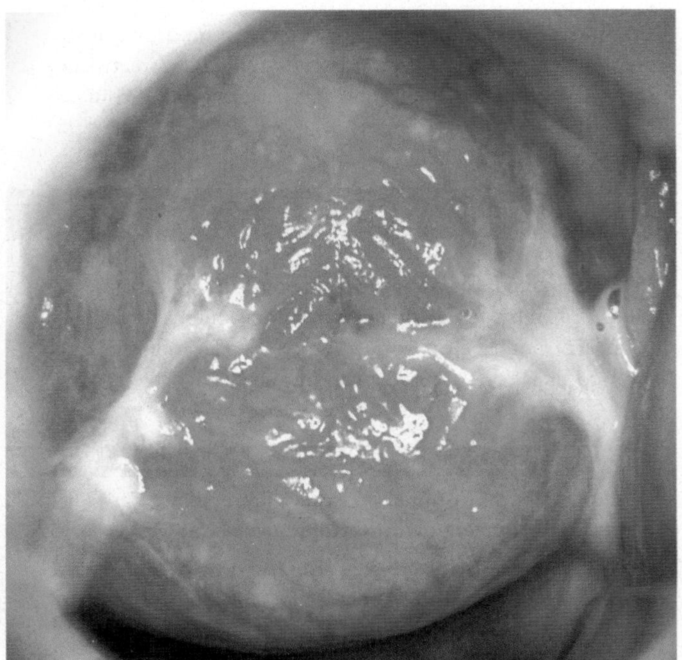

FIGURE 90-10 Colposcopic view of an ectropion. This patient was 22 years of age, but her cervix had the appearance of the cervix of a younger female. She was asymptomatic. (*Reproduced with permission from E.J. Mayeaux, Jr., MD.*)

MANAGEMENT

NONPHARMACOLOGIC

- Nabothian cysts do not require any treatment. If you tell patients that they have a Nabothian cyst, please tell them that this is a normal finding.

MEDICATIONS

- Atrophic vaginal or cervical epithelium can be treated with intravaginal estrogen for 2 to 4 weeks before colposcopy in order to "normalize" the epithelium. SOR Ⓒ This is generally safe, even if dysplasia or cancer is present, because the duration of therapy is short, and these lesions do not express any more estrogen receptors than a normal cervix.[7]
- Vaginocervicitis is treated with anti-infectives once the source is diagnosed.
- Treatment for cervical polyps is removal by twisting the polyp with ringed forceps. Smaller polyps may be removed with colposcopy biopsy forceps. Polyps with a thick stalk may require surgical or electrosurgical removal. If polyps are removed after a recently abnormal Pap test, the polyp should be sent for analysis, as dysplasia may be found on the polyp.[8]
- Cervical dysplastic changes should be handled according to national evidence-based guidelines (see Chapters 91, Colposcopy of Low-Grade Lesions; and 92, Colposcopy of High-Grade Lesions).[9]
- An ectropion may be treated with ablation (such as cervical cryotherapy) if significant discharge or postcoital bleeding is present, and after dysplasia and cancer have been ruled out.[2]

FOLLOW-UP

- If an infection coexists with an abnormal Pap smear or grossly abnormal-appearing cervix, the infection should be treated and the colposcopic assessment should be performed approximately 1 month later.

PATIENT EDUCATION

- Patients should be discouraged from douching, as it irritates the mucous membranes, disrupts normal flora, and makes acquisition of an STD more likely if exposed. Safer-sex education should be given to all patients at risk of acquiring an STD.

PATIENT RESOURCES

- National Cancer Institute. *Cervical Cancer: Patient Version*—**http://www.cancer.gov/cancertopics/screening/cervical.**
- WebMD. *What's a Colposcopy?*—**http://www.webmd.com/cancer/cervical-cancer/do-i-need-colposcopy-and-cervical-biopsy.**
- MedlinePlus. *Nabothian Cyst*—**http://www.nlm.nih.gov/medlineplus/ency/article/001514.htm.**
- MedlinePlus. *Cervical Polyps*—**https://medlineplus.gov/ency/article/001494.htm.**

PROVIDER RESOURCES

- ASCCP (formerly the American Society for Colposcopy and Cervical Pathology). Includes colposcopy and treatment algorithms—**http://www.asccp.org.**
- Medscape. *Colposcopy*—**http://emedicine.medscape.com/article/265097.**
- Merck Manual Professional Version. *Cervical Polyps*—**http://www.merckmanuals.com/professional/gynecology-and-obstetrics/benign-gynecologic-lesions/cervical-polyps.**

REFERENCES

1. Sirovich BE, Welch HG. The frequency of Pap smear screening in the United States. *J Gen Intern Med.* 2004;19:243-250.
2. Casey PM, Long ME, Marnach ML. Abnormal cervical appearance: what to do, when to worry? *Mayo Clin Proc.* 2011;86(2):147-150.
3. Aaro LA, Jacobson LJ, Soule EH. Endocervical polyps. *Obstet Gynecol.* 1963;21:659-665.
4. Schnatz PF, Ricci S, O'Sullivan DM. Cervical polyps in postmenopausal women: is there a difference in risk? *Menopause.* 2009;16(3):524-528.
5. Stafl A, Wilbanks GD. An international terminology of colposcopy: report of the nomenclature committee of the International federation of cervical pathology and colposcopy. *Obstet Gynecol.* 1991;77:313-314.
6. Goldacre MJ, Loudon N, Watt B, et al. Epidemiology and clinical significance of cervical erosion in women attending a family planning clinic. *Br Med J.* 1978;1(6115):748-750.
7. Sadan O, Frohlich RP, Driscoll JA, et al. Is it safe to prescribe hormonal contraception and replacement therapy to patients with premalignant and malignant uterine cervices? *Gynecol Oncol.* 1986;34:159-163.
8. Chin N, Platt AB, Nuovo GJ. Squamous intraepithelial lesions arising in benign endocervical polyps: a report of 9 cases with correlation to the Pap smears, HPV analysis, and immunoprofile. *Int J Gynecol Pathol.* 2008;27(4):582-590.
9. Massad LS, Einstein MH, Huh WK, et al.; 2012 ASCCP Consensus Guidelines Conference. 2012 updated consensus guidelines for the management of abnormal cervical cancer screening tests and cancer precursors. *J Low Genit Tract Dis.* 2013;17(5 suppl 1):S1-S27.

91 COLPOSCOPY OF LOW-GRADE LESIONS

E.J. Mayeaux, Jr., MD

PATIENT STORY

A 23-year-old woman has a low-grade squamous intraepithelial lesion on her Papanicolaou (Pap) test. One colposcopic view of her cervix shows acetowhite changes consistent with a cervical intraepithelial neoplasia grade 1 lesion (CIN 1) (**Figure 91-1**). She has no other suspicious findings and biopsy of the acetowhite area confirms CIN 1. The endocervical sampling is negative for neoplastic disease. During the follow-up visit, the doctor and patient together decide to proceed with watchful waiting and repeat Pap and human papillomavirus (HPV) co-testing at 12 and 24 months.

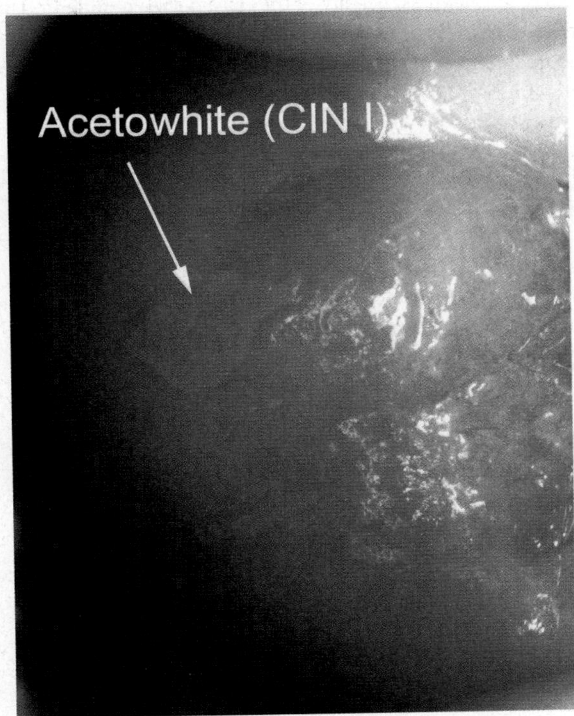

FIGURE 91-1 Colposcopic view of acetowhite changes on the cervix of cervical intraepithelial neoplasia grade 1 lesions after the application of acetic acid. Note the irregular geographic borders. (*Reproduced with permission from E.J. Mayeaux, Jr., MD.*)

INTRODUCTION

Our knowledge of the genesis and development of cervical cancer has grown greatly over the last 30 years. It was once believed that HPV infection and CIN 1 disease were the first steps in cancer formation. We now know that HPV infection and CIN 1 are essentially the same thing and will resolve without treatment in most immunocompetent women. Which women will progress to high-grade dysplasia or cancer is not completely understood.

EPIDEMIOLOGY

- In low-grade squamous intraepithelial lesion (LSIL) Pap tests, the abnormalities are typically associated with HPV infection and are histologically called CIN grade 1 lesions.[1] Overall rates of Pap test abnormalities are often estimated from regional studies. For example, in an observational cohort study of routine cervical tests in the northwestern United States, in women of all ages (n = 150,052), atypical squamous cells was diagnosed at a rate of 9.8 per 1000, LSIL was diagnosed at a rate of 3.5 per 1000, and negative routine tests occurred at a rate of 278.5 per 1000.[2]
- In HPV vaccine age groups, there have been significant reductions in the CIN incidence per 100,000 women screened for all grades of CIN. In female individuals 15 to 19 years old, the incidence of CIN 1 dropped from 3468.3 to 1590.6 per 100,000, for CIN 2 from 896.4 to 414.9, and for CIN 3 from 240.2 to 0 per 100,000.[3]

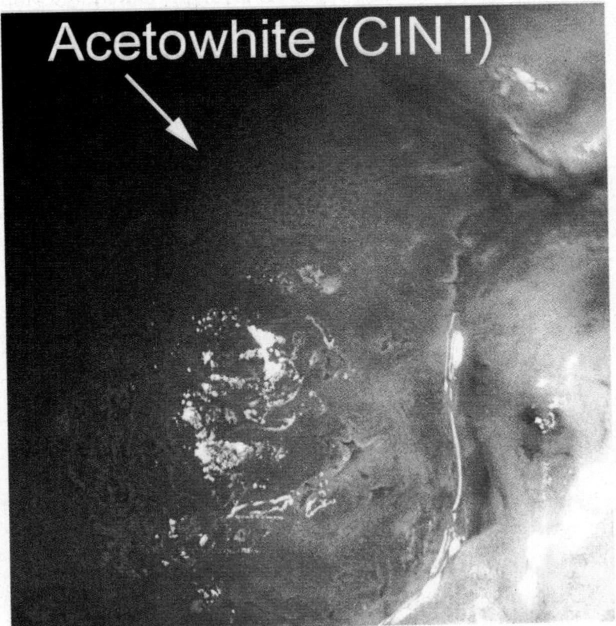

FIGURE 91-2 Another colposcopy view of acetowhite changes on the cervix of cervical intraepithelial neoplasia grade 1 lesions. (*Reproduced with permission from E.J. Mayeaux, Jr., MD.*)

ETIOLOGY AND PATHOPHYSIOLOGY

- Essentially all CIN is caused by HPV. Ten percent to 15% of CIN 1 lesions will also develop CIN 2-3, and 0.3% will eventually develop cervical cancer.[4]
- There is no way to determine which CIN 1 lesions (**Figures 91-1** to **91-3**) or simple HPV lesions (**Figures 91-4** and **91-5**) will develop high-grade disease.

- Colposcopy is the standard of care for assessing abnormal cervical cancer screening tests and cervical dysplasia. It entails the use of a field microscope to examine the cervix after acetic acid (see **Figures 91-1** to **91-4**) and sometimes Lugol iodine are applied (see **Figure 91-5**).
- An atypical transformation zone is defined as a transformation zone with findings suggesting cervical dysplasia or neoplasia. Differences in thickness, density of the cells, degree of differentiation, and keratin production determine the color and opacity of the epithelium and may produce the abnormal findings of leukoplakia and acetowhite epithelium.

RISK FACTORS

- Sexual intercourse.
- Other types of sexual activity including digital/anal, oral/anal, and digital/vaginal contact.
- Immunosuppression.

DIAGNOSIS

CLINICAL FEATURES

- The diagnosis of low-grade cervical abnormalities is made on colposcopic examination. Findings consistent with this diagnosis include[1]:
  - Acetowhite changes (see **Figures 91-1** to **91-4**). A transient, white-appearing epithelium following the application of 3%–5% acetic acid may be abnormal and correlates with higher nuclear density. The more sharp and angular the margin is, the likelier it is to be dysplastic. The margins of low-grade disease are usually feathery or geographic borders. Most low-grade lesions are snowy white with a shiny surface that rapidly fades. Condylomatous changes including a papillary surface are often indicative of low-grade or HPV disease.[4]
  - Punctation is a stippled appearance of small looped capillaries seen end-on, often found within an acetowhite area, appearing as fine-to-coarse red dots. Superficial bridging of these vessels produces a mosaic pattern. Fine punctation and mosaicism has fine-caliber vessels that are regularly spaced and is usually associated with benign conditions or low-grade disease (see **Figures 91-3** and **91-4**).[4]
  - Lack of iodine staining (Schiller test) may be used when further clarification of potential biopsy sites is necessary (see **Figure 91-5**). It need not be used in all cases. The sharp outlining afforded by Lugol solution can be dramatic and very helpful.

LABORATORY TESTING[5]

- Screening and management strategies provide similar management strategies for similar levels of risk of high-grade dysplasia.[6,7]
- Cervical cytology (Pap testing) is the time-tested standard for screening and prevention of cervical cancer.
- Pap test screening is not recommended for females younger than the age of 21 years.[6] Pap test screening is recommended with 3-year cytology intervals for women ages 21 to 29 years.[6]

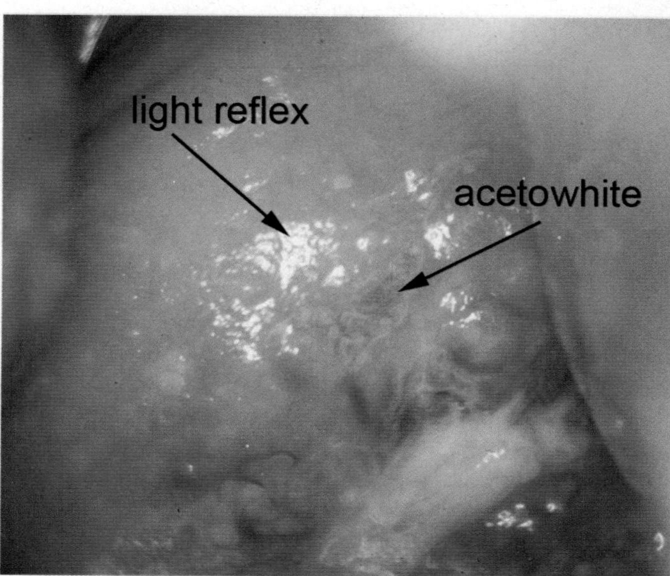

FIGURE 91-3 Colposcopy view of an indistinct acetowhite lesion on the anterior lip. Note the light reflex just above the lesion that may be confused with an actual lesion. (*Reproduced with permission from E.J. Mayeaux, Jr., MD.*)

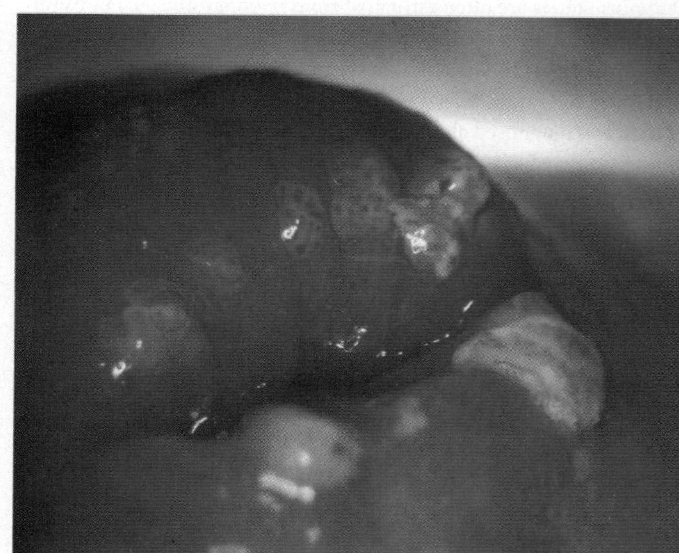

FIGURE 91-4 Colposcopy view of condyloma of the cervix. Note the bright acetowhite effect that is common on condyloma. (*Reproduced with permission from E.J. Mayeaux, Jr., MD.*)

- Cervical cancer screening is recommended for women ages 30 to 64 years with 3-year cytology intervals, 3-year high-risk human papillomavirus (HRHPV) intervals, or 5-year co-testing intervals.[6]
- Screening women ages 65 years and older is not recommended in low-risk women. Women who have a history of CIN 2+, VaIN 2+, AIN 2+, or VIN 2+ should continue cervical or vaginal screening for at least 20 years. Other risk factors include HIV infection and other immunosuppression.
- Women with an unsatisfactory cytology result should have repeat cytology in 2–4 months regardless of any HRHPV results. Colposcopy is recommended for women with two consecutive unsatisfactory Pap results. Women with cytology reported as negative but with absent or insufficient EC/transition zone do not have a higher risk for CIN 3+ over time and so are managed the same as women with negative results.[6]
- High-risk HPV testing (mainly HPV types 16, 18, 31, 33, 35, 39, 45, 51, 52, 56, 58, and 59) can be used to further define a patient's risk for dysplasia and cancer after an atypical squamous cell (ASC) Pap result. For women 30 years of age and older with HRHPV-positive but cytology-negative results should have repeat co-testing in 1 year. Patients with ASC and a positive high-risk HPV test should be triaged to immediate colposcopy and patients with a negative HPV test may be triaged to re-Pap in 3 years. Women ages 21–24 years with atypical squamous cells of undetermined significance (ASC-US) Pap results should have a repeat Pap test in 12 months.[6]

BIOPSY

- Biopsy is usually indicated to establish the histologic grade of the abnormalities present. The report of the ASCCP Colposcopy Standards Committee recommends multiple biopsies targeting all areas with acetowhitening, metaplasia, or higher abnormalities. Usually, at least 2 and up to 4 targeted biopsies from distinct acetowhite lesions should be taken. Nontargeted biopsies are not recommended for women referred to colposcopy at the lowest end of risk, that is, those with less than high-grade squamous intraepithelial lesion (HSIL) cytology, no evidence for HPV-16/-18, and a completely normal colposcopic impression (i.e., no acetowhitening, metaplasia, or other visible abnormality).[8]

DIFFERENTIAL DIAGNOSIS

- CIN 1 and HPV lesions must be differentiated from nonmalignant inflammatory lesions such as yeast vaginitis and sexually transmitted diseases, which usually present with vaginal itching, odor, and/or discharge (see Chapter 85, *Candida* Vulvovaginitis).
- High-grade dysplasia (CIN 2 and CIN 3) and cancer must also be ruled out, usually by colposcopic examination and biopsy (see Chapter 92, Colposcopy of High-Grade Lesions).

MANAGEMENT

NONPHARMACOLOGIC

- According to the 2012 consensus guidelines, women with CIN 1 or no lesion on colposcopy preceded by a screening test with lesser abnormalities (HPV-16 or HPV-18 positivity only, persistent

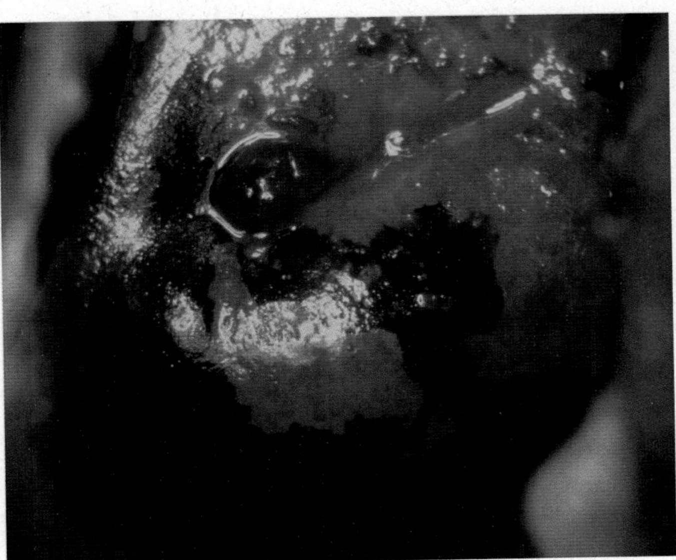

FIGURE 91-5 Colposcopic view of a cervix after Lugol solution is applied. The abnormal cervical intraepithelial neoplasia grade 1 lesion is the area on the cervix that does not stain brown with the iodine in the Lugol solution. The areas that do not stain can then be biopsied. This is called the Schiller test. (*Reproduced with permission from E.J. Mayeaux, Jr., MD.*)

untyped oncogenic HPV, ASC-US, and LSIL) should have co-testing at 1 year. If CIN 1 persists for at least 2 years, either continued follow-up or treatment is acceptable.[5,6] SOR B Most cases of CIN 1 spontaneously regress.

- Women with CIN 1 or no lesion preceded by ASC-H or HSIL should be managed with either a diagnostic excisional procedure or observation with co-testing at 12 months and 24 months if the colposcopic examination is adequate and the endocervical sampling is negative.[6]
- Observation without treatment is acceptable in pregnant women with CIN 1 and in women with unsatisfactory colposcopy.[4,5] SOR B
- If CIN 1 is detected on endocervical sampling after lesser abnormalities, management should follow ASCCP management guidelines for CIN 1, with the addition of repeat endocervical sampling in 12 months.[6]
- If someone younger than the age of 21 years is inappropriately screened, observation without treatment is the recommended follow-up for CIN 1 disease.[6]
- Cytology reported as negative for malignant cells but lacking endocervical cells can be managed without early repeat Pap testing.[6]
- CIN 1 on endocervical curettage should be managed as CIN 1, not as a positive ECC.[6]
- HPV genotyping triages HPV-positive women with HPV type 16 or type 18 to earlier colposcopy only after negative cytology; colposcopy is indicated for all women with ASC-US HPV+ regardless of genotyping result.[6]
- For ASC-US cytology, immediate colposcopy is not an option. The serial cytology option for ASC-US incorporates cytology at 12 months, not 6 months and 12 months, and then, if negative, cytology every 3 years.[6]
- ASC-US HPV-negative results should be followed with HRHPV co-testing at 3 years rather than 5 years.[6]
- Women with LSIL cytology and no HPV test or a positive HPV test should have colposcopy. If contesting shows HPV-negative LSIL, repeat co-testing at 1 year is preferred but colposcopy may be performed.[6] SOR A

COMPLEMENTARY AND ALTERNATIVE THERAPY

- In one study, oral supplements of indole-3-carbinol were shown to promote regression in high-grade cervical dysplasias when administered orally for 12 weeks.[9] SOR B Indole-3-carbinol occurs naturally in cruciferous vegetables, such as broccoli, cabbage, cauliflower, Brussels sprouts, collard greens, and kale, or can be purchased as a supplement.

SURGICAL

- Treatment options for CIN can be grouped into chemically destructive, surgical ablative, and surgical excisional methods. Cryotherapy, laser, and loop electrosurgical methods are commonly employed when treatment is selected.
- Candidates for outpatient cervical cryotherapy are patients with smaller lesions that do not enter the cervical os. Endocervical sampling is recommended before applying any ablative treatment.[4,6] SOR B
- Large lesions (more than 1 inch in diameter, more than 0.5 inch from the os, or involving more than 2 cervical quadrants) may be more appropriate for loop or laser therapy.[4,6] SOR B

PREVENTION

- The patient should also be counseled that an HPV vaccine may still be of benefit, if indicated. The U.S. Advisory Committee on Immunization Practices (ACIP) recommends giving the vaccine to girls and women in the indicated age group (11 to 26 years of age) even if they have had an abnormal Pap test; although it will not change the course of the current infection, it will protect from any HPV types to which the patient has not yet been exposed.[10]
- According to the National Cancer Institute, scientific evidence supports the following for prevention of HPV infection.[11]
  - Abstinence from sexual activity
  - Barrier protection and/or spermicidal gel during sexual intercourse
  - Vaccination against HPV-16/HPV-18

FOLLOW-UP

- Follow-up is in 6-month intervals until the patient has two serial normal examinations, with co-testing.[6] Recurrence is most common in the first 2 years after therapy. Recurrences are most common in the os and on the outside margins.
- After two consecutive negative Pap tests or one negative high-risk HPV DNA test, patients should continue to be routinely screened.

PATIENT EDUCATION

- Smoking cessation counseling is an important part of therapy for women who continue to smoke (see Chapter 248, Smoking and Tobacco Addiction).

PATIENT RESOURCES

- American Sexual Health Association. *HPV*—**http://www.ashasexualhealth.org/stdsstis/hpv/.**
- Centers for Disease Control and Prevention. *HPV Vaccine Information for Young Women—Fact Sheet*—**http://www.cdc.gov/std/hpv/stdfact-hpv-vaccine-young-women.htm.**
- Oncolink. *All About Cervical Cancer*—**https://www.oncolink.org/cancers/gynecologic/cervical-cancer/all-about-cervical-cancer.**

PROVIDER RESOURCES

- ASCCP (formerly American Society for Colposcopy and Cervical Pathology). *Guidelines for Managing Abnormal Cervical Cancer Screens and CIN/AIS*—**http://www.asccp.org/asccp-guidelines.**
- National Cancer Institute. *Cervical Cancer Prevention (PDQ)*—**http://www.cancer.gov/cancertopics/pdq/prevention/cervical/HealthProfessional.**
- Medscape. *Colposcopy*—**http://emedicine.medscape.com/article/265097.**

REFERENCES

1. Stafl A, Wilbanks GD. An international terminology of colposcopy: report of the nomenclature committee of the International Federation of Cervical Pathology and Colposcopy. *Obstet Gynecol.* 1991;77:313-314.
2. Insinga RP, Glass AG, Rush BB. Diagnoses and outcomes in cervical cancer screening: a population-based study. *Am J Obstet Gynecol.* 2004;191:105-113.
3. Benard VB, Castle PE, Jenison SA, et al. Population-based incidence rates of cervical intraepithelial neoplasia in the human papillomavirus vaccine era. *JAMA Oncol.* 2017;3(6):833-837.
4. Khan MJ, Werner CL, Darragh TM, et al. ASCCP Colposcopy Standards: role of colposcopy, benefits, potential harms, and terminology for colposcopic practice. *J Low Genit Tract Dis.* 2017;21(4):223-229.
5. Spitzer M, Apgar BS, Brotzman GL. Management of histologic abnormalities of the cervix. *Am Fam Physician.* 2006;73:105-112.
6. Massad LS, Einstein MH, Huh WK, et al.; 2012 ASCCP Consensus Guidelines Conference. 2012 updated consensus guidelines for the management of abnormal cervical cancer screening tests and cancer precursors. *J Low Genit Tract Dis.* 2013;17(5 suppl 1):S1-27.
7. Wentzensen N, Massad LS, Mayeaux EJ Jr, et al. Evidence-based consensus recommendations for colposcopy practice for cervical cancer prevention in the United States. *J Low Genit Tract Dis.* 2017;21(4):216-222.
8. Wentzensen N, Schiffman M, Silver MI, et al. ASCCP Colposcopy Standards: risk-based colposcopy practice. *J Low Genit Tract Dis.* 2017;21(4):230-234.
9. Bell MC, Crowley-Nowick P, Bradlow HL, et al. Placebo-controlled trial of indole-3-carbinol in the treatment of CIN. *Gynecol Oncol.* 2000;78(2):123-129.
10. Advisory Committee on Immunization Practices (ACIP). *ACIP Recommendations for the Use of Quadrivalent HPV Vaccine.* https://www.cdc.gov/mmwr/preview/mmwrhtml/rr56e312a1.htm.
11. National Cancer Institute. *Cervical Cancer Prevention (PDQ).* http://www.cancer.gov/cancertopics/pdq/prevention/cervical/HealthProfessional. Accessed March 2012.

92 COLPOSCOPY OF HIGH-GRADE LESIONS

E.J. Mayeaux, Jr., MD

PATIENT STORY

A 36-year-old woman presented for follow-up of a persistently abnormal Papanicolaou (Pap) test. She is a smoker and has had multiple new sexual partners in the past decade. Although she has had several "abnormal Pap tests" in the past, she states she has never needed treatment. She was found to have a dense acetowhite (AW) lesion on colposcopy that was biopsied (**Figure 92-1**). The pathology returned high grade consistent with cervical intraepithelial neoplasia grade 3 (CIN 3), and the patient was treated with loop electrosurgery. She had negative margins on the loop electrosurgical excision procedure specimen and remained recurrence-free at 3 years.

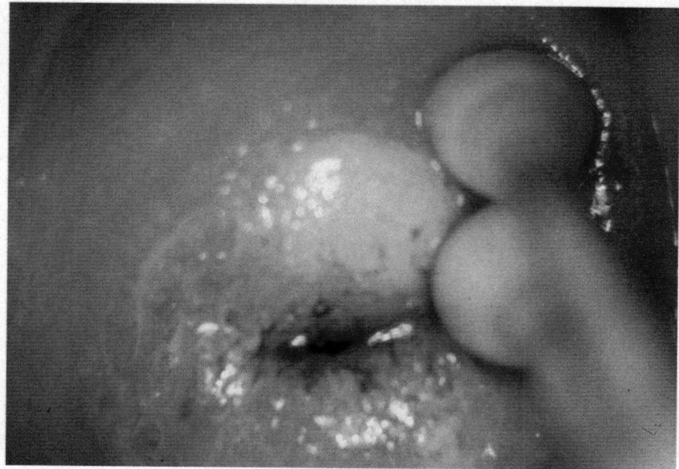

FIGURE 92-1 Dense acetowhite (white after application of vinegar) lesions with "rolled" edges in a patient with high-grade disease. Her colposcopically directed biopsies showed cervical intraepithelial neoplasia grade 3. (*Reproduced with permission from E.J. Mayeaux, Jr., MD.*)

INTRODUCTION

High-grade squamous intraepithelial lesions in adult women are considered true cancer precursors because if left untreated, they have a significant chance of developing into invasive cancer.

SYNONYMS

Cervical intraepithelial neoplasia (CIN 3 and CIN 2) are high-grade lesions.

EPIDEMIOLOGY

- Overall rates of Pap test abnormalities are usually estimated from local or regional studies. For example, in an observational cohort study of routine cervical tests in the northwestern United States, in women of all ages (n = 150,052), high-grade squamous intraepithelial lesion was diagnosed at a rate of 0.8 per 1000 compared to negative routine tests that were diagnosed at a rate of 278.5 per 1000.[1]
- In HPV vaccine age groups, there were significant reductions in the CIN incidence per 100,000 women screened for all grades of CIN. In female individuals 15 to 19 years old, the incidence dropped from 3468.3 to 1590.6 for CIN 1 per 100,000, from 896.4 to 414.9 for CIN 2, and from 240.2 to 0 for CIN 3 per 100,000.[2]

ETIOLOGY AND PATHOPHYSIOLOGY

- In high-grade squamous intraepithelial lesions, the abnormalities are immature parabasilar cell types. They have an increased nuclear-to-cytoplasmic ratio, enlarged hyperchromatic nucleoli, few nucleoli, and a reticular or granular appearance.
- On histology, abnormal maturation and nuclear atypia defines CIN. Koilocytosis (perinuclear cytoplasmic vacuolization) is

indicative of human papillomavirus (HPV) infection and may be found with high-grade CIN. High-grade CIN is diagnosed when immature basaloid cells with nuclear atypia occupy more than the lower one third of the epithelium. With increasing lesion severity there is also increased nuclear crowding, pleomorphism, normal and abnormal mitosis, and loss of polarity.[3]

- Traditionally, high-grade CIN had been thought to arise as a small focus within a larger area of low-grade CIN that expands and eventually replaces much of the low-grade lesion.
- It is now thought that high-grade CIN is a process that develops concurrently and somewhat independently from low-grade CIN. This theory is supported by the fact that CIN 3 can develop without a detectable preceding low-grade CIN lesion, and high-grade CIN is almost always found closer to the squamocolumnar junction than concomitant low-grade lesions. It has also been found that women who turned HPV-16/-18–positive had a 39% rate of high-grade CIN at 2 years compared to HPV-negative women.
- Schiffman et al. reported that both CIN 1 and CIN 2 or 3 lesions developed within the same time frame in a large group of women who turned HPV-positive and were followed for 4 years.[4]

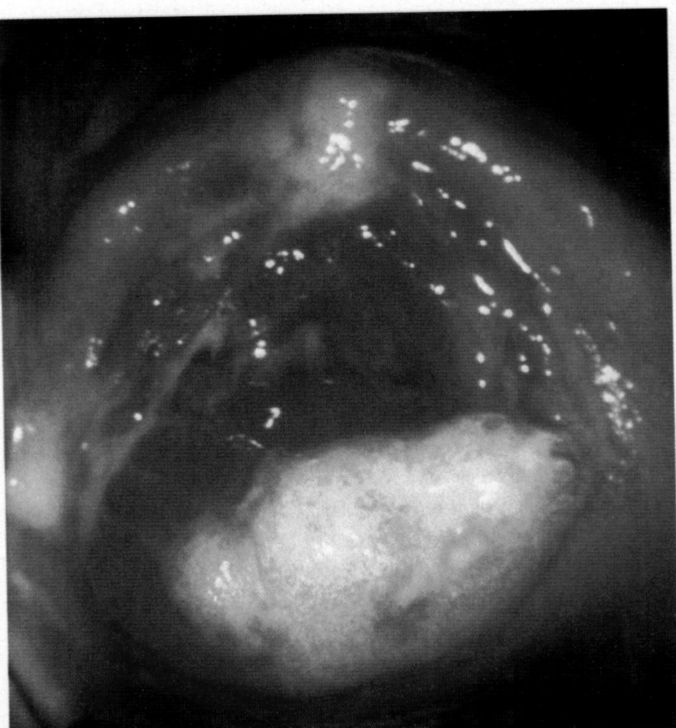

FIGURE 92-2 Leukoplakia (white lesion before application of vinegar) of the cervix seen with colposcopy in a patient with high-grade squamous intraepithelial lesion. (*Reproduced with permission from E.J. Mayeaux, Jr., MD.*)

RISK FACTORS[5]

- HPV infection.
- Nonuse of barrier protection and/or spermicidal gel during sexual intercourse.
- No Pap or HPV testing within the last 3–5 years in low-risk women with a cervix or within 1 year for high-risk women.
- Nonvaccination status for high-risk HPV types.
- Tobacco smoking.

DIAGNOSIS

CLINICAL FEATURES

- Leukoplakia, as shown in **Figure 92-2**, is typically an elevated, white plaque seen prior to the application of acetic acid. It is caused by a thick keratin layer that obscures the underlying epithelium and may signal severe dysplasia or cancer. Although it may be associated with benign findings, it always warrants a biopsy.
- AW epithelium following the application of acetic acid is typical for CIN 2 and 3 lesions (see **Figure 92-1**). The AW effect tends to develop more slowly than in lower-grade lesions and to persist longer. The margins of high-grade CIN are straighter and sharper compared to the vague, feathery, geographic borders of CIN 1 or HPV disease.
- With increasing levels of CIN, desmosomes (intracellular bridges) that attach the epithelium to the basement membrane are often lost, producing an edge that easily peels. This loss of tissue integrity should raise the suspicion of high-grade dysplasia. The extreme expression of this effect is the ulceration that sometimes forms with invasive disease.
- High-grade CIN lesions are usually proximal to or touch the squamocolumnar junction, even when contained in larger lesions (**Figures 92-1** to **92-5**).

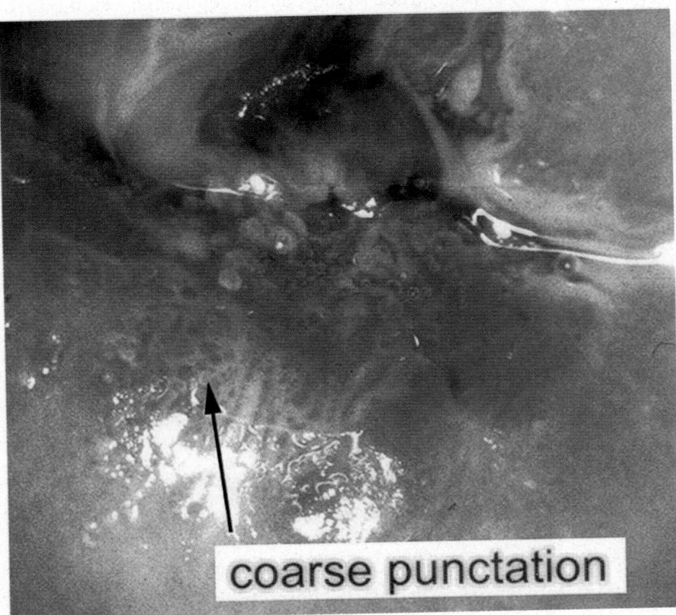

FIGURE 92-3 Coarse punctation of the cervix seen through the colposcope in a patient with high-grade disease. (*Reproduced with permission from E.J. Mayeaux, Jr., MD.*)

- Nodular elevations on the surface of lesions and ulceration are suspicious for high-grade or invasive cancer.
- Increases in local factors such as tumor angiogenesis factor or vascular endothelial growth factor, which are much more commonly produced by CIN 3 lesions, cause growth of abnormal surface vasculature, producing punctation (see **Figures 92-3** and **92-4**), mosaicism (**Figures 92-5** and **92-6**), and frankly abnormal vessels. However, most high-grade lesions do not develop any abnormal vessels.
- Punctation is a stippled appearance of small looped capillaries seen end-on, often found within AW area, appearing as fine-to-coarse red dots (see **Figures 92-3** and **92-4**). Coarse punctation represents increased-caliber vessels that are spaced at irregular intervals, and it is more highly associated with increasing levels of dysplasia.
- Mosaicism is an abnormal pattern of small blood vessels suggesting a confluence of "tiles" or a "chicken-wire pattern" with reddish borders. Mosaicism represents capillaries that grow on or near the surface of the lesion that form partitions between blocks of proliferating epithelium (see **Figures 92-5** and **92-6**). It develops in a manner very similar to punctation and is often found in the same lesions. Coarse mosaic forms a consistently irregular cobblestone effect with dilated coarse vessels that is highly associated with CIN 2 and 3.

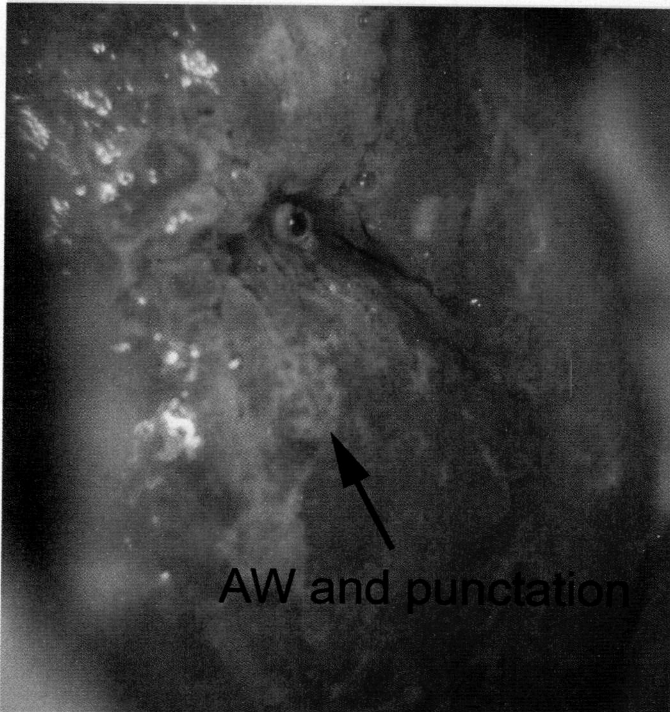

FIGURE 92-4 Acetowhite (AW) epithelium and coarse punctation on the same cervix (*arrow*). The biopsies of this area showed cervical intraepithelial neoplasia grade 3. (*Reproduced with permission from E.J. Mayeaux, Jr., MD.*)

TYPICAL DISTRIBUTION

- CIN 2 or 3 disease usually touches the active squamocolumnar junction (SCJ).
- When CIN 2 or 3 coexists in the same lesion with a lower-grade lesion, the higher-grade lesion often presents by an internal margin (also known as a border-within-a-border) separating the different-grade lesions (**Figure 92-7**). The higher-grade disease is usually proximal to the os.

LABORATORY TESTING

- Women with ASC-H (atypical squamous cells, cannot exclude high grade disease) or high-grade squamous intraepithelial lesion (HSIL) cytology should have colposcopy regardless of any HPV result. Reflex HPV testing is not recommended. In nonpregnant, nonadolescent women with HSIL cytology, immediate loop electrosurgical excision or colposcopy is acceptable.[6]
- Women with all subcategories of atypical glandular cells (AGCs) and adenocarcinoma in situ (AIS), except atypical endometrial cells, should have colposcopy with endocervical sampling regardless of HPV result.[6]

BIOPSY

- Biopsy is usually indicated to establish the histologic grade of the abnormalities present. Biopsies are performed under colposcopic direction. A minimum of two biopsies are recommended, although one biopsy may be replaced with an endocervical sampling.[7]

DIFFERENTIAL DIAGNOSIS

- CIN 2 and 3 lesions must be differentiated from nonmalignant inflammatory lesions, especially trichomoniasis and *Chlamydia* infections, which usually present with vaginal itching, odor, and/or discharge (see Chapters 86, *Trichomonas* Vaginitis; and 87, *Chlamydia* Cervicitis).

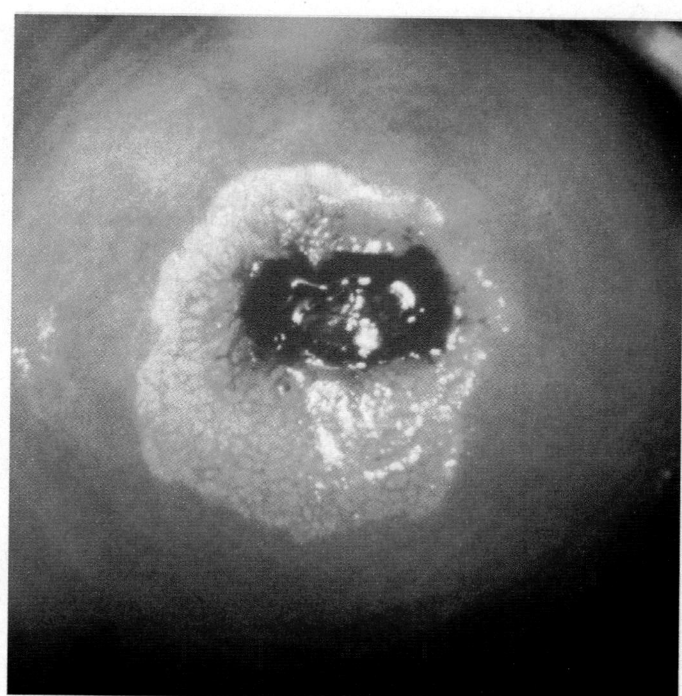

FIGURE 92-5 Colposcopy with findings of mosaicism in a patient with cervical intraepithelial neoplasia grade 3. (*Reproduced with permission from E.J. Mayeaux, Jr., MD.*)

- Flat HPV lesions may mimic the dense AW lesions of CIN 2 and 3.
- CIN 2 and 3 lesions must be differentiated from both CIN 1 and cancer (see Chapters 91, Colposcopy of Low-Grade Lesions; and 93, Colposcopy of Cervical Cancer).

MANAGEMENT

- Women with CIN 1 or no lesion preceded by ASC-H or HSIL should be managed with either a diagnostic excisional procedure or observation with co-testing at 12 months and 24 months if the colposcopic examination is adequate and the endocervical sampling is negative.[6]
- Except in special circumstances, women with biopsy-confirmed CIN 2 or 3 should be treated. CIN 2 may be followed with colposcopy and Pap tests in patients who have not attained their 21st birthday.[6]
- Effective treatment of CIN 2 and 3 requires the removal of the entire transformation zone rather than just the removal of the lesion. When colposcopy is satisfactory, any ablative or excisional modality will treat CIN effectively.[6,8] SOR Ⓐ However, because excisional modalities allow for the pathologic identification of unanticipated microinvasive or occult invasive cancer, some physicians prefer these methods to treat biopsy-confirmed CIN 2 and 3.[3] SOR Ⓒ
- Both excision and ablation are acceptable treatment choices for nonpregnant adult women with a histologic diagnosis of CIN 2 and 3 and satisfactory colposcopy.[6] For adolescents and young women with a histologic diagnosis of CIN 2, observation with colposcopy and cytology at 6-month intervals is preferred, but treatment is acceptable.[6] Treatment efficacy ranges from 90% to 95%, and most failures occur within 2 years.[9]
- Observation is unacceptable in women with CIN 2 except during pregnancy and in very compliant adolescents with satisfactory colposcopy and negative results on endocervical curettage.[10] SOR Ⓒ
- Immunosuppressed women with abnormal screening results should be managed in the same manner as immunocompetent women.[6]
- A randomized clinical trial demonstrated that condom use promotes regression of CIN and clearance of HPV after treatment.[11] SOR Ⓑ
- Because a small number of women with biopsy-confirmed CIN 2 or 3 and unsatisfactory colposcopy have occult invasive cancer, excisional procedures should be performed. Cold knife and loop electrosurgical excision procedure conizations effectively diagnose and treat these women.[10] SOR Ⓑ
- Hysterectomy is preferred for women who have completed childbearing and have a histologic diagnosis of AIS from a diagnostic excisional procedure. Excision is acceptable if future fertility is desired.[6]

COMPLEMENTARY AND ALTERNATIVE THERAPY

- In one study, oral supplements of indole-3-carbinol have been shown to promote regression in high-grade cervical dysplasias when administered orally for 12 weeks.[12] SOR Ⓑ Indole-3-carbinol occurs naturally in cruciferous vegetables, such as broccoli,

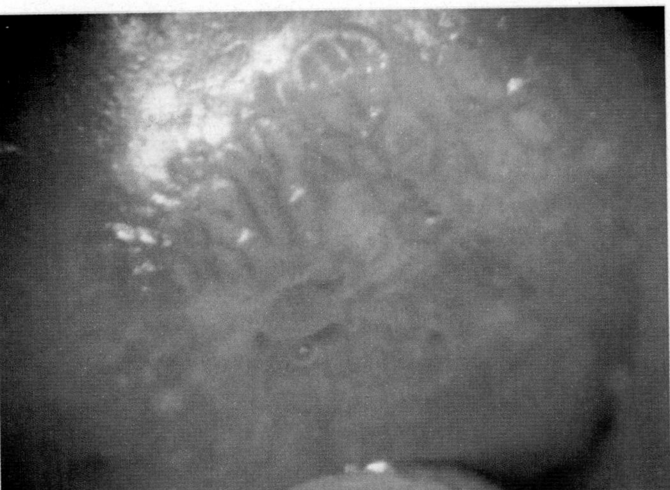

FIGURE 92-6 High-power colpophotograph of mosaicism in a patient with cervical intraepithelial neoplasia grade 3. Note the coarse pattern consisting of large-caliber vessels, irregular tile shapes, and irregular sizes. There are also a few punctations contained within the mosaic pattern, which is common. *(Reproduced with permission from E.J. Mayeaux, Jr., MD.)*

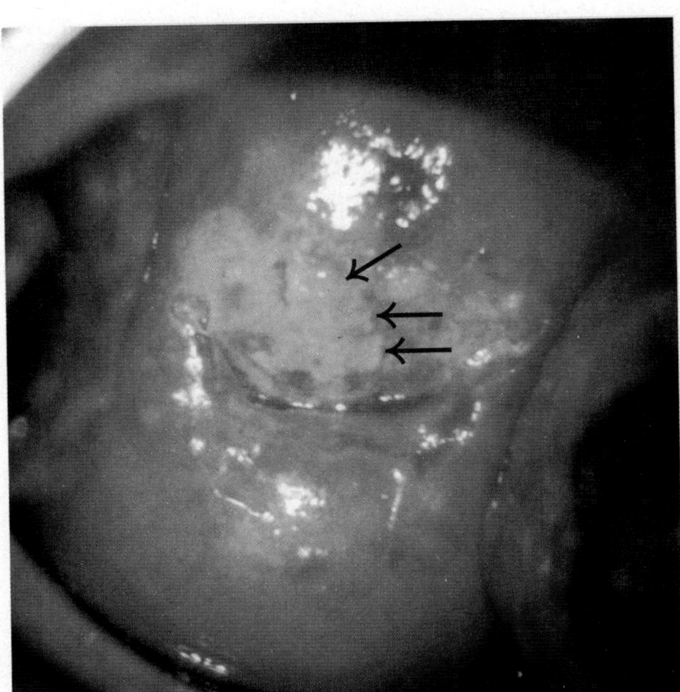

FIGURE 92-7 High-power colpophotograph of a cervical intraepithelial neoplasia grade 3 lesion. Note the internal margin *(arrows)*. *(Reproduced with permission from E.J. Mayeaux, Jr., MD.)*

cabbage, cauliflower, Brussels sprouts, collard greens, and kale, or can be purchased as a supplement.

PREVENTION

- The patient should also be counseled that an HPV vaccine may still be of benefit if indicated. The U.S. Advisory Committee on Immunization Practices (ACIP) recommends giving the vaccine to women in the indicated age group (11 to 26 years of age) even if they have had an abnormal Pap test. Although it will not change the course of the current infection, it will protect women from other HPV types to which they have not yet been exposed.[10]
- Vaccination with high-risk HPV L1 VLP vaccines that contain at least HPV-16 and HPV-18 prior to exposure to the corresponding viruses can prevent the majority of cervical cancers. Vaccines that contain more high-risk HPV types prevent a higher percentage of cancers.[13] The ASCCP Colposcopy Standards Project Colposcopy Quality Improvement Recommendations include an attempt should be made to contact a patient with suspected invasive disease within 2 week of receipt of report or referral and that they should be seen within 2 week of contact.[14]
- According to the National Cancer Institute (NCI), scientific evidence supports the following for prevention of cervical cancer[15]:
    - Prevention of HPV infection through abstinence from sexual activity and barrier protection and/or spermicidal gel during sexual intercourse
    - Vaccination against HPV-16/HPV-18, and potentially other high-risk HPV types
    - Screening via gynecologic examinations and cytologic screening
- Avoidance of all tobacco smoke.

PROGNOSIS

- For untreated CIN 2, approximately 43% will spontaneously regress, 35% will persist, and 22% will progress to carcinoma in situ or invasive cancer.[3] The regression rate of CIN 2 is higher in adolescents.
- For untreated CIN 3, approximately 32% will regress, 56% will persist, and 14% of CIN 3 will progress to carcinoma in situ or invasive cancer.[3]
- Most treatment failures will recur within 2 years, although cancers can develop years to decades later. Margin status is a predictor of recurrence but does not appear to be an independent risk factor for recurrence.[6]

FOLLOW-UP

- After treatment for CIN 2 or 3, acceptable management methods include contesting (cytology plus high-risk HPV testing) at 12-month intervals until two negative evaluations have been obtained. Then contesting is performed in 3 years, and if negative, the patient may return to routine screening.[6] SOR Ⓑ

PATIENT EDUCATION

- Tobacco smoking has been linked to the development and recurrence of CIN. Part of any treatment program should include smoking cessation.
- Studies on the effect of treatments on future pregnancy outcomes are conflicting, although many indicate an approximately twofold increase in preterm delivery risk.[6] This is generally considered to be much less risk than that of cervical cancer.

PATIENT RESOURCES

- National Cancer Institute. *What You Need to Know About cervical Cancer*—**http://www.cancer.gov/cancertopics/wyntk/cervix.**
- Oncolink. *All About Cervical Cancer*—**https://www.oncolink.org/cancers/gynecologic/cervical-cancer/all-about-cervical-cancer.**
- Centers for Disease Control and Prevention. *Cervical Cancer*—**https://www.cdc.gov/cancer/cervical/index.htm.**

PROVIDER RESOURCES

- National Cancer Institute. *Cervical Cancer Prevention (PDQ®)*—**http://www.cancer.gov/cancertopics/pdq/prevention/cervical/HealthProfessional.**
- ASCCP (formerly American Society for Colposcopy and Cervical Pathology) guidelines for abnormal screening tests and the management of women with CIN—**http://www.asccp.org/asccp-guidelines,**
- Medscape. *Colposcopy*—**http://emedicine.medscape.com/article/265097.**

REFERENCES

1. Insinga RP, Glass AG, Rush BB. Diagnoses and outcomes in cervical cancer screening: a population-based study. *Am J Obstet Gynecol.* 2004;191:105-113.
2. Benard VB, Castle PE, Jenison SA, et al. Population-based incidence rates of cervical intraepithelial neoplasia in the human papillomavirus vaccine era. *JAMA Oncol.* 2017;3(6):833-837.
3. Spitzer M, Apgar BS, Brotzman GL. Management of histologic abnormalities of the cervix. *Am Fam Physician.* 2006;73:105-112.
4. Schiffman MH, Bauer HM, Hoover RN, et al. Epidemiological evidence showing that human papillomavirus infection causes most cervical intraepithelial neoplasia. *J Natl Cancer Inst.* 1994;85:958-964.
5. National Cancer Institute. *Cervical Cancer Prevention.* https://www.cancer.gov/types/cervical/hp/cervical-prevention-pdq. Accessed June 8, 2018.
6. Massad LS, Einstein MH, Huh WK, et al.; 2012 ASCCP Consensus Guidelines Conference. 2012 updated consensus guidelines

for the management of abnormal cervical cancer screening tests and cancer precursors. *J Low Genit Tract Dis.* 2013;17(5 suppl 1): S1-S27.

7. Wentzensen N, Schiffman M, Silver MI, et al. ASCCP Colposcopy Standards: risk-based colposcopy practice. *J Low Genit Tract Dis.* 2017;21(4):230-234.
8. Wright TC Jr, Massad LS, Dunton CJ, et al. 2006 Consensus guidelines for the management of women with cervical intraepithelial neoplasia or adenocarcinoma in situ. *Am J Obstet Gynecol.* 2007;197(4):340-345.
9. Paraskevaidis E, Arbyn M, Sotiriadis A, et al. The role of HPV DNA testing in the follow-up period after treatment for CIN: a systematic review of the literature. *Cancer Treat Rev.* 2004;30:205-211.
10. Wright TC Jr, Massad LS, Dunton CJ, et al. 2006 Consensus guidelines for the management of women with abnormal cervical cancer screening tests. *Am J Obstet Gynecol.* 2007;197(4): 346-355.
11. Hogewoning CJ, Bleeker MC, van den Brule AJ, et al. Condom use promotes regression of cervical intraepithelial neoplasia and clearance of human papillomavirus: a randomized clinical trial. *Int J Cancer.* 2003;107:811-816.
12. Bell MC, Crowley-Nowick P, Bradlow HL, et al. Placebo-controlled trial of indole-3-carbinol in the treatment of CIN. *Gynecol Oncol.* 2000;78(2):123-129.
13. Huh WK, Joura EA, Giuliano AR, et al. Final efficacy, immunogenicity, and safety analyses of a nine-valent human papillomavirus vaccine in women aged 16–26 years: a randomized, double-blind trial. *Lancet.* 2017;390:2143-2159.
14. Mayeaux EJ Jr, Novetsky AP, Chelmow D, et al. ASCCP Colposcopy Standards: colposcopy quality improvement recommendations for the United States. *J Low Genit Tract Dis.* 2017;21(4):242-248.
15. National Institutes of Health—National Cancer Institute. *Cervical Cancer Prevention (PDQ).* http://www.cancer.gov/cancertopics/pdq/prevention/cervical/HealthProfessional. Accessed March 2017.

93 COLPOSCOPY OF CERVICAL CANCER

E.J. Mayeaux, Jr., MD

PATIENT STORY

A 51-year-old woman presents with postcoital bleeding. She has not had a period in 3 years, but has started spotting after intercourse. Her last Papanicolaou (Pap) test was after the birth of her last child 25 years ago and was normal. Other than an occasional mild hot flash, she has no other complaints. On colposcopy she was found to have a densely acetowhite lesion with abnormal vessel near the cervical os (**Figure 93-1**). Biopsy demonstrated invasive squamous cell carcinoma. The patient then had a radical hysterectomy with pelvic/paraaortic lymphadenectomy. Fortunately, her lymph nodes were all negative.

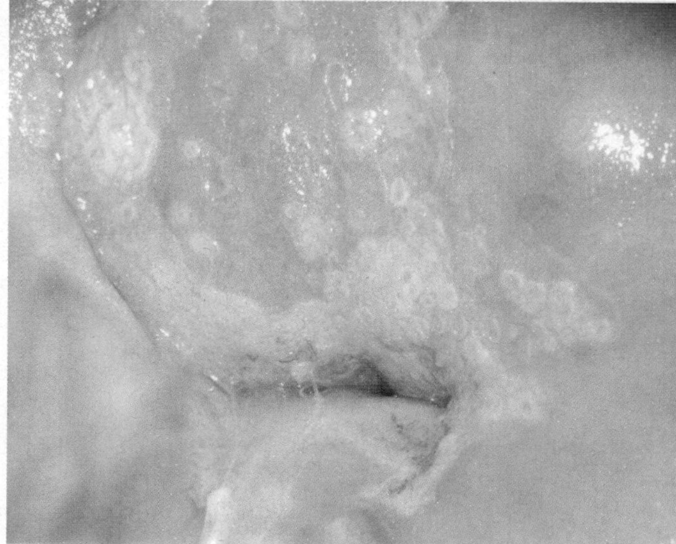

FIGURE 93-1 Colposcopic view of invasive squamous cell carcinoma. The lesion is densely acetowhite with abnormal vessels on the anterior lip just above the cervical os. (*Reproduced with permission from E.J. Mayeaux, Jr., MD.*)

INTRODUCTION

Colposcopy is an important visualization technique used to investigate abnormal Pap tests and to direct biopsies for histologic diagnosis of cervical cancer. Follow-up for abnormal cervical cancer screening tests and abnormal colposcopy results is now based on the estimated risk of cervical cancer development.[1] Because human papillomavirus (HPV) is present in 95% to 100% of all squamous cell cancers (SCCs), the International Agency for Research on Cancer proclaimed cervical cancer to be the first human cancer known to have a single necessary cause.[2,3]

EPIDEMIOLOGY

- Worldwide, carcinoma of the cervix is the fourth most common cancer in women, and the seventh most common cancer overall. There were an estimated 528,000 new cases worldwide in 2012, with around 85% of the global burden occurring in the less developed regions. There were an estimated 266,000 deaths from cervical cancer worldwide in 2012, which accounts for 7.5% of all female cancer deaths.[4]
- In the United States in 2014, 12,578 women were diagnosed with cervical cancer and 4115 women died from the disease.[5]
- In developed countries, roughly half of cases occur in women never screened and an additional 10% in women not screened within the past 5 years.[6]
- Ninety-three percent of invasive cervical cancers are SCCs (**Figures 93-1** to **93-4**). They almost all contain HPV DNA, and 90% are subtypes 16 or 18, which are the most virulent.[7]
- Approximately 7% of cases are adenocarcinomas, but these are on the rise[7] (**Figure 93-5**).
- It is rare to find invasive cancer of the uterine cervix in pregnancy. The incidence varies from 1 to 15 cases per 10,000 pregnancies, and the prognosis is similar to that of nonpregnant patients.[8]
- The peak prevalence of invasive cervical cancer is 40 to 50 years of age.[9]

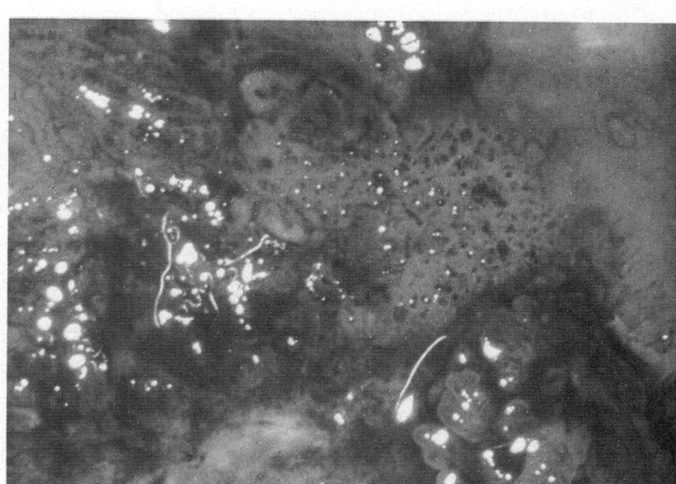

FIGURE 93-2 Colposcopic view of invasive squamous cell cancer with abnormal vessels. (*Reproduced with permission from E.J. Mayeaux, Jr., MD.*)

ETIOLOGY AND PATHOPHYSIOLOGY

- Oncogenic HPV serve as initiator, and other factors relating to immune status, such as cigarette smoking, nutrition, or other genital infections, may be promoters.[10]
- Cervical cancer is unique in that no other human cancer has been shown to have such a clearly identified cause, which are oncogenic strains of HPV.[1]

RISK FACTORS[11]

- HPV infection.
- Nonuse of barrier protection and/or spermicidal gel during sexual intercourse.
- No Pap testing within the last 3 years in low-risk women with a cervix or within 1 year for high-risk women.
- Nonvaccination status for high-risk HPV types, especially HPV-16 and HPV-18.
- Tobacco smoking.

DIAGNOSIS

CLINICAL FEATURES

- Leukoplakia is typically an elevated, white plaque seen prior to the application of acetic acid. It is caused by a thick keratin layer that obscures the underlying epithelium (**Figure 93-1**). It always warrants a biopsy.
- Early invasion often is associated with a decline in the acetowhite reaction with a gray-white color being more common. Yellow-hued color change is also a marker for early or frank invasive lesions (see **Figure 93-4**).
- With increasing levels of cervical intraepithelial neoplasia (CIN), desmosomes (intracellular bridges) that attach the epithelium to the basement membrane are often lost, producing an edge that easily peels. This loss of tissue integrity should raise the suspicion of high-grade dysplasia. The extreme expression of this effect is the ulceration that sometimes forms with invasive disease. The ulcer can have a rolled edge around it without vessels visible in the ulcer cavity.
- Nodular elevations and ulceration are suspicious for high-grade or invasive cancer.
- Coarse punctation and coarse mosaic patterns may be associated with high-grade dysplasia or cancer (see Chapter 92, Colposcopy of High-Grade Lesions).
- Abnormal blood vessels are atypical irregular surface vessels that have lost their normal arborization or branching pattern (see **Figures 93-1** and **93-2**). This represents an exaggeration of the abnormalities of punctation and mosaicism, and it usually represents increasing severity of the lesion. They can be indicative of invasive cancer, but can occasionally be seen with high-grade CIN. These vessels are often best seen before application of acetic

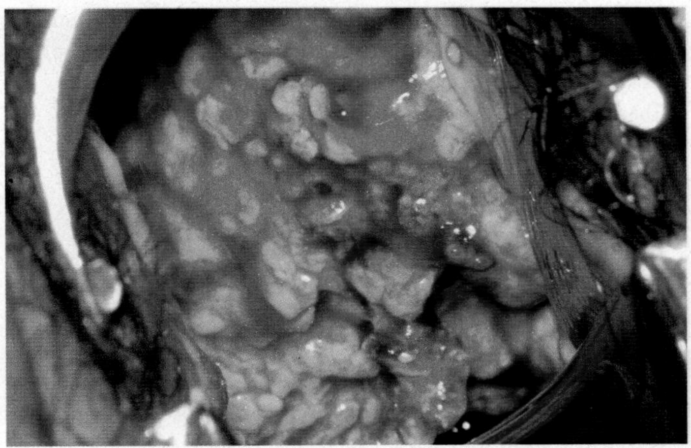

FIGURE 93-3 Colposcopic view of invasive squamous cell cancer. Note how the cancer has replaced the entire surface of the cervix with friable epithelium. (*Reproduced with permission from Daron Ferris, MD.*)

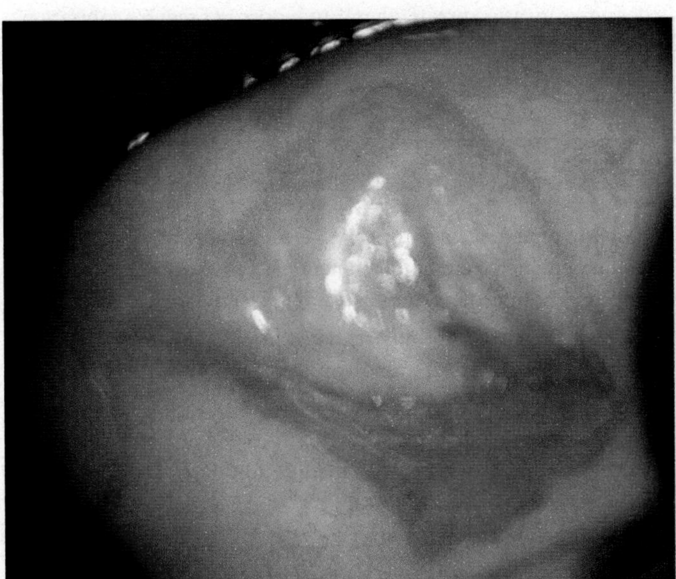

FIGURE 93-4 Colposcopic view of a rarer yellow-hued invasive squamous cell cancer of the cervix. (*Reproduced with permission from E.J. Mayeaux, Jr., MD.*)

acid. They are usually nonbranching, appear with abrupt courses and patterns, and often appear as commas, corkscrews, hairpins, or spaghetti. They may also appear as coarse parallel vessels. There is no definite repetitive pattern as with punctation or mosaicism.

- A thin watery vaginal discharge is the most common early complaint of a woman with cervical cancer. As the lesions progress or enlarge, complaints occur of postcoital bleeding or painless intermenstrual bleeding.
- More advanced lesions present with heavier and frequent bleeding until it may become continuous. Pain, hematuria, obstipation, and rectal bleeding are symptoms of late disease because of local direct invasion of surrounding paracervical structures. Lower-extremity edema may occur with pelvic sidewall involvement of tumor. Hemorrhage and uremia are preterminal events.
- Findings on speculum examination include an exophytic mass (see **Figures 93-3** and **93-5**), cervical ulcer, or barrel-shaped cervix.

LABORATORY TESTING

- Although HPV testing is used for screening for cervical cancer, it is not useful in the diagnosis of the disease.

IMAGING

- The staging of biopsy proven cervical cancer remains clinical. Physical examination with cystoscopy and proctoscopy usually starts the process. Routine X-ray studies are also used, including chest X-ray, intravenous pyelogram, and barium enema.

BIOPSY

- Colposcopy and biopsy or conization are needed to make the diagnosis. A histologic biopsy that is suspicious, but not confirmatory, of invasion requires cervical excision for definitive diagnosis. A biopsy of microinvasive carcinoma requires excision for definitive diagnosis and to rule out a more invasive lesion. A biopsy with definitive invasion greater than 5 mm does not require conization to plan therapy. Any frank lesion of the cervix requires biopsy for diagnosis.

DIFFERENTIAL DIAGNOSIS

- Because some cancers of the cervix ulcerate, cervical cancer must be differentiated from nonmalignant ulcerative diseases such as herpes virus infections (see Chapter 135, Herpes Simplex).
- Cervical cancer must be differentiated from CIN II and CIN III lesions (see Chapter 92, Colposcopy of High-Grade Lesions).
- Flat HPV lesions may mimic dense acetowhite lesions or leukoplakia (see Chapter 139, Genital Warts). A colposcopically directed biopsy can distinguish between these conditions.

MANAGEMENT

- **Table 93-1** shows the staging and treatment methods for cervical cancer.

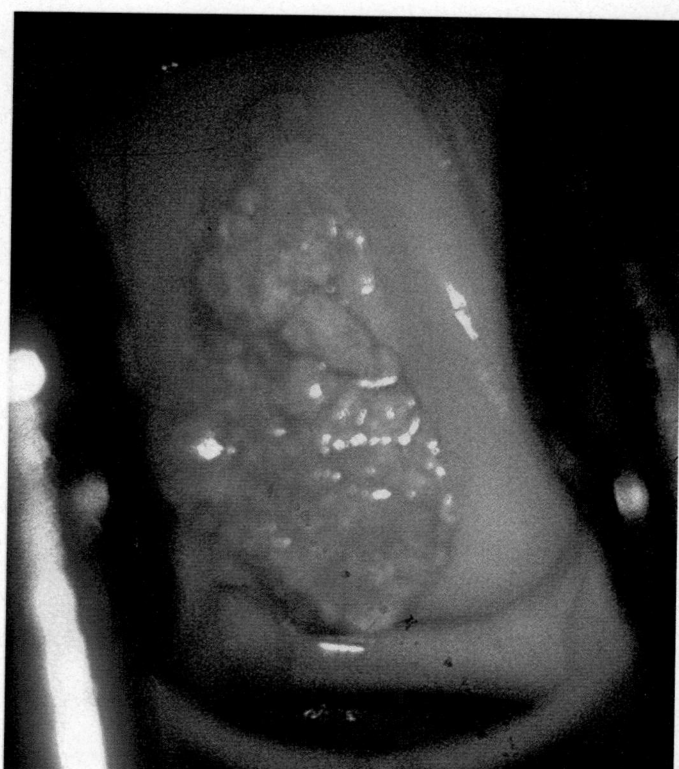

FIGURE 93-5 Adenocarcinoma of the cervix. (*Reproduced with permission from E.J. Mayeaux, Jr., MD.*)

TABLE 93-1 Staging and Treatment of Cervical Cancer*,†

Stage	Description	Treatment	5-Year Survival (%)
0	Carcinoma in situ	Surgical excision or ablation. Hysterectomy may be used for postreproductive patients and internal radiation therapy for medically inoperable patients.	
I	Tumor is confined to the cervix		91.3
IA	Invasive cancer identified only microscopically. Invasion is limited to measured stromal invasion with a maximum depth of 5 mm and no wider than 7 mm	Conization, total hysterectomy, modified radical hysterectomy with lymphadenectomy, radical trachelectomy, or intracavitary radiation therapy	98.1
IB	Clinical lesions confined to the cervix or preclinical lesions greater than stage IA	Radiation therapy with concomitant chemotherapy, radical hysterectomy and bilateral pelvic lymphadenectomy with or without total pelvic radiation therapy plus chemotherapy, radical trachelectomy, neoadjuvant chemotherapy, radiation therapy alone, or intensity-modulated radiation therapy (IMRT)	88.2
II	Extends beyond the cervix, but does not involve the pelvic sidewall or lowest third of the vagina		60.7
IIA	Involvement of the upper two-thirds of vagina, without lateral extension into the parametrium	Radiation therapy with concomitant chemotherapy, radical hysterectomy and bilateral pelvic lymphadenectomy with or without total pelvic radiation therapy plus chemotherapy, radical trachelectomy, neoadjuvant chemotherapy, radiation therapy alone, or intensity-modulated radiation therapy (IMRT)	67.2
IIB	Obvious parametrial involvement but not onto the pelvic sidewall	Radiation therapy with concomitant chemotherapy, interstitial brachytherapy, or neoadjuvant chemotherapy	57.9
III	Involves the lowest third of the vagina or pelvic sidewall or causes hydronephrosis		46.8
IIIA	Involvement of the lowest third of the vagina	Radiation therapy with concomitant chemotherapy, interstitial brachytherapy, or neoadjuvant chemotherapy	38.6
IIIB	Involvement of pelvic sidewall or hydronephrosis or nonfunctioning kidney	Radiation therapy with concomitant chemotherapy, interstitial brachytherapy, or neoadjuvant chemotherapy	47.7
IV	The carcinoma has extended beyond the true pelvis or has clinically involved the mucosa of the bladder and/or rectum		
IVA	Spread of the tumor onto adjacent pelvic organs	Radiation therapy with concomitant chemotherapy, interstitial brachytherapy, or neoadjuvant chemotherapy	15.5
IVB	Distant metastases	Palliative radiation therapy or palliative chemotherapy	14.6

*Staging system based on the Federation of International Gynecologists and Obstetricians. Treatment Option Overview. https://www.cancer.gov/types/cervical/hp/cervical-treatment-pdq#link/_405 and https://www.cancer.gov/types/cervical/hp/cervical-treatment-pdq#section/_85. Accessed September 2017.

†Survival data based on the *SEER Survival Monograph: Cancer Survival Among Adults: US SEER Program, 1988–2001, Patient and Tumor Characteristics*. Chapter 14: Cancer of the Cervix Uteri. http://seer.cancer.gov/publications/survival/surv_cervix_uteri.pdf.

PREVENTION

- Most cases are detected in the precancerous stages or as early disease in industrialized countries through the use of the Pap test and HPV testing.[12] The current death rate, however, is far higher than it should be because the Pap test and HPV testing are not performed on approximately 33% of eligible women. Vaccination with high-risk HPV L1 VLP vaccines that contain at least HPV-16 and HPV-18 prior to exposure to the corresponding viruses can prevent the majority of cervical cancers. Vaccines that contain more high-risk HPV types prevent a higher percentage of cancers.[13] The ASCCP Colposcopy Standards Project Colposcopy Quality Improvement Recommendations include that an attempt should be made to contact a patient with suspected invasive disease within 2 weeks of receipt of report or referral and that they should be seen within 2 weeks of contact.[14]

PROGNOSIS

- The prognosis for patients with cervical cancer is mostly defined by the extent of disease at the time of diagnosis (see **Table 93-1**).[11,15] Clinical stage, volume and grade of tumor, histologic type, lymphatic spread, and vascular invasion also affect prognosis. The factors that best predict decreased disease-free survival are clinical stage, depth of stromal invasion, capillary-lymphatic space involvement by tumor, and increased tumor size.

FOLLOW-UP

- Patients who recur are most likely to do so within the first 2 years after treatment.[16] Most guidelines recommend follow-up every 3 to 4 months for the first 2 years, followed by evaluations every 6 months. Most recurrences are diagnosed secondary to new signs and symptoms including abdominal pain, back pain, painful or swollen legs, and problems with urination, unexplained cough, and fatigue.[17] The usefulness of routine Pap testing and chest X-ray is unclear.[17,18] The follow-up visits should also screen for possible complications of previous treatment.

PATIENT EDUCATION

- Fertility-sparing surgery is available for very early stage cervical cancer. Menopausal symptoms are a common side effect of chemotherapy.

PATIENT RESOURCES

- Oncolink. *All About Cervical Cancer*—**https://www.oncolink.org/cancers/gynecologic/information-about-gynecologic-cancers/cervical-cancer/all-about-cervical-cancer.**
- National Cancer Institute. *Cervical Cancer Treatment (PDQ)—Patient Version*—**https://www.cancer.gov/types/cervical/patient/cervical-treatment-pdq.**
- National Cancer Institute. *What You Need to Know About Cervical Cancer*—**https://www.cancer.gov/publications/patient-education/wyntk-cervical-cancer.**

PROVIDER RESOURCES

- American Society for Colposcopy and Cervical Pathology. *Guidelines*—**http://www.asccp.org/asccp-guidelines.**
- National Cancer Institute. *Cervical Cancer Treatment (PDQ)–Health Professional Version*—**http://www.cancer.gov/cancertopics/pdq/treatment/cervical/HealthProfessional.**

REFERENCES

1. Massad LS, Einstein MH, Huh WK, et al.; 2012 ASCCP Consensus Guidelines Conference. 2012 updated consensus guidelines for the management of abnormal cervical cancer screening tests and cancer precursors. *J Low Genit Tract Dis.* 2013;17(5 suppl 1): S1-27.
2. Tjalma WA, Van Waes TR, Van den Eeden LE, Bogers JJ. Role of human papillomavirus in the carcinogenesis of squamous cell carcinoma and adenocarcinoma of the cervix. *Best Pract Res Clin Obstet Gynaecol.* 2005;19:469-483.
3. Bosch FX, Munoz N. The viral etiology of cervical cancer. *Virus Res.* 2002;89:183-190.
4. World Health Organization IARC Globocan. *Cervical Cancer—Estimated Incidence, Mortality and Prevalence Worldwide in 2012.* http://globocan.iarc.fr/old/FactSheets/cancers/cervix-new.asp. Accessed September 2017.
5. U.S. Cancer Statistics Working Group. *United States Cancer Statistics: 1999–2014 Incidence and Mortality Web-based Report.* Atlanta (GA): Department of Health and Human Services, Centers for Disease Control and Prevention, and National Cancer Institute; 2017. http://www.cdc.gov/uscs. Accessed June 21, 2018.
6. National Institutes of Health. *NIH Consensus Development Conference Statement—April 1–3, 1996.* http://consensus.nih.gov/1996/1996cervicalcancer102html.htm. Accessed August 2012.
7. Schiffman MH, Bauer HM, Hoover RN, et al. Epidemiological evidence showing that human papillomavirus infection causes most cervical intraepithelial neoplasia. *J Natl Cancer Inst.* 1994; 85:958-964.
8. Campion MJ, Sedlacek TV. Colposcopy in pregnancy. *Obstet Gynecol Clin North Am.* 1993;20(1):153-163.
9. Moscicki AB, Schiffman M, Kjaer S, Villa LL. Chapter 5: Updating the natural history of HPV and anogenital cancer. *Vaccine.* 2006;24 Suppl 3:S3:42-51.
10. Berrington DE, Gonzalez A, Green J. Comparison of risk factors for invasive squamous cell carcinoma and adenocarcinoma of the cervix: collaborative reanalysis of individual data on 8,097 women with squamous cell carcinoma and 1,374 women with adenocarcinoma from 12 epidemiological studies. *Int J Cancer.* 2007;120:885.
11. National Cancer Institute. *Cervical Cancer Prevention (PDQ)—Health Professional Version.* https://www.cancer.gov/types/cervical/hp/cervical-prevention-pdq. Accessed September 2017.
12. The 1988 Bethesda System for reporting cervical/vaginal cytological diagnoses. National Cancer Institute Workshop. *JAMA.* 1989;262(7):931-934.

13. Huh WK, Joura EA, Giuliano AR, et al. Final efficacy, immunogenicity, and safety analyses of a nine-valent human papillomavirus vaccine in women aged 16–26 years: a randomised, double-blind trial. *Lancet*. 2017;390:2143-2159.
14. Mayeaux EJ Jr, Novetsky AP, Chelmow D. ASCCP Colposcopy Standards: Colposcopy Quality Improvement Recommendations for the United States. *J Low Genit Tract Dis.* 2017;21(4):242-248.
15. Zaino RJ, Ward S, Delgado G, et al. Histopathologic predictors of the behavior of surgically treated stage IB squamous cell carcinoma of the cervix. A Gynecologic Oncology Group study. *Cancer*. 1992;69(7):1750-1758.
16. Ansink A, de Barros Lopes A, Naik R, et al. Recurrent stage IB cervical carcinoma: evaluation of the effectiveness of routine follow up surveillance. *Br J Obstet Gynaecol.* 1996;103(11): 1156-1158.
17. Duyn A, Van Eijkeren M, Kenter G, et al. Recurrent cervical cancer: detection and prognosis. *Acta Obstet Gynecol Scand.* 2002;81(4):351-355.
18. Morice P, Deyrolle C, Rey A, et al. Value of routine follow-up procedures for patients with stage I/II cervical cancer treated with combined surgery-radiation therapy. *Ann Oncol.* 2004;15(2): 218-223.

SECTION E BREAST

94 BREAST ABSCESS AND MASTITIS

E.J. Mayeaux, Jr., MD

PATIENT STORY

A 23-year-old woman who is currently breastfeeding and 6 weeks postpartum presents with a hard, red, tender, indurated area medial to her right nipple (**Figure 94-1**). She also has a low-grade fever. There is a local area of fluctuance, and so incision and drainage is recommended. The area is anesthetized with 1% lidocaine and epinephrine and drained with a #11 scalpel. A lot of purulence is expressed, and the wound is packed. The patient is started on cephalexin 500 mg qid for 10 days to treat the surrounding cellulitis and seen in follow-up the next day. The patient was already feeling better the next day and went on to full resolution in the following weeks.

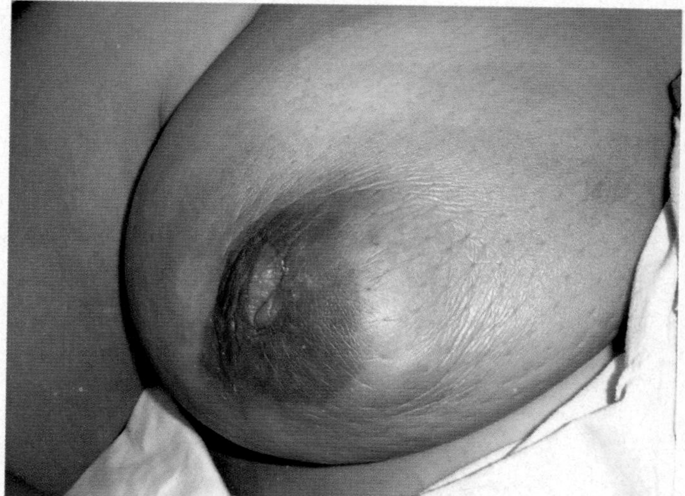

FIGURE 94-1 Localized cellulitis and breast abscess in a breastfeeding mother. Note the peau d'orange appearance of the edematous breast tissue. (*Reproduced with permission from Nicolette Deveneau, MD.*)

EPIDEMIOLOGY

- The prevalence of mastitis is estimated to be at least 2% to 10% of breastfeeding women.[1] Risk factors include partial blockage of the milk duct, pressure on the breast, oversupply of milk, infrequent feedings, rapid weaning, illness in mother or baby, maternal stress or excessive fatigue, maternal malnutrition, history of mastitis with a previous child, cracks and nipple sores, use of an antifungal nipple cream in the same month, and use of a manual breast pump.[2]
- Breast abscess is an uncommon problem in breastfeeding women, with an incidence of approximately 0.1%.[3] Risk factors include maternal age more than 30 years, primiparity, gestational age of 41 weeks, and mastitis.[3,4] Breast abscess develops in 5% to 11% of women with mastitis, often caused by inadequate therapy.[4]

ETIOLOGY AND PATHOPHYSIOLOGY

- Mastitis, defined as an infection of the breast, and breast abscesses are typically found in breastfeeding women (see **Figure 94-1**). A breast abscess can occur in older women unrelated to pregnancy and breastfeeding (**Figure 94-2**).
- Mastitis is most commonly caused by *Staphylococcus aureus*, *Streptococcus* species, and *Escherichia coli*.
- Recurrent mastitis can result from poor selection or incomplete use of antibiotic therapy, or failure to resolve underlying lactation management problems. Mastitis that repeatedly recurs in the same location, or does not respond to appropriate therapy, may indicate the presence of breast cancer.[4]

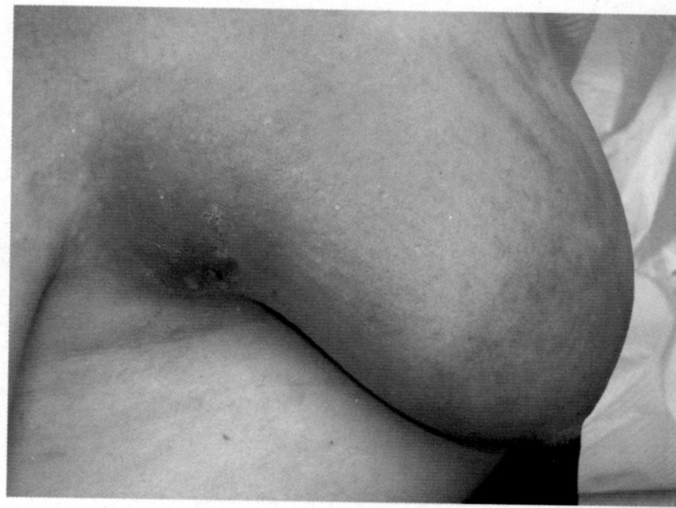

FIGURE 94-2 Breast abscess and cellulitis in a 40-year-old woman. Pus was already draining at the time of presentation, but a further incision and drainage through the openings yielded another 30 mL of pus. The patient was treated with oral antibiotics and scheduled to get a mammogram when the infection is cleared. (*Reproduced with permission from Richard P. Usatine, MD.*)

DIAGNOSIS

CLINICAL FEATURES

- Mastitis causes a hard, red, tender, swollen area on the breast (**Figures 94-1** to **94-3**).
- Fever is common.
- Pain usually extends beyond the indurated area.
- It is often associated with other systemic complaints including myalgia, chills, malaise, and flu-like symptoms.
- Breast abscess can occur with mastitis, except a fluctuant mass is palpable. (In **Figure 94-2**, the fluctuant mass is close to the midline with two openings of spontaneous drainage. The remainder of the erythema is cellulitis.)
- Breast abscesses, especially in the inframammary area, may also be associated with hidradenitis suppurativa **(Figure 94-4)**.[5]
- Typical distribution is usually unilateral.
- Biopsy is unnecessary, but in persistent cases, a midstream milk sample may be cultured and antibiotics prescribed based on the identification and sensitivity of the specific pathogen.

TYPICAL DISTRIBUTION

- The typical distribution is usually unilateral.

LABORATORY TESTING

- In persistent cases, a midstream milk sample may be cultured and antibiotics prescribed based on the identification and sensitivity of the specific pathogen.

IMAGING

- Ultrasonography may be used to distinguish abscesses from other types of lesions. Abscesses appear as ill-defined masses and have central hypoechoic areas with either septations or low-level internal echoes, and posterior enhancement.[6]

BIOPSY

- Biopsy is needed if a palpable mass remains after the infection is cleared.

DIFFERENTIAL DIAGNOSIS

- Mastitis should be distinguished from plugged milk ducts, which present as hard, locally tender, red areas without associated regional pain or fever.
- Severe engorgement occurs due to interstitial edema and may be distinguished from severe engorgement which is bilateral and not typically associated with systemic symptoms of fever.
- A galactocele (milk retention cyst) is a cystic collection of fluid that results from an obstructed milk duct. Galactoceles present as soft, nontender, cystic masses not associated with systemic symptoms. Ultrasonography may demonstrate a simple milk cyst or a complex mass. The diagnosis is made on the basis of the clinical history and needle aspiration.

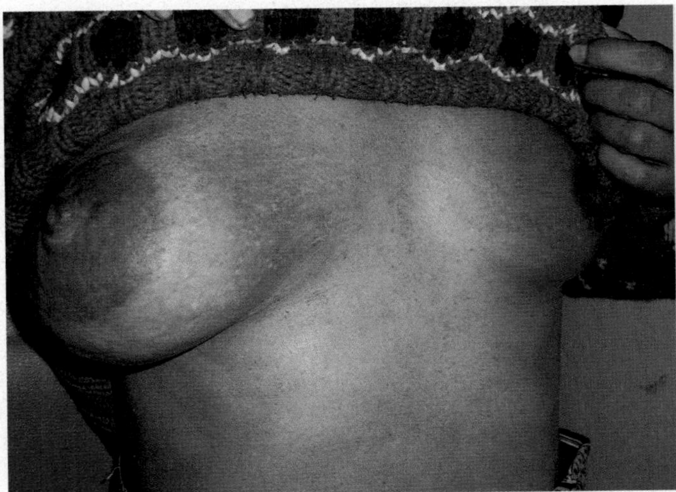

FIGURE 94-3 Mastitis in a postpartum breastfeeding woman. The right breast was warm, tender, enlarged, and painful. Erythema is barely visible on the areola because of the naturally darker pigmentation of the skin. (*Reproduced with permission from Richard P. Usatine, MD.*)

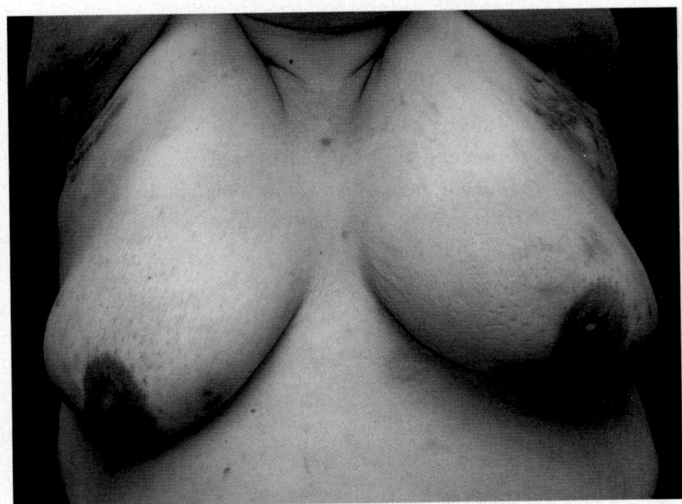

FIGURE 94-4 A breast abscess in the left breast of a 43-year-old women with hidradenitis suppurativa. Note the peau d'orange appearance of the left breast before the abscess was drained. Both breasts and axillae have multiple old scars from previous incisions to drain abscesses and hidradenitis in the past. Her axillae have active chronic disease, but her acute problem is the breast abscess. (*Reproduced with permission from Richard P. Usatine, MD.*)

- Inflammatory breast cancer (IBC) should be considered if mastitis does not resolve with appropriate treatment and is diagnosed with biopsy.
- Periductal mastitis is an inflammatory condition of the subareolar ducts seen in young nonlactating women who are smokers.
- An infected or inflamed epidermal inclusion cyst is a skin infection that may not involve the underlying breast tissue but still requires an incision and drainage (**Figure 94-5**).

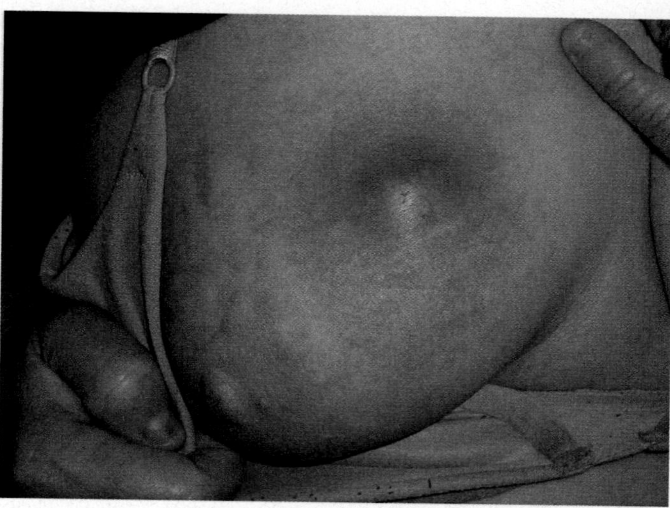

FIGURE 94-5 An inflamed and infected epidermal inclusion cyst on the breast but in the subcutaneous tissue. An incision and drainage was performed. (*Reproduced with permission from Richard P. Usatine, MD.*)

MANAGEMENT

- Management of mastitis includes supportive measures such as continued breastfeeding and bed rest. SOR Ⓒ If the infant cannot relieve breast fullness during nursing, breast massage during nursing or pumping afterwards may help reduce discomfort (see **Figure 94-3**).
- Acetaminophen or an anti-inflammatory agent such as ibuprofen may be used for pain control.
- Antibiotic treatment should be initiated with dicloxacillin or cephalexin (500 mg po 4 times daily) for 10 to 14 days.[7] SOR Ⓐ Consider clindamycin if the patient is allergic to penicillin and/or cephalosporins.[7] Clindamycin may be a good choice if methicillin-resistant *Staphylococcus aureus* (MRSA) is suspected. All of the antibiotics recommended are safe for the baby during pregnancy and lactation. Trimethoprim/sulfamethoxazole is an alternative for MRSA and/or penicillin-allergic patients, but it should be avoided near term in pregnancy and in the first 2 months of breastfeeding because of a risk to the baby of kernicterus. Shorter courses of antibiotic therapy may be associated with higher relapse rates. SOR Ⓒ
- The management of a breast abscess consists of drainage of the abscess.[7] SOR Ⓐ Antibiotic therapy should be considered and is especially important if there is surrounding cellulitis (see **Figure 94-2**).
- Drainage can usually be performed by needle aspiration, with the addition of ultrasound guidance if necessary. It appears to be equally as effective as incision and drainage with less morbidity.[8]
- If needle aspiration is not effective, incision and drainage should be performed. Incision and drainage is often preferred because it allows for continued drainage through the opening. In many cases a cotton wick is placed to keep the abscess open while the purulence drains in the following days.[8]
- Breastfeeding may continue on both breasts if the incision isn't too painful and it does not interfere with the baby latching on. Otherwise a breast pump may be used on the affected breast for 3 to 4 days until nursing can resume.

FOLLOW-UP

- If no response is seen within 48 hours or if MRSA is a possibility, antibiotic therapy should be switched to trimethoprim-sulfamethoxazole 1 double strength po twice a day, or clindamycin 300 mg orally q6h. Avoid trimethoprim/sulfamethoxazole near term pregnancy and in the first 2 months of breastfeeding.

- Hospitalization and intravenous antibiotics are rarely needed but should be considered if the patient is systemically ill and not able to tolerate oral antibiotics.

PATIENT EDUCATION

- The patient may take acetaminophen or ibuprofen for pain, since these medications are safe while breastfeeding and are indicated for use in children.
- Warm compresses applied before and after feedings can provide some pain relief. A warm bath may also help.
- Instruct the patient to finish the antibiotic prescription, even if she feels better in a few days, to lower the risk of bacterial resistance or relapse.
- Continue feedings and use a breast pump to completely empty the breast if necessary.
- Educate the parents that the mastitis or the antibiotics will not harm the baby, and that the source of the infection was probably the baby's own mouth.
- Continue to drink plenty of water and eat well-balanced meals.

PATIENT RESOURCES

- MedlinePlus. *Breast Infection*—**http://www.nlm.nih.gov/medlineplus/ency/article/001490.htm.**
- WebMD. *What Is Mastitis?*—**http://www.webmd.com/parenting/baby/tc/what-is-mastitis#1.**
- Mayo Clinic. *Mastitis*—**https://www.mayoclinic.org/diseases-conditions/mastitis/symptoms-causes/syc-20374829.**

PROVIDER RESOURCES

- eMedicine. *Abscesses and Masses*—**https://emedicine.medscape.com/article/781116-overview.**
- American Family Physician. *Management of Mastitis in Breast-feeding Women*—**http://www.aafp.org/afp/2008/0915/p727.html.**
- Andolsek KM, Copeland JA. Benign breast conditions and disease: mastitis. In: Taylor RB, ed. *Family Medicine Principles and Practice.* 6th ed. New York, NY: Springer, 2003:898.

REFERENCES

1. Committee on Health Care for Underserved Women, American College of Obstetricians and Gynecologists. ACOG Committee Opinion No. 361: Breastfeeding: maternal and infant aspects. Obstet Gynecol 2007; 109:479.
2. Foxman B, D'Arcy H, Gillespie B, et al. Lactation mastitis: Occurrence and medical management among 946 breastfeeding women in the United States. *Am J Epidemiol.* 2002;155:103.
3. Kvist LJ, Rydhstroem H. Factors related to breast abscess after delivery: a population-based study. *BJOG.* 2005;112:1070.
4. Berens PD. Prenatal, intrapartum, and postpartum support of the lactating mother. *Pediatr Clin North Am.* 2001;48:365.
5. Dixon JM. ABC of breast diseases. Breast infection. *BMJ.* 1994;309(6959):946-949.
6. Muttarak M, Chaiwun B. Imaging of giant breast masses with pathological correlation. *Singapore Med J.* 2004;45(3):132-139.
7. Stevens DL, Bisno AL, Chambers HF, et al. Practice guidelines for the diagnosis and management of skin and soft-tissue infections. *Clin Infect Dis.* 2005;41:1373-1406.
8. Irusen H, Rohwer AC, Steyn DW, Young T. Treatments for breast abscesses in breastfeeding women. *Cochrane Database Syst Rev.* 2015;(8):CD010490.

95 BREAST CANCER

E.J. Mayeaux, Jr., MD

PATIENT STORY

A 55-year-old woman presents for routine screening mammogram. The patient does not have any complaints but has a family history of breast cancer in a sister at the age of 40 years. Her mammogram demonstrates an irregular mass with possible local spread (**Figures 95-1** and **95-2**). She is referred to a breast surgeon, and the biopsy confirms the diagnosis of breast cancer.

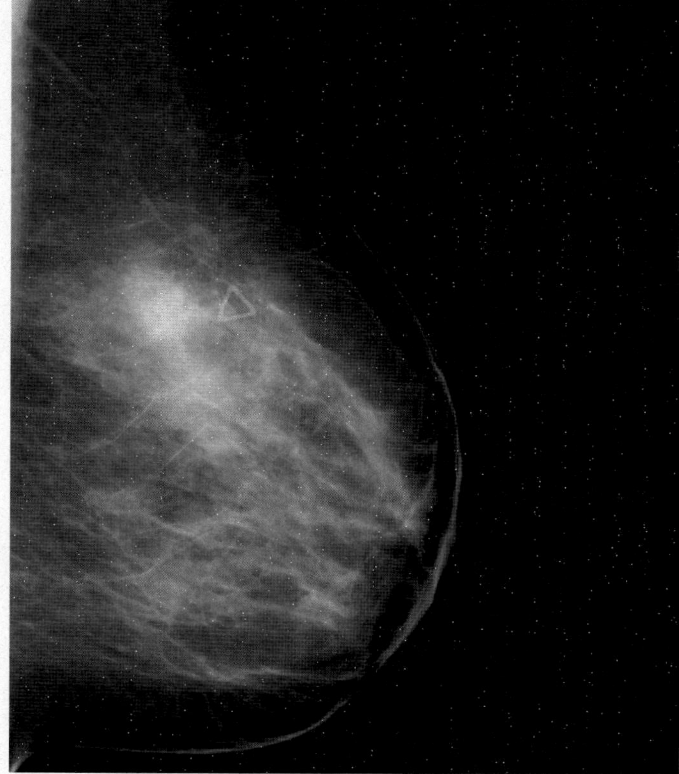

FIGURE 95-1 A mammogram that demonstrates an irregular mass with possible local spread. *(Reproduced with permission from John Braud, MD.)*

INTRODUCTION

Breast cancer is a major health concern for all women. It is the most common female cancer in the United States, and the second most common cause of cancer death in women after lung cancer.[1]

EPIDEMIOLOGY

- In 2012, approximately 250,000 women in the United States were diagnosed with breast cancer.[2] Breast cancer incidence in the United States has doubled over the past 60 years. Since the early 1980s, most of the increase has been in early stage and in situ cancers because of mammogram screening and better chemotherapy (**Figures 95-1** to **95-4**).
- Approximately 232,620 new cases of invasive breast cancer were expected to be diagnosed in the United States in 2011, and 39,970 were expected to die from the disease.[1]
- Globally, breast cancer is the most common cancer, and the leading cause of cancer death in females. Breast cancer incidence rates are highest in North America, Australia–New Zealand, and Europe, and lowest in Asia and sub-Saharan Africa.[2,3]
- Locally advanced breast cancer (LABC) has been decreasing in frequency over the past several decades, at least partially as a result of earlier diagnosis because of better screening (**Figures 95-5** to **95-8**). It represents 30% to 50% of newly diagnosed breast cancers in medically underserved populations.[4]
- Primary inflammatory breast cancer (IBC) is relatively rare, accounting for 0.5% to 2% of invasive breast cancers.[5] However, it accounts for a greater proportion of cases presenting with more advanced disease. IBC is a clinical diagnosis. At presentation, almost all women with primary IBC have lymph node involvement and approximately one third have distant metastases.[6]

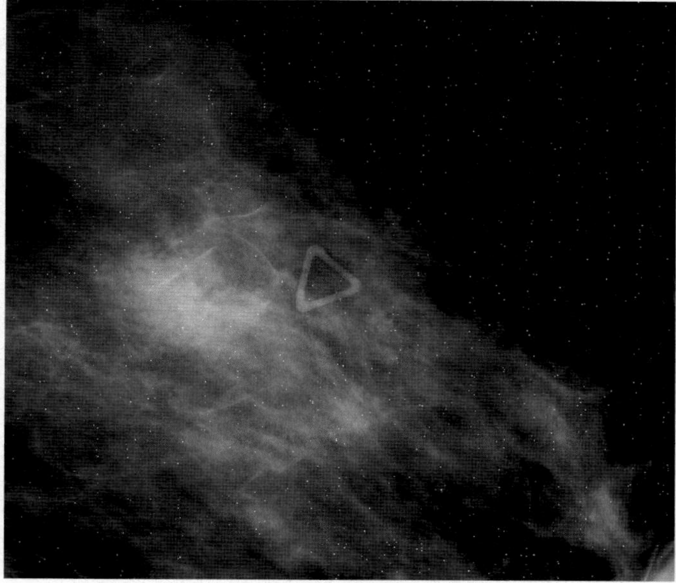

FIGURE 95-2 A close-up view of the lesion shown in **Figure 95-1**. *(Reproduced with permission from John Braud, MD.)*

ETIOLOGY AND PATHOPHYSIOLOGY

- The incidence of breast cancer increases with age. White women are more likely to develop breast cancer than black women. One percent of breast cancers occur in men.

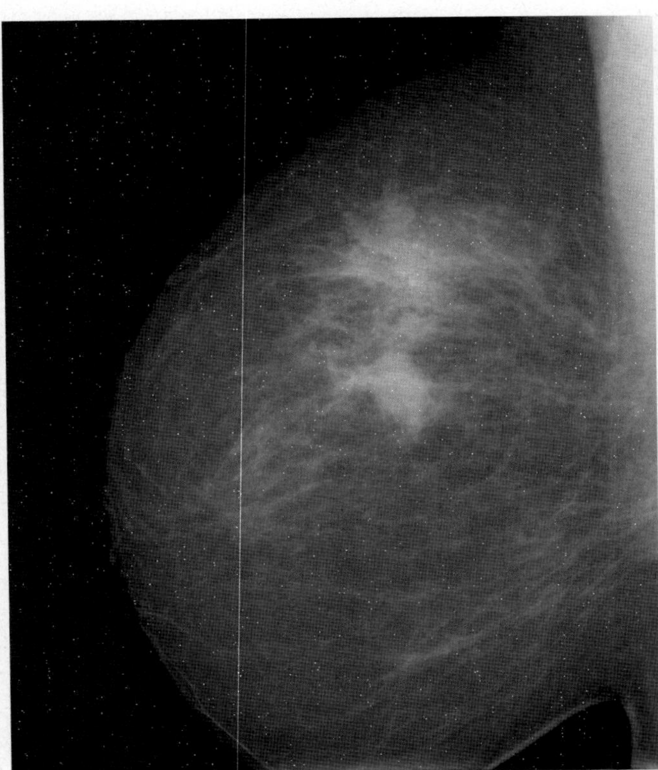

FIGURE 95-3 A screening mammogram of a 55-year-old woman who is without breast complaints. The mammogram demonstrates a significant mass with spiculations. (*Reproduced with permission from John Braud, MD.*)

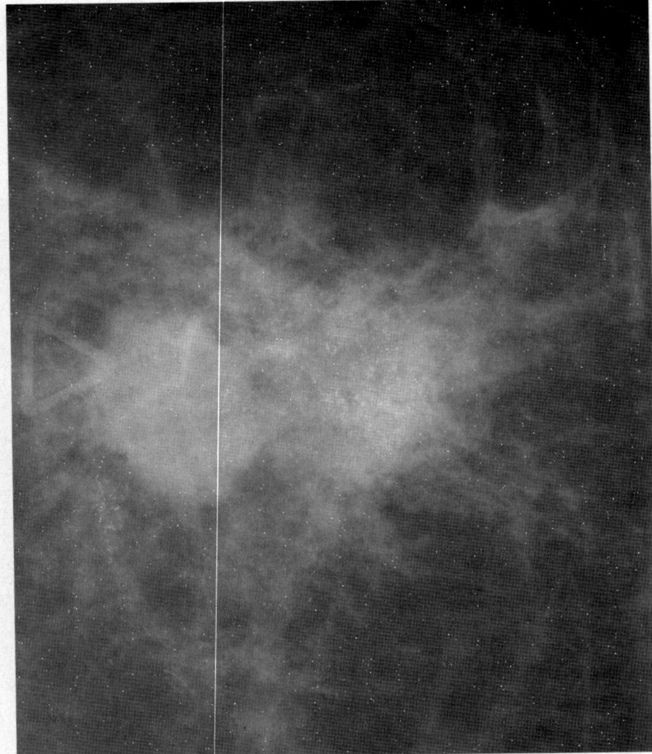

FIGURE 95-4 Close-up view of the mass shown in **Figure 95-3** demonstrating clear spiculations and microcalcifications. (*Reproduced with permission from John Braud, MD.*)

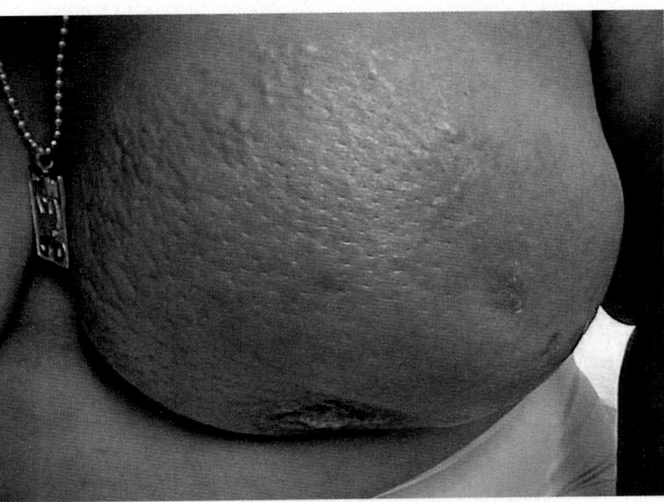

FIGURE 95-5 Woman with advanced breast cancer and peau d'orange sign. The skin looks like the skin of an orange as a consequence of lymphedema. (*Reproduced with permission from Richard P. Usatine, MD.*)

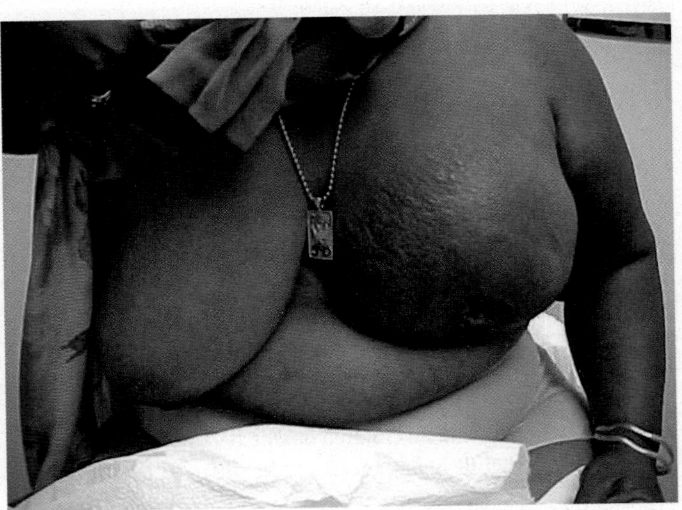

FIGURE 95-6 The patient in **Figure 95-5** showing breast retraction and brawny edema of the breast and arm. (*Reproduced with permission from Richard P. Usatine, MD.*)

- Primary risk factors for the development of breast cancer include age older than 50 years, female sex, increased exposure to estrogen (including early menarche and late menopause), and a family history in a first-degree maternal relative (especially if diagnosed premenopausally).
- Approximately 8% of breast cancers are hereditary, and half of these are associated with mutations in genes BRCA1 and BRCA2. It is more common in premenopausal women, multiple family generations, and bilateral breasts.[7] Typically, several family members are affected over at least three generations and can include women from the paternal side of the family.
- A history of a proliferative breast abnormality, such as atypical hyperplasia, may increase a woman's risk for developing breast cancer.
- The selective estrogen receptor modulator tamoxifen (and possibly raloxifene) reduces the risk of developing breast cancer.
- The American Cancer Society, American College of Radiology, American Medical Association, and American College of Obstetrics and Gynecology all recommend starting routine screening at age 40 years.[8]
- The United States Preventive Services Task Force and the 2002 statement by the American Academy of Family Physicians recommend screening mammography every 1 to 2 years for women ages 40 years and older.[9]
- Women who have a family history of BRCA mutation should begin annual mammography between 25 and 35 years of age.[10] SOR Ⓐ
- MRI screening is more sensitive for detecting breast cancers than mammography and is being used to screen women with BRCA mutations.[11] It is not proven that surveillance regimens that include MRI will reduce mortality from breast cancer in high-risk women.[11]
- Although the sensitivity of MRI is greater than that of conventional imaging, MRI has a lower specificity. One study suggests that unnecessary biopsies can be avoided with second-look ultrasound when MRI is positive and mammography is not. Second-look ultrasound can be used to recognize false-positive MRI results and guide biopsies.[12]

RISK FACTORS

- Positive family history of breast and/or ovarian cancer (especially with BRCA mutations).
- Personal history of breast cancer.
- Increasing age in women.
- Early age at menarche and late menopause.
- Prolonged exposure to and higher concentrations of endogenous or exogenous estrogen.
- Exposure to ionizing radiation.
- Dense breast tissue and atypical hyperplasia.
- Women who have had no children or who had their first child after age 30 have a slightly higher breast cancer risk.
- Low physical activity levels.
- High-fat diet.
- Alcohol intake of two or more drinks daily.

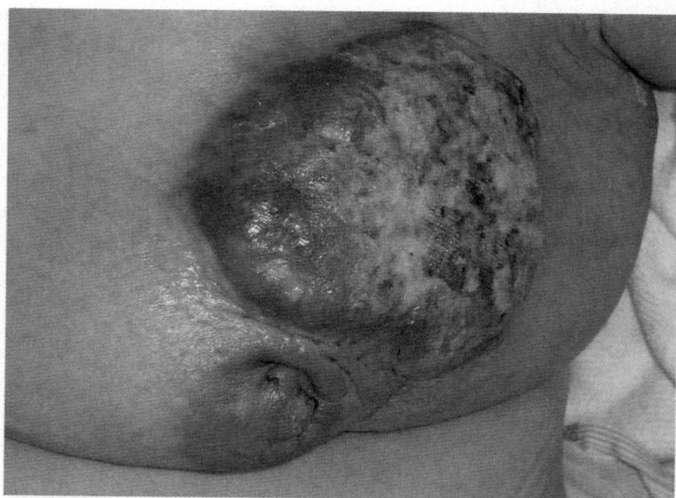

FIGURE 95-7 Advanced breast cancer with fungating mass and distortion of the normal breast anatomy. (*Reproduced with permission from Kristen Sorensen, MD.*)

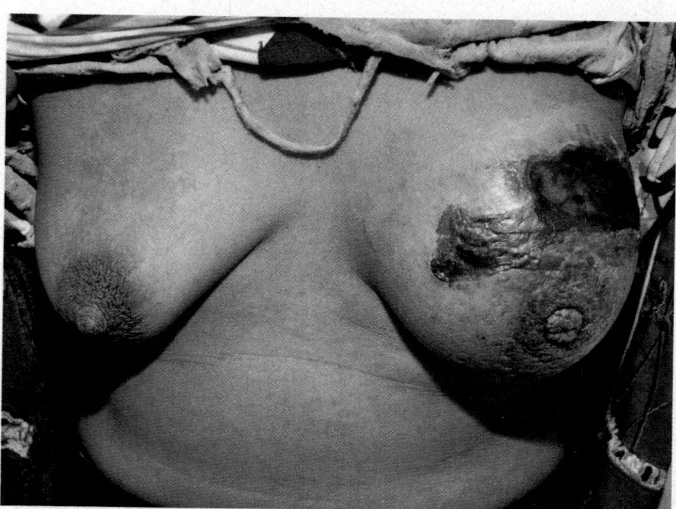

FIGURE 95-8 Ethiopian woman with breast cancer and five enlarged firm left axillary lymph nodes. Note the breast asymmetry and the peau d'orange skin on the left breast. The dark black area was caused by a "traditional healer" who burned the skin. Unfortunately the woman could not afford to get care at the local hospital, making her prognosis very grave. (*Reproduced with permission from Richard P. Usatine, MD.*)

DIAGNOSIS

CLINICAL FEATURES

- In countries with established breast cancer screening programs, most breast cancer is identified by abnormal mammogram.
- Detection of a breast mass is the most common patient presenting breast complaint. However, 90% of all breast masses are caused by benign lesions. Breast pain is also a common presenting problem. Physical examination of the breast should be performed in the upright (sitting) and supine positions. Inspect for differences in size, retraction of the skin or nipple (see **Figures 95-5** and **95-6**), prominent venous patterns, and signs of inflammation (see **Figures 95-5** and **95-6**). Palpate the breast tissue, axillary area, and supraclavicular areas for masses or adenopathy. The classic presentation is a hard, immovable, single dominant lesion with irregular borders. Gently squeeze the nipple to check for discharge.
- Most LABCs are both palpable and visible (see **Figures 95-7** and **95-8**). Careful palpation of the skin, breasts, and regional lymph nodes is the initial step in diagnosis. The patient in **Figure 95-8** had five palpable lymph nodes at the time of presentation.
- IBC usually presents clinically as a diffuse brawny induration of the skin of the breast with an erythematous edge, and usually without an underlying palpable mass. Patients with de novo IBC typically present with pain and a rapidly enlarging breast. The skin over the breast is warm and thickened, with a "peau d'orange" (skin of an orange) appearance (see **Figures 95-5** and **95-6**). The skin color can range from a pink flushed discoloration to a purplish hue.

TYPICAL DISTRIBUTION

- A mass that is suspicious for breast cancer is usually solitary, discrete, hard, unilateral, and nontender. It may be fixed to the skin or the chest wall.

IMAGING

- More than 90% of breast cancers are identified mammographically.[13] Classic mammographic findings of breast cancer include a soft tissue density and clustered microcalcifications. A spiculated soft tissue mass is the most specific feature of an invasive cancer. When an abnormality is found, supplemental mammographic views and possibly ultrasound are usually done. Diagnostic mammography is associated with higher sensitivity but lower specificity as compared to screening mammography.[14]
- Sonographic features of breast malignancy include spiculation, hypoechogenicity, microlobulation, internal calcifications, shadowing, and angular margins.[15]

BIOPSY

- Fine-needle aspiration biopsy generally uses a 20- to 23-gauge needle to obtain samples from a solid mass for cytology. Ultrasound or stereotactic guidance is used to assist in collecting a fine-needle aspiration from a nonpalpable lump. Core biopsy uses a 14-gauge or similar needle to remove cores of tissue from a mass. Excisional biopsy is done as the initial procedure or when needle biopsies are negative when the clinical suspicion is high. Guided biopsy and nonguided biopsy are also commonly used to make a definitive diagnosis.

DIFFERENTIAL DIAGNOSIS

- Fibroadenomas usually present as smooth, rounded, rubbery masses in women in their 20s and 30s. A clinically suspicious mass should be biopsied even if mammography findings are normal.
- Benign cysts are rubbery and hollow-feeling in women in their 30s and 40s. A cyst can be diagnosed by ultrasound imaging. A simple cyst can be aspirated, but a residual mass requires further evaluation. Ultrasound is useful to differentiate between solid and cystic breast masses, especially in young women with dense breast tissue.
- Bilateral mastalgia is rarely associated with breast cancer, but it does not eliminate the possibility. It is usually related to fibrocystic changes in premenopausal women that are associated with diffuse lumpy breasts. A unilateral breast lump with pain must be evaluated for breast cancer.
- Nipple discharge may be from infection, which is usually purulent, and from pregnancy, stimulation, or prolactinoma, which produces a thin, milky, often bilateral discharge. A pregnancy test may be helpful. A suspicious discharge from a single duct can be evaluated with a ductogram.
- Infectious mastitis and breast abscess, which typically occur in lactating women, appear similar to IBC but are generally associated with fever and leukocytosis (see Chapter 94, Breast Abscess and Mastitis).
- Ductal ectasia with inflammation appears similar but is usually localized.
- Leukemic involvement of the breast may mimic IBC, but the peripheral blood smear is typically diagnostic.

MANAGEMENT

FIRST LINE

- Surgical resection is required in all patients with invasive breast cancer. Oncologic outcomes are similar with mastectomy and breast-conserving therapy (lumpectomy plus breast radiation therapy) in appropriately selected patients. For women undergoing mastectomy, breast reconstruction may be performed at the same time as the initial breast cancer surgery, or deferred to a later date.[16] SOR Ⓐ Following surgical treatment, adjuvant systemic therapy may be offered based on tumor size, grade, number of involved lymph nodes, the status of estrogen (ER) and progesterone (PR) receptors, and expression of the human epidermal growth factor 2 (HER2) receptor.
- With the emergence of breast-conserving therapy (BCT), many women now have the option of preserving a cosmetically acceptable breast without sacrificing survival for early stage invasive breast cancer.
- Long-term survival can be achieved in approximately 50% of women with LABC who are treated with a multimodality approach.[17] Prognostic factors include age, menopausal status, tumor stage and histologic grade, clinical response to neoadjuvant therapy, and estrogen receptor status.

- In general, women with IBC are approached similarly to those with noninflammatory LABC except that BCT is generally considered inappropriate for these women.[18] SOR Ⓐ

SECOND LINE

- Adjuvant systemic therapy consists of administration of hormone therapy, chemotherapy, and/or trastuzumab (a humanized monoclonal antibody directed against HER-2/neu) after definitive local therapy for breast cancer. It benefits most women with early stage breast cancer, but the magnitude of benefit is greatest for those with node-positive disease.[19] SOR Ⓐ
- The most common approach for advanced breast cancer is preoperative chemotherapy followed by surgery and radiotherapy. Questions regarding sequencing and choice of specific chemotherapy regimens and extent of surgery (including the utility of the sentinel node biopsy) persist. SOR Ⓐ
- Preoperative (as opposed to postoperative) chemotherapy has several advantages for treatment of advanced breast cancer (see **Figure 95-7**). It can reduce the size of the primary tumor, thus allowing for breast-conserving surgery; it permits assessing an identified mass to determine the sensitivity of the tumor cells to drugs with discontinuation of ineffective therapy (thus avoiding unnecessary toxicity); and it enables drug delivery through an intact tumor vasculature.[20] SOR Ⓐ
- Tamoxifen and aromatase inhibitors may be used in selected patients as neoadjuvant hormone therapy to decrease overall tumor volume. SOR Ⓐ

REFERRAL

- Any patient presenting with obvious metastatic breast cancer needs referral to a medical oncologist along with a breast cancer surgeon (**Figure 95-9**).

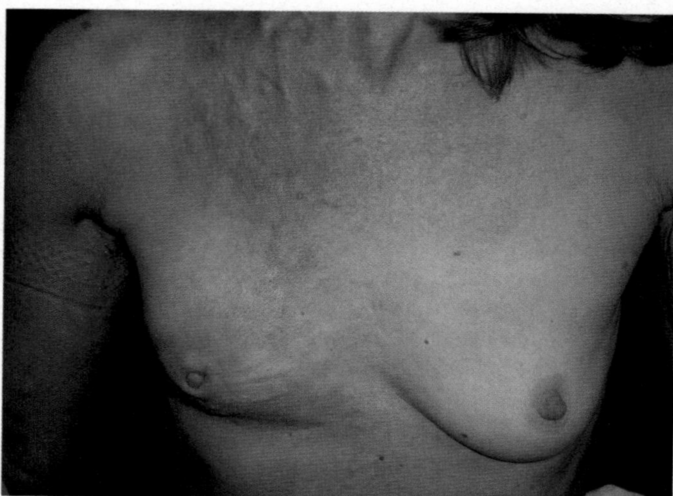

FIGURE 95-9 Metastatic breast cancer with firm palpable skin metastases on the chest, palpable lymph nodes, and lymphedema. The breast itself is rock hard and retracted, and there is nipple retraction as well. Chest X-ray showed large pleural effusions. *(Reproduced with permission from Richard P. Usatine, MD.)*

PREVENTION

- Healthy lifestyle choices can decrease the risk of breast cancer, including a low-fat diet, regular exercise, and no more than one drink daily.
- Having children before age 30 years and prolonged breastfeeding may be of help in primary prevention, but will not be a commonly used strategy for most women.
- Secondary prevention involves screening for breast cancer with physical exams and mammography. There is a strong consensus based on consistent findings from multiple randomized trials that routine screening mammography should be offered to women ages 50 to 69 years. Consensus is less strong for routine screening among women ages 40 to 49 years, women older than age 70 years, or for how frequently to screen.
    - The American Cancer Society,[21] the National Cancer Institute,[22] the American College of Obstetricians and Gynecologists,[23] and the National Comprehensive Cancer Network[24] recommend starting routine screening at age 40 years.
    - The U.S. Preventive Services Task Force (USPSTF)[25] and the Canadian Task Force on the Periodic Health Examination[26] recommend beginning routine screening at age 50 years.

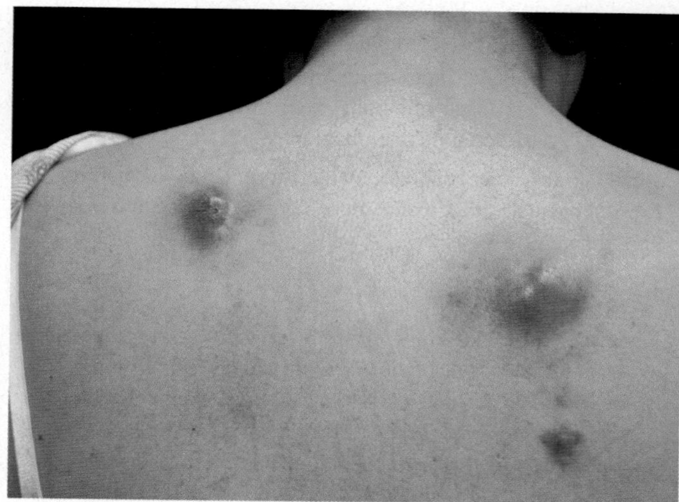

FIGURE 95-10 Metastatic breast cancer with firm palpable nodules on the back. *(Reproduced with permission from Richard P. Usatine, MD.)*

- Prophylactic mastectomy is an effective and accepted method for some BRCA-positive women after childbearing when their risk of lifetime breast cancer without this intervention is high (e.g., over 60%).
- Chemoprevention with tamoxifen or raloxifene is an option for women who are high risk for breast cancer.

FOLLOW-UP

- Regular follow-up will usually be maintained during treatment. After treatment, lifelong regular follow-up for surveillance should be maintained. Metastases can present in many ways, including difficulty breathing, back pain, or a new skin nodule (**Figure 95-10**). These complaints should be taken seriously and worked up carefully in any patient with a history of breast cancer.

PATIENT EDUCATION

- The contralateral breast is at increased risk of breast cancer and should be monitored. Patients on tamoxifen should be monitored for endometrial hyperplasia or cancer.

PATIENT RESOURCES

- Breast Cancer. American Cancer Society—**https://www.cancer.org/cancer/breast-cancer.html.**
- Breastcancer.org—**http://www.breastcancer.org.**

PROVIDER RESOURCES

- American Academy of Family Physicians. *Putting Prevention into Practice, An Evidence-Based Approach—Screening for Breast Cancer*—**http://www.aafp.org/afp/2016/0715/p143.html.**
- U.S. Preventive Services Task Force. *Breast Cancer: Screening*—**https://www.uspreventiveservicestaskforce.org/Page/Document/RecommendationStatementFinal/breast-cancer-screening1.**
- Breast Cancer Screening (PDQ®). *Health Professional Version*—**https://www.cancer.gov/types/breast/hp/breast-screening-pdq.**
- Centers for Disease Control and Prevention. *Breast Cancer*—**https://www.cdc.gov/cancer/breast/.**

REFERENCES

1. Siegel R, Ward E, Brawley O, Jemal A. Cancer statistics, 2011: the impact of eliminating socioeconomic and racial disparities on premature cancer deaths. *CA Cancer J Clin.* 2011;61(4):212-236.
2. Globocan 2012. *Fast Stats.* Most frequent cancers: both sexes. http://globocan.iarc.fr/Pages/fact_sheets_cancer.aspx. Accessed March 2017.
3. Siegel RL, Miller KD, Jemal A. Cancer statistics, 2017. *CA Cancer J Clin.* 2017;67:7.
4. Hortobagyi GN, Sinigletary SE, Strom EA. Treatment of locally advanced and inflammatory breast cancer. In: Harris JR, Lippman ME, Morrow M, Osborne CK, eds. *Diseases of the Breast*, 2nd ed. Philadelphia, PA: Lippincott Williams & Wilkins; 2000:645-660.
5. Hance KW, Anderson WF, Devesa SS, et al. Trends in inflammatory breast carcinoma incidence and survival: The Surveillance, Epidemiology, and End Results Program at the National Cancer Institute. *J Natl Cancer Inst.* 2005;97(13):966-975.
6. Kleer CG, van Golen KL, Merajver SD. Molecular biology of breast cancer metastasis: inflammatory breast cancer: clinical syndrome and molecular determinants. *Breast Cancer Res.* 2000;2(6):423-429.
7. Krainer M, Silva-Arrieta S, FitzGerald MG, et al. Differential contributions of BRCA1 and BRCA2 to early-onset breast cancer. *N Engl J Med.* 1997;336(20):1416-1421.
8. Smith RA, Saslow D, Sawyer KA, et al. American Cancer Society guidelines for breast cancer screening: update 2003. *CA Cancer J Clin.* 2003;53(3):141-169.
9. U.S. Preventive Services Task Force. *Guide to Clinical Preventive Services*, 3rd ed. http://www.ahrq.gov/clinic/uspstfix.htm. Accessed February 2012.
10. Burke W, Daly M, Garber J, et al. Recommendations for follow-up care of individuals with an inherited predisposition to cancer. II. BRCA1 and BRCA2. *JAMA.* 1997;277(12):997-1003.
11. Warner E, Plewes DB, Hill KA, et al. Surveillance of BRCA1 and BRCA2 mutation carriers with magnetic resonance imaging, ultrasound, mammography, and clinical breast examination. *JAMA.* 2004;292(11):1317-1325.
12. Trecate G, Vergnaghi D, Manoukian S, et al. MRI in the early detection of breast cancer in women with high genetic risk. *Tumori.* 2006;92(6):517-523.
13. Smart CR, Hartmann WH, Beahrs OH, Garfinkel L. Insights into breast cancer screening of younger women. Evidence from the 14-year follow-up of the Breast Cancer Detection Demonstration Project. *Cancer.* 1995;72(4 Suppl):1449-1456.
14. Barlow WE, Lehman CD, Zheng Y, et al. Performance of diagnostic mammography for women with signs or symptoms of breast cancer. *J Natl Cancer Inst.* 2002;94(15):1151-1159.
15. Stavros AT, Thickman D, Rapp CL, et al. Solid breast nodules: use of sonography to distinguish between benign and malignant lesions. *Radiology.* 1995;196:123.
16. Vandeweyer E, Hertens D, Nogaret JM, Deraemaecker R. Immediate breast reconstruction with saline-filled implants: no interference with the oncologic outcome? *Plast Reconstr Surg.* 2001;107(6):1409-1412.
17. Brito RA, Valero V, Buzdar AU, et al. Long-term results of combined-modality therapy for locally advanced breast cancer with ipsilateral supraclavicular metastases: The University of Texas M.D. Anderson Cancer Center experience. *J Clin Oncol.* 2001;19(3):628-633.
18. Lyman GH, Giuliano AE, Somerfield MR, et al.; American Society of Clinical Oncology. American Society of Clinical Oncology guideline recommendations for sentinel lymph node biopsy in early-stage breast cancer. *J Clin Oncol.* 2005;23(30):7703-7720.

19. Goldhirsch A, Glick JH, Gelber RD, et al. Meeting highlights: international expert consensus on the primary therapy of early breast cancer 2005. *Ann Oncol.* 2005;16(10):1569-1583.

20. Fisher B, Gunduz N, Saffer EA. Influence of the interval between primary tumor removal and chemotherapy on kinetics and growth of metastases. *Cancer Res.* 1983;43(4):1488-1492.

21. Smith RA, Cokkinides V, Brawley OW. Cancer screening in the United States, 2009: a review of current American Cancer Society guidelines and issues in cancer screening. *CA Cancer J Clin.* 2009; 59(1):27-41.

22. National Cancer Institute. *Breast Cancer Screening (PDQ).* http://www.cancer.gov/cancertopics/pdq/screening/breast/HealthProfessional/page2. Accessed March 2017.

23. American College of Obstetricians and Gynecologists. Practice Bulletin No. 122: Breast cancer screening. *Obstet Gynecol.* 2011; 118(2 Pt 1):372-382.

24. Bevers TB, Anderson BO, Bonaccio E, et al.; National Comprehensive Cancer Network. NCCN Clinical Practice Guidelines in Oncology: breast cancer screening and diagnosis. *J Natl Compr Canc Netw.* 2009;7(10):1060-1096.

25. U.S. Preventive Services Task Force. *Screening for Breast Cancer.* https://www.uspreventiveservicestaskforce.org/Page/Document/UpdateSummaryFinal/breast-cancer-screening1. Accessed March 2017.

26. Canadian Task Force on the Periodic Health Examination. *Screening for Breast Cancer.* http://canadiantaskforce.ca/guidelines/published-guidelines/breast-cancer/. Accessed March 2017.

96 PAGET DISEASE OF THE BREAST

E.J. Mayeaux, Jr., MD

PATIENT STORY

A 62-year-old woman presents with a 6-month history of an eczematous, scaly, rash near her nipple. It is mildly pruritic. On physical examination, the nipple and the areola are involved (**Figure 96-1**). Also, a hard mass is present in the lateral lower quadrant of the same breast. A 4-mm punch biopsy of the affected area including the nipple demonstrates Paget disease. The mammogram is suspicious for breast cancer at the site of the mass, and the patient is referred to a breast surgeon.

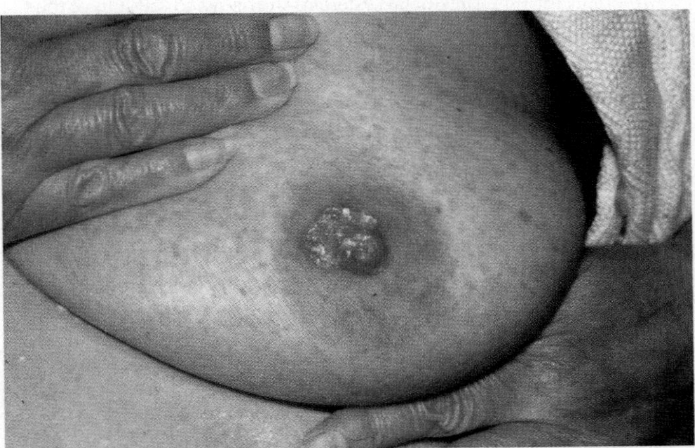

FIGURE 96-1 Paget disease of the breast of a 62-year-old woman that presented as a persistent eczematous lesion. *(Reproduced with permission from Richard P. Usatine, MD.)*

INTRODUCTION

Paget disease of the breast is a low-grade malignancy of the breast that is often associated with other malignancies. It is an important consideration when working up a chronic persistent abnormality of the nipple.

SYNONYMS

Paget's disease, mammary Paget disease.

EPIDEMIOLOGY

- The incidence of Paget disease of the breast is approximately 0.4% in women in the United States, according to National Cancer Institute Surveillance, Epidemiology, and End Results (SEER) data.[1] Paget disease, like all breast cancers, is rare in men.
- The peak incidence is between 50 and 60 years of age.[2]
- It is associated with underlying in situ and/or invasive breast cancer 85% to 88% of the time.[3]
- Some epidemiologic data suggest that the incidence of Paget disease of the breast is decreasing over time.[3]

ETIOLOGY AND PATHOPHYSIOLOGY

- Most patients delay presentation, assuming the abnormality is a benign condition of some sort. The median duration of signs and symptoms prior to diagnosis is 6 to 8 months.[2]
- Presenting symptoms are sometimes limited to persistent pain, burning, and/or pruritus of the nipple (**Figures 96-1** and **96-2**).
- A palpable breast mass is present in 50% of cases, but is often located more than 2 cm from the nipple–areolar complex.[4]
- Twenty percent of cases will have a mammographic abnormality without a palpable mass, and 25% of cases will have neither a mass nor abnormal mammogram, but will have an occult ductal carcinoma.

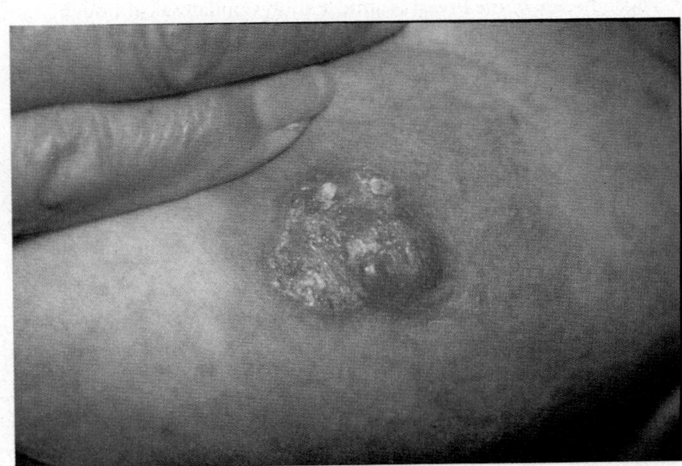

FIGURE 96-2 Close-up of Paget disease of the breast. Note the erythematous, eczematous, scaly appearance of the lesion. *(Reproduced with permission from Richard P. Usatine, MD.)*

- In less than 5% of cases, Paget disease of the breast is an isolated finding.[4]
- There are two theories regarding the pathogenesis of Paget disease of the breast, the choice of which affects treatment choices.
    - The more widely accepted epidermotropic theory proposes that the Paget cells arise from an underlying mammary adenocarcinoma that migrates through the ductal system of the breast to the skin of the nipple. It is supported by the fact that Paget disease is usually associated with an underlying ductal carcinoma, and both Paget cells and mammary ductal cells usually express similar immunochemical staining patterns and molecular markers. This could mean that there is a common genetic alteration and/or a common progenitor cell for both Paget cells and the underlying ductal carcinoma.
    - The less widely accepted transformation theory proposes that epidermal cells in the nipple transform into malignant Paget cells, and that Paget disease of the breast represents an independent epidermal carcinoma in situ. It is supported by the fact that there is no parenchymal cancer identified in a small percentage of cases, and underlying breast carcinomas are often located at some distance from the nipple. Most pathologists disagree with the transformation theory.

FIGURE 96-3 Paget disease of the breast of a 29-year-old woman that presented as a persistent eczematous lesion for 8 months prior to biopsy. The patient did not have a palpable breast mass. (*Reproduced with permission from Richard P. Usatine, MD.*)

DIAGNOSIS

CLINICAL FEATURES

- Paget disease of the breast presents clinically in the nipple–areolar complex as a dermatitis that may be erythematous, eczematous, scaly, raw, vesicular, or ulcerated (**Figures 96-1** to **96-4**). The nipple is usually initially involved, and the lesion then spreads to the areola. Spontaneous improvement or healing of the nipple dermatitis can occur and should not be taken as an indication that Paget disease is not present. The diagnosis is made by finding malignant, intraepithelial adenocarcinoma cells on pathology. Rarely, nipple retraction is found.
- Pain, burning, and/or pruritus may be present or even precede clinically apparent disease developing on the skin.

TYPICAL DISTRIBUTION

- Paget disease of the breast is almost always unilateral, although bilateral cases have been reported.
- Work-up must also be directed toward identifying any underlying breast cancer.

LABORATORY TESTING

- The diagnosis is made by finding intraepithelial adenocarcinoma cells (Paget cells) either singly or in small groups within the epidermis of the nipple complex.
- Approximately one-half of cases express hormone receptors, and when present, estrogen and/or progesterone receptor positivity is helpful in planning treatment.

IMAGING

- Bilateral mammography is mandatory to asses for associated cancers. MRI may disclose occult cancer in some women with Paget disease of the breast and normal mammography and/or physical examination.[5]

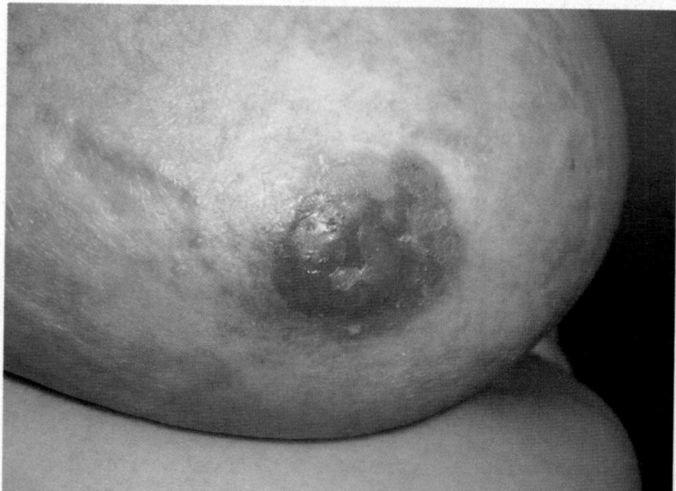

FIGURE 96-4 Close-up of Paget disease of the breast in the young woman in **Figure 96-3**. Note the erythematous, scaly, and ulcerated appearance of the lesion. (*Reproduced with permission from Richard P. Usatine, MD.*)

- Ultrasound may be useful to identify masses in cases with negative mammograms. However, findings are nonspecific.[6]
- Polarized dermoscopy may also be useful in diagnosis, especially in cases of pigmented mammary Paget disease.[7]

BIOPSY

- The diagnosis is usually made by full-thickness punch or wedge biopsy that shows Paget cells. The sample should contain part of the lactiferous duct and the areola if it is affected.[6] Nipple scrape cytology can diagnose Paget disease and may be considered for screening eczematous lesion of the nipple.

DIFFERENTIAL DIAGNOSIS

- Eczema of the areola is the most common cause of scaling of the breast (**Figure 96-5**). If the patient (see **Figure 96-5**) had new nipple inversion with the onset of skin changes, this would be more suspicious for Paget disease.
- Bowen disease is squamous cell carcinoma in situ and can differentiate from Paget disease by histology. Also, Bowen disease expresses high-molecular-weight keratins, whereas Paget disease expresses low-molecular-weight keratins (see Chapters 173, Actinic Keratosis and Bowen Disease, and 178, Squamous Cell Carcinoma).
- Superficial spreading malignant melanoma may be confused with Paget disease, but histologic study and immunohistochemical staining can separate the two (**Figure 96-6**) (see Chapter 179, Melanoma).
- Seborrheic keratoses and benign lichenoid keratoses can occur on and around the areola and be suspicious for Paget disease (**Figure 96-7**). A biopsy is the best way to make the diagnosis (see Chapter 164, Seborrheic Keratosis).
- Nipple adenoma, which usually presents as an isolated mass with redness, can be diagnosed with biopsy.
- Other inflammatory diseases including psoriasis (see Chapter 158, Psoriasis) and contact dermatitis (see Chapter 152, Contact Dermatitis) should be considered.

MANAGEMENT

SURGICAL

- The treatment and prognosis of Paget disease of the breast is first based on the stage of any underlying breast cancer. Simple mastectomy has traditionally been the standard treatment for isolated Paget disease of the breast, but breast-conserving treatment is being used more often. Breast-conserving surgery combined with breast irradiation is gaining wider acceptance. The surgically conservative approaches include excision of the complete nipple–areolar complex with margin evaluation. Sentinel lymph node biopsy should be performed to evaluate axillary lymph node status.[8] SOR Ⓑ

PROGNOSIS

- Patients with only noninvasive Paget disease of the nipple have excellent cancer outcome with conservative surgery, with survival

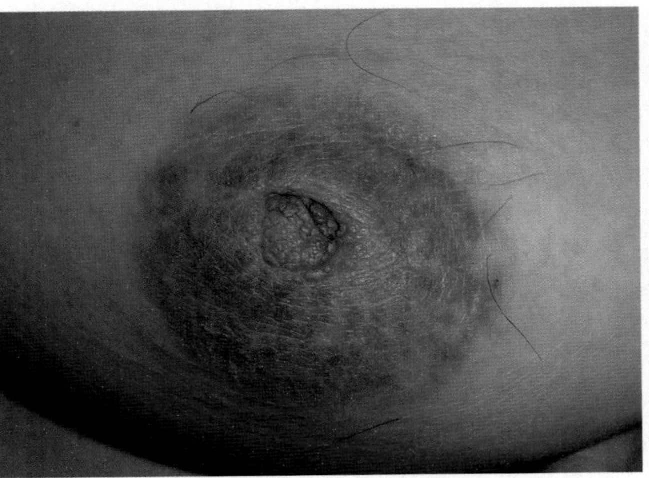

FIGURE 96-5 Eczema of the areola in a 43-year-old woman who has had an inverted nipple her whole adult life. She remembers having difficulty breastfeeding her children. The current eczema has been present on the areola on and off for more than 10 years and always responds to topical corticosteroids. Breast examination and mammography are negative. *(Reproduced with permission from Richard P. Usatine, MD.)*

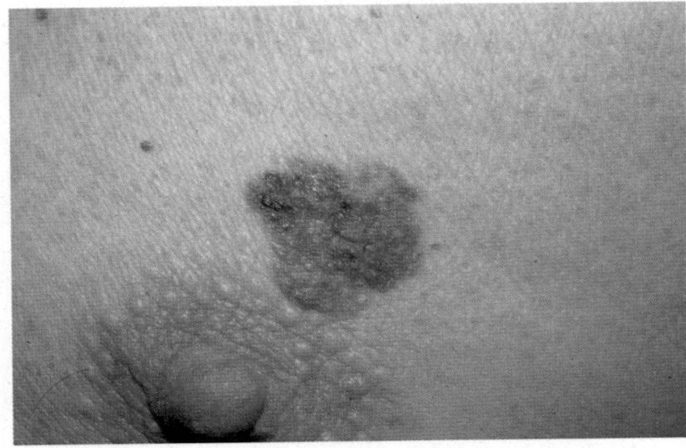

FIGURE 96-6 Superficial spreading melanoma adjacent to the areola. *(Reproduced with permission from Richard P. Usatine, MD.)*

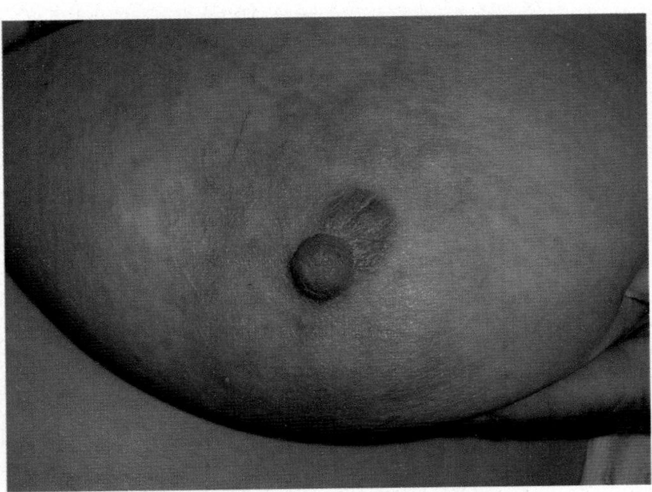

FIGURE 96-7 Benign lichenoid keratosis on the areola proven by biopsy. *(Reproduced with permission from Richard P. Usatine, MD.)*

rates similar to those achieved with mastectomy.[9,10] SOR Ⓑ The prognosis of Paget disease with synchronous cancer is dependent on the tumor stage of the underlying cancer. Factors indicating an unfavorable prognosis include the presence of a palpable breast tumor, enlarged lymph nodes, histologically unfavorable tumors, and patients younger than 60 years.[6]

PATIENT EDUCATION

- All lesions of the breast that do not heal should be checked for cancer.
- The patient's prognosis is based on the underlying cancer, if present, not the Paget disease itself.

PATIENT RESOURCES

- Breastcancer.org. *Paget's Disease of the Nipple*—**www.breastcancer.org/symptoms/types/pagets/.**
- Imaginis. *Paget's Disease of the Nipple*—**http://imaginis.com/breasthealth/pagets_disease.asp.**
- Macmillan Cancer Support. *Paget's Disease of the Breast*—**http://www.macmillan.org.uk/Cancerinformation/Cancertypes/Breast/Aboutbreastcancer/Typesandrelatedconditions/Pagetsdisease.aspx.**

PROVIDER RESOURCES

- Medscape. *Mammary Paget Disease*—**http://emedicine.medscape.com/article/1101235-overview.**
- National Cancer Institute. *Paget Disease of the Breast*—**http://www.cancer.gov/cancertopics/factsheet/Sites-Types/pagets-breast.**

REFERENCES

1. SEER Breast Cancer. *Cancer Statistics Review 1975–2013. Table 4.1 Cancer of the Female Breast (Invasive).* https://seer.cancer.gov/csr/1975_2013/results_merged/sect_04_breast.pdf. Accessed March 2017.
2. Chaudary MA, Millis RR, Lane EB, Miller NA. Paget's disease of the nipple: a ten year review including clinical, pathological, and immunohistochemical findings. *Breast Cancer Res Treat.* 1986; 8(2):139-146.
3. Chen CY, Sun LM, Anderson BO. Paget disease of the breast: changing patterns of incidence, clinical presentation, and treatment in the U.S. *Cancer.* 2006;107(7):1448-1458.
4. Ashikari R, Park K, Huvos AG, Urban JA. Paget's disease of the breast. *Cancer.* 1970;26(3):680-685.
5. Morrogh M, Morris EA, Liberman L, et al. MRI identifies otherwise occult disease in select patients with Paget disease of the nipple. *J Am Coll Surg.* 2008;206(2):316-321.
6. Lopes Filho LL, Lopes IM, Lopes LR, et al. Mammary and extramammary Paget's disease. *An Bras Dermatol.* 2015;90(2):225-231.
7. Crignis GS, Abreu Ld, Buçard AM, Barcaui CB. Polarized dermoscopy of mammary Paget disease. *An Bras Dermatol.* 2013; 88(2):290-292.
8. Caliskan M, Gatti G, Sosnovskikh I, et al. Paget's disease of the breast: the experience of the European Institute of Oncology and review of the literature. *Breast Cancer Res Treat.* 2008;112(3): 513-521. http://www.springerlink.com/content/6270v27346461v08/. Accessed February 2008.
9. Marshall JK, Griffith KA, Haffty BG, et al. Conservative management of Paget disease of the breast with radiotherapy: 10- and 15-year results. *Cancer.* 2003;97(9):2142-2149.
10. Pezzi CM, Kukora JS, Audet IM, et al. Breast conservation surgery using nipple-areolar resection for central breast cancers. *Arch Surg.* 2004;139(1):32-37.

PART XII

MUSCULOSKELETAL PROBLEMS

Strength of Recommendation (SOR)	Definition
A	Recommendation based on consistent and good-quality patient-oriented evidence.*
B	Recommendation based on inconsistent or limited-quality patient-oriented evidence.*
C	Recommendation based on consensus, usual practice, opinion, disease-oriented evidence, or case series for studies of diagnosis, treatment, prevention, or screening.*

*See Appendix A on pages 1603–1606 for further information.

97 ARTHRITIS OVERVIEW

Heidi S. Chumley, MD, MBA
Richard P. Usatine, MD

PATIENT STORY

A 50-year-old woman presents with new complaint of pain in several fingers. She has had psoriasis for many years; however, she only developed joint pain last year. Her examination is significant for swelling and tenderness at the distal interphalangeal (DIP) joints of her second, third, and fourth fingers (**Figure 97-1, *A***). She had an elevated erythrocyte sedimentation rate (ESR) and radiographs with erosive changes (**Figure 97-1, *B***). Choices for therapy include nonsteroidal anti-inflammatory drugs (NSAIDs) in conjunction with a conventional synthetic disease-modifying anti-rheumatic drug (csDMARD), such as methotrexate. Many other medications are now available for patients who do not respond to initial therapy.

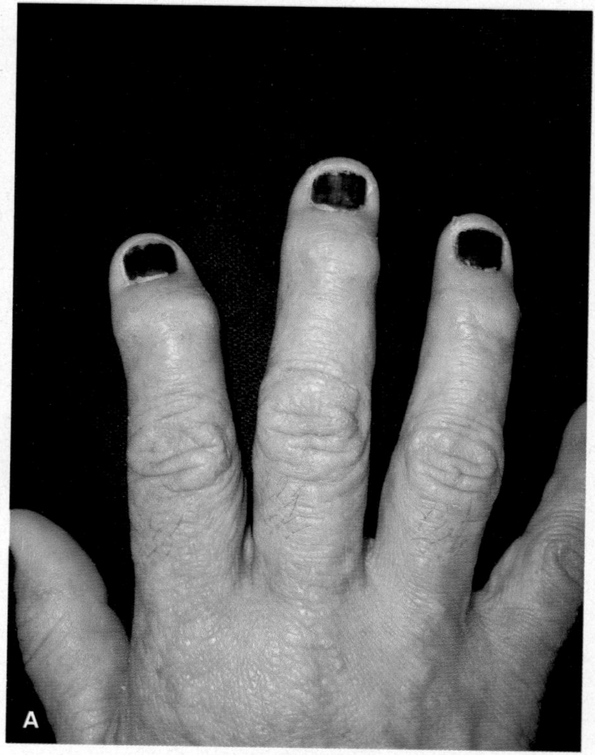

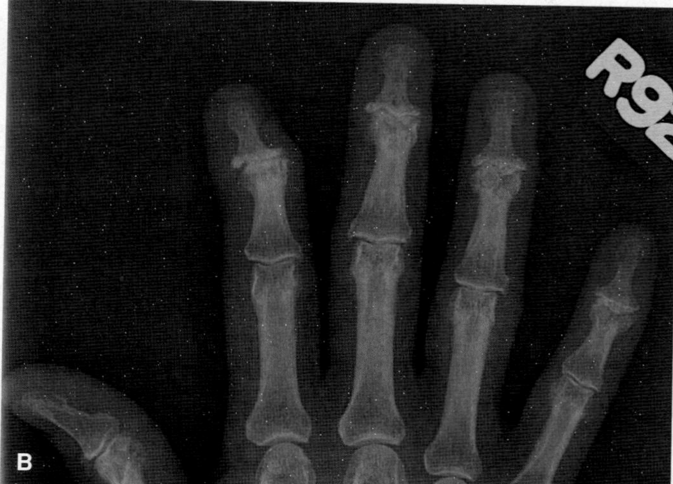

FIGURE 97-1 Psoriatic arthritis at initial presentation in a 50-year-old woman with psoriasis and new-onset hand pain. **A.** Note the prominent involvement of the distal interphalangeal joints. **B.** Radiography showing early psoriatic arthritis changes with periarticular erosions seen at the distal interphalangeal joints. *(Reproduced with permission from Richard P. Usatine, MD.)*

INTRODUCTION

Arthritis means joint inflammation; however, the term is used for any disease or condition that affects joints or the tissues around the joints. Joint pain can be classified as monoarticular or polyarticular and inflammatory or noninflammatory. Diagnosis is based on a combination of clinical presentation, synovial fluid analysis, other laboratory tests, and radiographic findings. Management goals include minimizing joint damage, controlling pain, maximizing function, and improving quality of life.

EPIDEMIOLOGY

- More than 50 million adults in the United States have been diagnosed with arthritis by a physician.
- Arthritis is more common in women than men with age-adjusted prevalence of 23.5% compared to 18.1%.[1]
- Arthritis is the most common cause of disability in the United States. Twenty-three million adults have functional limitations because of arthritis.[1]
- Fifty percent of adults age 65 years or older have been diagnosed with arthritis.[1]
- One in every 250 children younger than the age of 18 have some form of arthritis.[2]
- In 2003, the total cost attributable to arthritic conditions was $128 billion.[1]

ETIOLOGY AND PATHOPHYSIOLOGY

Arthritis can be caused by one of several mechanisms.

- Noninflammatory arthritis (i.e., osteoarthritis) is caused by bony overgrowth (osteophytes) and degeneration of cartilage and underlying bone (**Figures 97-2** and **97-3**).

- Autoimmune arthritis (i.e., rheumatoid arthritis, systemic lupus erythematosus [SLE], psoriatic arthritis) is caused by an inappropriate immune response.
- Crystalline arthritis (i.e., gout, calcium pyrophosphate dehydrate deposition disease) is caused by deposition of uric acid crystals (gout) or calcium pyrophosphate dehydrate crystals (CPPD) resulting in episodic flares with periods of remission.
- Septic arthritis can be caused by many types of infectious agents, but is most commonly caused by *Neisseria gonorrhoeae* (in the United States), *Staphylococcus*, or *Streptococcus*. *Kingella kingae* is the most common cause in children ages 6 to 36 months.
- About 1% of acute arthritis in adults is due to a viral illness.[3]
- Postinfectious (reactive) arthritis is caused by an immune reaction several weeks after a urethritis or enteric infection.

DIAGNOSIS

CLINICAL FEATURES

- Two features help limit the differential diagnosis: mono- or polyarticular and inflammatory or noninflammatory.
  - Monoarticular noninflammatory—Osteoarthritis, trauma, avascular necrosis (AVN).
  - Monoarticular inflammatory—Infectious (gonococcal, staphylococcal, Lyme disease) or crystalline (gout or CPPD).
  - Polyarticular noninflammatory—Osteoarthritis.
  - Polyarticular inflammatory—Rheumatologic (rheumatoid arthritis [RA], SLE, psoriatic, ankylosing spondylitis [AS], and others) or infectious (bacterial, viral, postinfectious) or crystalline later in the disease.

TYPICAL DISTRIBUTION

- Most commonly affected joints
  - Osteoarthritis (see Chapter 98, Osteoarthritis)—Knees, hips, hands (DIP and proximal interphalangeal [PIP]), and spine (**Figures 97-2** to **97-4**).
  - RA (see Chapter 99, Rheumatoid Arthritis)—Wrists, metacarpophalangeal (MCP), PIP, metatarsophalangeal (MTP) early in the disease with larger joints affected later in the disease (**Figures 97-5** and **97-6**). Rheumatoid nodules may be found over the fingers, hands, wrists, or elbows (**Figures 97-6** and **97-7**).
  - SLE—Hands, wrists, and knees (see Chapter 188, Lupus: Systemic and Cutaneous) (**Figure 97-8**).
  - AS—Lower back and hips, costosternal junctions, shoulders (see Chapter 100, Ankylosing Spondylitis).
  - Psoriatic arthritis (PsA)—Hands, feet, knees, spine, sacroiliac; typically with a personal or family history or psoriasis (**Figures 97-9** to **97-11**). The five types of psoriatic arthritis are
    1. Symmetric arthritis—Involves multiple symmetric pairs of joints in the hands and feet; resembles rheumatoid arthritis. Affects approximately 15% of patients with psoriatic arthritis.[4]
    2. Asymmetric arthritis—Involves only 1–3 joints in an asymmetric pattern and may affect any joint (e.g., knee, hip, ankle, and wrist). Hands and feet may have enlarged "sausage" digits due to dactylitis. Most common type found in approximately 80% of patients.[4]

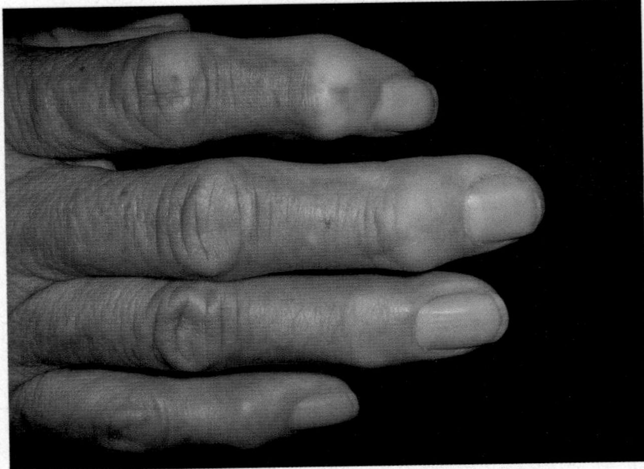

FIGURE 97-2 Osteoarthritis in an elderly woman with Heberden nodes at the distal interphalangeal joints. There is some swelling beginning at the proximal interphalangeal joints creating Bouchard nodes. *(Reproduced with permission from Richard P. Usatine, MD.)*

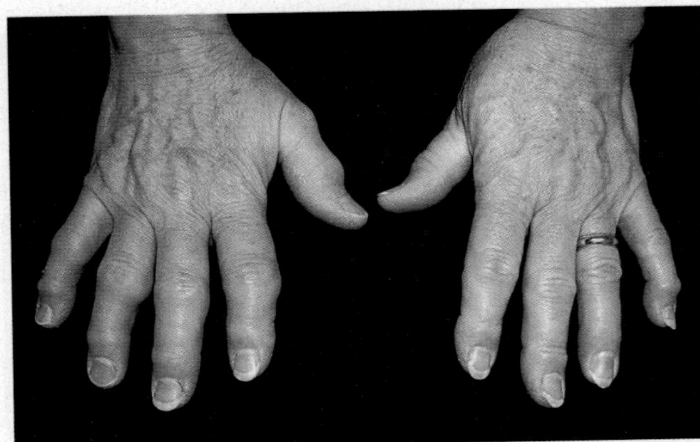

FIGURE 97-3 Osteoarthritis with visible Heberden (DIP) and Bouchard (PIP) nodes. *(Reproduced with permission from Ricardo Zuniga-Montes, MD.)*

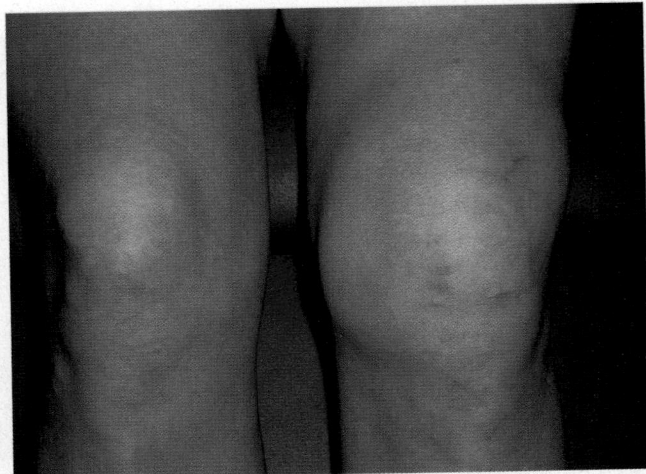

FIGURE 97-4 Osteoarthritis with visible unilateral knee effusion. The effusion was tapped and the synovial fluid was consistent with osteoarthritis. An intraarticular steroid injection was given and provided great relief to the pain and stiffness. *(Reproduced with permission from Richard P. Usatine, MD.)*

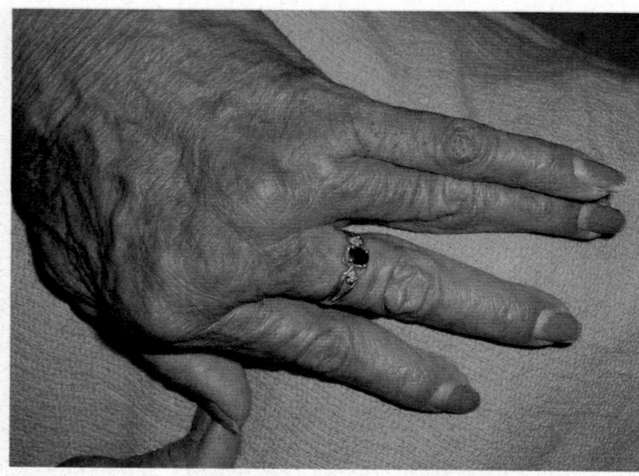

FIGURE 97-5 Rheumatoid arthritis showing typical ulnar deviation at the metacarpophalangeal joints. (*Reproduced with permission from Richard P. Usatine, MD.*)

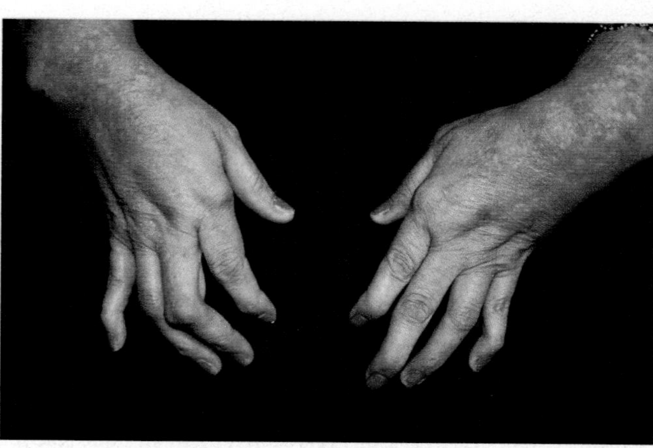

FIGURE 97-8 Longstanding lupus erythematosus has caused swan-neck deformities without bone erosions. This is called Jaccoud arthropathy and is caused by synovitis and inflammatory capsular fibrosis. (*Reproduced with permission from Everett Allen, MD.*)

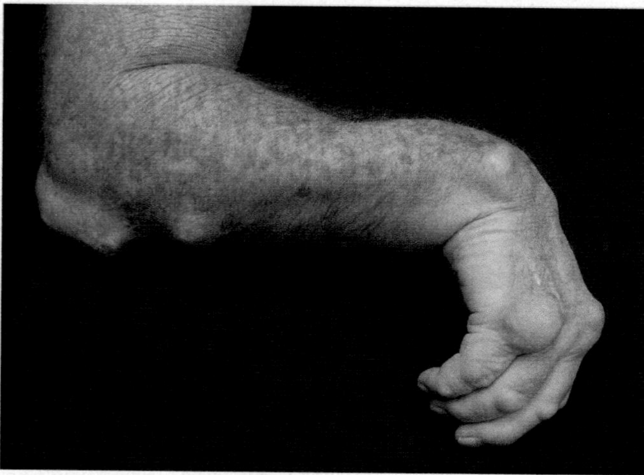

FIGURE 97-6 Rheumatoid arthritis involving the whole upper-extremity joints with nodules on the elbow, wrist, and hand joints. (*Reproduced with permission from Ricardo Zuniga-Montes, MD.*)

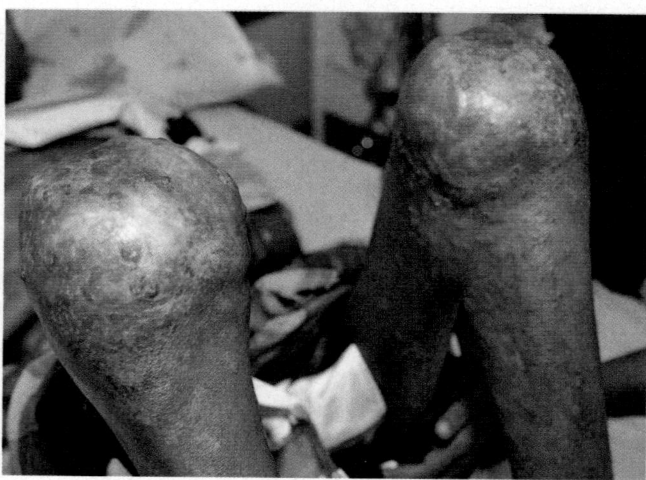

FIGURE 97-9 Psoriatic arthritis of both knees. This patient has asymmetric psoriatic arthritis in his hands. (*Reproduced with permission from Richard P. Usatine, MD.*)

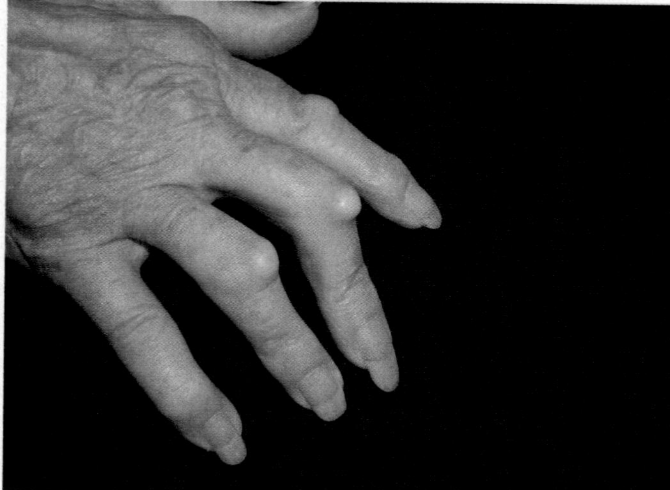

FIGURE 97-7 Rheumatoid arthritis with rheumatoid nodules over the PIP joints along with deformities of the digits. (*Reproduced with permission from Ricardo Zuniga-Montes, MD.*)

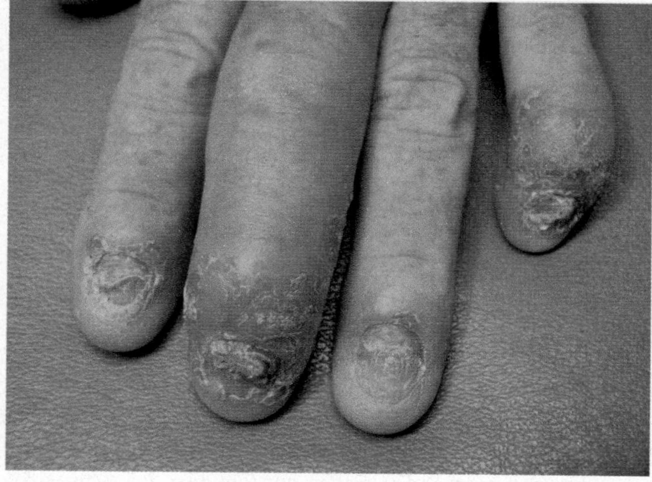

FIGURE 97-10 Psoriatic arthritis with dactylitis and significant distal interphalangeal joint involvement. Note the destruction of the nails. Almost all patients with psoriatic arthritis have nail involvement. (*Reproduced with permission from Ricardo Zuniga-Montes, MD.*)

3. Distal interphalangeal predominant (DIP)—Involves distal joints of the fingers and toes. It may be confused with osteoarthritis, but nail changes are common in this type of PsA. The fingers with DIP involvement are most likely to have psoriatic nail changes such as pitting. This "classic type" occurs in approximately 5% of patients.[4]
4. Spondylitis (axial)—Inflammation of the spinal column causing a stiff neck and pain in the lower back and sacroiliac area. The arthritis may involve peripheral joints in the hands, arms, hips, legs, and feet.[4]
5. Arthritis mutilans—A severe, deforming type of arthritis that usually affects a few joints in the hands and feet. It has been associated with pustular psoriasis. Affecting <5% of patients with PsA.[4]

- Gonococcal—Migratory with a single joint affected, such as knee, wrist, ankle, hand, or foot.
- Lyme disease—Knee and/or other large joints.
- Gout (see Chapter 102, Gout)—Begins as monoarticular with MTP joint of the first toe; hands, ankles, tarsal joints, and knee may also be affected (**Figures 97-12** to **97-14**); gout may present with tophi over any joint; olecranon bursitis can also be the result of gout (**Figure 97-15**).
- CPPD—Knee, but also seen in shoulder, elbow, wrist, hands, and ankle joints; most patients have polyarticular disease.
- Septic arthritis can involve any joint; acute onset of pain, swelling, and joint immobility; fever may be present; must be recognized and treated immediately as joint destruction occurs within days (**Figure 97-16**).

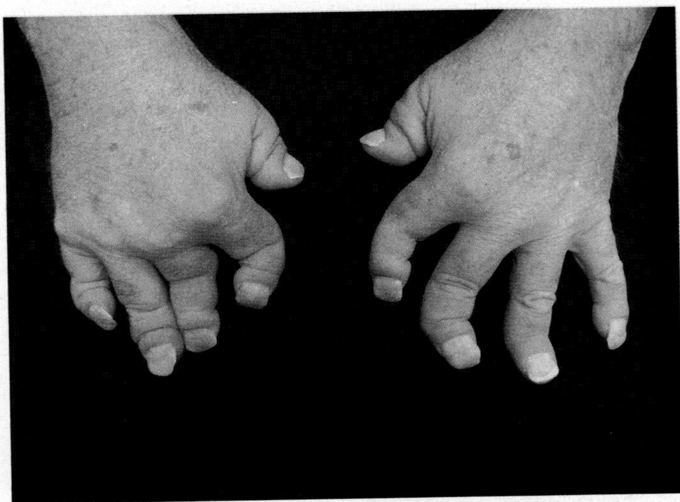

FIGURE 97-11 Psoriatic arthritis mutilans with severe destruction of the fingers. (*Reproduced with permission from Ricardo Zuniga-Montes, MD.*)

LABORATORY TESTING

- Not indicated for noninflammatory arthritis.
- Inflammatory polyarthritis: Use laboratory tests to supplement the clinical impression. Initial tests to consider include:
  - ESR or C-reactive protein as a nonspecific measure of inflammation.
  - Rheumatoid factor or anti-CCP (anti-cyclic citrullinated peptide) antibody when RA is expected. Anti-CCP antibody is more sensitive and specific than rheumatoid factor.
  - Antinuclear antibody (ANA), anti–double-stranded DNA (dsDNA) and anti-Ro when SLE is expected.
  - Human leukocyte antigen (HLA)-B27 when AS is expected.
  - Serum uric acid can be used, especially to follow hypouricemic therapy; levels can be normal or low during an attack.
- Joint aspiration:
  - Synovial fluid analysis is critical when septic or crystalline arthritis are suspected.
  - Assess for clarity/color, cell count, crystals, and culture. Gram stain may give quick information, but a culture should also be done. If there is clinical suspicion for septic arthritis, empiric antibiotics should be started even if the Gram stain is negative.
  - White blood cell (WBC)—Normal <200 cells/μL; noninflammatory arthritis <2000 cells/μL; inflammatory, crystalline, or septic arthritis >2000 cells/μL, often 30,000 to 50,000 cells/μL.
  - Crystals—Monosodium urate (gout) are needle-shaped and negatively birefringent; CPPD are rhomboid-shaped and positively birefringent.

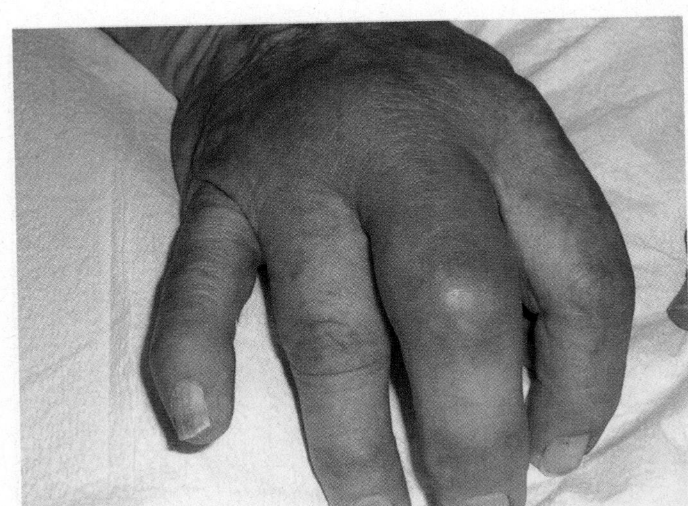

FIGURE 97-12 An acute gouty arthritis attack of multiple finger joints in a 75-year-old man with gout. His joints have been painful for 3 weeks. Erythema from the acute inflammation is evident. (*Reproduced with permission from Richard P. Usatine, MD.*)

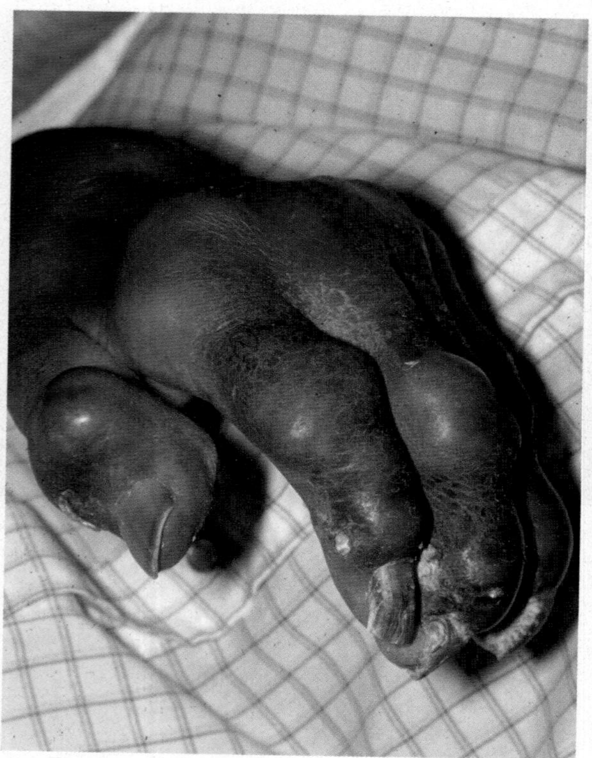

FIGURE 97-13 Severe tophaceous gout with chronic gouty arthritis causing hand deformities and disabilities. (*Reproduced with permission from Jack Resneck, Sr., MD.*)

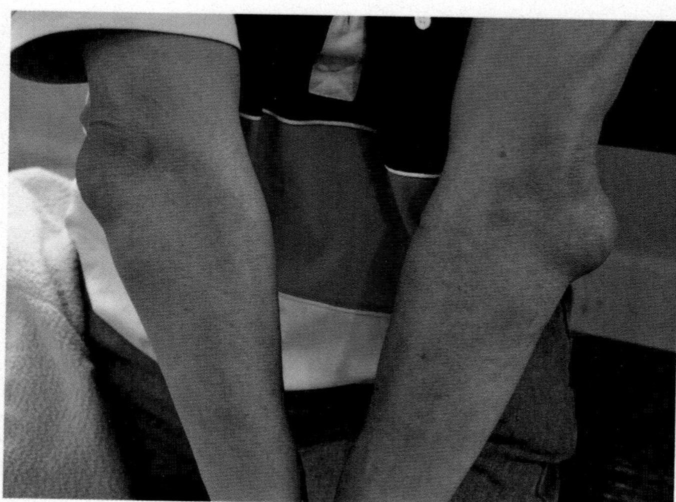

FIGURE 97-15 Olecranon bursitis bilaterally in a man with gout. (*Reproduced with permission from Richard P. Usatine, MD.*)

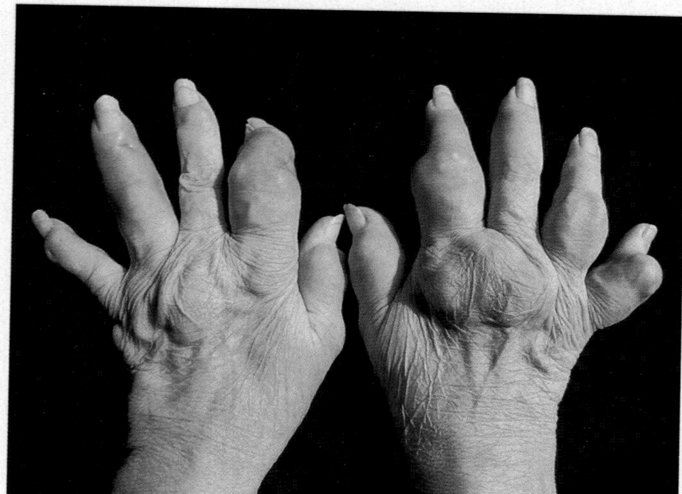

FIGURE 97-14 Severe tophaceous gout with large tophi and joint destruction of the hands. (*Reproduced with permission from Ricardo Zuniga-Montes, MD.*)

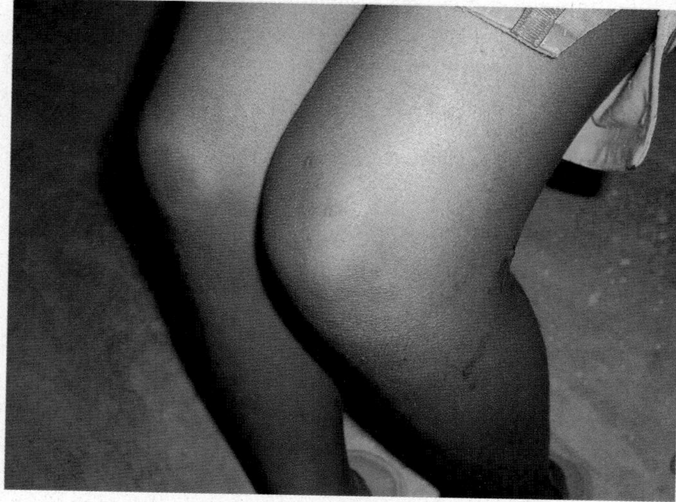

FIGURE 97-16 Septic left knee joint in a young girl who presented with knee pain, fever, and limited ability to ambulate. (*Reproduced with permission from Richard P. Usatine, MD.*)

- Culture—Gonococcal arthritis synovial fluid cultures can be negative in two-thirds of cases (synovial biopsy is positive); tuberculosis, fungal, and anaerobic infections may also be difficult to identify on culture.

IMAGING

- Osteoarthritis—Osteophytes, sclerosis, narrowed joint space (**Figure 97-17**).
- Rheumatoid arthritis—Soft-tissue swelling, erosions, and loss of joint space; severe destruction and subluxation in advanced disease. MRI changes may appear first and include synovitis, effusions, and bone marrow changes.
- SLE—Soft-tissue swelling; erosions are rare and joint deformities are uncommon.
- AS—Symmetric sacroiliitis, erosions, sclerosis; active sacroiliitis is best seen on MRI.
- Psoriatic arthritis—Erosions with adjacent proliferation, "pencil-in-cup" deformity, osteolysis, digit telescoping, asymmetric sacroiliitis.
- Gout—Only soft-tissue swelling until advanced disease when erosions with sclerotic margins may be present.
- CPPD—Can mimic other types of arthritis; chondrocalcinosis, linear or punctate radiodense deposits in cartilage or menisci may be present.

Table 97-1 provides a comparison of psoriatic arthritis with RA, osteoarthritis, and AS.

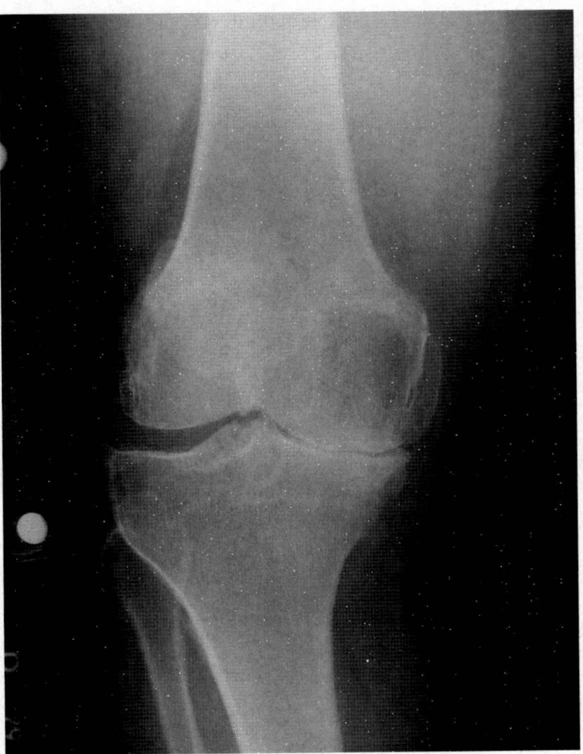

FIGURE 97-17 Radiograph showing osteoarthritis of the knee with asymmetric joint space narrowing. (*Reproduced with permission from Ricardo Zuniga-Montes, MD.*)

DIFFERENTIAL DIAGNOSIS

- Bursitis is inflammation of a bursa. Pain and tenderness is localized to the bursa. Common locations include subdeltoid, trochanteric, olecranon.

TABLE 97-1 Comparison of Psoriatic Arthritis with Rheumatoid Arthritis, Osteoarthritis, and Ankylosing Spondylitis

	PsA	RA	OA	AS
Peripheral disease	Asymmetric	Symmetric	Asymmetric	No
Sacroiliitis	Asymmetric	No	No	Symmetric
Stiffness	In morning and/or with immobility	In morning and/or with immobility	With activity	Yes
Female-to-male ratio	1:1	3:1	Hand/foot more common in female patients	1:3
Enthesitis	Yes	No	No	No
High-titer rheumatoid factor	No	Yes	No	No
HLA association	CW6, B27	DR4	No	B27
Nail lesions	Yes	No	No	No
Psoriasis	Yes	Uncommon	Uncommon	Uncommon

Abbreviations: AS, ankylosing spondylitis; *OA*, osteoarthritis; *PsA*, psoriatic arthritis; *RA*, rheumatoid arthritis.
Reproduced with permission from Gottlieb A, Korman NJ, Gordon KB, et al. Guidelines of care for the management of psoriasis and psoriatic arthritis: Section 2. Psoriatic arthritis: overview and guidelines of care for treatment with an emphasis on the biologics, J Am Acad Dermatol. 2008;58(5):851-864.

- Tendinitis is inflammation of a tendon that produces a localized pain aggravated by stretching of the affected tendon.
- Inflammatory myopathy or myositis is inflammation of the muscle most commonly caused by an autoimmune or infectious process. Pain is in the muscles instead of the joints.
- Polymyalgia rheumatica is a systemic inflammatory disease with aching and stiffness in the torso and proximal extremities. Pain is in the muscles, but synovitis or tenosynovitis may also be present. Passive joint range of motion is preserved. ESR is elevated. Normocytic anemia and thrombocytosis can be present.
- Fibromyalgia—Widespread pain not limited to joints. Joint swelling is absent. Laboratory tests and imaging if obtained are normal.

MANAGEMENT

The goals of treatment are to control pain, maximize function, improve quality of life, and, for inflammatory causes, minimize joint damage.

NONPHARMACOLOGIC

- Recommend an exercise program. Aerobic exercise, strength training, or both improves pain and function in arthritis and other rheumatic diseases.[4] SOR Ⓐ
- Splints or braces may be used to offload stress on a particular joint.
- Weight loss reduces joint load for weight-bearing joints.

MEDICATIONS

See specific chapters.

REFERRAL OR HOSPITALIZATION

- Hospitalize patients with suspected septic arthritis and begin empiric therapy with appropriate intravenous antibiotics.
- Refer patients in whom the diagnosis is unclear, especially if RA or PsA is suspected as early diagnosis and treatment improves outcomes.
- Refer patients in whom surgical management is indicated.

PROGNOSIS

Prognosis depends on the type of arthritis as well as psychosocial factors and socioeconomic status.

FOLLOW-UP

Acute arthritis should be followed closely until resolution. Chronic arthritis is managed like other chronic diseases, with the frequency of follow-up dependent on the type of arthritis and the severity of the disease.

PATIENT EDUCATION

For chronic arthritic conditions, the goals of treatment are to control pain, maximize function, improve quality of life, and minimize joint damage. Self-management is an important part of chronic arthritic conditions.

PATIENT RESOURCES

- Centers for Disease Control and Prevention. Information on the Arthritis Self-Management Program is available in English and Spanish—**http://www.cdc.gov/arthritis/interventions/self_manage.htm#1.**

PROVIDER RESOURCES

- Centers for Disease Control and Prevention. Information on arthritis and other rheumatologic conditions—**http://www.cdc.gov/arthritis/.**
- American College of Rheumatology. Clinical support, including practice guidelines, classification criteria, and clinical forms—**http://www.rheumatology.org/Practice-Quality/Clinical-Support/Clinical-Practice-Guidelines.**

REFERENCES

1. Centers for Disease Control and Prevention. *Arthritis.* Updated March 7, 2017. https://www.cdc.gov/arthritis/data_statistics/national-statistics.html. Accessed March 2017.
2. Sacks JJ, Helmick CG, Luo YH, et al. Prevalence of and annual ambulatory health care visits for pediatric arthritis and other rheumatologic conditions in the United States in 2001–2004. *Arthritis Rheum.* 2007;57:1439-1445.
3. Marks M, Marks JL. Viral arthritis. *Clin Med (Lond).* 2016;16(2):129-134.
4. Kelley GA, Kelley KS, Hootman JM, Jones DL. Effects of community-deliverable exercise on pain and physical function in adults with arthritis and other rheumatic diseases: a meta-analysis. *Arthritis Care Res (Hoboken).* 2011;63(1):79-93.

98 OSTEOARTHRITIS

Jana K. Zaudke, MD, MA
Heidi S. Chumley, MD, MBA

PATIENT STORY

A 70-year-old woman presents with pain and swelling in the joints of both hands, which impedes her normal activities. Her pain is better in the morning after resting and worse after she has been working with her hands. She denies stiffness. On examination, you find bony enlargement of some distal interphalangeal (DIP) and proximal interphalangeal (PIP) joints on both hands (**Figure 98-1**). Radiographs confirm the presence of Heberden and Bouchard nodes. She begins taking 1 g of acetaminophen twice a day and has significant improvement in her pain and function.

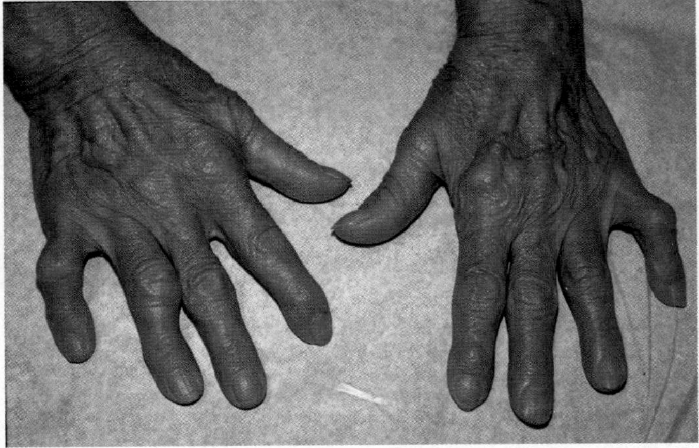

FIGURE 98-1 Bony enlargement of some distal interphalangeal (DIP) and proximal interphalangeal (PIP) joints consistent with Heberden (DIP) and Bouchard (PIP) nodes. (*Reproduced with permission from Richard P. Usatine, MD.*)

INTRODUCTION

Osteoarthritis is the most common type of arthritis. It involves degeneration of the articular cartilage accompanied by osteophytes (hypertrophic bone changes) around the joints. Osteoarthritis leads to pain in the joints with movement and relief with rest. Multiple non-pharmacologic and pharmacologic interventions can improve pain and function.

SYNONYMS

Degenerative joint disease.

EPIDEMIOLOGY

- Osteoarthritis is the most common type of arthritis, affecting 10% of men and 13% of women age 60 years or older.[1,2]
- Incidence and prevalence will likely increase given the obesity epidemic and the aging of the population.[2]
- Hip and knee osteoarthritis was ranked as the 11th highest contributor to global disability.[3]
- Globally, age-standardized prevalence of knee OA is 3.8% and hip OA is 0.85%. Prevalence of both knee and hip osteoarthritis is higher in females than males.[3]
- In the Framingham cohort (mean age 71 years at baseline) women and men developed symptomatic knee osteoarthritis at the rate of 1% and 0.7% per year, respectively.[1]
- Risk of developing osteoarthritis increases with knee injury in adolescence or adulthood (relative risk [RR] = 2.95) and obesity (RR = 1.51 to 2.07).[1]
- Occupational physical activity and abnormal joint loading also increase the risk.[1,2]

ETIOLOGY AND PATHOPHYSIOLOGY

- Recent evidence suggests that osteoarthritis should be considered as a systemic rather than focal musculoskeletal disease.[4]
- Biomechanical factors and inflammation upset the balance of articular cartilage biosynthesis and degradation.
- Chondrocytes attempt to repair the damage; eventually, however, enzymes produced by the chondrocytes digest the matrix and accelerate cartilage erosion.
- Inflammation plays a significant role in the progression of osteoarthritis.[4]

RISK FACTORS

- Advanced age.
- Female gender.
- Genetics.
- Obesity.
- Knee injury in adolescence and adulthood.
- Abnormal joint loading.
- Occupational history.

DIAGNOSIS

The American College of Rheumatology uses the following criteria for the most common joints involved in osteoarthritis.

- Knee—Knee pain, osteophytes on radiograph, and 1 of 3: age older than 50 years, stiffness less than 30 minutes, or crepitus on physical examination (sensitivity = 91%, specificity = 86%).[5]
- Hip—Hip pain and 2 of 3: erythrocyte sedimentation rate (ESR) less than 20 mm/h; femoral or acetabular osteophytes by radiograph; superior, axial, or medial joint space narrowing by radiograph (sensitivity = 89%, specificity = 91%).[5]
- Hand—Hand pain, aching, or stiffness and 3 of 4: hard tissue enlargement of 2 or more DIP joints, fewer than 3 swollen metacarpophalangeal (MCP) joints, hand tissue enlargement of 2 or more selected joints, deformity of 1 or more selected joints. Selected joints include second and third DIP, second and third PIP, first carpometacarpal (CMC) on both hands (sensitivity = 94%, specificity = 87%).[5]

CLINICAL FEATURES

- Typically, joint pain is worsened with movement and relieved by rest. A small subset may demonstrate inflammatory symptoms including prolonged stiffness.
- Loss of function (i.e., impaired gait with knee or hip osteoarthritis, impaired manual dexterity with hand osteoarthritis).
- Radicular pain when vertebral column osteophytes impinge nerve roots.
- Bony enlargement of the DIP joints (Heberden nodes) or PIP joints (Bouchard nodes) (see **Figure 98-1**).

TYPICAL DISTRIBUTION

Most common joints affected include knees, hands, hips, and back.

LABORATORY TESTING

- Not typically indicated. Normal ESR and synovial fluid white blood cell count (WBC) less than 2000/mm.[5]

IMAGING

- Loss of joint space or osteophytes on radiographs (**Figures 98-2** to **98-5**).

DIFFERENTIAL DIAGNOSIS

Musculoskeletal pain can also be caused by:

- Connective tissue diseases (scleroderma and lupus) that have other specific systemic signs.
- Fibromyalgia—Pain at trigger points instead of joints.
- Polyarticular gout—Erythematous joints and crystals in joint aspirate (see Chapter 102, Gout).
- Polymyalgia rheumatica—Proximal joint pain without deformity, elevated ESR.
- Seronegative spondyloarthropathies—Asymmetric joint involvement, spine often involved (see Chapter 100, Ankylosing Spondylitis).
- Reactive arthritis—History of infection, sexually transmitted disease, or bowel complaints. The patient may have conjunctivitis, iritis, urethritis in addition to joint pain and arthritis (see Chapter 161, Reactive Arthritis).
- Rheumatoid arthritis—Symmetric soft-tissue swelling in distal joints, stiffness after inactivity, positive rheumatoid factor. Ulnar deviation of the fingers at the MCP joints is a distinct finding in rheumatoid arthritis (**Figure 98-6**; see Chapter 99, Rheumatoid Arthritis).
- Bursitis—Pain at one site, often increased with direct pressure.

MANAGEMENT

NONPHARMACOLOGIC

Table 98-1 lists the nonpharmacologic options for management of osteoarthritis.

- Recommend therapeutic land-based or aquatic exercise to maintain range of motion and strengthen muscles surrounding affected joints.[6] SOR Ⓐ
- Recommend weight loss for knee or hip osteoarthritis. Weight loss may not improve current pain, but may slow progression and can be recommended for numerous other health reasons.[6] SOR Ⓒ
- In knee OA, consider mechanical interventions including patellar taping, medial wedged insoles (lateral compartment OA), or laterally wedged subtalar strapped insoles (medial compartment OA).[6] SOR Ⓒ

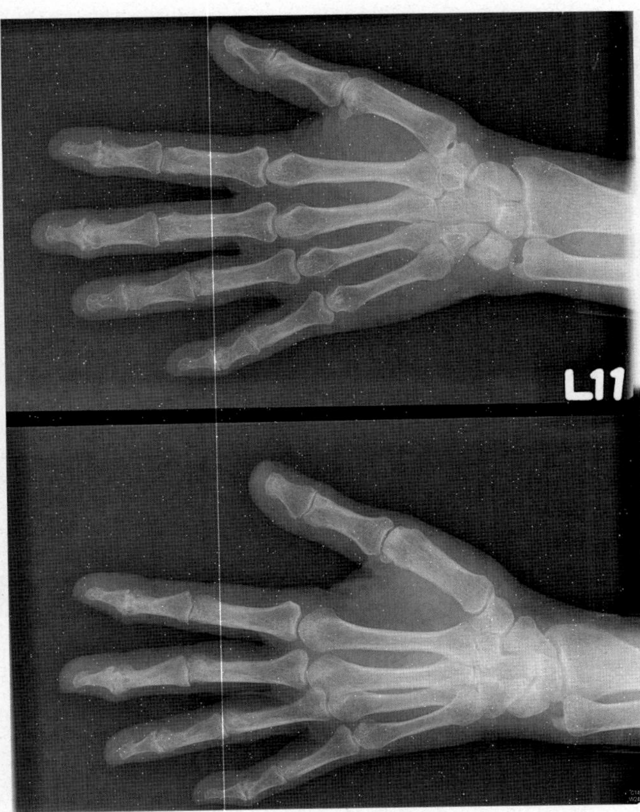

FIGURE 98-2 Joint space narrowing, marginal osteophytes, and Heberden nodes at the distal interphalangeal joints of the second through fifth fingers. (*Reproduced with permission from Heidi Chumley, MD.*)

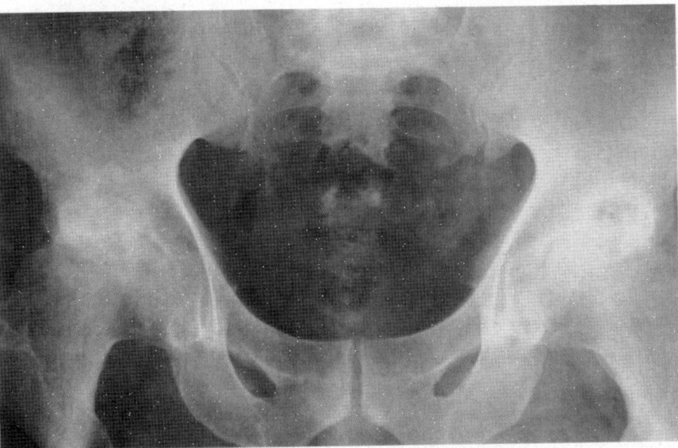

FIGURE 98-4 Articular space narrowing, sclerosis, and subchondral cyst formation of both hips because of osteoarthritis. (*Reproduced with permission from Chen MYM, Pope TL Jr, Ott DJ. Basic Radiology. New York, NY: McGraw-Hill Education; 2004.*)

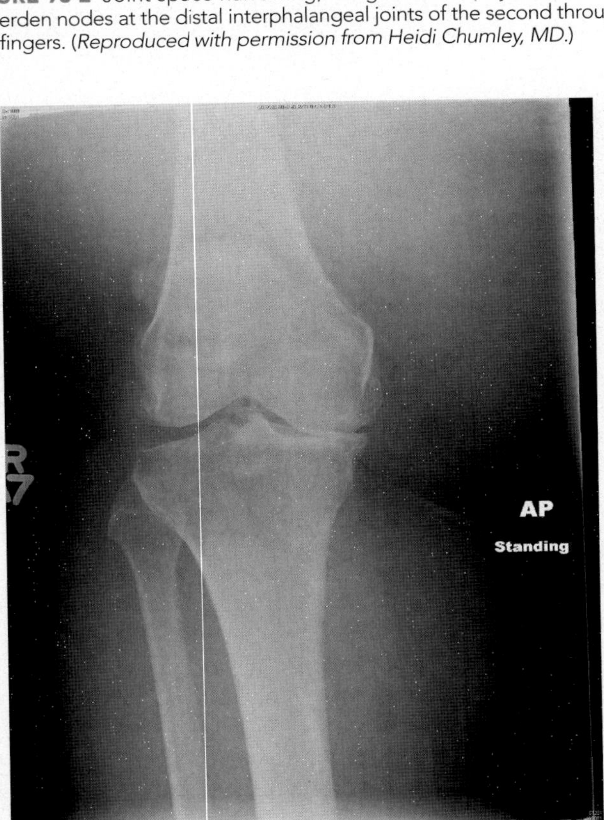

FIGURE 98-3 Osteoarthritis of the knee causing joint space narrowing, sclerosis, and bony spurring in all three compartments of the right knee, most pronounced in the medial compartment. (*Reproduced with permission from Heidi Chumley, MD.*)

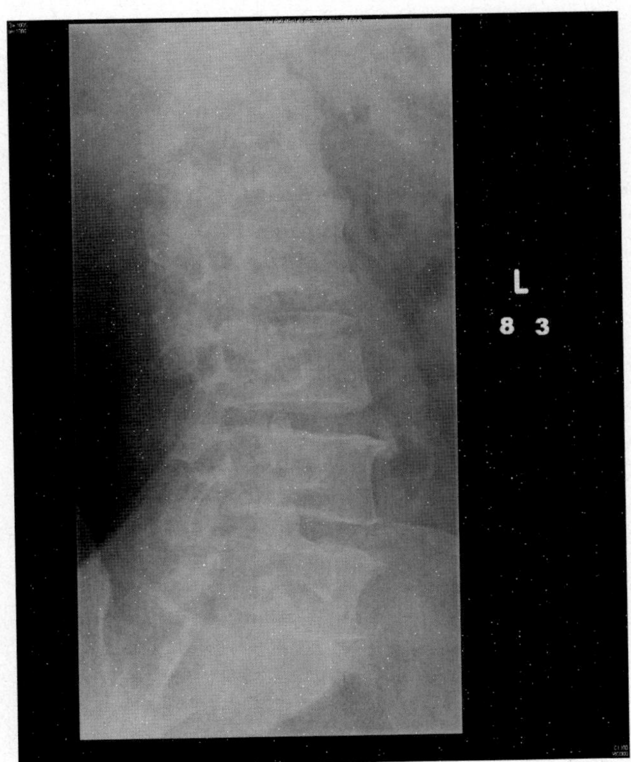

FIGURE 98-5 Loss of disc space and facet arthropathy at L5-S1 and small osteophytes, best seen on L4 and L5. These changes are caused by osteoarthritis. (*Reproduced with permission from Heidi Chumley, MD.*)

TABLE 98-1 Nonpharmacologic Options for Osteoarthritis

Weight loss (if overweight)
Aerobic exercise
Range-of-motion exercises
Muscle-strengthening exercises
Assistive devices for walking
Yoga and tai chi
Safe shoes
Lateral-wedged insoles (for genu varum bracing)
Physical and occupational therapy
Joint protection such as braces
Assistive devices for activities of daily living
Arthritis Foundation Self-Management Program
Social support

MEDICATIONS

Table 98-2 lists the pharmacologic therapy for osteoarthritis.

- Prescribe acetaminophen (2 to 4 g/day) for pain relief in patients at higher risk for GI complications. In a pooled analysis, acetaminophen improved pain by 5%, number needed to treat (NNT) 4 to 14.[7] SOR Ⓐ
- Prescribe an NSAID for moderate to severe hip or knee osteoarthritis in patients who are at low risk for GI complications. GI bleeding is a significant risk to many elderly patients with osteoarthritis (**Table 98-3**). A 2006 Cochrane review found NSAIDs were slightly more effective than acetaminophen, although more likely to produce adverse GI events.[7] SOR Ⓐ
- If NSAIDs are to be used in patients with risk factors (see **Table 98-3**), consider giving a misoprostol or a proton pump inhibitor for

TABLE 98-2 Pharmacologic Options for Osteoarthritis

Oral
• Acetaminophen
• COX-2-specific inhibitor
• NSAID plus a proton pump inhibitor
• Opioids (e.g., hydrocodone)
• Salsalate
• Tramadol
Topical
• Methylsalicylate
• Topical NSAID (e.g., diclofenac gel)
Intraarticular
• Glucocorticoids (e.g., triamcinolone)
• Hyaluronic acid

Abbreviations: COX-2, cyclooxygenase-2; *NSAID*, nonsteroidal anti-inflammatory drug.

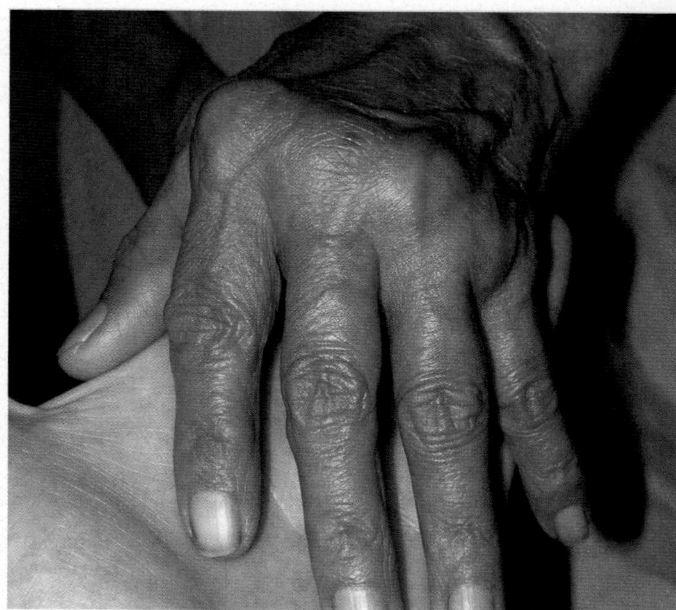

FIGURE 98-6 Rheumatoid arthritis showing ulnar deviation of the fingers at the metacarpophalangeal joints. (*Reproduced with permission from Chen MYM, Pope TL Jr, Ott DJ. Basic Radiology. New York, NY: McGraw-Hill Education; 2004.*)

TABLE 98-3 Risk Factors for Upper GI Adverse Effects in Persons Taking NSAIDs

• Age 65 years or older
• Anticoagulants
• Comorbid medical conditions
• History of peptic ulcer disease
• History of upper gastrointestinal bleeding
• Oral steroids
• Taking NSAIDs with an empty stomach

Abbreviation: NSAID, nonsteroidal anti-inflammatory drug.

protection.[6] Note that H_2-blockers may decrease gastric symptoms from NSAIDs but are not protective against GI bleeding.

- Consider opioid analgesics for patients with severe osteoarthritis who have not responded to NSAIDs (be careful to not prescribe narcotics to patients in recovery from substance abuse).[6] SOR C
- Consider a topical NSAID rather than an oral NSAID for hand or knee osteoarthritis, especially in patients 75 years of age or older. SOR C There is not yet enough data to recommend topical NSAID for hip osteoarthritis.[6]
- Consider topical capsaicin 0.025% cream 4 times a day for hand osteoarthritis.[6] SOR B
- Consider an intraarticular corticosteroid injection for acute pain related to knee or hip osteoarthritis.[6] SOR B

COMPLEMENTARY AND ALTERNATIVE THERAPY

- Glucosamine and chondroitin or glucosamine alone is effective in reducing pain and improving function in patients with knee OA.[8]
- Consider participation in tai chi programs for knee or hip osteoarthritis.[6]
- Consider traditional Chinese acupuncture or transcutaneous electrical stimulation for patients with knee osteoarthritis who choose not to have or are not candidates for a total-knee arthroplasty.[6]

REFERRAL

Refer patients who do not respond to conservative therapy to:

- Any physician with experience doing joint injections if this is not within your skill set.
- Rheumatologist for evaluation and treatment.
- Orthopedic surgeon for evaluation for arthroplasty or joint replacement.

FOLLOW-UP

There are no recommended intervals for follow-up; however, it is reasonable to see patients periodically to assess pain management and function.

PATIENT EDUCATION

Osteoarthritis is a chronic, progressive disease. Nonpharmacologic and pharmacologic therapies can reduce pain and preserve function.

PATIENT RESOURCES

- Arthritis Foundation. *Osteoarthritis*—**https://www.arthritis.org/about-arthritis/types/osteoarthritis/**
- PubMed Health. *Osteoarthritis*—**https://www.ncbi.nlm.nih.gov/pubmedhealth/PMHT0024679/.**

PROVIDER RESOURCES

- American College of Rheumatology 2012 *Recommendations for the Use of Nonpharmacologic and Pharmacologic Therapies in Osteoarthritis of the Hand, Hip, and Knee*—**http://mqic.org/pdf/2012_ACR_OA_Guidelines_FINAL.PDF**

REFERENCES

1. Sharma L, Kapoor D, Issa S. Epidemiology of osteoarthritis: an update [review]. *Curr Opin Rheumatol.* 2006;18(2):147-156.
2. Zhang Y, Jordan JM. Epidemiology of osteoarthritis. *Clin Geriatr Med.* 2010;26(3):355-369.
3. Cross M, Smith E, Hoy D, et al. The global burden of hip and knee osteoarthritis: estimates from the global burden of disease 2010 study. *Ann Rheum Dis.* 2014;73(7):1323-1330.
4. Malemud CJ. Biologic basis of osteoarthritis: state of the evidence. *Curr Opin Rheumatol.* 2015:27(3):289-294.
5. American College of Rheumatology. ACR Endorsed Criteria. https://www.rheumatology.org/Practice-Quality/Clinical-Support/Criteria/ACR-Endorsed-Criteria. Accessed November 2017.
6. Hochberg MC, Altman RD, April KT, et al. American College of Rheumatology 2012 recommendations for the use of nonpharmacologic and pharmacologic therapies in osteoarthritis of the hand, hip and knee. *Arthritis Care Res.* 2012;64(4):465-474.
7. Towheed TE, Maxwell L, Judd MG, et al. Acetaminophen for osteoarthritis. *Cochrane Database Syst Rev.* 2006;(1):CD004257.
8. Zeng C, Wei J, Li H, et al. Effectiveness and safety of glucosamine, chondroitin, the two in combination, or celecoxib in the treatment of osteoarthritis of the knee. *Sci Rep.* 2015;5:16827.

99 RHEUMATOID ARTHRITIS

Heidi S. Chumley, MD, MBA

PATIENT STORY

A 79-year-old woman with late-stage rheumatoid arthritis comes for routine follow-up (**Figures 99-1** to **99-4**). She began having hand pain and stiffness approximately 40 years ago. She took nonprescription medications for pain for approximately 10 years before seeing a physician. She was diagnosed with rheumatoid arthritis using a combination of clinical, laboratory, and radiographic findings. She was treated with prednisone and tried most of the disease-modifying agents as they became available; however, her disease progression continued. Approximately 10 years ago, she began having increased foot pain and difficulty walking. Today, she works with a multidisciplinary team to control pain and preserve hand function and independence.

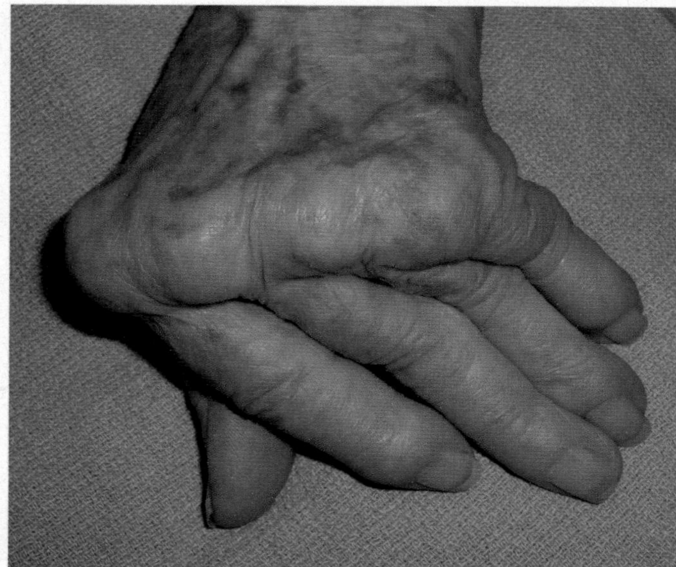

FIGURE 99-1 Ulnar deviation at metacarpophalangeal joints in advanced rheumatoid arthritis. Also note the swelling at the distal interphalangeal joints, seen best on the first finger. (*Reproduced with permission from Richard P. Usatine, MD.*)

INTRODUCTION

Rheumatoid arthritis (RA) is a progressive chronic illness that causes significant pain and disability. RA is a polyarticular inflammatory arthritis that causes symmetrical joint pain and swelling and typically involves the hands. Early recognition and treatment with nonbiologic and/or biologic disease-modifying anti-rheumatologic drugs (DMARDs) can induce remission and preserve function.

EPIDEMIOLOGY

- RA is found in 0.9% of the adult population.[1]
- RA is more common in women. Under the age of 50, incidence in women is four to five times higher than in men. After age 60, RA is twice as common in women.[2]
- Typical age of onset is 30 to 50 years.

ETIOLOGY AND PATHOPHYSIOLOGY

- Genetic predisposition coupled with an autoimmune or infection-triggering incident.
- Synovial macrophages and fibroblasts proliferate, leading to increased lymphocytes and endothelial cells.
- Increased cellular material occludes small blood vessels, causing ischemia, neovascularization, and inflammatory reactions.
- Inflamed tissue grows irregularly, causing joint damage.
- Damage causes further release of cytokines, interleukins, proteases, and growth factors, resulting in more joint destruction and systemic complications, including a higher risk for cardiovascular disease.

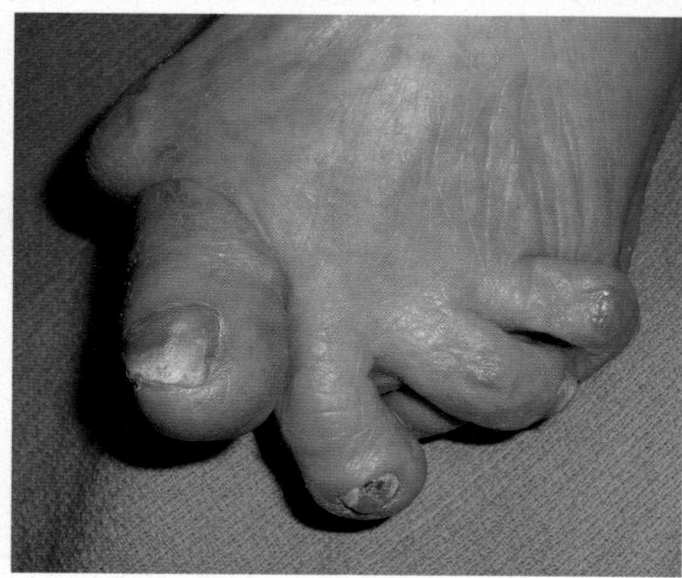

FIGURE 99-2 Rheumatoid arthritis in the foot of a 79-year-old woman with subluxation of the first metatarsophalangeal joint. (*Reproduced with permission from Richard P. Usatine, MD.*)

RISK FACTORS

Genetic predisposition signified by a positive family history.

DIAGNOSIS

The 2010 American College of Rheumatology/European League Against Rheumatism classification criteria uses a scoring system to designate patients as definite RA. A score of 6 or greater out of 10 meets criteria for definite RA.[3]

- Joint involvement—1 large joint (0 points); 2 to 10 large joints (1 point); 1 to 3 small joints with or without large joints (2 points); 4 to 10 small joints with or without large joints (3 points); more than 10 joints with at least 1 small joint (5 points).
- Serology—Negative rheumatoid factor (RF) and anticitrullinated protein antibody (ACPA) (0 points); low positive RF or ACPA (2 points); high positive RF or ACPA (3 points).
- Acute-phase reactants—Normal C-reactive protein (CRP) and erythrocyte sedimentation rate (ESR) (0 points); abnormal CRP or ESR (1 point).
- Duration of symptoms—Less than 6 weeks (0 points); 6 or more weeks (1 point).

Multiple studies in community populations demonstrate these criteria to have a sensitivity and specificity of 0.82 and 0.61, respectively.[4]

American Rheumatism Association criteria (with positive likelihood ratio abbreviated as LR+)[5]:

- Stiffness around joint for 1 hour after inactivity (LR+1.9).
- Three or more of these have soft-tissue swelling—Wrist, proximal interphalangeal (PIP), metacarpophalangeal (MCP), elbow, knee, ankle, metatarsophalangeal (MTP) (LR+1.4).
- Hand joints involved (LR+1.5) (see **Figures 99-1, 99-4,** and **99-5**).
- Symmetrical involvement of one of these: wrist, PIP, MCP, elbow, knee, ankle, MTP (LR+1.2).
- Subcutaneous nodules (LR+3.0) (**Figures 99-5** and **99-6**).
- Positive serum RF (LR+8.4).
- Osteopenia or erosion of surrounding joints on hand or wrist films (LR+11) (**Figures 99-7** and **99-8**).

CLINICAL FEATURES

Joint pain and swelling, polyarticular and symmetrical.

TYPICAL DISTRIBUTION

- Hands are typically involved (see **Figures 99-1, 99-4,** and **99-5**).
- Commonly involved joints include wrist, PIP, MCP, elbow, knee, ankle, MTP.
- Subcutaneous nodules (see **Figures 99-5** and **99-6**).

LABORATORY TESTING

- RF (negative in 30% of patients; positive in many connective tissue, neoplastic, and infectious diseases).

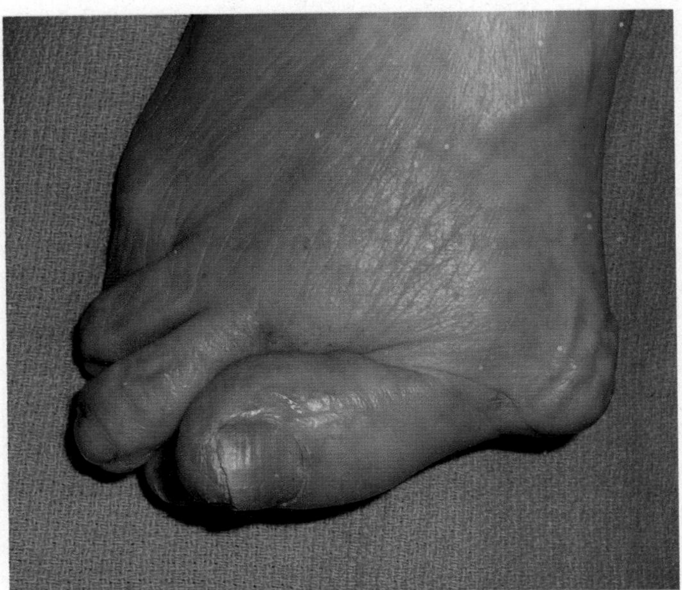

FIGURE 99-3 Deviation at the metatarsophalangeal joints from bony destruction in advanced rheumatoid arthritis. *(Reproduced with permission from Richard P. Usatine, MD.)*

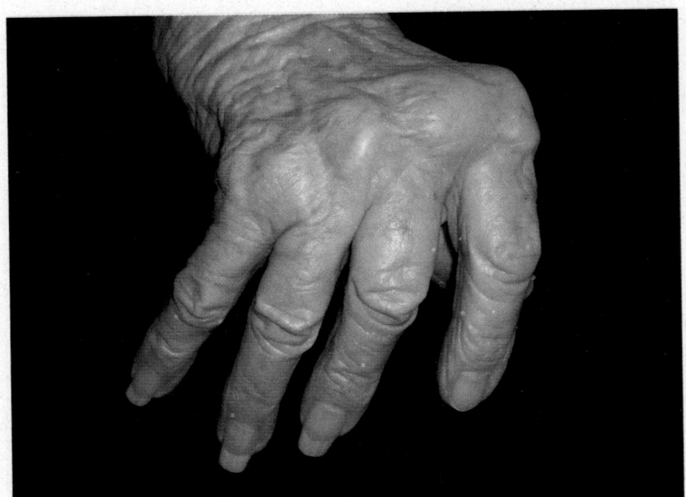

FIGURE 99-4 Ulnar deviation at metacarpophalangeal joints seen in a 79-year-old woman with advanced rheumatoid arthritis. Note one rheumatoid nodule just distal to the second MCP joint. *(Reproduced with permission from Richard P. Usatine, MD.)*

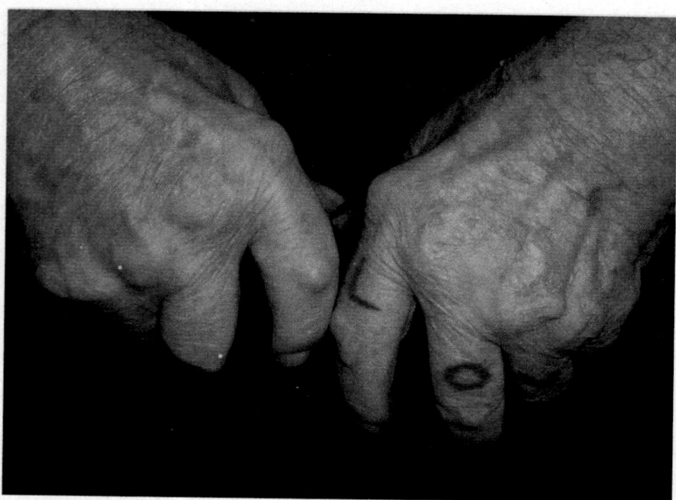

FIGURE 99-5 Rheumatoid nodules in the hands. (*Reproduced with permission from Richard P. Usatine, MD.*)

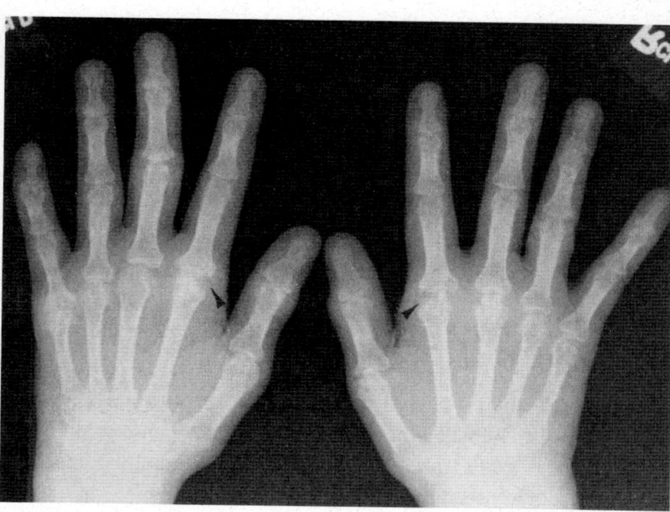

FIGURE 99-7 Hand radiographs in long-standing rheumatoid arthritis demonstrating carpal destruction, radiocarpal joint narrowing, bony erosion (*arrowheads*), and soft-tissue swelling. (*Reproduced with permission from Chen MYM, Pope TL Jr, Ott DJ. Basic Radiology. New York, NY: McGraw-Hill Education; 2004.*)

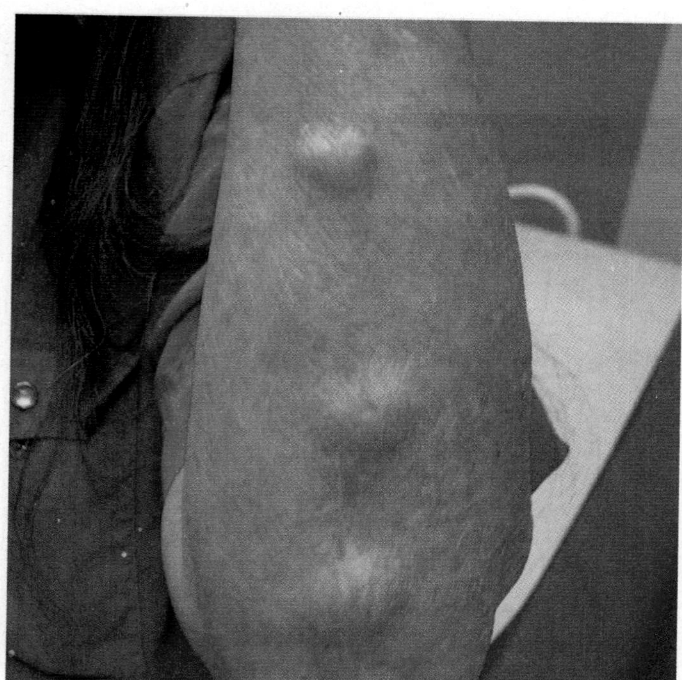

FIGURE 99-6 Rheumatoid nodules on the arm of a patient with rheumatoid arthritis. (*Reproduced with permission from Richard P. Usatine, MD.*)

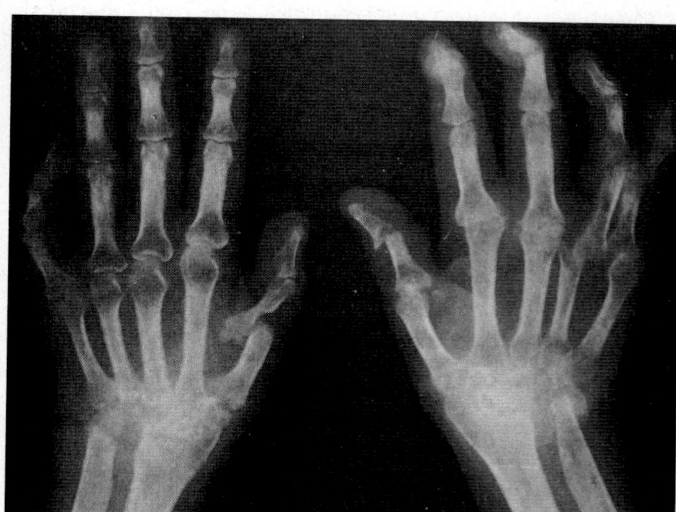

FIGURE 99-8 Severe changes of late rheumatoid arthritis including radiocarpal joint destruction, ulnar deviation, erosion of the ulnar styloid bilaterally, dislocation of the left thumb proximal interphalangeal (PIP) joint, and dislocation of the right fourth and fifth metacarpophalangeal (MCP) joints. (*Reproduced with permission from Brunicardi CF, Andersen DK, Billiar TR, et al. Schwartz's Principles of Surgery. New York, NY: McGraw-Hill Education; 2005.*)

- ACPA (anticitrullinated protein antibody), high specificity, often present before definitive diagnosis can be made; presence predicts arthritis development.
- CRP (>0.7 pg/mL) or ESR (>30 mm/h).
- Complete blood count (normocytic or microcytic anemia, thrombocytosis).
- Liver function tests and renal function tests are helpful in guiding therapy and avoiding toxic effects of various medications.[6]

IMAGING

- Hand or wrist radiographs may show soft tissue swelling, osteopenia, erosions, subluxations, and deformities (see **Figures 99-7** and **99-8**).

DIFFERENTIAL DIAGNOSIS

RA can mimic many systemic diseases and should be differentiated from the following:

- Connective tissue diseases (scleroderma and lupus), which have other specific systemic signs.
- Fibromyalgia—Pain at trigger points instead of joints.
- Hemochromatosis—Abnormal iron studies and skin changes.
- Infectious endocarditis—Heart murmurs, high fever, risk factors such as IV drug use.
- Polyarticular gout—Erythematous joints and crystals in joint aspirate.
- Polymyalgia rheumatica—Proximal joint pain without deformity.
- Seronegative spondyloarthropathies (including ankylosing spondylitis and psoriatic arthritis)—Asymmetric joint involvement, spine often involved.
- Reactive arthritis—History of infection, sexually transmitted disease, or bowel complaints.

MANAGEMENT

Target outcome is remission through use of disease-modifying agents.

Monitor for complications:

- Patients with RA are twice as likely to have serious GI complications; monitor carefully.
- Anemia—25% will respond to iron therapy.
- Cancer—Twofold increase risk of lymphomas and leukemias.
- Cardiac complications such as pericarditis or pericardial effusion (30% at diagnosis).
- Cervical spine disease—Atlas instability; careful with intubation and avoid flexion films after trauma until atlas visualized.

NONPHARMACOLOGIC

- Use of multidisciplinary team improves outcomes.[7] SOR Ⓑ
- Exercise improves aerobic capacity and strength without increases in pain or disease activity.[6] SOR Ⓑ

MEDICATIONS

- Nonbiologic DMARDs such as methotrexate, leflunomide, hydroxychloroquine, sulfasalazine, and minocycline reduce disease progression and should be considered in all patients without contraindications.[8] SOR Ⓐ
- Biologic DMARDs, such as antitumor necrosis factor (TNF) drugs (adalimumab, etanercept, and infliximab), rituximab, abatacept reduce disease progression and should be considered in patients with high disease activity and poor prognostic features.[8] SOR Ⓒ Abatacept affects T-cell function, and rituximab leads to selective killing of B-cells.
- Systemic corticosteroids relieve pain and slow progression, SOR Ⓐ but have serious side effects and should be used at lowest dose possible with added bone protection (e.g., calcium and vitamin D or a bisphosphonate).[8]
- NSAIDs can be used for pain control,[6] SOR Ⓐ but do not alter disease progression and should not be used alone.

COMPLEMENTARY AND ALTERNATIVE THERAPY

- Tai chi and yoga may have some beneficial effects.[6]
- Evening primrose or black currant seed oil contain gamma-linolenic acid and may have potential benefits.[9]
- Thunder god vine extract may reduce symptoms but has serious side effects.[9]

REFERRAL

- Refer patients with new diagnosis of or with a suspicion of RA to a physician experienced in the use of nonbiologic and biologic DMARDs.

Recommendations for initiating DMARDs are based on[8]:

- Disease duration.
- Presence of poor prognostic factors (high disease activity positive RF and/or ACPA, bony erosions) as well as functional limitations and extraarticular manifestations.
- Classification of low, moderate, or high disease activity, based on one of several validated instruments (e.g., Rheumatoid Arthritis Disease Activity Index).

DMARDs reduce disease progression, but have several contraindications and must be followed closely.

- Do not start nonbiologic or biologic DMARDs when the patient has an active bacterial infection, active or latent (before preventive therapy is initiated) tuberculosis (TB), acute hepatitis B or C, active herpes zoster, or a systemic fungal infection.[6]
- Avoid DMARDs if white blood cell count (WBC) is less than 3000/mm^3 or platelets are under 50,000/mm^3, New York Heart Association class III or IV heart failure, or liver transaminases more than twice the normal value.[6]
- Start methotrexate or leflunomide monotherapy for any disease duration, with or without poor prognostic factors, and any classification of disease activity.[8]
- Combination DMARD therapy (e.g., methotrexate [MTX] and sulfasalazine) may be used in patients with any duration of disease, poor prognostic features, and moderate or high disease activity.[8]

- Consider biologic DMARDs for patients with any disease duration, high disease activity, and poor prognostic features. Anti-TNF biologics such as etanercept, infliximab, and adalimumab improve function and quality of life as monotherapy or in combination with nonbiologic DMARDs.[8]

PROGNOSIS

- 10%–50% of RA patients achieve remission.[6]
- Poor prognostic features include high disease activity, positive RF and/or ACPA, and bony erosions.[10]
- RA patients have an increased risk of cardiovascular disease and lymphoma.[6]
- RA patients have higher mortality than the general population.[11]

FOLLOW-UP

Multidisciplinary follow-up with primary care, rheumatologist, occupational and physical therapists, and patient educators improves outcomes.

PATIENT EDUCATION

RA is a chronic illness. Ten percent to 50% of patients will have remission with therapy. Early treatment can prevent complications and allow the person to maintain function. It is best for patients to stay active and exercise to the best of their ability.

PATIENT RESOURCES

- Information on RA is available at **https://www.arthritis.com/.**
- American College of Rheumatology. *For Patients & Caregivers*—**https://www.rheumatology.org/I-Am-A/Patient-Caregiver.**

PROVIDER RESOURCES

- 2015 American College of Rheumatology Guideline for the Treatment of Rheumatoid Arthritis—**https://www.rheumatology.org/Portals/0/Files/ACR%202015%20RA%20Guideline.pdf.**

REFERENCES

1. Widdifield J, Paterson JM, Bernatsky S, et al. The epidemiology of rheumatoid arthritis in Ontario, Canada. *Arthritis Rheumatol.* 2014:66(4):786-793.
2. Kvien TK, Uhlig T, Ødegård S, Heiberg MS. Epidemiological aspects of rheumatoid arthritis: the sex ratio. *Ann N Y Acad Sci.* 2006;1069:212-222.
3. American College of Rheumatology/European League Against Rheumatism. 2010 rheumatoid arthritis classification criteria. *Arthritis Rheum.* 2010;62(9):2569-2581.
4. Radner H, Neogi T, Smolen JS, Aletaha D. Performance of the 2010 ACR/EULAR classification criteria for rheumatoid arthritis: a systematic literature review. *Ann Rheum Dis.* 2014;73(1):114-123.
5. Saraux A, Berthelot JM, Chales G, et al. Ability of the American College of Rheumatology 1987 criteria to predict rheumatoid arthritis in patients with early arthritis and classification of these patients two years later. *Arthritis Rheum.* 2001;44(11):2485-2491.
6. Wasserman AM. Diagnosis and management of rheumatoid arthritis. *Am Fam Phys.* 2011:84(11):1245-1252.
7. Vliet Vlieland TP, Breedveld FC, Hazes JM. The 2-year follow-up of a randomized comparison of in-patient multidisciplinary team care and routine out-patient care for active rheumatoid arthritis. *Br J Rheum.* 1997;36(1):82-85.
8. Singh JA, Saag KG, Bridges SL, et al. 2015 American College of Rheumatology guideline for the treatment of rheumatoid arthritis. *Arthritis Rheumatol.* 2016;68(1):1-25.
9. Cameron M, Gagnier JJ, Chrubasik S. Herbal therapy for treating rheumatoid arthritis. *Cochrane Database Syst Rev.* 2011(2): CD002948.
10. Albrecht K and Zink A. Poor prognostic factors guiding treatment decisions in rheumatoid arthritis patients: a review of data from randomized clinical trials and cohort studies. *Arthritis Res Ther.* 2017;19:68.
11. Dadoun S, Zeboulon-Ktorza N, Combescure C, et al. Mortality in rheumatoid arthritis over the last fifty years: systematic review and meta-analysis. *Joint Bone Spine.* 2013;80(1):29-33.

100 ANKYLOSING SPONDYLITIS

Heidi S. Chumley, MD, MBA

PATIENT STORY

A 43-year-old man falls and presents with acute back and diffuse abdominal pain. He has had back pain on and off for at over 5 years. Also, his wife notes that he has become "stooped" forward in the last few years. The radiographs show flowing ligamentous ossification and syndesmophyte formation about the cervical, thoracic, and lumbar spine consistent with ankylosing spondylitis (bamboo spine) (**Figure 100-1**). The KUB (kidneys, ureters, bladder) view film also shows fusion of the sacroiliac joints consistent with ankylosing spondylitis (**Figure 100-2**). No fracture, dislocation, or abdominal pathology is identified. The patient's symptoms are treated and nonsteroidal anti-inflammatory drugs (NSAIDs) are started. On follow-up a blood test reveals that he is human leukocyte antigen (HLA)-B27–positive.

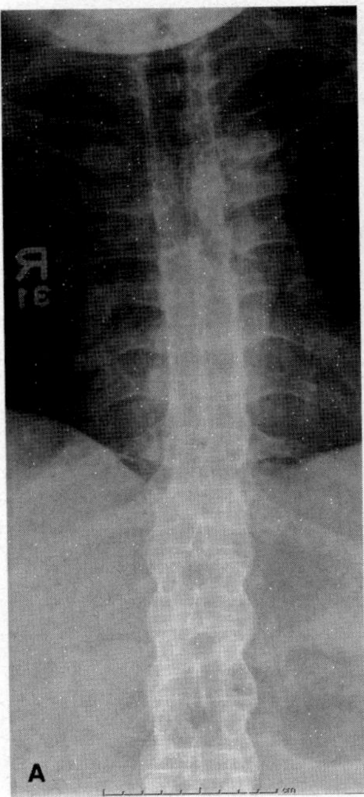

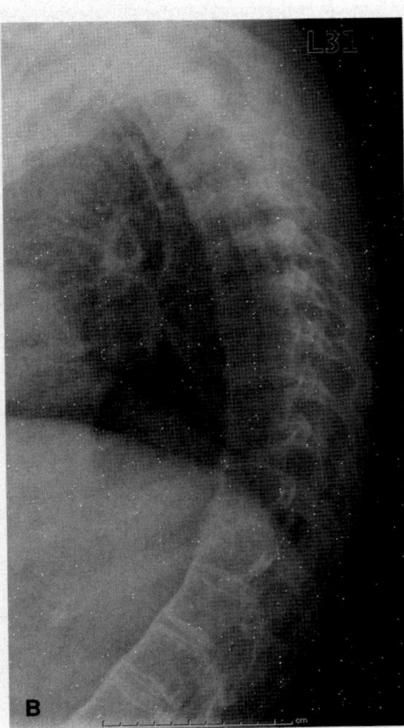

FIGURE 100-1 A. Fusion of the vertebral bodies and posterior elements gives the spine the classic "bamboo" appearance seen in ankylosing spondylitis. B. Note the marked kyphosis and the syndesmophytes that are the thin vertical connections between the anterior aspects of the vertebral bodies. They are located in the outer layers of the annulus fibrosis. *(Reproduced with permission from Richard P. Usatine, MD.)*

TERMINOLOGY

Axial spondyloarthritis is an umbrella term, which includes ankylosing spondylitis (AS) with radiographic findings suggestive of structural damage and patients with axial spine inflammation who do not have radiographic findings (non-radiographic axial spondyloarthritis).

INTRODUCTION

Ankylosing spondylitis is an inflammatory disease of the axial spine associated with the HLA-B27 genotype and radiographic findings. Symptoms of low back and/or hip pain begin in late adolescence or early adulthood. Diagnosis is based on clinical features and radiographic findings.

EPIDEMIOLOGY

- Prevalence varies by geographic region and is highest in North America and Europe (31.9 and 23.8 per 10,000) and lowest in Latin America and Africa (10.2 and 7.4 per 10,000).[1]
- 16% of primary care patients ages 18–45 with chronic low back pain for more than 3 months have ankylosing spondylitis (AS).[2]
- AS is more common in males than in females (approximate ratio: 2:1).[3]
- Ninety percent of patients are HLA-B27–positive.[4] However, many people with HLA-B27 do not develop the disease.

ETIOLOGY AND PATHOPHYSIOLOGY

- Inflammatory arthritis with a poorly understood pathology.
- Environment triggers and genetic factors result in inflammation.
- Chronic inflammation causes extensive new bone formation.

RISK FACTORS

- Male gender.
- HLA-B27–positive genotype.

DIAGNOSIS

- Mean delay of 8 years until diagnosis.[5]
- Consider referring/testing patients younger than 45 years of age with chronic low back pain with at least two of the following: inflammatory back pain, good response to nonsteroidal anti-inflammatory drugs, family history of spondyloarthritis (SpA) and low back pain duration longer than 5 years (sensitivity 75%, specificity 58%).[2]
- Criteria for axial SpA from the Spondyloarthritis International Society Classification[6]:
  - Sacroiliitis on imaging and at least one SpA feature or HLA-B27 and at least 2 SpA features
  - SpA features include:
    - Inflammatory back pain
    - Arthritis
    - Enthesitis
    - Uveitis
    - Dactylitis
    - Psoriasis
    - Crohn disease
    - Positive HLA-B27 and elevated C-reactive protein

CLINICAL FEATURES

- Younger patient (younger than 40 years of age at start of disease).
- Inflammatory back pain (pain and stiffness worsen with immobility and improve with motion; symptoms are worse at night or early morning) is seen in 90%.[4]
- Two-thirds have a good response to NSAIDs.[4]

PHYSICAL EXAMINATION

- Limited range of motion of the spine is seen in 50%.[4]
- Tenderness over the spine and sacroiliac joints.
- In the advanced stages, kyphosis may occur with a stooped posture (see **Figure 100-1**).
- Uveitis of the eye is the most common extraarticular manifestation occurring in 40% of patients.[4] This can present with a red painful eye along with photophobia. The involved eye may have an irregular pupil and a 360-degree perilimbal injection (see Chapter 20, Uveitis and Iritis).

TYPICAL DISTRIBUTION

- Pain in lower back and/or sacroiliac joints.

LABORATORY TESTING

- HLA-B27 is positive in 90% of patients with AS.[4]
- As back pain is common in primary care, consider ordering HLA-B27 for patients with inflammatory back pain only.

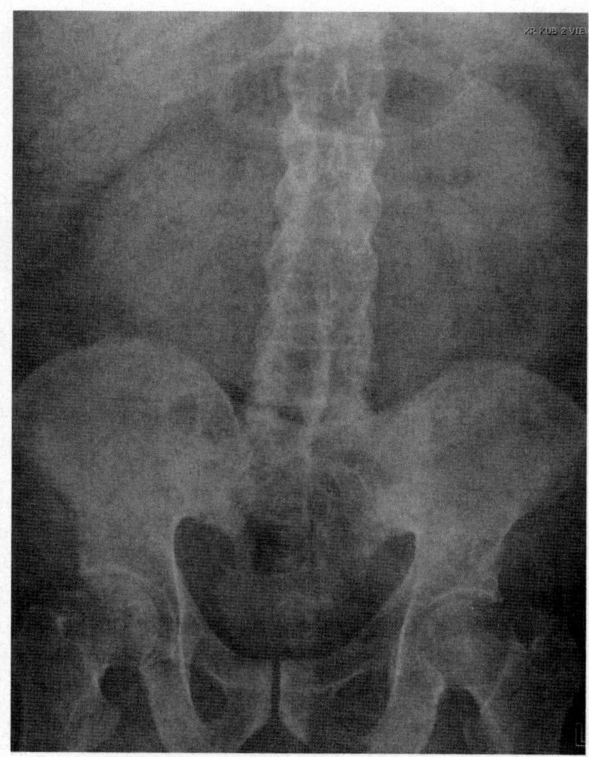

FIGURE 100-2 Kidney, ureter, bladder (KUB) view showing bamboo spine and fusion of both sacroiliac joints. (*Reproduced with permission from Richard P. Usatine, MD.*)

IMAGING

- Radiologic findings confirm the diagnosis; however, these may occur years after the onset of symptoms.
- Plain films—Typical spinal features include erosions, squaring, sclerosis, syndesmophytes, and fractures; may also see sacroiliac joint fusion (**Figure 100-3**). Flowing ligamentous ossification and syndesmophyte formation about the cervical, thoracic, and lumbar spine form the classic bamboo spine described in ankylosing spondylitis (see **Figures 100-1** and **100-2**).
- MRI—Detects inflammation, such as acute sacroiliitis, which occurs prior to bony change visible by radiographs.

FIGURE 100-3 Ankylosing spondylitis with near fusion of right sacroiliac (SI) joint and pseudowidening (from erosive changes) of the left SI joint. (*Reproduced with permission from Everett Allen, MD.*)

DIFFERENTIAL DIAGNOSIS

Causes of back pain in patients younger than age 45 years:

- Lumbar strain or muscle spasm—Acute onset often with precipitating event.
- Herniated disc—Acute onset with pain radiating below the knee into lower leg or foot with numbness, weakness, and/or loss of ankle jerk reflex.
- Vertebral fractures—Risk factors are osteoporosis or significant trauma.
- Abdominal pathology such as pancreatitis—Associated with GI symptoms.
- Kidney diseases—Nephrolithiasis (pain radiating into groin); pyelonephritis (fever, nausea, and urinary symptoms).
- Osteoarthritis—Worse after working; less commonly has inflammatory symptoms. (See Chapter 98, Osteoarthritis.)
- Other types of spondyloarthritis (SpA) include psoriatic spondyloarthritis (**Figure 100-4**), SpA associated with inflammatory bowel disease, reactive SpA, and undifferentiated SpA.

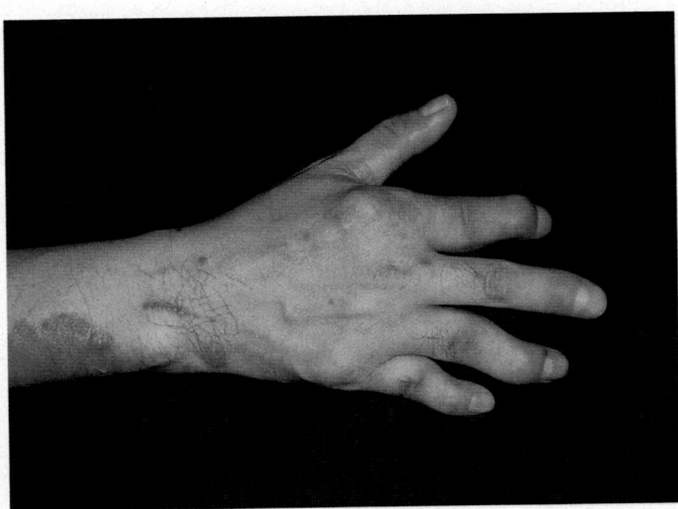

FIGURE 100-4 Psoriatic arthritis showing swan-neck deformities, involvement of proximal interphalangeal (PIP) and distal interphalangeal (DIP) joints, and skin plaques. (*Reproduced with permission from Richard P. Usatine, MD.*)

MANAGEMENT

FIRST LINE

- NSAIDs, including COX-2 inhibitors, reduce pain and improve function.[7] SOR Ⓐ
- Continuous NSAIDs may reduce radiographic progression in subsets of patients, including those with a high C-reactive protein (CRP).[7] SOR Ⓑ
- Refer for physical therapy.[8] SOR Ⓑ

SECOND LINE

- Tissue necrosis factor (TNF) inhibitors are recommended for patients who fail NSAIDs and physical therapy.[8] SOR Ⓐ Failure is lack of response (or intolerance) to two different NSAIDs over a month, or incomplete response to two different NSAIDs over 2 months.[8]
  - 50% of patients responded to the TNF inhibitors etanercept, adalimumab, or infliximab; however, 25% of patients discontinue therapy due to side effects.[9] SOR Ⓑ

- Concomitant use of sulfasalazine may increase continuation of TNF therapy,[9] but is currently not recommended by the American College of Rheumatology as primary therapy.[8]

PROGNOSIS

- Cardiovascular and cerebrovascular mortality is increased in patients with AS (adjusted hazard ratio 1.46 in men and 1.24 in women).[10]
- Risk factors for reduced survival include absence of NSAID use (odds ratio [OR] 4.35), work disability (OR 3.65), increased CRP (OR 2.68), and diagnostic delay (OR 1.05).[11]

FOLLOW-UP

Follow patients for progression of pain or decreased function using standard ankylosing spondylitis, such as the Ankylosing Spondylitis Disease Activity Score or the Bath Ankylosing Spondylitis Disease Activity Index or Functional Index.

PATIENT EDUCATION

Ankylosing spondylitis is a chronic disease. NSAIDs and physical therapy and exercise are important in controlling pain and slowing progression of disease. If these are ineffective, tissue necrosis factor blockers are effective; however, these have higher discontinuation rates, and pain recurs when they are stopped.

PATIENT RESOURCES

- American College of Rheumatology. Patient education handout: *Spondylarthritis*—**https://www.rheumatology.org/I-Am-A/Patient-Caregiver/Diseases-Conditions/Spondyloarthritis**
- The Spondylitis Association of America—**https://www.spondylitis.org.**
- PubMed Health. *Ankylosing Spondylitis*—**http://www.ncbi.nlm.nih.gov/pubmedhealth/PMH0001457/.**

PROVIDER RESOURCES

- Assessment of SpondyloArthritis International Society. *Ankylosing Spondylitis Disease Activity Score Information and Online Calculator*—**https://www.asas-group.org/.**
- American College of Rheumatology/Spondylitis Association of America/Spondyloarthritis Research and Treatment Network 2015 recommendations for treatment—**http://onlinelibrary.wiley.com/doi/10.1002/acr.22708/full.**
- Bath Ankylosing Spondylitis Disease Activity and Functional Indices—**http://basdai.com/select.htm.**
- Assessment of SpondyloArthritis International Society (ASAS) Ankylosing Spondylitis Disease Activity Score—**https://www.asas-group.org/clinical-instruments/asdas-calculator/.**

REFERENCES

1. Dean LE, Jones GT, MacDonald AG, et al. Global prevalence of ankylosing spondylitis. *Rheumatology (Oxford).* 2014;53(4):650-657.
2. van Hoeven L, Vergouwe Y, de Buck PD, et al. External validation of a referral rule for axial spondyloarthritis in primary care patients with chronic low back pain. *PLoS One.* 2015;10(7):e0131963.
3. Exarchou S, Lindström U, Askling J. The prevalence of clinically diagnosed ankylosing spondylitis and its clinical manifestations: a nationwide register study. *Arthritis Res Ther.* 2015:9(17):118.
4. Wright KA, Crowson CS, Michet CJ, Matteson EL. Time trends in incidence, clinical features, and cardiovascular disease in ankylosing spondylitis over three decades: a population-based study. *Arthritis Care Res (Hoboken).* 2015;67(6):836-841.
5. Seo MR, Baek HL, Yoon HH, et al. Delayed diagnosis is linked to worse outcomes and unfavourable treatment responses in patients with axial spondyloarthritis. *Clin Rheumatol.* 2015;34(8):1397-1405.
6. Rudwaleit M, van der Heijde D, Landewé R, et al. The development of assessment of SpondyloArthritis International Society classification criteria for axial spondyloarthritis (part II): validation and final selection. *Ann Rheum Dis.* 2009;68:777-783.
7. Kroon FP, van der Burg LR, Ramiro S, et al. Non-steroidal anti-inflammatory drugs (NSAIDs) for axial spondyloarthritis (ankylosing spondylitis and non-radiographic axial spondyloarthritis). *Cochrane Database Syst Rev.* 2015;(7):CD010952.
8. Ward MM, Deodhar A, Akl EA, et al. American College of Rheumatology/Spondylitis Association of America/Spondyloarthritis Research and Treatment Network 2015 recommendations for the treatment of ankylosing spondylitis and nonradiographic axial spondyloarthritis. *Arthritis Care Res.* 2016;68(2):282-298.
9. Heinonen AV, Aaltonen KJ, Joensuu JT, et al. Effectiveness and drug survival of TNF inhibitors in the treatment of ankylosing spondylitis: a prospective cohort study. *J Rheumatol.* 2015;42(12):2339-2346.
10. Haroon NN, Paterson JM, Li P, et al. Patients with ankylosing spondylitis have increased cardiovascular and cerebrovascular mortality: a population-based study. *Ann Intern Med.* 2015;163(6):409-416.
11. Bakland G, Gran JT, Nossent JC. Increased mortality in ankylosing spondylitis is related to disease activity. *Ann Rheum Dis.* 2011;70(11):1921-1925.

101 BACK PAIN

Heidi S. Chumley, MD, MBA

PATIENT STORY

A 60-year-old woman presents with chronic low back pain that began many years ago. Her back pain waxes and wanes, and she has taken acetaminophen and ibuprofen with some relief. About 3 months ago, she began to have daily pain. She recalls no trauma. Her examination is unremarkable other than some decreased flexion. Straight-leg raise test is negative. As the patient is older than 55 years of age, radiographs are ordered, and they demonstrate degenerative changes in her lumbar spine (**Figure 101-1**). She is started on an exercise program and yoga.

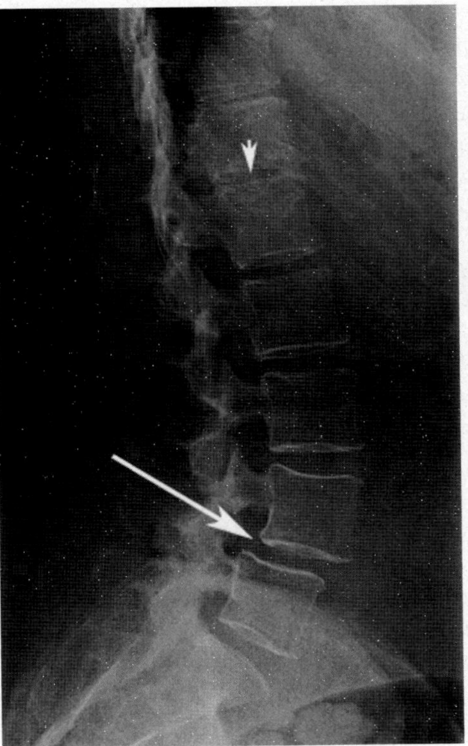

FIGURE 101-1 Lateral view shows grade 1 degenerative spondylolisthesis at L4-L5 (*arrow*), moderate facet osteoarthritis of L5-S1. Marked T12-L1 disc degeneration (*arrowhead*) and mild L4-L5 disc degeneration.

INTRODUCTION

Back pain is one of the most common reasons that adults see their physician. Most acute back pain is a result of mechanical causes. Serious pathology is rare and occurs in the presence of red flags. Acute back pain is treated with reassurance, returning to activities, and nonsteroidal anti-inflammatory drugs (NSAIDs). Psychological factors increase the risk of development of chronic pain. Chronic back pain is difficult to treat, and the best outcomes are typically achieved by an interprofessional team.

EPIDEMIOLOGY

- Six percent of visits to primary care physicians are for back pain.[1]
- 28.9% of community-living adults have had back pain in the last 3 months.[2]
- The incidence of low back pain (LBP) is 139 per 100,000 person years.[3]
- Thoracic back pain prevalence in working adults ages 20–59 is 10% in men and 20% in women.[4]
- Treatment for back and neck problems accounted for approximately $90 billion in health care expenditures in the United States per year; lost productivity is estimated to cost an additional $10 to $20 billion.[5]
- Prevalence of fracture in patients with LBP presenting to primary care is 1% to 4%[6]; less than 1% will have a malignancy.[7]

ETIOLOGY AND PATHOPHYSIOLOGY

- LBP can be caused by pain in the muscles, ligaments, joints, bones, discs, nerves, or blood vessels.[8]
- In 90% of cases, the specific cause of LBP is unclear.[8]
- In 10% of cases, a specific cause such as an infection, fracture, or cancer is identified.[8]

RISK FACTORS

- Older age—Prevalence of LBP increases with age into the sixth decade.[8]
- Low educational status.[8]
- Occupational factors—Manual labor, bending, twisting, and whole-body vibration.[8]
- Psychosocial factors increase the risk of transition from acute to chronic pain.[8]
- Risk factors for cancer—Previous history of cancer (positive likelihood ratio [LR+] 20.0, negative likelihood ratio [LR−] 0.46).[7]

DIAGNOSIS

The diagnosis can be classified into three categories:

1. Nonspecific back pain—Pain for less than 4 weeks (acute), 4 to 12 weeks (subacute), or more than 12 weeks (chronic); negative straight-leg raise test; absence of red flags.
2. Radicular syndrome—LBP with radiation down leg; positive straight-leg raise test; absence of red flags.
3. Serious pathology—Further work-up required for presence of red flags, including age younger than 20 or older than 55 years; significant trauma; prior history of cancer; fever; unexplained weight loss; neurologic signs of cauda equina; progressive neurologic deficit.

TYPICAL DISTRIBUTION

Lumbar pain is about twice as common as thoracic pain.

LABORATORY TESTING

Helpful in the presence of red flags:

- Complete blood count (CBC) to evaluate for anemia (malignancy) or leukocytosis (infection).
- Consider human leukocyte antigen (HLA)-B27 in younger patients with inflammatory symptoms.

IMAGING

- In acute back pain without red flags, imaging can be delayed for 6 weeks.
- Radiographs may show degenerative joint disease changes in osteoarthritis; vertebral fractures; malignancies; and findings of ankylosing spondylitis including erosions, sclerosis, syndesmophytes (see Chapter 100, Ankylosing Spondylitis).
- MRI is the best imaging test for disc herniation and imaging of the spinal cord. Emergent MRI is indicated in patients with suspected spinal cord compromise or cauda equina syndrome.
- CT myelogram is a useful alternative to evaluate disc herniation in patients who cannot undergo MRI.

DIFFERENTIAL DIAGNOSIS

- Osteoporotic vertebral fracture—Acute onset of pain, typically seen in older patients or those at risk for osteoporosis, point tenderness

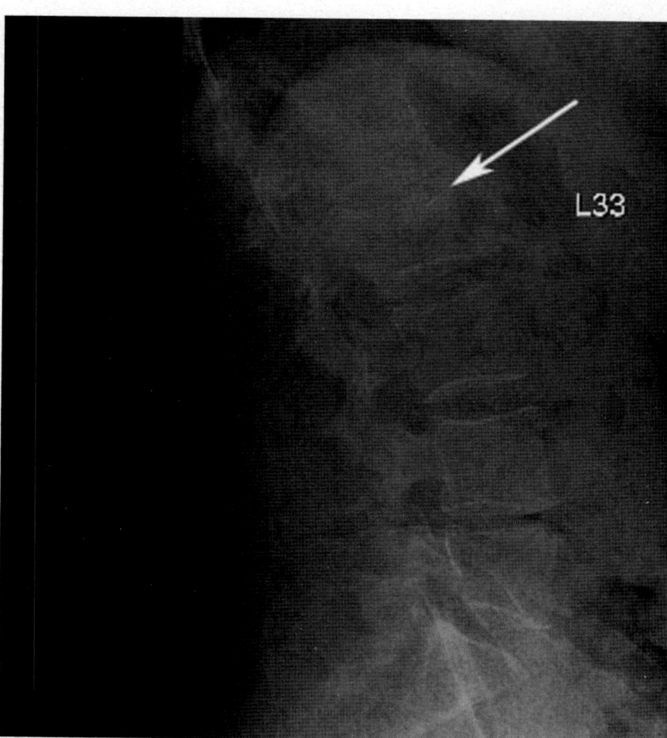

FIGURE 101-2 Lateral view demonstrating the loss of vertebral body height seen with a compression fracture deformity (*arrow*) of the superior end plate of the L2 vertebral body. There is also a mild concave compression deformity of the superior end plate of the L5 vertebral body.

at the level of the fracture, confirmation by plain radiographs demonstrating compression or burst fracture (**Figure 101-2**).

- Spinal stenosis—Pain worse with extension, presence of unilateral or bilateral leg symptoms worse with walking and better with sitting, confirmation by CT or MRI.
- Herniated disc—Radicular pain that is worse with flexion or sitting, may be accompanied by numbness or weakness of foot plantar flexion (L5/S1) or dorsiflexion (L4/L5), MRI confirms the level and shows the type of herniation (**Figures 101-3** and **101-4**).
- Spinal infection/abscess—Most commonly seen in patients who use IV drugs, have diabetes mellitus, have cancer, or have a transplant; symptoms include fever, night pain, night sweats, and elevated erythrocyte sedimentation rate (ESR). MRI is the study of choice. If neurologic deficit is present, obtain an urgent MRI to evaluate for an abscess, which would require hospitalization and consultation with a spinal surgeon.
- Ankylosing spondylitis (see Chapter 100, Ankylosing Spondylitis)—Pain, most commonly in the low back or sacroiliac joints, usually begins in late adolescence or early adulthood. Pain and stiffness worsen with immobility and improve with motion. HLA-B27 may be positive. Radiographic findings confirm the diagnosis, but occur years after symptoms.
- Malignancy—Typically seen in an older patient; symptoms of weight loss and night pain; significant anemia; history of cancer; nonresponse to therapy. Often seen on plain radiographs. Bone scan is the most sensitive test.
- Abdominal pathology such as pancreatitis, pyelonephritis, and cholecystitis can present as back pain or pain radiating to the back.

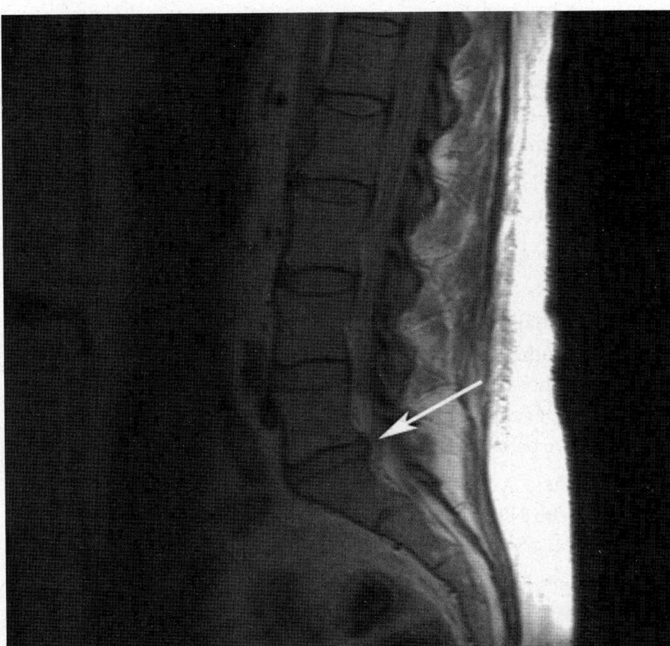

FIGURE 101-3 MRI showing herniated nucleus pulposus (*arrow*) at L5-S1 in a patient with radicular pain and a poor response to 6 weeks of conservative therapy.

MANAGEMENT

ACUTE BACK PAIN

Most national guidelines agree on the following[9]:

- Nonpharmacologic:
  - Reassure patients without red flags that they do not have a serious condition, advise them to remain active, discourage bed rest, and encourage an early return to work while back pain is still present.
  - Exercise is considered no more effective than return to normal activities for LBP within the first 4 to 6 weeks.[9]
- Medications:
  - Add NSAID if needed (ask about GI problems and protect against ulcers as needed).
  - Consider a short course of muscle relaxers if pain is severe and inadequately treated with NSAIDs.
  - Consider antidepressants (such as amitriptyline) or anticonvulsants (such as gabapentin) for radicular pain.
  - Acetaminophen is no longer recommended due to lack of effectiveness.[10]
- Complementary and alternative therapy:
  - National guidelines differ; American College of Physician guidelines recommend superficial heat, massage, acupuncture, or spinal manipulation.[11]

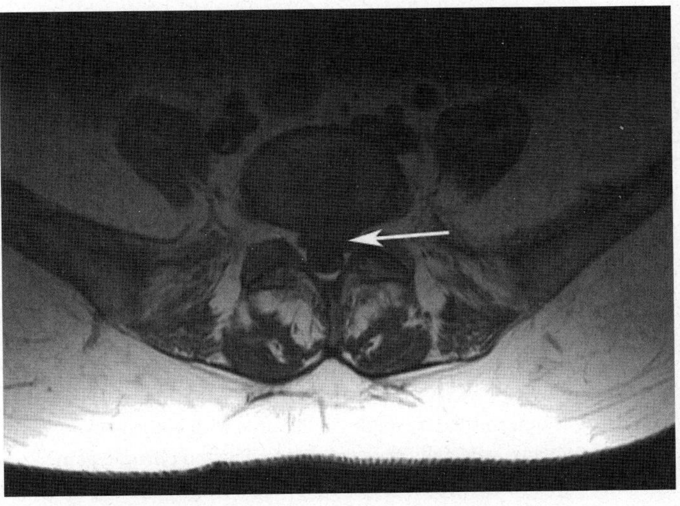

FIGURE 101-4 MRI cross section demonstrates that the herniated disc (*arrow*) is compressing S1 nerve root.

- Referral or hospitalization:
  - Patients with cauda equina syndrome should have expedient imaging and urgent referral to a spinal surgeon.
  - Refer patients with serious pathology such as infection, tumor, or fracture to appropriate consultants.

CHRONIC (>12 WEEKS) BACK PAIN

ACP recommendations include[11]:

- First line:
  - Treat initially with nonpharmacologic interventions. SOR Ⓐ
  - Use a multidisciplinary approach.
  - Commonly available options supported by evidence include[11-13]: exercise, acupuncture, yoga, stress reduction techniques, cognitive behavioral therapy, or spinal manipulation.
- Second line:
  - Treat with NSAIDs.
  - Consider tramadol or duloxetine if NSAIDs are not effective.
  - Acetaminophen is no longer recommended due to lack of effectiveness.[10]
- Third line:
  - Opioids should be used rarely when benefits clearly outweigh the risk for an individual patient. SOR Ⓒ
- Referral or hospitalization:
  - Chronic pain is difficult to treat (see Appendix B, Chronic Pain). Use an interdisciplinary team to maximize effectiveness if possible.
  - Consider referring patients who do not respond to conservative therapy to a pain management specialist or a spine surgeon.

PREVENTION

Good posture, appropriate lifting techniques, maintaining a healthy weight, and enjoying an active lifestyle may help prevent back pain. Adding yoga to an active lifestyle has the potential to prevent recurrent back pain and diminish the pain of chronic back pain.[12] SOR Ⓐ

PROGNOSIS

- Patients with nonradicular acute back pain—By 12 months, 40% recover fully.[14]
- Patients with acute back pain who have psychological factors at baseline are more likely to develop chronic LBP.[15]

FOLLOW-UP

Follow-up is determined by etiology. Patients with acute back pain, without red flags, especially those at risk to develop chronic pain, should be followed closely. Patients with chronic pain benefit from ongoing treatment by an interprofessional team.

PATIENT EDUCATION

- Reassure patients without red flags that most acute back pain is not a result of a serious cause and can be treated conservatively.
- Advise patients with chronic back pain that a comprehensive approach to pain management is more likely to result in pain improvement than medications alone.

PATIENT RESOURCES

- Written and auditory patient information is available in English and Spanish at Family Doctor.org—**http://familydoctor.org/familydoctor/condition/low-back-pain.html.**
- Gentle yoga routine for lower back relief on YouTube—**https://www.youtube.com/watch?v=pyFNz8zJSdw.**

PROVIDER RESOURCES

- A comprehensive list of red flags for back pain can be found in family practice notebook—**http://www.fpnotebook.com/Ortho/Sx/LwBckPnRdFlg.htm.**
- WebMD Back Pain Health Center. Useful for patients and providers—**http://www.webmd.com/back-pain/default.htm.**

REFERENCES

1. Jordan KP, Kadam UT, Hayward R, et al. Annual consultation prevalence of regional musculoskeletal problems in primary care: an observational study. *BMC Musculoskelet Disord.* 2010; 11:144.
2. National Center on Health Statistics. *United States, 2011: With Special Feature on Socioeconomic Status and Health.* Hyattsville, MD; Author. 2012.
3. Waterman BR, Belmont PJ, Jr., Schoenfeld AJ. Low back pain in the United States: incidence and risk factors for presentation in the emergency setting. *Spine J.* 2012;12(1):63-70.
4. Fouquet N, Bodin J, Descatha A, et al. Prevalence of thoracic spine pain in a surveillance network. *Occup Med (Lond).* 2015; 65(2):122-125.
5. Davis MA. Where the United States spends its spine dollars: expenditures on different ambulatory services for the management of back and neck conditions. *Spine.* 2012;37(19):1693-1701.
6. Williams CM, Henschke N, Maher CG, et al. Red flags to screen for vertebral fracture in patients presenting with low-back pain. *Cochrane Database Syst Rev.* 2013;(1):CD008643.
7. Henschke N, Maher CG, Ostelo RW, et al. Red flags to screen for malignancy in patients with low-back pain. *Cochrane Database Syst Rev.* 2013;(2):CD008686.
8. Hoy D, Brooks P, Blyth F, Buchbinder R. The epidemiology of low back pain. *Best Pract Res Clin Rheumatol.* 2010;24(6):769-781.
9. Koes BW, van Tulder M, Lin CW, et al. An updated overview of clinical guidelines for the management of non-specific low back pain in primary care. *Eur Spine J.* 2010;19(12):2075-2094.

10. Saragiotto BT, Machado GC, Ferreira ML, et al. Paracetamol for low back pain. *Cochrane Database Syst Rev.* 2016(6):CD012230.
11. Qaseem A, Wilt TJ, McLean RM, Forciea MA. Noninvasive treatments for acute, subacute, and chronic low back pain: a clinical practice guideline from the American College of Physicians. *Ann Intern Med.* 2017;166(7):514-530.
12. Cramer H, Lauche R, Haller H, Dobos G. A systematic review and meta-analysis of yoga for low back pain. *Clin J Pain.* 2013; 29(5):450-460.
13. Rubinstein SM, van Middelkoop M, Assendelft WJ, et al. Spinal manipulative therapy for chronic low-back pain. *Cochrane Database Syst Rev.* 2011;(2):CD008112.
14. Costa Lda C, Maher CG, McAuley JH, et al. Prognosis for patients with chronic low back pain: inception cohort study. *BMJ.* 2009; 339:b3829.
15. Mello M, Elfering A, Egli Presland C, et al. Predicting the transition from acute to persistent low back pain. *Occup Med (Lond).* 2011; 61(2):127-131.

102 GOUT

Heidi S. Chumley, MD, MBA
Mindy A. Smith, MD, MS

PATIENT STORY

A 91-year-old woman arrives by ambulance to the emergency department because she was experiencing severe pain in her right middle finger (**Figure 102-1**). History reveals that she has had swelling of her finger for approximately 1 year. Palpation of the distal interphalangeal joint demonstrated firmness rather than fluctuance. A radiograph of the finger was ordered (**Figure 102-2**). The radiograph and physical examination are consistent with acute gouty arthritis superimposed on tophaceous gout. The diagnosis was confirmed by an aspirate of the finger that demonstrated negatively birefringent, needle-like crystals, both intracellularly and extracellularly. She was given 1.2 mg of colchicine followed by a second dose of 0.6 mg after 1 hour. Her pain was markedly decreased in 4 hours. Her serum uric acid level was determined to be 10.7 mg/dL. Colchicine was used in this case because the risk of using nonsteroidal anti-inflammatory drugs (NSAIDs) was considered to be high because of her previous history of gastric bleeding secondary to NSAIDs.

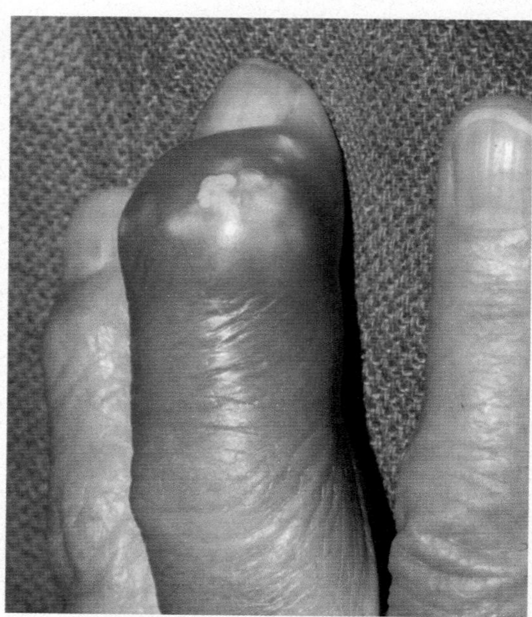

FIGURE 102-1 Acute gouty arthritis superimposed on tophaceous gout. (*Reproduced with permission from Geiderman JM. An elderly woman with a warm, painful finger, West J Med. 2000;172(1):51-52.*)

INTRODUCTION

Gout is an inflammatory crystalline arthritis. Elevated uric acid leads to deposition of monosodium urate (MSU) crystals in the joints resulting in a red, hot, swollen joint. Gout typically begins as a monoarthritis, but can become polyarthritic. Treatment of acute episodes includes NSAIDs, colchicine, or intraarticular steroids. Chronic therapy includes lowering the uric acid level using dietary modifications and urate-lowering drugs.

EPIDEMIOLOGY

- One-year prevalence of gout in many different countries is approximately 5 per 1000.[1]
- Incidence of gout is approximately 1–2 per 1000 person years.[1]
- Gout is four times more common in men than women until age 65; after age 65, gout is three times more common in men than women.[2]
- Gout usually begins after the age of 30 in men and after menopause in women.
- Several polymorphisms that regulate uric acid levels have been associated with increases in risk and severity of gout.[2]

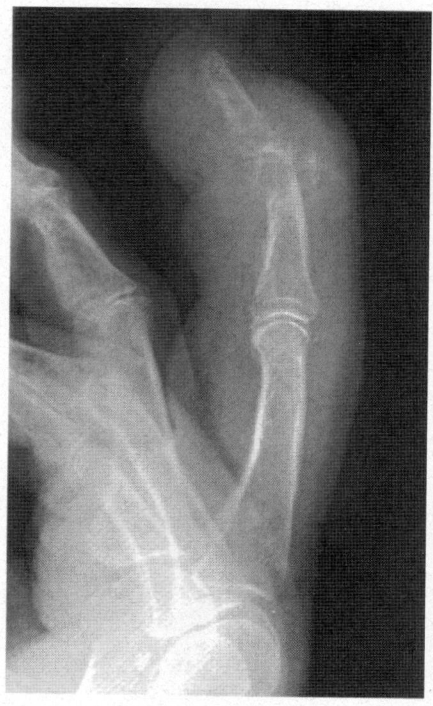

FIGURE 102-2 This X-ray of the finger in **Figure 102-1** shows several tophi (monosodium urate [MSU] deposits) in the soft tissue over the third distal interphalangeal joint. Note the typical punched-out lesions under the tophi. This is subchondral bone destruction. (*Reproduced with permission from Geiderman JM. An elderly woman with a warm, painful finger, West J Med. 2000;172(1):51-52.*)

ETIOLOGY AND PATHOPHYSIOLOGY

- Defective uric acid metabolism with inefficient renal urate excretion leads to underexcretion of uric acid and an elevated serum uric acid level.

- Overproduction of uric acid, instead of underexcretion, occurs in approximately 10% of patients with gout, and also leads to elevated serum uric acid levels.
- Elevated serum uric acid leads to deposition of MSU crystals in the joints and the kidneys.
- Crystals trigger proinflammatory cytokines, which cause local inflammation, tissue necrosis, fibrosis, and subchondral bone destruction.

RISK FACTORS

- Increasing age and male gender.[2]
- Race/ethnicity: more common in African American than in white persons; higher prevalence also reported in Maori, Hmong, and Filipino populations.[2]
- Genetic polymorphism that contribute to higher uric acid levels.
- Medications that cause hyperuricemia—Thiazide diuretics, cyclosporine, aspirin (<1 g/day).
- Conditions associated with gout—Insulin resistance, obesity, hypertension, hypertriglyceridemia, hypercholesterolemia, congestive heart failure, renal insufficiency, early menopause, organ transplant.
- Dietary—Increased intake of meat and seafood, alcohol (beer and liquor), soft drinks, and fructose.[2]

DIAGNOSIS

The American College of Rheumatology and the European League Against Rheumatism developed these diagnostic criteria in 2015.[3]

- Required: One or more episodes of swelling, pain, or tenderness in a joint or bursa
- Sufficient for diagnosis: MSU crystals in the synovial fluid of a symptomatic joint or bursa or in a tophus (**Figure 102-3**)
- If testing for crystals is not performed, a score of ≥8 on the following scoring system (sensitivity 92%, specificity 89%)[3]:
  - History
    - Location:
      - +1 point for mid-foot/ankle without first MTP involvement
      - +2 points for first MTP involvement (**Figure 102-4**)
    - Typical time course: (at least 2 of 3) time to maximal pain <24 hours, resolution in ≤14 days, complete resolution between episodes
      - +1 point for one typical time course
      - +2 points for recurrent typical time courses
    - Common presentation: 1 point for each of the following
      - +1 point for erythema over painful joint
      - +1 point for cannot bear touch or pressure
      - +1 point for great difficulty using joint (i.e., walking)
  - Physical examination
    - +4 points for tophus (**Figures 102-5** to **102-7**)
  - Laboratory
    - Serum urate
      - <BL4>–4 points for <4 mg/dL
      - +2, +3, +4 points for 6–7.9 mg/dL, 8–9.9 mg/dL, and ≥10 mg/dL, respectively
    - –2 points for absence of MSU crystals

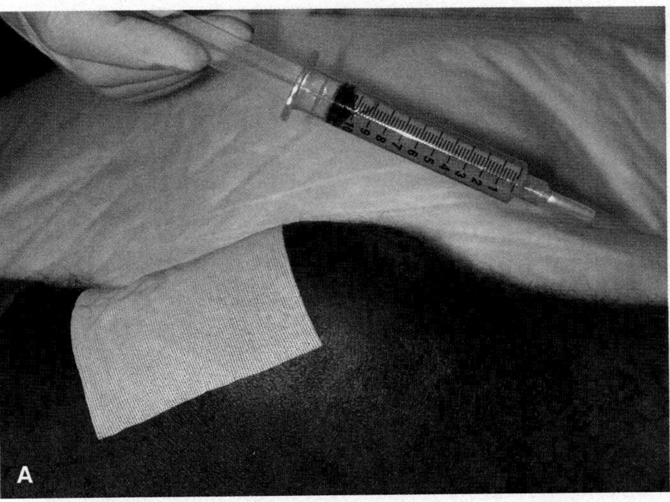

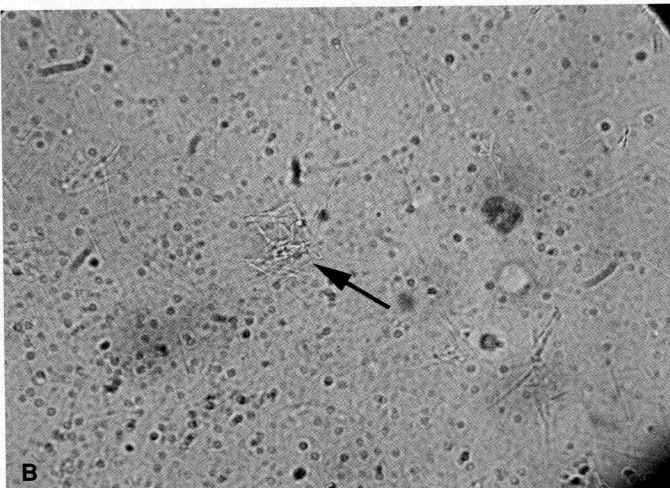

FIGURE 102-3 **A.** A 52-year-old homeless man with acute monoarticular gouty arthritis presenting with knee pain and swelling. Knee aspiration revealed a straw-colored effusion. **B.** With light microscopy numerous refractile needle-shaped crystals of uric acid were visualized in the joint fluid. The *arrow* points to a cluster of needle-shaped uric acid crystals. (*Reproduced with permission from Usatine RP, Sacks B, Sorci J. A swollen knee, J Fam Pract. 2003;52(1):53-55. Frontline Medical Communications. Inc.*)

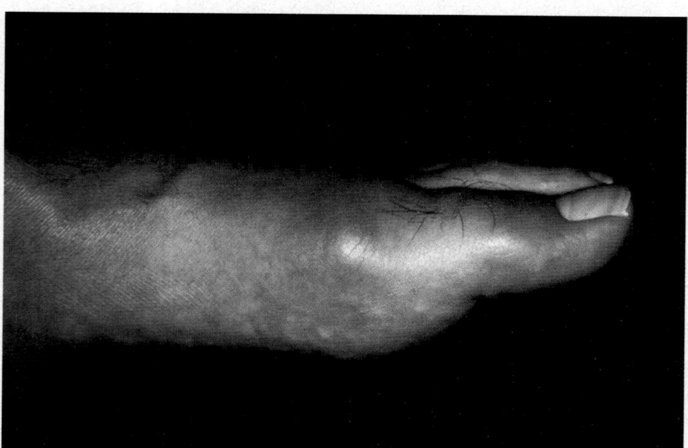

FIGURE 102-4 Podagra. Typical inflammatory changes of gout at first metatarsophalangeal (MTP) joint. (*Reproduced with permission from Richard P. Usatine, MD.*)

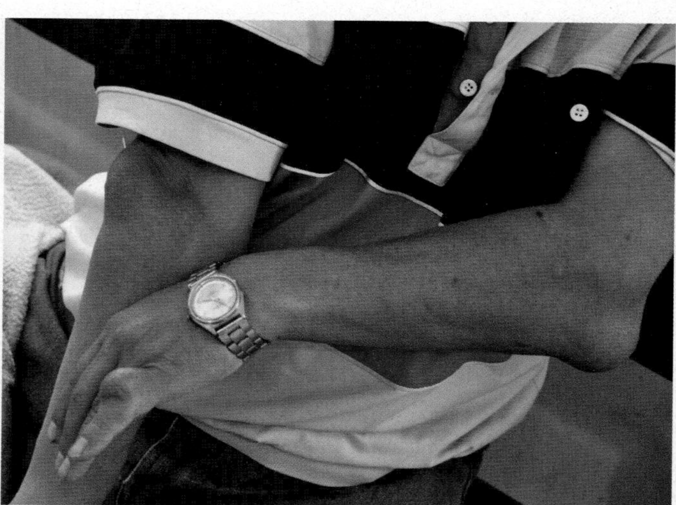

FIGURE 102-6 Tophaceous deposits on both elbows and one finger in a man with gout. (*Reproduced with permission from Richard P. Usatine, MD.*)

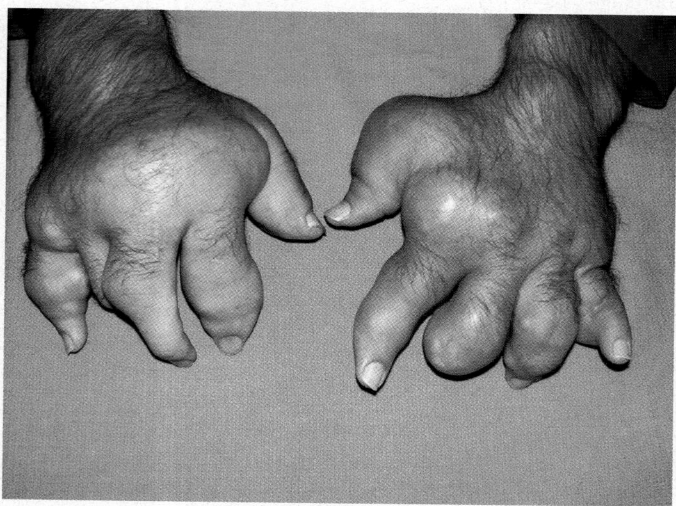

FIGURE 102-5 Severe tophaceous gout causing major deformities in the hands. (*Reproduced with permission from Eric Kraus, MD.*)

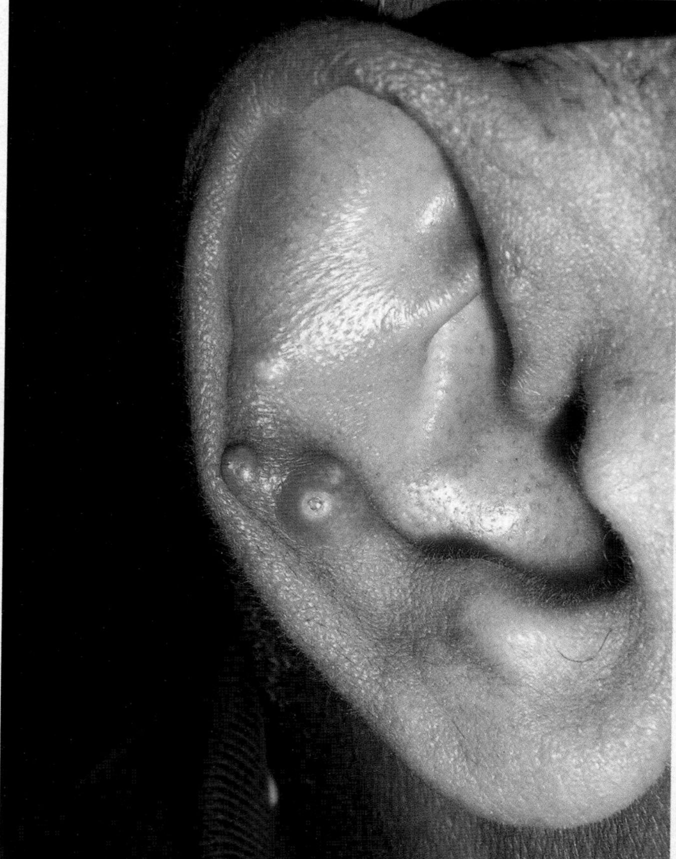

FIGURE 102-7 Tophaceous deposits in the pinna of black man with gout. (*Reproduced with permission from Richard P. Usatine, MD.*)

- Radiographic
  - +4 points for imaging evidence of urate deposition
  - +4 points for imaging evidence of gout-related joint damage

CLINICAL FEATURES

- Gout usually begins at night as an acute attack over several hours.
- Fever, chills, and arthralgias sometimes precede gout.
- The affected joint is swollen, red, hot, and painful to touch and movement (see **Figures 102-1**, **102-3**, and **102-4**). Symptoms subside in 3 to 10 days.
- Dietary or alcohol excess, trauma, surgery, and serious medical illness can precipitate gout attacks.

TYPICAL DISTRIBUTION

Initially, only one joint may be affected, but other joints commonly involved are fingers and toes (75%) and knees and ankles (50%).

- The most common site is the first MTP joint, and the name for gout at this site is podagra (see **Figure 102-4**).
- Joint involvement is often asymmetric.
- Tophi may be seen at the MTP joint, elbow, hands, and ears (**Figures 102-1**, **102-5** to **102-7**).

LABORATORY TESTING

- Serum uric acid is often elevated, but is variable from week to week and normal in 25% of patients with gout.
- On microscopy, the presence of MSU crystals from synovial fluid or a tophus that are negatively birefringent in polarized light (yellow against a red background) confirms the diagnosis.
- Even with light microscopy, refractile needle-shaped crystals of uric acid can be visualized in the joint fluid (see **Figure 102-3**).

IMAGING

Although radiographs are negative early in the disease, punched-out erosions ("rat bites") are seen later and contribute to the diagnosis, especially if seen adjacent to tophi (see **Figure 102-2**).

DIFFERENTIAL DIAGNOSIS

In addition to gout, the differential diagnosis of inflammatory monoarthritis includes the following:

- Cellulitis—Joint motion is not painful; synovial culture is negative (see Chapter 126, Cellulitis).
- Septic arthritis—Fever; painful motion; synovial fluid has many white blood cells and a positive culture.
- Rheumatic arthritis—Symmetric joint involvement (usually hands); slow onset; synovial culture is negative (see Chapter 99, Rheumatoid Arthritis).
- Pseudogout—Findings like gout; synovial fluid with short rods; crystal refraction blue on red background (calcium pyrophosphate dihydrate).

MANAGEMENT

ACUTE GOUT

- Mild to moderate attack: select one of the following:
  - NSAID or COX-2 at anti-inflammatory doses[4,5] SOR Ⓐ
  - 5- to 10-day course of oral glucocorticoids (e.g., prednisone) followed by a taper.[4,5] SOR Ⓐ
  - Colchicine 1.2 mg followed by 0.6 mg, start within 36 hours of symptom onset.[4,5] SOR Ⓐ
  - In monoarticular gout, consider an intraarticular injection with long-acting steroid (e.g., triamcinolone acetonide, 10 to 40 mg, depending on the size of the joint).[4,5] SOR Ⓒ
- Severe: consider combination therapy with anti-inflammatory agent and colchicine.[4,5]

CHRONIC GOUT

The treatment of chronic gout includes modifications in diet and existing medications (if possible) and lowering urate levels.

Treatment measures include[6]:

- Nonpharmacologic:
  - Encourage a healthy lifestyle: weight loss for obese patients, regular exercise, cessation of smoking, and adequate hydration. SOR Ⓒ
  - Reduce the intake of purine-rich foods (e.g., organ meats, red meats, and seafood). SOR Ⓑ
  - Avoid foods and beverages sweetened with high-fructose corn syrup. SOR Ⓒ
  - Limit alcohol intake to 2 drinks per day for men and 1 drink per day for women. SOR Ⓒ
  - Increase low- or non-fat dairy products, as these may be protective against gout. SOR Ⓒ
- Medications:
  - Re-evaluate the benefits of low-dose aspirin for cardioprotection, as low-dose aspirin raises the risk of recurrent gouty episodes. Consider using antihypertensive medications other than a thiazide diuretic.
  - Lower urate levels to <6 mg/dL (or <5 mg/dL if needed for symptom control) in patients with two or more attacks in a year, ≥stage 2 kidney disease, tophi, or history of urolithiasis.[6]
    - Xanthine oxidase inhibitors, allopurinol 100 mg/day (adjust for renal disease) titrated every 2 to 5 weeks up to 800 mg/day (for doses above 300 mg/day divide bid-qid); give with food
    - Uricosuric agents (e.g., probenecid) if unable to take xanthine oxidase inhibitor
    - Combination xanthine oxidase inhibitor and uricosuric agent if needed to reach target
    - Or uricase agents (e.g., pegloticase) for severe gout when other agents fail or are contraindicated
  - Use prophylactic treatment with low-dose colchicine or NSAIDs to prevent flares during initiation of urate-lowering therapy. Continue for a minimum of 6 months and longer if needed to reach target urate level. Then continue prophylactic treatment for another 3 months at target urate levels if no tophi and 6 months at target urate level if tophi present.[6]

- Complementary and alternative therapy:
  - A number of Chinese and Vietnamese medicinal plants and herbs have xanthine oxidase inhibitory activity, but few have been tested for clinical effectiveness.

PREVENTION

- Intake of dairy products, folate, and coffee lowers risk of gout.[2]
- In a patient with a prior episode of gout, avoid medications that cause hyperuricemia—thiazide diuretics, cyclosporine, aspirin (<1 g/day).

PROGNOSIS

- Recurrent attacks are common, with 19% of patients experiencing a recurrence in year 1 and 32% within 5 years.[7]

FOLLOW-UP

- Follow patients with an acute flare through resolution and initiation of prophylactic therapy if indicated.

PATIENT EDUCATION

Advise patients to lose weight, minimize alcohol use, eat less meat and seafood, and obtain more protein from dairy.[6]

PATIENT RESOURCES

- The Arthritis Foundation. *Gout*—**http://www.arthritis.org/about-arthritis/types/gout/.**
- MedlinePlus. *Gout*—**https://medlineplus.gov/gout.html.**
- The American College of Rheumatology. *Gout*—**https://www.rheumatology.org/I-Am-A/Patient-Caregiver/Diseases-Conditions/Gout.**

PROVIDER RESOURCES

- MD+Calc. *Gout Diagnosis Calculator*—**https://www.mdcalc.com/acr-eular-gout-classification-criteria.**

REFERENCES

1. Roddy E, Choi HK. Epidemiology of gout. *Rheum Dis Clin North Am.* 2014;40(2):155-175.
2. MacFarlane LA, Kim SC. Gout: a review of nonmodifiable and modifiable risk factors. *Rheum Dis Clin North Am.* 2014;40(4):581-604.
3. Neogi T, Jansen TL, Dalbeth N, et al. 2015 Gout classification criteria: an American College of Rheumatology/European League Against Rheumatism collaborative initiative. *Ann Rheum Dis.* 2015;74(10):1789-1798.
4. Khanna D, Fitzgerald JD, Khanna PP, et al. 2012 American College of Rheumatology guidelines for management of gout. Part 2: therapy and antiinflammatory prophylaxis of acute gouty arthritis. *Arthritis Care Res (Hoboken).* 2012;64(10):1447-1461.
5. Khanna PP, Gladue HS, Singh MK, et al. Treatment of acute gout: a systematic review. *Semin Arthritis Rheum.* 2014;44(1):31-38.
6. Khanna D, Fitzgerald JD, Khanna PP, et al. 2012 American College of Rheumatology guidelines for management of gout. Part 1: systematic nonpharmacologic and pharmacologic therapeutic approaches to hyperuricemia. *Arthritis Care Res (Hoboken).* 2012;64(10):1431-1446.
7. Trifirò G, Morabito P, Cavagna L, et al. Epidemiology of gout and hyperuricaemia in Italy during the years 2005-2009: a nationwide population-based study. *Ann Rheum Dis.* 2013;72(5):694-700.

103 OLECRANON BURSITIS

Emily Krodel, MD
Christopher G. Mazoue, MD

PATIENT STORY

A 50-year-old man presents with swelling in his posterior right elbow for the last 2 months. He does not have pain at rest but does have discomfort when he rests his elbows on his desk at work. He denies any trauma or fevers. **Figure 103-1** demonstrates a 5-cm fluctuant "goose egg" swelling over the olecranon process that is not warm and is mildly tender to palpation. He has full range of motion of 0–150 degrees. His olecranon bursitis was treated with ice, compression, nonsteroidal anti-inflammatory drugs (NSAIDs), and activity modification to avoid leaning on his elbow.

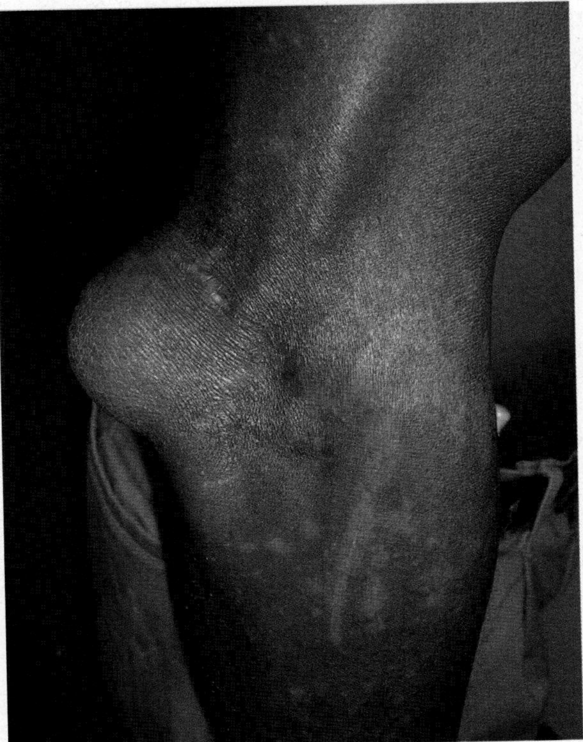

FIGURE 103-1 Chronic aseptic olecranon bursitis in a 60-year-old man showing typical swelling over the olecranon. There is no erythema or tenderness. (*Reproduced with permission from Richard P. Usatine, MD.*)

INTRODUCTION

An olecranon bursa is a subcutaneous synovial pouch which functions to reduce friction between the olecranon process and its overlying skin. Historically, enlargement of a bursa has been termed "bursitis," although a true inflammatory process doesn't always exist.[1] Olecranon bursitis can be broadly classified as acute or chronic and aseptic or septic. Differences in clinical presentation help distinguish aseptic from septic olecranon bursitis; however, analysis of fluid may be necessary. Aseptic olecranon bursitis is commonly treated with an elbow pad, NSAIDs, and ice. Septic olecranon bursitis may be treated with antibiotics only or may require surgical drainage in addition to antibiotics.

SYNONYMS

Popeye elbow, student's elbow, baker's elbow.

EPIDEMIOLOGY

The actual incidence of olecranon bursitis is unknown and difficult to quantify, but aseptic bursitis is estimated to be 3–4 times more common than septic bursitis.[2]

- Peak age of onset is 30 to 60 years.[3]
- Male predominance.
- 33%–77% have antecedent trauma.[2]

ETIOLOGY AND PATHOPHYSIOLOGY

Inflammation or degeneration of the bursal sac overlying the olecranon process from:

- Repetitive motion or microtrauma to the elbow.

- Systemic diseases such as gout, pseudogout, diabetes, alcoholism, and rheumatoid arthritis, either directly due to the comorbidity or secondary to immunosuppression from treating it.[2]
- Infection, typically by *Staphylococcus aureus* or another Gram-positive organism.

RISK FACTORS

- Acute bursitis—Direct trauma or prolonged pressure on bursa.
- Chronic bursitis—Multiple acute episodes, occupational activities, systemic disorders.
- Septic bursitis—Immunocompromised state, direct inoculation from nearby skin wound, cellulitis, or iatrogenic from an aspiration attempt.

DIAGNOSIS

The diagnosis of olecranon bursitis is made clinically by its typical appearance (**Figures 103-1** and **103-2**). When necessary, joint aspiration verifies the diagnosis and separates septic from aseptic bursitis.

CLINICAL FEATURES OF SEPTIC BURSITIS[2]

- Tenderness (88%).
- Erythema/cellulitis (83%).
- Warmth (84%).
- History of trauma or skin lesion (50%).
- Fever with temperature ≥37.8°C or 100. 4°F (38%).

CLINICAL FEATURES OF ASEPTIC BURSITIS

- Tenderness (36%).
- Erythema/cellulitis (27%).
- Warmth (56%).
- History of trauma or skin lesion (25%).
- Fever (0%).

LABORATORY TESTING

- The gold standard for septic bursitis is a positive bursal fluid culture.
- No single lab test is sensitive or specific enough to distinguish between septic and aseptic bursitis, but combining several laboratory tests with a good history and physical can be helpful.
- Bursal fluid tests: microbiologic culture, Gram stain, leukocyte (WBC) count with differential crystal analysis, glucose.[2]
    - Average WBC count is 63,000 in septic bursitis and 2000 in aseptic bursitis. However, there is very wide variation, and levels may be elevated in certain systemic conditions.
    - Neutrophil predominance >50% in septic bursitis; monocytes >50% in aseptic bursitis.
    - Glucose <50% of serum glucose in septic bursitis; >70% of serum glucose in aseptic bursitis.
    - Gram-positive organisms on gram stain in septic bursitis.

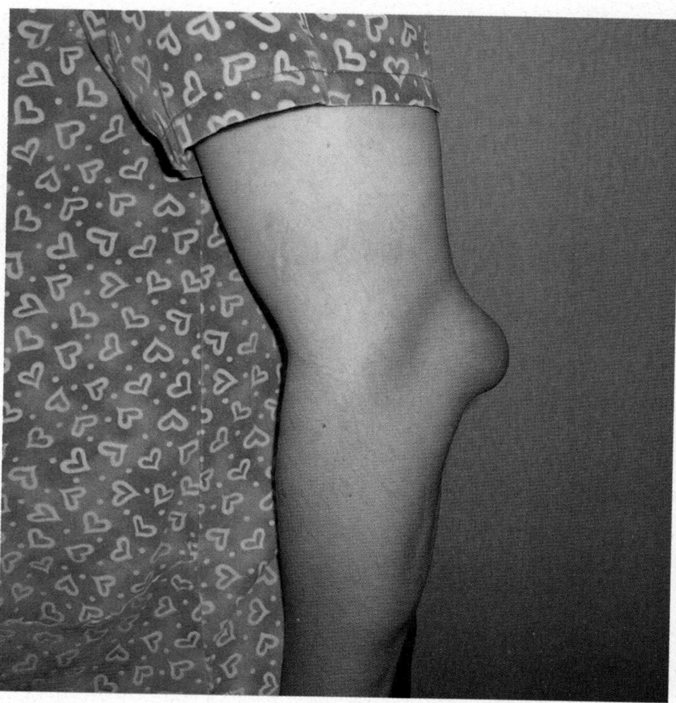

FIGURE 103-2 Aseptic olecranon bursitis secondary to repetitive elbow leaning in this computer programmer. There is some erythema and minimal tenderness. The aspirated fluid was clear. Most patients (70%) retain full extension in the elbow despite swelling over the olecranon. (*Reproduced with permission from Richard P. Usatine, MD.*)

- Peripheral blood tests: complete blood count with differential, glucose, erythrocyte sedimentation rate, and C-reactive protein.

IMAGING

- Usually not indicated.
- Bedside ultrasound may show a bursal fluid collection and features of synovial proliferation.
- In traumatic bursitis, radiographs may identify a foreign body or fracture.
- In atypical cases, MRI may be needed to determine the extent of soft-tissue involvement.

ASPIRATION

- Aspirate the lesion when there is suspicion of infection or crystal disease or for discomfort caused by extensive swelling, keeping in mind that aspiration could increase risk of infection or fistula formation.

When indicated, aspirate fluid as follows[4]:

- Place the patient supine with elbow flexed to 45 degrees.
- Mark the area of maximal fluctuance for skin entry.
- Using sterile technique, insert needle in the direction of the medial epicondyle. Consider using a 20- to 22-gauge needle. If an 18-gauge needle is used, administer a local anesthetic prior to aspirating. Also consider slightly displacing the overlying skin prior to needle entry to decrease risk of fistula formation.
- Aspirate fluid and send for bursal fluid tests mentioned above.
- Consider injecting steroid (see below) only if clear aspirate and not concerned for infection.
- Apply pressure dressing.

DIFFERENTIAL DIAGNOSIS

- Gout, pseudogout, or rheumatoid arthritis, especially if there is a prior history (see Chapter 102, Gout).
- Septic joint can occur simultaneously with bursitis; usually with decreased range of motion.
- Hemorrhage into the bursa (with history of trauma, bruising).

MANAGEMENT

ASEPTIC BURSITIS

- Elbow pad, compression, activity modification (no leaning on elbows).
- Ice, rest, NSAIDs as tolerated.
- Small-volume corticosteroid injection has been found to decrease symptom duration. Consider this in cases of severe pain or recurrent fluid accumulation. SOR C Because aspiration and steroid injection increase the risk of converting an aseptic olecranon bursitis to a septic one, the treatment options noted above should be exhausted prior to consideration of steroid injection.[2]
- Consider surgical referral for recalcitrant fluid accumulation.
- Open olecranon bursectomy is notoriously associated with wound healing problems. Arthroscopic bursectomy may decrease this risk and also allows for olecranon spur removal if indicated.[2]

SEPTIC BURSITIS

- Cornerstones of treatment have traditionally been drainage and initiating effective antibiotics. However, length of antibiotic treatment and route of administration are debated.
- Aspirate bursal fluid and send for culture and other studies prior to starting antibiotics.
- In mild to moderate cases (local inflammation, slightly elevated WBC count), treat empirically with oral antibiotics until culture results are available. First-generation cephalosporins and penicillinase-resistant penicillin are the first-line agents for *Staphylococcus* and *Streptococcus* species. In patients who are allergic to these antibiotics, clindamycin or trimethoprim/sulfamethoxazole can be used.[1] SOR C
- In severe cases (extensive local infection, systemic symptoms, significantly elevated WBC count), immunosuppressed patients, those not responding to oral treatment, or high suspicion of methicillin-resistant *S. aureus*, consider hospitalization and intravenous vancomycin.[1] SOR C
- Aspirate after several days of treatment, and continue antibiotics for 5 days after fluid is sterile. The average length of antibiotic treatment with this strategy is close to 10 days.[2] SOR C
- Refer to an orthopedic specialist if surgical debridement or bursectomy is needed. SOR C

PROGNOSIS

- Aseptic olecranon bursitis often resolves with conservative therapy, and many acute lesions subside spontaneously.
- Significantly immunocompromised patients have been found to require 3 times as long to achieve bursal fluid sterility as their immunocompetent counterparts.[2]
- Septic bursitis can lead to chronic bursal infection, osteomyelitis, and cutaneous fistula formation if not treated adequately.[2]

FOLLOW-UP

If managing septic bursitis as an outpatient, reevaluate on a daily basis after starting oral antibiotics.[1] Re-aspirate after several days of treatment. Once the fluid is sterile, continue antibiotics for an additional 5 days.

PATIENT EDUCATION

Prevention of recurrent olecranon bursitis is the best treatment. Limit bursa aggravation by not leaning on elbows or pushing off on elbows when arising. If the triggering activity cannot be avoided, a padded orthosis may be worn over the elbow. It is important that this does not significantly interfere with range of motion, as this can lead to contractures.[2]

PATIENT RESOURCES

- **http://orthoinfo.aaos.org/PDFs/A00028.pdf.**

PROVIDER RESOURCES

- Includes description of aspiration technique—**http://www.aafp.org/afp/2002/1201/p2097.html.**

REFERENCES

1. Khodaee M. Common superficial bursitis. *Am Fam Physician.* 2017;95(4):224-231.
2. Reilly D, Kamineni S. Olecranon bursitis. *J Shoulder Elbow Surg.* 2016;25:158-167.
3. Shikino K, Katsuyama Y, Ohira Y, Ikusaka M. Acute onset of elbow swelling. *Am Fam Physician.* 2016;94(3):243-244.
4. Cardone DA, Tallia AF. Diagnostic and therapeutic injection of the elbow region. *Am Fam Physician.* 2002;66(11):2097-2100.

104 CLAVICULAR FRACTURE

Tenley E. Murphy, MD
Jeffrey Guy, MD
Heidi S. Chumley, MD, MBA

PATIENT STORY

A 17-year-old girl presents after falling and landing directly on her lateral shoulder. She had immediate pain and swelling in the middle of her clavicle. Her examination revealed a painful bump in the middle of her clavicle. A radiograph confirmed a midshaft clavicle fracture (**Figure 104-1**). She was treated conservatively with a sling. The bump on her clavicle is still palpable at 6 weeks, but X-ray reveals a healing callus (**Figure 104-2**).

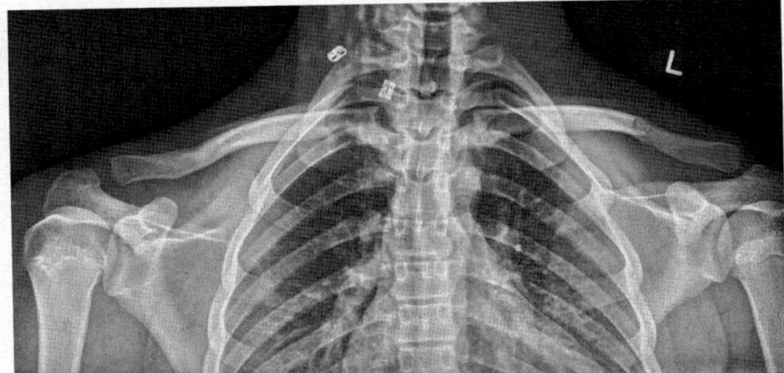

FIGURE 104-1 Midshaft clavicle fracture. Clavicle fractures are designated midshaft (in the middle third), distal (distal third), or medial (medial third). (*Reproduced with permission from E.J. Mayeaux, Jr., MD.*)

INTRODUCTION

Clavicular fractures are common in both children and adults and are most commonly caused by accidental trauma. The clavicle most commonly fractures in the midshaft (**Figures 104-1** to **104-3**), but can also fracture distally (**Figure 104-4**). Many fractures can be treated conservatively. Patients with significant displacement should be referred for surgical evaluation.

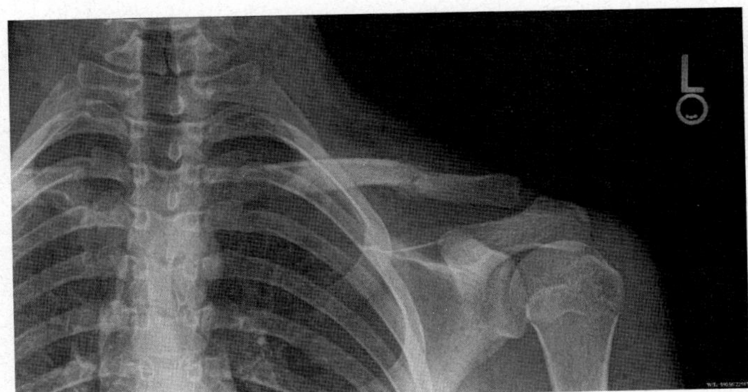

FIGURE 104-2 This is the same patient as in **Figure 104-1** after 6 weeks of conservative therapy. Note the bone callus forming over the break as she heals. (*Reproduced with permission from E.J. Mayeaux, Jr., MD.*)

EPIDEMIOLOGY

- Clavicular fractures account for 2.6% to 4% of all fractures in adults, with an overall incidence of 64 per 100,000 people per year. Midshaft fractures account for approximately 69% to 81% of all clavicle fractures, of which half are displaced.[1,2]
- Accounts for 10% to 15% of fractures in children; 90% are midshaft fractures.[3]

ETIOLOGY AND PATHOPHYSIOLOGY

- Most are caused by trauma from fall against the lateral shoulder or an outstretched hand or direct blow to the clavicle; however, stress fractures in gymnasts and divers have been reported.
- Pathologic fractures (uncommon) can result from bone tumors or radiation.
- Birth trauma (neonatal).
- Physical assaults and child abuse can cause clavicular fractures.

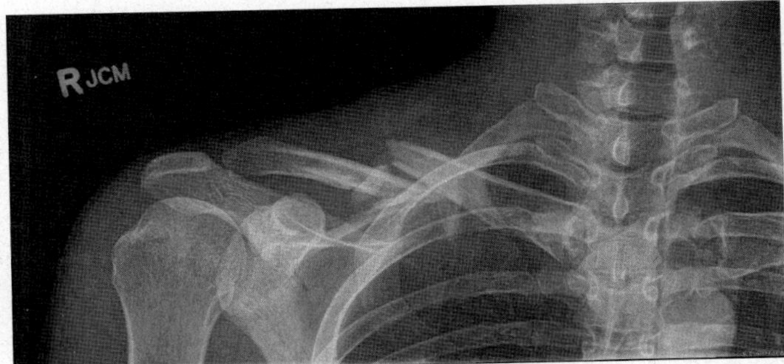

FIGURE 104-3 Midshaft clavicular fracture with proximal fragment displaced superiorly from the pull of the sternocleidomastoid muscle. (*Reproduced with permission from E.J. Mayeaux, Jr., MD.*)

DIAGNOSIS

CLINICAL FEATURES

- History of trauma with a mechanism known to result in clavicle fractures (i.e., fall on an outstretched hand or lateral shoulder, or direct blow).

TABLE 104-1 Typical Distribution/Classification

Group (Approx. %)	Fracture Location	Radiographic Appearance
Group I (80%)	Middle third	Upward displacement (**Figures 102-1 and 102-3**)
Group II (15%)	Distal third	Medial side of fragment is displaced upward (**Figure 102-4**)
Type I		Minimal displacement
Type II		Fracture medial to coracoclavicular ligaments; some overlapping of fragments
Type III		Fracture at the articular surface of the acromioclavicular (AC) joint; can look like AC separation
Group III (5%)	Medial third	Medial side of fragment up; distal side down

- Pain and swelling at the fracture site.
- Crepitus on palpation.
- Gross deformity at site of fracture.

TYPICAL DISTRIBUTION

- For the typical distribution and classification of clavicular fractures, see **Table 104-1**.

IMAGING

- Obtain plain films of the clavicle for radiographic evidence of fracture, including serendipity view. Films should be obtained upright, as over three times more patients meet operative indications when placed in the upright versus supine position.[4]

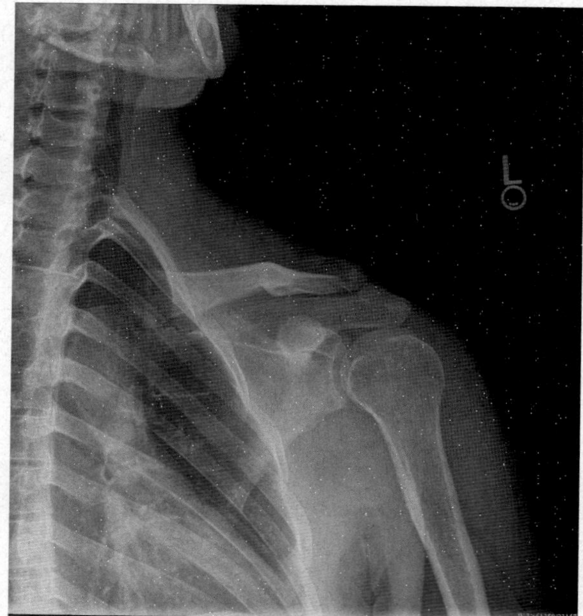

FIGURE 104-4 Distal clavicular fracture. (*Reproduced with permission from E.J. Mayeaux, Jr., MD.*)

DIFFERENTIAL DIAGNOSIS

- Acromioclavicular (AC) separation (**Figure 104-5**)—Fall directly on the "point" of the shoulder or a direct blow, pain with overhead movement, tenderness at the AC joint, and AC joint separation on radiographs.
- Sternoclavicular dislocation—Fall on the shoulder, chest and shoulder pain exacerbated by arm movement or when lying down, and a prominence from the superomedial displacement of the clavicle (uncommon).
- Pseudoarthrosis of the clavicle—Painless mass in the middle of the clavicle from failure of the central part of the clavicle to ossify (extremely rare).

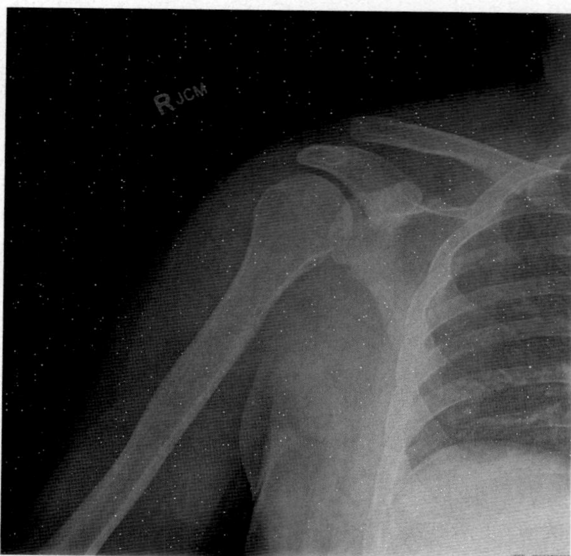

FIGURE 104-5 Acromioclavicular joint separation (third degree) with a wide AC joint and the clavicle displaced from the acromion. (*Reproduced with permission from E.J. Mayeaux, Jr., MD.*)

MANAGEMENT

For all adults and children:

- Assess neurovascular status of injured extremity.
- Assess for damage to lungs (pneumothorax or hemothorax).
- Determine the classification and amount of displacement by radiograph (see **Figure 104-1**; see also **Table 104-1**).

NONPHARMACOLOGIC

Most clavicular fractures can be treated nonoperatively; other options include internal fixation with plates and screws.

▶ Pediatric clavicle fracture

- Treat most children with any type of clavicle fracture conservatively, without immobilization.[3] SOR Ⓒ
- Treat children nonoperatively even with 90-degree displacement and several inches of overlap.[3] SOR Ⓒ

▶ Adult midclavicular fractures

- Treat adults with nondisplaced midshaft clavicular fractures nonoperatively. SOR Ⓑ
- Place adults in a sling instead of a figure-of-eight. Patients treated with a sling had higher treatment satisfaction than those treated with a figure-of-eight bandage.[5] SOR Ⓑ
- Midclavicular fractures are treated until radiographic evidence of healing has occurred. SOR Ⓒ
- Refer patients with initial fracture shortening over 2 cm to discuss operative and conservative options. SOR Ⓑ These patients have a higher risk of a nonunion associated with poor functional outcomes.[6]

▶ Adult distal clavicular fractures

- Treat patients with nondisplaced distal clavicle fractures conservatively.
- Distal clavicle fractures are commonly treated by wearing a sling for 6 weeks to minimize the weight of the arm pulling on the distal clavicle fragment.
- Some patients with displaced distal clavicle fracture may benefit from surgery. Refer patients, other than the very elderly, to discuss risks and benefits of operative and nonoperative options.[7]

MEDICATIONS

- Treat pain as needed with acetaminophen or nonsteroidal anti-inflammatory drugs (NSAIDs).

REFERRAL

- Refer for surgical evaluation: children with tenting of the skin, instability of shoulder girdle, displacement with skin perforation/necrosis, or risk to mediastinal structures.[3] SOR Ⓒ
- Refer patients with displaced mid-clavicular fractures for accelerated return to work or sport, decrease in malunion, and decrease in nonunion.[1] Nonoperative treatment has a 15.1% nonunion rate, whereas operative rates are 0% to 2%.[2]
- Consider consulting with a physician skilled in managing clavicular fractures in patients with a distal clavicle fracture. These fractures have a high rate of nonunion; however, only a portion of nonunions are painful or inhibit function. If the patient continues to have a symptomatic nonunion after many months, surgery may be considered.

PROGNOSIS

- Midclavicular displaced fractures treated nonoperatively have a nonunion rate of up to 15% and a poor functional outcome in up to 5%. Operative nonunion rates are 0% to 2%.[2]
- Patients with distal clavicle fractures treated nonoperatively had nonunion rates of 21%; however, there was no difference in function between those who healed and those with a nonunion.[8] SOR Ⓑ

FOLLOW-UP

- Monitor with examination and radiographs until pain has resolved, any lost function has returned, and there is radiographic evidence of healing. Initially, repeat X-ray every 1 to 2 weeks to evaluate for any change in alignment. If the fracture is stable, repeat X-ray every 4 to 6 weeks until the clavicle has healed. If there is no evidence of healing after 2 to 3 months, referral should be considered.

PATIENT EDUCATION

Most clavicle fractures heal without surgery, especially if the fracture is not displaced. Fractures in adults take 6 to 8 weeks to heal, and fractures in children take approximately 3 to 4 weeks to heal. Often, there will be a bump at the site of the healed fracture, which typically does not interfere with any activities.

PATIENT RESOURCES

- American Academy of Orthopedic Surgeons. Patient information handout under *Broken Collarbone*—**http://orthoinfo.aaos.org/topic.cfm?topic=A00072.**

PROVIDER RESOURCES

- **http://emedicine.medscape.com/article/1260953.**
- Duke University online. *Wheeless' Textbook of Orthopaedics*—**http://www.wheelessonline.com/ortho/clavicle_fractures.**

REFERENCES

1. Smeeing D, van der Ven D, Hietbrink F, et al. Surgical versus non-surgical treatment for midshaft clavicle fractures in patients aged 16 years and older. *Am J Sports Med.* 2017;45(8):1937-1945.
2. Zlowodzki M, Zelle BA, Cole PA, et al; Evidence-Based Orthopaedic Trauma Working Group. Treatment of acute midshaft clavicle fractures: systematic review of 2144 fractures: on behalf of the Evidence-Based Orthopaedic Trauma Working Group. *J Orthop Trauma.* 2005;19(7):504-507.
3. Kubiak R, Slongo T. Operative treatment of clavicle fractures in children: a review of 21 years. *J Pediatr Orthop.* 2002;22:736-739.
4. Backus JD, Merriman DJ, McAndrew CM, et al. Upright versus supine radiographs of clavicle fracture: does positioning matter? *J Orthop Trauma.* 2014;28(11):636-641.
5. Andersen K, Jensen PO, Lauritzen J. Treatment of clavicular fractures. Figure-of-eight bandage versus a simple sling. *Acta Orthop Scand.* 1987;58(1):71-74.
6. Preston CF, Egol KA. Midshaft clavicle fractures in adults. *Bull NYU Hosp Jt Dis.* 2009;67(1):52-57.
7. Khan LA, Bradnock TJ, Scott C, Robinson CM. Fractures of the clavicle. *J Bone Joint Surg Am.* 2009;91(2):447-460.
8. Robinson CM, Cairns DA. Primary nonoperative treatment of displaced lateral fractures of the clavicle. *J Bone Joint Surg Am.* 2004;86-A(4):778-782.

105 DISTAL RADIUS FRACTURE

Heidi S. Chumley, MD, MBA
Richard P. Usatine, MD

PATIENT STORY

A 65-year-old woman tripped on a rug in her home and fell on her outstretched hand with her wrist dorsiflexed (extended). She felt immediate pain in her wrist and has difficulty in moving her wrist or hand. She has been postmenopausal for 15 years and has never taken hormone replacement therapy or bisphosphonates. She presented with pain and swelling in her wrist. Her arm had a "dinner-fork" deformity. Radiographs showed a distal radius fracture with dorsal angulation on the lateral view (**Figure 105-1**).

INTRODUCTION

Distal radius fractures are common, especially in postmenopausal women. Patients present with wrist pain and a "dinner-fork" deformity. Diagnosis is confirmed by radiographs. Treatment is either operative or nonoperative, based on the degree of displacement and the age of the patient.

SYNONYMS

Colles fracture is the most common type. Other types of distal radius fractures include Smith fracture, Barton fracture, and Hutchinson fracture.

EPIDEMIOLOGY

- Bimodal distribution: more common under the age of 17, lowest between ages 18 and 39, then increasing with age.[1]
- More common in women compared to men at ages 40–64 (35 vs. 16 per 10,000), ages 65–79 (77 vs. 19 per 10,000), and over age 80 (110 vs. 31 per 10,000); less common in girls compared to boys under the age of 17 (42 vs. 64 per 10,000).[1] These differences are likely due to higher rates of osteoporosis in older women than age-matched men and higher risk-taking physical activities in boys than age-matched girls under the age of 17.

ETIOLOGY AND PATHOPHYSIOLOGY

- Classic history is a fall on an outstretched hand.
- 65% of patients older than 65 years of age who were seen with a distal radial fracture in an emergency room had osteoporosis.[2]
- Men and women over the age of 60 with distal radius fractures are more than five times as likely (85 vs. 15 per 10,000) to have a hip fracture within 1 year as age-/gender-matched controls. Most of these hip fractures occur within the first month after the radius fracture.[3] This is

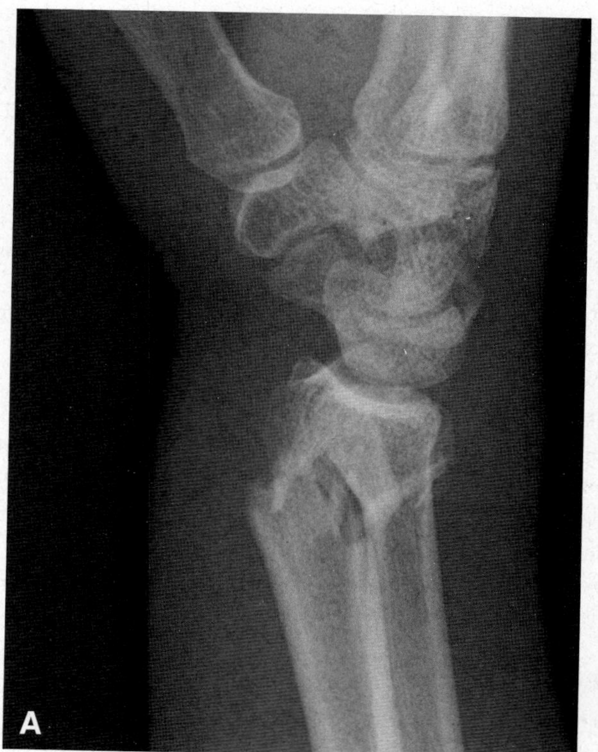

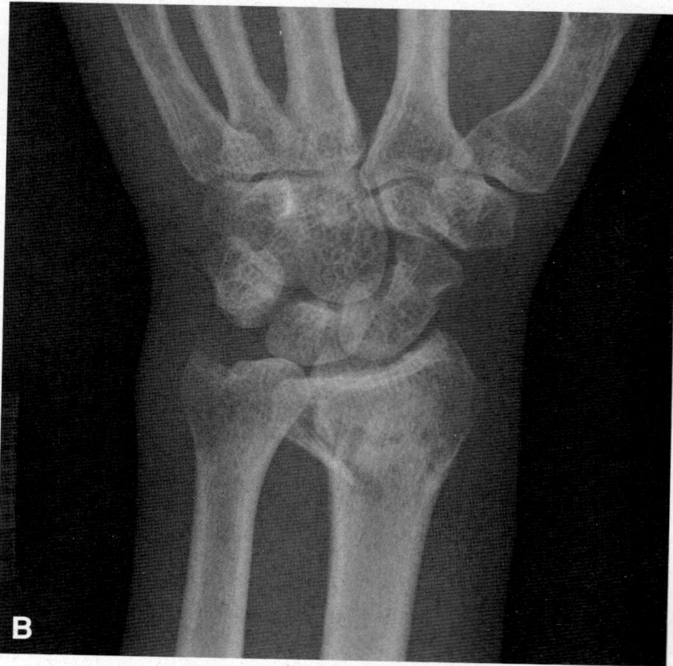

FIGURE 105-1 Colles fracture. This occurred after a fall on an extended wrist. **A.** Lateral view shows a distal radius fracture with dorsal angulation. **B.** Anterior–posterior view demonstrating a transverse distal radius fracture. (*Reproduced with permission from Rebecca Loredo-Hernandez, MD.*)

likely due to increased risk of falls and decreased bone density in the patients who have already suffered a distal radius fracture.

RISK FACTORS

- Osteoporosis.[4]
- Engaging in activities that increase the risk of falls on the wrist, such as skating, gymnastics, snowboarding, and skiing. (Many coaches and parents encourage wrist guards in an attempt to decrease the risk of wrist fractures.) Unfortunately, there are few data to support these observations.

DIAGNOSIS

Diagnosis is suspected by a compatible history, such as falling on a dorsiflexed wrist, and confirmed with a plain radiograph showing the fracture of the distal radius (see **Figure 105-1**).

CLINICAL FEATURES

Patients present with wrist pain and are not able to use the wrist or hand. The distal radius typically angles dorsally, creating the "dinner-fork" deformity (see **Figure 105-1**). Swelling is usually present.

IMAGING

Wrist radiographs (two views) confirm the fracture and demonstrate the degree of displacement and angulation.

While Colles fracture is the most common distal radius fracture, there are 3 other types that can be classified based on their radiographic appearance, history, and physical exam:

1. Smith fracture is a reverse Colles fracture in which the angulation is in the palmar direction. It usually occurs after a fall on a flexed wrist or a direct blow to the dorsal wrist. The distal radial metaphysis is displaced and angulated in the palmar direction, and an associated ulna styloid fracture may be seen (**Figure 105-2**).
2. Barton fracture is an intraarticular dorsal or volar rim fracture. It occurs with forced wrist dorsiflexion and pronation. A triangular fragment of the distal radial styloid occurs as seen in **Figure 105-3**.
3. Hutchinson fracture (chauffeur's fracture) is a fracture through the base of the radial styloid. It occurs with forced hyperextension of the wrist. There will be tenderness at the radial styloid on exam and the radiograph indicates a radial styloid fracture (**Figure 105-4**). It is also named a chauffeur's fracture from the past when a chauffeur would crank a car manually and the kickback could break the wrist in this pattern.

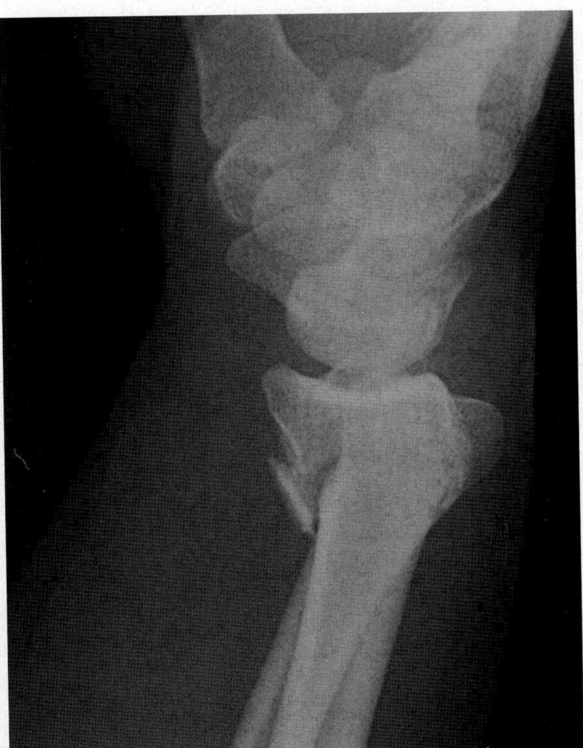

FIGURE 105-2 Smith fracture (reverse Colles fracture). Lateral view of a fracture of the distal radial metaphysis that is displaced and angulated in the palmar direction. This occurred after a fall on a flexed wrist. *(Reproduced with permission from Rebecca Loredo-Hernandez, MD.)*

DIFFERENTIAL DIAGNOSIS

Other causes of pain at the wrist include:

- Scaphoid fracture—Forced hyperextension, tenderness in anatomic snuffbox; radiograph demonstrates scaphoid fracture (70%).
- de Quervain tenosynovitis—No acute injury, pain on radial side of wrist from abductor pollicis longus and extensor pollicis brevis

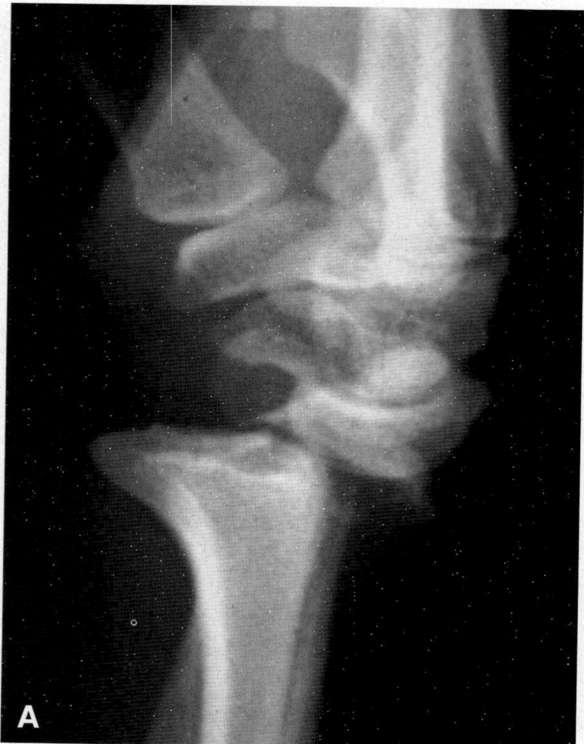

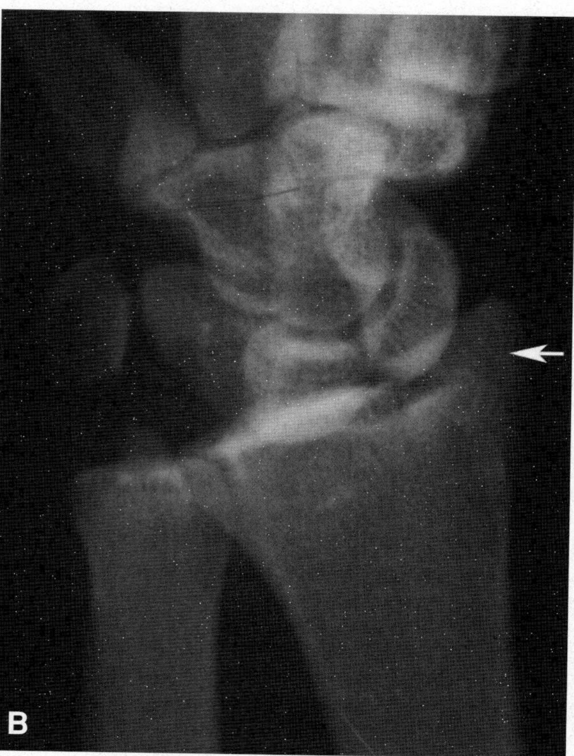

FIGURE 105-3 Barton fracture. **A.** Lateral view showing a marginal fracture of the dorsal rim of the radius that is displaced along with the carpus, producing a fracture-subluxation. **B.** AP view showing the triangular fragment of the radial styloid (*arrow*). (*Reproduced with permission from Rebecca Loredo-Hernandez, MD.*)

involvement, pain over the tendon when the thumb is placed into the patient's fist and the wrist is deviated to the ulnar side; radiographs (not usually done) are normal.

MANAGEMENT

Examine patients for the following associated complications:

- Flexor tendon injuries.
- Median and ulnar nerve injuries.

Examine radiographs for the following associated injuries:

- Ulnar styloid or neck fractures.
- Carpal fractures.
- Distal radioulnar subluxation.

Management is based on whether the fracture is nonarticular or articular, displaced or nondisplaced, reducible or irreducible (**Figure 105-5**). Although there are multiple accepted classification schemes, the Universal Classification of radial fractures, shown in **Table 105-1**, is simple, has moderate reliability and reproducibility, and provides straightforward management recommendations.[5] See **Figure 105-6** for a successful open reduction and internal fixation on a distal radial fracture. Note that this fracture was articular with displacement (see **Figure 105-5**).

- The patient's wrist in most cases is splinted for the first few days after injury to allow swelling to decrease prior to casting.

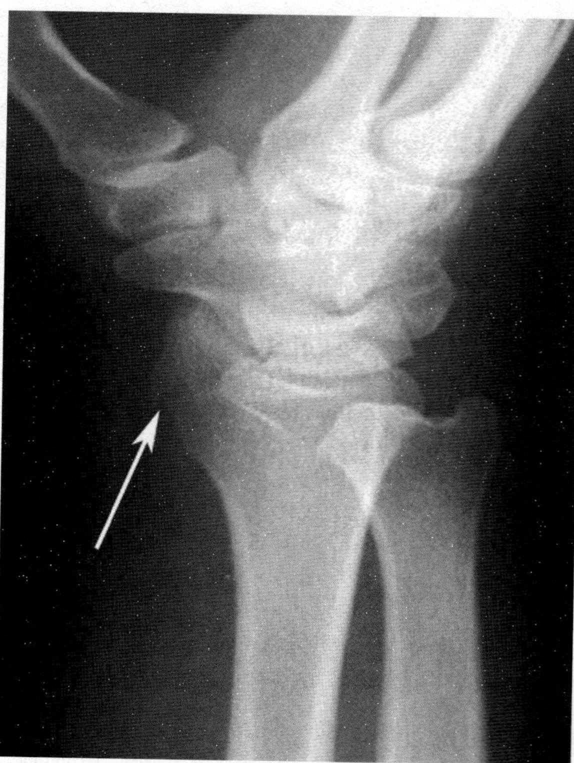

FIGURE 105-4 Hutchinson fracture or chauffeur's fracture. This oblique view demonstrates a fracture through the base of the radial styloid (*arrow*). (*Reproduced with permission from Rebecca Loredo-Hernandez, MD.*)

TABLE 105-1 Universal Classification of Radial Fracture

Fracture Classification	Management
I Nonarticular, nondisplaced	Immobilization with cast or splint[6] for 4 to 6 weeks
II Nonarticular, displaced	Reduction with cast or splint immobilization; surgical management if irreducible or unstable fracture
III Articular, nondisplaced	Immobilization; pinning if unstable
IV Articular, displaced	Surgical management (**Figures 105-5** and **105-6**)

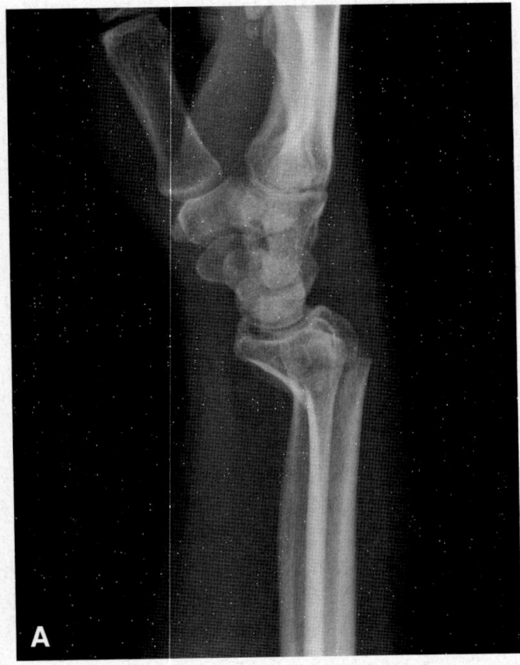

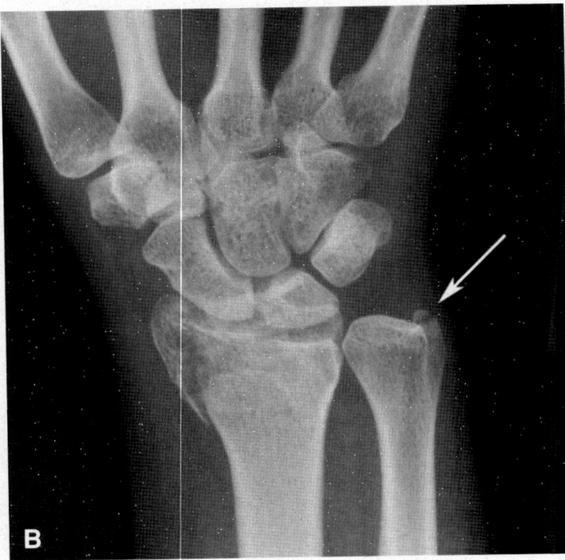

FIGURE 105-5 A 31-year-old woman fell on a flexed wrist. **A.** Lateral view shows a distal radius comminuted intraarticular fracture with palmar displacement and volar angulation occurred (Smith fracture). This Type IV fracture is best managed with surgery. **B.** PA view shows an associated ulna styloid process fracture that is mildly displaced (*arrow*). (*Reproduced with permission from Richard P. Usatine, MD.*)

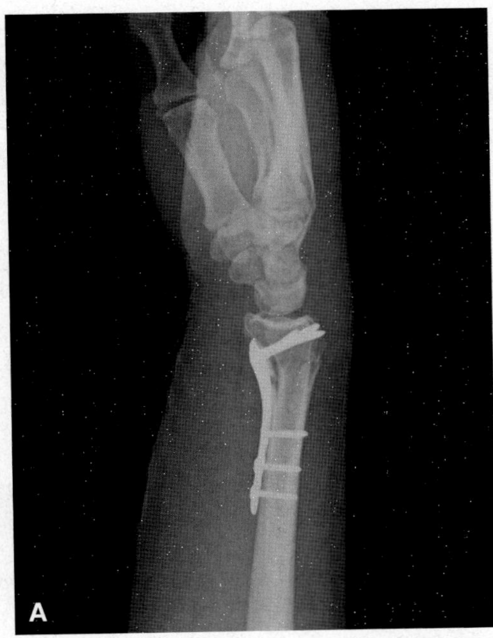

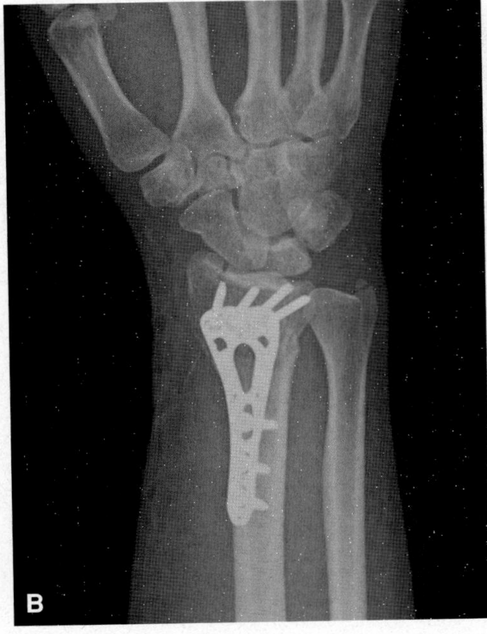

FIGURE 105-6 Open reduction and internal fixation of the distal radius fracture in **Figure 105-5**. Volar plate and screw fixation has placed the wrist in anatomic alignment for healing. **A.** Lateral view. **B.** Oblique view. (*Reproduced with permission from Richard P. Usatine, MD.*)

- On the basis of the type of fracture, the patient's wrist is typically cast from 4 to 6 weeks and followed with serial radiographs.
- The patient should be referred to a musculoskeletal or orthopedic specialist if a fracture requires reduction. Management of displaced fractures is controversial, with surgical and nonsurgical treatments demonstrating similar outcomes.
    - Surgical, compared to conservative, management reduces displacement but does not result in an improved functional outcome in adults.[6]
- All patients with a low-impact distal radius fracture are at a higher risk for osteoporosis, and clinicians should consider screening for osteoporosis.

PREVENTION

Screening for and treatment of osteoporosis may reduce fractures, including distal radial fractures.

PROGNOSIS

Most patients recover adequate function and do not have chronic pain, whether treated nonsurgically or surgically. In nonsurgically treated patients, a higher degree of displacement leads to increased risk of poor function or pain 10 years after fracture.[7]

FOLLOW-UP

- Management and follow-up often involve a physician with expertise in managing distal radial fractures.
- Evaluate for osteoporosis.

PATIENT EDUCATION

- Distal radial fractures may result in limitations of wrist function.
- Nontraumatic fractures, in patients older than 40 years of age, may indicate osteoporosis.

PATIENT RESOURCES

- WebMD has information on distal radial fractures—**https://www.webmd.com/a-to-z-guides/colles-fracture#1.**
- *Wheeless' Textbook of Orthopaedics* has additional information about the types of distal radius fractures, classification systems, and radiographic findings—**http://www.wheelessonline.com/ortho/12591.**

REFERENCES

1. Wilcke MK, Hammarberg H, Adolphson PY. Epidemiology and changed surgical treatment methods for fractures of the distal radius: a registry analysis of 42,583 patients in Stockholm County, Sweden, 2004–2010. *Acta Orthop.* 2013;84(3):292-296.
2. Jantzen C, Cieslak LK, Barzanji AF, et al. Colles' fractures and osteoporosis—a new role for the Emergency Department. *Injury.* 2016;47(4):930-933.
3. Chen CW, Huang TL, Su LT, et al. Incidence of subsequent hip fractures is significantly increased within the first month after distal radius fracture in patients older than 60 years. *J Trauma Acute Care Surg.* 2013;74(1):317-321.
4. Oyen J, Brudvik C, Gjesdal CG, et al. Osteoporosis as a risk factor for distal radial fractures: a case-control study. *J Bone Joint Surg Am.* 2011;93(4):348-356.
5. Shehovych A, Salar O, Meyer C, Ford DJ. Adult distal radius fractures classification systems: essential clinical knowledge or abstract memory testing? *Ann R Coll Surg Engl.* 2016;98(8):525-531.
6. Song J, Yu AX, Li ZH. Comparison of conservative and operative treatment for distal radius fracture: a meta-analysis of randomized controlled trials. *Int J Clin Exp Med.* 2015;8(10):17023-17035.
7. Foldhazy Z, Törnkvist H, Elmstedt E, et al. Long-term outcome of nonsurgically treated distal radial fractures. *J Hand Surg Am.* 2007;32(9):1374-1384.

106 METATARSAL FRACTURE

Heidi S. Chumley, MD, MBA

PATIENT STORY

A 37-year-old man inverted his ankle while playing basketball with his teenagers in their driveway. He felt a pop and had immediate pain. He had tenderness over the base of his fifth metatarsal. Having met the Ottawa ankle rules for radiographs (see later), a radiograph was obtained, which revealed a nondisplaced fracture at the base of the fifth metatarsal (**Figure 106-1**).

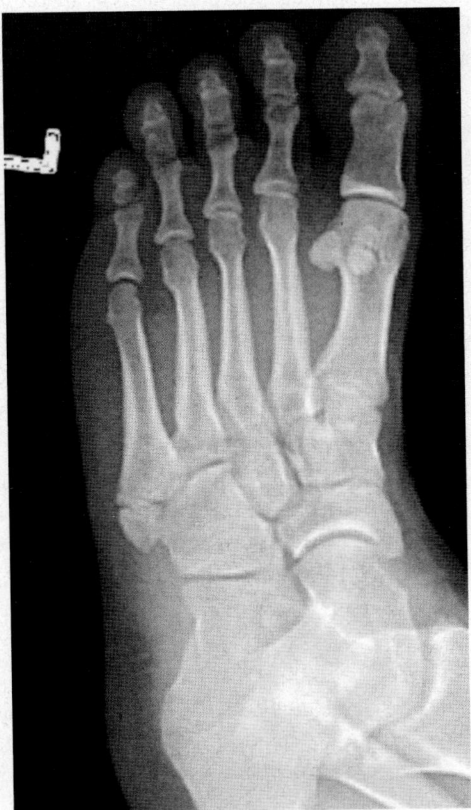

FIGURE 106-1 Fifth metatarsal tuberosity avulsion fracture (dancer fracture). *(Reproduced with permission from Simon RR, Sherman SC, Koenigsknecht SJ. Emergency Orthopedics, 5th ed. New York, NY: McGraw-Hill Education; 2007.)*

INTRODUCTION

Most metatarsal fractures involve the fifth metatarsal and include avulsion fractures at the base, acute diaphyseal fractures (Jones fracture), and diaphyseal stress fractures. Fractures of the first through fourth metatarsals are less common but can be associated with a Lisfranc injury. Diagnosis is based on the mechanism of injury or type of overuse activity and radiographic appearance. Treatment depends on the type of fracture. Most metatarsal fractures have a good prognosis; however, Jones fractures have a high rate of nonunion, and Lisfranc injuries can result in chronic symptoms.

SYNONYMS

Avulsion fracture at base of fifth metatarsal: fifth metatarsal tuberosity fracture, dancer fracture, pseudo-Jones fracture.

Jones fracture: acute diaphyseal fracture of the fifth metatarsal.

EPIDEMIOLOGY

- Foot fractures are common injuries among recreational and serious athletes; however, incidence and prevalence in most populations is unknown.
- In women older than age 70 years, the incidence of foot fractures is 3.1 per 1000 woman-years, and more than 50% of these are fifth metatarsal fractures.[1]
- Fifty percent of metatarsal fractures in adults ages 16 to 75 years involve the fifth metatarsal.[2]
- The majority of fifth metatarsal fractures are avulsion injuries (see **Figure 106-1**).
- Twenty-three percent of elite military personnel sustain metatarsal stress fractures; most of these occur after 6 months of training.[3]

ETIOLOGY AND PATHOPHYSIOLOGY

- Avulsion fractures result when the peroneus brevis tendon and the lateral plantar fascia pull off the base of the fifth metatarsal, typically during an inversion injury while the foot is in plantar flexion.

- Jones (acute diaphyseal) fracture results from landing on the outside of the foot with the foot plantar flexed.
- Diaphyseal stress fractures are caused by chronic stress from activities such as jumping and marching.
- Fractures of the first through fourth metatarsals are caused by direct blows or falling forward over a plantar-flexed foot. These fractures may be associated with a Lisfranc injury.

DIAGNOSIS

The diagnosis of avulsion or Jones fractures is made on plain radiographs in a patient with a history of injury and acute lateral foot pain. Diaphyseal stress fractures may require CT imaging.

CLINICAL FEATURES

- Avulsion injury—Sudden onset of pain (and tenderness on examination) at the base of the fifth metatarsal after forced inversion with the foot and ankle in plantar flexion.
- Acute Jones fracture—Sudden pain at the base of the fifth metatarsal, with difficulty bearing weight on the foot, after a laterally directed force on the forefoot during plantar flexion of the ankle.
- Stress fracture—History of chronic foot pain with repetitive motion.

IMAGING

- Avulsion fracture—Fracture line at base of fifth metatarsal oriented perpendicularly to the metatarsal shaft (**Figure 106-1**). May extend into joint with cuboid bone, but does not extend into the intermetatarsal joint.
- Acute Jones fractures (**Figure 106-2**) and stress fractures both have a fracture line through the proximal 1.5 cm of the fifth metatarsal shaft. These should be classified into type I, II, or III as below[4]:
  - Type I fractures have a sharp, narrow fracture line, no intramedullary sclerosis, and minimal cortical hypertrophy.
  - Type II fractures (delayed unions) have a widened fracture line with radiolucency, involve both cortices, and have intramedullary sclerosis.
  - Type III fractures (nonunions) have a wide fracture line, periosteal new bone and radiolucency, and obliteration of the medullary canal by sclerotic bone.
- Early stress fractures may have normal radiographs and can be seen on CT, MRI, or bone scan. Ultrasound may be a less expensive option—sensitivity 83%, specificity 76%, positive predictive value 59% and negative predictive value 92% in one small study.[5]

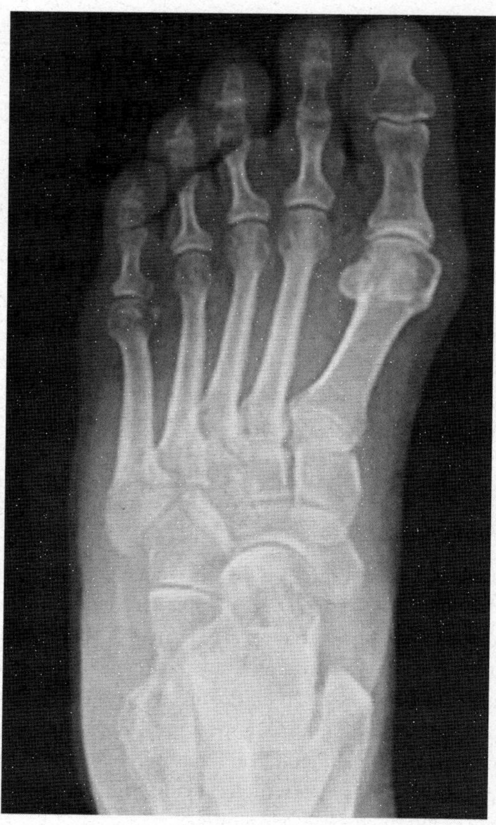

FIGURE 106-2 Jones fracture, a transverse fracture at the junction of the diaphysis and metaphysis. (*Reproduced with permission from Simon RR, Sherman SC, Koenigsknecht SJ. Emergency Orthopedics, 5th ed. New York, NY: McGraw-Hill Education; 2007.*)

DIFFERENTIAL DIAGNOSIS

Pain at the fifth metatarsal can also be caused by:

- Diaphyseal stress fracture—May be radiographically similar to Jones fracture but is often seen more distally in the shaft; occurs in patients with no injury and history of overuse (e.g., ballet dancing, marching).

- Lisfranc injury—Disruption of the tarsal metatarsal joints. This pain is typically in the midfoot and more commonly medial. May be associated with fractures in the first through fourth metatarsals.

X-ray findings that can be confused with foot fractures include:

- Apophysis, a secondary center of ossification at the proximal end of the fifth metatarsal seen in girls, ages 9 to 11 years, and boys, ages 11 to 14 years. The apophysis is oblique to the metatarsal shaft, whereas avulsion fractures are perpendicular.
- Accessory ossicles (i.e., os peroneum, located at the lateral border of the cuboid) have smooth edges, whereas avulsion fractures have rough edges.

MANAGEMENT

- Apply the Ottawa ankle rules to determine which patients with an injury and ankle/foot pain do not need an X-ray (sensitivity 99.4%, specificity 35.3%).[6] SOR Ⓐ
  - Obtain ankle radiographs: pain in the malleolar zone and localized tenderness over the lateral malleolus, tenderness over the medial malleolus or inability to walk four steps immediately after the injury and in the emergency room
  - Obtain foot radiographs: pain in the midfoot and bone tenderness at the base of the 5th metatarsal, bone tenderness at the navicular, or inability to walk four steps both immediately after the injury and in the emergency room.[7]
- Treat nondisplaced avulsion fractures with an ankle splint or walking boot with ambulation for 3 to 6 weeks.[8] SOR Ⓑ
- Refer displaced avulsion fractures.[8]
- Consider referring Jones fractures because of the high rate of nonunion caused by the poor blood supply. Type I or II may be treated with immobilization for at least 6 to 8 weeks. Type II can also be treated with surgery. Type III requires surgical repair. Elite athletes or patients needing a faster recovery are often surgically treated.[8] SOR Ⓑ
- Treat stress fractures with elimination of the causative activity for 4 to 8 weeks. Immobilization is often not required. If walking is painful, partial or non–weight bearing for 1 to 3 weeks may be necessary.[9]

Refer patients with[9]:

- Neurovascular compromise, compartment syndrome, or open fractures.
- First metatarsal fracture, multiple metatarsal fractures, displaced fracture, intraarticular fracture, or Lisfranc injury.
- Inadequate response to treatment.

PROGNOSIS

Metatarsal fractures have an excellent outcome, with most patients symptom free at 33 months. Patients with higher body mass index (BMI), diabetes mellitus, women, and a dislocation with the fracture have less-positive outcomes.[2]

FOLLOW-UP

Patients should be followed every 1 to 3 weeks to evaluate for appropriate clinical and radiographic response to treatment.

PATIENT EDUCATION

Patients with nondisplaced avulsion fractures require a splint or boot but can remain ambulatory. Jones fractures have a poor blood supply and often do not reconnect, even with immobilization. Surgery may result in a faster return to activities in some cases.

PATIENT RESOURCES

- Patient.co.uk has patient information on metatarsal fractures—**http://www.patient.co.uk/health/Metatarsal-Fractures.htm.**

PROVIDER RESOURCES

- The Ottawa ankle rules are available in several places online including—**https://www.mdcalc.com/ottawa-ankle-rule.**

REFERENCES

1. Hasselman CT, Vogt MT, Stone KL, et al. Foot and ankle fractures in elderly white women. Incidence and risk factors. *J Bone Joint Surg Am.* 2003;85-A(5):820-824.
2. Cakir H, Van Vliet-Koppert ST, Van Lieshout EM, et al. Demographics and outcome of metatarsal fractures. *Arch Orthop Trauma Surg.* 2011;131(2):241-245.
3. Finestone A, Milgrom C, Wolf O, et al. Epidemiology of metatarsal stress fractures versus tibial and femoral stress fractures during elite training. *Foot Ankle Int.* 2011;32(1):16-20.
4. Lehman RC, Torg JS, Pavlov H, Delee JC. Fractures of the base of the fifth metatarsal distal to the tuberosity: a review. *Foot Ankle.* 1987;7:245-252.
5. Banal F, Gandjbakhch F, Foltz V, et al. Sensitivity and specificity of ultrasonography in early diagnosis of metatarsal bone stress fractures: a pilot study of 37 patients. *J Rheumatol.* 2009;36(8):1715-1719.
6. Beckenkamp PR, Lin CC, Macaskill P, et al. Diagnostic accuracy of the Ottawa Ankle and Midfoot Rules: a systematic review with meta-analysis. *Br J Sports Med.* 2017;51(6):504-510.
7. Stiell I. *The Ottawa Ankle Rules.* http://www.theottawarules.ca/ankle_rules. Accessed December 2017.
8. Bowes J, Buckley R. Fifth metatarsal fractures and current treatment. *World J Orthop.* 2016;7(12):793-800.
9. Hatch RL, Alsobrook JA, Clugston JR. Diagnosis and management of metatarsal fractures. *Am Fam Physician.* 2007;76(6):817-826.

107 HIP FRACTURE

Heidi S. Chumley, MD, MBA

PATIENT STORY

A 60-year-old woman comes to the emergency room for hip pain. She felt a pop in her hip accompanied by the immediate onset of pain that prohibited her from walking. She had fallen 2 days prior. **Figure 107-1** shows a transcervical left femoral neck fracture with varus angulation and superior offset of the distal fracture fragment. She was evaluated by an orthopedic surgeon and underwent surgery the next day in a hospital that provides co-management by a geriatrician (**Figure 107-2**). After many months of rehabilitation, she was able to walk again.

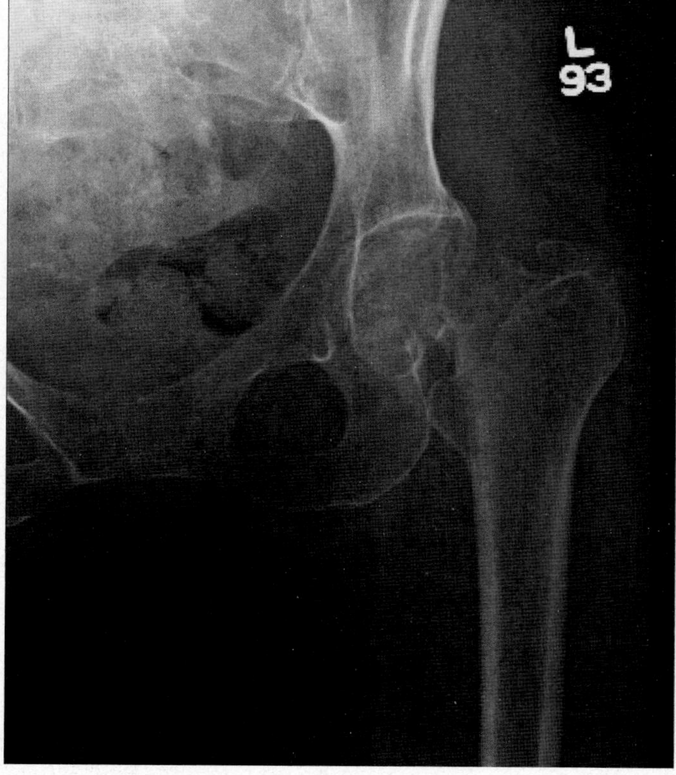

FIGURE 107-1 Transcervical left femoral neck fracture with varus angulation and superior offset of the distal fracture fragment. The femoral head is within the acetabular cup. Degenerative changes of the left hip are also present. *(Reproduced with permission from John E. Delzell, Jr., MD.)*

EPIDEMIOLOGY

- Approximately 300,000 hip fractures per year occur in the United States.[1]
- More common in the United States (554 per 100,000 women, 197 per 100,000 men) and North Europe; intermediate prevalence in Asian countries; lowest prevalence in Latin America and Africa.[2]
- 70% to 80% of hip fractures occur in women.[1]
- Average age is 77 years in women; risk increases with age.[3]
- Half of patients with a hip fracture have osteoporosis.[4]

ETIOLOGY AND PATHOPHYSIOLOGY

- In postmenopausal women, 68% to 83% of hip fractures are caused by a fall.[3]

RISK FACTORS

- Between the age of 60 and 80 years:
  - Women: lower body weight, prior osteoporotic fracture, hip fracture in first-degree relatives and lower plasma 25-hydroxyvitamin D (25OHD).[5]
  - Men: prior osteoporotic fracture and lower plasma 25OHD.[5]
- Over age 80 years, in both women and men, falls are the most important risk factor.[5]
- Short- and long-term use of a proton pump inhibitor is associated with an increased risk of fracture [RR = 1.26, 95% confidence intervals 1.16–1.36].[6]

DIAGNOSIS

CLINICAL FEATURES: HISTORY AND PHYSICAL

- History
  - Risk factors including older age, female gender
  - Recent fall

- Pain in the groin, which may be referred to the thigh or knee[7]
- Inability to walk is common; rarely patients are ambulating with an assistive device and experience increased pain with walking[7]

- Physical examination
  - Abducted and externally rotated hip; limp or refusal to walk[7]
  - Pain elicited with internal and external rotation while patient lies supine[7]
  - Groin pain elicited with an axial load[7]

TYPICAL DISTRIBUTION

- Hip fractures are classified according to anatomic location.[7]
  - Intracapsular (femoral head or femoral neck fracture; **Figures 107-1** and **107-3**).
  - Extracapsular (intertrochanteric or subtrochanteric fracture; **Figure 107-4**).

IMAGING

- Plain radiographs show most hip fractures. Order a lateral view of the hip and an anteroposterior view of the pelvis. Avoid the frogleg view because it is painful and can further displace a fracture.[7]
- Consider MRI or bone scan for indeterminate radiographs.

DIFFERENTIAL DIAGNOSIS

Hip pain can be caused by bone or joint pathology, soft-tissue injuries, or spine pathology, or it can be referred. Some causes include:

- Pelvic fractures, bone cancers, or metastases; osteoarthritis, inflammatory, crystal, or septic arthritis.
- Iliotibial band syndrome, trochanteric bursitis, iliopsoas bursitis, pyriformis syndrome, muscle strain.
- Lumbar disc herniation, lumbar spinal stenosis, sciatica.
- Hernia, abdominal or pelvic pathology.

MANAGEMENT

- Refer to an orthopedic surgeon skilled in management of hip fractures.
- In-hospital co-management by an orthopedic surgeon and a geriatrician reduces in-hospital mortality (relative risk 0.60; 95% confidence interval 0.43–0.84) and long-term mortality (relative risk 0.83; 95% confidence interval 0.74–0.94).[8]

PREVENTION

Preventing hip fracture is important; 50% of patients with a hip fracture do not regain previous level of function; 1-year mortality is 21%, which has not decreased in the last 30 years.[9]

Lower risk of hip fracture by:

- Screening for osteoporosis in women age 65 years or older and in younger women whose fracture risk is equal to or greater than that of a 65-year-old white woman.[10] SOR Ⓑ

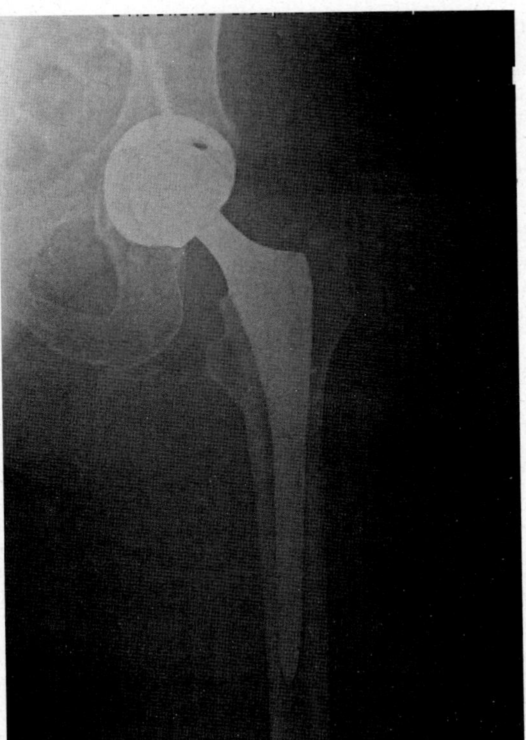

FIGURE 107-2 Postsurgical portable radiograph demonstrating good positioning of artificial hip. *(Reproduced with permission from John E. Delzell, Jr., MD.)*

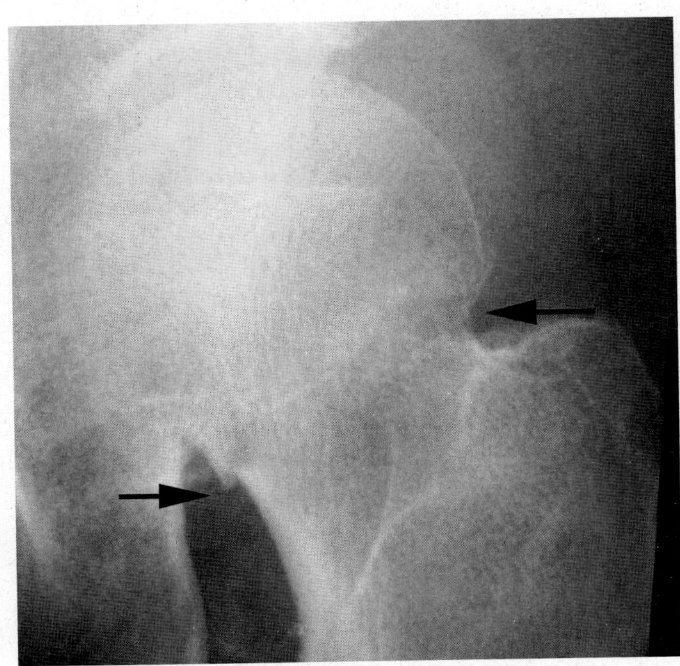

FIGURE 107-3 Nondisplaced, complete, femoral neck fracture (*black arrows*). Nondisplaced fractures can be incomplete (fracture through part of the femoral neck) or complete (fracture through the entire femoral neck). *(Reproduced with permission from Simon RR, Sherman SC, Koenigsknecht SJ. Emergency Orthopedics, 5th ed. New York, NY: McGraw-Hill Education; 2007.)*

- Treating osteoporosis with bisphosphonates. SOR Ⓐ
- Preventing falls by monitoring vision; assessing gait, strength, and balance; and minimizing the use of psychotropic medications in the elderly. SOR Ⓒ
- Encouraging exercise, such as tai chi, for lower-body strengthening and balance.
- Calcium and vitamin D supplementation slightly decreases risk of hip fracture (RR 0.84, 95% confidence interval 0.74 to 0.96) and should be part of an osteoporosis prevention and treatment strategy.[11] SOR Ⓐ
- Providing hip protectors to older residents of nursing home facilities may reduce the number of hip fractures; however, the clinical significance of the intervention is unclear.[12] SOR Ⓐ
- Use hypertensive medications (thiazide diuretics, beta-blockers, calcium channel blockers, angiotensin 2 receptor blockers, angiotensin-converting enzyme [ACE] inhibitor/thiazide combination products, and angiotensin 2 receptor blocker/thiazide combination products) associated with reduced risk of hip fracture.[13]
- Avoid loop diuretics or ACE inhibitors (single drug), which are associated with a higher risk of hip fracture.[13]
- Population interventions are effective. Kaiser Permanente decreased hip fractures by 40% by identifying patients who had not received recommended bone density screening and treating as appropriate.[14]

PROGNOSIS

- One-year mortality is 21%.[9]

FOLLOW-UP

Patients with hip fracture may benefit from multidisciplinary follow-up, including monitoring for complications such as avascular necrosis, identifying and treating osteoporosis, modifying risk factors for further falls, and maximizing function through therapy.

PATIENT EDUCATION

It is much easier to prevent hip fractures than to treat hip fractures. After a hip fracture, patients often need prolonged time (months) in a nursing care facility. Physical therapy is crucial in regaining as much function as possible.

PATIENT RESOURCES

- FamilyDoctor.org has written and auditory information in English and Spanish—**http://familydoctor.org/familydoctor/en/diseases-conditions/hip-fractures.html.**
- Mayo Health on hip fractures—**http://www.mayoclinic.com/health/hip-fracture/DS00185.**

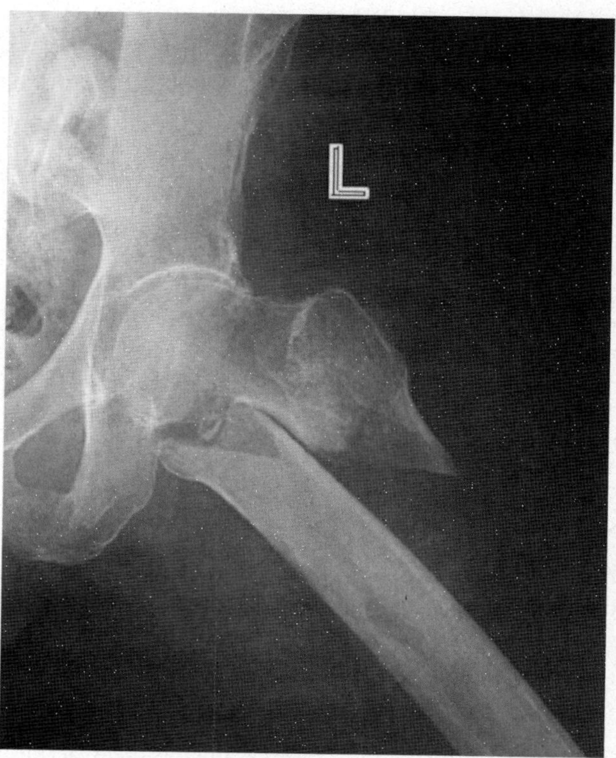

FIGURE 107-4 Unstable intertrochanteric fracture demonstrating displacement and a reverse oblique fracture line. Intertrochanteric fractures are unstable when there are multiple fracture lines, displacement between the femoral shaft and neck, or when the fracture line runs in an oblique reverse direction, with the most superior part of the fracture on the medial surface of the femur. The patient experiences severe pain, hip swelling, and shortening of the involved leg. (*Reproduced with permission from Simon RR, Sherman SC, Koenigsknecht SJ. Emergency Orthopedics, 5th ed. New York, NY: McGraw-Hill Education; 2007.*)

PROVIDER RESOURCES

- eMedicine article: Davenport M et al. *Hip Fracture in Emergency Medicine*—**http://emedicine.medscape.com/article/825363-overview.**
- FRAX, a fracture risk assessment too—**https://www.sheffield.ac.uk/FRAX/tool.jsp.**

REFERENCES

1. National Center for Health Statistics. Center for Disease Control. Department of Health and Human Services. *National Health and Nutrition Examination Survey (NHANES) 2005–2006*. http://www.cdc.gov/nchs. Accessed December 2017.
2. Dhanwal DK, Dennison EM, Harvey NC, Cooper C. Epidemiology of hip fracture: worldwide geographic variation. *Indian J Orthop*. 2011;45(1):15-22.
3. Costa AG, Wyman A, Siris ES, et al. When, where and how osteoporosis-associated fractures occur: an analysis from the Global Longitudinal Study of Osteoporosis in Women (GLOW). Harvey N, ed. *PLoS ONE*. 2013;8(12):e83306.
4. Robbins JA, Schott AM, Garnero P, et al. Risk factors for hip fracture in women with high BMD: EPIDOS study. *Osteoporos Int*. 2005;16(2):149-154.
5. Anpalahan M, Morrison SG, Gibson SJ. Hip fracture risk factors and the discriminability of hip fracture risk vary by age: a case-control study. *Geriatr Gerontol Int*. 2014;14(2):413-419.
6. Zhou B, Huang Y, Li H, Sun W, Liu J. Proton-pump inhibitors and risk of fractures: an update meta-analysis. *Osteoporos Int*. 2016;27(1):339-347.
7. LeBlanc KE, Muncie HL, LeBlanc LL. Hip fracture: diagnosis, treatment, and secondary prevention. *Am Fam Physician*. 2014;89(12):945-951.
8. Grigoryan KV, Javedan H, Rudolph JL. Ortho-geriatric care models and outcomes in hip fracture patients: a systematic review and meta-analysis. *J Orthop Trauma*. 2014;28(3):e49-55.
9. Mundi S, Pindiprolu B, Simunovic N, Bhandari M. Similar mortality rates in hip fracture patients over the past 31 years. *Acta Orthop*. 2014;85(1):54-59
10. US Preventive Services Task Force. *Osteoporosis: Screening*. https://www.uspreventiveservicestaskforce.org. Updated January 2011.
11. Avenell A, Mak JCS, O'Connell D. Vitamin D and vitamin D analogues for preventing fractures in post-menopausal women and older men. *Cochrane Database Syst. Rev*. 2014;(4): CD000227.
12. Gillespie WJ, Gillespie LD, Parker MJ. Hip protectors for preventing hip fractures in older people. *Cochrane Database Syst Rev*. 2010;(10):CD001255.
13. Ruths S, Bakken MS, Ranhoff AH, et al. Risk of hip fracture among older people using antihypertensive drugs: a nationwide cohort study. *BMC Geriatr*. 2015;15:153.
14. Dell R. Fracture prevention in Kaiser Permanente Southern California. *Osteoporos Int*. 2011;22(Suppl 3):457-460.

108 KNEE INJURY

Shaun Spielman, MD
Heidi S. Chumley, MD, MBA

PATIENT STORY

A 33-year-old woman felt a pop in her knee while skiing around a tree. She felt immediate pain and had difficulty walking when paramedics removed her from the slopes. Within a couple of hours, her knee was swollen. On examination the next day, she was able to walk 4 steps with pain. She had a moderate effusion without gross deformity and full range of motion. She had no tenderness at the joint line, the head of the fibula, over the patella, or over the medial or lateral collateral ligaments. She had a positive Lachman test, a negative McMurray test, and no increased laxity with valgus or varus stress. The physician suspected an anterior cruciate ligament (ACL) tear, placed her in a long-leg range-of-motion brace, and advised her to use crutches until an evaluation by her physician within the next several days. She was treated with acetaminophen for pain and advised to rest, apply ice, and keep her leg elevated. Later, an MRI confirmed an ACL tear (**Figure 108-1**).

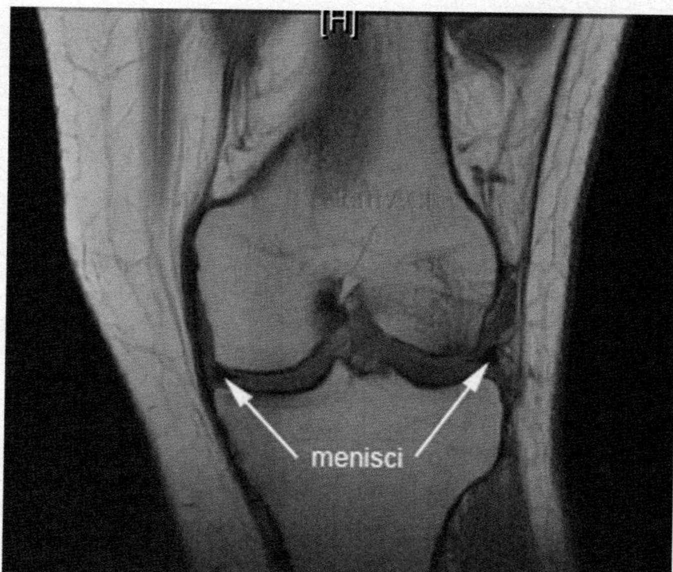

FIGURE 108-1 MRI of anterior cruciate ligament (ACL) tear in the frontal view. Note the normal menisci, which are black throughout. *(Reproduced with permission from John E. Delzell, Jr., MD, MSPH.)*

INTRODUCTION

Knee injuries are common, especially in adolescents. Women have a greater risk of knee injuries because of body mechanics. Most knee injuries involve the ACL or meniscus. Patellar subluxation/dislocation is becoming an increasingly recognized mechanism of injury, especially in young athletes. The mechanism of injury and physical examination findings suggest the type of injury, which can be confirmed by MRI. Treatment includes rest, ice, compression, elevation, and sometime requires referral to an orthopedic surgeon.

EPIDEMIOLOGY

- Knees were the most commonly injured body part in studies of high school[1] and collegiate athletes,[2] comprising one-third of injuries.
- In patients presenting with knee injuries with hemarthrosis, over 70% occurred during sports; 52% ACL rupture, 41% meniscal tear, and 17% lateral patella dislocation.[3]
- ACL injuries occur at an annual incidence of 77/100,000.[3] The annual incidence is higher in children and adolescents (121/100,000), peaking at 392/100,000 in 16-year-old girls and 422/100,000 in 17-year-old boys.[4]
- 88% of ACL tears are accompanied by another injury, most commonly a meniscal tear.[3]
- Meniscal tears are seen on MRI in 91% of patients with symptomatic osteoarthritis arthritis, but are also seen in 76% of age-matched controls without knee pain.[5]

- Patellar dislocations accounted for 36% of knee effusions in 10- to 14-year-olds and 28% of knee effusions in 15- to 18-year-olds in a series of 131 patients who presented to a pediatric emergency department.[6]

Figure 108-2 shows the normal anatomy of the knee.

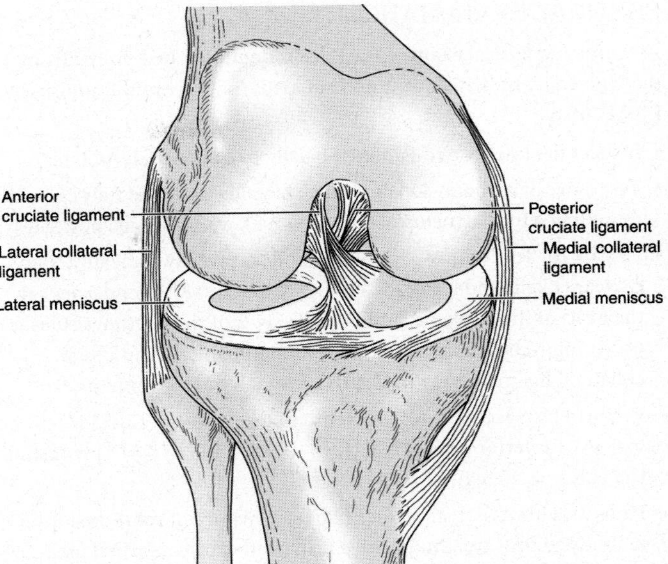

FIGURE 108-2 Anatomy of a normal knee. (*Reproduced with permission from Simon RR, Sherman SC, Koenigsknecht SJ. Emergency Orthopedics, 5th ed. New York, NY: McGraw-Hill Education; 2007.*)

ETIOLOGY AND PATHOPHYSIOLOGY

- ACL injuries occur with sudden deceleration with a rotational maneuver, usually without contact.
- ACL injuries are thought to occur more commonly in women because of decreased leg strength, increased ligamentous laxity, and differences in lumbopelvic core control.
- Acute meniscal injuries occur with a twisting motion on the weight-bearing knee.
- Chronic meniscal tears occur from mechanical grinding of osteophytes on the meniscus in older patients with osteoarthritis.
- Medial collateral and lateral collateral injuries occur from valgus and varus stress, respectively.
- Patellar dislocations occur from direct contact or a sudden change of direction.

RISK FACTORS

- Women are at higher risk for ACL injuries.
- Individuals engaging in sporting competitions are at a higher risk of acute knee injuries.

DIAGNOSIS

CLINICAL FEATURES ON HISTORY

ACL:

- Rotational injury.
- "Pop" reported by patient.
- Unable to bear full weight.
- Effusion within the first few hours.

Meniscal injury:

- Foot planted with femur rotated internally with valgus stress (medial) or femur rotated externally with varus stress (lateral).
- Joint line pain.
- Effusion over the first several hours.
- Usually ambulatory with instability or locking (mechanical) symptoms.

Collateral injury:

- Valgus or varus stress injury.
- Usually ambulatory without instability or locking symptoms.

Patellar dislocation:

- Pain on or around the patella; swelling with an acute dislocation.
- Patellar slipping or knee giving out.

PHYSICAL EXAMINATION

A complete physical exam of the knee is demonstrated online from the University of British Columbia at http://www.youtube.com/user/BJSMVideos.

- Inspect the knee for effusions—Usually present for an ACL tear.
- Test range of motion—Often normal; inability to extend fully can indicate either a medial meniscal tear or an ACL tear displaced posteriorly.
- Palpate for tenderness—Joint line tenderness may indicate a meniscal tear (likelihood ratio, LR+ = 1.1; LR− = 0.8).[7] Tenderness at the head of the fibula or at the patella are 2 of the 5 Ottawa rules for obtaining radiographs; tenderness along the medial or lateral collateral ligament may indicate damage to those ligaments.
- Perform tests for ACL tear—Lachman test (LR+ = 12.4; LR− = 0.14),[7] anterior drawer test (LR+ = 3.7; LR− = 0.6),[7] pivot shift test (LR+ = 20.3; LR− = 0.4).[7]
- Patients with ACL tears typically have a history of rotational injury; inability to bear weight; positive provocative tests; normal plain radiographs; and abnormal MRI.
- Perform tests for meniscal tears—McMurray test (LR+ = 17.3; LR− = 0.5).[7]
- Patients with meniscal tears typically have history of rotational injury with valgus/varus stress or history of osteoarthritis; able to bear weight, commonly with instability or locking; positive McMurray test; normal plain radiographs; and abnormal MRI.
- Perform varus and valgus stress to test the lateral and medial collateral ligaments.
- Patients with injuries to the collateral ligaments typically have a history of valgus/varus stress to extended knee; able to bear weight without instability or locking; laxity with valgus or varus stress testing; normal plain radiographs and abnormal MRI.
- Patients with patellar dislocations, even those that have spontaneously reduced, may have tenderness at or around the patella, and a positive patellar apprehension sign on exam.

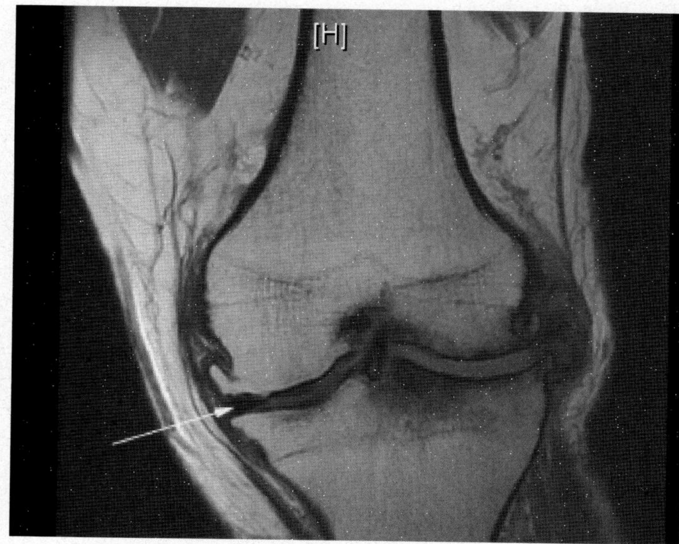

FIGURE 108-3 Medial meniscal tear on the frontal view, seen as a faint small white line through the black meniscus. (*Reproduced with permission from Heidi Chumley, MD.*)

IMAGING

- Determine whether or not to obtain plain radiographs (anteroposterior, lateral, intercondylar notch, and sunrise views) to assess for a fracture based on either the Pittsburgh or Ottawa knee rules (the Ottawa rules may be less sensitive in children):
  - Pittsburgh (99% sensitivity, 60% specificity; tested in population ages 6 to 96 years)[7]—Obtain X-ray for:
    - Recent significant fall or blunt trauma.
    - Age younger than 12 years or older than 50 years.
    - Unable to take 4 unaided steps.
  - Ottawa (98.5% sensitivity, 48.6% specificity; LR− = 0.05; tested in 6 studies of 4249 adult patients)[8]—Obtain X-ray for:
    - Age 55 years or older.
    - Tenderness at the head of the fibula.
    - Isolated tenderness of the patella.
    - Inability to flex knee to 90 degrees.
    - Inability to bear weight for 4 steps both immediately and in the examination room regardless of limping.
- MRI is 95% and 90% accurate in identifying ACL tears and meniscal injuries, respectively (**Figures 108-2** to **108-4**).[9]

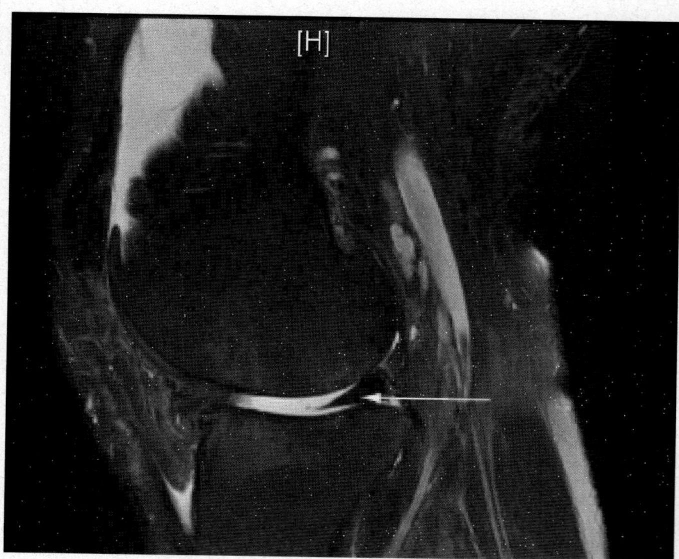

FIGURE 108-4 Lateral meniscal tear on a sagittal view, seen as a faint small white line in the black meniscus. (*Reproduced with permission from Heidi Chumley, MD.*)

- In patellar dislocation, plain radiographs may be normal or show a subtle fracture. MRI can show subtle fractures and possible rupture of the medial patellofemoral ligament.

DIFFERENTIAL DIAGNOSIS

Acute knee pain can be caused by trauma affecting structures of the knee other than ligaments and menisci, arthritis, infection, or tumors including:

- Intraarticular fractures (patella, femoral condyles, tibial eminence, tibial tuberosity, and tibial plateau)—History of trauma or chronic overuse; edema, ecchymosis, point tenderness, or deformity may be present; visible on plain radiographs (**Figures 108-5** and **108-6**).
- Patellar dislocation—Severe hyperextension (anterior dislocation), fall on a bent knee or knee hitting the dashboard (posterior dislocation), valgus or varus stress (medial or lateral dislocation); visible deformity; effusion and immobility; neurovascular complications (peroneal nerve and popliteal artery); visible on plain radiographs.
- Arthritis—No history of trauma.
- Reactive arthritis—Fever/malaise; oligoarthritis involving the knee, ankle, feet and/or wrist; urethritis; conjunctivitis or iritis; elevated C-reactive protein or erythrocyte sedimentation rate (ESR); arthritic changes on radiographs (see Chapter 161, Reactive Arthritis).
- Juvenile rheumatoid arthritis (JRA)—Children younger than age 16 years; acute pain and swelling without trauma; fever or skin rashes (systemic JRA); knee is commonly involved; arthritic changes on plain radiographs.
- Rheumatoid arthritis—Adults ages 30 to 50 years, more commonly women; polyarthritis involving hands, wrists, feet, and knees; fever/malaise; positive rheumatoid factor; erosive arthritis changes on radiographs (see Chapter 99, Rheumatoid Arthritis).
- Gout or pseudogout—Adults ages 30 to 60 years, more commonly men; single joint erythema, warmth and tenderness without trauma; abnormal joint fluid with elevated white blood cell count (WBC); radiographs may be normal or abnormal (sclerotic regions, degenerative changes, or soft tissue calcifications) (see Chapter 102, Gout).
- Osteoarthritis—Older adults; gradual onset; symptoms worse after use; radiographic osteophytes (see Chapter 98, Osteoarthritis).
- Infections such as cellulitis, septic arthritis (**Figure 108-7**), osteomyelitis—May have history of skin break by bite or puncture wound; fever; erythema, warmth with cellulitis; decreased range of motion, inability to walk, abnormal fluid aspirate with septic arthritis; chronic symptoms and abnormal radiograph with osteomyelitis.
- Malignant tumors (e.g., osteosarcoma, chondroblastoma) or benign tumors (e.g., bone cysts, osteochondroma)—No (or insignificant) history of trauma; chronic symptoms or acute symptoms caused by pathologic fracture; abnormal radiographs and MRI.

MANAGEMENT

Initial management for traumatic knee pain includes rest, ice, compression, and elevation.

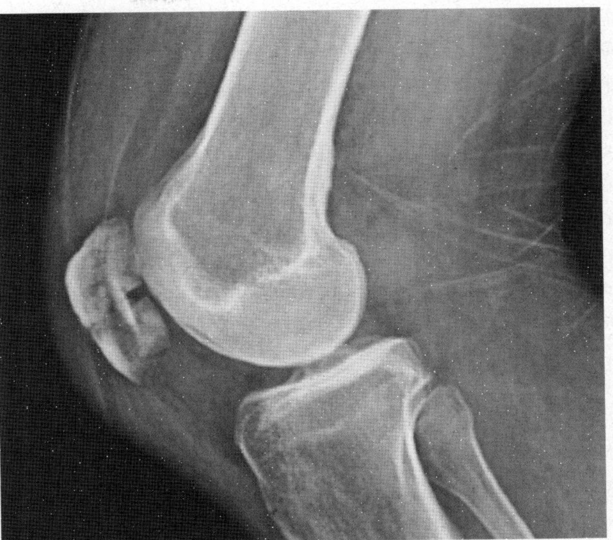

FIGURE 108-5 Nondisplaced patellar fracture seen best on the lateral view. (*Reproduced with permission from Simon RR, Sherman SC, Koenigsknecht SJ. Emergency Orthopedics, 5th ed. New York, NY: McGraw-Hill Education; 2007.*)

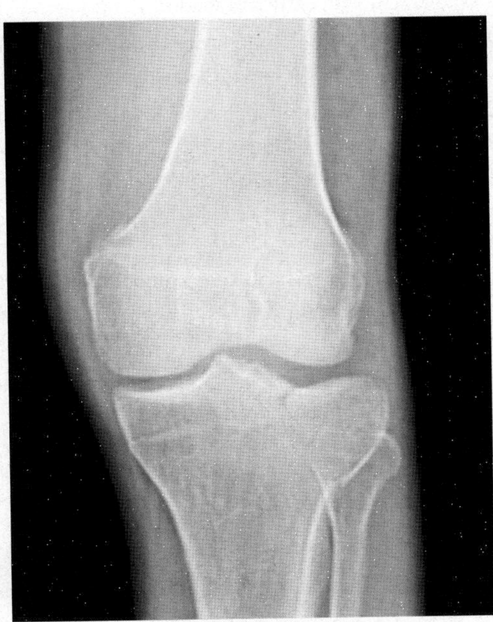

FIGURE 108-6 Lateral condylar split fracture (type 1) has no depression of the articular surface and is usually the result of low-impact trauma. More common in children. (*Reproduced with permission from Simon RR, Sherman SC, Koenigsknecht SJ. Emergency Orthopedics, 5th ed. New York, NY: McGraw-Hill Education; 2007.*)

- Provide pain relief with acetaminophen. Add a nonsteroidal anti-inflammatory medication if needed.[10] SOR Ⓒ
- Prevent further injury (e.g., limit activities to toe-touch weight bearing and place in a long-leg range-of-motion brace)[9] until evaluation by a provider trained to manage acute knee injuries. SOR Ⓒ
- Obtain plain radiographs if indicated by the Pittsburgh or Ottawa rules.[8] SOR Ⓐ
- Consider an MRI for suspected ACL, meniscal, or collateral ligament tear based on the mechanism of injury and physical examination findings.[9] SOR Ⓒ

FOR ACL TEARS

- Refer to a physician trained in surgical repair, as repair results in 80% to 95% return to normal activity in 4 to 6 months.[10] SOR Ⓒ
- Surgical repair is typically done at least 3 weeks after the injury. Repair within the first 3 weeks results in a high incidence of arthrofibrosis.
- Refer to physical therapy if available to institute early knee range of motion (before surgery).[10] SOR Ⓒ

FOR MENISCAL TEARS

- Refer to a physician for discussion of nonsurgical and surgical treatments as rates of healing vary by location of meniscal tear and associated injuries.[11] SOR Ⓒ

FOR COLLATERAL TEARS

- The treatment is based on the severity of the tear. SOR Ⓒ
- For all grades, instruct in early range-of-motion exercises (or refer to physical therapy).
- Grade I medial collateral ligament (MCL) or lateral collateral ligament (LCL) (≤5 cm laxity on valgus or varus stress), weight-bearing as tolerated with early ambulation.
- Grade II MCL or LCL (5 to 10 cm laxity), place in a brace blocking the last 20 degrees of flexion, weight-bearing as tolerated.
- Grade III MCL (>10 cm laxity), place in a hinged brace, initially non–weight bearing, advancing to weight bearing over 4 weeks. Grade III LCL tears often require surgery.

FOR PATELLAR DISLOCATIONS

- Initial treatment involves rest and knee immobilization in 20 degrees of flexion. Mobilization and weight bearing are permitted when symptoms allow.[12] SOR Ⓒ
- For recurrent dislocations, surgical intervention is associated with improved clinical outcomes in the first 5 years after injury. After 5 years, there is no difference between those treated conservatively and those treated surgically.[12] SOR Ⓐ

PREVENTION

- Neuromuscular retraining programs reduce the incidence of ACL injuries in female basketball, soccer, and basketball players.[13]
- The Prevent Injury, Enhance Performance Program achieved a 75% to 88% reduction in ACL injuries among female soccer players ages

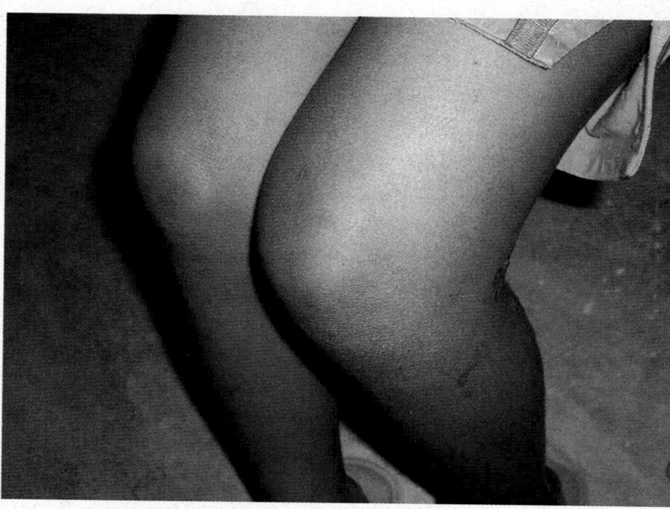

FIGURE 108-7 Septic arthritis in a young girl who presented with a painful swollen left knee, decreased range of motion, and difficulty walking. A knee aspiration revealed turbid fluid with elevated leukocytes. The joint fluid culture grew *Staphylococcus aureus*. (*Reproduced with permission from Richard P. Usatine, MD.*)

14 to 18 years. The program includes warm-up, stretching, strengthening, plyometrics, and agility exercises.[14]

- Structured warm-up program to improve cutting, jumping, balance and strength decreased acute knee injuries; number needed to treat was 43 over 8 months.[15]

PROGNOSIS

- Of children and adolescents who have had ACL surgery, 84.2% achieve excellent or good knee function.[16]
- Nonsurgical management of ACL tears has a good prognosis from 1 to 5 years, but patients reduce their activity level by 21%.[17]
- While as many as 92% of athletes with ACL tears return to some level of competitive sport by 13 months, as many as 66% do not return to their preinjury level of play.[18]

FOLLOW-UP

Timing of follow-up is determined by the orthopedic surgeon, sports medicine specialist, or other provider skilled in acute knee injury management.

PATIENT EDUCATION

- ACL tears often require surgery, take 4 to 6 months to heal, and require a commitment to rehabilitation for the best results.
- Meniscal tears may require surgery when mechanical symptoms are present. The location of the tear determines how likely surgical repair is to be effective because of the blood supply available for healing.
- Meniscal tears are commonly seen on MRI in patients with osteoarthritis who do not have pain, and meniscal tears seen on MRI may not be contributing to arthritic pain.
- Collateral tears can often be treated conservatively, while protecting the knee in a brace and preserving range of motion. Complete tears to the LCL often require surgery.
- Patellar dislocations are treated conservatively with bracing, a period of non–weight-bearing, physical therapy, and strengthening. Surgery may be required for associated fractures or recurrent instability.

PATIENT RESOURCES

- The American Academy of Family Physicians has a patient algorithm for knee pain—**https://familydoctor.org/symptom/knee-problems.**
- The National Institute of Health through the National Institute for Arthritis and Musculoskeletal and Skin Diseases has patient information on several types of knee problems—**http://www.niams.nih.gov/Health_Info/Knee_Problems/default.asp.**

PROVIDER RESOURCES

- The Ottawa and Pittsburgh Knee Rules are available in an online calculator—**Ottawa Knee Rule: https://www.mdcalc.com/ottawa-knee-rule.**
- Pittsburgh Knee Rules: **https://www.mdcalc.com/pittsburgh-knee-rules.**
- Dr. Hutchinson's Knee Exam from the University of British Columbia—**http://www.youtube.com/user/BJSMVideos.**

REFERENCES

1. Tirabassi J, Brou L, Khodaee M, et al. Epidemiology of high school sports-related injuries resulting in medical disqualification: 2005–2006 through 2013–2014 academic years. *Am J Sports Med.* 2016;44(11):2925-2932.
2. Kay MC, Register-Mihalik JK, Gray AD, et al. The epidemiology of severe injuries sustained by national collegiate athletic association student-athletes, 2009–2010 through 2014–2015. *J Athl Train.* 2017;52(2):117-128.
3. Olsson O, Isacsson A, Englund M, Frobell RB. Epidemiology of intra and peri-articular structural injuries in traumatic knee joint hemarthrosis—data from 1145 consecutive knees with subacute MRI. *Osteoarthritis Cartilage.* 2016;24(11):1890-1897.
4. Beck NA, Lawrence JT, Nordin JD, et al. ACL tears in school-aged children and adolescents over 20 years. *Pediatrics.* 2017;139(3): e20161877.
5. Bhattacharya T, Gale D, Dewire P, et al. The clinical importance of meniscal tears demonstrated by magnetic resonance imaging in osteoarthritis of the knee. *J Bone Joint Surg Am.* 2003;85-A:4-9.
6. Abbasi D, May MM, Wall EJ, et al. MRI findings in adolescent patients with acute traumatic knee hemarthrosis. *J Pediatr Orthop.* 2012;32(8):760-764.
7. Ebell MH. Evaluating the patient with a knee injury. *Am Fam Physician.* 2005;71(6):1169-1172.
8. Bachmann KM, Haberzeth S, Steurer J, Ter Riet G. The accuracy of the Ottawa knee rule to rule out knee fractures: a systematic review. *Ann Intern Med.* 2004;140(2):121-124.
9. David K, Frank B. Anterior cruciate ligament rupture. *Br J Sports Med.* 2005;39:324-329.
10. New Zealand Guidelines Group (NZGG). *The Diagnosis and Management of Soft Tissue Knee Injuries: Internal Derangements.* Wellington, NZ: New Zealand Guidelines Group (NZGG), 2003:100.
11. Greis PE, Bardana DD, Holmstrom MC, Burks RT. Meniscal injury I: basic science and evaluation. *J Am Acad Orthop Surg.* 2002;10(2):168-176.
12. Longo UG, Ciuffreda M, Locher J, et al. Treatment of primary acute patellar dislocation: systematic review and quantitative synthesis of the literature. *Clin J Sport Med.* 2017;27(6):511-523.
13. Barber-Westin SD, Noyes FR, Smith ST, Campbell TM. Reducing the risk of noncontact anterior cruciate ligament injuries in the female athlete. *Phys Sportsmed.* 2009;37(3):49-61.
14. Mandelbaum BR, Silvers HJ, Watanabe DS, et al. Effectiveness of a neuromuscular and proprioceptive training program in preventing

anterior cruciate ligament injuries in female athletes: 2-year follow-up. *Am J Sports Med.* 2005;33(7):1003-1010.

15. Olsen OE, et al. Exercises to prevent lower limb injuries in youth sports: cluster randomised controlled trial. *BMJ.* 2005;330(7489):449.
16. Frosch KH, Stengel D, Brodhun T, et al. Outcomes and risks of operative treatment of rupture of the anterior cruciate ligament in children and adolescents. *Arthroscopy.* 2010;26(11):1539-1550.
17. Muaidi QI, Nicholson LL, Refshauge KM, et al. Prognosis of conservatively managed anterior cruciate ligament injury: a systematic review. *Sports Med.* 2007;37(8):703-716.
18. Morris RC, Hulstyn MJ, Fleming BC, et al. Return to play following anterior cruciate ligament reconstruction. *Clin Sports Med.* 2016;35(4):655-668.

109 DUPUYTREN DISEASE

John E. Delzell, Jr, MD, MSPH
Heidi S. Chumley, MD, MBA

PATIENT STORY

A 53-year-old man presented with stiffness in his hands. He said his hands began to feel stiff several years ago, and now he finds that he cannot straighten many of his fingers (**Figure 109-1**). He delayed seeing a physician because he did not feel any pain in his hands. He recently began having difficulty holding his woodworking tools and wants to regain the function he has lost in his hands. The physician diagnosed him with Dupuytren contracture and discussed the disease with him along with his options for treatment.

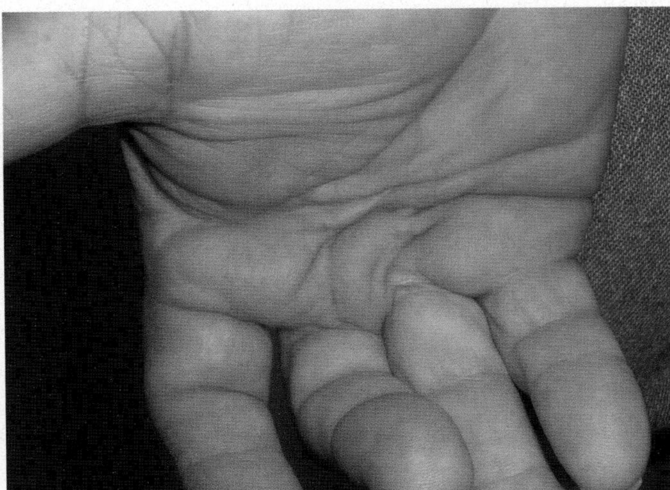

FIGURE 109-1 Dupuytren contracture in a 53-year-old man showing flexion contractures at the proximal interphalangeal joints of the third digit and a palmar cord. (*Reproduced with permission from Richard P. Usatine, MD.*)

INTRODUCTION

Dupuytren contracture is a flexion contracture of one or more of the fingers in the hand. Patients develop a progressive thickening of the palmar fascia, which causes the fingers to bend in toward the palm and limits extension. Diagnosis is clinical and the palpable nodules in the palm are considered diagnostic. Treatment has historically been surgical, but a new nonsurgical treatment with a collagenase has been approved.

SYNONYMS

Dupuytren disease, Dupuytren contractures, palmar fibromatosis, morbus Dupuytren, Ledderhose disease.

EPIDEMIOLOGY

- Dupuytren contracture is an autosomal dominant disease with incomplete penetrance (**Figure 109-2**).
- Higher prevalence among whites, particularly of northern European descent. There is an increasing incidence related to aging.[1]
- More common in men (approximately 6:1).[1,2]
- Incidence in the United States is estimated to be approximately 3 per 10,000 adults with an estimated prevalence of 7%.[1]
- Higher incidence in people who use tobacco and alcohol or who have diabetes mellitus or epilepsy.[1,3]

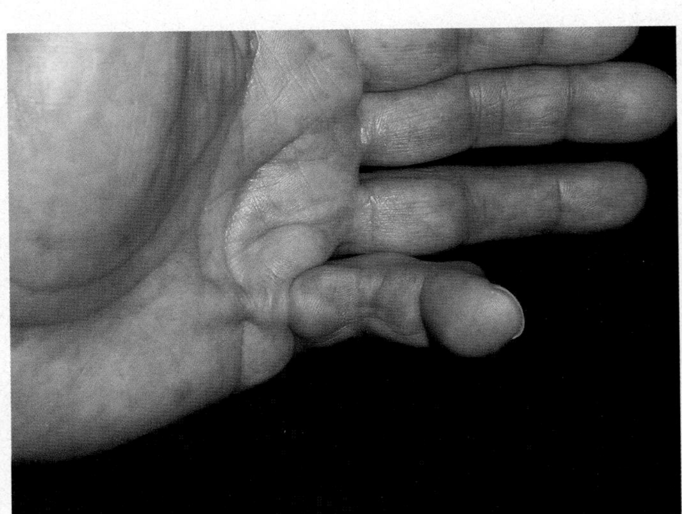

FIGURE 109-2 Dupuytren contracture in a 60-year-old man showing a flexion contracture of the fifth digit and a palmar cord. All of his brothers have Dupuytren contractures. (*Reproduced with permission from Richard P. Usatine, MD.*)

ETIOLOGY AND PATHOPHYSIOLOGY

Dupuytren contractures form in three stages:

- Myofibroblasts in the palmar fascia proliferate to form nodules.
- Myofibroblasts then align along the lines of tension, forming cords.
- Tissue becomes acellular, leaving thick cords of collagen that tighten, resulting in flexion contractures at the metacarpal

phalangeal joint, the proximal interphalangeal joint, and, occasionally, the distal interphalangeal joint.[4]

RISK FACTORS

- Tobacco use.
- Alcohol consumption.
- Epilepsy.
- Diabetes mellitus.
- Carpal tunnel syndrome.
- History of manual labor.
- History of hand injury.

DIAGNOSIS

CLINICAL FEATURES

- Clinical diagnosis that is based on the history and physical examination.
- Patients complain of a slowly progressive tightness in the hands and a lack of the ability to fully extend their fingers.
- Typically painless.
- Examination findings—Nodules with flexion contractures are considered diagnostic, particularly in older white males; however, nodules may disappear late in the disease.[3]

TYPICAL DISTRIBUTION

- Can be either hand.
- More commonly seen in the fourth and fifth digits (**Figure 109-3**).

LABORATORY TESTING

- Not indicated.

IMAGING

- MRI of the contractures may be helpful prior to surgical intervention, but is not needed to confirm a clinical diagnosis.

BIOPSY

- Not indicated.
- Diagnosis in atypical populations, such as children, may require histologic confirmation.

DIFFERENTIAL DIAGNOSIS

Consider the other causes of hand contractures and palmar nodules including:

- Intrinsic joint contractures—Loss of range of motion from any primary joint disease.
- Trigger finger, stenosing tenosynovitis—Localized swelling of the flexor tendon limits movement within the sheath with resulting "triggering"; digit catches, but can be straightened.

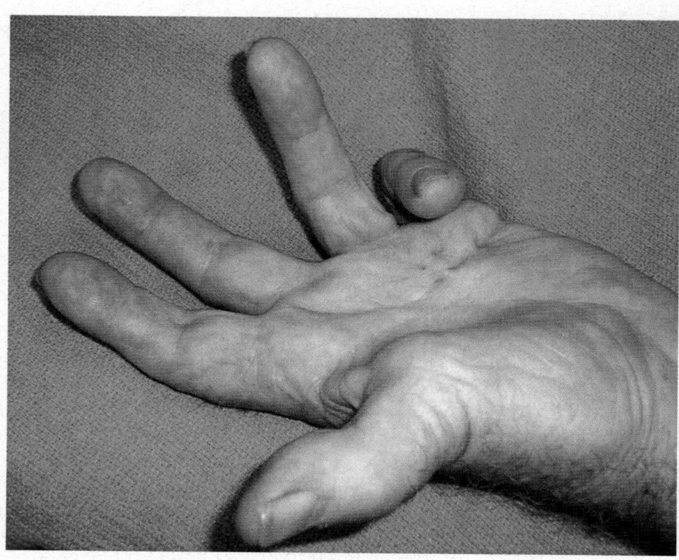

FIGURE 109-3 Dupuytren contracture in a 58-year-old man showing flexion contractures of the fourth and fifth digits and a palmar cord. *(Reproduced with permission from Richard P. Usatine, MD.)*

- Rheumatoid arthritis—Bony deformities resulting in ulnar deviation at the metacarpophalangeal joints and/or the wrist.
- Ganglion cysts and palmar nodules.
- Occupational hyperkeratosis and callous formation.
- Hand tumors including epithelioid sarcomas and soft-tissue giant cell tumors.

MANAGEMENT

The treatment goal of Dupuytren contracture is to maintain or restore hand function by increasing range of motion at involved joints.

NONPHARMACOLOGIC

- Physical therapy with splinting does not seem to be helpful as a sole treatment.[4,5] SOR C
- Radiation therapy has been used, but there is little evidence to support it and significant potential side effects of the treatment.[4] SOR C
- There is little evidence to support hyperbaric oxygen treatment.[4] SOR C

MEDICATIONS

- Intranodular injection of corticosteroids may reduce the size of the nodule with minimal change in contracture and may increase the risk for tendon rupture.[4] SOR C
- Intralesional collagenase injection, a nonsurgical treatment, is costly, but moderately effective and has minimal complications.[6,7] SOR B

REFERRAL FOR SURGERY

- Surgical correction should be considered when there is at least 30 degrees of contracture at the metacarpophalangeal (MCP) joint. SOR C
- Fasciotomy decreases the degree of flexion deformity and results in modest improvements in hand function. Intraoperative correction and complete correction at follow-up seems to be better in contracture of the metacarpal phalangeal joint, but improvement in function is better correlated with correction at the proximal interphalangeal joint.[7,8] SOR B
- Percutaneous needle aponeurotomy can be an effective treatment for initial correction but has a high recurrence rate.[7] SOR B

PROGNOSIS

- Recurrence rate is related to the amount of fascia that is removed on surgery.
- There is an increased risk for recurrence with time.

FOLLOW-UP

- Postoperative follow-up should include hand therapy with a goal of increasing extension in the affected digits.

PATIENT EDUCATION

- Modifying risk factors (e.g., smoking, alcohol intake) known to contribute to the development of Dupuytren contracture is prudent, but is not shown to alter the course of the disease.[3]
- After surgery, postoperative hand therapy may improve function and use of the hand. However, initial decreases in joint deformity and improvements in hand function may be lost over time.[4]

PATIENT RESOURCES

- PubMed Health. *Dupuytren Contracture*—**http://www.ncbi.nlm.nih.gov/pubmedhealth/PMH0002213/.**
- American Family Physician (AAFP). *Dupuytren's Disease: What You Should Know*—**http://www.aafp.org/afp/2007/0701/p90.html.**

PROVIDER RESOURCES

- Mayo Clinic. *Dupuytren's Contracture*—**http://www.mayoclinic.com/health/dupuytrens-contracture/DS00732.**
- American Family Physician (AAFP). Trojian TH, Chu SM. Dupuytren's disease: diagnosis and treatment. *Am Fam Physician.* 2007;76(1):86-89—**http://www.aafp.org/afp/2007/0701/p86.html.**
- Medscape. *Dupuytren Contracture*—**http://emedicine.medscape.com/article/329414.**

REFERENCES

1. Dibenedetti DB, Nguyen D, Zografos L, et al. Prevalence, incidence, and treatments of Dupuytren's disease in the United States: results from a population-based study. *Hand (N Y)* 2011;6(2):149-158.
2. Lanting R1, Broekstra DC, Werker PM, van den Heuvel ER. A systematic review and meta-analysis on the prevalence of Dupuytren disease in the general population of Western countries. *Plast Reconstr Surg.* 2014;133(3):593-603.
3. Trojian TH, Chu SM. Dupuytren's disease: diagnosis and treatment. *Am Fam Physician.* 2007;76(1):86-89.
4. Ball C, Izadi D, Verjee LS, et al. Systematic review of non-surgical treatments for early Dupuytren's disease. *BMC Musculoskelet Disord.* 2016;17:345.
5. Lo S, Pickford M. Current concepts in Dupuytren's disease. *Curr Rev Musculoskelet Med* 2013;6(1):26-34.
6. Lauritzson A, Atroshi I. Collagenase injections for Dupuytren's disease: prospective cohort study assessing 2-year treatment effect durability. *BMJ Open.* 2017;7(3):e012943.
7. Henry M. Dupuytren's disease: current state of the art. *Hand (N Y)* 2014;9(1):1-8.
8. Donaldson OW, Pearson D, Reynolds R, Bhatia RK. The association between intraoperative correction of Dupuytren's disease and residual postoperative contracture. *J Hand Surg Eur.* 2010;35(3):220-223.

PART XIII

DERMATOLOGY

Strength of Recommendation (SOR)	Definition
A	Recommendation based on consistent and good-quality patient-oriented evidence.*
B	Recommendation based on inconsistent or limited-quality patient-oriented evidence.*
C	Recommendation based on consensus, usual practice, opinion, disease-oriented evidence, or case series for studies of diagnosis, treatment, prevention, or screening.*

*See Appendix A on pages 1603–1606 for further information.

SECTION A FOUNDATIONS OF DERMATOLOGY

110 TERMINOLOGY OF SKIN DISORDERS

Richard P. Usatine, MD

It is important to have a shared common terminology for the description and diagnosis of skin disorders. While immediate pattern recognition may be available to those clinicians with the greatest experience and expertise, recognizing morphologic characteristics of skin disorders is a great first step to diagnosis. In these days of Google searches and excellent online dermatologic resources, being able to describe a lesion or rash may help clinicians arrive at an excellent differential diagnosis simply by putting the appropriate terms in a search engine. The terminology that we will define in this chapter includes morphology, pigmentation, shapes, other descriptors, and distribution.

MORPHOLOGY

Primary morphology are the terms we use to describe the initial changes of a skin lesion or eruption. Secondary morphology terms are based on what happens to lesions and eruptions over time. Although we present morphology terms divided into these two categories, the most important information is the terms themselves.

▶ Primary morphology:

- Macule—a nonpalpable, well-circumscribed change in skin color less than 1 cm
- Patch—a nonpalpable, well-circumscribed change in skin color greater than 1 cm
- Papule—a palpable, elevated, solid skin lesion less than 1 cm
- Plaque—a palpable, elevated skin lesion greater than 1 cm
- Wheal—a transient smooth papule or plaque seen in urticaria
- Vesicle—a small fluid-containing blister less than 1 cm
- Bulla—a large fluid-containing blister greater than 1 cm
- Pustule—a vesicle containing pus
- Nodule—a solid, nonsuperficial skin mass between 1 and 2 cm
- Tumor—a solid skin mass greater than 2 cm

▶ Secondary morphology:

- Scale—flaking off of the stratum corneum
- Crust—dried exudate
- Excoriation—areas of skin damage that are linear and secondary to scratching or scraping
- Lichenification—thickening of the skin with prominent skin lines secondary to repeated rubbing or scratching
- Erosions—loss of areas of the epidermis secondary to manipulation of the skin or popping of blistered areas
- Ulcers—deeper areas of skin loss that extend at least into the deeper dermis
- Fissures—cracking of the skin in a somewhat linear pattern
- Atrophy—thinning of the skin
- Hypertrophy—thickening of the skin

EXAMPLES OF SKIN CONDITIONS WITH THESE MORPHOLOGIC CHARACTERISTICS

▶ Primary morphology

- Macule—junctional nevus, labial melanotic macule. (**Figure 110-1**)
- Patch—large congenital nevus, dermal melanosis. (**Figure 110-2**)
- Papule—acne, intradermal nevus. (**Figure 110-3**)
- Plaque—psoriasis. (**Figure 110-4**)
- Wheal—urticaria. (**Figure 110-5**)
- Vesicle—varicella, zoster. (**Figure 110-6**)
- Bulla—bullous pemphigoid. (**Figure 110-7**)
- Pustule—folliculitis, pustular psoriasis. (**Figure 110-8**)
- Nodule—nodular basal cell carcinoma (BCC), dermatofibroma. (**Figure 110-9**)
- Tumor—melanoma. (**Figure 110-10**)

▶ Secondary morphology

- Scale—seborrheic dermatitis, psoriasis. (**Figure 110-11**)
- Crust—impetigo. (**Figure 110-12**)
- Excoriation—any condition such as psoriasis with pruritus. (**Figure 110-13**)
- Lichenification—lichen simplex chronicus. (**Figure 110-14**)
- Erosions—bullous pemphigoid with popped blisters. (**Figure 110-15**)
- Ulcers—pyoderma gangrenosum, stasis ulcers. (**Figure 110-16**)
- Fissures—hand dermatitis. (**Figure 110-17**)
- Atrophy—morphea, discoid lupus. (**Figure 110-18**)
- Hypertrophy—hypertrophic lichen planus. (**Figure 110-19**)

COLOR AND PIGMENTATION

There are special terms for color changes and pigmentary changes.

- Erythematous—pink to red in color with an increase in blood flow to the area

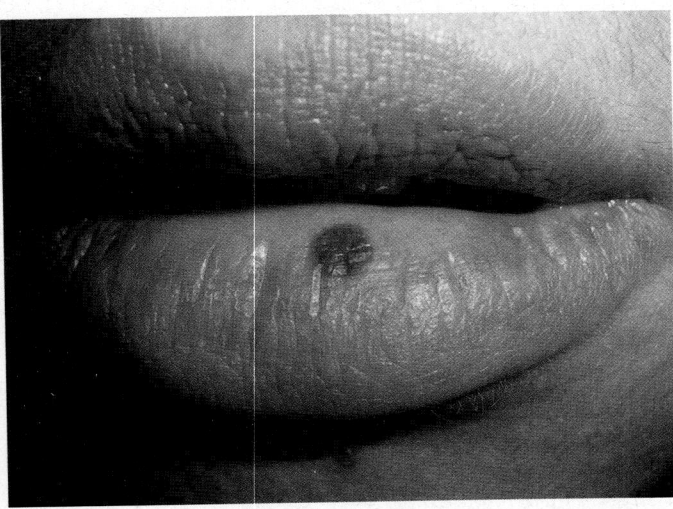

FIGURE 110-1 Macule—labial melanotic macule. (*Reproduced with permission from Richard P. Usatine, MD.*)

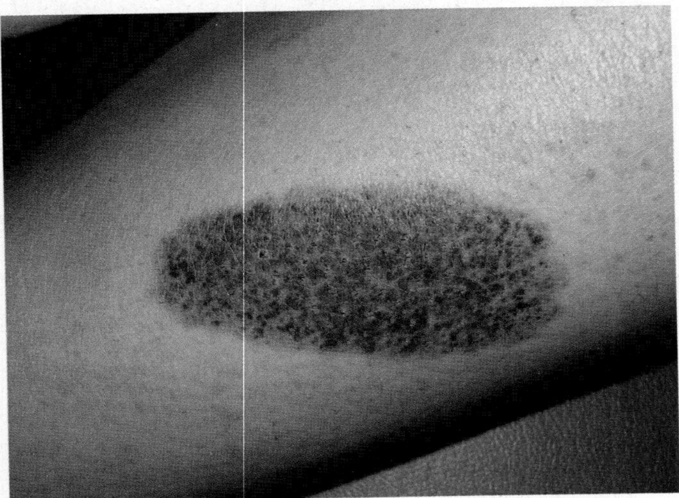

FIGURE 110-2 Patch—speckled nevus. (*Reproduced with permission from Richard P. Usatine, MD.*)

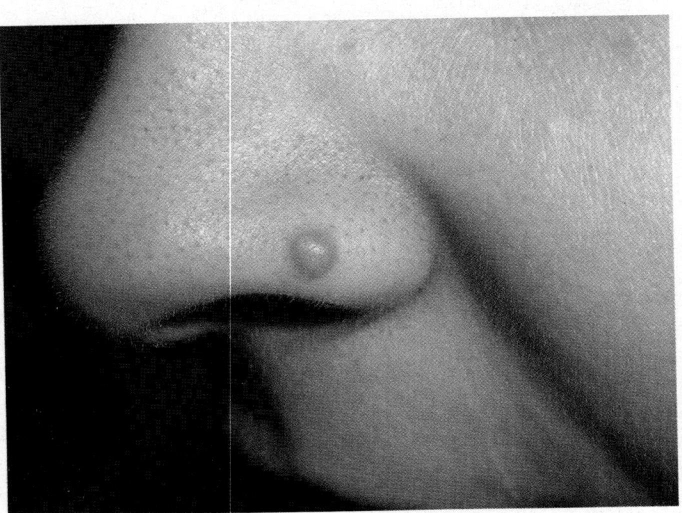

FIGURE 110-3 Papule—Spitz nevus. (*Reproduced with permission from Richard P. Usatine, MD.*)

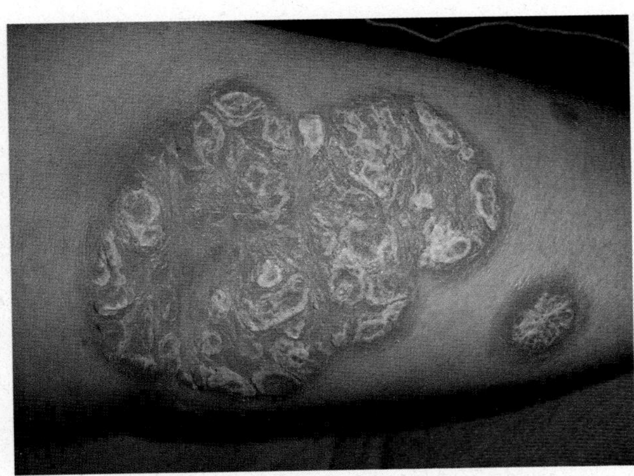

FIGURE 110-4 Plaque—psoriatic plaque. (*Reproduced with permission from Richard P. Usatine, MD.*)

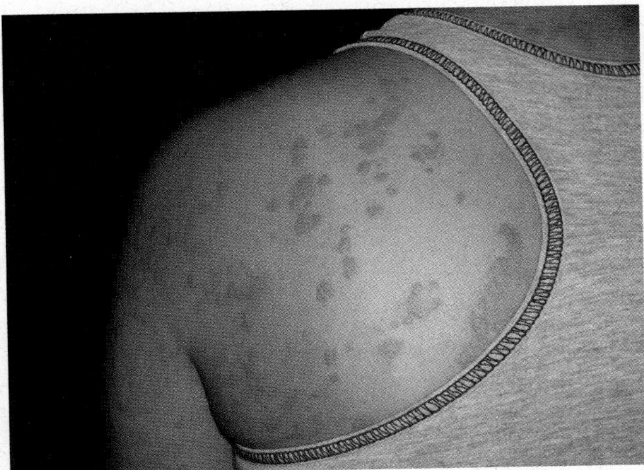

FIGURE 110-5 Wheal—the wheals of urticaria. (*Reproduced with permission from Richard P. Usatine, MD.*)

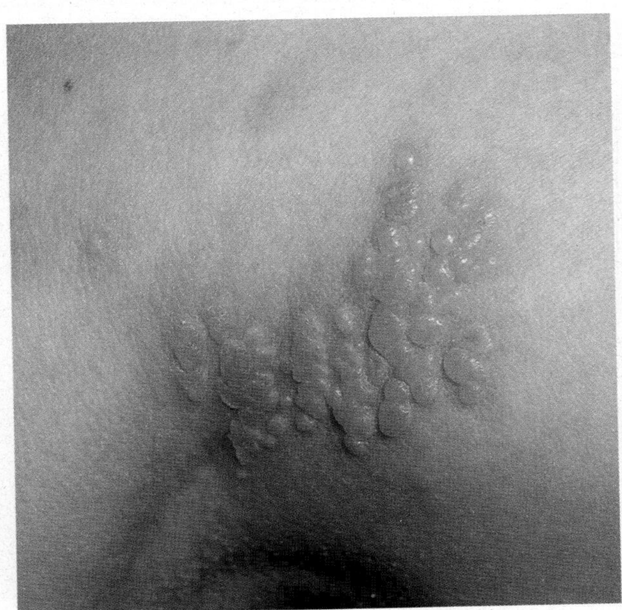

FIGURE 110-6 Vesicles—herpes zoster. (*Reproduced with permission from Richard P. Usatine, MD.*)

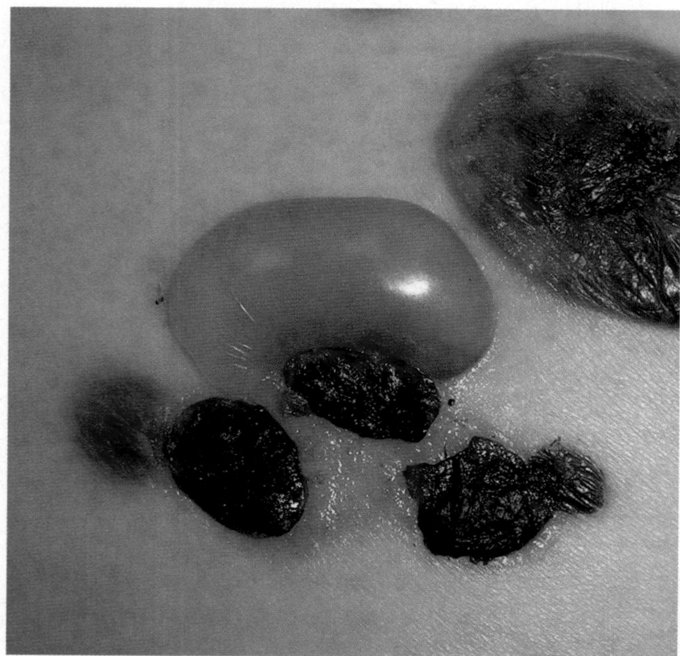

FIGURE 110-7 Bulla—bullous pemphigoid. (*Reproduced with permission from Richard P. Usatine, MD.*)

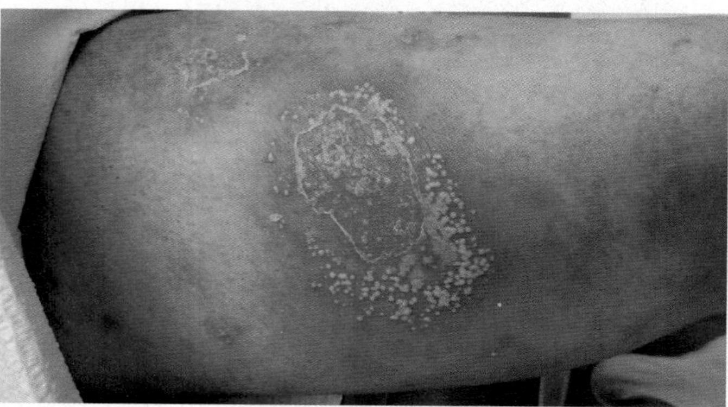

FIGURE 110-8 Pustules—pustular psoriasis. (*Reproduced with permission from Robert Gilson, MD.*)

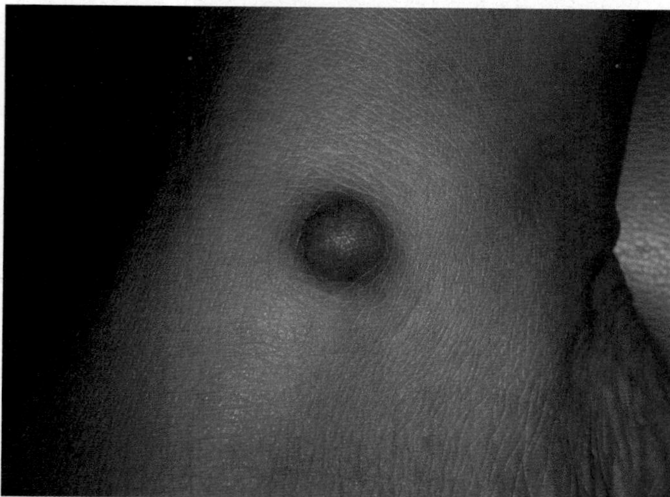

FIGURE 110-9 Nodule—large pigmented dermatofibroma. (*Reproduced with permission from Richard P. Usatine, MD.*)

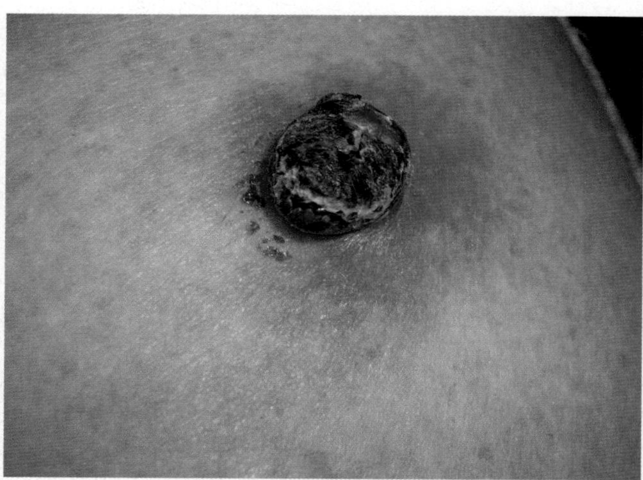

FIGURE 110-10 Tumor—melanoma. (*Reproduced with permission from Richard P. Usatine, MD.*)

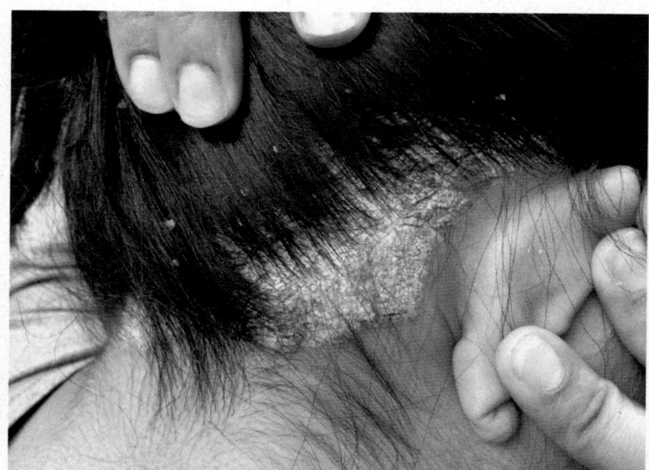

FIGURE 110-11 Scale—scalp psoriasis. (*Reproduced with permission from Richard P. Usatine, MD.*)

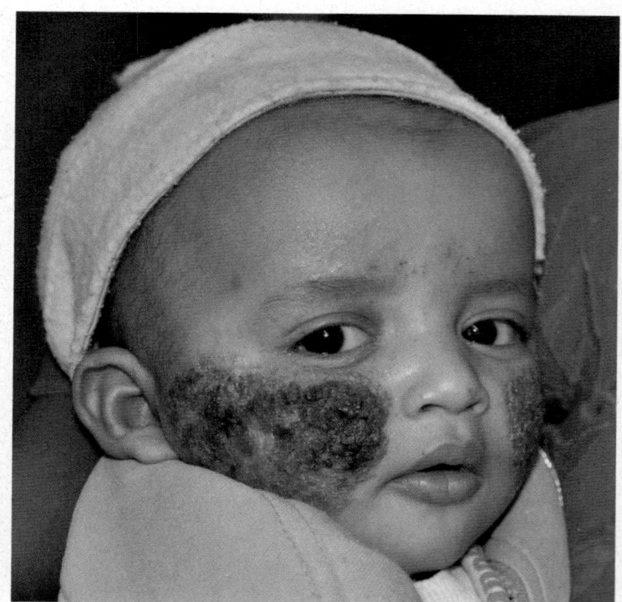

FIGURE 110-12 Crust—super infected atopic dermatitis. (*Reproduced with permission from Richard P. Usatine, MD.*)

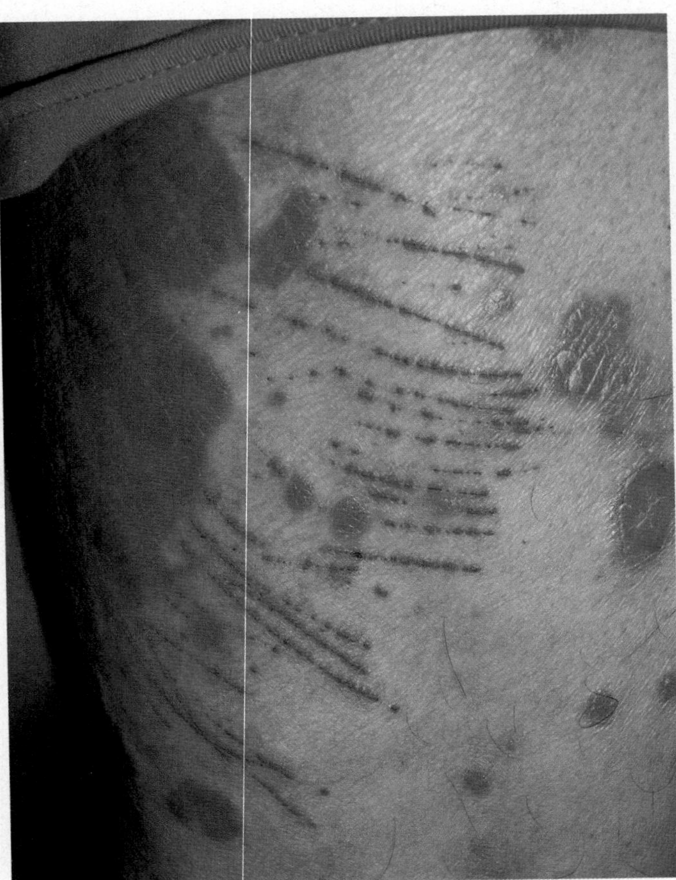

FIGURE 110-13 Excoriations—scratching the trunk due to itching of psoriasis. *(Reproduced with permission from Richard P. Usatine, MD.)*

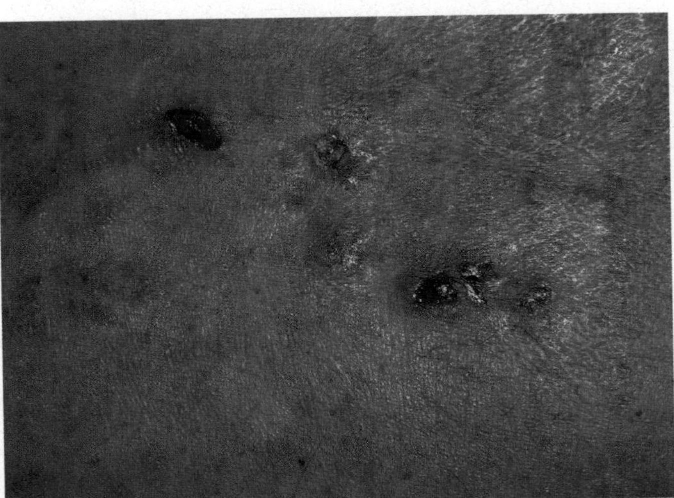

FIGURE 110-15 Erosions—bullous pemphigoid after blisters have been broken. *(Reproduced with permission from Richard P. Usatine, MD.)*

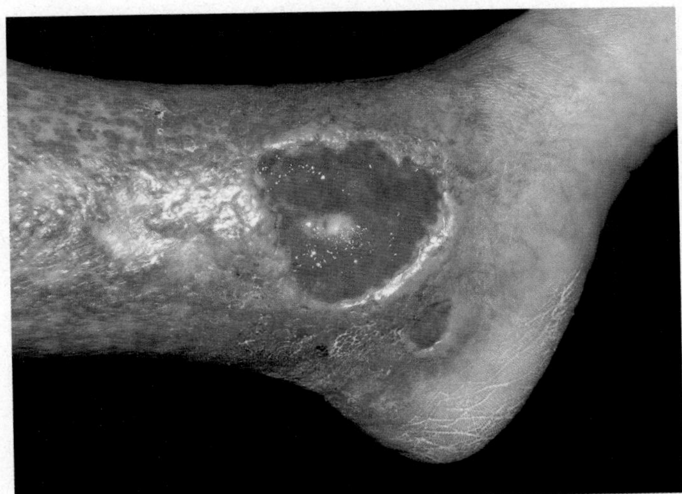

FIGURE 110-16 Ulcer—venous stasis ulcer. *(Reproduced with permission from Richard P. Usatine, MD.)*

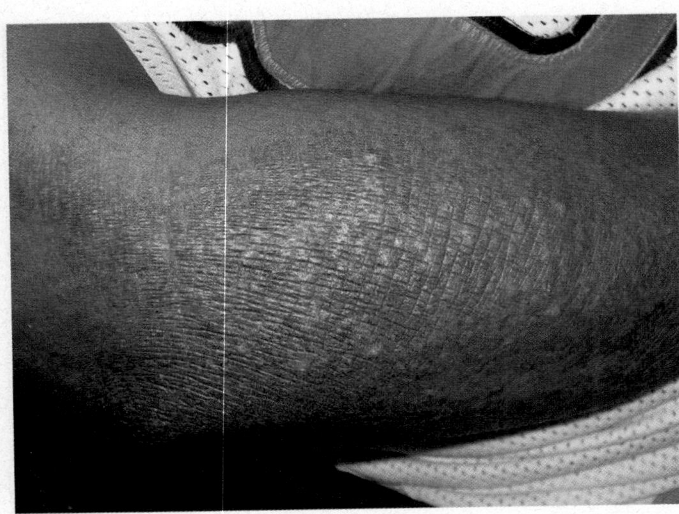

FIGURE 110-14 Lichenification—lichen simplex chronicus. *(Reproduced with permission from Richard P. Usatine, MD.)*

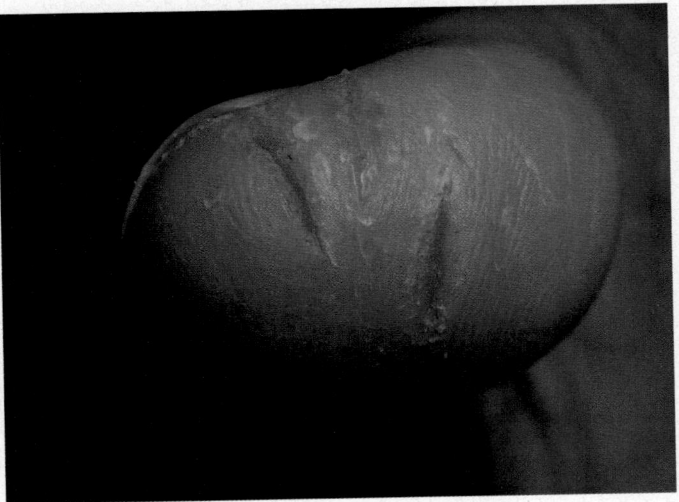

FIGURE 110-17 Fissures—hand dermatitis. *(Reproduced with permission from Richard P. Usatine, MD.)*

- Hypopigmented—a decrease in pigmentation from the surrounding skin
- Depigmented—complete lack of pigmentation
- Hyperpigmented—an increase in pigmentation from the surrounding skin

EXAMPLES OF COLOR/PIGMENTARY TERMS

- Erythematous—cellulitis, erythroderma. (**Figure 110-20**)
- Hypopigmented—postinflammatory hypopigmentation. (**Figure 110-21**)
- Depigmented—vitiligo. (**Figure 110-22**)
- Hyperpigmented—postinflammatory hyperpigmentation, acanthosis. (**Figure 110-23**)

VASCULAR TERMINOLOGY

- Ecchymosis—bruising from bleeding under the skin
- Petechiae—pinpoint bleeding in the skin
- Purpura—larger areas of bleeding or vascular inflammation
- Telangiectasias—small dilated vessels

EXAMPLES OF VASCULAR TERMINOLOGY

- Petechiae—thrombocytopenia or vasculitis. (**Figure 110-24**)
- Purpura—thrombocytopenic purpura. (**Figure 110-25**)
- Telangiectasias—basal cell carcinomas, CREST syndrome, rosacea. (**Figure 110-26**)

SURFACE CHARACTERISTICS

- Verrucous—wartlike with a rough surface—common warts. (**Figure 110-27**)
- Smooth or pearly—molluscum, BCC. (**Figure 110-28**)

SHAPES WITH EXAMPLES

- Nummular—coin shaped, nummular eczema. (**Figure 110-29**)
- Serpiginous—snakelike, cutaneous larva migrans. (**Figure 110-30**)
- Annular—bordered by a raised ring, granuloma annulare. (**Figure 110-31**)
- Reticular—netlike, confluent and reticulated papillomatosis. (**Figure 110-32**)
- Umbilicated—like an umbilicus, molluscum contagiosum. (**Figure 110-33**)

DISTRIBUTION TERMS

- Acral—hands and feet
- Intertriginous—in areas of skin folds. (**Figure 110-34**)
- Photo-distributed—in areas that are prone to sun exposure

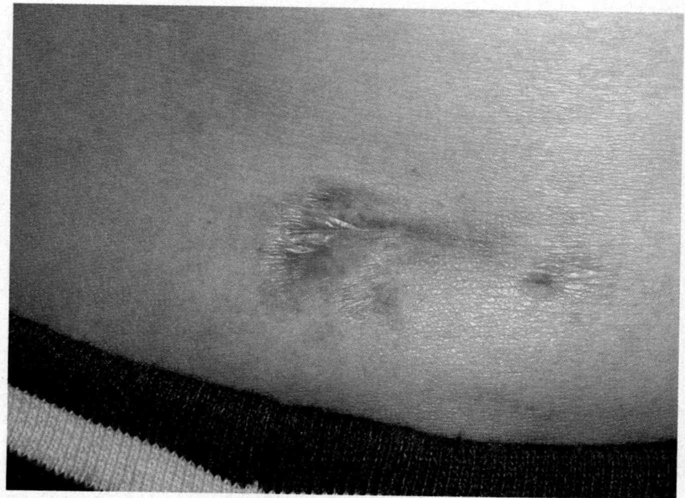

FIGURE 110-18 Atrophy—discoid lupus. (*Reproduced with permission from Richard P. Usatine, MD.*)

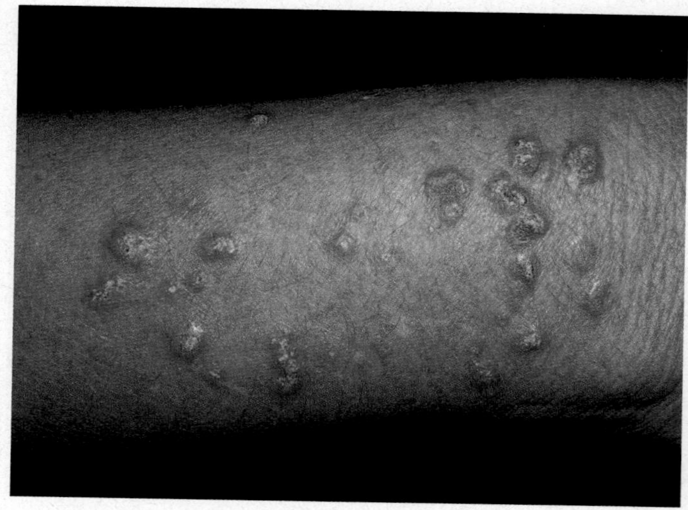

FIGURE 110-19 Hypertrophy—hypertrophic lichen planus. (*Reproduced with permission from Richard P. Usatine, MD.*)

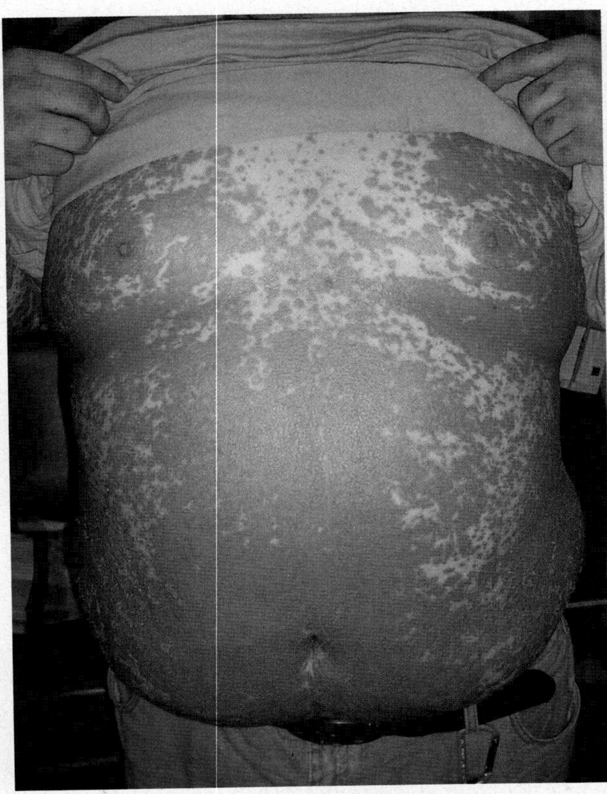

FIGURE 110-20 Erythematous—erythrodermic psoriasis. (*Reproduced with permission from Richard P. Usatine, MD.*)

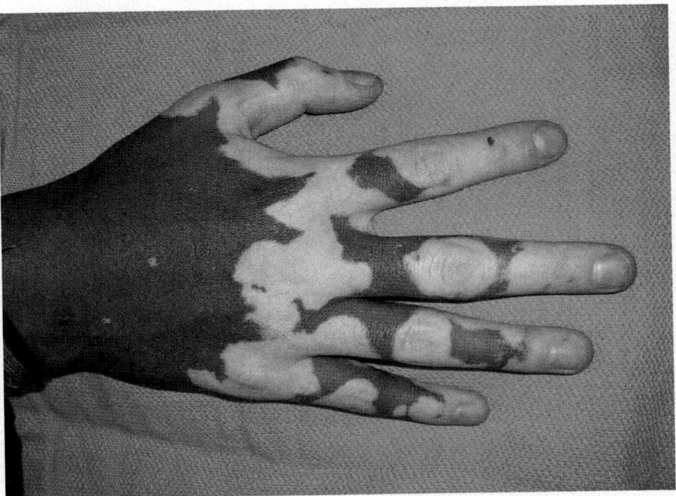

FIGURE 110-22 Depigmented—vitiligo. (*Reproduced with permission from Richard P. Usatine, MD.*)

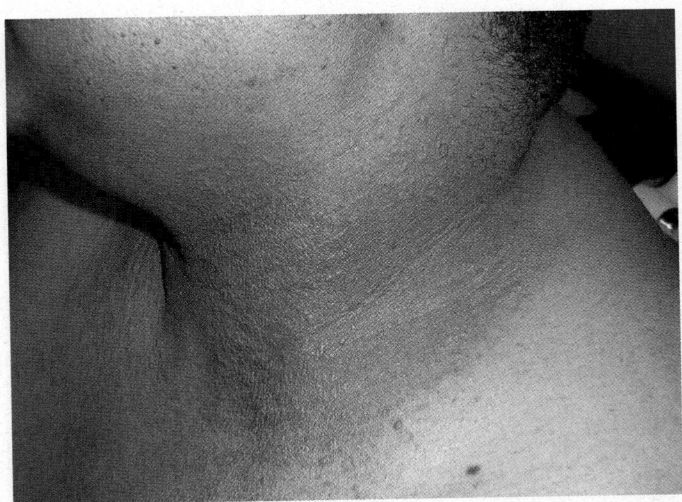

FIGURE 110-23 Hyperpigmented—postinflammatory hyperpigmentation and acanthosis nigricans. (*Reproduced with permission from Richard P. Usatine, MD.*)

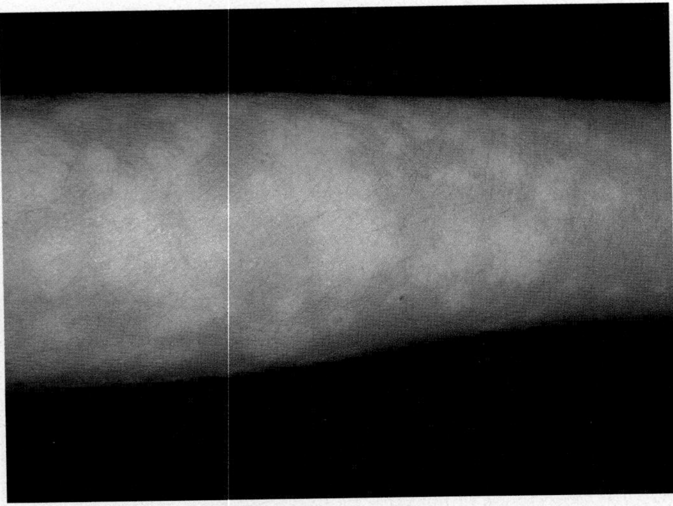

FIGURE 110-21 Hypopigmented—postinflammatory hypopigmentation with treatment of psoriasis. (*Reproduced with permission from Richard P. Usatine, MD.*)

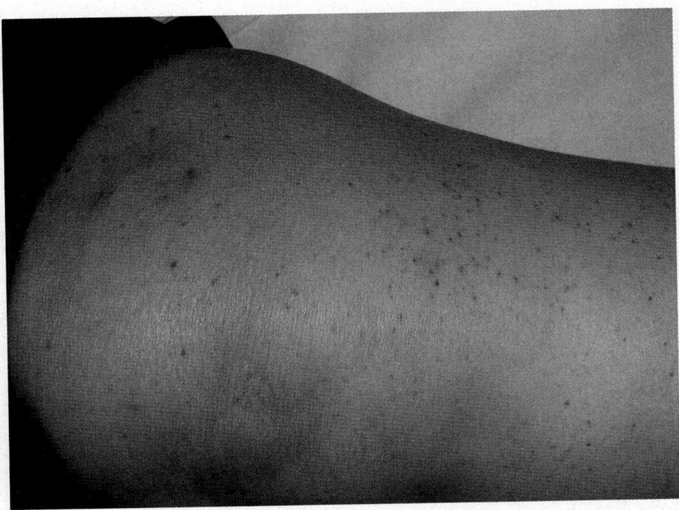

FIGURE 110-24 Petechiae—thrombocytopenia. (*Reproduced with permission from Richard P. Usatine, MD.*)

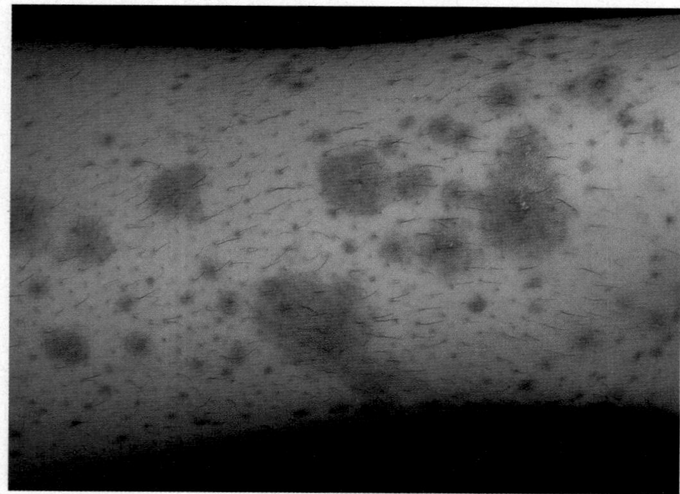

FIGURE 110-25 Purpura—palpable purpura in Henoch–Schönlein purpura. (*Reproduced with permission from Richard P. Usatine, MD.*)

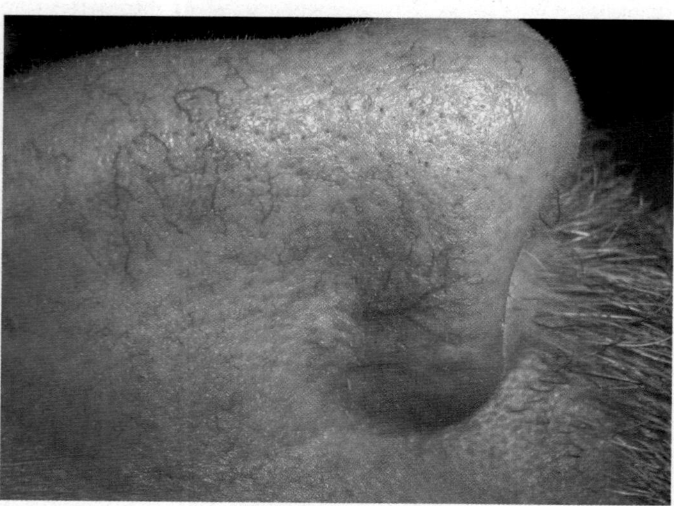

FIGURE 110-26 Telangiectasias—rosacea. (*Reproduced with permission from Richard P. Usatine, MD.*)

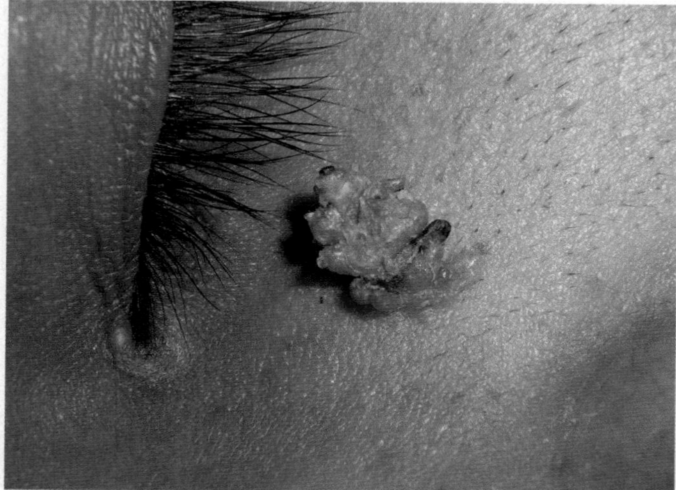

FIGURE 110-27 Verrucous—wart. (*Reproduced with permission from Richard P. Usatine, MD.*)

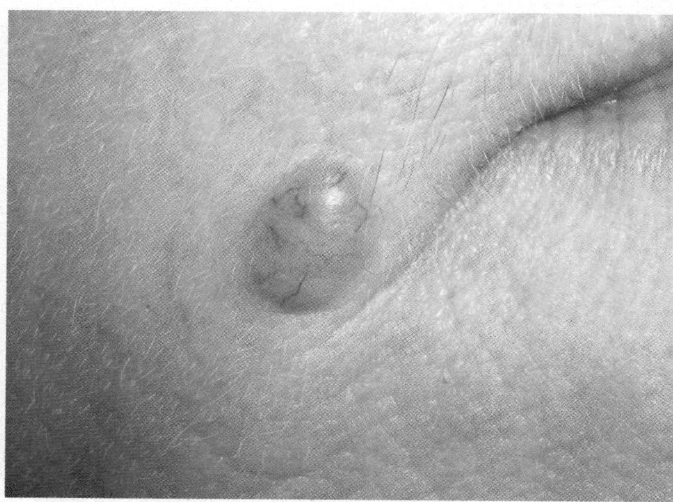

FIGURE 110-28 Pearly and smooth—basal cell carcinoma. (*Reproduced with permission from Richard P. Usatine, MD.*)

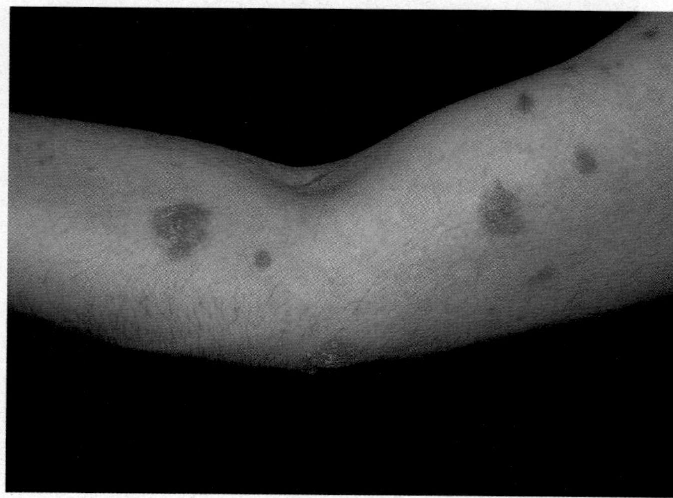

FIGURE 110-29 Nummular—nummular dermatitis. (*Reproduced with permission from Richard P. Usatine, MD.*)

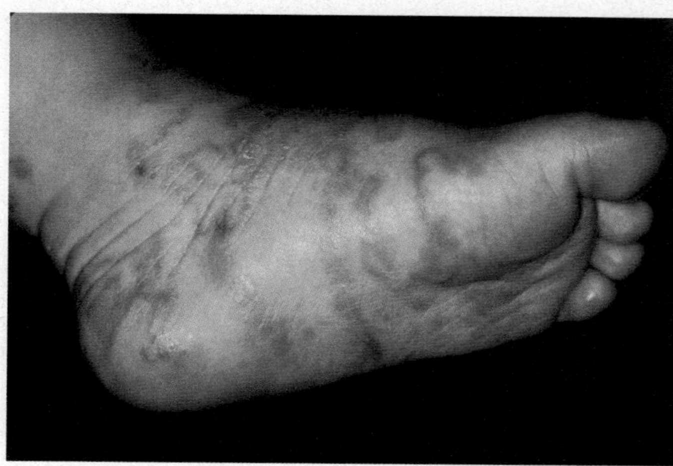

FIGURE 110-30 Serpiginous—cutaneous larva migrans. (*Reproduced with permission from Richard P. Usatine, MD.*)

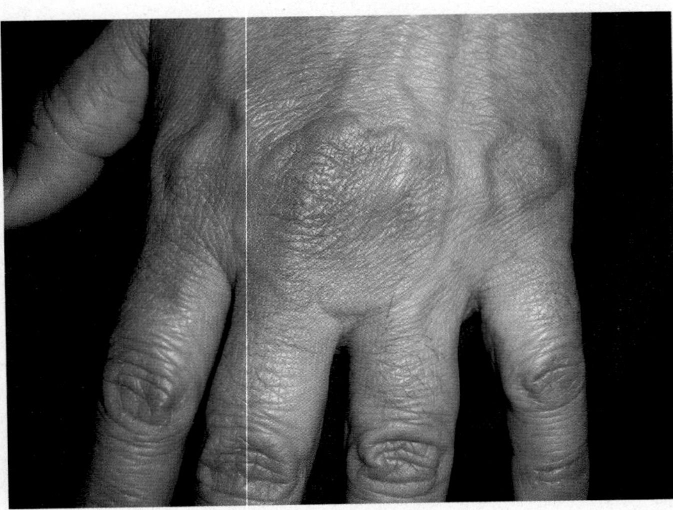

FIGURE 110-31 Annular—granuloma annulare. (*Reproduced with permission from Richard P. Usatine, MD.*)

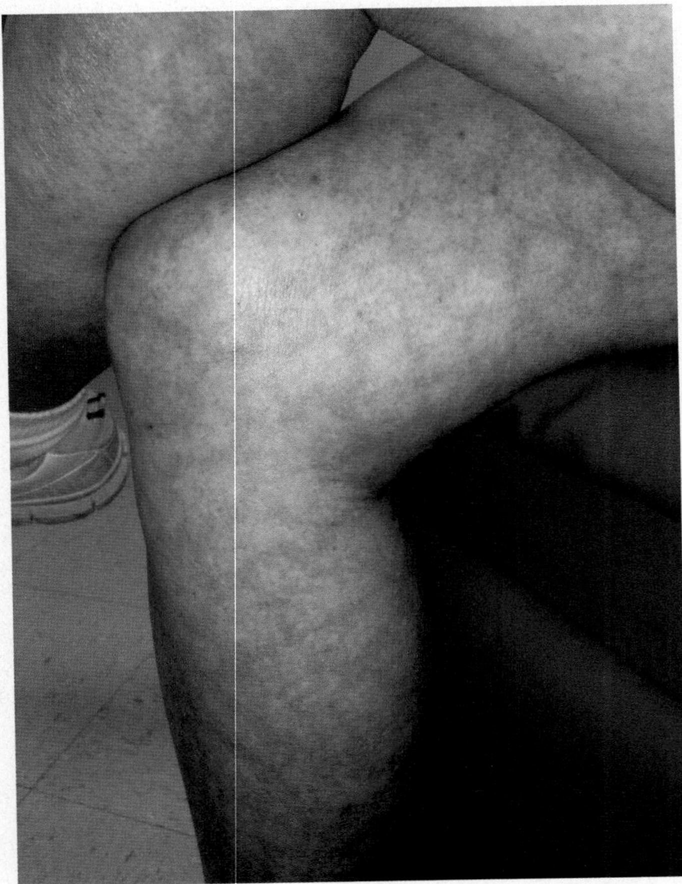

FIGURE 110-32 Reticular—livedo reticularis. (*Reproduced with permission from Richard P. Usatine, MD.*)

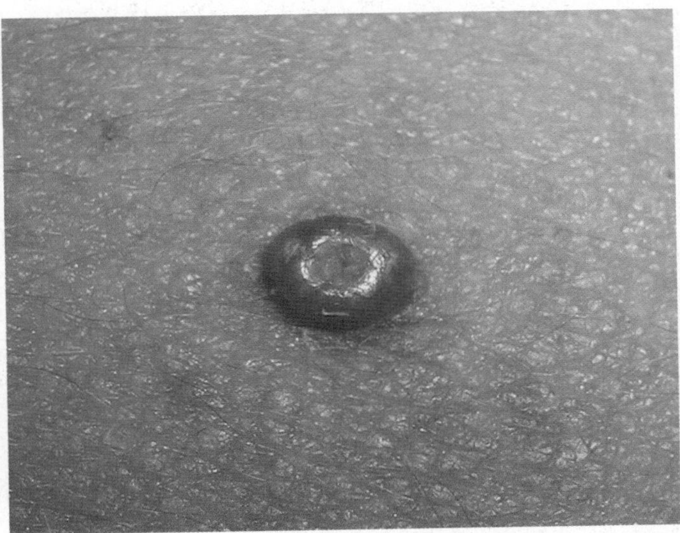

FIGURE 110-33 Umbilicated—molluscum. (*Reproduced with permission from Richard P. Usatine, MD.*)

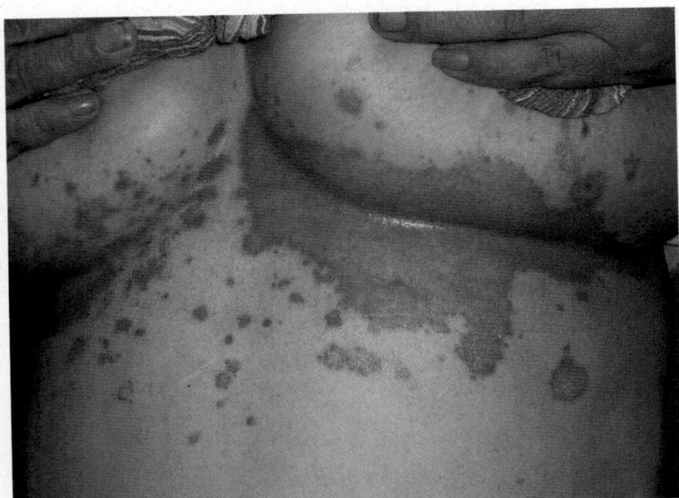

FIGURE 110-34 Intertriginous—inverse psoriasis. (*Reproduced with permission from Richard P. Usatine, MD.*)

CONCLUSION

Mastering these terms will lead to improved diagnosis in dermatology and an ability to discuss and document your patient's skin findings. The next time you do not recognize a rash or a skin lesion, open up a search engine such as Google, and type in the descriptive terms that apply to this unknown condition. More often than not, the results will contain helpful diagnoses and images that will lead to an excellent differential diagnosis. Of course, if there is a concern for malignancy, a biopsy will always be needed. If it appears to be a benign growth or self-limited rash, it is possible that a biopsy or referral can be avoided. Specific dermatology search engines such as VisualDx and the Interactive Dermatology Atlas (see resources below) are other options for searching for answers. The digital world has much to offer when you have mastered the terminology in this chapter. The following dermatology chapters will then help you to hone in on the diagnosis and treatment of the suspected condition.

PROVIDER RESOURCES

- VisualDx. Use dermatology terms within the differential builder on the mobile app or Internet site to build a differential diagnosis. Then evaluate the options to improve diagnostic accuracy. VisualDx has a vast image library including some of the world's best medical images—https://www.visualdx.com. (Personal or institutional subscription needed.)
- Interactive dermatology atlas. An online atlas created by Dr. Usatine that is free for all to use. There are more than 1400 images that can be searched using the terminology described in this chapter—http://www.dermatlas.net.

111 DERMOSCOPY

Konstantinos Liopyris, MD
Cristian Navarrete-Dechent, MD
Oriol Yélamos, MD
Zachary J. Wolner, MD
Ayelet Rishpon, MD
Richard P. Usatine, MD
Ashfaq A. Marghoob, MD

INTRODUCTION

The dermatoscope is to the skin as the otoscope is to the ear. Once you have examined the ear with an otoscope, it is hard to imagine examining the ear without one. The same is true for the dermatoscope and the skin. The dermatoscope allows you to see into the skin and make diagnoses with greater accuracy and confidence. The dermatoscope was originally used and studied to better diagnose skin cancers, but its use has been expanded into all aspects of dermatology including the diagnosis of scabies, alopecia, nail disorders, and inflammatory skin diseases.

SYNONYMS

The scope is called either the dermatoscope or dermoscope.
The process of using the dermatoscope is interchangeably called dermoscopy or dermatoscopy.

DERMOSCOPY

Dermoscopy is a technique that allows clinicians to evaluate subsurface structures within the skin with an instrument called a dermatoscope (**Figure 111-1**). Most of the light shining onto the skin is scattered at the air-skin interface, resulting in back-scattered light (glare). The dermatoscope is a handheld device consisting of a 10× magnification lens and a transilluminating polarized or non-polarized light source designed to diminish surface glare to see into the deeper layers of the skin.

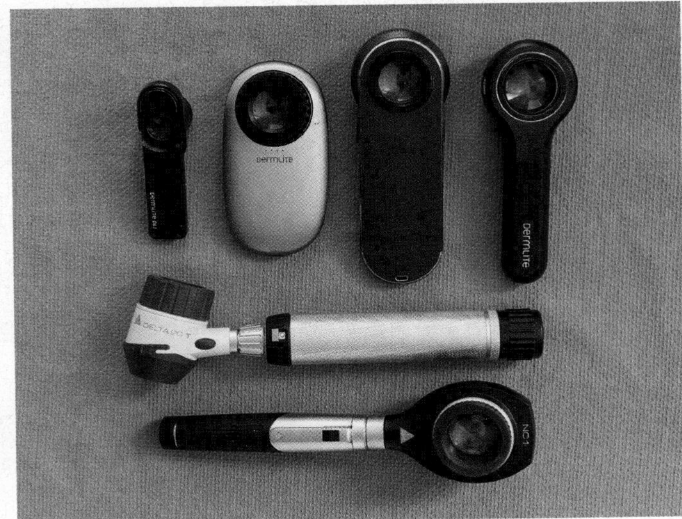

FIGURE 111-1 Various dermatoscopes. (*Reproduced with permission from Richard P. Usatine, MD.*)

NON-POLARIZED DERMOSCOPY (NPD)

Non-polarized dermatoscopes (NPDs) eliminate the air-skin interface with the glass faceplate of the dermatoscope and immersion fluid. The following liquids work well: ultrasound gel, mineral oil, and alcohol. Because of the lack of air bubbles and the clarity of the image, 70% alcohol is the preferred immersion liquid. For certain locations such as the nail, ultrasound gel is preferred, as it will not flow off the nail plate surface.[1] NPDs primarily allow for the observation of structures located between the stratum corneum and superficial papillary dermis, with the superficial structures being more conspicuous (**Figure 111-2**).

POLARIZED DERMOSCOPY (PD)

Polarized dermatoscopes (PDs) are similar to NPDs with the main difference between the two being that PD uses two polarized filters

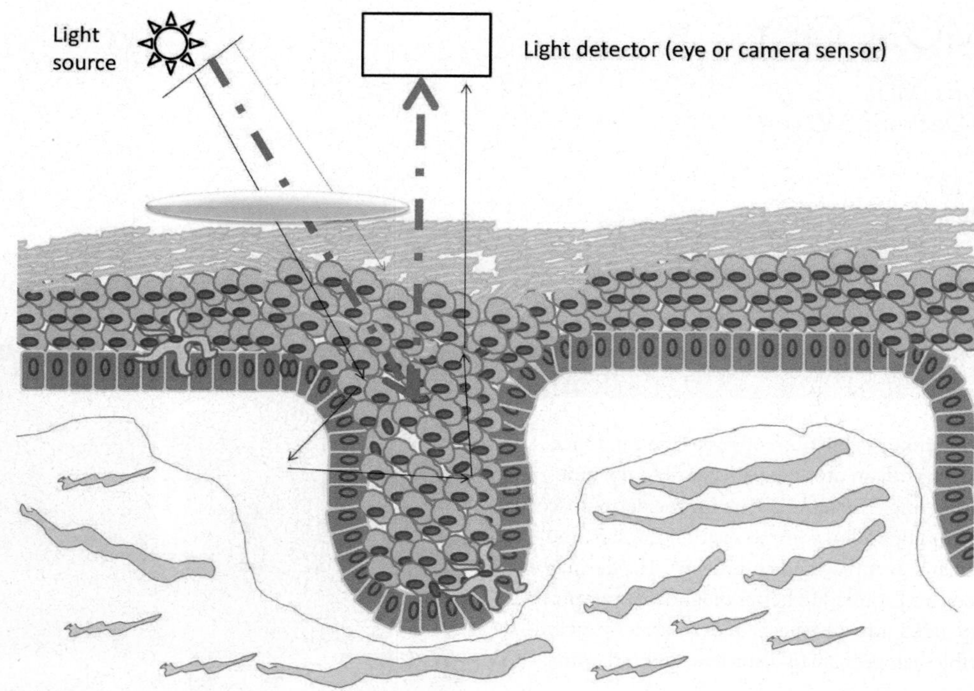

FIGURE 111-2 Non-polarized dermoscopy. Light is transmitted via the dermatoscope—light source (*blue, black,* and *red arrows*). The *red arrow* represents the superficial penetrating light, the main source of contrast using non-polarized dermoscopy, which undergoes minimal scattering events. The *black arrow* represents the deep penetrating light, contributing a small fraction of the back-reflected light due to multiple scattering events. The *blue arrow* represents the surface glare, eliminated by the use of the immersion fluid.

to achieve cross-polarization, which eliminates the glare off the skin.[2] One advantage of PDs is that they do not require direct contact with the skin, nor do they need an immersion fluid interface. More importantly, PDs allow the visualization of structures deeper in the skin as compared with NPDs, but this does come at the cost of making the features in the superficial layers more inconspicuous (**Figure 111-3**). For example, PD makes blood vessels and dermal changes more conspicuous but makes milia-like cysts and blue-white veil less prominent.[3,4] Of great importance, shiny white structures due to collagen deposition seen in many skin cancers are only visible with PD.[5,6]

STRUCTURES

The numerous structures and colors seen with dermoscopy can help users correctly diagnose and manage skin cancers and a multitude of other skin lesions. The structures most commonly encountered with dermoscopy are depicted in **Figure 111-4** and explained in the tables under the different steps of the 2-step algorithm.

ALGORITHMS

Multiple algorithms have been created to help users render a diagnosis or to triage lesions.[7-10] If the aim is to reach to a specific diagnosis, the 2-step algorithm is ideal, whereas, if the aim is to triage lesions to detect skin cancer for biopsy or not, the triage amalgamated dermoscopy algorithm (TADA) is a great option.

THE 2-STEP ALGORITHM

The 2-step algorithm was originally described in 2001 as a simplified approach to examine lesions with the dermatoscope and diagnose skin cancer.[11] The first step is intended to aid in the differentiation between melanocytic and non-melanocytic lesions. Melanocytic lesions are tumors (benign or malignant) composed of melanocytes, and these lesions can be pigmented or non-pigmented. Non-melanocytic lesions are tumors composed of cells other than melanocytes, and these lesions can also be pigmented or non-pigmented. The second step of the algorithm helps discriminate between benign melanocytic lesions (nevi) and melanoma.[11] Marghoob and Braun suggested a modified version of the 2-step algorithm in 2010 in order to include the different vascular patterns and hypopigmented melanocytic lesions that were difficult to diagnose with the classic 2-step algorithm.[12-14] This was further modified in 2017 in an attempt to simplify the algorithm by eliminating the need to first differentiate melanocytic from non-melanocytic lesions.[15] The revised 2-step algorithm is based on the rationale that the observer should first try to arrive at a specific diagnosis based on the most common dermoscopic patterns encountered in nevi and non-melanocytic lesions. If this is not possible, then in the second step the observer must exclude melanoma by looking for structures, colors, and patterns associated with melanoma.

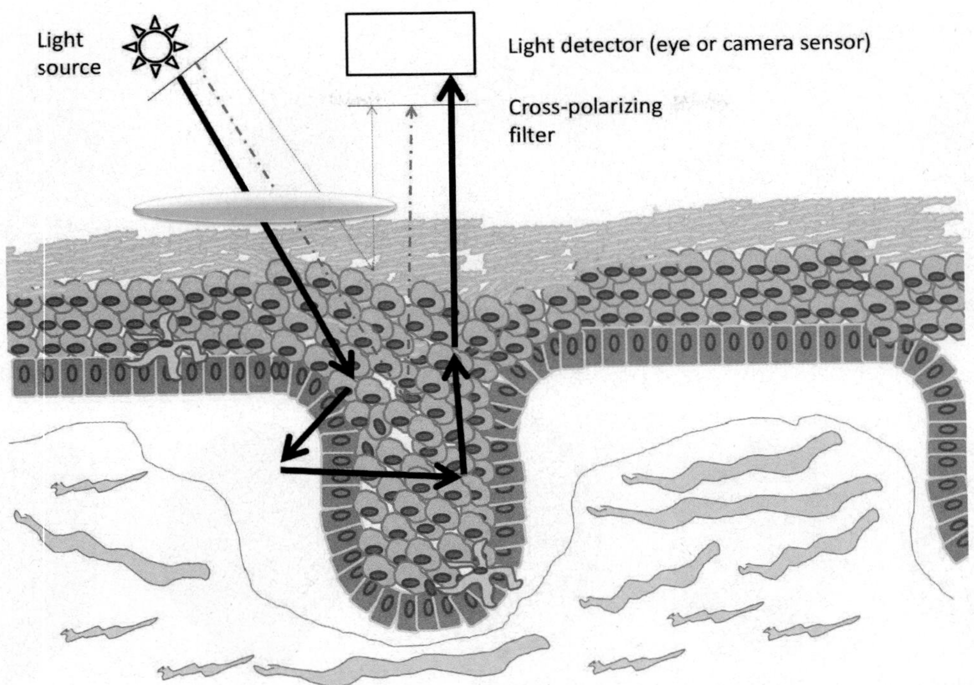

FIGURE 111-3 Polarized dermoscopy. Light is transmitted via the dermatoscope—light source (*blue, black*, and *red arrows*). Deep penetrating light (*black arrow*) is the main source of contrast with polarized dermoscopy. It undergoes multiple scattering events, resulting in randomization of polarization, and reaches our eyes allowing the visualization of dermoscopic structures from dermoepidermal junction and superficial dermis. Surface glare (*blue arrow*) and superficial light (*red arrow*) do not go through the randomization of polarization and cannot cross through the cross-polarized filter.

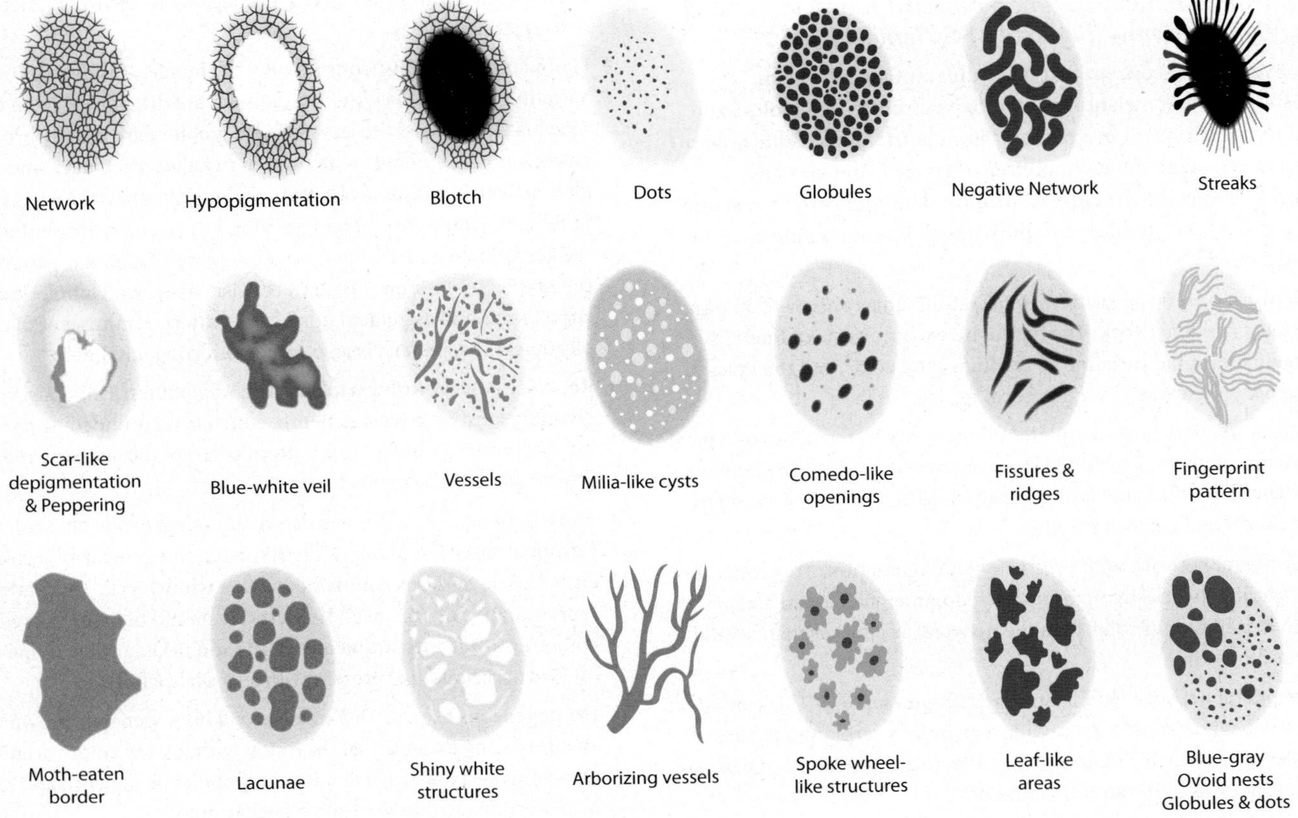

FIGURE 111-4 Structures commonly encountered with dermoscopy. (*Reproduced with permission from www.dermoscopedia.org.*)

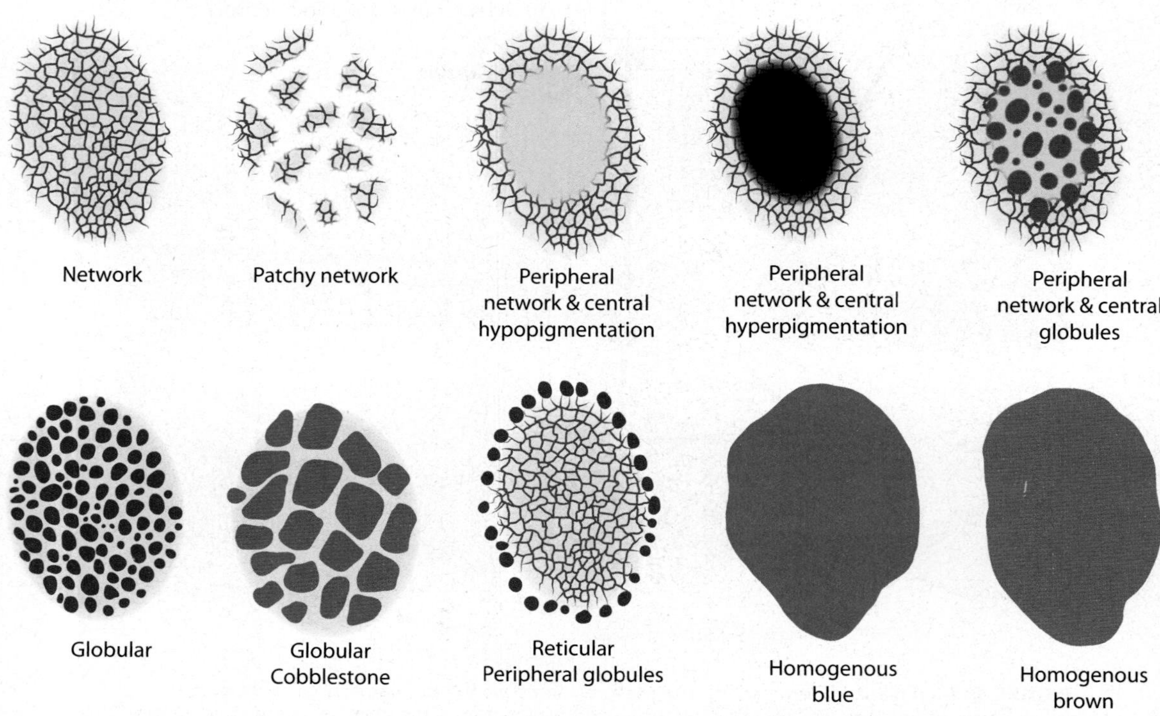

FIGURE 111-5 Common nevus patterns. (*Reproduced with permission from www.dermoscopedia.org.*)

▶ Step 1

Level 1a: The most common patterns found in flat and slightly raised nevi (**Figure 111-5, Table 111-1**)

The overarching concept that helps differentiate nevi from melanoma is that melanomas tend to be disorganized (colors and structures distributed in a random, asymmetric, and chaotic fashion) whereas nevi tend to be symmetric, organized, and lack any melanoma-specific structures. The most common patterns encountered in nevi that are flat to slightly raised, but not sessile or pedunculated, are[16-19]:

- Network or reticular pattern/reticulation: This consists of an organized, typical network. The typical network consists of lines displaying minimal variation in thickness and color, and the holes of the network are relatively uniform in size.
- Patchy network/reticular pattern: This consists of patches of typical network that are distributed in an organized fashion. The network patches have the same type of network with minimal variation in thickness and color of the lines.
- Peripheral network with central hypopigmentation: This consists of a typical network surrounding a hypopigmented central area, which is lighter in color than the network, yet darker than the surrounding skin.
- Peripheral network with central hyperpigmentation: This consists of a typical network surrounding a central hyperpigmented area, called a blotch. This blotch is often due to accumulation of pigment keratinocytes in the stratum corneum.
- Peripheral network with central globules: This consists of a typical network surrounding an area of homogeneous brown pigmentation with typical globules.
- Globular pattern: This consists only of globules, displaying minimal variation in size and color. The globules are distributed in an organized fashion across the lesion. These globules are usually brown in color, but white globules can be seen in balloon cell nevi, and blue globules can occasionally be seen in congenital nevi. However, the presence of multiple globules, varying in size and color should raise the suspicion for melanoma. A specific type of globular pattern called the "cobblestone" pattern consists of brown globules that are large in size and angulated, forming a pattern reminiscent of cobblestones. This pattern is associated with congenital nevi.
- Reticular pattern with peripheral rim of globules: This consists of a centrally located, typical network, which is surrounded by a rim of regular brown globules. This pattern corresponds with the radial growth phase of some nevi.
- Homogeneous blue: This consists of a homogeneous blue color (minimal variation of hues), distributed homogeneously across the entire lesion and is accompanied with a whitish veil. This pattern is representative of blue nevi. However, it should be underscored that epidermotropic melanoma metastasis and nodular melanoma can on rare occasions also present with a similar pattern.
- Homogeneous brown: This consists of a homogeneous brown color encompassing the entity of the lesion without any color variations. Occasionally a few scattered dots or globules or network areas may be discernible within the brown background.

TABLE 111-1 Common Benign Patterns of Nevi

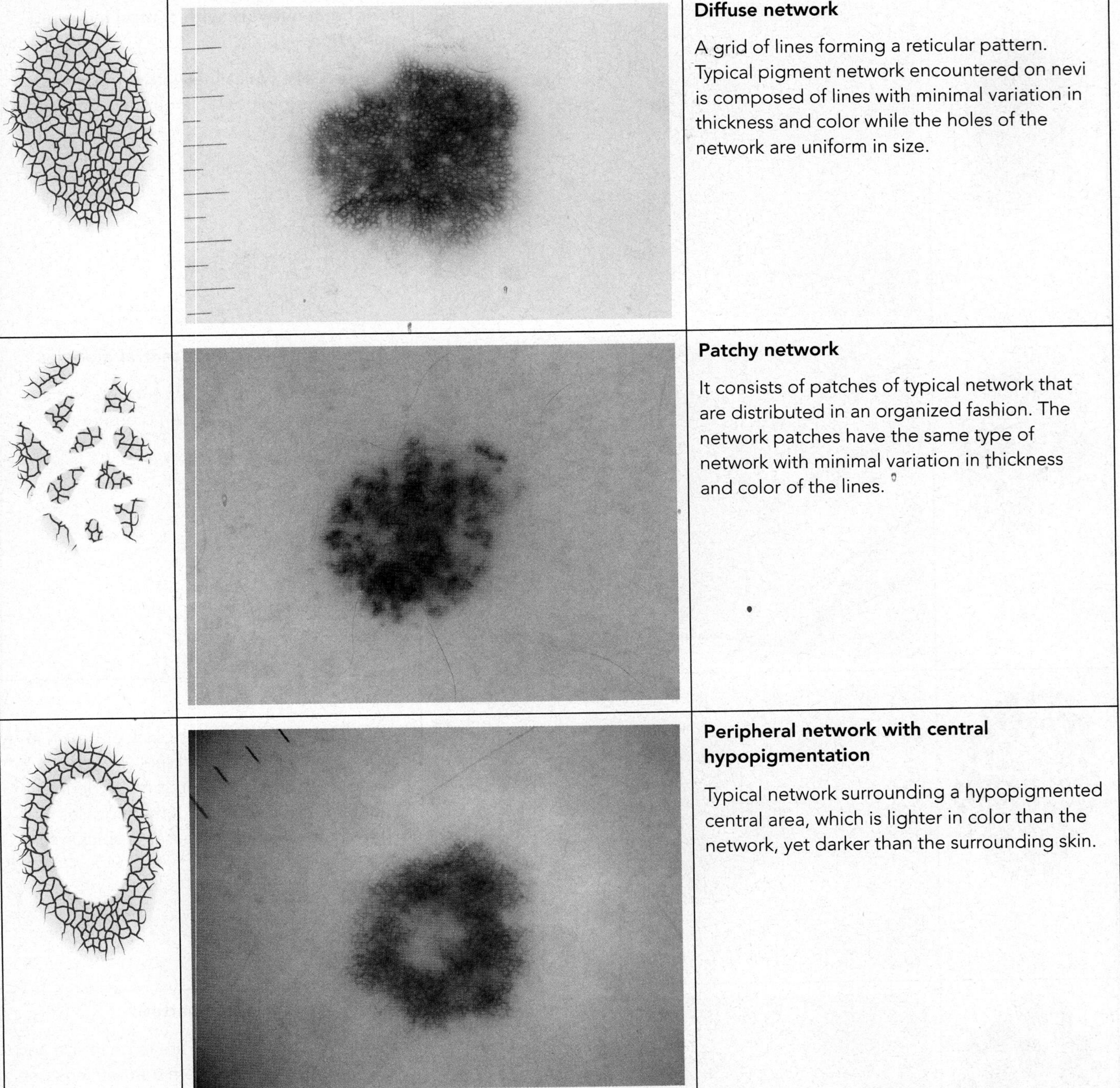

Diagram	Dermoscopy image	Description
		Diffuse network A grid of lines forming a reticular pattern. Typical pigment network encountered on nevi is composed of lines with minimal variation in thickness and color while the holes of the network are uniform in size.
		Patchy network It consists of patches of typical network that are distributed in an organized fashion. The network patches have the same type of network with minimal variation in thickness and color of the lines.
		Peripheral network with central hypopigmentation Typical network surrounding a hypopigmented central area, which is lighter in color than the network, yet darker than the surrounding skin.

(continued)

TABLE 111-1 Common Benign Patterns of Nevi (*Continued*)

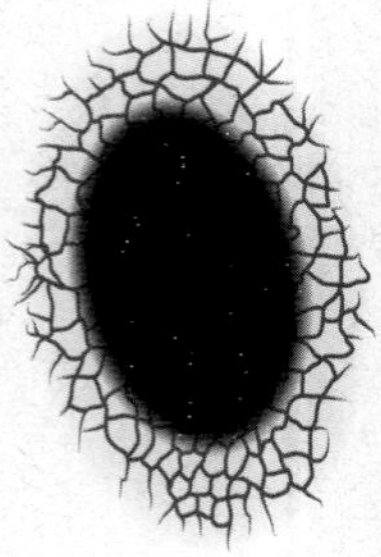	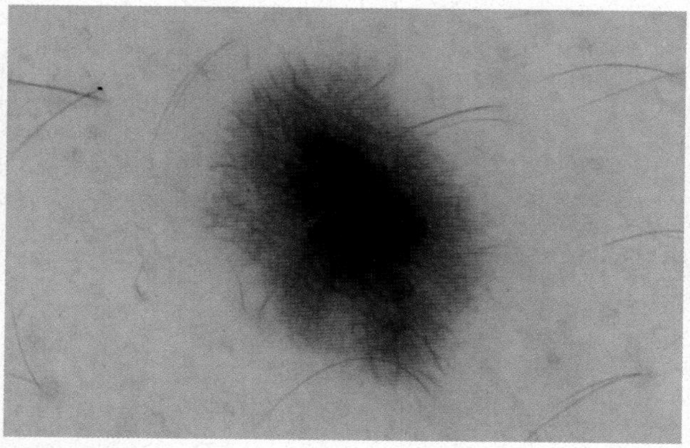	**Peripheral network with central hyperpigmentation** It consists of a typical network surrounding a central hyperpigmented area, called a blotch.
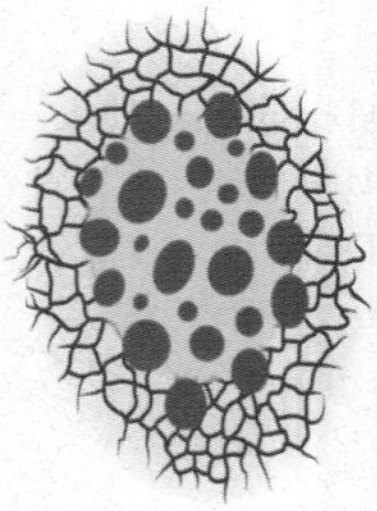	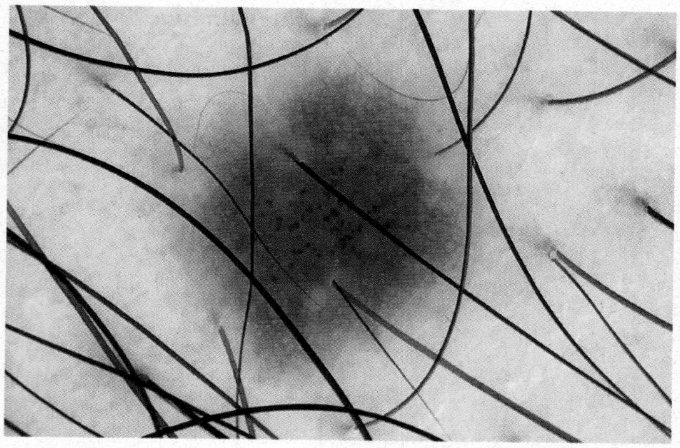	**Peripheral network with central globules** It consists of typical network surrounding an area of homogeneous brown pigmentation with typical globules.
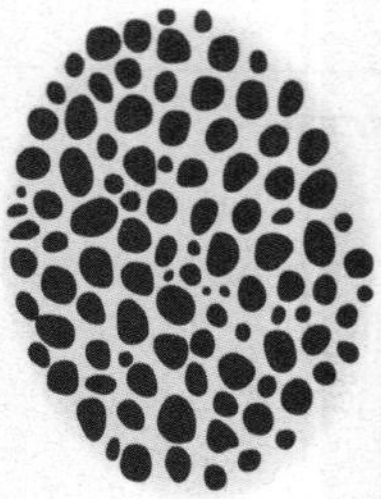	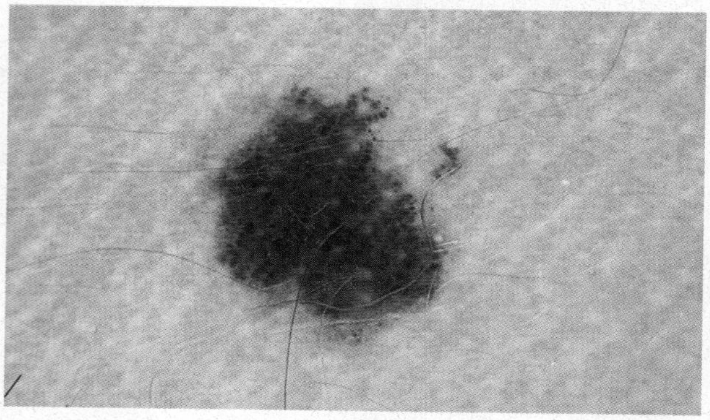	**Diffuse globules** Typical globules are usually black or brown in color, but they can appear blue when the melanocytic nests are located in the dermis. Variation in size and color of the globules makes them atypical and raises suspicion for malignancy.
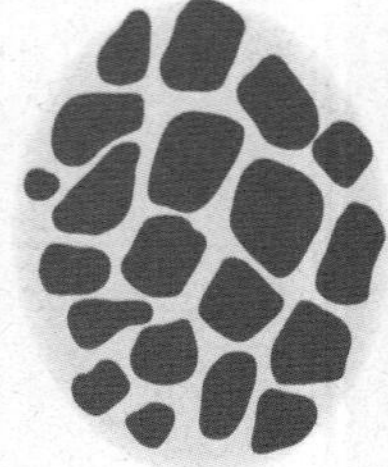	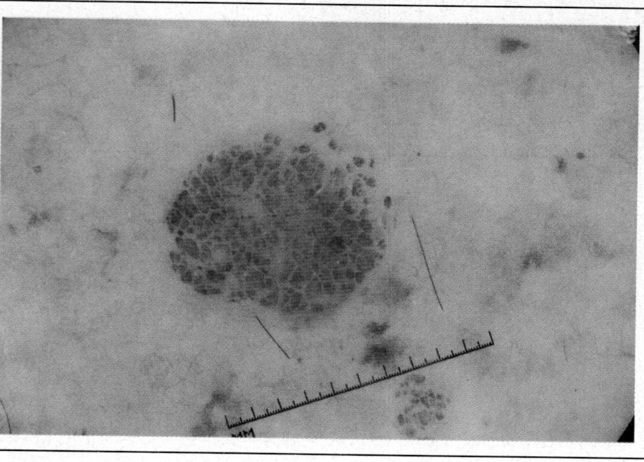	**Globular—cobblestone pattern** It consists of globules that are large in size and angulated, forming a pattern that reminds one of cobblestones. This pattern is associated with congenital nevi.

TABLE 111-1 Common Benign Patterns of Nevi (*Continued*)

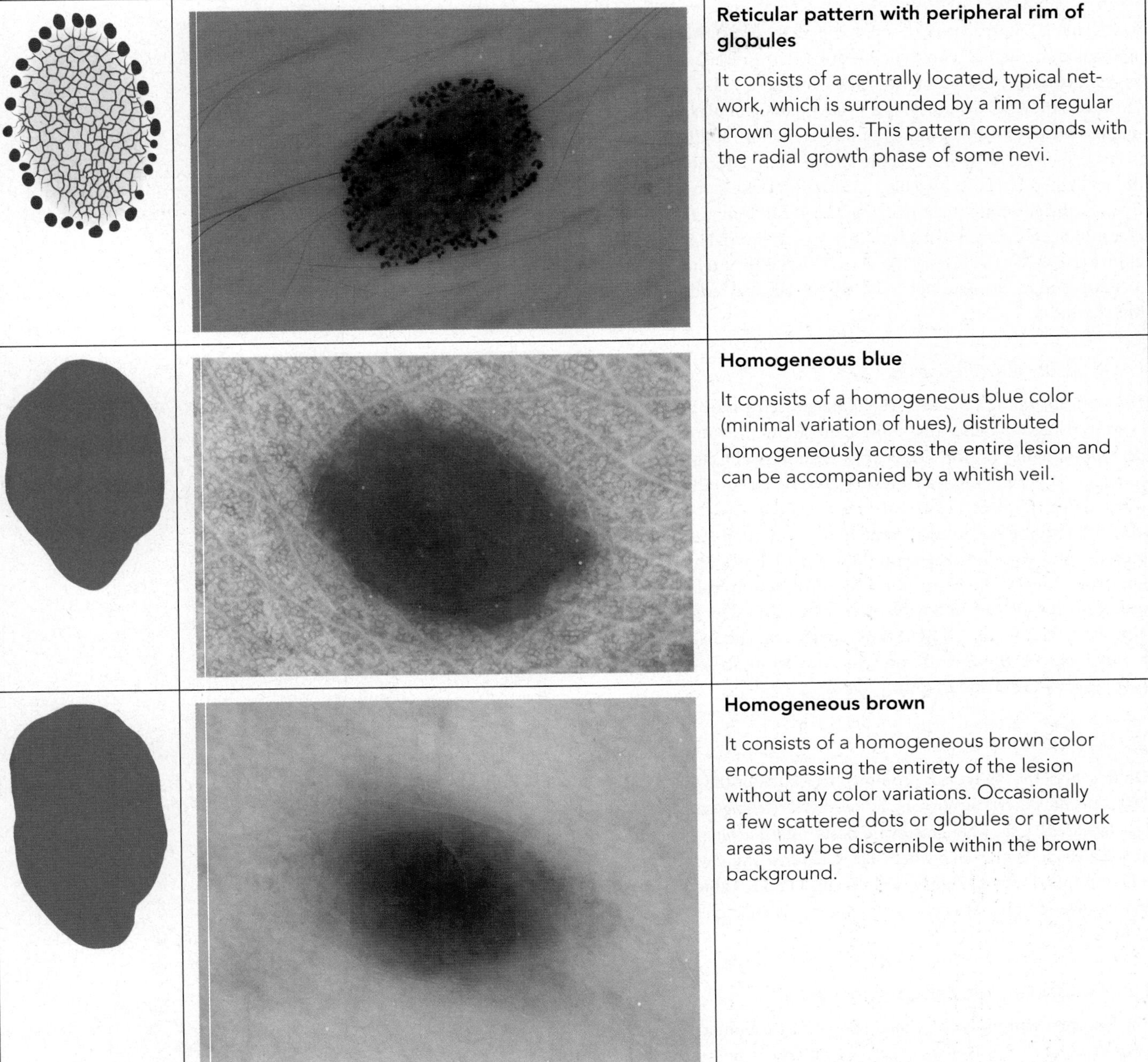

		Reticular pattern with peripheral rim of globules It consists of a centrally located, typical network, which is surrounded by a rim of regular brown globules. This pattern corresponds with the radial growth phase of some nevi.
		Homogeneous blue It consists of a homogeneous blue color (minimal variation of hues), distributed homogeneously across the entire lesion and can be accompanied by a whitish veil.
		Homogeneous brown It consists of a homogeneous brown color encompassing the entirety of the lesion without any color variations. Occasionally a few scattered dots or globules or network areas may be discernible within the brown background.

Reproduced from www.isic-archive.com, courtesy of Harold Rabinovitz, MD and Richard P. Usatine, MD.

Level 1b: Sessile to dome-shaped to pedunculated nevi; intradermal nevi (IDN)

Clinically, IDN present as raised dome-shaped papules or as sessile to pedunculated, mamillated lesions. The presence of multiple comma vessels is the hallmark of IDN (**Figures 111-6** and **111-7**). However, they can also display a brown halo, globules, hypopigmented areas, and small foci of tan pigmentation in the skin that is not associated with any specific structure. In addition, the dome-shaped IDN can also have arborizing vessels, making it difficult to differentiate them from basal cell carcinoma (BCC). The clues that can assist in differentiating BCC from IDN is that in contrast to BCC, the arborizing vessels in the IDN tend not to be as sharply in focus, tend not to be bright red, and tend to have a bluish hue.

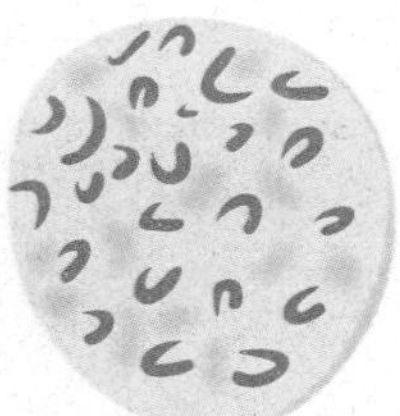

FIGURE 111-6 Schematics of intradermal nevus presenting with comma/curved vessels, brown halo, brown pigmentation, and globules. (*Reproduced with permission from www.dermoscopedia.org.*)

Level 2: Dermatofibromas

Dermatofibromas (DFs) are usually diagnosed clinically as symmetric firm papules that dimple on lateral pressure. On dermoscopy they typically appear as symmetrical lesions with a thin typical peripheral network surrounding a centrally located white patch **(Figures 111-8** and **111-9)**. At the border between the network and the central white patch, one can often see ring-like globules and vessels.[20] The central area of a DF will appear different depending on the light source used. With non-polarized dermoscopy, the central area will appear as a white structureless area. However, with polarized light the central area will display more of a pink hue and will also often reveal shiny white structures (see **Figures 111-8** and **111-9**).[21]

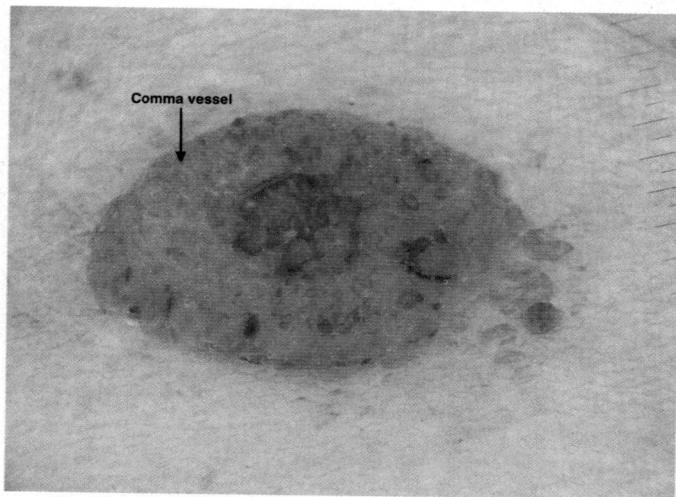

FIGURE 111-7 Typical intradermal nevus with multiple comma vessels. (*Reproduced with permission from www.isic-archive.com.*)

Level 3: BCC

On this level, the observer is prompted to search for the following BCC-specific criteria: arborizing blood vessels (telangiectasias), leaf-like areas, large blue-gray ovoid nests, multiple blue-gray non-aggregated globules, spoke-wheel-like structures, shiny white areas, add multiple erosions **(Figures 111-10** and **111-11, Table 111-2)**. In the absence of a pigment network, these criteria are highly suggestive of BCC.[22-25]

Level 4: Squamous cell carcinoma (SCC)

The features commonly associated with SCC are glomerular vessels, white circles, brown circles, brown dots radially arranged, and yellow scale (**Figures 111-12** and **111-13, Table 111-3**).[26,27] An additional feature called "rosette" is only visible with polarized light. In actinic keratosis (AK), the observer can encounter a strawberry pattern. This is a pink-to-red "pseudonetwork" surrounding the hair follicles, combined with white-to-yellow scale. Linear vessels surround the hair follicles and hair follicle openings and are filled with yellowish keratotic plugs and/or surrounded by a white halo. In keratoacanthoma, in contrast, one often sees hairpin vessels with a whitish halo.[28] These hairpin vessels are often located at the peripheral edge of the keratoacanthoma.[26]

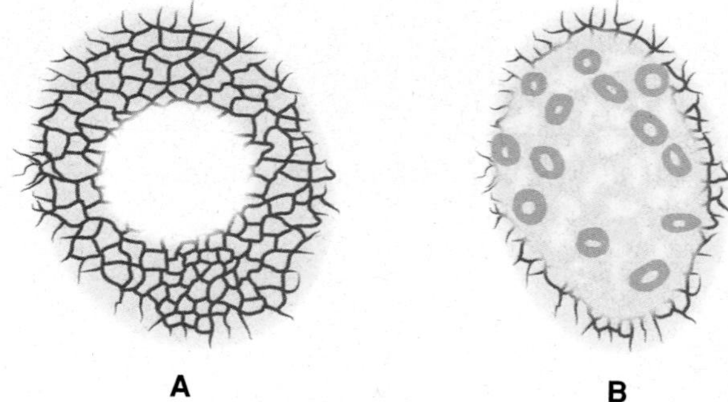

FIGURE 111-8 The two most common patterns seen in dermatofibromas: **A.** Network with central white patch. **B.** Network with ring-like globules, shiny white streaks, and pink hue. (*Reproduced with permission from www.dermoscopedia.org.*)

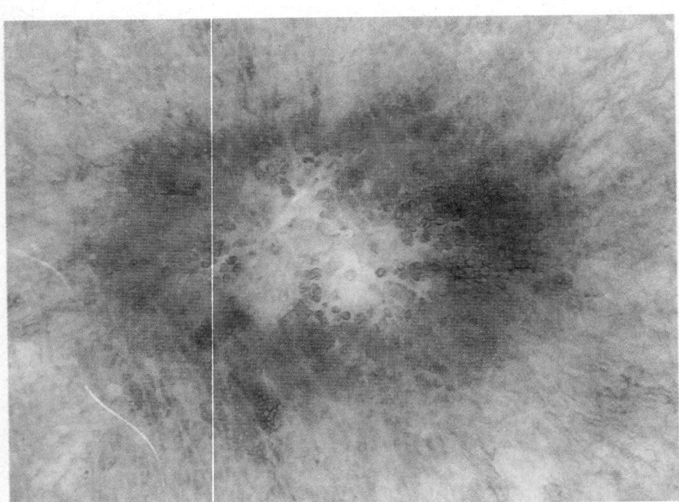

FIGURE 111-9 Dermatofibroma with central white patch, ring-like globules, and fine reticular peripheral network. (*Reproduced with permission from Richard P. Usatine, MD.*)

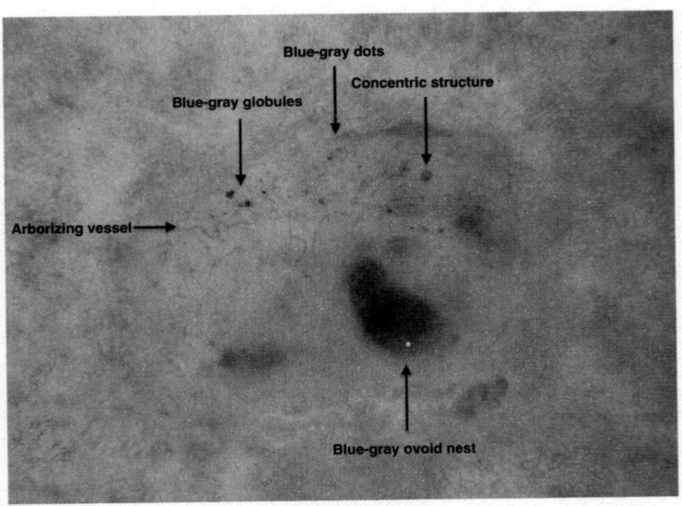

FIGURE 111-11 Basal cell carcinoma presenting with large blue-gray ovoid nests, blue-gray globules, multiple blue-gray dots in focus, concentric structures, and arborizing vessels. (*Reproduced from www.isic-archive.com, courtesy of Harold Rabinovitz, MD.*)

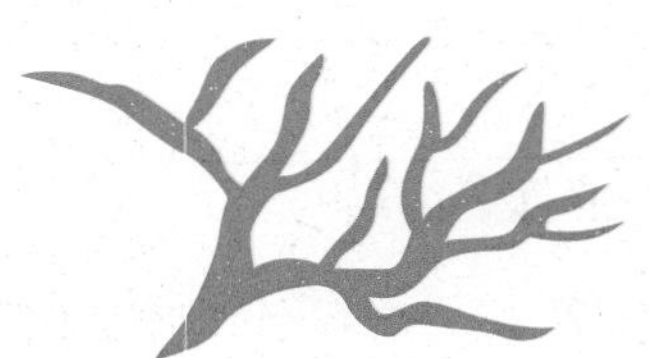

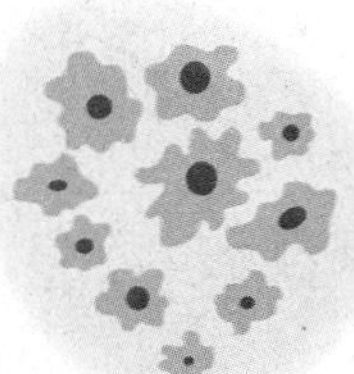

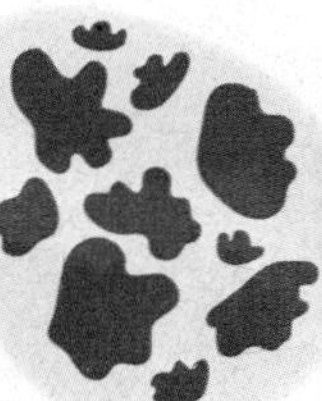

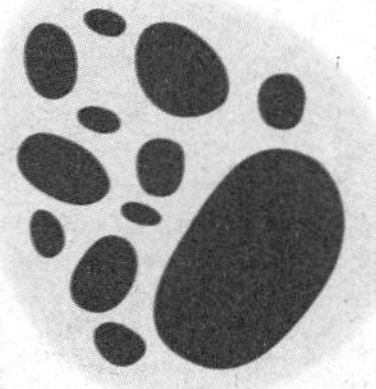

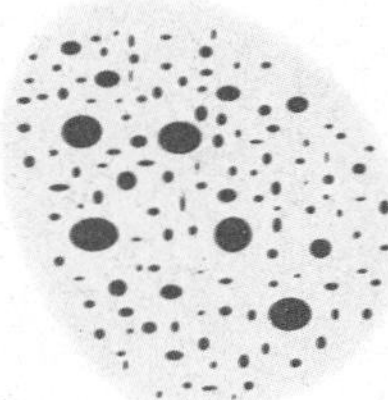

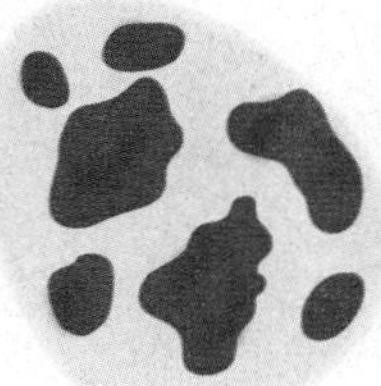

FIGURE 111-10 The most common dermoscopic features of basal cell carcinoma. (*Reproduced with permission from www.isic-archive.com.*)

TABLE 111-2 Basal Cell Carcinomas: Dermoscopic Features

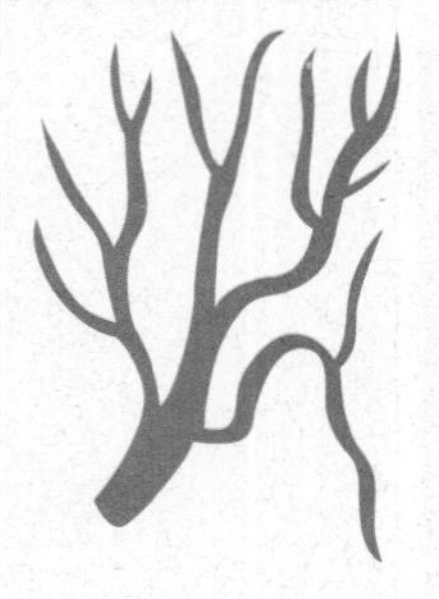	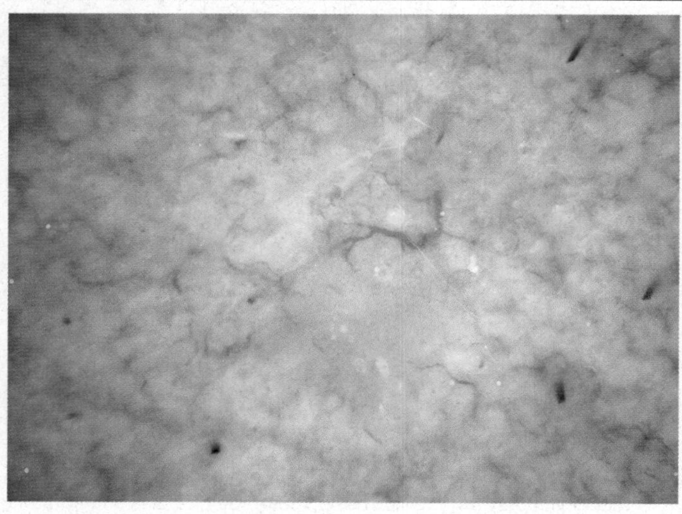	**Arborizing vessels** Vessels originating from a large base and subsequently branching into smaller calibers.
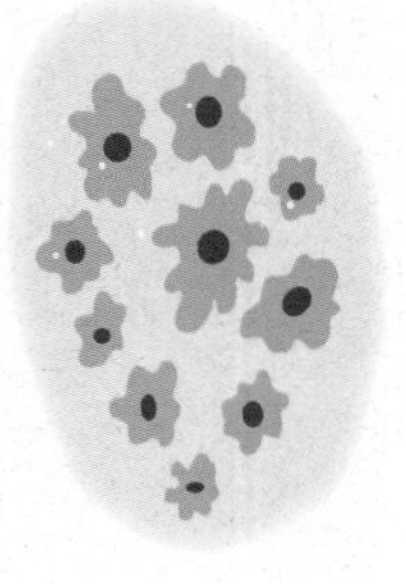	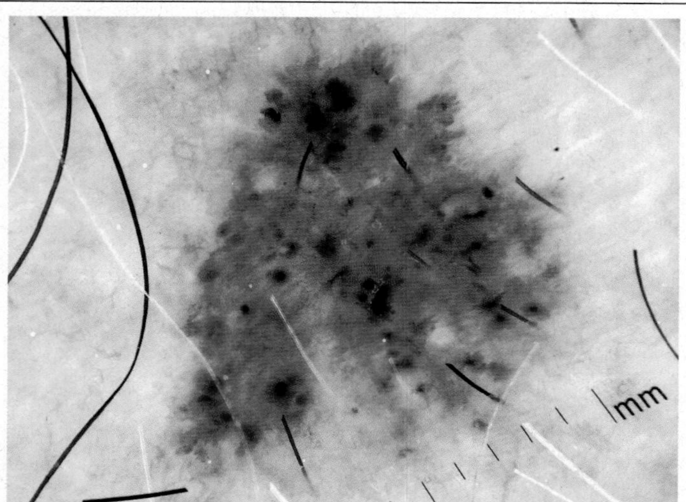	**Concentric structures and spoke-wheel areas** Radial projections surrounding a darker central spot. When the projections are ill-defined, surrounding the dark spot, these structures are called "concentric structures."
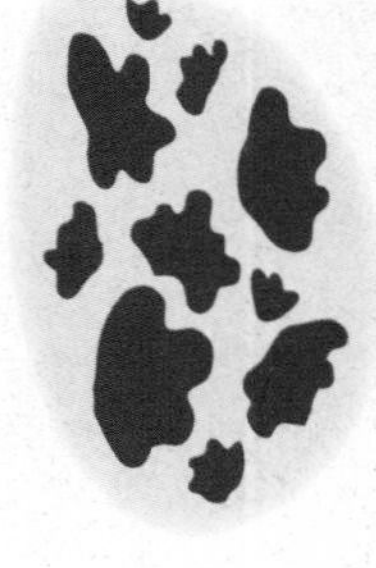	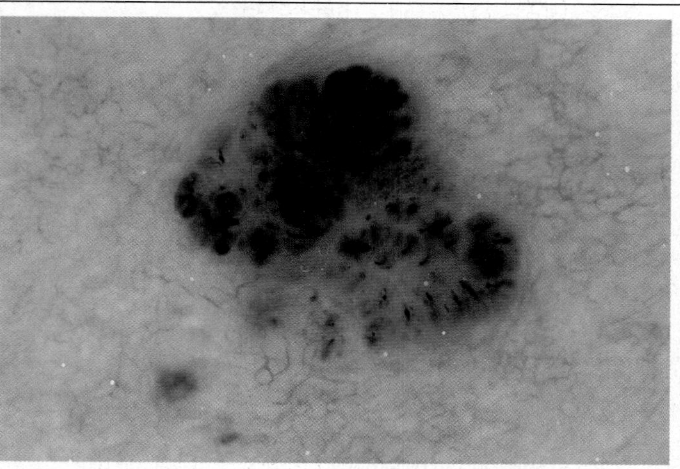	**Leaf-like areas** Brown to blue-gray projections arranged around a common base creating a structure that resemble maple leaves.

TABLE 111-2 Basal Cell Carcinomas: Dermoscopic Features (*Continued*)

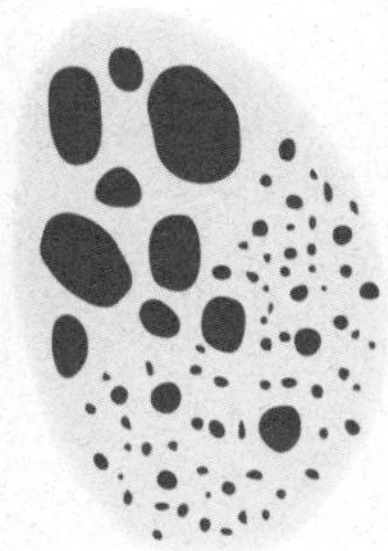	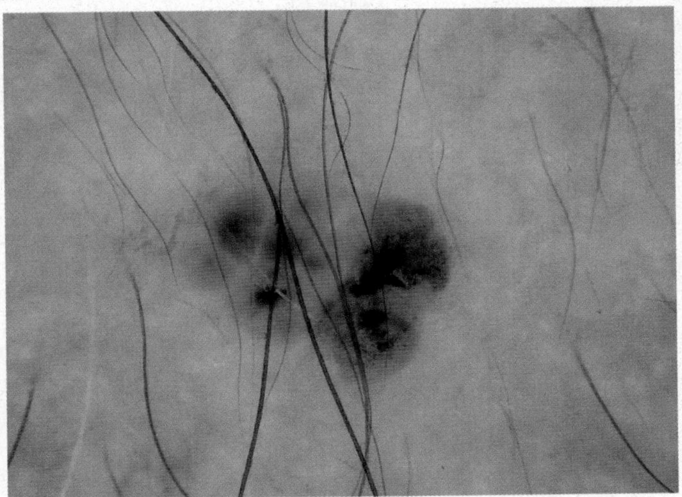	**Blue-gray ovoid nests, globules, and dots** Blue-gray ovoid nests are well-defined, large, ovoid areas within a lesion. Blue-gray globules are well-defined, round to oval structures, occupying less space than the ovoid nests, yet larger than the blue-gray dots, which can appear in a buckshot distribution.
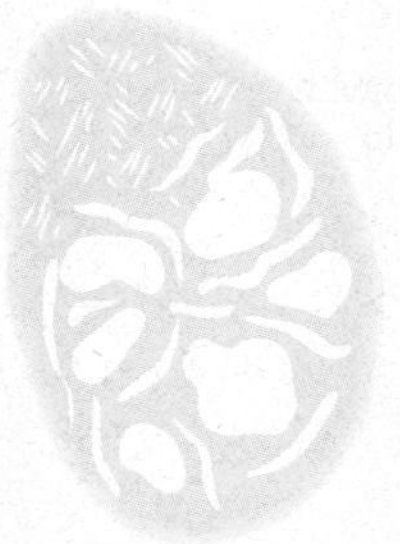	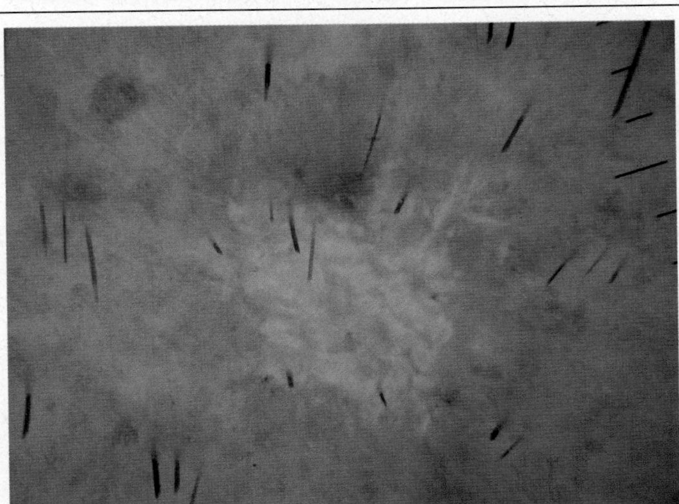	**Shiny white structures** Lines; white, perpendicular, or white structures in the form of circles; oval structures; or large structureless areas that are bright-white longer and less well-defined lines oriented parallel or distributed haphazardly or forming blotches (shiny white clods). Seen only under polarized dermoscopy.
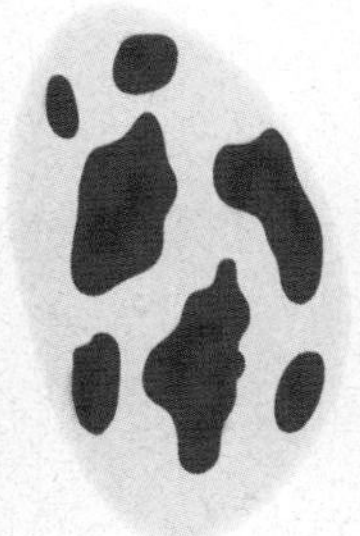	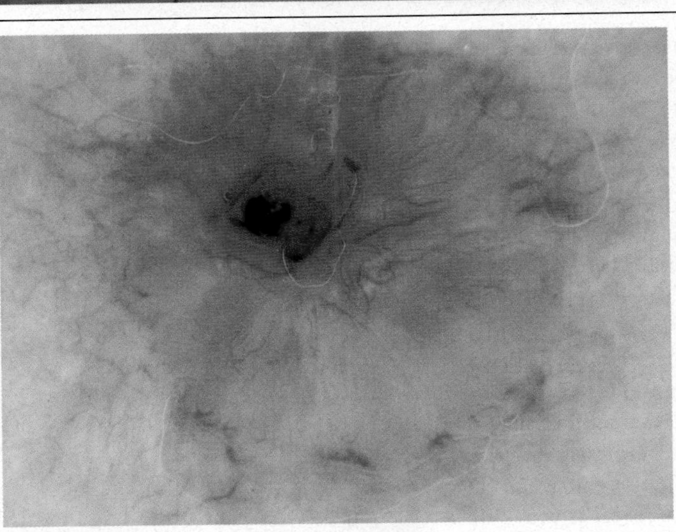	Ulcerations and erosions can appear once or multiple times in a single lesion. They most commonly appear red, covered with black/maroon to orange hue due to a serosanguinous crust. Multiple, small ulcerations are associated with superficial basal cell carcinoma (BCC), whereas the presence of large ulcerations, covering large areas of the lesion, is associated with nodular BCC.

Photos reproduced with permission from www.isic-archive.com, Harold Rabinovitz, MD and Richard P. Usatine, MD.

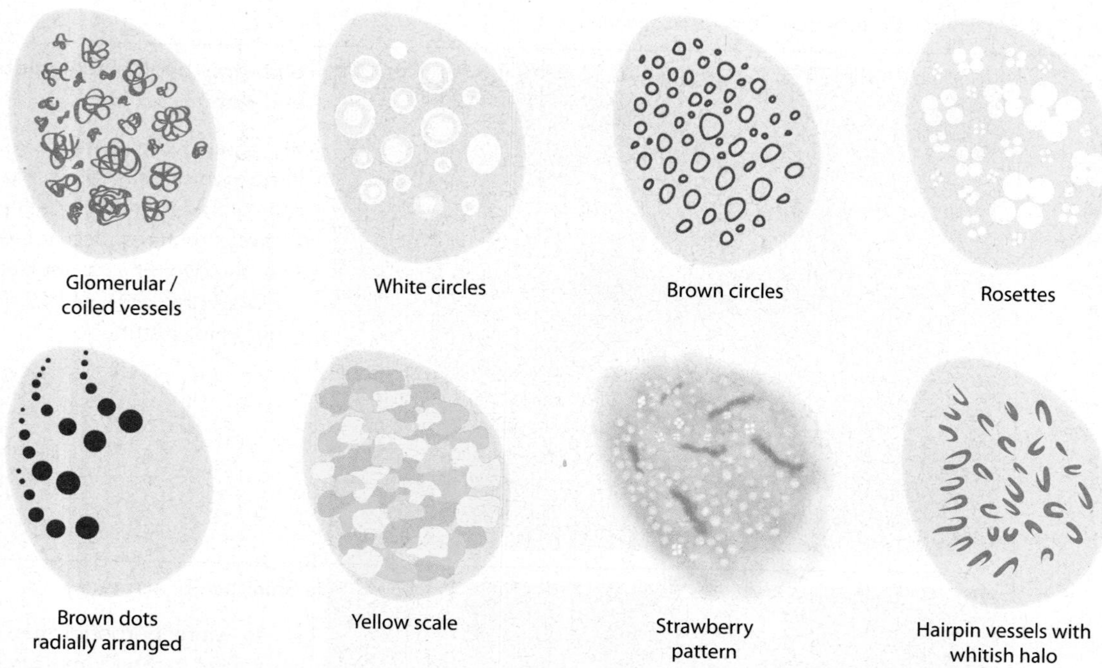

FIGURE 111-12 The most common dermoscopic features of squamous cell carcinoma. (*Reproduced with permission from www.dermoscopedia.org.*)

Level 5: Seborrheic keratosis and lentigo

On this next level the observer is asked to examine the lesion for the presence of any of the seborrheic keratosis (SK) or lentigo specific features. These include milia-like cysts, comedo-like openings, fissures (sulci), and ridges (gyri), which together can create a cerebriform pattern—fingerprint-like structures, moth-eaten borders, sharp demarcation of the lesions, and hairpin vessels with a whitish halo (**Figures 111-14** and **111-15, Table 111-4**).[29-31]

Level 6: Angioma/angiokeratoma

These lesions display red or red-purple to bluish lacunae. The lacunae represent dilated vascular spaces, and as such they usually appear as discrete clods that are separated from each other with intervening stroma. The intervening stroma or septae usually have a blue-whitish color. Thrombosed lacunae present with a black color. Angiokeratomas are benign vascular lesions that display red-maroon and black lacunae with a central blue-whitish veil and having an erythematous halo surrounding the lesion (**Figure 111-16, Table 111-5**).

Level 7: Sebaceous hyperplasia and clear cell acanthoma.

Sebaceous hyperplasia is the overgrowth of sebaceous glands that can mimic BCC on the face (**Figures 111-17** and **111-18**). Clear cell acanthoma is a benign erythematous epidermal tumor usually found on the leg (**Figure 111-19**). Sebaceous hyperplasias are papules that have white to yellowish globules that resemble popcorn or white clouds. These lesions will also reveal crown vessels, which are vessels that radiate towards the center of the lesion but do not cross the midline.[32] The dermoscopic pattern of sebaceous hyperplasia resembles the one seen in molluscum contagiosum. Clear cell acanthomas present as pink lesions that have dotted or glomerular vessels arranged in a serpiginous fashion resembling a string of pearls.[33]

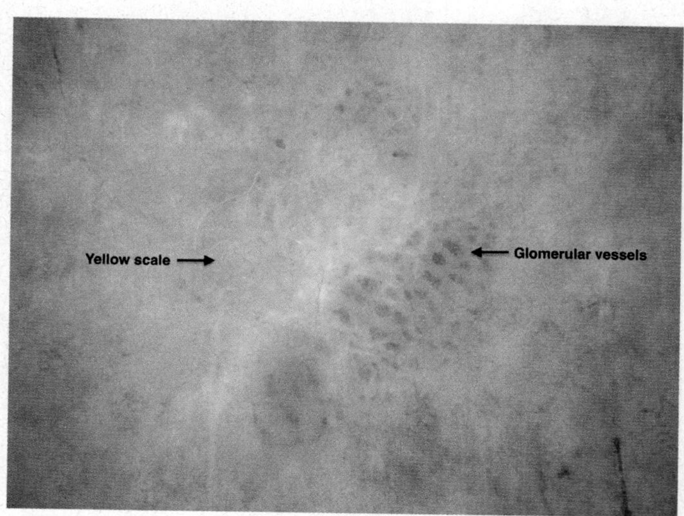

FIGURE 111-13 Squamous cell carcinoma exhibiting multiple glomerular vessels, yellow scale, and shiny white structures. (*Reproduced with permission from www.isic-archive.com.*)

TABLE 111-3 Squamous Cell Carcinomas: Dermoscopic Features

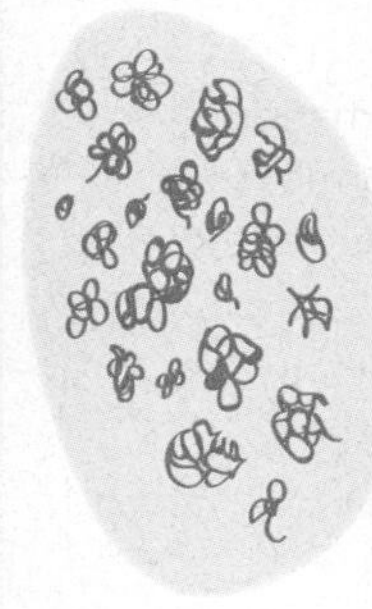	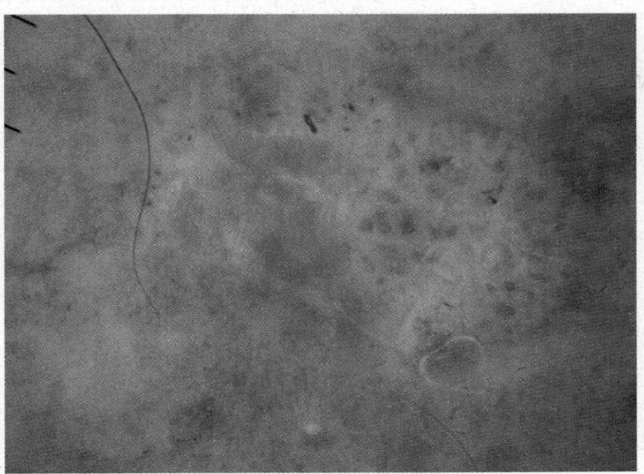	**Glomerular vessels** They are larger than dotted vessels and can be seen in grouped together in squamous cell carcinoma (SCC).
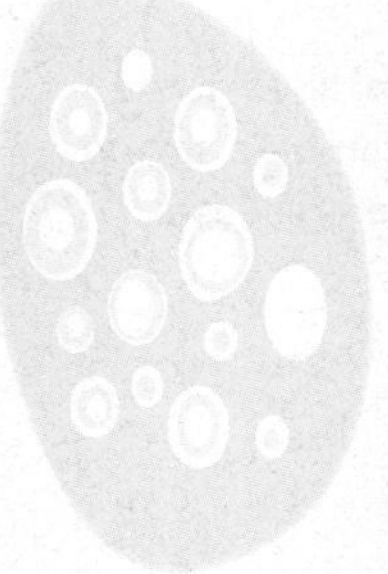	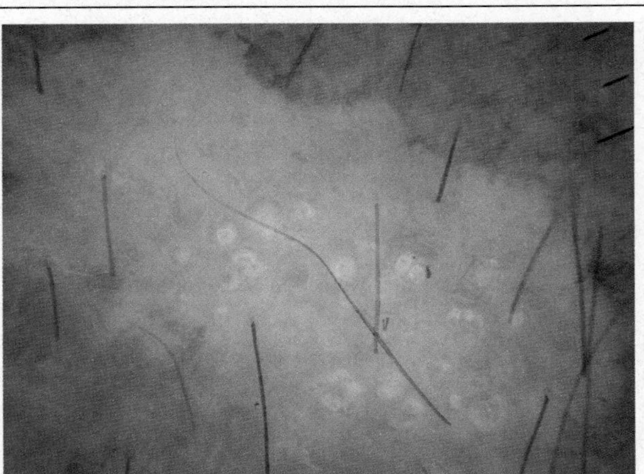	**White circles** White ring-like structures within the hair follicle. The follicle may have a targetoid appearance with central yellowish keratotic plug surrounded by a white halo. This feature is commonly encountered with pigmented actinic keratoses (AKs) and well-differentiated SCC.
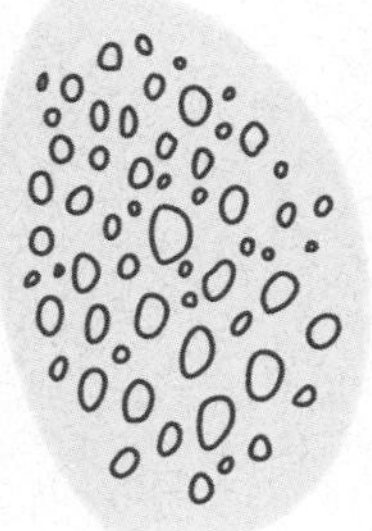	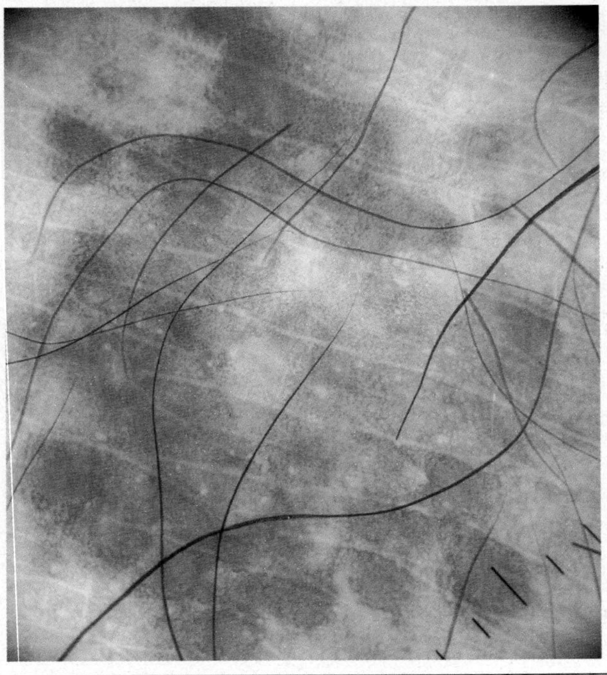	**Brown circles** These brown circles are usually encountered in pigmented SCC.

(continued)

TABLE 111-3 Squamous Cell Carcinomas: Dermoscopic Features (*Continued*)

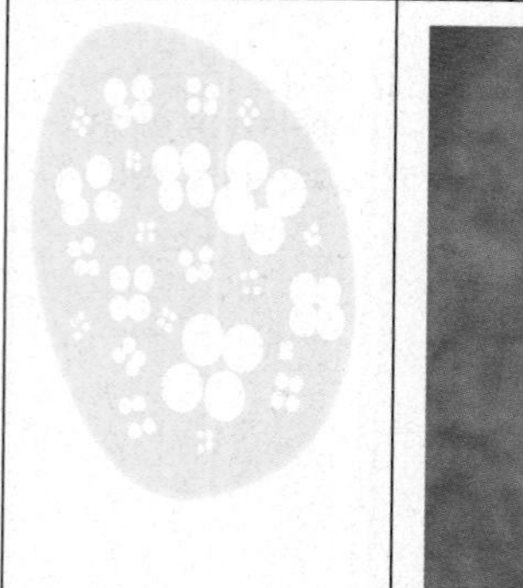	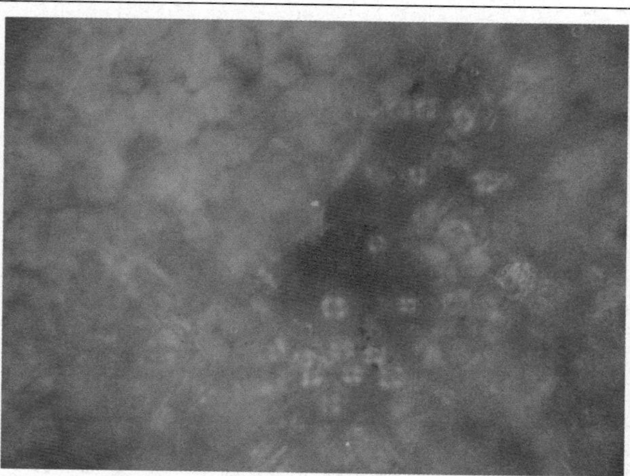	**Rosettes** A white, four-leaf-clover-like formation, apparent only with polarized dermoscopy. It can present as AK, BCC, SCC, and in actinic-damaged skin.
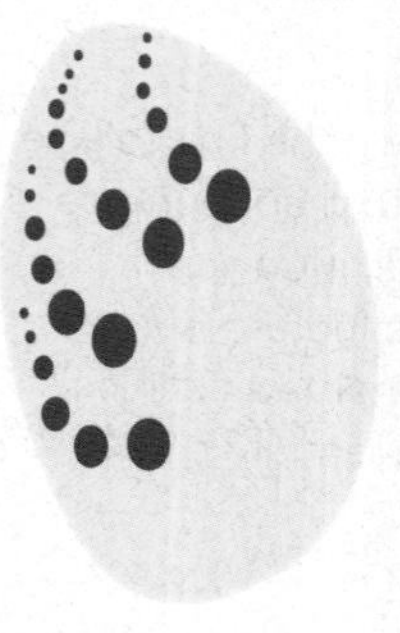	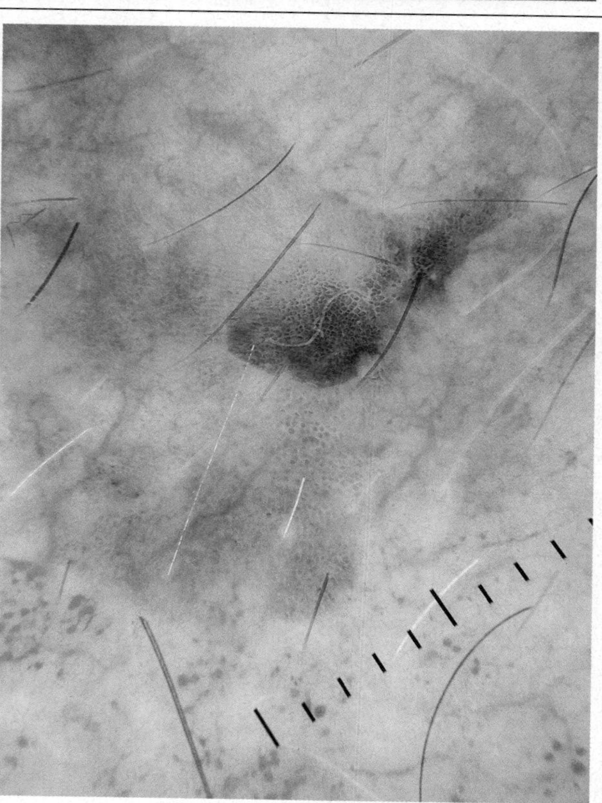	**Brown dots** When arranged as linear radial lines at the periphery of the lesion they can be a strong indicator for pigmented Bowen disease.

TABLE 111-3 Squamous Cell Carcinomas: Dermoscopic Features (*Continued*)

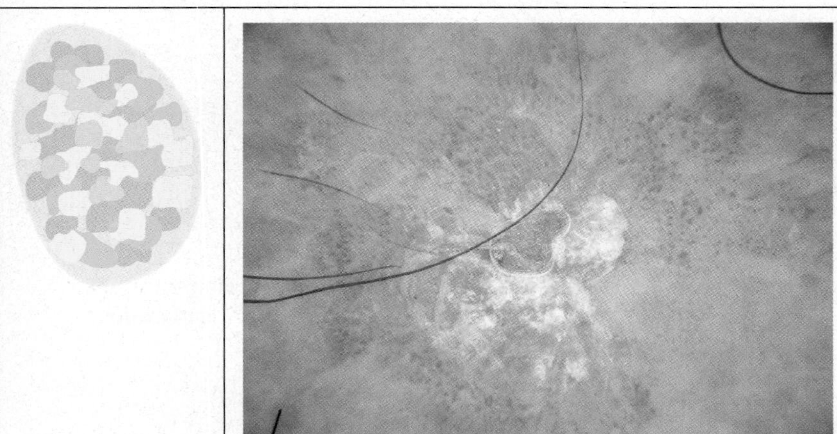		**Yellow scale** The concomitant presence of surface scale (hyperkeratosis) combined with other diagnostic features (i.e., rosettes, white circles, brown dots, brown circles) can lead to the diagnosis of Bowen disease (SCC in situ).
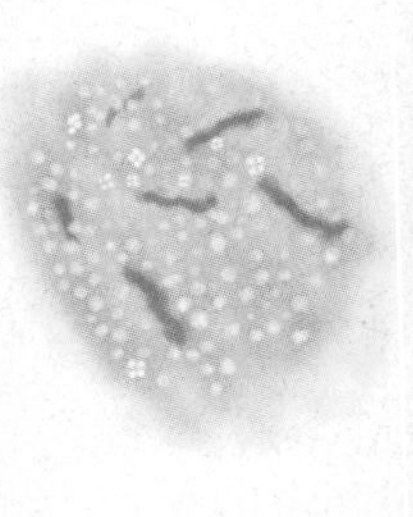	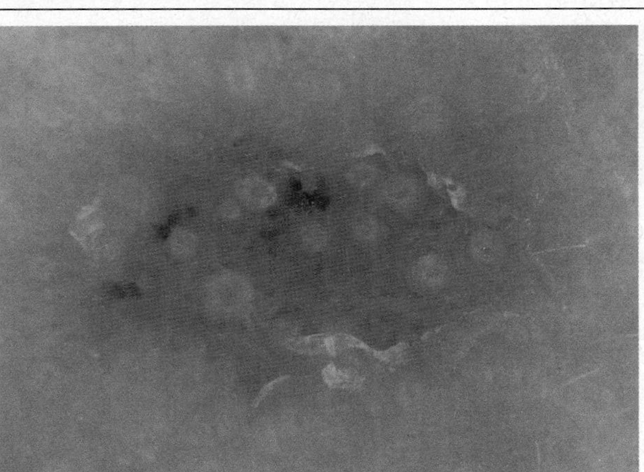	**Strawberry pattern** Pink-to-red "pseudonetwork" surrounding the hair follicles combined with white-to-yellow scale, and linear vessels surrounding the hair follicles and hair follicle openings filled with yellowish keratotic plugs (and/or surrounded by a white halo).
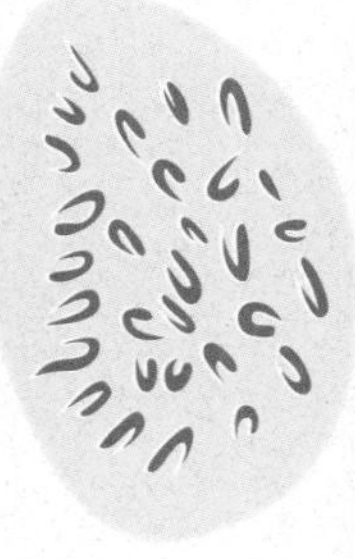	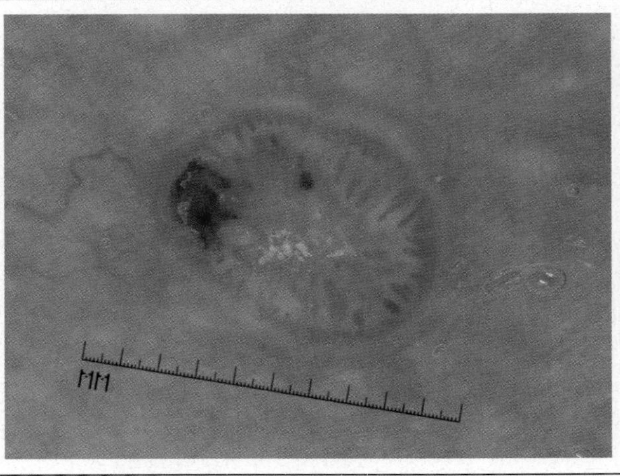	**Hairpin vessels** They have a U shape, resembling that of a hairpin, and they can present with a whitish halo surrounding them. They are typically present in seborrheic keratoses and peripherally in keratoacanthomas (KAs). However, they can also be present in melanocytic lesions and BCCs.

Reproduced from www.isic-archive.com, courtesy of Harold Rabinovitz, MD.

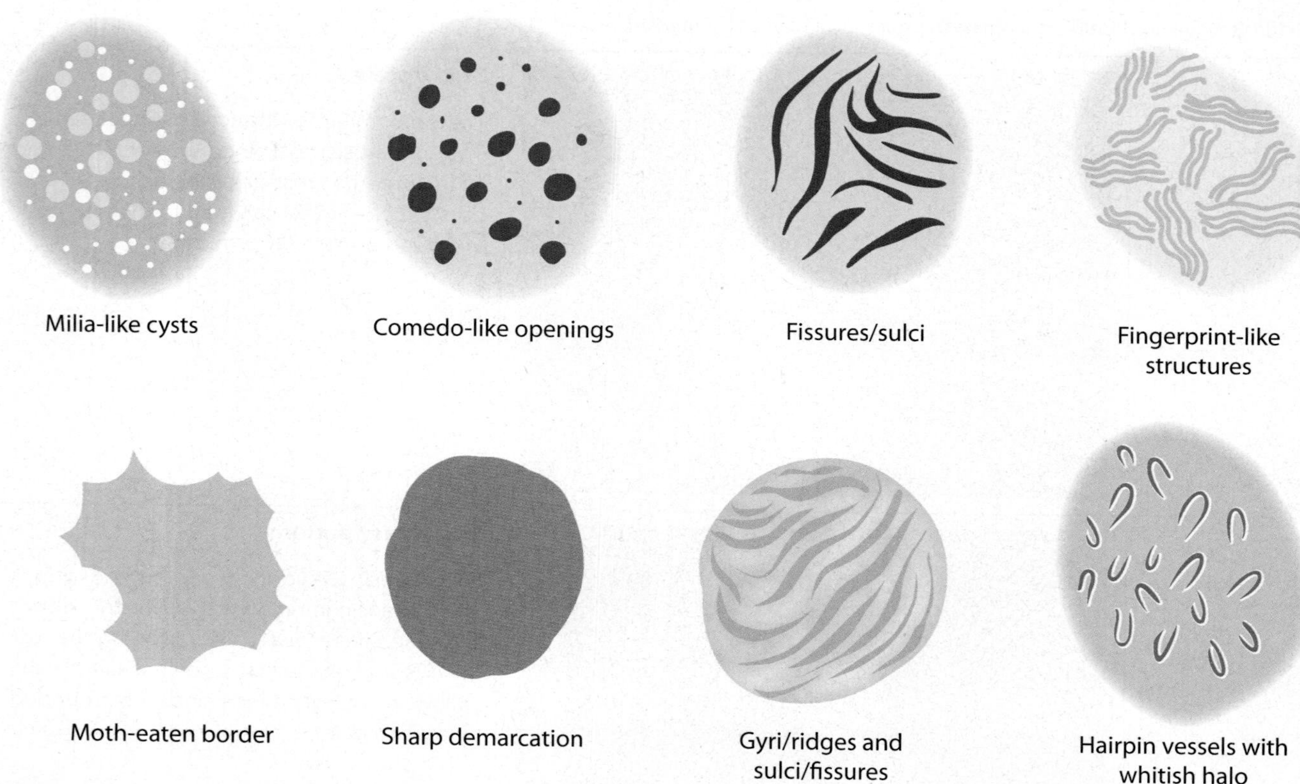

FIGURE 111-14 The most common dermoscopic features of seborrheic keratoses. (*Reproduced with permission from www.dermoscopedia.org.*)

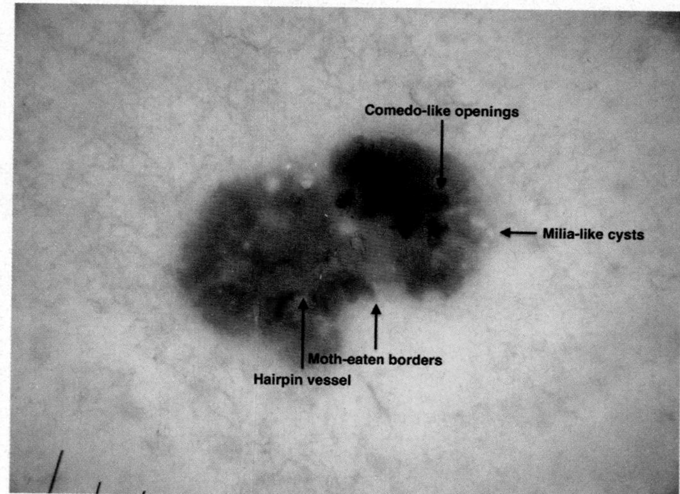

FIGURE 111-15 Seborrheic keratosis presenting with sharply demarcated borders and multiple milia-like cysts, comedo-like openings, hairpin vessels, moth-eaten borders. (*Reproduced from www.isic-archive.com, courtesy of Harold Rabinovitz, MD.*)

TABLE 111-4 Seborrheic Keratosis Dermoscopic Features

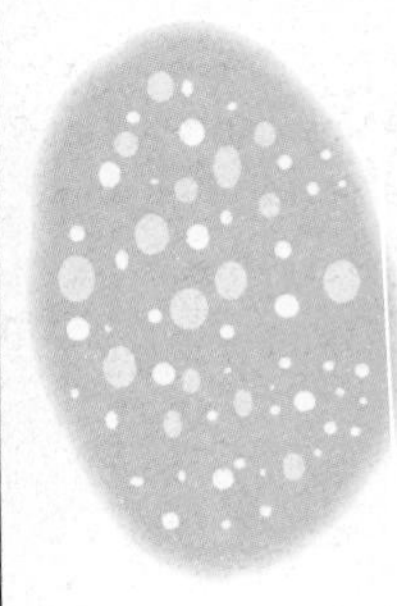	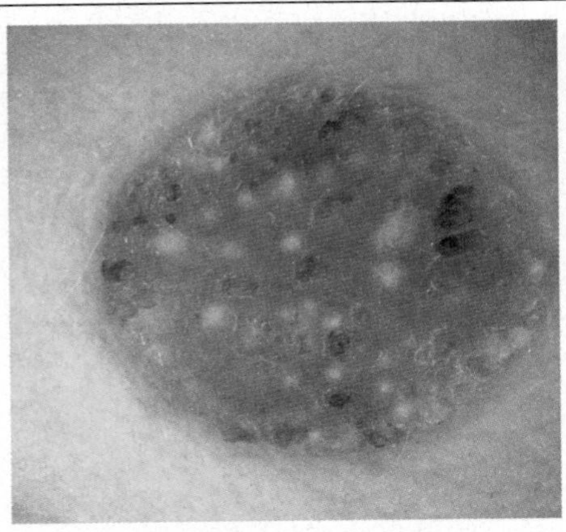	**Milia-like cysts** Round whitish to yellowish structures, typically encountered on seborrheic keratoses.
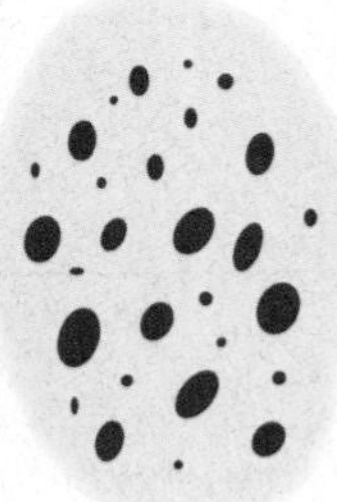	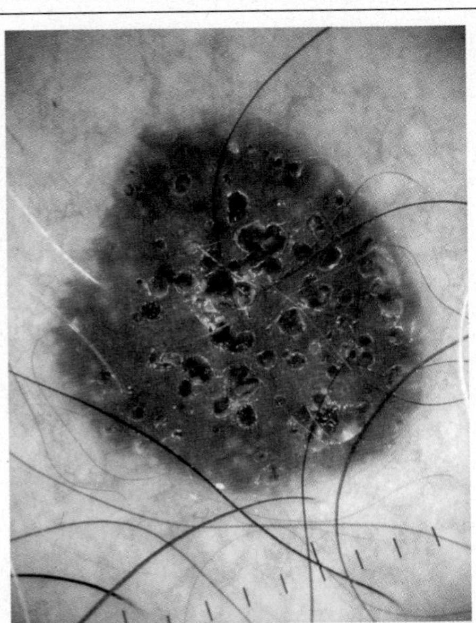	**Comedo-like openings** Dark, round to oval structures filled with keratin, corresponding to surface invaginations. Typically seen on seborrheic keratoses.
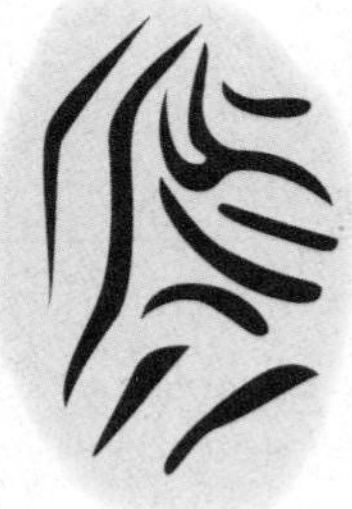	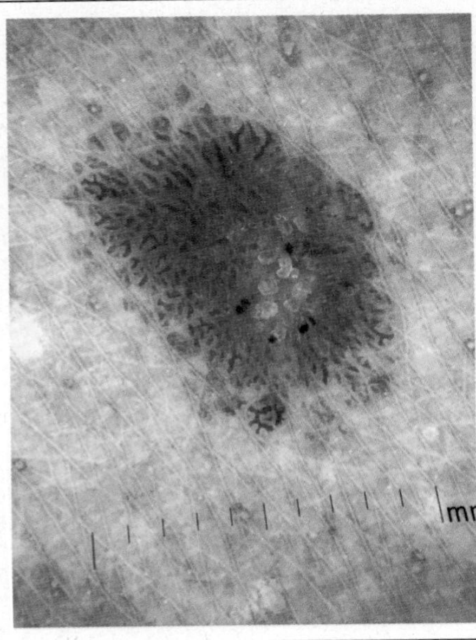	**Fissures and ridges** Dark, elongated surface invaginations filled with keratin. They are similar to comedo-like openings and can create a cerebriform appearance.

(*continued*)

TABLE 111-4 Seborrheic Keratosis Dermoscopic Features (*Continued*)

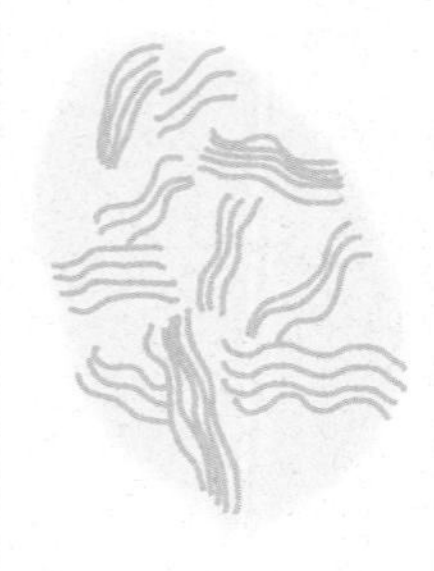	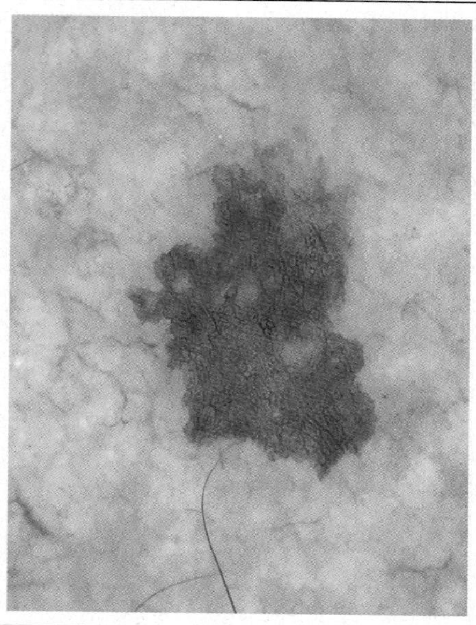	**Fingerprint pattern** Small, parallel ridges producing a pattern reminiscent of that of fingerprints. Typically encountered on solar lentigines and seborrheic keratoses.
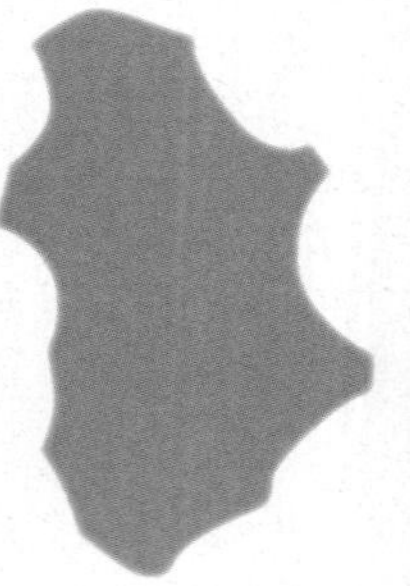	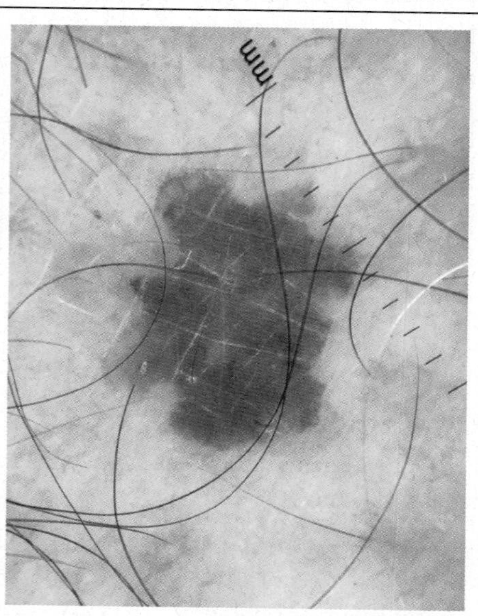	**Moth-eaten borders** Concave borders, ending in a semi-circular fashion resembling that of moth-eaten fabric. Typically presents on flat seborrheic keratoses and solar lentigines.
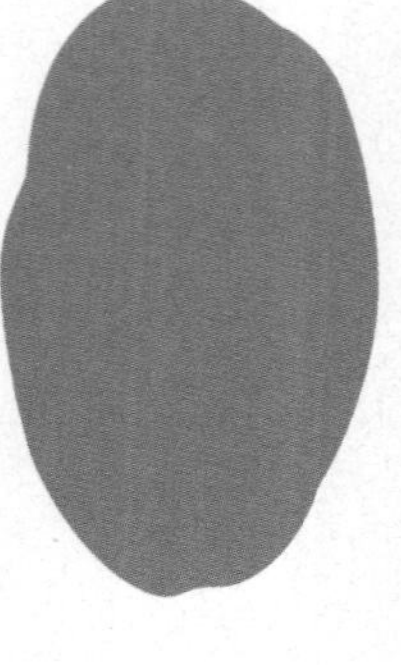	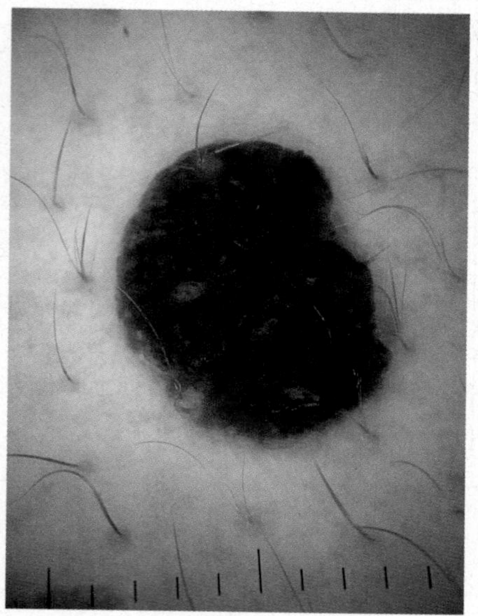	**Sharply demarcated borders** As noticed in clinical examination, seborrheic keratoses usually appear with edges that are sharply delineated.

TABLE 111-4 Seborrheic Keratosis Dermoscopic Features (*Continued*)

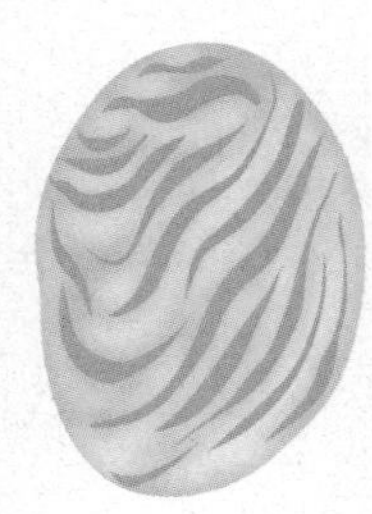	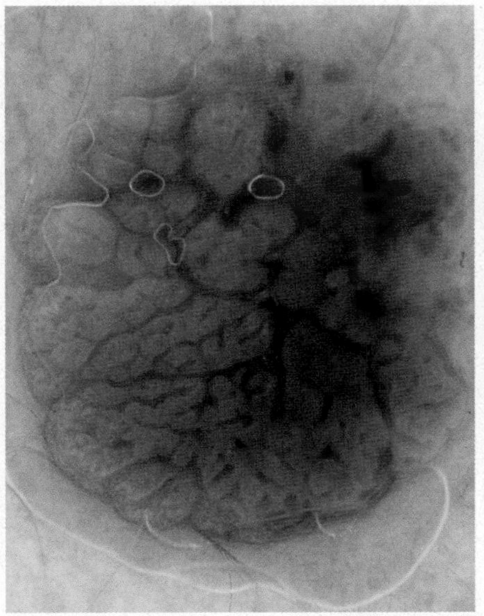	**Gyri/ridges and sulci/fissures creating a cerebriform appearance** The combination of fissures and ridges can lead to an appearance that resembles that of the brain, called a cerebriform appearance.
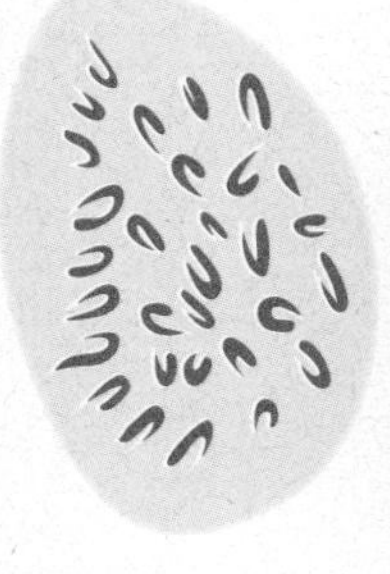	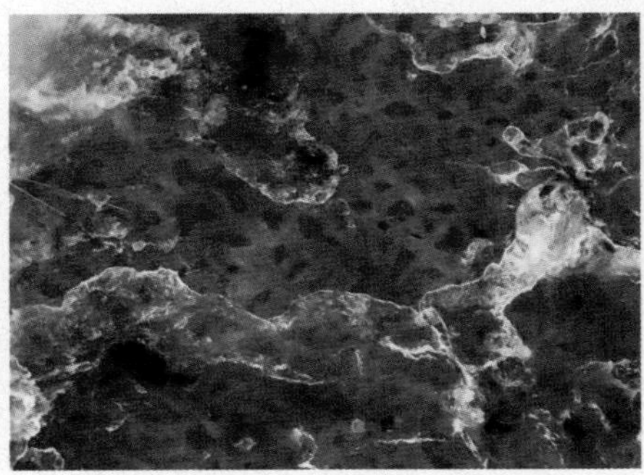	**Hairpin vessels** They have a U shape, resembling that of a hairpin, and they can present with a whitish halo surrounding them. They are typically present in seborrheic keratoses and peripherally in keratoacanthomas (KAs). However, they can also be present in melanocytic lesions and BCCs.

Photos reproduced with permission from Richard P. Usatine, MD.

▶Step 2

If the observer is unable to render a specific diagnosis based on the structures and patterns outlined in step one, then he/she is prompted to proceed to the second step of the algorithm. The main goal of this second step is to maximize the sensitivity for detecting melanoma.

▶Nevi requiring special attention

There are some patterns associated with nevi that require context for their interpretation (**Figure 111-20, Table 111-6**).

1. Two-component and symmetric multi-component nevi: These can be seen in patients with many nevi (atypical mole syndrome or AMS). They will usually have multiple nevi displaying a similar pattern. However, if the lesion is isolated or is an outlier, then melanoma should be ruled out.
2. Structureless tan/pink: If isolated or an outlier, then melanoma remains in differential. In addition, it is important to pay attention to the patient's skin type. These nevi are common in types I–II skin but are considered atypical in darker skin.
3. Peripheral globules/tiered globules: This is another nevus dermoscopic pattern that should be interpreted with caution and should

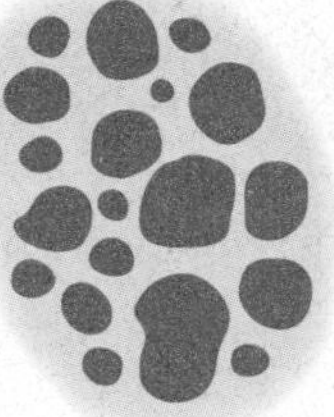

Angioma:
Red lacunae

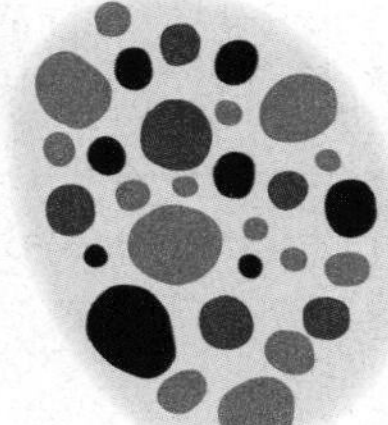

Angiokeratoma:
Red / blue / black lacunae

FIGURE 111-16 Typical dermoscopic presentations of angioma/angiokeratoma. (*Reproduced with permission from www.dermoscopedia.org.*)

TABLE 111-5 Dermoscopic Features of Angioma/Angiokeratoma

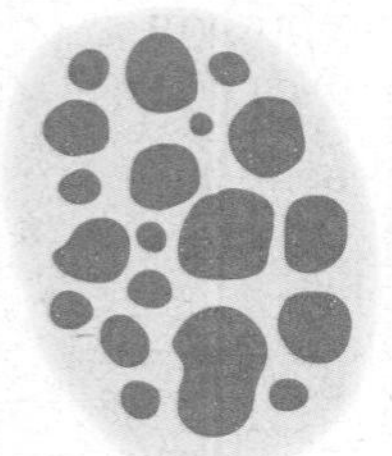 Red lacunae	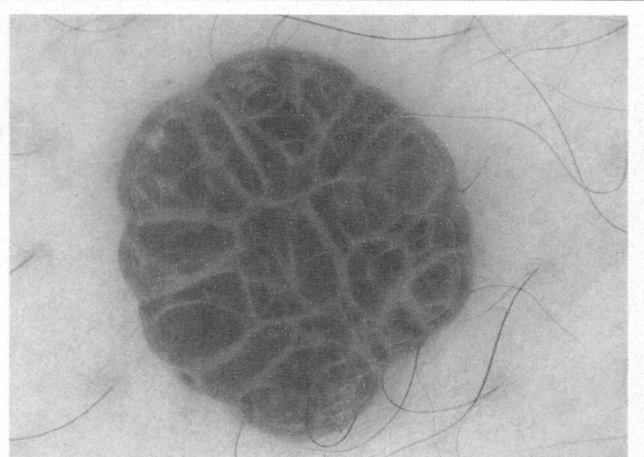 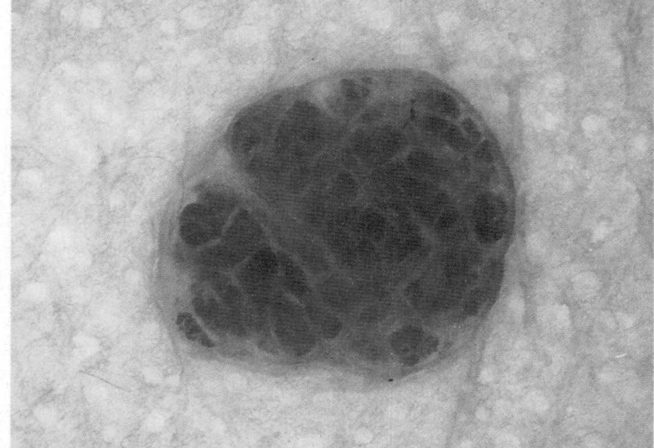	**Angioma** Well-demarcated, round to oval lacunae with red to reddish-blue color. The colored areas are separated by blue-whitish septae.
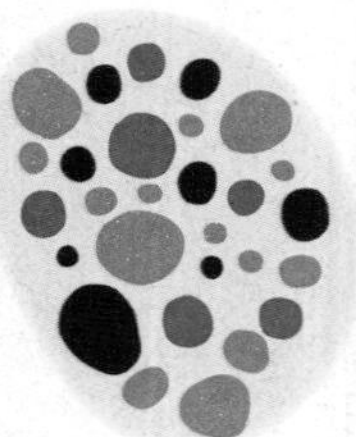 Red/blue/black lacunae	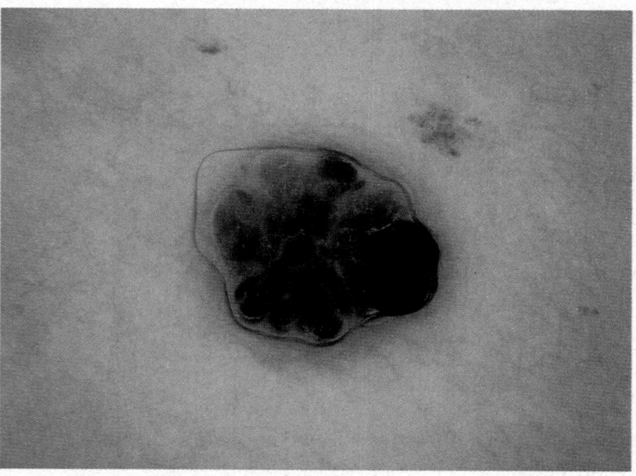	**Angiokeratoma** When vessels forming the lacunae are thrombosed, they can appear with a blue-black to black color.

Photos reproduced with permission from www.isic-archive.com and Richard P. Usatine, MD.

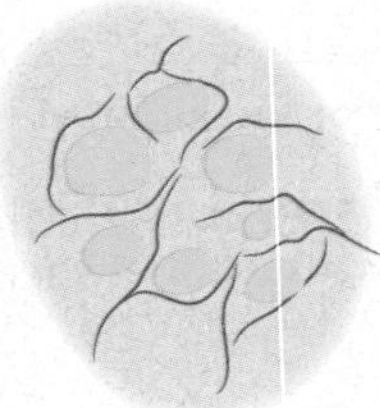

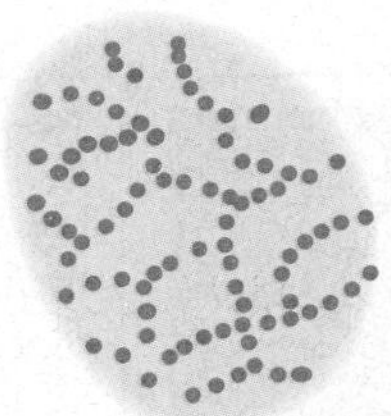

FIGURE 111-17 Typical dermoscopic presentations of sebaceous hyperplasia and clear cell acanthoma (CCA). (*Reproduced with permission from www.dermoscopedia.org.*)

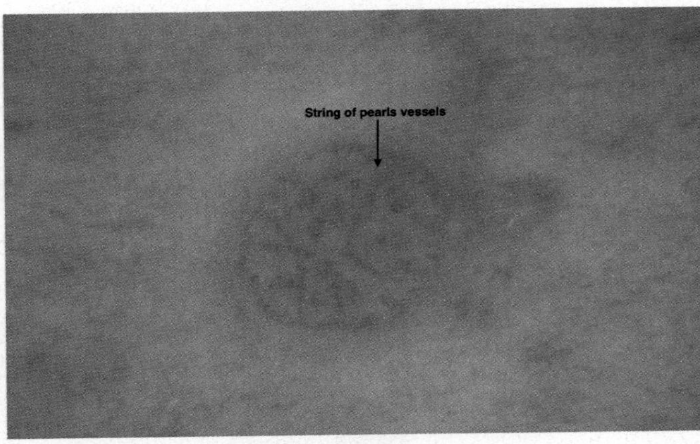

FIGURE 111-19 Typical dermoscopic presentation of clear cell acanthoma with multiple vessels arranged like a string-of-pearls. (*Reproduced from www.isic-archive.com, courtesy of Harold Rabinovitz, MD.*)

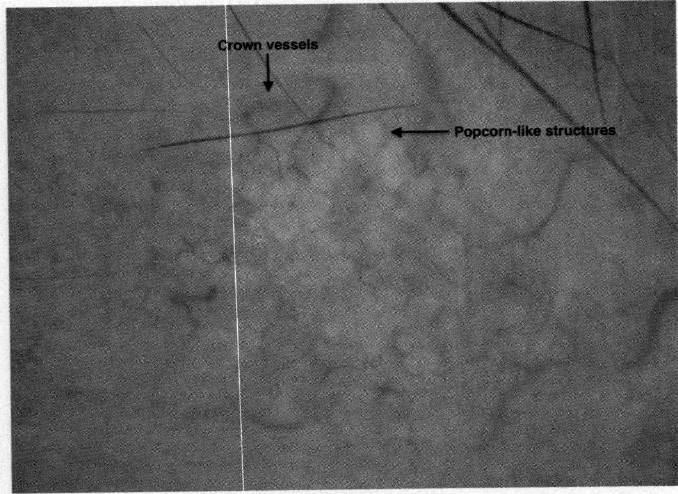

FIGURE 111-18 Sebaceous hyperplasia presenting with multiple vessels in a crown-like arrangement. Although the vessels resemble the arborizing vessels encountered in basal cell carcinomas, they do not cross the center of the lesion. Note the popcorn-like structures formed by the sebaceous glands. (*Reproduced from www.isic-archive.com, courtesy of Harold Rabinovitz, MD.*)

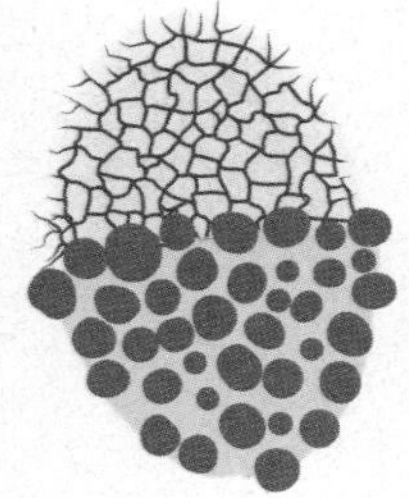

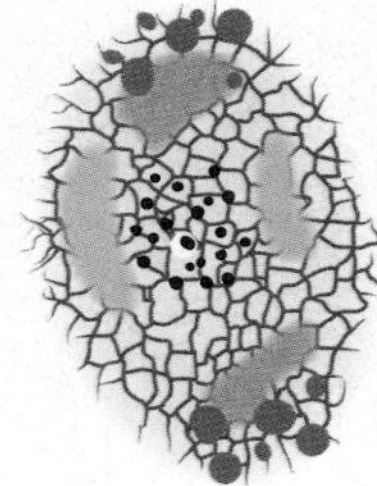

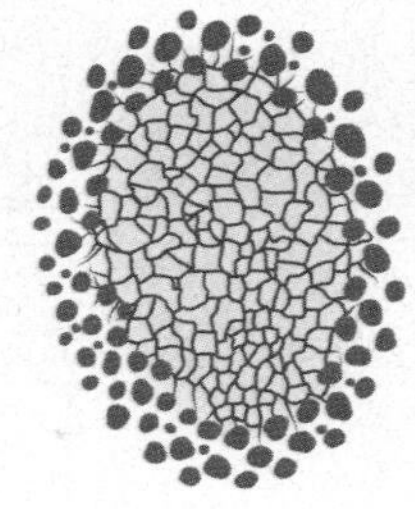

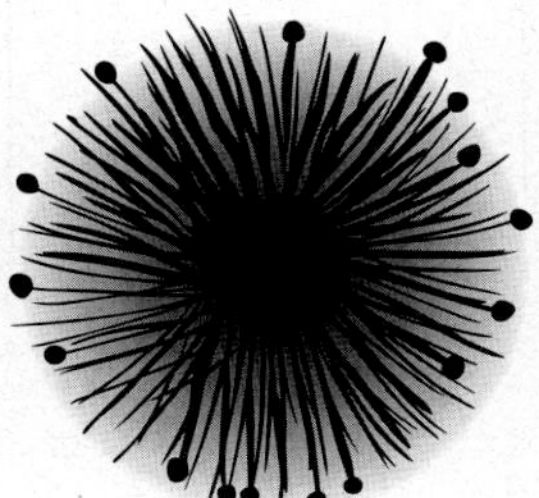

FIGURE 111-20 Dermoscopic nevus patterns requiring special attention to avoid missing melanoma. (*Reproduced with permission from www.dermoscopedia.org.*)

TABLE 111-6 Nevi Requiring Special Attention

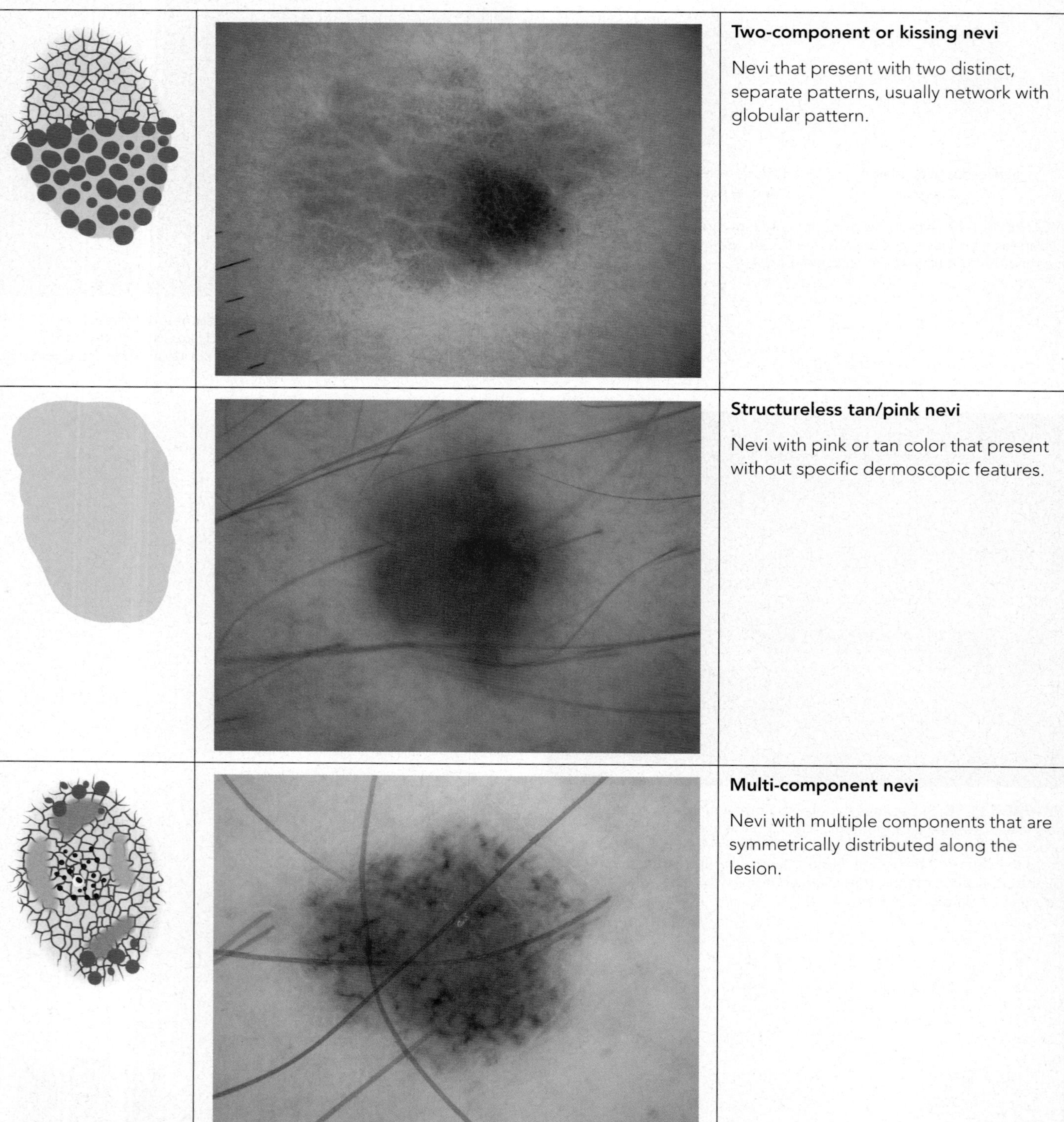

Type	Description
Two-component or kissing nevi	Nevi that present with two distinct, separate patterns, usually network with globular pattern.
Structureless tan/pink nevi	Nevi with pink or tan color that present without specific dermoscopic features.
Multi-component nevi	Nevi with multiple components that are symmetrically distributed along the lesion.

TABLE 111-6 Nevi Requiring Special Attention (*Continued*)

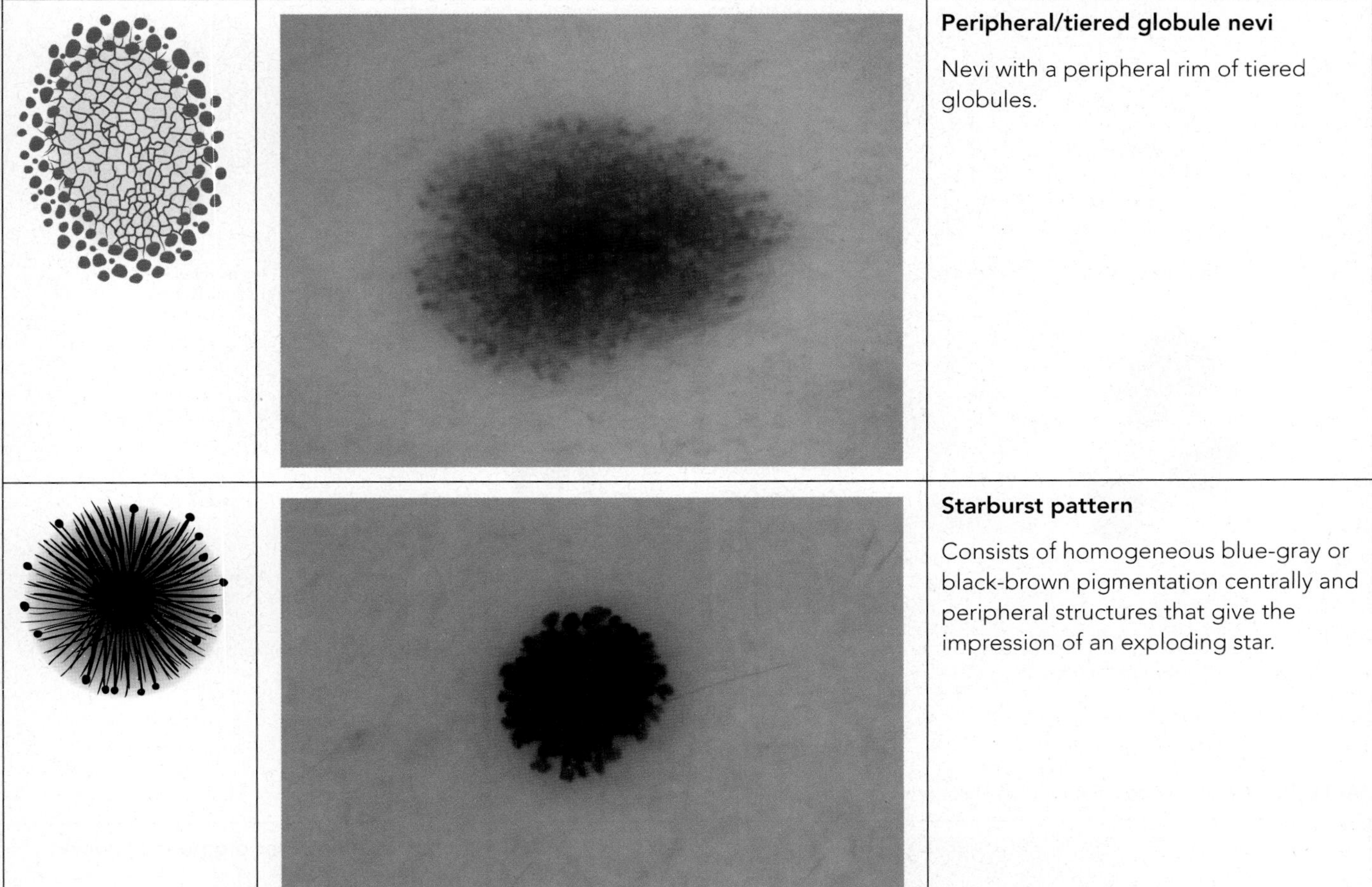

Pattern	Description
Peripheral/tiered globule nevi	Nevi with a peripheral rim of tiered globules.
Starburst pattern	Consists of homogeneous blue-gray or black-brown pigmentation centrally and peripheral structures that give the impression of an exploding star.

Photos reproduced with permission from www.isic-archive.com.

take the patient's age into consideration. Peripheral globules indicate a growing or evolving lesion, which can be expected in patients below 40 years of age but could be indicative of melanoma in older patients.

4. Starburst pattern: The typical presentation of a Spitz or Reed nevus consists of a starburst pattern, identified as homogeneous blue-gray or black-brown pigmentation centrally, and peripheral structures that give the impression of an exploding star may be regularly arranged streaks or radially streaming lines, pseudopods, or globules.[34,35] This presentation should always be evaluated with caution, because although it can be normal in children less than 12 years of age, in older patients it could be a spitzoid melanoma. Thus, a lesion with starburst pattern in people older than 12 years old should be biopsied, or closely monitored.[36]

▶ Final Step: Melanoma

At the final step, the lesion should be examined for the presence of any of the melanoma-specific structures and patterns. Differentiating some nevi from melanoma can be a challenging endeavor. The inclusion of dermoscopy can significantly aid clinicians in making this differentiation.[37-39] Dermoscopic structures that are more commonly associated with melanoma, the so-called melanoma-specific structures, are crucial in differentiating a nevus from a melanoma. The melanoma-specific structures include: atypical pigment network, angulated lines, negative pigment network, atypical dots, irregular globules, irregular streaks, shiny white lines, irregular blotch, blue-white veil, regression structures, polymorphous vasculature, and tan peripheral structureless areas (**Figure 111-21, Table 111-7**).[40] Also see images representative of each feature in Chapter 179, Melanoma.

Atypical/irregular pigment network

Pigment network corresponds to a grid of lines forming a reticular pattern. A pigment network is a common feature among all melanocytic lesions, but it becomes concerning when it is atypical. In an atypical pigment network, the network lines vary in size, color, thickness, and distribution.[41] Determination of what is atypical is often individualized in each patient, since a patient with an atypical nevus syndrome, for example, may have multiple nevi with atypical appearance without any of them being an outlier for the particular patient. When atypical, the rete ridges appear disarranged and there is a varying number of atypical melanocytes.[42]

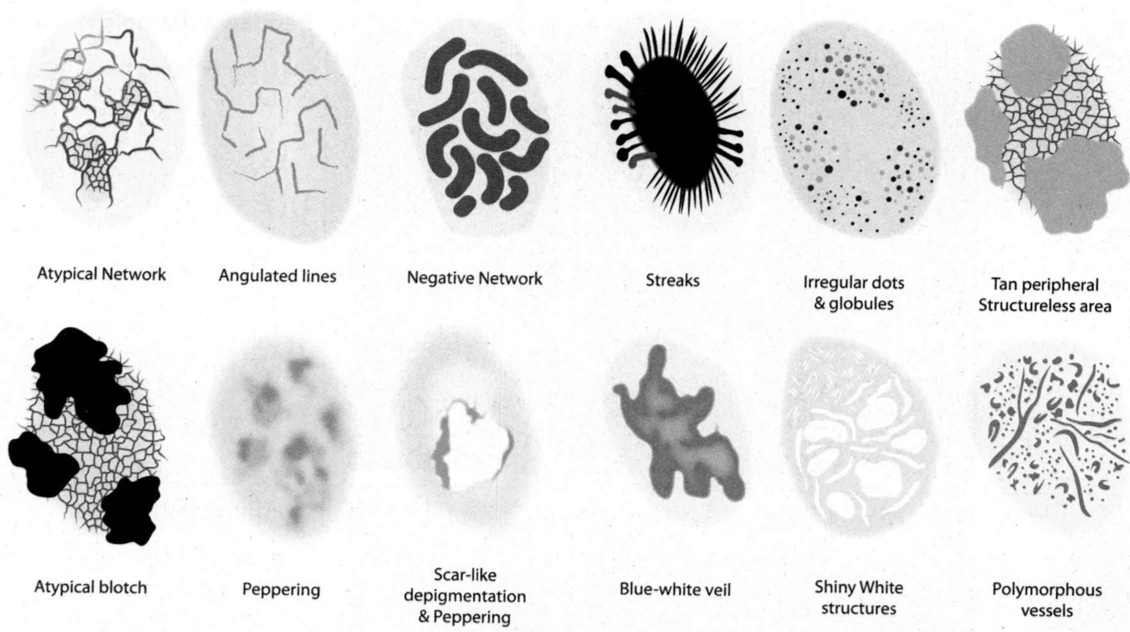

FIGURE 111-21 Schematics of dermoscopic melanoma-specific features. (*Reproduced with permission from www.dermoscopedia.org.*)

TABLE 111-7 Dermoscopic Features of Melanoma

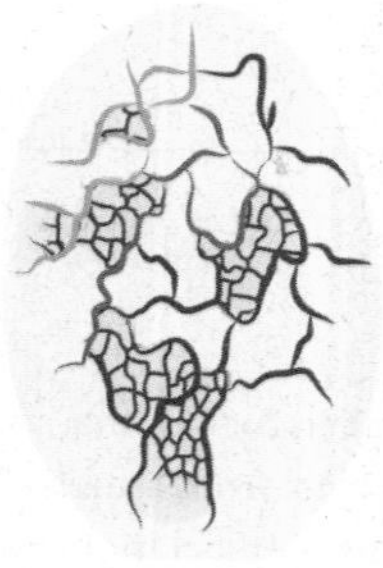	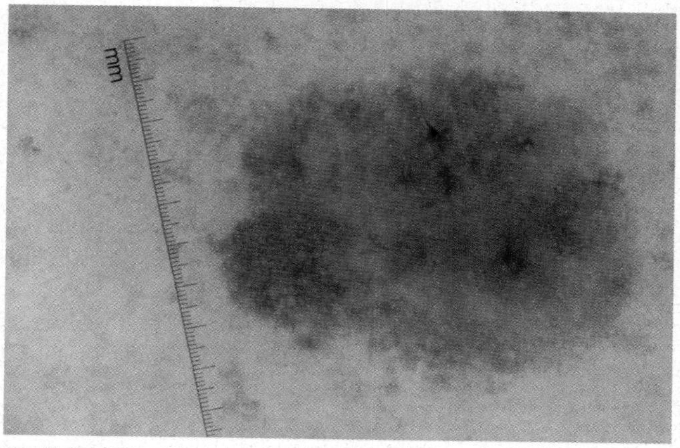	**Atypical/irregular pigment network** Network lines varying in size, color, thickness and distribution.
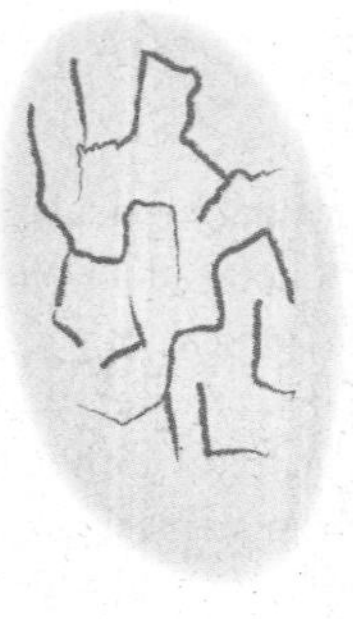	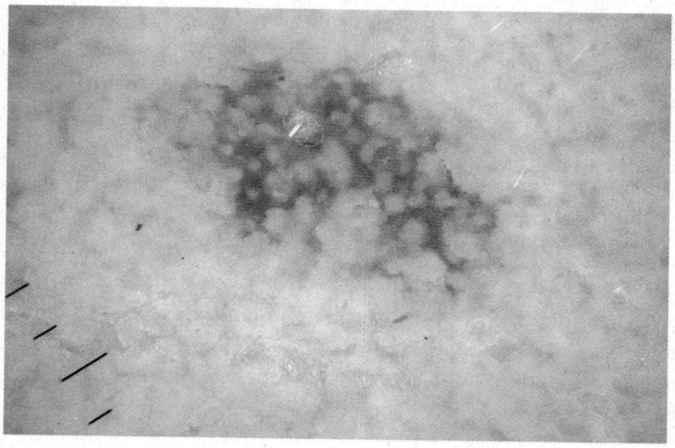	**Angulated lines** Linear brown/gray lines that intersect at acute angles forming a zigzag pattern or polygons, such as rhomboids.

TABLE 111-7 Dermoscopic Features of Melanoma (*Continued*)

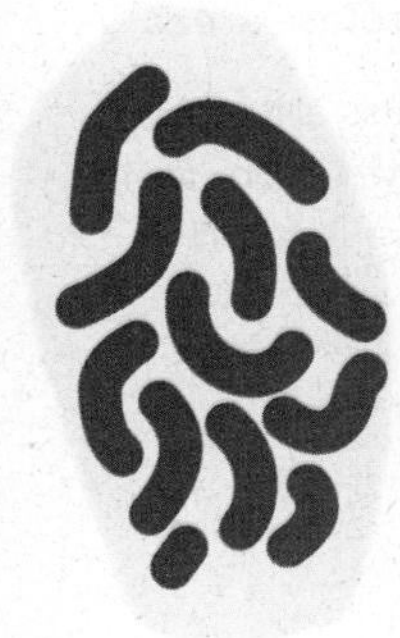	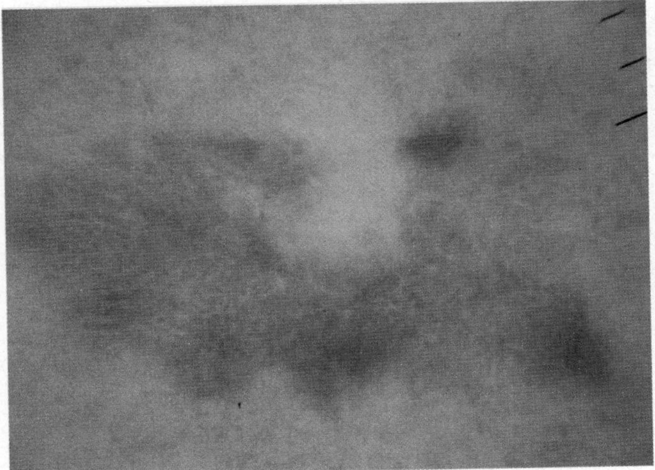	**Negative network** Hypopigmented lines connecting between pigmented structures in a serpiginous fashion.
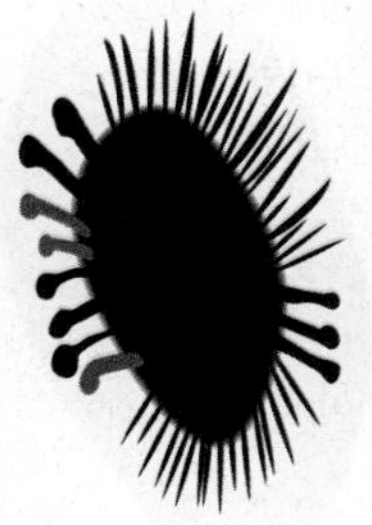	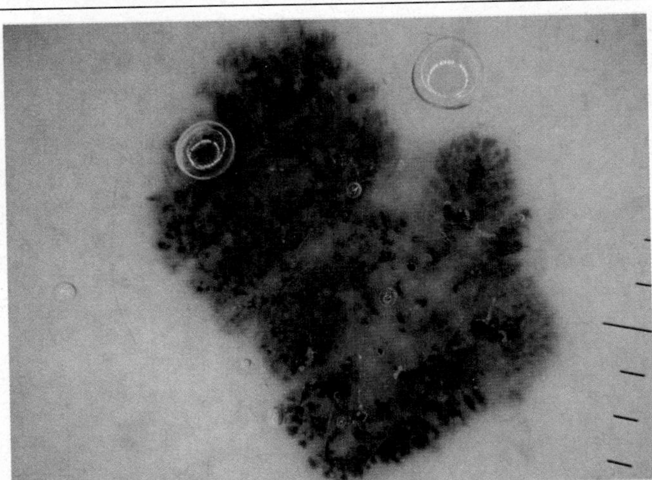	**Streaks (radial streaming and pseudopods)** Linear projections emerging from the periphery of a lesion and extending into surrounding skin.
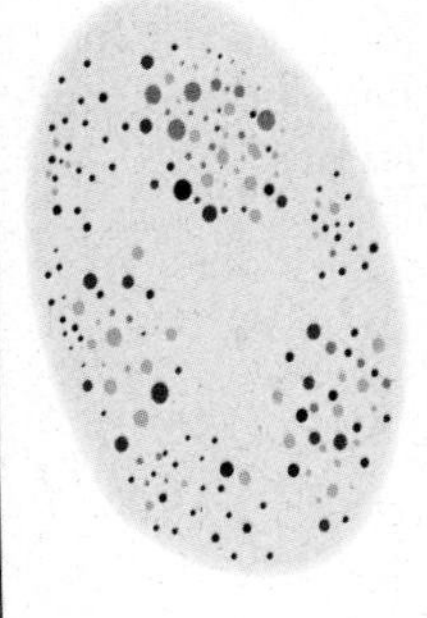		**Atypical/irregular globules** Globules varying in color, size, and/or shape.

(*continued*)

TABLE 111-7 Dermoscopic Features of Melanoma (*Continued*)

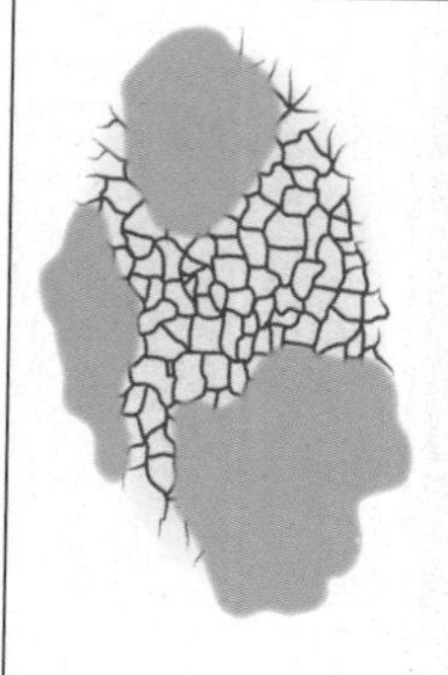	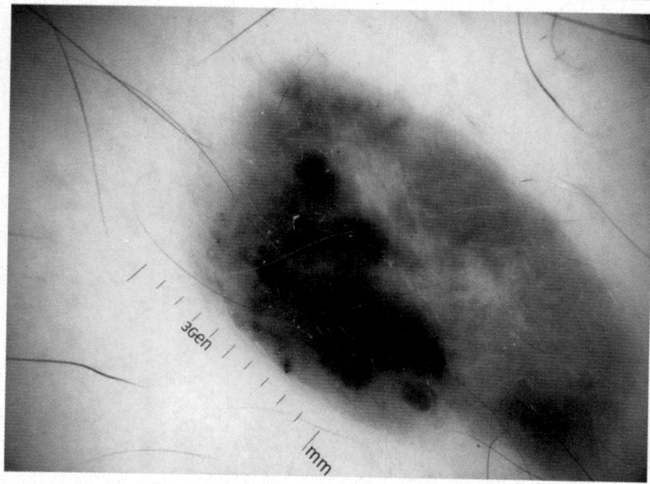	**Tan peripheral structureless areas** Tan or brown structureless areas are abnormal when they cover more than 10% of the lesion and are located on the periphery of the lesion.
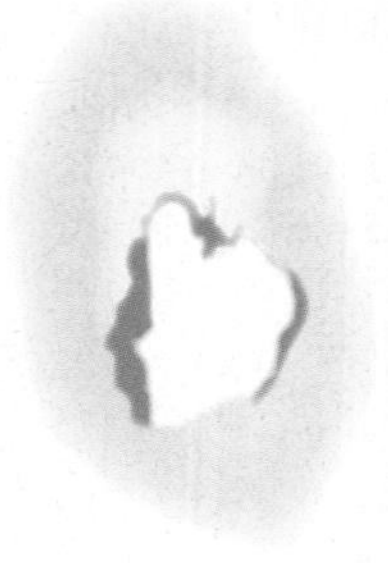	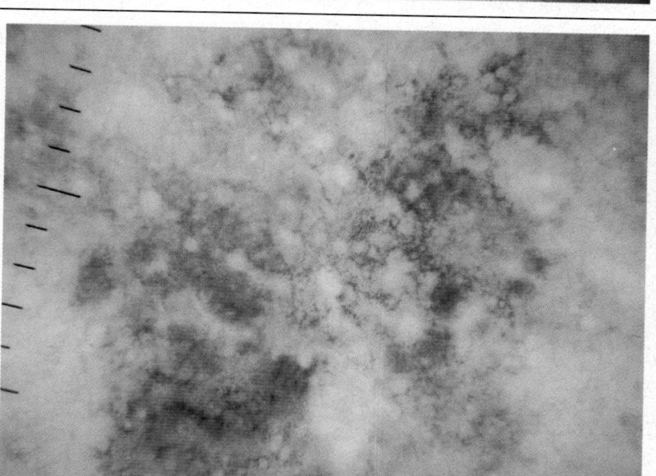	**Regression structures (scar-like depigmentation and peppering/granularity)** Scar-like depigmentation appears as white, structureless areas that are lighter in color when compared to the surrounding skin. Peppering/granularity consists of fine blue-gray dots.
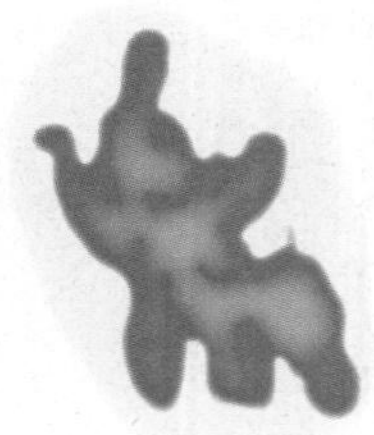	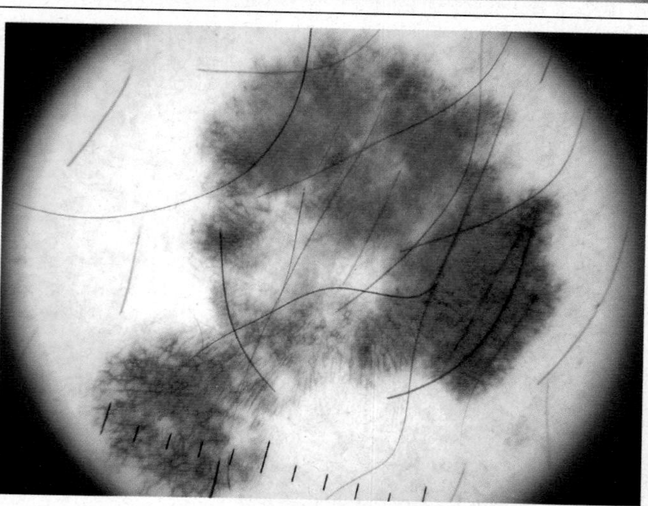	**Blue-whitish veil** A whitish ground-glass haze located over a blue, raised area of a lesion.

TABLE 111-7 Dermoscopic Features of Melanoma (*Continued*)

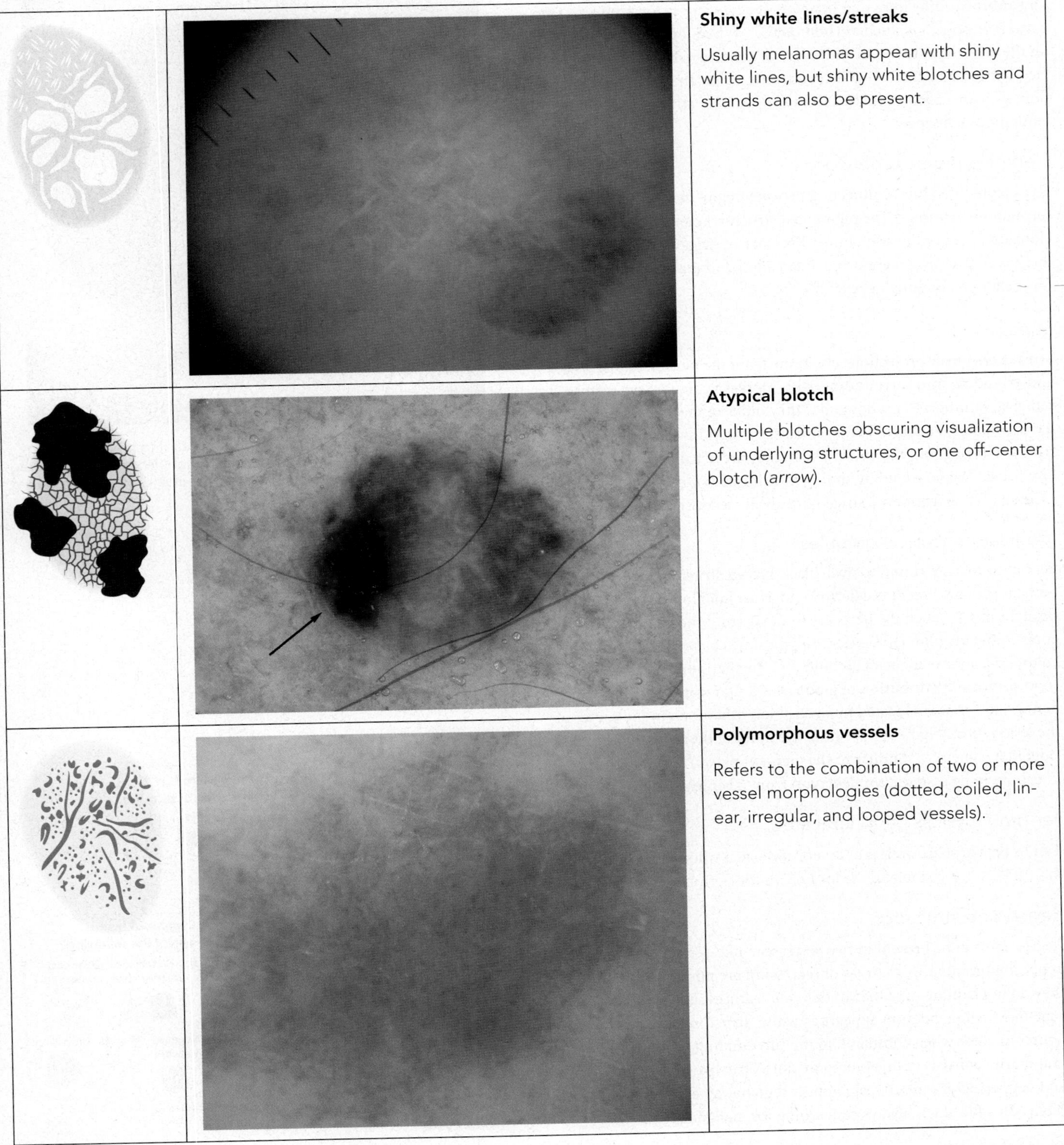

		Shiny white lines/streaks Usually melanomas appear with shiny white lines, but shiny white blotches and strands can also be present.
		Atypical blotch Multiple blotches obscuring visualization of underlying structures, or one off-center blotch (*arrow*).
		Polymorphous vessels Refers to the combination of two or more vessel morphologies (dotted, coiled, linear, irregular, and looped vessels).

Photos reproduced with permission from www.isic-archive.com, Harold Rabinovitz, MD.

Angulated lines

Linear brown/gray lines that intersect at acute angles forming a zigzag pattern or polygons, such as rhomboids.[43] When identified in lesions on the face, they are highly indicative of a melanoma common to the face, lentigo maligna.[44-47] When encountered on an extra-facial location, they are called angulated lines and are indicative of melanoma, lentiginous subtype.[15]

Negative pigment network

Hypopigmented lines connecting between pigmented structures in a serpiginous fashion.[48] The pigmented structures can be conceived as elongated to curvilinear globules. Presence of negative pigment network is almost always abnormal in an adult and is a good indicator for melanoma or Spitz nevus.[49,50]

Streaks

Streaks are linear projections emerging from the periphery of a lesion and extending into surrounding skin.[51] Streaks come in two forms: radial streaming and pseudopods. They differ in that pseudopods have a bulbous ending.[52] When streaks are found symmetrically distributed throughout the entire lesion, they are usually indicative of a Spitz/Reed lesion, a benign finding in children but more concerning in adults.[34-36] Asymmetric streaks are always a concerning finding.[41]

Irregular or atypical globules

Globules/dots are round to oval, black/brown structures representing nests of melanocytes at the dermoepidermal junction (DEJ) or superficial dermis.[42] When the nests are in the dermis, the globules will appear blue in color. Globules are atypical when there is variation in color, size, and/or shape of globules.[17,51] Furthermore, an asymmetric (non-uniform) distribution of globules is a sign worrisome for malignancy. Dots that are located in any fashion other than in the center of the lesion or on pigment lines or in the holes of the network are considered irregular.[41,53] Similar to the pigment network, globules and dots have to be assessed for deviation from a benign pattern.

Tan structureless peripheral area

Tan or brown structureless areas are abnormal when they cover more than 10% of the lesion and are located on the periphery of the lesion.

Regression structures

Regression can be present in two ways: scar-like depigmentation and peppering/granularity.[51] Areas of regression are non-palpable, and they do not exhibit any other underlying features such as vessels. Scar-like depigmentation appears as white, structureless areas that are lighter in color when compared to the surrounding skin. Peppering/granularity consists of fine blue-gray dots. Scar-like depigmentation and peppering/granularity can appear together on a lesion or separately. This finding is always concerning for malignancy.[54,55]

Blue-whitish veil

Blue-whitish veil, or blue-white veil, is a whitish ground-glass haze located over a blue, raised area of a lesion (**Figure 111-22**).[41,56] The white color is due to compact orthokeratosis, while the bluish color is attributed to melanocytes or melanin in the dermis.[54] Blue-whitish veil can appear covering the entire lesion in blue nevi and metastatic melanoma, but when focal, it is indicative of malignancy.[41,53,57]

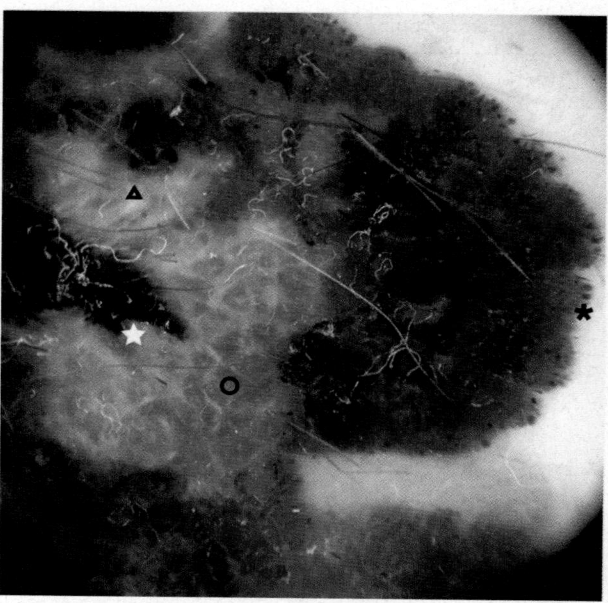

FIGURE 111-22 Example of a superficial spreading melanoma with blue-white veil (*triangle*), irregular dots and globules (*asterisk*), an irregular blotch (*white star*), and shiny white structures (*circle*). (*Reproduced with permission from www.isic-archive.com.*)

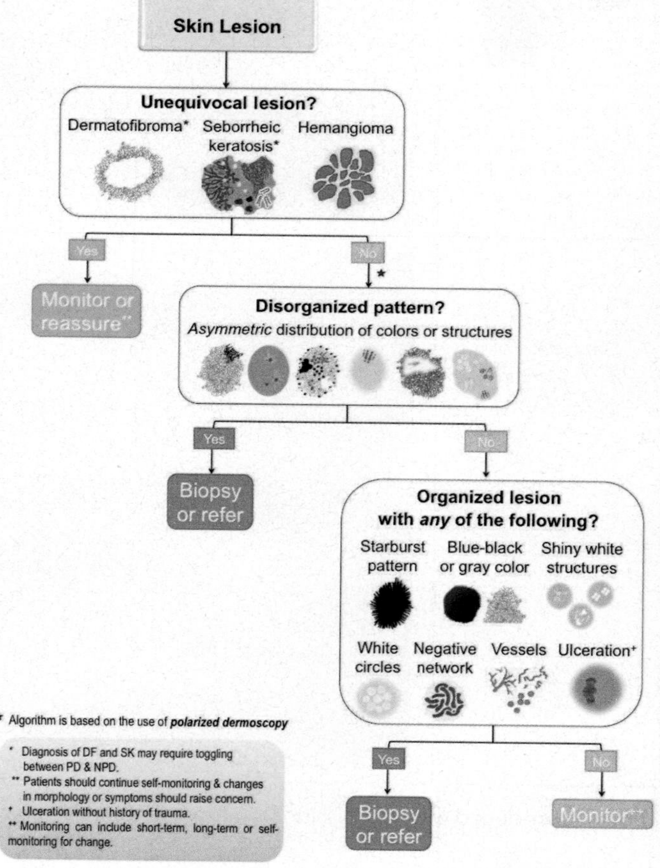

FIGURE 111-23 Triage amalgamated dermoscopy algorithm (TADA algorithm). *Abbreviations: DF*, dermatofibroma; *NPD*, non-polarized dermoscopy; *PD*, polarized dermoscopy; *SK*, seborrheic keratosis. (*Reproduced with permission from www.dermoscopedia.org.*)

Shiny white lines/streaks

As discussed earlier, shiny white lines can only be seen with polarized light and consist of discrete short white lines oriented in an orthogonal or parallel fashion.[50,58,59] In addition to malignancy, this feature also presents in Spitz nevi.[36,60]

Atypical blotch

Blotches are heavily pigmented areas obscuring the visualization of the underlying structures, such as a pigment network, and can be located anywhere on a lesion.[41,61] Atypical blotches consist of either multiple blotches or one, off-centered blotch.

Polymorphous vessels

The presence of multiple vessel morphologies in the same lesion is termed "polymorphous vessels." The combination of two or more vessel morphologies (dotted, coiled, linear irregular, and looped vessels) within a lesion is usually indicative of malignancy.[13]

TRIAGE AMALGAMATED DERMOSCOPY ALGORITHM (TADA)

TADA is an algorithm designed to triage the management of skin lesions (**Figure 111-23**). It serves as a relatively simple guide for the identification of lesions that are at risk for being malignant.[62] What differentiates TADA from other more extensive and complex algorithms is that the commonly encountered and diagnostically unequivocal benign lesions, namely, angiomas, DFs, and SK, are excluded from the algorithm. Thus, in the first step of the algorithm, unequivocal angiomas, DFs, or SKs based on clinical and dermoscopic examination are excluded from further analysis. The second step of the algorithm requires the observer to judge whether the lesion manifests architectural disorder. Architectural disorder can be defined as chaotic/disorganized distribution of colors and structures within the lesion. Architectural disorder is a powerful discriminator for skin cancer with an odds ratio of 6.6. In addition, architectural disorder had high interobserver agreement among the participants of the study by the International Dermoscopy Society (intraclass correlation coefficient of 0.43, where 0 corresponds to agreement by chance and 1 is perfect agreement).[10] If the lesion is considered to be disorganized, then the examining physician should biopsy or refer the patient to an expert dermatologist.

If the lesion is symmetric, then the observer moves to the third step of the algorithm. Because on rare occasions malignancy can present itself in an organized and symmetric fashion, these organized lesions need to be evaluated further for the presence of six sensitive features for malignancy. The six additional features include the starburst pattern (spitzoid melanomas), blue-black or gray color (nodular melanoma and melanoma on sun-damaged skin), shiny white structures (seen with polarized light in any skin cancer), negative network (melanoma), and vessels or ulceration (any skin cancer). Presence of any one of these six criteria should prompt biopsy or referral to an expert. Lesions that are not angiomas, SK, or DF, and lesions that are not disorganized and lesions that are organized but lack one of the six features mentioned above, can be safely monitored. The efficiency of the TADA algorithm was tested in a group of novices, experienced dermatologists, and family physicians. After only 1 day of training, the participants achieved sensitivity for skin cancer (BCC, squamous cell carcinoma, and melanoma) of 93.3% and specificity of 74.1%. There was no difference in sensitivity between novices and experts, and there was no difference in sensitivity between dermatologists and family physicians.[63]

HOW TO CHOOSE A DERMATOSCOPE

1. *Choose a hybrid dermatoscope:* NPDs and PDs provide different but complementary information (**Table 111-8**). PD enables users

TABLE 111-8 Differences in Structure Visualization between Non-polarized and Polarized Dermoscopy (PD)

	NPD	PD
	Requires skin contact	Does not require skin contact
	Requires liquid interface	Does not require liquid interface
Colors		
Melanin	+	Better visualized with PD
Red/Pink	+	Better visualized with PD
Blue-white due to orthokeratosis (blue-whitish veil)	+++	+
Blue-white due to regression	+++	++
Structures		
Peppering	+++	++
Shiny white structures	+/–	+++
Vessels	+	+++
Milia-like cysts	+++	+/–
Comedo-like opening	+++	+

Reproduced with permission from www.dermoscopedia.org.

to identify structures such as vessels and shiny white structures that are highly sensitive features for skin cancer. Because PDs have a high sensitivity for detecting skin cancer and do not require a liquid interface or direct skin contact, a PD is the ideal dermatoscope to use for skin cancer screening.[41,64] However, to maintain the highest specificity requires the complementary use of NPD, which identifies surface structures seen in seborrheic keratoses and other benign lesions. Thus, if the aim is to maintain the highest diagnostic accuracy, then the most ideal method to evaluate lesions is by using both NPD and PD. The preferred dermatoscope models are hybrids that permit the observer to toggle between PD and NPD in one device.

2. *Choose a dermatoscope that attaches to your smartphone and/or a camera:* This helps you to capture images that can be analyzed on the screen without having your face so close to the patient. With the image on the screen, you can blow up certain areas for in-depth analysis of structures and patterns. You can also share the image with the patient to explain why a biopsy is or is not needed. If you are teaching students or residents, these on-screen images are invaluable at the point of care as well as for future teaching. In addition, the dermoscopic images are the best way to follow lesions over time when monitoring is indicated. Finally, these images are one of the best ways to ensure your continued learning of dermoscopy. After each biopsy result comes back, we recommend going back to your dermoscopic image and correlating it with the biopsy report. If your suspected diagnosis was correct, this will reinforce your knowledge; if the pathology diagnosis is unexpected, you can learn by correlating the pathology result to the original image, seeing structures and patterns that you may have missed at first. Sometimes you might even question the pathology based on the dermoscopy, and this should prompt a call to the pathologist. You can only do all these activities to improve patient care and learning if you can capture your dermoscopic images digitally. Looking through the dermatoscope with your eye is the first step; however, digital dermoscopy with image capture takes dermoscopy to the highest level.

CONCLUSION

Family physicians can expand their diagnostic abilities in dermatology with the acquisition of a dermatoscope and the time invested in learning how to interpret dermoscopic patterns. Dermoscopy greatly improves the user's diagnostic accuracy through identification of the absence or presence of specific and sensitive dermoscopic features and patterns. Algorithms place these structures into an easy-to-follow framework to guide the observer in making a diagnosis or a management decision. Algorithms such as the 2-step algorithm are extensive with the intention of assisting the user in making a specific diagnosis. In contrast, triage algorithms such as TADA are narrower in scope but designed to guide the clinician's management.

Multiple studies have shown that indeed, the use of dermoscopy requires familiarization with the method, and there is a learning curve for the user to achieve high levels of competence. Fortunately, we live in an era when information and continuous training are widely and freely available.

RESOURCES FOR ADDITIONAL LEARNING

Free Dermoscopy apps

- Dermoscopy: Two Step Algorithm. Available on the iOS App Store and Google Play. Learn more at **www.usatinemedia.com**. This app is intended to help you interpret the dermoscopic patterns seen with your dermatoscope. You will be asked a series of questions that will lead you to the most probable diagnosis. This app also contains more than 80 photos and charts to help you in your diagnosis. There are 50 interactive cases to solve. Once the full app is downloaded, Internet connectivity is not needed to use it.
- YOUdermoscopy Training offers a fun game interface to test and expand your dermoscopy skills. Available on iOS App store and Google play.

Dermoscopy Internet Resources

- International Dermoscopy Society. Tutorials and podcasts—**http://www.dermoscopy-ids.org.**
- The Encyclopedia of Dermoscopy—**www.dermoscopedia.org.**
- A database of dermoscopy images available to all—**www.isic-archive.com.**

Dermoscopy Courses

Courses are a great way to get started and/or to advance your skills (the following courses are taught by some of the authors of this chapter):

- The American Dermoscopy Meeting is held yearly in the summer in a national park—**http://www.americandermoscopy.com.**
- Memorial Sloan Kettering Cancer Center holds a yearly dermoscopy workshop each fall in New York City—**http://www.mskcc.org/events/.**
- American Academy of Family Physicians (AAFP) yearly FMX offers dermoscopy workshops—**http://www.aafp.org/events/assembly.html.**

REFERENCES

1. Gewirtzman AJ, Saurat J-H, Braun RP. An evaluation of dermoscopy fluids and application techniques. *Br J Dermatol.* 2003;149(1):59-63.
2. Benvenuto-Andrade C, Dusza SW, Agero ALC, et al. Differences between polarized light dermoscopy and immersion contact dermoscopy for the evaluation of skin lesions. *Arch Dermatol.* 2007;143(3):329-338.
3. Wang SQ, Dusza SW, Scope A, et al. Differences in dermoscopic images from nonpolarized dermoscope and polarized dermoscope influence the diagnostic accuracy and confidence level: a pilot study. *Dermatol Surg.* 2008;34(10):1389-1395.
4. Pan Y, Gareau DS, Scope A, et al. Polarized and nonpolarized dermoscopy: the explanation for the observed differences. *Arch Dermatol.* 2008;144(6):828-829.
5. Marghoob AA, Cowell L, Kopf AW, Scope A. Observation of chrysalis structures with polarized dermoscopy. *Arch Dermatol.* 2009;145(5):618.

6. Liebman TN, Rabinovitz HS, Dusza SW, Marghoob AA. White shiny structures: dermoscopic features revealed under polarized light. *J Eur Acad Dermatol Venereol.* 2012;26(12):1493-1497.
7. Dolianitis C, Kelly J, Wolfe R, Simpson P. Comparative performance of 4 dermoscopic algorithms by nonexperts for the diagnosis of melanocytic lesions. *Arch Dermatol.* 2005;141(8): 1008-1014.
8. Annessi G, Bono R, Sampogna F, et al. Sensitivity, specificity, and diagnostic accuracy of three dermoscopic algorithmic methods in the diagnosis of doubtful melanocytic lesions: the importance of light brown structureless areas in differentiating atypical melanocytic nevi from thin melanomas. *J Am Dermatol.* 2007;56(5): 759-767.
9. Blum A. [Diagnostic dermoscopic algorithms]. *Hautarzt.* 2005; 56(1):81-93, quiz 94-5.
10. Carrera C, Marchetti MA, Dusza S, et al. Validity and reliability of dermoscopic criteria used to differentiate nevi from melanoma: a web-based International Dermoscopy Society study. *JAMA Dermatol.* 2016;152(7):798-806.
11. Argenziano G, Soyer HP, Chimenti S, et al. Dermoscopy of pigmented skin lesions: results of a consensus meeting via the Internet. *J Am Acad Dermatol.* 2003;48(5):679-693.
12. Argenziano G, Zalaudek I, Corona R, et al. Vascular structures in skin tumors: a dermoscopy study. *Arch Dermatol.* 2004;140(12): 1485-1489.
13. Menzies SW, Kreusch J, Byth K, et al. Dermoscopic evaluation of amelanotic and hypomelanotic melanoma. *Arch Dermatol.* 2008; 144(9):1120-1127.
14. Marghoob AA, Braun R. Proposal for a revised 2-step algorithm for the classification of lesions of the skin using dermoscopy. *Arch Dermatol.* 2010;146(4):426-428.
15. Marghoob DA, Lallas A, Braun R. *Revised 2-step Algorithm—Dermoscopedia.* 2018. https://dermoscopedia.org/Revised_two-step_algorithm. Accessed June 2018.
16. Braun RP, Rabinovitz HS, Oliviero M, et al. Pattern analysis: a 2-step procedure for the dermoscopic diagnosis of melanoma. *Clin Dermatol.* 2002;20(3):236-239.
17. Zalaudek I, Schmid K, Marghoob AA, et al. Frequency of dermoscopic nevus subtypes by age and body site: a cross-sectional study. *Arch Dermatol.* 2011;147(6):663-670.
18. Fonseca M, Marchetti MA, Chung E, et al. Cross-sectional analysis of the dermoscopic patterns and structures of melanocytic naevi on the back and legs of adolescents. *Br J Dermatol.* 2015;173(6):1486-1493.
19. Chen LL, Dusza SW, Jaimes N, Marghoob AA. Performance of the first step of the 2-Step Dermoscopy Algorithm. *JAMA Dermatol.* 2015;151(7):715-721.
20. Zaballos P, Puig S, Llambrich A, Malvehy J. Dermoscopy of dermatofibromas: a prospective morphological study of 412 cases. *Arch Dermatol.* 2008;144(1):75-83.
21. Navarrete-Dechent C, Bajaj S, Marchetti MA, et al. Association of shiny white blotches and strands with nonpigmented basal cell carcinoma. *JAMA Dermatol.* 2016;152(5):546-547.
22. Menzies SW, Westerhoff K, Rabinovitz H, et al. Surface microscopy of pigmented basal cell carcinoma. *Arch Dermatol.* 2000;136(8): 1012-1016.
23. Giacomel J, Zalaudek I. Dermoscopy of superficial basal cell carcinoma. *Dermatol Surg.* 2005;31(12):1710-1713.
24. Ahnlide I, Zalaudek I, Nilsson F, et al. Preoperative prediction of histopathological outcome in basal cell carcinoma: flat surface and multiple small erosions predict superficial basal cell carcinoma in lighter skin types. *Br J Dermatol.* 2016;175(4):751-761.
25. Lallas A, Tzellos T, Kyrgidis A, et al. Accuracy of dermoscopic criteria for discriminating superficial from other subtypes of basal cell carcinoma. *J Am Dermatol.* 2014;70(2):303-311.
26. Rosendahl C, Cameron A, Argenziano G, et al. Dermoscopy of squamous cell carcinoma and keratoacanthoma. *Arch Dermatol.* 2012;148(12):1386-1392.
27. Cameron A, Rosendahl C, Tschandl P, et al. Dermatoscopy of pigmented Bowen's disease. *J Am Dermatol.* 2010;62(4):597-604.
28. Zalaudek I, Giacomel J, Argenziano G, et al. Dermoscopy of facial nonpigmented actinic keratosis. *Br J Dermatol.* 2006;155(5):951-956.
29. Minagawa A. Dermoscopy-pathology relationship in seborrheic keratosis. *J Dermatol.* 2017;44(5):518-524.
30. Braun RP, Ludwig S, Marghoob AA. Differential diagnosis of seborrheic keratosis: clinical and dermoscopic features. *J Drugs Dermatol.* 2017;16(9):835-842.
31. Annessi G, Bono R, Abeni D. Correlation between digital epiluminescence microscopy parameters and histopathological changes in lentigo maligna and solar lentigo: a dermoscopic index for the diagnosis of lentigo maligna. *J Am Dermatol.* 2017;76(2): 234-243.
32. Zaballos P, Ara M, Puig S, Malvehy J. Dermoscopy of sebaceous hyperplasia. *Arch Dermatol.* 2005;141(6):808.
33. Tiodorovic-Zivkovic D, Lallas A, Longo C, et al. Dermoscopy of clear cell acanthoma. *J Am Dermatol.* 2015;72(1 Suppl):S47-9.
34. Marchell R, Marghoob AA, Braun RP, Argenziano G. Dermoscopy of pigmented Spitz and Reed nevi: the starburst pattern. *Arch Dermatol.* 2005;141(8):1060.
35. Argenziano G, Agozzino M, Bonifazi E, et al. Natural evolution of Spitz nevi. *Dermatology.* 2011;222(3):256-260.
36. Lallas A, Apalla Z, Ioannides D, et al. Update on dermoscopy of Spitz/Reed naevi and management guidelines by the International Dermoscopy Society. *Br J Dermatol.* 2017;177(3):645-655.
37. Argenziano G, Soyer HP. Dermoscopy of pigmented skin lesions—a valuable tool for early diagnosis of melanoma. *Lancet Oncol.* 2001;2(7):443-449.
38. Menzies SW, Zalaudek I. Why perform dermoscopy? The evidence for its role in the routine management of pigmented skin lesions. *Arch Dermatol.* 2006;142(9):1211-1212.
39. Argenziano G, Puig S, Zalaudek I, et al. Dermoscopy improves accuracy of primary care physicians to triage lesions suggestive of skin cancer. *J Clin Oncol.* 2006;24(12):1877-1882.
40. Wolner Z, Yélamos O, Liopyris K, et al. Enhancing Skin Cancer Diagnosis with Dermoscopy. *Dermatol Clin.* 2017;35(4):417-437.

41. Marghoob AA, Malvehy J, Braun RP. *An Atlas of Dermoscopy, Second Edition*. Boca Raton, FL: CRC Press; 2012.
42. Woltsche N, Schmid-Zalaudek K, Deinlein T, et al. Abundance of the benign melanocytic universe: dermoscopic-histopathological correlation in nevi. *J Dermatol*. 2017;44(5):499-506.
43. Jaimes N, Marghoob AA, Rabinovitz H, et al. Clinical and dermoscopic characteristics of melanomas on nonfacial chronically sun-damaged skin. *J Am Dermatol*. 2015;72(6):1027-1035.
44. Schiffner R, Schiffner-Rohe J, Vogt T, et al. Improvement of early recognition of lentigo maligna using dermatoscopy. *J Am Dermatol*. 2000;42(1 Pt 1):25-32.
45. Tschandl P, Rosendahl C, Kittler H. Dermatoscopy of flat pigmented facial lesions. *J Eur Acad Dermatol Venereol*. 2015;29(1):120-127.
46. Carbone A, Ferrari A, Paolino G, et al. Lentigo maligna of the face: a quantitative simple method to identify individual patient risk probability on dermoscopy. *Australas J Dermatol*. 2017;58(4):286-291.
47. Lallas A, Tschandl P, Kyrgidis A, et al. Dermoscopic clues to differentiate facial lentigo maligna from pigmented actinic keratosis. *Br J Dermatol*. 2016;174(5):1079-1085.
48. Pizzichetta MA, Talamini R, Marghoob AA, et al. Negative pigment network: an additional dermoscopic feature for the diagnosis of melanoma. *J Am Dermatol*. 2013;68(4):552-559.
49. Bassoli S, Ferrari C, Borsari S, et al. Negative pigment network identifies a peculiar melanoma subtype and represents a clue to melanoma diagnosis: a dermoscopic study of 401 melanomas. *Acta Derm Venereol*. 2013;93(6):650-655.
50. Pizzichetta MA, Canzonieri V, Soyer PH, et al. Negative pigment network and shiny white streaks: a dermoscopic-pathological correlation study. *Am J Dermatopathol*. 2014;36(5):433-438.
51. Kittler H, Marghoob AA, Argenziano G, et al. Standardization of terminology in dermoscopy/dermatoscopy: results of the third consensus conference of the International Society of Dermoscopy. *J Am Dermatol*. 2016;74(6):1093-1106.
52. Menzies SW, Ingvar C, McCarthy WH. A sensitivity and specificity analysis of the surface microscopy features of invasive melanoma. *Melanoma Res*. 1996;6(1):55-62.
53. Kittler H, Pehamberger H, Wolff K, Binder M. Diagnostic accuracy of dermoscopy. *Lancet Oncol*. 2002;3(3):159-165.
54. Massi D, De Giorgi V, Soyer HP. Histopathologic correlates of dermoscopic criteria. *Dermatol Clin*. 2001;19(2):259-268.
55. Braun RP, Kerl K. Histopathologic correlation of dermoscopic structures. *Dermoscopedia*. 2018. https://dermoscopedia.org/Histopathologic_correlation_of_dermoscopic_structures. Accessed June 2018.
56. Braun RP, Rabinovitz HS, Oliviero M, et al. Dermoscopy of pigmented skin lesions. *J Am Dermatol*. 2005;52(1):109-121.
57. Massi D, De Giorgi V, Carli P, Santucci M. Diagnostic significance of the blue hue in dermoscopy of melanocytic lesions: a dermoscopic-pathologic study. *Am J Dermatopathol*. 2001;23(5):463-469.
58. Shitara D, Ishioka P, Alonso-Pinedo Y, et al. Shiny white streaks: a sign of malignancy at dermoscopy of pigmented skin lesions. *Acta Derm Venereol*. 2014;94(2):132-137.
59. Di Stefani A, Campbell TM, Malvehy J, et al. Shiny white streaks: an additional dermoscopic finding in melanomas viewed using contact polarised dermoscopy. *Australas J Dermatol*. 2010;51(4):295-298.
60. Botella-Estrada R, Requena C, Traves V, et al. Chrysalis and negative pigment network in Spitz nevi. *Am J Dermatopathol*. 2012;34(2):188-191.
61. Stoecker WV, Gupta K, Stanley RJ, et al. Detection of asymmetric blotches (asymmetric structureless areas) in dermoscopy images of malignant melanoma using relative color. *Skin Res Technol*. 2005;11(3):179-184.
62. Rogers T, Marino ML, Dusza SW, et al. A clinical aid for detecting skin cancer: the Triage Amalgamated Dermoscopic Algorithm (TADA). *J Am Board Fam Med*. 2016;29(6):694-701.
63. Rogers T, Marino M, Dusza SW, et al. Triage amalgamated dermoscopic algorithm (TADA) for skin cancer screening. *Dermatol Pract Concept*. 2017;7(2):39-46.
64. https://dermoscopedia.org.

112 TOPICAL AND INTRALESIONAL STEROIDS

Richard P. Usatine, MD

One of the most important skills in the treatment of skin disorders is the use of topical and intralesional steroids. The number of allergic, inflammatory, and immunologic skin diseases that respond to topical and intralesional steroids is vast. However, the indiscriminate use of topical steroids on unknown skin disorders can result in problems such as skin atrophy, telangiectasias, or tinea incognito (a condition caused by the incorrect application of topical steroids to a fungal infection, allowing the tinea to worsen). (See Chapter 144, Tinea Corporis.) Some of the types of skin diseases in which topical steroids are effective include:

- Allergic skin diseases including atopic dermatitis, contact dermatitis, and hand eczema.
- Papulosquamous conditions including psoriasis, lichen planus, and seborrheic dermatitis.
- Connective tissue diseases of skin including lupus.
- Autoimmune bullous disease including pemphigus.
- Infiltrative and immunologic diseases including sarcoidosis and granuloma annulare.

Learning to use topical steroids effectively requires understanding the range of potencies, the vehicles available, and the amounts needed for acute and chronic skin conditions. It is also essential to understand the possible adverse reactions and to be able to balance those risks against the benefits of topical and intralesional steroids. The common side effects are listed in **Table 112-1.**

STEROID POTENCY

Topical steroids have a wide range of potency (**Table 112-2**). Choosing the correct potency is the first step in prescribing a topical steroid. The most important factors to consider are:

- Location—area of the skin involved. Skin atrophy is more likely in areas of thin skin such as the face, the genitalia, and the intertriginous areas. Therefore, lower potency steroids are preferentially used on the face and in the intertriginous areas.
- Diagnosis—some conditions such as seborrhea do well with low-potency steroids, whereas others such as psoriasis require high-potency steroids.
- Age—younger patients are more prone to skin atrophy and suppression of the hypothalamic–pituitary axis.
- History—find out if previous topical steroids have been used and the degree of response before writing a new prescription.

One exception to the caveat of avoiding high-potency steroids on the genitals is the condition lichen sclerosus (previously known as lichen sclerosus et atrophicus) (**Figure 112-1**). The evidence

TABLE 112-1 Common Side Effects of Topical Corticosteroids

Skin atrophy	Most common adverse effect Epidermal thinning may begin after only a few days Dermal thinning usually takes several weeks to develop Usually reversible within 2 months after stopping the corticosteroid
Telangiectasia	Most often occurs on the face, neck, and upper chest Tends to decrease when steroid discontinued, but may be irreversible
Striae	Usually occur around flexures (groin, axillary, and inner thigh areas) Usually permanent, but may fade with time
Purpura	Frequently occurs after minimal trauma Attributed to loss of perivascular supporting tissue in the dermis
Hypopigmentation	May be reversible upon discontinuing the corticosteroid
Acneform eruptions	Particularly common on the face, especially with the "potent" and "very potent" corticosteroids Usually reversible
Fine hair growth	Reversible upon discontinuation of the corticosteroid
Infections	May worsen viral, bacterial, or fungal skin infections May cause tinea incognito
Hypothalamic–pituitary–adrenal axis suppression	Rare with topicals >30 g/week of "very potent" corticosteroids should be limited to 3 to 4 weeks Children (>10 g/week) and elderly are at higher risk because of thinner skin

TABLE 112-2 Corticosteroid Potency Chart

Generic Name	U.S. Trade Name and Strength
Class 1—Superpotent	
Betamethasone dipropionate	Diprolene lotion/gel/ointment, 0.05%
Clobetasol propionate	Temovate cream/emollient base cream/gel/ointment, 0.05% Clobex ointment/lotion/shampoo/spray aerosol, 0.05% Cormax ointment/solution, 0.05% Olux foam aerosol, 0.05%
Diflorasone diacetate	Psorcon or ApexiCon ointment, 0.05%
Halobetasol propionate	Ultravate cream/ointment, 0.05%
Fluocinonide	Vanos cream, 0.1%
Flurandrenolide	Cordran Tape, 4 mcg/cm^2
Class 2—Potent	
Amcinonide	Cyclocort or Amcort ointment, 0.1%
Betamethasone dipropionate	Diprosone ointment/augmented cream, 0.05%
Desoximetasone	Topicort cream/ointment, 0.25%; gel, 0.05%
Diflorasone diacetate	ApexiCon cream/ointment, 0.05% Florone ointment, 0.05%; Psorcon cream/ointment, 0.05%
Fluocinonide	Lidex cream/ointment/gel/solution, 0.05%
Halcinonide	Halog cream/ointment/cream/solution, 0.1%
Class 3—Upper Mid-Strength	
Amcinonide	Amcort cream//lotion, 0.1%; Cyclocort cream, 0.1%
Betamethasone dipropionate	Diprosone cream or hydrophilic emollient, 0.05%
Betamethasone valerate	Valisone or Betatrex ointment, 0.1%; Luxiq foam, 0.12%
Diflorasone diacetate	Generic cream/ointment/lotion, 0.1%
Diflorasone diacetate	Maxiflor, Florone, Psorcon cream, 0.05% Generic cream/ointment, 0.05%
Fluticasone propionate	Cutivate ointment, 0.005%
Fluocinonide	Lidex-E cream, aqueous emollient, 0.05%
Mometasone furoate	Elocon cream/ointment, 0.1%
Class 4—Mid-Strength	
Clocortolone pivalate	Cloderm cream, 0.1%
Desoximetasone	Topicort LP cream, 0.05%
Fluocinolone acetonide	Synalar-HP, Synalar ointment, 0.025%
Flurandrenolide	Cordran ointment, 0.05%
Hydrocortisone valerate	Westcort ointment, 0.2%
Mometasone furoate	Elocon cream, lotion, solution, 0.1%
Triamcinolone acetonide	Kenalog cream, ointment, 0.1%
Class 5—Lower Mid-Strength	
Betamethasone dipropionate	Diprosone lotion, 0.05%
Betamethasone valerate	Valisone, Beta-Val, Betatrex cream, 0.1%
Desonide	DesOwen, Tridesilon ointment, 0.05% Desonate gel, 0.05%

(continued)

The largest container sizes available in the United States are:

- Hydrocortisone 1%, 2.5%—454 g tub (1 lb jar)
- Triamcinolone—80 g tube or 454 g tub (1 lb jar)
- Fluocinonide—120 g tube or 60 mL solution
- Clobetasol—60 g tube or 50 mL solution

This does not mean that topical steroids should be given without monitoring for side effects and making sure that patients are using them appropriately. The next section describes options for prescribing long-term topical steroids safely.

TOPICAL STEROIDS FOR LONG-TERM USE

Patients with psoriasis, eczema, or other chronic skin conditions often want to use high-potency steroids on a continuous basis because they are perceived to be more effective than other options. Patients with psoriasis rarely get skin atrophy from topical steroids,[10] since the plaques are often thick, whereas patients with eczema are more prone to get skin atrophy.

Here are methods to avoid side effects of chronic topical steroid use regardless of the diagnosis.

1. *Step-down approach:* Start with a potent preparation and then decrease to a lower potency preparation as the condition improves. Or start with twice daily and taper to once daily.
2. *Short burst therapy:* Periods of steroid use followed by another topical agent that is not a steroid.
3. *Pulse therapy:* One pattern of pulse therapy consists of using a high-potency steroid on the weekend only and some other medicine or no medicine at all on weekdays. Another option is to have the patient use the topical steroid twice weekly with an alternative topical in between.
4. *Combination therapy:* Use a steroid-sparing agent in one area or at one time of day and a topical steroid in another area or time.

ATOPIC DERMATITIS

Alternative topical agents for atopic dermatitis are:

- Emollients.
- Calcineurin inhibitors (pimecrolimus, tacrolimus).
- Crisaborole (Eucrisa)—very expensive new topical agent (see Chapter 151, Atopic Dermatitis).

These can be used intermittently in pulse therapy or daily in combination therapy.

STRATEGIES IN PSORIASIS

- Clobetasol or betamethasone for worst and thickest plaques.
- Triamcinolone for less severe areas.
- Topical vitamin D to be used in combination with steroid or alternating with a steroid.

METHODS TO INCREASE EFFECT OF TOPICAL STEROIDS

- Occlusion—Topical steroids can become more potent when occluded with plastic wrap or gloves. This is one strategy for lichen simplex chronicus or recalcitrant hand dermatitis.
- Wet wrap therapy—This is especially useful for erythrodermic conditions often caused by psoriasis or atopic dermatitis. This method can be used for any severe inflammatory skin condition:
    - Apply steroid ointment or cream to the inflamed skin.
    - Use pajamas or other cloth and soak in warm water.
    - Wring out excess water and apply to skin.
    - Put the "dry layer" such as a blanket over the "wet layer."
    - Leave in place overnight or 3 hours during the day but stop if patient becomes chilled.
    - Perform daily for up to 2 weeks, but do not use as long-term therapy.

INTRALESIONAL STEROIDS

Intralesional steroids are a powerful treatment tool for many dermatologic conditions including:

- Acne (**Figure 112-2**).
- Alopecia areata (**Figure 112-3**).
- Frontal fibrosing alopecia.
- Granuloma annulare.
- Psoriasis.
- Hypertrophic lichen planus.
- Prurigo nodularis.
- Hidradenitis suppurativa.
- Keloids and hypertrophic scars (**Figure 112-4**).

The most commonly used steroid for injection is triamcinolone acetonide (Kenalog) suspension. This is sold in concentrations of 10 mg/mL or 40 mg/mL. See **Table 112-4** for the recommended concentrations for injection. Steroid dilutions can be made with sterile saline for injection. This is less painful for the patient than diluting the steroid with lidocaine. Use a 27-gauge needle when injecting intralesional steroids to minimize pain. A Luer-Lok syringe is helpful to keep the needle from popping off during the injection. Wear eye protection for safety. Informed consent should emphasize the risks of skin atrophy and hypopigmentation **(Figure 112-5)**. These are more likely to occur with intralesional steroids than topical steroids and may not be reversible. This is the reason for following the dilution guide in **Table 112-4**. However, atrophy and/or hypopigmentation can occur even when everything is performed correctly. While the risks are real, the benefits of intralesional steroids can be both wonderful and rapid.

RESOURCES

- GoodRx. Website and mobile app (iOS and Android) for the best prices on topical steroids in the area, including discounts through coupons—**https://www.goodrx.com.**
- For further information on performing intralesional injections, see Usatine R, Pfenninger J, Stulberg D, Small R. *Dermatologic and Cosmetic Procedures in Office Practice.* Philadelphia, PA: Elsevier; 2012. This text and accompanying videos can also be purchased as an electronic application—**http://www.usatinemedia.com.**

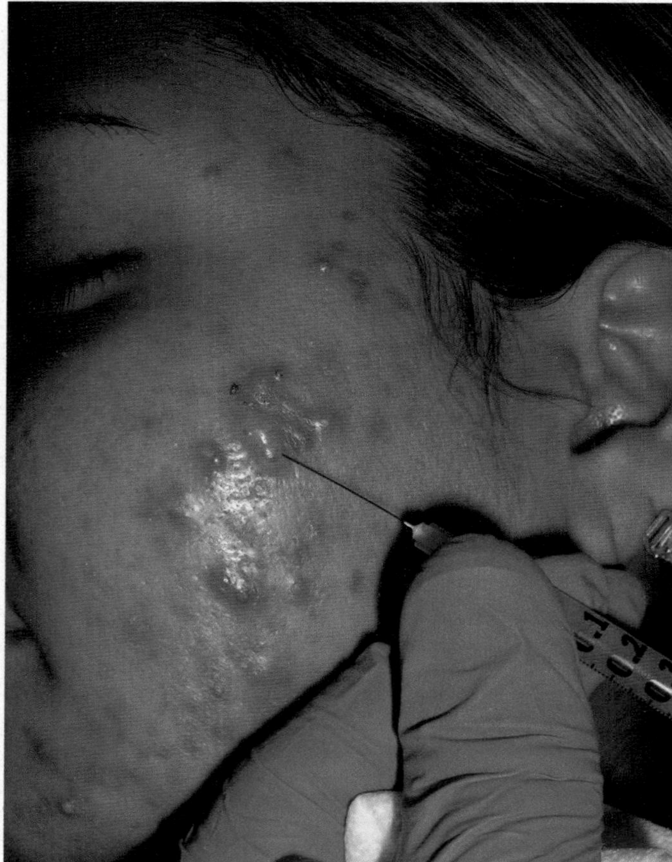

FIGURE 112-2 Injecting painful cystic acne with 2 mg/mL triamcinolone using a 30-gauge needle. (*Reproduced with permission from Richard P. Usatine, MD.*)

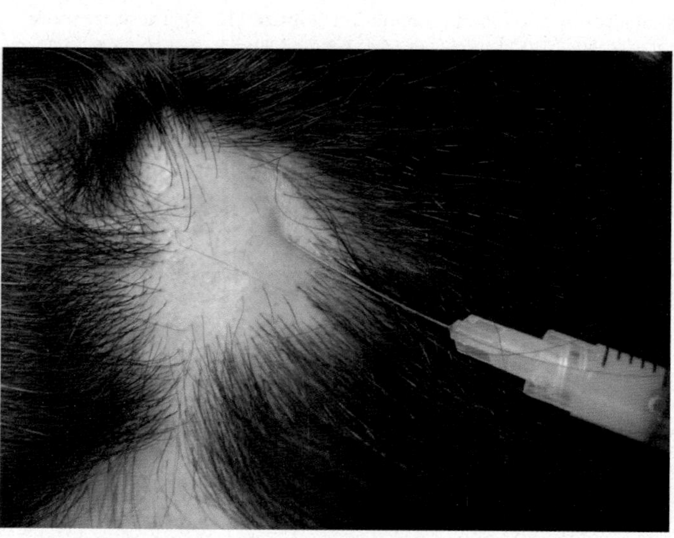

FIGURE 112-3 Injecting alopecia areata with 5 mg/mL triamcinolone using a 27-gauge needle on a Luer-Lok syringe. (*Reproduced with permission from Richard P. Usatine, MD.*)

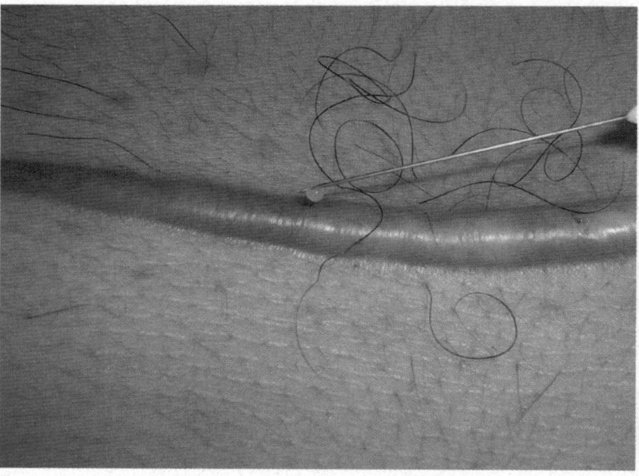

FIGURE 112-4 Injecting a hypertrophic scar with 10 mg/mL triamcinolone using a 27-gauge needle on a Luer-Lok syringe. (*Reproduced with permission from Richard P. Usatine, MD.*)

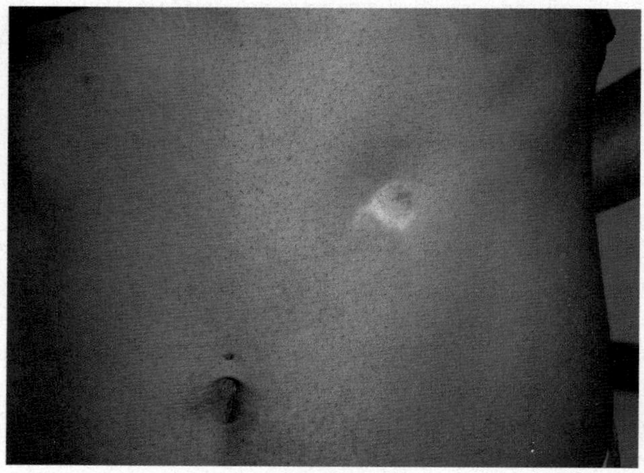

FIGURE 112-5 Hypopigmentation and skin atrophy that occurred after injecting a keloid with triamcinolone. (*Reproduced with permission from Richard P. Usatine, MD.*)

TABLE 112-4 Intralesional Steroids—Concentrations for Injection

Condition	Concentration of Triamcinolone Acetonide Solution (mg/mL)
Acne (see **Figure 112-2**)	2 to 2.5
Alopecia areata (see **Figure 112-3**)	5 to 10
Frontal fibrosing alopecia	5 to 10
Granuloma annulare	5
Psoriasis	5 to 10
Hypertrophic lichen planus	5 to 10
Prurigo nodularis	5 to 10
Hidradenitis suppurativa	10
Keloids and hypertrophic scars (see **Figure 112-4**)	10 to 40

REFERENCES

1. Chi CC, Kirtschig G, Baldo M, et al. Topical interventions for genital lichen sclerosus. *Cochrane Database Syst Rev.* 2011;7;(12):CD008240.

2. Freeman S, Howard A, Foley P, et al. Efficacy, cutaneous tolerance and cosmetic acceptability of desonide 0.05% lotion (Desowen) versus vehicle in the short-term treatment of facial atopic or seborrheic dermatitis. *Australas J Dermatol.* 2002;43(3):186-189.

3. Zivkovich AH, Feldman SR. Are ointments better than other vehicles for corticosteroid treatment of psoriasis? *J Drugs Dermatol.* 2009;8(6):570-572.

4. Lagos BR, Maibach HI. Frequency of application of topical corticosteroids: an overview. *Br J Dermatol.* 1998;139(5):763-766.

5. Green C, Colquitt JL, Kirby J, Davidson P. Topical corticosteroids for atopic eczema: clinical and cost effectiveness of once-daily vs. more frequent use. *Br J Dermatol.* 2005;152(1):130-141.

6. van de Kerkhof PC. Once daily vs. twice daily applications of topical treatments in psoriasis. *Br J Dermatol.* 2005;153(6):1245.

7. Hoare C, Li Wan Po A, Williams H. Systematic review of treatments for atopic eczema. *Health Technol Assess.* 2000;4(37):1-191.

8. van de Kerkhof PC. The impact of a two-compound product containing calcipotriol and betamethasone dipropionate (Daivobet/Dovobet) on the quality of life in patients with psoriasis vulgaris: a randomized controlled trial. *Br J Dermatol.* 2004;151(3):663-668.

9. van de Kerkhof PCM, de Hoop D, de Korte J, et al. Patient compliance in the treatment of psoriasis. *Dermatology.* 2000;200:292-298.

10. Mason AR, Mason J, Cork M, et al. Topical treatments for chronic plaque psoriasis. *Cochrane Database Syst Rev.* 2013;28(3):CD005028.

113 BIOPSY PRINCIPLES AND TECHNIQUES

Richard P. Usatine, MD

The most commonly performed skin biopsies are the shave biopsy, punch biopsy, and elliptical excisional biopsy. Other less common biopsy types that are rarely needed include incisional biopsy, which is performed like an elliptical excision but does not include the whole lesion, and biopsy by curettage. A deep shave biopsy is also called a saucerization. Most skin cancers can be biopsied using the shave or saucerization technique, and most rashes can be biopsied using a 4-mm punch biopsy.

SYNONYMS

Saucerization is synonymous with a deep shave biopsy. Elliptical excision is also called a fusiform excision.

ANESTHESIA

Anesthesia is needed before any biopsy is performed. The preferred anesthesia is 1% lidocaine with epinephrine. There is a myth that epinephrine should never be used when doing surgery on the fingers, toes, nose, and penis. This myth is taught in medical school and tested on the boards by those who still believe it is true. In reality, dermatologists, plastic surgeons, and head and neck surgeons use lidocaine with epinephrine safely every day in these areas, and the evidence supports this practice.[1-4]

There is no evidence to support that lidocaine with epinephrine can cause necrosis in areas with end-arteries, and no case of necrosis has been reported since the introduction of commercial lidocaine with epinephrine in 1948.[1] In addition, epinephrine supplementation results in a relatively bloodless operating field and longer effectiveness of local anesthesia. It also diminishes the chance for lidocaine toxicity, as it slows the lidocaine from being systemically distributed. Epinephrine-supplemented local anesthetics for ear and nose surgery were used without complications in more than 10,000 surgical procedures.[1] The relative absence of blood in the operating field significantly reduces the duration of surgery and increases the healing rate, as less electrosurgery is needed.[2] Both the nose and the ear have excellent blood supplies and can bleed profusely when surgeries are performed on them without epinephrine.

The addition of epinephrine in digital blocks minimizes the need for the use of tourniquets and large volumes of anesthetic and provides better and longer pain control during procedures.[3] Evidence also suggests that one can safely use epinephrine in digital blocks even in patients with vascular disease.[4] A Cochrane review in 2015 identified four randomized controlled trials studying the use of epinephrine in digital blocks.[5] In these studies, there were no reports of adverse events such as digital ischemia. Although some biopsies on the fingers can be performed with a local anesthetic at the biopsy site only, sometimes it is beneficial to perform a digital block only or first. Another method of providing local anesthetic to a finger or toe biopsy site is to perform the digital block using lidocaine without epinephrine and then use 1% lidocaine with epinephrine locally at the site of biopsy once the digital block is effective. It may take time to drop one's fear of using epinephrine on the digits, but the evidence is supportive. The use of epinephrine is beneficial when doing biopsies on the fingers, toes, nose, and penis.

There are a number of methods available to decrease the pain of local anesthesia:

- Use a small-gauge needle (27 or 30 gauge).
- Add sodium bicarbonate to the lidocaine and epinephrine.[6,7]
- Pinch or vibrate the skin as the needle enters the skin (based on the gate theory of pain).
- Distract the patient in conversation or with music.
- Inject very slowly because tissue distention hurts.
- Use only one injection site if possible and place subsequent injections into areas already anesthetized.

In most sites 3 mL of anesthesia should be sufficient for a shave biopsy and 5 mL should be sufficient for a punch biopsy. This is just a guideline for drawing up anesthesia, and the correct amount is determined by complete numbness at the biopsy site. Areas with less subcutaneous fat will need less volume of anesthesia.

Use 30-gauge needles on the most sensitive areas, including the face, the ears, the fingers, and the genitals. Although the needle should be inserted quickly, the injection will be less painful if the anesthesia is injected slowly. The more superficial the injection, the more painful it is. For example, an injection bleb similar to that of a tuberculin skin test is more painful than a deeper subcutaneous injection. It is usually less painful if the injection is done slowly and deeply at first, followed by redirecting the needle for a more superficial, dermal, blanching type of injection. In this manner, a volume of 5 mL can be given slowly through one injection site. Skin blanching and visible tissue distention helps determine the area that has been anesthetized. Also, tissue induration can be palpated to determine the distribution of the anesthesia. If need be, this area can be extended by reinjecting through another site that has already been anesthetized.

Adding sodium bicarbonate (8.4% for injection) in a 1:10 dilution to the lidocaine and epinephrine anesthetic solution markedly decreases the pain caused by injection (e.g., 1 mL of sodium bicarbonate can be added to 9 mL of lidocaine). The addition of sodium bicarbonate creates a solution with a neutral pH from the commercially available lidocaine-epinephrine solutions that have a pH of 4 to 6. Although this takes a bit more time to prepare, the patients will appreciate that the injection is less painful. In our office we use these mixtures:

- 3-mL syringes with 2.25 mL of lidocaine-epi and 0.25 mL bicarbonate for shave biopsies.
- 5- or 6-mL syringes with 4.5 mL of lidocaine-epi and 0.5 mL bicarbonate for punch biopsies.
- 10- or 12-mL syringes with 9 mL of lidocaine-epi and 1 mL bicarbonate for elliptical excisions.

The lidocaine will usually work within 1 minute, but the epinephrine will have its maximal effect after 10 minutes. If one is biopsying a suspected skin cancer, it does help to wait the 10 minutes, as skin cancers are more likely to bleed heavily when biopsied. To remain efficient, see another patient or complete some charting (including the pathology request) while waiting for the epinephrine to reach maximal effect.

SHAVE BIOPSY

The advantages of the shave biopsy include:

- Speed (because no sutures are required).
- Minimal risk of bleeding.
- Sterile gloves not needed (because a full-thickness wound is not created).
- Excellent cosmetic results.[8,9]

Shave equipment needed:

- Razor blade (favored over the scalpel).
- Aluminum chloride for hemostasis (favored over Monsel solution).
- Cotton-tip applicators (need not be sterile) to stabilize the final cut and apply aluminum chloride.
- Adson forceps (optional).

Shave biopsy can be performed with a razor blade or a scalpel. Razor blades are sharp and are preferred as they bend to fit the lesion and the depth of biopsy. Nonsterile clean razor blades can be purchased and broken in half as the most economical option. However, it is easier and safer to use a sterile razor blade with a plastic handle. The DermaBlade is one such option that allows for convenient superficial and deep shave biopsies (**Figure 113-1**).

In most cases it helps to mark the biopsy site with a surgical marker before injecting the lidocaine and epinephrine. This is especially true if the lesion is small and not pigmented. If a 2-mm margin is desired, it is easier to measure this and mark it before beginning the biopsy (**Figure 113-2**). It is easier to cut along the marked line than to estimate margins without clear marking.

If the lesion sticks up above the skin and the intent of the biopsy is to only remove the skin that is protruding, the blade should be held flat with the skin surface, and a gentle sawing motion is used to remove the lesion. In order to perform a saucerization (deep shave biopsy) it helps to hold the blade so it makes a 30- to 45-degree angle with the skin (**Figure 113-3**). With a sawing motion, the blade cuts under the pigmented lesion and the blade is then flattened out as additional cuts are made. If the lesion is suspected to be a melanoma, then the cut skin can be lifted with the end of a cotton-tipped applicator to make sure that the biopsy is below the pigment (**Figure 113-4**). Some aluminum chloride can be applied to the bleeding area if needed to see the tissue below the blade. If one sees pigment below, angle the blade deeper for the rest of the biopsy.

This method is easier to do if one waits at least 10 minutes for the epinephrine to reach maximal effect. Management of a melanoma changes when depths greater than 1 mm are found, as they suggest the need for a sentinel lymph node biopsy and consideration of larger margins for definitive surgery (2 cm rather than 1 cm). The saucerization

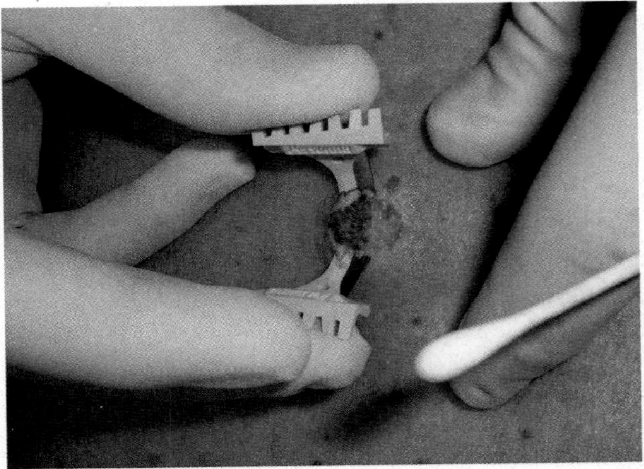

FIGURE 113-1 Saucerization of a suspected melanoma using a DermaBlade. The biopsy successfully sampled the full melanoma with clear peripheral and deep margins. The pathology showed invasive melanoma less than 1 mm in depth, and an elliptical excision with 1-cm margins was performed for definitive treatment. (*Reproduced with permission from Richard P. Usatine, MD.*)

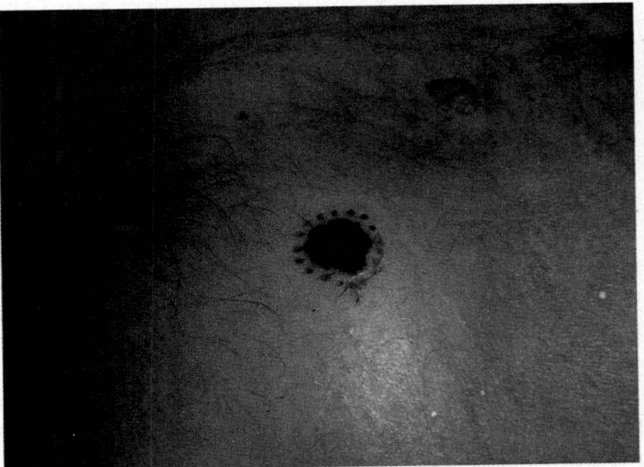

FIGURE 113-2 Preparing for deep shave biopsy of a suspected melanoma by drawing a 1- to 2-mm margin around the lesion. Pathology showed a melanoma in situ. The blanching is secondary to the injection of the lidocaine and epinephrine. (*Reproduced with permission from Richard P. Usatine, MD.*)

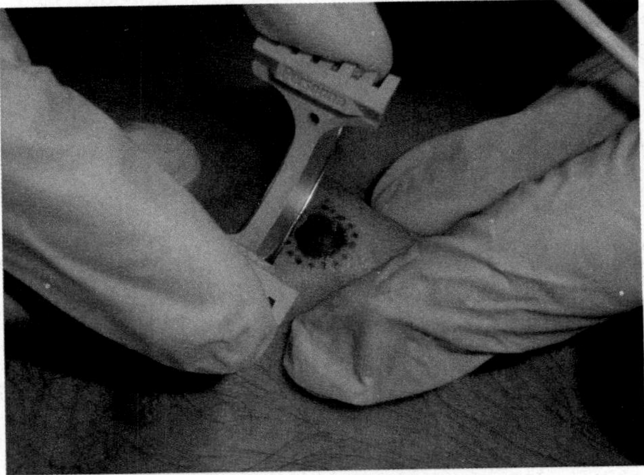

FIGURE 113-3 The DermaBlade is positioned to make a 30-degree angle with the skin in performing a saucerization. The nondominant hand is used to pinch the skin to stabilize it during the cutting. (*Reproduced with permission from Richard P. Usatine, MD.*)

is completed when the blade is directed upward and comes out of the skin.

Two technical challenges with the shave biopsy are:

1. The skin moving side to side as the blade moves back and forth, preventing the blade from cutting.
2. The skin flipping over at the end of the shave biopsy, making it hard to cut the last piece of skin off.

The first challenge can be overcome by stabilizing the skin with the nondominant hand while cutting with the blade in the dominant hand. Most of the time stabilization involves pinching the skin in front of the biopsy site (**Figure 113-3**). Once the blade is moving through the skin and getting close to the final edge, it is critical to move the nondominant hand far enough from the razor blade that no fingers are cut.

The second challenge is met by holding a cotton-tipped applicator in the nondominant hand and applying the wooden stick end to the skin so that the skin does not flip over (**Figure 113-5**). With practice, the cotton-tipped applicator can be held in the nondominant hand even while pinching the skin for stabilization. The skin is held in place for the final cut by pressure from the stick (**Figure 113-5**).

Hemostasis can be obtained with aluminum chloride and/or electrocoagulation. Aluminum chloride can be purchased as 20% in alcohol (Drysol) by prescription or in formulations in water up to 70%. Aluminum chloride 70% in water is available for purchase from www.delasco.com and is my preferred hemostatic agent. Avoid silver nitrate and Monsel's solution as they may stain/tattoo the skin.

The aluminum chloride is applied using a cotton-tipped applicator and a twisting motion (**Figure 113-6**). It helps if downward pressure is applied vertically while twisting the cotton-tipped applicator. It is best if the cotton-tipped applicator is not too wet with the aluminum chloride. If the applicator is very wet, a completely dry cotton-tipped applicator can be twisted onto the bleeding site with pressure to dry the site and complete the hemostasis. If this does not work, electrocoagulation is the next best step. If electrocoagulation is not available, continued pressure for minutes on the bleeding site will often be sufficient.

Place the shave biopsy into a bottle with formalin. If an assistant is available, he or she can help by pushing the specimen off the blade into the formalin using the stick end of a cotton-tipped applicator. Make sure that the specimen actually ends up in the bottle.

A free video of the shave procedure is available on the *Journal of Family Practice* website: https://www.mdedge.com/jfponline/article/80274/dermatology/shave-biopsy.

PUNCH BIOPSY

The advantages of a punch biopsy include:

- Faster and easier than an elliptical biopsy.
- Minimal risk of bleeding.
- Rapid healing as the cut is small.
- Excellent cosmetic results.
- Sterile gloves are not needed.

Punch equipment needed:

- Punch biopsy tool.
- Adson forceps.

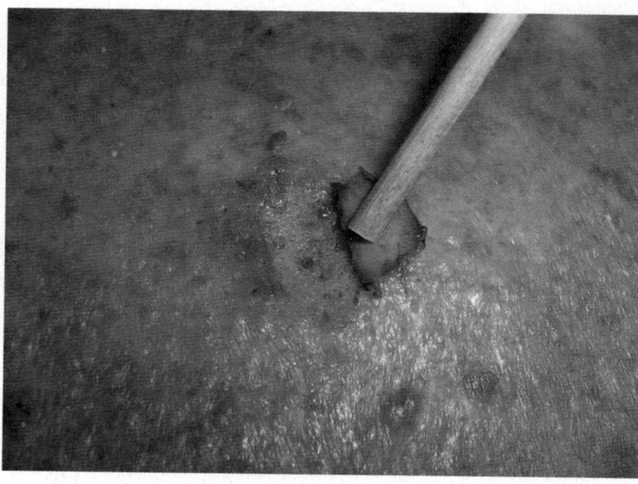

FIGURE 113-4 Pausing during a saucerization to look for pigment at the base of the specimen. The base was clear and the full pigmented lesion was biopsied with a clear deep margin. *(Reproduced with permission from Richard P. Usatine, MD.)*

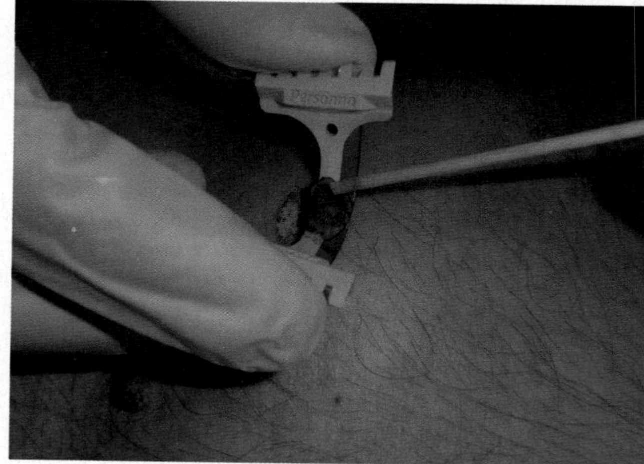

FIGURE 113-5 Using the stick end of a cotton-tipped applicator to stabilize the pigmented lesion at the end of a deep shave biopsy. This helps to keep the specimen from flipping over and makes it easier to remove. *(Reproduced with permission from Richard P. Usatine, MD.)*

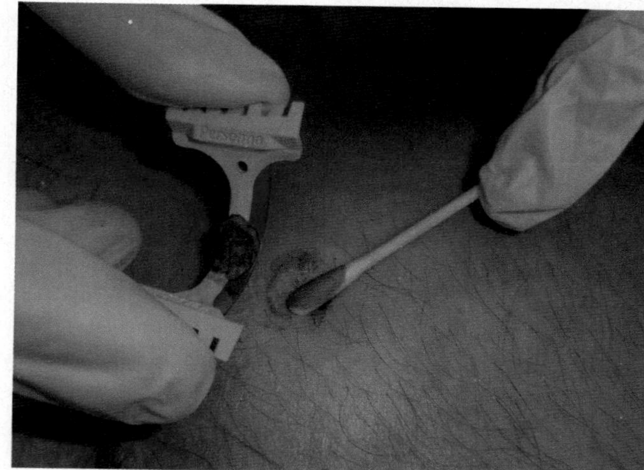

FIGURE 113-6 Applying aluminum chloride to the shave biopsy site to stop the bleeding. *(Reproduced with permission from Richard P. Usatine, MD.)*

- Iris scissor.
- Needle driver for suturing.
- Cotton-tip applicators (sterile) for temporary hemostasis.

After the shave biopsy, the punch biopsy is the next easiest and fastest biopsy to perform. It is usually the biopsy of choice to diagnose an unknown rash. While punch biopsy tools can range in diameter from 2 mm to 10 mm, the most useful size is 4 mm. The 4-mm punch is the optimal size for the diagnosis of most rashes. It gives enough tissue to the pathologist without creating a large scar for the patient. One study showed that a 4-mm punch biopsy can be left open to heal by second intention, but in that study the clinicians packed the wound with a clotting agent and had the patient return for a special appointment just to remove this clotting agent two days after the surgery.[10] We recommend closing a 4-mm punch biopsy with a single suture. In most cases nylon suture is sufficient. The suture helps to obtain quick hemostasis and a good cosmetic result. Electrosurgery and chemical hemostatic agents do not work well to stop the bleeding after a punch biopsy, and a suture works very well.

Just like the shave biopsy, it helps to mark the area for the punch. Obtain anesthesia with 1% lidocaine and epinephrine and wait 10 minutes if possible to minimize the bleeding during the procedure.

When a rash covers large parts of the skin, it is usually best to choose new lesions rather than old lesions. Also, a biopsy from an upper extremity is preferred over the lower extremity. If the rash is equal on the front and the back of the trunk, choose the front of the trunk so that the patient will be able to see and care for the healing wound more easily. Don't forget to mark the punch site before giving the anesthesia. Also, the biopsy should sample a lesion clearly representative of the affected skin. A margin of normal skin is only needed if the lesion is an ulcer or a bulla.

A free video of the punch procedure is available on the *Journal of Family Practice* website (https://www.mdedge.com/jfponline/article/79581/dermatology/punch-biopsy). In this video I used sterile gloves, but subsequently I have changed to clean gloves only. The data support the use of clean gloves even though a suture will be placed in most cases.[11] It is uncommon for punch biopsies to become infected regardless of glove type. We still prep the site with chlorhexidine and use a sterile fenestrated drape for the suturing.

Before starting to cut with the punch tool, make sure that your equipment is ready to go. This means having the forceps and scissors ready and easy to grab from your Mayo stand. It helps to have some sterile gauze on the field next to the intended biopsy site in the direction in which blood would run. Start the biopsy by holding the punch against the skin and twirling it back and forth while putting gentle pressure downward (**Figure 113-7**). The punch tool is a rounded blade and cuts best by rotating it rather than pushing it against the skin. Cut downward until the punch passes into the subcutaneous tissue. Often one can feel the difference as the punch passes from the firm dermis into the softer subcutaneous tissue below. If one is not sure if the punch tool is deep enough, it can be removed, and if adequate depth was obtained, the round biopsy core will be seen to separate and rise up from the skin around it (**Figure 113-8**). If the core is firmly in place, cut deeper until the core separates from the surrounding skin. Now lift the core gently with the forceps and cut it off as deep as possible with the iris scissors (**Figure 113-9**). Place the core sample into the formalin. Place a sterile cotton-tipped applicator into the

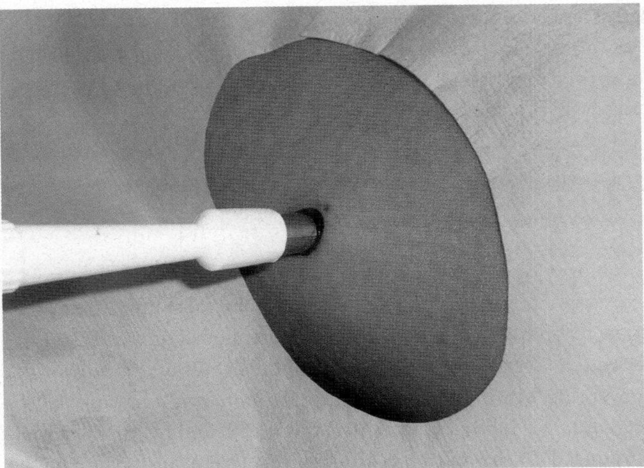

FIGURE 113-7 Performing a punch biopsy by rotating the punch tool back and forth while applying gentle downward pressure. (*Reproduced with permission from Richard P. Usatine, MD.*)

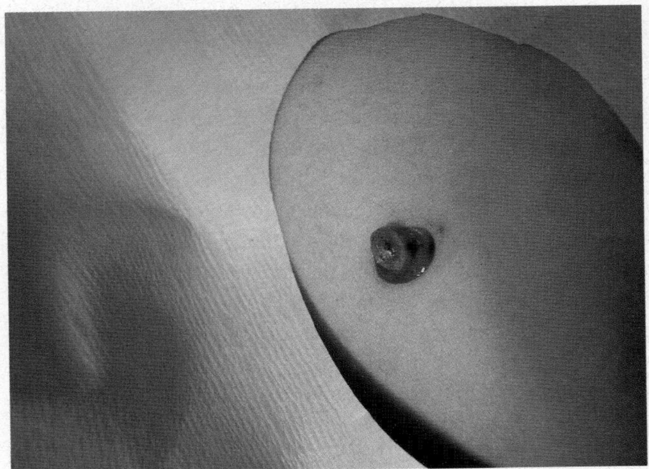

FIGURE 113-8 Note how the punch biopsy core is elevated from the surrounding tissue once the punch biopsy has cut through the dermis into the subcutaneous tissue. This is the proper depth for the biopsy. (*Reproduced with permission from Richard P. Usatine, MD.*)

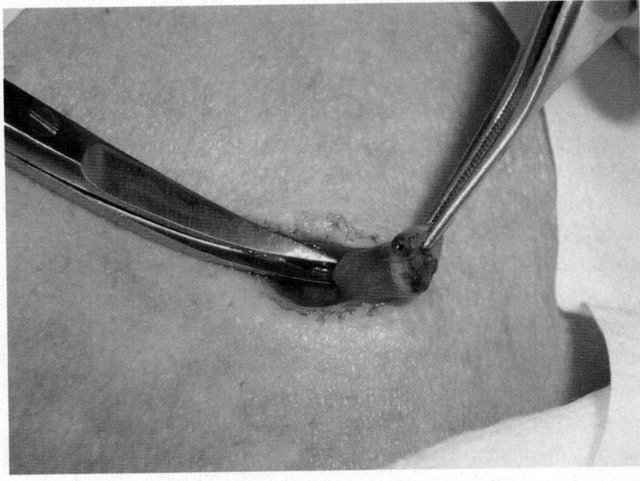

FIGURE 113-9 Using gentle pressure to elevate the punch biopsy specimen while snipping off the specimen at the base with as iris scissor. (*Reproduced with permission from Richard P. Usatine, MD.*)

defect and let it stand there to slow the bleeding (**Figure 113-10**). Place a single interrupted stitch to close the defect and provide hemostasis (**Figure 113-11**). If the bleeding is excessive, a figure-of-eight suture will provide better hemostasis (**Figure 113-12**).

ELLIPTICAL EXCISIONAL BIOPSY

This biopsy type is the most complex and time consuming. It is rarely needed as a biopsy, although the ellipse is the most important excisional technique for the definitive treatment of skin cancers. It is beyond the scope of this book to teach the details of this biopsy type. I cover this fully in my book entitled *Dermatologic and Cosmetic Procedures in Office Practice*. Also, the Watch and Learn video that I produced for the *Journal of Family Practice* is available free on the JFP website—http://www.mdedge.com/jfponline/article/82000/dermatology/elliptical-excision.

BIOPSY OF SKIN CANCERS

Many clinicians were taught that a punch biopsy is the preferred biopsy type for melanoma because it gets full depth. In reality, a deep shave biopsy (saucerization) is often the procedure of choice when biopsying a suspicious melanoma.[12] The National Comprehensive Cancer Network (NCCN) melanoma guidelines on the principles of biopsy state that an excisional biopsy (elliptical, punch, or saucerization) with 1- to 3-mm margins is the preferred method of biopsy for a melanoma.[12] Unless one can get a 1- to 3-mm margin around the melanoma with a punch, a saucerization or elliptical excision is preferred.[13] The saucerization technique allows for sampling both the breadth and depth of the growth and thus provides the pathologist with tissue from both the epidermis and dermis (see **Figure 113-1**).

Depth is important because it predicts prognosis and affects management of melanoma. For tumors greater than 1 mm in depth, a sentinel lymph node biopsy (SLNB) should be considered.[13,14] The goal should be to get the accurate tumor depth with the initial biopsy. In addition, surgical margins depend on primary tumor depth. To ensure a depth greater than 1 mm, the clinician should aim to get a tissue specimen that is at least as thick as a dime (1.3 mm).

Partial sampling of large melanocytic tumors with a punch biopsy can lead to sampling error.[15] Ng and colleagues found that there was a significant increase in histopathologic misdiagnosis with punch biopsy of part of a lesion (odds ratio [OR] 16.6) and a shallow shave biopsy (OR 2.6) compared with excisional biopsy (including saucerization). Punch biopsy of part of the lesion was also associated with increased odds of misdiagnosis with an adverse outcome (OR 20).[15] Partial biopsies of growths suspicious for melanoma should be avoided when possible.

With the goal of avoiding partial sampling, a challenge exists when the suspicious growth is quite large. Many melanomas are broader than a centimeter. Although punch biopsies ensure a depth of 1 mm or more, they risk missing the thickest portion of the tumor.[16] They, however, do offer a reasonable option when the melanoma is too large (broad) for a complete saucerization. Options include a large saucerization of the visibly deepest part of the melanoma or multiple 4- to 6-mm punch biopsies to reduce the risk of sampling error. Punch

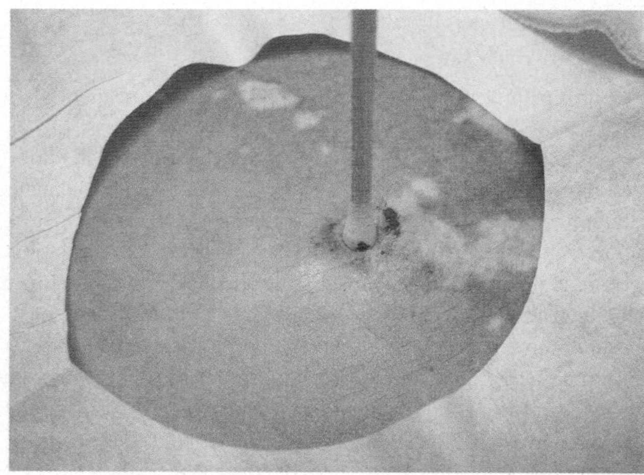

FIGURE 113-10 Note how the cotton-tipped applicator remains upright in the 4-mm punch defect to provide immediate hemostasis, allowing the operator to load the needle holder for suturing. (*Reproduced with permission from Richard P. Usatine, MD.*)

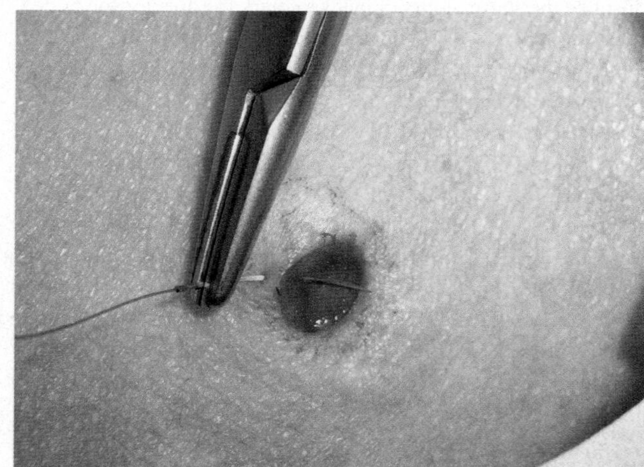

FIGURE 113-11 Suturing the punch biopsy closed with a single interrupted suture. This is usually adequate for a 4-mm punch biopsy. (*Reproduced with permission from Richard P. Usatine, MD.*)

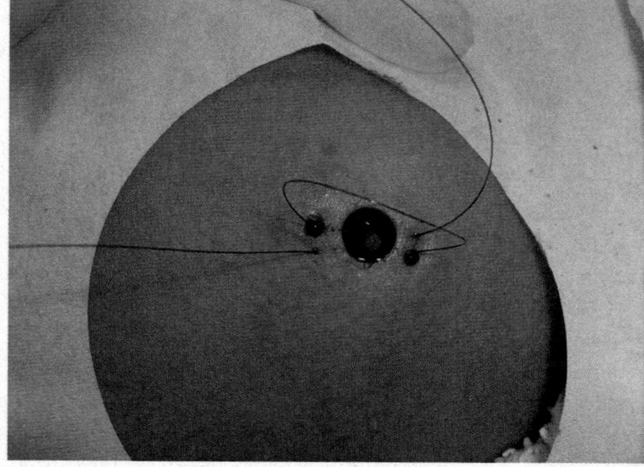

FIGURE 113-12 Figure-of-eight suture provides excellent hemostasis when needed and requires placing the needle twice through the skin before tying the knot. (*Reproduced with permission from Richard P. Usatine, MD.*)

biopsies smaller than 4 mm should be avoided, as the breadth of tissue is inadequate. For example, even with dermoscopy, facial lentigo maligna melanoma is often difficult to differentiate from pigmented actinic keratosis and solar lentigines. A broad shave biopsy is a preferred method of biopsy for lentigo maligna melanoma in situ according to the NCCN.[13]

If the biopsy confirmed a malignancy, a larger surgery with suturing will be needed. The most important issue to keep in mind is that if partial sampling leads to a benign diagnosis of a suspicious lesion, then the remainder of the lesion must be excised and sent for pathology.

Saucerization is also the preferred biopsy type for basal cell and squamous cell carcinoma. Studies have shown that tumor depth is the most important factor in predicting metastasis of SCC as well as tumor relapse rate, making identification of depth of the tumor important in both management and prognosis.[17] A saucerization should provide adequate depth when performed properly.

Family physicians can learn to do a saucerization quickly and easily in the office during a standard 15-minute visit. A quick saucerization avoids the time and inconvenience of setting up a designated surgery time to perform an elliptical excision. This also can prevent delays in diagnosis that can occur with long wait times to see a dermatologist and/or no-shows for a future appointment.

CONCLUSION

The information in this chapter should empower family physicians and other primary care clinicians to be on the front line of detecting skin cancers at their earliest stage. Most skin cancers including melanoma are curable when detected early. Avoiding delays in diagnosis by rapid high-quality skin biopsies can save lives and prevent physical deformities from large skin cancers.

Family physicians and other primary care clinicians can also use appropriate skin biopsies to detect challenging skin rashes. Although many rashes can be diagnosed by a good history and physical exam and collecting clues from multiple areas such as nails and feet, there are rashes that truly need biopsy for a definitive diagnosis. Being able to perform a good punch biopsy can avoid a referral to dermatology and provide a quick, reliable diagnosis for an accurate treatment plan.

RESOURCES

- Usatine R, Pfenninger J, Stulberg D, Small R. *Dermatologic and Cosmetic Procedures in Office Practice*. Philadelphia, PA: Elsevier; 2012.
- Free Watch and Learn videos on the *Journal of Family Practice* website—
https://www.mdedge.com/jfponline/article/80274/dermatology/shave-biopsy
https://www.mdedge.com/jfponline/article/79581/dermatology/punch-biopsy
http://www.mdedge.com/jfponline/article/82000/dermatology/elliptical-excision.

REFERENCES

1. Nielsen LJ, Lumholt P, Hölmich LR. [Local anaesthesia with vasoconstrictor is safe to use in areas with end-arteries in fingers, toes, noses and ears]. *Ugeskr Laeger*. 2014;176(44). http://www.ncbi.nlm.nih.gov/pubmed/25354008. Accessed June 2017.
2. Häfner H-M, Röcken M, Breuninger H. Epinephrine-supplemented local anesthetics for ear and nose surgery: clinical use without complications in more than 10,000 surgical procedures. *J Dtsch Dermatol Ges*. 2005;3(3):195-199. http://www.ncbi.nlm.nih.gov/pubmed/16372813. Accessed June 2017.
3. Krunic AL, Wang LC, Soltani K, et al. Digital anesthesia with epinephrine: an old myth revisited. *J Am Acad Dermatol*. 2004;51(5):755-759.
4. Ilicki J. Safety of epinephrine in digital nerve blocks: a literature review. *J Emerg Med*. 2015;49(5):799-809.
5. Prabhakar H, Rath S, Kalaivani M, Bhanderi N. Adrenaline with lidocaine for digital nerve blocks. *Cochrane Database Syst Rev*. 2015;(3):CD010645.
6. Colaric KB, Overton DT, Moore K. Pain reduction in lidocaine administration through buffering and warming. *Am J Emerg Med*. 1998;16:353-356.
7. Bartfield JM, Crisafulli KM, Raccio-Robak N, Salluzzo RF. The effects of warming and buffering on pain of infiltration of lidocaine. *Acad Emerg Med*. 1995;2:254-258.
8. Gambichler T, Senger E, Rapp S, et al. Deep shave excision of macular melanocytic nevi with the razor blade biopsy technique. *Dermatol Surg*. 2000;26(7):662-666.
9. Ferrandiz L, Moreno-Ramirez D, Camacho FM. Shave excision of common acquired melanocytic nevi: cosmetic outcome, recurrences, and complications. *Dermatol Surg*. 2005;31(9 Pt 1):1112-1115.
10. Christenson LJ, Phillips PK, Weaver AL, Otley CC. Primary closure vs second-intention treatment of skin punch biopsy sites: a randomized trial. *Arch Dermatol*. 2005;141(9):1093-1099.
11. Heal C, Sriharan S, Buttner PG, Kimber D. Comparing non-sterile to sterile gloves for minor surgery: a prospective randomised controlled non-inferiority trial. *Med J Aust*. 2015;202(1):27-31.
12. Zager JS, Hochwald SN, Marzban SS, et al. Shave biopsy is a safe and accurate method for the initial evaluation of melanoma. *J Am Coll Surg*. 2011;212(4):454-460.
13. Coit DG, Andtbacka R, Bichakjian CK, et al. Melanoma. *J Natl Compr Canc Netw*. 2009;7(3):250-275.
14. Gershenwald JE, Scolyer RA, Hess KR, et al. Melanoma of the skin. *AJCC Cancer Staging Man*. 2017;8:563-585.
15. Ng JC, Swain S, Dowling JP, et al. The impact of partial biopsy on histopathologic diagnosis of cutaneous melanoma: experience of an Australian tertiary referral service. *Arch Dermatol*. 2010;146(3):234-239.
16. Kaiser S, Vassell R, Pinckney RG, et al. Clinical impact of biopsy method on the quality of surgical management in melanoma. *J Surg Oncol*. 2014;109(8):775-779.
17. D'souza G, Carey TE, William WN, et al. Epidemiology of head and neck squamous cell cancer among HIV-infected patients. *J Acquir Immune Defic Syndr*. 2014;65(5):603-610.

SECTION B CHILDHOOD DERMATOLOGY

114 NORMAL SKIN CHANGES

Cathy M. Feller, MD
Brian Z. Rayala, MD

PATIENT STORY

A 2-week-old infant is brought to the office for her first well-baby check. The parents noticed a rash on the face. You diagnose the white spots on the bridge of the nose as milia and benign cephalic pustulosis (BCP) on the cheeks. The parents are happy to hear that BCP and milia will go away without treatment (**Figures 114-1** and **114-2**).

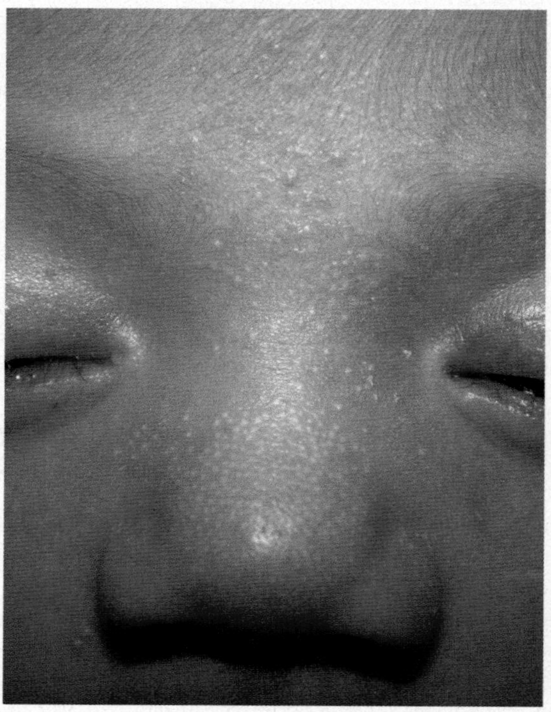

FIGURE 114-1 Milia on the face of a 2-week-old infant with greatest number of milia on the nose. *(Reproduced with permission from Richard P. Usatine, MD.)*

INTRODUCTION

- Rashes are common in newborns. Physicians will be consulted frequently, as they are a common parental concern. Most newborn rashes are benign; however, a few are associated with more serious conditions. A newborn's skin shows a variety of changes during the first 2 months of life, and most are self-limited. Physicians must be prepared to identify common rashes and advise parents.[1]
- Milia are inclusion cysts that appear as tiny white papules in the skin (see **Figure 114-1**) or on the roof of the mouth.
- BCP is an acneiform eruption appearing as noncomedonal papules or pustules with surrounding erythema on the skin of newborns (see **Figure 114-2**). BCP accounts for the vast majority of diagnosed neonatal acne. True neonatal acne, though, encompasses comedonal and papulopustular lesions.
- Congenital dermal melanocytosis (CDM) is a hereditary, congenital patch of bluish-black or bluish-gray pigment usually in the sacral area, back, and buttocks of infants (**Figures 114-3** and **114-4**).
- Erythema toxicum neonatorum (ETN) is a benign, self-limited skin eruption appearing as small yellow-white papules or vesicles with surrounding skin erythema (**Figures 114-5** and **114-6**).

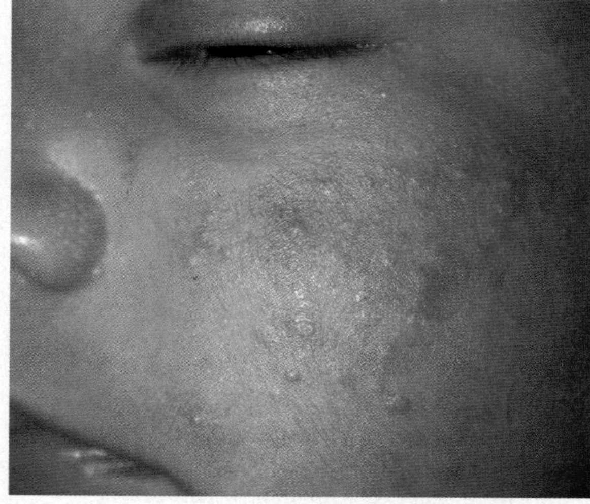

FIGURE 114-2 Benign cephalic pustulosis on the same infant. *(Reproduced with permission from Richard P. Usatine, MD.)*

SYNONYMS

- Milia are also called milk spots or oil seed.
- CDM is also known as Mongolian spots, Mongolian blue spots, slate grey patches, and dermal melanocytosis.
- ETN is also referred to as erythema toxicum, or toxic erythema of the newborn.

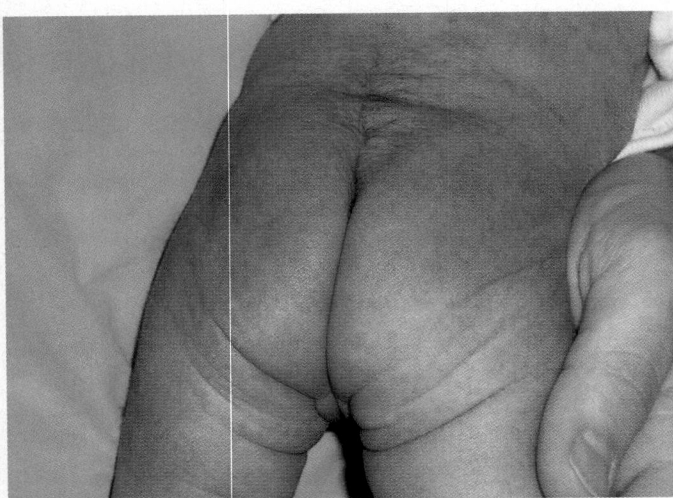

FIGURE 114-3 Congenital dermal melanocytosis (mongolian spots) covering the buttocks and back of a Hispanic infant. (*Reproduced with permission from Richard P. Usatine, MD.*)

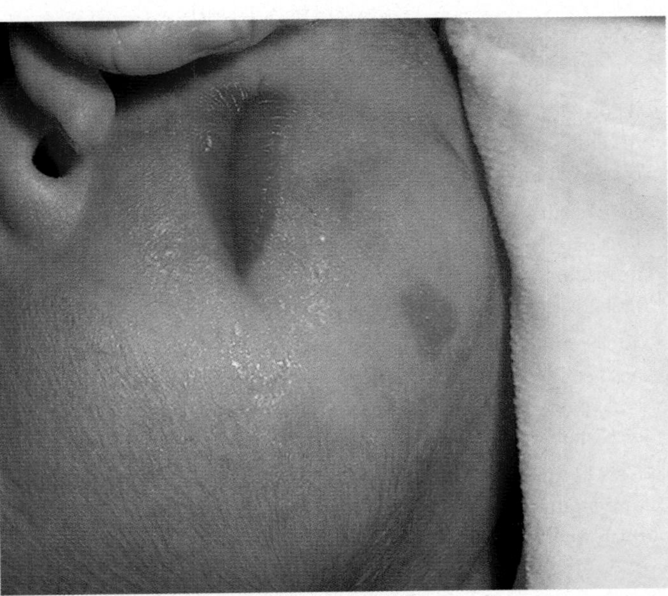

FIGURE 114-5 One small spot of erythema toxicum neonatorum on a 2-day-old infant. (*Reproduced with permission from Richard P. Usatine, MD.*)

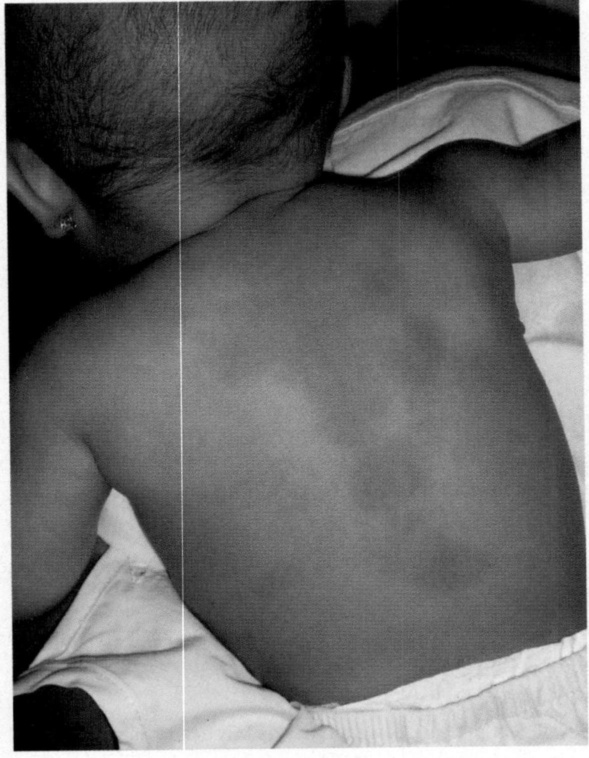

FIGURE 114-4 Congenital dermal melanocytosis (mongolian spots) on the back of a 1-year-old black child. (*Reproduced with permission from Richard P. Usatine, MD.*)

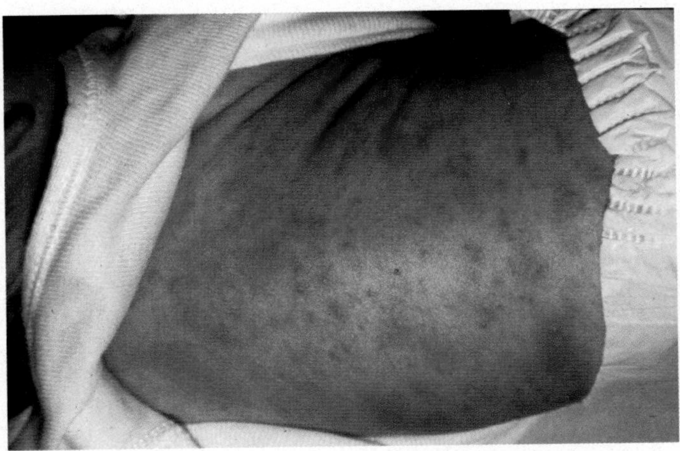

FIGURE 114-6 More widespread case of erythema toxicum neonatorum covering the infant. ETN is completely benign and will resolve spontaneously. (*Reproduced with permission from Richard P. Usatine, MD.*)

EPIDEMIOLOGY

- Approximately 40% to 50% of newborn infants in the United States develop milia.[2] This condition is mainly associated with newborns carried to full term or near term.
- BCP occurs in many newborns. It typically consists of erythematous papules and pustules but no comedones. BCP affects the forehead, chin, and cheeks. The eruption usually presents during the first 2 weeks of life.[3]
- The prevalence of CDM varies among different ethnic groups. It has been reported in approximately 96% of black infants, 90% of Native American infants, 81% to 90% of Asian infants, 46% to 70% of Hispanic infants, and 1% to 10% of white infants.[4,5]
- ETN occurs in 30% to 70% of full-term infants and in 5% of premature infants. The incidence rises with increasing gestational age and birth weight.[6,7]

ETIOLOGY AND PATHOPHYSIOLOGY

- Milia are inclusion cysts that contain trapped keratinized stratum corneum surrounded by a dense lymphocytic infiltrate. Milia are caused by retention of keratin within the dermis. They may rarely be associated with other abnormalities in syndromes such as epidermolysis bullosa and the orofacial digital syndrome (type 1).[2,8]
- BCP has been associated with *Malassezia* species acquired from normal parental skin flora.[3] Maternal androgenic hormones that stimulate sebaceous glands likely cause true neonatal acne.[9]
    - In true neonatal acne, histologic examination shows hyperplastic sebaceous glands with keratin-plugged orifices.
- CDM is a hereditary, congenital, developmental condition exclusively involving the skin. It results from entrapment of melanocytes in the dermis during their migration from the neural crest into the epidermis.
    - CDM is associated with cleft lip, spinal meningeal tumor, melanoma, and phakomatosis pigmentovascularis types 2 and 5.[10]
    - A few cases of extensive CDM have been reported with inborn errors of metabolism, the most common being Hurler syndrome, followed by gangliosidosis type 1, Niemann-Pick disease, Hunter syndrome, and mannosidosis.[3,4] In such cases, they are likely to persist rather than resolve.[4]
- The etiology of ETN is not known. ETN is thought to be an immune system reaction; the condition is associated with increased levels of immunologic and inflammatory mediators (e.g., interleukins, eotaxin).[3]
    - The eosinophilic infiltrate of ETN suggests an allergic-related or hypersensitivity-related etiology, but no allergens have been identified. Newborn skin appears to respond to any injury with an eosinophilic infiltrate.
    - Because ETN rarely is seen in premature infants, it is believed that mature newborn skin is required to produce this reaction pattern.

DIAGNOSIS

CLINICAL FEATURES

- Milia are characterized as tiny, pearly white papules (see **Figure 114-1**) that are actually small inclusion cysts ranging from 1 to 2 mm in diameter. No visible opening is present.[2]
    - Milia usually appear after 4 to 5 days of life in full-term newborns. Manifestations of milia may be delayed from days to weeks in infants born before term.[8,10]
- BCP is a noncomedonal papulopustular eruption. True neonatal acne (**Figure 114-2**) includes comedones (i.e., whiteheads), papules, and pustules.[3] Papules and pustules are the most frequent types of lesions (72.7%), followed by comedones only (22.7%).[2,9]
- CDM (**Figures 114-3** and **114-4**) is a bluish-black macule or patch typically a few centimeters in diameter, although much larger lesions also can occur. Lesions may be solitary or numerous.
    - Generalized CDM involving large areas covering the entire posterior or anterior trunk and the extremities have been reported.
    - Several variants exist, including[4,5]:
        - Persistent CDM—These are larger, have sharper margins, and persist for many years (**Figure 114-4**).
        - Aberrant CDM involve unusual sites such as the face or extremities.
        - Persistent aberrant CDM also are referred to as macular-type blue nevi.
- ETN commonly presents with a blotchy, evanescent, macular erythema (**Figures 114-5** and **114-6**).
    - The macules are irregular, blanchable, and vary in size.
    - In more severe cases (**Figure 114-6**), pale yellow or white wheals or papules on an erythematous base may follow. In approximately 10% of patients, 2- to 4-mm pustules develop.[1,7]
    - ETN occurs within the first 4 days of life in full-term infants, with the peak onset within the first 48 hours following birth. Rare cases have been reported at birth.
    - Delayed onset can rarely occur in full-term and preterm infants up to 14 days of age.
    - Infants with ETN otherwise are healthy and lack systemic symptoms.

TYPICAL DISTRIBUTION

- Milia are found on the forehead, nose, upper lip, cheeks, and scalp. They can, however, occur anywhere and may be present at birth or appear subsequently. The milia on the child in **Figure 114-1** were present at birth.
- BCP occurs on the face with a predilection for nose, cheeks, and chin (**Figure 114-2**).[3]
- CDM most commonly involve the lumbosacral area (**Figure 114-3**), but the buttocks, flanks, and shoulders (**Figure 114-4**) may be affected with extensive lesions.
- ETN sites of predilection include the forehead, face, trunk, and proximal extremities, typically sparing the genital and acral areas.[3] Involvement of the mucous membranes rarely occurs (**Figures 114-5** and **114-6**).

LABS AND IMAGING

- No laboratory studies are required.
- Severe or persistent neonatal acne may warrant further work-up for congenital adrenal hyperplasia, a virilizing tumor, or other endocrinopathy.[11]
- In extensive CDM involving the back, radiographic studies are needed to rule out a spinal meningeal tumor or anomaly.[4]
- ETN is often diagnosed clinically, based on history and physical examination, but a peripheral smear of intralesional contents can be done to confirm the diagnosis.[7]
    - A Tzanck smear or Gram stain shows inflammatory cells with greater than 90% eosinophils and variable numbers of neutrophils.
    - A complete blood count (CBC) may show eosinophilia in 7% to 18% of patients.[12] Eosinophilia may be more pronounced when the eruption shows a marked pustular component.

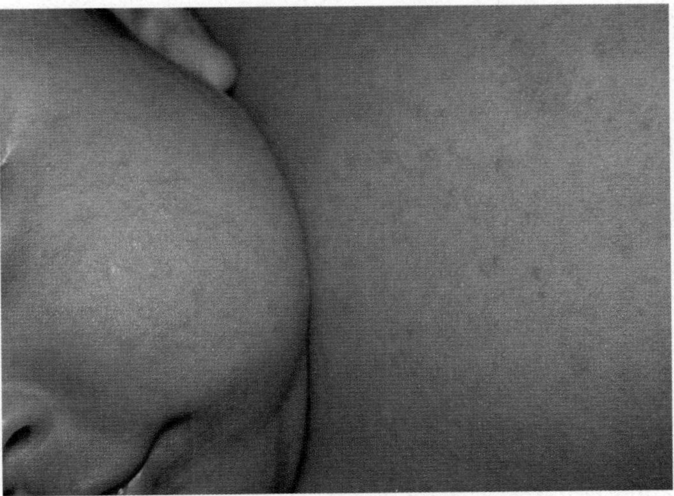

FIGURE 114-7 Miliaria (heat rash) in a 6-month-old infant on a warm summer day. *(Reproduced with permission from Richard P. Usatine, MD.)*

DIFFERENTIAL DIAGNOSIS

Other diagnoses that may be confused with milia, BCP, and ETN include:

- Miliaria—Heat rash (prickly heat) with tiny papules that can be red (miliaria rubra), clear (miliaria crystallina), or pustular (miliaria pustulosa) (**Figure 114-7**). Miliaria results from sweat retention caused by partial closure of eccrine structures. Both milia and miliaria result from immaturity of the skin structures, but they are clinically distinct entities.
- Neonatal pustular melanosis—This eruption, present at birth, consists of 2- to 4-mm nonerythematous vesicles filled with a milky fluid. This rash occurs in 5% of African-American newborns and in less than 1% of white newborns, and fades in the first 3 to 4 weeks of life (see Chapter 116, Pustular Diseases of Childhood).
- Sebaceous hyperplasia—Yellow papules present at birth, typically located on the nose, and resolve within two months (see Chapter 165, Sebaceous Hyperplasia). Attributed to fetal exposure to maternal androgen.[11]

CDM may be confused with the following lesions also present at birth or shortly after:

- Congenital melanocytic nevi—These lesions are much less common (1% to 2% of newborns). They are of variable color from tan or brown to red or black, often within a single lesion and the pigment may fade off into surrounding skin. The borders are often irregular and the lesion can appear slightly raised over time (although a macular portion is usually found at the edges). Most congenital melanocytic nevi have a darker color and more discrete borders than CDM. A biopsy is only needed if melanoma is suspected (see Chapter 169, Congenital Melanocytic Nevi).
- There are reports of CDM being confused for the bruising that occurs in child abuse. A good history and a clear knowledge of the pattern of CDM should help to differentiate between these two entities.

ETN can be confused with the following:

- Folliculitis—Primary lesion is a papule or pustule pierced by a central hair, although the hair may not always be visualized. Deeper lesions present as erythematous, often fluctuant nodules. Folliculitis rarely occurs in the first few days of life when ETN is most commonly seen (see Chapter 123, Folliculitis).

- Chickenpox—The characteristic rash appears in crops of lesions beginning with red macules and passing through stages of papule, vesicle (on an erythematous base), pustule, and crust. Simultaneous presence of different stages of the rash is a hallmark. Infants are mostly born with adequate maternal antibodies to varicella, so that timing should differentiate between these two conditions (see Chapter 129, Chickenpox).
- Cutis marmorata (**Figure 114-8**) is reticulated mottled skin with symmetric involvement of the trunk and extremities produced by a vascular response to cold; the change resolves with heat. This entity can persist for weeks or months. No treatment is indicated.
- Harlequin color change affects 10% of full-term babies and occurs when the newborn lies on one side and erythema develops on one side of the body, while blanching is seen on the contralateral side. The color change fades after 30 seconds to 20 minutes and resolves with increased muscle activity or crying. It begins between the second to fifth days of life and lasts up to 3 weeks.[13]
- Neonatal lupus is a rare syndrome in which maternal autoantibodies are passively transferred to the baby, producing well-demarcated, erythematous, scaling patches that are often annular, predominately on the scalp, neck, or face (**Figure 114-9**). The condition is self-limited and resolves without scarring by 6 to 7 months of age. It is associated with congenital heart block. Treatment includes photoprotection; mild topical steroids may be helpful.

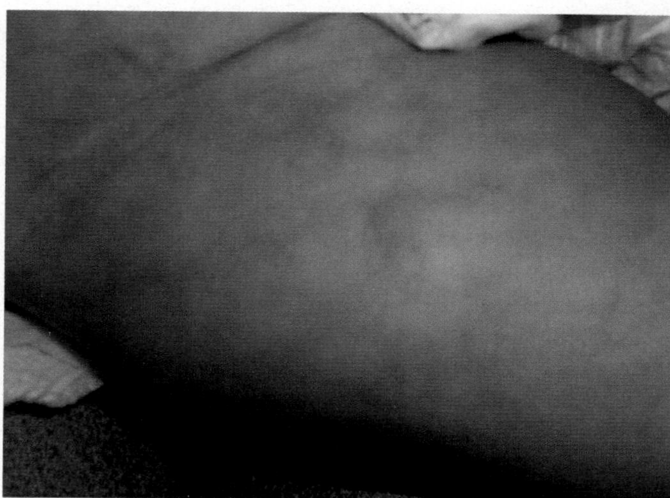

FIGURE 114-8 Cutis marmorata in a 4-month-old infant in a cold exam room. Notice the reticular pattern. This resolved when the infant was warmed. (*Reproduced with permission from Richard P. Usatine, MD.*)

MANAGEMENT

FIRST LINE

- Milia, BCP, CDM, and ETN are benign conditions and parents should be reassured that they resolve with time. SOR Ⓐ
- If treatment for BCP is pursued, topical azole creams will result in quick resolution of lesions.[3] SOR Ⓒ This includes OTC clotrimazole and miconazole.

SECOND LINE

- If treatment is chosen for severe neonatal acne, there is low-quality evidence for the following:
    - Comedones may be treated with azelaic acid cream 20% or tretinoin cream 0.025% to 0.05%.[14,15] SOR Ⓒ
    - For inflammatory lesions, erythromycin solution 2% and benzoyl peroxide gel 2.5% may be used.[14,16] SOR Ⓒ
    - Oral erythromycin is the preferred antibiotic if systemic therapy is pursued.[14] SOR Ⓒ

PROGNOSIS

- Milia usually disappear within a few weeks.
- BCP may persist for a few weeks to several months.
- CDM may persist for many years but usually disappear within 3 to 5 years and almost always by puberty.
- ETN usually lasts for several days but can change rapidly, with lesions appearing and disappearing in different areas over hours.

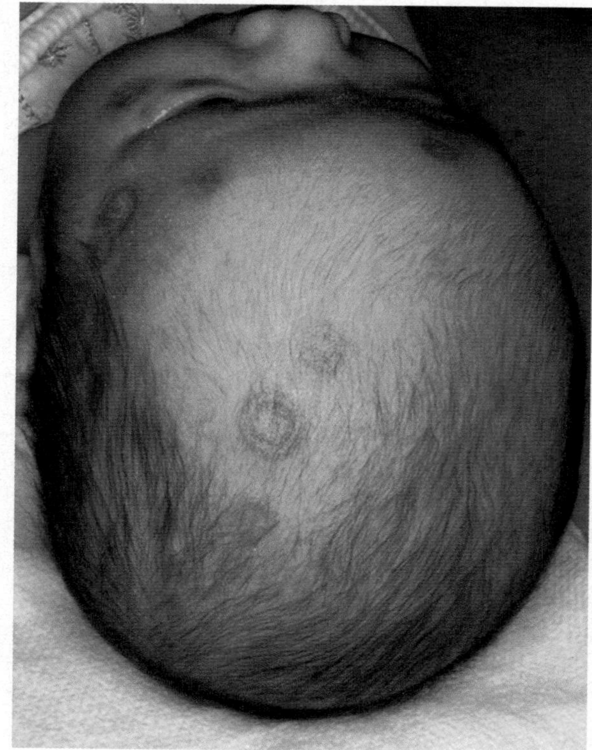

FIGURE 114-9 Neonatal lupus from acquired antibodies through transplacental transmission from the mother with active systemic lupus erythematosus (SLE). Note the annular patterns of scale. (*Reproduced with permission from Warner AM, Frey KA, Connolly S. Photo rounds: annular rash on a newborn, J Fam Pract. 2006;55(2):127-129. Frontline Medical Communications, Inc.*)

PARENT EDUCATION

- Milia is a benign self-limiting condition that disappears within a few weeks without leaving any scars. No drug therapy is required, and use of nonprescription rash medications is not recommended.
- BCP resolves on its own in weeks. Oils and lotions do not help and may actually aggravate the acne. An OTC azole cream may be used.
- CDM is likely to fade over time and may disappear by age 7 to 13 years.
- ETN will usually disappear within 2 weeks.

PATIENT RESOURCES

- Milia—**https://medlineplus.gov/ency/article/001367.htm.**
- BCP—**https://www.dermnetnz.org/topics/neonatal-cephalic-pustulosis.**
- Neonatal acne—**https://medlineplus.gov/ency/imagepages/19645.htm.**
- CDM—**https://medlineplus.gov/ency/article/001472.htm.**
- ETN—**https://medlineplus.gov/ency/article/001458.htm.**

PROVIDER RESOURCES

- **http://www.adhb.govt.nz/newborn/teachingresources/dermatology/BenignLesions.htm.**
- **http://www.aafp.org/afp/2008/0101/p47.html.**

REFERENCES

1. McLaughlin MR, O'Connor NR, Ham P. Newborn skin: part II. Birthmarks. *Am Fam Physician.* 2008;77(1):56-60.
2. Nguyen NV. *Pediatric Milia.* http://emedicine.medscape.com/article/910405-overview. Updated April 8, 2016. Accessed June 2017.
3. Rayala BZ, Morrell DS. Common skin conditions in children: neonatal skin lesions. *FP Essent.* 2017;453:11-17.
4. Ashrafi MR, Shabanian R, Mohammadi M, Kavusi S. Extensive Mongolian spots: a clinical sign merits special attention. *Pediatr Neurol.* 2006;34(2):143-145.
5. Cordova A. The Mongolian spot: a study of ethnic differences and a literature review. *Clin Pediatr (Phila).* 1981;20(11): 714-719.
6. Clemons RM. Issues in newborn care. *Prim Care.* 2000;27(1): 251-267.
7. Liu C, Feng J, Qu R. Epidemiologic study of the predisposing factors in erythema toxicum neonatorum. *Dermatology.* 2005; 210(4):269-272.
8. Johr RH, Schachner LA. Neonatal dermatologic challenges. *Pediatr Rev.* 1997;18(3):86-94.
9. Van Praag MC, Van Rooij RW, Folkers E, et al. Diagnosis and treatment of pustular disorders in the neonate. *Pediatr Dermatol.* 1997;14(2):131-143.
10. Mallory SB. Neonatal skin disorders. *Pediatr Clin North Am.* 1991; 38(4):745-765.
11. Katsambas AD, Katoulis AC, Stavropoulos P. Acne neonatorum: a study of 22 cases. *Int J Dermatol.* 1999;38:128-130.
12. Berg FJ, Solomon LM. Erythema neonatorum toxicum. *Arch Dis Child.* 1987;62(4):327-328.
13. Selmogul MA, Dilmen U, Karkelleoglu C, et al. Picture of the month. Harlequin color change. *Arch Pediatr Adolesc Med.* 1995; 149(10):1171-1172.
14. Jansen T, Burgdorf WH, Plewig G. Pathogenesis and treatment of acne in childhood. *Pediatr Dermatol.* 1997;14:17-21.
15. Antoniou C, Dessinioti C, Stratigo AJ, et al. Clinical and therapeutic approach to childhood acne: an update. *Pediatr Dermatol.* 2009;26:373-380.
16. Van Praag MC, Van Rooij RW, Folkers E, et al. Diagnosis and treatment of pustular disorders in the neonate. *Pediatr Dermatol.* 1997;14:131-143.

115 CHILDHOOD HEMANGIOMAS

Richard P. Usatine, MD
Megha Madhukar Kapoor, MD
Elbert M. Belk, MD

PATIENT STORY

A baby girl is brought to the office because her mother is concerned over the growing strawberry hemangioma on her face. Her mother is reassured that most of these childhood hemangiomas regress over time and that there is no need for immediate treatment (**Figure 115-1**).

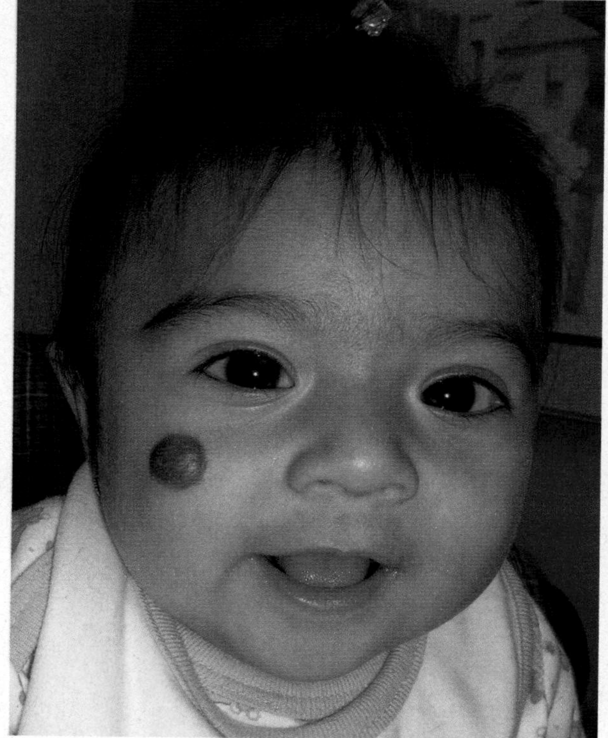

FIGURE 115-1 Strawberry hemangioma on the face causing no functional problems. Treatment is reassurance and watchful waiting. (*Reproduced with permission from Richard P. Usatine, MD.*)

INTRODUCTION

Hemangiomas are the most common benign tumors of infancy, affecting approximately 5% to 10% of children with Caucasian ethnicity.[1]

Up to 70% of hemangiomas are small and of cosmetic concern only and will resolve at the predictive rate of 10% per year, that is, 50% will have involuted by age 5; 90% by age 9.[2]

Segmental morphology, large size, and location on the face are predictive of poorer outcomes as measured by complication rates and suggest the need for further investigative study.[3]

SYNONYMS

Infantile hemangiomas, angiomas. Strawberry hemangiomas are also called superficial hemangiomas of infancy. Cavernous hemangiomas are also called deep hemangiomas of infancy.

EPIDEMIOLOGY

- Approximately 30% of hemangiomas are present at birth; the other 70% appear within the first few weeks of life.
- Although the most predictive condition involving infantile hemangioma is low birth weight, other factors to be considered are prematurity, fair-skinned infants, female sex (2.4:1), and even in some cases family history.[1,4]
- In one study, the mothers of children with hemangiomas are of higher maternal age, have a higher incidence of preeclampsia and placenta previa, and are more likely to have had multiple-gestation pregnancies.[5]

ETIOLOGY AND PATHOPHYSIOLOGY

- Hemangiomas consist of an abnormally dense group of dilated blood vessels.
- Hemangiomas are characterized by an initial phase of rapid proliferation, followed by spontaneous and slow involution, often leading to complete regression.

- Vascular malformations do not exhibit rapid proliferation but rather grow in proportion to the child and are considered a separate and distinct diagnosis with differing treatment regimens.
- Most childhood hemangiomas are small and innocuous, but some grow to threaten a particular function or even life.
- Rapid growth during the first month of life is the historical hallmark of hemangiomas, when rapidly dividing endothelial cells are responsible for the enlargement of these lesions. The hemangiomas become elevated and may take on numerous morphologies (dome-shaped, lobulated, plaque-like, and/or tumoral). The proliferation phase occurs during the first year, with most growth taking place during the first 6 months of life. Proliferation then slows and the hemangioma begins to involute.
- The involutional phase may be rapid or prolonged. No specific feature has been identified in explaining the rate or completeness of involution. However, in one type of hemangioma, the rapidly involuting congenital hemangioma, the proliferation phase occurs entirely in utero such that the lesion is fully developed at birth, followed by complete involution during the second year of life.
- Of the lesions that have involuted by age 6 years, 38% will leave residual evidence of the hemangioma in the form of a scar, telangiectasia, or redundant, "bag-like" skin. The chance of a permanent scar increases the longer it takes to involute. For example, of the lesions that involute after age 6 years, 80% may exhibit a cosmetic deformity requiring surgical intervention. Surgical intervention should only be performed by trained specialists because of the propensity for excessive bleeding from these vascular lesions.[6]

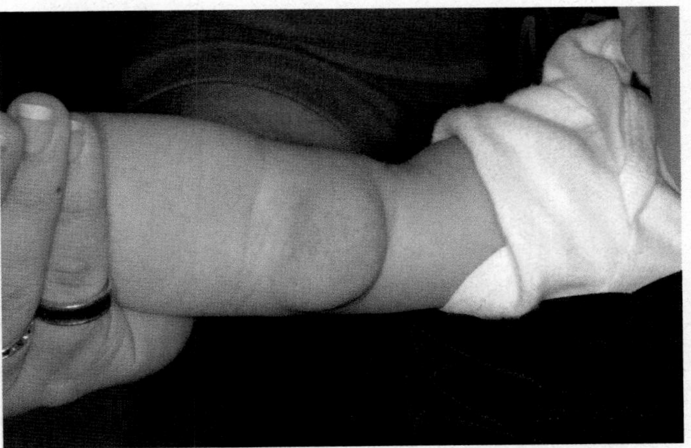

FIGURE 115-2 Deep (cavernous) hemangioma on the arm in a 9-month-old child. Treatment is watchful waiting. (*Reproduced with permission from Richard P. Usatine, MD.*)

DIAGNOSIS

CLINICAL FEATURES

Early lesions may be subtle, resembling a scratch or bruise, or alternatively may look like a small patch of telangiectasias or an area of hypopigmentation. A hemangioma can start off as a flat red mark, but as proliferation ensues, it grows to become a spongy mass protruding from the skin. The earliest sign of a hemangioma is blanching of the involved skin with a few fine telangiectasias followed by a red macule. Rarely, a shallow ulceration may be the first sign of an incipient hemangioma. Hemangiomas are typically diagnosed based on appearance, rarely warranting further diagnostic tests.[7]

Hemangiomas may be superficial, deep, or a combination of both. Superficial hemangiomas are well defined, are bright red, and appear as nodules or plaques located above clinically normal skin (see **Figure 115-1**). Deep hemangiomas are raised flesh-colored nodules, which often have a bluish hue and feel firm and rubbery (**Figure 115-2**).

Most are clinically insignificant unless they impinge on vital structures, ulcerate, bleed, incite a consumptive coagulopathy, or cause high-output cardiac failure or structural abnormalities. Blocking vision is a common reason needed for treatment (**Figures 115-3** and **115-4**).

TYPICAL DISTRIBUTION

Anywhere on the body, most often on the face, scalp, back, or chest.

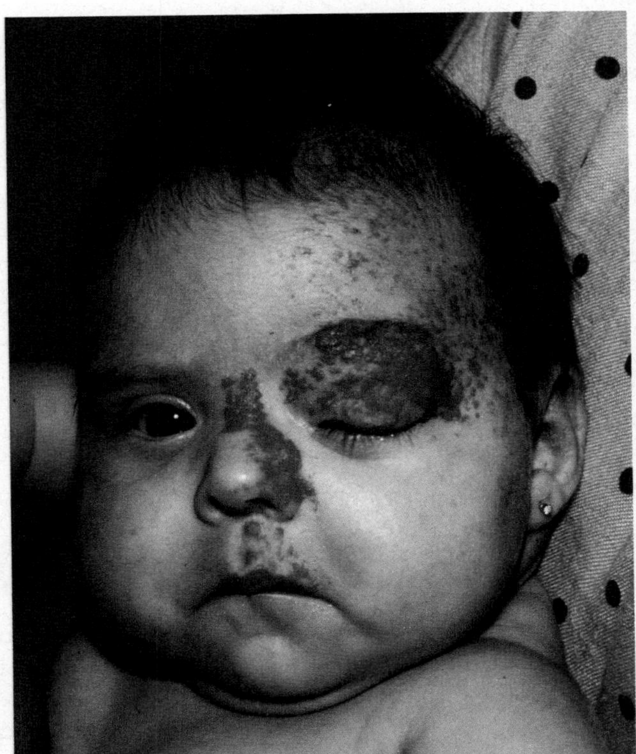

FIGURE 115-3 Large hemangioma on the face needing immediate treatment to prevent amblyopia in the left eye. Although this hemangioma follows the V1 dermatome, this is not a port-wine stain and the patient does not have Sturge-Weber syndrome. (*Reproduced with permission from Richard P. Usatine, MD.*)

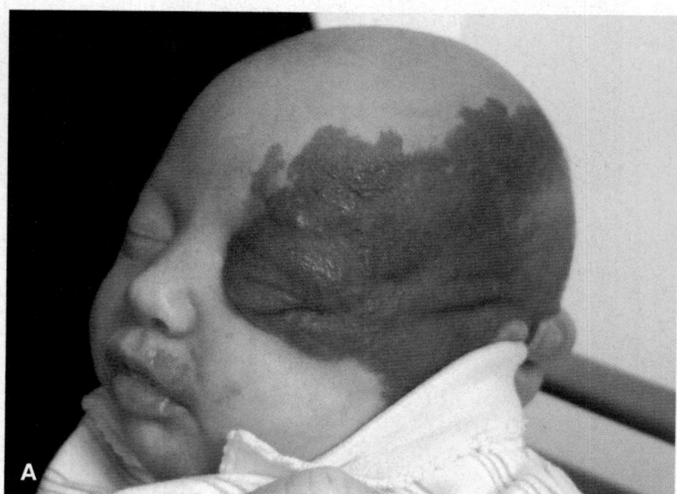

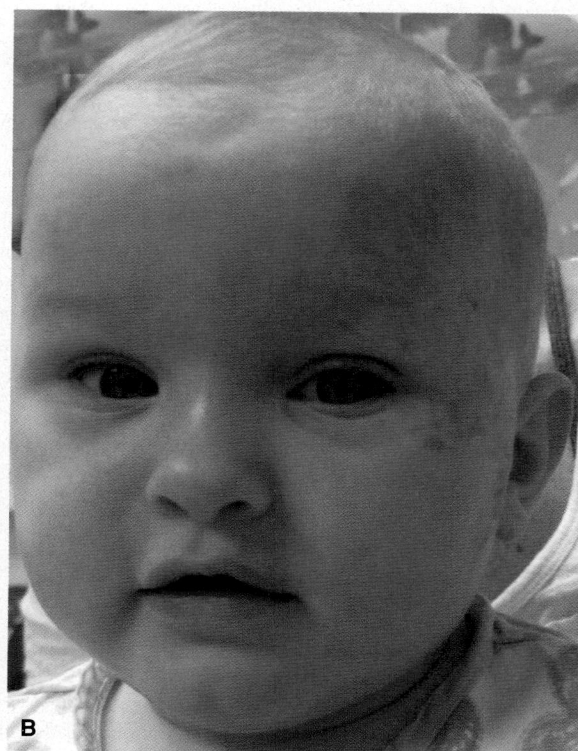

FIGURE 115-4 Large infantile hemangioma blocking vision. Propranolol was used to shrink this hemangioma. **A.** Before propranolol therapy. **B.** After propranolol therapy. (*Reproduced with permission from John Browning, MD.*)

IMAGING

Most hemangiomas of infancy do not need imaging. If the hemangioma is very large, deep, or undefined, MRI with and without IV gadolinium helps delineate the location and extent of hemangiomas while also differentiating them from high-flow vascular lesions, such as arteriovenous malformations.[7] Ultrasound is a useful tool to differentiate hemangiomas from other subcutaneous structures such as cysts and lymph nodes as well as from other soft-tissue masses but is limited in determining the depth or extent of the hemangioma.[8]

Plain radiography may be useful for evaluating hemangiomas that impinge on an airway.[7]

BIOPSY

Biopsies are rarely needed and can be risky because vascular lesions may bleed profusely. If a biopsy is being considered, referral is recommended.

DIFFERENTIAL DIAGNOSIS

- Superficial capillary malformations that are frequently seen in infants include those above the eyelids and nape of the neck. These are called salmon patches and are not dangerous. The "angel's kisses" on the eyelids (**Figure 115-5**) usually disappear by age 2 years. The "stork bites" may last into adulthood but are rarely an issue because they are often covered by hair (**Figure 115-6**). These capillary malformations are a variant of nevus flammeus or port-wine stain. They are macular, sharply circumscribed, pink to purple, and varied in size (see Chapter 211, Hereditary and Congenital Vascular Skin Lesions).

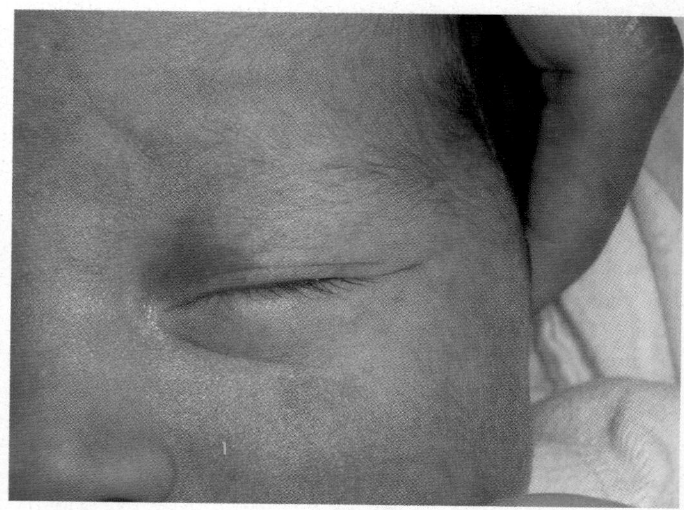

FIGURE 115-5 Salmon patch (a variant of nevus flammeus) on the upper eyelid called an "angel's kiss." These resolve by age 2 years. (*Reproduced with permission from Richard P. Usatine, MD.*)

- Blue rubber bleb nevus syndrome—Bluish cutaneous vascular malformations that empty with pressure; texture resembles rubbery nodules, similar to deep hemangiomas.[9]
- Maffucci syndrome—Rare congenital nonhereditary mesodermal dysplasia characterized by multiple enchondromata, cutaneous hemangiomas, and more recently spindle cell hemangiomas.[10] It is important to identify Maffucci syndrome early because it is associated with an increased risk of malignancy. May appear as multiple vascular malformations of the skin with a "grape-like" appearance (see Chapter 211, Hereditary and Congenital Vascular Skin Lesions).
- Angiosarcoma—Rare, malignant endothelial tumor characterized as ill-defined red patches, plaques, or nodules (see Chapter 210, Acquired Vascular Skin Lesions).[11]
- Arteriovenous malformation—Benign, single red papules on head or neck; may be cutaneous or mucosal.[11]
- Infantile fibrosarcoma—A rare and highly malignant tumor of childhood that may take on the form of a highly vascularized mass, resembling a hemangioma, especially after a hemangioma has ulcerated as a result of rapid proliferation.[12]

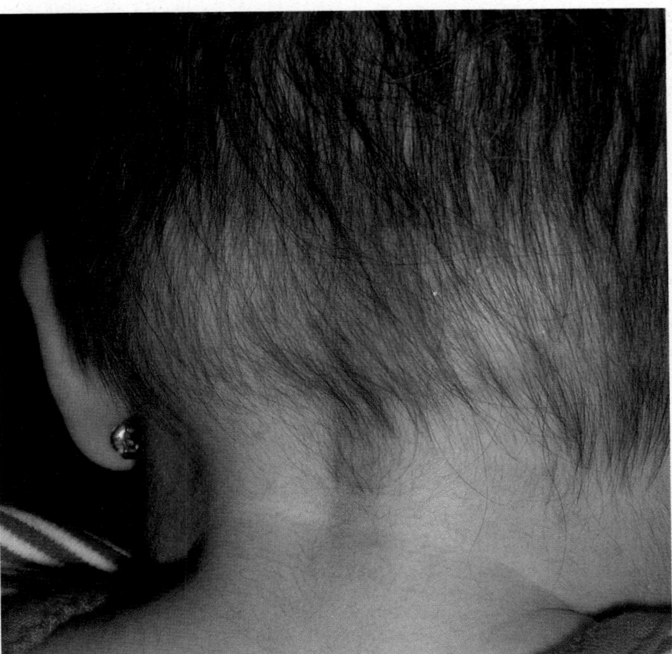

FIGURE 115-6 Salmon patch (a variant of nevus flammeus) on the neck of this young child called a "stork bite." These vascular malformations persist into adulthood. *(Reproduced with permission from Richard P. Usatine, MD.)*

MANAGEMENT

- The majority of hemangiomas will eventually involute without complications and require no treatment, but approximately 20% cause complications such as ulcerations or irreversible cutaneous expansion, or threaten vital structures such as the eyes, nose, or airways.[13]
- Hemangiomas in trauma-prone areas are the most likely to ulcerate. These include the diaper area (**Figure 115-7**) and the back of the head. Small ulcerations can be treated with topical mupirocin in morning and metronidazole gel in the evening. SOR Ⓒ
- Any lower face or beard area hemangioma can be a marker for laryngeal hemangiomatosis (**Figure 115-8**). Snoring or frequent cough in such a child should prompt a referral to a head and neck surgeon.
- Any large segmental hemangioma on the face could be part of the PHACE syndrome:

  P—Posterior fossa malformations

  H—Hemangiomas, usually large, segmental, "plaque-like" lesions (**Figure 115-9**)

  A—Arterial anomalies

  C—Cardiac anomalies and coarctation of the aorta

  E—Eye abnormalities, that is, microphthalmos, exophthalmos, colobomas, retinal vascular abnormalities, optic nerve atrophy, or iris hypertrophy or hypoplasia. A coloboma is a hole in one of the structures of the eye that can cause blindness (**Figure 115-10**).

Beta blockers are now the first-line therapy for cosmetically significant or function-impairing and rapidly proliferating infantile hemangiomas. Propranolol (FDA approved, 20 mg/5 mL) 1 mg/kg to 3 mg/kg dosages were used in the largest randomized controlled trial to date for treatment durations of 3 to 13 months, with the median length of treatment being 6 months (see **Figure 115-10**). The benefit of continuing treatment beyond 12 months is not clear.[14,15] SOR Ⓑ

- Propranolol treatment can cause side effects such as diarrhea, sleep disturbance, electrolyte abnormalities, and/or cold extremities.

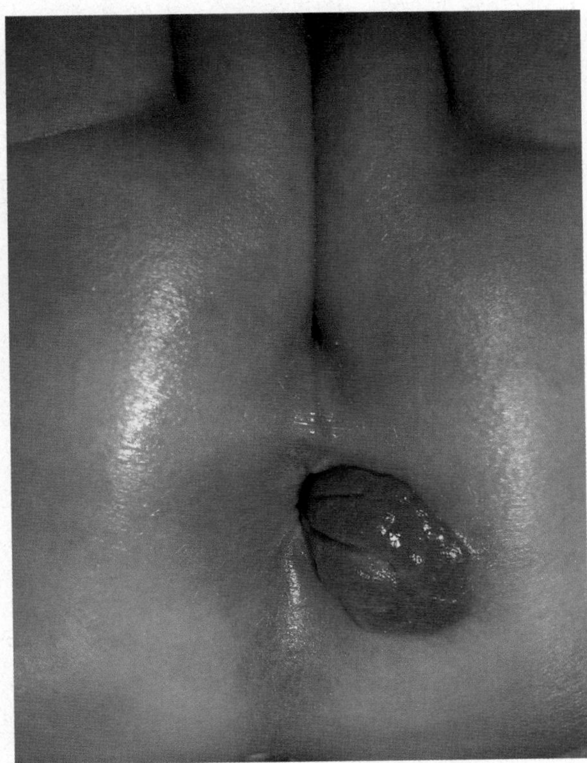

FIGURE 115-7 Strawberry hemangioma in the perianal area of a 5-month-old girl. This is at high risk of ulceration. *(Reproduced with permission from Richard P. Usatine, MD.)*

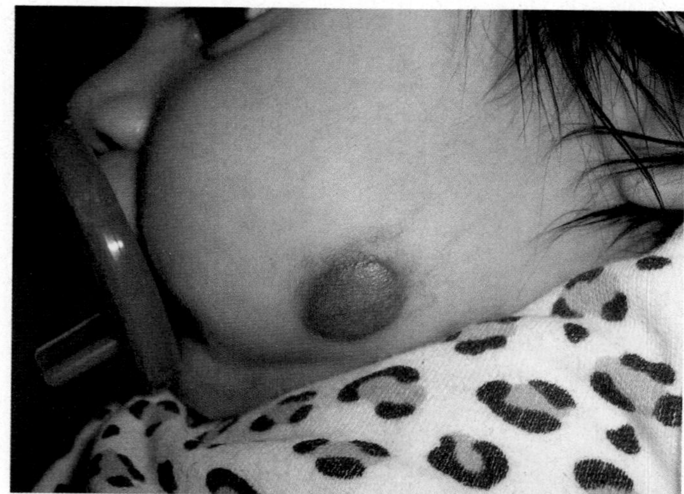

FIGURE 115-8 Strawberry hemangioma in the beard area of the face causing no functional problems in a 3-month-old girl. The parents requested treatment, and a course of topical timolol gel 0.5% was initiated. While the hemangioma was in the beard area, the child had no problems with breathing, coughing, or snoring. A referral to ENT was not needed to investigate for laryngeal hemangiomatosis. (*Reproduced with permission from Richard P. Usatine, MD.*)

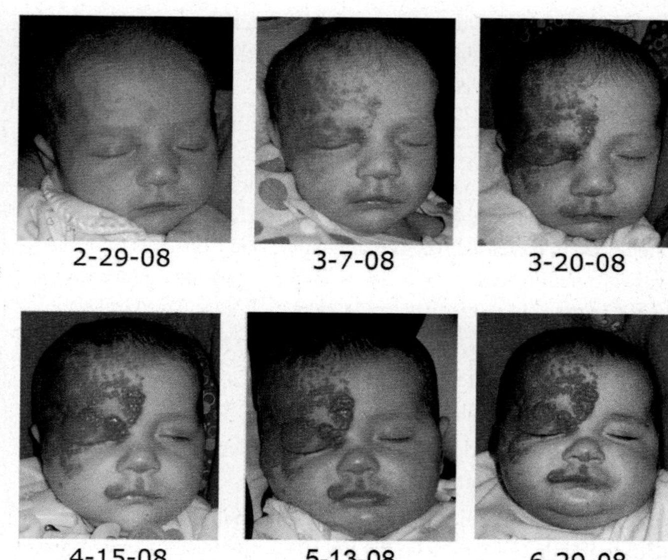

2-29-08
3-7-08
3-20-08
4-15-08
5-13-08
6-29-08
Progression of the hemangioma.

FIGURE 115-9 Progression of a large segmental hemangioma in an infant with PHACE syndrome. (*Reproduced with permission from AngelPHACE.com.*)

7-14-08
7-20-08
8-25-08
9-30-08
3-10-09
7-20-09
The difference in a year:
The difference in a year:

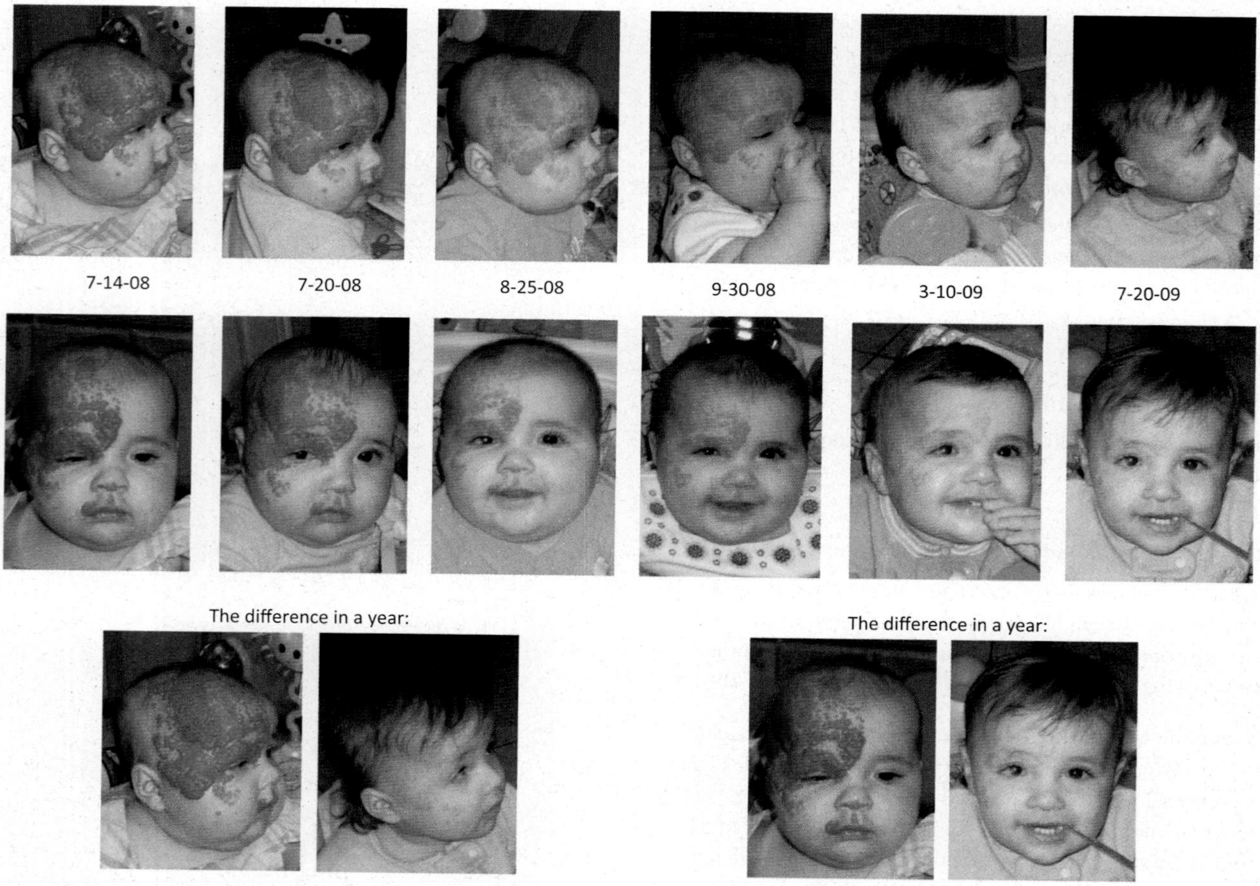

FIGURE 115-10 Regression of the same large segmental hemangioma in **Figure 115-9** with PHACE syndrome after nearly 8 months of propranolol therapy. Initially prednisolone was being used simultaneously, but that was stopped approximately halfway through the treatment with the propranolol. The coloboma of the right eye is seen best in the last photo and is part of the syndrome. (*Reproduced with permission from AngelPHACE.com.*)

Watch for the major side effects (which would warrant cessation of therapy), hypotension and hypoglycemia. Bronchial hyper-reactivity has also been reported. Monitoring the patient in the office after the first dose is advisable, although the treatment has been found to be safe in a number of studies.[14,15]

- Combined treatment with propranolol and 940-nm diode laser for particularly severe hemangiomas was shown to be more effective for cosmesis in one study.[16] Other studies have had differing results, with combined laser/propranolol treatment showing little to no advantage from the added laser therapy over propranolol alone.[17]
- For patients who cannot tolerate beta blocker therapy, prednisone 3 to 5 mg/kg per day had been shown to provide an effective and rapid way of treating hemangiomas, and in fact, was the treatment of choice prior to the discovery of beta blocker treatment for this condition.[18] SOR Ⓑ In a study, 68% of patients receiving systemic corticosteroid treatment with oral prednisone experienced rapid and virtually complete involution of hemangiomas.[18] Another 25% experienced significant regression, and treatment demonstrated no effect in 7% of patients. The authors recommended treating with oral prednisone for 6 to 8 weeks, and in more severe cases, for 12 weeks.
- Side effects of oral steroid therapy include Cushingoid facies, mood changes/irritability, hypertension and increased susceptibility to infection, and short-term growth retardation, all of which seem to be transient and resolve after cessation of the therapy.[18]
- Ultrapotent topical corticosteroids have been found especially helpful in the treatment of small hemangiomas, especially periocular hemangiomas and those at sites prone to ulceration and disfigurement. Seventy-four percent of patients demonstrated good or at least partial response to treatment, with the majority experiencing cessation of growth before what would have been expected for their age. Thinner, more superficial hemangiomas demonstrated better improvement than thicker, deeper lesions.[19] SOR Ⓑ
- Intralesional corticosteroid injections, composed of a mixture containing triamcinolone acetonide (20 mg average dose) and betamethasone acetate (3 mg average dose) with varying number of injections, have been found to successfully treat head and neck childhood hemangiomas in properly selected infants. In a research study, 13% of the hemangiomas treated with intralesional injections almost completely involuted, 32% showed greater than 50% reduction in volume, 32% showed definite but less than 50% reduction in volume, and 23% showed little to no decrease in size.[20] SOR Ⓑ Avoid intralesional steroids around the eye.
- Treatment with flashlamp-pumped pulsed-dye laser has been found to be an effective treatment method for superficial cutaneous hemangiomas at sites of potential functional impairment and on the face. In a study, 85% of patients were found to have excellent or good results with the flashlamp-pumped pulsed-dye laser. Hemangiomas with a deep component do not seem to benefit from flashlamp-pumped pulsed-dye laser therapy to the same degree as a truly superficial hemangioma, as the laser is limited by its depth of vascular injury.[21-23] SOR Ⓑ The pulsed-dye laser seems especially promising with its ability to selectively damage blood vessels with minimal damage to surrounding tissues. This procedure is also associated with decreased pain and increased healing.[24] SOR Ⓑ
- Facial hemangiomas causing severe functional disturbance and serious psychological distress are strong reasons to consider

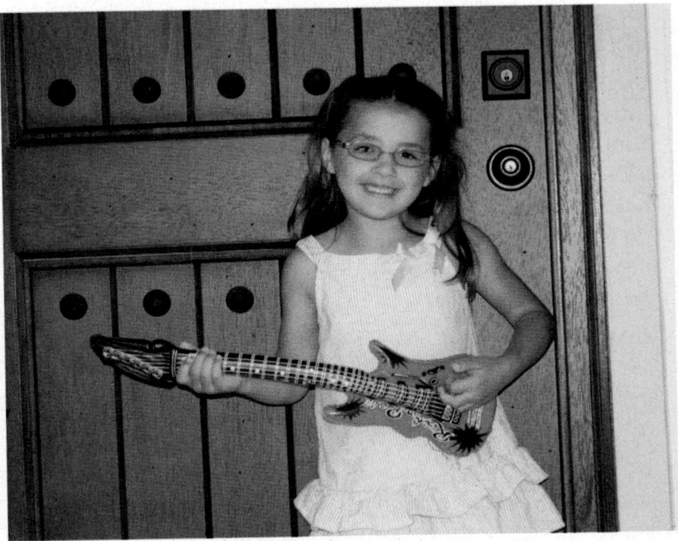

FIGURE 115-11 The girl from **Figures 115-9** and **155-10** on her first day of kindergarten, showing almost complete regression of the hemangioma. (*Reproduced with permission from AngelPHACE.com.*)

surgical excision before the child reaches the expected age of spontaneous regression. SOR C

- Large periocular hemangiomas demand prompt treatment to prevent debilitating consequences such as amblyopia (see **Figure 115-2**). Early treatment is also recommended for proliferative labial tumors because they not only have a tendency to bleed, but they also make eating difficult. Additionally, early treatment with a consideration for surgery is advised for hemangiomas located on the nasal tip, as they regress slowly and may ultimately result in distortion of the nasal framework.[23]
- Surgical excision of involuted hemangiomas is not uncommon to remove residual tissue that may be causing cosmetic or functional impairment. Excision is performed in late involution to reduce the risk of hemorrhage.
- Depending on the location and how complex the hemangioma is, consultations with pediatric dermatologists, ophthalmologists, otolaryngologists, plastic surgeons, and pediatric neurosurgeons may be necessary to ensure proper care.

TOPICAL THERAPY

- Topical timolol ophthalmic gel or solution has been shown in a number of studies to effectively treat infantile hemangiomas (**Figure 115-8**).[25-27] SOR B One of the studies noted that predictors of better response were superficial type of hemangioma ($p = 0.01$), 0.5% timolol concentration ($p = 0.01$), and duration of use longer than 3 months ($p = 0.04$).[16] SOR B Another study using 0.5% ophthalmic solution 3–4 times daily in patients with small superficial hemangiomas found that treatment was most effective in the early proliferative stage.[25] SOR B

FOLLOW-UP

Watchful waiting and serial observations during well-child examinations are recommended for uncomplicated hemangiomas of infancy. Hemangiomas with complicating factors need close follow-up on an individual basis.

PATIENT EDUCATION

Hemangiomas are benign and are not cancer. They are common, and up to 10% of lighter skinned infants will have one. Most hemangiomas will go away spontaneously and not need treatment. For those needing treatment, there are treatments that are safe and effective (oral propranolol and topical timolol). Feel free to show the great results of therapy of some of the largest and most worrisome hemangiomas in this chapter to the parents in your office (**Figures 115-9** to **115-11**).

PATIENT RESOURCES

- Vascular Birthmarks Foundation—**http://www.birthmark.org.**

PROVIDER RESOURCES

- National Organization of Vascular Anomalies (NOVA)—**http://www.novanews.org.**

REFERENCES

1. Munden A, Butschek R, Tom WL, et al. Prospective study of infantile hemangiomas: incidence, clinical characteristics and association with placental abnormalities. *Br J Dermatol.* 2014:170:907.
2. Metry DW, Herbert AA. Benign cutaneous vascular tumors of infancy: when to worry, what to do. *Arch Dermatol.* 2000; 136:905
3. Haggstrom AN, Drolet BA, Baselga E, et al. Prospective study of infantile hemangiomas: clinical characteristics predicting complications and treatment. *Pediatrics.* 2006;118:882.
4. Blei F, Walter J, Orlow SJ, Marchuk DA. Familial segregation of hemangiomas and vascular malformations as an autosomal dominant trait. *Arch Dermatol.* 1998;134:718.
5. Haggstrom AN, Drolet BA, Baselga E, et al. Prospective study of infantile hemangiomas: demographic, prenatal, and perinatal characteristics. *J Pediatr.* 2007;150(3):291-294.
6. Achauer BM, Chang CJ, Vander Kam VM. Management of hemangioma of infancy: review of 245 patients. *Plast Reconstr Surg.* 1997;99(5):1301-1308.
7. Antaya R. *Infantile Hemangioma.* http://emedicine.medscape.com/article/1083849. Accessed May 2017.
8. Dubois J, Patriquin HB, Garel L, et al. Soft-tissue hemangioma in infants and children: diagnosis using Doppler sonography. *AJR Am J Roentgenol.* 1998;171(1):247-252.
9. Elewski BE, Hughey LC, Parsons ME. *Differential Diagnosis in Dermatology.* St. Louis, MO: Elsevier; 2005:545.
10. McDermott AL, Dutt SN, Shavda SV, Morgan DW. Maffucci's syndrome: clinical and radiological features of a rare condition. *J Laryngol Otol.* 2001;115(10):845-847.
11. Barnhill RL. Vascular tumors. In: Hunt SJ, Santa Cruz DJ, Barnhill RL, eds. *Textbook of Dermatopathology.* New York: McGraw-Hill; 1998:821.
12. Yan AC, Chamlin SL, Liang MG, et al. Fibrosarcoma: a masquerader of ulcerated hemangioma. *Pediatr Dermatol.* 2006;23(4):330-334.
13. Anjolras O, Wassef M, Mazoyer E, et al. Infants with Kasabach-Merritt syndrome do not have "true" hemangiomas. *J Pediatr.* 1997;130(4):631-640.
14. Leaute-Labreze C, Hoeger P, Mazereeuw-Hautier J, et al. A randomized, controlled trial of oral propranolol in infantile hemangioma. *N Engl J Med.* 2015;372(8):735-746.
15. Drolet BA, Frommelt PC, Chamlin SL, et al. Initiation and use of propranolol for infantile hemangioma: report of a consensus conference. *Pediatrics.* 2013;131(1):128-140.
16. Deme T, Jones S. The treatment of problematic hemangiomas in children with propranolol and 940nm diode laser. *J Pediatr Surg.* 2016;51(5) 863-868.
17. Bin Y, Li L, Li-xin Z, et al. Clinical characteristics and treatment options of infantile vascular anomalies. *Medicine.* 2015;94:40.
18. Sadan N, Wolach B. Treatment of hemangiomas of infants with high doses of prednisone. *J Pediatr.* 1996;128(1):141-146.
19. Garzon MC, Lucky AW, Hawrot A, Frieden IJ. Ultrapotent topical corticosteroid treatment of hemangiomas of infancy. *J Am Acad Dermatol.* 2005;52:281-286.

20. Sloan G, Reinisch J, Nichter L, et al. Intralesional corticosteroid therapy for infantile hemangiomas. *Plast Reconstr Surg.* 1989;83:459-466.

21. Rizzo C, Brightman L, Chapas AM, et al. Outcomes of childhood hemangiomas treated with the pulsed-dye laser with dynamic cooling: a retrospective chart analysis. *Dermatol Surg.* 2009;35:1947.

22. Poetke M, Phillip C, Berlien HP. Flashlamp-pumped pulsed dye laser for hemangiomas in infancy: treatment of superficial vs. mixed hemangiomas. *Arch Dermatol.* 2000;136(5):628-632.

23. Demiri EC, Pelissier P, Genin-Etcheberry T, et al. Treatment of facial haemangiomas: the present status of surgery. *Br J Plast Surg.* 2001;54(8):665-674.

24. Eedy DJ, Breathnach SM, Walker NPJ. *Surgical Dermatology.* Oxford, UK: Blackwell Science; 1996:245.

25. Oranje AP, Janmohamed SR, Madern GC, de Laat PC. Treatment of small superficial haemangioma with timolol 0.5% ophthalmic solution: a series of 20 cases. *Dermatology*. 2011;223:330-334.

26. Chakkittakandiyil A, Phillips R, Frieden IJ, et al. Timolol maleate 0.5% or 0.1% gel-forming solution for infantile hemangiomas: a retrospective, multicenter, cohort study. *Pediatr Dermatol.* 2012;29:28-31.

27. Semkova K, Kazandjieva J. Topical timolol maleate for treatment of infantile haemangiomas: preliminary results of a prospective study. *Clin Exp Dermatol.* 2013;38(2):143-146.

Acknowledgment: We thank Mary Alice for the photographs of her daughter with PHACE syndrome. One can learn more about their family story at http://angelphace.com/. Also visit www.PHACEsyndromecommunity.org, the site for the organization that supports individuals with PHACE and their families.

116 PUSTULAR DISEASES OF CHILDHOOD

Andrew Shedd, MD
Richard P. Usatine, MD
Heidi S. Chumley, MD, MBA
Andrea L. Darby-Stewart, MD

PATIENT STORY

A 1-year-old boy is brought for a second opinion about the recurrent pruritic vesicles and pustules on his hands and feet. This is the third episode, and in both previous episodes, the physicians thought the child had scabies. The child was treated with permethrin both times, and within 2 to 3 weeks the skin cleared. No other family members have had lesions or symptoms. **Figures 116-1** to **116-3** demonstrate a typical case of infantile acropustulosis that is often misdiagnosed as scabies. Although the condition can be recurrent, it is ultimately self-limited and will resolve.

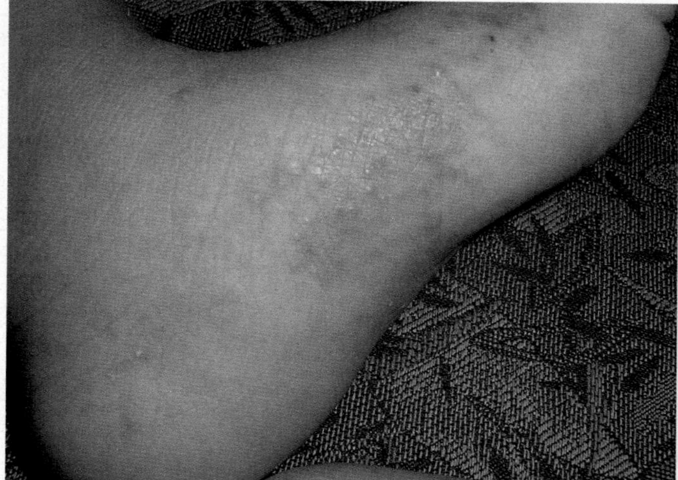

FIGURE 116-1 Infantile acropustulosis (acropustulosis of infancy) on the foot of a 1-year-old boy. (*Reproduced with permission from Richard P. Usatine, MD.*)

INTRODUCTION

Acropustulosis and transient neonatal pustular melanosis (TNPM) are pustular diseases that typically present in infancy. Acropustulosis is a pruritic vesiculopustular disease presenting between 2 and 10 months of age and remitting spontaneously by 36 months of age. TNPM is present at birth and characterized by 2- to 3-mm hyperpigmented macules and pustules. Acropustulosis may require symptomatic treatment of pruritus, but otherwise both illnesses are self-limiting.

EPIDEMIOLOGY

Acropustulosis:

- Rare, intensely pruritic, vesiculopustular disease of young children.[1]
- Typically begins in the second or third months[1] of life and as late as 10 months of age.[2]
- Occur slightly more often in darker-skinned patients and males.[1]
- Typically spontaneously remits by 6 to 36 months of life.[2]

Transient neonatal pustular melanosis:

- A disease of newborns.[3]
- Equal male-to-female ratio.[3]
- Seen in 4.4% of black infants and 0.6% of white infants.[4]
- Early, spontaneous remission.[3]

ETIOLOGY AND PATHOPHYSIOLOGY

Acropustulosis:

- The exact cause and mechanism have yet to be determined.[5]
- Some physicians speculate that it is a persistent reaction to scabies ("postscabies syndrome"). Suggestive of this infectious etiology,

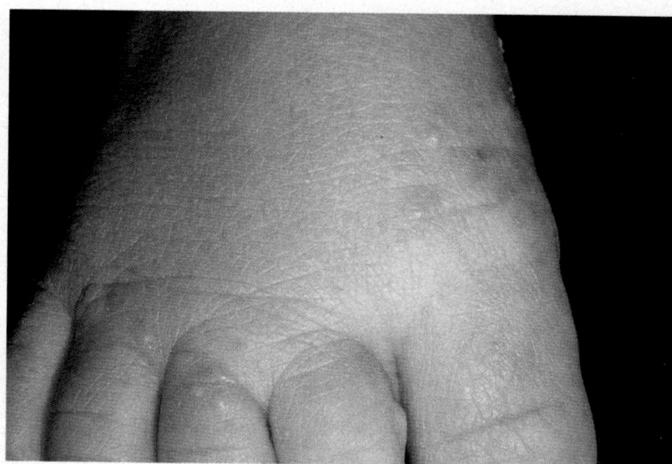

FIGURE 116-2 Acropustulosis with vesiculopustular eruption on the toes of the boy shown in **Figure 116-1**. (*Reproduced with permission from Richard P. Usatine, MD.*)

infantile acropustulosis will occasionally be concurrently present among siblings. Also, patients diagnosed with this disorder frequently have received prior treatment for scabies, which may either provide evidence of an infectious etiology or demonstrate the frequent misdiagnosis, as in the patient above. Odom et al. conclude that in some cases, this disease may represent a hypersensitivity reaction to *Sarcoptes scabiei.*[4]

Transient neonatal pustular melanosis:

- The etiology is uncertain[6]; however, it may result from an obstruction of the pilosebaceous orifice.[3]

DIAGNOSIS

- Acropustulosis—A work-up to rule out potentially serious infectious causes should be considered whenever confronted with a new pustular dermatosis early in a child's life. A work-up might include a scraping for scabies and KOH preparation as rapid diagnostic tests. If these studies are negative, the diagnosis may be made clinically as described below.
- TNPM—This diagnosis can be made clinically. However, if performed, a Wright stain of the exudate will reveal a predominance of neutrophils with an occasional eosinophil, and the Gram stain will be negative.[3]

CLINICAL FEATURES

Acropustulosis:

- These vesiculopustular lesions begin around the second or third months of life and are typically concentrated on the hands and feet (see **Figures 116-1** to **116-3**).[1]
- They begin acutely as small pink papules and progress within 24 hours to pustules[1] of less than 5 mm in diameter.[2]
- Recurrent episodes of these intensely pruritic lesions typically last 10 days and may recur every 2 to 5 weeks,[1,2] decreasing in frequency and severity[2] until spontaneous remission around 3 years of age.[1] Because of the pruritic nature of these lesions, infants may be irritable and appear uncomfortable during eruptions.[5]
- There may be a residual scale and postinflammatory hyperpigmentation.[2]

Transient neonatal pustular melanosis:

- This condition is characterized by the presence at birth of 2- to 3-mm macules and pustules[4] on a nonerythematous base (**Figures 116-4** and **116-5**).[7]
- The lesions probably evolve prenatally[7] and subsequently rupture postnatally in 1 to 2 days.
- They heal with hyperpigmented macules that fade by 3 months of age,[3] with lighter-skinned patients experiencing less hyperpigmentation.[7]
- Sometimes, the only evidence of the disease is the presence of small, brown macules with a rim of scale at birth.[7]
- Newborns with TNPM have no other systemic symptoms and are well appearing.[6]

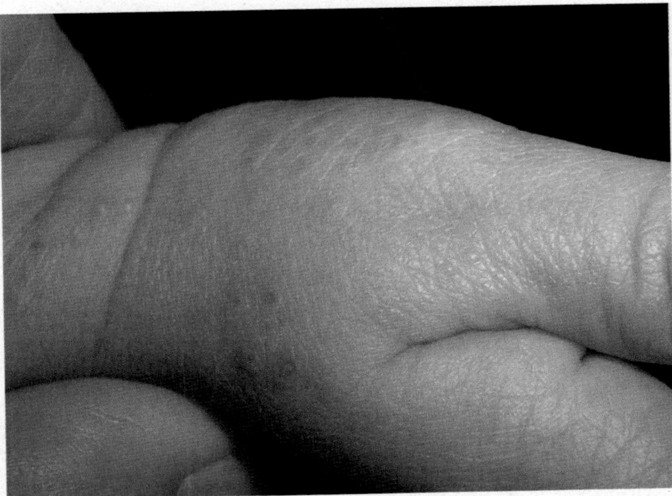

FIGURE 116-3 Acropustulosis with pruritic eruption on the hand and wrist of the boy shown in **Figures 116-1** and **116-2**. (*Reproduced with permission from Richard P. Usatine, MD.*)

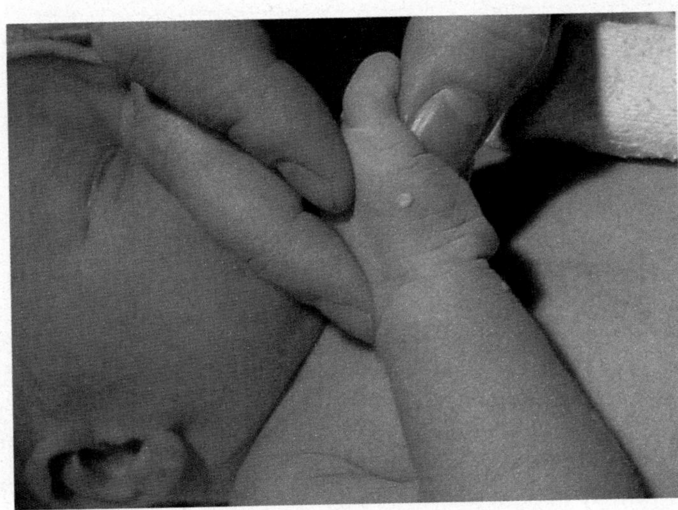

FIGURE 116-4 Neonatal pustular melanosis on the hand of a newborn. (*Reproduced with permission from Dan Stulberg, MD.*)

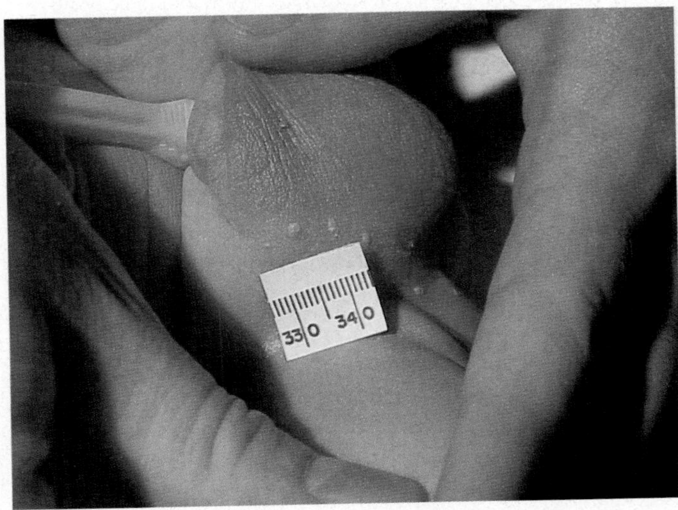

FIGURE 116-5 Neonatal pustular melanosis on scrotum of the same newborn. (*Reproduced with permission from Dan Stulberg, MD.*)

TYPICAL DISTRIBUTION

- Acropustulosis—Although most commonly found on the palms and soles, the pustules may also be found on the dorsal surfaces of the hands and feet and occasionally the face, scalp, and trunk.[5]
- TNPM—They are most common on the face and chin; however, they may also be present on the neck, chest, sacrum, abdomen, and thighs.[7]

LABORATORY TESTING

- Acropustulosis—A blood count is not needed but might reveal a slight leukocytosis and frequently an eosinophilia. Stained smears of the lesions are also not needed but will demonstrate many neutrophils,[1] with some eosinophils possible early in the course.[2]
- TNPM—A Wright stain will reveal numerous neutrophils and some eosinophils, with a negative Gram stain.[3] Blood counts should be normal, and no laboratory work-up is generally indicated.

DIFFERENTIAL DIAGNOSIS

- Scabies infestation—Characterized by pruritic, intraepidermal burrows and vesicles with scale and crust, most commonly found in the web spaces of the digits, wrists, elbow, genitals, and lower extremities. May be present in other family members and is not present at birth. Microscopic examination of the scrapings of the burrows may reveal mites, feces, eggs, or all of the above.[3] Acropustulosis will be refractory to all scabies therapies, but scabies therapy may appear to work because each episode of acropustulosis is self-limited (see Chapter 149, Scabies).
- Erythema toxicum neonatorum—Appearing on the neonate 1 to 2 days after birth, this disease of unknown etiology causes 2- to 3-cm diffuse blotchy macules with 1- to 4-mm central vesicles. The lesions, which spare the palms and soles, contain a predominance of eosinophils and resolve spontaneously by 2 weeks of age (see Chapter 114, Normal Skin Changes).[3]
- Impetigo—A superficial infection of the skin with vesicles, bullae, and honey-colored crusts, caused by group A *Streptococcus*, or *Staphylococcus aureus*. Gram stain and culture should be positive (see Chapter 122, Impetigo).[3]
- Cutaneous candidiasis—Slightly pruritic areas of intensely erythematous papules, pustules, and plaques, possibly with white exudate, found around the genitals and folds of skin. *Candida* yeast forms present on KOH preparation or culture (see Chapter 142, Candidiasis).[3]
- Varicella—Characteristic "dewdrops on a rose petal" that develop in childhood. Uniformly distributed, pruritic, with known contacts likely. Now less common because of immunization (see Chapter 129, Chickenpox).
- Herpes—Grouped, painful vesicles on an erythematous base. May occur as gingivostomatitis in young children but rarely seen in the distribution of the pustular diseases of childhood. More likely to be vesicular rather than pustular (see Chapter 135, Herpes Simplex).
- Hand, foot, and mouth disease—This illness is caused by the coxsackievirus and produces papules and macules of the hands and feet that progress to flat vesicles before ulceration and eventual resolution. They typically affect the dorsum of the hands and feet and are also accompanied by painful oral lesions (see Chapter 134, Hand Foot Mouth Syndrome).[3]
- Psoriasis, pustular—This severe form of psoriasis is rare in children and is characterized by the acute appearance of diffuse, painful, pinpoint pustules with high fever, fatigue, and anorexia (see Chapter 158, Psoriasis).[1]

MANAGEMENT

Acropustulosis:

- Oral corticosteroids generally are not effective[1] and not necessary in management.[5] SOR Ⓒ
- Topical corticosteroids have been shown to be effective in case series; no randomized controlled trials are available to verify efficacy. If corticosteroids are prescribed, use the lowest effective potency for the lowest amount of time to avoid side effects such as hypopigmentation and skin thinning.[8,9] SOR Ⓒ
- Oral antihistamines may be helpful in controlling pruritus.[1] SOR Ⓒ
- Pramoxine, lotion or cream, may be used topically for control of itching as it works by a different mechanism than antihistamines.[5] SOR Ⓒ
- Dapsone (1 to 2 mg/kg per day, maximum dose of 100 mg/day)[5] has been used with good results. However, the risks of complications are generally considered to outweigh the benefits, unless the pruritus is debilitating.[1] SOR Ⓒ

Transient neonatal pustular melanosis:

- No treatment is necessary. The parents should be reassured that the condition is benign and will resolve spontaneously with eventual normalization of any hyperpigmented macules.[6] SOR Ⓑ

PROGNOSIS

- Acropustulosis resolves spontaneously by 6 to 36 months of age.
- TNPM resolves spontaneously by 3 months of age.

FOLLOW-UP

Acropustulosis may require initial follow-up for control of symptoms and assurance of a stable disease course. With symptoms controlled, follow-up may be unnecessary as the child ages and the disease decreases in severity and frequency. If dapsone is prescribed, proper monitoring is indicated.

TNPM needs no specific follow-up other than normal well-child care.

PATIENT EDUCATION

Once other conditions have been ruled out, reassurance that these diseases are self-limited is the most important piece of information to communicate to the family.

PATIENT AND PROVIDER RESOURCES

- Medscape. *Acropustulosis of Infancy*—**http://emedicine.medscape.com/article/1109935.**
- Medscape. *Transient Neonatal Pustular Melanosis*—**http://emedicine.medscape.com/article/1112258.**

REFERENCES

1. Ruggero C, Gelmetti C. *Pediatric Dermatology and Dermatopathology: A Concise Atlas*. London, UK: Martin Dunitz; 2002.
2. Weinberg S, Prose NS, Leonard K. *Color Atlas of Pediatric Dermatology*, 3rd ed. New York, NY: McGraw-Hill; 1998.
3. Kane KS, Bissonette J, Baden HP, et al. *Color Atlas and Synopsis of Pediatric Dermatology*. New York, NY: McGraw-Hill; 2002.
4. Odom RB, James WD, Timothy GB. *Andrews' Diseases of the Skin, Clinical Dermatology*, 9th ed. Philadelphia, PA: Saunders; 2000.
5. Andreychik C. *Acropustulosis of Infancy.* http://emedicine.medscape.com/article/1169935.htm. Accessed May 2017.
6. Sorrell J. *Transient Neonatal Pustular Melanosis.* http://emedicine.medscape.com/article/1112258.htm. Accessed May 2017.
7. Cohen BA. *Pediatric Dermatology*, 3rd ed. Philadelphia, PA: Elsevier Mosby; 2005.
8. Pielop J. *Benign Skin and Scalp Lesions in the Newborn and Young Infant*. UpToDate. https://www.uptodate.com/contents/benign-skin-and-scalp-lesions-in-the-newborn-and-young-infant?source=machineLearning&search=acropustulosis&selectedTitle=1~2§ionRank=1&anchor=H8#H25. Accessed May 2017.
9. Mancini AJ, Frieden IJ, Paller AS. Infantile acropustulosis revisited: history of scabies and response to corticosteroids. *Pediatr Dermatol.* 1998;15(5):337-341.

117 DIAPER RASH AND PERIANAL DERMATITIS

Bridget Godwin, MD
Julie Scott Taylor, MD, MSc

PATIENT STORY

A 2-month-old baby girl was brought to the office with a severe diaper rash that was not getting better with Desitin. Upon examination, the physician noted a white coating on the tongue and buccal mucosa. The diaper area was red with skin erosions and satellite lesions (**Figure 117-1**). History and physical are consistent with candidiasis of the mouth (thrush) and the diaper region. The child was treated with oral nystatin suspension and topical clotrimazole cream in the diaper area with good results.

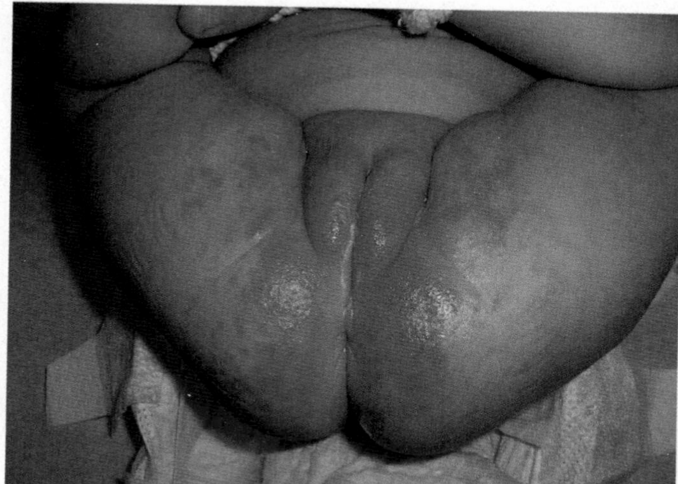

FIGURE 117-1 *Candida* diaper dermatitis in an infant who has oral thrush. *(Reproduced with permission from Richard P. Usatine, MD.)*

INTRODUCTION

Diaper rash is a general term used to describe any type of red or inflammatory skin rash that is located in the diaper area.

SYNONYMS

Diaper dermatitis, napkin dermatitis.

EPIDEMIOLOGY

- Diaper dermatitis is the most common dermatitis of infancy.
- Variability in prevalence of 4% to 35% among children in their first 2 years of life in different studies.[1]
- Diaper rash is thought to be present in 25% of children presenting for outpatient visits.[2]
- No differences in prevalence between genders or among ethnic groups.
- One study showed an incidence of 19.4% in children ages 3 to 6 months.[1]
- Higher incidence among formula-fed compared with breastfed infants.[1]
- Condition typically begins around age 3 weeks, peaks at age 9 to 12 months, and then decreases with age until it resolves completely with toilet training.[3]
- Individual episodes last from 1 day to 2 weeks.
- Aggravating factors include poor skin care, diarrhea, recent antibiotic use, and urinary tract abnormalities.
- Perianal streptococcal dermatitis occurs in children between 6 months and 10 years of age (**Figures 117-2** and **117-3**).

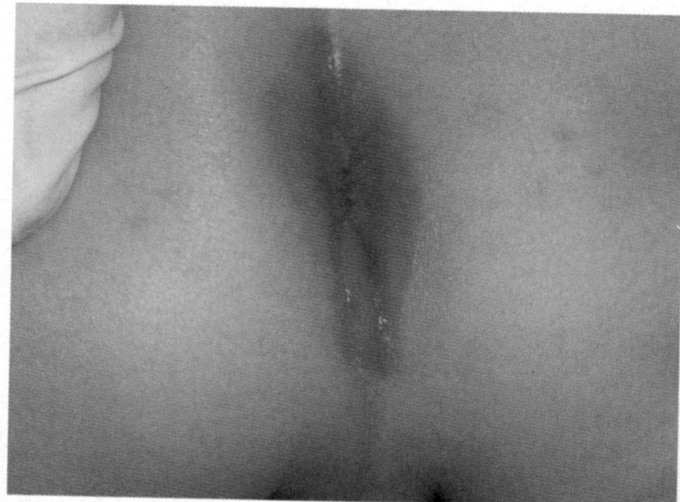

FIGURE 117-2 Perianal dermatitis caused by group A β-hemolytic streptococci. *(Reproduced with permission from Sheth S, Schechtman AD. Itchy perianal erythema. J Fam Pract. 2007;56(12):1025-1027. Frontline Medical Communications, Inc.)*

ETIOLOGY AND PATHOPHYSIOLOGY

- Primary diaper dermatitis—An acute skin inflammation in the diaper area with a multifactorial etiology.[4] The main cause is irritation of thin skin as a result of prolonged contact with moisture including feces and urine. The multiple factors involved are:

1. Occlusion/lack of exposure to air.
2. Friction and mechanical trauma.
3. Local irritants—Fecal proteases and lipases.
4. Increased pH.
5. Maceration of the stratum corneum with loss of the protective barrier function of skin.

- Irritant diaper dermatitis (IDD) is a combination of intertrigo (wet skin damaged from chafing) and miliaria (heat rash) when eccrine glands become obstructed from excessive hydration. It is a noninfectious, nonallergic, often asymptomatic contact dermatitis that typically lasts for less than 3 days after a change in diaper practices.
- Candidal diaper dermatitis—Within 3 days, 45% to 75% of diaper rashes are colonized with *Candida albicans* of fecal origin.
- Bacterial diaper dermatitis may be a secondary infection caused by *Staphylococcus aureus* or *Streptococcus pyogenes*.[5] Other common bacterial isolates include *Escherichia coli, Peptostreptococcus,* and *Bacteroides*. Usually occurs during the warm summer months.
- Perianal streptococcal dermatitis is caused by group A b-hemolytic streptococci (see **Figures 117-2** and **117-3**).

RISK FACTORS

- Diarrhea.
- Formula-fed infants.
- Recent antibiotic use.
- Oral thrush.
- Poor skin care, including infrequent diaper changes and lack of barrier cream use.

DIAGNOSIS

CLINICAL FEATURES

- IDD begins with shiny erythema with or without scale and poorly demarcated margins on the convex skin surfaces in areas covered by diapers. Moderate cases can have papules, plaques, vesicles, and small superficial erosions that can progress to well-demarcated ulcerated nodules, typically with sparing of skin folds (**Figure 117-4**).
- Pustules or papules beyond the rash border (called "satellite lesions"), involvement of the skin folds, and white scaling all indicate a fungal infection with *Candida* (**Figure 117-5**).
- Secondary bacterial infections can have redness, honey-colored crusting, swelling, red streaking, and/or purulent discharge. With impetigo in the diaper area, bullae are not usually intact but instead present as superficial erosions.
- Perianal streptococcal dermatitis is a bright red, sharply demarcated rash sometimes associated with blood-streaked stools (see **Figure 117-2**).

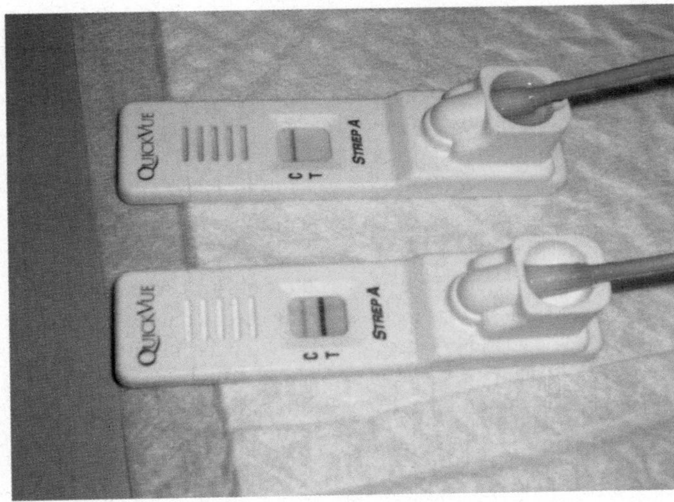

FIGURE 117-3 A positive rapid strep test taken from a swab of the perianal area of the infant in the previous photo. (*Reproduced with permission from Sheth S, Schechtman AD. Itchy perianal erythema. J Fam Pract. 2007;56(12):1025-1027. Frontline Medical Communications, Inc.*)

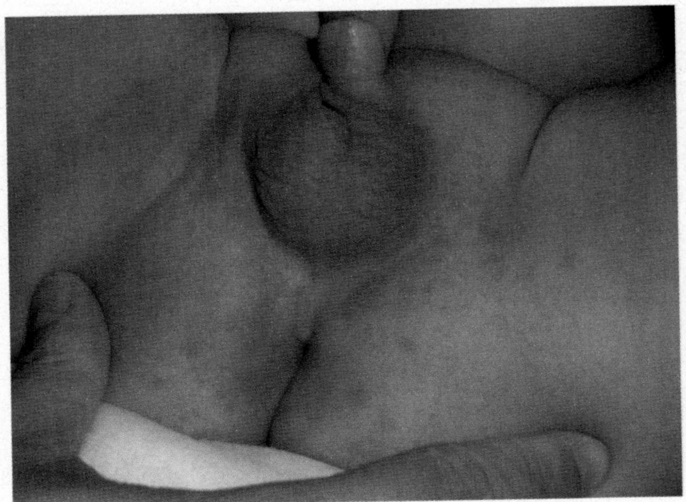

FIGURE 117-4 Irritant diaper dermatitis precipitated by diarrhea secondary to amoxicillin-clavulanate prescribed to treat otitis media. Note the absence of satellite lesions. (*Reproduced with permission from Richard P. Usatine, MD.*)

TYPICAL DISTRIBUTION

Diaper dermatitis is primarily found on the buttocks, the genitalia, the mons pubis and lower abdomen, and the medial thighs. Be sure to evaluate for rashes outside of the diaper area as well. If *Candida* is suspected, the oropharynx should be inspected for signs of thrush, such as adherent white plaques on the mucosa.

LABORATORY STUDIES

Clinical diagnosis is based primarily on the physical examination. Rarely indicated tests that are occasionally used in more complicated cases include potassium hydroxide preparation for fungal elements, mineral oil preparation for scabies, complete blood count with differential, zinc level, or skin biopsy (**Figure 117-6**). A rapid strep test can be used to diagnose perianal streptococcal dermatitis (see **Figures 117-2** and **117-3**).

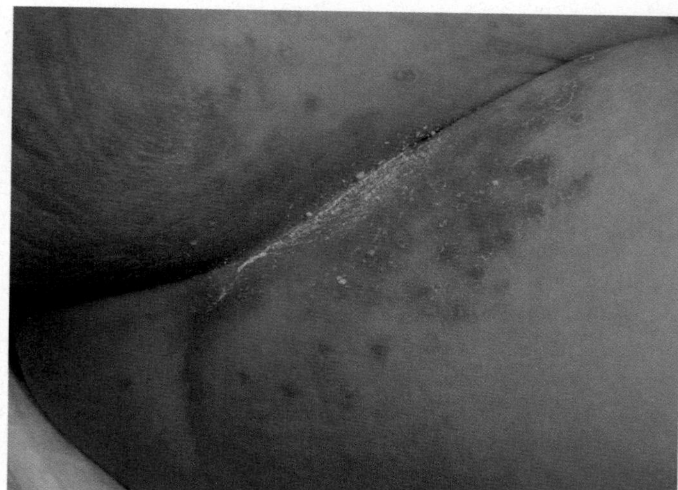

FIGURE 117-5 Close-up of a *Candida* diaper dermatitis in a 5-month-old infant. Note the superficial scaling around the satellite lesions. *(Reproduced with permission from Richard P. Usatine, MD.)*

DIFFERENTIAL DIAGNOSIS

There are two distinctive severe variants of IDD. Jacquet's diaper dermatitis (dermatitis syphiloides posterosiva or erosive variant) is a term used to describe severe, slow-healing, noduloerosive lesions with heaped-up borders seen in children with persistent diarrhea.[6] Granuloma gluteale infantum is a rare and poorly understood primary diaper dermatitis that presents with granulomatous nodules that can have large, raised, purple erosions with rolled margins. It resolves spontaneously over the course of a few months once the causative agent is discovered and removed, often with residual scarring and hyperpigmentation.[7]

Perianal pseudoverrucous papules are shiny, smooth, red, moist, flat-topped lesions that are commonly confused with the genital warts that occur in the context of Hirschsprung disease.

Secondary diaper dermatitis is an eruption in the diaper area with a defined etiology. Atopic dermatitis, seborrheic dermatitis, and psoriasis are examples of rashes that can appear anywhere on the body and can be exaggerated in the groin as a result of wearing diapers. Family history of atopy or psoriasis and rash in other locations besides the groin can be helpful.

Congenital syphilis, scabies, HIV, Langerhans cell histiocytosis, and acrodermatitis enteropathica are examples of rashes in the diaper area unrelated to the diaper. Allergic contact dermatitis as a result of an allergen in the diaper itself is possible but rare.

Suspect acrodermatitis enteropathica caused by zinc deficiency when the diaper dermatitis is severe and accompanied by perioral dermatitis (see **Figure 117-6**). The serum zinc level will be low and zinc supplementation will be needed.

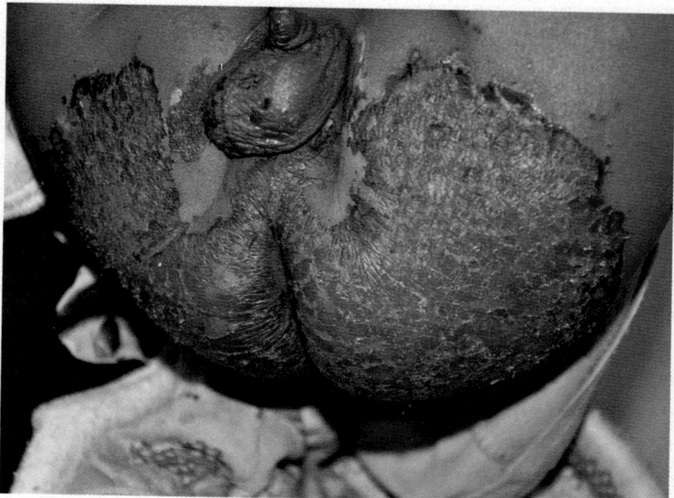

FIGURE 117-6 Acrodermatitis enteropathica caused by zinc deficiency. The child also had perioral dermatitis that appeared similar to the diaper dermatitis. *(Reproduced with permission from Richard P. Usatine, MD.)*

MANAGEMENT

FIRST LINE

- Parental behavior change to keep the skin as exposed and dry as possible. SOR B Frequent diaper changes (as soon as they are wet or soiled and at least every 3 to 4 hours); use disposable diapers. SOR B Frequent gentle cleaning of the affected area with lukewarm tap water instead of commercial wipes containing alcohol and pat dry. A squeeze bottle with lukewarm water can be used to avoid rubbing the delicate skin.

- Superabsorbent diapers that pull moisture away from the skin are helpful.[1] SOR Ⓑ
- Apply barrier preparations, including zinc oxide paste, petroleum jelly, vitamin A & D ointment, or Burow solution, to affected area after each diaper change.[1] SOR Ⓑ A 2015 study demonstrated improvement with use of a 2% magnesium cream.[8] Pastes are better than ointments, which, in turn, are better than creams or lotions. Avoid products with fragrances or preservatives to minimize allergic potential. Apply thickly like "icing on a cake." These barrier preparations should be used *on top* of other indicated therapies.
- For moderate to severe inflammation, consider a nonfluorinated, low-potency topical steroid such as 1% hydrocortisone ointment (up to 3 times daily) to the affected area until the dermatitis is gone. To avoid skin erosions, atrophy, and striae, it is best to not go beyond 2 weeks of therapy with any topical steroid on a baby's bottom.
- Avoid combination antifungal–steroid agents that contain steroids stronger than hydrocortisone (e.g., Lotrisone). Potent topical steroids can cause striae and skin erosions, hypothalamus–pituitary–adrenal axis suppression, and Cushing syndrome.[1]
- For *Candida*, use topical nonprescription antifungal creams such as clotrimazole, miconazole after every diaper change until the rash resolves. SOR Ⓑ For concomitant oral thrush, treat with oral nystatin swish and swallow 4 times daily.
- For mild bacterial infections, use topical antibiotic ointments such as bacitracin or mupirocin after every diaper change until the rash resolves. SOR Ⓑ
- Recommend dye-free diapers for allergic contact dermatitis. SOR Ⓑ

SECOND LINE

- Ciclopirox 0.77% topical suspension (Loprox), a broad-spectrum agent with antifungal, antibacterial, and anti-inflammatory properties, was used safely and effectively in 1 trial of 44 children to treat diaper dermatitis caused by *Candida*.[1] SOR Ⓑ
- For more severe bacterial infections, consider a broad-spectrum oral antibiotic such as amoxicillin-clavulanate. Perianal bacterial dermatitis has been reported to be predominantly caused by *S. aureus*.[6] Oral cephalexin is a good choice because it covers *S. aureus* and group A b-hemolytic streptococcus. If methicillin-resistant *S. aureus* (MRSA) is suspected, consider trimethoprim-sulfamethoxazole. SOR Ⓑ

PREVENTION AND ROUTINE SKIN CARE

- Keep the diaper region as dry and clean as possible.
- Promote the use of barrier preparations daily to maintain skin integrity.
- There is no evidence to suggest that topical vitamin A prevents diaper dermatitis.[9] SOR Ⓑ
- Disposable diapers—Although many individual trials show benefits, a 2006 Cochrane review found that there is not enough evidence from good-quality randomized controlled trials to support or refute the use and type of disposable diapers for the prevention of diaper dermatitis in infants.[10] SOR Ⓑ

PROGNOSIS

Diaper dermatitis has an excellent prognosis when treated as above.

FOLLOW-UP

No follow-up needed unless the rash worsens or persists. The exception is severe bacterial infection where follow-up is recommended because recurrences are common.

PATIENT (PARENT) EDUCATION

Prevention and early treatment are the best strategies. Keep the child's diaper area as clean, cool, and dry as possible with frequent diaper changes. Do *not* use creams that contain boric acid, camphor, phenol, methyl salicylate, compound of benzoin, or talcum powder or cornstarch. Reassure parents that, although this common condition is sometimes distressing for parents and uncomfortable for children, it is rarely dangerous.

PATIENT RESOURCES

- FamilyDoctor.org. *Diaper Rash*—**http://familydoctor.org/familydoctor/en/diseases-conditions/diaper-rash.html.**
- WebMD. *Understanding Diaper Rash—the Basics*—**http://children.webmd.com/tc/diaper-rash-topic-overview.**

PROVIDER RESOURCES

- Medscape. *Diaper Rash*—**http://emedicine.medscape.com/article/801222.**

REFERENCES

1. Dib R. *Diaper Rash*. http://emedicine.medscape.com/article/801222-overview#a0199. Updated November 17, 2016.
2. Adalat S, Wall D, Goodyear H. Diaper dermatitis—frequency and contributory factors in hospital attending children. *Pediatr Dermatol.* 2007;24(5):483-488.
3. Blume-Peytavi U, Hauser M, Lunnemann L, et al. Prevention of diaper dermatitis in infants—a literature review. *Pediatr Dermatol.* 2014;31(4):413-429.
4. Adam R. Skin care of the diaper area. *Pediatr Dermatol.* 2008;25(4):427-433.
5. Heath C, Desai N, Silverberg N. Recent microbiological shifts in perianal bacterial dermatitis: *Staphylococcus aureus* predominance. *Pediatr Dermatol.* 2009;26(6):696-700.
6. Ricci F, Paradisi A, Perino F, et al. Jacquet erosive diaper dermatitis: a not-so-rare syndrome. *Eur J Dermatol.* 2014;24(2):252-253.

7. Al-Faraidy N, Al-Natour S. A forgotten complication of diaper dermatitis: granuloma gluteale infantum. *J Family Community Med.* 2010;17(2):107-109.
8. Nourbakhsh S, Rouhi-Boroujeni H, Kheiri M, et al. Effect of topical application of the cream containing magnesium 2% on treatment of diaper dermatitis and diaper rash in children: a clinical trial study. *J Clin Diagnos Res.* 2016;10(1):WC04-6.
9. Davies MW, Dore AJ, Perissinotto KL. Topical vitamin A, or its derivatives, for treating and preventing napkin dermatitis in infants. *Cochrane Database Syst Rev.* 2005;(4):CD004300.
10. Baer EL, Davies MW, Easterbrook KJ. Disposable nappies for preventing napkin dermatitis in infants. *Cochrane Database Syst Rev.* 2006;(3):CD004262.

SECTION C ACNEIFORM AND FOLLICULAR DISORDERS

118 ACNE VULGARIS

Richard P. Usatine, MD
Pavela G. Bambekova, BS
Valerie Fisher Shiu, MD

PATIENT STORY

A 16-year-old boy (**Figure 118-1**) with severe nodulocystic acne and scarring presents for treatment. After trying oral antibiotics, topical retinoids, and topical benzoyl peroxide with no significant benefit, the patient and his mother requested isotretinoin (Accutane). After 4 months of isotretinoin, the nodules and cysts cleared, and only a few papules remained (**Figure 118-2**). He is much happier and more confident with his appearance. His skin cleared fully after 6 months of isotretinoin.

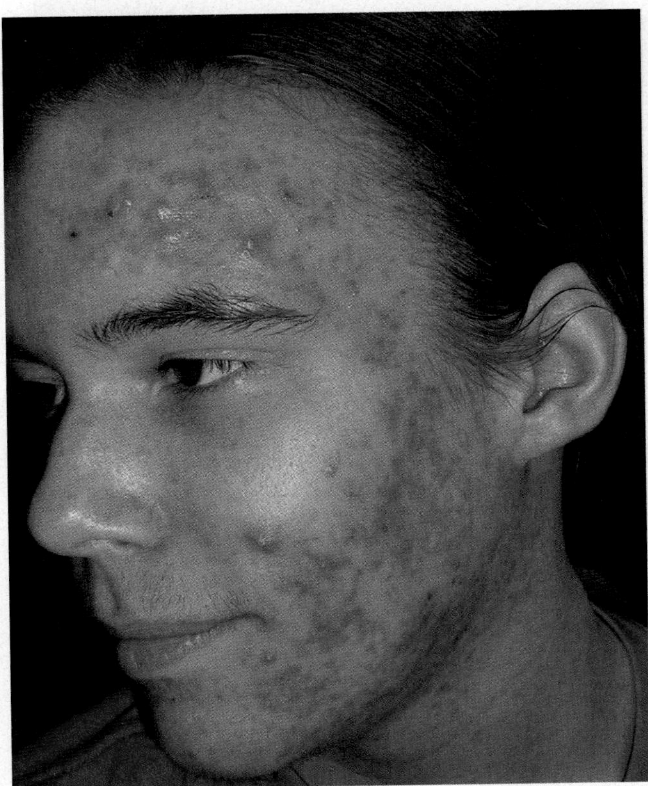

FIGURE 118-1 Severe nodulocystic acne with scarring in a 16-year-old boy. *(Reproduced with permission from Richard P. Usatine, MD.)*

INTRODUCTION

Acne is an obstructive and inflammatory disease of the pilosebaceous unit predominantly found on the face, but it may also involve the trunk. It can occur at any age, but it is most common during adolescence.

EPIDEMIOLOGY

Acne vulgaris affects more than 80% of teenagers and persists beyond the age of 25 in 3% of men and 12% of women.[1] Neonatal acne is most often benign cephalic pustulosis. It is temporary and thought to be related to *Malassezia* species (**Figure 118-3**) (see Chapter 114, Normal Skin Changes).

ETIOLOGY AND PATHOPHYSIOLOGY

The four most important steps in acne pathogenesis are:

1. Sebum overproduction related to androgenic hormones and genetics
2. Abnormal desquamation of the follicular epithelium (keratin plugging)
3. *Propionibacterium acnes* proliferation
4. Follicular obstruction, which can lead to inflammation and follicular disruption

Acne can be precipitated by mechanical pressure such as a helmet strap (**Figure 118-4**) and medications such as phenytoin and lithium (**Figure 118-5**).

Some studies suggest that consumption of large quantities of milk (especially skim milk) and foods with a high glycemic index increase the risk for acne.[2] SOR Ⓑ However, a systematic review did not find sufficient evidence to support diet changes for acne.[3]

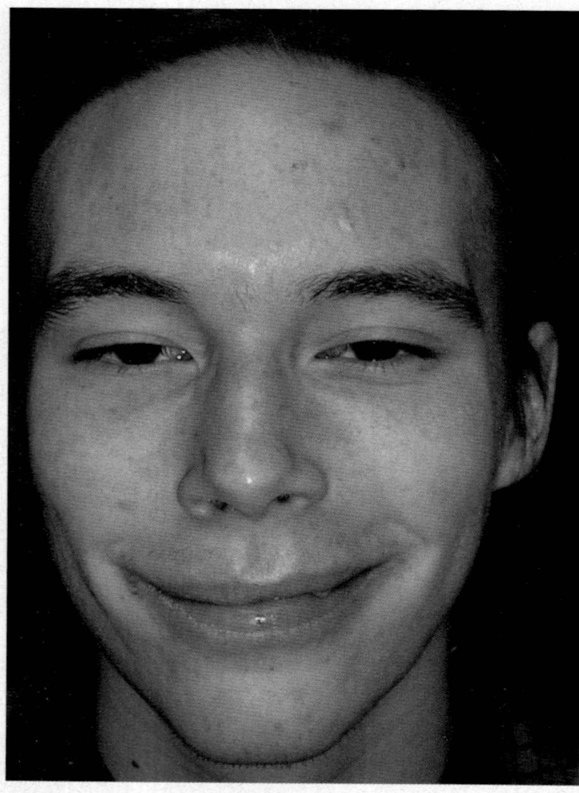

FIGURE 118-2 A happier boy now that his nodules and cysts have cleared at the start of the fifth month of isotretinoin treatment. (*Reproduced with permission from Richard P. Usatine, MD.*)

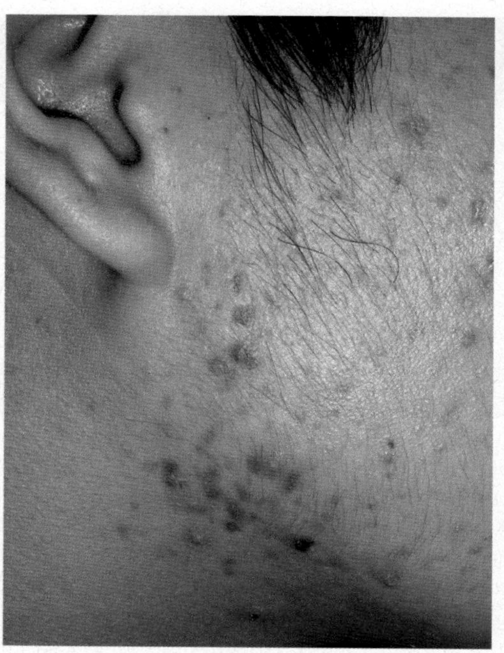

FIGURE 118-4 Inflammatory acne showing pustules and nodules in a 17-year-old boy who uses a helmet while playing football in high school. (*Reproduced with permission from Richard P. Usatine, MD.*)

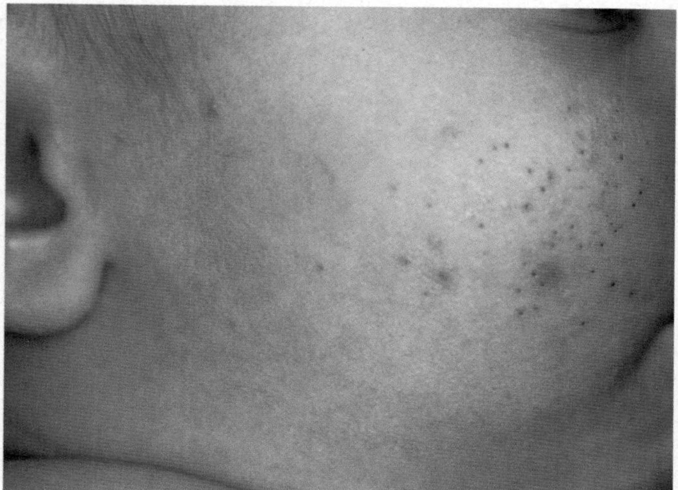

FIGURE 118-3 Neonatal acne in a healthy 2-week-old infant that resolved without treatment. (*Reproduced with permission from Richard P. Usatine, MD.*)

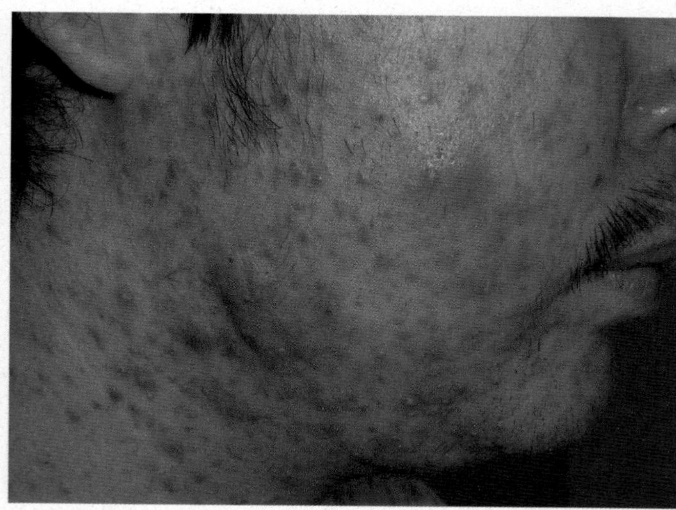

FIGURE 118-5 Severe inflammatory acne in a young adult. His acne worsened when he was started on phenytoin for his seizure disorder. (*Reproduced with permission from Richard P. Usatine, MD.*)

DIAGNOSIS

CLINICAL FEATURES

Morphology of acne includes comedones, papules, pustules, nodules, and cysts.

- Obstructive acne = comedonal acne = noninflammatory acne consisting only of comedones (**Figure 118-6**).
- Open comedones are called blackheads, and closed comedones are called whiteheads and look like small pink papules.
- Inflammatory acne consists of papules, pustules, nodules, and cysts in addition to comedones (see **Figure 118-5**).

TYPICAL DISTRIBUTION

Face, back, chest, and neck.

LABORATORY STUDIES

None, unless suspecting androgen excess and/or polycystic ovarian syndrome (PCOS).[4] SOR Ⓑ Obtain testosterone and DHEA-S levels if you suspect androgen excess and/or PCOS. Consider also adding follicle-stimulating hormone (FSH) and luteinizing hormone (LH) levels if suspecting PCOS.

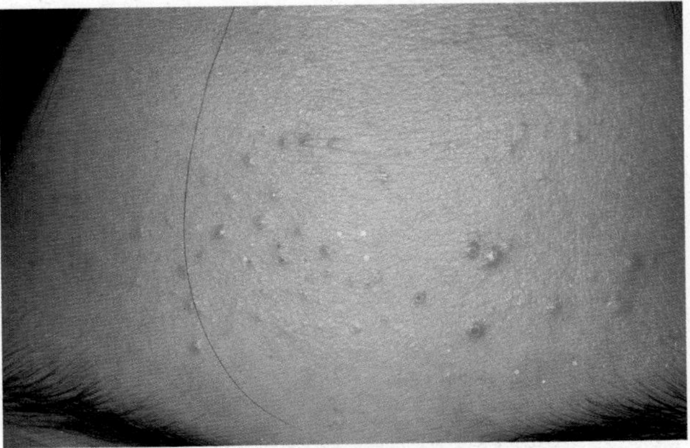

FIGURE 118-6 Comedonal acne in a 15-year-old girl. Open comedones (blackheads) and closed comedones (whiteheads) are visible on her forehead. *(Reproduced with permission from Richard P. Usatine, MD.)*

DIFFERENTIAL DIAGNOSIS

- *Acne conglobata* is an uncommon and unusually severe form of acne characterized by multiple comedones, cysts, sinus tracts, and abscesses. The inflammatory lesions and scars can lead to significant disfigurement.[5] Sinus tracks can form with multiple openings that drain foul-smelling purulent material (**Figures 118-7 to 118-9**). The comedones and nodules are usually found on the chest, shoulders, back, buttocks, and face. In some cases, acne conglobata is part of a follicular occlusion triad along with hidradenitis and dissecting cellulitis of the scalp (**Figure 118-9**).
- *Acne fulminans* is characterized by sudden onset ulcerative crusting cystic acne found mostly on the chest and back (**Figures 118-10 and 118-11**).[6] Fever, malaise, nausea, arthralgia, myalgia, and weight loss are common. Leukocytosis and elevated erythrocyte sedimentation rate are usually present. There may also be focal osteolytic lesions. The term *acne fulminans* may also be used in cases of severe aggravation of acne without systemic features.[5]
- *Rosacea* can resemble acne due to the presence of papules and pustules on the face. It is usually seen in older adults with prominent erythema and telangiectasias. Rosacea does not include comedones and may have ocular or nasal manifestations (Chapter 119, Rosacea). *Rosacea fulminans* or *pyoderma faciale* has features of severe acne and rosacea (**Figure 118-12**).
- *Folliculitis* on the back may be confused with acne. Look for hairs centrally located in the inflammatory papules to help distinguish it from acne. Acne on the back usually accompanies acne on the face (Chapter 123, Folliculitis).
- *Acne keloidalis nuchae* consists of papules, pustules, nodules, and keloidal tissue found at the posterior hairline. It is most often seen

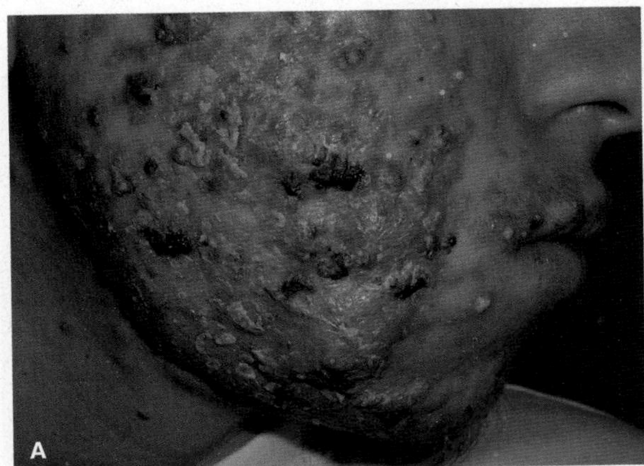

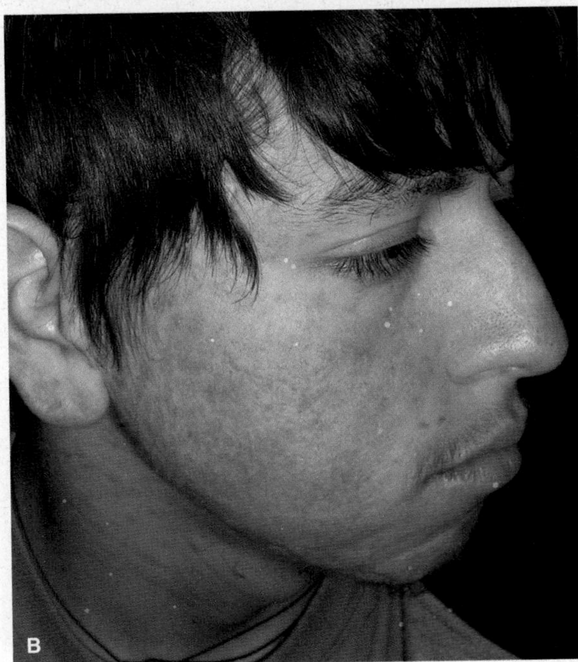

FIGURE 118-7 **A.** Acne conglobata in a 16-year-old boy. He has severe cysts on his face with sinus tracts between them. He required many weeks of oral prednisone before isotretinoin was started. His acne cleared completely with his treatment. **B.** Acne conglobata cleared with minimal scarring after oral prednisone and 5 months of isotretinoin therapy. *(Reproduced with permission from Richard P. Usatine, MD.)*

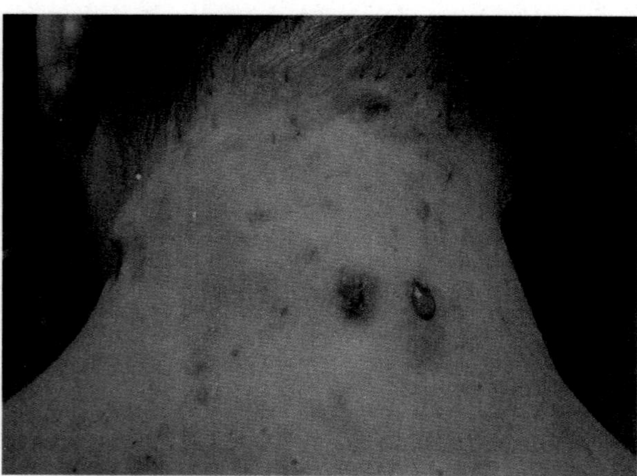

FIGURE 118-8 Acne conglobata in a 42-year-old woman showing communicating sinus tracts between cysts. There is pus draining from one of the sinus tracts on the right side of the neck. (*Reproduced with permission from Richard P. Usatine, MD.*)

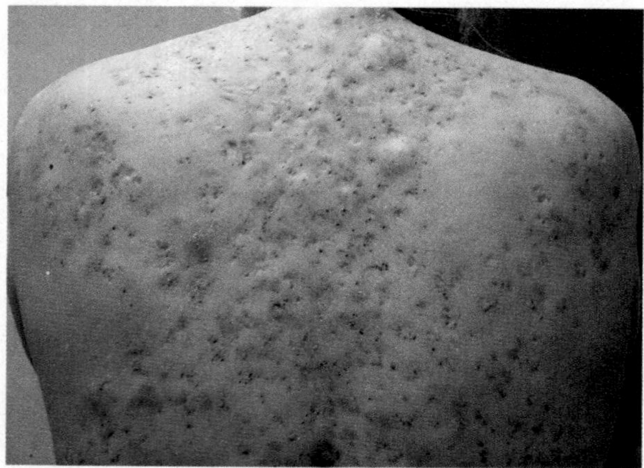

FIGURE 118-9 Acne conglobata in a 53-year-old man covered with open comedones and cysts on his back. He has the follicular occlusion triad including hidradenitis, dissecting cellulitis of the scalp, and acne conglobata. (*Reproduced with permission from Richard P. Usatine, MD.*)

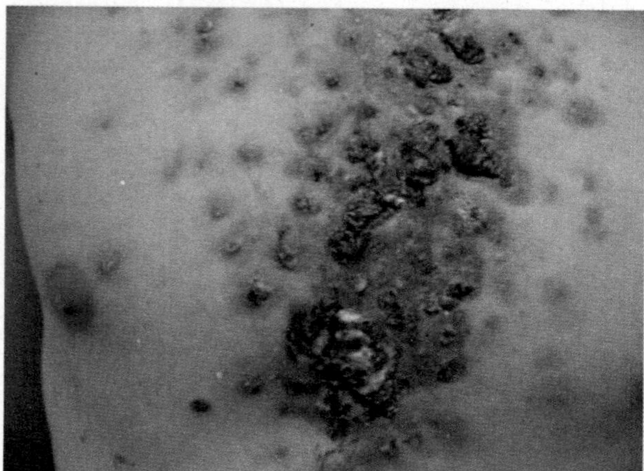

FIGURE 118-10 Acne fulminans in a 17-year-old boy. He was on isotretinoin when he developed worsening of his acne with polymyalgia and arthralgia. He presented with numerous nodules and cysts covered by hemorrhagic crusts on his chest and back. (*Reproduced with permission from Grunwald MH, Amichai B. Nodulo-cystic eruption with musculoskeletal pain. J Fam Pract. 2007;56:205-206. Frontline Medical Communications, Inc.*)

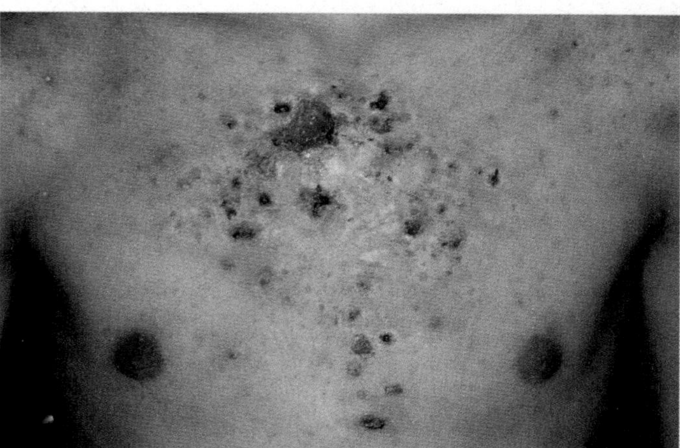

FIGURE 118-11 Acne fulminans with severe rapidly worsening truncal acne in a 15-year-old boy. He did not have fever or bone pain but had a white blood cell count of 17,000. He responded rapidly to prednisone and was started on isotretinoin. The ulcers and granulation tissue worsened initially on isotretinoin, but prednisone helped to get this under control. (*Reproduced with permission from Richard P. Usatine, MD.*)

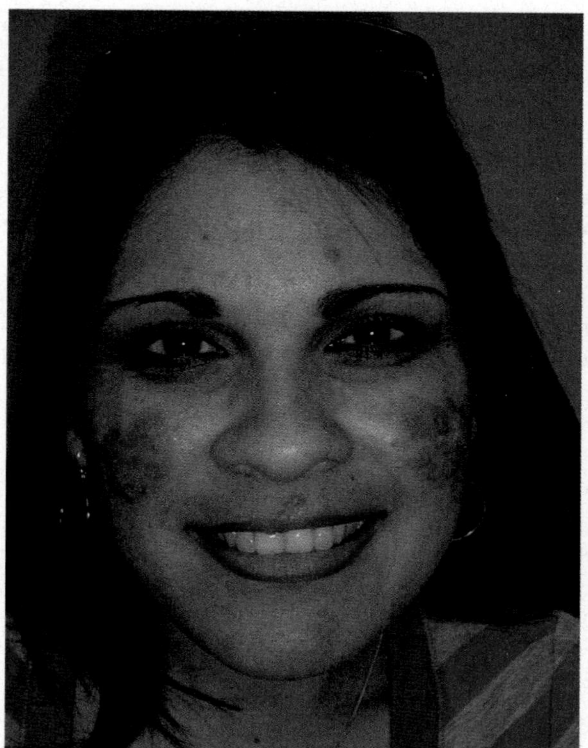

FIGURE 118-12 Pyoderma faciale is almost exclusively seen in adult women. It can present with severe cystic facial acne often in a malar distribution. It also is called rosacea fulminans. It started abruptly 6 months before, and is not related to cutaneous lupus. (*Reproduced with permission from Richard P. Usatine, MD.*)

in men of color after shaving the hair at the nape of the neck (Chapter 120, Pseudofolliculitis and Acne Keloidalis Nuchae).

- *Actinic comedones* (blackheads, Favre and Racouchot disease) are related to sun exposure and are seen later in life (**Figure 118-13**).

MANAGEMENT

Treatment is based on acne type and severity. Therapies include topical retinoids, topical antimicrobials, systemic antimicrobials, hormonal therapy, oral isotretinoin, and injection therapy.

FIRST LINE

TOPICAL

- Benzoyl peroxide (2.5%, 5%, 10%)—Antimicrobial effect (gel, cream, lotion), available over the counter (OTC); 10% benzoyl peroxide causes more irritation and is not more effective.[1] SOR Ⓐ
- Topical antibiotics—Clindamycin and erythromycin are the mainstays of treatment. SOR Ⓐ
- Erythromycin—Solution, gel.[3] SOR Ⓐ
  - Clindamycin—Solution, gel, lotion.[3] SOR Ⓐ
  - Benzamycin gel—Erythromycin 3%, benzoyl peroxide 5%.[3] SOR Ⓐ
  - BenzaClin gel—Clindamycin 1%, benzoyl peroxide 5%.[3] SOR Ⓐ
  - Dapsone 5% gel.[7] SOR Ⓐ
- Azelaic acid—Useful to treat post-inflammatory hyperpigmentation and acne (**Figure 118-14**).[3] SOR Ⓐ

RETINOIDS

- Tretinoin (Retin-A) gel, cream, liquid, micronized.[1] SOR Ⓐ
- Adapalene gel (Differin)—Less irritating than tretinoin.[1] SOR Ⓐ Now available OTC. The OTC 0.1% adapalene gel is less expensive than generic and brand-name tretinoin, and this is a game changer for acne therapy in patients without health insurance.
- Tazarotene (Tazorac)—Strongest topical retinoid with greatest risk of irritation.[8] SOR Ⓐ

Topical retinoids will often result in skin irritation during the first 2 to 3 months of treatment, but new systematic reviews do not demonstrate that they worsen acne lesion counts during the initial period of use.[2]

ORAL ANTIBIOTICS

- Doxycycline 40 to 100 mg qd-bid—Well tolerated, can take with food (but not foods high in calcium), and increases sun sensitivity.[3] SOR Ⓐ
- Minocycline 50 to 100 mg qd-bid—Not proven to be better than other systemic antibiotics, including tetracycline.[3,9] SOR Ⓐ
- Tetracycline 500 mg qd-bid—Absorbed best on an empty stomach.[3] SOR Ⓐ
- Erythromycin 250 to 500 mg bid—Frequent gastrointestinal (GI) disturbance but can be used in pregnancy.[3] SOR Ⓐ
- Trimethoprim/sulfamethoxazole DS bid—Effective but poses risk of Stevens-Johnson syndrome. Reserve for short courses in particularly severe and resistant cases.[3] SOR Ⓑ

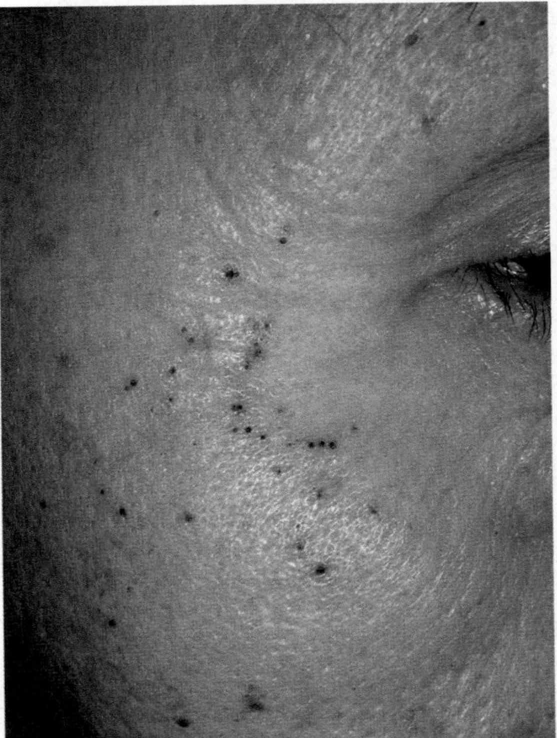

FIGURE 118-13 Actinic comedones related to sun exposure in an older man. These are typically seen on the side of the face clustering around the eyes. (*Reproduced with permission from Richard P. Usatine, MD.*)

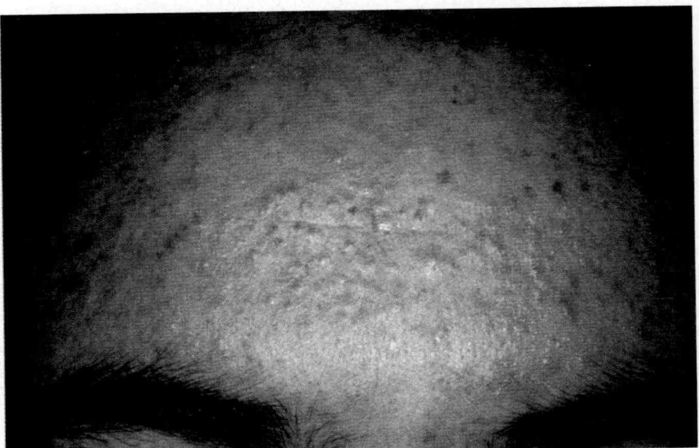

FIGURE 118-14 Obstructive or comedonal acne with spotty hyperpigmentation. Azelaic acid was helpful to treat the acne and the hyperpigmentation. (*Reproduced with permission from Richard P. Usatine, MD.*)

- Oral azithromycin has been prescribed in pulse dosing for acne in a number of small studies and has not been found to be inferior to oral doxycyline.[10] The two most common dosing variations are 500 mg daily for 3 days each month or 250 mg every other day on an ongoing basis. It is a viable alternative to doxycycline, as the price for generic azithromycin has come down and it does not cause photosensitivity. SOR Ⓒ

SECOND LINE

- Isotretinoin (originally known as Accutane, but this brand name has been discontinued) is the most powerful treatment for acne. It is especially useful for cystic and scarring acne that has not responded to other therapies.[3] SOR Ⓐ Dosed at approximately 1 mg/kg per day for 6 months. Women of childbearing age must be completely abstinent from sex or use two forms of contraception. Monitor for dry skin, muscle aches, dry eyes, depression, and GI side effects.[11] Patients should have baseline comprehensive metabolic profile and lipid panel, then repeat 1 month after being on isotretinoin to monitor for elevated liver enzymes and triglycerides. Monthly lab tests are no longer recommended.[12] SOR Ⓑ
    - The U.S. Food and Drug Administration requires that prescribers of isotretinoin, patients who take isotretinoin, and pharmacists who dispense isotretinoin all must register with the iPLEDGE system (www.ipledgeprogram.com).
- Hormonal treatments
    - Oral contraceptives only for females—Choose ones with low androgenic effect.[3] SOR Ⓐ FDA-approved oral contraceptives for acne include Ortho Tri-Cyclen, Yaz, and Estrostep. Other oral contraceptives with similar formulations also help to treat acne in women even though these have not received FDA approval for this indication. Note that Yaz and Yasmin have the progestin drospirenone,[13] which is derived from 17α-spironolactone. It shares an antiandrogenic effect with spironolactone.
    - Spironolactone is another systemic option in females over the age of 12 years.[3,14] This may be especially useful if the patient has hirsutism but this is not a requirement for use. Start with 25 mg daily and go to 50 mg daily as needed. It is best absorbed with food. Sometimes 50 mg bid is needed (max dose is 100 mg bid). The risk of hyperkalemia increases with a higher dose, but there is no proven value to monitoring for hyperkalemia in healthy young women not taking other potassium-sparing medications.[15] Monitor potassium if the woman is over age 45 years if using higher doses. Titrate up as needed and tolerated.[3] SOR Ⓑ The most common side effects are diuresis, breast tenderness, and menstrual irregularities, which are dose dependent. One systematic review failed to show a benefit for spironolactone in acne even though it was found to decrease hirsutism.[16] Despite the lack of published data, relying on available evidence, experience, and expert opinion, the American Academy of Dermatology work group supports the use of spironolactone in the management of acne in select women (American Academy of Dermatology Acne Clinical Guideline: https://www.aad.org/practice-tools/quality-care/clinical-guidelines/acne).
    - One small prospective study of 27 women with severe papular and nodulocystic acne used a combination of EE/DRSP (Yasmin) and spironolactone 100 mg daily. Eighty-five percent of subjects were entirely clear of acne lesions or had excellent improvement with no significant elevation of serum potassium.[17]
- Steroid injection therapy—For painful nodules and cysts. SOR Ⓒ Be careful to avoid producing skin atrophy. Dilute 0.1 mL of 10 mg/mL triamcinolone acetonide (Kenalog) with 0.4 mL of sterile saline for a 2 mg/mL suspension. Inject 0.1 mL with a 1-mL tuberculin syringe into each nodule using a 30-gauge needle (**Figure 112-15**).

COMPLEMENTARY AND ALTERNATIVE THERAPY

- Tea tree oil 5% gel.[18] SOR Ⓑ
- Other herbal agents.[19] SOR Ⓑ

ACNE THERAPY BY SEVERITY

Comedonal acne (Figure 118-6)

- Topical retinoid or azelaic acid. Benzoyl peroxide may also help.
- No need for antibiotics or antimicrobials—do not need to kill *P. acnes*.

Mild papulopustular acne

- Topical antibiotics and benzoyl peroxide.
- Topical retinoid or azelaic acid.
- May add oral antibiotics if topical agents are not working.

Papulopustular or nodulocystic acne—moderate to severe—inflammatory

- Topical retinoid, benzoyl peroxide, and oral antibiotic.
- Oral antibiotics or hormonal therapy for women are often essential at this stage.
- Azelaic acid if simultaneously treating unwanted hyperpigmentation.
- Steroid injection therapy—for painful nodules and cysts.

Severe cystic or scarring acne

- Isotretinoin if there are no contraindications.
- Steroid injection therapy—for painful nodules and cysts.

Acne fulminans (see Figures 118-9 to 118-11)

- Start with systemic steroids (prednisone 40 to 60 mg/day—approximately 1 mg/kg per day).[20] SOR Ⓒ
- Systemic steroid treatment rapidly controls the skin lesions and systemic symptoms. The duration of steroid treatment in one Finnish series was 2 to 4 months to avoid relapses.[20] SOR Ⓒ
- Therapy with isotretinoin, antibiotics, or both was often combined with steroids.[20] SOR Ⓒ
- One British series used oral prednisolone 0.5 to 1 mg/kg daily for 4 to 6 weeks (thereafter slowly reduced to zero).[21] SOR Ⓒ
- Oral isotretinoin was added to the regimen at the fourth week, initially at 0.5 mg/kg daily and gradually increased to achieve complete clearance.[21] SOR Ⓒ
- Consider introducing isotretinoin at approximately 4 weeks in addition to the oral prednisone if there are no contraindications. SOR Ⓒ
- Acne conglobata and pyoderma faciale may be treated like acne fulminans, but the course of oral prednisone does not need to be as long. SOR Ⓒ

COMBINATION THERAPIES

- Combination therapy with multiple topical agents can be more effective than single agents.[3] SOR Ⓐ
- Topical retinoids and topical antibiotics are more effective when used in combination than when either are used alone.[3] SOR Ⓐ
- Benzoyl peroxide and topical antibiotics used in combination are effective treatment for acne by helping to minimize antibiotic resistance.[3] SOR Ⓐ
- The adjunctive use of clindamycin/benzoyl peroxide gel with tazarotene cream promotes greater efficacy and may also enhance tolerability.[3] SOR Ⓐ
- Combination therapy with topical retinoids and oral antibiotics can be helpful at the start of acne therapy. However, maintenance therapy with combination tazarotene and minocycline therapy showed a trend for greater efficacy but no statistical significance compared to tazarotene alone.[22]

MEDICATION COST

The most affordable medications for acne include OTC topical benzoyl peroxide and OTC topical adapalene gel 0.1%. Even generic tretinoin has become very expensive. The most expensive acne medications are the brand-name combination products of existing topical medications. These medications are convenient for those with insurance that covers them (Epiduo contains benzoyl peroxide and adapalene; Ziana contains clindamycin and tretinoin). Unfortunately, previously affordable oral antibiotics in the tetracycline family have become more expensive. While they continue to play an important role in acne therapy, they are often only affordable to those patients fortunate enough to have medical insurance without large deductibles. Isotretinoin is also very expensive even though it has been generic for many years. Using the smartphone app GoodRx is one method to find the best price for a particular prescription acne medication in the local area.

NEWER EXPENSIVE MODES OF THERAPY

Intense pulsed light (IPL) and photodynamic therapy (PDT) are options for people in whom using oral and topical treatment is ineffective, inconvenient, poorly tolerated, or harmful.[21] However, these therapies are often expensive, and data do not suggest that these should be first-line therapies at this time. Light and laser treatments have been shown to be of short-term benefit if patients can afford therapy and tolerate some discomfort, but the usefulness of red light or blue light as standard therapy for patients with moderate to severe acne carries low certainty.[23] Thus, these therapies have not been shown to be better than simple topical treatments.[2] One comparative trial demonstrated that PDT was less effective than topical adapalene in the short-term reduction of inflammatory lesions.[2] Chemical peels with glycolic acid or salicylic acid can also be used to treat acne. Studies have demonstrated that chemical peels are well tolerated despite some mild discomfort.[24]

FOLLOW-UP

Isotretinoin requires monthly follow-up visits, but other therapies can be monitored every few months at first and then once to twice per

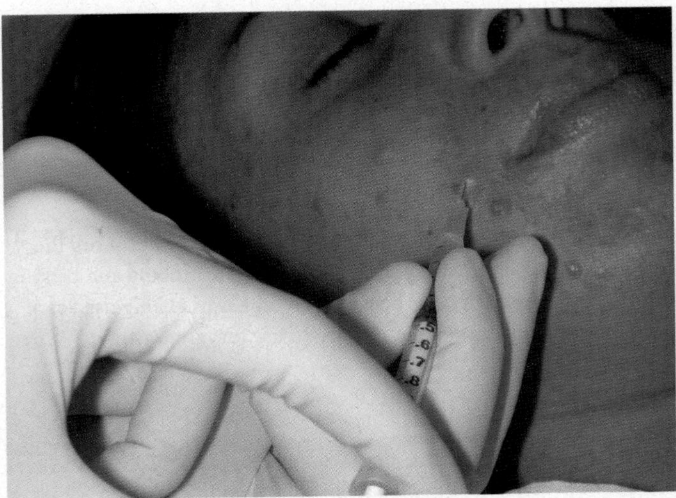

FIGURE 118-15 Injection of acne nodules with 2 mg/mL triamcinolone acetonide. *(Reproduced with permission from Richard P. Usatine, MD.)*

year. Keep in mind that many treatments for acne take months to work, so quick follow-up visits may be disappointing.

PATIENT EDUCATION

Adherence to medication regimens is crucial for therapy success. Adequate face washing twice per day is sufficient. Do not scrub the face with abrasive physical or chemical agents. Scrubbing and picking the skin can worsen acne. If benzoyl peroxide is not being used as a leave-on product, it can be purchased to use for face washing.

PATIENT RESOURCES

- PubMed Health has good patient education information—**http://www.ncbi.nlm.nih.gov/pubmedhealth/PMH0001876/.**

PROVIDER RESOURCES

- American Academy of Dermatology. *Acne Clinical Guideline*—**https://www.aad.org/practice-tools/quality-care/clinical-guidelines/acne.**
- Usatine R, Pfenninger J, Stulberg D, Small R. *Dermatologic and Cosmetic Procedures in Office Practice*. Philadelphia: Elsevier; 2012. Covers how to do acne surgery, steroid injections for acne, chemical peels, PDT and laser treatment for acne. It is also available as an app—**www.usatinemedia.com.**

REFERENCES

1. Purdy S, de Berker D. Acne vulgaris. *Clin Evid (Online)*. 2011; 2011.
2. Smith EV, Grindlay DJ, Williams HC. What's new in acne? An analysis of systematic reviews published in 2009–2010. *Clin Exp Dermatol.* 2011;36:119-122.
3. Fiedler F, Stangl GI, Fiedler E, Taube KM. Acne and nutrition: a systematic review. *Acta Derm Venereol.* 2017;97(1):7-9.
4. Legro RS, Arslanian SA, Ehrmann DA, et al. Diagnosis and treatment of polycystic ovary syndrome: an Endocrine Society clinical practice guideline. *J Clin Endocrinol Metab.* 2013;98:4565-4592.
5. Shirakawa M, Uramoto K, Harada FA. Treatment of acne conglobata with infliximab. *J Am Acad Dermatol.* 2006;55:344-346.
6. Grunwald MH, Amichai B. Nodulo-cystic eruption with musculoskeletal pain. *J Fam Pract.* 2007;56:205-206.
7. Tanghetti E, Harper JC, Oefelein MG. The efficacy and tolerability of dapsone 5% gel in female vs male patients with facial acne vulgaris: gender as a clinically relevant outcome variable. *J Drugs Dermatol.* 2012;11:1417-1421.
8. Gregoriou S, Kritsotaki E, Katoulis A, Rigopoulos D. Use of tazarotene foam for the treatment of acne vulgaris. *Clin Cosmet Investig Dermatol.* 2014;7:165-170.
9. Garner SE, Eady A, Bennett C, et al. Minocycline for acne vulgaris: efficacy and safety. *Cochrane Database Syst Rev.* 2012;(8):CD002086.
10. Maleszka R, Turek-Urasinska K, Oremus M, et al. Pulsed azithromycin treatment is as effective and safe as 2-week-longer daily doxycycline treatment of acne vulgaris: a randomized, double-blind, noninferiority study. *Skinmed.* 2011;9:86-94.
11. Vallerand IA, Lewinson RT, Farris MS, et al. Efficacy and adverse events of oral isotretinoin for acne: a systematic review. *Br J Dermatol.* 2018;178(1):76-85.
12. Lee JW, Yoo KH, Park KY, et al. Effectiveness of conventional, low-dose and intermittent oral isotretinoin in the treatment of acne: a randomized, controlled comparative study. *Br J Dermatol.* 2011;164:1369-1375.
13. Maloney JM, Dietze P Jr, Watson D, et al. A randomized controlled trial of a low-dose combined oral contraceptive containing 3 mg drospirenone plus 20 microg ethinylestradiol in the treatment of acne vulgaris: lesion counts, investigator ratings and subject self-assessment. *J Drugs Dermatol.* 2009;8:837-844.
14. Trivedi MK, Shinkai K, Murase JE. A review of hormone-based therapies to treat adult acne vulgaris in women. *Int J Womens Dermatol.* 2017;3(1):44-52.
15. Plovanich M, Weng QY, Mostaghimi A. Low usefulness of potassium monitoring among healthy young women taking spironolactone for acne. *JAMA Dermatol.* 2015;151(9):941–944.
16. Brown J, Farquhar C, Lee O, et al. Spironolactone versus placebo or in combination with steroids for hirsutism and/or acne. *Cochrane Database Syst Rev.* 2009;(2):CD000194.
17. Krunic A, Ciurea A, Scheman A. Efficacy and tolerance of acne treatment using both spironolactone and a combined contraceptive containing drospirenone. *J Am Acad Dermatol.* 2008;58:60-62.
18. Enshaieh S, Jooya A, Siadat AH, Iraji F. The efficacy of 5% topical tea tree oil gel in mild to moderate acne vulgaris: a randomized, double-blind placebo-controlled study. *Indian J Dermatol Venereol Leprol.* 2007;73:22-25.
19. Fouladi RF. Aqueous extract of dried fruit of *Berberis vulgaris* L. in acne vulgaris, a clinical trial. *J Diet Suppl.* 2012;9:253-261.
20. Karvonen SL. Acne fulminans: report of clinical findings and treatment of twenty-four patients. *J Am Acad Dermatol.* 1993; 28:572-579.
21. Seukeran DC, Cunliffe WJ. The treatment of acne fulminans: a review of 25 cases. *Br J Dermatol.* 1999;141:307-309.
22. Leyden J, Thiboutot DM, Shalita AR, et al. Comparison of tazarotene and minocycline maintenance therapies in acne vulgaris: a multicenter, double-blind, randomized, parallel-group study. *Arch Dermatol.* 2006;142:605-612.
23. Barbaric J, Abbott R, Posadzki P, et al. Light therapies for acne: abridged Cochrane systematic review including GRADE assessments. *Br J Dermatol.* 2018;178(1):61-75.
24. Al-Talib H, Al-khateeb A, Hameed A, Murugaiah C. Efficacy and safety of superficial chemical peeling in treatment of active acne vulgaris. *An Bras Dermatol.* 2017;92(2):212-216.

119 ROSACEA

Richard P. Usatine, MD
Cynthia M. Villanueva Ramos, MD

PATIENT STORY

A 34-year-old woman with extensive papulopustular rosacea (**Figures 119-1** to **119-3**) has a history of easy facial flushing since her teen years. Her face has been persistently redder in the past 5 years and she is bothered by this. She acknowledges that her mom has similar redness in her face and that she is from northern European heritage. In the last 6 months, since her daughter was born, she has developed many "pimples." Physical examination reveals papules, pustules, and telangiectasias. No comedones are seen. She knows that the sun makes it worse but finds that many sunscreens are irritating to her skin. The patient is started on oral tetracycline daily and 0.75% metronidazole cream to use once daily. She agrees to wear a hat and stay out of the sun during the middle of the day. She will continue to look for a sunscreen she can tolerate. She knows that precipitating factors for her include hot and humid weather, alcohol, hot beverages, and spicy foods. She will do her best to avoid those factors.

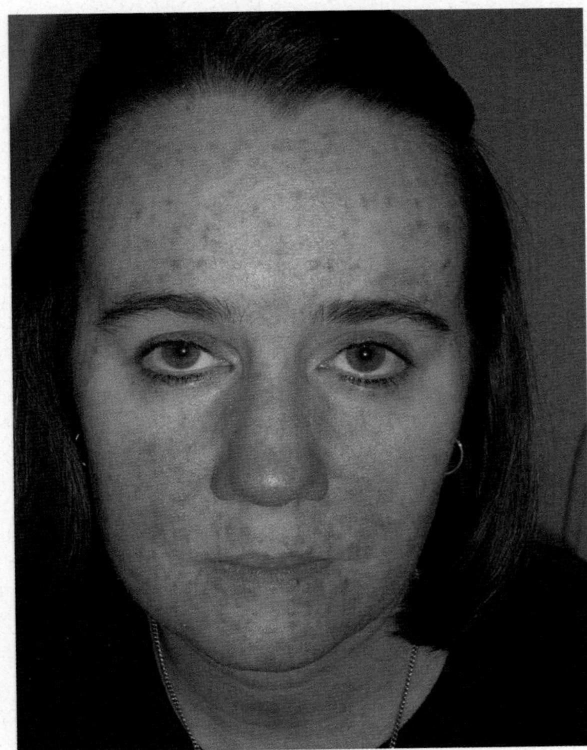

FIGURE 119-1 Rosacea in a 34-year-old woman showing erythema, papules, and pustules covering much of the face. Note her fair skin and blue eyes from her northern European heritage. *(Reproduced with permission from Richard P. Usatine, MD.)*

INTRODUCTION

Rosacea is an inflammatory condition of the face and eyes that mostly affects adults. Most commonly the face becomes reddened over the cheeks and nose, and this is often accompanied by telangiectasias and a papulopustular eruption.

SYNONYMS

Rosacea is also called acne rosacea but is not a type of acne.

EPIDEMIOLOGY

- Common in fair-skinned people of Celtic and northern European heritage.
- Women are more often affected than men.
- Men are more prone to the extreme forms of hyperplasia, which causes rhinophymatous rosacea (**Figures 119-4** and **119-5**).

ETIOLOGY AND PATHOPHYSIOLOGY

- Although the exact etiology is unknown, the pathophysiology involves nonspecific inflammation followed by dilation around follicles and hyperreactive capillaries. These dilated capillaries become telangiectasias (**Figures 119-6** and **119-7**). Neurovascular dysregulation and innate immune responses are involved.[1]

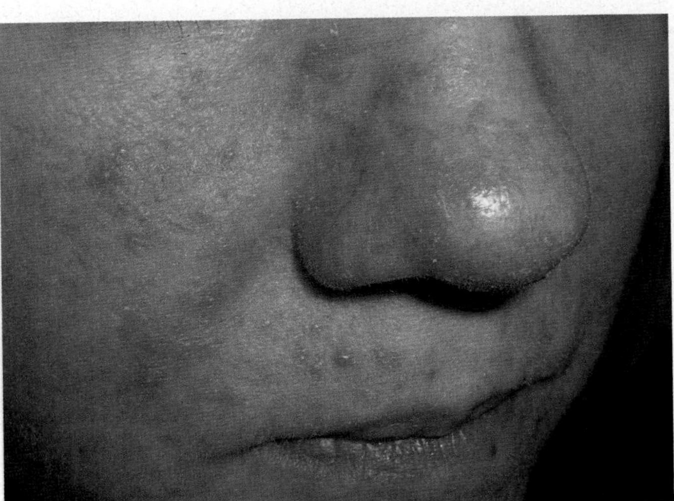

FIGURE 119-2 Close-up of papules and pustules in the same woman. Note the absence of comedones. This is not acne. This is papulopustular rosacea. *(Reproduced with permission from Richard P. Usatine, MD.)*

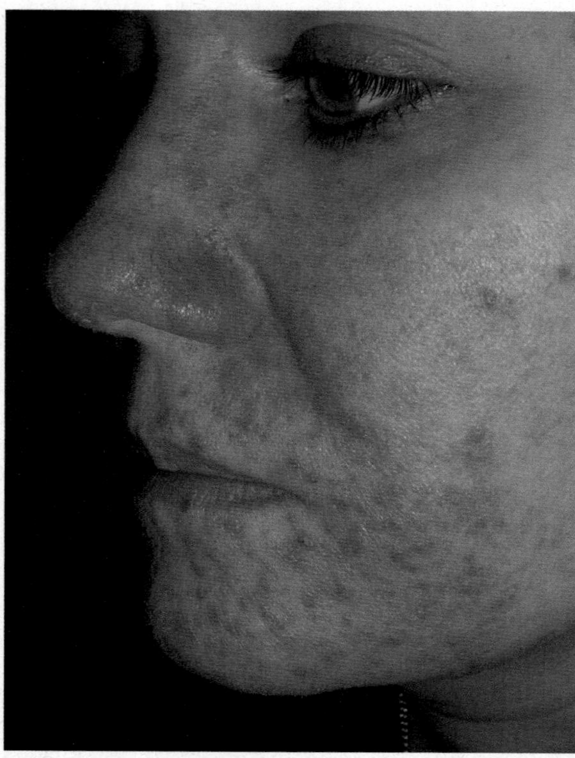

FIGURE 119-3 Close-up showing telangiectasias on the nose and papules around the mouth and chin. (*Reproduced with permission from Richard P. Usatine, MD.*)

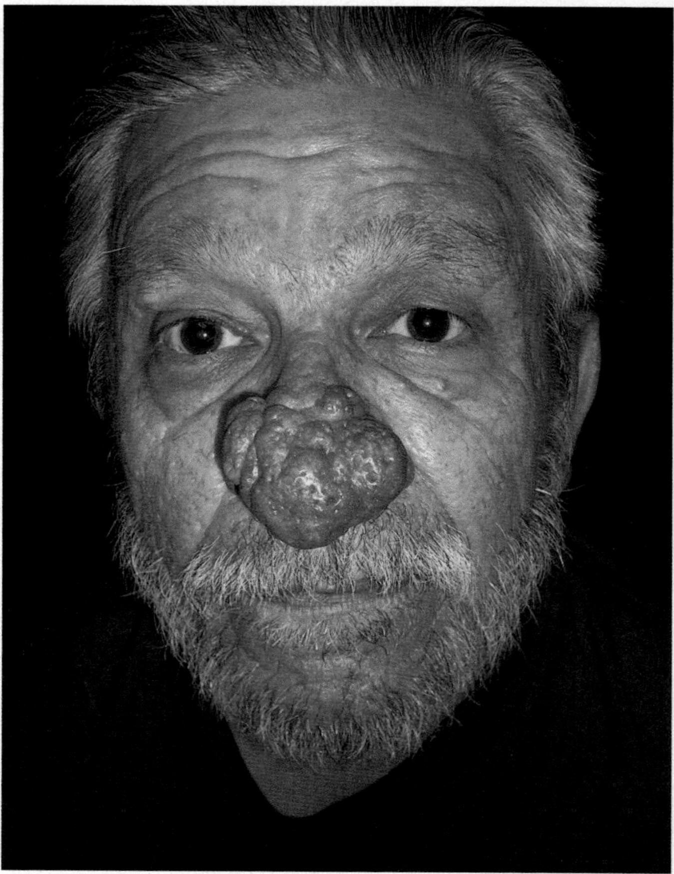

FIGURE 119-5 Rhinophymatous rosacea in an older man who does not drink alcohol. Although this is often called a W. C. Fields nose, it is not necessarily related to heavy alcohol use. (*Reproduced with permission from Richard P. Usatine, MD.*)

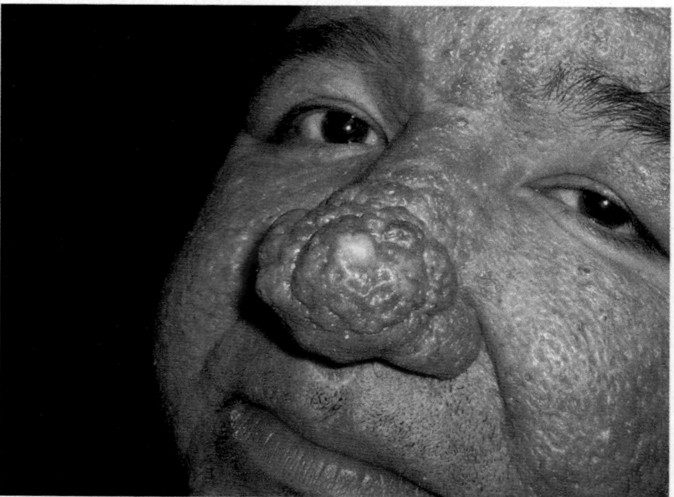

FIGURE 119-4 Rhinophymatous rosacea with skin thickening, glandular hyperplasia, and a bulbous appearance of the nose in this young Hispanic man. The cheeks and forehead also show erythema and papules. The patient acknowledges current heavy alcohol intake. (*Reproduced with permission from Richard P. Usatine, MD.*)

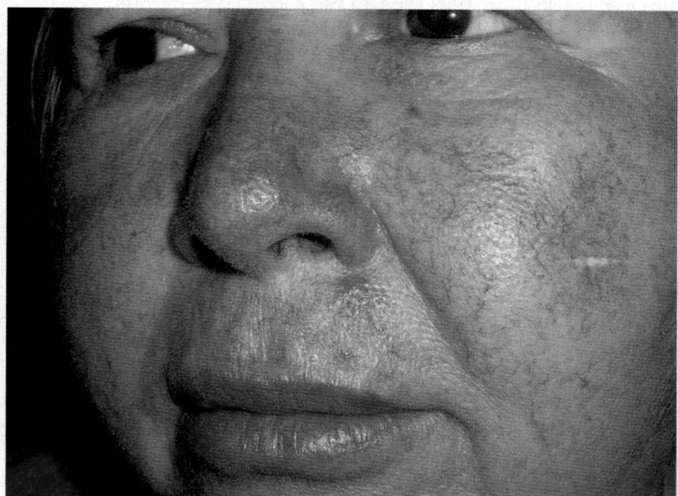

FIGURE 119-6 Erythematotelangiectatic subtype of rosacea in a middle-aged Hispanic woman. Note that she does have papules under the nose, as there is overlap in subtypes. (*Reproduced with permission from Richard P. Usatine, MD.*)

- Phymatous changes involve diffuse hypertrophy of the connective tissue and sebaceous gland hyperplasia (see **Figures 119-4** and **119-5**).
- Alcohol may accentuate erythema, but does not cause the disease. Rosacea runs in families.
- Sun exposure may precipitate an acute rosacea flare, but flare-ups can happen without sun exposure.
- A significant increase in the hair follicle mite *Demodex folliculorum* is sometimes found in rosacea.[2] It is theorized that these mites play a role because they incite an inflammatory or allergic reaction by mechanical blockage of follicles.

RISK FACTORS

Genetics, *Demodex* infestation,[2] sun exposure.

DIAGNOSIS

- Diagnosis is now based on the new classification schema for rosacea in **Table 119-1**.[1]
- A patient with fixed centrofacial erythema in a characteristic pattern that may periodically intensify and/or phymatous changes automatically meets criteria for rosacea (these are the 2 diagnostic phenotypes).[1]
- Without one of the 2 diagnostic phenotypes, the presence of 2 or more major features may be considered diagnostic for rosacea[1]:
  - Flushing
  - Papules and pustules
  - Telangiectasia
  - Ocular manifestations

CLINICAL FEATURES

The standard rosacea subtypes are still helpful in considering the diagnosis of rosacea (note that there is often overlap for each patient):

1. ***Erythematotelangiectatic rosacea*** (see **Figures 119-6** and **119-7**)—This stage is characterized by frequent mild to severe flushing with persistent central facial erythema.

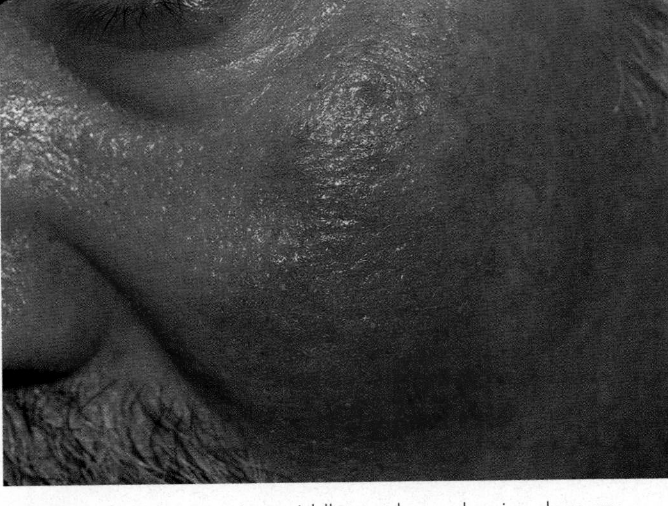

FIGURE 119-7 Rosacea in a middle-aged man showing deep erythema and many telangiectasias. (*Reproduced with permission from Richard P. Usatine, MD.*)

TABLE 119-1 Phenotypes of Rosacea

Diagnostic*	Major†	Secondary
Fixed centrofacial erythema in a characteristic pattern that may periodically intensify	Flushing	Burning sensation
	Papules and pustules	Stinging sensation
Phymatous changes	Telangiectasia	Edema
	Ocular manifestations • Lid margin telangiectasia • Interpalpebral conjunctival injection • Spade-shaped infiltrates in the cornea • Scleritis and sclerokeratitis	Dryness Ocular manifestations • "Honey crust" and collarette accumulation at the base of the lashes • Irregularity of the lid margin • Evaporative tear dysfunction (rapid tear breakup time)

*These features by themselves are diagnostic of rosacea.
†Two or more major features may be considered diagnostic.
Reproduced with permission from Gallo RL, Granstein RD, Kang S, et al: Standard classification and pathophysiology of rosacea: The 2017 update by the National Rosacea Society Expert Committee, J Am Acad Dermatol. 2018;78(1):148-155.

2. ***Papulopustular rosacea*** (**Figures 119-1** to **119-3, 119-8,** and **119-9**)—This is a highly vascular stage that involves longer periods of flushing than the first stage, often lasting from days to weeks. Minute telangiectasias and papules start to form by this stage, and some patients begin having very mild ocular complaints such as ocular grittiness or conjunctivitis. These patients may have many unsightly pustules with severe facial erythema. They are more prone to develop a hordeolum (stye) (see Chapter 15, Hordeolum and Chalazion).
3. ***Phymatous or Rhinophymatous rosacea*** (see **Figures 119-4** and **119-5**)—Characterized by hyperplasia of the sebaceous glands that form thickened confluent plaques on the nose known as rhinophyma. This hyperplasia can cause significant disfigurement to the forehead, eyelids, chin, and nose. The nasal disfiguration is seen more commonly in men than women. W. C. Fields is famous for his rhinophyma and intake of alcohol. Rhinophyma can occur without any alcohol use, as seen in the patient in **Figure 119-5**.
4. ***Ocular rosacea*** (**Figures 119-10** to **119-12**)—An advanced subtype of rosacea that is characterized by impressive, severe flushing with persistent telangiectasias, papules, and pustules. The patient may complain of watery eyes, a foreign-body sensation, burning, dryness, vision changes, and lid or periocular erythema. The eyelids are most commonly involved with telangiectasias, blepharitis, and recurrent hordeola and chalazia (**Figures 119-10** and **119-11**). Conjunctivitis may be chronic. Although corneal involvement is least common, it can have the most devastating consequences. Corneal findings may include punctate erosions, corneal infiltrates, and corneal neovascularization. In the most severe cases, blood vessels may grow over the cornea and lead to blindness (**Figure 119-12**).

Note that many patients have a combination of these subtypes. This is one factor that has led to a new classification schema for rosacea based on pathophysiology (see **Table 119-1**).[1]

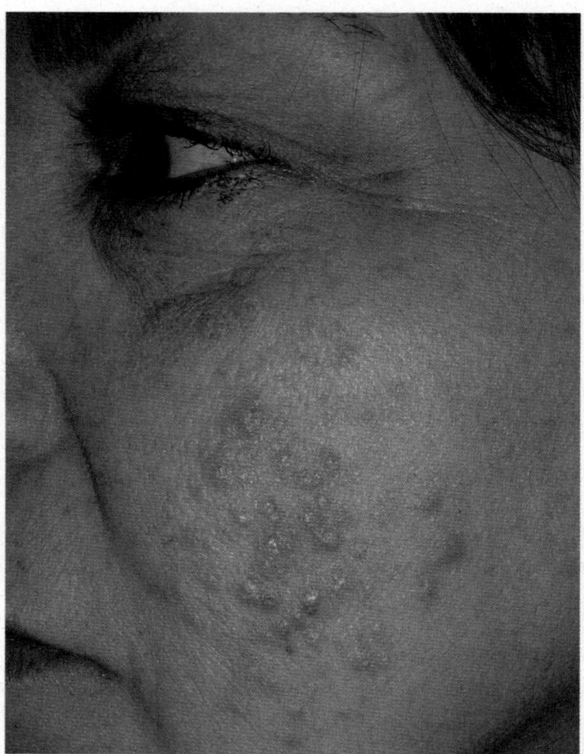

FIGURE 119-8 Papulopustular rosacea in a middle-aged woman. (*Reproduced with permission from Richard P. Usatine, MD.*)

TYPICAL DISTRIBUTION

Rosacea occurs on the face, especially on the cheeks and nose. However, the forehead, eyelids, and chin can also be involved (**Figure 119-13**).

LABORATORY STUDIES

Not needed when the clinical picture is clear. If you are considering lupus or sarcoid, an antinuclear antibody (ANA), chest X-ray, or punch biopsy may be needed.

DIFFERENTIAL DIAGNOSIS

- Acne—The age of onset for rosacea tends to be 30 to 50 years, much later than the onset for acne vulgaris. Comedones are prominent in most cases of acne and generally absent in rosacea (see Chapter 118, Acne Vulgaris).
- Sarcoidosis on the face is much less common than rosacea, but the inflamed plaques can be red and resemble the inflammation of rosacea (see Chapter 184, Sarcoidosis).
- Seborrheic dermatitis tends to produce scale, whereas rosacea does not. Although both cause central facial erythema, papules and telangiectasias are present in rosacea and are not part of seborrheic dermatitis (see Chapter 157, Seborrheic Dermatitis).

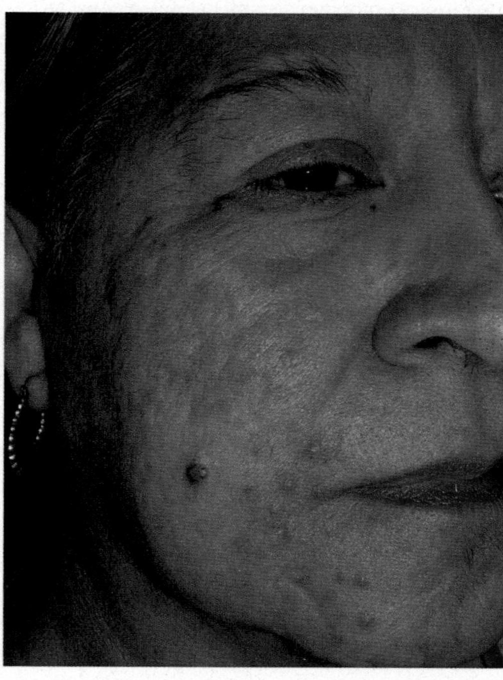

FIGURE 119-9 Papulopustular rosacea in a woman who has a history of recurrent hordeola. (*Reproduced with permission from Richard P. Usatine, MD.*)

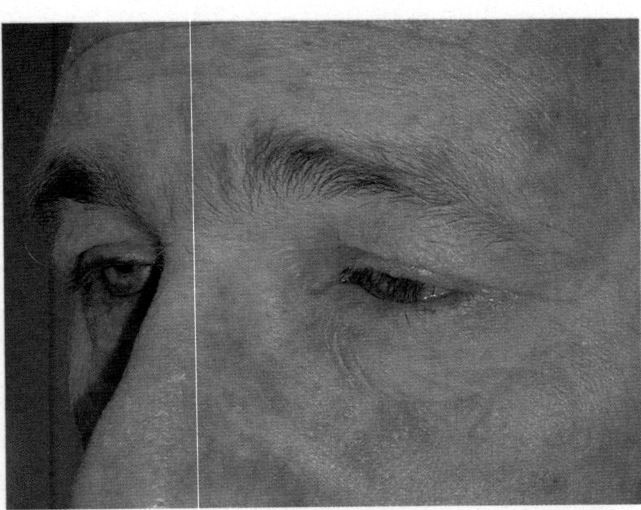

FIGURE 119-10 Ocular rosacea showing blepharitis, conjunctival hyperemia, and telangiectasias of the lid. (*Reproduced with permission from Richard P. Usatine, MD.*)

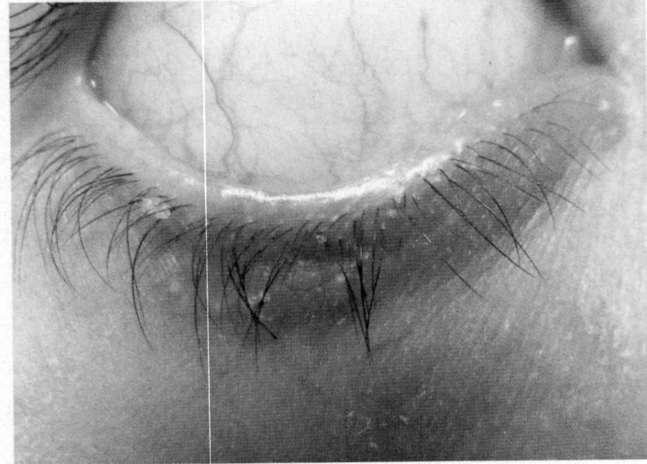

FIGURE 119-11 Ocular rosacea with blepharitis, conjunctivitis, and crusting around the eyelashes. This patient has meibomian gland dysfunction. (*Reproduced with permission from Richard P. Usatine, MD.*)

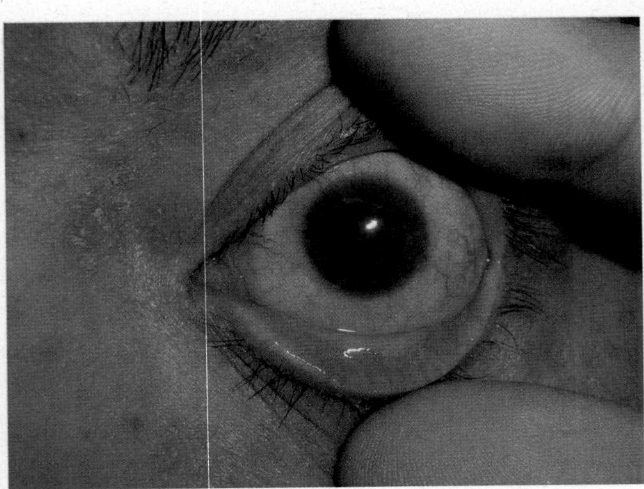

FIGURE 119-12 Severe ocular rosacea in a young woman showing vascularization of the cornea. This type of corneal involvement can lead to blindness. (*Reproduced with permission from Richard P. Usatine, MD.*)

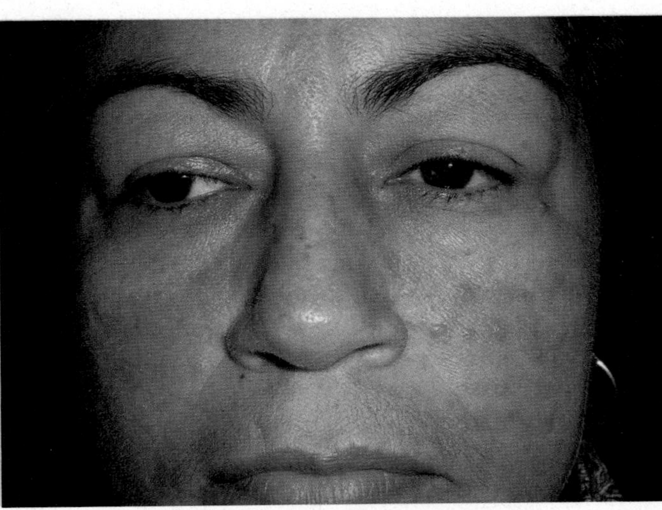

FIGURE 119-13 Rosacea in a young woman with a butterfly pattern. This is not lupus. (*Reproduced with permission from Richard P. Usatine, MD.*)

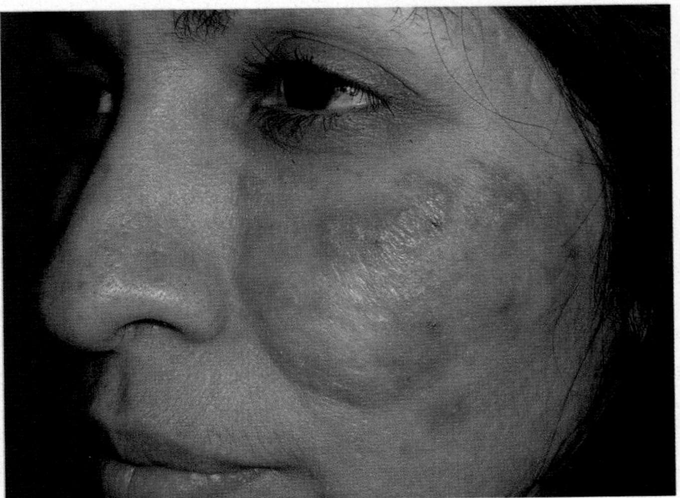

FIGURE 119-14 Rosacea fulminans (known as pyoderma faciale) is characterized by the sudden appearance of papules, pustules, and nodules, along with fluctuating and draining sinuses that may be interconnecting. (*Reproduced with permission from Richard P. Usatine, MD.*)

- Systemic lupus erythematosus (SLE) can be scarring, does not usually produce papules or pustules, and spares the nasolabial folds and nose (see Chapter 188, Lupus—Systemic and Cutaneous). The patient in **Figure 119-13** has a butterfly distribution of her rosacea, but her right nasolabial fold is involved along with her chin.

The following three diagnoses were once considered variants of rosacea, but a recent classification system identified these as separate entities[3]:

- Rosacea fulminans (known as pyoderma faciale) is characterized by the sudden appearance of papules, pustules, and nodules, along with fluctuating and draining sinuses that may be interconnecting. The condition appears primarily in women in their 20s, and intense redness and edema also may be prominent (**Figure 119-14**).[3]
- Steroid-induced acneiform eruption is not a variant of rosacea and can occur as an inflammatory response in any patient during or after chronic corticosteroid use. The same inflammatory response may also occur in patients with rosacea (**Figure 119-15**).
- Perioral dermatitis without rosacea symptoms should not be classified as a variant of rosacea. Perioral dermatitis is characterized by microvesicles, scaling, and peeling around the mouth (**Figure 119-16**).

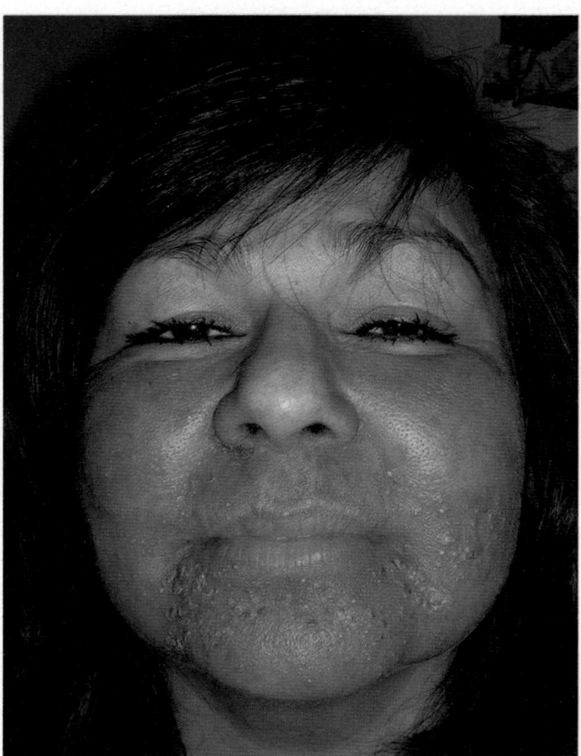

FIGURE 119-15 Steroid-induced acneiform eruption caused by the use of topical fluocinonide daily in this woman who probably had some underlying rosacea. (*Reproduced with permission from Richard P. Usatine, MD.*)

MANAGEMENT

FIRST LINE

- The topical medications that are first line for papulopustular rosacea are azelaic acid, ivermectin, and metronidazole. According to a Cochrane Database systematic review, the highest quality evidence supports azelaic acid applied twice daily as a 15% gel or 20% cream and topical ivermectin 1% cream applied daily.[4] SOR Ⓐ
- The evidence for topical metronidazole (gel or cream—1% or 0.75%) is moderate quality.[4] SOR Ⓑ
- Topical ivermectin 1% cream (Soolantra) has been approved for once-daily application to the inflammatory lesions of acne rosacea. It was developed based on the theory that *Demodex* mite overgrowth is part of the pathophysiology of rosacea, and ivermectin kills mites. It has demonstrated efficacy in patients with moderate to severe papulopustular rosacea.[5] SOR Ⓑ
- In comparative studies, topical ivermectin 1% cream applied once daily appeared to be slightly more effective than metronidazole 0.75% twice daily.[4,6] SOR Ⓑ
- When there are a limited number of papules and pustules, start with topical medication rather than an oral antibiotic.
  - There are no substantial differences between topical metronidazole of 0.75% and 1%, or between once-daily and twice-daily regimens.[7] Metronidazole cream, gel, and lotion have similar efficacies as well.[7]
- Azelaic acid in a 15% gel applied bid appeared to offer some modest benefits over 0.75% metronidazole gel in a manufacturer-sponsored study.[4] Azelaic acid was not as well tolerated, so both medications are reasonable options, with the choice depending on patient preference and tolerance.[4] SOR Ⓑ One study found that once-daily azelaic acid 15% gel was as effective as twice-daily application, which can translate into a significant cost saving.[4]

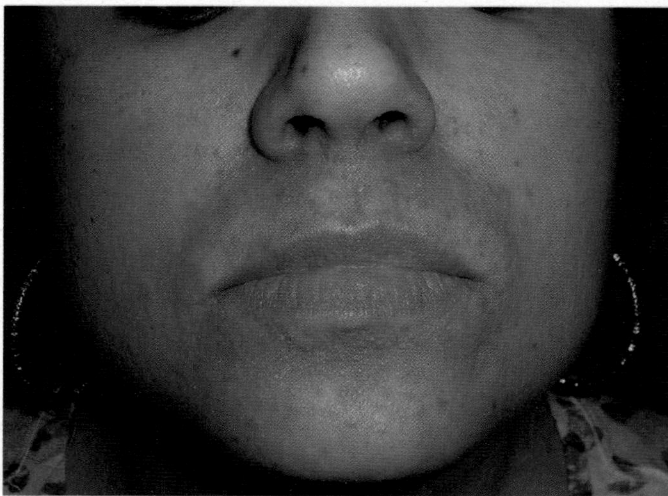

FIGURE 119-16 Perioral (periorificial) dermatitis in a young woman with tiny papules, scaling, and erythema around the mouth and nasal orifices. (*Reproduced with permission from Richard P. Usatine, MD.*)

- Topical brimonidine 0.33% has been FDA approved for persistent facial erythema related to rosacea. It is to be applied once daily. Some cases of transient rebound erythema hours after application have been reported.[8]
- Topical oxymetazoline 1% cream was FDA approved in January 2017 but has been available as OTC Afrin for decades. The studies show modest efficacy for facial erythema.[9]
- If the skin lesions are more extensive, oral antibiotics such as doxycycline (40 mg or 100 mg once to twice daily) are recommended.[4] SOR Ⓐ When attempting to avoid the photosensitivity side effects of doxycycline, it is reasonable to prescribe oral minocycline (50 mg or 100 mg once to twice daily) or oral metronidazole (250 mg to 500 mg daily). SOR Ⓒ
- Oral doxycycline appeared to be significantly more effective than placebo, and there was no statistically significant difference in effectiveness between the 100-mg and 40-mg doses.[4] SOR Ⓐ There is evidence to support the effectiveness of topical metronidazole (0.75% or 1%) or azelaic acid (15% or 20%) for the treatment of moderate to severe rosacea.[4] SOR Ⓐ
- Patients who are started on oral antibiotics alone and improve may be switched to topical agents such as metronidazole or azelaic acid for maintenance.

SECOND LINE

- Severe papulopustular disease refractory to antibiotics and topical treatments can be treated with oral isotretinoin at a low dose of 0.3 mg/kg per day.[10] SOR Ⓑ
- Before topical ivermectin was available, one study found permethrin 5% cream to be as effective as metronidazole 0.75% gel and superior to placebo in the treatment of rosacea.[11] SOR Ⓑ
- Simple electrosurgery or light-based therapies without anesthesia can be used to treat the telangiectasias associated with rosacea. SOR Ⓒ
- Rhinophyma can be excised with radiofrequency electrosurgery or laser. Isotretinoin is also used to treat rhinophyma.[10] SOR Ⓑ

Ocular rosacea:

- Traditional therapies for mild ocular rosacea include oral tetracyclines, lid hygiene, and warm compresses.[4] SOR Ⓒ
- Consider oral doxycycline 100 mg once to twice daily for ocular rosacea not responding to local measures.[4,12] In a prospective trial of oral doxycycline 100 mg daily for 12 weeks, signs and symptoms of ocular rosacea improved.[11] SOR Ⓑ
- Topical ophthalmic cyclosporine 0.05% (Restasis) is more effective than artificial tears for the treatment of rosacea-associated lid and corneal changes.[13] SOR Ⓑ
- Cyclosporine ophthalmic emulsion was significantly more effective than artificial tears for treating ocular rosacea (for all outcomes).[4] SOR Ⓐ
- Ocular rosacea that involves the cornea should be immediately referred to an ophthalmologist to prevent blindness (see **Figure 119-12**).

FOLLOW-UP

Follow-up can be in 1 to 3 months as needed.

PATIENT EDUCATION

Sun protection, including use of a hat and daily application of sunscreen, and gentle skin care should be emphasized. Choose a sunscreen that is nonirritating and protects against UVA and UVB rays. Advise patients to keep a diary to identify and avoid precipitating factors such as hot and humid weather, alcohol, hot beverages, spicy foods, medications, and large, hot meals.

PATIENT RESOURCES

- National Rosacea Society. Its mission is to improve the lives of people with rosacea by raising awareness, providing public health information, and supporting medical research—**http://www.rosacea.org.**

PROVIDER RESOURCES

- The National Rosacea Society also has an excellent set of materials that are geared for physicians—**http://www.rosacea.org.**
- Standard classification and pathophysiology of rosacea: The 2017 update by the National Rosacea Society Expert Committee—**http://www.jaad.org/article/S0190-9622(17)32297-1/fulltext.**

REFERENCES

1. Gallo RL, Granstein RD, Kang S, et al. Standard classification and pathophysiology of rosacea: The 2017 update by the National Rosacea Society Expert Committee. *J Am Acad Dermatol.* 2018; 78(1):148-55.
2. Zhao YE, Wu LP, Peng Y, Cheng H. Retrospective analysis of the association between *Demodex* infestation and rosacea. *Arch Dermatol.* 2010;146:896-902.
3. Wilkin J, Dahl M, Detmar M, et al. Standard classification of rosacea: report of the National Rosacea Society Expert Committee on the Classification and Staging of Rosacea. *J Am Acad Dermatol.* 2002;46:584-7.
4. Van Zuuren EJ, Fedorowicz Z, Carter B, et al. Interventions for rosacea. *Cochrane Database Syst Rev.* 2015;(4):CD003262.
5. Stein L, Kircik L, Flowler J, et al. Efficacy and safety of ivermectin 1% cream in treatment of papulopustular rosacea: results of two randomized, double blind, vehicle-controlled pivotal studies. *J Drugs Dermatol.* 2014;13(3):316-23.
6. Taieb A, Khemis A, Ruzicka T, et al. Maintenance of remission following successful treatment of papulopustular rosacea with ivermectin 1% cream vs. metronidazole 0.75% cream; 36 extension of the ATTRACT randomized study. *J Eur Acad Dermatol Venereol.* 2016;30(5):829-36.
7. Yoo J, Reid DC, Kimball AB. Metronidazole in the treatment of rosacea: do formulation, dosing, and concentration matter? *J Drugs Dermatol.* 2006;5:317-9.
8. Ilkovitch D, Pomerantz RG. Brimonidine effective but may lead to significant rebound erythema. *J Am Acad Dermatol.* 2014;70(5): e109-10.

9. Patel NU, Shukla S, Zaki J, Feldman SR. Oxymetazoline hydrochloride cream for facial erythema associated with rosacea. *Expert Rev Clin Pharmacol.* 2017;10(10):1049-54.
10. Gollnick H, Blume-Peytavi U, Szabo EL, et al. Systemic isotretinoin in the treatment of rosacea doxycycline- and placebo-controlled, randomized clinical study. *J Dtsch Dermatol Ges.* 2010;8:505-15.
11. Kocak M, Yagli S, Vahapoglu G, Eksioglu M. Permethrin 5% cream versus metronidazole 0.75% gel for the treatment of papulopustular rosacea. A randomized double-blind placebo-controlled study. *Dermatology.* 2002;205:265-70.
12. Quarterman MJ, Johnson DW, Abele DC, et al. Ocular rosacea. Signs, symptoms, and tear studies before and after treatment with doxycycline. *Arch Dermatol.* 1997;133(1):49-54.
13. Schechter BA, Katz RS, Friedman LS. Efficacy of topical cyclosporine for the treatment of ocular rosacea. *Adv Ther.* 2009;26:651-9.

120 PSEUDOFOLLICULITIS AND ACNE KELOIDALIS NUCHAE

E.J. Mayeaux, Jr., MD

PATIENT STORY

A young African-American man comes to the office because he has been bothered by the uncomfortable bumps on the back of his neck and lower scalp (**Figure 120-1**). He likes to wear his hair short but notices that every times he shaves his scalp, the bumps on his scalp get irritated. He is diagnosed with acne keloidalis nuchae. It was suggested that he minimize shaving the scalp and let the hair grow out a bit longer. Additional treatment consisted of 0.025% tretinoin cream and 0.1% triamcinolone cream once to twice daily to the involved area.

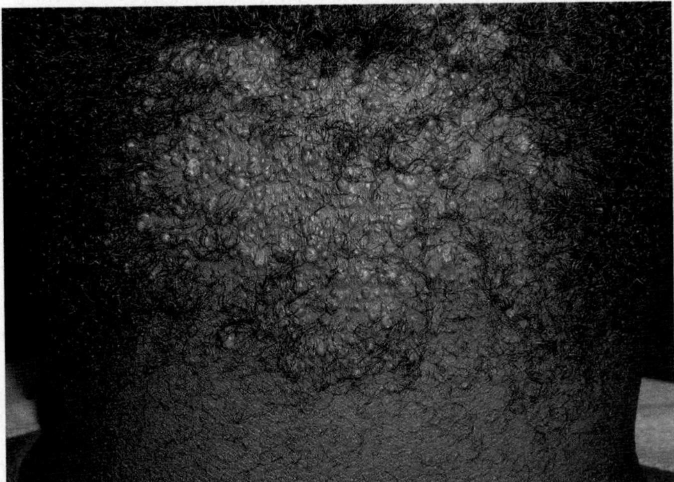

FIGURE 120-1 Acne keloidalis nuchae in a young African-American man. He likes to wear his hair short but notices that every times he shaves his scalp, the bumps on his scalp get irritated. (*Reproduced with permission from Richard P. Usatine, MD.*)

INTRODUCTION

Pseudofolliculitis is a common skin condition affecting the hair-bearing areas of the body that are shaved (**Figures 120-2** to **120-4**). Potential complications include postinflammatory hyperpigmentation, bacterial superinfection, and keloid formation. Acne keloidalis is a chronic disorder involving inflammation and scarring of hair follicles with development of keloid-like papules and plaques with scarring alopecia.

SYNONYMS

- Pseudofolliculitis—Razor bumps, shave bumps, ingrown hairs.
- Acne keloidalis nuchae—Folliculitis keloidalis, sycosis framboesiformis, dermatitis papillaris capillitii.

EPIDEMIOLOGY

- Pseudofolliculitis is most common in black men, with 45% to 83% of black men and 3% of white men who shave their facial hair developing pseudofolliculitis barbae.[1,2] In the beard area it is called *pseudofolliculitis barbae*, and when it occurs after pubic hair is shaved, it is referred to as *pseudofolliculitis pubis*. It may also occur in any hair-bearing area.[2]
- Acne keloidalis nuchae occurs most often in black men but can be seen in all ethnicities (**Figures 120-1**, **120-5**, and **120-6**). The lesions are often painful and cosmetically disfiguring.
- Both conditions are seen in women, but far less often than in men (**Figure 120-7**).

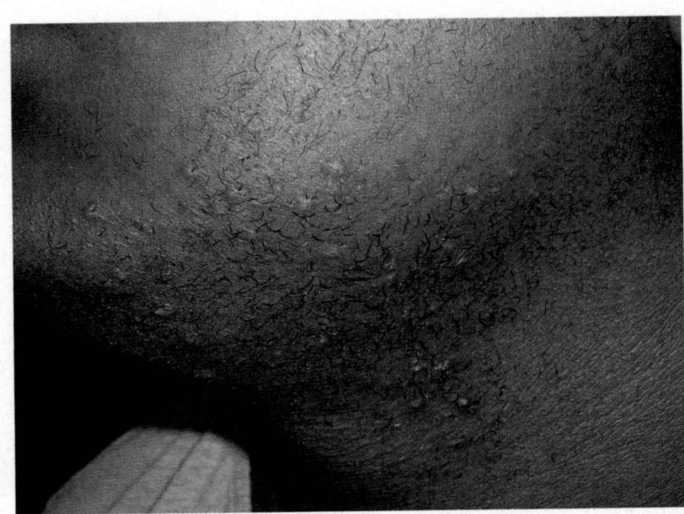

FIGURE 120-2 Pseudofolliculitis barbae along the jawline and neck in a young man. (*Reproduced with permission from Richard P. Usatine, MD.*)

ETIOLOGY AND PATHOPHYSIOLOGY

- Pseudofolliculitis develops when, after shaving, the free end of tightly coiled hair reenters the skin, causing a foreign-body–like

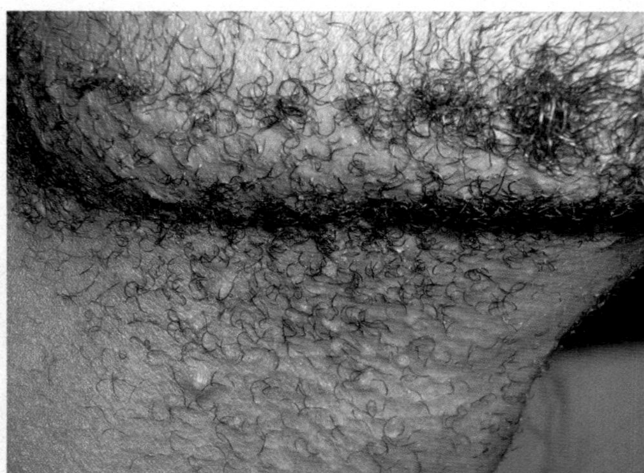

FIGURE 120-3 Pseudofolliculitis barbae in a Latin American man. Note the active pustules on the neck. *(Reproduced with permission from Richard P. Usatine, MD.)*

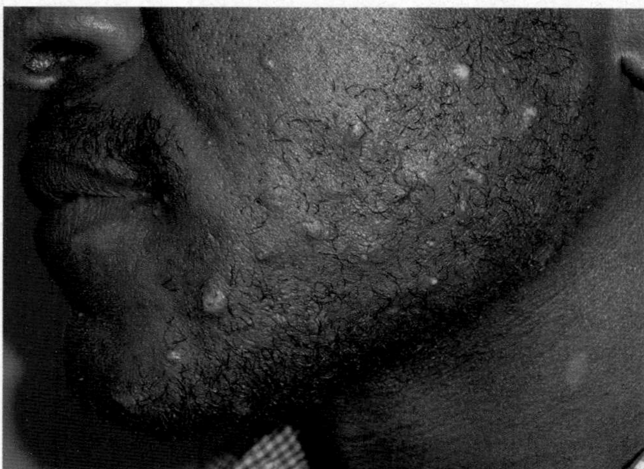

FIGURE 120-4 Pseudofolliculitis barbae on the face of a 28-year-old African man who works providing aid to Darfur refugees. The painful nodules become worse every time he shaves. *(Reproduced with permission from Richard P. Usatine, MD.)*

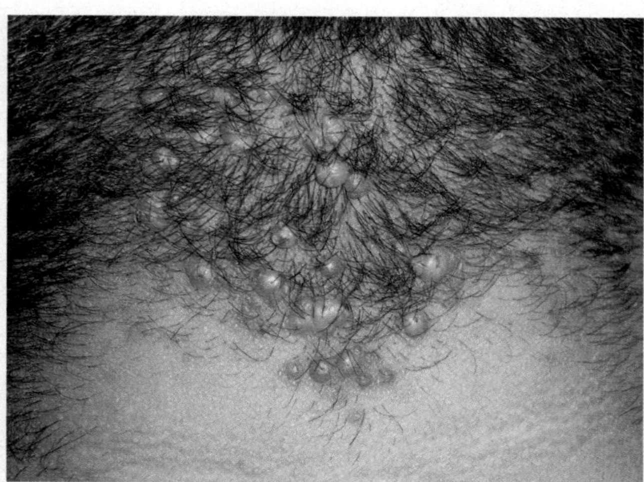

FIGURE 120-5 Acne keloidalis with multiple firm keloidal papules in a Hispanic man who prefers to keep his hair short. *(Reproduced with permission from Richard P. Usatine, MD.)*

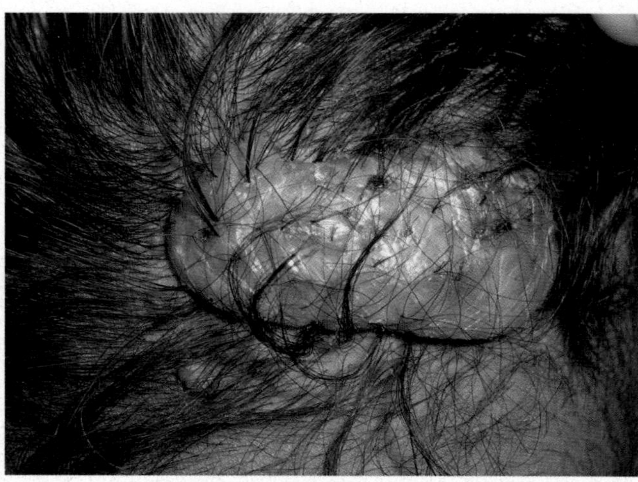

FIGURE 120-6 Acne keloidalis nuchae with large keloidal mass in a Hispanic man. Note that multiple hairs can be seen growing from single follicles (hair tufts). Surgery is the only treatment that can remove this keloidal mass. *(Reproduced with permission from Richard P. Usatine, MD.)*

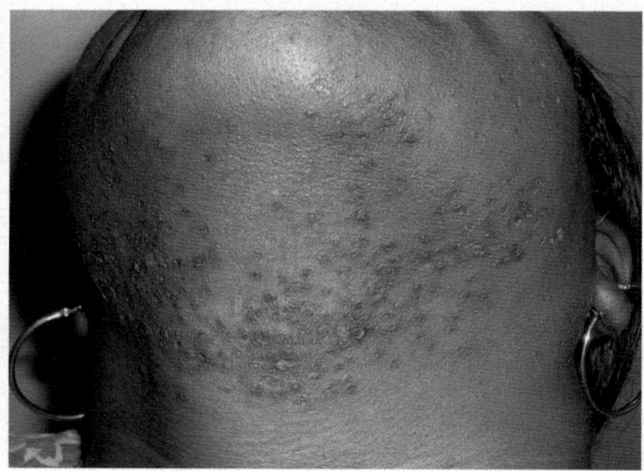

FIGURE 120-7 Pseudofolliculitis barbae in a black woman with hirsutism. The scarring is related to plucking and shaving the hairs on the neck. *(Reproduced with permission from Richard P. Usatine, MD.)*

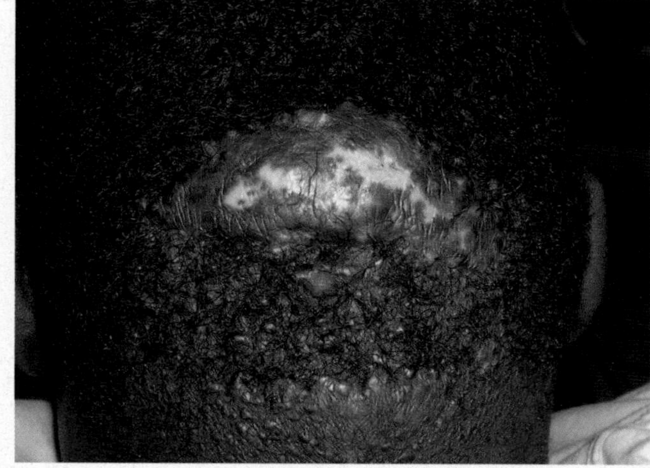

FIGURE 120-8 Acne keloidalis nuchae after injection with intralesional triamcinolone. Although the keloid is smaller and softer, some hypopigmentation has occurred. *(Reproduced with permission from Richard P. Usatine, MD.)*

inflammatory reaction. Shaving produces a sharp free end below the skin surface. Tightly curled hair has a greater tendency for the tip to pierce the side of the follicle and form ingrown hairs. This explains the relative predominance of this condition in patients of African ethnicity. The hair eventually forms a loop, and if the embedded tip is pulled out, there may be spontaneous resolution of symptoms. Another mechanism involves the distal end of a hair curving back into the interfollicular skin after it has already exited the follicular orifice.[2] Although shaving is most commonly associated with pseudofolliculitis barbae, other hair removal techniques may result in this condition.[2]

- The exact cause of acne keloidalis is uncertain. It often develops in areas of pseudofolliculitis or folliculitis. It may be associated with haircuts where the posterior hairline is shaved with a razor and with tightly curved hair shafts. Other possible etiologies include irritation from shirt collars, sporting equipment, chronic bacterial infections, and an autoimmune process. It is a form of primary scarring alopecia.[3] As such, multiple hairs can be seen growing from single follicle (hair tufts) in the midst of the keloidal scarring (see **Figure 120-6**).

RISK FACTORS

- Pseudofolliculitis:
  - African ethnicity
  - Curly hair
- Acne keloidalis nuchae:
  - Shaving the hair on the neck
  - Pseudofolliculitis

DIAGNOSIS

CLINICAL FEATURES

- The diagnosis of pseudofolliculitis is based on clinical appearance. A piece of hair often may be identified protruding from a lesion. Inflammation results in the formation of firm, skin-colored, erythematous or hyperpigmented papules that occur after shaving (see **Figures 120-2 to 120-4**). The lesions are often pruritic. Pustules may develop secondarily. The severity varies from a few papules or pustules to hundreds of lesions.
- Patients with acne keloidalis initially develop a folliculitis or pseudofolliculitis, which heals with keloid-like lesions, sometimes with discharging sinuses. It starts after puberty as 2- to 4-mm firm, follicular papules (see **Figure 120-2**). More papules appear and enlarge over time (see **Figure 120-5**). Papules may coalesce to form keloid-like plaques, which are usually arranged in a bandlike distribution along the posterior part of the hairline (see **Figures 120-6** and **120-8**).

TYPICAL DISTRIBUTION

- Pseudofolliculitis affects the hair-bearing areas of the body that are shaved, especially the face, neck, and pubic area (see **Figures 120-2 to 120-4**).
- Acne keloidalis occurs on the occipital scalp and the posterior part of the neck (see **Figures 120-1**, **120-5**, and **120-6**).

BIOPSY

- Histologic evaluation of a biopsy may confirm either diagnosis but is usually not necessary.

DIFFERENTIAL DIAGNOSIS

- True folliculitis, which is an acute pustular infection of a hair follicle with more localized inflammation (see Chapter 123, Folliculitis).
- Impetigo, which presents with yellowish pustules or bullae that rupture and develop honey crusts, sometimes with adenopathy (see Chapter 122, Impetigo).
- Acne vulgaris, which presents with comedones and pustules usually including the forehead (see Chapter 118, Acne Vulgaris).
- Tinea barbae, which is a dermatophyte infection, involves the beard area. Patients may present with pustules, papules, nodules, or scaly erythematous plaques.

MANAGEMENT

NONPHARMACOLOGIC

- Avoid close shaving, avoid all shaving, or permanently remove hair.[4] Some occupations, however, such as the military and law enforcement, require facial shaving. Occasionally, a doctor's note will allow these men to go without shaving. In mild cases, shaving should be discontinued for a month. The beard can be coarsely trimmed with scissors or electric clippers during this time.
- Shaving should not resume until all inflammatory lesions have resolved. Use generous amounts of a highly lubricating shaving cream or gel prior to shaving, use a single-blade razor rather than a multiple-bladed razor, and shave only in the direction of hair growth. Specialized razors that use a guard system to prevent a very close shave (e.g., Bump Fighter razor) may also be helpful. Avoid stretching the skin during shaving.
- Warm Burow solution compresses may be applied to the lesions for 10 minutes, 2 times per day. Instruct the patient to search for ingrown hairs each day using a magnifying mirror and release them gently using a sterilized needle or tweezers. The hairs should not be plucked, as this may cause recurrence of symptoms with hair regrowth (see **Figure 120-7**). SOR Ⓒ
- Chemical depilatories (Nair, VEET, Magic Shave, and others) cause fewer symptoms than shaving.[5] SOR Ⓑ However, these creams can cause severe irritation, so testing a small amount on the forearm is important. They work by breaking the disulfide bonds in hair, which results in the hair being bluntly broken at the follicular opening instead of sharply cut below the surface. They should be used every second or third day to avoid skin irritation, although this can be controlled with hydrocortisone cream. Calcium thioglycolate preparations are left on 10 to 15 minutes, but the fragrances can cause an allergic reaction, and chemical burns can result if it is left for too long.
- People who have acne keloidalis nuchae should avoid anything that causes folliculitis or pseudofolliculitis, such as getting their neck or

hairline shaved with a razor or irritation from tight-fitting hats, helmets, or high-collared shirts.

MEDICATIONS

- Topical eflornithine HCl 13.9% cream (Vaniqa) may be used to inhibit hair growth. It decreases the rate of hair growth and may make the hair finer and lighter. Unfortunately, this medication is expensive and requires daily application for continued efficacy. SOR C
- Twice-daily treatment with a mid-potency corticosteroid may be sufficient to shrink pseudofolliculitis lesions and relieve symptoms (see Chapter 112: Topical and Intralesional Corticosteroids). SOR C
- When pustules, crust formation, or drainage is present, use topical clindamycin or erythromycin. Unresponsive patients may be changed to a systemic antibiotic. SOR C
- Topical erythromycin, clindamycin, or combination clindamycin–benzoyl peroxide or erythromycin–benzoyl peroxide may be used once or twice daily.[6] SOR B
- Oral doxycycline 100 mg bid or erythromycin 500 mg bid may be used for patients with more severe secondary inflammation. SOR C
- Tretinoin cream, 0.025%, may be useful in patients with mild acne keloidalis, but is rarely helpful in moderate to severe cases.[7] It is applied nightly for a week, then reduced to every second or third night. Tretinoin may be used in conjunction with a mid-potency topical corticosteroid applied each morning. The mechanism of action is thought to be by relieving hyperkeratosis and "toughening" the skin. Topical combination cream (tretinoin 0.05%, fluocinolone acetonide 0.01%, and hydroquinone 4%) (Tri-Luma) adds an additional postinflammatory hyperpigmentation treatment. SOR C
- For mild acne keloidalis, high-potency topical corticosteroids may be effective for small inflammatory papules. Intralesional steroid injections (2.5 to 20 mg/mL) may be used to soften and shrink inflamed scars. Warn patients that this therapy may cause hypopigmentation (see **Figure 120-8**). SOR C Topical antibiotics should be started when signs of infection are present.

SURGICAL

- The only definitive cure for pseudofolliculitis is permanent hair removal. Electrolysis is expensive, painful, and sometimes unsuccessful. Laser hair removal is fairly successful for treating pseudofolliculitis.[8] SOR B Diode laser (810 nm) treatments have been proven safe and effective in patients with skin phototypes I to IV.[9]
- Excision of acne keloidalis lesions may be attempted. Recalcitrant keloidal lesions may be treated with removing individual papules with a small punch, or large keloids (see **Figure 120-9**) with an elliptical excision closed with sutures. After removal, the wound edges should be injected with a mixture of equal amount of triamcinolone acetonide 40 mg/mL and sterile saline. Remove the sutures in 1 to 2 weeks and inject the edges every month with the above mixture for 3 to 4 months. SOR C Excision should extend into the subcutaneous tissue, and the wound edges can be injected with 10 to 40 mg/mL of triamcinolone acetonide and be reapproximated. SOR C Recurrence is common, especially with shallow excisions or not treating with steroids.

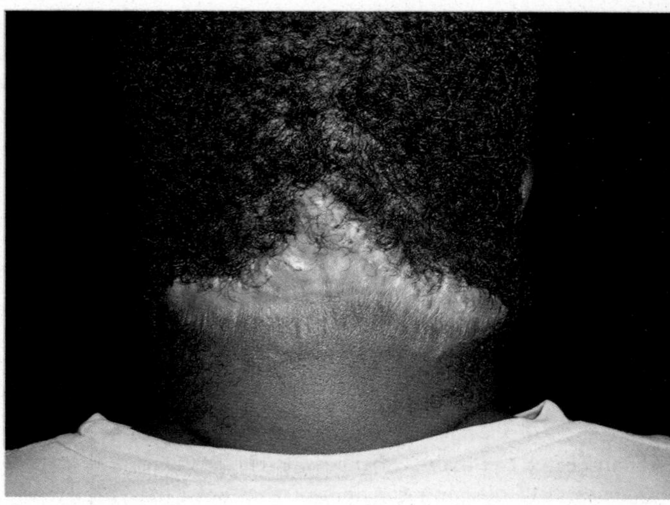

FIGURE 120-9 Hypertrophic scarring after the excision of acne keloidalis nuchae. (*Reproduced with permission from Richard P. Usatine, MD.*)

- Other therapies that may be considered are laser therapy (carbon dioxide or Nd:YAG [neodymium:yttrium-aluminum-garnet]) followed by intralesional triamcinolone injections or cryotherapy for two 20-second bursts that are allowed to thaw and are then applied again a minute later. These methods may produce more pain and hypopigmentation. SOR Ⓒ

PREVENTION

- Termination of shaving may prevent the development of new lesions of pseudofolliculitis.

PROGNOSIS

- No specific cure exists. If the patient is able to stop shaving, the problem usually lessens or disappears (except for any scar formation).

FOLLOW-UP

- Instruct patients to return if any complications occur. Otherwise have them return for possible initiation of intralesional steroid injections or topical steroid/retinoic acid therapy once the area has healed.

PATIENT EDUCATION

- For those who must shave, have the patient clip hairs no shorter than needed for maintenance. Use fine scissors or facial hair clippers if possible. When shaving, have the patient rinse with warm tap water for several minutes, use generous amounts of a highly lubricating shaving gel, and allow it to soften the skin for 5 to 10 minutes before shaving. The patient should always use sharp razors and shave in the direction of hair growth. Specialized guarded razors (e.g., PFB Bump Fighter) are available in pharmacies and by mail order. After shaving, rinse the face with tap water, and then apply cold water compresses.
- With acne keloidalis, instruct males who play football to make sure their helmets fit properly and do not cause irritation on the posterior part of the scalp. They should avoid having the posterior part of the hairline shaved with a razor as part of a haircut, and discontinue wearing garments that rub or irritate the posterior parts of the scalp and the neck.

PATIENT RESOURCES

- American Osteopathic College of Dermatology. *Pseudofolliculitis Barbae*—**http://aocd.org/skin/dermatologic_diseases/pseudofolliculitis.html.**
- DermNet NZ. *Folliculitis barbae and pseudofolliculitis barbae.* **https://www.dermnetnz.org/topics/folliculitis-barbae?utm_source=TrendMD&utm_medium=cpc&utm_campaign=DermNet_NZ_TrendMD_0**

PROVIDER RESOURCES

- eMedicine. *Pseudofolliculitis of the Beard*—**http://emedicine.medscape.com/article/1071251.**
- eMedicine. *Acne Keloidalis Nuchae*—**http://emedicine.medscape.com/article/1072149.**
- DermNet NZ. *Folliculitis Keloidalis*—**http://dermnetnz.org/acne/keloid-acne.html.**
- DermNet NZ. *Folliculitis Barbae and Pseudofolliculitis Barbae*—**http://www.dermnetnz.org/topics/folliculitis-barbae/.**

REFERENCES

1. Coquilla BH, Lewis CW. Management of pseudofolliculitis barbae. *Mil Med.* 1995;160(5):263-269.
2. Perry PK, Cook-Bolden FE, Rahman Z, et al. Defining pseudofolliculitis barbae in 2001: a review of the literature and current trends. *J Am Acad Dermatol.* 2002;46:S113.
3. Sperling LC, Homoky C, Pratt L, Sau P. Acne keloidalis is a form of primary scarring alopecia. *Arch Dermatol.* 2000;136(4):479-484.
4. Chui CT, Berger TG, Price VH, Zachary CB. Recalcitrant scarring follicular disorders treated by laser-assisted hair removal: a preliminary report. *Dermatol Surg.* 1999;25(1):34-37.
5. Hage JJ, Bowman FG. Surgical depilation for the treatment of pseudofolliculitis or local hirsutism of the face: experience in the first 40 patients. *Plast Reconstr Surg.* 1991;88:446-451.
6. Cook-Bolden FE, Barba A, Halder R, Taylor S. Twice-daily applications of benzoyl peroxide 5% clindamycin 1% gel versus vehicle in the treatment of pseudofolliculitis barbae. *Cutis.* 2004;73(6 Suppl):18-24.
7. Brown LA Jr. Pathogenesis and treatment of pseudofolliculitis barbae. *Cutis.* 1983;32(4):373-375.
8. Ross EV, Cooke LM, Timko AL, et al. Treatment of pseudofolliculitis barbae in skin types IV, V, and VI with a long-pulsed neodymium: yttrium aluminum garnet laser. *J Am Acad Dermatol.* 2002;47(2): 263-270.
9. Kauvar AN. Treatment of pseudofolliculitis with a pulsed infrared laser. *Arch Dermatol.* 2000;136(11):1343-1346.

121 HIDRADENITIS SUPPURATIVA

Richard P. Usatine, MD
Daniel Wallis, MD
Vineet Mishra, MD

PATIENT STORY

A 25-year-old woman presents with new tender lesions in her axilla (**Figure 121-1**). She admits to years of similar outbreaks in both axillae and occasional painful bumps in the groin. She states that it is painful to have them opened and just wants to get some relief without surgery. We elected to inject the nodules with triamcinolone and start the patient on doxycycline 100 mg twice daily. Smoking cessation was emphasized, and the patient agreed to start on a nicotine patch that evening. She had relief within 24 hours from the steroid injection.

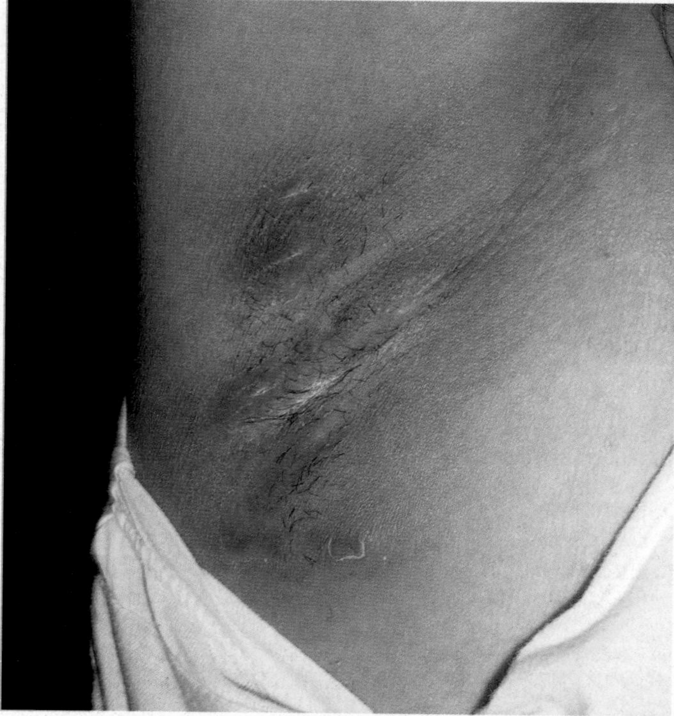

FIGURE 121-1 Mild hidradenitis suppurativa in the axilla of a young woman. She has a history of recurrent lesions in her axilla. *(Reproduced with permission from Richard P. Usatine, MD.)*

INTRODUCTION

Hidradenitis suppurativa (HS) is an inflammatory disease of the pilosebaceous unit in the apocrine gland-bearing skin, specifically the terminal hair. HS is most common in the axilla and inguinal area, but may be found in the inframammary, buttock, and perianal areas as well. It produces painful inflammatory nodules, cysts, and sinus tracts with mucopurulent discharge and progressive scarring. The disease can severely impact quality of life due to pain, odoriferous drainage, and complications such as large abscesses and fistulas.[1]

SYNONYMS

It is called acne inversa because it involves intertriginous areas and not the regions affected by acne (similar to inverse psoriasis).

EPIDEMIOLOGY

- Occurs after puberty in approximately 1% of the population.[2]
- Incidence is higher in females, in the range of 4:1 to 5:1. Flare-ups may be associated with menses.[2]

ETIOLOGY AND PATHOPHYSIOLOGY

- Disorder of the terminal follicular epithelium in the apocrine gland-bearing skin.[2]
- Starts with occlusion of hair follicles via hyperkeratosis that leads to occlusion of surrounding apocrine glands and subsequent rupture of the follicular epithelium, releasing sebum, keratin, hairs, and bacteria into the dermis.[1]
- Chronic relapsing inflammation and secondary bacterial infection with mucopurulent discharge result.

- Can lead to sinus tracts, draining fistulas, progressive scarring, and large abscesses (**Figures 121-2** to **121-7**).

RISK FACTORS

- Obesity, smoking, and tight-fitting clothing.
- Certain autosomal dominant gamma-secretase gene mutations (NCSTN, PSENEN, and PSEN1) have particularly severe and early onset disease.[1]

DIAGNOSIS

CLINICAL FEATURES

- Most common presentation is painful, tender, firm, nodular lesions in axillae (see **Figures 121-1** to **121-3**).
- Nodules may open and drain purulent fluid spontaneously and heal slowly, with or without drainage, over 10 to 30 days.[2]
- Nodules may recur several times yearly, or in severe cases new lesions form as old ones heal.
- Surrounding cellulitis may be present and require systemic antibiotic treatment.
- Chronic recurrences result in thickened sinus tracts, which may become draining fistulas (see **Figures 121-3** to **121-7**).
- HS can cause disabling pain, diminished range of motion, and social isolation (see **Figure 121-5**). It can affect sexual function, especially if the groin areas are involved.
- Although rare, cutaneous malignancy is another possible complication, with squamous cell carcinoma occurring in 3.2% of perineal HS.[3]

TYPICAL DISTRIBUTION

- Axillary, inguinal, periareolar, intermammary zones; pubic area; infraumbilical midline; gluteal folds; top of the anterior thighs; and the perianal region.[2]

LABORATORY STUDIES

Culture of purulence is likely to yield staphylococci and streptococci and is usually unnecessary to determine treatment. Culture may be useful if you suspect methicillin-resistant *Staphylococcus aureus*.

DIFFERENTIAL DIAGNOSIS

- Bacterial infections, including folliculitis, carbuncles, furuncles, abscess, and cellulitis may resemble HS but are less likely to be recurrent in the intertriginous areas.
- Epidermal cysts in the intertriginous regions may resemble HS. Theses cysts contain malodorous keratin contents.
- Granuloma inguinale and lymphogranuloma venereum are sexually transmitted infections that can produce inguinal ulcers and adenopathy that could be mistaken for HS.

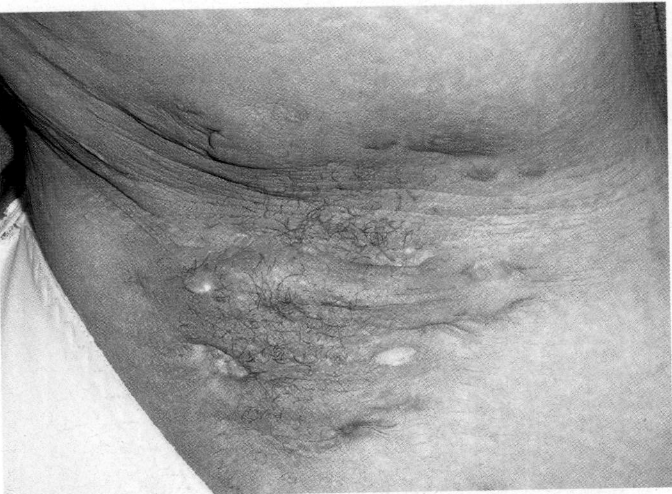

FIGURE 121-2 Moderate HS in a young woman. The lesions are deeper, and there have been some chronic changes with scarring and fibrosis from previous lesions. (*Reproduced with permission from Richard P. Usatine, MD.*)

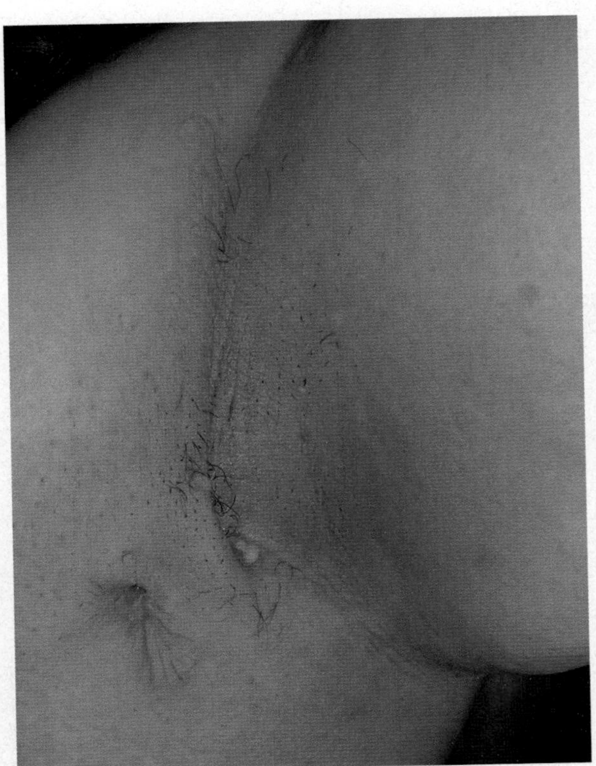

FIGURE 121-3 A 33-year-old Hispanic woman with sinus tracts, draining fistulas, and scarring secondary to her chronic HS. Note the mucopurulent discharge. (*Reproduced with permission from Richard P. Usatine, MD.*)

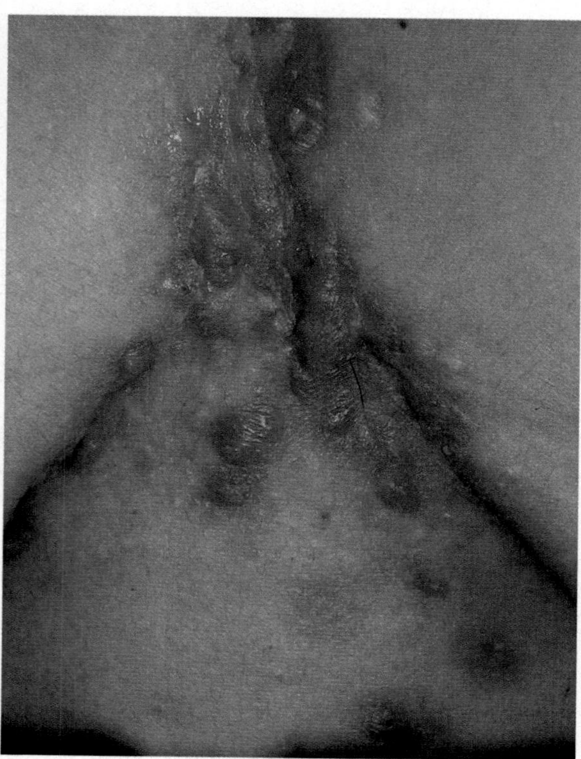

FIGURE 121-4 Long-standing painful severe HS between the breasts of a 45-year-old woman. (*Reproduced with permission from Richard P. Usatine, MD.*)

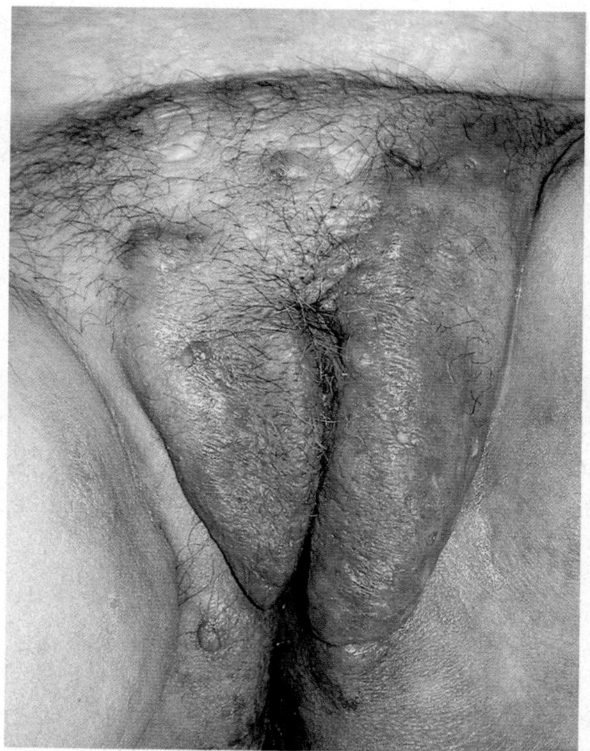

FIGURE 121-6 Severe HS in the vulva and on the mons pubis. The skin is thickened and hyperpigmented from the ongoing inflammatory lesions present in the area. (*Reproduced with permission from Suraj Reddy, MD.*)

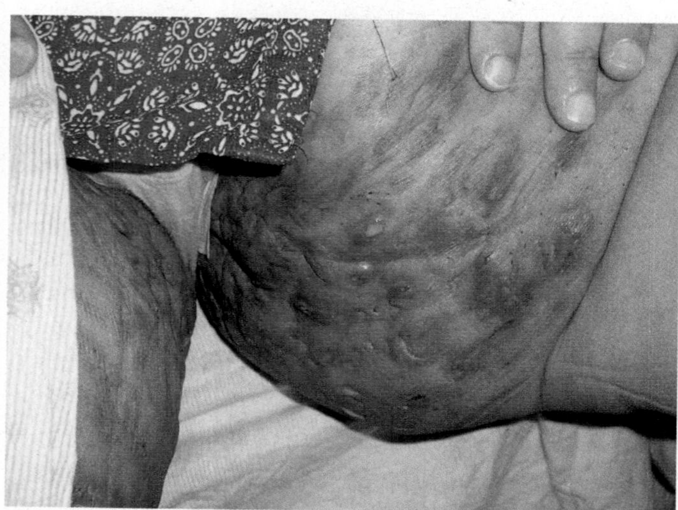

FIGURE 121-5 Severe hidradenitis in the groin and upper thighs of a woman suffering from obesity. This makes it painful to walk. (*Reproduced with permission from Richard P. Usatine, MD.*)

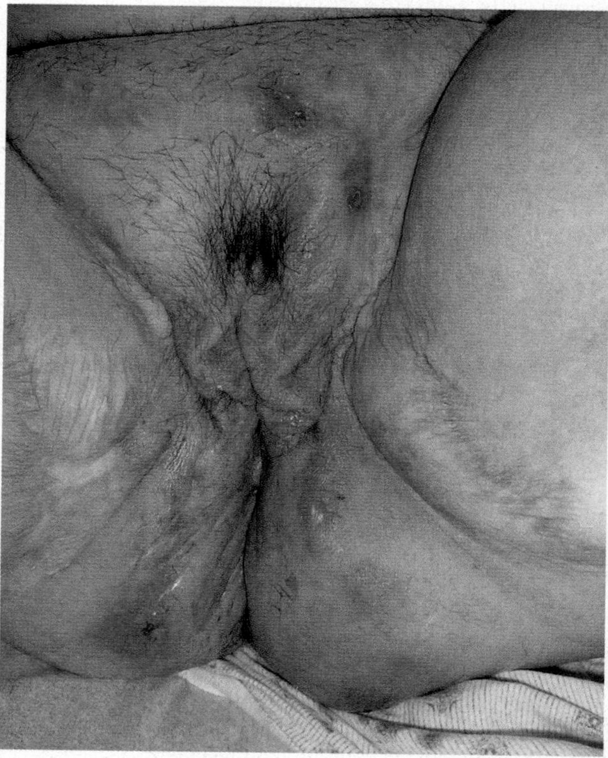

FIGURE 121-7 Thirty-year history of severe hidradenitis in a 54-year-old woman. Note the scars from previous plastic surgeries. Note the draining cysts, fistulas, and the acute abscess on her right buttock. (*Reproduced with permission from Richard P. Usatine, MD.*)

MANAGEMENT

FIRST LINE

- Lifestyle changes are recommended, including weight loss if obesity is present. SOR C
  - Smoking is a risk factor for HS and cessation is highly recommended for many reasons.[2] See SOR B for HS and SOR A for other health reasons.
- Frequent bathing, dilute bleach baths, and wearing loose-fitting clothing may help.

First-line medical treatments include:

- Oral antibiotics are used in acute and chronic treatment. Oral tetracyclines, clindamycin, rifampin, ofloxacin, and dapsone have been touted as beneficial. If methicillin-resistant *S. aureus* is present, trimethoprim/sulfamethoxazole or clindamycin should be used.
- Tetracycline 500 mg bid and doxycycline 100 mg bid can be used acutely and to prevent new lesions in the mildest of cases. Many patients do not find these antibiotics to be of great help. In one small randomized controlled trial (RCT), oral tetracycline showed statistically significant improvement in participants' global assessment when compared with topical clindamycin; however, this RCT was limited by attrition bias.[4] SOR C
- Topical clindamycin bid may be helpful in the mildest of cases; however, in one trial of 30 patients, topical clindamycin did not show a statistically significant benefit when compared to placebo.[4] SOR C
- Combination of systemic clindamycin (300 mg twice daily) and rifampin (600 mg daily) is recommended for patients with more severe HS.[5,6] In a series of 116 patients, parameters of severity improved, as did the quality-of-life score.[5] In another study, 28 of 34 patients (82%) experienced at least partial improvement, and 16 (47%) showed a total remission.[6] The maximum effect of treatment appeared within 10 weeks. Following total remission, 8 of 13 (61.5%) patients experienced a relapse after a mean period of 5 months. Nonresponders were predominantly patients with severe disease. The most frequent side effect is diarrhea.[5,6] SOR C
  - As an alternative to the above regimen, systemic clindamycin (600 mg to 1800 mg/day) can be combined with systemic ofloxacin (200 mg to 400 mg/day).[7] SOR C
- One antitumor necrosis factor (anti-TNF) agent has been FDA approved for HS (**Figure 121-8**). Adalimumab subcutaneously weekly (160 mg at week 0, 80 mg at week 2, and 40 mg at weeks 4–15) improved patients' dermatology life quality index when compared to placebo, but every-other-week dosing was not effective.[8] More recent phase 3 trials have supported weekly adalimumab's effectiveness, and the newest European guidelines suggest it as a first-line agent for patients with moderate to severe disease in whom oral antibiotics are ineffective.[9,10] SOR A
- Oral dapsone may be considered in milder cases. In one study, only 38% of patients experienced improvement.[11] SOR B Rapid recurrence after stopping treatment suggests that anti-inflammatory effects may predominate over antimicrobial effects. The total effect appears to be smaller than that reported with combination therapy using clindamycin and rifampicin. Dapsone causes hemolysis, so requires careful monitoring.

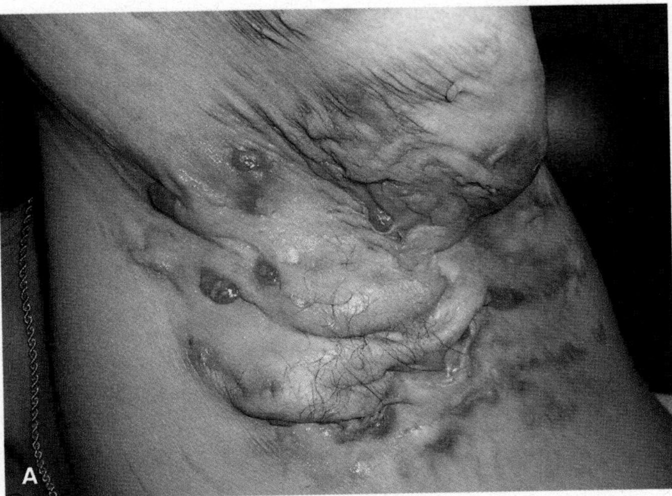

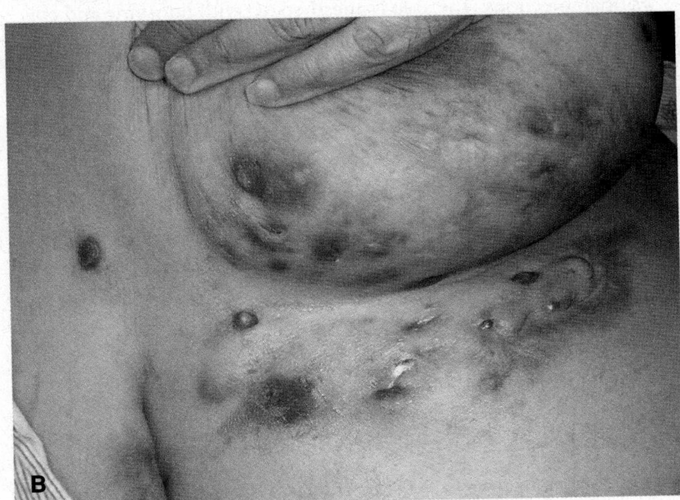

FIGURE 121-8 Severe recalcitrant hidradenitis in this 42-year-old woman with sinus tracts and scarring. **A.** Axillary involvement. **B.** Inframammary involvement. She was started on adalimumab with some benefit. *(Reproduced with permission from Richard P. Usatine, MD.)*

- Intralesional steroids with 5 to 10 mg/mL of triamcinolone may help to decrease inflammation and pain in particularly painful lesions within 24 to 48 hours (**Figure 121-10**).[10] SOR C These can be repeated as often as every month in patients with severe disease who are not getting sufficient relief from all the other treatment modalities.

SECOND LINE (SURGICAL AND MEDICAL)

- Incision and drainage of acute lesions may occasionally be of benefit for the largest fluctuant lesions that can occur in HS. Although this may give some relief of the pressure, the surgical treatment and repacking of the wound is painful. Lancing small nodules is more painful than helpful and is not recommended. Intralesional steroids should be attempted before approaching inflamed lesions with a scalpel. SOR C
- Surgical unroofing (deroofing) is being used more frequently to treat recalcitrant inflammatory lesions and sinus tracts. It can be more effective and long lasting than incision and drainage or intralesional injections. The area is anesthetized with lidocaine and epinephrine, and the lesion is opened with a scalpel. The top of the lesion is cut off with scissors, including any sinus tracts. The gelatinous material below is wiped away with gauze and/or a skin curette. Bleeding can be controlled with chemical hemostasis or electrosurgery. The area is covered with petrolatum and gauze and allowed to heal by second intention. SOR C
- Surgical excision of affected area with or without skin grafting is used for recalcitrant disabling disease and should be individualized based on the stage and location of the disease.[12] SOR B One surgical group has been using a medial thigh lift for immediate defect closure after radical excision of localized inguinal hidradenitis.[13] A primary factor in therapeutic outcome after excision is width of excision.[10] It may be best to decrease the inflammatory disease with systemic medication before the surgery to maximize the results. SOR C
- IPL, Nd:YAG, and neosomal methylene blue gel photodynamic therapy have been studied and have been shown to be of benefit. However, their evidence quality is generally lower due to performance bias and imprecision.[14] Intense pulsed light (IPL) with laser may be worth considering for patients who can afford the cost and time for treatment. In one study of 18 patients who were randomized to treatment of one axilla, groin, or inframammary area with IPL 2 times per week for 4 weeks, there was a significant improvement in the mean examination score, which was maintained at 12 months. Patients reported high levels of satisfaction with the IPL treatment.[12] SOR B
- Isotretinoin can reduce the severity of attacks in some patients, particularly for mild to moderate disease and younger female patients with a history of acne. It is less efficacious in patients with severe HS.[15,16] SOR C
- Acitretin can be an effective treatment for refractory HS. In one study, all 12 patients achieved remission and experienced a significant decrease in pain. Long-lasting improvement was observed in 9 patients, with no recurrence of lesions after 6 months (n = 1), 1 year (n = 3), more than 2 years (n = 2), more than 3 years (n = 2), and more than 4 years (n = 1).[16] SOR B
- Infliximab (biologic anti-TNF agent given by intravenous infusions) has been found helpful for HS (see **Figure 121-8**). In one RCT study of 38 patients, infliximab therapy (weight based) improved pain and physician's global assessment when compared

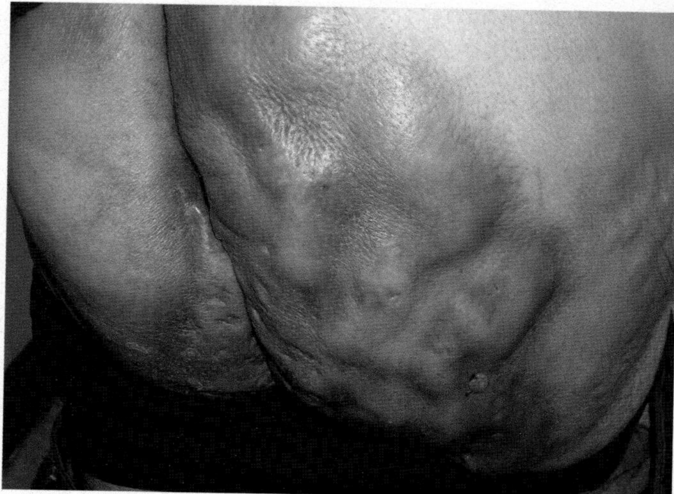

FIGURE 121-9 Severe recalcitrant hidradenitis of the buttocks that makes it painful to sit for this patient. After this photo, regular infliximab infusions and intralesional steroid injections as needed have improved the quality of life for this patient. (*Reproduced with permission from Richard P. Usatine, MD.*)

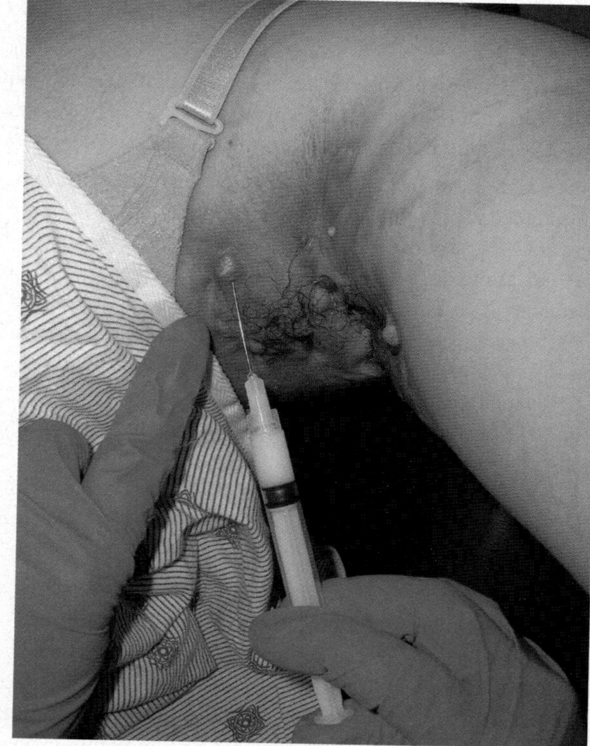

FIGURE 121-10 Intralesional injections using triamcinolone can give rapid relief to patients with painful hidradenitis lesions. (*Reproduced with permission from Richard P. Usatine, MD.*)

to placebo (**Figure 121-9**).[17] SOR B Other literature supports its use in patients with HS who were resistant to previous therapy.[18] This is in agreement with preexisting literature showing that 52 of 60 patients (87%) were improved after infliximab therapy.[18] More recently, infliximab has been shown to be effective long term in the treatment of HS; however, relapse after 8 months is common in patients with severe disease.[19] SOR B While infliximab is used at 5 mg/kg for psoriasis, some experts will use up to 10 mg/kg for HS as often as every 4 weeks. Low-dose weekly methotrexate may then be employed to prevent blocking antibodies and extend the long-term effectiveness of infliximab. SOR C

- Etanercept (another anti-TNF agent) 50 mg SQ twice weekly for 12 weeks was found to have no relative effect vs. placebo in a small RCT of 17 participants.[20]
- Metformin has been shown to improve Hidradenitis Suppurativa Severity Index scores in a group of 25 patients, most of whom were women.[21]
- Hormonal therapy has been used in women in an analogous method for treating acne with anti-androgenic therapy. Spironolactone and estrogen-dominant oral contraceptive pills have been used for HS. SOR C

PAIN MANAGEMENT

- It is important to remember that pain from lesions of HS can significantly affect a patient's quality of life, and thus should be treated (see Appendix B, Chronic Pain). The following pain management strategies are options:
  - Topical analgesics such as ice packs, xylocaine, and diclofenac.
  - Oral analgesics such as acetaminophen and nonsteroidal anti-inflammatory drugs (NSAIDs).
  - For neuropathic pain, gabapentin and low-dose tricyclic antidepressants (TCAs) such as nortriptyline or amitriptyline.
  - Opioids in low doses for breakthrough pain are one option, but should be prescribed with caution given the potential for addiction.[22]

COMPLEMENTARY AND ALTERNATIVE THERAPY

A few small studies have provided limited evidence for the use of over-the-counter (OTC) zinc gluconate in the treatment of mild to moderate HS. In one study using 90 mg per day, there were 8 complete remissions and 14 partial remissions.[23] Since the most common side effect is GI discomfort, it is reasonable to start with low doses of 30 mg daily with food and increase that to 2–3 times a day as tolerated. SOR C

FOLLOW-UP

If there is cellulitis or a large abscess was drained, follow-up should be within days. Chronic relapsing disease can ultimately be managed with appointments every 1 to 6 months depending on the treatment and its success.

PATIENT EDUCATION

Smoking cessation, weight loss if overweight, and avoidance of tight-fitting clothes.

PATIENT RESOURCES

- Patient education materials at MedlinePlus—**http://www.nlm.nih.gov/medlineplus/hidradenitissuppurativa.html.**
- Hidradenitis Suppurativa Foundation—**http://www.hs-foundation.org/**

PROVIDER RESOURCES

- **http://emedicine.medscape.com/article/1073117-overview.**
- Danby FW, Hazen PG, Boer J. New and traditional surgical approaches to hidradenitis suppurativa. *J Am Acad Dermatol.* 2015;73(5 Suppl 1):S62-S65.

REFERENCES

1. James WD, Elston DM, Berger TG. Acne. In: *Andrews Diseases of the Skin: Clinical Dermatology*, 12th ed. Philadelphia, PA: Elsevier; 2016:236-238.
2. Jemec GB, Wendelboe P. Topical clindamycin versus systemic tetracycline in the treatment of hidradenitis suppurativa. *J Am Acad Dermatol.* 1998;39:971-974.
3. Makris GM, Poulakaki N, Papnota AM, et al. Vulvar, perianal and perineal cancer after hidradenitis suppurativa. *Dermatol Surg.* 2017;43(1):107-115.
4. Clemmensen OJ. Topical treatment of hidradenitis suppurativa with clindamycin. *Int J Dermatol.* 1983;22:325-328.
5. Gener G, Canoui-Poitrine F, Revuz JE, et al. Combination therapy with clindamycin and rifampicin for hidradenitis suppurativa: a series of 116 consecutive patients. *Dermatology.* 2009;219:148-154.
6. van der Zee HH, Boer J, Prens EP, Jemec GBE. The effect of combined treatment with oral clindamycin and oral rifampicin in patients with hidradenitis suppurativa. *Dermatology.* 2009;219:143-147.
7. Delaunay J, Villani A, Guillem P, et al. Oral ofloxacin and clindamycin as an alternative to the classic rifampicin/clindamycin in hidradenitis suppurativa: retrospective analysis of 65 patients. *Br J Dermatol.* 2018;178(1):e15-16.
8. Kimball AB, Kerdel F, Adams D, et al. Adalimumab for the treatment of moderate to severe hidradenitis suppurativa: a parallel randomized trial. *Ann Intern Med.* 2012;157:846-855.
9. Kimball AB, Okun MM, Williams DA, et al. Two phase 3 trials of adalimumab for hidradenitis suppurativa. *N Engl J Med.* 2016; 375(5):422-434.
10. Gulliver W, Zouboulis CC, Prens E, et al. Evidence-based approach to the treatment of hidradenitis suppurativa/acne inversa, based on the European guidelines for hidradenitis suppurativa. *Rev Endocr Metab Disord.* 2016;17(3):343-351.
11. Yazdanyar S, Boer J, Ingvarsson G, et al. Dapsone therapy for hidradenitis suppurativa: a series of 24 patients. *Dermatology.* 2011;222(4):342-346.
12. Kagan RJ, Yakuboff KP, Warner P, Warden GD. Surgical treatment of hidradenitis suppurativa: a 10-year experience. *Surgery.* 2005; 138:734-740.

13. Rieger UM, Erba P, Pierer G, Kalbermatten DF. Hidradenitis suppurativa of the groin treated by radical excision and defect closure by medial thigh lift: aesthetic surgery meets reconstructive surgery. *J Plast Reconstr Aesthet Surg*. 2009;62:1355-1360.
14. Ingram JR, Woo PN, Chua SL, et al. Interventions for hidradenitis suppurativa: a Cochrane systemic review incorporating GRADE assessment of evidence quality. *Br J Dermatol*. 2016;174:976-977.
15. Huang CM, Kirchhof MG. A new perspective on isotretinoin treatment of hidradenitis suppurativa: a retrospective chart review of patient outcomes. *Dermatology*. 2017;233(2-3) 120-125.
16. Boer J, Nazary M. Long-term results of acitretin therapy for hidradenitis suppurativa. Is acne inversa also a misnomer? *Br J Dermatol*. 2011;164:170-175.
17. Grant A, Gonzalez T, Montgomery MO, et al. Infliximab therapy for patients with moderate to severe hidradenitis suppurativa: a randomized, double-blind, placebo-controlled crossover trial. *J Am Acad Dermatol*. 2010; 62:205-217.
18. Delage M, Samimi M, Atlan M, et al. Efficacy of infliximab for hidradenitis suppurativa: assessment of clinical and biological inflammatory markers. *Acta Derm Venereol*. 2011;91:169-171.
19. Paradela S, Rodriguez-Lojo R, Fernandez-Torrez R, et al. Long-term efficacy of infliximab in hidradenitis suppurativa. *J Dermatolog Treat*. 2012;23(4):278-283.
20. Adams DR, Yankura JA, Fogelberg AC, Anderson BE. Treatment of hidradenitis suppurativa with etanercept injection. *Arch Dermatol*. 2010;146:501-504.
21. Alhusayen R, Shear NH. Scientific evidence for the use of current traditional systemic therapies in patients with hidradenitis suppurativa. *J Am Acad Dermatol*. 2015;73(5):S42-46.
22. Horvath B, Jance IC, Sibbald GR. Pain management in patients with hidradenitis suppurativa. *J Am Acad Dermatol*. 2015;73(5): S47-51.
23. Brocard A, Knol AC, Khammari A, Dréno B. Hidradenitis suppurativa and zinc: a new therapeutic approach. A pilot study. *Dermatology*. 2007;214(4):325-327.

SECTION D BACTERIAL

122 IMPETIGO

Richard P. Usatine, MD

PATIENT STORIES

A young woman presented to the office with a 3-day history of an uncomfortable rash on her lip and chin (**Figure 122-1**). She denied any trauma or previous history of oral herpes. This case of impetigo resolved quickly with oral cephalexin.

An 11-year-old child presented with a 5-day history of a skin lesion that started after a hiking trip (**Figure 122-2**). This episode of bullous impetigo was found to be secondary to methicillin-resistant *Staphylococcus aureus* (MRSA). The lesion was rapidly progressive and was developing a surrounding cellulitis. She was admitted to a hospital and treated with intravenous clindamycin with good results.[1]

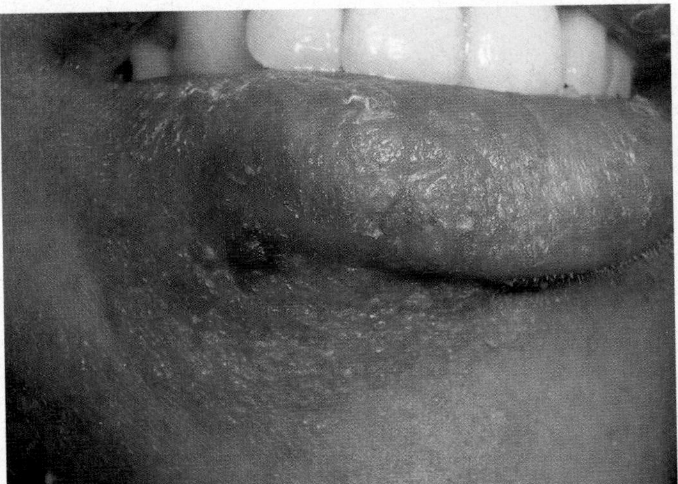

FIGURE 122-1 Typical honey-crusted plaque on the lip of an adult with impetigo. (*Reproduced with permission from Richard P. Usatine, MD.*)

INTRODUCTION

Impetigo is the most superficial of bacterial skin infections. It causes honey crusts, bullae, and erosions.

EPIDEMIOLOGY

- Most frequent in children ages 2 to 6 years, but it can be seen in patients of any age.
- Common among homeless people living on the streets.
- Seen often in third world countries in persons living without easy access to clean water and soap.
- Contagious and can be spread within a household.

ETIOLOGY AND PATHOPHYSIOLOGY

- Impetigo is caused by *Staphylococcus aureus (S. aureus)* and/or a β-hemolytic *Streptococcus (S. pyogenes)*.[2]
- Bullous impetigo is almost always caused by *S. aureus* and is less common than the typical crusted impetigo.
- Impetigo may occur after minor skin injury, such as an insect bite, abrasion, or dermatitis.

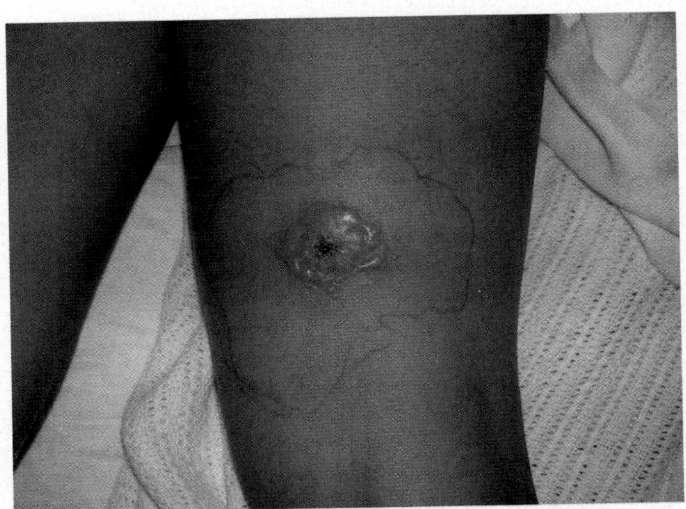

FIGURE 122-2 Bullous impetigo secondary to methicillin-resistant *Staphylococcus aureus* (MRSA) on the leg of an 11-year-old child. Note the surrounding cellulitis. (*Reproduced with permission from Studdiford J, Stonehouse A. Bullous eruption on the posterior thigh 1. J Fam Pract. 2005;54:1041-1044. Frontline Medical Communications, Inc.*)

DIAGNOSIS

CLINICAL FEATURES

- Vesicles, pustules, honey-colored (see **Figure 122-1**), brown or dark crusts, erythematous erosions (**Figure 122-3**), ulcers in ecthyma (**Figure 122-4**), bullae in bullous impetigo (**Figures 122-5** to **122-7**).

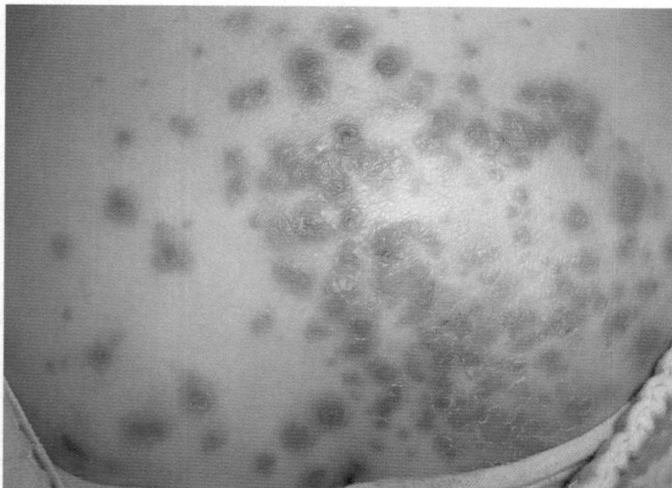

FIGURE 122-3 Widespread impetigo with honey-crusted erythematous lesions on the back of a 7-year-old child. (*Reproduced with permission from Richard P. Usatine, MD.*)

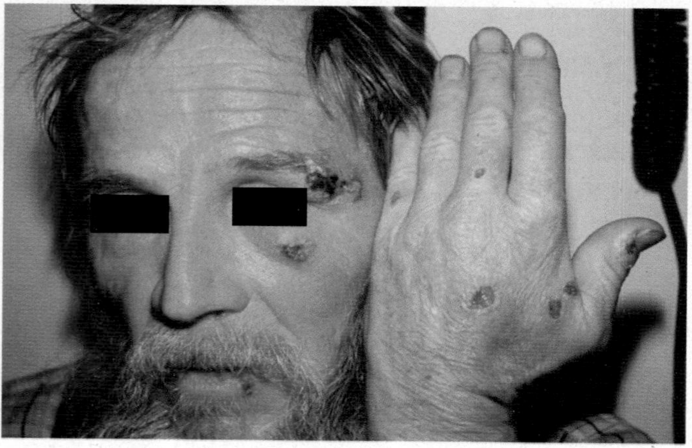

FIGURE 122-4 Impetigo on the face and hand of a homeless man. Note the ecthyma (ulcerated impetigo) on the dorsum of the hand. (*Reproduced with permission from Richard P. Usatine, MD.*)

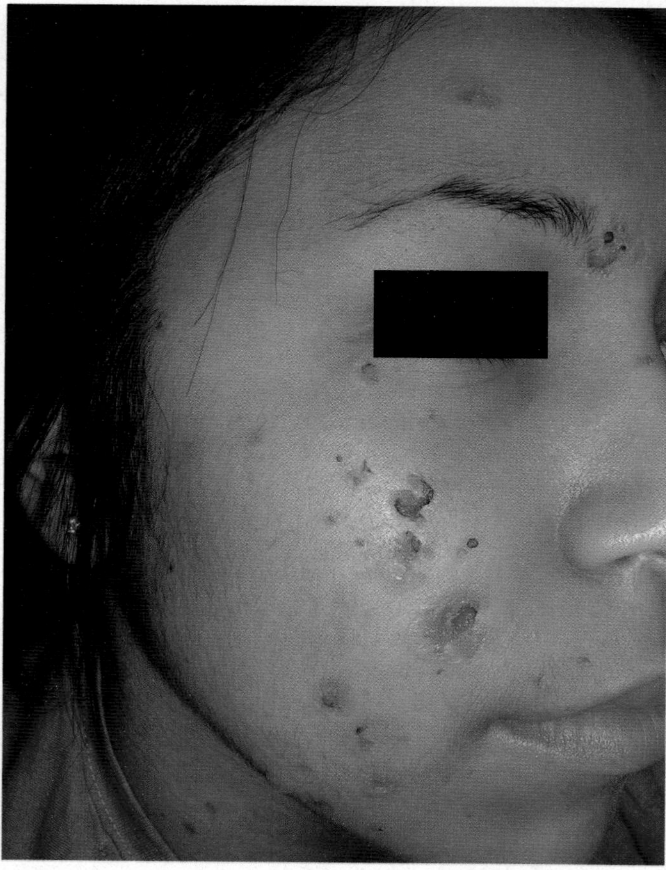

FIGURE 122-6 Bullous impetigo on the face of a 14-year-old girl. Methicillin-resistant *Staphylococcus aureus* was cultured from the impetigo. (*Reproduced with permission from Richard P. Usatine, MD.*)

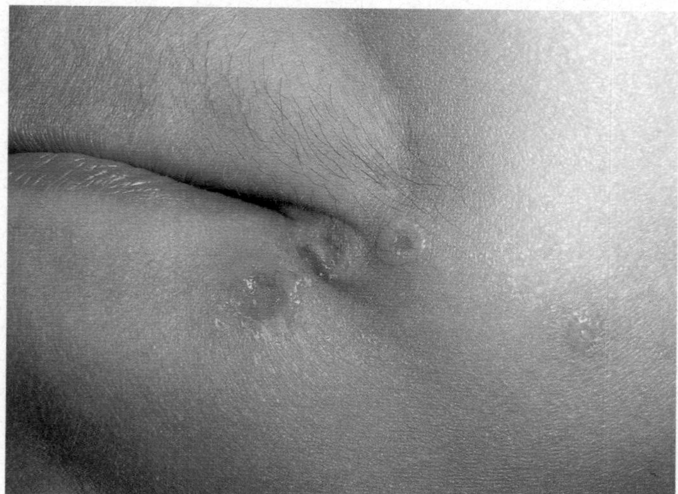

FIGURE 122-5 Bullous impetigo around the mouth of a young boy that progressed to desquamation of the skin on his hands and feet. (*Reproduced with permission from Richard P. Usatine, MD.*)

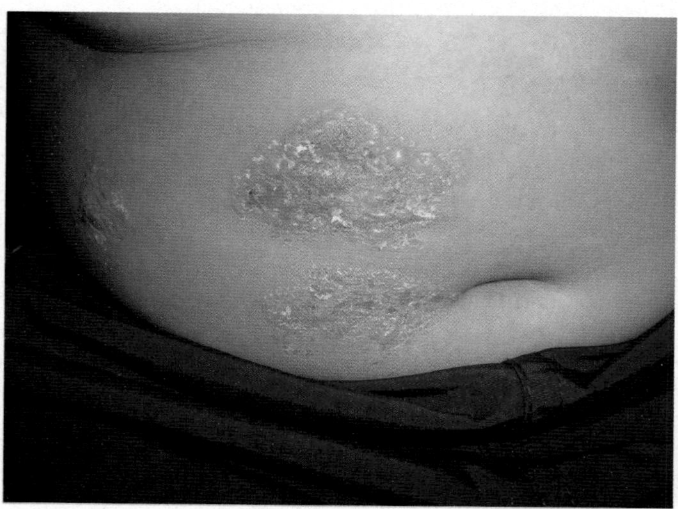

FIGURE 122-7 Bullous impetigo on the abdomen of an 8-year-old boy. (*Reproduced with permission from Richard P. Usatine, MD.*)

TYPICAL DISTRIBUTION

- Face (**Figures 122-1, 122-4** to **122-6**, and **122-8**) is most common, followed by hands, legs (**Figures 122-2** and **122-9**), trunk, and buttocks.

CULTURE

- Culture should be considered in more severe cases because of the risk of MRSA-causing impetigo.

DIFFERENTIAL DIAGNOSIS

Many of the conditions below can become impetigo after being secondarily infected (**Figures 122-10** and **122-11**) with bacteria. This process is called impetiginization.

- Atopic dermatitis—A common inflammatory skin disorder characterized by itching and inflamed skin. It can become secondarily infected with bacteria (see **Figure 122-11**) (see Chapter 151, Atopic Dermatitis).
- Herpes simplex virus infection anywhere on the skin or mucous membranes can become secondarily infected (see Chapter 135, Herpes Simplex).
- Eczema herpeticum is eczema superinfected with herpes rather than bacteria (see **Figure 145-4**).
- Scabies—Pruritic contagious disease caused by a mite that burrows in skin (see Chapter 149, Scabies).
- Folliculitis—Inflammation and/or infection of hair follicles that may be bacterial (see Chapter 123, Folliculitis).
- Tinea corporis—A cutaneous fungal infection caused by dermatophytes, frequently with ring-like scale (see Chapter 144, Tinea Corporis).
- Pemphigus vulgaris—Somewhat rare bullous autoimmune condition with flaccid vesicles and bullae that rupture easily, affecting people between 40 and 60 years of age (see Chapter 193, Pemphigus).
- Bullous pemphigoid—An autoimmune condition with multiple tense bullae that primarily affects people older than 60 years of age (see Chapter 192, Bullous Pemphigoid).
- Acute allergic contact dermatitis—Dermatitis from direct cutaneous exposure to allergens such as poison ivy. Acute lesions are erythematous papules and vesicles in a linear pattern (see Chapter 152, Contact Dermatitis).
- Insect bites—Scratched, open lesions can become secondarily infected with bacteria (impetiginized) (**Figure 122-9**).
- Second-degree burn or sunburn—The blisters when opened leave the skin susceptible to secondary infection (**Figure 122-10**).
- Staphylococcal scalded skin syndrome—Life-threatening syndrome of acute exfoliation of the skin caused by an exotoxin from a staphylococcal infection. This condition is seen almost entirely in infants and young children (**Figure 122-12**).

MANAGEMENT

FIRST LINE

(Recommendations by the Infectious Diseases Society of America.[3])

- Gram stain and culture of the pus or exudates from skin lesions of impetigo and ecthyma are recommended to help identify whether

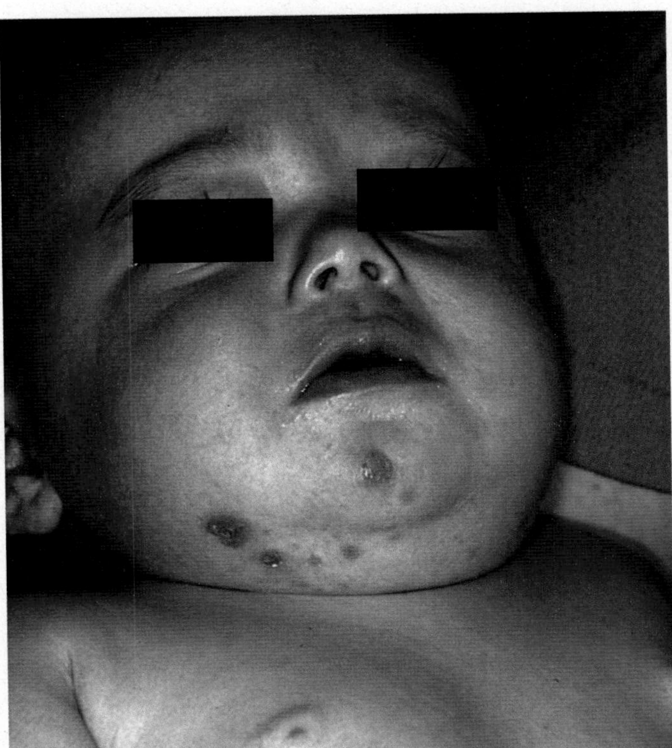

FIGURE 122-8 Impetigo on the face and neck of an infant. (*Reproduced with permission from Richard P. Usatine, MD.*)

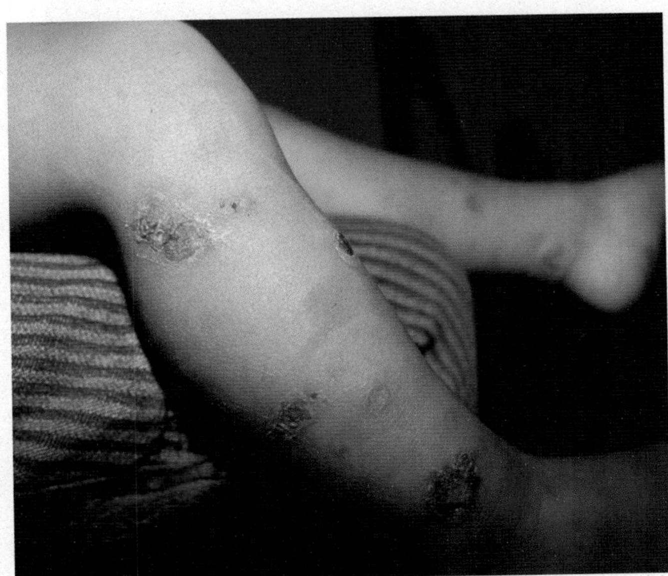

FIGURE 122-9 Impetigo secondary to flea bites on the legs of a young girl. (*Reproduced with permission from Richard P. Usatine, MD. Previously published in the Western Journal of Medicine.*)

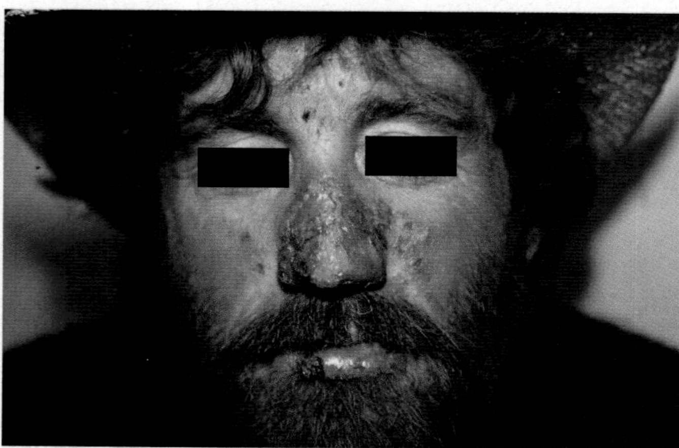

FIGURE 122-10 Secondary impetiginization of a second-degree sunburn in a man experiencing homelessness. (*Reproduced with permission from Richard P. Usatine, MD.*)

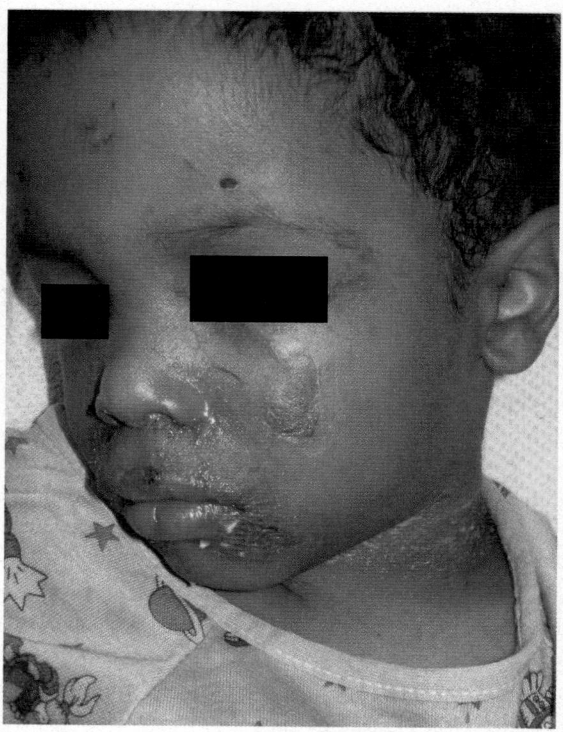

FIGURE 122-12 Staphylococcal scalded skin syndrome in a young child. A severe form of bullous impetigo with large areas of skin exfoliation. Note the prominent involvement of the neck, as this condition tends to involve areas with skin folds. (*Reproduced with permission from Deborah Henderson, MD.*)

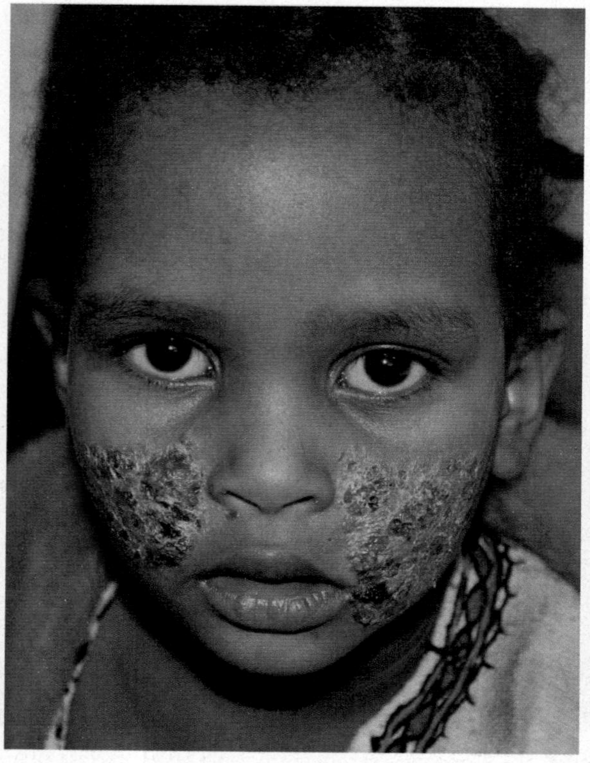

FIGURE 122-11 Atopic dermatitis complicated by secondary impetiginization. (*Reproduced with permission from Richard P. Usatine, MD.*)

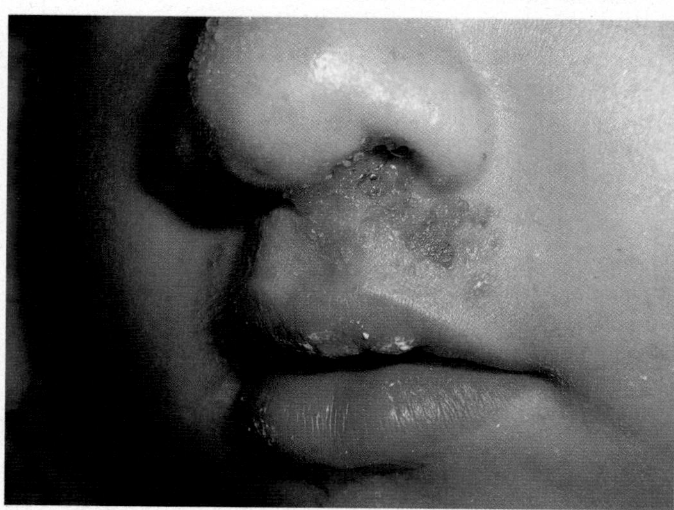

FIGURE 122-13 Impetigo around the nares in a 4-year-old child in Central America who has just chewed a dose of albendazole to treat intestinal parasitosis. (*Reproduced with permission from Richard P. Usatine, MD.*)

Staphylococcus aureus and/or a β-hemolytic *Streptococcus* is the cause, but treatment without these studies is reasonable in typical cases.[3] SOR Ⓐ

- Bullous and nonbullous impetigo can be treated with oral or topical antimicrobials, but oral therapy is recommended for patients with numerous lesions or in outbreaks affecting several people to help decrease transmission of infection. Treatment for ecthyma should be an oral antimicrobial.
  - Bullous and nonbullous impetigo should be treated with either mupirocin or retapamulin twice daily for 5 days.[3] SOR Ⓐ
  - Oral therapy for ecthyma or impetigo should be a 7-day regimen with an agent active against *S. aureus,* unless cultures yield streptococci alone (when oral penicillin is the recommended agent).[3] SOR Ⓐ
  - Because *S. aureus* isolates from impetigo and ecthyma are usually methicillin susceptible, dicloxacillin or cephalexin is recommended.[3] SOR Ⓐ
  - When MRSA is suspected or confirmed, doxycycline, clindamycin, or sulfamethoxazole-trimethoprim (SMX-TMP) is recommended (strong, moderate).[3] SOR Ⓐ
- Note that trimethoprim-sulfamethoxazole achieved 100% clearance in the treatment of impetigo in children cultured with MRSA and *S. pyogenes* in one small randomized controlled trial (RCT).[4]

SECOND LINE

- If there are recurrent MRSA infections, one might choose to prescribe intranasal mupirocin ointment and chlorhexidine bathing to decrease MRSA colonization.[5] SOR Ⓑ Note how impetigo can frequently be seen around the nares (**Figure 122-13**).
- Treat scabies or any other underlying cause of the impetigo.[6] SOR Ⓐ
- Systemic antibiotics should be used for infections during outbreaks of poststreptococcal glomerulonephritis to help eliminate nephritogenic strains of *S. pyogenes* from the community.[3] SOR Ⓐ

PREVENTION

Practice good hygiene with soap and water. Avoid sharing towels, and wash clothes.

FOLLOW-UP

Arrange follow-up based on severity of case and the age and immune status of the patient.

PATIENT EDUCATION

Discuss hygiene issues and how to avoid spread within the household or other living situations such as homeless shelters.

PATIENT RESOURCE

- **https://www.ncbi.nlm.nih.gov/pubmedhealth/PMH0072721/**

PROVIDER RESOURCES

- Practice guidelines for the diagnosis and management of skin and soft tissue infections: 2014 update by the Infectious Diseases Society of America.—**http://cid.oxfordjournals.org/content/59/2/e10.full#sec-61.**
- Shim J, Lanier J, Qui MK. Clinical inquiry: what is the best treatment for impetigo? *J Fam Pract.* 2014;63(6):333-335.—**http://www.mdedge.com/jfponline/article/82698/dermatology/what-best-treatment-impetigo/page/0/2.**

REFERENCES

1. Studdiford J, Stonehouse A. Bullous eruption on the posterior thigh 1. *J Fam Pract.* 2005;54:1041-1044.
2. Koning S, Verhagen AP, van-Suijlekom-Smit LWA, et al. Interventions for impetigo. *Cochrane Database Syst Rev.* 2012;(1):CD003261.
3. Stevens DL, Bisno AL, Chambers HF, et al.; Infectious Diseases Society of America. Practice guidelines for the diagnosis and management of skin and soft tissue infections: 2014 update by the Infectious Diseases Society of America. *Clin Infect Dis.* 2014;59(2):e10-52.
4. Tong SY, Andrews RM, Kearns T, et al. Trimethoprim-sulfamethoxazole compared with benzathine penicillin for treatment of impetigo in aboriginal children: a pilot randomised controlled trial. *J Paediatr Child Health.* 2010;46(3):131-133.
5. Wendt C, Schinke S, Württemberger M, et al. Value of whole-body washing with chlorhexidine for the eradication of methicillin-resistant *Staphylococcus aureus:* a randomized, placebo-controlled, double-blind clinical trial. *Infect Control Hosp Epidemiol.* 2007;28(9):1036-1043.
6. Bowen AC, Tong SY, Chatfield MD, Carapetis JR. The microbiology of impetigo in indigenous children: associations between *Streptococcus pyogenes, Staphylococcus aureus,* scabies, and nasal carriage. *BMC Infect Dis.* 2014;14:727.

123 FOLLICULITIS

Richard P. Usatine, MD

PATIENT STORY

A 42-year-old woman is seen for multiple papules and pustules on her back (**Figure 123-1**). Further questioning demonstrates that she was in a friend's hot tub twice over the previous weekend. The outbreak on her back started after she went into the hot tub the second time. This is a case of *Pseudomonas* folliculitis or "hot tub" folliculitis. The patient avoided this hot tub and the folliculitis disappeared spontaneously. Another option is to treat with an oral fluoroquinolone that covers *Pseudomonas*.

INTRODUCTION

Folliculitis is an inflammation of hair follicles, usually from an infectious etiology. Multiple species of bacteria have been implicated, as well as fungal organisms.

EPIDEMIOLOGY

- Folliculitis is a cutaneous disorder that affects all age groups and races, and both genders.
- It can be infectious or noninfectious. It is most commonly of bacterial origin (**Figures 123-2** and **123-3**).
- Pseudofolliculitis barbae is most frequently seen in men of color and is made worse by shaving (**Figure 123-4**).[1]
- Acne keloidalis nuchae is commonly seen in black men or men of color but can also be seen in women (**Figures 123-5** and **123-6**).[2]
- Eosinophilic folliculitis is described in patients with HIV infection (**Figure 123-7**).
- Methicillin-resistant *Staphylococcus aureus* (MRSA) can pose a challenge to the treatment of folliculitis (**Figure 123-8**).

ETIOLOGY AND PATHOPHYSIOLOGY

- Folliculitis is an infection of the hair follicle and can be superficial, in which it is confined to the upper hair follicle, or deep, in which inflammation spans the entire depth of the follicle.
- Infection can be of bacterial, viral, or fungal origin. *S. aureus* is by far the most common bacterial causative agent.
- The noninfectious form of folliculitis is often seen in adolescents and young adults who wear tight-fitting clothes. Folliculitis can also be caused by chemical irritants or physical injury.
- Topical steroid use, ointments, lotions, or makeup can swell the opening to the pilosebaceous unit and cause folliculitis.
- Bacterial folliculitis or *Staphylococcus* folliculitis typically presents as infected pustules most prominent on the face, buttocks, trunk, or

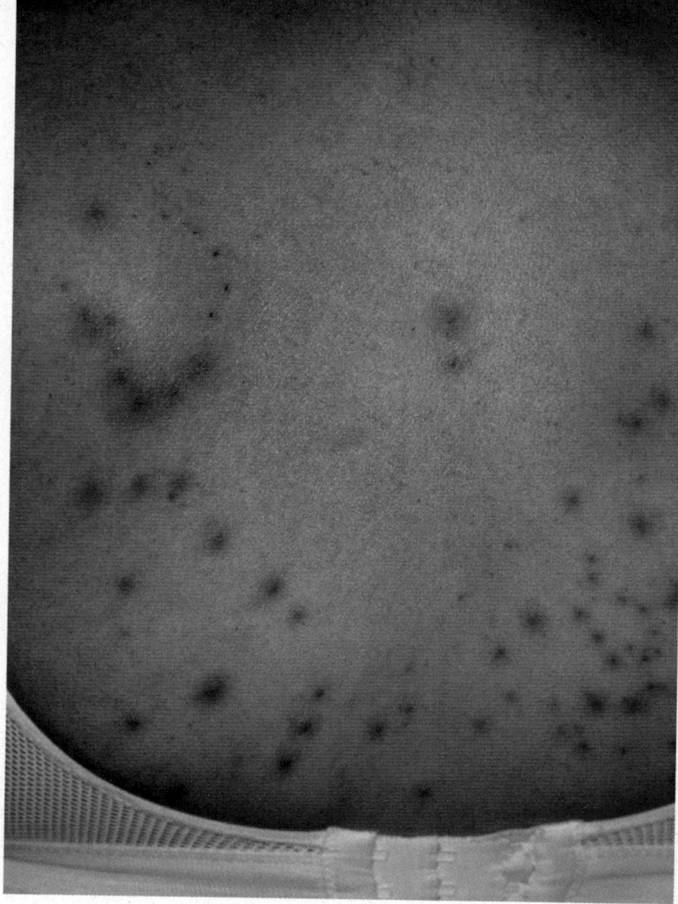

FIGURE 123-1 "Hot-tub" folliculitis from *Pseudomonas aeruginosa* in a hot tub. *(Reproduced with permission from Richard P. Usatine, MD.)*

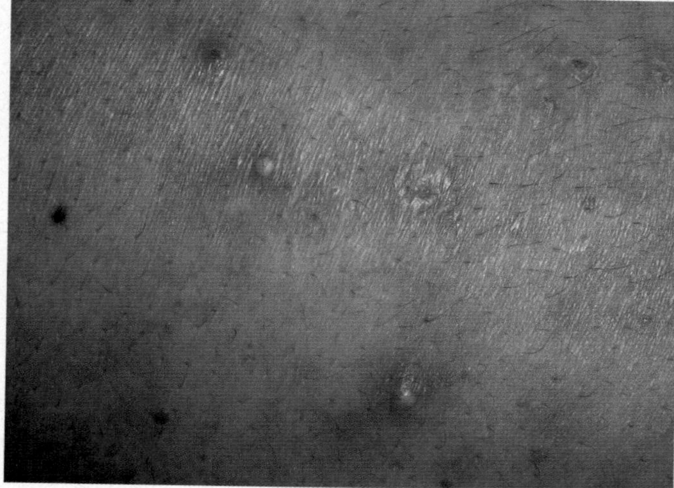

FIGURE 123-2 Close-up of bacterial folliculitis showing hairs coming through pustules. *(Reproduced with permission from Richard P. Usatine, MD.)*

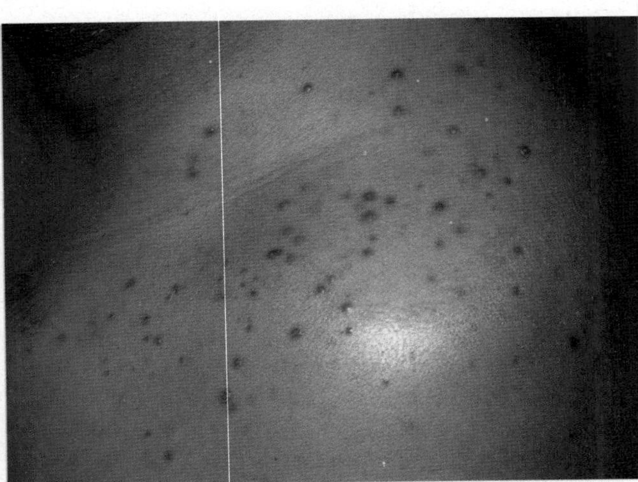

FIGURE 123-3 Chronic bacterial folliculitis (biopsy proven) on the shoulders and back with scarring and hyperpigmentation. (*Reproduced with permission from Richard P. Usatine, MD.*)

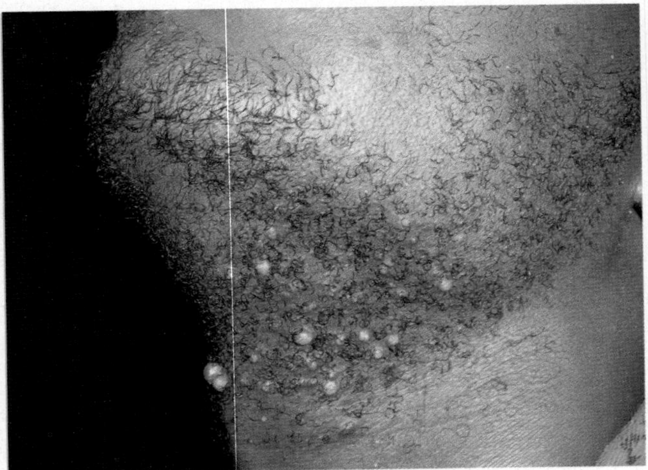

FIGURE 123-4 Pseudofolliculitis barbae in a black man. Shaving makes it worse and he notes many problems with ingrown hairs. (*Reproduced with permission from Richard P. Usatine, MD.*)

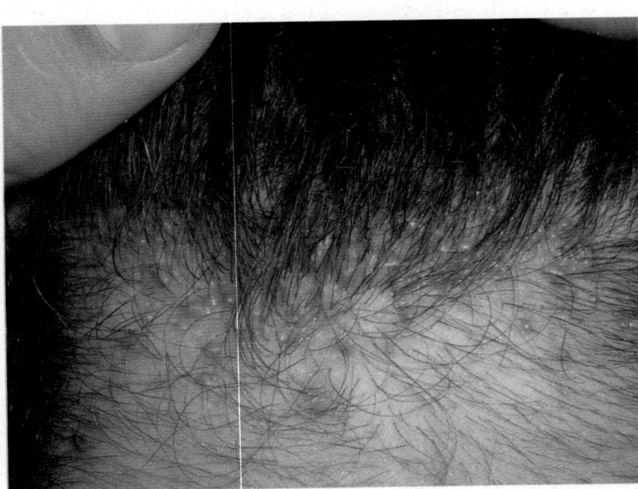

FIGURE 123-5 Acne keloidalis nuchae with inflamed papules and pustules on the neck of a young Hispanic man. (*Reproduced with permission from Richard P. Usatine, MD.*)

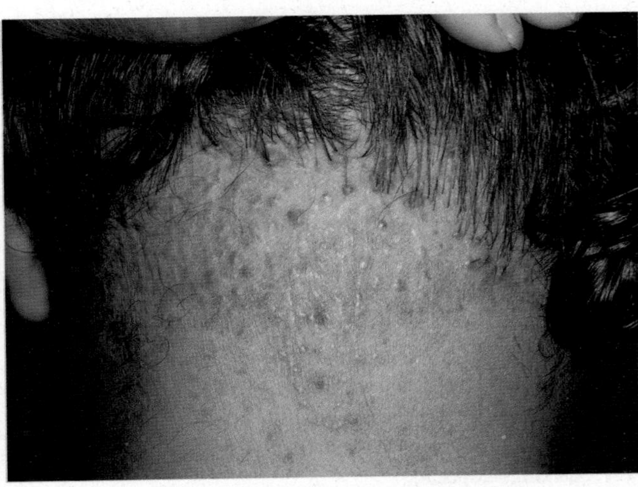

FIGURE 123-6 Acne keloidalis nuchae in a woman, demonstrating the folliculitis around the hair follicles and the scarring alopecia that has occurred. (*Reproduced with permission from Richard P. Usatine, MD.*)

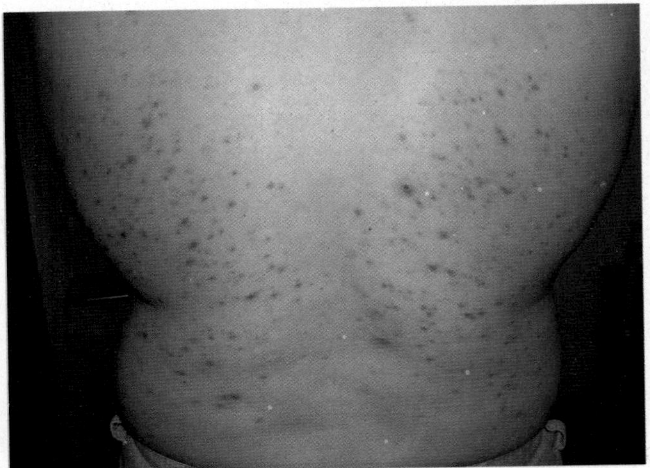

FIGURE 123-7 Eosinophilic folliculitis on the back of an HIV-positive man. (*Reproduced with permission from Richard P. Usatine, MD.*)

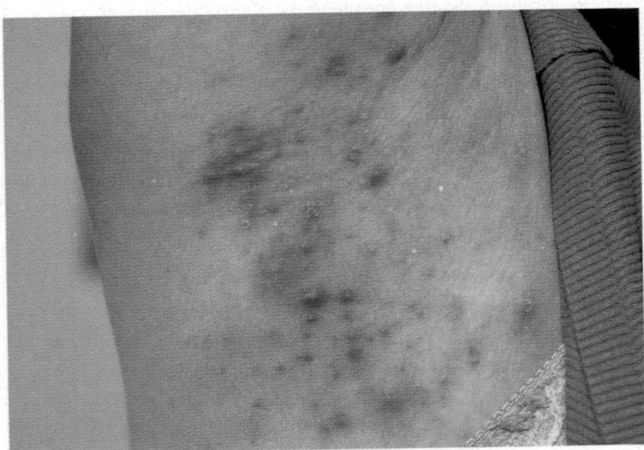

FIGURE 123-8 MRSA folliculitis in the axilla of a 29-year-old woman. The lesions were present for 4 weeks in the axilla, left forearm, and right thigh. The MRSA was sensitive to tetracyclines and resolved with oral doxycycline. (*Reproduced with permission from Plotner AN, Brodell RT. Bilateral axillary pustules, J Fam Pract. 2008;57(4):253-255. Frontline Medical Communications, Inc.*)

extremities. It can progress to a deeper infection with the development of furuncles or boils (**Figure 123-9**). Infection can occur as a result of mechanical injury or via local spread from nearby infected wounds. An area of desquamation is frequently seen surrounding infected pustules in *S. aureus* folliculitis.[1-3]

- Parasitic folliculitis usually occurs as a result of mite infestation (*Demodex*). These are usually seen on the face, nose, and back and typically cause an eosinophilic pustular-like folliculitis.[1]
- Folliculitis decalvans is a chronic form of folliculitis involving the scalp, leading to hair loss or alopecia (**Figure 123-10**). Staphylococcal infection is the usual causative agent, but a genetic component to this condition has also been suggested.[1] It is also called tufted folliculitis because some of the hair follicles will have many hairs growing from them simultaneously (**Figure 123-11**) (see Chapter 197, Scarring Alopecia).
- Acne keloidalis nuchae is a chronic form of folliculitis found on the posterior neck that can be extensive and lead to keloidal tissue and alopecia.[1-3] Although it is often thought to occur almost exclusively in black men, it can be seen in men of all ethnic backgrounds and occasionally in women (see **Figures 123-5** and **123-6**; also see Chapter 120, Pseudofolliculitis and Acne Keloidalis Nuchae).
- Fungal folliculitis is epidermal fungal infections that are seen frequently. Tinea capitis infections are a form of dermatophytic folliculitis (see Chapter 143, Tinea Capitis). *Malassezia (Pityrosporum)* folliculitis is caused by the same yeast that causes tinea versicolor and is seen in a distribution similar to those of tinea versicolor and bacterial folliculitis. This is a capelike distribution that may include the upper back, chest, and shoulders (**Figure 123-12**) (see Chapter 147, Tinea Versicolor).
- *Pseudomonas* folliculitis or "hot tub" folliculitis is usually a self-limited infection that follows exposure to water or objects that are contaminated with *Pseudomonas aeruginosa* (**Figure 123-13**). This occurs when hot tubs are inadequately chlorinated or brominated. This also occurs when loofah sponges or other items used for bathing become a host for pseudomonal growth. Onset of symptoms is usually within 6 to 72 hours after exposure, with the complete resolution of symptoms in a couple of days, provided that the individual avoids further exposure.[4]
- Gram-negative folliculitis is an infection with Gram-negative bacteria that most typically occurs in individuals who have been on long-term antibiotic therapy, usually those taking oral antibiotics for acne. The most frequently encountered infective agents include *Klebsiella, Escherichia coli, Enterobacter,* and *Proteus.*[5]
- Pseudofolliculitis barbae (razor bumps) is most commonly seen in black males who shave. Papules develop when the sharp edge of the hair shaft reenters the skin (ingrown hairs) and is seen on the cheeks and neck as a result of curled ingrown hair.[2] It can also occur in women with hirsutism who shave or pluck their hairs (see **Figure 120-7**) (see Chapter 120, Pseudofolliculitis and Acne Keloidalis Nuchae).[6]
- Viral folliculitis seen is primarily caused by herpes simplex virus and molluscum contagiosum.[4] Herpetic folliculitis is seen primarily in individuals with a history of herpes simplex infections type I or II. But most notably, it may be a sign of immunosuppression, as is the case with HIV infection.[7] The expression of herpes folliculitis in

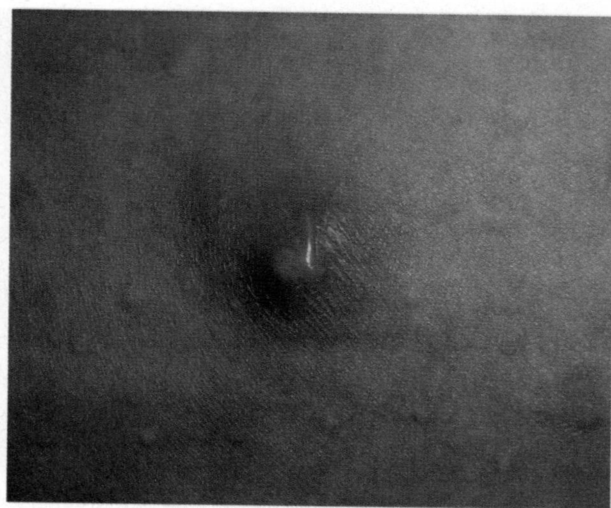

FIGURE 123-9 Isolated single furuncle in an adult woman. (*Reproduced with permission from Richard P. Usatine, MD.*)

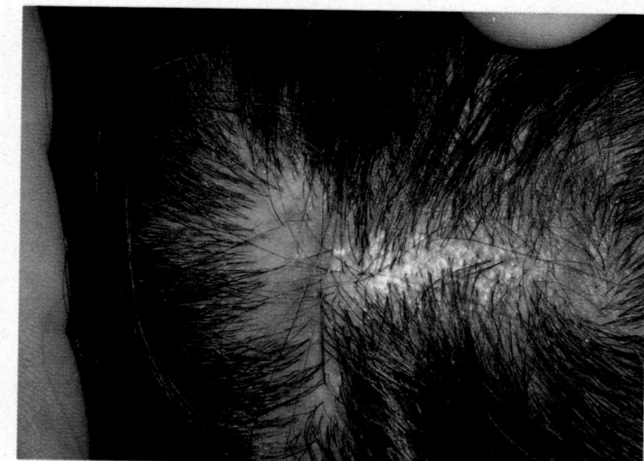

FIGURE 123-10 Early folliculitis decalvans showing scalp inflammation, pustules around hair follicles, and scarring alopecia. (*Reproduced with permission from Richard P. Usatine, MD.*)

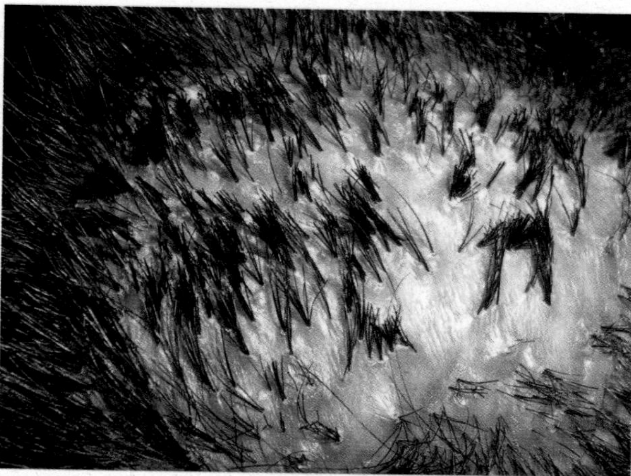

FIGURE 123-11 Tufted folliculitis with visible tufts of hair (multiple hairs from one follicle) growing from a number of abnormal follicles. This is one example of scarring alopecia. (*Reproduced with permission from Richard P. Usatine, MD.*)

HIV infection ranges from simple to necrotizing folliculitis and ulcerative lesions. Molluscum is a pox virus, and molluscum contagiosum has been well documented in similar patient populations (i.e., HIV and AIDS) and in children (see Chapters 135, Herpes Simplex, and 136, Molluscum Contagiosum).[7-9]

- Actinic superficial folliculitis is a sterile form of folliculitis seen predominantly in warm climates or during hot or summer months. Pustules occur primarily on the neck, over the shoulders, upper trunk, and upper arms, usually within 6 to 36 hours after sun exposure.[10]
- Eosinophilic folliculitis is associated with HIV infection and can occur as a result of the viral infection itself, in which case the exact mechanism by which this occurs is uncertain (though it is thought to be auto-immune) (see **Figure 123-7**).[9,11,12,13,14] It is associated with diminished CD4 cell counts. Eosinophilic folliculitis generally improves with the initiation of highly active antiretroviral therapy (HAART), but can occur during the restoration of immune function with HAART.[12]

DIAGNOSIS

Often the diagnosis of folliculitis is based on a good history and physical.

CLINICAL FEATURES

Folliculitis has its characteristic presentation as the development of papules or pustules that are thin-walled and surrounded by a margin of erythema or inflammation. Look for a hair at the center of the lesions (see **Figure 123-2**). There is usually an absence of systemic signs, and patients' symptoms range from mild discomfort and pruritus to severe pain with extensive involvement.

TYPICAL DISTRIBUTION

Any area of the skin may be affected, and often location may be related to the pathogen or cause of folliculitis. The face, scalp, neck, trunk, axillae, extremities, and groin are some of the more common areas affected.

LABORATORY TESTS

Laboratory testing may be unnecessary in simple superficial folliculitis and where the history is clear and quick resolution occurs. Clinical diagnosis of herpes and fungal folliculitis may be difficult, and diagnosis may be made based on strong clinical suspicion or as a result of failed antimicrobial therapy. A KOH prep can be used to look for *Malassezia* if the infected follicle is opened with a needle or tip of a scalpel. If *Malassezia* is detected it will most likely be the oval type. Herpes genetic probe testing can be used when herpes is suspected.[1] SOR Ⓐ

DIFFERENTIAL DIAGNOSIS

- *Grover disease* is a very pruritic condition of unknown cause that produces reddish papules and slight scale on the backs of middle-aged men. It is also called "transient acantholytic dermatosis" and may resolve spontaneously in a period of years. It resembles folliculitis, but the papules are not centered on hair follicles (**Figure 123-14**).

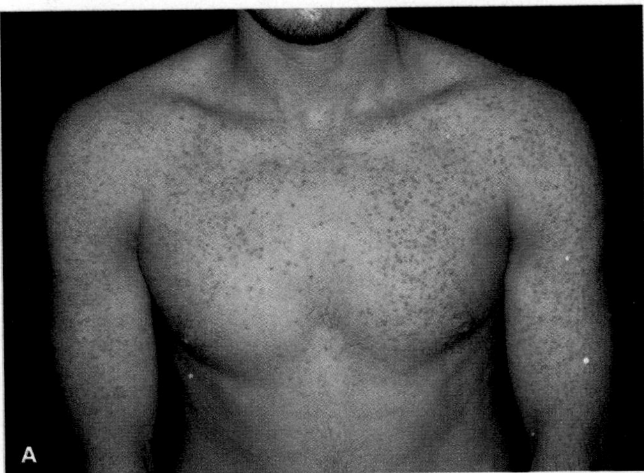

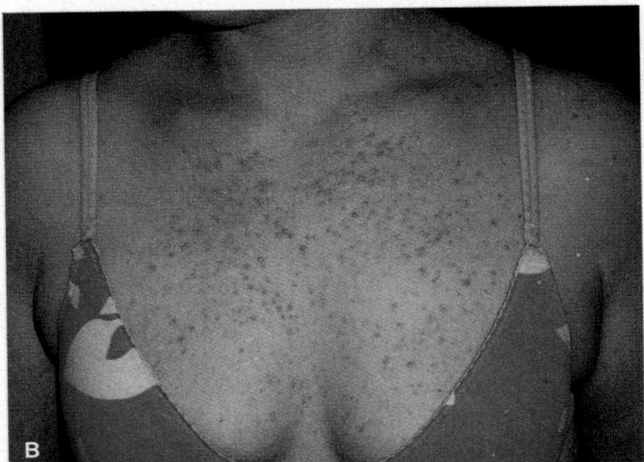

FIGURE 123-12 **A.** *Pityrosporum* folliculitis on the chest, shoulders, and arms of a young man; biopsy proven. **B.** *Pityrosporum* folliculitis on the chest of a young woman. KOH preparation showed *Pityrosporum* looking like ziti and meatballs. *(Reproduced with permission from Richard P. Usatine, MD.)*

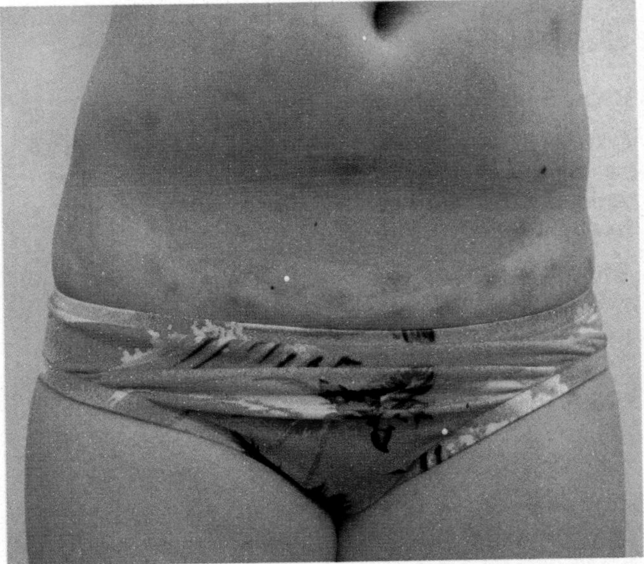

FIGURE 123-13 "Hot-tub" folliculitis from *Pseudomonas aeruginosa* in a hot tub. The folliculitis tends to be distributed under or around the bathing suit. *(Reproduced with permission from Daniel Stulberg, MD.)*

- *Perforating collagenosis* is a disorder that can occur around hair follicles and be known as perforating folliculitis. It is most likely to be seen in connection with end-stage renal disease inpatients who have diabetes and are on dialysis (**Figure 123-15**).
- *Miliaria* is blockage of the sweat glands that can resemble the small papules of folliculitis. The eccrine sweat glands become blocked so that sweat leaks into the dermis and epidermis. Clinically, skin lesions may range from clear vesicles to pustules. These skin lesions primarily occur in times of increased heat and humidity and are self-limited (see Chapter 114, Normal Skin Changes).[1]
- *Keratosis pilaris* consists of papules that occur as a result of a buildup of keratin in the openings of hair follicles, especially on the lateral upper arms and thighs. It is not an infection but can develop into folliculitis if lesions become infected (see Chapter 151, Atopic Dermatitis).[1,6]
- *Acne vulgaris* is characterized by the presence of comedones, papules, pustules, and nodules that are a result of follicular hyperproliferation and plugging with excessive sebum. Inflammation occurs when *Propionibacterium acnes* and other inflammatory substances get extruded from the blocked pilosebaceous unit.[15] Although acne on the face is rarely confused with folliculitis, acne on the trunk can resemble folliculitis. To distinguish between them, look for facial involvement and comedones seen in acne (see Chapter 118, Acne Vulgaris).

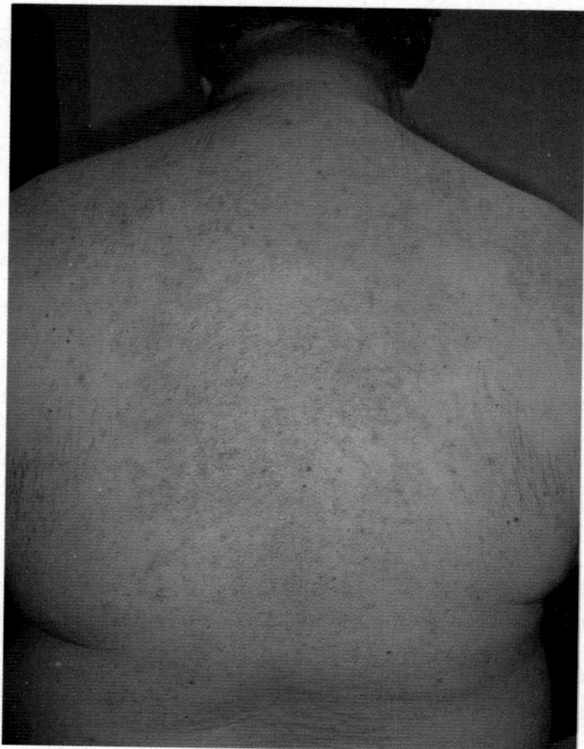

FIGURE 123-14 Grover disease on the back of a middle-aged man. This is also called "transient acantholytic dermatosis." It is very pruritic with reddish papules and slight scale. *(Reproduced with permission from Richard P. Usatine, MD.)*

MANAGEMENT

FIRST LINE

- Management of folliculitis must be specific to the causative agent.
- With superficial bacterial folliculitis, treatment with topical preparations such as mupirocin (Bactroban) or fusidic acid may be sufficient.[1] SOR Ⓐ Additionally, topical clindamycin may be considered in the mildest cases in which MRSA is involved.[1] SOR Ⓐ
- Deep or extensive bacterial folliculitis warrants oral therapy with first-generation cephalosporins (cephalexin), penicillins that cover *S. aureus* (amoxicillin/clavulanate and dicloxacillin), macrolides, or fluoroquinolones.[1,4,6] SOR Ⓐ

SECOND LINE

- *Pseudomonas* or "hot tub" folliculitis usually resolves untreated within a week of onset (see **Figure 123-13**). For severe cases, treatment with ciprofloxacin provides adequate antipseudomonal coverage.[1,4] SOR Ⓑ
- *Malassezia* (*Pityrosporum*) folliculitis may be treated with systemic antifungals, topical azoles, and/or with shampoos containing azoles, selenium, or zinc (see **Figure 123-12**) (see Chapter 147, Tinea Versicolor). Evidence is scanty for treatment but does support oral fluconazole and topical 2% ketoconazole shampoo.[16]
- *Demodex* folliculitis can be treated with ivermectin or topically with 5% permethrin cream.[4] SOR Ⓑ
- Herpes folliculitis can be treated with acyclovir, valacyclovir, and famciclovir. Acyclovir 400 mg twice daily for 5 days is one option (see Chapter 135, Herpes Simplex).[1] SOR Ⓑ
- Eosinophilic folliculitis associated with HIV is treated with HAART, topical steroids, antihistamines, itraconazole,

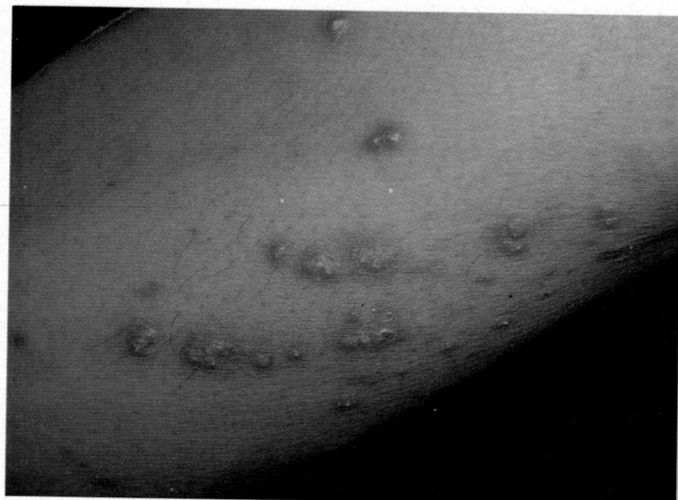

FIGURE 123-15 Perforating folliculitis (perforating collagenosis) in a 60-year-old man on dialysis secondary to end-stage renal disease (from his diabetes). *(Reproduced with permission from Richard P. Usatine, MD.)*

metronidazole, oral retinoids, and UV light therapy.[11] Topical steroids, nonsteroidal anti-inflammatory drugs (NSAIDs), and isotretinoin are treatments of choice for HIV-associated eosinophilic folliculitis.[9-12,17] SOR B Relief with systemic antihistamines is variable, and UV therapy is time-consuming and expensive.[11,12] SOR C

- Treatment of folliculitis decalvans is covered in the chapter on scarring alopecia (Chapter 197), and pseudofolliculitis barbae and acne keloidalis nuchae are covered in Chapter 120.
- Perforating folliculitis is somewhat rare other than in patients on dialysis. Treatment options include topical and oral retinoids. SOR C

FOLLOW-UP

Follow-up is dependent on the severity, cause, and chronicity of the folliculitis.

PATIENT EDUCATION

Prevention is most important and centers on good personal hygiene and proper laundering of clothing. Patients should be encouraged to avoid tight-fitting clothing. Hot tubs should be properly cleaned, and the chemicals should be maintained appropriately. The best way to prevent pseudofolliculitis barbae and acne keloidalis nuchae is to avoid shaving the hair in the involved areas.

PATIENT RESOURCE

- **http://www.webmd.com/skin-problems-and-treatments/tc/folliculitis-topic-overview#1.**

PROVIDER RESOURCE

- **http://www.dermnetnz.org/topics/folliculitis/.**

REFERENCES

1. Luelmo-Aguilar J, Santandreu MS. Folliculitis recognition and management. *Am J Clin Dermatol.* 2004;5(5):301-310.
2. Habif, T. *Clinical Dermatology: A Color Guide to Diagnosis and Therapy*, 5th ed. Philadelphia, PA: Elsevier; 2009.
3. Levy AL, Simpson G, Skinner RB Jr. Medical pearl: circle of desquamation, a clue to the diagnosis of folliculitis and furunculosis caused by *Staphylococcus aureus. J Am Acad Dermatol.* 2006; 55(6):1079-1080.
4. Stulberg DL, Penrod MA, Blatny RA. Common bacterial skin infections. *Am Fam Physician.* 2002;66(1):119-124.
5. Neubert U, Jansen T, Plewig G. Bacteriologic and immunologic aspects of Gram-negative folliculitis: a study of 46 patients. *Int J Dermatol.* 1999;38(4):270-274.
6. Ferri F, et al, eds. *Ferri's Clinical Advisor 2012*. Philadelphia, PA: Elsevier/Saunders; 2011.
7. Boer A, Herder N, Winter K, Falk T. Herpes folliculitis: clinical histopathological, and molecular pathologic observations. *Br J Dermatol.* 2006;154(4):743-746.
8. Weinberg JM, Mysliwiec A, Turiansky GW, et al. Viral folliculitis. Atypical presentations of herpes simplex, herpes zoster, and molluscum contagiosum. *Arch Dermatol.* 1997;133(8):983-986.
9. Fearfield LA, Rowe A, Francis N, et al. Itchy folliculitis and human immunodeficiency virus infection: clinicopathological and immunological features, pathogenesis and treatment. *Br J Dermatol.* 1999;141(1):3-11.
10. Labandeira J, Suarez-Campos A, Toribio J. Actinic superficial folliculitis. *Br J Dermatol.* 1998;138(6):1070-1074.
11. Nervi SJ, Schwartz RA, Dmochowski M. Eosinophilic pustular folliculitis: a 40 year retrospect. *J Am Acad Dermatol.* 2006;55(2): 285-289.
12. Rajendran PM, Dolev JC, Heaphy MR Jr, Maurer T. Eosinophilic folliculitis: before and after the introduction of antiretroviral therapy. *Arch Dermatol.* 2005;141(10):1227-1231.
13. Nomura T, Katoh M, Yamamoto Y, Miyachi Y, Kabashima K. Eosinophilic pustular folliculitis: A proposal of diagnostic and therapeutic algorithms. *J Dermatol.* 2016 Nov;43(11):1301-1306.
14. Toutous-Trellu L, Abraham S, Pechère M, et al. Topical tacrolimus for effective treatment of eosinophilic folliculitis associated with human immunodeficiency virus infection. *Arch Dermatol.* 2005; 141(10):1203-1208.
15. Strauss JS, Krowchuk DP, Leyden JJ, et al. Guidelines of care for acne vulgaris management. *J Am Acad Dermatol.* 2007;56(4):651-663.
16. Hald M, Arendrup MC, Svejgaard EL, et al. Danish Society of Dermatology. Evidence-based Danish guidelines for the treatment of *Malassezia*-related skin diseases. *Acta Derm Venereol.* 2015; 95(1):12-19.
17. Jang KA, Kim SH, Choi JH, et al. Viral folliculitis on the face. *Br J Dermatol.* 2000;142(3):555-559.

124 PITTED KERATOLYSIS

Richard P. Usatine, MD
Michael J. Babcock, MD

PATIENT STORY

A 34-year-old man comes to the office with a terrible foot odor problem. He is wearing cowboy boots and he says that his feet are always sweaty. He is embarrassed to remove his boots, but when the physician convinces him to do so the odor is overwhelming. While breathing through the mouth, the physician sees the typical pits of pitted keratolysis. His socks are moist and the skin is somewhat macerated from the hyperhidrosis. His foot has many crateriform pits on the heel (**Figure 124-1**). He is prescribed topical erythromycin solution for the pitted keratolysis and topical aluminum chloride for the hyperhidrosis. It is suggested that he wear a lighter and more breathable shoe until this problem improves.

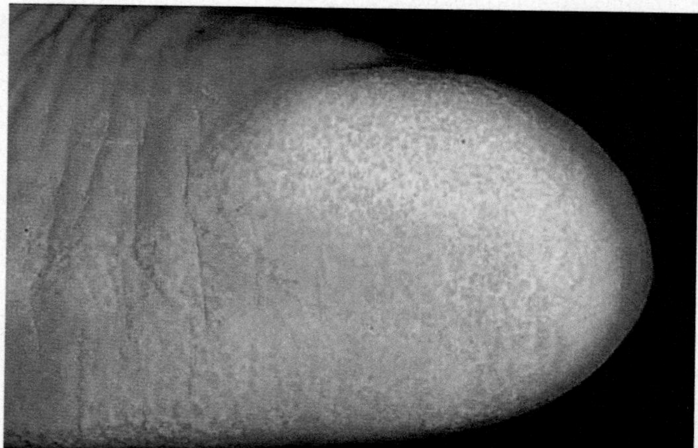

FIGURE 124-1 Many crateriform pits on the heel of a foot in a man with pitted keratolysis and hyperhidrosis. (*Reproduced with permission from Richard P. Usatine, MD.*)

INTRODUCTION

Pitted keratolysis is a superficial foot infection caused by Gram-positive bacteria. These bacteria degrade the keratin of the stratum corneum, leaving visible pits on the soles of the feet.

EPIDEMIOLOGY

- Seen more commonly in men.
- Often a complication of hyperhidrosis.
- Seen more often in hot and humid climates.
- Prevalence can be as high as 42.5% among paddy field workers.[1]
- May be common in athletes with moist, sweaty feet.[2]

ETIOLOGY AND PATHOPHYSIOLOGY

- *Kytococcus sedentarius* (formerly *Micrococcus* spp.), *Corynebacterium* species, and *Dermatophilus congolensis* have all been shown to cause pitted keratolysis.[3]
- Proteases produced by the bacteria degrade keratins to give the clinical appearance.[4]
- The associated malodor is likely secondary to the production of sulfur by-products.[3]

DIAGNOSIS

CLINICAL FEATURES

Pitted keratolysis usually presents as painless, malodorous, crateriform pits coalescing into larger superficial erosions of the stratum corneum (**Figures 124-1** to **124-4**). It may be associated with itching and a burning sensation in some patients (**Figure 124-3**).

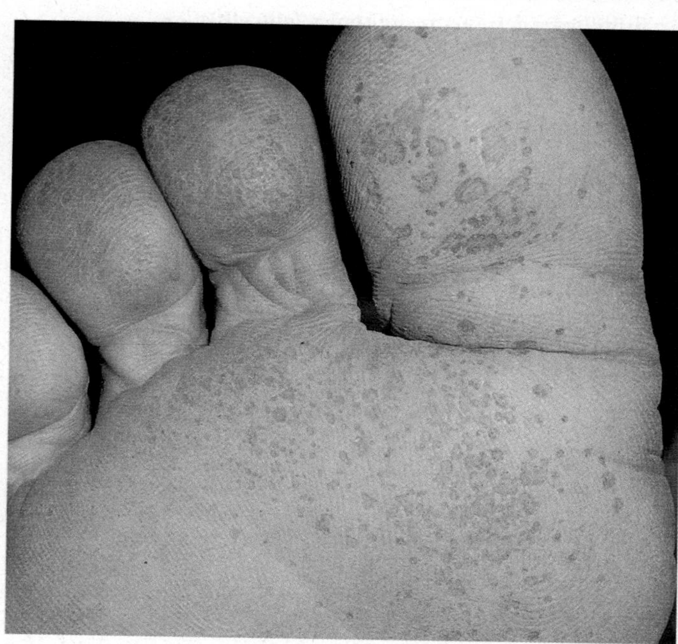

FIGURE 124-2 Pitted keratolysis on the pressure-bearing areas of the toes and the ball of the foot. (*Reproduced with permission from Richard P. Usatine, MD.*)

TYPICAL DISTRIBUTION

Pitted keratolysis usually involves the callused pressure-bearing areas of the foot, such as the heel, ball of the foot, and plantar great toe. It can also be found in friction areas between the toes.[5]

LABORATORY STUDIES

Typically a clinical diagnosis, but biopsy will reveal keratin pits lined by bacteria.

DIFFERENTIAL DIAGNOSIS

- Characteristic clinical features make the diagnosis easy, but it is possible to have other diseases causing plantar pits, which can be included in the differential. These other diseases include plantar warts, basal cell nevus syndrome, and arsenic toxicity.
- Plantar warts are typically not as numerous. They have a firm callus ring around a soft core with small black dots from thrombosed capillaries (see Chapter 140, Plantar Warts).
- Basal cell nevus syndrome typically has pits involving the palms and soles, bone abnormalities, a history of many basal cell carcinomas, and a characteristic facies with frontal bossing, hypoplastic maxilla, and hypertelorism (wide-set eyes) (see Chapter 177, Basal Cell Carcinoma).
- Arsenic toxicity can result in pits on the palms and soles, but it can also have hyperpigmentation, many skin cancers, Mees lines (white lines on the fingernails), or other nail disorders.

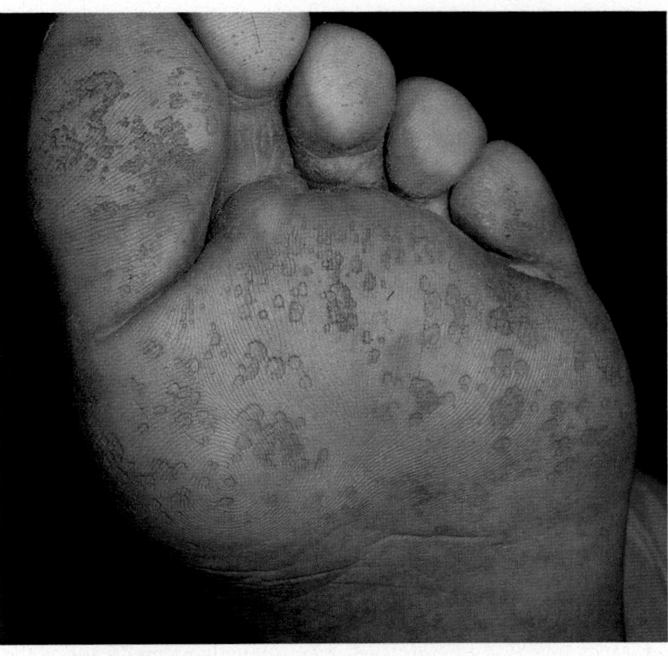

FIGURE 124-3 Pitted keratolysis with hyperpigmented crateriform pits on the pressure-bearing areas of the foot. The patient complained of itching and burning on the feet. *(Reproduced with permission from Richard P. Usatine, MD.)*

MANAGEMENT

FIRST LINE

- Treatment is based on bacterial elimination and reducing the moist environment in which the bacteria thrive. Attention to foot hygiene including the use of clean, dry socks may be helpful for prevention and treatment. SOR Ⓒ
- Topical 2% erythromycin or 1% clindamycin solution or gel may be applied twice daily until the condition resolves. SOR Ⓒ It may take 3 to 4 weeks to clear the odor and skin lesions.
- Topical 2% mupirocin ointment is also effective.[6,7] SOR Ⓒ In one case report, resolution of pitted keratolysis occurred with twice-daily applications of 2% mupirocin ointment for 3 weeks. Eight weeks later there was no recurrence.[6] SOR Ⓒ
- Treat underlying hyperhidrosis. This can be done with topical aluminum chloride solution of varying concentrations. SOR Ⓒ *Drysol* is a 20% aluminum chloride solution that comes with an applicator top.

SECOND LINE

- It is questionable if oral antibiotics are effective. It is best to focus on treating the hyperhidrosis, improving foot hygiene, and relying on topical antibiotics.[7] SOR Ⓒ
- Botulinum toxin injection is an expensive, painful and effective treatment for hyperhidrosis and pitted keratolysis.[8] SOR Ⓒ In one case report, 2 patients were successfully treated and returned without any sign of disease between 6 and 10 months.[8]

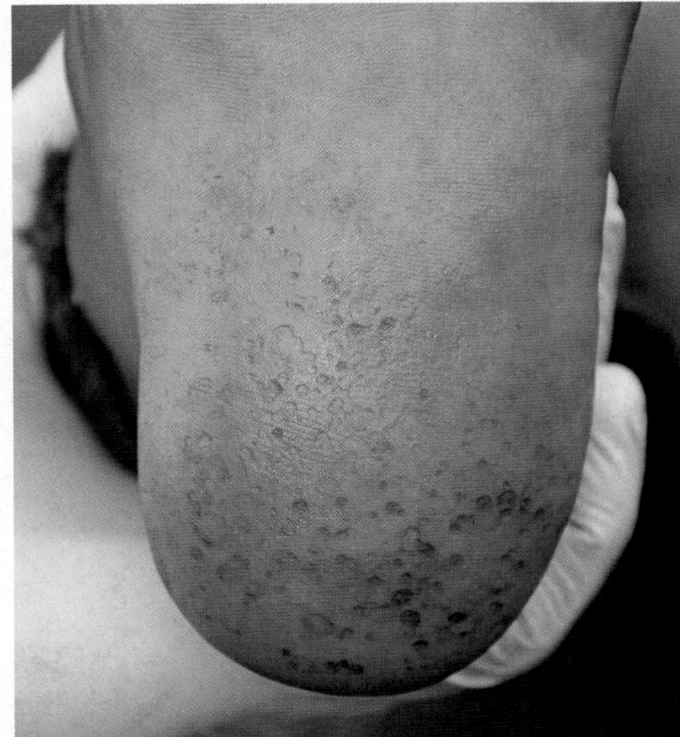

FIGURE 124-4 Pitted keratolysis with many crateriform pits on the heel. *(Reproduced with permission from Richard P. Usatine, MD.)*

FOLLOW-UP

Follow-up is needed for treatment failures, recurrences, and the treatment of underlying hyperhidrosis if present.

PATIENT EDUCATION AND PREVENTION

Teach patients about connections between hyperhidrosis, foot hygiene issues, and pitted keratolysis. Helpful preventive strategies include avoiding occlusive footwear and using moisture-wicking socks (wool socks may be preferable to cotton socks). Clean socks should be used daily and may need to be changed more frequently in severe cases of plantar hyperhidrosis.

PATIENT RESOURCES

- International Hyperhidrosis Society—**http://www.sweathelp.org.**

PROVIDER RESOURCES

- Medscape. *Pitted Keratolysis*—**http://emedicine.medscape.com/article/1053078-overview.**

REFERENCES

1. Shenoi SD, Davis SV, Rao S, et al. Dermatoses among paddy field workers—a descriptive, cross-sectional pilot study. *Indian J Dermatol Venereol Leprol.* 2005;71:254-258.
2. Conklin RJ. Common cutaneous disorders in athletes. *Sports Med.* 1990;9:100-119.
3. Bolognia J, Jorizzo J, Rapini R. *Dermatology*, 2nd ed. Philadelphia, PA: Mosby; 2008:1088-1089.
4. Takama H, Tamada Y, Yano K, et al. Pitted keratolysis: clinical manifestations in 53 cases. *Br J Dermatol.* 1997;137(2):282-285.
5. Longshaw C, Wright J, Farrell A, et al. *Kytococcus sedentarius*, the organism associated with pitted keratolysis, produces two keratin-degrading enzymes. *J Appl Microbiol.* 2002;93(5):810-816.
6. Greywal T, Cohen PR. Pitted keratolysis: successful management with mupirocin 2% ointment monotherapy. *Dermatol Online J.* 2015;21(8).
7. Bristow IR, Lee YL. Pitted keratolysis: a clinical review. *J Am Podiatr Med Assoc.* 2014;104(2):177-182.
8. Tamura BM, Cucé LC, Souza RL, Levites J. Plantar hyperhidrosis and pitted keratolysis treated with botulinum toxin injection. *Dermatol Surg.* 2004;30(12 Pt 2):1510-1514.

125 ERYTHRASMA

Richard P. Usatine, MD
Mindy A. Smith, MD, MS

PATIENT STORY

A 59-year-old woman (with obesity and type 2 diabetes) presents with a 6-month history of a brown somewhat pruritic rash in both axillae (**Figure 125-1A**). She had been seen by multiple physicians and received many antifungal creams and topical steroids with no improvement. She had stopped wearing deodorant for fear that she was allergic to all deodorants. The rash demonstrated the classic coral red fluorescence of erythrasma (**Figure 125-1B**). The patient was given a prescription for oral erythromycin, and to her great delight the erythrasma cleared.

INTRODUCTION

Erythrasma is a chronic superficial bacterial skin infection that usually occurs in a skin fold.

EPIDEMIOLOGY

- The incidence of erythrasma is approximately 4%.[1]
- Both sexes are equally affected.
- The inguinal location is more common in men.

ETIOLOGY AND PATHOPHYSIOLOGY

- *Corynebacterium minutissimum*, a lipophilic Gram-positive non–spore-forming rod-shaped organism, is the causative agent.
- Under favorable conditions, such as heat and humidity, this organism invades and proliferates the upper one-third of the stratum corneum.
- The organism produces porphyrins that result in the coral red fluorescence seen under a Wood's lamp (**Figures 125-1** and **125-2**).

RISK FACTORS[1]

- Warm climate.
- Diabetes mellitus.
- Immunocompromised states.
- Obesity.
- Hyperhidrosis.
- Poor hygiene.
- Advanced age.

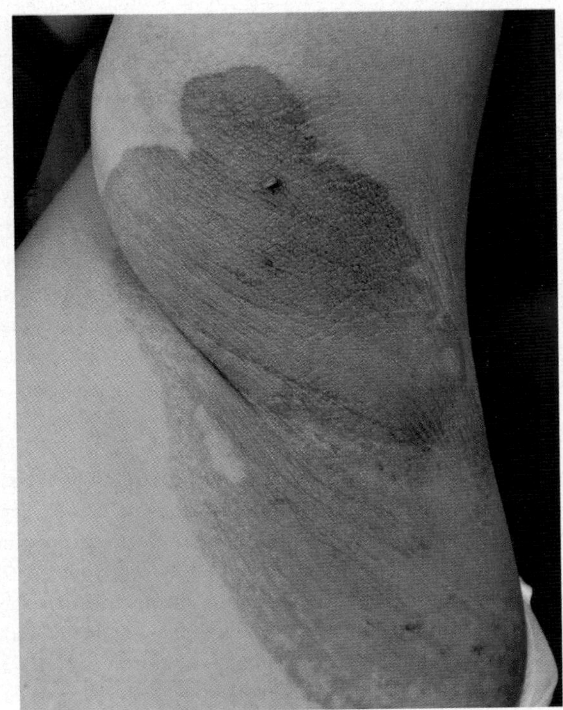

A

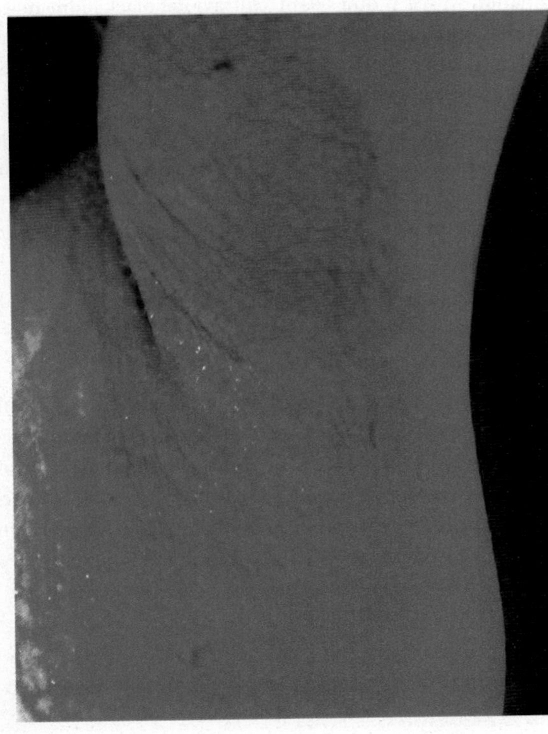

B

FIGURE 125-1 **A.** Erythrasma in the axilla of a 59-year-old woman with obesity and diabetes. **B.** Coral red fluorescence seen with a Wood's lamp. (*Reproduced with permission from Richard P. Usatine, MD.*)

DIAGNOSIS

CLINICAL FEATURES

- Erythrasma is a sharply delineated, dry, red-brown patch with slightly scaling patches. Some lesions appear redder, whereas others have a browner color (**Figures 125-3** and **125-4**).
- In a study of 151 patients, the reported signs and symptoms included pruritus in 81 patients (53.6%), erythema in 109 patients (72.2%), scaling in 145 patients (96%), and hyperhidrosis in 45 patients (29.8%).[2]
- It may appear as maceration between the toes and be mistaken for tinea pedis or coexisting with tinea pedis (**Figures 125-5** and **125-6**).[3] In a study of 182 patients with interdigital lesions in a podiatry clinic, 40% were diagnosed as having erythrasma. Diagnoses were made by Wood's lamp examination, Gram stain, and KOH preparations. The authors stated that simple and rapid diagnosis can be made with the Wood's lamp examination alone.[3]

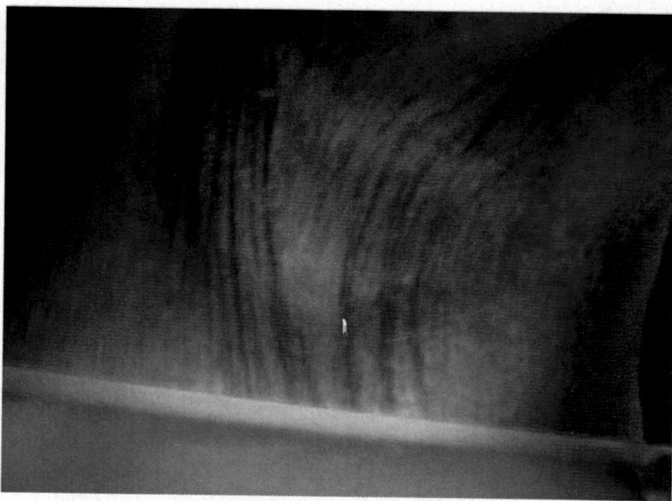

FIGURE 125-2 Coral red fluorescence seen with a Wood's lamp held in the axilla of a patient with erythrasma. (*Reproduced with permission from Richard P. Usatine, MD.*)

TYPICAL DISTRIBUTION

Erythrasma is characteristically found in the intertriginous areas, especially the axilla and the groin (**Figures 125-6** and **125-7**). Erythrasma may also be found in the interspaces of the toes, intergluteal cleft, perianal skin, and inframammary area.[2,3] In one study of 151 patients with erythrasma, the most common site noted was in the toe webs (64.9%), which was followed by the inguinal region (17.9%), the axillary region (14.6%), and the inframammary region (2.6%).[2]

LABORATORY STUDIES

- Illumination with a Wood's lamp (ultraviolet black light) reveals coral red fluorescence (**Figure 125-8**). If patients wash the area before examination, it may eliminate the fluorescence by washing away the porphyrins produced by the bacteria.
- The diagnosis may be confirmed by applying Gram stain or methylene blue stain to scrapings from the skin to reveal Gram-positive rods and dark blue granules, respectively. This is rarely performed or needed in a time when most family physicians don't have access to a microscope.
- Microscopic examination is useful if erythrasma is suspected, but the plaque does not fluoresce. The specimen can be sent to the laboratory for Gram stain and culture.
- Bacterial culture should be considered in treatment-resistant cases. In a study stimulated by erythromycin-resistant cases noted in Turkey, 40 patients with erythrasma had their lesions cultured for *C. minutissimum*.[4] They found that 95% of the cultured organisms were resistant to erythromycin. Amoxicillin/clavulanate was the most potent antibiotic in vitro, with 95% susceptibility.[4] This study suggests the value of a culture if a treatment failure occurs.

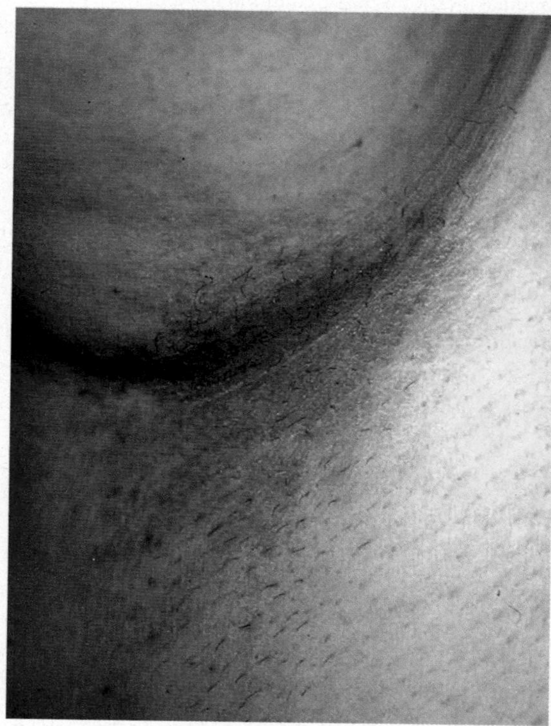

FIGURE 125-3 Reddish brown erythrasma in the axilla of an obese woman with diabetes. (*Reproduced with permission from Richard P. Usatine, MD.*)

DIFFERENTIAL DIAGNOSIS

- Psoriasis—Inverse psoriasis occurs in the same areas as erythrasma and also causes pink to red plaques with well-demarcated borders. The best way to distinguish psoriasis from erythrasma is to look for

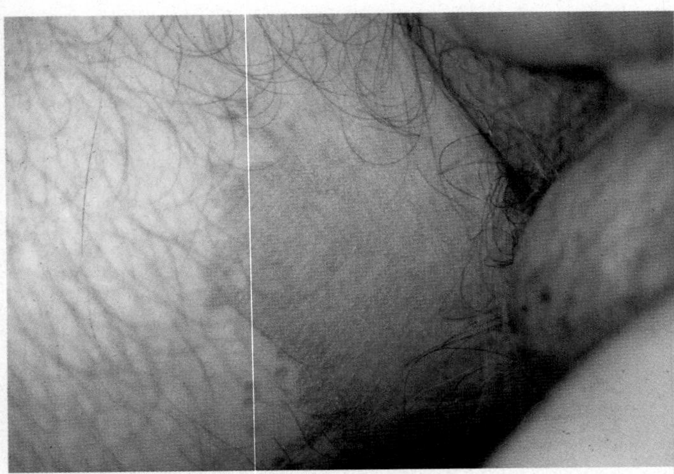

FIGURE 125-4 Brown erythrasma in the groin of a man with diabetes. (*Reproduced with permission from Richard P. Usatine, MD.*)

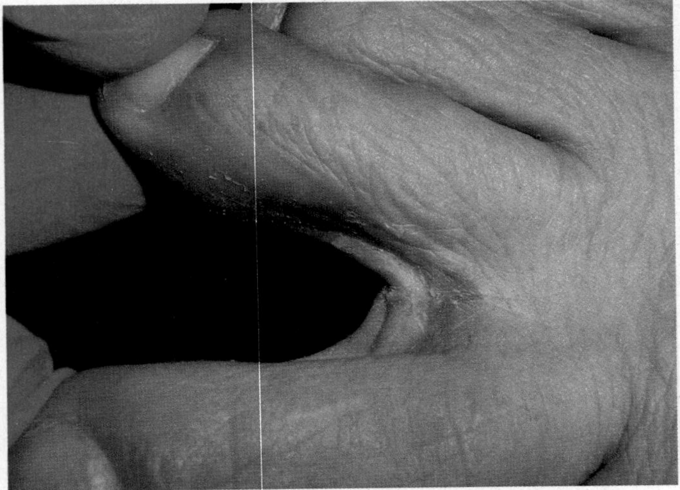

A

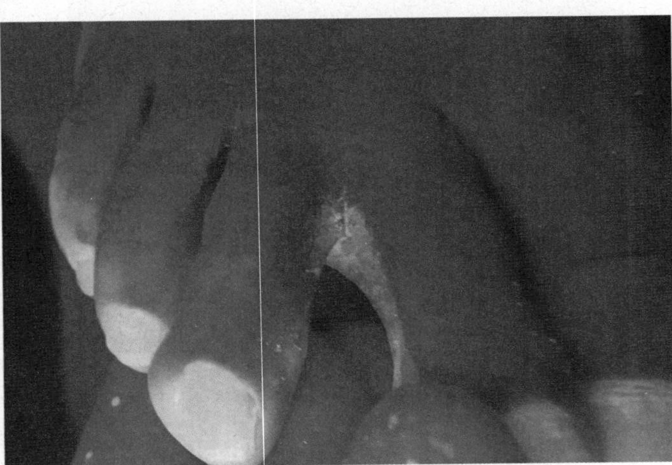

B

FIGURE 125-5 **A.** Erythrasma in the interdigital spaces of the feet in this 49-year-old woman. She presented with foot odor. **B.** Diagnosis was made by this classic coral red fluorescence seen with a Wood's lamp. (*Reproduced with permission from Richard P. Usatine, MD.*)

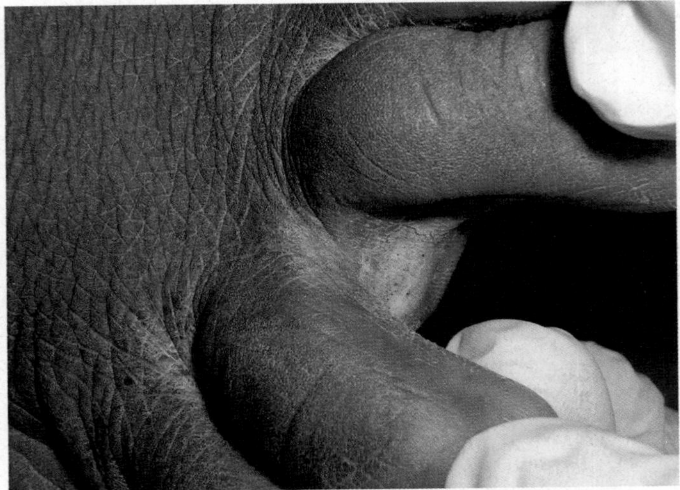

A

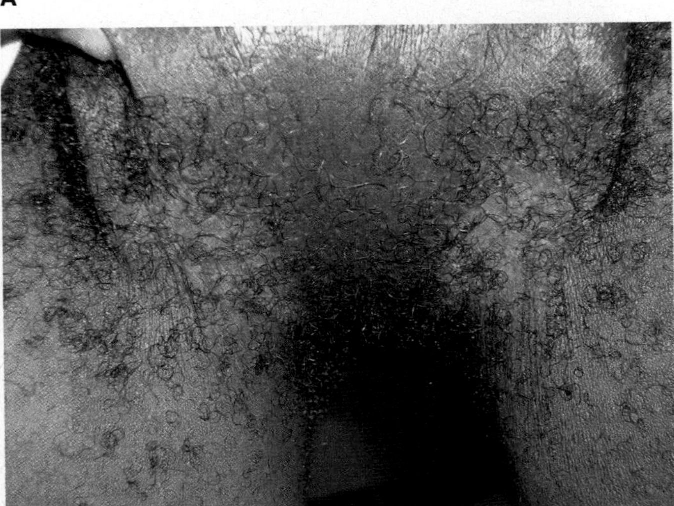

B

FIGURE 125-6 **A.** Erythrasma and tinea pedis in the interdigital spaces of the feet in this African man. This was diagnosed with a positive KOH preparation and coral red fluorescence with the Wood's lamp. **B.** His initial complaint was a pruritic rash in the groin that was also erythrasma with tinea cruris. (*Reproduced with permission from Richard P. Usatine, MD.*)

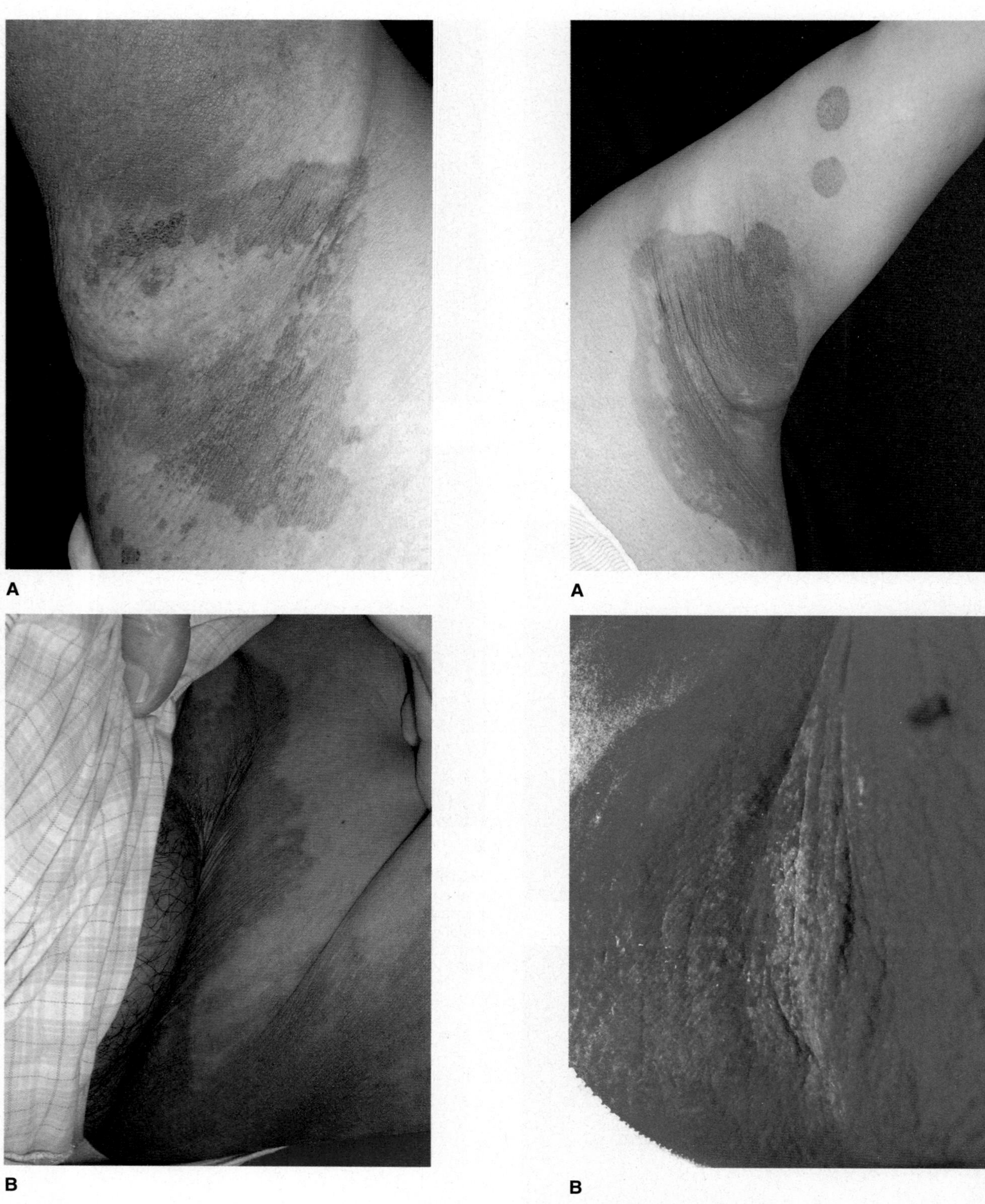

FIGURE 125-7 Erythrasma in the axilla and groin of a middle-aged woman with diabetes. **A.** Axilla. **B.** Groin. (*Reproduced with permission from Richard P. Usatine, MD.*)

FIGURE 125-8 **A.** Erythrasma in the axilla with 2 satellite areas of involvement on the upper arm. **B.** Close-up of coral red fluorescence with Wood's lamp in the same patient. (*Reproduced with permission from Richard P. Usatine, MD.*)

other clues of psoriasis in the patient, including nail pitting or onycholysis and hyperkeratotic plaques on the elbows, knees, or scalp. Also, inverse psoriasis may be seen in the intergluteal cleft as well as below the breasts or pannus in overweight individuals (see Chapter 158, Psoriasis). The Wood's lamp may help differentiate between these diagnoses.

- Dermatophytosis—Cutaneous fungal infections also closely resemble erythrasma when they occur in the axillary, inguinal areas and interdigital areas of the feet. Wood's lamp examination, KOH preparations, Gram stain, and bacterial and/or fungal cultures can help to distinguish between tinea and erythrasma. Start with Wood's lamp and a KOH preparation to minimize cost and time delays. Note that tinea and erythrasma can coexist, especially in the interdigital spaces of the feet.[3] Also, examination of the feet will frequently show tinea pedis and onychomycosis when there are tinea infections elsewhere on the body (see Chapters 144, Tinea Corporis, and 145, Tinea Cruris).
- Candidiasis—Look for satellite lesions to help distinguish candidiasis from erythrasma. Candidiasis will not fluoresce coral red, and a KOH preparation for suspected *Candida* infection should show branching pseudohyphae (see Chapter 142, Candidiasis).
- Intertrigo—This is a term for inflammation in intertriginous areas (skin folds). It is caused or exacerbated by heat, moisture, maceration, friction, and lack of air circulation. It is frequently caused by or made worse from infection with *Candida*, bacteria, or dermatophytes. Obesity and diabetes especially predispose to this condition. All efforts should be made to find coexisting infections and treat them. Patients should be counseled about the benefits of weight loss.
- Contact dermatitis to deodorants may mimic erythrasma in the axilla. The history and Wood's lamp should help to differentiate between the two conditions (see Chapter 152, Contact Dermatitis).

MANAGEMENT

FIRST LINE

NONPHARMACOLOGIC

- Good hygiene should help treat and prevent erythrasma. Bathing with soap and water should decrease some of the bacterial load. SOR C
- Consider loose-fitting cotton undergarments during treatment and to help prevent recurrence. SOR C

MEDICATIONS

- Clarithromycin 1 g (2 tabs of 500 mg) once orally has shown to have greater effectiveness (at 48 hours) than 1 g of erythromycin orally daily (either 500 mg bid or 250 mg qid) for 14 days.[2] SOR B
  - Please note there is a new FDA safety warning on clarithromycin in patients with heart disease.[5,6] The major study was based on patients with heart disease who took clarithromycin for 2 weeks.[6] While this cannot be extrapolated to a single dose, the FDA safety warning is not dose dependent, and care should be taken with patients that have pre-existing heart disease. SOR B
- Because of the new exorbitant prices of many older generic antibiotics, the cost of 2 weeks of oral erythromycin is over $300 while 2 tabs of clarithromycin can be purchased for less than $10 (GoodRx 2018). Check to make sure there will be no drug interactions with either of these oral macrolides, and take a history for heart disease.
- While topical fusidic acid had the best results in a number of studies, unfortunately it is not approved for use in the United States.[2,7,8] SOR B
- For years the treatment of choice has been reported to be oral erythromycin 250 mg 4 times a day for 14 days.[1,9] SOR B Current data in one study showed that *Corynebacterium minutissimum* has significant resistance to erythromycin.[3] However, in another study, while 1 g of clarithromycin as a single dose was better than 1 g of erythromycin daily for 14 days (when observed at 48 hours), there was no difference in outcomes at 7 and 14 days.[2]
- Topical miconazole cream has shown clearance rates as high as 88% after twice-daily application for 2 weeks.[8] While the two studies that provide this evidence are from the 1970s, this is a very reasonable choice because topical miconazole cream is over-the-counter, very affordable, and virtually side-effect free.[10,11] Also, there is no need to worry about the drug interactions that might occur with an oral macrolide antibiotic. Topical miconazole especially makes sense when it appears that the erythrasma is coexisting with tinea. This is not uncommon in the interdigital spaces between the toes and in the groin (see **Figure 125-6**). Using one OTC inexpensive cream to treat erythrasma with or without tinea is a very smart first-line treatment. SOR B

SECOND LINE

- Amoxicillin/clavulanate was the most potent antibiotic in vitro with 95% susceptibility in one study and should be considered for oral treatment if there is a treatment failure.[4] SOR B
- Topical 1% clindamycin and 2% erythromycin solution or gel applied twice daily for 2 weeks has been advocated for use by expert opinion.[1,9] SOR C While there is strong evidence for topical fusidic acid, the evidence for the available topical antibiotics in the United States is lacking.
- Topical erythromycin and clindamycin are significantly more expensive than OTC miconazole or 2 tabs of clarithromycin and have no proven benefit over these treatments.[4,5] SOR B

PROGNOSIS

- Erythrasma tends to recur if the predisposing conditions are not addressed.

FOLLOW-UP

Have the patient follow-up in 2 to 4 weeks to determine if the erythrasma has resolved.

PATIENT EDUCATION

Reassure the patient that erythrasma is curable with antibiotic treatment.

PATIENT RESOURCES

- Skinsight. *Erythrasma*—**https://www.skinsight.com/skin-conditions/adult/erythrasma**
- Dermnet NZ. *Erythrasma*—**http://www.dermnetnz.org/bacterial/erythrasma.html.**

PROVIDER RESOURCES

- Medscape. *Erythrasma*—**http://emedicine.medscape.com/article/1052532.**

REFERENCES

1. Kibbi AG, Sleiman M. *Erythrasma.* http://emedicine.medscape.com/article/1052532-overview#a0199. Updated May 2016. Accessed December 2017.
2. Avci O, Tanyildizi T, Kusku E. A comparison between the effectiveness of erythromycin, single-dose clarithromycin and topical fusidic acid in the treatment of erythrasma. *J Dermatolog Treat.* 2013;24(1):70-74.
3. Polat M, İlhan MN. The prevalence of interdigital erythrasma: a prospective study from an outpatient clinic in Turkey. *J Am Podiatr Med Assoc.* 2015;105(2):121-124.
4. Turk BG, Turkmen M, Aytimur D. Antibiotic susceptibility of *Corynebacterium minutissimum* isolated from lesions of Turkish patients with erythrasma. *J Am Acad Dermatol.* 2011;65(6):1230-1231.
5. FDA Drug Safety Communication: FDA review finds additional data supports the potential for increased long-term risks with antibiotic clarithromycin (Biaxin) in patients with heart disease. Posted February 22, 2018. https://www.fda.gov/Drugs/DrugSafety/ucm597289.htm. Accessed April 2018.
6. Winkel P, Hilden J, Fischer Hansen J, et al. Clarithromycin for stable coronary heart disease increases all-cause and cardiovascular mortality and cerebrovascular morbidity over 10 years in the CLARICOR randomised, blinded clinical trial. *Int J Cardiol.* 2015;182:459-465.
7. Chodkiewicz HM, Cohen PR. Erythrasma: successful treatment after single-dose clarithromycin. *Int J Dermatol.* 2013;52(4):516-518.
8. Hamann K, Thorn P. Systemic or local treatment of erythrasma? A comparison between erythromycin tablets and Fucidin cream in general practice. *Scand J Prim Health Care.* 1991;9(1):35-39.
9. Holdiness MR. Management of cutaneous erythrasma. *Drugs.* 2002;62(8):1131-1141.
10. Pitcher DG, Noble WC, Seville RH. Treatment of erythrasma with miconazole. *Clin Exp Dermatol.* 1979;4(4):453-456.
11. Clayton YM, Knight AG. A clinical double-blind trial of topical miconazole and clotrimazole against superficial fungal infections and erythrasma. *Clin Exp Dermatol.* 1976;1(3):225-232.

126 CELLULITIS

Richard P. Usatine, MD

PATIENT STORY

A 4-year-old child presents with a fever and a red and swollen foot (**Figure 126-1**). The patient injured her foot 3 days ago by catching it in a door. On physical examination, the foot is warm, tender, red, and swollen, and the child's temperature is 39.4°C (103°F). The clinician diagnoses cellulitis and admits the child for IV antibiotics.

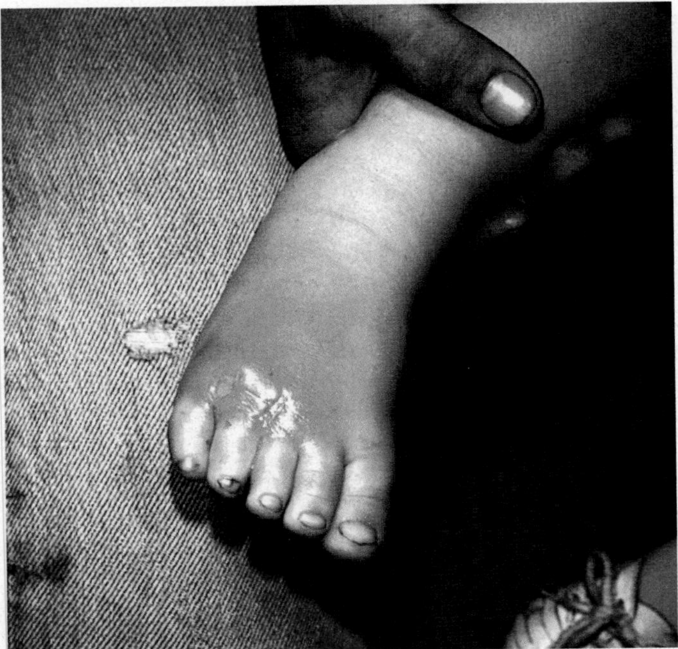

FIGURE 126-1 Cellulitis of the foot after an injury with a door in a 4-year-old girl. (*Reproduced with permission from Richard P. Usatine, MD.*)

INTRODUCTION

Cellulitis is an acute infection of the skin that involves the dermis and subcutaneous tissues. Cellulitis causes erythema, swelling, warmth, and tenderness of the involved skin. Erysipelas is a specific type of superficial cellulitis with prominent lymphatic involvement leading to a sharply defined and elevated border (see **Figure 126-6**). Purulent cellulitis is defined as the presence of pustules, purulent drainage or an abscess within or adjacent to the cellulitis.

EPIDEMIOLOGY

Cellulitis is a common skin infection, with more than 650,000 admissions per year in the United States alone.[1,2]

In the United States, an estimated 14.5 million cases annually of cellulitis account for $3.7 billion in ambulatory care costs.[1,3]

ETIOLOGY AND PATHOPHYSIOLOGY

- Cellulitis often begins with a break in the skin caused by trauma, excoriations, a bite, or an underlying skin disease (e.g., psoriasis, eczema, tinea pedis, stasis dermatitis) (**Figures 126-2** to **126-4**).

The most common causative organisms are *Streptococcus* species and *Staphylococcus aureus*.[1]

Unfortunately, cellulitis is difficult to culture from the skin, so we have few reliable data about the organisms based on direct culture of the cellulitis. If there is coexisting purulence, *S. aureus* is likely to be involved.

Data from blood cultures can be used to help us understand the microbiology of the most severe cases of cellulitis. That is because most routine cases of cellulitis do not result in bacteremia.

From a systematic review of bacteremia in cellulitis and erysipelas, the following data are available[4]:

- For cellulitis, 7.9% of 1578 patients had positive blood cultures, of which 19% were *Streptococcus pyogenes*, 38% were other β-hemolytic streptococci, 14% were *S. aureus*, and 28% were Gram-negative organisms.[4]
- For erysipelas, 4.6% of 607 patients had positive blood cultures, of which 46% were *S. pyogenes*, 29% were other β-hemolytic streptococci, 14% were *S. aureus*, and 11% were Gram-negative organisms.[4]

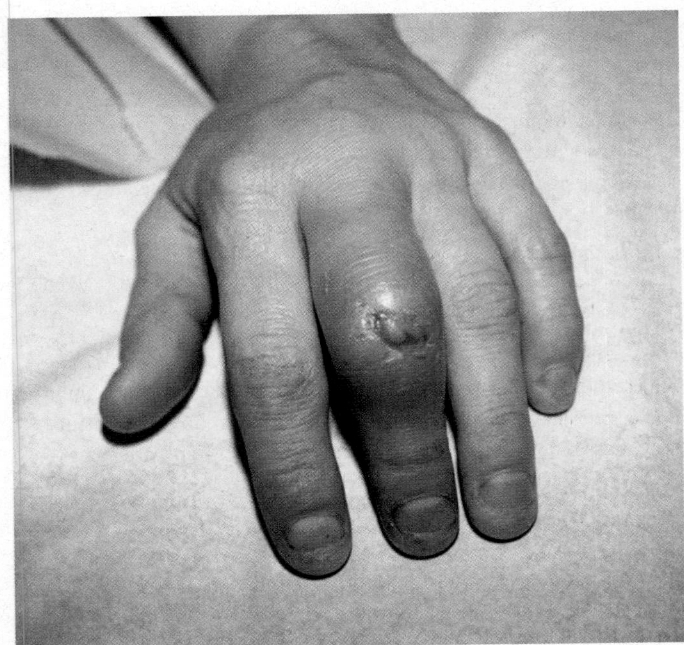

FIGURE 126-2 Cellulitis and abscess of the finger after a clenched fist injury in which the patient cut his finger on the tooth of the man he assaulted. (*Reproduced with permission from Richard P. Usatine, MD.*)

The high proportion of Gram-negative bacteria might be due to inclusion of immunocompromised patients and those with cirrhosis, exposure to aquatic injuries, or animal bites.[4]

- After a cat or dog bite, cellulitis may be caused by *Pasteurella multocida*.
- After saltwater exposure, cellulitis can be secondary to *Vibrio vulnificus* in warm climates (**Figure 126-5**). A *Vibrio vulnificus* infection can be especially deadly.
- *S. aureus* is more likely to be the causative organism in purulent cellulitis. This was demonstrated in a study of 422 patients who presented with "purulent skin and soft tissue infections" to 11 emergency departments, in which skin surface swab cultures revealed methicillin-resistant *S. aureus* (MRSA) in 59% of patients, methicillin-sensitive *S. aureus* in 17%, and β-hemolytic streptococci in 2.6%.[1,5]
- MRSA should be considered as the potential causative organism for purulent cellulitis in known high-risk populations, such as athletes, children, men who have sex with men, prisoners, military recruits, residents of long-term care facilities, individuals with previous MRSA exposure, and injection drug users.[1,6]

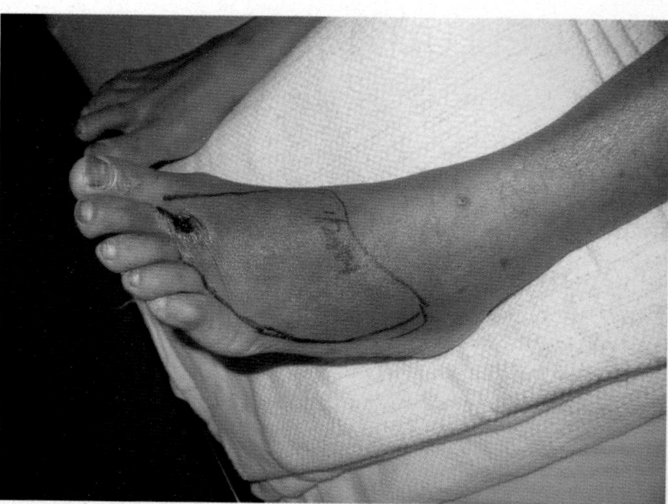

FIGURE 126-3 Cellulitis of the foot of a diabetic person in which there is possible necrosis and gangrene of the second toe, requiring hospitalization and a podiatry consult. (*Reproduced with permission from Richard P. Usatine, MD.*)

RISK FACTORS

In one meta-analysis, risk of non-purulent cellulitis of the leg was associated with[7]:

- Previous cellulitis odds ratio (OR) 40
- Coexisting wound OR 19
- Current leg ulcers OR 14
- Lymphedema/chronic leg edema OR 7
- Excoriating skin diseases OR 4
- Tinea pedis OR 3
- Body mass index > 30 OR 2.4[7]

Diabetes, smoking, and alcohol consumption were not found to be associated with an increased risk of cellulitis.[7]

In other studies, risk factors for acute and recurrent cellulitis include[8,9]:

- Psoriasis OR 4
- Diabetes OR 1.7
- Cirrhosis[9]

In a smaller case control study of recurrent lower extremity cellulitis in U.S. veterans, two physical factors—lower extremity edema and body mass index, one behavioral factor—smoking, and one demographic factor—homelessness, were significantly and independently associated with recurrent cellulitis.[10]

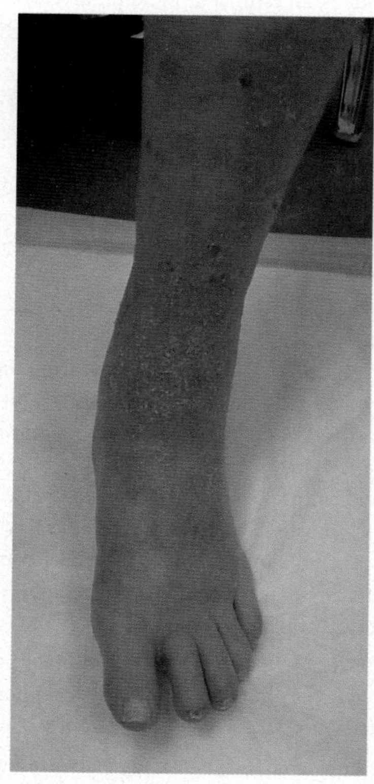

FIGURE 126-4 Cellulitis in an older man with venous stasis dermatitis. (*Reproduced with permission from Richard P. Usatine, MD.*)

DIAGNOSIS

CLINICAL FEATURES

Rubor (red), calor (warm), tumor (swollen), and dolor (painful).

TYPICAL DISTRIBUTION

Can occur on any part of the body, but is most often seen on the extremities and face (**Figures 126-1** to **126-8**). Periorbital cellulitis can be life-threatening (**Figure 126-9**). Perianal cellulitis can occur in children or adults (**Figure 126-10**).

LABORATORY TESTS

▶ Blood culture

- Cultures of blood or cutaneous aspirates, biopsies, or swabs are not routinely recommended.[11] SOR Ⓑ
- Cultures of blood and cutaneous aspirates should be considered in patients with malignancy on chemotherapy, neutropenia, severe cell-mediated immunodeficiency, immersion injuries, or animal bites.[11] SOR Ⓒ

▶ Ultrasound

- Point-of-care ultrasound is useful in identifying abscess in ED patients with skin and soft tissue infections. In cases where physical examination is equivocal, ultrasound can help physicians to distinguish abscess from cellulitis.[12] SOR Ⓑ

DIFFERENTIAL DIAGNOSIS

- Abscess—An abscess with surrounding erythema can look like cellulitis or in fact be what we call "purulent cellulitis." The red and swollen area should be palpated for fluctuance and aspiration, and/or incision and drainage should be performed to determine if an abscess is present (**Figure 126-11**).
- Deep vein thrombosis (DVT) can cause a red and swollen lower extremity. While it is rare for a patient with cellulitis or erysipelas to have a DVT as well, the diagnosis of DVT should be considered in patients with thromboembolic risk factors (e.g., hypercoagulable state from pregnancy, oral contraceptives, malignancy). If a DVT is under consideration, Doppler studies of the red and swollen lower leg should be ordered.
- Venous stasis and lymphedema—both conditions lead to swelling and erythema of the lower extremities, and both can be associated with cellulitis. In this case, venous stasis dermatitis appears like cellulitis (see **Figure 126-4**) (see Chapter 54, Venous Insufficiency).
- Allergic reactions—Allergic reactions to vaccines or bug bites may resemble cellulitis because of the erythema and swelling (**Figure 126-12**).
- Acute gout—May resemble cellulitis if there is significant cutaneous inflammation beyond the involved joint (see Chapter 102, Gout).
- Necrotizing fasciitis—Deep infection of the subcutaneous tissues and fascia with diffuse swelling, severe pain, and bullae in a toxic-appearing patient. It is important to recognize the difference between standard cellulitis and necrotizing fasciitis. Imaging procedures can detect gas in the soft tissues. Rapid progression from mild erythema to violaceous or necrotic lesions and/or bullae in a number of hours is a red flag for necrotizing fasciitis. The toxicity of the patient and the other physical findings should encourage rapid surgical consultation (see Chapter 128, Necrotizing Fasciitis).

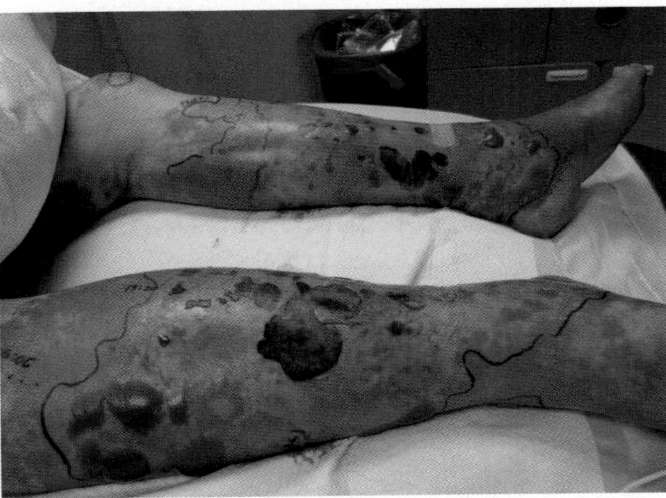

FIGURE 126-5 Fatal *Vibrio vulnificus* infection with widespread cellulitis and bullae. The violaceous bullae should be a red flag for this infection and/or necrotizing fasciitis. Even though the infection was identified early, the overwhelming sepsis resulted in death. (*Reproduced with permission from Donna Nguyen, MD.*)

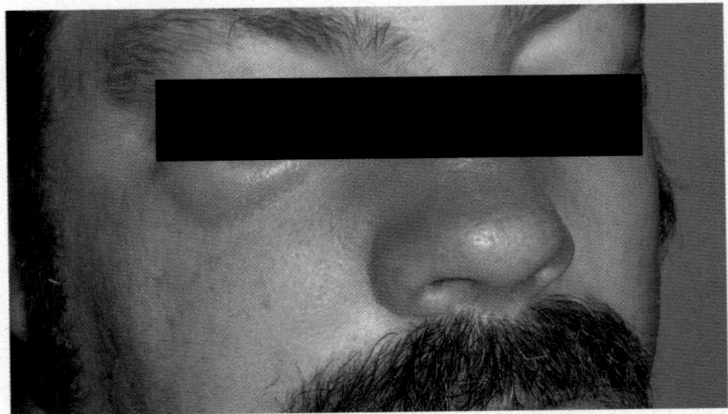

FIGURE 126-6 Erysipelas of the central face that responded well to oral antibiotic therapy. (*Reproduced with permission from Ernesto Samano Ayon, MD.*)

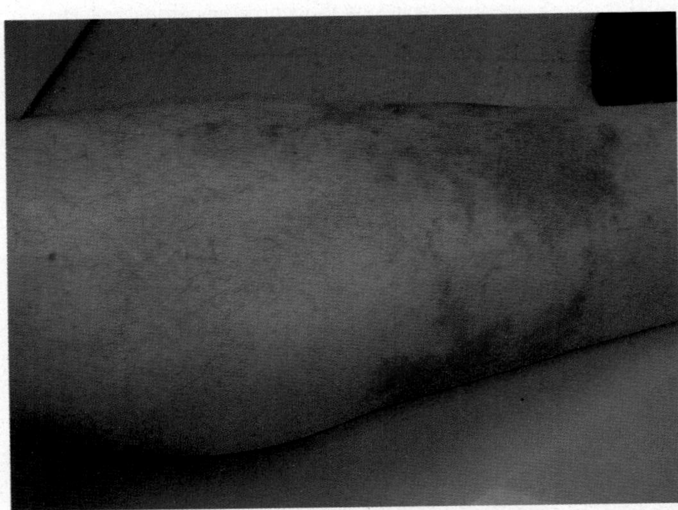

FIGURE 126-7 Cellulitis of the leg in a 55-year-old man that developed after a minor abrasion and a long plane flight. Petechiae and ecchymoses are visible and not infrequently seen in cellulitis. (*Reproduced with permission from Richard P. Usatine, MD.*)

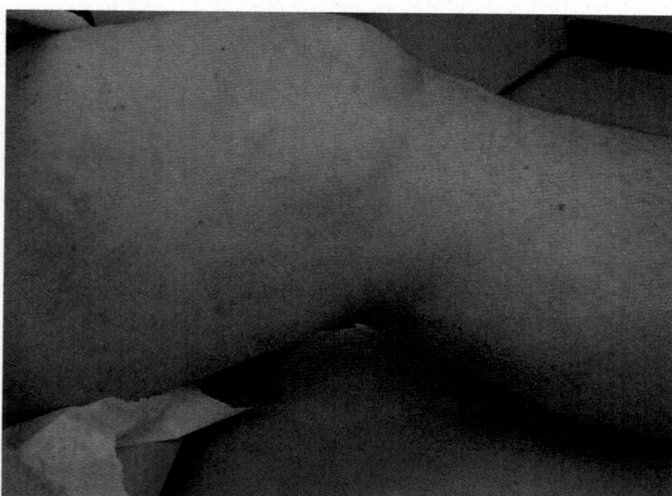

FIGURE 126-8 Ascending lymphangitis characterized by lymphatic streaking up the leg in a 55-year-old man with cellulitis. (*Reproduced with permission from Richard P. Usatine, MD.*)

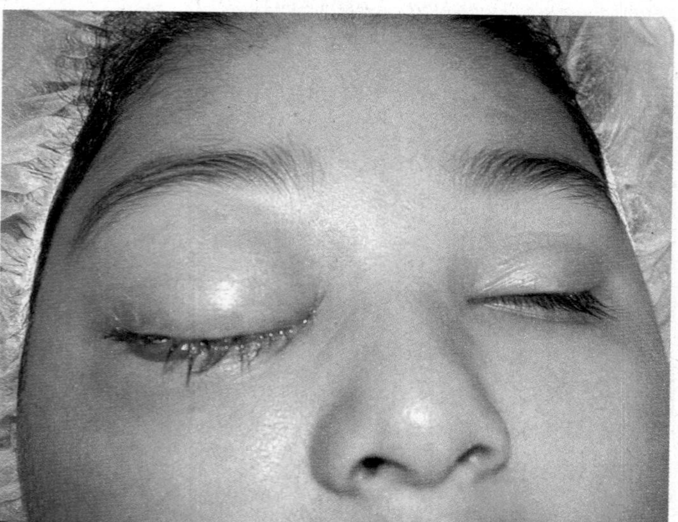

FIGURE 126-9 Life-threatening staphylococcal periorbital cellulitis requiring operative intervention. (*Reproduced with permission from Frank Miller, MD.*)

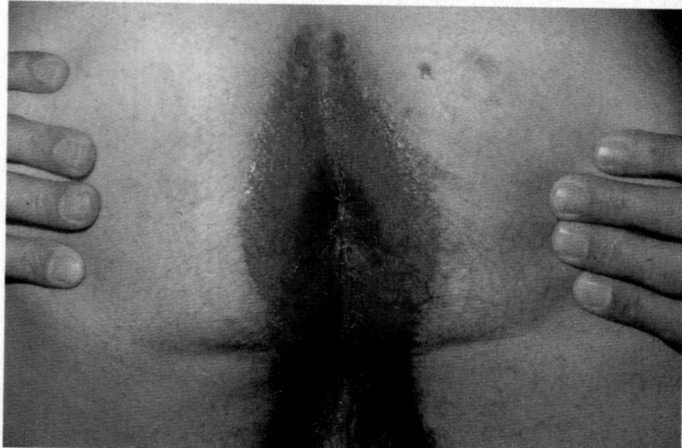

FIGURE 126-10 Severe perianal cellulitis in an adult man. (*Reproduced with permission from Jack Resneck Sr., MD.*)

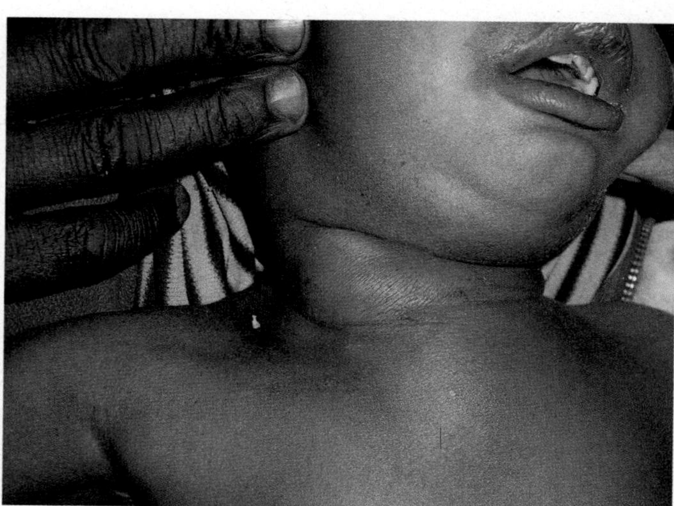

FIGURE 126-11 Cellulitis and abscess of the neck and chest in a 2-year-old girl in Ethiopia. Incision and drainage of the fluctuance over the neck revealed pus. A drain was placed to allow the pus to continue to drain from the incision site. She was treated with IV ceftriaxone, and she survived. (*Reproduced with permission from Richard P. Usatine, MD.*)

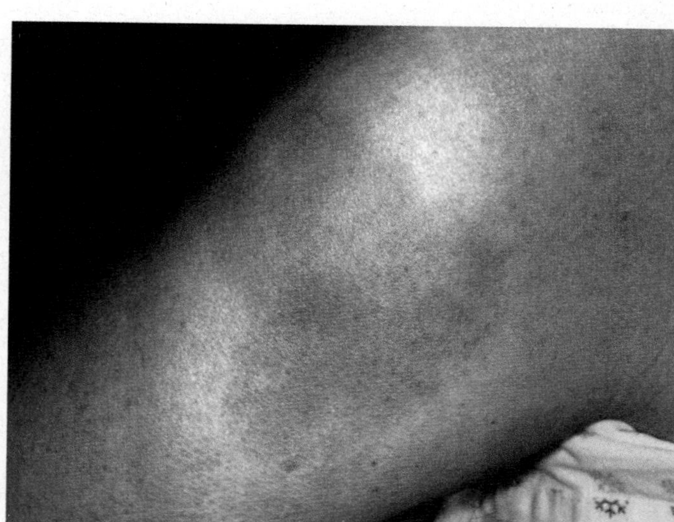

FIGURE 126-12 Redness and swelling after a pneumococcal vaccine the day before in a 66-year-old woman. This allergic reaction looks like bacterial cellulitis. It resolved with oral diphenhydramine. (*Reproduced with permission from Richard P. Usatine, MD.*)

MANAGEMENT

FIRST LINE

- Outpatient therapy is recommended for patients who do not have sepsis, altered mental status, or hemodynamic instability.[11] SOR B
- Hospitalization is recommended if there is concern for a deeper or necrotizing infection, for patients with poor adherence to therapy, for infection in a severely immunocompromised patient, or if outpatient treatment is failing.[11] SOR B
- Patients with non-purulent cellulitis without systemic signs of infection should receive an antimicrobial agent that is active against streptococci and methicillin-susceptible *S. aureus* (MSSA), such as oral cephalexin or oral dicloxacillin 500 mg four times a day for a minimum of 5 days.[11] SOR B
- The recommended duration of antimicrobial therapy is 5 days, but treatment should be extended if the infection has not improved within this time period.[11] SOR B
- Patients with cellulitis and systemic signs of infection such as fever should receive systemic antibiotics such as ceftriaxone IM and should be considered for hospitalization for IV antibiotics.[11] SOR B
- If there is significant purulence, incision and drainage should be performed.[11] SOR B Consider oral antibiotics if there is an extension of the erythema and swelling beyond the abscess; then coverage against MSSA may be sufficient.[11] SOR C
- For patients whose cellulitis is associated with penetrating trauma, evidence of MRSA infection elsewhere, nasal colonization with MRSA, injection drug use, or sepsis, IV vancomycin in the hospital may be the treatment of choice.[11] SOR B
- If MRSA is suspected and the patient is stable for outpatient treatment, appropriate oral antibiotics include trimethoprim-sulfamethoxazole (TMP-SMX), doxycycline, minocycline, and clindamycin.[11] SOR B
- One randomized controlled trial (RCT) found no significant difference between clindamycin and TMP-SMX, with respect to either efficacy or side-effect profile, for the treatment of uncomplicated skin infections, including both cellulitis and abscesses. The study involved 524 patients including 155 children (29.6%). One hundred sixty patients (30.5%) had an abscess, 280 (53.4%) had cellulitis, and 82 (15.6%) had mixed infection, defined as at least one abscess lesion and one cellulitis lesion. *S. aureus* was isolated from the lesions of 217 patients (41.4%); the isolates in 167 (77.0%) of these patients were MRSA.[13]

SECOND LINE

- In severely compromised patients, broad-spectrum intravenous antimicrobial coverage may be considered.[11] SOR C Vancomycin plus either piperacillin-tazobactam or imipenem/meropenem is recommended as an empiric regimen for such severe infections. SOR C
- Identify and treat predisposing conditions such as edema, obesity, eczema, psoriasis, lymphedema, venous insufficiency, and interdigital infections.[11] SOR B
- Elevation of the affected area and treatment of predisposing factors, such as edema or underlying cutaneous disorders, are recommended.[11] SOR B
- In lower-extremity cellulitis, clinicians should carefully examine the interdigital toe spaces for fissuring, scaling, or maceration, which may be caused by tinea pedis (see Chapter 146) and/or erythrasma (see Chapter 125). Treating these pathogens may reduce the incidence of recurrent infection. SOR A
- Systemic corticosteroids (e.g., prednisone 40 mg daily for 7 days) could be considered in nondiabetic adult patients with cellulitis.[11] SOR C
- Clinicians should consider the treatment of modifiable risk factors including leg edema, wounds, ulcers, areas of skin breakdown, and tinea pedis while administering antibiotic treatment for non-purulent cellulitis of the leg.[7] SOR B
- Given the low reported overall incidence of DVT, neither routine prophylactic anticoagulation nor systematic paraclinical investigation for DVT is indicated in low-risk patients with erysipelas or cellulitis of the lower extremities. DVT should still be considered in patients with high pretest probability or other thromboembolic risk factors.[14] SOR B

PREVENTION

Preventing cellulitis and recurrent cellulitis:

- Identify and treat predisposing conditions such as edema, obesity, eczema, psoriasis, lymphedema, venous insufficiency, and interdigital infections to prevent cellulitis and recurrent cellulitis.[7,8,11] SOR A
- When patients have recurrent cellulitis despite attempts to treat or control predisposing factors, then prophylactic antibiotics should be considered. A systematic review supports the use of oral penicillin VK or erythromycin twice daily in patients with recurrent cellulitis.[15] Meta-analysis of 5 RCTs showed that antibiotic prophylaxis reduced the risk of recurrent cellulitis by approximately 50%.[15] Antibiotics should be continued as long as the predisposing factors persist.[11,15] SOR A

PROGNOSIS

If the patient is immunocompetent without major risk factors and the case is uncomplicated, the prognosis for rapid and full recovery is excellent. However, patients who are immunocompromised and bacteremic with less common organisms are at risk for severe and fatal outcomes without rapid and aggressive treatment. Be careful to not miss necrotizing fasciitis, as this is life and limb threatening (see Chapter 128).

FOLLOW-UP

If prescribing oral outpatient therapy, consider follow-up in 2 days to assess response to the antibiotic and to determine the adequacy of outpatient therapy. If cultures are performed, make sure that the patient is on an appropriate antibiotic.

PATIENT EDUCATION

During treatment for cellulitis of an extremity, patients should elevate the involved extremity. If outpatient therapy is pursued, make sure the patient understands that an inability to tolerate the oral antibiotic is indication for seeking immediate care. Explain to the patient what their risk factors for cellulitis include. Include them in the treatment plan so that they may attempt to alter modifiable risk factors for the prevention of recurrent cellulitis. This often involves weight loss through a healthy lifestyle with good diet and exercise.

PATIENT RESOURCES

- MedlinePlus for patients—**http://www.nlm.nih.gov/medlineplus/cellulitis.html.**

PROVIDER RESOURCES

- Executive Summary: Practice Guidelines for the Diagnosis and Management of Skin and Soft Tissue Infections: 2014 Update by the Infectious Diseases Society of America—**http://cid.oxfordjournals.org/content/59/2/147.long.**
- A predictive model for diagnosis of lower extremity cellulitis: A cross-sectional study. *J Am Acad Dermatol.* 2017;76(4):618-625.

REFERENCES

1. Raff AB, Kroshinsky D. Cellulitis: a review. *JAMA.* 2016;316(3): 325-337.
2. Christensen KLY, Holman RC, Steiner CA, et al. Infectious disease hospitalizations in the United States. *Clin Infect Dis.* 2009;49(7): 1025-1035.
3. Hersh AL, Chambers HF, Maselli JH, Gonzales R. National trends in ambulatory visits and antibiotic prescribing for skin and soft-tissue infections. *Arch Intern Med.* 2008;168(14):1585-1591.
4. Gunderson CG, Martinello RA. A systematic review of bacteremias in cellulitis and erysipelas. *J Infect.* 2012;64(2):148-155.
5. Moran GJ, Krishnadasan A, Gorwitz RJ, et al. Methicillin-resistant *S. aureus* infections among patients in the emergency department. *N Engl J Med.* 2006;355:666-674.
6. Daum RS. Clinical practice. Skin and soft-tissue infections caused by methicillin-resistant *Staphylococcus aureus*. *N Engl J Med.* 2007; 357(4):380-390.
7. Quirke M, Ayoub F, McCabe A, et al. Risk factors for nonpurulent leg cellulitis: a systematic review and meta-analysis. *Br J Dermatol.* 2017;177(2):382-394.
8. Karppelin M, Siljander T, Huhtala H, et al. Recurrent cellulitis with benzathine penicillin prophylaxis is associated with diabetes and psoriasis. *Eur J Clin Microbiol Infect Dis.* 2013;32(3):369-372.
9. Hamza RE, Villyoth MP, Peter G, et al. Risk factors of cellulitis in cirrhosis and antibiotic prophylaxis in preventing recurrence. *Ann Gastroenterol.* 2014;27(4):374-379.
10. Lewis SD, Peter GS, Gómez-Marín O, Bisno AL. Risk factors for recurrent lower extremity cellulitis in a U.S. Veterans Medical Center population. *Am J Med Sci.* 2006;332(6):304-307.
11. Stevens DL, Bisno AL, Chambers HF, et al; Infectious Diseases Society of America. Practice guidelines for the diagnosis and management of skin and soft tissue infections: 2014 update by the Infectious Diseases Society of America. *Clin Infect Dis.* 2014; 59(2):e10-52.
12. Subramaniam S, Bober J, Chao J, Zehtabchi S. Point-of-care ultrasound for diagnosis of abscess in skin and soft tissue infections. *Acad Emerg Med.* 2016;23(11):1298-1306.
13. Miller LG, Daum RS, Creech CB, et al; DMID 07-0051 Team. Clindamycin versus trimethoprim-sulfamethoxazole for uncomplicated skin infections. *N Engl J Med.* 2015;372(12):1093-1103.
14. Mortazavi M, Samiee MM, Spencer FA. Incidence of deep vein thrombosis in erysipelas or cellulitis of the lower extremities. *Int J Dermatol.* 2013;52(3):279-85; quiz 284-285.
15. Oh CC, Ko HC, Lee HY, et al. Antibiotic prophylaxis for preventing recurrent cellulitis: a systematic review and meta-analysis. *J Infect.* 2014;69(1):26-34.

127 ABSCESS

Richard P. Usatine, MD

PATIENT STORY

A young man is seen in a shelter in San Antonio after being evacuated from New Orleans after the devastating floods of Hurricane Katrina (**Figure 127-1**). He has facial pain and swelling and noticeable pus near the eye. His vision is normal. The area is anesthetized with lidocaine and epinephrine. The abscess is drained with a #11 blade. The patient is started on oral trimethoprim/sulfamethoxazole double-strength, two tablets twice daily, because of the proximity to the eye and the local erythema and swelling that could represent early cellulitis. A culture to look for methicillin-resistant *Staphylococcus aureus* (MRSA) was not available in the shelter, but close follow-up was set for the next day, and the patient was doing much better.

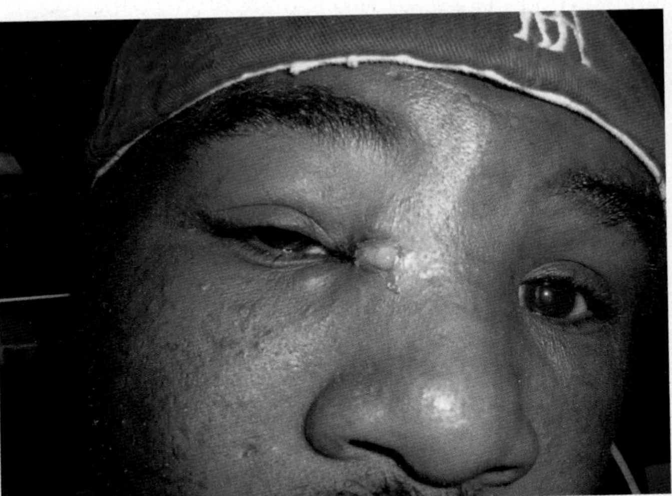

FIGURE 127-1 Abscess seen on the face of a man after evacuation from the floodwaters of New Orleans following Hurricane Katrina. *(Reproduced with permission from Richard P. Usatine, MD.)*

INTRODUCTION

An abscess is a collection of pus in infected tissues. The abscess represents a walled-off infection in which there is a pocket of purulence. In abscesses of the skin, the offending organism is almost always *S. aureus*.[1]

EPIDEMIOLOGY

- MRSA was the most common identifiable cause of skin and soft-tissue infections (including abscesses) among patients presenting to emergency departments in 11 U.S. cities. *S. aureus* was isolated from 76% of these infections, and 59% were community-acquired MRSA.[2]

ETIOLOGY AND PATHOPHYSIOLOGY

- Most cutaneous abscesses are caused by *S. aureus*.[1,3]
- MRSA is the most common type of *S. aureus* found in abscesses (**Figures 127-2** and **127-3**).
- One study that evaluated management of skin abscesses drained in the emergency department showed that there was no significant association between amount of surrounding cellulitis or abscess size and the likelihood of MRSA-positive cultures.[4]
- A dental abscess can spread into tissue outside the mouth, as in the person experiencing homelessness in **Figure 127-4**.

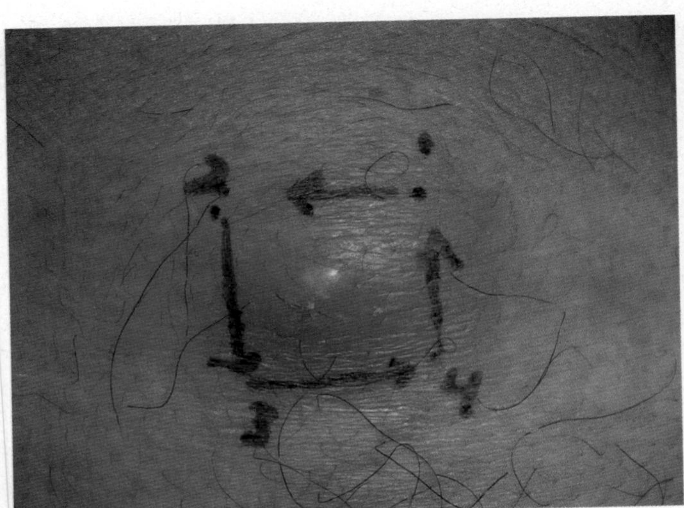

FIGURE 127-2 MRSA abscess on the back of the neck that patient thought was a spider bite. Note that a ring block was drawn around the abscess with a surgical marker to demonstrate how to perform this block. *(Reproduced with permission from Richard P. Usatine, MD.)*

RISK FACTORS

- Intravenous drug use.
- Homelessness (**Figure 127-4**).

- Dental disease (**Figure 127-4**).
- Contact sports.
- Incarceration.
- Previous MRSA infection and colonization.
- Recent hospitalization.[4]

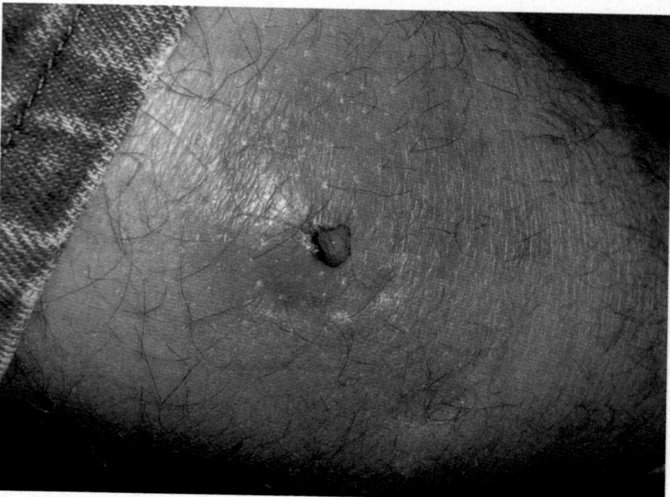

FIGURE 127-3 Large MRSA abscess on the leg in a 62-year-old man beginning to drain spontaneously. The abscess cavity was large, and patient was placed on trimethoprim-sulfamethoxazole (TMP-SMX) to cover the surrounding cellulitis. (*Reproduced with permission from Richard P. Usatine, MD.*)

DIAGNOSIS

CLINICAL FEATURES

Collection of pus in or below the skin. Patients often feel pain and have tenderness at the involved site. There is swelling, erythema, warmth, and fluctuance in most cases (**Figures 127-1** to **127-5**). Determine if the patient is febrile and if there is surrounding cellulitis.

TYPICAL DISTRIBUTION

Skin abscesses can be found anywhere from head to feet. Frequent sites include the hands, feet, extremities, head, neck, buttocks, and breast (**Figure 127-5**).

LABORATORY STUDIES

Clinical cure is often obtained with incision and drainage (I&D) alone, so the benefits of pathogen identification and sensitivities are low in low-risk patients.[2] Most clinical studies have excluded patients who were immunocompromised, diabetic, or had other significant comorbidities.[2] Consequently, it may be reasonable to obtain wound cultures in high-risk patients, those with signs of systemic infection, and in patients with history of high recurrence rates.[2,3]

The Infectious Diseases Society of America (IDSA) states:

1. Gram stain and culture of pus from carbuncles and abscesses are recommended, but treatment without these studies is reasonable in typical cases.[3]
2. Gram stain and culture of pus from inflamed epidermoid cysts are not recommended.[3]

DIFFERENTIAL DIAGNOSIS

- Epidermal inclusion cyst with inflammation/infection—These cysts (also known as epidermoid cysts) can become inflamed, swollen, and superinfected. Although the initial erythema may be sterile inflammation, these cysts can become infected with *S. aureus*. The treatment consists of I&D and antibiotics if cellulitis is also present. If these are removed before they become inflamed, the cyst may come out intact (**Figure 127-6**).
- Cellulitis with swelling and no pocket of pus—When it is unclear if an area of infected skin has an abscess, needle aspiration with a large-gauge needle may be helpful to determine whether to incise the skin. Cellulitis alone should have no area of fluctuance (see Chapter 126, Cellulitis).
- Hidradenitis suppurativa—Recurrent inflammatory cysts surrounding the pilosebaceous units of the axilla, inguinal areas, breasts, and buttocks (see Chapter 121, Hidradenitis Suppurativa). These often respond better to intralesional injection with

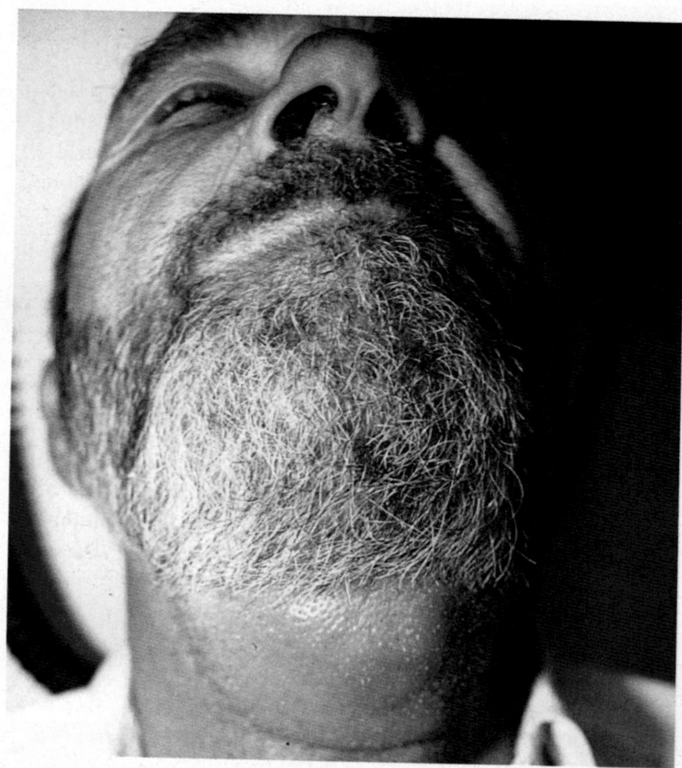

FIGURE 127-4 Neck abscess secondary to dental abscess in a homeless man. This was drained in the operating room by an ear, nose, and throat (ENT) surgeon. (*Reproduced with permission from Richard P. Usatine, MD.*)

triamcinolone than to I&D.[5] Incision of these areas of purulence can be painful and not better than intralesional injections.

- Furuncles and carbuncles—A furuncle or boil is an abscess that starts in a hair follicle or sweat gland. A carbuncle is larger and occurs when the furuncle extends into the subcutaneous tissue.
- Acne cysts—More sterile inflammation than true abscess; often better to inject with triamcinolone rather than incise and drain (see Chapter 118, Acne Vulgaris).
- Pilonidal disease—This consists of cysts, abscesses, and/or sinus tracts around the coccygeal area that may begin with ingrown hairs. It may start like an epidermal cyst but can become an abscess and develop sinus tracts to the skin. Although this disease may involve an abscess, it is more complex to treat than a simple abscess. Definitive treatment to prevent recurrence requires surgery by an experienced surgeon in the operating room (**Figure 127-7**).

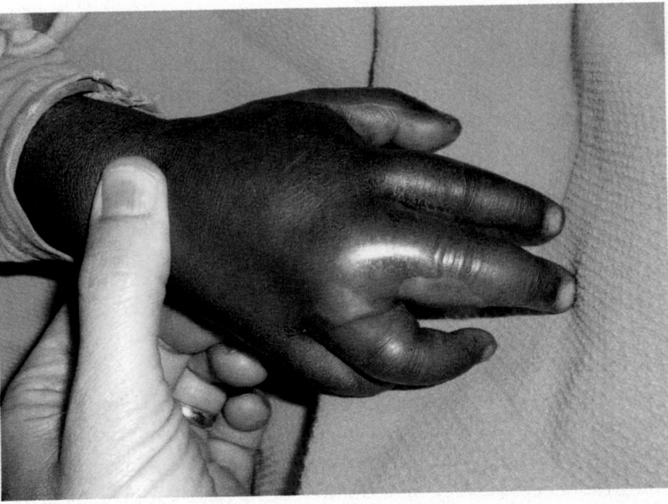

FIGURE 127-5 A large abscess of the hand in a 2-year-old girl in Ethiopia. Incision and drainage was performed, and antibiotics were given to cover the surrounding cellulitis and any deeper infections. (*Reproduced with permission from Richard P. Usatine, MD.*)

MANAGEMENT

FIRST LINE

- The evidence strongly supports I&D of an abscess.[3,4,6] SOR Ⓐ Using a 27-gauge needle, inject 1% lidocaine with epinephrine into the skin at the site you plan to open. A ring block can be helpful rather than injecting into the abscess itself (see **Figure 127-3**). Open the abscess with a linear incision using a #11 blade scalpel, following skin lines if possible.[7]

Based on the recommendations of the Infectious Diseases Society of America (IDSA) in their evidence-based review of the literature, the following management recommendations are made:

- I&D is the recommended treatment for abscesses, inflamed epidermoid cysts, carbuncles, and large furuncles.[3] SOR Ⓐ
- The decision to administer antibiotics directed against *S. aureus* as an adjunct to I&D should be made based on the presence or absence of systemic inflammatory response syndrome (SIRS), such as temperature >38°C or <36°C, tachypnea >24 breaths per minute, tachycardia >90 beats per minute, or white blood cell count >12,000 or <400 cells/μL.[3] SOR Ⓐ
- An antibiotic active against MRSA is recommended for patients with carbuncles or abscesses who have failed initial antibiotic treatment or have markedly impaired host defenses or in patients with SIRS and hypotension.[3] SOR Ⓐ

After the IDSA published its recommendations, a new, somewhat revolutionary study was published in the *New England Journal of Medicine* in 2016 which concluded that in settings in which MRSA was prevalent, trimethoprim-sulfamethoxazole treatment resulted in a higher cure rate among patients with a drained cutaneous abscess than placebo.[8] This was a randomized trial performed at five U.S. emergency departments with over a thousand participants. Clinical cure occurred in 92.9% of the trimethoprim-sulfamethoxazole group versus 85.7% in the placebo group (number needed to treat [NNT] =14). The trimethoprim-sulfamethoxazole group was superior to placebo in lower rates of subsequent surgical drainage procedures (3.4% vs. 8.6%) and skin infections at new sites (3.1% vs. 10.3%).[8]

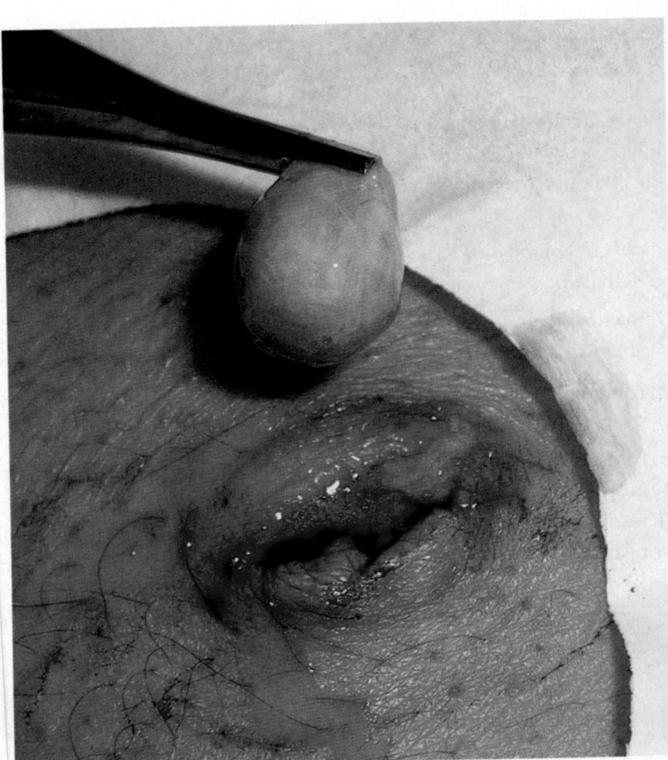

FIGURE 127-6 Epidermal inclusion cyst removed intact. There is no need for antibiotics in this case. (*Reproduced with permission from Richard P. Usatine, MD.*)

SECOND LINE

Although many physicians still pack a drained abscess with ribbon gauze, there is limited data on whether or not packing of an abscess cavity improves outcomes. A small study concluded that routine packing of simple cutaneous abscesses is painful and probably unnecessary.[9] SOR Ⓒ The author of this chapter often packs abscesses lightly to provide hemostasis and has the patient remove the packing in the shower 2 days later, avoiding additional visits and painful repacking of the healing cavity. SOR Ⓒ However, if a large abscess is not packed, it can seal over and the pus may reaccumulate. A large abscess may do better with multiple episodes of repacking with return visits to monitor the treatment progress. SOR Ⓒ

An alternative to open I&D for community-acquired soft tissue abscesses in children is the placement of a subcutaneous drain.[10] All of these procedures were done with conscious sedation or in the operating room because they were children being cared for in hospital by a surgical team. Stab incisions were made at each end of the abscess cavity, and the skin bridge overlying the abscess was left intact. A subcutaneous drain (Penrose catheter) was placed into one of the stab incisions and pulled through the counter incision, traversing the entire abscess cavity. The ends of the drains were secured by tying the two ends together. The wounds were irrigated with normal saline either through the incision or via the stab incisions using angiocaths. The results were as good as the I&D cases and were reported to have a better cosmetic appearance once healed and thought to be less painful for the children.[10] SOR Ⓑ However, the children in the I&D group had daily repacking of their wounds and this is truly painful, traumatic and probably unnecessary. This procedure is being performed in adults as well but probably has no real benefit over an I&D.

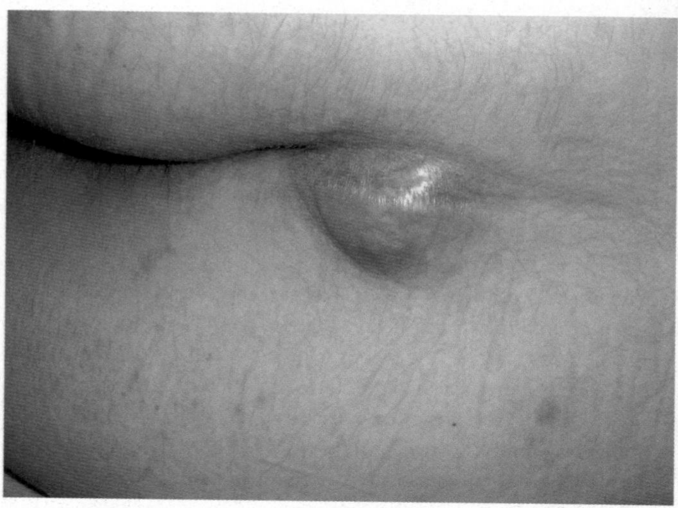

FIGURE 127-7 Recurrent pilonidal cyst in a 30-year-old pregnant woman. (*Reproduced with permission from Richard P. Usatine, MD.*)

PREVENTION

For recurrent skin abscesses, based on the recommendations of the Infectious Diseases Society of America in their evidence-based review of the literature, the following management recommendations are made[3]:

- A recurrent abscess at a site of previous infection should prompt a search for local causes such as a pilonidal cyst (see **Figure 127-7**), hidradenitis suppurativa (see Chapter 121), or foreign material.[3] SOR Ⓐ
- Recurrent abscesses should be drained and cultured early in the course of infection.[3] SOR Ⓐ
- After obtaining cultures of recurrent abscess, treat with a 5- to 10-day course of an antibiotic active against the pathogen isolated.[3] SOR Ⓒ
- Consider a 5-day decolonization regimen twice daily of intranasal mupirocin, daily chlorhexidine washes, and frequent hot water washing of personal items such as towels, sheets, and clothes for recurrent *S. aureus* infection.[3] SOR Ⓒ
- Adult patients should be evaluated for neutrophil disorders if recurrent abscesses began in early childhood.[3] SOR Ⓐ

PROGNOSIS

The prognosis for a simple abscess is generally excellent, and even in MRSA-prevalent areas a simple I&D results in cure rates of over 85%.[8] Some abscesses will need to be treated with adjunct antibiotics or need a second surgical drainage.[8] When an abscess does not heal as expected, consider other diagnoses including hidradenitis and pilonidal cysts, depending on the location of the disease.[3]

FOLLOW-UP

In patients or wounds at higher risk for complications, follow-up should be scheduled in 24 to 48 hours. If packing was placed, the patient or a family member can remove it if follow-up is not needed.

PATIENT EDUCATION

Patients may shower daily 24 to 48 hours after I&D and then reapply dressings. Patients should be given return precautions for worsening of symptoms and if there is continued redness, pain, or purulent drainage.

PATIENT RESOURCES

- **http://www.skinsight.com/adult/abscess.htm.**

PROVIDER RESOURCES

- Executive Summary: Practice Guidelines for the Diagnosis and Management of Skin and Soft Tissue Infections: 2014 Update by the Infectious Diseases Society of America—**http://cid.oxfordjournals.org/content/59/2/147.long#content-block.**

REFERENCES

1. Johnson RC, Ellis MW, Schlett CD, et al. Bacterial etiology and risk factors associated with cellulitis and purulent skin abscesses in military trainees. Seleem MN, ed. *PLoS One*. 2016;11(10):e0165491.
2. Moran GJ, Krishnadasan A, Gorwitz RJ, et al. Methicillin-resistant *S. aureus* infections among patients in the emergency department. *N Engl J Med*. 355(7):666-674.
3. Stevens DL, Bisno AL, Chambers HF, et al. Practice guidelines for the diagnosis and management of skin and soft tissue infections: 2014 update by the Infectious Diseases Society of America. *Clin Infect Dis*. 2014;59(2):e10-52.
4. Gillian R. How do you treat an abscess in the era of increased community-associated methicillin-resistant *Staphylococcus aureus* (MRSA)? *J Emerg Med*. 41(3):276-281.
5. Riis PT, Boer J, Prens EP, et al. Intralesional triamcinolone for flares of hidradenitis suppurativa (HS): a case series. *J Am Acad Dermatol*. 2016;75(6):1151-1155.
6. Sorensen C, Hjortrup A, Moesgaard F, Lykkegaard-Nielsen M. Linear incision and curettage vs. deroofing and drainage in subcutaneous abscess. A randomized clinical trial. *Acta Chir Scand*. 153(11-12):659-660.
7. Usatine R, Stulberg D, Pfenninger J, Small R. *Dermatologic and Cosmetic Procedures in Office Practice*. Philadelphia, PA: Elsevier/Saunders; 2012.
8. Talan DA, Mower WR, Krishnadasan A, et al. Trimethoprim-sulfamethoxazole versus placebo for uncomplicated skin abscess. *N Engl J Med*. 2016;374(9):823-832.
9. O'Malley GF, Dominici P, Giraldo P, et al. Routine packing of simple cutaneous abscesses is painful and probably unnecessary. *Acad Emerg Med*. 2009;16(5):470-473.
10. McNamara WF, Hartin CW Jr., Escobar MA, et al. An alternative to open incision and drainage for community-acquired soft tissue abscesses in children. *J Pediatr Surg*. 2011;46(3):502-506.

128 NECROTIZING FASCIITIS

Richard P. Usatine, MD

PATIENT STORY

A 54-year-old woman with diabetes was brought to the emergency department with right leg swelling, fever, and altered mental status.[1] The patient noted a pimple in her groin 5 days earlier and over the past few days had increasing leg pain. Her right leg was tender, red, hot, and swollen (**Figure 128-1**). Large bullae were present. Her temperature was 38.9°C (102°F) and her blood sugar was 573. The skin had a "woody" feel, and a radiograph of her leg showed gas in the muscles and soft tissues (**Figure 128-2**). She was taken to the operating room for debridement of her necrotizing fasciitis. Broad-spectrum antibiotics were also started, but the infection continued to advance quickly. The patient died the following day; her wound culture later grew *Escherichia coli, Proteus vulgaris, Corynebacterium, Enterococcus, Staphylococcus* sp., and *Peptostreptococcus.*[1]

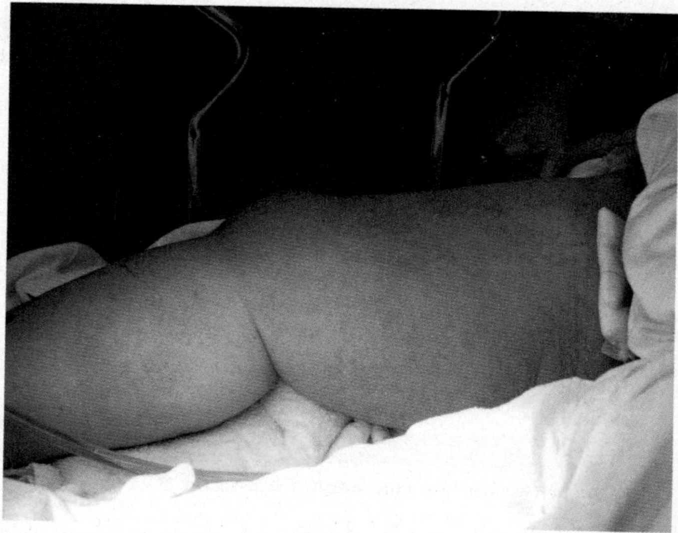

FIGURE 128-1 Necrotizing fasciitis on the leg and groin showing erythema, swelling, and bullae. *(Reproduced with permission from Dufel S, Martino M. Simple cellulitis or a more serious infection? J Fam Pract. 2006;55(5):396-400. Frontline Medical Communications, Inc.)*

INTRODUCTION

Necrotizing fasciitis (NF) is a rapidly progressive infection of the deep fascia, with necrosis of the subcutaneous tissues. It usually occurs after surgery or trauma. Patients have erythema and pain disproportionate to the physical findings. Immediate surgical debridement and antibiotic therapy should be initiated.[2]

SYNONYMS

- Flesh-eating bacteria, necrotizing soft-tissue infection (NSTI), suppurative fasciitis, hospital gangrene, and necrotizing erysipelas. Fournier gangrene is a type of NF or NSTI in the genital and perineal region.[3]

EPIDEMIOLOGY

- Incidence in adults is 0.40 cases per 100,000 population.[4]
- NF caused by *Streptococcus pyogenes* is the most common form of NF.[4]

ETIOLOGY AND PATHOPHYSIOLOGY

- Type I NF is a polymicrobial infection with aerobic and anaerobic bacteria:
  - Frequently caused by enteric Gram-negative pathogens including Enterobacteriaceae organisms and *Bacteroides*.
  - Can occur with Gram-positive organisms such as non–group A streptococci and *Peptostreptococcus.*[5]
  - Saltwater variant can occur with penetrating trauma or an open wound contaminated with saltwater containing marine vibrios. *Vibrio vulnificus* is the most virulent.[6]
  - Up to 15 pathogens have been isolated in a single wound.
  - Average of five different isolates per wound.[7]

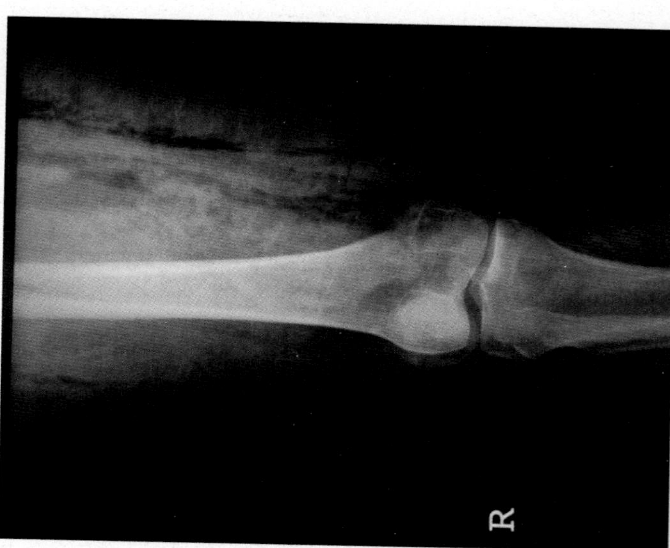

FIGURE 128-2 Radiograph of the patient's leg showing gas in the soft tissues and muscles. *(Reproduced with permission from Dufel S, Martino M. Simple cellulitis or a more serious infection? J Fam Pract. 2006;55(5):396-400. Frontline Medical Communications, Inc.)*[1]

- Type II NF occurs from common skin organisms:
  - Generally a monomicrobial infection caused by *S. pyogenes*:
    - May occur in combination with *Staphylococcus aureus*.
    - Methicillin-resistant *S. aureus* is no longer a rare cause of NF.[5]
    - *S. pyogenes* strains may produce pyrogenic exotoxins, which act as superantigens to stimulate production of tumor necrosis factor (TNF)-α, TNF-β, interleukin (IL)-1, IL-6, and IL-2.[7]

RISK FACTORS

- Risk factors for type I NF (polymicrobial):
  - Diabetes mellitus.
  - Severe peripheral vascular disease.
  - Obesity.
  - Alcoholism and cirrhosis.
  - Intravenous drug use.
  - Decubitus ulcers.
  - Poor nutritional status.
  - Postoperative patients or those with penetrating trauma.
  - Abscess of the female genital tract.
- Risk factors of type II NF (group A β-hemolytic *Streptococcus* [GABHS] and *S. aureus*):
  - Diabetes mellitus.
  - Severe peripheral vascular disease.
  - Recent parturition (**Figure 128-3**).
  - Trauma.
  - Varicella.[5]

DIAGNOSIS

Early recognition based on signs and symptoms is potentially lifesaving. Although lab tests and imaging studies can confirm one's clinical impression, rapid treatment with antibiotics and surgery is crucial to improving survival.

CLINICAL FEATURES

- Rapid progression of erythema to violaceous skin and bullae (**Figures 128-4** and **128-5**), necrosis and gangrene (**Figures 128-6** and **128-7**).
- The skin can become gangrenous and develop a black eschar.[2]
- Edematous, wooden feel of subcutaneous tissues extending beyond the margin of erythema.
- High fevers and severe systemic toxicity.
- Unrelenting intense pain out of proportion to cutaneous findings.
- Pain progresses to cutaneous anesthesia as disease evolves. Anesthesia of the skin develops as a result of infarction of cutaneous nerves.[2]
- Crepitus occurs when there is gas in the soft tissues.
- Unresponsive to empiric antimicrobial therapy.

TYPICAL DISTRIBUTION

- May occur at any anatomic location.
- Majority of cases occur on the lower extremities (see **Figures 128-5** and **128-7**) but can occur on the upper extremities.

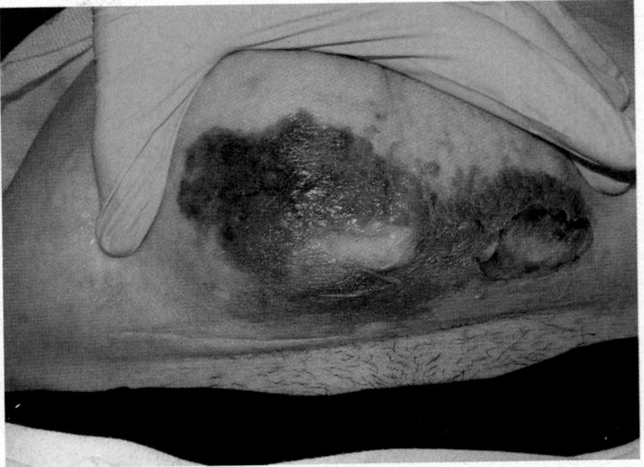

FIGURE 128-3 Necrotizing fasciitis with violaceous color of the skin on the affected skin above the C-section. (*Reproduced with permission from Michael Babcock, MD.*)

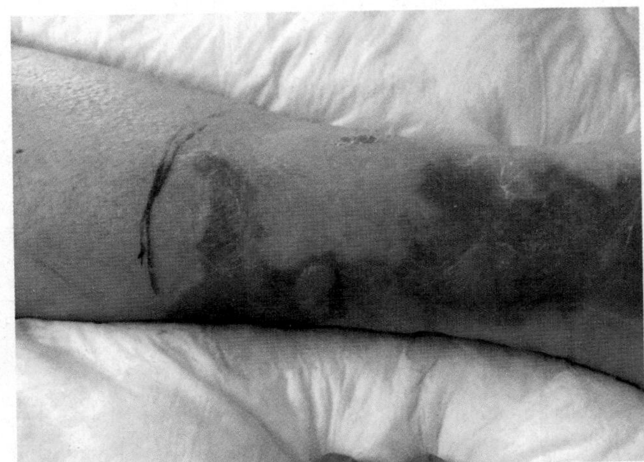

FIGURE 128-4 Necrotizing fasciitis with violaceous color and large bullae of the skin on the affected leg. (*Reproduced with permission from Milton Moore, MD.*)

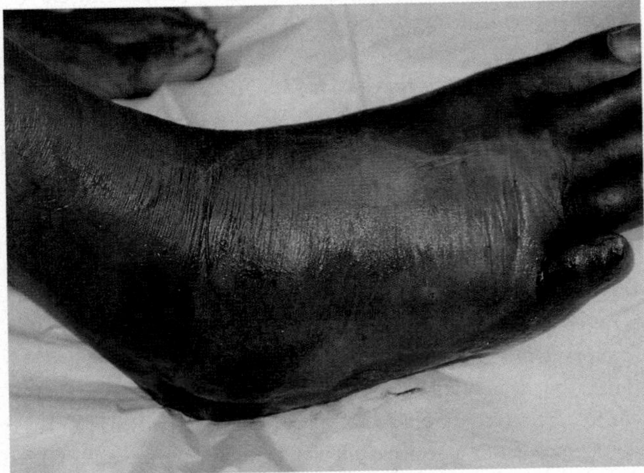

FIGURE 128-5 Necrotizing fasciitis that started when patient stepped on a nail. A large flaccid bulla is visible along with swelling and erythema. A rapid below the knee amputation allowed this patient to survive. (*Reproduced with permission from Subramaniam R, Shirley OB. Oozing puncture wound on foot. J Fam Pract. 2009 Jan;58(1):37-39. Frontline Medical Communications, Inc.*)

- Also common on abdominal wall (see **Figure 128-4**) and in perineum (Fournier gangrene).

LABORATORY AND IMAGING

- Routine laboratory tests are nonspecific but common findings include an elevated white blood cell count (WBC), a low serum sodium, and a high blood urea nitrogen (BUN).
- Histology and culture of deep tissue biopsy are essential; surface cultures cannot be relied on alone. Gram staining of the exudate may provide clues about the pathogens while the physician awaits culture results.[2]
- Standard radiographs are of little value unless air is demonstrated in the tissues (see **Figure 128-2**).
- Radiography, CT, ultrasonography, and MRI can be used to detect gas within soft tissues or muscles.[2]
- Although imaging may help delineate the extent of disease, it should not delay surgical consultation.

BIOPSY

- Gross examination reveals swollen, dull, gray fascia with stringy areas of necrosis.[6]
- Necrosis of superficial fascia and fat produces watery, foul-smelling "dishwater pus."[2]
- Histology demonstrates subcutaneous fat necrosis, vasculitis, and local hemorrhage.[2]

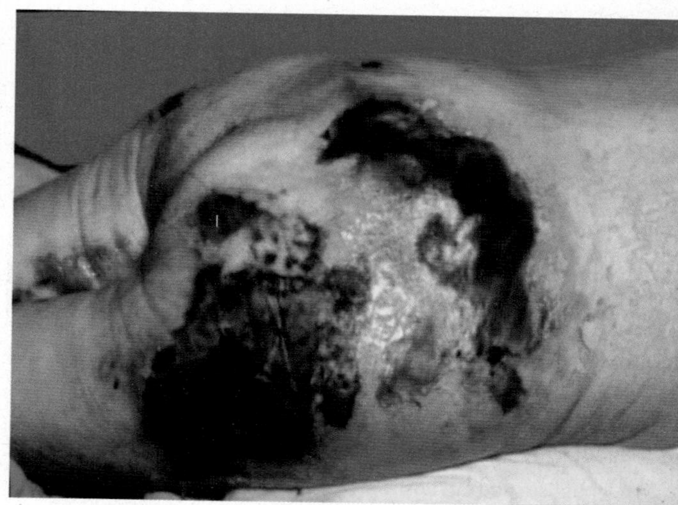

FIGURE 128-6 Necrotizing fasciitis with gangrene. Even with a radical hemipelvectomy this patient did not survive. (*Reproduced with permission from Fred Bongard, MD.*)

DIFFERENTIAL DIAGNOSIS

- Cellulitis—Acute spreading infection of skin and soft tissues characterized by erythema, edema, pain, and calor. Rapid progression of disease despite antibiotics, systemic toxicity, intense pain, and skin necrosis suggest NF rather than cellulitis (see Chapter 126, Cellulitis).
- Pyomyositis—Suppuration within individual skeletal muscle groups. Synergistic necrotizing cellulitis is an NSTI that involves muscle groups in addition to superficial tissues and fascia.[7] Although pyomyositis may occur with NF, it can occur independent of cutaneous and soft-tissue infections. Imaging of the muscle confirms the diagnosis.
- Clostridial myonecrosis—Acute necrotizing infection of muscle tissue caused by clostridial organisms. Surgical exploration and cultures are required to differentiate from NF.
- Erythema induratum—Tender, erythematous subcutaneous nodules occurring on the lower legs (especially the calves). Lack of fever, systemic toxicity, and skin necrosis suggest erythema induratum rather than NF. Lesions of erythema induratum may have a chronic, recurrent course, and the patient frequently has a history of tuberculosis or a positive purified protein derivative (PPD) test.
- Streptococcal or staphylococcal toxic shock syndrome—Systemic inflammatory response to a toxin-producing bacteria characterized by fever, hypotension, generalized erythroderma, myalgia, and multisystem organ involvement. NF may occur as part of the toxic shock syndrome.

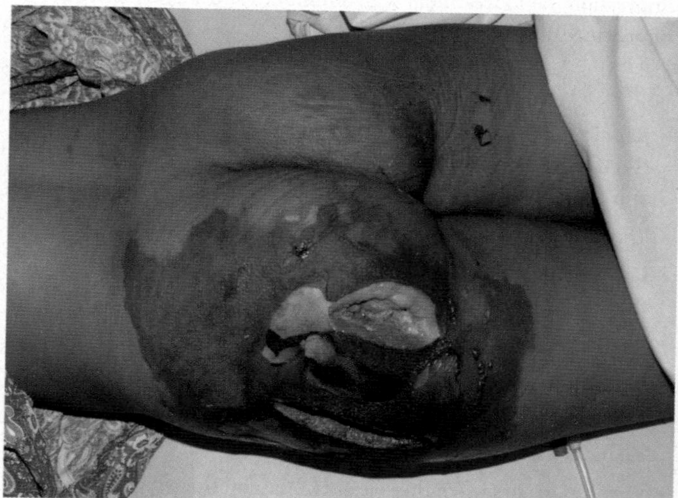

FIGURE 128-7 Necrotizing fasciitis of the left gluteal region following an intramuscular injection received in rural India. This 16-year-old female was febrile and in septic shock. The entire left gluteal region had full-thickness necrosis and was emitting a foul odor. The skin was violaceous with purple bullae and areas of exfoliation. Previous attempts at incision and drainage were not helpful. (*Reproduced with permission from Dr. N. Jithendran and http://diabeticfootsalvage.blogspot.in/2012/11/post-intramuscular-injection-soft.html.*)

MANAGEMENT

FIRST LINE

Start by maintaining a high index of suspicion for NF. If the first debridement occurs within 24 hours from the onset of symptoms, there is a significantly improved chance of survival.[8]

- Surgical debridement is the primary therapeutic modality.[2,3,5,7-10] SOR A
    - Extensive, definitive debridement should be the goal with the first surgery. This may require amputation of an extremity to control the disease. Surgical debridement is repeated until all infected devitalized tissue is removed.
- Antibiotics are the main adjunctive therapy to surgery. Broad-spectrum empiric antibiotics should be started immediately when NF is suspected and should include coverage of Gram-positive, Gram-negative, and anaerobic organisms.[7] SOR A

Recommendations of the Infectious Diseases Society of America:

1. Prompt surgical consultation is recommended for patients with aggressive infections associated with signs of systemic toxicity or suspicion of necrotizing fasciitis or gas gangrene.[7] SOR A
2. Empiric antibiotic treatment should be broad (e.g., vancomycin or linezolid plus piperacillin-tazobactam or a carbapenem; or plus ceftriaxone and metronidazole), as the etiology can be polymicrobial (mixed aerobic–anaerobic microbes) or monomicrobial (group A streptococci, community-acquired MRSA).[7] SOR B
3. Penicillin plus clindamycin is recommended for treatment of documented group A streptococcal necrotizing fasciitis.[7] SOR B

SECOND LINE

- Aggressive fluid resuscitation is often necessary because of massive capillary leak syndrome. Supplemental enteral nutrition is often necessary for patients with NSTIs.
- Vacuum-assisted closure devices may be helpful in secondary wound management after debridement of NSTIs.[10]
- Hyperbaric oxygen (HBO_2) may have beneficial effects when used postoperatively in NSTIs. One recent study demonstrated decreased morbidity (amputations 50% vs. 0%) and mortality (34% vs. 11.9%) with the use of postoperative HBO_2.[11] SOR B

PROGNOSIS AND FOLLOW-UP

- Overall case fatality rate remains 20% to 47% despite aggressive, modern therapy.[5,6]
    - However, in a retrospective chart review of patients with NSTIs treated at six academic hospitals in Texas between 2004 and 2007, mortality rates varied between hospitals from 9% to 25% (n = 296).[12]
- Early diagnosis and treatment can reduce case fatality rate to 12%.[5]
- Carrying out the first fasciotomy and radical debridement within 24 hours of symptom onset is associated with significantly improved survival.[8]

PATIENT EDUCATION

The serious life-threatening nature of NF should be explained to the patient and family when informed consent is given prior to surgery. The risk of losing life and limb should be explained while giving hope for recovery. For those patients who survive but have lost a limb, counseling should be offered to help them deal with the psychological effects of the amputation.

PATIENT RESOURCES

- **http://www.pamf.org/health/healthinfo/index.cfm?A=C&hwid=hw140405.**

PROVIDER RESOURCES

- Executive Summary: Practice Guidelines for the Diagnosis and Management of Skin and Soft Tissue Infections: 2014 Update by the Infectious Diseases Society of America—**http://cid.oxfordjournals.org/content/59/2/147.long#content-block.**

REFERENCES

1. Dufel S, Martino M. Simple cellulitis or a more serious infection? *J Fam Pract.* 2006;55:396-400.
2. Usatine RP, Sandy N. Dermatologic emergencies. *Am Fam Physician.* 2010;82:773-780.
3. Koukouras D, Kallidonis P, Panagopoulos C, et al. Fournier's gangrene, a urologic and surgical emergency: presentation of a multi-institutional experience with 45 cases. *Urol Int.* 2011;86:167-172.
4. Trent JT, Kirsner RS. Diagnosing necrotizing fasciitis. *Adv Skin Wound Care.* 2002;15:135-138.
5. Cheng NC, Chang SC, Kuo YS, et al. Necrotizing fasciitis caused by methicillin-resistant *Staphylococcus aureus* resulting in death. A report of three cases. *J Bone Joint Surg Am.* 2006;88:1107-1110.
6. Horseman MA, Surani S. A comprehensive review of *Vibrio vulnificus*: an important cause of severe sepsis and skin and soft-tissue infection. *Int J Infect Dis.* 2011;15:e157-166.
7. Stevens DL, Bisno AL, Chambers HF, et al. Practice guidelines for the diagnosis and management of skin and soft tissue infections: 2014 update by the Infectious Diseases Society of America. *Clin Infect Dis.* 2014;59(2):e10-52.
8. Cheung JP, Fung B, Tang WM, Ip WY. A review of necrotising fasciitis in the extremities. *Hong Kong Med J.* 2009;15:44-52.
9. Angoules AG, Kontakis G, Drakoulakis E, et al. Necrotising fasciitis of upper and lower limb: a systematic review. *Injury.* 2007;38 Suppl 5:S19-26.
10. Endorf FW, Cancio LC, Klein MB. Necrotizing soft-tissue infections: clinical guidelines. *J Burn Care Res.* 2009;30:769-775.
11. Escobar SJ, Slade JB Jr, Hunt TK, Cianci P. Adjuvant hyperbaric oxygen therapy (HBO2) for treatment of necrotizing fasciitis reduces mortality and amputation rate. *Undersea Hyperb Med.* 2005;32:437-443.
12. Kao LS, Lew DF, Arab SN, et al. Local variations in the epidemiology, microbiology, and outcome of necrotizing soft-tissue infections: a multicenter study. *Am J Surg.* 2011;202:139-145.

SECTION E VIRAL

129 CHICKENPOX

E.J. Mayeaux, Jr., MD
Jan Hood, MD
Sujatha Gubbala, MD

PATIENT STORY

A 12-year-old girl presents with a 3-day history of an extensive vesicular and pruritic rash (**Figure 129-1**). The episode started 24 hours before the rash with fever and malaise. The patient is diagnosed with varicella, and no antiviral medications are given. Acetaminophen and/or ibuprofen are recommended for fever and discomfort.

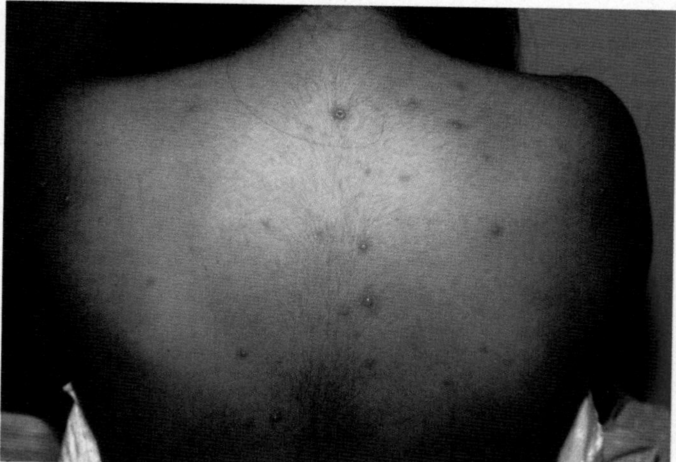

FIGURE 129-1 Chickenpox in a child. Note lesions in various stages (papules, intact vesicles, pustules, and crusted papules) caused by multiple crops of lesions. The vesicles are on a red base. *(Reproduced with permission from Richard P. Usatine, MD.)*

INTRODUCTION

Primary varicella, commonly known as chickenpox, is a highly contagious viral infection characterized by a distinctive rash with the potential to cause serious acute illness and to manifest later as zoster. The epidemiology of chickenpox has changed markedly since 1995 in the United States and other countries with high varicella vaccine coverage.

EPIDEMIOLOGY

- Varicella-zoster virus (VZV) is distributed worldwide. Humans are the only natural reservoir.
- Incidence is seasonal, except in tropical climates, with most cases occurring during the winter and early spring. Peak incidence in the United States is between March and May.[1]

United States epidemiology before the vaccination program:

- Estimated incidence of about 4 million/year.
- Essentially everyone acquired varicella before adulthood, most as young children (**Figure 129-2**).
- Most experienced the illness as a painful but benign and self-limited rash.
- Household infection rate was more than 90% of susceptible individuals[1] (**Figure 129-3**).
- Complications from varicella accounted for approximately 11,000 hospital admission and 100 deaths annually.[1]
- Complications were more prevalent in babies, older adults, and immunocompromised persons; most deaths actually occurred in immunocompetent children and adults.

United States epidemiology since the vaccination program:

- The incidence of chicken pox abruptly declined by 97%.
- A high percentage of remaining cases are breakthrough varicella (infection with wild-type VZV more than 42 days after vaccination).[1]

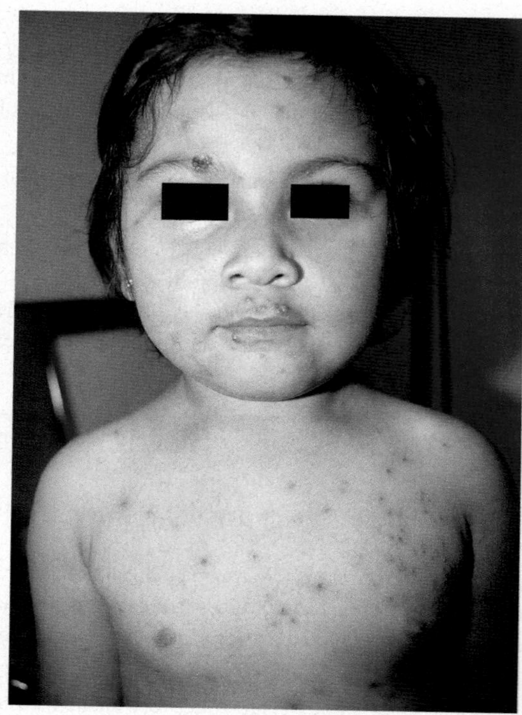

FIGURE 129-2 Chickenpox in a child. Note the widespread distribution of the lesions. The honey-crusted lesion on the eyebrow suggests a secondary bacterial infection (impetigo). *(Reproduced with permission from Richard P. Usatine, MD.)*

- Complications, including death, also declined dramatically—especially in children and young adults, where it decreased by 99%.[2]
- Current groups vulnerable to morbidity and mortality include[2,3]:
  - Persons living with natural and/or medically induced immunodeficiency
  - Susceptible immigrants from the tropics

ETIOLOGY AND PATHOPHYSIOLOGY

- Chickenpox is caused by a primary infection with the varicella-zoster virus (VZV), a double-stranded, linear DNA herpesvirus.
- VZV is primarily transmitted through the desquamation of vesicular skin lesions, which releases fully infectious viral particles into the air. Current evidence questions the long-held supposition of spread through infected respiratory secretions, although most sources continue to report this and to report infectivity up to 48 hours prior to the formation of the rash.[3]
- Infectivity, enhanced by scratching, lasts until skin lesions are fully crusted.
- Incubation is approximately 15 days.
- The VZV enters the susceptible host through the respiratory mucosa and conjunctiva.
- The virus replicates locally and in regional lymph nodes, leading to an initial viremia 4–6 days later. Multiple organs are seeded, including the sensory ganglia (important for latent infection), and viral production continues. A second viremia involving the skin occurs about 15 days after exposure and results in the typical skin lesions.[1]
- The most frequent complication in healthy children is bacterial skin superinfection (**Figure 129-4**). Less-common skin complications (seen more frequently in immunosuppressed hosts) include bullous varicella, purpura fulminans, and necrotizing fasciitis.
- Encephalitis is a serious potential complication of chickenpox. One form, acute cerebellar ataxia, occurs mostly in children and is generally followed by complete recovery. The more severe form occurs primarily in adults and may produce delirium, seizures, focal neurologic signs, long-term neurologic sequelae, and death.
- Pneumonia is rare in healthy children but accounts for a majority of serious complications in adults, including pregnant women; mortality rate approaches 30%.[1] VZV pneumonia usually develops insidiously a few days after the initial lesions and presents with progressive tachypnea, dyspnea, and dry cough. Chest x-rays reveal diffuse bilateral infiltrates.
- Immunocompromised patients are at risk for complications with VZV, most commonly encephalitis and pneumonia. Disseminated disease is relatively common in this cohort and can lead to a more fulminant course with multi-organ failure.
- Congenital varicella syndrome, although rare in the United States even before the routine use of the vaccine, can lead to an array of congenital problems. Mortality of this potentially devastating complication has been significantly reduced in recent times through the availability of VZV immune globulin and intensive supportive care.[4]
- Reactivation of latent VZV results in herpes zoster or shingles (see Chapter 130, Zoster).

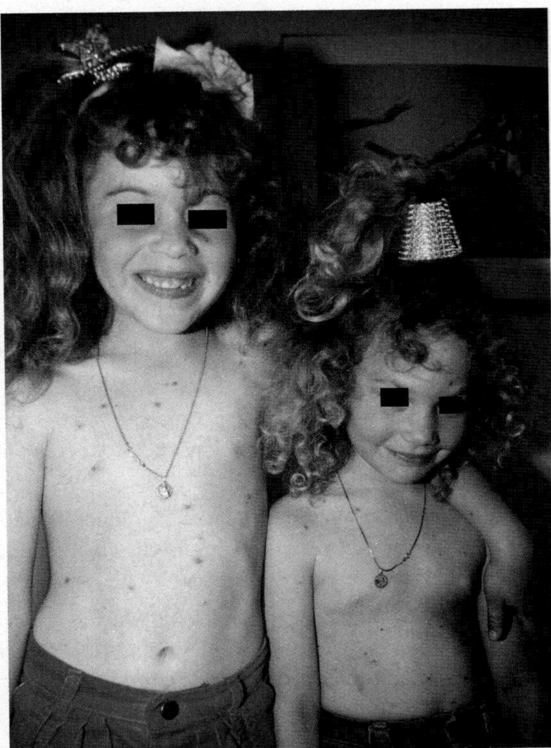

FIGURE 129-3 Chickenpox in sisters seen before the varicella vaccine was available. The girls are feeling better now that the disease is resolving. (*Reproduced with permission from Richard P. Usatine, MD.*)

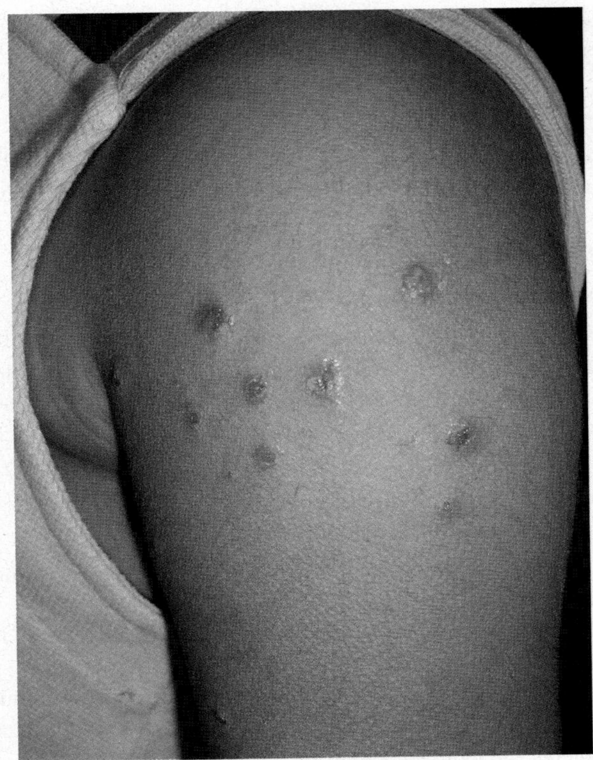

FIGURE 129-4 Honey-crusted lesions of superinfected varicella. This is impetiginized chickenpox caused by a secondary bacterial infection (impetigo). (*Reproduced with permission from Richard P. Usatine, MD.*)

DIAGNOSIS

CLINICAL FEATURES

- The typical clinical manifestations of chickenpox include a prodrome of fever, malaise, and pharyngitis, followed by the development of a generalized vesicular rash in approximately 24 hours.
- A prodrome of fever and malaise is more common in adults than children and may precede the rash by 1 to 2 days.
- Fever and malaise often accompany the rash for 2–3 days even in healthy children.
- The characteristic pruritic, vesicular rash appears in crops for several days, resulting in lesions of various stages of development throughout its distribution.
- Natural infection in a healthy child generally produces about 200–500 lesions, whereas breakthrough varicella often produces less than 50 and is less likely to cause fever.
- Lesions typically start as vesicle on a red base, which is classically described as a dewdrop on a rose petal (**Figure 129-5**). The lesions gradually develop a pustular component (**Figure 129-6**) followed by the evolution of crusted papules (**Figure 129-7**).
- Breakthrough varicella lesions may present only as papules, without a vesicular component.
- The lesions are pruritic and appear as successive crops of vesicles over 3 to 4 days.
- Coexisting lesions in different stages of development on the face, trunk, and extremities are common (**Figure 129-8**).
- New lesions stop forming in approximately 4 days, and most lesions have crusted completely by day 7.

TYPICAL DISTRIBUTION

- Body wide: Lesions typically appear first on the head and trunk followed by the extremities. Mucosal membranes may be involved.

LABORATORY TESTING

- Diagnosis is usually based on classic presentation.
- Laboratory testing is helpful when the presentation is atypical, including cases of possible breakthrough varicella; for infection control purposes; and for patients with potentially severe illness, including immunocompromised individuals (**Figure 129-9**).
- Viral isolation is no longer considered the gold standard for diagnosis, but may be helpful if resistance to antivirals is suspected.[3]
- Polymerase chain reaction (PCR) is now the diagnostic procedure of choice.[3]
  - Results are available within 1–2 days, are highly accurate, and are relatively inexpensive.
  - VZV can be readily detected from a variety of bodily sites and fluids, including skin and throat swabs, cerebrospinal fluid and blood, and biopsy or autopsy specimens.
  - The assay may be available at no charge through surveillance laboratories.

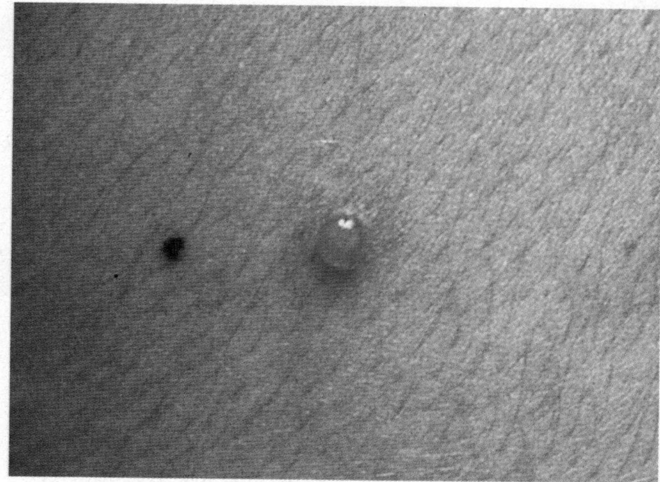

FIGURE 129-5 Dewdrop on a rose petal is the classic description of a varicella vesicle on a red base. (*Reproduced with permission from Richard P. Usatine, MD.*)

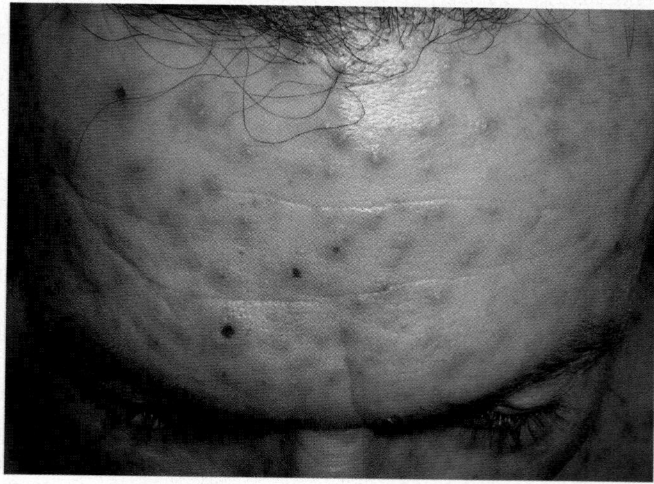

FIGURE 129-6 Pustules and crusted lesions on the face of a homeless man with varicella. Note how varicella has lesions simultaneously visible at different stages. (*Reproduced with permission from Richard P. Usatine, MD.*)

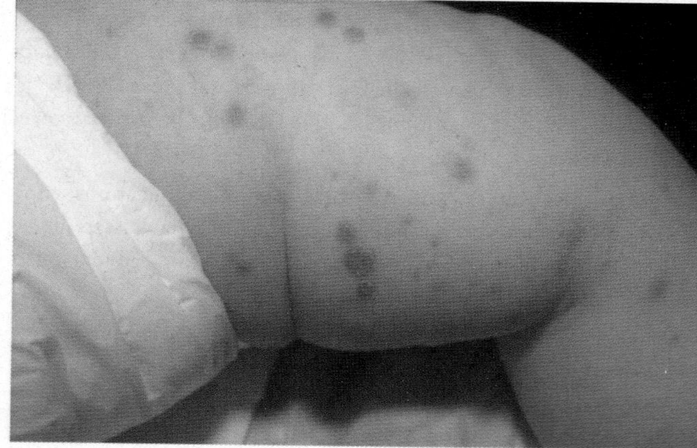

FIGURE 129-7 Varicella on the leg of an infant after the lesions have crusted over. The patient is probably not contagious at this time. (*Reproduced with permission from Richard P. Usatine, MD.*)

- Use of restriction enzyme treatment of PCR can differentiate between infection from wild-type (WT) VZV and breakthrough infections caused by the vaccine (vOka).
- Interesting note: Saliva is often positive for VZV DNA in persons under stress, even without disease. Unlike herpes simplex virus, VZV in saliva is not considered infectious.
- Indirect immunofluorescence can rapidly detect VZV in skin vesicles with reasonable sensitivity, but is less sensitive than PCR and cannot differentiate between WT VZV and vOka.[3]

- Serologic testing is sometimes used in an attempt to confirm recent illness with VZV or to assess immunologic protection from infection, but problems with this testing limit its utility.
- Humoral immunity does not protect against reactivation of the VZV as zoster.

DIFFERENTIAL DIAGNOSIS

- Herpes simplex infection presents with similar lesions, but is generally restricted to the genital and oral areas. The vesicles of herpes simplex tend to be more clustered in a group rather than the wide distribution of varicella (see Chapter 135, Herpes Simplex).
- Herpes zoster, the manifestation of latent VZV, is classically unilateral and follows dermatomal distribution (see Chapter 130, Zoster).
- Pemphigus and bullous pemphigoid occur most often in adults and are usually not febrile conditions. The bullae are usually larger than the vesicles of varicella (see Chapters 192, Bullous Pemphigoid, and 193, Pemphigus).
- Dermatitis herpetiformis, seen with gluten-induced enteropathy, is characterized by a chronic and intensely pruritic papulovesicular rash over the extremities and on the trunk. There is no fever, and the patient is not systemically ill other than possible symptoms from the enteropathy (see Chapter 194, Other Bullous Disease).
- Impetigo can have bullous or crusted lesions anywhere on the body. The lesions often have mild erythema and a yellowish color to the crusts. Varicella lesions can be secondarily infected, causing a superimposed picture (see Chapter 122, Impetigo).
- The vesicular lesions of hand, foot, and mouth disease (HFMD) are typically flat and painful without the characteristic dew-drop appearance and pruritus of varicella. Atypical HFMD with Coxsackie A6 may be more difficult to differentiate from varicella, as both conditions cause systemic illness (see Chapter 134, Hand Foot Mouth Syndrome).
- Atypical and breakthrough VZV may present similarly to a wide variety of relatively common dermatologic conditions including as miliaria, insect bites, infestations, papular urticaria, guttate psoriasis, secondary syphilis, and contact dermatitis (see respective chapters.)
- VZV should also be considered on the differential diagnosis of acutely ill patients with skin findings (see Chapter 185, Erythema Multiforme, Stevens-Johnson Syndrome, and Toxic Epidermal Necrolysis, and Chapter 187, Vasculitis, which includes Henoch–Schönlein purpura).

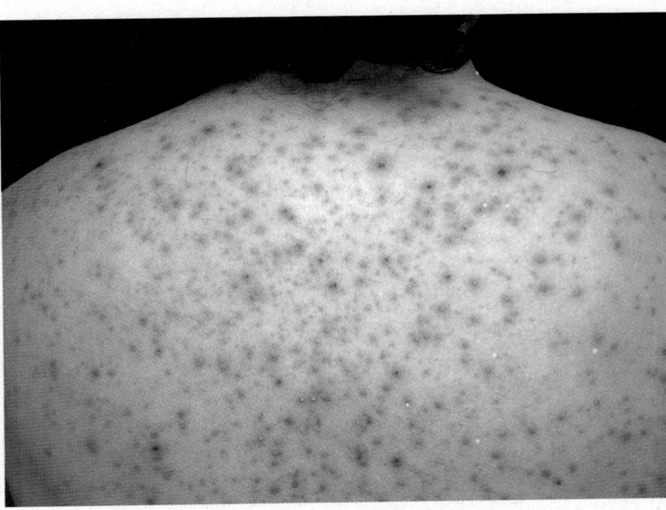

FIGURE 129-8 Varicella on the trunk of a nonimmunized man demonstrating the simultaneous appearance of papules, pustules and crusted lesions. *(Reproduced with permission from Richard P. Usatine, MD.)*

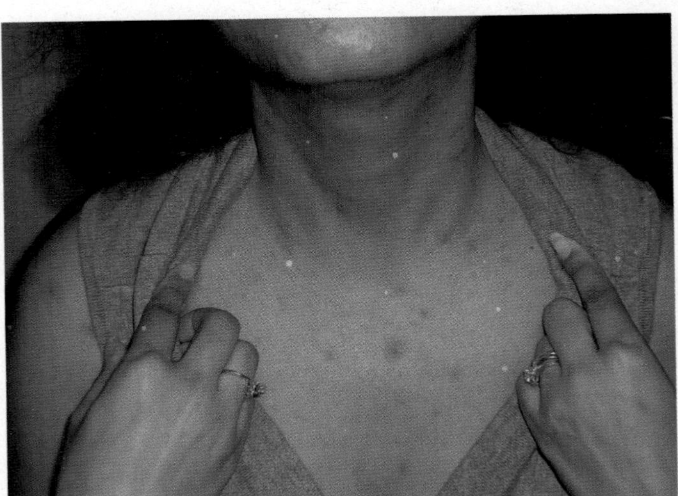

FIGURE 129-9 A 29-year-old woman with a mild case of varicella. Her previous history of varicella in childhood was uncertain, so a direct scraping of a lesion was performed and the varicella virus was identified quickly with a direct fluorescent antibody test. *(Reproduced with permission from Richard P. Usatine, MD.)*

MANAGEMENT

FIRST LINE

- Antihistamines are helpful in the symptomatic treatment of pruritus.
- Acetaminophen should be used to treat fever in children, as aspirin use is associated with Reye syndrome in the setting of viral infections.[5] SOR Ⓐ
- Superinfection may be treated with topical or oral antibiotics.
- Treatment with acyclovir 20 mg/kg PO 4 times daily (max 3200 mg/day) started within the first 24 hours and continued for 5 days should be considered for children at risk for moderate to severe illness; this includes children over the age of 12, those with chronic cutaneous and pulmonary disorders, and patients receiving chronic salicylates or steroids.
- Acyclovir 800 mg PO 4–5 times daily for 5–7 days, ideally started within the first 24 hours of the rash, should be considered for all adults, including both immunocompetent and immunocompromised patients. SOR Ⓐ

SECOND LINE

- Although acyclovir is approved for treatment of varicella in healthy children, the Committee on Infectious Disease of the American Academy of Pediatrics does not consider the routine administration of acyclovir to all healthy children with varicella to be justified. SOR Ⓒ
- Valacyclovir 20 mg/kg PO every 8 hours for 5 days and famciclovir 250 mg PO every 8 hours for 7 to 10 days are considered alternative agents to the more frequently dosed oral acyclovir in adults.
- Early treatment with intravenous acyclovir 10 mg/kg IV every 8 hours given for 7 to 10 days may be effective for treatment of varicella complications, including hepatitis and pneumonia, and may also be useful in the treatment of immunosuppressed patients. SOR Ⓑ Ensure adequate hydration and monitor for adverse reactions.
- IV foscarnet at 90 mg/kg every 12 hours is indicated for acyclovir-resistant varicella in ill patients. Adequate hydration is encouraged.
- Pruritus can be treated with calamine lotion, pramoxine gel, or powdered oatmeal baths.
- Fingernails should be closely cropped to avoid significant excoriation and secondary bacterial infection.

POST EXPOSURE PROPHYLAXIS

- Varicella vaccine is recommended to healthy, non-pregnant persons without immunity who are exposed to VZV. The vaccine may prevent infection and/or substantially modify the risk of severe disease when given within 3–5 days. SOR Ⓑ
- Even after 5 days, susceptible individuals should be vaccinated to protect against future exposures. **This live vaccine should not be given to pregnant women or most immunocompromised individuals.**
- Varicella zoster immune globulin (VariZIG) dosed by weight in recently exposed susceptible individuals (maximum efficacy within 96 hours) can attenuate the disease. Access to this product is limited in the United States and is primarily reserved for exposed individuals who are immunocompromised or pregnant, and for neonates and preterm infants.[6]
- Antivirals are not typically indicated for prophylaxis, but some experts recommend oral acyclovir to prevent secondary cases (which tend to be more severe) within a household.

PREVENTION

- All immunocompetent children younger than 13 years of age should receive 2 doses of varicella-containing vaccine, with the first dose administered at 12 to 15 months of age and the second dose at 4 to 6 years of age (i.e., before first grade). SOR Ⓐ The second dose can be administered at an earlier age, provided the interval between the first and second dose is at least 3 months.[1]
- All adolescents and adults without evidence of immunity to varicella should receive 2 doses of varicella separated by 4–6 weeks.[1] Particular effort should be expended to identify and immunize susceptible non-pregnant women of childbearing age and family members of immunocompromised individuals.
- Varicella vaccine is contraindicated in individuals allergic to gelatin or neomycin, in immunosuppressed individuals, and in pregnancy.
- Varicella vaccine is available alone (Varivax, Merck) and in combination with live-attenuated measles-mumps-rubella (ProQuad, Merck). The combination is only licensed for use in children aged 12 months through 12 years. When both vaccines are indicated, the combined vaccine is preferred.[1]
- Both vaccines contain the live attenuated Oka strain of VZV and produce an equivalent antibody response.[1]

FOLLOW-UP

- Follow-up is unnecessary for immunocompetent children and adults without complications.

PATIENT EDUCATION

- Avoid scratching the blisters and keep fingernails short. Scratching may lead to superinfection.
- Calamine lotion, pramoxine gel, and oatmeal (Aveeno) baths may help relieve itching.
- Do not use aspirin or aspirin-containing products to relieve fever. The use of aspirin is associated with development of Reye syndrome, which may cause death.
- Emergency precautions should be given to all persons, especially those at high risk of complications.
- Isolate infected patients until all lesions are fully crusted and advise prophylaxis for all susceptible exposed persons.

PATIENT RESOURCES

- KidsHealth. *Chickenpox*—**http://www.kidshealth.org/parent/infections/skin/chicken_pox.html.**
- MedlinePlus. *Chickenpox*—**https://medlineplus.gov/chickenpox.html.**

PROVIDER RESOURCES

- Centers for Disease Control and Prevention. *Chickenpox/ Varicella Vaccination*—**https://www.cdc.gov/vaccines/vpd/varicella/index.html.**
- Case-based varicella surveillance is ongoing in 40 states. For state-specific reporting requirements, contact the state health department. Information also available through the Council of State and Territorial Epidemiology—**http://www.cste2.org/izenda/entrypage.aspx.**

REFERENCES

1. Centers for Disease Control and Prevention. Varicella. In: Hamborsky J, Kroger A, Wolfe S, eds. *Epidemiology and Prevention of Vaccine-Preventable Diseases.* 13th ed. Washington D.C. Public Health Foundation, 2015:353-375.
2. Leung J, Bialek SR, Marin M. Trends in varicella mortality in the United States: data from vital statistics and the national surveillance system. *Hum Vaccin Immunother.* 2015;11(3):662-668.
3. Gershon AA, Gershon MD. Pathogenesis and current approaches to control of varicella-zoster virus infections. *Clin Microbiol Rev.* 2013;26(4):728-743.
4. Centers for Disease Control and Prevention. *Chickenpox: People at High Risk for Complications.* https://www.cdc.gov/chickenpox/hcp/high-risk.html. Accessed February 2017.
5. Belay ED, Bresee JS, Holman RC, et al. Reye's syndrome in the United States from 1981 through 1997. *N Engl J Med.* 1999;340(18): 1377-1382.
6. Centers for Disease Control and Prevention. Updated recommendations for use of VariZIG—United States, 2013. *MMWR Morb Mortal Wkly Rep.* 2013;62:574-576.

130 ZOSTER

E.J. Mayeaux, Jr., MD
Richard P. Usatine, MD

PATIENT STORY

A 75-year-old woman presented with a severely painful case of herpes zoster in a lower abdominal/lower extremity distribution. Groups of vesicles were becoming bullae and leading to erosions (**Figure 130-1**). The woman was treated with oral analgesics and an oral antiviral medication. Her primary care physician treated her zoster aggressively in an attempt to prevent postherpetic neuralgia (PHN).

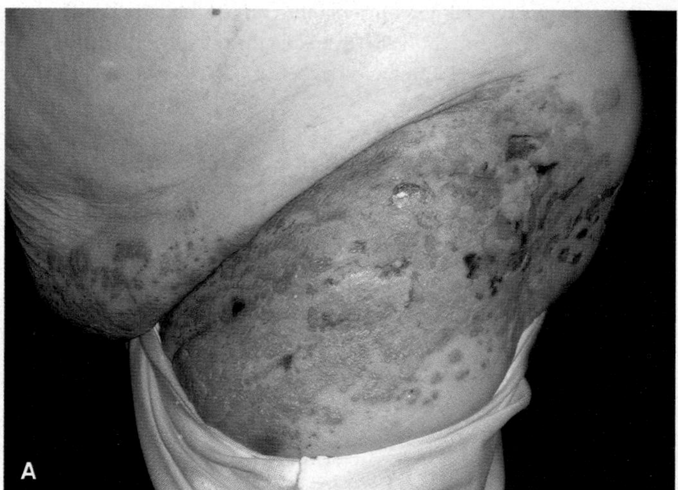

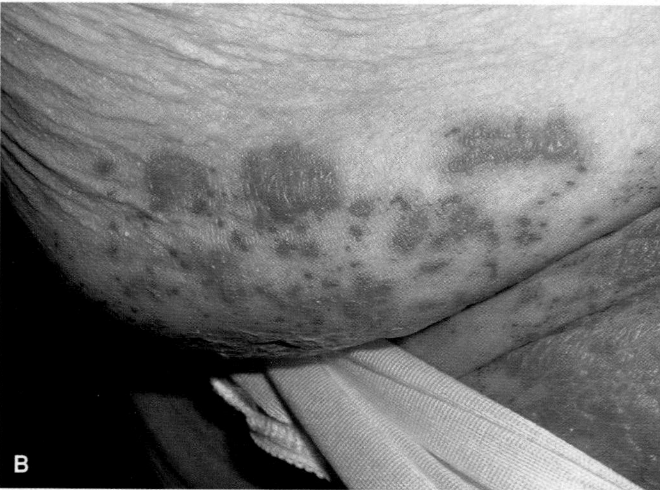

FIGURE 130-1 A 75-year-old woman with severe case of herpes zoster in a lower abdominal/lower extremity distribution. **A.** Note the erosions on the upper thighs in addition to the vesicles and bullae. **B.** Close-up of the zoster lesions showing grouped vesicles and bullae on a red base. (*Reproduced with permission from Richard P. Usatine, MD.*)

INTRODUCTION

Herpes zoster (shingles) is a syndrome characterized by a painful, usually unilateral vesicular eruption that develops in a restricted dermatomal distribution (**Figures 130-1** and **130-2**).[1-3]

SYNONYMS

Shingles.

EPIDEMIOLOGY

- According to the Centers for Disease Control and Prevention (CDC), 32% of persons in the United States will experience zoster during their lifetimes, accounting for about 1 million cases annually.[4] Older age groups account for the highest incidence of zoster. Approximately 4% of patients will experience a second episode of herpes zoster.[5]
- More zoster cases have been observed among women, even when controlling for age.[6]
- Herpes zoster occurs more frequently and more severely in immunosuppressed patients, including transplantation patients.

ETIOLOGY AND PATHOPHYSIOLOGY

- After primary infection with either chickenpox or vaccine-type varicella-zoster virus (VZV), a latent infection is established in the sensory dorsal root ganglia. Reactivation of this latent VZV infection results in herpes zoster (shingles).
- Both sensory ganglia neurons and satellite cells surrounding the neurons serve as sites of VZV latent infection. During latency, the virus expresses only a small number of viral proteins.
- How the virus emerges from latency is not clearly understood. Once reactivated, virus spreads to other cells within the ganglion. The dermatomal distribution of the rash corresponds to the sensory fields of the infected neurons within the specific ganglion.[3]

- Loss of VZV-specific cell-mediated immune response is responsible for reactivation.[3]
- The pain associated with zoster infections and PHN is thought to result from injury to the peripheral nerves and altered central nervous system processing.
- The most common complications are PHN and bacterial superinfection that can delay healing and cause scarring of the zoster lesions.
- Approximately 19% of patients develop complications that may include[7]:
  - PHN—The most common complication is seen in 10% at 90 days[7] (see below).
  - Ocular complications, including uveitis and keratitis (seen in 4%)[7] (see Chapter 131, Zoster Ophthalmicus).
  - Bell palsy and other motor nerve plastic (seen in 3%).[7]
  - Bacterial skin infection (seen in 2%).[7]
  - Meningitis caused by central extension of the infection.
  - Herpes zoster oticus (Ramsay Hunt syndrome) (**Figure 130-3**) includes the triad of ipsilateral facial paralysis, ear pain, and vesicles in the auditory canal and auricle.[8] Disturbances in taste perception, hearing (tinnitus, hyperacusis), lacrimation, and vestibular function (vertigo) may occur.
  - Other rare complications may include acute retinal necrosis, transverse myelitis, encephalitis, leukoencephalitis, contralateral thrombotic stroke syndrome, and granulomatous vasculitis.[9]
- Immunosuppressed patients are at increased risk for complications, including severe complications such as broader dermatomal involvement, disseminated infection, visceral involvement, pneumonitis, and/or meningoencephalitis.
- PHN is the persistence of pain, numbness, and/or dysesthesias precipitated by movement or in response to stimuli in the affected dermatome for more than 1 month after the onset of zoster. The incidence of PHN in the general population is 1.38 per 1000 person-years, and it occurs more commonly in individuals older than age 60 years and in immunosuppressed individuals.[3]
- In a large study, rates of zoster-associated pain (PHN) persisting at least 90 days were:
  - 10% overall; 12% in women and 7% in men.
  - Ages 22 to 59 years—5% overall; 6% in women and 5% in men.
  - Ages 60 to 69 years—10% overall; 14% in women and 5% in men.
  - Ages 70 to 79 years—17% overall; 18% in women and 15% in men.
  - Age 80 years and older—20% overall; 23% in women and 13% in men.[7]

RISK FACTORS

ZOSTER[3]

- Older age.
- Underlying malignancy.
- Disorders of cell-mediated immunity.
- Chronic lung or kidney disease.
- Autoimmune disease.
- Female sex.[10]

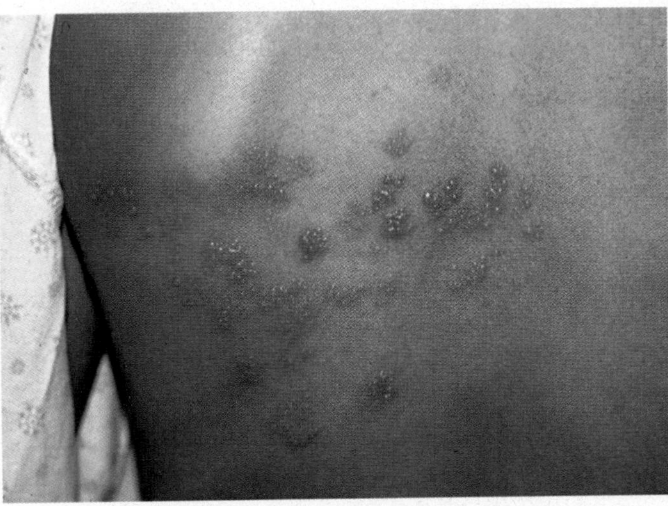

FIGURE 130-2 Herpes zoster on the back of a young woman. Note the grouped vesicles on a red base. Some of the vesicles cross the midline as there is some cross-innervation of the spinal sensory nerves on the back. (*Reproduced with permission from Richard P. Usatine, MD.*)

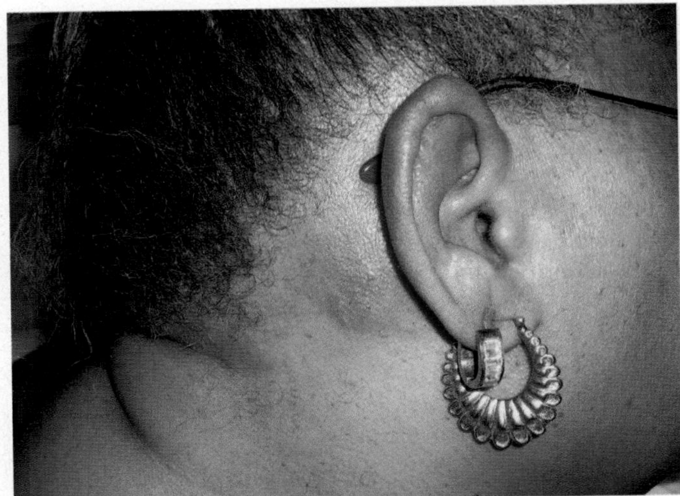

FIGURE 130-3 Herpes zoster with redness and vesicles on the auricle. Fortunately, she did not have the Ramsay Hunt syndrome with facial paralysis. (*Reproduced with permission from Richard P. Usatine, MD.*)

PHN

- Age older than 60 years.
- Negative vaccine status.

DIAGNOSIS

CLINICAL FEATURES

- A deep burning pain and sometimes redness in a dermatomal pattern is the most common first symptom and can precede the rash by days to weeks (**Figure 130-4**). A prodrome of fever, dysesthesias, malaise, and headache leads in several days to a dermatomal vesicular eruption.
- The rash may start as erythematous papules but usually quickly becomes grouped vesicles or bullae which evolve into pustular or hemorrhagic lesions within 3 to 4 days (**Figures 130-1** to **130-6**). The lesions typically crust in approximately a week, with complete resolution within 3 to 4 weeks.[5]

TYPICAL DISTRIBUTION

- The rash is generally limited to one dermatome in immunocompetent patients, but sometimes affects neighboring dermatomes. Rarely, a few scattered vesicles are located away from the involved dermatome as a result of release of VZV from the infected ganglion into the bloodstream.[3] If there are more than 20 lesions distributed outside the dermatome affected, the patient has disseminated zoster. The thoracic and lumbar dermatomes are the most commonly involved. Occasionally zoster will be seen on the extremities (see **Figure 130-5**).
- Approximately 80% of patients have significant systemic symptoms such as headache, fever, malaise, or fatigue.[11]
- Rarely, the dermatomal pain may be related to herpes zoster but without the typical rash, which is known as zoster sine herpete.[12]

LABORATORY TESTING

- Meningitis associated with VZV infection can be diagnosed by cerebrospinal fluid showing pleocytosis.

DIFFERENTIAL DIAGNOSIS

- Pemphigus and other bullous diseases present with blisters, but not the classic dermatomal distribution (see Chapters 191, Overview of Bullous Disease and 193, Pemphigus).
- Molluscum contagiosum presents with white or yellow flat-topped papules with central umbilication caused by a pox virus. The lesions are more firm and, unless irritated, do not have a red base as seen with zoster (see Chapter 136, Molluscum Contagiosum).
- Scabies may present as a pustular rash that is not confined to dermatomes and usually has characteristic lesions in the webs of the fingers (see Chapter 149, Scabies).
- Insect bites are often suspected by history and can occur over the entire body.
- Folliculitis presents with characteristic pustules arising from hair shafts (see Chapter 123, Folliculitis).

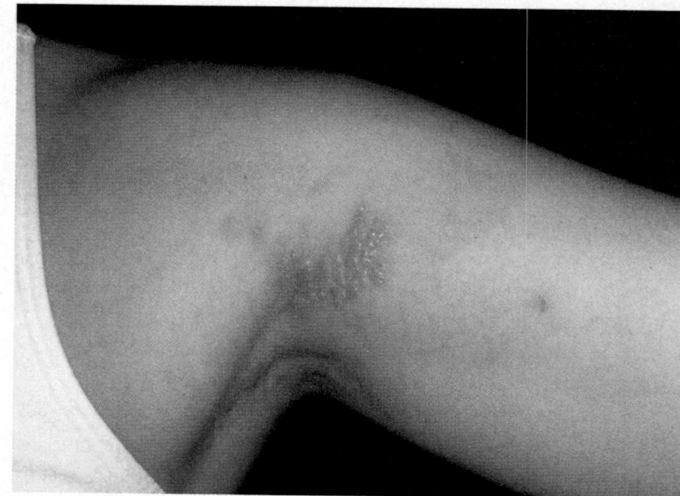

FIGURE 130-4 Herpes in the axilla of a young woman. Notice the redness in the dermatome that has started producing blisters. *(Reproduced with permission from Richard P. Usatine, MD.)*

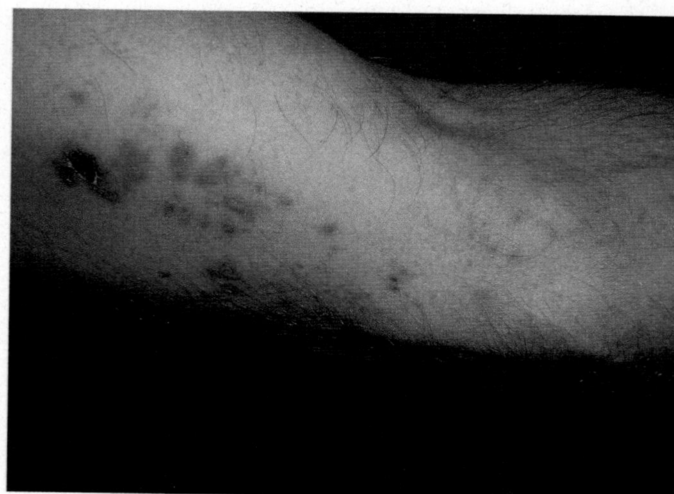

FIGURE 130-5 Herpes zoster on the arm that follows a dermatomal pattern. *(Reproduced with permission from E.J. Mayeaux, Jr., MD.)*

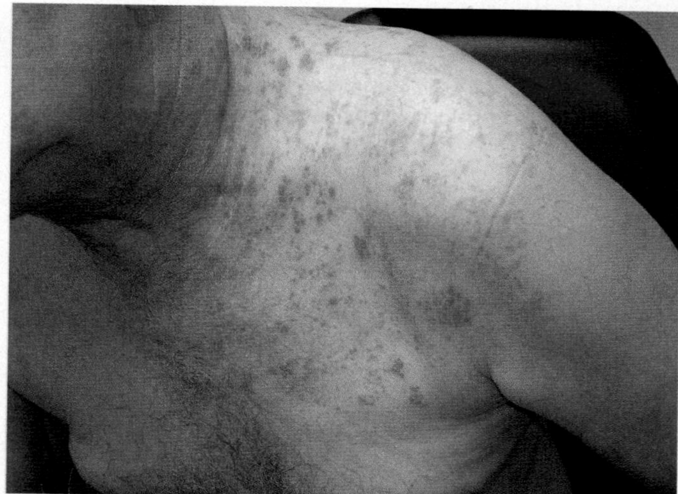

FIGURE 130-6 Herpes zoster of the C4-C5 dermatomal distribution. *(Reproduced with permission from Richard P. Usatine, MD.)*

- Zoster mimics coronary artery disease when it presents with chest pain before the vesicles are visible.
- Herpes simplex infection presents with similar lesions but is usually restricted to the perioral region, genital area, buttocks, and fingers (see Chapter 135, Herpes Simplex).

MANAGEMENT

NONPHARMACOLOGIC

- Calamine lotion and topically administered lidocaine may be used to reduce pain and itching. SOR Ⓒ

MEDICATIONS

FIRST LINE

- The objectives of treatment of herpes zoster include (a) hastening the resolution of the acute viral infection, (b) treatment of the associated pain, and (c) prevention of PHN.
- Antiviral agents used in the treatment of herpes zoster include acyclovir (Zovirax), famciclovir (Famvir), and valacyclovir (Valtrex), all started within 72 hours of the onset of the rash (**Table 130-1**).[13] SOR Ⓐ

SECOND LINE

- Adding corticosteroids to acyclovir therapy may accelerate times to crusting and healing, return to uninterrupted sleep, resumption of full activity, and discontinuation of analgesic. Data are lacking for combining corticosteroids with other antivirals.
- Pain can be managed with nonprescription analgesics or narcotics. Pain should be treated aggressively. This may actually prevent or lessen the severity of PHN. Narcotic analgesics with hydrocodone are appropriate when needed. SOR Ⓒ
- Treatment of herpes zoster with steroids does not reduce the prevalence of PHN.
- Treatment of PHN includes tricyclic antidepressants, gabapentin (Neurontin), pregabalin (Lyrica), glucocorticoids, and/or opioid analgesics (**Table 130-2**).
- Treatment of herpes zoster early with valacyclovir, famciclovir, or amitriptyline does reduce pain of PHN at 6 months.

TABLE 130-1 Treatments for Herpes Zoster

Medication	Dosage
Acyclovir (Zovirax)	800 mg orally 5 times daily for 7 days or 10 mg/kg intravenously every 8 hours for 7 to 10 days
Famciclovir (Famvir)	500 mg orally 3 times daily for 7 days
Valacyclovir (Valtrex)	1000 mg orally 3 times daily for 7 days
Prednisone (Deltasone)	30 mg orally twice daily for 1 week followed by a tapering dose for approximately 2 weeks

TABLE 130-2 Effective Treatments for Postherpetic Neuralgia

Treatment	Benefit/Risk	Risks	NNT for ≥50% Pain Reduction	Dose/Duration
Lidocaine patch 5%	Reduces pain and acts as mechanical barrier	Application site sensitivity	2	Apply up to 3 patches for up to 12 hours
Tricyclic antidepressants (including amitriptyline) (strongest evidence)	Reduce pain, better sleep, decreases anxiety and depression	Multiple side effects, including sedation and dry mouth	2.7	25 to 150 mg qhs
Gabapentin (Neurontin) (strongest evidence)	Reduces pain, improves sleep, mood, and quality of life	Somnolence, dizziness, decreased memory	2.8–5.3	300 to 600 mg tid (can go as high as 1200 mg tid)
Pregabalin (Lyrica)	May reduce pain	Peripheral edema and weight gain	5	75 mg bid
Opioids (morphine, oxycodone, methadone)	Reduce pain	Somnolence, constipation, tolerance	Variable	Start low and titrate to effective dose
Tramadol	Reduces pain and is not a true narcotic	Dizziness, nausea, somnolence, constipation	4.8	50 to 100 mg qid

Abbreviation: NNT, number needed to treat.
Data from Garroway N, Chhabra S, Landis S, Skolnik DC. Clinical inquiries: what measures relieve postherpetic neuralgia? *J Fam Pract.* 2009;58(7):384, and Tyring SK. Management of herpes zoster and postherpetic neuralgia. *J Am Acad Dermatol.* 2007;57 (6 Suppl):S136-142.

PREVENTION

- During its October 2017 meeting, the Advisory Committee on Immunization Practices (ACIP) voted to recommend preferential use of the herpes zoster subunit (HZ/su; Shingrix) vaccine over the previously recommended herpes zoster live (Zostavax) vaccine for adults 50 and older, even if they previously received the Zostavax immunization. The HZ/su is a non-live, recombinant subunit glycoprotein vaccine given intramuscularly in a series of two 0.5-mL doses, with the second dose given 2 to 6 months after the first. Clinical trials on the HZ/su vaccine showed it was more effective and provided longer-lasting protection than the one-dose Zostavax vaccine.[14]
- Use of varicella (chickenpox) vaccine has not led to an increase in vaccine-associated herpes zoster in immunized patients or in the general population, and has led to an overall decrease in herpes zoster.[8]

PROGNOSIS

- Recurrence of clinical zoster is uncommon in immunocompetent patients.[15] Recurrences are much more common in the immunocompromised patients.[16]

FOLLOW-UP

- Follow-up is based on the severity of the case and the immune status of the patient.

PATIENT EDUCATION

- Herpes zoster in an immunocompetent host is contagious from contact with open lesions and possible airborne particles.[17] The lesions are no longer infectious once they become dry and crust over.
- Patients with disseminated zoster or with zoster and who are immunocompromised should be isolated from nonimmune individuals.
- Individuals who have not had varicella and are exposed to a patient with herpes zoster are only at risk of developing primary varicella and not herpes zoster.

PATIENT RESOURCES

- Centers for Disease Control and Prevention. *Vaccine Information Statements*—**http://www.cdc.gov/vaccines/hcp/vis/index.html.**
- CDC. *Shingles (Herpes Zoster)*—**https://www.cdc.gov/shingles/.**
- Medinfo UK. *Shingles (Herpes Zoster)*—**http://www.medinfo.co.uk/conditions/shingles.html.**
- The Skin Site. *Herpes Zoster (Shingles)*—**http://www.skinsite.com/info_herpes_zoster.htm.**
- MedlinePlus. *Shingles*—**http://www.nlm.nih.gov/medlineplus/ency/article/000858.htm.**

PROVIDER RESOURCES

- MedlinePlus. *Herpes Zoster*—**http://emedicine.medscape.com/article/218683.**
- Stankus SJ, Dlugopolski M, Packer D. Management of herpes zoster (shingles) and postherpetic neuralgia. *Am Fam Physician.* 2000;61:2437-2444—**http://www.aafp.org/afp/20000415/2437.html.**
- CDC. *Shingles (Herpes Zoster) for Health Care Professionals*—**https://www.cdc.gov/shingles/hcp/index.html.**

REFERENCES

1. Usatine RP, Clemente C. Is herpes zoster unilateral? *West J Med.* 1999;170(5):263.
2. Gnann JW Jr, Whitley RJ. Clinical practice. Herpes zoster. *N Engl J Med.* 2002;347(5):340-346.
3. Oxman MN. Immunization to reduce the frequency and severity of herpes zoster and its complications. *Neurology.* 1995;45 (12 Suppl 8):S41-46.
4. Harpaz R, Ortega-Sanchez IR, Seward JF; Advisory Committee on Immunization Practices (ACIP) Centers for Disease Control and Prevention (CDC). Prevention of herpes zoster: recommendations of the Advisory Committee on Immunization Practices (ACIP). *MMWR Recomm Rep.* 2008;57(RR-5):1-30.
5. Stankus SJ, Dlugopolski M, Packer D. Management of herpes zoster (shingles) and postherpetic neuralgia. *Am Fam Physician.* 2000;61(18):2437-44, 2447-2448.
6. Opstelten W, Van Essen GA, Schellevis F, et al. Gender as an independent risk factor for herpes zoster: a population-based prospective study. *Ann Epidemiol.* 2006;16(9):692-695.
7. Yawn BP, Saddier P, Wollan PC, et al. A population-based study of the incidence and complication rates of herpes zoster before zoster vaccine introduction. *Mayo Clin Proc.* 2007;82(11): 1341-1349.
8. Adour KK. Otological complications of herpes zoster. *Ann Neurol.* 1994;35 Suppl:S62-64.
9. Arvin AM, Pollard RB, Rasmussen LE, Merigan TC. Cellular and humoral immunity in the pathogenesis of recurrent herpes viral infections in patients with lymphoma. *J Clin Invest.* 1980;65(4): 869-878.
10. Opstelten W, Van Essen GA, Schellevis F, et al. Gender as an independent risk factor for herpes zoster: a population-based prospective study. *Ann Epidemiol.* 2006;16:692.
11. Dworkin RH, Johnson RW, Breuer J, et al. Recommendations for the management of herpes zoster. *Clin Infect Dis.* 2007;44 Suppl 1:S1.
12. Gilden DH, Kleinschmidt-DeMasters BK, LaGuardia JJ, et al. Neurologic complications of the reactivation of varicella-zoster virus. *N Engl J Med.* 2000;342:635.
13. Tyring SK, Beutner KR, Tucker BA, et al. Antiviral therapy for herpes zoster: randomized, controlled clinical trial of valacyclovir and famciclovir therapy in immunocompetent patients 50 years and older. *Arch Fam Med.* 2000;9(9):863-869.

14. Centers for Disease Control and Prevention (CDC). *October 2017 ACIP Meeting—Herpes Zoster Vaccine.* https://www.youtube.com/watch?v=3HtrqrQaeLg. Accessed January 2018.
15. Tseng HF, Chi M, Smith N, et al. Herpes zoster vaccine and the incidence of recurrent herpes zoster in an immunocompetent elderly population. *J Infect Dis.* 2012;206:190.
16. Yawn BP, Wollan PC, Kurland MJ, et al. Herpes zoster recurrences more frequent than previously reported. *Mayo Clin Proc.* 2011; 86:88.
17. Centers for Disease Control and Prevention. *Shingles (Herpes Zoster).* http://www.cdc.gov/shingles/hcp/clinical-overview.html. Accessed July 2017.

131 ZOSTER OPHTHALMICUS

E.J. Mayeaux, Jr., MD
Richard P. Usatine, MD

PATIENT STORY

A 44-year-old HIV-positive Hispanic man presented with painful herpes zoster of his right forehead (**Figure 131-1**). He was particularly worried because his right eye was red, painful, and very sensitive to light (**Figure 131-2**). On physical examination, there was significant conjunctival injection, corneal punctate epithelial erosions, and clouding, and a small layer of blood in the anterior chamber (hyphema). The pupil was somewhat irregular. Along with the hyphema and ciliary flush, this indicated an anterior uveitis. The patient had a unilateral ptosis on the right side with limitations in elevation, depression, and adduction of the eye secondary to cranial nerve III palsy from the zoster. The patient was immediately referred to ophthalmology and the anterior uveitis, corneal involvement, and cranial nerve III palsy were confirmed. The ophthalmologist started the patient on topical ophthalmic preparations of erythromycin, moxifloxacin, prednisolone, and atropine. Oral acyclovir was also prescribed. Unfortunately, the patient did not return for follow-up until 6 months later, when he returned to the ophthalmologist with significant corneal scarring (**Figure 131-3**). The patient is currently on a waiting list for a corneal transplantation.

INTRODUCTION

Herpes zoster is a common infection caused by varicella-zoster virus, the same virus that causes chickenpox. Reactivation of the latent virus in neurosensory ganglia produces the characteristic manifestations of herpes zoster (shingles). Herpes zoster outbreaks may be precipitated by aging, poor nutrition, immunocompromised status, physical or emotional stress, and excessive fatigue. Although zoster most commonly involves the thoracic and lumbar dermatomes, reactivation of the latent virus in the trigeminal ganglia may result in herpes zoster ophthalmicus (HZO) (**Figures 131-1** to **131-7**).

SYNONYMS

Ocular herpes zoster.

EPIDEMIOLOGY

- Incidence rates of HZO complicating herpes zoster range from 8% to 56%.[1]
- In the United States, there are an estimated incidence of 3.2 cases per 1000 person-years and a male-to-female ratio of 4:1. The peak incidence is between the ages of 50 and 79 years, with the highest rates in patients over age 80 years.[2]
- Ocular involvement is not correlated with age, gender, or severity of disease.

FIGURE 131-1 A 44-year-old HIV-positive Hispanic man with painful herpes zoster of his right forehead.

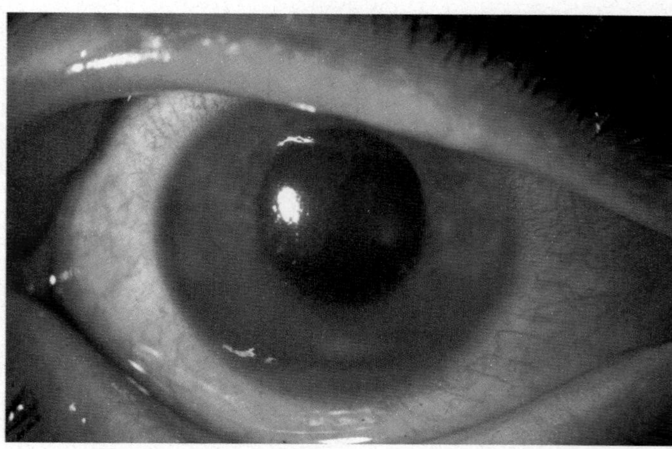

FIGURE 131-2 Acute zoster ophthalmicus of the same patient with conjunctival injection, corneal punctation (keratitis), and a small layer of blood in the anterior chamber (hyphema). A diagnosis of anterior uveitis was suspected based on the irregularly shaped pupil, the hyphema, and ciliary flush. A slit-lamp examination confirmed the anterior uveitis (iritis).

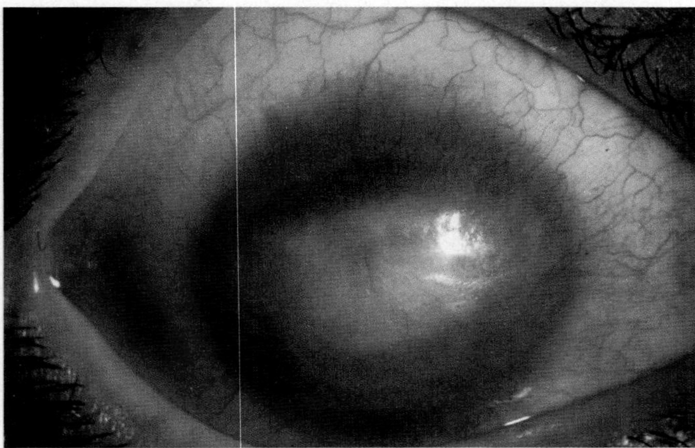

FIGURE 131-3 Corneal scarring and conjunctival injection of the same patient 6 months later after being lost to follow-up.

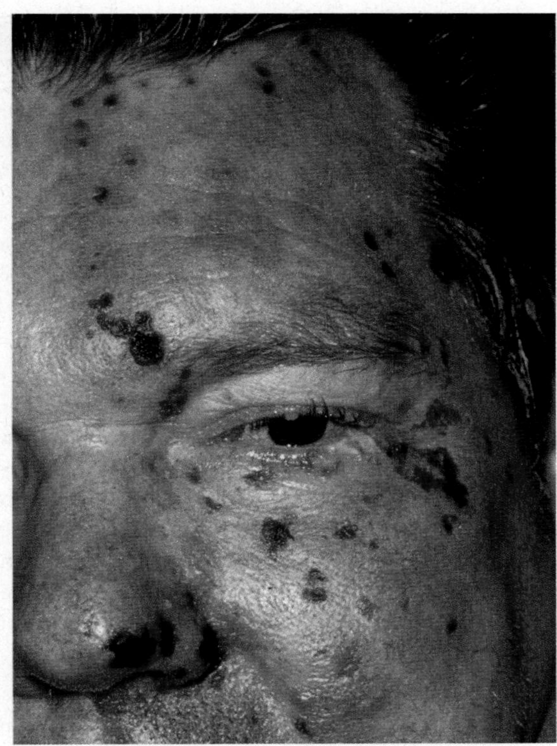

FIGURE 131-5 Herpes zoster ophthalmicus involving the first and second branch of the trigeminal nerve and the eyelids. There is conjunctival hyperemia and purulent left eye discharge. The nasociliary branch of the ophthalmic branch of the trigeminal nerve is involved, producing the black crusting on the tip of the nose. (*Reproduced with permission from Richard P. Usatine, MD.*)

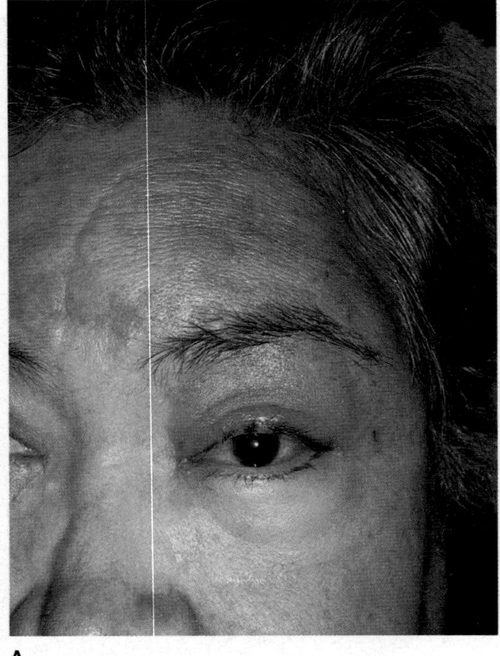

A

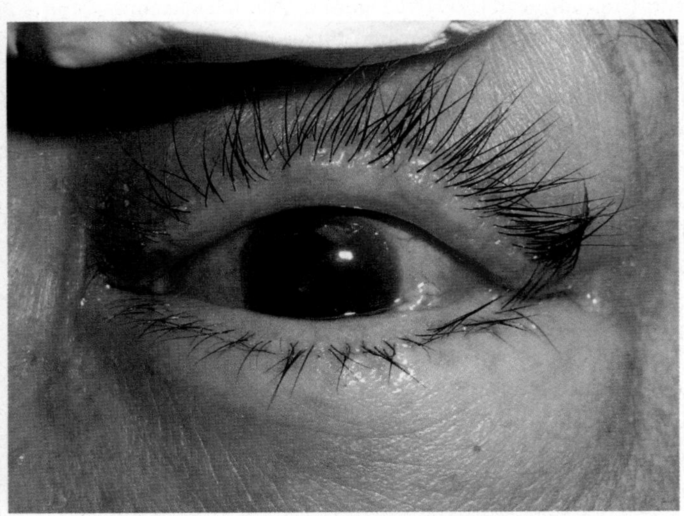

B

FIGURE 131-4 **A.** Herpes zoster ophthalmicus showing a V1 distribution in this 55-year-old woman who is immunosuppressed with prednisone and azathioprine for her dermatomyositis. She had tremendous eye and facial pain and developed significant blepharospasm secondary to this pain. **B.** It began with eye pain with no findings evident to the ophthalmologist. A few days later there were vesicles on the upper lid and conjunctival injection with discharge. In this photograph the fluorescein staining is still visible after seeing the ophthalmologist earlier that day. There is no corneal damage and the material at 1:00 is just fluorescein and discharge on the surface of the cornea. (*Reproduced with permission from Richard P. Usatine, MD.*)

ETIOLOGY AND PATHOPHYSIOLOGY

- Serious sequelae may occur, including chronic ocular inflammation, vision loss, and disabling pain. Early diagnosis is important to prevent progressive corneal involvement and potential loss of vision.[3]
- Because the nasociliary branch of the first (ophthalmic) division of the trigeminal (fifth cranial) nerve innervates the globe (see **Figure 131-7**), the most serious ocular involvement develops if this branch is involved.
- Classically, involvement of the side of the tip of the nose (Hutchinson sign) has been thought to be a clinical predictor of ocular involvement via the external nasal nerve (see **Figures 131-5** and **131-6**). The Hutchinson sign is a powerful predictor of ocular inflammation and corneal denervation with relative risks of 3.35 and 4.02, respectively. In one study, the manifestation of herpes zoster skin lesions at the dermatomes of both nasociliary branches (at the tip, the side, and the root of the nose) was invariably associated with the development of ocular inflammation.[4]
- Epithelial keratitis is the earliest potential corneal finding (see **Figure 131-2**). On slit-lamp examination, it appears as multiple, focal, swollen spots on the cornea that stain with fluorescein dye. They may either resolve or progress to dendrite formation. Herpes zoster virus dendrites form branching or frondlike patterns that have tapered ends and stain with fluorescein dye. These lesions can lead to anterior stromal corneal infiltrates.
- Stromal keratitis occurs in 25% to 30% of patients with HZO and is characterized by multiple fine granular infiltrates in the anterior corneal stroma. The infiltrates probably arise from antigen–antibody reaction and may be prolonged and recurrent.[5]
- Anterior uveitis evolves to inflammation of the iris and ciliary body and occurs frequently with HZO (see **Figure 131-2**). The inflammation is usually mild, but may cause a mild intraocular pressure elevation. The course of disease may be prolonged, especially without timely treatment, and may lead to glaucoma and cataract formation.
- Herpes zoster virus is the most common cause of acute retinal necrosis. Symptoms include blurred vision and/or pain in one or both eyes, and signs include peripheral patches of retinal necrosis that rapidly coalesce, occlusive vasculitis, and vitreous inflammation. It commonly causes retinal detachment. Bilateral involvement is observed in one-third of patients, but may be as high as 70% in patients with untreated disease. Treatment includes long courses of oral and intravenous acyclovir (Zovirax), and corticosteroids.[6]
- Varicella-zoster virus is a member of the same family (Herpesviridae) as herpes simplex virus, Epstein-Barr virus, and cytomegalovirus.
- The virus damages the eye and surrounding structures by neural and secondary perineural inflammation of the sensory nerves. This often results in corneal anesthesia.
- Conjunctivitis, usually with *Staphylococcus aureus*, is a common complication of HZO.

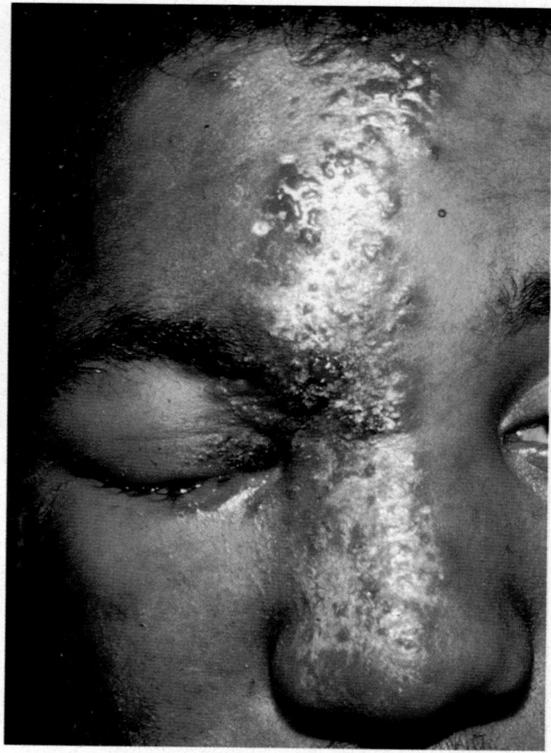

FIGURE 131-6 Herpes zoster ophthalmicus causing eyelid swelling and ptosis. Note the positive Hutchinson sign. (*Reproduced with permission from Richard P. Usatine, MD.*)

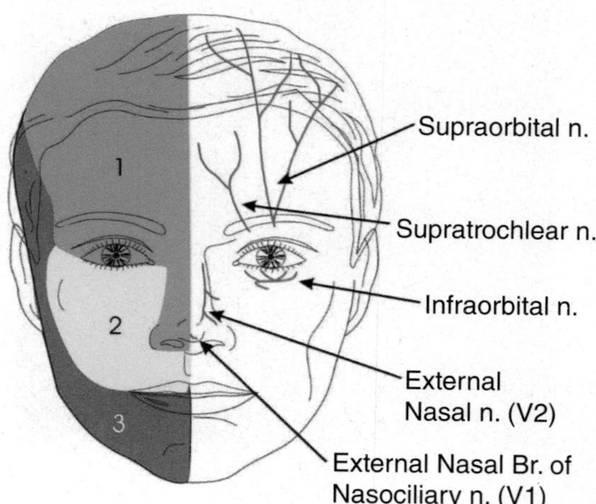

FIGURE 131-7 Diagram demonstrating the sensory distribution of the trigeminal (fifth cranial) nerve, and major peripheral nerves of the first (ophthalmic) division that may be involved with herpes zoster ophthalmicus. The infraorbital nerve from the second division is also shown. (*Reproduced with permission from E.J. Mayeaux, Jr., MD.*)

RISK FACTORS

- Immunocompromised persons, especially those with human immunodeficiency virus infection, have a much higher risk of developing zoster complications, including HZO.

DIAGNOSIS

CLINICAL FEATURES

- The syndrome usually begins with a prodrome of low-grade fever, headache, and malaise that may start up to 1 week before the rash appears.
- Unilateral pain or hypesthesia in the affected eye, forehead, top of the head, and/or nose may precede or follow the prodrome. The rash starts with erythematous macules along the involved dermatome, then rapidly progresses over several days to papules, vesicles, and pustules (see **Figures 131-4** to **131-6**). The lesions rupture and typically crust over, requiring several weeks to heal completely.
- With the onset of a vesicular rash along the trigeminal dermatome, hyperemic conjunctivitis, episcleritis, and lid droop (ptosis) can occur (see **Figure 131-6**).
- Approximately two-thirds of patients with HZO develop corneal involvement (keratitis).[1] The epithelial keratitis may feature punctate or dendritiform lesions (see **Figure 131-2**). Complications of corneal involvement can lead to corneal scarring (see **Figure 131-3**).[7]
- Iritis (anterior uveitis) occurs in approximately 40% of patients and can be associated with hyphema and an irregular pupil (see **Figure 131-2**).[1]
- Rarely, zoster can be associated with cranial nerve palsies.

TYPICAL DISTRIBUTION

- The frontal branch of the first division of the trigeminal nerve (which includes the supraorbital, supratrochlear, and external nasal branch of the anterior ethmoidal nerve) is most frequently involved, and 50% to 72% of patients experience direct eye involvement (see **Figure 131-7**).[1]
- Although HZO most often produces a classic dermatomal rash in the trigeminal distribution, a minority of patients may have only cornea findings.

DIFFERENTIAL DIAGNOSIS

- Bacterial or viral conjunctivitis presents as eye pain and foreign body sensation associated with discharge but no rash (see Chapter 18, Conjunctivitis).
- Trigeminal neuralgia presents with facial pain but without the rash or conjunctival findings.
- Glaucoma presents as inflammation, pain, and injection, but without the rash or conjunctival findings (see Chapter 21, Glaucoma).
- Traumatic abrasions usually present with a history of trauma and corneal findings but no other zoster findings (see Chapter 17, Corneal Foreign Body and Corneal Abrasion).
- Pemphigus and other bullous diseases present with blisters, but not in a dermatomal distribution (see Chapter 191, Overview of Bullous Disease).

MANAGEMENT

MEDICATIONS

- The standard treatment for HZO is to initiate antiviral therapy with acyclovir (800 mg, 5 times daily for 7 to 10 days), valacyclovir (1000 mg 3 times daily for 7 or 14 days), or famciclovir (500 mg orally 3 times a day for 7 days), as soon as possible so as to decrease the incidence of dendritic and stromal keratitis as well as anterior uveitis.[8] SOR Ⓐ Therapy should be initiated within 72 hours of presentation to maximize the potential benefits.
- Oral acyclovir, valacyclovir, and famciclovir in patients with ophthalmic involvement have comparable outcomes. Treatment is most commonly oral acyclovir, but intravenous acyclovir (10 mg/kg 3 times daily for 7 days) may be considered in immunocompromised patients or the rare patient who is extremely ill.[9] SOR Ⓐ
- Topical steroid ophthalmic drops are applied to the involved eye, after examination by the ophthalmologist, to reduce the inflammatory response and control immune keratitis and iritis.[1,3] SOR Ⓑ
- The ophthalmologist may prescribe a topical cycloplegic (such as atropine) to treat the ciliary muscle spasm that is painful in iritis. SOR Ⓒ
- Topical ophthalmic antibiotics may also be prescribed to prevent secondary infection of the eye. SOR Ⓒ
- As in all cases of zoster, pain should be treated effectively with oral analgesics and other appropriate medications. Early and effective treatment of pain may help to prevent postherpetic neuralgia (see Chapter 130, Zoster).
- Topical anesthetics should never be used with ocular involvement because of their corneal toxicity. SOR Ⓑ
- Secondary infection, usually *S. aureus*, may develop and should be treated with broad-spectrum topical and/or systemic antibiotics.

REFERRAL OR HOSPITALIZATION

- Referral to an ophthalmologist urgently should be initiated when eye involvement is seen or suspected.
- Hospital admission should be considered for patients with loss of vision, severe symptoms, immunosuppression, or involvement of multiple dermatomes, or for those with significant facial bacterial superinfection.

PREVENTION

- The herpes zoster vaccine reduces the incidence of herpes zoster by 51% compared with placebo.[10] In those who do develop zoster, the duration of pain and discomfort is shorter and the incidence of postherpetic neuralgia (PHN) is greatly reduced. It reduces the incidence of PHN from 1.38 to 0.46 per 1000 person-years.[10]

PROGNOSIS

- Approximately 50% of patients with HZO develop complications. Systemic antiviral therapy can lower the emergence of complications.[11,12]
- HZO can become chronic or relapsing. The overall 1-, 3-, and 5-year recurrence rates for either recurrent eye disease or rash is 8%, 17%, and 25%, respectively. Ocular hypertension and uveitis are associated with an increased risk of recurrent and chronic HZO.[13]

FOLLOW-UP

- Early diagnosis is critical to prevent progressive corneal involvement and potential loss of vision. Patients with herpes zoster should be informed that they should present for medical care with any zoster involving the first (ophthalmic) division of the trigeminal nerve or the eye itself.

PATIENT EDUCATION

- Zoster of the eye is a very serious vision-threatening illness that requires strict adherence to medical therapy and close follow-up.
- Viral transmission to nonimmune individuals from patients with herpes zoster can occur, but it is less frequent than with chickenpox. Virus can be transmitted through contact with secretions.

PATIENT RESOURCES

- Merck Manual—**https://www.merckmanuals.com/home/eye-disorders/corneal-disorders/herpes-zoster-ophthalmicus.**

PROVIDER RESOURCES

- Shaikh S, Ta CN. Evaluation and management of herpes zoster ophthalmicus. *Am Fam Physician.* 2002;66(9):1723-1730—**https://www.aafp.org/afp/2002/1101/p1723.html.**
- Touch Ophthalmology. *Herpes Zoster Ophthalmicus—Diagnosis and Management*—**http://www.touchophthalmology.com/articles/herpes-zoster-ophthalmicus-diagnosis-and-management.**
- Catron T, Hern HG. Herpes zoster ophthalmicus. *West J Emerg Med.* 2008;9(3):174-176.—**https://www.ncbi.nlm.nih.gov/pmc/articles/PMC2672268/.**
- Merck Manual. *Herpes Zoster Ophthalmicus*—**http://www.merckmanuals.com/professional/eye-disorders/corneal-disorders/herpes-zoster-ophthalmicus.**

REFERENCES

1. Pavan-Langston D. Herpes zoster ophthalmicus. *Neurology.* 1995;45(12 Suppl 8):S50-51.
2. Tran KD, Falcone MM, Choi DS, et al. Epidemiology of herpes zoster ophthalmicus: recurrence and chronicity. *Ophthalmology.* 2016;123(7):1469-1475.
3. Severson EA, Baratz KH, Hodge DO, Burke JP. Herpes zoster ophthalmicus in Olmsted County, Minnesota: have systemic antivirals made a difference? *Arch Ophthalmol.* 2003;121(3):386-390.
4. Zaal MJ, Völker-Dieben HJ, D'Amaro J. Prognostic value of Hutchinson's sign in acute herpes zoster ophthalmicus. *Graefes Arch Clin Exp Ophthalmol.* 2003;241(3):187-191.
5. Liesegang TJ. Corneal complications from herpes zoster ophthalmicus. *Ophthalmology.* 1985;92(3):316-324.
6. Liesegang TJ. Herpes zoster ophthalmicus natural history, risk factors, clinical presentation, and morbidity. *Ophthalmology.* 2008;115(2 Suppl):S3-12.
7. Albrecht Ma. *Clinical Features of Varicella-Zoster Virus Infection: Herpes Zoster.* http://www.uptodate.com/contents/clinical-manifestations-of-varicella-zoster-virus-infection-herpes-zoster. Accessed September 2012.
8. McGill J, Chapman C, Mahakasingam M. Acyclovir therapy in herpes zoster infection. A practical guide. *Trans Ophthalmol Soc U K.* 1983;103(Pt 1):111-114.
9. Gnann JW Jr, Whitley RJ. Clinical practice. Herpes zoster. *N Engl J Med.* 2002;347(5):340-346.
10. Oxman MN. Immunization to reduce the frequency and severity of herpes zoster and its complications. *Neurology.* 1995;45 (12 Suppl 8):S41-46.
11. Miserocchi E, Waheed NK, Dios E, et al. Visual outcome in herpes simplex virus and varicella zoster virus uveitis: a clinical evaluation and comparison. *Ophthalmology.* 2002;109(8):1532-1537.
12. Zaal MJ, Volker-Dieben HJ, D'Amaro J. Visual prognosis in immunocompetent patients with herpes zoster ophthalmicus. *Acta Ophthalmol Scand.* 2003;81(3):216-220.
13. Tran KD, Falcone MM, Choi DS, et al. Epidemiology of herpes zoster ophthalmicus: recurrence and chronicity. *Ophthalmology.* 2016Jul;123(7):1469-1475.

132 MEASLES

E.J. Mayeaux, Jr., MD
Luke M. Baudoin, MD
Francis J. DeMarco, MD

PATIENT STORY

An 18-month-old boy, who is visiting family in San Antonio with his parents from Central America, presents with a 3-day history of fever, malaise, conjunctivitis, coryza, and cough. He had been exposed to a child with similar symptoms approximately 2 weeks prior. A day before, he developed a maculopapular rash that blanches under pressure (**Figures 132-1** and **132-2**). His shot records are unavailable, but his mother states that his last vaccine was before age 1 year. He is diagnosed with measles and supportive care is provided.

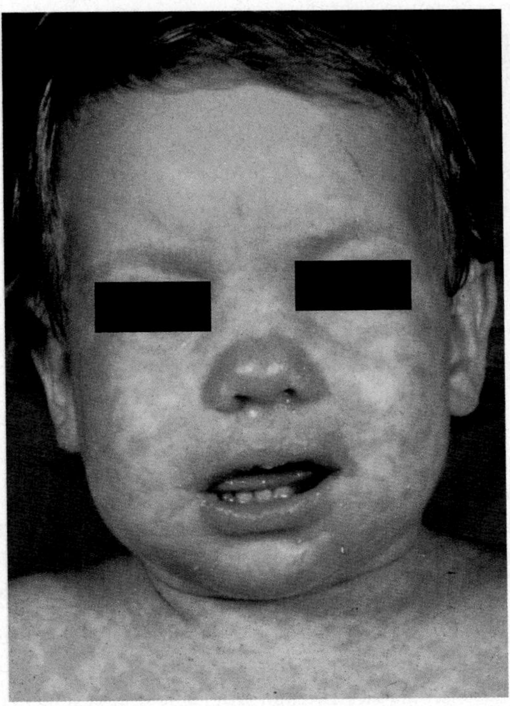

FIGURE 132-1 Typical measles rash that began on the face and became confluent. (*Reproduced with permission from Richard P. Usatine, MD.*)

INTRODUCTION

Measles is a highly communicable, acute, viral illness that is still one the most serious infectious diseases in human history. Until the introduction of the measles vaccination, it was responsible for millions of deaths worldwide annually. Although the epidemiology of this disease makes eradication a possibility, the ease of transmission and the low percentage of nonimmunized population that is required for disease survival have made eradication of measles extremely difficult.

EPIDEMIOLOGY

- A major outbreak in the United States from 1989 to 1991 prompted changes in immunization policies which led to the initiation of two measles, mumps, rubella (MMR) vaccines administered prior to kindergarten.
- This change in practice led to all-time lows in cases reported, and in 2000 the CDC declared that the United States had achieved measles elimination (defined as interruption of year-round endemic measles transmission).[1]
- Despite the declaration of elimination, measles cases continue to be reported in the United States, with most cases being linked to incomplete vaccinations. In 2015, an outbreak was noted when 110 patients in California were diagnosed with measles in association with a theme park. Of those patients, 45% were unvaccinated, 43% had unknown or undocumented vaccination status, and 5% had only one dose of measles-containing vaccination.[2] Among 37 vaccine-eligible patients, 28 (76%) were intentionally unvaccinated because of personal beliefs.[2]
- The worldwide incidence of measles was reduced from 280,525 cases in 2014 to 195,762 in 2015 according to WHO Global and Regional Immunization Profile. In 2015, approximately 85% of the world's target population received one dose of measles vaccine, up from 84% in 2014, and 61% received 2 doses, up from 58% in 2014.[3]

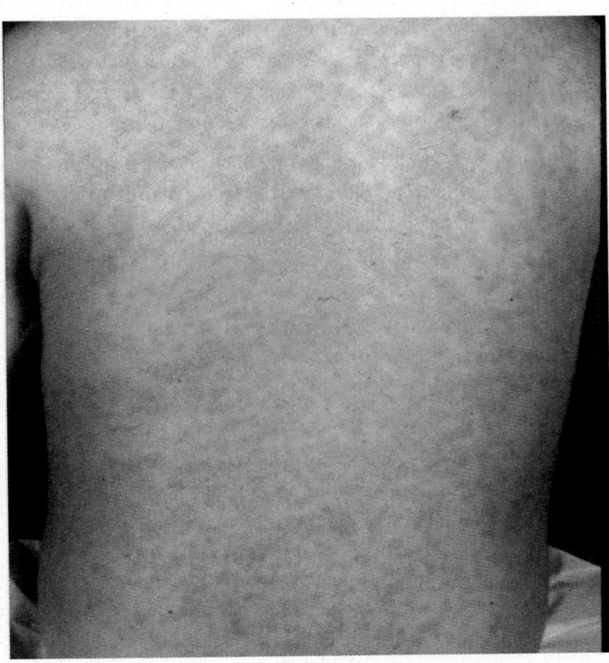

FIGURE 132-2 The typical measles rash on the trunk. (*Reproduced with permission from Richard P. Usatine, MD.*)

ETIOLOGY AND PATHOPHYSIOLOGY

- Measles is caused by the measles virus, a member of the family Paramyxoviridae, genus *Morbillivirus* (hence the name morbilliform rash).
- It is highly contagious, is transmitted by airborne droplets, and commonly causes outbreaks.
- Classic measles infection starts with the incubation phase, which is usually asymptomatic and lasts for 10 to 14 days. It starts after entry of the virus into the respiratory mucosa with local viral replication. The infection then spreads to regional lymphatic tissues, and then throughout the body through the bloodstream.
- The prodrome phase starts with the appearance of systemic symptoms including fever, malaise, anorexia, conjunctivitis, coryza, and cough (**Figure 132-3**). The respiratory symptoms are caused by mucosal inflammation from viral infection of epithelial cells. Patients may develop Koplik spots, which are small whitish, grayish, or bluish papules with erythematous bases that develop on the buccal mucosa, usually near the molar teeth (**Figure 132-4**). The prodrome usually lasts for 2 to 3 days.
- The classic measles rash (**Figures 132-1**, **132-2**, and **132-5**) is maculopapular and blanches under pressure. Clinical improvement in symptoms typically ensues within 2 days. Three to 4 days after the rash first appears, it begins to fade to a brownish color, which is followed by fine flaking. The cough may persist for up to 2 weeks.
- Fever persisting beyond the third day of rash suggests a measles-associated complication.
- Immunity after measles infection is thought to be lifelong in most cases. Measles reinfection occasionally occurs, but it is extremely rare.
- Atypical measles is a measles variant that occurs in previously vaccinated persons. Patients develop high fever and headache 7 to 14 days after exposure and often present with a dry cough and pleuritic chest pain. Two to 3 days later, a rash develops that spreads from the extremities to the trunk. The rash may be vesicular, petechial, purpuric, or urticarial. Patients may develop respiratory distress, peripheral edema, hepatosplenomegaly, paresthesias, or hyperesthesia.
- The measles virus can cause a variety of clinical syndromes, including the classic childhood illness and a less intense form in persons with suboptimal levels of antimeasles antibodies.
- Measles virus infection can also result in more severe illness, including lymphadenopathy, splenomegaly, laryngotracheobronchitis (croup), giant cell pneumonia, and measles inclusion body encephalitis in immunocompromised patients.[4] This form occurs in the very old and young, in those with vitamin A deficiency, and in pregnant women.
- Postinfection neurologic syndromes can occur. Postinfectious encephalomyelitis is a demyelinating disease that presents during the recovery phase and is thought to be caused by a postinfectious autoimmune response.[5] The major manifestations include fever, headache, neck stiffness, ataxia, mental status changes, and seizures. Cerebrospinal fluid (CSF) analysis demonstrates lymphocytosis and elevated proteins. Postinfectious encephalomyelitis has a 10% to 20% mortality rate, and residual neurologic abnormalities are common.[5]

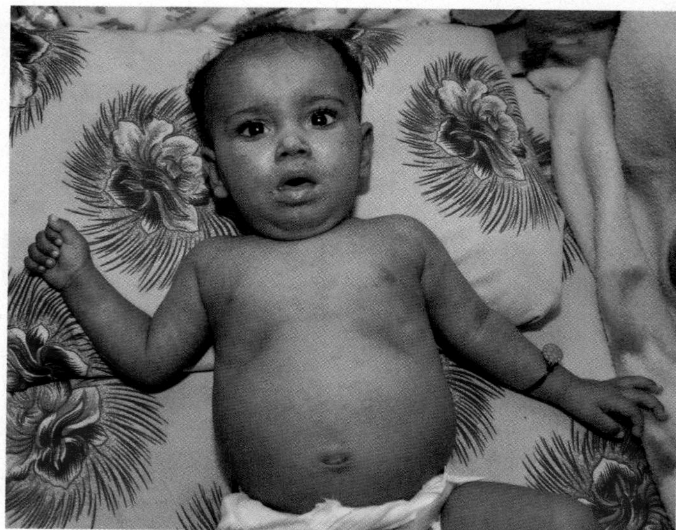

FIGURE 132-3 Measles in an Ethiopian infant during a measles outbreak. The rash is faint but her cough is prominent, and subcostal retractions are seen during this cough. She also has rhinorrhea and conjunctivitis. (*Reproduced with permission from Richard P. Usatine, MD.*)

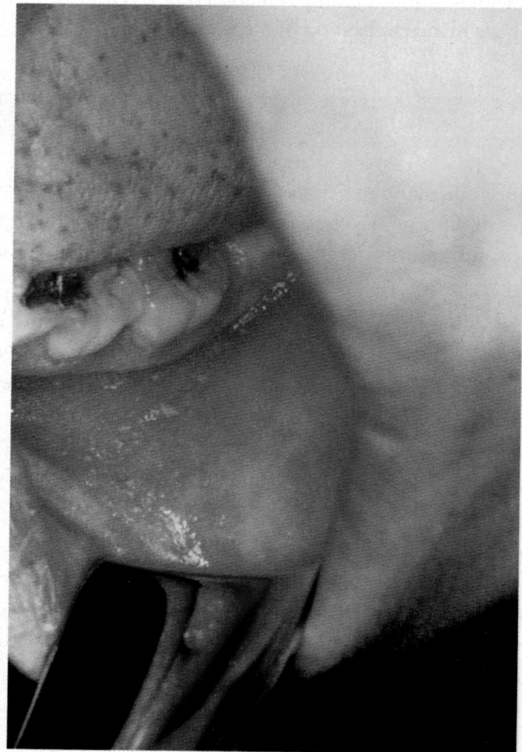

FIGURE 132-4 Koplik spots occur 1 to 2 days before to 1 to 2 days after the cutaneous rash. Their presence is considered to be pathognomonic for measles, and they appear as punctate blue-white spots on the bright red background of the oral buccal (cheek) mucosa. (*Reproduced with permission from the Centers for Disease Control and Prevention.*)

- Subacute sclerosing panencephalitis (SSPE) is a progressive, fatal, neurologic degenerative disease that may represent a persistent infection of the central nervous system with a variant of the virus. It usually occurs in patients younger than 20 years of age and 7 to 10 years after natural measles.[6] Patients develop neurologic symptoms, myoclonus, dementia, and eventually flaccidity or decorticate rigidity.
- Measles in pregnancy is a rare entity in areas that practice vaccination. Premature births may be more common in gravid women with measles, but there is no clear evidence of teratogenicity.[7]

RISK FACTORS

For developing measles:

- Failure to receive immunization.
- Failure to receive second immunization dose.
- Travel to endemic areas.
- Exposure to travelers from endemic areas.

For developing severe measles or for developing complications:

- Immunodeficiency.
- Malnutrition.
- Pregnancy.
- Vitamin A deficiency.
- Age younger than 5 years or older than 20 years.

DIAGNOSIS

Measles is a distinct disease characterized by fever, malaise, conjunctivitis, coryza, cough, rash, and Koplik spots.

CLINICAL FEATURES

Koplik spots appear during the prodrome phase and are pathognomonic for measles infection; they occur approximately 48 hours before the characteristic measles exanthem. The classic blanching rash is usually adequate to make a tentative diagnosis. The most rapid and accurate test to confirm acute measles is a blood test for measles-specific immunoglobulin (Ig) M antibodies. By waiting until the third day of the rash, a false-negative IgM result can be avoided.[8]

TYPICAL DISTRIBUTION

The rash begins on the face and spreads centrifugally to involve the neck, trunk, and, finally, the extremities. The lesions may become confluent, especially on the face. This cranial-to-caudal rash progression is characteristic of measles.

DIFFERENTIAL DIAGNOSIS

- Upper respiratory tract infections—The prodrome stage of measles can be confused with an upper respiratory infection (URI), except that significant fever is typically present with measles infection.

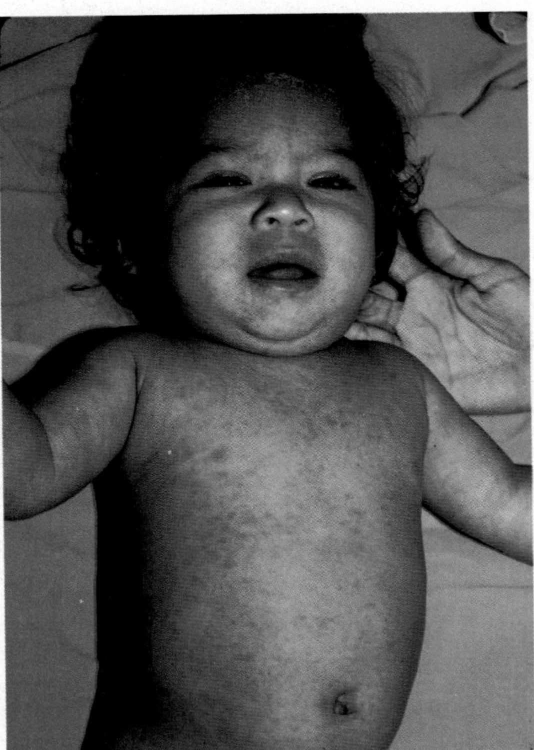

FIGURE 132-5 A South American child with a measles exanthem that has spread down the trunk. (*Reproduced with permission from Eric Kraus, MD.*)

- Fordyce spots—Tiny yellow-white granules on the buccal or lip mucosa caused by benign ectopic sebaceous glands that may be mistaken for Koplik spots. Fordyce spots do not have an erythematous base.
- Alternative diagnoses that may be confused with the measles rash include Rocky Mountain spotted fever, infectious mononucleosis, scarlet fever, Kawasaki disease, toxic shock syndrome, dengue fever, and simple drug eruption (see Chapter 212, Cutaneous Drug Reactions).
- Measles can usually be distinguished clinically from rubella, erythema infectiosum (parvovirus B19 infection), roseola, and enteroviral infection by the intensity of the measles rash, its subsequent brownish coloration, and the disease course.

MANAGEMENT

NONPHARMACOLOGIC

- The treatment of measles is mostly supportive. Suspected cases of measles should be immediately reported to the local or state department of health.

MEDICATIONS

- Measures to control spread of infection should not be delayed for laboratory confirmation. Vaccine should be promptly administered to all susceptible persons, or they should be removed from the outbreak setting for a minimum of 3 weeks. SOR C
- Giving serum immune globulin 0.25 mL/kg of body weight to a maximum dose of 15 mL to a susceptible person within 6 days of exposure to measles can prevent or modify disease. This is especially important in patients in whom the risk of complications of measles is higher, such as pregnant women, children younger than 1 year of age, and immunocompromised patients. SOR C
- Vitamin A reduces morbidity and mortality and is recommended by the World Health Organization (WHO) for children in areas where vitamin A deficiency is prevalent or where the mortality from measles exceeds 1%.[7] SOR B

REFERRAL OR HOSPITALIZATION

Consider hospitalization in the following scenarios:

- Difficulty breathing or noisy breathing—Bronchopneumonia occurs in 5% to 10% of patients.
- Changes in behavior, confusion—May be a harbinger of acute disseminated encephalomyelitis.
- There is dehydration, which can be the result of diarrhea, vomiting, and poor oral intake.

Refer to ophthalmology if there are changes in vision, as measles keratitis can lead to permanent scarring and blindness.

PREVENTION

- Measures to control spread of infection should not be delayed for laboratory confirmation. Vaccine should be promptly administered to all susceptible persons, or they should be removed from the outbreak setting for a minimum of 3 weeks.
- Initial and booster immunization.
- Avoidance of endemic areas without being fully immunized.
- Adequate nutrition and handwashing.

PROGNOSIS

- The disease is typically self-limited. Measles typically lasts approximately 10 to 14 days from the beginning of the prodrome to the fading of the eruption.
- Approximately 30% of measles cases have one or more complications. Complications of measles are more common among patients younger than 5 years of age and adults 20 years of age and older. Centers for Disease Control and Prevention (CDC)–reported measles complications include[9]:
  - Diarrhea—8%.
  - Otitis media—7%.
  - Pneumonia—6%.
  - Encephalitis—0.1%.
  - Seizures—0.6% to 0.7%.
  - Death—0.2%.

FOLLOW-UP

- Have patients watched for changes that indicate more severe disease or complications and follow up if these occur.
- Make sure return appointments for full vaccination are scheduled.

PATIENT EDUCATION

- Drink plenty of fluids to avoid dehydration. Use antipyretics/analgesics to control fever and discomfort. Avoid aspirin to prevent Reye syndrome.
- Avoid exposure to other individuals, particularly unimmunized children and adults, pregnant women, and immunocompromised persons, until at least 4 days after rash onset.

PATIENT RESOURCES

- KidsHealth. *Measles*—**http://kidshealth.org/parent/infections/bacterial_viral/measles.html#cat20028.**
- Centers for Disease Control and Prevention. *Two Options for Protecting Your Child Against Measles, Mumps, Rubella, and Varicella*—**https://www.cdc.gov/vaccines/vpd/mmr/public/vacopt-factsheet-parent.html.**
- Centers for Disease Control and Prevention. *Measles Vaccination*—**https://www.cdc.gov/vaccines/vpd/measles/index.html.**
- Centers for Disease Control and Prevention. Who should NOT get vaccinated with the MMRV (measles, mumps, rubella, and varicella) vaccine—**https://www.cdc.gov/vaccines/vpd/should-not-vacc.html#mmr.**
- World Health Organization. *Measles*—**http://www.who.int/topics/measles/en/.**

PROVIDER RESOURCES

- MedlinePlus. *Measles*—**http://www.nlm.nih.gov/medlineplus/measles.html.**
- Centers for Disease Control and Prevention. *Measles*—**http://www.cdc.gov/measles/index.html.**
- Centers for Disease Control and Prevention. *Manual for the Surveillance of Vaccine-Preventable Diseases,* 4th ed. (2008). *Chapter 7: Measles*—**http://www.cdc.gov/vaccines/pubs/surv-manual/chpt07-measles.html.**
- Centers for Disease Control and Prevention. *Epidemiology and Prevention of Vaccine-Preventable Diseases, The Pink Book: Course Textbook,* 12th ed. (April 2011): *Measles*—**http://www.cdc.gov/vaccines/pubs/pinkbook/meas.html.**

REFERENCES

1. Katz SL, Hinman AR. Summary and conclusions: measles elimination meeting, 16–17 March 2000. *J Infect Dis.* 2004;189(Suppl 1):S43-47.
2. Zipprich J, Winter K, Hacker J, et al. Measles outbreak—California, December 2014–February 2015. *MMWR Morb Mortal Wkly Rep.* 2015;64(6):153-154.
3. *WHO 2018 Global and regional immunization profile data.* http://www.who.int/immunization/monitoring_surveillance/data/gs_gloprofile.pdf?ua=1.
4. Kaplan LJ, Daum RS, Smaron M, McCarthy CA. Severe measles in immunocompromised patients. *JAMA.* 1992;267:1237-1241.
5. Johnson RT, Griffin DE, Hirsch RL, et al. Measles encephalomyelitis—clinical and immunologic studies. *N Engl J Med.* 1984;310:137-141.
6. Bellini WJ, Rota JS, Lowe LE, et al. Subacute sclerosing panencephalitis: more cases of this fatal disease are prevented by measles immunization than was previously recognized. *J Infect Dis.* 2005;192:1686-1693.
7. Siegel M, Fuerst HT. Low birth weight and maternal virus diseases. A prospective study of rubella, measles, mumps, chickenpox, and hepatitis. *JAMA.* 1966;197:680-684.
8. Centers for Disease Control and Prevention. *Manual for the Surveillance of Vaccine-Preventable Diseases,* 4th ed. (2008). Chapter 7: Measles. http://www.cdc.gov/vaccines/pubs/surv-manual/chpt07-measles.html. Accessed November 2011.
9. Hamborsky J, Kroger A, Wolfe S, eds. *Epidemiology and Prevention of Vaccine-Preventable Diseases, 13th Edition: The Pink Book.* Washington, DC: Public Health Foundation; 2015.

133 FIFTH DISEASE

Khaled Z. Aqeel, MD, MBA
Anisha R. Turner, MD
E.J. Mayeaux, Jr., MD

PATIENT STORY

A 2-year-old boy presents with mild flu-like symptoms and a rash. He had erythematous malar rash and a "lace-like" erythematous rash on the trunk and extremities (**Figures 133-1** and **133-2**). The "slapped cheek" appearance made the diagnosis easy for fifth disease. The parents were reassured that this would go away on its own. The child returned to daycare the next day.

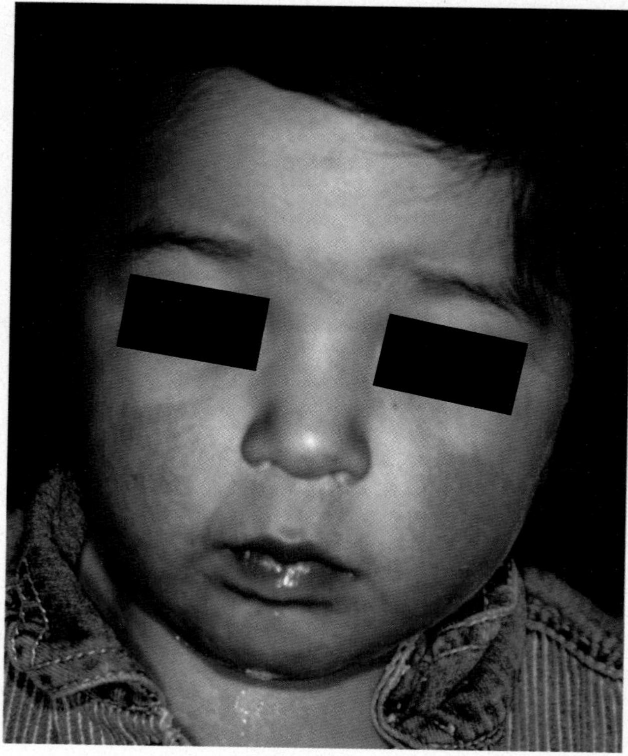

FIGURE 133-1 Classic erythematous malar rash with "slapped cheek" appearance of fifth disease (erythema infectiosum). (*Reproduced with permission from Richard P. Usatine, MD.*)

INTRODUCTION

Fifth disease is also commonly referred to as erythema infectiosum or slapped cheek syndrome. The name derives from the fact that it represents the fifth of the six common childhood viral exanthems described. Transmission occurs through respiratory secretions, possibly through fomites, and parenterally via vertical transmission from mother to fetus and by transfusion of blood or blood products.

SYNONYMS

Erythema infectiosum, parvovirus B19 infections, slapped cheek syndrome.

EPIDEMIOLOGY

- Fifth disease is common throughout the world, with antiparvovirus B19 immunoglobulin (Ig) G reported in approximately 50% to 70% of the United States, Asia, or Europe depending on the geographic location.[1] The only known host for B19 is humans.[2]
- Most individuals become infected during their school years, with the peak incident rates occurring in 6- to 14-year-old children and the age-specific risk being highest in children 7 to 9 years old.[1,3]
- Fifth disease is very contagious via the respiratory route and occurs more frequently between late winter and early summer, specifically between December and July, with April accounting for 16% of infections.[3] Up to 50% of the population is seropositive for antiparvovirus B19 IgG by age 18 years.[3] In some communities, there are cycles of local epidemics every 4 to 7 years lasting up to 6 months at a time.[1,4,5]
- Most cases of infection in pregnant women seem to occur in late spring and summer.[6] Thirty percent to 40% of pregnant women lack measurable IgG to the infecting agent and are, therefore, presumed to be susceptible to infection.[7] About 1% to 16% of susceptible pregnant women will develop serologic evidence in pregnancy.[6,8] The risk of infection increases with increased exposure,

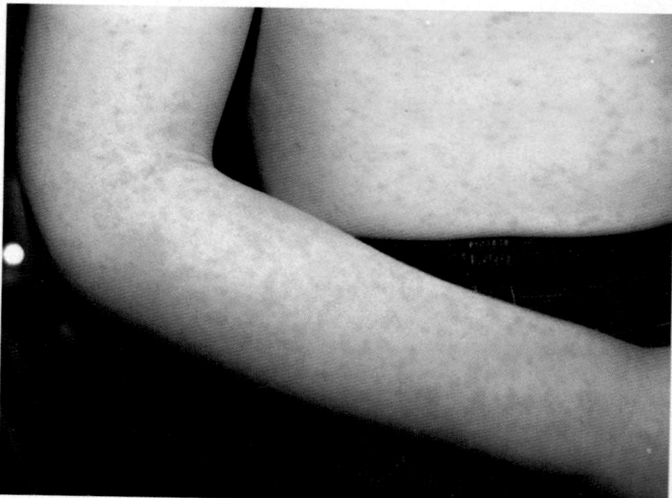

FIGURE 133-2 Classic fifth disease "lace-like" erythematous rash on the trunk and extremities. (*Reproduced with permission from Richard P. Usatine, MD.*)

such as working in nursery schools, after-school clubs, or daycare centers; having serious medical conditions; having stressful jobs; or having a first child or more than three children.[6] Infection during pregnancy can in some cases lead to fetal death, although most fetuses infected with parvovirus have spontaneous resolution with no adverse long-term developmental sequelae.[6,8] SOR B

ETIOLOGY AND PATHOPHYSIOLOGY

- Fifth disease is a mild viral febrile illness with an associated rash caused by parvovirus B19 (**Figure 133-3**).
- Most persons with parvovirus B19 infection never develop the clinical picture of fifth disease.
- Parvovirus B19 infects rapidly dividing cells and is cytotoxic for erythroid progenitor cells.
- After initial infection, a viremia occurs with an associated precipitous drop in the reticulocyte count and anemia. The anemia is rarely clinically apparent in healthy patients, but can cause serious anemia if the red blood cell count is already low. Patients with a chronic anemia such as sickle cell or thalassemia may experience a transient aplastic crisis.[1]
- Vertical transmission can result in congenital infection if a woman becomes infected during her pregnancy, with the transmission rate being 17% to 33%.[6] Transplacental transmission occurs in as many as 33% of cases, with the highest risk of fetal infection occurring between the 9th and 20th weeks of gestation and within 2 to 4 weeks of maternal infection.[8] The risk of a fetal loss (loss rate of 13%) or hydrops fetalis is greatest (loss rate of 4.7%) when the infection occurs within the first 20–25 weeks of gestation, compared to 0.5% and 2.3% after 20 weeks of gestation, respectively.[6]

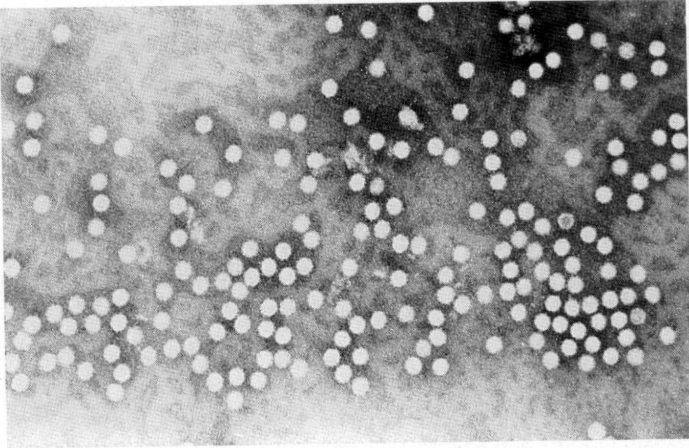

FIGURE 133-3 Transmission electron microscopy of parvovirus B19. *(Reproduced with permission from the Centers for Disease Control and Prevention.)*

RISK FACTORS

- Exposure to infected children.
- Reception of blood products.

DIAGNOSIS

- Diagnosis is typically made based on the patient's clinical features.
- The diagnosis of parvovirus B19 infection can also be made by IgG and IgM antibody testing, although polymerase chain reaction assays may also be helpful in certain situations. Nevertheless, it is recommended that serologic testing be reserved for pregnant women or patients with chronic hemolytic conditions or severe or persistent arthropathy.[9]
- The diagnosis of fetal parvovirus B19 infection relies primarily on PCR on amniotic fluid or fetal blood for B19 IgM.

CLINICAL FEATURES

- Fifth disease is usually a biphasic illness, starting with upper respiratory tract symptoms that may include headache, fever, sore throat, pruritus, coryza, abdominal pain, diarrhea, and/or arthralgias. These constitutional symptoms coincide with onset of viremia, and they usually resolve for about a week before the next stage begins.

- The second stage is characterized by a classic erythematous malar rash with relative circumoral pallor or "slapped cheek" appearance in children (**Figures 133-1** and **133-4**) followed by a "lace-like" erythematous rash on the trunk and extremities (**Figures 133-2** and **133-5**). Arthropathy affecting the hands, wrists, knees, and ankles may precede the development of a rash in adults. The course is usually self-limited.

TYPICAL DISTRIBUTION

- The rash starts with the classic slapped cheek appearance (see **Figures 133-1** and **133-4**). Then an erythematous macular rash occurs on the extremities. After several days, the extremities rash fades into a lacy pattern (see **Figures 133-2** and **133-5**). The lacy rash/exanthem may wax and wane for up to 3 weeks, with flaring triggered by exercise, sun exposure, bathing in hot water, or stress.[9]

LABORATORY TESTING

- Laboratory studies are not usually needed, as the diagnosis can be made by history and physical exam. Serum B19-specific IgM may be ordered in pregnant women exposed to fifth disease. Serum B19-specific IgM can usually be detected 10 days after infection and can persist for 3 months, while serum B19-specific IgG is produced 2 weeks after inoculation and presumably lasts for life.[9] After 3 weeks, infection is also indicated by a fourfold or greater rise in serum B19-specific IgG antibody titers.
- Patients with symptoms of anemia, a history of increased red blood cell (RBC) destruction (e.g., sickle cell disease, hereditary spherocytosis), or with decreased RBC production (e.g., iron-deficiency anemia) should be tested for anemia.
- Pregnant women who are exposed to or have symptoms of parvovirus infection should have serologic testing to assess maternal immunity and determine whether evaluation for fetal hydrops is necessary.[8] SOR C Prior to 20 weeks' gestation, women testing positive for acute infection (i.e., positive IgM and negative IgG) should be counseled concerning the low risk of fetal loss and congenital anomalies.

IMAGING

- If serologic testing in pregnant women is positive, some experts recommend that the patient should receive serial ultrasounds to look for signs of fetal hydrops.[6] SOR C Intrauterine transfusion is currently the only effective treatment to alleviate fetal anemia.[6]

DIFFERENTIAL DIAGNOSIS

- Acute rheumatic fever presents as a fine papular (sandpaper) rash in association with a *Streptococcus* infection (see Chapter 36, Scarlet Fever and Strawberry Tongue).
- Allergic-hypersensitivity reactions (erythema multiforme, erythema nodosum, and cutaneous vasculitis) often involve the arms and legs but rarely affect the face (see Hypersensitivity Syndromes section).

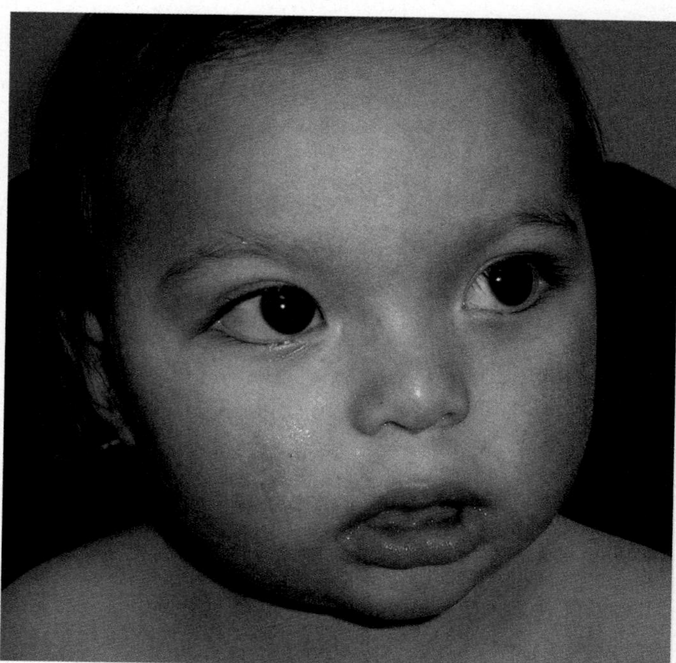

FIGURE 133-4 Classic erythematous malar rash with "slapped cheek" appearance of fifth disease in an 18-month-old child. (*Reproduced with permission from Richard P. Usatine, MD.*)

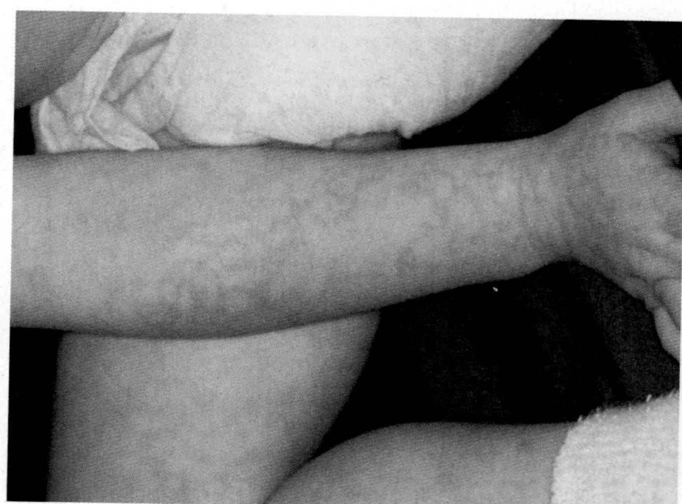

FIGURE 133-5 Classic reticular eruption on the extremities. (*Reproduced with permission from Jeffrey Meffert, MD.*)

- Lyme disease presents with an expanding rash with central clearing (see Chapter 227, Lyme Disease).
- Measles produces a blanching rash that begins on the face and spreads centrifugally to involve the neck, trunk, and finally the extremities. It tends to become more confluent instead of lacy with time (see Chapter 132, Measles).

MANAGEMENT

NONPHARMACOLOGIC

- Fifth disease is usually self-limited and requires no specific therapy.
- See "Patient Education" below for further information about parvovirus B19 infections in pregnancy.

MEDICATIONS

FIRST LINE

- Nonsteroidal anti-inflammatory drug (NSAID) or acetaminophen therapy may alleviate fevers and arthralgias. SOR Ⓒ

SECOND LINE

- If needed, a low-dose oral corticosteroid can be used without prolonging the viral illness.[9] SOR Ⓒ
- Rarely, an immunocompromised patient with hematologic complications may require intravenous immunoglobulin treatment or, in severe cases, bone marrow transplantation.[9] SOR Ⓒ
- Transient aplastic anemia is very rare but may be severe enough to require transfusion until the patient's red cell production recovers. SOR Ⓒ

PREVENTION

- Because it is spread through respiratory secretions and possibly through fomites, good hand sanitation and infection-control techniques are recommended.
- Infected individuals should avoid excessive heat or sunlight, which can cause rash flare-ups.
- Excluding pregnant women from the workplace is unwarranted (SOR Ⓒ, expert opinion), as infection rates are similar in a variety of maternal workplace environments (SOR Ⓐ, prospective cohort studies).[8]

PROGNOSIS

- The rash of erythema infectiosum usually is self-limiting, but may last weeks to months with exacerbations.
- Aplastic anemia usually lasts up to 2 weeks but may become chronic. The onset of erythema infectiosum rash usually indicates that reticulocytosis has returned and aplastic crisis will not occur.
- Studies of the long-term effects on children of maternal parvovirus B19 infection suggest most infants do not have long-term adverse sequelae.[5]

PATIENT EDUCATION

- Explain to parents that the disease is usually self-limited. Normal activities may be pursued as tolerated with sun protection or avoidance.
- Children who present with the classic findings of fifth disease are past the infectious state and can attend school and daycare.
- During pregnancy, a woman who has an acute infection prior to 20 weeks' gestation should be counseled concerning the low risks of fetal loss and congenital anomalies. Beyond 20 weeks' gestation, some physicians recommend repeated ultrasounds to look for signs of fetal hydrops.

PATIENT RESOURCES

- Centers for Disease Control and Prevention (CDC). *Parvovirus B19 and Fifth Disease*—**http://www.cdc.gov/parvovirusb19/.**
- Centers for Disease Control and Prevention (CDC). *Pregnancy and Fifth Disease*—**http://www.cdc.gov/parvovirusb19/pregnancy.html.**

PROVIDER RESOURCES

- Medscape. *Parvovirus B19 Infection*—**http://emedicine.medscape.com/article/961063-overview.**
- Merck Manual. *Erythema Infectiosum*—**http://www.merckmanuals.com/professional/pediatrics/miscellaneous-viral-infections-in-infants-and-children/erythema-infectiosum.**

REFERENCES

1. Obeid OE. Molecular and serological assessment of parvovirus B19 infections among sickle cell anemia patients. *J Infect Dev Ctries.* 2011;5(07):535-539.
2. Gallinella G. Parvovirus B19 achievements and challenges. *ISRN Virol.* 2013;2013:898730. https://www.hindawi.com/journals/isrn/2013/898730/, Accessed December 2016.
3. Valentin M, Cohen P. Pediatric parvovirus B19: spectrum of clinical manifestations. *Cutis.* 2013;92(4):179-184.
4. de Jong EP, Walther FJ, Kroes AC, Oepkes D. Parvovirus B19 infection in pregnancy: new insights and management. *Prenat Diagn.* 2011;31:419-425.
5. Dijkmans AC, de Jong EP, Dijkmans BA, et al. Parvovirus B19 in pregnancy: prenatal diagnosis and management of fetal complications. *Curr Opin Obstet Gynecol.* 2012;24:95-101.
6. Crane J, Mundle W, Boucoiran I, et al. Parvovirus B19 infection in pregnancy. *J Obstet Gynaecol Can.* 2014;36:1107-1116.
7. Temesgen Z, Baddour LM, Steckelberg JM. *Mayo Clinic Infectious Diseases Board Review.* Rochester, MN: Mayo Clinic Scientific Press; 2012.
8. Wallace R, Snyder M. What should you tell pregnant women about exposure to parvovirus? *J Fam Pract.* 60(12):765-766.
9. O'Grady J. Fifth and sixth diseases: more than a fever and a rash. *Clin Rev.* 24(10):E1-5.

134 HAND FOOT MOUTH SYNDROME

Theresa Thuy Vo, MD
E.J. Mayeaux, Jr., MD
Steven N. Bienvenu, MD

PATIENT STORY

A 1-year-old boy presents to the clinic with lesions on his face, trunk and extremities **(Figure 134-1)**. Two days ago, the patient had a fever of 103°F and was very irritable. No one in the family has this rash. On exam, a flat oval vesicle was seen on the hand following skin lines **(Figure 134-2)**. The physician diagnosed hand, foot, and mouth disease. She suspected that it was caused by Coxsackievirus A6 because of the high fever and the wide distribution of lesions. The physician recommended fluid and antipyretics as needed, and the disease resolved without complications.

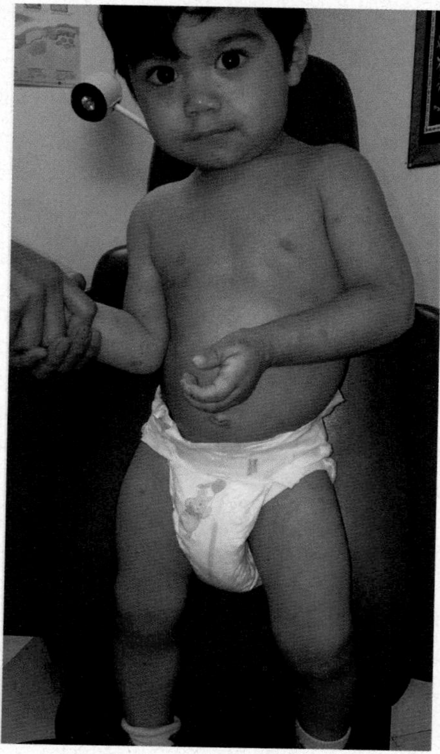

FIGURE 134-1 A 1-year-old boy with hand-foot-mouth disease likely to be caused by Coxsackievirus A6. PCR confirmed presence of enterovirus. (*Reproduced with permission from Richard P. Usatine, MD.*)

INTRODUCTION

Hand, foot, and mouth disease (HFMD) is a viral illness that may affect humans and some animals and has a distinct clinical presentation. The disease occurs worldwide and was typically caused by Coxsackievirus A16. Worldwide outbreaks with a more virulent Coxsackievirus A6 started as early as 2008.[1]

EPIDEMIOLOGY

- In temperate climates, the peak incidence is in summer and early fall. Outbreaks and sporadic episodes have occurred during winter months.[2]
- Typical HFMD caused by Coxsackievirus A16 generally has a mild course. It mostly occurs in infants and children up to 8 years old.[3]
- Atypical HFMD caused by Coxsackievirus A6 (CVA6) has a more severe course and affects young children and adults.[1,2]
- There is no racial or gender predilection.

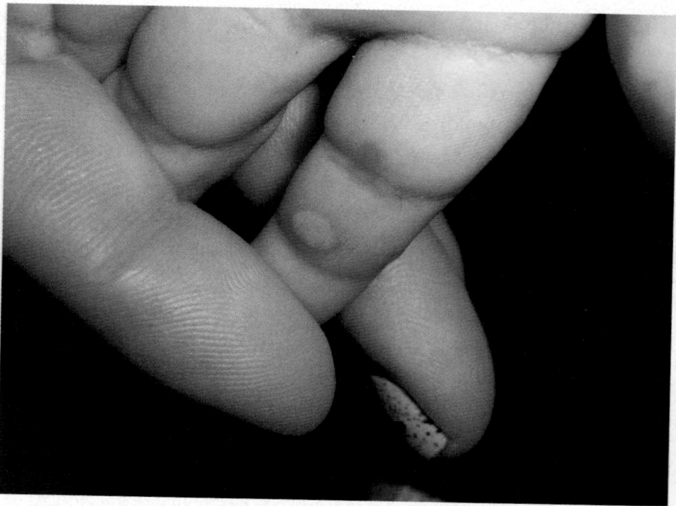

FIGURE 134-2 A single flat, gray, oval vesicular lesion on ventral finger of the child in **Figure 134-1**. (*Reproduced with permission from Richard P. Usatine, MD.*)

ETIOLOGY AND PATHOPHYSIOLOGY

- HFMD is most commonly caused by members of the enterovirus genus, especially Coxsackievirus. Epidemic infections in the United States were usually caused by Coxsackievirus A16 and enterovirus 71 before Coxsackievirus A6 began to appear.
- Outbreaks of strains of EV71 enterovirus producing large epidemics of HFMD with significant morbidity and mortality have occurred in east and southeast Asia. Enterovirus 71 was first isolated in California, USA, in 1969.[4]
- Atypical presentations of HFMD caused by Coxsackievirus A6 have been reported in Asian and Europe since 2008 and in the United

States since 2011.[5-8] In the fall of 2011 and early winter of 2012, 63 cases of apparent but more severe HFMD from four U.S. states were reported to the Centers for Disease Control and Prevention (CDC). Polymerase chain reaction (PCR) and gene sequencing detected an A6 strain of coxsackievirus in 74% of clinical specimens from 34 cases.[5]

- Coxsackievirus infections are highly contagious. For example, an outbreak of 53 cases of HFMD was caused by CVA6 in military training base in Texas.[9] Transmission occurs via aerosolized droplets of nasal and/or oral secretions via the fecal–oral route, or from contact with skin lesions. During epidemics, the virus is spread from child to child and from mother to fetus.
- The incubation period averages 3 to 6 days. Initial viral implantation is in the GI tract mucosa, and it then spreads to lymph nodes within 24 hours. Viremia rapidly ensues, with spread to the oral mucosa and skin. Rarely, aseptic meningitis may occur. Usually by day 7, a neutralizing antibody response develops, and the virus is cleared from the body.
- HFMD may also result in neurologic problems such as a polio-like syndrome, aseptic meningitis, encephalitis, acute cerebellar ataxia, acute transverse myelitis, Guillain-Barré syndrome, and benign intracranial hypertension. Rarely, cardiopulmonary complications such as myocarditis, interstitial pneumonitis, and pulmonary edema may occur.[10-12]
- Infection in the first trimester of pregnancy may lead to spontaneous abortion or intrauterine growth retardation.

RISK FACTORS

- Attendance at childcare centers.
- Contact with HFMD.

DIAGNOSIS

CLINICAL FEATURES—HISTORY AND PHYSICAL

- A prodrome lasting 12 to 36 hours is usually the first sign of HFMD, and it usually consists of typical general viral infection symptoms with anorexia, abdominal pain, fever, emesis, and diarrhea.[2] In typical HFMD, a fever, if present, is generally below 101°F.[12,13]
- Skin and mucosal findings include an oral enanthem and skin exanthem, which can occur together or separately.[13-15] Lesions heal spontaneously in 7 to 10 days.
- Each lesion in typical HFMD begins as a 2- to 10-mm erythematous macule, which develops a gray, oval, football-shaped vesicle (**Figure 134-3**) that parallels the skin tension lines in its long axis (**Figure 134-4**). The oral lesions (**Figure 134-5**) begin as erythematous macules, evolve into 2- to 3-mm vesicles on an erythematous base, and then rapidly become ulcerated. The oral lesions are painful and may interfere with eating. The skin lesions are not generally pruritic.
- Atypical, severe HFMD (CVA6) may be associated with fever as high as 103° to 105°F and may produce much more extensive, denser rash in more locations, with greater malaise and likelihood of anorexia, dehydration, and pain.[5]

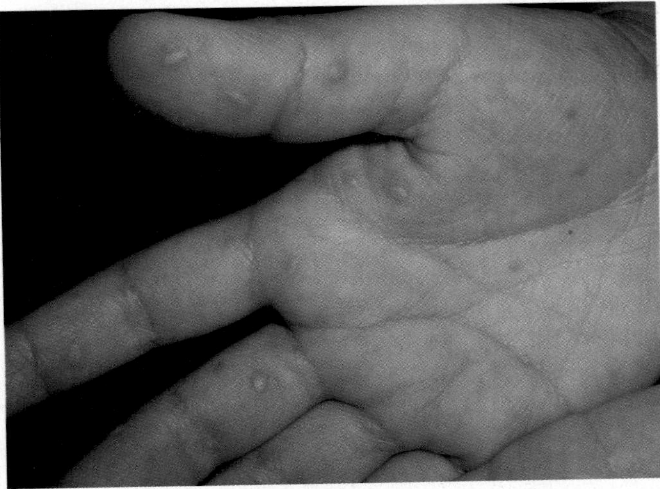

FIGURE 134-3 Typical flat, gray, oval vesicular lesions on the ventral hand and fingers of a 3-year-old boy with hand, foot, and mouth disease. (*Reproduced with permission from Richard P. Usatine, MD.*)

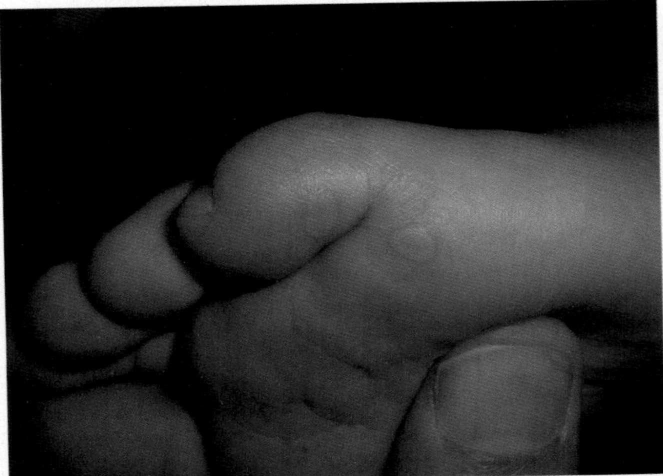

FIGURE 134-4 Flat, gray, oval vesicular lesions on plantar foot of the boy in **Figure 134-3**. (*Reproduced with permission from Richard P. Usatine, MD.*)

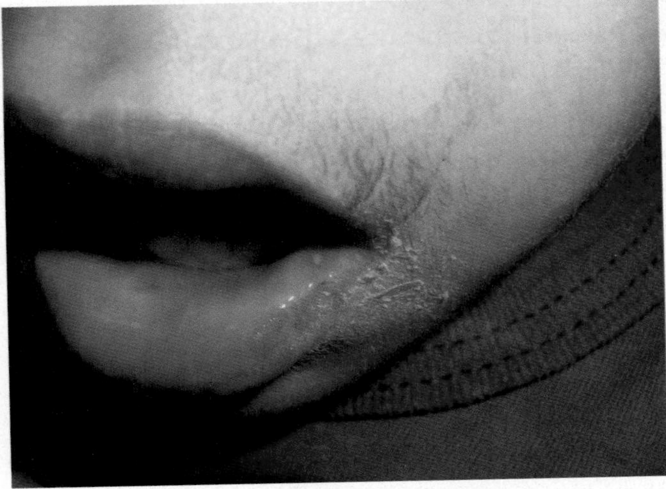

FIGURE 134-5 Mouth lesions in the boy in **Figure 134-3** appear as small ulcers on the lips and oral mucosa. (*Reproduced with permission from Richard P. Usatine, MD.*)

- **Atypical** (CVA6) HFMD may produce lesions that are very protean in their character and evolution. Early lesions are usually maculovesicular as with the milder A16 form, but may coalesce (**Figure 134-6**). Others may be vesiculobullous and may drain, or simply papular (**Figure 134-7)** and ulcerative (**Figure 134-8**).[4,6,7]
- Cervical or submandibular lymphadenopathy may be present.

TYPICAL DISTRIBUTION

- Skin lesions of the milder form (A16) develop on the hands, feet, and/or buttocks, and oral lesions may involve the palate, buccal mucosa, gingiva, and/or tongue. Lesions on the hands and feet are largely limited to the palmar and plantar surfaces (**Figures 134-3** and **134-4**).
- Atypical, severe HFMD (A6) produces a much more extensive rash, and may include the lips and perioral area of the face (**Figure 134-6**), arms, legs, knees genitalia, trunk, buttocks, perianal area, and distinctively the *dorsal* areas of the hands (**Figure 134-8**) and feet as well as palmar and plantar surfaces The lesions may concentrate in areas of active or dormant eczema, known as "eczema coxsackium."[2,5]

LABORATORY TESTING

- Laboratory tests are usually not needed for diagnosis. Diagnosis is typically made clinically, based on history and appearance/location of enanthem and exanthem. If there is diagnostic uncertainty and a change in management based on diagnosis (e.g., CVA6 vs. HSV in eczema herpeticum), viral testing can be performed.[16] It is much easier, less expensive, and faster to get amplified probe testing for HSV than to get viral testing for Coxsackieviruses. If HSV is the cause, antivirals are available, whereas there are no antivirals that affect the course of HFMD.
- For epidemiologic research, genotyping to determine the specific virus causing the HFMD is offered by the CDC. Guidelines for specimen collection can be found on the CDC website—https://www.cdc.gov/laboratory/specimen-submission/cdc-lab-tests.pdf. Because turnaround time is 14 days, this testing is not valuable for clinical management.

DIFFERENTIAL DIAGNOSIS

- Aphthous stomatitis presents as single or multiple painful ulcers in the mouth without skin eruptions (see Chapter 43, Aphthous Ulcer).
- Chickenpox presents with body-wide vesicular lesions in multiple crops (see Chapter 129, Chickenpox).
- Erythema multiforme demonstrates body-wide target lesions that also involve the skin of the palms and soles (see Chapter 185, Erythema Multiforme, Stevens-Johnson Syndrome, and Toxic Epidermal Necrolysis).
- Herpes simplex presents with painful recurrent ulcerations of the lips or genitals without simultaneous hand or foot lesions unless there is a herpetic whitlow on the hand (see Chapter 135, Herpes Simplex).
- Eczema herpeticum (HSV in persons with atopic dermatitis) lesions may resemble eczema coxsackium (CVA6 in patients with atopic dermatitis). Careful exam usually reveals the typical perioral/intraoral

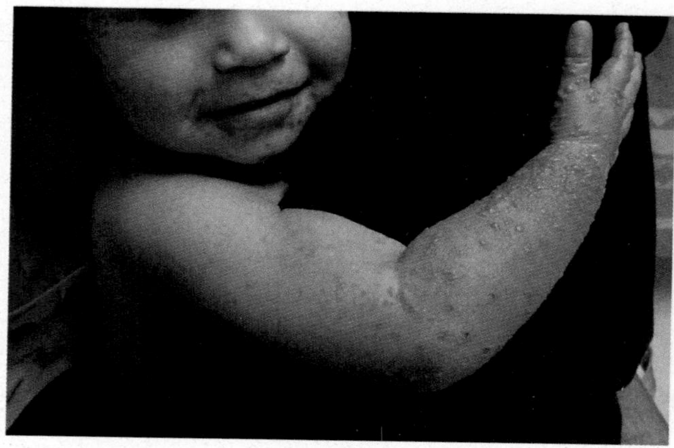

FIGURE 134-6 Hand, foot, and mouth disease in a 1-year-old boy. It is likely caused by Coxsackievirus A6. His temperature reached 103.8°F, and there are many lesions covering the forearms, dorsal hands, and face as seen with the CVA6. Some lesions have coalesced on the forearm. (*Reproduced with permission from Ann Petru, MD and Julie Kulhanjian, MD.*)

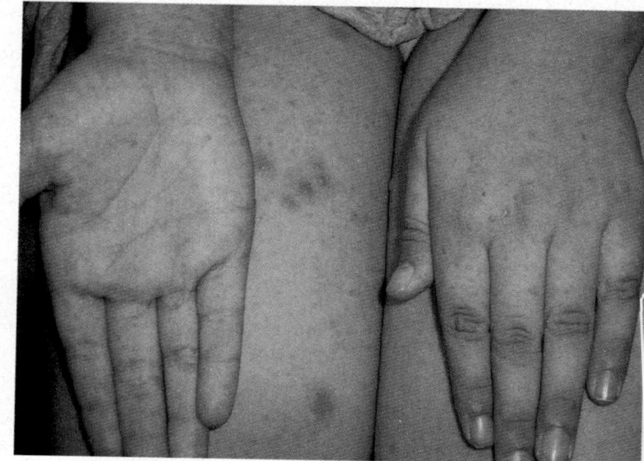

FIGURE 134-7 Hand, foot, and mouth disease in a 6-year-old girl. The clinical picture suggests this was caused by Coxsackievirus A6. (*Reproduced with permission from Richard P. Usatine, MD.*)

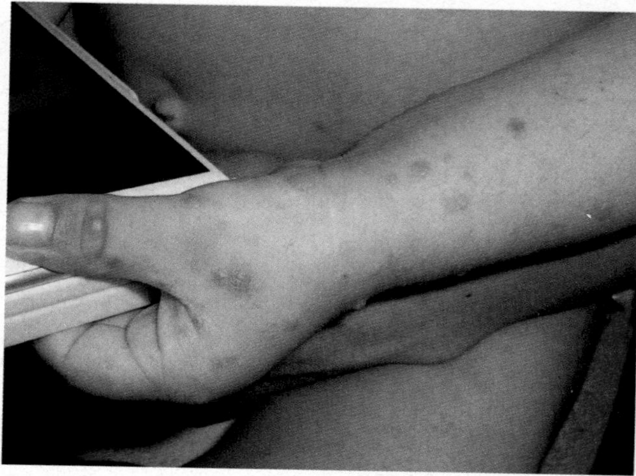

FIGURE 134-8 Hand, foot, and mouth disease in a 1-year-old boy. The vesicles on dorsal and plantar sides of hand along with the wide distribution of lesions suggests this was caused by Coxsackievirus A6. Same child as in **Figure 134-1**. (*Reproduced with permission from Richard P. Usatine, MD.*)

lesions and concurrent hand and foot distribution of HFMD. Unfortunately, some cases of eczema coxsackium have not manifested intraoral lesions, or lesions on hands or feet.[2] Then it helps to get rapid amplified probe testing for HSV to determine the virus involved. This is crucial, as specific antiviral therapy is available for HSV.[17]

- Id reaction (autoeczematization) occurs as a pruritic, papulovesicular eruption due to hypersensitivity response to fungal antigens. This rash is particularly pruritic, and the fungal infection is often on the feet. The papulovesicles are usually smaller in size than those in HFMD, and the presence of a fungal infection points toward an Id reaction.
- Gianotti–Crosti syndrome (papular acrodermatitis of childhood) presents as papules and/or papulovesicles on the extremities and buttocks in children during or within a few weeks after a viral infection (**Figure 134-9**). The child does not usually appear ill, and the parents bring the child for evaluation because the papular eruption can be frightening. The papulovesicles are very similar in appearance and distribution to atypical HFMD. Look for flat oblong vesicles on the palmar and plantar regions along with lesions in the mouth to differentiate HFMD from Gianotti–Crosti syndrome.

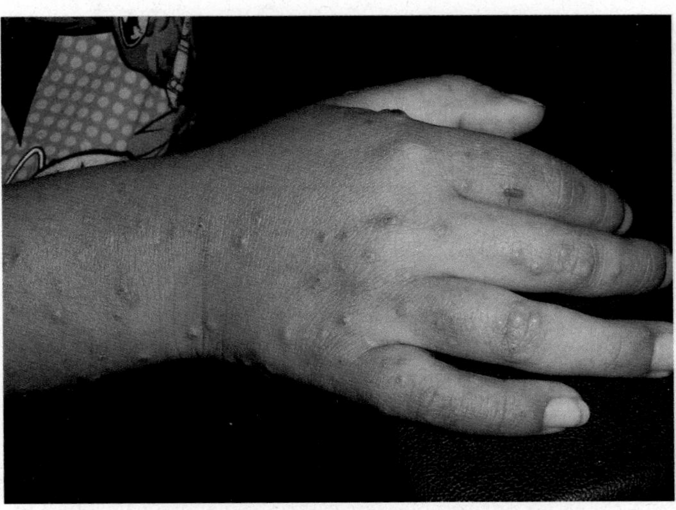

FIGURE 134-9 Gianotti-Crosti syndrome (papular acrodermatitis of childhood) in a 4-year-old boy after an upper respiratory infection. Note how the papules and vesicles can easily be mistaken for those caused by atypical hand, foot, and mouth disease. (*Reproduced with permission from Richard P. Usatine, MD.*)

MANAGEMENT

FIRST LINE

- The treatment of HFMD is supportive therapy.[18] Usually the mouth lesions are not as painful as in herpes gingivostomatitis. If there is a lot of mouth pain leading to poor oral intake, the following medications may be considered. Topical oral anesthetics such as 2% lidocaine gel by prescription or 20% topical benzocaine (Orabase) nonprescription may be used to treat painful oral ulcers, but are not routinely recommended given lack of evidence of benefit from clinical trials[19] and potential harm (e.g. systemic absorption, allergic reaction[20,21]). Benzocaine is not safe in children under 2 years of age because of the risk of methemoglobinemia.[22] SOR Ⓒ
- Acetaminophen or NSAIDs may be used to manage fever and treat arthralgias. SOR Ⓒ Aspirin should not be used in viral illnesses in children younger than 12 years of age to prevent Reye syndrome. SOR Ⓒ

SECOND LINE

Studies are being conducted in Asia for alternative treatment modalities including interferon-α,[23,24] ribavirin aerosol,[25,26] low-level laser,[27] and immunoglobulin.[28]

REFERRAL OR HOSPITALIZATION

- Indications for hospitalization include: (1) inability to maintain adequate hydration, (2) development of neurologic or cardiovascular complications, and (3) inability to differentiate eczema coxsackium from eczema herpeticum.[29]

PREVENTION

- Good handwashing is critical to reduce the spread of disease, both at home and at daycare facilities experiencing cases. Virus may be shed in stool for at least several weeks.

- Infants and children with active skin lesions of HFMD should be excused from daycare facilities. Adults with active lesions should stay out of work.
- A vaccine against enterovirus 71 has entered phase III clinical trials in Asia and has shown efficacy of 95.1% for up to 2 years.[30,31] Currently, there are still obstacles for mass production.

PROGNOSIS

- HFMD caused by coxsackievirus A16 is generally a mild self-limited illness that resolves in around 7 to 10 days. Typical HFMD may rarely recur, persist, or cause serious complications.
- CVA6 resulted in a high rate of hospitalization (about 1 in 5 cases) in 63 cases reported to the CDC. Fortunately, there were no deaths. CVA6 may also cause palmar plantar desquamation 1 to 2 weeks afterwards. Lesions tend to heal completely if not complicated.
- Beau's lines (see Chapter 198, Normal Nail Variants) and onychomadesis (loss of nail) may occur many weeks later, followed by complete healing.[5,15]
- HFMD is usually followed by complete recovery without scarring.
- Uncommon CNS involvement (meningitis, encephalitis) has been the cause of rare morbidity and mortality associated with HFMD.

PATIENT EDUCATION

- Educate parents of young children to watch for signs of dehydration owing to decreased oral intake secondary to mouth pain.
- To reduce viral spreading, do not rupture blisters.
- The patient may attend school once fever and symptoms subside, no new lesions have appeared, and all lesions have dried or scabbed over.[32]
- The virus that causes HFMD may be shed in the patient's stool for weeks.
- Report any neurologic symptoms to healthcare providers immediately.
- Good handwashing and contact precautions are critical to preventing spread to others.

PATIENT RESOURCES

- Centers for Disease Control and Prevention. *CDC Feature: Hand, Foot & Mouth Disease*—**http://www.cdc.gov/Features/HandFootMouthDisease/.**
- Centers for Disease Control and Prevention. *About Hand, Foot, and Mouth Disease (HFMD)*—**http://www.cdc.gov/hand-foot-mouth/about/.**
- eMedicine Health. *Hand, Foot, and Mouth Disease*—**http://www.emedicinehealth.com/hand_foot_and_mouth_disease/article_em.htm.**

PROVIDER RESOURCES

- Centers for Disease Control and Prevention. *Hand, Foot, and Mouth Disease (HFMD)*—**http://www.cdc.gov/hand-foot-mouth/index.html.**
- WebMD. *Facts About Hand-Foot-and-Mouth Disease*—**https://www.webmd.com/children/guide/hand-foot-mouth-disease#1.**

REFERENCES

1. Downing C, Ramirez-Fort MK, Doan HQ, et al. Coxsackievirus A6 associated hand, foot and mouth disease in adults: clinical presentation and review of the literature. J Clin Virol 2014; 60:381.
2. Flett K, Youngster I, Huang J, et al. Hand, foot, and mouth disease caused by coxsackievirus A6. *Emerg Infect Dis.* 2012;18(10):1702-1704.
3. Hongyan G, Chengjie M, Qiaozhi Y, et al. Hand, foot and mouth disease caused by coxsackievirus A6, Beijing, 2013. *Pediatr Infect Dis J.* 2014;33:1302.
4. Solomon T, Lewthwaite P, Perera D, et al. Virology, epidemiology, pathogenesis, and control of enterovirus 71. *Lancet Infect Dis.* 2010;10:778.
5. Centers for Disease Control and Prevention (CDC). Notes from the field: severe hand, foot, and mouth disease associated with coxsackievirus A6—Alabama, Connecticut, California, and Nevada, November 2011–February 2012. *MMWR Morb Mortal Wkly Rep.* 2012;61:213.
6. Feder HM Jr, Bennett N, Modlin JF. Atypical hand, foot, and mouth disease: a vesiculobullous eruption caused by Coxsackie virus A6. *Lancet Infect Dis.* 2014;14:83.
7. Han JF, Xu S, Zhang Y, et al. Hand, foot, and mouth disease outbreak caused by coxsackievirus A6, China, 2013. *J Infect.* 2014;69:303.
8. Buttery VW, Kenyon C, Grunewald S, et al. Atypical presentations of hand, foot, and mouth disease caused by coxsackievirus A6—Minnesota, 2014. *MMWR Morb Mortal Wkly Rep.* 2015;64:805.
9. Banta J, Lenz B, Pawlak M, et al. Notes from the field: outbreak of hand, foot, and mouth disease caused by coxsackievirus a6 among basic military trainees—Texas, 2015. *MMWR Morb Mortal Wkly Rep.* 2016;65:678-680.
10. Chan KP, Goh KT, Chong CY, et al. Epidemic hand, foot and mouth disease caused by human enterovirus 71, Singapore. *Emerg Infect Dis.* 2003;9(1):78-85.
11. Chen SC, Chang HL, Yan TR, et al. An eight-year study of epidemiologic features of enterovirus 71 infection in Taiwan. *Am J Trop Med Hyg.* 2007;77(1):188-191.
12. Alsop J, Flewett TH, Foster JR. "Hand-foot-and-mouth disease" in Birmingham in 1959. *BMJ* 1960;2:1708.
13. Froeschle JE, Nahmias AJ, Feorino PM, et al. Hand, foot, and mouth disease (Coxsackievirus A16) in Atlanta. *Am J Dis Child.* 1967;114:278.
14. Adler JL, Mostow SR, Mellin H, et al. Epidemiologic investigation of hand, foot, and mouth disease. Infection caused by coxsackievirus A 16 in Baltimore, June through September 1968. *Am J Dis Child.* 1970;120:309.

15. Sinclair C, Gaunt E, Simmonds P, et al. Atypical hand, foot, and mouth disease associated with coxsackievirus A6 infection, Edinburgh, United Kingdom, January to February 2014. *Euro Surveill.* 2014;19:20745.
16. Stellrecht KA, Lamson DA, Romero JR. Enteroviruses and parechoviruses. In: Jorgensen JH, Pfaller MA, Carroll KC, et al., eds. *Manual of Clinical Microbiology*. 11th ed. Washington, DC: American Society for Microbiology; 2015:1536.
17. Fang Y, Wang S, Zhang L, et al. Risk factors of severe hand, foot and mouth disease: a meta-analysis. *Scand J Infect Dis.* 2014;46:515.
18. Omaña-Cepeda C, Martínez-Valverde A, del Mar Sabater-Recolons M, et al. A literature review and case report of hand, foot and mouth disease in an immunocompetent adult. *BMC Res Notes.* 2016;9:165.
19. Hopper SM, McCarthy M, Tancharoen C, et al. Topical lidocaine to improve oral intake in children with painful infectious mouth ulcers: a blinded, randomized, placebo-controlled trial. *Ann Emerg Med.* 2014;63:292.
20. Hess GP, Walson PD. Seizures secondary to oral viscous lidocaine. *Ann Emerg Med.* 1988;17:725.
21. U.S. Food and Drug Administration. *Questions & Answers: Reports of a Rare, but Serious and Potentially Fatal Adverse Effect with the use of Over-the-Counter (OTC) Benzocaine Gels and Liquids Applied to the Gums or Mouth.* https://www.fda.gov/Drugs/DrugSafety/ucm250024.htm. Accessed December 2016.
22. U.S. Food and Drug Administration. *Drug Safety Communication.* http://www.fda.gov/drugs/drugsafety/ucm250024.htm. Accessed December 2016.
23. Huang X, Zhang X, Wang F, et al. Clinical Efficacy of therapy with recombinant human interferon α1b in hand, foot, and mouth disease with enterovirus 71 infection. *PLoS One.* 2016;11(2): e0148907.
24. Lin H, Huang L, Zhou J, et al. Efficacy and safety of interferon-α2b spray in the treatment of hand, foot, and mouth disease: a multicenter, randomized, double-blind trial. *Arch Virol.* 2016; 161(11):3073-3080.
25. Zhang HP, Wang L, Qian JH, et al. Efficacy and safety of ribavirin aerosol in children with hand-foot-mouth disease. *Zhongguo Dang Dai Er Ke Za Zhi.* 2014;16(3):272-276. Chinese.
26. Pan S, Qian J, Gong X, Zhou Y. Effects of ribavirin aerosol on viral exclusion of patients with hand-foot-mouth disease. *Zhonghua Yi Xue Za Zhi.* 2014;94(20):1563-1566. Chinese.
27. Toida M, Watanabe F, Goto K, Shibata T. Usefulness of low-level laser for control of painful stomatitis in patients with hand-foot-and-mouth disease. *J Clin Laser Med Surg.* 2003;21(6):363-367.
28. Jiang M, Wang XC. Clinical research of early, enough methylprednisone combined with immunoglobulin in treatment of severe hand-foot-mouth disease. *Zhonghua Shi Yan He Lin Chuang Bing Du Xue Za Zhi.* 2013;27(5):363-365.
29. World Health Organization Regional Office for the Western Pacific Region. News Release: Severe hand, foot and mouth disease killed Cambodian children. 12 July 2012. http://www.wpro.who.int/mediacentre/releases/2012/20120713/en/. Accessed December 2017.
30. Li JX, Song YF, Wang L, et al. Two-year efficacy and immunogenicity of Sinovac Enterovirus 71 vaccine against hand, foot and mouth disease in children. *Expert Rev Vaccines.* 2016;15(1): 129-137.
31. Li R, Liu L, Mo Z, et al. An inactivated enterovirus 71 vaccine in healthy children. *N Engl J Med.* 2014;370(9):829-837.
32. Inyo County Health and Human Services, Public Health Division. *Inyo County Health Brief: Atypical Hand, foot, and Mouth Disease Circulating.* http://www.nih.org/docs/ICPHB_hand_foot_7_18_12.pdf. 2012. Accessed December 2017.

135 HERPES SIMPLEX

E.J. Mayeaux, Jr., MD

PATIENT STORY

A 32-year-old man presents with complaints of a 1-week history of multiple painful vesicles on the shaft of his penis associated with tender groin adenopathy (**Figure 135-1**). The vesicles broke 2 days ago and the pain has increased. He had similar lesions 1 year ago but never went for a healthcare examination at that time. He has had 3 different female sexual partners in the past 2 years but has no knowledge of them having any sores or diseases. He was given the presumptive diagnosis of genital herpes and a course of acyclovir. His herpes polymerase chain reaction (PCR) came back positive, and his rapid plasma reagin (RPR) and HIV tests were negative.

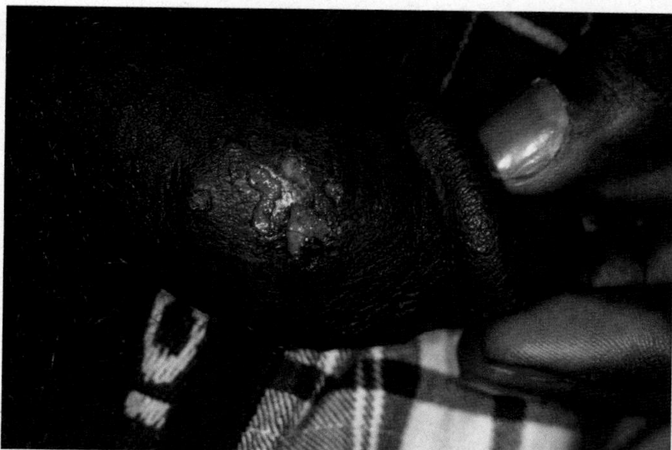

FIGURE 135-1 Recurrent genital herpes simplex virus on the penis showing grouped ulcers (deroofed vesicles). (*Reproduced with permission from Richard P. Usatine, MD.*)

INTRODUCTION

Herpes simplex virus (HSV) infection can involve the skin, mucosa, eyes, and central nervous system. HSV establishes a latent state followed by viral reactivation and recurrent local disease. Perinatal transmission of HSV can lead to significant fetal morbidity and mortality.

EPIDEMIOLOGY

HSV affects more than one-third of the world's population, with the 2 most common cutaneous manifestations being genital (**Figures 135-1** to **135-4**) and orolabial herpes (**Figures 135-5** to **135-7**).[1]

The Centers for Disease Control and Prevention (CDC) reports that at least 50 million persons in the United States have genital HSV-2 infection. Over the past decade, the percentage of Americans with genital herpes infection in the United States has remained stable. Most persons infected with HSV-2 have not been diagnosed with genital herpes.[2]

Genital HSV-2 infection is more common in women (approximately 1 of 5 women 14 to 49 years of age) than in men (approximately 1 of 9 men 14 to 49 years of age). Transmission from an infected male to his female partner is believed to be more likely than from an infected female to her male partner.

Orolabial herpes is the most prevalent form of herpes infection and often affects children younger than 5 years of age (**Figure 135-7**), although all age groups are affected. The duration of the illness is 2 to 3 weeks, and oral shedding of virus may continue for as long as 23 days.[1]

Herpetic whitlow is an intense painful infection of the hand involving the terminal phalanx of one or more digits. In the United States, the estimated annual incidence is 2.4 cases per 100,000 persons.[3]

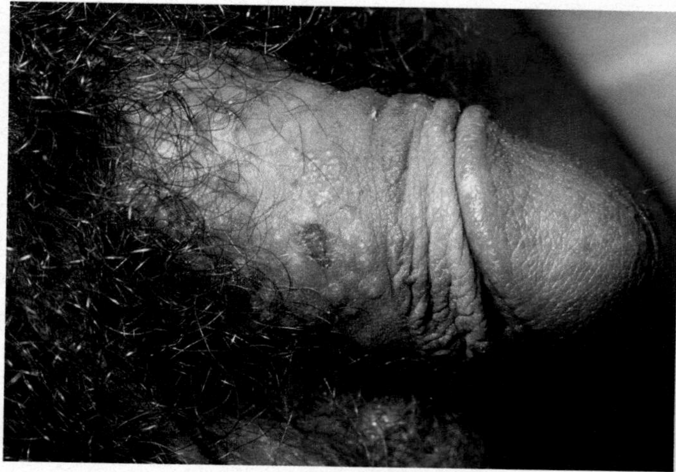

FIGURE 135-2 Herpes simplex on the penis with intact vesicles and visible crusts. (*Reproduced with permission from Eric Kraus, MD.*)

ETIOLOGY AND PATHOPHYSIOLOGY

- HSV belongs to the family Herpesviridae and is a double-stranded DNA virus.

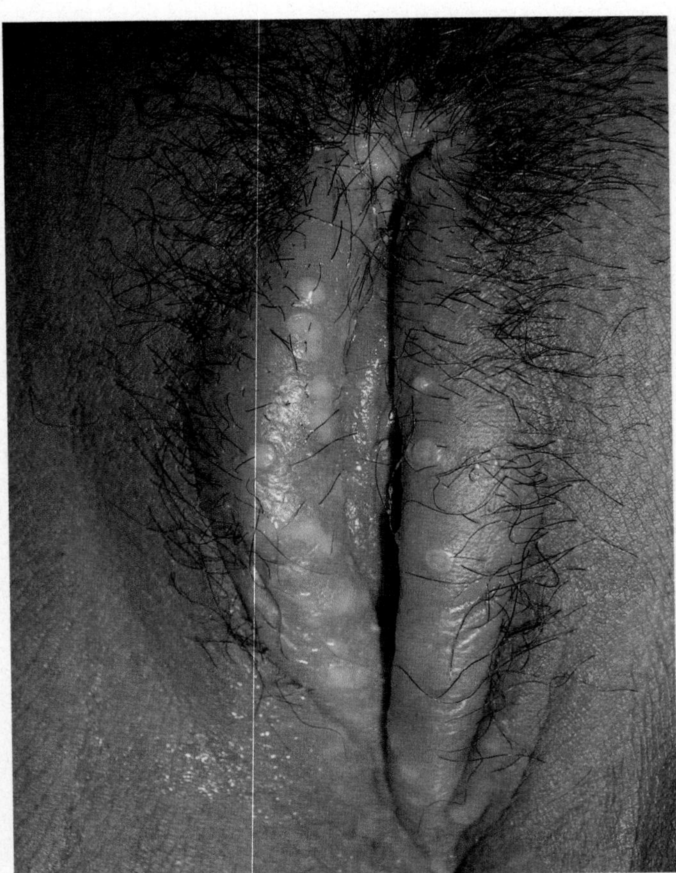

FIGURE 135-3 Vulvar primary herpes simplex virus at the introitus showing vesicles, pustules, and ulcers in this pregnant woman. (*Reproduced with permission from Richard P. Usatine, MD.*)

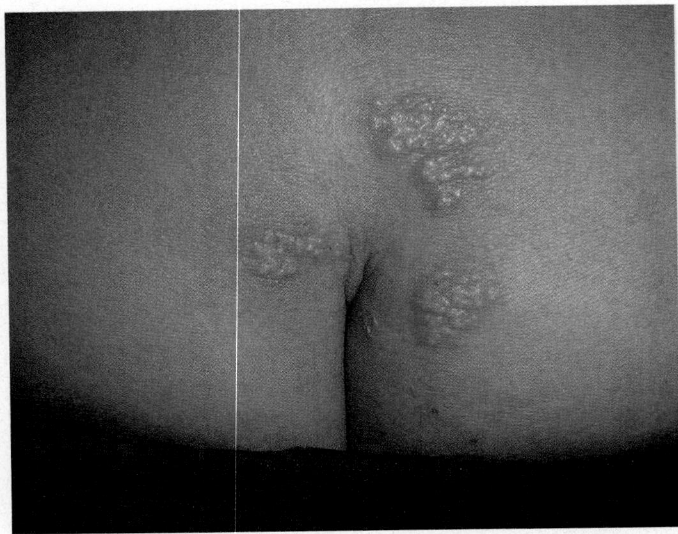

FIGURE 135-4 Recurrent herpes simplex virus on the buttocks of a woman with clusters of vesicles. Women are prone to getting buttocks involvement owing to sleeping with partners who have genital involvement. (*Reproduced with permission from Flowers H, Brodell RT. Recurrent vesicular rash over the sacrum. J Fam Pract. 2015 Sep;64(9):577-579.*)

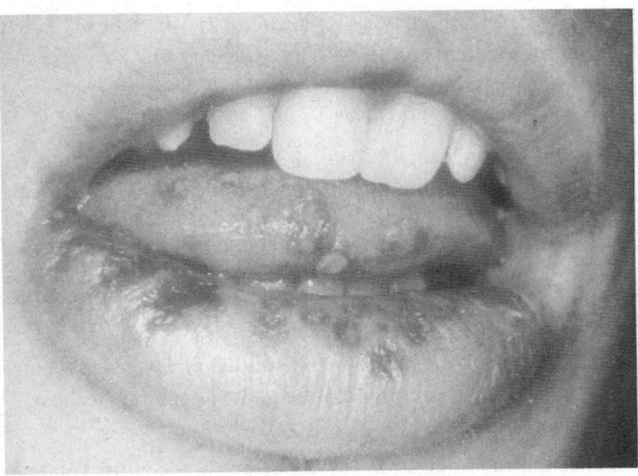

FIGURE 135-5 Primary herpes gingivostomatitis presenting with multiple ulcers on the tongue and lower lip. (*Reproduced with permission from Richard P. Usatine, MD.*)

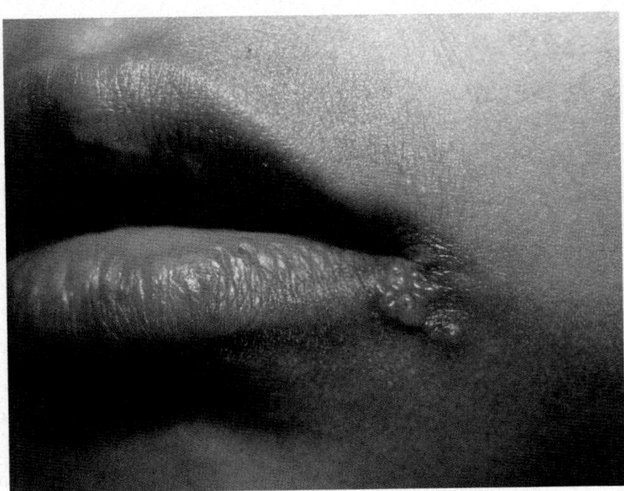

FIGURE 135-6 Close-up of recurrent herpes simplex virus-1 showing vesicles at the vermilion border. (*Reproduced with permission from Richard P. Usatine, MD.*)

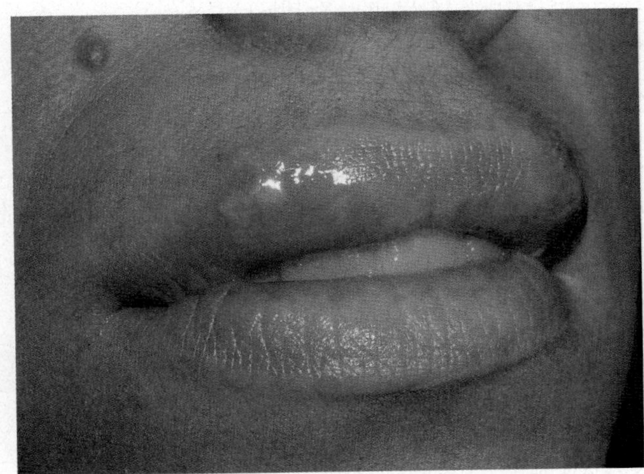

FIGURE 135-7 Orolabial herpes simplex virus in an adult woman showing deroofed blisters (ulcer). (*Reproduced with permission from Richard P. Usatine, MD.*)

- HSV exists as 2 separate types (types 1 and 2), which have affinities for different epithelia.[3] Ninety percent of HSV-2 infections are genital, whereas 90% of those caused by HSV-1 are oral–labial.
- HSV enters through abraded skin or intact mucous membranes. Once infected, the epithelial cells die, forming vesicles and creating multinucleated giant cells.
- Retrograde transport into sensory ganglia leads to lifelong latent infection.[1] Reactivation of the virus may be triggered by immunodeficiency, trauma, fever, and UV light.
- Genital HSV infection is usually transmitted through sexual contact. When it occurs in a preadolescent, the possibility of abuse must be considered.
- Evidence indicates that 21.9% of all persons in the United States 12 years or older have serologic evidence of HSV-2 infection, which is more commonly associated with genital infections.[4]
- As many as 90% of those infected are unaware that they have herpes infection and may unknowingly shed virus and transmit infection.[5]
- Primary genital herpes has an average incubation period of 4 days, followed by a prodrome of itching, burning, or erythema (**Figure 135-8**).
- With both types, systemic symptoms are common in primary disease and include fever, headache, malaise, abdominal pain, and myalgia.[6] Recurrences are usually less severe and shorter in duration than the initial outbreak.[1,6]
- Maternal–fetal transmission of HSV is associated with significant morbidity and mortality. Manifestations of neonatal HSV include localized infection of the skin, eyes, and mouth, central nervous system (CNS) disease, or disseminated multiple organ disease. The CDC and the American College of Obstetricians and Gynecologists recommend that cesarean delivery should be offered as soon as possible to women who have active HSV lesions or, in those with a history of genital herpes, symptoms of vulvar pain or burning at the time of delivery.
- Herpetic whitlow occurs as a complication of oral or genital HSV infection and in medical personnel who have contact with oral secretions (**Figures 135-9** and **135-10**).
- Toddlers and preschool children are susceptible to herpetic whitlow if they have herpes labialis and engage in thumb-sucking or finger-sucking behavior.
- Like all HSV infections, herpetic whitlow usually has a primary infection, which may be followed by subsequent recurrences. The virus migrates to the peripheral ganglia and Schwann cells where it lies dormant. Recurrences observed in 20% to 50% of cases are usually milder and shorter in duration.

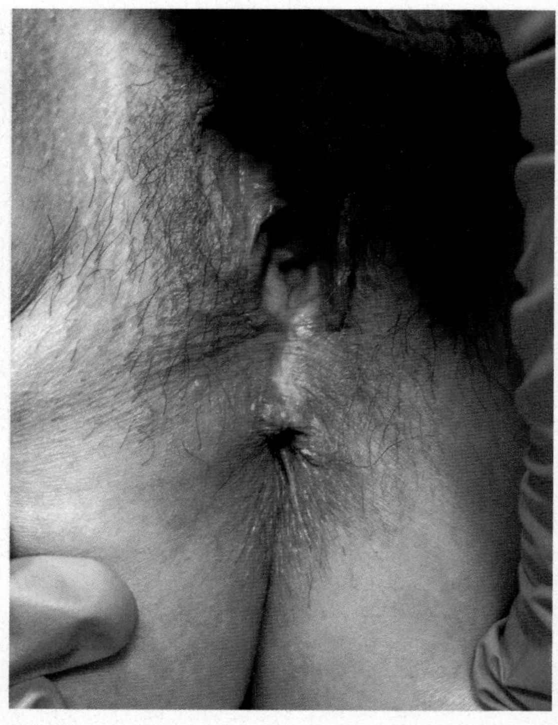

FIGURE 135-8 Primary genital herpes in a 51-year-old woman with prominent erythema and very small vesicles. The woman was in a great deal of pain. (*Reproduced with permission from Richard P. Usatine, MD.*)

RISK FACTORS

- Multiple sexual partners.
- Female gender.
- Low socioeconomic status.
- HIV infection.

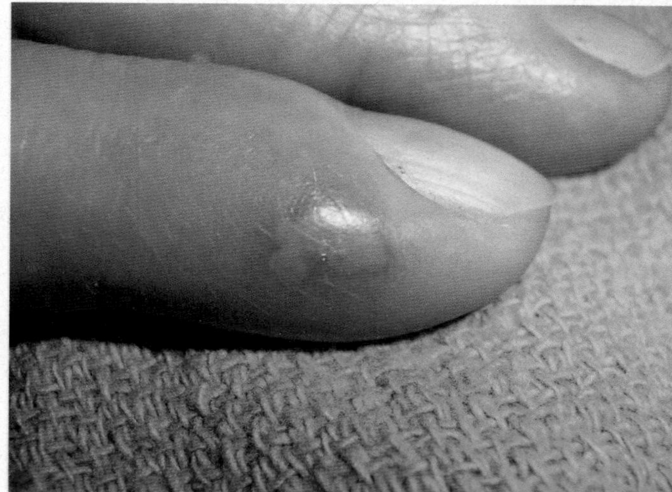

FIGURE 135-9 Herpetic whitlow lesion on distal index finger. (*Reproduced with permission from Richard P. Usatine, MD.*)

DIAGNOSIS

CLINICAL FEATURES

- The diagnosis of HSV infection may be made by clinical appearance. Many patients have systemic symptoms, including fever, headache, malaise, and myalgias. Nontypical cases should be confirmed with laboratory testing.[2]
- Orolabial herpes typically takes the form of painful vesicles and ulcerative erosions on the tongue, palate, gingiva, buccal mucosa, and lips (see **Figures 135-5** to **135-7**).
- Genital herpes presents with multiple transient, painful vesicles that appear on the penis (see **Figures 135-1** and **135-2**), vulva (see **Figure 135-3**), buttocks (**Figures 135-4** and **135-11**), perineum, vagina or cervix, and tender inguinal lymphadenopathy.[6] The vesicles break down and become ulcers that develop crusts while these are healing.
- Recurrences typically occur 2 to 3 times a year. The duration is shorter and less painful than in primary infections. The lesions are often single, and the vesicles heal completely by 8 to 10 days.
- UV radiation in the form of sunlight may trigger outbreaks, another reason to use sun protection when outdoors. Sunlight triggers recurrence of orolabial HSV-1, an effect that is not fully suppressed by acyclovir.

LABORATORY STUDIES

- The gold standard of diagnosis is viral isolation by tissue culture and PCR testing.[2]
  - PCR is extremely sensitive (96%) and specific (99%) and is preferred for all testing.[2] It is used for cerebrospinal fluid (CSF) testing in suspected HSV encephalitis or meningitis.[2]
  - The culture sensitivity rate is only 50% and depends upon the stage at which the specimen is collected. The sensitivity is highest at first in the vesicular stage and declines with ulceration and crusting. The tissue culture assay can be positive within 48 hours but may take longer.
- HSV-specific glycoprotein G2 (HSV-2) and glycoprotein G1 (HSV-1) type-specific HSV serologic assays are 80%–98% specific. Because nearly all HSV-2 infections are sexually acquired, the presence of type-specific HSV-2 antibody implies anogenital infection. Type-specific HSV serologic assays might be useful in patients with recurrent symptoms and negative HSV cultures and an asymptomatic patient with a partner with genital herpes. Screening for HSV-1 and HSV-2 in the general population is not indicated.[2]
- The Tzanck test and antigen detection tests have lower sensitivity rates than viral culture and should not be relied on for diagnosis.[2]
- The CDC does not currently recommend routine type 2 HSV testing in someone with no symptoms suggestive of herpes infection (i.e., for the general population).[7]
- If the herpes was acquired by sexual contact, screening should be performed for other sexually transmitted diseases (STDs), such as syphilis and HIV.
- Biopsy is usually unnecessary unless no infectious etiology is found for a genital lesion and a malignancy is suspected.

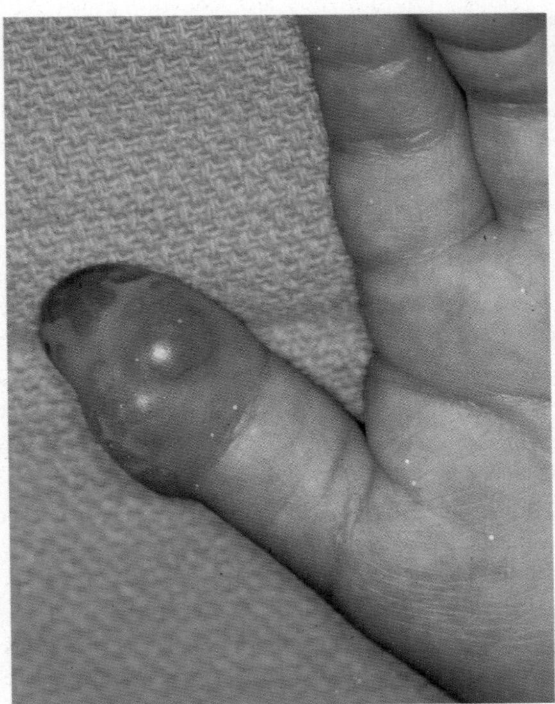

FIGURE 135-10 Severely painful herpetic whitlow on the thumb. *(Reproduced with permission from Eric Kraus, MD.)*

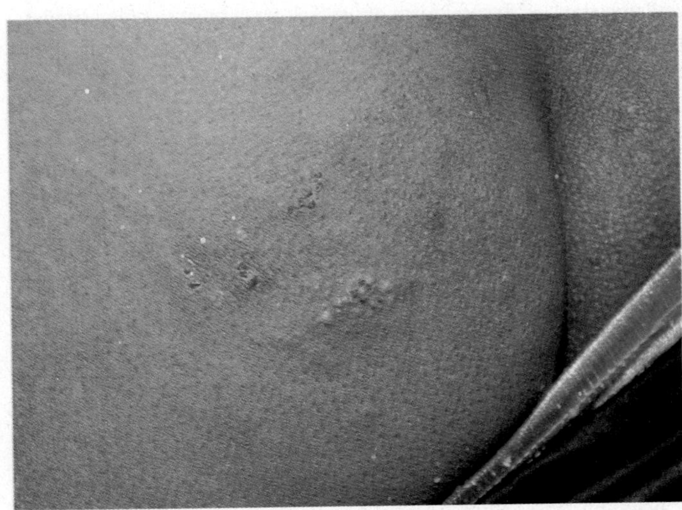

FIGURE 135-11 Recurrent herpes simplex virus on the buttocks of a woman. Note the vesicles and crusts in a unilateral cluster. *(Reproduced with permission from Richard P. Usatine, MD.)*

DIFFERENTIAL DIAGNOSIS

- Syphilis produces a painless or mildly painful, indurated, clean-based ulcer (chancre) at the site of exposure. It is best to investigate for syphilis or coexisting syphilis in any patient presenting for the first time with a genital ulcer of unproven etiology (see Chapter 225, Syphilis).
- Chancroid produces a painful deep, undermined, purulent ulcer that may be associated with painful inguinal lymphadenitis (see Chapter 225, Syphilis).
- Drug eruptions produce pruritic papules or blisters without associated viral symptoms (see Chapter 212, Cutaneous Drug Reactions).
- Behçet disease produces ulcerative disease around the mouth and genitals, possibly before onset of sexual activity (**Figure 135-12**).
- Acute paronychia presents as a localized abscess in a nail fold and is the main differential diagnosis in the consideration of herpetic whitlow (see Chapter 202, Paronychia).
- Felon—A red, painful infection, usually bacterial, of the fingertip pulp. It is important to distinguish whitlow from a felon (where the pulp space usually is tensely swollen), as incision and drainage of a felon is needed, but should be avoided in herpetic whitlow because it may lead to an unnecessary secondary bacterial infection.

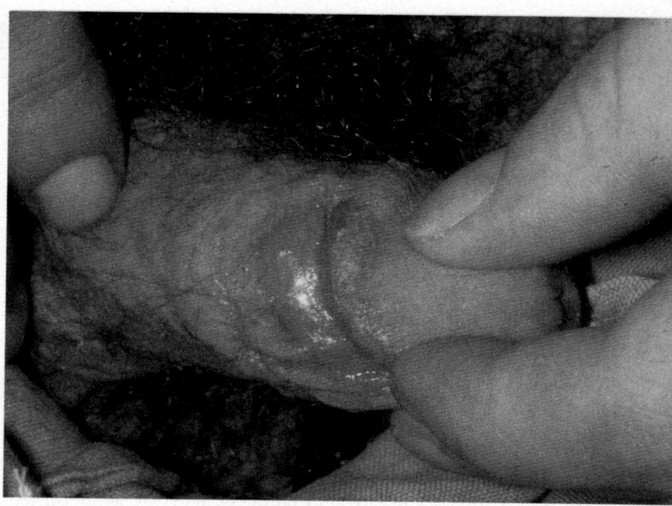

FIGURE 135-12 Young man with Behçet syndrome presenting with a painful penile ulcer and aphthous ulcers in his mouth. (*Reproduced with permission from Richard P. Usatine, MD.*)

MANAGEMENT

NONPHARMACOLOGIC

- Women with active primary or recurrent genital herpetic lesions at the onset of labor should deliver by cesarean section to lower the chance of neonatal HSV infection.[2] SOR Ⓐ

MEDICATIONS

- Acyclovir is a guanosine analog that acts as a DNA chain terminator which, when incorporated, ends viral DNA replication. Valacyclovir is the l-valine ester prodrug of acyclovir that has enhanced absorption after oral administration and high oral bioavailability. Famciclovir is the oral form of penciclovir, a purine analog similar to acyclovir. They must be administered early in the outbreak to be effective, but are safe and extremely well-tolerated.[6] SOR Ⓐ

Genital herpes:

- Antiviral therapy is recommended for an initial genital herpes outbreak. **Table 135-1** shows the dosages for antiherpes drugs. Although systemic antiviral drugs can partially control the signs and symptoms of herpes episodes, no therapy eradicates latent virus.[8]
- Acyclovir, famciclovir, and valacyclovir are equally effective for episodic treatment of genital herpes, but famciclovir appears somewhat less effective for suppression of viral shedding.[2] SOR Ⓑ
- Effective episodic treatment of herpes requires initiation of therapy during the prodrome period or within 1 day of lesion onset. Providing the patient with a prescription for the medication with instructions to initiate treatment immediately when symptoms begin improves efficacy.[2] SOR Ⓑ
- IV acyclovir therapy at 5 to 10 mg/kg IV every 8 hours for 2 to 7 days followed by oral antiviral therapy to complete at least

TABLE 135-1 Dosages of Treatments for Genital Herpes Infection[2]

Drug	Primary Infection Dosage	Recurrent Infection Dosage	Chronic Suppressive Therapy
Acyclovir (Zovirax)	400 mg 3 times daily for 7 to 10 days or 200 mg 5 times daily	400 mg 3 times daily for 5 days or 800 mg twice daily for 5 days or 800 mg 3 times daily for 2 days	400 mg twice daily
Famciclovir (Famvir)	250 mg 3 times daily for 7 to 10 days	125 mg twice daily for 5 days or 1 g twice daily for 1 day or 500 mg once, followed by 250 mg twice daily for 2 days	250 mg PO twice daily
Valacyclovir (Valtrex)	1 g twice daily for 7 to 10 days	500 mg twice daily for 3 days or 1 g daily for 5 days	500 mg to 1 g once daily

10 days of total therapy should be provided for patients who have severe HSV disease or complications.[2] SOR Ⓒ

- HSV strains resistant to acyclovir have been detected in immunocompromised patients, so other antivirals (e.g., famciclovir) need to be considered in these patients. SOR Ⓒ
- Topical medication for HSV infection is generally not effective. Topical penciclovir applied every 2 hours for 4 days reduces clinical healing time by approximately 1 day.[1,2]
- All patients with a first episode of genital herpes should receive antiviral therapy, as even with mild clinical manifestations initially, they can develop severe or prolonged symptoms.
- Toxicity of these 3 antiviral drugs is rare, but in patients who are dehydrated or who have poor renal function, the drug can crystallize in the renal tubules, leading to a reversible creatinine elevation or, rarely, acute tubular necrosis. Adverse effects, usually mild, include nausea, vomiting, rash, and headache. Lethargy, tremulousness, seizures, and delirium have been reported rarely in studies of renally impaired patients.[9]

Oral herpes:

Table 135-2 provides an overview of treatments for herpes labialis.

- In the treatment of primary orolabial herpes, oral acyclovir (200 mg 5 times daily for 5 days) accelerates healing by 1 day and can reduce the mean duration of pain by 36%.[10] SOR Ⓐ
- The oral lesions in primary herpes gingivostomatitis can lead to poor oral intake especially in children and the elderly (**Figure 135-13**). To prevent dehydration, the following medications may be considered. Topical oral anesthetics such as 2% viscous lidocaine by prescription or 20% topical benzocaine over the counter (OTC) may be used to treat painful oral ulcers. SOR Ⓒ A solution combining aluminum and magnesium hydroxide (liquid antacid) and 2% viscous lidocaine has been reported as helpful when swished and spit out several times a day as needed for pain. SOR Ⓒ

TABLE 135-2 Treatments for Herpes Labialis

Drug	Dose or Dosage	Evidence Rating†
Episodic oral treatment for recurrences‡		
Acyclovir (Zovirax)	200 mg 5 times per day or 400 mg 3 times per day for 5 days	A
Famciclovir (Famvir)	1500 mg once for 1 day	B
Valacyclovir (Valtrex)	2 g twice for 1 day	B
Episodic topical treatment for recurrences‡		
Acyclovir cream	Apply 5 times per day for 4 days	B
Docosanol cream (Abreva)	Apply 5 times per day until healed	B
Penciclovir cream (Denavir)	Apply every 2 hours while awake for 4 days	B
Treatment to prevent recurrences		
Acyclovir	400 mg twice per day (ongoing)	A
Valacyclovir	500 mg once per day (ongoing)	B

Abbreviation: NA, not available.
†*A*, Consistent, good-quality, patient-oriented evidence; *B*, inconsistent or limited-quality, patient-oriented evidence; *C*, consensus, disease-oriented evidence, usual practice, expert opinion, or case series.
‡Most effective if treatment is started at the onset of symptoms.
Reproduced with permission from with permission from Usatine RP, Tinitigan R. Nongenital herpes simplex virus, Am Fam Physician. 2010;82(9):1075-1082.

- Docosanol cream (Abreva) is available without prescription for oral herpes. One randomized controlled trial (RCT) of 743 patients with herpes labialis showed a faster healing time in patients treated with docosanol 10% cream compared with placebo cream (4.1 vs. 4.8 days), as well as reduced duration of pain symptoms (2.2 vs. 2.7 days).[11] More than 90% of patients in both groups healed completely within 10 days.[11] Treatment with docosanol cream, when applied 5 times per day and within 12 hours of episode onset, is safe and somewhat effective.[12]

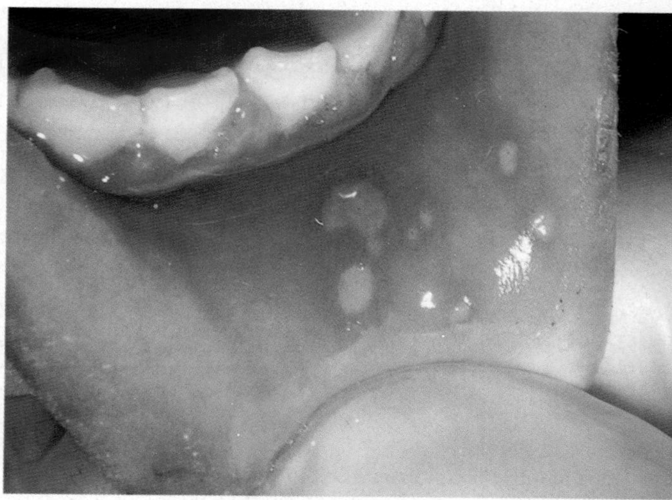

FIGURE 135-13 Primary herpes gingivostomatitis in a 4-year-old girl. Note the cluster of ulcers inside the lower lip typical of herpes simplex virus. The patient also had involvement of her gingiva, which were swollen and painful. (*Reproduced with permission from Richard P. Usatine, MD.*)

PREVENTION

- Barrier protection using latex condoms is recommended to minimize exposure to genital HSV infections (see "Patient Education" below).
- Suppressive therapy with antiviral drugs reduces the frequency of genital herpes recurrences by 70% to 80% in patients with frequent recurrences.[2] SOR Ⓐ Traditionally this is reserved for use in patients who have more than 4 to 6 outbreaks per year (see **Table 135-1**).
- Short-term prophylactic therapy with acyclovir for orolabial HSV may be used in patients who anticipate intense exposure to UV light. Early treatment of recurrent orolabial HSV infection with famciclovir 250 mg 3 times daily for 5 days can markedly decrease the size and duration of lesions.[13] SOR Ⓐ

FOLLOW-UP

The patient should return for follow-up if pain is uncontrolled or superinfection is suspected. The patient should be periodically evaluated for the need for suppressive therapy based on the number of recurrences per year.

PATIENT EDUCATION

Measures to prevent genital HSV infection:

- Abstain from sexual activity or limit number of sexual partners to prevent exposure to the disease.
- Use condoms to protect against transmission, but this is not foolproof as ulcers can occur on areas not covered by condoms.
- Prevent autoinoculation by patting dry affected areas, not rubbing with towel.
- Studies show that patients may shed virus when they are otherwise asymptomatic. A link between HSV genital ulcer disease and sexual transmission of HIV has been established. Safer sex practices should be strongly encouraged to prevent transmission of HSV to others and acquiring HIV by the patient.

PATIENT RESOURCES

- Centers for Disease Control and Prevention. *Genital Herpes–CDC Fact Sheet*—**http://www.cdc.gov/std/Herpes/STDFact-Herpes.htm.**

- Skinsight. *Herpetic Whitlow–Information for Adults*—**http://www.skinsight.com/adult/herpeticWhitlow.htm.**

PROVIDER RESOURCES

- Medscape. *Herpes Simplex*—**http://emedicine.medscape.com/article/218580.**
- Medscape. *Dermatologic Manifestations of Herpes Simplex*—**http://emedicine.medscape.com/article/1132351.**
- Usatine RP, Tinitigan R. Nongenital HSV. *Am Fam Physician.* 2010;82(9):1075-1082—**http://www.aafp.org/afp/2010/1101/p1075.html.**
- Emmert DH. Treatment of common cutaneous HSV infections. *Am Fam Physician.* 2000;61(6):1697-1704—**http://www.aafp.org/afp/2000/0315/p1697.html.**

REFERENCES

1. Whitley RJ, Kimberlin DW, Roizman B. Herpes simplex viruses. *Clin Infect Dis.* 1998;26:541-555.
2. Workowski KA, Bolan GA; Centers for Disease Control and Prevention. Sexually transmitted diseases treatment guidelines, 2015. *MMWR Recomm Rep.* 2015;64(RR-03):1-137.
3. Gill MJ, Arlette J, Buchan K. Herpes simplex virus infection of the hand. A profile of 79 cases. *Am J Med.* 1988;84:89-93.
4. Fleming DT, McQuillan GM, Johnson RE, et al. Herpes simplex virus type 2 in the United States, 1976 to 1994. *N Engl J Med.* 1997;337:1105-1111.
5. Mertz GJ. Epidemiology of genital herpes infections. *Infect Dis Clin North Am.* 1993;7:825-839.
6. Clark JL, Tatum NO, Noble SL. Management of genital herpes. *Am Fam Physician.* 1995;51:175-182, 187-188.
7. Centers for Disease Control and Prevention (CDC). Seroprevalence of herpes simplex virus type 2 among persons aged 14–49 years—United States, 2005–2008. *MMWR Morb Mortal Wkly Rep.* 2010;59(15):456-459.
8. Heslop R, Roberts H, Flower D, Jordan V. Interventions for men and women with their first episode of genital herpes. *Cochrane Database Syst Rev* 2016(8):CD010684.
9. Emmert DH. Treatment of common cutaneous herpes simplex virus infections. *Am Fam Physician.* 2000;61(6):1697-1706, 1708.
10. Spruance SL, Stewart JC, Rowe NH, et al. Treatment of recurrent herpes simplex labialis with oral acyclovir. *J Infect Dis.* 1990;161:185-190.
11. Sacks SL, Thisted RA, Jones TM, et al; Docosanol 10% Cream Study Group. Clinical efficacy of topical docosanol 10% cream for herpes simplex labialis: a multi-center, randomized, placebo-controlled trial. *J Am Acad Dermatol.* 2001;45(2):222-230.
12. Usatine RP, Tinitigan R. Nongenital herpes simplex virus. *Am Fam Physician.* 2010;82(9):1075-1082.
13. Spruance SL, Rowe NH, Raborn GW, et al. Perioral famciclovir in the treatment of experimental ultraviolet radiation-induced herpes simplex labialis: a double-blind, dose-ranging, placebo-controlled, multicenter trial. *J Infect Dis.* 1999;179:303-310.

136 MOLLUSCUM CONTAGIOSUM

E.J. Mayeaux, Jr., MD

PATIENT STORY

An 8-year-old girl is brought to the office because of an outbreak of bumps on her face for the past 3 months (**Figure 136-1**). Occasionally she scratches them, but she is otherwise asymptomatic. The mother and child are unhappy with the appearance of the molluscum contagiosum and chose to try topical therapy. A topical treatment was chosen to avoid the risk of hypopigmentation that can occur in dark-skinned individuals with cryotherapy.

An 11-year-old girl was also seen with molluscum on her face. The child and her mother decided to try cryotherapy as her treatment. She tolerated the treatment with liquid nitrogen in a Cryogun (**Figure 136-2**). The molluscum disappeared without scarring or hypopigmentation after 2 treatments.

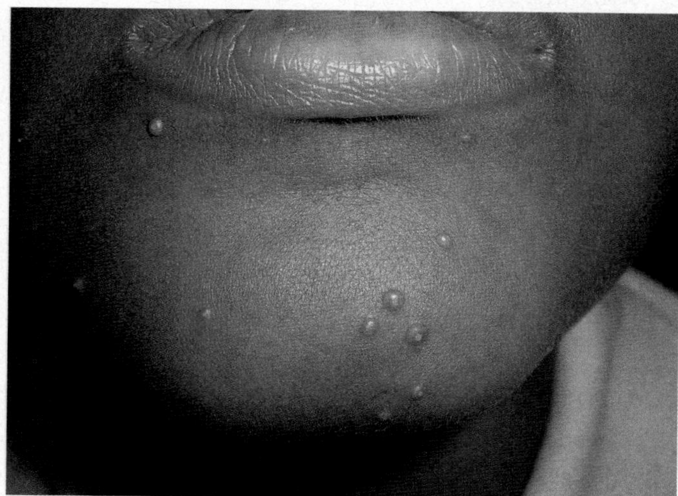

FIGURE 136-1 Molluscum contagiosum on the face of an 8-year-old girl. (*Reproduced with permission from Richard P. Usatine, MD.*)

INTRODUCTION

Molluscum contagiosum is a viral skin infection that produces pearly papules that often have a central umbilication. It is seen most commonly in children, but can also be transmitted sexually among adults.

EPIDEMIOLOGY

- Molluscum contagiosum infection has been reported worldwide. An Australian seroepidemiology study found a seropositivity rate of 23%.[1]
- Up to 5% of children in the United States have clinical evidence of molluscum contagiosum infection.[2] It is a common, nonsexually transmitted condition in children (see **Figures 136-1** to **136-4**).
- The number of cases of molluscum in U.S. adults increased in the 1980s with the onset of the HIV/AIDS epidemic. Since the introduction of highly active antiretroviral therapy (HAART), the number of molluscum contagiosum cases in HIV/AIDS patients has decreased.[3] However, the prevalence of molluscum contagiosum in patients who are HIV-positive may still be as high as 5% to 18% (**Figures 136-5**).[4,5]

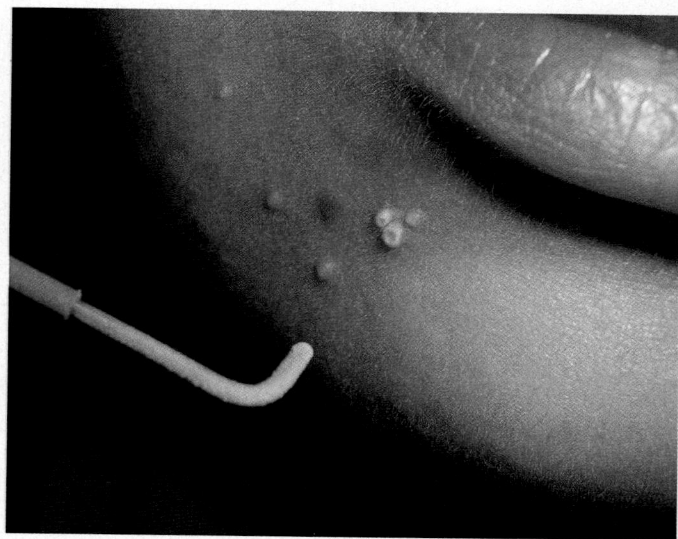

FIGURE 136-2 Cryotherapy of molluscum on the face of an 11-year-old girl. The central umbilication is easily seen in the 2 papules that were just frozen. (*Reproduced with permission from Richard P. Usatine, MD.*)

ETIOLOGY AND PATHOPHYSIOLOGY

- Molluscum contagiosum is a benign condition that is often transmitted through close contact in children and through sexual contact in adults.
- It is a large DNA virus of the Poxviridae family of poxvirus. It is related to the orthopoxviruses (variola, vaccinia, smallpox, and monkeypox viruses).

- Molluscum replicates in the cytoplasm of infected epithelial cells. It causes a chronic localized skin infection consisting of dome-shaped pearly papules on the skin.
- Like most of the viruses in the poxvirus family, molluscum is spread by direct skin-to-skin contact. It can also spread by autoinoculation when scratching, touching, or treating lesions. Any single lesion is usually present for approximately 2 months, but autoinoculation often causes continuous crops of lesions.

RISK FACTORS

- Common childhood disease.
- Molluscum contagiosum may be more common in patients with atopic dermatitis based on reported prevalence rates for atopic dermatitis of 18% to 45% in patients with molluscum, which exceeds the prevalence of 10% to 20% in the general pediatric population (**Figure 136-6**).[2,6]
- The disease also may be spread by participation in contact sports.[2]
- It is also associated with immunodeficient states such as in HIV infection (see **Figure 136-5**) and with immunosuppressive drug treatment.

DIAGNOSIS

CLINICAL FEATURES—HISTORY AND PHYSICAL

- Firm, multiple, 2- to 5-mm dome-shaped papules with a characteristic shiny surface and umbilicated center (**Figure 136-7**). Not all the papules have a central umbilication, so it helps to take a moment and look for a papule that has this characteristic morphology. If all features point to molluscum and no single lesion has central umbilication, do not rule out molluscum as the diagnosis.
- The lesions range in color from pearly white, to flesh-colored, to pink or yellow.
- Pruritus may be present or absent.

TYPICAL DISTRIBUTION

- The lesions may appear anywhere on the body except the palms and soles. The number of lesions may be greater in an HIV-infected individual.
- Typically in adults and occasionally in children, they are found around the genitalia, inguinal area, buttocks, or inner thighs. In children, the lesions are often on the trunk or face.
- If a child is found to have molluscum contagiosum in the genital area, a history and physical exam should be directed at looking for other clues that might indicate sexual abuse (see Chapter 10, Child Sexual Abuse). Not all cases of molluscum in this area will be secondary to sexual abuse (**Figure 136-8**).

LABORATORY TESTING

- Sexually active adolescents and adults with genital lesions should be evaluated for other sexually transmitted diseases, including HIV and syphilis.

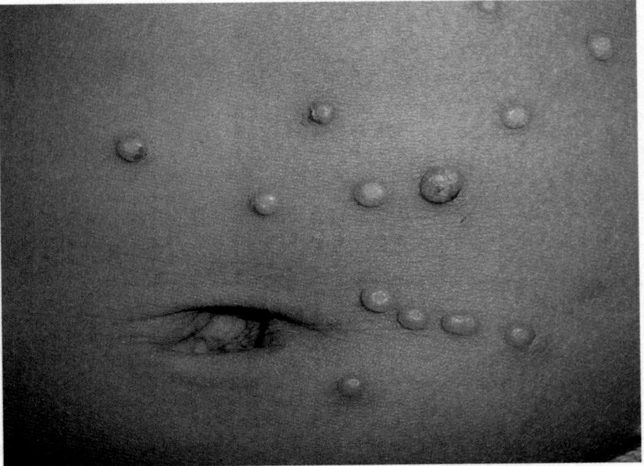

FIGURE 136-3 A group of molluscum contagiosum lesions on the abdomen of a 4-year-old boy. (*Reproduced with permission from Richard P. Usatine, MD.*)

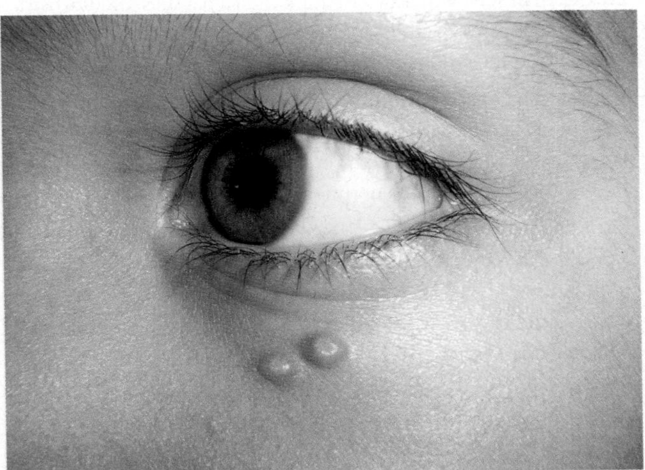

FIGURE 136-4 Molluscum contagiosum under the eye of a young girl with central umbilication. (*Reproduced with permission from Richard P. Usatine, MD.*)

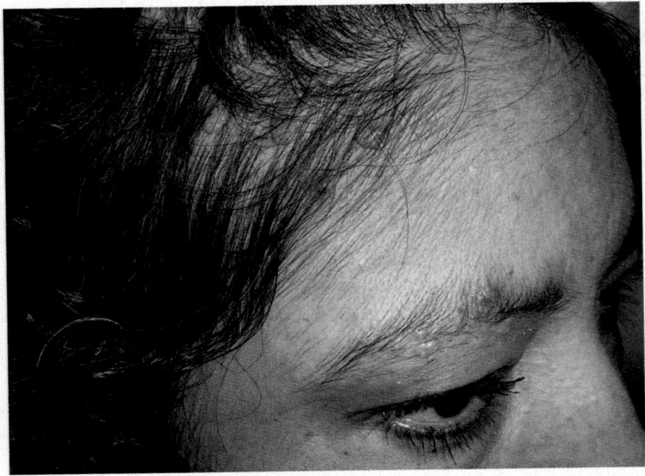

FIGURE 136-5 Molluscum contagiosum on the face of a woman with HIV. Note the large molluscum on the scalp. (*Reproduced with permission from Richard P. Usatine, MD.*)

DERMOSCOPY/BIOPSY

- The typical dermoscopic appearance of a molluscum lesion is a round pearly papule with crown-like vessels surrounding central oval globules (**Figure 136-9**).
- If confirmation is needed, smears of the caseous material expressed from the lesions can be examined directly under the microscope looking for molluscum bodies (enlarged keratinocytes that are engorged with viral inclusion bodies).
- Hematoxylin and eosin (H&E) staining from a shave biopsy usually reveals keratinocytes that contain eosinophilic cytoplasmic inclusion bodies.[5] If a single lesion is suspicious for basal cell carcinoma (BCC), perform a shave biopsy.

DIFFERENTIAL DIAGNOSIS

- Scabies is caused by *Sarcoptes scabiei* mite and can be transmitted through close or sexual contact. The itching and excoriations are greater than seen with molluscum. Scabies papules and burrows differ in appearance from the stuck-on pearly umbilicated papules of molluscum (see Chapter 149, Scabies).
- Dermatofibromas—Firm to hard nodules ranging in color from flesh to black that typically dimple downward when compressed laterally. Usually not seen in crops as in molluscum. These nodules are deeper in the dermis and do not appear stuck on like molluscum.
- BCCs are also pearly and raised but are rarely found in pediatric populations. Usually not seen in crops as in molluscum. If a single lesion could be a BCC or molluscum, a biopsy is warranted (see Chapter 177, Basal Cell Carcinoma).
- Genital warts may be flat and grossly resemble molluscum but they lack the characteristic shiny surface and central umbilication (see Chapter 139, Genital Warts).

MANAGEMENT

FIRST LINE

NONPHARMACOLOGIC

- Treatment of nongenital lesions is usually not medically mandatory as the infection is usually self-limited and spontaneously resolves after a few months. Treatment may be performed in an attempt to decrease autoinoculation and hasten resolution. Patients and parents of children often want treatment for cosmetic reasons and when watchful waiting fails.
- A 2017 Cochrane Database systematic review investigated the efficacy of treatments for nongenital molluscum contagiosum in healthy individuals and found insufficient evidence to conclude that any treatment was definitively effective.[7] SOR Ⓐ
- In the HIV-infected patient, molluscum may resolve after control of HIV disease with HAART.[3] SOR Ⓑ
- Immunocompromised patients should have a full-body skin examination to ensure that all lesions are identified. Treatment is still optional but should proceed in patients whose parents desire intervention.

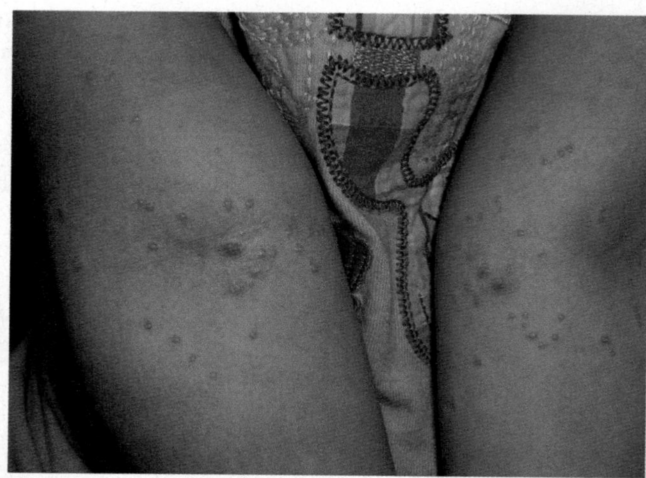

FIGURE 136-6 Molluscum contagiosum in the antecubital fossa of a 6-year-old girl with atopic dermatitis. *(Reproduced with permission from Richard P. Usatine, MD.)*

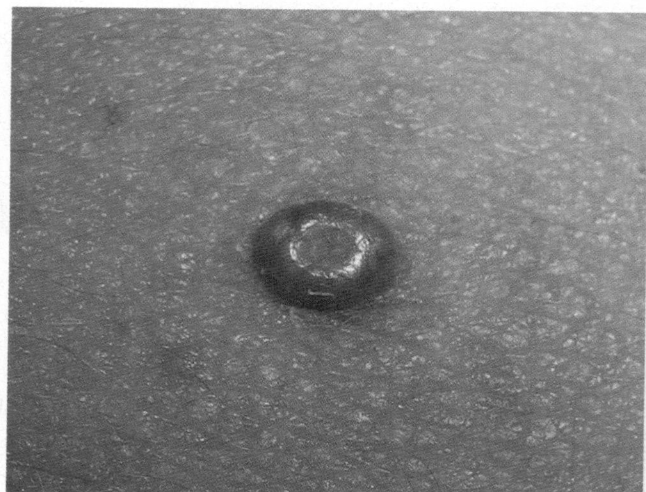

FIGURE 136-7 Close-up of a molluscum lesion on the back of a child showing a dome-shaped pearly papule with a characteristic umbilicated center. *(Reproduced with permission from Richard P. Usatine, MD.)*

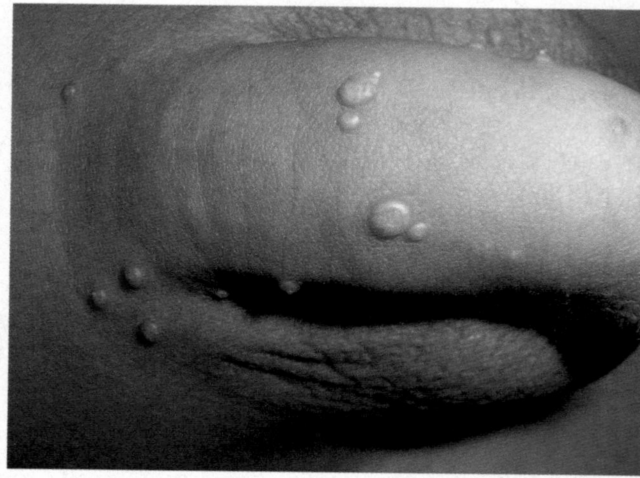

FIGURE 136-8 Molluscum contagiosum on and around the penis of a young boy. There was no evidence for sexual abuse. *(Reproduced with permission from Richard P. Usatine, MD.)*

SURGICAL

- Cryotherapy applied by cotton-tipped applicator or sprayer is a physical method used to eradicate molluscum.[8-10] SOR Ⓐ Hypopigmentation (which may be permanent) is a potential side effect, especially in skin of color. Cryotherapy is painful and scary to most young children. For older children and brave younger children, it is an easy treatment. Some parents are so upset with the molluscum they will ask the physician to proceed with treatment despite the child's screaming protestations. It is best to offer topical therapy under those circumstances. Other choices involve using topical anesthetic cream and distractions such as smartphones to keep children happy while treating their molluscum.
- Curettage is another physical method.[8] SOR Ⓑ It can be performed with or without anesthesia in adults and brave children. Some patients state that the lidocaine injections hurt more than the curettage and prefer no anesthesia. Topical anesthesia with anesthetic creams or sprays is another option.

MEDICATIONS

- Cantharidin is a topical blistering agent that was studied in 300 children for molluscum, and the parents reported 90% of children experienced lesion clearing and 8% experienced lesion improvement (**Figure 136-10**). SOR Ⓑ Furthermore, 95% of parents stated they would use cantharidin therapy again.[11] Local erythema, burning, pruritus, and inflammation were reported side effects. Fortunately, the application is painless because the blistering occurs after the child leaves the office (see **Figure 136-10**). It can be a good choice for children if one can get the cantharidin compounded in a nearby pharmacy.
- Podophyllotoxin 0.5% (Condylox) is an antimitotic agent that is indicated for the treatment of genital warts. The efficacy of podophyllotoxin was established in a randomized trial of lesions located on the thighs or genitalia. SOR Ⓐ Local erythema, burning, pruritus, inflammation, and erosions can occur with the use of this agent. The safety and efficacy of this drug has not been established in young children.[12] In a randomized trial of 150 males (ages 10 to 26 years), the patients applied 0.5% podophyllotoxin cream, 0.3% podophyllotoxin cream, or placebo twice daily for three consecutive days per week for up to 4 weeks. The 0.5% podophyllotoxin was group had 92% clearance (16% for placebo).[12]

SECOND LINE

- Tretinoin cream[11] 0.1% or gel 0.025% applied daily is commonly used but not FDA-approved for this indication. SOR Ⓑ
- Trichloroacetic acid and salicylic acid[13] are topical keratolytic chemicals that can be applied by the physician in the office. SOR Ⓑ Local irritation is common.
- Topical imiquimod 5% was found in small trials to be effective, but a recent systematic review found that it was no more effective than vehicle alone.[6]

COMPLEMENTARY/ALTERNATIVE THERAPY

- ZymaDermis is a nonprescription, topical, homeopathic agent that is marketed for the treatment of molluscum contagiosum, but no published studies have evaluated its efficacy or safety.

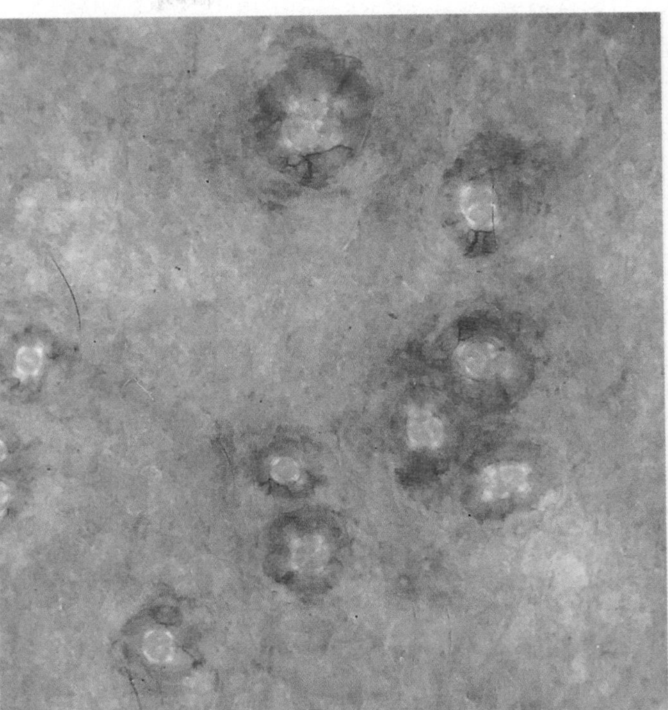

FIGURE 136-9 Dermoscopy of multiple molluscum lesions showing round pearly papules with crown-like vessels surrounding central oval globules. (*Reproduced with permission from Richard P. Usatine, MD.*)

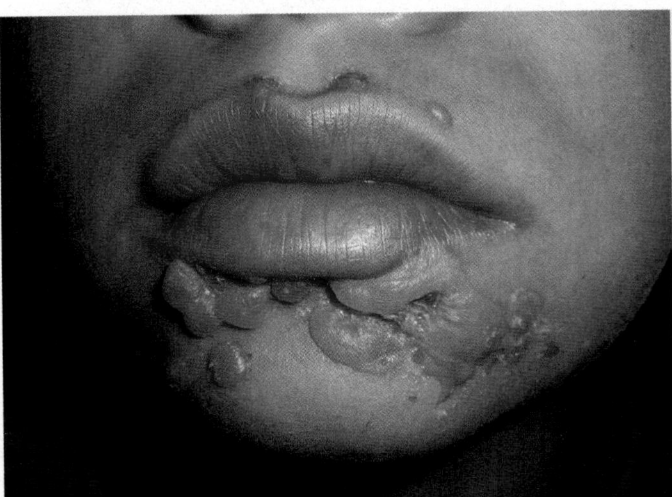

FIGURE 136-10 Blisters that formed the next day after treating molluscum contagiosum with cantharidin. The blisters are not always so large but are supposed to form, as the cantharidin is derived from the blister beetle and helps eradicate the molluscum. (*Reproduced with permission from Richard P. Usatine, MD.*)

- Potassium hydroxide has been used for molluscum but has not proved to be statistically significant when compared to placebo.[14]
- Pulsed dye lasers have shown to be safe and effective in case reports and small uncontrolled studies. One prospective study of 19 children between 2 and 13 concluded that all patients tolerated the 585 nm laser well and 84.3% had complete lesion resolution with one treatment.[15]

PREVENTION

- Molluscum contagiosum is a common childhood disease.
- Limiting sexual exposure or number of sexual contacts may help prevent exposure in adults.
- Genital lesions should be treated to prevent spread by sexual contact (**Figure 136-11**).

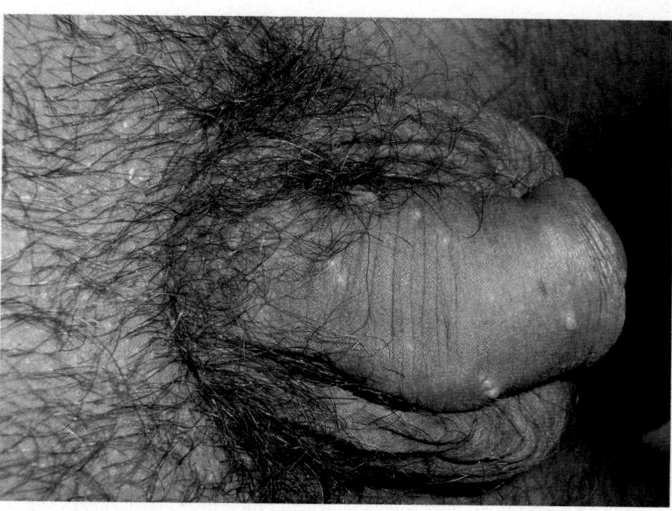

FIGURE 136-11 Molluscum contagiosum on and around the penis. His girlfriend has them on the buttocks. (*Reproduced with permission from Richard P. Usatine, MD.*)

PROGNOSIS

- In immunocompetent patients, lesions usually spontaneously resolve within several months. In a minority of cases, disease persists for a few years.[16]

FOLLOW-UP

- Have patients watch for complications that may include irritation, inflammation, and secondary infections. Lesions on eyelids may be associated with follicular or papillary conjunctivitis, so eye irritation should prompt a visit to an eye care specialist.

PATIENT EDUCATION

- Instruct patients to avoid scratching to prevent autoinoculation.

PATIENT RESOURCES

- Centers for Disease Control and Prevention. *Molluscum Contagiosum*—**http://www.cdc.gov/ncidod/dvrd/molluscum/.**
- Pubmed Health. *Treatments for Molluscum Contagiosum*—**https://www.ncbi.nlm.nih.gov/pubmedhealth/PMH0013007/.**
- American Academy of Dermatology. *Molluscum Contagiosum*—**https://www.aad.org/public/diseases/contagious-skin-diseases/molluscum-contagiosum.**
- eMedicine. *Molluscum Contagiosum*—**http://www.emedicinehealth.com/molluscum_contagiosum/article_em.htm.**
- MedlinePlus. *Molluscum Contagiosum*—**http://www.nlm.nih.gov/medlineplus/ency/article/000826.htm.**

PROVIDER RESOURCES

- eMedicine. *Molluscum Contagiosum*—**http://emedicine.medscape.com/article/910570.**

- eMedicine. *Molluscum Contagiosum in ED*—**http://emedicine.medscape.com/article/762548.**
- Centers for Disease Control and Prevention. *Clinical Information: Molluscum Contagiosum*—**http://www.cdc.gov/ncidod/dvrd/molluscum/clinical_overview.htm.**

REFERENCES

1. Konya J, Thompson CH. Molluscum contagiosum virus: antibody responses in persons with clinical lesions and seroepidemiology in a representative Australian population. *J Infect Dis.* 1999;179(3):701-704.
2. Dohil MA, Lin P, Lee J, et al. The epidemiology of molluscum contagiosum in children. *J Am Acad Dermatol.* 2006;54(1):47-54.
3. Calista D, Boschini A, Landi G. Resolution of disseminated molluscum contagiosum with highly active anti-retroviral therapy (HAART) in patients with AIDS. *Eur J Dermatol.* 1999;9(3):211-213.
4. Schwartz JJ, Myskowski PL. Molluscum contagiosum in patients with human immunodeficiency virus infection. *J Am Acad Dermatol.* 1992;27(4):583-588.
5. Cotell SL, Roholt NS. Images in clinical medicine. Molluscum contagiosum in a patient with the acquired immunodeficiency syndrome. *N Engl J Med.* 1998;338(13):888.
6. Berger EM, Orlow SJ, Patel RR, Schaffer JV. Experience with molluscum contagiosum and associated inflammatory reactions in a pediatric dermatology practice: the bump that rashes. *Arch Dermatol.* 2012;148:1257.
7. van der Wouden JC, van der Sande R, Kruithof EJ, et al. Interventions for cutaneous molluscum contagiosum. *Cochrane Database Syst Rev.* 2017;(5):CD004767.
8. Hanna D, Hatami A, Powell J, et al. A prospective randomized trial comparing the efficacy and adverse effects of four recognized treatments of molluscum contagiosum in children. *Pediatr Dermatol.* 2006;23(6):574-579.
9. Wetmore SJ. Cryosurgery for common skin lesions. Treatment in family physicians' offices. *Can Fam Physician.* 1999;45:964-974.
10. Al-Mutairi N, Al-Doukhi A, Al-Farag S, Al-Haddad A. Comparative study on the efficacy, safety, and acceptability of imiquimod 5% cream versus cryotherapy for molluscum contagiosum in children. *Pediatr Dermatol.* 2010;27:388.
11. Silverberg NB, Sidbury R, Mancini AJ. Childhood molluscum contagiosum: experience with cantharidin therapy in 300 patients. *J Am Acad Dermatol.* 2000;43(3):503-507.
12. Syed TA, Lundin S, Ahmad M. Topical 0.3% and 0.5% podophyllotoxin cream for self-treatment of molluscum contagiosum in males. A placebo-controlled, double-blind study. *Dermatology.* 1994;189(1):65-68.
13. Yoshinaga IG, Conrado LA, Schainberg SC, Grinblat M. Recalcitrant molluscum contagiosum in a patient with AIDS: combined treatment with CO(2) laser, trichloroacetic acid, and pulsed dye laser. *Lasers Surg Med.* 2000;27(4):291-294.
14. Romiti R, Ribeiro AP, Romiti N. Evaluation of the effectiveness of 5% potassium hydroxide for the treatment of molluscum contagiosum. *Pediatr Dermatol.* 2000;17:495.
15. Binder B, Weger W, Komericki P, Kopera D. Treatment of molluscum contagiosum with a pulsed dye laser: Pilot study with 19 children. J Dtsch Dermatol Ges 2008; 6:121
16. Lee R, Schwartz RA. Pediatric molluscum contagiosum: reflections on the last challenging poxvirus infection, part 1. *Cutis.* 2010;86(5):230-236.

137 COMMON WARTS

E.J. Mayeaux, Jr., MD
Jonathan B. Karnes, MD

PATIENT STORY

An 11-year-old girl presents with multiple warts on the fingertips that have been present for 3 months (**Figure 137-1**). She occasionally bites at the warts. Mom has tried over-the-counter freezing, but it was very uncomfortable for her daughter. Although the family is anxious about them spreading, you recommend watchful waiting, and in 6 months all warts have completely resolved.

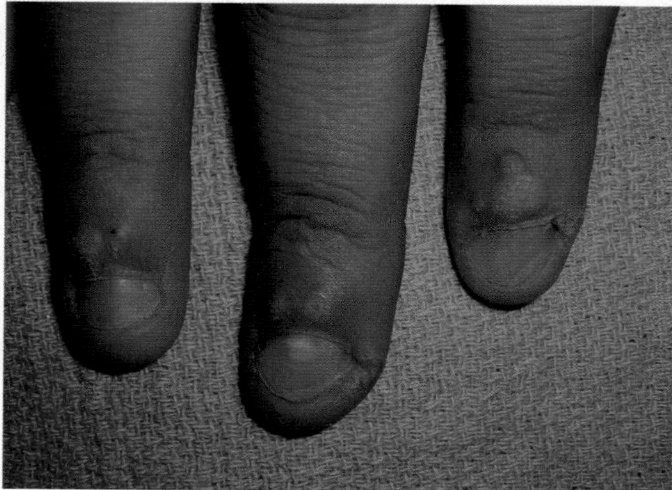

FIGURE 137-1 Common warts on the hands of an 11-year-old girl. *(Reproduced with permission from Richard P. Usatine, MD.)*

INTRODUCTION

Human papillomaviruses (HPVs) are DNA viruses that infect skin and mucous membranes. Infection is usually confined to the epidermis and does not result in disseminated systemic infection. The most common clinical manifestation of these viruses is warts (verrucae). There are more than 200 distinct HPV subtypes based on DNA testing. Some tend to infect specific body sites or types of epithelium. Some types have potential to cause malignant change, but this is rare on keratinized skin.

SYNONYMS

Verrucae, verruca vulgaris, common warts.

EPIDEMIOLOGY

- Nongenital cutaneous warts are widespread worldwide and are more common in children, with a peak incidence in the teenage years and a sharp decline thereafter.[1]
- They are most commonly caused by HPV types 1 to 5, 7, 27, 29.[1]
- High-risk HPV has been isolated in warts but the significance is unclear.[2]
- Common warts account for approximately 70% of non-genital cutaneous warts.[3]
- Common warts occur most commonly in children and young adults (**Figures 137-1** and **137-2**).[4]

ETIOLOGY AND PATHOPHYSIOLOGY

- Infection with HPV occurs by skin-to-skin contact. It starts with a break in the integrity of the epithelium caused by maceration or trauma that allows the virus to infect the basal layers.
- Warts may infect the skin on opposing digits, causing "kissing warts" (**Figure 137-3**).

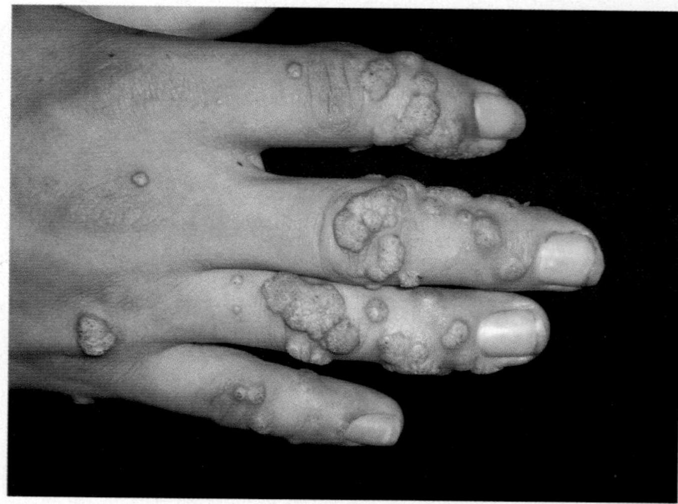

FIGURE 137-2 Many common warts on the hand of an HIV-negative young adult. *(Reproduced with permission from Richard P. Usatine, MD.)*

- Individuals with subclinical infection may serve as a reservoir for HPVs.
- An incubation period following inoculation lasts for approximately 2 to 6 months.

RISK FACTORS[1]

- Young age.
- Disruption to the normal epithelial barrier.
- More common among meat handlers.[5]
- Atopic dermatitis.
- Nail biters more commonly have multiple periungual warts.
- Conditions that decrease cell-mediated immunity such as HIV (**Figure 137-4**) and immunosuppressant drugs (**Figure 137-5**).

DIAGNOSIS

CLINICAL FEATURES

- The diagnosis of warts is based on clinical appearance. The wart will interrupt normal skin markings.
- Common warts are well-demarcated, rough, hard papules with irregular papillary surface. They are usually asymptomatic unless located on a pressure point.
- Warts may form cylindrical or filiform projections (**Figure 137-6**).

TYPICAL DISTRIBUTION

- Common anatomic locations include the dorsum of the hand, between the fingers, flexor surfaces, and periungual fingertips (see **Figures 137-1** and **137-2**).

LABORATORY TESTING

- HPV testing may reflect resistance to treatment but is not the standard of care at this time.[6]
- HIV testing may be useful if the warts are severe and there are risk factors present (see **Figure 137-4**).

DERMOSCOPY/BIOPSY

- Dermoscopy of a common wart may show the same subsurface structures without the need to pare off the surface. Magnification and polarization show densely packed papillae with a central vascular structure that may appear as a red dot, black dot, or capillary loop, surrounded by a whitish keratin halo (**Figure 137-7**).
- Paring the surface with a surgical blade may expose punctate hemorrhagic capillaries, or black dots, which are thrombosed capillaries. If the diagnosis is in doubt, a shave biopsy is indicated to confirm the diagnosis.[4]

DIFFERENTIAL DIAGNOSIS

- Seborrheic keratoses are usually more darkly pigmented, have a stuck-on appearance, and demonstrate comedo-like openings and milia-like cysts on dermoscopy (see Chapter 111, Dermoscopy).

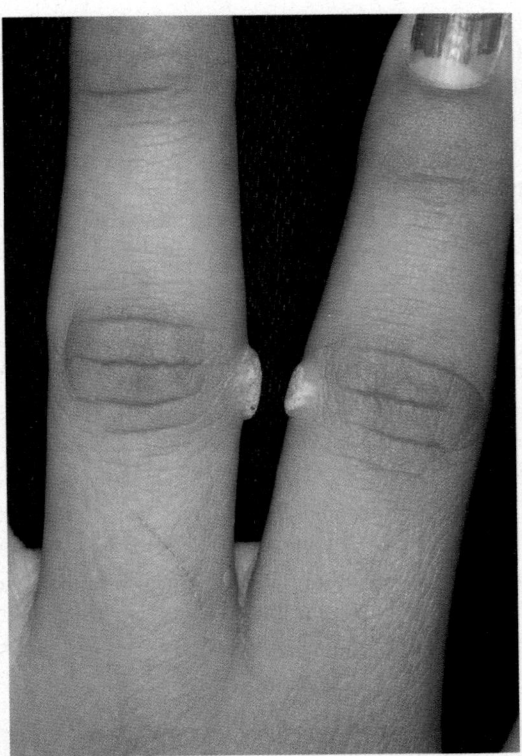

FIGURE 137-3 Warts may infect the skin on opposing digits, causing "kissing warts." (*Reproduced with permission from Richard P. Usatine, MD.*)

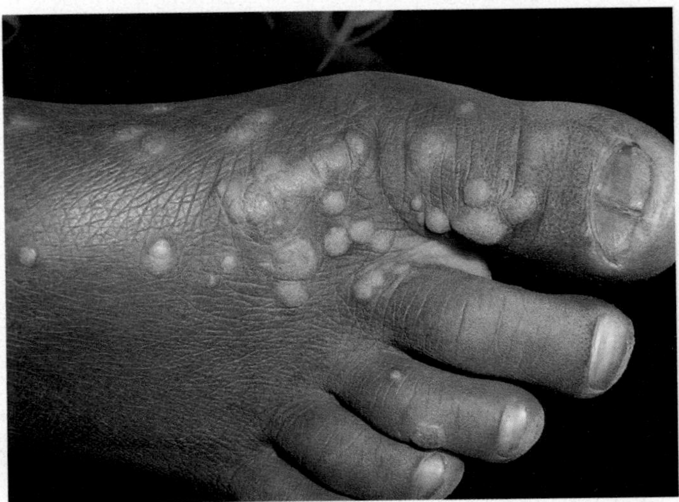

FIGURE 137-4 Large cluster of warts on the foot of a child in Africa found to be HIV-positive. (*Reproduced with permission from Richard P. Usatine, MD.*)

- Acrochordon (skin tags) are pedunculated flesh-colored papules that are more common in obese persons and in skin folds. They lack the surface roughness of common warts. Filiform warts also may be pedunculated, but are firm with finger-like projections (see Chapter 163, Skin Tag).
- Squamous cell carcinoma (SCC) should be considered when lesions have irregular growth, pigmentation, or ulceration, or resist therapy, particularly in sun-exposed areas; in immunosuppressed patients; and for recalcitrant lesions on the fingers of adults (see Chapter 178, Squamous Cell Carcinoma). The patient in **Figure 137-8** had a wart that was not going away, and a biopsy demonstrated SCC in situ within an HPV-induced lesion.
- Amelanotic melanoma—Though extremely rare, melanoma may present without pigment as a de novo pink papule[7] (see Chapter 179, Melanoma).
- Early warts may appear similar to actinic keratosis in sun-exposed areas (see Chapter 173, Actinic Keratosis and Bowen Disease).
- Advanced warts may appear similar to a keratoacanthoma to casual inspection. The characteristic findings of the keratoacanthoma and biopsy will separate the two conditions (see Chapter 174, Keratoacanthoma).

MANAGEMENT

FIRST LINE

- Many treatment options are listed below, but the highest quality evidence supports observation without treatment, topical salicylic acid, or cryotherapy as the most effective choices.[8] SOR Ⓐ

NONPHARMACOLOGIC

- Because spontaneous regression occurs in two-thirds of warts within 2 years and 80% in 4 years, observation without treatment is a good option.[9]
- Treatment does not decrease transmissibility of the virus.[10]
- Therapies for common warts do not specifically treat the HPV virus. They work by destruction of virus-containing skin while preserving uninvolved tissue. This usually exposes the immune system to the virus, promoting a response.
- The least-painful methods should be used first, especially in children. SOR Ⓒ
- Topical salicylic acid is more effective than placebo and safe in children and adults with minimal side effects.[11] SOR Ⓐ Combined results from 5 randomized controlled trials (RCTs) showed a 52% cure rate compared with 23% for placebo at 12 weeks.[11] A number of preparations are available without a prescription. Topical 17% salicylic acid is applied overnight and is the most commonly used form of treatment. Soak the wart with warm water for 5 minutes and gently file down any thick skin with a dedicated pumice stone or emery board. Apply salicylic acid and cover with tape occlusion. Repeat until the wart has cleared, or for up to 12 weeks. Discontinue treatment if severe redness or pain occurs. Do not use salicylic acid on the face because of an increased risk of hypopigmentation.[1]
- Forty percent salicylic acid plasters (Mediplast and others) are available over the counter and can be cut to accommodate larger or thicker

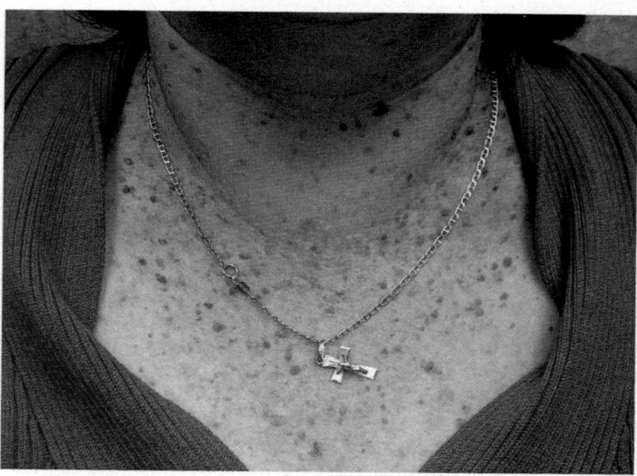

FIGURE 137-5 Biopsy-proven warts on the neck and chest of a woman on azathioprine after a renal transplantation. Human papillomavirus lesions can proliferate as a result of immunosuppressive medications. This patient is also being monitored for squamous cell carcinoma, as this is a more significant risk in posttransplantation patients. (*Reproduced with permission from Richard P. Usatine, MD.*)

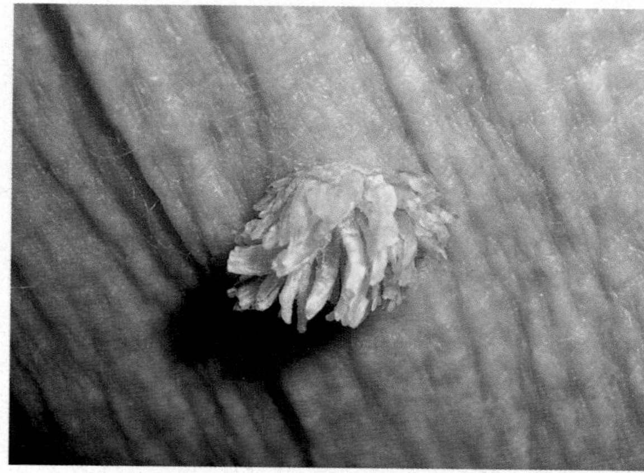

FIGURE 137-6 Filiform warts are identified by their multiple projections as opposed to a unified papule. This wart was on the face of an elderly woman and was removed by shave excision and sent for pathology. It was proven to be a wart and not squamous cell carcinoma. (*Reproduced with permission from Richard P. Usatine, MD.*)

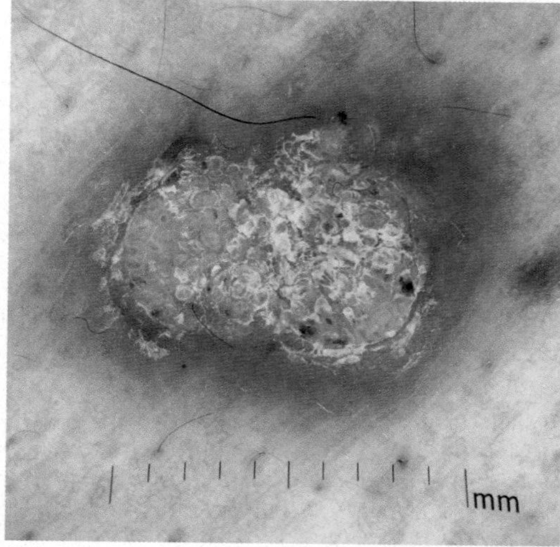

FIGURE 137-7 Dermoscopy of a common wart showing densely packed papillae with a central vascular structure that may appear as a red dot, black dot or capillary loop, surrounded by a whitish keratin halo. (*Reproduced with permission from Richard P. Usatine, MD.*)

warts. Cut the plaster a few millimeters larger than the wart and apply for 48 hours. After removing the patch, pare the wart with a pumice stone or emery board and repeat the process for up to 12 weeks.

- Cryotherapy, most commonly with liquid nitrogen, is another good first-line therapy but is painful and often unsuitable for young children. Though cure rates are similar to those for salicylic acid, patients may have a preference for cryotherapy, based on one well-designed trial.[12] SOR Ⓐ Chemical cryogens are now available over the counter but are not as cold or effective as liquid nitrogen. Most trials comparing cryotherapy with salicylic acid found similar effectiveness, with overall cure rates of 50% to 70% after 3 or 4 treatments.[1] Aggressive cryotherapy (10 to 30 seconds) is more effective than less-aggressive cryotherapy, but may increase complications.[1] SOR Ⓑ Anesthesia is rarely necessary but may be achieved with 1% lidocaine or EMLA (eutectic mixture of local anesthetics) cream applied under occlusion for an hour. Liquid nitrogen is applied for 10 seconds via a spray canister or cotton swab so that a freeze ball extends 2 mm beyond the lesion (**Figure 137-9**). Two freeze cycles may improve resolution. Patients will tolerate two 10-second freeze cycles better than one 20-second freeze, as the pain starts increasing exponentially at 10 seconds for many people. Avoid overfreezing, which may lead to permanent scarring and hypopigmentation (especially in skin of color). Treatments are often repeated every 2–3 weeks. There is no therapeutic benefit beyond 3 months.[1] SOR Ⓑ Because HPV can survive in liquid nitrogen, cotton swabs and residual liquid nitrogen should be properly discarded to avoid spreading the virus to other patients or contaminating the liquid nitrogen reservoir.[1] After cryotherapy, the skin shows erythema and may progress to hemorrhagic blistering. Healing occurs in approximately a week, and hypopigmentation may occur. Ring warts may result from an inadequate margin of treatment of a common wart. Common adverse effects of cryotherapy include pain, blistering, and hypo- or hyperpigmentation. Cryotherapy must be used cautiously where nerves are located superficially (such as on the fingers) to prevent pain and neuropathy. Overfreezing in the periungual region can result in permanent nail dystrophy.
- Simple excision is effective for small or filiform warts. The area is injected with lidocaine and the wart is excised with sharp scissors or a scalpel blade. SOR Ⓒ

SECOND LINE

- Intralesional injections with *Candida* antigen induces a localized, cell-mediated, and HPV-specific response that may target the injected wart as well as more distant warts (**Figure 137-10**). Nonrandomized trials suggest a clearance rate of 39%–70%.[11] SOR Ⓑ The *Candida* antigen must be diluted before used (**Table 137-1**). Inject 0.1 to 0.3 mL into the largest warts using a 30-gauge needle and up to 1 mL per treatment. Warn the patient to expect itching in the area, occasional erythema, burning, or peeling. Repeat every 4 weeks, up to 3 treatments or until warts are gone.
- Imiquimod 5% is an expensive topical immunomodulator that is indicated for treatment of anogenital warts. Open studies of imiquimod applied under occlusion suggested up to an 80% cure rate, but pharmaceutical-company sponsored RCTs demonstrated a cure rate of 10%–12.8% compared with 2.9% in the vehicle groups.[8,13]
- Cantharidin 0.7% is an extract of the blister beetle that is applied to the wart, after which blistering occurs on the following day.

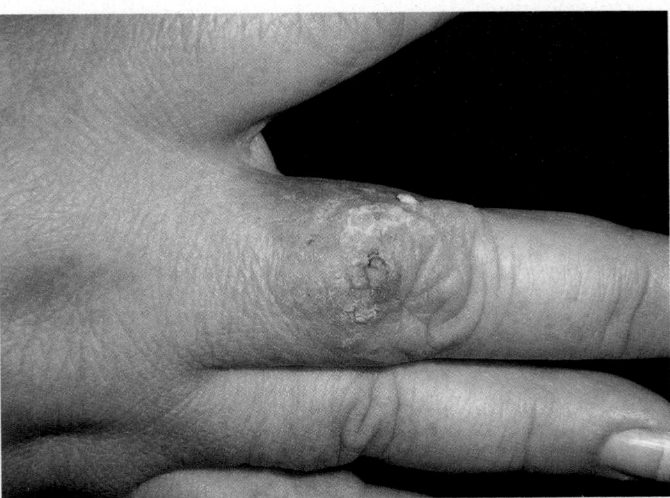

FIGURE 137-8 Squamous cell carcinoma in situ that started from a human papillomaviruses–positive lesion. When cryotherapy is not working on what appears to be a wart, consider performing a biopsy. (*Reproduced with permission from Richard P. Usatine, MD.*)

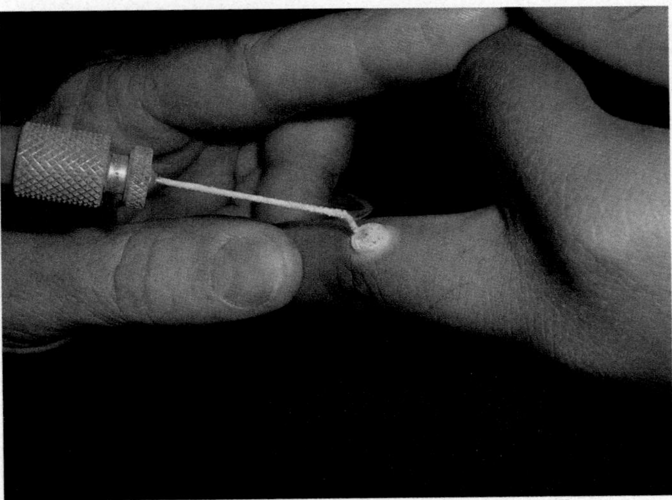

FIGURE 137-9 Cryotherapy showing an adequate free zone (halo) around the wart. (*Reproduced with permission from Richard P. Usatine, MD.*)

TABLE 137-1 *Candida* Dilutions

Creating 1.0 mL for Injection	*Candida* Antigen (mL)	Normal Saline (mL)
Generic 1:1000	0.25	0.75
Candin 1:500	0.5	0.5

Reprinted with permission from: Usatine R, Pfenninger J, Stulberg D, Small R. *Dermatologic and Cosmetic Procedures in Office Practice.* Philadelphia, PA: Elsevier; 2012.

Unfortunately, it is hard to get, and some regulations prevent using it for multiple patients. It may be used in resistant cases. It is also useful in young children because application is painless in the office. However, painful blisters often occur within a day after application. Be careful not to overtreat with cantharidin because the blistering can be quite severe. Carefully apply to multiple lesions using the wooden end of a cotton-tipped applicator (**Figure 137-11**). SOR Ⓒ

- Contact immunotherapy using dinitrochlorobenzene, squaric acid dibutylester, or diphenylcyclopropenone may be applied to the skin to sensitize the patient and then to the lesion to induce an immune response. SOR Ⓒ
- Early open-label, uncontrolled studies indicated that cimetidine might be useful in treating warts. However, three placebo-controlled, double-blind studies and two open-label comparative trials demonstrate that its efficacy is equal to placebo.[14] SOR Ⓐ
- Although preliminary studies were promising, duct tape is likely no better than placebo.[8] SOR Ⓑ
- Photodynamic therapy (PDT) with aminolevulinic acid with and without salicylic acid has been evaluated in small studies of low quality demonstrating efficacy of 42%–72%. SOR Ⓑ It is expensive and often requires referral.[8]
- Pulsed-dye laser can be considered for treatment of recalcitrant warts, although its effectiveness is unproven.[8] SOR Ⓑ

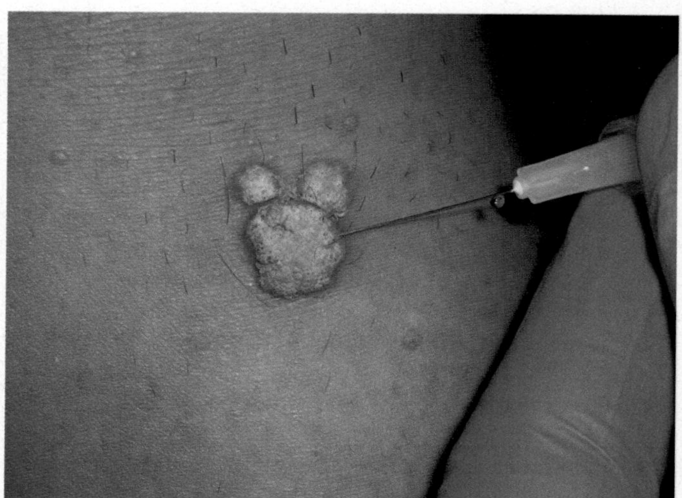

FIGURE 137-10 *Candida* antigen is being injected into a cluster of warts on the knee of a teenage boy. His warts did not respond to multiple therapies, including topical salicylic acid and cryotherapy. (*Reproduced with permission from Richard P. Usatine, MD.*)

PREVENTION

- Tools used for paring down warts, such as nail files and pumice stones, should not be used on normal skin or by other people.
- Hair-bearing areas with warts should be shaved with depilatories, electric razors, or not at all to help limit spread of warts.

PROGNOSIS

- Two-thirds of warts resolve in 2 years and 80% resolve in 4 years.[11]
- New warts may appear while others are regressing. This is not a treatment failure but part of the natural disease process with HPV.

FOLLOW-UP

- Schedule patients for return visits after treatment to limit loss of follow-up and to assess therapy.

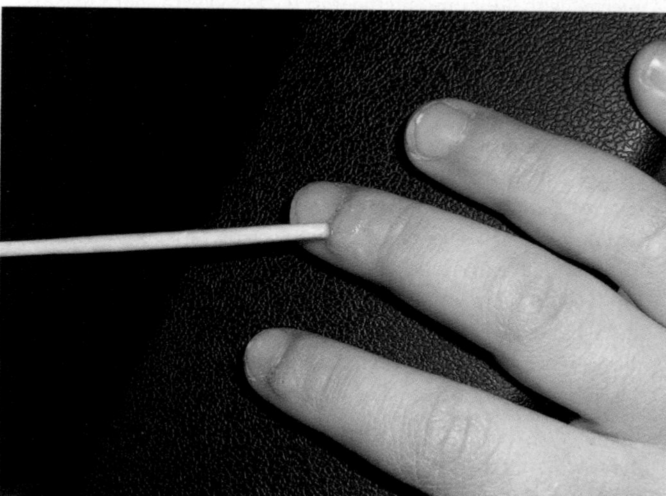

FIGURE 137-11 Cantharidin is being applied to periungual warts on the fingers of a 5-year-old child. Note the use of the wooden stick of a cotton-tipped applicator. If the cotton tip is used, the cantharidin stays within the cotton and the application is insufficient. (*Reproduced with permission from Richard P. Usatine, MD.*)

- Follow-up visits can be left to the patient's discretion when self-applied therapy is being used.

PATIENT EDUCATION

- Therapy can take weeks to months and warts may resolve spontaneously. Set reasonable expectations and never make the treatment worse than the problem.

PATIENT RESOURCES

- AFP Patient Information. *Am Fam Physician*. 2011;84(3):296.—**http://www.aafp.org/afp/2011/0801/p288.html.**
- DermNet New Zealand—**http://www.dermnetnz.org/topics/viral-warts.**
- FamilyDoctor.org. American Academy of Family Physicians. *Warts*—**https://familydoctor.org/condition/warts/.**
- MayoClinic.com. *Common Warts*—**http://www.mayoclinic.com/health/common-warts/DS00370.**

PROVIDER RESOURCES

- Cochrane review. *Topical Treatments for Skin Warts*—**http://www.cochrane.org/CD001781/SKIN_topical-treatments-for-skin-warts.**
- DermNet New Zealand—**http://www.dermnetnz.org/topics/viral-warts.**
- For information on treating warts including how to dilute *Candida* antigen:

  Usatine R, Pfenninger J, Stulberg D, Small R. *Dermatologic and Cosmetic Procedures in Office Practice*. Philadelphia, PA: Elsevier; 2012. This can also be purchased as an app at **www.usatinemedia.com.**

REFERENCES

1. Mulhem E, Pinelis S. Treatment of nongenital cutaneous warts. *Am Fam Physician*. 2011;84(3):288-293.
2. Giannaki M, Kakourou T, Theodoridou M, et al. Human papillomavirus (HPV) genotyping of cutaneous warts in Greek children. *Pediatr Dermatol*. 2013;30(6):730-735.
3. Micali G, Dall'Oglio F, Nasca MR, Tedeschi A. Management of cutaneous warts: an evidence-based approach. *Am J Clin Dermatol*. 2004;5(5):311-317.
4. Sterling JC, Gibbs S, Hussain SSH, et al. British Association of Dermatologists' guidelines for the management of cutaneous warts 2014. *Br J Dermatol*. 2014;171(4):696-712.
5. Keefe M, al-Ghamdi A, Coggon D, et al. Cutaneous warts in butchers. *Br J Dermatol*. 1994;130(1):9-14.
6. Bruggink SC, Gussekloo J, Bavinck JNB. HPV type in plantar warts influences natural course and treatment response: Secondary analysis of a randomised controlled trial. *J Clin Virol*. 2013; 57(3):227-232.
7. Cordoro KM, Gupta D, Frieden IJ, et al. Pediatric melanoma: results of a large cohort study and proposal for modified ABCD detection criteria for children. *J Am Acad Dermatol*. 2013;68(6): 913-925.
8. Kwok CS, Gibbs S, Bennett C, et al. Topical treatments for cutaneous warts. *Cochrane Database Syst Rev*. 2012;(9):CD001781.
9. Kuwabara AM, Rainer BM, Basdag H, Cohen BA. Children with warts: a retrospective study in an outpatient setting. *Pediatr Dermatol*. 2015;32(5):679-683.
10. Rivera A, Tyring SK. Therapy of cutaneous human Papillomavirus infections. *Dermatol Ther*. 2004;17(6):441-448.
11. Sterling J. Treatment of warts and molluscum: what does the evidence show? *Curr Opin Pediatr*. 2016;28(4):490-499.
12. Bruggink S, et al. Cryotherapy with liquid nitrogen versus topical salicylic acid application for cutaneous warts in primary care: randomized controlled trial. *CMAJ*. 2010;182(15):1624.
13. Micali G, Dall'Oglio F. An open label evaluation of the efficacy of imiquimod 5% cream in the treatment of recalcitrant subungual and periungual cutaneous warts. *J Dermatolog Treat*. 2003; 14(4):233.
14. Yilmaz E, Alpsoy E, Basaran E. Cimetidine therapy for warts: a placebo-controlled, double-blind study. *Arch Dermatol*. 1996; 34(6):1005-1007.

138 FLAT WARTS

E.J. Mayeaux, Jr., MD
Theresa Thuy Vo, MD

PATIENT STORY

A 16-year-old girl presents with multiple flat lesions on her forehead (**Figure 138-1**). It started with just a few lesions but has spread over the past 3 months. She is diagnosed with flat warts, and topical imiquimod is prescribed as the initial treatment.

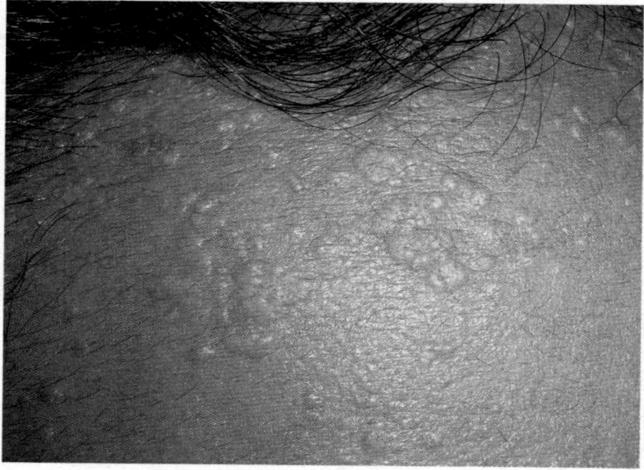

FIGURE 138-1 Flat warts on a patient's forehead. (*Reproduced with permission from Richard P. Usatine, MD.*)

INTRODUCTION

Flat warts are one of the three cutaneous manifestations of warts caused by human papillomavirus (HPV). Flat warts are characterized as flat or slightly elevated flesh-colored papules. Ranging from a few to hundreds of lesions, these warts occur most commonly on the face, hands, and shins and can cause significant patient distress (**Figure 138-2**).

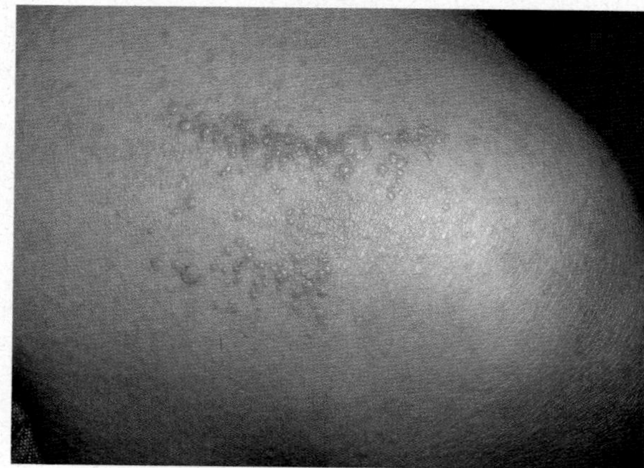

FIGURE 138-2 Flat warts just above the knee of a young woman. Probably spread by shaving. (*Reproduced with permission from Richard P. Usatine, MD.*)

SYNONYMS

Plane warts, verruca plana, verruca plana juvenilis.

EPIDEMIOLOGY

- Flat warts (verruca plana) are most commonly found in children and young adults (**Figures 138-1** to **138-5**).
- Flat warts are the least common variety of wart but are generally numerous on an individual.[1] They represent up to 4% of all cutaneous warts, while common and plantar warts represent 71% and 34%, respectively.[2]
- Flat warts are usually caused by HPV types 3, 10, 28, and 29.[3]

ETIOLOGY AND PATHOPHYSIOLOGY

- Like all warts, flat warts are caused by HPV.[3] Infection with HPV can occur by coming in direct contact with intact, macerated, or traumatized skin.
- Flat warts may spread in a linear pattern secondary to spread by scratching or trauma, such as shaving (Koebner phenomenon) (**Figure 138-2**).
- Flat warts present a special treatment problem because they persist for a long time, they are generally located in cosmetically important areas, and they are resistant to therapy.

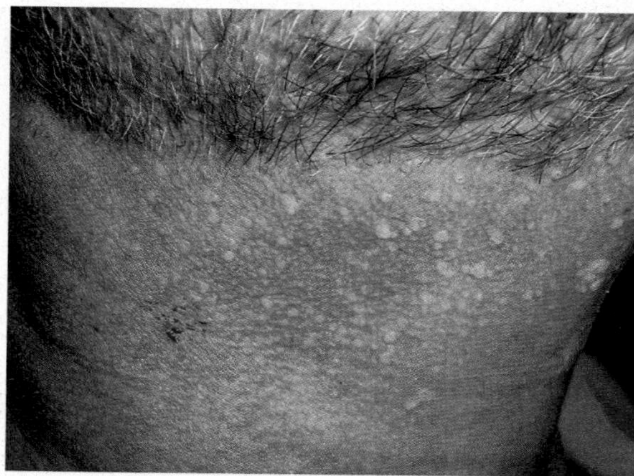

FIGURE 138-3 Flat warts on the neck of an HIV-positive man. The warts have been spread by shaving. Cryotherapy and imiquimod were not successful, but intralesional *Candida* antigen injections cleared all the warts. (*Reproduced with permission from Richard P. Usatine, MD.*)

RISK FACTORS

- Direct skin contact.
- Shaving next to infected areas (**Figures 138-2** and **138-3**).
- HIV infection or other types of immunosuppression (see **Figure 138-3**).

DIAGNOSIS

CLINICAL FEATURES

- Flat warts appear as multiple small, flat-topped papules that may be pink, light brown, or light yellow. They may be polygonal in shape, smooth, or slightly hyperkeratotic. They range in size from 1 to 5 mm or more (**Figure 138-4**).

TYPICAL DISTRIBUTION

- Flat warts typically appear on the forehead (see **Figure 138-1**), around the mouth (**Figure 138-5**), on the backs of the hands, and in shaved areas, such as the lower face and neck in men (see **Figure 138-3**) and the lower legs in women (see **Figure 138-2**).

LABORATORY TESTING

- HPV testing is not useful for flat warts.[4]

BIOPSY

- Although usually not necessary, a shave biopsy can confirm the diagnosis.

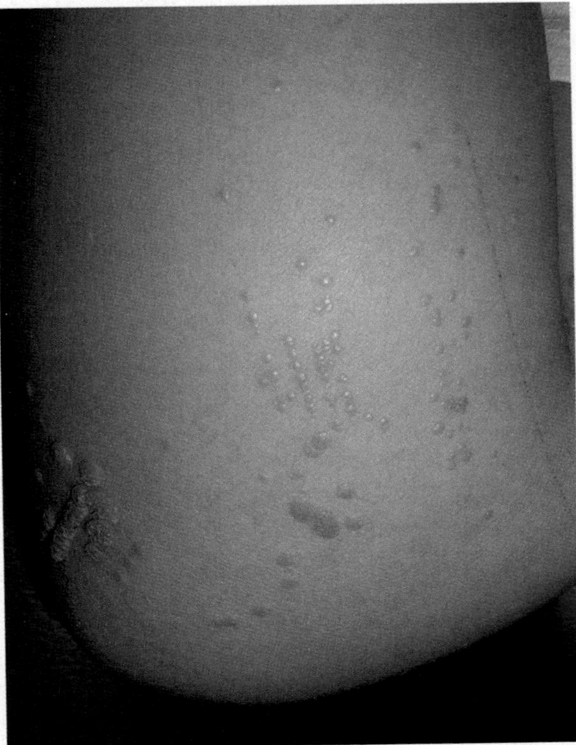

FIGURE 138-4 Flat warts and the common warts on the arm of a young boy. Note how the flat warts are truly flatter and follow a linear pattern due to Koebnerization. (*Reproduced with permission from Richard P. Usatine, MD.*)

DIFFERENTIAL DIAGNOSIS

- Lichen planus produces flat-topped papules that may be confused with flat warts. Look for characteristic signs of lichen planus such as symmetric distribution, purplish coloration, and oral lacy lesions. (Wickham striae are white, fine, reticular scale seen on the lesions.) The distribution of lichen planus is different, with the most common sites being the ankles, wrists, and back (see Chapter 160, Lichen Planus).
- Seborrheic keratoses are often more darkly pigmented and have a stuck-on appearance; "horn cysts" may be visible on close examination (see Chapter 164, Seborrheic Keratosis).
- Squamous cell carcinoma should be considered when lesions have irregular growth or pigmentation, ulceration, or resist therapy, particularly in sun-exposed areas and in immunosuppressed patients (see Chapter 178, Squamous Cell Carcinoma).
- Corns are thickenings of skin over the pressure points on the feet or areas of friction. Although a corn may obscure normal skin lines just like a wart, no thrombosed capillaries would be seen after scraping with a #15 blade.
- Acrochordons, or skin tags, can be filiform and resemble warts.
- Epidermodysplasia verruciformis is an extremely rare inherited or acquired disease characterized by a high susceptibility to infection of HPV and disseminated polymorphic lesions, including flat-topped, wart-like papules (**Figure 138-6**).

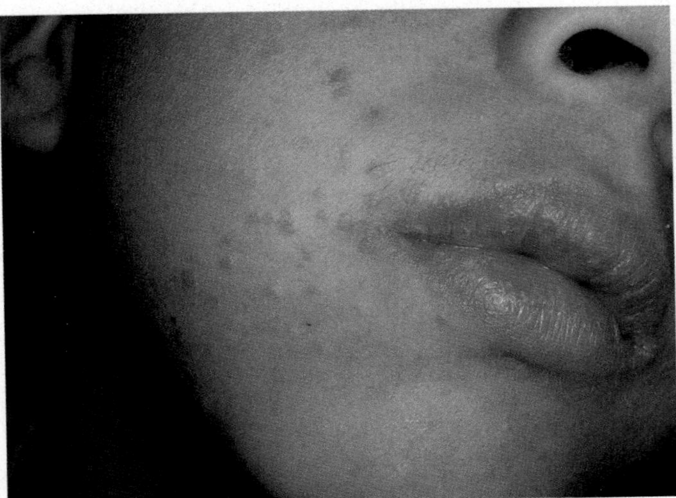

FIGURE 138-5 Flat warts around the mouth and cheeks of a 5-year-old boy. (*Reproduced with permission from Richard P. Usatine, MD.*)

MANAGEMENT

FIRST LINE

NONPHARMACOLOGIC

- Watchful waiting is a reasonable option for management. Spontaneous remission of warts occurs in up to two-thirds of children within 2 years. Spontaneous resolution in adults may take several years.[5]

- There are no current therapies for HPV that are virus specific.

MEDICATIONS OR SURGICAL

- A 2012 meta-analysis of randomized trials found that topical salicylic acid significantly increased the chance of clearance of warts (RR [risk ratio] 1.56, 95% CI [confidence interval] 1.20 to 2.03).[6] SOR Ⓐ Reported likelihoods of wart clearance following salicylic therapy have ranged from 0% to more than 80%, with higher efficacy suggested for warts on hands than feet.[6] Salicylic acid of concentrations ranging from 17% to 50% are typically used in treatment. Seventeen percent salicylic acid is found over the counter; while 40% to 50% is reserved for areas with thick stratum corneum such as palms or soles.
- Cryotherapy with liquid nitrogen is a commonly used modality of treatment. Although a 2012 meta-analysis did not find a statistically significant outcome difference for liquid nitrogen cryosurgery compared with placebo (RR 1.45, 95% CI 0.65–3.23), there was no difference in efficacy between cryotherapy and salicylic acid, the latter of which is more effective than placebo. SOR Ⓐ Liquid nitrogen is applied for 5 to 10 seconds via a Cryogun or a cotton swab so that the visibly frozen area includes wart and a 2-mm rim of normal tissue surrounding the wart. Two freeze–thaw cycles increased probability of resolution. Although aggressive cryotherapy can be more effective than gentle cryotherapy (RR 1.90, 95% CI 1.15 to 3.15), there is increased risk of adverse effects including pain, scarring, or hyper- or hypopigmentation. Because HPV can survive in liquid nitrogen, cotton swabs and residual liquid nitrogen should be properly discarded to avoid contaminating the communal liquid nitrogen reservoir. There was no significant difference in cure rates between cryotherapy at 2-, 3-, and 4-weekly intervals; thus, patients are normally seen back at 2- to 3-week intervals.
- Intralesional immunotherapy with skin test antigens (i.e. mumps, *Candida*, or *Trichophyton* antigens) aids in resolution of both the injected and neighboring untreated warts by inducing a localized, cell-mediated, and HPV-specific response.[7] A single-blind study of 201 patients showed that patients treated with skin test antigens had greater resolution of the injected wart than those injected with interferon alone or saline (60% versus 26% and 22%, respectively).[8] In addition, patients with multiple warts had resolution of at least one wart other than the injected wart (49% versus 9% and 19%).[8] The *Candida* antigen is most frequently used and must be diluted before used (see **Table 137-1**). Inject 0.1 to 0.3 mL into the largest warts using a 30-gauge needle and up to 1 mL per treatment. Using formulations of skin test antigens that are stable to be diluted with lidocaine, instead of normal saline, is helpful in reducing pain experienced during and after cryotherapy as well. Injections can be repeated every 3–4 weeks. SOR Ⓑ

SECOND LINE

- Cantharidin 0.7% is a clinician-administered blistering agent used for molluscum contagiosum and warts. Cantharidin is painless to apply on individual or multiple warts, which is an advantage when treating young children. Blistering will occur within 2 to 24 hours. Reapplication of cantharidin can be done every 3 weeks.[5] Although

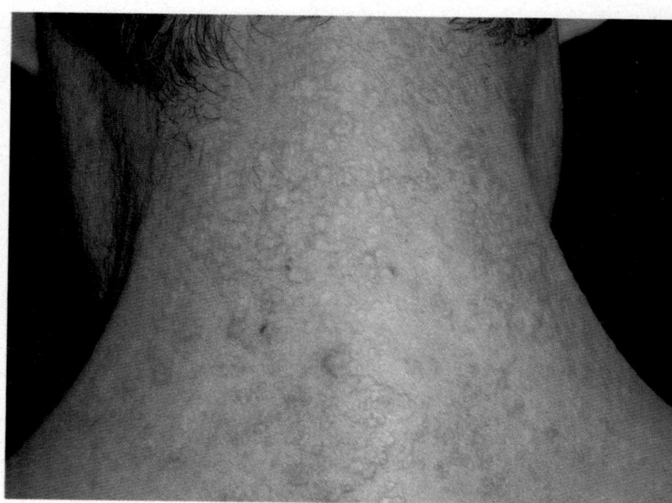

FIGURE 138-6 Epidermodysplasia verruciformis (EDV) caused by uncontrolled HPV in a patient with AIDS. It appears like flat warts but can become squamous cell carcinoma. *(Reproduced with permission from Richard P. Usatine, MD.)*

cantharidin is not commercially available in the United States, compounded cantharidin is sometimes available through compounding pharmacies. SOR C

- Tretinoin cream, 0.025%, 0.05%, or 0.1%, applied at bedtime over the entire involved area is one accepted treatment. The frequency of application is then adjusted so as to produce a mild, fine scaling and erythema. Sun protection is important. Treatment may be required for weeks or months and may not be effective. No published studies were found to support this treatment. SOR C
- Fluorouracil (Efudex 5% cream, Fluoroplex 1%) may be used topically or intralesionally to treat flat warts in adults. There is limited evidence available for efficacy.[6] Clinical trials have been highly variable in methods and quality, and the evidence from these studies was weak.[9] While the efficacy is not determined clearly and future studies are needed, topical treatment with 5-FU does have a therapeutic effect and should be considered in recalcitrant warts. Apply the cream to affected areas twice daily for 3 to 4 weeks. Sun protection is essential because the drug is photosensitizing. Persistent hypo- or hyperpigmentation may occur following use, but applying it with a cotton-tipped applicator to individual lesions instead of to the area may minimize this adverse reaction.[10,11] SOR B
- Imiquimod 5% cream is an expensive topical immunomodulatory that can be helpful, particularly when treating anogenital warts. Although there are uncontrolled studies and a right-left comparison study, randomized controlled trial data are limited.[6] It is nonscarring and painless to apply. There are rare reports of systemic side effects. As the optimal regimen is unclear, clinicians often instruct patients to apply imiquimod 5% to lesions 3 times a week (every other day). The cream may be applied to the affected area, not strictly to the lesion itself. It can be used on all external HPV-infected sites, but not on occluded mucous membranes. Imiquimod has the advantage of having almost no risk of scarring.[12,13] SOR B A lower concentration of imiquimod (3.75% cream) is also available, but data for its use with flat or common warts are lacking. The U.S. Food and Drug Administration (FDA) has approved it only for ages 12 and older.

THIRD LINE

- Other treatments, including intralesional 5-fluorouracil,[14,15] oral cimetidine,[16,17] intralesional bleomycin,[6] immunotherapy with contact allergens,[6] photodynamic therapy,[18] and duct tape treatments,[19,20] are not used commonly, even by skin specialists. Although these modes of treatment have limited evidence for their effectiveness, they may be considered for warts that are recalcitrant to simpler, safer treatments, such as salicylic acid or cryotherapy.

PREVENTION

- Hair-bearing areas with warts should be shaved with depilatories, or electric razors, or not at all, to help limit spread of warts.

FOLLOW-UP

- Schedule patients for a return visit in 2 to 3 weeks after therapy to assess efficacy.

PATIENT EDUCATION

- To help avoid spreading warts, patients should avoid touching or scratching the lesions.
- Razors that are used in areas where warts are located should not be used on unaffected skin or by other people to prevent spread.

PATIENT RESOURCES

- KidsHealth—**https://kidshealth.org/en/kids/warts.html.**
- American Academy of Dermatology—**https://www.aad.org/public/diseases/contagious-skin-diseases/warts.**
- MedlinePlus. *Warts*—**http://www.nlm.nih.gov/medlineplus/ency/article/000885.htm.**

PROVIDER RESOURCES

- Bacelieri R, Johnson SM. Cutaneous warts: an evidence-based approach to therapy. *Am Fam Physician.* 2005;72:647-652—**http://www.aafp.org/afp/20050815/647.html.**
- Cochrane Review. *Topical Treatments for Skin Warts*—**http://www.cochrane.org/CD001781/SKIN_topical-treatments-for-skin-warts.html.**
- Treatment of warts is covered extensively in: Usatine R, Pfenninger J, Stulberg D, Small R. *Dermatologic and Cosmetic Procedures in Office Practice*. Philadelphia, PA: Elsevier; 2012. This can also be purchased as an app at **www.usatinemedia.com.**

REFERENCES

1. Williams H, Pottier A, Strachan D. Are viral warts seen more commonly in children with eczema? *Arch Dermatol.* 1993;129:717-720.
2. Bonnez W, Reichman RC. Papillomaviruses. In: Mandell GL, Bennett JE, Dolin R, eds. *Principles and Practice of Infectious Diseases.* 5th ed. Philadelphia, PA: Churchill Livingstone; 2000:1630.
3. Mulhem E, Pinelis S. Treatment of nongenital cutaneous warts. *Am Fam Physician.* 2011;84(3):288-293.
4. Gibbs S, Harvey I. Topical treatments for cutaneous warts. *Cochrane Database Syst Rev.* 2006;(3):CD001781.
5. Sterling JC, Gibbs S, Haque Hussain SS, et al. British Association of Dermatologists' guidelines for the management of cutaneous warts 2014. *Br J Dermatol.* 2014;171:696.
6. Kwok CS, Gibbs S, Bennett C, et al. Topical treatments for cutaneous warts. *Cochrane Database Syst Rev.* 2012;(9):CD001781.
7. Johnson SM, Roberson PK, Horn TD. Intralesional injection of mumps or *Candida* skin test antigens: a novel immunotherapy for warts. *Arch Dermatol.* 2001;137:451.
8. Horn TD, Johnson SM, Helm RM, Roberson PK. Intralesional immunotherapy of warts with mumps, *Candida*, and *Trichophyton* skin test antigens: a single-blinded, randomized, and controlled trial. *Arch Dermatol.* 2005;141:589.

9. Batista CS, Atallah AN, Saconato H, da Silva EM. 5-FU for genital warts in non-immunocompromised individuals. *Cochrane Database Syst Rev.* 2010;(4):CD006562.
10. Lockshin NA. Flat facial warts treated with fluorouracil. *Arch Dermatol.* 1979;115:929-1030.
11. Lee S, Kim J-G, Chun SI. Treatment of verruca plana with 5% 5-fluorouracil ointment. *Dermatologica.* 1980;160:383-389.
12. Cutler K, Kagen MH, Don PC, et al. Treatment of facial verrucae with topical imiquimod cream in a patient with human immunodeficiency virus. *Acta Derm Venereol.* 2000;80:134-135.
13. Kim MB. Treatment of flat warts with 5% imiquimod cream. *J Eur Acad Dermatol Venereol.* 2006;20(10):1349-1350.
14. Isçimen A, Aydemir EH, Göksügür N, Engin B. Intralesional 5-fluorouracil, lidocaine and epinephrine mixture for the treatment of verrucae: a prospective placebo-controlled, single-blind randomized study. *J Eur Acad Dermatol Venereol.* 2004;18:455.
15. Yazdanfar A, Farshchian M, Fereydoonnejad M, Farshchian M. Treatment of common warts with an intralesional mixture of 5-fluorouracil, lidocaine, and epinephrine: a prospective placebo-controlled, double-blind randomized trial. *Dermatol Surg.* 2008; 34:656.
16. Yilmaz E, Alpsoy E, Basaran E. Cimetidine therapy for warts: a placebo-controlled, double-blind study. *J Am Acad Dermatol.* 1996; 34:1005.
17. Rogers CJ, Gibney MD, Siegfried EC, et al. Cimetidine therapy for recalcitrant warts in adults: is it any better than placebo? *J Am Acad Dermatol.* 1999;41:123.
18. Robson KJ, Cunningham NM, Kruzan KL, et al. Pulsed-dye laser versus conventional therapy in the treatment of warts: a prospective randomized trial. *J Am Acad Dermatol.* 2000;43:275.
19. de Haen M, Spigt MG, van Uden CJ, et al. Efficacy of duct tape vs placebo in the treatment of verruca vulgaris (warts) in primary school children. *Arch Pediatr Adolesc Med.* 2006;160:1121.
20. Wenner R, Askari SK, Cham PM, et al. Duct tape for the treatment of common warts in adults: a double-blind randomized controlled trial. *Arch Dermatol.* 2007;143:309.

139 GENITAL WARTS

E.J. Mayeaux, Jr., MD
Matthew J. Lenhard, MD
Richard P. Usatine, MD

PATIENT STORY

An 18-year-old woman presents with a concern that she might have genital warts (**Figure 139-1**). She has never had a sexually transmitted disease (STD) but admits to two new sexual partners in the last 6 months. She has not been vaccinated against human papillomavirus (HPV). The patient is told that her concern is accurate and she has condyloma caused by HPV (an STD). The treatment options are discussed and she chooses to have cryotherapy with liquid nitrogen followed by imiquimod self-applied beginning 2 weeks after cryotherapy. A urine test for gonorrhea and *Chlamydia* is performed and the patient is sent to the lab to have blood tests for syphilis and HIV. Fortunately, all the additional tests are negative. Further patient education is performed and follow-up is arranged.

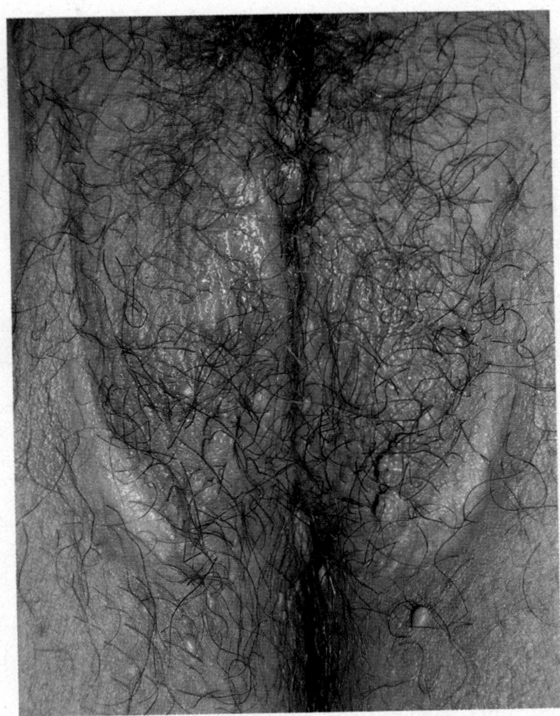

FIGURE 139-1 Multiple vulvar exophytic condyloma in an 18-year-old woman. (*Reproduced with permission from Richard P. Usatine, MD.*)

INTRODUCTION

More than 100 types of HPV exist, with more than 40 that can infect the human genital area. Most HPV infections are asymptomatic, unrecognized, or subclinical. Low-risk HPV types (e.g., HPV types 6 and 11) cause genital warts, although coinfection with HPV types associated with squamous intraepithelial neoplasia (e.g., HPV types 16, 18, 31, 45) can occur. Asymptomatic genital HPV infection is common and usually self-limited.[1]

SYNONYMS

Condyloma acuminata.

EPIDEMIOLOGY

- Anogenital warts are the most common viral STD in the United States. Incidence can vary, as there is no requirement to report the disease. Current data suggests that there are approximately 350,000 new cases of genital warts diagnosed per year in the United States, although that can range up to 1 million.[1] Worldwide, incidence may vary from 100 to 200 new cases (per 100,000 general population), with peak incidence in young males and females.[2,3]
- Some warts are transient and may clear within 1 year. There appears to be a time delay when patient first notices warts and seeks a healthcare opinion—on average, 76 days for men and 30 days for women.[1,2]
- Infections may persist and recur, causing much distress for the patient.

ETIOLOGY AND PATHOPHYSIOLOGY

- Genital warts are caused by HPV infection. HPV encompasses a family of primarily sexually transmitted double-stranded DNA viruses. The incubation period after exposure is variable and ranges from 3 weeks to 8 months.

RISK FACTORS[4]

- Penetrative intercourse (penis-vaginal, digital-vaginal, digital-anal).
- Oral intercourse (oral-vaginal and oral-anal).
- Immunosuppression, especially HIV (**Figure 139-2**).

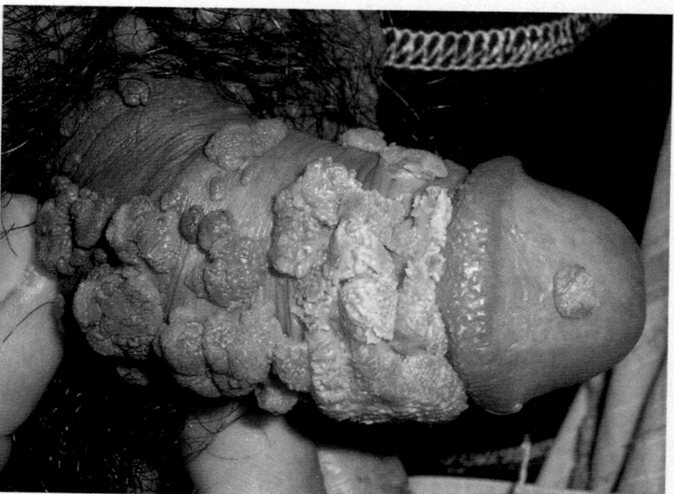

FIGURE 139-2 Multiple exophytic condyloma on the penis of a man with AIDS. (*Reproduced with permission from Richard P. Usatine, MD.*)

DIAGNOSIS

CLINICAL FEATURES

- Diagnosis of genital warts is usually clinical based on visual inspection.[1]
- Genital warts are usually asymptomatic and typically present as flesh-colored, exophytic lesions on the genitalia, including the penis, vulva, vagina, scrotum, perineum, and perianal skin.
- External warts can appear as small bumps, or they may be flat, verrucous, or pedunculated (**Figures 139-2** to **139-4**).
- Less commonly, warts can appear as reddish or brown, smooth, raised papules, or as dome-shaped lesions on keratinized skin.

TYPICAL DISTRIBUTION

- In women, the most common sites of infection are the vulva (85%) (see **Figure 139-1**), perianal area (58%), and the vagina (42%) (see **Figure 139-3**).
- In men, the most common sites of infection are the penis (**Figures 139-4** and **139-5**) and scrotum.
- Perianal warts (**Figure 139-6**) can occur in men or women, with or without a history of anal intercourse (**Figure 139-7**).[1]
- Condyloma acuminata may be seen on the abdomen or upper thighs in conjunction with genital warts (**Figure 139-8**).
- Condyloma caused by HPV can be seen in obese individuals within the folds of the pannus (**Figure 139-9**).
- A rapid plasma reagin (RPR) or Venereal Disease Research Laboratory (VDRL) test should be ordered to screen for syphilis, and an HIV test should be ordered as well. Genital warts are a sexually transmitted disease, and patients who have one STD should be screened for others.

LABORATORY TESTING

- HPV viral typing is not recommended because test results would not alter clinical management of the condition. The application of 3% to 5% acetic acid to detect mucosal changes attributed to HPV infection is not recommended.[1]

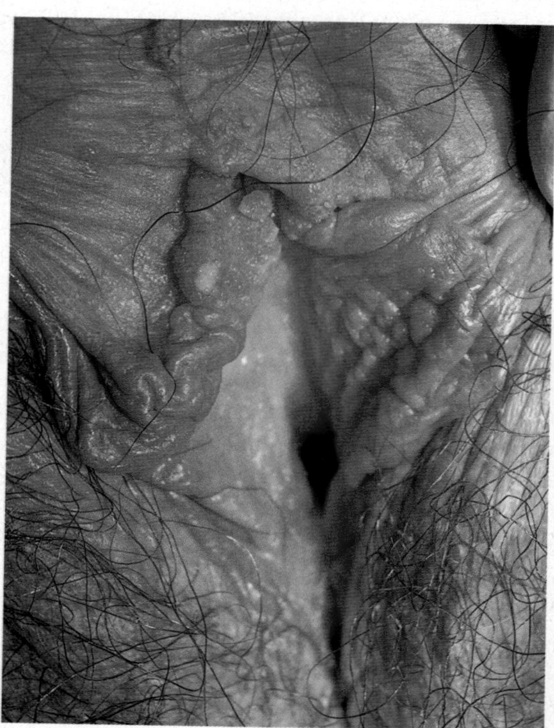

FIGURE 139-3 Condyloma around the clitoris, labia minor, and opening of the vagina. (*Reproduced with permission from Richard P. Usatine, MD.*)

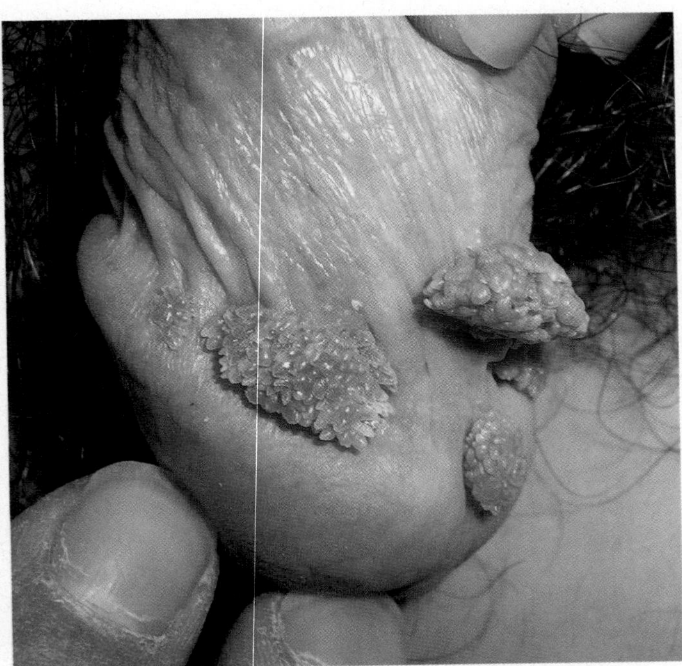

FIGURE 139-4 Condyloma acuminata demonstrating a cauliflower appearance with typical papillary surface seen when the foreskin is retracted in an uncircumcised man. Note that the top wart is pedunculated with a narrow base. (*Reproduced with permission from Richard P. Usatine, MD.*)

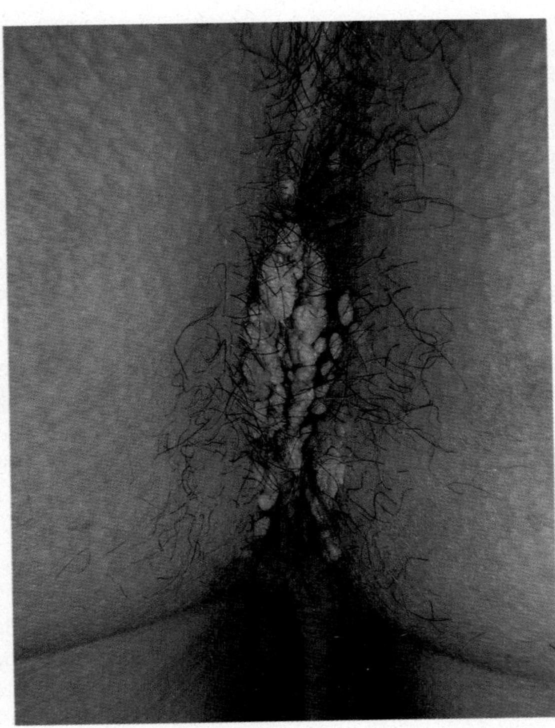

FIGURE 139-6 Perianal warts in an HIV-positive man with history of anal-receptive intercourse. These lesions responded to cryotherapy. (*Reproduced with permission from Richard P. Usatine, MD.*)

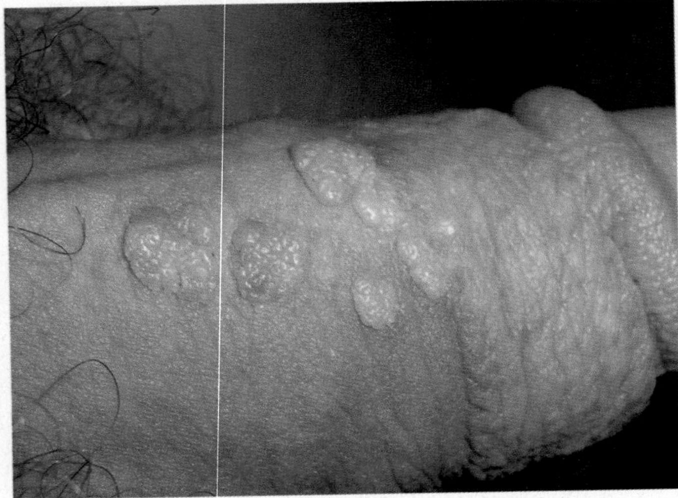

FIGURE 139-5 Smooth-topped condyloma on the well-keratinized skin of a circumcised man. (*Reproduced with permission from Richard P. Usatine, MD.*)

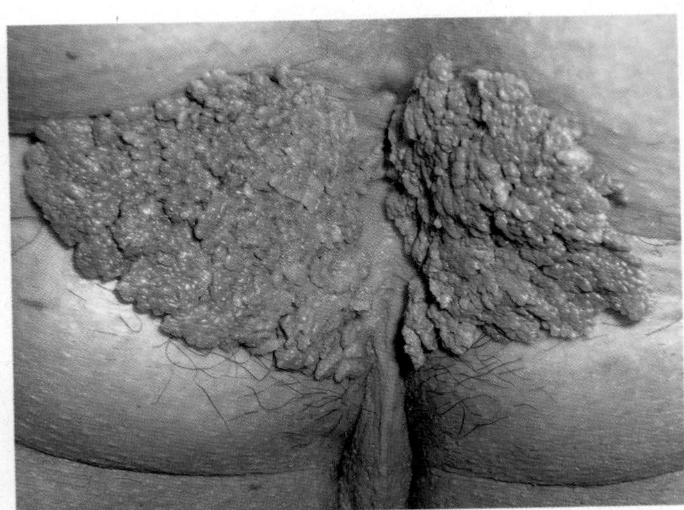

FIGURE 139-7 Extensive perianal warts in a 17-year-old boy who denies sexual abuse and anal intercourse. Patient failed imiquimod therapy and was referred to surgery. (*Reproduced with permission from Richard P. Usatine, MD.*)

BIOPSY

- Diagnosis may be confirmed by shave or punch biopsy if necessary.[1] Biopsy is indicated if:
  - The diagnosis is uncertain.
  - The patient has a poor response to appropriate therapy.
  - Warts are atypical in appearance (unusually pigmented, indurated, fixed, or ulcerated).
  - The patient has compromised immunity and/or squamous cell carcinoma is suspected (one type of HPV-related malignancy).

DIFFERENTIAL DIAGNOSIS

- Pearly penile papules, which are small papules around the edge of the glans penis (**Figure 139-10**).
- Common skin lesions, such as seborrheic keratoses and nevi—these are rare in the genital area (**Figure 139-11**) (see Chapters 164, Seborrheic Keratosis, and 168, Benign Nevi).
- Giant condyloma or Buschke-Lowenstein tumor is a low-grade, locally invasive malignancy that can appear as a fungating condyloma (**Figure 139-12**). Persons with HIV/AIDS have a higher risk of giant condyloma and malignant transformation (**Figure 139-13**).
- Molluscum contagiosum—Waxy umbilicated papules around the genitals and lower abdomen (see Chapter 136, Molluscum Contagiosum).
- Malignant neoplasms, such as basal cell carcinoma and squamous cell carcinomas (see Chapters 177, Basal Cell Carcinoma, and 178, Squamous Cell Carcinoma).
- Condyloma lata is caused by secondary syphilis infection; lesions appear flat and velvety (see Chapter 225, Syphilis). A full work-up for other STDs, including syphilis, should be done for any patient with genital warts (**Figure 139-14**).
- Micropapillomatosis of the vulva is a normal variant and appears as distinct individual papillary projections from the labia in a symmetrical pattern.

MANAGEMENT

- The primary reason for treating genital warts is the amelioration of symptoms and ultimately removal of the warts.[1]
- Choice of therapy is based on the number, size, site, and morphology of lesions, as well as patient preference, treatment cost, convenience, adverse effects, and physician experience.
- While currently available therapies for genital warts are likely to reduce HPV infectivity, they probably do not eradicate transmission.[1]

MEDICATIONS AND SURGICAL METHODS

- Treatments for external genital warts include topical medications, cryotherapy (**Figure 139-15**), and surgical methods, and are shown in **Table 139-1**.
- Cryotherapy is best applied with a bent-tipped spray applicator that allows for precise application with a less painful attenuated flow

FIGURE 139-8 Condyloma that started on the penis and spread up the abdomen and on to the thighs. Note how these warts are hyperpigmented in this Latino man. *(Reproduced with permission from Richard P. Usatine, MD.)*

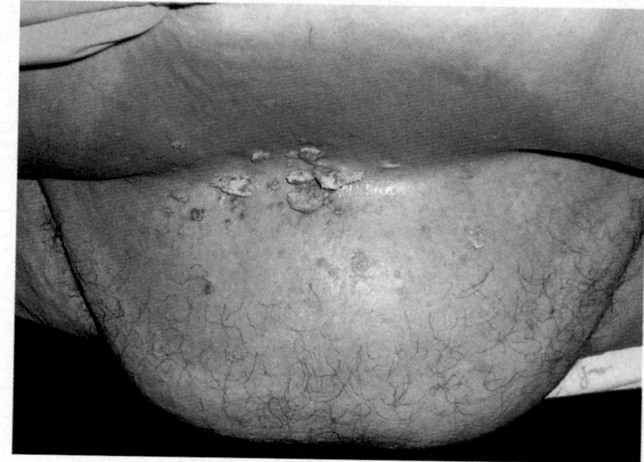

FIGURE 139-9 Pannus condyloma from HPV growing between the folds of heavy adipose tissue in this obese woman. *(Reproduced with permission from Richard P. Usatine, MD.)*

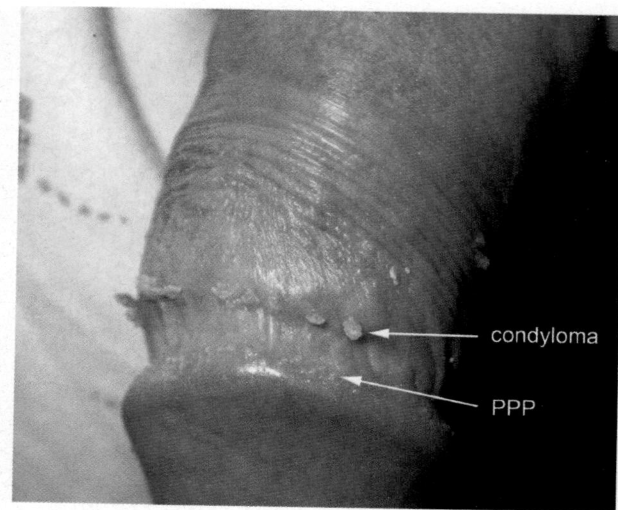

FIGURE 139-10 Condyloma coexisting with pearly penile papules (PPPs), which are a normal variant on the edge of the corona. *(Reproduced with permission from Richard P. Usatine, MD.)*

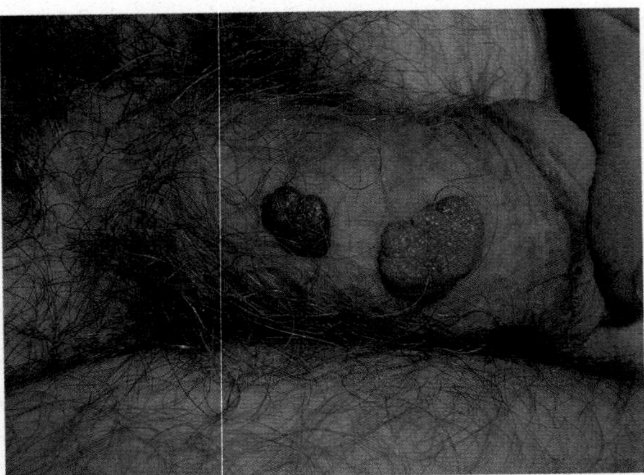

FIGURE 139-11 Two large condylomas that resemble seborrheic keratoses. Shave biopsy was positive for HPV. *(Reproduced with permission from Richard P. Usatine, MD.)*

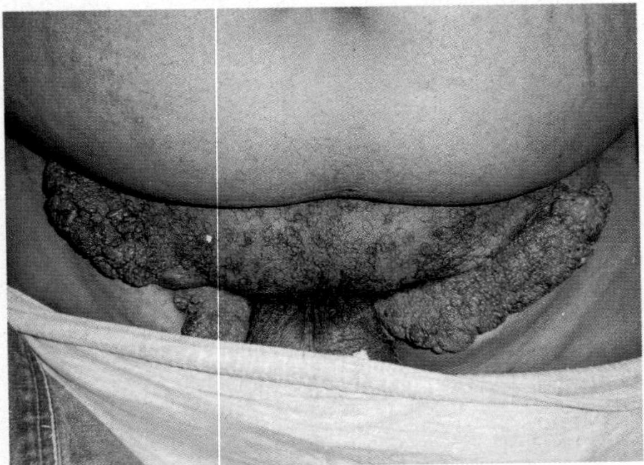

FIGURE 139-12 Buschke-Lowenstein tumors (giant condylomata acuminata) in the inguinal and genital regions. A biopsy did not show squamous cell carcinoma, but the patient was referred to surgery for full surgical excisions. *(Reproduced with permission from Richard P. Usatine, MD.)*

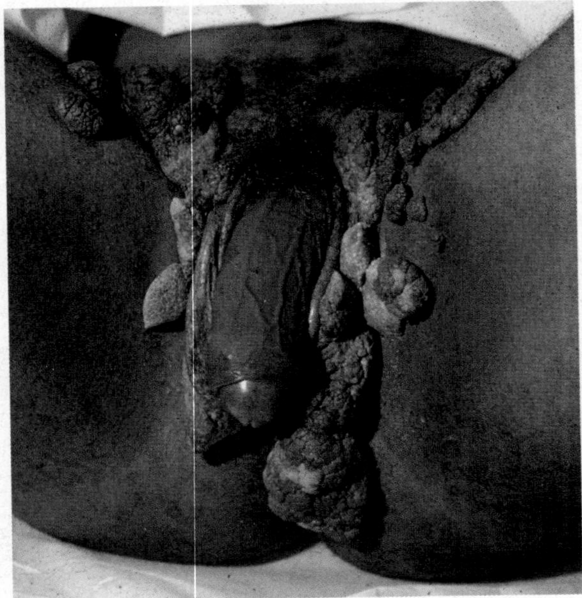

FIGURE 139-13 Giant condylomata acuminata in a man with AIDS. *(Reproduced with permission from Jack Resneck, Sr., MD.)*

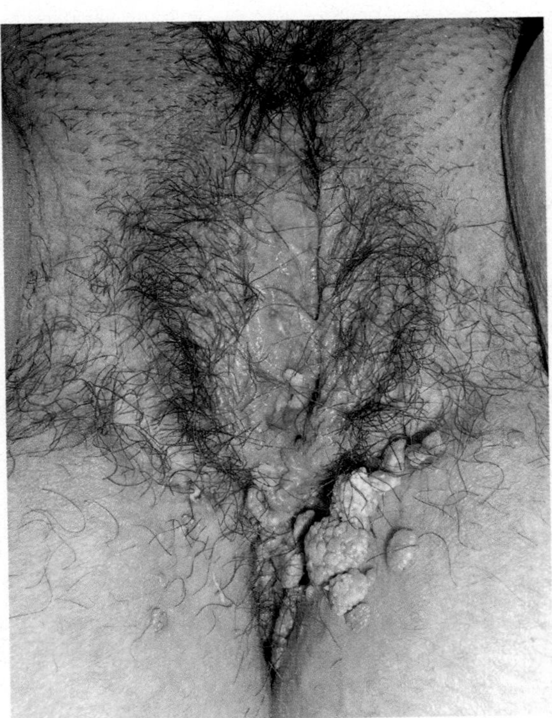

FIGURE 139-14 This 22-year-old woman with an addiction to heroin presented with many condyloma in the anogenital region. A rapid plasma reagin (RPR) was positive for syphilis. The patient was treated with penicillin as well as cryotherapy. The visible condyloma in this image are most likely HPV and not condyloma lata based on their verrucous morphology. *(Reproduced with permission from Richard P. Usatine, MD.)*

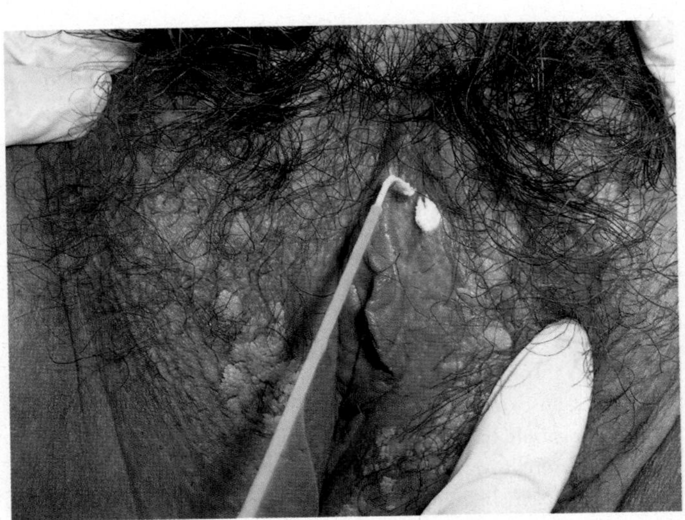

FIGURE 139-15 Cryotherapy of vulvar warts using a liquid nitrogen spray technique and a bent-tipped applicator. *(Reproduced with permission from Richard P. Usatine, MD.)*

TABLE 139-1 Treatments for External Genital Warts

Treatment	Possible Adverse Effects	Clearance (%)	Recurrence (%)
Patient-Applied Therapy			
Imiquimod (Aldara) is applied at bedtime for 3 days, then rest 4 days; alternatively, apply every other day for 3 applications; may repeat weekly cycles for up to 16 weeks[7] SOR Ⓐ	Erythema, irritation, ulceration, pain, and pigmentary changes; minimal systemic absorption	30 to 50	15
Sinecatechins 15% ointment—apply a 0.5-cm strand of ointment to each wart 3 times daily[8] SOR Ⓐ	Erythema, pruritus/burning, pain, ulceration, edema, induration, and vesicular rash	53 to 57	3.7
Podofilox (Condylox) is applied twice daily for 3 days, then rest 4 days; may repeat for 4 cycles[9] SOR Ⓐ	Burning, pain, inflammation; low risk for systemic toxicity unless applied to occluded membranes	45 to 80	5 to 30
Provider-Applied Therapy			
Cryotherapy performed with liquid nitrogen or a cryoprobe[8] SOR Ⓑ	Pain or blisters at application site, scarring	60 to 90	20 to 40
Podophyllin resin is applied to each wart and allowed to dry, and is repeated weekly as needed[8,9] SOR Ⓐ	Local irritation, erythema, burning, and soreness at application site; neurotoxic and oncogenic if absorbed	30 to 80	20 to 65
Surgical treatment for warts involves removal to the dermal–epidermal junction; options include scissor excision, shave excision, laser vaporization, and loop electrosurgical excision procedure (LEEP) excision[8] SOR Ⓑ	Pain, bleeding, scarring; risk for burning and allergic reaction from local anesthetic; laser and LEEP have risk for spreading HPV in plume	35 to 70	5 to 50
Trichloroacetic acid (TCA) and bichloracetic acid (BCA) are applied to each wart and allowed to dry; repeated weekly[8] SOR Ⓑ	Local pain and irritation; no systemic side effects	50 to 80	35

(see **Figure 139-15**).[5] Application may be repeated every 2 weeks if necessary.

- Treatment with 5% fluorouracil cream (Efudex) is no longer recommended because of severe local side effects and teratogenicity.[1]

REFERRAL OR HOSPITALIZATION

- Consider consultation for patients with very large or recalcitrant lesions.

PREVENTION

- HPV vaccination is recommended for females and males ages 9 to 26 years. The newest vaccine is nine-valent (9vHPV), thereby protecting persons against the 7 HPV types with the highest risk for cancer and the 2 types that cause the majority of genital warts. For persons 9 through 14 years of age, this HPV vaccine can be given using a 2-dose or 3-dose schedule. For the 2-dose schedule, the second shot should be given 6–12 months after the first shot. For persons 15 through 26 years of age, the nine-valent vaccine is given using a 3-dose schedule; the second shot should be given 2 months after the first shot and the third shot should be given 6 months after the first shot. The 9vHPV vaccine induced a very robust immune response against all vaccine types, with seroconversion rates close to 100%. These 9 HPV types in the vaccine are responsible for about 95.5% of all cervical lesions in North America.[10]
- A bivalent vaccine (Cervarix) containing HPV types 16 and 18 and a quadrivalent vaccine (Gardasil) vaccine containing HPV types 6, 11, 16, and 18 are also licensed in the United States. The quadrivalent HPV vaccine protects against the HPV types that cause 90% of genital warts (i.e., types 6 and 11) in males and females when given prophylactically.
- Both vaccines offer protection against the HPV types that cause 70% of cervical cancers (i.e., types 16 and 18). In the United States, the 9-valent (Gardasil) HPV vaccine can also be used in males and females ages 9 to 26 years to prevent genital warts.[6]

PROGNOSIS

- Many genital warts will eventually resolve without treatment. Therapy can hasten resolution (see **Table 139-1**).

FOLLOW-UP

- Patients should be offered a follow-up evaluation 2 to 3 months after treatment to check for new lesions.[1] SOR Ⓒ

PATIENT EDUCATION

- HPV is transmitted mainly by skin-to-skin contact. Although condoms may decrease the levels of transmission, they are imperfect barriers at best as they can fail, and they do not cover the scrotum or vulva, where infection may reside.

PATIENT RESOURCES

- eMedicineHealth. *Genital Warts (HPV Infection)*—**http://www.emedicinehealth.com/genital_warts/article_em.htm.**
- PubMed Health. *About Genital Warts*—**https://www.ncbi.nlm.nih.gov/pubmedhealth/PMHT0027103/.**
- American Academy of Dermatology. *Genital Warts*—**http://www.aad.org/skin-conditions/dermatology-a-to-z/genital-warts.**
- MedlinePlus. *Genital Warts*—**http://www.nlm.nih.gov/medlineplus/ency/article/000886.htm.**
- Centers for Disease Control and Prevention. *Human Papillomavirus (HPV)*—**https://www.cdc.gov/std/hpv/stdfact-hpv.htm.**

PROVIDER RESOURCES

- Centers for Disease Control and Prevention. *Anogenital Warts*—**https://www.cdc.gov/std/tg2015/warts.htm.**
- Medscape. *Human Papillomavirus*—**http://emedicine.medscape.com/article/219110-overview#showall.**
- Medscape. *Genital Warts*—**http://emedicine.medscape.com/article/763014-overview#showall.**

REFERENCES

1. Frieden TR, Jaffe HW, Cono J, et al. Sexually Transmitted Diseases Treatment Guidelines, 2015. *MMWR Recomm Rep.* 2015; 64(No. 63):84-89.
2. Patel H, Wagner M, Singhal P, et al. Systematic review of the incidence and prevalence of genital warts. *BMC Infect Dis.* 2013;13:39.
3. Chesson HW, Ekwueme DU, Saraiya M, et al. Estimates of the annual direct medical costs of the prevention and treatment of disease associated with human papillomavirus in the United States. *Vaccine.* 2012;30:6016-6019.
4. Palefsky JM. Cutaneous and genital HPV-associated lesions in HIV-infected patients. *Clin Dermatol.* 1997;15:439-447.
5. Usatine R, Stulberg D. Cryosurgery. In: Usatine R, Pfenninger J, Stulberg D, Small R, eds. *Dermatologic and Cosmetic Procedures in Office Practice.* Philadelphia, PA: Elsevier; 2012:182-198.
6. Centers for Disease Control and Prevention (CDC). FDA licensure of quadrivalent human papillomavirus vaccine (HPV4, Gardasil) for use in males and guidance from the Advisory Committee on Immunization Practices (ACIP). *MMWR Morb Mortal Wkly Rep.* 2010;59(20):630-632.
7. Gotovtseva EP, Kapadia AS, Smolensky MH, Lairson DR. Optimal frequency of imiquimod (Aldara) 5% cream for the treatment of external genital warts in immunocompetent adults: a meta-analysis. *Sex Transm Dis.* 2008;35(4):346-351.
8. Mayeaux EJ Jr, Dunton C. Modern management of external genital warts. *J Low Genit Tract Dis.* 2008;12:185-192.
9. Langley PC, Tyring SK, Smith MH. The cost effectiveness of patient-applied versus provider-administered intervention strategies for the treatment of external genital warts. *Am J Manag Care.* 1999;5(1):69-77.
10. Yang DY, Bracken K. Update on the new 9-valent vaccine for human papillomavirus prevention. *Can Fam Physician.* 2016; 62(5):399-402.

140 PLANTAR WARTS

E.J. Mayeaux, Jr., MD
Jonathan C. Banta, MD

PATIENT STORY

A 15-year-old boy presents with painful growths on his right heel for approximately 6 months (**Figure 140-1**). It is painful to walk on and he would like it treated. He was diagnosed with multiple large plantar warts called *mosaic warts*. The lesions were treated with gentle paring with a #15 blade scalpel and liquid nitrogen therapy over a number of sessions. He and his mother were instructed on how to use salicylic acid plasters on the remaining warts.

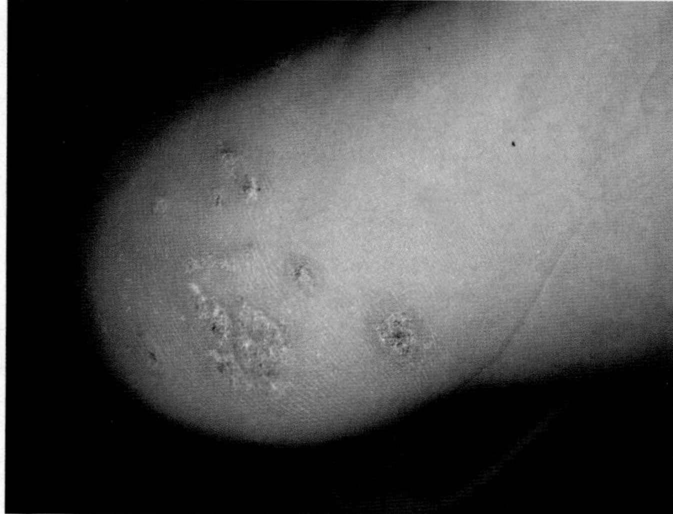

FIGURE 140-1 Plantar warts. Note small black dots in the warts that represent thrombosed vessels. Large plantar warts such as these are called mosaic warts. *(Reproduced with permission from Richard P. Usatine, MD.)*

INTRODUCTION

Plantar warts (verruca plantaris) are human papillomavirus (HPV) lesions that occur on the soles of the feet (**Figures 140-1** to **140-5**) and palms of the hands (**Figure 140-6**).

SYNONYMS

Palmoplantar warts, myrmecia.

EPIDEMIOLOGY

- Plantar warts affect mostly adolescents and young adults, affecting up to 10% of people in these age groups.[1]
- Prevalence studies demonstrate a wide range of values, from 0.84% in the United States,[2] to 3.3% to 4.7% in the United Kingdom,[3] to 24% in 16- to 18-year-olds in Australia.[4]

ETIOLOGY AND PATHOPHYSIOLOGY

- Plantar warts are caused by HPV.
- They usually occur at points of maximum pressure, such as on the heels (**Figures 140-1** to **140-4**) or over the heads of the metatarsal bones (**Figure 140-5**), but may appear anywhere on the plantar surface including the tips of the fingers (**Figure 140-7**).
- A thick, painful callus forms in response to the pressure that is induced as the size of the lesion increases. Even a minor wart can cause a lot of pain.
- A cluster of many warts that appear to fuse is referred to as a *mosaic wart* (see **Figures 140-1** and **140-4**).

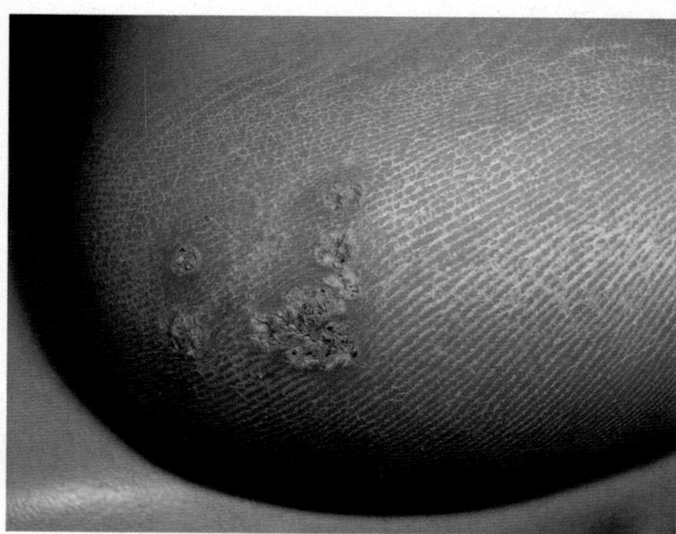

FIGURE 140-2 Close-up of plantar wart on the side of the heel. Note the disruption of skin lines and black dots. *(Reproduced with permission from Richard P. Usatine, MD.)*

RISK FACTORS

- Young age.
- Decreased immunity.
- Occupational exposure to meat, poultry, or fish.

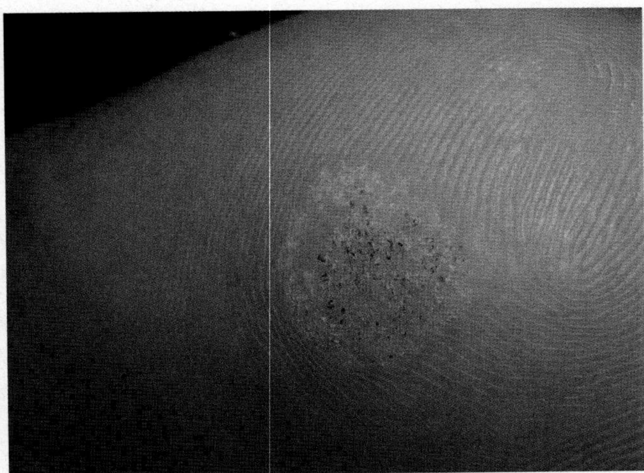

FIGURE 140-3 Close-up of a plantar wart demonstrating disruption of normal skin lines. Corns and callus do not disrupt normal skin lines. The black dots are thrombosed vessels, which are frequently seen in plantar warts. (*Reproduced with permission from Richard P. Usatine, MD.*)

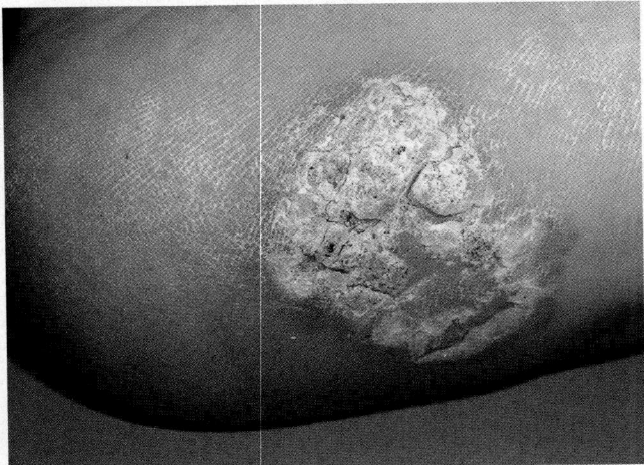

FIGURE 140-4 A mosaic wart is formed when several plantar warts become confluent. This patient is HIV positive and the thrombosed vessels are visible in some of this large wart. (*Reproduced with permission from Richard P. Usatine, MD.*)

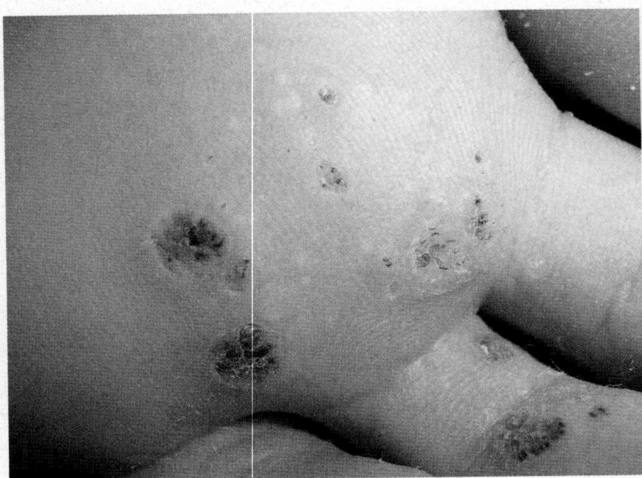

FIGURE 140-5 Multiple plantar warts on the ball of the foot and toes. The thrombosed vessels within the warts appear as black dots. (*Reproduced with permission from Richard P. Usatine, MD.*)

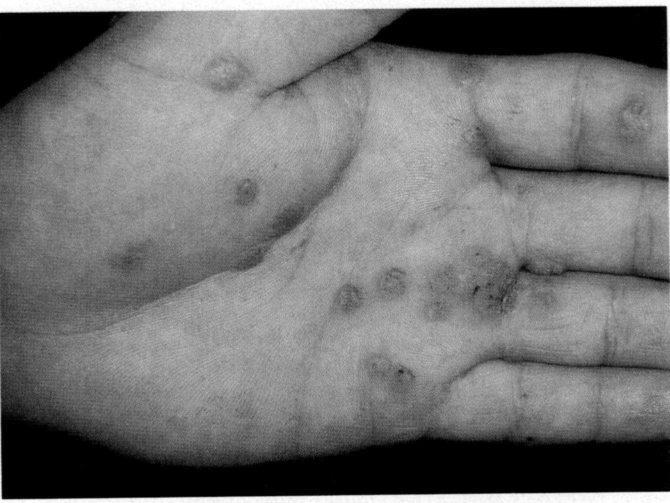

FIGURE 140-6 Multiple plantar warts on the palms of an HIV-positive man. (*Reproduced with permission from Richard P. Usatine, MD.*)

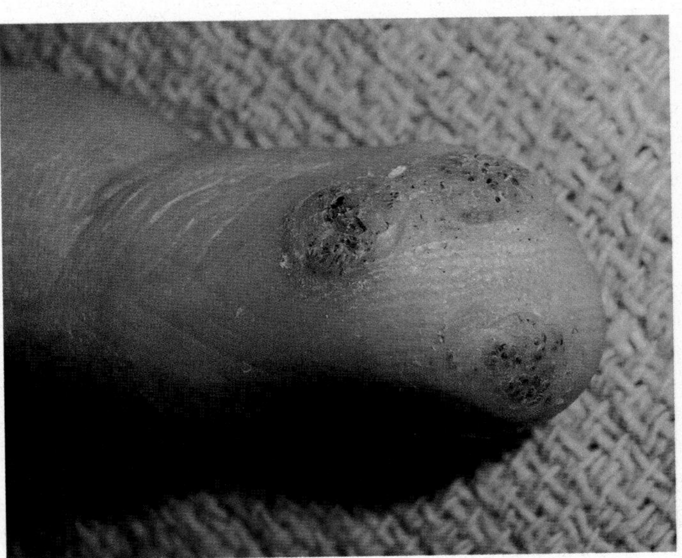

FIGURE 140-7 Close up of plantar wart on a finger that also shows disruption of skin lines and black dots. (*Reproduced with permission from Richard P. Usatine, MD.*)

DIAGNOSIS

CLINICAL FEATURES

Plantar warts present as thick, painful endophytic plaques located on the soles and/or palms. Warts have the following features:

- Begin as small shiny papules.
- Lack skin lines crossing their surface (see **Figure 140-3**).
- Have a highly organized mosaic pattern on the surface when examined with a hand lens.
- Have a rough keratotic surface surrounded by a smooth collar of callused skin.
- Are painful when compressed laterally.
- May have centrally located black dots (thrombosed vessels) that may bleed with paring (see **Figures 140-1** to **140-7**).

TYPICAL DISTRIBUTION

- They occur on the palms of the hands and soles of the feet. They are more commonly found on weight-bearing areas, such as under the metatarsal heads or on the heel.[5]

DERMOSCOPY/BIOPSY

- Examining the suspected wart with a dermatoscope can show the disrupted skin lines and thrombosed capillaries even on very small warts due to the magnification and lighting (**Figure 140-8**).
- If the diagnosis is not certain, a shave biopsy is indicated to confirm the diagnosis.[6]

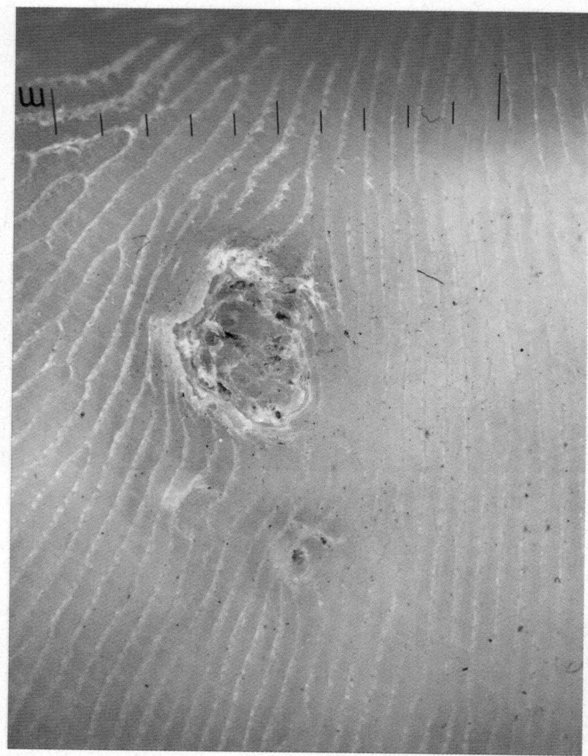

FIGURE 140-8 Dermoscopy of a plantar wart showing the disruption of skin lines and the thrombosed capillaries. (*Reproduced with permission from Richard P. Usatine, MD.*)

DIFFERENTIAL DIAGNOSIS

- Corns and calluses are pressure-induced skin thickenings that occur on the feet and can be mistaken for plantar warts. Calluses are generally found on the sole, and corns are usually found on the toes. Calluses and corns have skin lines crossing the surface and are painless with lateral pressure (see Chapter 216, Corn and Callus).
- Porokeratosis (punctate) of the foot is a focal hyperkeratosis on the plantar aspect of the foot that also disrupts the skin lines but does not have the thrombosed capillaries seen in plantar warts (**Figure 140-9**) . Factors that are believed to cause these are mechanical stressors from walking and the blockage of eccrine sweat ducts. These focal hyperkeratoses are not uncommon and are usually under 5 mm in size. They may appear as one isolated lesion or occur as a few simultaneously. The easiest treatment is to pare them down with a #15 scalpel (or curette) to remove the central keratosis. Anesthesia is not needed, and this can be followed by home use of a pumice stone. Walking on these porokeratoses can be like walking on small pebbles in the shoe, and patients will have immediate relief of pain on walking after the paring has been completed.
- Black heel (talon noir) presents as a cluster of blue-black dots that result from ruptured capillaries. They appear on the plantar surface of the heel following the shearing trauma of sports that involve sudden stops or position changes. Examination reveals normal skin lines, and paring does not cause additional bleeding. The condition resolves spontaneously in a few weeks.

FIGURE 140-9 Porokeratosis (punctate) of the foot is a focal hyperkeratosis on the plantar aspect of the foot that also disrupts the skin lines but does not have the thrombosed capillaries seen in plantar warts. These porokeratoses are small and usually have a small keratin core that is painful to walk on. (*Reproduced with permission from Richard P. Usatine, MD.*)

- Black warts are plantar warts undergoing spontaneous resolution, which may turn black and feel soft when pared with a blade.[7]
- Squamous cell carcinoma should be considered when lesions have irregular growth or pigmentation, ulceration, or resist therapy, particularly in immunosuppressed patients (see Chapter 178, Squamous Cell Carcinoma).
- Amelanotic melanoma, although extremely rare, can look similar to HPV lesions. Lesions that are treatment resistant or atypical, particularly on the palms or soles, should be monitored closely. A biopsy is required to establish the diagnosis (see Chapter 179, Melanoma).
- Palmoplantar keratoderma describes a rare heterogeneous group of disorders characterized by thickening of the palms and the soles that can also be an associated feature of different syndromes. They can be classified as having uniform involvement versus focal hyperkeratosis located mainly on pressure points and sites of recurrent friction (**Figure 140-10**). This latter type can be differentiated from plantar warts by the more diffuse locations on the palmoplantar surfaces, the mainly epidermal involvement, the lack of thrombosed capillaries, and biopsy, if necessary (**Figure 140-11**).

MANAGEMENT

FIRST LINE

NONPHARMACOLOGIC

- Painless plantar warts do not require therapy. Minimal discomfort can be relieved by periodically removing the hyperkeratosis with a blade or pumice stone. Painful warts should be treated using a technique that causes minimal scarring, as scars on the soles of the feet are usually permanent and painful. Patients with diabetes must be treated with the utmost care to minimize complications.
- Cryotherapy (cryosurgery) with liquid nitrogen is commonly used; however, plantar warts are more resistant than other cutaneous HPV lesions. The liquid nitrogen is sprayed on the warts to form a freeze ball that covers the lesion with 2 mm of surrounding normal tissue. Freeze each plantar wart for approximately 10 seconds, allow it to thaw, and then refreeze for another 10 seconds. It is always better to underfreeze than to overfreeze in areas where scarring can produce permanent disability. SOR Ⓑ

PHARMACOLOGIC

- Topical salicylic acid solutions are available in nonprescription form and provide conservative keratolytic therapy. These preparations are non-scarring, minimally painful, and relatively effective, but require persistent application of medication once each day for weeks to months. The wart is first pared with a blade, pumice stone, or emery board, and the area soaked in warm water. The solution or gel is then applied each evening, allowed to dry, reapplied, and occluded with adhesive tape.[8] White, pliable keratin forms and should be pared away carefully between applications until pink skin is exposed.[9] SOR Ⓐ
- Seventeen percent to 50% salicylic acid solution, gel, and plasters are available in nonprescription and prescription forms. However, the 17% solutions are more prevalent and easier to find in nonprescription form. The treatment is similar to the previous process, except that with plasters the salicylic acid has been incorporated into a pad.

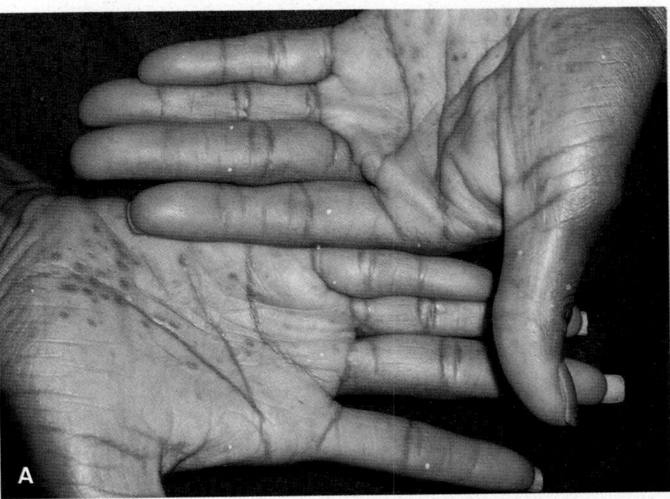

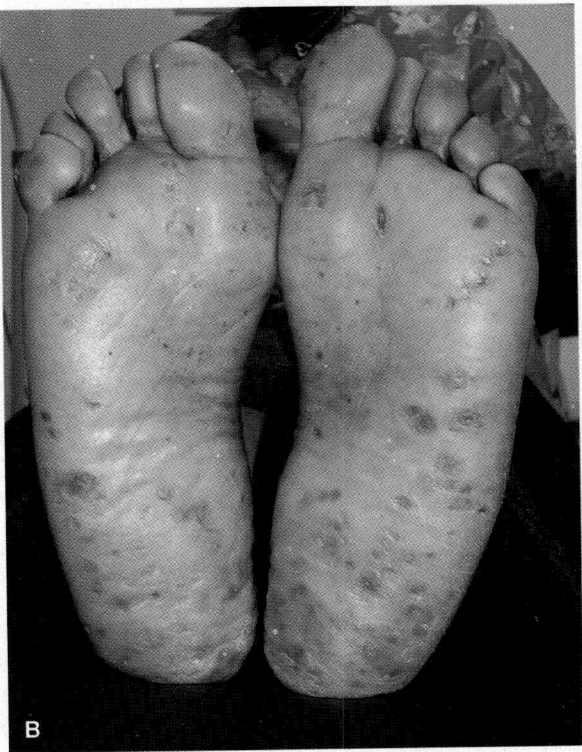

FIGURE 140-10 Focal palmoplantar keratoderma of the palms (**A**) and soles (**B**). This is an inherited genodermatosis. Note lesions are located mainly on higher pressure areas. (*Reproduced with permission from Richard P. Usatine, MD.*)

They are particularly useful in treating mosaic warts covering a large area. Pain is quickly relieved in plantar warts, because a large amount of keratin is removed during the first few days of treatment.[9] SOR Ⓑ A recent multicenter, open-label, randomized, controlled trial found that 50% salicylic acid and cryotherapy were equally effective for clearance of plantar warts.[10] SOR Ⓐ

SECOND LINE

NONPHARMACOLOGIC

- Laser treatment of plantar warts with CO_2, KTP, or pulse dye lasers has been well documented in medical literature. The same principle applies no matter which approach is taken—they all result in controlled thermal destruction of the lesion. However, special training is mandatory for the use of lasers, and the cost of the equipment can be prohibitive in primary care.[11] SOR Ⓒ

PHARMACOLOGIC

- Acid chemotherapy with trichloroacetic acid (TCA) or bichloracetic acid (BCA) may be used to treat plantar warts in the office. This is considered safe during pregnancy for external lesions. The excess keratin is first pared with a scalpel, then the entire lesion is coated with acid, and the acid is worked into the wart with a sharp toothpick. The process is repeated every 7 to 10 days. SOR Ⓒ
- Intralesional immunotherapy with skin-test antigens (i.e., *Candida*, MMR, PPD, MWC, BCG, or *Trichophyton* antigens) may lead to the resolution of both the injected wart and other warts that were not injected. Intralesional antigen therapy is thought to work by inducing a systemic T-cell response that helps the body clear the causal virus. The exact mechanism of action remains unknown. The best results are normally seen after 3 to 5 treatments 2 to 4 weeks apart. Resolution of recalcitrant warts treated with intralesional skin-test antigens has been reported as high as 80%.[11-13] In fact, in one randomized controlled trial that directly compared MMR, PPD, and normal saline, 90% of patients were responsive to treatment, with 80% of the MMR group having complete resolution compared to 60% in the PPD group. Combination therapy employing multiple antigens may further improve outcomes by generating a response through multiple immune pathways.[14] SOR Ⓑ
- Cantharidin is an extract of the blister beetle that has been used for decades as a form of office-based treatment of recalcitrant warts. Cantharidin extract is applied to the wart, after which blistering occurs 48–72 hours later. Application of cantharidin is painless and is something to consider when treating young children.[16] In 2015, cantharidin was placed on the FDA's bulk drug substances list, which means that it can be used to compound drug products even though the drug itself is not approved by the FDA. This is a promising vote of confidence in a therapy that has been safely used to treat warts since the 1950s.[15] SOR Ⓒ
- Contact immunotherapy using dinitrochlorobenzene, squaric acid dibutylester, and diphenylcyclopropenone may be applied to the skin to sensitize the patient and then to the lesion to induce an immune response.[17] Like cantharidin, both squaric acid dibutylester and diphenylcyclopropenone were added to the FDA's bulk drug substances list in 2015 because of their long history of successful use in the treatment of warts.[15] SOR Ⓒ

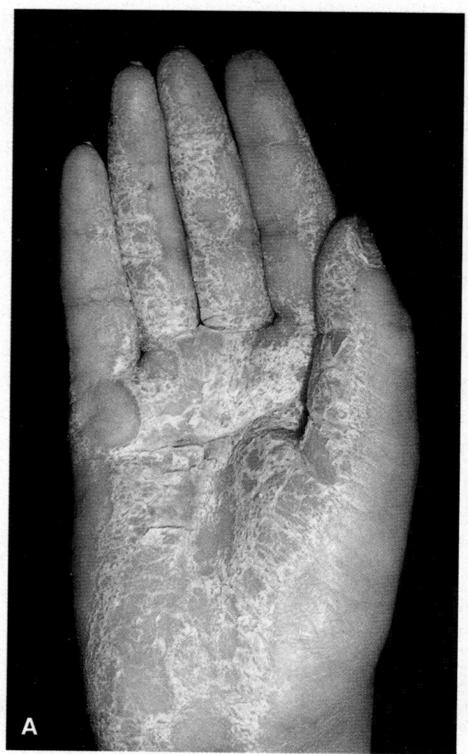

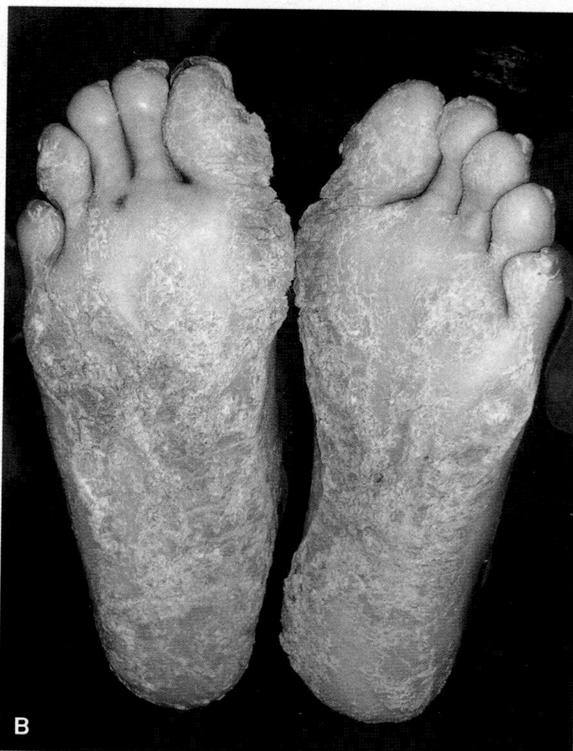

FIGURE 140-11 Diffuse palmoplantar keratoderma of the palms (**A**) and soles (**B**) in an 11-year-old girl. This is a rare inherited genodermatosis with severe functional consequences. (*Reproduced with permission from Richard P. Usatine, MD.*)

COMPLEMENTARY AND ALTERNATIVE THERAPY

- Although many complementary and alternative therapies are promoted for wart therapy, there is no significant data supporting their use in the treatment of plantar warts.

PREVENTION

- Infection with HPV occurs through direct skin-to-skin contact with an incubation period of 2 to 6 months. Although transmission through fomites (inanimate objects) has been theorized, this mode of transmission has yet to be proven. Sites of skin maceration or trauma predispose to inoculation with the virus.

PROGNOSIS

- In children, most plantar warts will spontaneously disappear without treatment within 2 years.
- In adults, spontaneous resolution of plantar warts tends to be slower and may take several years.
- In all demographics, treatment often hastens resolution of lesions.

FOLLOW-UP

- Regular follow-up to assess treatment efficacy, adverse reactions, and patient tolerance is recommended to minimize treatment dropouts.

PATIENT EDUCATION

- Because spontaneous regression occurs, observation of painless lesions without treatment is preferable.
- Therapy often takes weeks to months, so patience and perseverance are essential for success.

PATIENT RESOURCES

- Mayo Clinic. *Plantar Warts*—**http://www.mayoclinic.org/diseases-conditions/plantar-warts/symptoms-causes/syc-20352691.**
- MedlinePlus. *Warts*—**https://medlineplus.gov/warts.html.**
- Cleveland Clinic. *Warts*—**http://my.clevelandclinic.org/health/diseases/15045-warts.**

PROVIDER RESOURCES

- Bacelieri R, Johnson SM. Cutaneous warts: an evidence-based approach to therapy. *Am Fam Physician.* 2005;72(4):647-652—**http://www.aafp.org/afp/20050815/647.html.**
- Medscape. *Nongenital Warts*—**http://emedicine.medscape.com/article/1133317.**

REFERENCES

1. Laurent R, Kienzler JL. Epidemiology of HPV infections. *Clin Dermatol.* 1985;3(4):64-70.
2. Johnson ML, Roberts J. *Skin Conditions and Related Need for Medical Care among Persons 1-74 Years.* Rockville, MD: US Department of Health, Education, and Welfare; 1978:1-26.
3. Williams HC, Pottier A, Strachan D. The descriptive epidemiology of warts in British schoolchildren. *Br J Dermatol.* 1993;128:504-511.
4. Kilkenny M, Merlin K, Young R, Marks R. The prevalence of common skin conditions in Australian school students: 1. Common, plane and plantar viral warts. *Br J Dermatol.* 1998;138:840-845.
5. Holland TT, Weber CB, James WD. Tender periungual nodules. Myrmecia (deep palmoplantar warts). *Arch Dermatol.* 1992;128(1):105-106, 108-109.
6. Beutner, KR. Nongenital human papillomavirus infections. *Clin Lab Med.* 2000;20:423-430.
7. Berman A, Domnitz JM, Winkelmann RK. Plantar warts recently turned black. *Arch Dermatol.* 1982;118:47-51.
8. Landsman MJ, Mancuso JE, Abramow SP. Diagnosis, pathophysiology, and treatment of plantar verruca. *Clin Podiatr Med Surg.* 1996;13(1):55-71.
9. Gibbs S, Harvey I. *Cochrane Summaries. Topical Treatments for Cutaneous Warts.* http://www.cochrane.org/reviews/en/ab001781.html. Accessed April 2008.
10. Cockayne S, Hewitt C, Hicks K, et al. Cryotherapy versus salicylic acid for the treatment of plantar warts (verrucae): a randomized controlled trial. *BMJ.* 2011;342:d3271.
11. Leung L. Recalcitrant nongenital warts. *Aust Fam Physician.* 2011;40(1-2):40-42.
12. Shaheen MA, Salem SA, Fouad DA, El-fatah AA. Intralesional tuberculin (PPD) versus measles, mumps, rubella (MMR) vaccine in treatment of multiple warts: a comparative clinical and immunological study. *Dermatol Ther.* 2015;28(4):194-200.
13. Na CH, Choi H, Song SH, et al. Two-year experience of using the measles, mumps and rubella vaccine as intralesional immunotherapy for warts. *Clin Exp Dermatol.* 2014;39(5):583-589.
14. Aldahan AS, Mlacker S, Shah VV, et al. Efficacy of intralesional immunotherapy for the treatment of warts: a review of the literature. *Dermatol Ther.* 2016;29(3):197-207.
15. Brown, T. FDA Panel Backs Updates to Bulk Drugs List for Compounding. *Medscape.* February 25, 2015. https://www.medscape.com/viewarticle/840363. Accessed July 2018.
16. Torbeck R, Pan M, Demoll E, Levitt J. Cantharidin: a comprehensive review of the clinical literature. *Dermatol Online J.* 2014;20(6).
17. Word AP, Nezafati KA, Cruz PD. Treatment of warts with contact allergens. *Dermatitis.* 2015;26(1):32-37.

SECTION F FUNGAL

141 FUNGAL OVERVIEW

Richard P. Usatine, MD

PATIENT STORY

A 55-year-old woman presents with a red pruritic area on her face for 3 months (**Figure 141-1**). The annular distribution immediately is suspicious for a dermatophyte infection. Further investigation demonstrates that the patient has severe tinea pedis in a moccasin distribution. The patient is treated with an oral terbinafine 250 mg daily for 1 month and her fungal infection clears completely.

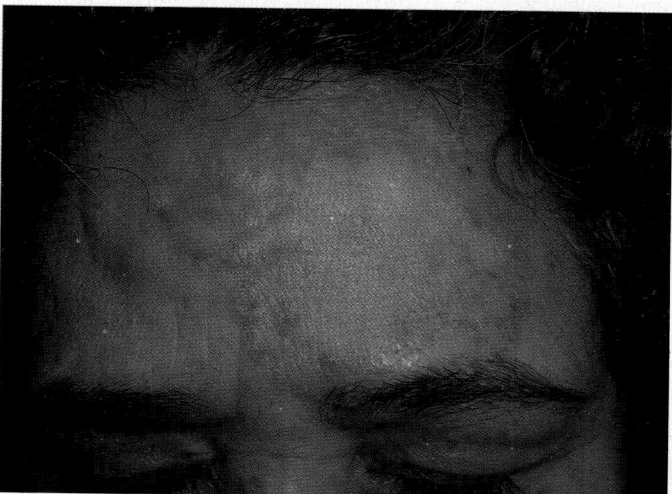

FIGURE 141-1 Tinea faciei on the face of a 55-year-old woman with typical scaling and ringlike pattern (ringworm). Note the well-demarcated raised border and central clearing. (*Reproduced with permission from Richard P. Usatine, MD.*)

INTRODUCTION

Fungal infections of the skin and mucous membranes are ubiquitous and common. There are many types of fungus that grow on humans, but they all share a predilection for warm and moist areas. Consequently, hot and humid climates promote fungal infections, but many areas of the skin can get warm and sweaty even in cold climates, such as the feet and groin.

SYNONYMS

Pityriasis versicolor equals tinea versicolor.

PATHOPHYSIOLOGY

Mucocutaneous fungal infections are caused by:

- Dermatophytes in three genera: *Microsporum*, *Epidermophyton*, and *Trichophyton*. There are approximately 40 species in the three genera, and these fungi cause tinea pedis and manus, tinea capitis, tinea corporis, tinea cruris, tinea faciei, and onychomycosis (**Figures 141-1** to **141-6**).
- Yeasts in the genera of *Candida* and *Pityrosporum* (*Malassezia*)—There are also multiple types of *Candida* species. *Pityrosporum* is the cause of seborrhea and tinea versicolor (**Figures 141-7** and **141-8**). Although tinea versicolor has the name tinea in it, it is not a true dermatophyte and may be best called pityriasis versicolor.

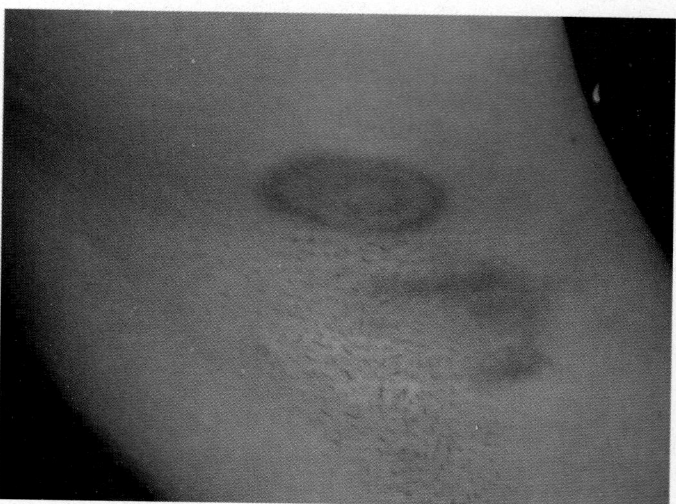

FIGURE 141-2 Annular pruritic lesion with concentric rings in the axilla of a young woman caused by tinea corporis. The concentric rings have a high specificity for tinea infections. (*Reproduced with permission from Richard P. Usatine, MD.*)

DIAGNOSIS

CLINICAL FEATURES OF TINEA INFECTIONS

Scaling, erythema, pruritus, central clearing, concentric rings, and maceration (**Table 141-1**). Changes in pigmentation are not uncommon in various types of tinea, especially tinea versicolor.

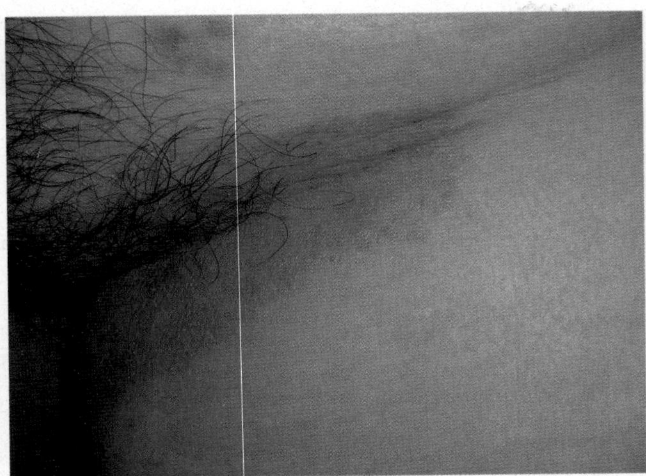

FIGURE 141-3 Tinea cruris with well-demarcated raised border and no central clearing. (*Reproduced with permission from Richard P. Usatine, MD.*)

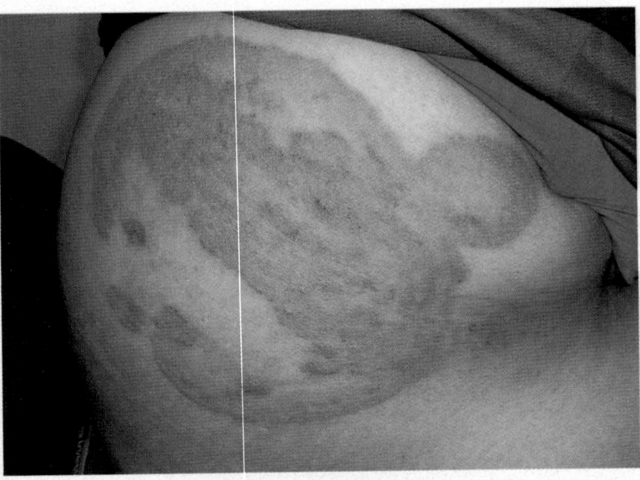

FIGURE 141-4 Tinea corporis on the right flank of a woman bending forward. Note that post-inflammatory hyperpigmentation is seen in the skin affected by the tinea corporis. (*Reproduced with permission from Richard P. Usatine, MD.*)

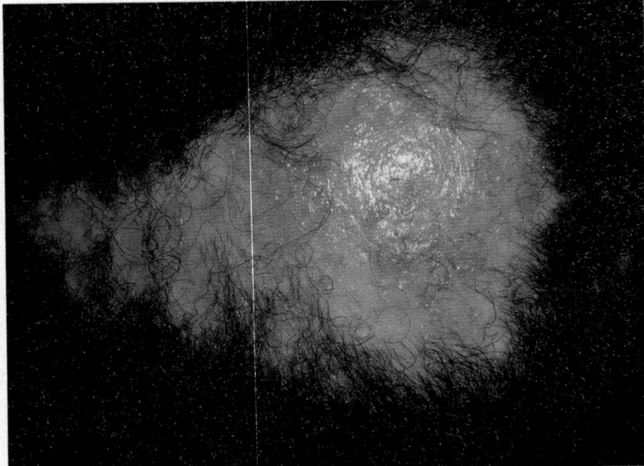

FIGURE 141-5 Tinea capitis in a 5-year-old black girl with hair loss and an inflammatory response. Her kerion is healing after initiating oral griseofulvin. (*Reproduced with permission from Richard P. Usatine, MD.*)

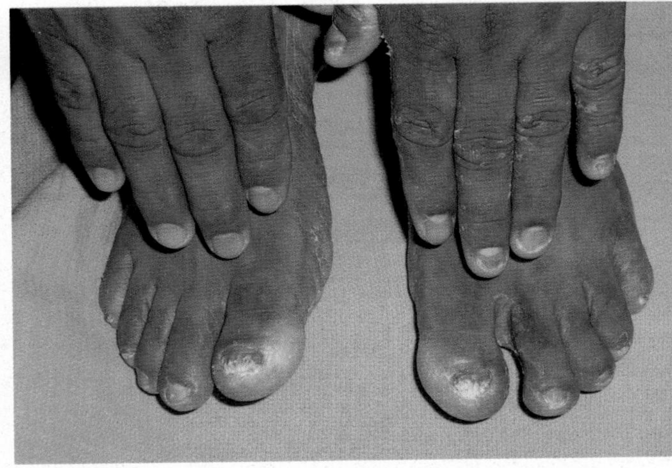

FIGURE 141-6 Two-foot, one-hand syndrome with tinea manus of one hand and tinea pedis of both feet. (*Reproduced with permission from Richard P. Usatine, MD.*)

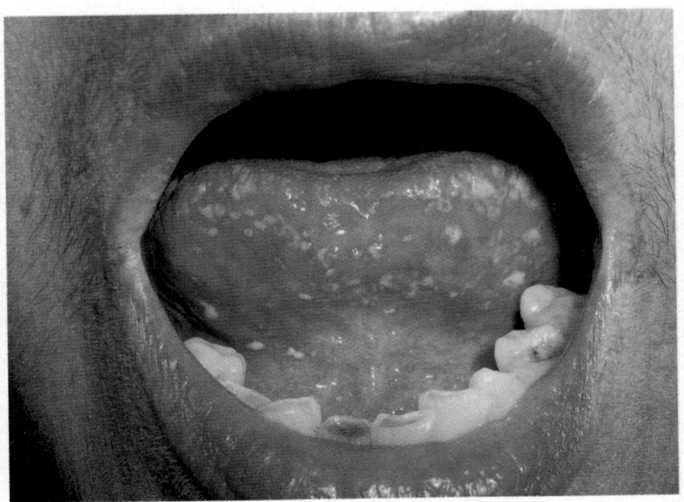

FIGURE 141-7 Thrush in the mouth of an immunosuppressed woman caused by *Candida*. The *Candida* is also coating the buccal mucosa. (*Reproduced with permission from Richard P. Usatine, MD.*)

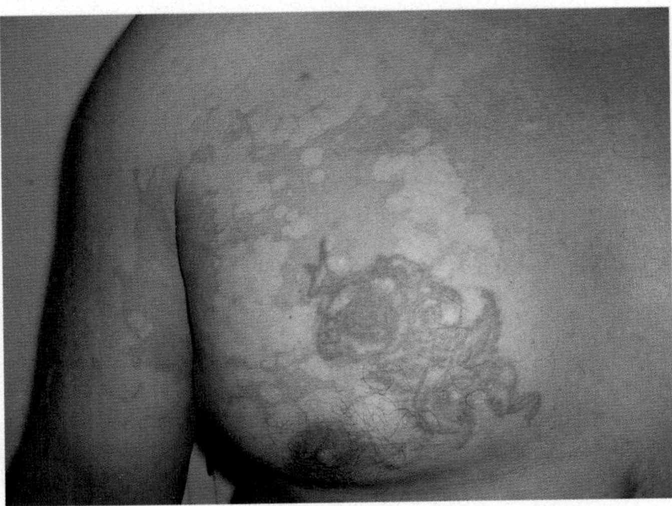

FIGURE 141-8 Tinea versicolor showing hypopigmentation on the chest. (*Reproduced with permission from Richard P. Usatine, MD.*)

TABLE 141-1 Diagnostic Value of Selected Signs and Symptoms in Tinea Infection*

Sign/Symptom	Sensitivity (%)	Specificity (%)	PV+ (%)	PV– (%)	LR+	LR–
Scaling	77	20	17	80	0.96	1.15
Erythema	69	31	18	83	1.00	1.00
Pruritus	54	40	16	80	0.90	1.15
Central clearing	42	65	20	84	1.20	0.89
Concentric rings	27	80	23	84	1.35	0.91
Maceration	27	84	26	84	1.69	0.87

*Signs and symptoms were compiled by 27 general practitioners prior to submission of skin for fungal culture. Specimens were taken from 148 consecutive patients with erythematosquamous lesions of glabrous skin. Culture results were considered the gold standard; level of evidence = 2b.
Abbreviations: LR–, negative likelihood ratio; LR+, positive likelihood ratio; PV–, negative predictive value; PV+, positive predictive value.
Reproduced with permission from Lousbergh D, Buntinx F, Piérard G. Diagnosing dermatomycosis in general practice, Fam Pract. 1999;16(6):611-615. Frontline Medical Communications. Inc..

- **Figure 141-1** shows tinea faciei on the face with typical scaling and ringlike pattern; hence the name ringworm. There is also erythema and central clearing. The patient was experiencing pruritus.
- **Figure 141-2** shows annular pruritic lesion with concentric rings in the axilla of a young woman caused by tinea corporis. The concentric rings have a high specificity (80%) for tinea infections.
- Note that tinea infections will not show central clearing in 58% of cases, as in **Figure 141-3** in which tinea cruris has no central clearing.
- Post-inflammatory hyperpigmentation is common in skin of color, as seen in **Figure 141-4**. Note that the hyperpigmentation is seen within the area affected by the tinea corporis.
- Hypopigmentation is frequently seen in tinea versicolor (**Figure 141-8**).

TYPICAL DISTRIBUTION

Literally found from head to toes:

- **Figure 141-5** shows tinea capitis in a 5-year-old black girl with hair loss and an inflammatory response. Her kerion (inflammatory response to tinea) is healing with oral griseofulvin.
- The two-foot, one-hand syndrome is a curious phenomenon with tinea manus of one hand and tinea pedis of both feet (**Figure 141-6**). It is not clear why only one hand is involved in these cases. In this case it was the nondominant hand, but either hand can be involved.

LABORATORY STUDIES

Creating a KOH prep:

- Scrape the leading edge of the lesion on to a slide using the side of another microscope slide or a #15 scalpel (**Figure 141-9**). (Online video by Dr. Usatine https://www.youtube.com/watch?v=LUwNQI_0BWU&t=2s.)
- Use your coverslip to push the scale into the center of the slide.
- Add one to two drops of KOH (or fungal stain) to the slide and place coverslip on top.

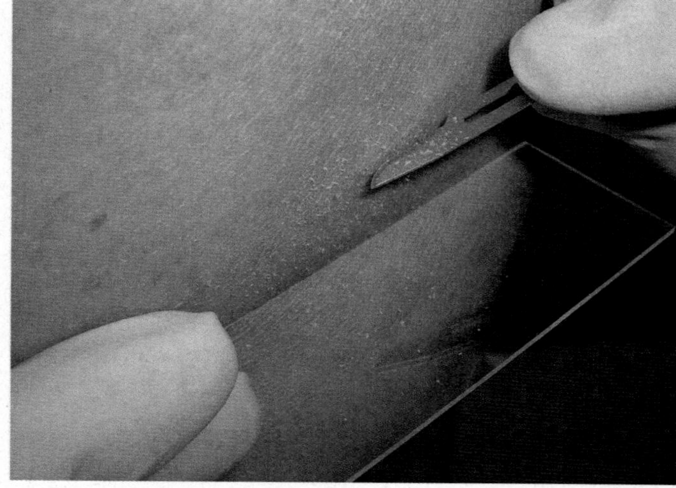

FIGURE 141-9 Making a KOH preparation by scraping in area of scale with a #15 blade. This was a case of tinea versicolor. *(Reproduced with permission from Richard P. Usatine, MD.)*

- Fungal stains that come with KOH and a surfactant in the solution are very simple to use. These inexpensive stains come in small plastic squeeze bottles that have a shelf life of 1 to 3 years. Two useful stains that can that make it easier to identify fungus are chlorazol and Swartz Lamkins stains. Swartz Lamkins stain has a longer shelf life and is my preferred stain.
- Consider also gently heating with flame from a lighter. Avoid boiling. This helps to speed up the dissolution of the human cells and make the fungal elements visible more rapidly. This is not always needed and is most beneficial in KOH preparations done from nails and when the skin scrapings are thicker.
- Examine with microscope starting with 10× power to look for the cells and hyphae and then switch to 40× power to confirm your findings (**Figures 141-10** to **141-13**). The fungal stain helps the hyphae stand out among the epithelial cells.
- It helps to start with 10× power to find the clumps of cells and look for groups of cells that appear to have fungal elements within them (see **Figure 141-10**).
- Don't be fooled by cell borders that look linear and branching. True fungal morphology at 40× power should confirm that you are looking at real fungus and not artifact. The fungal stains bring out these characteristics, including septae and nuclei (see **Figures 141-11** to **141-13**).
- KOH test characteristics (without fungal stains)—Sensitivity 77% to 88%, specificity 62% to 95% (**Table 141-2**).[1] The sensitivity and specificity should be higher with fungal stains and the experience of the person performing the test.

OTHER LABORATORY STUDIES

- Fungal culture—Send skin scrapings, hair, or nail clippings to the laboratory in a sterile urine cup. These will be plated out on fungal agar and the laboratory can report the species if positive.
- Biopsy specimens (or nail clippings) can be sent in formalin for periodic acid–Schiff (PAS) staining when KOH and fungal cultures seem to be falsely negative.
- UV light (Wood lamp), looking for fluorescence. The *Microsporum* species are most likely to fluoresce. However, the majority of tinea infections are caused by *Trichophyton* species that do not fluoresce.

MANAGEMENT

There is a wide variety of topical antifungal medications (**Table 141-3**). A Cochrane systematic review of 70 trials of topical antifungals for tinea pedis showed good evidence for efficacy compared to placebo[2] for:

- Allylamines (naftifine, terbinafine, butenafine).
- Azoles (clotrimazole, miconazole, econazole).
- Allylamines cure slightly more infections than azoles but are more expensive.[2]
- No differences in efficacy found between individual topical allylamines or individual azoles.[2] SOR Ⓐ

There is some evidence that topical ciclopirox olamine and butenafine may help treat onychomycosis, but they both need to be applied daily for at least 1 year.[3]

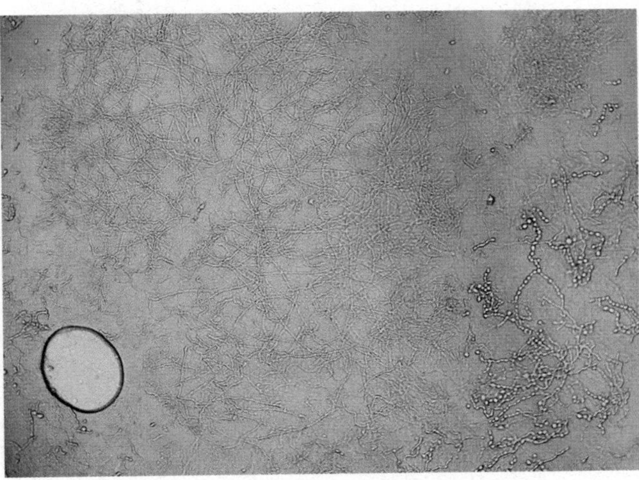

FIGURE 141-10 *Trichophyton rubrum* from tinea cruris visible among skin cells using light microscopy at 10× power and Swartz-Lamkins fungal stain. Start your search on 10× power and move to 40× power to confirm your findings. (*Reproduced with permission from Richard P. Usatine, MD.*)

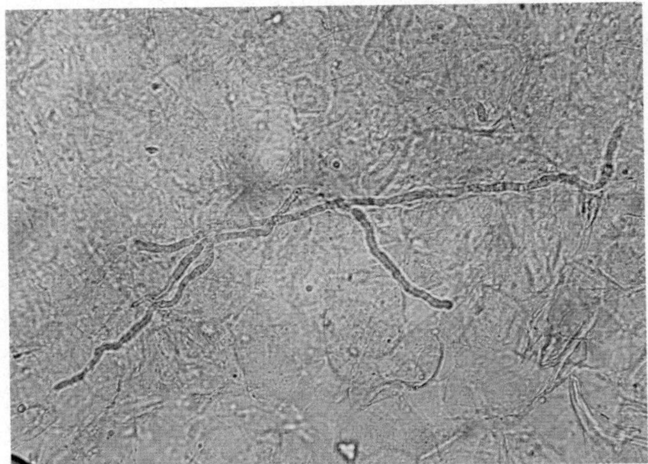

FIGURE 141-11 *Trichophyton rubrum* from tinea cruris using Swartz Lamkins fungal stain at 40× power. Note the hyphae with visible septae. (*Reproduced with permission from Richard P. Usatine, MD.*)

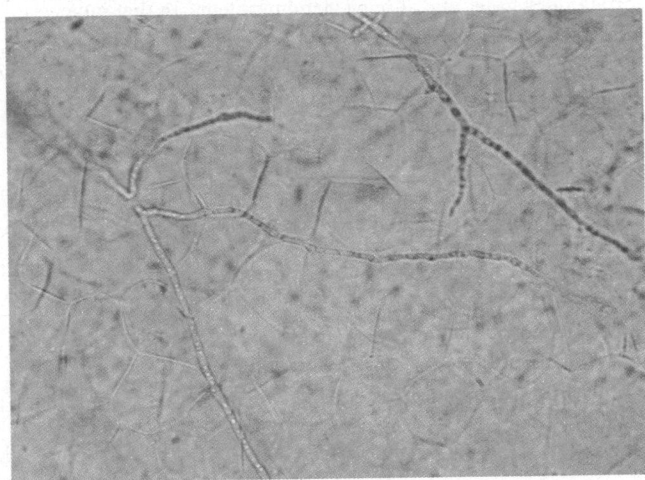

FIGURE 141-12 Prominently visible nuclei in hyphae using Swartz Lamkins fungal stain at 40× power. Note the branching human cell borders that are not caused by hyphae. (*Reproduced with permission from Richard P. Usatine, MD.*)

TABLE 141-2 Diagnostic Value of Clinical Diagnosis and KOH Prep in Tinea Infection

Test	Sensitivity (%)	Specificity (%)	PV+ (%)	PV– (%)	LR+	LR–
Clinical diagnosis*	81	45	24	92	1.47	0.42
KOH prep (study one)†	88	95	73	98	17.6	0.13
KOH prep (study two)†	77	62	59	79	2.02	0.37

*The clinical diagnosis set was compiled by 27 general practitioners prior to submission of skin for fungal culture. Specimens were taken from consecutive patients with erythrosquamous lesions. Culture results were considered the gold standard; study quality = 2b.
†Both studies of KOH preps were open analyses of patients with suspicious lesions. Paired fungal culture was initiated simultaneously with KOH prep and was considered the gold standard; study quality = 2b.
Abbreviations: LR–, negative likelihood ratio; LR+, positive likelihood ratio; PV–, negative predictive value; PV+, positive predictive value.
Reproduced with permission from Thomas B. Clear choices in managing epidermal tinea infections, J Fam Pract. 2003;52(11): 850-862. Frontline Medical Communications. Inc.

Oral antifungals are needed for all tinea capitis infections and for more severe infections of the rest of the body.[4,5] True dermatophyte infections that do not respond to topical antifungals may need an oral agent.

- A Cochrane systematic review of 15 trials of oral antifungals for tinea pedis showed oral terbinafine more effective than oral griseofulvin.[6] SOR Ⓐ
- Terbinafine and itraconazole are more effective than no treatment for tinea pedis.[6] SOR Ⓐ
- There were no significant differences in comparisons between a number of other oral agents.[6]

Oral antifungals used for fungal infections of the skin, nails, or mucous membranes:

- Itraconazole (Sporanox).
- Fluconazole (Diflucan).
- Griseofulvin.
- Ketoconazole (Nizoral). FDA recommended limited use of oral ketoconazole in 2013 due to potentially fatal liver injury, risk of drug interactions, and adrenal gland problems. In that same year Australia and Europe removed oral ketoconazole from their markets due to concerns over increased liver toxicity, drug interactions, and endocrinologic side effects. These concerns do not apply to topical ketoconazole.[7-9]

Given that there are better, safer, and less expensive alternatives to oral ketoconazole, we do not recommend its use in the treatment of fungal skin infections.

- Terbinafine (Lamisil).

A number of studies and meta-analyses suggest that terbinafine is more efficacious than griseofulvin in treating tinea capitis caused by *Trichophyton* species, whereas griseofulvin is more efficacious than terbinafine in treating tinea capitis caused by *Microsporum* species.[4,10] SOR Ⓐ

Details of treatments for multiple types of fungal skin infections are supplied in the subsequent chapters.

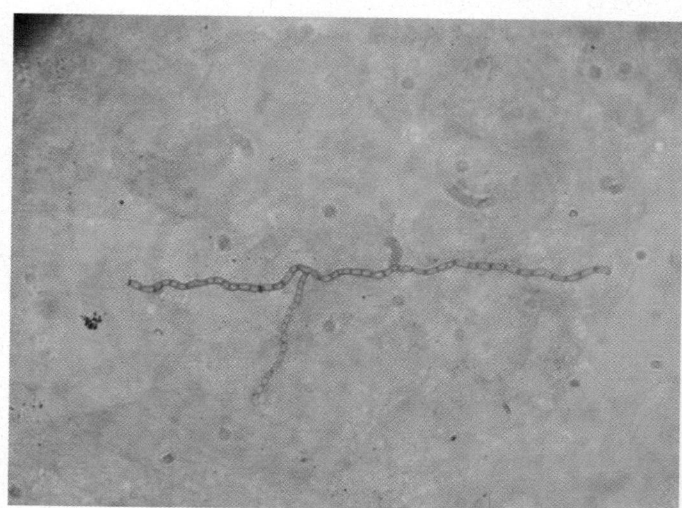

FIGURE 141-13 Prominently visible septate hyphae using Swartz Lamkins fungal stain at 40× power. (*Reproduced with permission from Richard P. Usatine, MD.*)

TABLE 141-3 Topical Antifungal Preparations

Generic Name	Brand Name	OTC or R_x	Class
Butenafine	Mentax Lotrimin Ultra	R_x OTC	Allylamine
Ciclopirox	Loprox	R_x	Pyridone
Clotrimazole	Lotrimin AF Cream Lotrimin AF Spray	OTC	Azole
Econazole	Spectazole	R_x	Azole
Ketoconazole	Nizoral	2% R_x	Azole
Miconazole	Micatin Generic	OTC	Azole
Naftifine	Naftin	R_x	Allylamine
Oxiconazole	Oxistat	R_x	Azole
Sertaconazole	Ertaczo	R_x	Azole
Terbinafine	Lamisil AT	OTC	Allylamine
Tolnaftate*	Tinactin cream Lamisil AF defense and Tinactin powder spray Generic cream	OTC	Miscellaneous

*All the above antifungals will treat dermatophytes and *Candida*. Tolnaftate is effective only for dermatophytes and not *Candida*. Nystatin is effective only for *Candida* and not dermatophytes.
Abbreviation: OTC, over-the-counter.

PATIENT RESOURCES

- **http://www.webmd.com/skin-problems-and-treatments/guide/fungal-infections-skin#1.**

PROVIDER RESOURCES

- KOH preparation and interpretation video (4 minutes by Dr. Usatine)—**https://www.youtube.com/watch?v=LUwNQI_0BWU&t=2s.**
- From New Zealand. *Fungal Skin Infections*—**http://www.dermnetnz.org/fungal/.**
- World of dermatophytes from Canada—**http://www.provlab.ab.ca/mycol/tutorials/derm/dermhome.htm.**
- Swartz Lamkins fungal stain can be purchased online at—**http://www.delasco.com/pcat/1/Chemicals/Swartz_Lamkins/dlmis023/.**

REFERENCES

1. Thomas B. Clear choices in managing epidermal tinea infections. *J Fam Pract.* 2003;52(11):850-862.
2. Crawford F, Hart R, Bell-Syer S, et al. Topical treatments for fungal infections of the skin and nails of the foot. *Cochrane Database Syst Rev.* 2000;(2):CD001434.
3. Crawford F, Hollis S. Topical treatments for fungal infections of the skin and nails of the foot. *Cochrane Database Syst Rev.* 2007;(3):CD001434.
4. Chen X, Jiang X, Yang M, et al. Systemic antifungal therapy for tinea capitis in children. *Cochrane Database Syst Rev.* 2016;(5):CD004685.
5. Gupta AK, Adam P, Dlova N, et al. Therapeutic options for the treatment of tinea capitis caused by *Trichophyton* species: griseofulvin versus the new oral antifungal agents, terbinafine, itraconazole, and fluconazole. *Pediatr Dermatol.* 18(5):433-438.
6. Bell-Syer SEM, Khan SM, Torgerson DJ. Oral treatments for fungal infections of the skin of the foot. Bell-Syer SE, ed. *Cochrane Database Syst Rev.* 2012;(10):CD003584.
7. Greenblatt HK, Greenblatt DJ. Liver injury associated with ketoconazole: review of the published evidence. *J Clin Pharmacol.* 2014;54(12):1321-1329.
8. Gupta AK, Daigle D, Foley KA. Drug safety assessment of oral formulations of ketoconazole. *Expert Opin Drug Saf.* 2015;14(2):325-334.
9. Gupta AK, Lyons DCA. The rise and fall of oral ketoconazole. *J Cutan Med Surg.* 2015;19(4):352-357.
10. Gupta AK, Drummond-Main C. Meta-analysis of randomized, controlled trials comparing particular doses of griseofulvin and terbinafine for the treatment of tinea capitis. *Pediatr Dermatol.* 2013;30(1):1-6.

142 CANDIDIASIS

Richard P. Usatine, MD

PATIENT STORY

A 42-year-old man (**Figure 142-1**) was admitted to the hospital for community-acquired pneumonia and type 2 diabetes out of control. On the second day of admission, when he was feeling a bit better, he asked about the itching he was having on his penis. Physical examination revealed an uncircumcised penis with white discharge on the glans and inside the foreskin consistent with *Candida* balanitis. KOH prep was positive for the pseudohyphae of *Candida*. The patient was treated with a topical azole and the balanitis resolved.

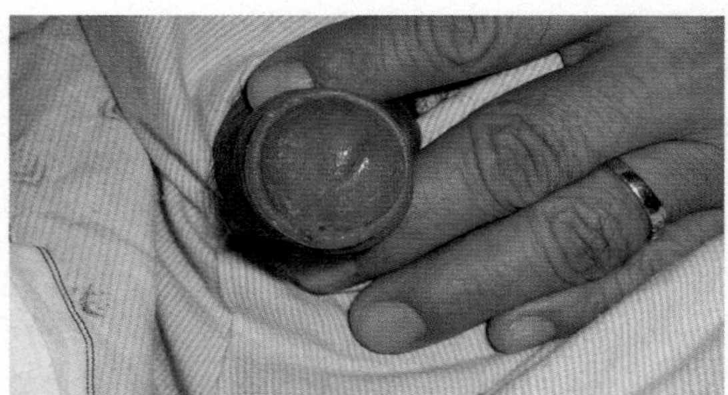

FIGURE 142-1 *Candida* balanitis in a man with uncontrolled diabetes. *(Reproduced with permission from Richard P. Usatine, MD.)*

INTRODUCTION

Cutaneous and mucosal *Candida* infections are seen commonly in persons with obesity, diabetes, hyperhidrosis, and/or immunodeficiency.

SYNONYMS

Perlèche = angular cheilitis.

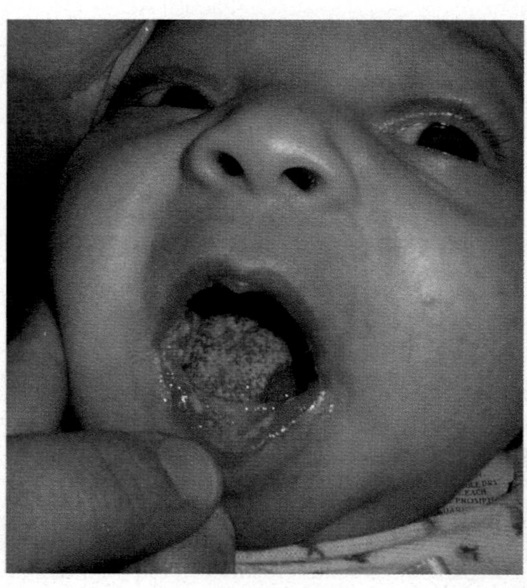

FIGURE 142-2 Thrush in an otherwise healthy infant. *(Reproduced with permission from Richard P. Usatine, MD.)*

EPIDEMIOLOGY

Candida thrush is common in normal infants and in adults may be a sign of immunosuppression (**Figure 142-2**).

Candida balanitis is more common in uncircumcised men than in those who have been circumcised (**Figure 142-1**).

ETIOLOGY AND PATHOPHYSIOLOGY

- Infections caused by *Candida* species are primarily *Candida albicans*.[1]
- *C. albicans* has the ability to exist in both hyphal and yeast forms (termed *dimorphism*). If pinched cells do not separate, a chain of cells is produced and is termed *pseudohyphae*.[1]

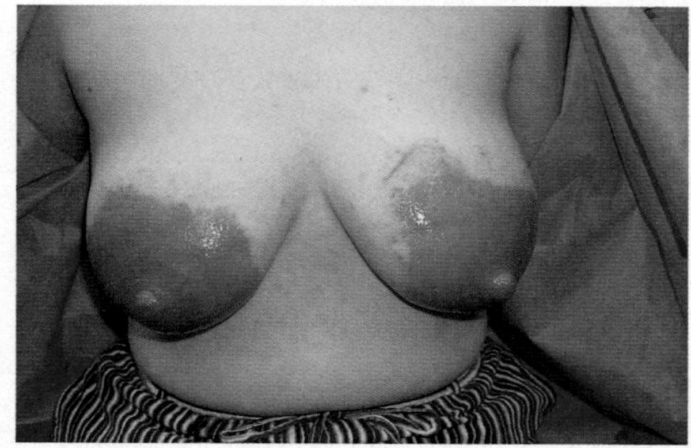

FIGURE 142-3 *Candida* rash with superimposed contact dermatitis in a breastfeeding woman. Her baby has thrush and both need treatment to eradicate the infection. The contact dermatitis was to the neomycin-containing topical antibiotic she applied to her sore breasts. *(Reproduced with permission from Jack Resneck, Sr., MD.)*

RISK FACTORS

Obesity, diabetes, hyperhidrosis, immunodeficiency, HIV, heat, use of oral antibiotics, and use of inhaled or systemic steroids.[1]

DIAGNOSIS

CLINICAL FEATURES

- Typical distribution—Groin, glans penis, vulva, inframammary, under abdominal pannus, between fingers, in the creases of the neck, corners of mouth, nail folds in chronic paronychia.
- Morphology—Macules, patches, plaques that are pink to bright red with small peripheral satellite lesions.
- Candidiasis of the nipple in the nursing mother is associated with infantile thrush (**Figures 142-2** and **142-3**). Nipple candidiasis is almost always bilateral, with the nipples appearing bright red and inflamed. In this case, the inflammation was made worse by the application of a topical antibiotic that caused a secondary contact dermatitis.
- *Candida* infection in the corners of the mouth is called perlèche or angular cheilitis (**Figure 142-4**). When accompanied by thrush it may be a sign of HIV/AIDS.
- Thrush can be caused be *Candida* growing on the upper plate of a denture and the roof of the mouth (**Figure 142-5**).
- Ask about recent antibiotic use if there is a new onset of a rash with satellite lesions. In **Figure 142-6**, the man with diabetes had a course of antibiotics before he developed a *Candida* infection in his groin.

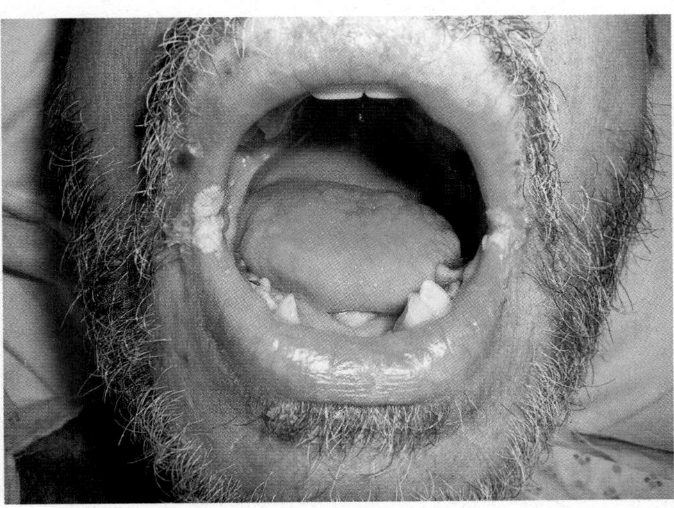

FIGURE 142-4 Thrush and perlèche in a man with AIDS. The *Candida* infection in the corners of the mouth are called perlèche or angular cheilitis. (*Reproduced with permission from Richard P. Usatine, MD.*)

LABORATORY STUDIES

Scrape involved area and add to a slide with KOH (DMSO optional). *C. albicans* exists in both hyphal and yeast forms (dimorphism). Look for pseudohyphae and/or budding yeast (**Figure 142-7**).

DIFFERENTIAL DIAGNOSIS

- Intertrigo is a nonspecific inflammatory condition of the skin folds. It is induced or aggravated by heat, moisture, maceration, and friction. The condition frequently is worsened by infection with *Candida* or dermatophytes (**Figures 142-8** and **142-9**). In **Figure 142-8** there is significant hyperpigmentation secondary to the inflammation.
- Tinea corporis or cruris—Can be distinguished from *Candida* when you see an annular pattern or concentric circles in the tinea (**Figure 142-9**). There is no scrotal involvement in tinea cruris. *Candida* intertrigo may have scrotal involvement (see Chapters 144, Tinea Corporis, and 145, Tinea Cruris).
- Erythrasma—May be brown and glows a coral red with UV light (see Chapter 125, Erythrasma).
- Inverse psoriasis—Psoriasis in the intertriginous areas as seen in **Figure 142-10** (see Chapter 158, Psoriasis).
- Seborrhea—Inflammation related to overgrowth of *Pityrosporum*, a yeast-like organism (see Chapter 157, Seborrheic Dermatitis).

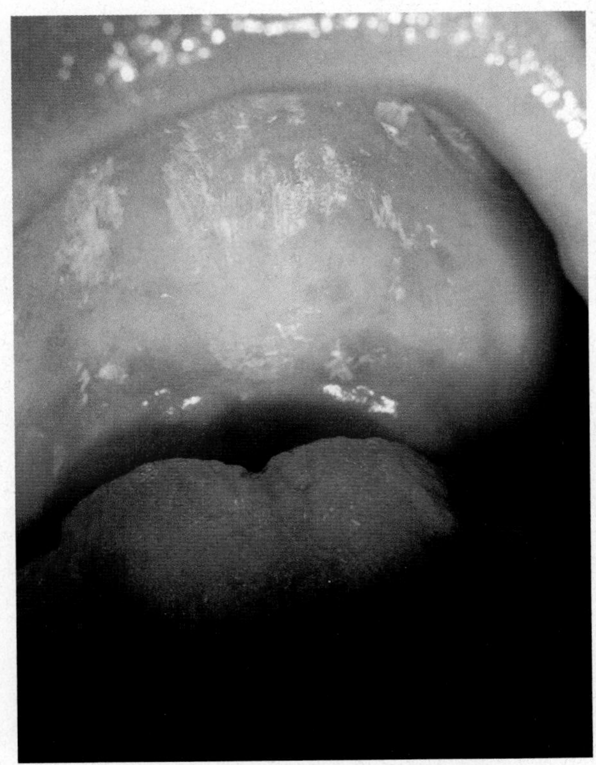

FIGURE 142-5 *Candida* on the roof of the mouth in an elderly woman using dentures. This is a common complication of denture use and should be suspected if a patient presents with new-onset pain under the dentures. (*Reproduced with permission from Richard P. Usatine, MD.*)

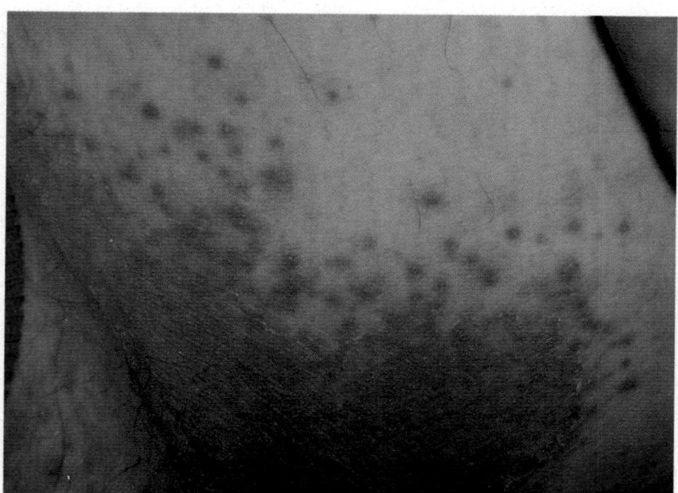

FIGURE 142-6 *Candida* inguinal eruption in a 61-year-old man after a course of antibiotics for bronchitis. Note the satellite lesions. (*Reproduced with permission from Richard P. Usatine, MD.*)

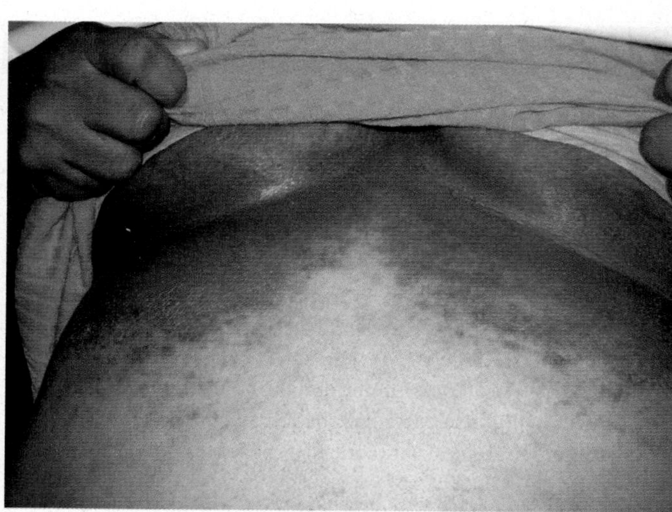

FIGURE 142-8 *Candida* under the breasts of an overweight Hispanic woman showing hyperpigmentation. The border is not well-demarcated and there are satellite lesions. (*Reproduced with permission from Richard P. Usatine, MD.*)

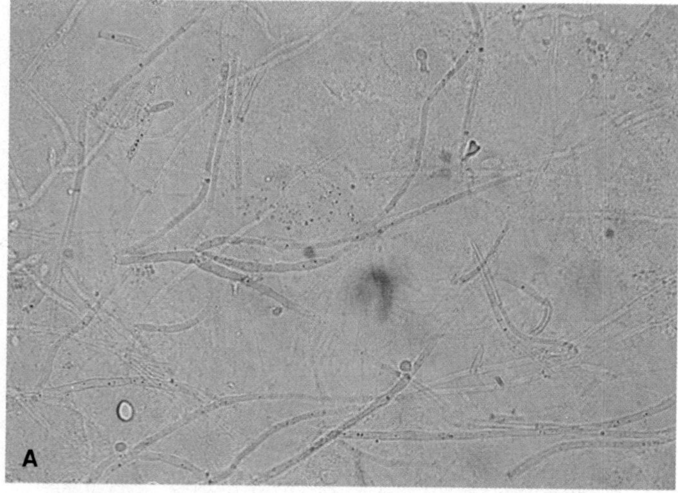

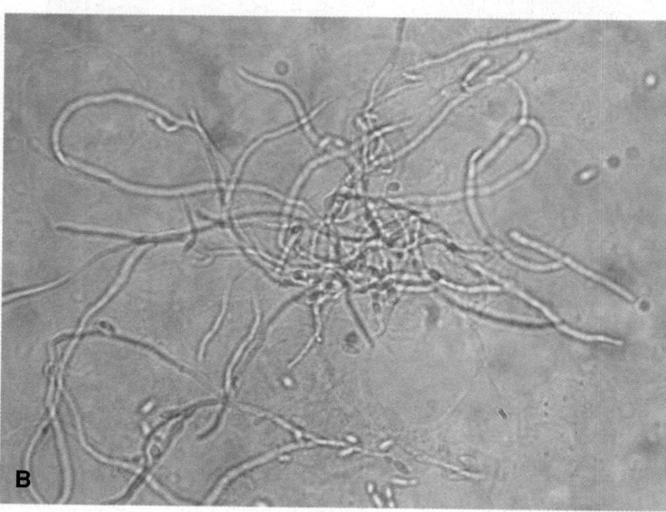

FIGURE 142-7 The branching pseudohyphae and budding yeast of *Candida* under high power. **A.** *Candida* from thrush. **B.** *Candida* from vaginitis. (*Reproduced with permission from Richard P. Usatine, MD.*)

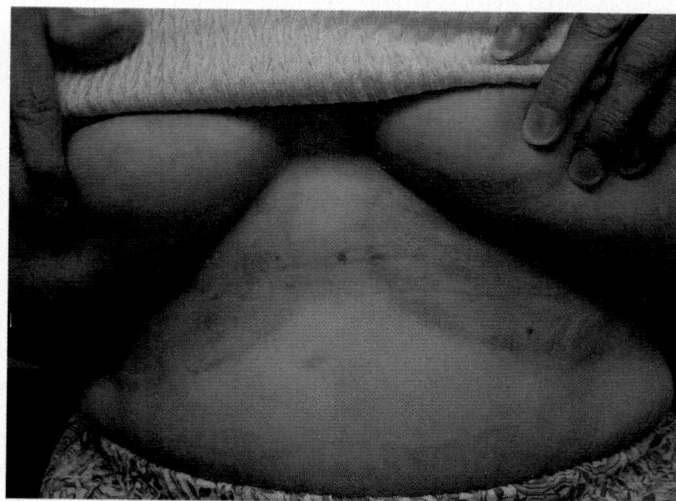

FIGURE 142-9 Tinea corporis under the breasts of a 55-year-old woman. Note the annular pattern with well-demarcated borders. KOH was positive for dermatophytes and not *Candida*. (*Reproduced with permission from Richard P. Usatine, MD.*)

MANAGEMENT

PRIMARY CANDIDAL SKIN INFECTIONS

- Topical azoles, including clotrimazole, miconazole, and nystatin (polyenes), are effective.[2] SOR Ⓑ
- Keeping the infected area dry is important.[3] SOR Ⓒ
- For more details of the topical antifungals, see **Table 141-3** in Chapter 141, Fungal Overview.
- In one study, miconazole ointment was well tolerated and significantly more effective than the zinc oxide/petrolatum vehicle control for treatment of diaper dermatitis complicated by candidiasis.[2]
- Do not use tolnaftate, which is active against dermatophytes but not *Candida*.
- If recurrent or recalcitrant, consider fluconazole 150 mg/wk for 2 weeks.

OROPHARYNGEAL CANDIDIASIS

- Treat initial episodes with clotrimazole troches (one 10-mg troche 5 times per day for adults) or nystatin (available as a suspension of 100,000 U/mL [dosage, 4 to 6 mL qid] or as flavored 200,000 U pastilles [dosage, 1 or 2 pastilles 4 to 5 times per day for 7 to 14 days]).[3] SOR Ⓑ
- Oral fluconazole (100–200 mg/day for 7 to 14 days) is as effective as—and, in some studies, superior to—topical therapy.[3] SOR Ⓐ
- Itraconazole solution (200 mg/day for 7 to 14 days) is as effective as fluconazole.[3] SOR Ⓐ
- Ketoconazole and itraconazole capsules are less effective than fluconazole, because of variable absorption.[3] SOR Ⓐ
- Fluconazole-refractory oropharyngeal candidiasis will respond to oral itraconazole therapy (>200 mg/day, preferably in solution form) approximately two thirds of the time.[3] SOR Ⓐ
- Children with thrush are usually treated with oral nystatin suspension.[3] SOR Ⓑ
- HIV/AIDS patients with oral candidiasis may be treated with clotrimazole troches. If unresponsive to topical therapy, fluconazole may be needed.[3] SOR Ⓐ
- Denture-related disease may require extensive and aggressive disinfection of the denture for definitive cure.[3] SOR Ⓒ

MAMMARY CANDIDIASIS IN BREASTFEEDING

- Most mammary candidiasis does not present with the red breasts seen in **Figure 142-3**.
- Nipple pain and discomfort along with thrush are adequate data to treat the mother and child.
- Topical nystatin and oral fluconazole are safe for infants and the mother.[3]

CHRONIC MUCOCUTANEOUS CANDIDIASIS

- Chronic mucocutaneous candidiasis (**Figure 142-11**) requires a long-term approach that is analogous to that used in patients with AIDS.[3]

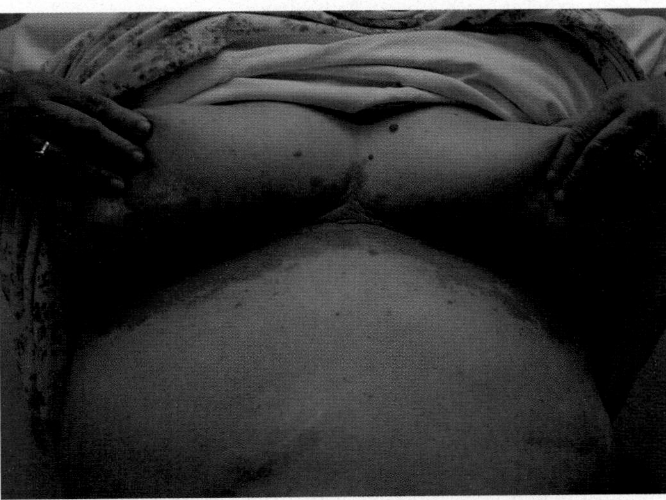

FIGURE 142-10 Inverse psoriasis that closely resembles *Candida* intertrigo in the submammary folds. This patient did not improve with topical antifungals, and finally a biopsy showed that this was inverse psoriasis. Inverse psoriasis is often mistaken for a fungal infection unless the physician is aware of this condition. Frequently there are other clues to the diagnosis of psoriasis in the skin and nails so that a biopsy is not needed. (*Reproduced with permission from Richard P. Usatine, MD.*)

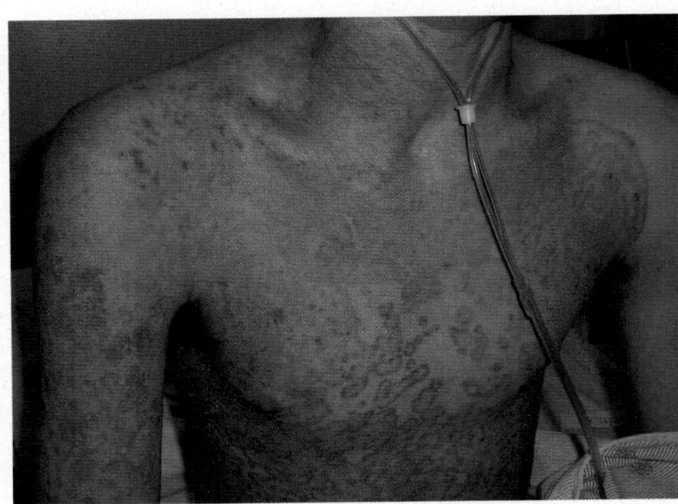

FIGURE 142-11 Severe chronic cutaneous candidiasis in a 22-year-old man with immunosuppression. (*Reproduced with permission from Richard P. Usatine, MD.*)

- Systemic therapy is needed, and azole antifungal agents (fluconazole and itraconazole) have been used successfully.[3]
- As with HIV-infected patients, development of resistance to these agents has been described.[3]

PATIENT EDUCATION

Keep the infected area clean and dry. For thrush in a baby, treat sources of infection such as the mother's breasts and bottle nipples. If the baby is bottle fed, boil the nipples between uses.

PATIENT AND PROVIDER RESOURCES

- *Clinical Practice Guideline for the Management of Candidiasis: 2016 Update by the Infectious Diseases Society of America*—**https://academic.oup.com/cid/article/62/4/409/2462633**
- *Cutaneous Candidiasis*—**http://emedicine.medscape.com/article/1090632.**
- *Intertrigo*—**http://emedicine.medscape.com/article/ 1087691.**

REFERENCES

1. Scheinfeld N. *Cutaneous Candidiasis*. Updated May 22, 2018. https://emedicine.medscape.com/article/1090632-overview. Accessed August 2, 2018.
2. Spraker MK, Gisoldi EM, Siegfried EC, et al. Topical miconazole nitrate ointment in the treatment of diaper dermatitis complicated by candidiasis. *Cutis*. 2006;77(2):113-120.
3. Pappas PG, Kauffman CA, Andes DR, et al. Executive summary: clinical practice guideline for the management of candidiasis: 2016 update by the infectious diseases society of America. *Clin Infect Dis*. 2016;62(4):409-417.

143 TINEA CAPITIS

Richard P. Usatine, MD

PATIENT STORY

An 11-year-old boy has a history of 2 months of progressive patchy hair loss (**Figure 143-1**). He has some itching of the scalp, but his mother is worried about his hair loss. Physical examination reveals alopecia with scaling of the scalp and broken hairs looking like black dots in the areas of hair loss. A KOH preparation is created by using a #15 scalpel to scrape some scale and small broken hairs onto a slide. With the help of a fungal stain and KOH, branching septate hyphae are seen under the microscope. The most likely cause of this tinea capitis is *Trichophyton tonsurans*; therefore 4 weeks of oral terbinafine is prescribed. The tinea capitis fully resolves and the hair does grow back over time.

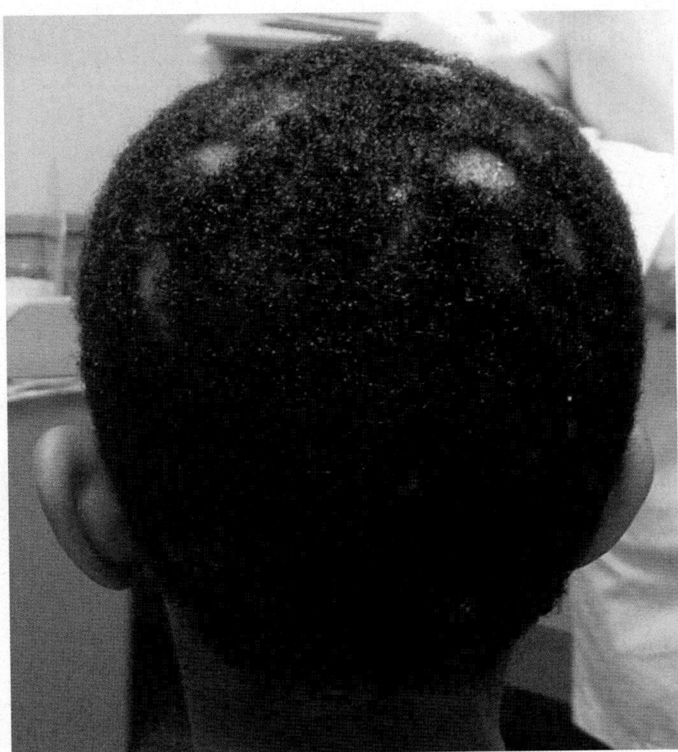

FIGURE 143-1 Tinea capitis in a young black boy. The most likely organism is *Trichophyton tonsurans*. (*Reproduced with permission from Richard P. Usatine, MD.*)

INTRODUCTION

Tinea capitis is a fungal infection involving the scalp and hair. Common signs include hair loss, scaling, black dots, erythema, and impetigo-like plaques.

SYNONYMS

Ringworm of the scalp.

EPIDEMIOLOGY

- Tinea capitis is the most common type of dermatophytoses in children younger than 10 years (**Figures 143-1** to **143-5**). It is much less common after puberty or in adults. The infection has a worldwide distribution.
- Tinea capitis is more common in young African-American children.[1] Boys are infected more often than girls.[1]
- Combs, brushes, couches, and sheets may harbor the live dermatophyte for a long period of time.
- Spread from person to person with direct contact or through fomites (especially *Trichophyton tonsurans*).
- Occasionally spread from cats and dogs to humans (especially *Microsporum* species).

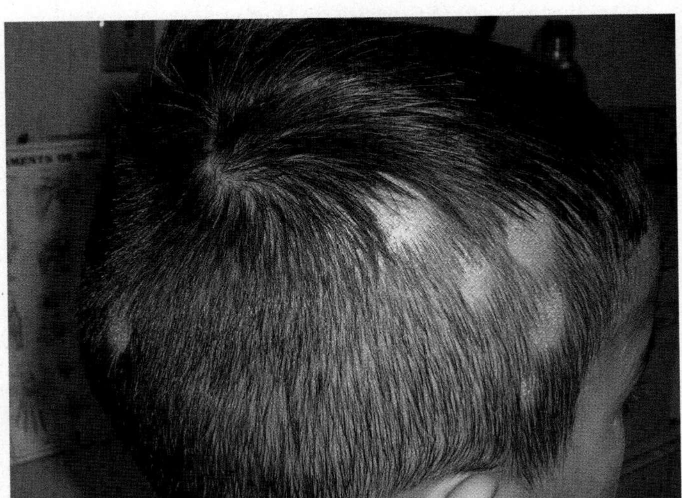

FIGURE 143-2 Tinea capitis with patchy hair loss and scaling of the scalp in a young boy. (*Reproduced with permission from Richard P. Usatine, MD.*)

ETIOLOGY AND PATHOPHYSIOLOGY

- Tinea capitis is a superficial fungal infection affecting hair shafts and follicles on the scalp.
- Caused by *Trichophyton* and *Microsporum* dermatophytes. The most common organism in the United States is *Trichophyton*

tonsurans, which is associated with black dot alopecia.[1] *Microsporum canis* is less common in the United States now than decades ago. *M. canis* is still highly prevalent in developing countries and parts of Europe.[2] The natural reservoir of *M. canis* is dogs and cats.

RISK FACTORS

- Lack of access to clean water and soap, especially in developing countries.[2]
- Poverty—rural and urban.[1]
- African descent, as the dermatophytes grow well in the follicles of short curly hairs.[1]
- Crowded living arrangements in which infected individuals spread the tinea to others.
- Sharing combs, brushes, and hair ornaments.
- Wrestling (tinea capitis gladiatorum).

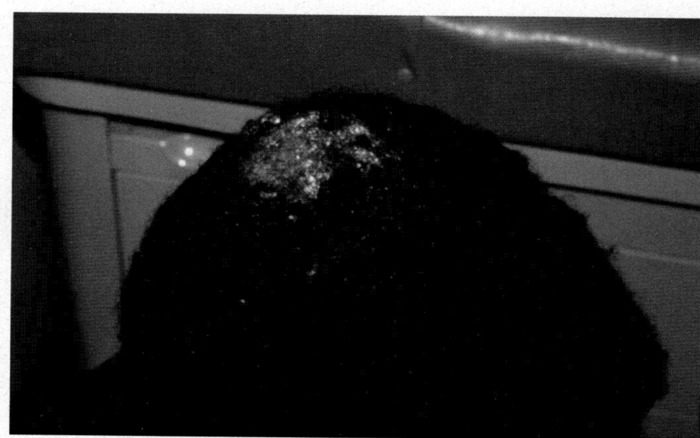

FIGURE 143-3 A kerion resulting from inflammation of the tinea capitis on this young boy. The kerion looks superinfected, but it is nothing more than an exuberant inflammatory response to the dermatophyte. (*Reproduced with permission from Richard P. Usatine, MD.*)

DIAGNOSIS

- The clinical appearance may be classic, but consider looking at the scalp with an ultraviolet light (Wood lamp), looking for fluorescence (see more detail under Laboratory).
- A positive KOH prep can confirm the diagnosis within a setting that has access to a microscope. A KOH preparation is created by using a #15 scalpel or the edge of another slide to scrape some scale and broken hairs onto a slide. Apply 1 to 2 drops of KOH (preferably with a fungal stain) to the slide and add a coverslip (see online video by Dr. Usatine under Provider Resources). Look for septate hyphae and arthroconidia (fungal spores) (**Figure 143-6**). Look for invasion of the hair shaft with fungus.

CLINICAL FEATURES

- Alopecia and scaling of the scalp (see **Figures 143-1** and **143-2**).
- A kerion occurs when there is an inflammatory response to the tinea. The scalp gets red, swollen, and boggy. There may be serosanguinous discharge and some crusting as this dries (see **Figure 143-3**).
- There may be broken hairs that look like black dots in the areas of hair loss (see **Figure 143-4**). This is especially common with *T. tonsurans.*
- Cervical lymphadenopathy occurs commonly with tinea capitis (see **Figure 143-5**).
- Tinea capitis can even be annular, as the name "ringworm" of the scalp implies (see **Figure 143-6**).

TYPICAL DISTRIBUTION

By definition it occurs on the head, but usually is found on the scalp. Rarely involves the eyebrows and eyelashes.

LABORATORY STUDIES

Whenever possible it is very important to confirm or dispel one's clinical suspicion with mycologic evidence before starting weeks of oral antifungal medicines.

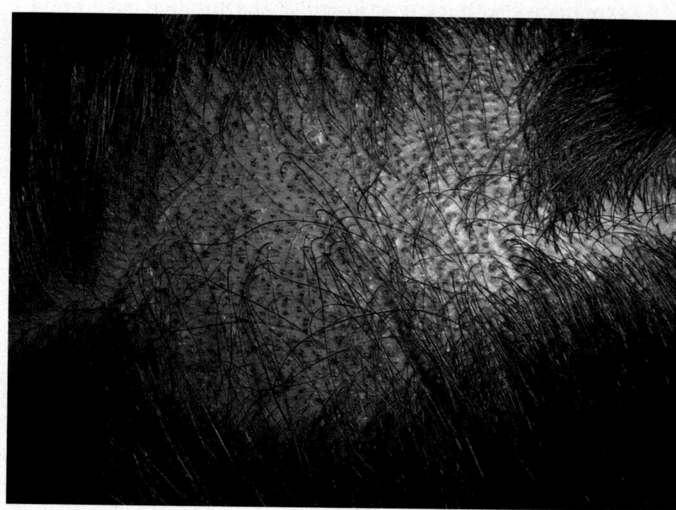

FIGURE 143-4 Close-up of black dot alopecia in a 7-year-old girl showing the black dots where infected hairs have broken off. (*Reproduced with permission from Richard P. Usatine, MD.*)

- KOH preparation—Scrape the scale and infected hairs using a #15 blade. Apply KOH or a fungal stain to the slide. Use the microscope to look for septate, branching hyphae under 10× and 40× power (**Figure 143-7**). The hyphae or arthroconidia (fungal spores) of *Microsporum* may be found on the exterior of the hair (ectothrix) while the hyphae or arthroconidia of *Trichophyton tonsurans* and *T. violaceum* are found in the interior of the hair (endothrix) (**Figure 143-8**).
- Fungal culture—If the diagnosis is uncertain or the species is desired for therapeutic decisions, send a few loose hairs and a scraping of the scalp scale for a fungal culture. A specimen for culture may be obtained using a #15 scalpel, the edge of the slide, a cytobrush, or a sterile gauze rubbed across the infected area.[2] The specimen should be placed in a sterile urine cup and sent to the laboratory for culture.
- Wood lamp examination—Only the *Microsporum* species demonstrate bright green/blue fluorescence of infected hairs (**Figure 143-9**) because of their ectothrix pattern. *Trichophyton tonsurans* and *T. violaceum* are endothrix infections so do not fluoresce. However, *T. schoenleinii* can fluoresce dull green.[2] As the majority of tinea capitis in the United States and United Kingdom is caused by *T. tonsurans*, one should not rule out tinea capitis in these countries when fluorescence is absent.[2] in general, the presence of fluorescence is helpful but the absence is not.

DERMOSCOPY

Dermoscopy of the hair is called trichoscopy. Dermoscopy may help visualize black dot hair stubs, comma hairs, and corkscrew hairs in tinea capitis (**Figure 143-10**). One small study suggests that these features are seen more often in *T. tonsurans* and that "elbow" shaped hairs may be seen with *Microsporum* as the hairs break off at a higher level from the scalp.[3]

DIFFERENTIAL DIAGNOSIS

- Alopecia areata—Produces areas of hair loss with no scaling, inflammation, or scarring in the underlying scalp. It is an autoimmune process in which the immune system attacks the person's own hair follicles (see Chapter 195, Alopecia Areata).
- Seborrhea of the scalp (dandruff)—Is caused by the *Pityrosporum* yeast, resulting in scaling and inflammation but rarely causing hair loss. The scalp involvement tends to be more widespread than patchy and localized as seen in tinea capitis (see Chapter 157, Seborrheic Dermatitis).
- Scalp psoriasis—Rarely causes alopecia. There are mild cases with slight, fine scaling on the scalp, or severe cases with silvery, thick, crusted plaques covering the majority of the scalp. Often psoriatic plaques are seen elsewhere on the body and nail changes are visible.
- Trichotillomania—Self-inflicted alopecia caused when the patient pulls and twists her/his own hair (see Chapter 196, Traction Alopecia and Trichotillomania).
- Traction alopecia—Alopecia that occurs when the patient or parent pulls the hair to style it into braids or ponytails. There should be no scaling of the scalp (unless there is coexisting seborrhea) and the pattern of hair loss should match the hairstyle (see Chapter 196, Traction Alopecia and Trichotillomania).

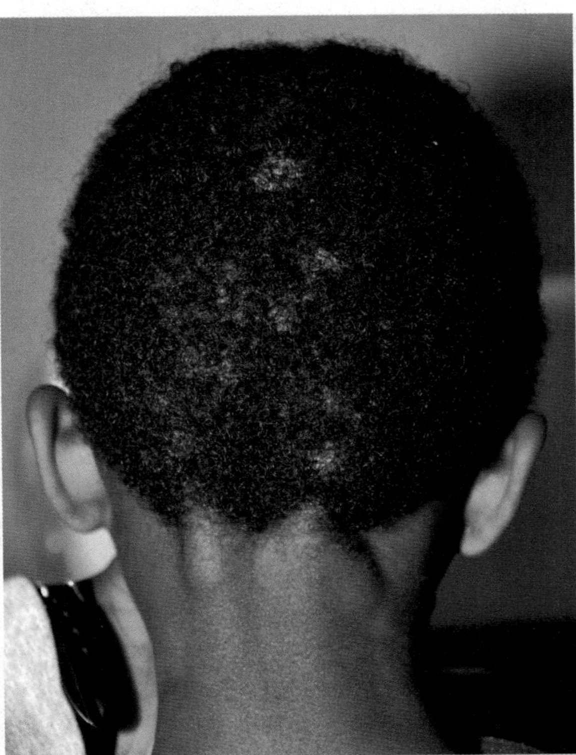

FIGURE 143-5 Lymphadenopathy visible in the neck of this young boy with tinea capitis. The fungal infection shows more scaling and crusting than actual hair loss. The lymphadenopathy is a reaction to the tinea and not a bacterial superinfection. (*Reproduced with permission from Richard P. Usatine, MD.*)

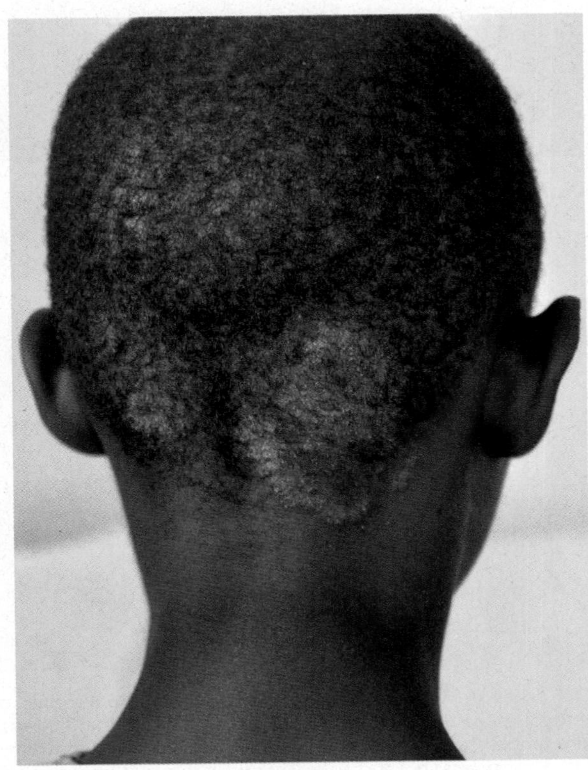

FIGURE 143-6 Tinea capitis with an annular configuration. (*Reproduced with permission from Richard P. Usatine, MD.*)

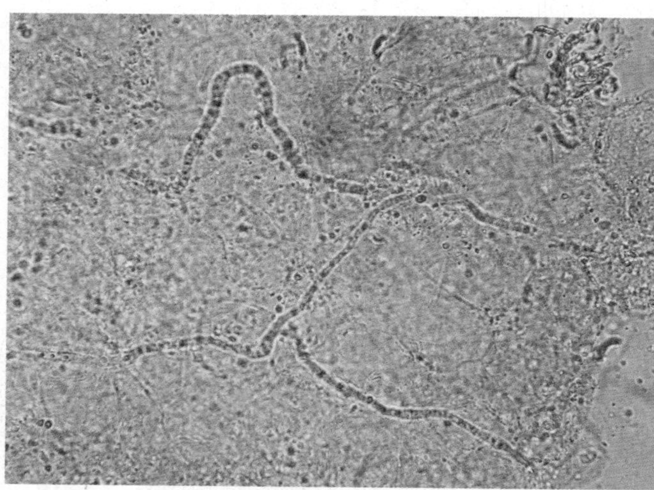

FIGURE 143-7 *T. tonsurans* from tinea capitis visible among skin cells at 40× power after adding Swartz Lamkins fungal stain. (*Reproduced with permission from Richard P. Usatine, MD.*)

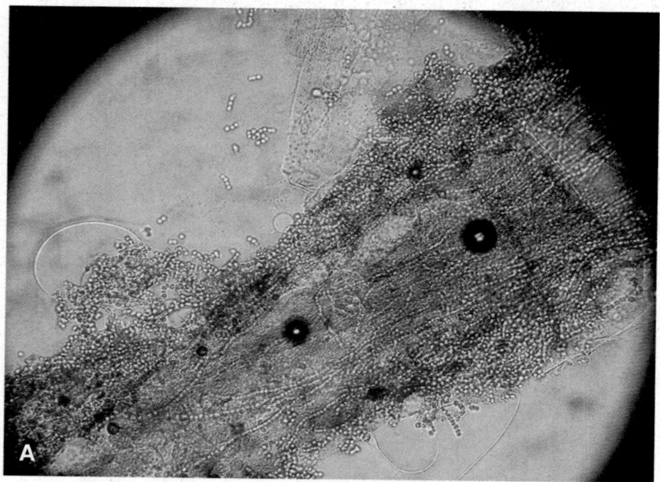

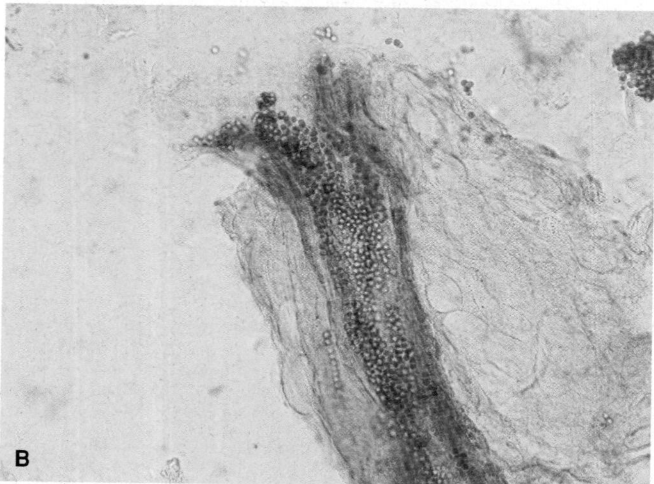

FIGURE 143-8 A. *M. canis* showing arthroconidia (fungal spores) on the exterior of the hair (ectothrix) at 40× power after adding Swartz Lamkins fungal stain. (*Reproduced with permission from Eric Kraus, MD.*) B. *T. tonsurans* showing arthroconidia in the interior of the hair (endothrix) at 40× power after adding Swartz-Lamkins fungal stain. (*Reproduced with permission from Patrick E. McCleskey, MD.*)

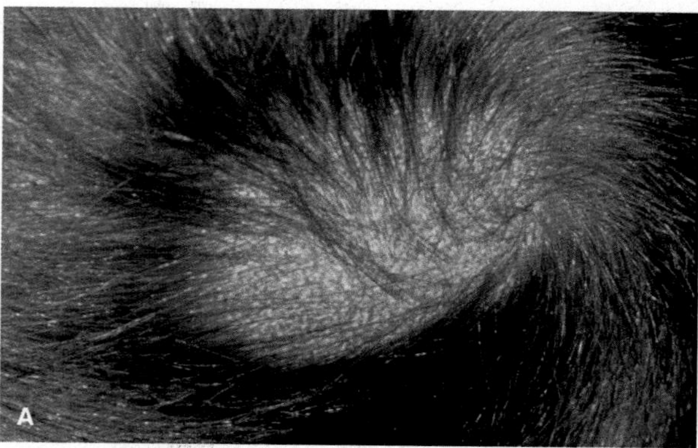

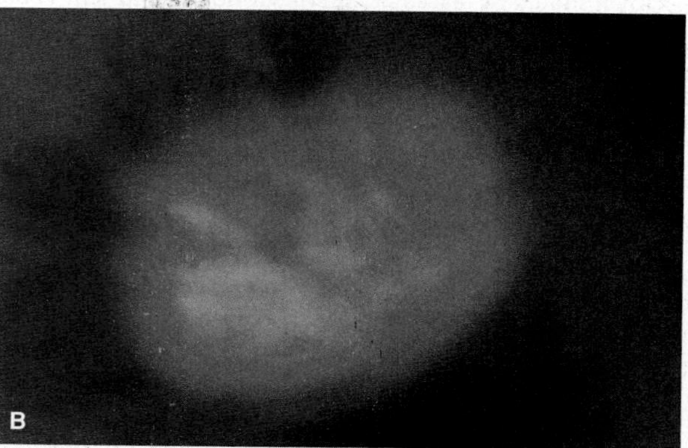

FIGURE 143-9 A. Tinea capitis in a young boy. B. Fluorescence with an ultraviolet light indicating that this is a *Microsporum* species causing the tinea capitis. (*Reproduced with permission from Jeff Meffert, MD.*)

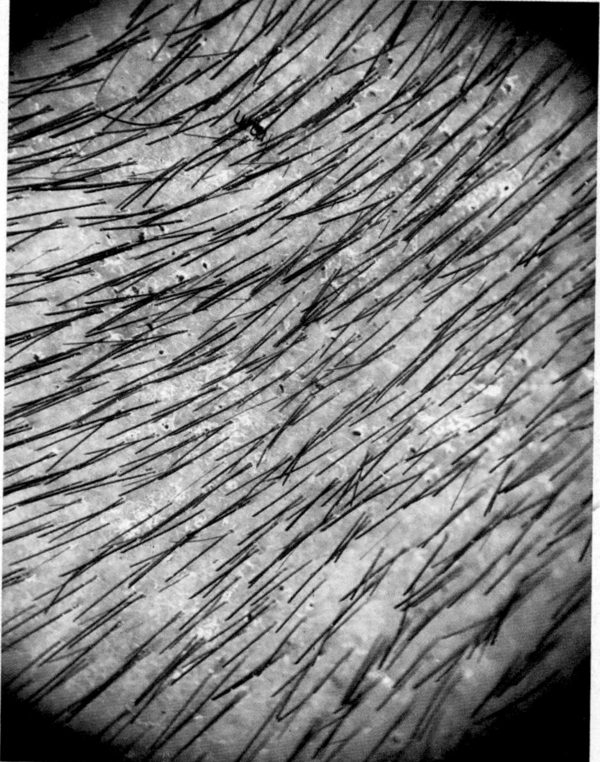

FIGURE 143-10 Dermoscopy of tinea capitis. Note the black dot hair stubs, comma hairs, and scale. (*Reproduced with permission from Richard P. Usatine, MD.*)

MANAGEMENT

FIRST LINE

- Oral antifungal therapy is needed and topical therapy alone is insufficient.[4] SOR Ⓐ
- A new Cochrane meta-analysis confirms that terbinafine is more effective than griseofulvin in children with *T. tonsurans* infection and griseofulvin is better than terbinafine in children with *Microsporum* infections.[4,5] SOR Ⓐ
- For *Microsporum* infections in children, a meta-analysis of two studies found that the complete cure was lower for terbinafine (6 weeks) than for griseofulvin (6–12 weeks) (34.7% vs. 50.9%).[4] SOR Ⓐ
- For *T. tonsurans* infections in children, terbinafine was better than griseofulvin (52.1% vs. 35.4%).[4] SOR Ⓐ
- Given the data above, all efforts should be made to distinguish between infections caused by *Trichophyton* or *Microsporum* species. First it helps to know the relative prevalence of the dermatophytes causing tinea capitis in your community or nation. Then the Wood lamp and dermatoscope may help. A KOH preparation in which an endothrix or exothrix pattern is seen may also help. This information can be used to choose the best oral antifungal agent initially. Fungal cultures are not always available and may take 1 to 2 weeks for results. However, they can confirm the diagnosis and influence the choice of ongoing oral antifungal therapy. In the United States where *T. tonsurans* is most common, oral terbinafine is often the best choice as the initial therapy (see cost data below).
- Other oral antifungals including itraconazole and fluconazole are at least as effective as griseofulvin in children with tinea capitis caused by *Trichophyton* species.[4] SOR Ⓐ
- Ketoconazole is less effective than griseofulvin and should be avoided because of higher risks for liver toxicity and drug interactions.[4,6]
- Fluconazole daily for 3 weeks was as similarly effective as 6 weeks of fluconazole in one study of 491 patients infected with *T. tonsurans* and *M. canis* (cure rates of 30.2% vs. 34.1%).[4] SOR Ⓐ
- Adverse event frequency for terbinafine and griseofulvin (9.2% vs. 8.3%) was similar, and severe adverse events were rare (0.6% vs. 0.6%).[4] SOR Ⓐ
- Adverse events for terbinafine, griseofulvin, itraconazole, and fluconazole were all mild and reversible.[4] SOR Ⓐ

PRACTICAL CONSIDERATIONS

Forms available:

- Griseofulvin and fluconazole are available in liquid suspensions for children. Terbinafine is not available in a liquid form and comes as a scored 250 mg tablet. There is a terbinafine brand-name (Lamisil) granule formulation that comes in packets of 125 mg and 187.5 mg. Griseofulvin comes as microsize and ultramicrosize tablets, too. Fluconazole also comes as 50 mg, 100 mg, 150 mg, and 200 mg tablets. Itraconazole is available as a 100 mg capsule only, which limits dosing flexibility.

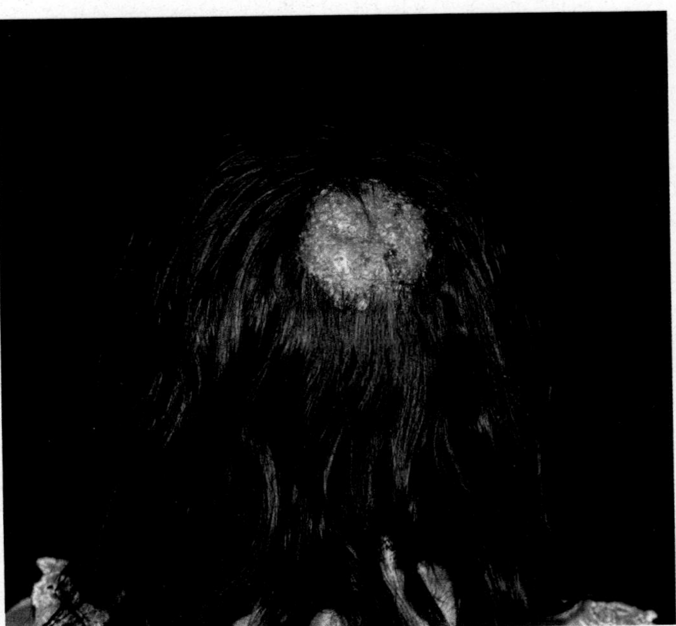

FIGURE 143-11 A kerion in a 5-year-old girl infected with *Trichophyton rubrum*. *(Reproduced with permission from Eric Kraus, MD.)*

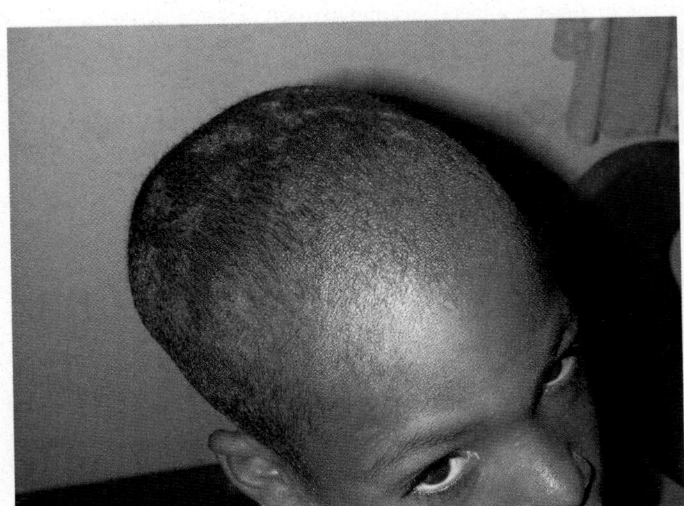

FIGURE 143-12 Tinea capitis in a schoolboy in Panama. Many of his classmates also had tinea capitis. An antifungal shampoo was prescribed for the children while waiting to get access to a systemic antifungal agent. *(Reproduced with permission from Richard P. Usatine, MD.)*

Recommended doses:

- Terbinafine—recommended dosage for children less than 25 kg is 125 mg daily (one half a tablet); and for children who weigh more than 35 kg, one 250 mg tablet daily. Children between 25 to 35 kg should receive 187.5 mg daily (accomplished with compounding or breaking tablets into pieces).
- Microsize griseofulvin suspension is 20–25 mg/kg per day and ultramicrosize griseofulvin tablets is 10–15 mg/kg per day. Ultramicrosize preparations are stronger per mg than the microsize, but do not come in liquid form.
- Fluconazole—recommended dosage is 5 to 6 mg/kg per day.

Length of treatment:

- Griseofulvin—8 weeks, and consider up to 12 weeks
- Terbinafine—6 weeks for *Trichophyton*, and 8 to 12 weeks may be needed for *Microsporum*.
- Fluconazole—3 to 6 weeks.

Cost:

- Oral terbinafine has become very affordable in the United States and appears on most $4 and $5 lists. Terbinafine granules (Lamisil brand name only) were expensive and were discontinued. Oral griseofulvin suspension or tablets may easily cost hundreds of dollars to the patient or healthcare system. Fluconazole and itraconazole are more expensive than terbinafine.

Other considerations:

- Oral antifungal therapy does not require laboratory monitoring at the recommended lengths of treatment for tinea capitis in an otherwise healthy child.[7] SOR C
- A kerion will resolve with oral antifungal treatment alone. If it is severe and painful, some would consider a short pulse of oral steroids in addition (**Figure 143-11**). However, current evidence does not support the benefit of oral steroids for treatment of a kerion.[2] SOR C While a kerion appears similar to an abscess, an incision and drainage is unnecessary and harmful.

SECOND LINE

- Topical treatment can be used as adjuvant therapy: 1% to 2.5% selenium sulfide or 1% ciclopirox should be applied to the scalp and hair for 5 minutes 2 or 3 times a week for 8 weeks.[8] SOR B
- Shampoos with selenium sulfide or ciclopirox have been shown to be of equal efficacy.[8] SOR B
- Another use for antifungal shampoo is empirical treatment while waiting for a culture to come back in an equivocal case. Topical antifungal shampoo may decrease the spread of the tinea in crowded living environments while waiting for the oral therapy to work (**Figure 143-12**). SOR C

PREVENTION

Family members or playmates should be screened, and asymptomatic carriers should be treated. Close physical contact and sharing of toys or combs/hairbrushes should be avoided.[2] SOR B

PROGNOSIS

With some oral antifungal treatments, studies showed that complete clinical cure was greater than 90% (e.g., one study of terbinafine or griseofulvin for *Trichophyton* infections). In other comparison studies, the proportion cured was much lower, in the range of 50%.[4]

PATIENT EDUCATION

Patients and parents need to exercise care to avoid spreading the infection to others. Explain the importance of not sharing combs, brushes, and towels.

FOLLOW-UP

Follow-up appointments should be scheduled to make sure that the patient is taking the medication as prescribed and not suffering any adverse effects. Because the course for overall antifungal medicines is typically 4 to 8 weeks, a follow-up in 1 month provides for an opportunity to check on medication adherence and clinical response. With cure rates in many studies as low as 50%, it makes sense to follow the patient until there is full clinical and mycologic cure. Scale and inflammation should resolve initially and hair should regrow in most cases.

PATIENT RESOURCE

- MedlinePlus article for patients—**http://www.nlm.nih.gov/medlineplus/ency/article/000878.htm.**

PROVIDER RESOURCES

- KOH preparation and interpretation video (4 minutes by Dr. Usatine)—**https://www.youtube.com/watch?v=LUwNQI_0BWU&t=2s.**
- Systemic antifungal therapy for tinea capitis in children. *Cochrane Database Syst Rev.* 2016;(5):CD004685.—**https://www.ncbi.nlm.nih.gov/pubmed/27169520.**

REFERENCES

1. Mirmirani P, Tucker L. Epidemiologic trends in pediatric tinea capitis: a population-based study from Kaiser Permanente Northern California. *J Am Acad Dermatol.* 2013;69(6):916-921.
2. Fuller LC, Barton RC, Mohd Mustapa MF, et al. British Association of Dermatologists' guidelines for the management of tinea capitis 2014. *Br J Dermatol.* 2014;171(3):454-463.
3. Schechtman RC, Silva NDV, Quaresma MV, et al. Dermatoscopic findings as a complementary tool in the differential diagnosis of the etiological agent of tinea capitis. *An Bras Dermatol.* 2015;90(3):13-15.
4. Chen X, Jiang X, Yang M, et al. Systemic antifungal therapy for tinea capitis in children. *Cochrane Database Syst Rev.* 2016;(5):CD004685.

5. Gupta AK, Drummond-Main C. Meta-analysis of randomized, controlled trials comparing particular doses of griseofulvin and terbinafine for the treatment of tinea capitis. *Pediatr Dermatol.* 2013;30(1):1-6.
6. Gupta AK, Daigle D, Foley KA. Drug safety assessment of oral formulations of ketoconazole. *Expert Opin Drug Saf.* 2015;14(2): 325-334.
7. Pride HB, Tollefson M, Silverman R. What's new in pediatric dermatology? *J Am Acad Dermatol.* 2013;68(6):899.e1-899.e11.
8. Chen C, Koch LH, Dice JE, et al. A randomized, double-blind study comparing the efficacy of selenium sulfide shampoo 1% and ciclopirox shampoo 1% as adjunctive treatments for tinea capitis in children. *Pediatr Dermatol.* 2010;27(5):459-462.

144 TINEA CORPORIS

Richard P. Usatine, MD
Adeliza S. Jimenez, MD

PATIENT STORY

A 30-year-old woman presents to a family physician with a rash on most of her forearm that is now encroaching on her hand. She states that it has been going on for 6 months and that 2 months ago she went to an urgent care where she was given two creams to apply to the rash. Fortunately, she had the creams with her, and **Figure 144-1** shows the two creams adjacent to the eruption. The physician diagnosed tinea incognito. The urgent care provider recognized the original eruption as fungal but did not know that nystatin only treats *Candida* and not the dermatophytes that cause tinea corporis. Therefore, the nystatin was useless and the triamcinolone contributed to the rapid growth of this "fungus on steroids." The patient was given 4 weeks of oral terbinafine 250 mg daily, and the tinea incognito cleared completely.

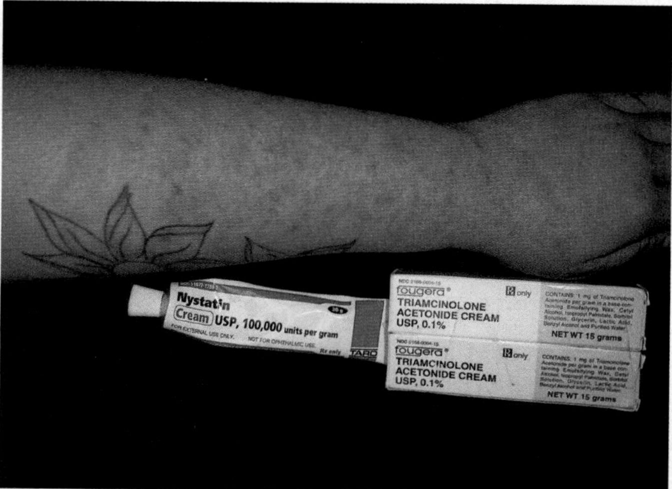

FIGURE 144-1 Tinea corporis on the arm that was incorrectly treated with topical nystatin and topical triamcinolone. As neither agent is effective against *T. rubrum*, the dermatophyte grew to cover most of the forearm. Nystatin treats *Candida* and not dermatophytes, so the missed treatment was similar to a misdiagnosis and the steroid allowed this simple tinea infection to become tinea incognito. (*Reproduced with permission from Richard P. Usatine, MD.*)

INTRODUCTION

Tinea corporis is a common superficial fungal infection of the body, characterized by well-demarcated, annular lesions with central clearing, erythema, and scaling of the periphery.

SYNONYMS

Ringworm, dermatophytosis.

EPIDEMIOLOGY

- It is estimated that 10% to 20% of the world population is affected by fungal skin infections.[1]
- Dermatophytes are the most prevalent agents causing fungal infections of the skin.[2]
- *Trichophyton rubrum* causes the majority of cases of tinea corporis.[2]
- The prevalence of tinea corporis gladiatorum (in wrestlers) ranges from 20% to 77%.[3]
- Most reported cases of tinea corporis gladiatorum have been caused by *T. tonsurans*.[3]

ETIOLOGY AND PATHOPHYSIOLOGY

- Tinea corporis is caused by fungal species from any one of the following three dermatophyte genera: *Trichophyton*, *Microsporum*, and *Epidermophyton*.
- Dermatophytes produce enzymes such as keratinase that penetrate keratinized tissue. Their hyphae invade the stratum corneum and spread centrifugally outward.

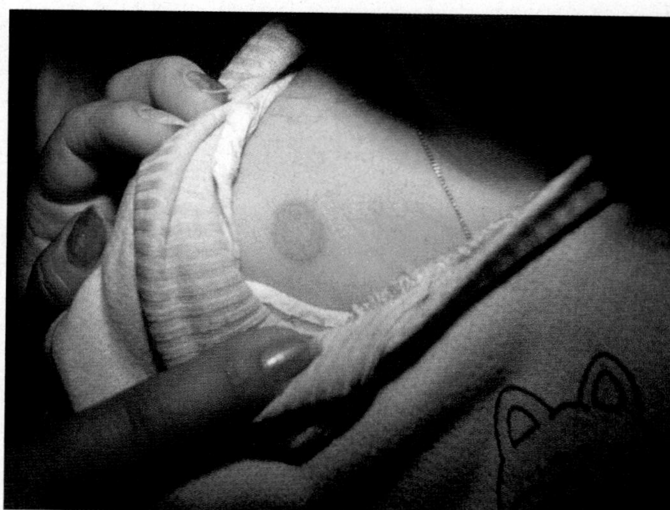

FIGURE 144-2 Tinea corporis with two concentric rings and central sparing. The child probably acquired this from the new family cat, making *Microsporum canis* the most likely causative organism. Her sweatshirt is a clue to her love of cats.

RISK FACTORS

- Participation in daycare centers.
- Wrestling (tinea corporis gladiatorum).[3]
- Living in a nursing home.
- Poor personal hygiene.
- Living conditions with poor sanitation.
- Warm, humid environments.
- Conditions that cause weakening of the immune system (e.g., AIDS, cancer, organ transplantation, diabetes).

DIAGNOSIS

The diagnosis can be made from history, clinical presentation, culture, and direct microscopic observation of hyphae and spores in infected tissue and hairs after KOH preparation. An ultraviolet light (Wood lamp) is helpful only in cases with *Microsporum* species. Since almost all tinea corporis is caused by *Trichophyton rubrum* or *Trichophyton tonsurans* (in wrestlers), the Wood lamp is rarely positive in current-day tinea corporis.

CLINICAL FEATURES

- Pruritus of affected area.
- Well-demarcated, annular lesions with central clearing, erythema, and scaling of the periphery. Concentric rings are highly specific for tinea infections (**Figure 144-2**).
- Central clearing is not always present (**Figure 144-3**).
- Tinea corporis is frequently pink to red in white skin but can be silver (**Figure 144-3**) or hyperpigmented in darker skin (**Figure 144-4**).
- Tinea incognito is a type of tinea infection that was previously unrecognized by the physician or patient, and topical steroids were used on the site. While the steroid is being used, the dermatophyte continues to grow and may form concentric rings (**Figures 144-1, 144-5,** and **144-6**).
- Although scale is the most prominent morphologic characteristic, some tinea infections will actually cause pustules from the inflammatory response (**Figure 144-7**).
- Majochi granuloma (**Figure 144-8**) is a type of tinea in which the fungus has gone deep into the hair follicles and creates a granulomatous appearance. This may be caused by the application of topical steroids so that this is a deep type of tinea incognito in some cases. Shaving or occlusion of the skin may be involved in the pathophysiology as well. It is a deep and persistent suppurative folliculitis so that pustules and nodules may be present along with the superficial erythema and scale visible in typical tinea corporis.

TYPICAL DISTRIBUTION

Any part of the body including the face, known as tinea faciei (**Figure 144-9**).

Tinea corporis can cover large parts of the body as in **Figure 144-10**.

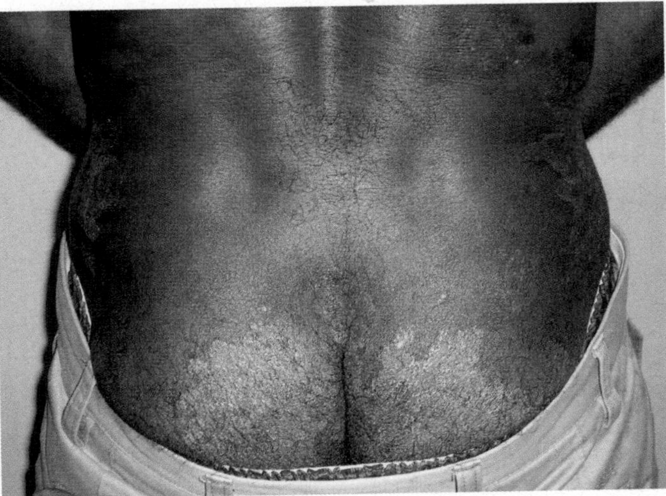

FIGURE 144-3 Tinea corporis covering the buttocks and not showing areas of central clearing. Note how the color is silver rather than pink in this dark skinned individual. The differential diagnosis includes psoriasis, so a KOH prep was performed, and it was positive to confirm the diagnosis of tinea. (*Reproduced with permission from Richard P. Usatine, MD.*)

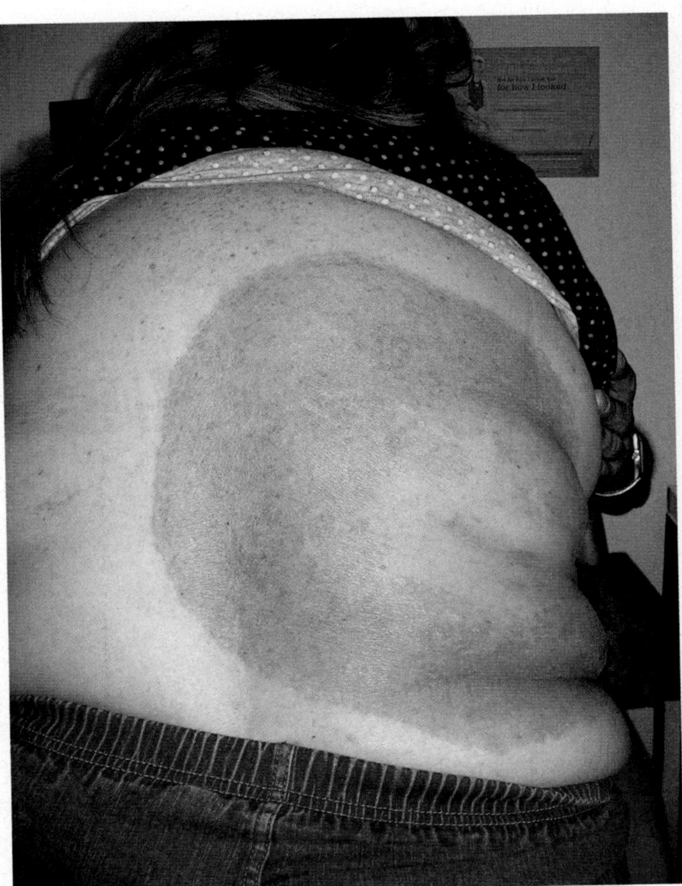

FIGURE 144-4 Tinea corporis covering the back and showing well-demarcated borders. (*Reproduced with permission from Richard P. Usatine, MD.*)

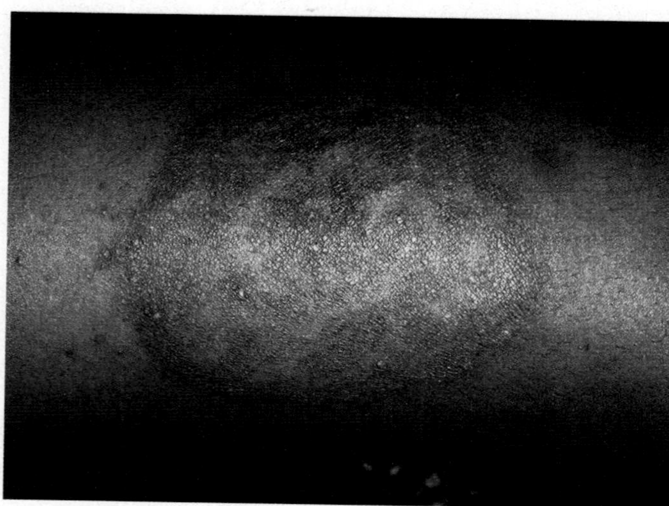

FIGURE 144-5 Tinea incognito on the arm of this woman. This tinea infection continued to grow as the patient applied the topical steroids given to her by her physician. There is postinflammatory hyperpigmentation with concentric rings. (*Reproduced with permission from Richard P. Usatine, MD.*)

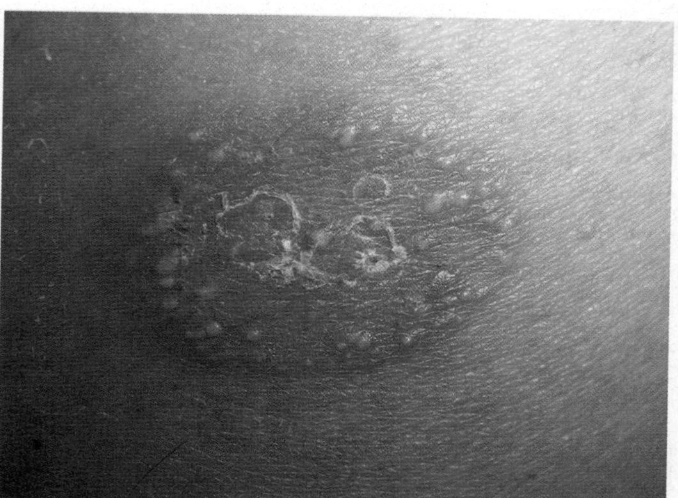

FIGURE 144-7 Tinea corporis with pustules and scale. KOH preparation was positive for branching hyphae. The pustules are a manifestation of an inflammatory response to the dermatophyte infection. (*Reproduced with permission from Richard P. Usatine, MD.*)

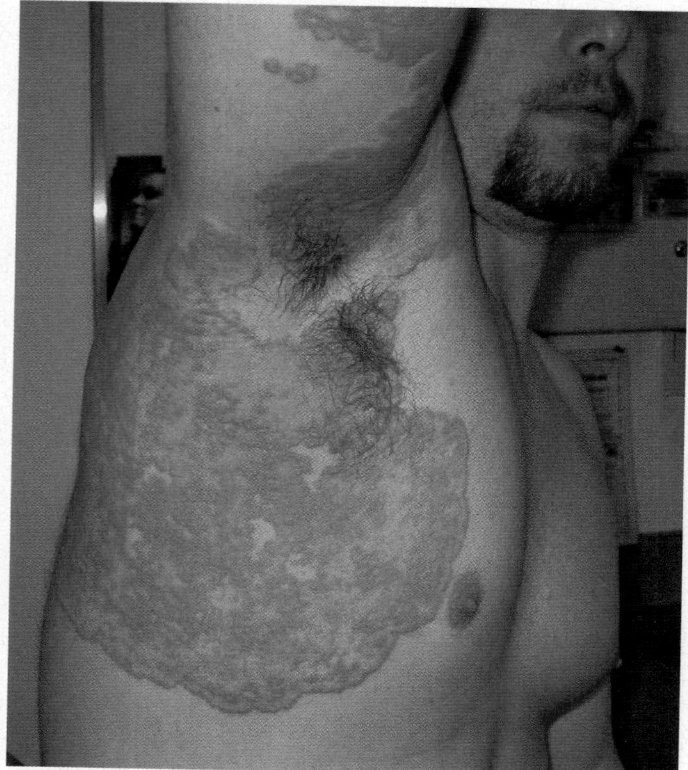

FIGURE 144-6 Tinea incognito in a young man who was incorrectly prescribed topical steroids for a tinea infection. Note the well-demarcated borders and multiple annular structures. Although there is some hyperpigmentation, erythema is most prominent. (*Reproduced with permission from Chris Wenner, MD.*)

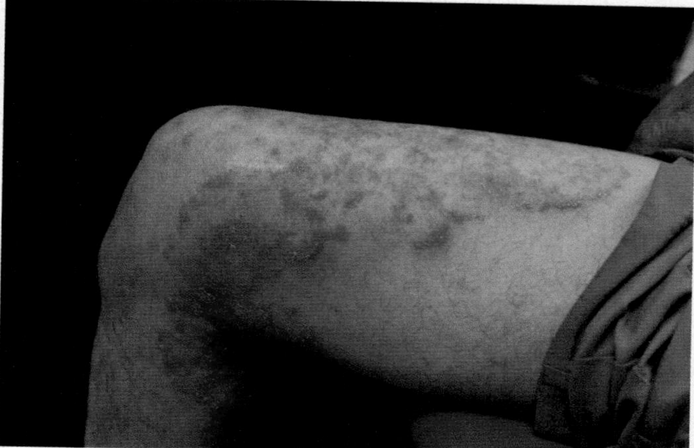

FIGURE 144-8 Majochi granuloma in which the tinea has gone deep into the hair follicles and has created a granulomatous appearance. This deep and suppurative folliculitis has persisted even after 1 month of oral terbinafine. The KOH prep was positive before treatment and at this stage during treatment. It took 3 months of oral terbinafine to clear this infection completely. (*Reproduced with permission from Richard P. Usatine, MD.*)

LABORATORY STUDIES

- KOH preparation of skin scraping can be very useful to confirm a clinical impression or when the diagnosis is not certain. Scrape the skin with the side of a slide or scalpel, making sure to scrape the periphery and the erythematous part. Scrape hard enough to get some stratum corneum without causing significant bleeding. False negatives can occur secondary to inadequate scraping, patient using topical antifungals, or an inexperienced microscopist.
- Use KOH (plain, with dimethyl sulfoxide [DMSO], or in a fungal stain) to break up the epithelial cells more rapidly without heating (**Figure 144-11**). It is easy to purchase a small bottle of Swartz Lamkins fungal stain that includes KOH, a surfactant, and blue ink. The blue ink allows the hyphae to stand out, thereby saving time and decreasing the chance of a false-negative result (**Figure 144-12**). If the epithelial cells are not breaking up sufficiently, use a flame under the slide for approximately 5 seconds to speed up the process.
- Skin scraping and culture—Gold standard, but more costly and may take up to 2 weeks for the culture to grow. Consider culture if the KOH is negative but tinea is still suspected, or when a microscope is not available.
- Skin biopsy sent in formalin for periodic acid–Schiff (PAS) staining when the KOH and culture remain negative but the clinical picture is consistent with a fungal infection.

DIFFERENTIAL DIAGNOSIS

- Granuloma annulare—Inflammatory, benign dermatosis of unknown cause, characterized by both dermal and annular papules (**Figure 144-13**) (see Chapter 182, Granuloma Annulare).
- Psoriasis—Plaque with scale on extensor surfaces and trunk. Occasionally, the plaques can have an annular appearance (**Figure 144-14**). Inverse psoriasis in intertriginous areas can also mimic tinea corporis (see Chapter 158, Psoriasis).
- Erythema annulare centrifugum (EAC)—Scaly red rings with normal skin in the center of the rings. The scale is trailing the erythema as the ring expands while the scale is leading in tinea corporis (**Figure 144-15**) (see Chapter 215, Erythema Annulare Centrifugum).
- Cutaneous larva migrans has serpiginous burrows made by the hookworm larvae, and these burrows can look annular and be confused with tinea corporis (see Chapter 150, Cutaneous Larva Migrans).
- Nummular eczema—Round coin-like red scaly plaques without central clearing (see Chapter 151, Atopic Dermatitis).
- Erythrasma—Found in the axilla and groin without an annular configuration and central clearing. Fluoresces coral red under UV lamp (see Chapter 125, Erythrasma).

MANAGEMENT

FIRST LINE

- Use topical antifungal medications for tinea corporis that involves small areas of the body such as seen in **Figure 144-2**.

FIGURE 144-9 Tinea faciei with prominent involvement of the nose. There is a subtle annular pattern and the KOH preparation was positive for branching hyphae. It resolved with a topical antifungal medicine. (*Reproduced with permission from Richard P. Usatine, MD.*)

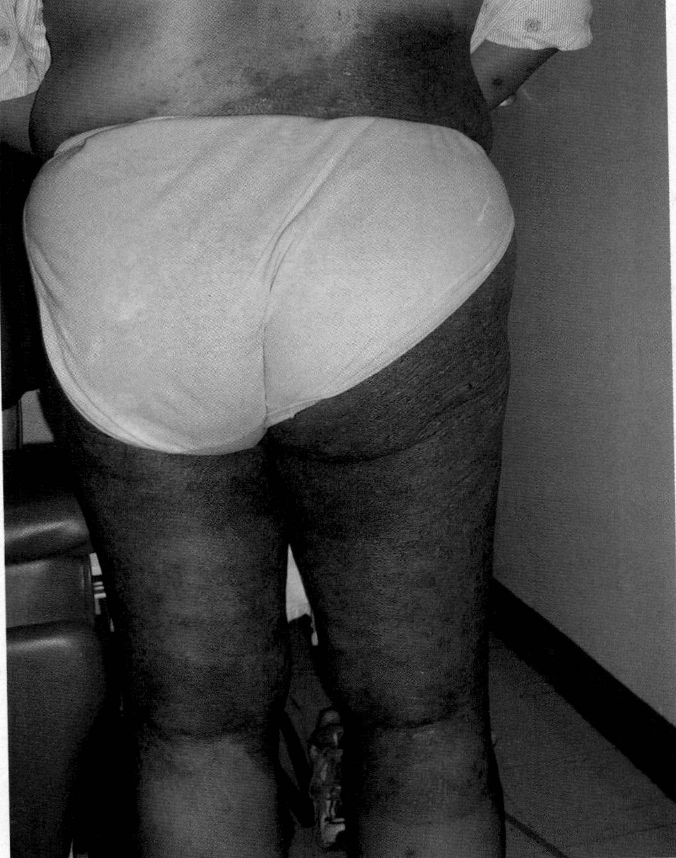

FIGURE 144-10 Tinea corporis from the trunk down both legs with significant hyperpigmentation. (*Reproduced with permission from Richard P. Usatine, MD.*)

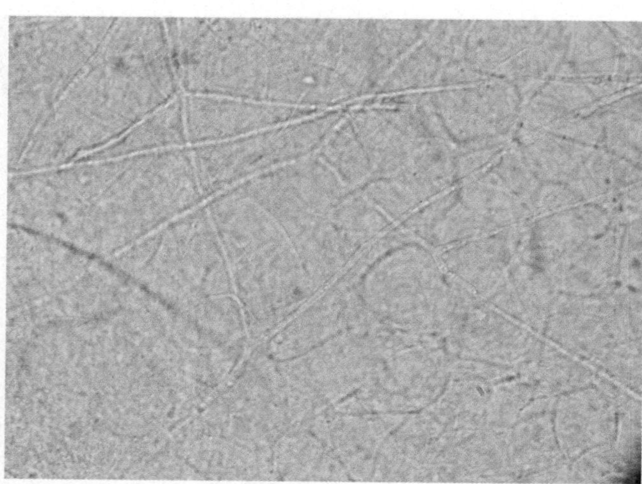

FIGURE 144-11 Branching hyphae at 40× power from a KOH preparation of tinea corporis without using a fungal stain. (*Reproduced with permission from Richard P. Usatine, MD.*)

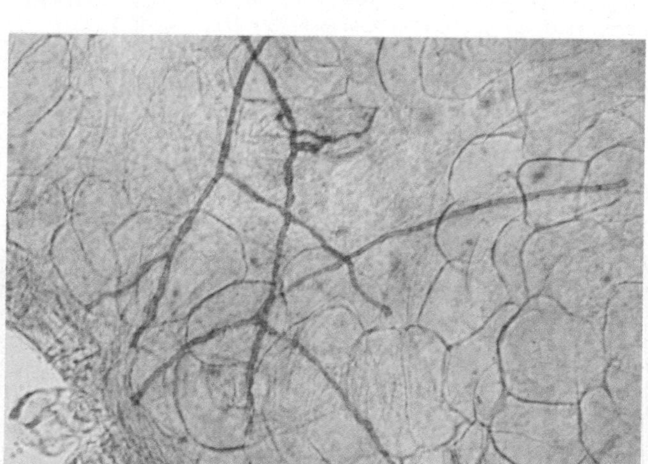

FIGURE 144-12 Branching hyphae easily seen at 40× power using fungal stain (Swartz Lamkins) from a scraping of tinea corporis. Note how the hyphae stand out with the blue ink color. (*Reproduced with permission from Richard P. Usatine, MD.*)

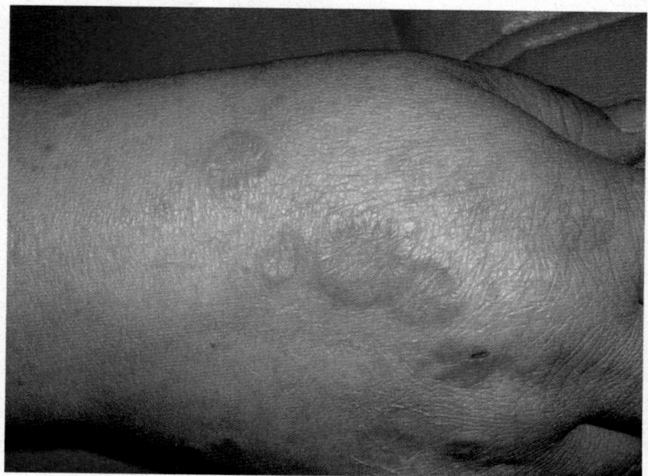

FIGURE 144-13 Multiple annular lesions caused by granuloma annulare. No scale is visible. (*Reproduced with permission from Richard P. Usatine, MD.*)

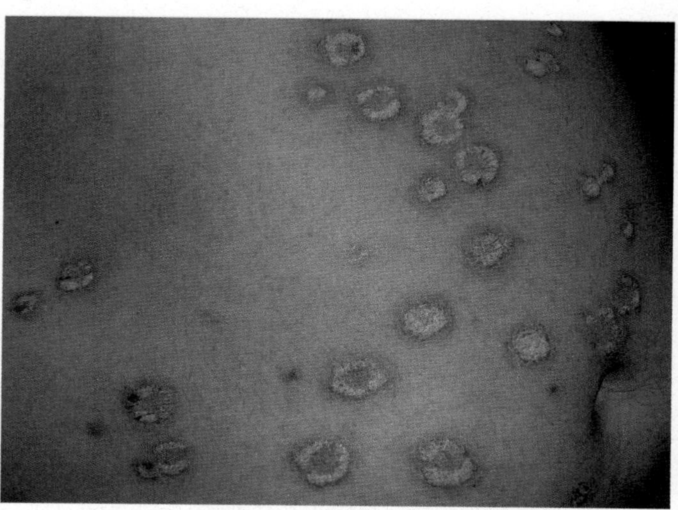

FIGURE 144-14 Widespread annular lesions caused by psoriasis. Not all lesions that are annular with scale are tinea corporis. (*Reproduced with permission from Richard P. Usatine, MD.*)

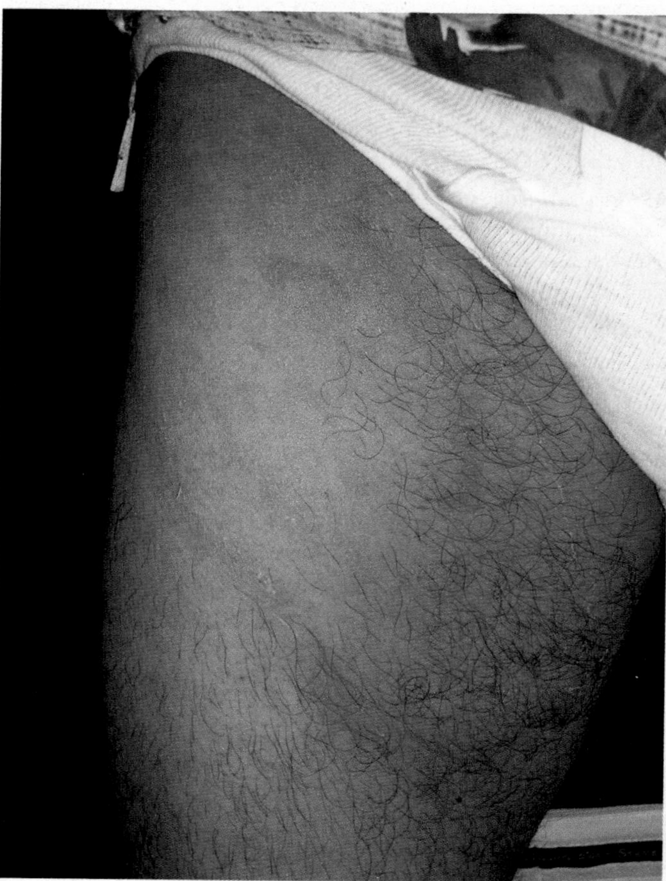

FIGURE 144-15 Erythema annulare centrifugum (EAC) on the leg of this man. A punch biopsy showed this to be EAC. Note the trailing scale rather than leading scale seen in tinea corporis. (*Reproduced with permission from Richard P. Usatine, MD.*)

- Across five of the best studies identified in a Cochrane review, significantly higher clinical cure rates were seen in tinea infected individuals treated with topical terbinafine compared to placebo (number needed to treat [NNT] 3).[1]
- Although all the topical antifungal agents may be effective, the evidence supports the greater effectiveness of the allylamines (terbinafine) over the less-expensive azoles for tinea pedis and corporis. Allylamines cure slightly more infections than azoles and are now available over the counter.[4,5] SOR Ⓐ
- Studies show that terbinafine 1% cream or solution applied once daily for 7 days is highly effective for tinea corporis/cruris.[6,7] The 1% cream (which is available over the counter as Lamisil AF) produced a mycologic cure of 84.2% versus 23.3% with placebo. NNT = 1.6.[6] SOR Ⓐ
- Oral antifungal agents should be considered for first-line therapy for tinea corporis covering large areas of the body. However, it is not wrong to attempt topical treatment if the size of the area infected is on the borderline.
- One randomized controlled trial (RCT) showed that oral itraconazole 200 mg daily for 1 week is similarly effective, equally well tolerated, and at least as safe as itraconazole 100 mg for 2 weeks in the treatment of tinea corporis or cruris.[8] SOR Ⓑ
- In one study, patients with mycologically diagnosed tinea corporis and tinea cruris were randomly allocated to receive either 250 mg of oral terbinafine once daily or 500 mg of griseofulvin once daily for 2 weeks. The cure rates were higher for terbinafine at 6 weeks.[9] SOR Ⓑ
- Majochi granuloma can be especially difficult to treat and requires oral antifungals just like tinea capitis. It might actually require months of terbinafine 250 mg daily with monthly follow-up until the infection is fully cleared.
    - Terbinafine 250 mg daily for 2 weeks.[9] SOR Ⓑ (Terbinafine is available as an inexpensive generic prescription on the $4 and $5 plans in the United States. It also has fewer drug interactions than itraconazole. For these reasons it is usually the preferred treatment when an oral agent is needed.)

SECOND LINE

- Itraconazole 200 mg daily for 1 week.[8] SOR Ⓑ (More expensive with more drug interactions than terbinafine.)
    - Itraconazole 100 mg daily for 2 weeks.[8] SOR Ⓑ
- Fluconazole 200 mg weekly for 4 weeks produced a 100% cure in the study of tinea corporis in wrestlers.[10]

PREVENTION

Tinea corporis and cruris are dermatophyte infections that are particularly common in areas of excessive heat and moisture. A dry, cool environment may play a role in reducing infection. In addition, avoiding contact with farm animals and other individuals infected with tinea corporis and cruris may help in preventing infection. Preventative measures for tinea infections include practicing good personal hygiene; keeping the skin dry and cool at all times; and avoiding sharing towels, clothing, or hair accessories with infected individuals.[11]

In individuals involved in contact sports such as wrestling, a comprehensive skin disease prevention protocol includes some combination of the following: washing of wrestling mats before and after each practice and competition; showers before and after each practice; use of clean clothing before each practice; and exclusion of infected athletes.[12]

For wrestling teams, consider giving fluconazole 100 mg daily for 3 days twice per season to each wrestler.[13] In the study that supports this recommendation, the incidence rate of tinea gladiatorum dropped from 67.4% to 3.5% over a 10-year study.[13] SOR Ⓑ

PATIENT EDUCATION

Keep the skin clean and dry. Use the topical or oral antifungal according to directions. If the rash persists after the treatment, schedule an appointment for further evaluation. Infected pets should be treated.

FOLLOW-UP

Consider follow-up appointments in 4 to 6 weeks for difficult and more widespread cases. If there are concerns about bacterial superinfection, follow-up should be sooner.

PATIENT RESOURCES

- Skinsight. *Ringworm*—**http://www.skinsight.com/skin-conditions/adult/tinea-corporis-ringworm-of-body.htm.**
- MedlinePlus Medical Encyclopedia—**http://medlineplus.gov/ency/article/000877.htm.**

PROVIDER RESOURCES

- KOH preparation and interpretation video (4 minutes by Dr. Usatine)—**https://www.youtube.com/watch?v=LUwNQI_0BWU&t=2s.**
- Swartz Lamkins fungal stain can be purchased online at: **http://www.delasco.com/pcat/1/Chemicals/Swartz_Lamkins/dlmis023/.**

REFERENCES

1. El-Gohary M, van Zuuren EJ, Fedorowicz Z, et al. Topical antifungal treatments for tinea cruris and tinea corporis. *Cochrane Database Syst Rev*. 2014;(8):CD009992.
2. Foster KW, Ghannoum MA, Elewski BE. Epidemiologic surveillance of cutaneous fungal infection in the United States from 1999 to 2002. *J Am Acad Dermatol*. 2004;50(5):748-752.
3. Adams BB. Tinea corporis gladiatorum. *J Am Acad Dermatol*. 2002;47(2):286-290.
4. Crawford F, Hollis S. Topical treatments for fungal infections of the skin and nails of the foot. *Cochrane Database Syst Rev*. 2007;(3):CD001434.

5. Thomas B. Clear choices in managing epidermal tinea infections. *J Fam Pract.* 52(11):850-862.
6. Budimulja U, Bramono K, Urip KS, et al. Once daily treatment with terbinafine 1% cream (Lamisil) for one week is effective in the treatment of tinea corporis and cruris. A placebo-controlled study. *Mycoses.* 2001;44(7-8):300-306.
7. Lebwohl M, Elewski B, Eisen D, Savin RC. Efficacy and safety of terbinafine 1% solution in the treatment of interdigital tinea pedis and tinea corporis or tinea cruris. *Cutis.* 2001;67(3):261-266.
8. Boonk W, De GD, De KE, et al. Itraconazole in the treatment of tinea corporis and tinea cruris: comparison of two treatment schedules. *Mycoses.* 2008;41(11-12):509-514.
9. Voravutinon V. Oral treatment of tinea corporis and tinea cruris with terbinafine and griseofulvin: a randomized double blind comparative study. *J Med Assoc Thai.* 1993;76(7):388-393.
10. Kohl TD, Martin DC, Nemeth R, et al. Fluconazole for the prevention and treatment of tinea gladiatorum. *Pediatr Infect Dis J.* 2000;19(8):717-722.
11. Gupta AK, Chaudhry M, Elewski B. Tinea corporis, tinea cruris, tinea nigra, and piedra. *Dermatol Clin.* 2003;21(3):395-400, v.
12. Hand JW, Wroble RR. Prevention of tinea corporis in collegiate wrestlers. *J Athl Train.* 1999;34(4):350-352.
13. Brickman K, Einstein E, Sinha S, et al. Fluconazole as a prophylactic measure for tinea gladiatorum in high school wrestlers. *Clin J Sport Med.* 2009;19(5):412-414.

145 TINEA CRURIS

Richard P. Usatine, MD
Mindy A. Smith, MD, MS

PATIENT STORY

A 59-year-old man presents with itching in the groin (**Figure 145-1**). On examination, he was found to have scaly erythematous plaques in the inguinal area. A KOH preparation was performed with Swartz Lamkins stain, and the dermatophyte was highly visible under the microscope (**Figure 145-2**). He was treated with a topical antifungal medicine until his tinea cruris resolved.

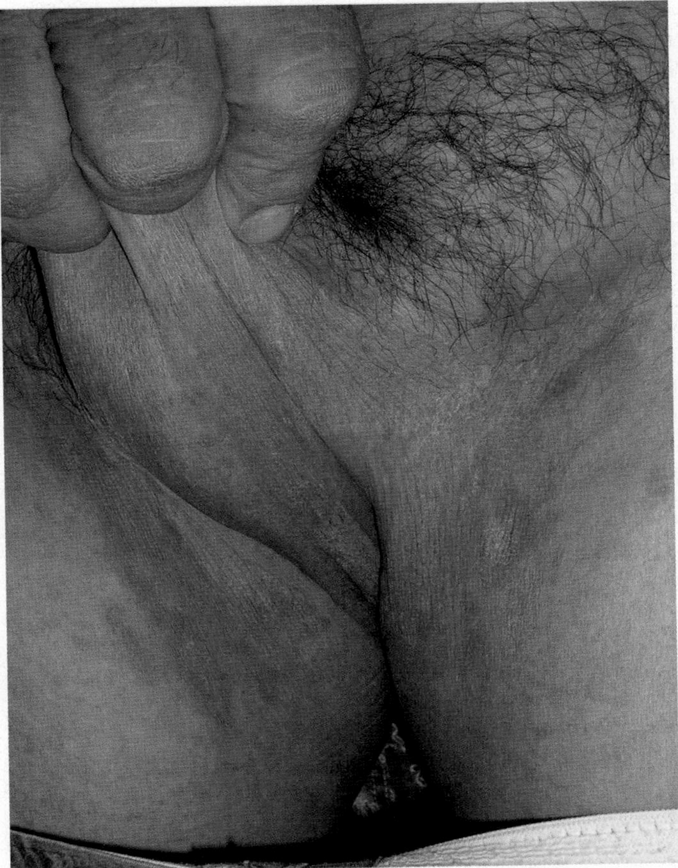

FIGURE 145-1 Tinea cruris in a 59-year-old Hispanic man present for 1 year. (*Reproduced with permission from Richard P. Usatine, MD.*)

INTRODUCTION

Tinea cruris is a pruritic superficial infection of the groin and adjacent skin caused by a dermatophyte fungus.

SYNONYMS

Common names: Crotch rot and jock itch.

EPIDEMIOLOGY

- It is estimated that 10% to 20% of the world population is affected by fungal skin infections.[1]
- Dermatophytes are the most prevalent agents causing fungal infections of the skin.[2]
- *Trichophyton rubrum* causes the majority of cases of tinea cruris.[2]
- Tinea cruris is more common in men than women (threefold) and rare in children.

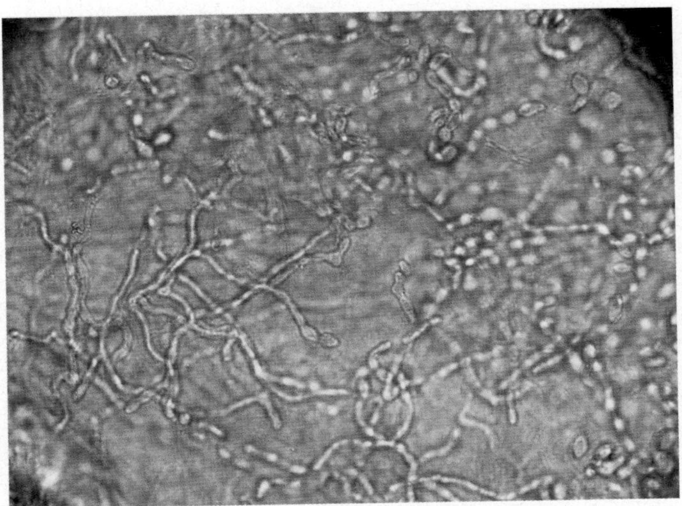

FIGURE 145-2 Microscopic view of the scraping of the groin in a man with tinea cruris. The hyphae are easy to see under 40× power with Swartz Lamkins stain. (*Reproduced with permission from Richard P. Usatine, MD.*)

ETIOLOGY AND PATHOPHYSIOLOGY

- Caused by the dermatophytes *Trichophyton rubrum, Epidermophyton floccosum, Trichophyton mentagrophytes,* and *Trichophyton verrucosum.*
- Can be spread by fomites, such as contaminated towels.
- The dermatophytes release keratinases, which allow invasion of the cornified cell layer of the epidermis.
- Autoinoculation can occur from fungus on the feet or hands.

RISK FACTORS

- Wearing tight-fitting or wet clothing or underwear has traditionally been suggested; however, in a study of Italian soldiers, none of the risk factors analyzed (e.g., hyperhidrosis, swimming pool attendance) were significantly associated with any fungal infection.[3]

- Obesity and diabetes mellitus may be risk factors.[4]

DIAGNOSIS

CLINICAL FEATURES

The cardinal features are scale and signs of inflammation. In light-skinned persons inflammation often appears pink or red, and in dark-skinned persons the inflammation often leads to hyperpigmentation (**Figures 145-3** and **145-4**). Occasionally, tinea cruris may show central sparing with an annular pattern as in **Figure 145-5**, but most often is homogeneously distributed as in **Figures 145-3** and **145-4**.

TYPICAL DISTRIBUTION

By definition tinea cruris is in the inguinal area. However, the fungus can grow outside of this area to involve the abdomen and thighs (**Figures 145-4** and **145-6**). Tinea can be present in multiple locations, as in the patient in **Figure 145-7,** who had tinea in the groin, on her feet and face, and under her breasts.

LABORATORY STUDIES

Diagnosis is often made based on clinical presentation, but a skin scraping treated with KOH and a fungal stain analyzed under the microscope can be helpful (see **Figure 145-2**). False negatives may occur if scraping is inadequate, the patient is using topical antifungals, or the viewer is inexperienced.

Skin scraping and culture is definitive but expensive and may take up to 2 weeks for the culture to grow.

UV lamp can be used to look for the coral red fluorescence of erythrasma (see Chapter 125, Erythrasma). Since most tinea cruris is caused by *T. rubrum*, it will not fluoresce.

DIFFERENTIAL DIAGNOSIS

- Cutaneous *Candida* in the groin can become red and have scaling that extends to the thigh and scrotum. Tinea cruris does not often involve the scrotum. *Candida* often has satellite lesions (see Chapter 142, Candidiasis).
- Erythrasma in the groin appears similar to tinea cruris but has a less well demarcated border. It is less common than tinea cruris and may show coral red fluorescence with a UV light (**Figure 145-8**) (see Chapter 125, Erythrasma). If the KOH preparation is negative, consider using a UV light to examine the groin and interdigital spaces of the toes (erythrasma may be found between the toes just as in tinea pedis).
- Contact dermatitis can occur anywhere on the body. If the contact is near the groin this can be mistaken for tinea cruris (see Chapter 152, Contact Dermatitis).
- Inverse psoriasis causes inflammation in the intertriginous areas of the body. It does not have the thick plaques of plaque psoriasis. Inverse psoriasis is frequently misdiagnosed as a fungal infection until an astute clinician recognizes the pattern or does a biopsy (**Figure 145-9**; see Chapter 158, Psoriasis). However, even patients with psoriasis can get tinea cruris (**Figure 145-10**).

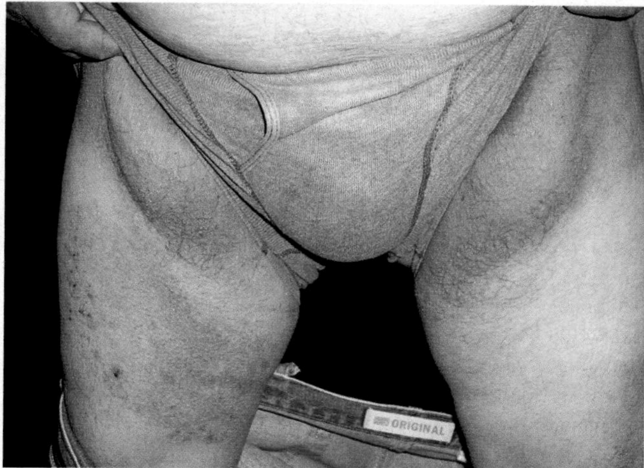

FIGURE 145-3 Tinea cruris and tinea corporis in a Hispanic man with hyperpigmentation secondary to the inflammatory response. KOH positive. (*Reproduced with permission from Richard P. Usatine, MD.*)

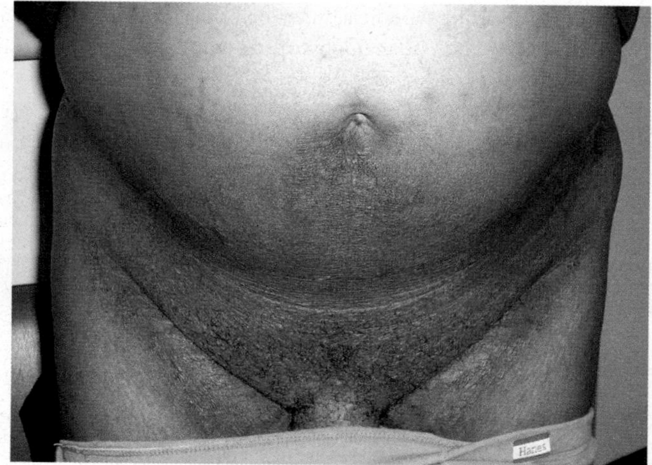

FIGURE 145-4 Tinea cruris that has expanded beyond the inguinal area in this 35-year-old black man. Postinflammatory hyperpigmentation is visible throughout the infected area. (*Reproduced with permission from Richard P. Usatine, MD.*)

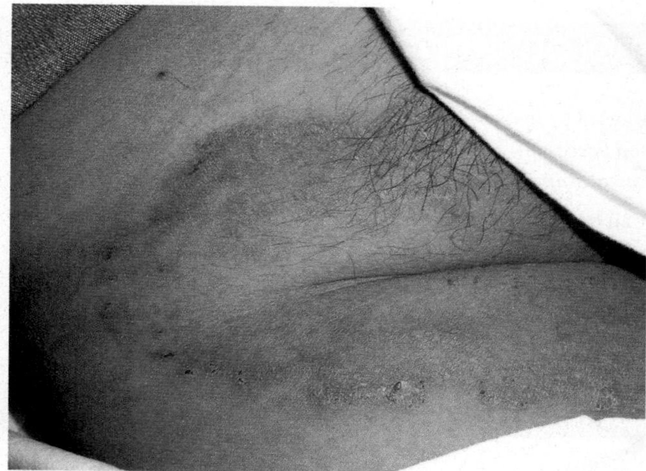

FIGURE 145-5 An 18-year-old woman with tinea cruris showing erythema and scale in an annular pattern. Central clearing is less common in tinea cruris than tinea corporis but can occur. (*Reproduced with permission from Richard P. Usatine, MD.*)

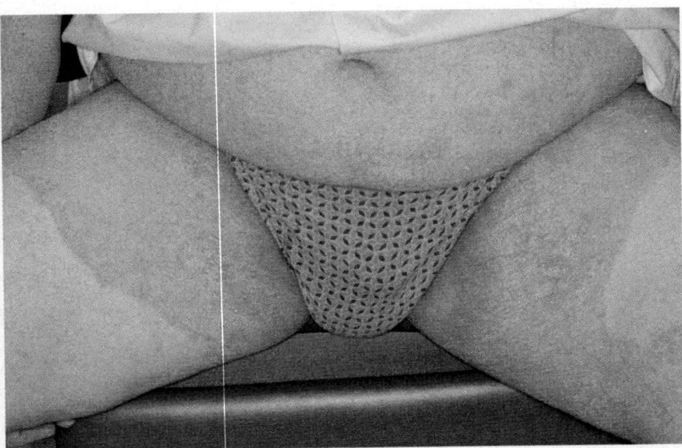

FIGURE 145-6 A 54-year-old man with tinea cruris and corporis for decades despite multiple treatments with oral antifungal medications. His cultures show *T. rubrum* sensitive to all the typical oral antifungal medications, but his tinea never completely clears. He does not have a known immunodeficiency but his immune system appears not to recognize the *T. rubrum* as foreign. *(Reproduced with permission from Richard P. Usatine, MD.)*

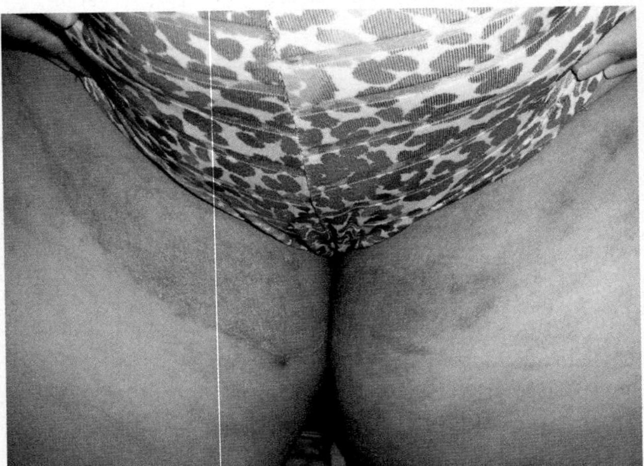

FIGURE 145-7 A 56-year-old woman with tinea cruris showing erythema and scale with well-demarcated borders. Although less common in women, women do get tinea cruris. This patient has had tinea cruris in the past. Despite being treated with oral terbinafine with clinical clearance, this is a recurrence of her tinea cruris. *(Reproduced with permission from Richard P. Usatine, MD.)*

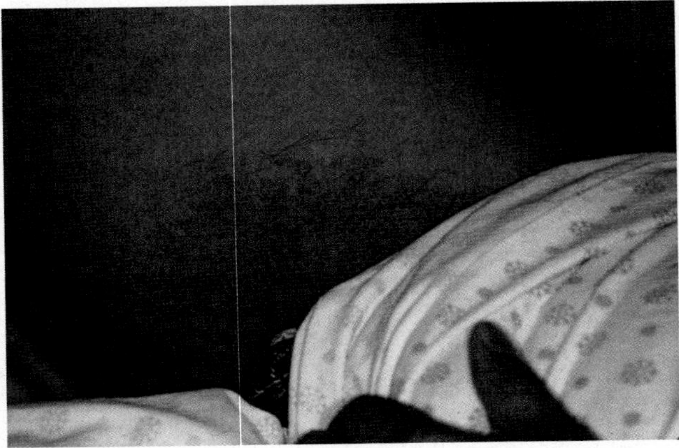

FIGURE 145-8 Erythrasma in the groin can be mistaken for tinea cruris. This erythrasma fluoresced coral red with an ultraviolet light. *(Reproduced with permission from Richard P. Usatine, MD.)*

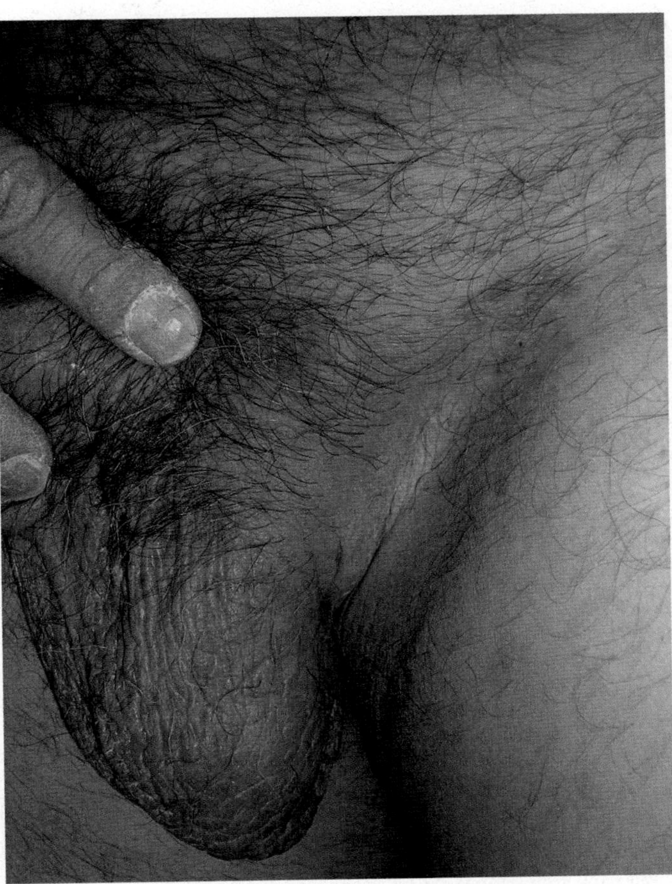

FIGURE 145-9 Inverse psoriasis in a man who also has the nail changes of psoriasis. *(Reproduced with permission from Richard P. Usatine, MD.)*

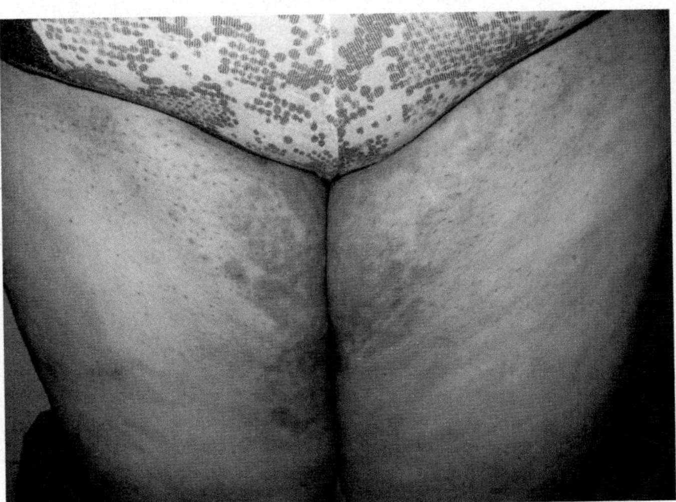

FIGURE 145-10 Tinea cruris presenting as tinea incognito in a young woman with psoriasis who applied her high-potency steroid to a new rash in her groin and thighs assuming that it was psoriasis. It continued to worsen until she presented to the office and a KOH preparation was positive for branching hyphae. It resolved with 2 weeks of oral terbinafine. *(Reproduced with permission from Richard P. Usatine, MD.)*

- Majochi granuloma (**Figure 145-11**) is a type of tinea in which the fungus has gone deep into the hair follicles and creates a granulomatous appearance. This may be caused by the application of topical steroids so that this is a deep type of tinea incognito in some cases. It is a deep and persistent suppurative folliculitis so that pustules and nodules may be present along with the superficial erythema and scale.
- Intertrigo is an inflammatory condition of the skin folds. It is induced or aggravated by heat, moisture, maceration, and friction. It is a nonspecific diagnosis, and the condition frequently is worsened by infection with *Candida* or dermatophytes.[5] It is best to look for an etiology and reserve this diagnosis for cases where no etiology is found.

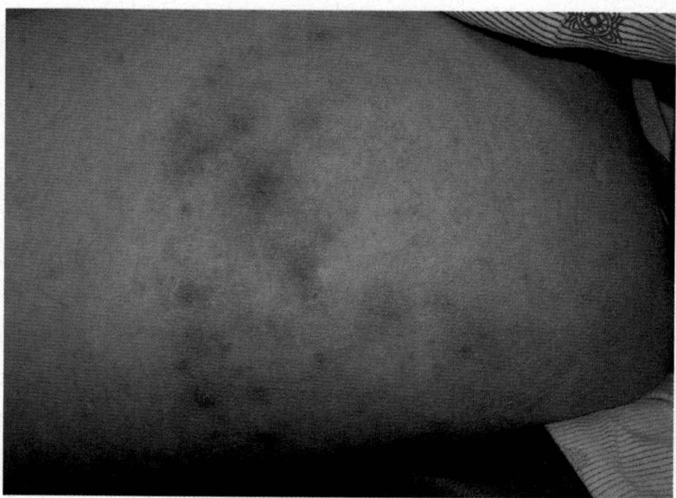

FIGURE 145-11 Majochi granuloma in an HIV-positive man who has been applying a topical steroid to a case of tinea cruris. He has painful and deep nodules where the dermatophyte has penetrated the skin surrounding his hair follicles. Months of oral terbinafine were needed to clear this fungal infection. (*Reproduced with permission from Richard P. Usatine, MD.*)

MANAGEMENT

FIRST LINE

- Tinea cruris is best treated with a topical allylamine or an azole antifungal (SOR Ⓐ, based on multiple randomized controlled trials [RCTs]).[6] Differences in current comparison data are insufficient to stratify the two groups of topical antifungals.[7] In one RCT, cure rates were higher at 1 week with butenafine (once daily for 2 weeks) versus clotrimazole (twice daily for 4 weeks) (26.5% vs. 2.9%, respectively), but were not significantly different at 4 or 8 weeks.[8]
- The fungicidal allylamines (naftifine and terbinafine) and butenafine (allylamine derivative) are more convenient as they allow for a shorter duration of treatment compared with fungistatic azoles (clotrimazole, econazole, ketoconazole, oxiconazole, miconazole, and sulconazole).[7]
- Topical azoles should be continued for 4 weeks and topical allylamines for 2 weeks or until clinical cure.[6-8] SOR Ⓐ
- Azole and steroid combination creams were slightly more effective in achieving clinical cure compared to azoles alone immediately at the end of treatment (relative risk [RR] 0.67, number needed to treat [NNT] 6), but there was no difference in mycologic cure rate (RR 0.99). The quality of evidence for these two outcomes was rated as low.[1] SOR Ⓑ

SECOND LINE

- Systemic treatment with oral antifungals is second line when topical antifungal agents fail but are first-line therapy in widespread cases of tinea cruris in which large areas are involved (see **Figures 145-4** and **145-6**). Of course, it is important to make sure that the failure of topical antifungal agents is not due to a missed diagnosis of inverse psoriasis, which is a common look-alike condition with tinea cruris.
- Oral terbinafine 250 mg daily for 2 weeks is the oral treatment of choice. Patients with mycologically diagnosed tinea cruris were randomly allocated to receive either 250 mg of oral terbinafine once daily or 500 mg of griseofulvin once daily for 2 weeks. The cure rates were higher for terbinafine at 6 weeks.[9] SOR Ⓑ
- Fluconazole 150 mg once weekly for 2 to 4 weeks appears to be effective in the treatment of tinea cruris.[10] SOR Ⓑ
- One RCT showed that itraconazole 200 mg for 1 week is similarly effective, equally well tolerated, and at least as safe as itraconazole 100 mg for 2 weeks in the treatment of tinea corporis or cruris

(clinical response: 73% and 80% at the end of follow-up, respectively).[11] SOR B

- Majochi granuloma (which involves hair follicles) can be especially difficult to treat and requires oral antifungals just like tinea capitis. It might actually require months of terbinafine 250 mg daily with monthly follow-up until the infection is fully cleared.
- If there are multiple sites infected with fungus, treat all active areas of infection simultaneously to prevent reinfection of the groin from other body sites.

FOLLOW-UP

As needed.

PATIENT EDUCATION

- Advise patients with tinea pedis to put on their socks before their undershorts to reduce the possibility of direct contamination. SOR C
- Dry the groin completely after bathing. SOR C

PATIENT RESOURCES

- Medscape Family Medicine. *Tinea Cruris in Men: Bothersome but Treatable*—**http://www.medscape.com/viewarticle/512992.**
- MedlinePlus. *Jock Itch*—**http://medlineplus.gov/ency/article/000876.htm.**

PROVIDER RESOURCES

- DermNet NZ. *Fungal Skin Infections*—**http://www.dermnetnz.org/fungal-skin-infection/.**
- KOH preparation and interpretation video (4 minutes by Dr. Usatine)—**https://www.youtube.com/watch?v=LUwNQI_0BWU&t=2s.**
- Medscape. *Tinea Cruris*—**http://emedicine.medscape.com/article/1091806.**

REFERENCES

1. El-Gohary M, van Zuuren EJ, Fedorowicz Z, et al. Topical antifungal treatments for tinea cruris and tinea corporis. *Cochrane Database Syst Rev.* 2014;(8):CD009992.
2. Foster KW, Ghannoum MA, Elewski BE. Epidemiologic surveillance of cutaneous fungal infection in the United States from 1999 to 2002. *J Am Acad Dermatol.* 2004;50(5):748-752.
3. Ingordo V, Naldi L, Fracchiolla S, Colecchia B. Prevalence and risk factors for superficial fungal infections among Italian Navy cadets. *Dermatology.* 2004;209(3):190-196.
4. Patel GA, Wiederkehr M, Schwartz RA. Tinea cruris in children. *Cutis.* 2009;84(3):133-137.
5. Selden ST. *Intertrigo*, http://emedicine.medscape.com/article/1087691-overview, accessed September 2017.
6. Drake LA, Dinehart SM, Farmer ER, et al. Guidelines of care for superficial mycotic infections of the skin: tinea corporis, tinea cruris, tinea faciei, tinea manuum, and tinea pedis. Guidelines/Outcomes Committee. American Academy of Dermatology. *J Am Acad Dermatol.* 1996;34(2 Pt 1):282-286.
7. Nadalo D, Montoya C, Hunter-Smith D. What is the best way to treat tinea cruris? *J Fam Pract.* 2006;55:256-258.
8. Singal A, Pandhi D, Agrawal S, Das S. Comparative efficacy of topical 1% butenafine and 1% clotrimazole in tinea cruris and tinea corporis: a randomized, double-blind trial. *J Dermatolog Treat.* 2005;16(506):331-335.
9. Voravutinon V. Oral treatment of tinea corporis and tinea cruris with terbinafine and griseofulvin: a randomized double blind comparative study. *J Med Assoc Thai.* 1993;76:388-393.
10. Nozickova M, Koudelkova V, Kulikova Z, et al. A comparison of the efficacy of oral fluconazole, 150 mg/week versus 50 mg/day, in the treatment of tinea corporis, tinea cruris, tinea pedis, and cutaneous candidosis. *Int J Dermatol.* 1998;37:703-705.
11. Boonk W, de Geer D, de Kreek E, et al. Itraconazole in the treatment of tinea corporis and tinea cruris: comparison of two treatment schedules. *Mycoses.* 1998;41:509-514.

146 TINEA PEDIS

Richard P. Usatine, MD
Catherine Reppa, MD

PATIENT STORY

A 34-year-old woman presents with an itching rash on both feet for the past 6 months (**Figure 146-1**). She is in otherwise good health and has occasionally tried some over-the-counter (OTC) athlete's foot medicine for this rash with slight improvement. On physical exam, the patient has erythema and scale in the moccasin distribution as well as some of her interdigital spaces. A KOH preparation is positive for branching hyphae with visible nuclei enhanced by the Schwartz Lamkins stain (**Figure 146-2**). Patient denies a history of hepatitis or heavy alcohol use and would like to try an oral medication because she is tired of the itching. The patient is given oral terbinafine 250 mg daily for 2 weeks.

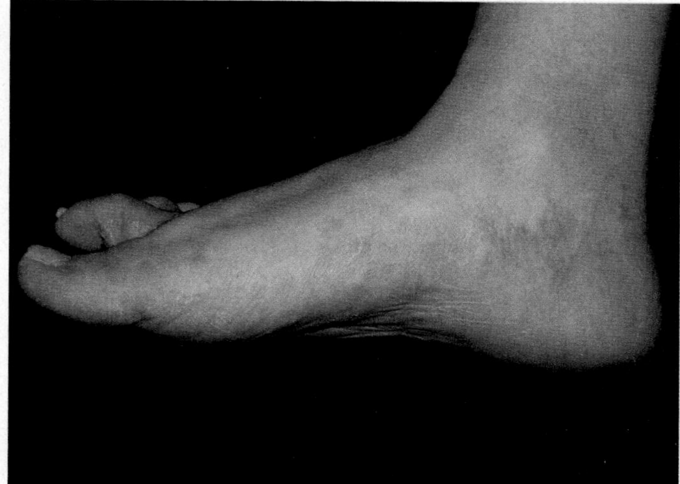

FIGURE 146-1 Tinea pedis in the moccasin and interdigital distribution. *(Reproduced with permission from Richard P. Usatine, MD.)*

INTRODUCTION

Tinea pedis is a common cutaneous infection of the feet caused by dermatophyte fungus. The clinical manifestation presents in 1 of 3 major patterns: interdigital, moccasin, and inflammatory/vesicular. Concurrent fungal infection of the nails (onychomycosis) occurs frequently.

SYNONYMS

Athlete's foot.

EPIDEMIOLOGY

- Tinea pedis is the most common human dermatophytosis.[1]
- 70% of the population will be infected with tinea pedis at some time.[1]
- Prevalence increases with age and it is less common before adolescence.[1]

ETIOLOGY AND PATHOPHYSIOLOGY

- A cutaneous fungal infection most commonly caused by *Trichophyton rubrum*.[1]
- *Trichophyton mentagrophytes* and *Epidermophyton floccosum* follow in that order.
- *T. rubrum* causes most tinea pedis and onychomycosis.

RISK FACTORS

- Use of public showers, baths or pools—especially if protective footwear is not used.[2]
- Household member with tinea pedis infection.[2]

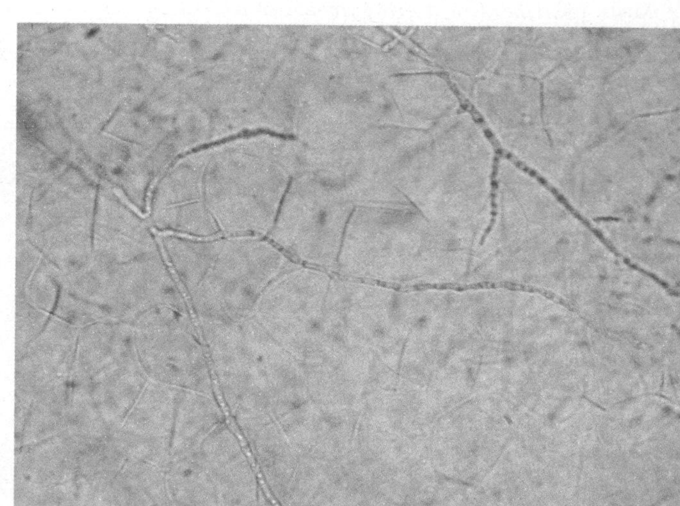

FIGURE 146-2 Microscopic view of the KOH preparation showing branching hyphae with nuclei that are easy to see under 40× power with Swartz Lamkins stain. *(Reproduced with permission from Richard P. Usatine, MD.)*

- Certain occupations (miners, farmers, soldiers, meat factory workers)—especially where there is use of heavy boots and the feet are warm and sweaty.[2]
- Persons experiencing homelessness.[3]

DIAGNOSIS

TYPICAL DISTRIBUTION AND MORPHOLOGY

Three types of tinea pedis:

- Interdigital type (intertriginous type)—very common (**Figure 146-3**).
- Moccasin type—very common (**Figures 146-1** and **146-4**).
- Vesiculobullous type—least common (**Figures 146-5** and **146-6**).

However, many persons have both the interdigital and moccasin type simultaneously, as seen in **Figure 146-1**. In one prospective study of 135 patients presenting consecutively with tinea pedis, lesions were suggestive of the intertriginous type in 24 patients, moccasin type in 50 patients, and both intertriginous and moccasin type in 58 patients. Among the remaining patients, 1 had the vesiculobullous type and another had both the vesiculobullous and intertriginous types.[4]

In another larger study of 1174 persons, 674 had only interdigital tinea pedis while 500 subjects had a moccasin distribution in addition to the interdigital presentation.[5]

Some authors describe an ulcerative type (**Figure 146-7**).

CLINICAL FEATURES

- Interdigital—white or green fungal growth between toes with erythema, maceration, cracks, and fissures—especially between fourth and fifth digits (see **Figure 146-3**). The dry type has more scale, and the moist type becomes macerated.
- Moccasin—scale on sides and soles of feet (see **Figures 146-1** and **146-4**).
- Vesiculobullous—vesicles and bullae on feet (see **Figures 146-5** and **146-6**).
- Ulcerative tinea pedis is characterized by rapidly spreading vesiculopustular lesions, ulcers, and erosions, typically in the web spaces (see **Figure 146-7**). It is accompanied by a secondary bacterial infection. This can lead to cellulitis or lymphangitis. Tinea pedis is a proven risk factor for nonpurulent leg cellulitis.[6]
- Examine nails for evidence of onychomycosis—fungal infections of nails may include subungual keratosis, yellow or white discolorations, dysmorphic nails (Chapter 201, Onychomycosis).
- Autoeczematization (dermatophytid reaction; Id reaction) is an uncommon hypersensitivity response to a fungal infection causing papules on the skin (**Figure 146-8**).

TYPICAL DISTRIBUTION

Between the toes, on the soles, and lateral aspects of the feet.

LABORATORY STUDIES

The most rapid method to confirm a clinical diagnosis is the KOH preparation. The involved skin is scraped with side of the microscope slide or a scalpel onto another slide. The slide is then prepared with

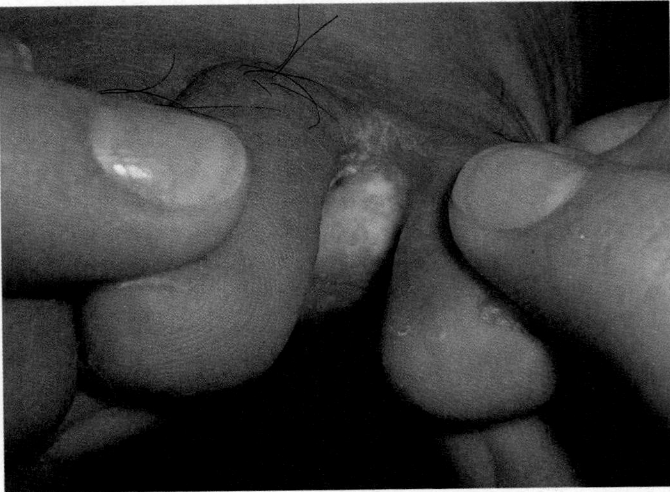

FIGURE 146-3 Tinea pedis seen in the interdigital space between the fourth and fifth digits. This is the most common area to see tinea pedis. *(Reproduced with permission from Richard P. Usatine, MD.)*

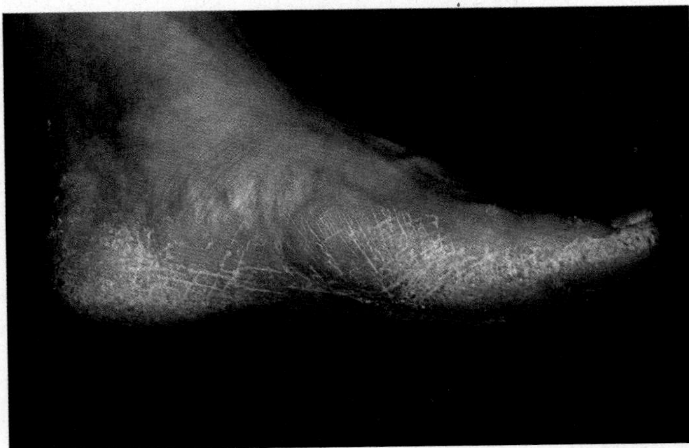

FIGURE 146-4 Tinea pedis in the moccasin distribution. *(Reproduced with permission from Richard P. Usatine, MD.)*

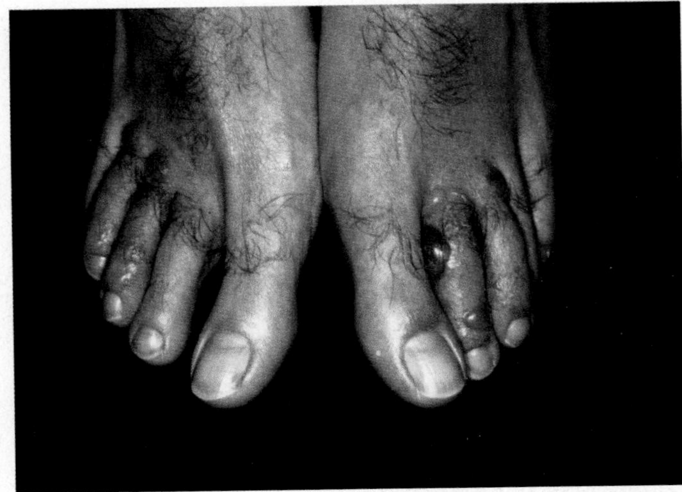

FIGURE 146-5 Vesiculobullous tinea pedis with bullae present. This is an inflammatory reaction to the tinea pedis. *(Reproduced with permission from Richard P. Usatine, MD.)*

KOH or KOH and a fungal stain. The slide is examined for hyphal elements (video https://www.youtube.com/watch?v=LUwNQI_0BWU) (see **Figure 146-2**). One study showed that the use of two KOH preparations from different parts of the suspected tinea pedis provided a substantial increase in diagnostic sensitivity.[4]

In a patient with tinea incognito on his foot and lower leg, the topical steroid masked the symptoms while the tinea spread up his leg (**Figure 146-9**). It took a KOH preparation to demonstrate that this was tinea and not lupus to get the patient the antifungal treatment he needed.

A fungal culture is sometimes needed if one does not have the microscope to do a KOH preparation or if the KOH prep is negative but fungus is still suspected. A fungal culture may take up to 2 weeks for an answer, but the lab can often provide a KOH result within 1–2 days from the same sample. Just scrape the suspected tinea into a sterile urine cup and send to the lab.

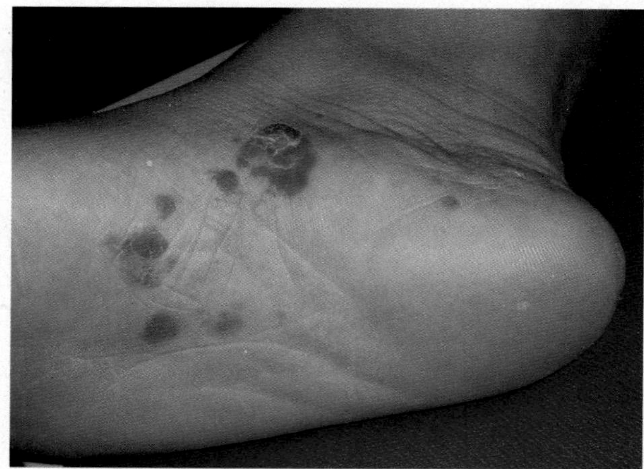

FIGURE 146-6 Vesiculobullous tinea pedis with vesicles and bullae over the arch region of the foot. The arch is a typical location for vesiculobullous tinea pedis. (*Reproduced with permission from Richard P. Usatine, MD.*)

DIFFERENTIAL DIAGNOSIS

- Erythrasma is a bacterial infection found in intertriginous areas. It may appear as maceration between the toes and be mistaken for tinea pedis or coexist with tinea pedis (see **Figures 125-5** and **125-6**). In a study of 182 patients with interdigital lesions in a podiatry clinic, 40% were diagnosed as having erythrasma.[7] Look for coral red fluorescence with a Wood lamp to diagnose erythrasma between the toes. A KOH preparation is helpful to confirm tinea. Fortunately, topical miconazole can treat both erythrasma and interdigital tinea pedis simultaneously[8] (see Chapter 125, Erythrasma).
- Pitted keratolysis: well-demarcated pits or erosions in the sole of the foot caused by bacteria (**Figure 146-10**) (see Chapter 124, Pitted Keratolysis).
- Contact dermatitis tends to be seen on the dorsum and sides of the foot (**Figure 146-11**) (Chapter 152, Contact Dermatitis).
- Keratodermas: thickening of the soles of the feet that can be caused by a number of etiologies, including genetics and menopause (**Figure 146-12**). This condition may look like tinea pedis in the moccasin distribution.
- Dyshidrotic eczema is characterized by scale and tapioca-like vesicles on the hands and feet (**Figure 146-13**) (Chapter 153, Hand Eczema).
- Friction blisters: blisters on the feet of persons leading an active athletic lifestyle.
- Psoriasis can mimic tinea pedis but will usually be present in other areas as well (**Figure 146-14**) (Chapter 158, Psoriasis). Especially on the palms if this is palmarplantar psoriasis.

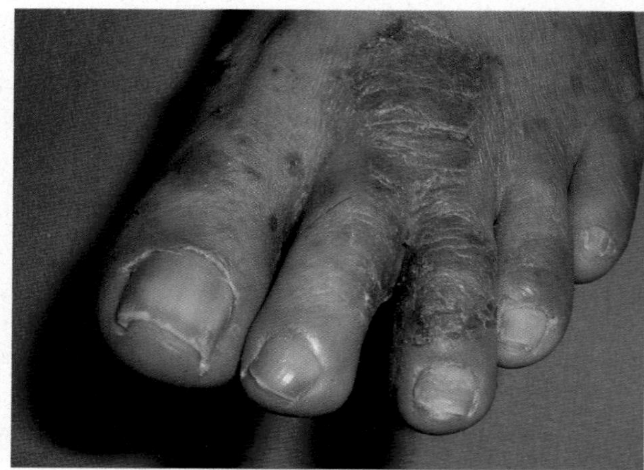

FIGURE 146-7 Ulcerative tinea pedis with spreading vesicles related to a bacterial superinfection. The patient was treated with antifungals and antibiotics. (*Reproduced with permission from Richard P. Usatine, MD.*)

MANAGEMENT

See **Table 146-1** for management of tinea pedis.

FIRST LINE

TOPICAL ANTIFUNGALS

- Systematic review of 70 trials of topical antifungals showed good evidence for efficacy compared to placebo for the following:

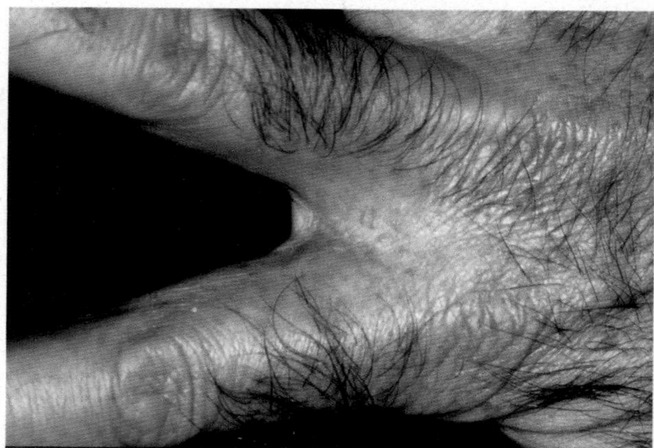

FIGURE 146-8 The hand shows an autoeczematization reaction to the inflammatory tinea pedis in the **Figure 146-5**. The vesicles between the fingers are typical of an autoeczematization reaction, also known as an Id reaction. (*Reproduced with permission from Richard P. Usatine, MD.*)

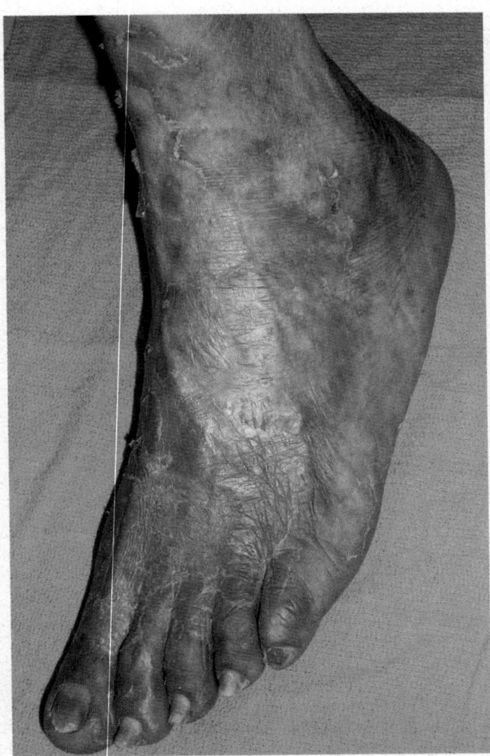

FIGURE 146-9 Tinea incognito on the foot of a 63-year-old black man with lupus. He was given topical steroids that allowed this fungus to spread and thrive. (*Reproduced with permission from Richard P. Usatine, MD.*)

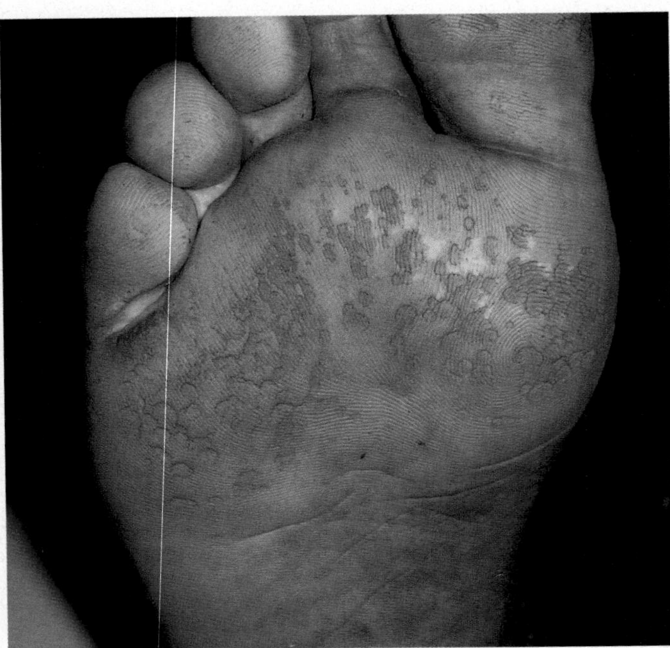

FIGURE 146-10 Pitted keratolysis on the sole of the foot with some interdigital tinea pedis. The pits are caused by bacteria and if not treated with an antibiotic will not resolve. (*Reproduced with permission from Richard P. Usatine, MD.*)

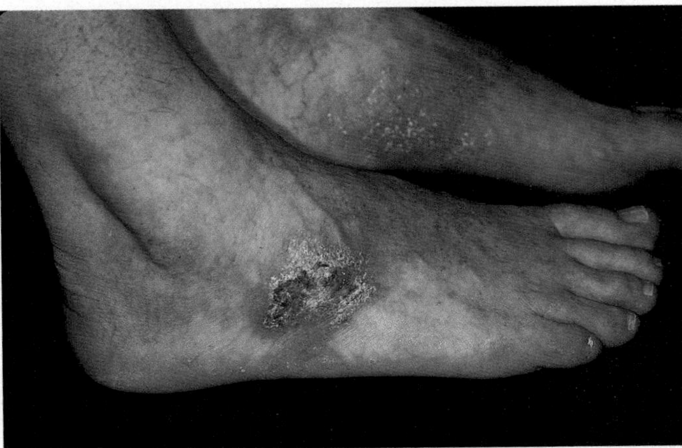

FIGURE 146-11 Contact dermatitis to an allergen in tennis shoes with typical distribution that crosses the dorsum of the foot. (*Reproduced with permission from Richard P. Usatine, MD.*)

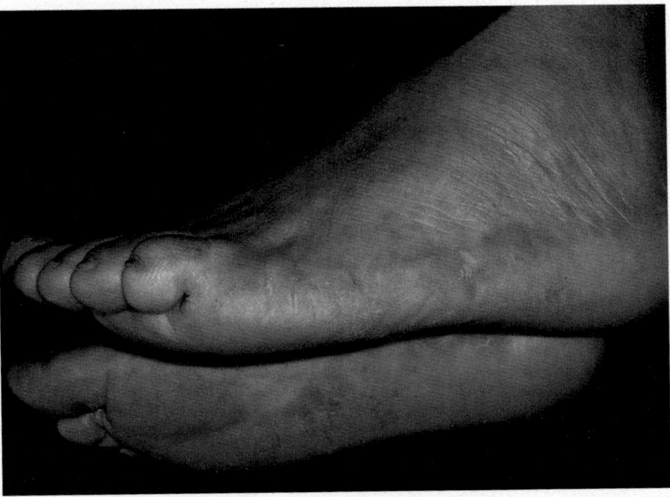

FIGURE 146-12 Keratoderma climactericum, which started when this woman entered menopause. (*Reproduced with permission from Richard P. Usatine, MD.*)

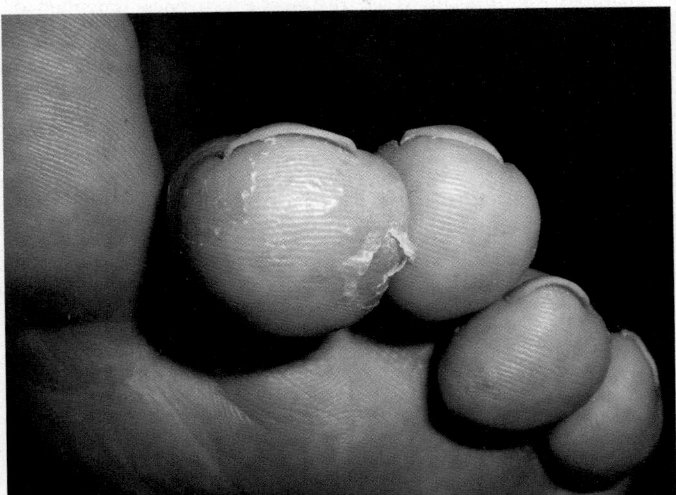

FIGURE 146-13 Dyshidrotic eczema on the foot showing tapioca vesicles with peeling of skin on the tip of the second toe. The patient also has typical tapioca vesicles between the fingers. (*Reproduced with permission from Richard P. Usatine, MD.*)

TABLE 146-1 Management of Tinea Pedis

Tinea Pedis Type	Treatment for Mild Cases	Treatment for Recalcitrant Cases	SOR
Interdigital type	Topical antifungal	Another topical antifungal or an oral antifungal	A
Moccasin type	Topical antifungal	Oral antifungal	A
Vesiculobullous type	Oral antifungal	Oral antifungal	A

Adapted with permission from Thomas B. Clear choices in managing epidermal tinea infections, J Fam Pract. 2003;52(11): 850-862. Frontline Medical Communications Inc.

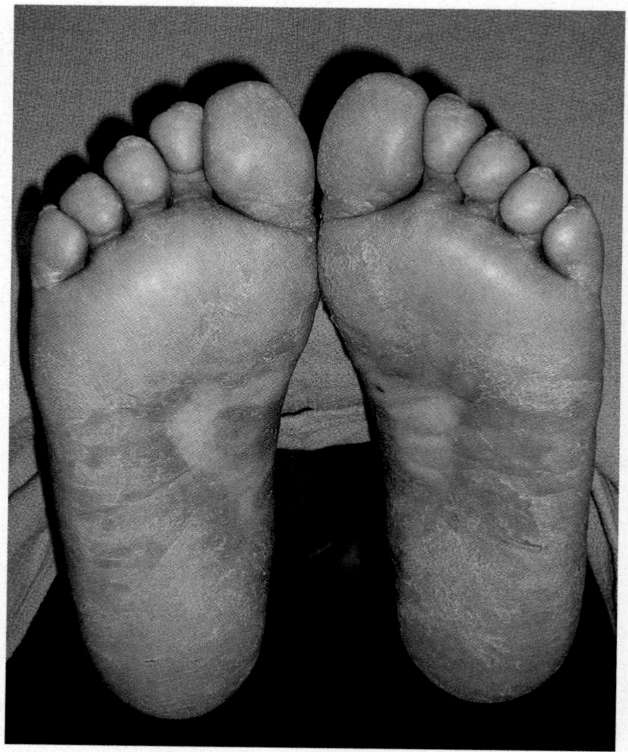

FIGURE 146-14 Plantar psoriasis in a patient with other areas of psoriasis also present. (*Reproduced with permission from Richard P. Usatine, MD.*)

    - Allylamines (naftifine, terbinafine, butenafine)[9] SOR Ⓐ
    - Azoles (clotrimazole, miconazole, econazole)[9] SOR Ⓐ
    - Allylamines cure slightly more infections than azoles[9] SOR Ⓐ
    - No differences in efficacy found between individual allylamines or individual azoles (**Table 146-2**) SOR Ⓐ
- In one meta-analysis, topical terbinafine was found to be equally effective as other topical antifungals, but the average duration of treatment was shorter (1 week instead of 2 weeks).[10] SOR Ⓐ
- Topical terbinafine is a great first-line choice for tinea pedis because of its affordable cost as an OTC cream. SOR Ⓒ
- The moccasin distribution is more challenging to treat topically. In one large study, Naftifine gel 2% (Rx only) and vehicle treatment were applied once daily for 2 weeks.[5] Then at week 6, the cure rates in the naftifine arm vs. the vehicle were statistically higher for mycologic cure rate (65.8% vs. 7.8%), treatment effectiveness (51.4% vs 4.4%), and complete cure rate (19.2% vs. 0.9%) for moccasin-type tinea pedis.[5] Note that mycologic cure is defined as a negative dermatophyte culture and KOH, treatment effectiveness is defined as mycologic cure and symptom severity scores of 0 or 1, and complete cure is defined as mycologic cure and symptoms severity scores of 0. While naftifine gel was much better than vehicle, the data demonstrate that there may be significant failure to cure this type of tinea pedis and one should then consider oral antifungal treatment.
- Luliconazole cream has recently been FDA approved for interdigital tinea pedis. It requires a prescription, and one tube is over $400. There are currently no data to recommend it over the inexpensive OTC topical antifungals.

SECOND LINE

ORAL ANTIFUNGALS

- In a Cochrane systematic review of 15 trials involving 1438 participants, the evidence suggests that terbinafine is more effective than griseofulvin.[11] SOR Ⓐ
- In the same review, terbinafine or itraconazole are more effective than no treatment.[11] SOR Ⓐ

TABLE 146-2 Topical Antifungal Medications

Agent	Formulation	Frequency*	Duration* (weeks)	NNT†
Imidazoles				
Clotrimazole	1% cream 1% solution 1% swabs	Twice daily	2 to 4	2.9
Econazole	1% cream	Twice daily	2 to 4	2.6
Ketoconazole	2% cream	Once daily	2 to 4	No data available
Luliconazole	1% cream	Once daily	2	No data available
Miconazole	2% cream 2% spray 2% powder	Twice daily	2 to 4	2.8 (at 8 weeks)
Oxiconazole	1% cream 1% lotion	Once to twice daily	2 to 4	2.9
Sulconazole	1% cream 1% solution	Once to twice daily	2 to 4	2.5
Allylamines				
Naftifine	1% cream 1% gel	Once to twice daily	1 to 4	1.9
Terbinafine	1% cream 1% solution	Once to twice daily	1 to 4	1.6
Benzylamine				
Butenafine	1% cream	Once to twice daily	1 to 4	1.9
Other				
Ciclopirox	0.77% cream 0.77% lotion	Twice daily	2 to 4	2.1
Tolnaftate	1% powder 1% spray 1% swabs	Twice daily	4	3.6 (at 8 weeks)

*Manufacturer guidelines.
†NNT, number needed to treat. NNT is calculated from systematic review of all randomized controlled trials for tinea pedis at 6 weeks after the initiation of treatment except where otherwise noted.
Adapted with permission from Thomas B. Clear choices in managing epidermal tinea infections, J Fam Pract. 2003;52(11):850-862. Frontline Medical Communications Inc..

- No significant difference was detected between terbinafine and itraconazole, fluconazole and itraconazole, fluconazole and ketoconazole, or griseofulvin and ketoconazole, although the trials were generally small.[11] SOR Ⓐ
- Terbinafine is the oral treatment of choice, as it is very affordable being on the $4 and $5 lists at many pharmacies. It is at least as effective as other oral agents and more effective than griseofulvin. It has no more side effects or precautions than other oral antifungal agents. The dosing is 250 mg PO daily for 2 weeks. Avoid use if there is hepatic impairment, absolute neutrophil count (ANC) <1000, or creatinine clearance less than 50.

Patients with onychomycosis may have recurrences of the skin infection related to the fungus that remains in the nails and, therefore, may need oral treatment for 3 months to achieve better results.

Topical ammonium lactate (6% or 12%) and urea (10% to 40%) may be useful to decrease scaling in patients with hyperkeratotic soles in addition to treating their tinea pedis.

ALTERNATIVE THERAPY

One small pilot study with 56 participants showed significant improvement or resolution of symptoms in patients treated by wearing socks containing copper-oxide fibers daily for a minimum of 8 to 10 days.[12] SOR Ⓑ

PATIENT EDUCATION

- Do not go barefoot in public showers and locker rooms. Shower shoes may prevent tinea pedis. SOR Ⓒ

- Keep feet dry and clean, and use clean socks and shoes that allow the feet to get fresh air. SOR Ⓒ
- Use the topical antifungal medication again if recurrence occurs. SOR Ⓒ

PATIENT RESOURCES

- eMedicineHealth. *Athlete's Foot*—**http://www.emedicinehealth.com/athletes_foot/article_em.htm.**

PROVIDER RESOURCES

- Video on KOH preparation by Dr. Usatine—**https://www.youtube.com/watch?v=LUwNQI_0BWU.**
- Medscape. *Tinea Pedis*—**http://emedicine.medscape.com/article/1091684.**

REFERENCES

1. Robbins C. *Tinea Pedis*. http://emedicine.medscape.com/article/1091684. Accessed September 2017.
2. Seebacher C, Bouchara JP, Mignon B. Updates on the epidemiology of dermatophyte infections. *Mycopathologia*. 2008;166(5-6):335-352.
3. To MJ, Brothers TD, Van Zoost C. Foot Conditions among homeless persons: a systematic review. *PLoS One*. 2016;11(12):e0167463.
4. Karaman B, Topal S, Aksungur V, et al. Successive potassium hydroxide testing for improved diagnosis of tinea pedis. *Cutis*. 2017;100:110-114.
5. Stein Gold LF, Vlahovic T, Verma A, et al. Naftifine hydrochloride gel 2%: an effective topical treatment for moccasin-type tinea pedis. *J Drugs Dermatol*. 2015;14(10):1138-1144.
6. Quirke M, Ayoub F, McCabe A, et al. Risk factors for nonpurulent leg cellulitis: a systematic review and meta-analysis. *Br J Dermatol*. 2017;177(2):382-394.
7. Polat M, İlhan MN. The prevalence of interdigital erythrasma: a prospective study from an outpatient clinic in Turkey. *J Am Podiatr Med Assoc*. 2015;105(2):121-124.
8. Clayton YM, Knight AG. A clinical double-blind trial of topical miconazole and clotrimazole against superficial fungal infections and erythrasma. *Clin Exp Dermatol*. 1976;1(3):225-232.
9. Crawford F, Hollis S. Topical treatments for fungal infections of the skin and nails of the foot. *Cochrane Database Syst Rev*. 2007;(3):CD001434.
10. Kienke P, Korting HC, Nelles S, Rychlik R. Comparable efficacy and safety of various topical formulations of terbinafine in tinea pedis irrespective of the treatment regimen: results of a meta-analysis. *Am J Clin Dermatol* 2007;8(6):357-364.
11. Bell-Syer SE, Khan SM, Torgerson DJ. Oral treatments for fungal infections of the skin of the foot. *Cochrane Database Syst Rev*. 2012;10:CD003584.
12. Zatcoff RC, Smith MS, Borkow G. Treatment of tinea pedis with socks containing copper-oxide impregnated fibers. *Foot (Edinb)*. 2008;18(3):136-141.

147 TINEA VERSICOLOR

Richard P. Usatine, MD
Phyllis D. MacGilvray, MD

PATIENT STORY

A young black man presents to the office with a 5-year history of white spots on his trunk (**Figure 147-1**). He denies any symptoms but worries if this could spread to his girlfriend. These spots get worse during the summer months but never go away completely. He was relieved to receive a treatment for his tinea versicolor and to find out that it is not spread to others through contact.

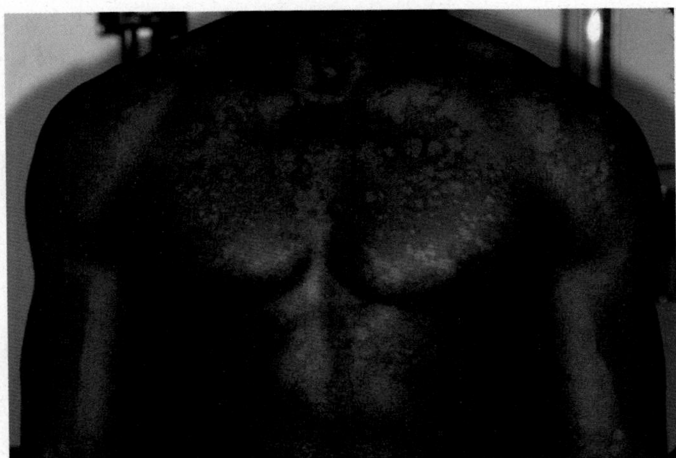

FIGURE 147-1 Tinea versicolor showing areas of hypopigmentation. *(Reproduced with permission from Usatine RP. What is in a name? West J Med. 2000;173(4):231-232.)*

INTRODUCTION

Tinea versicolor is a common superficial skin infection caused by the dimorphic lipophilic yeast in the genus *Malassezia*, formerly known as *Pityrosporum*. The most typical presentation is a set of hypopigmented macules and patches with fine scale over the trunk and proximal upper extremities in a capelike distribution.[1]

SYNONYMS

Pityriasis (from *Pityrosporum*) versicolor is actually a more accurate name, as "tinea" implies a dermatophyte infection. Tinea versicolor is caused by yeast in the genus *Malassezia* and not a dermatophyte.[1,2]

EPIDEMIOLOGY

- Seen more commonly in men than in women.
- Seen more commonly in adolescents and young adults.
- Seen more often during the summer and is especially common in warm and humid climates.

ETIOLOGY AND PATHOPHYSIOLOGY

- Tinea versicolor is caused by yeast in the genus *Malassezia* which is a lipid-dependent, dimorphic fungus that is a component of normal human cutaneous flora.[2,3]
- *Malassezia* lipophilic yeasts are causative agents in tinea versicolor, seborrheic dermatitis, and *Malassezia* folliculitis and can even exacerbate atopic dermatitis.[2] In one microbiology study using polymerase chain reaction (PCR), the authors were able to determine the prevalence of various *Malassezia* species on patients with *Malassezia* associated skin conditions.[2] The two most common species isolated from humans were *M. globosa* and *M. furfur*.[2]
- Transformation of *Malassezia* from yeast to the pathogenic mycelial form followed by invasion into the stratum corneum precedes the development of the classic appearance of tinea versicolor.[4]

- Versicolor refers to the variable changes in pigmentation noted in this condition.[2-4]
- Hypopigmentation changes are secondary to melanocytic damage caused by azelaic acid produced by the genus *Malassezia*, while the hyperpigmented and erythematous lesions are a result of an inflammatory reaction to the organism.[4]
- *Malassezia* is lipid dependent and thrives on sebum and moisture. The lesions are more common in areas of greater sebum production, such as the upper trunk and proximal upper extremities.[2,3]

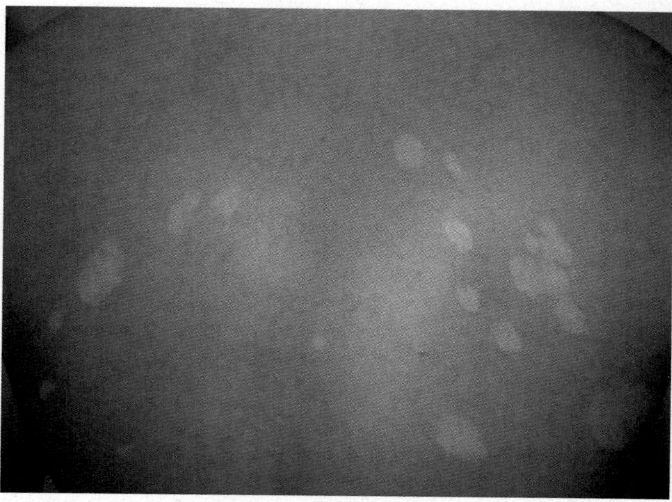

FIGURE 147-2 Patches of hypopigmentation across the back caused by tinea versicolor in a young Latino man. Vitiligo is on the differential diagnosis in this case. A KOH preparation confirmed tinea versicolor. (*Reproduced with permission from Richard P. Usatine, MD.*)

DIAGNOSIS

CLINICAL FEATURES

Tinea versicolor consists of hypopigmented, hyperpigmented, or pink macules and patches on the trunk and proximal upper extremities that are finely scaled and well-demarcated. Versicolor means a variety of or variation in colors; tinea versicolor tends to come in white, pink, and brown colors (**Figures 147-1** to **147-5**).

TYPICAL DISTRIBUTION

Tinea versicolor is found on the chest, abdomen, upper arms, and back.

LABORATORY STUDIES

A scraping of the scaling portions of the skin may be placed onto a slide using the side of another slide or a scalpel. KOH (with or without a fungal stain) is placed on the slide and covered with a coverslip. Microscopic examination reveals the typical "spaghetti-and-meatballs" pattern of tinea versicolor. The "spaghetti," or more accurately "ziti," is the short mycelial form and the "meatballs" are the round yeast form (**Figures 147-6** and **147-7**). Fungal stains such as the Swartz Lamkins stain help make the identification of the fungal elements easier.[3]

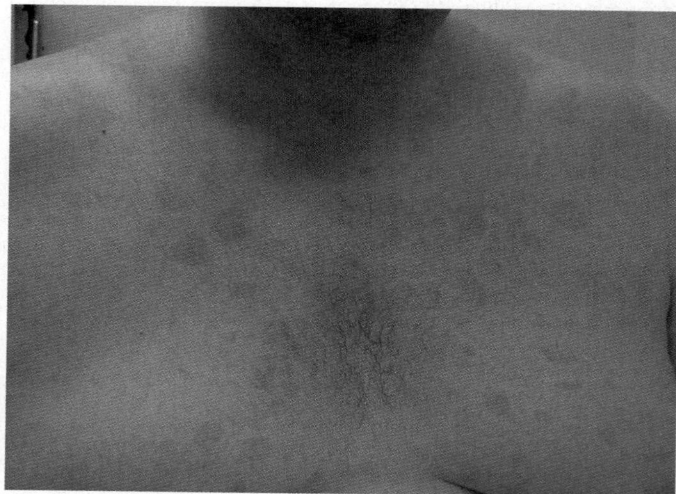

FIGURE 147-3 Pink scaly patches caused by tinea versicolor. Seborrhea may be seen in this location, but tends to be worse in the presternal region. (*Reproduced with permission from Richard P. Usatine, MD.*)

DIFFERENTIAL DIAGNOSIS

- Seborrheic dermatitis on the trunk typically is more erythematous, has a thicker scale, and is located in the central chest. Patients usually have other lesions in the scalp, eyebrows, and nasolabial folds.
- Pityriasis rosea has a fine collarette scale around the border of the lesions and is frequently seen with a herald patch. Negative KOH (see Chapter 159, Pityriasis Rosea).
- Secondary syphilis is usually not scaling and tends to have macules on the palms and soles. Negative KOH (see Chapter 225, Syphilis).
- Tinea corporis is rarely as widespread as tinea versicolor, and each individual lesion usually has central clearing and a well-defined, raised, scaling border. The KOH preparation in tinea corporis shows hyphae with multiple branch points and not the "ziti-and-meatballs" pattern of tinea versicolor (see Chapter 144, Tinea Corporis).
- Vitiligo—The degree of hypopigmentation is greater and the distribution is frequently different with vitiligo involving the hands and face (see Chapter 206, Vitiligo and Hypopigmentation).

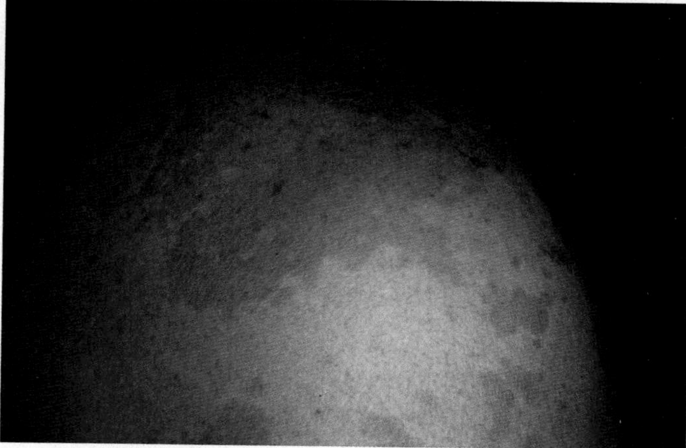

FIGURE 147-4 Large areas of pink tinea versicolor on the shoulder in a capelike distribution. (*Reproduced with permission from Richard P. Usatine, MD.*)

- Pityriasis alba—Lightly hypopigmented areas with slight scale that tend to be found on the face and trunk of children with atopy. These patches are frequently smaller and rounder than tinea versicolor (see Chapter 151, Atopic Dermatitis).
- *Pityrosporum* (*Malassezia*) folliculitis is caused by the same organism but presents with pink or brown papules on the back. The patient complains of itchy rough skin, and there is evidence of perifollicular inflammation (**Figure 147-8**).

MANAGEMENT

FIRST LINE

- Because tinea versicolor is usually asymptomatic, the treatment is mostly for cosmetic reasons.
- The mainstay of treatment has been topical therapy using antidandruff shampoos, because the same *Malassezia* species that cause seborrhea and dandruff also cause tinea versicolor.[1,2]
- Patients may apply selenium sulfide 2.5% lotion or shampoo or zinc pyrithione shampoo to the involved areas daily for 2 weeks. Various amounts of time are suggested to allow the preparations to work, but there are no studies that compare exposure times. Although 5 minutes has been used in some studies, 2 minutes may be more realistic. A typical regimen involves applying the lotion or shampoo to the involved areas for 2–5 minutes and then washing it off in the shower.[3] SOR Ⓒ
- One study used ketoconazole 2% shampoo as a single application or daily for 3 days and found it safe and highly effective with greater than 80% cure in treating tinea versicolor.[3,5] SOR Ⓑ
- A single-dose 400-mg oral fluconazole provides excellent clinical and mycologic cure rates, with no relapse during 12 months of follow-up.[6-8] SOR Ⓑ

SECOND LINE

- A single dose of 300 mg of oral fluconazole repeated weekly for 2 weeks was equal to 400 mg of ketoconazole in a single dose repeated weekly for 2 weeks. No significant differences in efficacy, safety, and tolerability between the two treatment regimens were found.[7-10] SOR Ⓑ
- However, in 2016, the FDA advised against the use of oral ketoconazole for tinea versicolor due to life-threatening hepatotoxicity, adrenal insufficiency, and multiple adverse drug-drug interactions.[11,12] SOR Ⓑ
- Topical antifungal creams for smaller areas of involvement can include ketoconazole, clotrimazole, terbinafine, and ciclopirox.[13] SOR Ⓒ
- There is no evidence that establishes the need to sweat after taking oral antifungals to treat tinea versicolor.[3]

PREVENTION

- Prophylaxis with topical ketoconazole 2% shampoo applied to the entire body for 5 minutes once per month is an effective therapy.[5] SOR Ⓑ

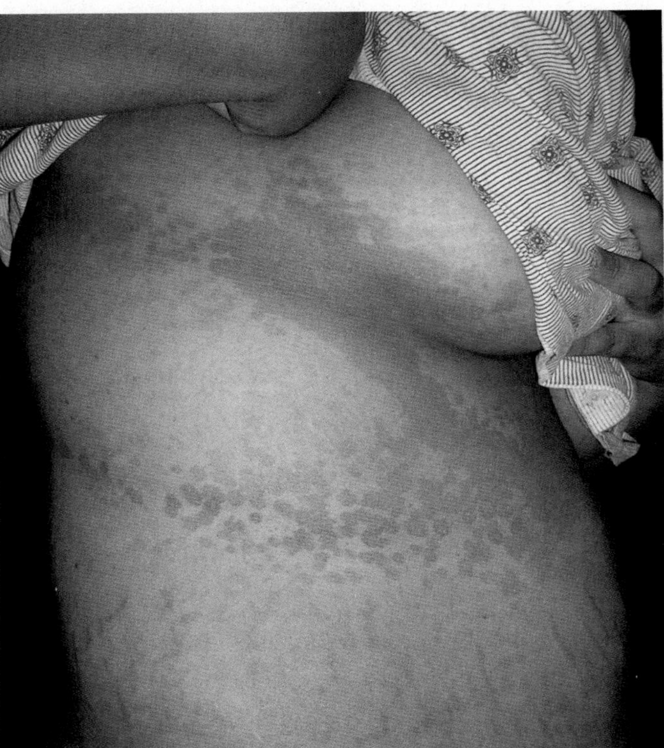

FIGURE 147-5 Hyperpigmented variant of tinea versicolor in a Hispanic woman. (*Reproduced with permission from Richard P. Usatine, MD.*)

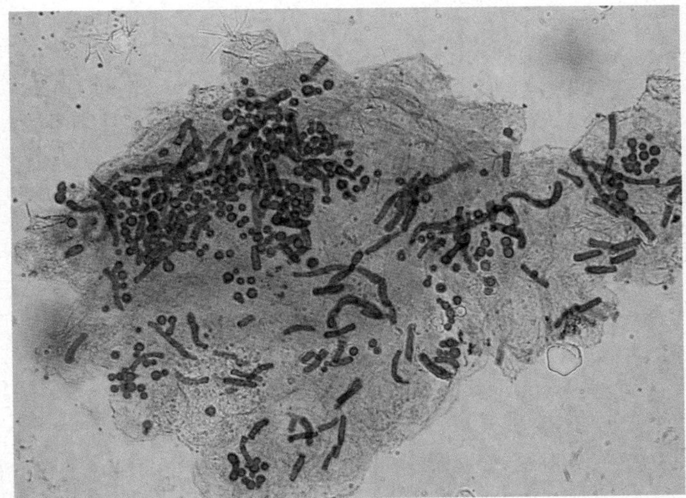

FIGURE 147-6 Microscopic examination of scrapings done from previous patient with tinea versicolor showing short mycelial forms and round yeast forms suggestive of spaghetti and meatballs. Swartz Lamkins stain was used. (*Reproduced with permission from Richard P. Usatine, MD.*)

- Oral itraconazole 200 mg given twice a day for one day a month has been shown to be safe and effective as a prophylactic treatment for tinea versicolor.[14,15] SOR Ⓑ

PATIENT EDUCATION

Patients should be told that the change in skin color will not reverse immediately. The first sign of successful treatment is the lack of scale. The yeast acts like a sunscreen in the hypopigmented macules. Sun exposure will hasten the normalization of the skin color in patients with hypopigmentation.

FOLLOW-UP

None needed unless it is a stubborn or recurrent case. Recurrent cases can be treated with monthly topical or oral therapy.

PATIENT RESOURCES

- **http://www.skinsight.com/skin-conditions/adult/tinea-versicolor.htm.**

PROVIDER RESOURCES

- **https://emedicine.medscape.com/article/1091575-overview.**

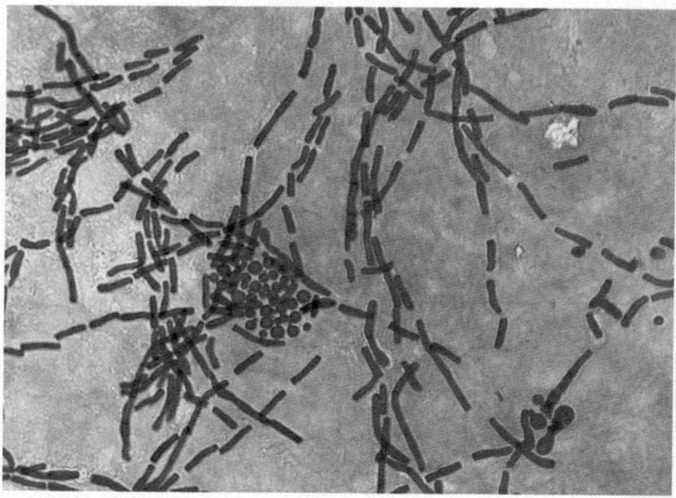

FIGURE 147-7 Close-up of *Malassezia* (*Pityrosporum*) showing the ziti-and-meatball appearance after Swartz Lamkins stain was applied to the scraping of tinea versicolor in a young woman. (*Reproduced with permission from Richard P. Usatine, MD.*)

FIGURE 147-8 *Pityrosporum* (*Malassezia*) folliculitis on the back of a man with pruritus. (*Reproduced with permission from Richard P. Usatine, MD.*)

REFERENCES

1. Gupta AK, Batra R, Bluhm R, Faergemann J. Pityriasis versicolor. *Dermatol Clin.* 2003;21:413.
2. Ilahi A, Hadrich I, Neji S, et al. Real-time PCR identification of six *Malassezia* species. *Curr Microbiol.* 2017;74(6):671-677.
3. Schwartz RA. Superficial fungal infections. *Lancet.* 2004;364:1173.
4. Galadari I, Komy M, Mousa A, et al. Tinea versicolor: histologic and ultrastructural investigation of pigmentary changes. *Int J Dermatol.* 1992;31:253.
5. Lange DS, Richards HM, Guarnieri J, et al. Ketoconazole 2% shampoo in the treatment of tinea versicolor: a multicenter, randomized, double-blind, placebo-controlled trial. *J Am Acad Dermatol.* 1998;39(6):944-950.
6. Hu SW, Bigby M. Pityriasis versicolor: a systematic review of interventions. *Arch Dermatol.* 2010;146(10):1132-1140.
7. Gupta AK, Lane D, Paquet M. Systematic review of systemic treatments for tinea versicolor and evidence-based dosing regimen recommendations. *J Cutan Med Surg.* 2014;18:79.
8. Bhogal CS, Singal A, Baruah MC. Comparative efficacy of ketoconazole and fluconazole in the treatment of pityriasis versicolor: a one year follow-up study. *J Dermatol.* 2001;28(10):535-539.
9. Farschian M, Yaghoobi R, Samadi K. Fluconazole versus ketoconazole in the treatment of tinea versicolor. *J Dermatolog Treat.* 2002;13(2):73-76.
10. Gupta AK, Del Rosso JQ. An evaluation of intermittent therapies used to treat onychomycosis and other dermatomycoses with the oral antifungal agents. *Int J Dermatol.* 2000;39(6):401-411.

11. http://www.fda.gov/Drugs/DrugSafety/ucm362415.htm. Accessed January 2018.
12. http://www.fda.gov/Safety/MedWatch/SafetyInformation/SafetyAlertsforHumanMedicalProducts/ucm502073.htm. Accessed January 2018.
13. Faergemann J. Management of seborrheic dermatitis and pityriasis versicolor. *Am J Clin Dermatol.* 2000;1:75-80.
14. Faergemann J, Gupta AK, Mofadi AA, et al. Efficacy of itraconazole in the prophylactic treatment of pityriasis (tinea) versicolor. *Arch Dermatol.* 2002;138:69-73.
15. Wahab MA, Ali ME, Rahman MH, et al. Single dose (400 mg) versus 7 day (200 mg) daily dose itraconazole in the treatment of tinea versicolor: a randomized clinical trial. *Mymensingh Med J.* 2010;19(1):72-76.

SECTION G INFESTATIONS

148 LICE

E.J. Mayeaux, Jr., MD
Richard P. Usatine, MD
Jonathan C. Banta, MD

PATIENT STORY

A 64-year-old homeless woman with schizophrenia presented to a homeless clinic for itching all over her body. She stated that she could see creatures feed on her and move in and out of her skin. The physical examination revealed that she was unwashed and had multiple excoriations over her body (**Figure 148-1**). Body lice and their progeny were visible along the seams of her pants (**Figure 148-2**). Treatment of this lousy infestation required giving her new clothes and a shower.[1]

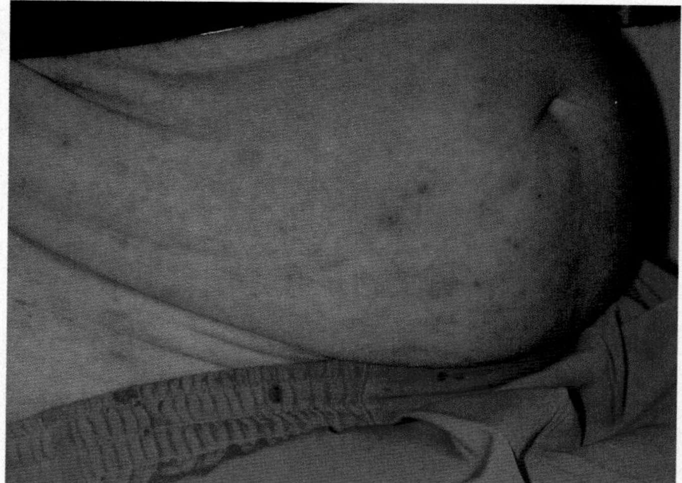

FIGURE 148-1 Body lice in a 64-year-old homeless woman with schizophrenia. (*Reproduced with permission from Usatine RP, Halem L. A terrible itch, J Fam Pract. 2003;52(5):377-379. Frontline Medical Communications. Inc.*)

INTRODUCTION

Lice are ectoparasites that live on or near the body. They will die of starvation within 10 days of removal from their human host. Lice have coexisted with humans for at least 10,000 years.[2] Lice are ubiquitous and remain a major problem throughout the world.[3]

SYNONYMS

Pediculosis, crabs (pubic lice).

EPIDEMIOLOGY

- Human lice (pediculosis corporis, pediculosis pubis, and pediculosis capitis) are found in all countries and climates.[3]
- Head lice are most common among school-age children. Each year, approximately 6 to 12 million children, ages 3 to 12 years, are infested.[4]
- Head lice infestation is seen across all socioeconomic groups and is not a sign of poor hygiene.[5]
- In the United States, black children are affected less often as a result of their oval-shaped hair shafts that are difficult for lice to grasp.[4]
- Body lice infest the seams of clothing (see **Figure 148-2**) and bed linen. Infestations are associated with poor hygiene and conditions of crowding.
- Pubic lice are most common in sexually active adolescents and adults. Young children with pubic lice typically have infestations of the eyelashes. Although infestations in this age group may be an indication of sexual abuse, children generally acquire the crab lice from their parents.[6]

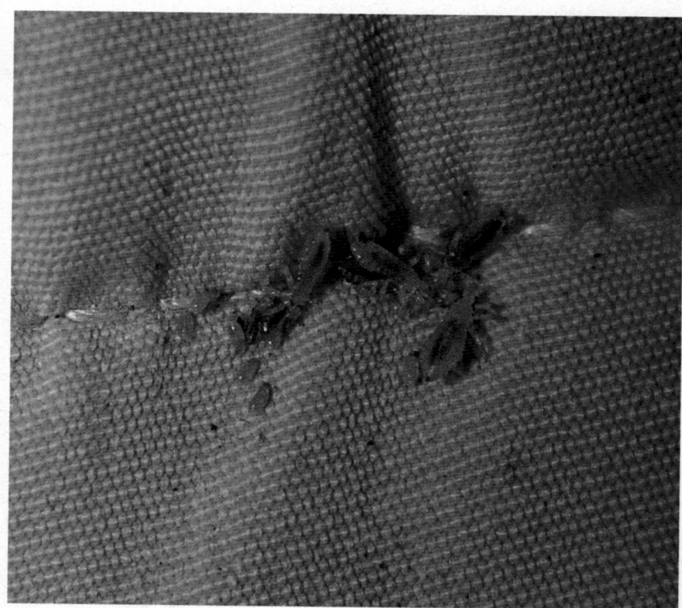

FIGURE 148-2 Adult body lice and eggs visible along the pant seams of the woman in **Figure 148-1**. (*Reproduced with permission from Richard P. Usatine, MD.*)

ETIOLOGY AND PATHOPHYSIOLOGY

- Lice are parasites that have six legs with terminal claws that enable them to attach to hair and clothing. There are three types of lice responsible for human infestation. All three kinds of lice must feed daily on human blood and can only survive 1 to 2 days away from the host. The three types of lice are as follows:
  - Head lice (*Pediculus humanus capitis*)—Measure 2 to 4 mm in length and are uniquely adapted to living on human hair (**Figure 148-3**).
  - Body lice (*Pediculus humanus corporis*)—Body lice similarly measure 2 to 4 mm in length and live on clothing between feeding on the human body (**Figure 148-4**).
  - Pubic or crab lice (*Phthirus pubis*)—Pubic lice are shorter, with a broader body, and have an average length of 1 to 2 mm (**Figure 148-5**).
- Female lice have a lifespan of approximately 30 days and can lay approximately 10 eggs (nits) a day.[4]
- Nits are firmly attached to the hair shaft or clothing seams by a gluelike substance produced by the louse (**Figures 148-6** to **148-8**).
- Nits are incubated by the host's body heat.
- The incubation period from laying eggs to hatching of the first nymph is 7 to 14 days.
- Mature adult lice capable of reproducing appear 2 to 3 weeks later.[5]
- Transmission of head lice occurs through direct contact with the hair of infested individuals. The role of fomites (e.g., hats, combs, brushes) in transmission is negligible.[6] Head lice do not serve as vectors for transmission of disease among humans.
- Transmission of body lice occurs through direct human contact or contact with infested material. Unlike head lice, body lice are well-recognized vectors for transmission of the pathogens responsible for epidemic typhus, trench fever, and relapsing fever.[5]
- Pubic or crab lice are transmitted primarily through sexual contact. In addition to pubic hair (**Figure 148-9**), infestations of eyelashes, eyebrows, beard, and upper-thigh, abdominal, and axillary hairs may also occur.

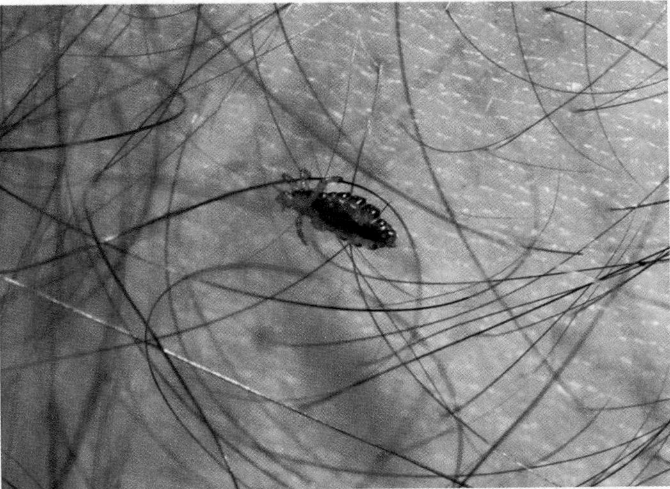

FIGURE 148-3 Adult head louse with elongated body. (*Reproduced with permission from Richard P. Usatine, MD.*)

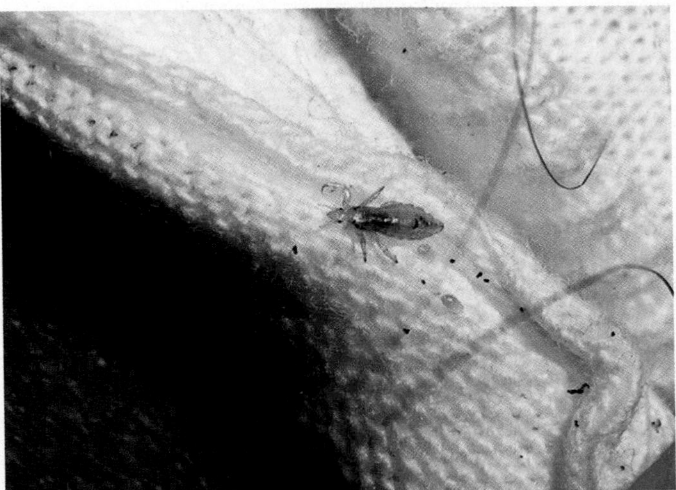

FIGURE 148-4 A body louse. (*Reproduced with permission from Richard P. Usatine, MD.*)

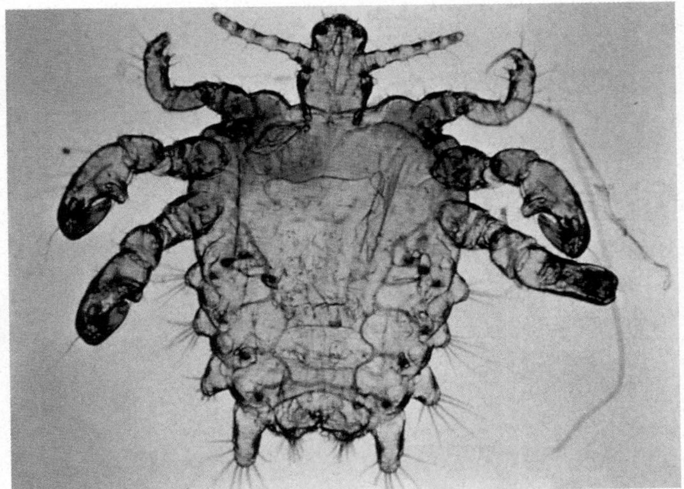

FIGURE 148-5 The crab louse has a short body, and its large claws are responsible for the "crab" in its name. (*Reproduced with permission from Centers for Disease Control and Prevention and World Health Organization.*)

RISK FACTORS

- Contact with an infected individual.
- Living in crowded quarters such as homeless shelters (**Figure 148-10**).
- Poor hygiene and mental illness.

DIAGNOSIS

CLINICAL FEATURES

- Nits can be seen in active disease or treated disease. Nits closer to the base of the hairs are generally newer and more likely to be live and unhatched. Unfortunately, nits that were not killed by pediculicides can hatch and start the infestation cycle over again. Note that nits are glued to the hairs and are hard to remove, whereas flakes of dandruff can be easily brushed off.

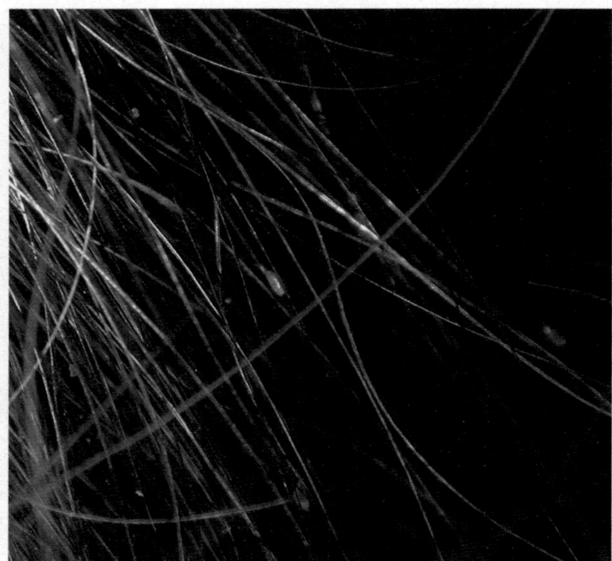

FIGURE 148-6 Pearly nits on the hair of a schoolgirl. (*Reproduced with permission from Richard P. Usatine, MD.*)

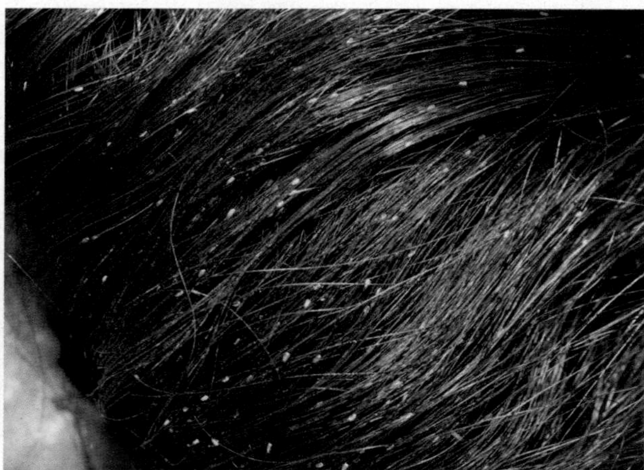

FIGURE 148-7 Massive infestation of head lice with many nits on a man experiencing mental health problems. (*Reproduced with permission from Richard P. Usatine, MD.*)

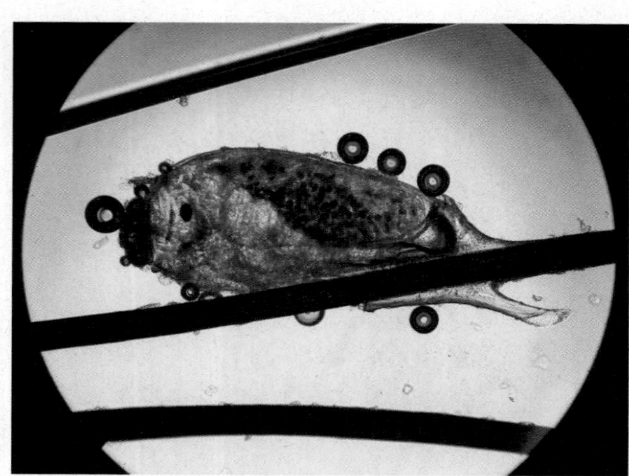

FIGURE 148-8 Microscopic view of a nit cemented to the hair and about to hatch. (*Reproduced with permission from Richard P. Usatine, MD.*)

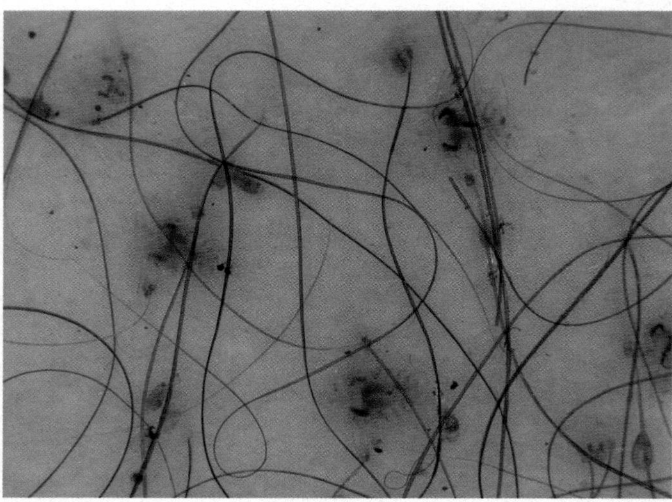

FIGURE 148-9 Crab lice infesting pubic hair seen through a dermatoscope. The bodies are translucent and their claws are holding on to the pubic hairs. (*Reproduced with permission from Luis Dehesa, MD.*)

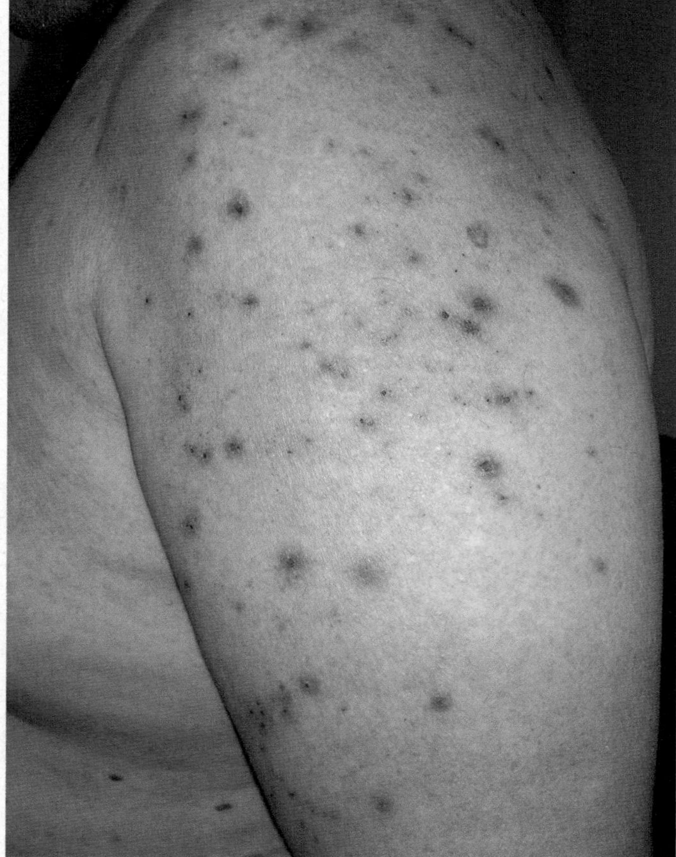

FIGURE 148-10 A homeless man infested with body lice and living in a shelter in which other persons are also infested. Note the multiple excoriations from the pruritus. He presented with a rash and did not know that body lice were living on his clothing. Examination of the seams led to the diagnosis. (*Reproduced with permission from Richard P. Usatine, MD.*)

- Pruritus is the hallmark of lice infestation. It is the result of an allergic response to louse saliva.[7] Head lice are associated with excoriated lesions that appear on the scalp, ears, neck, and back.
- Occipital and cervical adenopathy may develop, especially when lesions become super-infected.
- Body lice result in small maculopapular eruptions that are predominantly found on the trunk (see **Figure 148-1**) and the clothing (see **Figure 148-2**). Also, the pruritus leads to excoriations (**Figure 148-10**).
- Chronic infestations often result in hyperpigmented, lichenified plaques known as "vagabond's skin."[8]
- Pubic lice produce bluish-gray spots (macula cerulea) that can be found on the chest, abdomen, and thighs.[8]

TYPICAL DISTRIBUTION

- Head lice—Look for nits and lice in the hair, especially above the ears, behind the ears, and at the nape of the neck. There are many more nits present than live adults. Finding nits without an adult louse does not mean that the infestation has resolved (see **Figures 148-6** and **148-7**). Systematically combing wet or dry hair with a fine-toothed nit comb (teeth of comb are 0.2 mm apart) better detects active louse infestation than visual inspection of the hair and scalp alone.[9]
- Body lice—Look for the lice and larvae in the seams of the clothing (see **Figures 148-2** and **148-4**).
- Pubic lice—Look for nits and lice on the pubic hairs (see **Figure 148-9**). These lice and their nits may also be seen on the hairs of the upper thighs, abdomen, axilla, beard, eyebrows, and eyelashes. Little specks of dried blood may be seen in the underwear as a clue to the infestation.

LABORATORY TESTING

- Direct visualization and identification of live lice or nits are sufficient to make a diagnosis (see **Figures 148-2** to **148-7** and **148-9**).
- The use of a magnification lens or dermatoscope may aid in the detection or confirmation of lice infestation (see **Figure 148-9**).
- Under Wood light, the head lice nits fluoresce a pale blue.
- If you find an adult louse, put it on a slide with a coverslip loosely above it. Look at it under the microscope on the lowest power (see **Figure 148-5**). You will see the internal workings of the live organs. If the louse was not found in a typical location, you can use the morphology of the body and legs to determine the type of louse causing the infestation.
- In cases of pubic lice infestations, individuals should be screened for other sexually transmitted diseases.[5]

DIFFERENTIAL DIAGNOSIS

- Dandruff, hair casts, and debris should be ruled out in cases of suspected lice infestations. Unlike nits, these particles are easily removed from the hair shaft. In addition, adult lice are absent.
- Scabies is also characterized by intense pruritus and papular eruptions. Unlike lice infestations, scabies may be associated with vesicles, and the presence of burrows is pathognomonic. Diagnosis is confirmed by microscopic examination of the scrapings from lesions for the presence of mites or eggs (see Chapter 149, Scabies).

MANAGEMENT

NONPHARMACOLOGIC

FIRST LINE

- In young children or others who wish to avoid topical pediculicides for head lice, mechanical removal of lice by wet combing is an alternative therapy. A 1:1 vinegar:water rinse (left under a conditioning cap or towel for 15 to 20 minutes) or 8% formic acid crème rinse may enhance removal of tenacious nits.[8] Combing is performed until no lice are found for 2 weeks. SOR Ⓑ
  - Nits are also removed with a fine-toothed comb following the application of all treatments. This step is critical in achieving resolution.
  - Combs and hairbrushes should be discarded, soaked in hot water (at a temperature of at least 55°C [130°F]) for 5 minutes, or treated with pediculicides.[10]

SECOND LINE

- The natural substances of tea tree oil and nerolidol were shown in 2012 to have promising results as a natural alternative to pediculosis resistant cases. In the study, a compound ratio of 1:2 (tree oil 0.5% plus nerolidol 1.0%) when applied to head lice and their eggs resulted in 100% death of all head lice after 30 minutes and an ovicidal effect on louse eggs after 5 days.[11] SOR Ⓑ

MEDICATIONS

Pediculus humanus capitis (head lice):

FIRST LINE

- Nonprescription 1% permethrin cream rinse (Nix), pyrethrins with piperonyl butoxide (which inhibits pyrethrin catabolism; RID) shampoo, or permethrin 1% is applied to the hair and scalp and left on for 10 minutes, then rinsed out.[12]
- Pyrethrins are only pediculicidal, whereas permethrin is both pediculicidal and ovicidal. It is important to note that treatment failure is common with these agents owing to the emergence of resistant strains of lice. After 7 to 10 days, repeating the application is optional when permethrin is used, but is a necessity for pyrethrin. Lice persisting after treatment with a pyrethroid may be an indication of resistance.[13] SOR Ⓐ
- Malathion 0.5% (Ovide) is available by prescription only and is a highly effective pediculicidal and ovicidal agent for resistant lice. Malathion may have greater efficacy than pyrethrins.[14] It is approved for use in children age 6 years and older. The lotion is applied to dry hair for 8 to 12 hours and then washed. Repeat application is recommended after 7 to 10 days if live lice are still present. When used appropriately, malathion is 78% to 95% effective.[14] SOR Ⓐ
- Hair conditioners should not be used prior to the application of pediculicides; these products may result in reduced efficacy.[15]
- A Cochrane review found no evidence that any one pediculicide was better than another; permethrin, synergized pyrethrin, and malathion were all effective in the treatment of head lice.[16] SOR Ⓐ

SECOND LINE

- Benzyl alcohol 5% lotion (Ulesfia) is a newer treatment option in patients 6 months of age and older. It works by asphyxiating the parasite. It is applied for 10 minutes with saturation of the scalp and hair, and then rinsed off with water. The treatment is repeated after 7 days.[17] SOR Ⓐ
- Spinosad (Natroba) is a topical prescription medication approved by the U.S. Food and Drug Administration (FDA) in 2011 for the treatment of lice. Spinosad is a fermentation product of the soil bacterium *Saccharopolyspora spinosa* that compromises the central nervous system of lice. It is approximately 85% effective in lice eradication, usually after one application. It is applied to completely cover the dry scalp and hair, and rinsed off after 10 minutes. Treatment should be repeated if live lice remain 7 days after the initial application.[18] SOR Ⓐ
- In February 2012, the FDA approved ivermectin 0.5% lotion for the treatment of head lice. It is applied as a single 10-minute topical application. The safety of ivermectin in infants younger than age 6 months has not been established. SOR Ⓐ
- Permethrin 5% is conventionally used to treat scabies; however, it is anecdotally recommended for treatment of recalcitrant head lice.[5] SOR Ⓒ
- Oral therapy options include a 10-day course of trimethoprim-sulfamethoxazole or 2 doses of ivermectin (200 mcg/kg) 7 to 10 days apart. SOR Ⓒ Trimethoprim-sulfamethoxazole is postulated to kill the symbiotic bacteria in the gut of the louse.[4] Combination therapy with 1% permethrin and trimethoprim-sulfamethoxazole is recommended in cases of multiple treatment failure or suspected cases of resistance to therapy.[5,10] SOR Ⓒ
- Abametapir is a new therapy that, in two randomized, double-blind, phase 3 clinical trials published in 2016, was shown to effectively kill both lice and their eggs with one application. Abametapir works by inhibiting metalloproteinases, which are enzymes that are necessary for both egg development and the survival of living lice. The compound comes in a lotion and is applied to dry hair and left to sit for 10 minutes. It is subsequently washed out with warm water and requires no further treatments.[19] Abametapir has yet to be approved by the FDA at the time of writing, but an application is pending.

Pediculus humanus corporis (body lice):

- Improving hygiene and laundering clothing and bed linen at temperatures of 65°C (149°F) for 15 to 30 minutes will eliminate body lice.[8]
- In settings where individuals cannot change clothing (e.g., those who are homeless), a monthly application of 10% lindane powder can be used to dust the lining of all clothing.[8]
- Additionally, lindane lotion or permethrin cream may be applied to the body for 8 to 12 hours to eradicate body lice.

Phthirus pubis (pubic lice):

- Pubic lice infestations are treated with a 10-minute application of the same topical pediculicides used to treat head lice.
- Retreatment is recommended 7 to 10 days later.
- Petroleum ointment applied 2 to 4 times a day for 8 to 10 days will eradicate eyelash infestations.
- Clothing, towels, and bed linen should also be laundered to eliminate nit-bearing hairs.[8]

PREVENTION

- Washing clothing and linen used by the head or pubic lice-infested person during the 2 days prior to therapy in hot water and/or drying the items on a high-heat dryer cycle (54.5°C [130°F]). Items that cannot be washed may be dry cleaned or stored in a sealed plastic bag for 2 weeks.

FOLLOW-UP

- Patients should be reexamined upon completion of therapy to confirm eradication of lice.

PATIENT EDUCATION

- Patients should be instructed to wash potentially contaminated articles of clothing, bed linen, combs, brushes, and hats.
- Nit removal is important in preventing continued infestation as a result of new progeny. Careful examination of close contacts, with appropriate treatment for infested individuals, is important in avoiding recurrence.
- In cases of pubic lice, all sexual contacts should be treated.

PATIENT RESOURCES

- eMedicineHealth. *Lice*—**http://www.emedicinehealth.com/lice/article_em.htm.**
- Centers for Disease Control and Prevention. *Parasites–Lice*—**http://www.cdc.gov/parasites/lice/index.html.**

PROVIDER RESOURCES

- Centers for Disease Control and Prevention. *Parasites*—**http://www.cdc.gov/ncidod/dpd/parasites/lice/default.htm.**
- Medscape. *Pediculosis and Pthiriasis (Lice Infestation)*—**http://emedicine.medscape.com/article/225013.**

REFERENCES

1. Usatine RP, Halem L. A terrible itch. *J Fam Pract.* 2003;52(5):377-379.
2. Araujo A, Ferreira LF, Guidon N, et al. Ten thousand years of head lice infection. *Parasitol Today.* 2000;16(7):269.
3. Roberts RJ. Clinical practice. Head lice. *N Engl J Med.* 2002;346:1645.
4. Frankowski BL, Weiner LB. Head lice. *Pediatrics.* 2002;110(3):638-643.
5. Pickering LK, Baker CJ, Long SS, McMillan JA. *Red Book: 2006 Report of the Committee on Infectious Diseases*, 27th ed. Elk Grove Village, IL: American Academy of Pediatrics; 2006:488-493.

6. Maguire JH, Pollack RJ, Spielman A. Ectoparasite infestations and arthropod bites and stings. In: Kasper DL, Fauci AS, Longo DL, et al., eds. *Harrison's Principles of Internal Medicine*, 16th ed. New York, NY: McGraw-Hill; 2005:2601-2602.

7. Flinders DC, De Schweinitz P. Pediculosis and scabies. *Am Fam Physician*. 2004;69(2):341-348.

8. Darmstadt GL. Arthropod bites and infestations. In: Behrman RE, Kliegman RM, Jenson HB, eds. *Nelson Textbook of Pediatrics*, 16th ed. Philadelphia, PA: Saunders; 2000:2046-2047.

9. Jahnke C, Bauer E, Hengge UR, Feldmeier H. Accuracy of diagnosis of pediculosis capitis: visual inspection vs wet combing. *Arch Dermatol.* 2009;145(3):309-313.

10. Hipolito RB, Mallorca FG, Zuniga-Macaraig ZO, et al. Head lice infestation: single drug versus combination therapy with one percent permethrin and trimethoprim/sulfamethoxazole. *Pediatrics.* 2001;107(3):E30.

11. Di Campli E, Di Bartolomeo S, Delli Pizzi P, et al. Activity of tea tree oil and nerolidol alone or in combination against *Pediculus capitis* (head lice) and its eggs. *Parasitol Res.* 2012;111(5):1985-1992.

12. Meinking TL, Clineschmidt CM, Chen C, et al. An observer-blinded study of 1% permethrin creme rinse with and without adjunctive combing in patients with head lice. *J Pediatr.* 2002;141(5):665-670.

13. Koch E, Clark JM, Cohen B, et al. Management of head louse infestations in the United States—a literature review. *Pediatr Dermatol.* 2016;33(5):466-472.

14. Meinking TL, Serrano L, Hard B, et al. Comparative in vitro pediculicidal efficacy of treatments in a resistant head lice population in the United States. *Arch Dermatol.* 2002;138(2):220-224.

15. Lebwohl M, Clark L, Levitt J. Therapy for head lice based on life cycle, resistance, and safety considerations. *Pediatrics.* 2007;119(5):965-974.

16. Dodd CS. Interventions for treating head lice. *Cochrane Database Syst Rev.* 2006;(4):CD001165.

17. Meinking TL, Villar ME, Vicaria M, et al. The clinical trials supporting benzyl alcohol lotion 5% (Ulesfia): a safe and effective topical treatment for head lice (pediculosis humanus capitis). *Pediatr Dermatol.* 2010;27(1):19-24.

18. Stough D, Shellabarger S, Quiring J, Gabrielsen AA Jr. Efficacy and safety of spinosad and permethrin creme rinses for pediculosis capitis (head lice). *Pediatrics.* 2009;124(3):e389-e395.

19. Harrison, L. (2016, November 2). Abametapir kills lice and eggs in phase 3 trials. http://www.medscape.com/viewarticle/871279. Accessed July 2018.

149 SCABIES

Richard P. Usatine, MD
Vineet Mishra, MD
Kaley K. El-Arab, BS

PATIENT STORY

A 17-year-old young man is seen with severe itching of his hands and feet. He has no lesions between his fingers and no one else in the family is itching. He has seen multiple clinicians in the past 5 months and has been given many types of topical steroids and antihistamines. The last clinician referred him for psychotherapy, thinking that this must be psychogenic. On close examination, there are multiple burrows on the hands (**Figure 149-1**). Dermatoscopy shows the typical pattern of a "jet plane with a contrail," clinching the diagnosis of scabies (**Figure 149-2**). The patient is treated with permethrin cream overnight and repeated in 7 days. At the following visit his itching is gone, and he is so thankful. This case demonstrates the importance of looking for burrows as the morphologic manifestation of the mite under the skin. Although it was nice to have a dermatoscope to confirm the diagnosis, this diagnosis could easily have been made clinically just by careful observation. Not every patient with scabies has lesions between the fingers and contacts at home with pruritus.

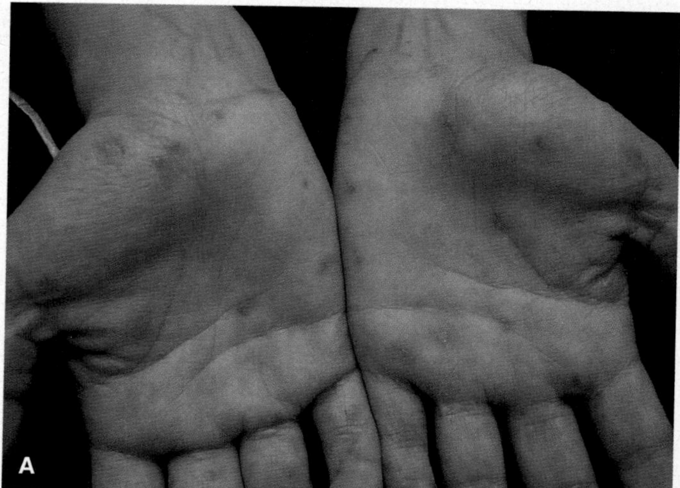

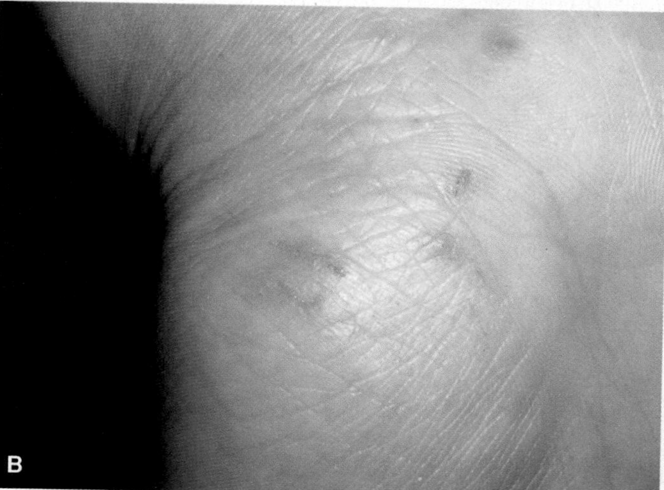

FIGURE 149-1 **A.** Scabies on the hands of a 17-year-old young man. **B.** Close-up of the right thenar eminence showing two obvious burrows caused by the mites. (*Reproduced with permission from Richard P. Usatine, MD.*)

INTRODUCTION

Scabies may be one of the most overdiagnosed and underdiagnosed conditions in medicine. Not every patient with a pruritic rash has scabies, and the patterns of scabies are multiple and variable. Scabies may present with papules, pustules, nodules, and/or crusts, and while there are typical patterns of distribution, each case does not read the textbook (not even this textbook). Looking for burrows is always worthwhile, as it is the pathognomonic feature of scabies. Although there may be nodules in the axilla or on the penis, there probably will be some burrows somewhere, such as on the wrist or between the first and second interspace of the hand. Having a dermatoscope to see the real mite is a great advance in the diagnosis of this potentially elusive condition (see **Figure 149-2**).

SYNONYMS

Crusted scabies has been called Norwegian scabies. The preferred term is now crusted scabies.

EPIDEMIOLOGY

- Three hundred million cases per year are estimated worldwide.[1] In some tropical countries, scabies is endemic.
- The incidence of scabies in a study performed in general practices in England and Wales was 351 per 100,000 person-years in men and 437 per 100,000 person-years in women.[2]

- Data from the Royal Infirmary in Edinburgh show that 5% of patients with skin disease between 1815 and 2000 had scabies; the prevalence during wartime reached over 30%.[3]

ETIOLOGY AND PATHOPHYSIOLOGY

- Human scabies is caused by the mite *Sarcoptes scabiei*, an obligate human parasite: without contact with human skin, the scabies mite can live only 24–36 hours (**Figure 149-3**).[1,4]
- Adult mites spend their entire life cycle, around 30 days, within the epidermis. After copulation the male mite dies and the female mite burrows through the superficial layers of the skin, excreting feces (**Figure 149-4**) and laying eggs (**Figure 149-5**), which then hatch and repeat the cycle.[5]
- Mites move through the superficial layers of skin by secreting proteases that degrade the stratum corneum.
- Infected individuals usually have fewer than 100 mites. In contrast, immunocompromised hosts, those with HIV, older patients, and people affected with Down syndrome[5] can have up to 1 million mites and are susceptible to crusted scabies (**Figures 149-6** to **149-9**).[1]
- Transmission usually occurs via direct skin contact. Scabies in adults is frequently sexually transmitted.[6] Scabies mites can also be transmitted from animals to humans.[1]
- Mites can also survive for 3 days outside of the human epidermis, allowing for infrequent transmission through bedding and clothing.
- The incubation period is on average 3 to 4 weeks for an initial infestation. Sensitized individuals can have symptoms within hours of reexposure.

FIGURE 149-2 Dermatoscopy of a scabies mite showing a jet plane (delta wing) with a contrail-type appearance. The jet plane is the anterior portion of the mite that is darker because of the front legs and mouthparts. The contrail is the burrow that the mite has produced while eating through the epidermis. (*Reproduced with permission from Richard P. Usatine, MD.*)

RISK FACTORS

- Scabies is more common in young children, healthcare workers, homeless and impoverished persons, and individuals who are immunocompromised or suffering from dementia.[1]
- Institutionalized individuals and those living in crowded conditions also have a higher incidence of the infestation.[1]

DIAGNOSIS

CLINICAL FEATURES

- Pruritus is a hallmark of the disease.[1]
- Skin findings include papules (see **Figure 149-9**), burrows (**Figures 149-10** and **149-11**), nodules (**Figure 149-12**), and vesiculopustules (**Figure 149-13**).
- Burrows are the classic morphologic finding in scabies and the best location to find the mite (see **Figures 149-10** and **149-11**).
- Infants and young children can also exhibit irritability and poor feeding.
- Pruritic papules/nodules around the axillae (see **Figure 149-12**) or umbilicus, or on the penis and scrotum (**Figures 149-14** and **149-15**), are highly suggestive of scabies.

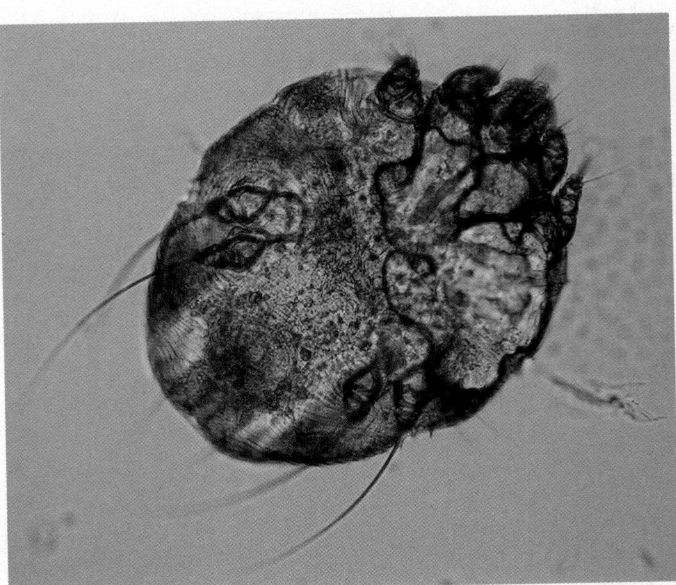

FIGURE 149-3 Microscopic view of the scabies mite. Note how the anterior portion of the mite is darker because of the front legs and mouthparts. This is what causes the jet plane or triangular formation visible on dermatoscopy. (*Reproduced with permission from Richard P. Usatine, MD.*)

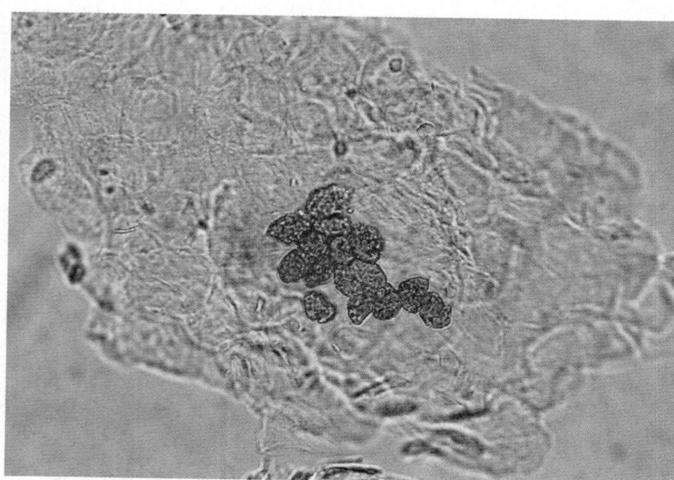

FIGURE 149-4 Scraping of the patient's hand produced a good view of the scybala (the mites' feces). (*Reproduced with permission from Richard P. Usatine, MD.*)

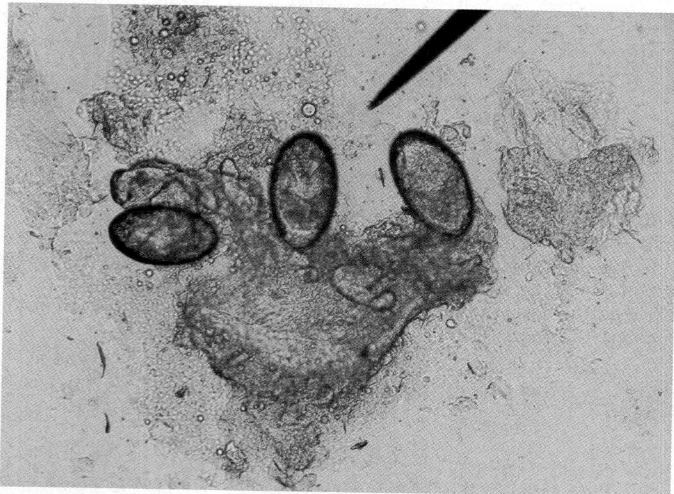

FIGURE 149-5 Scabies eggs from a scraping. (*Reproduced with permission from Richard P. Usatine, MD.*)

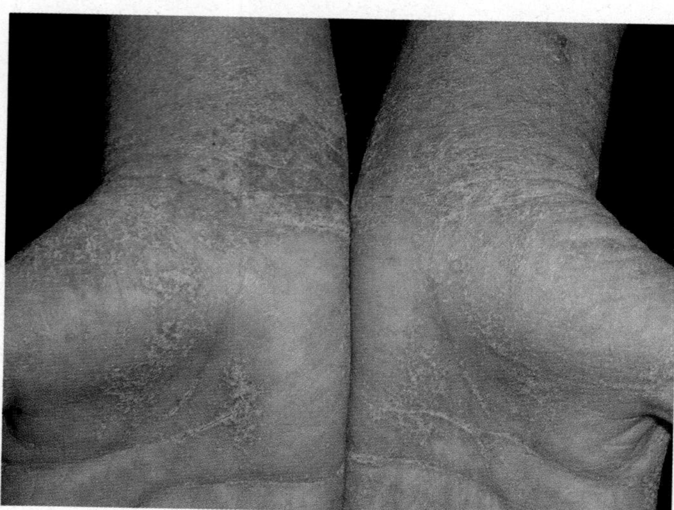

FIGURE 149-6 Crusted scabies on the hands and wrists of a 22-year-old man who has been HIV-positive since birth. (*Reproduced with permission from Richard P. Usatine, MD.*)

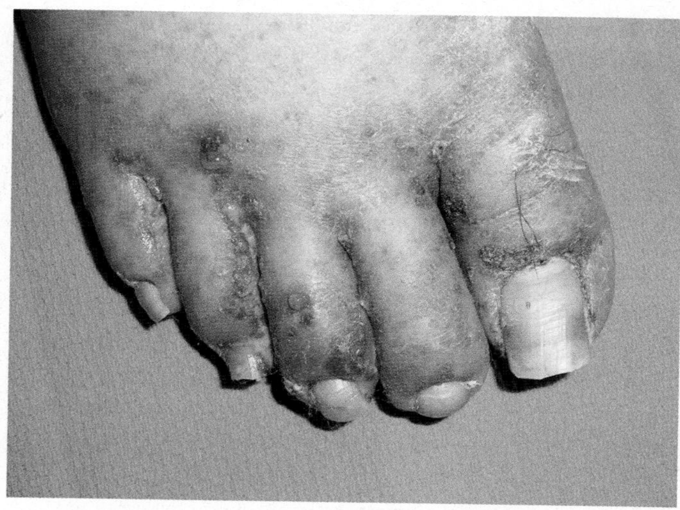

FIGURE 149-7 Crusted scabies on the foot that has also become superinfected. Notice the yellow exudate that suggests a bacterial superinfection. (*Reproduced with permission from Richard P. Usatine, MD.*)

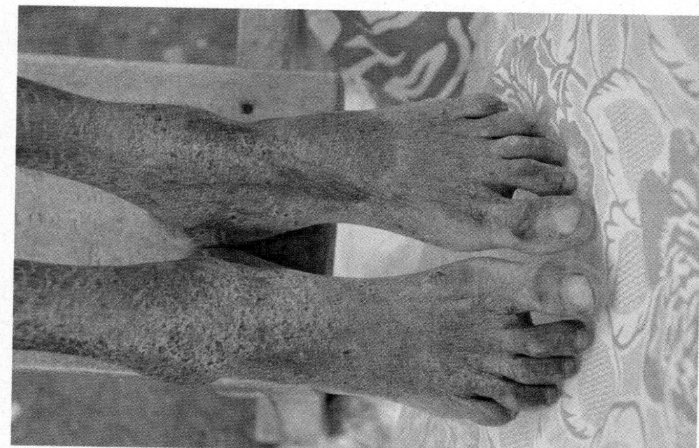

FIGURE 149-8 Crusted scabies on the foot of a 5-year-old boy with Down syndrome. (*Reproduced with permission from Richard P. Usatine, MD.*)

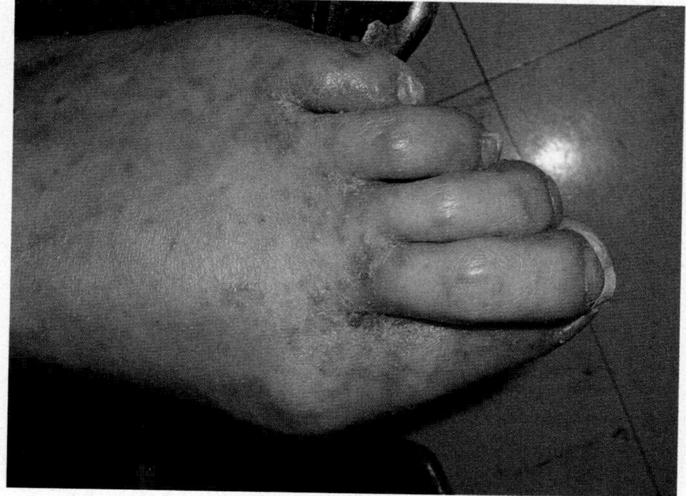

FIGURE 149-9 Crusted scabies on the foot of a disabled man who had experienced a stroke previously. (*Reproduced with permission from Richard P. Usatine, MD.*)

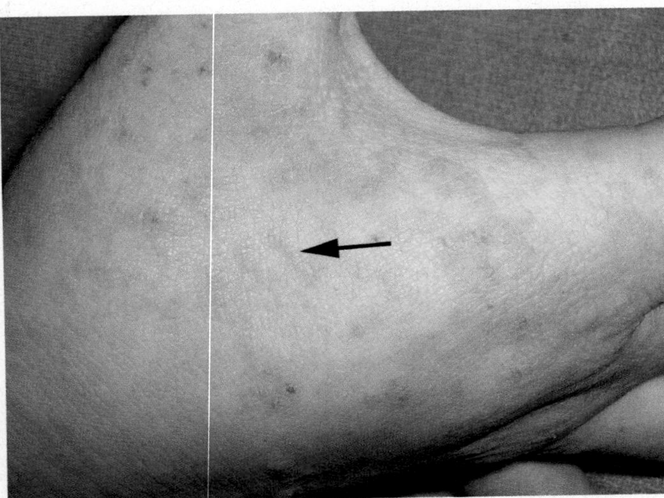

FIGURE 149-10 Scabies infestation on the hand and interdigital web space of an incarcerated woman. *Arrow* points to 1 burrow. (*Reproduced with permission from Richard P. Usatine, MD.*)

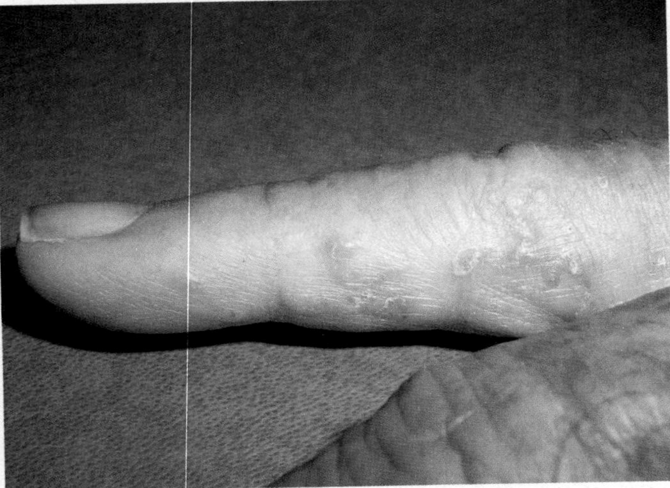

FIGURE 149-11 Burrows prominently visible between the fingers of this homeless man with scabies. Burrows are a classic manifestation of scabies. (*Reproduced with permission from Richard P. Usatine, MD.*)

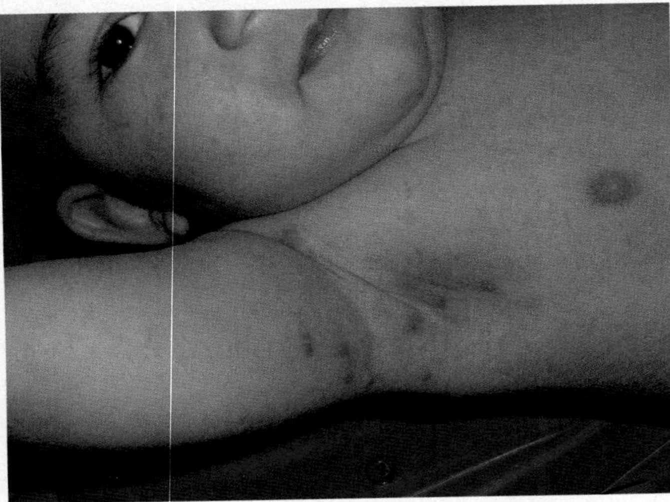

FIGURE 149-12 Scabetic nodules in the axilla of a toddler with scabies. (*Reproduced with permission from Richard P. Usatine, MD.*)

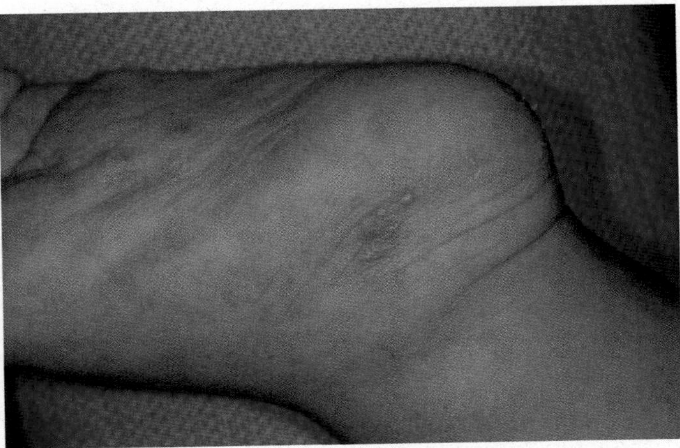

FIGURE 149-13 Scabies on the foot of a 9-month-old infant with pustules. Although this also looks like acropustulosis, the mother also had scabies. (*Reproduced with permission from Richard P. Usatine, MD.*)

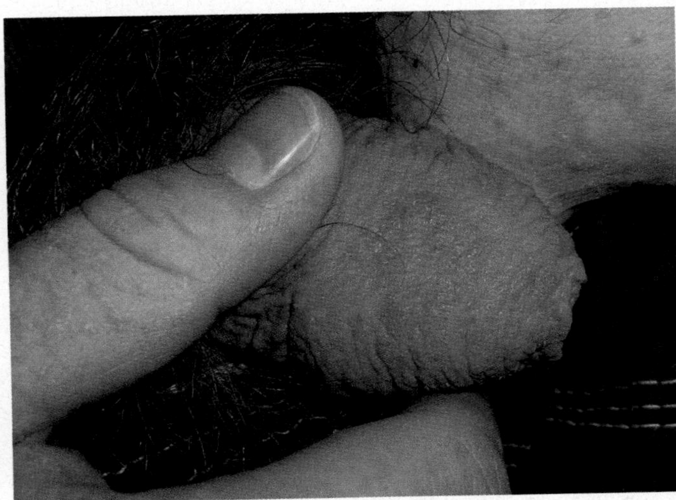

FIGURE 149-14 Pruritic papules on the foreskin of the penis, hands, and groin acquired as a sexually transmitted disease. (*Reproduced with permission from Richard P. Usatine, MD.*)

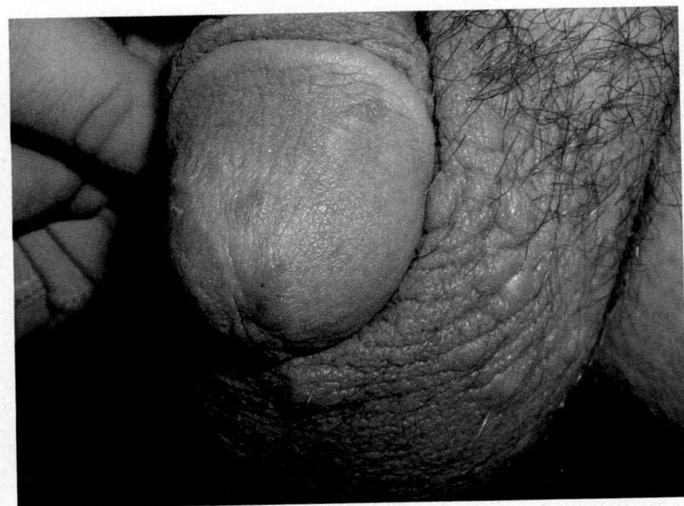

FIGURE 149-15 Pruritic papules and nodules on the glans penis and scrotum caused by scabies. Dermatoscopy demonstrated scabies mites in these lesions. (*Reproduced with permission from Richard P. Usatine, MD.*)

TYPICAL DISTRIBUTION

- Classic distribution in scabies includes the interdigital spaces (see **Figures 149-10** and **149-11**), wrists (see **Figure 149-6**), ankles, waist (**Figure 149-16**), groin, axillae, palms, and soles.
- Genital involvement can also occur. Especially on the penis (see **Figures 149-14** and **149-15**).
- In young children, the face and head can also be involved (**Figure 149-17**).

LABORATORY STUDIES AND IMAGING

- Light microscopy of skin scrapings provides a definitive diagnosis when mites, eggs, or feces are identified (see **Figures 149-3** to **149-5**). This can be challenging and time-consuming, even when mites, eggs, or feces are present. Packing-tape stripping of skin has also been used instead of a scalpel to find mites for examination under the microscope.[7]
- Dermatoscopy is a useful and rapid technique for identifying a scabies mite at the end of a burrow. The mite has been described as a jet plane (delta wing) with a contrail (**Figure 149-18**). The advantage of the dermatoscope is that multiple burrows can be examined quickly without causing any pain to the patient. Children are more likely to stay still for this than scraping with a scalpel or skin stripping with tape.
- If a dermatoscope is available, start with this noninvasive examination.[8] If the findings are typical, then a microscopic examination is not needed. If the findings are not convincing, or a dermatoscope is not available, perform a scraping. It is best to scrape the skin at the end of a burrow. Use a #15 scalpel that has been dipped into mineral oil or microscope immersion oil. Scrape holding the blade perpendicular to the skin until the burrow (or papule) is opened (some slight bleeding is usual). Transfer the material to a slide and add a coverslip.
- Tips for microscopic examination—Start by examining the slide with the lowest power available, as mites may be seen under 4× power, and the slide can be scanned most quickly with the lowest power. If no mites are seen switch to 10× power and scan the slide again looking for mites, eggs, and feces. Forty power may be used to confirm findings under 10× power.
- One study comparing dermatoscopic mite identification with microscopic examination of skin scrapings found the former technique to be of comparable sensitivity (91% and 90%, respectively) with specificity of 86% vs. 100%, even in inexperienced hands.[9] Another study reported sensitivity of dermatoscopy at 83%.[10] In this study, the negative predictive value was identical for dermatoscopy and the adhesive tape test (0.85), making the latter a good screening test as long as a microscope is available.
- Video dermatoscopy can also be used to diagnose scabies.[11] Video dermatoscopy allows for higher skin magnification than standard dermatoscopy but at a much greater cost for equipment.
- *S. scabiei* recombinant antigens have diagnostic potential and are under investigation for identifying antibodies in individuals with active scabies.[12]

BIOPSY

Rarely necessary unless there are reasons to suspect another diagnosis.

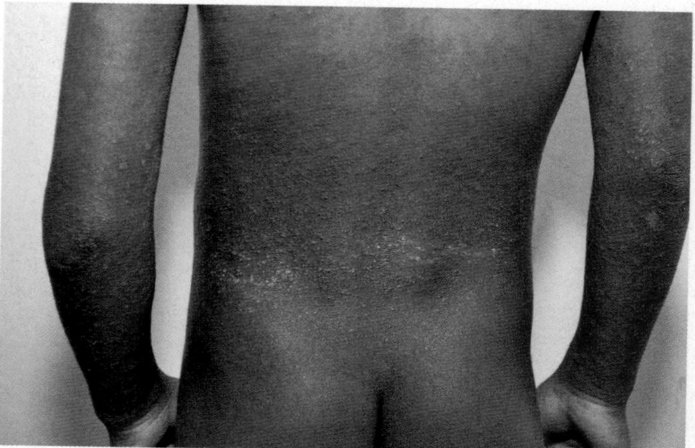

FIGURE 149-16 Scabies around the waist showing postinflammatory hyperpigmentation along with multiple papules and some crusting. (*Reproduced with permission from Richard P. Usatine, MD.*)

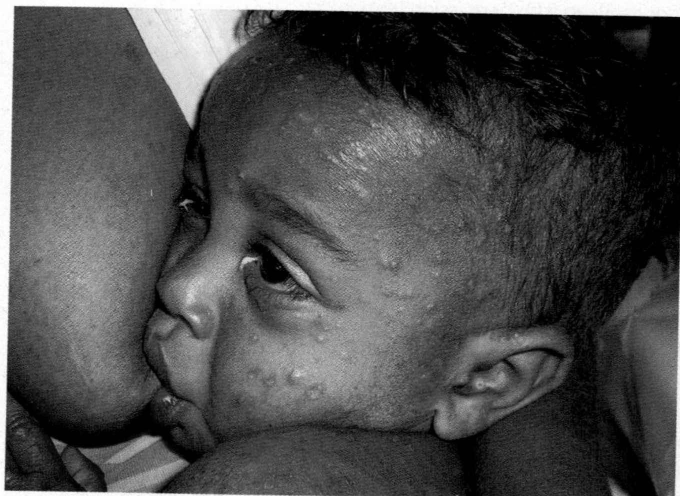

FIGURE 149-17 Scabies on the head and face of a young breastfeeding boy. (*Reproduced with permission from Richard P. Usatine, MD.*)

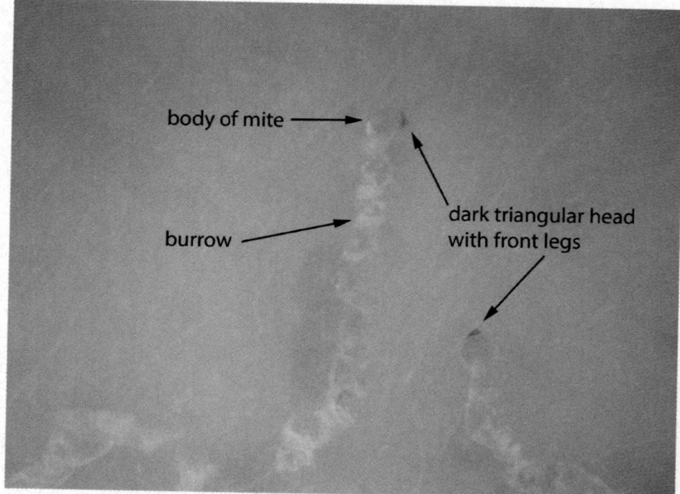

FIGURE 149-18 Two scabies mites visible with dermatoscopy. Note how the darkest, most visible aspect of the mite looks like a jet plane. In this case the oval bodies of the mites are also visible. (*Reproduced with permission from Richard P. Usatine, MD.*)

DIFFERENTIAL DIAGNOSIS

- Bed bugs live in the sleeping area and feed on people sleeping in their beds (**Figure 149-19**). Therefore, the pruritic papules of bed bug bites tend to appear in the morning. The skin manifestations of these bites can appear anywhere on the body, especially in skin not covered by pajamas. The bites may occur in a linear pattern of 3 bites in a row (**Figure 149-20**). The mnemonic for this is breakfast, lunch, and dinner. However, bed bug bites do not have to follow this pattern. Bed bug bites do not follow the typical scabetic pattern and will not show burrows in the skin. If bed bugs are suspected, it is best to have a professional come out to investigate for their presence.
- Arthropod bites—Bites may exhibit puncta that allow for differentiation from scabies. They usually don't follow the typical scabies distribution. Consider body lice as a possible diagnosis if the patient is living on the streets or in a homeless shelter. Look for the lice in the seams of the clothing rather than on the skin (see Chapter 148, Lice).
- Acropustulosis of infancy—A vesiculopustular recurrent eruption limited to the hands, wrists, feet, and ankles. It is rare after 2 years of age (see Chapter 116, Pustular Diseases of Childhood).
- Cutaneous larva migrans (CLM)—The serpiginous burrows of CLM may be mistaken for scabies burrows. CLM tends to have longer serpiginous lesions than does scabies. Also, the lesions of CLM are found in areas of the skin that have contacted soil contaminated by feces containing hookworm larvae (see Chapter 150, Cutaneous Larva Migrans).
- Dermatitis—All kinds of dermatitis (atopic dermatitis, contact dermatitis, seborrheic dermatitis, and drug eruptions) with pruritus can be mistaken for scabies. A good history and physical exam should help to distinguish the various patterns of dermatitis from scabies.

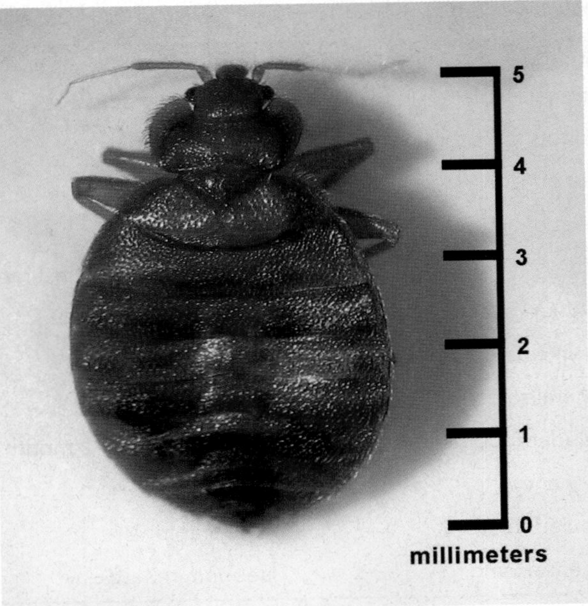

FIGURE 149-19 Adult bed bugs are on average 5 mm long, oval-shaped, and dorsoventrally flattened. They possess piercing-sucking mouthparts and are virtually wingless. Nymphs look like smaller, paler versions of the adults. (*Reproduced with permission from CDC/Blaine Mathison.*)

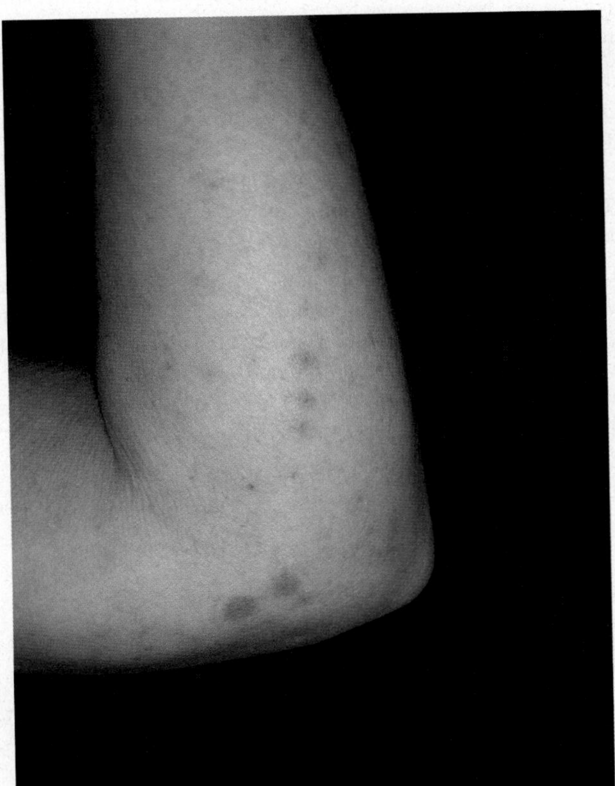

FIGURE 149-20 Bed bug bites on the arm of a 42-year-old woman. Note there is a linear pattern of 3 bites on the forearm. One way to remember this pattern is to think of the bedbug eating breakfast, lunch, and dinner. However, bed bug bites don't have to come in patterns of three. Scabies does not create this pattern. (*Reproduced with permission from Richard P. Usatine, MD.*)

MANAGEMENT

FIRST LINE

- Treatment consists of administration of a scabicide and an antipruritic.[1,13] The two most commonly used scabicidal medications are permethrin and ivermectin (see **Table 149-1** comparing these two medications). Antipruritic medications are typically oral antihistamines as needed.
- All household or family members living in the infested home and their sexual contacts should be simultaneously treated. SOR C Failure to treat all involved individuals often results in recurrent infestation within the family. Use of insecticide sprays and fumigants is not recommended.
- Environmental decontamination is a standard component of all therapies. SOR B Clothing, bed linens, and towels should be machine washed in hot water. Clothing or other items (e.g., stuffed animals) that cannot be washed may be dry cleaned or stored in sealed bags for at least 72 hours.
- Topical permethrin—First-line therapy often begins with topical permethrin 5% cream. Permethrin 5% cream is the most effective

TABLE 149-1 Comparison of Topical Permethrin to Oral Ivermectin in Treatment of Scabies

	Permethrin	Ivermectin
Form available	5% topical cream overnight	Oral tablets (3 or 6 mg) (0.2 mg/kg)
Strength of recommendation	A level evidence	B level evidence
Ease of use	Messy and cumbersome to apply	Easy to swallow—take with food
Onset of action	Quick	Delayed
Cost	Expensive without insurance	Relatively inexpensive
FDA approval for scabies	Yes	No
Use in crusted scabies	Acceptable	Preferred
General safety	Safe	Safe
Excluded populations	Avoid under age 2 months	Avoid under 15 kg weight
Pregnancy	Category B	Category C—Avoid use
Population use	Acceptable	Preferred
Repeat dosing	Needed in 7–10 days	May not be needed but often recommended in 7–10 days

treatment based on a systematic review in the Cochrane database.[13] SOR A It has the advantages of having a quick onset of action and FDA approval for scabies. The cream should be applied before bed to all areas from neck down in adults and children and head to toe in infants. Make sure to get under all fingernails and toenails, while sparing the eyes and mouth if applied to the face. The cream should be washed off 8 to 14 hours later. Repeat treatment is often recommended in 7 to 10 days. In patients with crusted scabies, use of a keratolytic cream may facilitate the breakdown of skin crusts and improve penetration of the cream.[14] Unfortunately, scabies resistance to permethrin is increasing. Although permethrin is now available generically, the prescription cost is still high.

- Oral ivermectin is available in 3 and 6 mg tablets and is prescribed as a single dose based on weight (0.2 mg/kg).[13] SOR B Dosing often needs to be rounded up to accommodate the use of whichever tablets are available. The need for a second dose at 7–10 days is debated, and the evidence for this is not strong. It is recommended that the tablets be taken with food to enhance absorption.[14] Although ivermectin is routinely prescribed for scabies, it is not FDA approved for this indication. It is not recommended in children weighing less than 15 kg.

SECOND LINE

- Other topical treatments include crotamiton, benzyl benzoate, malathion, and sulfur in petrolatum.[13]
- Lindane is no longer used in the United States. It is contraindicated for infants because of high risk for neurotoxicity, seizures, and aplastic anemia. It is also contraindicated in pregnancy.
- Symptomatic treatment with antipruritics such as diphenhydramine, hydroxyzine, and mid-potency steroid creams can be used for symptom management. SOR C
- Antibiotics are needed if there is evidence of a bacterial superinfection (see **Figure 149-7**). SOR C

Special populations:

- Infants—First-line therapy in infants is topical permethrin 5% cream. However, in infants younger than 2 months of age, a sulfur preparation is recommended as safe.[14,15] It is used as 5% to 10% precipitated sulfur in petrolatum and applied as described earlier for permethrin. Unfortunately, it has a bad odor.
- Elderly—First-line treatment for geriatric patients with scabies is either oral ivermectin or topical 5% permethrin cream. In elderly patients topical permethrin should also be applied to the scalp and face, as mites can infest the hairline and forehead in these patients. Patients should be advised to avoid applying cream to the eyes and mouth.[15]
- Pregnant women—First-line treatment in pregnancy is permethrin 5% cream, which is classified as category B in pregnancy; no category A treatments are available. Second-line treatments include topical sulfur and benzyl benzoate. Ivermectin is not recommended in pregnancy as it is category C.
- Breastfeeding women—Permethrin 5% cream is the drug of choice for breastfeeding women because there is no known risk to infant safety. Ivermectin is not recommended due to inadequate data on infant safety.
- Crusted scabies (severe scabies with crusting especially on the hands and feet)—The patient may be immunosuppressed and there are many more mites present, so the CDC recommends the use of both oral ivermectin and topical permethrin together.[15] SOR C Depending on the severity of the crusted scabies, the oral ivermectin may be prescribed in three doses (approximately days 1, 2, and 8), five doses (approximately days 1, 2, 8, 9, and 15), or seven doses (approximately days 1, 2, 8, 9, 15, 22, and 29).[15] SOR C The CDC also recommends prescribing the topical permethrin to be applied overnight every 2–3 days for 1–2 weeks to treat crusted scabies.[15] SOR C

COMPLEMENTARY AND ALTERNATIVE THERAPY

- Tea tree oil contains oxygenic terpenoids, found to have rapid scabicidal activity.[5]

- Anise seed oil displays antibacterial and scabicidal activity and is used topically, but should not be used in pregnancy.[16]

PREVENTION

- Avoid direct skin-to-skin contact with an infested person or with items such as clothing or bedding used by an infested person.
- Treat members of the same household and other potentially exposed persons at the same time as the infested person to prevent possible reexposure and reinfestation.
- Prophylactic treatment to prevent infestation of those with skin-to-skin contact has been shown by Cochrane database to have unknown outcomes.[17]
- Oral ivermectin may reduce the prevalence of scabies at 1 year in populations with endemic disease more than topical permethrin.[18] SOR B

PROGNOSIS

- The prognosis with proper diagnosis and treatment is excellent unless the patient is immunocompromised; reinfestation, however, often occurs if environmental risk factors continue.[1]
- Postinflammatory hyper- or hypopigmentation can occur.[1]

FOLLOW-UP

- Routine follow-up is indicated when symptoms do not resolve.
- Consider an immunologic work-up for individuals with crusted scabies.

PATIENT EDUCATION

- Patients should avoid direct contact including sleeping with others until they have completed the first application of the medicine.
- Patients may return to school and work 24 hours after first treatment.
- Patients should be warned that itching may persist for 1 to 2 weeks after successful treatment but that if symptoms are still present by the third week, the patient should return for further evaluation.

PATIENT RESOURCES

- **http://www.cdc.gov/parasites/scabies/.**
- **https://www.skinsight.com/skin-conditions/adult/scabies.**

PROVIDER RESOURCES

- What is the most effective treatment for scabies? *J Fam Pract.* 2017 August;66(8):E11-E12—**https://www.mdedge.com/jfponline/article/143068/dermatology/what-most-effective-treatment-scabies.**
- **http://emedicine.medscape.com/article/1109204.**
- **http://dermnetnz.org/arthropods/scabies.html.**

REFERENCES

1. Hengge UR, Currie B, Jäger G, et al. Scabies: a ubiquitous neglected skin disease. *Lancet Infect Dis.* 2006;6(12):769-779.
2. Pannell RS, Fleming DM, Cross KW. The incidence of molluscum contagiosum, scabies and lichen planus. *Epidemiol Infect.* 2005; 133(6):985-991.
3. Savin JA. Scabies in Edinburgh from 1815 to 2000. *J R Soc Med.* 2005;98(3):124-129.
4. Paller AS, Mancini AJ. Scabies. In: Paller AS, Mancini AJ, eds. *Hurwitz Clinical Pediatric Dermatology: A Textbook of Skin Disorders of Childhood and Adolescence.* Philadelphia, PA: Saunders; 2006:479-488.
5. Carson CF, Hammer KA, Riley TV. *Melaleuca alternifolia* (Tea Tree) oil: a review of antimicrobial and other medicinal properties. *Clin Microbiol Rev.* 2006;19(1):50-62.
6. Centers for Disease Control and Prevention. *Scabies: Epidemiology and Risk Factors.* http://www.cdc.gov/parasites/scabies/epi.html. Accessed November 2017.
7. Albrecht J, Bigby M. Testing a test. Critical appraisal of tests for diagnosing scabies. *Arch Dermatol.* 2011;147(4):494-497.
8. Fox GN, Usatine RP. Itching and rash in a boy and his grandmother. *J Fam Pract.* 2006;55(8):679-684.
9. Dupuy A, Dehen L, Bourrat E, et al. Accuracy of standard dermoscopy for diagnosing scabies. *J Am Acad Dermatol.* 2007; 56(1):53-62.
10. Walter B, Heukelbach J, Fengler G, et al. Comparison of dermoscopy, skin scraping, and the adhesive tape test for the diagnosis of scabies in a resource-poor setting. *Arch Dermatol.* 2011;147(4):468-473.
11. Lacarrubba F, Musumeci ML, Caltabiano R, et al. High-magnification videodermatoscopy: a new noninvasive diagnostic tool for scabies in children. *Pediatr Dermatol.* 2001;18(5):439-441.
12. Walton SF, Currie BJ. Problems in diagnosing scabies, a global disease in human and animal populations. *Clin Microbiol Rev.* 2007;20(2):268-279.
13. Strong M, Johnstone PW. Interventions for treating scabies. *Cochrane Database Syst Rev.* 2007;(3):CD000320.
14. Currie BJ, McCarthy JS. Permethrin and ivermectin for scabies, *N Engl J Med.* 2010;362(8):717-725.
15. Centers for Disease Control and Prevention. *Scabies—Resources for Health Professionals.* https://www.cdc.gov/parasites/scabies/health_professionals/meds.html. Accessed November 2017.
16. McGuffin M, Hobbs C, Upton R, Goldberg A, eds. *Botanical Safety Handbook.* Boca Raton, FL: CRC Press; 1997.
17. FitzGerald D, Grainger RJ, Reid A. Interventions for prevention the spread of infestation in close contacts of people with scabies. *Cochrane Database Syst Rev.* 2014;(2):CD009943.
18. Romani L, Whitfeld MJ, Koroivueta J, et al. Mass drug administration for scabies control in a population with endemic disease. *N Engl J Med.* 2015;373:2305-2313.

150 CUTANEOUS LARVA MIGRANS

Jennifer Tickal Keehbauch, MD

PATIENT STORY

A mother brought her 18-month-old son to the physician's office for an itchy rash on his feet and buttocks (**Figures 150-1** and **150-2**).[1] The first physician examined the child and made the incorrect diagnosis of tinea corporis. The topical clotrimazole cream failed. The child was unable to sleep because of the intense itching and was losing weight secondary to his poor appetite. He was taken to an urgent care clinic, where the physician learned that the family had returned from a trip to the Caribbean prior to the visit to the first physician. The child had played on beaches that were frequented by local dogs. The physician recognized the serpiginous pattern of cutaneous larva migrans (CLM) and successfully treated the child with oral ivermectin. The child was 15 kg, so the dose was 3 mg (0.2 mg/kg), and the tablet was ground up and placed in applesauce.

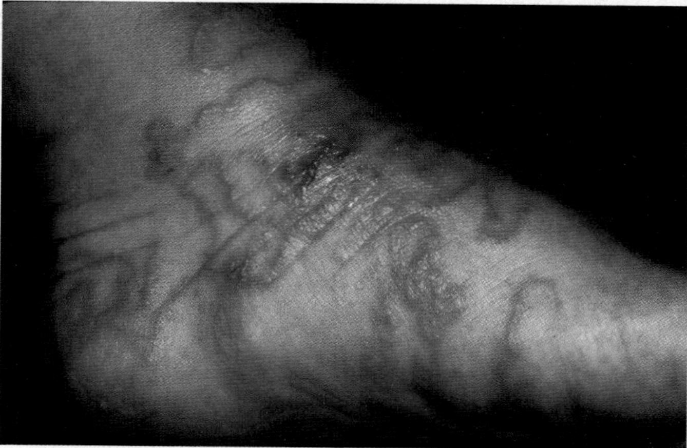

FIGURE 150-1 The serpiginous rash of cutaneous larva migrans on the foot of an 18-month-old boy after a family trip to the beaches of the Caribbean. (*Reproduced with permission from Richard P. Usatine, MD. Usatine RP. A rash on the feet and buttocks. West J Med. 1999;170(6):344-335.*)

SYNONYMS

Creeping eruption, plumber's itch.

EPIDEMIOLOGY

- Endemic in developing countries, particularly Brazil, India, South Africa, Somalia, Malaysia, Indonesia, and Thailand.[2,3]
- Peak incidence in the rainy seasons.[3]
- During peak rainy seasons, the prevalence in children is as high as 15% in resource-poor areas, but much less common in affluent communities in these same countries with only 1 to 2 per 10,000 individuals per year.[4]
- In the United States, it is found predominantly in Florida, southeastern Atlantic states, and the Gulf Coast.[2]
- Children are more frequently affected than adults.[4]

ETIOLOGY AND PATHOPHYSIOLOGY

- Caused most commonly by dog and cat hookworms (i.e., *Ancylostoma braziliense, Ancylostoma caninum, Uncinaria stenocephala*).[4]
- Eggs are passed in cat or dog feces.[2]
- Larvae are hatched in moist, warm sand/soil.[2]
- Infective-stage larvae penetrate the skin.[2]

DIAGNOSIS

The diagnosis is based on history and clinical findings.

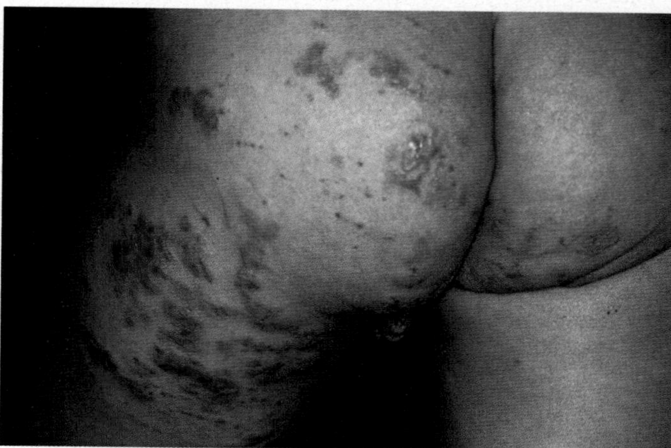

FIGURE 150-2 Cutaneous larva migrans on the buttocks and thigh of the same boy showing significant excoriations. (*Reproduced with permission from Richard P. Usatine, MD. Usatine RP. A rash on the feet and buttocks. West J Med. 1999;170(6):344-335.*)

CLINICAL FEATURES

- Elevated, serpiginous, or linear reddish-brown tracks 1 to 5 cm long (**Figures 150-1** to **150-3**).[2,5]
- Intense pruritus, which often disrupts sleep.[3]
- Symptoms last for weeks to months, and, rarely, years. Most cases are self-limiting.[5]

TYPICAL DISTRIBUTION

- Feet and lower extremities (73%), buttocks (13% to 18%), and abdomen (16%).[6,7]
- Areas that come in contact with contaminated skin.
  - Most commonly the feet, buttocks, and thigh.[3]

LABORATORY AND IMAGING

- Not indicated, but rarely blood tests shows eosinophilia or elevated immunoglobulin E levels.[5]

DIFFERENTIAL DIAGNOSIS

May be confused with the following conditions:

- Cutaneous fungal infections—Lesions are typically scaling plaques and annular macules with central clearing. If the serpiginous track of CLM is circular, this can lead to the incorrect diagnosis of "ringworm." The irony is that ringworm is a dermatophyte fungus whereas CLM really is a worm (see Chapter 144, Tinea Corporis).
- Contact dermatitis—Differentiate by distribution of lesions, presence of vesicles, and absence of classical serpiginous tracks (see Chapter 152, Contact Dermatitis).
- Erythema migrans of Lyme disease—Lesions are usually annular macules or patches and are not raised and serpiginous (see Chapter 227, Lyme Disease).
- Phytophotodermatitis—The acute phase of phytophotodermatitis is erythematous with vesicles; this later develops into postinflammatory hyperpigmented lesions. This may be acquired while preparing drinks with lime on the beach and not from the sandy beach infested with larvae (see Chapter 208, Photosensitivity).

MANAGEMENT

- Ivermectin (Stromectol) lacks FDA indication, but has been well studied and is the current drug of choice.[3]
  - A single dose of ivermectin 0.2 mg/kg is recommended.[3] SOR Ⓑ
  - Cure rates of 77% to 100% with a single dose.[8]
  - Ivermectin has been used worldwide on millions with an excellent safety profile.[3]
  - Ivermectin is contraindicated in pregnancy, in breastfeeding mothers, and in children weighing less than 15 kg.[3]
- Albendazole has been successfully prescribed for more than 25 years and is the Centers for Disease Control and Prevention (CDC) drug of choice.[5]
  - Albendazole also lacks FDA indication, and the recommended dose is 400 mg daily for 3 to 7 days.[3,5]

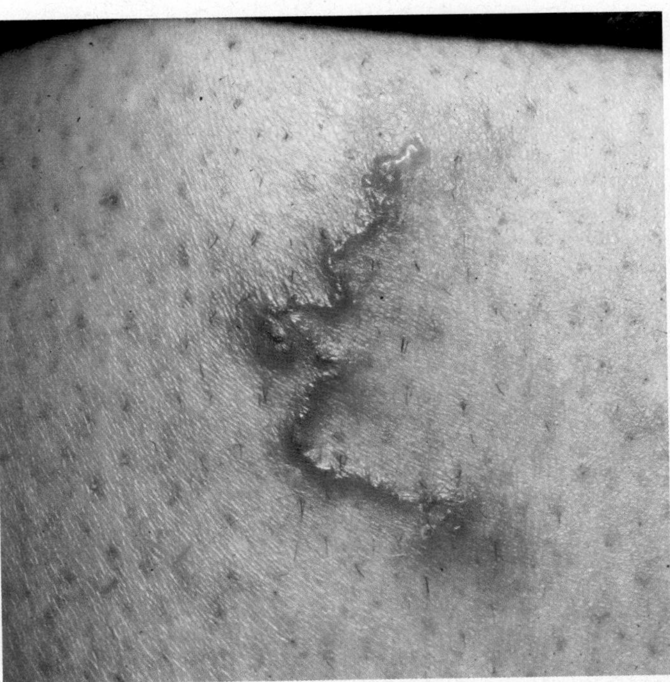

FIGURE 150-3 Close-up of a serpiginous burrow from cutaneous larva migrans on the leg. The actual larva is 2 to 3 cm beyond the visible tracks. (*Reproduced with permission from John Gonzalez, MD.*)

- Cure rates with albendazole exceed 92%, but it is less with single dosage.[3]
- Studies on compounded ivermectin and albendazole for topical use are limited, but promising for use in children.[3]

- Oral thiabendazole was the first proven therapy with FDA approval. It was removed from the U.S. market in 2010 but continues to be used outside the United States.

ADJUNCT THERAPY

- Antihistamines may relieve itching.
- Antibiotics may be used if secondary infection occurs.

PATIENT EDUCATION

- Wear shoes on beaches where animals are allowed.
- Keep covers on sand boxes.
- Pet owners should keep pets off the beaches, deworm pets, and dispose of feces properly.

FOLLOW-UP

- Follow up if lesions persist.

PATIENT AND PROVIDER RESOURCES

- eMedicine. *Cutaneous Larva Migrans*—**http://emedicine.medscape.com/article/1108784.**
- eMedicine. *Pediatric Cutaneous Larva Migrans*—**http://emedicine.medscape.com/article/998709.**
- Centers for Disease Control and Prevention (CDC). *Parasites–Zoonotic Hookworm*—**http://www.cdc.gov/parasites/zoonotichookworm/health_professionals/index.html.**

REFERENCES

1. Usatine RP. A rash on the feet and buttocks. *West J Med.* 1999;170(6):334-335.
2. Bowman D, Montgomery S, Zajac A, et al. Hookworms of dogs and cats as agents of cutaneous larva migrans. *Trends Parasitol.* 2010;26(4):162-167.
3. Heukelbach J, Feldmeier H. Epidemiological and clinical characteristics of hookworm-related cutaneous larva migrans. *Lancet Infect Dis.* 2008;8(5):302-309.
4. Feldmeier H, Heukelbach J. Epidermal parasitic skin diseases: a neglected category of poverty-associated plagues. *Bull World Health Organ.* 2009;87(2):152-159.
5. Montgomery S. Cutaneous larva migrans. In: *Infectious Disease Related to Travel. CDC Yellow Book.* 2012. http://wwwnc.cdc.gov/travel/yellowbook/2012/chapter-3-infectious-diseases-related-to-travel/cutaneous-larva-migrans.htm. Accessed October 2012.
6. Hotez P, Brooker S, Bethony J, et al. Hookworm infection. *N Engl J Med.* 2004;351(8):799-807.
7. Jelinek T, Maiwald H, Nothdurft H, Loscher T. Cutaneous larva migrans in travelers: synopsis of histories, symptoms and treating 98 patients. *Clin Infect Dis.* 1994;19:1062-1066.
8. Veraldi S, Angileri L, Parducci BA, Nazzaro G. Treatment of hookworm-related cutaneous larva migrans with topical ivermectin. *J Dermatol Treat.* 2017;28(3):263.

SECTION H DERMATITIS/ALLERGIC

151 ATOPIC DERMATITIS

Richard P. Usatine, MD
Lindsey B. Finklea, MD

PATIENT STORY

A 1-year-old Asian American girl is brought to her family physician for a new rash on her face and legs (**Figures 151-1** and **151-2**). The child is scratching both areas but is otherwise healthy. There is a family history of asthma, allergic rhinitis, and atopic dermatitis (AD) on the father's side. The child responded well to low-dose topical corticosteroids and emollients.

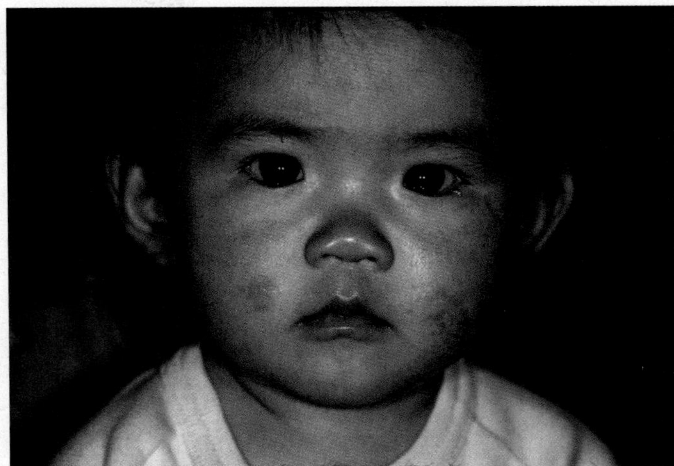

FIGURE 151-1 Atopic dermatitis on the cheeks of an infant. (*Reproduced with permission from Milgrom EC, Usatine RP, Tan RA, et al: Practical Allergy. Philadelphia, PA: Elsevier; 2004.*)

INTRODUCTION

AD is a chronic and relapsing inflammatory skin disorder characterized by itching and inflamed skin that is triggered by the interplay of genetic, immunologic, and environmental factors.

SYNONYMS

Eczema, atopic eczema.

EPIDEMIOLOGY

- AD is the most frequent inflammatory skin disorder in the United States and the most common skin condition in children.[1]
- Worldwide prevalence in children is 15% to 20% and is increasing in industrialized nations.[2]
- Sixty percent of cases begin during the first year of life and 90% by 5 years of age.[1] One third will persist into adulthood.[2]
- Sixty percent of adults with AD have children with AD (**Figure 151-3**).[1]
- It is estimated that 2% to 3% of the adult population is affected.[3]

ETIOLOGY AND PATHOPHYSIOLOGY

- Strong familial tendency, especially if atopy is inherited from the maternal side.
- Associated with elevated T-helper (Th) 2 cytokine response, elevated serum immunoglobulin (Ig) E, hyperstimulatory Langerhans cells, defective cell-mediated immunity, and loss of function mutation in filaggrin, an epidermal barrier protein.
- Exotoxins of *Staphylococcus aureus* act as superantigens and stimulate activation of T cells and macrophages, worsening AD without

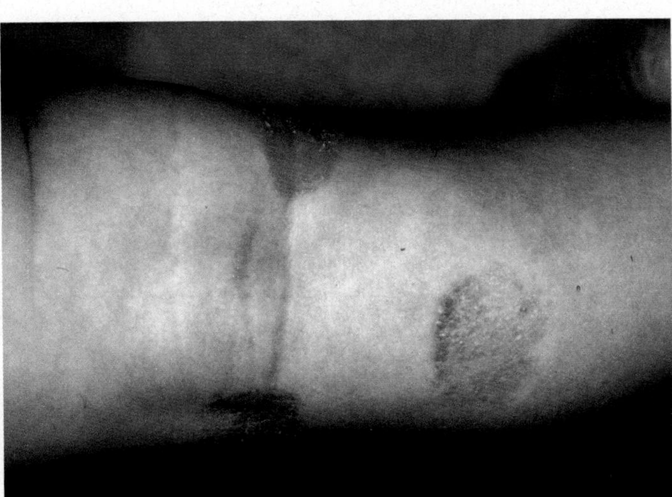

FIGURE 151-2 Atopic dermatitis on the leg of the infant in **Figure 151-1**. The coinlike pattern is that of nummular eczema. (*Reproduced with permission from Milgrom EC, Usatine RP, Tan RA, et al: Practical Allergy. Philadelphia, PA: Elsevier; 2004.*)

actually showing signs of superinfection. This bacterium has been found on more than 90% of adults with the disease, and only 5% of nonaffected adults.[4]

- Patients may have a primary T-cell defect. This may be why they can get more severe skin infections caused by herpes simplex virus (eczema herpeticum as seen in **Figure 151-4**) or bacteria (widespread impetigo). They are also at risk of a bad reaction to the smallpox vaccine with dissemination of the attenuated virus beyond the vaccination site. Eczema vaccinatum is a potentially deadly complication of smallpox vaccination (**Figure 151-5**).

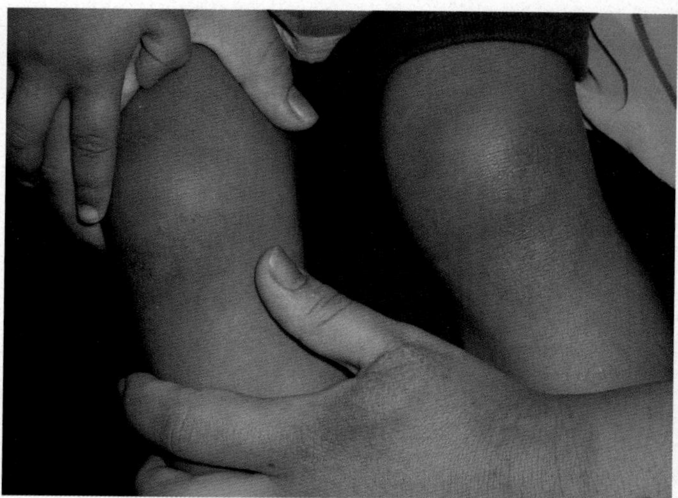

FIGURE 151-3 The child and his mother both have atopic dermatitis, but not in the most typical distribution. (*Reproduced with permission from Richard P. Usatine, MD.*)

DIAGNOSIS

- History—Pruritus is the hallmark symptom of AD. It is referred to as "the itch that rashes" as patients will often feel the need to scratch before a primary lesion appears. If it does not itch, it is not AD. Persons with AD often have a personal or family history of other allergic conditions, namely asthma and allergic rhinitis.
- The atopic triad is AD, allergic rhinitis, and asthma. Atopic persons have an exaggerated inflammatory response to factors that irritate the skin.
- Physical examination—Primary lesions include vesicles, scale, papules, and plaques.
- Secondary (or sequential) lesions include linear excoriations from scratching or rubbing that may result in lichenification (thickened skin with accentuation of skin lines), fissuring, and prurigo nodularis. Crust may indicate that a secondary infection has occurred. Postinflammatory hyperpigmentation and follicular hyperaccentuation (more prominent hyperkeratotic follicles) (**Figure 151-6**) may also be identified.

TYPICAL DISTRIBUTION

- AD often starts on the face in infancy and childhood (**Figures 151-1** and **151-7**) and then appears in the flexural folds, especially the antecubital and popliteal fossa (**Figures 151-8** to **151-10**).
- Involvement of the neck, wrists, and ankles also may occur (**Figures 151-11** and **151-12**).
- AD in adults can occur on the hands, around the mouth, or eyelids as well as all the other areas (**Figures 151-13** and **151-14**).
- In one series, the prevalence of hand involvement in patients with active AD was 58.9%. There was a significant trend toward an increasing prevalence of hand involvement with increasing age.[5]

OTHER FEATURES OR CONDITIONS ASSOCIATED WITH ATOPIC DERMATITIS

- Keratosis pilaris (**Figure 151-15**).
- Ichthyosis (**Figure 151-16**).
- Pityriasis alba (**Figures 151-17** and **151-18**).
- Palmar or plantar hyperlinearity.
- Dennie-Morgan lines (infraorbital fold) (see **Figure 151-14**).
- Hand or foot dermatitis (see Chapter 153, Hand Eczema).
- Cheilitis (see Chapter 34, Angular Cheilitis).

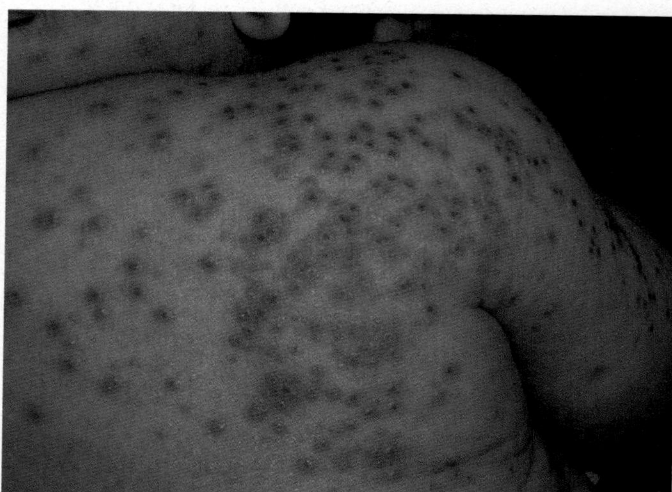

FIGURE 151-4 An 8-month-old infant with atopic dermatitis superinfected by herpes (eczema herpeticum). The father had an active case of herpes labialis (HSV1) before the outbreak began. (*Reproduced with permission from Buccolo LS. Severe rash after dermatitis. J Fam Pract. 2004;53(8):613-615. Frontline Medical Communications. Inc.*)

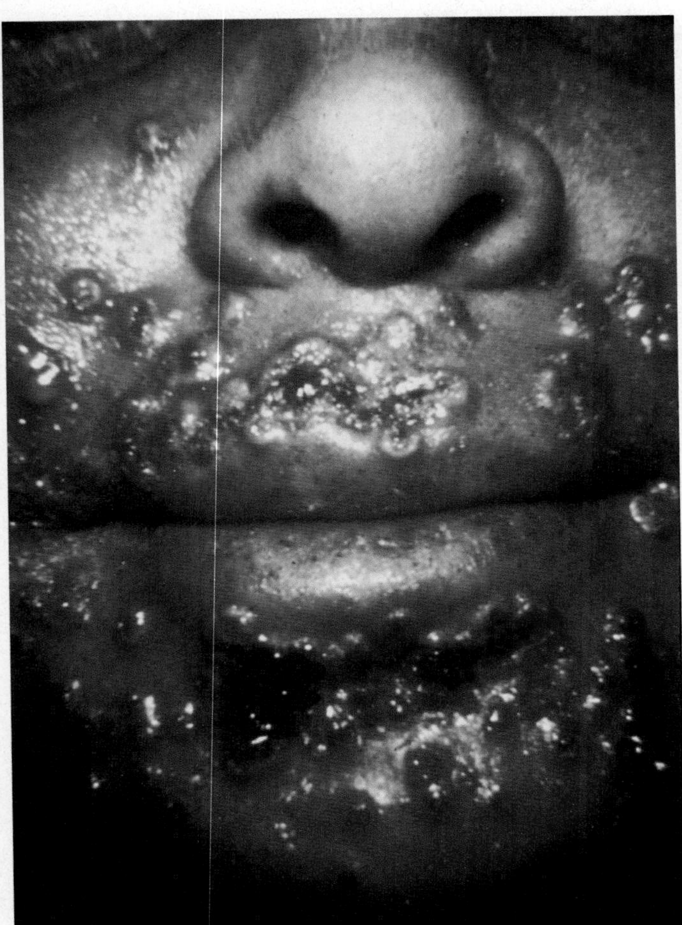

FIGURE 151-5 Eczema vaccinatum in a 17-year-old woman with atopic dermatitis who was given the smallpox vaccine. This eruption became this severe 8 days after her vaccination. (*Reproduced with permission from CDC and Arthur E. Kaye.*)

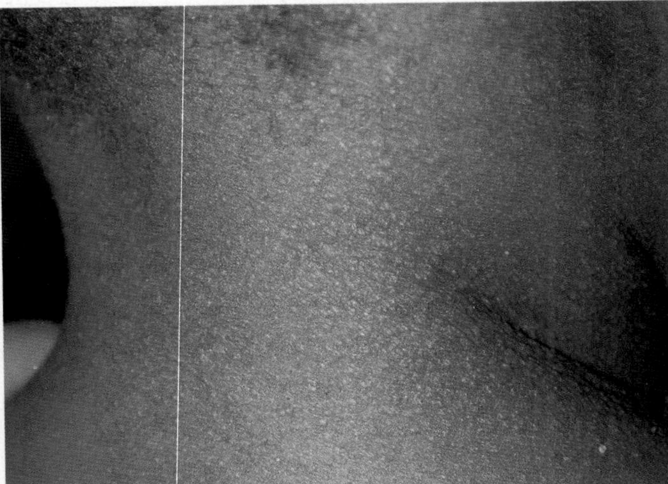

FIGURE 151-6 A young black girl with atopic dermatitis showing follicular hyperaccentuation on the neck. This pattern of atopic dermatitis is more common in persons of color. (*Reproduced with permission from Richard P. Usatine, MD.*)

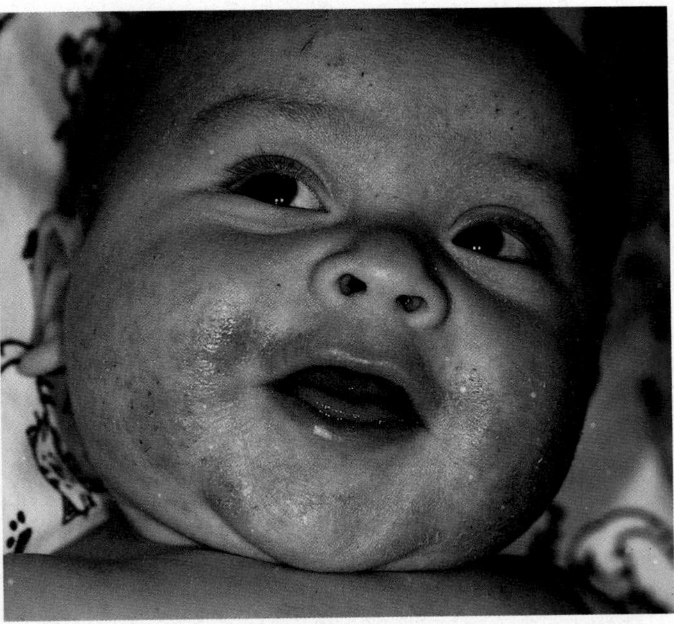

FIGURE 151-7 An infant with atopic dermatitis on the face that has become superinfected. (*Reproduced with permission from Milgrom EC, Usatine RP, Tan RA, Spector SL. Practical Allergy. Philadelphia, PA: Elsevier; 2004.*)

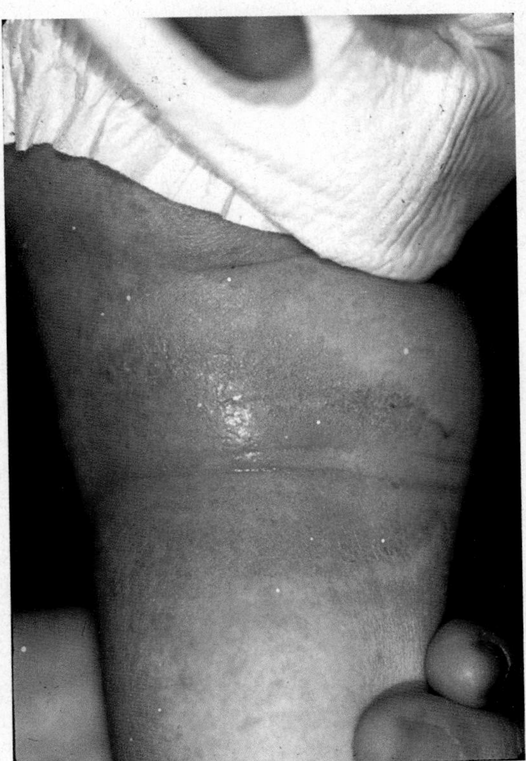

FIGURE 151-8 The same infant with superinfected atopic dermatitis of the popliteal fossa. (*Reproduced with permission from Milgrom EC, Usatine RP, Tan RA, et al: Practical Allergy. Philadelphia, PA: Elsevier; 2004.*)

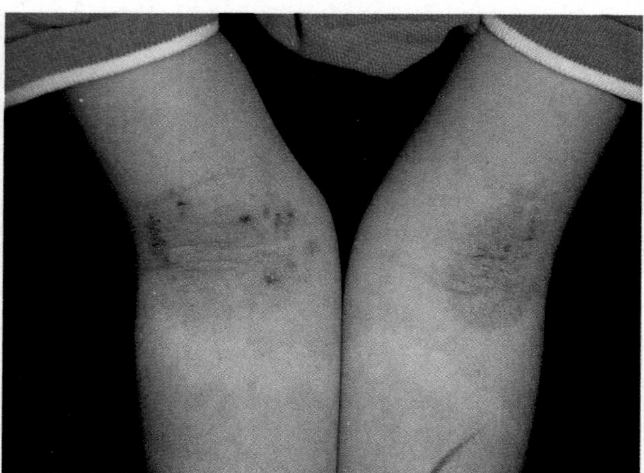

FIGURE 151-9 Atopic dermatitis in the antecubital fossae of a 6-year-old boy. Note the erythematous plaques with excoriations. (*Reproduced with permission from Richard P. Usatine, MD.*)

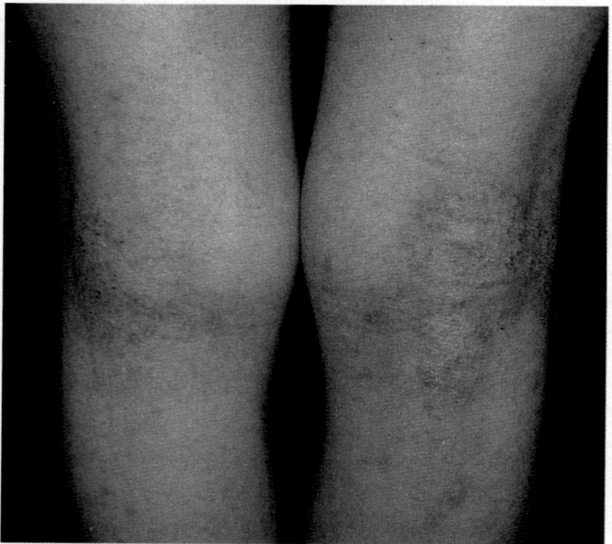

FIGURE 151-10 A 20-year-old young woman with severe chronic atopic dermatitis showing lichenification and hyperpigmentation in the popliteal fossa. (*Reproduced with permission from Richard P. Usatine, MD.*)

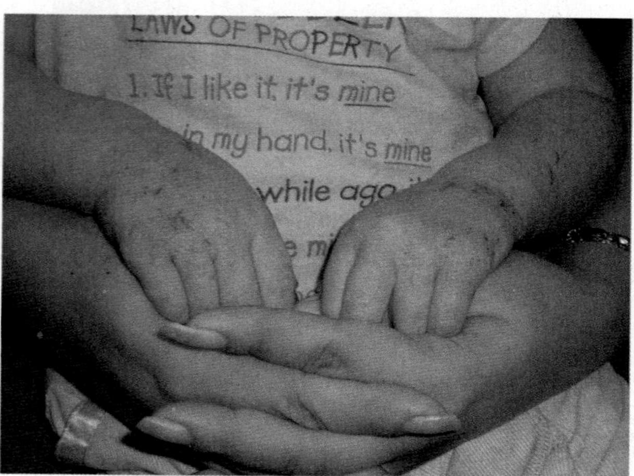

FIGURE 151-11 A 2-year-old girl with atopic dermatitis visible on her hands, wrists, and arms. (*Reproduced with permission from Richard P. Usatine, MD.*)

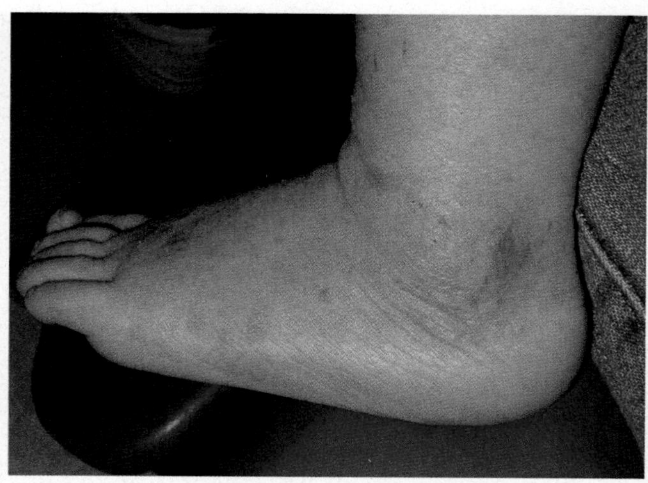

FIGURE 151-12 The girl in **Figure 151-11** with an exacerbation of her atopic dermatitis on the ankle showing many excoriations. (*Reproduced with permission from Richard P. Usatine, MD.*)

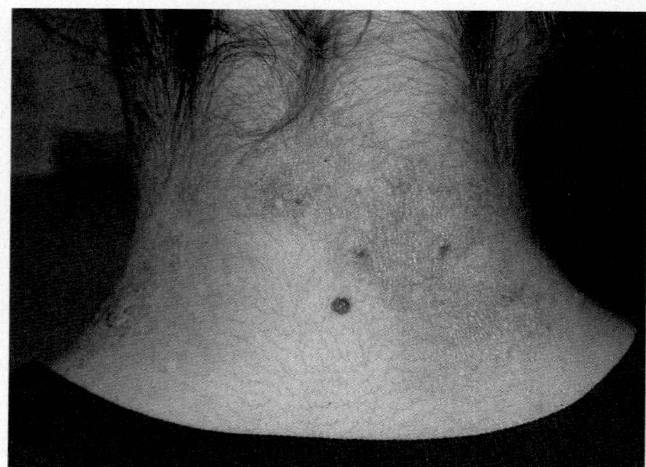

FIGURE 151-13 A young nurse with atopic dermatitis made worse by wearing the stethoscope around her neck. (*Reproduced with permission from Milgrom EC, Usatine RP, Tan RA, et al: Practical Allergy. Philadelphia, PA: Elsevier; 2004.*)

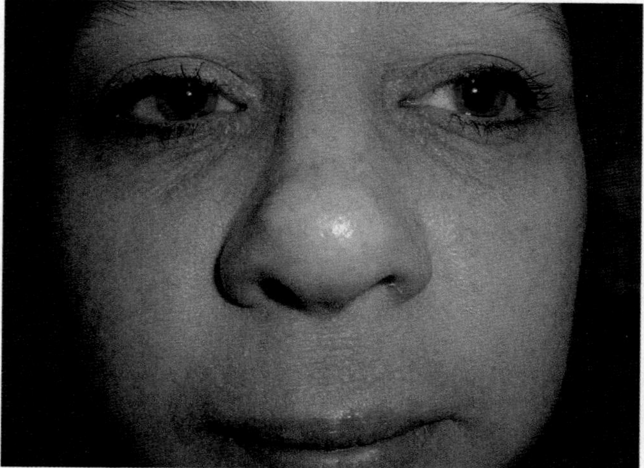

FIGURE 151-14 A young woman with chronic atopic dermatitis around her eyes and mouth. In addition to the eyelid involvement, the patient has Dennie-Morgan lines visible on the lower eyelids. (*Reproduced with permission from Richard P. Usatine, MD.*)

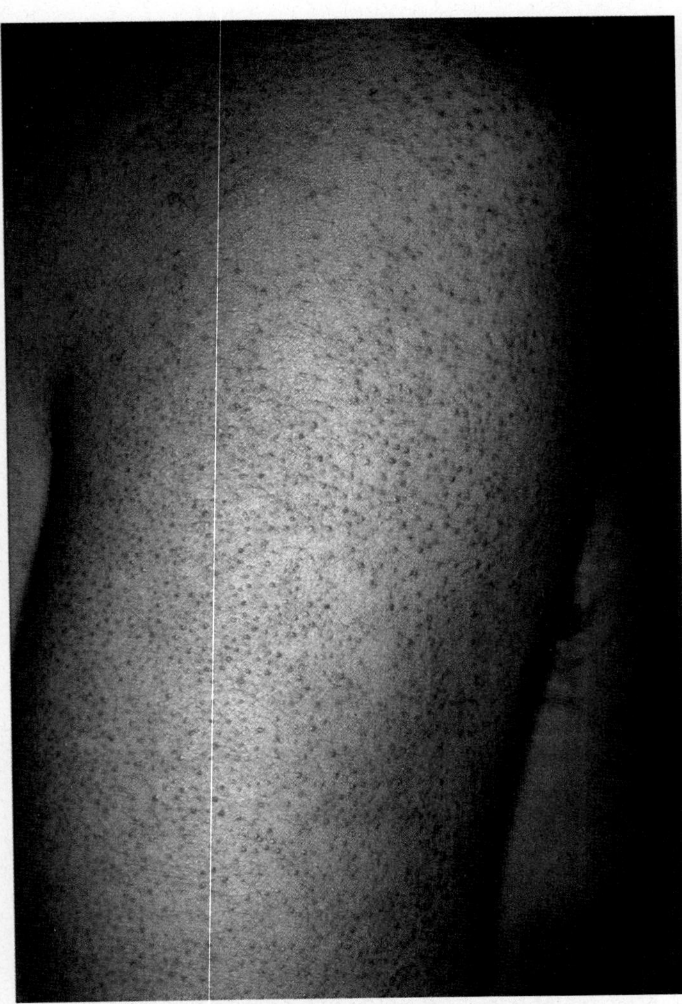

FIGURE 151-15 Keratosis pilaris on the lateral upper arm. Note how the papules can vary in color from pink to brown to white depending on the skin color of the person. (*Reproduced with permission from Richard P. Usatine, MD.*)

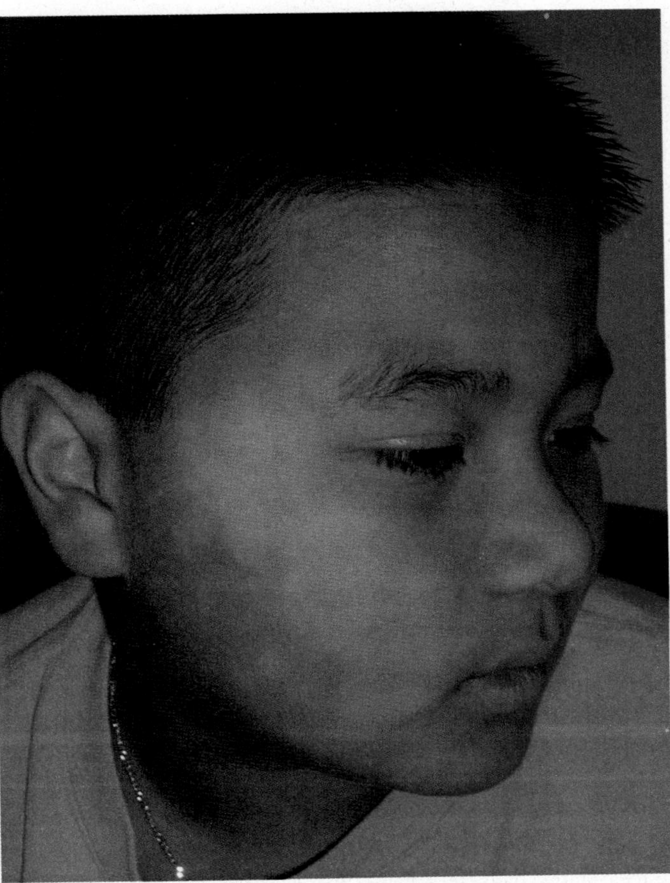

FIGURE 151-17 Pityriasis alba on the face of a young boy. (*Reproduced with permission from Richard P. Usatine, MD.*)

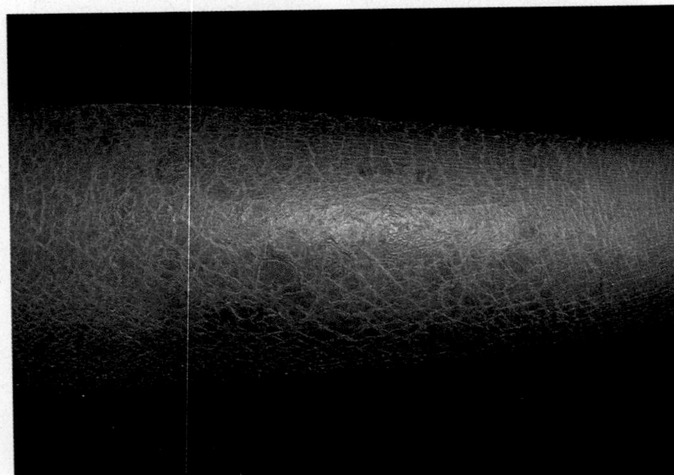

FIGURE 151-16 Acquired ichthyosis on the leg of a 9-year-old boy with atopic dermatitis. Note the fish-scale appearance along with the dry skin. (*Reproduced with permission from Richard P. Usatine, MD.*)

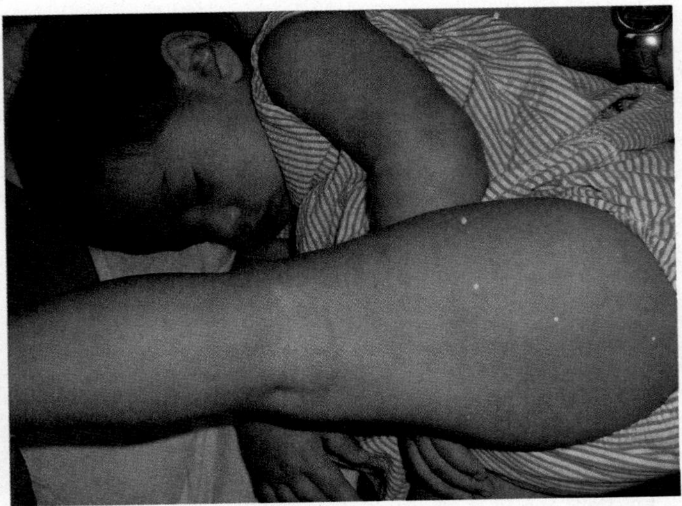

FIGURE 151-18 An 18-month-old girl with atopic dermatitis visible in her popliteal fossa and pityriasis alba on her arm. (*Reproduced with permission from Richard P. Usatine, MD.*)

- Susceptibility to cutaneous infections (see **Figures 151-4** and **151-5**).
- Xerosis (dry skin) (**Figure 151-19**).
- Eye findings—Recurrent conjunctivitis, keratoconus (**Figure 151-20**), cataracts, orbital darkening.
- A horizontal nasal crease may be seen over the bridge of the nose in a patient with allergic rhinitis prone to performing the allergic salute. In some patients this crease may become hyperpigmented (**Figure 151-21**).

LABORATORY STUDIES

Labs are rarely needed if the history and physical examination support the diagnosis. Occasionally, a KOH preparation may be needed to rule out tinea or a skin scraping to rule out scabies. Of course, both of these conditions can occur on top of AD. RAST (radioallergosorbent test) testing for food allergies and serum IgE levels are not of proven benefit.

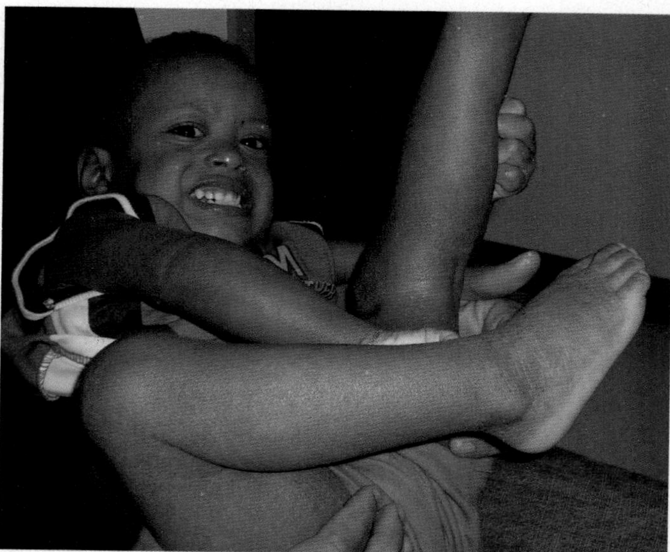

FIGURE 151-19 Severe atopic dermatitis in a 2-year-old black boy with very dry (xerotic) skin. He is spontaneously scratching and crying out in discomfort. (*Reproduced with permission from Richard P. Usatine, MD.*)

DIFFERENTIAL DIAGNOSIS

- Dyshidrotic eczema—Dry inflamed scaling skin on the hands and feet with tapioca-like vesicles, especially seen between the fingers (see Chapter 153, Hand Eczema).
- Seborrheic dermatitis—Greasy, scaly lesions on scalp, face, and chest (see Chapter 157, Seborrheic Dermatitis).
- Psoriasis—Thickened plaques on extensor surfaces, scalp, and buttocks; pitted nails (see Chapter 158, Psoriasis).
- Lichen simplex chronicus (sometimes called neurodermatitis)—Usually, a single patch in an area accessible to scratching such as the ankle, wrist, and neck (see Chapter 155, Psychocutaneous Disorders).
- Contact dermatitis—Positive exposure history, rash in area of exposure; absence of family history. Patch testing may be helpful in distinguishing from AD (see Chapter 152, Contact Dermatitis).
- Scabies—Papules, burrows, finger web involvement, positive skin scraping (see Chapter 149, Scabies).
- Dermatophyte infection—On the hands or feet, can look just like hand or foot dermatitis; a positive KOH preparation for hyphae can help make the diagnosis (see Chapter 146, Tinea Pedis).

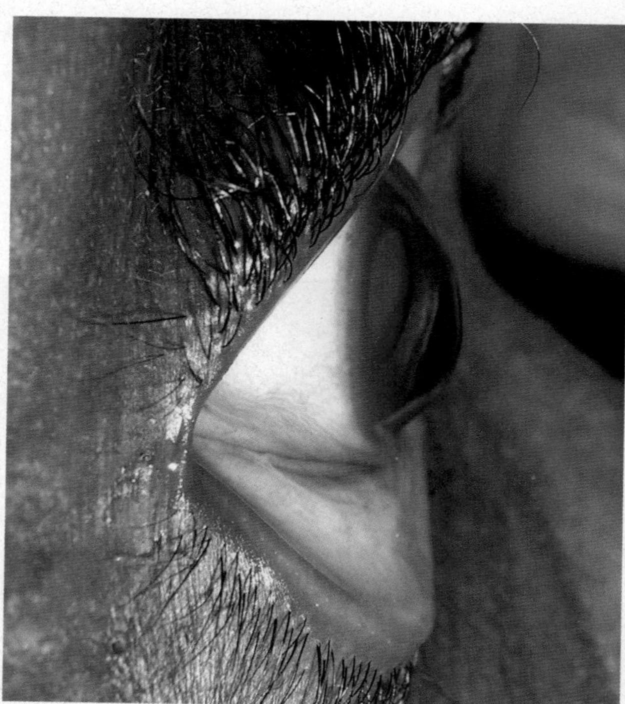

FIGURE 151-20 Keratoconus in a young woman with severe atopic dermatitis. She admits to rubbing her eyes frequently. In keratoconus the cornea bulges out in the middle like a cone and can adversely affect the health of the eye. (*Reproduced with permission from Richard P. Usatine, MD.*)

MANAGEMENT

FIRST LINE

TOPICAL THERAPIES

- Topical steroids and emollients have been proven to work for AD and are the mainstay of treatment.[1] SOR Ⓐ
- Over-the-counter emollients are recommended two to three times daily. Prescription-strength emollient devices are available and contain distinct ratios of lipids that repair the skin's barrier function.[6] SOR Ⓐ
- Vehicle selection and steroid strength area based on age, body location, and lesion morphology. The ointments are best for dry and

cracked skin and are more potent. Creams are easier to apply and are better tolerated by some patients.

- Use stronger steroids for thicker skin, severe outbreaks, or lesions that have not responded to weaker steroids. Avoid strong steroids on face, genitals, and armpits and in infants and small children.
- To avoid adverse effects, the highest potency steroids (e.g., clobetasol) should not be used for longer than 2 weeks continuously. However, they can be used intermittently for recurring AD in a pulse-therapy mode (e.g., apply every weekend, with no application on weekdays).
- Topical calcineurin inhibitors (immunomodulators, such as pimecrolimus and tacrolimus) reduce the rash severity and symptoms in children and adults.[1] SOR Ⓐ These work by suppressing antigen-specific T-cell activation and inhibiting inflammatory cytokine release. These are steroid-sparing medications that are helpful for eyelid eczema and in other areas when steroids may thin the skin (**Figure 151-22**).
- Topical phosphodiesterase 4 inhibitor (crisaborole) is a newer compound shown to regulate inflammation and decrease pruritus in preliminary studies. It is indicated for mild to moderate atopic dermatitis and has a favorable safety profile.[7] SOR Ⓑ However, its very high cost makes it available only to patients with insurance that will cover it. It will most likely require prior authorization and proof that other agents have failed.
- Dilute bleach baths (0.5 cup of 6% bleach in tub of bath water) lower the *S. aureus* burden on the skin, decreasing severity of AD.[8] SOR Ⓑ
- Short-term adjunctive use of topical doxepin may aid in the reduction of pruritus.[1] Its use should be limited to small body surface areas, as systemic absorption may cause drowsiness. SOR Ⓐ
- Topical and systemic antibiotics are used for AD that has become secondarily infected with bacteria. The most common infecting organism is *S. aureus*. Weeping fluid and crusting during an exacerbation should prompt consideration of antibiotic use[1] (**Figures 151-7**, **151-8**, and **151-23**). SOR Ⓐ
- The evidence that wet wrap therapy is more effective than conventional treatment with topical steroids in AD is of low quality.[9]

SECOND LINE

ORAL/SYSTEMIC THERAPIES

- For extensive flares, consider oral prednisone or an IM shot of triamcinolone (40 mg in 1 mL of 40 mg/mL suspension for adults). However, reliance on systemic steroids is not advised.[1] SOR Ⓒ
- The value of antihistamines in AD is controversial. If antihistamines are to be used, the sedating agents are most effective and can be given at night.[1] SOR Ⓑ
- UV phototherapy may also be used in refractory AD with some success.[1] SOR Ⓐ
- Cyclosporine, methotrexate, mycophenolate mofetil, and azathioprine for severe, refractory AD can be used in long-term maintenance therapy to treat and avoid relapse.[1] Cyclosporine is approved

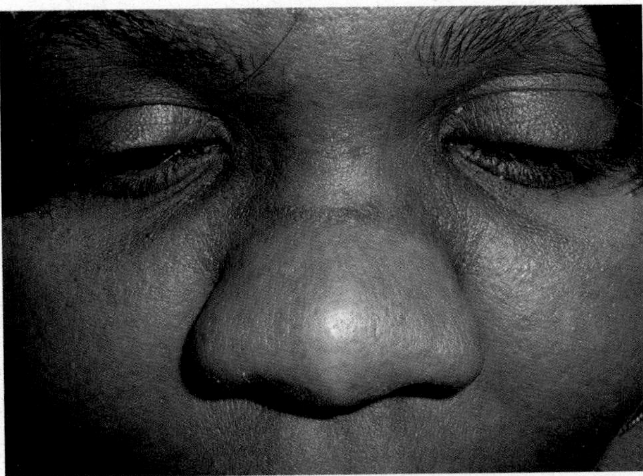

FIGURE 151-21 Hyperpigmented horizontal nasal crease in a patient with the atopic triad who repeatedly performs the allergic salute when her nose is feeling itchy. *(Reproduced with permission from Richard P. Usatine, MD.)*

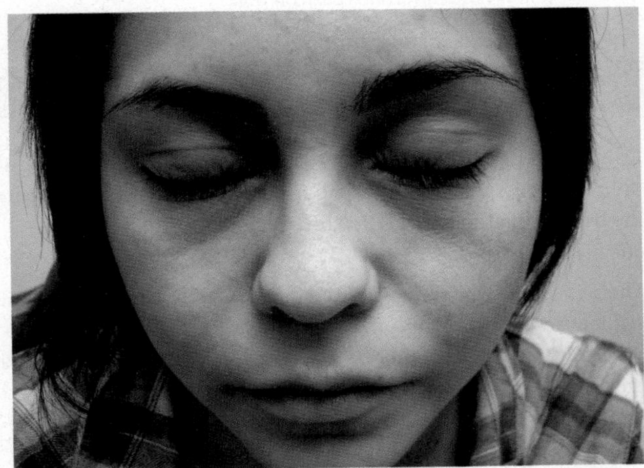

FIGURE 151-22 Atopic dermatitis involving the eyelids in this 19-year-old woman with relatively severe atopic dermatitis since infancy. A topical calcineurin inhibitor helped to get the eyelid eczema under control. *(Reproduced with permission from Richard P. Usatine, MD.)*

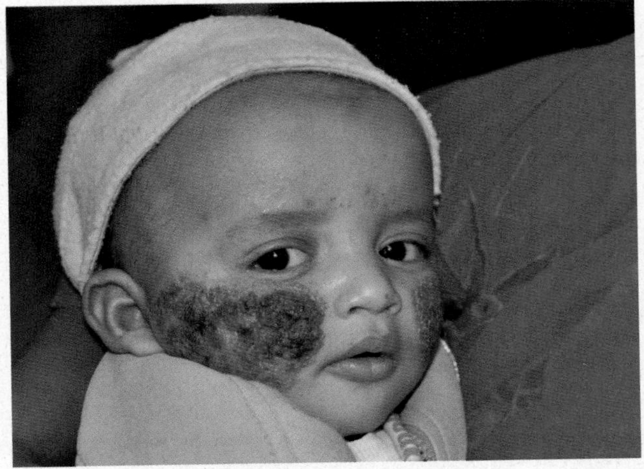

FIGURE 151-23 Superinfected atopic dermatitis on the cheeks. The crusting is a sign of secondary infection usually caused by *Staphylococcus aureus* or *Streptococcus pyogenes*. *(Reproduced with permission from Richard P. Usatine, MD.)*

for 1 year of lifetime therapy for skin diseases in the United States and 2 years in Europe (**Figure 151-24**). These medications require lab monitoring. SOR Ⓐ

- The biologic medication for chronic urticaria known as omalizumab decreased IgE levels in atopic dermatitis but this has not shown to consistently improve disease severity.[10] SOR Ⓒ
- The new biologic medication dupilumab is a monoclonal antibody that received U.S. Food and Drug Administration (FDA) approval for adults with moderate to severe atopic dermatitis in 2017. It inhibits IL-4 and IL-13 and has shown efficacy in improving the signs and symptoms of atopic dermatitis in adults during phase 2 and 3 studies.[11,12] SOR Ⓑ Injection-site reactions and conjunctivitis were more frequent in the dupilumab groups than in the placebo groups.[11,12] It is priced at over $30,000 per year. It will certainly require prior authorization and proof that other agents have failed.
- There are insufficient data to recommend for or against probiotics, vitamin or oil supplements, Chinese herbal therapy, and other complementary and alternative medicine.[13]

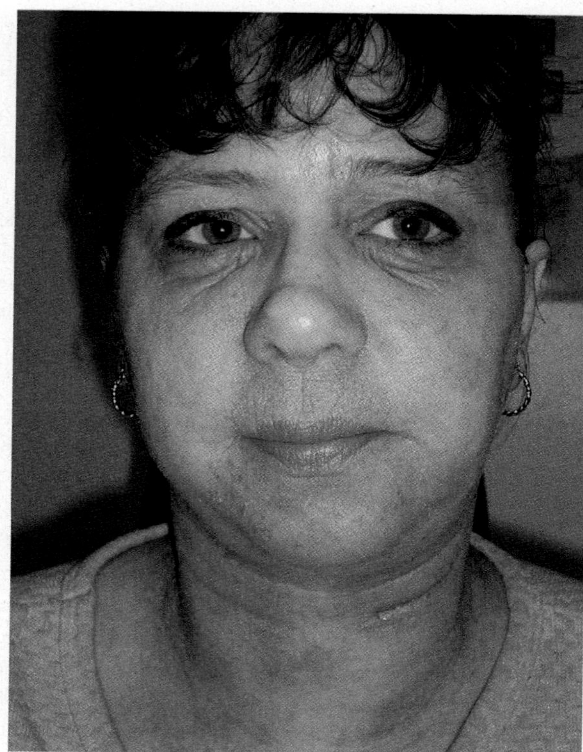

FIGURE 151-24 Atopic dermatitis was so flared up that this woman was started on oral cyclosporine 2 days ago. Her response to cyclosporine over the ensuing months was excellent. (*Reproduced with permission from Richard P. Usatine, MD.*)

PREVENTION

- Daily moisturization from birth to age 6 months (in high-risk children) may represent a cost-effective, preventative strategy to reduce the burden of atopic dermatitis. Petrolatum was the most cost-effective.[14]
- There is some evidence suggesting that controlling house dust mites reduces severity of symptoms in patients with the atopic triad. Bedding covers were found to be the most effective method to control dust mites and AD symptoms in this subgroup of AD patients. Unfortunately, dust mite interventions are not proven to be effective for patients with AD who do not have the full atopic triad.[1] SOR Ⓑ
- Dietary restriction is controversial but may be useful for true immunoglobulin E–mediated allergy. Common allergens include milk, egg, peanut, wheat, and soy. SOR Ⓑ There is insufficient evidence that dietary manipulation in children or adults without true allergy reduces symptom severity, and it may cause iatrogenic malnourishment.[13]
- One meta-analysis showed that serum vitamin D level was lower in the AD patients, and vitamin D supplementation could be a new therapeutic option for AD.[15]
- Patient education, avoidance of possible triggers (enzyme-rich detergents, wool clothing), and dry skin care should be optimized.
- There is some evidence suggesting that probiotic treatment of the pregnant mother and prolonged nursing of the child may delay onset of AD.[1] SOR Ⓑ

PROGNOSIS

The median duration of disease is 3 years. Factors portending a poorer prognosis include female gender, onset between 0 and 2 years

TABLE 151-1 Written Action Plan to Be Given to Patients (or Their Parents)

No skin lesions or dry skin	Prevention: Emollients, dry skin care, fragrance-free detergent, no drier sheets, once-weekly bleach bath
Mild flare	Prevention plus low- to mid-potency topical steroid and/or calcineurin inhibitors (e.g., hydrocortisone 2.5% or tacrolimus 0.1% to affected areas of face, axillae, genitals; triamcinolone 0.1% to extremities and body)
Moderate flare	Prevention plus mid- to high-potency topical steroids and/or calcineurin inhibitor (e.g., short course of triamcinolone under wet pajamas and/or stronger steroids such as betamethasone or fluocinonide)
Severe flare	Make an appointment ASAP to be evaluated for systemic therapy. This could be a short course of systemic corticosteroid as a bridge to a steroid-sparing systemic agent (e.g., cyclosporine, methotrexate or dupilumab)

Data from Rance F, Boguniewicz M, Lau S,[2] and from Chisolm SS, Taylor SL, Balkrishnan R, et al.[15]

of age, and more severe disease at time of onset. Twenty percent of children with atopic dermatitis will continue to have persistent disease beyond 8 years of age, and only 5% will have disease beyond 20 years of age.[17]

PATIENT EDUCATION

Patients need to know that scratching their AD makes is worse. Behavior modification is especially challenging in young children and may involve cutting fingernails short and occluding hands/body at night with cotton gloves or clothing. Because of its chronicity and cyclic nature, AD patients may have poor adherence. In one recent study, overall adherence was 32%. A written action plan may be employed to improve adherence (**Table 151-1**).

FOLLOW-UP

Regular follow-up should be given to patients with chronic and difficult-to-control AD. Establishing a good regimen is crucial to good control, and then visits may be adjusted to longer intervals between visits.

PATIENT RESOURCES

- Excellent patient education from Rady Children's Hospital in San Diego—**http://eczemacenter.org.**
- American Academy of Dermatology. Patient portal with tips and videos—**https://www.aad.org/public/diseases/eczema/atopic-dermatitis.**
- Baylor College of Medicine. Patient handout with explanation of wet-wrap protocol—**https://www.texaschildrens.org/sites/default/files/uploads/documents/atopic%20dermatitis%20%28eczema%29.pdf.**

PROVIDER RESOURCES

- **https://www.aad.org/practicecenter/quality/clinical-guidelines/atopic-dermatitis.**
- **http://emedicine.medscape.com/article/1049085-guidelines.**

REFERENCES

1. Hanifin JM, Cooper KD, Ho VC, et al. Guidelines of care for atopic dermatitis. *J Am Acad Dermatol.* 2004;50:391-404.
2. Rance F, Boguniewicz M, Lau S. New visions for atopic eczema: an iPAC summary and future trends. *Pediatr Allergy Immunol.* 2008;19 Suppl 19:17-25.
3. Sidburry R, Davis DM, Cohen DE, et al. Guidelines of care for the management of atopic dermatitis: Section 3. Management and treatment with phototherapy and systemic agents. *J Am Acad Dermatol.* 2014;71(2):327-349.
4. Boguniewicz M, Sampson H, Leung SB, et al. Effects of cefuroxime axetil on *Staphylococcus aureus* colonization and superantigen production in atopic dermatitis. *J Allergy Clin Immunol.* 2001;108:651-652.
5. Simpson EL. Prevalence and morphology of hand eczema in patients with atopic dermatitis. *Dermatitis.* 2006;17:123-127.
6. Eichenfield LF, Wynnis TL, Berger TG, et al. Guidelines of care for the management of atopic dermatitis: Section 2. Management and treatment of atopic dermatitis with topical therapies. *J Am Acad Dermatol.* 2014;71(1):116-132.
7. Paller AS, Tom WL, Lebwohl MG, et al. Efficacy and safety of crisaborole ointment, a novel, nonsteroidal phosphodiesterase 4 (PDE4) inhibitor for the topical treatment of atopic dermatitis (AD) in children and adults. *J Am Acad Dermatol.* 2016;75(3): 494-503.e6.
8. Huang JT, Abrams M, Tlougan B, et al. Dilute bleach baths for *Staphylococcus aureus* colonization in atopic dermatitis to decrease disease severity. *Pediatrics.* 2009;123(5):e808-e814.
9. Gonzalez-Lopez G, Ceballos-Rodriguez RM, Gonzalez-Lopez JJ, et al. Efficacy and safety of wet wrap therapy for patients with atopic dermatitis: a systematic review and meta-analysis. *Br J Dermatol.* 2017;177(3):688-695.
10. Heil PM, Maurer D, Klein B, et al. Omalizumab therapy in atopic dermatitis: depletion of IgE does not improve the clinical course—a randomized, placebo-controlled and double blind pilot study. *J Dtsch Dermatol Ges.* 2010;8:990-998.
11. Simpson EL, Bieber T, Guttman-Yassky E, et al.; SOLO 1 and SOLO 2 Investigators. Two phase 3 trials of dupilumab versus placebo in atopic dermatitis. *N Engl J Med.* 2016;375(24): 2335-2348.

12. Simpson EL, Gadkari A, Worm M, et al. Dupilumab therapy provides clinically meaningful improvement in patient-reported outcomes (PROs): a phase IIb, randomized, placebo-controlled, clinical trial in adult patients with moderate to severe atopic dermatitis (AD). *J Am Acad Dermatol.* 2016;75(3):506-515.
13. Sidbury R, Tom WL, Bergman JN, et al. Guidelines of care for the management of atopic dermatitis: Section 4. Prevention of disease flares and use of adjunctive therapies and approaches. *J Am Acad Dermatol.* 2014;71(6):1218-1233.
14. Xu S, Immaneni S, Hazen GB, et al. Cost-effectiveness of prophylactic moisturization for atopic dermatitis. *JAMA Pediatr.* 2017;171(2):e163909.
15. Kim MJ, Kim SN, Lee YW, et al. Vitamin D status and efficacy of vitamin D supplementation in atopic dermatitis: a systematic review and meta-analysis. *Nutrients.* 2016;8(12):789.
16. Chisolm SS, Taylor SL, Balkrishnan R, et al. Written action plans: potential for improving outcomes in children with atopic dermatitis. *J Am Acad Dermatol.* 2008;59:677-683.
17. Kim PH, Chao LX, Simpson EL, et al. Persistence of atopic dermatitis (AD): a systematic review and meta-analysis. *J Am Acad Dermatol.* 2016;75(4):681-687.

152 CONTACT DERMATITIS

Richard P. Usatine, MD
Sahand Rahnama-Moghadam, MD, MS

PATIENT STORY

A 38-year-old woman twisted her right ankle and applied a Chinese medicine patch to relieve the pain. The following day the patient developed a severe contact dermatitis (CD) with many small vesicles (<5 mm) and bullae (>5 mm) (**Figure 152-1**). The erythema had a well-demarcated border and was traced by the doctor's pen. Cold compresses and a high-potency topical steroid were prescribed. When the patient showed little improvement, a 2-week course of oral prednisone was given, starting with 60 mg daily and tapering down to 5 mg daily. The patient responded rapidly and the CD fully resolved.[1,2]

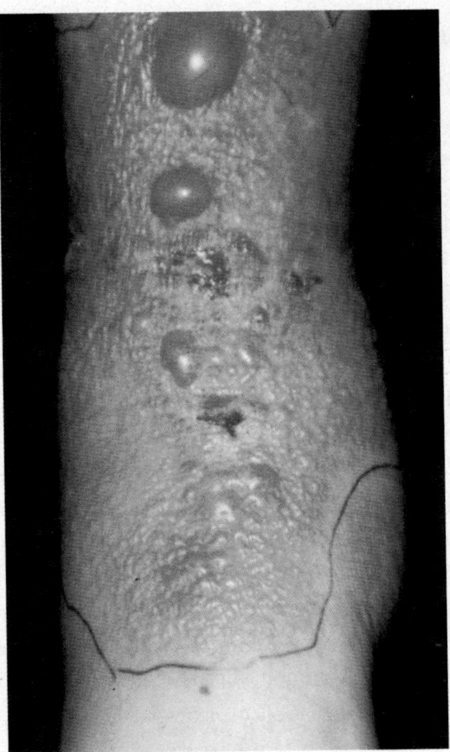

FIGURE 152-1 Severe acute allergic contact dermatitis on the ankle of a woman after application of a Chinese topical medicine for a sprained ankle. *(Reproduced with permission from Milgrom EC, Usatine RP, Tan RA, Spector SL. Practical Allergy. Philadelphia, PA: Elsevier; 2004.)*

INTRODUCTION

CD is a common inflammatory skin condition characterized by erythematous and pruritic skin lesions resulting from the contact of skin with a foreign substance. Irritant contact dermatitis (ICD) is caused by the non–immune-modulated irritation of the skin by a substance, resulting in a skin changes. Allergic contact dermatitis (ACD) is a delayed-type (type-IV) hypersensitivity reaction in which a foreign substance comes into contact with the skin and, upon reexposure, skin changes occur.[3]

EPIDEMIOLOGY

- Some of the most common types of CD are secondary to exposures to poison ivy, nickel, preservatives, and fragrances.[4,5]
- Patch testing data indicate that the five most prevalent contact allergens of more than 3700 known are nickel (20.1% of patients tested), fragrance mix (11.9%), the preservative methylisothiazolinone (MI) (10.9%), neomycin (8.4%), and a three-way tie (7.4%) between bacitracin, cobalt, and balsam of Peru.[6]
- Occupational skin diseases (chiefly CD) rank second only to traumatic injuries as the most common type of occupational disease. Chemical irritants such as solvents and cutting fluids account for most ICD cases. In occupational skin diseases, 80% of the cases are related to ICD.[5] Hands were primarily affected in 64% of ACD and 80% of ICD[4] (**Figure 152-2**).

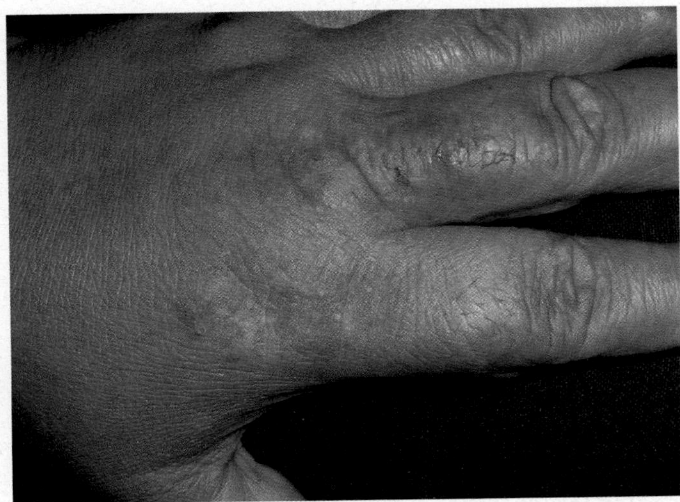

FIGURE 152-2 Occupational irritant contact dermatitis in a woman whose hands are exposed to onions while cooking in her family restaurant. *(Reproduced with permission from Richard P. Usatine, MD.)*

ETIOLOGY AND PATHOPHYSIOLOGY

- CD is a common inflammatory skin condition characterized by erythematous and pruritic skin lesions resulting from the contact of skin with a foreign substance.
- ICD is caused by the non–immune-modulated irritation of the skin by a substance, resulting in a skin rash.

- ACD is a delayed-type hypersensitivity reaction in which a foreign substance comes into contact with the skin and is linked to skin protein forming an antigen complex that leads to sensitization. Upon reexposure of the epidermis to the antigen, the sensitized T cells initiate an inflammatory cascade, leading to the skin changes seen in ACD.

DIAGNOSIS

HISTORY

Ask about contact with known allergens (i.e., nickel, fragrances, preservatives, neomycin, and poison ivy/oak).

- Nickel exposure is often related to the wearing of rings, jewelry (especially costume jewelry), and metal belt buckles (**Figures 152-3** through **152-6**).
- Fragrances in the forms of deodorants and perfumes, whether applied to the skin or the clothes (**Figure 152-7**).
- Neomycin applied as a triple antibiotic ointment by patients (**Figure 152-8**).
- Poison ivy/oak in outdoor settings. Especially ask when the distribution of the reaction is linear (**Figure 152-9**).
- Ask about occupational exposures, especially wet work and solvents. For example, chemicals used in shoes can cause ACD on the hands of someone working in a shoe store (**Figure 152-10**).
- Tapes applied to skin after cuts or surgery are frequent causes of CD.
- If the CD is on the feet, ask about new shoes, as adhesives and rubber accelerators are common culprits (**Figures 152-11** and **152-12**).
- Preservatives in the forms of cosmetics, wet wipes, and personal care products.
- Wet wipes for the skin of the face, body, and anogenital area are becoming a more common cause of CD, often to isothiazolinone (**Figures 152-13** and **152-14**).
  - In **Figure 152-15**, this truck driver was using baby wipes to clean his skin during long drives. Patch testing ultimately revealed that he was allergic to one of the ingredients in those wipes.

Thus a detailed history of products used on the skin may reveal a suspected allergen.

CLINICAL FEATURES

All types of CD have erythema. Although it is not always possible to distinguish between ICD and ACD, here are some features that might help:

- ICD:
  - Location—usually the hands.
  - Symptoms—burning, pruritus, pain.
  - Dry and fissured skin (see **Figure 152-2**).
  - Indistinct borders.
- ACD:
  - Location—usually exposed area of skin, often the hands.
  - Pruritus is the dominant symptom.
  - Vesicles and bullae (see **Figures 152-1** and **152-8**).
  - Patterned angles, lines, and borders (see **Figures 152-8** through **152-12**).

Both ICD and ACD may be complicated by bacterial superinfection showing signs of exudate, weeping, and crusts.

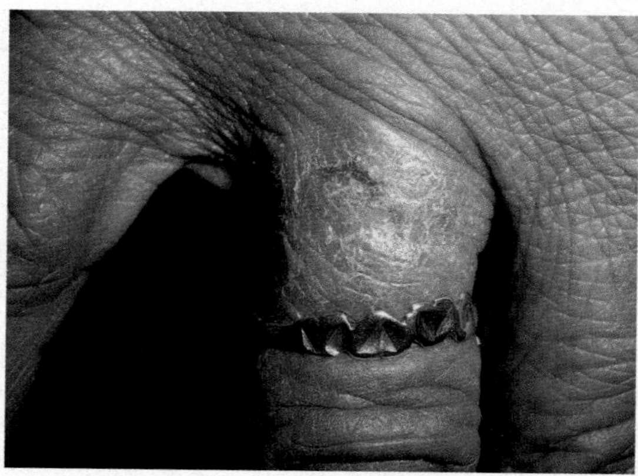

FIGURE 152-3 Patient moved up her ring to show the allergic contact dermatitis secondary to a nickel allergy to the ring. Patch testing showed she was allergic to nickel, bacitracin, and neomycin. (*Reproduced with permission from Richard P. Usatine, MD.*)

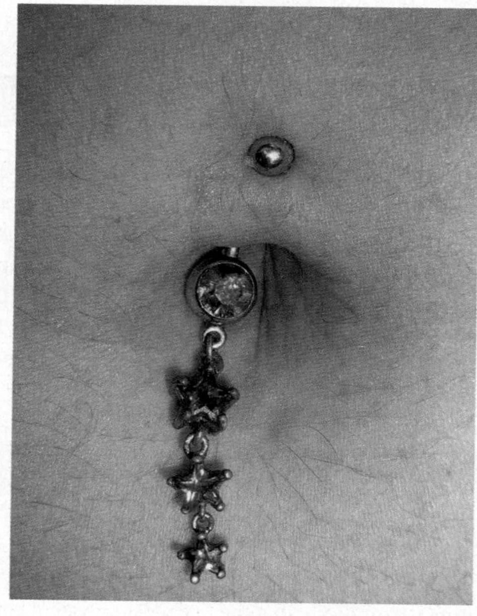

FIGURE 152-4 Allergic contact dermatitis to the metal in the bellybutton ring of a young woman. (*Reproduced with permission from Richard P. Usatine, MD.*)

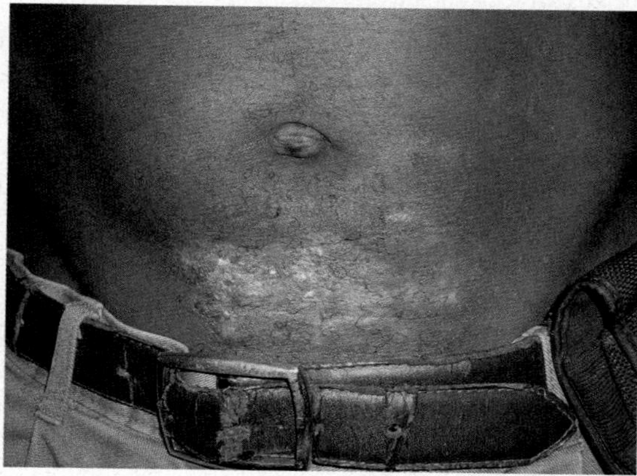

FIGURE 152-5 Allergic contact dermatitis to the metal in the belt buckle causing erythema, scaling, and hyperpigmentation. (*Reproduced with permission from Richard P. Usatine, MD.*)

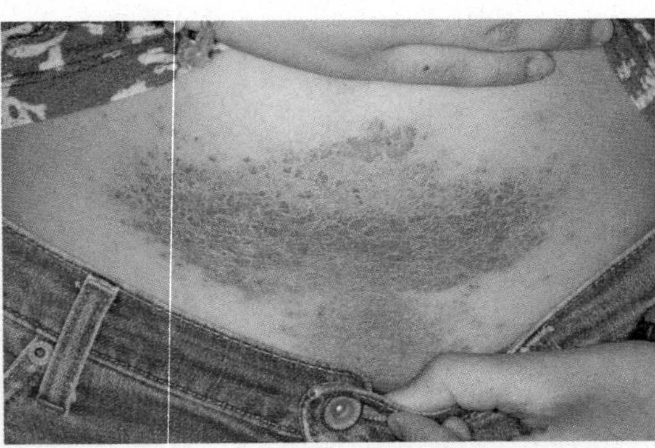

FIGURE 152-6 A 12-year-old girl with atopic dermatitis and allergy to the metal in her pants' fastener and metal belts when she wears them. (*Reproduced with permission from Richard P. Usatine, MD.*)

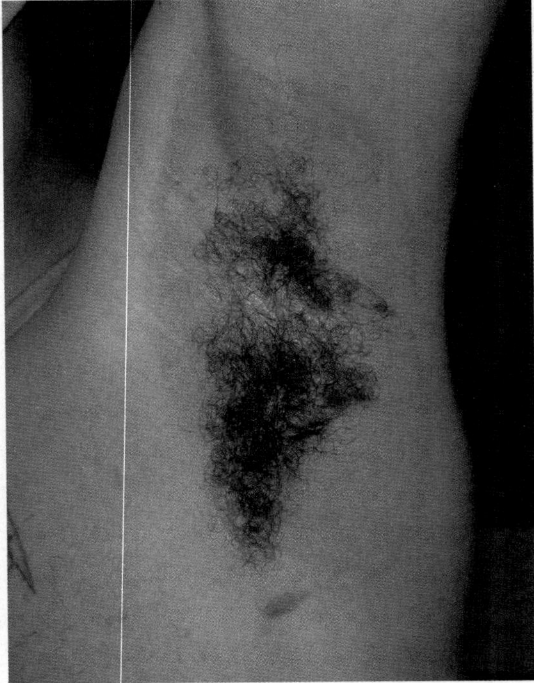

FIGURE 152-7 Allergic contact dermatitis to the fragrance in a new deodorant. (*Reproduced with permission from Milgrom EC, Usatine RP, Tan RA, et al: Practical Allergy. Philadelphia, PA: Elsevier; 2004.*)

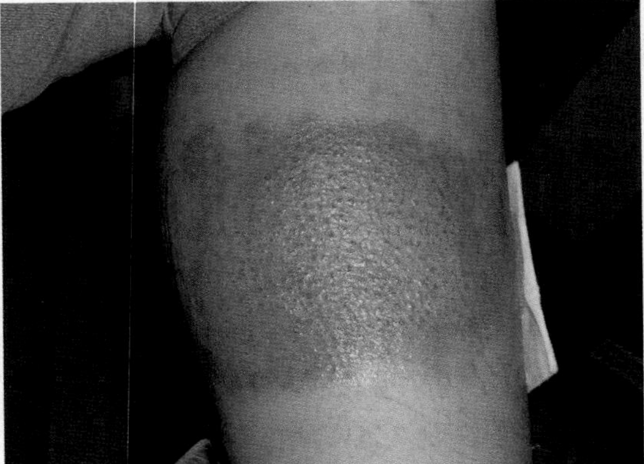

FIGURE 152-8 Allergic contact dermatitis to neomycin applied to the leg of a young woman. Her mom gave her triple antibiotic ointment to place over a bug bite with a large nonstick pad. The contact allergy follows the exact size of the pad and only occurs where the antibiotic was applied. (*Reproduced with permission from Richard P. Usatine, MD.*)

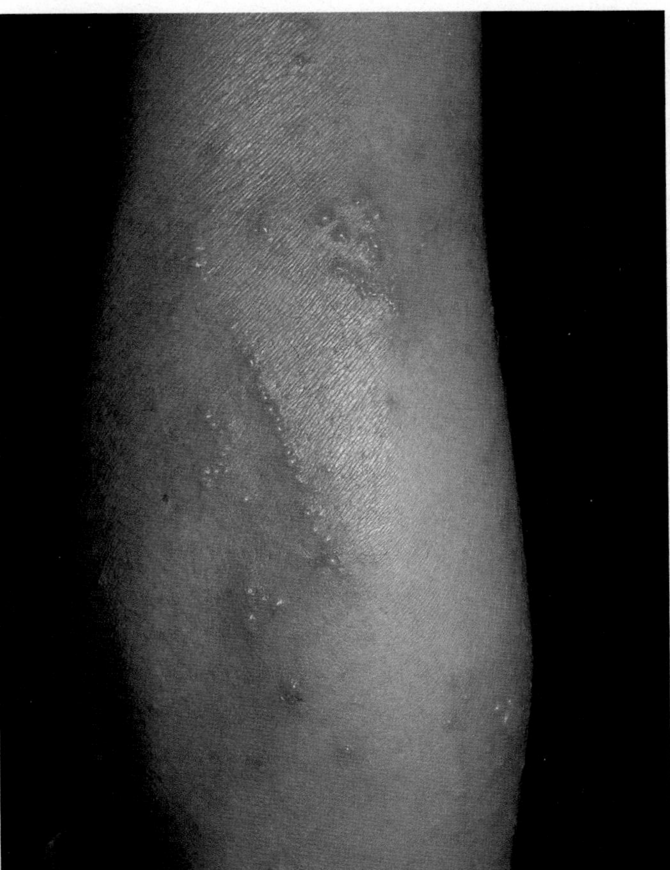

FIGURE 152-9 A linear pattern of allergic contact dermatitis from poison ivy. Note the impressive line of vesicles where the leaf brushed the skin. (*Reproduced with permission from Richard P. Usatine, MD.*)

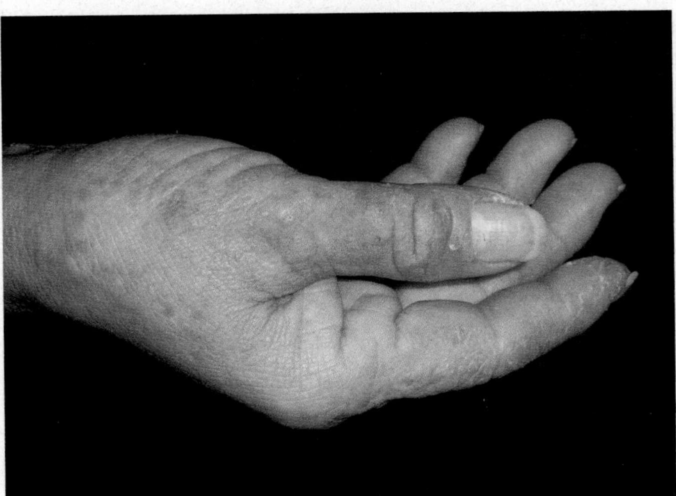

FIGURE 152-10 Occupation-related contact dermatitis on the hands of a shoe store employee. Her patch test was positive to thiurams used in processing the rubber of shoes. (*Reproduced with permission from Richard P. Usatine, MD.*)

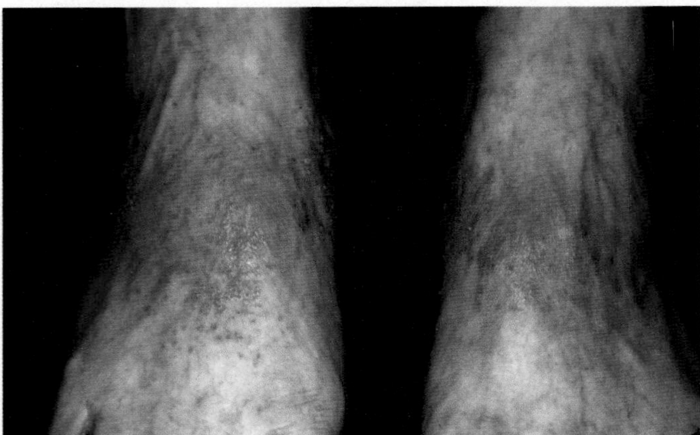

FIGURE 152-11 Allergic contact dermatitis from new shoes. This is the typical distribution found on the dorsum of the feet. (*Reproduced with permission from Milgrom EC, Usatine RP, Tan RA, et al: Practical Allergy. Philadelphia, PA: Elsevier; 2004.*)

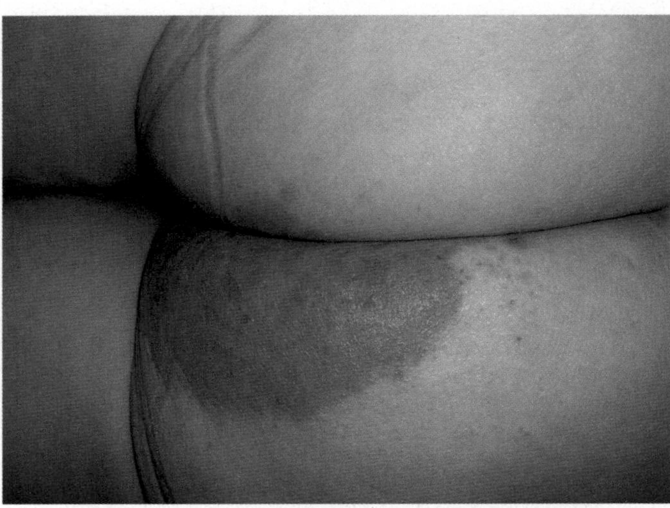

FIGURE 152-13 Contact dermatitis on the buttocks to isothiazolinone in baby wipes. Note that she is right-handed, accounting for the asymmetric pattern and explaining the eruption that was on her right hand as well. (*Reproduced with permission from Richard P. Usatine, MD.*)

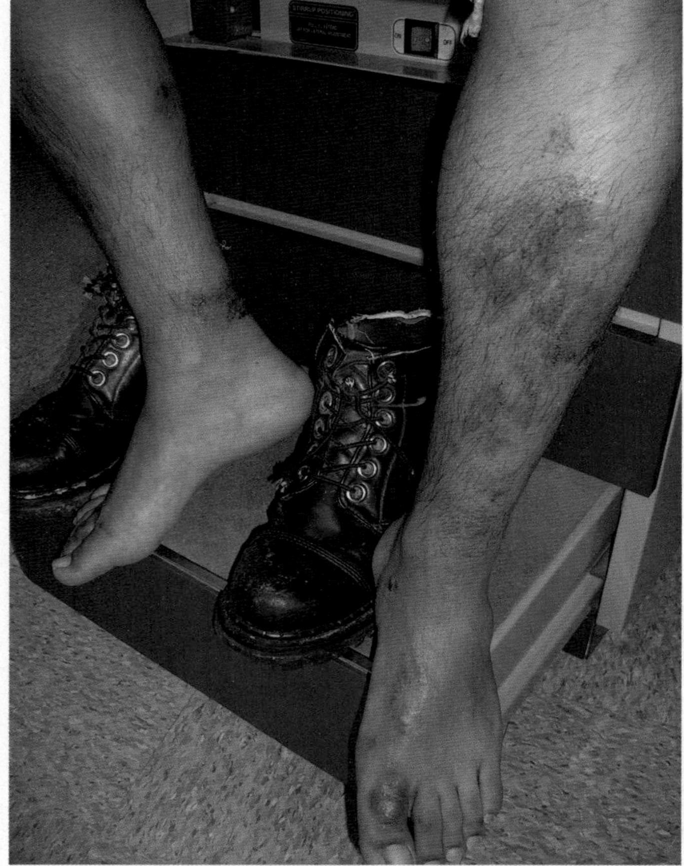

FIGURE 152-12 A 25-year-old man with allergic contact dermatitis to a chemical in his boots. His boots were higher but he cut them down to try to alleviate the discomfort coming from the boots higher on his leg. (*Reproduced with permission from Richard P. Usatine, MD.*)

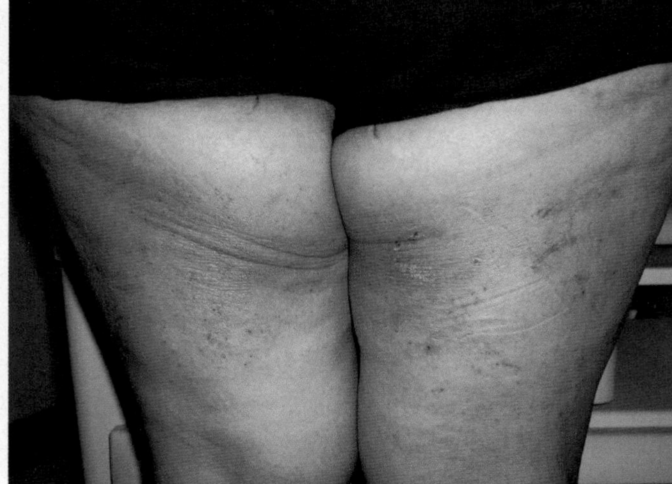

FIGURE 152-14 Contact dermatitis on the upper thighs to isothiazolinone in baby wipes. The patient was wiping the toilet seats in a public shelter for cleanliness but developed dermatitis where her skin touched the seat. (*Reproduced with permission from Richard P. Usatine, MD.*)

Toxicodendron (Rhus) dermatitis (poison ivy, poison oak, and poison sumac) is caused by urushiol, which is found in the saps of this plant family. Clinically, a line of vesicles can occur from brushing against one of the plants. Also, the linear pattern occurs from scratching oneself and dragging the oleoresin across the skin with the fingernails (**Figures 152-9** and **152-16**).

Systemic CD is a rare form of CD seen after the systemic administration of a substance, usually a drug, to which topical sensitization has previously occurred.[7]

LABORATORY STUDIES

The diagnosis is most often made by history and physical examination. Consider culture if there are signs of superinfection and there is a concern for methicillin-resistant *Staphylococcus aureus* (MRSA). The following tests may be considered when the diagnosis is not clear.

- KOH preparation and/or fungal culture if tinea is suspected.
- Microscopy for scabies mites and eggs.
- Latex allergy testing—This type of reaction is neither ICD (nonimmunologic) nor ACD. The latex allergy type of reaction is a type I, or immunoglobulin (Ig)E-mediated response to the latex allergen.
- Patch testing—Common antigens are placed on the skin of a patient. The T.R.U.E. Test, which has been approved by the U.S. Food and Drug Administration (FDA), comes in three tape strips that are easy to apply to the back (**Figure 152-17**). There is no preparation needed to test for the 35 common allergens embedded into these strips (see **Table 152-1** for a list of the 35 allergens and one control). The strips are removed in 2 days and read at that time and again in 2 more days (**Figure 152-18**). The T.R.U.E. Test website provides detailed information on how to perform the testing and how to counsel patients about the meaning of their results. Any clinician with an interest in patch testing can easily perform this service in the office.
    - A meta-analysis of the T.R.U.E. Test shows that nickel (14.7% of tested patients), thimerosal (5.0%), cobalt (4.8%), fragrance mix (3.4%), and balsam of Peru (3.0%) (**Figure 152-19**) are the most prevalent allergens detected using this system.[7]
    - Critics of the T.R.U.E. Test state that it misses other important antigens. A number of dermatologists create their own more extensive panels in their offices. If the suspected allergen is not in the T.R.U.E. Test, refer to a specialist who will customize the patch testing. Also, personal products, such as cosmetics and lotions, can be diluted for special patch testing.
    - A meta-analysis of children patch tested for ACD showed the top five allergens to be nickel, ammonium persulfate, gold sodium thiosulfate, thimerosal, and toluene-2,5-diamine (*p*-toluenediamine).[8] Three of these five allergens are in the T.R.U.E. Test, which is now FDA-approved for the diagnosis of allergic contact dermatitis in persons 6 years of age and older.
    - Once the patch test results are known, it is important to determine if the result is "relevant" to the patient's dermatitis. One method for classifying clinical relevance of a positive patch test reaction is: (a) current relevance—the patient has been exposed to the allergen during the current episode of dermatitis and improves when the exposure ceases; (b) past relevance—past episode of dermatitis from exposure to the allergen; (c) relevance not known—not sure if exposure is current or old; (d) cross-reaction—the positive test is a result of cross-reaction with

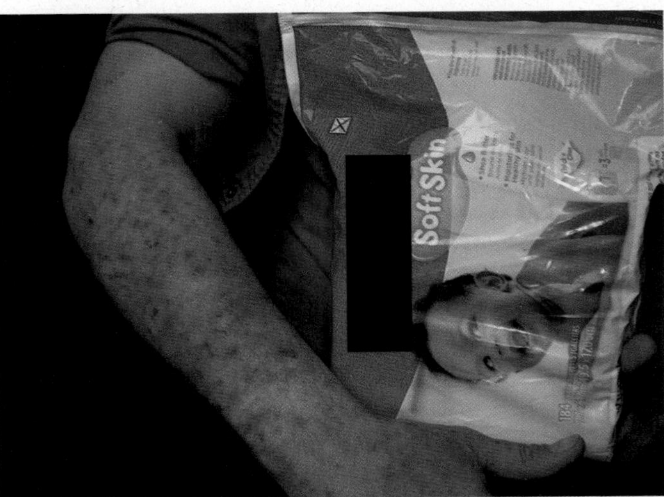

FIGURE 152-15 A 49-year-old truck driver developed pruritic erythematous eruption on his arms and trunk that persisted for 1 year despite various treatments. Patch testing ultimately revealed that he was allergic to isothiazolinone. He went home and discovered this was one of the ingredients in the baby wipes he used to clean his skin during long drives. His allergic contact dermatitis resolved once he stopped using the wipes. (*Reproduced with permission from Richard P. Usatine, MD.*)

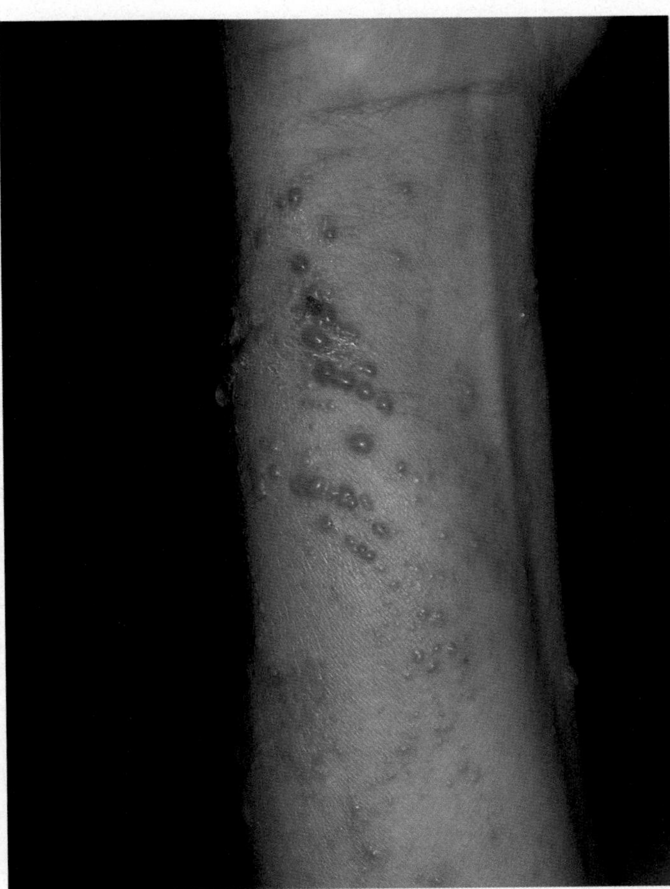

FIGURE 152-16 Multiple lines of vesicles from poison ivy on the arm. Patterns like this should suggest contact dermatitis. (*Reproduced with permission from Richard P. Usatine, MD.*)

another allergen; and (e) exposed—a history of exposure but not resulting in dermatitis from that exposure, or no history of exposure but a definite positive allergic patch test.[6]

- Punch biopsy—When another underlying disorder is suspected that is best diagnosed with histology (e.g., psoriasis).

DIFFERENTIAL DIAGNOSIS

- Atopic dermatitis is usually more widespread than CD. There is often a history of other atopic conditions, such as allergic rhinitis and asthma. There may be family history of allergies. However, persons with atopic dermatitis are more prone to CD (see **Figure 152-6**; Chapter 151, Atopic Dermatitis).
- Dyshidrotic eczema—Seen on the hands and feet with deep-seated "tapioca-like" vesicles, erythema, and scale. Although this is not primarily caused by contact to allergens, various irritating substances can make it worse (see Chapter 153, Hand Eczema).
- Immediate IgE contact reaction (e.g., latex glove allergy)—Immediate erythema, itching, and possibly systemic reaction after contact with a known (or suspected) allergen.
- Fungal infections—A dermatophyte infection can closely resemble CD when it occurs on the hands and feet. Tinea pedis is usually seen between the toes, on the soles, or on the sides of the feet. CD of the feet is often on the dorsum of the foot and related to rubber or other chemicals in the shoes (see **Figures 152-11** and **152-12**; Chapter 146, Tinea Pedis).
- Scabies on the hands can be mistaken for CD. Look for burrows and for the typical distribution of the scabies infestation to distinguish this from CD (see Chapter 149, Scabies).
- Allergies to the dyes used in tattoos can occur. Although this is not strictly a CD because the dye is injected below the skin, the allergic process is similar (**Figure 152-20**).

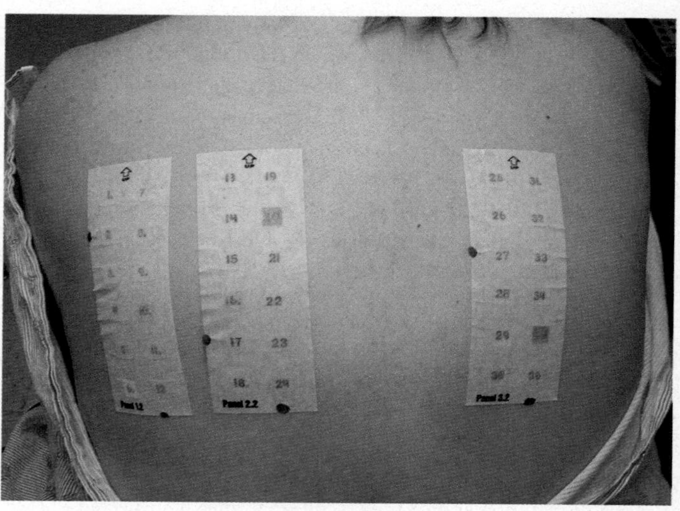

FIGURE 152-17 The T.R.U.E. Test is an easy-to-use standardized patch test that is applied to the back using 3 tape strips to test for 35 common allergens. The skin is marked at the notches on the tapes. The next step involves adding additional hypoallergenic tape to keep the strips from peeling off for 2 days. (*Reproduced with permission from Richard P. Usatine, MD.*)

TABLE 152-1 Allergens in T.R.U.E. Test (Patch Test for Contact Dermatitis)

Panel 1.2	Panel 2.2	Panel 3.2
1. Nickel sulfate	13. *p-tert*-Butylphenol formaldehyde resin	25. Diazolidinyl urea
2. Wool alcohols	14. Epoxy resin	26. Quinoline mix
3. Neomycin sulfate	15. Carba mix	27. Tixocortol-21-pivalate
4. Potassium dichromate	16. Black rubber mix	28. Gold sodium thiosulfate
5. Caine mix	17. Cl^+ Me^- isothiazolinone (MCI/MI)	29. Imidazolidinyl urea
6. Fragrance mix	18. Quaternium-15	30. Budesonide
7. Colophony	19. Methyldibromo glutaronitrile	31. Hydrocortizone-17-butyrate
8. Paraben mix	20. *p*-Phenylenediamine	32. Mercaptobenzothiazole
9. Negative control	21. Formaldehyde	33. Bacitracin
10. Balsam of Peru	22. Mercapto mix	34. Parthenolide
11. Ethylenediamine dihydrochloride	23. Thimerosal	35. Disperse blue 106
12. Cobalt dichloride	24. Thiuram mix	36. 2-Bromo-2-nitropropane-1,3-diol (Bronopol)

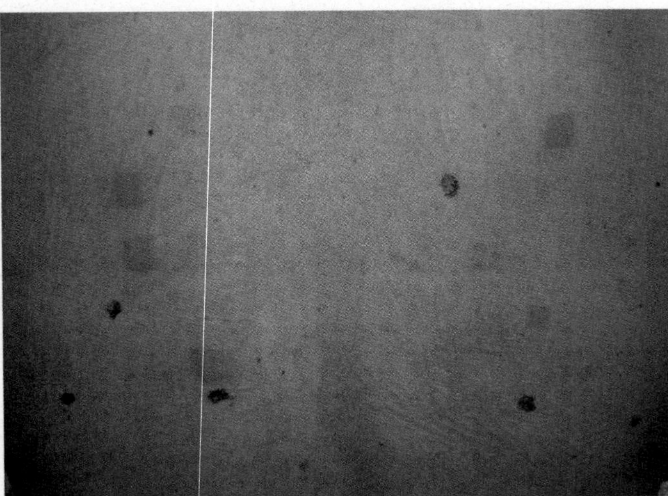

FIGURE 152-18 Positive patch tests are visible as erythematous squares with small vesicles at the sites where the allergen touched the skin. The T.R.U.E. Test reading strips are held against the skin to identify the positive antigens. (*Reproduced with permission from Richard P. Usatine, MD.*)

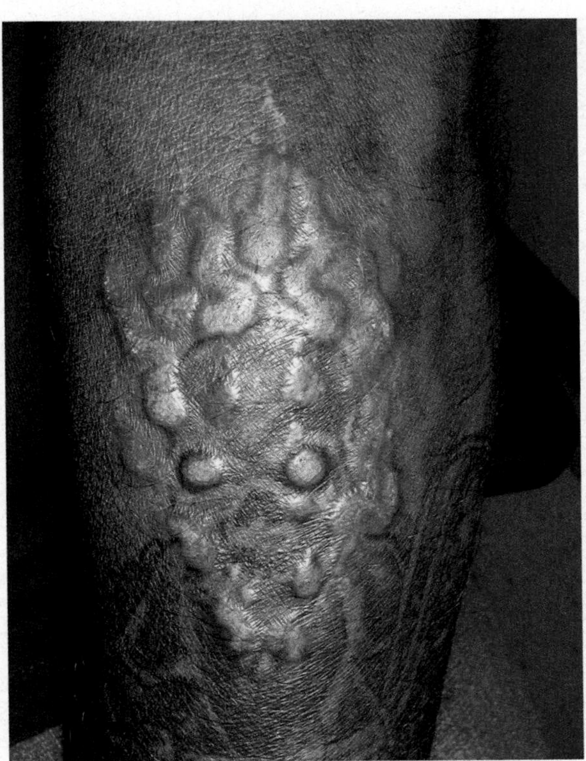

FIGURE 152-20 Man with allergy to red dye in tattoo. Everywhere that the red dye was used, the patient developed pain and swelling. (*Reproduced with permission from Richard P. Usatine, MD.*)

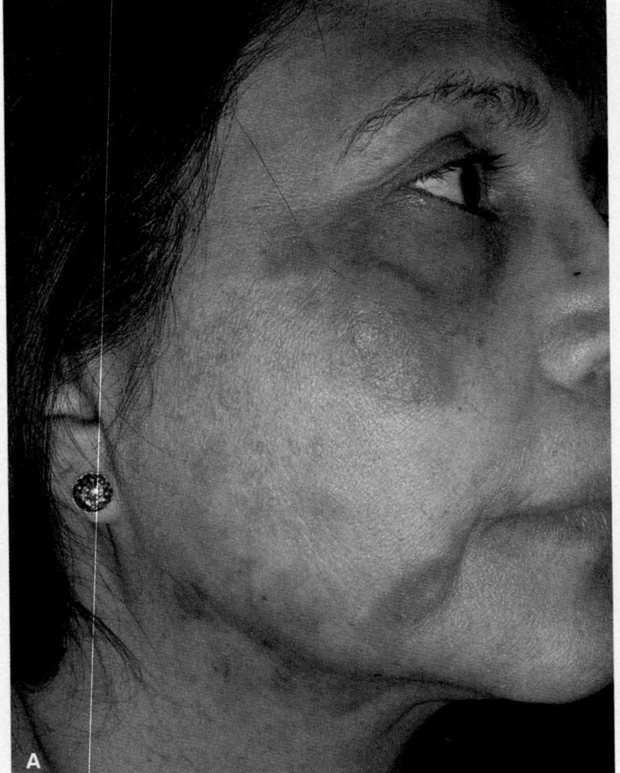

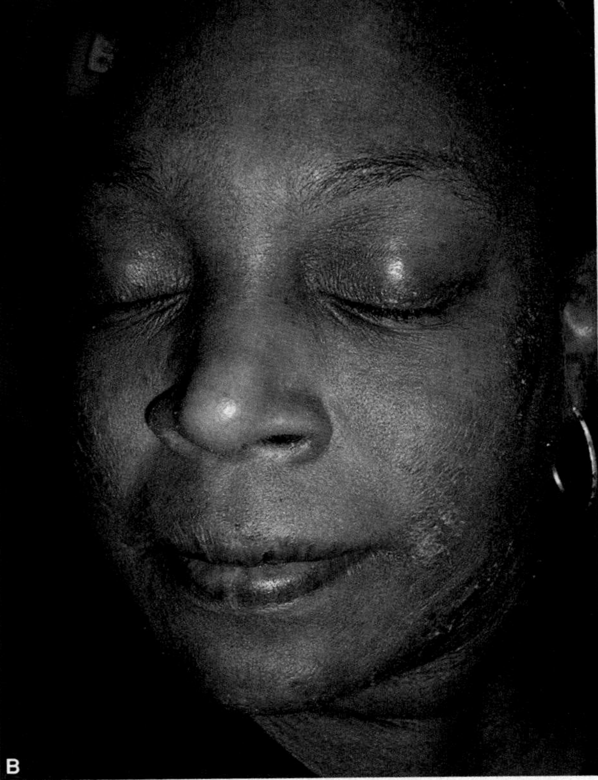

FIGURE 152-19 **A.** Contact dermatitis to Balsam of Peru and formaldehyde showing erythematous patches on the face. The eruption resolved when the products with the offending agents were stopped. **B.** Contact dermatitis to Balsam of Peru and isothiazolinone in a young woman applying new moisturizer to the face. Note how the erythema is less visible in skin of color. (*Reproduced with permission from Richard P. Usatine, MD.*)

MANAGEMENT

FIRST LINE

- Stop the exposure to the offending agent. In **Figure 152-21**, the woman developed a contact dermatitis to lip licking and then made it worse with Carmex application. Although a topical steroid was used to treat the inflammation, she will not get better until she stops licking her lips and applying Carmex.
- Localized acute ACD lesions respond best with mid-potency to high-potency topical steroids such as 0.1% triamcinolone to 0.05% clobetasol, respectively.[4] SOR Ⓐ
- On areas of thinner skin (e.g., flexural surfaces, eyelids, face, anogenital region), lower-potency steroids such as hydrocortisone or desonide can minimize the risk of skin atrophy.[3,4] SOR Ⓑ
- There are insufficient data to support the use of topical steroids for ICD, but because it is difficult to distinguish clinically between ACD and ICD, these agents are frequently tried. SOR Ⓒ
- If ACD involves extensive skin areas (>20%), systemic steroid therapy is often required and offers relief within 12 to 24 hours. The recommended dose is 0.5 to 1 mg/kg daily for 5 to 7 days, and if the patient is comfortable at that time, the dose may be reduced by 50% for the next 7 days. The rate of reduction of steroid dosage depends on factors such as severity, duration of ACD, and how effectively the allergen can be avoided.[4] SOR Ⓑ
- Oral steroids should be prescribed for 2 to 3 weeks (including a tapered dosing) because rapid discontinuance of steroids can result in rebound dermatitis. Severe poison ivy/oak is often treated with oral prednisone for 2 to 3 weeks. Avoid using a Medrol dose-pack, which has insufficient dosing and duration.[4] SOR Ⓑ
- Though widely used, the efficacy of topical immunomodulators (tacrolimus and pimecrolimus) in ACD or ICD has not been well established.[4] However, one randomized controlled trial (RCT) did demonstrate that tacrolimus ointment is more effective than vehicle in treating chronically exposed, nickel-induced ACD.[10] SOR Ⓑ

SECOND LINE

- Although antihistamines are generally not effective for pruritus associated with ACD, they are commonly used. Sedation from more soporific antihistamines may offer some degree of symptom relief (diphenhydramine, hydroxyzine).[4] SOR Ⓒ
- Bacterial superinfection should be treated with an appropriate antibiotic that will cover *Streptococcus pyogenes* and *S. aureus*. Treat for MRSA if suspected.

NONPHARMACOLOGIC THERAPY

- Cool compresses can soothe the symptoms of acute cases of CD.[4] SOR Ⓒ
- Calamine and colloidal oatmeal baths may help to dry and soothe acute, oozing lesions.[3,4] SOR Ⓒ
- Once the diagnosis of any CD is established, emollients and moisturizers may help soothe irritated skin.[4] SOR Ⓒ

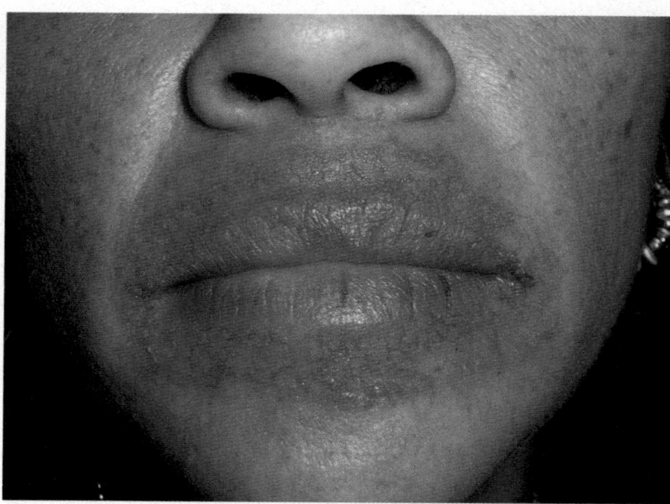

FIGURE 152-21 Contact dermatitis to lip licking which worsened with Carmex application. (*Reproduced with permission from Richard P. Usatine, MD.*)

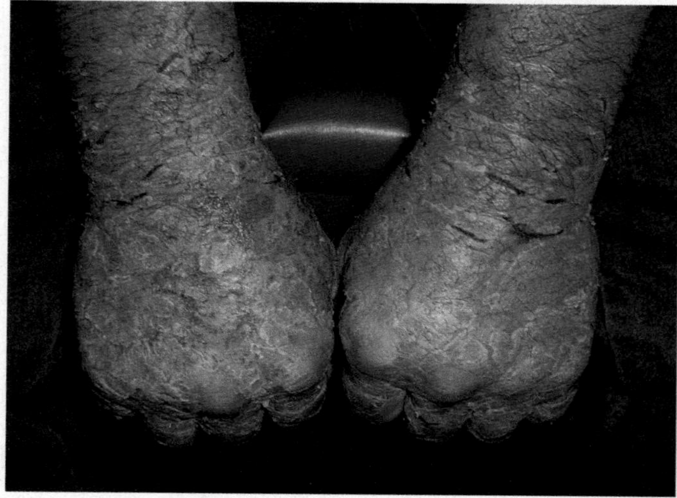

FIGURE 152-22 Severe occupational contact dermatitis to petroleum products in a man who works as a car mechanic. (*Reproduced with permission from Richard P. Usatine, MD.*)

PREVENTION

- Identify and avoid the offending agent(s).[4] SOR Ⓐ
  - Be aware that some patients are actually allergic to topical steroids. This unfortunate situation can be diagnosed with patch testing.
  - In cases of nickel ACD, there are ways to avoid purchasing nickel products. Costco sells nickel-free eyeglass frames; Calvin Klein and Levis sell nickel-free jeans; EyeCareCosmetics and RMS Beauty sell nickel-free makeup. https://nonickel.com/ sells belts, buckles, watches, and jewelry free of nickel.

For ICD and occupational CD of the hands:

- Wear protective gloves when working with known allergens or potentially irritating substances such as solvents, soaps, and detergents.[6,11] SOR Ⓐ
- Use cotton liners under the gloves for both comfort and the absorption of sweat. Wearing cotton glove liners can prevent the development of an impaired skin barrier function caused by prolonged wearing of occlusive gloves.[9,10] SOR Ⓑ
  - There is insufficient evidence to promote the use of barrier creams to protect against contact with irritants.[6,9] SOR Ⓐ
  - After work, conditioning creams can improve skin condition in workers with damaged skin.[9] SOR Ⓐ
- Keep hands clean, dry, and well-moisturized whenever possible.
- Petrolatum applied twice a day is a great way to moisturize dry and cracked skin without exposing the patient to new irritants.

If the CD is severe enough (**Figure 152-22**), the patient may need to change work to completely avoid the offending irritant or antigen.

FOLLOW-UP

May need frequent follow-up if the offending substance is not found, if the rash does not resolve, and if patch testing will be needed.

PATIENT EDUCATION

Avoid the offending agent and take the medications as prescribed to relieve symptoms.

PATIENT RESOURCES

- PubMed Health. *Allergic Contact Dermatitis*—**http://www.ncbi.nlm.nih.gov/pubmedhealth/PMH0096287/.**
- Dermatitis Academy. Resources for patients and providers—**https://www.dermatitisacademy.com.**
- The T.R.U.E. Test website has a wealth of information on reading labels, common allergens and patch testing for patients—**http://www.truetest.com.**

PROVIDER RESOURCES

- American Family Physician. *Diagnosis and Management of Contact Dermatitis*—**http://www.aafp.org/afp/2010/0801/p249.html.**
- The T.R.U.E. Test website has a wealth of information on patch testing for healthcare professionals—**http://www.truetest.com.**
- Dermatitis Academy. Resources for providers—**https://www.dermatitisacademy.com.**
- The American Contact Dermatitis Society's website has information on patch testing, specific allergens, and providers who patch test—**http://www.contactderm.org.**

REFERENCES

1. Usatine RP. A red twisted ankle. *West J Med.* 1999;171:361-362.
2. Halstater B, Usatine RP. Contact dermatitis. In: Milgrom E, Usatine RP, Tan R, Spector S, eds. *Practical Allergy*. Philadelphia, PA: Elsevier; 2004.
3. Usatine RP, Riojas M. Diagnosis and management of contact dermatitis. *Am Fam Physician.* 2010;82:249-255.
4. Beltrani VS, Bernstein IL, Cohen DE, Fonacier L. Contact dermatitis: a practice parameter. *Ann Allergy Asthma Immunol.* 2006;97:S1-S38.
5. Fonacier L, Bernstein BI, Pacheco K. Contact dermatitis: a practice parameter—update 2015. *J Allergy Clin Immunol Pract.* 2015; 3:S1-S39.
6. DeKoven JG, Warshaw EM, Belsito DV, et al. North American Contact Dermatitis Group patch test results 2013–2014. *Dermatitis* 2017;28:33-46.
7. Bourke J, Coulson I, English J. Guidelines for the management of contact dermatitis: an update. *Br J Dermatol.* 2009;160:946-954.
8. Krob HA, Fleischer AB Jr, D'Agostino R Jr, et al. Prevalence and relevance of contact dermatitis allergens: a meta-analysis of 15 years of published T.R.U.E. test data. *J Am Acad Dermatol.* 2004; 51:349-353.
9. Bonitsis NG, Tatsioni A, Bassioukas K, Ioannidis JP. Allergens responsible for allergic contact dermatitis among children: a systematic review and meta-analysis. *Contact Dermatitis.* 2011; 64:245-257.
10. Belsito D, Wilson DC, Warshaw E, et al. A prospective randomized clinical trial of 0.1% tacrolimus ointment in a model of chronic allergic contact dermatitis. *J Am Acad Dermatol.* 2006; 55:40-46.
11. Nicholson PJ, Llewellyn D, English JS. Evidence-based guidelines for the prevention, identification and management of occupational contact dermatitis and urticaria. *Contact Dermatitis.* 2010; 63:177-186.

153 HAND ECZEMA

Richard P. Usatine, MD
Anoop Patel, MD

PATIENT STORY

An Asian American physician presents with dry scaling on her hands. Frequent handwashing makes it worse, and it sometimes cracks. She has allergic rhinitis, and she had more widespread atopic dermatitis in her youth. This is a case of chronic atopic hand dermatitis (**Figure 153-1**). Her physician recommended she use Cetaphil (or equivalent non-soap cleanser) instead of soap and water for handwashing. Triamcinolone 0.1% ointment was prescribed for use twice daily, including use of cotton gloves overnight over the ointment. Her hands improved greatly with this treatment, and she was pleased with the results.

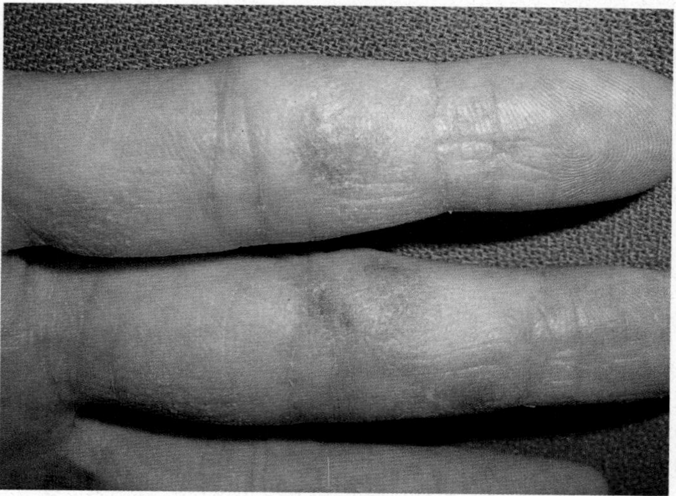

FIGURE 153-1 An Asian American physician with chronic atopic hand dermatitis. She has allergic rhinitis and she had more widespread atopic dermatitis in her youth. (*Reproduced with permission from Richard P. Usatine, MD.*)

INTRODUCTION

Hand eczema refers to a wide spectrum of inflammatory skin diseases of the hands, including atopic dermatitis, contact dermatitis, pompholyx, and dyshidrotic eczema.

SYNONYMS

Hand dermatitis, pompholyx, dyshidrotic eczema, vesicular palmoplantar eczema. Although some people use pompholyx and dyshidrotic eczema synonymously, others reserve pompholyx for hand eczema with vesicles and bullae on the palms and dyshidrotic eczema for conditions with smaller vesicles between the fingers and toes.

EPIDEMIOLOGY

- The prevalence of hand dermatitis is estimated at approximately 2% to 8.9% in the general population, with only a fraction of adults with hand eczema seeking medical care.[1,2]

ETIOLOGY AND PATHOPHYSIOLOGY

- There are many clinical variants of hand dermatitis and a number of different classification schemas. Here is one accepted classification scheme:
  1. Contact (i.e., allergic and irritant) (**Figure 153-2**).
  2. Hyperkeratotic (i.e., psoriasiform) (**Figure 153-3**).
  3. Frictional (**Figure 153-4**).
  4. Nummular (**Figure 153-5**).
  5. Atopic (**Figure 153-6**).
  6. Pompholyx (i.e., dyshidrosis) (**Figures 153-7** and **153-8**).
  7. Chronic vesicular hand dermatitis[1] (**Figure 153-9**).

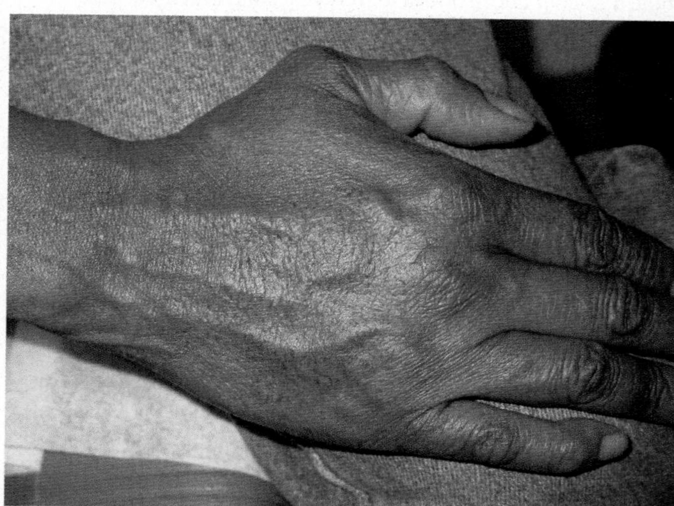

FIGURE 153-2 Contact dermatitis to fragrance mix on the dorsum of the hand secondary to using the back of the hand to apply perfume to neck. (*Reproduced with permission from Usatine RP. New rash on the right hand and neck, J Fam Pract. 2003;52(11):863-865. FrontlineMedical Communications, Inc.*)

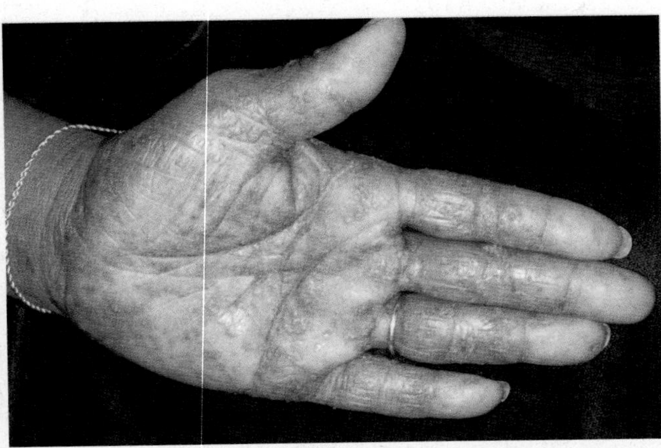

FIGURE 153-3 Hyperkeratotic hand dermatitis in a black woman. (*Reproduced with permission from Richard P. Usatine, MD.*)

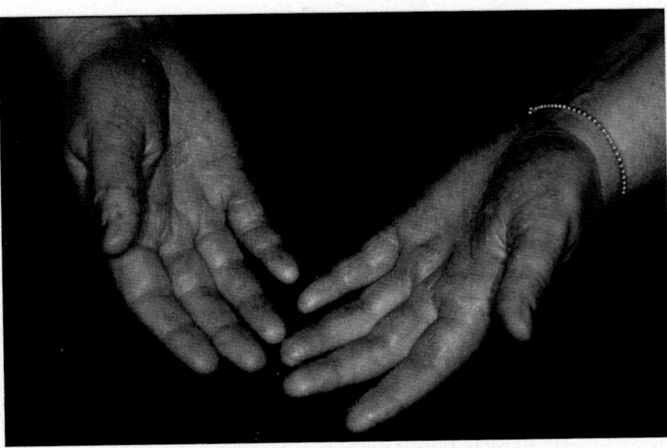

FIGURE 153-6 Atopic hand dermatitis on palms in an Asian American woman with long history of atopic dermatitis. (*Reproduced with permission from Richard P. Usatine, MD. Previously published in Practical Allergy.*)

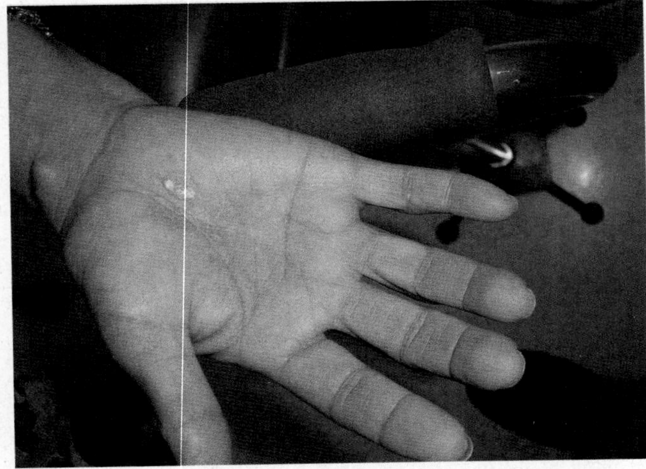

FIGURE 153-4 Frictional hand eczema that is worse on the hand that is used for the cane. The other side was affected by a stroke, so only one hand is usable for ambulating with a cane. (*Reproduced with permission from Richard P. Usatine, MD.*)

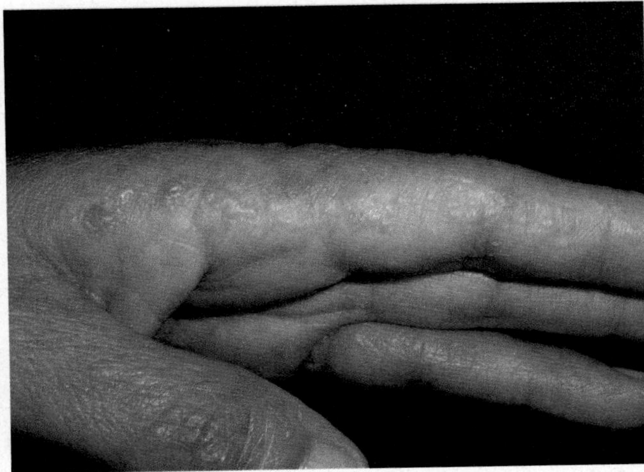

FIGURE 153-7 Dyshidrotic eczema with acute outbreak of tapioca vesicles on the sides of the fingers. (*Reproduced with permission from Richard P. Usatine, MD.*)

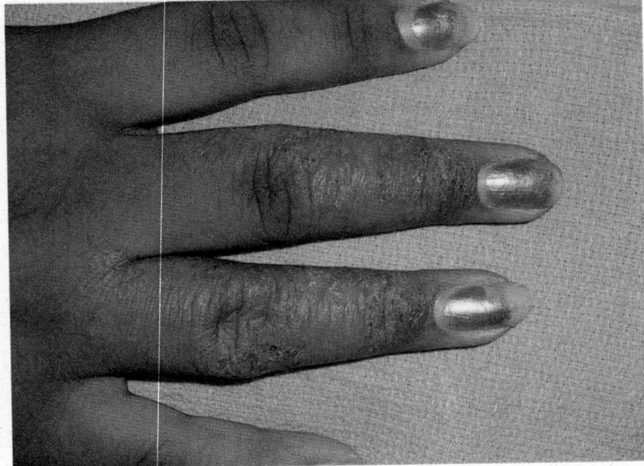

FIGURE 153-5 Nummular hand dermatitis with tiny papules, papulovesicles, and "coin-shaped" eczematous plaques on the distal fingers of a 14-year-old girl. (*Reproduced with permission from Richard P. Usatine, MD.*)

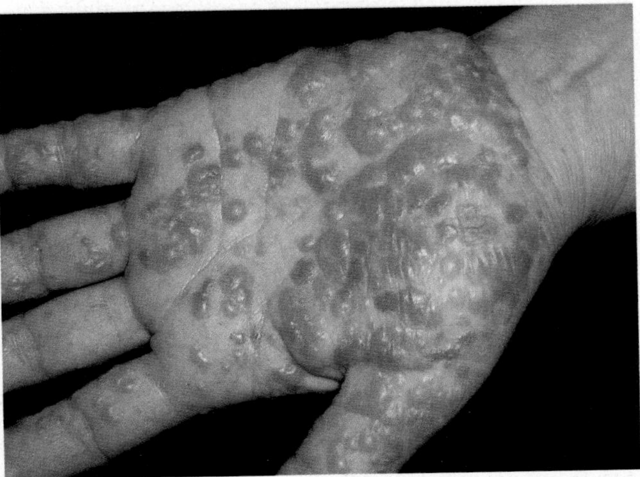

FIGURE 153-8 Severe pompholyx worsening with topical steroids. Patch testing showed she was allergic to topical steroids. Her hands finally cleared with oral cyclosporine and avoidance of all topical and oral steroids. (*Reproduced with permission from Richard P. Usatine, MD.*)

- Another way of looking at hand dermatitis is to break it down into three categories[3]:
  1. Endogenous—Atopic, psoriasis, pompholyx, dyshidrotic (we do not include psoriasis as a type of hand eczema in this chapter).
  2. Exogenous—Allergic and irritant contact dermatitis.
  3. Infectious—Tinea, *Candida*, and/or superimposed *Staphylococcus aureus* (**Figure 153-10**).
- Most contact dermatitis of the hands is secondary to irritants such as soap, water, solvents, and other chemicals.
- Allergic contact dermatitis (ACD) is a type IV, delayed-type, cell-mediated, hypersensitivity reaction.
- The nine most frequent allergens related to hand contact dermatitis were identified by patch testing from 1994 to 2004.[4] These are quaternium-15 (16.5%), formaldehyde (13.0%), nickel sulfate (12.2%), fragrance mix (11.3%), thiuram mix (10.2%), balsam of Peru (9.6%), carba mix (7.8%), neomycin sulfate (7.7%), and bacitracin (7.4%).[4]
- Rubber allergens were commonly associated with occupation. One third of patients with ACD had identifiable relevant irritants.[4]
- Acrylates and methacrylates were found to be good screening allergens for occupational exposure.[5]
- Most common allergens are preservatives, metals, fragrances, topical antibiotics, or rubber additives.[4]
- Although dyshidrotic eczema had been thought to be related to sweating, histologic examination has revealed no sweat duct abnormalities.[6]

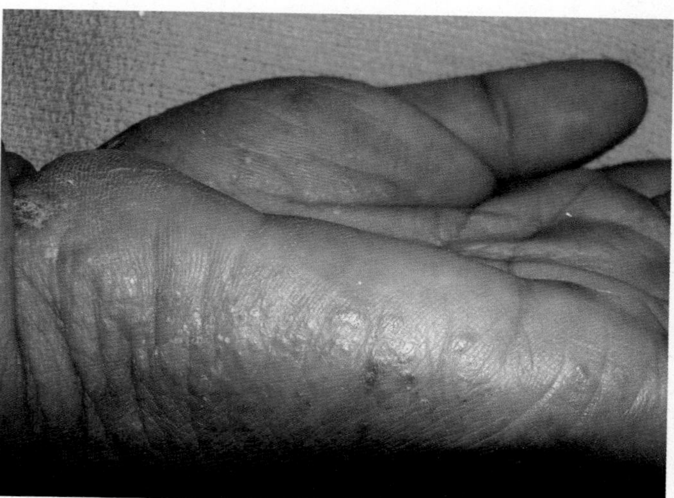

FIGURE 153-9 Chronic vesicular hand dermatitis going on for decades in this 51-year-old Hispanic woman. It is particularly bad in the hypothenar area. (*Reproduced with permission from Richard P. Usatine, MD.*)

DIAGNOSIS

CLINICAL FEATURES[1]

Contact (i.e., allergic and irritant) (see **Figure 153-2**).

- Symptoms include burning, stinging, itching, and tenderness at the site of exposure to the irritant or allergen.[1]
- Acute signs include papules, vesicles, bullae, and edema.
- Weeping and crusting can occur with or without superinfection.
- Chronic signs include plaques with fissuring, hyperpigmentation, and/or lichenification.
- Irritant contact dermatitis may predispose to ACD.

Hyperkeratotic (i.e., psoriasiform) (see **Figure 153-3**).

- Symmetric hyperkeratotic plaques.
- May be localized to the proximal or middle part of the palms.
- Painful fissures are common.

Frictional (see **Figure 153-4**).

- Mechanical factors, often from work, such as trauma, friction, pressure, and vibration, induce skin changes with erythema and scale.
- "Wear-and-tear dermatitis."[1]
- Can be caused by contact with paper and fabrics.

Nummular (see **Figure 153-5**).

- Nummular hand dermatitis (also called discoid hand dermatitis).

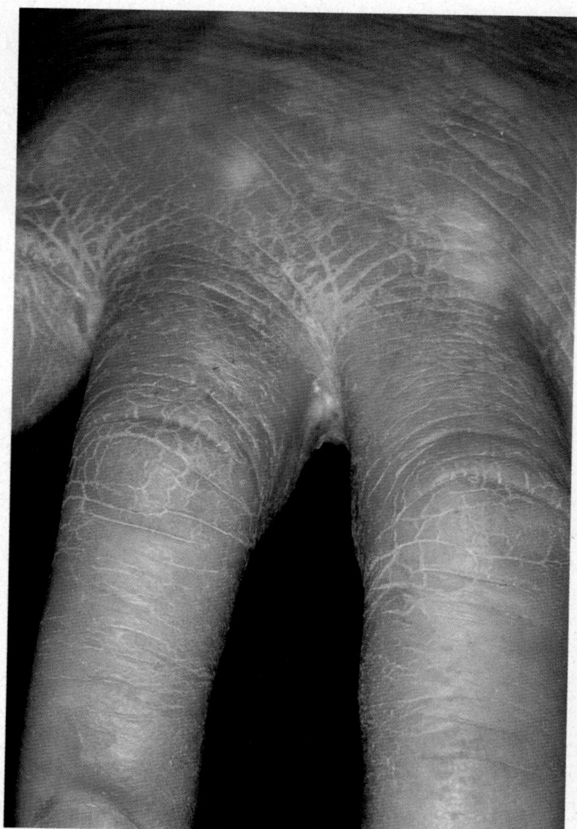

FIGURE 153-10 Contact hand dermatitis in a Chinese cook superinfected with *Candida*. See white scale between the fingers. The *Candida* in the interdigital space is also called erosio interdigitalis blastomycetica and is seen in patients with diabetes. (*Reproduced with permission from Richard P. Usatine, MD.*)

- Tiny papules, papulovesicles, or "coin-shaped" eczematous plaques.
- Dorsal hands and distal fingers are often involved.

Atopic.

- Patients with childhood atopic dermatitis are predisposed to develop hand dermatitis as adults (see **Figure 153-6**).
- There is no characteristic pattern, and it can occur on any part of the hand.
- Extension to or involvement of the wrist is common (**Figure 153-11**).

Pompholyx (i.e., dyshidrosis, dyshidrotic eczema).

- Has recurrent crops of papules, vesicles, and bullae on the lateral aspects of the fingers, as well as the palms and soles, on a background of nonerythematous skin (see **Figures 153-7** and **153-8**).
- These are described as tapioca vesicles, as they look like the small spheres in tapioca. The vesicles open and the skin then peels (mild desquamation).
- There may be pruritus or pain.
- Although some use the terms pompholyx and dyshidrotic eczema interchangeably, others only use the term pompholyx to describe an explosive onset of large bullae, usually on the palms (see **Figure 153-8**) and dyshidrotic eczema to mainly describe chronic small tapioca vesicles on the sides of the fingers (see **Figure 153-7**).
- Both conditions may last 2 to 3 weeks and resolve, leaving normal skin, only to recur again at varying intervals.
- Both conditions are idiopathic and closely related, if not identical.
- Symptoms may be associated with exogenous factors (e.g., nickel or hot weather) or endogenous factors (e.g., atopy or stress).

Chronic vesicular hand dermatitis (see **Figure 153-9**).

- Chronic vesicles that are mostly palmar and pruritic.
- Differentiated from pompholyx by a more chronic course and the presence of vesicles with an erythematous base.
- The soles of the feet may also be involved.
- Poorly responsive to treatments.
- In one series, 55% of patients with this type of hand dermatitis were found to have positive patch test results.[7]

TYPICAL DISTRIBUTION

Of course, hand dermatitis is on the hands, but both hands and feet can be involved in dyshidrotic eczema and chronic vesicular hand dermatitis.

LABORATORY STUDIES

Scraping and using microscopy with KOH (with or without a fungal stain) to look for dermatophytes is helpful (see Chapter 141, Fungal Overview).

Patch testing can be crucial to the diagnosis and treatment of hand eczema. Patch testing is described in detail in the previous chapter (Chapter 152, Contact Dermatitis). The patient in **Figure 153-8** had severe pompholyx worsening with topical steroids. Patch testing showed she was allergic to topical steroids (**Figure 153-12**). Her hands finally cleared with oral cyclosporine and avoidance of all topical and oral steroids.

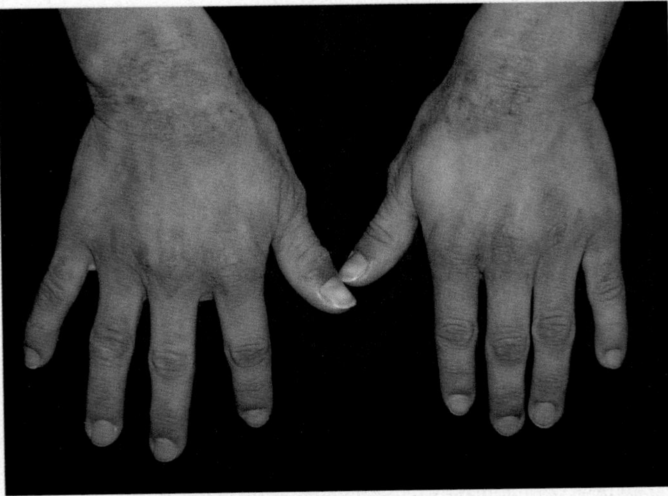

FIGURE 153-11 Hand dermatitis with prominent wrist involvement in a 20-year-old Hispanic woman with moderately severe widespread atopic dermatitis. (*Reproduced with permission from Richard P. Usatine, MD.*)

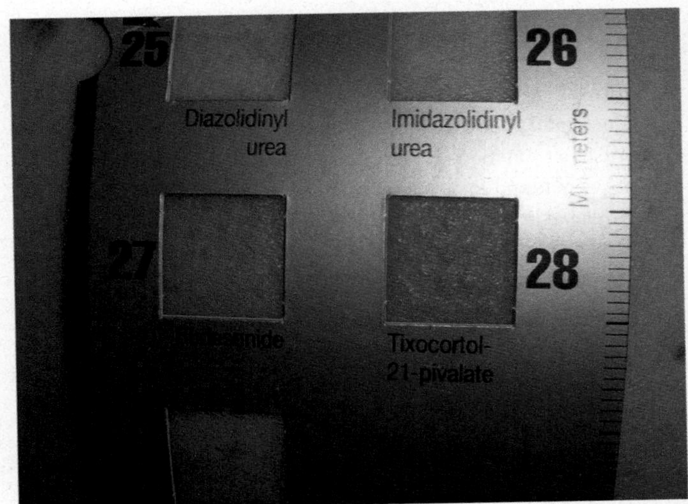

FIGURE 153-12 Patch testing positive to two types of topical steroids in a patient with severe pompholyx and topical steroid allergic contact dermatitis. Reading of T.R.U.E. test. (*Reproduced with permission from Richard P. Usatine, MD.*)

DIFFERENTIAL DIAGNOSIS

- Tinea manus is often found as part of the two-foot, one-hand syndrome in which both feet have scaling tinea pedis and one hand has scale as well (**Figure 153-13**) (see Chapter 146, Tinea Pedis).
- *Candida* can be seen in between the fingers with erythema and scale over the fingers and hand (see **Figure 153-10**) (see Chapter 142, Candidiasis).
- Psoriasis often involves the hand. It can present with plaques on the dorsum of hand and over the knuckles of the fingers or on the palm of the hand. Palmoplantar psoriasis will involve the hands and feet (see Chapter 158, Psoriasis).
- Knuckle pads are thickening of the skin over the knuckles. These can be accompanied by hyperpigmentation (**Figure 153-14**).

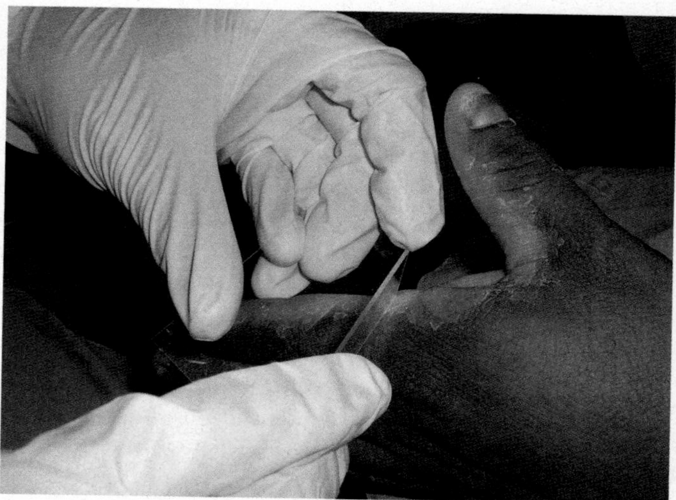

FIGURE 153-13 Tinea manus in a patient with two-foot, one-hand syndrome. The scraping showed hyphae under the microscope with a KOH preparation. (*Reproduced with permission from Richard P. Usatine, MD.*)

MANAGEMENT

FIRST LINE

GENERAL MEASURES

- Lifestyle modifying factors, as listed in **Table 153-1**, are essential.
- Avoid irritants and "wet work" at home and at work as much as possible. SOR Ⓒ
- Wear protective gloves when working with known allergens or potentially irritating substances such as solvents, soaps, and detergents.[8,9] SOR Ⓐ
- Use cotton liners under the gloves for both comfort and the absorption of sweat. Wearing cotton glove liners can prevent the development of an impaired skin barrier function caused by prolonged wearing of occlusive gloves.[8,9] SOR Ⓑ

There is insufficient evidence to promote the use of barrier creams to protect against contact with irritants.[8,9] SOR Ⓐ

Applying conditioning creams after work can improve skin condition in workers with damaged skin on the hands.[9] SOR Ⓐ

- Avoid latex gloves because of a high risk of latex allergy among patients with hand dermatitis. SOR Ⓒ
- Frequent and liberal use of emollients can help restore normal skin-barrier function. Simple, inexpensive, petrolatum-based emollients were found to be just as effective as an emollient containing skin-related lipids in a 2-month study of 30 patients with mild to moderate hand dermatitis.[10] SOR Ⓑ
- For patients with very dry skin that is not irritated by water, it may help to soak hands 3 to 5 minutes in warm water at night, apply triamcinolone 0.1% ointment, and cover with cotton gloves overnight. The cotton gloves may be used repeatedly even though they will soak up some of the ointment. SOR Ⓒ
- Do not wash hands with soap. Use Cetaphil or another non-soap cleanser. SOR Ⓒ

See **Table 153-2** for a summary of the recommended therapeutic agents for different types of hand dermatitis.

- Avoid smoking, as it may worsen hand eczema.[11] SOR Ⓑ

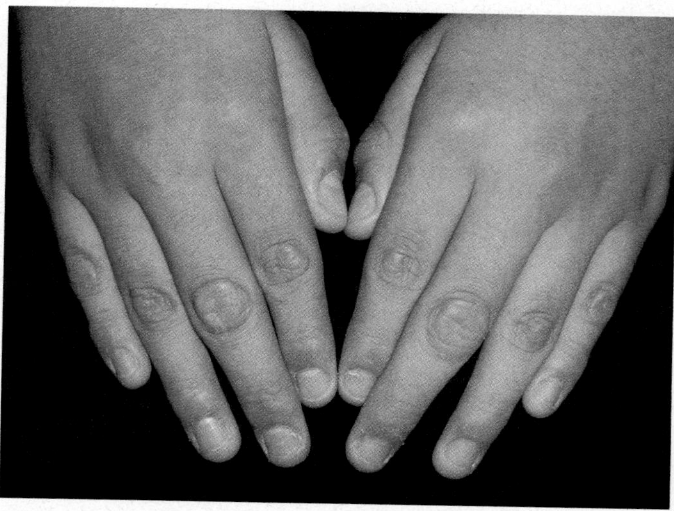

FIGURE 153-14 Knuckle pads in 15-year-old boy. These are idiopathic but the patient picks at them, which worsens the condition. (*Reproduced with permission from Richard P. Usatine, MD.*)

TABLE 153-1 Sample Patient Handout on Lifestyle Management of Hand Dermatitis

Handwashing and moisturizing:
- Use lukewarm or cool water, and mild cleansers without perfume, coloring, or antibacterial agents, and with minimal preservatives. In general, bar soaps tend to have fewer preservatives than liquid soaps (Cetaphil or Aquanil liquid cleansers or generic equivalents are exceptions to this statement).
- Pat hands dry, especially between fingers.
- Immediately following partial drying of hands (e.g., within 3 minutes), apply a generous amount of a heavy cream or ointment (not lotion); petroleum jelly, a one-ingredient lubricant, works well.
- It is helpful to have containers of creams or ointments next to every sink in your home (next to the bed, next to the TV, in the car, and at multiple places at work).
- Moisturizing should be repeated as often as possible throughout the day, ideally 15 times per day.
- Avoid using washcloths, rubbing, scrubbing, or overuse of soap or water.

Occlusive therapy at night for intensive therapy:
- Apply a generous amount of your doctor's recommended emollient or prescribed medicine on your hands.
- Then put on cotton gloves and wear overnight.

When performing "wet work":
- Wear cotton gloves under vinyl or other non-latex gloves.
- Try not to use hot water, and decrease exposure to water to less than 15 minutes at a time, if possible.
- Use running water rather than immersing hands, if possible.
- Remove rings before wet or dry work.

Wear protective gloves in cold weather and for dusty work. For frictional exposures, wear tight-fitting leather gloves (e.g., riding or golfing gloves).

Avoid direct contact with the following, if possible:
- Peeling fruits and vegetables, especially citrus fruits and onions;
- Polishes of all kinds;
- Solvents (e.g., white spirit, thinners, and turpentine);
- Hair lotions, creams, and dyes;
- Detergents and strong cleansing agents;
- Fragranced chemicals;
- "Unknown" chemicals.

Heavy-duty vinyl gloves are better than rubber, nitrile, or other synthetic gloves because vinyl is less likely to cause allergic reactions.

Adapted with permission from Warshaw E, Lee G, Storrs FJ. Hand dermatitis: a review of clinical features, therapeutic options, and long-term outcomes, Am J Contact Dermat. 2003;14(3):119-137.

MEDICATIONS—TOPICAL AGENTS

- Topical steroids are first-line agents for inflammatory hand dermatitis.[12] Ointments are considered more effective and contain fewer preservatives and additives than creams. Some patients will prefer a cream vehicle, so patient preference should be considered in prescribing topical steroids. It is better to have a patient use a cream than not use an ointment.
- Start with 0.1% triamcinolone ointment bid, as it is inexpensive and effective. SOR Ⓒ Cut back on use when possible to avoid skin atrophy, striae, and telangiectasias.
- Topical calcineurin inhibitors, tacrolimus and pimecrolimus, are effective in the treatment of atopic and other allergic types of hand dermatitis.[13,14] SOR Ⓑ Skin burning or an unpleasant sensation of warmth is reported by approximately 50% of patients using topical tacrolimus and 10% with pimecrolimus.[15]

SECOND LINE

PHOTOTHERAPY AND IONIZING RADIATION

- Psoralen and UVA irradiation (PUVA) has been used to treat patients with all forms of hand dermatitis.[15] SOR Ⓒ This combination is more frequently used for hyperkeratotic hand eczema as a first-line treatment compared to vesicular eczema, where corticosteroids are preferred as first-line treatment.[16]
- Grenz rays (ionizing radiation with ultra-soft X-rays or Bucky rays) usually requires 200 to 400 rad (2 to 4 grays or Gy) every 1 to 3 weeks for up to a total of 6 treatments, followed by a 6-month hiatus.[15] SOR Ⓒ

SYSTEMIC STEROIDS AND IMMUNOMODULATORS

- Intramuscular triamcinolone or oral prednisone may be used to treat the most severe and recalcitrant cases of hand dermatitis. Pulse dosing of prednisone 40 to 60 mg daily for 3 to 4 days may

TABLE 153-2 Recommended Therapies for Hand Dermatitis Variants

	Hand Dermatitis Variant						
Therapeutic Agent	Irritant Contact	Allergic Contact	Hyperkeratotic	Nummular	Pompholyx (Dyshidrosis)	Frictional	Chronic Vesicular
Corticosteroids:							
Topical	✓	✓		✓	✓	✓	✓
Oral		✓			✓*		✓
Cyclosporine		✓			✓		✓
Methotrexate		✓	✓		✓		✓
Mycophenolate mofetil		✓		✓	✓		✓
Tacrolimus or pimecrolimus (topical)	✓	✓		✓	✓		✓
Phototherapy (UVB, psoralen UVA, and Grenz)	✓	✓	✓	✓	✓	✓	✓
Retinoids (topical and/or oral)			✓			✓	✓
Calcipotriene (topical)			✓			✓	✓

*Acute flares.

Reproduced with permission from Warshaw E, Lee G, Storrs FJ. Hand dermatitis: a review of clinical features, therapeutic options, and long-term outcomes, *Am J Contact Dermat.* 2003;14(3):119-137.

be valuable.[15] An IM injection of 40–60 mg triamcinolone acetonide is a very effective temporary treatment for all types of hand dermatitis. SOR C Systemic steroids work so well that patients often want this treatment to be repeated every time they have flares of their hand eczema. The goal is to find other effective treatments to avoid repeating the injections or the oral prednisone.

- Cyclosporine is a potent immunomodulating agent used to treat severe and recalcitrant cases of atopic dermatitis and hand dermatitis. In a systematic review, cyclosporine consistently decreased the severity of atopic dermatitis. The decrease in disease severity was greater at 2 weeks with dosages greater than or equal to 4 mg/kg. After 6 to 8 weeks the relative effectiveness was 55%.[17] For patients with severe functional problems, this can be a great relief (see **Figure 153-8**). Unfortunately, relapse rates are high after discontinuation of the cyclosporine.[15] SOR B Also, the recommendation in the United States is to not continue the cyclosporine for longer than 1 year to avoid renal damage.
- Mycophenolate mofetil and methotrexate have been reported to be beneficial for hand dermatitis in case reports.[15] SOR C
- Alitretinoin (9-*cis*-retinoic acid) is an effective treatment for severe chronic hand eczema.[18,19] SOR B Like all systemic retinoids it is teratogenic and requires careful monitoring. However, compared to other retinoids, it is less likely to be discontinued due to adverse events.[20,21] This medication is not yet available for oral use in the United States for treatment of chronic hand eczema, but is being used in Canada and the United Kingdom. The closest oral retinoid option in the United States is acitretin, which should not be given to women of childbearing potential.

COMPLEMENTARY/ALTERNATIVE THERAPY

- Oxybutynin has been reported to be an alternative treatment for hyperhidrosis and beneficial in relapsing dyshidrotic eczema.[22]

PATIENT EDUCATION

- See **Table 153-1**.

FOLLOW-UP

Patients with chronic hand dermatitis are often desperately looking for help and often appreciate frequent follow-up until the dermatitis is controlled. Patch testing requires three visits within a 1-week period. KOH preparation, bacterial culture, and skin biopsy may be included.

PATIENT RESOURCES

- DermNet New Zealand—**http://www.dermnetnz.org/topics/hand-dermatitis.html.**

PROVIDER RESOURCES

- *Dyshidrotic Eczema*—**http://emedicine.medscape.com/article/1122527.**
- *Vesicular Palmoplantar Eczema*—**http://emedicine.medscape.com/article/1124613.**

REFERENCES

1. Warshaw E, Lee G, Storrs FJ. Hand dermatitis: a review of clinical features, therapeutic options, and long-term outcomes. *Am J Contact Dermat.* 2003;14:119-137.

2. Crane M, Webb D, Watson E, et al. Hand eczema and steroid-refractory chronic hand eczema in general practice: prevalence and initial treatment. *Br J Dermatol.* 2017;176(4):955-964.
3. Bolognia J. *Dermatology.* St. Louis, MO: Mosby; 2003.
4. Warshaw EM, Ahmed RL, Belsito DV, et al; North American Contact Dermatitis Group. Contact dermatitis of the hands: cross-sectional analyses of North American Contact Dermatitis Group Data, 1994–2004. *J Am Acad Dermatol.* 2007;57(2):301-314.
5. Ramos L, Cabral R, Gonçalo M. Allergic contact dermatitis caused by acrylates and methacrylates—a 7-year study. *Contact Dermatitis.* 2014;71(2):102-107.
6. Nishizawa A. Dyshidrotic eczema and its relationship to metal allergy. *Curr Probl Dermatol.* 2016;51:80-85.
7. Li LF, Wang J. Contact hypersensitivity in hand dermatitis. *Contact Dermatitis.* 2002;47:206-209.
8. Bourke J, Coulson I, English J. Guidelines for the management of contact dermatitis: an update. *Br J Dermatol.* 2009;160:946-954.
9. Nicholson PJ, Llewellyn D, English JS. Evidence-based guidelines for the prevention, identification and management of occupational contact dermatitis and urticaria. *Contact Dermatitis.* 2010;63:177-186.
10. Kucharekova M, Van De Kerkhof PC, Van Der Valk PG. A randomized comparison of an emollient containing skin-related lipids with a petrolatum-based emollient as adjunct in the treatment of chronic hand dermatitis. *Contact Dermatitis.* 2003;48:293-299.
11. Lukács J, Schliemann S, Elsner P. Association between smoking and hand dermatitis—a systematic review and meta-analysis. *J Eur Acad Dermatol Venereol.* 2015;29(7):1280-1284.
12. Das A, Panda S. An evidence based approach of use of topical corticosteroids in dermatology. *Indian J Dermatol.* 2017;62(3): 237-250.
13. Belsito DV, Fowler JF Jr, Marks JG Jr, et al; Multicenter Investigator Group. Pimecrolimus cream 1%: a potential new treatment for chronic hand dermatitis. *Cutis.* 2004;73(1):31-38.
14. Belsito D, Wilson DC, Warshaw E, et al. A prospective randomized clinical trial of 0.1% tacrolimus ointment in a model of chronic allergic contact dermatitis. *J Am Acad Dermatol.* 2006; 55:40-46.
15. Warshaw EM. Therapeutic options for chronic hand dermatitis. *Dermatol Ther.* 2004;17:240-250.
16. Smith I, Brown S, Nixon J, et al. Using results from a UK-wide survey to justify choice of comparator for the treatment of severe chronic hand eczema. *Clin Exp Dermatol.* 2017;42(2): 185-188.
17. Schmitt J, Schmitt N, Meurer M. Cyclosporin in the treatment of patients with atopic eczema—a systematic review and meta-analysis. *J Eur Acad Dermatol Venereol.* 2007;21:606-619.
18. Ruzicka T, Lynde CW, Jemec GBE, et al. Efficacy and safety of oral alitretinoin (9-*cis*-retinoic acid) in patients with severe chronic hand eczema refractory to topical corticosteroids: results of a randomized, double-blind, placebo-controlled, multicentre trial. *Br J Dermatol.* 2008;158:808-817.
19. Thaçi D, Augustin M, Westermayer B, et al. Effectiveness of alitretinoin in severe chronic hand eczema: PASSION, a real-world observational study. *J Dermatolog Treat.* 2016;27(6):577-583.
20. Bissonnette R, Diepgen TL, Elsner P, et al. Redefining treatment options in chronic hand eczema (CHE). *J Eur Acad Dermatol Venereol.* 2010;24:1-20.
21. Politiek K, Christoffers WA, Coenraads P-J, Schuttelaar M-LA. Alitretinoin and acitretin in severe chronic hand eczema: results from a retrospective daily practice study. *Dermatol Ther.* 2016;29(5):364-371.
22. Markantoni V, Kouris A, Armyra K, et al. Remarkable improvement of relapsing dyshidrotic eczema after treatment of coexistant hyperhidrosis with oxybutynin. *Dermatol Ther.* 2014;27(6): 365-368.

154 NUMMULAR ECZEMA

Yu Wah, MD
Richard P. Usatine, MD

PATIENT STORY

A 2-year-old Hispanic boy presents to the clinic with erythematous, round, moist, crusted lesions on the left thigh (**Figure 154-1**) and right arm. His mother noted several small bumps initially, which developed into coin-shaped lesions over the next few weeks. The child is scratching them but is otherwise healthy. A KOH preparation of the scraping from the lesions did not show fungal structures. The child responds well to treatment with topical midpotency corticosteroids, emollients, and dressing in long-sleeved clothes to prevent scratching the lesions. His nummular eczema resolved in 6 weeks.

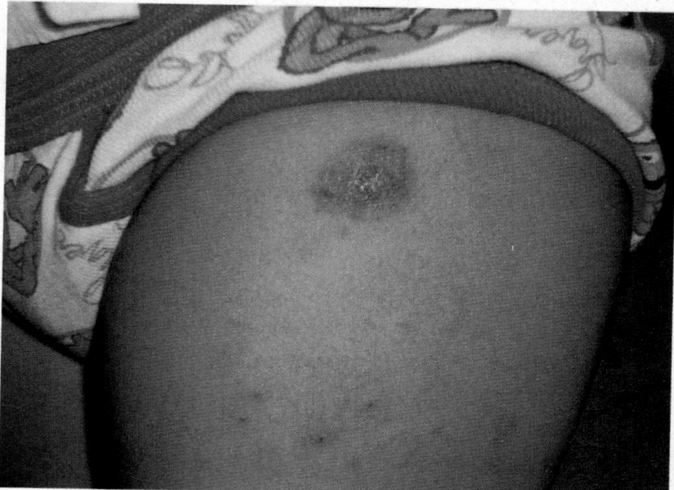

FIGURE 154-1 A 2-year-old child with nummular eczema on the left thigh. The lesion shows abrasions and excoriations from scratching. He has another similar lesion on the right arm. *(Reproduced with permission from Yu Wah, MD.)*

INTRODUCTION

Nummular eczema (NE) is a type of eczema characterized by circular or oval-shaped scaling plaques with well-defined borders. The term *nummular* refers to the shape of a coin (Latin for coin is *nummus*). The lesions are typically multiple and most commonly found on the dorsa of the hands, arms, and legs. It often overlaps with other clinical types of eczema: atopic dermatitis, stasis dermatitis, and asteatotic eczema.[1,2]

SYNONYMS

Nummular dermatitis, discoid eczema, microbial eczema, and orbicular eczema.

EPIDEMIOLOGY

- Prevalence is reported to range widely from 0.1% to 9.1%.[1]
- It is slightly more common in males than in females.[1]
- Males are also affected at a later age (peak older than age 50 years) than females (peak younger than age 30 years).[1]
- It is less common in children.

ETIOLOGY AND PATHOPHYSIOLOGY

Many factors have been reported in association with NE, but their role in the etiology and pathogenesis is not well established:

- NE has been viewed as microbial in origin, secondary either to bacterial colonization or to hematogenous spread of bacterial toxins,[1,3] but an infectious source is not identified in most cases of NE.

- NE is reported to be associated with xerosis of the skin that subsequently weakens the skin barrier function and sensitizes it to environmental allergens.[4]
- NE is frequently reported in association with contact sensitization to various agents, including nickel, chromate, balsam of Peru, and fragrances. Allergic or chronic contact dermatitis has been frequently reported to manifest as NE on the dorsa of the hands.[1,5]
- Onset of NE has been reported in association with various medications, including interferon and ribavirin therapy for hepatitis C[6,7] and isotretinoin.[8] Most of these reports are based on single or limited number of cases.
- Mercury in the dental amalgam was reported to induce NE in two cases with relapsing NE.[9]

DIAGNOSIS

HISTORY

- Onset is reported to be within days to weeks. Simultaneous or subsequent development of multiple lesions is often reported.
- Intense pruritus or burning is common.
- Lesions may last months to years without treatment and may be recurrent.
- History of medications, atopy, and exposure to allergens may be helpful to tailor the management of NE.

PHYSICAL EXAMINATION

- Primary morphology includes small papules and vesicles that coalesce to form circular to oval-shaped patches and plaques (**Figures 154-2** and **154-3**).
- Secondary morphology includes abrasion and excoriations from scratching (see **Figure 154-1**), weeping and crusting after the vesicles leak (**Figures 154-2** to **154-4**), and scaling and lichenification in more chronic lesions (**Figures 154-5** and **154-6**). Excessive weeping and crusting may indicate secondary bacterial infection.

TYPICAL DISTRIBUTION

- Dorsal hand is most commonly affected (**Figures 154-2** and **154-7**). The extensor aspects of the forearm (see **Figures 154-3** and **154-6**), the lower leg (see **Figure 154-5**), the thighs (see **Figure 154-1**), and the flanks are frequently involved, but NE may be seen in any part of the body (**Figures 154-4**, **154-8**, and **154-9**).

LABORATORY TESTING

- Diagnosis in most cases is made from clinical features.
- KOH preparation is helpful to investigate for tinea corporis.
- Patch testing may be considered if contact allergy is suspected.

BIOPSY

- Biopsy is rarely needed, but should be performed if there is suspicion of other serious clinical entities (e.g., mycosis fungoides, psoriasis) or if the diagnosis is uncertain.

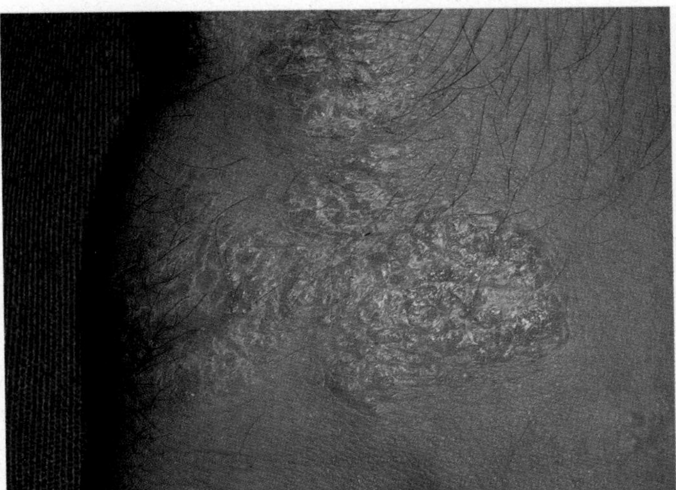

FIGURE 154-2 Multiple nummular lesions on the dorsum of the hand, a common site of nummular eczema. The lesions show multiple papules and vesicles that coalesce to form coin-shaped plaques; oozing and crusting can be seen from ruptured vesicles. *(Reproduced with permission from Richard P. Usatine, MD.)*

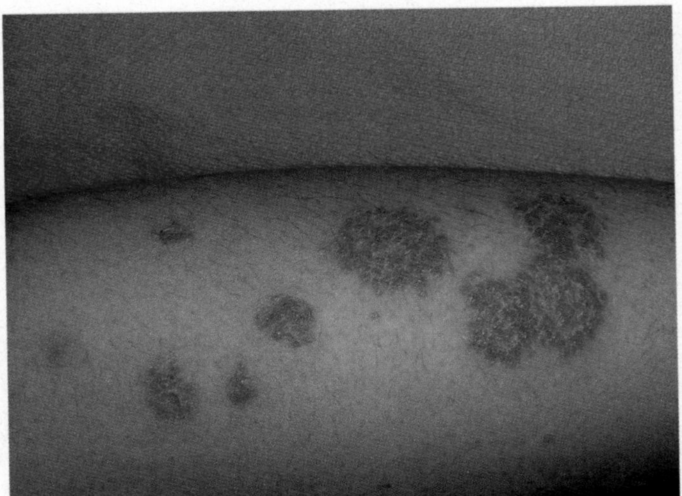

FIGURE 154-3 Nummular eczema on the forearm of a 22-year-old man. The lesions show multiple papules and vesicles that coalesce to form coin-shaped plaques; oozing and crusting can be seen from ruptured vesicles. *(Reproduced with permission from Richard P. Usatine, MD.)*

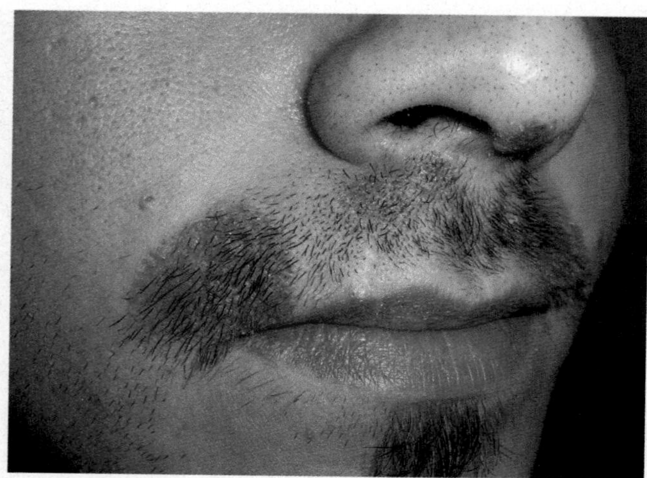

FIGURE 154-4 Nummular eczema on the face of a young man. (*Reproduced with permission from Richard P. Usatine, MD.*)

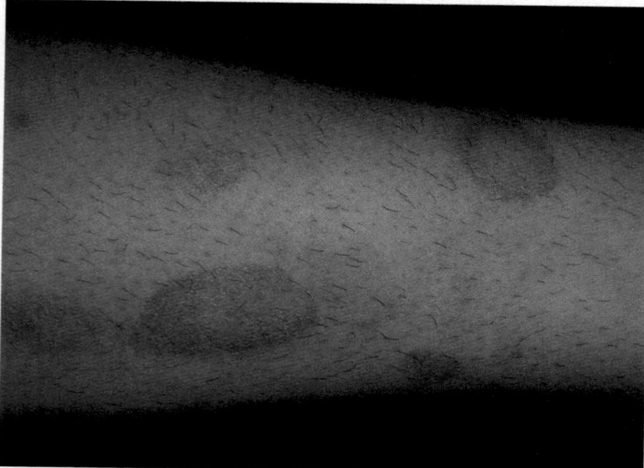

FIGURE 154-5 Multiple nummular lesions on the lower leg of a 15-year-old girl. Lesions of nummular eczema can be dry and scaly. The lesions prevented the patient from shaving her legs. (*Reproduced with permission from Richard P. Usatine, MD.*)

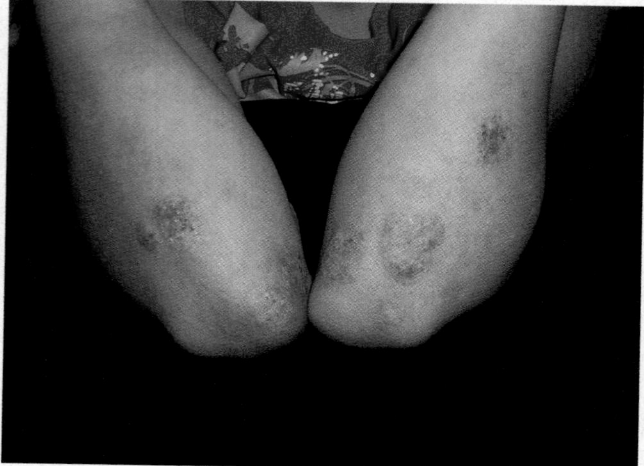

FIGURE 154-6 Nummular eczema on the extensor surface of the forearms and elbows. Thickened, scaly lesions resemble psoriatic plaques. A biopsy was performed to confirm the diagnosis of nummular eczema. (*Reproduced with permission from Richard P. Usatine, MD.*)

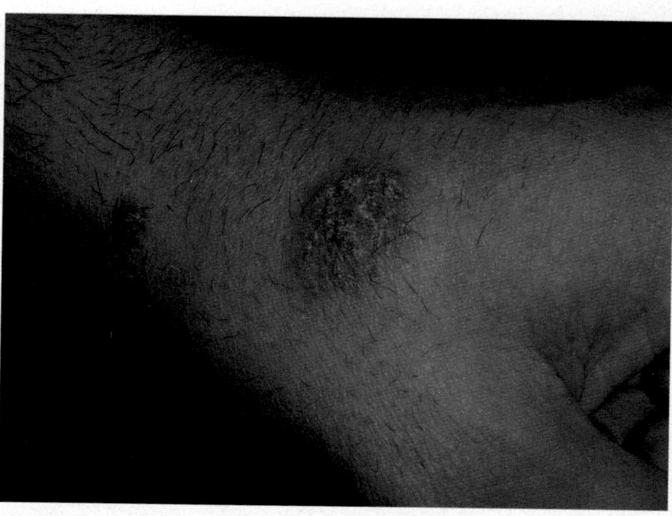

FIGURE 154-7 Nummular eczema on the dorsum of the hand and wrist. (*Reproduced with permission from Richard P. Usatine, MD.*)

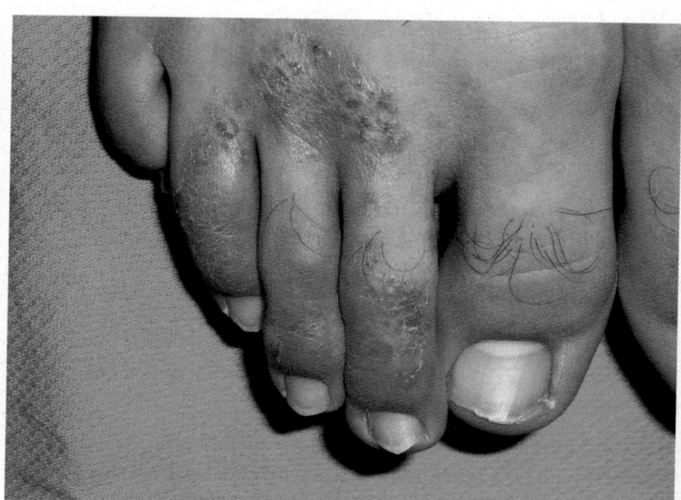

FIGURE 154-8 Nummular eczema on the dorsum of the foot. Contact dermatitis and tinea pedis were also in the differential diagnosis. (*Reproduced with permission from Richard P. Usatine, MD.*)

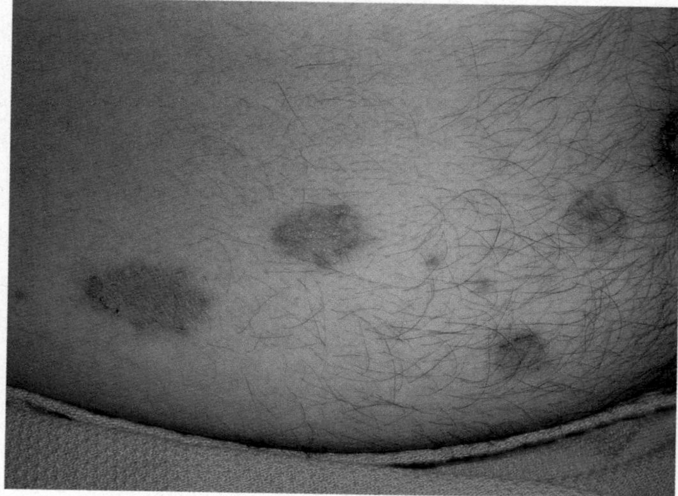

FIGURE 154-9 Nummular eczema on the abdomen of a 27-year-old man. (*Reproduced with permission from Richard P. Usatine, MD.*)

DIFFERENTIAL DIAGNOSIS

- Tinea corporis may present as pruritic annular lesions with scales and vesicles. Vesicles are typically at the periphery of the lesion compared to NE, where they are also seen in the center. A positive KOH preparation for hyphae can help with the diagnosis (see Chapter 144, Tinea Corporis).
- Psoriasis typically presents with thickened plaques on the extensor surfaces of arms and legs, scalp and sacral areas. Nail changes may be present (see Chapter 158, Psoriasis).
- Lichen simplex chronicus usually presents as a single plaque in an area easily accessible to scratching such as the ankle, wrist, and neck (see Chapter 155, Psychocutaneous Disorders).
- Mycosis fungoides is a type of cutaneous T-cell lymphoma, which may present with scaly patches or plaques that are often pruritic and usually erythematous. A biopsy can help make the diagnosis (see Chapter 180, Cutaneous T-Cell Lymphoma).
- Nummular lesions of atopic dermatitis may have features similar to NE. Presence of other lesions typically on flexural surfaces and a history of atopy, asthma, or seasonal allergies may help make the diagnosis (see Chapter 151, Atopic Dermatitis).
- Contact dermatitis (CD) may present with nummular lesions. History of exposure to contact allergens at the affected areas can raise the suspicion for CD. Patch testing may be used to confirm the clinical suspicion (see Chapter 152, Contact Dermatitis).
- Asteatotic dermatitis may have overlapping features with NE but has a less-well-defined margin.

MANAGEMENT

FIRST LINE

- Emollients are beneficial to help restore and maintain normal skin barrier function. SOR Ⓒ
- Hydration by bathing before bedtime followed by ointment application to wet skin is reported as an effective method of skin care in patients with eczema.[10] SOR Ⓑ
- A medium- to high-potency topical corticosteroid ointment is the first line of treatment.[10-12] SOR Ⓑ A cream preparation may be prescribed if the patient has a strong preference for cream over ointment.
- Oral antihistamines are often used to treat pruritus. Topical doxepin is reported to be effective in treatment of pruritus associated with eczematous conditions.[13] SOR Ⓑ However, topical doxepin is very expensive and can cause local burning or discomfort upon application.
- Topical antibiotics (such as mupirocin) and/or systemic antibiotics may be needed to treat secondary or associated bacterial infection. SOR Ⓒ It helps to be aware that the inflammatory process in nummular eczema frequently looks like a bacterial superinfection in the absence of secondary infection.

SECOND LINE

- Topical calcineurin inhibitors such as topical tacrolimus and pimecrolimus have the benefit of not causing skin atrophy and have been shown to be effective in many types of eczema.[1] SOR Ⓑ They have a higher cost compared to topical corticosteroids and have a black box warning because of a reported risk of malignancies.
- Short courses of systemic corticosteroids may be necessary in severe or acute cases. SOR Ⓒ
- Methotrexate is reported to be safe, effective, and well-tolerated in treatment of moderate to severe childhood NE.[14] This was reported in a case series of 25 pediatric patients with refractory NE treated with 5 or 10 mg of methotrexate per week. Sixty-four percent had total clearance after an average of 10.5 months. No serious adverse events were observed in this study.[14] SOR Ⓑ
- Phototherapy may be used in generalized, severe, or refractory cases.[1,2] Narrow-band UVB is commonly used, and psoralen UVA has been used in more severe cases.[2] SOR Ⓒ

FOLLOW-UP

Regular follow-up is needed for the patient with chronic, refractory, or relapsing nummular dermatitis until remission or resolution is achieved.

PATIENT EDUCATION

Hydration and protection of skin from irritants is important. Apply moisturizer or topical medications immediately after bathing while the skin is still moist. Avoid strong soaps and use mild fragrance-free soap, or soap alternatives. Avoid tight clothing and fabrics that irritate the skin.

PATIENT RESOURCES

- American Academy of Dermatology. *Nummular Dermatitis*—**http://www.aad.org/public/diseases/eczema/nummular-dermatitis.**
- British Association of Dermatologists. *Discoid Eczema*—**http://www.bad.org.uk/shared/get-file.ashx?id=80&itemtype=document.**

PROVIDER RESOURCES

- Medscape. *Nummular Dermatitis*—**http://emedicine.medscape.com/article/1123605.**

REFERENCES

1. Bolognia J. *Dermatology*. Elsevier Saunders; 2012.
2. Miller J. *Nummular Dermatitis*. http://emedicine.medscape.com/article/1123605, updated March 25, 2016. Accessed February 2017.
3. Tanaka T, Satoh T, Yokozeki H. Dental infection associated with nummular eczema as an overlooked focal infection. *J Dermatol*. 2009;36(8):462-465.

4. Aoyama H, Tanaka M, Hara M, et al. Nummular eczema: an addition of senile xerosis and unique cutaneous reactivities to environmental aeroallergens. *Dermatology*. 1999;199(2):135-139.
5. Wilkinson DS. Discoid eczema as a consequence of contact with irritants. *Contact Dermatitis.* 1979;5(2):118-119.
6. Moore MM, Elpern DJ, Carter DJ. Severe, generalized nummular eczema secondary to interferon alfa-2b plus ribavirin combination therapy in a patient with chronic hepatitis C virus infection. *Arch Dermatol.* 2004;140(2):215-217.
7. Shen Y, Pielop J, Hsu S. Generalized nummular eczema secondary to peginterferon alfa-2b and ribavirin combination therapy for hepatitis C infection. *Arch Dermatol.* 2005;141(1):102-103.
8. Bettoli V, Tosti A, Varotti C. Nummular eczema during isotretinoin treatment. *J Am Acad Dermatol.* 1987;16(3 Pt 1):617.
9. Adachi A, Horikawa T, Takashima T, Ichihashi M. Mercury-induced nummular dermatitis. *J Am Acad Dermatol.* 2000;43(2):383-385.
10. Gutman AB, Kligman AM, Sciacca J, James WD. Soak and smear: a standard technique revisited. *Arch Dermatol.* 2005;141(12): 1556-1569.
11. Yawalkar SJ, Macarol V, Montanari C. An overview of international clinical trials with halometasone ointment in chronic eczematous dermatoses. *J Int Med Res.* 1983;11 Suppl 1:13-20.
12. Belknap BS, Dobson RL. Efficacy of halcinonide cream, 0.1 percent, in the treatment of moderate and severe dermatoses. *Cutis.* 1981;27(4):433-435.
13. Drake LA, Millikan LE. The antipruritic effect of 5% doxepin cream in patients with eczematous dermatitis. Doxepin Study Group. *Arch Dermatol.* 1995;131(12):1403-1408.
14. Roberts H, Orchard D. Methotrexate is a safe and effective treatment for paediatric discoid (nummular) eczema: a case series of 25 children. *Australas J Dermatol.* 2010;51(2): 128-130.

155 PSYCHOCUTANEOUS DISORDERS

Anne E. Johnson, MD
Bettina Suzanne Fehr, MD
Richard P. Usatine, MD

PATIENT STORY

A 55-year-old woman presents with severe itching on her arms and legs. The itching disrupts her sleep, and she sometimes scratches her arms and legs until exhaustion (**Figures 155-1** and **155-2**).[1] She had used moisturizers, emollients, and topical corticosteroids, but they only alleviated the itching temporarily. The itching began 10 months earlier after finalizing the divorce from her husband of 20 years. The patient's right leg had been amputated above the knee after a car accident, and she now wore a prosthetic leg. The patient readily admitted to a great deal of psychological distress. She described feeling depressed since her divorce, and the loss of her leg further aggravated her situation. She has had difficulty securing a job and had high anxiety about being able to pay for rent and bills. The physician diagnosed an "excoriation disorder," and the patient understood that she was doing this to her own skin. The patient improved with nail cutting, topical clobetasol, and acknowledging the self-inflicted nature of her excoriations. One year later, the patient was working in the hospital laboratory with a tremendous improvement in her skin condition (**Figure 155-3**).

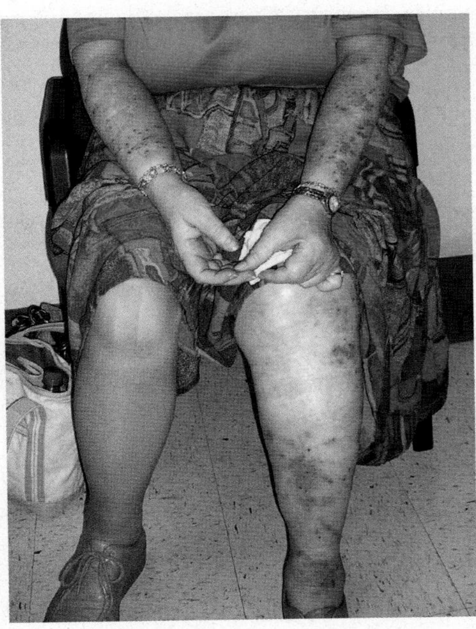

FIGURE 155-1 Excoriation disorder (neurodermatitis) seen on 3 of 4 extremities. The fourth extremity is a prosthetic leg. *(Reproduced with permission from Usatine RP, Saldana-Arregui MA. Excoriations and ulcers on the arms and legs. J Fam Pract. 2004;53(9):713-716. Frontline Medical Communications. Inc.)*

INTRODUCTION

Psychocutaneous disorders (sometimes referred to as "self-inflicted dermatoses" or "psychogenic dermatoses") include excoriation disorder, lichen simplex chronicus, and prurigo nodularis. In these conditions, repeated scratching, skin-picking, rubbing, or other self-inflicted damage to the skin occurs for psychiatric reasons, without evidence of a primary medical or dermatologic disorder. Psychocutaneous disorders can present a challenge to the clinician, as multiple underlying medical etiologies must be ruled out to arrive at their diagnosis and the pathophysiology of these diseases is not well understood. In addition, these disorders may be difficult to treat successfully. There is no clear standard of care for treatment, although a vast array of treatments targeting different etiologies has been tried clinically, and many have some amount of research to support them. As with other psychosomatic conditions, nonpharmacologic interventions, including the physician–patient relationship itself, are important to treatment.

Excoriation (skin-picking) disorder was established as a separate psychiatric diagnosis in the *Diagnostic and Statistical Manual of Mental Disorders, Fifth Edition* (DSM-5)[2] in 2013. It is grouped under obsessive–compulsive and related disorders. In addition to the presence of recurrent, time-consuming skin picking, essential features of the diagnosis include repeated attempts to stop or decrease the skin picking, impairment in functioning or clinically significant distress, and that other conditions do not account for the skin picking

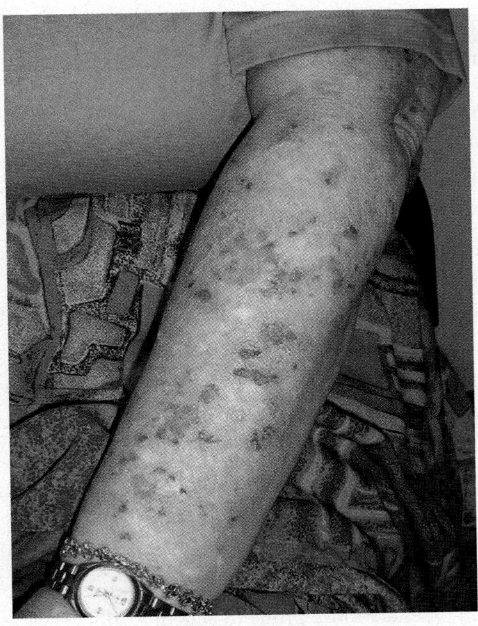

FIGURE 155-2 Excoriation disorder with close-up of arm. *(Reproduced with permission from Usatine RP, Saldana-Arregui MA. Excoriations and ulcers on the arms and legs. J Fam Pract. 2004;53(9):713-716. Frontline Medical Communications. Inc.)*

(including delusional parasitosis, tactile hallucinations, nonsuicidal self-injury, or the presence of scabies).

SYNONYMS

- Excoriation disorder—Skin-picking disorder; neurotic excoriations; neurodermatitis.
- Lichen simplex chronicus—Neurodermatitis circumscripta; neurodermatitis.
- Prurigo nodularis—Picker's nodules; lichen simplex chronicus, prurigo nodularis type; atypical nodular form of neurodermatitis circumscripta; skin-picking disorder.

EPIDEMIOLOGY

- Excoriation disorder primarily affects females, with onset usually occurring during adolescence[2] (**Figures 155-1** to **155-5**).
- Excoriation disorder is present in 2% of patients seen in dermatologic clinics,[3] and lifetime prevalence in the general population may be as high as 5.4%.[4]
- Lichen simplex chronicus (LSC) is observed more commonly in females than in males[5] (**Figures 155-6** to **155-9**). Lichen nuchae is a form of lichen simplex that occurs on the midposterior neck (**Figures 155-8** and **155-9**).
- LSC occurs mostly in mid-to-late adulthood, with highest prevalence in persons ages 30 to 50 years.[5,6]
- For prurigo nodularis (PN) there is no documented difference in frequency between males and females. PN most often occurs in middle-aged and older persons[7] (**Figures 155-10** to **155-15**).

ETIOLOGY AND PATHOPHYSIOLOGY

- All 3 conditions are found on the skin in regions accessible to scratching.
- Excoriation disorder is considered a psychiatric diagnosis on the obsessive–compulsive spectrum. It often begins with benign picking either of normal skin or of mild skin diseases, such as acne, before becoming pathologic.[2-4]
- Negative affective states such as tension, anxiety, or boredom may directly trigger neurotic picking and excoriations.[4]
- In all three disorders, pruritus may occur, provoking scratching that produces clinical lesions. This is particularly true in LSC and PN.
- The underlying pathophysiology is unknown for all 3 conditions. Central nervous system (CNS)[8] and peripheral nervous system[9,10] dysfunction have been implicated in the pathogenesis of the pruritus underlying psychocutaneous disorders.
- Some skin types are more prone to lichenification, such as skin that tends toward eczematous conditions (i.e., atopic dermatitis).[6]
- The pathogenesis of PN is still unknown. PN shares some histologic features (epidermal proliferation) with psoriasis and ichthyosis, but

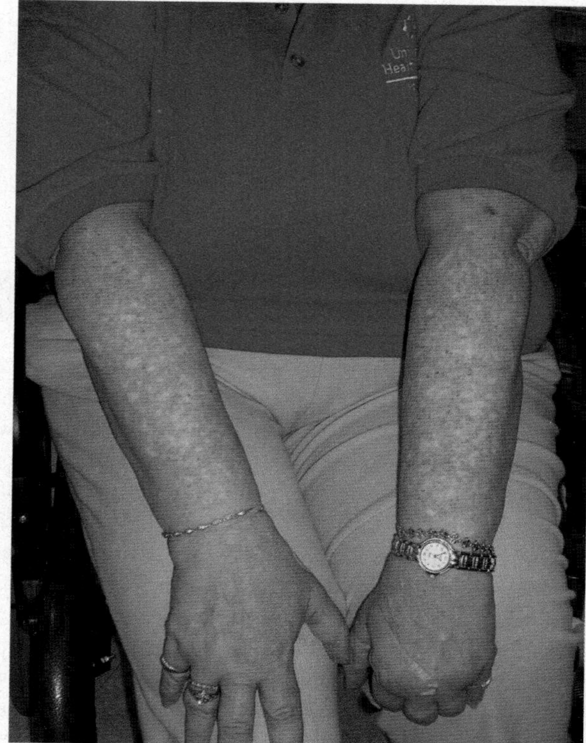

FIGURE 155-3 Same patient with excoriation disorder 1 year later after successful therapy. Hypopigmented scarring remains. (*Reproduced with permission from Richard P. Usatine, MD.*)

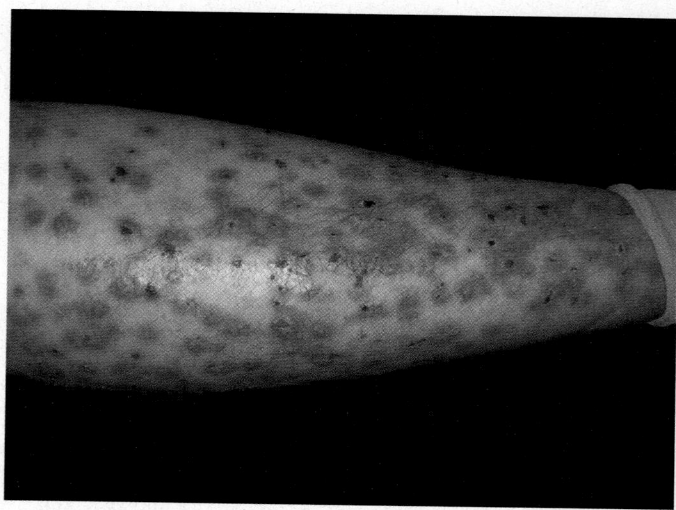

FIGURE 155-4 Excoriation disorder on the leg with significant postinflammatory hyperpigmentation. (*Reproduced with permission from Richard P. Usatine, MD.*)

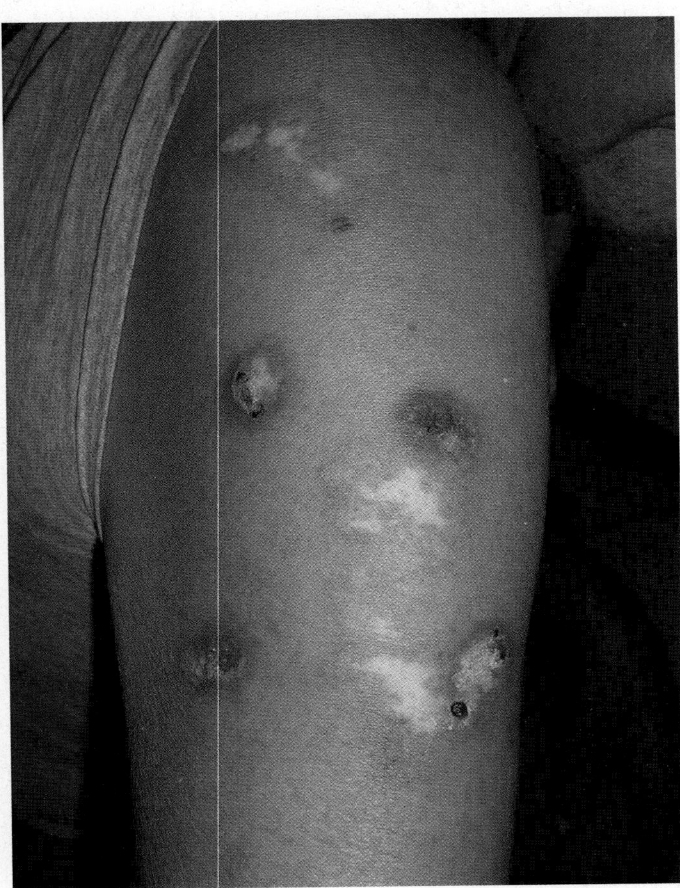

FIGURE 155-5 Excoriation disorder (skin-picking) on the upper arm with hypopigmented scarring. (*Reproduced with permission from Richard P. Usatine, MD.*)

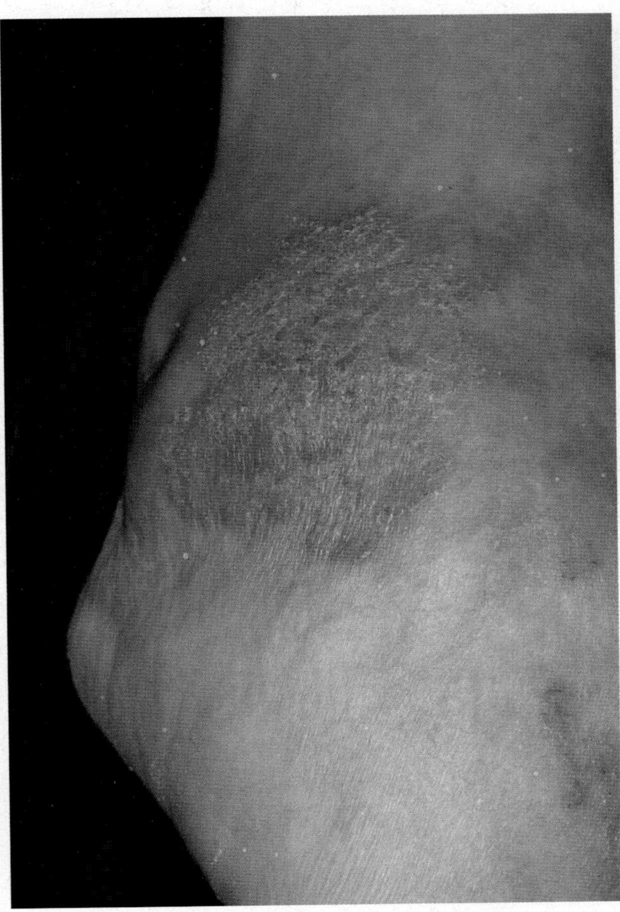

FIGURE 155-7 Lichen simplex chronicus on the ankle. (*Reproduced with permission from Richard P. Usatine, MD.*)

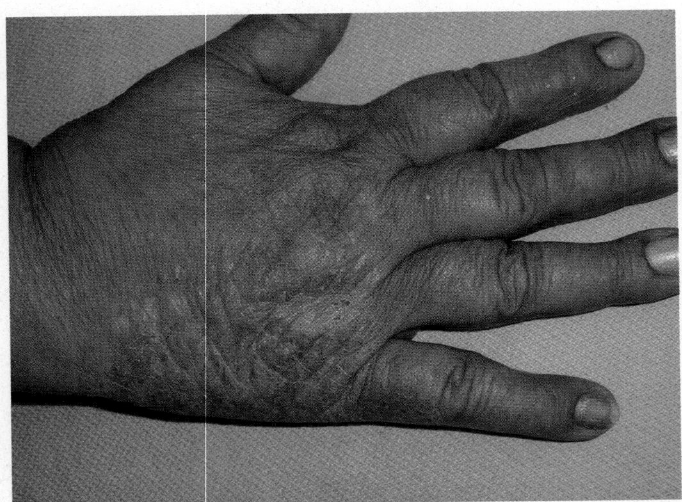

FIGURE 155-6 Lichen simplex chronicus on the hand of a middle-aged woman with thick lichenification, erythema, and hyperpigmentation. She was continually scratching at her hand. (*Reproduced with permission from Richard P. Usatine, MD.*)

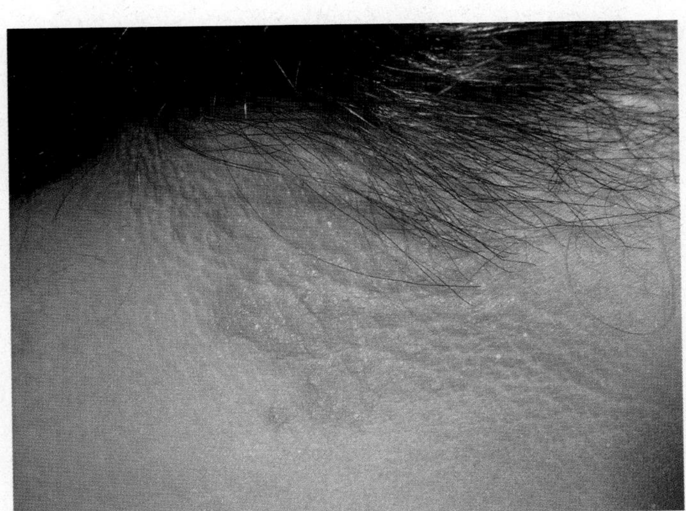

FIGURE 155-8 Lichen simplex chronicus on the neck of a Hispanic woman who also has acanthosis nigricans. (*Reproduced with permission from Richard P. Usatine, MD.*)

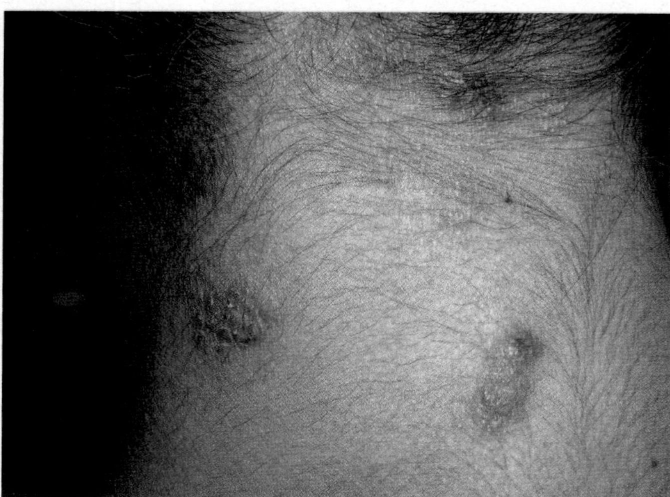

FIGURE 155-9 Lichen simplex chronicus on the neck of a Hispanic woman with thick plaque formation that resembles prurigo nodularis. (*Reproduced with permission from Richard P. Usatine, MD.*)

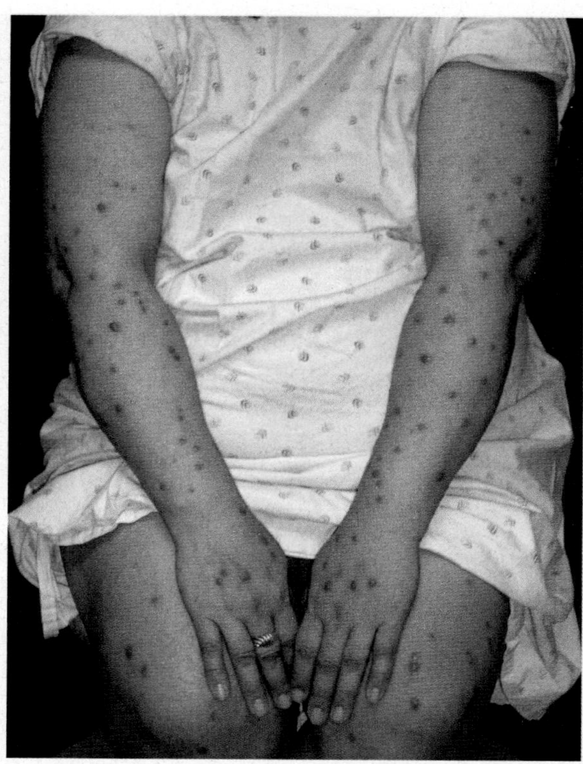

FIGURE 155-11 Prurigo nodularis on the arms and legs after 9 months of unsuccessful treatment in the patient in **Figure 155-10**. (*Reproduced with permission from Richard P. Usatine, MD.*)

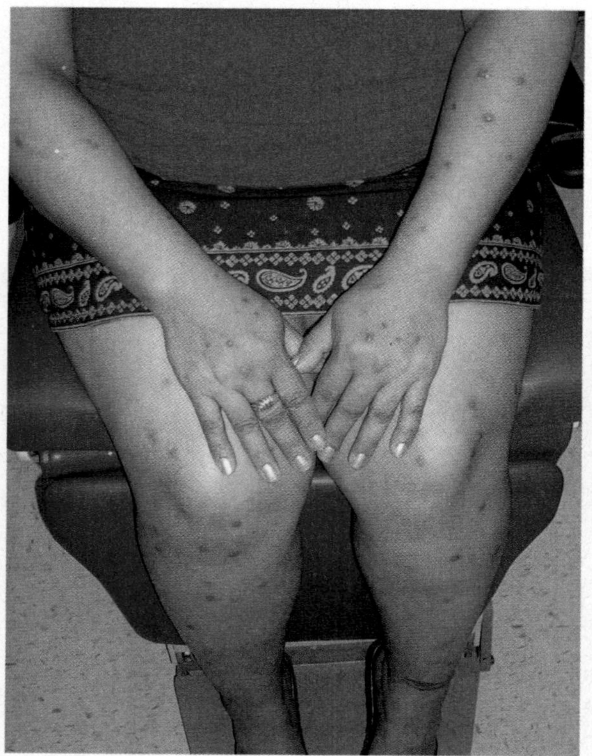

FIGURE 155-10 Prurigo nodularis on the arms and legs of a 42-year-old Hispanic woman. (*Reproduced with permission from Richard P. Usatine, MD.*)

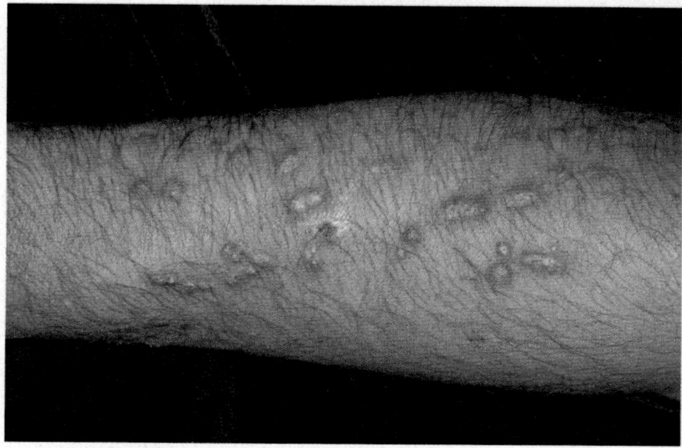

FIGURE 155-12 Severe prurigo nodularis on the arm. The nodules are somewhat linear from years of scratching. (*Reproduced with permission from Richard P. Usatine, MD.*)

is largely self-inflicted.[7] There is some evidence to suggest that immune dysregulation is involved, as PN is more common in patients with HIV/AIDS (pruritic papular eruption) and other forms of immunosuppression than in the general population.[7] Some histologic studies have shown changes in intraepidermal nerve fibers, suggesting the presence of a subclinical small-fiber neuropathy.[11]

DIAGNOSIS

CLINICAL FEATURES

Self-inflicted damage to the skin by repeated scratching, rubbing, or picking—which the patient readily admits to—is a typical finding for these psychocutaneous disorders. The patient will often complain of intense itching. Common psychiatric problems associated with these disorders include significant social stress, depression, anxiety, and obsessive–compulsive disorder. Patients are often observed scratching and rubbing their skin. This results in:

- Lichenification of the skin (skin thickening with exaggerated skin lines) (see **Figures 155-6** and **155-9**).
- Pigmentary changes (especially hyperpigmentation) (see **Figures 155-4, 155-5, 155-9, 155-11,** and **155-15**).
- Excoriations, erosions, and ulcerations.

Common physical examination findings for all three disorders include:

- Excoriation disorder—Skin lesions may vary from dug-out erosions, to ulcers covered with crusts and surrounded by erythema, to areas receding into hypopigmented depressed scars (see **Figure 155-5**).
- Lichen simplex chronicus—One or more slightly erythematous, scaly, well-demarcated, lichenified, firm, rough plaques (see **Figures 155-6** to **155-9**).
- Prurigo nodularis—Raised nodules from 2 to 20 mm, colors vary from shades of red to brown (see **Figures 155-10** to **155-15**). Excoriations are almost always present on initial presentation. With treatment the excoriations may subside and the nodules may remain.

TYPICAL DISTRIBUTION

- Excoriation disorder occurs on areas easily reached by the patient, such as the arms, legs, and upper back (see **Figures 155-1** to **155-5**).
- LSC occurs on:
  - Hands, wrists, extensor forearms, and elbows (see **Figure 155-6**).
  - Knees, lower legs, and ankles (see **Figure 155-7**).
  - Nape of neck (see **Figures 155-8** and **155-9**).
  - Vulva and scrotum.
- In PN, nodules occur on the extensor surfaces of the arms, the legs, and sometimes the trunk (see **Figures 155-10** to **155-15**).

LABORATORY STUDIES

A comprehensive medical profile may be useful to make sure that the pruritus is not related to renal or hepatic disease.

Punch biopsy may be helpful when the diagnosis is uncertain.

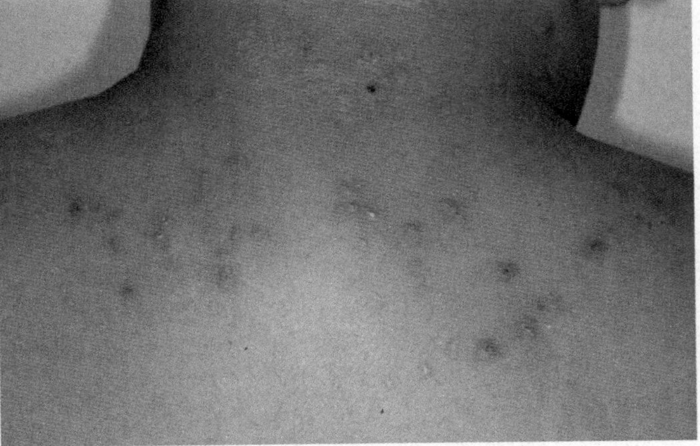

FIGURE 155-13 Prurigo nodularis on the upper back of a man. *(Reproduced with permission from Richard P. Usatine, MD.)*

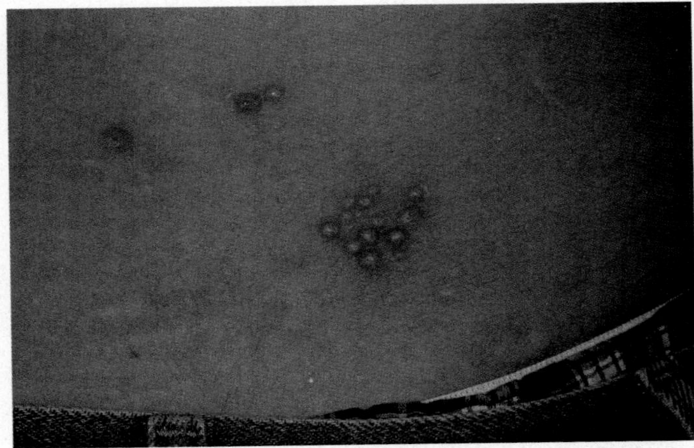

FIGURE 155-14 A cluster of nodules on the back of the same patient with prurigo nodularis. *(Reproduced with permission from Richard P. Usatine, MD.)*

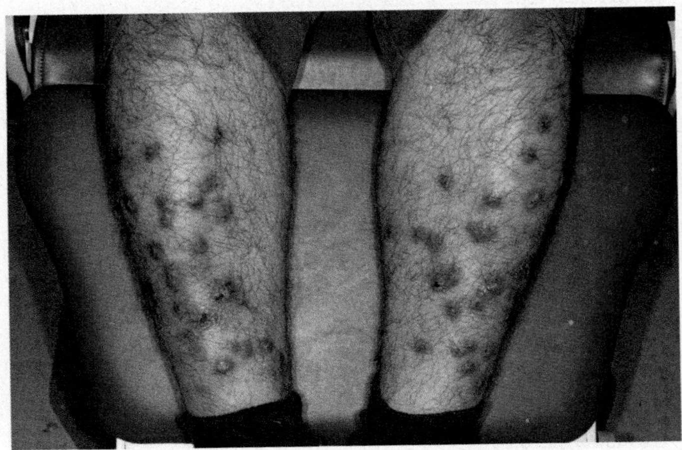

FIGURE 155-15 Severe prurigo nodularis on the legs with prominent hyperpigmentation of the nodules and some secondary infection. *(Reproduced with permission from Richard P. Usatine, MD.)*

DIFFERENTIAL DIAGNOSIS

- Acne keloidalis nuchae—Acneiform eruption at the hairline from ingrown hairs, worse with shaving and short haircuts (see Chapter 120, Pseudofolliculitis and Acne Keloidalis Nuchae).
- Atopic dermatitis—An allergic skin disorder in patients with a personal or family history of atopic conditions. Patients with atopic dermatitis are more likely to get LSC (see Chapter 151, Atopic Dermatitis).
- Contact dermatitis—A common inflammatory skin condition characterized by erythematous and pruritic skin lesions resulting from the contact of skin with a toxic substance or a contact allergen (see Chapter 152, Contact Dermatitis).
- Delusions of parasitosis (Delusional parasitosis or delusional infestation)—Delusions that tiny bugs or parasites are living on or below the patient's skin, leading them to try to dig them out with their fingernails and other devices. This condition may look just like excoriation disorder; however, the patient believes there are parasites causing the pruritus, and it is very difficult to convince them otherwise.
- Dermatitis artefacta (factitious dermatitis)—A condition in which individuals deliberately damage their skin in order to receive medical care.
- Nonsuicidal self-injury—Self-inflicted harm (such as cutting) that is not intended to produce death. The person may cut their skin to self-punish or relieve extreme emotional distress. This psychological distress is more acute in nature than the anxiety and tension that may trigger habitual skin picking.
- Nummular eczema—Eczematous lesions in the shape of coins, seen most often on the legs.
- Scabies—Look for burrows between the fingers and other typical distribution sites of scabies on the hands, feet, wrists, waist, and axillae to differentiate scabies from a psychocutaneous disorder. Scraping lesions and finding evidence of the scabies mite is the best way to confirm a true scabies infestation. Often family members have itching and lesions as well when the real diagnosis is scabies (see Chapter 149, Scabies).

MANAGEMENT

Get a good psychosocial history and offer the patient treatment for any problems uncovered. It may help for patients to understand the connection between their self-inflicted lesions and their stressors. Some patients will have anxiety disorders or depression, whereas others will be suffering with great psychosocial stressors like loss of work, homelessness, or grief. Offer pharmacotherapy (including selective serotonin reuptake inhibitors [SSRIs]) and counseling if indicated. Refer as needed for these therapies. Other specific treatments to consider are listed below for each disorder.

EXCORIATION DISORDER

FIRST LINE

- Nonpharmacologic:
  - Psychotherapy is generally recommended as a first-line treatment and has been shown in meta-analyses to be effective for excoriation disorder.[12,13] SOR Ⓐ
    - The types of psychotherapy that have been most studied in excoriation disorder are standard cognitive behavioral therapy (CBT) and habit reversal therapy (HRT). There is currently insufficient evidence to recommend one of these types of psychotherapy over the other.
- Medications:
  - SSRIs as a class have been reported in one meta-analysis to be effective for excoriation disorder with a large effect size.[12] However, another meta-analysis concluded there was insufficient evidence that SSRIs were superior to non-treatment control conditions.[13] Given their efficacy in several psychiatric disorders that may be comorbid with excoriation disorder and the existence of positive randomized controlled trials for SSRIs in excoriation disorder, we recommend that SSRIs be considered early in treatment, either in combination with psychotherapy or if there is insufficient response with psychotherapy alone. SOR Ⓑ
    - SSRIs can also have an anti-pruritic effect independent of mood effects.[1,3]
  - Topical or oral antibiotics should be prescribed if secondary infection is present. SOR Ⓒ
  - If pruritus is present:
    - Topical corticosteroids—use mid-potency to high-potency steroids except in areas of thin skin. Steroid creams are usually used, but steroid ointments are preferred if deeper excoriations or ulcers are present.[1] SOR Ⓒ
    - Oral antihistamines such as hydroxyzine. SOR Ⓒ
    - Oral low-dose doxepin, a tricyclic antidepressant with sedating properties (10–25 mg at night).[3] SOR Ⓒ

SECOND LINE

- Nonpharmacologic:
  - Physical barriers to scratching, such as occlusive dressings—alone or with topical medication.[3] SOR Ⓒ
- Medications:
  - *N*-Acetylcysteine (NAC) has growing evidence in excoriation disorder, including a positive randomized controlled trial with doses of 1200–3000 mg per day.[14] SOR Ⓑ
  - Lamotrigine has been studied in excoriation disorder, with mixed results, and may be considered for treatment-resistant cases.[12] SOR Ⓒ
  - Atypical antipsychotics, either alone or as an augmentation of antidepressants, may be helpful in treatment-resistant cases. SOR Ⓒ
- Complementary/alternative therapy:
  - Hypnosis has a small amount of evidence in treating psychocutaneous disorders, including excoriation disorder.[15] SOR Ⓒ

LICHEN SIMPLEX CHRONICUS

FIRST LINE

- Nonpharmacologic:
  - Psychotherapy.[5] SOR Ⓒ
  - Physical barriers to scratching such as occlusive dressings, typically in combination with topical medication.[6] SOR Ⓒ
- Medications:
  - In general, topical glucocorticoid creams or ointments are the first-line treatment.[5,6,16,17] SOR Ⓑ High- or ultrahigh-potency topical steroids may be used for short (i.e., up to 6 weeks) courses

and may need to be tapered. For longer term use, midpotency steroids may be used.

- Recommendations differ according to source for topical steroid use in vulvar LSC, with some authors recommending an initial 2- to 6-week course of high- or ultrahigh-potency steroids (or midpotency for mild symptoms)[18] and other authors recommending low-potency steroids.[6] SOR C

SECOND LINE

- Nonpharmacologic:
  - In one uncontrolled study of 22 patients with LSC, transcutaneous electrical nerve stimulation (TENS) reduced pruritus by greater than 50% in 80% of the patients.[19] SOR C
- Medications:
  - The topical calcineurin inhibitors tacrolimus and pimecrolimus have some evidence to support them in vulvar and nonvulvar LSC.[5,18,20,21] SOR C
  - Intralesional steroids, such as triamcinolone acetonide.[5,6,18] SOR C
  - Oral antihistamines such as diphenhydramine or hydroxyzine.[6] SOR C
  - Oral low-dose doxepin.[6] SOR C
  - Doxepin 5% cream has been studied in patients with LSC, nummular eczema, and contact dermatitis. Applied four times a day for a period of 7 days, it led to an 84% response rate in reduction of pruritus (not lesions).[21] SOR B
  - Gabapentin has some reported successes in reducing pruritus in patients with PN and LSC.[9] SOR C This is a very affordable option and may be especially beneficial in patients who have other reasons for neuropathy (i.e., diabetes).
- Complementary/alternative therapy:
  - Hypnosis[15] SOR C

PRURIGO NODULARIS

FIRST LINE

- Nonpharmacologic:
  - Psychotherapy.[5] SOR C
- Medications:
  - Topical glucocorticoid creams or ointments.[22] SOR C
  - Oral antihistamines.[23] SOR C
  - Intralesional steroids such as triamcinolone[5,7,22-24]—start with 5–10 mg/mL; some authors recommend increasing as needed, up to 40 mg/mL.[22] SOR C
  - Topical capsaicin is recommended by some experts.[22-25] SOR C Explain to the patient that this stings and burns the skin and mucus membranes before it works.

SECOND LINE

- Nonpharmacologic:
  - Cryotherapy—applied to each nodule to flatten the nodules and decrease pruritus.[22,24] SOR C
  - Phototherapy—Several modalities have some evidence to support them, either alone or in combination with one another. Modalities studied in PN include UVB (both broadband and narrowband), UVA, PUVA (psoralens + UVA), and monochromatic excimer light (308 nm). A review of phototherapy in PN concluded that there is insufficient evidence to recommend one phototherapy modality over the others.[26] SOR C Narrowband UVB is generally safest and most affordable. It is usually prescribed 2–3 times weekly for at least 3–4 months.
- Medications
  - Topical vitamin D, such as calcipotriol ointment.[27] SOR C
  - Gabapentin[9] or pregabalin.[28] SOR C Generic gabapentin is most affordable, and dosing should be at least 300 mg three times daily to see any benefit.
  - SSRIs.[24] SOR C
  - Oral low-dose doxepin.[22] SOR C
  - A short course of oral corticosteroids.[23] SOR C
- Complementary/alternative therapy:
  - Hypnosis.[15] SOR C

REFER OR HOSPITALIZE

For all 3 disorders:

- Referral to dermatology, psychotherapy, and/or psychopharmacology should be considered in any of these disorders that do not respond to treatment in the primary care setting. Hospitalization is rarely needed.

PATIENT EDUCATION

Help patients to understand that they are unintentionally hurting their own skin. Patients need to minimize touching, scratching, and rubbing affected areas. Suggest that patients gently apply their medication or a moisturizer instead of scratching the pruritic areas. Give patients hope and show them **Figures 155-1** to **155-3** to demonstrate that even the most severe cases can heal if they stop manipulating their skin.

FOLLOW-UP

Follow-up is essential because these problems are chronic and difficult to treat. Patients need to know that you will not abandon them but will continue to work with them to get relief. This is especially important when the patient is suffering from anxiety, depression, or other psychological problems.

PATIENT RESOURCES

- Neurodermatitis—**http://www.mayoclinic.org/diseases-conditions/neurodermatitis/basics/definition/con-20027919.**
- *Prurigo Nodularis*—**http://www.aocd.org/?page=PrurigoNodularis.**
- *Excoriation Disorder*—**http://www.webmd.com/mental-health/skin-picking-disorder.**

PROVIDER RESOURCES

- *Lichen Simplex Chronicus*—**http://emedicine.medscape.com/article/1123423.**
- *Prurigo Nodularis*—**http://emedicine.medscape.com/article/1088032.**

- *Excoriation Disorder*—**http://emedicine.medscape.com/article/1122042.**
- Kuhn H, Mennella C, Magid M, et al. Psychocutaneous disease: pharmacotherapy and psychotherapy. *J Am Acad Dermatol.* 2017 May;76(5):795-808.

REFERENCES

1. Usatine RP, Saldana-Arregui MA. Excoriations and ulcers on the arms and legs. *J Fam Pract.* 2004;53(9):713-716.
2. American Psychiatric Association. *Diagnostic and Statistical Manual of Mental Disorders.* 5th ed. Arlington, VA: American Psychiatric Association; 2013.
3. Scheinfeld, N. *Neurotic Excoriations.* http://emedicine.medscape.com/article/1122042. Updated January 26, 2016. Accessed January 2017.
4. Abramowitz JS, Jacoby RJ. Pickers, pokers, and pullers: obsessive-compulsive and related disorders in dermatology. In: *Practical Psychodermatology.* West Sussex, UK: John Wiley and Sons; 2014:134-141.
5. Lotti T, Buggiani G, Prignano F. Prurigo nodularis and lichen simplex chronicus. *Dermatol Ther.* 2008;21(1):42-46.
6. Schoenfeld J. *Lichen Simplex Chronicus.* http://emedicine.medscape.com/article/1123423. Updated March 30, 2016. Accessed January 2017.
7. Hogan, D. *Prurigo Nodularis.* http://emedicine.medscape.com/article/1088032. Updated August 25, 2016. Accessed January 2017.
8. Krishnan A, Koo J. Psyche, opioids, and itch: therapeutic consequences. *Dermatol Ther.* 2005;18(4):314-322.
9. Gencoglan G, Inanir I, Gunduz K. Therapeutic hotline: treatment of prurigo nodularis and lichen simplex chronicus with gabapentin. *Dermatol Ther.* 2010;23(2):194-198.
10. Solak O, Kulac M, Yaman M, et al. Lichen simplex chronicus as a symptom of neuropathy. *Clin Exp Dermatol.* 2009;34(4):476-480.
11. Schuhknecht B, Marziniak M, Wissel A, et al. Reduced intraepidermal nerve fibre density in lesional and nonlesional prurigo nodularis skin as a potential sign of subclinical cutaneous neuropathy. *Br J Dermatol.* 2011;165(1):85-91.
12. Selles RR, McGuire JF, Small BJ, Storch EA. A systematic review and meta-analysis of psychiatric treatments for excoriation (skin-picking) disorder. *Gen Hosp Psychiatry.* 2016;41:29-37.
13. Schumer MC, Bartley CA, Bloch MH. Systematic review of pharmacological and behavioral treatments for skin picking disorder. *J Clin Psychopharmacol.* 2016;36(2):147-152.
14. Grant JE, Chamberlain SR, Redden SA, et al. *N*-Acetylcysteine in the treatment of excoriation disorder: a randomized clinical trial. *JAMA Psychiatry.* 2016;73(5):490-496.
15. Shenefelt PD. Biofeedback, cognitive-behavioral methods, and hypnosis in dermatology: is it all in your mind? *Dermatol Ther.* 2003;16(2):114-122.
16. Brunner N, Yawalkar S. A double-blind, multicenter, parallel-group trial with 0.05% halobetasol propionate ointment versus 0.1% diflucortolone valerate ointment in patients with severe, chronic atopic dermatitis or lichen simplex chronicus. *J Am Acad Dermatol.* 1991;25(6 Pt 2):1160-1163.
17. Datz B, Yawalkar S. A double-blind, multicenter trial of 0.05% halobetasol propionate ointment and 0.05% clobetasol 17-propionate ointment in the treatment of patients with chronic, localized atopic dermatitis or lichen simplex chronicus. *J Am Acad Dermatol.* 1991;25(6 Pt 2):1157-1160.
18. Thorstensen KA, Birenbaum DL. Recognition and management of vulvar dermatologic conditions: lichen sclerosus, lichen planus, and lichen simplex chronicus. *J Midwifery Womens Health.* 2012; 57(3):260-275.
19. Engin B, Tufekci O, Yazici A, Ozdemir M. The effect of transcutaneous electrical nerve stimulation in the treatment of lichen simplex: a prospective study. *Clin Exp Dermatol.* 2009;34(3):324-328.
20. Goldstein AT, Thaci D, Luger T. Topical calcineurin inhibitors for the treatment of vulvar dermatoses. *Eur J Obstet Gynecol Reprod Biol.* 2009;146(1):22-29.
21. Drake LA, Millikan LE. The antipruritic effect of 5% doxepin cream in patients with eczematous dermatitis. Doxepin Study Group. *Arch Dermatol.* 1995;131(12):1403-1408.
22. Lee MR, Shumack S. Prurigo nodularis: a review. *Australas J Dermatol.* 2005;46(4):211-218; quiz 219-220.
23. Saco M, Cohen G. Prurigo nodularis: picking the right treatment. *J Fam Pract.* 2015;64(4):221-226.
24. Tan WS, Tey HL, Tang MBY. Nodular prurigo. In: *Practical Psychodermatology.* West Sussex, UK: John Wiley and Sons; 2014:134-141.
25. Stander S, Luger T, Metze D. Treatment of prurigo nodularis with topical capsaicin. *J Am Acad Dermatol.* 2001;44(3):471-478.
26. Nakamura M, Koo JY. Phototherapy for the treatment of prurigo nodularis: a review. *Dermatol Online J.* 2016;22(4).
27. Wong SS, Goh CL. Double-blind, right/left comparison of calcipotriol ointment and betamethasone ointment in the treatment of Prurigo nodularis. *Arch Dermatol.* 2000;136(6):807-808.
28. Mazza M, Guerriero G, Marano G, et al. Treatment of prurigo nodularis with pregabalin. *J Clin Pharm Ther.* 2013;38(1):16-18.

156 URTICARIA AND ANGIOEDEMA

Richard P. Usatine, MD
Paige M. Seeker, MD
Holly H. Volz, MD

PATIENT STORY

A 26-year-old man was prescribed trimethoprim-sulfamethoxazole for sinusitis and broke out in hives 1 week later. The hives were all over his trunk and arms (**Figures 156-1** and **156-2**). He denied throat tightening, trouble breathing, and lip or periorbital swelling. His sinus symptoms were mostly resolved, so he was told to stop the antibiotic and take an oral antihistamine. The H_1-blocker gave him relief of symptoms, and the urticaria disappeared over the next 2 days.

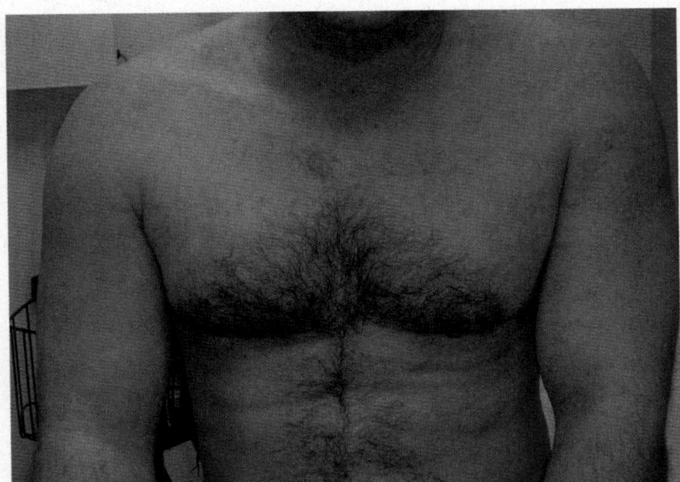

FIGURE 156-1 A 26-year-old man with acute urticaria due to trimethoprim-sulfamethoxazole. (*Reproduced with permission from Richard P. Usatine, MD.*)

INTRODUCTION

Urticaria is a common disorder characterized by transient skin or mucosal swellings that develop secondary to plasma leakage. The clinical presentation is determined by the depth of swelling. Superficial dermal swellings present as transient, pink, pruritic swellings known as wheals. Deeper swellings of the dermis, subcutaneous, or mucosal tissue present as flesh-colored to pink, painful, less well-defined swellings known as angioedema.[1] Urticaria and angioedema result from a large variety of underlying causes, are elicited by a great diversity of factors, and present clinically in a highly variable way.[2] Standard hives with transient wheals is the most common manifestation of urticaria.

SYNONYMS

Hives.

EPIDEMIOLOGY

- It is estimated that 15% to 25% of the population may have urticaria sometime during their lifetime.[2]
- Urticaria affects 6% to 7% of preschool children and 17% of children with atopic dermatitis.[3] Viral infections are a common cause of urticaria in children.
- Among all affected age groups, approximately 50% have both urticaria and angioedema, 40% have isolated urticaria, and 10% have angioedema alone.[3]
- Acute urticaria is defined as less than 6 weeks' duration. A specific cause is more likely to be identified in acute urticaria.[3]
- The cause of chronic urticaria (>6 weeks' duration) is determined in less than 20% of cases.[3]
- Chronic urticaria is twice as common in women as in men.[4]
- Chronic urticaria predominantly affects adults, with peak incidence occurring between ages 20 and 40.[4]

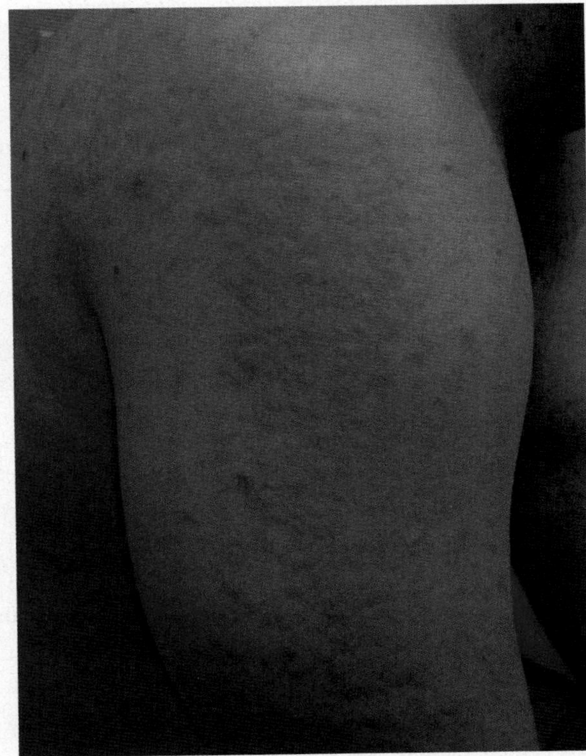

FIGURE 156-2 Note the confluence of wheals with a well-demarcated border on the arm of the man with acute urticaria due to trimethoprim-sulfamethoxazole. (*Reproduced with permission from Richard P. Usatine, MD.*)

- Up to 40% of patients with chronic urticaria of more than 6 months' duration still have urticaria 10 years later.[4]
- Chronic urticaria is more prevalent in those with autoimmune disorders.[5,6] Hashimoto thyroiditis is the most commonly associated autoimmune disease.[6]

ETIOLOGY AND PATHOPHYSIOLOGY

- The pathophysiology of angioedema and urticaria can be immunoglobulin (Ig) E mediated, complement mediated, related to physical stimuli, autoantibody mediated, or idiopathic.
- These mechanisms lead to mast cell degranulation resulting in the release of histamine. The histamine and other inflammatory mediators produce the wheals, edema, and pruritus.
- Urticaria is a dynamic process in which new wheals evolve as old ones resolve. These wheals result from localized capillary vasodilation, followed by transudation of protein-rich fluid into the surrounding skin. The wheals resolve when the fluid is slowly reabsorbed.
- Angioedema is an edematous area that involves transudation of fluid into the dermis and subcutaneous tissue (**Figures 156-3** and **156-4**).

The following etiologic types exist:

- Immunologic—IgE mediated, complement mediated. Occurs more often in patients with an atopic background. Antigens are most commonly foods or medications. The most common foods are milk, nuts, wheat, and shellfish.
- Physical urticaria—Dermatographism, cold, cholinergic, solar, pressure, vibratory urticaria (**Figures 156-5** and **156-6**).
- Urticaria caused by mast cell-releasing agents—Mastocytosis, urticaria pigmentosa (**Figures 156-7** and **156-8**).
- Urticaria associated with vascular/connective tissue autoimmune disease.
- Hereditary angioedema is a potentially life-threatening disorder that is inherited in an autosomal dominant manner. In this disease, angioedema occurs without urticaria (**Figure 156-9**).

DIAGNOSIS

CLINICAL FEATURES

- Symptoms include itching, burning, and stinging.
- Wheals vary in size from small, 2-mm papules of cholinergic urticaria (see **Figure 156-6**) to giant hives where a single wheal may cover a large portion of the trunk.
- The wheal may be all red or white, or the border may be red with the remainder of the surface white.
- Wheals may be annular (**Figures 156-10** and **156-11**).
- If dermatographism is present, one can write on the skin and be able to see the resulting words or shapes (see **Figure 156-5**).
- Wheals associated with chronic urticaria are typically present for 4 to 36 hours, whereas hives associated with primary dermatographism usually resolve within 2 hours.[5]

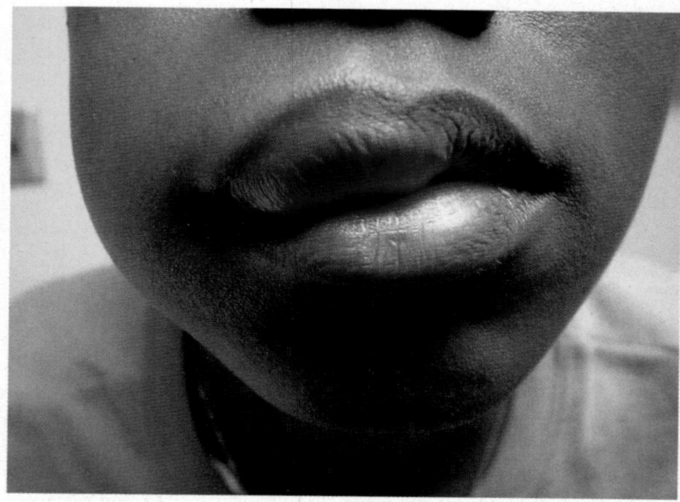

FIGURE 156-3 Young black woman with angioedema after being started on an angiotensin-converting enzyme (ACE) inhibitor for essential hypertension. (*Reproduced with permission from Adrian Casillas, MD.*)

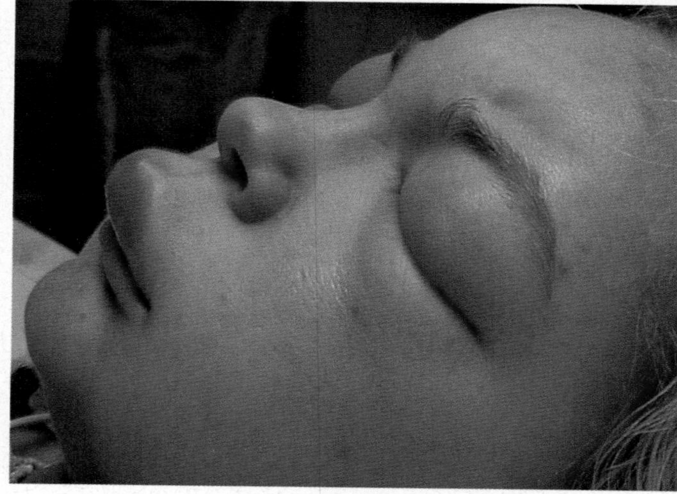

FIGURE 156-4 Severe angioedema around the eyes and mouth in a high school girl. (*Reproduced with permission from Daniel Stulberg, MD.*)

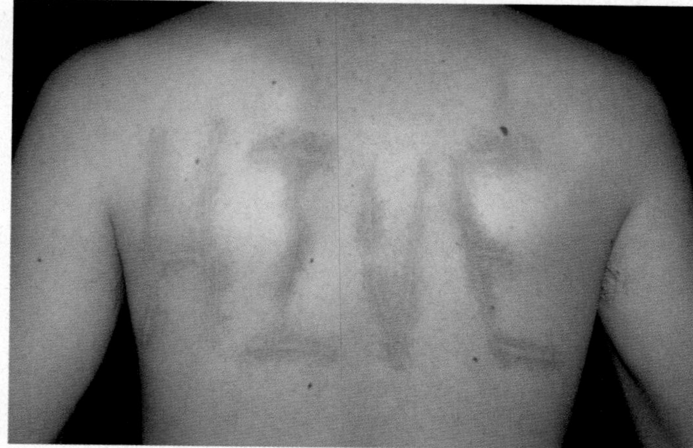

FIGURE 156-5 Dermatographism in a 21-year-old man with chronic urticaria. Note the exaggerated triple reaction. (*Reproduced with permission from Richard P. Usatine, MD.*)

FIGURE 156-6 Cholinergic urticaria showing small wheals. The patient would get this urticaria after exercising. (*Reproduced with permission from Philip C. Anderson, MD.*)

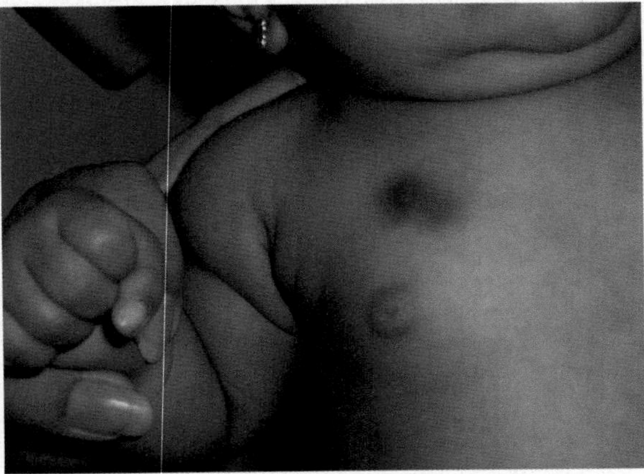

FIGURE 156-7 Urticaria pigmentosa on the chest of this 9-month-old girl. She has a positive Darier sign in which stroking the lesion results in edema. (*Reproduced with permission from Richard P. Usatine, MD.*)

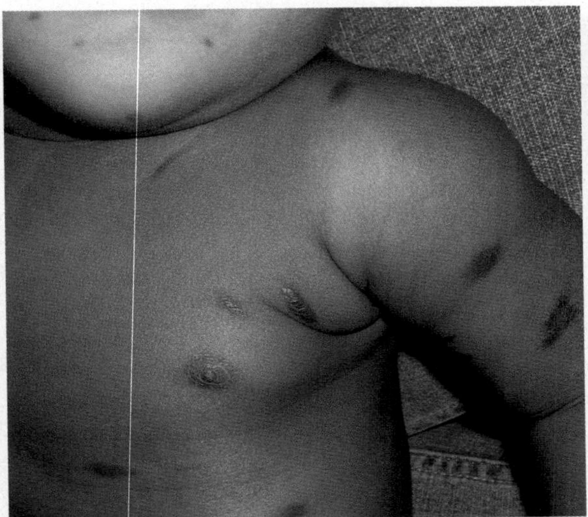

FIGURE 156-8 Urticaria pigmentosa in a 4-month-old black boy. His lesions started on day 2 of life and have proliferated. (*Reproduced with permission from Richard P. Usatine, MD.*)

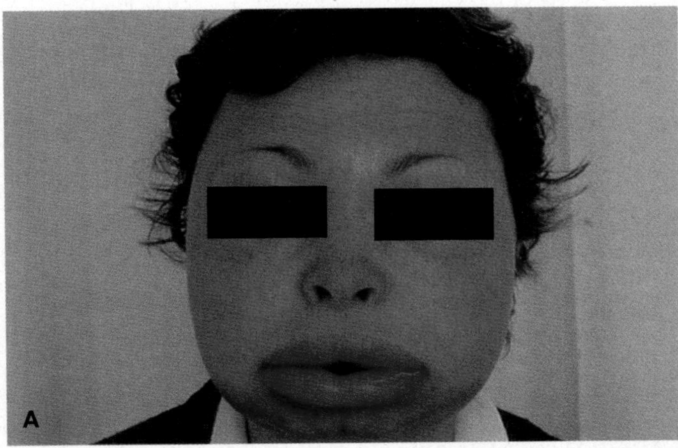

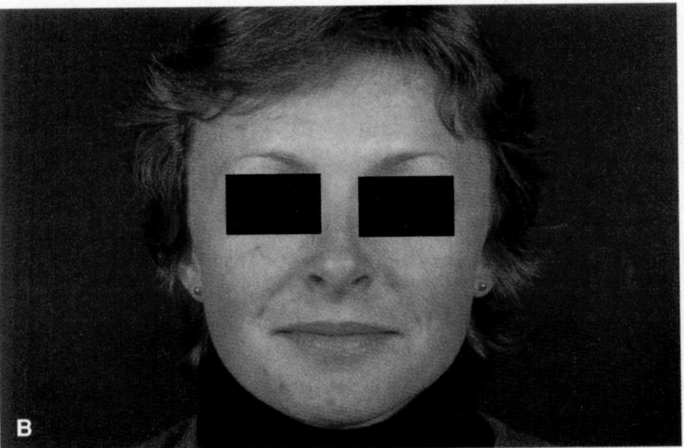

FIGURE 156-9 Hereditary angioedema. **A.** Severe edema of the face during an episode, leading to grotesque disfigurement. **B.** Angioedema will subside within hours. The patient had a positive family history and had multiple similar episodes including colicky abdominal pain. (*Reproduced with permission from Wolff K, Johnson R, Suurmond R: Fitzpatrick's Color Atlas and Synopsis of Clinical Dermatology, 5th ed. New York, NY: McGraw-Hill Education; 2005.*)

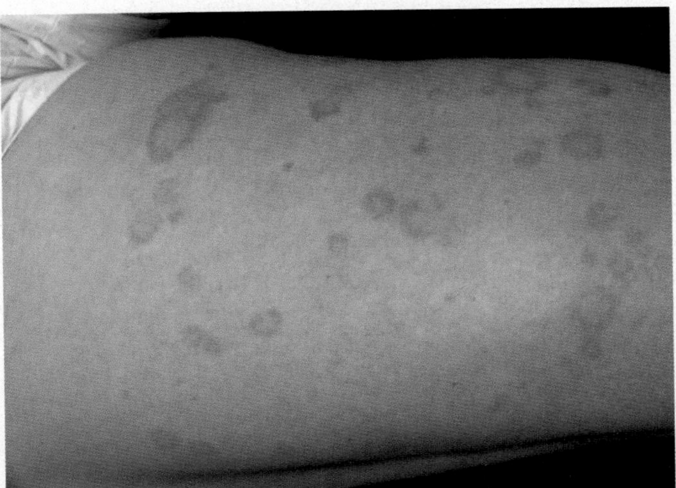

FIGURE 156-10 Chronic urticaria with annular urticarial plaques. (*Reproduced with permission from Wolff K, Johnson R, Suurmond R: Fitzpatrick's Color Atlas and Synopsis of Clinical Dermatology, 5th ed. New York, NY: McGraw-Hill Education; 2005.*)

- If you suspect urticaria pigmentosa, stroke a lesion with the wooden end of a cotton-tipped applicator. This induces erythema of the plaque, and the wheal is confined to the stroke site. This is called Darier sign (**Figure 156-12**).

TYPICAL DISTRIBUTION

- Angioedema is seen more often on the face and is especially common around the mouth and eyes (see **Figures 156-3** and **156-4**). Sometimes angioedema can occur on the genitals or the trunk (**Figure 156-13**).
- Urticaria can be found anywhere on the body and is often on the trunk and extremities (see **Figures 156-1** and **156-2**).

LABORATORY STUDIES

Urticaria can be diagnosed by clinical presentation. Extensive laboratory work-up without clinical suspicion of underlying cause is unnecessary. Consider tests that might help reveal the underlying cause of the urticaria and/or angioedema.

- In chronic urticaria, consider complete blood count (CBC) with differential, erythrocyte sedimentation rate (ESR) and/or C-reactive protein (CRP), liver enzymes, and thyroid-stimulating hormone (TSH) to investigate for underlying causes.
- Thyroid antibodies should be considered in those who develop chronic urticaria, especially in cases with suspected autoimmune etiology.[6]
- Punch biopsy of the involved area may be used to diagnose urticarial vasculitis or mastocytosis.
- Order complement studies (C4, C1, and C1 inhibitor levels) to investigate for hereditary or acquired C1 esterase inhibitor deficiency when angioedema occurs repeatedly without urticaria (see **Figure 156-9**).
- Allergen skin testing is not recommended for routine evaluation of chronic idiopathic urticaria.[7] SOR Ⓑ

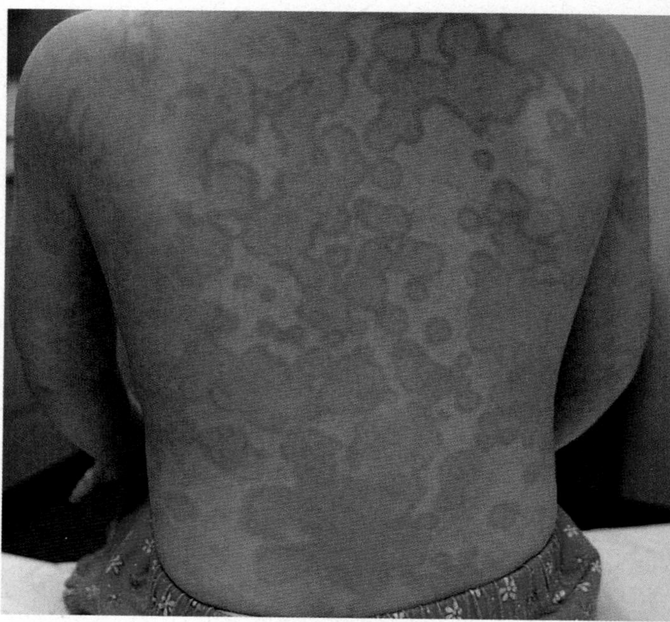

FIGURE 156-11 Giant urticaria (urticaria multiforme). Although this appears to have targets, the real target lesions of erythema multiforme have a central lesion and have a scaling or bullous component affecting the epidermis. The history suggests that this may have been a serum sickness type reaction. (*Reproduced with permission from Milgrom EC, Usatine RP, Tan RA, et al: Practical Allergy. Philadelphia, PA: Elsevier; 2003. Photo contributor: Daniel Stulberg, MD.*)

DIFFERENTIAL DIAGNOSIS

- Insect bites—A good history and physical examination should help to distinguish between insect bites and urticaria.
- Erythema multiforme, like urticaria, can occur in response to an allergic/immunologic reaction to medications, infections, and neoplasms. The classic lesion of erythema multiforme is the target lesion, in which there is disruption of the epithelium in the center. This disruption may be a vesicle, bulla, or erosion. Do not confuse annular lesions or concentric rings with erythema multiforme if the epidermis is intact (**Figure 156-11** is *not* erythema multiforme) (see Chapter 185, Erythema Multiforme, Stevens-Johnson Syndrome, and Toxic Epidermal Necrolysis).
- Urticarial vasculitis typically has lesions that last longer than 24 hours. The lesions are found more commonly on the lower extremities, and when they heal, they often leave hyperpigmented areas. Causes range from a hypersensitivity vasculitis, such as Henoch-Schönlein purpura, to underlying connective tissue disease (**Figure 156-14**).[3]

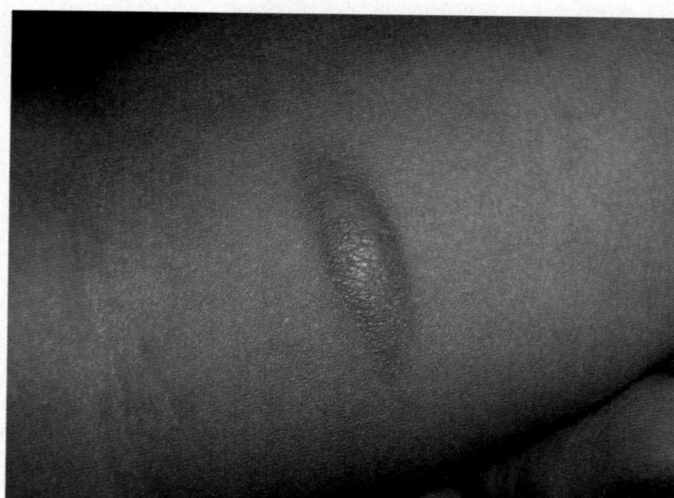

FIGURE 156-12 Positive Darier sign in which stroking the lesion of urticaria pigmentosum results in edema. (*Reproduced with permission from Richard P. Usatine, MD.*)

- Mast cell releasability syndromes are syndromes in which there are too many mast cells in the skin or other organs of the body. These include cutaneous mastocytosis and urticaria pigmentosa (see **Figures 156-5**, **156-6**, and **156-11**).
- Pruritic urticarial papules and plaques of pregnancy can be differentiated from urticaria in pregnancy because the eruption remains fixed and increases in intensity until delivery (**Figure 156-15**) (see Chapter 77, Pruritic Urticarial Papules and Plaques of Pregnancy).
- Pemphigoid gestationis can have lesions that are urticarial. However, it also has bullae that distinguish it from urticaria, and of course the patient is pregnant or postpartum (see Chapter 78, Pemphigoid Gestationis).

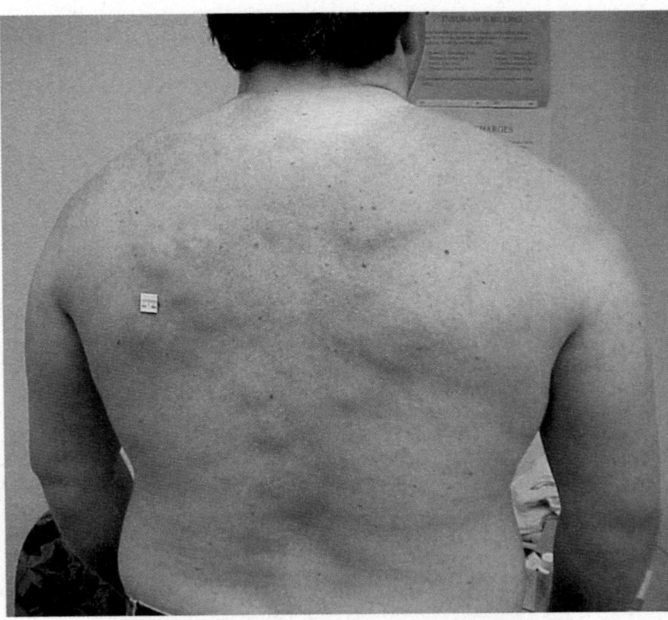

FIGURE 156-13 Angioedema and urticaria of the back. The thicker, deeper wheals are angioedema. (*Reproduced with permission from Milgrom EC,Usatine RP, Tan RA, et al: Practical Allergy. Philadelphia, PA: Elsevier; 2003. Photo contributor: Daniel Stulberg, MD.*)

MANAGEMENT

ACUTE URTICARIA

- Nonpharmacologic therapy:
  - The first step in evaluation of acute urticaria is to rule out anaphylaxis by conducting a thorough cardiovascular and pulmonary exam.
  - Avoid any known causative agent, medication, stimulus, or antigen. SOR Ⓑ
- Pharmacologic therapy:
  - Second-generation H_1 antihistamines are the first-line therapy for acute urticaria. SOR Ⓑ The dosage can be increased up to four times the normal amount to achieve symptom control.[8]
  - If control is not achieved with H_1 antihistamines, H_2 antihistamines may be added.
  - In severe acute angioedema a 3- to 10-day course of oral corticosteroids may be prescribed.[8]

CHRONIC URTICARIA

Table 156-1 is a stepwise approach to therapy.

- Nonpharmacologic therapy:
  - Avoid any known causative agent, medication, stimulus, or antigen. SOR Ⓑ
  - Patients may benefit from avoidance of potential urticarial precipitants such as aspirin, NSAIDs (**Figure 156-16**), opiates, and alcohol.[2] SOR Ⓑ
  - Infections may be a cause, an aggravating factor, or an unassociated bystander.[2] Look for sources of chronic infections such as parasitic infections, dental infections, GI infections, respiratory infections, and tinea pedis. Consider treatment of these infections, as it is possible, though unproven, that they may contribute to the chronic urticaria. SOR Ⓒ
  - Stop all unnecessary medications, supplements, and vitamins. SOR Ⓒ
  - Avoidance of physical stimuli for the treatment of physical urticaria is desirable, but not always possible (observational studies only).[2] SOR Ⓑ
  - Stress reduction techniques may help in chronic urticaria, but this is unproven. SOR Ⓒ
  - Phototherapy is sometimes helpful for pruritus, although it does not improve whealing.[4] SOR Ⓒ

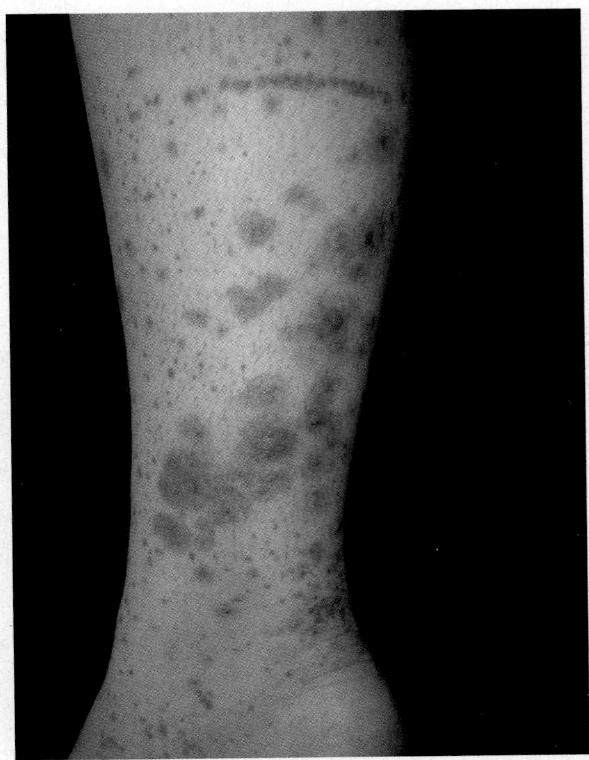

FIGURE 156-14 Henoch-Schönlein purpura on the leg of a 20-year-old woman. This is a type of urticarial vasculitis. (*Reproduced with permission from Milgrom EC, Usatine RP, Tan RA, et al: Practical Allergy. Philadelphia, PA: Elsevier; 2003. Photo contributor: Richard P. Usatine, MD.*)

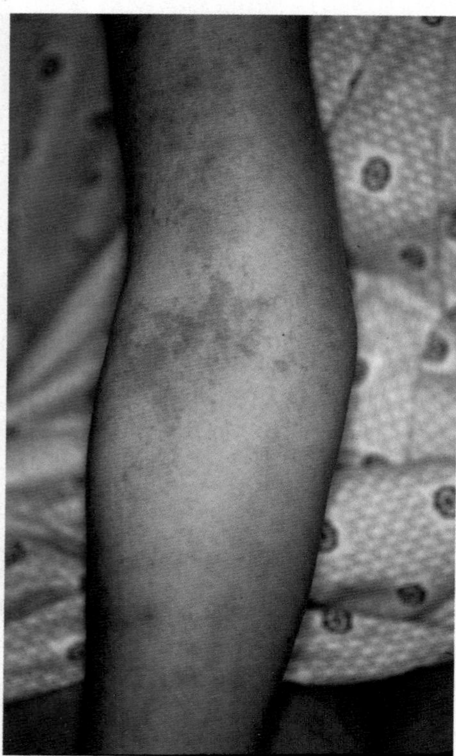

FIGURE 156-15 Pruritic urticarial papules and plaques of pregnancy on the arm of a pregnant woman. The wheals are indistinguishable from other types of urticaria. (*Reproduced with permission from Milgrom EC, Usatine RP, Tan RA, et al: Practical Allergy. Philadelphia, PA: Elsevier; 2003. Photo contributor: Richard P. Usatine, MD.*)

TABLE 156-1 Stepwise Management of Chronic Urticaria

STEP 1

Avoid possible allergic triggers
Start second-generation H_1 antihistamine
(cetirizine or loratadine 10 mg once to twice daily)
Increase cetirizine or loratadine up to 20 mg twice daily

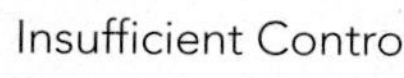

STEP 2

Add a first-generation antihistamine at night
(hydroxyzine or diphenhydramine)
Add an H_2 antihistamine such as ranitidine 150 mg bid
Try a different second-generation H_1 antihistamine

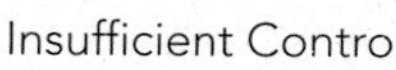

STEP 3

Add a leukotriene receptor antagonist (montelukast)
Add a high-potency antihistamine (doxepin before bed)
Add a short course of low-dose oral steroids (0.5 to 1 mg prednisone for 3–10 days) if symptoms are severe

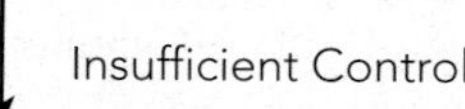

STEP 4

Refer for immunomodulatory therapy
(e.g., cyclosporine, omalizumab)

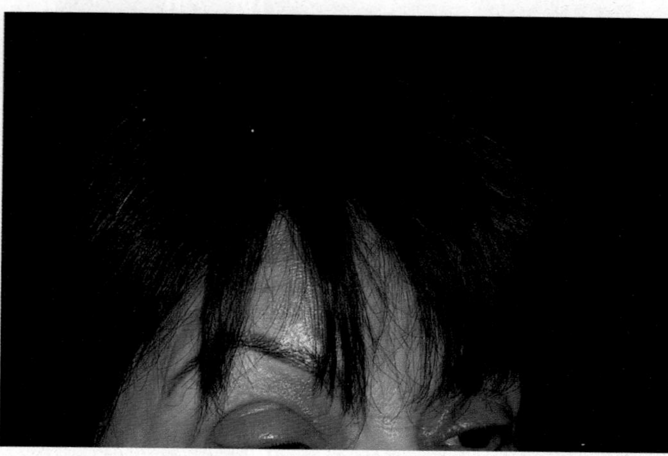

FIGURE 156-16 Urticaria that occurred within an hour after a boy was given ibuprofen to treat a high fever. (*Reproduced with permission from Richard P. Usatine, MD.*)

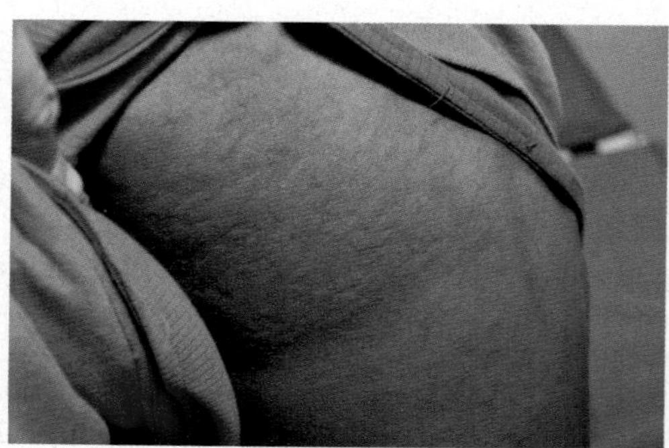

FIGURE 156-17 Angioedema secondary to an angiotensin receptor blocker given for hypertension. The angioedema resolved and did not return once the patient stopped the offending medication. (*Reproduced with permission from Richard P. Usatine, MD.*)

FIRST LINE

- Second-generation H_1 antihistamines (cetirizine, loratadine) should be prescribed as first-line treatment for chronic urticaria.[5,7] SOR Ⓐ
- Increasing the dose of H_1 antihistamines is often helpful in severe cases of chronic urticaria.[4] Increasing the dose of cetirizine from 10 mg to 20 mg daily produced a significant improvement in the severity of wheal and itching in urticaria refractory to the standard doses of antihistamines.[9] SOR Ⓑ
- The British guidelines suggest using second-generation antihistamines at up to quadruple the manufacturers' recommended dosages (e.g., cetirizine 20 mg bid) before changing to an alternative therapy. They also recommend waiting up to 4 weeks to allow full effectiveness of the antihistamines before considering referral to a specialist.[2] SOR Ⓒ
- Second-generation antihistamines seem to be effective in the treatment of acquired cold urticaria by significantly reducing the presence of wheals and pruritus after cold exposure.[4] SOR Ⓐ
- Topical antipruritic emollients such as calamine lotion or 1% menthol cream are helpful for symptomatic relief.[4] SOR Ⓐ
- The addition of an H_2 antagonist may give better control of urticaria than H_1 antagonists alone, although a benefit is not always seen.[4] In one study, adding H_2 blockers to H_1 antagonists resulted in improvement of certain cutaneous outcomes for patients presenting with acute allergic syndromes to an emergency department.[10] SOR Ⓑ

SECOND LINE

- Oral corticosteroids should be restricted to short courses for severe acute urticaria or angioedema affecting the mouth (e.g., prednisone 60 mg/day for 3 to 4 days in adults).[4,11] SOR Ⓑ
- Long-term oral corticosteroids should not be used in chronic urticaria. It is better to use oral cyclosporine if needed, as it has a far better risk-to-benefit ratio compared with steroids.[2,4]
- When initial antihistamines are not working, consider doxepin, an antidepressant and potent H_1 antagonist.[12] SOR Ⓑ Its use is limited by the side effects of sedation and dry mouth. Start with 10 mg doxepin in the evening and titrate up as needed and tolerated.
- Nifedipine has been shown effectively reduce pruritus in some cases of chronic urticaria.[4] SOR Ⓒ
- The evidence for leukotriene modifiers in the treatment of chronic idiopathic urticaria is poor, although some studies have demonstrated their efficacy in chronic urticaria associated with aspirin, food additives, or autoreactivity to intradermal serum injection.[13] SOR Ⓒ
- Anti-IgE Antibody (omalizumab) was licensed in 2014 for the treatment of antihistamine-refractory chronic idiopathic urticaria. It has been shown to reduce symptom severity most effectively at a dose of 300 mg as a subcutaneous monthly injection.[14] SOR Ⓑ As there is a risk of anaphylaxis, this new high-cost medication needs to be given by a specialist (often allergist) with experience in its administration.
- Anti-inflammatory drugs, such as colchicine, dapsone, and sulfasalazine, have been reported as helpful in uncontrolled trials or case series.[2] SOR Ⓒ
- Short tapering courses of oral steroids over 3 to 4 weeks may be necessary for severe delayed pressure urticaria.
- Immunosuppressive therapies for autoimmune urticaria should be restricted to patients with disabling disease who have not responded to optimal conventional treatments.[7]
- A retrospective study of methotrexate in 8 patients with recalcitrant chronic urticaria indicated that methotrexate was both safe and effective, with a mean dose of 15 mg methotrexate/week. Seven of eight patients achieved a complete response, and five of eight remained disease-free after methotrexate was stopped.[15] SOR Ⓑ
- Cyclosporine, plasmapheresis, and intravenous immunoglobulin have been used in severe recalcitrant cases.[2] SOR Ⓒ
- Thyroxine treatment in euthyroid patients with antithyroid antibodies has been found to occasionally result in improvement of symptoms.[4] SOR Ⓒ
- A randomized controlled trial showed that clobetasol 0.05% in a foam formulation was safe and effective in the short-term treatment of patients with delayed pressure urticaria.[16] SOR Ⓑ

ANGIOEDEMA

FIRST LINE

- Epinephrine is valuable in severe acute angioedema, especially if there is a suspicion of airway compromise or anaphylaxis. Immediate airway assessment and early intubation are recommended in cases of laryngeal swelling. SOR Ⓒ Patients with history of airway compromise should be prescribed epinephrine autoinjectors.[8]
- Epinephrine is not helpful for patients with C1 inhibitor deficiency.[3]
- Corticosteroids and antihistamines are used to control symptom severity in acute idiopathic angioedema.[8] SOR Ⓑ
- Angiotensin-converting enzyme inhibitors (ACEIs) are especially prone to causing angioedema so should be stopped as soon as possible when suspected to be the cause of angioedema or urticaria (see **Figure 156-3**).[2] SOR Ⓐ Even an angiotensin receptor blocker (ARB) can cause angioedema and should be suspected in a patient on this class of medication (see **Figure 156-17**).

SECOND LINE

- The medications for hereditary angioedema require referral to an allergist. These medications are very costly and beyond the scope of primary care.

REFERRAL OR HOSPITALIZATION

- Acute urticaria and/or angioedema may present with respiratory distress and shock as part of an anaphylactic reaction. These patients should be treated immediately with epinephrine and be transported to the hospital with a call to 9-1-1 if they are in your office.
- Chronic urticaria and/or chronic angioedema may be very complex to work up and treat, so that a referral to an allergist or dermatologist is a very appropriate consideration. Many of the new medications available to treat these conditions are extraordinarily costly and beyond the scope of primary care.

PATIENT EDUCATION

In most cases, the cause of chronic urticaria will remain unknown. Fortunately, most chronic urticaria will subside over time, and there are medicines to treat the condition until it runs its course. If one medication doesn't work, schedule follow-up visits to try other medications. Carefully observe for causative agents.

FOLLOW-UP

Follow-up is especially needed when the urticaria/angioedema persists or recurs.

PATIENT RESOURCES

- eMedicineHealth.com is a consumer health site with information and support groups—**http://www.emedicinehealth.com/hives_and_angioedema/article_em.htm.**

PROVIDER RESOURCES

- Practice parameters by various allergy specialty groups:
- Bernstein J, Lang D, Khan D. The Diagnosis and Management of Acute and Chronic Urticaria: 2014 Update. *J Allergy Clin Immunol.* 2015;133(5):1270-1277.—**http://www.jacionline.org/article/S0091-6749(14)00335-2/fulltext.**
- Acute and Chronic Urticaria: Evaluation and Treatment. Published in the *American Family Physician*—**http://www.aafp.org/afp/2017/0601/p717.html.**

REFERENCES

1. Bolognia JL, Jorizzo JL, Shaffer JV. Urticaria and angioedema. In: Grattan CEH, ed. *Dermatology*. 3rd ed. Philadelphia, PA: Elsevier Saunders; 2014.
2. Zuberbier T, Asero R, Bindslev-Jensen C, et al. EAACI/GA(2) LEN/EDF/WAO guideline: management of urticaria. *Allergy.* 2009;64:1427-1443.
3. Baxi S, Dinakar C. Urticaria and angioedema. *Immunol Allergy Clin North Am.* 2005;25:353-367, vii.
4. Usatine RP. Urticaria and angioedema. In: Milgrom E, Usatine RP, Tan R, Spector S, eds. *Practical Allergy*. Philadelphia, PA: Elsevier; 2003:78-96.
5. Grattan C, Powell S, Humphreys F. Management and diagnostic guidelines for urticaria and angio-oedema. *Br J Dermatol.* 2007; 157:1116-1123.
6. Kolkhir P, Metz M, Altrichter S, Maurer M. Comorbidity of chronic spontaneous urticaria and autoimmune thyroid diseases: a systematic review. *Allergy.* 2017;72(10):1440-1460.
7. Ortonne JP. Chronic urticaria: a comparison of management guidelines. *Expert Opin Pharmacother.* 2011;12(17):2683-2693.
8. Schaefer, P. Acute and chronic urticaria: evaluation and treatment. *Am Fam Physician.* 2017;95(11):717-724.
9. Okubo Y, Shigoka Y, Yamazaki M, Tsuboi R. Double dose of cetirizine hydrochloride is effective for patients with urticaria resistant: a prospective, randomized, non-blinded, comparative clinical study and assessment of quality of life. *J Dermatolog Treat.* 2013;24(2):153-160.
10. Lin RY, Curry A, Pesola GR, et al. Improved outcomes in patients with acute allergic syndromes who are treated with combined H1 and H2 antagonists. *Ann Emerg Med.* 2000;36:462-468.
11. Pollack CV Jr, Romano TJ. Outpatient management of acute urticaria: the role of prednisone. *Ann Emerg Med.* 1995;26: 547-551.
12. Goldsobel AB, Rohr AS, Siegel SC, et al. Efficacy of doxepin in the treatment of chronic idiopathic urticaria. *J Allergy Clin Immunol.* 1986;78:867-873.
13. Gabriele Di L, Alberto D, Manfredi R, et al. Leukotriene receptor antagonists in monotherapy or in combination with antihistamines in the treatment of chronic urticaria: a systematic review. *J Asthma Allergy, Vol 2009, Iss Default, Pp9-16 (2008),* (default), 9.
14. Zhao ZT, Ji CM, Yu WJ, Meng L, Hawro T, Wei JF, Maurer M. Omalizumab for the treatment of chronic Spontaneous Urticaria: A Meta-Analysis of Randomized Clinical Trials. *J Allergy Clin Immunol.* 2016 Jun;137 (6):1742-1750.
15. Sagi L, Solomon M, Baum S, et al. Evidence for methotrexate as a useful treatment for steroid-dependent chronic urticaria. *Acta Derm Venereol.* 2011;91:303-306.
16. Vena GA, Cassano N, D'Argento V, Milani M. Clobetasol propionate 0.05% in a novel foam formulation is safe and effective in the short-term treatment of patients with delayed pressure urticaria: a randomized, double-blind, placebo-controlled trial. *Br J Dermatol.* 2006;154:353-356.

SECTION I PAPULOSQUAMOUS CONDITIONS

157 SEBORRHEIC DERMATITIS

Edward Bae, MD
Meredith M. Hancock, MD
Yoon-Soo Cindy Bae, MD
Richard P. Usatine, MD

PATIENT STORY

A 59-year-old man presents with a 3-month history of an itchy rash on his face (**Figures 157-1** and **157-2**). He states that he has had this rash intermittently for many years, but that it had recently worsened. He denies any major risk factors for HIV and does not have Parkinson disease. He has been under more stress lately and has noticed that this exacerbates his rash. There was scale visible on the forehead, under the eyebrows, and in the beard. There is also some mild erythema on the cheeks and around the nasolabial folds. The diagnosis of seborrheic dermatitis was made and treatment began with appropriate topical agents to treat the inflammation and the *Malassezia*. On the following visit, the patient had complete clearance of his seborrheic dermatitis.

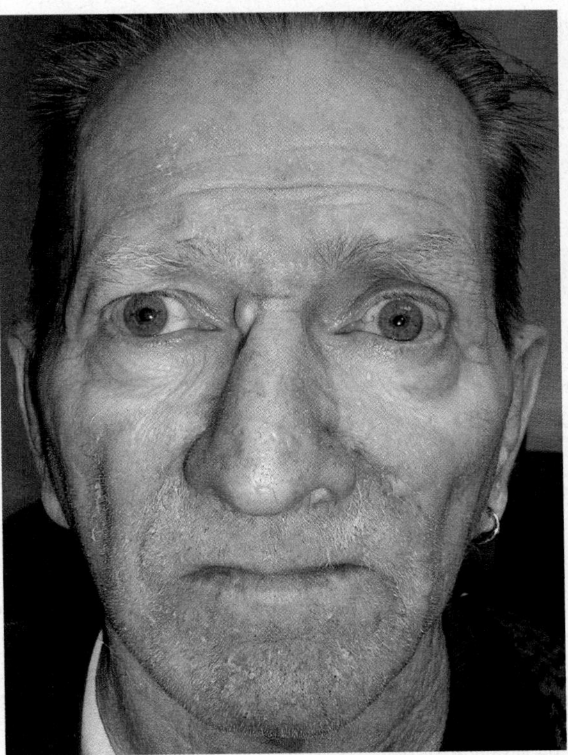

FIGURE 157-1 Seborrheic dermatitis following the typical distribution on the face of a 59-year-old man. Note the prominent scale and erythema on his forehead, glabella, and beard region. *(Reproduced with permission from Richard P. Usatine, MD.)*

INTRODUCTION

Seborrheic dermatitis is a common, chronic, relapsing dermatitis affecting sebum-rich areas of the body. Presentation may vary from mild erythema to greasy scale to, rarely, erythroderma. Treatment goals include reducing inflammation and irritation.

SYNONYMS

Seborrhea, seborrheic eczema, dandruff, and cradle cap.

EPIDEMIOLOGY

- Seborrheic dermatitis is most commonly seen in male patients between the ages of 20 to 50 years, though it can affect women, infants, and the elderly as well.
- The prevalence is approximately 3% to 5% in healthy young adults who are HIV-negative.[1] The statistics may be underrepresented, as many do not seek medical attention for mild cases.
- The prevalence is higher in immunocompromised persons (e.g., HIV-positive/AIDS); however, the vast majority of affected persons have a normal immune system.
- More common in persons with underlying neurologic disease including Parkinson disease and tardive dyskinesia.[2]

ETIOLOGY AND PATHOPHYSIOLOGY

- The actual cause of seborrheic dermatitis is not well understood. It appears to be related to the interplay between host factors including hormonal expression, environmental factors, and local immune response to antigens.[2-5]
- Patients with seborrheic dermatitis may be colonized with certain species of lipophilic yeast of the genus *Malassezia* (also called *Pityrosporum)*. However, *Malassezia* is considered normal skin flora, as it is also found in unaffected persons.
- Some evidence suggests that *Malassezia* may produce different irritants or metabolites on affected skin.[5]
- Genomic analyses of the *Malassezia* genus has revealed genetic sequences for lipases and phospholipases, which could be involved in compromising the barrier function of the skin.[2,3]
- It is postulated that an overgrowth of *Malassezia* leads to the inflammatory dermatitis in seborrhea.

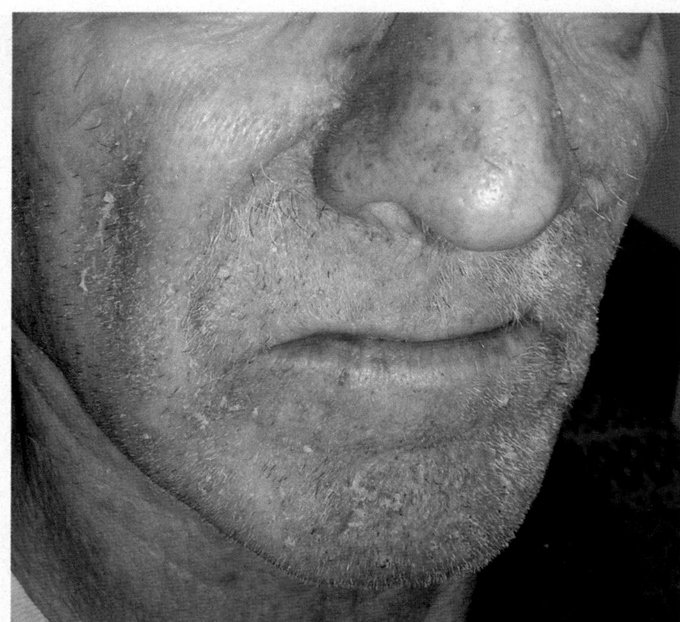

FIGURE 157-2 Close-up of seborrheic dermatitis showing the flaking scale and erythema around the beard region. (*Reproduced with permission from Richard P. Usatine, MD.*)

RISK FACTORS

- Male gender.
- Immunocompromised state (HIV/AIDS).
- Neurologic diseases such as Parkinson disease.
- Stress.
- Environmental factors (cold, dry weather).
- Certain medications, including captopril, cimetidine, interleukin-2, isotretinoin, nicotine, and psoralens, may cause seborrheic dermatitis to flare.[6-10]

DIAGNOSIS

The clinical diagnosis is made by history and physical examination. Biopsy is not generally indicated unless ruling out other possibilities (see Differential Diagnosis below).

CLINICAL FEATURES

- Chronic skin condition characterized by remissions and exacerbations.
- Poorly demarcated, erythematous plaques of greasy, yellow scale (**Figure 157-3**) in the characteristic seborrheic distribution (see description below) that can be very pruritic.
- Common precipitating factors are stress, immunosuppression, and cold weather.
- May be the presenting sign of HIV seropositivity.
- In dark-skinned individuals, the involved skin and scale may become hyperpigmented (**Figure 157-4**).

TYPICAL DISTRIBUTION

In adults, the scalp (i.e., dandruff), eyebrows (**Figures 157-5** and **157-6**), nasolabial creases, forehead, cheeks, around the nose, behind the ears (**Figure 157-7**), external auditory meatus, and under facial hair for men (**Figure 157-8**) are common areas affected. Seborrheic dermatitis

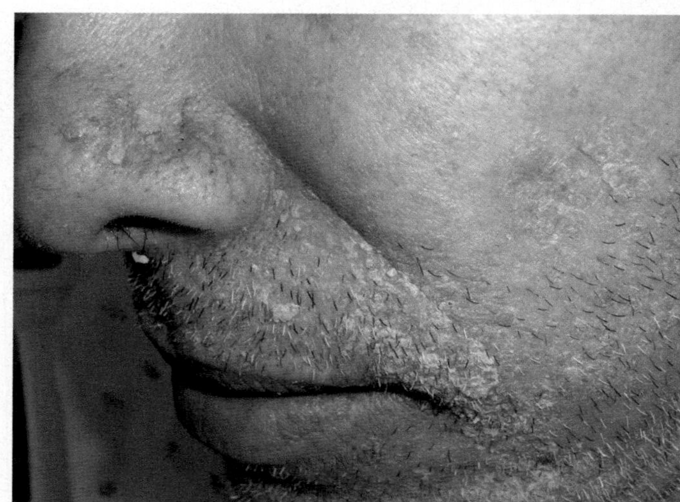

FIGURE 157-3 Severe seborrheic dermatitis on the face of a hospitalized man. The stress of his illness has worsened his otherwise mild seborrhea. (*Reproduced with permission from Richard P. Usatine, MD.*)

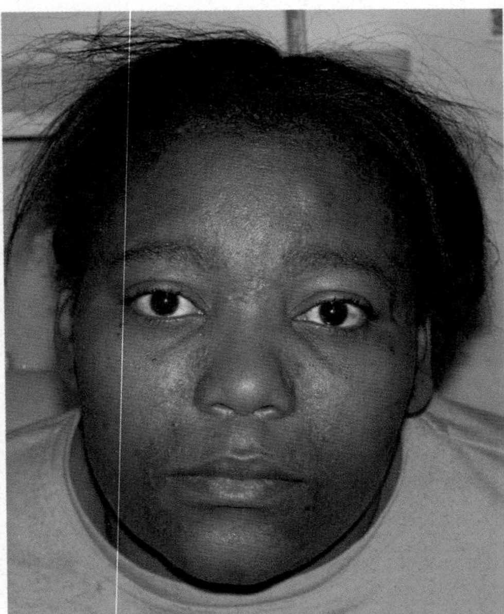

FIGURE 157-4 Seborrhea in a black woman with hyperpigmentation related to the inflammation. Note the prominent involvement in the nasolabial folds. (*Reproduced with permission from Richard P. Usatine, MD.*)

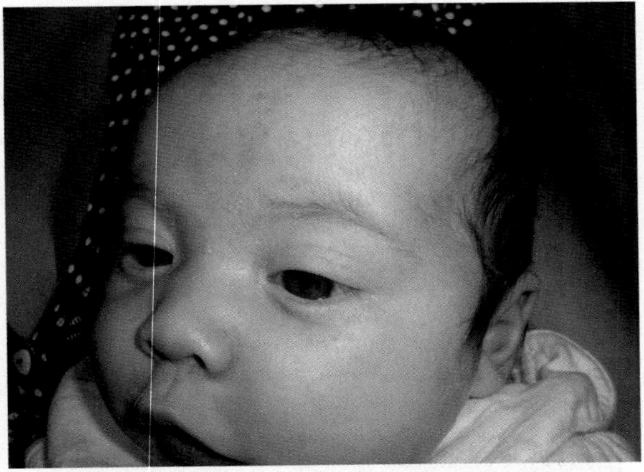

FIGURE 157-5 Mild seborrheic dermatitis with subtle flaking around the eyebrows of a 2-month-old girl who also has cradle cap. (*Reproduced with permission from Richard P. Usatine, MD.*)

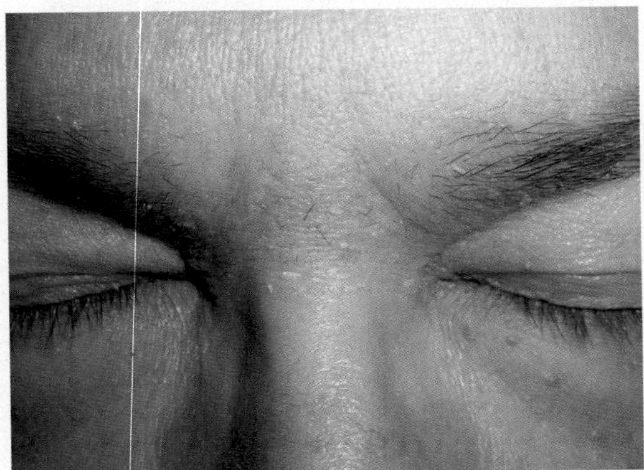

FIGURE 157-6 Seborrheic dermatitis with erythema and scale under the eyebrows and in the glabella region on a young man. (*Reproduced with permission from Richard P. Usatine, MD.*)

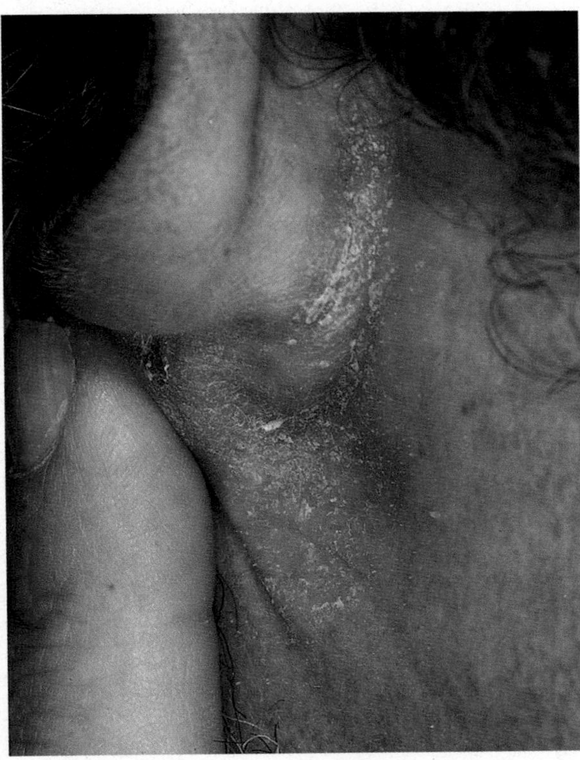

FIGURE 157-7 Seborrheic dermatitis behind the ear in a young woman. This is a good place to look for evidence of seborrhea. (*Reproduced with permission from Richard P. Usatine, MD.*)

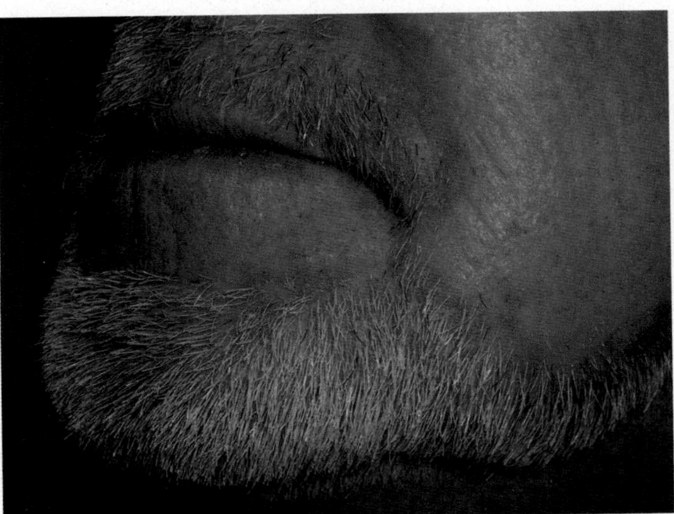

FIGURE 157-8 Seborrhea of the beard and mustache distribution with prominent erythema. (*Reproduced with permission from Richard P. Usatine, MD.*)

can also occur over the sternum and in the axillae, inframammary folds, umbilicus, groin, and gluteal cleft.

- Infants may develop scale on the scalp, known as "cradle cap" (**Figure 157-9**). The eyebrows may also be affected (**Figure 157-5**). In addition to the areas that affect adults, infants can have involvement of the diaper area. Some infants have a wider distribution involving the neck creases, armpits, or groin.

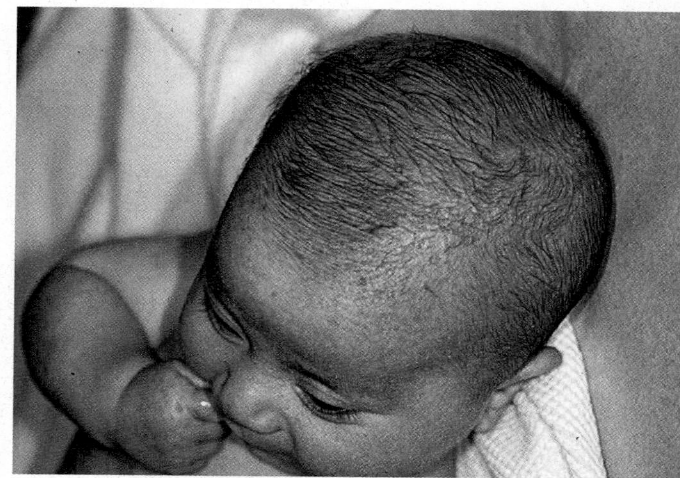

FIGURE 157-9 Cradle cap in an infant who also has atopic dermatitis. *(Reproduced with permission from Richard P. Usatine, MD.)*

LABORATORY STUDIES

- Test for HIV and/or syphilis if patient has risk factors (**Figures 157-10** and **157-11**).
- Consider KOH preparation of the scale to rule out a true dermatophyte.
- Consider zinc level or alkaline phosphatase (low) to rule out nutritional/zinc deficiency.

DIFFERENTIAL DIAGNOSIS[11]

- Psoriasis—The plaques on the scalp tend to be thicker and well-demarcated. Look for signs of nail involvement that may support the diagnosis of psoriasis (see Chapter 158, Psoriasis).
- Sebopsoriasis—A diagnosis sometimes given when the scalp has features of both psoriasis and seborrhea. A biopsy can sometimes distinguish between them. However, treatments with topical steroids and various shampoos can work for this entity and each of the distinct diagnoses.
- Systemic lupus erythematosus (SLE) with butterfly rash—Rash across nasal bridge with associated systemic symptoms and abnormal blood tests (see Chapter 188, Lupus—Systemic and Cutaneous).
- Rosacea—The erythema on the face is often associated with papules, pustules, telangiectasia, and an absence of scales. May also present with eye involvement (see Chapter 119, Rosacea).
- Tinea capitis—Scale and erythema commonly with associated hair loss. More often in children but can rarely be seen in adults. KOH and/or culture can help make the distinction (see Chapter 143, Tinea Capitis).
- Secondary syphilis—Skin presentation may rarely mimic seborrheic dermatitis. Examine patient for mucosal or palmar involvement. Lab testing for syphilis may be necessary.
- Periorificial dermatitis—Usually restricted to skin around the mouth, nose, and eyes with papules, pustules, and minimal to no scale.
- Tinea versicolor—The scale of tinea versicolor tends to be fine with a white color. In addition, the scale is less adherent when scraping. It is related to the same as *Malassezia* furfur but is seen on the trunk, neck and upper arms with a cape-like distribution. Seborrheic dermatitis is usually in the suprasternal region when below the neck.
- Candidiasis—May be found in intertriginous areas, but often presents as bright red rash with satellite lesions.
- Erythrasma—Usually manifests in between the toes, groin, and axillae with brown-colored scale and has a coral red fluorescence with an ultraviolet light.

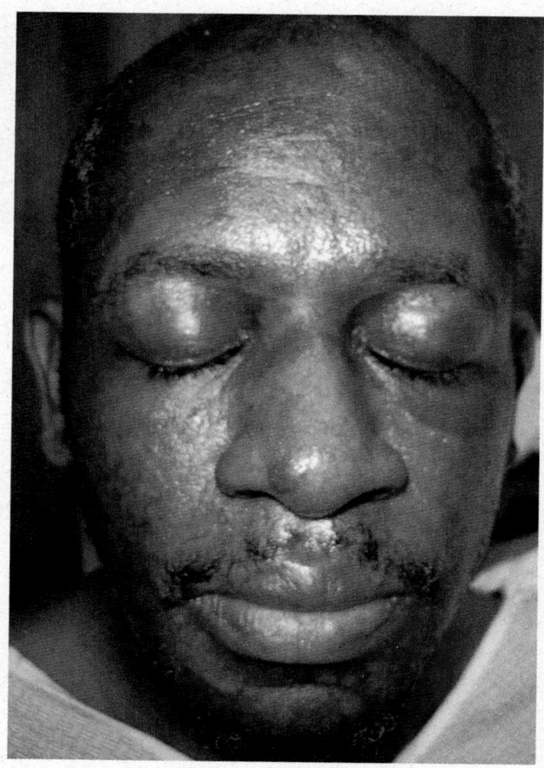

FIGURE 157-10 Seborrheic dermatitis on the face of a man with acquired immune deficiency syndrome. Note the involvement of the forehead, cheeks, and chin causing hypopigmentation and scaling. *(Reproduced with permission from Yoon-Soo Cindy Bae-Harboe, MD.)*

- Impetigo—Lesions are caused by bacterial infection (*Staphylococcus* and/or *Streptococcus*) and begin as fragile vesicles that ooze fluid, eventually turning into yellow-brown crusts.
- Lichen simplex chronicus—This condition is more common in adults and is the result of persistent scratching leading to lichenification of the skin. When this is seen on the posterior neck hairline, it could be confused with seborrhea of the scalp. However, it is more well-demarcated and the plaques are thicker.
- Pityriasis rosea—Onset usually begins with a herald patch with subsequent lesions sometimes in a "Christmas tree" pattern of distribution on the trunk and proximal extremities. The lesions should show a collarette scale.
- Nutritional deficiency (e.g., zinc, vitamin A)—May present with facial lesions and acral rash.

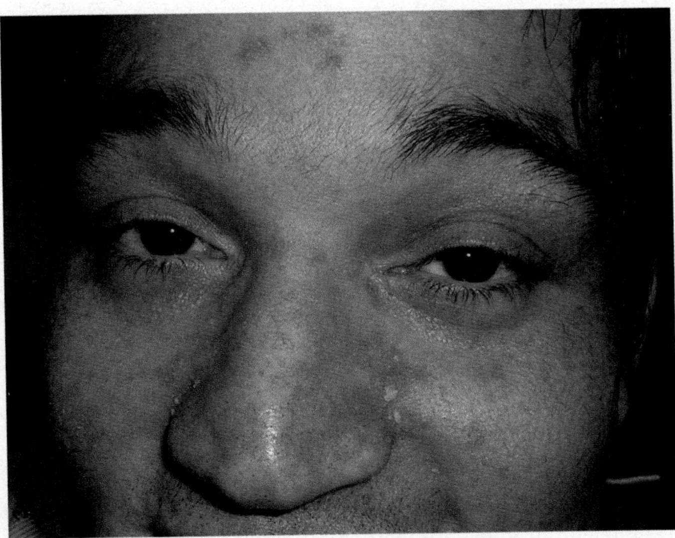

FIGURE 157-11 Seborrheic dermatitis on the face of a man with acquired immune deficiency syndrome. Note erythema and scale on the forehead, nose, and cheeks. (*Reproduced with permission from Richard P. Usatine, MD.*)

MANAGEMENT

FIRST LINE

As seborrheic dermatitis is a recurrent, chronic condition, repeated and/or maintenance therapy is often required. The goal of treatment is to diminish the fungal overgrowth and to treat the inflammatory response. The mainstay of treatment is ongoing topical antifungals in shampoos and other preparations, along with a topical steroid at first to treat the inflammation.

- For seborrheic dermatitis of the scalp, patients should wash their hair with antifungal shampoos (containing selenium sulfide, ketoconazole, zinc pyrithione [ZPT] or ciclopirox) daily or at least several times per week, each time leaving the lather on the affected areas for several minutes; this should be repeated until remission is attained. Patients should continue to use antifungal shampoo as maintenance therapy.[4]
- Shampoos containing ketoconazole, selenium sulfide, or ZPT are active against *Malassezia* and are effective in the treatment of moderate to severe dandruff.[12,13] SOR Ⓐ
- Ketoconazole 2% shampoo was found to be superior to ZPT 1% shampoo when used twice weekly. Ketoconazole led to a 73% improvement in the total dandruff severity score compared with 67% for ZPT 1% at 4 weeks.[13] SOR Ⓑ
- Ciclopirox shampoo 1% is effective and safe in the treatment of seborrheic dermatitis of the scalp.[14,15] SOR Ⓐ
- Ketoconazole 2% cream, gel, or emulsion is safe and effective for facial seborrheic dermatitis.[16-18] SOR Ⓑ
- Ciclopirox 1% cream is also safe and effective for facial seborrheic dermatitis and is equivalent to ketoconazole 2% cream.[16,19] SOR Ⓑ
- Topical corticosteroids are useful in treating erythema and pruritus associated with the condition.[4] However, long-term use may lead to skin atrophy[4] on the face, but less likely on the scalp.
- Lotion or solution is preferable on hair-covered area for patient comfort and usability. Cream is still a viable option and may be more affordable.
- Hydrocortisone 1% cream or lotion can be used twice a day on the face, scalp, and other affected areas.[18,20] SOR Ⓑ

- Desonide 0.05% lotion is safe and effective for short-term treatment of seborrheic dermatitis of the face.[21] SOR B It is a nonfluorinated low- to midpotency steroid that is higher in potency than hydrocortisone 1%.
- For moderate to severe seborrheic dermatitis on the scalp.
  - Fluocinonide 0.05% solution once daily is beneficial. SOR C
  - Clobetasol 0.05% shampoo, solution, spray, or foam works well but is often more costly. SOR C

SECOND LINE

- Oral terbinafine 250 mg daily for 4 weeks is effective for moderate to severe seborrhea.[22,23] SOR A However, because of the potential for harmful side effects of oral antifungals and the limited study of their efficacy, they are not first-line treatments.[4] Oral terbinafine may be considered in erythroderma caused by seborrhea.
- Pimecrolimus cream 1% is an effective and well-tolerated treatment for facial seborrheic dermatitis.[20,24,25] SOR B In one study, there was more burning noted with the pimecrolimus than with the betamethasone 17-valerate 0.1% cream.[24]
- Tacrolimus 0.1% ointment has shown similar efficacy to hydrocortisone 1% cream but required fewer applications for similar results. The adverse effects reported in this study included flushing and irritation at the site of application.[26]
- In another study, use of tacrolimus 0.1% applied 2 times per week (after stabilization was achieved) showed successful remission of the disease over the course of 10 weeks.[27]
- Metronidazole gel has shown variable results in two small studies in the treatment of seborrheic dermatitis of the face. One suggests it works better than the vehicle alone, and the other found no statistically significant difference from placebo.[28,29] SOR B

COMPLEMENTARY AND ALTERNATIVE THERAPY

- Tea tree oil 5% shampoo showed a 41% improvement in the quadrant-area-severity score compared with 11% in the placebo. Statistically significant improvements were also observed in the total area of involvement score, the total severity score, and the itchiness and greasiness components of the patients' self-assessments.[30] SOR B
- One small randomized controlled trial using homeopathic medication consisting of potassium bromide, sodium bromide, nickel sulfate, and sodium chloride for 10 weeks showed significant improvement over placebo.[31] SOR C

FOLLOW-UP

- Patients with long-standing and severe seborrhea will appreciate a follow-up visit in most cases.
- Milder cases can be followed as needed.

PATIENT EDUCATION

For improved treatment results, encourage patients to wash the hair and scalp daily with an antifungal shampoo. Some patients fear that washing their hair too often will cause a "dry" scalp and need to understand that the scaling and flaking will improve rather than worsen with more frequent hair washing.

PATIENT RESOURCES

- PubMed Health. *Seborrheic Dermatitis*—**http://www.ncbi.nlm.nih.gov/pubmedhealth/PMH0001959/.**

PROVIDER RESOURCES

- Medscape. *Seborrheic Dermatitis*—**http://emedicine.medscape.com/article/1108312.**

REFERENCES

1. Usatine RP. A red rash on the face. *J Fam Pract*. 2003;52:697-699.
2. Dessinioti C, Katsambas A. Seborrheic dermatitis: etiology, risk factors, and treatments: facts and controversies. *Clin Dermatol*. 2013;31(4):343-351.
3. Gaitanis G, Magiatis P, Hantschke M, et al. The *Malassezia* genus in skin and systemic diseases. *Clin Microbiol Rev*. 2012;25(1):106-141.
4. Naldi L, Alfredo Rebora A. Seborrheic dermatitis. *N Engl J Med*. 2009;360;4:387-396.
5. Hay RJ. *Malassezia*, dandruff and seborrheic dermatitis: an overview. *Br J Dermatol*. 2011;165(Suppl 2):2-8.
6. Yamamoto T, Tsuboi R. Interleukin-2-induced seborrheic dermatitis-like eruption. *J Eur Acad Dermatol Venereol*. 2008;22(2):244-245.
7. Sudan BJ, Brouillard C, Sterboul J, Sainte-Laudy J. Nicotine as a hapten in seborrheic dermatitis. *Contact Dermatitis*. 1984;11(3):196-197.
8. Kitamura K, Aihara M, Osawa J, et al. Sulfhydryl drug-induced eruption: a clinical and histological study. *J Dermatol*. 1990;17(1):44-51.
9. Tegner E. Seborrheic dermatitis of the face induced by PUVA treatment. *Acta Derm Venereol*. 1983;63(4):335-339.
10. Barzilai A, David M, Trau H, Hodak E. Seborrheic dermatitis-like eruption in patients taking isotretinoin therapy for acne: retrospective study of five patients. *Am J Clin Dermatol*. 2008;9(4):255-261.
11. Clark GW, Pope SM, Jaboori KA. Diagnosis and treatment of seborrheic dermatitis. *Am Fam Physician*. 2015;91(3):185-190.
12. Danby FW, Maddin WS, Margesson LJ, Rosenthal D. A randomized, double-blind, placebo-controlled trial of ketoconazole 2% shampoo versus selenium sulfide 2.5% shampoo in the treatment of moderate to severe dandruff. *J Am Acad Dermatol*. 1993;29:1008-1012.
13. Pierard-Franchimont C. A multicenter randomized trial of ketoconazole 2% and zinc pyrithione 1% shampoos in severe dandruff and seborrheic dermatitis. *Skin Pharmacol Appl Skin Physiol*. 2002;15(6):434-441.
14. Aly R. Ciclopirox gel for seborrheic dermatitis of the scalp. *Int J Dermatol*. 2003;42(Suppl 1):19-22.
15. Lebwohl M, Plott T. Safety and efficacy of ciclopirox 1% shampoo for the treatment of seborrheic dermatitis of the scalp in the US population: results of a double-blind, vehicle-controlled trial. *Int J Dermatol*. 2004;43(Suppl 1):17-20.

16. Chosidow O, Maurette C, Dupuy P. Randomized, open-labeled, non-inferiority study between ciclopiroxolamine 1% cream and ketoconazole 2% foaming gel in mild to moderate facial seborrheic dermatitis. *Dermatology*. 2003;206:233-240.

17. Pierard GE, Pierard-Franchimont C, Van CJ, et al. Ketoconazole 2% emulsion in the treatment of seborrheic dermatitis. *Int J Dermatol*. 1991;30:806-809.

18. Katsambas A, Antoniou C, Frangouli E, et al. A double-blind trial of treatment of seborrheic dermatitis with 2% ketoconazole cream compared with 1% hydrocortisone cream. *Br J Dermatol*. 1989; 121:353-357.

19. Dupuy P, Maurette C, Amoric JC, Chosidow O. Randomized, placebo-controlled, double-blind study on clinical efficacy of ciclopiroxolamine 1% cream in facial seborrheic dermatitis. *Br J Dermatol*. 2001;151:1033-1037.

20. Firooz A, Solhpour A, Gorouhi F, et al. Pimecrolimus cream, 1%, vs hydrocortisone acetate cream, 1%, in the treatment of facial seborrheic dermatitis: a randomized, investigator-blind, clinical trial. *Arch Dermatol*. 2006;142:1066-1067.

21. Freeman SH. Efficacy, cutaneous tolerance and cosmetic acceptability of desonide 0.05% lotion (Desowen) versus vehicle in the short-term treatment of facial atopic or seborrheic dermatitis. *Australas J Dermatol*. 2002;43(3):186-189.

22. Vena GA, Micali G, Santoianni P, et al. Oral terbinafine in the treatment of multi-site seborrheic dermatitis: a multicenter, double-blind placebo-controlled study. *Int J Immunopathol Pharmacol*. 2005;18:745-753.

23. Scaparro E, Quadri G, Virno G, et al. Evaluation of the efficacy and tolerability of oral terbinafine (Daskil) in patients with seborrheic dermatitis. A multicentre, randomized, investigator- blinded, placebo-controlled trial. *Br J Dermatol*. 2001;151(4):854-857.

24. Rigopoulos D, Ioannides D, Kalogeromitros D, et al. Pimecrolimus cream 1% vs. betamethasone 17-valerate 0.1% cream in the treatment of seborrheic dermatitis. A randomized open-label clinical trial. *Br J Dermatol*. 2004;151:1071-1075.

25. Warshaw EM, Wohlhuter RJ, Liu A, et al. Results of a randomized, double-blind, vehicle-controlled efficacy trial of pimecrolimus cream 1% for the treatment of moderate to severe facial seborrheic dermatitis. *J Am Acad Dermatol*. 2007;57(2): 257-264.

26. Papp KA, Papp A, Dahmer B, Clark CS. Single-blind, randomized controlled trial evaluating the treatment of facial seborrheic dermatitis with hydrocortisone 1% ointment compared with tacrolimus 0.1% ointment in adults. *J Am Acad Dermatol*. 2012;67(1):e11-e15.

27. Kim TW, Mun JH, Jwa SW, et al. Proactive treatment of adult facial seborrhoeic dermatitis with 0.1% tacrolimus ointment: randomized, double-blind, vehicle-controlled, multi-centre trial. *Acta Derm Venereol*. 2013;93(5):557-561.

28. Parsad D, Pandhi R, Negi KS, Kumar B. Topical metronidazole in seborrheic dermatitis—a double-blind study. *Dermatology*. 2001;202:35-37.

29. Koca R. Is topical metronidazole effective in seborrheic dermatitis? A double-blind study. *Int J Dermatol*. 2003;42(8):632-635.

30. Satchell AC, Saurajen A, Bell C, Barnetson RS. Treatment of dandruff with 5% tea tree oil shampoo. *J Am Acad Dermatol*. 2002;47(6):852-855.

31. Smith SA, Baker AE, Williams JH. Effective treatment of seborrheic dermatitis using a low dose, oral homeopathic medication consisting of potassium bromide, sodium bromide, nickel sulfate, and sodium chloride in a double-blind, placebo-controlled study. *Altern Med Rev*. 2002;7(1):59-67

158 PSORIASIS

Richard P. Usatine, MD
Jennifer L. Wipperman, MD, MPH

PATIENT STORY

A 33-year-old woman presents with uncontrolled psoriasis for 20 years. In addition to the plaque psoriasis (**Figure 158-1**), she has inverse psoriasis (**Figure 158-2**). Topical ultrahigh-potency steroids and topical calcipotriene have not controlled her psoriasis. The options for phototherapy and systemic therapy were discussed. The patient chose to try narrowband UVB treatment in addition to her topical therapy.

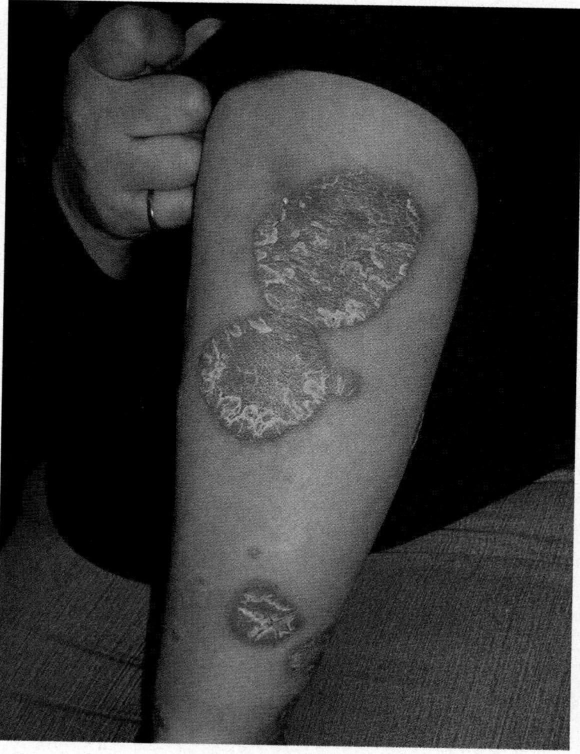

FIGURE 158-1 Typical plaque psoriasis on the elbow and arm. *(Reproduced with permission from Richard P. Usatine, MD.)*

INTRODUCTION

Psoriasis is a chronic inflammatory papulosquamous and immune-mediated skin disorder. It is also associated with joint and cardiovascular comorbidities. Psoriasis can present in many different patterns from the scalp to the feet and cause psychiatric distress and physical disabilities. It is crucial to be able to identify psoriasis in all its myriad presentations so that patients receive the best possible treatments to improve their quality of life and avoid comorbidities.

EPIDEMIOLOGY

Psoriasis affects approximately 1% to 8% of the world population.[1] In the United States, 3.7% of non-Hispanic white patients have psoriasis compared to 2.0% of African American patients and 1.6% of Hispanic patients.[2] Psoriasis affects men and women equally, but occurs earlier in women. While psoriasis can begin at any age, it has two peak incidences: ages 20–29 and 50–59 among women and ages 30–39 and 60–69 among men.[1]

ETIOLOGY AND PATHOPHYSIOLOGY

Psoriasis is an immune-mediated disease in which T cells play a pivotal role. Evidence suggests that foreign antigens in the skin first trigger antigen-presenting cells to release cytokines, including interleukin (IL)-23 and IL-1β. These cytokines trigger dermal T cells and helper T cells that release more cytokines, including IL-17 and tumor necrosis factor (TNF)-α, promoting keratinocyte hyperproliferation. This inflammatory immune response attracts more immune cells to the skin, which release further cytokines and chemokines. An escalated positive feedback loop results in psoriatic plaques. Greater understanding of the pathophysiology has led to the development of effective treatments targeted at TNF-α, IL-17, and IL-23.

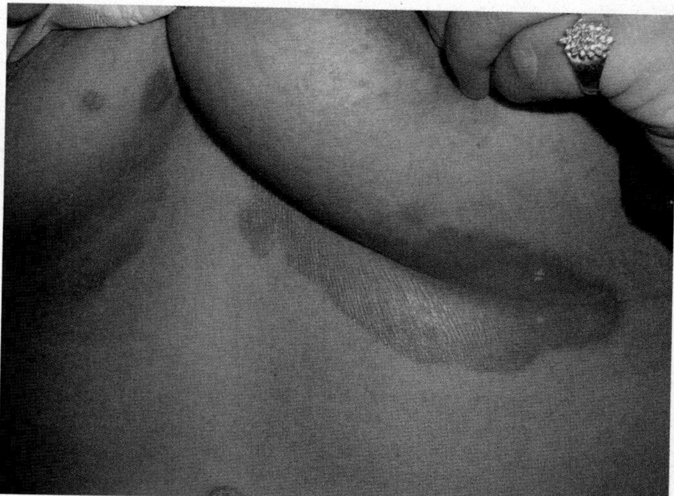

FIGURE 158-2 Inverse psoriasis in the inframammary folds of the patient in **Figure 158-1**. This is not a *Candida* infection. *(Reproduced with permission from Richard P. Usatine, MD.)*

TABLE 158-1 Factors that Trigger and Exacerbate Psoriasis

- Stress
- Physical trauma to the skin (Koebner phenomenon)
- Cold dry weather
- Sun or hot weather
- Infections (including strep throat and HIV)
- Medications (e.g., biologics, ACE-inhibitors, corticosteroids, lithium, antimalarials, β-blockers, NSAIDs)

RISK FACTORS

Table 158-1 lists the factors that trigger and exacerbate psoriasis.

- Family history: 60% of patients report a family history of psoriasis.[3] The psoriasis-susceptibility (PSORS) locus on chromosome 6p21 is a major genetic source of susceptibility to psoriasis.[4] Other identified loci include IL-12 and IL-23 related genes, which code for the interleukin receptors. Mutations in the IL36RN gene have been found in patients with generalized pustular psoriasis.
- Obesity: Obesity is associated with more severe psoriasis (odds ratio [OR] mild psoriasis 1.46 (95% confidence index [CI] 1.17–1.82) vs severe psoriasis 2.23 (95% CI 1.63–3.05).[5]
- Smoking and environmental smoke: Current and former smoking are associated with psoriasis (OR 1.78, 95% CI 1.52–2.06) with a dose-dependent effect on incidence.[6]
- Alcohol use: A large, prospective study found an increased risk of developing psoriasis among women who regularly drank alcohol (relative risk [RR] 1.72, 95% CI 1.15–2.57).[7] Alcohol use is associated with increased risk of psoriasis among both women and men.

Medications: Many medications are associated with worsening psoriasis or a psoriasis-like skin changes, including beta-blockers, lithium, and anti-malarial drugs.

DIAGNOSIS

Psoriasis manifests in many forms and locations. These nine categories were used to describe psoriasis in a consensus statement of the American Academy of Dermatology (AAD)[8]:

1. Plaque (80% of patients with psoriasis)[9] (**Figures 158-1** and **158-3**).
2. Scalp psoriasis (**Figure 158-4**).
3. Guttate psoriasis (**Figure 158-5**).
4. Inverse psoriasis (**Figures 158-2** and **158-6**).
5. Palmar-plantar psoriasis (**Figure 158-7**). Also known as palmoplantar psoriasis.
6. Erythrodermic psoriasis (**Figure 158-8**).
7. Pustular psoriasis—localized and generalized (**Figure 158-9**).
8. Nail psoriasis (**Figure 158-10**) (see Chapter 203, Psoriatic Nails).
9. Psoriatic arthritis (**Figure 158-11**).

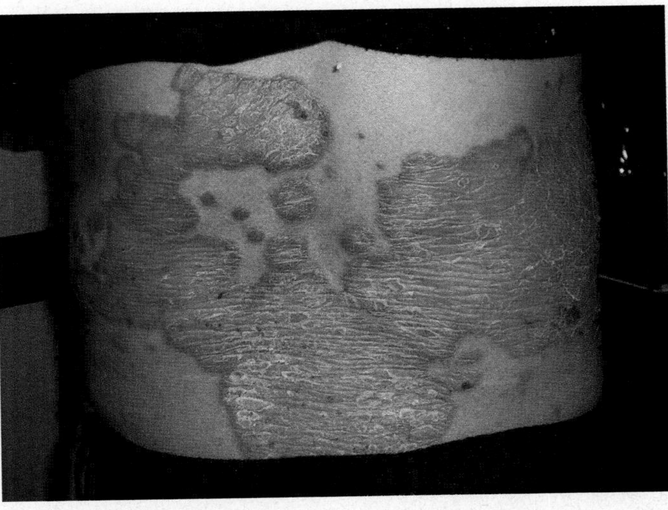

FIGURE 158-3 Well-demarcated plaques of plaque psoriasis in a 44-year-old man with severe psoriasis and psoriatic arthritis. (*Reproduced with permission from Richard P. Usatine, MD.*)

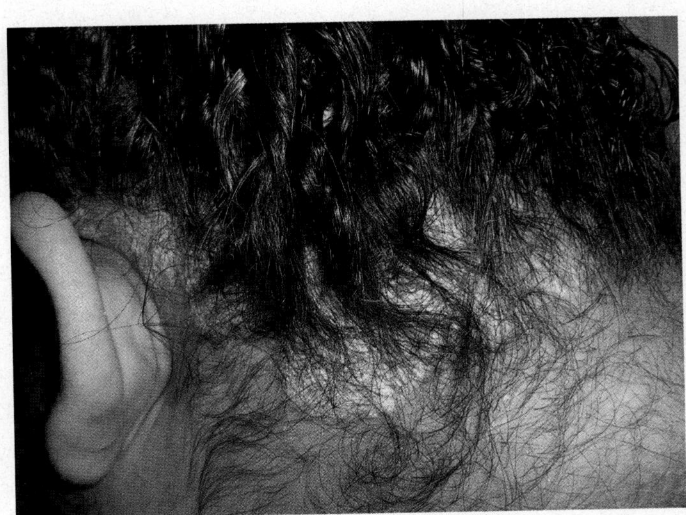

FIGURE 158-4 Scalp psoriasis visible at the hairline. (*Reproduced with permission from Richard P. Usatine, MD.*)

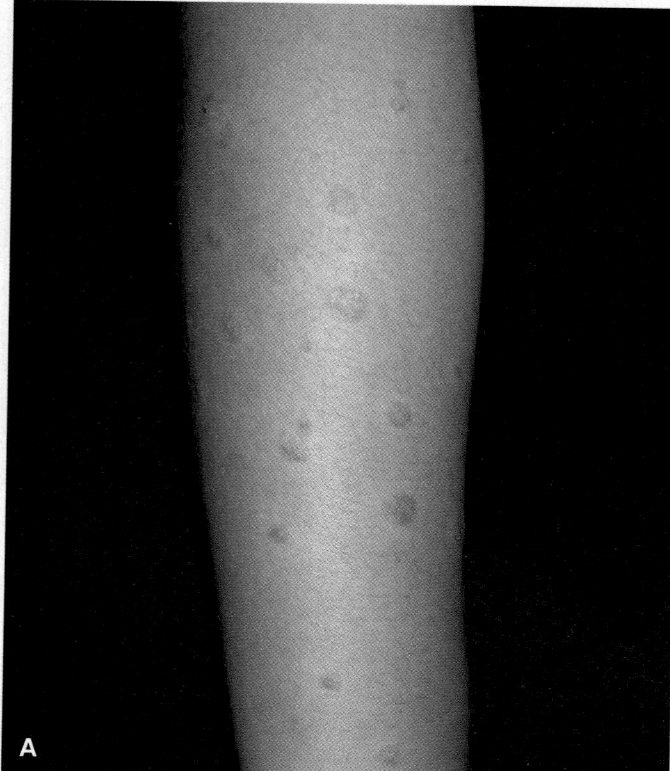

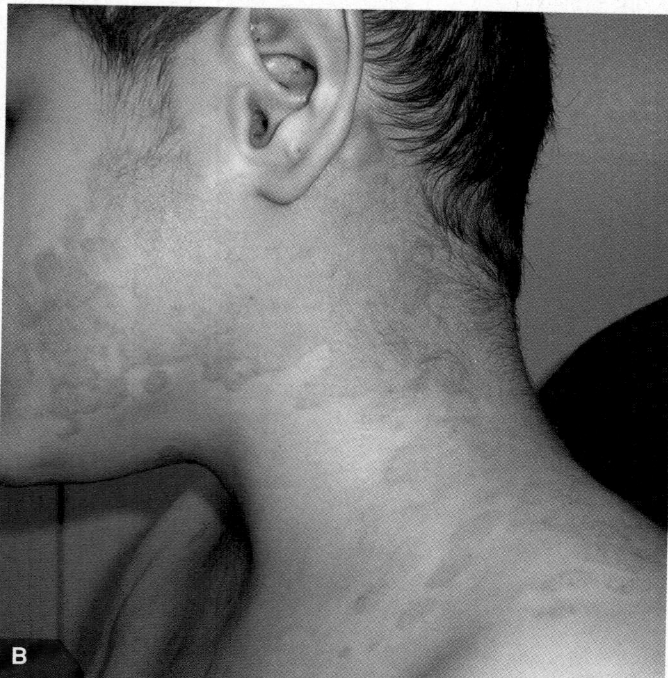

FIGURE 158-5 Two cases of guttate psoriasis that started 2 weeks after strep pharyngitis. **A.** Note the typical drop-like (guttate) lesions on the arm of this 11-year-old girl. **B.** The salmon patches of guttate psoriasis in a 7-year-old boy with prominent neck, ear, and scalp involvement. *(Reproduced with permission from Richard P. Usatine, MD.)*

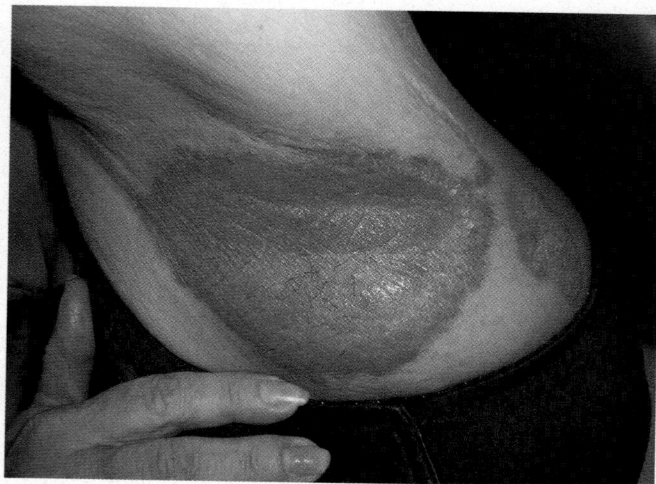

FIGURE 158-6 Inverse psoriasis in the axilla of this middle-aged woman. There is considerable erythema and very little scale. Prior to this visit her condition was misdiagnosed as fungal in origin. *(Reproduced with permission from Richard P. Usatine, MD.)*

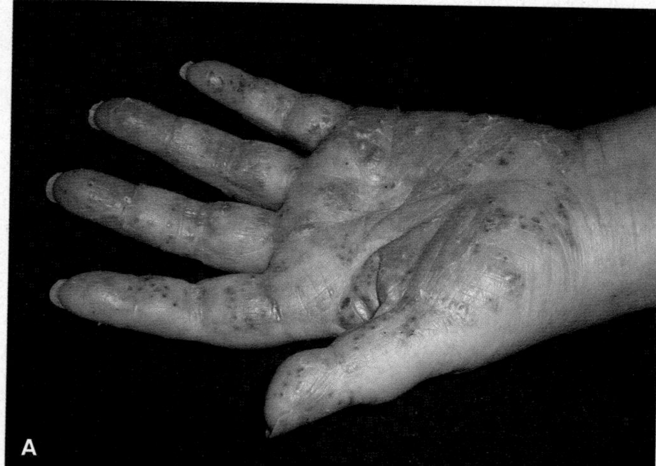

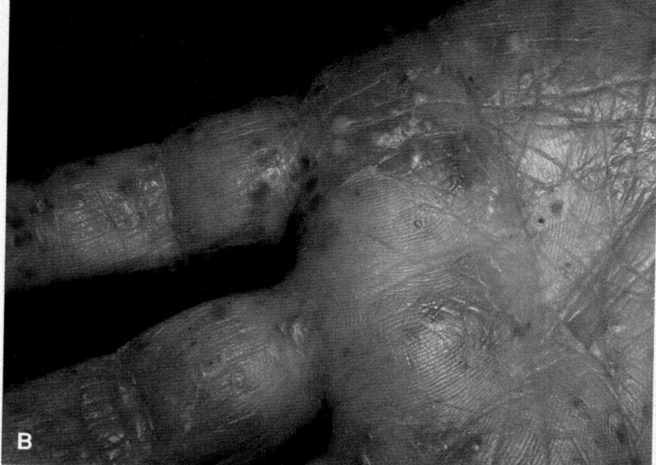

FIGURE 158-7 **A.** Palmoplantar psoriasis with pustulosis that started 3 months ago on the hands of a 62-year-old woman. **B.** Note the erythema, scale, brown macules (mahogany spots), and pustules that are typical of this condition. This is considered to be a localized form of pustular psoriasis. *(Reproduced with permission from Richard P. Usatine, MD.)*

FIGURE 158-8 Erythrodermic psoriasis covering most of the body surface. (*Reproduced with permission from Richard P. Usatine, MD.*)

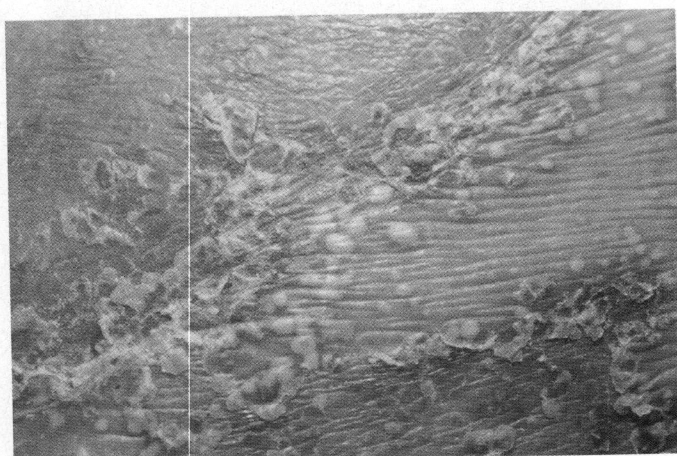

FIGURE 158-9 Pustular psoriasis on the back that occurred when oral prednisone was stopped. (*Reproduced with permission from Jack Resneck, Sr., MD.*)

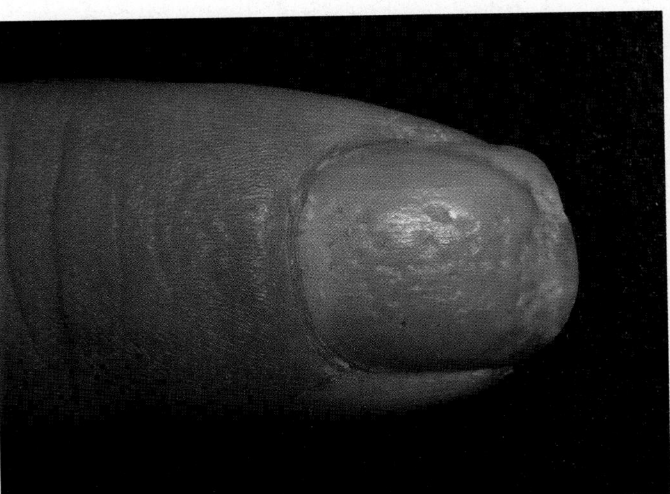

FIGURE 158-10 Nail pitting from psoriasis. (*Reproduced with permission from Richard P. Usatine, MD.*)

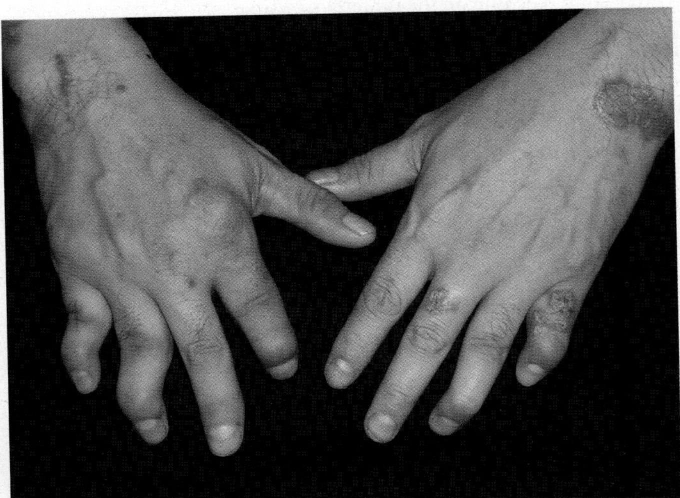

FIGURE 158-11 Psoriatic arthritis that has become crippling to this 44-year-old man. The shortening of the fingers fits the psoriatic arthritis mutilans subtype.(*Reproduced with permission from Richard P. Usatine, MD.*)

TABLE 158-2 The Most Common Locations of Lesions in Patients with Psoriasis[9]

Location	% of Psoriasis Patients
Scalp	42
Elbows and/or knees	35
Limbs and/or legs	35
Trunk	19
Face	11
Intragluteal/perianal	10
Genital	7
Palms and/or soles	7
Groin	3

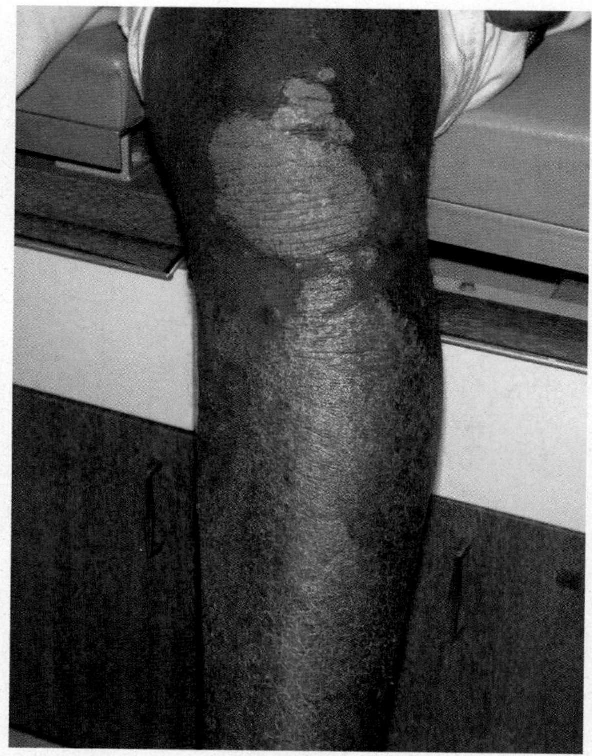

FIGURE 158-12 Plaque psoriasis with silvery scale on a black man. *(Reproduced with permission from Richard P. Usatine, MD.)*

The most common areas involved are listed in **Table 158-2**. Patients frequently present with more than one subtype.

Plaque psoriasis:

- Plaques tend to be symmetrically distributed along the elbows, knees, and other extensor surfaces. Extent can vary from localized to widespread involvement. Most patients experience some pruritus.
- White scale on an erythematous raised base with well-demarcated borders (see **Figures 158-1** and **158-3**).
- Silvery scale with hyperpigmentation may be seen in patients with darker skin (**Figures 158-12** and **158-13**).
- Plaques can appear in different colors including hypopigmented (**Figure 158-14**) and silvery gray (**Figure 158-15**). A tricolored presentation occurs when the inflammation leads to leukoderma or when there is coexisting vitiligo (**Figure 158-16**).
- The thickness and extent of the scale is variable (see **Figure 158-15**).
- A positive Auspitz sign is when peeling of a plaque's scale produces pinpoint bleeding on the underlying skin.
- The plaques can be found from head to toe including the penis (**Figure 15-17**).
- Plaques can be annular with central clearing (**Figure 158-18**).
- When plaques occur at a site of skin trauma, it is known as the Koebner phenomenon (**Figure 158-19**).

Scalp psoriasis:

- Plaque on the scalp that may be seen at the hairline and around the ears (see **Figure 158-4**).
- The thickness and extent of the plaques are variable, as seen in plaque psoriasis.

Guttate psoriasis:

- Small round plaques that resemble water drops (guttate means like a water drop) (**Figure 158-20**).
- Classically described as occurring after strep pharyngitis or another bacterial infection. More often occurs in children and young adults without a prior history of psoriasis.

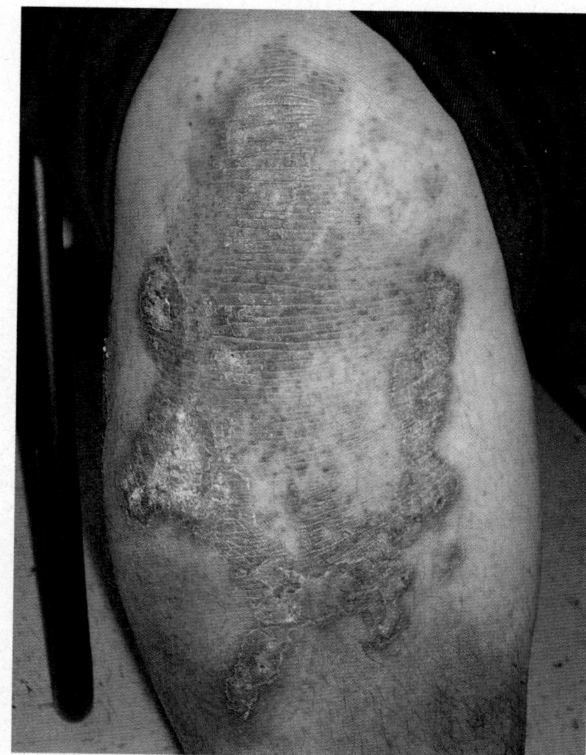

FIGURE 158-13 Psoriasis on the knee of a Hispanic man showing postinflammatory hyperpigmentation. *(Reproduced with permission from Richard P. Usatine, MD.)*

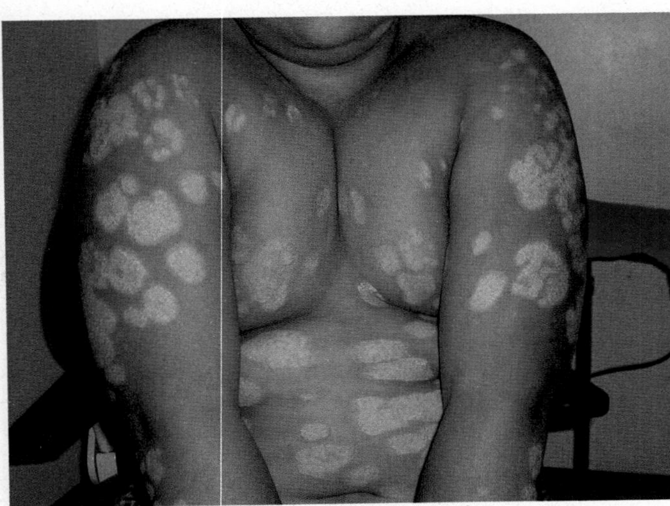

FIGURE 158-14 Plaque psoriasis with hypopigmentation in this 12-year-old obese boy. (*Reproduced with permission from Richard P. Usatine, MD.*)

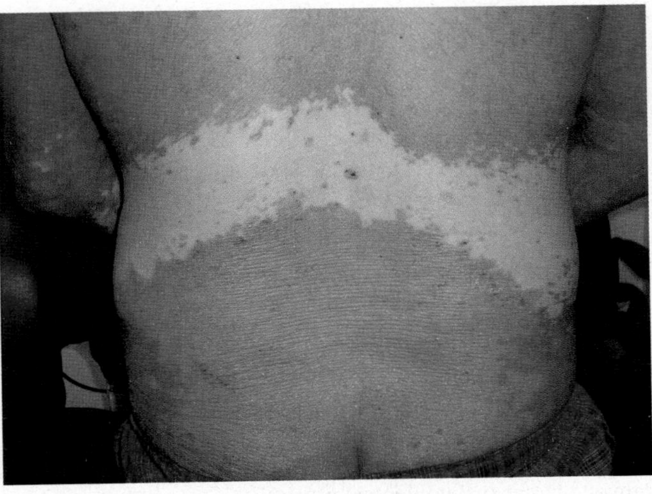

FIGURE 158-16 Plaque psoriasis that has caused hypopigmentation in a band across the back. His original skin color is brown so that the brown, white, and pink colors produce the appearance of Neapolitan ice cream. (*Reproduced with permission from Richard P. Usatine, MD.*)

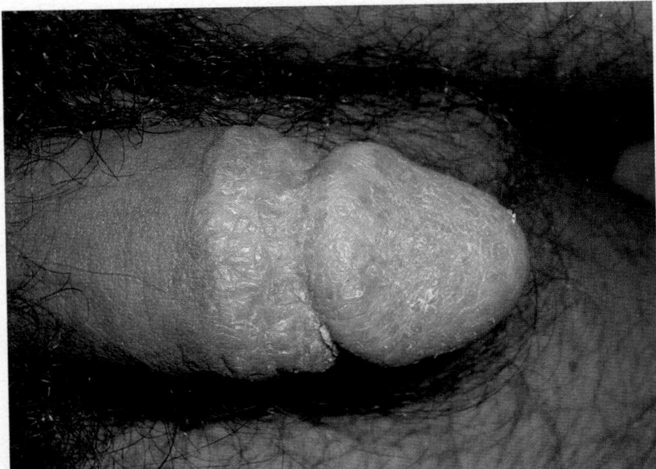

FIGURE 158-17 Plaque psoriasis on the penis, covering the glans and part of the shaft. (*Reproduced with permission from Richard P. Usatine, MD.*)

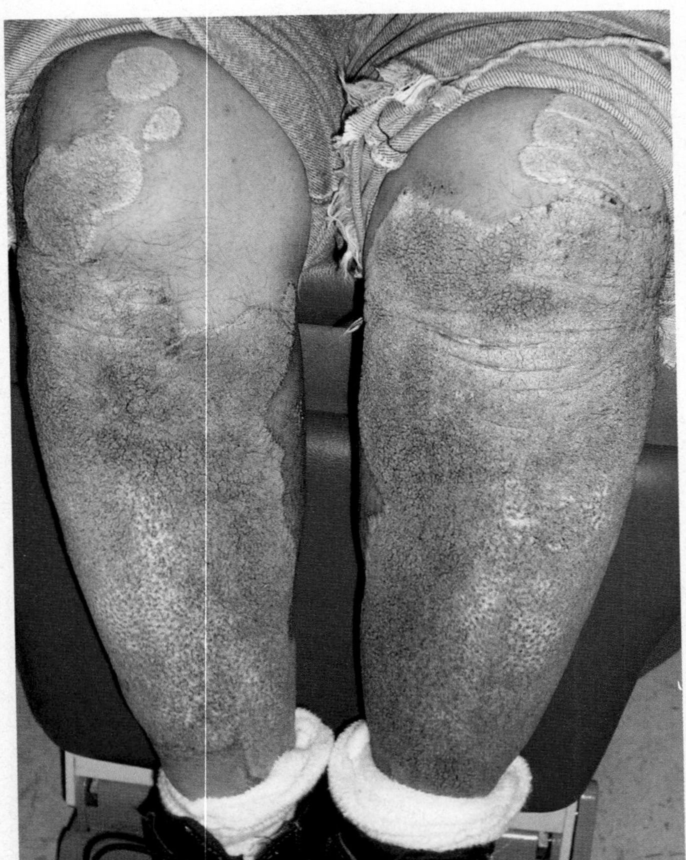

FIGURE 158-15 Thick plaque psoriasis covering the lower legs of this obese man. Note the silver gray color to his plaques. (*Reproduced with permission from Richard P. Usatine, MD.*)

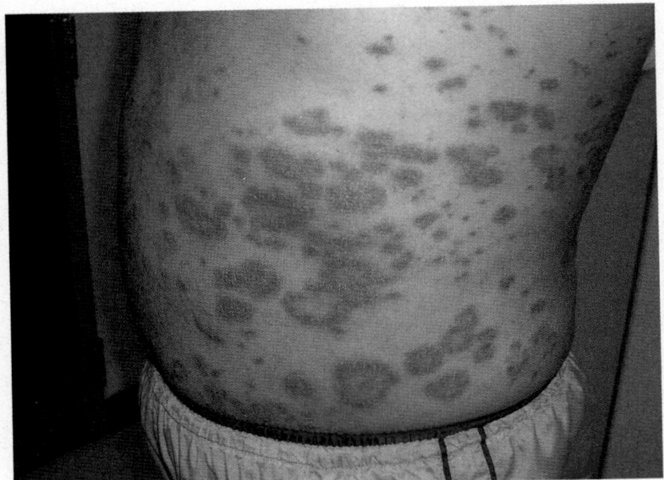

FIGURE 158-18 Plaque psoriasis with an annular configuration. (*Reproduced with permission from Richard P. Usatine, MD.*)

- Typical distribution includes the trunk and extremities, but may include the face and neck (**Figure 158-21**).

Inverse psoriasis:

- Found in the intertriginous areas of the axilla, groin, and inframammary and intergluteal folds (**Figures 158-2**, **158-6**, and **158-22**). It can also be seen below the pannus or within adipose folds in obese individuals.
- The term *inverse* refers to the fact that the distribution is not on extensor surfaces but in areas of body folds.
- Lesions are flat and well-demarcated and have little to no visible scale.
- Color is generally pink to red but can be hyperpigmented in dark-skinned individuals.

Palmar-plantar (palmoplantar) psoriasis:

- Psoriasis that mainly occurs on the plantar aspects of the hands and feet (palms and soles) (**Figure 158-23**), but can involve other parts of the hands and feet.
- Patients with this type of psoriasis often experience severe foot and hand pain that can impair walking and other daily activities of living. Hand involvement can result in pain with many types of work.
- Lesions may be plaque-like, vesicular, or pustular (**Figure 158-24**). Brown macules or flat papules ("mahogany spots") are characteristic of palmar-plantar psoriasis, but not uniformly present. Exfoliation of the skin can occur.

Erythrodermic psoriasis:

- Erythrodermic psoriasis is widespread and erythematous, covering most of the skin (**Figure 158-25**).
- Morphologically, it can have plaques and erythema or the erythroderma can appear with the desquamation of pustular psoriasis.
- Widespread distribution can impair the important functions of the skin, and this can be a dermatologic urgency requiring hospitalization and IV fluids. Chills, fever, tachycardia, and orthostatic hypotension are all signs that the patient may need hospitalization.

Pustular psoriasis:

- Pustular psoriasis comes in localized and generalized types. One example of the local type is pustular psoriasis on the feet (see **Figure 158-24**).
- In the generalized type, the skin initially becomes fiery red and tender and the patient experiences constitutional signs and symptoms such as headache, fever, chills, arthralgia, malaise, anorexia, and nausea (**Figure 158-26**). The desquamation that occurs in the generalized form can impair the important functions of the skin, predisposing to dehydration and sepsis. This is a dermatologic emergency requiring hospitalization and IV fluids, preferably in an ICU or monitored bed with good nursing care.
- Typical distribution: Flexural and anogenital (**Figure 158-27**). Less often, facial lesions occur. Pustules may occur on the tongue and subungually, resulting in dysphagia and nail shedding, respectively.
- Time course: Within hours, clusters of non-follicular, superficial 2- to 3-mm pustules may appear in a generalized pattern. These pustules coalesce within 1 day to form lakes of pus that dry and

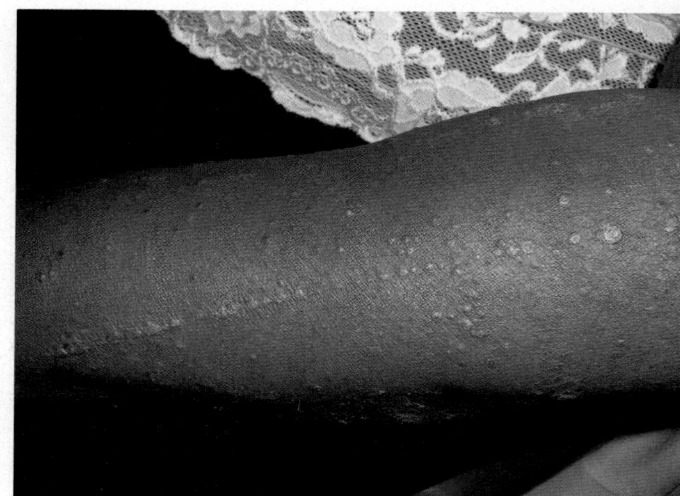

FIGURE 158-19 Linear distribution of psoriasis on the arm secondary to the Koebner phenomenon. (*Reproduced with permission from Richard P. Usatine, MD.*)

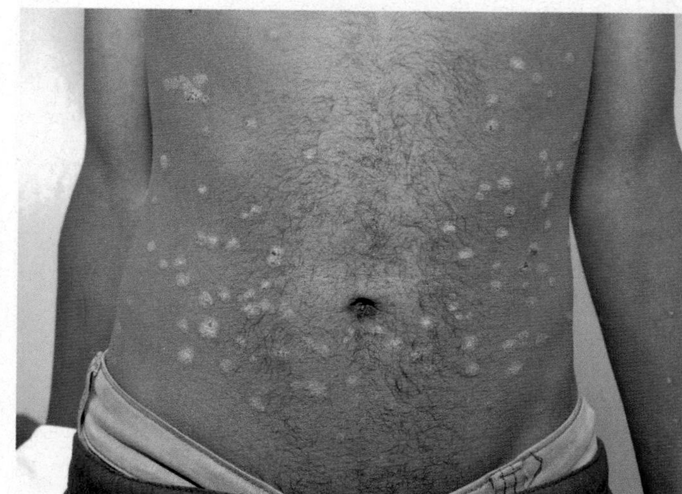

FIGURE 158-20 Guttate psoriasis in a 17-year-old young man following an episode of strep pharyngitis. (*Reproduced with permission from Richard P. Usatine, MD.*)

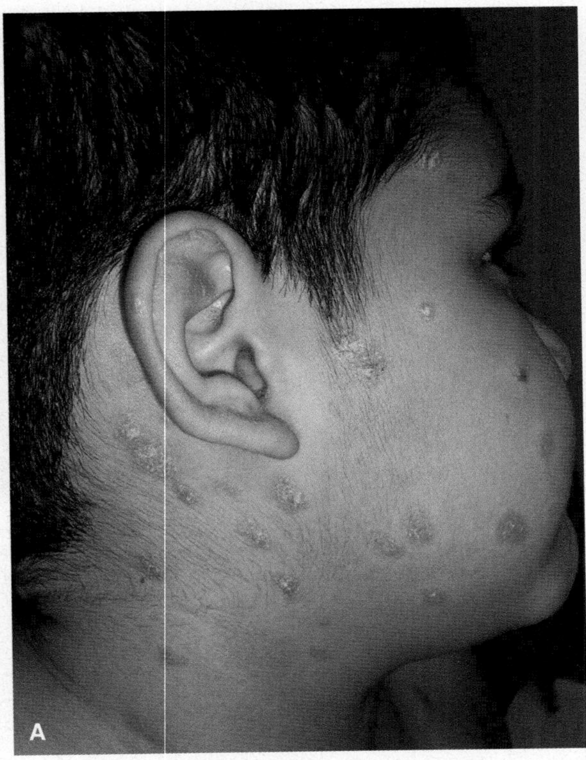

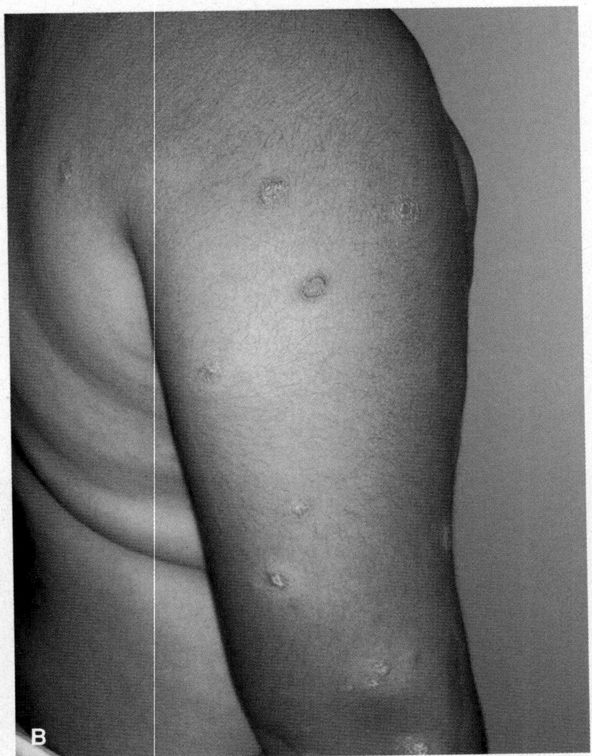

FIGURE 158-21 This young boy developed guttate psoriasis after an upper respiratory infection. **A.** Note the droplike pink plaques on the face and neck. **B.** Droplike plaques on the arms and trunk. (*Reproduced with permission from Richard P. Usatine, MD.*)

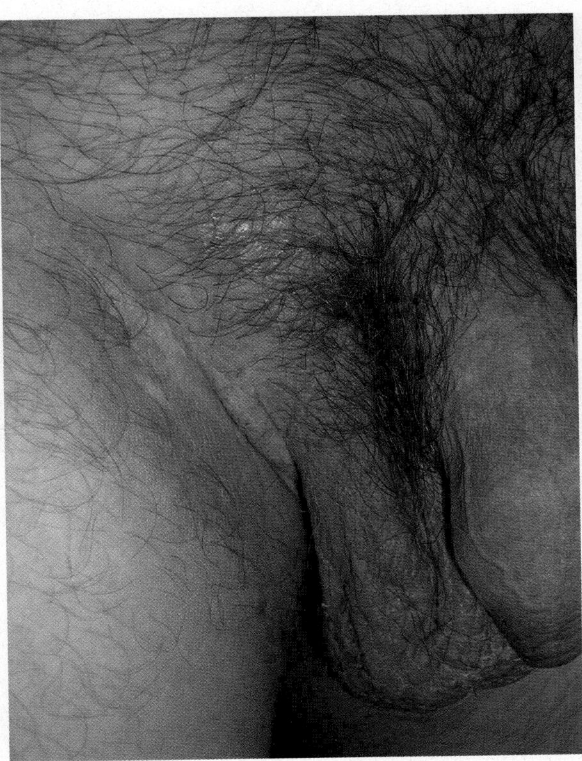

FIGURE 158-22 Inverse psoriasis in the inguinal area. This was mistaken for tinea cruris for a long time. (*Reproduced with permission from Richard P. Usatine, MD.*)

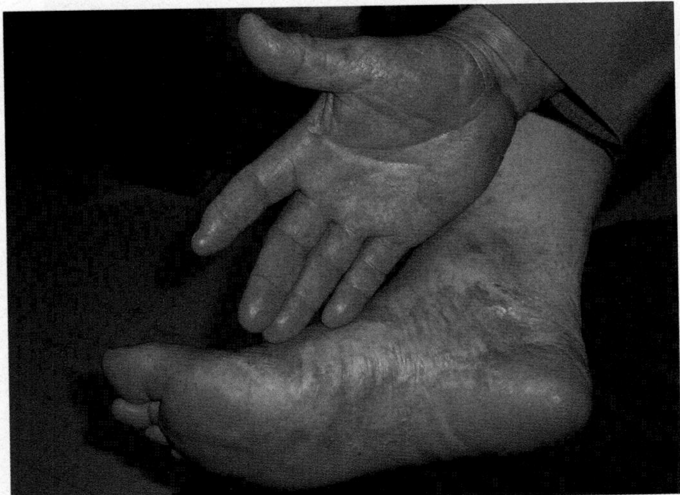

FIGURE 158-23 Palmar-plantar psoriasis that was biopsy proven. Note the widespread erythema and scale that could be mistaken for tinea pedis and tinea manus. The patient does not have pustules or mahogany spots, but those lesions are often not present in palmar-plantar psoriasis. (*Reproduced with permission from Richard P. Usatine, MD.*)

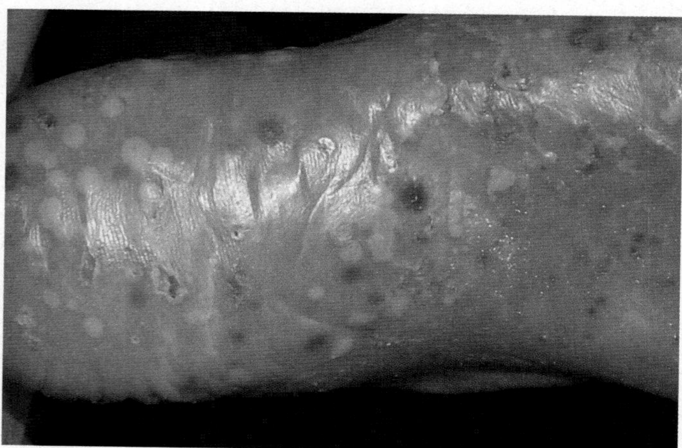

FIGURE 158-24 Palmar-plantar psoriasis with extensive pustules and mahogany spots. (*Reproduced with permission from UTHSCSA dermatology.*)

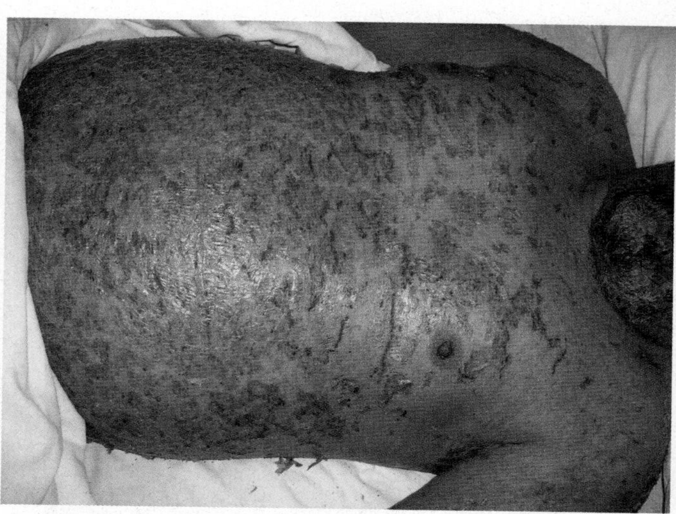

FIGURE 158-26 Generalized pustular psoriasis in a 47-year-old man with fever, exfoliation, and dehydration. This is the twentieth time for this patient in his life. His siblings also get severe generalized pustular psoriasis. (*Reproduced with permission from Richard P. Usatine, MD.*)

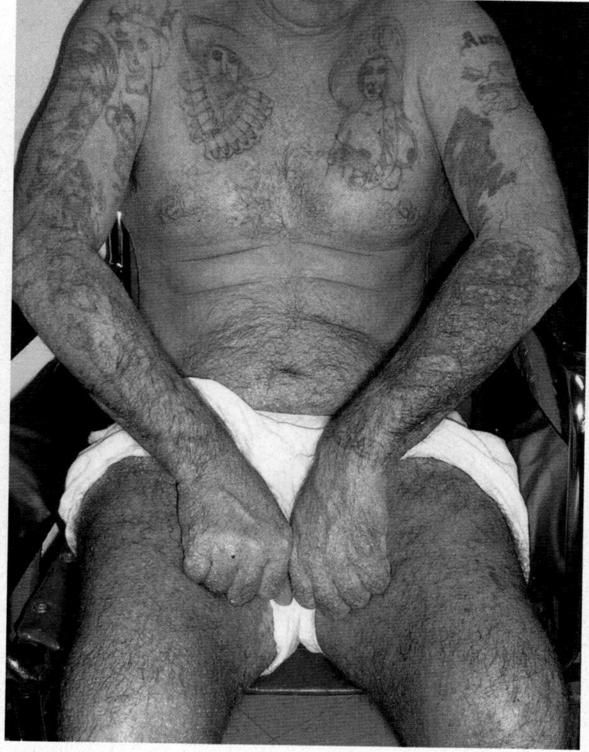

FIGURE 158-25 Erythrodermic psoriasis in a 45-year-old man. Note the extensive exfoliation of the skin along with the deep erythema. (*Reproduced with permission from Richard P. Usatine, MD.*)

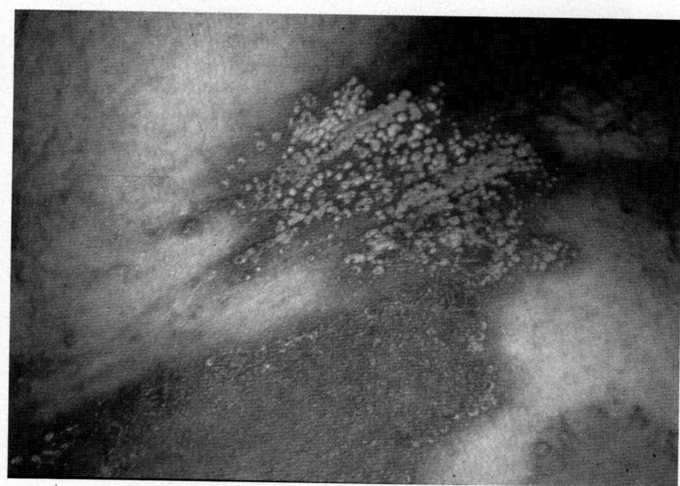

FIGURE 158-27 Localized pustular psoriasis in the groin. (*Reproduced with permission from Jeffrey Meffert, MD.*)

desquamate in sheets, leaving behind a smooth erythematous surface on which new crops of pustules may appear. These episodes of pustulation may occur for days to weeks, causing the patient severe discomfort and exhaustion. Upon remission of the pustular component, most systemic symptoms disappear; however, the patient may be in an erythrodermic state or may have residual lesions.[1]

Nail psoriasis:

- Nail involvement in psoriasis can lead to pitting, onycholysis, subungual keratosis, splinter hemorrhages, oil spots, and nail loss (see **Figure 158-10** and Chapter 203, Psoriatic Nails).

Psoriatic arthritis:

- Psoriatic arthritis (PsA) is an inflammatory seronegative spondyloarthropathy that presents as stiffness, pain, and swelling of the joints and surrounding soft tissues. Stiffness is worse in the morning and after prolonged inactivity, lasting more than 30 minutes. Most patients have a polyarticular arthritis involving the hands, feet, and knees, which can resemble rheumatoid arthritis.[10] However, the spectrum of PsA is variable and can involve axial to peripheral disease. Distal interphalangeal joint (DIP) involvement is a classic finding, but DIP predominance is present in the minority of cases. The fingers may be swollen like sausages, which is called dactylitis (**Figure 158-28**). See **Table 97-1** in Chapter 97, Arthritis Overview, for a description of the five types of psoriatic arthritis.
- Hand involvement can be disabling (see **Figure 158-11**). X-rays should be ordered when a person with psoriasis has joint pains suggesting psoriatic arthritis. Typical findings are juxtaarticular erosions, bony proliferation, and osteolysis, including the "pencil in cup" deformity (**Figure 158-29**).
- There may be inflammation at the insertion of tendons onto bone (enthesopathy). This may occur at the Achilles tendon.
- Nail involvement is common and correlates with the severity of arthritis.
- Patients with psoriatic arthritis need to be treated earlier with systemic agents (methotrexate or biologics) to prevent permanent joint damage and disability, often in conjunction with a rheumatologist.

DISEASE SEVERITY

- Moderate-to-severe disease is defined by psoriasis of the palms, soles, head and neck, or genitalia, and in patients with more than 5% body surface area (BSA) involvement.[11] A person's palm with fingers extended and abducted is approximately 1% BSA.
- Another grading system for severity uses percent BSA:
  - Mild: Up to 3% BSA
  - Moderate: 3% to 10% BSA
  - Severe: >10% BSA
- Patients with psoriatic arthritis may have limited skin disease but require more aggressive systemic therapies.
- Note that palmoplantar psoriasis is considered moderate-to-severe even if the BSA involved is not above 5% (**Figure 158-30**).

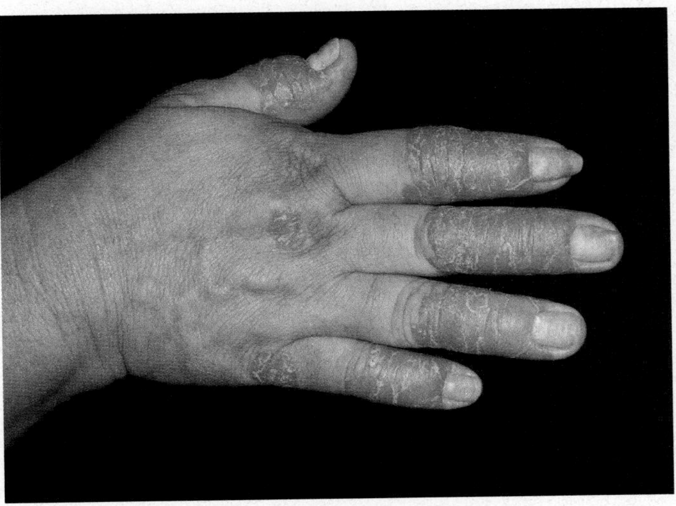

FIGURE 158-28 Dactylitis with sausage-shaped fingers in this middle-aged woman with plaque psoriasis and psoriatic arthritis. Note the nail involvement along with distal interphalangeal joint involvement. *(Reproduced with permission from Richard P. Usatine, MD.)*

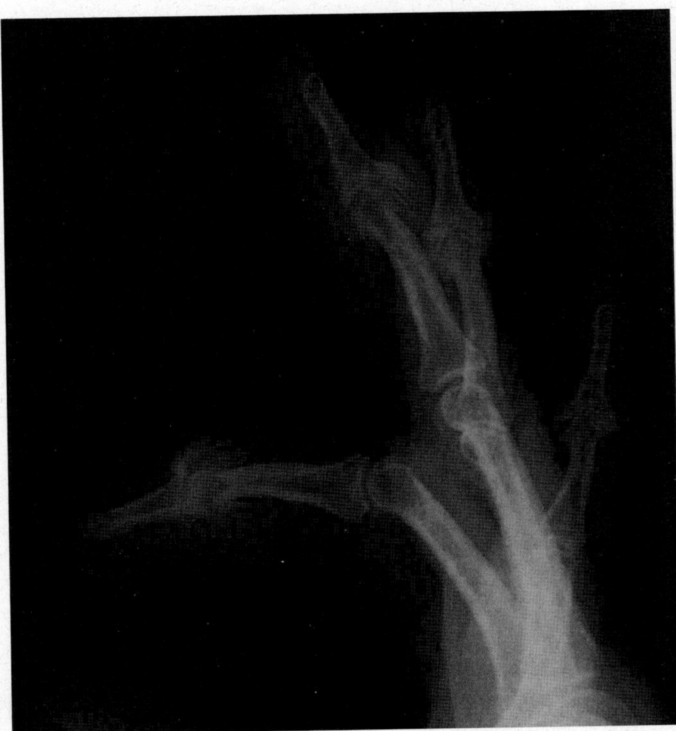

FIGURE 158-29 Radiograph showing the pencil-in-cup deformity at the distal interphalangeal joint of the second and third digits. *(Reproduced with permission from Richard P. Usatine, MD.)*

LABORATORY STUDIES

Laboratory studies are rarely needed for diagnosis. A punch biopsy or scoop shave is used for evaluating atypical cases. For pustular psoriasis, a 4-mm punch around an intact pustule is preferred (**Figure 158-31**). A KOH prep is useful for ruling out tinea. A complete blood count (CBC) with differential, renal and hepatic function testing, electrolytes, and blood and skin cultures should be obtained in cases of erythroderma or acute generalized pustular psoriasis.

IMAGING

Plain films should be ordered when a person with psoriasis has joint symptoms suggesting psoriatic arthritis (see **Figure 158-29**). Early psoriatic arthritis often has no findings on plain films, but if history and physical exam suggest the diagnosis, one should not wait for irreversible visible joint damage to initiate therapy.

DIFFERENTIAL DIAGNOSIS

- Cutaneous T-cell lymphoma (CTCL) can have plaques that resemble psoriasis. In most cases of psoriasis, the distribution and nail changes will help to differentiate between these diseases. Plaque-type CTCL tends to be more central and truncal, whereas psoriasis often involves the extremities along with the trunk. If needed, a punch biopsy can help to differentiate between these two conditions (see Chapter 180, Cutaneous T- Cell Lymphoma).
- Lichen planus is another papulosquamous disease. Classic findings include polygonal purple and pink pruritic papules/plaques. Patients may have fine white lines on the buccal mucosa ("Wickham striae"). Lichen planus occurs on flexor surfaces and around the wrists and ankles rather than the elbows and knees. (see Chapter 160, Lichen Planus).
- Lichen simplex chronicus is the end result of repeated scratching from a variety of causes, manifesting as a hyperkeratotic plaque with lichenification. It is typically found on the posterior neck, ankle, wrist, or lower leg where the patient can reach and scratch. There is usually more lichenification than thick scale, and it is always pruritic (see Chapter 155, Psychocutaneous Disorders).
- Nummular eczema presents with coinlike plaques ranging from 1 to 10 cm in diameter, typically on the legs. Lesions are usually not as thick as the plaques of psoriasis, have less scale, and are more pruritic. Nummular eczema may have vesicles and bullae. The face and scalp are spared (see Chapter 151, Atopic Dermatitis).
- Pityriasis rosea is a self-limited process that has papulosquamous plaques and may be confused with guttate psoriasis. These plaques are less keratotic, have a fine collarette of scale, and follow skin lines. Pityriasis rosea frequently has a herald patch (see Chapter 159, Pityriasis Rosea).
- Seborrheic dermatitis of the scalp can closely resemble psoriasis of the scalp, especially when it is severe. Psoriasis generally has thicker plaques on the scalp, and the plaques often cross the hairline. Seborrhea and psoriasis can both involve the ear. Both conditions respond to topical steroids (see Chapter 157, Seborrheic Dermatitis).
- Syphilis is the great imitator, and secondary syphilis can have a papulosquamous eruption similar to guttate psoriasis. Secondary

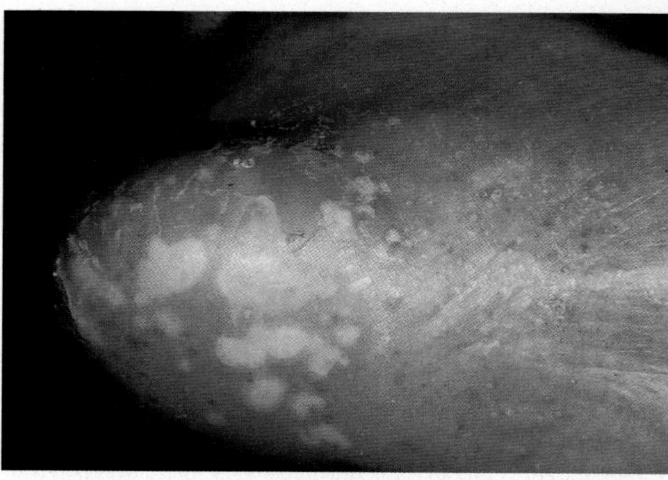

FIGURE 158-30 Palmoplantar psoriasis in a 31-year-old man with erythema, pustules, and lakes of pus. Note the typical brown macules that are called mahogany spots. High-potency topical steroids did not help at all. It is painful for him to walk and systemic therapy has just been started. This is a localized form of pustular psoriasis. (*Reproduced with permission from Jeff Meffert, MD.*)

syphilis often involves the palms and soles, and the rapid plasma reagin (RPR) will be positive (see Chapter 225, Syphilis).

- Tinea corporis or cruris can resemble inverse psoriasis in the intertriginous areas, as both conditions tend to have erythema and thinner plaques without central clearing in these regions. Tinea corporis in non-intertriginous areas presents with annular plaques with central clearing and peripheral scale. Psoriasis can do this, as seen in **Figure 158-18**. Tinea corporis usually does not have as many plaques as psoriasis, but a KOH preparation can be obtained if needed (see Chapter 144, Tinea Corporis). Onychomycosis can be confused with psoriatic nail changes, and a nail clipping may be sent for fungal culture to distinguish this from psoriasis (see Chapter 201, Onychomycosis). However, it is possible to have a fungal infection in nails affected by psoriasis.
- Cutaneous candidiasis appears similar to inverse psoriasis when found in intertriginous areas, but often has satellite lesions (see Chapter 142, Candidiasis).
- Reactive arthritis (see Chapter 161, Reactive Arthritis) is a noninfectious acute oligoarthritis that occurs in response to an infection, most commonly in the GI or urogenital tract. Patients present 1 to 4 weeks after the triggering infection, with joint pain in asymmetric large joints, eye disease such as conjunctivitis, and skin changes including erythema nodosum, keratoderma blennorrhagicum, and circinate balanitis. Diagnosis is based on the clinical presentation plus evidence of associated infection. The skin lesions closely resemble psoriasis, so the diagnosis depends on the constellation of the clinical involvement and the history.

MANAGEMENT

When caring for a patient with psoriasis, physicians should consider goals of treatment, disease severity, disease pattern, response to prior treatments, patient comorbidities, family planning, and individual preferences. Patients' perception of their disease and expectations for improvement are as important as the following evidence-based recommendations. Some patients are willing to live with some continued skin changes rather that start systemic treatment, whereas others desire maximal therapy with a goal of 100% clearance. Further, patients may prefer different vehicles of topical treatment or the convenience of some regimens compared to others. One of the most important factors in successful treatment is patient adherence. The most effective treatment is often the one that is most acceptable to the patient.

NONPHARMACOLOGIC

All patients should apply daily emollients to keep skin soft, thereby limiting pruritus and irritation. Address lifestyle changes that can affect psoriasis, including:

- Smoking cessation.
- Avoid or minimize alcohol use.
- Weight loss for obese patients.
- Address depression and offer stress management techniques.
- Avoid known precipitants.

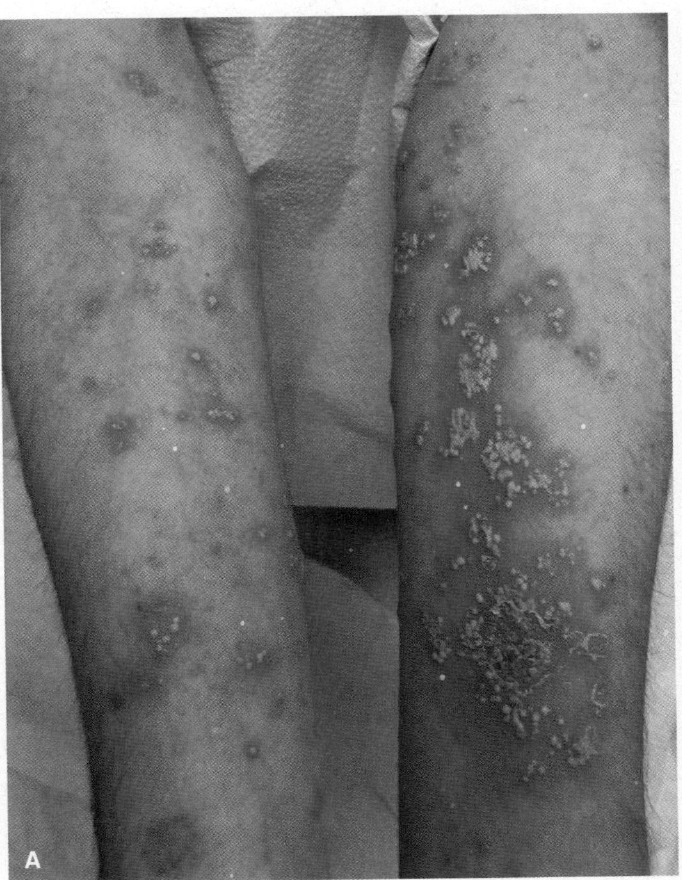

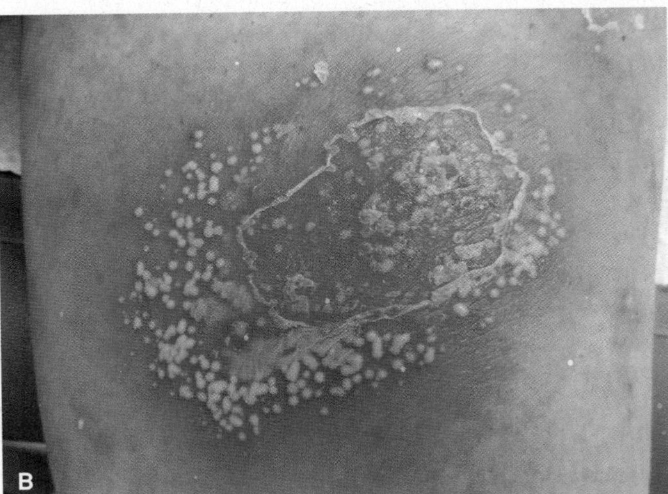

FIGURE 158-31 Pustular psoriasis in a 41-year-old woman. A 4-mm punch biopsy including at least one pustule helped to confirm the clinical diagnosis. The patient was stable for outpatient treatment and was started on cyclosporine and acitretin together with the plan to stop the cyclosporine once the pustules have cleared. **A.** Arm involvement. **B.** Close-up of pustules on the leg. (*Reproduced with permission from Robert T. Gilson, MD.*)

TABLE 158-3 Strength of Recommendations for the Treatment of Psoriasis Using Topical Therapies

Agent	Strength of Recommendation	Level of Evidence
Class I corticosteroids (highest potency)	A	I
Class II corticosteroids	B	II
Classes III/IV corticosteroids (medium potency)	A	I
Classes V/VI/VII corticosteroids (lowest potency)	A	I
Vitamin D analogs	A	I
Tazarotene	A	I
Tacrolimus and pimecrolimus	B	II
Anthralin	C	III
Coal tar	B	II
Combination corticosteroid and salicylic acid	B	II
Combination corticosteroid and vitamin D analog	A	I
Combination corticosteroid and tazarotene	A	I
Combination tacrolimus and salicylic acid	B	II

Adapted with permission from Menter A, Korman NJ, Elmets CA, et al; American Academy of Dermatology. Guidelines of care for the management of psoriasis and psoriatic arthritis. Section 3. Guidelines of care for the management and treatment of psoriasis with topical therapies. *J Am Acad Dermatol.* 2009;60(4):643-659.

Choice of topical vehicles:

- An ointment has a petrolatum base and will penetrate thick scale best.
- An emollient cream has some of the advantages of an ointment but is cosmetically more appealing to patients who find a basic ointment to be too greasy.
- Some patients prefer cream to avoid the oily feel of ointment. The most effective vehicle is the one the patient will use.
- Lotions and foams are good for hair-bearing areas when some moisturizing is desired.
- Steroid solutions work well for psoriasis of the scalp.
- New foam and spray preparations have rapid absorption and are cosmetically appealing. These tend to be more expensive at this time.

FIRST LINE

Topical treatments:

- Very potent topical corticosteroids are the single most effective topical agent for psoriasis. A meta-analysis of 34 randomized controlled trials (RCTs) found that very potent corticosteroids applied twice daily resulted in 78.2% of patients reporting clear or nearly clear disease.[12] SOR Ⓐ
- Topical vitamin D analogs available include calcipotriene, calcitriol, and tacalcitol. They are as effective as potent corticosteroids, but are more likely to cause side effects including irritation and burning.[13] SOR Ⓐ Calcitriol may be less irritating than calcipotriene.
- Topical vitamin D analogs have slower onset of action compared to topical corticosteroids, but result in longer disease-free periods after cessation.[14]
- Combined treatment with topical vitamin D and potent corticosteroid is more effective than either alone and is as well tolerated as potent corticosteroids.[13] SOR Ⓐ Although this is available in combination products, it is less expensive to prescribe each component separately in their generic formulations.
- Tazarotene is a topical retinoid applied once daily with comparable efficacy to vitamin D analogs.[13] SOR Ⓑ Applying in combination with a corticosteroid is recommended to improve efficacy and reduce irritation. A double-blind RCT comparing a combination of halobetasol propionate 0.01% and tazarotene 0.045% lotion to either component alone found increased efficacy and reduced irritation with the combination compared to tazarotene alone.[15]
- Topical calcineurin inhibitors are less effective than potent topical steroids, but are useful for sensitive areas such as the face and skin folds due to increased risk of irritation and skin atrophy from topical vitamin D and corticosteroids, respectively.[11,13] SOR Ⓑ
- Maintenance with weekend potent corticosteroid use, with or without weekday topical vitamin D, increases likelihood of remission.[16] SOR Ⓑ

SECOND LINE

Phototherapy:

- UV-based treatment with narrow-band UVB (NB-UVB) or psoralen-UVA (PUVA) are highly effective, safe treatments for widespread psoriasis or psoriasis not responding to topical therapy. A meta-analysis of UV-based therapies found that PUVA resulted in clearance rates of 79% (95% CI 69–88) and NB-UVB resulted in clearance rates of 68% (95% CI 57–78).[17] SOR Ⓐ
- Narrow-band UVB is more effective than broadband UVB with fewer side effects.[17,18] SOR Ⓑ

- Evidence is controversial regarding the relative efficacy of NB-UVB directly compared to PUVA.[18] A systematic review of 5 low-quality, head-to-head RCTs found that oral PUVA resulted in longer-lasting clearance and required fewer treatments compared to NB-UVB, but had similar relapse rates at 6 months.[18] SOR Ⓑ
- NB-UVB offers several advantages over PUVA, including lack of need for pretreatment with a photosensitizing medication, lower long-term risk of skin cancer, and safety in pregnancy.[11] Therefore, it may be considered as a first choice, with PUVA reserved for treatment failures.
- PUVA is associated with increased risk of squamous (SCC) and basal cell carcinomas. A 30-year prospective cohort study of 1380 patients treated with PUVA found that undergoing more than 350 treatments greatly increased risk of developing SCC (incidence rate ratio 20.9, 95% CI 14.0–31.1).[19]
- Targeted phototherapy, with high energy 308-nm excimer laser, delivers UV radiation to localized areas of skin. A trial of 124 patients receiving twice weekly treatments for 10 weeks found that 84% of patients (95% CI 79%-87%) reported 75% or better improvement in their psoriasis.[20] SOR Ⓑ
- Combining systemic agents with UV-based therapy can increase response rates, improve tolerance, and reduce UV exposure. Effective combinations include methotrexate and acitretin.[17] SOR Ⓑ Cyclosporine should not be combined with UV treatments because of increased risk of skin cancer.[11]

Systemic agents:

When topical agents and/or phototherapy fail, systemic agents are the next step (**Table 158-4**). Systemic agents include acitretin, apremilast, cyclosporine, methotrexate, and the biologics. Systemic agents

TABLE 158-4 Systemic Drugs Used in Treatment of Psoriasis[41]

Drug Name	Classification/Mechanism of Action	Comments
Acitretin	Oral retinoid	First-line systemic drug for chronic palmoplantar or pustular psoriasis in patients of non-childbearing potential. Limited benefit for plaque psoriasis.
Cyclosporine	Oral calcineurin inhibitor	Fast-acting systemic drug that is often used first-line for pustular psoriasis or erythrodermic psoriasis. For intermittent use in periods up to 12 wk as a short-term agent to control a flare of psoriasis.
Methotrexate sodium	Inhibitor of folate biosynthesis	May be used as a first-line systemic drug for plaque psoriasis and psoriatic arthritis. Compared with cyclosporine, has a more modest effect, but can be used continuously for years or decades.
Adalimumab	TNF inhibitor	May be used as first-line systemic treatment of plaque psoriasis and psoriatic arthritis. Has higher efficacy and lower rate of adverse effects compared with methotrexate.
Etanercept	TNF inhibitor	Commonly used as a first-line systemic drug for chronic plaque psoriasis and psoriatic arthritis.
Infliximab	TNF inhibitor	Intravenous infusion with high rates of effectiveness. Fast-acting drug that is often used as a second- or third-line biological for chronic plaque psoriasis.
Ustekinumab	Monoclonal antibody that binds the shared p40 protein subunit of IL-12 and IL-23	Favorable results when compared with etanercept in terms of efficacy and safety. May be used as first-line systemic treatment for chronic plaque psoriasis.
Secukinumab	Monoclonal antibody targeting IL-17A	Effective for moderate-severe psoriasis, greater efficacy compared to ustekinumab
Ixekizumab	Monoclonal antibody targeting IL-17A	Recently approved for moderate-severe psoriasis, highest efficacy of all the biologics
Apremilast	PDE-4 inhibitor	Oral medication taken twice daily. Similar in efficacy to methotrexate, similar in cost to biologics. Second-line for moderate-severe psoriasis. May be used in psoriatic arthritis.

Abbreviations: IL, interleukin; TNF, tumor necrosis factor; PDE-4, phosphodiesterase-4.

(excluding acitretin and apremilast) have immunosuppressant effects and therefore require baseline evaluation, including:

- CBC with differential, renal and hepatic function testing.
- Tuberculosis screening with purified protein derivative (PPD) or QuantiFERON-TB Gold.
- Hepatitis and HIV serologies to exclude chronic hepatitis B, C and HIV.
- Vaccination status, preferably completing required vaccinations prior to treatment.
- Pregnancy test in women of childbearing age (methotrexate and cyclosporine).
- Psoriasis Area and Severity Index (PASI) is the most widely used tool for the measurement of severity of psoriasis. PASI combines the assessment of the severity of lesions and the area affected into a single score in the range 0 (no disease) to 72 (maximal disease)
- A 75% reduction in the PASI score (PASI-75) is the current benchmark of primary endpoints for most clinical trials

Methotrexate:

- Methotrexate has been used for over 50 years in the treatment of psoriatic skin, nail and arthritic disease. A meta-analysis of 11 RCTs found that 45.2% (95% CI 34.1–60.0) of patients achieve PASI-75 after 16 weeks of treatment.[21] SOR Ⓐ
- Methotrexate (MTX) is given as a weekly dose of 5 to 25 mg/week depending on response and side effects. The starting dose is between 5 and 10 mg/week for the first week, then escalated with monitoring to obtain a therapeutic target dose of 15 to 25 mg/week. Oral dosing is preferred, but intravenous, intramuscular, and subcutaneous delivery is available in cases of intolerable GI side effects (same dosing as oral).
- Major side effects include hepatotoxicity, pulmonary fibrosis, bone marrow suppression, and fetal malformations. Folic acid 1 mg daily helps mitigate hepatotoxic and hematologic side effects. Women of childbearing age should be counseled and use effective contraception. A CBC and complete metabolic panel (CMP) should be monitored regularly. Expert consensus recommends liver biopsy after a cumulative dose of 3.5 g in low-risk patients and 1.5 g in high-risk patients.[22] SOR Ⓒ Risk factors for hepatotoxicity include diabetes mellitus, obesity, excessive alcohol use, and history of liver disease such as chronic hepatitis B or C. Noninvasive markers of liver fibrosis include the serum tests FibroSURE and procollagen III peptide, and transient elastography (FibroScan). One small study suggested that 2 of these 3 tests be abnormal before requiring liver biopsy.[23] SOR Ⓑ Still, the question of whether or when to do a liver biopsy and/or stop MTX is controversial.
- Methotrexate is less effective than biologic agents.[24] An RCT of 271 patients comparing methotrexate to adalimumab found that 36% vs. 80%, respectively, reached PASI-75 after 16 weeks of treatment.[25]

Cyclosporine:

- Cyclosporine is a T-cell inhibitor and is an effective, rapid treatment for psoriasis. The recommended starting dose is 2.5 to 5 mg/kg/day orally divided twice a day.[11] SOR Ⓑ
- Major side effects include renal toxicity and hypertension, which are dose-related. Serum creatinine and blood pressure should be measured monthly, along with CBC, uric acid, potassium, lipids, liver function tests (LFTs), and magnesium. Cyclosporine is associated with increased risk of premature birth but not major fetal malformations, and it may be used in pregnancy.
- Cyclosporine is very effective for treating psoriasis flares, but can be used for maintenance with up to a 1-year maximum per U.S. guidelines and 2-year maximum per European guidelines.[26,27]
- Cyclosporine is comparable in efficacy to methotrexate doses of 15 mg/week.[28] SOR Ⓑ

Acitretin:

- Acitretin is a potent oral retinoid used for psoriasis. As monotherapy, acitretin may be particularly effective in pustular psoriasis, including palmoplantar, compared with plaque-type psoriasis.[29] SOR Ⓑ
- Major side effects include hepatotoxicity and hypertriglyceridemia; therefore lipid levels and LFTs should be monitored. Because acitretin is a known teratogenic medication than can remain in the body for 3 years after cessation, it contraindicated in women of childbearing age. Low-dose acitretin (25 mg/day) is better tolerated with fewer adverse effects than 50 mg/day.[30] SOR Ⓑ
- Acitretin may be added to phototherapy to improve clearance and reduce UV exposure.[18] SOR Ⓑ

Biologics:

Biologic agents have become a mainstay of treatment for moderate to severe psoriasis in the past 10 years, and several new agents are available. Treatments approved by the U.S. Food and Drug Administration (FDA) include the TNF-α inhibitors (etanercept, adalimumab, and infliximab) and the anti-interleukin monoclonal antibodies (ustekinumab—IL-12/23, secukinumab—IL-17A, and ixekizumab—IL-17A) (**Table 158-5**).

- Biologic agents are administered either via the subcutaneous route or as an intravenous infusion at regular intervals, ranging from twice a week to every 12 weeks (see **Table 158-5**).
- Safety concerns for biologics include risk of serious infection and cytopenia. TNF-a inhibitors have been associated with increased risk of autoimmune conditions (lupus, demyelinating disease), congestive heart failure, and malignancy (lymphoma).[10] Therefore, in addition to the baseline evaluation discussed, a CBC with differential, LFTs, creatinine, and electrolytes should be monitored every 6 months and tuberculosis (TB) screening yearly. Patients should be offered participation in long-term safety registries (Psoriasis Longitudinal Assessment and Registry [PSOLAR]). An observational study of more than 12,000 patients from PSOLAR found no increased risk of death, malignancy, or major cardiovascular events among patients treated with biologic compared to nonbiologic agents.[31]
- A meta-analysis of 27 RCTs found that infliximab was the most effective short-term biologic for psoriasis, followed by secukinumab and ustekinumab (PASI-75 95.9%, 90.9%, and 73.6%, respectively). Ustekinumab had the best safety profile.[32] SOR Ⓐ
- Infliximab has a faster onset of action than other biologic agents, but the highest incidence of serious infection.[32,33] SOR Ⓐ
- Interleukin-17A antibody. 300 mg SQ weekly × 5 weeks then every 4 weeks. Comparable to ustekinumab in efficacy and tolerability.

TABLE 158-5 FDA-Approved Biologic Agents for Treating Psoriasis

	Adalimumab (Humira)	Etanercept (Enbrel)	Infliximab (Remicade)	Ixekizumab (Taltz)	Secukinumab (Cosentyx)	Ustekinumab (Stelara)
Mechanism of Action	TNF-α inhibitor	TNF-α inhibitor	TNF-α inhibitor	Monoclonal antibody targeting IL-17A	Monoclonal antibody targeting IL-17A	Monoclonal antibody targeting IL-12 and IL-23
Dose	SQ every 2 weeks	SQ 1-2 times a week	IV infusion every 8 weeks	SQ every 2 weeks for three months, then every 4 weeks	SQ every 4 weeks	SQ every 12 weeks
Clear/nearly clear (PASI 90) at 12–16 weeks[24] (95% CI)	34% (23–46)	23% (17–29)	45% (30–61)	68% (58–77)	58% (48–68)	41% (34–39)

Abbreviations: CI, confidence index; IL, Interleukin; TNF, tumor necrosis factor; SQ, subcutaneous; IV, intravenous; PASI, Psoriasis Area and Severity Index.

PASI is used to express the severity of psoriasis. It combines the severity (erythema, induration, and desquamation) and percentage of affected area (lower number is better and the highest number for worst disease is 72); PASI 90 = 90% reduction in PASI score—excellent improvement.

Jabbar-Lopez ZK, et al. Quantitative Evaluation of Biologic Therapy Options for Psoriasis: A Systematic Review and Network Meta-Analysis. *J Invest Dermatol.* 2017.[24]

- Ixekizumab is a recently approved IL-17A antibody with high levels of efficacy. Two large RCTs found that at 12 weeks of treatment, PASI-75 rates of ixekizumab vs etanercept were 87–90% and 42–53%, respectively.[34] Up to 75% of patients maintained PASI-75 at 60 weeks of continued treatment with ixekizumab.[35] SOR Ⓐ A recent meta-analysis of 41 RCTs found that ixekizumab was the highest ranked in terms of efficacy and tolerability compared to all other biologic therapies.[24] SOR Ⓐ
- Biologic agents are effective for psoriatic arthritis and should be considered early for patients with severe, erosive PsA.[11] SOR Ⓐ
- Although the biologic agents are all very expensive, insurance often pays, and there are patient assistance programs for uninsured patients with limited resources. Prior authorization forms may require the prescribing physician to be a dermatologist.

Apremilast

- Apremilast is a phosphodiesterase-4 (PDE-4) inhibitor recently approved for psoriasis, given as an oral dose of 30 mg twice daily.[36] SOR Ⓐ Its theoretical mechanism of action is to block cytokine production, thereby improving psoriasis.
- Diarrhea is a common side effect, and it is recommended to titrate up the dose during the first week. Patients may also experience weight loss, nausea, headaches, and depression.
- Apremilast is similar in cost to the biologics, but similar in efficacy to methotrexate with one study reporting 28.8% of patients reaching PASI-75 at 16 weeks.[36,37] SOR Ⓐ It is useful for patients with PsA who are not candidates for methotrexate, but do not require biologics.

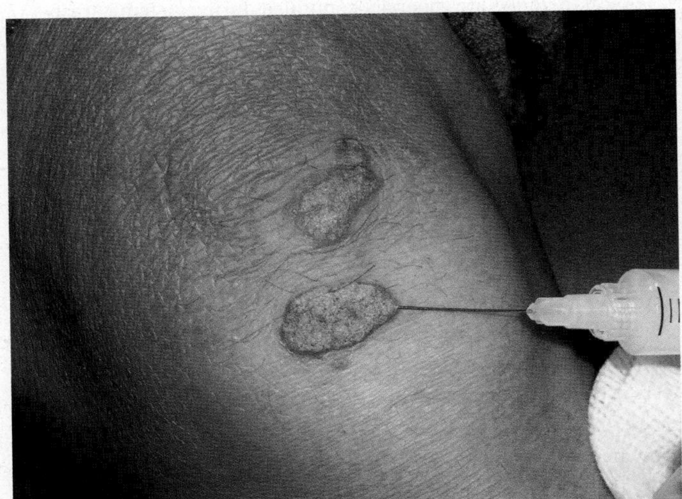

FIGURE 158-32 Intralesional injection of small plaques over the knee that were resistant to treatment with high-potency topical steroids. A 27-gauge needle was employed with 5 mg/mL triamcinolone. *(Reproduced with permission from Richard P. Usatine, MD.)*

THERAPY BY TYPE OF PSORIASIS

▶ Plaque type

Mild plaque psoriasis:

First-line options include the following topical treatments: corticosteroids, vitamin D analogs, tazarotene, calcineurin inhibitor (flexures and face), and targeted phototherapy (see **Table 158-3**).[11]

- Most patients may be started with a very potent topical corticosteroid, such as clobetasol, twice daily for 2–4 weeks. Once controlled, topical vitamin D can be applied twice daily during the week and corticosteroid on the weekend for maintenance.
- Another option is to apply a very potent topical corticosteroid in the morning and topical vitamin D in the evening.

Second-line treatment includes the short-term use of a systemic agent and older agents such as anthralin and coal tar.[11]

- Systemic agent may be considered for patients who fail topical treatments, or who wish to gain rapid control (for example, who have an upcoming wedding).[11]
- Intralesional steroids may be effective for small plaques (**Figure 158-32**). Typically, triamcinolone acetonide 5 to 10 mg/mL is injected using a 27-gauge needle directly into the plaque. SOR Ⓒ

Moderate to severe plaque psoriasis:

First-line options for patients with more significant disease include UV-based and systemic treatments. Additional indications include failed topical treatment; those with affected vulnerable areas, such as the face, hands, feet, or genitals; and those with poor quality of life.

- Patients with access to UV-based therapy should be offered UV treatment.[11]
- NB-UVB therapy may be combined with methotrexate or acitretin,[11] and PUVA may be combined with acitretin.
- Patients without access to UV treatment may be offered systemic agents.
- Topical therapies are generally continued during systemic treatment for symptomatic relief.
- Biologics should be considered if methotrexate and cyclosporine have failed, are not tolerated, or are contraindicated.[11]

Second-line treatments of moderate to severe disease include infliximab, acitretin monotherapy, and apremilast.

▶ Scalp

A recent meta-analysis of nearly 12,000 patients found that potent topical corticosteroids are the most effective treatment for scalp psoriasis.[38] SOR Ⓐ Topical vitamin D preparations are less effective than corticosteroids and cause more irritation. Although combination corticosteroid–vitamin D products are available, the benefit is small compared to potent corticosteroids alone.

First-line therapies:

- Fluocinonide solution applied daily
- Derma-smooth, a combination product of a high-potency steroid and peanut oil

Second-line therapies alone or in combination with a first-line therapy:

- Shampoos with tar and/or salicylic acid (Neutrogena T-Gel and T-Sal) have a keratolytic effect to dissolve and wash away scale
- Systemic treatments

▶ Guttate psoriasis

UV therapy is the first-line treatment for guttate psoriasis, mainly based on experience with plaque psoriasis and the widespread nature of disease.[8] SOR Ⓒ NB-UVB is preferred because of its safety and efficacy profile, especially in children and young adults.[11] SOR Ⓒ Topical therapies can be used if phototherapy is not available.[8] SOR Ⓒ Although there is an association between recent streptococcal pharyngitis and guttate psoriasis, evidence is lacking to support routine antibiotics.[39]

▶ Inverse psoriasis

Effective topical treatments for inverse psoriasis include mid- to high-potency steroids, vitamin D analogs, and calcineurin inhibitors.[13] SOR Ⓑ Topical corticosteroids should be limited because of increased penetration in skin folds and risk of skin atrophy. Topical calcineurin inhibitors have similar efficacy to vitamin D analogs.[13] SOR Ⓑ Patients may find topical vitamin D preparations irritating, especially in the skin folds. Topical calcineurin inhibitors may cause a warm sensation or pruritus with initial application, and patients should be counseled that this may improve with time. Applying an emollient to affected areas after bathing may also be beneficial.[11] SOR Ⓒ

▶ Palmar-plantar psoriasis

All patients should be encouraged to quit smoking because of the strong association of palmar-plantar psoriasis with smoking.[40] SOR Ⓒ Topical treatments, as in plaque psoriasis, are a first-line treatment for mild disease and should be applied under occlusion.[11] For moderate to severe cases, first-line options include acitretin and PUVA, alone or in combination. Second-line options cases include MTX and the biologics.

▶ Erythrodermic/generalized psoriasis

Treatment considerations include hospitalization for dehydration, close monitoring, and broad-spectrum antibiotics for secondary infection and sepsis. Cyclosporine is a first-line treatment option that is very effective in rapidly treating the most severe erythrodermic psoriasis (see **Figure 158-25**).[41] SOR Ⓒ Other options include MTX, acitretin, and the biologics—in particular infliximab due to its rapid onset of action.[11,42] Topical corticosteroids and emollients applied under occlusion provide symptomatic relief and restore the skin barrier.[11]

▶ Pustular psoriasis

Acitretin is the preferred first-line treatment for relatively stable pustular psoriasis.[43] SOR Ⓑ Additional options include MTX and cyclosporine. For patients with severe, acute flares of pustular psoriasis, hospitalization may be required. Cyclosporine has a long history as an effective, rapid treatment of acute pustular psoriasis, with marked improvement occurring within a few days of initiating treatment. SOR Ⓒ Infliximab may also be used in acute flares. SOR Ⓒ One strategy is to start cyclosporine and acitretin together and to stop the cyclosporine once the pustules have cleared. Second-line options include the other biologics, PUVA + acitretin or cyclosporine, or a combination of a first-line agent and biologic.[43] Systemic corticosteroid therapy should be avoided in all patients with psoriasis, as it can provoke life-threatening pustular flares (see **Figure 158-26**). SOR Ⓒ

SPECIAL CIRCUMSTANCES

- Pregnancy. Approximately 50% of women will note spontaneous improvement of their psoriasis during pregnancy, and others will note no change or worsening.[44] Topical emollients and corticosteroids are the mainstay of treatment, and potent corticosteroids should be limited because of association with low birth weight. NB-UVB is preferred for women who need additional control. Biologic agents have shown safety in pregnancy, with the most data for anti-TNF-a agents and cyclosporine.[45] Pustular psoriasis of pregnancy is a generalized pustular psoriasis that occurs in pregnant women, usually without a prior history of psoriasis, and is associated with poor fetal outcomes. Prompt systemic treatment and close fetal monitoring are required.
- Hepatitis C. UVB is preferred in patients with moderate to severe disease, in additional to topical therapies.[46] Methotrexate should be avoided due to the potential for liver toxicity.
- Tonsillectomy. A systematic review of 20 low-quality trials found that 70% of patients reported improvement in psoriasis after tonsillectomy.[47] Because of the low quality of the studies, tonsillectomy should be considered only for patients with recalcitrant psoriasis in association with episodes of tonsillitis.

PROGNOSIS

Prognosis depends on several factors, including psoriasis subtype. Palmar-plantar psoriasis is the most difficult to treat. Although erythrodermic and generalized pustular psoriasis are the most immediately dangerous types, the response to treatment may vary from excellent to disappointing. Widespread plaque psoriasis is challenging—the prognosis is not easily predictable, and patient adherence is a very important factor. New biologic agents have the potential to control previously severe, recalcitrant disease.

FOLLOW-UP

Patients with moderate to severe psoriasis should be followed initially at 3 months after treatment initiation and then every 6 months. Patients should be assessed for adequate treatment response, medication side effects, and appropriate laboratory monitoring. A recent expert consensus panel defined an adequate treatment response as <3% BSA or 75% improvement in BSA involvement from baseline, with a target response of <1% BSA.[48] Patients should be asked about joint symptoms, including morning stiffness lasting more than 30 minutes, to screen for PsA. Well-controlled psoriasis on topical agents does not require frequent follow-up.

PATIENT EDUCATION

Patients should be counseled that psoriasis cannot be cured, but can be managed effectively. Time should be taken to listen to patients, develop shared treatment goals, and educate patients so that they feel empowered to take control of their disease. Physicians should emphasize skin care, importance of adherence to topical medications, and lifestyle changes such as smoking cessation and weight management. Patients need to develop a trusting relationship with a family physician or dermatologist to control the psoriasis for maximum quality of life. **Table 158-6** lists discussion points.

TABLE 158-6 Discussion Points for Healthcare Provider and Patient at Initial Visits

- Hereditary aspects
- Systemic manifestations
- Exacerbating and ameliorating factors
- Past treatment responses
- Range of therapeutic options
- Chronic long-term disease
- Psychological issues
- Optimism for tomorrow based on rapid research developments
- Support/services available from the National Psoriasis Foundation

PATIENT RESOURCES

- The National Psoriasis Foundation—**www.psoriasis.org.**

PROVIDER RESOURCES

- Hsu S, Papp KA, Lebwohl MG, et al. Consensus guidelines for the management of plaque psoriasis. *Arch Dermatol.* 2012;148(1):95-102—**http://archderm.ama-assn.org/cgi/content/short/148/1/95.**
- Guidelines of Care for the Management of Psoriasis and Psoriatic Arthritis: 6 parts published in *Journal of the American Academy of Dermatology* from 2008 to 2011.
- The National Psoriasis Foundation. This includes a Pocket Guide that can be downloaded as a PDF. This excellent pocket guide includes treatment algorithms for specific patient types, combination therapies, and transitional strategies for switching meds. By joining the NPF you can get this printed guide for your pocket—**http://www.psoriasis.org/health-care-providers/treating-psoriasis.**
- Medscape. *Psoriasis*—**http://emedicine.medscape.com/article/1943419.**

REFERENCES

1. Parisi R, Symmons DP, Griffiths CE, et al. Global epidemiology of psoriasis: a systematic review of incidence and prevalence. *J Invest Dermatol.* 2013;133(2):377-385.
2. Helmick CG, Lee-Han H, Hirsch SC, et al. Prevalence of psoriasis among adults in the U.S.: 2003-2006 and 2009-2010 National Health and Nutrition Examination Surveys. *Am J Prev Med.* 2014; 47(1):37-45.

3. Di Lernia V, Ficarelli E, Lallas A, Ricci C. Familial aggregation of moderate to severe plaque psoriasis. *Clin Exp Dermatol.* 2014; 39(7):801-805.
4. Harden JL, Krueger JG, Bowcock AM. The immunogenetics of psoriasis: a comprehensive review. *J Autoimmun.* 2015;64:66-73.
5. Armstrong AW, Harskamp CT, Armstrong EJ. The association between psoriasis and obesity: a systematic review and meta-analysis of observational studies. *Nutr Diabetes.* 2012;2:e54.
6. Armstrong AW, Harskamp CT, Dhillon JS, Armstrong EJ. Psoriasis and smoking: a systematic review and meta-analysis. *Br J Dermatol.* 2014;170(2):304-314.
7. Qureshi AA, Dominguez PL, Choi HK, et al. Alcohol intake and risk of incident psoriasis in US women: a prospective study. *Arch Dermatol.* 2010;146(12):1364-1369.
8. Callen JP, Krueger GG, Lebwohl M, et al. AAD consensus statement on psoriasis therapies. *J Am Acad Dermatol.* 2003;49(5):897-899.
9. Icen M, Crowson CS, McEvoy MT, et al. Trends in incidence of adult-onset psoriasis over three decades: a population-based study. *J Am Acad Dermatol.* 2009;60(3):394-401.
10. Gottlieb A, Korman NJ, Gordon KB, et al. Guidelines of care for the management of psoriasis and psoriatic arthritis: Section 2. Psoriatic arthritis: overview and guidelines of care for treatment with an emphasis on the biologics. *J Am Acad Dermatol.* 2008; 58(5):851-864.
11. American Academy of Dermatology Work G, Menter A, Korman NJ, et al. Guidelines of care for the management of psoriasis and psoriatic arthritis: section 6. Guidelines of care for the treatment of psoriasis and psoriatic arthritis: case-based presentations and evidence-based conclusions. *J Am Acad Dermatol.* 2011;65(1): 137-174.
12. Samarasekera EJ, Sawyer L, Wonderling D, et al. Topical therapies for the treatment of plaque psoriasis: systematic review and network meta-analyses. *Br J Dermatol.* 2013;168(5):954-967.
13. Mason AR, Mason J, Cork M, Dooley G, Hancock H. Topical treatments for chronic plaque psoriasis. *Cochrane Database Syst Rev.* 2013(3):CD005028.
14. Camarasa JM, Ortonne JP, Dubertret L. Calcitriol shows greater persistence of treatment effect than betamethasone dipropionate in topical psoriasis therapy. *J Dermatolog Treat.* 2003;14(1):8-13.
15. Sugarman JL, Gold LS, Lebwohl MG, et al. A phase 2, multicenter, double-blind, randomized, vehicle controlled clinical study to assess the safety and efficacy of a halobetasol/tazarotene fixed combination in the treatment of plaque psoriasis. *J Drugs Dermatol.* 2017;16(3):197-204.
16. Castela E, Archier E, Devaux S, et al. Topical corticosteroids in plaque psoriasis: a systematic review of efficacy and treatment modalities. *J Eur Acad Dermatol Venereol.* 2012;26 Suppl 3:36-46.
17. Almutawa F, Alnomair N, Wang Y, et al. Systematic review of UV-based therapy for psoriasis. *Am J Clin Dermatol.* 2013;14(2):87-109.
18. Chen X, Yang M, Cheng Y, et al. Narrow-band ultraviolet B phototherapy versus broad-band ultraviolet B or psoralen-ultraviolet A photochemotherapy for psoriasis. *Cochrane Database Syst Rev.* 2013(10):CD009481.
19. Stern RS, Study PF-U. The risk of squamous cell and basal cell cancer associated with psoralen and ultraviolet A therapy: a 30-year prospective study. *J Am Acad Dermatol.* 2012;66(4):553-562.
20. Feldman SR, Mellen BG, Housman TS, et al. Efficacy of the 308-nm excimer laser for treatment of psoriasis: results of a multicenter study. *J Am Acad Dermatol.* 2002;46(6):900-906.
21. West J, Ogston S, Foerster J. Safety and efficacy of methotrexate in psoriasis: a meta-analysis of published trials. *PLoS One.* 2016; 11(5):e0153740.
22. Kalb RE, Strober B, Weinstein G, Lebwohl M. Methotrexate and psoriasis: 2009 National Psoriasis Foundation Consensus Conference. *J Am Acad Dermatol.* 2009;60(5):824-837.
23. Lynch M, Higgins E, McCormick PA, et al. The use of transient elastography and FibroTest for monitoring hepatotoxicity in patients receiving methotrexate for psoriasis. *JAMA Dermatol.* 2014;150(8):856-862.
24. Jabbar-Lopez ZK, Yiu ZZN, Ward V, et al. Quantitative evaluation of biologic therapy options for psoriasis: a systematic review and network meta-analysis. *J Invest Dermatol.* 2017;137(8):1646-1654.
25. Saurat JH, Stingl G, Dubertret L, et al. Efficacy and safety results from the randomized controlled comparative study of adalimumab vs. methotrexate vs. placebo in patients with psoriasis (CHAMPION). *Br J Dermatol.* 2008;158(3):558-566.
26. Nast A, Kopp I, Augustin M, et al. German evidence-based guidelines for the treatment of psoriasis vulgaris (short version). *Arch Dermatol Res.* 2007;299(3):111-138.
27. Rosmarin DM, Lebwohl M, Elewski BE, Gottlieb AB, National Psoriasis Foundation. Cyclosporine and psoriasis: 2008 National Psoriasis Foundation Consensus Conference. *J Am Acad Dermatol.* 2010;62(5):838-853.
28. Schmitt J, Rosumeck S, Thomaschewski G, et al. Efficacy and safety of systemic treatments for moderate-to-severe psoriasis: meta-analysis of randomized controlled trials. *Br J Dermatol.* 2014;170(2):274-303.
29. Sbidian E, Maza A, Montaudie H, et al. Efficacy and safety of oral retinoids in different psoriasis subtypes: a systematic literature review. *J Eur Acad Dermatol Venereol.* 2011;25 Suppl 2:28-33.
30. Haushalter K, Murad EJ, Dabade TS, et al. Efficacy of low-dose acitretin in the treatment of psoriasis. *J Dermatolog Treat.* 2012;23(6):400-403.
31. Papp K, Gottlieb AB, Naldi L, et al. Safety surveillance for ustekinumab and other psoriasis treatments from the Psoriasis Longitudinal Assessment and Registry (PSOLAR). *J Drugs Dermatol.* 2015;14(7):706-714.
32. Gomez-Garcia F, Epstein D, Isla-Tejera B, et al. Short-term efficacy and safety of new biological agents targeting the interleukin-23-T helper 17 pathway for moderate-to-severe plaque psoriasis: a systematic review and network meta-analysis. *Br J Dermatol.* 2017;176(3):594-603.
33. Nast A, Sporbeck B, Rosumeck S, et al. Which antipsoriatic drug has the fastest onset of action? Systematic review on the rapidity of the onset of action. *J Invest Dermatol.* 2013;133(8): 1963-1970.

34. Griffiths CE, Reich K, Lebwohl M, et al. Comparison of ixekizumab with etanercept or placebo in moderate-to-severe psoriasis (UNCOVER-2 and UNCOVER-3): results from two phase 3 randomised trials. *Lancet.* 2015;386(9993):541-551.
35. Gordon KB, Blauvelt A, Papp KA, et al. Phase 3 trials of ixekizumab in moderate-to-severe plaque psoriasis. *N Engl J Med.* 2016;375(4):345-356.
36. Paul C, Cather J, Gooderham M, et al. Efficacy and safety of apremilast, an oral phosphodiesterase 4 inhibitor, in patients with moderate-to-severe plaque psoriasis over 52 weeks: a phase III, randomized controlled trial (ESTEEM 2). *Br J Dermatol.* 2015; 173(6):1387-1399.
37. Armstrong AW, Betts KA, Sundaram M, et al. Comparative efficacy and incremental cost per responder of methotrexate versus apremilast for methotrexate-naive patients with psoriasis. *J Am Acad Dermatol.* 2016;75(4):740-746.
38. Schlager JG, Rosumeck S, Werner RN, et al. Topical treatments for scalp psoriasis. *Cochrane Database Syst Rev.* 2016;2: CD009687.
39. Owen CM, Chalmers RJ, O'Sullivan T, Griffiths CE. A systematic review of antistreptococcal interventions for guttate and chronic plaque psoriasis. *Br J Dermatol.* 2001;145(6):886-890.
40. Brunasso AM, Puntoni M, Aberer W, et al. Clinical and epidemiological comparison of patients affected by palmoplantar plaque psoriasis and palmoplantar pustulosis: a case series study. *Br J Dermatol.* 2013;168(6):1243-1251.
41. Hsu S, Papp KA, Lebwohl MG, et al. Consensus guidelines for the management of plaque psoriasis. *Arch Dermatol.* 2012;148(1): 95-102.
42. Rosenbach M, Hsu S, Korman NJ, et al. Treatment of erythrodermic psoriasis: from the medical board of the National Psoriasis Foundation. *J Am Acad Dermatol.* 2010;62(4):655-662.
43. Robinson A, Van Voorhees AS, Hsu S, et al. Treatment of pustular psoriasis: from the Medical Board of the National Psoriasis Foundation. *J Am Acad Dermatol.* 2012;67(2):279-288.
44. Murase JE, Chan KK, Garite TJ, et al. Hormonal effect on psoriasis in pregnancy and post partum. *Arch Dermatol.* 2005;141(5):601-606.
45. Porter ML, Lockwood SJ, Kimball AB. Update on biologic safety for patients with psoriasis during pregnancy. *Int J Womens Dermatol.* 2017;3(1):21-25.
46. Frankel AJ, Van Voorhees AS, Hsu S, et al. Treatment of psoriasis in patients with hepatitis C: from the Medical Board of the National Psoriasis Foundation. *J Am Acad Dermatol.* 2009;61(6):1044-1055.
47. Rachakonda TD, Dhillon JS, Florek AG, Armstrong AW. Effect of tonsillectomy on psoriasis: a systematic review. *J Am Acad Dermatol.* 2015;72(2):261-275.
48. Armstrong AW, Siegel MP, Bagel J, et al. From the Medical Board of the National Psoriasis Foundation: Treatment targets for plaque psoriasis. *J Am Acad Dermatol.* 2017;76(2):290-298.

159 PITYRIASIS ROSEA

Lina M. Cardona, MD
David Henderson, MD
Richard P. Usatine, MD

PATIENT STORY

A 17-year-old young woman is brought to the office by her mom because of a rash that appeared 3 weeks ago for no apparent reason (**Figures 159-1** to **159-3**). She was feeling well and the rash is only occasionally pruritic. With and without mom in the room, the young woman denied sexual activity. The diagnosis of pityriasis rosea was made by the clinical appearance even though there was no obvious herald patch. The collarette scale was visible and the distribution was consistent with pityriasis rosea. The young woman and her mom were reassured that this would resolve spontaneously. At a subsequent visit for a college physical, the skin was found to be completely clear with no scarring.

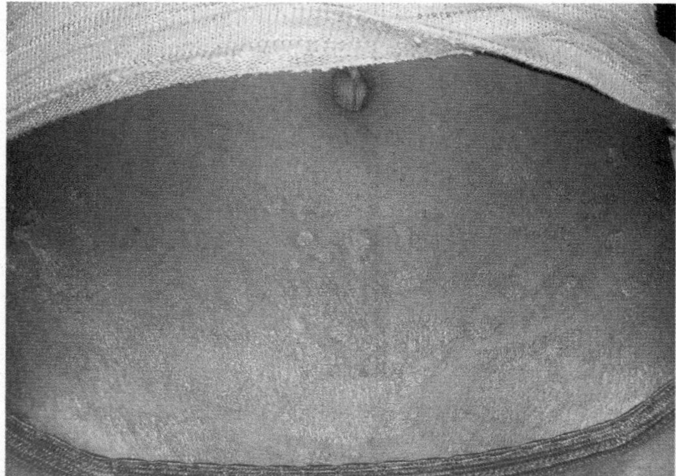

FIGURE 159-1 Pityriasis rosea in a 17-year-old young woman. Lesions are often concentrated in the lower abdominal area. (*Reproduced with permission from Richard P. Usatine, MD.*)

INTRODUCTION

Pityriasis rosea (PR) is a common, self-limited, papulosquamous skin condition originally described in the 19th century. It is seen in children and adults. Despite the long history, its etiology remains elusive. A number of infectious etiologies have been proposed, but at present, supporting evidence is inconclusive. Pityriasis rosea has unique features, including a herald patch that is present in approximately 90% of cases[1] and collarette scale, that are useful in distinguishing it from other papulosquamous eruptions.

EPIDEMIOLOGY

- Pityriasis rosea is a papulosquamous eruption of unknown etiology.
- It occurs throughout the life cycle. It is most commonly seen between the ages of 10 and 35 years.[1-4]
- The peak incidence is between 20 and 29 years of age.[1-4]
- The gender distribution is essentially equal.[1,2,4]
- The rash is most prevalent in winter months.[1,2,4]

ETIOLOGY AND PATHOPHYSIOLOGY

- The cause of pityriasis rosea is unknown, although numerous causes have been proposed.
- It has long been suspected that it may have a viral etiology because a viral-like prodrome often occurs prior to the onset of the rash. Human herpesviruses 6 and 7 have been proposed as causes, but studies have failed to demonstrate conclusive supportive evidence.[1-5] Acyclovir has been successfully used to treat PR based on the premise that it is caused by human herpesviruses 6 and 7.[1-5]

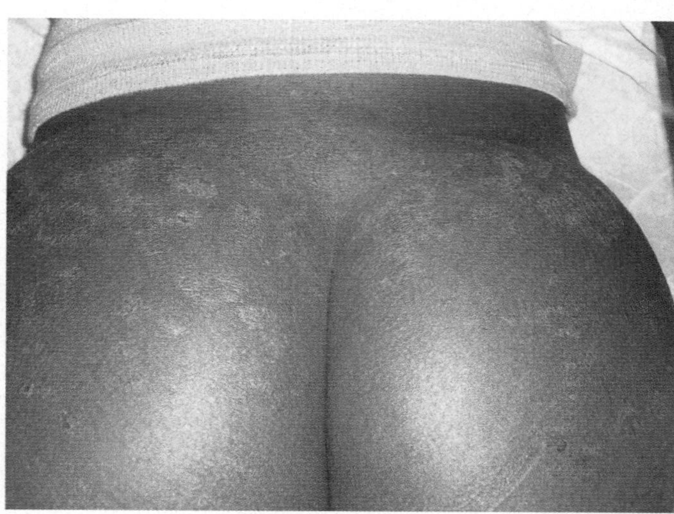

FIGURE 159-2 Scaling lesions seen on the buttocks of the same young woman. Note how some of the lesions are annular. (*Reproduced with permission from Richard P. Usatine, MD.*)

- *Chlamydia, Mycoplasma, Legionella, Epstein-Barr virus, cytomegalovirus,* and *parvovirus B19* have also been proposed as potential etiologic agents, but studies have not demonstrated any significant rise in antibody levels against any of these pathogens in patients with pityriasis rosea.[4]
- Pityriasis rosea has also been associated with negative pregnancy outcomes, particularly premature birth. The risk seems to be greatest when the condition occurs in the first 15 weeks of gestation.[1,2]
- Pityriasis rosea may rarely occur as the result of a drug reaction. Documented drug reactions that have produced a pityriasis rosea-like eruption include angiotensin-converting enzyme inhibitors (ACEIs), beta blockers, diuretics, tumor necrosis factor (TNF) inhibitors, oral retinoids, proton pump inhibitors, metronidazole, anticonvulsants, terbinafine, nonsteroidal anti-inflammatory drugs, clonidine, interferon, bismuth, gold, and vaccines such as hepatitis B and influenza.[1,2,4]

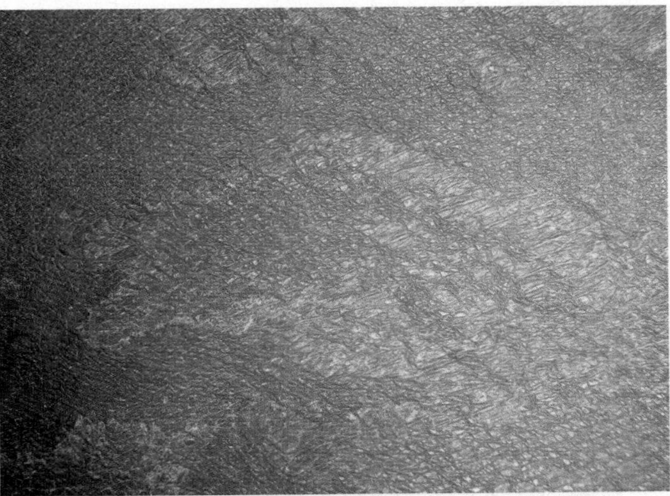

FIGURE 159-3 Close-up of lesion showing collarette scale. Note how the lesions can be annular with some central clearing. (*Reproduced with permission from Richard P. Usatine, MD.*)

DIAGNOSIS

CLINICAL FEATURES

- Pityriasis rosea is accompanied by a viral-like prodrome (fever, malaise, arthralgias, sore throat, nausea, headache, adenopathies) in 69% of cases.[1-4]
- This is followed by the appearance of a *herald patch* in 50% to 90% of cases (**Figures 159-4** to **159-6**).[1-4]
- The herald patch is a solitary, oval, flesh-colored to salmon-colored lesion with scaling at the border. It often occurs on the trunk and is generally 2 to 10 cm in diameter (see **Figures 159-4** and **159-5**).
- One to 2 weeks after the appearance of the herald patch, other papulosquamous lesions appear on the trunk and sometimes on the extremities.
- These lesions vary from oval macules to slightly raised plaques, 0.5 to 2 cm in size. They are salmon colored (or hyperpigmented in individuals with dark skin) and typically have a collarette of scaling at the border (see **Figure 159-3**). It is common for some of the lesions to appear annular with central clearing.
- In many cases, the herald patch has resolved by the time the rest of the exanthem erupts, which can make the diagnosis more difficult.
- There are no systemic symptoms.[1,2]
- Itching occurs in approximately 50% of patients.[1]
- Pityriasis rosea has been reported in closed groups (dormitories, military), favoring an infectious etiology.[1,2]
- Pityriasis rosea can relapse, usually without a herald patch, within 5–18 months after initial presentation in approximately 1% to 3% of patients.[1,2]
- The exanthem resolves in 8 weeks in the majority of patients.[1,2] However, it can last up to 3 to 5 months.[1,2]

TYPICAL DISTRIBUTION

- The rash is bilaterally symmetrical, generally most dense on the trunk, but also involves the upper and lower extremities.
- The lesions follow the cleavage, or Langer lines, and may create the typical *fir* or *Christmas tree* pattern over the back (**Figure 159-7**). Do not expect to always see a Christmas tree pattern.

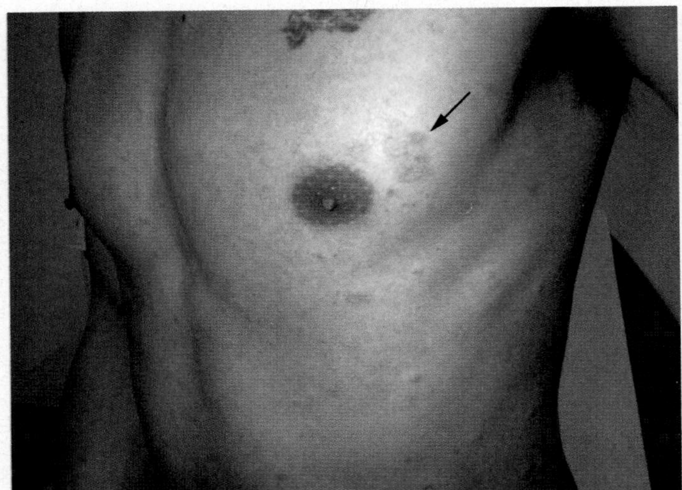

FIGURE 159-4 Pityriasis rosea in a 25-year-old Hispanic man. *Arrow points to herald patch. (Reproduced with permission from Scott Youngquist, MD. Previously published in Youngquist S, Usatine R. It's beginning to look a lot like Christmas. West J Med. 2001;175(4):227-228.)*

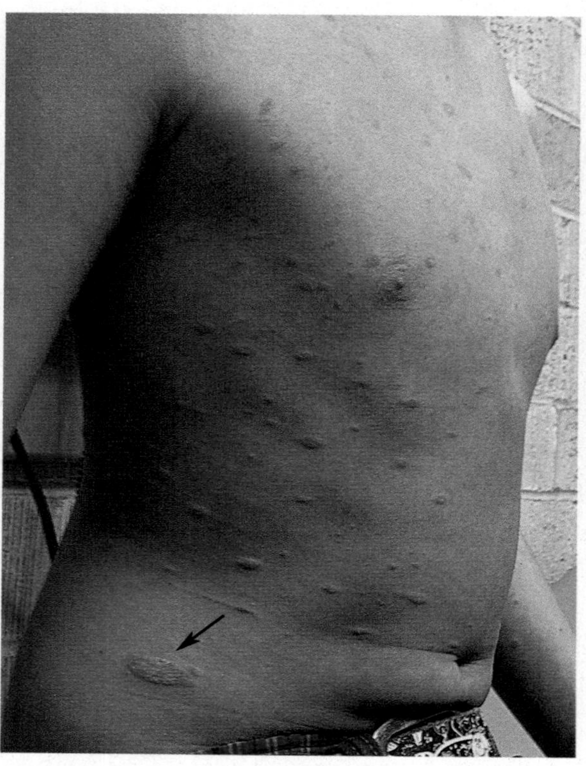

FIGURE 159-5 Pityriasis rosea in a 13-year-old boy. Arrow points to herald patch. (*Reproduced with permission from Richard P. Usatine, MD.*)

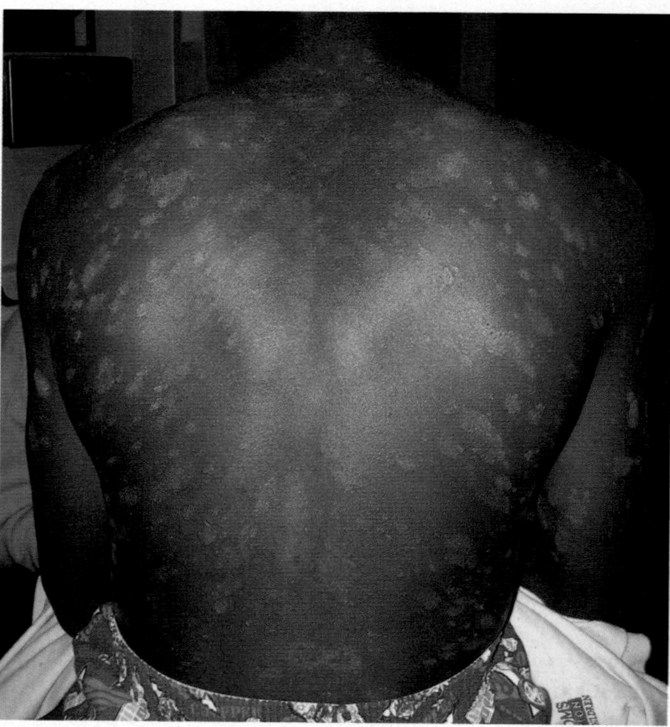

FIGURE 159-7 Pityriasis rosea in a 16-year-old boy. The scaling lesions follow skin lines and resemble a Christmas tree. (*Reproduced with permission from E.J. Mayeaux, Jr., MD.*)

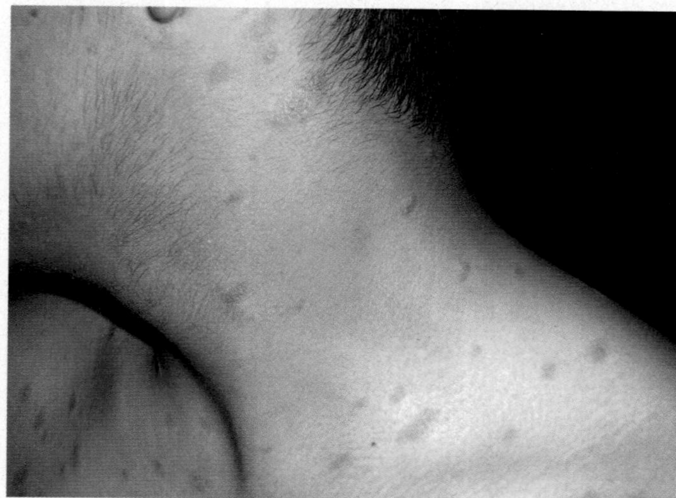

FIGURE 159-6 Pityriasis rosea in a 15-year-old boy with the herald patch on the neck near the hairline. (*Reproduced with permission from Richard P. Usatine, MD.*)

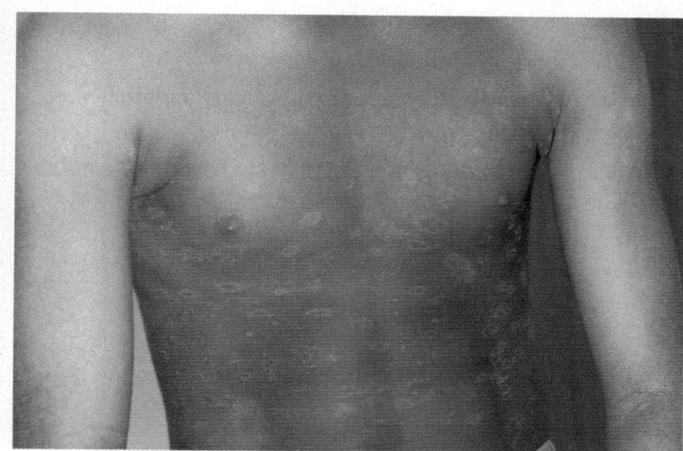

FIGURE 159-8 Pityriasis rosea in a 12-year-old boy showing classic scaling lesions across the chest and abdomen. Small annular lesions are visible. (*Reproduced with permission from Jeffrey Meffert, MD.*)

- Other rare forms of pityriasis rosea have been reported: inverse, oral, papular, vesicular, urticarial, pustular, and purpuric.[4]
- Over the chest, the lesions create a V-shaped pattern and run transversely over the abdomen (**Figures 159-8** and **159-9**).
- An inverse form has been described, characterized by more intense involvement of the extremities and relative sparing of the trunk (**Figures 159-10** and **159-11**).

LABORATORY STUDIES

- Pityriasis rosea is a clinical diagnosis. There are no laboratory tests that aid in the diagnosis.
- Biopsy of lesions typically reveals only nonspecific inflammatory changes such as interface dermatitis. It is usually performed to rule out other conditions (guttate psoriasis, lichen planus, subacute cutaneous lupus erythematosus, cutaneous T-cell lymphoma).[4,5]
- Blood test for syphilis should be considered because secondary syphilis is also a papulosquamous eruption and can be difficult to distinguish from pityriasis rosea on clinical grounds. Taking a sexual history is important when a diagnosis of pityriasis rosea is being considered (see **Figures 159-9** and **159-10**) (see Chapter 225, Syphilis).
- A KOH preparation is helpful to detect tinea corporis (see Chapter 144, Tinea Corporis).
- Dermoscopy shows irregularly distributed or focal dotted vessels with white scaling. Sometimes, yellowish structureless areas are also seen.[6]

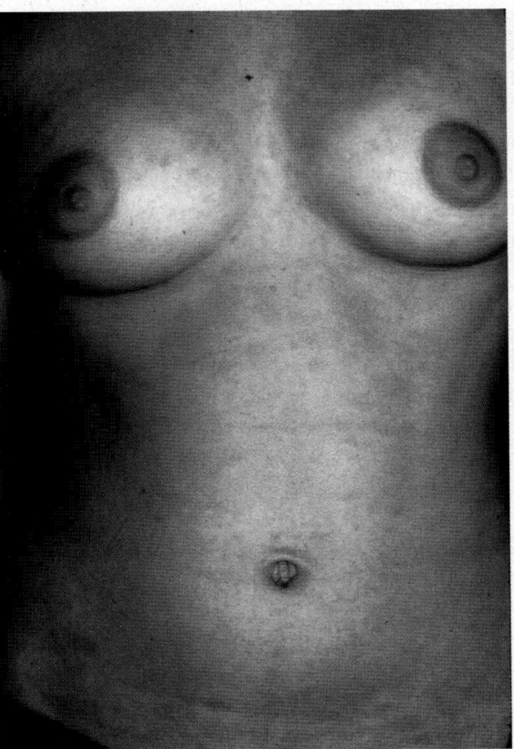

FIGURE 159-9 Pityriasis rosea on the chest and abdomen of a young woman. Blood test for syphilis was negative. (*Reproduced with permission from Richard P. Usatine, MD.*)

DIFFERENTIAL DIAGNOSIS

- Tinea corporis is usually more localized than pityriasis rosea. However, the annular patterns, scale, and central clearing of some lesions in pityriasis rosea can mislead the clinician to misdiagnose tinea corporis. Tinea corporis tends to have fewer annular lesions and may have concentric circles rather than a single ring. Microscopy with KOH usually demonstrates branching hyphae (see Chapter 144, Tinea Corporis).
- Tinea versicolor has a distribution similar to pityriasis rosea but is not associated with a herald patch. The pattern of scaling noted is generally more diffuse and not annular. Microscopy with KOH demonstrates the *spaghetti-and-meatball* pattern typical of *Pityrosporum* (see Chapter 147, Tinea Versicolor).
- Secondary syphilis is also a papulosquamous eruption. Lesions are often found on the palms and soles, which is not the case in pityriasis rosea; however, because the two conditions cannot always be accurately distinguished on clinical grounds, a blood test for syphilis is indicated if there is a significant doubt in the diagnosis (see Chapter 225, Syphilis).
- Nummular eczema has coinlike areas of scale that can resemble pityriasis rosea. The scale is not collarette and nummular eczema has a predilection for the legs, an area that is less often involved with pityriasis rosea (see Chapter 151, Atopic Dermatitis).
- Guttate psoriasis generally presents as oval to round, scaly macules on the trunk and so can be confused with pityriasis rosea. However, the scaling is generally thicker and more adherent than in pityriasis rosea (see Chapter 158, Psoriasis).

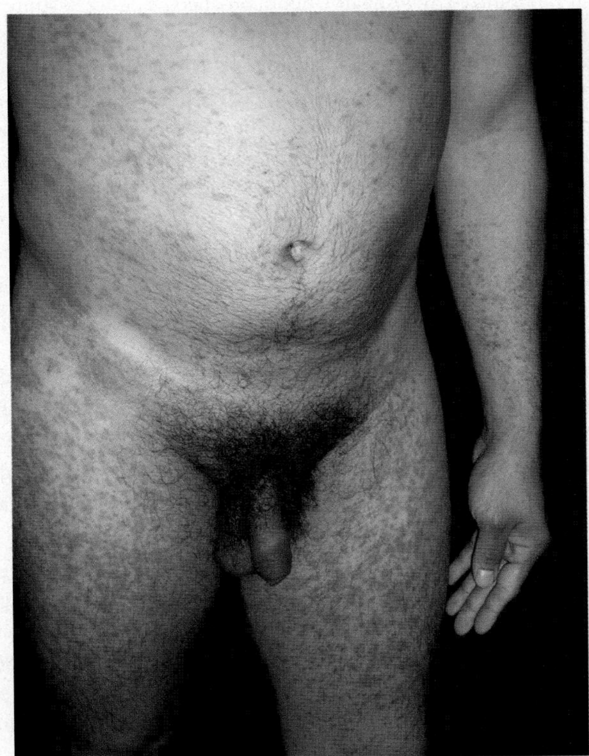

FIGURE 159-10 Pityriasis rosea in a 40-year-old man with an inverse pattern. Note how there is a higher density of lesions on the legs. Rapid plasma reagin (RPR) was negative, and the diagnosis was confirmed with a punch biopsy. (*Reproduced with permission from Richard P. Usatine, MD.*)

MANAGEMENT

FIRST LINE

- Pityriasis rosea may require no treatment at all other than reassurance that it will resolve on its own over 4–8 weeks.
- However, many patients either have symptoms or are worried about waiting 8 weeks for resolution of an extensive rash. The treatment with the current best evidence is acyclovir.[7-13] SOR Ⓑ The evidence for acyclovir is generally supportive, with 5 of the 6 best studies to date supporting the use of acyclovir in PR. Here they are in chronological order to help determine if acyclovir is a good option for your patient:
    - Eighty-seven patients were treated for 1 week with either oral acyclovir (800 mg 5 times daily) or placebo. At 2 weeks, 79% of treated patients fully regressed compared with 4% of the placebo group. The lesions cleared in 18.5 days in treated patients and in 37.9 days in the placebo group. Clearance was achieved in 17.2 days in patients treated in the first week from onset and in 19.7 days in the patients treated later. On the 7th day, there were significantly fewer new lesions in patients treated in the first week than in those treated later. Unfortunately, this trial was neither randomized nor double blind. Objectivity was achieved by counting the lesions. The authors concluded that acyclovir may be effective in the treatment of pityriasis rosea, especially in patients treated in the first week from onset.[7]
    - This next study compared lower dose acyclovir (400 mg five times a day for a week) with follow-up for the treatment of PR. A randomized, investigator-blind, prospective, 4-week study was designed, and 64 patients with PR presenting at the outpatient clinic were randomly allocated to acyclovir or follow-up group. Statistically, acyclovir was more effective than follow-up in reducing erythema and scaling at the end of weeks 1–3 of treatment. The authors concluded that acyclovir may be more effective than follow-up in reducing erythema and shortening of duration of PR even in lower doses.[8]
    - In a randomly assigned comparison between acyclovir and erythromycin, acyclovir was faster in the healing of lesions and the improvement of pruritus in the treatment of PR.[9] This study included some children, and acyclovir dosing was adults: 800 mg five times a day; children: 20 mg/kg/day in five divided doses; maximum dose: 4 g/day; duration: 7 days. Oral erythromycin dosing was adults: 500 mg qid; children: 40 mg/ kg/day in four divided doses; maximum dose: 2 g/day; duration: 7 days. However, in this study all patients received oral cetirizine daily and topical fluocinolone twice daily even if they had no pruritus.[9]
- In another randomized controlled trial (RCT), acyclovir 800 mg five times was compared with placebo and found to be effective in the treatment of PR. The results showed that 53.33% and 86.66% of the patients belonging to the acyclovir group had complete resolution on the 7th day and 14th day, respectively, following the first visit compared to 10% and 33.33% of patients from the placebo group.[10]
- An observer-blind, randomized trial was conducted on 24 adult patients with PR. All patients received oral cetirizine 10 mg daily and topical calamine. Group A received acyclovir 400 mg 3 times

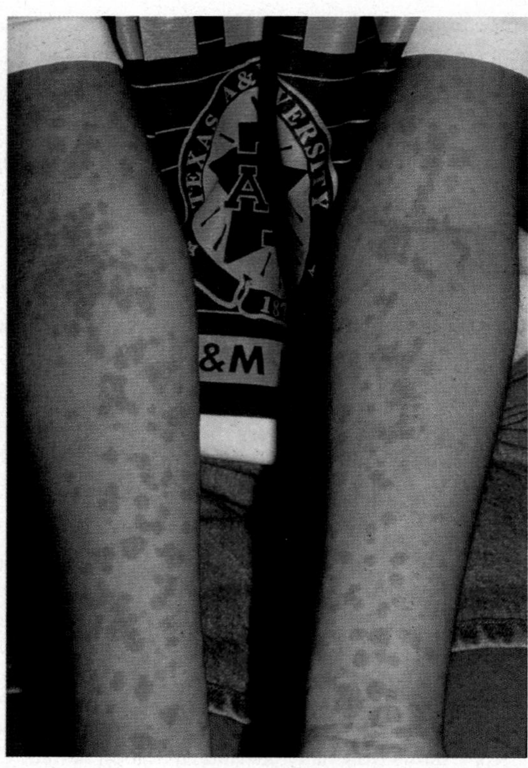

FIGURE 159-11 Pityriasis rosea on the arms with prominent erythematous lesions. (*Reproduced with permission from Richard P. Usatine, MD.*)

daily for 7 days. Group A complained of significantly fewer new lesions than group B (P = 0.046). A complete response was obtained in all patients of group A and 83% patients of group B at the end of the 4 weeks. Acyclovir decreased clinical severity from second week onward as compared to supportive therapy alone.[11]
   - In an RCT that was triple-blinded, acyclovir was not effective for PR. The acyclovir group received 800 mg five times per day for 1 week. The number of days (mean ± standard deviation) for skin clearance was not significantly different between the two groups (placebo 26.5 ± 9.1 days vs. acyclovir 33.2 ± 9.4 days; P = 0.07).[12] This was the only study that did not show some benefit of acyclovir in the treatment of PR.
- A European position statement on the management of patients with pityriasis rosea endorsed the use of acyclovir for patients with severe PR or PR in early pregnancy.[13] SOR B Their statement includes:
   - PR is a self-limiting disease, and most patients do not need any treatment.
   - For patients needing active treatment, oral acyclovir as 400 mg three times daily for 7 days can be considered.
   - When PR occurs in early pregnancy, oral acyclovir could be considered.
   - Inadequate information exists in the use of acyclovir to treat PR in children and breastfeeding women.[13]
- Topical steroids, topical calamine, and oral antihistamines may be used to relieve itching when there is pruritus involved. As noted in 2 studies above, oral cetirizine 10 mg daily was the antihistamine of choice. There are no studies comparing antihistamines versus placebo or comparing one antihistamine versus another. In the one study above that used a topical steroid, a midpotency steroid was chosen. SOR C

SECOND LINE

- One study found oral erythromycin to be effective in treating patients with pityriasis rosea, although a subsequent study did not find erythromycin to be better than placebo.[1,2,4,9,14] SOR B
- Oral steroids have been used in severe cases: prednisolone or prednisone 40 mg daily for 1–2 weeks to alleviate symptoms.[2] Given the safety and effectiveness of acyclovir and the risks of systemic steroids, this is not generally recommended. SOR C
- Azithromycin did not cure pityriasis rosea in a study of children with this condition and is not recommended.[15] SOR B
- Low-dose UVA and UVB phototherapy may improve the eruption and pruritus, but not the clinical course of the disease.[1,2,4] SOR C

FOLLOW-UP

- Patients should be instructed to follow up if the rash persists for longer than 3 months, as reevaluation and consideration of an alternative diagnosis may be prudent.

PATIENT EDUCATION

- Patients are often concerned about the duration of the rash and whether they are contagious. They should be reassured that pityriasis rosea is self-limited and not truly contagious. Although there have been reported clusters of pityriasis rosea in settings where people are living in close quarters (e.g., dormitories, the military), it is not considered to be contagious. It has a reported recurrence rate of only 1% to 3%.[1,2,4]

PATIENT RESOURCES

- Mayo Clinic. *Pityriasis Rosea*—**https://www.mayoclinic.org/diseases-conditions/pityriasis-rosea/symptoms-causes/syc-20376405.**
- WebMD. *What Is Pityriasis Rosea?*—**http://www.webmd.com/skin-problems-and-treatments/whats-pityriasis-rosea#1.**
- American Academy of Dermatology. *Pityriasis Rosea*—**https://www.aad.org/public/diseases/rashes/pityriasis-rosea.**

PROVIDER RESOURCES

- Medscape. *Pityriasis Rosea*—**https://emedicine.medscape.com/article/1107532-overview.**
- American Family Physician. *Pityriasis Rosea: Diagnosis and Treatment*—**https://www.aafp.org/afp/2018/0101/p38.html.**

REFERENCES

1. Villalon-Gomez J. Pityriasis rosea: diagnosis and treatment. *Am Fam Physician.* 2018;97(1):38-44.
2. Habif TP. *Clinical Dermatology: a Color Guide to Diagnosis and Therapy.* 6th ed. St. Louis, MO: Saunders; 2016:263-328.
3. Drago F, Ciccarese G, Broccolo F, et al. Pityriasis rosea in children: clinical features and laboratory investigations. *Dermatology.* 2015;231(1):9-14.
4. Drago F, Ciccarese G. Pityriasis rosea: an update on etiopathogenesis and management of difficult aspects—a reply. *Indian J Dermatol.* 2017;62(1):95.
5. Robera A, Drago F, Broccolo F. Pityriasis rosea and herpesviruses: facts and controversies. *Clin Dermatol.* 2010;28(5):497-501.
6. Errichetti E, Stinco G. Dermoscopy in general dermatology: a practical overview. *Dermatol Ther (Heidelb).* 2016;6(4):471-507.
7. Drago F, Vecchio F, Rebora A. Use of high-dose acyclovir in pityriasis rosea. *J Am Acad Dermatol.* 2006;54(1):82-85.
8. Rassai S, Feily A, Sina N, Abtahian S. Low dose of acyclovir may be an effective treatment against pityriasis rosea: a random investigator-blind clinical trial on 64 patients. *J Eur Acad Dermatol Venereol.* 2011;25(1):24-26.
9. Amatya A, Rajouria EA, Karn DK. Comparative study of effectiveness of oral acyclovir with oral erythromycin in the treatment of pityriasis rosea. *Kathmandu Univ Med J (KUMJ).* 2012;10(37):57-61.
10. Ganguly S. A randomized, double-blind, placebo-controlled study of efficacy of oral acyclovir in the treatment of pityriasis rosea. *J Clin Diagn Res.* 2014;8(5):YC01-YC04.
11. Das A, Sil A, Das NK, et al. Acyclovir in pityriasis rosea: an observer-blind, randomized controlled trial of effectiveness, safety, and tolerability. *Indian Dermatol Online J.* 2015;6:181-184.

12. Singh S, Anurag, Tiwary NK. Acyclovir is not effective in pityriasis rosea: results of a randomized, triple-blind, placebo-controlled trial. *Indian J Dermatol Venereol Leprol.* 2016;82(5):505-509.
13. Chuh A, Zawar V, Sciallis G, Kempf W. A position statement on the management of patients with pityriasis rosea. *J Eur Acad Dermatol Venereol.* 2016;30(10):1670-1681.
14. Rasi A, Tajziehchi L, Savabi-Nasab S. Oral erythromycin is ineffective in the treatment of pityriasis rosea. *J Drugs Dermatol.* 2008;7(1):35-38.
15. Pandhi D, Singal A, Verma P, Sharma R. The efficacy of azithromycin in pityriasis rosea: a randomized, double-blind, placebo-controlled trial. *Indian J Dermatol Venereol Leprol.* 2014;80(1):36-40.

160 LICHEN PLANUS

Robert L. Kraft, MD
Richard P. Usatine, MD

PATIENT STORY

A 38-year-old Hispanic woman presents with a rash on her forearms, wrists, ankle, and back (**Figures 160-1** to **160-4**). She states the rash is mildly itchy and she does not like the way it looks. She would like some medication to make this better. Lichen planus (LP) was diagnosed and clobetasol was prescribed to keep the LP under better control.

INTRODUCTION

LP is a self-limited, recurrent, or chronic autoimmune disease affecting the skin, oral mucosa, and genitalia. LP is generally diagnosed clinically with lesions classically described using the six Ps (planar, purple, polygonal, pruritic, papules, and plaques).

EPIDEMIOLOGY

- LP is an inflammatory dermatosis of skin or mucous membranes that occurs in approximately 1% of all new patients seen at health-care clinics.[1]
- Although most cases occur between ages 30 and 60 years, LP can occur at any age.[1,2]
- There may be a slight female predominance.[2-4]

ETIOLOGY AND PATHOPHYSIOLOGY

- Usually idiopathic, thought to be a cell-mediated immune response to an unknown antigen.[2,3,5]
- Possible human leukocyte antigen (HLA)-associated genetic predisposition.[2]
- Lichenoid-type reactions may be associated with medications (e.g., angiotensin-converting enzyme inhibitors [ACEIs], thiazide-type diuretics, tetracycline, chloroquine), metals (e.g., gold, mercury), or infections (e.g., secondary syphilis).[2,5]
- Associated with liver disease, especially related to hepatitis C virus.[2,5,6]
- LP may be found with other diseases of altered immunity (e.g., ulcerative colitis, alopecia areata, myasthenia gravis).[1]
- Malignant transformation has been reported in ulcerative oral lesions in men.[1]

RISK FACTORS

- Possible HLA-associated genetic predisposition.

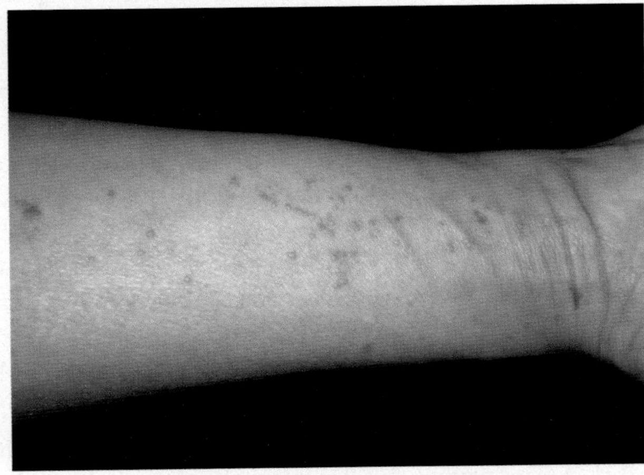

FIGURE 160-1 A 38-year-old Hispanic woman with lichen planus on her wrist. (*Reproduced with permission from Richard P. Usatine, MD.*)

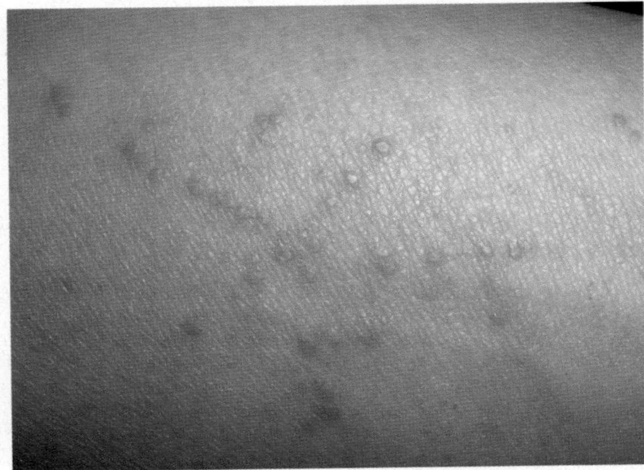

FIGURE 160-2 Close-up of wrist showing linearity of the lesions on the flexor surface. Lesions may be pink rather than purple. (*Reproduced with permission from Richard P. Usatine, MD.*)

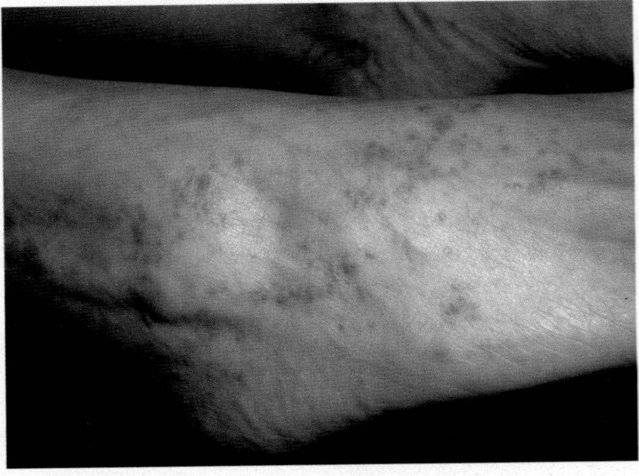

FIGURE 160-3 Ankle of the woman in **Figure 160-1** with typical lichen planus eruption. (*Reproduced with permission from Richard P. Usatine, MD.*)

- Hepatitis C virus infection, although causal relationship is not established.[6]
- Certain drugs (see "Etiology and Pathophysiology" above).

DIAGNOSIS

CLINICAL FEATURES[2,5]

- Classically, the six Ps of LP are planar, purple, polygonal, pruritic, papules, and plaques (**Figures 160-1** to **160-5**).
- These well-demarcated flat-topped violaceous lesions are often covered by lacy, reticular white lines (called Wickham striae or Wickham lines) (see **Figure 160-4B**).
- An initial lesion is usually located on the flexor surface of the limbs, such as the wrists, followed by a generalized eruption with maximal spreading within 2 to 16 weeks.[1]
- Lesions may demonstrate the Koebner phenomenon (linear distribution) from scratching (see **Figure 160-2**).
- Lesions are more often hyperpigmented rather than purple or pink in dark-skinned persons, and skin may remain hyperpigmented after lesions resolve (**Figures 160-6** and **160-7**).
- Skin variants
  - Hypertrophic—Typical papules develop into thicker reddish-brown to purple plaques (see **Figures 160-5** and **160-7**), most commonly on the foot and shins. Seen more often in black men with hyperpigmented and hypertrophic lesions (see **Figure 160-7**).
  - Follicular—Pinpoint hyperkeratotic projections often on scalp, may lead to cicatricial alopecia.
  - Vesicular—Vesicles or bullae occur alongside the more typical LP lesions (**Figure 160-8**).
  - Actinic—Typical lesions in sun-exposed areas, such as the face, back of hands, and arms (**Figure 160-9**).
  - Atrophic—The lesions are atrophic rather than standard plaques (**Figure 160-10**).
  - Ulcerative—Ulcers develop within typical lesions or start as waxy semitranslucent plaques on palms and soles; may require skin grafting.
- Mucous membrane variants
  - May be reticular (netlike; **Figure 160-11**), atrophic, erosive (**Figures 160-12** and **160-13**), or bullous. It is almost always bilateral.
  - Oral lesions may be asymptomatic or have a burning sensation; pain occurs with ulceration.[1,4]
  - Oral LP is often associated with extraoral LP.[7,8]
- Genitalia variants
  - Reticular, annular (**Figure 160-14**), papular (**Figure 160-15**), or erosive lesions on penis, scrotum, vulva (**Figure 160-16**) or vagina.
  - Vulvar/vaginal lesions may be associated with dyspareunia, a burning sensation, and/or pruritus.[1,7]
  - Vulvar and urethral stenosis can also be present.[1,7]
- Hair and nail variants; the latter present in 10% of patients.[1]
  - Violaceous, scaly, pruritic papules on the scalp can progress to scarring alopecia. Lichen planopilaris (LP of the scalp) can cause widespread hair loss (see Chapter 197, Scarring Alopecia).[9]

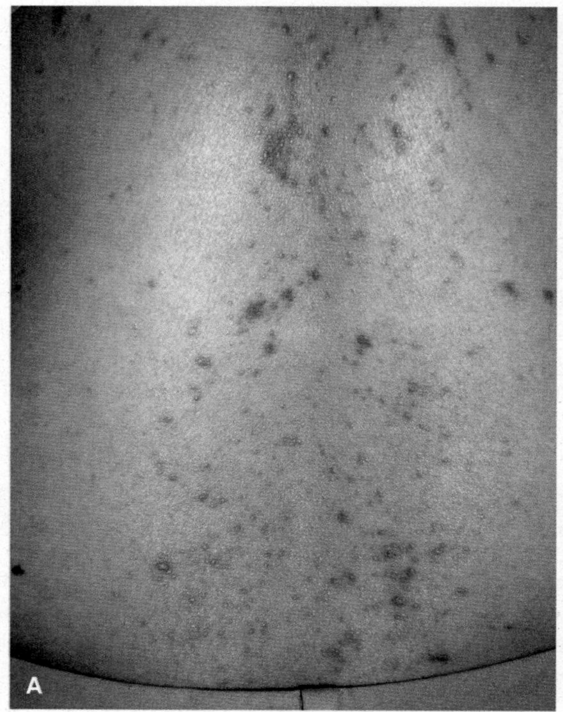

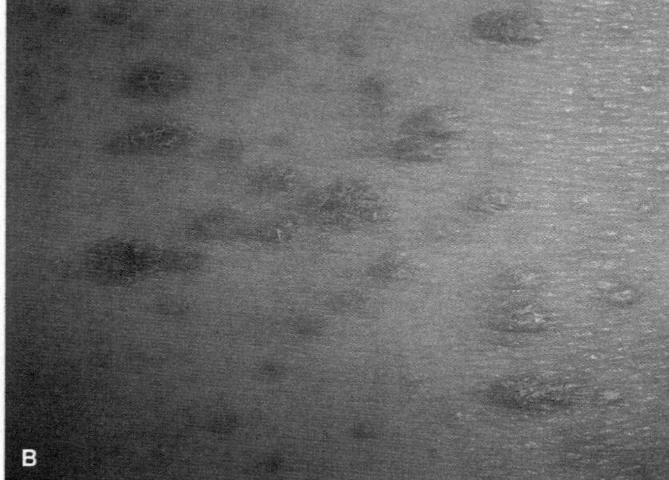

FIGURE 160-4 **A.** Lichen planus on the back of the woman in **Figure 160-1**. **B.** Close-up of lesions on the back showing Wickham striae crossing the flat papules of lichen planus. These lines are white and reticular like a net. (*Reproduced with permission from Richard P. Usatine, MD.*)

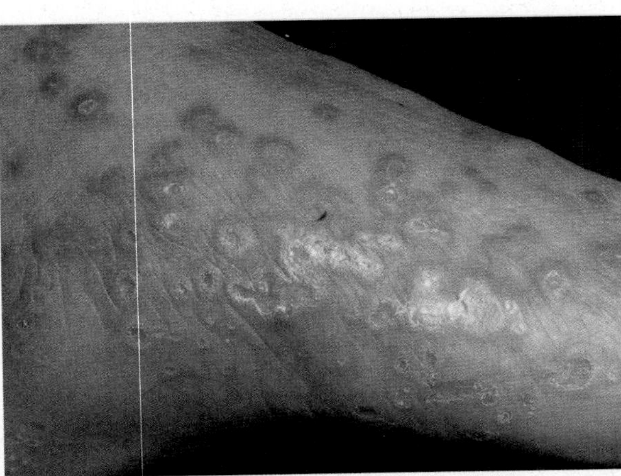

FIGURE 160-5 Hypertrophic lichen planus on the foot of a man. Purple polygonal papules and plaques are visible. *(Reproduced with permission from M. Craven, MD.)*

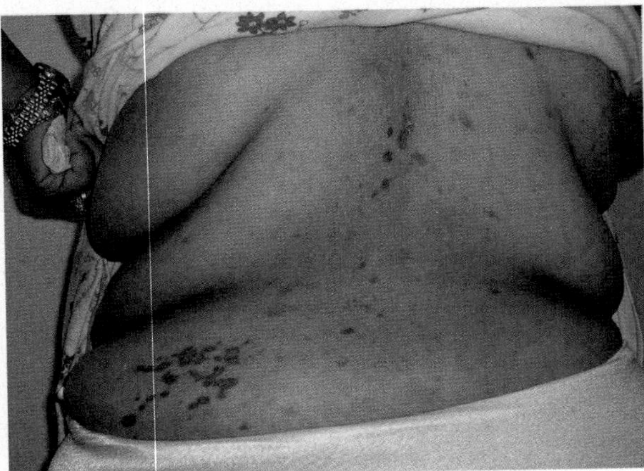

FIGURE 160-6 Hyperpigmented lichen planus on the back proven by punch biopsy. *(Reproduced with permission from Richard P. Usatine, MD.)*

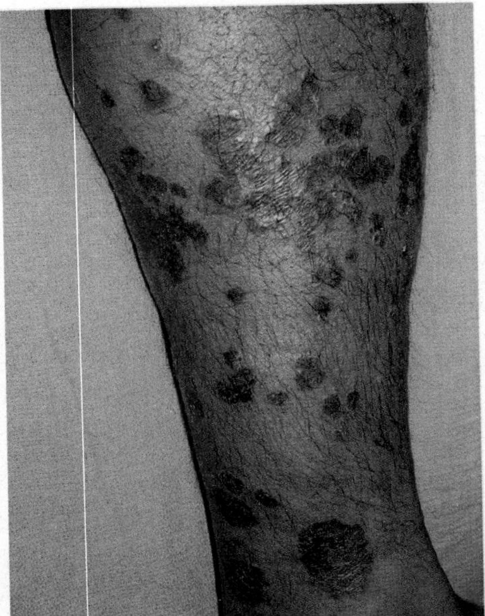

FIGURE 160-7 Hypertrophic lichen planus on the leg of a black man. Note the hyperpigmentation that is common when lichen planus occurs in a person with dark skin. *(Reproduced with permission from Richard P. Usatine, MD.)*

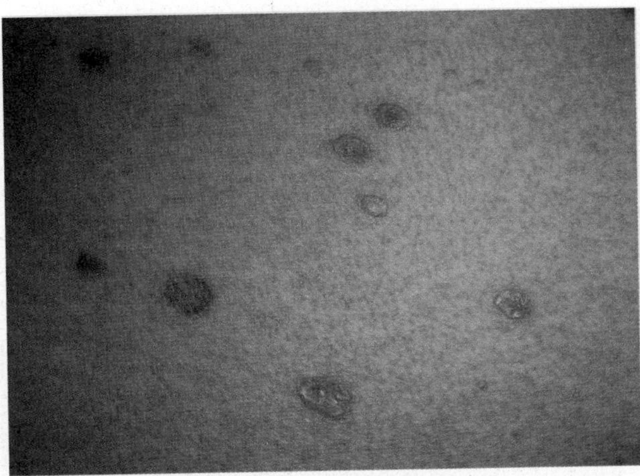

FIGURE 160-8 Bullous lichen planus on the buttocks. *(Reproduced with permission from Richard P. Usatine, MD.)*

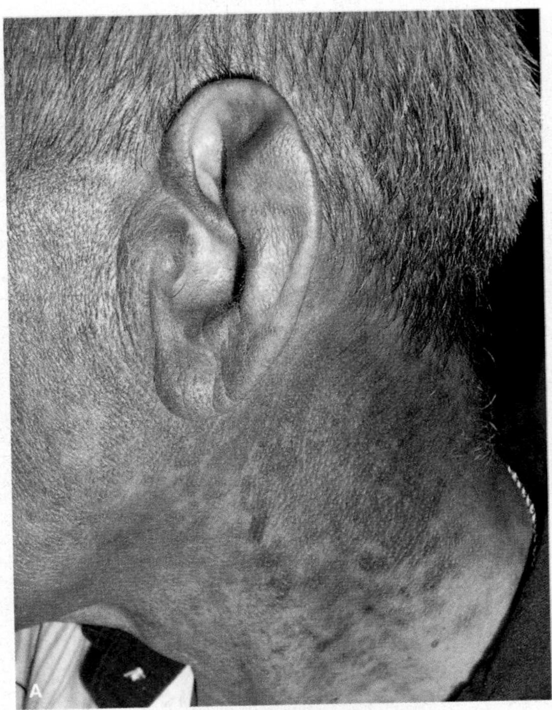

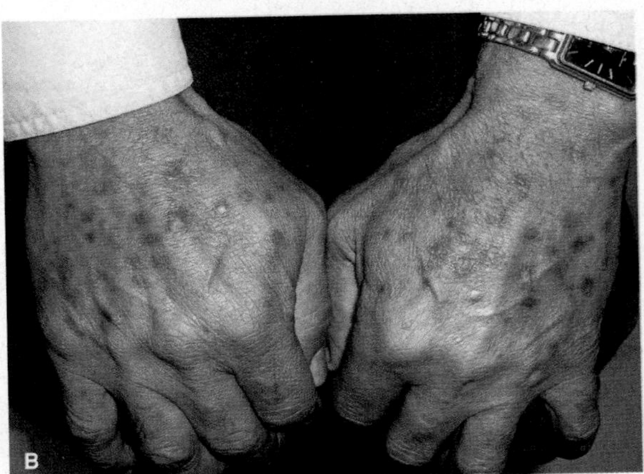

FIGURE 160-9 **A.** Actinic lichen planus on the face and neck. **B.** Actinic LP on the back of the hand. *(Reproduced with permission from Richard P. Usatine, MD.)*

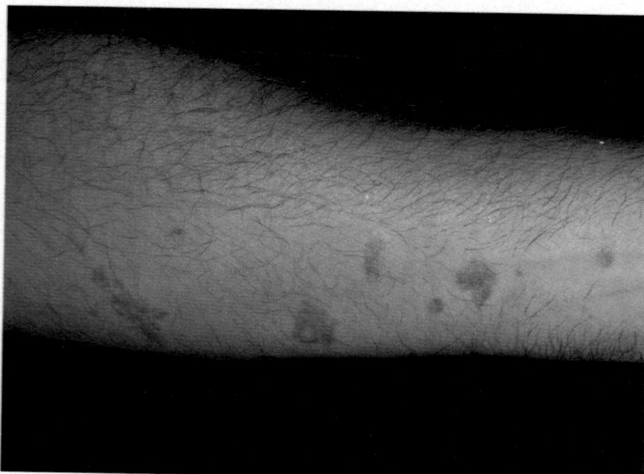

FIGURE 160-10 Atrophic lichen planus (biopsy proven) on the forearm showing multiple colors within the atrophic lesions. (*Reproduced with permission from Richard P. Usatine, MD.*)

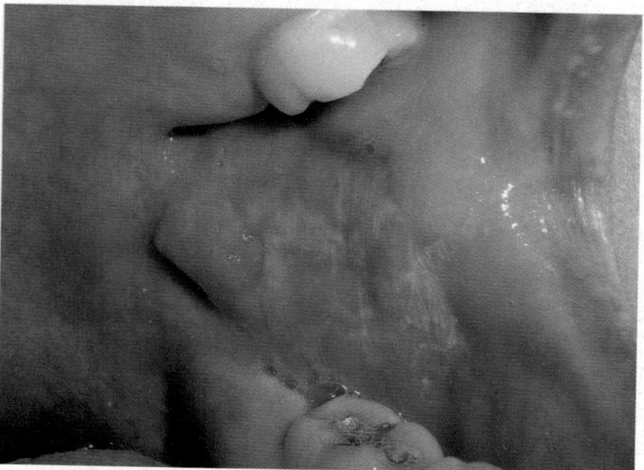

FIGURE 160-11 Asymptomatic white keratotic striae of lichen planus on left buccal mucosa of a 56-year-old woman. The patient had similar involvement of the right buccal mucosa and gingivae. Lichen planus in the mouth is bilateral. (*Reproduced with permission from Richard P. Usatine, MD.*)

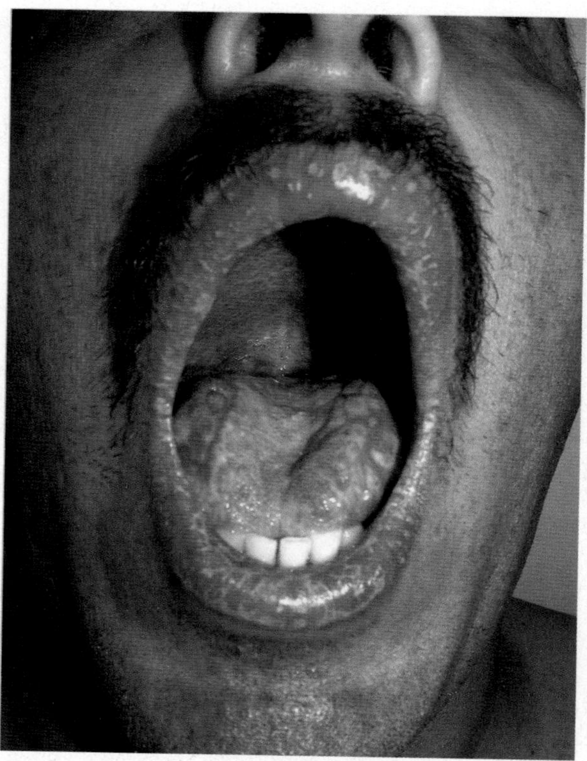

FIGURE 160-13 Lichen planus in the mouth with erosions. The lips, tongue, and palate are all involved. (*Reproduced with permission from Eric Kraus, MD.*)

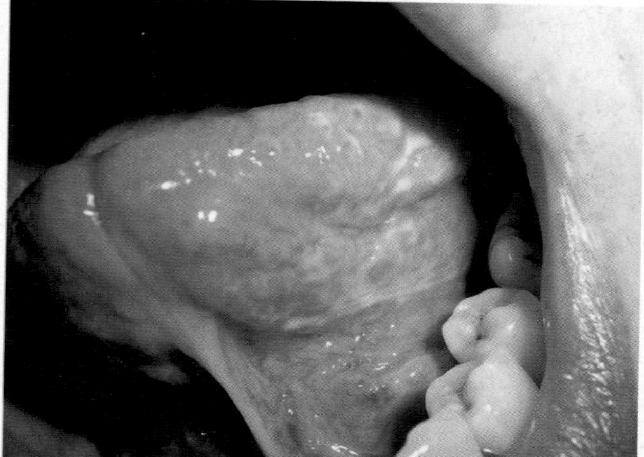

FIGURE 160-12 Erosive lichen planus, lateral surface of the tongue. This 52-year-old woman experiences tongue discomfort while eating acidic or spicy foods. (*Reproduced with permission from Richard P. Usatine, MD.*)

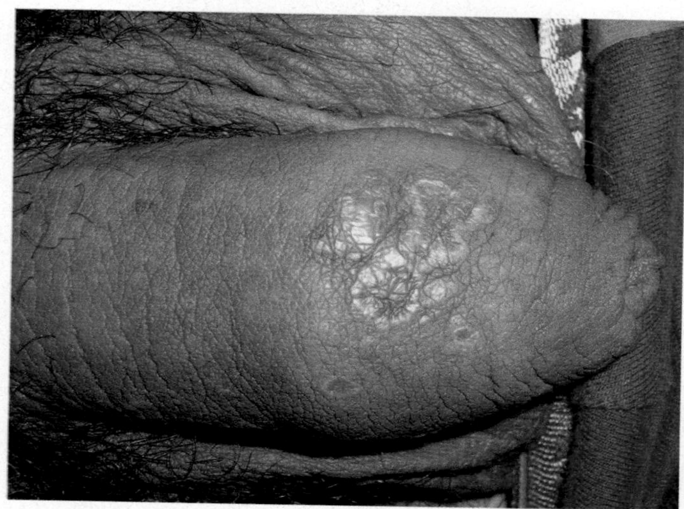

FIGURE 160-14 Lichen planus on the penis showing an annular pattern. (*Reproduced with permission from Richard P. Usatine, MD.*)

- Nail plate thinning results in longitudinal grooving and ridging; rarely destruction of nail fold and nail bed with splintering (**Figure 160-17**).
- Hyperpigmentation, subungual hyperkeratosis, onycholysis, and longitudinal melanonychia can result from LP.[1]

TYPICAL DISTRIBUTION

Wrists (**Figure 160-18**), ankles, lower back, eyelids, shins, scalp, penis, mouth (i.e., buccal mucosa, lateral tongue, and gingiva).[2,5]

LABORATORY STUDIES

- Wickham striae can be accentuated by a drop of oil on the skin plaque and magnification.[5] Not all LP has visible Wickham striae. Dermoscopy provides magnification to see the Wickham striae. If the diagnosis is uncertain, a punch biopsy should be performed.

BIOPSY

- A punch biopsy is a valuable method to make an initial diagnosis if the clinical picture is not certain. A biopsy is rarely needed to evaluate for malignant transformation.[5,10]
- Mainly lymphocytic immunoinflammatory infiltrate with hyperkeratosis, increased granular layer, and liquefaction of basal cell layer.[2,5]
- Linear fibrin and fibrinogen deposits along basement membrane.[2,5]
- Direct immunofluorescence on biopsy specimen reveals globular deposits of immunoglobulin (Ig) G, IgM, IgA, and complement at dermal–epidermal junction.[5]

DIFFERENTIAL DIAGNOSIS

Skin lesions that may be confused with LP:

- Eczematous dermatitis—"The itch that rashes:" dry skin, itching, often excoriations and lichenification of skin with predilection for flexor surfaces (see Chapter 151, Atopic Dermatitis).
- Psoriasis has more prominent silvery scale and is generally located on extensor surfaces.[5] A punch biopsy can be used to distinguish between these two when the clinical picture is not clear (see Chapter 158, Psoriasis).
- Stasis dermatitis—Lower-extremity eczematous dermatitis with inflammatory papules and often ulceration, in the setting of chronic venous insufficiency with dependent edema (see Chapter 54, Venous Insufficiency).
- Pityriasis rosea—Herald patch and subsequent pink papules and plaques with long axes along skin lines (Christmas tree pattern) (see Chapter 159, Pityriasis Rosea).
- Chronic cutaneous lupus erythematosus—Bright red sharply demarcated papules with adherent scale. Tend to regress centrally and can be light induced. Generally located on face, scalp, or forearms, and hands. Biopsy may be necessary to differentiate (see Chapter 188, Lupus: Systemic and Cutaneous).[5]
- Bowen disease—Sharply demarcated pink, red, brown, or black scaling or hyperkeratotic macule, papule, or plaque, usually mistaken for eczema or psoriasis, associated with ultraviolet radiation,

FIGURE 160-15 Lichen planus on the penis with pink papules on the glans. *(Reproduced with permission from Richard P. Usatine, MD.)*

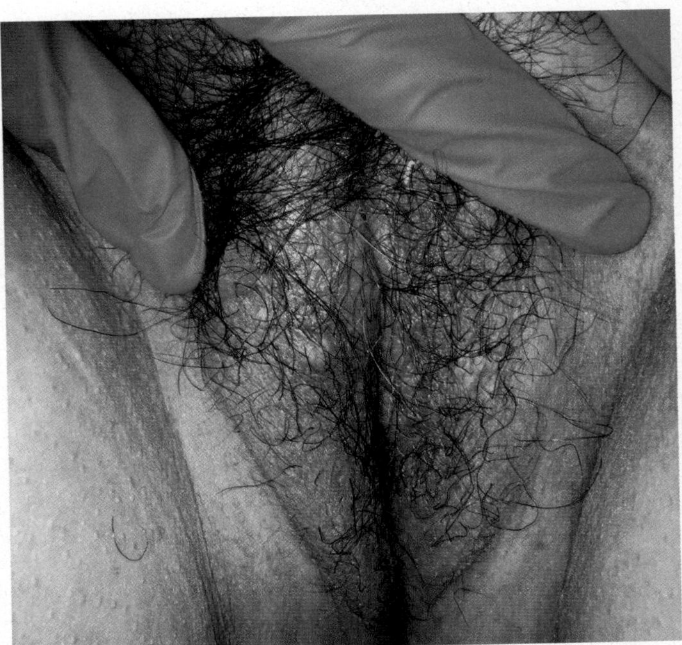

FIGURE 160-16 Vulvar lichen planus in a patient who also has typical LP on the wrists and in the mouth. *(Reproduced with permission from Richard P. Usatine, MD.)*

human papillomavirus (HPV), chemicals, and chronic heat exposure. Biopsy is needed to make the diagnosis (see Chapter 173, Actinic Keratosis and Bowen Disease).

- Lichen simplex chronicus—Localized confluence of lichenification from excoriation; patients have a strong urge to scratch their skin (see Chapter 149, Psychocutaneous Disorders).
- Prurigo nodularis—Nodular form of lichen simplex chronicus, brown to red hard, domed nodules from scratching and picking of intense pruritus. LP is not usually so pruritic (see Chapter 155, Psychocutaneous Disorders).

Other mucous membrane lesions that may appear similar[5]:

- Leukoplakia—White adherent patch or plaque to oral mucosa. Less netlike pattern. Biopsy warranted because of the risk of malignancy (see Chapter 44, Leukoplakia).
- Thrush—Removable whitish plaques over an erythematous mucosal surface caused by *Candida* infection, confirmed by KOH preparation (see Chapter 142, Candidiasis).
- Bite trauma in the mouth—May result in white areas of the lip or buccal mucosa; persons may have a white bite line where the upper and lower molars occlude, and this can be confused with oral LP. If in doubt, a biopsy may be needed.

Genital lesions that may be differentiated from LP[5]:

- Psoriasis on the penis can look like LP on the penis. A shave biopsy can be used to differentiate between these two diagnoses (see Chapter 158, Psoriasis).
- Syphilis—Primary infection manifests as painless shallow ulcer (chancre) at site of inoculation, if untreated, secondary syphilis presents with macular and then papular, pustular, or acneiform eruption on trunk, neck, palms, and soles, and condyloma lata (soft, moist, flat-topped pink to tan papules) in the anogenital region (see Chapter 225, Syphilis).

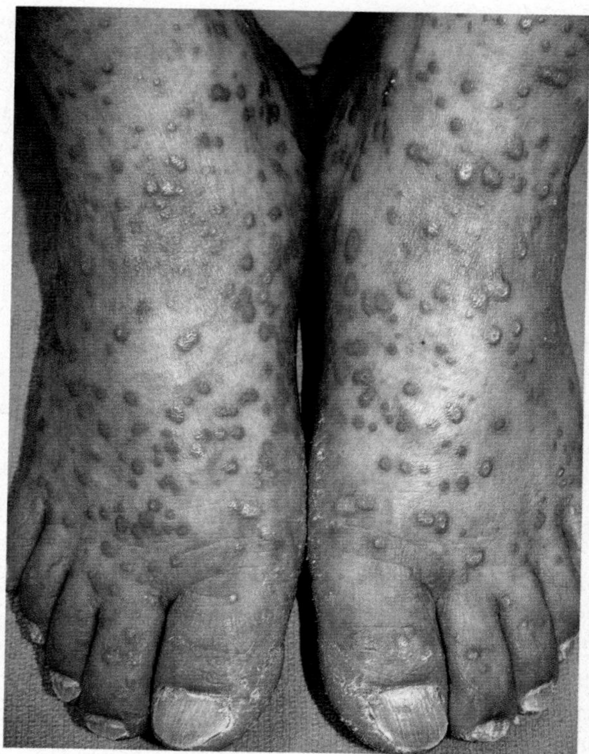

FIGURE 160-17 Hypertrophic lichen planus covering the dorsum of both feet with nail splintering. Note the purple color and Wickham lines. (*Reproduced with permission from Eric Kraus, MD.*)

MANAGEMENT

LP may persist for months to years. Hypertrophic LP and oral LP can last for decades.[2] Any type of LP can recur. Antihistamines can be used for symptomatic pruritus.[5] SOR Ⓒ Symptomatic and severe cases can be treated as follows.

FIRST LINE

- Localized/topical treatment.
  - Topical corticosteroids twice a day.[11-13] SOR Ⓑ Mid- to high-potency steroids are usually needed. Clobetasol cream or ointment may be used on the skin, and clobetasol cream or gel may be used in the mouth. Topical corticosteroids have also been found effective for vulvar LP.[14,15] SOR Ⓑ
- Systemic treatment may be needed even in first-line therapy, as LP can often be widespread and symptomatic.
  - Oral metronidazole is a relatively benign systemic off-label treatment for lichen planus that has been shown to be effective in a few non-randomized trials.[16,17] SOR Ⓑ
  - In one study patients were given metronidazole 250 mg three times daily for up to 3 months, and the overall treatment

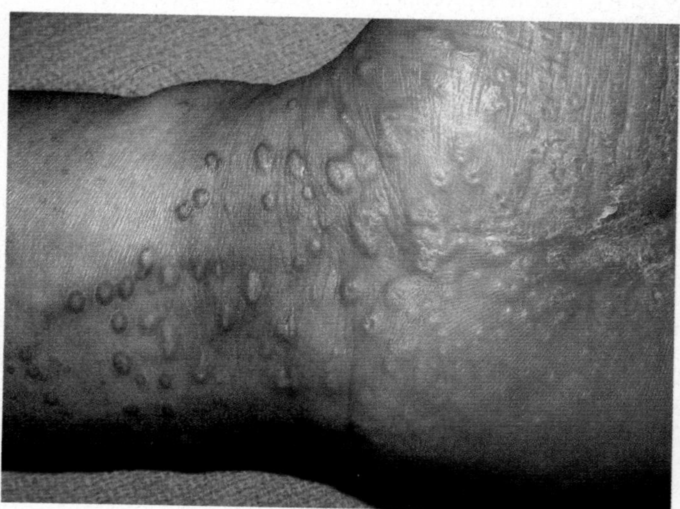

FIGURE 160-18 Thick hypertrophic papules and plaques on the wrist of the man in **Figure 160-17.** (*Reproduced with permission from Eric Kraus, MD.*)

response rate was 74% for skin lesions, 67% for mucosal lesions, and 75% for diminished itching.[16]
  - In a second study, 19 patients with LP who were free from protozoal infections were treated with oral metronidazole, 500 mg twice daily, for 20 to 60 days. Fifteen patients (79%) improved with metronidazole treatment; complete response was observed in 13 patients and partial response in 2 patients.[17]
  - Oral steroids may be used starting with a 3-week tapered course of oral prednisone (60 mg/day starting dose × 1 week, then 40 mg/day × 1 week, then 20 mg/day × 1 week).[2,10,11,18,19] SOR B This can be very effective, and the effect may persist beyond the treatment period. Prednisone can also be started at 40 mg/day × 1 week and tapered down by 10 mg/week for 4 weeks with a final dose of 10 mg/day in the last week.

SECOND LINE

- Localized/topical
  - Intralesional triamcinolone (3 to 5 mg/mL) for hypertrophic or mucous membrane lesions; may repeat every 3 to 4 weeks.[2,5,10,11] SOR B
  - Topical aloe vera gel has demonstrated efficacy against oral LP.[20,21] SOR B
  - Tacrolimus, pimecrolimus, retinoids, or cyclosporine in mouthwash or adhesive base for oral disease unresponsive to topical corticosteroids.[3,4,10,12,22-25] SOR B
  - Tacrolimus and aloe vera gel have demonstrated efficacy for vulvar LP.[14,15] SOR B
- Systemic treatment can be considered for resistant, widespread, or severe cases (all systemic treatments are off-label).
  - Systemic retinoids: acitretin (25 mg/day). Monitor serum creatinine, liver function tests (LFTs), lipids.[3,10,19,26] SOR B In one double-blind, placebo-controlled study of 65 patients, 64% to 83% responded favorably to 30 mg daily.[27] Contraindicated in women of childbearing potential and preexisting liver disease.
  - Mycophenolate mofetil (MMF): In one study, this was step 3 in an algorithmic approach to mucosal LP.[28] If the patients failed 1 month of oral prednisone, they were started on mycophenolate 500 mg twice daily for 1 week, 500 mg 3 times daily for the second week, and 1000 mg twice daily thereafter. A complete blood cell count with differential was monitored weekly at first and then every 3 months. Of the 22 patients treated with MMF, 15 improved with less pain and fewer lesions.[27]
  - Cyclosporine--modified (5 mg/kg per day). Monitor complete blood count, serum creatinine, LFTs, uric acid, magnesium, and blood pressure.[2] SOR B Contraindicated in renal disease and uncontrolled hypertension.
  - Azathioprine may be used as a steroid-sparing agent (25 to 50 mg PO daily to start and titrate to 100 to 200 mg PO in twice-daily dosing). Monitor complete blood count and LFTs.[5,10] SOR C An initial thiopurine methyltransferase (TPMT) level is helpful to identify patients who are poor metabolizers and should either not receive azathioprine or be given only the lowest dose. If the test is not available, start with 25 mg and titrate up slowly. Poor metabolizers will have side effects early and azathioprine can be stopped.
- Light therapy
  - Psoralen with UVA (PUVA) and narrow-band UVB phototherapy may be considered in widespread LP. Typically narrow-band UVB is preferred, as PUVA can cause phototoxic reactions and increase the risk of skin cancers.[29,30] SOR C

PROGNOSIS

- Generally self-limiting, and spontaneous resolution may occur in 12 to 18 months.
- Recurrences are common.
- Mucosal LP is generally more persistent than cutaneous forms.
- Malignant transformation of LP is rare, but patients with vulvar LP should be monitored for this possibility.

FOLLOW-UP

- Follow-up depends on severity and treatment course.
- Oral and vaginal disease may be most challenging to treat.
- Follow oral or vaginal/vulvar lesions for possible malignant transformation. Because of low risk of transformation even with oral LP (best estimate: 0.2% per year), routine screening and biopsy is not recommended.[10] Biopsy if suspecting malignancy; lesion becomes larger, ulcerated, or nodular, or loses reticular pattern.

PATIENT EDUCATION

- Patients should understand that LP is often self-limiting and may resolve in 12 to 18 months.
- There is a significant chance of recurrence.

PATIENT RESOURCES

- Handout—**https://familydoctor.org/condition/lichen-planus/.**
- Online support group for LP—**http://www.mdjunction.com/lichen-planus.**
- Online support group for oral LP—**https://dentistry.tamhsc.edu/olp/.**

PROVIDER RESOURCES

- Usatine RP, Tinitigan M. Diagnosis and treatment of lichen planus. *Am Fam Physician.* 2011;84(1):53-60—**http://www.aafp.org/afp/2011/0701/p53.html#afp20110701p53-b14.**

REFERENCES

1. Chuang T-Y, Stitle L. http://emedicine.medscape.com/article/1123213-overview. Accessed February 2017.
2. Wolff K, Johnson RA. *Fitzpatrick's Color Atlas and Synopsis of Clinical Dermatology.* 6th ed. New York, NY: McGraw-Hill; 2009;128-133.

3. Zakrzewska JM, Chan ES-Y, Thornhill MH. A systematic review of placebo-controlled randomized clinical trials of treatments used in oral lichen planus. *Br J Dermatol.* 2005;153:336-341.
4. Laeijendecker R, Tank B, Dekker SK, Neumann HA. A comparison of treatment of oral lichen planus with topical tacrolimus and triamcinolone acetonide ointment. *Acta Derm Venereol.* 2006; 86(3):227-229.
5. Habif TP. *Clinical Dermatology: A Color Guide to Diagnosis and Therapy.* 5th ed. Philadelphia, PA: Mosby; 2010.
6. Alaizari NA, Al-Maweri SA, Al-Shamiri HM, et al. Hepatitis C virus infections in oral lichen planus: a systematic review and meta-analysis. *Aust Dent J.* 2016;61(3)282-287.
7. Di Fede O, Belfiore P, Cabibi D, et al. Unexpectedly high frequency of genital involvement in women with clinical and histological features of oral lichen planus. *Acta Derm Venereol.* 2006; 86(5):433-438.
8. Imail SB, Kumar SK, Zain RB. Oral lichen planus and lichenoid reactions: etiopathogenesis, diagnosis, management and malignant transformation. *J Oral Sci.* 2007;49(2):89-106.
9. Cevacso NC, Bergfeld WF, Remzi BK, de Knott HR. A case-series of 29 patients with lichen planopilaris: the Cleveland Clinic Foundation experience on evaluation, diagnosis, and treatment. *J Am Acad Dermatol.* 2007;57(1):47-53.
10. Lodi G, Scully C, Carrozzo M, et al. Current controversies in oral lichen planus: report of an international consensus meeting, part 2. Clinical management and malignant transformation. *Oral Surg Oral Med Oral Pathol Oral Radiol Endod.* 2005;100:164-178.
11. Cribier B, Frances C, Chosidow O. Treatment of lichen planus. An evidence-based medicine analysis of efficacy. *Arch Dermatol.* 1998;134(12):1521-1530.
12. Corrocher G, Di Lorenzo G, Martinelli N, et al. Comparative effect of tacrolimus 0.1% ointment and clobetasol 0.05% ointment in patients with oral lichen planus. *J Clin Periodontol.* 2008;35(3):244-249.
13. Carbone M, Arduino PG, Carrozzo M, et al. Topical clobetasol in the treatment of atrophic-erosive oral lichen planus: a randomized controlled trial to compare two preparations with different concentrations. *J Oral Pathol Med.* 2009;38(2):227-233.
14. Rajar UD, Majeed R, Parveen N, et al. Efficacy of aloe vera gel in the treatment of vulval lichen planus. *J Coll Physicians Surg Pak.* 2008;18(10):612-614.
15. McPherson T, Cooper S. Vulval lichen sclerosis and lichen planus. *Dermatol Ther.* 2010;23(5):523-532.
16. Rasi A, Behzadi AH, Davoudi S, et al. Efficacy of oral metronidazole in treatment of cutaneous and mucosal lichen planus. *J Drugs Dermatol.* 2010;9(10):1186-1190.
17. Büyük AY, Kavala M. Oral metronidazole treatment of lichen planus. *J Am Acad Dermatol.* 2000;43(2 Pt 1):260-262.
18. Thongprasom K, Dhanuthai K. Steroids in the treatment of lichen planus: a review. *J Oral Sci.* 2008;50(4):377-385.
19. Asch S, Goldenberg G. Systemic treatment of cutaneous lichen planus: an update. *Cutis.* 2011;87(3):129-134.
20. Nair GR, Naidu GS, Jain S, et al. Clinical effectiveness of aloe vera in the management of oral mucosal diseases—a systematic review. *J Clin Diagn Res.* 2016; 10(8):ZE01-ZE07.
21. Salazar SN. Efficacy of topical *Aloe vera* in patients with oral lichen planus: a randomized double-blind study. *J Oral Pathol Med.* 2010;39(10):735-740.
22. Conrotto D, Carbone M, Carrozzo M, et al. Ciclosporine vs. clobetasol in the topical management of atrophic and erosive oral lichen planus: a double-blind, randomized controlled trial. *Br J Dermatol.* 2006;160(1):139-145.
23. Guo CL, Zhao JZ, Zhang J, Dong HT. Efficacy of topical tacrolimus for erosive oral lichen planus: a meta-analysis. *Chin Med Sci J.* 2015;30(4):210-217.
24. Volz T, Caroli U, Ludtke H, et al. Pimecrolimus cream 1% in erosive oral lichen planus—a prospective randomized double-blind vehicle-controlled study. *Br J Dermatol.* 2008;159(4):936-941.
25. Thongprasom K, Carrozzo M, Furness S, Lodi G. Interventions for treating oral lichen planus. *Cochrane Database Syst Rev.* 2011;(7):CD001168.
26. Atzmony L, Reiter O, Hodak E, et al. Treatments for cutaneous lichen planus: a systematic review and meta-analysis. *Am J Clin Dermatol.* 2016;17(1):11-22.
27. Laurberg G, Geiger JM, Hjorth N, et al. Treatment of lichen planus with acitretin. A double-blind, placebo-controlled study in 65 patients. *J Am Acad Dermatol.* 1991;24(3):434-437.
28. Ashack KA, Haley LL, Luther CA, et al. Assessing the clinical effectiveness of an algorithmic approach for mucosal lichen planus (MLP): a retrospective review. *J Am Acad Dermatol.* 2016; 74(6):1073-1076.e2.
29. Wackernagel A, Legat FJ, Hofer A, et al. Psoralen plus UVA vs. UVB-311 nm for the treatment of lichen planus. *Photodermatol Photoimmunol Photomed.* 2007;23(1):15-19.
30. Habib F, Stoebner PE, Picot E, et al. Narrow band UVB phototherapy in the treatment of widespread lichen planus. *Ann Dermatol Venereol.* 2005;132(1):17-20.

161 REACTIVE ARTHRITIS

Barbara Kiersz-Mueller, DO
Heidi S. Chumley, MD, MBA
Angela D. Shedd, MD
Suraj G. Reddy, MD
Richard P. Usatine, MD

PATIENT STORY

A 29-year-old man presented with concerns about an extensive rash that had developed over the previous month. The rash was reported to involve the scalp, abdomen, penis, hands, and feet (**Figures 161-1** to **161-5**). He also complained of severe joint pain, involving the back, knees, and feet. He denied ocular, GI, or genitourinary complaints, but was prescribed a course of antibiotics last month when his partner was diagnosed with *Chlamydia*.

The patient's young age, rapid onset of symptoms, dermatologic findings, and arthritis were suggestive of reactive arthritis. The patient's joint pain was treated with nonsteroidal anti-inflammatory drugs (NSAIDs), and skin lesions were treated with topical corticosteroids. No antibiotics were prescribed because no current infectious agent was identified. In conjunction with a dermatologist, acitretin 25 mg daily was started to treat his psoriasiform lesions.

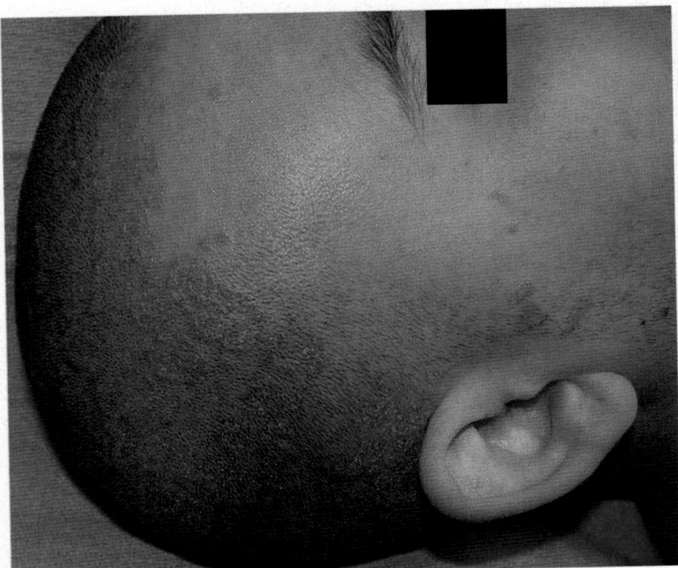

FIGURE 161-1 Reactive arthritis in a young man showing annular scalp lesions (circinate plaques). (*Reproduced with permission from Shedd AD, Reddy SG, Meffert JJ, Kraus EW. Acute onset of rash and oligoarthritis, J Fam Pract. 2007;56(10):811-814. Frontline Medical Communications. Inc..*)

INTRODUCTION

Reactive arthritis is a noninfectious acute oligoarthritis that occurs in response to an infection, most commonly in the GI or urogenital tract.[1] Patients present 1 to 4 weeks after the infection with joint pain in asymmetric large joints, eye disease (such as conjunctivitis), and skin changes including erythema nodosum, keratoderma blennorrhagicum, and circinate balanitis. A smaller number of patients may present with arthritis in the small joints and axial skeleton, and enthesitis (most commonly around the Achilles tendon). The diagnosis is clinical and based on all three of the following: characteristic musculoskeletal findings, evidence of preceding infection, and lack of evidence of a more likely diagnosis. Treatment includes anti-inflammatory medications and treatment of triggering infection.

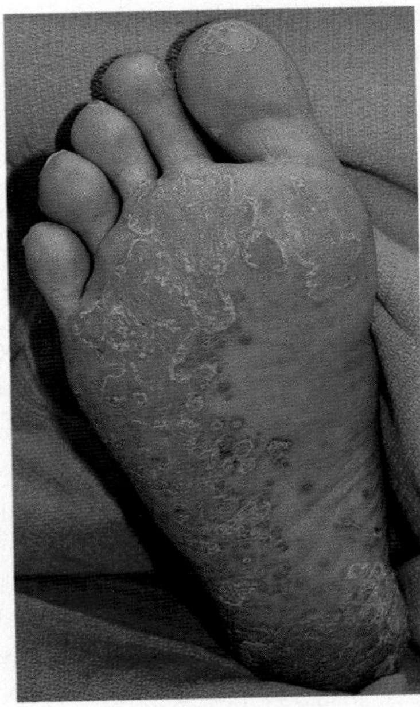

FIGURE 161-2 Keratoderma blennorrhagicum with hyperkeratotic papules, plaques, and pustules that have coalesced to form circular borders. (*Reproduced with permission from Shedd AD, Reddy SG, Meffert JJ, Kraus EW. Acute onset of rash and oligoarthritis. J Fam Pract. 2007;56(10):811-814. Frontline Medical Communications.*)

SYNONYMS

Reiter syndrome is no longer the preferred name, as Dr. Reiter was a Nazi physician who performed unethical experimentation on human subjects.

EPIDEMIOLOGY

- Incidence is 0.6 to 27 per 100,000 people.[2]
- Most common in young adults ages 30 to 40 years; rare in children.[2]

- Reactive arthritis after a genitourinary (GU) infection is more common in young men; reactive arthritis after a GI infection is equally common in men and women.[2]

ETIOLOGY AND PATHOPHYSIOLOGY

- Follows a GI (*Yersinia, Salmonella, Shigella, Campylobacter*, or rarely *Escherichia coli* or *Clostridium difficile*) or GU (*Chlamydia trachomatis, Ureaplasma urealyticum*) infection; less commonly follows a respiratory infection with *Chlamydia* pneumonia.
- Mechanism by which the triggering agent leads to development of arthritis is not fully understood.

RISK FACTORS

- Infection with a triggering agent.
- Presence of human leukocyte antigen (HLA)-B27 is associated with an increased risk of chronic disease and a more severe arthritis.[3]
- HLA-B27 has been found in a high percentage of patients with severe disease, but there is no increase in HLA-B27 prevalence in population studies.[4]

DIAGNOSIS

Definite reactive arthritis: Both major criteria and one minor criterion.

Probable reactive arthritis: One major criterion and one minor criterion.

Major criteria:

- Arthritis with two of three features: Asymmetric, mono- or oligoarthritis, lower limbs predominately affected.
- Preceding enteritis or urethritis.

Minor criteria:

- Evidence of triggering infection.
- Evidence of synovial infection.

CLINICAL FEATURES

- The classic triad consists of urethritis, conjunctivitis (**Figure 161-6**), and arthritis[2]; however, few patients present with the classic triad.
- Tendinitis, bursitis or enthesitis, or low back pain may be present.
- Skin findings (psoriasiform) typically involve the palms, the soles (keratoderma blennorrhagicum) (**Figures 161-2** and **161-7**), and the glans penis (balanitis circinata). Nail dystrophy, thickening, and destruction may occur (**Figures 161-3** and **161-8**). Many other body surfaces may be affected, including the scalp (see **Figure 161-1**), intertriginous areas (see **Figure 161-4**), and oral mucosa (**Figure 161-9**). Erosive lesions on the tongue and hard palate may be seen.
- Rarely, carditis and atrioventricular conduction disturbances are present.

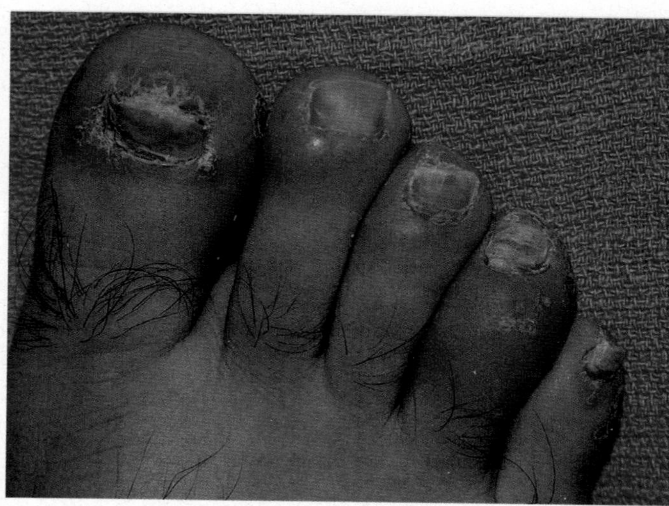

FIGURE 161-3 Erythema and scale seen on the toes of the patient in **Figure 161-1**. Note the nail involvement with subungual keratosis and onycholysis. The fourth toe is red and swollen; this is called dactylitis. *(Reproduced with permission from Shedd AD, Reddy SG, Meffert JJ, Kraus EW. Acute onset of rash and oligoarthritis. J Fam Pract. 2007;56(10):811-814. Frontline Medical Communications.)*

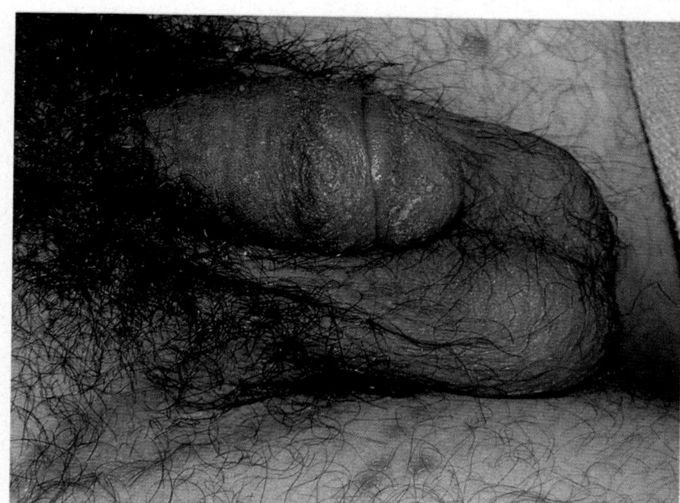

FIGURE 161-4 The patient in **Figure 161-1** with psoriasiform lesions on the corona and glans. The patient also has erythema in the inguinal area that resembles inverse psoriasis. This particular case does not exemplify classic balanitis circinata, which is characterized by annular or arcuate thin scaly plaques, as opposed to the nonspecific scaly plaques found on this patient. *(Reproduced with permission from Suraj Reddy, MD.)*

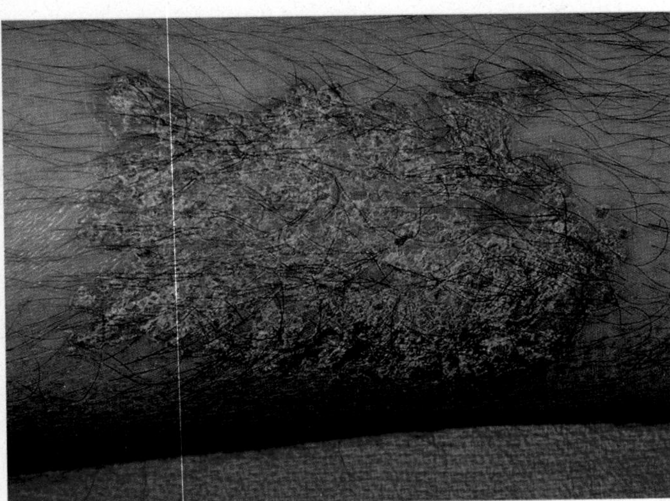

FIGURE 161-5 Psoriatic-appearing plaque on the leg in the same patient with reactive arthritis in **Figure 161-1**. *(Reproduced with permission from Shedd AD, Reddy SG, Meffert JJ, Kraus EW. Acute onset of rash and oligoarthritis, J Fam Pract. 2007;56(10):811-814. Frontline Medical Communications. Inc.)*

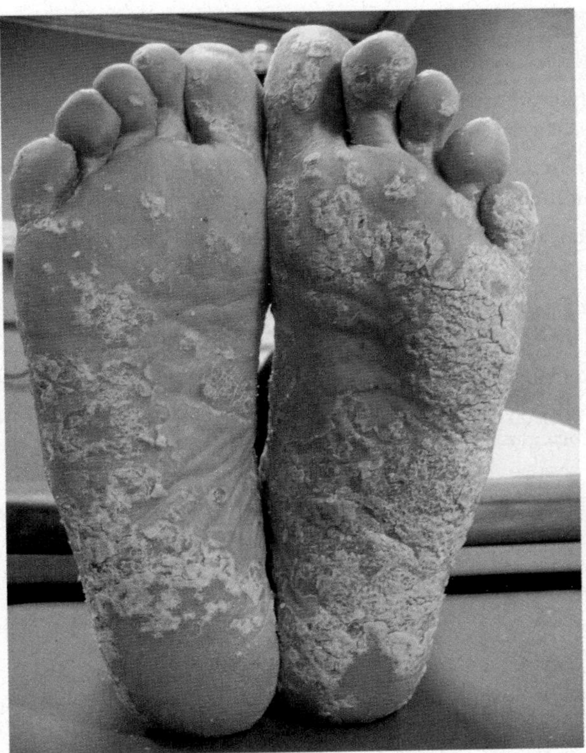

FIGURE 161-7 *Keratoderma blennorrhagicum* on the soles of the foot of a man with reactive arthritis. *(Reproduced with permission from Ricardo Zuniga-Montes, MD.)*

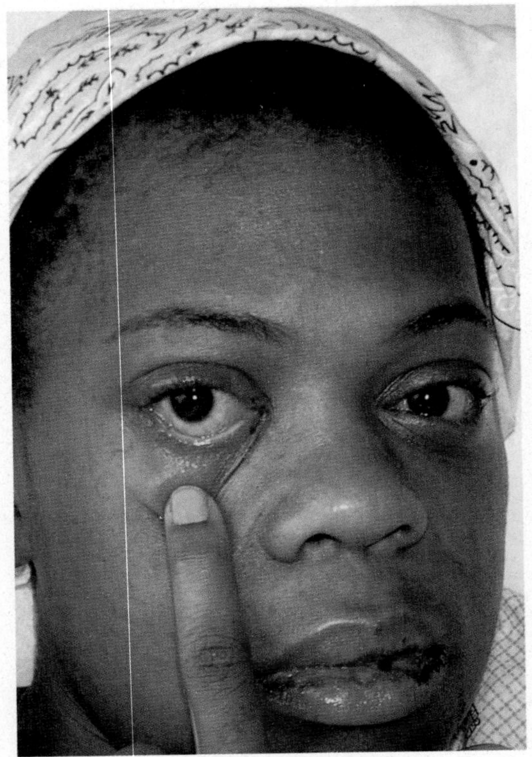

FIGURE 161-6 Reactive arthritis with conjunctivitis as a result of chlamydial pelvic inflammatory disease in a 42-year-old woman. She presented with fever, chills, and generalized pain in her joints, abdomen, and pelvis. *(Reproduced with permission from Mazziotta JM, Ahmed N. Conjunctivitis and cervicitis, J Fam Pract. 2004;53(2):121-123. Frontline Medical Communications. Inc.)*

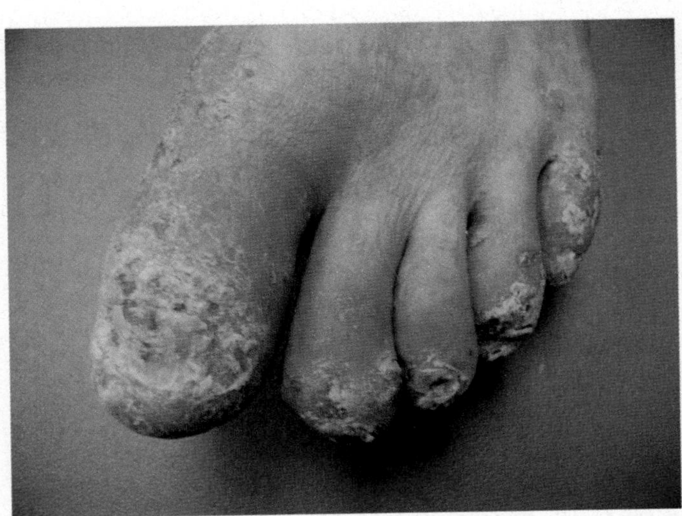

FIGURE 161-8 Nail dystrophy, thickening, and nail destruction in a man with reactive arthritis. *(Reproduced with permission from Ricardo Zuniga-Montes, MD.)*

LABORATORY TESTING

- No specific laboratory test is used to confirm reactive arthritis.
- Erythrocyte sedimentation rate (ESR) and C-reactive protein are usually elevated.
- Urethral/cervical swab or urine test for *C. trachomatis* when a GU infection precedes the onset of symptoms.
- Stool culture may detect an enteric pathogen when GI infection precedes the onset of symptoms.
- *Salmonella*, *Yersinia*, and *Campylobacter* antibodies can be detected in the serum after microbes are no longer detectable in the stool.
- Skin biopsy, if performed, resembles that of psoriasis with acanthosis of the epidermis, a neutrophilic perivascular infiltrate, and spongiform pustules.

DIFFERENTIAL DIAGNOSIS

- Spondyloarthropathies and reactive arthropathies may present with acute joint pain but often lack the skin findings seen with reactive arthritis (see Chapter 100, Ankylosing Spondylitis).
- Psoriatic arthritis may be easily confused, especially in immunocompromised patients. Lack of constitutional symptoms and a more chronic course help differentiate from reactive arthritis.
- Gonococcal arthritis is characterized by migratory polyarthralgia that settles in one or more joints. Often erythematous macules or hemorrhagic papules on acral sites help distinguish from reactive arthritis.
- Rheumatoid arthritis often presents with a progressive, symmetric polyarthritis of the small joints of the hands and wrists. Females are affected more often than males (see Chapter 99, Rheumatoid Arthritis).

MANAGEMENT

FIRST LINE

- Treat patients with acute *C. trachomatis* with 1 g azithromycin single dose or 100 mg doxycycline twice a day for 10 days. SOR Ⓐ Treat partners when possible.[5]
- The current recommendation no longer calls for long-term antibiotics, as studies do not support this previous treatment.[6,7] SOR Ⓑ
- GI-triggering infections are typically self-limiting and do not require antibiotics.
- Treat inflammation with NSAIDs. SOR Ⓑ
- Consider glucocorticoid joint injections in patients with severe joint pain.
- For refractory arthritic disease, immunosuppressive agents, such as sulfasalazine at 2000 mg/day, have demonstrated some benefit.[8] SOR Ⓑ
- Treat mucosal and skin lesions with topical corticosteroids.
- Psoriasiform skin lesions may be treated with some of the same medications used to treat psoriasis (including acitretin). SOR Ⓒ

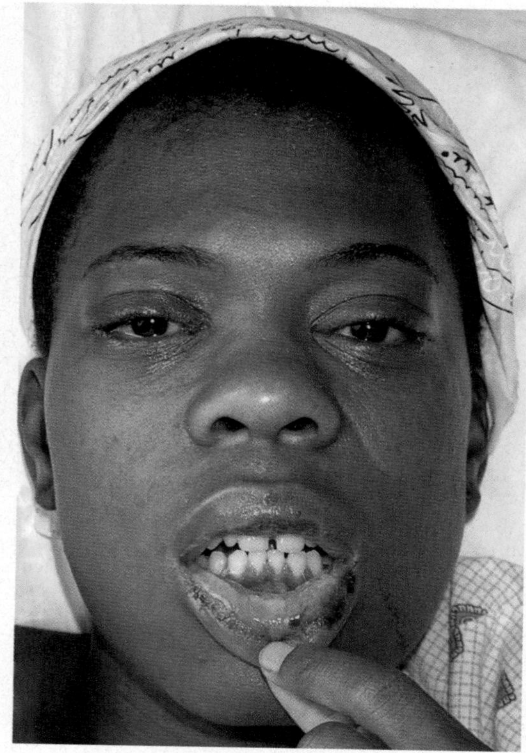

FIGURE 161-9 Oral mucosal inflammation with reactive arthritis secondary to chlamydial pelvic inflammatory disease. The cervix was also inflamed on examination. (*Reproduced with permission from Mazziotta JM, Ahmed N. Conjunctivitis and cervicitis, J Fam Pract. 2004;53(2): 121-123. Frontline Medical Communications. Inc.*)

SECOND LINE

- Systemic steroids are indicated for patients with systemic symptoms (fever) or in those who develop carditis.
- Current evidence demonstrates that chronic antimicrobial therapy should not be recommended in most cases. However, one double-blind, triple-placebo, prospective trial revealed that in patients with *Chlamydia* infection, 22% achieved remission after 6 months of combination antibiotics with doxycycline plus rifampin OR azithromycin and rifampin (versus 0% remission in the placebo group).[9,10]

REFERRAL

- Refer patients with severe or nonresponsive joint pain to a rheumatologist.
- Refer patients who develop cardiac manifestations to a cardiologist.

PROGNOSIS

- Arthritic symptoms typically resolve in 3 to 5 months.[1] Most patients achieve complete remission by 6–12 months. Persistent symptoms that last longer than 6 months are associated with the development of chronic symptoms.
- Twenty percent to 50% of patients developed chronic symptoms across several studies.
- *Yersinia*, *Salmonella*, *Chlamydia*, and *Shigella* are associated with chronic symptoms.[1]

FOLLOW-UP

- Follow patients closely at the time of diagnosis to ensure response to therapy and timely referral for nonresponders.

PATIENT EDUCATION

There is no curative treatment. Symptoms may resolve permanently, relapse, or persist. Medications and physical/occupational therapy can help relieve pain and preserve function. Seek medical care for extraarticular symptoms, especially those involving the eye.

PATIENT RESOURCES

- American College of Rheumatology—**https://www.rheumatology.org/I-Am-A/Patient-Caregiver/Diseases-Conditions/Reactive-Arthritis**

PROVIDER RESOURCES

- Medscape. *Reactive Arthritis*—**http://emedicine.medscape.com/article/331347.**

REFERENCES

1. Stavropoulos PG, Soura E, Kanelleas A, et al. Reactive arthritis. *J Eur Acad Dermatol Venereol.* 2015;29:415.
2. Ajene AN, Fischer Walker CL, Black RE. Enteric pathogens and reactive arthritis: a systematic review of *Campylobacter*, *Salmonella* and *Shigella*-associated reactive arthritis. *J Health Popul Nutr.* 2013;31:299.
3. Colmegna I, Cuchacovich R, Espinoza LR. HLA-B27-associated reactive arthritis: pathogenetic and clinical considerations. *Clin Microbiol Rev.* 2004;17(2):348-369.
4. Hannu T. Reactive arthritis. *Best Pract Res Clin Rheumatol.* 2011;25(3):347-357.
5. Putschky N, Pott HG, Kuipers JG, et al. Comparing 10-day and 4-month doxycycline courses for treatment of *Chlamydia trachomatis*–reactive arthritis: a prospective, double-blind trial. *Ann Rheum Dis.* 2006;65(11):1521-1524.
6. Barber CE, Kim J, Inman RD, et al. Antibiotics for treatment of reactive arthritis: a systematic review and metaanalysis. *J Rheumatol.* 2013;40:916.
7. Kuuliala A, Julkunen H, Paimela L, et al. Double-blind, randomized, placebo-controlled study of three-month treatment with the combination of ofloxacin and roxithromycin in recent-onset reactive arthritis. *Rheumatol Int.* 2013;33(11):2723-2729.
8. Clegg DO, Reda DJ, Weisman MH, et al. Comparison of sulfasalazine and placebo in the treatment of reactive arthritis (Reiter's syndrome). A Department of Veterans Affairs Cooperative Study. *Arthritis Rheum.* 1996;39(12):2021-2027.
9. Carter JD, Espinoza LR, Inman RD, et al. Combination antibiotics as a treatment for chronic *Chlamydia*-induced reactive arthritis: a double-blind, placebo-controlled, prospective trial. *Arthritis Rheum.* 2010;62(5):1298-1307.
10. Kvien TK, Gaston JS, Bardin I, et al. Three months treatment of reactive arthritis with azithromycin: a EULAR double blind, placebo controlled study. *Ann Rheum Dis.* 2004;63(9):1113-1119.

162 ERYTHRODERMA

David Henderson, MD
Tiffanie C. Wong, DO

PATIENT STORY

A 34-year-old man presented with red skin from his neck to his feet for the last month (**Figure 162-1**). He was having a lot of itching, and his skin was shedding so that wherever he would sit, there would be a pile of skin that would remain. He denied fever and chills. He admitted to smoking and drinking heavily. The patient's vital signs were stable with normal blood pressure, and he preferred not to be hospitalized. He had some nail pitting but no personal or family history of psoriasis. The presumed diagnosis was erythrodermic psoriasis, but a punch biopsy was performed to confirm this. A complete blood count (CBC) and chemistry panel were ordered in anticipation of the patient requiring systemic medications. A purified protein derivative (PPD) was also placed at this time. The patient was then started on total body 0.1% triamcinolone under wet wrap overnight and given a follow-up appointment for the next day. The patient was also counseled to quit smoking and drinking. The following day his labs only revealed mild elevation in his liver function tests (LFTs). Two days following initial presentation, his PPD was negative and he was already feeling a bit better from the topical triamcinolone. Cyclosporine was promptly initiated, and the patient improved rapidly as a result.

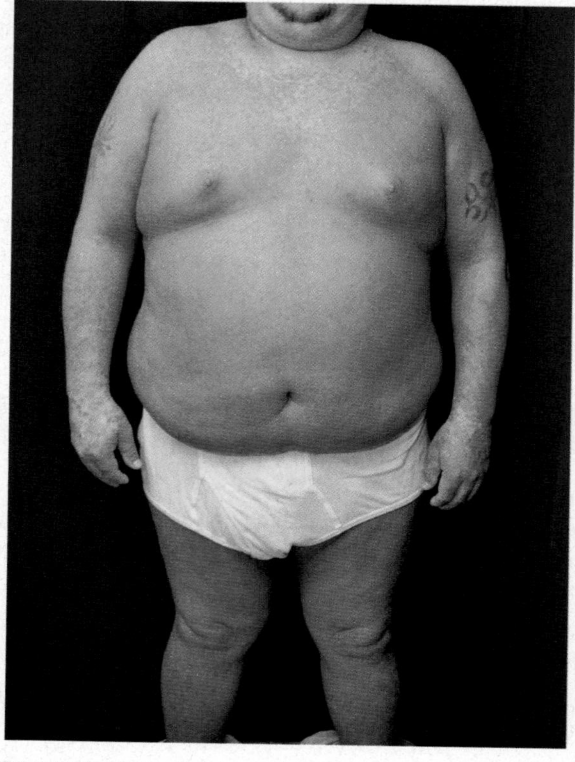

FIGURE 162-1 Erythrodermic psoriasis in a 34-year-old man. *(Reproduced with permission from Richard P. Usatine, MD.)*

INTRODUCTION

Erythroderma is an uncommon condition that affects all age groups. It is characterized by a generalized erythematous rash with associated scaling, affecting greater than 90% of the body's surface area. It is generally a manifestation of another underlying dermatosis or systemic disorder. It is associated with a range of morbidity and can have life-threatening metabolic and cardiovascular complications. Therapy is usually focused on treating the underlying disease, as well as addressing the systemic complications.

EPIDEMIOLOGY

Erythroderma is an uncommon condition that is generally a manifestation of underlying systemic or cutaneous disorders.

- It affects all age groups, from infants to the elderly.
- In adults, the average age of onset is 41 to 61 years of age, with a male-to-female ratio ranging from 2:1 to 4:1.[1]
- It accounts for approximately 1% of all dermatologic hospital admissions.[2]
- It can be a very serious condition resulting in metabolic, infectious, cardiorespiratory, and thermoregulatory complications.[3]
- Mortality rate of 11.3 per 1000 patient years.[4]

ETIOLOGY AND PATHOPHYSIOLOGY

In almost 50% of cases, erythroderma occurs in the setting of a preexisting dermatosis; however, it may also occur secondary to underlying systemic disease, malignancy, and drug reactions. It is classified as idiopathic in 9% to 47% of cases.[3]

- The pathophysiology is not fully understood, but it is related to the pathophysiology of the underlying disease. However, the factors that promote the development of erythroderma are not well defined.
- The rapid maturation and migration of cells through the epidermal layer results in excessive scaling. The rapid turnover of the epidermis may also result in fluid, electrolyte, and protein losses that may have severe metabolic consequences, including heart failure and acute respiratory distress syndrome.[5]
- The underlying pathogenesis may be an interaction of immunologic modulators, including interleukins 1, 2, and 8, as well as tumor necrosis factor.[2]

Dermatologic conditions associated with erythroderma include[1-3,5]:

- Psoriasis (**Figures 162-1** to **162-4**). The most common cause.
- Atopic dermatitis (**Figure 162-5**).[2,3]
- Contact dermatitis.
- Seborrhea.
- Pityriasis rubra pilaris.
- Bullous pemphigoid.[5]
- Impetigo herpetiformis.[5]
- Photosensitivity reaction.[5]

Erythroderma may also occur secondary to a number of infectious diseases, including:

- Crusted scabies (**Figure 162-6**).
- HIV (see **Figure 162-6**).
- Tuberculosis.
- Hepatitis.
- Human herpesvirus 6.[5]
- Toxic shock syndrome.[5]
- Staphylococcal scalded skin syndrome.[5]
- Histoplasmosis.[3]

Systemic diseases associated with erythroderma include the following:

- Sarcoidosis.
- Thyrotoxicosis.
- Graft-versus-host reaction.
- Dermatomyositis.[3,5]

The exact incidence of erythroderma in association with underlying malignancy is not known, but reticuloendothelial neoplasms are the most common, most notably T-cell lymphomas.[1,2] It may precede or follow the diagnosis of cutaneous T-cell lymphoma, and chronic idiopathic erythroderma carries a high risk of development of cutaneous T-cell lymphoma over time (**Figure 162-7**).[6] In addition, solid

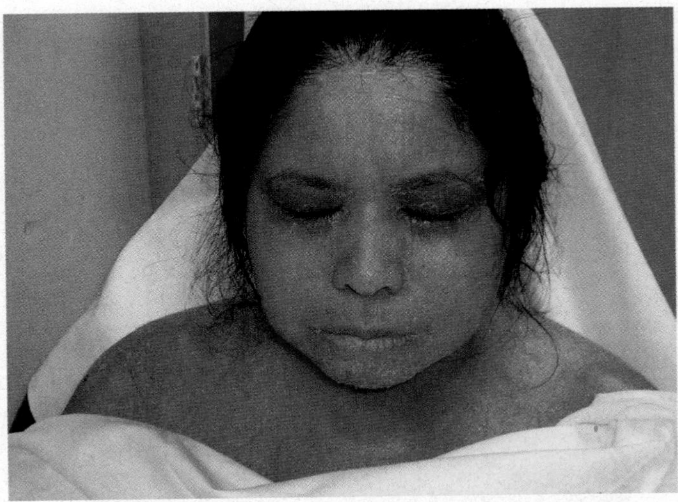

FIGURE 162-2 Erythrodermic psoriasis in a 39-year-old woman as her initial presentation of psoriasis. She was red from head to toe and had extensive exfoliation. She was dehydrated and tachycardic. Her skin was hot and painful. She was hospitalized for fluids and urgent treatment. *(Reproduced with permission from Richard P. Usatine, MD.)*

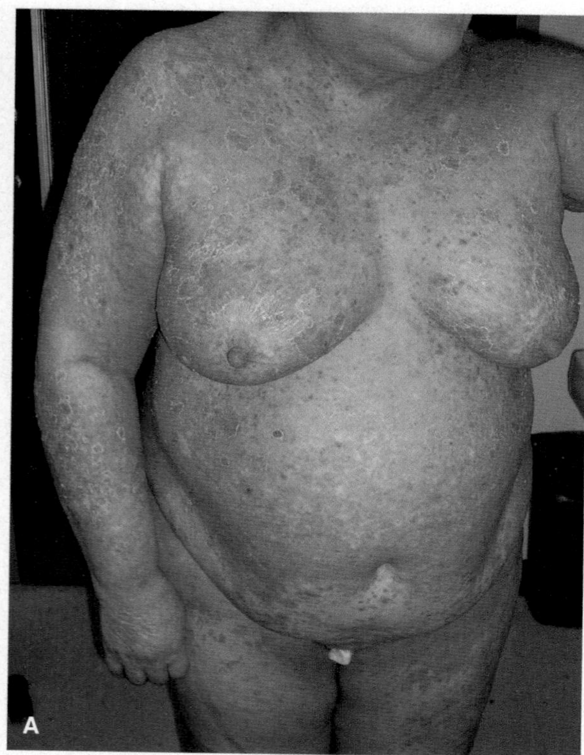

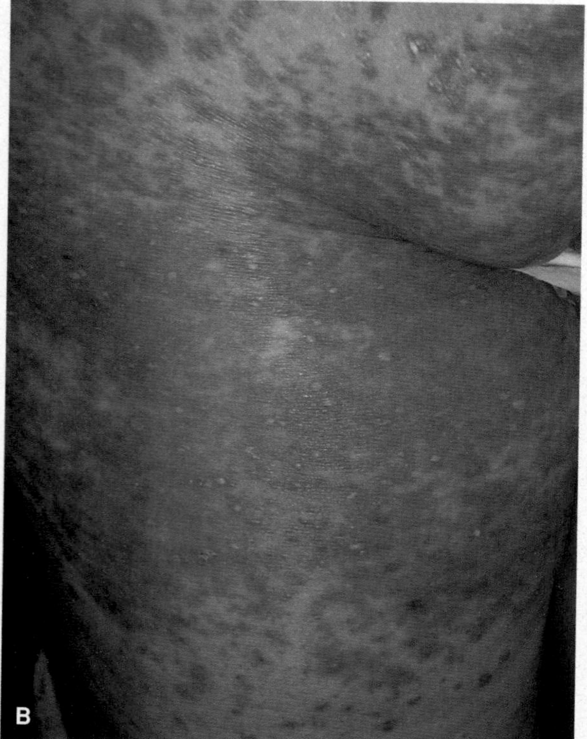

FIGURE 162-3 **A.** Generalized pustular psoriasis causing a life-threatening case of erythroderma in a 67-year-old woman. This all started 3 weeks before presentation, and she had no previous history of psoriasis. Patient was hospitalized and treated with topical steroids and oral acitretin with good results. **B.** Close-up of posterior thigh showing pustules on an erythematous plaque in a new case of erythroderma from generalized pustular psoriasis. (*Reproduced with permission from Richard P. Usatine, MD.*)

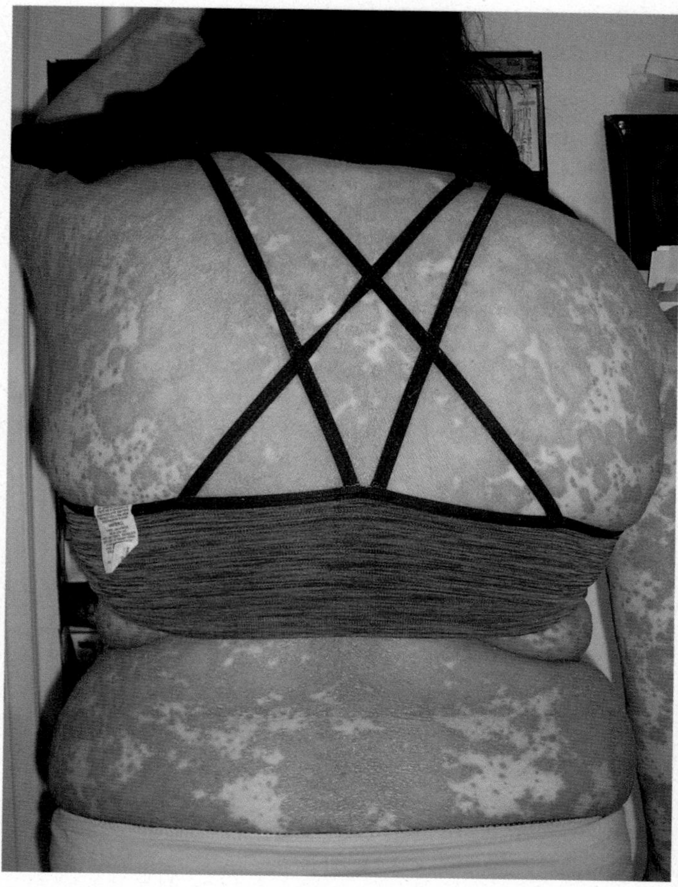

FIGURE 162-4 Erythrodermic psoriasis in a young woman. (*Reproduced with permission from Richard P. Usatine, MD.*)

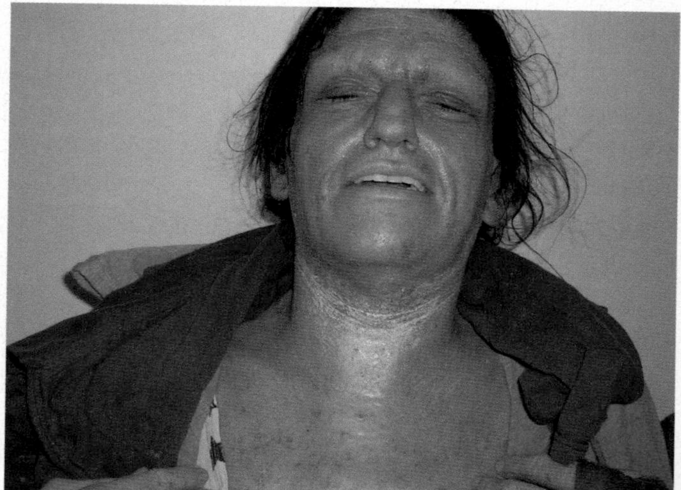

FIGURE 162-5 Erythroderma atopic dermatitis in a woman without health insurance. Note all the excoriations in addition to the deep erythema. Her young son has severe atopic dermatitis that was finally controlled with cyclosporine. (*Reproduced with permission from Richard P. Usatine, MD.*)

organ cancers such as colon, lung, prostate, and thyroid malignancies account for 1% of cases of erythroderma.[2] Specifically in children, it may be associated with:

- Kwashiorkor.
- Cystic fibrosis.
- Amino acid disorders.[1-3,5,6]

Drug reactions are a common cause of erythroderma, accounting for up to 20% of cases.[7]

The list of drugs associated with erythroderma is extensive and includes both systemic and topical medications, many of which are very commonly used, including a number of herbal, homeopathic, and ayurvedic medications.[6] The list of most commonly involved medications includes the following:

- Antibiotics (i.e., penicillins, sulfonamides, tetracycline derivatives, sulfonylureas, etc.).
- Antituberculosis medications (i.e., isoniazid, rifampin).
- Antiepileptic drugs (i.e., phenobarbital, carbamazepine, phenytoin, etc.).
- Allopurinol.
- Calcium channel blockers.
- Captopril.
- Thiazides.
- Nonsteroidal anti-inflammatory drugs (NSAIDs).
- Barbiturates.
- Lithium.[2,3,5]

In children, an association with topical boric acid has been identified.[6]

The cause of erythroderma may not always be identified. The onset of erythroderma due to drug reactions is typically sudden, and resolution occurs more quickly than erythroderma attributed to other causes. There is an exception when erythroderma is due to systemic drug hypersensitivity reactions due to antibiotics, anticonvulsants, or allopurinol. In such cases, hypersensitivity develops within 2–5 weeks after the medication is started and may persist for several weeks despite discontinuation of the medication.[3]

DIAGNOSIS

CLINICAL FEATURES

- The clinical presentation of erythroderma may be variable depending on the underlying cause. In association with drug reactions, the onset tends to be more abrupt and the resolution more rapid.
- Cutaneous manifestations begin with pruritic, erythematous patches that spread and coalesce into areas of erythema that cover the body. Scaling eventually develops. Large scales are seen more often in acute settings; in chronic erythroderma smaller scales predominate.
- Although the red color of erythroderma is very evident in light skin, erythroderma may be only light pink to brown in darker-skinned individuals (**Figure 162-8**).
- Symptoms common in long-standing erythroderma of any etiology include lichenification, diffuse alopecia, dermatographic lymphadenopathy, keratoderma, nail dystrophy, and ectropion.[3]

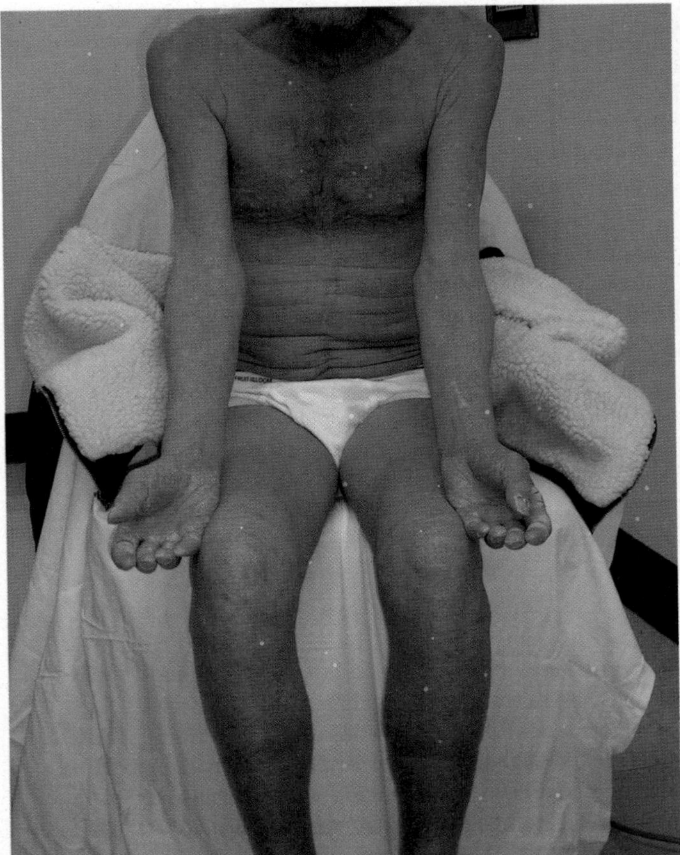

FIGURE 162-6 Erythroderma in an HIV positive man with crusted scabies. He was tachycardic and required hospitalization for fluids and treatment. (*Reproduced with permission from Richard P. Usatine, MD.*)

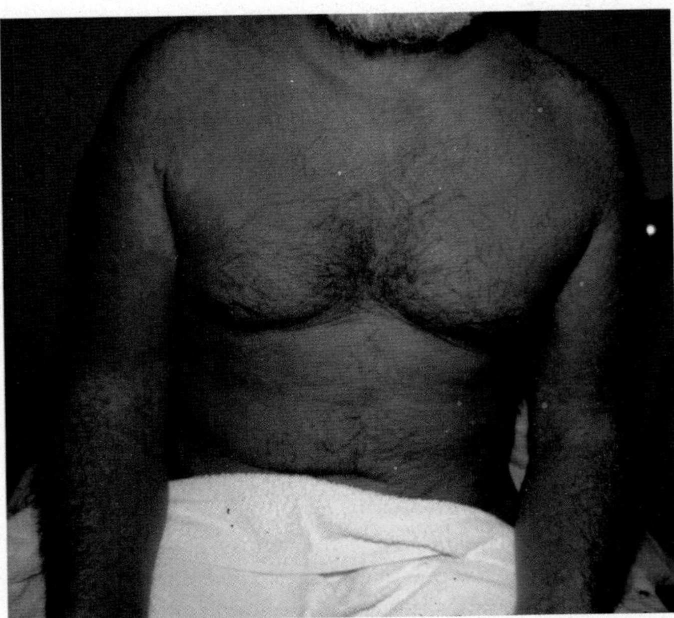

FIGURE 162-7 Erythema secondary to new-onset mycosis fungoides. (*Reproduced with permission from Richard P. Usatine, MD.*)

- Scalp involvement is very common, with alopecia occurring in 25% of patients.[2]
- Pitting pretibial and pedal edema has been reported to have been observed in up to 50% of erythrodermic patients.[3]
- Systemic manifestations associated with compromise of the protective cutaneous barrier and loss of vasoconstriction of vessels in the dermis that occurs in erythroderma include loss of fluid and electrolytes.
- Protein losses can be as high as 25% to 30% in psoriatic erythroderma, resulting in hypoalbuminemia and edema.[3] Increased perfusion to denuded inflamed skin may result in thermoregulatory disturbances and high-output cardiac failure. In addition, there is an increased risk of staphylococcal infection and sepsis.[2,3] Any of these complications can be life threatening.

TYPICAL DISTRIBUTION

The distribution is variable, but there is usually sparing of mucous membranes, the palms, and the soles of the feet. Sparing of the nose and nasolabial region has also been reported.[2]

LABORATORY STUDIES

Skin biopsy is useful to narrow the differential diagnosis, but may often be nondiagnostic, making clinical and pathological correlation a troublesome task. This occurs because the specific features of dermatoses can be masked by the nonspecific features of erythroderma.[4] However, studies show that multiple biopsies of an erythrodermic patient suggest a higher diagnostic accuracy from 53% to 66%.[8]

In addition to conventional histopathologic evaluation, direct immunofluorescence may be helpful in immunobullous disease (e.g., pemphigus). T-cell receptor gene rearrangement studies may aid in the diagnosis of lymphoproliferative disorders.[3] Laboratory tests are often nonspecific; however, common findings include:

- Leukocytosis.
- Lymphocytosis.
- Mild anemia.
- Eosinophilia.
- Elevated sedimentation rate.
- Polyclonal gammopathy.
- Elevated immunoglobulin (Ig) E level (reported in cases of psoriatic erythroderma).[9]
- Hypoalbuminemia.
- Elevated serum creatinine.
- Elevated uric acid levels.[1-3,5,6]

HIV testing should be considered in those with risk factors.[6] In children a sweat test, zinc, amino acid, and lipid levels should be considered.[6]

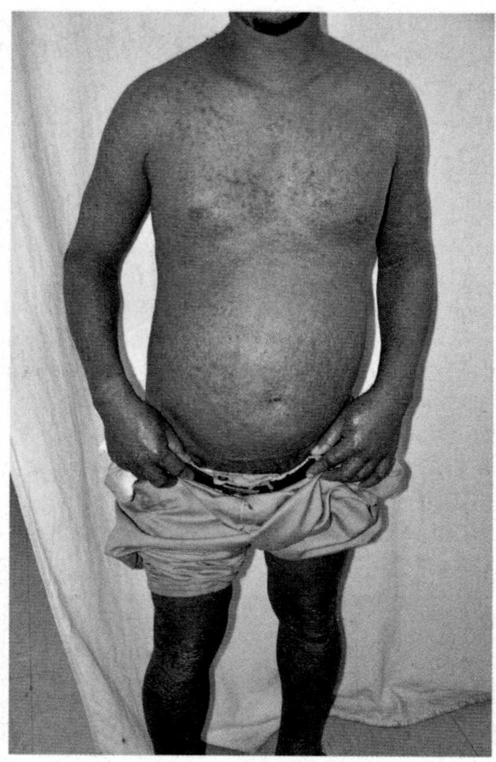

FIGURE 162-8 Erythrodermic psoriasis in a black man showing visible scaling but less obvious erythema secondary to the darker skin color. *(Reproduced with permission from Richard P. Usatine, MD.)*

DIFFERENTIAL DIAGNOSIS

Erythroderma is the dermatologic manifestation of a number of underlying disease processes, including infectious diseases, lymphoproliferative disorders, malignancies, dermatoses, acquired and inborn metabolic disorders, and drug reactions. The key to proper diagnosis and treatment is contingent on identification of the underlying cause.[1-3,5,6] (For a list of underlying conditions, see Etiology and Pathophysiology above.)

MANAGEMENT

FIRST LINE

Hospitalization and urgent dermatologic referral should be considered for patients presenting with erythroderma acutely, as the metabolic, infectious, thermoregulatory, and cardiovascular complications can be life threatening.[2,6]

Therapeutic interventions include:

- Topical skin care measures such as emollients, oatmeal baths, and wet dressings.[1-3,5,6] SOR C
- Placing the patient in a warm and humidified environment often increases patient comfort, prevents hypothermia, and improves moisturization of the skin.[3]
- Oral antihistamines can be prescribed to relieve pruritis.
- Midpotency topical steroid ointments such as 0.1% triamcinolone applied to all the affected areas.[1-3,5,6] SOR C Using the wet wrap technique (see Chapter 151, Atopic Dermatitis) can help promote quicker absorption and faster onset of action. SOR C
- High-potency topical steroids and topical immunomodulators should be avoided owing to risk of increased cutaneous absorption.[3] SOR C
- Systemic steroids are useful in drug reactions and eczema, but should be avoided in psoriasis.[2,3,6] SOR C
- Consider methotrexate or cyclosporine for cases secondary to psoriasis. The biologics infliximab, etanercept, and adalimumab have also been used.[2,4,10] SOR C Cyclosporine acts most rapidly in cases caused by psoriasis or atopic dermatitis. SOR C
- Immunosuppressive agents (methotrexate, azathioprine, infliximab, etanercept, and adalimumab).[2,3,5] SOR C
- Discontinuation of all nonessential medications.[2,3] SOR C
- Close monitoring of fluid, electrolyte, and nutritional status and replacement of deficits.[1-3,5,6] SOR C

SECOND LINE

- Antibiotic therapy when infection is suspected.[2,3] SOR C

FOLLOW-UP

The prognosis in erythroderma is very much dependent on the underlying cause. Most deaths occur in malignancy-associated erythroderma. Drug-induced erythroderma carries the best prognosis and the lowest risk of recurrence. Relapses occur in 15% of patients with psoriatic erythroderma. Fifty percent of patients with idiopathic erythroderma experience partial remission, and one third complete remission.[3]

PATIENT EDUCATION

Patients should be advised that erythroderma can be life-threatening because of the infectious, thermoregulatory, metabolic, and cardiovascular complications. This is important when it might be necessary to hospitalize a patient who does not appreciate the seriousness of the condition. They should also be advised that with certain underlying etiologies, the condition may recur.

PATIENT RESOURCES

- Health-Disease—a Family Medical Guide. *Erythroderma*—**http://www.health-disease.org/skin-disorders/erythroderma.htm.**

PROVIDER RESOURCES

- Medscape. *Erythroderma (Generalized Exfoliative Dermatitis)*—**https://search.medscape.com/search/?q=erythroderma.**
- DermNet NZ. *Erythroderma*—**https://www.dermnetnz.org/topics/erythroderma/.**
- DermIS. Images of *congenital ichthyosiform and psoriatic erythroderma*—**http://www.dermis.net/dermisroot/en/list/erythroderma/search.htm.**

REFERENCES

1. Rothe MJ, Bialy TL, Grant-Kels JM. Erythroderma. *Dermatol Clin.* 2000;18:405-415.
2. Karakayli G, Beckham G, Orengo I, Rosen T. Exfoliative dermatitis. *Am Fam Physician.* 1999;59(3):625-630.
3. Rothe JH, Bernstein ML, Grant-Kels JM. Life-threatening erythroderma: diagnosing and treating the "red man." *Clin Dermatol.* 2005;23(2):206-217.
4. Khaled A, Sellami A, Fazaa B, et al. Acquired erythroderma in adults: a clinical and prognostic study. *J Eur Acad Dermatol Venereol.* 2010;24(7):781-788.
5. Grant-Kels JM, Bernstein ML, Rothe MJ. Exfoliative dermatitis. In: Wolff K, Goldsmith LA, Katz SI, et al., eds. *Fitzpatrick's Dermatology in General Medicine*, 7th ed. New York, NY: McGraw-Hill; 2006.
6. Sehgal VN, Srivastava G. Erythroderma/generalized exfoliative dermatitis in pediatric practice: an overview. *Int J Dermatol.* 2006;45:831-839.
7. Rowe CJ, Robertson I, James D, McMeniman E. Warfarin-induced erythroderma. *Australas J Dermatol.* 2015;56(1):e15-e17.
8. Megna M, Sidikov AA, Zaslavsky DV, et al. The role of histological presentation in erythroderma. *Int J Dermatol.* 2017 Apr;56(4):400-404.
9. Li LF, Sujan SA, Yang H, Wang WH. Serum immunoglobulins in psoriatic erythroderma. *Clin Exp Dermatol.* 2005;30(2):125-127.
10. Mistry N, Gupta A, Alavi A, et al. A review of the diagnosis and management of erythroderma (generalized red skin). *Adv Skin Wound Care.* 2015;28:228-236.

SECTION J BENIGN NEOPLASMS

163 SKIN TAG

Mindy A. Smith, MD, MS
Richard P. Usatine, MD

PATIENT STORY

A 55-year-old man requests removal of multiple skin tags around his neck. He is overweight and has diabetes and acanthosis nigricans. Although some of his skin tags occasionally get caught on his clothing, he just doesn't like the way they look. The patient chose to have many of them removed by the snip excision method.

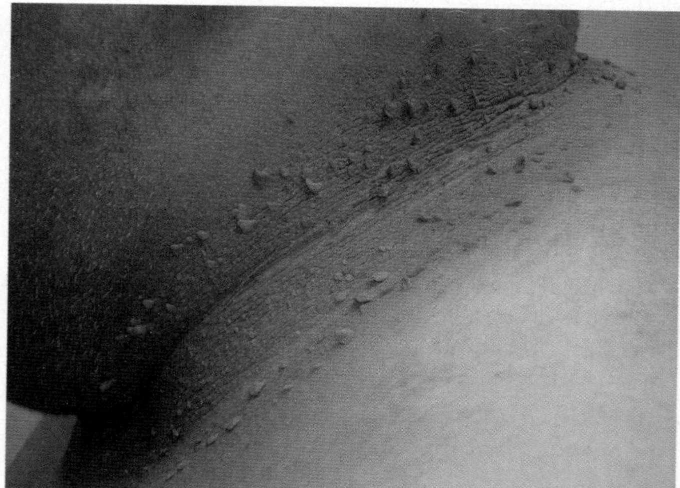

FIGURE 163-1 Many skin tags and acanthosis nigricans on the neck of a man with diabetes. (*Reproduced with permission from Richard P. Usatine, MD.*)

INTRODUCTION

Skin tags (acrochordons) are flesh-colored, pedunculated lesions that tend to occur in areas of skin folds, especially around the neck and in the axillae.

SYNONYMS

Acrochordons, fibroepithelial polyps.

EPIDEMIOLOGY

- In an unselected population study, skin tags were found in 46% of adults, particularly in persons who were obese.[1]
- Skin tags increase in frequency through the fifth decade of life so that as many as 59% of individuals have them by the time they are 70 years old; however, the increase slows after age 50 years.[1]

ETIOLOGY AND PATHOPHYSIOLOGY

- Three types of skin tags are described[1]:
  - Small, furrowed papules of approximately 1 to 2 mm in width and height, located mostly on the neck and the axillae (**Figure 163-1**).
  - Single or multiple filiform lesions of approximately 2 mm in width and 5 mm in length occurring elsewhere on the body (**Figure 163-2**).
  - Large, pedunculated tumor or nevoid, baglike, soft fibromas that occur on the lower part of the trunk (**Figure 163-3**).
- Etiology is unknown, but it is theorized that skin tags occur in localized areas with a paucity of elastic tissue resulting in sessile or atrophic lesions. In addition, hormone imbalances appear to facilitate their development (e.g., high levels of estrogen and

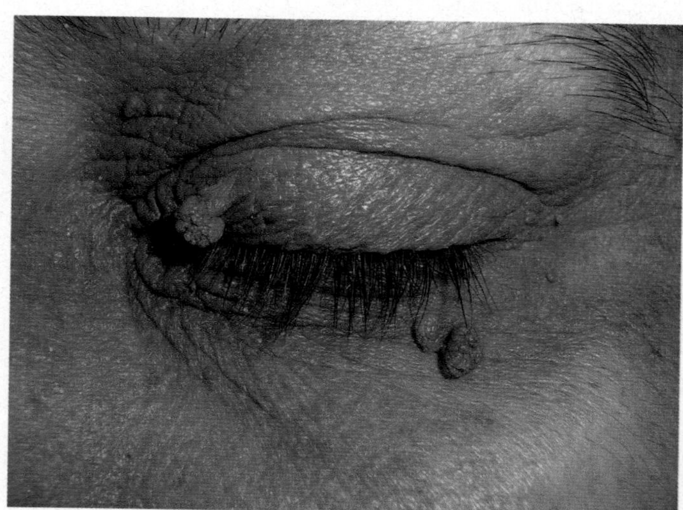

FIGURE 163-2 Filiform pedunculated skin tags on the eyelids. These were removed with a radiofrequency loop after local anesthesia with lidocaine and epinephrine to minimize bleeding. (*Reproduced with permission from Richard P. Usatine, MD.*)

progesterone seen during pregnancy) and other factors including epidermal growth factor, tissue growth factor-α, and infection have been implicated as cofactors.

- Mast cells were found in higher density in skin tags than in normal skin in one study, suggesting a possible role in promoting fibrosis and skin tag development.[2]
- Acrochordons also appear to be associated with impaired carbohydrate metabolism and diabetes[3] (see **Figure 163-1**), as well as colon polyps (odds ratio [OR] 7.07).[4]
- Very rarely, neoplasms are found at the base of skin tags. In a study of consecutive cutaneous pathology reports, 5 of 1335 clinically diagnosed fibroepithelial polyp specimens were malignant (i.e., 4 were basal cell carcinomas and 1 was squamous cell carcinoma in situ).[5] There is a large selection bias in this study because most skin tags are not sent to the pathologist (nor should they be sent unless there is a suspicious feature).

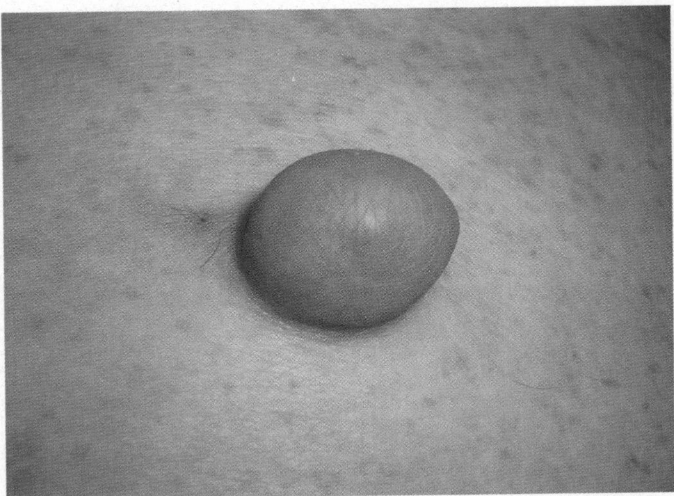

FIGURE 163-3 Large pedunculated baglike soft fibroma on the trunk. This is a large acrochordon or fibroepithelial polyp. Local anesthetic was given prior to excision. (*Reproduced with permission from Richard P. Usatine, MD.*)

DIAGNOSIS

CLINICAL FEATURES

- Small, soft, usually pedunculated lesions.
- Skin colored or hyperpigmented.
- Most vary in size from 2 to 5 mm, but larger ones do occur.
- Usually asymptomatic, but can be pruritic or become painful and inflamed by catching on clothing or jewelry.

TYPICAL DISTRIBUTION

- Most typically seen on the neck and in the axillae (see **Figure 163-1**), but any skin fold may be affected. They are also seen on the trunk (see **Figure 163-3**), the abdomen, and the back.

BIOPSY

- Not usually indicated unless the diagnosis is not clear. Typical skin tags do not need to be sent to pathology upon removal. Skin tags, on histology, are characterized by acanthotic, flattened, or frondlike epithelium. A papillary-like dermis is composed of loosely arranged collagen fibers and dilated capillaries and lymphatic vessels.

DIFFERENTIAL DIAGNOSIS

Lesions that can be confused with skin tags include:

- Warts—Cutaneous neoplasm caused by papillomavirus. There are common warts, flat warts, plantar warts, and condyloma acuminatum. Filiform common warts resemble skin tags more than most other warts. The typical distribution of warts on the hands, feet, and genitalia helps to differentiate these from skin tags.
- Neurofibromas—These benign Schwann cell tumors are soft pedunculated masses (**Figure 163-4**). These can be solitary tumors in persons who do not have neurofibromatosis. It is relatively easy to differentiate these from skin tags in persons who do have neurofibromatosis.
- Nevi—Any small benign pedunculated nevus may resemble a skin tag, but usually their larger size, location, and pigment pattern

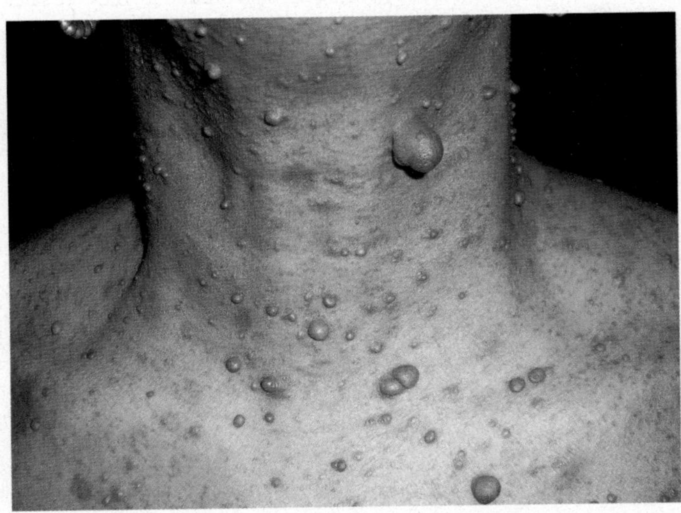

FIGURE 163-4 Multiple soft neurofibromas on the neck of a patient with neurofibromatosis. (*Reproduced with permission from Richard P. Usatine, MD.*)

differentiate them from skin tags. Epidermal hyperplasia in melanocytic nevi (also called keratotic melanocytic nevus [KMN]) may have overlying hyperplastic epidermis resembling skin tags. In a study of melanocytic nevi submitted for pathology over an 8-month period, 6% were KMN, most often located on the trunk (76%).[6] Intradermal nevi can be pedunculated and sparsely pigmented, but they are usually larger than skin tags and are often found on the face.

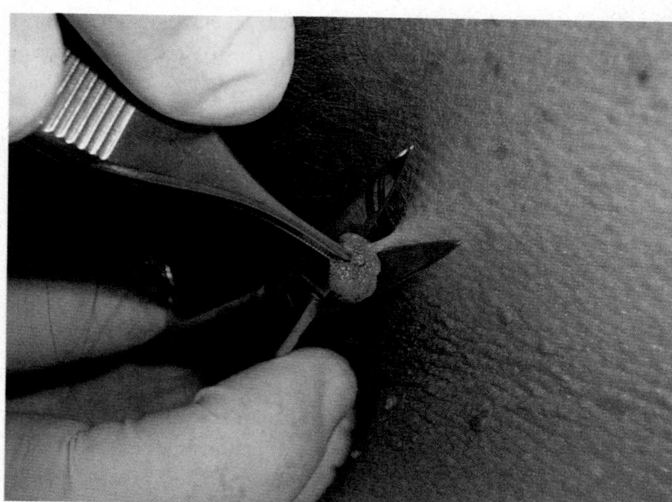

FIGURE 163-5 Snip excision of skin tag with iris scissors and no anesthesia. (*Reproduced with permission from Richard P. Usatine, MD.*)

MANAGEMENT

FIRST LINE

- Give the patient a choice between snip excisions and cryotherapy. Snip excisions are fast and provide immediate results. Cryotherapy is also rapid and does not cause bleeding in the office. The downside of cryotherapy is that it may take 2 weeks for the skin tags to fall off and there is no guarantee that 100% of them will fall off. Both methods are well tolerated. Some patients may fear the snip excision more than the freezing method; others may want to try both methods to see which one hurts least. Ultimately the best method is a matter of patient preference.
- Snip excision—Small lesions may be snipped with a sharp iris scissor with or without anesthesia (**Figure 163-5**). The advantage of this method is that it works immediately and is 100% effective. If there is any bleeding, aluminum chloride on a cotton-tipped applicator is applied for hemostasis. It is unnecessary to use anesthesia for the smallest skin tags unless the patient requests it. It helps to use 1% lidocaine with epinephrine injected with a 30-gauge needle under the skin tag when skin tags are large or have a wide base. This makes the snip painless and decreases the bleeding (especially if one waits for the epinephrine to take effect).
- Cryotherapy with liquid nitrogen can be applied directly to the skin tag with a spray from a cryogun or direct application with forceps or Cryo Tweezers. Cryo Tweezers are manufactured by Brymill, Inc. They have a large metal end to hold the cold longer (**Figure 163-6**). The Cryo Tweezers are usually less painful because the skin tag can be frozen without the spray freezing the skin around it. They are safer for skin tags on the eyelids than the spray method. This is a very efficient way to treat multiple skin tags (approximately 10–15 with a single dip into the liquid nitrogen). Standard forceps require redipping into the liquid nitrogen for every 1 to 2 skin tags. Although cryotherapy is easy to perform and some patients find it less painful, it is not uncommon for some of the skin tags to not fall off.
- Larger skin tags and fibromas may be removed with a snip or shave excision after injecting the base with 1% lidocaine and epinephrine.
- Most insurance companies will not pay for the cosmetic removal of skin tags.
- To avoid large healthcare costs, send only suspicious-looking skin tags to the pathologist.

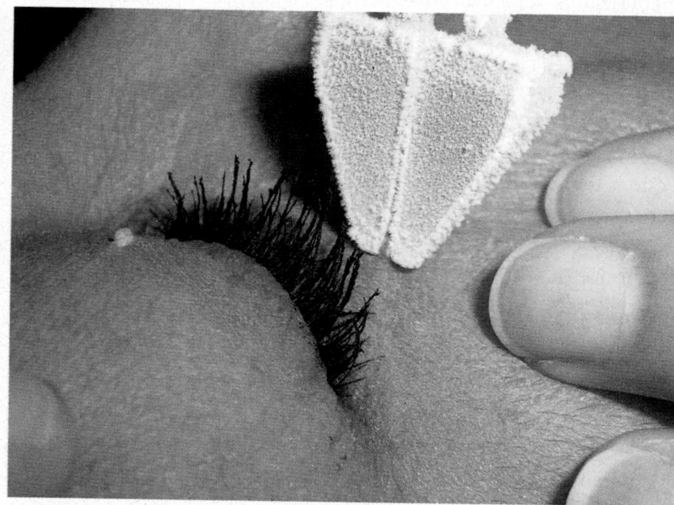

FIGURE 163-6 Cryotherapy using Cryo Tweezers to grasp the skin tag without freezing the skin around it. This is especially helpful on the eyelids. (*Reproduced with permission from Richard P. Usatine, MD.*)

SECOND LINE

- Ethyl chloride spray anesthesia has been described as one method to decrease pain during snip excision with microscissors and microforceps.[7] The spray itself is somewhat uncomfortable and jarring when it hits the skin, and the effect lasts for a few seconds. It can also produce intoxication through inhalation. In our experience there is insufficient benefit to outweigh the risks, time, and costs of ethyl chloride. When anesthesia is needed, injectable lidocaine with epinephrine is most reliable.

- Cryotherapy using liquid nitrogen applied with a cotton-tipped applicator is an option in practices that do not have a cryogun or Cryo Tweezers.
- Cryotherapy with cryogens other than liquid nitrogen provides additional options. As these cryogens are not as cold as liquid nitrogen, they are considered second-line therapy.
- An adhesive patch that applies pressure to the base of a skin tag was found effective in 65% of skin tags in one case series.[8]
- Electrodesiccation with or without anesthesia works for very tiny skin tags too small to grab with the forceps.

FOLLOW-UP

- Follow-up is not usually necessary.

PATIENT EDUCATION

- Advise patients that these are benign growths that can be removed if irritation occurs or for cosmetic purposes. Patients who are overweight should be encouraged to lose weight for their general health and to avoid new skin tags.

PATIENT RESOURCES

- **http://www.nlm.nih.gov/medlineplus/ency/article/000848.htm.**

PROVIDER RESOURCES

- For quick cryosurgery of skin tags, the Cryo Tweezer can be ordered from: **http://www.brymill.com.**

REFERENCES

1. Banik R, Lubach D. Skin tags: localization and frequencies according to sex and age. *Dermatologica.* 1987;174(4):180-183.
2. Abdou AG, Maraee AH, Antar AG, Fareed S. Role of mast cells in skin tag development: an immunohistochemical study. *Anal Quant Cytopathol Histopathol.* 2014;36(4):222-230.
3. Demir S, Demir Y. Acrochordon and impaired carbohydrate metabolism. *Acta Diabetol.* 2002;39(2):57-59.
4. Oran M, Ergan G, Mete R, et al. Association of colon adenomas and skin tags: coincidence or coexistence? *Eur Rev Med Pharmacol Sci.* 2014;18(7):1073-1077.
5. Eads TJ, Chuang TY, Fabre VC, et al. The utility of submitting fibroepithelial polyps for histological examination. *Arch Dermatol.* 1996;132(12):1459-1462.
6. Horenstein MG, Prieto VG, Burchette JL Jr, Shea CR. Keratotic melanocytic nevus: a clinicopathologic and immunohistochemical study. *J Cutan Pathol.* 2000;27(7):344-350.
7. Fredriksson CH, Ilias M, Anderson CD. New mechanical device for effective removal of skin tags in routine health care. *Dermatol Online J.* 2009;15(2):9.
8. Görgülü T, Torun M, Güler R, et al. Fast and painless skin tag excision with ethyl chloride. *Aesthetic Plast Surg.* 2015;39(4):644-645.

164 SEBORRHEIC KERATOSIS

Mindy A. Smith, MD, MS
Richard P. Usatine, MD

PATIENT STORY

An elderly woman noted growth of a lesion on her chest (**Figure 164-1**). She was afraid that it might be melanoma. Her family physician recognized the typical features of a seborrheic keratosis (SK) (stuck on with visible horn cysts) and attempted to reassure her. Dermoscopy was performed, and the features were typical of an SK; the physician was able to convince the patient to not have a biopsy (**Figure 164-2**). The black comedo-like openings and white milia-like cysts are typical of an SK and can be seen with the naked eye in this case, and even better with a dermatoscope.

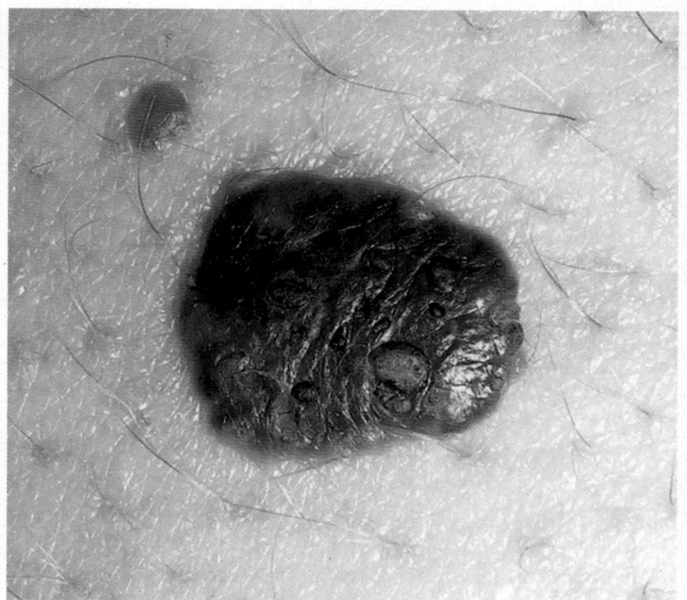

FIGURE 164-1 Seborrheic keratosis with associated horn cysts. *(Reproduced with permission from Richard P. Usatine, MD.)*

INTRODUCTION

- An SK is a benign skin tumor and a form of localized hyperpigmentation as a result of epidermal alteration; it develops from the proliferation of epidermal cells, although the cause is unknown.

SYNONYMS

Senile keratoses, age spots.

EPIDEMIOLOGY

- Most common benign tumor in older individuals; frequency increases with age.
- In a study of individuals older than age 64 years in North Carolina, 88% had at least one SK. Ten or more SKs were found in 61% of the black men and women, 38% of the white women, and 54% of the white men in the study.[1]
- In an Australian study preformed in 2 general practices, 23.5% (40 of 170) of individuals between ages 15 and 30 years had at least 1 SK; prevalence and size increased with age.[2]
- Approximately half of cases of multiple SKs occur within families, with an autosomal dominant mode of inheritance.[3]

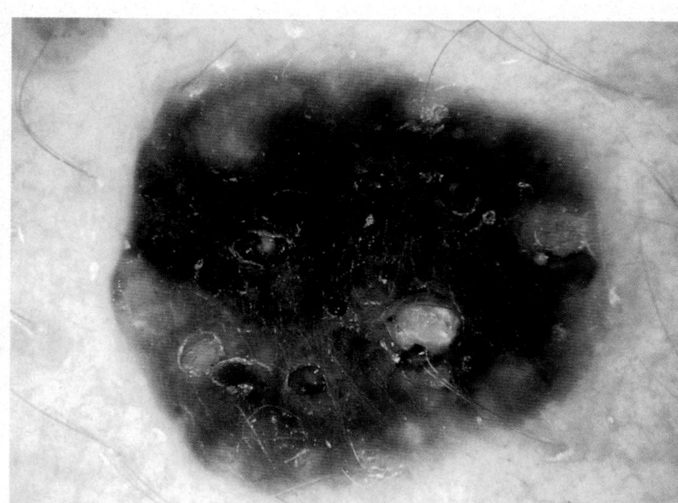

FIGURE 164-2 Dermoscopy of the seborrheic keratosis in the previous figure showing comedo-like openings (black, like blackheads) and milia-like cysts (white, like milia). *(Reproduced with permission from Richard P. Usatine, MD.)*

ETIOLOGY AND PATHOPHYSIOLOGY

- In pigmented SKs, the proliferating keratinocytes secrete melanocyte-stimulating cytokines, triggering activation of neighboring melanocytes.[3]
- A high frequency of mutations has been found in certain types of SKs in the gene encoding the tyrosine kinase receptor fibroblast growth factor receptor 3 (FGFR3).[3] One study found that FGFR3 and transcription factor forkhead box N1 (FOXN1) were highly

expressed in SKs but close to undetectable in squamous cell skin cancer.[4] This may represent a positive regulatory loop between FGFR3 and FOXN1 that underlies a benign versus malignant skin tumor phenotype.

- Reticulated SKs, usually found on sun-exposed skin, may develop from solar lentigines.[3]
- Multiple eruptive SKs (the sign of Leser-Trélat) have been associated with internal malignancy in case reports (see **Figure 164-3**),[5] although this association has been questioned.[6,7]
- An eruption of SKs may develop after an inflammatory dermatosis such as severe sunburn or eczema.[3]

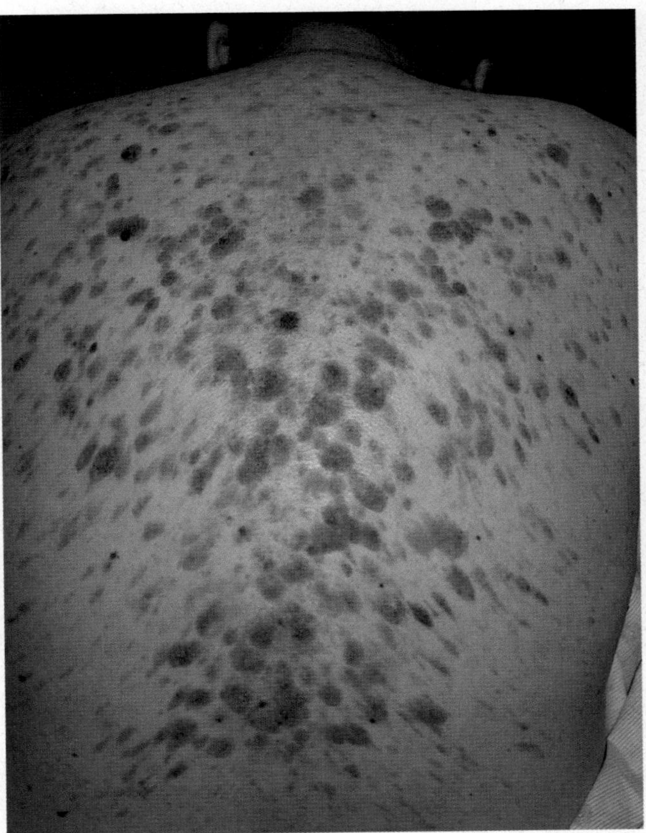

FIGURE 164-3 Many seborrheic keratoses appeared within a short period of time on this 49-year-old man's back. While this may be called the sign of Leser-Trélat, this patient did not have any evidence of malignancy. The patient is cancer free over 5 years later, and no major work-up was needed. (*Reproduced with permission from Richard P. Usatine, MD.*)

DIAGNOSIS

SKs have a variety of appearances. They are all superficial with an abundance of keratin on the surface causing various patterns.

CLINICAL FEATURES

- Typically oval or round brown plaques with adherent greasy scale (**Figure 164-4**).
- Color can be black, brown, tan, pink, or a combination of these colors (**Figures 164-4** to **164-6**).
- Most often have a velvety to finely verrucous surface and appear to be "stuck on."
- Some are so verrucous they can appear to be warty (**Figure 164-6**).
- SKs may be large, pigmented, and have irregular borders (**Figure 164-5**).
- Early SKs may be flat like a solar lentigo (**Figure 164-7**).
- Many lesions show keratin plugging of the surface (**Figures 164-1** and **164-2**).
- May have surface ridges of keratin and associated horn cysts (keratin-filled cystic structures). The dermoscopy terms for the horn cysts are comedo-like openings and milia-like cysts (**Figure 164-2**, see Chapter 111, Dermoscopy). The keratin ridges give many SKs the cerebriform appearance.
- Occasionally, lesions become irritated and can itch, grow, and bleed. These lesions should be considered for biopsy as these features are also suggestive of melanoma.
- Variants of SKs include:
  - Dermatosis papulosa nigra—Consists of multiple brown-black dome-shaped or pedunculated SKs on the face in persons of color (**Figures 164-8** and **164-9**).
  - Stucco keratosis—Consists of superficial gray-to-light brown flat keratotic lesions usually on the tops of the feet, the ankles, and the back of the hands and forearms (**Figure 164-10**). They resemble a stucco wall, and that is the origin of the name.

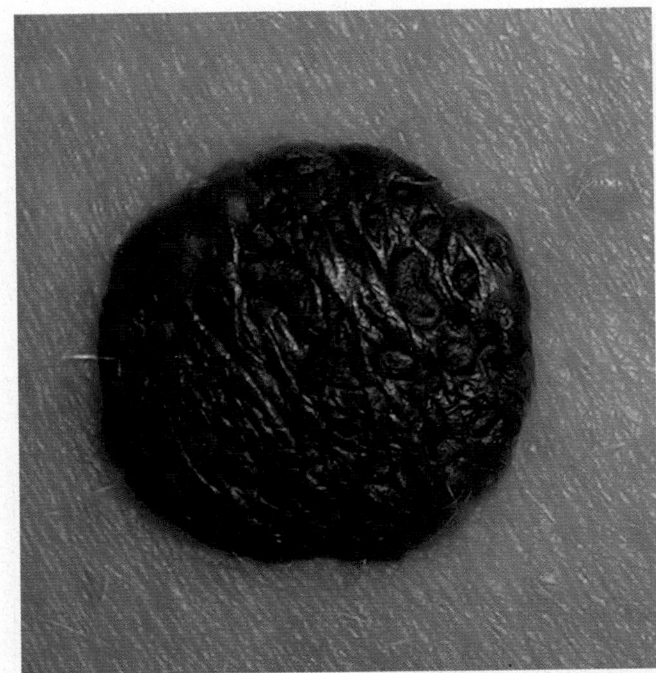

FIGURE 164-4 Round elevated seborrheic keratosis with very visible horn cysts (comedo-like openings of keratin). (*Reproduced with permission from Richard P. Usatine, MD.*)

DERMOSCOPIC FEATURES

- Multiple milia-like cysts and comedo-like openings.
- Fissures and ridges of keratin create cerebriform patterns and fat finger-like structures.

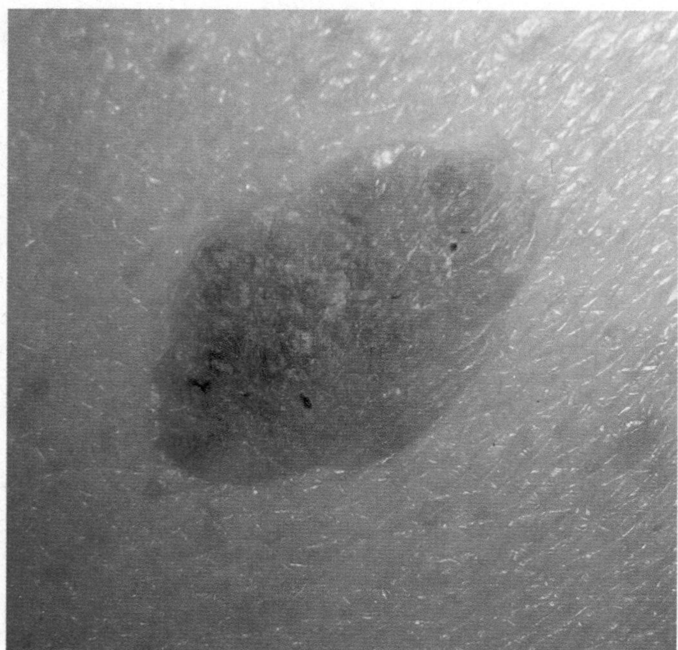

FIGURE 164-5 Seborrheic keratosis that is lightly pigmented, waxy, and appears stuck on. (*Reproduced with permission from Richard P. Usatine, MD.*)

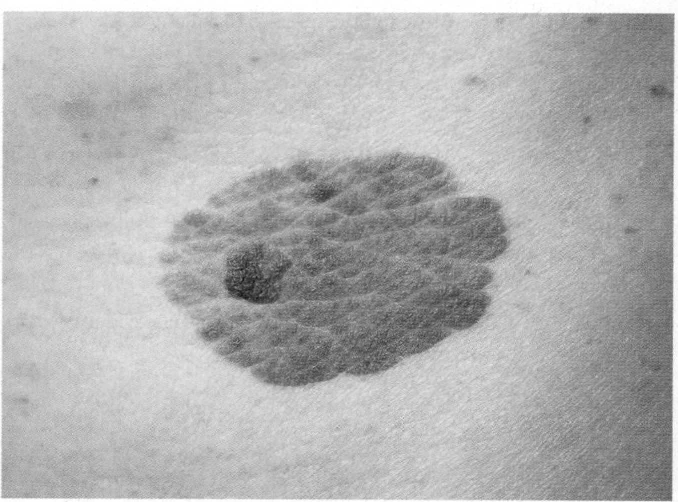

FIGURE 164-7 Seborrheic keratosis with irregular borders and variation in color that might suggest a possible melanoma using the ABCDE criteria. Dermoscopically it was completely benign and a biopsy was not needed. (*Reproduced with permission from Richard P. Usatine, MD.*)

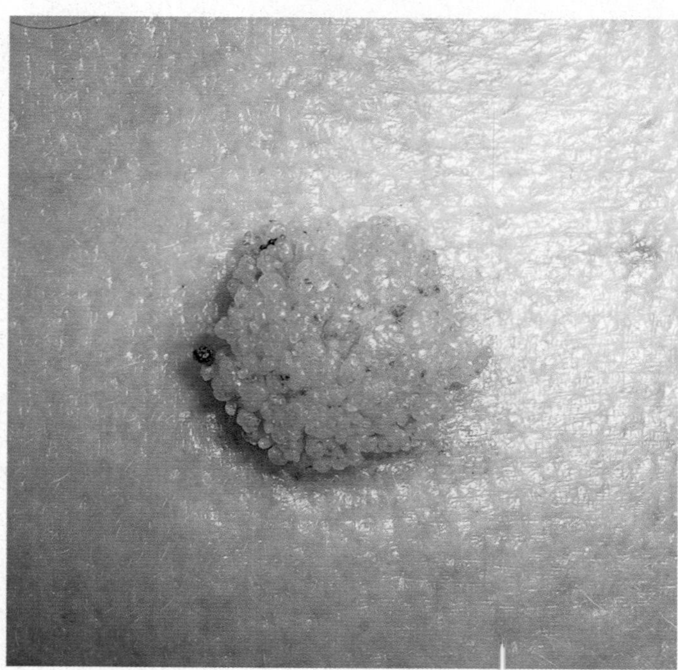

FIGURE 164-6 Seborrheic keratosis with verrucous appearance on the forehead. (*Reproduced with permission from Richard P. Usatine, MD.*)

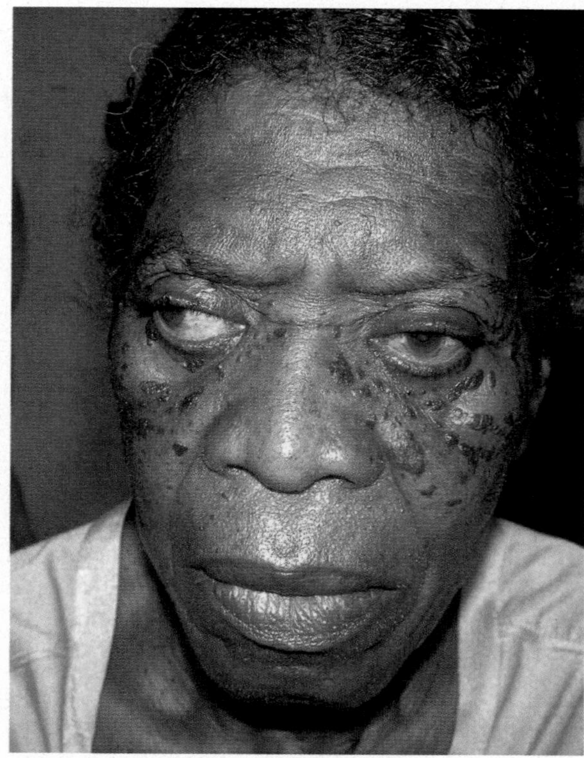

FIGURE 164-8 Dermatosis papulosa nigra with multiple seborrheic keratoses on the face of a Central American woman. (*Reproduced with permission from Richard P. Usatine, MD.*)

- Flatter SKs may have fingerprint-like structures and moth-eaten borders (like solar lentigines).
- Hairpin shaped vessels (other keratinizing tumors such as squamous cell carcinoma may also have hairpin vessels) (see Chapter 111, Dermoscopy).

TYPICAL DISTRIBUTION

- Trunk, face, back, abdomen, extremities; not present on the palms and soles or on mucous membranes. May be present on the areola and breasts (**Figures 164-11** and **164-12**).
- Dermatosis papulosa nigra is found on the face, especially the upper cheeks and lateral orbital areas (see **Figures 164-8** and **164-9**).

IMAGING

- No imaging studies are needed even if there is a sudden appearance of multiple seborrheic keratoses as described in the sign of Leser-Trélat (see **Figure 164-3**). The relationship between malignancy and Leser-Trélat sign is conflicting, and no evidence other than multiple case reports supports the presence of the sign as a predictor of malignancy.[3,7,8] Most likely these are coincidental, and to date there is no scientific mechanism to explain the connection observed by Leser and Trélat. A work-up for malignancy should be based on other signs or symptoms of disease (and age-appropriate screening) and not on the number or rapid appearance of SKs alone.

BIOPSY

- Should be performed if there is a suspicion of melanoma (**Figure 164-13**). Some melanomas resemble SKs, and a biopsy is needed to avoid missing the diagnosis of melanoma. Do not freeze or curette a suspicious SK; these need a biopsy (usually a shave under the lesion such as a saucerization or deep shave) to send tissue to the pathologist.[9-11] An elliptical excision is not needed in most cases, and a punch biopsy increases the risk of misdiagnosis by incomplete sampling.[9]

DIFFERENTIAL DIAGNOSIS

- Melanoma—When many keratin plugs are visible in the surface of the SK, this helps to distinguish it from a melanoma. However, some melanomas have these same features as part of their morphology. **Figure 164-7** is an SK that has the ABCDE features (Asymmetry, Border irregular, Color variation, Diameter >6 mm, Evolving) of melanoma (Chapter 179, Melanoma). A biopsy was performed and the lesion was proven to be benign. In **Figure 164-13**, a possible SK turned out to be a melanoma in situ. **Figure 164-14** is a melanoma on the vulva that had appeared similar to an SK, and it was only because dermoscopy revealed the blue-white veil that a biopsy was done and the melanoma was not missed.
- Solar lentigo—Flat, uniformly medium or dark brown lesion with sharp borders (Chapter 175, Lentigo Maligna). These are flat and seen in sun-exposed areas, typically on the face or back of the hands. Also called liver spots, these hyperpigmented areas are not palpable, whereas an SK is a palpable plaque even when the SK is thin (**Figure 164-7**). Flat solar lentigines can evolve into seborrheic keratoses. While most SKs do not start as solar lentigines, some SKs do start as a solar lentigo (**Figure 164-15**).

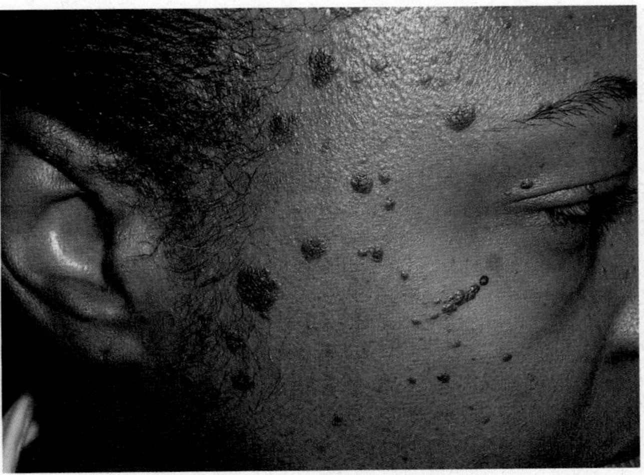

FIGURE 164-9 Dermatosis papulosa nigra on the cheeks and in the hairline. The patient was treated effectively with cryotherapy and had a great cosmetic result. (*Reproduced with permission from Richard P. Usatine, MD.*)

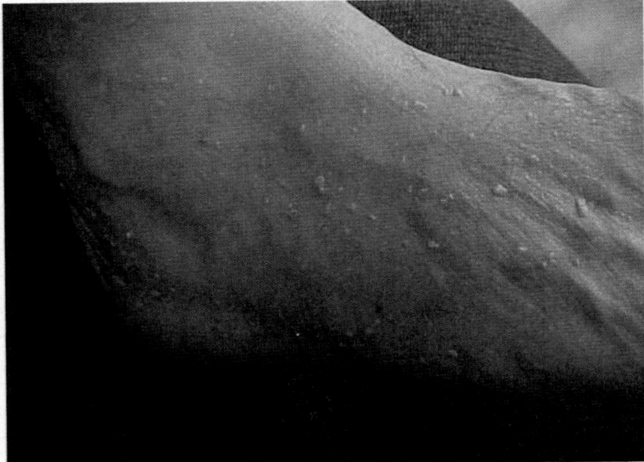

FIGURE 164-10 Stucco keratosis on the foot of an elderly man. (*Reproduced with permission from Richard P. Usatine, MD.*)

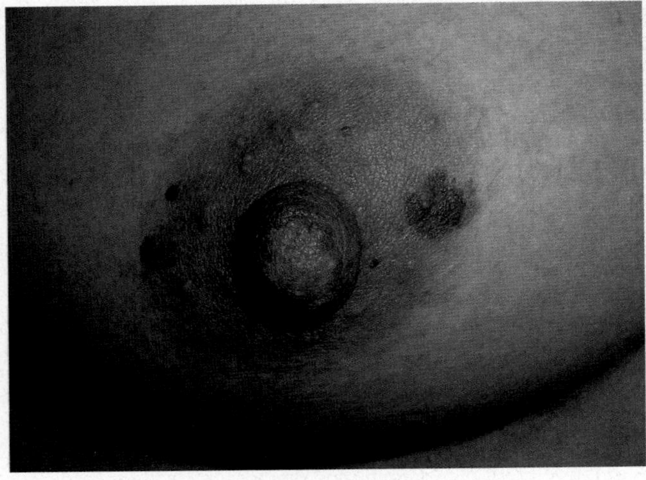

FIGURE 164-11 Multiple seborrheic keratoses on the areola of a 46-year-old woman. Cryotherapy cleared the seborrheic keratoses easily. (*Reproduced with permission from Richard P. Usatine, MD.*)

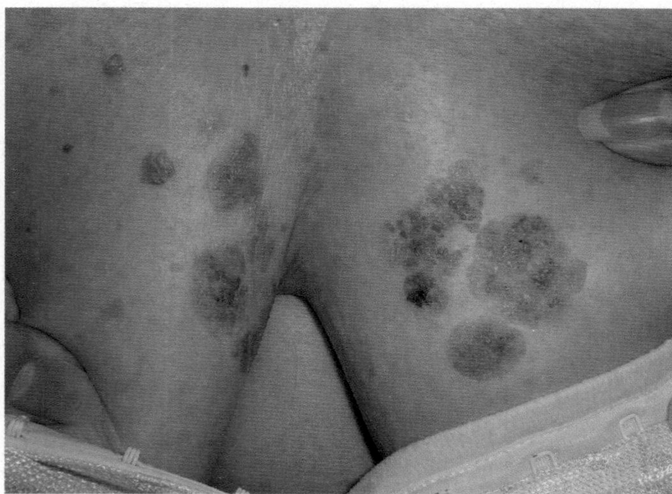

FIGURE 164-12 Waxy large seborrheic keratoses on the breasts of this 70-year-old woman. (*Reproduced with permission from Richard P. Usatine, MD.*)

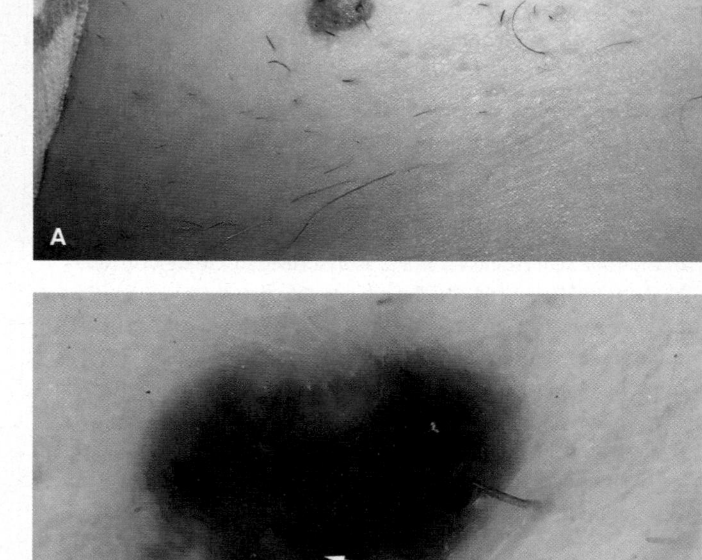

FIGURE 164-14 **A.** Melanoma in the inguinal area of a 57-year-old woman that resembled a seborrheic keratosis with visible horn cysts. **B.** Fortunately, dermoscopy revealed a blue-white veil suspicious for melanoma. A deep shave biopsy was performed and the melanoma was not missed. (*Reproduced with permission from Richard P. Usatine, MD.*)

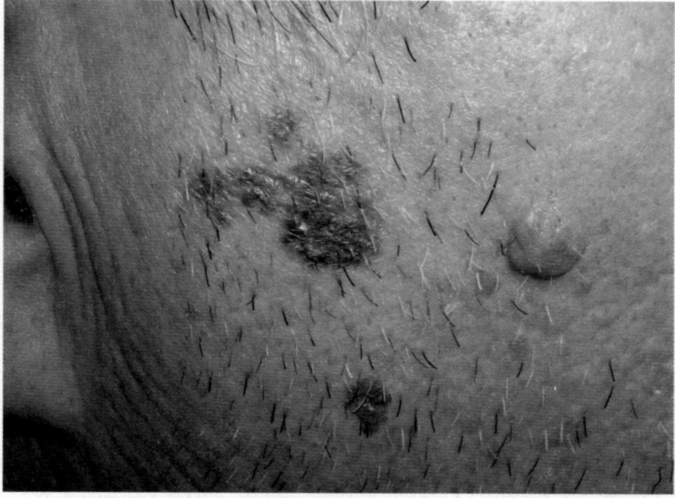

FIGURE 164-13 Melanoma in situ on the lateral face of a 55-year-old man. This resembles a seborrheic keratosis, but this large lesion also has all the ABCDEs of melanoma and dermoscopy features suspicious for a lentigo maligna. A saucerization biopsy of the most suspicious area provided the diagnosis. (*Reproduced with permission from Richard P. Usatine, MD.*)

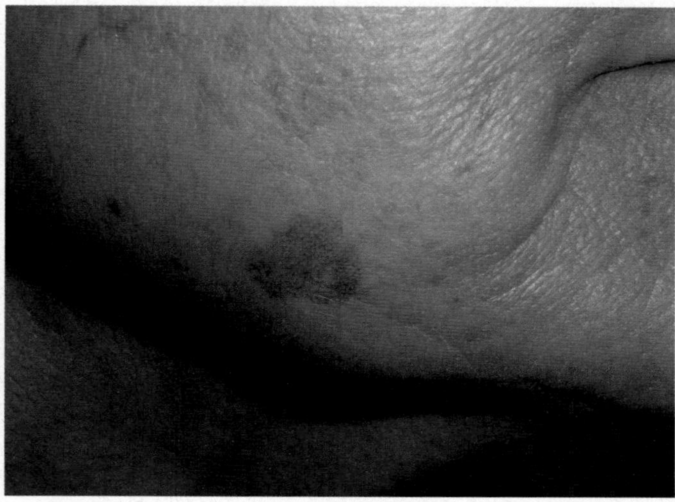

FIGURE 164-15 Early flat seborrheic keratosis that started as a solar lentigo on the face. (*Reproduced with permission from Richard P. Usatine, MD.*)

- Lichen planus–like keratosis (LPLK) is a regressing SK. With regression these lesions will show blue-gray granules and dots on dermoscopy, reflecting melanophage activity. These can be confused with melanomas and should be biopsied to rule out melanoma.
- Wart—Cutaneous neoplasm caused by HPV (Chapter 137, Common Warts). Warts also have a hyperkeratotic surface like an SK. They tend to be papillomatous with thrombosed vessels and disruption of skin lines. As both warts and SKs are benign, cryotherapy is appropriate for both lesions when treatment is desired.
- Pigmented actinic keratosis (AK)—Although most AKs are nonpigmented and don't look like an SK, occasionally a biopsy of an unknown pigmented plaque will be a pigmented AK secondary to sun damage (Chapter 173, Actinic Keratosis and Bowen Disease).
- An inflamed SK may be confused with a malignant melanoma or a squamous cell carcinoma and should be biopsied to determine the diagnosis. Inflamed SKs show more hairpin vessels under dermoscopy (**Figure 164-16**).
- Even a basal cell carcinoma (BCC) can have features that suggest an SK. If the SK is atypical with BCC-like features, a biopsy is warranted (Chapter 177, Basal Cell Carcinoma).

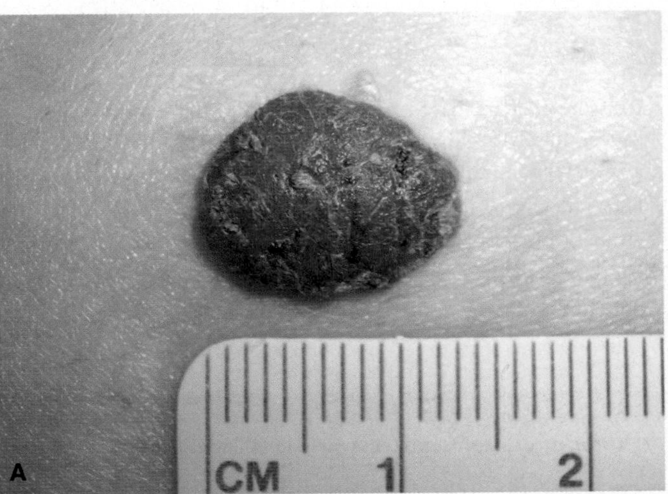

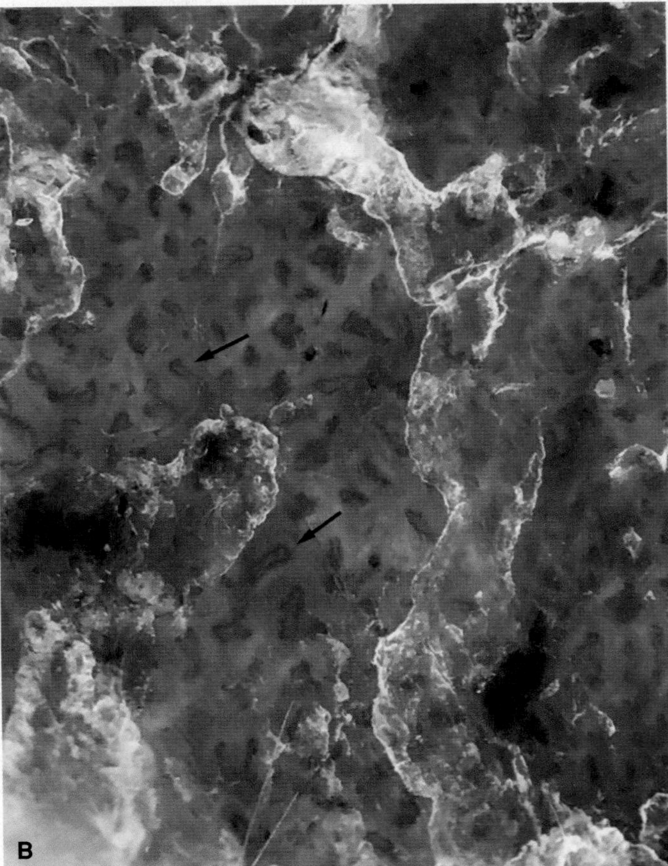

FIGURE 164-16 **A.** Inflamed seborrheic keratosis showing a pinker coloration. **B.** Dermoscopy of part of the lesion showing hairpin vessels (arrows). Note that some of the other hairpin vessels are twisted. *(Reproduced with permission from Richard P. Usatine, MD.)*

MANAGEMENT

FIRST LINE

- Cryosurgery with liquid nitrogen, with a 1-mm halo, is a quick and easy treatment. The risks include pigmentary changes, incomplete resolution, and scarring. Hypopigmentation is the most common complication of this treatment, especially in dark-skinned individuals.
- Shave biopsy—If melanoma or another skin cancer is suspected, perform a shave excision or saucerization just deep enough to get under the lesion and send to pathology (see Chapter 113, Biopsy Principles and Techniques).

SECOND LINE

- Removal of a benign-appearing SK by curettage is one option if one is certain of the diagnosis. After local anesthesia with lidocaine and epinephrine, light electrofulguration can make the curettage easier, and sometimes the SK may be rubbed off with a wet gauze pad. A skin curette works well for this procedure. This is second line because it is more work than a shave excision and does not provide as good a tissue sample for histology. As long as one is not freezing the SK and is using a local anesthetic, it is safest to send the tissue for pathology.
- A new highly concentrated hydrogen peroxide solution, A-101, is being studied for topical treatment of SKs of the face.[12]

FOLLOW-UP

- Follow-up as needed. Patients with multiple SKs do not need special monitoring unless there are other risk factors for skin or internal malignancy.

PATIENT EDUCATION

- Reassure patients that SKs are benign lesions that do not become cancer. Rarely, a skin cancer can arise in an SK. Although SKs may grow larger and thicker with time, this is not usually dangerous.
- Unless the SK is suspicious for cancer or inflamed, removal is for cosmetic purposes only and is often not covered by insurance.
- Although SKs may resolve on occasion, spontaneous resolution does not ordinarily occur.

PATIENT RESOURCES

- **http://medlineplus.gov/ency/article/000884.htm.**

PROVIDER RESOURCES

- **http://emedicine.medscape.com/article/1059477-overview.**

REFERENCES

1. Tindall JP, Smith JG. Skin lesions of the aged and their association with internal changes. *JAMA*. 1963;186:1039-1042.
2. Gill D, Dorevitch A, Marks R. The prevalence of seborrheic keratoses in people aged 15 to 30 years. *Arch Dermatol.* 2000;136: 759-762.
3. Balin AK. *Seborrheic Keratosis*. http://emedicine.medscape.com/article/1059477-overview#a0104. Accessed January 2017.
4. Mandinova A, Kolev V, Neel V, et al. A positive FGFR3/FOXN1 feedback loop underlies benign skin keratosis versus squamous cell carcinoma formation in humans. *J Clin Invest.* 2009;119(10): 3127-3137.
5. Ponti G, Luppi G, Losi L. Leser-Trélat syndrome in patients affected by six multiple metachronous primitive cancers. *J Hematol Oncol.* 2010;3:2.
6. Lindelof B, Sigurgeirsson B, Melander S. Seborrheic keratoses and cancer. *J Am Acad Dermatol.* 1992;26(6):947-950.
7. Turan E, Gurel MS, Erdemir AT. Leser-Trélat sign: a paraneoplastic process? *Cutis*. 2014;94(5):E14-E15.
8. Cascajo CD, Reichel M, Sanchez JL. Malignant neoplasms associated with seborrheic keratoses. An analysis of 54 cases. *Am J Dermatopathol.* 1996;18(3):278-282.
9. Ng JC, Swain S, Dowling JP, et al. The impact of partial biopsy on histopathologic diagnosis of cutaneous melanoma: experience of an Australian tertiary referral service. *Arch Dermatol.* 2010;146(3): 234-239.
10. Coit DG, Andtbacka R, Bichakjian CK, et al. NCCN Melanoma Panel. Melanoma. *J Natl Compr Canc Netw.* 2009;7(3):250-275.
11. Zager JS, Hochwald SN, Marzban SS, et al. Shave biopsy is a safe and accurate method for the initial evaluation of melanoma. *J Am Coll Surg.* 2011;212(4):454-460.
12. DuBois JC, Jarratt M, Beger BB, et al. A-101, a proprietary topical formulation of high-concentration hydrogen peroxide solution: a randomized, double-blind, vehicle-controlled, parallel group study of the dose-response profile in subjects with seborrheic keratosis of the face. *Dermatol Surg.* 2018;44(3):330-340.

165 SEBACEOUS HYPERPLASIA

Mindy A. Smith, MD, MS
Richard P. Usatine, MD

PATIENT STORY

A 65-year-old man noted a new growth on his face for 1 year (**Figure 165-1A**). On close examination, the growth was pearly with a few telangiectasias. The donut shape and presence of sebaceous hyperplasia scattered on other areas of the face were reassuring that this is likely a benign sebaceous hyperplasia. To confirm our clinical impression, the lesion was examined with a dermatoscope (**Figure 165-1B**). Vessels extending toward the center of the lesion from the periphery but not crossing the center (like the shape of a crown) were seen. This along with the yellow color of the sebaceous glands strongly supported the diagnosis. Because the patient wanted the lesion to be removed, a shave biopsy was performed to completely rule out basal cell carcinoma (BCC). The patient was happy with the cosmetic result and relieved that the pathology showed sebaceous hyperplasia.

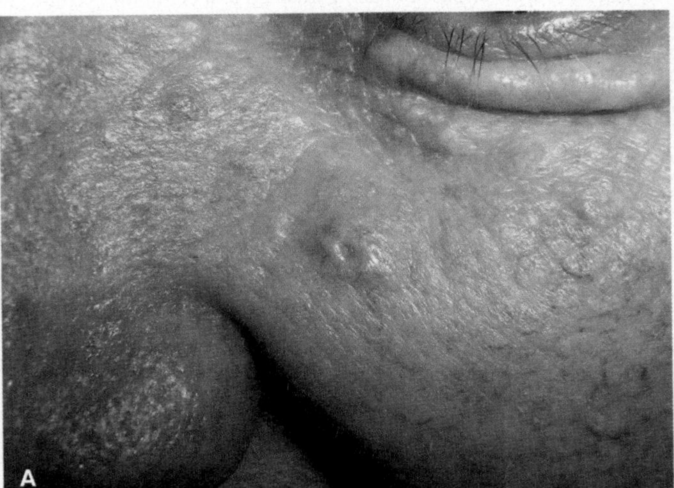

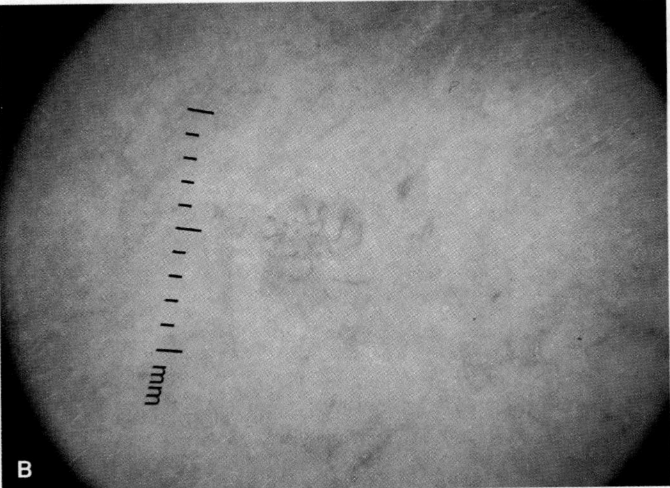

FIGURE 165-1 **A.** Large single lesion of sebaceous hyperplasia that was examined by dermoscopy to confirm that it was not a basal cell carcinoma. **B.** Typical features of sebaceous hyperplasias were seen (crown vessels among yellow sebaceous glands). (*Reproduced with permission from Richard P. Usatine, MD.*)

INTRODUCTION

Sebaceous hyperplasia (SH) is a common, benign condition of sebaceous glands consisting of multiple asymptomatic small yellow papules with a central depression. The sebaceous lobules of SH are greater in number and higher in the dermis than normal sebaceous glands, and only 1 gland appears enlarged.[1] Consequently, the term *hyperplasia* appears to be a misnomer, and SH is more accurately classified as a hamartoma (disorganized overgrowth of tissue normally found at that site).[1]

EPIDEMIOLOGY

- SH occurs in approximately 1% to 26% of the adult population; the latter number is from a population study of hospitalized patients with a mean age of 82 years.[1]
- The prevalence of SH is increased in those with immunosuppression by 10-fold to 30-fold[1]; for example, 10% to 30% of patients receiving long-term immunosuppression with cyclosporine have SH.[2,3]
- SH has also been reported in infants, where they are considered physiologic,[4] and in young adults who may have a family history of SH.[1]
- SH has been reported overlying other skin lesions including neurofibromas, melanocytic nevi, verruca vulgaris, and skin tags.[1]
- Rare forms of SH include giant linear (up to 5 cm in diameter) and functional familial (also called premature or diffuse SH); the latter occur typically around puberty as thick plaque-like lesions with pores resembling an orange peel.[1]

ETIOLOGY AND PATHOPHYSIOLOGY

- Sebaceous glands, a component of the pilosebaceous unit, are found throughout the skin, everywhere that hair is found. The greatest number is found on the face, chest, back, and upper outer arms.
- The glands are composed of acini attached to a common excretory duct. In some areas, these ducts open directly onto the epithelial surface, including the lips and buccal mucosa (i.e., Fordyce spots), glans penis or clitoris (i.e., Tyson glands), female areolae (i.e., Montgomery glands), and eyelids (i.e., meibomian glands).[1]
- Sebaceous glands are highly androgen sensitive, become increasingly active at puberty, and reach their maximum by the third decade of life.
- The cells that form the sebaceous gland, sebocytes, accumulate lipid material as they migrate from the basal layer of the gland to the central duct, where they release the lipid content as sebum. In younger individuals, turnover of sebocytes occurs approximately every month.
- With aging, the turnover of sebocytes slows; this results in crowding of primitive sebocytes within the sebaceous gland, causing a benign hamartomatous enlargement called SH.[1]
- Genetic factors include overexpression of the aging-associated gene Smad7 and parathormone-related protein.[5] In a small case series, activating HRAS, KRAS, and EGFR mutations were found in 60% of 43 sebaceous gland hyperplasia lesions.[6]
- There is no known potential for malignant transformation, but SH may be associated with nonmelanoma skin cancer in patients following organ transplantation.

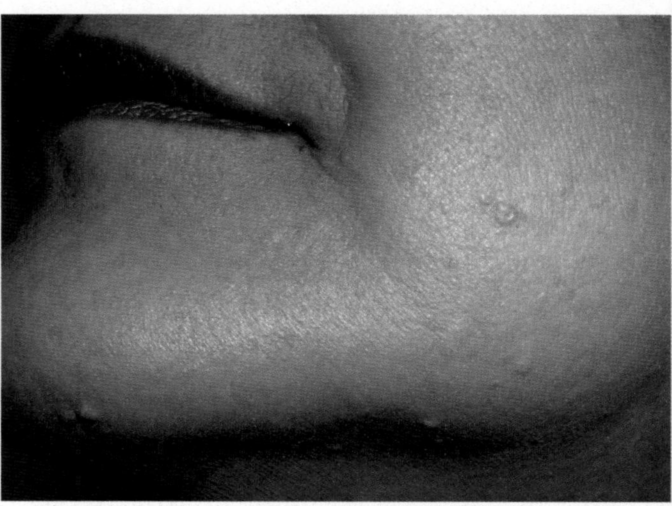

FIGURE 165-2 Multiple lesions of sebaceous hyperplasia on the cheek and chin. Simultaneous appearance of multiple lesions makes them less likely to be basal cell carcinoma. (*Reproduced with permission from Richard P. Usatine, MD.*)

RISK FACTORS

- Associated with Muir-Torre syndrome (concurrent or sequential development of a sebaceous neoplasm and an internal malignancy or multiple keratoacanthomas, an internal malignancy, and a family history of Muir-Torre syndrome).
- Immunosuppression.
- Ultraviolet radiation.

DIAGNOSIS

CLINICAL FEATURES

- Lesions appear as yellowish, soft, small papules ranging in size from 2 to 9 mm (**Figures 165-1** to **165-3**).[1]
- Surface varies from smooth to slightly verrucous.
- Lesions can be single or multiple.
- Increasing number of lesions with aging; higher frequencies after 40 to 50 years of age.[1]
- In functional familial SH, lesions may appear thick and plaque-like, with pores that resemble an orange peel; the skin in these patients is quite oily.[1]

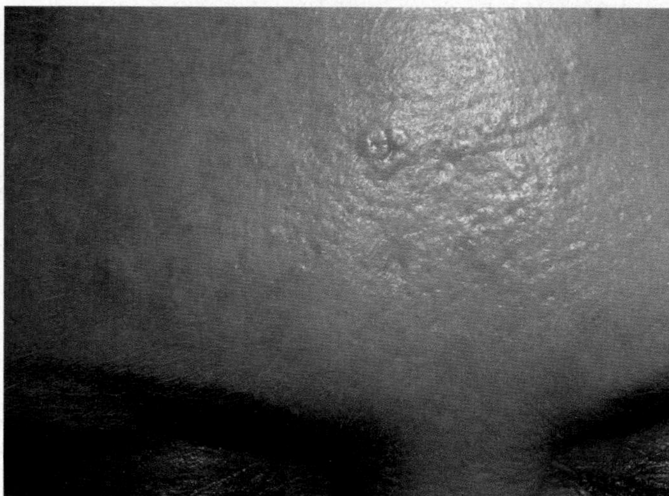

FIGURE 165-3 Large sebaceous hyperplasia on the forehead with telangiectasias. Donut shape visible. (*Reproduced with permission from Richard P. Usatine, MD.*)

- Lesions may become red and irritated and bleed after scratching, shaving, or other trauma; they may be associated with telangiectasias.
- Central umbilication (donut shape) from which a small amount of sebum can sometimes be expressed (**Figures 165-1** to **165-3**).

TYPICAL DISTRIBUTION

- Most commonly located on the face, particularly the nose, cheeks, and forehead. May also be found on the chest, areola, mouth, and, rarely, the vulva.[1,7]

IMAGING

- Dermoscopy can aid in distinguishing between nodular BCC and SH; a vascular pattern with orderly winding, scarcely branching vessels extending toward the center of the lesion is specific for SH. These are described as crown vessels that extend through the yellow sebaceous glands (see **Figure 165-1B**).[8]

BIOPSY

- Not usually necessary unless concerned about BCC.

DIFFERENTIAL DIAGNOSIS

- Nodular BCC—These lesions can appear as waxy papules with a central depression that may ulcerate, most commonly located on the head, neck, and upper back. They may have a pearly appearance, surface telangiectases, and bleed easily (**Figures 165-4** and **165-5**).
- Fibrous papule of the face is a benign, firm, papule of 1 to 5 mm that is usually dome-shaped and indurated with a shiny, skin-colored appearance. Most lesions are located on the nose and, less commonly, on the cheeks, chin, neck, and, rarely, the lip or forehead.
- Milia are common, benign, keratin-filled cysts (histologically identical to epidermoid cysts) that occur in persons of all ages. They are 1 to 2 mm, superficial, uniform, pearly white to yellowish, domed lesions usually occurring on the face (**Figure 165-6**).
- Molluscum contagiosum are firm, smooth, usually 2- to 6-mm umbilicated papules that may be present in groups or widely disseminated on the skin and mucosal surfaces. The lesions can be flesh colored, white, translucent, or even yellow in color. Lesions generally are self-limited but can persist for several years (Chapter 136, Molluscum Contagiosum).
- Syringoma is a benign adnexal neoplasm formed by well-differentiated ductal elements. They are 1- to 3-mm skin-colored or yellowish dermal papules with a rounded or flat top arranged in clusters, and symmetrically distributed primarily on the upper parts of the cheeks and lower eyelids (see **Figure 165-6**).
- Xanthomas are deposits of lipid in the skin or subcutaneous tissue that manifest clinically as yellowish papules, nodules, or tumors. They are usually a consequence of primary or secondary hyperlipidemia and occur in patients older than age 50 years. The lesions are soft, velvety, yellow, flat, polygonal papules that are asymptomatic and usually bilateral and symmetric (Chapter 232, Hyperlipidemia and Xanthomas).

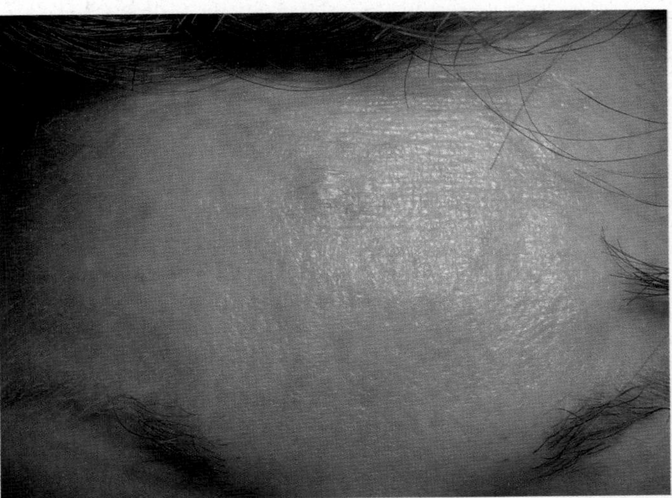

FIGURE 165-4 Basal cell carcinoma on the forehead that could be mistaken for sebaceous hyperplasia. (*Reproduced with permission from Richard P. Usatine, MD.*)

FIGURE 165-5 Close-up of same basal cell carcinoma on the forehead that shows irregular distribution of telangiectasias and lack of the donut shape. (*Reproduced with permission from Richard P. Usatine, MD.*)

MANAGEMENT

SH does not require treatment but can be removed for cosmetic purposes or if it becomes irritated. Evidence supporting treatment comes primarily from case series.

- Options for removal include cryotherapy, electrodesiccation, topical chemical treatments (e.g., with bichloracetic acid or trichloroacetic acid), oral isotretinoin (10 to 40 mg a day for 2 to 6 weeks), laser treatment (e.g., with argon, carbon dioxide, or pulsed-dye laser), photodynamic therapy (PDT; i.e., combined use of 5-aminolevulinic acid and visible light),[9] shave excision, and punch excision.[1] Complications of these therapies include atrophic scarring and changes in pigmentation.

FIRST LINE

- The easiest and most effective method in the family physician's office is to lightly electrodesiccate the SH with electrosurgery using 2 to 2.3 watts with a blunt-tip electrode. This can be done without anesthesia and provides a good cosmetic result. The electrode is moved in a circular or linear fashion around or across the SH until the tissue turns gray (**Figure 165-7**).
- If there is any suspicion that what appears to be sebaceous hyperplasia may be a BCC, perform a shave biopsy as treatment and send the tissue for histology.

SECOND LINE

- In one case series of 20 patients with sebaceous hyperplasia, use of isotretinoin at 1 mg/kg/day significantly decreased the number of lesions from an average of 24 lesions per patient to 2 per patient at 2 months and 4 per patient at 2 years.[10] Discontinuation is associated with high relapse rates.[11]
- Authors of a systematic review of laser treatment and PDT for sebaceous hyperplasia found that use of wavelength-specific laser of 1720 nm had better outcomes with minimal damage.[11] In addition, pretreatment with carbon dioxide laser ablation or pulsed-dye laser before PDT offered higher cure rates over stand-alone laser or PDT treatments using fewer sessions with similar transient side effects.

FOLLOW-UP

No follow-up is needed.

PATIENT RESOURCES

- **https://www.skinsight.com/skin-conditions/adult/sebaceous-hyperplasia.**

PROVIDER RESOURCES

- **http://emedicine.medscape.com/article/1059368-overview.**

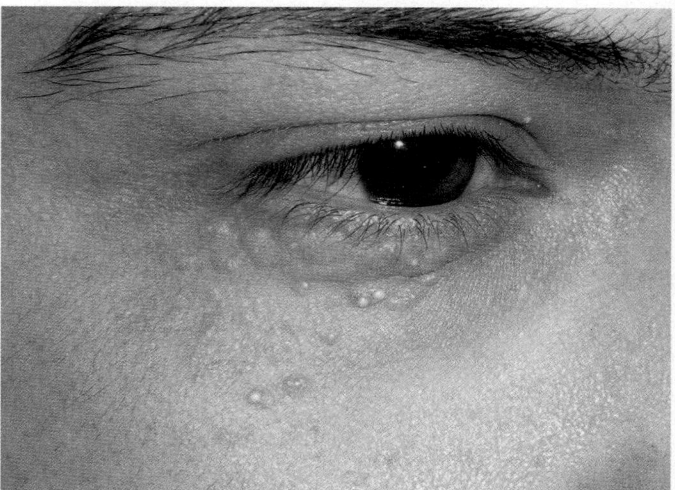

FIGURE 165-6 Syringomas and milia on the lower eyelid of a 23-year-old man. The milia are the white round epidermal cysts, and the syringomas are flesh colored and larger. (*Reproduced with permission from Richard P. Usatine, MD.*)

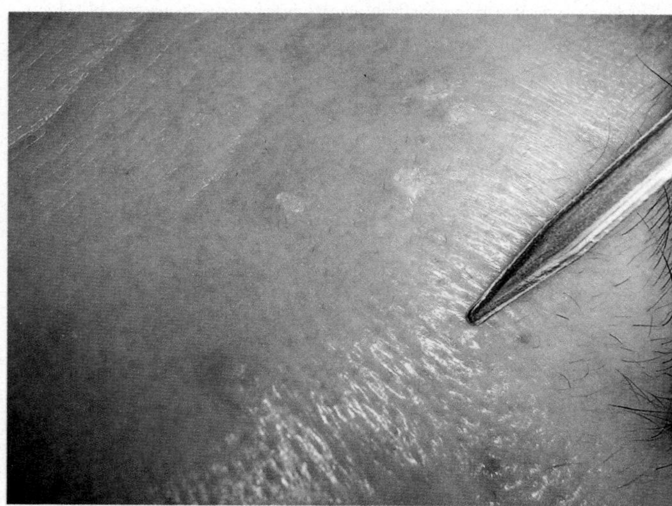

FIGURE 165-7 Electrosurgery of sebaceous hyperplasia using a blunt-tip electrode. Four lesions of sebaceous hyperplasia have already been treated and show the gray coloration found after treatment, and two areas remain to be treated. (*Reproduced with permission from Richard P. Usatine, MD.*)

REFERENCES

1. Eisen DB, Michael DJ. Sebaceous lesions and their associated syndromes: part 1. *J Am Acad Dermatol.* 2009;61:549-560.
2. Boschnakow A, May T, Assaf C, et al. Ciclosporin A-induced sebaceous gland hyperplasia. *Br J Dermatol.* 2003;149(1):198-200.
3. Wilken R, Fung MA, Shi VY, et al. Cyclosporine-induced sebaceous hyperplasia in a hematopoetic stem cell transplant patient: delayed onset of a common adverse event. *Dermatol Online J.* 2016;22(1). pii: 13030/qt4865202s.
4. Oh ST, Kwon HJ. Premature sebaceous hyperplasia in a neonate. *Pediatr Dermatol.* 2007;24:443-445.
5. Zouboulis CC, Boschnakow A. Chronological ageing and photoageing of the human sebaceous gland. *Clin Exp Dermatol.* 2001;26(7):600-607.
6. Groesser L, Singer S, Peterhof E, et al. KRAS, HRAS and EGFR mutations in sporadic sebaceous gland hyperplasia. *Acta Derm Venereol.* 2016;96(6):737-741.
7. Al-Daraji WI, Wagner B, Ali RBM, McDonagh AJG. Sebaceous hyperplasia of the vulva: a clinicopathological case report with a review of the literature. *J Clin Pathol.* 2007;60(7):835-837.
8. Zaballos P, Ara M, Puig S, Malvehy J. Dermoscopy of sebaceous hyperplasia. *Arch Dermatol.* 2005;141:808.
9. Gold MH, Bradshaw WL, Boring MM, et al. Treatment of sebaceous hyperplasia by photodynamic therapy with 5-aminolevulinic acid and a blue light source or intense pulsed light source. *J Drugs Dermatol.* 2004;3(6 Suppl):S6-S9.
10. Tagliolatto S, Santos Neto Ode O, Alchorne MM, et al. Sebaceous hyperplasia: systemic treatment with isotretinoin. *An Bras Dermatol.* 2015;90(2):211-215.
11. Simmons BJ, Griffith RD, Falto-Aizpurua LA, et al. Light and laser therapies for the treatment of sebaceous gland hyperplasia a review of the literature. *J Eur Acad Dermatol Venereol.* 2015;29(11):2080-2087.

166 DERMATOFIBROMA

Mindy A. Smith, MD, MS
Richard P. Usatine, MD

PATIENT STORY

A 25-year-old woman reports a firm nodule on her leg that gets in the way of shaving her leg (**Figure 166-1**). Upon questioning, the nodule may have appeared in that location after she cut her leg shaving 1 year ago. She is worried it could be a cancer and wants it removed. Close observation showed a brown halo and a firm nodule that dimpled down when pinched. A diagnosis of a dermatofibroma (DF) was made and the choices for treatment were discussed.

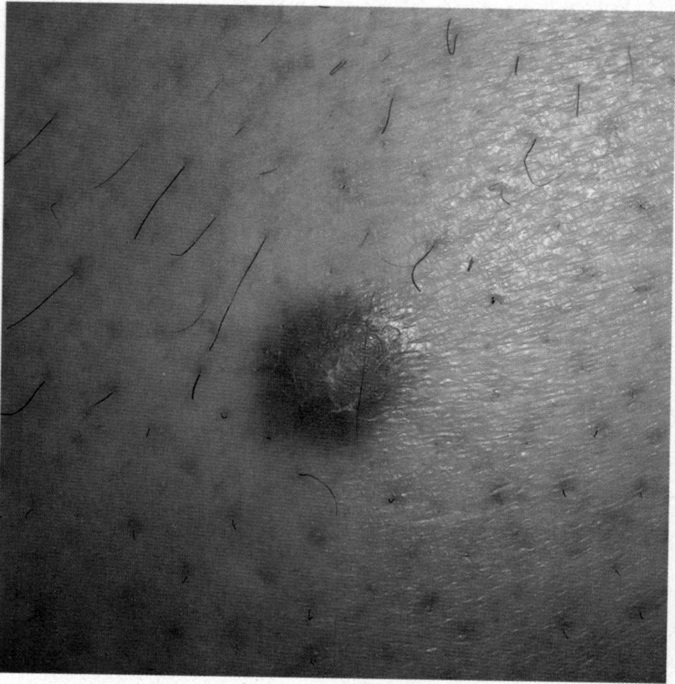

FIGURE 166-1 Dermatofibroma on the leg of a 25-year-old woman that may have begun after she cut her leg shaving 1 year ago. Note the brown halo, pink hue, and raised center. (*Reproduced with permission from Richard P. Usatine, MD.*)

INTRODUCTION

DF is a benign fibrohistiocytic tumor, usually found in the mid dermis, composed of a mixture of fibroblastic and histiocytic cells. These scarlike nodules are most commonly found on the legs and arms of adults.

SYNONYMS

Also called benign fibrous histiocytoma.

EPIDEMIOLOGY

- Occurs more often in women (male-to-female ratio is 1:2).[1]
- Found in patients of all races.
- Approximately 20% occur in patients younger than age 20 years.[1] In one case series, 80% occurred in people between the ages of 20 and 49 years.[2]

ETIOLOGY AND PATHOPHYSIOLOGY

- Uncertain etiology—Nodule may represent a fibrous reaction triggered by trauma, a viral infection, or insect bite; however, DFs show clonal proliferative growth seen in both neoplastic and inflammatory conditions.[3]
- The epidermal regions of DFs are similar to seborrheic keratosis in terms of histologic features and activation of fibroblast growth factor receptor 3 and forkhead box N1.[4]
- Multiple DFs (i.e., >15 lesions) have been reported associated with systemic lupus erythematosus, HIV infection, Down syndrome, Graves disease, or leukemia and may represent a worsening of immune function.[1] A case of familial eruptive DFs has also been reported associated with atopic dermatitis.[5]

DIAGNOSIS

CLINICAL FEATURES

- Firm to hard nodule; skin is freely movable over the nodule, except for the area of dimpling.
- Color of the overlying skin ranges from flesh to gray, pink, red, blue, brown, or black (**Figures 166-2** and **166-3**), or a combination of hues (**Figure 166-4**).
- Dimples downward when compressed laterally because of tethering of the overlying epidermis to the underlying nodule (see **Figure 166-3**).
- Usually asymptomatic but may be tender or pruritic.
- Size ranges from 0.3 to 10 mm; usually less than 6 mm. Rarely, DFs grow to larger than 5 cm.[6]
- May have a hyperpigmented halo and a scaling surface (see **Figure 166-4**).
- DFs can rarely be located entirely within subcutaneous tissue.[7]

DERMOSCOPY

- Dermoscopy is a useful diagnostic technique for DF (**Figure 166-5**). Although the most common finding is a peripheral pigment network with a central white area (34.7% of cases), 10 dermoscopic patterns have been identified; in a large case series, pigment network was observed in 71.8% (3% atypical pigment network).[8] (See Chapter 111, Dermoscopy.) Another common pattern contains ringlike globules in the central scar like area (**Figure 166-6**).

TYPICAL DISTRIBUTION

- May be found anywhere, but usually on the legs and arms, especially the lower legs. In one case series, 70% were on the lower extremities.[2]

BIOPSY

- A punch biopsy can be both diagnostic and therapeutic. DFs have been reported with overlying basal cell carcinoma and associated melanoma[9,10]; rarely, DFs are malignant.[11]
- Histologically, DFs are classified as fibrous histiocytomas (80%) followed by aneurysmal (5.7%), hemosiderotic (5.7%), epithelioid (2.6%), cellular (2.1%), lipidized (2.1%), atrophic (1.0%), and clear cell (0.5%) variants.[12] It is recommended to fully excise cellular DFs with clear margins, as these tend to be more aggressive and may be malignant.[11,13]

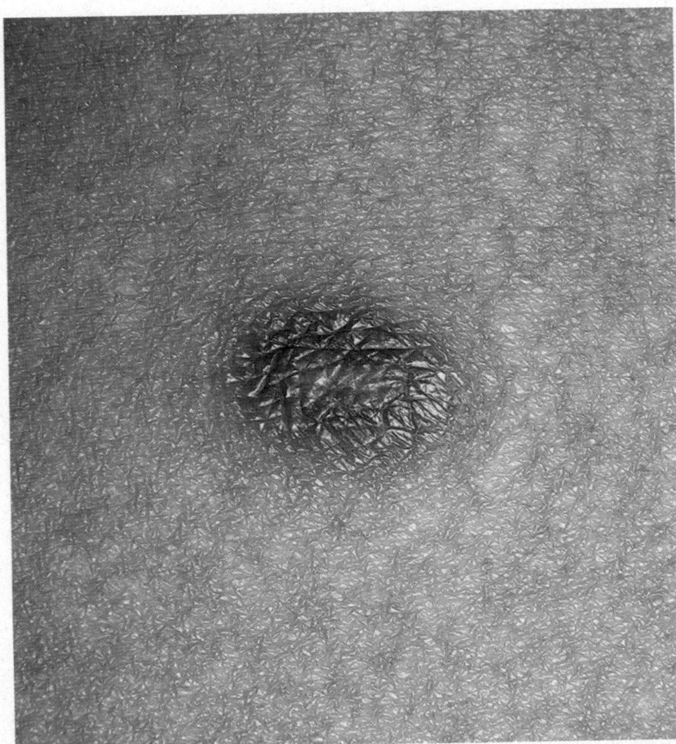

FIGURE 166-2 Dermatofibroma on the thigh of a black woman. Note the darker brown halo around the lighter center. *(Reproduced with permission from Richard P. Usatine, MD.)*

DIFFERENTIAL DIAGNOSIS

DFs can be confused with the following malignant tumors; diagnosis based on histology and excision should be undertaken for enlarging or ulcerating tumors:

- Dermatofibrosarcoma protuberans—A malignant fibrotic tumor of the skin and subcutaneous tissues (**Figure 166-7**). A punch biopsy may provide adequate tissue to make the diagnosis, but a larger incisional biopsy may be needed. These are dangerous tumors with a high risk of recurrence, so they should be referred to Mohs

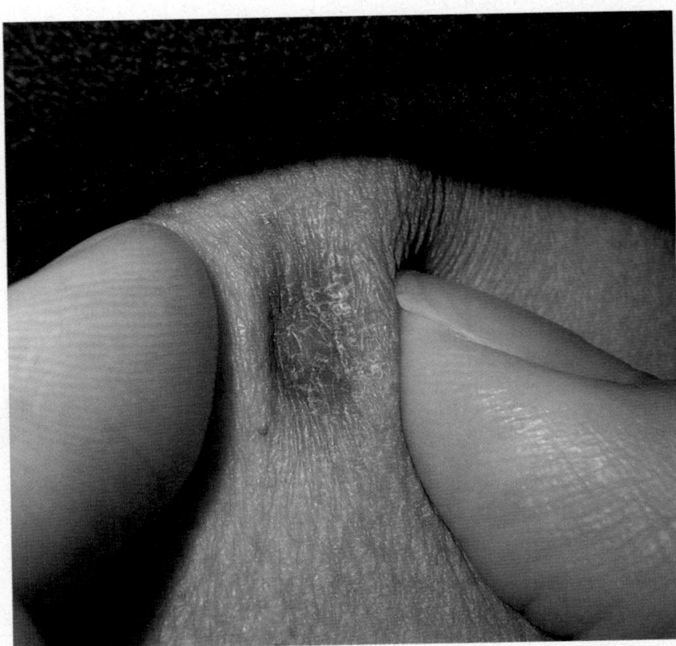

FIGURE 166-3 Pinch test showing a deep dimpling of this dermatofibroma. Ask for the patient's permission before pinching. *(Reproduced with permission from Richard P. Usatine, MD.)*

surgery for complete excision. They resemble a large irregular DF, but a DF is not a precursor to this. It is a separate malignant tumor, not the result of a DF growing out of control.

- Pseudosarcomatous DF—A rare connective tissue tumor arising on the trunk and limbs in young adults.
- Malignant fibrous histiocytoma—A common soft-tissue sarcoma occurring in the extremities. Presentation as a primary cutaneous lesion is rare; more often presents as a metastasis from another location such as the breast.

Many benign lesions have a similar appearance, including:

- Pigmented seborrheic keratosis—May be macular and often larger than DF. Distinguished by surface cracks, verrucous features, stuck-on appearance, and adherent greasy scale (Chapter 164, Seborrheic Keratosis).
- Hypertrophic scar—Occurs within previous wounds or lacerations.
- Neurofibroma—Benign Schwann cell tumors; single lesions are seen in normal individuals. Cutaneous tumors tend to form multiple, soft, pedunculated masses, whereas subcutaneous nodules are skin-colored soft nodules attached to peripheral nerves. The latter show invagination similar to that in DF (Chapter 245, Neurofibromatosis).

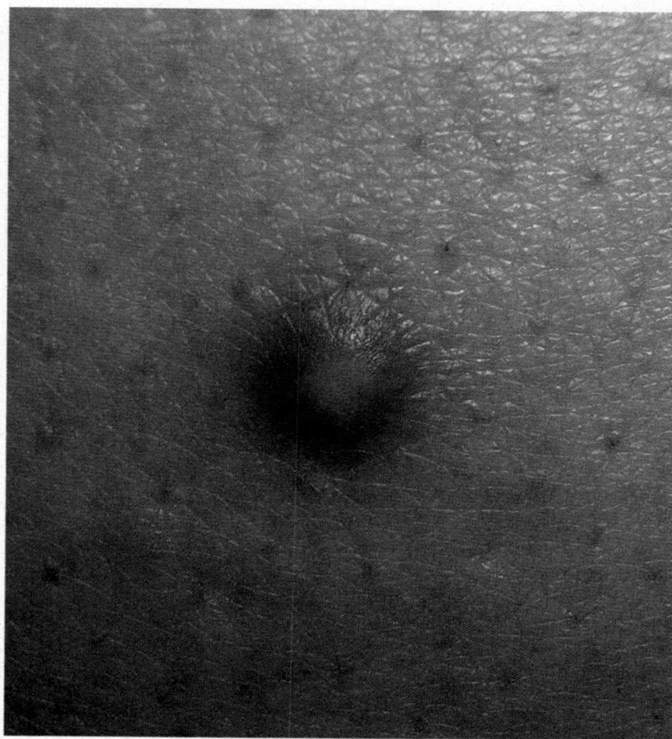

FIGURE 166-4 Dermatofibroma on the back. Note the brown halo around the lighter central nodule. (*Reproduced with permission from Richard P. Usatine, MD.*)

MANAGEMENT

FIRST LINE

- No treatment is necessary unless the diagnosis is questioned or symptoms warrant.
- Punch excision or shave excision may be used for small lesions; with the latter technique, the healed area may remain hard as a result of remaining fibrous tissue.
- Larger lesions may require an elliptical (fusiform) excision, down to the subcutaneous fat.
- One author noted that DFs occurring on the face often have involvement of deeper structures and an increased rate of local recurrences, and therefore recommended excision with wider margins in comparison with DFs occurring on the extremities.[14]

SECOND LINE

- Cryotherapy has also been used, but the cure rate is lower and lesions may recur.
- Several case reports found success in treating multiple DFs with carbon dioxide laser.[15]

PROGNOSIS

- Although DFs are usually unchanging and persist indefinitely, there are reports of spontaneous regression.[16]
- Following excision, DFs have a low recurrence rate of less than 2%, with higher recurrence believed to occur in cellular, aneurysmal, and atypical types.[8,13]
- A higher rate of recurrence has been noted in the subcutaneous and deep types, and in lesions located on the face, in which a recurrence rate of 15% to 19% has been reported.[17,18]

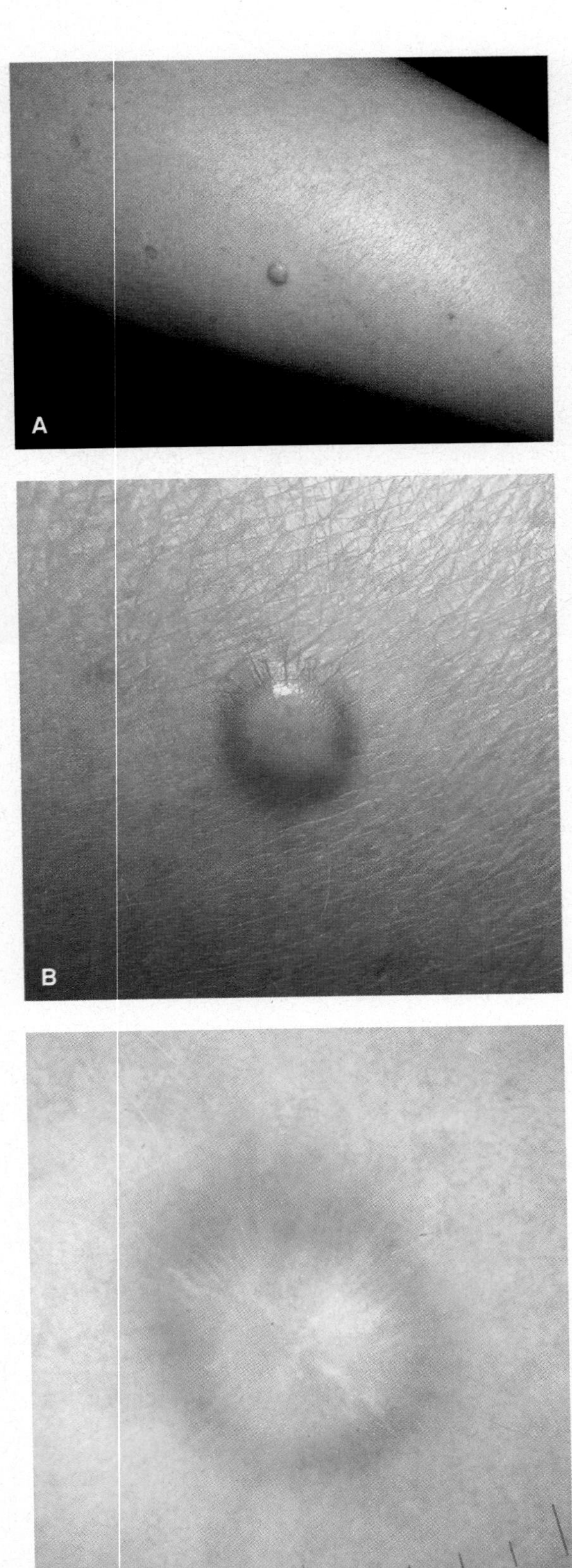

FIGURE 166-5 **A.** Dermatofibroma on the leg that has a pink center and a light brown halo. **B.** Close-up of the dermatofibroma showing the pink center and brown halo. **C.** Dermoscopic view of the dermatofibroma showing the typical pattern with a radially streaking brown halo and a pink center with white stellate scar. (*Reproduced with permission from Richard P. Usatine, MD.*)

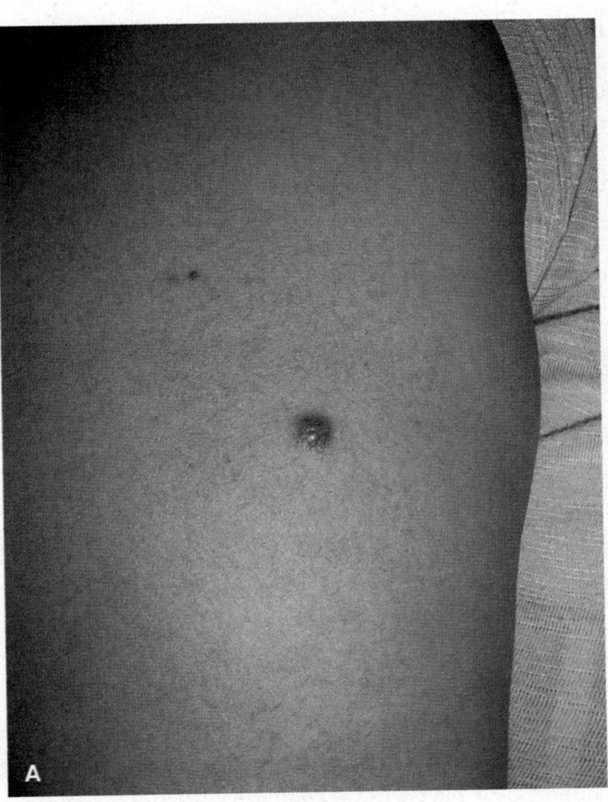

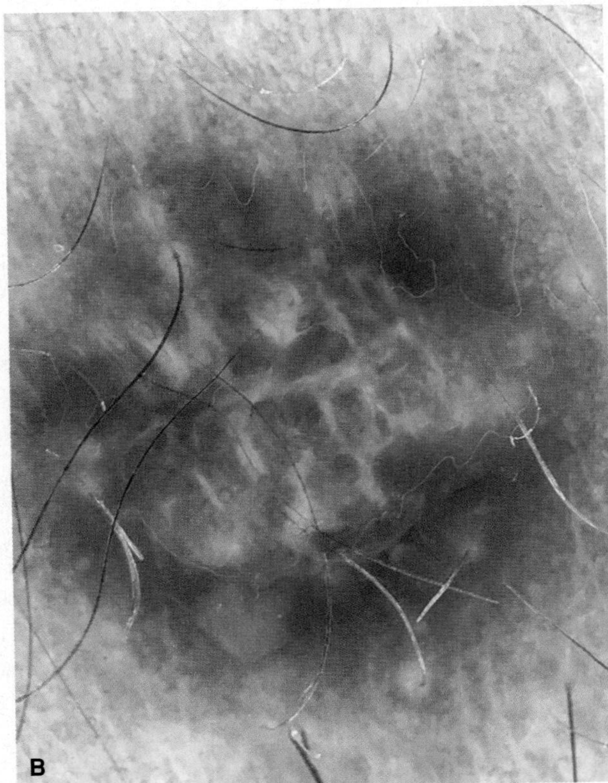

FIGURE 166-6 **A.** Dermatofibroma on the arm of a 26-year-old Hispanic woman. **B.** Note the ringlike globules in the central scar seen with dermoscopy. (*Reproduced with permission from Richard P. Usatine, MD.*)

- In a report of 7 cases of clinically aggressive DFs arising in various locations, mean size of the lesions was 3 cm (range 1–9 cm) and infiltration of the subcutis was seen in 5 of 7 cases.[11] Local recurrences were seen in 6 cases and metastases in 6 cases (identified between 3 months and 8 years after diagnosis); 2 patients died of the disease. Histology of the primary tumor was more often the cellular type (4 of 7 cases). Five neoplasms showed chromosomal aberrations by array-comparative genomic hybridization, which may be helpful in identifying cases with metastatic potential.

PATIENT EDUCATION

- DFs are best left alone if they are relatively asymptomatic and stable.

PATIENT RESOURCES

- **http://www.aocd.org/?page=Dermatofibroma&hhSearchTerms=%22dermatofibroma%22.**
- **https://www.skinsight.com/skin-conditions/adult/dermatofibroma.**

PROVIDER RESOURCES

- **http://emedicine.medscape.com/article/1056742-overview.**

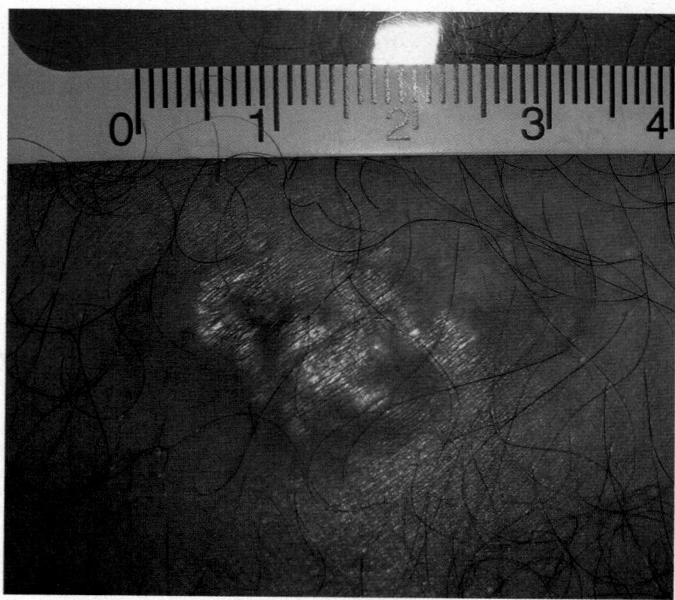

FIGURE 166-7 Large dermatofibrosarcoma protuberans growing on the thigh of this 55-year-old man. The first punch biopsy was read as a benign dermatofibroma. Continued growth prompted a second biopsy that detected the malignancy. The first excision did not achieve clear margins, so the final treatment consisted of Mohs surgery. Note the shiny surface and multilobular look that can be characteristic of a dermatofibrosarcoma protuberans. (*Reproduced with permission from Richard P. Usatine, MD.*)

REFERENCES

1. Pierson JC. *Dermatofibroma.* http://emedicine.medscape.com/article/1056742-overview (updated March 3, 2016). Accessed January 2017.
2. Han TY, Chang HS, Lee JH, et al. A clinical and histopathological study of 122 cases of dermatofibroma (benign fibrous histiocytoma). *Ann Dermatol.* 2011;23(2):185-192.
3. Chen TC, Kuo T, Chan HL. Dermatofibroma is a clonal proliferative disease. *J Cutan Pathol.* 2000;27:36-39.
4. Ishigami T, Hida Y, Matsudate Y, et al. The involvement of fibroblast growth factor receptor signaling pathways in dermatofibroma and dermatofibrosarcoma protuberans. *J Med Invest.* 2013;60(1-2):106-113.
5. Yazici AC, Baz K, Ikizoglu G, et al. Familial eruptive dermatofibromas in atopic dermatitis. *J Eur Acad Dermatol Venereol.* 2006;20(1):90-92.
6. Lang KJ, Lidder S, Hofer M, et al. Rapidly evolving giant dermatofibroma. *Case Report Med.* 2010;2010:620910.
7. Jung KD, Lee DY, Lee JH, et al. Subcutaneous dermatofibroma. *Ann Dermatol.* 2011;23(2):254-257.
8. Zaballos P, Puig S, Llambrich A, Malvehy J. Dermoscopy of dermatofibromas: a prospective morphological study of 412 cases. *Arch Dermatol.* 2008;144(1):75-83.
9. Rosmaninho A, Farrajota P, Peixoto C, et al. Basal cell carcinoma overlying a dermatofibroma: a revisited controversy. *Eur J Dermatol.* 2011;21(1):137-138.

10. Kovach BT, Boyd AS. Melanoma associated with dermatofibroma. *J Cutan Pathol.* 2007;34(5):420-492.

11. Mentzel T, Wiesner T, Cerroni L, et al. Malignant dermatofibroma: clinicopathological, immunohistochemical, and molecular analysis of seven cases. *Mod Pathol.* 2013;26(2):256-267.

12. Alves JV, Matos DM, Barreiros HF, Bártolo EA. Variants of dermatofibroma—a histopathological study. *An Bras Dermatol.* 2014;89(3):472-477.

13. Doyle LA, Fletcher CD. Metastasizing "benign" cutaneous fibrous histiocytoma: a clinicopathologic analysis of 16 cases. *Am J Surg Pathol.* 2013;37(4):484-495.

14. Mentzel T, Kutzner H, Rutten A, Hugel H. Benign fibrous histiocytoma (dermatofibroma) of the face: clinicopathologic and immunohistochemical study of 34 cases associated with an aggressive clinical course. *Am J Dermatopathol.* 2001;23(5):419-426.

15. Sardana K, Garg VK. Multiple dermatofibromas on face treated with carbon dioxide laser: the importance of laser parameters. *Indian J Dermatol Venereol Leprol.* 2008;74(2):170.

16. Niemi KM. The benign fibrohistiocytic tumours of the skin. *Acta Derm Venereol Suppl (Stockh).* 1970;50(63):Suppl 63:1-66.

17. Fletcher CD. Benign fibrous histiocytoma of subcutaneous and deep soft tissue: a clinicopathologic analysis of 21 cases. *Am J Surg Pathol.* 1990;14:801-809.

18. Mentzel T, Kutzner H, Rütten A, Hügel H. Benign fibrous histiocytoma (dermatofibroma) of the face: clinicopathologic and immunohistochemical study of 34 cases associated with an aggressive clinical course. *Am J Dermatopathol.* 2001;23:419-426.

167 PYOGENIC GRANULOMA

Harry Colt, MD
Richard P. Usatine, MD

PATIENT STORY

A 22-year-old woman comes in to the clinic for a new growth that has evolved over the past 3 months on her finger (**Figure 167-1**). It started at the end of her pregnancy and she is now postpartum. The growth is painless, but bleeds easily. She was diagnosed with a probable pyogenic granuloma (PG) and treatment options were discussed. She opted for shave excision, followed by curettage and electrodesiccation (**Figure 167-2**). The tissue was sent for pathology and confirmed the diagnosis of PG. On follow-up the site was healing well and the patient was very happy with the result.

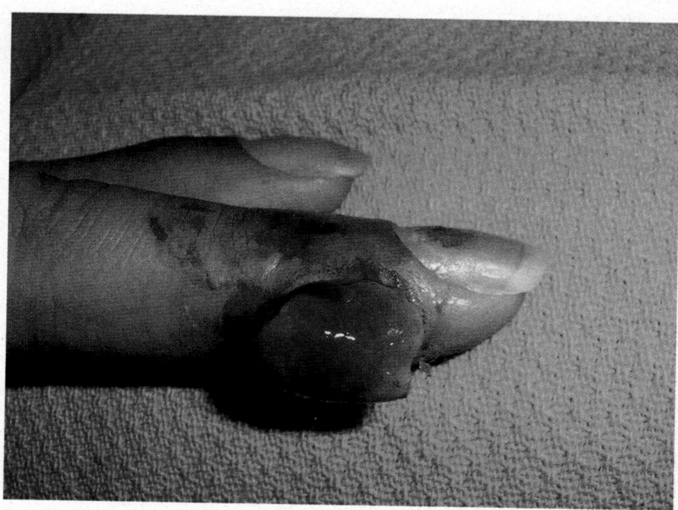

FIGURE 167-1 Pyogenic granuloma on the finger that started in pregnancy.

INTRODUCTION

Pyogenic granuloma (PG) is a relatively common benign acquired vascular growth of the skin and mucous membranes.

SYNONYMS

PG is also known as lobular capillary hemangioma (LCH) due to its histologic appearance. PG is a misnomer as it is neither pyogenic nor granulomatous. However, it often has a purulent-appearing exudate that explains how it got its name (**Figure 167-3**).

EPIDEMIOLOGY

- Seen most commonly in children, teens, and young adults. Mean onset in children is age 6.7, but can occur throughout childhood. Generally acquired, but 1% are present at birth.[1]
- Oral lesions are more common in women, particularly in the 2nd and 3rd decades of life, and in pregnancy.[1]
- PGs have also rarely been reported in the GI tract, nose, conjunctiva, and subcutaneous and intravenous locations.

ETIOLOGY AND PATHOPHYSIOLOGY

- Etiology is unknown. PGs may be associated with prior trauma (see **Figure 167-3**), wound, and hormonal changes, but a direct relationship has not been proven.
- It is hypothesized that pro-angiogenic growth factors play a role in development of PG. This may account for the reported response of pediatric PGs to beta blockers.[2]
- Histopathology demonstrates proliferation of capillaries and venules with neutrophilic infiltrates, in a lobular pattern.[3,4]

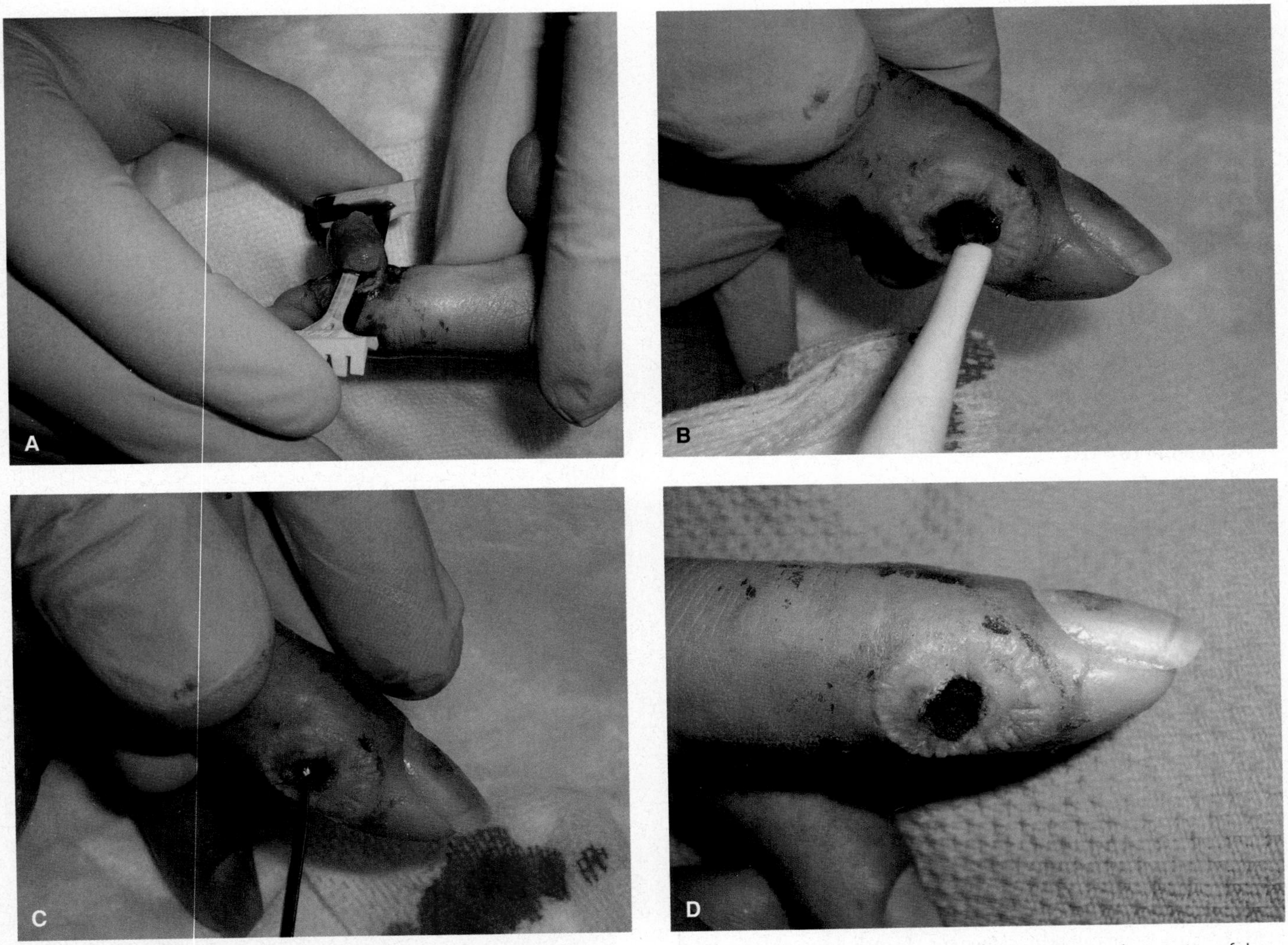

FIGURE 167-2 Pyogenic granuloma treatment. **A.** Shave excision to be sent for pathology. **B.** Curettage of the base. **C.** Electrodesiccation of the base. **D.** Immediate final result. Note how the stalk was much narrower than the lesion itself. *(Reproduced with permission from Richard P. Usatine, MD.)*

RISK FACTORS

- Prior local trauma (in a minority of patients).[1]
- Pregnancy (**Figure 167-4**) and oral contraceptives may be risk factors, possibly due to the effect of hormones on angiogenesis.
- Medications (including retinoids, protease inhibitors, and antineoplastic agents).[3]
- *Bartonella*—associated with increased *Bartonella* seropositivity in one report.[1]
- Manipulation—infrequently, satellite PG lesions can occur.

DIAGNOSIS

CLINICAL FEATURES

- Painless red papule or nodule that is friable and bleeds easily even with minor trauma. Several millimeters to several centimeters in size.

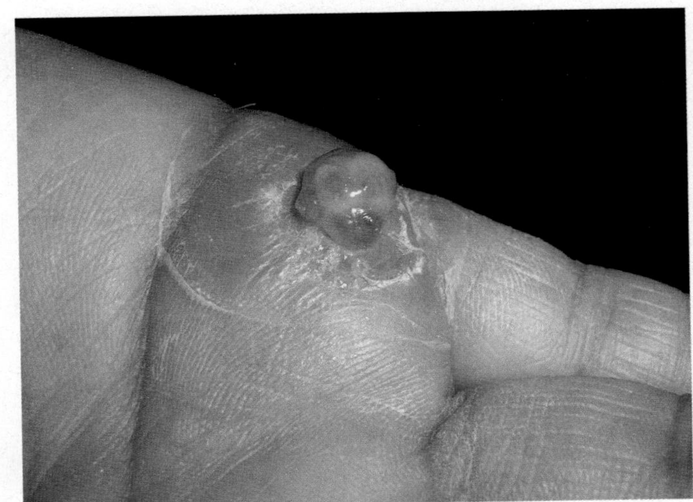

FIGURE 167-3 Pyogenic granuloma that started with trauma from a three-ring binder. Note how it appears purulent, explaining how it got named "pyogenic" despite the fact that it is not a bacterial infection. *(Reproduced with permission from Richard P. Usatine, MD.)*

- Usually singular, but occasionally multiple lesions.
- Develops rapidly over several weeks.
- May ulcerate (**Figure 167-5**) or crust over.

TYPICAL DISTRIBUTION

- Most commonly found on the head, neck, trunk, and upper limbs. Hands and fingers are the most frequent sites on the upper limb (**Figure 167-6**). PGs are also found on the scalp (see **Figure 167-5**).
- In pregnant women, PG found most frequently on the oral mucosa.
- Rarely, lesions may be subcutaneous, IV, or visceral.

DERMOSCOPY

- Dermoscopy reveals reddish homogenous areas, white collarettes, "white rail" lines and ulceration, all of which are associated with PGs (**Figure 167-7**).[5]
- Multiple patterns or combinations of the above can be seen in PGs.[5]
- Reddish homogeneous area, white collarettes, and white rail lines together had a specificity for PG of 100%.[5]

BIOPSY

- Capillaries in edematous stroma with associated neutrophilic infiltrate. Over time, develops an increasingly lobular pattern. Often the lesion has a surrounding epidermal collarette. Develops increasing fibrosis before regressing.[1,3,4,6]
- It is crucial to send the specimen to pathology to rule out amelanotic melanoma (**Figure 167-8**).

DIFFERENTIAL DIAGNOSIS

- Malignancies that can be mistaken for PG include basal cell cancer, squamous cell cancer, keratoacanthoma, amelanotic melanoma (see **Figure 167-8**), cutaneous metastatic lesions, and Kaposi sarcoma. Therefore, every PG that is excised should be sent to pathology.
- Benign tumors that can resemble PG include hemangiomas (**Figure 167-9**), angiokeratomas, and fibrous papules.
- Bacillary angiomatosis may be confused with PG, and its histopathology has similar features (see **Figure 226-10**). It is a rare infection seen more commonly in patients in patients with AIDS or advanced immunosuppression.[4]

MANAGEMENT

PGs eventually resolve slowly over time. However, patients often opt for treatment for cosmetic reasons or due to bleeding. Treatment options include both pharmacologic and surgical approaches. If clinicians have any diagnostic uncertainty, the lesion should be removed and sent to pathology.

Treatment choice is usually driven by the patient's age, location of the lesion, cosmetic concerns, and whether there is any diagnostic uncertainty. Younger pediatric patients with typical PG lesions may be treated with topical agents or cryotherapy.

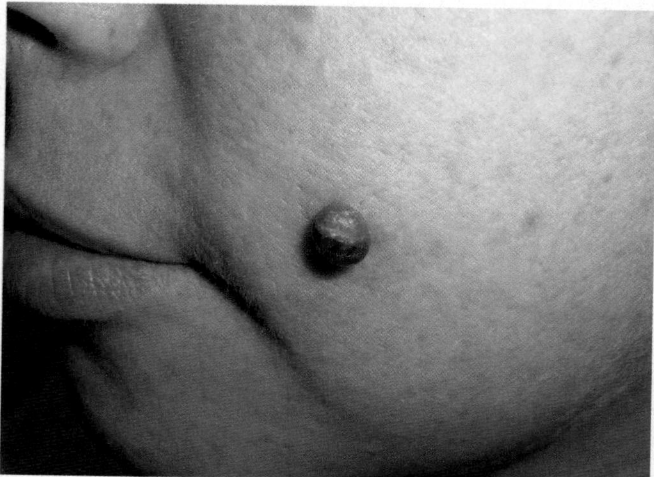

FIGURE 167-4 Pyogenic granuloma on the face of a 25-year-old woman who is 32 weeks pregnant. (*Reproduced with permission from Richard P. Usatine, MD.*)

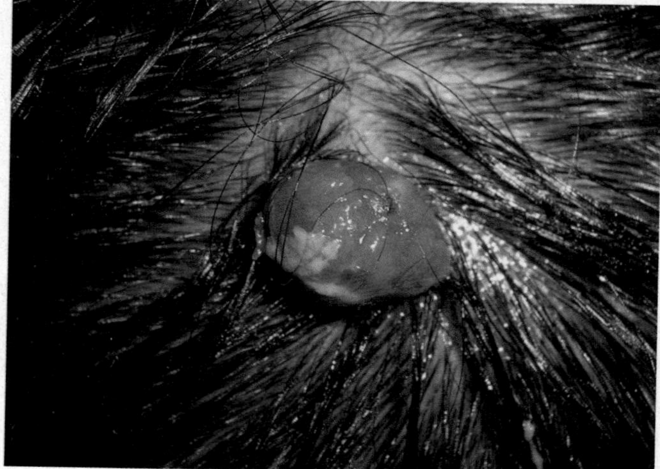

FIGURE 167-5 Pyogenic granuloma on the scalp of a 31-year-old man with significant ulcerations. It is very friable and bleeds easily. (*Reproduced with permission from Richard P. Usatine, MD.*)

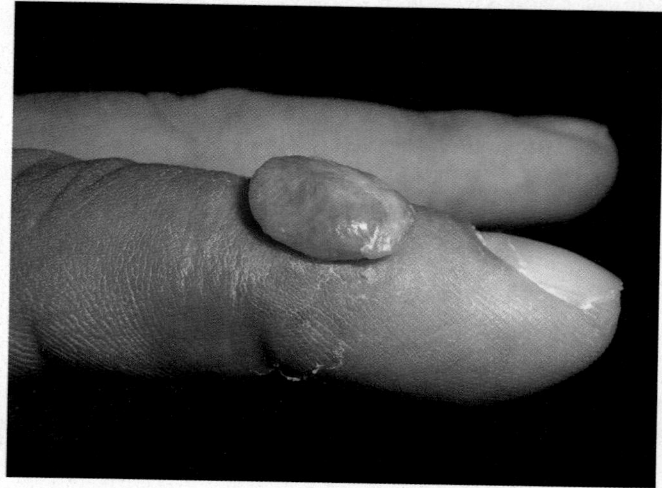

FIGURE 167-6 Large pyogenic granuloma on the finger of a man present for 2 months. Note how the base is narrower than the lesion. This is very typical. (*Reproduced with permission from Richard P. Usatine, MD.*)

OBSERVATION

- Untreated PGs become increasingly fibrotic and eventually resolve over months to years. Most patients want treatment because of the frequent bleeding.

PHARMACOLOGIC

- A number of small series of patients have been treated successfully with topical imiquimod 5% cream. The frequency of application has varied from three times a week to twice daily for periods ranging from 2 to 8 weeks.[7] SOR Ⓒ
- Topical timolol 0.5% gel is frequently used for treatment of superficial infantile hemangiomas. Recently, case reports indicate that PG may be treated successfully with topical timolol two to three times a day for weeks or months.[2] SOR Ⓒ

PROCEDURES

- Surgical excision has the lowest recurrence rate (3.7%), but has a higher incidence of scarring (55%).[8] SOR Ⓒ It is not uncommon for PGs of the lip to recur unless treated with surgical excision (**Figure 167-10**).
- Shave excision followed by curetting and electrodesiccation of the base has a recurrence rate of 10%, with scarring in approximately 30%.[8] SOR Ⓒ PGs bleed extensively when manipulated or cut. It is important to use lidocaine with epinephrine, wait 10 minutes for the epinephrine to work, and have an electrosurgery device to control bleeding. Cut the PG off with a blade and send to pathology. Curetting the base will also help stop the bleeding and prevent recurrence. The base is curetted and electrodesiccated until the bleeding stops. SOR Ⓒ
- Laser surgery often requires more than one treatment session, and scarring and recurrence rates are variable.[8] SOR Ⓒ
- Cryotherapy has low recurrence rates but often requires more than one treatment, and it is often associated with scarring (42%) (**Figure 167-11**).[8,9] SOR Ⓒ

PROGNOSIS

- PGs usually develop over several weeks. They are generally present for months and sometimes years. Over time, they become increasingly fibrotic and involute.[1]

FOLLOW-UP

- In 2 to 3 weeks to check on resolution of the lesion, wound healing, and pathology findings.

PATIENT EDUCATION

- Inform patients that these lesions are benign and will often resolve spontaneously over months to years. However, there are several effective treatment options available if desired for cosmetic reasons or to prevent bleeding.
- If the lesion recurs, early follow-up is appropriate, as small lesions are generally easier to treat than large ones.

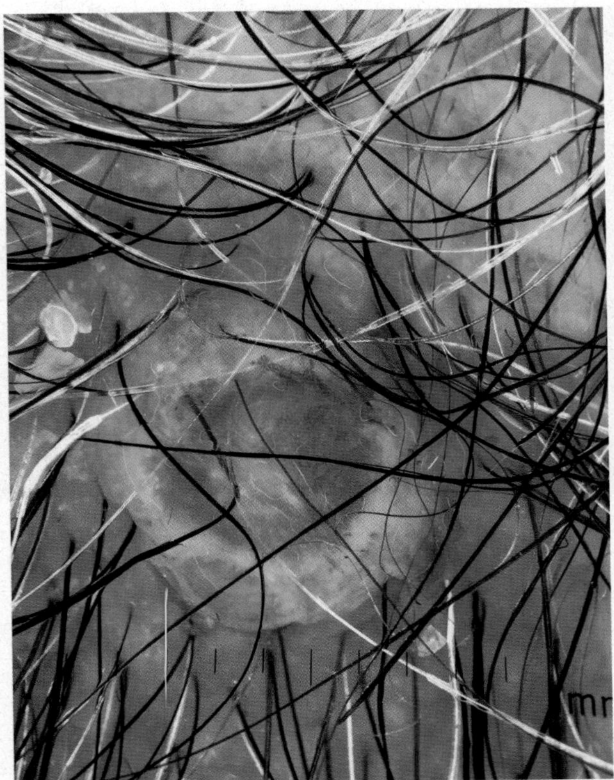

FIGURE 167-7 Dermoscopy of a pyogenic granuloma showing a white collarette pattern around the edge with white rail lines inside the lesion. (*Reproduced with permission from Richard P. Usatine, MD.*)

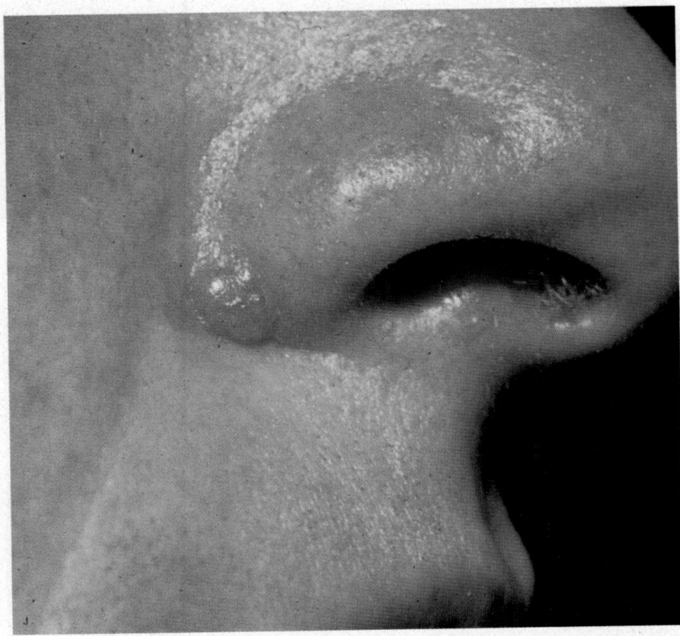

FIGURE 167-8 Amelanotic melanoma on the nose that could be confused with a pyogenic granuloma. Always send what you suspect to be a PG to the pathologist. (*Reproduced with permission from Richard P. Usatine, MD.*)

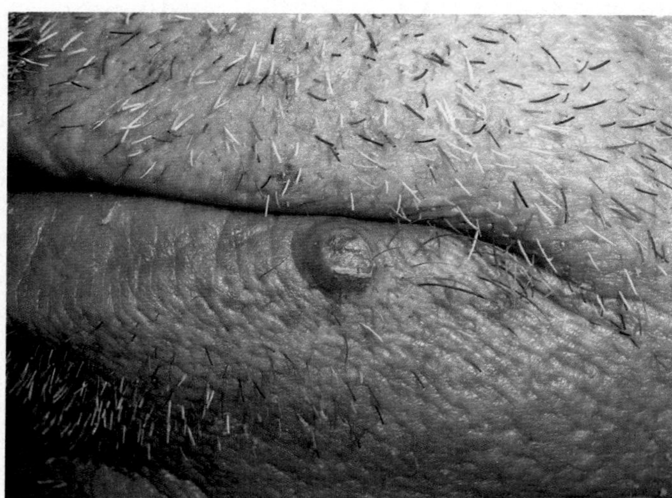

FIGURE 167-9 Hemangioma on the lip of a 67-year-old man. By appearance alone this is hard to differentiate from a pyogenic granuloma (lobular capillary hemangioma). This did not bleed extensively at time of excision, and the pathology result confirmed that this was a hemangioma. (*Reproduced with permission from Richard P. Usatine, MD.*)

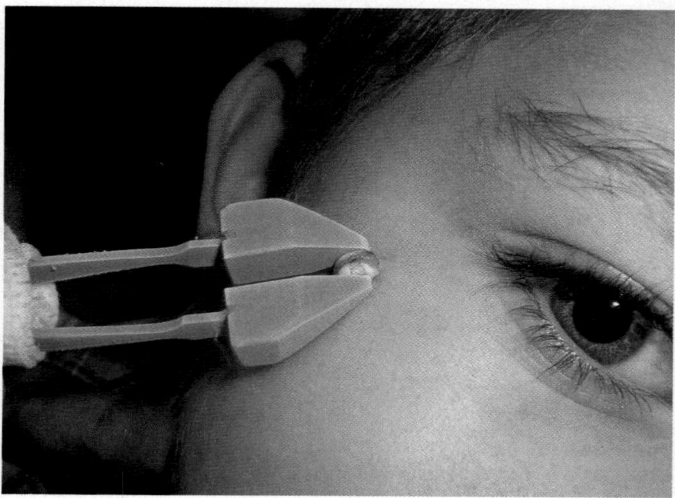

FIGURE 167-11 Cryotherapy of a pyogenic granuloma using a Cryo Tweezer. The young girl was afraid of needles so would not permit excision but did tolerate the cryotherapy well. (*Reproduced with permission from Richard P. Usatine, MD.*)

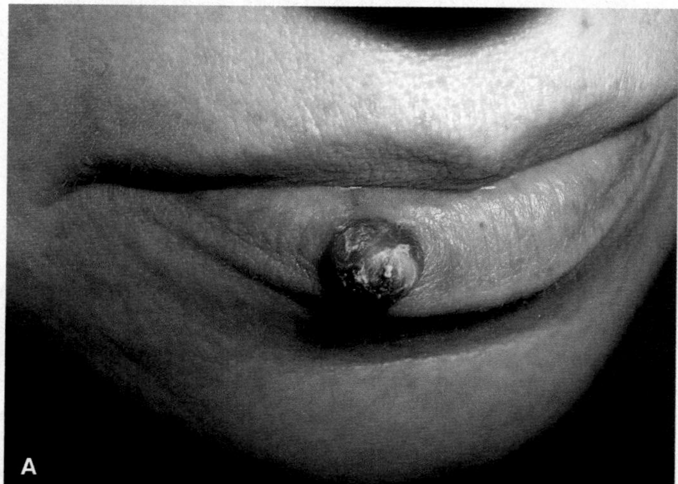

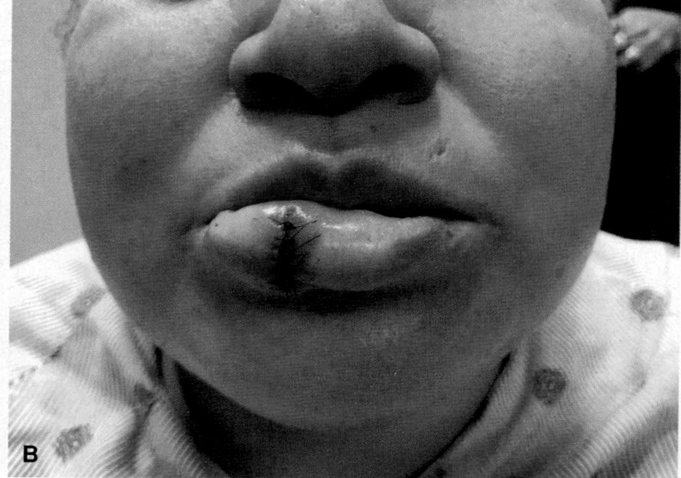

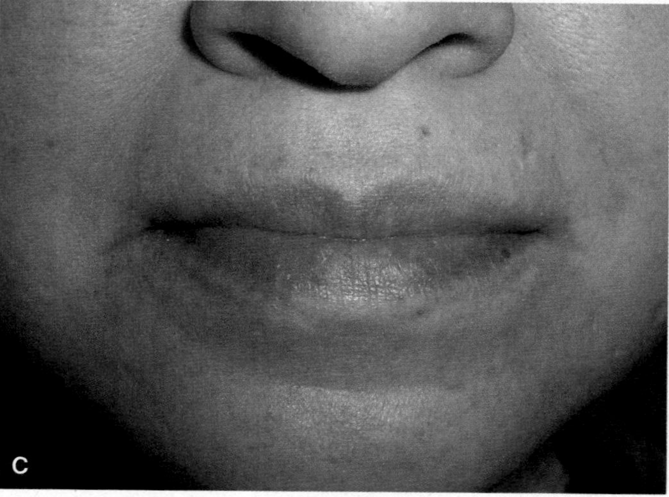

FIGURE 167-10 **A.** Recurrent pyogenic granuloma on the lip of a 33-year-old woman. The original lesion was treated with shave excision, curettage, and electrodesiccation 1 month ago. **B.** Swollen lip and sutured incision after the excision of a pyogenic granuloma. A chalazion clamp was used to assist with the surgery and help control the bleeding. The lip is swollen from the lidocaine and epinephrine needed to perform the surgery. **C.** The lip has healed beautifully 1 month after surgery, and any faint signs of surgery will fade over time. (*Reproduced with permission from Richard P. Usatine, MD.*)

PATIENT RESOURCES

- **https://www.skinsight.com/skin-conditions/adult/pyogenic-granuloma.**

PROVIDER RESOURCES

- Pyogenic Granuloma—**https://emedicine.medscape.com/article/1084701-overview.**
- Usatine R, Pfenninger J, Stulberg D, Small R. *Dermatologic and Cosmetic Procedures in Office Practice*. Philadelphia, PA: Elsevier; 2012. This text focuses on the dermatologic procedural skills helpful in removing pyogenic granuloma and other skin lesions. It is also available in electronic app forms through **www.usatinemedia.com.**

REFERENCES

1. Lin RL, Janninger CK. Pyogenic Granuloma. *Cutis*. 2004;74(4): 229-233.
2. Lee LW, Goff KL, Lam JM, et al. Treatment of pediatric pyogenic granulomas using beta-adrenergic receptor antagonists. *Pediatr Dermatol*. 2014;31(2):203-207.
3. Piraccini BM, Bellavista S, Misciali C, et al. Periungual and subungual pyogenic granuloma. *Br J Dermatol*. 2010;163:941-953.
4. Fortna RR, Junkins-Hopkins JM. A case of lobular hemangioma (pyogenic granuloma), localized to the subcutaneous tissue, and a review of the literature. *Am J Dermatopathol*. 2007;(29)4: 408-411.
5. Zaballos P, Carulla M, Ozdemir F, et al. Dermoscopy of pyogenic granuloma: a morphologic study. *Br J Dermatol*. 2010;163: 1229-1237.
6. Giblin AV, Clover AJP, Athanassopoulos A, Budny PG. Pyogenic granuloma—the quest for optimum treatment: audit of 408 cases. *J Plast Aest Surg*. 2007;60:1030-1035.
7. Musumeci ML, Lacarrubba R, Anfuso R, et al. Two pediatric cases of pyogenic granuloma treated with imiquimod 5% cream: combined clinical and dermatoscopic evaluation and review of the literature. *G Ital Dermatol Venereol*. 2013;148:147-152.
8. Gilmore A, Kelsberg G, Safranek MLS. Clinical Inquiries. What's the best treatment for pyogenic granuloma? *J Fam Pract*. 2010;59(1):40-42.
9. Lee J, Sinno H, Tahiri Y, Gilardio MS. Treatment options for cutaneous pyogenic granulomas: a review. *Plast Reconstr Surg*. 2011; 64:1216-1220.

SECTION K NEVI

168 BENIGN NEVI

Mindy A. Smith, MD, MS
Richard P. Usatine, MD

PATIENT STORY

A young woman comes to the office because her husband has noted that the moles on her back are changing **(Figure 168-1)**. A few have white halos around the brown pigmentation, and some have lost their pigment completely, with a light area remaining. She has no symptoms but wants to make sure these are not skin cancers. Halo nevi are an uncommon variation of common nevi. These appear benign, and the patient is reassured.

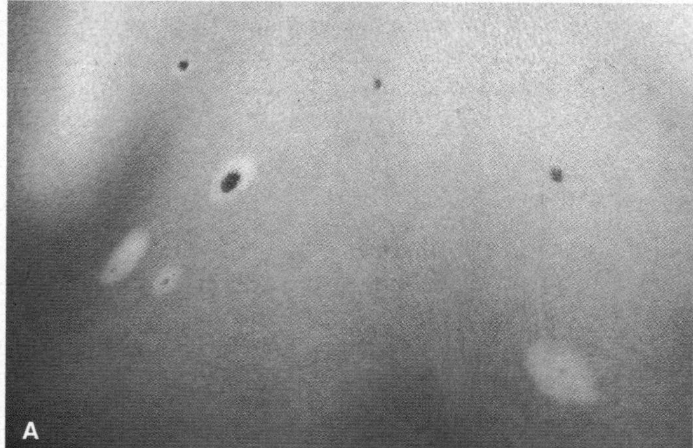

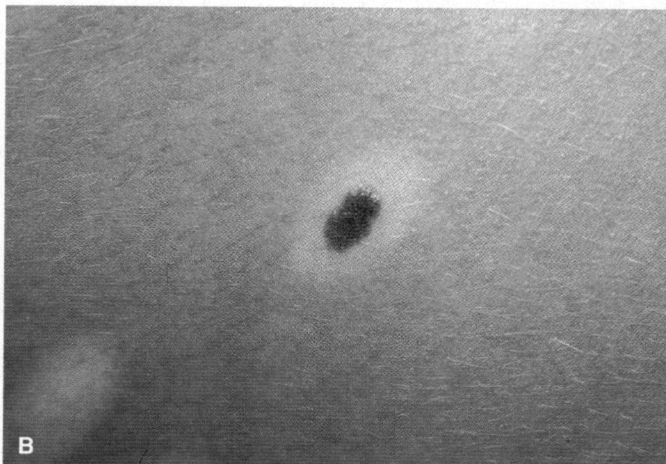

FIGURE 168-1 **A.** Multiple halo nevi on the back. **B.** Close-up of a halo nevus in transition. *(Reproduced with permission from Richard P. Usatine, MD.)*

INTRODUCTION

Most nevi are benign tumors caused by the aggregation of melanocytic cells in the skin. However, nevi can occur on the conjunctiva, sclera, and other structures of the eye. There are also nonmelanocytic nevi that are produced by other cells, as seen in Becker nevi and comedonal nevi. Although most nevi are acquired, many nevi are present at birth.

SYNONYMS

Moles.

EPIDEMIOLOGY

- Acquired nevi are common lesions, forming during early childhood; few adults have none.
- Prevalence appears to be lower in dark-skinned individuals.
- Present in 1% to 2% of neonates. In a case series of 594 infants in San Diego, 1.3% had small congenital melanocytic nevi (CMN) and 1% had medium-sized lesions.[1] CMNs were most common among African-American (17.9%) and Caucasian (2.6%) infants; none were identified among Hispanic infants.
- Prevalence increases through childhood, peaking at puberty; new nevi may continue to appear in adulthood. In a population study of children (N = 180, ages 1 to 15 years) in Barcelona, the mean number of nevi was 17.5.[2]
- Adults typically have 10 to 40 nevi scattered over the body. In a population study in Germany, 60.3% of 2823 adults (mean age: 49 years; 50% women) exhibited 11 to 50 common nevi and 5.2% had at least 1 atypical nevus.[3]
- The peak incidence of melanocytic nevi (MN) is in the fourth to fifth decades of life; the incidence decreases with each successive decade.[4]

ETIOLOGY AND PATHOPHYSIOLOGY

- Benign tumors composed of nevus cells derived from melanocytes, pigment-producing cells that colonize the epidermis.
- MN represent proliferations of melanocytes that are in contact with each other, forming small collections of cells known as nests. Genetic mutations present in common nevi as well as in melanomas include BRAF, NRAS, and *c*-kit.[5]
- Sun (UV) exposure, skin-blistering events (e.g., sunburn), and genetics play a role in the formation of new nevi.[4]
- Nevi commonly darken and/or enlarge during pregnancy. Melanocytes have receptors for estrogens and androgens, and melanogenesis is responsive to these hormones.[4]
- Three broad categories of MN are based on location of nevus cells[3]:
    - Junctional nevi—Composed of nevus cells located in the dermal–epidermal junction; may change into compound nevi after childhood (except when located on the palms, soles, or genitalia) (**Figure 168-2**).
    - Compound nevi—A nevus in which a portion of nevus cells have migrated into the dermis (**Figure 168-3**).
    - Dermal nevi—Composed of nevus cells located within the dermis (usually found only in adults). These are usually raised and have little to no visible hyperpigmentation (**Figures 168-4** and **168-5**).
- Special categories of nevi:
    - Halo nevus—Compound or dermal nevus that develops a symmetric, sharply demarcated, depigmented border (see **Figure 168-1**). Most commonly occurs on the trunk and develops during adolescence. Repigmentation may occur.
    - Blue nevus—A dermal nevus that contains large amounts of pigment so that the brown pigment absorbs the longer wavelengths of light and scatters blue light (Tyndall effect) (**Figure 168-6**). Blue nevi are not always blue and color varies from tan to blue, black, and gray. Types of blue nevi include amelanotic, desmoplastic, atypical, and malignant variants; genetic mutations seen in blue nevi are often different from those seen in common nevi.[5] The nodules are firm because of associated stromal sclerosis. Usually appear in childhood on the extremities, dorsum of the hands, and face. In a case series of blue nevi in older adults (mean age 62.8 years, primarily men), most had been present for less than 10 years and were located on the arm, back, scalp, or face; all were benign.[6] A rare variant, the cellular blue nevus is large (>1 cm), frequently located on the buttocks, and may become melanoma. While a typical blue nevus is benign, any variation of typical should be excised, as a nodular melanoma may be masquerading as a blue nevus.
    - Nevus spilus (speckled nevus)—Hairless, oval, or irregularly shaped brown lesion with darker brown to black dots containing nevus cells (**Figure 168-7**). May appear at any age or be present at birth; unrelated to sun exposure. Melanoma can arise in a nevus spilus.
    - Spitz nevus (formerly called benign juvenile melanoma because of its clinical and histologic similarity to melanoma)—A typical benign Spitz nevus may be a hairless, brown, black, red, or reddish-brown dome-shaped papule (**Figures 168-8** and **168-9**). These are generally found in children but can occur in adults. They can be atypical, and some of these lesions are Spitzoid melanomas.

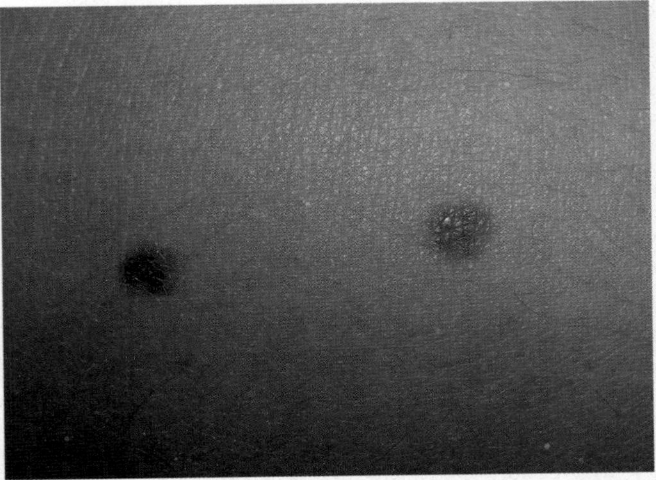

FIGURE 168-2 Two benign junctional nevi on the arm of a 19-year-old woman. Note how these are flat macules. (*Reproduced with permission from Richard P. Usatine, MD.*)

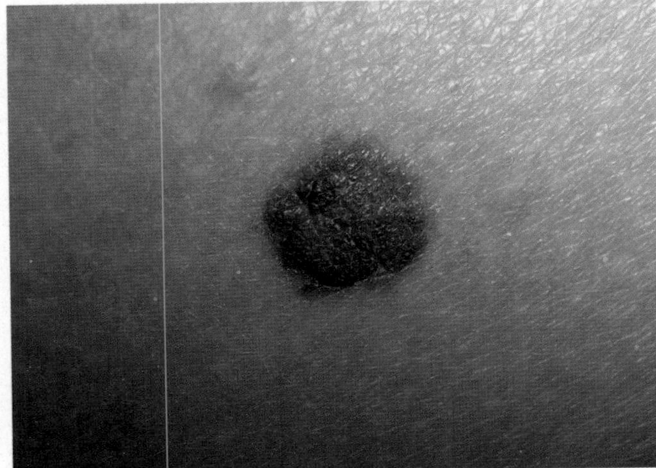

FIGURE 168-3 Benign compound nevus proven by biopsy on the back of a 35-year-old woman. (*Reproduced with permission from Richard P. Usatine, MD.*)

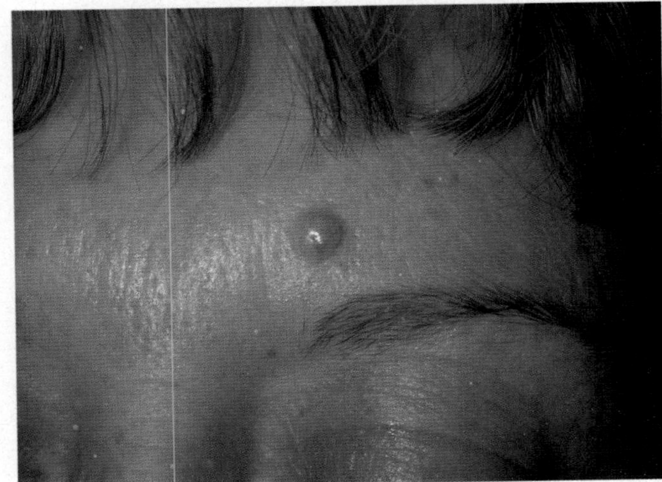

FIGURE 168-4 Dermal nevus (intradermal melanocytic nevus)—dome shaped with some scattered pigmentation. (*Reproduced with permission from Richard P. Usatine, MD.*)

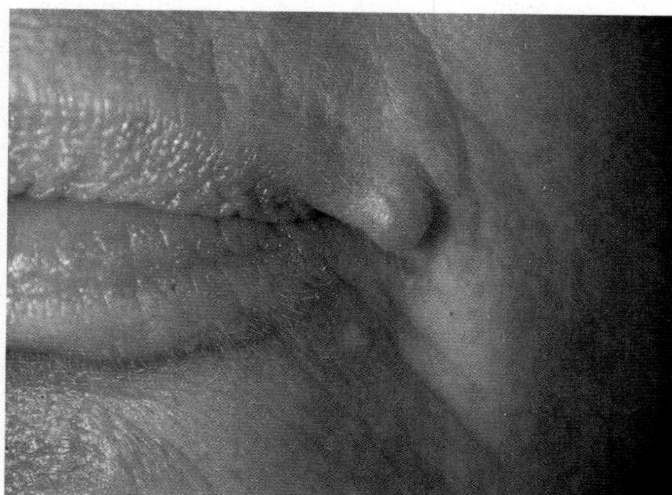

FIGURE 168-5 Dermal nevus pedunculated with small telangiectasias. (*Reproduced with permission from Richard P. Usatine, MD.*)

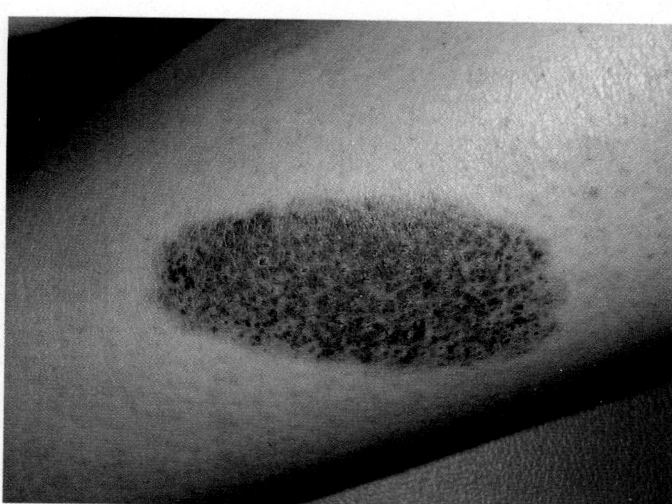

FIGURE 168-7 Nevus spilus on the leg of a young woman from birth. It appears benign and needs no intervention. (*Reproduced with permission from Richard P. Usatine, MD.*)

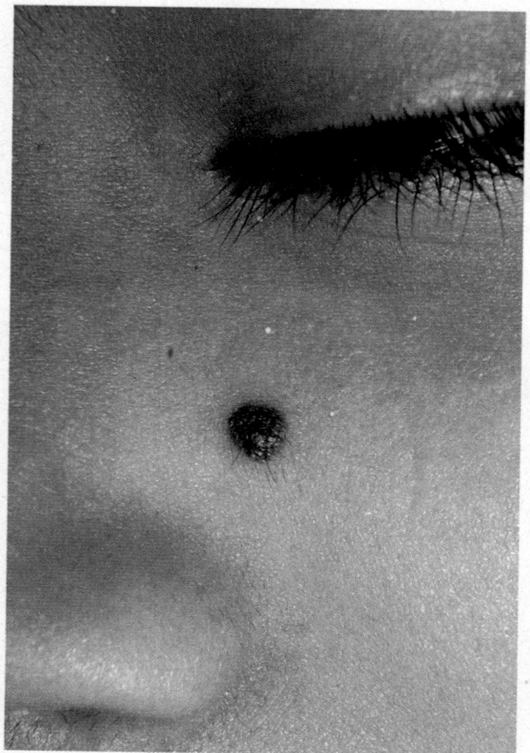

FIGURE 168-6 Blue nevus on the left cheek that could resemble a melanoma with its dark color. In this case it was fully excised with a 5-mm punch with a good cosmetic result. Blue nevi are benign and do not need to be excised unless there are suspicious changes. (*Reproduced with permission from Richard P. Usatine, MD.*)

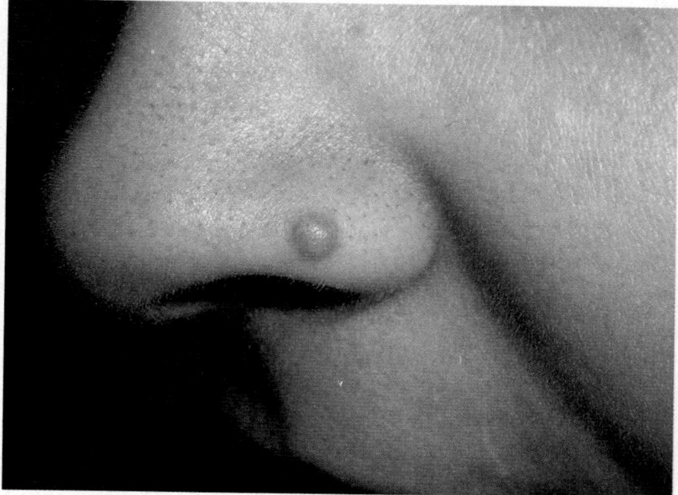

FIGURE 168-8 Spitz nevus on the nose of an 18-year-old woman. It was biopsied and then excised with no complications. (*Reproduced with permission from Richard P. Usatine, MD.*)

Most importantly, these should be fully excised with clear margins (see Chapter 171, Dysplastic Nevus and Spitz Nevus).
  - Nevus of Ota—Dark brown nevus that occurs most commonly around the eye and can involve the sclera (**Figure 168-10**).
- Both acquired and CMN hold some risk for the development of melanoma; the number of MN, especially more than 100, is an important independent risk factor for cutaneous melanoma.[7] In a 20-year follow-up study of children from families with familial melanoma, the total number of atypical nevi, particularly located on the buttocks, were associated with risk of melanoma.[8]

NONMELANOCYTIC NEVI

- Becker nevus—A brown patch often with hair located on the shoulder, back, or submammary area, most often in adolescent men (**Figures 168-11** and **168-12**). The lesion may enlarge to cover an entire shoulder or upper arm. Although it is called a nevus, it does not actually have nevus cells and has no malignant potential. It is a type of hamartoma, an abnormal mixture of cells and tissues normally found in the body where the growth occurs.
- Nevus depigmentosus is usually present at birth or starts in early childhood. There is a decreased number of melanosomes within a normal number of melanocytes. It typically has a serrated or jagged edge (**Figure 168-13**).
- Nevus anemicus—A congenital hypopigmented macule or patch that is stable in relative size and distribution. It is due to localized hypersensitivity to catecholamines and not a decrease in melanocytes. On diascopy (pressure with a glass slide) the skin is indistinguishable from the surrounding skin (**Figure 168-14**).
- Nevus comedonicus (comedonal nevus) is a rare congenital hamartoma characterized by an aggregation of comedones in one region of the skin (**Figure 168-15**).
- Epidermal nevi are congenital hamartomas of ectodermal origin classified based on their main component: sebaceous, apocrine, eccrine, follicular, or keratinocytic. See Chapter 169, Congenital Melanocytic Nevi, for a full discussion of this type of nevus.

Note that nevus comedonicus and epidermal nevi tend to follow Blaschko lines, which come from embryologic development.

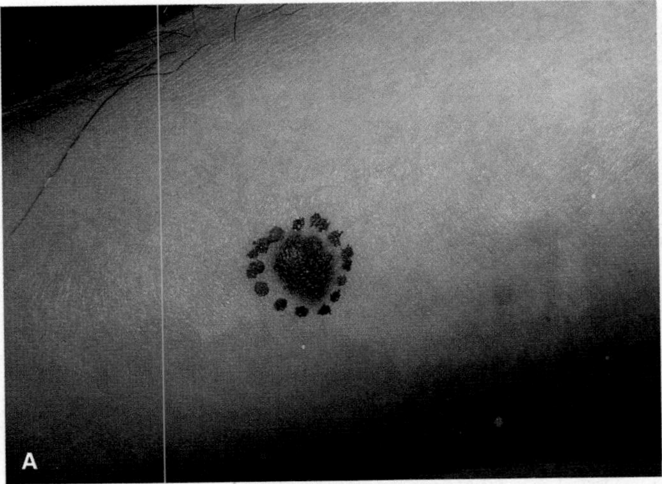

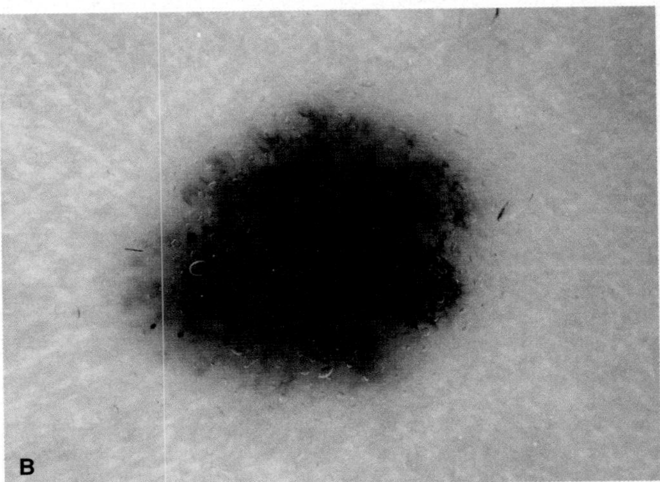

FIGURE 168-9 **A.** Spitz nevus that grew over the past year on the foot of this 25-year-old man. A 2-mm margin was marked for a saucerization biopsy. **B.** Dermoscopy with asymmetric streaks and globules indicating growth in the bottom left-hand corner made this suspicious for melanoma. *(Reproduced with permission from Richard P. Usatine, MD.)*

RISK FACTORS

- In the Barcelona study of children, male gender, history of sunburns, facial freckling, and family history of breast cancer were independent risk factors for having a higher number of nevi.[2]
- In one study among very light-skinned (and not darker skinned) children without red hair, children who develop tans had greater numbers of nevi.[9]

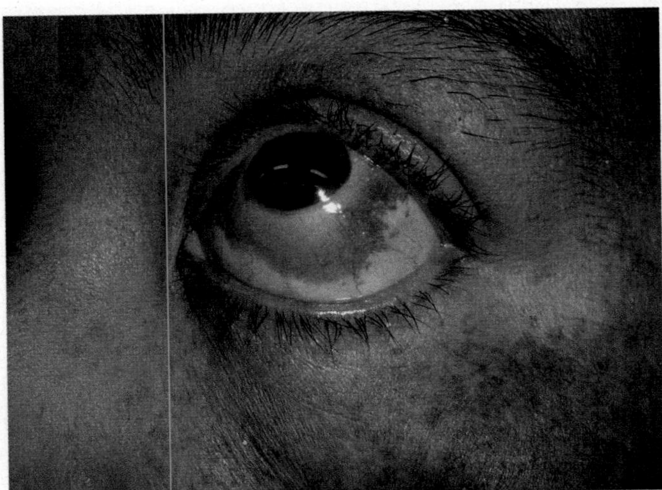

FIGURE 168-10 Nevus of Ota on the face of this young woman since early childhood. It involved both eyes and the skin around both eyes. The scleral pigmentation looks blue. *(Reproduced with permission from Richard P. Usatine, MD.)*

DIAGNOSIS

CLINICAL FEATURES

Most benign MN are skin colored, tan to brown, usually less than 6 mm, with round shape and distinct borders. Nevi in redheads may be pink. The clinical features of the most common acquired MN are:

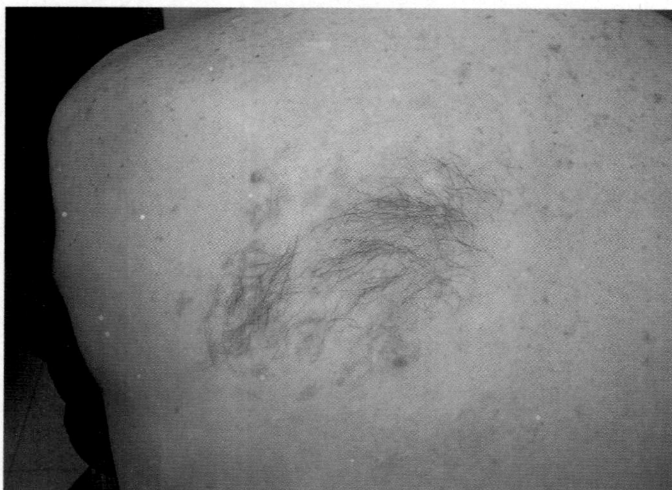

FIGURE 168-11 Becker nevus that developed during adolescence. Hair is frequently seen on this type of nonmelanocytic nevus. (*Reproduced with permission from Richard P. Usatine, MD.*)

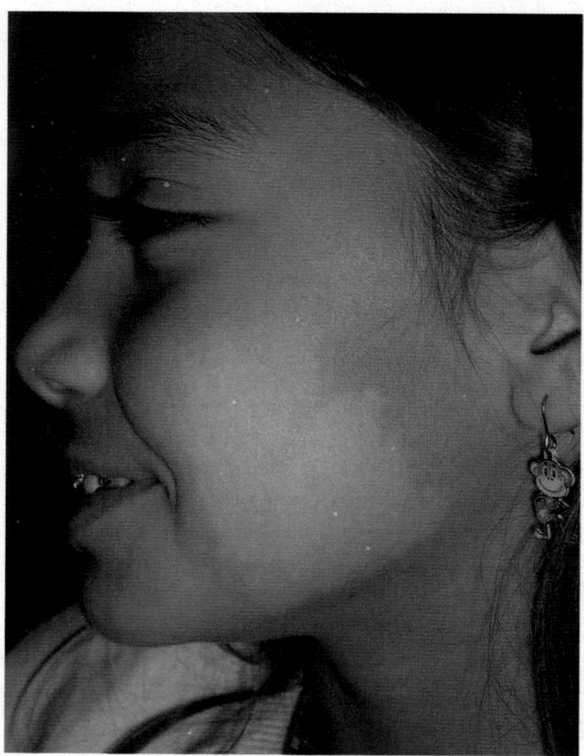

FIGURE 168-13 Nevus depigmentosus on the face of this young girl since birth. (*Reproduced with permission from Richard P. Usatine, MD.*)

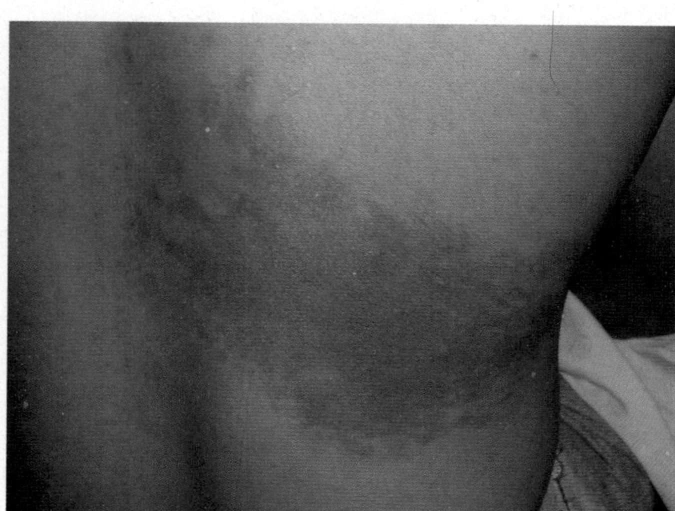

FIGURE 168-12 Becker nevus on the back of a 16-year-old Hispanic boy for 2 years. While this nevus did not have hair, it did have increased acne within the area—another feature of the Becker nevus. (*Reproduced with permission from Richard P. Usatine, MD.*)

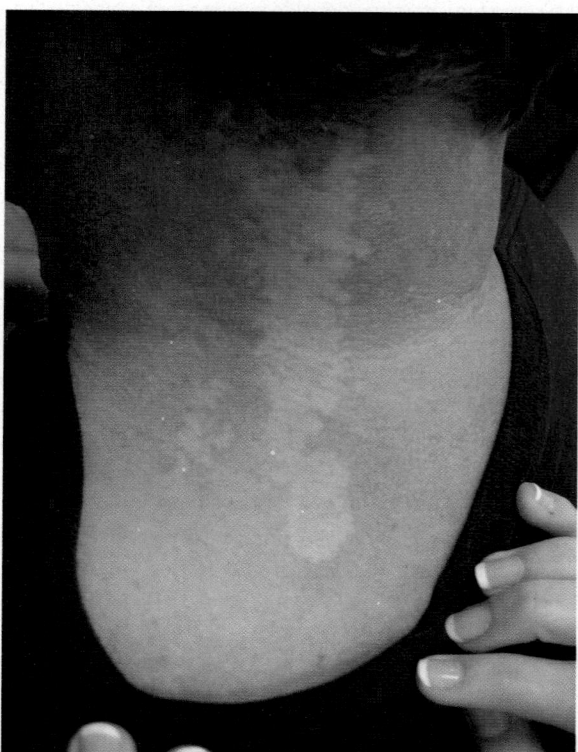

FIGURE 168-14 Nevus anemicus on the posterior neck. The localized hypersensitivity to catecholamines causes the area to stay lighter than the surrounding skin. (*Reproduced with permission from Richard P. Usatine, MD.*)

- Junctional nevi—Macular or slightly elevated mole of uniform brown to black pigmentation, smooth surface, and a round or oval border (see **Figure 168-2**). Most are hairless and vary from 1 to 6 mm.
- Compound nevi—Slightly elevated, symmetric, uniformly flesh colored or brown with a round or oval border, often becoming more elevated with age (see **Figure 168-3**). Hair may be present and a white halo may form.
- Dermal nevi (same as intradermal nevi)—Skin color or brown color that may fade with age; dome shaped is most common, but shapes vary, including polypoid, warty, and pedunculated. Often found on the face and may have telangiectasias (see **Figures 168-4** and **168-5**). Size ranges from 1 to 10 mm.

TYPICAL DISTRIBUTION

- Most often above the waist on sun-exposed areas, but may appear anywhere on the cutaneous surface; less commonly found on the scalp, breasts, or buttocks.
- Among the children in the Barcelona study, 61.1% had nevi on the face and neck, 17.2% on the buttocks, and 11.7% on the scalp; approximately one-third had CMN (Chapter 169, Congenital Melanocytic Nevi).[1]
- In an Australian study of white children, MN of all sizes were highest on the outer forearms, followed by the outer upper arms, neck, and face.[10] Boys had higher densities of MN of all sizes on the neck than girls, and girls had higher densities of MN of 2 mm or greater on the lower legs and thighs than boys. Habitually sun-exposed body sites had higher densities of small MN and highest prevalence of larger MN.

DERMOSCOPY

- Dermoscopy is a useful technique for distinguishing benign nevi from melanoma. For MN, dermoscopic diagnosis relies on color; pattern (i.e., globular, reticular, starburst, and homogeneous blue pattern); pigment distribution (i.e., multifocal, central, eccentric, and uniform); and special sites (e.g., face, acral areas, nail, and mucosa), in conjunction with patient factors (e.g., history, pregnancy).[11] (See Chapter 111, Dermoscopy.)
- In the Barcelona study, the most frequent dominant dermoscopic pattern was the globular type, with the homogeneous pattern predominating in the youngest children and the reticular pattern predominating in adolescents.[1] The reticular pattern is more common in adults as well, but some adults do have a globular pattern if the nevus is still growing. A globular pattern in older adults is suspicious for melanoma, as nevi should not be growing after young adulthood.
- There are 10 benign patterns of nevi described in the dermoscopy chapter (see Chapter 111, Dermoscopy). Deviations from these patterns warrant evaluation for melanoma.

BIOPSY

A biopsy is needed if a skin lesion is suspicious for melanoma or Spitz nevus (see Chapter 171, Dysplastic Nevus and Spitz Nevus). A biopsy that cuts below the pigmented area is preferred if there is a suspicion for melanoma. This can be done with a saucerization (deep shave), a punch that includes the whole lesion if it is small, or an elliptical excision (see Chapter 113, Biopsy Principles and Techniques). If the

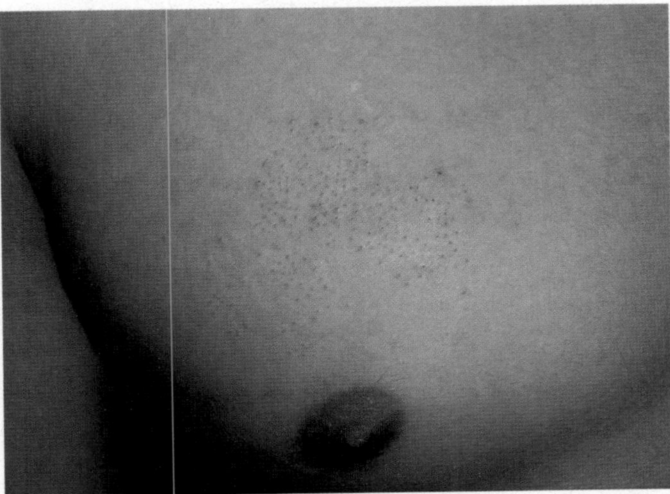

FIGURE 168-15 Nevus comedonicus on the chest of this 15-year-old boy since birth. This is a congenital hamartoma with open comedones. It is not acne. (*Reproduced with permission from Richard P. Usatine, MD.*)

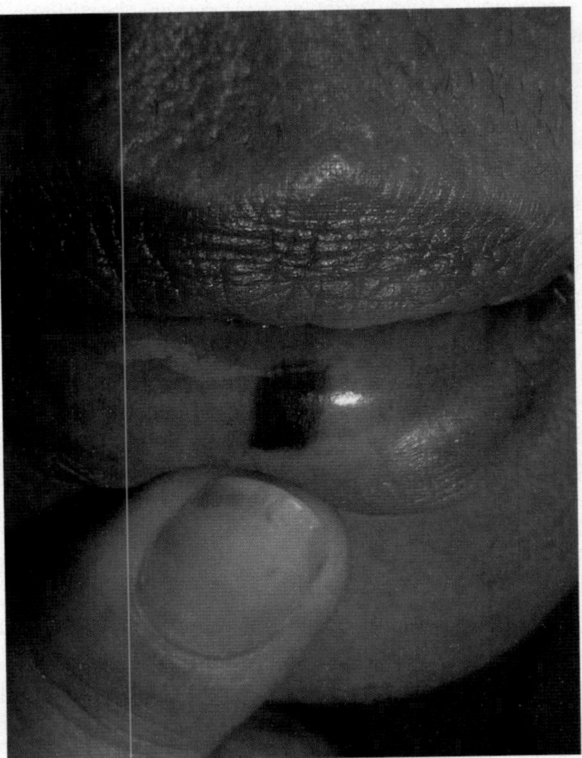

FIGURE 168-16 Labial melanotic macule. These are benign but are not nevi. (*Reproduced with permission from Richard P. Usatine, MD.*)

patient wants a raised, benign-appearing nevus excised for cosmetic reasons, a shave excision may be adequate. Send all lesions (except skin tags) to the pathologist for examination, even when they appear benign, to avoid missing a melanoma.

DIFFERENTIAL DIAGNOSIS

Benign nevi may rarely develop into a melanoma. However, most melanomas develop de novo (not from a pre-existing lesion). The skill needed is to distinguish benign lesions such as nevi, seborrheic keratoses, solar lentigines, dermatofibromas, and vascular lesions from melanoma using the naked eye and dermoscopy (when available). The old ABCDE approach (asymmetry, border irregularity, color irregularity, diameter >6 mm, evolution) is a good start but will miss many melanomas if this is relied on as the only method of evaluation. Any lesion that becomes symptomatic (e.g., itchy, painful, irritated, or bleeding), or develops a loss or increase in pigmentation, should be evaluated and biopsied if needed. Dermoscopy is extremely useful to increase one's accuracy in distinguishing among benign nevi, other benign lesions, and melanoma (see Chapter 111, Dermoscopy).

- Melanomas are skin cancers that may develop from a preexisting nevus but usually develop de novo. It is critical to know the patterns of all types of melanoma to avoid missing this dangerous skin cancer (see Chapter 179, Melanoma).
- Dysplastic nevi (atypical moles) are benign nevi that have a flat component and are larger than 6 mm. Often, the lesions exhibit target-like or fried egg–like morphology, with a central papular zone and a macular surrounding area with differing pigmentation (see Chapter 171, Dysplastic Nevus and Spitz Nevus). If suspicious for melanoma, a saucerization or excision should be performed for pathology. If the pathology is read as severely dysplastic, then the lesion should be managed like a melanoma in situ.
- Seborrheic keratoses (SKs) are benign growths that appear more with increasing age and are often hyperpigmented. These are more superficial and stuck-on in their appearance (Chapter 164, Seborrheic Keratosis). Unfortunately, they sometime mimic melanoma and melanoma sometimes appears like an SK, so care should be taken in their evaluation.
- Labial melanotic macules are benign dark macules on the lip that are not nevi or melanomas (**Figure 168-16**). They can be removed for cosmetic purposes or left alone.

MANAGEMENT

Nevi are generally removed only for cosmetic reasons or because of concern over features of or changes in the lesion that are suggestive of melanoma.

- A full excisional biopsy with a sutured closure or a deep shave is usually the best means to diagnose a lesion if concern exists regarding the possibility of melanoma. If the lesion is found to be benign, no further treatment is usually required.
  - If a Spitz nevus is suspected, either biopsy it now or schedule the patient for a full excision. The histopathology is too close to a melanoma to just watch it.
- Punch excision can be used to excise smaller lesions.
- Deep shave (saucerization)—Unfortunately, if a punch biopsy is used to sample a larger lesion, it may miss a melanoma in another part of the lesion. A broad deep shave is better than a punch biopsy when a full elliptical excision is not possible or desirable (e.g., a large flat pigmented lesion on the face).
  - Nevi removed for cosmesis are often removed by shave excision.
- Argon laser photoablation has been successfully used for removal of superficial conjunctival nevi in one case series.[12]

Becker nevi and comedonal nevi do not become melanoma because they lack melanocytes. Therefore, there is no reason to excise them. Generally, these are large, and the risks of excision for cosmetic reasons outweigh the benefits.

PREVENTION

- Sun protection to limit sunburn may help reduce the appearance of nevi. In a trial of 209 white children, children randomized to the sunscreen group, especially those with freckles, had significantly fewer new nevi on the trunk than did children in the control group at 3-year follow-up.[13] Sunscreens can partially prevent ultraviolet-B effects on nevi, but not quite as effectively as physical barriers.[14]

PROGNOSIS

- Degeneration of common nevi into melanoma is very rare. However, in one large Brazilian study, nevus-associated melanomas represented one-third of the identified melanomas; these were associated with intermittent sun exposure, superficial spreading melanomas, and lower Breslow thickness.[15]
- Patients with multiple or large MN appear to have an increased risk of melanoma.[4] In a cohort study of patients at high risk for melanoma, of whom 13.6% developed melanoma during 15-year follow-up, just over half were associated with MN; high nevus count was a risk factor.[16]
- Nevi may recur or persist following removal; in one study, dysplastic MN were the most likely to persist.[17] In another study, of 61 benign nevi biopsy sites reexamined, two (3.3%) recurred.[18]

FOLLOW-UP

- Patients with multiple or sizable MN should be followed by an experienced clinician because they appear to have an increased lifetime risk of melanoma, with the risk increasing in rough proportion to the size and/or number of lesions.[4]

PATIENT EDUCATION

- Patients should be encouraged to use sunscreen to prevent skin cancer as well as to reduce the development of new nevi.
- Patients with multiple or sizable MN should be taught to look for and report asymmetry, border irregularity, new symptoms, and color and size changes.

PATIENT RESOURCES

- Skinsight—**https://www.skinsight.com/skin-conditions/adult/common-acquired-nevus-mole.**
- MedlinePlus—**http://www.nlm.nih.gov/medlineplus/moles.html.**
- American Osteopathic College of Dermatology—**http://www.aocd.org/page/moles?.**
- American Academy of Dermatology—**https://www.aad.org/public/diseases/bumps-and-growths/moles.**

PROVIDER RESOURCES

- **http://emedicine.medscape.com/article/1058445-overview.**

REFERENCES

1. Kanada KN, Merin MR, Munden A, Friedlander SF. A prospective study of cutaneous findings in newborns in the United States: correlation with race, ethnicity, and gestational status using updated classification and nomenclature. *J Pediatr.* 2012;161(2):240-245.
2. Aguilera P, Puig S, Guilabert A, et al. Prevalence study of nevi in children from Barcelona. Dermoscopy, constitutional and environmental factors. *Dermatology.* 2009;18(3):203-214.
3. Schafer T, Merkl J, Klemm E, et al. The epidemiology of nevi and signs of skin aging in the adult general population: results of the KORA-Survey 2000. *J Invest Dermatol.* 2006;126(7):1490-1496.
4. McCalmont T. *Melanocytic Nevi.* http://emedicine.medscape.com/article/1058445-overview. Accessed February 2017.
5. Zembowicz A, Phadke PA. Blue nevi and variants: an update. *Arch Pathol Lab Med.* 2011;135(3):327-336.
6. Cabral ES, Chen FW, Egbert BM, Swetter SM. Acquired blue nevi in older individuals: retrospective case series from a Veterans Affairs population, 1991 to 2013. *JAMA Dermatol.* 2014;150(8):873-876.
7. Gandini S, Sera F, Cattaruzza MS, et al. Meta-analysis of risk factors for cutaneous melanoma: I. Common and atypical nevi. *Eur J Cancer.* 2005;41(1):28-44.
8. Vredenborg A, Böhringer S, Boonk SE, et al. Acquired melanocytic nevi in childhood and familial melanoma. *JAMA Dermatol.* 2014 Jan;150(1):35-40.
9. Aalborg J, Morelli JG, Mokrohisky ST, et al. Tanning and increased nevus development in very-light-skinned children without red hair. *Arch Dermatol.* 2009;145(9):989-996.
10. Harrison SL, Buettner PG, MacLennan R. Body-site distribution of MN in young Australian children. *Arch Dermatol.* 1999;135(1):47-52.
11. Zalaudek I, Docimo G, Argenziano G. Using dermoscopic criteria and patient-related factors for the management of pigmented melanocytic nevi. *Arch Dermatol.* 2009;145(7):816-826.
12. Chen FW, Tseng D, Reddy S, et al. Involution of eruptive melanocytic nevi on combination BRAF and MEK inhibitor therapy. *JAMA Dermatol.* 2014;150(11):1209-1212.
13. Lee TK, Rivers JK, Gallagher RP. Site-specific protective effect of broad-spectrum sunscreen on nevus development among white schoolchildren in a randomized trial. *J Am Acad Dermatol.* 2005;52(5):786-792.
14. Carrera C, Puig-Butillè JA, Aguilera P, et al. Impact of sunscreens on preventing UVR-induced effects in nevi: in vivo study comparing protection using a physical barrier vs sunscreen. *JAMA Dermatol.* 2013;149(7):803-813.
15. Shitara D, Nascimento MM, Puig S, et al. Nevus-associated melanomas: clinicopathologic features. *Am J Clin Pathol.* 2014;142(4):485-491.
16. Haenssle HA, Mograby N, Ngassa A, et al. Association of patient risk factors and frequency of nevus-associated cutaneous melanomas. *JAMA Dermatol.* 2016;152(3):291-298.
17. Sommer LL, Barcia SM, Clarke LE, Helm KF. Persistent melanocytic nevi: a review and analysis of 205 cases. *J Cutan Pathol.* 2011;38(6):503-507.
18. Goodson AG, Florell SR, Boucher KM, Grossman D. Low rates of clinical recurrence after biopsy of benign to moderately dysplastic melanocytic nevi. *J Am Acad Dermatol.* 2010;62(4):591-596.

169 CONGENITAL MELANOCYTIC NEVI

Mindy A. Smith, MD, MS

PATIENT STORY

A small congenital nevus (**Figure 169-1**) was noted on this 6-month-old child by his new family physician during a routine examination. The parents acknowledged that it was present from birth and asked if it needed to be removed. They were reassured that nothing needs to be done about it now.

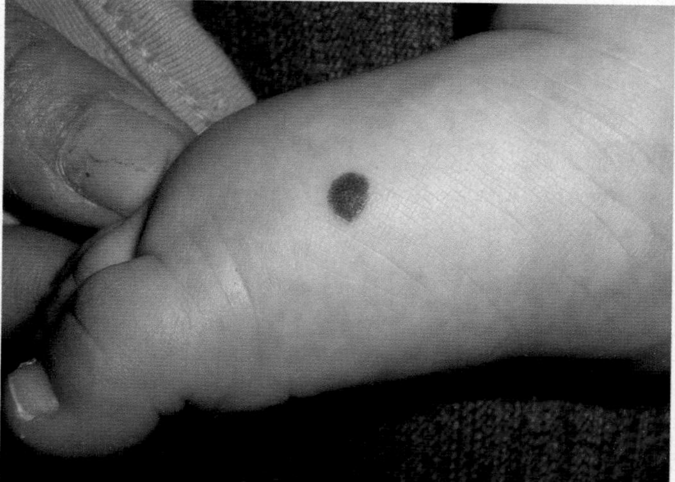

FIGURE 169-1 Small congenital nevus found on the foot of a 6-month-old child. The parents were counseled that this nevus does not need to be excised for the prevention of melanoma. (*Reproduced with permission from Richard P. Usatine, MD.*)

INTRODUCTION

Congenital melanocytic nevi (CMN) are benign pigmented lesions that have a wide variation in presentation and are composed of melanocytes, the pigment-forming cells in the skin (**Figures 169-1** to **169-7**).

SYNONYMS

- Garment nevus, bathing trunk nevus, giant hairy nevus, giant pigmented nevus, pigmented hairy nevus, nevus pigmentosus, nevus pigmentosus et pilosus, and Tierfell nevus.[1]
- Tardive congenital nevus refers to a nevus that has similar features to congenital nevi, but appears at age 1 to 2 years.

EPIDEMIOLOGY

- CMN develop in 1% to 6% of newborns and are present at birth or develop during the first year of life.[1]
- In a study of 594 newborns in San Diego examined within the first 48 hours of life, CMN were found in 2.4%.[2]
- In an Italian prevalence study of more than 3000 children ages 12 to 17 years, CMN or congenital nevus-like nevi were found in 17.5%; most (92%) were small (<1.5 cm).[3]
- CMN are also seen in neurocutaneous melanocytosis, a rare syndrome characterized by the presence of congenital melanocytic nevi and melanotic neoplasms of the central nervous system.[4] CMN are also associated with congenital brain and spinal cord malformations.[5]
- The development of melanoma within CMN (**Figure 169-8**) is believed to occur at a higher rate than in normal skin. Estimates range from 4% to 10%, with smaller lesions having lowest risk.[1]
    - In a systematic review, 46 of 6571 patients with CMN (0.7%), who were followed for 3.4 to 23.7 years, developed melanomas, representing a 465-fold increased relative risk of developing melanoma during childhood and adolescence.[6] The mean age at diagnosis of melanoma was 15.5 years (median: 7 years).

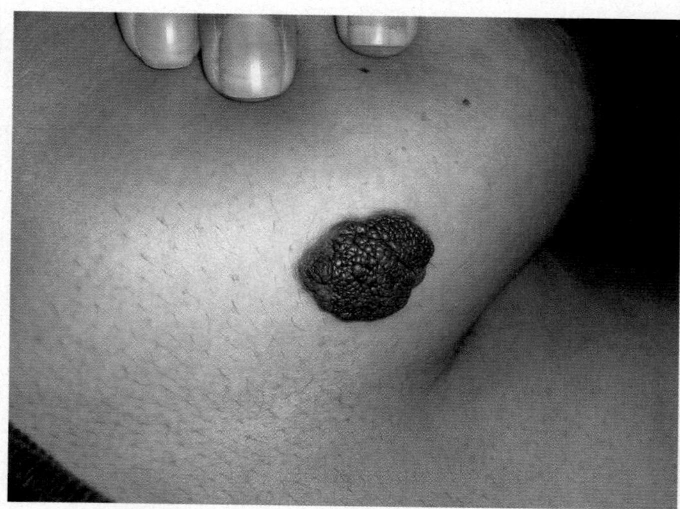

FIGURE 169-2 Congenital nevus on the breast of a 24-year-old woman. It is verrucous, but entirely benign. (*Reproduced with permission from Richard P. Usatine, MD.*)

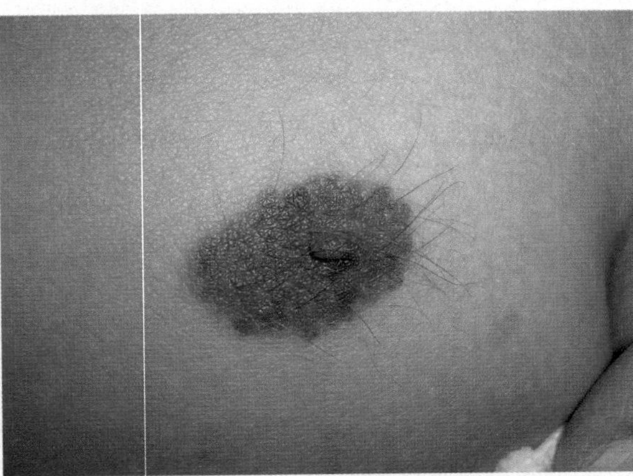

FIGURE 169-3 A benign hairy congenital nevus on the upper buttocks of a 7-year-old boy. The parents requested a consult with plastic surgery to discuss removal. (*Reproduced with permission from Richard P. Usatine, MD.*)

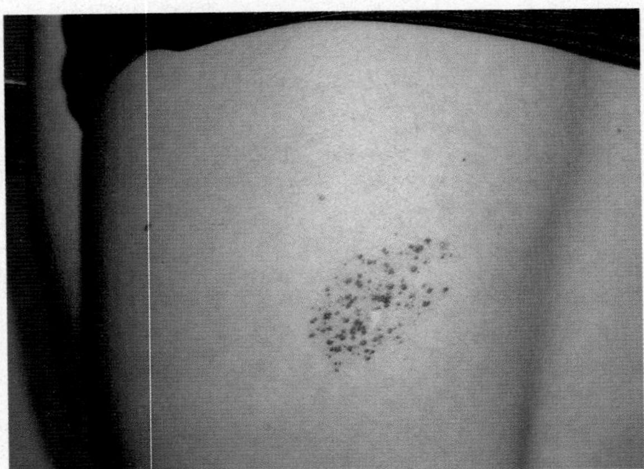

FIGURE 169-4 A speckled congenital nevus (nevus spilus) on the back of a young woman. (*Reproduced with permission from Richard P. Usatine, MD.*)

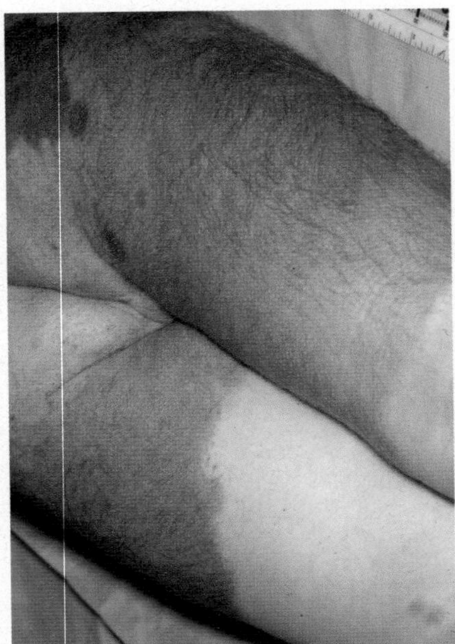

FIGURE 169-5 Large bathing trunk nevus seen on the legs of this older child. (*Reproduced with permission from Jack Resneck, Sr., MD.*)

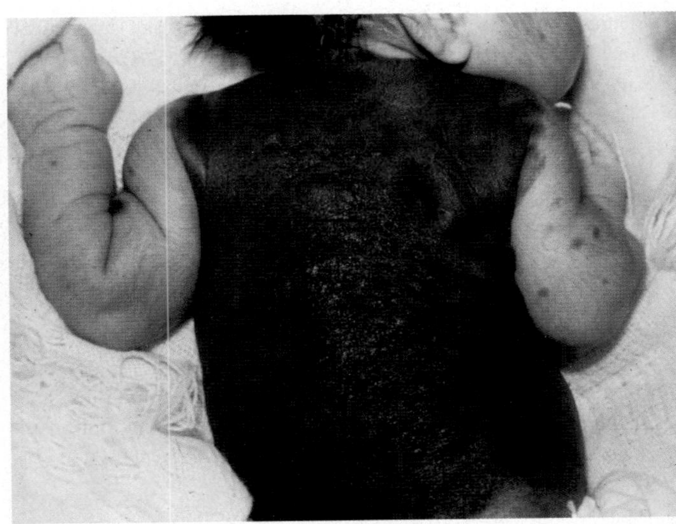

FIGURE 169-6 Infant born with large bathing trunk nevus covering most of the back and chest. (*Reproduced with permission from Richard P. Usatine, MD.*)

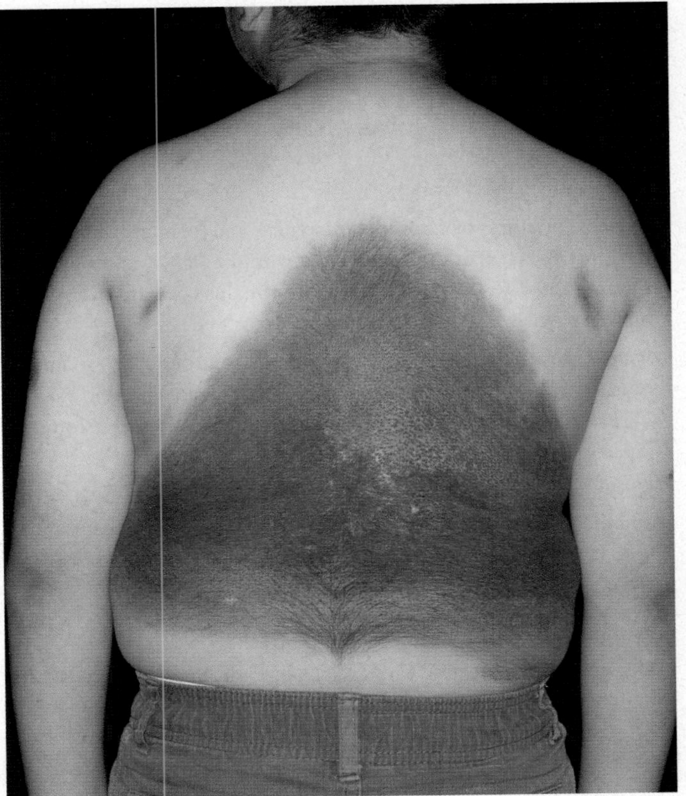

FIGURE 169-7 Giant congenital bathing trunk nevus surrounded by satellite nevi in a 7-year-old Hispanic boy. The patient was referred to plastic surgery so that his parents might consider a staged removal of this large nevus. (*Reproduced with permission from Richard P. Usatine, MD.*)

- Patients with giant CMN appear to be at highest risk—subsequent melanoma occurs in about 2%.[7] In this study of 2578 patients, age at melanoma diagnosis ranged from birth to 58 years (mean 12.6 years). Most CMNs in patients developing melanomas were >40 cm (74%) and had satellite nevi (94%). Melanomas were mostly cutaneous (82%) and located on the trunk (68%); 7 were visceral. About half (55%) were fatal, with a mean age at death of 10 years.
- In a prospective study of 230 medium-size CMN (1.5 to 19.9 cm) in 227 patients from 1955 to 1996, no melanomas occurred. The average follow-up period was 6.7 years to an average age of 25.5 years.[8]
- Other risk factors for melanoma include personal or family history of melanoma or other skin cancer, presence of multiple nevi, red hair, blue eyes, freckling, and history of radiation (see Chapter 179, Melanoma).[1]

ETIOLOGY AND PATHOPHYSIOLOGY

- The etiology of CMN is unknown.
- CMN result from a proliferation of benign melanocytes in the dermis, epidermis, or both. Melanocytes of the skin originate in the neuroectoderm and migrate vertically to the skin and other locations such as the central nervous system and eye.[1] Defects in migration or maturation are hypothesized as causal.

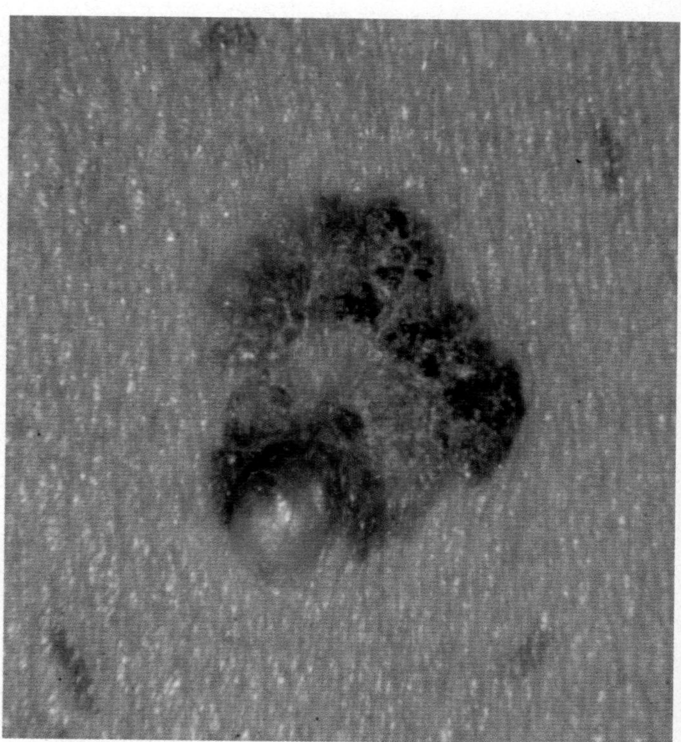

FIGURE 169-8 Melanoma arising in an acquired nevus showing features of central regression and a new elevated nodule. These are the same features that make a congenital nevus suspicious for melanoma. *(Reproduced with permission from Richard P. Usatine, MD.)*

DIAGNOSIS

Diagnosis is usually made based on clinical features and the history of the nevus being present at birth or developing during the first year of life.

CLINICAL FEATURES[1]

- Variable mixtures of color including pink-red (primarily at birth), tan, brown, black, or multiple shades within a single lesion (see **Figures 169-1** to **169-7**); color usually remains constant over time, but the nevus will grow as the person grows.
- Shapes are also highly variable, including oval, round, linear, and random; lesions have irregular but well-demarcated borders (see **Figures 169-1** to **169-8**). The pigment may fade off into surrounding skin (see **Figures 169-3** and **169-4**).
- Nevi may become raised over time (see **Figures 169-2** and **169-3**), and the skin surface ranges from smooth to pebbly to hyperkeratotic (eczema-like appearance).
- Macular portion usually found at edges.
- Frequently exhibit hypertrichosis (see **Figure 169-5**).
- Heavily pigmented large CMN over a limb may be associated with underdevelopment of the limb.[1]
- Lesions are classified by size in adulthood as[1]:
  - Small (<1.5 cm) (see **Figure 169-1**).
  - Medium (1.5 cm to 19 cm) (see **Figures 169-2** and **169-3**).
  - Large (>20 cm) (see **Figures 169-5** to **169-7**). Giant nevi (>40–60 cm) are often surrounded by several smaller satellite nevi (see **Figures 169-5** to **169-7**).

- Lesions on a child's head of less than 9 cm or body of greater than 6 cm are considered large based on likely eventual growth.[1]
- A new classification scheme including projected adult size, location, satellite nevus counts, and morphologic characteristics (color heterogeneity, rugosity, nodularity, and hypertrichosis) has been proposed and appears descriptively useful, but its predictive ability for neurocutaneous melanocytosis or melanoma remains unknown.[9]

IMAGING

- Dermoscopy findings depend on the age and location. In one study, the globular pattern was most common in children younger than age 11 years and on the trunk.[10] Most reticular lesions were located on the limbs, and the variegated pattern was the most specific for CMN.
- MRI of the central nervous system can be a useful diagnostic tool in patients suspected of having neurocutaneous melanocytosis; one author recommended a screening MRI for patients with giant CMN.[11]

TYPICAL DISTRIBUTION

- CMN can be found anywhere on the body.

BIOPSY

- Although there are many histologic subtypes, distinguishing histologic features of congenital nevi include[1]:
  - Involvement by nevus cells of deep dermal appendages and neurovascular structures (e.g., hair follicles, sebaceous glands, arrector pili muscles, and within walls of blood vessels).
  - Infiltration of nevus cells between collagen bundles.

DIFFERENTIAL DIAGNOSIS

- Becker nevus—A brown macule, patch of hair, or both on the shoulder, back, or submammary area that develops in adolescence. The border is irregular, and the lesion may enlarge to cover an entire shoulder or upper arm. It is a type of hamartoma and is not a melanocytic nevus (see Chapter 168, Benign Nevi).
- Café-au-lait spots—Coffee-and-milk-colored patch that can be present at birth or develop during early childhood. Although large café-au-lait spots are associated with neurofibromatosis, a few of them can occur in completely unaffected children. These light-brown patches have increased melanin but are not nevi (see Chapter 245, Neurofibromatosis).

MANAGEMENT

The management of CMN depends on size and location of the lesion (difficulty in monitoring), associated symptoms, the age of the patient, the effect on cosmesis, and the potential for malignant transformation.

- For small and medium-size CMN, the risk of malignant transformation is small and prophylactic removal is not recommended. For cosmesis, treatments include surgical excision or laser treatment.
  - For facial lesions, a multidirectional vector excision may reduce wound length and dogear deformity.[12]
- Larger CMN can be surgically removed but may require tissue expanders, tissue grafts, and tissue flaps to close large defects. Excisions can also be staged. Because the melanocytes may extend deep into underlying tissues (including muscle, bone, and central nervous system), removing the cutaneous component may not eliminate the risk of malignancy.
- Laser treatment of the lesions has been performed with different types of lasers. Based on a case series of 52 patients with 314 CMN, use of UCO2 laser and FDQS Nd:YAG lasers resulted in minimal visible pigmentation in 77% and high satisfaction (87% satisfied).[13] Because of the lack of penetrance to deeper tissue levels, long-term recurrence or malignant transformation is also an issue with these techniques.
- Careful lifelong follow-up with photographs is an acceptable approach.
- Garment or bathing trunk nevi (see **Figures 169-5** to **169-7**):
  - Approximately half of the melanomas that develop in bathing trunk nevi do so before age 5 years.[14] These melanomas can be missed by observation because they can have nonepidermal origins.
  - Surgical excision is recommended by some experts to prevent melanoma.[14] SOR C
- Changes to watch for that call for a biopsy include:
  - Partial regression (depressed white areas).
  - Inflammation.
  - Rapid growth or color change.
  - Development of a firm nodule (see **Figure 169-8**).

FOLLOW-UP

- Patients with giant CMN or multiple CNM may benefit from consultation with a neurologist, pediatrician, or both, because of the risk of neurocutaneous melanocytosis and its neurologic manifestations or obstructive hydrocephalus.
- Bathing trunk nevi can also be associated with spina bifida, meningocele, and neurofibromatosis.[14]
- Because patients with all forms of CMN, especially giant CMN, have an increased risk of developing melanoma, physicians should consider baseline photography and regular follow-up with an experienced clinician for these patients.

PATIENT EDUCATION

- All patients should be told about the importance of protection from UV light exposure. This is especially important in people with giant CMN, because they are at a significantly increased risk of melanoma.
- Patients (or their parents) should be taught to look for signs of melanoma (ABCDE) (asymmetry, border irregularity, color irregularity, diameter >6 mm, evolution).

PATIENT RESOURCES

- Giant congenital nevi—**http://medlineplus.gov/ency/article/001453.htm.**
- Genetics Home Reference—**https://ghr.nlm.nih.gov/condition/giant-congenital-melanocytic-nevus.**
- Support group—**http://www.nevus.org.**

PROVIDER RESOURCES

- **http://emedicine.medscape.com/article/1118659.**

REFERENCES

1. Lyon VB. Congenital melanocytic nevi. *Pediatr Clin North Am.* 2010;57:1155-1176.
2. Kanada KN, Merin MR, Munden A, Friedlander SF. A prospective study of cutaneous findings in newborns in the United States: correlation with race, ethnicity, and gestational status using updated classification and nomenclature. *J Pediatr.* 2012;161(2):240-245.
3. Gallus S, Naldi L; Oncology Study Group of the Italian Group for Epidemiologic Research in Dermatology. Distribution of congenital melanocytic naevi and congenital naevus-like naevi in a survey of 3406 Italian schoolchildren. *Br J Dermatol.* 2008;159(2):433-438.
4. Price HN, Schaffer JV. Congenital melanocytic nevi—when to worry and how to treat: facts and controversies. *Clin Dermatol.* 2010;28(3):293-302.
5. Dias M, Partington M; Section on Neurologic Surgery. Congenital brain and spinal cord malformations and their associated cutaneous markers. *Pediatrics.* 2015;136(4):e1105-1119.
6. Krengel S, Hauschild A, Schafer T. Melanoma risk in congenital melanocytic naevi: a systematic review. *Br J Dermatol.* 2006;155(1):1-8.
7. Vourc'h-Jourdain M, Martin L, Barbarot S; aRED. Large congenital melanocytic nevi: therapeutic management and melanoma risk: a systematic review. *J Am Acad Dermatol.* 2013;68(3):493-8.e1-14.
8. Sahin S, Levin L, Kopf AW, et al. Risk of melanoma in medium-sized congenital melanocytic nevi: a follow-up study. *J Am Acad Dermatol.* 1998;39:428-433.
9. Price HN, O'Haver J, Marghoob A, et al. Practical application of the new classification scheme for congenital melanocytic nevi. *Pediatr Dermatol.* 2015;32(1):23-27.
10. Seidenari S, Pellacani G, Martella A, et al. Instrument-, age- and site-dependent variations of dermoscopic patterns of congenital melanocytic naevi: a multicentre study. *Br J Dermatol.* 2006;155(1):56-61.
11. Arneia JS, Gosain AK. Giant congenital melanocytic nevi. *Plast Reconstr Surg.* 2009;124(1 Suppl):1e-13e.
12. Oh SI, Lee YH. Multidirectional vector excision leads to better outcomes than traditional elliptical excision of facial congenital melanocytic nevus. *Arch Plast Surg.* 2013;40(5):570-574.
13. Al-Hadithy N, Al-Nakib K, Quaba A. Outcomes of 52 patients with congenital melanocytic naevi treated with UltraPulse Carbon Dioxide and Frequency Doubled Q-Switched Nd:YAG laser. *J Plast Reconstr Aesthet Surg.* 2012;65(8):1019-1028.
14. Habif T. *Clinical Dermatology: A Color Guide to Diagnosis and Therapy.* 4th ed. St. Louis, MO: Mosby; 2003.

170 EPIDERMAL NEVUS AND NEVUS SEBACEUS

Mindy A. Smith, MD, MS

PATIENT STORY

A 15-year-old boy is brought in by his mother with a concern about growth of his birthmark. It has become somewhat more raised and bumpy in the past year (**Figure 170-1**). The adolescent reports no symptoms and is not worried about the appearance. He is otherwise healthy with no neurologic symptoms. The joint decision of the family and the doctor was to not excise the epidermal nevus at this time. He may choose to have this removed by a plastic surgeon in the future.

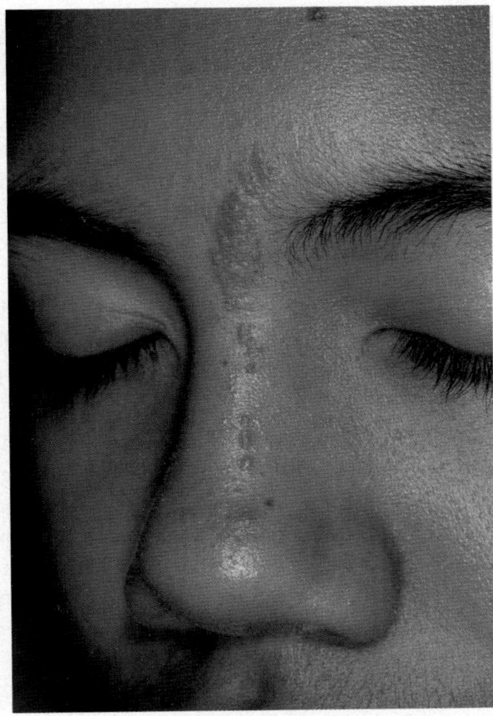

FIGURE 170-1 Epidermal nevus on the face of a teenager. This nevus has been present since birth, and the patient is otherwise healthy. *(Reproduced with permission from Richard P. Usatine, MD.)*

INTRODUCTION

- Epidermal nevi (EN) are congenital hamartomas of ectodermal origin classified based on their main component: sebaceous, apocrine, eccrine, follicular, or keratinocytic.
- Nevus sebaceus (NS) is a hamartoma of the epidermis, hair follicles, and sebaceous and apocrine glands. A hamartoma is the disordered overgrowth of benign tissue in its area of origin.

SYNONYMS

- EN syndrome is also called Solomon syndrome and is a neurocutaneous disorder characterized by EN and an assortment of neurologic and visceral manifestations.
- NS is also called sebaceous nevus and nevus sebaceus of Jadassohn (**Figure 170-2**).
- An inflammatory linear verrucous epidermal nevus (ILVEN) (**Figure 170-3**) can be part of an epidermal nevus syndrome, but some affected persons have only the cutaneous EN.

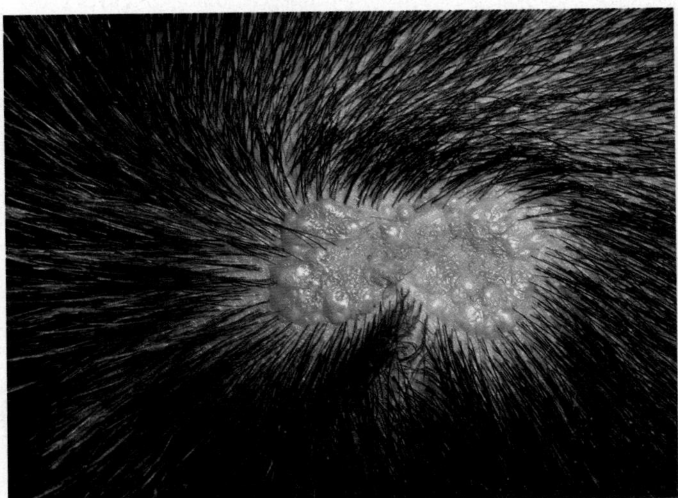

FIGURE 170-2 Nevus sebaceus on the scalp of a 14-year-old boy. *(Reproduced with permission from Richard P. Usatine, MD.)*

EPIDEMIOLOGY

- EN are uncommon (approximately 1% to 3% of newborns and children), sporadic, and usually present at birth, although they can appear in early childhood (**Figure 170-4**).
- EN are associated with disorders of the eye and nervous and musculoskeletal systems in 10% to 30% of patients; in one study, 7.9% of patients with EN had 1 of the 9 syndromes—an estimated 1 per 11,928 pediatric patients.[1]
- In another review of 131 cases of EN, most (60%) had noninflammatory EN, one-third had NS, and 6% had ILVEN.[2]
- NS is usually present at birth or noted in early childhood (**Figure 170-5**).[3] Most cases are sporadic, but familial cases have been reported.[2]

- Linear NS is estimated to occur in 1 per 1000 live births.[4]
- Linear NS syndrome includes a range of abnormalities, including the central nervous system (CNS); patients with CNS involvement typically have cognitive impairment and seizures[3]; other organ systems, including the cardiovascular, skeletal, ophthalmologic, and urogenital systems, may be involved.

ETIOLOGY AND PATHOPHYSIOLOGY

- EN histologically display hyperkeratosis and papillomatosis, similar microscopically to seborrheic keratosis (see Chapter 164, Seborrheic Keratosis).[2] Also similar to seborrheic keratosis, some EN of keratinocyte differentiation (approximately one third) have been found to have a mutation in the fibroblast growth factor receptor 3 (FGFR3) gene.
- Nine EN syndromes have been reported and are described in the referenced article.[5] It is likely that the varied clinical manifestations of these EN syndromes are linked to functional effects of specific genetic defects.[6]
- EN frequently have a linear pattern that follows Blaschko lines (see **Figures 170-1, 170-3**, and **170-4**), which are believed to represent epidermal migration during embryogenesis. Most systemic anomalies that are part of EN syndromes (skeletal, ocular, cardiovascular, endocrine, genitourinary, and orodental tissues) are due to defective neural crest.[6] The most frequent brain anomaly in all forms of epidermal nevus syndromes, and the principal cause of neurologic manifestations, is hemimegalencephaly.[7]
- EN tend to become thicker, verrucous (see **Figure 170-4**), and hyperpigmented at puberty.[2]
- Similarly, NS demonstrates stages of evolution paralleling the histologic differentiation of normal sebaceous gland[8]:
  - Infancy and young children—Smooth to slightly papillated, waxy, hairless thickening (see **Figure 170-5**).
  - Puberty—Epidermal hyperplasia resulting in verrucous irregularity of the surface covered with numerous closely aggregated yellow-to-brown papules (**Figure 170-6**).
  - Development of secondary appendageal tumors (**Figures 170-7** and **170-8**) occurs in 20% to 30% of patients, most are benign (most commonly basal cell epithelioma or trichoblastoma), but single (most commonly basal cell carcinoma) or multiple malignant tumors of both epidermal and adnexal origins may be seen, and metastases have been reported.[2] Rarely, these malignancies are seen in childhood.
- NS was shown to have a high prevalence of human papillomavirus DNA, and authors postulate that human papillomavirus (HPV) infection of fetal epidermal stem cells could play a role in the pathogenesis.[9]

DIAGNOSIS

Clinical features of EN:

- EN are linear, round, or oblong; well-circumscribed; elevated; and flat-topped (see **Figures 170-1** and **170-4**).
- Color is yellow-tan to dark brown; can be white.

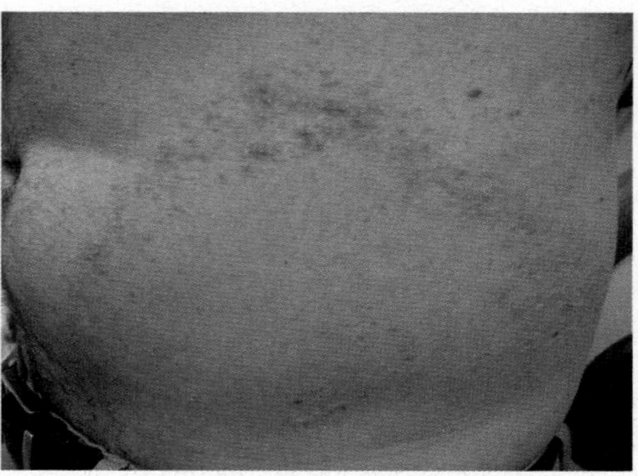

FIGURE 170-3 Inflammatory linear verrucous epidermal nevus (ILVEN) on the trunk of an adult man. Topical steroids were not helpful in diminishing his pruritus. (*Reproduced with permission from Robert T. Gilson, MD.*)

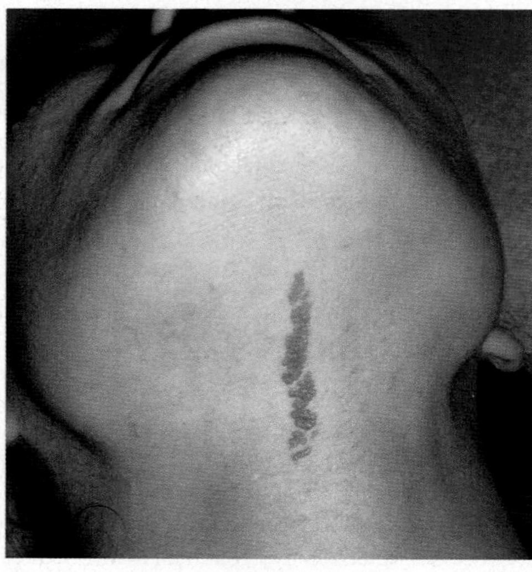

FIGURE 170-4 Linear epidermal nevus on the neck that appeared in early childhood. The patient had no neurologic, musculoskeletal, or vision problems. (*Reproduced with permission from Richard P. Usatine, MD.*)

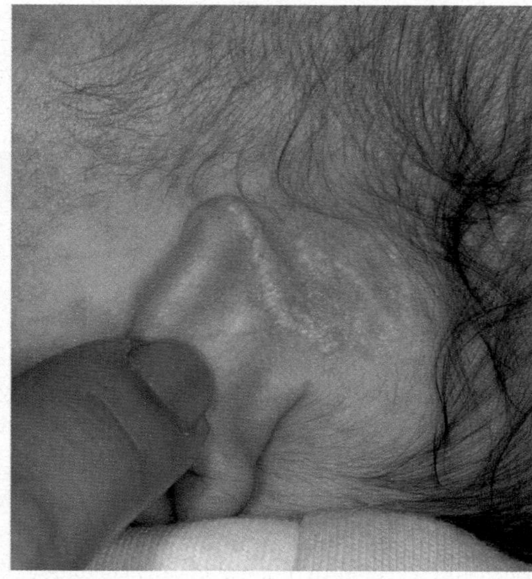

FIGURE 170-5 Nevus sebaceus behind the ear of an infant. Note the light color and the subtle presentation. (*Reproduced with permission from Richard P. Usatine, MD.*)

- Surface is uniform velvety or warty (see **Figures 170-4** and **170-5**).
- ILVEN, a less common type of EN, is pruritic and erythematous (see **Figure 170-3**).

Clinical features of NS:

- NS has an oval to linear shape ranging from 0.5 × 1 cm to 7 × 9 cm.
- NS is usually a solitary, smooth, waxy, hairless thickening noted on the scalp at birth or in early childhood (see **Figures 170-2** and **170-6**).
- Early NS may be pink, orange, yellow, or tan; later lesions can appear verrucous and nodular (see **Figure 170-5**).

TYPICAL DISTRIBUTION

- EN occur most commonly on the head and neck followed by the trunk and proximal extremities; only 13% have widespread lesions (**Figure 170-9**). Lesions may spread beyond their original distribution with age.
- NS are commonly found on the scalp followed by forehead and retroauricular region (see **Figures 170-2** and **170-5** to **170-8**) and rarely involve the neck, trunk, or other areas.

BIOPSY

- Biopsy is the most definitive method for diagnosing these nevi. A biopsy is not needed if the clinical picture is clear and no operative intervention is planned. A shave biopsy should provide adequate tissue for diagnosis because the pathology is epidermal and in the upper dermis.
    - Histologic features of epidermolytic hyperkeratosis within an EN are associated with mutations in the keratin gene that may be transmitted to offspring; widespread cutaneous involvement may be seen.[2]

DIFFERENTIAL DIAGNOSIS

- Linear lichen planus (**Figure 170-10**)—Discrete, pruritic, violaceous papules are arranged in a linear fashion, usually extending along an entire limb.
- Syringoma (**Figure 170-11**)—Benign adnexal tumor derived from sweat gland ducts. Autosomal dominant transmission; soft, small, skin-colored to brown papules develop during childhood and adolescence, especially around the eyes, but may be found on the face, neck, and trunk.
- Lichen striatus—Discrete pink, tan, or skin-colored asymptomatic papules in a linear band that suddenly appear. The papules may be smooth, scaly, or flat topped. It is mostly seen in children. Although it is most commonly seen on an extremity, it can appear on the trunk (**Figure 170-12**). It can resemble a linear EN, but lichen striatus will spontaneously regress within 1 year.
- Linear porokeratosis—Characterized by small, annular, hypertrophic verrucous plaques with a linear morphology usually limited to a single extremity. The annular morphology and dermatomal distribution should help distinguish this condition from EN and NS.

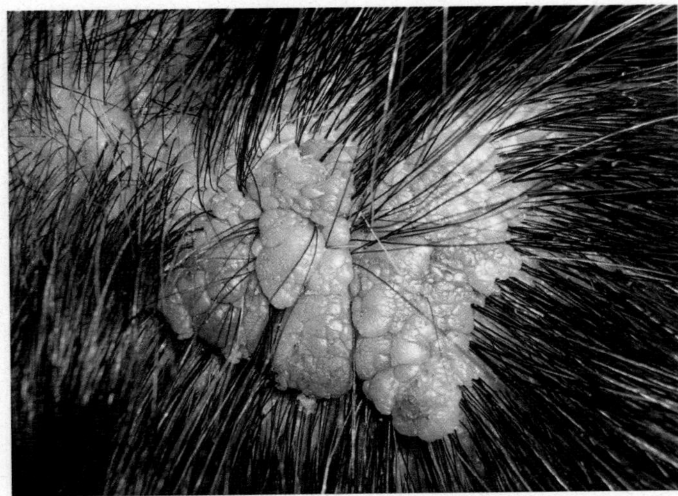

FIGURE 170-6 Nevus sebaceus on the scalp of a teenage female that is verrucous and brown. (*Reproduced with permission from Richard P. Usatine, MD.*)

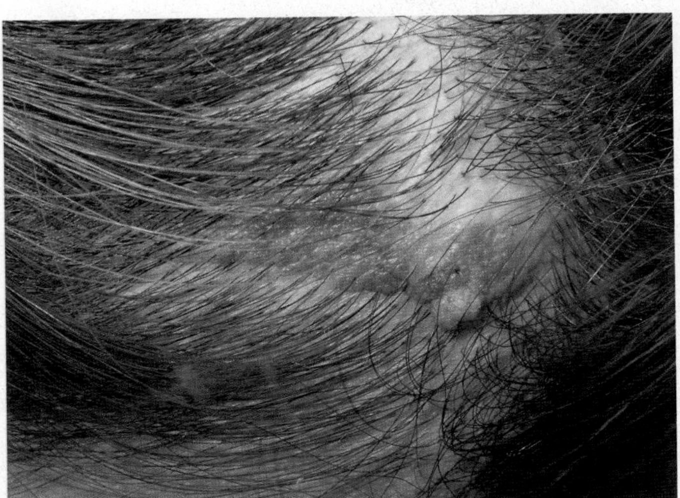

FIGURE 170-7 Nevus sebaceus on the scalp of a young woman. The patient reported a new area of elevation and bleeding. A biopsy showed no malignant transformation. It was most likely inadvertantly traumatized. (*Reproduced with permission from Richard P. Usatine, MD.*)

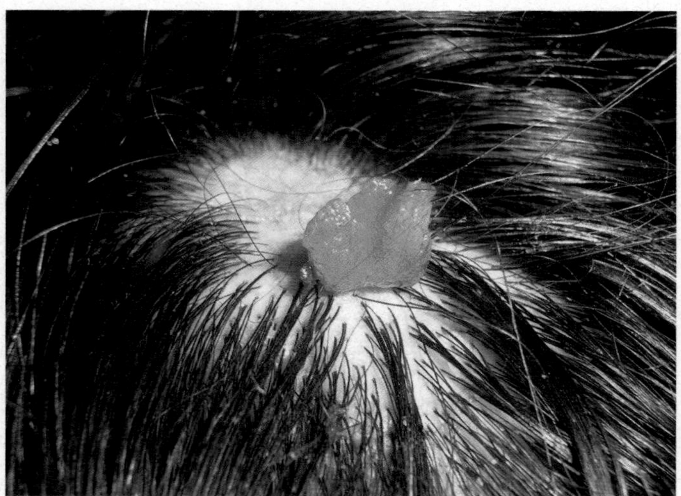

FIGURE 170-8 Nevus sebaceus with a benign tumor identified as a syringocystadenoma papilliferum by shave biopsy. Patient was referred for full removal of the nevus sebaceus. (*Reproduced with permission from Richard P. Usatine, MD.*)

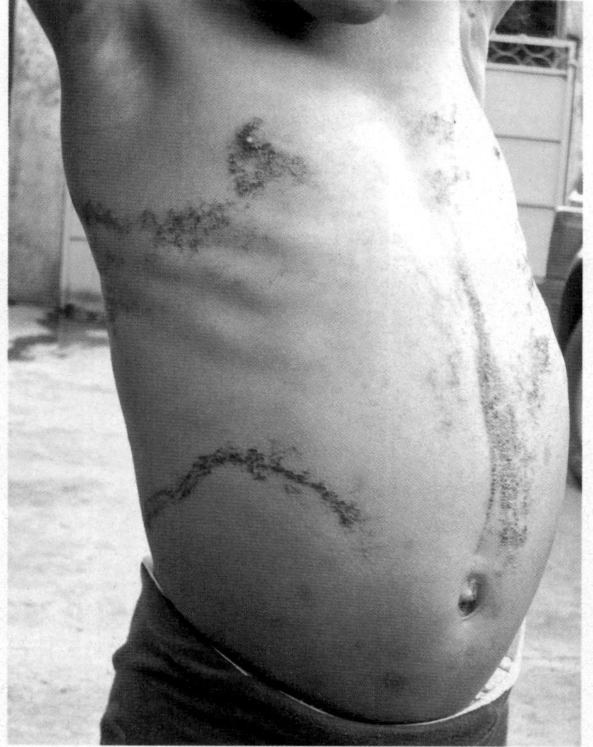

FIGURE 170-9 Extensive epidermal nevus following Blaschko lines on the trunk of this boy. Note how the lines are similar to the patient with inflammatory linear verrucous epidermal nevus (ILVEN) in **Figure 170-2**. (*Reproduced with permission from Rick Hodes, MD.*)

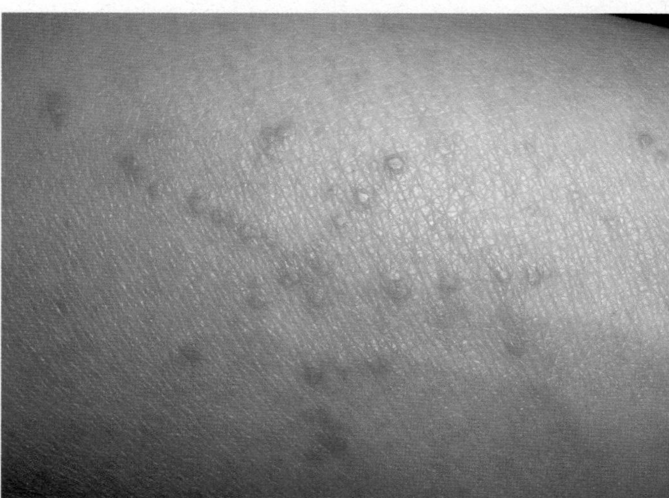

FIGURE 170-10 Lichen planus on the flexor aspect of the forearm in a linear pattern resembling a linear epidermal nevus. (*Reproduced with permission from Richard P. Usatine, MD.*)

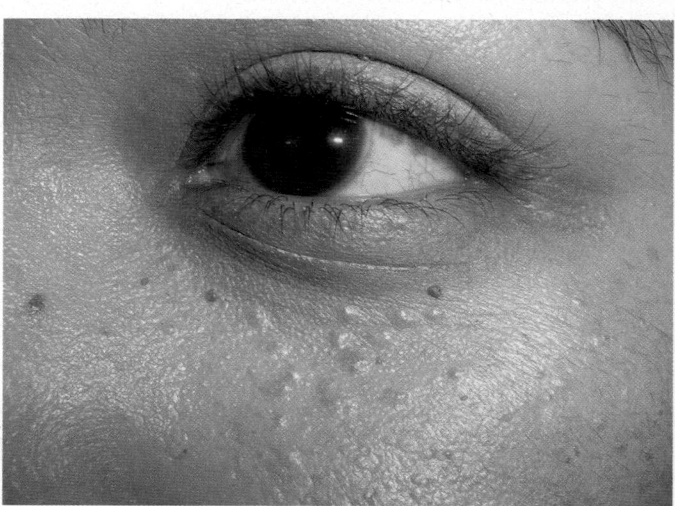

FIGURE 170-11 Syringoma on the lower eyelid. (*Reproduced with permission from Richard P. Usatine, MD.*)

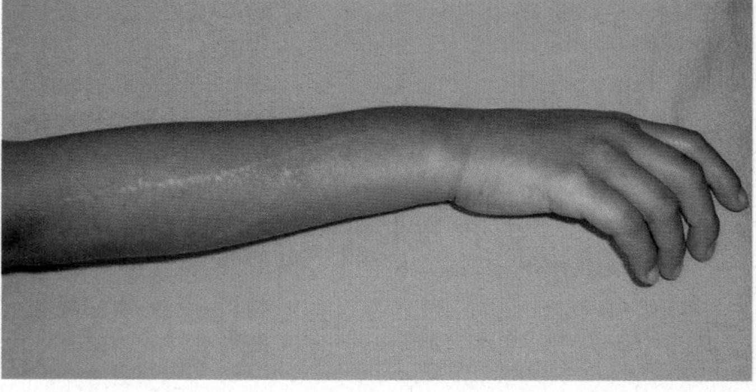

FIGURE 170-12 Lichen striatus that appeared suddenly on the arm of a young boy. (*Reproduced with permission from Richard P. Usatine, MD.*)

MANAGEMENT

FIRST LINE

PROCEDURES

- Destructive modalities for EN, such as electrodesiccation and cryotherapy, may temporarily improve the appearance of the lesion, but recurrence is frequent.[2]
- Carbon dioxide (CO_2) laser is an alternative option for EN; however, scarring and pigment changes are potential permanent complications, especially in patients with darker skin types.[10] This treatment does not completely remove NS, and there is recurrence risk.[2]
  - In a case series of 15 patients with EN and 5 with ILVEN treated with CO_2 laser, initial response rate was excellent (>75% reduction in lesion size) in 30 patients and good (>50% reduction) in half.[11] The recurrence rate at a minimum of 18 months, however, was 30%; hypopigmentation occurred in 25% of patients and scarring in 20%.
- Surgical excision is an option that may be complicated by scarring.
- Because of the potential for malignant transformation, particularly following puberty, some authors recommend early complete plastic surgical excision for NS; SOR C reconstructive surgery may be needed.
- Excision of large lesions may require reconstructive surgery with tissue expansion or grafting.[12]

SECOND LINE

MEDICATIONS

- There are no proven topical methods for treatment of these lesions. Topical retinoids may improve lesion appearance, but recurrence is common.[2]
- With the identification of epidermal signaling abnormalities underlying the cell proliferation in NS, medical treatments may be developed that target these aberrant pathways.[13]

PROGNOSIS

- There are reports of spontaneous improvement in patients with widespread involvement of EN.
- Malignant potential is low in EN.[2]
- Malignant potential in NS is uncertain. Reports range from 0% to 2.7%.[2]
  - Early reports suggested a high rate of developing basal cell carcinomas, whereas more recent studies identified trichoblastoma and syringocystadenoma papilliferum in NS, usually in adulthood.[2]
  - Data pooled from six large retrospective institutional studies with 2520 patients with NS demonstrated a cumulative incidence of benign and malignant tumors of 6.1% and 0.5%, respectively.[12]
  - In a retrospective analysis of 757 cases of NS from 1996 to 2002 in children age 16 years or younger, investigators found no malignancies and question the need for prophylactic surgical removal.[14]
  - Squamous cell carcinoma has also been described in an NS.[15]

FOLLOW-UP

- Patients with NS should be examined for other associated findings. Consider a consultation with a neurologist and/or ophthalmologist.
  - In a study of 196 subjects with NS examined for clinical neurologic abnormalities, only 7% had abnormalities.[16] Abnormal exams were more frequent in individuals with extensive nevi (21% vs. 5%) and a centrofacial location (21% vs. 2%). The patients depicted in this chapter had no neurologic abnormalities.

PATIENT RESOURCES

- Nevus Outreach—**http://www.nevus.org.**
- Genetics Home Reference. *Epidermal Nevus*—**http://ghr.nlm.nih.gov/condition/epidermal-nevus.**

PROVIDER RESOURCES

- Medscape. *Nevus Sebaceus*—**http://emedicine.medscape.com/article/1058733-overview.**
- Medscape. *Epidermal Nevus Syndrome*—**http://emedicine.medscape.com/article/1117506-overview.**

REFERENCES

1. Vidaurri-de la Cruz H, Tamayo-Sanchez L, Duran-McKinster C, et al. Epidermal nevus syndromes: clinical findings in 35 patients. *Pediatr Dermatol.* 2004;21(4):432-439.
2. Rogers M, McCrossin I, Commens C. Epidermal nevi and the epidermal nevus syndrome. A review of 131 cases. *J Am Acad Dermatol.* 1989;20(3):476-488.
3. Brandling-Bennett HA, Morel KD. Epidermal nevi. *Pediatr Clin North Am.* 2010;57:1177-1198.
4. Menascu S, Donner EJ. Linear nevus sebaceous syndrome: case reports and review of the literature. *Pediatr Neurol.* 2008;38(3):207-210.
5. Happle R. The group of epidermal nevous syndromes. Part I. Well-defined phenotypes. *J Am Acad Dermatol.* 2010;63:1-22.
6. Arch S, Sugarman JL. Epidermal nevus syndromes. *Handb Clin Neurol.* 2015;132:291-316.
7. Laura FS. Epidermal nevus syndrome. *Handb Clin Neurol.* 2013;111:349-368.
8. Hammadi AA. *Nevus Sebaceus.* Last updated May 2, 2016. http://emedicine.medscape.com/article/1058733-overview. Accessed March 2017.
9. Carlson JA, Cribier B, Nuovo G, et al. Epidermodysplasia verruciformis-associated and genital-mucosal high-risk human papillomavirus DNA are prevalent in nevus sebaceus of Jadassohn. *J Am Acad Dermatol.* 2008;59(2):279-294.
10. Boyce S, Alster TS. CO_2 laser treatment of epidermal nevi: long-term success. *Dermatol Surg.* 2002;28(7):611-614.
11. Alonso-Castro L, Boixeda P, Reig I, et al. Carbon dioxide laser treatment of epidermal nevi: response and long-term follow-up. *Actas Dermosifiliogr.* 2012;103(10):910-918.

12. Chepla KJ, Gosain AK. Giant nevus sebaceus: definition, surgical techniques, and rationale for treatment. *Plast Reconstr Surg.* 2012;130(2):296e-304e.
13. Aslam A, Salam A, Griffiths CE, McGrath JA. Naevus sebaceus: a mosaic RASopathy. *Clin Exp Dermatol.* 2014;39(1):1-6.
14. Santibanez-Gallerani A, Marshall D, Duarte AM, et al. Should nevus sebaceus of Jadassohn in children be excised? A study of 757 cases, and literature review. *J Craniofac Surg.* 2003;14(5):658-660.
15. Aguayo R, Pallarés J, Casanova JM, et al. Squamous cell carcinoma developing in Jadassohn's sebaceous nevus: case report and review of the literature. *Dermatol Surg.* 2010;36(11):1763-1768.
16. Davies D, Rogers M. Review of neurological manifestations in 196 patients with sebaceous naevi. *Australas J Dermatol.* 2002;43(1):20-23.

171 DYSPLASTIC NEVUS AND SPITZ NEVUS

Isac P. Simpson, DO
Mindy A. Smith, MD, MS
Richard P. Usatine, MD

PATIENT STORY

A 44-year-old man presents with concern over a mole on his back that his wife says is growing larger and more variable in color. The edges are irregular, and the color almost appears to be "leaking" into the surrounding skin. He reports no symptoms related to this lesion. On physical exam, the nevus is 9 mm in diameter with asymmetry and variations in color and an irregular border (**Figure 171-1**). A full-body skin exam demonstrated no other suspicious lesions. Dermoscopy showed an irregular network with multiple asymmetrically placed dots off the network (**Figure 171-2**). A saucerization (deep shave) was performed with a DermaBlade taking 2-mm margins of clinically normal skin (**Figure 171-3**). Pathology showed a completely excised compound dysplastic nevus with no signs of malignancy. No further treatment was needed except yearly skin exams to monitor for melanoma.

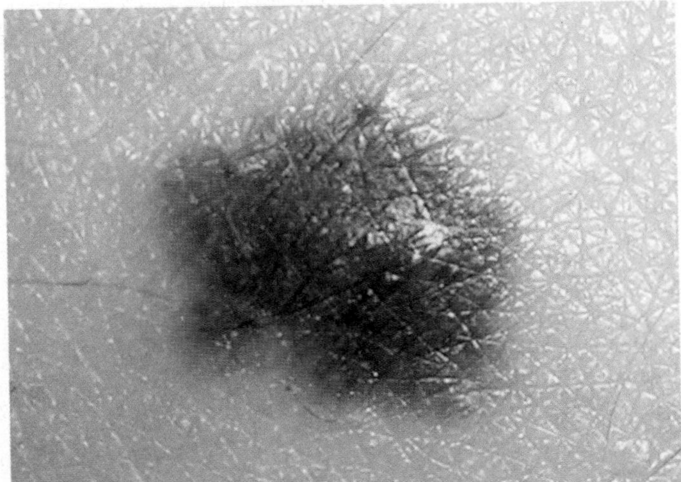

FIGURE 171-1 Growing 9-mm compound dysplastic nevus on the back of a 44-year-old man. There is asymmetry and variations in color and an irregular border. (*Reproduced with permission from Richard P. Usatine, MD.*)

INTRODUCTION

Dysplastic nevi (DN) (atypical moles) and Spitz nevi are irregular-appearing nevi with clinical and histologic definitions that are controversial and still evolving. Both DN and Spitz nevi have clinical, dermoscopic, and histologic features that overlap with melanoma. Patients with multiple DN or an atypical Spitz nevus have an increased risk for melanoma.[1] The presence of multiple DN is a marker for increased melanoma risk just as red hair is, and, analogously, cutting off the red hair or cutting out all the DN does not change that risk of melanoma. DN are not precursor lesions of melanoma; they are markers for an increased risk of melanoma. The problem with DN is that any one lesion that is suspicious for melanoma must be biopsied to avoid missing melanoma, not to prevent melanoma from occurring in that nevus in the future.

Spitz nevi (**Figures 171-4** and **171-5**) are uncommon solitary pink to black dome-shaped papules that usually appear in the first 2 decades of life. They have features histologically similar to melanoma, and some may in fact be spitzoid melanomas. Lesions suspected to be Spitz nevi should be biopsied for histopathologic diagnosis, and in the majority of cases complete excision with clear margins is recommended. Children less than 12 years of age with a typical Spitz nevus may be considered for close monitoring, but an atypical Spitz nevus at any age should be biopsied.[2,3]

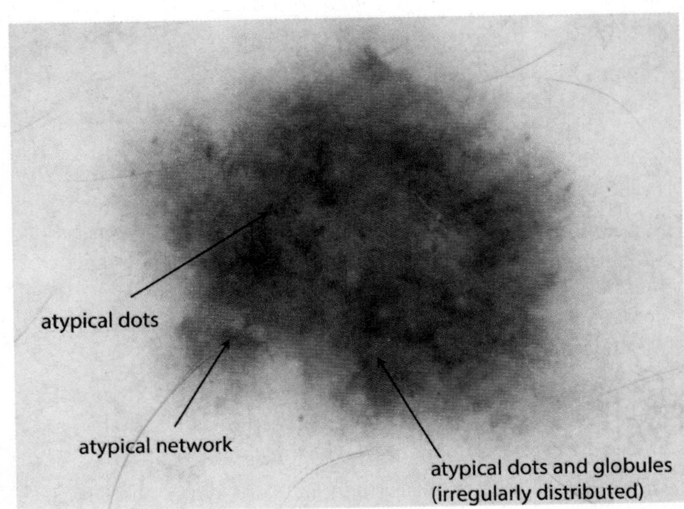

FIGURE 171-2 Dermoscopy of this compound dysplastic nevus shows an irregular network with multiple asymmetrically placed dots off the network. (*Reproduced with permission from Richard P. Usatine, MD.*)

SYNONYMS

Dysplastic nevus: atypical nevus, atypical mole, Clark nevus, nevus with architectural disorder, and melanocytic atypia.[1]

Spitz nevus: Spitz tumor, spindle-cell nevus, epithelioid cell nevus. A Reed nevus is a pigmented Spitz nevus. The term *benign juvenile melanoma* should be avoided as it is misleading.

EPIDEMIOLOGY

- Two to 9% of the population has atypical moles (AMs).[4,5] In a Swedish case-control study, 56% of cases (121 patients with melanoma) and 19% of 310 control subjects had nevi fulfilling the clinical criteria for DN.[6] Among patients with melanoma, the rate of DN ranges from 34% to 59%.[5] DN are uncommon in children; in a study of Swedish children (N = 524), none had DN.[7] In another study of pathology reports from nevi removed from patients younger than 18 years old, 3 of 199 nevi submitted for histologic analysis met the histologic criteria for DN.[8]
- Individuals with fair skin types are at higher risk of DN.[5]
- The sudden eruption of benign and atypical melanocytic nevi has been reported and is associated with blistering skin conditions and a number of disease states, including immunosuppression. Subsets of patients with immunosuppression have increased numbers of nevi on the palms and soles.[9]
- The National Institute of Health Consensus Conference on the diagnosis and treatment of early melanoma defined a syndrome of familial atypical mole and melanoma (FAMM). The criteria of FAMM syndrome are[10]:
  - The occurrence of malignant melanoma in one or more first- or second-degree relatives.
  - The presence of numerous (often >50) melanocytic nevi, some of which are clinically atypical.
- Approximately 70% of Spitz nevi will present in the first 2 decades of life.[11]
- There is no male-to-female predominance of Spitz nevi in children less than 15 years old. Above the age of 15 there is a 1:3 male-to-female ratio of occurrence.[12]
- Incidence of Spitz nevus is rare and is approximately 1.4 in 100,000.[13]

ETIOLOGY AND PATHOPHYSIOLOGY

- Most DN are compound nevi (see **Figure 171-1**) possessing a junctional and intradermal component (see Chapter 168, Benign Nevi).[1] The junctional component is highly cellular and consists of an irregular distribution of melanocytes arranged in nests and lentiginous patterns along the dermal–epidermal junction. The dermal component, located at the center, consists of nests and strands of melanocytes with distinct sclerotic changes.[1]
- DN exhibit a host response consisting of irregular rete ridge elongation, subepidermal sclerosis, proliferation of dermal capillaries, and a perivascular, lymphohistiocytic inflammatory infiltrate.[1]
- Individuals with DN may have deficient DNA repair, and DN lesions are associated with overexpression of pheomelanin (pigment produced by melanocytes), which may lead to increased oxidative DNA damage and tumor progression.[14]

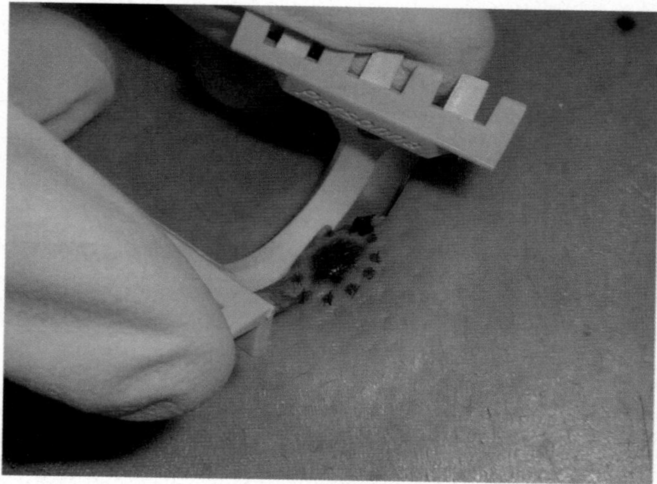

FIGURE 171-3 A saucerization was performed with a DermaBlade taking 2-mm margins of clinically normal skin. The pathology showed a completely excised benign compound dysplastic nevus. *(Reproduced with permission from Richard P. Usatine, MD.)*

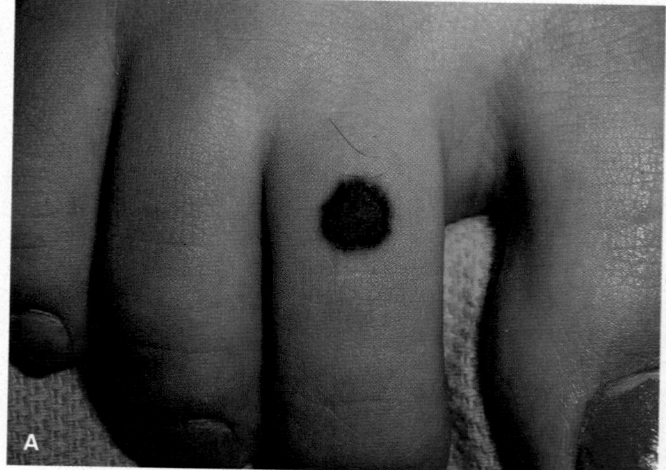

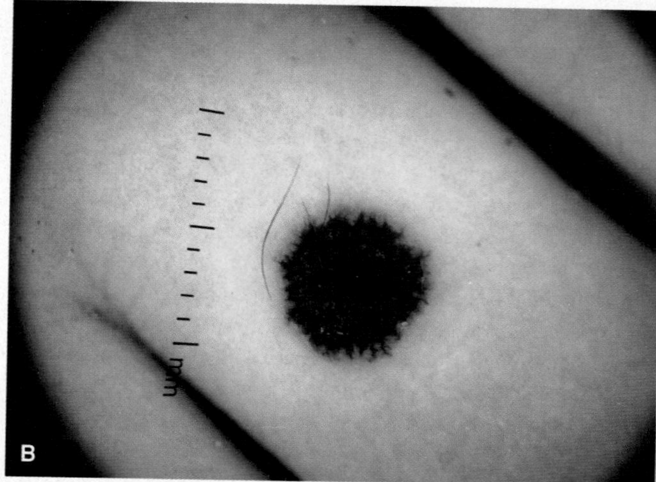

FIGURE 171-4 **A.** Spitz nevus growing on the foot of a 13-year-old girl. **B.** Dermoscopy shows a starburst pattern. The whole lesion was biopsied with a saucerization to make sure there was no melanoma present. When the pathology revealed a Spitz nevus, a conservative elliptical excision was performed. *(Reproduced with permission from Richard P. Usatine, MD.)*

- Spitz nevi contain histologic features of melanoma, which include asymmetric proliferation of large, atypical epithelioid and/or spindle-shaped melanocytes.
- Spitz nevus and melanoma are separate and distinct lesions, but the presence of spitzoid melanomas does muddy the waters.[15]

DIAGNOSIS

CLINICAL FEATURES

▶ Dysplastic nevus

- Variable mixtures of color including tan, brown, black, and red within a single lesion (**Figures 171-6** and **171-7**).
- Irregular, notched borders; pigment may fade off into surrounding skin (see **Figure 171-6**).
- Flat or slightly raised with the macular portion at edge. Not verrucous or pendulous.
- Usually larger than 6 mm (see **Figure 171-7**); may be larger than 10 mm.
- Patients with FAMM syndrome may have more than 100 lesions, far greater than the average number of common moles (<50) in most individuals.

▶ Spitz nevus

- Pink or flesh-colored dome-shaped papules, typically in young persons[15] (see **Figure 171-5**).
- Pigmented Spitz nevi (Reed nevi) are more common than the pink types[1,2,15] (see **Figure 171-4**).

TYPICAL DISTRIBUTION

- DN are usually on sun-exposed areas, especially the back (see **Figure 171-1**); may be found on sites where nevi are usually absent or rare such as the scalp, breasts (**Figure 171-8**), genital skin, buttocks, palm, and dorsa of feet.
- Spitz nevus is most commonly located on the lower extremities (see **Figures 171-4** and **171-5**), followed by the trunk in both children and adults.[12]

DERMOSCOPY

- Dermoscopy is an important part of the evaluation of pigmented lesions and can assist in the diagnosis of DN, Spitz nevi, and melanoma[16] (see Chapters 111 and 181).
- DN—The goal of dermoscopy is to be able to distinguish DN from melanoma. Various dermoscopic classifications of DN have been developed to help accomplish this.[17] This is an advanced aspect of dermoscopy and can be learned with study and experience (see Chapters 111 and 181). Some examples of dermoscopic images of DN are seen in **Figures 171-2**, **171-6B**, and **171-8B**. When in doubt, cut it out, or refer to a dermatologist.
- Spitz nevi may contain distinct dermoscopic features, some of which may include peripheral pseudopods, peripheral streaking, or a combination pseudopods and streaking. These typically

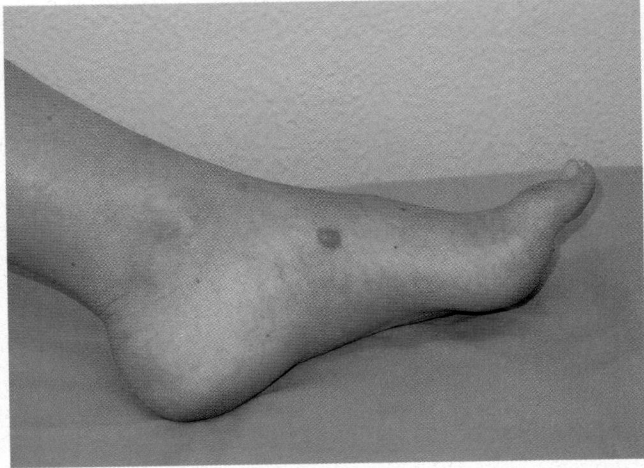

FIGURE 171-5 Spitz nevus on the foot of a young woman. Note how pink it is. It was biopsied because melanoma in young people can appear as a pink bump like this. (*Reproduced with permission from Giuseppe Argenziano, MD.*)

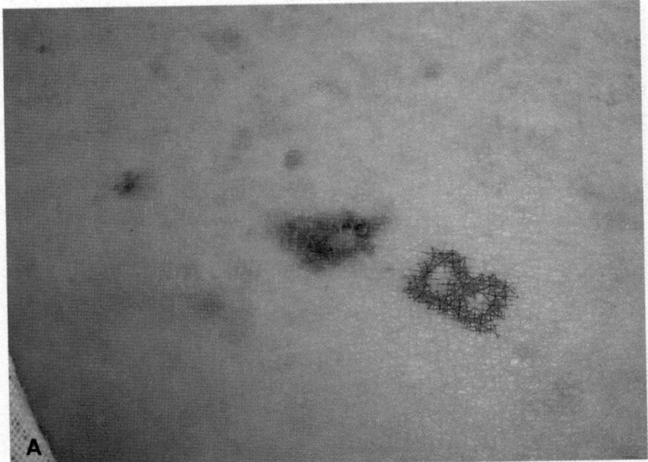

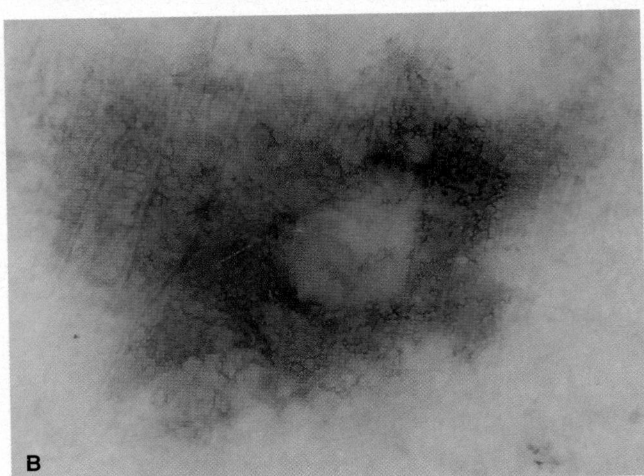

FIGURE 171-6 **A.** Dysplastic nevus on the breast of a 69-year-old woman. It has the typical fried-egg appearance of some dysplastic nevi, with the central raised area and flat pigmented periphery. It had many of the ABCDE characteristics of melanoma, so a saucerization was performed. Pathology showed a compound dysplastic nevus with mild atypia. **B.** Dermoscopy reveals an irregular network. (*Reproduced with permission from Richard P. Usatine, MD.*)

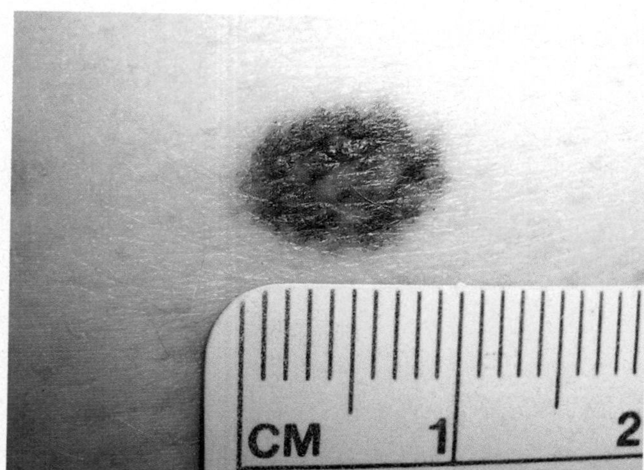

FIGURE 171-7 Dysplastic nevus greater than 6 mm in diameter with variation in color. This was fully excised with a saucerization to make sure there was no melanoma present. The result showed a compound dysplastic nevus with mild atypia. (*Reproduced with permission from Richard P. Usatine, MD.*)

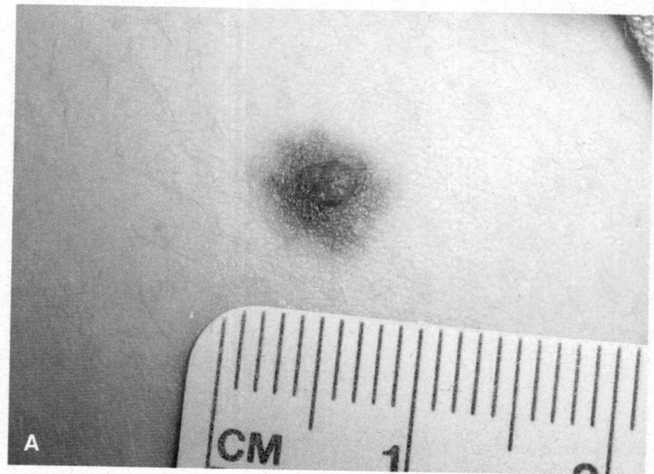

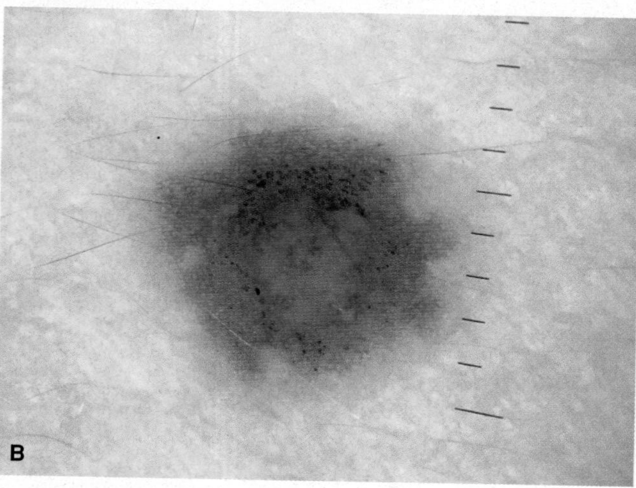

FIGURE 171-8 **A.** Dysplastic nevus on the breast of a 13-year-old girl with a central raised portion and a flat peripheral area. **B.** Dermoscopy showed asymmetric dots and globules. The patient was concerned about its growth and requested its removal. Excision revealed a compound dysplastic nevus. (*Reproduced with permission from Richard P. Usatine, MD.*)

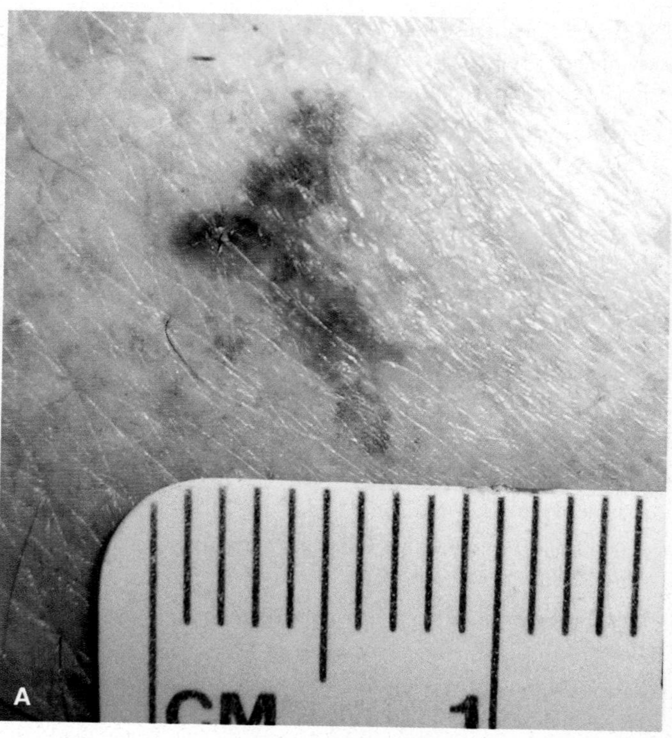

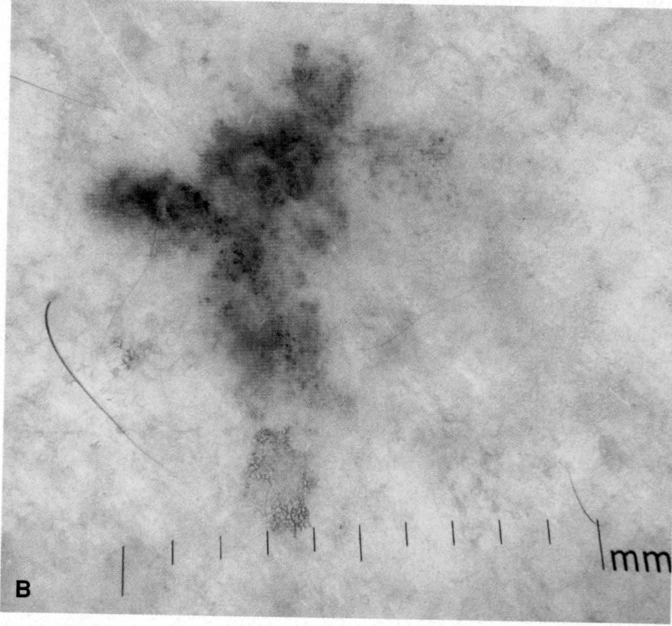

FIGURE 171-9 **A.** Dysplastic nevus with severe atypia on the back of a 64-year-old HIV-positive man. The lesion was very suspicious for melanoma based on its chaotic appearance, asymmetry, irregular borders, multiple colors and large diameter. **B.** Dermoscopy showed a number of melanoma-specific structures including irregular network, asymmetric dots and globules and white lines. Considering the clinical appearance, the histology with severe atypia, and the immunocompromised host, the lesion was excised with 5-mm margins just like removing melanoma in situ. (*Reproduced with permission from Richard P. Usatine, MD.*)

form a starburst pattern, which is present in >50% of Spitz nevi (see **Figure 171-4**).[18] Other dermoscopic features may include white lines, blue-white veil, and other melanoma-specific structures.

BIOPSY

- A full excisional biopsy should be performed on any suspicious DN or Spitz nevus to rule out melanoma.
- In a patient with many DN, biopsy of the most suspicious lesions is reasonable to rule out melanoma. Also, referral for total body photography can be helpful to determine which DN are changing and need biopsy.
- As any Spitz nevus may be a spitzoid melanoma, it is best to perform an excisional biopsy of any suspected Spitz nevus. This is especially true after age 12 years, when the risk for melanoma within a Spitz nevus increases.[19]
- A full excisional biopsy is most easily performed as a saucerization (deep shave biopsy with a DermaBlade or razor blade) including a 1- to 3-mm margin of clinically normal skin (see Chapter 113, Biopsy Principles and Techniques)[5] (see **Figure 171-3**).
- Partial biopsies with a punch biopsy technique are not recommended, as they may lead to a misdiagnosis.

DIFFERENTIAL DIAGNOSIS

- Melanocytic nevi—Most common nevi are tan to brown, smaller than 6 mm, round in shape, and with sharp borders (see Chapter 168, Benign Nevi).
- Melanoma—Skin cancer is often asymmetric, with irregular border and varied colors. It is usually chaotic in its clinical and dermoscopic appearance (see Chapter 179, Melanoma).

MANAGEMENT

FIRST LINE

- If melanoma is detected on biopsy, refer to a dermatologist or surgical oncologist for further surgery and staging.
- Management of a DN that has been biopsied is based on its degree of atypia. DN are graded into the 3 categories of mild, moderate, and severe.
- If a DN is fully excised clinically and the pathology shows only mild to moderate atypia, the evidence suggests that observation is reasonable rather than further surgery even if the histologic margins are not 100% clear.[20-23] SOR B
- In a cohort study of 115 patients, rates of clinical recurrence after biopsy of DN and benign nevi were extremely low even with positive margins. The authors concluded that reexcision of nevi, including mildly to moderately DN with a positive margin, may not be necessary.[20]
- In a large study of 1809 DN, reexcising mildly and moderately atypical DN resulted in a low histopathologic yield and rarely resulted in a clinically significant change in diagnosis. The authors concluded that clinical monitoring of margin-positive mildly and moderately atypical DN may be warranted.[21]
- In another cohort study, 498 patients with mild or moderate DN and positive histologic margins were clinically observed or reexcised with negative margins. They concluded that cases of mild and moderate DN with microscopically positive margins and no concerning clinical residual lesion may reasonably be observed rather than undergo reexcision.[22] They also found that partial biopsies of pigmented lesions suspicious for melanoma (e.g., punch biopsies) led to delayed melanoma diagnosis, and this should be discouraged.[22]
- If severe atypia is reported, many would treat the lesion as a melanoma in situ, and a reexcision with 5- to 9-mm margins would be performed (**Figure 171-9**). SOR C
- However, one study of 426 DN with moderate or severe atypia and clear histologic margins found that the DN were most likely removed by the shave procedure with a 98.4% negative predictive value (NPV). The authors concluded that routine excision of DN showing moderate or severe atypia with clear margins on saucerization is not necessary and that regular surveillance is sufficient.[23] SOR B
- Complete excision of Spitz nevi with either atypical features or initial presentation after the first 2 decades of life is recommended.[15] Therefore, if the original margins were not clear, a conservative reexcision to obtain completely clear margins is warranted. Close monitoring after excision is recommended, as there are documented cases of histopathologic error and/or melanoma transformation.[15]

PREVENTION

- Avoid direct sunlight and use sun protection measures (see Chapter 172, Sun Damage and Skin Cancer Prevention).
- Because of the low risk of any one DN developing malignant transformation, the prophylactic removal of all DN is not recommended. SOR C

PROGNOSIS

- DNs appear to be dynamic throughout adulthood. In a study of the natural history of DN, investigators found that 51% of all evaluated nevi (297 of 593) showed clinical signs of change during an average follow-up of 89 months.[24] New nevi were common in adulthood, continuing to form in more than 20% of patients older than age 50 years, and some nevi disappeared.
- The risk of a melanoma arising within a DN is estimated at 1:3000 per year.[1] However, there is also an increased risk of melanoma arising elsewhere on the skin in patients with DN; the actual incidence rate is uncertain and ranges from 0.5% to 46%.[5] There is also a substantially increased risk of melanoma associated with the number of atypical nevi (relative risk [RR] = 6.36; 95% confidence interval [CI]: 3.80, 10.33; for 5 versus 0).[25]
- In one case-control study, the estimated 10-year cumulative risk for developing melanoma in patients with AM syndrome was 10.7% (vs. 0.62% in a control population).[26]

- The prognosis for a patient with a benign Spitz nevus is excellent, as it is a benign neoplasm. The prognosis of a spitzoid melanoma is based on depth of the lesion, nodal metastasis, ulceration, and number of mitotic figures.[27]

FOLLOW-UP

- Patients with DN or a Spitz nevus should have regular skin examinations with biopsies performed of any suspicious lesions. Regrowth at previous biopsy sites should be excised based on the original pathology, the clinical and dermoscopic appearance, and timing of the regrowth (see **Figure 171-8**).[5]
- Consider photographs for monitoring patients with many DN (**Figure 171-10**).[5] In a study of 50 patients with 5 or more DN, the use of baseline digital photographs improved the diagnostic accuracy of skin self-examination on the back, chest, and abdomen and improved detection of changing and new moles.[28] Individual DN can be monitored more precisely with digital dermoscopic photos added to the skin photographs (see **Figure 171-10**). One can refer for full total-body photography, which is an even greater level of monitoring and should be considered in patients with FAMM.
- Patients with numerous DN and who have a family history of melanoma are at a higher risk of developing melanoma and should be encouraged to have regular follow-up with a provider skilled in detecting melanoma and be followed with total body photography.
- Patients with FAMM should also consider a baseline ophthalmologic examination because of a possible association between uveal melanoma and FAMM syndrome.[5]
- First-degree relatives of patients diagnosed with FAMM syndrome should be encouraged to be examined for DN and melanoma.

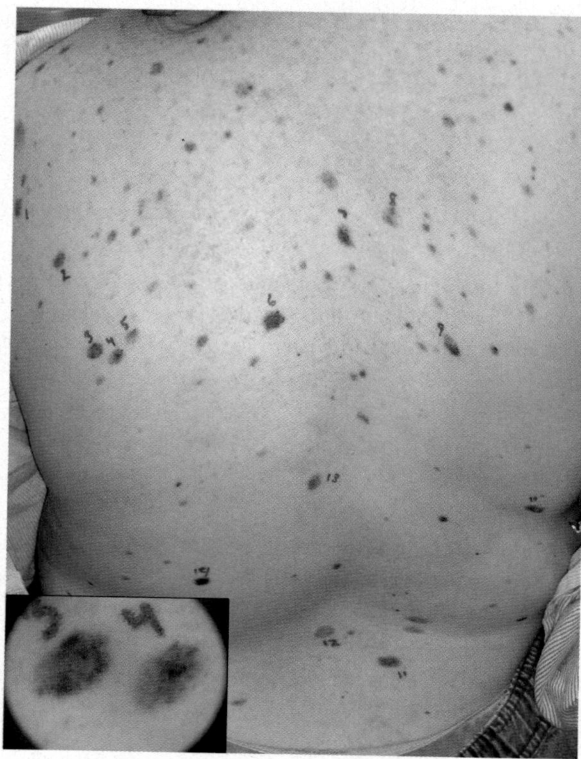

FIGURE 171-10 More than 14 dysplastic nevi are seen on the back of this 35-year-old woman with a history of 2 basal cell carcinomas on her back. She has never had a melanoma and has no family history of melanoma. Multiple biopsies so far have only shown dysplastic nevi, so she is being followed with serial digital photography of her nevi along with corresponding dermoscopic photographs. Note the dermoscopic images of nevi 3 and 4 in the bottom left corner. (*Reproduced with permission from Richard P. Usatine, MD.*)

PATIENT EDUCATION

- Patients with DN should avoid excessive exposure to natural or artificial UV light and routinely use a broad-spectrum sunscreen with a sun-protective factor of 30 or greater and/or sun-protective clothing.
- Patients should be taught self-examination to detect changes in existing moles and to recognize clinical features of melanomas. Patients should be taught to look for and report asymmetry, border irregularity, new symptoms (e.g., pain, pruritus, bleeding, or ulceration), and color and size changes.

PATIENT RESOURCES

- **http://www.nlm.nih.gov/medlineplus/moles.html.**
- **http://www.cancer.gov/types/skin/moles-fact-sheet.**

PROVIDER RESOURCES

- **http://emedicine.medscape.com/article/1056283-overview.**
- **http://www.aocd.org/page=Spitznevus?**

REFERENCES

1. Clarke LE. Dysplastic nevus. *Clin Lab Med.* 2011;31:255-265.
2. Ferrara G, Gianotti R, Cavicchini S, et al. Spitz nevus, Spitz tumor, and spitzoid melanoma: a comprehensive clinicopathologic overview. *Dermatol Clin.* 2013;31(4):589-598.
3. Tlougan BE, Orlow SJ, Schaffer JV. Spitz nevi beliefs, behaviors, and experiences of pediatric dermatologists. *JAMA Dermatol.* 2013;149(3):283-291.
4. Mooi WJ. The dysplastic naevus. *J Clin Pathol.* 1997;50:711-715.
5. Friedman RJ, Farber MJ, Warycha MA, et al. The "dysplastic" nevus. *Clin Dermatol.* 2009;27:103-115.
6. Stierner U, Augustsson A, Rosdahl I, Suurküla M. Regional distribution of common and dysplastic naevi in relation to melanoma site and sun exposure. A case-control study. *Melanoma Res.* 1992;1(5-6):367-375.
7. Synnerstad I, Nilsson L, Fredrikson M, Rosdahl I. Frequency and distribution pattern of melanocytic naevi in Swedish 8-9-year-old children. *Acta Derm Venereol.* 2004;84(4):271-276.
8. Haley JC, Hood AF, Chuang TY, Rasmussen J. The frequency of histologically dysplastic nevi in 199 pediatric patients. *Pediatr Dermatol.* 2000;17(4):266-269.
9. Woodhouse J, Maytin EV. Eruptive nevi of the palms and soles. *J Am Acad Dermatol.* 2005;52(5 Suppl 1):S96-S100.
10. Friedman RJ, Farber MJ, Warycha MA, et al. The "dysplastic" nevus. *Clin Dermatol.* 2009;27:103-115.
11. Weedon D, Little JH. Spindle and epithelioid cell nevi in children and adults. A review of 211 cases of the Spitz nevus. *Cancer.* 1977; 40(1):217-225.
12. Requena C, Requena L, Kutzner H, Sánchez Yus E. Spitz nevus: a clinicopathological study of 349 cases. *Am J Dermatopathol.* 2009;31(2):107-116.
13. Ko CB, Walton S, Wyatt EH, Bury HP. Spitz nevus. *Int J Dermatol.* 1993;32(5):354-357.
14. Elder DE. Dysplastic naevi: an update. *Histopathology.* 2010;56(1):112-120.
15. Kapur P, Selim MA, Roy LC, Yegappan M, et al. Spitz nevi and atypical Spitz nevi/tumors: a histologic and immunohistochemical analysis. *Mod Pathol.* 2005;18(2):197-204.
16. Marghoob AA, Usatine RP, Jaimes N. Dermoscopy for the family physician. *Am Fam Physician.* 2013 Oct 1;88(7):441-450.
17. Hofmann-Wellenhof R, Blum A, Wolf IH, et al. Dermoscopic classification of atypical melanocytic nevi (Clark nevi). *Arch Dermatol.* 2001;137(12):1575-1580.
18. Marchell R, Marghoob AA, Braun RP, Argenziano G. Dermoscopy of pigmented Spitz and Reed nevi: the starburst pattern. *Arch Dermatol.* 2005;141(8):1060.
19. Lallas A, Moscarella E, Longo C, et al. Likelihood of finding melanoma when removing a Spitzoid-looking lesion in patients aged 12 years or older. *J Am Acad Dermatol.* 2015;72(1):47-53.
20. Goodson AG, Florell SR, Boucher KM, Grossman D. Low rates of clinical recurrence after biopsy of benign to moderately dysplastic melanocytic nevi. *J Am Acad Dermatol.* 2010;62(4):591-596.
21. Strazzula L, Vedak P, Hoang MP, et al. The utility of reexcising mildly and moderately dysplastic nevi: a retrospective analysis. *J Am Acad Dermatol.* 2014;71(6):1071-1076.
22. Fleming NH, Egbert BM, Kim J, Swetter SM. Reexamining the threshold for reexcision of histologically transected dysplastic nevi. *JAMA Dermatol.* 2016;152(12):1327-1334.
23. Maghari A. Dysplastic (or atypical) nevi showing moderate or severe atypia with clear margins on the shave removal specimens are most likely completely excised. *J Cutan Med Surg.* 2017;21(1): 42-47.
24. Trock B, Synnestvedt M, Humphreys T. Natural history of dysplastic nevi. *J Am Acad Dermatol.* 1993;29(1):51-57.
25. Gandini S, Sera F, Cattaruzza MS, et al. Meta-analysis of risk factors for cutaneous melanoma: I. Common and atypical naevi. *Eur J Cancer.* 2005;41(1):28-44.
26. Marghoob AA, Kopf AW, Rigel DS, et al. Risk of cutaneous malignant melanoma in patients with "classic" atypical-mole syndrome. A case-control study. *Arch Dermatol.* 1994;130:993-998.
27. Troxel DB. Pitfalls in the diagnosis of malignant melanoma: findings of a risk management panel study. *Am J Surg Pathol.* 2003;27(9): 1278-1283.
28. Oliveria SA, Chau D, Christos PJ, et al. Diagnostic accuracy of patients in performing skin self-examination and the impact of photography. *Arch Dermatol.* 2004;140(1):57-62.

SECTION L SUN DAMAGE AND EARLY SKIN CANCER

172 SUN DAMAGE AND SKIN CANCER PREVENTION

Maria J. LaPlante, MD
Richard P. Usatine, MD

PATIENT STORY

A 63-year-old fair-skinned woman with a history of basal cell carcinoma presents for a screening skin exam. She has extensive sun damage to her skin from years of working outdoors without sun protection **(Figure 172-1)**. She would like to know what she can do to prevent development of new skin cancers.

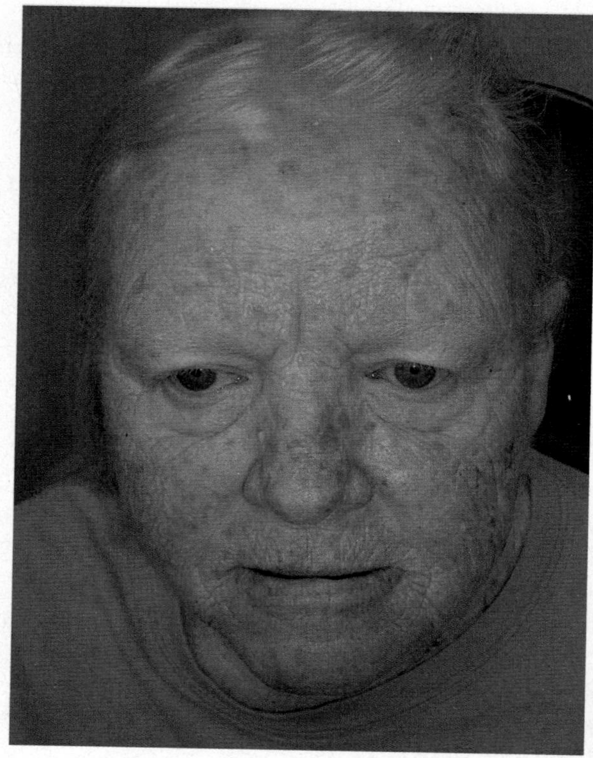

FIGURE 172-1 Extensive sun damage on the face of a 63-year-old woman from years of working outdoors without sun protection. *(Reproduced with permission from Richard P. Usatine, MD.)*

INTRODUCTION

Prolonged sun exposure has destructive effects on the skin and increases risk of skin cancer. It is the most common cancer in the United States: skin cancer affects an estimated 3.3 million Americans annually, and 1 in 5 Americans in their lifetime.[1,2] Prevention for many of these skin cancers is simple—sun protection. Educating our patients about sun protection has the potential to reduce morbidity and mortality from skin cancer.

SYNONYMS

Sun-damaged skin is also known as actinic elastosis, solar elastosis, chronic actinic damage of the skin, dermatoheliosis, and photoaging.

Nonmelanoma skin cancers are also known as keratinocyte carcinomas.

EPIDEMIOLOGY

In the United States, the incidence of nonmelanoma skin cancer is highest among the elderly, non-Hispanic white population. According to a 2010 study, 20% of non-Hispanic white 70-year-olds have had at least one nonmelanoma skin cancer, and most of that 20% have had several.[2]

The incidence of melanoma in the United States is also highest in non-Hispanic whites, with an incidence rate of 30.8 of 100,000 white men and 19.3 of 100,000 white women reported by the Centers for Disease Control and Prevention (CDC) in 2014.[3] For comparison, the next highest incidence rates are in American Indian/Alaskan native men and Hispanic women, occurring in 6.2 of 100,000, and 4.4 of 100,000, respectively.[3]

In people of color the incidence of both melanoma and nonmelanoma skin cancer is much lower than in non-Hispanic whites, occurring in about 5% of Hispanics, 4% of Asians, and 2% in people of African descent. Although the incidence of skin cancer is lower in people of color, it is more likely to present at a more advanced stage and have a poorer prognosis.[4,5]

Although the link between skin cancer and sun exposure is widely known and publicized, sunburn is still a common occurrence. National surveys from 2004 and 2005 show 1 in 3 adults in the United States reported sunburn in the past 12 months.[6] The incidence of sunburn for U.S. children is also high, with an estimate of 29% to 83% over the summer season.[7] The potential impact of sun protection in the pediatric population could be immense in preventing sun-damaged skin and skin cancer—an estimated 40% to 50% of cumulative UV radiation exposure to age 60 occurs before the age of 20.[8]

ETIOLOGY AND PATHOPHYSIOLOGY

Ultraviolet radiation (UVR) from the sun in both the ultraviolet A (320-400nm) and ultraviolet B (290-320nm) wavelengths cause skin damage through complex molecular mechanisms.[9-13] These include direct damage as it is absorbed by epidermal DNA as well as the generation of reactive oxygen species (ROS).[9,10] As the DNA absorbs the UV radiation, mutated lesions develop within the helix. The most common and toxic of these lesions are cyclobutenepyrimidine dimers (CPDs), which interfere with DNA transcription and replication.[9] A large amount of these mutations can be seen even in low, suberythemal doses of UVB radiation.[10] CPDs are repaired through nucleotide excision, a slow process which takes more than 24 hours for completion, allowing DNA distortion to accumulate with repeated daily exposure.[10]

Reactive oxygen species (ROS) also cause direct damage to DNA and play a role in the destruction of cellular proteins and extracellular connective tissue. Reactive oxygen species activate matrix metalloproteinases (MMPs). These MMPs degrade collagen and elastin, weakening the structural integrity of the skin.[9,11]

UV radiation also induces cutaneous immunosuppression. It suppresses cell-mediated immunity primarily through disruption of Langerhans cell migration, lymphocyte activity, and inflammatory cytokines. These immunosuppressive effects impair early recognition and destruction of neoplastic cells.[9,11-13]

All together these effects lead to inhibition of DNA repair mechanisms and impaired tumor suppression, which contribute to both photoaging and an increased risk of carcinogenesis.[9,11-13]

RISK FACTORS

- Fair skin.[14]
- Number of lifetime sunburns. A history of more than 5 sunburns doubles the lifetime risk of melanoma, regardless of the age the sunburns occurred.[15,16]
- Total lifetime UV radiation exposure, including ambient, occupational, recreational, and tanning beds. Importantly, chronic suberythemal exposure to UV radiation causes skin damage, even in the absence of sunburns.[14,17]
- History of previous skin cancer.
- Immunosuppression.[18]

Additionally, risk factors specific for melanoma include family history of melanoma, more than 5 dysplastic nevi, and presence of multiple (>100) nevi.[19]

DIAGNOSIS

CLINICAL FEATURES

Physical examination of sun-exposed skin may reveal the following features of chronic sun damage:

- Solar lentigines (solar lentigo—singular): irregularly shaped brown macules on sun-exposed skin, most commonly on the face and the backs of hands **(Figure 172-2)**.[9,12]
- Nodular elastosis (Favre-Racouchot disease): yellow, thickened skin with nodular texture and open comedones, around the lateral aspect of the eyes and upper cheekbones **(Figure 172-3)**.[9,13,20]
- Cutis rhomboidalis nuchae: thickened skin with deep furrows forming polygonal shapes on the back of the neck **(Figure 172-4)**.[9,20]
- Poikiloderma of Civatte: chronically erythematous and mottled-appearing skin of the lateral neck and chest with sparing of the shaded skin under the chin **(Figure 172-5)**. Additional features of this condition include prominent telangiectasias and the appearance of follicular papules from the sparing of perifollicular skin.[13]
- Idiopathic guttate hypomelanosis: hypopigmented round "drop-like" macules on sun-exposed skin **(Figure 172-6)**.[9,13]
- Telangiectasias.[12,13]
- Solar purpura: red or purple-red patches on sun-exposed skin that develop after skin trauma, including even minor skin trauma **(Figure 172-7)**. Chronic sun damage thins the skin and increases its fragility, predisposing to the development of these lesions. Solar purpura are commonly seen in the elderly population, particularly on the forearms and dorsal aspect of the hands. They may leave residual brown hyperpigmented patches from hemosiderin deposition in the dermis.[12,13]
- Actinic keratosis (AK), basal cell carcinoma (BCC), squamous cell carcinoma (SCC), and melanoma.

LABORATORY STUDIES

Biopsy is recommended if there is clinical suspicion of malignancy. Other nonmalignant skin lesions associated with sun damage are typically diagnosed by observation. Biopsy could be considered for confirmation if the diagnosis is in doubt.

DIFFERENTIAL DIAGNOSIS

Listed below is a differential diagnosis for sunburn-like erythema affecting sun-exposed skin. If chronic or recurrent, the following conditions may also present with associated poikiloderma or dyspigmentation:

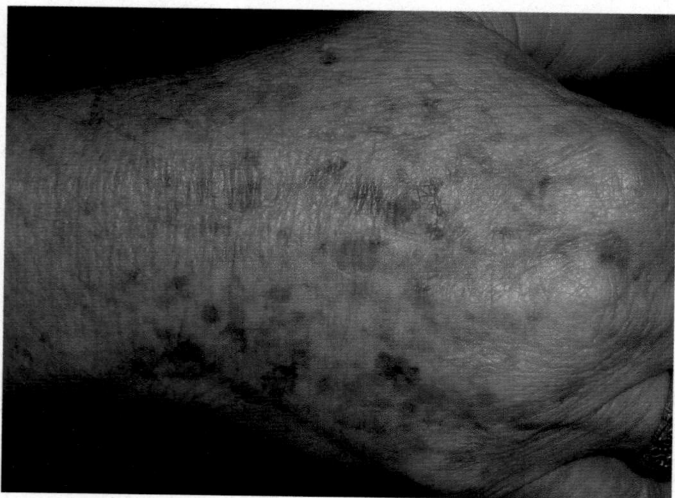

FIGURE 172-2 Many solar lentigines on the dorsum of the hand of a 52-year-old woman with a history of extensive sun exposure. *(Reproduced with permission from Richard P. Usatine, MD.)*

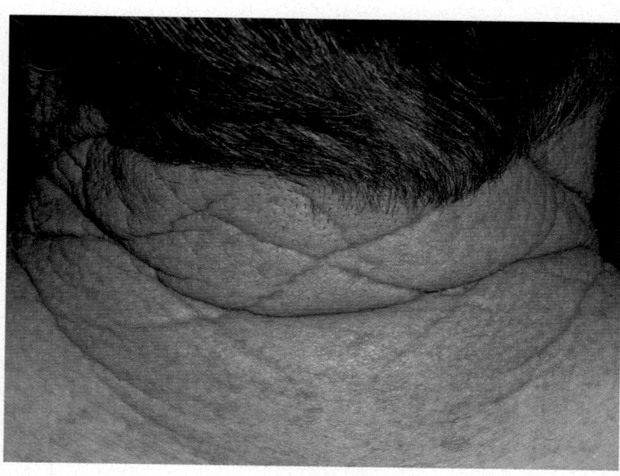

FIGURE 172-4 Cutis rhomboidalis nuchae is thickened skin with deep furrows forming polygonal shapes on the posterior neck secondary to extensive sun exposure. *(Reproduced with permission from Richard P. Usatine, MD.)*

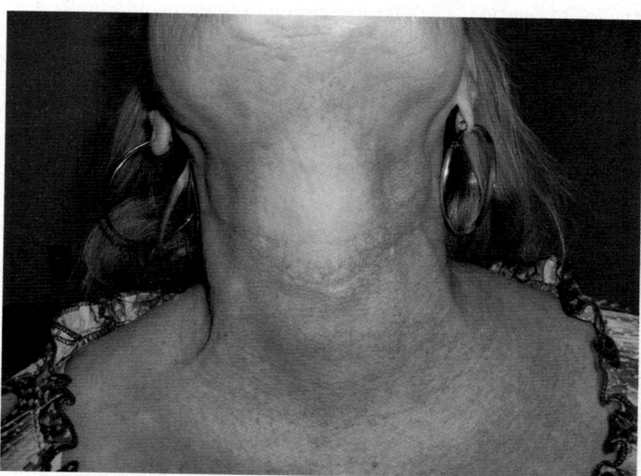

FIGURE 172-5 Poikiloderma of Civatte is chronically erythematous and mottled-appearing skin of the lateral neck and chest with sparing of the shaded skin under the chin. *(Reproduced with permission from Richard P. Usatine, MD.)*

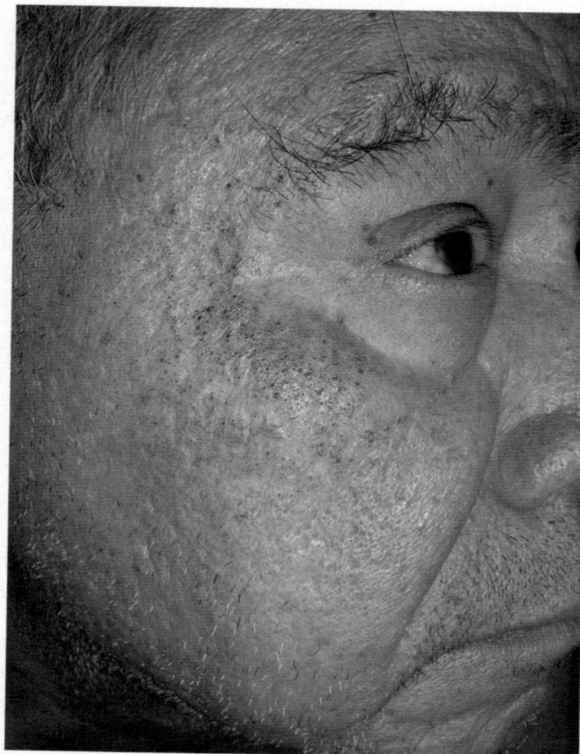

FIGURE 172-3 Actinic open comedones with nodular elastosis around the lateral aspect of the eyes and upper cheekbones (Favre-Racouchot disease) from cumulative sun exposure. *(Reproduced with permission from Richard P. Usatine, MD.)*

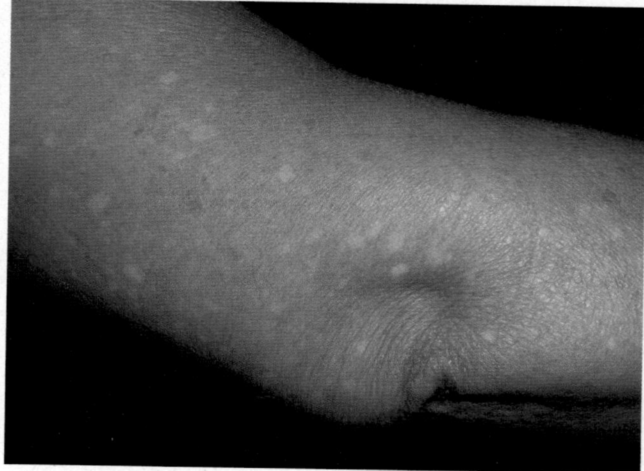

FIGURE 172-6 Idiopathic guttate hypomelanosis presents as hypopigmented round "droplike" macules on sun-exposed skin. As seen here it is often on the sun-exposed areas of the arms and legs. *(Reproduced with permission from Richard P. Usatine, MD.)*

- Dermatomyositis—An autoimmune connective tissue disease with additional features such as heliotrope rash, and proximal muscle weakness[13] (see Chapter 189, Dermatomyositis).
- Drug-induced photosensitivity reaction—Presents with a history of sun exposure and medication known to cause phototoxic or photoallergic reactions (see Chapter 208, Photosensitivity). Common medications include doxycycline and other tetracyclines, quinolones, diuretics such as furosemide and thiazides, amiodarone, and nonsteroidal anti-inflammatory drugs (NSAIDs), among others.[13]
- Phytophotodermatitis—A phototoxic reaction produced by the interaction of furocoumarins contained in some plants with ultraviolet radiation from the sun (see Chapter 208, Photosensitivity). Presents as an irregular or linear-shaped patch of erythema on the exposed skin, often with visible drip marks or handprints. Fades into hyperpigmented patches. Common agents are lime juice, celery, parsley, and figs.[13]
- Subacute cutaneous lupus erythematosus (SCLE): an autoimmune connective tissue disease that presents with annular plaques or scaly papules and plaques limited to sun-exposed skin (see Chapter 188, Lupus – Systemic and Cutaneous). About 10% to 15% will develop systemic lupus erythematosus (SLE).[13]
- Polymorphous light eruption (PMLE): erythematous papules, vesicles or plaques that develop within minutes to hours on sun-exposed skin after sunlight exposure (see Chapter 208, Photosensitivity). The eruption begins to fade over several days. It is most common in spring and early summertime.[13]

MANAGEMENT

Sun protection is essential for both management and prevention of sun-damaged skin and skin cancer.

- Daily use of sunscreen in adults reduces the risk of melanoma. SOR Ⓑ This was demonstrated by a randomized study in Australia in which daily application of a broad-spectrum sunscreen for 4 years in 1621 adult participants was compared to discretionary use. Daily sunscreen decreased the risk of melanoma by 50% (11 vs. 22 new primary melanomas) 10 years after the trial treatment phase had ended.[21]
- Daily use of sunscreen in adults reduces the risk of AKs and SCC, but has not been shown to significantly reduce the risk of BCC.[22-25] SOR Ⓑ A community-based trial in Australia of 1383 participants randomly assigned to daily sunscreen use versus discretionary use for 4.5 years demonstrated a reduction of 39% in SCC tumors.[25] Additional follow-up 8 years after the trial concluded showed an additional 40% reduction in SCC tumors in the daily sunscreen use group compared to discretionary use. There was no significant reduction in BCC tumors at the end of the trial or subsequent follow-up; however, there was a trend toward decline in BCC in the daily sunscreen use group.[25] Further studies and longer-term follow-up are needed to examine the correlation between BCC and sun protection.
- Daily use of sunscreen in adults has been shown to reduce the development of SCC in immunosuppressed patients with history of organ transplantation.[18] SOR Ⓑ

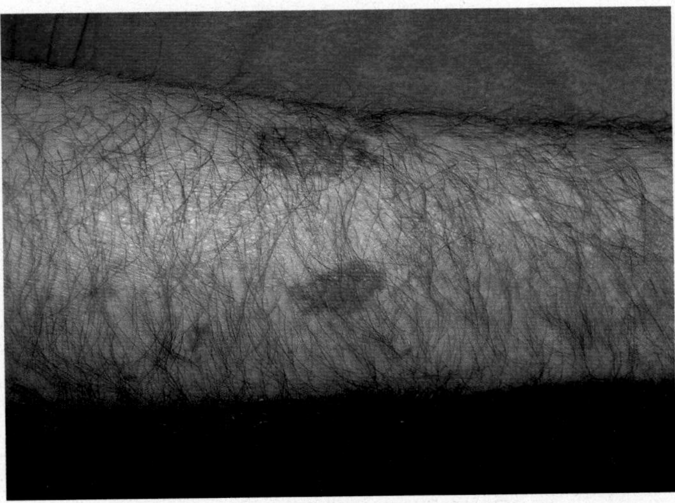

FIGURE 172-7 Solar purpura presenting as red to purple patches on the heavily sun-exposed skin of the forearm that developed spontaneously without the patient being aware of any significant skin trauma. *(Reproduced with permission from Richard P. Usatine, MD.)*

- Daily use of sunscreen can reduce clinical signs of photoaging.[26] SOR Ⓐ
- Clothing, particularly with tightly woven fibers, wool or polyester fabrics, and dark colors, and use of UV-absorbing additives to clothing can reduce UV radiation exposure.[11] Wearing a wide-brimmed hat can provide additional UVR protection.[11] SOR Ⓒ
- Appropriate treatment of AKs can prevent SCC (see Chapter 173).
- Treatment of BCC, SCC, and melanoma is discussed separately (in chapters 177, 178 and 179).

MEDICATIONS

▶ Prevention of skin cancer

The current data support sun protection as the first-line intervention for skin cancer prevention. Nevertheless, chemoprevention of skin cancer with systemic treatments is an area of growing interest and study. Its present-day use is targeted to specific high-risk patient populations in which the benefits outweigh the side-effect risks.

- Nicotinamide (vitamin B_3, niacinamide) has been shown to reduce the number of new nonmelanoma skin cancers in patients with a prior history of nonmelanoma skin cancer.[27] In a randomized placebo-controlled study, participants were randomized to nicotinamide 500 mg twice daily for 1 year or placebo. Those taking the nicotinamide developed 23% fewer new nonmelanoma skin cancers compared to placebo, and 3 to 5 fewer AKs compared to baseline. Nicotinamide does not carry the vasodilatory side effects (e.g., flushing, headache) that niacin does and is available for purchase over the counter. The beneficial effects of the nicotinamide are not maintained once the medication is discontinued, so patients should continue it on an ongoing basis.[27] SOR Ⓑ Tell patients to look for niacinamide, as it appears to be easier to find and is a very inexpensive OTC product.
- Acitretin, a systemic retinoid, has been shown in several small randomized controlled trials (RCTs) to significantly reduce the number of SCCs in immunosuppressed patients with history of solid organ transplantation.[28] SOR Ⓑ
- Systemic retinoid treatment with isotretinoin has been proven to prevent the development of nonmelanoma skin cancers in patients with xeroderma pigmentosum, a genetic condition that carries a 1000-fold increased risk of nonmelanoma skin cancer.[29] SOR Ⓑ
- Topical retinoids are not effective in prevention of nonmelanoma skin cancer.[30] SOR Ⓑ
- There are no systemic or topical medications that have been consistently proven to prevent melanoma.[31] SOR Ⓑ

▶ Treatment of sun-damaged skin and photoaging

- Topical tretinoin creams in concentrations of 0.025% to 0.1% are effective in reducing appearance of fine lines, wrinkles, and mottled hyperpigmentation associated with photoaging. The U.S. Food and Drug Administration (FDA) has approved tretinoin creams for this indication.[32] SOR Ⓐ
- Topical adapalene gel has also been shown to be effective in reducing signs of photoaging, including actinic keratoses, solar lentigo, wrinkles, and dyspigmentation, and is now available over the counter.[33] SOR Ⓑ
- Topical tazarotene is another alternative proven to be effective for improving signs of photodamage.[34] SOR Ⓐ Women of childbearing age should be counseled that this is a category X medication.

NONPHARMACOLOGIC

Physical modalities for cosmetic treatment of photoaging include chemical peels, photodynamic therapy, laser therapy, injectable botulinum toxin, and injectable fillers.[12]

COMPLEMENTARY/ALTERNATIVE THERAPY

- *Polypodium leucotomos*—A fern-leaf extract with antioxidant and anti-inflammatory properties that has been shown to significantly reduce photosensitivity in multiple small studies. Studied dosages included a range from 480 mg to 1200 mg daily.[35-37] SOR Ⓑ This is a promising option for systemic photoprotection.
- Beta-carotene—An antioxidant micronutrient present in plants that may have photoprotective effects with long-term supplementation or in a carotenoid-rich diet. Several small trials showed that beta-carotene supplementation over 12–24 weeks significantly increased the minimal erythemal dose (MED), or the amount of UV radiation required to create minimal sunburn erythema.[27,38,39] SOR Ⓑ In spite of this, two randomized controlled studies found that oral intake of beta-carotene did not prevent the development of nonmelanoma skin cancers.[25,27] SOR Ⓑ
- Polyphenols—Naturally occurring plant products found in green tea, honey, wine, chocolate, fruits, and vegetables. They have antioxidant and anti-inflammatory properties. A small, double-blind, placebo-controlled study showed that daily consumption of a beverage containing green tea polyphenols reduced UV-induced erythema in women.[40] SOR Ⓑ Furthermore, several small studies suggest that consumption of green tea polyphenols may help prevent nonmelanoma skin cancer.[41,42] SOR Ⓑ Further studies are needed to replicate and confirm these findings.

SKIN CANCER SCREENING

The USPTF has issued the following guidelines for skin cancer screening and counseling[19,43]:

- There is insufficient evidence to recommend for or against *general* screening skin exams.
- Children, adolescents, and young adults with fair skin should be counseled on sun protection.

However, there are some data to warrant regular skin cancer screening for patients who have already had one or more skin cancers:

- In a meta-analysis of 17 studies, 44% of patients diagnosed with a basal cell carcinoma developed a new one within 3 years.[44]
- In one study, patients with a history of melanoma and their partners were reliably taught to perform partner-assisted skin self-exams.[45] These patients and their partners performed skin self-exam more often than those patients in the control group. More importantly, patients in the intervention group identified new melanomas more often than those in the control group.[45]

PATIENT EDUCATION

Protecting the skin from the sun is fundamental in the prevention of sun-damaged skin and skin cancer. All ages and all skin types are susceptible to damage from ultraviolet radiation. The American Academy of Dermatology (AAD) provides the following general recommendations for skin photoprotection[46]:

- Avoid direct sunlight exposure by staying in the shade when possible.
- Use clothing for photoprotection. Wear a wide-brimmed hat, lightweight pants, and lightweight long-sleeved shirts.
- Wear sunglasses with UV protection.
- Avoid or limit outdoor activities during times of peak-intensity UV radiation, typically between 10 AM and 2 PM.
- Use a broad-spectrum sunscreen (protects against UVA and UVB) with at least SPF 50–100 on exposed skin. Reapply every 2 hours and after sweating or swimming. A new RCT with natural sunlight in actual use showed that SPF 100 sunscreen is more protective against sunburn than SPF 50.[47] This provides data to recommend high-SPF sunscreens.[47] SOR B
- Do not use indoor tanning beds or lamps.
- Take caution in water, sand, or snow. These surfaces reflect UV rays, and sunburns may develop more quickly.

In addition to the above, the AAD provides recommendations for specific populations as follows:

- Infants and children[48,49]:
  - Infants under 6 months should avoid direct sunlight exposure when possible, relying mainly on shade or clothing for photoprotection over sunscreen.
  - When it is not possible to stay in the shade or cover the infant's skin sufficiently with clothing, use a sunscreen with SPF 15 (we suggest higher SPF)[47] or higher on small areas of sun-exposed skin, such as the face and the back of the neck. Wash off sunscreen after outdoor activities are completed.
  - For children 6 months and older, supplement with 400 IU of vitamin D daily to prevent vitamin D deficiency.
- People of color[4,49]:
  - To prevent vitamin D deficiency while following guidelines for sun protection, take a vitamin D supplement: 400 IU daily for infants less than 2 years old, 600 IU daily for ages 1–70 years old, and 800 IU daily for adults age 70 years or more.
  - Perform regular skin self-examinations with close attention to palms, soles, fingernails, mucous membranes, groin, and perianal skin.
- The Australian motto is SLIP, SLOP, SLAP! Slip on a shirt, slop on some sunscreen, and slap on a hat. This can be taught to patients around the world.

PATIENT RESOURCES

- American Academy of Dermatology. *How to Prevent Skin Cancer*—**https://www.aad.org/public/kids/skin/skin-cancer/how-to-prevent-skin-cancer.**
- American Academy of Dermatology. *Sunscreen FAQs*—**https://www.aad.org/media/stats/prevention-and-care/sunscreen-faqs.**
- American Academy of Pediatrics. *Swim Safety Tips*—**https://www.healthychildren.org/English/safety-prevention/at-play/Pages/Sun-and-Water-Safety.aspx.**
- Skin Cancer Foundation. *Prevention Guidelines*—**http://www.skincancer.org/prevention/sun-protection/prevention-guidelines.**

PROVIDER RESOURCES

- U.S. Preventive Services Task Force. *Skin Cancer: Counseling*—**https://www.uspreventiveservicestaskforce.org/Page/Document/UpdateSummaryFinal/skin-cancer-counseling.**
- U.S. Preventive Services Task Force. *Skin Cancer: Screening*—**https://www.uspreventiveservicestaskforce.org/Page/Document/RecommendationStatementFinal/skin-cancer-screening2.**
- American Academy of Dermatology. Basic Derm Curriculum. Sun Protection Module—**https://www.aad.org/education/basic-derm-curriculum/suggested-order-of-modules/sun-protection.**

REFERENCES

1. Robinson JK. Sun exposure, sun protection, and vitamin D. *JAMA*. 2005;294:1541-1543.
2. Rogers HW, Weinstock MA, Feldman SR, Coldiron BM. Incidence estimate of nonmelanoma skin cancer (keratinocyte carcinomas) in the U.S. population, 2012. *JAMA Dermatol.* 2015;151(10):1081-1086.
3. Agbai ON, Buster K, Sanchez M, et al. Skin cancer and photoprotection in people of color: a review and recommendations for physicians and the public. *J Am Acad Dermatol.* 2014;70(4):748-762.
4. Gloster HM Jr, Neal K. Skin cancer in skin of color. *J Am Acad Dermatol.* 2006;55(5):741-760.
5. Centers for Disease Control and Prevention. *Skin Cancer Rates by Race and Ethnicity*. https://www.cdc.gov/cancer/skin/statistics/race.htm. Accessed November 2017.
6. Buller DB, Cokkinides V, Hall H, et al. Prevalence of sunburn, sun protection, and indoor tanning behaviors among Americans: review from national surveys and case studies of 3 states. *J Am Acad Dermatol.* 2011;65(5 Suppl 1):S114-S123.
7. Davis KJ, Cokkinides VE, Weinstock MA, et al. Summer sunburn and sun exposure among US youths ages 11 to 18: national prevalence and associated factors. *Pediatrics.* 2002;110(1 pt 1):27-35.
8. Green AC, Wallingford SC, McBride P. Childhood exposure to ultraviolet radiation and harmful skin effects: epidemiological evidence. *Prog Biophys Mol Biol.* 2011;107(3):349-355.
9. Bilac C, Sahin MT, Ozturkcan S. Chronic actinic damage of facial skin. *Clin Dermatol.* 2014;32(6):752-762.
10. Young AR, Claveau J, Rossi AB. Ultraviolet radiation and the skin: photobiology and sunscreen photoprotection. *J Am Acad Dermatol.* 2017;76(3S1):S100-S109.

11. Jansen R, Wang SQ, Burnett M, et al. Photoprotection, part I. Photoprotection by naturally occurring, physical, and systemic agents. *J Am Acad Dermatol.* 2013;69:853.e1-12.
12. Rapaport MJ, Rapaport V. Preventive and therapeutic approaches to short- and long-term sun damaged skin. *Clin Dermatol.* 1998;16(4):429-439.
13. Lim HW, Hawk JLM: Photodermatologic disorders. In: Bolognia JL, Jorizzo JL, Schaffer JV. *Dermatology*. 3rd ed, vol 2. Philadelphia, PA: Elsevier; 2012:1467-1485.
14. Armstrong BK, Kricker A. The epidemiology of UV induced skin cancer. *J Photochem Photobiol B.* 2001;63(1-3):8-18.
15. Dennis LK, Vanbeek MJ, Beane Freeman LE, et al. Sunburns and risk of cutaneous melanoma: does age matter? A comprehensive meta-analysis. *Ann Epidemiol.* 2008;18(8):614-627.
16. Pfahlberg A, Kolmel KF, Gefeller O. Timing of excessive ultraviolet radiation and melanoma: epidemiology does not support the existence of a critical period of high susceptibility to solar ultraviolet radiation-induced melanoma. *Br J Dermatol.* 2001;144(3): 471-475.
17. Seite S, Fourtanier A, Moyal D, Young AR. Photodamage to human skin by suberythemal exposure to solar ultraviolet radiation can be attenuated by sunscreens: a review. *Br J Dermatol.* 2010;163(5):903-914.
18. Ulrich, C, Jurgensen JS, Degen A, et al. Prevention of non-melanoma skin cancer in organ transplant patients by regular use of a sunscreen: a 24 months, prospective, case-control study. *Br J Dermatol.* 2009;161 Suppl 3:78-84.
19. U.S. Preventive Services Task Force. *Skin Cancer: Screening.* https://www.uspreventiveservicestaskforce.org/Page/Document/UpdateSummaryFinal/skin-cancer-screening2. Accessed January 2017.
20. Calderone DC, Fenske NA. The clinical spectrum of actinic elastosis. *J Am Acad Dermatol.* 1995;32(6):1016-1024.
21. Green AC, Williams GM, Logan V, et al. Reduced melanoma after regular sunscreen use: randomized trial follow-up. *J Clin Oncol.* 2011;29(3):257.
22. van der Pols JC, Williams GM, Pandeya N, et al. Prolonged prevention of squamous cell carcinoma of the skin by regular sunscreen use. *Cancer Epidemiol Biomarkers Prev.* 2006;15(12): 2546-2548.
23. Thompson SC, Jolley D, Marks R. Reduction of solar keratoses by regular sunscreen use. *N Engl J Med.* 1993;329(16):1147-1151.
24. Darlington S, Williams G, Neale R, et al. A randomized controlled trial to assess sunscreen application and beta carotene supplementation in the prevention of solar keratoses. *Arch Dermatol.* 2003; 139(4):451-455.
25. Green A, Williams G, Neale R, et al. Daily sunscreen application and betacarotene supplementation in prevention of basal-cell and squamous-cell carcinomas of the skin: a randomized controlled trial. *Lancet.* 1999;354(9180):723-729.
26. Hughes MC, Willias GM, Baker P, Green AC. Sunscreen and prevention of skin aging: a randomized trial. *Ann Intern Med.* 2013;158(11):781-790.
27. Chen AC, Martin AJ, Choy B, et al. A phase 3 randomized trial of nicotinamide for skin-cancer chemoprevention. *N Engl J Med.* 2015;373:1618-1626.
28. Chen K, Craig JC, Shuack S. Oral retinoids for the prevention of skin cancers in solid organ transplant recipients: a systematic review of randomized controlled trials. *Br J Dermatol.* 2005; 152(3):518-523.
29. Kraemer KH, DiGiovanna JJ, Peck GL. Chemoprevention of skin cancer in xeroderma pigmentosum. *J Dermatol.* 1992;19(11):715-718.
30. Weinstock MA, Bingham SF, DiGiovanna JJ, et al. Tretinoin and the prevention of keratinocyte carcinoma (basal and squamous cell carcinoma of the skin): a Veterans Affairs randomized chemoprevention trial. *J Invest Dermatol.* 2012;132(6):1583-1590.
31. Chhabra G, Ndiaye MA, Garcia-Peterson LM, Ahmad N. Melanoma chemoprevention: Current status and future prospects. *Photochem Photobiol.* 2017;93(4):975-989.
32. Weiss, JS, Ellis CN, Headington JT, et al. Topical tretinoin improves photoaged skin: a double-blind vehicle-controlled study. *JAMA.* 1988; 259:527-532.
33. Kang S, Goldfarb MT, Weiss JS, et al. Assessment of adapalene gel for the treatment of actinic keratoses and lentigines: a randomized trial. *J Am Acad Dermatol.* 2003;49(1):83-90.
34. Phillips TJ, Gottlieb AB, Leyden JJ, et al. Efficacy of 0.1% tazarotene cream for the treatment of photodamage: a 12-month multicenter, randomized trial. *Arch Dermatol.* 2002;138(11):1486-1493.
35. Aguilera P, Carrera C, Puig-Butille JA, et al. Benefits of oral polypodium leucotomos extract in MM high-risk patients. *J Eur Acad Dermatol Venereol.* 2013;27:1095-1100.
36. Caccialanza M, Recalcati S, Piccino R. Oral polypodium leucotomos extract photoprotective activity in 57 patients with idiopathic photodermatoses. *G Ital Dermatol Venereol.* 2011;146:85-87.
37. Kohli I, Shafi R, Isedeh P, et al. The impact of oral polypodium leucotomos extract on Soultraviolet B response: a human clinical study. *J Am Acad Dermatol.* 2017;77(1):33-41.
38. Lee J, Jiang S, Levine N, Watson RR. Carotenoid supplementation reduces erythema in human skin after simulated solar radiation exposure. *Proc Soc Exp Biol Med.* 2000;223(2):170-174.
39. Stahl W, Heinrich U, Jungmann H, et al. Carotenoids and carotenoids plus vitamin E protect against ultraviolet light-induced erythema in humans. *Am J Clin Nutr.* 2000;71(3):795-798.
40. Heinrich U, Moore CE, De Spirt S, et al. Green tea polyphenols provide photoprotection, increase microcirculation, and modulate skin properties of women. *J Nutr.* 2011;141:1202-1208.
41. Rees J, Stukel T, Perry A. Tea consumption and basal cell and squamous cell skin cancer: results of a case-control study. *J Am Acad Dermatol.* 2007;56(5):781-785.
42. Honigbaum A, Vivar K, Vera N, et al. Green tea and nonmelanoma skin cancer: is there an association? *J Am Acad Dermatol.* 2017;76(6S1):AB149.
43. U.S. Preventive Services Task Force. *Skin Cancer: Counseling.* https://www.uspreventiveservicestaskforce.org/Page/Document/UpdateSummaryFinal/skin-cancer-counseling. Accessed January 2017.

44. Marcil I, Stern RS. Risk of developing a subsequent nonmelanoma skin cancer in patients with a history of nonmelanoma skin cancer. A critical review of the literature and meta-analysis. *Arch Dermatol.* 2000;136(12):1524-1530.
45. Robinson JK, et al. Early detection of new melanomas by patients with melanoma and their partners using a structured skin self-examination skills training intervention: a randomized clinical trial. *JAMA Dermatol.* 2016;152(9):979-985.
46. American Academy of Dermatology. *Sunscreen FAQs.* https:www.aad.org/media/stats/prevention-and-care/sunscreen-faqs. Accessed January 2017.
47. Williams JD, Maitra P, Atillasoy E, et al. SPF 100+ sunscreen is more protective against sunburn than SPF 50+ in actual use: results of a randomized, double-blind, split-face, natural sunlight exposure clinical trial. *J Am Acad Dermatol.* 2018;78(5):902-910.e2.
48. American Academy of Pediatrics. *Sun and Water Safety Tips.* https://www.aap.org/en-us/about-the-aap/aap-press-room/news-features-and-safety-tips/Pages/Sun-and-Water-Safety-Tips.aspx. Accessed January 2017.
49. Cestari T, Buster K. Photoprotection in specific populations: children and people of color. *J Am Acad Dermatol.* 2017;76(3S1):S110-S121.

173 ACTINIC KERATOSIS AND BOWEN DISEASE

Yu Wah, MD
Richard P. Usatine, MD

PATIENT STORY

A 57-year-old woman presented with red and scaling skin on both arms (**Figure 173-1**) and a request for a prescription for 5-fluorouracil (5-FU). The patient had blue eyes and white hair and was found to have 2 basal cell carcinomas (BCCs) on her face and shoulder. The patient stated that 5-FU had helped her arms in the past, but that the scaly lesions had returned. She avoids sun exposure now, but acknowledges receiving too much sun exposure while growing up. Another course of 5-FU was prescribed for her arms to prevent new skin cancers from forming.

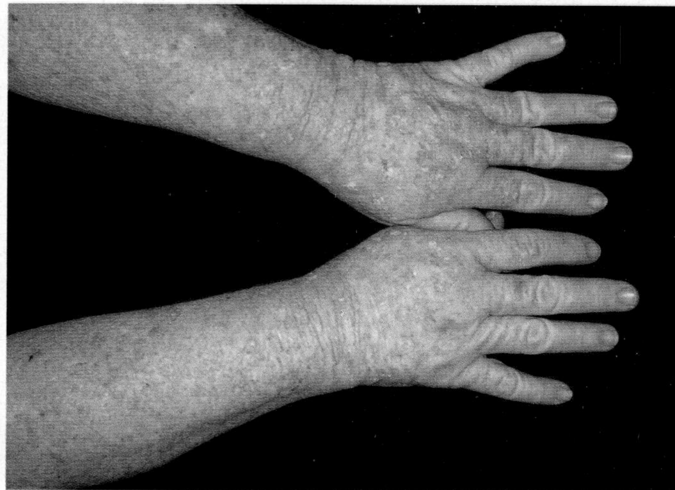

FIGURE 173-1 Actinic keratoses covering both arms and the dorsum of both hands in a fair-skinned woman who had significant sun exposure. Note that her left arm and hand are worse from driving a car and receiving more sun on the left arm. (*Reproduced with permission from Richard P. Usatine, MD.*)

INTRODUCTION

Actinic keratoses (AKs) are precursors on the continuum of carcinogenesis toward squamous cell carcinomas (SCCs). However, each AK has a low risk of progression to malignancy and a high probability of spontaneous regression.[1] Bowen disease (BD) is SCC in situ confined to the epidermis.

SYNONYMS

AK is also known as solar keratosis. AK on the lips is known as actinic cheilitis (**Figure 173-2**). BD is also known as SCC in situ of the skin. SCC in situ involving the penis is known as erythroplasia of Queyrat (**Figure 173-3**).

EPIDEMIOLOGY

- AKs and BD are seen frequently in light-skinned individuals who have had significant sun exposure.
- The prevalence of AK is estimated at 11% to 25% in adults older than age 40 years in the northern hemisphere, and increases with age.[1] AKs are so common that they account for more than 10% of visits to dermatologists.
- The prevalence of BD is unknown.[1]

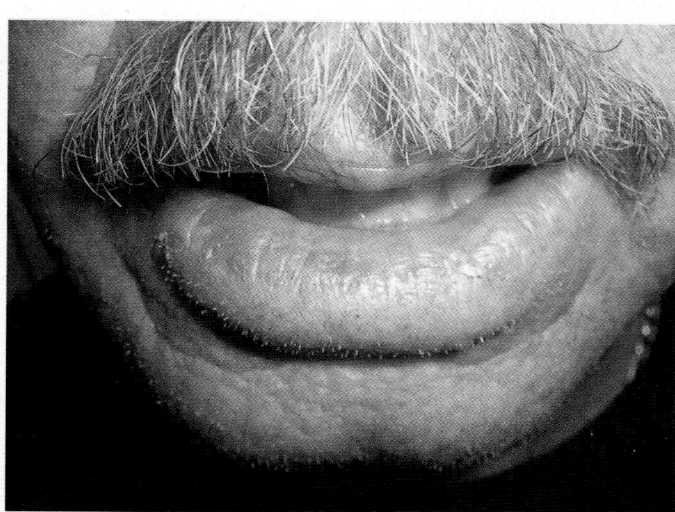

FIGURE 173-2 Actinic cheilitis involving lower lips. Note the erythema and scale caused by the sun damage. (*Reproduced with permission from Richard P. Usatine, MD.*)

ETIOLOGY AND PATHOPHYSIOLOGY

AKs and BD are both caused by cumulative UV exposure, most commonly from sunlight.

UV rays induce mutation of the tumor-suppressor gene P53. Subsequent proliferation of mutated atypical epidermal keratinocytes give rise to the clinical lesion of AK.[2] Multiple clinical and subclinical lesions may exist in an area of sun-damaged skin, a concept known as "field cancerization."

AKs have the potential to become SCCs. The rate of malignant transformation has been variably estimated, but is probably no greater than 6% per AK over a 10-year period.[3]

Although spontaneous regression of single AK lesions was overall seen between 20% to 30% (and up to 63% in one study), regression of complete fields of AK were reported in only 0% to 7.2% of patients.[4,5]

On a spectrum of malignant transformation, BD is SCC in situ before the SCC becomes invasive.

RISK FACTORS

- Total lifetime dose of UV radiation (natural sunlight, UV from tanning beds, and radiation).[1]
- Fair skin.[1]
- Site-specific risk factors include tobacco for actinic cheilitis and human papillomavirus for genital and anal lesions.[1]
- Exposure to immunosuppressive drugs, especially organ transplant recipients.
- Personal or family history of skin cancers.

DIAGNOSIS

CLINICAL FEATURES

AKs are rough scaly spots seen on sun-exposed areas (**Figures 173-1** to **173-6**). They may be found by touch, as well as close visual inspection of the patient's skin. BD appears similar to an AK, but tends to be larger in size and thicker with a well-demarcated border (**Figures 173-7** and **173-8**).

TYPICAL DISTRIBUTION

Both lesions are seen in areas with greatest sun exposure, such as the face, forearms, dorsum of hands, lower legs of women, and the balding scalp (see **Figure 173-5**) and tops of the ears in men.

LABORATORY STUDIES AND IMAGING

AKs that appear premalignant may be diagnosed by observation only and treated with destructive methods (e.g., excision, electrosurgery, or cryosurgery) without biopsy. BD requires a biopsy for diagnosis. BD or SCC should be biopsied prior to treatment. A shave biopsy should produce enough tissue for histopathology. Pigmented AKs on the face are more problematic as they can appear similar to lentigo maligna, and a biopsy may be preferential to treating blindly with cryosurgery.

Reflectance confocal microscopy (RCM), a noninvasive technique for in vivo skin imaging, may be used to detect AK, BD, and invasive SCC, as well as for monitoring treatments of AK with good accuracy. Overall sensitivity and specificity of RCM for diagnosing AK, BD, SCC, and keratoacanthoma were 79%–100% and 78%–100%, respectively.[6]

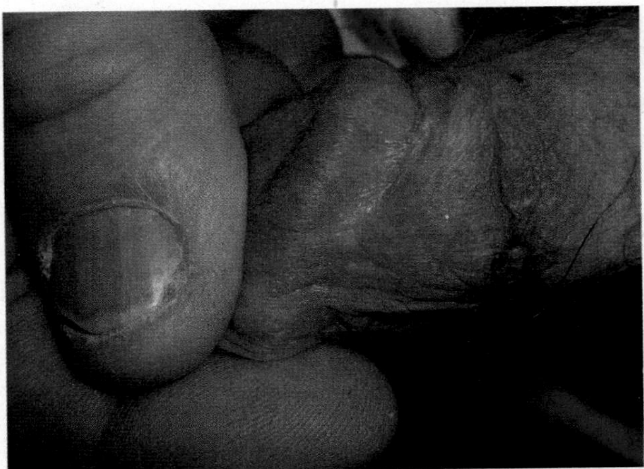

FIGURE 173-3 Bowen disease of the penis, also known as erythroplasia of Queyrat. Human papillomavirus is a risk factor in this location. *(Reproduced with permission from Richard P. Usatine, MD.)*

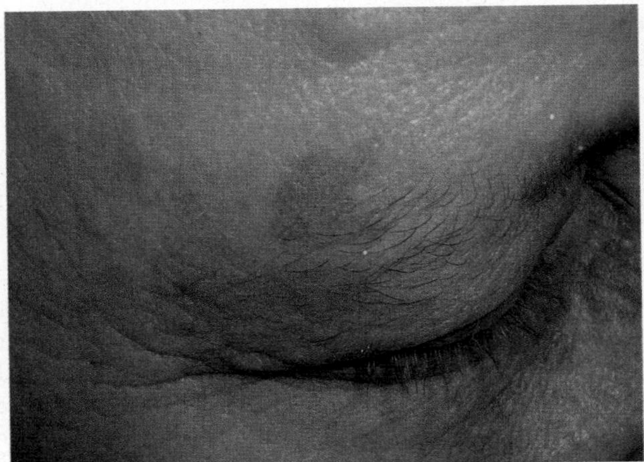

FIGURE 173-4 Large actinic keratoses over the eyebrow of an older adult. A biopsy was performed to make sure this was not already Bowen disease or squamous cell carcinoma. *(Reproduced with permission from Richard P. Usatine, MD.)*

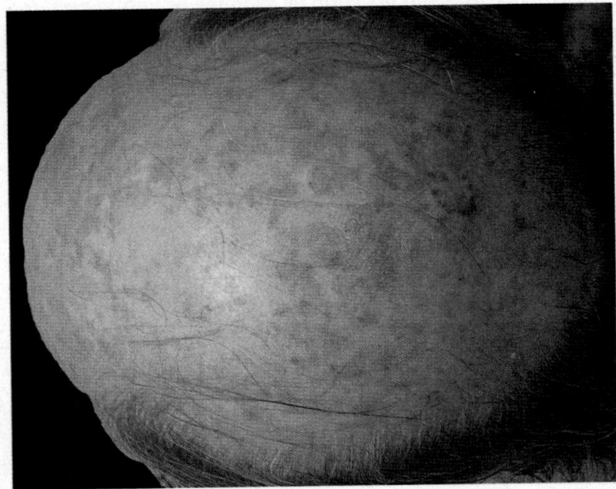

FIGURE 173-5 Actinic keratoses on the balding head of an older man. Hair loss results in less natural sun protection and is a risk factor for skin cancers on the scalp. The visible and palpable actinic keratoses were treated with cryotherapy and then the full scalp was treated with topical 5-fluorouracil. *(Reproduced with permission from Richard P. Usatine, MD.)*

DIFFERENTIAL DIAGNOSIS

- Nummular eczema—A type of eczema in which the scaly patches are coin-shaped. The patches are often seen in patients who have already had some eczema or atopic conditions. The patches usually respond well to topical corticosteroids and are not related to sun damage (see Chapter 151, Atopic Dermatitis).
- Seborrheic keratoses—Occur in aging adults but do not have any malignant potential. Typical seborrheic keratoses are brown in color and have a stuck-on appearance. Seborrheic keratoses may look greasy or verrucous and have surface cracks. Their borders tend to be more well demarcated than AKs, and their color is usually more brown than pink (see Chapter 164, Seborrheic Keratosis).
- Superficial BCCs—Can look like an AK or BD. Look for the pearly and thready border that may distinguish a superficial BCC from an AK or BD. Histopathology is the proven method to diagnose (see Chapter 177, Basal Cell Carcinoma).
- When in doubt, perform a shave biopsy to differentiate between an AK, BD, SCC, and superficial BCC.

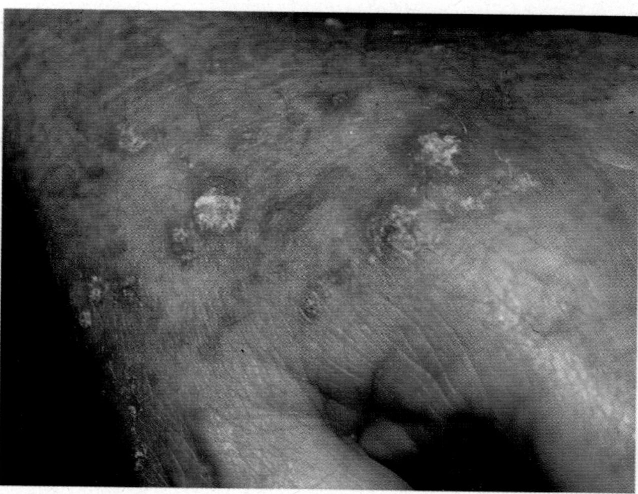

FIGURE 173-6 Actinic keratoses on the dorsum of the hand with some lesions suspicious for Bowen disease (squamous cell carcinoma in situ). *(Reproduced with permission from Usatine RP, Moy RL, Tobinick EL, et al: Skin Surgery: A Practical Guide. St. Louis, MO: Mosby; 1998.)*

MANAGEMENT

ACTINIC KERATOSES

- Presence of AK is a chronic and dynamic condition. Without adequate treatment, the rate of sustained complete spontaneous regression is low. Because of potential progression to invasive SCC and lack of reliable prognostic tools to determine the risk, an adequate treatment of either AK lesions or the affected field is recommended.[4] SOR C

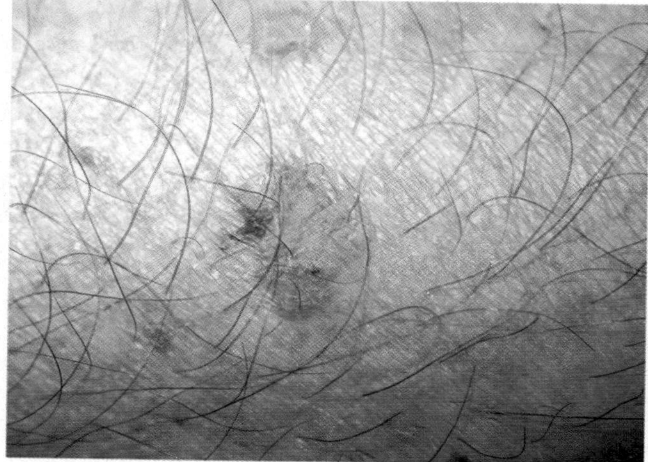

FIGURE 173-7 Lesions on the arm of an older man with Bowen disease in the central lesion and actinic keratosis on the upper lesion. *(Reproduced with permission from Richard P. Usatine, MD.)*

FIRST LINE

- Protection from sunlight is the best method of prevention. This include behavioral modification by avoiding or limiting sun exposure between 10 AM and 4 PM, use of sunscreens with a sun protection factor rating 30 and higher, and wearing protective gear including clothing, a wide-brimmed hat, and sunglasses.[4,7] SOR A
- Sunscreen applied twice daily for 7 months may protect against development of AKs.[2] SOR A
- AKs are most often treated by cryosurgery using liquid nitrogen (**Figure 173-9**). It is simple, rapid, and inexpensive.[1] SOR C One meta-analysis showed a 2-month cure rate of 97.0% with 2.1% recurrences in 1 year.[8]
- Treating AKs with liquid nitrogen using a 1-mm halo freeze demonstrated complete response of 39% for freeze times of less than 5 seconds, 69% for freeze times greater than 5 seconds, and 83% for freeze times greater than 20 seconds.[9] There is considerably more hypopigmentation caused by 20 seconds of freeze time. Determine the length of the freeze time based on the size and thickness of the lesion, using sufficient time for clearance while attempting to avoid hypopigmentation and scarring. SOR B
- Treat multiple AKs of the face, scalp, forearms, and hands topically with 5-FU, imiquimod, or diclofenac.[1,7,10] SOR A (**Table 173-1**).

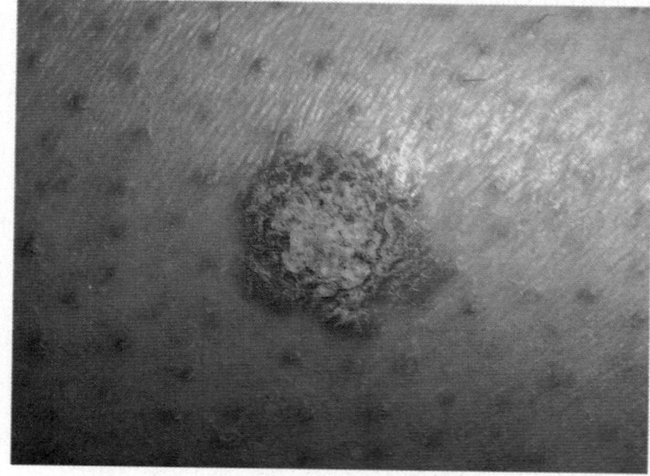

FIGURE 173-8 Bowen disease on the leg of an older woman. *(Reproduced with permission from Richard P. Usatine, MD.)*

TABLE 173-1 Comparison of Generic Topical Agents for the Treatment of AK

Topical Agent for AK	Duration of Treatment	Irritation	Cost
5-Fluorouracil 5% cream	3 to 4 weeks	Moderate to high	Less than $100
Diclofenac 3% gel	10 to 12 weeks	Moderate	More than $200
Imiquimod 5% cream	16 weeks	Moderate to high	Less than $100

- Topical 5-FU is an efficient therapeutic method and may be used for treatment of isolated, as well as large, areas of AK. It may be applied by the patient and is inexpensive compared with other topical modalities.[1] SOR Ⓐ
- 5-FU cream used twice daily for 3 to 6 weeks is effective for up to 12 months in clearance of the majority of AKs (**Figure 173-10**).[10] SOR Ⓐ Because of side effects of soreness, less aggressive regimens are often used. One such regimen involves using the 5-FU bid for one week, then take 4 weeks off and then continue bid for 2–3 weeks. SOR Ⓒ
- Imiquimod 5% cream has been demonstrated to be effective over a 16-week course of treatment, but studies have only measured 8 weeks of follow-up.[10] SOR Ⓑ
- One meta-analysis comparing imiquimod to 5-FU showed average complete clearance of AKs for each drug was 5-FU, 52 ± 18% and imiquimod, 70 ± 12%.[11]
- Imiquimod applied topically for 12 to 16 weeks produced complete clearance of AKs in 50% of patients compared to 5% with vehicle (number needed to treat [NNT] = 2.2). Adverse events included erythema (27%), scabbing or crusting (21%), flaking

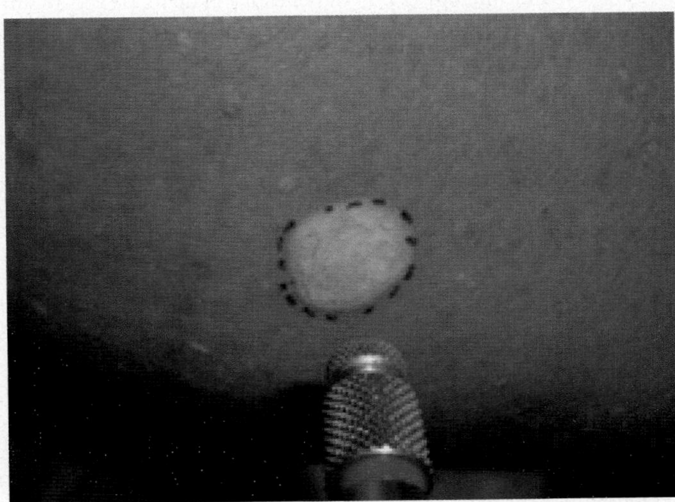

FIGURE 173-9 Cryosurgery of large actinic keratosis. The outside border was marked with a 1- to 2-mm margin. *(Reproduced with permission from Richard P. Usatine, MD.)*

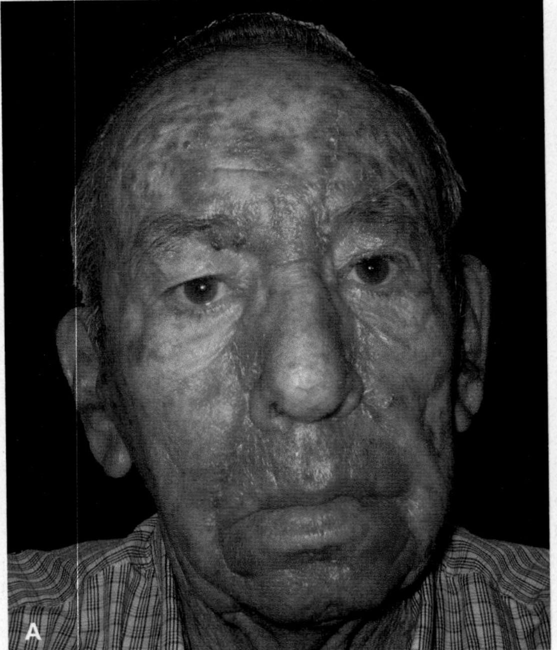

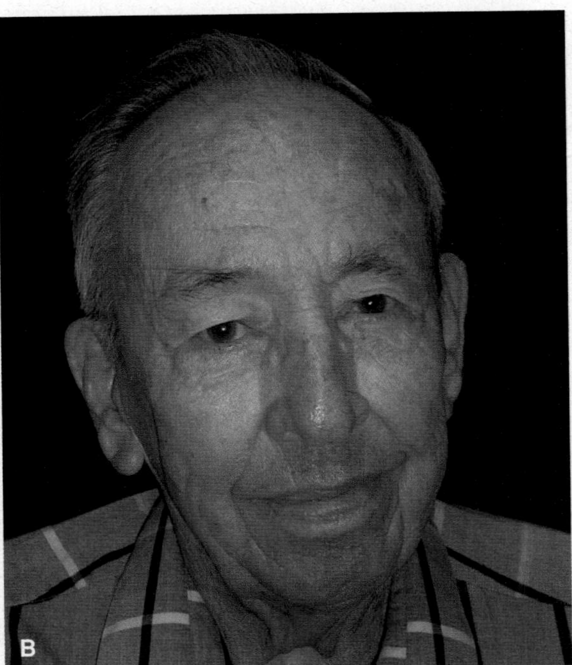

FIGURE 173-10 **A.** Actinic keratoses reddened and crusted by the application of 5-fluorouracil topically twice daily. **B.** Face healed months after the course of 5-fluorouracil was completed. *(Reproduced with permission from Richard P. Usatine, MD.)*

(9%), and erosions (6%) (number needed to harm [NNH] = 3.2 to 5.9).[12]

- Because of its immunostimulatory properties, imiquimod cream must be used with caution in transplant patients on immunosuppression therapy.[1] SOR Ⓒ
- Cryosurgery was effective for up to 75% of lesions in trials comparing it with photodynamic therapy. It may be particularly superior for thicker lesions, but may leave scars.[10] SOR Ⓐ
- Photodynamic therapy (PDT) was effective in up to 91% of AKs in trials comparing it with cryotherapy, with consistently good cosmetic results. It may be particularly good for superficial and confluent AKs, but is likely to be more expensive than most other therapies. It is of particular value where AKs are numerous or when located at sites of poor healing, such as the lower leg.[10] SOR Ⓑ

SECOND LINE

- Diclofenac gel applied twice daily for 10 to 12 weeks has moderate efficacy with low morbidity in mild AKs.[2] SOR Ⓑ There are few follow-up data to indicate the duration of benefit.[2] In one study, diclofenac 3% gel was as effective as 5-FU cream for AK of the face and scalp, and diclofenac produced fewer signs of inflammation.[13]
- Topical tretinoin has some efficacy on the face, with partial clearance of AKs, but may need to be used for up to a year at a time to optimize benefit.[10] SOR Ⓑ
- Ingenol mebutate (Picato)—A short 2 to 3 days of treatment with daily topical ingenol mebutate, from the sap of the *Euphorbia peplus* plant, showed promising efficacy with a favorable safety profile in several randomized controlled trials (RCTs). One multicenter RCT showed 34.1% to 42.2% complete clearance of AKs with 0.05% ingenol mebutate gel for trunk and extremities, and 0.015% gel for the face.[14] Another RCT with 0.05% gel showed a complete clearance of 71% of treated lesions.[15] Ingenol mebutate appears to have a dual mechanism of action by rapid lesion necrosis and subsequent immune-mediated cellular cytotoxicity, providing efficacy with a short treatment period.[16]
- Other less accessible and expensive methods include lasers, dermabrasion, and chemical peels.

BOWEN DISEASE

- **Table 173-2** compares and summarizes the main treatment options.[17]
- The risk of progression to invasive cancer is approximately 3%. This risk is greater in genital BD, and particularly in perianal BD. A high

TABLE 173-2 Summary of the Main Treatment Options for Bowen Disease[17]

Lesion Characteristics	Topical 5-FU	Topical Imiquimod*	Cryotherapy	Curettage	Excision	PDT	Radiotherapy	Laser†
Small, single/few, good healing site‡	3	3	2	1	3	3	5	4
Large, single, good healing site‡	3	3	3	4	5	2	4	7
Multiple, good healing site‡	2	3	2	3	5	3	4	4
Small, single/few, poor healing site‡	2	2	3	2	2	2	5	7
Large, single, poor healing site‡	3	2	5	4	5	1	6	7
Facial	3	3	4	2	4§	3	4	7
Digital	3	7	3	5	2	3	3	3
Nail bed	7	4	7	7	2§	3	4	4
Penile	3	3	4	5	4§	3	3	3
Lesions in immunocompromised patients	5	4	3	3	4	3	7	7

Abbreviations: 5-FU, 5-fluorouracil; PDT, photodynamic therapy; *1,* probably treatment of choice; *2,* generally good choice; *3,* generally fair choice; *4,* reasonable but not usually required; *5,* generally poor choice; *6,* probably should not be used; *7,* insufficient evidence available. The suggested scoring of the treatments listed takes into account the evidence for benefit, ease of application or time required for the procedure, wound healing, cosmetic result, and current availability/costs of the method or facilities required. Evidence for interventions based on single studies or purely anecdotal cases is not included.

*Does not have a product license for Bowen disease.

†Depends on site.

‡Refers to the clinician's perceived potential for good or poor healing at the affected site.

§Consider micrographic surgery for tissue sparing or if poorly defined/recurrent.

risk of recurrence, including late recurrence, is a particular feature of perianal BD, and prolonged follow-up is recommended for this variant.[18] SOR Ⓐ

- There is reasonable evidence to support use of 5-FU.[18] SOR Ⓑ It is more practical than surgery for large lesions, especially at potentially poor healing sites, and has been used for "control" rather than cure in some patients with multiple lesions.[13]
- Topical imiquimod may be used off-label for BD for larger lesions or difficult/poor healing sites.[18] SOR Ⓑ However, it is costly and the optimum regimen has yet to be determined.[18]
- One prospective study suggests a superiority of curettage and electrodesiccation (**Figure 173-11**) over cryotherapy in treating BD, especially for lesions on the lower leg (**Figure 173-11**).[19] Curettage was associated with a significantly shorter healing time, less pain, fewer complications, and a lower recurrence rate when compared with cryotherapy.[20]
- A Cochrane review found that significantly more lesions cleared with methyl aminolevulinate–photodynamic therapy compared to photodynamic therapy alone (risk ratio 1.68, 95%, confidence interval 1.12–2.52, n = 148) or cryotherapy (risk ratio 1.17, 95% confidence interval 1.01–1.37; n = 215).[21]

PREVENTION

- Protect from UV exposure by limiting outdoor activities and using sunscreens and protective gears (hat, umbrella, long sleeve garments, etc.).
- Avoid artificial tanning beds and tobacco.

PROGNOSIS

Prognosis of treated AK and BD is excellent.

FOLLOW-UP

Patients need skin examinations every 6 to 12 months to identify new pre-cancers and cancers. SOR Ⓒ More frequent examinations may be needed for those who have continued exposure to offending agents (e.g., organ transplant recipients on immunosuppressant therapy) and those with history of recurrent skin malignancies.

PATIENT EDUCATION

Patients must understand that they acquired these conditions through cumulative sun damage, and they need to avoid further sun damage to minimize the likelihood of additional pre-cancers and cancers. The sun damage is often from childhood and early adulthood, so the lesions are likely to form even with future sun protection. Self skin examination is recommended.

All topical treatments for AKs and BD will make the lesions look worse before they get better (see **Figure 173-10**). The 5-FU treatments are often given with topical corticosteroid preparations to use after the treatment is over so as to minimize the symptoms of the inflammation.

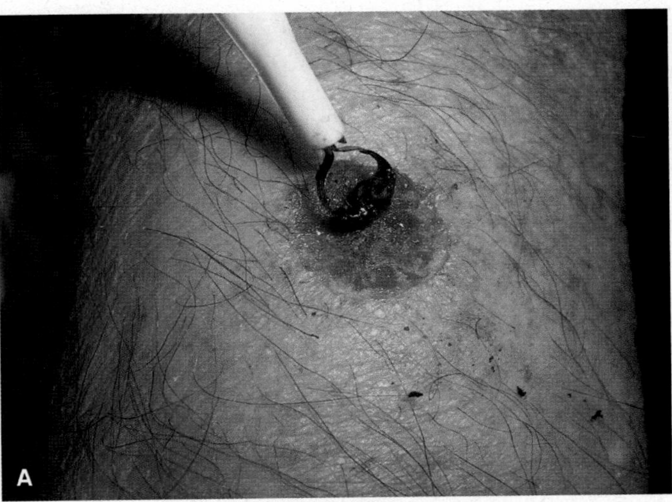

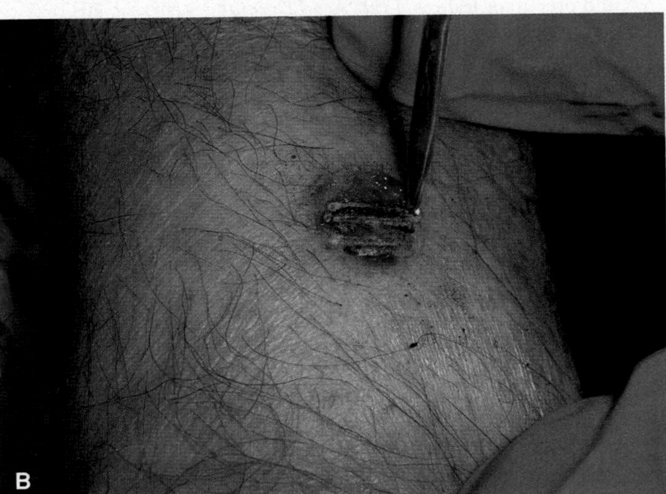

FIGURE 173-11 **A.** Curettage of Bowen disease on the arm. Each cycle begins with curettage and ends with electrodesiccation. **B.** Electrodesiccation of Bowen disease on the same leg. Three cycles were performed to complete the procedure. (*Reproduced with permission from Richard P. Usatine, MD.*)

PATIENT RESOURCES

- Skin Cancer Foundation has an excellent website with photos and patient information—**http://www.skincancer.org/ak/index.php.**

PROVIDER RESOURCE AND GUIDELINES

- Morton CA, Birnie AJ, Eedy DJ. British Association of Dermatologists' guidelines for the management of squamous cell carcinoma in situ (Bowen's disease) 2014. *Br J Dermatol.* 2014; 170(2):245-260.

REFERENCES

1. Bonerandi JJ, Beauvillain C, Caquant L, et al. Guidelines for the diagnosis and treatment of cutaneous squamous cell carcinoma and precursor lesions. *J Eur Acad Dermatol Venereol.* 2011;25 Suppl 5:1-51.
2. Leffell DJ. The scientific basis of skin cancer. *J Am Acad Dermatol.* 2000;42(1 Pt 2):18-22.
3. Anwar J, Wrone DA, Kimyai-Asadi A, Alam M. The development of actinic keratosis into invasive squamous cell carcinoma: evidence and evolving classification schemes. *Clin Dermatol.* 2004; 22(3):189-196.
4. Werner RN, Stockfleth E, Connolly SM, et al; International League of Dermatological Societies; European Dermatology Forum. Evidence- and consensus-based (S3) guidelines for the treatment of actinic keratosis—International League of Dermatological Societies in cooperation with the European Dermatology Forum—short version. *J Eur Acad Dermatol Venereol.* 2015;29(11):2069-2079.
5. Werner RN, Sammain A, Erdmann R, et al. The natural history of actinic keratosis: a systematic review. *Br J Dermatol.* 2013;169(3): 502-518.
6. Nguyen KP, Peppelman M, Hoogedoorn L, et al. The current role of in vivo reflectance confocal microscopy within the continuum of actinic keratosis and squamous cell carcinoma: a systematic review. *Eur J Dermatol.* 2016;26(6):549-565.
7. Gupta AK, Paquet M, Villanueva E, Brintnell W. Interventions for actinic keratoses. *Cochrane Database Syst Rev.* 2012;(12):CD004415.
8. Zouboulis CC, Röhrs H. [Cryosurgical treatment of actinic keratoses and evidence-based review]. *Hautarzt.* 2005;56(4):353-358.
9. Thai K-E, Fergin P, Freeman M, et al. A prospective study of the use of cryosurgery for the treatment of actinic keratoses. *Int J Dermatol.* 2004;43(9):687-692.
10. de Berker D, McGregor JM, Hughes BR. Guidelines for the management of actinic keratoses. *Br J Dermatol.* 2007;156(2):222-230.
11. Gupta AK, Davey V, McPhail H. Evaluation of the effectiveness of imiquimod and 5-fluorouracil for the treatment of actinic keratosis: critical review and meta-analysis of efficacy studies. *J Cutan Med Surg.* 2005;9(5):209-214.
12. Hadley G, Derry S, Moore RA. Imiquimod for actinic keratosis: systematic review and meta-analysis. *J Invest Dermatol.* 2006; 126(6):1251-1255.
13. Smith SR, Morhenn VB, Piacquadio DJ. Bilateral comparison of the efficacy and tolerability of 3% diclofenac sodium gel and 5% 5-fluorouracil cream in the treatment of actinic keratoses of the face and scalp. *J Drugs Dermatol.* 2006;5(2):156-159.
14. Lebwohl M, Swanson N, Anderson LL, et al. Ingenol mebutate gel for actinic keratosis. *N Engl J Med.* 2012;366(11):1010-1019.
15. Siller G, Gebauer K, Welburn P, et al. PEP005 (ingenol mebutate) gel, a novel agent for the treatment of actinic keratosis: results of a randomized, double-blind, vehicle-controlled, multicentre, phase IIa study. *Australas J Dermatol.* 2009;50(1):16-22.
16. Rosen RH, Gupta AK, Tyring SK. Dual mechanism of action of ingenol mebutate gel for topical treatment of actinic keratoses: rapid lesion necrosis followed by lesion-specific immune response. *J Am Acad Dermatol.* 2012;66(3):486-493.
17. Morton CA, Birnie AJ, Eedy DJ. British Association of Dermatologists' guidelines for the management of squamous cell carcinoma in situ (Bowen's disease) 2014. *Br J Dermatol.* 2014;170(2):245-260.
18. Cox NH, Eedy DJ, Morton CA. Guidelines for management of Bowen's disease: 2006 update. *Br J Dermatol.* 2007;156(1):11-21.
19. Hadley G, Derry S, Moore RA. Imiquimod for actinic keratosis: systematic review and meta-analysis. *J Invest Dermatol.* 2006; 126(6):1251-1255.
20. Ahmed I, Berth-Jones J, Charles-Holmes S, et al. Comparison of cryotherapy with curettage in the treatment of Bowen's disease: a prospective study. *Br J Dermatol.* 2000;143(4):759-766.
21. Bath-Hextall FJ, Matin RN, Wilkinson D, Leonardi-Bee J. Interventions for cutaneous Bowen's disease. *Cochrane Database Syst Rev.* 2013;(6):CD007281.

174 KERATOACANTHOMA

Lina M. Cardona, MD
Alfonso Guzman, Jr., MD
Richard P. Usatine, MD

PATIENT STORY

A 71-year-old woman presented with a rapidly growing lesion on her face over the past 4 months (**Figure 174-1**). The lesion had features of a basal cell carcinoma with a pearly border and telangiectasias (**Figure 174-2**). Also, the central crater with keratin gave it the appearance of a keratoacanthoma (KA). A shave biopsy was performed, and the pathology showed squamous cell carcinoma (SCC)–KA type. A full elliptical excision with 4-mm margins was then performed.

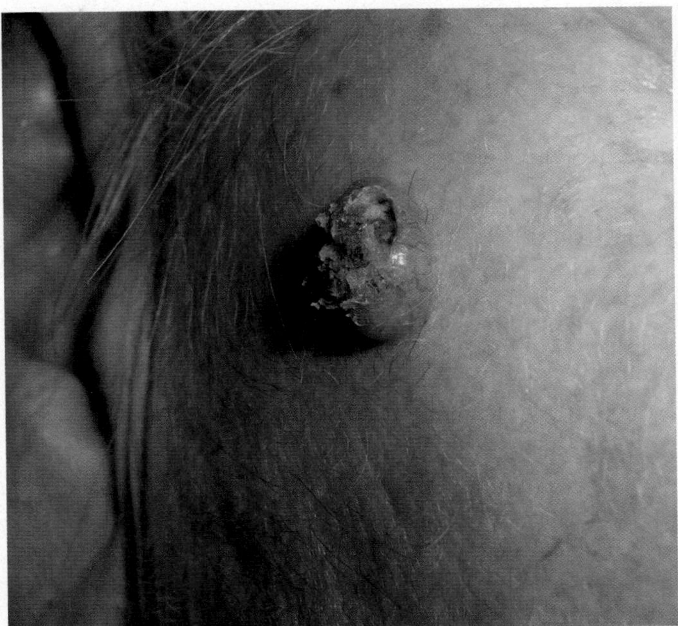

FIGURE 174-1 Pearly keratoacanthoma with telangiectasias and a central keratin core on the face of a 71-year-old woman. *(Reproduced with permission from Richard P. Usatine, MD.)*

INTRODUCTION

The KA is a unique epidermal tumor characterized by rapid, abundant growth and a spontaneous resolution, with the classic presentation in middle-aged, light-skinned individuals in hair-bearing, sun-exposed areas. In the late 1940s, Freudenthal of Wroclaw coined the term *keratoacanthoma*, owing to the considerable acanthosis observed in the tumor. Controversies have arisen since the 1950s about the real nature of the tumor; some KAs may metastasize, and there is still debate over the relationship to SCC.[1,2] With the current genetic and immunohistochemical data, many authors classify this tumor as a subtype of SCC.[3]

SYNONYMS[1]

Self-healing squamous cell carcinoma.

EPIDEMIOLOGY

- KA develops as a solitary nodule in sun-exposed areas.
- Seen more commonly later in life with a predilection for males.[1]
- Develops rapidly within 6 to 8 weeks.
- May spontaneously regress after 3 to 6 months or may continue to grow and rarely metastasize.
- It is commonly underdiagnosed due to rapid growth and spontaneous regression.[1]

ETIOLOGY AND PATHOPHYSIOLOGY

- KAs share features such as infiltration and cytologic atypia with SCCs.
- KAs have been reported to metastasize.[4]
- KA is considered to be a variant of SCC, called SCC-KA type.

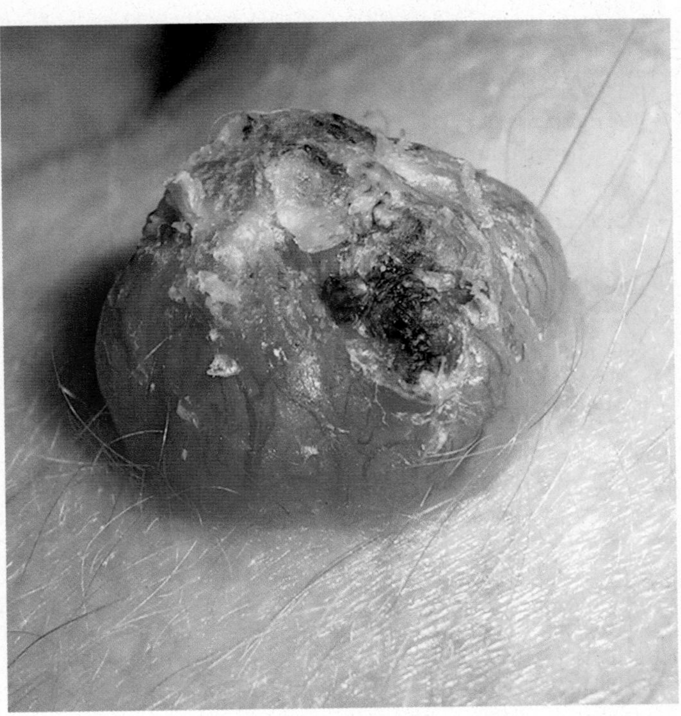

FIGURE 174-2 Close-up of the keratoacanthoma with telangiectasias and a central keratin core on the face of the woman in **Figure 174-1**. *(Reproduced with permission from Richard P. Usatine, MD.)*

- Current histologic criteria categorized KA as well-differentiated SCC[5]; needs to correlate with clinical presentation.
- In the majority of cases, KA originates from hair follicles, mainly from isthmus and infundibulum portion.[1,6] This factor in part explains why KAs behave in a triphasic pattern: rapid growth, stabilization, and regression.[1,6,7]

RISK FACTORS

- Age greater than 40.
- Sun-exposed skin.
- Light complexion.
- Male gender.
- Tattoos. KAs can develop in a new tattoo. Case reports reveal red ink is the most common cause.[8]
- Medications such as azathioprine, cyclophosphamide, and anti–tumor necrosis factor alpha[1] have been linked to KAs.
- Skin trauma (surgical, ablative lasers, cryotherapy, photodynamic therapy) due to Koebner phenomenon.
- Genetic skin disorders such as xeroderma pigmentosum[9] and incontinentia pigmenti.[10]
- Medications for metastatic or advanced melanoma. Cases have been reported linking the use of pembrolizumab (PD-1 receptor blocker),[11] and vemurafenib,[12] drabafenib[13] (both BRAF protein kinase inhibitors) with eruptive KAs.
- Human papillomavirus (HPV) infection.[14,15]

DIAGNOSIS

CLINICAL FEATURES

- The most common type is the solitary nodule in sun-exposed areas. Often have a central keratin plug that resembles a volcano (**Figures 174-1** to **174-5**). KAs may grow rapidly (**Figure 174-6**).
- Other rare types of keratoacanthomas have been reported: generalized eruptive KAs, mucosal KAs, subungual KA, multiple familial KA[1] and KAs as part of the Muir-Torre syndrome (genodermatosis with internal malignancy—usually colon cancer associated with KA and/or sebaceous tumor).

TYPICAL DISTRIBUTION

Sun-exposed areas, face, arms, hands, and trunk (see **Figures 174-3** and **174-5**). KAs can be found anywhere on the head and neck, including the ears (**Figures 174-6** and **174-7**).

DERMOSCOPY AND BIOPSY

Dermoscopic features of KA overlap with the dermoscopic features of SCC. Features that are most likely seen with SCC of the KA type include long twisted looped vessels on the periphery and a central yellow keratin core **(Figure 174-8)**. Biopsy is the only reliable method to make the diagnosis. Frequently a shave biopsy is sufficient as long as the base is included.

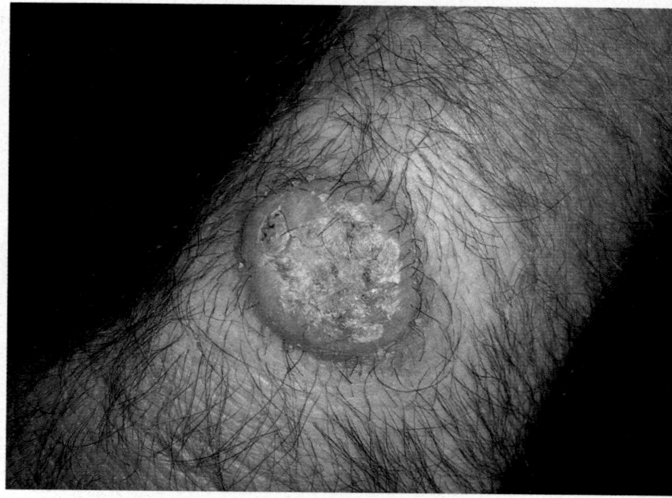

FIGURE 174-3 Keratoacanthoma on the arm with central scaling. *(Reproduced with permission from Richard P. Usatine, MD.)*

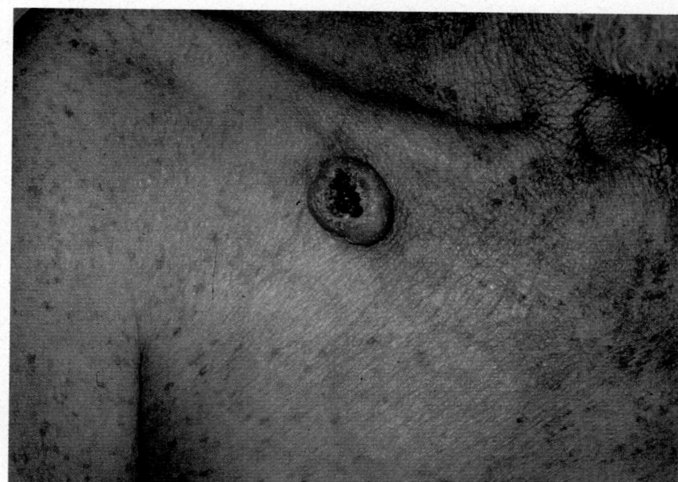

FIGURE 174-4 Giant keratoacanthoma under the clavicle. *(Reproduced with permission from Usatine RP, Moy RL, Tobinick EL, et al: Skin Surgery: A Practical Guide. St. Louis, MO: Mosby; 1998.)*

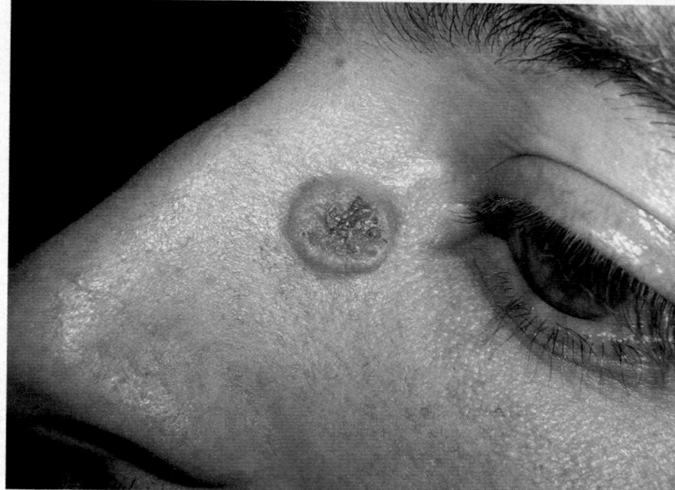

FIGURE 174-5 Keratoacanthoma with a central keratin core on the nose of a 29-year-old HIV-positive man. *(Reproduced with permission from Richard P. Usatine, MD.)*

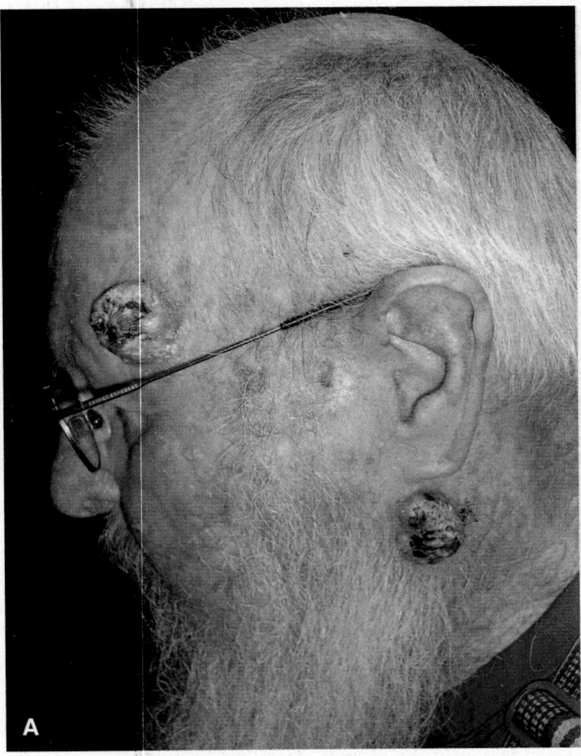

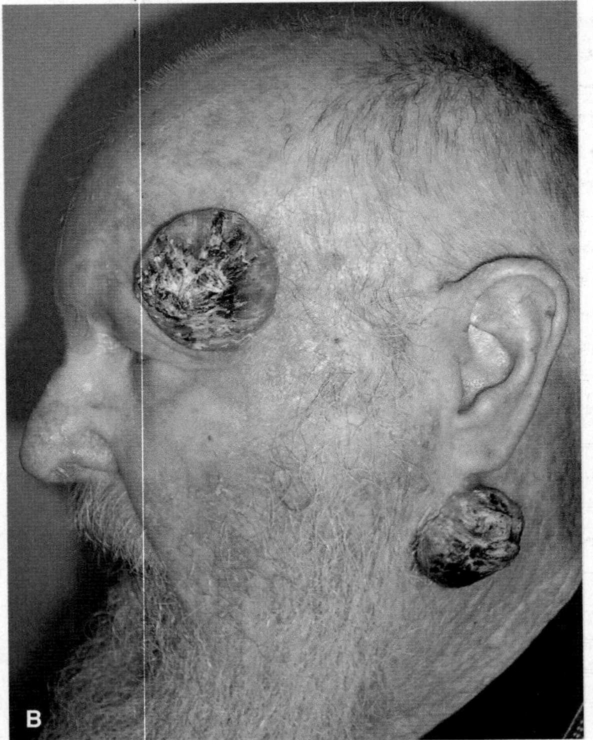

FIGURE 174-6 Two SCCs in a 65-year-old man. **A.** The SCC over the temple was a keratoacanthoma type, whereas the SCC on the neck was a well-differentiated SCC. **B.** Rapid growth occurred in both tumors over the 6-week period that the patient waited to have head and neck surgery. (*Reproduced with permission from Richard P. Usatine, MD.*)

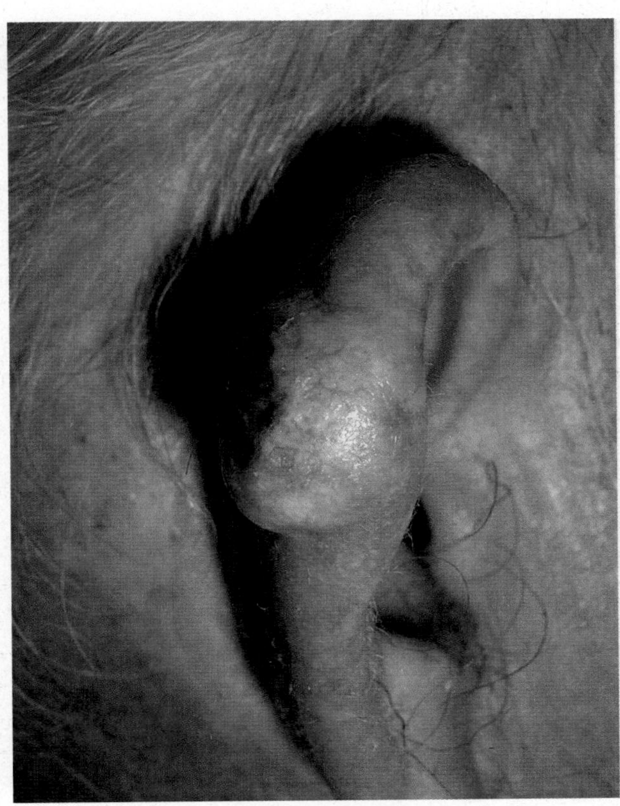

FIGURE 174-7 Keratoacanthoma on the ear. (*Reproduced with permission from Richard P. Usatine, MD.*)

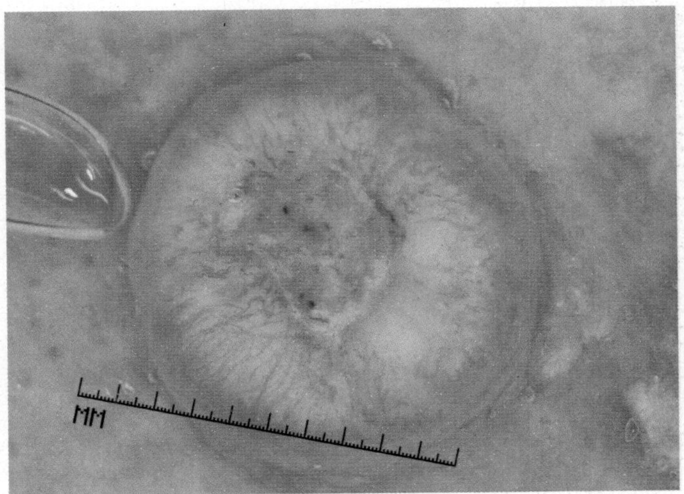

FIGURE 174-8 Dermoscopy of a keratoacanthoma showing long twisted looped vessels on the periphery and a central yellow keratin core. (*Reproduced with permission from Ash Marghoob, MD.*)

DIFFERENTIAL DIAGNOSIS

- SCCs of the skin have many forms, and KA is one type of SCC (see Chapter 178, Squamous Cell Carcinoma).
- Cutaneous horn is a raised keratinaceous lesion that can arise in warts, actinic keratoses, and SCC. It generally does not have pearly raised skin around the keratin horn and therefore does not have the crater appearance of a KA (see Chapter 176, Cutaneous Horn).
- Amelanotic melanoma, especially if exophytic, can be mistaken for KA clinically. Fortunately a biopsy should provide the correct diagnosis (see Chapter 179, Melanoma).
- Hypertrophic lichen planus (LP) can resemble eruptive KA. In this case the first biopsy was misread as a KA, and a second biopsy was needed to correctly identify this case of hypertrophic LP **(Figure 174-9)** (see Chapter 160, Lichen Planus).
- Ulcerative and exophytic in--fectious tumors can be mistaken as KAs. Deep fungal and mycobacterial infections are most likely to resemble KA, and biopsy for pathology and tissues cultures can help distinguish between these conditions

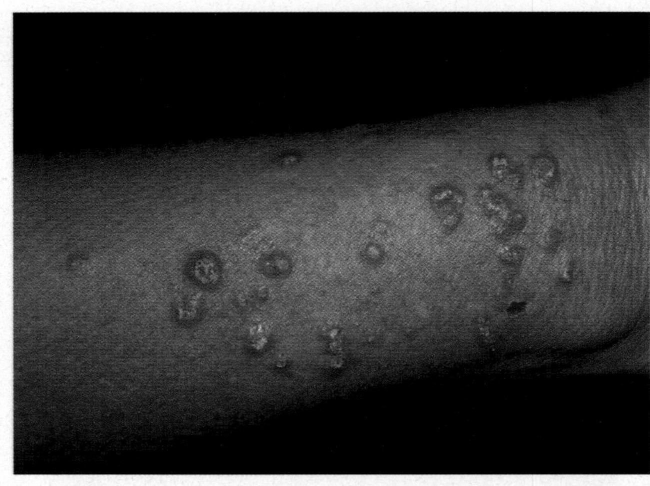

FIGURE 174-9 Hypertrophic lichen planus resembling eruptive keratoacanthomas. (*Reproduced with permission from Richard P. Usatine, MD.*)

MANAGEMENT

FIRST LINE

- A shave biopsy may be used for diagnosis but is not an adequate final treatment. Options for definitive treatment should be discussed with the patient.
- Although some KAs may regress spontaneously, there is no way to distinguish between these and the ones that may go on to become locally destructive and/or metastasize. Therefore, the standard of care is to excise or destroy the remaining tumor. SOR Ⓒ
- Elliptically excise a KA with margins of 5 mm to achieve >95% clearance.[16] SOR Ⓒ
- Smaller, less-aggressive KAs diagnosed with shave biopsy may be destroyed with curettage and desiccation or cryotherapy with 3- to 5-mm margins. SOR Ⓒ
- Mohs surgery may be indicated for large or recurrent KAs or KAs located in anatomic areas with cosmetic or functional considerations.[16] SOR Ⓒ

SECOND LINE

- Multiple eruptive KAs have been treated with oral retinoids, oral methotrexate, topical 5-fluorouracil, and topical imiquimod. SOR Ⓒ
- Intralesional chemotherapy with methotrexate,[17,18] 5-fluorouracil, bleomycin, or interferon has been used as a second line of therapy. These medications can be used before the excision to reduce the size of the tumor.[19]
- For resistant, aggressive, and/or recalcitrant KAs, treatment with erlotinib (an epidermal growth factor receptor inhibitor) has been reported.[20]

PROGNOSIS

When compared to other skin cancers, the prognosis is good. Excision is typically the first line of treatment, with high rates of cure and pathologic confirmation of clear margins.

FOLLOW-UP

Patients should perform their own skin exams and have yearly clinical skin examinations to examine for recurrence and the development of new skin cancers.

PATIENT EDUCATION

KA is similar to other nonmelanoma skin cancers in that it occurs on sun-exposed areas, and patients who have had one are at increased risk of developing new skin cancers. Therefore, sun avoidance and sun protection should be emphasized.

Patients should be advised to avoid chemical peels, microdermabrasion, lasers, and tattoos to diminish the risk of developing a new KA.

PATIENT RESOURCES

- Skinsight. *Keratoacanthoma*—**https://www.skinsight.com/skin-conditions/adult/keratoacanthoma.**

PROVIDER RESOURCES

- Medscape. *Keratoacanthoma*—**http://emedicine.medscape.com/article/1100471.**

REFERENCES

1. Kwiek B, Schwartz RA. Keratoacanthoma (KA): an update and review. *J Am Acad Dermatol.* 2016;74(6):1220-3123.
2. Ko CJ. Keratoacanthoma: facts and controversies. *Clin Dermatol.* 2010;28(3):254-261.
3. Savage JA, Maize JC Sr. Keratoacanthoma clinical behavior: a systematic review. *Am J Dermatopathol.* 2014;36(5):422-429.
4. Rossi AM, Park B, Qi B, et al. Solitary large keratoacanthomas of the head and neck: an observational study. *Dermatol Surg.* 2017;43(6):810-816.
5. Paolino G, Donati M, Didona D, et al. Histology of non-melanoma skin cancers: an update. *Biomedicines.* 2017;20;5(4).
6. Kossard S. The role of the follicular isthmus in the evolution of keratoacanthoma. *J Cutan Pathol.* 2015;42(4):299-300.
7. Misago N. The distinction of keratoacanthoma from various types of squamous cell carcinoma with crateriform architecture. *J Cutan Pathol.* 2016;43(12):1234-1237.
8. Kluger N, Douvin D, Dupuis-Fourdan F, et al. Keratoacanthomas on recent tattoos: two cases. *Ann Dermatol Venereol.* 2017;144(12):776-783.
9. Zheng JF, Mo HY, Wang ZZ. Clinicopathological characteristics of xeroderma pigmentosum associated with keratoacanthoma: a case report and literature review. *Int J Clin Exp Med.* 2014;7(10):3410-3414.
10. Barros B, Helm K, Zaenglein A, Seiverling E. Keratoacanthoma-like growths of incontinentia pigmenti successfully treated with intralesional methotrexate. *Pediatr Dermatol.* 2017;34(4): e203-e204.
11. Freites-Martinez A, Kwong BY, Rieger KE, et al. Eruptive keratoacanthomas associated with pembrolizumab therapy. *JAMA Dermatol.* 2017;153(7):694-697.
12. Furudate S, Fujimura T, Kambayashi Y, et al. Keratoacanthoma, palmoplantar keratoderma developing in an advanced melanoma patient treated with vemurafenib regressed by blockade of mitogen-activated protein kinase kinase signaling. *J Dermatol.* 2017; 44(9):e226-e227.
13. Lacroix JP, Wang B. Prospective case series of cutaneous adverse effects associated with dabrafenib and trametinib. *J Cutan Med Surg.* 2017;21(1):54-59.
14. Göktay F, Kaynak E, Güneş P, et al. Relationship between human papilloma virus and subungual keratoacanthoma: two case reports and the outcomes of surgical treatment. *Skin Appendage Disord.* 2017;2(3-4):92-96.
15. Norgauer J, Rohwedder A. Human papillomavirus and Grzybowski's generalized eruptive keratoacanthomas. *J Am Acad Dermatol.* 2003;49:771-772
16. Schell AE, Russell MA, Park SS. Suggested excisional margins for cutaneous malignant lesions based on Mohs micrographic surgery. *JAMA Facial Plast Surg.* 2013;15(5):337-343.
17. Yoo MG, Kim IH. Intralesional methotrexate for the treatment of keratoacanthoma retrospective study and review of the Korean literature. *Ann Dermatol.* 2014;26(2):172-176.
18. Aubut N, Alain J, Claveau J. Intralesional methotrexate treatment for keratoacanthoma tumors: a retrospective case series. *J Cutan Med Surg.* 2012;16(3):212-217.
19. Kirby JS, Miller CJ. Intralesional chemotherapy for nonmelanoma skin cancer: a practical review. *J Am Acad Dermatol.* 2010;63(4):689-702.
20. Bulj TK, Krunic AL, Cetner AS, Villano JL. Refractory aggressive keratoacanthoma centrifugum marginatum of the scalp controlled with the epidermal growth factor receptor inhibitor erlotinib. *Br J Dermatol.* 2010;163(3):633-637.

175 LENTIGO MALIGNA

Jonathan B. Karnes, MD
E.J. Mayeaux, Jr., MD
Richard P. Usatine, MD

PATIENT STORY

A 67-year-old man noted that a brown spot on his face was growing larger and darker (**Figure 175-1**). Dermoscopy was performed, and polygonal lines and rhomboidal structures were seen around the follicular openings (**Figure 175-2**). A broad shave biopsy of the whole lesion showed lentigo maligna (LM) (melanoma in situ). The patient had a long history of multiple skin cancers including multiple thin melanomas on his back. He also had cardiac problems and was on Coumadin. The options for treatment were presented, and he chose to try topical imiquimod. He was instructed to apply the imiquimod daily to the involved area and was seen monthly. After 2 months it was obvious that he was having an exuberant inflammatory response to the imiquimod as desired (**Figure 175-3**). He completed the 3-month course. Three months after completion his face appeared completely clear (**Figure 175-4**) clinically and dermoscopically.

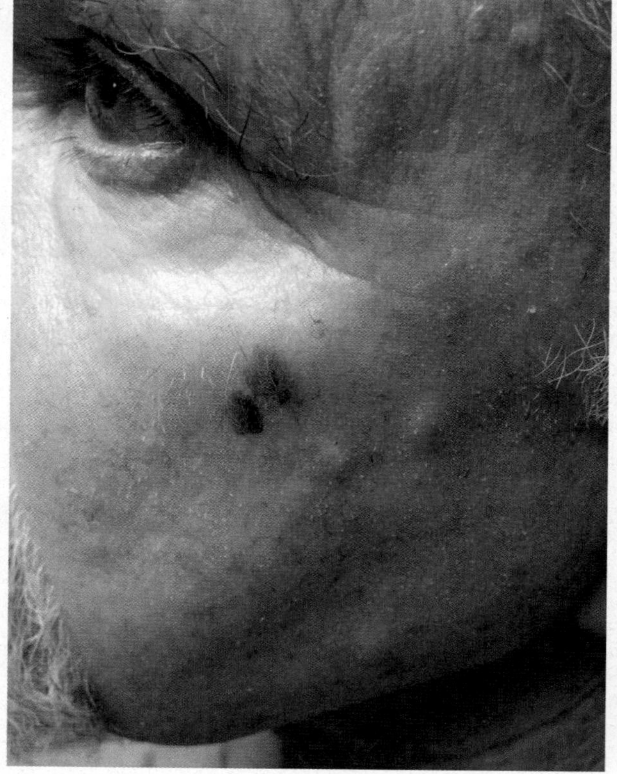

FIGURE 175-1 Lentigo maligna (melanoma in situ) on the face of a 67-year-old man. (*Reproduced with permission from Richard P. Usatine, MD.*)

INTRODUCTION

Lentigo maligna is a subtype of melanoma in situ that begins as a tan-brown macule, most often on sun-damaged areas of fair-skinned older individuals.

SYNONYMS

Hutchinson melanotic freckle.

EPIDEMIOLOGY

- The incidence of LM is directly related to sun exposure.
- Generally, patients with LM are older than age 40 years and fair skinned, with a peak incidence between the ages of 65 and 80.[1]
- LM may represent as much as 25% of all melanomas on the head and neck.[2]
- Melanoma in situ (of all types) is increasing at up to 10% per year, faster than any other cancer.[3]

ETIOLOGY AND PATHOPHYSIOLOGY

- LM is a subtype of melanoma in situ, a preinvasive lesion confined to the epidermis (**Figure 175-5**).
- It is caused by cumulative sun exposure and, therefore, seen later in life.
- Lentigo maligna melanoma (LMM) occurs when the lesion extends into the dermis (**Figure 175-6**).

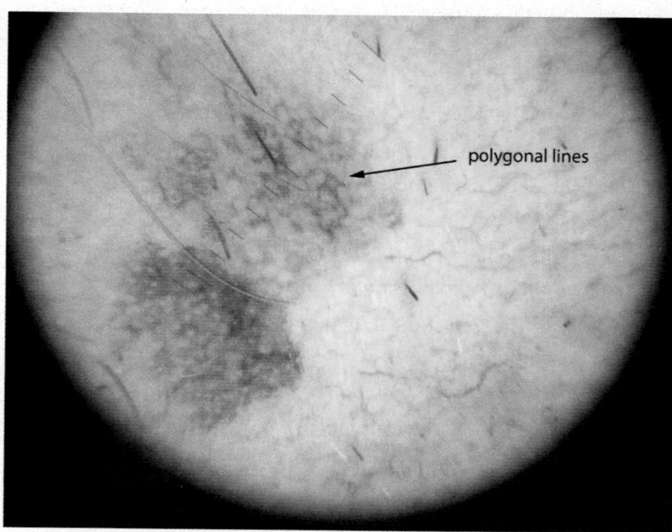

FIGURE 175-2 Dermoscopy of lentigo maligna on the cheek showing polygonal lines that make rhomboid structures around the follicular openings. (*Reproduced with permission from Richard P. Usatine, MD.*)

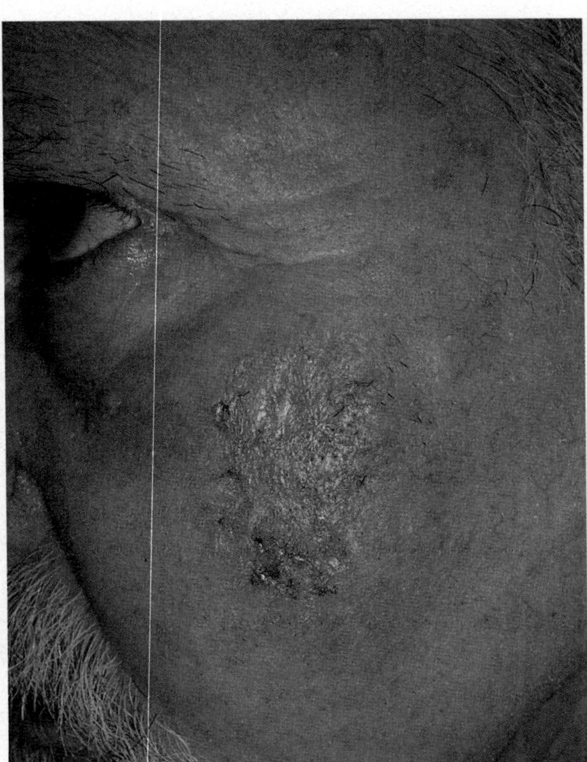

FIGURE 175-3 An exuberant inflammatory reaction to imiquimod applied daily to any remaining lentigo maligna on the cheek after a broad saucerization of the lesion. (*Reproduced with permission from Richard P. Usatine, MD.*)

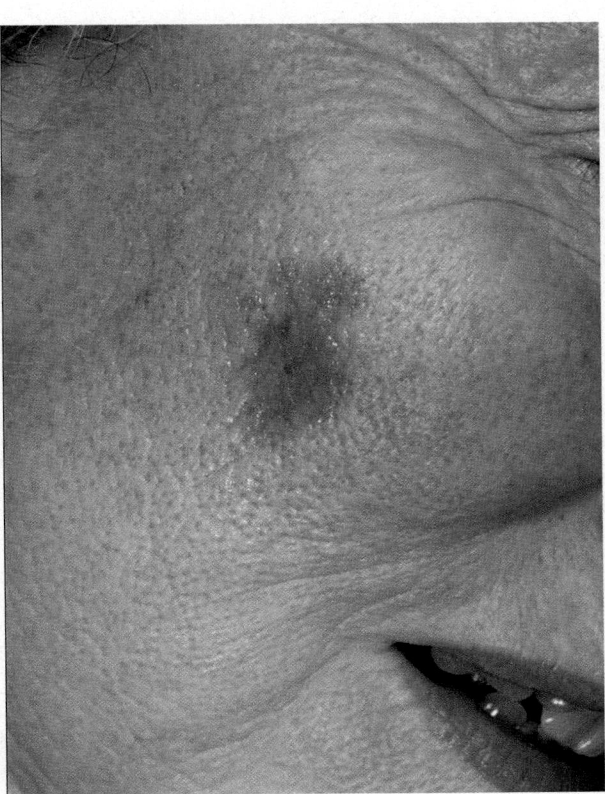

FIGURE 175-5 Lentigo maligna (melanoma in situ) on the cheek. (*Reproduced with permission from Usatine RP, Moy RL, Tobinick EL, et al: Skin Surgery: A Practical Guide. St. Louis, MO: Mosby; 1998.*)

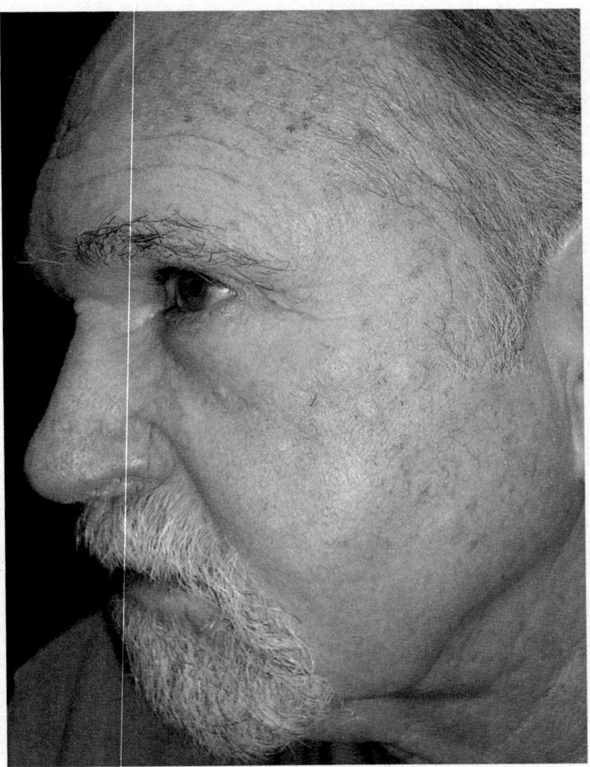

FIGURE 175-4 The face is clinically and dermoscopically clear of lentigo maligna 3 months after completing the treatment with imiquimod. Through years of follow-up the patient never had a clinical relapse of this LM. (*Reproduced with permission from Richard P. Usatine, MD.*)

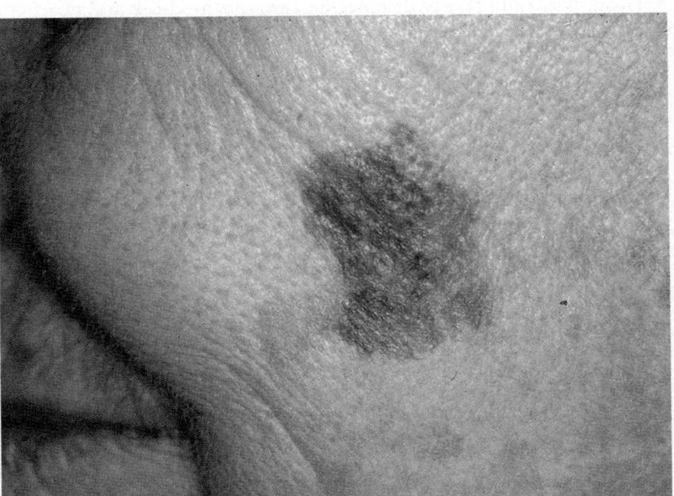

FIGURE 175-6 Lentigo maligna melanoma on the cheek. This lesion is invasive and no longer melanoma in situ. A partial broad scoop shave biopsy is a good way to make this diagnosis, as a full-depth complete excisional biopsy would be prohibitively large and a punch biopsy might miss the diagnosis. (*Reproduced with permission from the Skin Cancer Foundation. For more information www.skincancer.org.*)

- LM can be present for long periods (5 to 15 years) before invasion occurs, although rapid progression within months has been described.[4]
- The risk for progression to LMM appears to be proportional to the size of the lesion of LM.[4]

RISK FACTORS

- UV radiation exposure: risk increases with increased hours of exposure to sunlight, with the amount of actinic damage, and with a history of nonmelanoma skin cancer.
- Increased number of melanocytic nevi, including large or giant congenital nevi.
- Fair skin.
- History of severe sunburns.
- Porphyria cutanea tarda.
- Oculocutaneous albinism.
- Xeroderma pigmentosum.
- Occupational risk with sun exposure.

DIAGNOSIS

CLINICAL FEATURES

- Large pigmented patch with multiple colors, including brown, black, pink, and white (signifying regression).
- May have ill-defined borders with occult microscopic extension, presenting a challenge for achieving clear margins.
- Up to 29% may have upstaging to invasive disease at the time of excision.[5]

TYPICAL DISTRIBUTION

- Head, neck, and face with a predilection for the cheek and nose (**Figures 175-5** and **175-7**).

DERMOSCOPY

- Important dermoscopic features of LM include asymmetric pigmented follicular openings, rhomboidal structures, slate-gray globules, and slate-gray dots.[6] Rhomboidal structures are also described as polygonal lines and zigzag lines when the full rhomboid is not completed around the follicular opening (see **Figure 175-2**) (see Chapters 111 and 181 on dermoscopy).

BIOPSY

- LM may be quite heterogeneous, and broad scoop shave biopsies of the most clinically concerning areas are ideal to provide both full depth and breadth for microscopic assessment.
- A lesion suspicious for LM or LMM can be biopsied using a broad scoop shave biopsy approach with a DermaBlade or sharp razor blade.[7] The goal is to sample the dermal–epidermal junction and still produce a good cosmetic result (especially if the lesion turns out to be benign).
- An alternative approach is to biopsy samples of each morphologically distinct region of the lesion.[7]

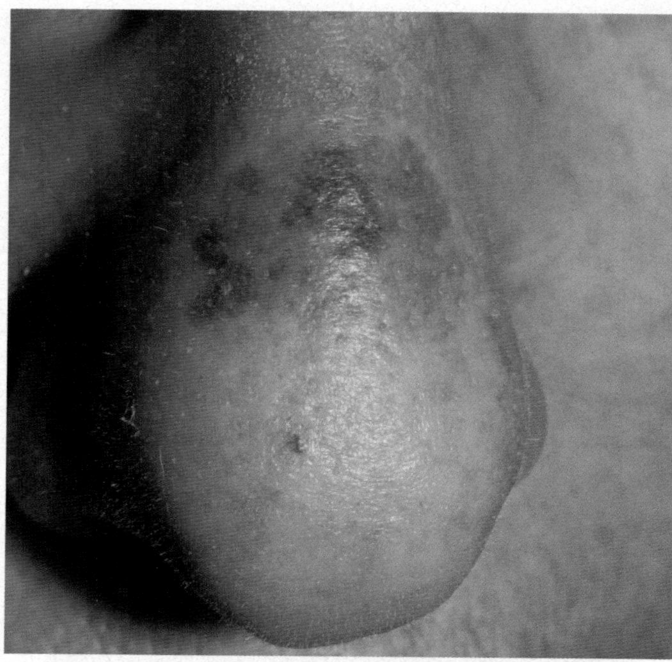

FIGURE 175-7 Lentigo maligna on the nose of a 65-year-old woman with adjacent actinic keratosis superiorly. Differentiating LM from pigmented actinic keratoses can be challenging, and both occur frequently on the face. *(Reproduced with permission from Jonathan B. Karnes, MD.)*

- If an area suspicious for invasion is noted, or if there is an area of induration suspicious for associated desmoplastic melanoma, a deeper scoop shave or incisional biopsy is warranted.[7]
- If sampling is incomplete, the presence of a solar lentigo, pigmented actinic keratosis, or reticulated seborrheic keratosis (SK) could lead the pathologist and clinician to the wrong conclusion that the incisional specimen is representative of the whole, and that no LM is present.[7]
- In a study of LM, contiguous pigmented lesions were present in 48% of the specimens obtained by broad shave biopsy or Mohs surgery. The most common lesion was a benign solar lentigo (30%), followed by pigmented actinic keratosis (24%).[7] This should be kept in mind when interpreting biopsy results to avoid false negatives.

DIFFERENTIAL DIAGNOSIS

- Solar lentigo (plural solar lentigines)—These hyperpigmented patches are very common on the faces and the dorsum of the hands of persons with significant sun exposure, and the incidence increases with age. A possible solar lentigo is more suspicious for LM or LMM when it is larger, more asymmetric, has irregular borders and has more variation in colors. Pigmented lesions with these characteristics should be biopsied to determine the correct diagnosis. Many fair-skinned individuals have a number of solar lentigines, making this a challenge. The use of dermoscopy and judicious biopsies is necessary to avoid missing LM and LMM.
- Seborrheic keratoses (SK) are ubiquitous benign growths that occur more frequently with age. An early SK can be flat and easily resemble LM. SKs on the back are less likely to be confused for LM, but a large flat SK on the face can easily be mistaken for an LM. More importantly, avoid missing an LM because it is assumed to be a flat early SK. When in doubt, biopsy the lesion with a quick and easy shave biopsy. Do not freeze a possible SK unless you are sure that it is truly benign (see Chapter 164, Seborrheic Keratosis).
- Invasive LMM is the feared outcome of missing an LM and not treating it properly. Any suspicious lesion requires biopsy. Early diagnosis does. LMM accounts for about 15% of cutaneous melanoma (see **Figure 175-5**) (see Chapter 179, Melanoma).[8]

MANAGEMENT

- Therapy is directed toward preventing progression to invasive LMM.

NONSURGICAL

- Nonsurgical therapy for primary cutaneous melanomas should be considered when surgical excision is not possible.
- Alternatives to surgery includes radiation, topical imiquimod, cryosurgery, and observation. There is a lack of well-designed trials to guide best therapy for LM.[9] SOR C

MEDICATIONS

- Topical imiquimod 5% cream applied 5–7 times per week for 3 months has been described in multiple studies to be effective in treating LM, especially in patients who are not surgical candidates.[9-13] SOR A
- In a systematic review of 347 tumors from 45 studies, imiquimod offers a 76% histologic and 78% clinical clearance rate for lentigo maligna. Both cumulative dose and treatment intensity affect tumor clearance. Daily applications produced higher histologic clearance than 5 applications per week.[10]
- Relapse rate over a median follow-up of 4.8 years was 18% in one study[11] and 23.5% in another study at 2–3 years.[12] The highest relapse rates were when LM was on the nose (33%).[12]
- In another study in which 67% were clear on biopsy after the imiquimod, 0% of these patients who were clear had signs of LM on confocal microscopy at 5- to 10-year follow-up.[13]
- Imiquimod can be an effective long-term treatment for LM. Its use avoids potentially disfiguring surgical resection, but it does require surveillance, especially if the LM is on the nose.[10-13]

RADIATION

- Radiation therapy protocols using either superficial radiotherapy or Grenz rays have the advantage of improved cosmetic outcomes compared to surgery and a recurrence rate of about 5% in published studies over a 3-year average follow-up. This is a more widely used therapy in Australia than in the United States but is an option for patients unable to undergo surgical intervention.[14]

SURGICAL

- For melanoma in situ, wide excision with 0.5- to 1.0-cm margins is recommended. For LM, histologic subtype may require larger than 0.5-cm margins to achieve histologically negative margins, because of characteristically broad subclinical extension.[15] SOR A
- Standard therapy is margin-controlled surgical excision with Mohs surgery (only special centers perform Mohs on pigmented lesions) or rush permanent sections.[15] SOR B
- The perimeter technique is a method of margin-controlled excision of LM with rush permanent sections. The main advantage is that all margins are examined with permanent sections. The main drawback is that multiple operative sessions days apart are required to complete the procedure.[16]
- A prospective trial of 1120 patients with melanoma in situ treated by Mohs surgery showed a 99% clearance rate with a 9-mm margin and an 86% clearance rate with 6-mm margins. Consequently, margin-controlled excision of LM is recommended.[15] SOR B
- Cryosurgery may be used in patients who are not good surgical candidates. In a study of 18 such patients with LM, the lesions resolved clinically in all cases, with no recurrence or metastasis detected during a mean follow-up of 75.5 months.[17] SOR C These patients were treated with two freeze–thaw cycles of liquid nitrogen under local anesthesia in a single sitting.

PREVENTION

- Because LMM is related to a lifetime of exposure to UV radiation, patients should limit sun exposure, especially between 10 a.m. and 4 p.m. When in the sun, make sure to wear sunscreen with a high sun-protection factor (SPF) that blocks both UVA and UVB. It's also a good idea to protect skin by wearing a broad-brim hat and clothing that covers your arms and legs.

PROGNOSIS

- There is a 5% estimated lifetime risk of developing LMM in patients diagnosed with LM at age 45 years.[4]

FOLLOW-UP

- The National Comprehensive Cancer Network recommends that patients with a history of LM have regular clinical skin examinations at least yearly by their family physician or a dermatologist with a focus on recurrence, new lesions, and lymph nodes.[15]

PATIENT EDUCATION

- Patients diagnosed with LM need to minimize sun exposure and do regular self-skin examinations.

PATIENT RESOURCES

- MedlinePlus. *Melanoma*—**http://www.nlm.nih.gov/medlineplus/melanoma.html.**

PROVIDER RESOURCES

- DermnetNZ—**https://www.dermnetnz.org/topics/lentigo-maligna-and-lentigo-maligna-melanoma/.**
- Dermoscopy. A website on dermoscopy to learn how to improve early diagnosis of melanoma—**http://www.dermoscopy.org.**

REFERENCES

1. Cohen LM. Lentigo maligna and lentigo maligna melanoma. *J Am Acad Dermatol.* 1995;33(6):923-936.
2. Cox NH, Aitchison TC, Sirel JM, et al. Comparison between lentigo maligna melanoma and other histogenetic types of malignant melanoma of the head and neck. *Br J Cancer.* 1996;73:940-944.
3. Higgins HW, Lee KC, Galan A, et al. Melanoma in situ. Part I. Epidemiology, screening and clinical features. *J Am Acad Dermatol.* 2015;73:181-190.
4. Weinstock MA, Sober AJ. The risk of progression of lentigo maligna to lentigo maligna melanoma. *Br J Dermatol.* 1987; 116(3):303-310.
5. Hawkey S, Affleck A. Diagnosis and management of lentigo maligna: an observational study comparing 2005 with 2014 data in one institution. *Clin Exp Dermatol.* 2017;42:320-323.
6. Schiffner R, Schiffner-Rohe J, Vogt T, et al. Improvement of early recognition of lentigo maligna using dermatoscopy. *J Am Acad Dermatol.* 2000;42(1 Pt 1):25-32.
7. Dalton SR, Gardner TL, Libow LF, Elston DM. Contiguous lesions in lentigo maligna. *J Am Acad Dermatol.* 2005;52:859-862.
8. Wang Y, Zhao Y, Shuangge M. Racial differences in six major subtypes of melanoma: descriptive epidemiology. *BMC Cancer.* 2016:16:691.
9. Tzellos T, Kyrgidis A, Mocellin S, et al. Interventions for melanoma in situ, including lentigo maligna. *Cochrane Database Syst Rev.* 2014;(12):CD010308.
10. Mora AN, Karia PS, Nguyen BM. A quantitative systematic review of the efficacy of imiquimod monotherapy for lentigo maligna and an analysis of factors that affect tumor clearance. *J Am Acad Dermatol.* 2015;73(2):205-212.
11. Gautschi M, Oberholzer PA, Baumgartner M, et al. Prognostic markers in lentigo maligna patients treated with imiquimod cream: a long-term follow-up study. *J Am Acad Dermatol.* 2016; 74(1):81-87.e1.
12. Greveling K, de Vries K, van Doorn MB, Prens EP. A two-stage treatment of lentigo maligna using ablative laser therapy followed by imiquimod: excellent cosmesis, but frequent recurrences on the nose. *Br J Dermatol.* 2016 May;174(5):1134-1136.
13. Kai AC, Richards T, Coleman A, et al. Five-year recurrence rate of lentigo maligna after treatment with imiquimod. *Br J Dermatol.* 2016;174(1):165-168.
14. Fogarty GB, Hong A, Scolyer RA, et al. Radiotherapy for lentigo maligna: a literature review and recommendations for treatment. *Br J Dermatol.* 2014;170(1):52-58.
15. Coit DG, Thompson JA, Albertini MR, et al. NCCN Clinical Practice Guidelines in Oncology: Melanoma. *NCCN Guidelines.* Version 2.2018. 2018.
16. Mahoney MH, Joseph M, Temple CL. The perimeter technique for lentigo maligna: an alternative to Mohs micrographic surgery. *J Surg Oncol.* 2005;91(2):120-125.
17. de Moraes AM, Pavarin LB, Herreros F, et al. Cryosurgical treatment of lentigo maligna. *J Dtsch Dermatol Ges.* 2007;5(6): 477-480.

176 CUTANEOUS HORN

Jonathan B. Karnes, MD

PATIENT STORY

A 90-year-old woman presents with a hard keratotic papule on the right cheek that has grown over 6 months. It is tender to the touch and has a pink base (**Figure 176-1**). A shave biopsy through the base is consistent with a cutaneous horn derived from a well-differentiated squamous cell carcinoma (SCC). The patient undergoes an elliptical excision at the base of the horn in the office for definitive therapy.

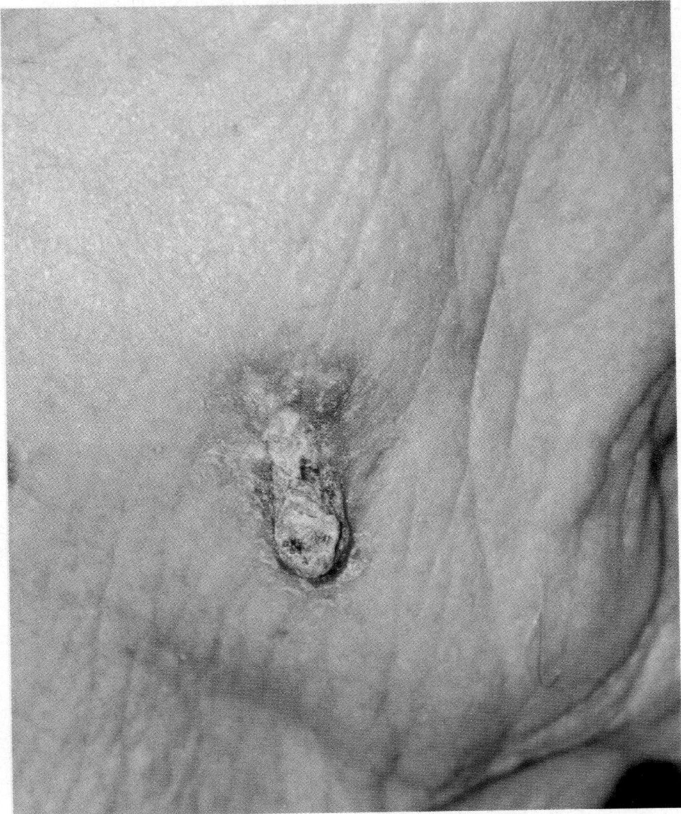

FIGURE 176-1 Cutaneous horn on the right cheek of a 90-year-old woman arising from a well-differentiated squamous cell carcinoma. (*Reproduced with permission from Jonathan B. Karnes, MD.*)

INTRODUCTION

Cutaneous horn is the descriptive morphologic term given to firm keratotic papules that arise from various benign and malignant underlying pathologies and have an appearance similar to an animal horn.

EPIDEMIOLOGY

- Cutaneous horns are found in both men and women, most commonly in white patients older than 50. The head, neck, and upper extremities are the most common location, following patterns of sun damage.[1]

ETIOLOGY AND PATHOPHYSIOLOGY

- Multiple benign, premalignant, and malignant causes including wart, seborrheic keratosis, actinic keratosis, Bowen disease, and squamous cell carcinoma lead to a final common pathway of retained stratum corneum rich with the keratin responsible for the firm hornlike quality.
- A large case series demonstrated premalignant or malignant causes in 39% of cases.[2]
- Likelihood of underlying malignancy increases with patient age and location on sun-damaged skin.[1]
- Associated with many types of skin neoplasms that can retain keratin and produce horns including actinic keratosis, warts (**Figures 176-4 to 176-6**), seborrheic keratosis (**Figure 176-7**), keratoacanthoma (**Figure 176-3**), sebaceous gland, and basal or squamous cell carcinoma (**Figures 176-1 to 176-3, 176-8**). In a case series, actinic keratosis was found in 83.8% of the premalignant cases and squamous cell carcinoma was found in 93.75% of the malignant cases.[3]
- Rare cases have been described in association with metastatic renal cell carcinoma, lymphoma, dermatofibroma, pyogenic granuloma (**Figure 176-9**), Kaposi sarcoma, and melanoma.[4,5]

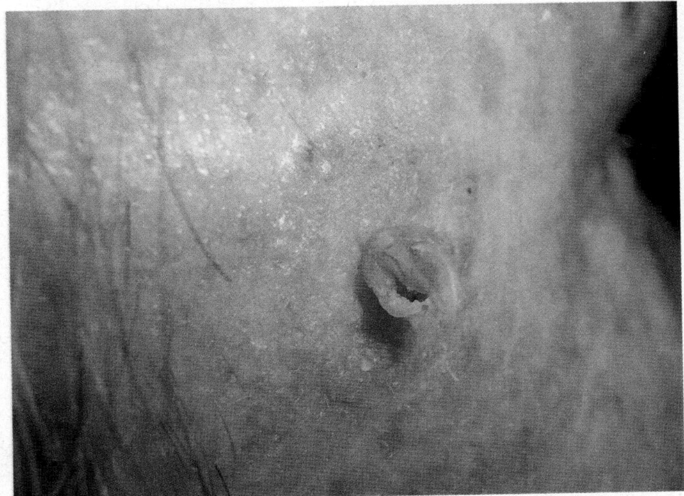

FIGURE 176-2 Cutaneous horn in a squamous cell carcinoma in situ just lateral to the eye. (*Reprodued with permission from Richard P. Usatine, MD*)

RISK FACTORS

- Advanced age (>70 years).
- Sun/radiation exposure.

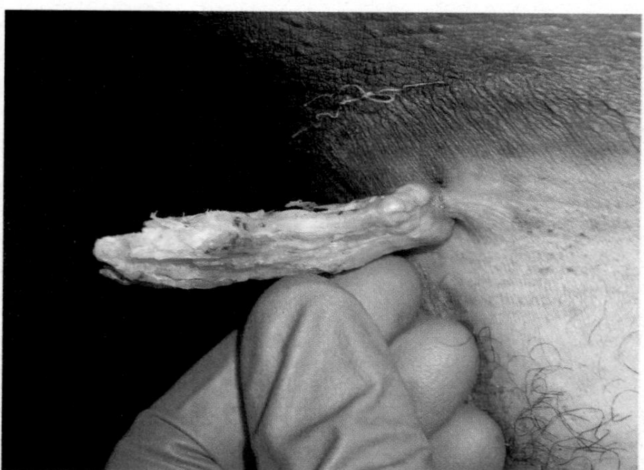

FIGURE 176-3 Cutaneous horn on the neck of a 43-year-old black man, which grew over several years. The pathologist first read it as a verruca with cutaneous horn, but when it was reviewed by the dermatopathologist the diagnosis was changed to keratoacanthoma with cutaneous horn. (*Reproduced with permission from Richard P. Usatine, MD.*)

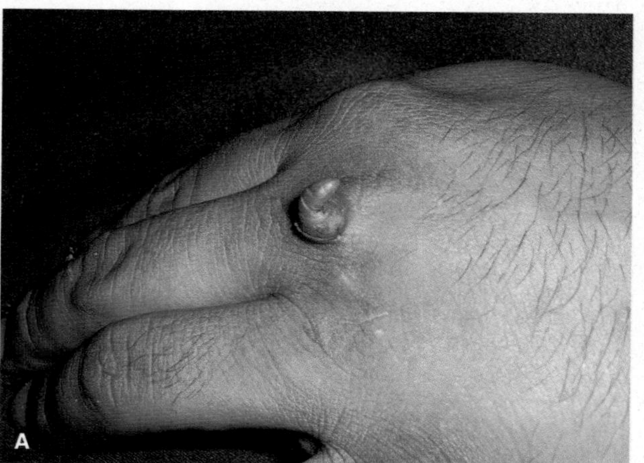

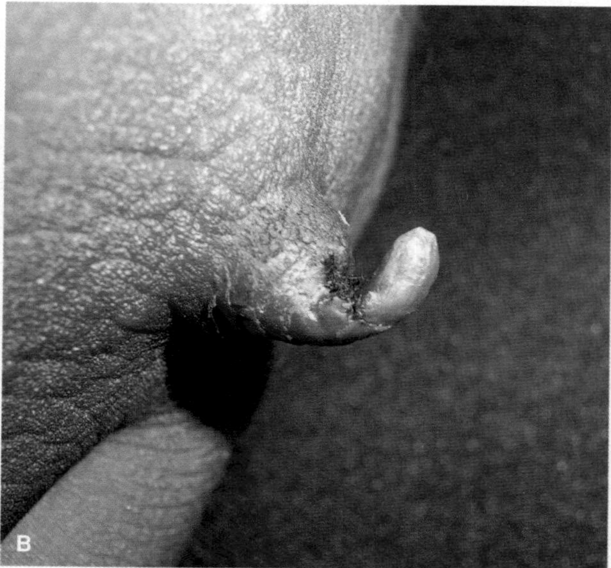

FIGURE 176-4 **A.** Cutaneous horn on the hand of a 33-year-old man for 8 years. He clipped it with nail clippers many times, but it always grew back. A shave excision successfully removed it and the pathology showed a viral wart at the base. **B.** Close-up of the cutaneous horn. (*Reproduced with permission from Richard P. Usatine, MD.*)

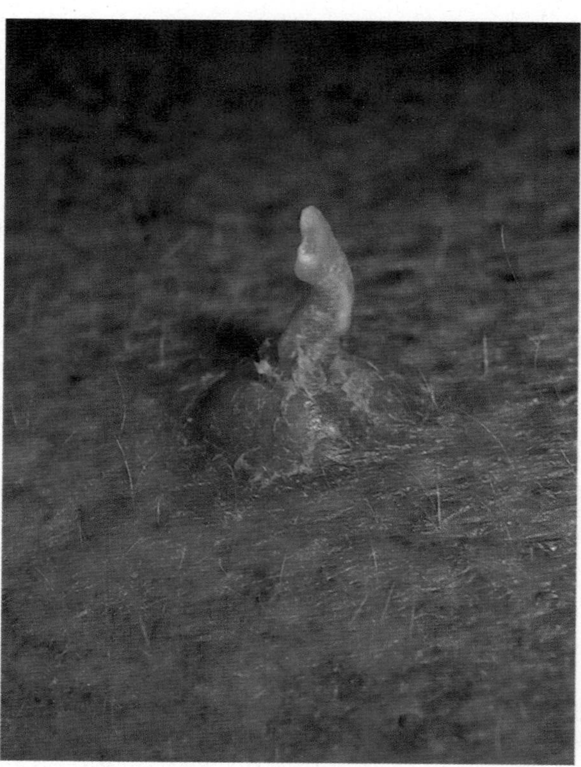

FIGURE 176-5 Cutaneous horn on the back of a 73-year-old woman within an endophytic wart. (*Reproduced with permission from Richard P. Usatine, MD.*)

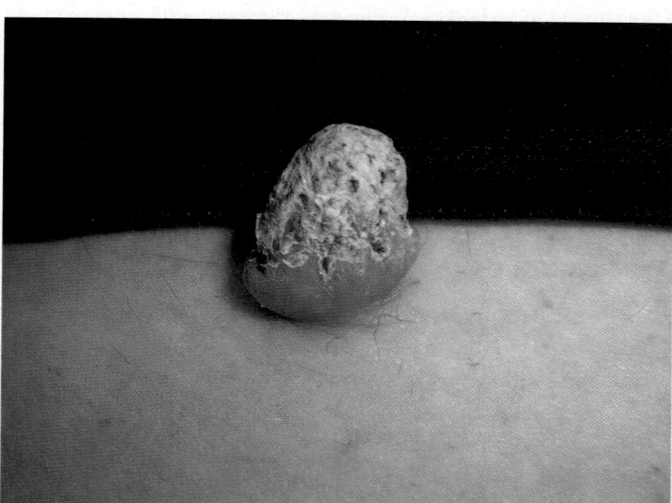

FIGURE 176-6 Cutaneous horn with a biopsy-proven wart at the base. (*Reproduced with permission from Richard P. Usatine, MD.*)

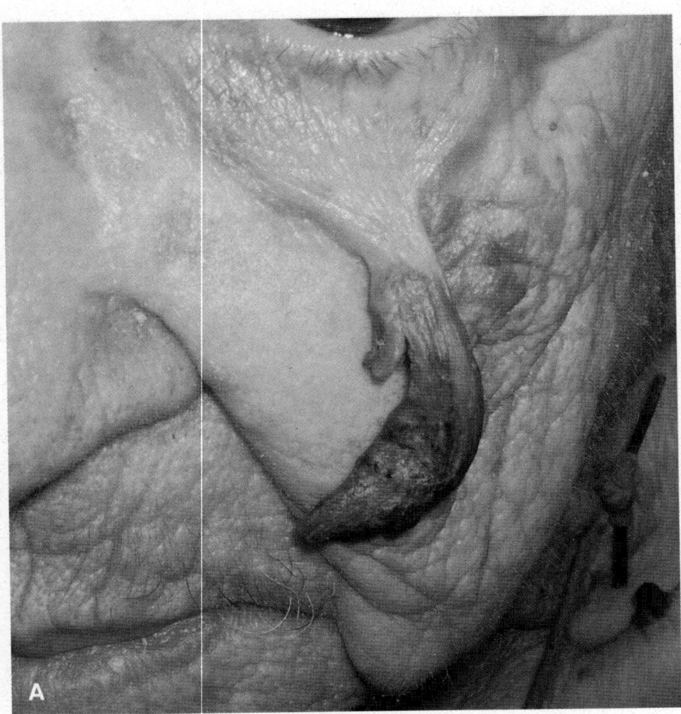

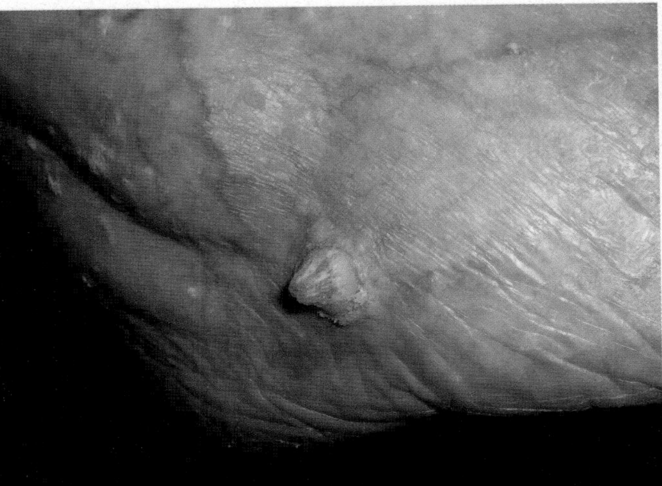

FIGURE 176-8 Cutaneous horn arising in a well-differentiated SCC on the foot. This 65-year-old woman has had multiple SCCs related to her immunosuppressive medication to prevent renal transplant rejection. (*Reproduced with permission from Richard P. Usatine, MD.*)

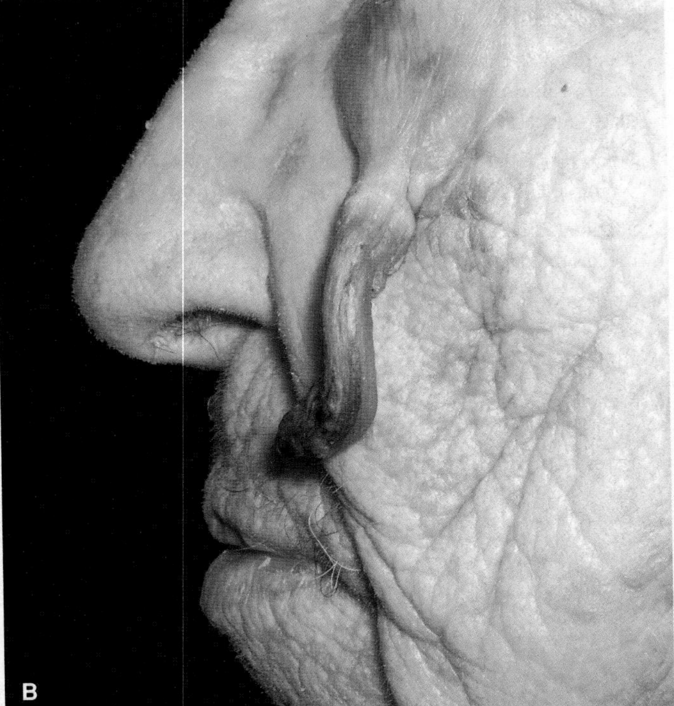

FIGURE 176-7 **A.** Large cutaneous horn on the face of an 88-year-old woman. After shave removal, the pathology showed seborrheic keratosis with chronic inflammation and cutaneous horn formation. **B.** Another view of this amazing cutaneous horn. The patient had had the lesion since her early 30s and attributed it to hot grease popping on her face. She had shown it to other physicians who declined to remove it. Patient stated it "made her feel 16 again" to have it removed. (*Reproduced with permission from Scott Bergeaux, MD.*)

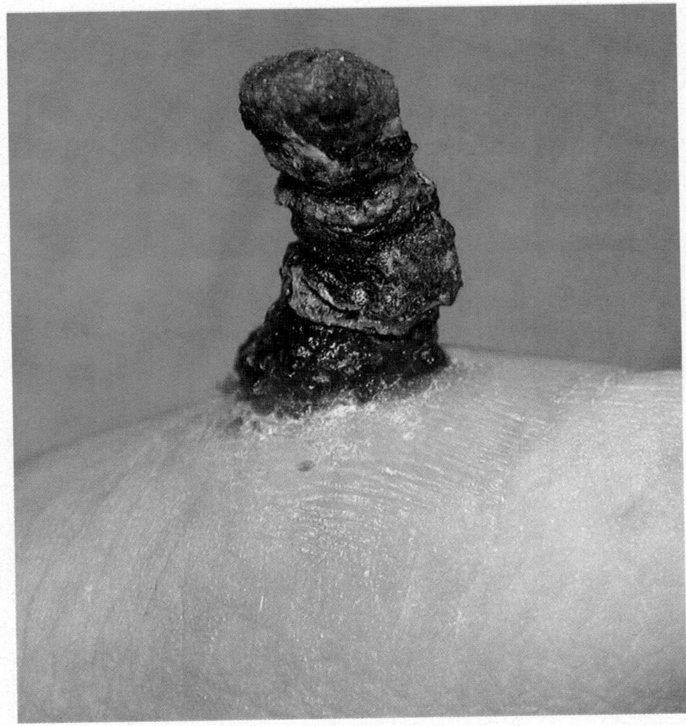

FIGURE 176-9 Cutaneous horn arising in a pyogenic granuloma. (*Reproduced with permission from Suraj Reddy, MD.*)

DIAGNOSIS

CLINICAL FEATURES

- Hornlike protuberance.
- Lesions are usually firm; have been described as flat, keratotic, nodular, pedunculated, and ulcerated.[2]
- Size may vary from a few millimeters to several centimeters; gigantic cutaneous horns (17 to 25 cm length and up to 2.5 cm width) have been reported, and in one series of 4 cases, all were benign.[6]
- Because of their height, cutaneous horns may be traumatized, causing bleeding or pain.

TYPICAL DISTRIBUTION

- May occur on any area of the body; approximately 30% are found on the face (see **Figures 176-2**, **176-6**, and **176-7**) and scalp and another 30% on the upper limbs.[3]

BIOPSY

- A scoop shave (deep shave) adequately deep to sample the underlying tissue is diagnostic (see Chapter 113, Biopsy Principles and Techniques). The horn material alone is insufficient, and too superficial a biopsy will be both challenging and nondiagnostic.

DIFFERENTIAL DIAGNOSIS

- Common warts are well-demarcated, rough, hard papules with an irregular papillary surface. Although they may form cylindrical projections, these often fuse to form a surface mosaic pattern; paring the surface exposes punctate hemorrhagic capillaries (see Chapter 137, Common Warts).

MANAGEMENT

- Management depends on the underlying etiology. An underlying wart may be treated with liquid nitrogen or simply observed, whereas an underlying malignancy frequently requires excision according to standard practices for tumor type and location.

FOLLOW-UP

- Routine follow-up is not needed, provided complete removal is accomplished for malignant and premalignant lesions; in one case series of 48 eyelid cutaneous horns, there was no recurrence over a mean of 21 months.[7]
- Patients with underlying skin cancer should be seen for skin surveillance in accordance with the underlying diagnosis. SOR C

PATIENT AND PROVIDER RESOURCES

- **http://emedicine.medscape.com/article/1056568-overview.**
- **https://www.dermnetnz.org/topics/cutaneous-horn/.**

REFERENCES

1. Phulari RG, Rathore R, Talegaon TP, et al. Cutaneous horn: a mask to underlying malignancy. *J Oral Maxillofac Pathol.* 2018;22:S87-S90.
2. Yu RC, Pryce DW, Macfarlane AW, Stewart TW. A histopathological study of 643 cutaneous horns. *Br J Dermatol.* 1991;124:499-452.
3. Mantese SA, Diogo PM, Rocha A, et al. Cutaneous horn: a retrospective histopathological study of 222 cases. *An Bras Dermatol.* 2010;85(2):157-163.
4. Onak KN, Gun BD, Barut F, et al. Cutaneous horn-related Kaposi's sarcoma: a case report. *Case Report Med.* 2010;2010. pii: 825949.
5. Nishida H, Daa T, Kashima K, et al. Cutaneous horn malignant melanoma. *Dermatol Rep.* 2013;5(1):e3.
6. Michal M, Bisceglia M, Di Mattia A, et al. Gigantic cutaneous horns of the scalp: lesions with a gross similarity to the horns of animals: a report of four cases. *Am J Surg Pathol.* 2002;26:789-794.
7. Mencia-Gutiérrez E, Gutiérrez-Diaz E, Redondo-Marcos I, et al. Cutaneous horns of the eyelid: clinicopathological study of 48 cases. *J Cutan Pathol.* 2004;31:539-543.

SECTION M SKIN CANCER

177 BASAL CELL CARCINOMA

Jonathan B. Karnes, MD
Richard P. Usatine, MD

PATIENT STORY

A 70-year-old man presented with a small ulcer on the nasal tip that he noticed while washing his face. The lesion bled easily, and on occasion the bleeding was hard to stop (**Figure 177-1**). He noticed it first about 6 months ago, and at times it seemed to almost heal. A photograph was taken to document the location of the lesion. Histology from a shave biopsy confirmed an infiltrative basal cell carcinoma (BCC), and he was referred for Mohs microsurgery for excellent margin control.

FIGURE 177-1 Ulcer on the nasal tip is the most obvious warning sign for this infiltrative BCC. (*Reproduced with permission from Richard P. Usatine, MD.*)

INTRODUCTION

Basal cell carcinoma is the most common cancer in humans. Usually found on the head and neck, it tends to grow slowly and almost never kills or metastasizes when treated in a timely fashion. However, the treatment necessary is often surgical, and this may cause scarring and changes in function.

EPIDEMIOLOGY

- BCC is the most common skin cancer, with more than 2 million cases diagnosed annually.[1]
- Incidence increases with age, related to cumulative sun exposure.
- Nodular BCCs—Most common type (70%) (**Figures 177-2** to **177-4**).
- Superficial BCCs—Next most common type (**Figures 177-5** and **177-6**).
- Sclerosing (or morpheaform) BCCs—The least common type (**Figures 177-1, 177-7** and **177-8**).

Other clinical variants including pigmented, polypoid, giant, keloidal, linear, and fibroepithelioma of Pinkus have been recognized, but are less common to very rare.[2]

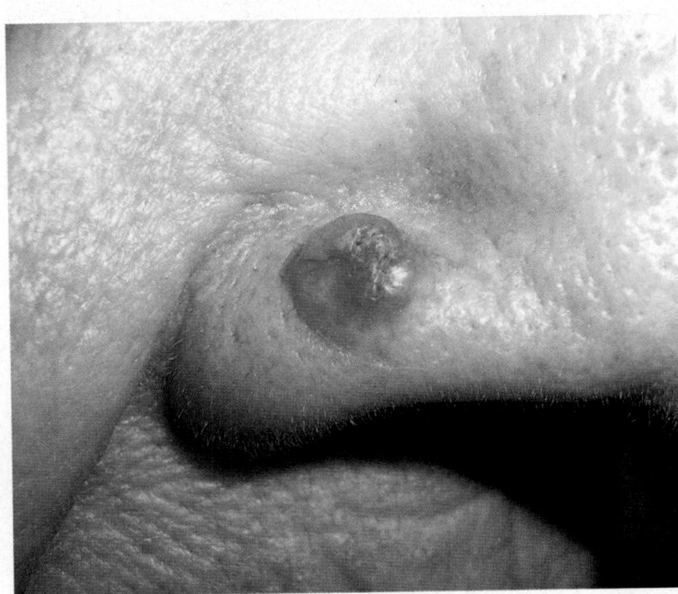

FIGURE 177-2 Nodular BCC on the nasal ala of an 82-year-old woman. The nose is a very common location for a basal cell carcinoma. (*Reproduced with permission from Richard P. Usatine, MD.*)

ETIOLOGY AND PATHOPHYSIOLOGY

- BCCs spread locally and very rarely metastasize.
- Basal cell nevus syndrome, also known as Gorlin syndrome, is a rare autosomal dominant condition in which affected individuals have multiple BCCs that may clinically mimic nevi (**Figure 177-9**).

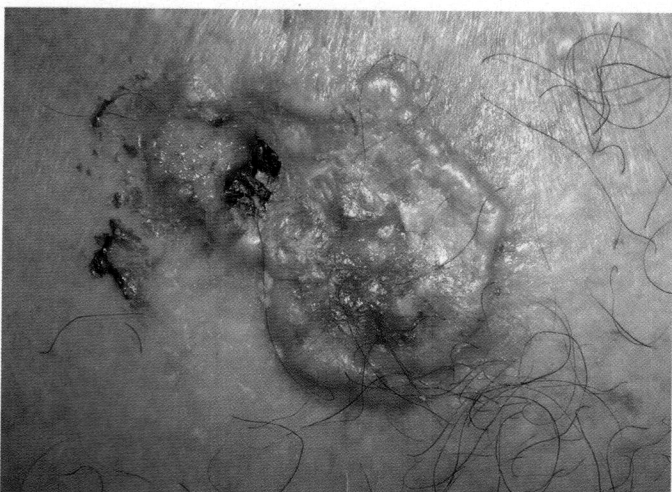

FIGURE 177-3 Large ulcerated nodular BCC on the mid-chest of a homeless man. The authors excised this in a free clinic located in a church basement. (*Reproduced with permission from Richard P. Usatine, MD.*)

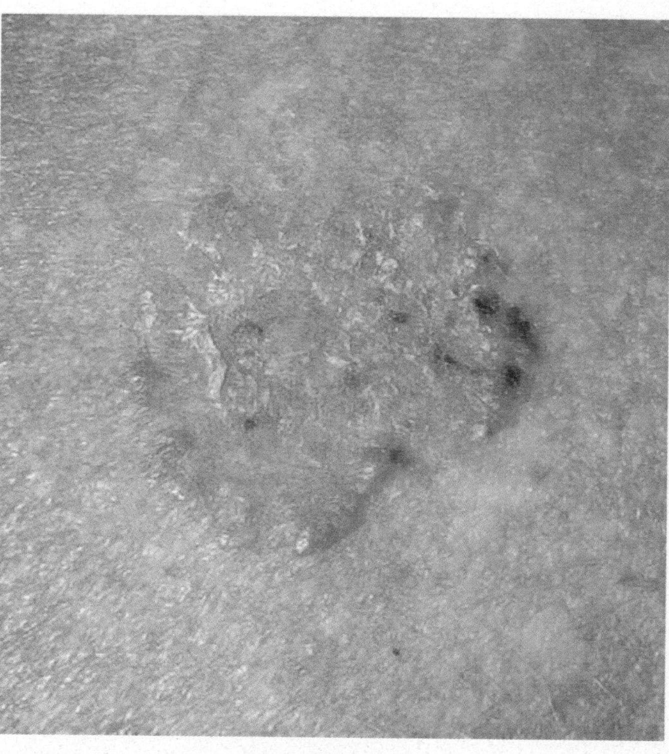

FIGURE 177-5 Superficial basal cell carcinoma on the back of a 45-year-old man who enjoys running in the California sun without his shirt. Note the diffuse scaling, thready border (slightly raised and pearly), and spotty hyperpigmentation on the edges. (*Reproduced with permission from Richard P. Usatine, MD.*)

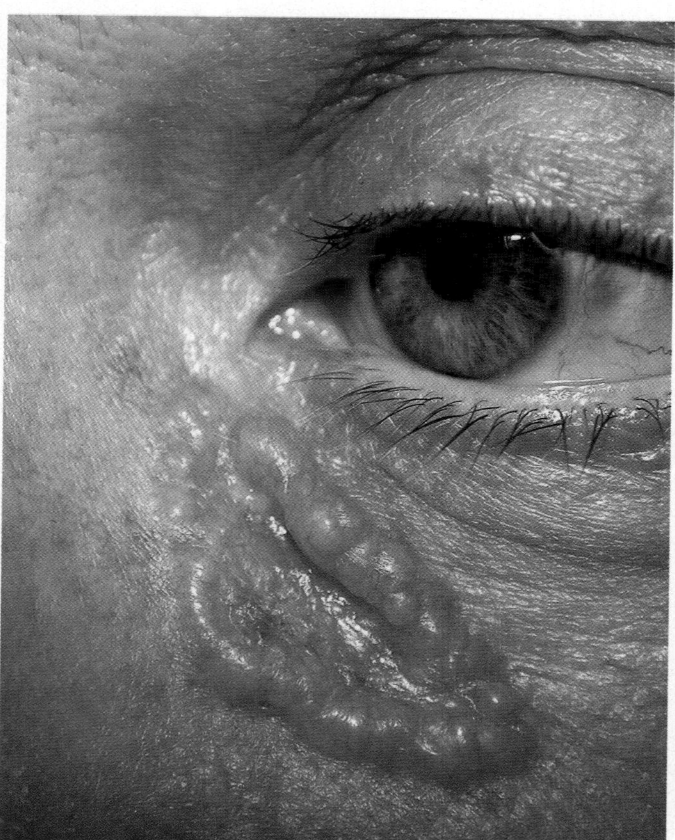

FIGURE 177-4 Large nodular basal cell carcinoma with an annular appearance on the face of a homeless woman. (*Reproduced with permission from Richard P. Usatine, MD.*)

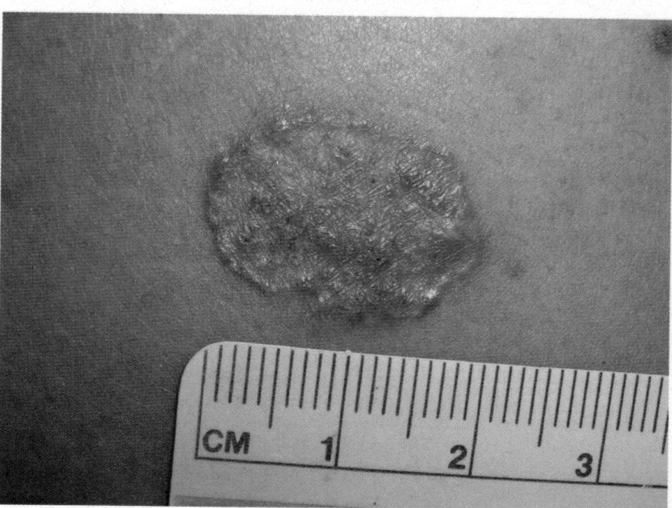

FIGURE 177-6 Large superficial BCC located on the back. Note the thready pearly border and small areas of pigmentation—both common features in superficial BCCs. (*Reproduced with permission from Richard P. Usatine, MD.*)

RISK FACTORS

- Advanced age.
- Cumulative sun exposure.
- Radiation exposure.
- Latitude.
- Immunosuppression.
- Genetic predisposition.
- Family history.
- Skin type.[3]

DIAGNOSIS

CLINICAL FEATURES

Common clinical features of the three most common morphologic types are listed below.

▶ Nodular BCC

- Raised pearly pink to white papule, often with telangiectasias.
- Smooth translucent surface with loss of the normal pore pattern (**Figures 177-2** to **177-4**).
- May be moderately to deeply pigmented (**Figures 177-10** to **177-12**).
- May ulcerate (**Figures 177-1, 177-3, 177-6, 177-13** to **177-16**) and leave a bloody crust.
- Micronodular types grow deeper and are more aggressive.

▶ Superficial BCC

- Red or pink patches to plaques often with mild scale and a thready border (slightly raised and pearly) (see **Figure 177-5**).
- More commonly on the trunk and upper extremities than the face.

▶ Sclerosing (morpheaform) and infiltrating (infiltrative) BCCs

- Ivory or colorless, flat or atrophic, indurated, may resemble scars (see **Figures 177-7** and **177-8**).
- Called morpheaform because of their resemblance to localized scleroderma (morphea).
- The border is not well defined and tumor may extend far beyond the clinical border (**Figure 177-17**).
- Infiltrating BCCs are also aggressive but may not appear morpheaform.
- These BCCs are the most dangerous and have the worst prognosis.

TYPICAL DISTRIBUTION

Most appear on face, ears, and head, with some found on the trunk and upper extremities (especially the superficial type).

Some may occur in relatively sun-protected areas.

Recently lesions on the ears have been associated with a more aggressive behavior (**Figure 177-18**).[4]

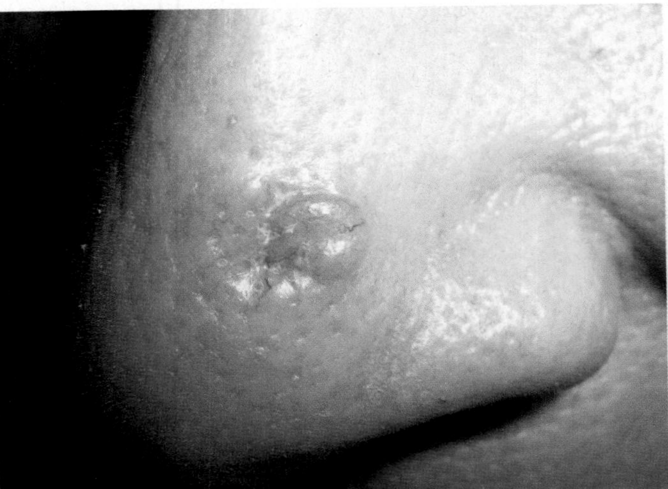

FIGURE 177-7 Sclerosing BCC on the nose. Note the ivory white tumor that extends beyond the pearly pink segment. This took 4 stages of Mohs surgery to remove. *(Reproduced with permission from Richard P. Usatine, MD.)*

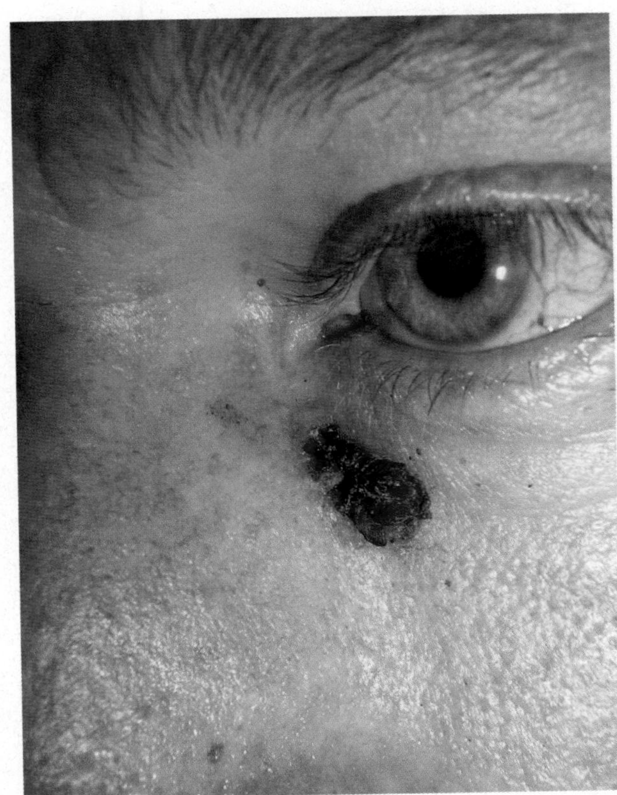

FIGURE 177-8 Sclerosing and infiltrative basal cell carcinoma in a 45-year-old man diagnosed with a shave biopsy. The patient was sent for Mohs surgery because the BCC was aggressive and encroaching on the lower eyelid. *(Reproduced with permission from Richard P. Usatine, MD.)*

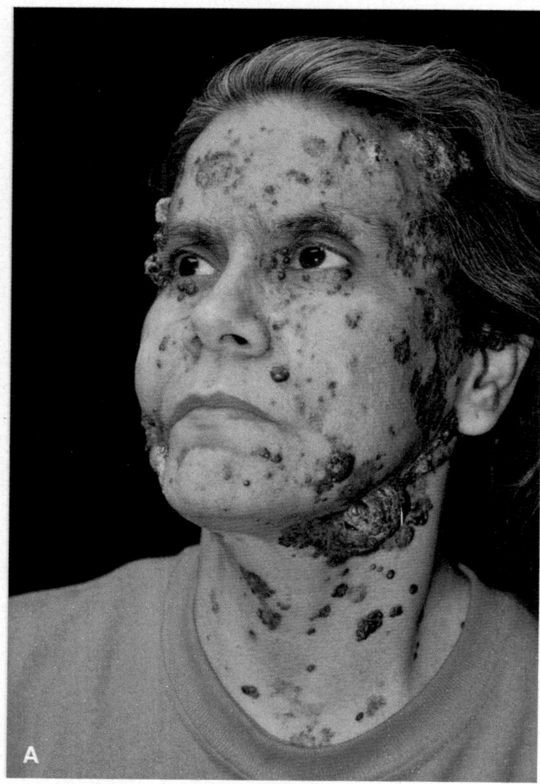

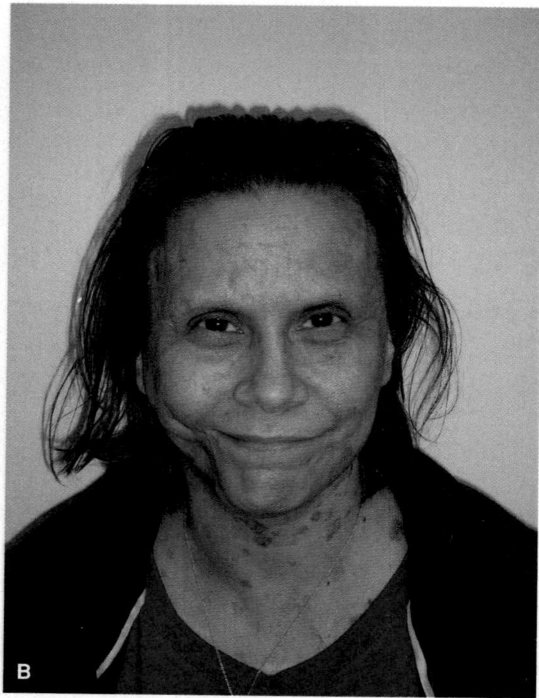

FIGURE 177-9 **A.** Basal cell nevus syndrome with multiple pigmented basal cell carcinomas on the face and neck before vismodegib. **B.** After being on vismodegib for 4 years. (*Reproduced with permission from Richard P. Usatine, MD.*)

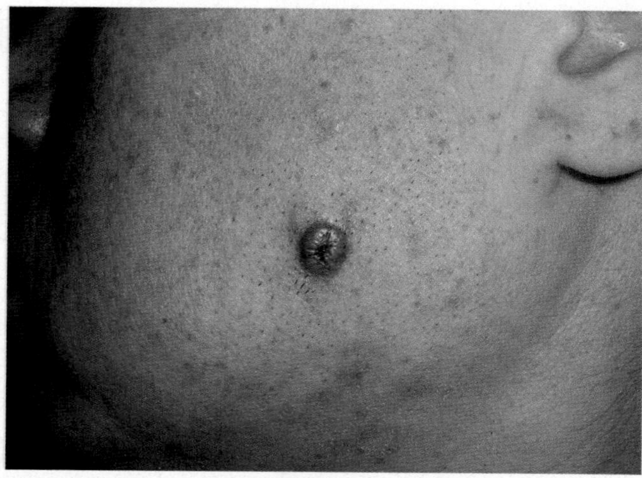

FIGURE 177-10 Pigmented nodular basal cell carcinoma on the face with ulceration mimicking melanoma in a 37-year-old HIV-positive man. (*Reproduced with permission from Richard P. Usatine, MD.*)

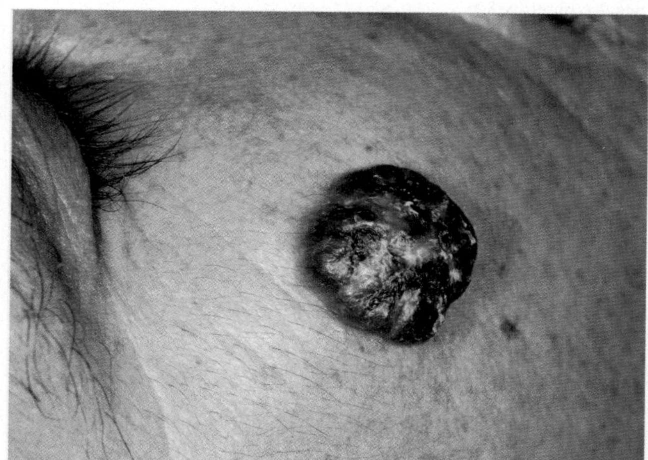

FIGURE 177-11 Darkly pigmented large basal cell carcinoma with raised borders and some ulceration in a 53-year-old Hispanic man. A biopsy was performed to rule out melanoma before this was excised. (*Reproduced with permission from Richard P. Usatine, MD.*)

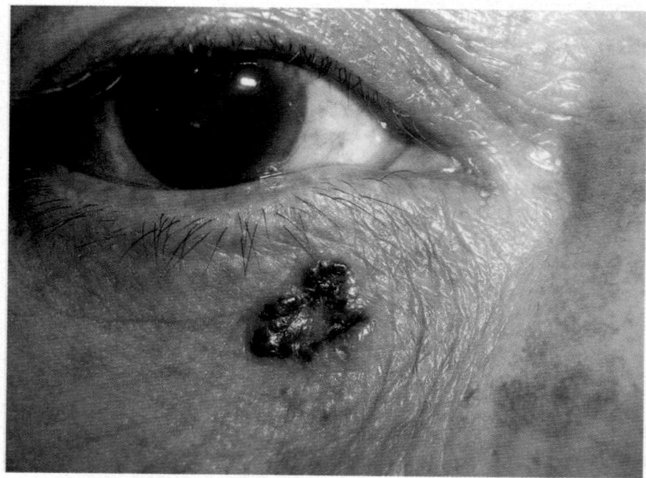

FIGURE 177-12 Darkly pigmented basal cell carcinoma with pearly surface on the lower eyelid. (*Reproduced with permission from Richard P. Usatine, MD.*)

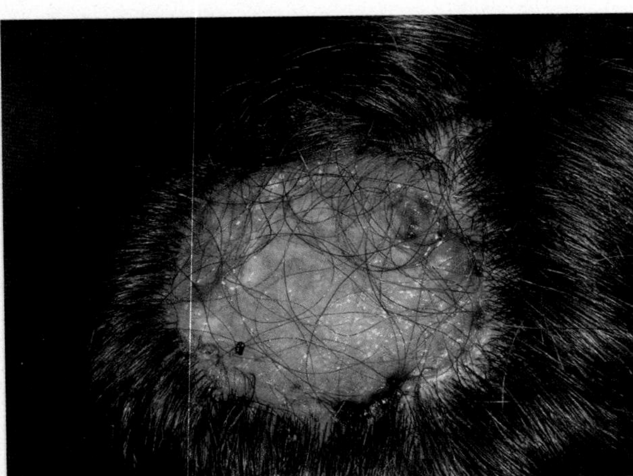

FIGURE 177-13 Ulcerated basal cell carcinoma on the scalp of a 35-year-old woman. (*Reproduced with permission from Richard P. Usatine, MD.*)

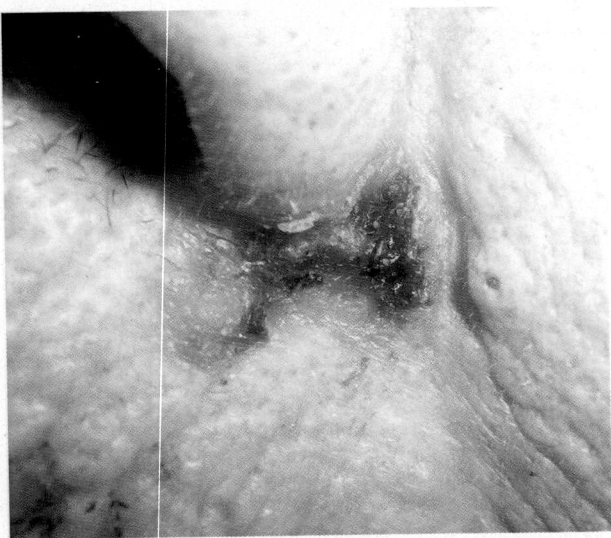

FIGURE 177-14 Basal cell carcinoma in the nasal alar groove. There is a high risk of recurrence at this site, so Mohs surgery is indicated for removal. (*Reproduced with permission from Richard P. Usatine, MD.*)

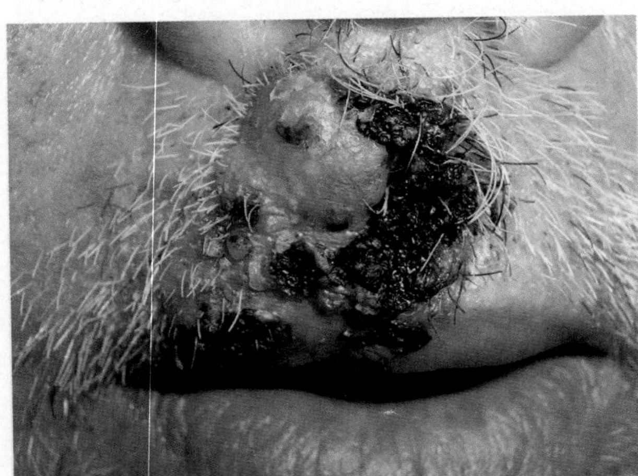

FIGURE 177-15 Large advanced basal cell carcinoma with ulcerations and bloody crusting infiltrating the upper lip. The patient was referred for Mohs surgery. (*Reproduced with permission from Richard P. Usatine, MD.*)

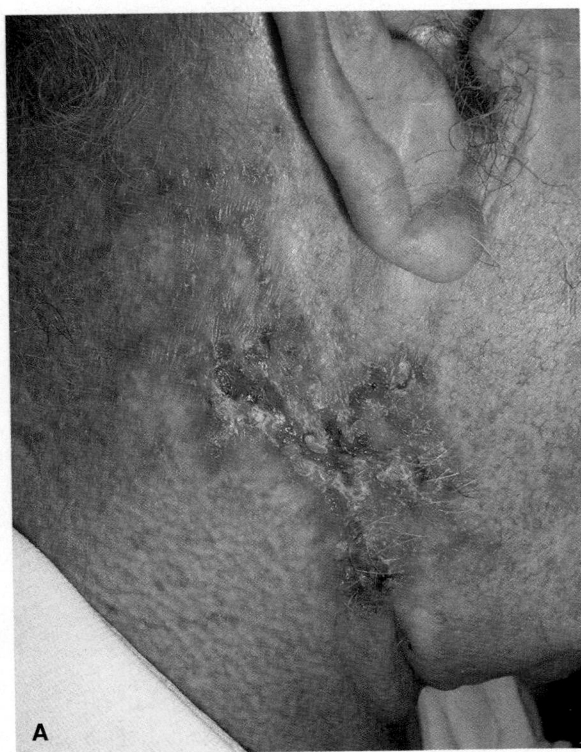

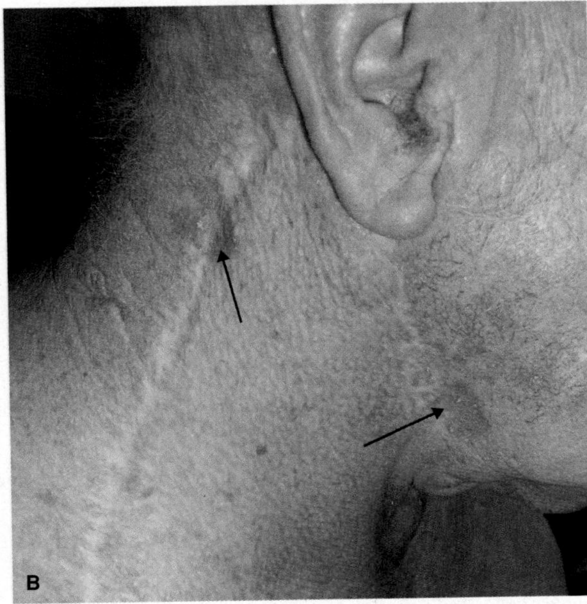

FIGURE 177-16 **A.** Very large ulcerating basal cell carcinoma on the neck of a 65-year-old white man, which has been growing there for 6 years. It was excised in the operating room with a large flap from his chest used to close the big defect. **B.** The same man showing recurrence within the scar a few years later. (*Reproduced with permission from Richard P. Usatine, MD.*)

DERMOSCOPY

Common dermoscopic characteristics of BCCs (**Figures 177-19** and **177-20**) include:

- Arborizing "treelike" telangiectasias.
- Leaf-like areas.
- Brown dots in focus.
- Shiny white structures (see Chapter 181, Advanced Dermoscopy of Skin Cancer).

BIOPSY

- A shave biopsy is adequate to diagnose a nodular BCC or a superficial BCC.
- A deeper scoop shave or punch biopsy is preferred if a sclerosing BCC is suspected.
- In some instances, excision at the time of definitive treatment reveals a different morphologic type in deeper tissue.[5]

DIFFERENTIAL DIAGNOSIS

▶ Nodular BCC

- Intradermal (dermal) nevi may look very similar to nodular BCCs with telangiectasias and smooth pearly borders (**Figure 177-21**). A history of stable size and lack of ulceration may be helpful in distinguishing them from a nodular BCC. A simple shave biopsy is diagnostic and produces a good cosmetic result. Excisional biopsy is usually unnecessary. It is remarkable how similar **Figure 177-21** may appear to a small nodular BCC (see Chapter 168, Benign Nevi).
- Sebaceous hyperplasia is a benign adnexal tumor common on the face in adults and usually presents with multiple lesions (**Figure 177-22**). These are characterized as small waxy yellow to pink papules with telangiectasias. Dermoscopy may show vessels that radiate out from the center like spokes on a wheel and a central dell (see Chapter 165, Sebaceous Hyperplasia).
- Fibrous papule of the face is a benign condition with small papules that can be firm, vascular, and smooth.
- Trichoepitheliomas/trichoblastomas/trichilemmomas are benign tumors of the midface. They may lack vascular markings. These are best diagnosed with a shave biopsy, but trichoepitheliomas can even mimic a BCC on histology.
- Keratoacanthoma is a type of squamous cell carcinoma that is raised, nodular, and may be pearly with telangiectasias. A central keratin-filled crater or horn may help to distinguish this from a BCC (see Chapter 174, Keratoacanthoma).

▶ Superficial BCC

- Actinic keratoses are precancers that are generally flat, pink, and scaly. They lack the pearly or thready border of the superficial BCC (see Chapter 173, Actinic Keratosis and Bowen Disease).
- Bowen disease is a squamous cell carcinoma in situ that appears like a larger and thicker actinic keratosis. It lacks the pearly and thready border of the superficial BCC (see Chapter 173, Actinic Keratosis and Bowen Disease).

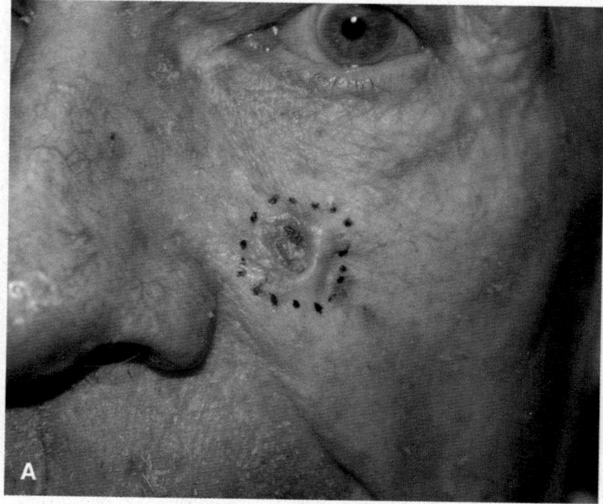

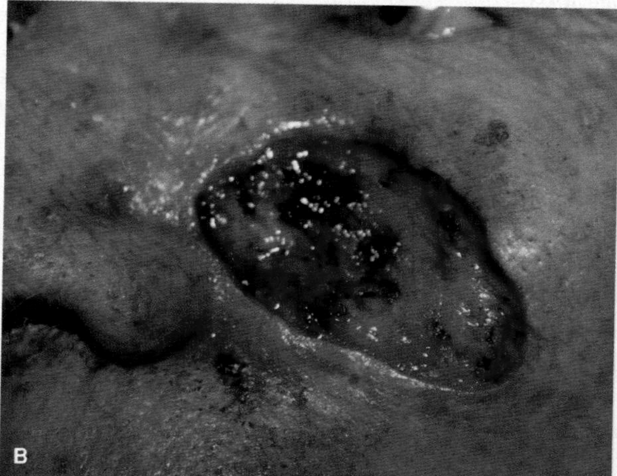

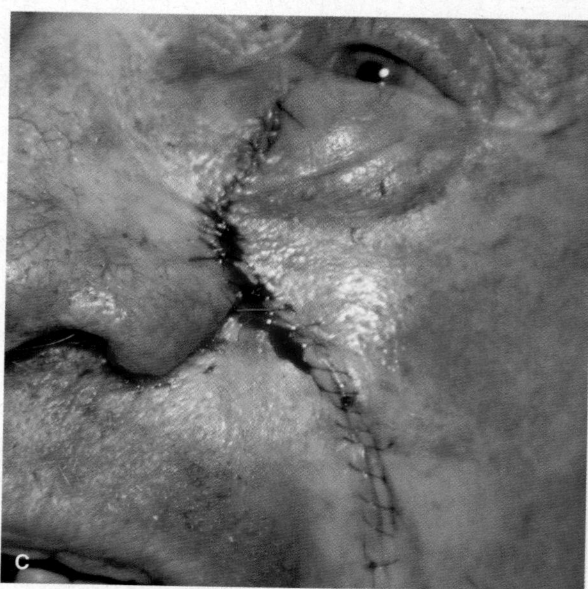

FIGURE 177-17 **A.** Sclerosing basal cell carcinoma in an elderly man. The size of the basal cell carcinoma did not appear large by clinical examination. **B.** Mohs surgery of the same sclerosing basal cell carcinoma. This took four excisions to get clean margins. Usual 4- to 5-mm margins with an elliptical excision would not have removed the full tumor. **C.** Repair by Mohs surgery to close the large defect. The cure rate should be close to 99%. *(Reproduced with permission from Ryan O'Quinn, MD.)*

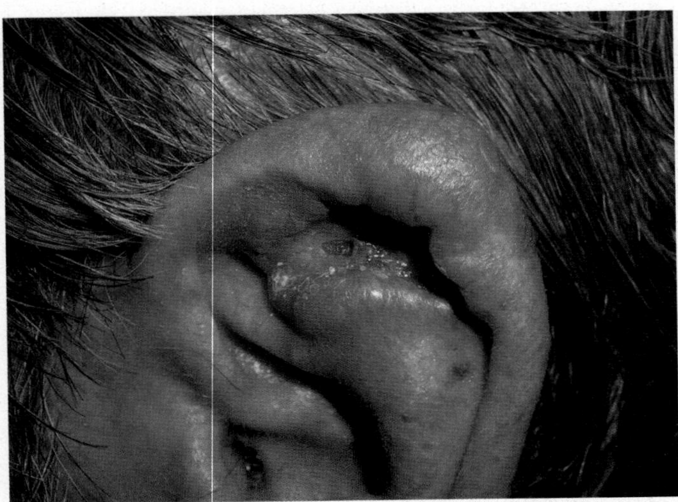

FIGURE 177-18 Ulcerated nodular basal cell carcinoma of the ear in a 67-year-old man. These may have more aggressive behavior. (*Reproduced with permission from Richard P. Usatine, MD.*)

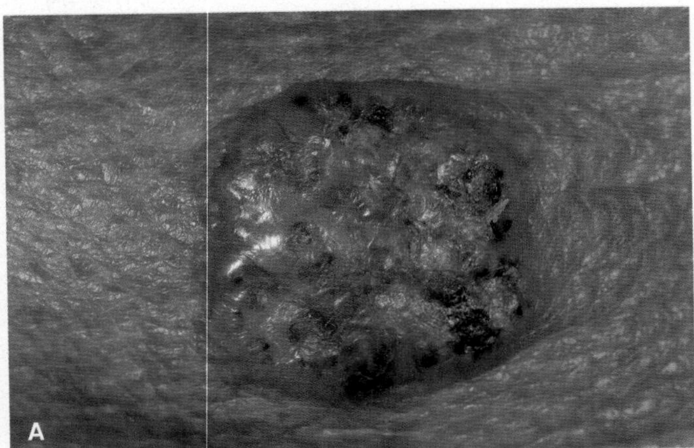

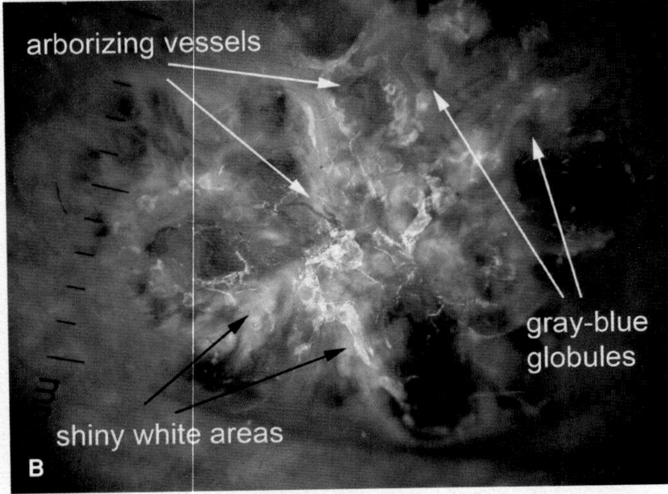

FIGURE 177-19 A. Large nodular basal cell carcinoma on the cheek of a 52-year-old man. There is a loss of normal pore pattern, pearly appearance, telangiectasias, and some areas of dark pigmentation. B. Dermoscopy of the nodular basal cell carcinoma. There are visible arborizing "treelike" telangiectasias, ulcerations, shiny white areas, and gray-blue globules, all consistent with a basal cell carcinoma. (*Reproduced with permission from Richard P. Usatine, MD.*)

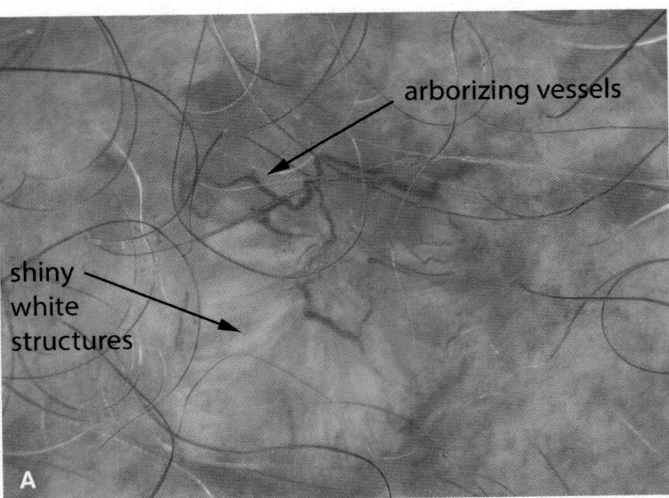

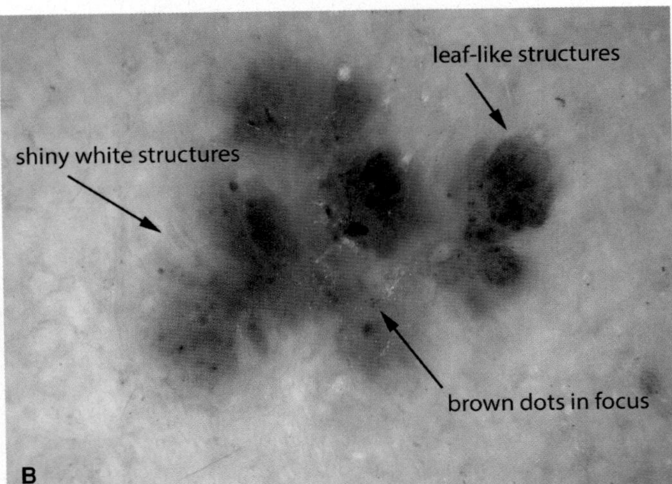

FIGURE 177-20 Dermoscopy of two different basal cell carcinomas. A. Characteristic findings of nodular nonpigmented basal cell carcinomas include arborizing vessels and shiny white structures. B. This pigmented BCC also shows leaflike structures and brown dots in focus. (*Reproduced with permission from Richard P. Usatine, MD.*)

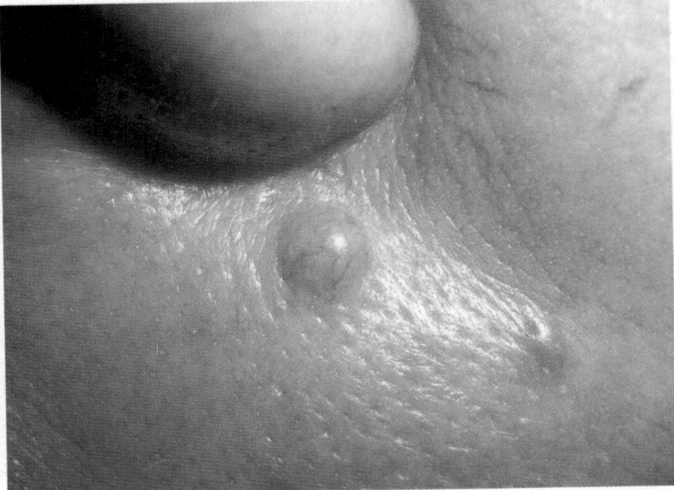

FIGURE 177-21 Pearly dome-shaped intradermal nevus near the nose with telangiectasias closely resembling a basal cell carcinoma. A shave biopsy proved that this was an intradermal nevus. (*Reproduced with permission from Richard P. Usatine, MD.*)

- Nummular eczema can usually be distinguished by its multiple coin-like shapes, transient nature, and rapid response to potent topical steroids. These lesions are pruritic, and most patients will have other signs and symptoms of atopy (see Chapter 151, Atopic Dermatitis).

▶ Sclerosing (morpheaform) and infiltrating (infiltrative) BCC

- Scars may look like a sclerosing BCC. Ask about previous trauma to the area. If the so-called scar is flat, shiny, and enlarging, a biopsy may be needed to rule out a sclerosing BCC.
- Infiltrating BCCs may appear as nonhealing ulcers with bloody crusts. Any nonhealing ulcer on the face or other sun-exposed areas should be biopsied to rule out skin cancer.

MANAGEMENT

- Mohs micrographic surgery (3 studies, $n = 2660$) is the gold standard but is not needed for all BCCs. Recurrence rate is 0.8% to 1.1% (see **Figure 177-17B**). Mohs micrographic surgery (pioneered by Dr. Frederick Mohs) involves surgical removal of tumors near the clinical margin with immediate histologic processing in sequential horizontal layers preserving a continuous peripheral margin that is mapped to the clinical lesion. Gradually larger surgical margins are taken until all margins are clear (see **Figure 177-17**). This is the treatment of choice for large and recurrent BCCs as well as those with poorly defined clinical margins or in areas of significant cosmetic or functional importance such as the face.[6] SOR Ⓐ
- A clinical photograph locating the lesion at the time of biopsy eliminates wrong-site surgery, which is a risk when the surgeon performing the definitive procedure is different from the physician performing the biopsy. A study of 271 surgical sites referred to a Mohs clinic showed that the physician and patient incorrectly identified the biopsy site 4.4% of the time when a clinical photograph was not available.[7]
- Surgical excision of small (<2 cm) nodular and superficial BCCs results in clearance rates of 85% with 3-mm margins and 95% with 5-mm margins.[8] However, with morpheaform BCCs, the cure rate drops to 66% with 3-mm margins, 82% with 4- to 5-mm margins, and >95% with 13- to 15-mm margins, emphasizing the importance of a biopsy prior to definitive treatment.[8] SOR Ⓐ
- Cryosurgery (4 studies, $n = 796$)—Recurrence rate was 3.0% to 4.3%. Cumulative 5-year recurrence rate (3 studies) ranged from 0% to 16.5%.[6] SOR Ⓐ Recommended freeze times are 30 to 60 seconds with a 5-mm halo. This can be divided up into two 30-second freezes with a thaw in between. For such long freeze times, most patients will prefer a local anesthetic (**Figure 177-23**). SOR Ⓒ
- Curettage and desiccation (6 studies, $n = 4212$): Recurrence rate ranged from 4.3% to 18.1%; cumulative 5-year rate ranged from 5.7% to 18.8%. Three cycles of curettage and desiccation can produce higher cure rates than one cycle (**Figure 177-24**).[6] SOR Ⓐ
- Imiquimod is approved by the U.S. Food and Drug Administration (FDA) for the treatment of superficial BCCs less than 2 cm in diameter.[9] SOR Ⓑ Confirm diagnosis with biopsy and use when surgical methods are contraindicated. A recent small study combining cryotherapy with imiquimod improved the recurrence rate.[10]

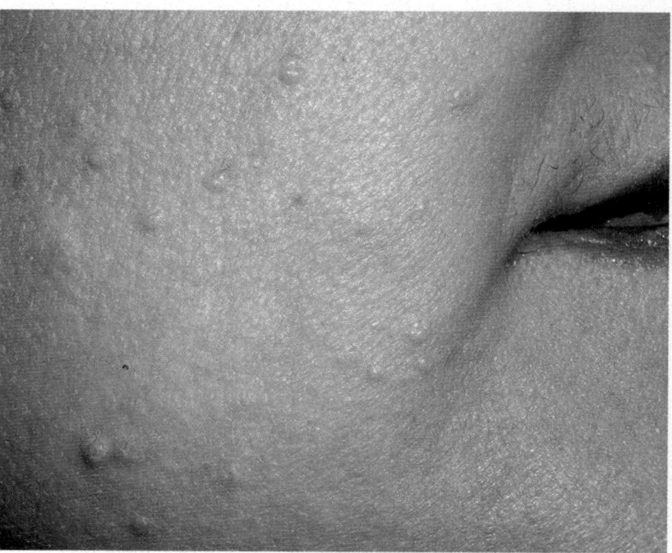

FIGURE 177-22 Extensive sebaceous hyperplasia on the cheek of a 52-year-old woman. The largest one has visible telangiectasias and could be mistaken for a basal cell carcinoma. *(Reproduced with permission from Richard P. Usatine, MD.)*

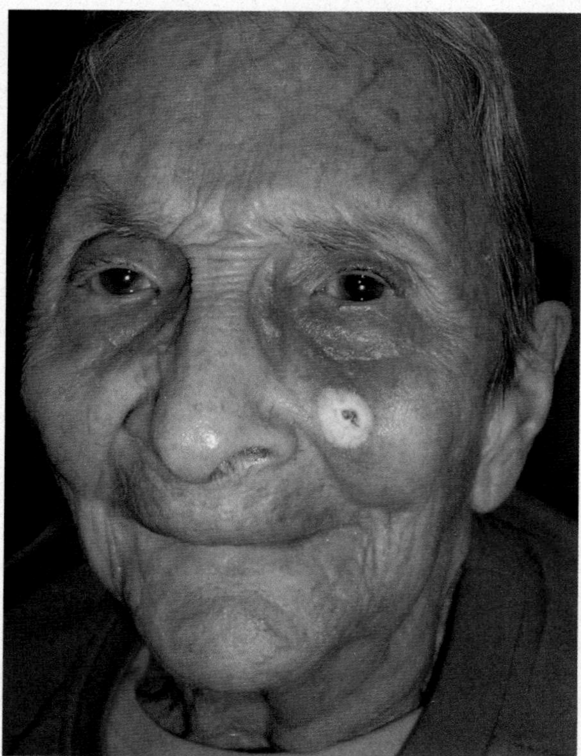

FIGURE 177-23 Cryosurgery was a favored treatment modality in a 94-year-old female patient with Alzheimer dementia with a basal cell carcinoma on the cheek. The family appreciated how easy this was to complete and how well it healed. *(Reproduced with permission from Richard P. Usatine, MD.)*

- Vismodegib and sonidegib are an FDA-approved targeted chemotherapies for the treatment of metastatic, locally advanced, or nonresectable BCCs that cannot be treated with radiation. It targets the smoothened pathway, which is mutated in basal cell nevus syndrome and altered in most BCCs.[11] SOR Ⓑ These hedgehog inhibitors may also be used to treat basal cell nevus syndrome (see **Figure 177-9**).

PREVENTION AND SCREENING

- All skin cancer prevention starts with sun protection.
- While it is known that UV causes BCCs and sunscreen blocks UV, high-quality studies showing real-world use of sunscreen preventing BCCs are lacking.[12]
- Most experts recommend SPF 30 or greater sunscreen applied and reapplied every 2 hours. SOR Ⓑ
- Sun protection should include sun avoidance, especially during peak hours of UV transmission, and protective clothing. SOR Ⓑ
- The U.S. Preventive Services Task Force has found insufficient evidence to recommend regular screening for any skin cancer in the general population.[13]
- Most experts believe that persons at high risk for BCC (including previous personal history of BCC, family history, and fair skin types with significant sun exposure) should be screened regularly for skin cancer by a physician trained in screening. SOR Ⓒ
- Evidence for the value of self-screening is lacking, but persons at high risk for skin cancer should also be encouraged to observe their own skin and to come in for evaluation if they see any suspicious changes or growths. SOR Ⓒ
- Nicotinamide 500 mg twice daily for 1 year reduced the incidence of BCCs by 20% compared to placebo in patients with a history of at least 2 nonmelanoma skin cancers in the previous 2 years.[14]

PROGNOSIS

The prognosis for basal cell carcinoma is generally excellent, with high cure rates with surgery and destructive modalities. The rate of metastasis has been estimated between 0.0028% and 0.55%. Large lesions on the face or lesions locally invading to deeper tissues have a poorer prognosis.[15]

FOLLOW-UP

Patients should be seen at least yearly after the diagnosis and treatment of a BCC. The 3-year risk of BCC recurrence after having a single BCC is 44%.[16]

PATIENT EDUCATION

Patients should practice skin cancer prevention by sun-protective behaviors such as avoiding peak sun, covering up, and using sunscreen.

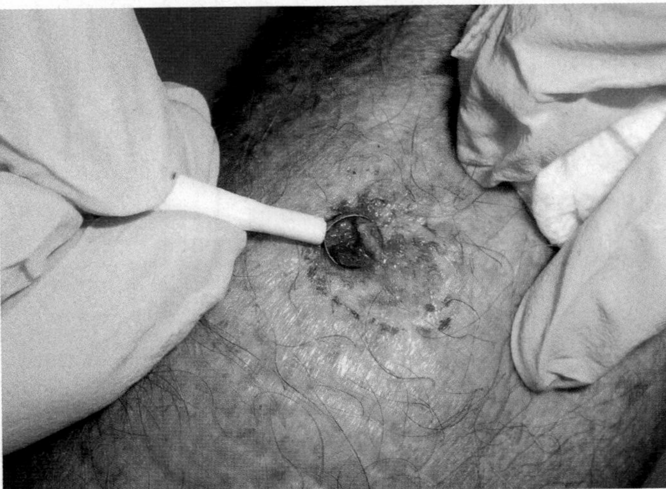

FIGURE 177-24 Curettage and electrodesiccation of a superficial basal cell carcinoma on the extremity is a rapid and effective treatment. The abnormal tumor tissue is softer than the surrounding normal skin and scoops out easily. (*Reproduced with permission from Richard P. Usatine, MD.*)

PATIENT RESOURCES

- The Skin Cancer Foundation—**http://www.skincancer.org/skin-cancer-information/basal-cell-carcinoma.**
- **http://medlineplus.gov/ency/article/000824.htm.**
- DermNet New Zealand—**http://www.dermnetnz.org/topics/basal-cell-carcinoma/.**

PROVIDER RESOURCES

- DermNet New Zealand—**http://www.dermnetnz.org/topics/basal-cell-carcinoma/.**
- Chapters and videos on diagnosing and surgically managing melanoma can be found in the following book/DVD or electronic application—Usatine R, Pfenninger J, Stulberg D, Small R. *Dermatologic and Cosmetic Procedures in Office Practice.* Philadelphia, PA: Elsevier; 2012.
- Information about smartphone and tablet apps of this resource can be viewed at—**www.usatinemedia.com.**

REFERENCES

1. Rogers HW, Weinstock MA, Feldman SR. Incidence estimate of nonmelanoma skin cancer (keratinocyte carcinomas) in the US population, 2012. *JAMA Dermatol.* 2015;151(10):1081.
2. Jackson S, Nesbitt LT. *Differential Diagnosis for the Dermatologist.* Springer Science & Business Media; 2012.
3. Madan V, Hoban P, Strange RC, et al. Genetics and risk factors for basal cell carcinoma. *Br J Dermatol.* 2006;154 Suppl 1:5-7.
4. Jarell AD, Mully TW. Basal cell carcinoma on the ear is more likely to be of an aggressive phenotype in both men and women. *J Am Acad Dermatol.* 2012;66(5):780-784.
5. Welsch MJ, Troiani BM, Hale L, et al. Basal cell carcinoma characteristics as predictors of depth of invasion. *J Am Acad Dermatol.* 2012;60(1):47-53.
6. Thissen MR, Neumann MH, Schouten LJ. A systematic review of treatment modalities for primary basal cell carcinomas. *Arch Dermatol.* 1999;135(10):1177-1183.
7. McGinness JL, Goldstein G. The value of preoperative biopsy-site photography for identifying cutaneous lesions. *Dermatol Surg.* 2010;36(2):194.
8. Telfer NR, Colver GB, Morton CA; British Association of Dermatologists. Guidelines for the management of basal cell carcinoma. *Br J Dermatol.* 2008;159(1):35-48.
9. Geisse J, Caro I, Lindholm J, et al. Imiquimod 5% cream for the treatment of superficial basal cell carcinoma: results from two phase III, randomized, vehicle-controlled studies. *J Am Dermatol.* 2004;50(5):722-733.
10. MacFarlane DF, Tal El AK. Cryoimmunotherapy: superficial basal cell cancer and squamous cell carcinoma in situ treated with liquid nitrogen followed by imiquimod. *Arch Dermatol.* 2011; 147(11):1326-1327.
11. Hoff Von DD, LoRusso PM, Rudin CM, et al. Inhibition of the hedgehog pathway in advanced basal-cell carcinoma. *N Engl J Med.* 2009;361(12):1164-1172.
12. Sánchez G, Nova J, Rodriguez-Hernandez AE, et al. Sun protection for preventing basal cell and squamous cell skin cancers. *Cochrane Database Syst Rev.* 2016;(7):CD011161.
13. Bibbins-Domingo K, Grossman DC, Curry SJ, et al. Screening for skin cancer: US Preventive Services Task Force Recommendation Statement. *JAMA.* 2016;316(4):429-435.
14. Chen AC, Martin AJ, Choy B, et al. A phase 3 randomized trial of nicotinamide for skin-cancer chemoprevention. *N Engl J Med.* 2015;373(17):1618-1626.
15. Alonso V, Revert A, Monteagudo C, et al. Basal cell carcinoma with distant multiple metastases to the vertebral column. *J Eur Acad Dermatol Venereol.* 2006;20(6):748-749.
16. Marcil I, Stern RS. Risk of developing a subsequent nonmelanoma skin cancer in patients with a history of nonmelanoma skin cancer: a critical review of the literature and meta-analysis. *Arch Dermatol.* 2000;136(12):1524-1530.

178 SQUAMOUS CELL CARCINOMA

Jonathan B. Karnes, MD
Richard P. Usatine, MD

PATIENT STORY

A 75-year-old man presents with a 2.6-cm enlarging inflamed tumor on the right cheek (**Figure 178-1**). He has a history of many actinic keratoses and grew up with significant sun exposure. Scoop shave biopsy is consistent with squamous cell carcinoma (SCC), and he undergoes Mohs surgery. **Figure 178-2** shows a shave biopsy of a smaller lesion on the scalp. Following excision, he follows up regularly for skin exams in order to detect any skin cancers or recurrence at an early stage.

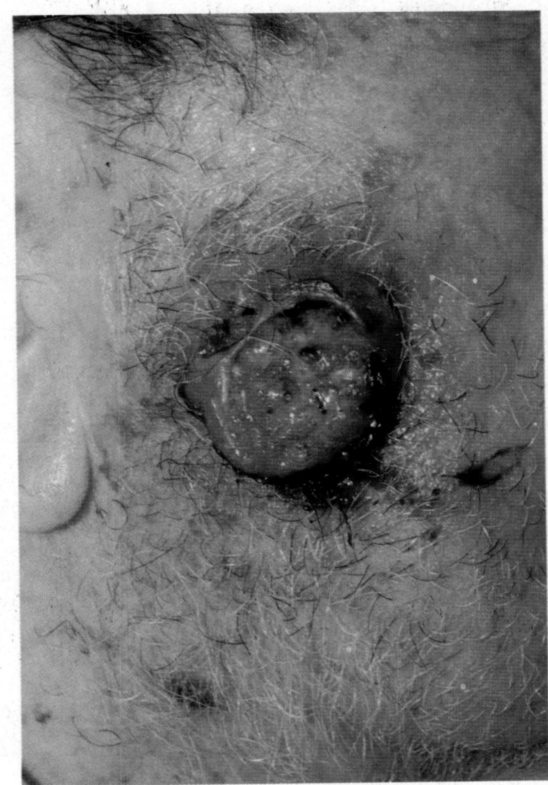

FIGURE 178-1 A large squamous cell carcinoma on the cheek of an elderly man, resembling a ruptured cyst. *(Reproduced with permission from Jonathan B. Karnes, MD.)*

INTRODUCTION

Cutaneous SCC is the second most common cancer in humans and arises most often as a result of cumulative sun damage. Incidence of cutaneous SCC (cSCC) in U.S. Medicare patients has been shown to have reached an incidence equal to that of basal cell carcinoma.[1] Although the mortality is declining, incidence is increasing in all populations, making this cancer a common and significant burden on patients.

EPIDEMIOLOGY

- Mortality from SCC has been observed as 0.29 per 100,000 population.[2]
- Metastasis from SCC occurs in 2% to 9.9% of cases.[3]
- The incidence is increasing in all age groups and populations at a rate of 3% to 10%.[3]
- In the United States, at least 200,000 to 400,000 new cases of cutaneous SCC are expected per year. Disease-related death occurs in more than 3000 people yearly.[4,5]
- SCC is the second most common skin cancer and accounts for at least 25% of nonmelanoma skin cancers.[4]
- SCC is the most common skin cancer in Hispanic, black, and Asian patients.[6]

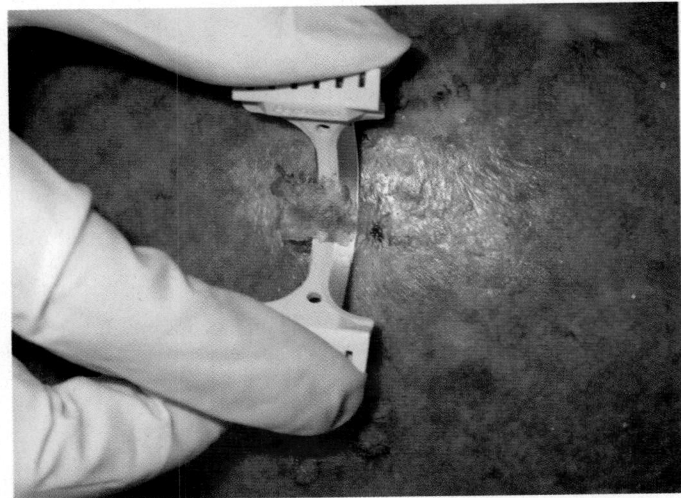

FIGURE 178-2 Shave biopsy of a squamous cell carcinoma on the scalp. *(Reproduced with permission from Richard P. Usatine, MD.)*

PATHOPHYSIOLOGY

SCC is a malignant tumor of keratinocytes. Most SCCs arise from precursor lesions called actinic keratoses. SCCs usually spread by local extension but are capable of regional lymph node metastasis and distant metastasis. Human papillomavirus (HPV)-related lesions may be found on the penis, labia, and perianal mucosa, or in the periungual region or elsewhere associated with immunosuppression.[7]

SCCs that metastasize most often start on mucosal surfaces and sites of chronic inflammation.

RISK FACTORS

- Long-term cumulative UV exposure is the greatest risk factor.
- Childhood sunburns.
- Occupational exposure.
- Other UV exposure including psoralen and UVA (PUVA) therapy and tanning beds.
- Smoking.
- HPV exposure.
- Exposure to ionizing radiation.
- Arsenic exposure.
- Fair skin.
- Age older than 60 years.
- Male gender.
- Living at lower latitude and higher altitude.
- Nonhealing ulcers.
- Chronic or severe immunosuppression, including posttransplant[8] immunosuppression, HIV, and long-term steroid use.
- Genetic syndromes, including Muir Torre, xeroderma pigmentosum, dystrophic epidermolysis bullosa, epidermodysplasia verruciformis, and oculocutaneous albinism.[4]

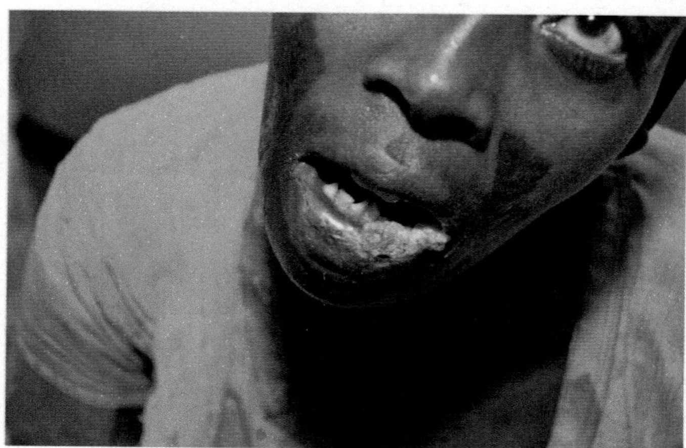

FIGURE 178-3 Marjolin ulcer (squamous cell carcinoma) arising in a burn that occurred years before on the face. (*Reproduced with permission from Richard P. Usatine, MD.*)

DIAGNOSIS

- Diagnosis is best made by shave, punch, or incisional biopsy.

CLINICAL FEATURES

SCC frequently presents as a rough keratotic papule, plaque, or tumor on chronically sun-damaged skin. SCC can partially ulcerate or present as a nonhealing ulcer.

Less common types of SCC:

- Marjolin ulcer—SCC of the extremities found in chronic skin ulcers or burn scars. This is a more common risk in darker pigmented individuals (**Figure 178-3**).
- Erythroplasia of Queyrat—SCC in situ on the penis or vulva related to HPV infection (**Figure 178-4**). This can progress to invasive SCC of the penis (**Figure 178-5**).

TYPICAL DISTRIBUTION

SCC is found in all sun-exposed areas and on mucous membranes. The most common sites are:

- Face (**Figures 178-6** and **178-7**).
- Lower lip (**Figures 178-8** and **178-9**).
- Ears (**Figure 178-10**).
- Scalp (**Figures 178-1** and **178-11**).
- Extremities—arm—(**Figures 178-12** and **178-13**).

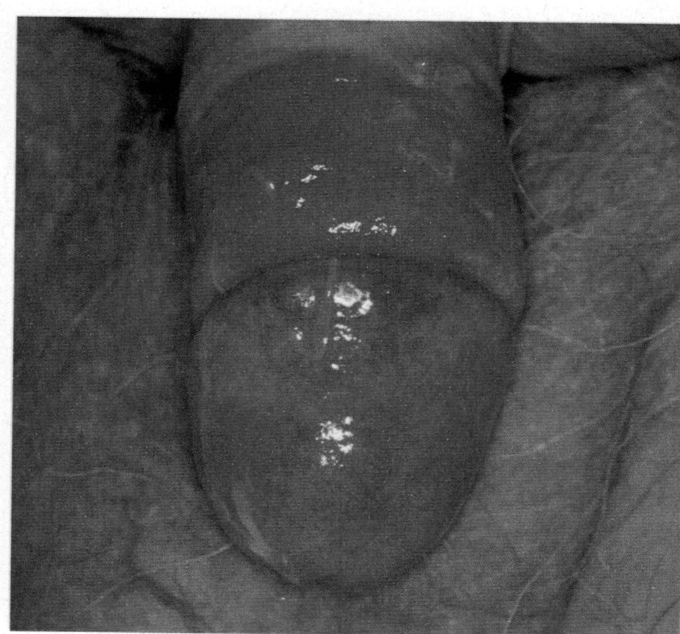

FIGURE 178-4 Erythroplasia of Queyrat (squamous cell carcinoma in situ) under the foreskin of an uncircumcised man. This is related to human papillomavirus infection, as is cervical cancer. (*Reproduced with permission from John Pfenninger, MD.*)

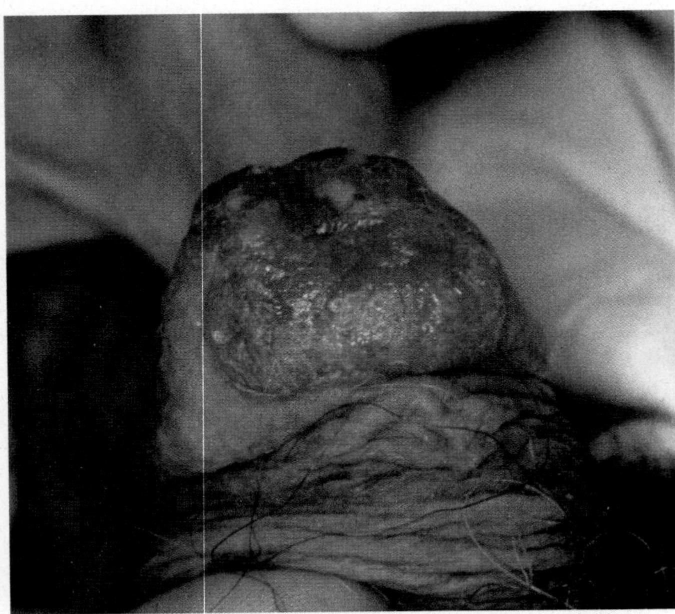

FIGURE 178-5 Squamous cell carcinoma of the glans penis. (*Reproduced with permission from Jeff Meffert, MD.*)

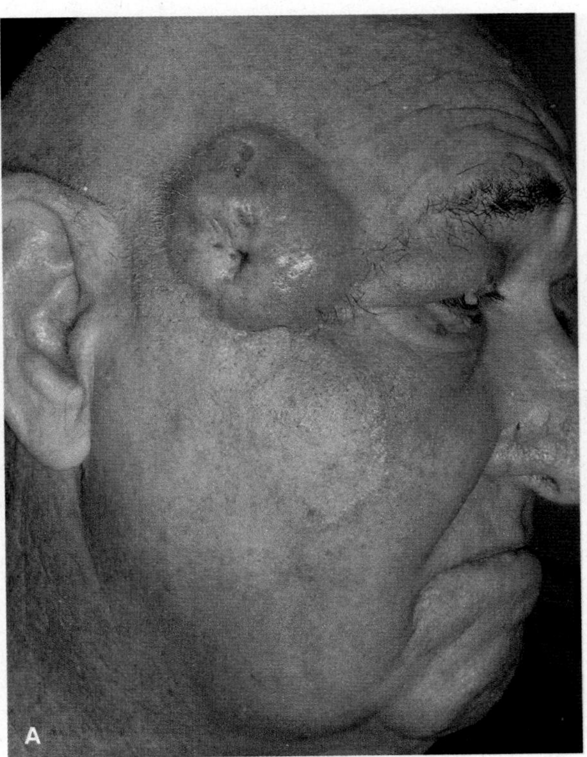

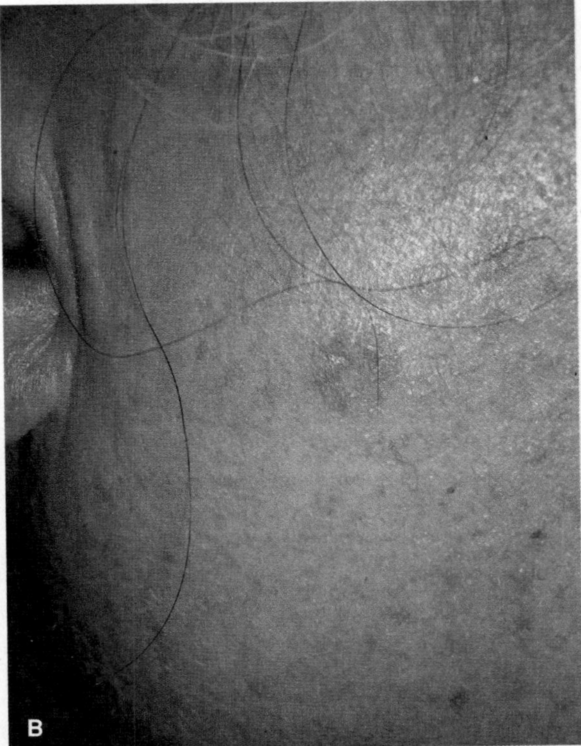

FIGURE 178-7 **A.** Large cystic-appearing squamous cell carcinoma on the face. Although this could have been a basal cell carcinoma, it definitely required a biopsy and excision. **B.** Small subtle invasive squamous cell carcinoma on the face that could have been overlooked or treated as an actinic keratosis. Any scaling lesion on the face that persists should be biopsied. (*Reproduced with permission from Richard P. Usatine, MD.*)

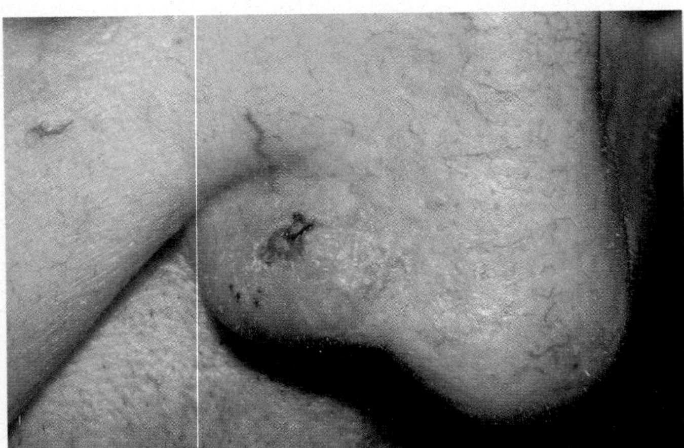

FIGURE 178-6 Squamous cell carcinoma on the nose of a 65-year-old man, which required a second biopsy to confirm the diagnosis. (*Reproduced with permission from Jonthan B. Karnes, MD.*)

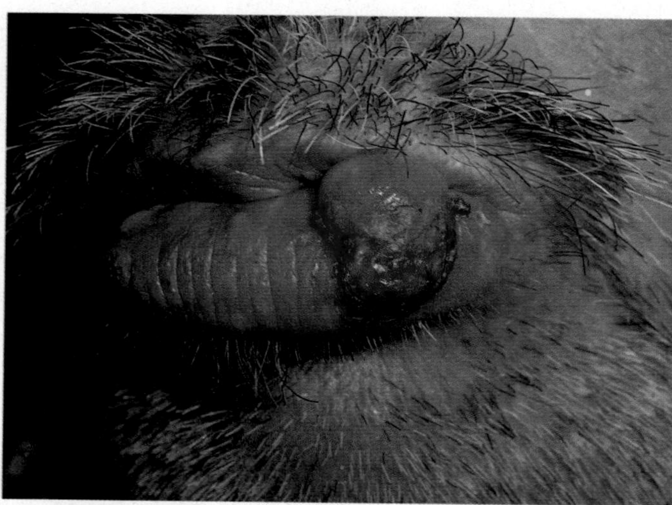

FIGURE 178-8 Squamous cell carcinoma on the lower lip growing rapidly in a patient who was taking an immunosuppressive medication after a renal transplant. (*Reproduced with permission from Richard P. Usatine, MD.*)

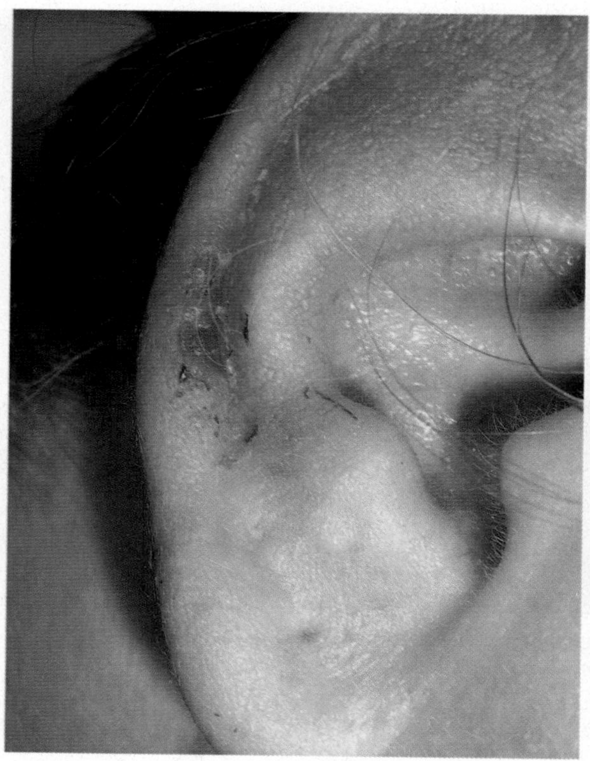

FIGURE 178-10 Squamous cell carcinoma arising in an actinic keratosis on the helix of a 33-year-old woman. (*Reproduced with permission from Richard P. Usatine, MD.*)

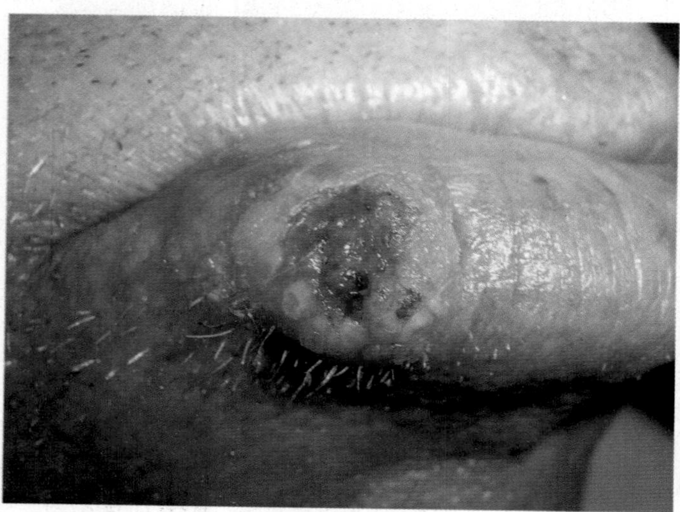

FIGURE 178-9 Squamous cell carcinoma showing ulceration on the lower lip of a man who was a smoker. (*Reproduced with permission from Richard P. Usatine, MD.*)

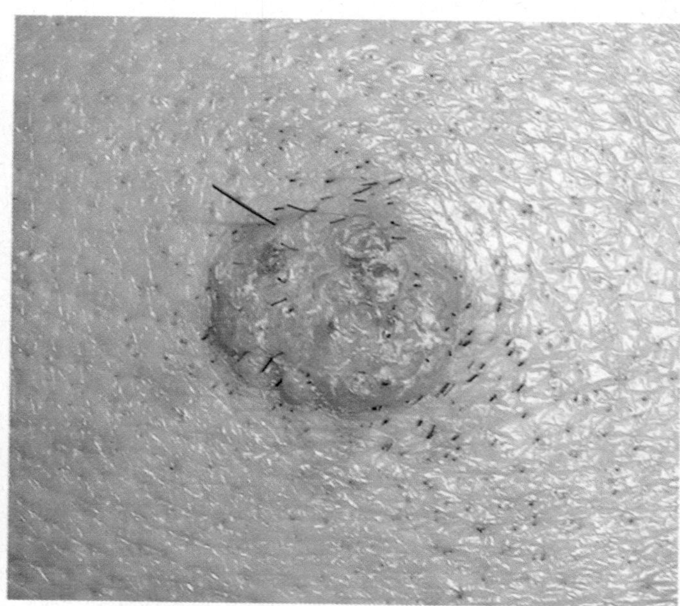

FIGURE 178-11 Squamous cell carcinoma on the shaven scalp of a 35-year-old man, which was formerly mistaken for a wart. (*Reproduced with permission from Richard P. Usatine, MD.*)

- Hands (**Figure 178-14**).
- Fingers (**Figure 178-15**).
- Mucous membranes (**Figure 178-16**) (see Chapter 43, Aphthous Ulcer).

DERMOSCOPY

There are many dermoscopic features that are helpful to diagnose SCC. See Chapters 111, Dermoscopy, and 181, Advanced Dermoscopy of Skin Cancer, for details on how dermoscopy helps make the diagnosis of SCC.

BIOPSY

- Deep shave biopsy is adequate to make the diagnosis of most SCCs.
- Punch biopsy or incisional biopsy is an alternative and useful for pigmented lesions or lesions with an unclear depth of involvement.

FACTORS AFFECTING METASTATIC POTENTIAL OF CUTANEOUS SQUAMOUS CELL CARCINOMA[9]

▶ Site

Tumor location influences prognosis: sites are listed in order of increasing metastatic potential.[2]

1. SCC arising at sun-exposed sites excluding lip and ear.
2. SCC of the lip (see **Figures 178-8** and **178-9**).
3. SCC of the ear (see **Figure 178-10**).
4. Tumors arising in non–sun-exposed sites (e.g., perineum, sacrum, sole of foot) (see **Figures 178-4, 178-5**, and **178-16**).
5. SCC arising in areas of radiation or thermal injury, chronic draining sinuses, chronic ulcers, chronic inflammation, or Bowen disease, such as the SCC arising in a burn site (see **Figure 178-3**).

▶ Size: diameter

Tumors larger than 2 cm in diameter double the risk of recurrence and triple the risk of metastasis compared with smaller tumors[6] (**Figure 178-17**).

▶ Size: depth

Depth is the most important factor associated with recurrence and metastasis. Tumors greater than 2 mm thick have 10 times the risk of recurrence. Tumors that extend beyond the subcutaneous fat recur and metastasize in 28% and 27% of cases, respectively.[10]

▶ Histologic differentiation

Poorly differentiated tumors have a worse prognosis, with more than double the local recurrence rate and triple the metastatic rate of better-differentiated SCC.[11] Tumors with significant perineural involvement have very high rates of local recurrence (47%) and metastasis (35%) with standard excision alone. Mohs microsurgery and radiation reduce this risk.[10]

▶ Host immunosuppression

Tumors arising in patients who are immunosuppressed have a poorer prognosis. Host cellular immune response may be important in determining both the local invasiveness of SCC and the host's response to metastases. **Figures 178-16, 178-17**, and **178-18** are SCCs in patients who are HIV-positive.[9]

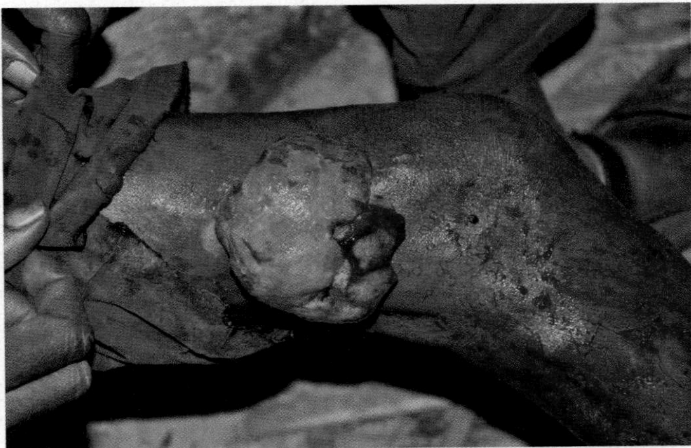

FIGURE 178-12 Large squamous cell carcinoma on the leg of a homeless man. (*Reproduced with permission from Richard P. Usatine, MD.*)

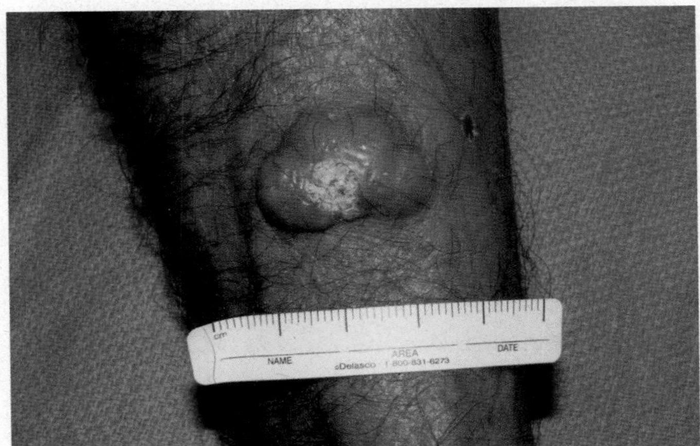

FIGURE 178-13 Large ulcerating squamous cell carcinoma on arm. (*Reproduced with permission from Jonathan B. Karnes, MD.*)

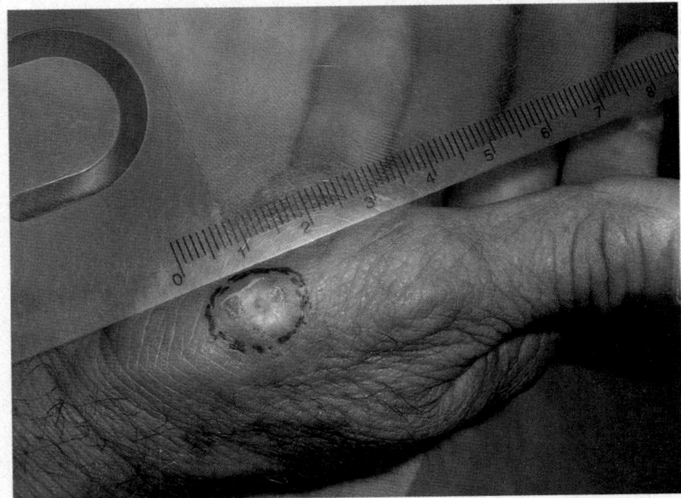

FIGURE 178-14 Squamous cell carcinoma in situ on the thenar eminence of the hand. (*Reproduced with permission from Richard P. Usatine, MD.*)

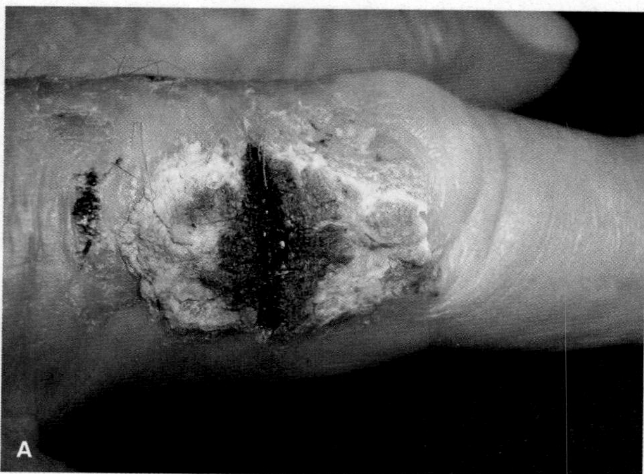

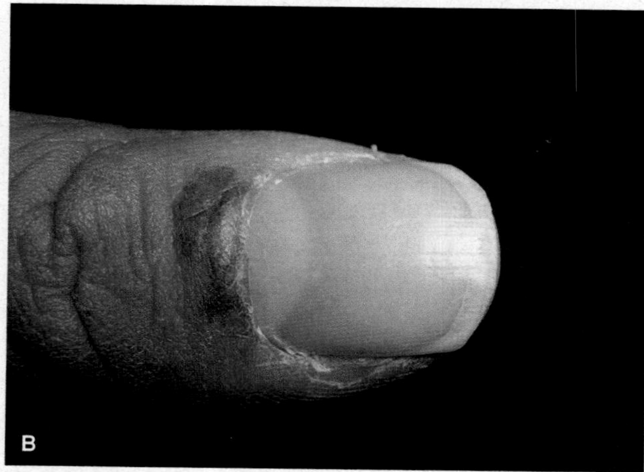

FIGURE 178-15 Two different-appearing cases of squamous cell carcinoma on the finger. **A.** It took 2 shave biopsies to establish the correct diagnosis in this case. **B.** Squamous cell carcinoma in situ with human papillomavirus changes and pigment incontinence in a 35-year-old woman. The irregular hyperpigmented lesion on the proximal nail fold was originally suspicious for melanoma. (*Reproduced with permission from Richard P. Usatine, MD.*)

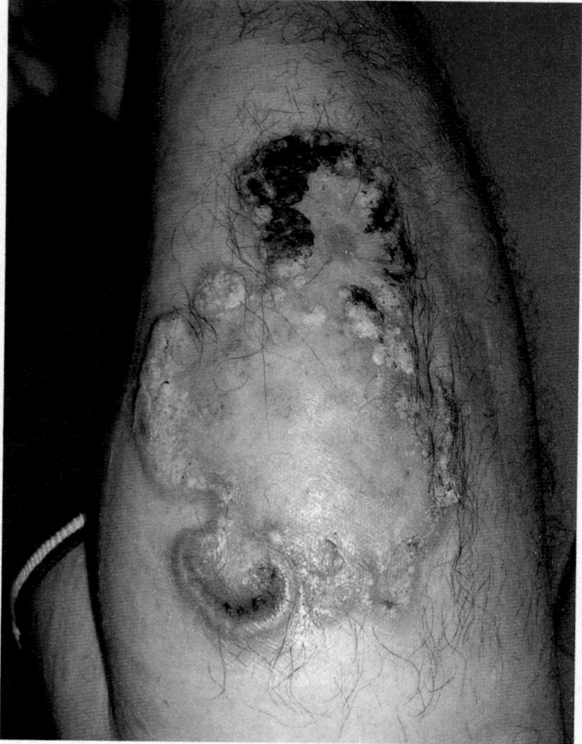

FIGURE 178-17 Large squamous cell carcinoma on the arm of a human immunodeficiency virus–positive 51-year-old man. It grew to this size in 1 year and took 2 biopsies to get a definitive diagnosis. Differential diagnosis includes mycosis fungoides. (*Reproduced with permission from Richard P. Usatine, MD.*)

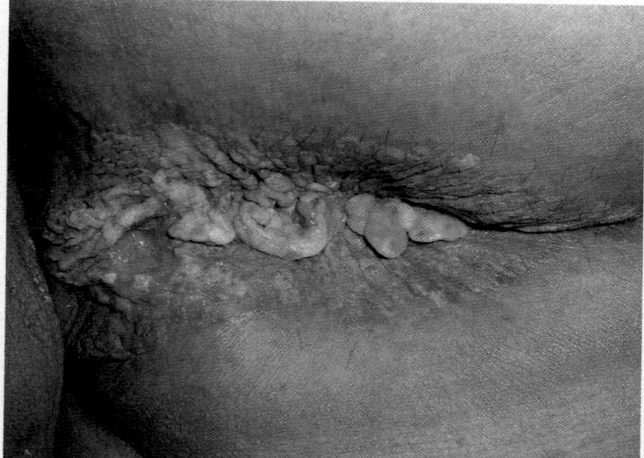

FIGURE 178-16 Perianal invasive squamous cell carcinoma in a human immunodeficiency virus–positive man who had engaged in anal intercourse and was infected with human papillomavirus. The ulcerations were suspicious for invasive squamous cell carcinoma and not typical of condyloma acuminata. (*Reproduced with permission from Richard P. Usatine, MD.*)

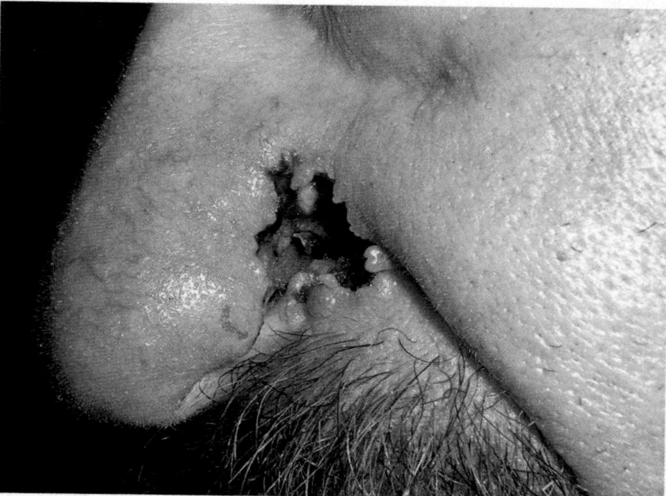

FIGURE 178-18 Squamous cell carcinoma invading the internal nasal structures in a human immunodeficiency virus–positive man who was afraid of having a biopsy done earlier. Patient referred to ear, nose, and throat specialist. (*Reproduced with permission from Richard P. Usatine, MD.*)

▶ Previous treatment and treatment modality

The risk of local recurrence depends on the treatment modality. Locally recurrent disease itself is a risk factor for metastatic disease. Local recurrence rates are considerably less with Mohs micrographic surgery than with any other treatment modality.

DIFFERENTIAL DIAGNOSIS

- Actinic keratoses are precancers on sun-exposed areas, which can progress to SCC (see Chapter 173, Actinic Keratosis and Bowen Disease).
- Bowen disease is SCC in situ before it invades the basement membrane (see Chapter 173, Actinic Keratosis and Bowen Disease).
- Keratoacanthoma is a subtype of SCC that may resolve spontaneously but is generally treated as a low-risk SCC. **Figure 178-19** shows an invasive SCC resembling a lower-risk keratoacanthoma subtype (see Chapter 174, Keratoacanthoma).
- Basal cell carcinoma (BCC) cannot always be distinguished from SCC by clinical appearance alone. **Figure 178-19** could be a BCC by appearance but was proven to be SCC by biopsy (see Chapter 177, Basal Cell Carcinoma).
- Merkel cell carcinoma (neuroendocrine carcinoma of the skin) is a rare aggressive malignancy. It is most commonly seen on the heads of elderly fair-skinned patients. It resembles an SCC, and the diagnosis is made by biopsy (**Figure 178-20**).
- Nummular eczema can usually be distinguished by the multiple coin-like shapes, transient nature, and pruritus (Chapter 151, Atopic Dermatitis).

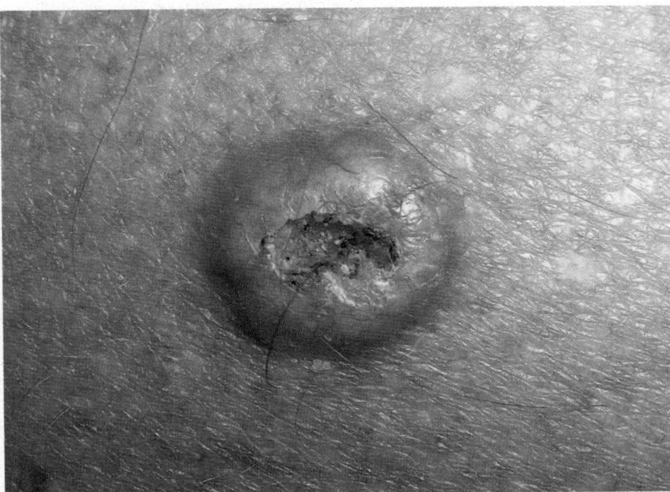

FIGURE 178-19 Squamous cell carcinoma on the shoulder of a human immunodeficiency virus–positive man. Note that the pearly borders and telangiectasias resemble a basal cell carcinoma and the central crater suggests that this could be a keratoacanthoma. (*Reproduced with permission from Richard P. Usatine, MD.*)

MANAGEMENT

Table 178-1 provides a summary of treatment options.

Surgical resection for definitive treatment should include margins as given below:

- 4-mm margin—Adequate for well-defined, low-risk tumors less than 2 cm in diameter; such margins are expected to remove the primary tumor mass completely in 95% of cases.[12] SOR Ⓐ
- 6-mm margin—Recommended for larger tumors, high-risk tumors, tumors extending into the subcutaneous tissue, and those in high-risk locations (ear, lip, scalp, eyelids, nose).[12]
- The tumor should be cut out to the deep subcutaneous fat and submitted for pathologic confirmation of complete excision.

MOHS MICROGRAPHIC SURGERY

Frederic Mohs pioneered the technique of excising skin cancers and immediately assessing the continuous margin via mapped en face sectioning—which involves sectioning the tumor like a bagel rather than standard breadboard sectioning, which cuts the tumor like a loaf of bread. Sequential mapped stages are removed until all margins are clear. Mohs surgery offers superior cure rates compared with standard excision or destructive techniques, spares uninvolved tissue, and allows for reconstruction at the time of excision.

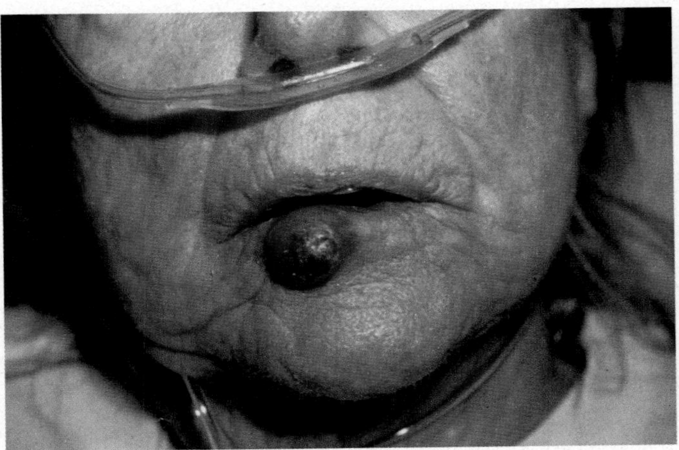

FIGURE 178-20 Merkel cell carcinoma on the lower lip of an elderly woman. This is an aggressive cancer with a high mortality rate. (*Reproduced with permission from Jeff Meffert, MD.*)

TABLE 178-1 Summary of Treatment Options for Primary Cutaneous Squamous Cell Carcinoma

Treatment	Indications	Contraindications	Notes
Surgical excision	All resectable tumors	Where surgical morbidity is likely to be unreasonably high	Generally treatment of choice for SCC High-risk tumors need wide margins or histologic margin control
Mohs micrographic surgery/excision with histologic control	High-risk tumors, recurrent tumors	Where surgical morbidity is likely to be unreasonably high	Treatment of choice for high-risk tumors
Radiotherapy	Nonresectable tumors	Where margins are ill defined	
Curettage and cautery	Small, well-defined, low-risk tumors	High-risk tumors	Curettage may be helpful prior to surgical excision
Cryotherapy	Small, well-defined, low-risk tumors	High-risk tumors, recurrent tumors	Only suitable for experienced practitioners

Reproduced with permission from Motley R, Kersey P, Lawrence C. Multiprofessional guidelines for the management of the patient with primary cutaneous squamous cell carcinoma, Br J Plast Surg. 2003;56(2):85-91.

Mohs surgery is specifically indicated for lesions larger than 2 cm, lesions with ill-defined clinical borders, lesions with aggressive histologic subtypes, recurrent lesions, and lesions on or near the eye, nose, ear, mouth, hair-bearing scalp, or chronic ulcers. Patients with chronic immunosuppression or genetic tumor syndromes may also benefit from Mohs surgery compared to standard excision.[12]

CURETTAGE AND ELECTRODESICCATION

Excellent cure rates have been reported in several case series, and small (<1 cm), well-differentiated, primary, slow-growing tumors arising on sun-exposed sites can be removed by experienced physicians with electrodesiccation and curettage (EDC).[5] EDC should be avoided on terminal hair-bearing areas such as scalp, pubis, axilla, and bearded area in men because of the risk of deep follicular invasion.

The experienced clinician undertaking EDC can detect tumor tissue by its soft consistency, which allows detection of clinically invisible tumor extension and ensures adequate treatment. Electrodesiccation is applied to the curetted wound, and the curettage-cautery cycle is then repeated twice.[12]

CRYOSURGERY

Good short-term cure rates have been reported for small, histologically confirmed SCC treated by cryosurgery in experienced hands. Prior biopsy is necessary to establish the diagnosis histologically. There is great variability in the use of liquid nitrogen for cryotherapy. Start by drawing a 4- to 6-mm margin around the SCC and then apply two 30-second freezes with a thaw in between. It is best to use local anesthesia with lidocaine first, because these long freeze times are quite painful. SOR Ⓒ

Cryosurgery and curettage and electrodesiccation are not appropriate for locally recurrent disease but may be useful in patients presenting with multiple or eruptive low-grade SCCs who may have a number of tumors effectively treated at a single visit.

RADIOTHERAPY

Primary treatment with radiation therapy alone offers short- and long-term cure rates for SCC that are comparable with other treatments, but radiation therapy is usually reserved for special situations where surgical therapies are contraindicated. Certain very advanced tumors, where surgical morbidity would be unacceptably high, may also be best treated by radiotherapy. SOR Ⓒ

PREVENTION AND SCREENING

- All skin cancer prevention starts with sun protection.
- There is good evidence from multiple randomized controlled trials (RCTs) that daily sunscreen use decreases the risk of developing sun-related SCCs.[13,14] SOR Ⓐ In the longest RCT, sunscreen was applied regularly to the head, neck, hands, and forearms for 4.5 years with a decrease in SCC during the study period.[13] At the end of the trial, the participants were followed for another 8 years and SCC tumor rates decreased by almost 40% during the follow-up period.[14]
- Sun protection should include sun avoidance, especially during peak hours of UV transmission; protective clothing; and sunscreen use.
- Indoor tanning is not safe and should be avoided.
- The U.S. Preventive Services Task Force has not found sufficient evidence to recommend regular screening for any skin cancer in the general population.[15]
- Most experts believe that persons at high risk for SCC (including previous personal history of any skin cancer, high-risk family history, high-risk skin types with significant sun exposure, or immunosuppression after an organ transplant) should be screened regularly for skin cancer by a physician trained in such screening.
- Evidence for the value of self-screening is lacking, but persons at high risk for skin cancer should also be encouraged to observe their own skin and to come in for evaluation if they see any suspicious changes or growths.
- A recent RCT of nicotinamide, 500 mg BID, showed a 30% reduction in the development of cutaneous SCC and a 23% reduction in nonmelanoma skin cancer over a 12-month period.[16]

PROGNOSIS

Prognosis is excellent for small, thin lesions less than 2 mm thick that are removed with clear margins in immunocompetent patients. In these patients, the risk of metastasis is near zero. The risk of metastasis increases markedly with thicker lesions, and lesions with thicknesses greater than 6 mm metastasize to the regional nodes 16% of the time.[11]

FOLLOW-UP

Patients should be seen at least yearly for skin examinations after the diagnosis and treatment of an SCC. The 3-year risk of recurrence of a new SCC after having a single SCC is 18%.[17]

PATIENT EDUCATION

Includes use of a hat and sunscreen on a regular basis with frequent follow-up for early recognition of new skin cancers.

PATIENT RESOURCES

- The Skin Cancer Foundation. *Squamous Cell Carcinoma*—**http://www.skincancer.org/skin-cancer-information/squamous-cell-carcinoma.**
- Skinsight. *Squamous Cell Carcinoma*—**https://www.skinsight.com/skin-conditions/adult/squamous-cell-carcinoma-scc.**
- MedlinePlus. *Squamous Cell Carcinoma*—**http://medlineplus.gov/ency/article/000829.htm.**

PROVIDER RESOURCES

- Medscape. *Cutaneous Squamous Cell Carcinoma*—**http://emedicine.medscape.com/article/1965430-overview.**
- DermNet NZ. *Cutaneous Squamous Cell Carcinoma*—**https://www.dermnetnz.org/topics/squamous-cell-carcinoma-of-the-skin.**
- Chapters and videos on diagnosing and surgically managing SCC can be found in the following book/DVD or electronic app: Usatine R, Pfenninger J, Stulberg D, Small R. *Dermatologic and Cosmetic Procedures in Office Practice*. Philadelphia, PA: Elsevier; 2012. Information about smartphone and tablet apps of this resource can be viewed at **www.usatinemedia.com.**

REFERENCES

1. Rogers HW, Weinstock MA, Coldiron BM, et al. Incidence estimate of nonmelanoma skin cancer (keratinocyte carcinomas) in the U.S. population, 2012. *JAMA Dermatol.* 2015;151:1081-1086.
2. Lewis KG, Weinstock MA. Nonmelanoma skin cancer mortality (1988–2000): the Rhode Island follow-back study. *Arch Dermatol.* 2004;140(7):837-842.
3. Weinberg AS, Ogle CA, Shim EK. Metastatic cutaneous squamous cell carcinoma: an update. *Dermatol Surg.* 2007;33(8):885-899.
4. Karia PS, Han J, Schmults CD. Cutaneous squamous cell carcinoma: estimated incidence of disease, nodal metastasis, and deaths from disease in the United States, 2012. *J Am Acad Dermatol.* 2013;68:957-966.
5. Karia PS, Jambusaria-Pahlajani A, Harrington DP, et al. Evaluation of American Joint Committee on Cancer, International Union Against Cancer, and Brigham and Women's Hospital tumor staging for cutaneous squamous cell carcinoma. *J Clin Oncol.* 2014;32:327-334.
6. Rowe DE, Carroll RJ, Day CL. Prognostic factors for local recurrence, metastasis and survival rates in squamous cell carcinoma of the skin, ear and lip. *J Am Acad Dermatol.* 1992;26:976-990.
7. Bolognia JL, Jorizzo JL, Schaffer JV. *Dermatology*, 3rd ed. Philadelphia, PA: Saunders; 2012:2776.
8. Berg D, Otley CC. Skin cancer in organ transplant recipients: epidemiology, pathogenesis, and management. *J Am Acad Dermatol.* 2002;47(1):1-17; quiz 18-20.
9. Motley R, Kersey P, Lawrence C; British Association of Dermatologists, British Association of Plastic Surgeons. Multiprofessional guidelines for the management of the patient with primary cutaneous squamous cell carcinoma. *Br J Plast Surg.* 2003;56(2):85-91.
10. Que SK, Zwald FO, Schmults CD. Cutaneous squamous cell carcinoma: incidence, risk factors, diagnosis, and staging. *J Am Acad Dermatol.* 2018;59:237-247.
11. Brantsch KD, Meisner C, Schönfisch B, et al. Analysis of risk factors determining prognosis of cutaneous squamous-cell carcinoma: a prospective study. *Lancet Oncol.* 2008;9(8):713-720.
12. Alam M, Armstrong A, Baum C, et al. Guidelines of care for the management of cutaneous squamous cell carcinoma. *J Am Acad Dermatol.* 2017;78:560-578.
13. Green A, Williams G, Neale R, et al. Daily sunscreen application and betacarotene supplementation in prevention of basal-cell and squamous-cell carcinomas of the skin: a randomised controlled trial. *Lancet.* 1999;354:723-729. Erratum: *Lancet.* 1999;354:1038.
14. van der Pols JC, Williams GM, Pandeya N, et al. Prolonged prevention of squamous cell carcinoma of the skin by regular sunscreen use. *Cancer Epidemiol Biomarkers Prev.* 2006;15(12):2546-2548.
15. Screening for Skin Cancer: US Preventive Services Task Force Recommendation Statement. *JAMA.* 2016;316(4):429-435.
16. Chen AC, et al. A phase 3 randomized trial of nicotinamide for skin-cancer chemoprevention. *N Engl J Med.* 2015;373:1618-1626.
17. Marcil I, Stern RS. Risk of developing a subsequent nonmelanoma skin cancer in patients with a history of nonmelanoma skin cancer: a critical review of the literature and metaanalysis. *Arch Dermatol.* 2000;136(12):1524-1530.

179 MELANOMA

Jonathan B. Karnes, MD
Richard P. Usatine, MD

PATIENT STORIES

A 51-year-old woman noticed a rapidly growing black lesion on the upper arm (**Figure 179-1**) and presented to her doctor. A narrow-margin biopsy confirmed an 8-mm-thick nodular melanoma. She was referred to surgical oncology for sentinel lymph-node biopsy, and one node was positive. She underwent a course of chemotherapy, and though she remains disease-free 2 years later, she is carefully monitored for metastasis and new primary lesions by a multidisciplinary team including family medicine, dermatology, and medical and surgical oncology.

A 60-year-old man underwent a skin exam as part of his regular physical exam. His family doctor noticed an irregular brown black patch on the back (**Figure 179-2**) and performed a narrow-margin scoop shave, which was diagnostic for melanoma in situ. The patient underwent wide local excision in the office with 5-mm margins and follows up regularly for skin exams with a cure rate very near 100%.

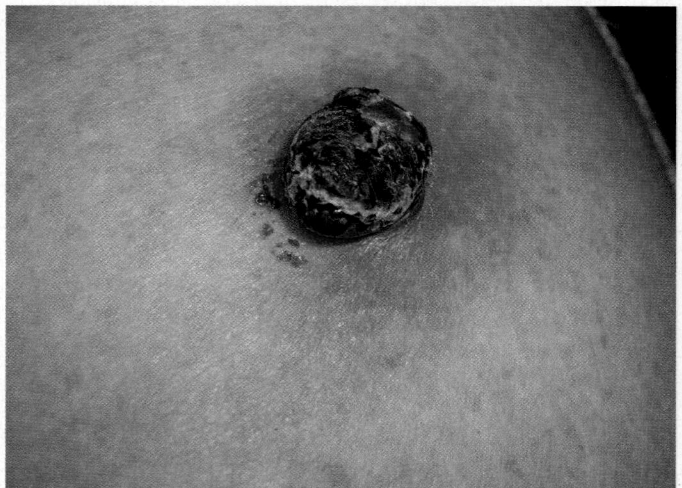

FIGURE 179-1 An 8 mm thick nodular melanoma on the arm of a middle-aged woman. (*Reproduced with permission from Richard P. Usatine, MD.*)

INTRODUCTION

Melanoma is the third most common skin cancer and the most deadly. The incidence of melanoma and the mortality from it are rising. Most lesions are found by clinicians on routine examination. When discovered early, surgical treatment is almost always curative. However, as depth increases, so does the risk of metastasis and mortality. New chemotherapy regimens are more promising than ever, but the best prognosis comes with prevention and early detection.

EPIDEMIOLOGY

- In 2018, the American Cancer Society estimates that 91,270 people in the United States will be diagnosed with melanoma, and 9320 will die from it.[1]
- Melanoma incidence has increased in every age group and in every thickness over the course of 1992 to 2006 among non-Hispanic whites, with death rates increasing in those older than age 65 years.[2]
- Incidence continues to increase worldwide at approximately 4% to 8% per year.[3]
- In the United States, the death rate for melanoma is decreasing among persons younger than age 65 years.[2]
- Deaths from thin melanomas account for more than 30% of total deaths.
- The lifetime risk of developing melanoma is 2.6%.[1]

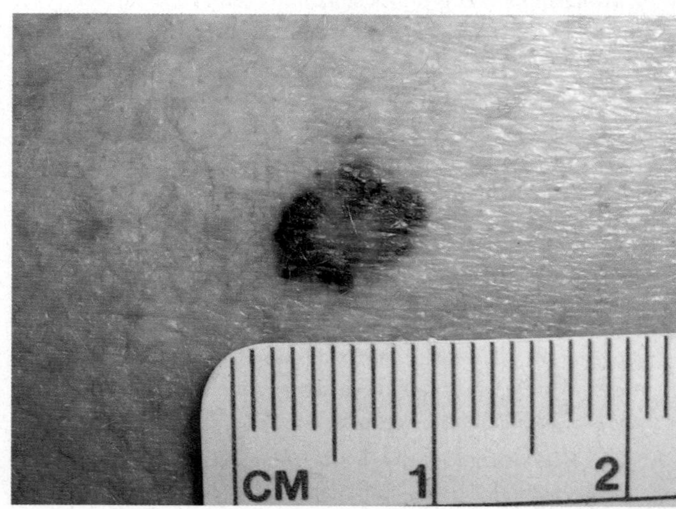

FIGURE 179-2 A melanoma in situ on the back. With appropriate margins, the cure rate after excision approaches 100%. (*Reproduced with permission from Richard P. Usatine, MD.*)

RISK FACTORS

Risk factors can be broadly thought of as genetic risks, environmental risks, and phenotypic risks arising from a combination of genetic and environmental risks. For example, a fair-skinned child (genetic) who gets a sunburn (environmental) is much more likely to develop freckles (phenotypic) and melanoma.

ENVIRONMENTAL RISKS

- Exposure to sunlight.
    - History of sunburn doubles the risk of melanoma and is worse at a young age.
- Living closer to the equator.
- Indoor tanning.
- History of immunosuppression.
- Higher socioeconomic status (likely associated with more frequent opportunity for sunburns).

GENETIC RISKS

- Fair skin, blue or green eyes, red or blonde hair.
- Male sex.
- Melanoma in a first-degree relative.
- History of xeroderma pigmentosum or familial atypical mole melanoma syndrome.

PHENOTYPIC RISKS

- Many nevi.
- Multiple dysplastic nevi.
- Increased age.
- Personal history of any skin cancer.

DIAGNOSIS

CLINICAL FEATURES

Remember the *ABCDE* guidelines for diagnosing melanoma (**Figure 179-3**).[4]

A = *Asymmetry*. Most early melanomas are asymmetric: a line through the middle will not create matching halves. Benign nevi are usually round and symmetric.

B = *Border*. The borders of early melanomas are often uneven and may have scalloped or notched edges. Benign nevi have smoother, more even borders.

C = *Color* variation. Benign nevi are usually a single shade of brown. Melanomas are often in varied shades of brown, tan, or black, but may also exhibit red, white, or blue.

D = *Diameter* greater than or equal to 6 mm. Early melanomas tend to grow larger than most nevi. (Note: Congenital nevi are often large.)

E = *Evolving*. Any evolving or enlarging nevus should make you suspect melanoma. Evolving could be in size, shape, symptoms (itching, tenderness), surface (especially bleeding), and shades of color.

- A prospective controlled study compared 460 cases of melanoma with 680 cases of benign pigmented tumors and found significant differences for all individual ABCDE criteria ($p < 0.001$) between melanomas and benign nevi.[4]

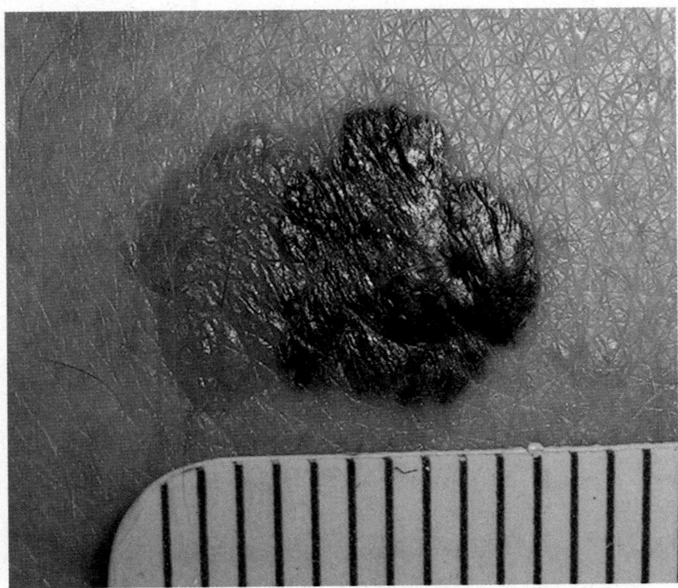

FIGURE 179-3 Superficial spreading melanoma on the back with ABCDE features of melanoma. *(Reproduced with permission from Richard P. Usatine, MD.)*

- Sensitivity of each criterion: A 57%, B 57%, C 65%, D 90%, E 84%; specificity of each criterion: A 72%, B 71%, C 59%, D 63%, E 90%.[4]
- Sensitivity of ABCDE criteria varies depending on the number of criteria needed: using 2 criteria it was 89.3%; with 3 criteria, it was 65.5%. Specificity was 65.3% using 2 criteria and 81% using 3.[4]
- The number of criteria present was different between benign nevi (1.24 ± 1.26) and melanomas (3.53 ± 1.53; $p < 0.001$). Unfortunately, no significant difference was found between melanomas and atypical nevi.[4]

There are 4 major categories of melanomas. With the exception of nodular melanoma, the growth patterns of the 3 other subtypes are characterized by a radial growth phase prior to dermal invasion. At the present time, the thickness of the lesion, ulceration, and lymphovascular invasion histologically are used for tumor staging and prognosis regardless of the morphologic subtype. Here are the major categories of melanomas:

1. *Superficial spreading melanoma* is the most common type, representing about 69% of all melanoma (**Figures 179-3** to **179-6**). This melanoma has the radial growth pattern before dermal invasion occurs. The first sign is the appearance of a flat macule or slightly raised discolored plaque that has irregular borders and is somewhat geometric in form. The color varies, with areas of tan, brown, black, red, blue, or white. These lesions can arise in an older nevus. The melanoma can be seen almost anywhere on the body, but is most likely to occur on the trunk in men, the legs in women, and the upper back in both. Superficial spreading melanoma is the most common type identified in young non-Hispanic white adults.[6]
2. *Nodular melanoma* occurs in 14% of cases (**Figures 179-1, 179-7** to **179-9**).[6] It is usually invasive at the time it is first diagnosed, and the malignancy is recognized when it becomes raised. The color is often black, but occasionally blue, gray, white, brown, tan, red, or nonpigmented. The nodule in **Figure 179-9** is multicolored.
3. *Lentigo maligna melanoma* occurs in about 15% of cutaneous melanoma.[6] It is similar to the superficial spreading type and appears as a flat or mildly elevated mottled tan, brown, or dark brown discoloration on sun-damaged skin (**Figures 179-10** and **179-11**). This type of melanoma is found most often in 50- to 80-year-olds and occurs on the head 90% of the time. Although it is most often found on the face and scalp, it can occur in other areas of sun-damaged skin. These grow slowly over 3–15 years, arising from the precursor lesion, lentigo maligna, which is melanoma in situ (**Figure 179-10**). The in situ precursor lesion may be quite large and has often existed for years or over a decade (see Chapter 175, Lentigo Maligna).
4. *Acral lentiginous melanoma* is the least common major subtype of melanoma and accounts for about 2% of all melanomas; however, it is one of the most frequent subtypes seen in African Americans (37%) though it actually occurs even more often in Hispanic and non-Hispanic whites.[6] It may occur under the nail plate or on the soles or palms (**Figures 179-12** to **179-16**). This subtype often carries a worse prognosis because of delays in diagnosis and the accompanying thickness at the time of diagnosis. Subungual melanoma may manifest as diffuse nail discoloration or a longitudinal pigmented band within the nail plate. When subungual pigment spreads to the proximal or lateral nail fold, it is referred to as the Hutchinson sign and is highly suggestive of acral lentiginous melanoma (**Figure 179-14**) (see Chapter 199, Pigmented Nail Disorders).

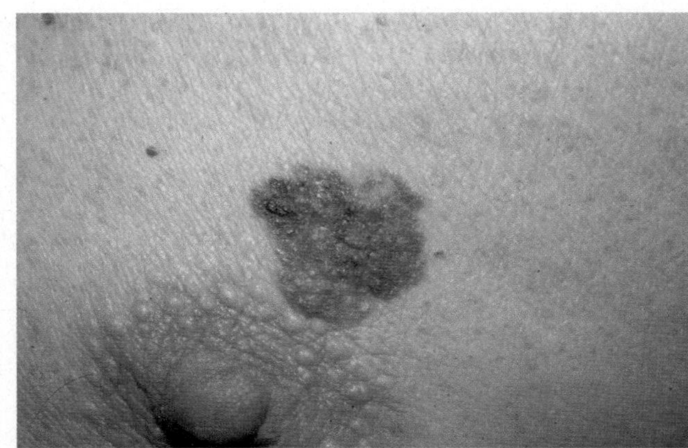

FIGURE 179-4 Superficial spreading melanoma near the areola. It is important to not mistake this for a seborrheic keratosis. Note the area of pigment regression near the top of the lesion. (*Reproduced with permission from Richard P. Usatine, MD.*)

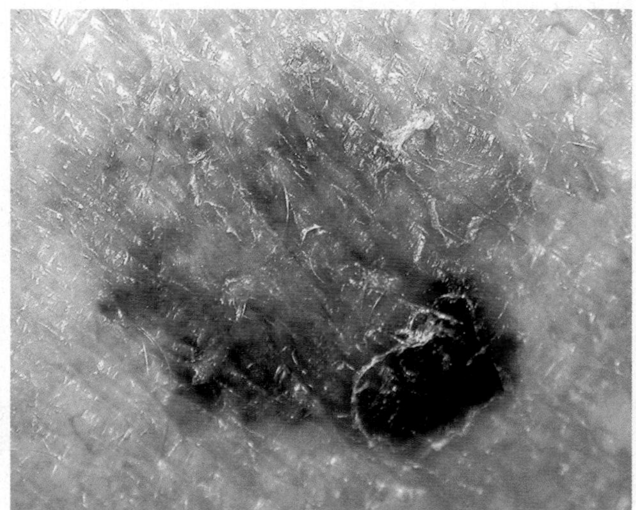

FIGURE 179-5 Superficial spreading melanoma on the arm with depth of 0.25 mm. Note the pale pink coloration along with the black area with some erosion. (*Reproduced with permission from Eric Kraus, MD.*)

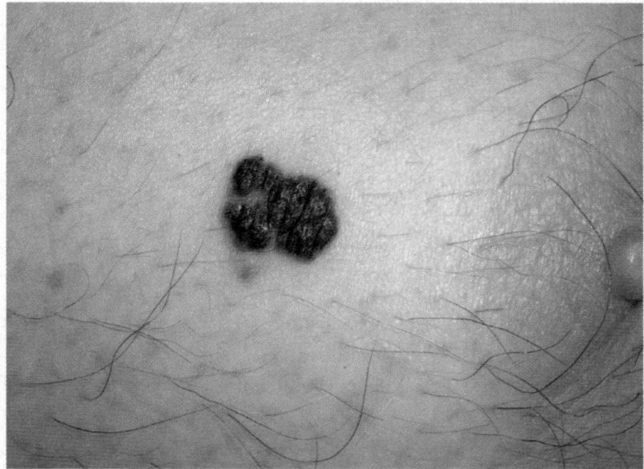

FIGURE 179-6 Superficial spreading melanoma with multiple colors and ABCDE features of melanoma. (*Reproduced with permission from Jonathan B. Karnes, MD.*)

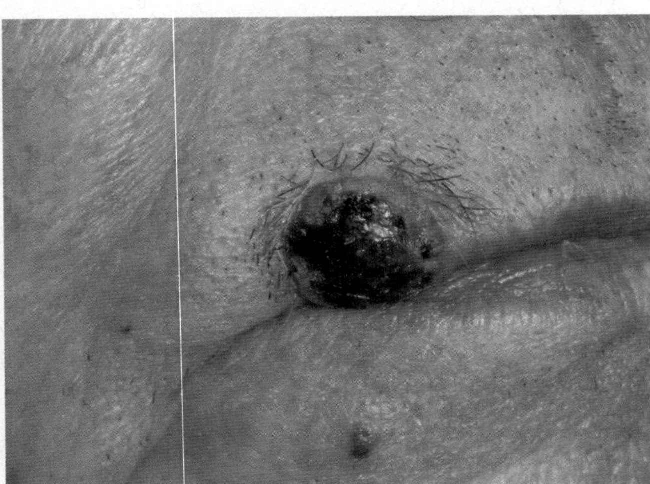

FIGURE 179-7 Thick nodular melanoma on the lip. (*Reproduced with permission from Jonathan B. Karnes, MD.*)

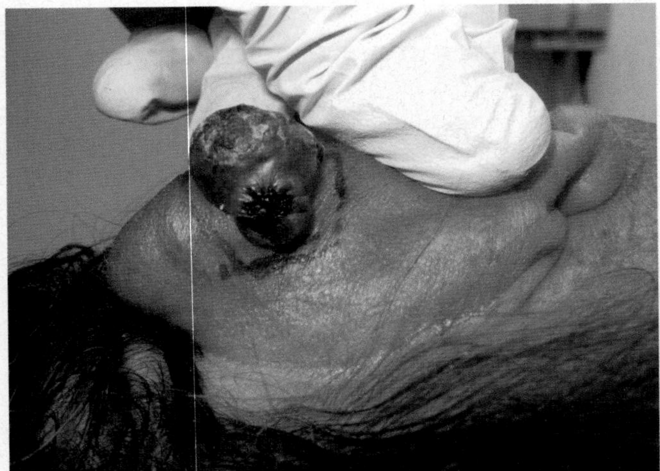

FIGURE 179-8 Large nodular melanoma on the posterior helix of the ear. Depth was 8 mm. (*Reproduced with permission from Jonathan B. Karnes, MD.*)

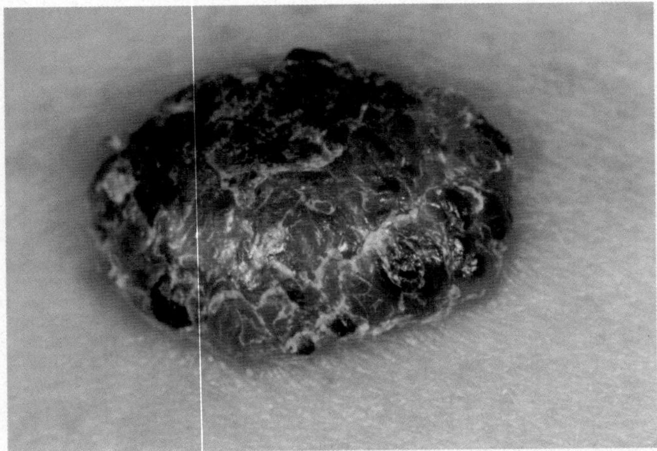

FIGURE 179-9 Raised, thick, nodular melanoma on the shoulder of a 37-year-old white woman with history of multiple sunburns from childhood. Note the multiple colors visible in the nodule. The Breslow depth is 8.5 mm. The sentinel node was negative and the patient underwent chemotherapy after wide excision. (*Reproduced with permission from Richard P. Usatine, MD.*)

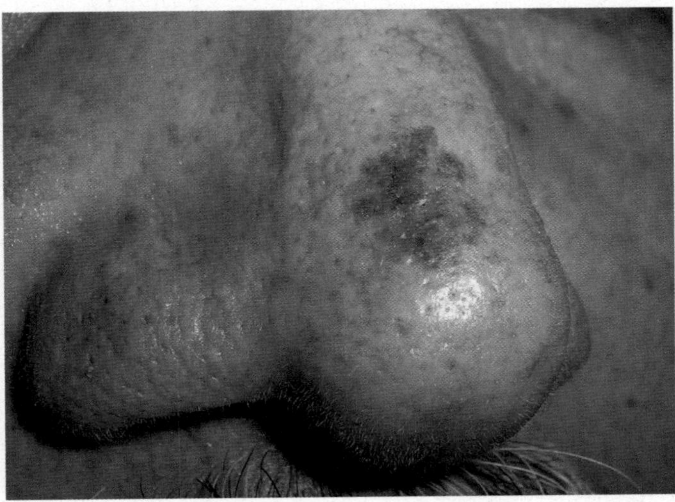

FIGURE 179-10 Lentigo maligna melanoma in situ on the nose of a 66-year-old man. This lesion was biopsied successfully with a scoop shave (saucerization) that completely cut under the lesion for full prognostic information. (*Reproduced with permission from Richard P. Usatine, MD.*)

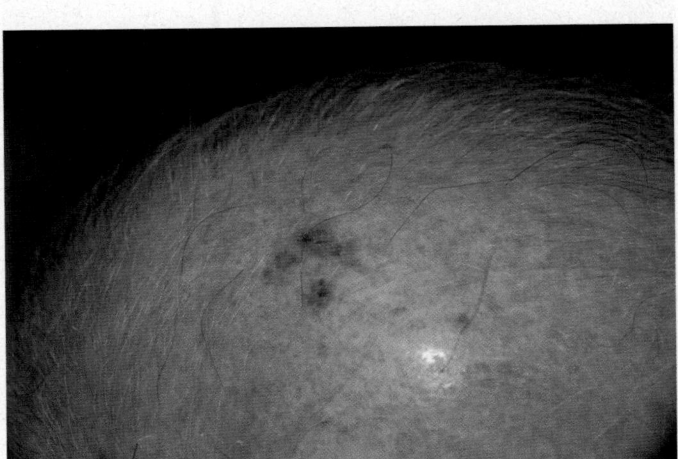

FIGURE 179-11 Lentigo maligna melanoma slowly growing on the scalp. At 2.0 mm thick, it is much deeper than clinical appearance may suggest. (*Reproduced with permission from Jonathan B. Karnes, MD.*)

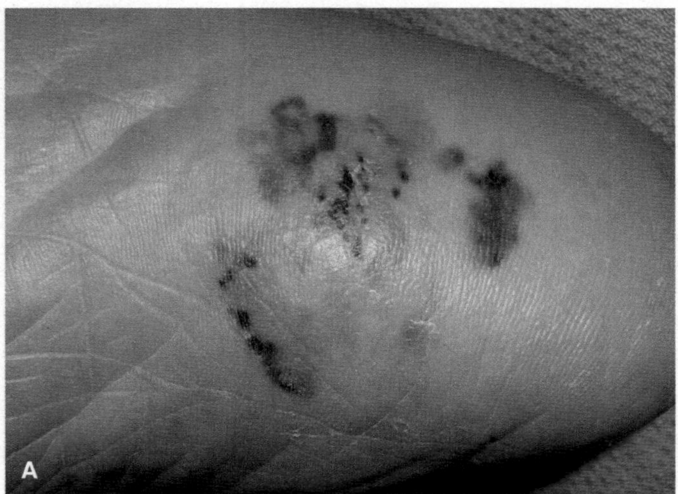

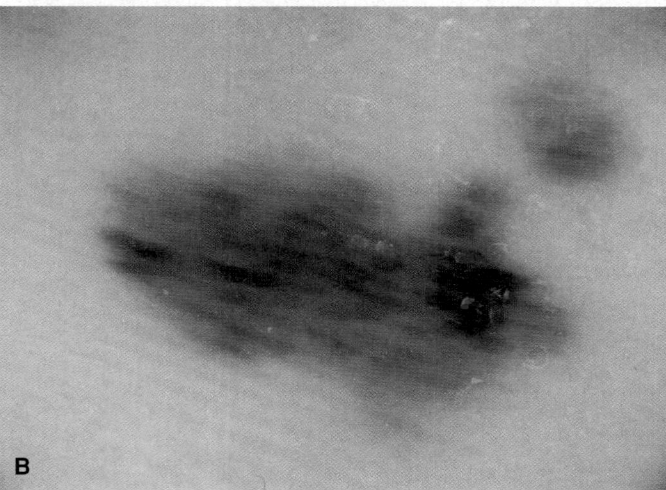

FIGURE 179-12 **A.** Acral lentiginous melanoma on the bottom of the foot, where it went undetected for years. **B.** Dermoscopy showing the parallel ridge pattern typical of a melanoma on the sole. (*Reproduced with permission from Richard P. Usatine, MD.*)

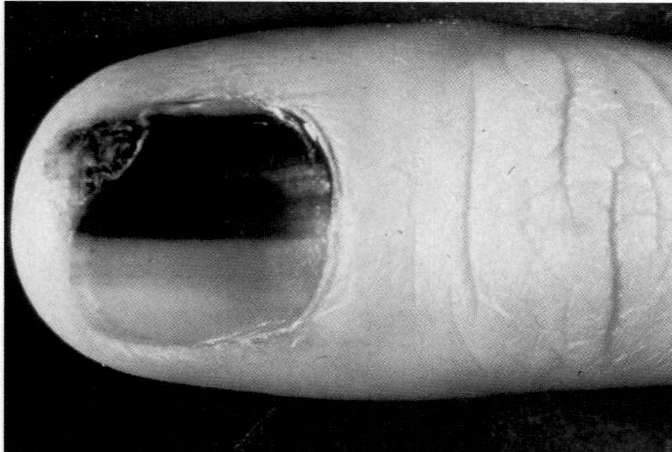

FIGURE 179-13 Subungual melanoma in a white man showing hyperpigmentation of the nail and nail bed. (*Reproduced with permission from the Skin Cancer Foundation. For more information www.skincancer.org*)

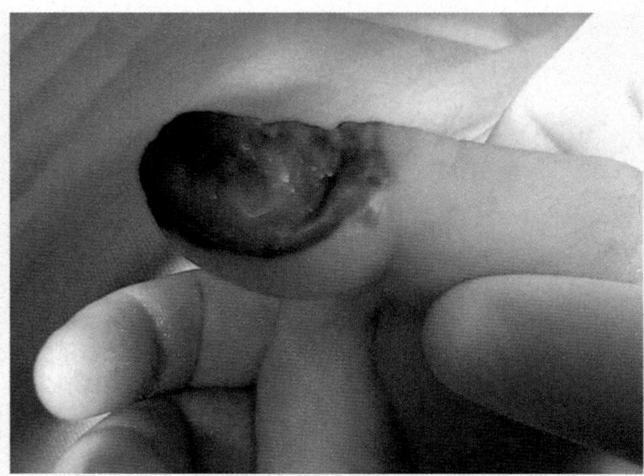

FIGURE 179-14 Acral lentiginous melanoma that started after trauma to the thumb, which led to a delay in diagnosis. Note the destruction of the nail bed and the hyperpigmentation around the nail fold. (*Reproduced with permission from Journal of Family Practice and Adam Leight, MD.*)

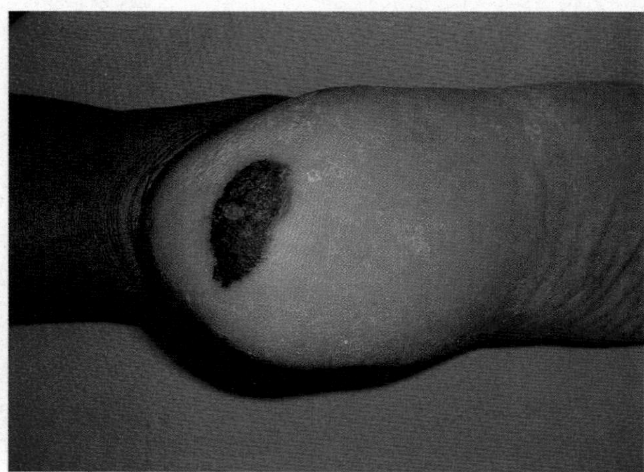

FIGURE 179-15 Nodular and acral lentiginous melanoma of the foot in a 30-year-old black woman. There is ulceration, and the depth was 5.5 mm. Sentinel node biopsy was positive for 2 of 2 nodes sampled. Stage IIIC (pT4b N2a MO). (*Reproduced with permission from Richard P. Usatine, MD.*)

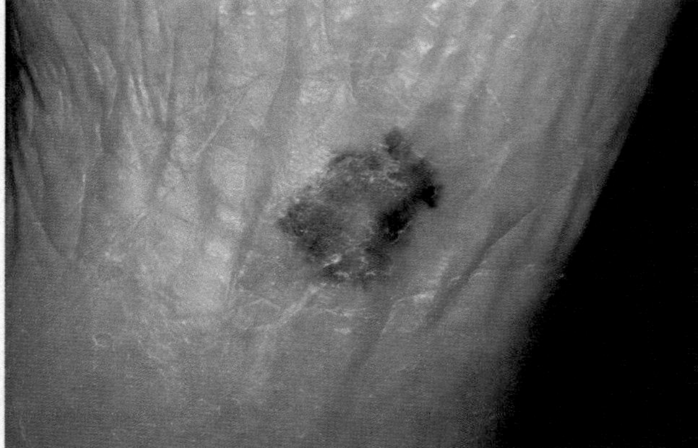

FIGURE 179-16 Acral lentiginous melanoma on the foot of an elderly woman. Although ALM is one of the most frequent subtypes in African Americans, it is still more common in Hispanic and non-Hispanic whites, who have the highest burden of melanoma overall. Disease burden is much more common in patients over 65.[6] (*Reproduced with permission from Jonathan B. Karnes, MD.*)

Less common types of melanomas include:

- *Amelanotic melanoma* (<5% of melanomas) is nonpigmented and appears pink or flesh-colored, often mimicking basal cell or squamous cell carcinoma or a ruptured hair follicle. Any of the 4 principal subtypes may present as an amelanotic variant, but nodular melanomas are highly represented. These may be intrinsically more aggressive and often present with a thicker Breslow depth than similarly pigmented melanomas (**Figures 179-17** to **179-19**).[7]
- Other rare melanoma variants include (a) nevoid melanomas, (b) malignant blue nevus, (c) desmoplastic/spindled/neurotropic melanoma, (d) clear cell sarcoma (in fact a melanoma), (e) animal-type melanoma, (f) ocular melanoma, and (g) mucosal (lentiginous) melanoma.[8]

TYPICAL DISTRIBUTION

Melanoma occurs most commonly on the trunk in white males and the lower legs and back in white females, but may occur in any location where melanocytes exist. The most common site in African Americans, Hispanics, and Asians is the plantar foot, followed by the subungual, palmar, and mucosal sites.

DERMOSCOPY

Dermoscopy can be used to determine if a pigmented lesion has features suspicious for a melanoma, and it can also help determine when a biopsy is needed.[9] In a prospective study of 401 lesions evaluated for melanoma by experts in dermoscopy, the sensitivity of 66.6% with ABCDE criteria improved to 80%, and specificity rose from 79.3% to 89.1% (**Figure 179-20**).[9]

In a study of dermoscopy done by 60 physicians (35 general practitioners, 10 dermatologists, and 16 dermatology trainees) on unaided photos of 40 lesions using the ABCD rule, the Menzies method, a 7-point checklist, and pattern analysis, the sensitivity rose over the unaided eye.[10] Physicians were instructed in each of the dermoscopy methods using a CD-ROM. The unaided eye using a standard photo of the lesion was 61% sensitive and 85% specific with a 73% diagnostic accuracy. The dermoscopic photo increased sensitivity (68% for

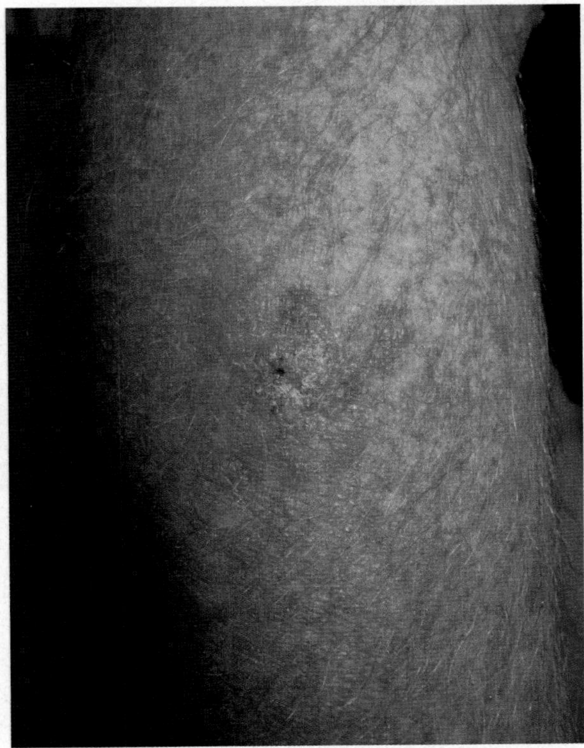

FIGURE 179-17 Amelanotic melanoma on the arm of a middle-aged man with marked sun damage. Breslow depth was 1.5 mm. (*Reproduced with permission from Jonathan B. Karnes, MD.*)

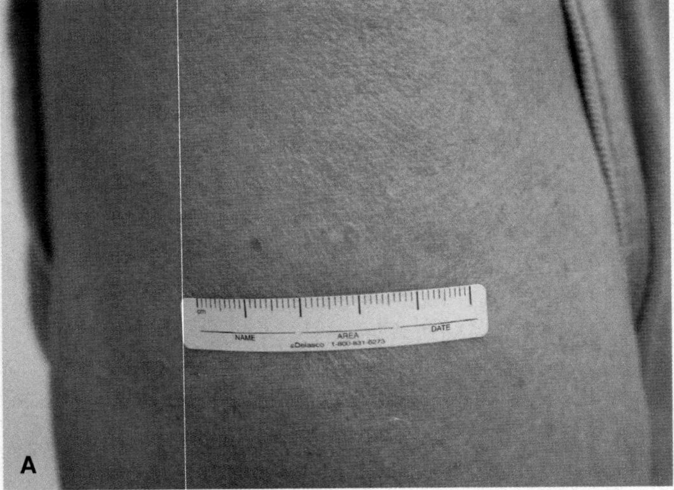

FIGURE 179-18 **A.** Amelanotic melanoma on the arm easily missed because of its small size and lack of dark pigmentation. **B.** Dermoscopy of the same melanoma showing white central area, peripheral pigment network, and linear vessels. (*Reproduced with permission from Jonathan B. Karnes, MD.*)

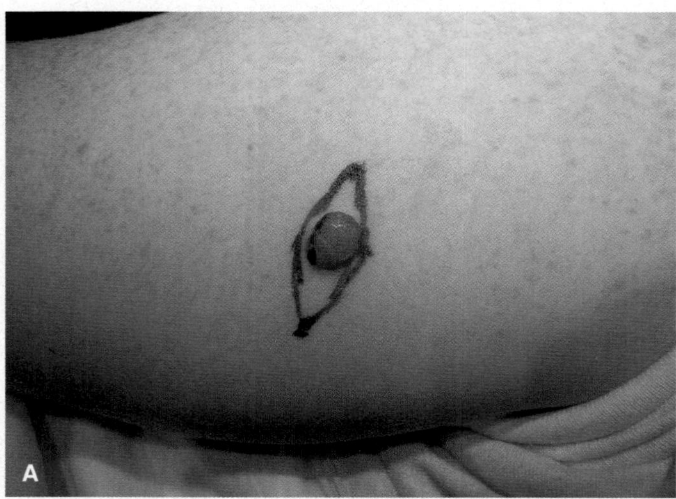

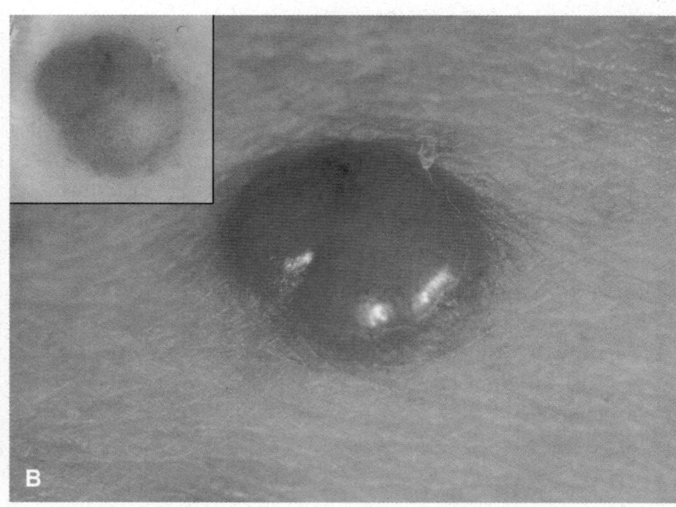

FIGURE 179-19 **A.** Amelanotic melanoma on the arm of a young woman prior to elliptical excision. The diagnosis was unexpected and shows the importance of excising suspicious lesions even when they are not pigmented. (*Reproduced with permission from E.J. Mayeaux, Jr., MD.*) **B.** Amelanotic melanoma with a dermoscopy insert in upper corner. The use of the dermatoscope and the recognition of the abnormal vascular pattern led to a high suspicion for amelanotic melanoma that was confirmed on excision. (*Reproduced with permission from Ashfaq Marghoob, MD.*)

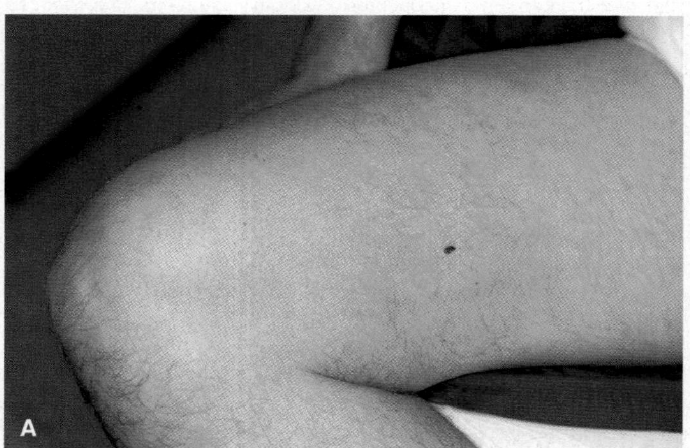

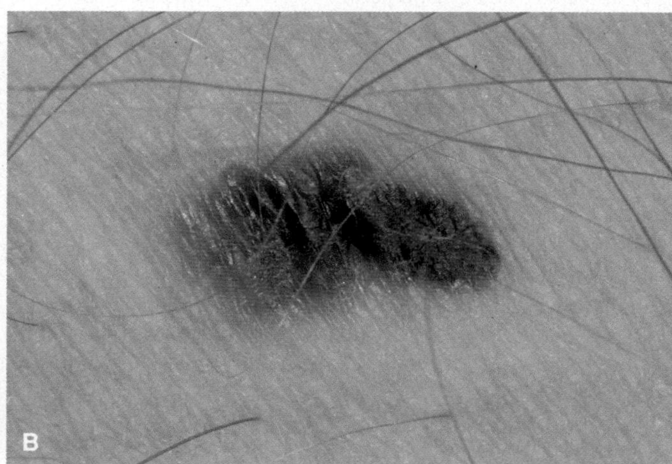

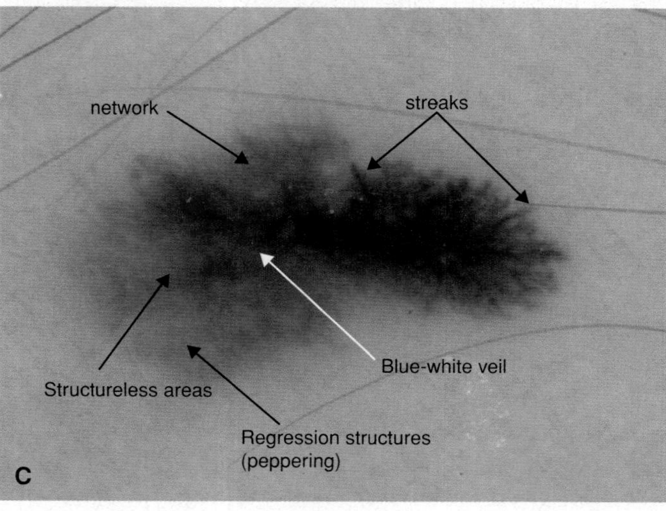

FIGURE 179-20 **A.** A melanoma on the leg that could be missed because of its small size (7 mm long). **B.** Close-up of that melanoma showing the asymmetry, irregular borders, and a variation in color. **C.** Dermoscopy of a melanoma showing a blue-white veil, radial streaks, pigment network, structureless areas, and regression structures with peppering. This early superficial-spreading melanoma was proven to be 0.55 mm at the time of excision. (*Reproduced with permission from Ashfaq Marghoob, MD.*)

pattern analysis, 77% for the ABCD rule, 81% for the 7-point checklist, and 85% for the Menzies method). The specificity did not improve. Sensitivity is more important than specificity to avoid missing melanoma. Although the number of biopsies could increase with some drop in specificity, the biopsy itself is the most specific test to differentiate melanoma from benign pigmented lesions.[10]

Accepted dermoscopic features of melanoma include:

- Atypical network (includes branched streaks).
- Streaks: pseudopods and radial streaming.
- Atypical dots and globules.
- Negative pigment network.
- Blotch (off center).
- Blue-white veil/peppering over macular areas (regression).
- Blue-white veil over raised areas.
- Atypical vascular structures.
- Peripheral tan/brown structureless areas.

Figure 179-20 demonstrates a number of these features. (See Chapters 111, Dermoscopy, and 181, Advanced Dermoscopy of Skin Cancer.)

BIOPSY

A full-thickness skin biopsy remains the gold standard for diagnosing melanoma. Narrow-margin (1–3 mm) biopsy by shave saucerization, punch, or elliptical excision is ideal for histologic diagnosis and tumor staging (**Box 179-1**). Wider margins are avoided to preserve accurate subsequent lymphatic mapping. Although there is evidence that a partial biopsy of a portion of a melanoma does not worsen the prognosis, this should only be performed when a lesion is too large to excise in the office. If the clinical impression differs markedly from the pathology report, discuss with the pathologist and share clinical photos if you haven't done so already. You may need to have the pathologist prepare "deeper sections" or "step sections"—meaning more slices from the same loaf of bread. Additionally, if the diagnosis of melanoma was expected and the result of an incisional biopsy does not meet the expectation, go forward with a complete excision or refer to a colleague who can.

Saucerization (scoop or deep shave biopsy) leads to an accurate diagnosis and staging 97% of the time (**Figure 179-21**).[11] This is because it provides breadth of sampling in addition to depth when performed correctly. The goal of the saucerization is to get under the lesion, especially in the region with the greatest depth. In most cases this is about the depth of a dime, and the visible pigment depth can be the guide (see Chapter 113, Biopsy Principles and Techniques). If pigment is seen at the base of the biopsy, a second saucerization can be added to the first pass to provide the pathologist with more tissue. Too shallow of a biopsy may miss important staging information. For very large lesions, such as a suspected lentigo maligna, a saucerization should provide better tissue to the pathologist than a single or several punch biopsies (see **Figure 179-10**).[12]

The impact of partial biopsy on histopathologic diagnosis of cutaneous melanoma has been studied extensively by Ng and colleagues in Australia. They found that increased odds of histopathologic misdiagnosis were associated with punch biopsy of part of the melanoma (odds ratio [OR] 16.6) and shallow shave biopsy (OR 2.6) compared with excisional biopsy (including saucerization). Punch biopsy of part of the melanoma was also associated with increased odds of misdiagnosis with an adverse outcome (OR 20).[13]

BOX 179-1 The National Comprehensive Cancer Network (NCCN) Melanoma Guidelines on the Principles of Biopsy of a Suspicious Pigmented Lesion[5]

- Excisional biopsy (elliptical, punch, or saucerization/deep shave) with 1- to 3-mm margins is preferred. Avoid wider margins to permit accurate subsequent lymphatic mapping.
- The orientation of an elliptial/fusiform excisional biopsy should be planned with definitive wide excision in mind (eg, vertically/parallel to underlying lymphatics on the extremities).
- Full-thickness incisional or punch biopsy of clinically thickest portion of the lesion is acceptable in certain anatomic areas (e.g., palm/sole, digit, face, and ear) or for very large lesions.
- Superficial shave biopsy may compromise pathologic diagnosis and complete assessment of Breslow thickness, but is acceptable when the index of suspicion is low.
  - For lentigo maligna melanoma in situ, lentigo maligna type broad shave biopsy may help to optimize diagnostic sampling.
  - If clinical evaluation of incisional biopsy suggests that microstaging is inadequate, consider narrow margin excisional biopsy.
- Repeat narrow-margin excisional biopsy is recommended if an initial partial biopsy is inadequate for diagnosis or microstaging but should not generally be performed if the initial specimen meets criteria for Sentinel lymph node staging.

DIFFERENTIAL DIAGNOSIS

Nevi of all types can mimic melanoma. Congenital nevi can be especially large and asymmetric. Therefore, it is important to ask the patient if the pigmented area has been there from birth. Because some melanomas arise in congenital nevi, a changing congenital nevus needs to be biopsied to rule out melanoma.

- Dysplastic nevi, also called atypical nevi, can mimic melanoma. When an atypical nevus is suspicious for melanoma, perform a narrow-margin biopsy. Only the less-suspicious and flat dysplastic nevi should be monitored with photography or serial exams (see Chapter 171, Dysplastic Nevus and Spitz Nevus).
- Spitz nevi can mimic melanoma or actually be a spitzoid melanoma. If a lesion appears to be a Spitz nevus, it should be biopsied. The only exceptions are typical Spitz nevi in children under age 12. However, if the lesion is atypical, a biopsy is always needed (see Chapter 171, Dysplastic Nevus and Spitz Nevus).
- Seborrheic keratoses (SKs) usually look like they are stuck on, with surface cracks and a verrucous (wartlike) appearance. These are benign and not precancerous. SKs can be darkly pigmented or asymmetric with irregular borders and can have varied colors. Perform a biopsy if the diagnosis is uncertain. Be careful to not

mistake a melanoma for an SK (**Figure 179-4**) (see Chapter 164, Seborrheic Keratosis). Do not perform cryosurgery on an SK with any atypical features. These should be biopsied. A number of malpractice lawsuits have been filed against physicians who froze a melanoma thought to be an SK.

- Solar lentigines appear as light brown macules on the face and the dorsum of the hands. Many patients call them liver spots, but they are unrelated to the liver. A large isolated solar lentigo on the face can mimic lentigo maligna melanoma. In this case, perform a broad scoop shave of the most suspicious area or the whole lesion. Dermoscopy is helpful to guide selecting the area to biopsy (see Chapters 111 and 181 on dermoscopy).
- Dermatofibromas are fibrotic nodules that occur most frequently on the legs and arms. They can be any color from skin color to black and often have a brown halo surrounding them. A pinch test will produce a dimpling of the skin in most cases (see Chapter 166, Dermatofibroma).
- Pyogenic granulomas can resemble an amelanotic melanoma, and sending for pathologic exam will ensure that the clinical diagnosis is correct (**Figure 179-22**) (see Chapter 167, Pyogenic Granuloma).
- Pigmented basal cell carcinomas (BCCs) may resemble a melanoma. However, the pigment in the BCC is often scattered throughout the lesion, and it has other features of a BCC, such as a pearly appearance with a rolled border (**Figure 179-23**) (see Chapter 177, Basal Cell Carcinoma). Dermoscopy can be very helpful, as a pigmented BCC has a number of specific dermoscopic structures to look for (see Chapters 111 and 181 on dermoscopy).
- Merkel cell carcinoma (see **Figure 178-20**) is a rare cutaneous neuroendocrine malignancy that is most common on the head and neck of elderly individuals as an enlarging pink to dark purple nodule that may mimic amelanotic or nodular melanoma.

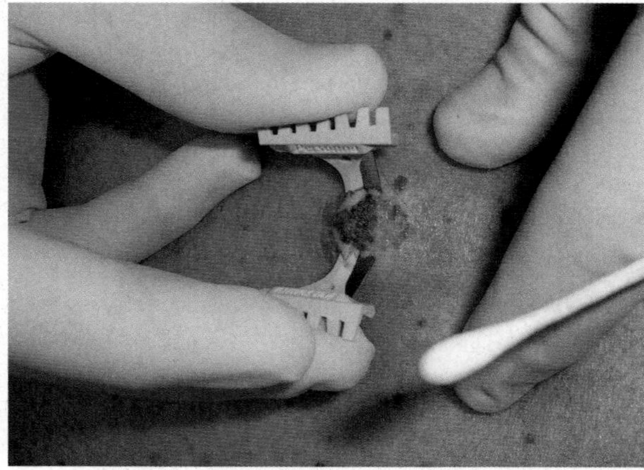

FIGURE 179-21 Saucerization (scoop or deep shave) of the entire pigmented lesion suspected to be a superficial spreading melanoma was performed successfully with a DermaBlade. Breslow thickness was 0.6 mm, and the patient then underwent a full surgical excision with 1-cm margins. (*Reproduced with permission from Richard P. Usatine, MD.*)

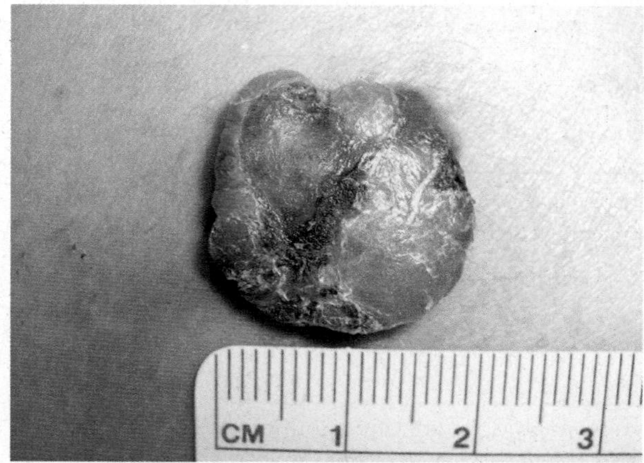

FIGURE 179-22 Thick ulcerated nodular mostly amelanotic on the back of a young woman that could be mistaken for a pyogenic granuloma or basal cell carcinoma. Most importantly, a full-depth biopsy was performed. The melanoma depth was greater than 1 mm, and the patient was sent for a complete excision with a sentinel node biopsy. (*Reproduced with permission from Richard P. Usatine, MD.*)

MANAGEMENT

- Cutaneous melanoma is surgically treated with complete full-skin-depth excision using margins determined by the Breslow depth. This depth is a measure of tumor thickness from the granular layer of the epidermis to the point of deepest invasion using an ocular micrometer.
- Current recommendations for excision margins range from 5 mm for in situ lesions to 1 to 2 cm for invasive lesions. **Table 179-1** shows a comparison of world recommendations.[14] SOR Ⓐ
- Mohs micrographic surgery, performed by specially trained physicians, may prove useful in completely removing subclinical tumor extension in certain subtypes of melanoma in situ, such as lentigo maligna, desmoplastic melanoma, and acral lentiginous melanoma in situ.[15]
- Sentinel lymph node biopsy (SLNB) is not recommended when the risk of a positive node is less than 5%. This includes tumors less than 0.8 mm without ulceration. SLNB should be discussed and considered when there is a 5%–10% chance of a positive node. This includes tumors >0.8 mm thick with ulceration, mitotic index of ≥2 mitoses per square millimeter, or the

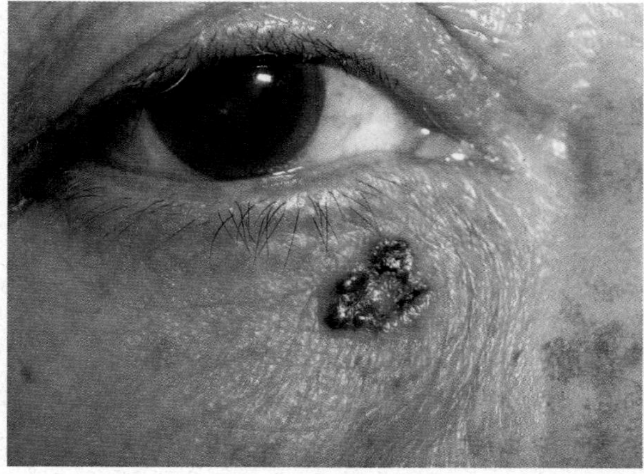

FIGURE 179-23 A pigmented basal cell carcinoma on the lower eyelid that has rolled pearly borders even though the color is black. A shave biopsy allowed a diagnosis of a basal cell carcinoma to be made. (*Reproduced with permission from Richard P. Usatine, MD.*)

TABLE 179-1 Currently Recommended Excision Margins for Primary Melanoma

Tumor Thickness	Excision Margin			
	UK MSG	WHO	Australian	Dutch MSG
In situ	2–5 mm	5 mm	5 mm	2 mm
<1 mm	1 cm	1 cm	1 cm	1 cm
1–2 mm	1–2 cm	1 cm*	1 cm	1 cm
2.1–4 mm	2–3 cm (2 cm preferred)	2 cm	1 cm	2 cm
>4 mm	2–3 cm	2 cm	2 cm	2 cm

Abbreviations: MSG, Melanoma Study Group; WHO, World Health Organization.
*For melanomas thicker than 1.5 mm, recommended excision margin is 2 cm.
Modified with permission from Bishop JA, Corrie PG, Evans J, et al: UK guidelines for the management of cutaneous melanoma, Br J Plast Surg. 2002 Jan;55(1):46-54.

presence of lymphovascular invasion. Rare cases with microsatellitosis within the original specimen upstage the tumor to stage III in transit, and SLNB is recommended regardless of the tumor thickness.

- Patients with advanced melanoma (**Figure 179-24**) should be referred to medical oncology and may receive combination therapy with multiple chemotherapeutic agents and immunotherapy. Many trials are ongoing, and new chemotherapy regimens are emerging rapidly. Consideration should be given to consulting palliative care early to improve quality of life (see Chapter 5, End of Life).
- Systemic therapy options for metastatic or unresectable disease are complex and evolving rapidly based on trial data and include immunotherapy with pembrolizumab, nivolumab, combination nivolumab/ipilimumab, and targeted BRAF therapy with dabrafenib/trametinib or vemurafenib/cobimetinib as well as conventional chemotherapy options.

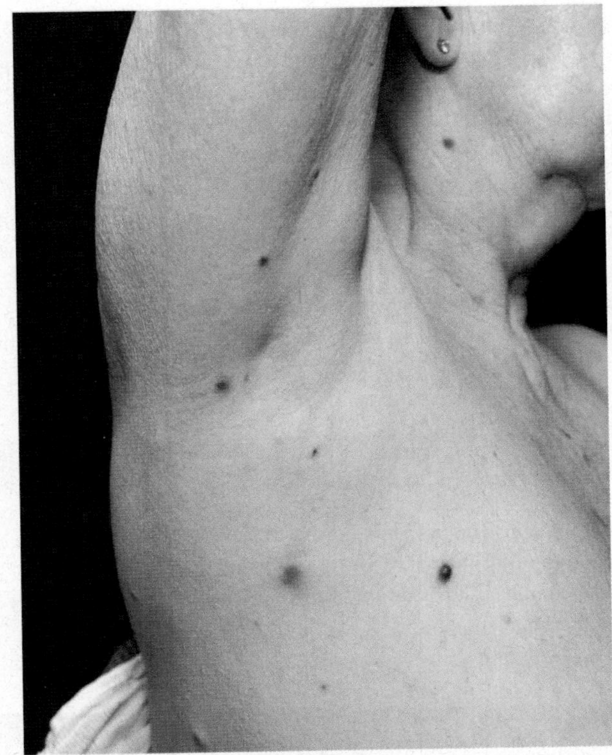

FIGURE 179-24 Metastatic melanoma with dark black nodules scattered over the body and neck. (*Reproduced with permission from Richard P. Usatine, MD.*)

PREVENTION AND SCREENING

- Melanoma prevention starts with sun protection.
- Sunscreen use has been shown in a randomized controlled trial to reduce the number of melanomas by roughly half.[16]
- Sun protection should include sun avoidance, protective clothing, and sunscreen.
- Indoor tanning is not safe and should be avoided.
- The U.S. Preventive Services Task Force has not found sufficient evidence to recommend regular screening for melanoma or skin cancer in the general population.[17]
- Most experts believe that persons at high risk for melanoma (including previous personal history of melanoma, high-risk family history, and high-risk skin types with significant sun exposure) should be screened regularly for melanoma by a physician trained in such screening.
- Evidence for the value of self-screening is lacking, but persons at high risk for melanoma should also be encouraged to observe their own skin and to come in for evaluation if they see any suspicious changes or growths.

PROGNOSIS

Prognosis depends on tumor depth, mitotic rate, the presence of ulceration, positive lymph nodes, and metastases. In stage 0 disease, surgical excision is almost always curative. Five-year survival in patients by tumor thickness is almost 100% for in situ lesions, 92% for lesions less than 0.8 mm thick, 81% for lesions between 1 and 2 mm thick, 70% for lesions 2 to 4 mm thick, and 53% for lesions thicker than 4 mm. When accounting for nodal and distant metastasis, stage III disease carries a 40% to 78% 5-year survival, depending on the number of nodal metastases, and stage IV disease carries a 15% to 20% 5-year survival.[18]

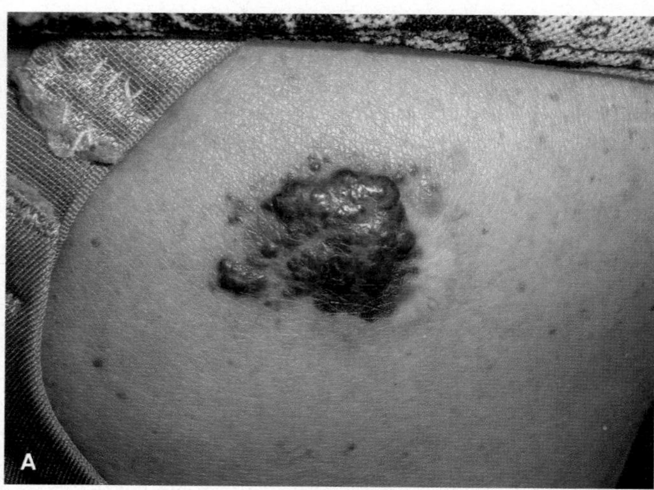

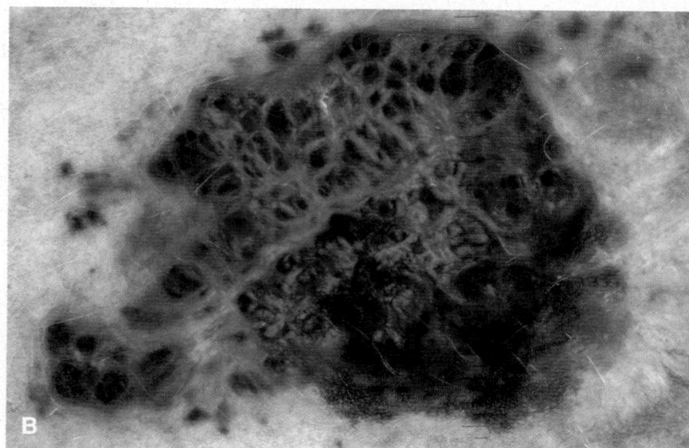

FIGURE 179-25 A. Large nodular melanoma on the right shoulder of a 63-year-old Hispanic woman that arose in a nevus and has in-transit metastases/satellites visible. Breslow depth of 5.5 mm. It was excised with 2 cm margins and the sentinel lymph node biopsy was positive. Note the multiple colors. The patient was uninsured and waited 3 years before seeking care. B. Dermoscopy showing pigment network of the original nevus at 5-6 o'clock and in-transit metastases/satellites visible especially in the top right and left corners. Note the shiny white lines with polarized dermoscopy. (*Reproduced with permission from Richard P. Usatine, MD.*)

FOLLOW-UP

The need for follow-up is largely determined by the stage of the disease (**Figure 179-25**). The prognosis is worsened by increasing depth, mitotic rate, presence of ulceration, positive lymph nodes, and metastases.

Follow-up for stages 0 and I cutaneous melanoma includes regular skin examinations by a physician trained in skin cancer screening. Total body photography may be of benefit in monitoring patients with multiple nevi (**Figure 179-26**). The rate of subsequent cutaneous melanomas among persons with a history of melanoma was found to be more than 10 times the rate of a first cutaneous melanoma, and the highest incidence of recurrence was in the first 3 to 5 years after initial diagnosis.[19,20]

PATIENT EDUCATION

Advise patients who have had melanoma to avoid future sun exposure and monitor their skin for new and changing moles. Recommend a complete skin examination yearly by a physician trained to detect early melanoma.

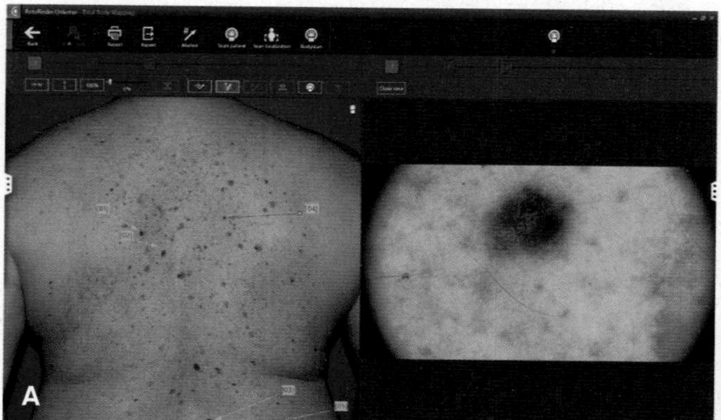

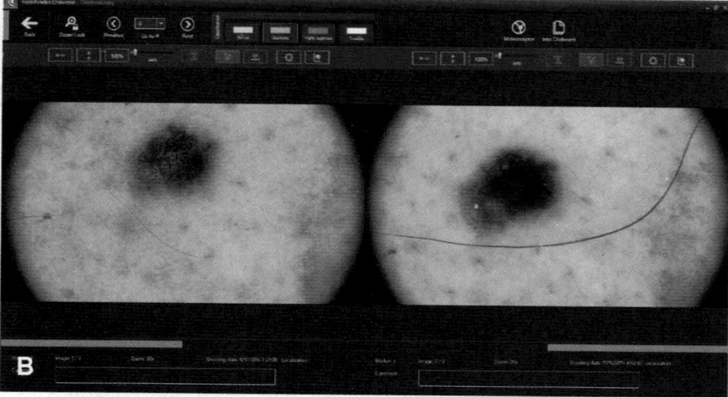

FIGURE 179-26 A. Total body photography for a 57-year-old man with multiple atypical nevi. He is followed with skin exams and serial photographs in 20 standardized poses that allow easy visual and computer aided assessment of changes. Lesions of concern may be marked for follow up and serial dermoscopic photos. The brown papule labeled 4 (with red arrow) is seen in a dermoscopic view on the right. A set of photos can be completed in about 15 minutes. B. Comparison of dermoscopic images of the same lesion reveals changes over time. A biopsy demonstrated a severely atypical nevus that required a full excision with margins. (*Reproduced with permission from Jonathan B. Karnes, MD.*)

PATIENT RESOURCES

- MedlinePlus. *Melanoma*—**http://medlineplus.gov/melanoma.html.**
- The Skin Cancer Foundation. *Melanoma*—**http://www.skincancer.org/skin-cancer-information/melanoma.**
- American Cancer Society. *Skin Cancer—Melanoma*—**http://www.cancer.org/cancer/melanoma-skin-cancer.html.**

PROVIDER RESOURCES

- DermNet NZ. *Melanoma*—**https://www.dermnetnz.org/topics/melanoma.**
- National Cancer Institute. *Melanoma Treatment*—**https://www.cancer.gov/types/skin/hp/melanoma-treatment-pdq/.**
- Chapters and videos on diagnosing and surgically managing melanoma can be found in the following book/DVD or electronic application: Usatine R, Pfenninger J, Stulberg D, Small R. *Dermatologic and Cosmetic Procedures in Office Practice*. Philadelphia, PA: Elsevier; 2012.
- Information about smartphone and tablet apps of this resource can be viewed at **www.usatinemedia.com.**

REFERENCES

1. American Cancer Society website. *Key Statistics for Melanoma Skin Cancer*. https://www.cancer.org/cancer/melanoma-skin-cancer/about/key-statistics.html. January 4, 2018. Accessed March 2018.
2. Jemal A, Saraiya M, Patel P, et al. Recent trends in cutaneous melanoma incidence and death rates in the United States, 1992-2006. *J Am Acad Dermatol*. 2011;65(5 Suppl 1):S17-S25.
3. Rigel DS. Trends in dermatology: melanoma incidence. *Arch Dermatol*. 2010;146(3):318.
4. Thomas L, Tranchand P, Berard F, et al. Semiological value of ABCDE criteria in the diagnosis of cutaneous pigmented tumors. *Dermatology*. 1998;197(1):11-17.
5. Coit DG, Thompson JA, Albertini MR, et al. NCCN Clinical Practice Guidelines in Oncology: Melanoma. *NCCN Guidelines*. Version 3.2018. 2018.
6. Wang Y, Zhao Y, Shuangge M. Racial differences in six major subtypes of melanoma: descriptive epidemiology. *BMC Cancer*. 2016;16:691.
7. Gualandri L, Betti R, Crosti C. Clinical features of 36 cases of amelanotic melanomas and considerations about the relationship between histologic subtypes and diagnostic delay. *J Eur Acad Dermatol Venereol*. 2009;23(3):283-287.
8. Jackson S, Nesbitt LT. *Differential Diagnosis for the Dermatologist*. Berlin, Germany: Springer; 2008:930-931.
9. Benelli C, Roscetti E, Pozzo VD, et al. The dermoscopic versus the clinical diagnosis of melanoma. *Eur J Dermatol*. 1999;9(6):470-476.
10. Dolianitis C, Kelly J, Wolfe R, Simpson P. Comparative performance of 4 dermoscopic algorithms by nonexperts for the diagnosis of melanocytic lesions. *Arch Dermatol*. 2005;141(8):1008-1014.
11. Zager JS, Hochwald SN, Marzban SS, et al. Shave biopsy is a safe and accurate method for the initial evaluation of melanoma. *J Am Coll Surg*. 2011;212(4):454-460; discussion 460-462.
12. Dalton SR, Gardner TL, Libow LF, Elston DM. Contiguous lesions in lentigo maligna. *J Am Acad Dermatol*. 2005;52(5):859-862.
13. Ng JC, Swain S, Dowling JP. The impact of partial biopsy on histopathologic diagnosis of cutaneous melanoma: experience of an Australian tertiary referral service. *Arch Dermatol*. 2010;146(3):234-239.
14. Lens MB, Dawes M, Goodacre T, Bishop JAN. Excision margins in the treatment of primary cutaneous melanoma: a systematic review of randomized controlled trials comparing narrow vs wide excision. *Arch Surg*. 2002;137(10):1101-1105.
15. Chang KH, Dufresne R, Cruz A, Rogers GS. The operative management of melanoma: where does Mohs surgery fit in? *Dermatol Surg*. 2011;37(8):1069-1079.
16. Green AC, Williams GM, Logan V, Strutton GM. Reduced melanoma after regular sunscreen use: randomized trial follow-up. *J Clin Oncol*. 2011;29(3):257-263.
17. U.S. Preventive Services Task Force; Bibbins-Domingo K, Grossman DC, Curry SJ, et al. Screening for Skin Cancer: U.S. Preventive Services Task Force Recommendation Statement. *JAMA*. 2016;316(4):429-435.
18. American Cancer Society website. *Survival Rates for Melanoma Skin Cancer by Stage*. https://www.cancer.org/cancer/melanoma-skin-cancer/detection-diagnosis-staging/survival-rates-for-melanoma-skin-cancer-by-stage.html. May 19, 2016. Accessed March 2018.
19. Tsao H, Atkins MB, Sober AJ. Management of cutaneous melanoma. *N Engl J Med*. 2004;351(10):998-1012.
20. Levi F, Randimbison L, Te V-C, La Vecchia C. High constant incidence rates of second cutaneous melanomas. *Int J Cancer*. 2005;117(5):877-879.

180 CUTANEOUS T-CELL LYMPHOMA

Gina Chacon, MD
Anjeli Nayar, MD
Richard P. Usatine, MD
Mindy A. Smith, MD, MS

PATIENT STORY

A 52-year-old black woman presented with a 7-month history of a hypopigmented rash in a symmetric distribution on her upper thighs and arms (**Figures 180-1** and **180-2**). She had been evacuated from New Orleans following Hurricane Katrina. She had waded through polluted waters for hours before being rescued by boat. Four days passed before she had access to a shower, at which time she noticed a single erythematous spot the size of a silver dollar on her left thigh. Over the next several weeks, it faded to hypopigmented macules and plaques and eventually spread to both thighs and arms. The physical examination revealed no lymphadenopathy. A hematoxylin and eosin (H&E) stain of a full-thickness punch biopsy revealed "cerebriform" lymphocytes at the dermal–epidermal junction characteristic of mycosis fungoides (MF), a type of cutaneous T-cell lymphoma (CTCL). Her blood tests were essentially normal, and she was HIV-negative. The patient reported no improvement with topical high-potency generic steroid to affected areas and was started on narrow-band UVB treatment twice weekly.

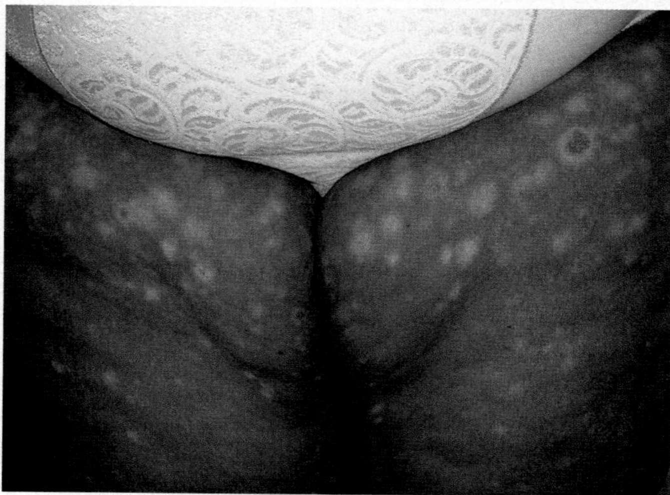

FIGURE 180-1 The hypopigmented patches of mycosis fungoides on the thighs of a 52-year-old black woman. This is the patch stage of the disease. Although this mimicked vitiligo, the distribution and appearance warranted a biopsy that provided a definitive diagnosis of mycosis fungoides. (*Reproduced with permission from Richard P. Usatine, MD.*)

INTRODUCTION

CTCL clinically and biologically represent a heterogeneous group of non-Hodgkin lymphomas.[1]

EPIDEMIOLOGY

- The annual incidence of CTCL in the United States increased from 2.8 per 1 million (1973–1977) to 10.2 per 1 million (2005–2009).[2] The incidence appears to have stabilized over the past 20 years, with an annual percentage change of only 0.1%.[2]
- CTCL is a rare disease, with about 3000 new cases per year in the United States.
- The most common types of CTCL are MF (50% to 72%), which is generally indolent in behavior (**Figures 180-1** to **180-5**); primary cutaneous CD30+ lymphoproliferative disorders (LPD; about 30%); and Sézary syndrome (SS; 1% to 3%), an aggressive leukemic form of the disease.[3] LPDs include lymphomatoid papulosis (12%) and cutaneous anaplastic large-cell lymphoma (C-ALCL, 9%) (**Figure 180-6**).[3,4]
- CTCL is more common in African Americans than in whites, with an incidence rate ratio of 1.3:1 (2005–2009).[2]
    - African-American and Hispanic individuals have an earlier onset of disease; in one study database, the mean age at diagnosis was 60.0 ± 14.8 years for Caucasian, 49.3 ± 16.9 years for

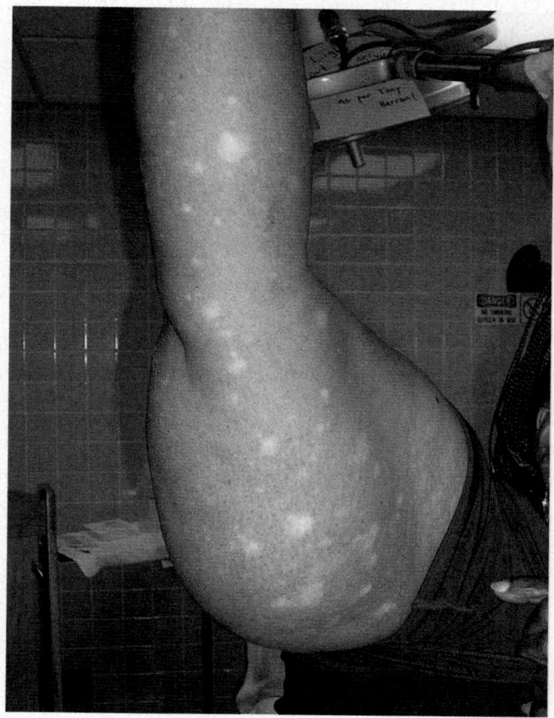

FIGURE 180-2 Hypopigmented patches on the arm of the woman in **Figure 180-1** with mycosis fungoides. (*Reproduced with permission from Richard P. Usatine, MD.*)

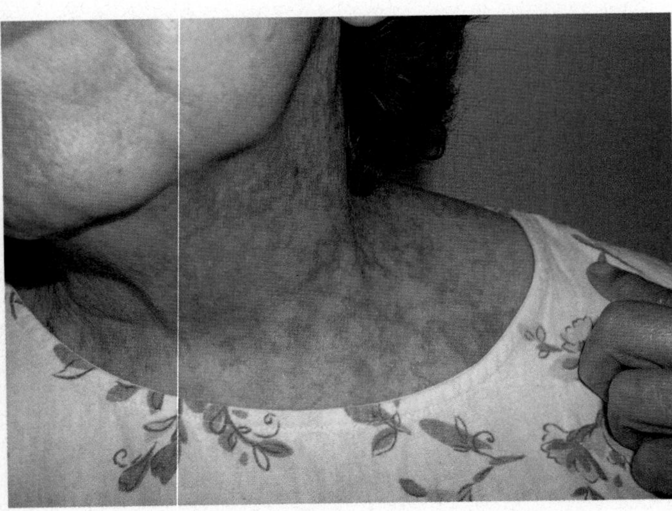

FIGURE 180-3 Reticulated mycosis fungoides (MF). This netlike pattern of mycosis fungoides is also called *parapsoriasis variegata*. (*Reproduced with permission from Heather Wickless, MD.*)

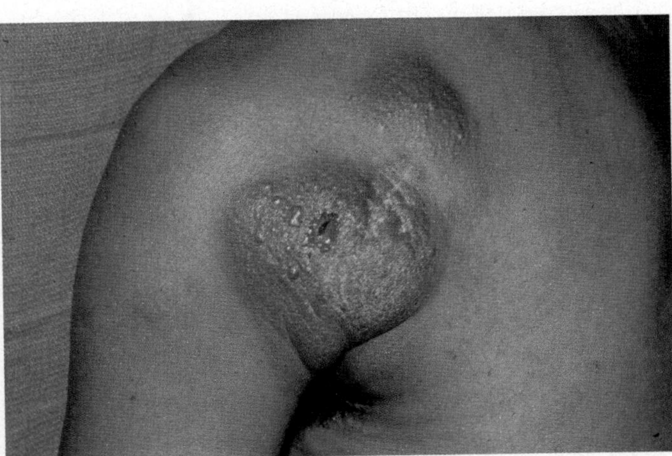

FIGURE 180-5 Tumor stage of mycosis fungoides (MF). (*Reproduced with permission from Richard P. Usatine, MD.*)

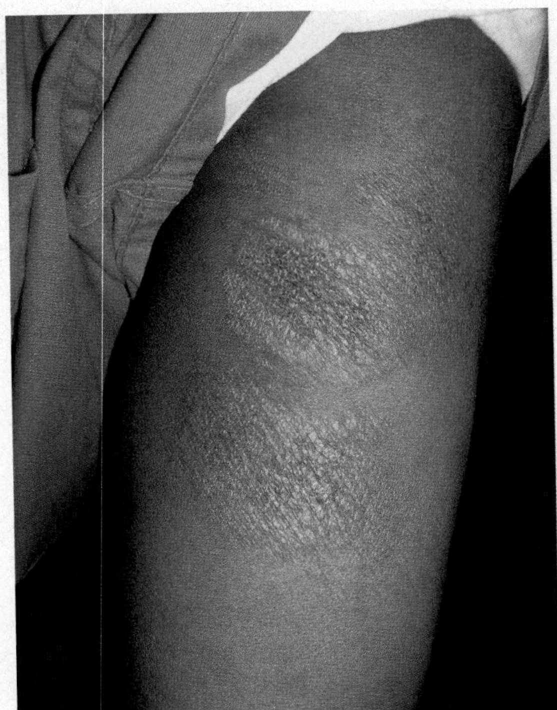

FIGURE 180-4 Plaque stage of mycosis fungoides (MF) on the arm of a 57-year-old nurse. She has had mycosis fungoides for 8 years and has intermittently been on chemotherapy. Recently, her mycosis fungoides has worsened and she was started on nitrogen mustard. (*Reproduced with permission from E.J. Mayeaux, Jr., MD.*)

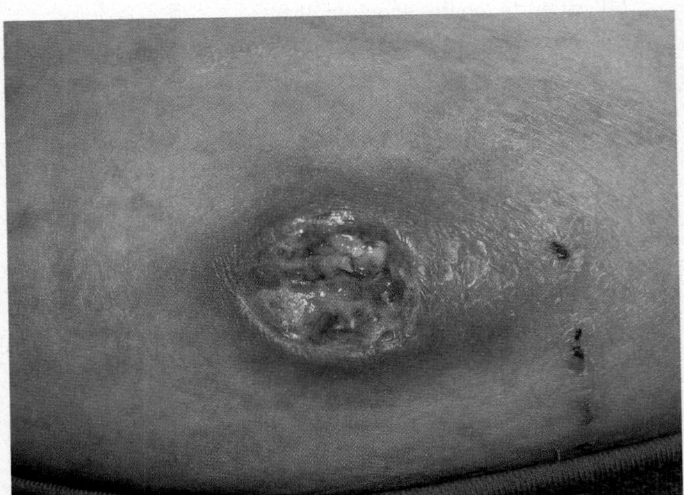

FIGURE 180-6 Anaplastic large cell cutaneous T-cell lymphoma that presented looking like cellulitis, then an abscess in a 17-year-old woman. When antibiotics and an incision and drainage failed, a punch biopsy revealed the surprising diagnosis. (*Reproduced with permission from Richard P. Usatine, MD.*)

African-American, and 47.4 ± 17.8 years for Hispanic patients.[5] In addition, more CTCLs among African Americans were diagnosed at a more advanced clinical stage compared to Caucasians or Hispanics (36.1% vs. 23% and 21.2%, respectively; odds ratio 2.83; 95% confidence interval 1.81, 4.42).[5]

- CTCL is more common in males, with a male-to-female ratio of 2:1; although the most recent data (2005–2009) show a ratio of 1.6:1.[2]
- Median age at presentation is between 50 and 70 years, although pediatric and young adult cases do occur.[1]

ETIOLOGY AND PATHOPHYSIOLOGY

- MF is a malignant lymphoma of helper T cells that usually remain confined to skin and lymph nodes (LNs)[3] and are named for the mushroom-like skin tumors seen in severe cases (**Figure 180-7**).[6]
- Lesions of primary cutaneous CD30+ LPD are defined by the variable number of atypical CD30+ lymphocytes that express the CD30 antigen in most of the tumor cells.[3]
- The exact etiology of CTCL is unknown, but environmental, infectious, and genetic causes have been suggested.
    - In one study in Texas, there was a clustering of cases in 3 communities with incidence rates 5- to 22-fold higher than the overall Texas population, suggesting an external etiologic factor.[5] Environmental exposure to Agent Orange may be responsible for some cases.[6]
    - Human T-lymphocytic virus (HTLV) types 1 and 2, HIV-1, cytomegalovirus (CMV), Epstein-Barr virus (EBV), and *Borrelia burgdorferi* have been suggested, but unproven, infectious causes of MF.[7] There is one case report of possible conjugal transmission of MF between a heterosexual couple who developed advanced MF within 14 months of one another.[7]
    - MF and SS are associated with specific human leukocyte antigen (HLA) types, and prognosis appears to correspond to certain HLA alleles.[8] Genetic predisposition is also suggested by detection of HLA class II alleles DRB1*11 and DQB1*03 in association with sporadic and familial malignancy and familial clustering among Israeli Jews.[9] PLCG1 mutations have also been reported in CTCLs.[10]
- Abnormal cytokine expression in interleukin-13 and its receptors, among others, may be responsible for the enhanced proliferation of malignant cells and/or depression of the antitumor immune response seen in CTCLs.[11] Defective apoptosis is also believed to play a central role in pathogenesis.[4]
- Metastasis to the liver, spleen, lungs, GI tract, bone marrow, and the central nervous system (CNS) may occur via T-cell spread through the lymphatic system.[7]
- The reduction of T-cell receptor complexity contributes to immunosuppression in advanced MF and SS and may manifest clinically as herpes simplex or zoster.[12] Death is usually due to systemic infection, especially from *Staphylococcus aureus* and *Pseudomonas aeruginosa*.
- Host antitumor immunity also deteriorates, and patients have an increased risk for secondary malignancies including Hodgkin lymphoma, lymphomatoid papulosis, and non-hematologic malignancies.[4]

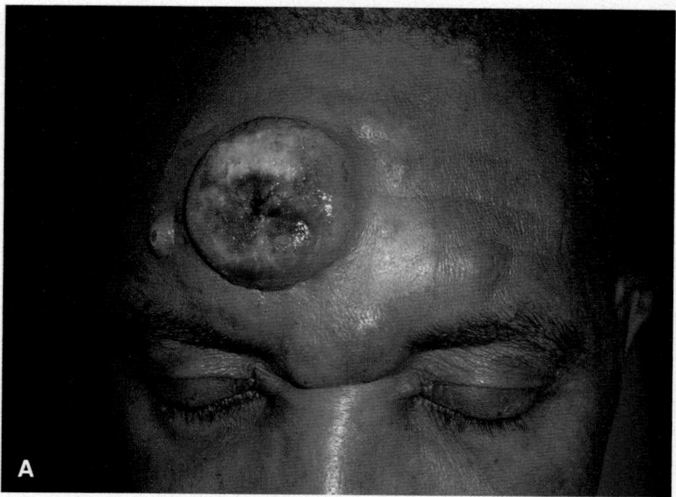

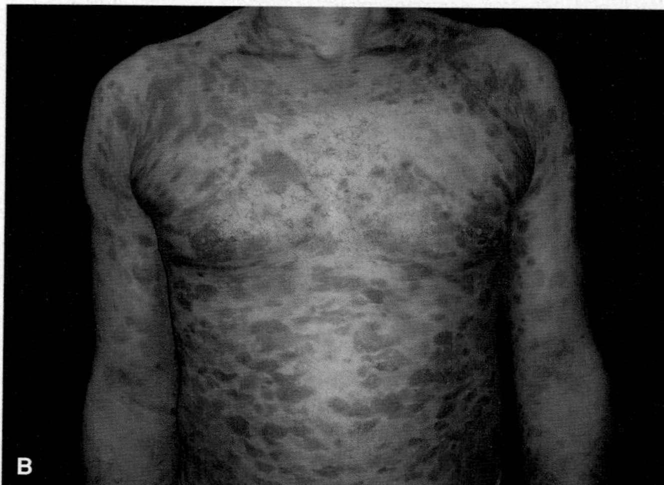

FIGURE 180-7 Tumor stage of mycosis fungoides (MF) in a 63-year-old black man. **A.** The large fungating tumor on the face resembles a mushroom, and this is the kind of lesion that led to the name of mycosis fungoides. **B.** Widespread hyperpigmented plaques from head to feet. (*Reproduced with permission from Richard P. Usatine, MD.*)

DIAGNOSIS

CLINICAL FEATURES

- The most common initial presentation of MF involves patches or scaly plaques with a persistent rash that is often pruritic and usually erythematous (see **Figures 180-1** to **180-4**).[4,7] Patches may evolve to generalized, infiltrated plaques or to ulcerated, exophytic tumors (see **Figures 180-5** to **180-7**).[3]
- Hypo- or hyperpigmented lesions, petechiae, poikiloderma (skin atrophy with telangiectasia), and alopecia with or without mucinosis are other findings. The folliculotropic variant of MF presents with spotty alopecia (**Figure 180-8**).
- A "premycotic" phase may precede definitive diagnosis for months to decades, which involves nonspecific, slightly scaling skin lesions that intermittently appear and may eventually resolve with topical steroids.
- Of the LPDs, lymphomatoid papulosis appears as recurring papules and nodules over the trunk and extremities that disappear in 3–12 weeks, sometimes leaving scars.[3] C-ALCL presents with solitary or localized nodular lesions of 1.5 cm or larger that may ulcerate (see **Figure 180-6**). In 20% of patients with C-ALCL, multifocal lesions are present, which may partially or completely regress; 10% develop extracutaneous dissemination, primarily to regional lymph nodes.[3]
- SS usually arises de novo and is characterized by generalized exfoliative erythroderma, lymphadenopathy, severe pruritus, and atypical Sézary cells in the peripheral blood.[4] Diffuse infiltration of atypical T cells in SS may exaggerate facial lines, creating a leonine facies.

TYPICAL DISTRIBUTION

- Lesions of MF may affect any skin surface, but typically initially develop on non–sun-exposed "bathing suit" areas, such as the trunk below the waistline, breasts, buttocks, and the groin areas (**Figure 180-9**).[4] Lesions of C-ALCL can be found on the face, trunk, extremities, and buttocks.[3]
- If there is follicular involvement, lesions may be found on the face or scalp (**Figures 180-10** and **180-11**).
- MF occasionally presents as a refractory dermatosis of the palms or soles.

BIOPSY AND LABORATORY STUDIES

- A full-thickness punch biopsy of the lesion is the most important diagnostic tool. If the initial biopsy is negative but the rash persists, the biopsy should be repeated.[7] Topical treatments and systemic immunosuppressants should be discontinued 2 to 4 weeks before the biopsy.[13]
- If the LNs are palpable or lymphadenopathy is suspected, also known as "dermatopathic lymphadenitis," biopsies should be performed (**Figure 180-12**).
- A bone marrow biopsy should be performed if there is proven nodal or blood involvement.
- Histology—Classic MF is characterized by a proliferation of mature CD4+CD45RO+ memory T lymphocytes. The skin biopsy may

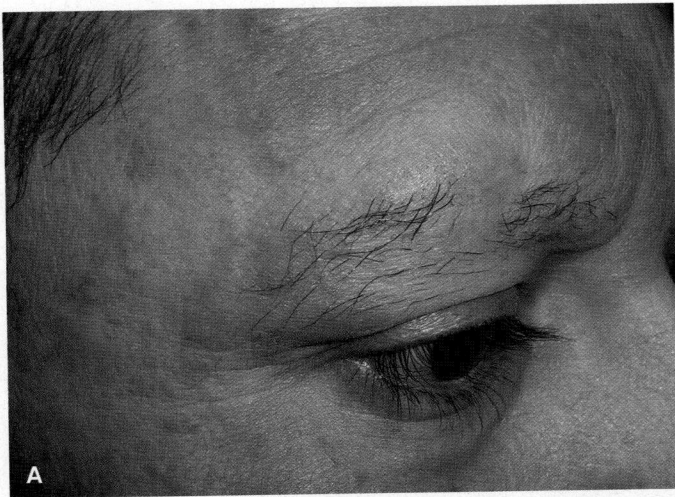

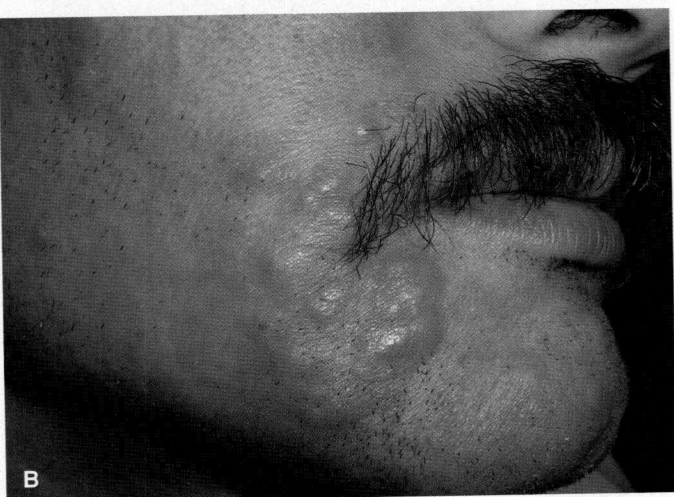

FIGURE 180-8 **A.** Folliculotropic variant of mycosis fungoides (MF) with visible alopecia in the eyebrow region of this 38-year-old man. **B.** Note the absence of hair growth in parts of the beard where there is follicular involvement. (*Reproduced with permission from Richard P. Usatine, MD.*)

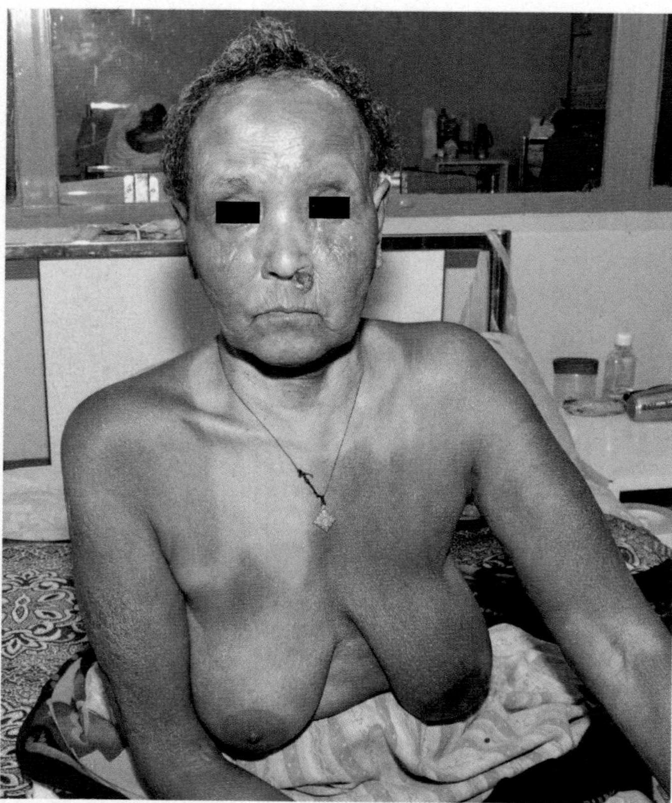

FIGURE 180-9 Mycosis fungoides (MF) causing hyperpigmented patches over the face, trunk, breasts, and upper extremities. (*Reproduced with permission from Richard P. Usatine, MD.*)

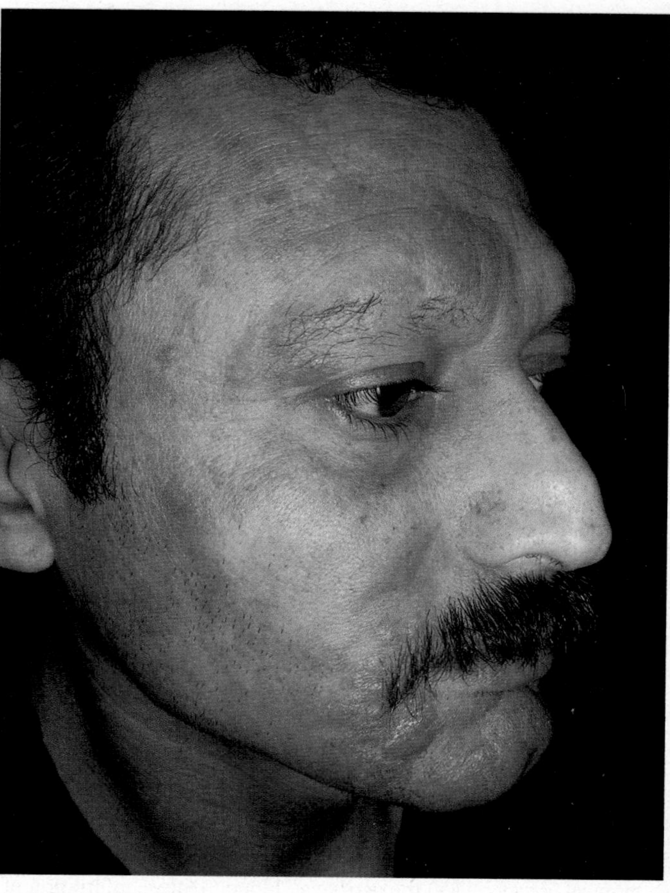

FIGURE 180-11 Facial predominance of this folliculotropic variant of mycosis fungoides (MF). Aside from the facial plaques, the only other area involved presented as alopecia in 1 area of the left forearm. (*Reproduced with permission from Richard P. Usatine, MD.*)

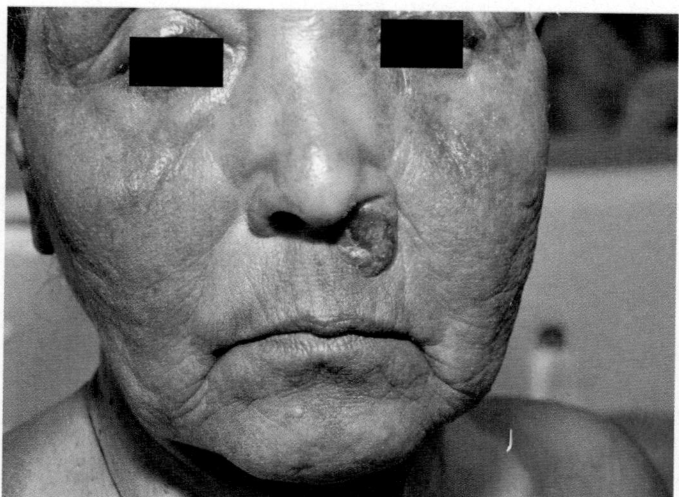

FIGURE 180-10 Mycosis fungoides (MF) on the face with an ulcerated tumor under the nose. (*Reproduced with permission from Richard P. Usatine, MD.*)

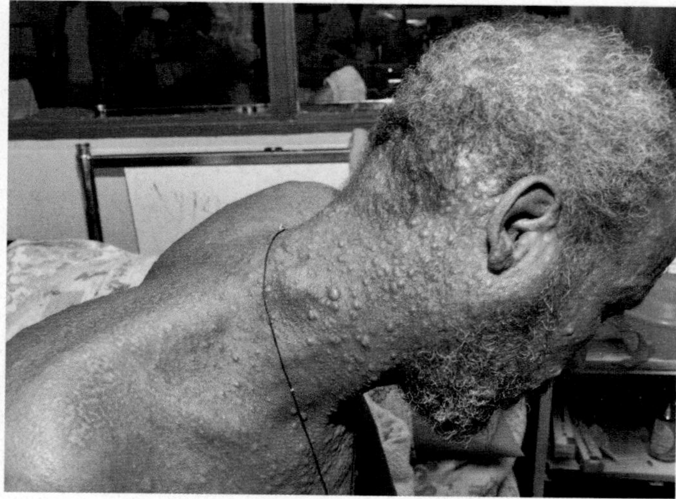

FIGURE 180-12 Tumor stage of mycosis fungoides (MF) with a large posterior cervical node visible. (*Reproduced with permission from Richard P. Usatine, MD.*)

reveal Pautrier microabscesses or an inflammatory cell bandlike infiltrate lining the basal layer or in the upper dermis ("mononuclear epidermotropism"). Malignant lymphocytes have hyperchromatic and convoluted or "cerebriform" nuclei.[4]

- Radiography—A chest radiograph and CT scan of the abdomen and pelvis are recommended for advanced stages IIB to IIIB, or if visceral disease is suspected.[14] Positron emission tomography (PET) scans offer more sensitive detection of LN involvement and can be considered in individual cases.[14]
- Serology and blood tests—A complete blood cell count with differential, a buffy coat smear to screen for Sézary cells, lactic dehydrogenase and uric acid as markers for bulky or aggressive disease, and liver function tests to detect hepatic involvement should be measured.[14] Peripheral eosinophilia is an independent marker for poor prognosis and disease progression.[15,16]
- Flow cytometry—This test may be used to detect malignant clones and to quantify CD8+ lymphocytes to assess immunocompetence.
- Immunophenotyping may be used to support histology results.
- Polymerase chain reaction (PCR) and Southern blot testing are recommended to detect T-cell rearrangements, if histology and immunophenotyping results are equivocal and to detect abnormal cells in LNs.[14]
- The International Society for Cutaneous Lymphoma proposed criteria for diagnosing MF and Sézary syndrome by incorporating clinical, histopathologic, molecular biologic, and immunopathologic features, including the percentage of skin coverage with lesions or erythema, presence of clinically abnormal peripheral lymph nodes, visceral organ involvement, and blood involvement (high tumor blood burden defined as absolute Sézary cell count of greater than 1000/mm^3).[17]

DIFFERENTIAL DIAGNOSIS

- "Premycotic" period preceding diagnosis of MF may resemble parapsoriasis en plaque or nonspecific dermatitis.[13]
- MF with erythroderma must be distinguished from generalized atopic dermatitis, contact dermatitis, photodermatitis, drug eruptions, erythrodermic psoriasis, and idiopathic hyper-eosinophilic syndrome (see Chapter 162, Erythroderma).[8]
- Unilesional MF may resemble nummular eczema, lichen simplex chronicus, erythema chronicum migrans, tinea corporis, or digitate dermatosis (a variant of small plaque parapsoriasis).[13]
- Vitiligo typically involves discrete, hypopigmented macules on the hands and face that coalesce into larger areas.[6] However, some MF may mimic vitiligo, as seen in **Figures 180-1** and **180-2**. The distribution of the hypopigmented macules in this case is atypical for vitiligo and this prompted a biopsy that led to the diagnosis of MF (see Chapter 206, Vitiligo and Hypopigmentation).
- Idiopathic guttate hypomelanosis is a benign condition involving smaller hypopigmented macules than those seen in MF.[6]
- In patients with HIV, histopathology resembling MF may represent a reactive inflammatory condition instead. Nonepidermotrophic large T-cell cutaneous lymphoma and B-cell diffuse cutaneous lymphoma are more frequent complications than MF in these patients.[18]

MANAGEMENT

- In addition to symptomatic treatments such emollients and antipruritics (Doxepin cream 5%), treatments for CTCL can be divided into skin-directed therapy and systemic therapy. Of the skin-directed therapies, topical corticosteroids are widely used in all stages of CTCL in the hopes that they will help control the disease and palliate any cutaneous symptoms of itch.[15] SOR Ⓑ
- For stage I disease localized to the skin, topical high-potency steroids (clobetasol cream) on an outpatient basis are recommended.[14] SOR Ⓒ Topical retinoids and topical chemotherapy (nitrogen mustard, bischloroethylnitrosourea, or carmustine) are treatment alternatives for localized disease and effective adjuvants in generalized disease.[6,14,19] SOR Ⓑ
  - Bexarotene 1% topical gel or alemtuzumab may be tried if disease persists despite treatment or if other medication is not tolerated.[14] When used in combination with psoralen-enhanced UV light (PUVA), bexarotene decreases the total UVA dosage needed and, if used as maintenance therapy, increases the duration of remission.[20] SOR Ⓒ
  - Alternatively, PUVA may also be used concurrently with interferon (IFN), 3 times weekly, or retinoids until skin lesions clear, then continued as maintenance therapy at a reduced frequency.[14,20] SOR Ⓒ
  - Tazarotene, low-dose oral etoposide, and imiquimod may be considered in the treatment of early CTCL.[14]
  - For a plaque recalcitrant to PUVA and retinoid combination therapy, 1 case study showed that imiquimod 5% topical cream effectively cleared the lesion.[12] SOR Ⓒ Topical mechlorethamine can also be considered for refractory, stage IA to IIA MF[14]; in one trial, both the gel and ointment formulation were safe and effective with a response at 1 year seen in 58.5% and 47.7%, respectively, using the Composite Assessment of Index Lesion Severity.[21]
  - Phototherapy is a safe, effective, and well-tolerated first-line therapy in patients with early-stage CTCL, with prolonged disease-free remissions being achieved. Narrow-band UVB is at least as effective as PUVA for treatment of early stage MF.[22,23] SOR Ⓒ
  - Narrow-band UVB light has proven effective in early MF and prolongs remission, although an optimal maintenance protocol still needs to be established.[14,24] SOR Ⓒ
  - The therapeutic effects of PUVA and UVB in immune-mediated skin diseases have been attributed to the direct apoptosis of lymphocytes, modification of cell surface receptors, and alteration in production of certain mediators.[22]
  - Photodynamic therapy with 5-aminolevulinic acid (PDT-ALA) was found to effectively eradicate localized infiltrates better than topical steroids, but more studies are needed before it becomes standardized treatment.[19] SOR Ⓒ In general, photodynamic therapy works via direct cytotoxicity, vascular damage, and immune host response.[25]
- Stage II disease involves the regional LNs and may be treated the same as for stage I. For stage IIB, the most recommended therapy is total-skin electron-beam therapy (EBT) followed by nitrogen mustard treatment for 6 or more months.[20] SOR Ⓒ For disease relapse after EBT, PUVA may be used in combination with IFN or a systemic retinoid.[20] SOR Ⓒ Other systemic therapies include fusion toxins, monoclonal antibody treatment, oral retinoids, and

single-agent chemotherapy.[14] For recalcitrant tumors, there is no evidence that combination systemic chemotherapy regimens offer survival outcome superior to that for single agents.[14] SOR Ⓒ

- Stage III, or erythrodermic disease without extracutaneous disease or with limited LN involvement, should be treated with chemotherapy or photophoresis for 4 weeks.[20] SOR Ⓒ Extracorporeal photochemotherapy involves irradiation of white blood cells with PUVA after leukapheresis before reinfusing the blood cells intravenously. If the response is delayed, photophoresis may be combined with IFN or systemic retinoids.
- Stage IV extracutaneous disease should be treated with systemic chemotherapy. Although response rates are improved with combination chemotherapy, the response duration is less than 1 year. Regimens include cyclophosphamide, vincristine, and prednisone (CVP), CVP plus doxorubicin, CVP plus methotrexate, or cyclophosphamide, vincristine, doxorubicin, and etoposide. Adjuvants treatments may include IFN, systemic retinoids, and photophoresis. Single-agent chemotherapy includes methotrexate, liposomal doxorubicin, gemcitabine, etoposide, cyclophosphamide, and purine analogs.[20] SOR Ⓒ The patient should be referred to a dermatologist, and to medical and radiation oncologists.[14]
- In patients with Sézary syndrome, risk of death from infection is high and consideration should be given to treatment with combination systemic and skin-directed immunomodulatory therapy before chemotherapy, unless disease burden or therapeutic failure dictates otherwise.[14]

PROGNOSIS AND FOLLOW-UP

- Overall 5-year survival for patients with CTCL is as follows: MF 88%, (follicular MF 80%, others 100%), CD30+ LPD 95%–100%, and SS 24%.[4]
- Patient age and stage are the most important clinical prognostic factors.[26]
- Patients have a normal life expectancy, if diagnosed early during stage IA, in which the patch or plaque is limited to less than 10% of the skin surface area.[6,14]
- MF and SS are otherwise difficult to cure and have a prognosis of 3.2 years for stage IIB cutaneous tumors (10-year survival 42%), 4 to 6 years for stage III generalized erythroderma (10-year survival 83%), and less than 1.5 years for stage IVA and stage IVB with LN and visceral involvement, respectively.[14]
- The patient should be monitored for development of secondary malignancies.

POTENTIAL COMPLICATIONS

- Infection, particularly from indwelling intravenous catheters or from lymph node biopsy sites.
- High-output cardiac failure.
- Anemia of chronic disorders.
- Edema.
- Secondary malignancies (e.g., skin cancer, melanoma).

PATIENT EDUCATION

- Avoid sun exposure, stay in a cool environment, and keep skin lubricated.
- See your physician if any new skin symptoms and signs appear or the medication is not working.
- Avoid smoking and secondhand smoke.

PATIENT RESOURCES

- Cutaneous Lymphoma Foundation. *About Cutaneous Lymphoma*—**http://www.clfoundation.org/about-cutaneous-lymphoma.**
- National Cancer Institute. *Mycosis Fungoides (Including Sézary Syndrome)*—**http://www.cancer.gov/types/lymphoma/patient/mycosis-fungoides-treatment-pdq.**

PROVIDER RESOURCES

- National Cancer Institute. *Mycosis Fungoides and the Sézary Syndrome Treatment*—**http://www.cancer.gov//types/lymphoma/patient/mycosis-fungoides-treatment-pdq.**
- Skin Cancer Foundation—**http://www.skincancer.org.**
- American Cancer Society—**http://www.cancer.org.**
- Medscape. *Cutaneous T-Cell Lymphoma*—**http://emedicine.medscape.com/article/2139720.**

REFERENCES

1. Li JY, Horwitz S, Moskowitz A, et al. Management of cutaneous T cell lymphoma: new and emerging targets and treatment options. *Cancer Manag Res.* 2012;4:75-89.
2. Korgavkar K, Xiong M, Weinstock M. Changing incidence trends of cutaneous T-cell lymphoma. *JAMA Dermatol.* 2013;149(11):1295-1299.
3. Sidiropoulos KG, Martinez-Escala ME, Yelamos O, et al. Primary cutaneous T-cell lymphomas: a review. *J Clin Pathol.* 2015;68(12):1003-1010.
4. Jawed SI, Myskowski PL, Horwitz S, et al. Primary cutaneous T-cell lymphoma (mycosis fungoides and Sézary syndrome). Part I. Diagnosis: clinical and histopathologic features and new molecular and biologic markers. *J Am Acad Dermatol.* 2014;70(2):205.e1-16.
5. Litvinov IV, Tetzlaff MT, Rahme E, et al. Demographic patterns of cutaneous T-cell lymphoma incidence in Texas based on two different cancer registries. *Cancer Med.* 2015;4(9):1440-1447.
6. Mahan RD, Usatine RP. Hurricane Katrina evacuee develops a persistent rash. *J Fam Pract.* 2007;56(6):454-457.
7. Adriana N, Schmidt AN, Jason B, et al. Conjugal transformed mycosis fungoides: the unknown role of viral infection and environmental exposures in the development of cutaneous T-cell lymphoma. *J Am Acad Dermatol.* 2006;54(5):S202-S205.
8. Brazzelli V, Rivetti N, Badulli C, et al. Immunogenetic factors in mycosis fungoides: can the HLA system influence the susceptibility and prognosis of the disease? Long-term follow-up study of 46 patients. *J Eur Acad Dermatol Venereol.* 2014;28(12):1732-1737.

9. Hodak E, Klein T, Gabay B, et al. Familial mycosis fungoides: report of 6 kindreds and a study of the HLA system. *J Am Acad Dermatol.* 2005;52(3):393-402.

10. Vaqué JP, Gómez-López G, Monsálvez V, et al. PLCG1 mutations in cutaneous T-cell lymphomas. *Blood.* 2014;123(13):2034-2043.

11. Geskin LJ, Viragova S, Stolz DB, Fuschiotti P. Interleukin-13 is overexpressed in cutaneous T-cell lymphoma cells and regulates their proliferation. *Blood.* 2015;125(18):2798-2805.

12. Navi D, Huntley A. Imiquimod 5 percent cream and the treatment of cutaneous malignancy. *Dermatol Online J.* 2004;10(1):4.

13. Pimpinelli N, Olsen EA, Santucci M, et al. Defining early mycosis fungoides. *J Am Acad Dermatol.* 2005;53(6):1053-1063.

14. Pinter-Brown LC. *Cutaneous T-Cell Lymphoma.* Updated June 23, 2017. http://emedicine.medscape.com/article/2139720-overview. Accessed December 2017.

15. Querfeld C, Rosen ST, Guitart J, et al. Phase II trial of subcutaneous injections of human recombinant interleukin-2 for the treatment of mycosis fungoides and Sézary syndrome. *J Am Acad Dermatol.* 2007;56(4):580-583.

16. Zampella JG, Hinds GA. Racial differences in mycosis fungoides: a retrospective study with a focus on eosinophilia. *J Am Acad Dermatol.* 2013;68(6):967-971.

17. Olsen E, Vonderheid E, Pimpinelli N, et al. Revisions to the staging and classification of mycosis fungoides and Sezary syndrome: a proposal of the International Society for Cutaneous Lymphomas (ISCL) and the cutaneous lymphoma task force of the European Organization of Research and Treatment of Cancer (EORTC). *Blood.* 2007;110(6):1713-1722.

18. Honda KS. HIV and skin cancer. *Dermatol Clin.* 2006;24(4): 521-530.

19. Blume JE, Oseroff AR. Aminolevulinic acid photodynamic therapy for skin cancers. *Dermatol Clin.* 2007;25(1):5-14.

20. Hoppe RT, Kim YH. *Treatment of Early Stage (IA to IIA) Mycosis Fungoides and Sézary Syndrome.* Updated February 23, 2012. http://www.uptodate.com/contents/treatment-of-advanced-stage-iib-to-iv-mycosis-fungoides-and-sezary-syndrome. UpToDate® www.uptodate.com. Accessed April 2012.

21. Lessin SR, Duvic M, Guitart J, et al. Topical chemotherapy in cutaneous T-cell lymphoma: positive results of a randomized, controlled, multicenter trial testing the efficacy and safety of a novel mechlorethamine, 0.02%, gel in mycosis fungoides. *JAMA Dermatol.* 2013;149(1):25-32.

22. Ahern K, Gilmore ES, Poligone B. Pruritus in cutaneous T-cell lymphoma: a review. *J Am Acad Dermatol.* 2012;26:1-9.

23. Ponte P, Serrao V, Apetato M. Efficacy of narrowband UVB vs. PUVA in patients with early-stage mycosis fungoides. *J Eur Acad Dermatol Venereol.* 2010;24(6):716-721.

24. Boztepe G, Sahin S, Ayhan M, et al. Narrowband ultraviolet B phototherapy to clear and maintain clearance in patients with mycosis fungoides. *J Am Acad Dermatol.* 2005;53(2):242-246.

25. Nayak CS. Photodynamic therapy in dermatology. *Indian J Dermatol Venereol Leprol.* 2005;71(3):155-160.

26. Suzuki SY, Ito K, Ito M, Kawai K. Prognosis of 100 Japanese patients with mycosis fungoides and Sézary syndrome. *J Dermatol Sci.* 2012; 57(1):37-43.

181 ADVANCED DERMOSCOPY OF SKIN CANCER

Konstantinos Liopyris, MD
Cristian Navarrete-Dechent, MD
Oriol Yélamos, MD
Zachary J. Wolner, MD
Ayelet Rishpon, MD
Richard P. Usatine, MD
Ashfaq A. Marghoob, MD

This chapter is an advanced dermoscopy guide to the 3 most common skin cancers: basal cell carcinoma (BCC), squamous cell carcinoma (SCC), and melanoma. The basic dermoscopic patterns of these skin cancers have been covered in Chapter 111 on dermoscopy (an overall introduction) and in the other chapters devoted to each skin cancer. This chapter provides further information and examples of dermoscopy for the various subtypes of these skin cancers.

BASAL CELL CARCINOMA (SUBTYPES)

BCCs have many recognizable dermoscopic features described in **Table 111-2**. They can be subdivided into pigmented and nonpigmented BCCs depending on the presence or absence of pigment clinically, dermoscopically, and histologically. See Chapter 177 (Basal Cell Carcinoma) for examples.

BCC is also subdivided into the following histologic categories, and each of these histologic types may present with different dermoscopic features:

1. Superficial BCC (**Figures 181-1** to **181-3**)
2. Nodular BCC (**Figure 181-4**)
3. Morpheaform BCC (**Figure 181-5**)
4. Sclerosing BCC (**Figure 181-6**)
5. Infiltrative BCC (**Figure 181-7**)

The features most predictive of superficial BCC are:

1. Leaflike structures
2. Spoke wheel-like structures
3. Concentric structures
4. Short, fine telangiectasias
5. Multiple small erosions
6. Shiny white blotches and strands (see **Figures 181-1** to **181-3**).

The evidence supports these features with odds ratio ranging between 2.7 and 7.7.[1-4]

Features that support BCCs that are not superficial BCCs are:

1. Arborizing vessels (negative OR 2.1) (see **Figures 181-5** and **181-7**)
2. Blue-gray ovoid nests (negative OR 3.2) (see **Figure 181-4**)
3. Ulceration (negative OR 2.1)[2] (see **Figure 181-4**)

SQUAMOUS CELL CARCINOMA (SUBTYPES)

The most common features of SCC are described and depicted in **Table 111-3**. Bowen disease (SCC in situ) can present as pigmented

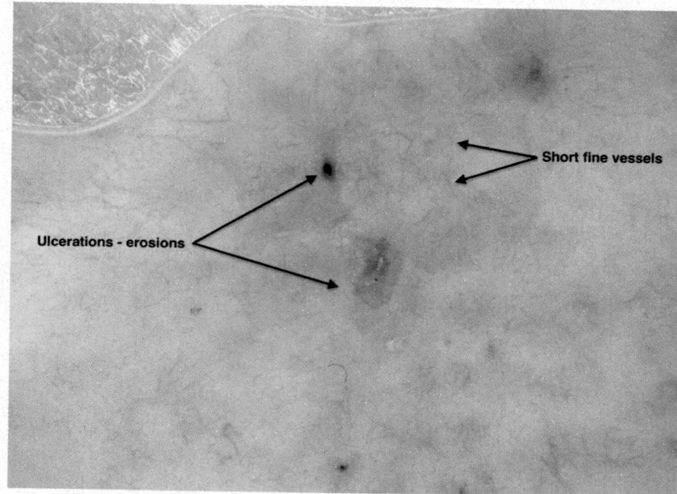

FIGURE 181-1 Non-pigmented, superficial basal cell carcinoma displaying two small erosions and short fine telangiectasias. *(Reproduced with permission from the International Skin Imaging Collaboration. Courtesy Harold Rabinovitz, MD.)*

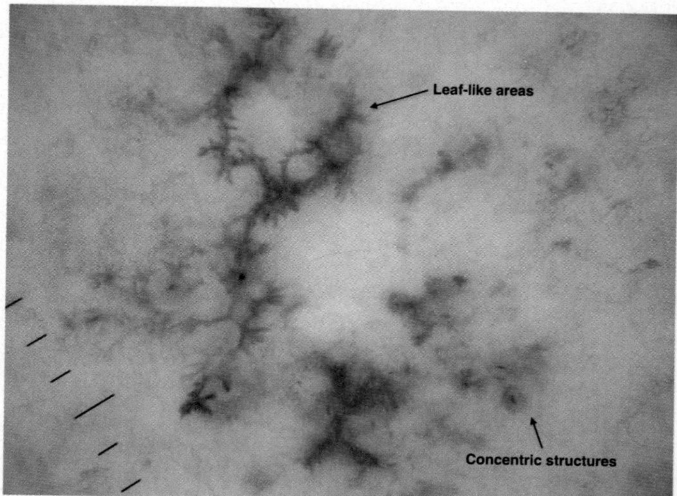

FIGURE 181-2 Pigmented superficial basal cell carcinoma presenting with leaflike areas and concentric structures. *(Reproduced with permission from the International Skin Imaging Collaboration. Courtesy Harold Rabinovitz, MD.)*

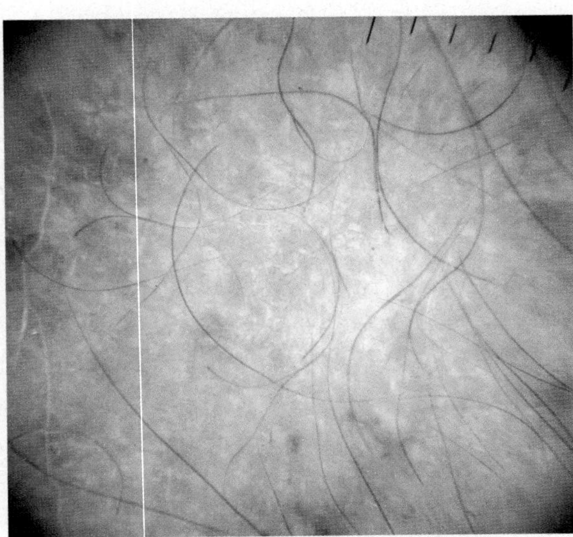

FIGURE 181-3 Nonpigmented, superficial basal cell carcinoma presenting only with shiny white blotches and strands. (*Reproduced with permission from the International Skin Imaging Collaboration. Courtesy Harold Rabinovitz, MD.*)

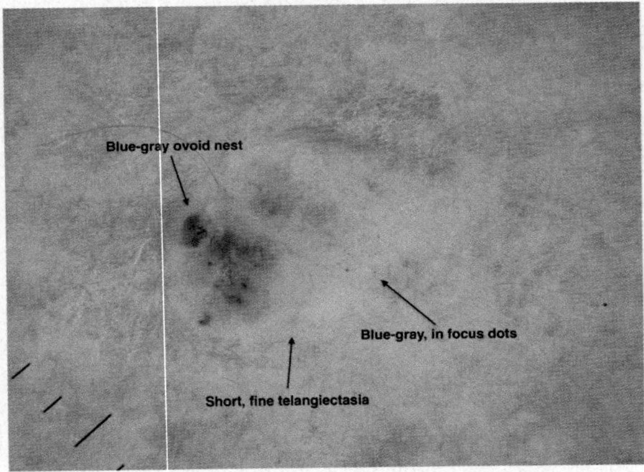

FIGURE 181-4 Nodular basal cell carcinoma displaying blue-gray ovoid nests, a short fine telangiectasia, and multiple in-focus, blue-gray dots. (*Reproduced with permission from the International Skin Imaging Collaboration. Courtesy Harold Rabinovitz, MD.*)

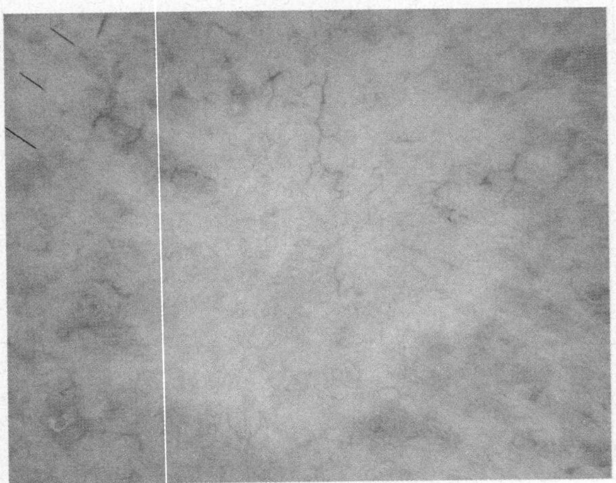

FIGURE 181-5 Morpheaform basal cell carcinoma on the cheek presenting with multiple arborizing vessels on a whitish background. (*Reproduced with permission from the International Skin Imaging Collaboration. Courtesy Harold Rabinovitz, MD.*)

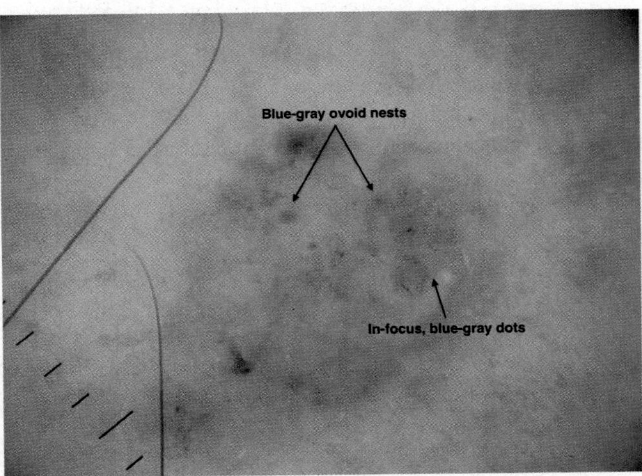

FIGURE 181-6 Sclerosing basal cell carcinoma displaying blue-gray ovoid nests and multiple in-focus, blue-gray dots. (*Reproduced with permission from the International Skin Imaging Collaboration. Courtesy Harold Rabinovitz, MD.*)

FIGURE 181-7 Infiltrative basal cell carcinoma presenting with multiple arborizing vessels on a whitish background. (*Reproduced with permission from the International Skin Imaging Collaboration. Courtesy Harold Rabinovitz, MD*)

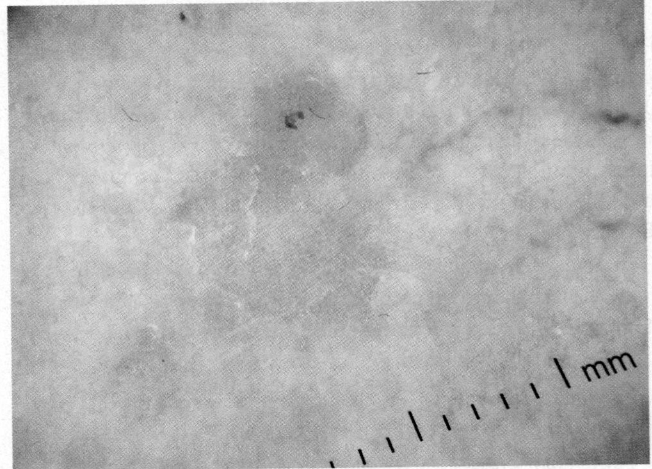

FIGURE 181-8 SCC in situ—Bowen disease, nonpigmented with a multitude of glomerular and dotted vessels throughout the lesion. Note the white scale and red ulceration. (*Reproduced with permission from Richard P. Usatine, MD.*)

or nonpigmented (see Chapter 173, Actinic Keratosis and Bowen Disease). Nonpigmented Bowen disease typically presents with a glomerular vascular pattern and scale (**Figure 181-8**). Pigmented Bowen disease presents typically on individuals of dark skin type, and the hallmark of diagnosis is brown circles and brown dots in a linear pattern on the periphery of the lesion (**Figure 181-9**).[5]

Keratoacanthoma is a well-differentiated variant of SCC which presents with a central keratin core within a raised tumor (see Chapter 174, Keratoacanthoma). On dermoscopy, it has a central structureless yellow keratin mass surrounded by hairpin (looped), linear irregular, and glomerular vessels (**Figure 181-10**).[5]

Finally, invasive SCC (see Chapter 178, Squamous Cell Carcinoma) presents with yellow keratin, ulcerations, scale, and hairpin and linear irregular vessels (**Figure 181-11**).[5]

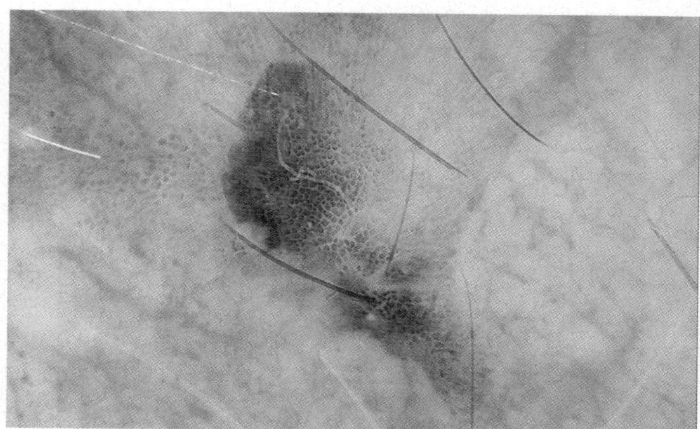

FIGURE 181-9 Pigmented Bowen disease with multiple brown circles and dots. *(Reproduced with permission from the International Skin Imaging Collaboration.)*

MELANOMA OF SPECIAL LOCATIONS

MELANOMA ON THE FACE AND SCALP

The most common features of melanoma in general are described and depicted in **Table 111-7**.

Lentigo maligna melanoma (LMM) is a subtype of melanoma that arises on the face, scalp, and other areas of sun-damaged skin (see Chapter 179, Melanoma). Lentigo maligna is the in-situ version of LMM (see Chapter 175, Lentigo Maligna). Angulated lines (polygonal lines) is a melanoma-specific structure that can be found in LMM arising on the face, scalp, or other area of sun-damaged skin.[6]

LMMs present as flat pigmented patches to plaques, light brown to black with color variation and asymmetric shape. They enlarge slowly in size and can cover a wide area of the face or scalp. Dermoscopically LMM is diagnosed by using the classic dermoscopic criteria introduced by Schiffner (**Table 181-1**).[7] Pralong and colleagues added red rhomboidal structures, darkening at dermoscopic examination, and increased density of vascularity as additional structures suggestive of LMM[8] (see **Table 181-1**). Two examples of LMM on the face are seen in **Figures 181-12** and **181-13**.

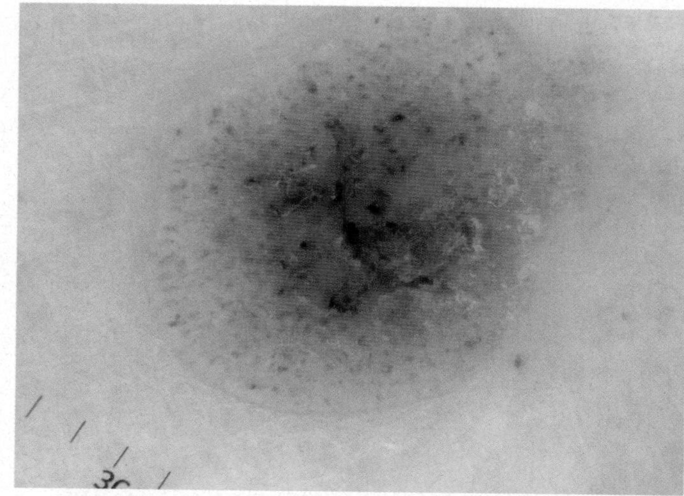

FIGURE 181-10 Well-differentiated SCC, keratoacanthoma type. Dermoscopically there are hairpin vessels in the periphery, surrounding a central keratin plug. *(Reproduced with permission from the International Skin Imaging Collaboration.)*

ACROLENTIGINOUS MELANOMA (ALM) (MELANOMA OF HANDS AND FEET)

The dermatoglyphic pattern of the skin at the palms and soles is due to the unique anatomy, specific for these regions, caused by the alteration between ridges and furrows. This anatomy can help us differentiate between nevi and melanoma, since the location of pigmentation differs among the two entities. In nevi, the pigmentation tends to favor the furrows of the lesions, while in melanoma it tends to favor the ridges (**Figure 181-14**).[9]

In order to distinguish benign acral nevi from ALM, one must know the most common dermoscopy patterns seen in acral nevi[10] (**Figure 181-15**) and acrolentiginous melanomas[11] (**Figure 181-16**).

Benign acral nevi have these patterns:

1. Parallel furrow pattern—Pigmentation located mainly on and around the furrows (**Figure 181-17**).
2. Lattice-like pattern—A parallel furrow pattern with the addition of parallel lines crossing over the ridges like a lattice (**Figure 181-18**).
3. Fibrillar pattern—Composed of multiple, transversely oriented, thin parallel lines that cross both furrows and ridges on areas of

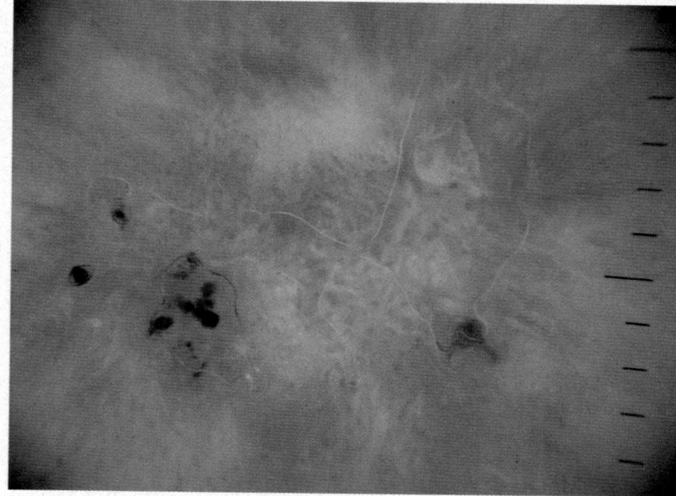

FIGURE 181-11 Invasive SCC with ulcerations, yellow keratin, scale, white structures, and vasculature with hairpin and linear irregular vessels. *(Reproduced with permission from the International Skin Imaging Collaboration.)*

TABLE 181-1 Lentigo Maligna Melanoma Dermoscopic Features and Definitions

Hyperpigmented follicular openings: They can appear symmetric or asymmetric, dark in color with a grayish hue. The patterns are fine circle, semicircle, signet ring–like circle, irregular circle, and double circle (circle within a circle). 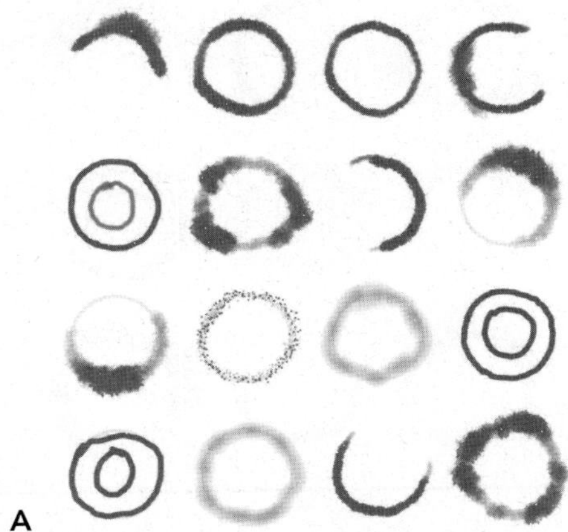 A	**Short and polygonal lines around and between adnexal openings:** Dots coalescing, forming short pigmented lines around and between follicular openings. When presenting in a polygonal fashion, they are also called zigzag patterns and rhomboidal structures. 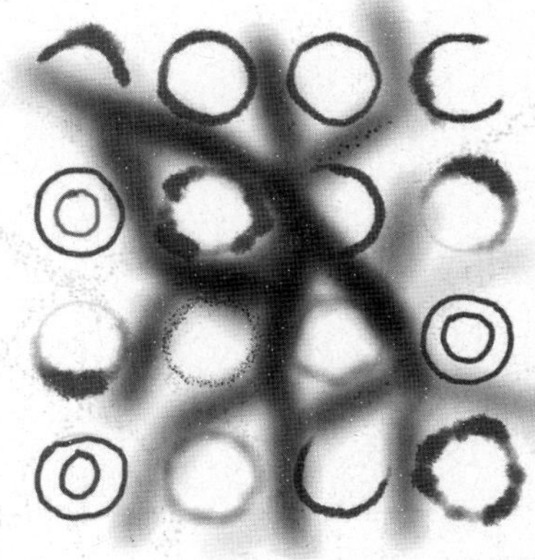 D
Annular-granular pattern: Consists of fine dots aggregated around follicular openings and /or short polygonal lines around and in between follicular openings. They can appear separately or in combination. 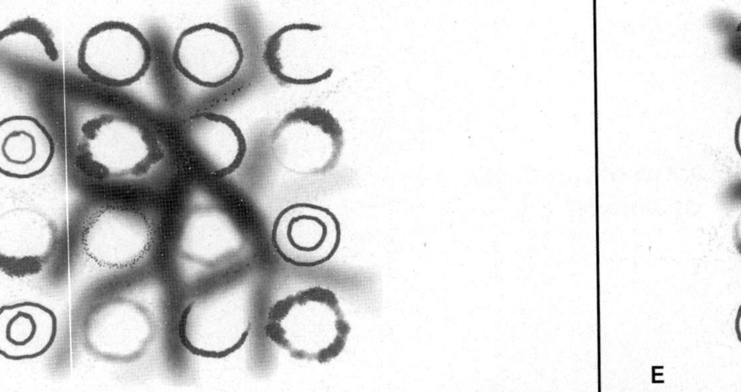 B	**Dark blotches and obliterated hair follicles:** Dark brown or black blotches initially spare the follicular openings, but as LMM progresses, the hair follicles becomes obliterated. 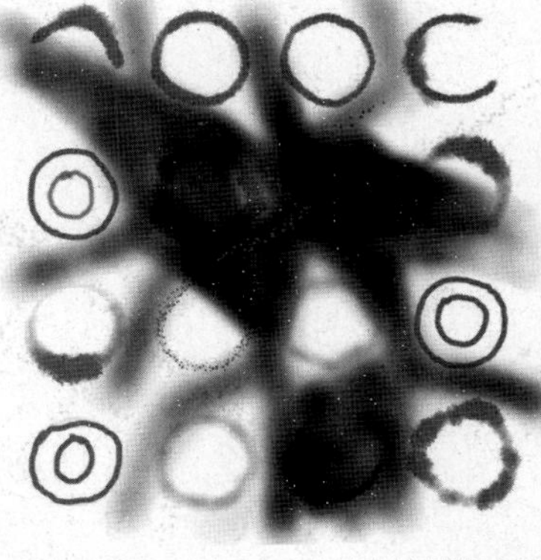 E
Dots aggregated around follicular openings: Vary in color and range from brown to black or blue-gray. They may be apparent throughout the lesion but usually cluster around follicular openings. 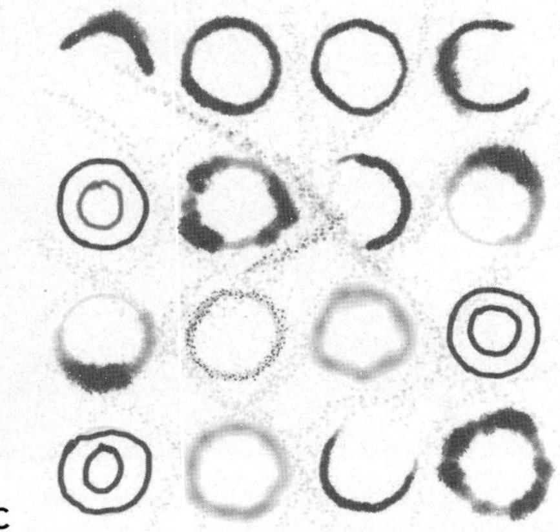 C	**Red rhomboidal structures:** A vascular pattern forming rhomboid structures and separating hair follicles. 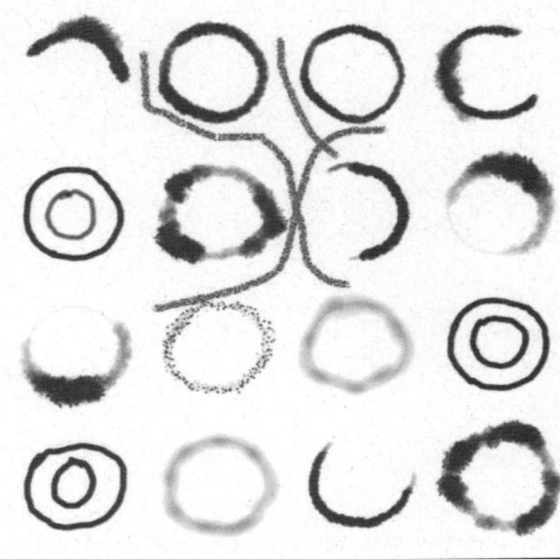 F

(continued)

TABLE 181-1 Lentigo Maligna Melanoma Dermoscopic Features and Definitions (*Continued*)

Darkening at dermoscopic examination: Or target-like pattern, is defined as the presence of a dark dot (not a hair) in the center of a hyperpigmented hair follicle.	G

*All schematics are adapted with permission from dermoscopedia.org.

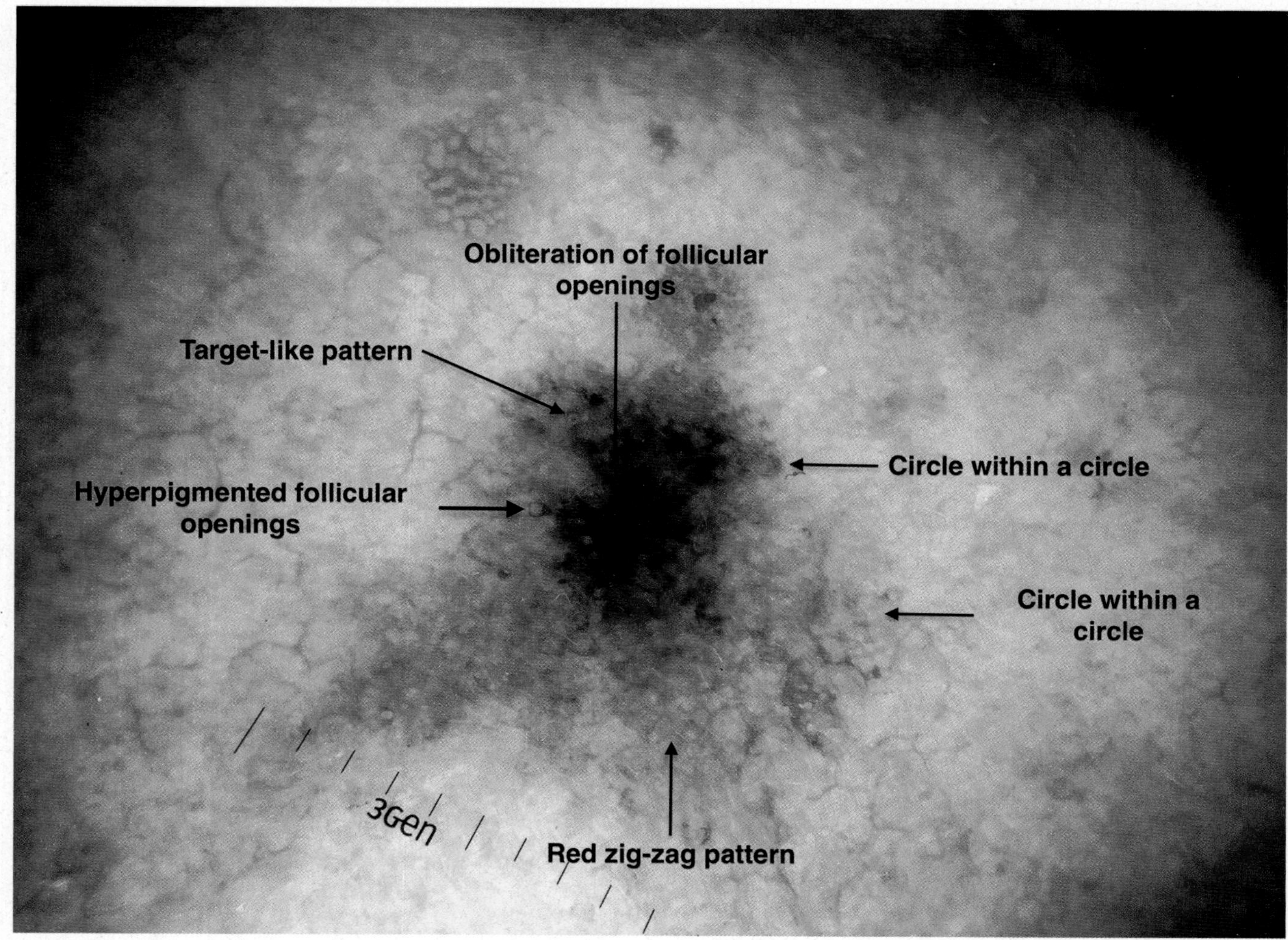

FIGURE 181-12 LMM on the face displaying hyperpigmented follicular openings, circle within a circle, dark blotches with obliterated hair follicles, red rhomboidal structures, darkening at dermoscopic examination (target-like pattern), and increased density of vascularity. (*Reproduced with permission from the International Skin Imaging Collaboration.*)

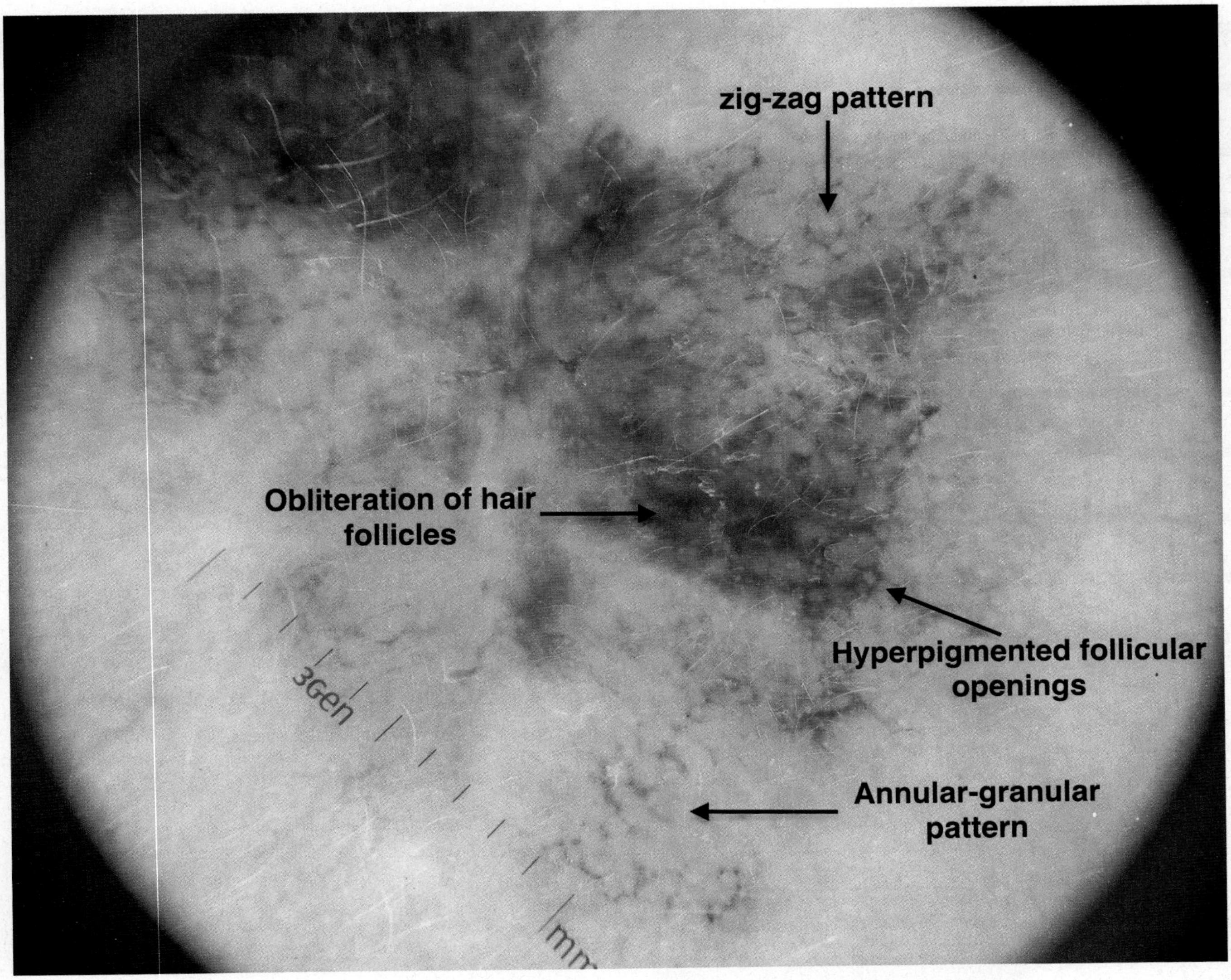

FIGURE 181-13 LMM on the face exhibiting hyperpigmented follicular openings, annular granular pattern, (zigzag pattern), and dark blotches with obliterated hair follicles. (*Reproduced with permission from the International Skin Imaging Collaboration.*)

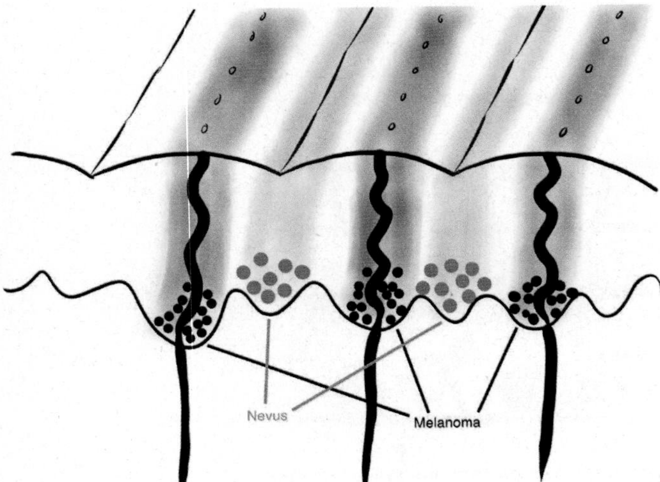

FIGURE 181-14 Anatomy of the acral skin, and the origination of pigment in nevi versus melanomas related to melanocyte location. (*Reproduced with permission from www.dermoscopedia.org.*)

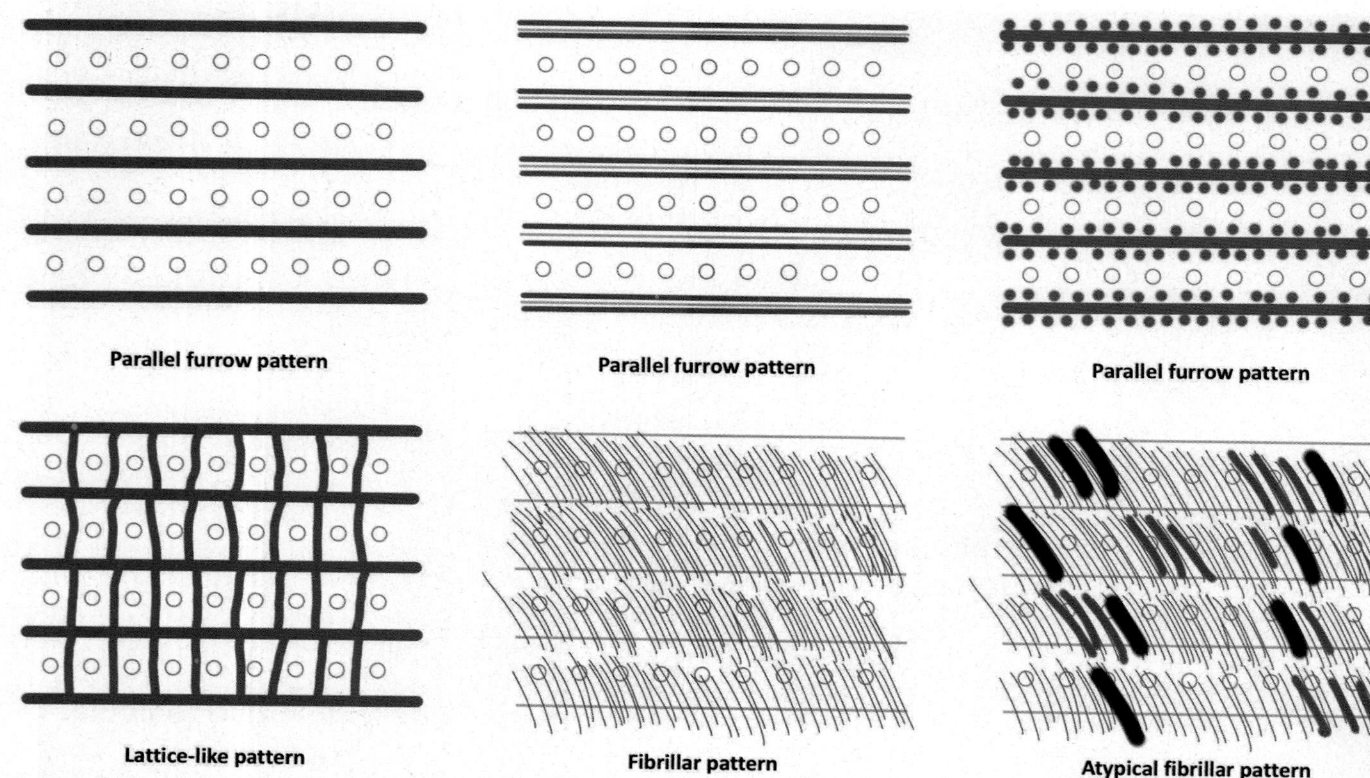

FIGURE 181-15 Benign dermoscopy patterns of acral nevi including the variations of parallel furrow pattern, lattice-like pattern, and fibrillar pattern. The atypical fibrillar pattern is very heterogeneous and should be considered with caution. (*Reproduced with permission from www.dermoscopedia.org.*)

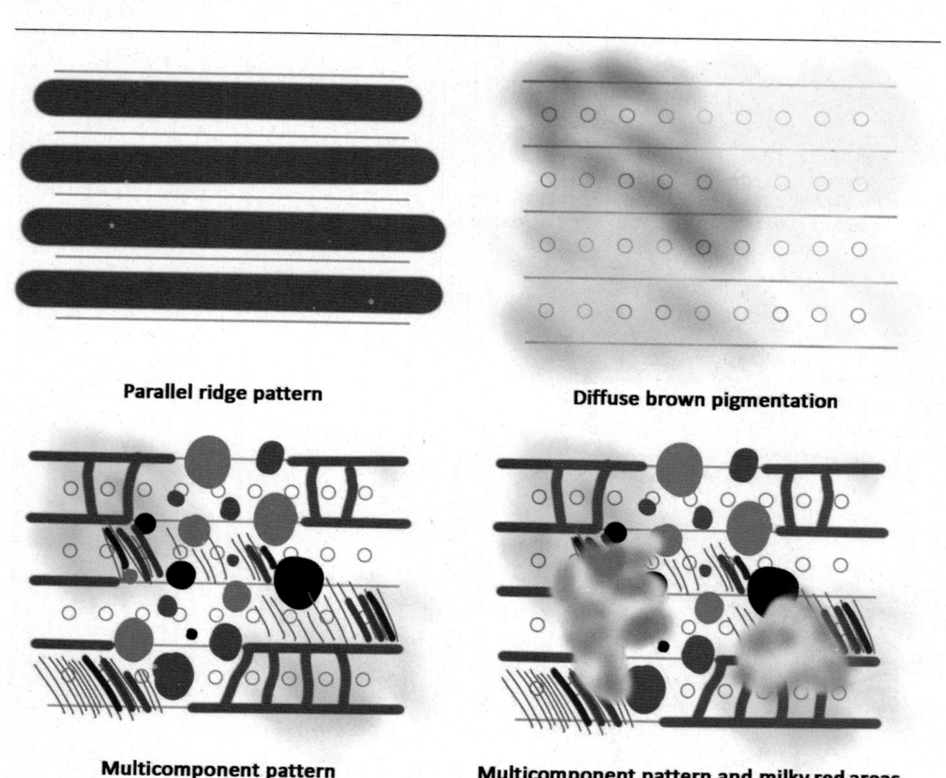

FIGURE 181-16 Dermoscopic patterns encountered in acrolentiginous melanomas including parallel ridge pattern, diffuse brown pigmentation, multicomponent pattern, and multicomponent pattern with milky red areas. (*Reproduced with permission from www.dermoscopedia.org.*)

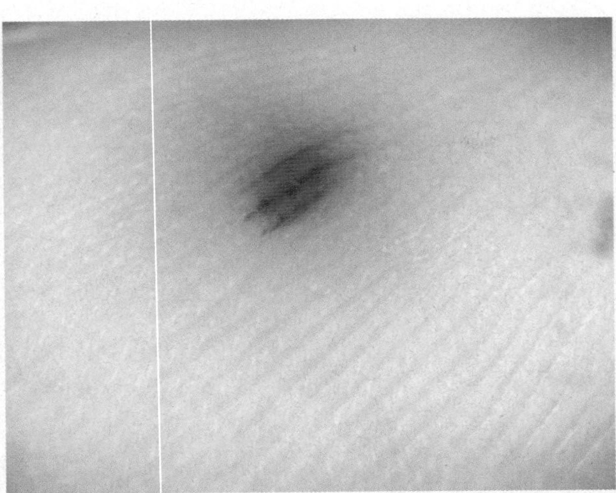

FIGURE 181-17 Acral nevus displaying parallel furrows pattern; the pigmentation is (mainly) confined on the furrows. (*Reproduced with permission from the International Skin Imaging Collaboration.*)

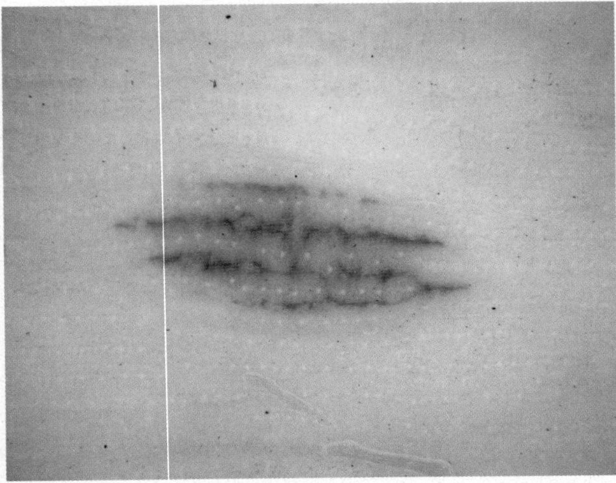

FIGURE 181-18 Acral nevus displaying a lattice-like pattern; pigmentation resides (mainly) in the furrows with the addition of parallel bands crossing over the ridges. (*Reproduced with permission from the International Skin Imaging Collaboration.*)

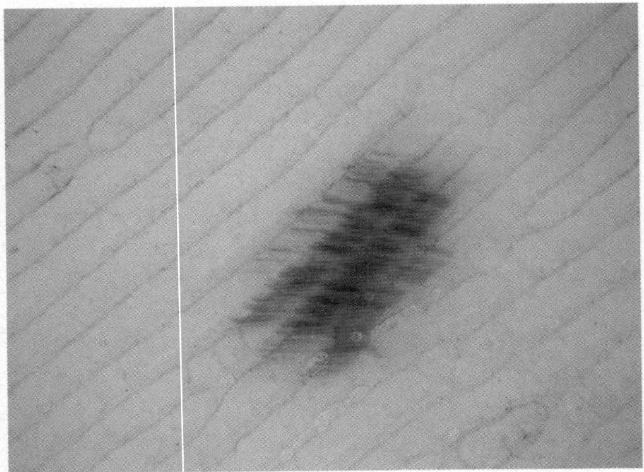

FIGURE 181-19 Acral nevus displaying a fibrillar pattern; dense fibrillar pigmentation crossing both the furrows and ridges on the weight-bearing area of the foot. (*Reproduced with permission from the International Skin Imaging Collaboration.*)

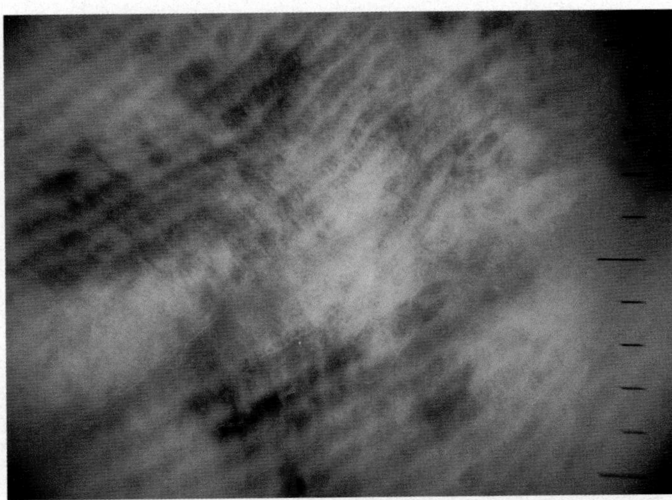

FIGURE 181-20 Acral melanoma displaying a parallel ridge pattern; pigmentation is located mainly along the ridges. (*Reproduced with permission from the International Skin Imaging Collaboration.*)

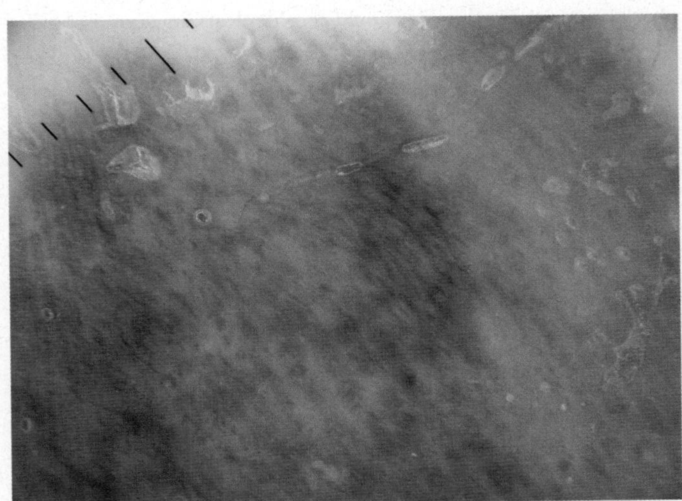

FIGURE 181-21 Acral melanoma displaying diffuse brown and gray pigmentation, expanding to both furrows and ridges. (*Reproduced with permission from the International Skin Imaging Collaboration.*)

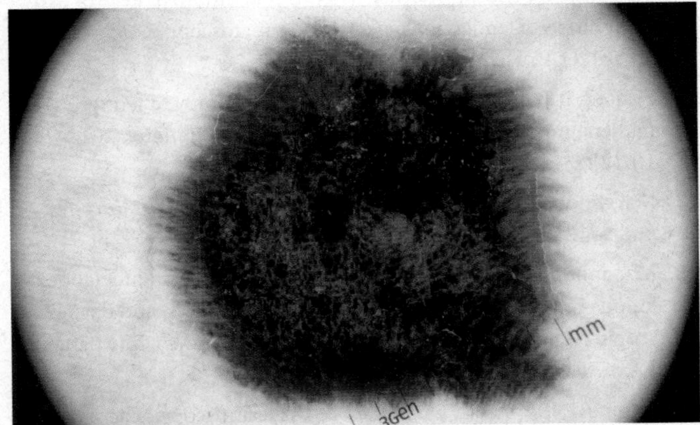

FIGURE 181-22 Acral melanoma displaying a multicomponent pattern. (*Reproduced with permission from the International Skin Imaging Collaboration.*)

weight bearing on the feet (**Figure 181-19**). When a fibrillar pattern has darker multicolored lines or occurs on the palms or non–weight-bearing areas of the feet, it is considered atypical, and a biopsy is warranted.

Acrolentiginous melanomas display these patterns:

1. Parallel ridge patterns—Pigmentation located predominantly on the ridges with hypopigmented furrows (**Figure 181-20**).
2. Diffuse pigmentation—Pigmentation of variable shades of brown and gray dispersed both on the ridges and furrows (**Figure 181-21**).
3. Multicomponent pattern—Combination of any pigmentation pattern (**Figure 181-22**).
4. Milky red areas—Red-whitish areas, which usually are a sign of invasion and nodularity (**Figure 181-23**).

CONCLUSION

Early diagnosis of skin cancer can save lives. Dermoscopy is an important tool for recognizing skin cancers from head to toe. Every physician caring for the skin should consider learning dermoscopy.

REFERENCES

1. Popadic M. Dermoscopic features in different morphologic types of basal cell carcinoma. *Dermatol Surg.* 2014;40(7):725-732.
2. Lallas A, Tzellos T, Kyrgidis A, et al. Accuracy of dermoscopic criteria for discriminating superficial from other subtypes of basal cell carcinoma. *J Am Dermatol.* 2014;70(2):303-311.
3. Puig S, Cecilia N, Malvehy J. Dermoscopic criteria and basal cell carcinoma. *G Ital Dermatol Venereol.* 2012;147(2):135-140.
4. Giacomel J, Zalaudek I. Dermoscopy of superficial basal cell carcinoma. *Dermatol Surg.* 2005;31(12):1710-1713.
5. Rosendahl C, Cameron A, Argenziano G, et al. Dermoscopy of squamous cell carcinoma and keratoacanthoma. *Arch Dermatol.* 2012;148(12):1386-1392.
6. Jaimes N, Marghoob AA, Rabinovitz H, et al. Clinical and dermoscopic characteristics of melanomas on nonfacial chronically sun-damaged skin. *J Am Dermatol.* 2015;72(6):1027-1035.
7. Schiffner R, Schiffner-Rohe J, Vogt T, et al. Improvement of early recognition of lentigo maligna using dermatoscopy. *J Am Dermatol.* 2000;42(1 Pt 1):25-32.
8. Pralong P, Bathelier E, Dalle S, et al. Dermoscopy of lentigo maligna melanoma: report of 125 cases. *Br J Dermatol.* 2012; 167(2):280-287.
9. Marghoob AA, Malvehy J, Braun RP. *An Atlas of Dermoscopy*, 2nd ed. Boca Raton, FL: CRC Press; 2012.
10. Madankumar R, Gumaste PV, Martires K, et al. Acral melanocytic lesions in the United States: prevalence, awareness, and dermoscopic patterns in skin-of-color and non-Hispanic white patients. *J Am Acad Dermatol.* 2016;74(4):724-730.e1.
11. Braun RP, Thomas L, Dusza SW, et al. Dermoscopy of acral melanoma: a multicenter study on behalf of the International Dermoscopy Society. *Dermatology.* 2013;227(4):373-380.

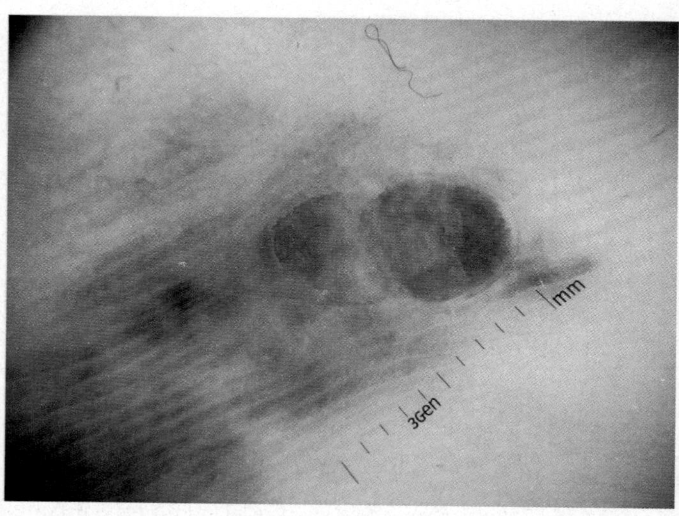

FIGURE 181-23 Acral melanoma displaying a multicomponent pattern with milky red areas. (*Reproduced with permission from the International Skin Imaging Collaboration.*)

SECTION N INFILTRATIVE IMMUNOLOGIC

182 GRANULOMA ANNULARE

Melissa M. Mauskar, MD
Richard P. Usatine, MD

PATIENT STORY

A 39-year-old woman presents with raised rings on her right hand. Not knowing the correct diagnosis, another physician prescribed topical steroids and antifungal medicines with no benefit. The diagnosis of granuloma annulare (GA) was made by the typical clinical appearance, and the patient was offered intralesional steroids. Triamcinolone acetonide was injected as seen in **Figure 182-1A**. The patient noted improvement over the subsequent weeks, but within a month new lesions began to appear on her other hand (**Figure 182-1B**). Additional injections were provided and 1 month later the patient had regression of the treated lesions but had new lesions on the right arm (**Figure 182-2A**). At the next visit, the patient had new lesions on her feet as well (**Figure 182-2B**). The diagnosis of disseminated GA was made and systemic treatment was started.

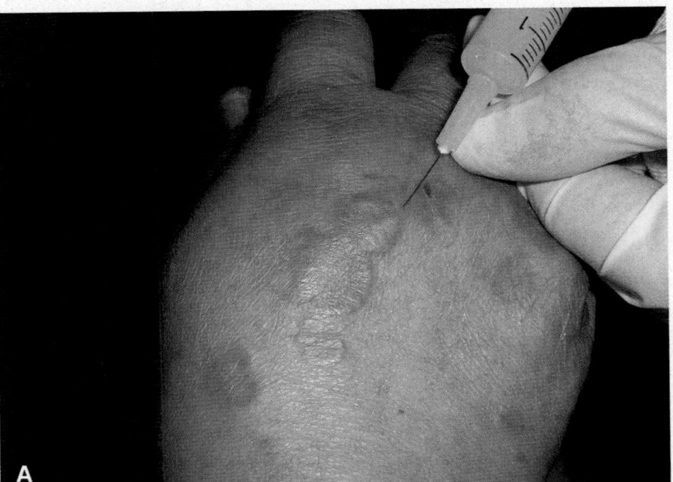

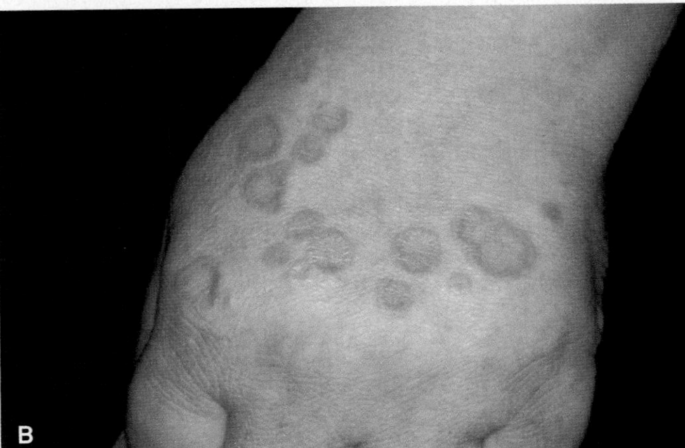

FIGURE 182-1 **A.** GA in a 42-year-old woman. Intralesional steroids were administered on the first visit with resolution of the injected lesions. **B.** Same patient months later with new annular lesions on the opposite hand. She requested additional injections. (*Reproduced with permission from Richard P. Usatine, MD.*)

INTRODUCTION

GA is a common dermatologic condition that presents as small, light-red, dermal papules coalescing into annular plaques without scale. As in the above vignette, it is often mistaken for nummular eczema or tinea corporis. Distribution, pattern, and lack of scale are important diagnostic clues.

EPIDEMIOLOGY

- GA affects twice as many women as men.[1]
- The four presentations of GA are localized, disseminated/generalized, perforating, and subcutaneous.
- Of the four variations, the localized form is seen most often.[1]

ETIOLOGY AND PATHOPHYSIOLOGY

- Benign cutaneous, inflammatory disorder of unknown origin.[1]
- Disease may be self-limiting, but may persist for many years.
- Reported associations include diabetes mellitus, viral infections (including HIV), *Borrelia* and streptococcal infections, insect bites, lymphoma, tuberculosis, and trauma.[2,3]

- One proposed mechanism for GA is a delayed-type hypersensitivity reaction as a result of T-helper–type cell (Th)-1 lymphocytic differentiation of macrophages. These macrophages become effector cells that express tumor necrosis factor (TNF)-α and matrix metalloproteinases. The activated macrophages are responsible for dermal collagen matrix degradation.[4]
- An association between high expression of gil-1 oncogene and granulomatous lesions of the skin, including GA, has been established.[5]

RISK FACTORS

The only identifiable risk factor is being a woman. There are several associations, but nothing has been shown to be causative.

DIAGNOSIS

CLINICAL FEATURES

Annular lesions have raised borders that are skin-colored to erythematous (see **Figures 182-1** and **182-2**). The rings may become hyperpigmented or violaceous (see **Figure 182-2B).** There is often a central depression within the ring. These lesions range from 2 mm to 5 cm. Although the classical appearance of GA is annular, the lesions may be arcuate instead of forming a complete ring (**Figure 182-3**). Most importantly, there should be no scaling as seen in tinea corporis (ringworm).

TYPICAL DISTRIBUTION

Each of the four types of GA has a different distribution. Localized and disseminated GA differ only in that disseminated lesions can spread to the trunk and neck and may be more pronounced in sun-exposed areas.[6]

- Localized—This is the most common form of GA, affecting 75% of GA patients.[1] It typically presents as solitary lesions on the dorsal surfaces of extremities, especially of hands and feet (**Figure 182-4**).
- Disseminated or generalized—Adults are most affected by this form, which begins in the extremities and can spread to the trunk and neck (**Figure 182-5**).
- Perforating—Children and young adults present with 1 to hundreds of 1- to 4-mm annular papules that may coalesce to form a typical annular plaque. Although this form can appear anywhere on the body, it has an affinity for extremities, especially the hands and fingers.[7] The papules may exude a thick and creamy or clear and viscous fluid.
- Subcutaneous—These lesions present as rapidly growing, nonpainful, subcutaneous or dermal nodules on the extremities, scalp, and forehead. Subcutaneous GA mainly affects children, with a mean age of 3.9 years (**Figure 182-6**).[6] These lesions are often ill defined and less discrete.

LABORATORY STUDIES

Often a diagnosis of GA is made on clinical presentation alone, without the need for biopsy. Subcutaneous GA may be an exception, as

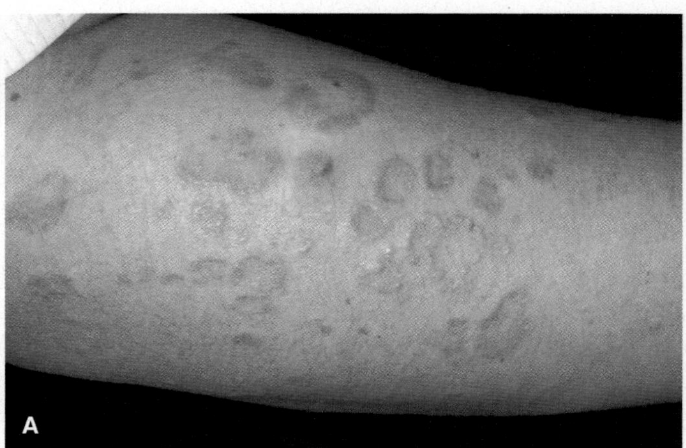

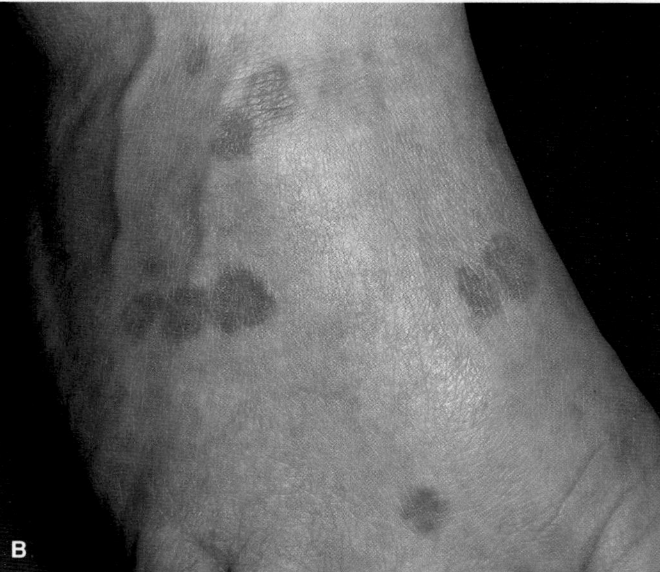

FIGURE 182-2 **A.** Same patient as in Figure 182-1 1 month later with new crops of lesions on the arms and feet. She has disseminated GA. Note the area of hypopigmentation secondary to a previous steroid intralesional steroid injection. **B.** Disseminated GA on the foot of the same patient. The rings are flatter and many are conjoined. (*Reproduced with permission from Richard P. Usatine, MD.*)

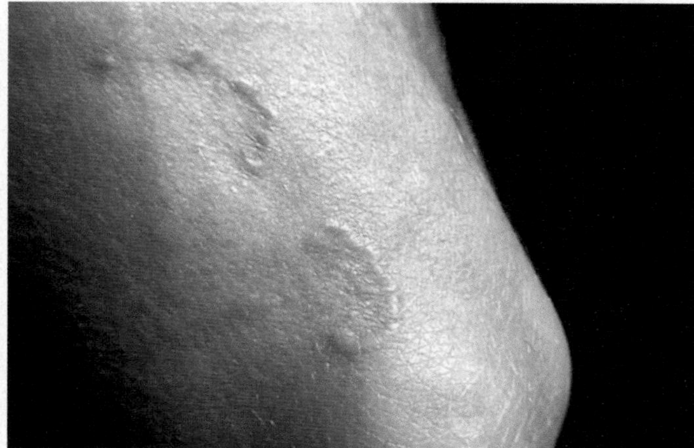

FIGURE 182-3 GA on the elbow showing how the rings may not be complete. This patient is in her fifties and has had new crops of lesions over the past 10 years. (*Reproduced with permission from Richard P. Usatine, MD.*)

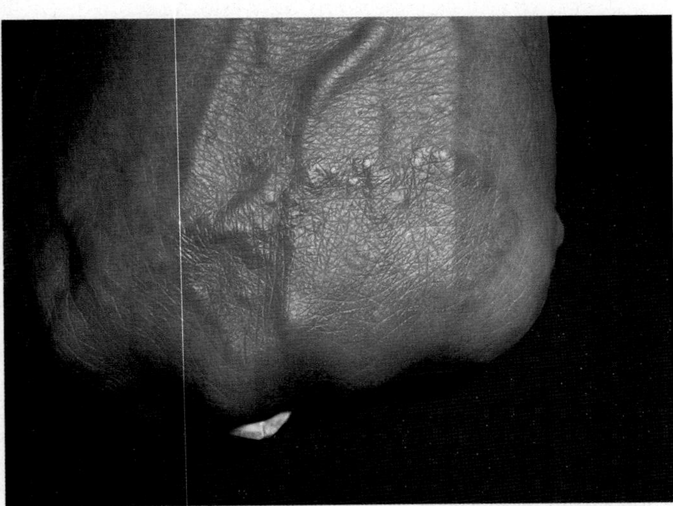

FIGURE 182-4 One single large irregular annular lesion of GA. This ring is also incomplete. (*Reproduced with permission from Richard P. Usatine, MD.*)

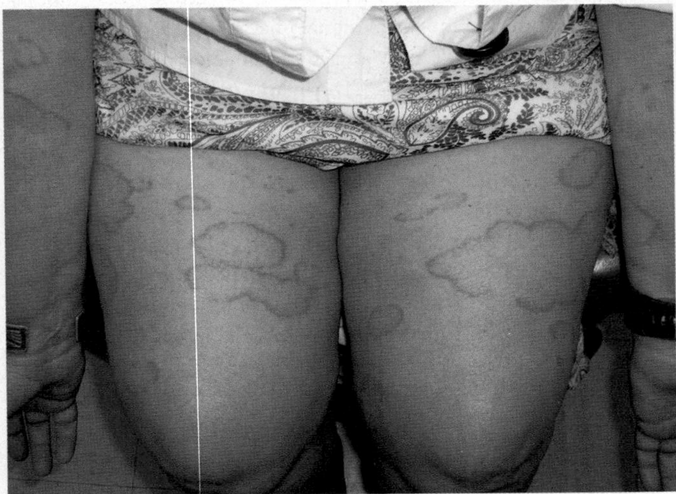

FIGURE 182-5 Disseminated GA in a middle-aged woman with diabetes. Her GA resolved after she was started on oral pentoxyfylline. (*Reproduced with permission from Richard P. Usatine, MD.*)

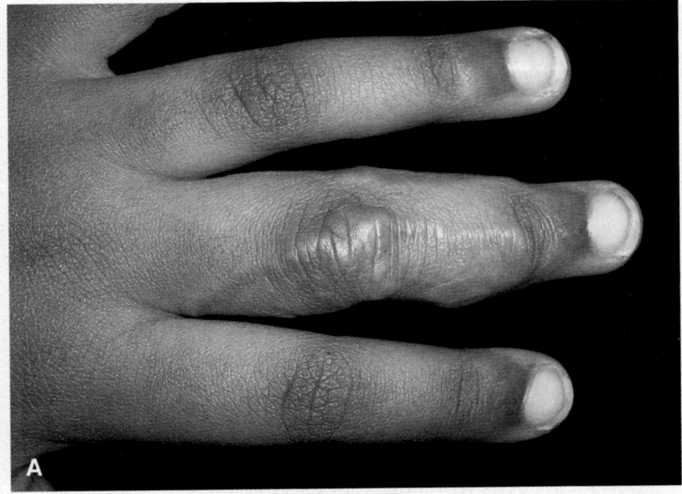

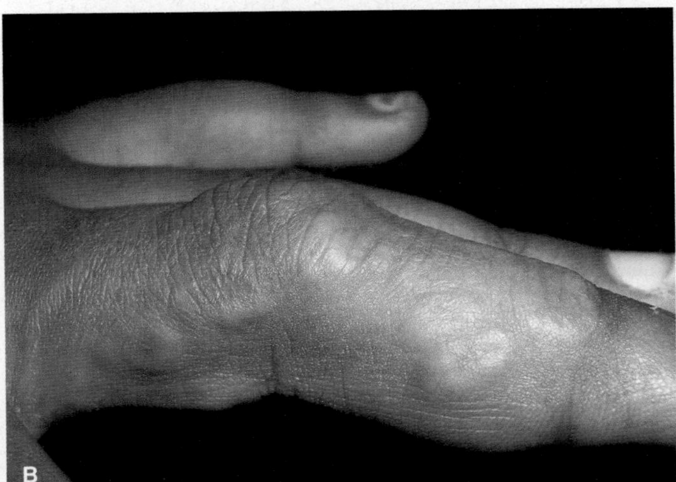

FIGURE 182-6 **A.** Subcutaneous GA in a 7-year-old girl showing one large ring on the dorsum of the finger with soft-tissue infiltration. **B.** Subcutaneous GA in a 7-year-old girl showing thickening of the involved finger along with the small annular patterns. Note the soft-tissue infiltration that has distorted the finger anatomy. (*Reproduced with permission from Richard P. Usatine, MD.*)

the unusual appearance may be mistaken for a rheumatoid nodule. Histologic examination reveals an increase of mucin, which is a hallmark of GA. There is also a dense infiltrate of histiocytes in the mid-dermis and sparse perivascular lymphocytic infiltrate. The histiocytes are either organized as palisading cells lining a collection of mucin or as a diffuse interstitial pattern. There are no signs of epidermal change.[3]

DIFFERENTIAL DIAGNOSIS

- Tinea corporis has a raised, scaling border and can present on any body surface. KOH preparation reveals hyphae with multiple branches (see Chapter 144, Tinea Corporis).
- Erythema annulare centrifugum has an affinity for thighs and legs. The diameter of these lesions can expand at a rate of 2 to 5 mm/day and may present with a trailing scale inside the advancing border.[2] Biopsy is helpful to differentiate this condition from GA, but may be made on clinical findings alone as GA does not have scale (see Chapter 215, Erythema Annulare Centrifugum).
- Sarcoidosis—Often presents as red-brown dermal papules without scale on the head and neck. Biopsy will help distinguish sarcoidosis from GA (see Chapter 184, Sarcoidosis).
- Nummular eczema presents commonly on extremities, but is almost always associated with scaling plaques and intense itching (see Chapter 154, Nummular Eczema).
- Pityriasis rosea often has oval lesions with a trailing collarette of scale. The lesions are minimally raised and have scale that is absent in GA (see Chapter 159, Pityriasis Rosea).
- Rheumatoid nodules may mimic appearance of subcutaneous GA. These nodules are often seen over the elbows, fingers, and other joints in a patient with joint pains and other clinical signs of arthritis (see Chapter 99, Rheumatoid Arthritis). Rheumatoid nodules have fibrin deposition on histologic examination, in contrast to mucin in GA.

MANAGEMENT

The evidence for various treatments is at best a small series of cases that are not randomized controlled trials. This disease is asymptomatic, and treatments only improve cosmetic appearance. Many patients may want intervention, as diffuse lesions can cause psychological distress. Although GA will eventually resolve, some treatments may cause pigment change or atrophy that might be permanent. Several of the treatments below have shown promise, but these treatments may appear to work when in fact the resolution was natural.

LOCALIZED GA

FIRST LINE

- In a retrospective study of children with localized GA (mean age: 8.6 years), 39 of 42 presented with complete clearance within 2 years. The average duration was 1 year. Researchers of this study consider most treatments unnecessary because of the self-limiting nature of this variation.[7] One treatment option is watchful waiting.[8] SOR B
- Intralesional corticosteroids can be injected into GA lesions with resolution of the area injected (see **Figure 182-1**). Inject directly into the ring itself with 3 to 5 mg/mL triamcinolone acetonide (Kenalog) using a 27-gauge needle. SOR C A large completed ring may take 4 injections to reach 360 degrees of the circle. The major complications include hypopigmentation (see **Figure 182-2A**) and skin atrophy at the injected sites.

SECOND LINE

- Cryotherapy was studied using nitrous oxide for 9 patients and liquid nitrogen for 22 patients. The results showed 80% clearing after a single freeze; however, 4 of 19 patients treated with liquid nitrogen developed atrophic scars when lesions were larger than 4 cm. All patients developed blisters.[9] Cryoatrophy may possibly be prevented by avoiding freeze–thaw cycles greater than 10 seconds and not overlapping treatment areas.[10] SOR C
- A 53-year-old Hispanic woman with GA on the dorsal surface of both hands agreed to treatment with cryotherapy on the right hand and intralesional steroids on the left hand (**Figure 182-7**). Cryotherapy was performed using a 9- to 10-second freeze time and a single freeze. The intralesional injections were performed with a 30-gauge needle and 5 mg/mL triamcinolone (10 mg/mL diluted 1:1 with 1% lidocaine). During the treatment the patient rated the pain from cryotherapy as 9 out of 10 and intralesional steroid 2 out of 10. **Figure 182-7** shows the initial lesions and final results after 1 month. The patient was happy with the results of intralesional steroid and disappointed with the results of the cryotherapy. The lesion treated with cryotherapy did not resolve, and spotted areas of hyperpigmentation and hypopigmentation occurred. Upon questioning, the patient states that the lesion treated with cryotherapy was painful for many days, whereas she had no residual pain from the lesion treated with intralesional steroid. The patient then asked for the two remaining lesions on her right hand to be injected with steroid. Although this is a single case example, we could find no published studies of a head-to-head comparison between these commonly used methods for local treatment of GA.

GENERALIZED/DISSEMINATED GA

- This variant is more difficult to treat and often has a longer duration than localized GA. Many treatments have been claimed to be effective, but the studies touting these treatments have small sample sizes and were not randomized.

FIRST LINE

- Recent case reports show that generalized disease responds well to antimalarial treatment. In a retrospective review of patients treated for generalized granuloma annulare, 10 of 18 patients improved after 3 months of treatment with hydroxychloroquine therapy 400 mg daily; by 6 months of therapy most lesions had resolved.[11] SOR C
- Pentoxifylline, a phosphodiesterase inhibitor, has been used to treat generalized GA with good results.[12,13] Although the mechanism of action on treatment is unknown, it may be related to the TNF-α

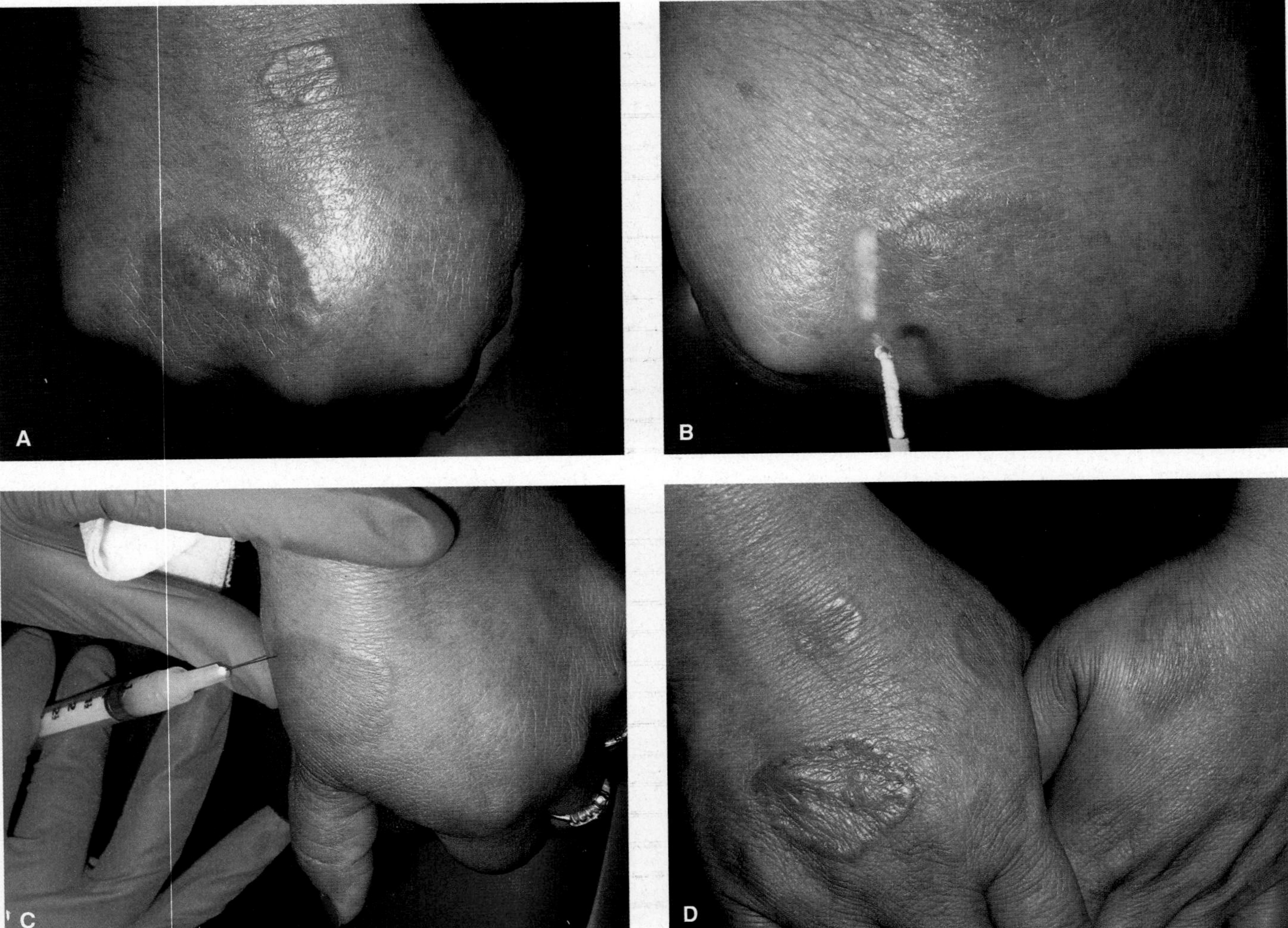

FIGURE 182-7 A. GA on the dorsum of the right hand of a 53-year-old Hispanic woman. B. Cryotherapy of the largest annular lesion. C. Intralesional triamcinolone being injected with a 30-gauge needle of a different GA lesion on the left hand. D. One month later the lesion on the left hand treated with intralesional steroid has flattened and begun to fade while the lesion on the right hand continues to be elevated and now has areas of hyperpigmentation and hypopigmentation secondary to the cryotherapy. At the time of therapy the patient stated the injection hurt less than the cryotherapy. (*Reproduced with permission from Richard P. Usatine, MD.*)

inhibition. Treatment with 400 mg three times a day provided impressive improvement in three months.[13] SOR Ⓒ

- The combination of rifampin 600 mg, ofloxacin 400 mg, and minocycline 100 mg successfully treated 6 patients with granuloma annulare. All patients had complete clearance after 3 to 5 months of treatment.[14] SOR Ⓒ
- Successful treatment of 6 patients with GA was achieved with 100 mg of dapsone, once a day. Complete clearance in all patients took between 4 weeks and 3 months.[15] SOR Ⓒ
- UVA1 phototherapy provided good or excellent results in 10 of 20 patients with disseminated GA. In patients with only a satisfactory treatment response, the disease reappeared soon after phototherapy was discontinued.[16] SOR Ⓒ
- Adalimumab resulted in rapid improvement of granuloma annulare lesions in 7 patients.[17] Three patients remained in remission after discontinuing therapy, while 2 patients had recurrence. When the patients with recurrent disease were placed back on adalimumab, their lesions cleared again within 11 weeks. SOR Ⓒ

SECOND LINE

- In a study of 4 patients, topical 5% imiquimod cream was effective when used once daily for an average of 2 months. After discontinuing treatment, 3 patients went an average of 12 months without recurrence; the fourth patient had a recurrence 10 days after treatment stopped, but after an additional 6 weeks of applying cream once daily, he was lesion-free for 18 months.[18] SOR Ⓒ
- Four patients were treated with twice-daily topical application of 0.1% tacrolimus ointment for 6 weeks; all reported improvement after 10 to 21 days. At treatment conclusion, two patients had complete clearance and the other two had marked improvement.[19] SOR Ⓒ
- Treatment with 0.5 to 1 mg/kg of isotretinoin daily has produced some positive results across multiple small studies; however, because of the potential for adverse effects, this option should be reserved for the most severe, nonresponsive cases in patients who are at low risk for the adverse effects of isotretinoin.[20] SOR Ⓒ

- Three patients were treated with vitamin E 400 IU daily and zileuton 2400 mg daily. All responded within 3 months with complete clinical clearing.[21] SOR Ⓒ

PERFORATING, SUBCUTANEOUS

- Although we could find no specific data to inform the treatment of these less-common types of GA, treatments for both localized and disseminated GA could be applied based on clinical judgment along with patient's severity and preferences.

PROGNOSIS

In 50% of cases there is spontaneous resolution within 2 years; however, recurrence rate is as high as 40%.[22] Patients with skin of color may have postinflammatory hyperpigmentation once the papules and plaques resolve.

FOLLOW-UP

Follow-up visits should be offered to patients who want active treatment.

PATIENT EDUCATION

It is important to reassure patients that this disease is self-limiting. Despite a displeasing appearance, the best treatment may be to let lesions resolve naturally. Numerous individual case studies and treatments have been attempted without consistent success. Treatments may produce side effects that are equally as unwanted, but more permanent, than the GA.

PATIENT RESOURCES

- Skinsight. *Granuloma Annulare: Information for Adults*—**http://www.skinsight.com/skin-conditions/adult/granuloma-annulare.htm.**

PROVIDER RESOURCES

- Medscape. *Granuloma Annulare*—**http://emedicine.medscape.com/article/1123031.**

REFERENCES

1. Cyr PR. Diagnosis and management of granuloma annulare. *Am Fam Physician*. 2006;74(10):1729-1824.
2. Ghadially R, Garg A. *Granuloma Annulare*. http://emedicine.medscape.com/article/ 1123031-overview. Accessed May 2012.
3. Ko CJ, Glusac EJ, Shapiro PE. Noninfectious granulomas. In: Elder DE, ed. *Lever's Histopathology of the Skin*, 10th ed. Philadelphia, PA: Lippincott Williams & Wilkins; 2009:361-364.
4. Fayyazi A, Schweyer S, Eichmeyer B, et al. Expression of IFN-gamma, coexpression of TNF-alpha and matrix metalloproteinases and apoptosis of T lymphocytes and macrophages in granuloma annulare. *Arch Dermatol Res*. 2000;292:384-390.
5. Macaron NC, Cohen C, Chen SC, Arbiser JL. gli-1 Oncogene is highly expressed in granulomatous skin disorders, including sarcoidosis, granuloma annulare, and necrobiosis lipoidica diabeticorum. *Arch Dermatol*. 2005;141:259-262.
6. Habif TP. *Clinical Dermatology*, 4th ed. St Louis, MO: Mosby; 2004.
7. Smith MD, Downie JB, DiCostanzo D. Granuloma annulare. *Int J Dermatol*. 1997;36:326-333.
8. Martinón-Torres F, Martinón-Sánchez JM, Martinón-Sánchez F. Localized granuloma annulare in children: a review of 42 cases. *Eur J Pediatr*. 1999;158(10):866.
9. Blume-Peytavi U, Zouboulis CC, Jacobi H, et al. Successful outcome of cryosurgery in patients with granuloma annulare. *Br J Dermatol*. 1994;130(4):494-497.
10. Lebwohl MG, Berth-Jones M, Coulson I. *Treatment of Skin Disease, Comprehensive Therapeutic Strategies*, 2nd ed. St. Louis, MO: Mosby; 2006:251.
11. Grewal SK, Rubin C, Rosenbach M. Antimalarial therapy for granuloma annulare: results of a retrospective analysis. *J Am Acad Dermatol*. 2017:76(4):765-767.
12. Lukács J, Schliemann S, Elsner P. Treatment of generalized granuloma annulare—a systematic review. *J Eur Acad Dermatol Venereol*. 2015;29(8):1467-1480.
13. Nambiar KG, Jagadeesan S, Balasubramanian P, Thomas J. Successful treatment of generalized granuloma annulare with pentoxifylline. *Indian Dermatol Online J*. 2017;8(3):218-220.
14. Marcus DV, Mahmoud BH, Hamzavi IH. Granuloma annulare treated with rifampin, ofloxacin, and minocycline combination therapy. *Arch Dermatol*. 2009;145(7):787-789.
15. Czarnecki DB, Gin D. The response of generalized granuloma annulare to Dapsone. *Acta Derm Venereol (Stockh)*. 1986;66: 82-84.
16. Schnopp C, Tzaneva S, Mempel M, et al. UVA1 phototherapy for disseminated granuloma annulare. *Photodermatol Photoimmunol Photomed*. 2005;21(2):68-71.
17. Min MS, Lebwohl M. Treatment of recalcitrant granuloma annulare (GA) with adalimumab: a single-center, observational study. *J Am Acad Dermatol*. 2016;74(1):127.
18. Badavanis G, Monastirli A, Pasmatzi E, Tsambaos D. Successful treatment of granuloma annulare with imiquimod cream 5%: a report of four cases. *Acta Derm Venereol*. 2005;85(6): 547-548.
19. Jain S, Stephens CJM. Successful treatment of disseminated granuloma annulare with topical tacrolimus. *Br J Dermatol*. 2004; 150:1042-1043.
20. Looney M. Isotretinoin in the treatment of granuloma annulare. *Ann Pharmacother*. 2004;38(3):494-497.
21. Smith KJ, Norwood C, Skelton H. Treatment of disseminated granuloma annulare with a 5-lipoxygenase inhibitor and vitamin E. *Br J Dermatol*. 2002;146(4):667-670.
22. Reisenauer A, White KP, Korcheva V, White CR. Non-infectious granulomas. In: Bolognia JL, Jorizzo JL, Schaffer JV, eds. *Dermatology*, 2nd ed. Philadelphia, PA: Elsevier; 2012.

183 PYODERMA GANGRENOSUM

E.J. Mayeaux, Jr., MD
Richard P. Usatine, MD

PATIENT STORY

A 32-year-old man was diagnosed with Crohn disease 10 years prior to his visit for these nonhealing leg ulcers (**Figure 183-1**). The patient experienced minor trauma to his lower leg 1 year ago and these ulcers developed (pathergy). Multiple treatments have been tried with partial success, but the ulcers persist.

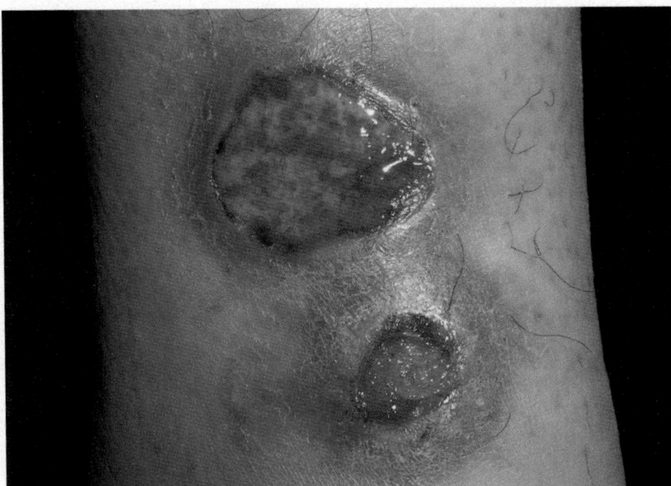

FIGURE 183-1 Classic pyoderma gangrenosum on the leg of a 32-year-old man with Crohn disease. This ulcer started with minor trauma (pathergy) and has been there for 1 year. *(Reproduced with permission from Richard P. Usatine, MD.)*

INTRODUCTION

Pyoderma gangrenosum (PG) is an uncommon ulcerative disease of the skin of unknown origin. It is a type of neutrophilic dermatosis—an inflammatory neutrophilic dermatosis—and is frequently associated with other systemic diseases.[1]

EPIDEMIOLOGY

- PG occurs in approximately 1 person per 100,000 each year.[2]
- A published case series reported a mean age between 50 and 63 years.[3] All ages may be affected.
- No racial predilection is apparent.
- A slight female predominance may exist.

ETIOLOGY AND PATHOPHYSIOLOGY

- Etiology is poorly understood. It has no infectious etiology and no tissue-related vascular gangrene.[1]
- Pathergy (initiation at the site of trauma or injury) is a common process, and it is estimated that 30% of patients with PG experienced pathergy.[2]
- Associated systemic diseases such as inflammatory bowel disease (IBD), hematologic malignancy, and rheumatoid arthritis and solid tumors have been documented in 33% to 75% of patients. The rest are idiopathic.[1,4]
- It associated with ulcerative colitis (5%–12%) and to a lesser extent Crohn disease (1%–2%) (**Figures 183-2** and **183-3**).[1]
- PG is thought to be autoimmune resulting from defects in cell-mediated immunity, neutrophil and monocyte function, and humoral immunity. Biopsies usually show a polymorphonuclear cell infiltrate with features of ulceration, infarction, and abscess formation.[1]
- PG also can be induced by drugs such as isotretinoin, propylthiouracil, granulocyte colony-stimulating factor, sunitinib, and cocaine.[5]

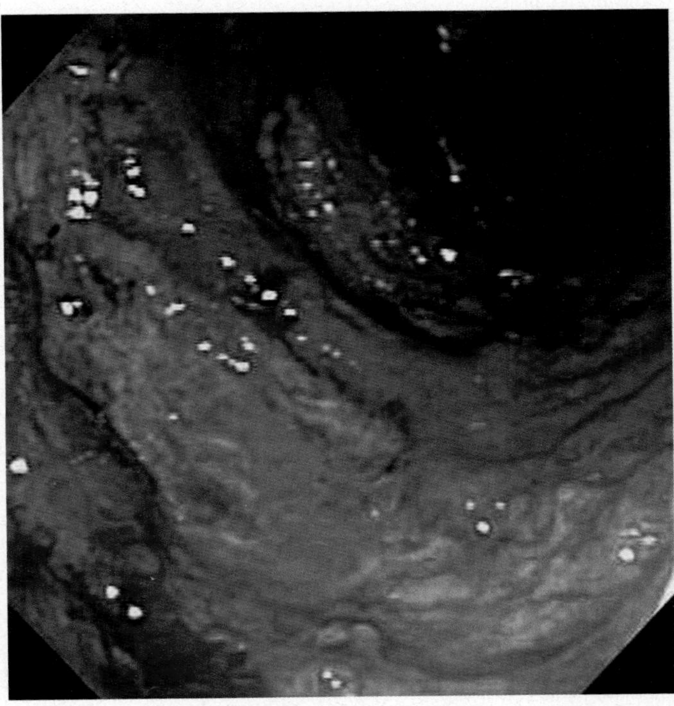

FIGURE 183-2 Friable inflamed mucosa of the colon in Crohn disease. *(Reproduced with permission from Shashi Mittal, MD.)*

RISK FACTORS[4,6]

- Ulcerative colitis.
- Crohn disease.
- Polyarthritis (seronegative or seropositive).
- Hematologic diseases/disorders such as leukemia (predominantly myelocytic).
- Monoclonal gammopathies (primarily immunoglobulin A).
- Psoriatic arthritis and rheumatoid arthritis (**Figure 183-4**).
- Hepatic diseases (hepatitis and primary biliary cirrhosis).
- Immunologic diseases (lupus erythematosus and Sjögren syndrome).

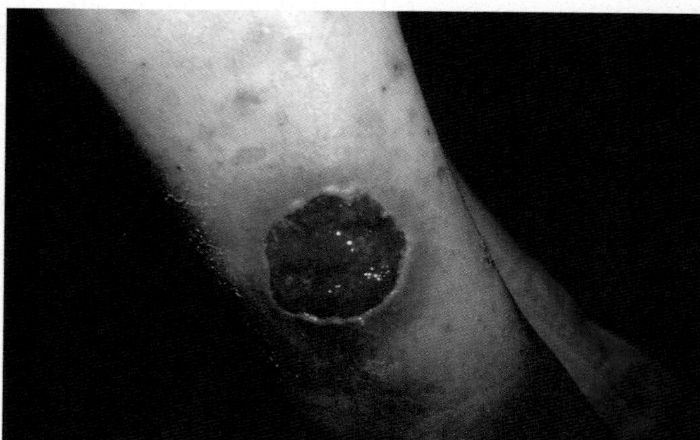

FIGURE 183-3 Classic pyoderma gangrenosum on the leg of a 35-year-old woman with Crohn disease. This ulcer started with minor trauma (pathergy) and has been there for 2 years. (*Reproduced with permission from Richard P. Usatine, MD.*)

DIAGNOSIS

CLINICAL FEATURES

- Typically classical PG presents with a deep painful ulcer with a well-defined border, which is usually violet or blue. The color has also been described as the color of gunmetal (**Figure 183-5**). The ulcer edge is often undermined, and the surrounding skin is erythematous and indurated (**Figure 183-6**). It usually starts as a pustule with an inflammatory base, an erythematous nodule, or a hemorrhagic bulla on a violaceous base. The central area then undergoes necrosis to form a single ulcer.[6] Classic PG is characterized by a deep ulceration with a violaceous border that overhangs the ulcer bed. These lesions of PG most commonly occur on the legs (see **Figures 183-1**, **183-3**, and **183-4**).[4] The lesions are painful and the pain can be severe.[4] Patients may have malaise, arthralgia, and myalgia.
- Vesicular-bullous PG variant most commonly presents on the face and the upper extremities, especially the dorsum of the hands. It occurs most often in association with infections, drug use, or acute myelogenous leukemia.[1]
    - Superficial granulomatous/vegetative PG has a vesiculopustular component (**Figure 183-7**). It is more benign and is erosive or superficially ulcerated, and most often occurs on the dorsal surface of the hands, the extensor parts of the forearms, or the face.[4]
- Other variants:
    - Peristomal PG may occur around stoma sites. This form is often mistaken for a wound infection or irritation from the appliance.[7]
    - Vulvar or penile PG occurs on the genitalia and must be differentiated from ulcerative sexually transmitted diseases (STDs) such as chancroid and syphilis.[4]
    - Intraoral PG is known as pyostomatitis vegetans. It occurs primarily in patients with IBD.[4]

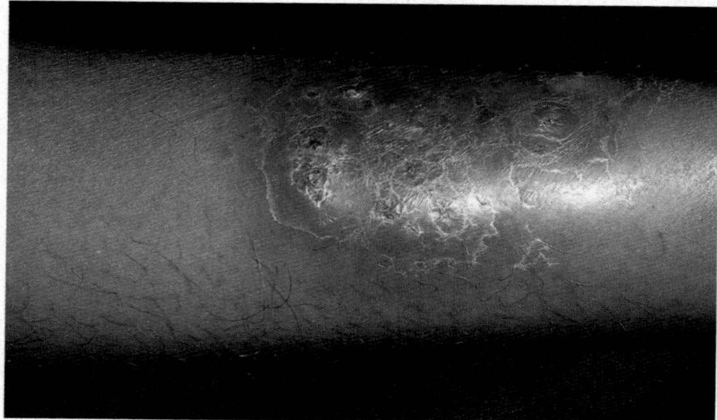

FIGURE 183-4 Pyoderma gangrenosum on the leg of a 56-year-old woman with rheumatoid arthritis. (*Reproduced with permission from Richard P. Usatine, MD.*)

TYPICAL DISTRIBUTION

- Most commonly seen on the legs and hands, but can occur on any skin surface including the genitalia, and around a stoma. PG can also be seen on the face and trunk (**Figures 183-5** and **183-8**).

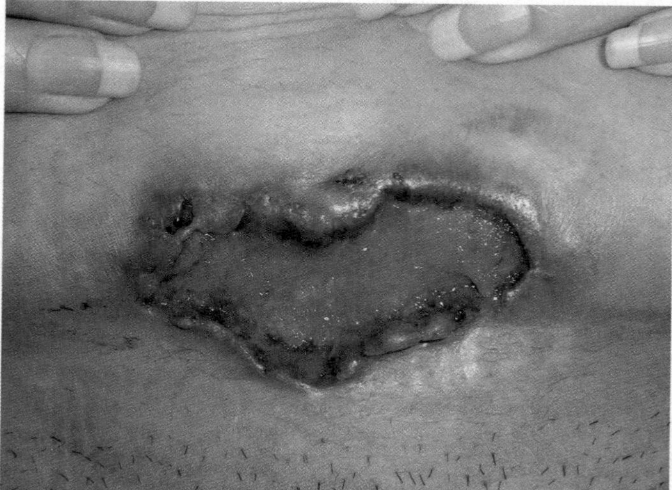

FIGURE 183-5 Pyoderma gangrenosum in the suprapubic area with classic gunmetal undermined borders. (*Reproduced with permission from Richard P. Usatine, MD.*)

LABORATORY TESTING

- Complete blood count (CBC), urinalysis (UA), and liver function tests (LFTs) should be obtained. Order a hepatitis profile to rule out hepatitis.[4] Systemic disease markers may be elevated if associated conditions exist, that is, erythrocyte sedimentation rate (ESR), antinuclear antibody (ANA), and rheumatoid factor. Obtain rapid plasma reagin (RPR), protein electrophoresis, and skin cultures as indicated. Consider culturing the ulcer/erosion for bacteria, fungi, atypical *Mycobacteria*, and viruses.[4]
- If GI symptoms exist, perform or refer for colonoscopy to look for IBD.

BIOPSY

- Biopsy an active area of disease along with the border. A punch biopsy is preferred (4-mm punch is adequate). Although there are no specific pathologic signs of PG, the biopsy can be used to rule out other causes of ulcerative skin lesions.[1]
- The pathologist may be able to confirm your clinical impression. Biopsy of the earliest lesions reveal a neutrophilic vascular reaction. Fully developed lesions exhibit dense neutrophilic infiltrate, and some lymphocytes and macrophages surrounding marked tissue necrosis. Ulceration, infarction of tissue, and abscess formation with fibrosing inflammation at the edge of the ulcer may be seen.[1,8]

DIFFERENTIAL DIAGNOSIS[1]

- PG is sometimes a diagnosis of exclusion, diagnosed with successful wound healing following immunosuppressant therapy.[9] When misdiagnosed it is often confused for vascular occlusive or venous disease, vasculitis, cancer, primary infection, drug-induced or exogenous tissue injury, and other inflammatory disorders.[10] Biopsy of a questionable lesion may be the only way to ultimately distinguish PG as the cause of ulcerative skin lesions.
- Ulcerative STDs, such as chancroid and syphilis, can resemble vulvar or penile PG. These STDs are more common than PG and should be diagnosed with appropriate tests, including RPR and bacterial culture for *Haemophilus ducreyi*. If these tests are negative, then PG should be considered. RPR should also be repeated in 2 weeks if it is initially negative at the start of a chancre—it takes some weeks to become positive and syphilis is easily treatable (see Chapter 225, Syphilis).
- Acute febrile neutrophilic dermatosis (Sweet syndrome) is a neutrophilic dermatosis like PG, but the patients are generally febrile with systemic symptoms (**Figure 183-9**). The diagnosis of Sweet syndrome is made when the patient fulfills 2 of 2 major criteria and 2 of 4 minor criteria. The 2 major criteria are (a) an abrupt onset of tender or painful erythematous plaques or nodules occasionally with vesicles, pustules, or bullae, and (b) predominantly neutrophilic infiltration in the dermis without leukocytoclastic vasculitis. Minor criteria include specific preceding or concurrent medical conditions, fever, abnormal lab values including leukocytosis and an elevated sedimentation rate, and a rapid response to systemic steroids.

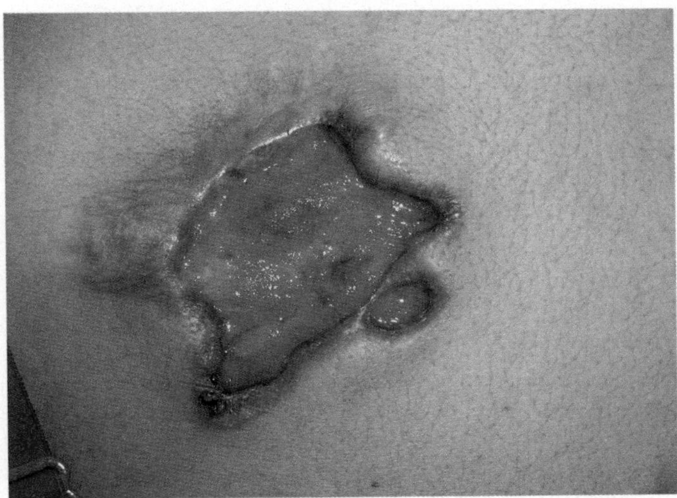

FIGURE 183-6 Pyoderma gangrenosum on the shoulder of a young woman that has recurred after healing leaving scarred borders. The current active borders have erythema and a gunmetal coloration. They are also undermined. (*Reproduced with permission from Richard P. Usatine, MD.*)

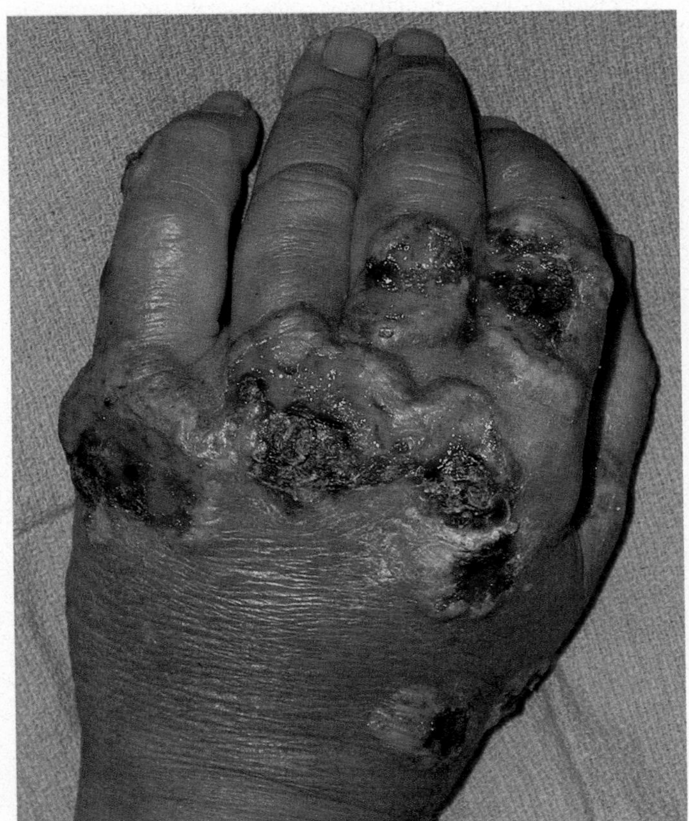

FIGURE 183-7 Atypical pyoderma gangrenosum with a vesiculopustular "juicy" component on the dorsal surface of the hand. Bullae were previously present before the ulcerations developed. The lesions are "juicy," resemble those seen in Sweet syndrome, and have occurred at sites of minor trauma (pathergy). (*Reproduced with permission from Eric Kraus, MD.*)

- Systemic vasculitis is perhaps the most difficult to differentiate, but history of minor trauma in the area preceding lesion formation (pathergy) and undermining of the violaceous border should lead one toward the diagnosis of PG.[10]
- Ecthyma is a type of impetigo in which ulcers form. Bacterial cultures will be positive and this disease should respond to cephalexin or other oral antibiotics (see Chapter 122, Impetigo).
- Brown recluse spider bites can easily resemble PG when they ulcerate. Any spider bite can ulcerate and become necrotic like PG (**Figure 183-10**). The history of a spider bite can help differentiate this from PG.
- Sporotrichosis is a fungal infection that often starts from an injury while gardening with roses. It is usually on the arm or hand and can resemble PG. Use fungal culture to diagnose this when the history suggests this as the diagnosis. Oral antifungal medications can treat this (**Figure 183-11**).
- Squamous cell carcinoma with ulcerations may look like PG. Its diagnosis requires a biopsy. If the ulcer is on sun-exposed area, squamous cell carcinoma should be considered. A shave or punch biopsy can be used to diagnose this malignancy (see Chapter 178, Squamous Cell Carcinoma).
- Venous insufficiency ulcers are typically seen around the medial malleolus, and the most severe of these ulcers resemble PG (**Figure 183-12**). The presence of signs and symptoms of vascular insufficiency should help differentiate this from PG (see Chapter 54, Venous Insufficiency).
- Mycosis fungoides is a cutaneous T-cell lymphoma that can ulcerate and resemble PG. Use tissue biopsy to differentiate these two conditions (see Chapter 180, Cutaneous T-Cell Lymphoma).

MANAGEMENT

FIRST LINE

- Perform appropriate wound care including cleansing, preventing secondary infections (mainly to prevent deeper infection), and providing moist wound healing.[1]
- At each visit, measure and document the lesion's depth, length, and width to track treatment progression.[11]
- Surgical debridement is contraindicated, as pathergy occurs in 25% to 50% of cases and surgery will make the lesions worse. SOR B
- Patients frequently are in pain from the lesions, so treatment is aimed at pain relief as well as healing the skin lesions.
- Therapy directed at the underlying disease (often IBD), when present, that usually results in healing. Treatment with steroids is also often necessary.[11] SOR B
- Topical medications are first-line therapy in cases of localized PG that are not severe. Start with potent corticosteroid ointments or tacrolimus ointment.[11,12] SOR B
- Small or indolent ulcers can be managed with topical steroid creams. SOR C
- Intralesional injections with corticosteroids are also an option.[11,12] SOR B

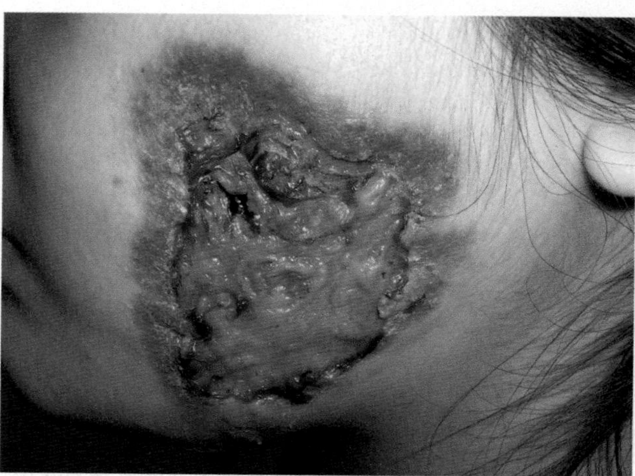

FIGURE 183-8 Pyoderma gangrenosum on the face of a young woman on and off for 4 years. The purulent-appearing base explains the term "pyoderma" in the name. (*Reproduced with permission from Richard P. Usatine, MD.*)

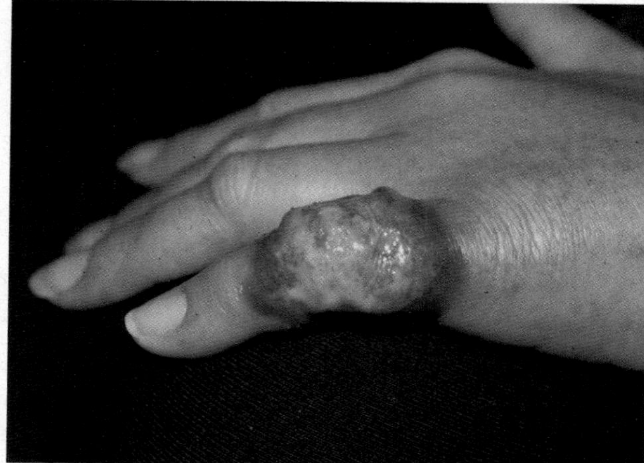

FIGURE 183-9 Sweet syndrome is the eponym for acute febrile neutrophilic dermatosis. The lesion looks like pyoderma gangrenosum and occurs at sites of minor trauma (pathergy). However, this patient has a fever and is systemically ill. (*Reproduced with permission from John Gonzalez, MD.*)

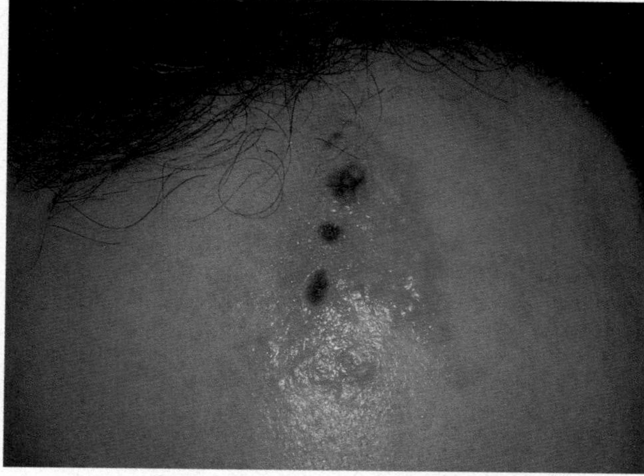

FIGURE 183-10 Necrotic ulcers on the forehead of a young man after probable brown recluse spider bites. He was working in the yard when he felt a sharp sting on the forehead. The following day three ulcers developed with significant erythema and swelling. Although the spider was never seen, it is most likely the cause of the ulcers. They resolved over time. (*Reproduced with permission from Richard P. Usatine, MD.*)

- Systemic treatment with oral corticosteroids, such as methylprednisolone (1 g/day IV for 3 days) or prednisone (0.5 to 1 mg/kg per day) or oral cyclosporine (e.g., 5 mg/kg per day) alone or together appears to be effective (in the absence of controlled trials) in many cases and should be considered first-line therapy.[7,12] SOR B Response is usually rapid, with stabilization of the PG within 24 hours.[13]

SECOND LINE

- In steroid-refractory PG associated with IBD, infliximab was effective in case series and a small placebo-controlled trial.[14,15] SOR B Other biologic therapies reported include alefacept, etanercept, efalizumab, and adalimumab.[11] SOR C
- Cyclosporine (2.5–5.0 mg/kg per day) is used as second-line and steroid-sparing treatment.[16] SOR A
- To date, case reports have been published that show therapeutic efficacy of dapsone (100 mg/day), azathioprine (50 to 150 mg/day), 6-mercaptopurine, mycophenolate mofetil (1 to 2 g twice daily), cyclophosphamide (2 to 3 mg/kg per day), and tacrolimus (0.1 mg/kg per day).[12,17] SOR C
- The TNF-α antagonists (etanercept, adalimumab, infliximab) have been reported effective in case reports. SOR C One small randomized controlled infliximab study showed benefit in 70% of patients.[18] SOR C

REFERRAL

In many cases, referral to a dermatologist is needed.

PROGNOSIS

- The prognosis of PG is variable, with residual scarring and recurrences being common.
- Although many patients improve with initial immunosuppressive therapy, patients may follow a refractory course and require multiple therapies.

FOLLOW-UP

- All patients suspected of having PG need close and frequent follow-up to obtain a definitive diagnosis and treat this challenging condition.

PATIENT EDUCATION

- PG is a rare ulcerative skin condition that is poorly understood.
- A skin biopsy is needed to rule out other diagnoses.
- Most treatments are empirical and based on small studies.
- The risks and benefits of steroids and/or other immunosuppressive medications need to be explained.
- Surgical treatments are contraindicated.

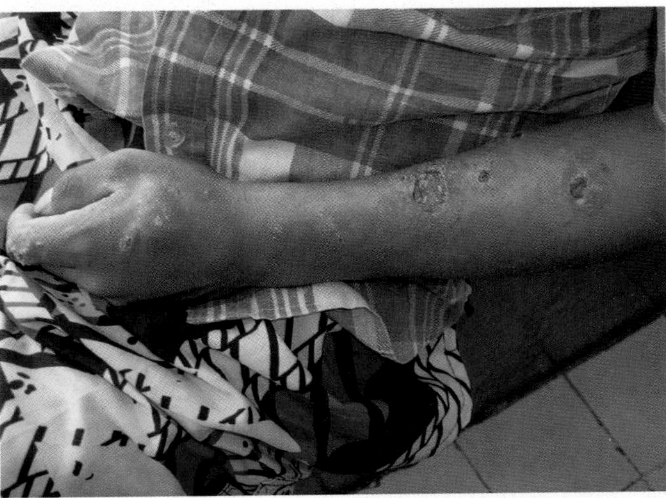

FIGURE 183-11 Sporotrichosis (fungal infection) with the typical sporotrichoid spread up the arm from an inoculation of the hand. Note how the ulcers resemble pyoderma gangrenosum. *(Reproduced with permission from Richard P. Usatine, MD.)*

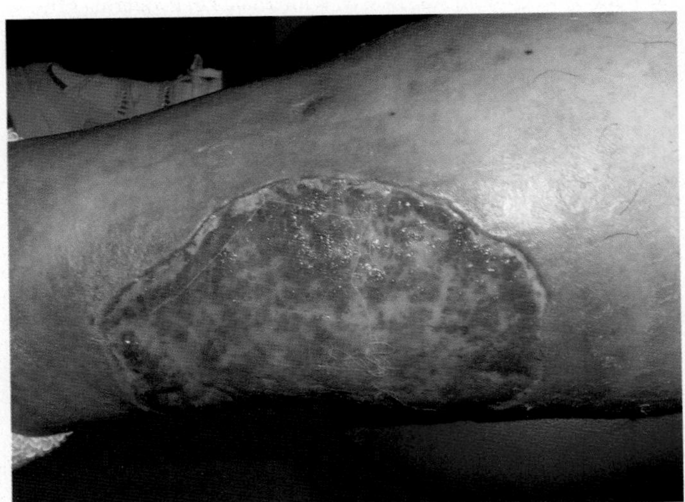

FIGURE 183-12 A large venous stasis ulcer on the lower leg not healing with intensive wound care and compression stockings. A punch biopsy on the edge was performed to make sure this was not pyoderma gangrenosum. *(Reproduced with permission from Richard P. Usatine, MD.)*

PATIENT RESOURCES

- American Autoimmune Related Diseases Association, Inc. Tel: 800-598-4668. *Pyoderma Gangrenosum*—**https://www.aarda.org/diseaseinfo/pyoderma-gangrenosum/.**
- Crohn's and Colitis Foundation of America. Tel: 800-932-2423—**http://www.crohnscolitisfoundation.org.**
- *Patient: Pyoderma Gangrenosum*—**https://patient.info/doctor/pyoderma-gangrenosum-pro**
- National Organization for Rare Disorders. *Pyoderma Gangrenosum*—**https://rarediseases.org/rare-diseases/pyoderma-gangrenosum/.**
- NIH Genetic and Rare Diseases Information Center (GARD). *Pyoderma Gangrenosum*—**https://rarediseases.info.nih.gov/diseases/7510/pyoderma-gangrenosum.**

PROVIDER RESOURCES

- Gameiro A, Pereira N, Cardoso JC, et al. Pyoderma gangrenosum: challenges and solutions. *Clin Cosmet Investig Dermatol.* 2015;8:285-293—**https://www.ncbi.nlm.nih.gov/pmc/articles/PMC4454198/.**
- **http://emedicine.medscape.com/article/1123821.**
- Mayo Clinic. *Pyoderma Gangrenosum*—**https://www.mayoclinic.org/diseases-conditions/pyoderma-gangrenosum/symptoms-causes/syc-20350386.**
- Wollina U. PG—a review. *Orphanet J Rare Dis.* 2007;2:19—**http://www.ncbi.nlm.nih.gov/pmc/articles/PMC1857704/.**

REFERENCES

1. Shavit E, Alavi A, Sibbald RG. Pyoderma gangrenosum: a critical appraisal. *Adv Skin Wound Care.* 2017;30(12):534-542.
2. Brooklyn T, Brooklyn T, Dunnill G, Probert C. Diagnosis and treatment of pyoderma gangrenosum. *BMJ.* 2006;333(7560):181-184.
3. Binus AM, Qureshi AA, Li VW, Winterfield LS. Pyoderma gangrenosum: a retrospective review of patient characteristics, comorbidities and therapy in 103 patients. *Br J Dermatol.* 2011;165(6):1244-1250.
4. Jackson JM, Callen JP. *Pyoderma Gangrenosum.* http://emedicine.medscape.com/article/1123821-overview. Accessed March 2012.
5. Wang JY, French LE, Shear NH, et al. Drug-induced pyoderma gangrenosum: a review. *Am J Clin Dermatol.* 2018;19(1):67-77.
6. Habif T. *Clinical Dermatology*, 4th ed. Philadelphia, PA: Mosby; 2004:653-654.
7. Keltz M, Lebwohl M, Bishop S. Peristomal pyoderma gangrenosum. *J Am Acad Dermatol.* 1992;27(2 Pt 2):360-364.
8. Su WP, Schroeter AL, Perry HO, Powell FC. Histopathologic and immunopathologic study of pyoderma gangrenosum. *J Cutan Pathol.* 1986;13(5):323-330.
9. Banga F, Schuitemaker N, Meijer P. Pyoderma gangrenosum after caesarean section: a case report. *Reprod Health.* 2006;3:9.
10. Weenig RH, Davis MD, Dahl PR, Su WP. Skin ulcers misdiagnosed as pyoderma gangrenosum. *N Engl J Med.* 2002;347(18): 1412-1418.
11. Miller J, Yentzer BA, Clark A, et al. Pyoderma gangrenosum: a review and update on new therapies. *J Am Acad Dermatol.* 2010;62(4):646-654.
12. Reichrath J, Bens G, Bonowitz A, Tilgen W. Treatment recommendations for pyoderma gangrenosum: an evidence-based review of the literature based on more than 350 patients. *J Am Acad Dermatol.* 2005;53(2):273-283.
13. Chow RK, Ho VC. Treatment of pyoderma gangrenosum. *J Am Acad Dermatol.* 1996;34(6):1047-1060.
14. De la Morena F, Martín L, Gisbert JP, et al. Refractory and infected pyoderma gangrenosum in a patient with ulcerative colitis: response to infliximab. *Inflamm Bowel Dis.* 2007;13(4): 509-510.
15. Brooklyn TN, Dunnill MG, Shetty A, et al. Infliximab for the treatment of pyoderma gangrenosum: a randomised, double blind, placebo controlled trial. *Gut.* 2006;55(4):505-509.
16. Ormerod AD, Thomas KS, Craig FE, et al. Comparison of the two most commonly used treatments for pyoderma gangrenosum: results of the STOP GAP randomized controlled trial. *BMI.* 2015;350:h2958.
17. Eaton PA, Callen JP. Mycophenolate mofetil as therapy for pyoderma gangrenosum. *Arch Dermatol.* 2009;145(7):781-785.
18. Brooklyn TN. Infliximab for the treatment of pyoderma gangrenosum: a randomised, double blind, placebo controlled trial. *Gut.* 2006;55(4):505-509.

184 SARCOIDOSIS

Edward Bae, MD
Yoon-Soo Cindy Bae, MD
Khashayar Sarabi, MD
Amor Khachemoune, MD

PATIENT STORY

A 42-year-old man presents with "multiple bumps" that had been growing on his scalp, the back of the neck, and on preexisting scars (**Figure 184-1**). These lesions started developing slowly over a period of 1 year. The differential diagnosis of these lesions included cutaneous sarcoidosis, acne keloidalis nuchae, and pseudofolliculitis barbae. A punch biopsy was performed and the diagnosis of sarcoidosis was made.

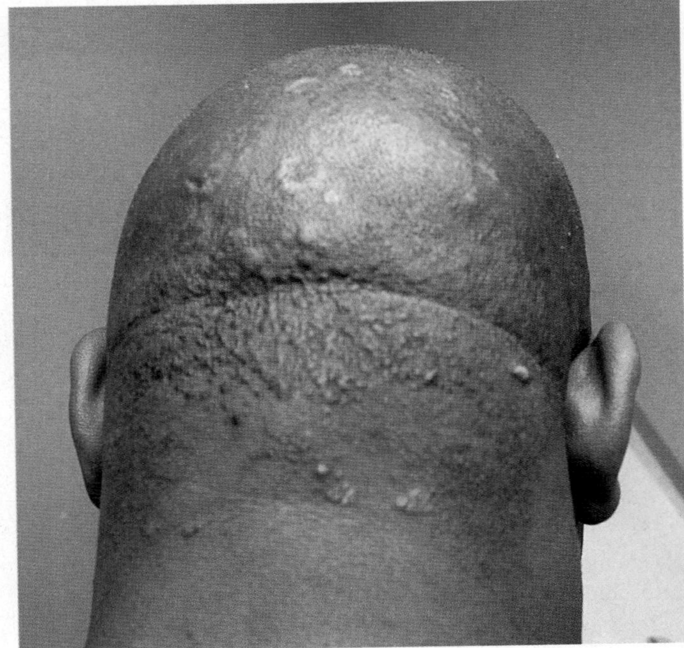

FIGURE 184-1 Papular and annular lesions of sarcoid on the scalp and neck of a 42-year-old black man. (*Reproduced with permission from Amor Khachemoune, MD.*)

INTRODUCTION

Sarcoidosis is a multisystem granulomatous disease most commonly involving the skin, lungs, lymph nodes, liver, and eyes. The condition more commonly affects patients of African descent compared to Caucasian patients. Diagnosing cutaneous sarcoidosis is critical, as 30% of these patients are later found to have systemic involvement. In addition, recent evidence has shown that approximately 25% of autopsies performed on patients with sarcoidosis revealed cardiac involvement.[1] Nevertheless, the diverse presentations of cutaneous sarcoidosis in addition to variants of specific sarcoidosis syndromes can make for a diagnostic challenge.

SYNONYMS

- Lupus pernio (cutaneous sarcoidosis).
- Darier-Roussy disease (subcutaneous sarcoidosis).
- Löfgren syndrome (erythema nodosum, hilar adenopathy, fever, arthritis).

EPIDEMIOLOGY

- Cutaneous manifestations occur in approximately 25% of systemic sarcoidosis patients.
- In approximately one third of cases, cutaneous lesions are the first signs of systemic sarcoidosis.[2]
- In the United States, the annual incidence is estimated at 35.5 per 100,000 persons of African descent and 10.9 per 100,000 Caucasians.[3]
- The ratio of patients with only cutaneous sarcoidosis versus multisystem involvement is 1:3.
- Specific cutaneous involvement is most common in older, female patients of African descent (**Figures 184-2** and **184-3**).
- Common types of cutaneous lesions seen in sarcoidosis include erythema nodosum (EN); papular or plaque type, lupus pernio, cutaneous or subcutaneous nodules, and infiltrative scars.

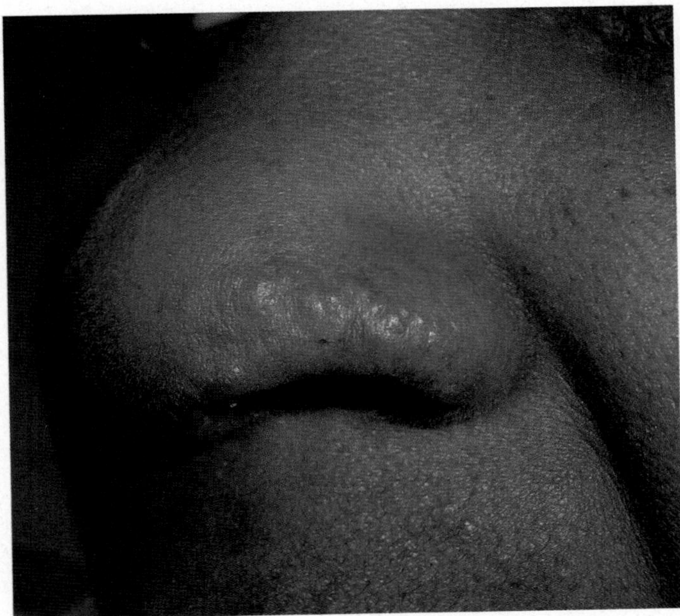

FIGURE 184-2 Lupus pernio in a 45-year-old black woman with sarcoid involving the nasal rim. (*Reproduced with permission from Richard P. Usatine, MD.*)

- EN occurs in 3% to 34% of patients with sarcoidosis and is the most common associated skin finding (see Chapter 186, Erythema Nodosum).
- Sarcoidosis-related EN is more prevalent in Caucasians, especially Scandinavians. EN also has a predilection for Irish and Puerto Rican populations.
- EN occurs between the second and fourth decades of life, more commonly in women.
- Other nonspecific lesions of sarcoidosis reported include erythema multiforme, calcinosis cutis, prurigo, and lymphedema. Nail changes can include clubbing, onycholysis, subungual keratosis, and dystrophy, with or without underlying changes in the bone (cysts).

ETIOLOGY AND PATHOPHYSIOLOGY

- Sarcoidosis is a granulomatous disease of unknown etiology involving multiple organ systems.
- It is thought that a combination of environmental exposures and host genetic factors affecting immune response are involved in the pathophysiology of sarcoidosis.[3]
- Microscopically, sarcoid lesions are characterized by the presence of circumscribed granulomas of epithelioid cells with little or no caseating necrosis, although fibrinoid necrosis is not uncommon.
- Granulomas are usually in the superficial dermis but may involve the thickness of dermis and extend to the subcutaneous tissue. These granulomas are called "naked" because they have only a sparse lymphocytic infiltrate at their margins.

RISK FACTORS

- Positive family history.
- African descent.
- Obesity.[4]

DIAGNOSIS

There is no singular definitive diagnostic test for sarcoidosis because of the myriad presentations of the disease. Rather, diagnosis is dependent on the constellation of clinical features, laboratory studies, imaging, and pathology via lesion biopsy.

CLINICAL FORMS OF DISEASE

Cutaneous lesions of the disease are either "specific" to sarcoidosis or "nonspecific," denoting a systemic immunologic response to a sarcoidosis lesion found elsewhere in the body.

- Specific:
  - These lesions are typically noncaseating granulomas, with no evidence of infection, foreign body, or other causes.
  - May be disfiguring, but usually are nontender and rarely ulcerate.
  - Maculopapular type is most common with red-brown or purplish papules on the face, neck, upper back, and limbs (**Figure 184-4**).

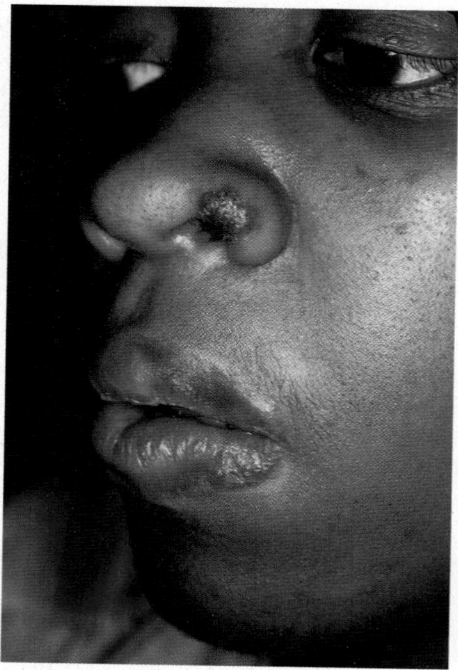

FIGURE 184-3 Lupus pernio with red to violaceous sarcoid papules and plaques on the nose and lips. *(Reproduced with permission from Amor Khachemoune, MD.)*

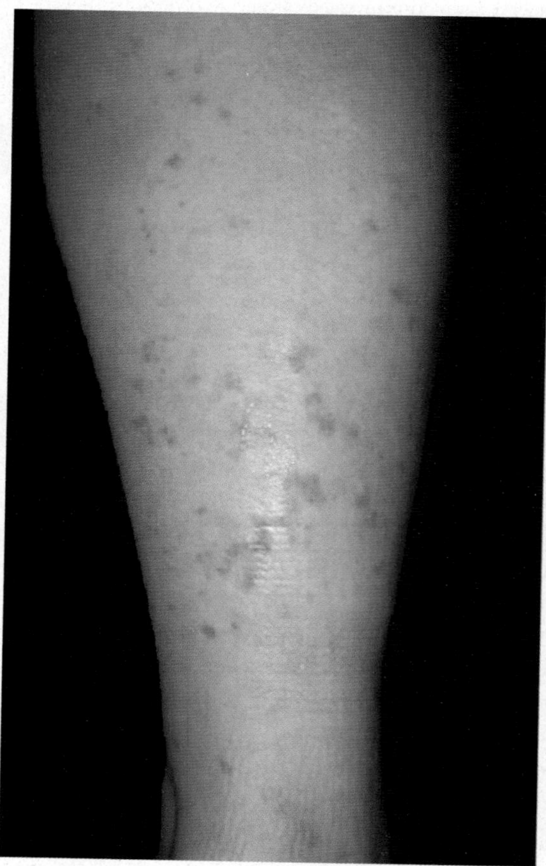

FIGURE 184-4 Maculopapular sarcoidosis on the leg of a 46-year-old white woman. *(Reproduced with permission from Amor Khachemoune, MD.)*

- Lupus pernio is distinctive as it presents as purplish lesions resembling frostbite (or lupus) covered with shiny skin, typically affecting nose, cheeks, ears, and lips and distal extremities (**Figures 184-2, 184-3,** and **184-5**).
- Lupus pernio may occur as a syndrome involving upper respiratory tract with pulmonary fibrosis, or may be associated with chronic uveitis and bone cysts.
- Annular or circinate type sarcoidosis lesions appear ribbon-like, with mild scaling, yellowish-red in color, centrifugal progression, and central healing and depigmentation (see **Figure 184-1**).
- Plaque sarcoidosis is typically chronic, occurring over the forehead, extremities, and trunk (**Figure 184-6**). It may be hypopigmented and can heal without scarring.
- Advanced systemic sarcoidosis typically presents with nodular cutaneous and subcutaneous plaques that are skin-colored or violaceous without epidermal involvement (**Figure 184-7**).
- Sarcoid granulomas may also infiltrate areas of old scars damaged by trauma, radiation, surgery, or tattoo (**Figures 184-8** and **184-9**). Lesions may be tender and appear indurated with red or purple discoloration.

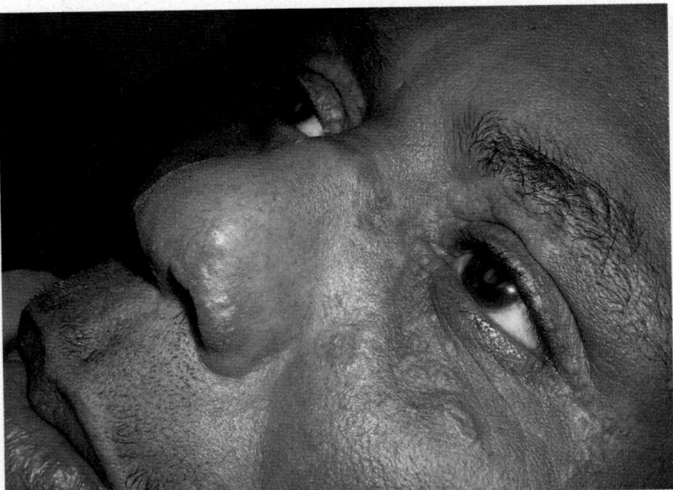

FIGURE 184-5 Lupus pernio in a 48-year-old black man with sarcoid lesions on the nose and around the eyes. (*Reproduced with permission from Richard P. Usatine, MD.*)

- Nonspecific:
  - EN lesions are the most common nonspecific lesions of sarcoidosis.
  - EN lesions are not usually disfiguring, but tender to touch, especially when they occur with fever, polyarthralgias, and sometimes arthritis and acute iritis.
  - EN appears abruptly with warm, tender, reddish nodules on the lower extremities, most commonly the anterior tibial surfaces, ankles, and knees.
  - EN nodules are 1 to 5 cm, usually bilateral, and evolve through color stages: first bright red, then purplish, and last a bruiselike yellow or green appearance.
  - EN bouts occur with fatigue, fever, symmetrical polyarthritis, and skin eruptions that typically last 3 to 6 weeks, with more than 80% of cases resolving within 2 years.[4]
  - EN is seen in the setting of Löfgren syndrome, appearing with hilar lymphadenopathy (most often bilaterally), and occasionally anterior uveitis and/or polyarthritis.
  - Löfgren syndrome is associated with right paratracheal lymph node involvement seen on X-ray.
  - Ulceration is typically not observed in EN, which heals without scarring.
  - Other nonspecific lesions of sarcoidosis include lymphedema, calcinosis cutis, prurigo, and erythema multiforme.
  - Nail changes seen in sarcoidosis include clubbing, onycholysis, and subungual keratosis.

LABORATORY STUDIES

- Complete blood count (CBC) count with differential:
  - Leukopenia (5%–10%) and/or thrombocytopenia may be seen.
  - Eosinophilia occurs in 24% of patients, and anemia occurs in 5% of patients.
  - Hypergammaglobulinemia (30%–80%), positive rheumatoid factor, and decreased skin test reactivity.
  - Autoimmune hemolytic anemia and hypersplenism can occur in some patients, although rare.

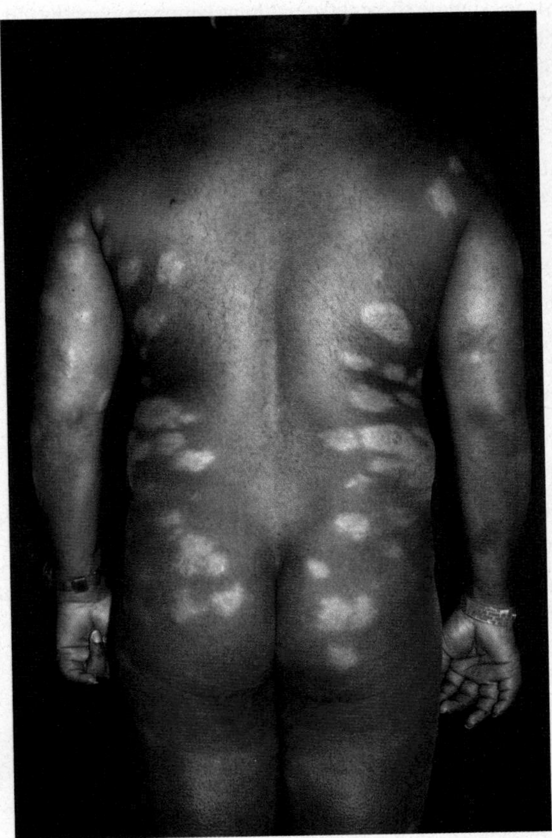

FIGURE 184-6 Hypopigmented widespread cutaneous plaque sarcoidosis predominantly on the back of a black man. (*Reproduced with permission from Eric Kraus, MD.*)

   - Hypocapnia and hypoxemia may be present in certain patient populations and may become worse with exercise.
- Serum calcium and 24-hour urine calcium levels:
   - Hypercalciuria has been found in 49% of patients in some studies, whereas 13% of patients had hypercalcemia.
   - Hypercalcemia occurs in sarcoidosis because of increased intestinal absorption of calcium that results from overproduction of a metabolite of vitamin D by pulmonary macrophages.
- Serum angiotensin-converting enzyme (ACE) level is elevated in 60% of patients:
   - Serum ACE levels are helpful in monitoring disease activity and treatment response. ACE is derived from epithelioid cells of the granulomas; therefore, it reflects granuloma load in the patient.
- Serum chemistries, such as alanine aminotransferase, aspartate aminotransferase, alkaline phosphatase, blood urea nitrogen (BUN), and creatinine levels. These levels may be elevated with hepatic and renal involvement.
- Other—Elevated erythrocyte sedimentation rate, elevated antinuclear antibodies (30%), diabetes insipidus, and renal failure may be noted.

IMAGING STUDIES

- Chest X-ray (CXR):
   - Radiographic involvement of the chest is seen in almost 90% of patients.
   - Stage I disease shows bilateral hilar lymphadenopathy (BHL).
   - Stage II disease shows BHL plus pulmonary infiltrates.
   - Stage III disease shows pulmonary infiltrates without BHL.
   - Stage IV disease shows pulmonary fibrosis.
- CT of the thorax may demonstrate lymphadenopathy or granulomatous infiltration. Other findings may include small nodules with a bronchovascular and subpleural distribution, thickened interlobular septae, honeycombing, bronchiectasis, and alveolar consolidation.
- Pulmonary function tests—Evidence of both restrictive abnormalities and obstructive abnormalities may be found.

BIOPSY

- A 4-mm punch biopsy is adequate to obtain a sample of skin that includes dermis.
- If EN nodules are deep, a deep punch biopsy should also include subcutaneous fat.
- Biopsy specimens are sent for histologic examination. If an infection (deep fungal, mycobacterium) is suspected, some tissue should be sent in a sterile urine cup for tissue cultures.

DIFFERENTIAL DIAGNOSIS

- Granulomatous skin disease (**Figure 184-10**).
   - Granuloma annulare (GA) is also a granulomatous skin disease, which appears in single or multiple rings in adults and children (see Chapter 182, Granuloma Annulare).

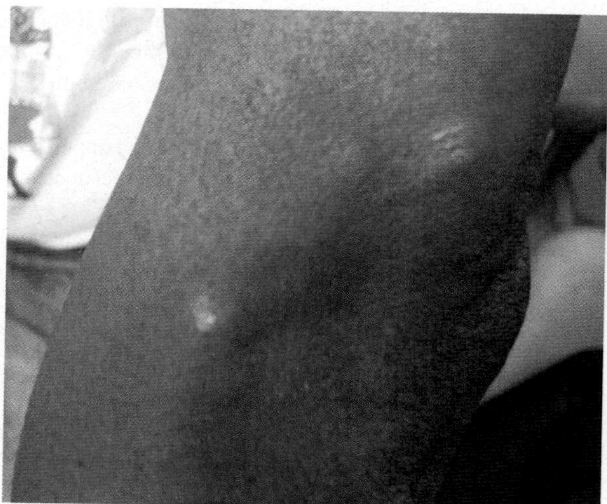

FIGURE 184-7 Subcutaneous sarcoid (Darier-Roussy syndrome) in a patient with advanced systemic sarcoidosis. (*Reproduced with permission from Amor Khachemoune, MD.*)

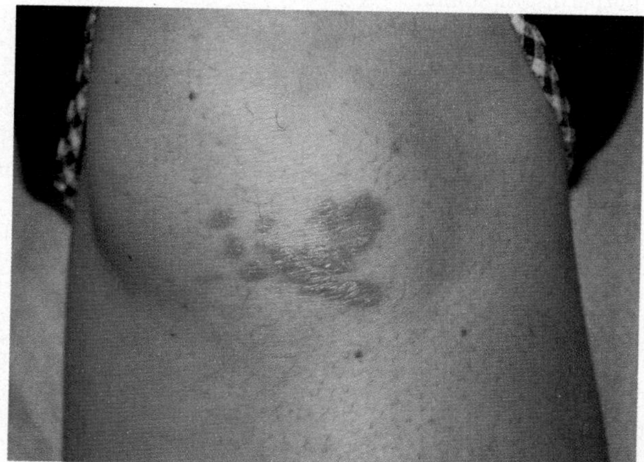

FIGURE 184-8 Sarcoidal plaque of the knee, which appeared after a trauma to the knee. (*Reproduced with permission from Amor Khachemoune, MD.*)

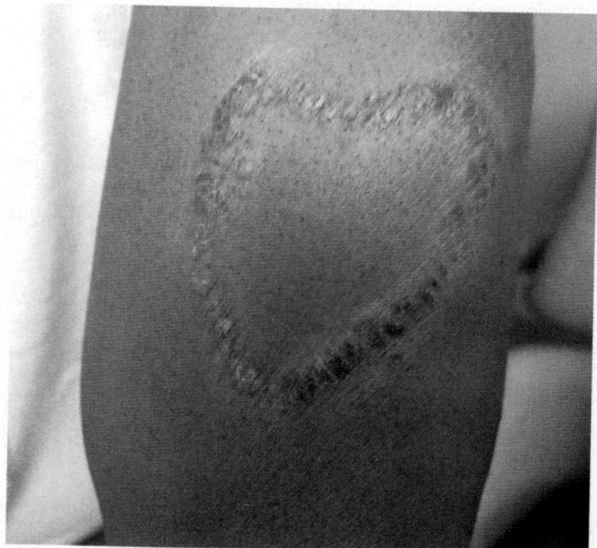

FIGURE 184-9 Sarcoid on a heart-shaped homemade tattoo over the knee. (*Reproduced with permission from Amor Khachemoune, MD.*)

- Rheumatoid nodules—These usually appear in the context of a diagnosed rheumatoid arthritis with joint disease present (see Chapter 99, Rheumatoid Arthritis).
- Granulomatous mycosis fungoides—This is a type of cutaneous lymphoma with many clinical forms including granuloma formation (see Chapter 180, Cutaneous T-Cell lymphoma).

- Maculopapular type:
  - Lupus vulgaris—This is a type of cutaneous involvement with *Mycobacterium tuberculosis*.
  - Syringoma—These are small firm benign adnexal tumors usually appearing around the upper cheeks and lower eyelids.
  - Xanthelasma—These are the most common type of xanthomas. They are benign yellow macules, papules, or plaques often appearing on the eyelids. Approximately half of patients with xanthelasma have a lipid disorder (see Chapter 232, Hyperlipidemia and Xanthomas).
  - Lichen planus—This is a very pruritic skin eruption with pink to violaceous papules and plaques. It may present in different body locations, but the most common areas are the wrists and ankles (see Chapter 160, Lichen Planus).
  - Granulomatous rosacea—This is a variant of rosacea made of uniform papules involving the face.
  - Acne keloidalis nuchae—This is commonly seen in dark-skinned patients. It presents with multiple perifollicular papules and nodules. The most common location is the back of the neck at the hairline (see Chapter 120, Pseudofolliculitis and Acne Keloidalis Nuchae).
  - Pseudofolliculitis barbae—This is most commonly seen in patients with darker skin color, triggered by ingrown hair involving the beard area (see Chapter 120, Pseudofolliculitis and Acne Keloidalis Nuchae).
- Annular or circinate type of sarcoidosis (**Figure 184-11**):
- Granuloma annulare—Annular type (previously described above; see Chapter 182, Granuloma Annulare).
- Annular form of necrobiosis lipoidica—A granulomatous disease with areas of necrobiosis. This is usually seen on the pretibial areas of patients with diabetes. But not all patients have diabetes (see Chapter 231, Necrobiosis Lipoidica).
- These two entities may be differentiated histologically.
- Nodular cutaneous and subcutaneous type:
  - Morphea—Also known as localized scleroderma caused by excessive collagen deposition in the dermis or subcutaneous tissue leading to the formation of nodules (see Chapter 190, Scleroderma and Morphea).
  - Epidermal inclusion cyst—This is an encapsulated keratin-filled nodule of different sizes often found in the subcutaneous tissue. A central pore or punctum is often noted on examination of the overlying epidermis.
  - Lipoma—These are soft nodules of different sizes composed of mature fat cells and often found in the subcutaneous tissue.
  - Metastatic carcinoma—These nodular lesions often present in the context of a diagnosed primary carcinoma of other internal organs.
  - Foreign-body granuloma—This is usually localized to the area of introduction of the foreign body into the skin.

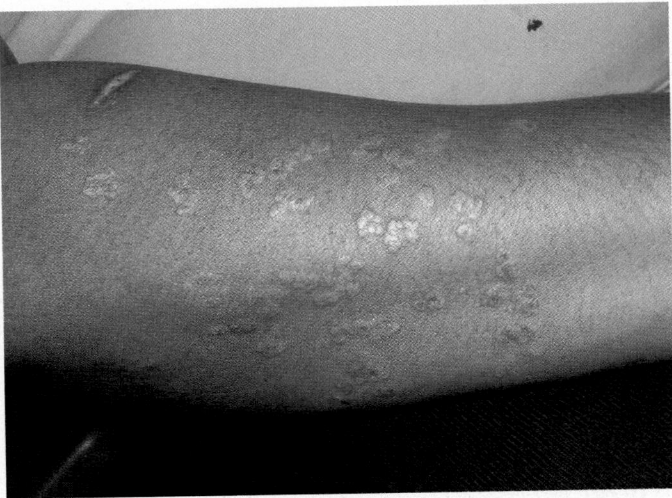

FIGURE 184-10 Granulomatous plaques of biopsy-proven sarcoidosis on the arm of a woman. She also has sarcoidosis of the lung. *(Reproduced with permission from Richard P. Usatine, MD.)*

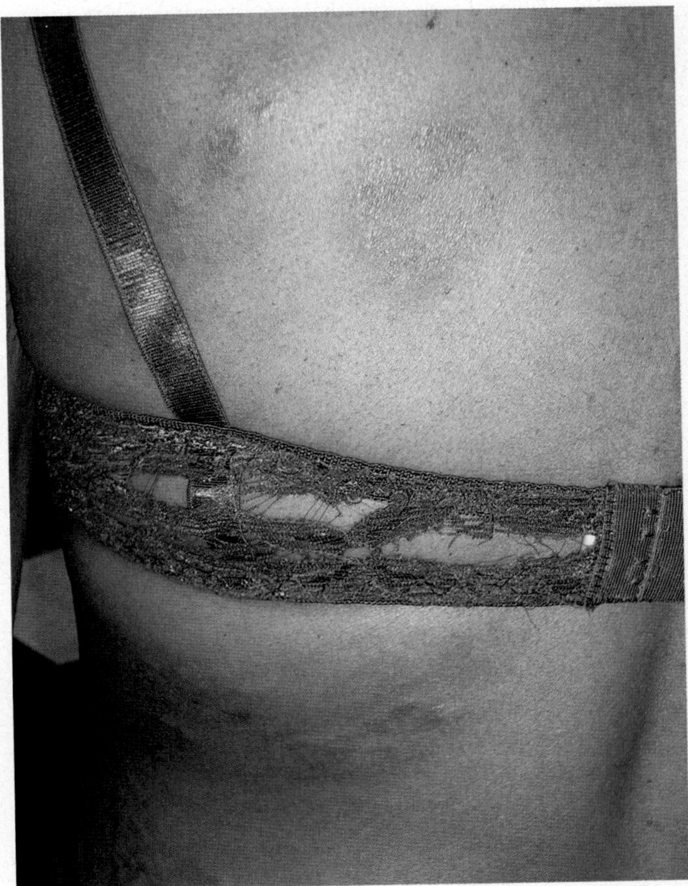

FIGURE 184-11 Violaceous sarcoidal papules coalescing into annular plaques on the back. *(Reproduced with permission from Richard P. Usatine, MD.)*

MANAGEMENT

FIRST LINE

- Cutaneous involvement of sarcoidosis is not life-threatening, so the major rationale for treatment is to prevent or minimize disfigurement. Cosmetic issues are particularly important on the face (**Figure 184-12A**). Also, the lesions can be painful.
- Corticosteroids are the mainstay of treatment.[3,5-10] SOR Ⓑ
- Limited cutaneous disease responds to very high-potency topical corticosteroids, or intralesional triamcinolone (repeated monthly as needed).[5,9] SOR Ⓑ

SECOND LINE

- Photochemotherapy (psoralen UVA) is successful in erythrodermic and hypopigmented lesions. SOR Ⓒ
- Patients with lupus pernio may benefit from pulsed-dye or carbon dioxide laser treatments. SOR Ⓒ
- Resistant lesions to topical therapy or large and diffuse lesions require prednisone.[7,8,10] SOR Ⓑ
- To prevent complications from long-term treatment by steroids, hydroxychloroquine or chloroquine can be used as a steroid-sparing agent.[10] SOR Ⓒ
- Other combinations that have been successful in chronic cutaneous disease and lung disease are methotrexate or azathioprine with low-dose prednisone.[10] SOR Ⓒ

THIRD LINE

- Agents such as cyclophosphamide and cyclosporin are also used, but with caution because of severe drug toxicity.[11] SOR Ⓒ
- Tumor necrosis factor (TNF)-α monoclonal antibody therapy has shown a response rate of up to 79% after 1 year of therapy for patients with cutaneous sarcoidosis (**Figure 184-13**).[12] SOR Ⓒ
- In addition, evidence has shown that infliximab is efficacious for sarcoidosis with pulmonary,[13] neurologic, hepatic, muscular, ocular, and cardiac involvement as well.[14]
- Adalimumab is another TNF-α monoclonal antibody agent that has shown efficacy especially in manifestations of sarcoidosis of the eye. In addition, this agent has shown efficacy for lung, skin, and bone involvement of the disease.[14]
- Both infliximab and adalimumab are considered third-line agents (after steroids and disease-modifying antisarcoid drugs such as methotrexate) for refractory cases of sarcoidosis. However, before starting any of these biologic agents, any infections including latent tuberculosis must be ruled out for fear of reactivation.[14]
- Etanercept, another anti-TNF-α biologic agent, is not useful for sarcoidosis given its history of treatment failure in several studies.[14]

REFERRAL

- A multidisciplinary approach is imperative in patients with systemic sarcoidosis.
- Patients with eye symptoms should be referred to an ophthalmologist (**Figure 184-12B**).

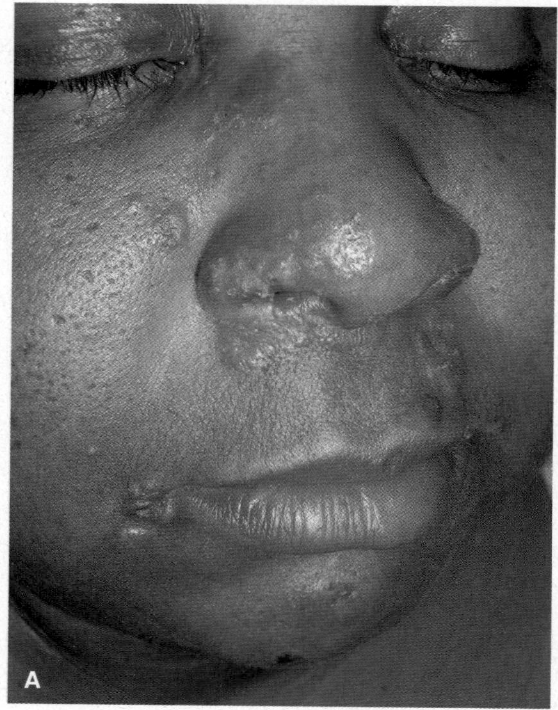

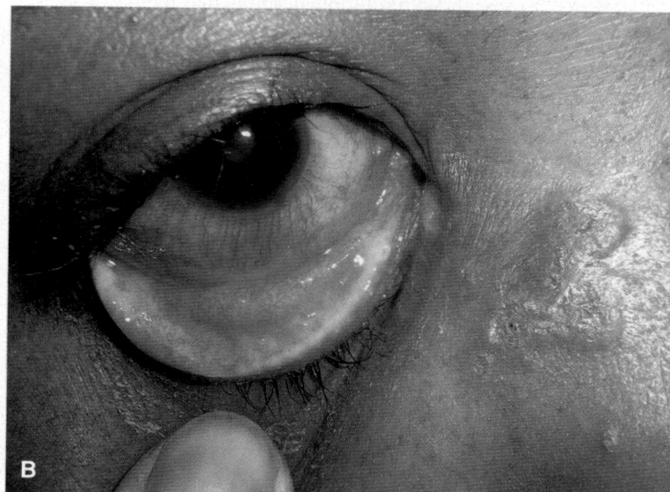

FIGURE 184-12 **A.** Sarcoidosis flare in a 50-year-old woman involving the face (lupus pernio), especially around the nose. **B.** She also has sarcoidosis of the eye with involvement of the conjunctiva and infiltration of the inner lower eyelid. (*Reproduced with permission from Richard P. Usatine, MD.*)

- Patients with lung involvement should be referred to a pulmonologist.
- Patients with possible cardiac involvement (a positive history of cardiac symptoms, abnormal ECG or echocardiogram) should be referred to a cardiologist.[1]
- Patients with lupus pernio should be referred to ENT for potential airway involvement.
- Results from laboratory work-up may help direct appropriate referral.

PREVENTION AND SCREENING

There are currently no preventative measures established, as the cause remains to be elucidated. Patients presenting with cutaneous sarcoidosis should be screened as clinically indicated depending on concomitant signs and symptoms. Patients placed on long-term oral steroids should be treated appropriately to prevent osteoporosis.

PROGNOSIS

- Patients of African descent tend to have more severe lung disease compared to Caucasian patients at presentation and an overall poorer long-term prognosis.[15]
- The presence of EN has been associated with a decreased frequency of respiratory involvement.[15] In addition, EN is associated with an acute course with better prognosis.[3]
- Lupus pernio, more commonly seen in patients of African descent, indicates a chronic disease course with upper respiratory or nasal mucosa involvement (**Figures 184-12** and **184-13**).[3,15]
- The prognostic value of cutaneous lesions alone remains unclear.[15]

FOLLOW-UP

Patients with cutaneous sarcoidosis should be monitored for possible systemic involvement. Regular follow-up is necessary, especially if biologic medications are used.

PATIENT EDUCATION

Inform patients about the risk that systemic sarcoidosis can occur even if the skin is the only area currently involved.

PATIENT RESOURCES

- National Heart, Lung, and Blood Institute. *What Is Sarcoidosis?*—**http://www.nhlbi.nih.gov/health-topics/sarcoidosis.**

PROVIDER RESOURCES

- Medscape. *Dermatologic Manifestations of Sarcoidosis*—**https://emedicine.medscape.com/article/1123970-overview**

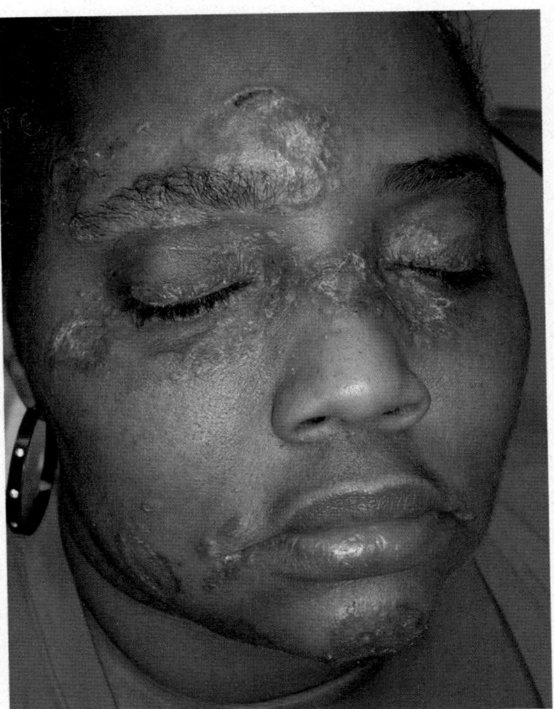

FIGURE 184-13 A 47-year-old African-American woman with widespread cutaneous sarcoidosis on face (lupus pernio), trunk, and extremities. She also has pulmonary involvement. Her sarcoidosis has improved since starting infliximab by IV infusion. (*Reproduced with permission from Richard P. Usatine, MD.*)

REFERENCES

1. Kron J, Ellenbogen KA. Cardiac sarcoidosis: contemporary review. *J Cardiovasc Electrophysiol.* 2015;26:104-109.
2. Yanardag H, Tetikkurt C, Bilir M, et al. Diagnosis of cutaneous sarcoidosis; clinical and the prognostic significance of skin lesions. *Multidiscip Respir Med.* 2013;8:26.
3. Wanat KA, Rosenbach M. A practical approach to cutaneous sarcoidosis. *Am J Clin Dermatol.* 2014;15:283-297.
4. Ungprasert P, Crowson CS, Matteson EL. Smoking, obesity and risk of sarcoidosis: a population-based nested case-control study. *Respir Med.* 2016;120:87-90.
5. Yeager H, Sina B, Khachemoune A. Dermatologic disease. In: Baughman RP, ed. *Sarcoidosis.* New York, NY: Taylor & Francis; 2006:593-604.
6. Grutters JC, van den Bosch JM. Corticosteroid treatment in sarcoidosis. *Eur Respir J.* 2006;28(3):627-636.
7. Haimovic A, Sanchez M, Judson MA, Prystowsky S. Sarcoidosis: a comprehensive review and update for the dermatologist: part II. Extracutaneous disease. *J Am Acad Dermatol.* 2012;66:719 e1-10; quiz 29-30.
8. Haimovic A, Sanchez M, Judson MA, Prystowsky S. Sarcoidosis: a comprehensive review and update for the dermatologist: part I. Cutaneous disease. *J Am Acad Dermatol.* 2012;66:699 e1-18; quiz 717-718.
9. Khatri KA, Chotzen VA, Burrall BA. Lupus pernio: successful treatment with a potent topical corticosteroid. *Arch Dermatol.* 1995;131(5):617-618.
10. Mosam A, Morar N. Recalcitrant cutaneous sarcoidosis: an evidence-based sequential approach. *J Dermatolog Treat.* 2004; 15(6):353-359.
11. Kouba DJ, Mimouni D, Rencic A, Nousari HC. Mycophenolate mofetil may serve as a steroid-sparing agent for sarcoidosis. *Br J Dermatol.* 2003;148(1):147-148.
12. Heidelberger V, Ingen-Housz-Oro S, Marquet A, et al. Efficacy and tolerance of anti–tumor necrosis factor α agents in cutaneous sarcoidosis: a French study of 46 cases. *JAMA Dermatol.* 2017; 153(7):681-685.
13. Baughman RP. Infliximab for refractory sarcoidosis. *Sarcoidosis Vasc Diffuse Lung Dis.* 2001;18(1):70-74; erratum in: *Sarcoidosis Vasc Diffuse Lung Dis.* 2001;18(3):310.
14. Drent M, Cremers JP, Jansen TL , Baughman RP. Practical eminence and experience-based recommendations for use of TNF-alpha inhibitors in sarcoidosis. *Sarcoidosis Vasc Diffuse Lung Dis.* 2014;31:91-107.
15. Heath CR, David J, Taylor SC. Sarcoidosis: are there differences in your skin of color patients? *J Am Acad Dermatol.* 2012;66(1):121. e1-e14.

SECTION O HYPERSENSITIVITY SYNDROMES

185 ERYTHEMA MULTIFORME, STEVENS-JOHNSON SYNDROME, AND TOXIC EPIDERMAL NECROLYSIS

Carolyn Milana, MD
Mindy A. Smith, MD, MS

PATIENT STORY

A 14-year-old boy presents to the emergency department with a 1-day history of fever associated with lip swelling and peeling **(Figure 185-1A)**. Within 48 hours he developed involvement of his ocular **(Figure 185-1B)** and urethral mucosa along with an erythematous papular rash on his trunk that spread to his extremities. In **Figure 185-1C**, target lesions can be seen on his back. He was diagnosed with Stevens-Johnson syndrome and admitted to the hospital.

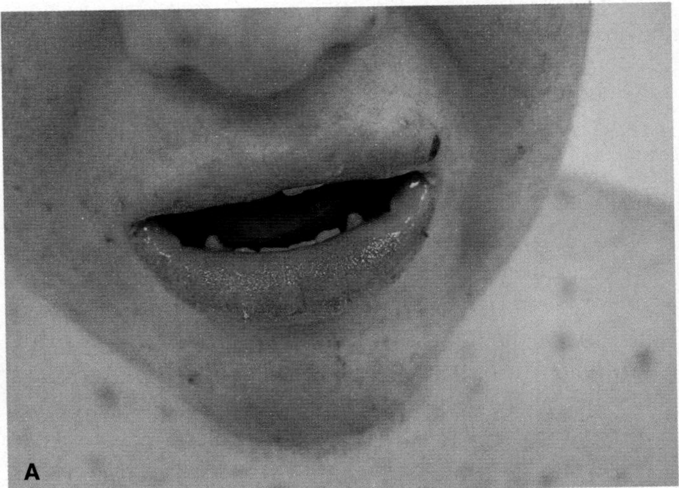

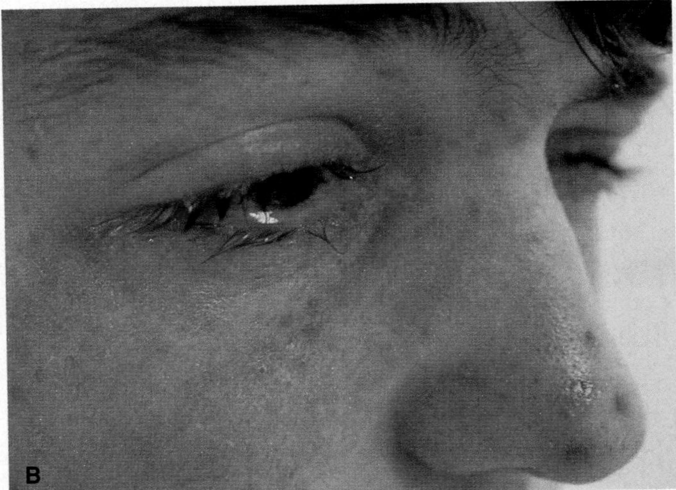

FIGURE 185-1 Stevens-Johnson syndrome in a 14-year-old boy who received penicillin for pneumonia. **A.** Lips and mouth are involved. **B.** Eye involvement. (*continued*)

INTRODUCTION

Erythema multiforme (EM), Stevens-Johnson syndrome (SJS), and toxic epidermal necrolysis (TEN) are skin disorders thought to be types of hypersensitivity reactions (undesirable reactions produced by a normal immune system in a presensitized host) that occur in response to medication, infection, or illness. Both SJS and TEN are severe cutaneous reactions thought to describe the same disorder, differing only in severity (TEN more severe); however, there is debate as to whether these three fall into a spectrum of disease that includes EM.

SYNONYMS

- EM has also been called EM minor.
- SJS has been called EM major in the past but is now thought to be a distinct entity different from all types of EM.
- TEN is also known as Lyell syndrome.

EPIDEMIOLOGY

- The incidence of EM has been estimated to range from 1 in 1000 persons to 1 in 10,000 persons.[1] The true incidence is unknown.[1]
- SJS and TEN are rare severe cutaneous reactions often caused by drugs. Reports of incidence vary from 1.2 to 6 per 1 million for SJS and from 0.4 to 1.2 per 1 million for TEN.[2-4]

- EM is rare in children under age 3 years and adults over age 50 years: 20% of cases occur in children and adolescents.[5]
- With respect to EM, males are affected more often than females (3:2 to 2:1).[5]

ETIOLOGY AND PATHOPHYSIOLOGY

Numerous factors have been identified as causative agents for EM:

- Herpes simplex virus (HSV) I and HSV II are the most common causative agents, having been implicated in at least 60% of cases (**Figure 185-2**).[6,7] The virus has been found in circulating blood,[8] as well as on skin biopsy of patients with EM minor.[6]
- Bacterial causes are numerous and include cat-scratch disease, chlamydial infections, hemolytic streptococci, legionellosis, *Neisseria meningitidis, Mycoplasma pneumoniae,* pneumococci, and rickettsial infections.[5]
- Other causes include foods and food preservatives, immunologic disorders, mechanical factors (e.g., tattooing), and malignancy.[5] Some cases are thought to be related to medications (e.g., sulfa drugs), although no test reliably proves the link to a specific drug, and half of EM cases are considered idiopathic.[5]

For SJS and TEN, most cases are drug induced.

- Drugs most commonly known to cause SJS and TEN are sulfonamide antibiotics, allopurinol, NSAIDs, amine antiepileptic drugs (phenytoin and carbamazepine), and lamotrigine.[9]
- *Mycoplasma pneumoniae* has been identified as the most common infectious cause for SJS[7]; in 2013, an outbreak of 8 pediatric cases of SJS was reported at Children's Hospital Colorado associated with *M. pneumoniae* infection.[10] Clinical presentation of cases of SJS following mycoplasma infection were different from non-associated SJS cases in having less extensive skin disease, an elevated erythrocyte sedimentation rate, and preceding respiratory symptoms.

Other less-common causative agents for EM, SJS, and TEN include:

- Infectious agents such as *Mycobacterium tuberculosis*, group A streptococci, hepatitis B, Epstein-Barr virus, *Francisella tularensis, Yersinia*, enteroviruses, *Histoplasma*, and *Coccidioides*.[1]
- Neoplastic processes, such as leukemia and lymphoma.[1]
- Antibiotics, such as penicillin, isoniazid, tetracyclines, cephalosporins, and quinolones.
- Anticonvulsants, such as phenobarbital and valproic acid.[1,7]
- Other drugs including captopril, etoposide, aspirin, and allopurinol.
- Immunizations such as bacillus Calmette-Guérin, diphtheria-tetanus toxoid, hepatitis B, measles-mumps-rubella, and poliomyelitis.[6]
- Other agents or triggers including radiation therapy, sunlight, pregnancy, connective tissue disease, and menstruation.[1]

Although the pathogenesis of EM, SJS, and TEN remains unknown, recent studies show that it may be as a result of a host-specific cell-mediated immune response to an antigenic stimulus that activates cytotoxic T cells and results in damage to keratinocytes.[6,9]

- The epidermal detachment (skin peeling) seen in SJS and TEN appears to result from epidermal necrosis in the absence of substantial dermal inflammation.

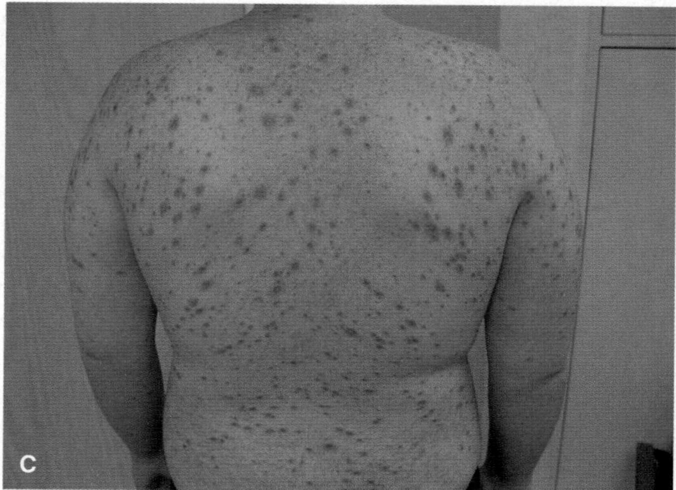

FIGURE 185-1 (*Continued*) **C.** Target lesions on his back. (*Reproduced with permission from Dan Stulberg, MD.*)

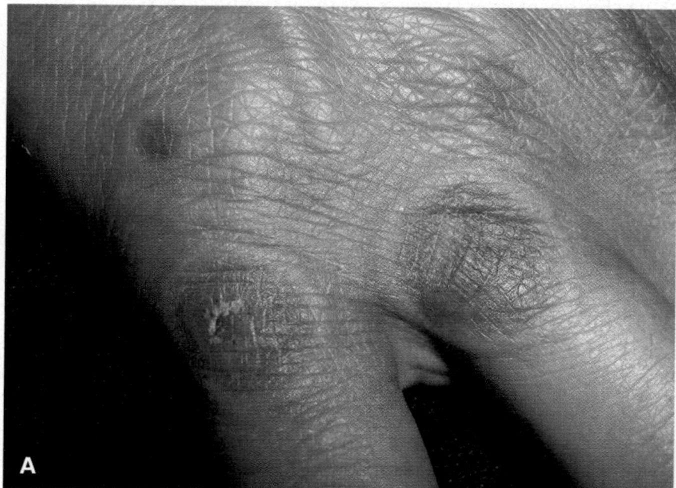

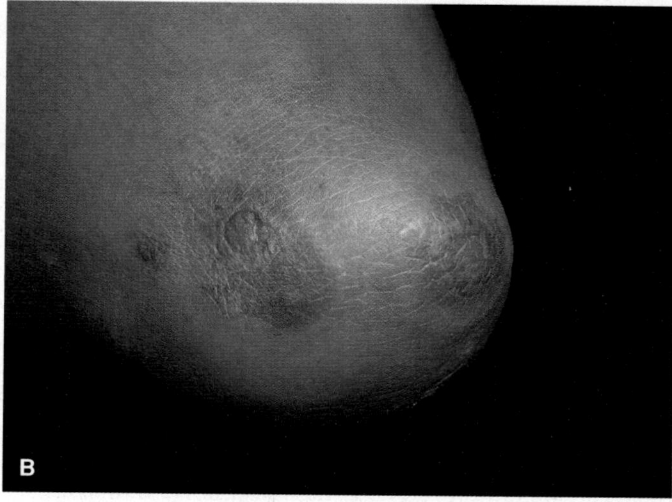

FIGURE 185-2 Erythema multiforme in a 43-year-old woman that recurs every time she breaks out with genital herpes. **A.** Target lesions on hand. **B.** Target lesions on elbow. (*Reproduced with permission from Richard P. Usatine, MD.*)

RISK FACTORS

- Recent evidence shows individuals with certain human leukocyte antigen (HLA) alleles may be predisposed to developing SJS/TEN, and to SJS-associated ocular involvement, when taking certain drugs.[2,11] In addition, IKZF1 has been identified as a susceptibility gene for cold medicine–induced SJS/TEN with severe mucosal involvement in Japanese, Korean, and Indian subjects.[12]
- Certain diseases such as HIV/AIDS (**Figure 185-3**), malignancy, or autoimmune disease, also predispose individuals to SJS/TEN.[2,13]

DIAGNOSIS

CLINICAL FEATURES

In these conditions, there is a rapid onset of skin lesions. EM is a disease in which patients present with the following lesions:

- Classic lesions begin as red macules and expand centrifugally to become target-like papules or plaques with an erythematous outer border and central clearing (iris or bull's-eye lesions) (**Figures 185-4** to **185-7**). Target lesions, although characteristic, are not necessary to make the diagnosis. The center of the lesions should have some epidermal disruption, such as vesicles or erosions.
- Lesions can coalesce and form larger lesions up to 2 cm in diameter with centers that can become dusky purple or necrotic.
- Unlike urticarial lesions, the lesions of EM do not appear and fade; once they appear they remain fixed in place until healing occurs many days to weeks later.
- Patients are usually asymptomatic, although a burning sensation or pruritus may be present.
- Lesions typically resolve without any permanent sequelae within 2 weeks.
- Recurrent outbreaks are often associated with HSV infection (see **Figure 185-2**).[6,7]

In both SJS and TEN, patients may have blisters that develop on dusky or purpuric macules. SJS is diagnosed when less than 10% of the body surface area is involved, SJS/TEN overlap when 10% to 30% is involved, and TEN when greater than 30% is involved.

- Lesions may become more widespread and rapidly progress to form areas of central necrosis, bullae, and areas of denudation (see **Figure 185-1**).
- Fever higher than 39°C (102.2°F) is often present.
- In addition to skin involvement, there is involvement of at least 2 mucosal surfaces, such as the eyes, oral cavity, upper airway, esophagus, GI tract, or the anogenital mucosa (see **Figures 185-1** and **185-3**).
- New lesions occur in crops and may take 4 to 6 weeks to heal.
- Large areas of epidermal detachment occur (**Figures 185-8** to **185-10**).
- Severe pain can occur from mucosal ulcerations, but skin tenderness is minimal.
- Skin erosions lead to increased insensible blood and fluid losses, as well as an increased risk of bacterial superinfection and sepsis.
- These patients are at high risk for ocular complications (e.g., conjunctivitis, lid-margin and conjunctival ulceration, corneal opacification) that may lead to blindness. Additional risks include bronchitis, pneumonitis, myocarditis, hepatitis, enterocolitis, polyarthritis, hematuria, and acute tubular necrosis.

TYPICAL DISTRIBUTION

- The distribution of the rash in EM can be widespread.
- The distal extremities, including the palms and soles, are most commonly involved.
- Extensor surfaces are favored.
- Oral lesions may be present, especially in SJS (see **Figures 185-1** and **185-3**).
- Severe lesions with exfoliation and extensive mucosal lesions occur in SJS and TEN (see **Figures 185-8** to **185-10**).

LABORATORY AND IMAGING

- There are no consistent laboratory findings with these conditions. The diagnosis is usually made based on clinical findings.
- Routine blood work may show leukocytosis, elevated liver transaminases, and an elevated erythrocyte sedimentation rate.
- In TEN, leukopenia may occur.

BIOPSY

- A cutaneous punch biopsy can be performed to confirm the diagnosis or to rule out other diseases.
- Histologic findings of EM will show a lymphocytic infiltrate at the dermal–epidermal junction. There is a characteristic vacuolization of the epidermal cells and necrotic keratinocytes within the epidermis.[1]

DIFFERENTIAL DIAGNOSIS

- Bullous pemphigoid—Can be either subacute or acute with tense widespread blisters that can occur after persistent urticaria; mucosal involvement is rare. Significant pruritus can be present. As with EM, SJS, and TEN, bullous pemphigoid can occur after certain exposures such as UV radiation or certain drugs (Chapter 192, Bullous Pemphigoid).
- Urticaria—A skin reaction characterized by red wheals that are usually pruritic. Unlike EM, individual lesions rarely last more than 24 hours (Chapter 156, Urticaria and Angioedema).
- Kawasaki disease—Fever persists at least 5 days and there must be at least four of the five following features to diagnose complete (or classic) Kawasaki disease.[14]
    - Changes in extremities—*Acute:* erythema and edema of the hands and feet; or *subacute:* periungual desquamation (peeling of fingers and toes).
    - Rash: maculopapular, diffuse erythroderma, or erythema multiforme–like.
    - Bilateral bulbar conjunctival injection without exudate.
    - Changes in lips and oral cavity—Erythema, lips cracking, strawberry tongue (see Chapter 36, Scarlet Fever and Strawberry Tongue), and/or erythema of the oral and pharyngeal mucosae.
    - Cervical lymphadenopathy (>1.5 cm diameter), usually unilateral.

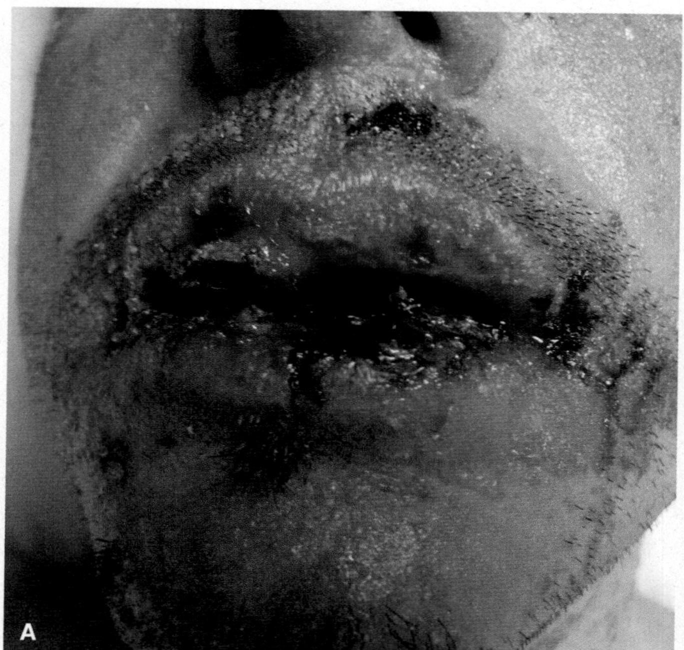

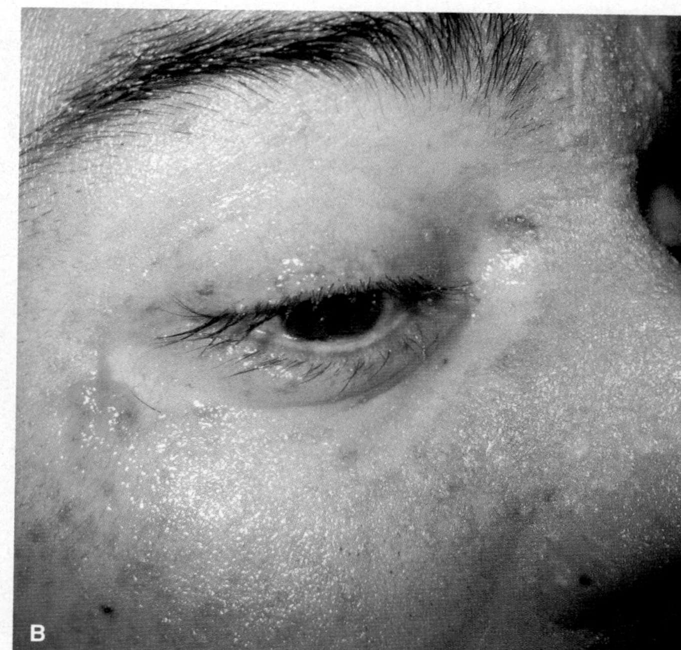

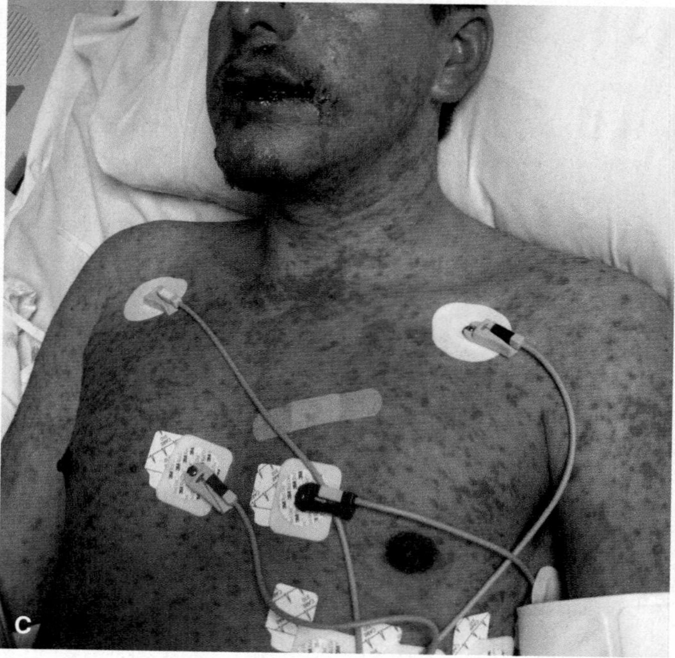

FIGURE 185-3 Stevens-Johnson syndrome that evolved into toxic epidermal necrolysis in a human immunodeficiency virus–positive man with a CD4 of 6. He presented to the emergency department with fever and rash on face, eyes, and mouth. Chest X-ray suggested pneumonia, so he was started on azithromycin, ceftriaxone, and trimethoprim-sulfamethoxazole. He developed bullae on skin, and a skin biopsy confirmed toxic epidermal necrolysis, possibly secondary to one of the antibiotics. He was transferred to a burn unit and given intravenous gamma-globulin 1 g/kg for 3 days. The patient survived. **A.** Oral lesions. **B.** Eye and facial involvement. **C.** Trunk and upper extremities involved so that greater than 30% of the skin was affected. (*Reproduced with permission from Robert T. Gilson, MD.*)

- Cutaneous vasculitis—Also caused by a hypersensitivity reaction, lesions are palpable papules or purpura. Blisters, hives, and necrotic ulcers can occur on the skin. Lesions are usually located on the legs, trunk, and buttocks (see Chapter 187, Vasculitis).
- Erythema annulare centrifugum—A hypersensitivity reaction caused by a variety of agents. Lesions look similar with erythematous papules of a few to several centimeters that enlarge and clear centrally and may be vesicular. Lesions tend to appear on the legs and thighs, but may occur on upper extremities, trunk, and face; palms and soles are spared (see Chapter 215, Erythema Annulare Centrifugum).
- Staphylococcal scalded skin syndrome—Rash may also follow a prodrome of malaise and fever but is macular, brightly erythematous, and initially involves the face, neck, axilla, and groin. Skin is markedly tender. Like SJS and TEN, large areas of the epidermis peel away. Unlike TEN, the site of the staphylococcal infection is usually extracutaneous (e.g., otitis media, pharyngitis) and not the skin lesions themselves (Chapter 122, Impetigo).

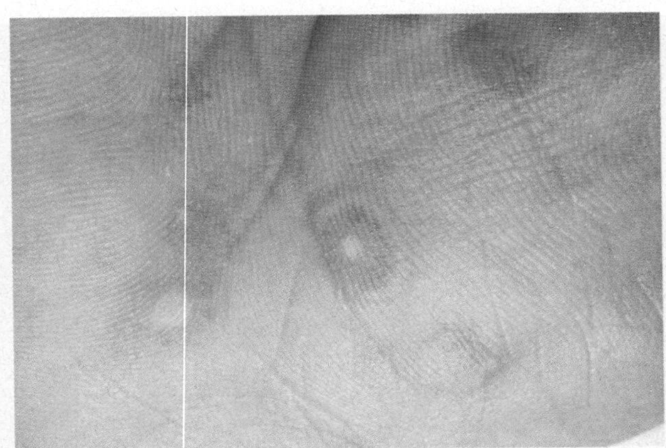

FIGURE 185-4 Erythema multiforme on the palm with target lesions that have a dusky red and white center. (*Reproduced with permission from Richard P. Usatine, MD.*)

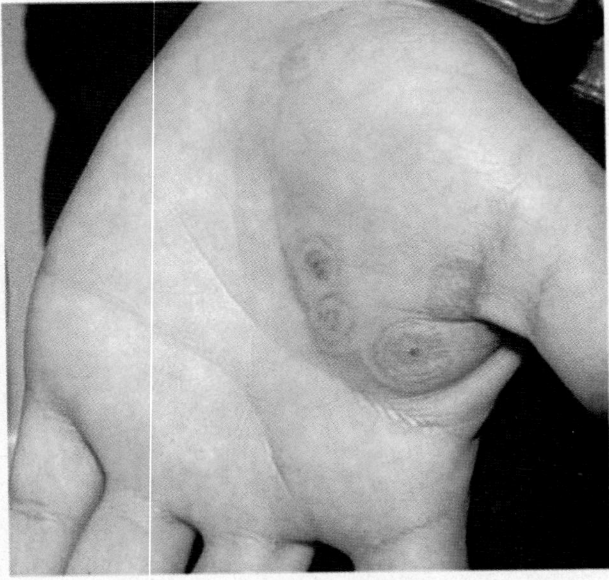

FIGURE 185-5 Erythema multiforme with target lesions on the palms secondary to an outbreak of oral herpes. (*Reproduced with permission from Richard P. Usatine, MD.*)

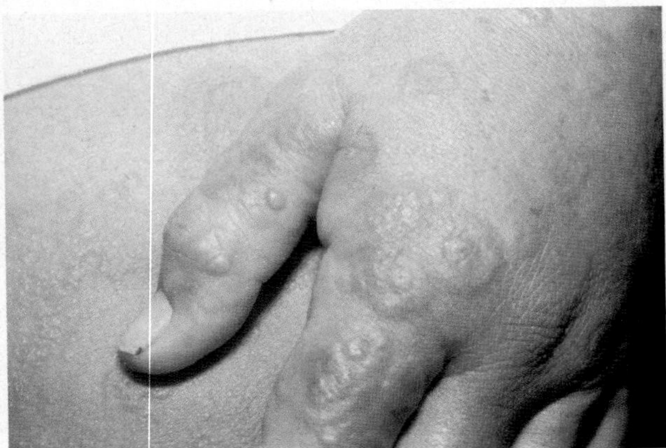

FIGURE 185-6 Erythema multiforme with vesicles and blistering of the target lesions on the hand. (*Reproduced with permission from Richard P. Usatine, MD.*)

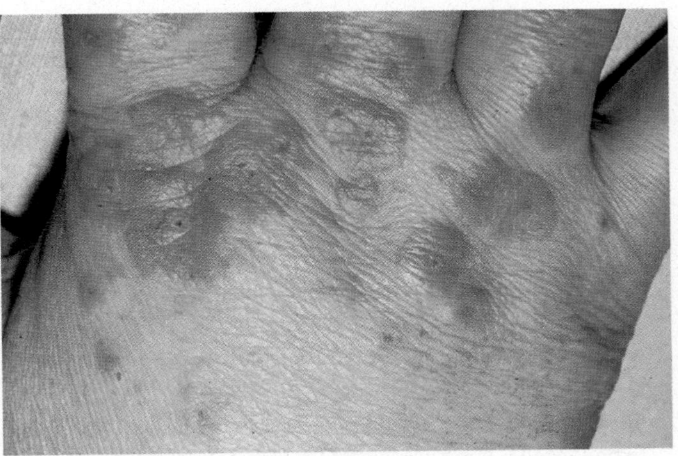

FIGURE 185-7 Erythema multiforme on the dorsum of the hand showing targets with small, eroded centers. There should be some epidermal erosion to diagnose erythema multiforme. (*Reproduced with permission from Richard P. Usatine, MD.*)

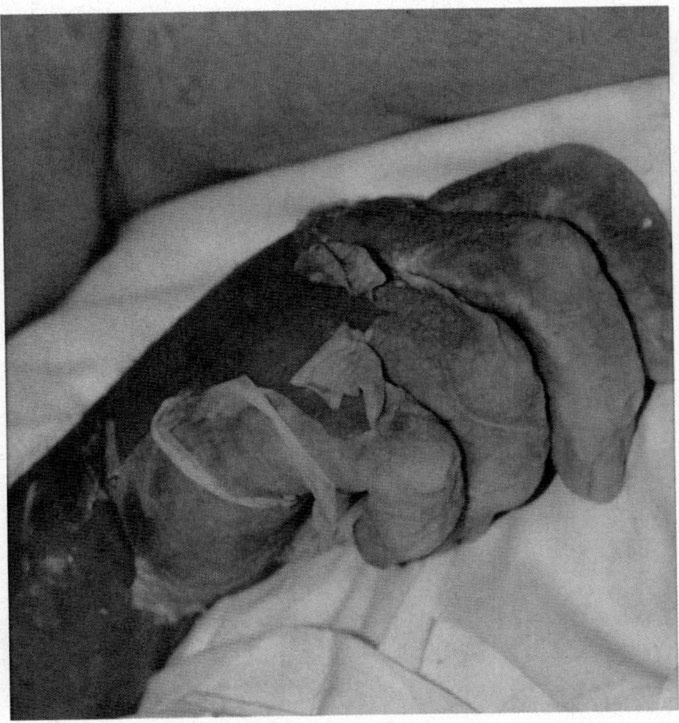

FIGURE 185-8 Toxic epidermal necrolysis with desquamation of skin on the hand. (*Reproduced with permission from Richard P. Usatine, MD.*)

MANAGEMENT

FIRST LINE

EM:

- Treat the infectious cause if known (e.g., herpes or mycoplasma).
- Withdraw the suspected drug (new medication within 2 months of onset).[5]
- Treatment is mainly supportive. Symptomatic relief may be provided with topical emollients and eye lubricants, mouthwashes (e.g., xylocaine), systemic oral antihistamines, and acetaminophen. These do not, however, alter the course of the illness.
- The use of corticosteroids has not been well studied but is thought to prolong the course or increase the frequency of recurrences in HSV-associated cases.[7]
- Prophylactic acyclovir has been used to control recurrent HSV-associated EM with some success.[7]

SJS and TEN:

- Treatment is mainly supportive and may require intensive care or placement in a burn unit. Early diagnosis is imperative so that triggering agents can be discontinued.
- Oral lesions can be managed with mouthwashes and glycerin swabs.
- Skin lesions should be cleansed with saline or Burow solution (aluminum acetate in water).
- IV fluids should be given to replace insensible losses.
- Daily examinations for secondary infections should occur, and systemic antibiotics should be started as needed.
- Consultation with an ophthalmologist is important because of the high risk of ocular sequelae.
- Pharmacologic therapy is widely debated in the literature. Intravenous immunoglobulin (IVIG) at doses of 2 to 3 g/kg may help shorten the course and improve outcome if started early during the disease.[15]
- Systemic corticosteroids have been the mainstay of treatment for SJS/TEN. Authors of a meta-analysis found that glucocorticosteroids and cyclosporine were the most promising therapies, although steroids were of statistically significant survival benefit in only one analysis, and cyclosporine was of significant benefit only in a feasible analysis of individual patient data.[16] In this review, IVIGs were not found to be helpful.

SECOND LINE

SJS and TEN:

- Agents that have been tried with limited success include thalidomide, tumor necrosis factor α inhibitors, cyclophosphamide, granulocyte colony-stimulating factors, and plasmapheresis.[16]
- A tear-exchangeable limbal contact lens was found to improve vision and quality of life in patients with ocular sequelae.[17]

PREVENTION

Screening populations known to carry HLA alleles prior to starting medications with higher risks for SJS/TEN has been suggested by some researchers[2] but, in one study, was not found to be cost effective.[18]

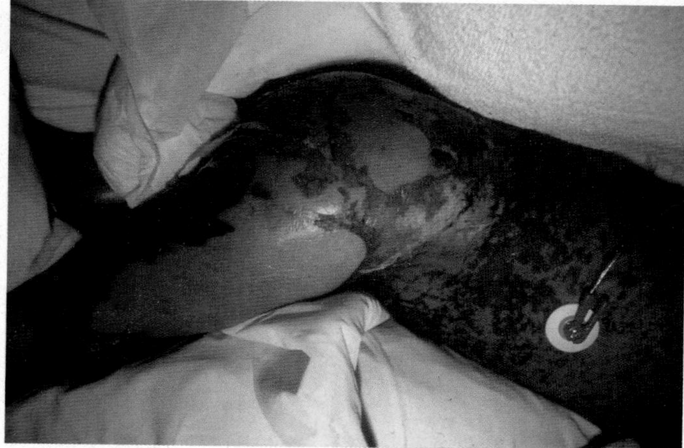

FIGURE 185-9 Toxic epidermal necrolysis with large areas of desquamation on the leg. (*Reproduced with permission from Richard P. Usatine, MD.*)

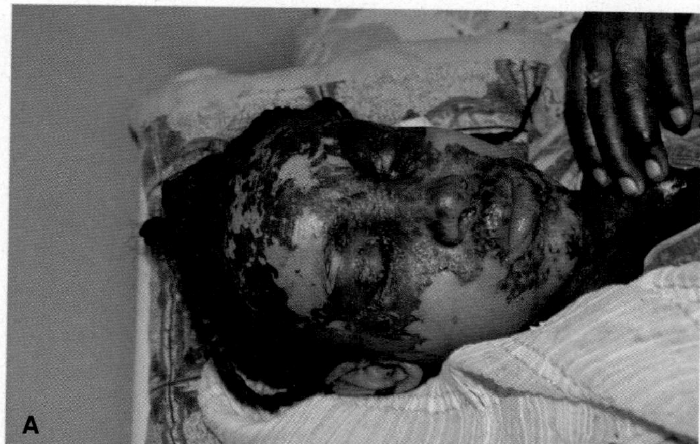

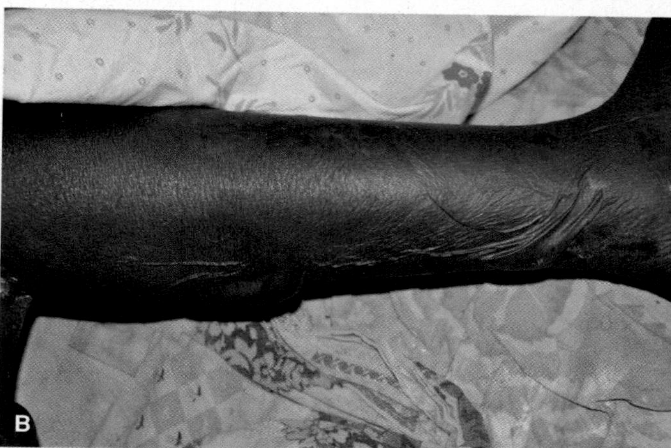

FIGURE 185-10 Toxic epidermal necrolysis secondary to amoxicillin. **A.** Face with large areas of desquamation and loss of pigmentation. **B.** Skin detaching from leg in large sheets and bullae. (*Reproduced with permission from Richard P. Usatine, MD.*)

PROGNOSIS

- EM usually resolves spontaneously within 1 to 2 weeks.
- Recurrence of EM is common, especially when preceded by HSV infection.
- Prognosis is poorer for patients with SJS and TEN, especially if they are older, have a large percentage of body surface area involved, or have intestinal or pulmonary involvement.
- About one quarter of patients with TEN require ventilator assistance; in one study, the need for a ventilator was associated with a higher percentage of epidermal-detached body surface area (especially greater than 30%), serum bicarbonates less than 20 mmol/L, serum urea greater than 10 mmol/L, WBCs more than 12,000/mm^3, and hemoglobin less than 8 g/dL, in addition to more extensive pulmonary infiltrates.[19]
- Mortality for SJS/TEN can be predicted based on the severity of illness score for TEN (SCORTEN).[20] One point is given for each of the following: serum blood urea nitrogen greater than 10 mmol/L; serum bicarbonate less than 20 mmol/L; serum glucose greater than 14 mmol/L; age older than 40 years; malignancy present; heart rate greater than 120 beats per minute; percentage of body surface area involved greater than 10%. Scores of 0 to 1 are associated with a mortality rate of 3.2%, whereas scores of 5 or higher are associated with a mortality rate of 90%.
- For patients with SJS, mortality rates have been reported of 5% to 10% and up to 30% for TEN.[9,21]

FOLLOW-UP

- For uncomplicated cases, no specific follow-up is needed.
- For patients with EM major and any of the complications listed above, follow-up should be arranged with the appropriate specialist.

PATIENT EDUCATION

- If an offending drug is found to be the cause, it should be discontinued immediately.
- Patients with HSV-associated EM should be made aware of the risk of recurrence.

PATIENT RESOURCES

- *Erythema Multiforme*—**https://medlineplus.gov/ency/article/000851.htm.**

PROVIDER RESOURCES

- Medscape. *Erythema Multiforme*—**http://emedicine.medscape.com/article/1122915.**
- Medscape. *Stevens-Johnson Syndrome*—**http://emedicine.medscape.com/article/1197450.**

REFERENCES

1. Shaw JC. Erythema multiforme. In: Noble J, Green H, Levinson W, et al, eds. *Textbook of Primary Care Medicine*, 3rd ed. St. Louis, MO: Mosby; 2001:815-816.
2. Tan SK, Tay YK. Profile and pattern of Stevens-Johnson syndrome and toxic epidermal necrolysis in a general hospital in Singapore: treatment outcomes. *Acta Derm Venereol.* 2012;92(1):62-66.
3. Finkelstein Y, Soon GS, Acuna P, et al. Recurrence and outcomes of Stevens-Johnson syndrome and toxic epidermal necrolysis in children. *Pediatrics.* 2011;128(4):723-728.
4. Del Pozzo-Magana BR, Lazo-Langner A, Carleton B. A systematic review of treatment of drug-induced Stevens-Johnson syndrome and toxic epidermal necrolysis in children. *J Popul Ther Clin Pharmacol.* 2011;18:e121-e133.
5. Plaza JA. *Erythema Multiforme.* Updated May 24, 2016. http://emedicine.medscape.com/article/1122915-overview. Accessed July 2017.
6. Darmstadt GL. Erythema multiforme. In: Long S, Pickering L, Prober C, eds. *Principles and Practice of Pediatric Infectious Diseases*, 2nd ed. New York, NY: Churchill Livingstone; 2003: 442-444.
7. Morelli JG. Vesiculobullous disorders. In: Behrman R, Kliegman RM, Jenson HB, eds. *Nelson Textbook of Pediatrics*, 19th ed. Philadelphia, PA: Saunders; 2011:2241-2249.
8. Weston WL. Herpes associated erythema multiforme. *J Invest Dermatol.* 2005;124(6):xv-xvi.
9. Chosidow OM, Stern RS, Wintroub BU. Cutaneous drug reactions. In: Kasper DL, Fauci AS, Longo DL, et al, eds. *Harrison's Principles of Internal Medicine*, 16th ed. New York, NY: McGraw-Hill; 2005:318-324.
10. Olson D, Watkins LK, Demirjian A, et al. Outbreak of mycoplasma pneumoniae-associated Stevens-Johnson syndrome. *Pediatrics.* 2015;136(2):e386-394.
11. Ueta M. Genetic predisposition to Stevens-Johnson syndrome with severe ocular surface complications. *Cornea.* 2015;34 (Suppl 11):S158-S165.
12. Ueta M, Sawai H, Sotozono C, et al. IKZF1, a new susceptibility gene for cold medicine-related Stevens-Johnson syndrome/toxic epidermal necrolysis with severe mucosal involvement. *J Allergy Clin Immunol.* 2015;135(6):1538-1545.e17.
13. Sanmarkan AD, Tukaram S, Thappa DM, et al. Retrospective analysis of Stevens-Johnson syndrome and toxic epidermal necrolysis over a period of 10 years. *Indian J Dermatol.* 2011;56(1):25-29.
14. McCrindle BW, Rowley AH, Newburger JW, et al. Diagnosis, treatment, and long-term management of Kawasaki disease: a scientific statement for health professionals from the American Heart Association. *Circulation.* 2017;135(17):e927-e999.
15. Worswick S, Cotliar J. Stevens-Johnson syndrome and toxic epidermal necrolysis: a review of treatment options. *Dermatol Ther.* 2011;24(2):207-218.
16. Zimmermann S, Sekula P, Venhoff M, et al. Systemic immunomodulating therapies for Stevens-Johnson syndrome and toxic

epidermal necrolysis: a systematic review and meta-analysis. *JAMA Dermatol.* 2017;153(6):514-522.

17. Sotozono C, Yamauchi N, Maeda S, Kinoshita S. Tear exchangeable limbal rigid contact lens for ocular sequelae resulting from Stevens-Johnson syndrome or toxic epidermal necrolysis. *Am J Ophthalmol.* 2014;158(5):983-993.
18. Chen Z, Liew D, Kwan P. Real-world cost-effectiveness of pharmacogenetic screening for epilepsy treatment. *Neurology.* 2016;86(12):1086-1094.
19. de Prost N, Mekontso-Dessap A, Valeyrie-Allanore L, et al. Acute respiratory failure in patients with toxic epidermal necrolysis: clinical features and factors associated with mechanical ventilation. *Crit Care Med.* 2014;42(1):118-128.
20. Bastuji-Garin S, Fouchard N, Bertocchi M, et al. SCORTEN: a severity of illness score for toxic epidermal necrolysis. *J Invest Dermatol.* 2000;115(2):149-153.
21. The Stevens-Johnson syndrome/toxic epidermal necrolysis spectrum of disease. In: Habif T, ed. *Clinical Dermatology*, 4th ed. Philadelphia, PA: Elsevier; 2004:627-631.

186 ERYTHEMA NODOSUM

E.J. Mayeaux, Jr., MD
Lucia Diaz, MD

PATIENT STORY

A young woman presented to the office with several days of overall malaise, fever, and sore throat. At the time of presentation she noted some painful bumps on her lower legs, and denied trauma (**Figure 186-1**). No history of recent cough or change in bowel habits has been reported. The patient had no chronic medical problems, took no medications, and had no known drug allergies. Her temperature was slightly elevated, but other vitals were normal. On examination, her oropharynx revealed tonsillar erythema and exudates. Bilateral lower extremities were spotted with slightly raised, tender, erythematous nodules that varied in size from 2 to 6 cm. Rapid strep test was positive, and she was diagnosed clinically with erythema nodosum (EN) secondary to group A β-hemolytic *Streptococcus*. She was treated with penicillin and nonsteroidal anti-inflammatory drugs (NSAIDs) and was advised temporary bed rest. She experienced complete resolution of the EN within 4 weeks.

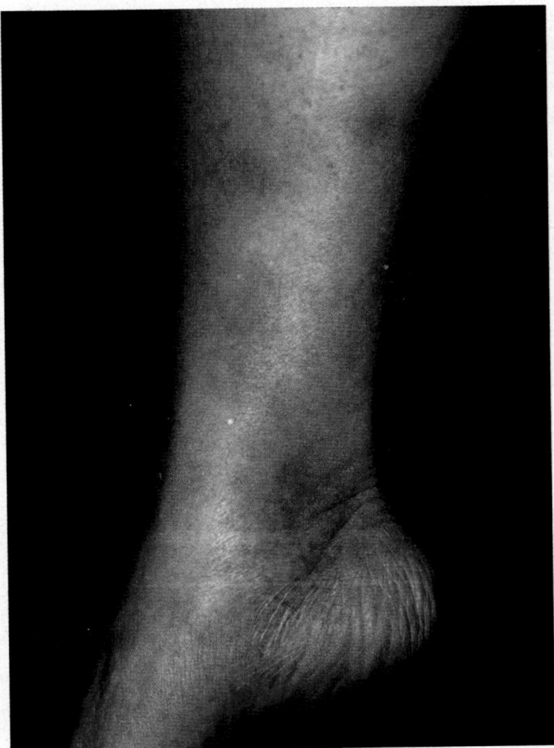

FIGURE 186-1 Erythema nodosum secondary to group A β-hemolytic *Streptococcus* in a young woman. (*Reproduced with permission from Richard P. Usatine, MD.*)

INTRODUCTION

EN is a common inflammatory panniculitis characterized by ill-defined, erythematous patches with underlying tender, subcutaneous nodules. It is a reactive process caused by chronic inflammatory states, infections, medications, malignancies, and unknown factors.

SYNONYMS

Löfgren syndrome (with hilar adenopathy).

EPIDEMIOLOGY

- Erythema nodosum occurs in approximately 1 to 5 per 100,000 persons.[1] It is the most frequent type of septal panniculitis (inflammation of the septa of fat lobules in the subcutaneous tissue).[2]
- EN tends to occur more often in women, with a male-to-female ratio of 1:4.5 in the adult population, generally during the second and fourth decades of life (**Figures 186-1** to **186-3**).[3]
- In 1 study, an overall incidence of 54 million people worldwide was cited in patients older than 14 years of age.[4]
- In the childhood form, the female predilection is not seen.

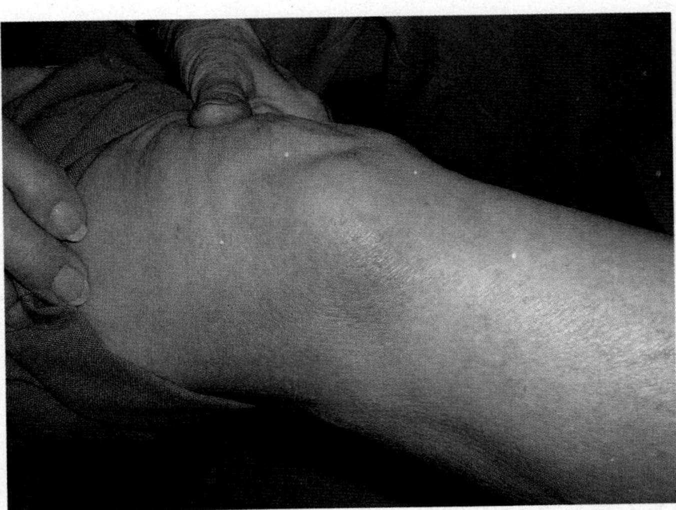

FIGURE 186-2 EN in a middle-aged woman around the knee secondary to sarcoidosis. (*Reproduced with permission from Richard P. Usatine, MD.*)

ETIOLOGY AND PATHOPHYSIOLOGY

- Most EN is idiopathic (**Figures 186-3** and **186-4**). Although the exact percentage is unknown, 1 study estimated that 55% of EN is idiopathic.[5] This may be influenced by the fact that EN may precede the underlying illness. The distribution of etiologic causes may be seasonal.[6] Identifiable causes can be infectious, reactive, pharmacologic, or neoplastic.

- Histologic examination is most useful in defining EN. Defining characteristics of EN are a septal panniculitis without presence of vasculitis. That this pattern develops in certain areas of skin may be linked to local variations in temperature and efficient blood drainage.
- Septal panniculitis begins with polymorphonuclear cells infiltrating the septa of fat lobules in the subcutaneous tissue. It is thought that this is in response to existing immune complex deposition in these areas.[7] This inflammatory change consists of edema and hemorrhage which is responsible for the nodularity, warmth, and erythema.
- The infiltrate progresses from predominantly polymorphonuclear cells, to lymphocytes, and then histiocytes where fibrosis occurs around the lobules. There may be some necrosis, although minimal as complete resolution without scarring is the typical course.
- The histopathologic hallmark of EN is the Miescher radial granuloma. This is a small, well-defined nodular aggregate of small histiocytes around a central stellate or banana-shaped cleft.

RISK FACTORS

- Group A β-hemolytic streptococcal pharyngitis has been linked to EN (see **Figure 186-1**). A retrospective study of 129 cases of EN over several decades reports that 28% had streptococcal infection.[5]
- Nonstreptococcal upper respiratory tract infections may also play a role.[1]
- Historically, tuberculosis (TB) was a common underlying illness with EN, but TB is now a rare cause of EN in developed countries. There are reports of EN occurring in patients receiving the bacille Calmette-Guérin vaccination.[8] In developed countries, sarcoidosis is more commonly found. One study estimates sarcoidosis as being the cause of 11% of EN cases (see **Figure 186-2**).[5,7]
- EN occurs in 3% of all patients with coccidiomycosis[9] and approximately 4% of patients with histoplasmosis.[10]
- EN is less frequently associated with other infections agents, including *Yersinia* gastroenteritis, *Salmonella*, *Campylobacter*, toxoplasmosis, syphilis, amebiasis, giardiasis, brucellosis, leprosy, *Chlamydia*, *Mycoplasma*, *Brucella*, hepatitis B (infection and vaccine), Epstein-Barr virus, and *Bartonella*.[4,11]
- When the EN rash occurs with hilar adenopathy, the entity is called Löfgren syndrome. Löfgren syndrome in TB represents primary infection. A more common cause of Löfgren syndrome is sarcoidosis.[7]
- The literature reports that EN is seen in patients with inflammatory bowel diseases. It is usually prominent around the time of GI flare-ups, but may occur before a flare. Most sources report a greater association between Crohn disease and EN than between ulcerative colitis and EN. Other chronic diseases associated with EN include Behçet disease and Sweet syndrome.[11]
- EN can be associated with pregnancy and oral contraceptive use.
- Besides oral contraceptives, medications implicated as causing EN are antibiotics including sulfonamides, penicillins, and bromides.

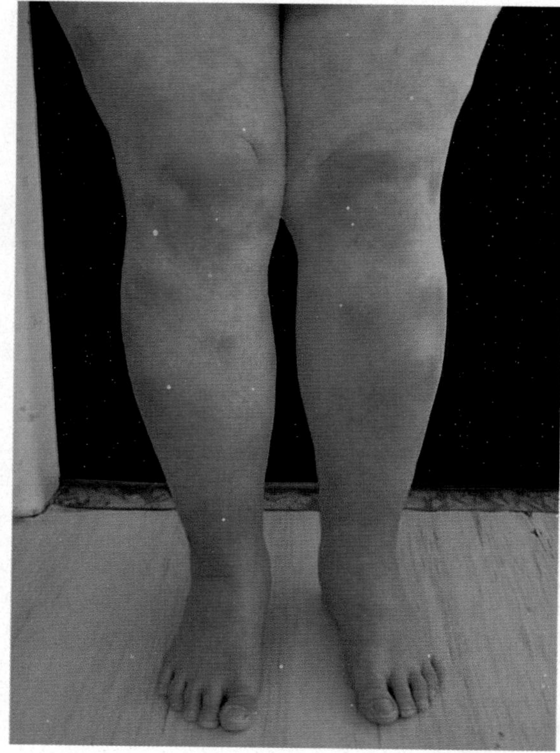

FIGURE 186-3 EN in a middle-aged woman with no known cause. These lesions are bright red, warm, and painful. (*Reproduced with permission from Hanuš Rozsypal, MD.*)

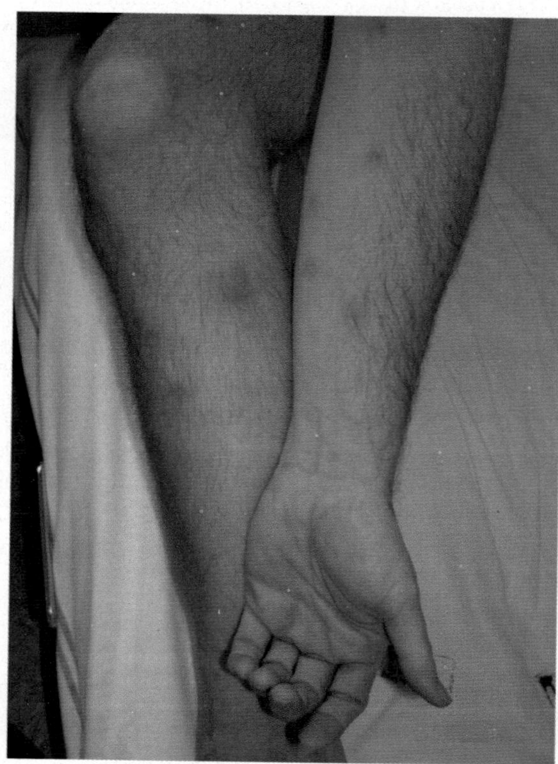

FIGURE 186-4 EN of unknown cause on the arms and legs in a young man. (*Reproduced with permission from Hanuš Rozsypal, MD.*)

However, the antibiotics may have been prescribed for the underlying infection that had caused EN.[11]

- Lymphomas, acute myelogenous leukemia, carcinoid tumor, and pancreatic carcinoma are associated with EN and should be considered in cases of persistent or recurrent EN.[11,12]

DIAGNOSIS

CLINICAL FEATURES

- The diagnosis is usually clinical.
- The lesions of EN are deep-seated nodules that may be more easily palpated than visualized.
- Lesions are initially firm, are round or oval, and are poorly demarcated.
- Lesions may be bright red, warm, and painful (see **Figure 186-3**).
- Lesions number from 1 to more than 10.5 and vary in size from 1 to 15 cm.
- Over their course, the lesions begin to flatten and change to a purplish color before eventually taking on the yellowish hue of a bruise.
- A characteristic of EN is the complete resolution of lesions with no ulceration or scarring.
- EN is associated with systemic occurrence of fever, malaise, and polyarthralgia sometime near eruption.

TYPICAL DISTRIBUTION

- Lesions appear on the anterior/lateral aspect of both lower extremities (see **Figures 186-1** to **186-3**).
- Although lesions may appear in other regions such as the arms, absence in the lower legs is unusual (see **Figure 186-4**).[1]
- Sarcoidosis, in particular, may present with lesions on the ankles and knees (see **Figure 186-2**).
- Lesions may appear in dependent areas in bedridden patients.

LABORATORY TESTING

- Blood tests may help to identify the underlying cause. Typical tests include complete blood count, chemistries, liver function tests, and erythrocyte sedimentation rate. Erythrocyte sedimentation rate may be elevated.
- For suspected *Streptococcus* cases, rapid strep test or throat cultures are best during acute illness, whereas antistreptolysin O titers may be used in the convalescent phase.[4]
- In sarcoidosis, angiotensin-converting enzyme levels may be helpful but are not 100% sensitive.[2] A chest X-ray and/or skin biopsy of a suspected sarcoid lesion can help make this diagnosis (see Chapter 184, Sarcoidosis).

BIOPSY

- The diagnosis of EN is mostly made on physical examination. When the diagnosis is uncertain, a biopsy that includes subcutaneous fat is performed. This can be a deep punch biopsy or a deep incisional biopsy sent for standard histology.

DIFFERENTIAL DIAGNOSIS

- Cellulitis should be considered and not missed. These patients tend to have more fever and systemic symptoms. EN tends to appear in multiple locations, whereas cellulitis is usually in one localized area (see Chapter 126, Cellulitis).
- Nodular cutaneous and subcutaneous sarcoid is skin-colored or violaceous without epidermal involvement. The lack of surface involvement makes this resemble EN. Subcutaneous sarcoidosis may be seen in advanced systemic sarcoidosis that can also be the cause of EN. Skin biopsy is the best method to distinguish between these two conditions. Either way, treatment is directed toward the sarcoidosis (see Chapter 184, Sarcoidosis).
- Erythema induratum of Bazin is a lobular panniculitis that occurs on the posterior lower extremity of women with tendency of lesions to ulcerate with residual scarring.[7] This condition is typically caused by TB and is more chronic in nature than EN.[2]
- Erythema nodosum leprosum may occur in patients with leprosy and probably represents an immune complex or hypersensitivity reaction (**Figures 186-5** and **186-6**). Erythema nodosum leprosum is typically seen as a type 2 reaction to standard leprosy therapy.[13] It is more common in multibacillary lepromatous leprosy. Although the lesions often look like standard EN, the lesions may also ulcerate.
- An infectious panniculitis should also be considered in the differential, especially in immunocompromised patients. These lesions are often asymmetric, and the patient may be febrile. If suspected, a punch biopsy of a lesion should be sent for tissue culture (bacteria, fungus, and *mycobacteria*).

MANAGEMENT

- Look for and treat the underlying cause. There is limited evidence to guide treatment unless an underlying cause is found.

FIRST LINE

NONPHARMACOLOGIC

- Cool, wet compresses, elevation of the involved extremities, bed rest, gradient support stockings, or pressure bandages may help alleviate the pain.[11] SOR Ⓒ

MEDICATIONS

- Treat the pain and discomfort of the nodules with NSAIDs and/or other analgesics.[14] SOR Ⓒ

SECOND LINE

MEDICATIONS

- The value of oral prednisone is controversial, and it should be avoided unless it is being used to treat the underlying cause (such as sarcoidosis) and if underlying infection, risk of bacterial dissemination or sepsis, and malignancy have been excluded.[1] SOR Ⓒ
- Oral potassium iodide (**Figure 186-7**) is an old therapy that has led to resolution of EN in several small studies.[6,7] SOR Ⓑ It is now available over the counter but is contraindicated in pregnancy.

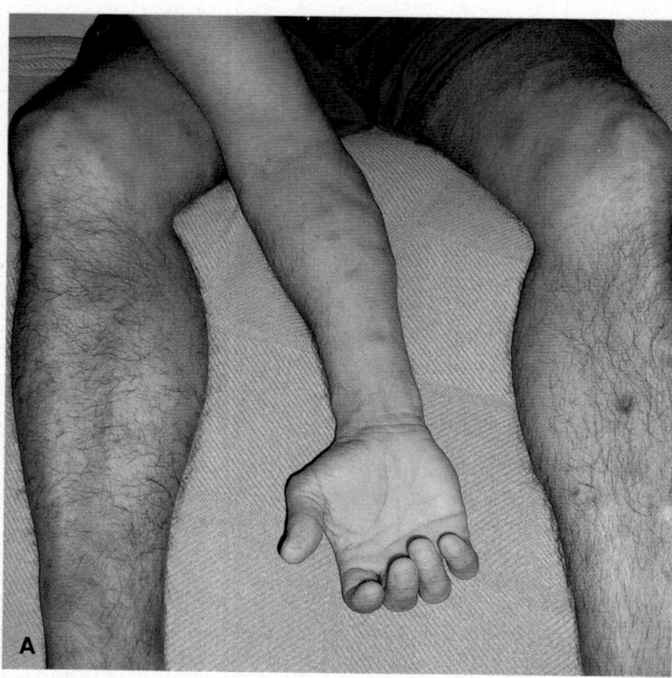

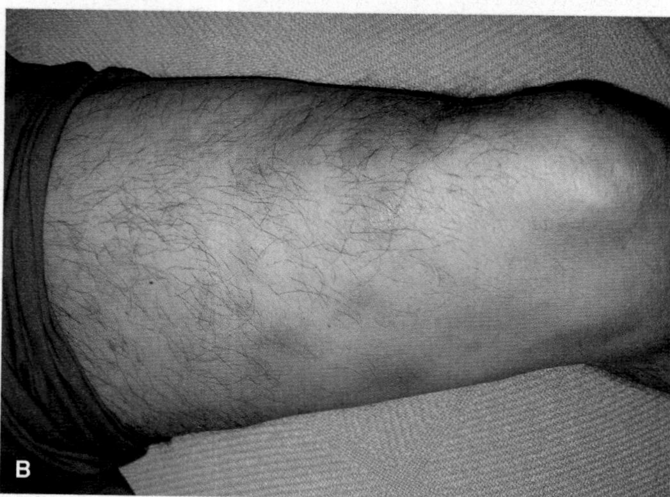

FIGURE 186-5 Erythema nodosum leprosum (ENL) in a Texas man who acquired multibacillary leprosy from handling and eating armadillos. His ENL started when he started the antibacterial treatment. **A.** Note the many subcutaneous nodules on his arms and legs. **B.** Close-up of the ENL lesions. (*Reproduced with permission from Richard P. Usatine, MD.*)

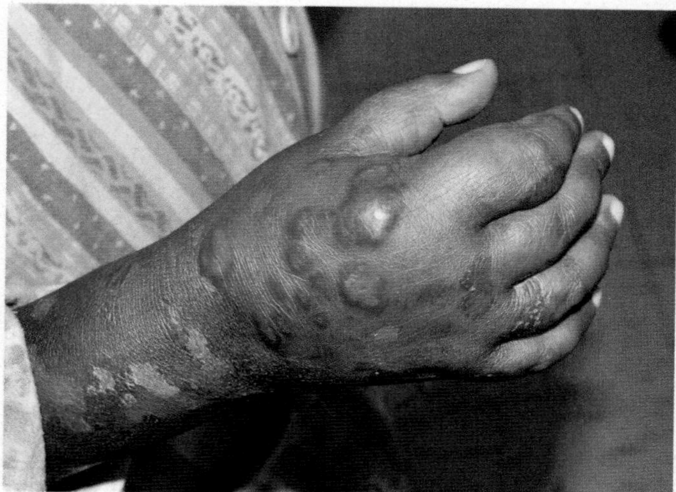

FIGURE 186-6 Erythema nodosum leprosum (ENL) on the hand and arm of an Ethiopian woman being treated with three antileprosy drugs for multibacillary lepromatous leprosy. (*Reproduced with permission from Richard P. Usatine, MD.*)

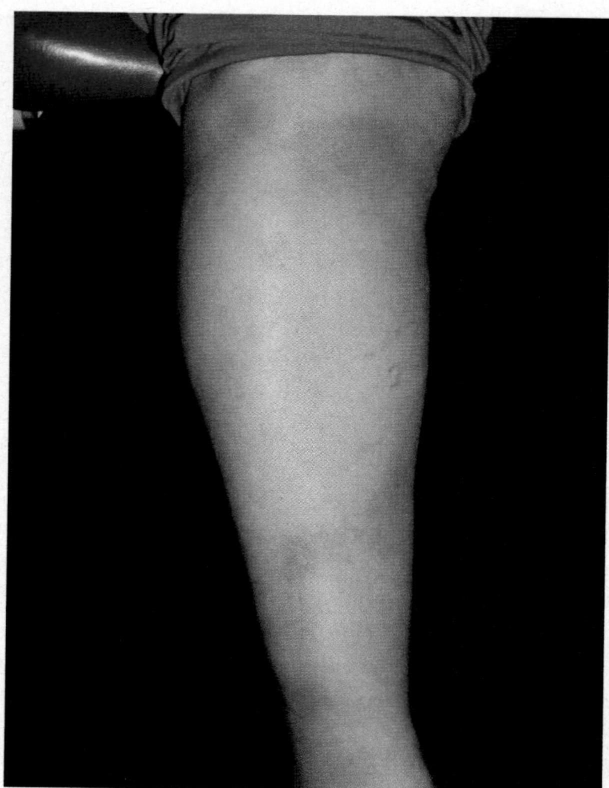

FIGURE 186-7 Erythema nodosum on the leg of a 76-year-old woman. Her EN was painful and did not respond to first-line therapies. She did well with potassium iodide. Her EN flared up like this when she stopped the potassium iodide because of the taste. (*Reproduced with permission from Richard P. Usatine, MD.*)

Potassium iodide can be mixed in orange juice to make it more palatable. It is available in many different concentrations, so it is important to pay close attention to the dosage.

- Colchicine, hydroxychloroquine, and dapsone have been used as well.[2,7] SOR ©
- There are a few case reports of EN treated with penicillin, erythromycin, adalimumab, etanercept, infliximab, mycophenolate mofetil, cyclosporine, thalidomide, and extracorporeal monocyte granulocytapheresis.[1,15,16] SOR ©
- There are a few case reports and one small study of minocycline and tetracycline leading to EN and erythema nodosum leprosum improvement.[17,18] SOR ©

PREVENTION

- Good handwashing and general health measures may prevent respiratory infections that may predispose to EN.

PROGNOSIS

- EN is usually self-limited or resolves with treatment of the underlying disorder.
- Patients may continue to develop nodules for a few weeks.
- The course depends on the etiology but usually lasts only 6 weeks.
- Lesions completely resolve with no ulceration or scarring.
- Recurrences occur in 33% to 41% of cases, usually when the etiology is unknown.[16]

FOLLOW-UP

- Follow-up is needed to complete the work-up for an underlying cause and to make sure that the patient is responding to symptomatic treatment.

PATIENT EDUCATION

Reassure the patient that there is complete resolution in most cases within 3 to 6 weeks. Inform the patient that some EN outbreaks may persist for up to 12 weeks, and some cases are recurrent.[6]

PATIENT RESOURCES

- MedicineNet. *Erythema Nodosum*—**http://www.medicinenet.com/erythema_nodosum/article.htm.**

PROVIDER RESOURCES

- Medscape. *Erythema Nodosum*—**http://emedicine.medscape.com/article/1081633-overview.**
- Schwartz RA, Nervi SJ. Erythema nodosum: a sign of systemic disease. *Am Fam Physician.* 2007;75(5):695-700—**http://www.aafp.org/afp/2007/0301/p695.html.**

REFERENCES

1. Schwartz RA, Nervi SJ. Erythema nodosum: a sign of systemic disease. *Am Fam Physician.* 2007;75(5):695-700.
2. Atzeni F, Carrabba M, Davin JC, et al. Skin manifestations in vasculitis and erythema nodosum. *Clin Exp Rheumatol.* 2006;24 (1 Suppl 40):S60-S66.
3. García-Porrua C, González-Gay MA, Vázquez-Caruncho M, et al. Erythema nodosum: etiologic and predictive factors erythema nodosum and erythema induratum in a defined population. *Arthritis Rheum.* 2000:43:584-592.
4. Gonzalez-Gay MA, Garcia-Porrua C, Pujol RM, Salvarani C. Erythema nodosum: a clinical approach. *Clin Exp Rheumatol.* 2001; 19(4):365-368.
5. Cribier B, Caille A, Heid E, Grosshans E. Erythema nodosum and associated diseases. A study of 129 cases. *Int J Dermatol.* 1998; 37(9):667-672.
6. Hannuksela M. Erythema nodosum. *Clin Dermatol.* 1986;4(4): 88-95.
7. Requena L, Requena C. Erythema nodosum. *Dermatol Online J.* 2002;8(1):4.
8. Fox MD, Schwartz RA. Erythema nodosum. *Am Fam Physician.* 1992;46(3):818-822.
9. Body BA. Cutaneous manifestations of systemic mycoses. *Dermatol Clin.* 1996;14:125-135.
10. Ozols II, Wheat LJ. Erythema nodosum in an epidemic of histoplasmosis in Indianapolis. *Arch Dermatol.* 1981;117:709-712.
11. Gilchrist H, Patterson JW. Erythema nodosum and erythema induratum (nodular vasculitis): diagnosis and management. *Dermatol Ther.* 2010;23(4):320-327.
12. Cho KH, Kim YG, Yang SG, et al. Inflammatory nodules of the lower legs: a clinical and histological analysis of 134 cases in Korea. *J Dermatol.* 1997;24:522-529.
13. Van Brakel WH, Khawas IB, Lucas SB. Reactions in leprosy: an epidemiological study of 386 patients in west Nepal. *Lepr Rev.* 1994;65(3):190-203.
14. Ubogy Z, Persellin RH. Suppression of erythema nodosum by indomethacin. *Acta Derm Venereol.* 1982;62:265.
15. Allen RA, Spielvogel RL. Erythema nodosum. In: Lebwohl MG, Heymann WR, Berth-Jones J, Coulson I, eds. *Treatment of Skin Disease*, 3rd ed. Philadelphia, PA: Saunders; 2010:223-225.
16. Gilchrist H, Patterson JW. Erythema nodosum and erythema induratum (nodular vasculitis): diagnosis and management. *Dermatol Ther.* 2010;23(4):320-327.
17. Davis MD. Response of recalcitrant erythema nodosum to tetracyclines. *J Am Acad Dermatol.* 2011;64(6):1211-1212.
18. Narang T, Sawatkar GU, Kumaran MS, et al. Minocycline for recurrent and/or chronic erythema nodosum leprosum. *JAMA Dermatol.* 2015;151(9):1026-1028.

187 VASCULITIS

E.J. Mayeaux, Jr., MD
Richard P. Usatine, MD
Nathan S. Martin, MD
Leah T. Williams, MD

PATIENT STORY

A 21-year-old woman presented with a 3-day history of a painful purpuric rash on her lower extremities (**Figures 187-1** and **187-2**). The lesions had appeared suddenly, and the patient had experienced no prior similar episodes. The patient had been diagnosed with a case of pharyngitis earlier that week and was given a course of clindamycin. She had not experienced any nausea or vomiting, fever, abdominal cramping, or gross hematuria. Urine dipstick revealed blood in her urine, but no protein. The typical palpable purpura on the legs is consistent with Henoch-Schönlein purpura (HSP), also known as IgA vasculitis.

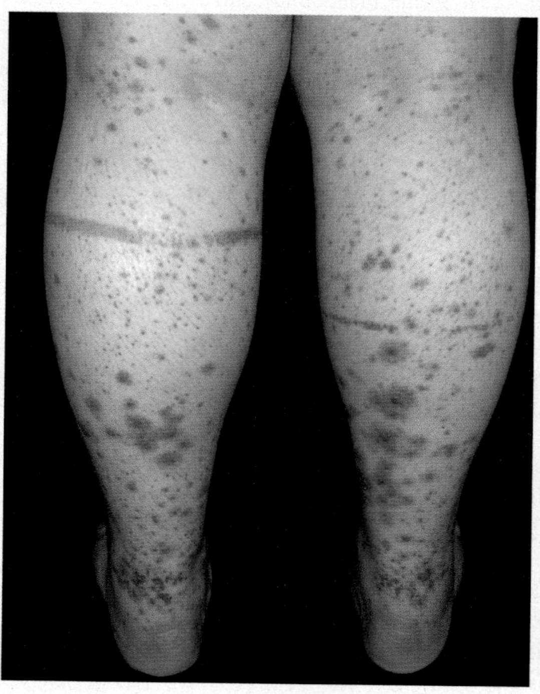

FIGURE 187-1 Henoch-Schönlein purpura presenting as palpable purpura on the lower extremity. The visible sock lines are from lesions that formed where the socks exerted pressure on the legs. (*Reproduced with permission from Richard P. Usatine, MD.*)

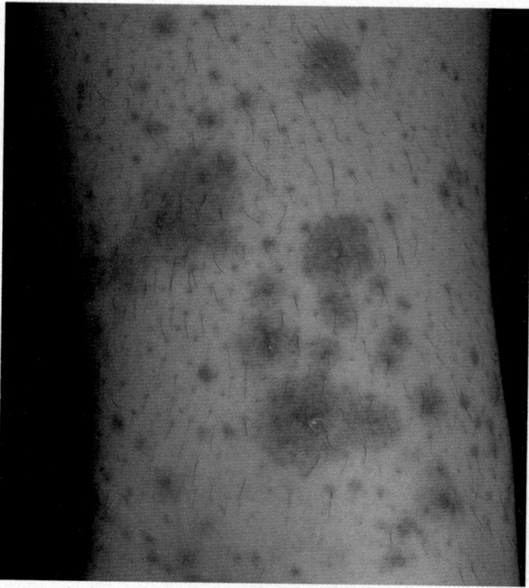

FIGURE 187-2 Close-up of palpable purpura from the patient in Figure 187-1. Some lesions look like target lesions, but this is Henoch-Schönlein purpura and not erythema multiforme. (*Reproduced with permission from Richard P. Usatine, MD.*)

INTRODUCTION

Vasculitis refers to a group of disorders characterized by inflammation and damage in blood vessel walls. They may be limited to skin or may be a multisystem disorder. Cutaneous vasculitic diseases are classified according to the size (small vs. medium to large vessel) and type of blood vessel involved (venule, arteriole, artery, or vein). Small- and medium-size vessels are found in the dermis and deep reticular dermis, respectively. While the classifications have not changed, the nomenclature has in an effort to characterize lesions based on the pathologic findings and underlying disease process. The most notable changes during the Chapel Hill Consensus Conference of 2012 changed HSP to IgA vasculitis (IgAV), Wegener's granulomatosis to granulomatosis with polyangitis (GPA), and Churg-Strauss to eosinophilic granulomatosis with polyangitis (EGPA).[1] The clinical presentation varies with the intensity of the inflammation and the size and type of blood vessel involved.[2]

SYNONYMS

Hypersensitivity vasculitis is also known as leukocytoclastic vasculitis.
HSP (IgAV) is a type of leukocytoclastic vasculitis.

EPIDEMIOLOGY

- HSP (IgAV) (**Figures 187-1** to **187-3**) occurs mainly in children with an incidence of approximately 1 in 5000 children annually.[3] It results from immunoglobulin (Ig) A–containing immune complexes in blood vessel walls in the skin, kidney, and GI tract. HSP (IgAV) is usually benign and self-limiting and tends to occur in the springtime. A streptococcal or viral upper respiratory infection often precedes the disease by 1 to 3 weeks. Prodromal symptoms include anorexia and fever. Most children with HSP (IgAV) also have joint pain and swelling with the knees and ankles being most

commonly involved (**Figure 187-3**). In half of cases there are recurrences, typically in the first 3 months. Recurrences are more common in patients with nephritis and are milder than the original episode. To make the diagnosis of HSP (IgAV), establish the presence of 3 or more of the following[4]:
  - Palpable purpura
  - Bowel angina (pain)
  - GI bleeding
  - Hematuria
  - Onset ≤20 years
  - No new medications
- Some patients with systemic lupus erythematosus (SLE) (**Figures 187-4** and **187-5**), rheumatoid arthritis (RA), relapsing polychondritis, and other connective tissue disorders develop an associated necrotizing vasculitis. It most frequently involves the small muscular arteries, arterioles, and venules. The blood vessels can become blocked, leading to tissue necrosis (see **Figures 187-4** and **187-5**). The skin and internal organs may be involved.
- Leukocytoclastic vasculitis (**Figures 187-6** to **187-8**) is the most commonly seen form of small vessel vasculitis. Prodromal symptoms include fever, malaise, myalgia, and joint pain. The palpable purpura begins as asymptomatic localized areas of cutaneous hemorrhage that become palpable. Few or many discrete lesions are most commonly seen on the lower extremities but may occur on any dependent area. Small lesions itch and are painful, but nodules, ulcers, and bullae may be very painful. Lesions appear in crops, last for 1 to 4 weeks, and may heal with residual scarring and hyperpigmentation. Patients may experience 1 episode (drug reaction or viral infection) or multiple episodes (RA or SLE). The disease is usually self-limited and confined to the skin. To make the diagnosis, look for presence of 3 or more of the following[5]:
  - Age older than 16 years
  - Use of a possible offending drug in temporal relation to the symptoms
  - Palpable purpura
  - Maculopapular rash
  - Biopsy of a skin lesion showing neutrophils around an arteriole or venule
- Systemic manifestations of leukocytoclastic vasculitis may include kidney disease, heart, nervous system, GI tract, lungs, and joint involvement.

ETIOLOGY AND PATHOPHYSIOLOGY

- Vasculitis is defined as inflammation of the blood vessel wall. The mechanisms of vascular damage consist of a humoral response, immune complex deposition, or cell-mediated T-lymphocyte response with granuloma formation.[6]
- Vasculitis-induced injury to blood vessels may lead to increased vascular permeability, vessel weakening, aneurysm formation, hemorrhage, intimal proliferation, and thrombosis that result in obstruction and local ischemia.[6]
- Small-vessel vasculitis is initiated by hypersensitivity to various antigens (drugs, chemicals, microorganisms, and endogenous antigens), with formation of circulating immune complexes that are deposited

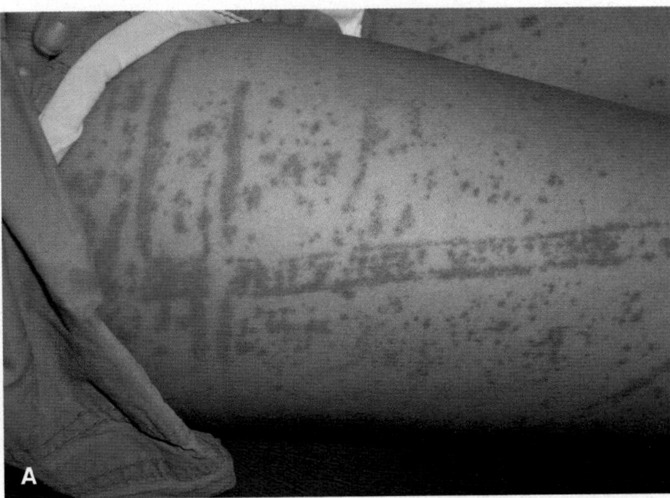

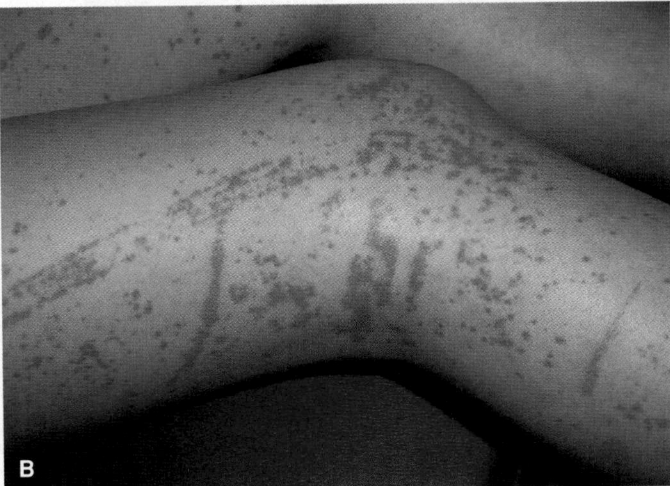

FIGURE 187-3 Henoch-Schönlein purpura in an 11-year-old girl. **A.** In addition to the palpable purpura, this patient also had abdominal pain. Note how the seam of her jeans is visible in the purpuric pattern. **B.** She also had knee pain and swelling and was walking with a limp. *(Reproduced with permission from Richard P. Usatine, MD.)*

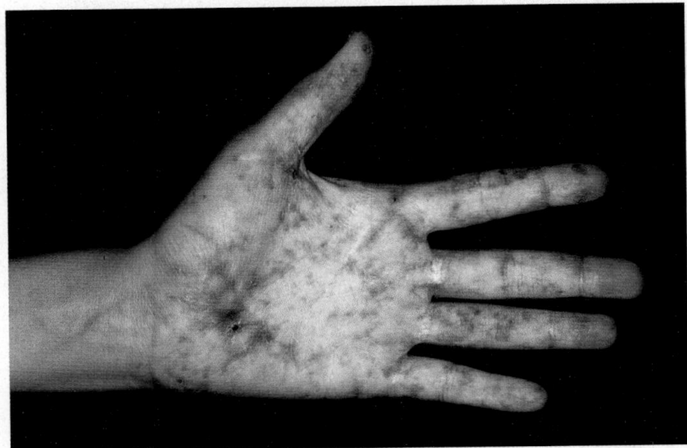

FIGURE 187-4 Necrotizing vasculitis in a young Asian woman with systemic lupus erythematosus. The circulation to the fingertips was compromised, and the woman was treated with high-dose intravenous steroids and intravenous immunoglobulins to prevent tissue loss. *(Reproduced with permission from Richard P. Usatine, MD.)*

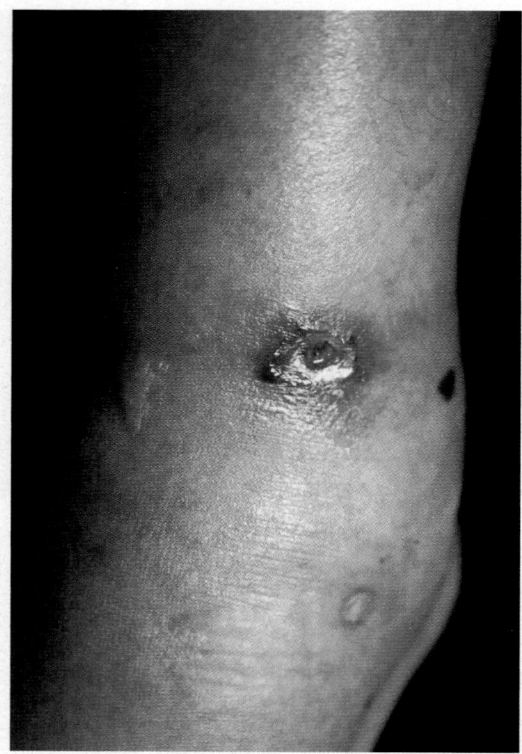

FIGURE 187-5 Vasculitis ulcer on the leg of a woman with systemic lupus erythematosus. (*Reproduced with permission from Everett Allen, MD.*)

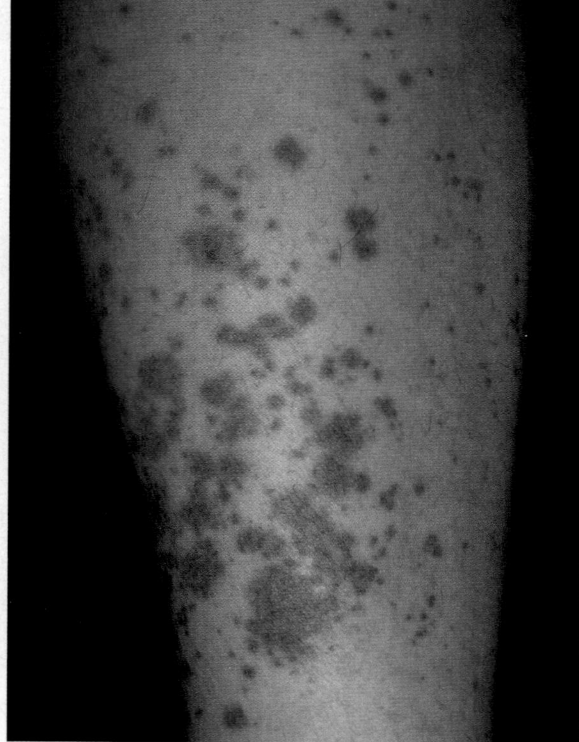

FIGURE 187-6 Leukocytoclastic vasculitis on the leg of a woman. (*Reproduced with permission from Richard P. Usatine, MD.*)

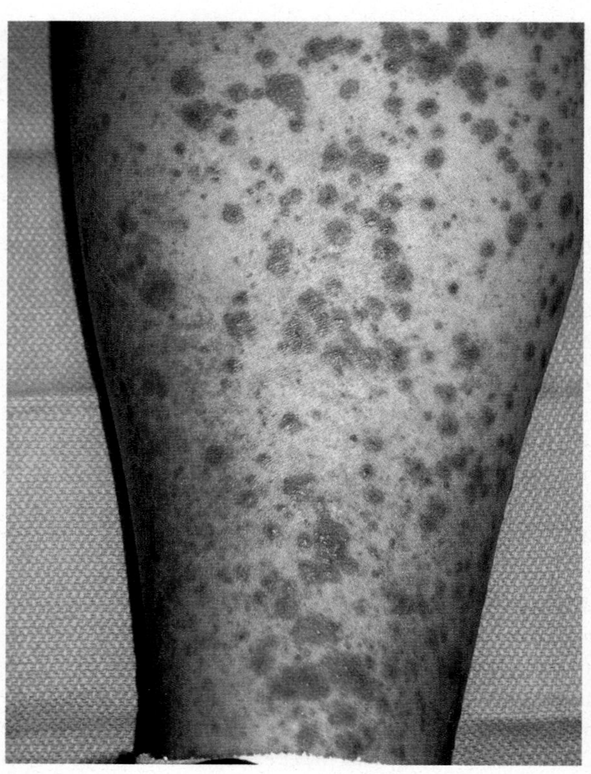

FIGURE 187-7 Very palpable purpura on the leg of a middle-aged woman with leukocytoclastic vasculitis. (*Reproduced with permission from Eric Kraus, MD.*)

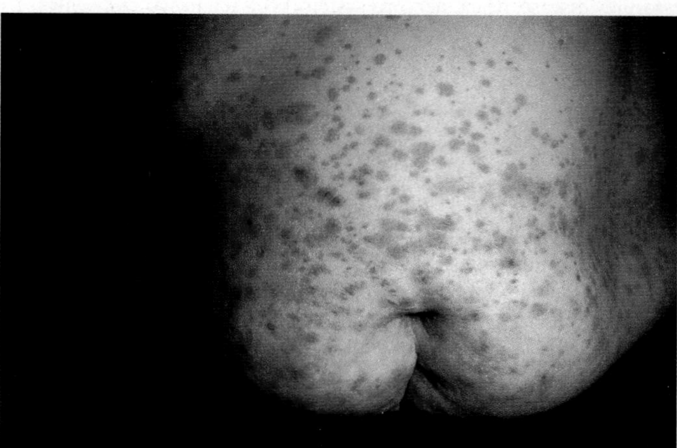

FIGURE 187-8 Vasculitis on the abdomen of a middle-aged woman who also has the vasculitis on her legs. (*Reproduced with permission from Everett Allen, MD.*)

in walls of postcapillary venules. The vessel-bound immune complexes activate complement, which attracts polymorphonuclear leukocytes. They damage the walls of small veins by release of lysosomal enzymes. This causes vessel necrosis and local hemorrhage.

- Small-vessel vasculitis most commonly affects the skin and rarely causes serious internal organ dysfunction, except when the kidney is involved. Small-vessel vasculitis is associated with leukocytoclastic vasculitis, HSP (IgAV), essential mixed cryoglobulinemia, connective tissue diseases or malignancies, serum sickness and serum sickness–like reactions, chronic urticaria, and acute hepatitis B or C infection.
- Hypersensitivity (leukocytoclastic) vasculitis causes acute inflammation and necrosis of venules in the dermis. The term *leukocytoclastic vasculitis* describes the histologic pattern produced when leukocytes fragment.

RISK FACTORS

- Viral infections.
- Autoimmune disorders.
- Drug hypersensitivity.
- Cocaine (adulterated with levamisole) (**Figure 187-9**) (see Chapter 251, Cocaine, for additional images and information).

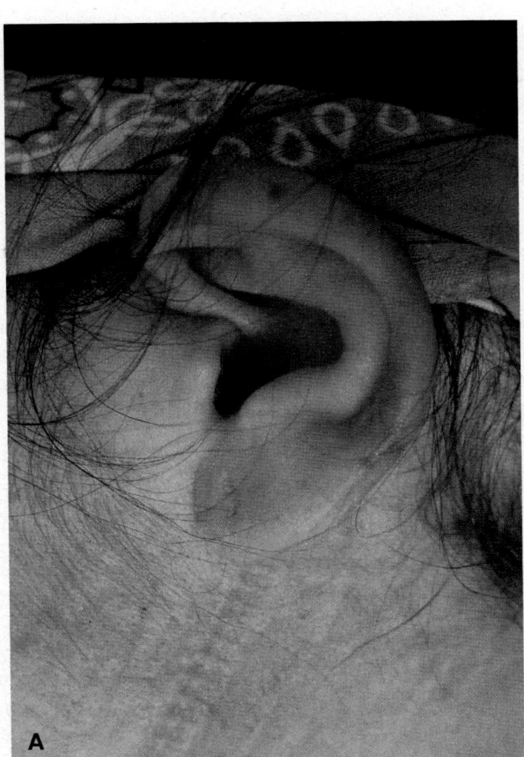

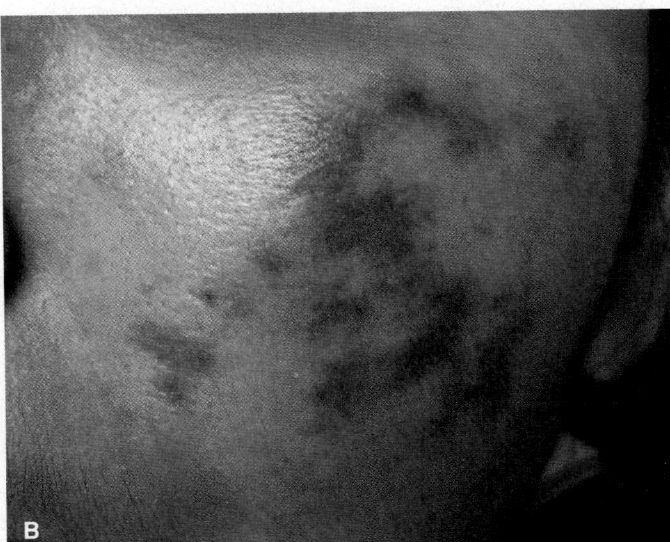

FIGURE 187-9 A. Cutaneous vasculitis of the ear caused by levamisole-adulterated cocaine. (*Reproduced with permission from Jonathan Karnes, MD.*) B. Cutaneous vasculitis in a retiform (netlike) pattern caused by the use of levamisole-adulterated cocaine. This is called *retiform purpura*. (*Reproduced with permission from John M. Martin IV, MD.*)

DIAGNOSIS

- Initially, determining the extent of visceral organ involvement is more important than identifying the type of vasculitis, so that organs at risk of damage are not jeopardized by delayed or inadequate treatment. In addition to the dermatologic findings, the physical examination may be useful in determining if large vessels are involved. Examination findings of a blood pressure difference of greater than 10 mm Hg in the arms, auscultation of bruits, and diminished peripheral pulses may indicate large vessel involvement.[7] It is critical to distinguish vasculitis occurring as a primary autoimmune disorder from vasculitis secondary to infection, drugs, malignancy, or connective tissue disease such as SLE or RA.[6]

CLINICAL FEATURES

- Small-vessel vasculitis is characterized by necrotizing inflammation of small blood vessels and may be identified by the finding of "palpable purpura." The lower extremities typically demonstrate "palpable purpura," varying in size from a few millimeters to several centimeters (**Figures 187-2, 187-6, 187-7,** and **187-10**). In its early stages leukocytoclastic vasculitis may not be palpable.
- The clinical features of HSP (IgAV) include nonthrombocytopenic palpable purpura mainly on the lower extremities and buttocks (see **Figures 187-1, 187-2** to **187-3**), GI symptoms, arthralgia, and nephritis.

TYPICAL DISTRIBUTION

- Cutaneous vasculitis is found most commonly on the legs but may be seen on the hands and abdomen (see **Figures 187-3, 187-8,** and **187-10**).

LABORATORY TESTING

- Laboratory evaluation is geared to finding the antigenic source of the immunologic reaction. Consider throat culture, antistreptolysin-*O* titer, erythrocyte sedimentation rate, platelets, complete blood count (CBC), serum creatinine, urinalysis, antinuclear antibody, serum protein electrophoresis, circulating immune complexes, hepatitis B surface antigen, hepatitis C antibody, cryoglobulins, and rheumatoid factor. The erythrocyte sedimentation rate is almost always elevated during active vasculitis. Immunofluorescent studies are best done within the first 24 hours after a lesion forms. The most common immunoreactants present in and around blood vessels are IgM, C3, and fibrin. The presence of IgA in blood vessels of a child with vasculitis suggests the diagnosis of HSP (IgAV).
- Basic laboratory analysis to assess the degree and types of organs affected should include serum creatinine, creatinine kinase, liver function studies, hepatitis serologies, urinalysis, and possibly chest X-ray and ECG.

BIOPSY

- The clinical presentation is so characteristic that a biopsy is generally unnecessary. In doubtful cases, a punch biopsy should be taken from the center of an active (nonulcerated) lesion or, if necessary, from the edge of an ulcer (see **Figure 187-4**). A 4-mm punch biopsy from a well-developed purpuric lesion (ideally 3 days old—or within 1 to 7 days) is best sent in formalin for hematoxylin–eosin-stained analysis.[8] If the specimen is to be sent for direct immunofluorescence to find out the type of antibodies present, the lesion should ideally be less than 24 hours old and sent in special Michelle media (or on a saline-soaked gauze in a sterile urine container to be transferred to the Michelle media in the lab).

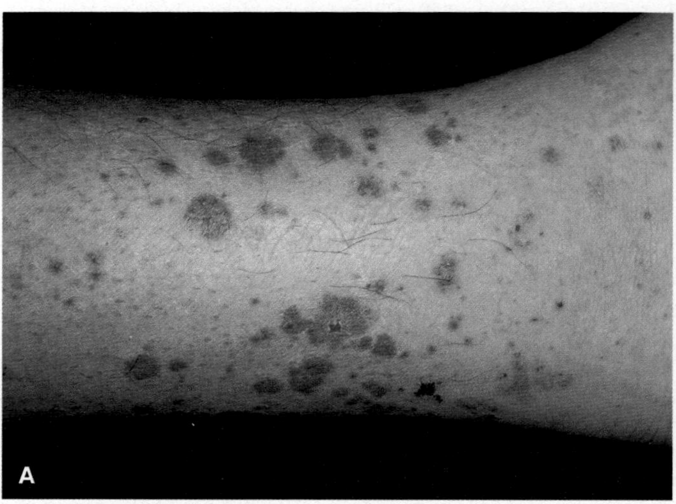

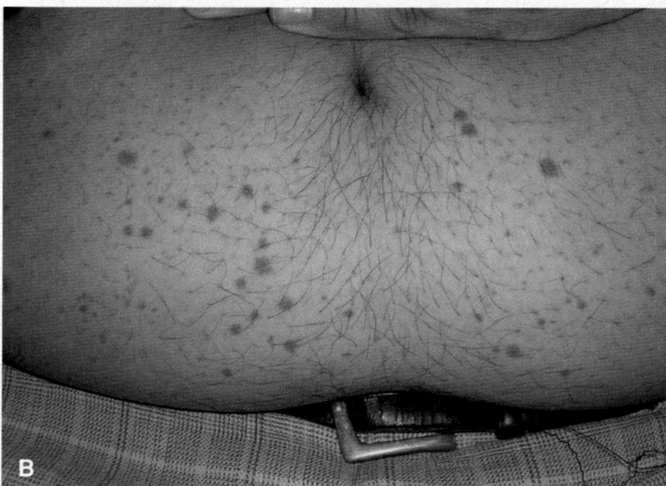

FIGURE 187-10 Leukocytoclastic vasculitis in a 26-year-old man. **A.** Palpable purpura on the lower leg. **B.** Involvement of the lower abdomen. (*Reproduced with permission from Richard P. Usatine, MD.*)

DIFFERENTIAL DIAGNOSIS

- Pigmented purpuric dermatosis is a capillaritis characterized by extravasation of erythrocytes in the skin with marked hemosiderin deposition. It is not palpable. Schamberg disease is a type of pigmented purpuric dermatosis found most often on the lower legs in older persons (**Figures 187-11** and **187-12**). It is described as a cayenne pepper–like appearance. Lichen aureus is a localized pigmented purpuric dermatosis seen in younger persons that may occur on the leg or in other parts of the body (**Figure 187-13**). The color may be yellow brown or golden brown. There is also a pigmented purpuric dermatosis of the Majocchi type that has an annular appearance with prominent elevated erythematous borders that may have telangiectasias (**Figure 187-14**). A dermatoscope can help to visualize the red or pink dots that represent inflamed capillaries in these conditions.
- Meningococcemia that presents with purpura in severely ill patients with central nervous system symptoms (**Figures 187-15** and **187-16**).
- Rocky Mountain spotted fever is a rickettsial infection that presents with pink to bright red, discrete 1- to 5-mm macules that blanch with pressure and may be pruritic. The lesions start distally and spread to the soles and palms (**Figure 187-17**).

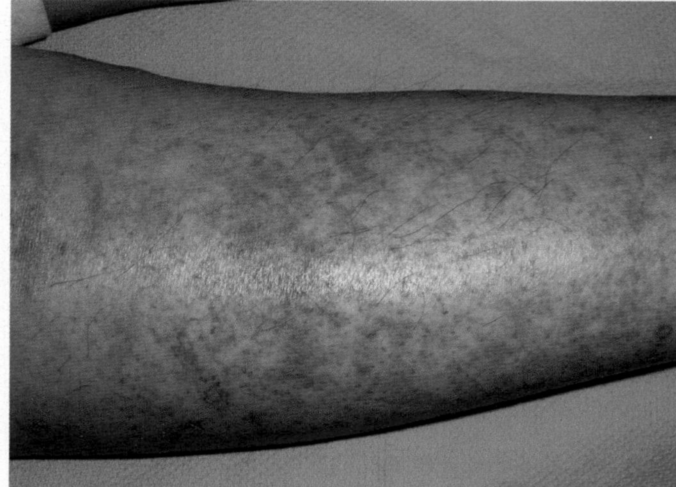

FIGURE 187-11 Schamberg disease (pigmented purpuric dermatosis) of the lower leg showing hemosiderin deposits and a cayenne pepper capillaritis. (*Reproduced with permission from Richard P. Usatine, MD.*)

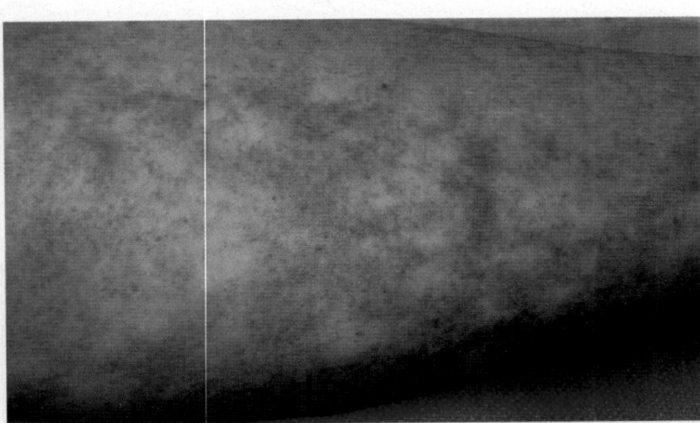

FIGURE 187-12 Schamberg disease with prominent petechiae and hemosiderin deposits. Note that this condition is not palpable. (*Reproduced with permission from Richard P. Usatine, MD.*)

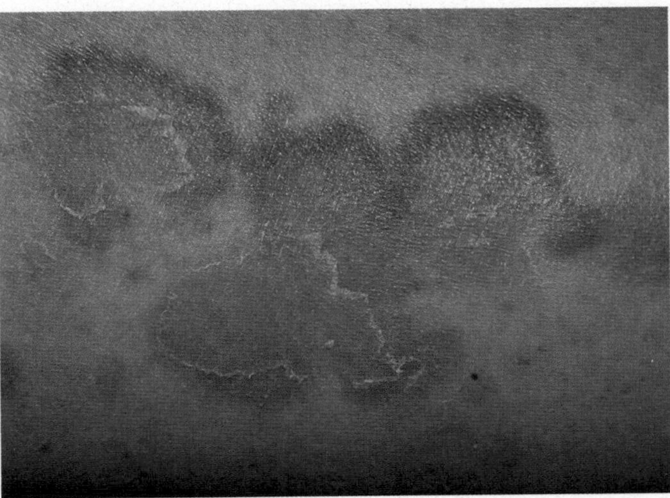

FIGURE 187-14 Pigmented purpuric dermatosis of the Majocchi type. Note the annular appearance and the prominent elevated erythematous borders. (*Reproduced with permission from Suraj Reddy, MD.*)

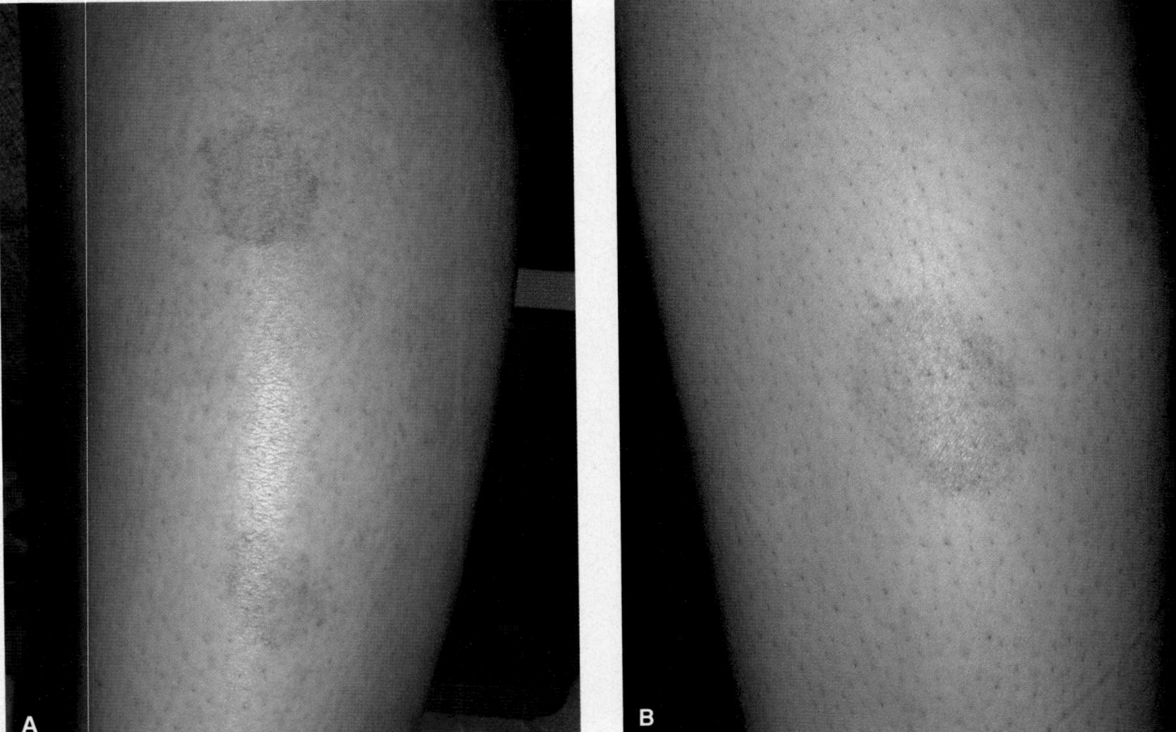

FIGURE 187-13 Lichen aureus. **A.** On the leg of a 27-year-old woman. **B.** On the leg of a 16-year-old girl. (*Reproduced with permission from Richard P. Usatine, MD.*)

- Malignancies, such as cutaneous T-cell lymphoma (mycosis fungoides) (see Chapter 180, Cutaneous T-Cell Lymphoma).
- Stevens-Johnson syndrome and toxic epidermal necrolysis (see Chapter 185, Erythema Multiforme, Stevens-Johnson Syndrome, and Toxic Epidermal Necrolysis).
- Idiopathic thrombocytopenia purpura can be easily distinguished from vasculitis by measuring the platelet count. Also, the purpura is usually not palpable and the petechiae can be scattered all over the body (**Figure 187-18**).
- Wegener granulomatosis (GPA) is an unusual multisystem disease characterized by necrotizing granulomatous inflammation and vasculitis of the respiratory tract, kidneys, and skin.
- Churg-Strauss syndrome (EGPA) presents with a systemic vasculitis associated with asthma, transient pulmonary infiltrates, and hypereosinophilia.
- Cutaneous manifestations of cholesterol embolism, which are leg pain, livedo reticularis (blue-red mottling of the skin in a netlike pattern), and/or blue toes in the presence of good peripheral pulses.

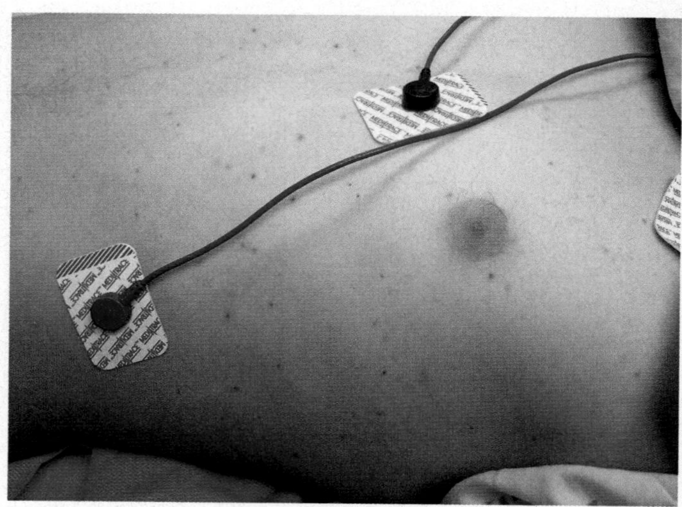

FIGURE 187-15 Petechiae of meningococcemia on the trunk of a hospitalized adolescent. (*Reproduced with permission from Tom Moore, MD.*)

MANAGEMENT

NONPHARMACOLOGIC

- The offending antigen should be identified and removed whenever possible. With a mild hypersensitivity vasculitis that is due to a drug, discontinuing the offending drug may be all the treatment that is necessary. SOR Ⓒ

MEDICATIONS

- An antihistamine might be used for itching. SOR Ⓒ
- Oral prednisone is used to treat visceral involvement and more severe cases of vasculitis of the skin. Short courses of prednisone (60 to 80 mg/day) are effective and should be tapered slowly. SOR Ⓑ
- Colchicine (0.6 mg twice daily for 7 to 10 days) and dapsone (100 to 150 mg/day) may be used to inhibit neutrophil chemotaxis.[9] SOR Ⓑ They are tapered and discontinued when lesions resolve. Azathioprine, cyclophosphamide, and methotrexate have also been studied. SOR Ⓒ
- In HSP (IgAV) and prolonged hypersensitivity vasculitis, treatment with nonsteroidal anti-inflammatory drugs is usually preferred. Treatment with corticosteroids may be of more benefit in patients with more severe disease such as more pronounced abdominal pain and renal involvement.[10] SOR Ⓑ Adding cyclophosphamide to the steroids may also be effective. SOR Ⓒ Azathioprine also may be used.[11] In children with persistent proteinuria a trial of angiotensin-converting enzyme inhibitors or angiotensin receptor blockers may be used; patients with rapidly progressive nephritis may benefit from plasmapheresis to prevent long-term renal dysfunction.[12] SOR Ⓒ

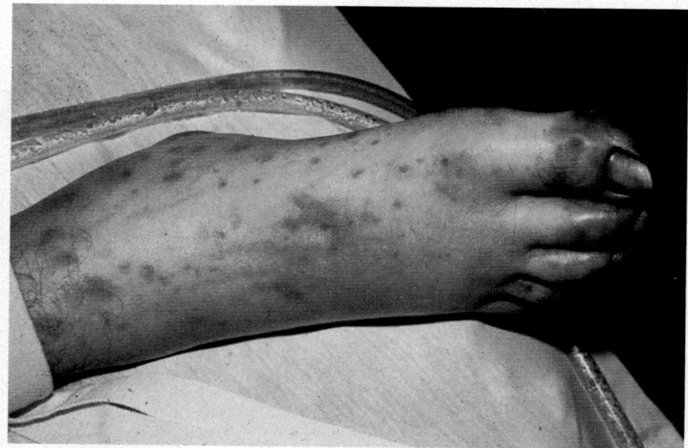

FIGURE 187-16 Petechiae, purpura, and acrocyanosis in a severely ill patient with meningococcemia. (*Reproduced with permission from Richard P. Usatine, MD.*)

REFER OR HOSPITALIZE

- Refer or hospitalize with significant internal organ involvement or prolonged disease course.

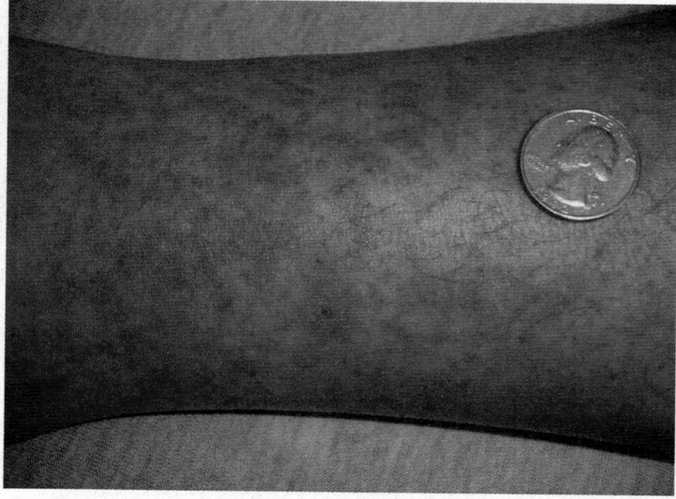

FIGURE 187-17 Rocky Mountain spotted fever with many petechiae visible around the original tick bite. This rickettsial disease looks similar to vasculitis. (*Reproduced with permission from Tom Moore, MD.*)

PROGNOSIS

- In leukocytoclastic (hypersensitivity) vasculitis, the cutaneous lesions usually resolve without sequelae. Visceral involvement (such as kidney and lung) most commonly occurs in HSP (IgAV), cryoglobulinemia and vasculitis associated with SLE.[13] Extensive internal organ involvement should prompt an investigation for coexistent medium-size vessel disease and referral to a rheumatologist.

FOLLOW-UP

- Relapses may occur, especially when the precipitating factor is an autoimmune disease. Regular monitoring is necessary.

PATIENT EDUCATION

- Reassure patients and parents that most cases of acute cutaneous vasculitis resolve spontaneously.

PATIENT RESOURCES

- MedicineNet. *Vasculitis*—**http://www.medicinenet.com/vasculitis/article.htm.**
- National Kidney and Urologic Diseases Information Clearinghouse. *Henoch-Schönlein Purpura*—**http://kidney.niddk.nih.gov/health-information/kidney-disease/henoch-schonlein-purpura.**
- National Heart Blood and Lung Institute. *What Is Vasculitis?*—**http://www.nhlbi.nih.gov/health/health-topics/vasculitis.**

PROVIDER RESOURCES

- Roane DW, Griger DR. An approach to diagnosis and initial management of systemic vasculitis. *Am Fam Physician.* 1999:60:1421-1430—**http://www.aafp.org/afp/1999/1001/p1421.html.**
- Sharma P, Sharma S, Baltaro R, Hurley J. Systemic vasculitis. *Am Family Physician.* 2011;83(5):556-565—**http://www.aafp.org/afp/2011/0301/p556.html.**
- Reamy BV, Williams PM, Lindsay TJ. Henoch-Schönlein purpura. *Am Fam Physician.* 2009;80(7):697-704—**http://www.aafp.org/afp/2009/1001/p697.html.**

REFERENCES

1. Jennette JC, Falk RJ, Bacon PA, et al. 2012 Revised International Chapel Hill Consensus Conference Nomenclature of Vasculitides. *Arthritis Rheum.* 2013;65(1):1-11.
2. Stone JH, Nousari HC. "Essential" cutaneous vasculitis: what every rheumatologist should know about vasculitis of the skin. *Curr Opin Rheumatol.* 2001;13(1):23-34.
3. Gardner-Medwin JM, Dolezalova P, Cummins C, Southwood TR. Incidence of Henoch-Schönlein purpura, Kawasaki disease, and

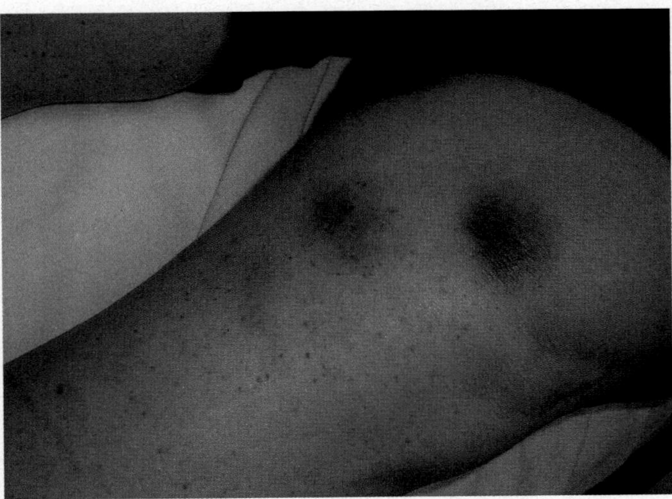

FIGURE 187-18 Petechiae and purpura in a patient with idiopathic thrombocytopenic purpura and a platelet count of 3000. Note that this purpura is not palpable. (*Reproduced with permission from Richard P. Usatine, MD.*)

rare vasculitides in children of different ethnic origins. *Lancet.* 2002;360(9341):1197-1202.

4. Michel BA, Hunder GG, Bloch DA, Calabrese LH. Hypersensitivity vasculitis and Henoch-Schönlein purpura: a comparison between the 2 disorders. *J Rheumatol.* 1992;19:721.
5. Calabrese LH, Michel BA, Bloch DA, et al. The American College of Rheumatology 1990 criteria for the classification of hypersensitivity vasculitis. *Arthritis Rheum.* 1990;33:1108.
6. Sharma P, Sharma S, Baltaro R, Hurley J. Systemic vasculitis. *Am Fam Physician.* 2011;83(5):556-565.
7. Weiss PF. Pediatric vasculitis. *Pediatr Clin North Am.* 2012;59(2): 407-423.
8. Elston DM, Stratman EJ, Miller SJ. Skin biopsy: biopsy issues in specific diseases. *J Am Acad Dermatol.* 2016;74(1):1-16; quiz 17-18.
9. Sais G, Vidaller A, Jucgla A, et al. Colchicine in the treatment of cutaneous leukocytoclastic vasculitis. Results of a prospective, randomized controlled trial. *Arch Dermatol.* 1995;131:1399-1402.
10. Weiss PF, Feinstein JA, Luan X, et al. Effects of corticosteroid on Henoch-Schönlein purpura: a systematic review. *Pediatrics.* 2007;120:1079-1087.
11. Chen JY, Mao JH. Henoch-Schönlein purpura nephritis in children: incidence, pathogenesis and management. *World J Pediatr.* 2015;11(1):29-34.
12. Saulsbury FT. Henoch-Schönlein purpura. *Curr Opin Rheumatol.* 2001;13:35-40.
13. Roane DW, Griger DR. An approach to diagnosis and initial management of systemic vasculitis. *Am Fam Physician.* 1999;60: 1421-1430.

SECTION P CONNECTIVE TISSUE DISEASE

188 LUPUS: SYSTEMIC AND CUTANEOUS

Allison Pye, MD
E.J. Mayeaux, Jr., MD
Vineet Mishra, MD
Richard P. Usatine, MD

PATIENT STORY

A 22-year-old woman presents with a red rash on her face, chest, upper arms, and thighs for the past 6 days (**Figures 188-1** and **188-2**). She had been diagnosed with systemic lupus erythematosus (SLE) 5 years ago but has never had a skin rash like this before. This rash had some itching associated with it but was otherwise asymptomatic. Her original SLE diagnosis was made at age 17 when she presented with a deep venous thrombosis. Six days ago she was in the sun for an extended period of time while cycling. Later that day the rash became very red on her face and upper arms. She was given a Medrol Dosepak in a local urgent care without any benefit. She was experiencing fatigue but no fever or other systemic symptoms. Laboratory testing showed a very high antinuclear antibody (ANA) with a white blood cell count of 1.1. The patient was referred to rheumatology and dermatology. They started her on prednisone 60 mg daily, as a Medrol Dosepak has insufficient prednisolone for this severe flare of acute cutaneous lupus. The hydroxychloroquine of 400 mg daily was continued, but her azathioprine was discontinued to make sure it was not responsible for the low white blood cell count. The following week the patient's skin and fatigue were much improved. In reviewing her SLE diagnosis, she met 8 of 11 criteria for SLE (see **Table 188-1**).

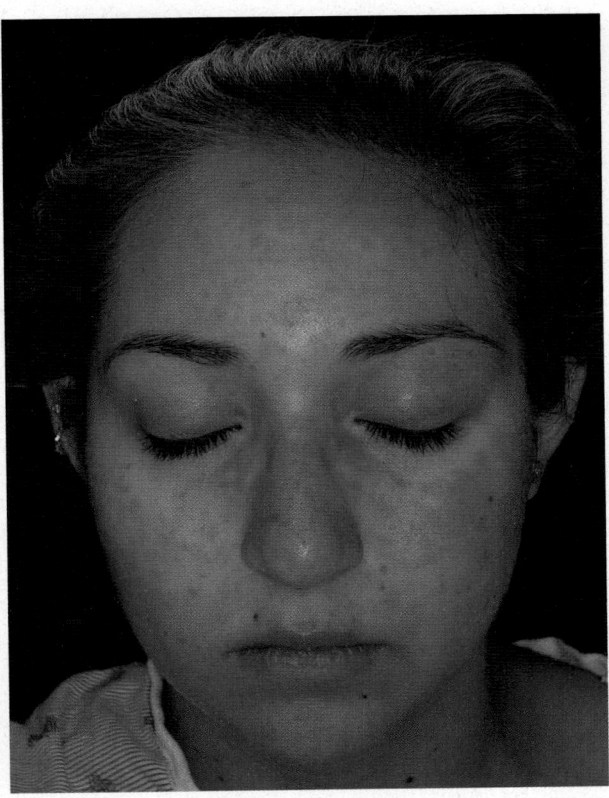

FIGURE 188-1 Malar and facial erythema and scale in a 22-year-old woman with a flare of acute cutaneous lupus. This patient has had SLE since age 17 and the flare occurred after extended sun exposure. Note how the flare is not just on the malar area. (*Reproduced with permission from Richard P. Usatine, MD.*)

INTRODUCTION

SLE is a chronic inflammatory disease that can affect many organs of the body, including the skin, joints, kidneys, lungs, nervous system, and mucous membranes. Cutaneous lupus can occur in one of three forms: chronic cutaneous lupus erythematosus/discoid lupus erythematosus (DLE), subacute cutaneous lupus erythematosus (SCLE), and acute cutaneous lupus erythematosus.

SYNONYMS

- Chronic cutaneous lupus erythematosus = discoid lupus = DLE.
- Lupus profundus = lupus panniculitis.

EPIDEMIOLOGY

- In the United States, the prevalence of SLE varies and is estimated to be 161,000 persons with definite SLE and 322,000 persons with

TABLE 188-1 American College of Rheumatology Criteria for Diagnosis of Systemic Lupus Erythematosus

Criterion	Definition
1. Malar rash	Fixed erythema, flat or raised, over the malar eminences, tending to spare the nasolabial folds
2. Discoid rash	Erythematosus-raised patches with adherent keratotic scaling and follicular plugging and later atrophic scarring
3. Photosensitivity	Skin rash as a result of unusual reaction to sunlight, by history or physician observation
4. Oral ulcers	Oral or nasopharyngeal ulceration, usually painless, observed by a physician
5. Arthritis	Nonerosive arthritis involving 2 or more peripheral joints, characterized by tenderness, swelling, or effusion
6. Serositis	Pleuritis—convincing history of pleuritic pain or rub heard by a physician or evidence of pleural effusion *or* pericarditis documented by ECG, rub, or evidence of pericardial effusion
7. Renal disorder	Persistent proteinuria greater than 0.5 g/day or greater than 3+ if quantitation not performed *or* red cell, hemoglobin, granular, tubular, or mixed cellular casts
8. Neurologic disorder	Seizures *or* psychosis—in the absence of offending drugs or known metabolic derangements (uremia, ketoacidosis, or electrolyte imbalance)
9. Hematologic disorder	Hemolytic anemia with reticulocytosis *or* leukopenia ($<4,000/mm^3$ on 2 or more occasions) *or* lymphopenia ($<1,500/mm^3$ on 2 or more occasions) *or* thrombocytopenia ($<100,000/mm^3$) in the absence of offending drugs
10. Immunologic disorders	Positive antiphospholipid antibody *or* anti-DNA antibody to native DNA in abnormal titer *or* anti-Smith antibody—presence of antibody to Smith nuclear antigen *or* false-positive serologic test for syphilis known to be positive for at least 6 months and confirmed by *Treponema pallidum* immobilization or fluorescent treponemal antibody absorption test
11. Antinuclear antibody	An abnormal titer of antinuclear antibody by immunofluorescence or an equivalent assay at any point in time and in the absence of drugs known to be associated with "drug-induced lupus" syndrome

SLE can be diagnosed if any 4 or more of the 11 criteria are present, serially or simultaneously, during any interval of observation.
Modified with permission from Callahan LF, Pincus T: Mortality in the rheumatic diseases, Arthritis Care Res. 1995;8(4):229-241.

indefinite or probable SLE.[1] Lupus more commonly affects women and patients with African-American ancestry.[1] Worldwide, SLE is thought to develop more frequently with more organ damage and higher mortality rates in Asian, Aboriginal, and African populations when compared to white individuals.[2]

- Discoid lupus erythematosus (DLE) develops in up to 25% of patients with SLE but can also occur in the absence of any other clinical feature of SLE.[3] Patients with disease limited to DLE have a 5% to 10% risk of developing SLE, which tends to follow a mild course in these cases.[4] DLE lesions usually slowly expand, with active inflammation at the periphery, and then heal, leaving depressed central scars, atrophy, telangiectasias, and hypopigmentation.[5] The female-to-male ratio of DLE is 2:1.

ETIOLOGY AND PATHOPHYSIOLOGY

- SLE is a multisystem autoimmune disease with variable presentations. A proposed mechanism for the etiology of SLE involves the development of autoantibodies that result from a defect in apoptosis. The specific defect involves the "find-me" (adenosine triphosphate [ATP]/uridine triphosphate [UTP]) or "eat-me" (phosphatidylserine) signals activated upon release of red cell nuclei. In the absence of apoptosis, the nuclei break down causing inflammation

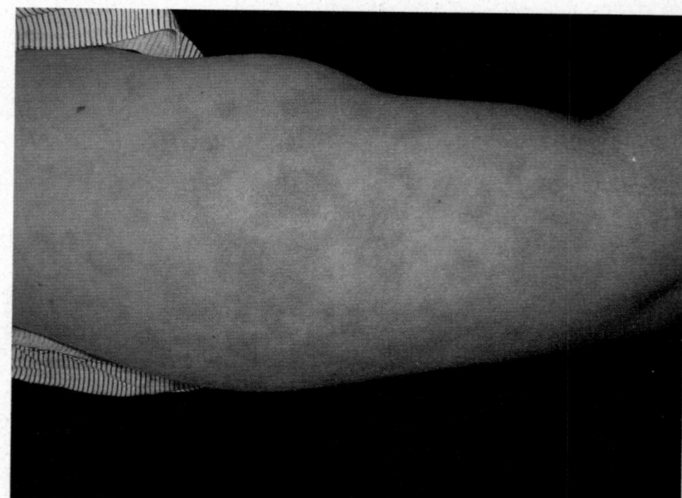

FIGURE 188-2 Reticular erythematous eruption on the upper arm of a 22-year-old woman experiencing acute cutaneous lupus. She had a similar eruption on the chest and upper thighs. (*Reproduced with permission from Richard P. Usatine, MD.*)

and contributing to the development of autoimmunity.[6] Many signs and symptoms of lupus erythematosus (LE) are caused by either circulating immune complexes or direct effects of antibodies on cells.

- A genetic predisposition for SLE exists. The concordance rate in monozygotic twins is between 25% and 70%. If a mother has SLE, her daughter's risk of developing the disease is 1:40 and her son's risk is 1:250.[7]
- The course of SLE consists of intermittent remissions punctuated by disease flares. Organ damage often progresses over time.
- Rarely, neonates may develop a lupus rash from antibodies acquired by transplacental transmission from a mother with active SLE (**Figure 188-3**).

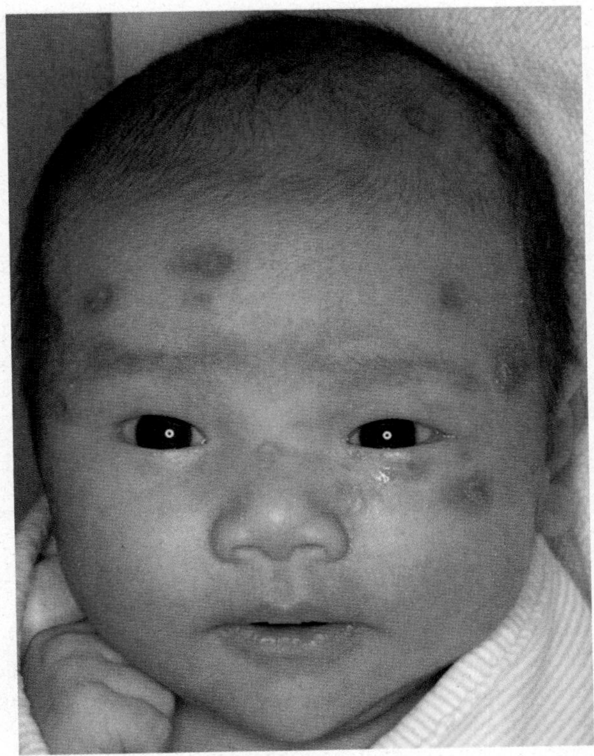

FIGURE 188-3 Neonatal lupus from acquired antibodies through transplacental transmission from a mother with active SLE. *(Reproduced with permission from Warner AM, Frey KA, Connolly S. Annular rash on a newborn. J Fam Pract. 2006;55(2):127-129. Frontline Medical Communications.*

RISK FACTORS

Precipitating factors for SLE include:

- Sun exposure (UV light, especially UVB).
- Infections.
- Stress.
- Trauma or surgery.
- Pregnancy (especially in the postpartum period).

Precipitating factors for cutaneous lupus include:

- Sun exposure (UV light, especially UVB).

DIAGNOSIS

CLINICAL FEATURES OF SYSTEMIC LUPUS ERYTHEMATOSUS

- SLE is a chronic, recurrent, and potentially fatal inflammatory disorder that can be difficult to diagnose. It is an autoimmune disease associated with antibodies directed against cell nuclei and can involve multiple organ systems. The disease has no single diagnostic sign or marker. Accurate diagnosis is important, as treatment can reduce morbidity and mortality.[8]
- SLE most often presents with a mixture of constitutional symptoms including fatigue, fever, myalgia, anorexia, nausea, and weight loss. Patients can present with symptoms so variable and nonspecific that diagnosis is often delayed for months to years.[9]
- The disease is characterized by exacerbations and remissions as well as intermittent aforementioned symptoms.
- The diagnosis of SLE is made if four or more of the manifestations mentioned below (and categorized in **Table 188-1**) have been present at some point or are present at time of presentation. Symptoms can occur serially or simultaneously. If two to three manifestations are present, some clinicians refer to the syndrome as "incomplete lupus."[10]
- Fatigue is the most common complaint of lupus patients and occurs in 80% to 100% of patients. It does not correlate with disease severity.[11]
- Over 50% of patients with SLE have fever, which can be a manifestation of active disease.[12] Fever of SLE must be distinguished from other causes of fever such as infection, drug reaction, or malignancy. Lupus related fever usually responds to nonsteroidal anti-inflammatory drugs (NSAIDs), acetaminophen, and/or glucocorticoids.

- Arthralgias are often the initial complaint and are usually disproportionate to physical findings. The polyarthritis is symmetric, nonerosive, and nondeforming. Long-standing disease can lead to rheumatoid-like deformities with swan-neck fingers.
- Fixed erythema, coined the "malar rash" or "butterfly rash," can occur over the cheeks and the bridge of the nose and spares the nasolabial folds (**Figures 188-2, 188-4,** and **188-5**). It may also involve the chin and ears. More severe malar rashes may cause severe atrophy, scarring, and hypopigmentation (see **Figure 188-5**).
- Patients can develop a rash associated with photosensitivity to UV light.
- A discoid rash consisting of erythematous plaques with adherent keratotic scaling and follicular plugging can occur. Atrophic scarring may occur in older lesions.
- Ulcers (usually painless) in the nose, mouth, or vagina are frequent complaints.
- Pleuritis, as evidenced by a convincing history of pleuritic chest pain/rub or evidence of pleural effusion, can also occur.
- Pericarditis is another manifestation and can be documented by ECG, auscultation of a friction rub, or evidence of pericardial effusion.
- Patients can develop renal impairment, characterized by cellular casts or persistent proteinuria greater than 0.5 g/day or greater than 3+ if quantitation is not performed.
- Central nervous system (CNS) symptoms of SLE range from mild cognitive dysfunction to psychosis or seizures. Any region of the CNS can be involved. The most common features of neurologic disease in patients with lupus are intractable headaches and difficulties with memory/reasoning.
- Lupus patients may also have hematologic disorders such as hemolytic anemia, leukopenia ($<4000/mm^3$ total on two or more occasions), lymphopenia ($<1500/mm^3$ on two or more occasions), or thrombocytopenia ($<100{,}000/mm^3$ in the absence of precipitating drugs).
- GI symptoms may include abdominal pain, diarrhea, and vomiting. Intestinal perforation and vasculitis are important diagnoses to exclude.
- Vasculitis (**Figures 188-6** to **188-8**) is a severe symptom and can include retinal vasculitis.
- Patients can have immunologic findings such as positive antiphospholipid antibodies, anti-DNA antibodies, anti-Smith antigens, or a false-positive serologic test for syphilis (known to be positive for at least 6 months and confirmed by a negative *Treponema*-specific test).
- An abnormal titer of ANA at any point in time, in the absence of drugs associated with "drug-induced lupus," is another manifestation of lupus.

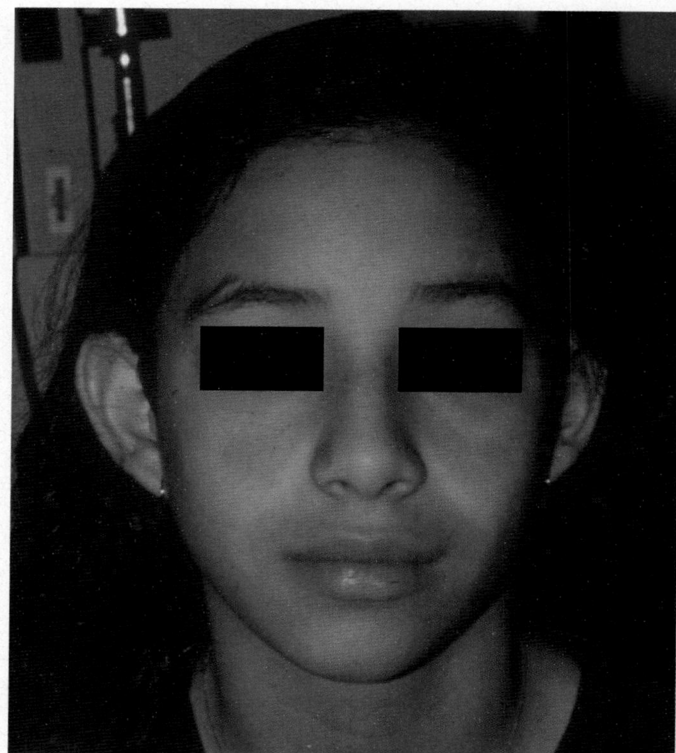

FIGURE 188-4 Malar rash in an adolescent Hispanic girl with SLE. Note the relative sparing of the nasolabial folds. (*Reproduced with permission from Richard P. Usatine, MD.*)

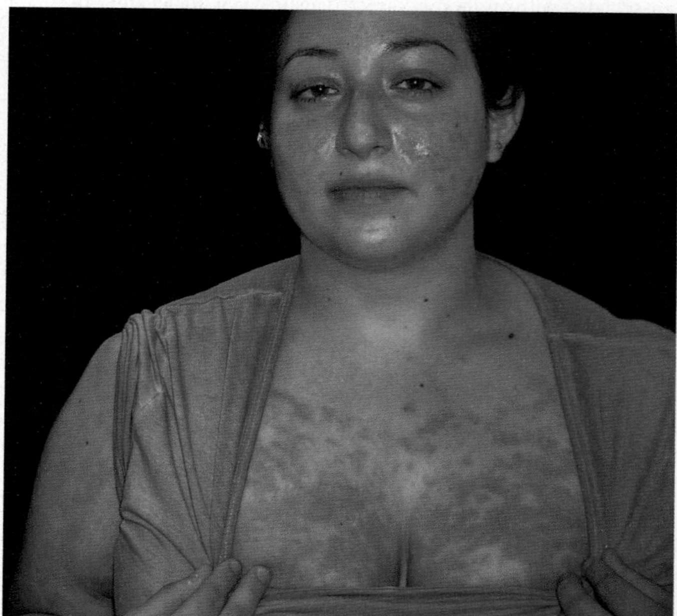

FIGURE 188-5 Malar rash and extensive skin erythema in a flare-up of acute cutaneous lupus in a young woman with SLE and active glomerulonephritis. (*Reproduced with permission from Richard P. Usatine, MD.*)

CLINICAL FEATURES OF CUTANEOUS LUPUS

Cutaneous lupus can be divided into three types:

1. Chronic cutaneous lupus (discoid lupus or DLE).
2. Subacute cutaneous lupus.
3. Acute cutaneous lupus (one of the criteria for SLE flare).

- Chronic cutaneous lupus (DLE) lesions are characterized by discrete, erythematous, slightly infiltrated papules or plaques covered by a well-formed adherent scale (**Figures 188-9** to **188-15**). As the

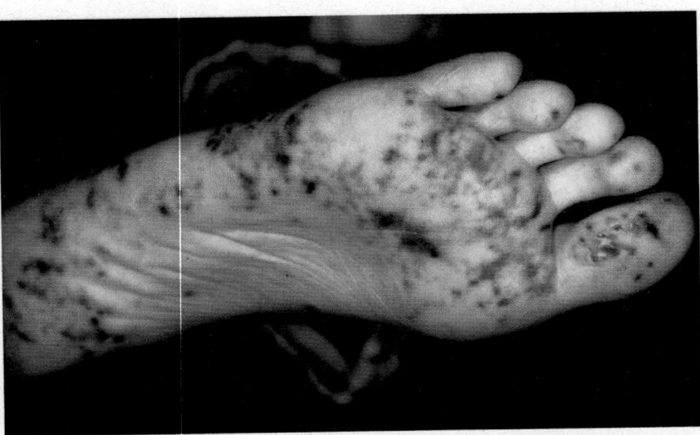

FIGURE 188-6 Necrotizing angiitis in a 28-year-old Japanese American woman with a severe lupus flare. Palpable purpura were evident on both feet and hands. (*Reproduced with permission from Richard P. Usatine, MD.*)

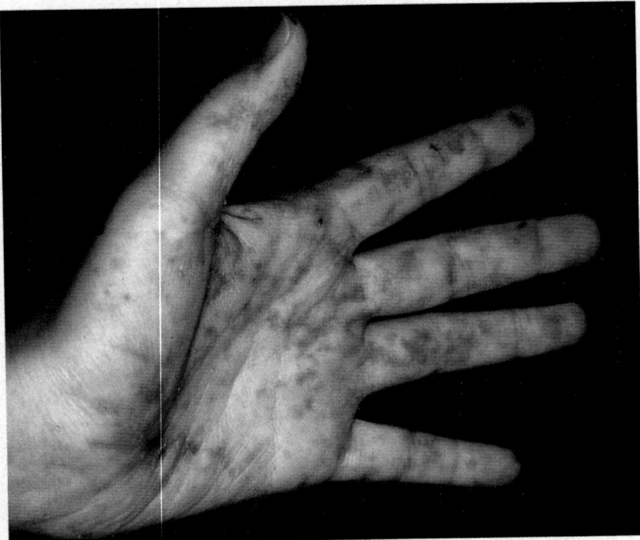

FIGURE 188-7 Necrotizing angiitis on the hand of the patient in **Figure 188-6** with lupus. (*Reproduced with permission from Richard P. Usatine, MD.*)

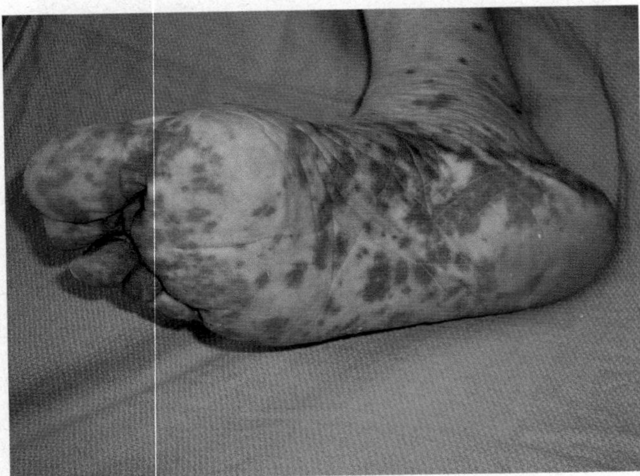

FIGURE 188-8 Leukocytoclastic vasculitis on the foot of a 69-year-old woman with systemic lupus. (*Reproduced with permission from Richard P. Usatine, MD.*)

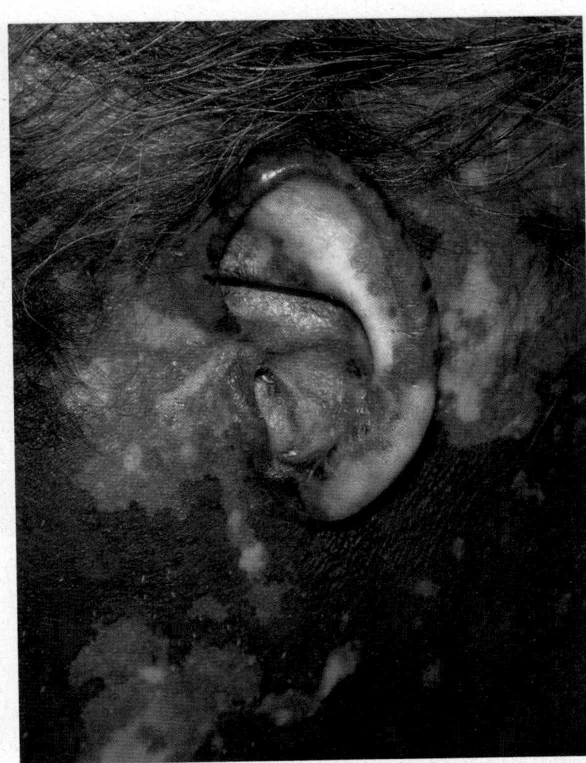

FIGURE 188-9 Discoid lupus in a middle-aged black man with hypopigmentation and scarring of the pinna. (*Reproduced with permission from Richard P. Usatine, MD.*)

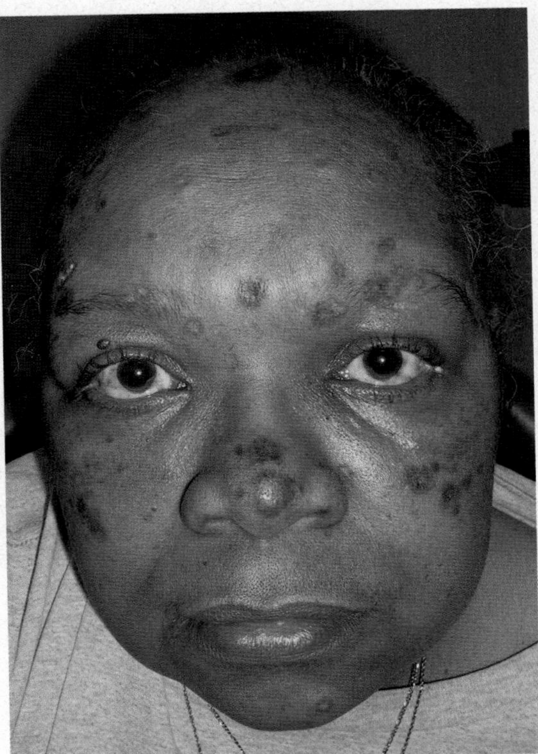

FIGURE 188-10 Discoid lupus on the face and scalp of a 56-year-old woman with hyperpigmented lesions that are indurated and atrophic. She also has similar lesions on the back and associated scarring alopecia. (*Reproduced with permission from Richard P. Usatine, MD.*)

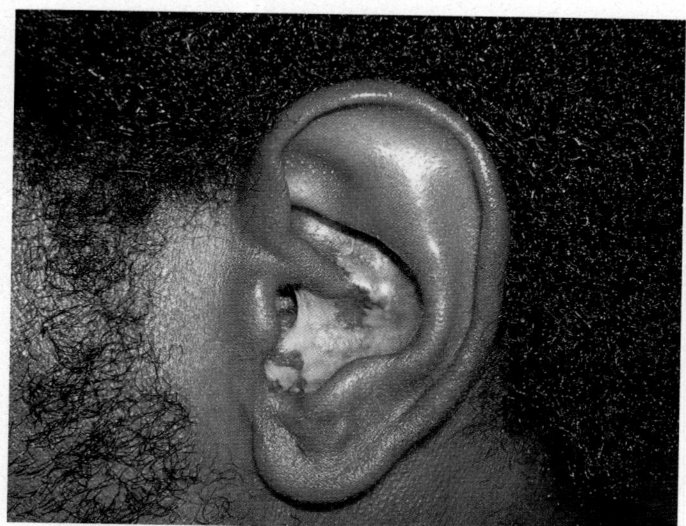

FIGURE 188-11 Discoid lupus with hypopigmentation and scarring inside the pinna. (*Reproduced with permission from E.J. Mayeaux, Jr., MD.*)

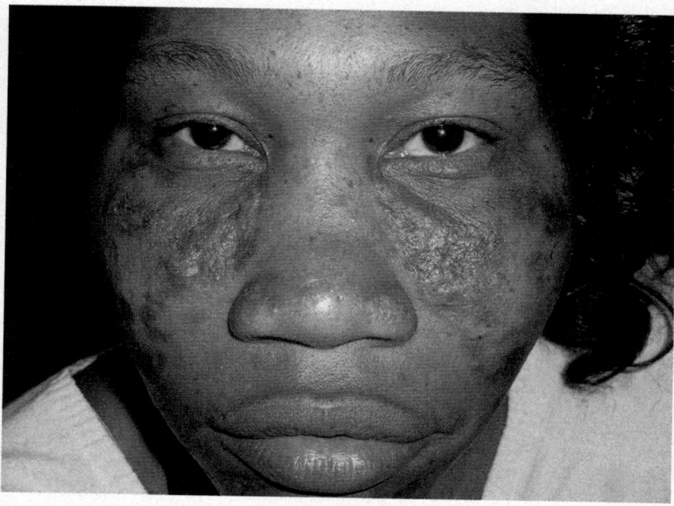

FIGURE 188-13 Severe discoid lupus in a malar distribution on the face of a 30-year-old woman. Note that this chronic cutaneous lupus has caused permanent scarring. (*Reproduced with permission from Richard P. Usatine, MD.*)

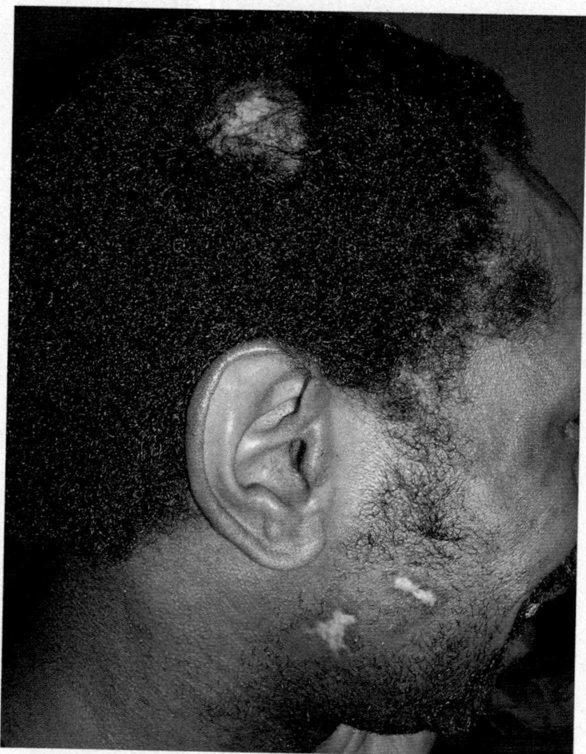

FIGURE 188-12 Discoid lupus with scarring alopecia and hypopigmentation on the scalp and face. (*Reproduced with permission from E.J. Mayeaux, Jr., MD.*)

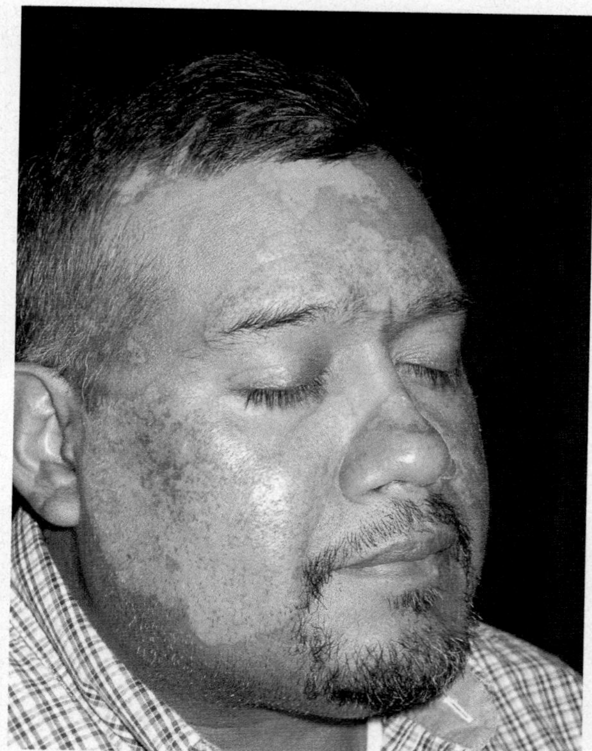

FIGURE 188-14 Chronic cutaneous lupus on the face of this Hispanic man with significant erythema and changes of skin coloration. (*Reproduced with permission from Richard P. Usatine, MD.*)

lesion progresses, the scale often thickens and adheres to the lesion. Hypopigmentation develops in the central area of the lesion and hyperpigmentation develops at the active border. Resolution of the active lesion results in atrophy and scarring. When lesions occur in the scalp, they often result in scarring alopecia (hair loss) (see **Figures 188-12** and **188-15**). Removing hair on the scalp may leave a "carpet tack sign" from follicular plugging.

- Subacute cutaneous lupus occurs most commonly in sun-exposed areas. Lesions can be erythematous with overlying scale and distinct borders, or lesions may be annular in shape (**Figure 188-16**). Photosensitivity explains the distribution of the lesions. These lesions do not scar or itch; however, they may leave postinflammatory hyperpigmentation upon healing.
- Acute cutaneous lupus is a term for the cutaneous manifestations of systemic lupus, such as the malar rash (also called the "butterfly rash"; see **Figure 188-4**). This rash may heal without scarring.
- Raynaud phenomenon, libido reticularis, and palmar erythema also occur in persons with lupus (**Figure 188-17**). Cold weather can exacerbate all three conditions.

TYPICAL DISTRIBUTION

- Discoid lesions are most often seen on the face, neck, and scalp. They also occur on the ears and infrequently on the upper torso.
- DLE lesions may be localized or widespread. Localized DLE occurs only in the head and neck area, whereas widespread DLE occurs anywhere. Patients with widespread involvement are more likely to develop SLE.
- Subacute cutaneous lupus lesions are most commonly found in the sun-exposed areas of the face, neck, and arms (see **Figure 188-16**).
- Acute cutaneous lupus is generally seen in the malar distribution, sparing the nasolabial folds, but it can occur on other parts of the body.
- Lupus panniculitis, or lupus profundus, is a lupus variant that primarily affects subcutaneous fat. It usually involves the proximal extremities, trunk, breasts, buttocks, and face (**Figure 188-18**).

LABORATORY TESTING

- The American College of Rheumatology recommends ANA testing in patients who have two or more unexplained signs or symptoms suggestive of lupus. Elevation of the ANA titer to or above 1:80 is the most sensitive of the American College of Rheumatology diagnostic criteria. Although many patients may have a negative ANA titer early in the disease, more than 99% of SLE patients will eventually have an elevated ANA titer.[13] The ANA test is not specific for lupus, and the most common reason for a positive ANA test without SLE (usually at titers <1:80) is the presence of another connective tissue disease. ANA titers are useful in screening and diagnosis but not in monitoring disease activity. Specific antibodies used in confirming the diagnosis include anti–double-stranded DNA (anti-dsDNA) and anti-Smith antibodies.
- Active SLE is often signaled by a rise in immunoglobulin (Ig) G anti-dsDNA titers and/or a fall in complement levels.[14]
- Patients with only discoid lupus erythematosus generally have negative or low-titer ANA titers, but approximately 70% of these patients have low-titer anti-Ro/SSA antibodies.[15]

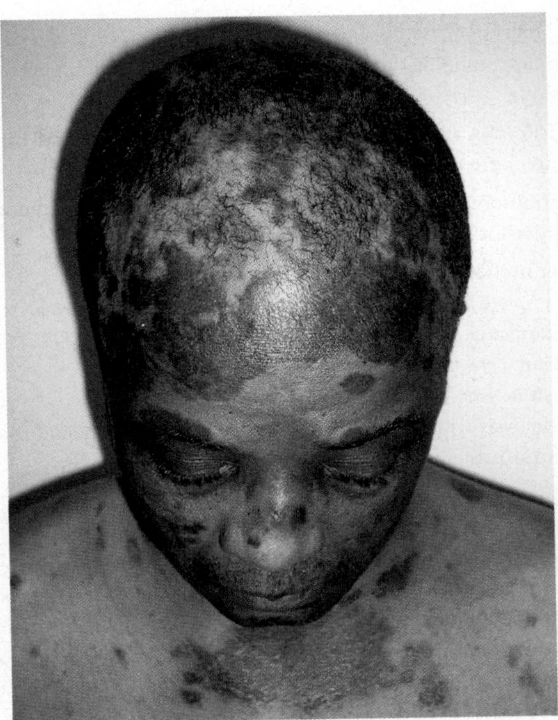

FIGURE 188-15 Severe chronic cutaneous lupus with hyperpigmentation, hypopigmentation, and scarring alopecia. Sun-exposed areas of the face and neck are heavily involved. (*Reproduced with permission from Richard P. Usatine, MD.*)

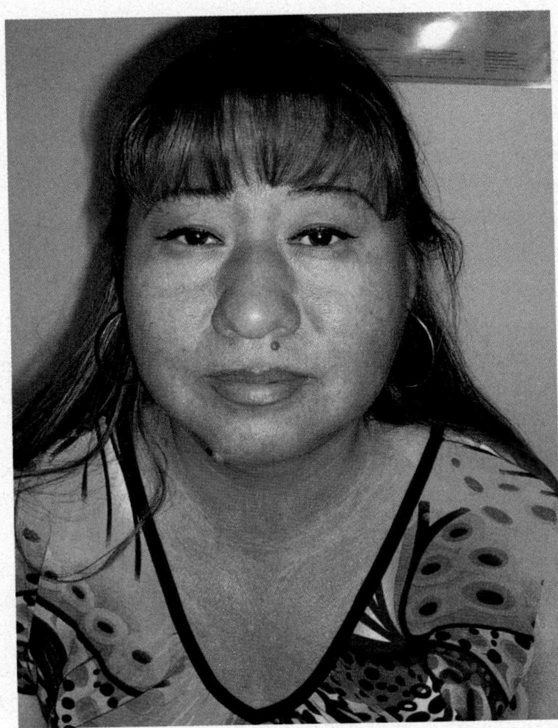

FIGURE 188-16 Subacute cutaneous lupus in a 47-year-old woman in sun-exposed areas of the face and V-neck. This all started after hydrochlorothiazide was initiated for hypertension. Biopsy revealed the diagnosis; the differential diagnosis includes a photosensitivity reaction related to the hydrochlorothiazide. (*Reproduced with permission from Richard P. Usatine, MD.*)

- Anti-dsDNA antibodies are highly specific and sensitive for SLE.
- Anti-Sm antibodies are highly specific for SLE but not highly sensitive.
- Anti-Ro/SSA and anti-La/SSB antibodies may be present with SLE but are more commonly associated with Sjögren syndrome.
- Antiribosomal P-protein antibodies are highly specific but not very sensitive for SLE.
- Other useful lab tests include:
  - Complete blood count and differential, which may reveal leukopenia, anemia, and/or thrombocytopenia
  - Serum creatinine, which may be suggestive of renal dysfunction
  - Urinalysis with urine sediment, which may reveal hematuria, pyuria, proteinuria, and/or cellular casts

BIOPSY

A biopsy is warranted to confirm the diagnosis even if the pattern seems typical, and a 4-mm punch biopsy provides adequate tissue for pathology. Biopsy confirmation is particularly helpful before initiation of potentially toxic medications. Common histopathologic features of most forms of cutaneous lupus include hyperkeratosis, epidermal atrophy, degeneration of the basal layer of the epidermis, superficial, perivascular and perifollicular mononuclear cell infiltrates, basement membrane thickening, and pigment incontinence.[16]

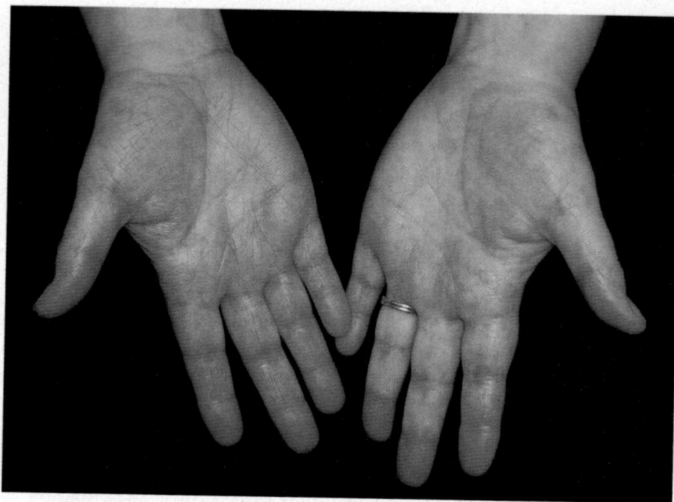

FIGURE 188-17 Palmar erythema in this young woman with SLE and an ANA of 1:640. (*Reproduced with permission from Richard P. Usatine, MD.*)

DIFFERENTIAL DIAGNOSIS

- Drug-induced lupus is a lupus-like syndrome most strongly associated with procainamide, hydralazine, isoniazid, chlorpromazine, methyldopa, and quinidine.
- Scleroderma presents with thickening of the skin and multisystem sclerosis (see Chapter 190, Scleroderma and Morphea).
- Actinic keratosis on the face may become confluent but lacks the systemic symptoms of lupus (see Chapter 173, Actinic Keratosis and Bowen Disease).
- Dermatomyositis presents with facial swelling, a "heliotrope" rash around the eyes, Gottron papules, periungual erythema in the hands, and proximal muscle "limb-girdle" weakness. It is often associated with internal malignancy (see Chapter 189, Dermatomyositis).
- Lichen planus produces a rash associated with the "Ps": polygonal, pruritic, purple, and papular (see Chapter 160, Lichen Planus).
- Psoriasis exhibits silver-white plaques that cover the elbows, knees, scalp, back, or vulva. Psoriasis may also involve the scalp and nails (see Chapter 158, Psoriasis).
- Rosacea is associated with midfacial erythema, papules, and pustules without the systemic symptoms of SLE and usually involves the nasolabial folds (see Chapter 119, Rosacea).
- Sarcoidosis may produce skin plaques—without the central clearing and atrophy of DLE (see Chapter 184, Sarcoidosis).
- Syphilis can present with a plaque-like rash often confused with DLE. The short course of the disease and serologic testing can

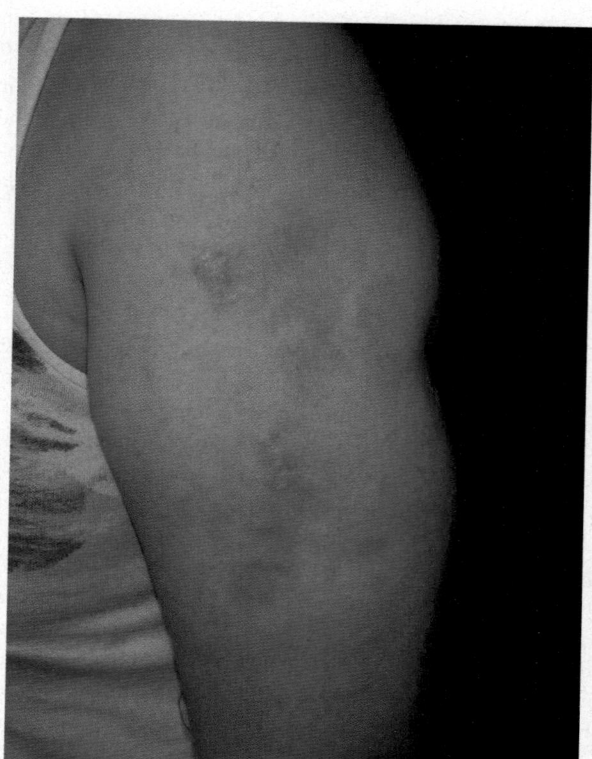

FIGURE 188-18 Lupus profundus showing localized atrophic changes of the arm secondary to panniculitis. This young woman also has lupus profundus on her face and other arm. The atrophy has been present for more than 1 year despite treatment. (*Reproduced with permission from Richard P. Usatine, MD.*)

distinguish these diseases; however, lupus autoantibodies may produce a false-positive screening test for syphilis (see Chapter 225, Syphilis).

MANAGEMENT

NONPHARMACOLOGIC

- Because UV light can flare SLE, use of sunscreen that blocks both UVA and UVB light should be encouraged (SOR A).

MEDICATIONS

▶ Topical

FIRST LINE

- Topical and intralesional corticosteroids are the mainstay of therapy for skin manifestations and avoid the side effects of systemic corticosteroids; however, cutaneous side effects can occur. High-potency steroids are often necessary, and their use on the face may be warranted in discoid lupus. Patients need to be cautioned and instructed to monitor for development of cutaneous side effects. Intralesional triamcinolone acetonide injections can be very effective for active discoid lupus lesions and can be repeated monthly while lesions are active (Grade B).[17]
- Intralesional triamcinolone acetonide should be diluted to match the area of involvement, with lower concentrations for the face. For example, an intralesional injection on the face may call for concentrations of 3–5 mg/mL, whereas one on the scalp could require a concentration of 5–10 mg/mL.

SECOND LINE

- Patients may benefit from trials of topical calcineurin inhibitors or topical retinoids if corticosteroids fail (Grade C).[17]

▶ Systemic

FIRST LINE

- Conservative management with NSAIDs or cyclooxygenase-2 selective inhibitors is recommended for arthritis, arthralgias, and myalgias of SLE (Grade B).[18]
- Antimalarial drugs (hydroxychloroquine [Plaquenil] 200 mg bid, maximum 5 mg/kg of real weight per day)[19] are recommended for skin manifestations and musculoskeletal complaints that do not adequately respond to NSAIDs. They may also prevent major damage to the kidneys and CNS and reduce the risk of disease flares (Grade B).[20] The maximum recommended dose of hydroxychloroquine is 400 mg per day to prevent retinopathy. If the patient tolerates the hydroxychloroquine, an ophthalmology referral should be made for a baseline retinal exam. Yearly screening for retinopathy should start after 5 years of therapy or sooner if there are any risk factors for earlier disease.[19]

SECOND LINE

- Systemic glucocorticoids (1 to 2 mg/kg per day of prednisone or equivalent) are helpful alone or with immunosuppressive agents in patients with significant renal and CNS disease or any other organ-threatening manifestation (Grade B). Lower doses of glucocorticoids (prednisone 10 to 20 mg/day) assist with symptomatic relief of severe or unresponsive musculoskeletal symptoms. In severe, life-threatening situations, methylprednisolone boluses (1 g IV/day) can be given for 3 consecutive days.[21] The goal is to avoid using prednisone long term or to use doses lower than 7.5 mg daily to avoid osteoporosis.
- Immunosuppressive medications (e.g., methotrexate, cyclophosphamide, azathioprine, mycophenolate, sulfasalazine, clofazimine, or rituximab) are generally reserved for patients with significant organ involvement or for those patients who have had an inadequate response to glucocorticoids (Grade B).[17,22]
- Belimumab (10 mg/kg IV every 2 weeks for 3 doses, then every 4 weeks) may be used in patients with active SLE who are not responding to standard therapy, such as NSAIDs, glucocorticoids, antimalarials, and/or immunosuppressives.[23]

OTHER TREATMENTS

- Patients with thrombosis, usually associated with the presence of antiphospholipid antibodies, require anticoagulation with warfarin (target international normalized ratio [INR] of 3–3.5 for arterial thrombosis and 2–3 for venous thrombosis).[24]
- DLE therapy includes corticosteroids (topical or intralesional) and antimalarials (Grade C). Other therapeutic options include auranofin, oral or topical retinoids, and immunosuppressive agents.[25]

PREVENTION

- There are no known methods for preventing discoid or systemic lupus. Avoiding precipitating factors such as sun exposure may decrease exacerbations and flares.

PROGNOSIS

- SLE can have a varied clinical course, ranging from a relatively benign illness to a rapidly progressive disease with organ failure and death. Most patients have a relapsing and remitting course.
- Poor prognostic factors for survival in SLE include[12]:
  - Renal disease (especially diffuse proliferative glomerulonephritis)
  - Hypertension
  - Male sex
  - Young age
  - Older age at presentation
  - Poor socioeconomic status
  - Black race
  - Presence of antiphospholipid antibodies
  - Antiphospholipid syndrome
  - High overall disease activity

FOLLOW-UP

- Patients should have regular follow-up appointments to monitor for and attempt to prevent end-organ damage. These visits are needed to monitor medication benefits and side effects and to coordinate the patient's overall care.

PATIENT EDUCATION

- Educate the patient on the necessity of protection from the sun, as UV exposure can cause lupus flares. Patients should use sunscreen, preferably one that blocks both UVA and UVB, with a minimum skin protection factor (SPF) of 30.
- Because cigarette smoking may increase the risk of developing SLE and smokers generally have more active disease, smokers with SLE should receive counseling on smoking cessation. Smoking has also been shown to decrease the effectiveness of hydroxychloroquine in patients with cutaneous lupus.[26]
- Patients should report any signs of superinfection of SLE-associated skin rashes or manifestations, as superinfections require antibiotic therapy.
- Sulfa drugs, which can cause lupus flares, should be avoided when possible.

PATIENT RESOURCES

- PubMed Health. *Systemic Lupus Erythematosus*—**http://www.ncbi.nlm.nih.gov/pubmedhealth/PMHT0024510/.**
- Mayo Clinic. *Lupus*—**http://www.mayoclinic.org/diseases-conditions/lupus/symptoms-causes/syc-20365789.**
- Womenshealth.gov. *Lupus Fact Sheet*—**https://www.womenshealth.gov/lupus.**
- Lupus Foundation—**http://www.lupus.org.**

PROVIDER RESOURCES

- Medscape. *Systemic Lupus Erythematosus (SLE)*—**http://emedicine.medscape.com/article/332244.**
- Medscape. *Discoid Lupus Erythematosus*—**http://emedicine.medscape.com/article/1065529.**

REFERENCES

1. Lawrence RC, Felson DT, Helmick CG, et al. Estimates of the prevalence of arthritis and other rheumatic conditions in the United States: Part II. *Arthritis Rheum.* 2008;58(1):26-35.
2. Carter EE, et al. The global burden of SLE: prevalence, health disparities and socioeconomic impact. *Nat Rev Rheumatol.* 2016; 12(10):605-620.
3. Pistiner M, Wallace DJ, Nessim S, et al. Lupus erythematosus in the 1980s: a survey of 570 patients. *Semin Arthritis Rheum.* 1991; 21(1):55-64.
4. Healy E, Kieran E, Rogers S. Cutaneous lupus erythematosus—a study of clinical and laboratory prognostic factors in 65 patients. *Ir J Med Sci.* 1995;164(2):113-115.
5. Rowell NR. Laboratory abnormalities in the diagnosis and management of lupus erythematosus. *Br J Dermatol.* 1971;84(3):210-216.
6. Nagata S, Hanayama R, Kawane K. Autoimmunity and the clearance of dead cells. *Cell.* 2010;140(5):619-630.
7. Lamont DW. Systemic lupus erythematosus. *eMedicine* . www.emedicine.com/emerg/topic564.htm. Accessed January 2017.
8. Gill JM, Quisel AM, Rocca PV, Walters DT. Diagnosis of systemic lupus erythematosus. *Am Fam Physician.* 2003;68(11):2179-2186. Accessed January 2017.
9. Bartels CM, et al. Systemic lupus erythematosus (SLE) treatment & management. *Medscape.* http://emedicine.medscape.com/article/332244-treatment#d1.
10. Hochberg MC. Updating the American College of Rheumatology revised criteria for the classification of SLE [letter]. *Arthritis Rheum.* 1997;40(9):1725.
11. Iaboni A, Ibanez D, Gladman DD, et al. Fatigue in systemic lupus erythematosus: contributions of disordered sleep, sleepiness, and depression. *J Rheumatol.* 2006;33:2453.
12. Cervera R, Khamashta MA, Font J, et al; European Working Party on Systemic Lupus Erythematosus. Morbidity and mortality in systemic lupus erythematosus during a 10-year period: a comparison of early and late manifestations in a cohort of 1,000 patients. *Medicine (Baltimore).* 2003;82(5):299-308.
13. Tan EM, Cohen AS, Fries JF, et al. The 1982 revised criteria for the classification of systemic lupus erythematosus. *Arthritis Rheum.* 1982;25(11):1271-1277.
14. Kao AH, Navratil JS, Ruffing MJ, et al. Erythrocyte C3d and C4d for monitoring disease activity in systemic lupus erythematosus. *Arthritis Rheum.* 2010;62(3):837-844.
15. Provost TT. The relationship between discoid and systemic lupus erythematosus. *Arch Dermatol.* 1994;130(10):1308-1310.
16. Lee HJ, Sinha AA. Cutaneous lupus erythematosus: understanding of clinical features, genetic basis, and pathobiology of disease guides therapeutic strategies. *Autoimmunity.* 2006; 39:433.
17. Lee LA, Werth VP: Lupus erythematosus. In: *Dermatology*, 3rd ed, vol 1. Philadelphia, PA: Elsevier Saunders; 2012:615-629.
18. Lander SA, Wallace DJ, Weisman MH. Celecoxib for systemic lupus erythematosus: case series and literature review of the use of NSAIDs in SLE. *Lupus.* 2002;11(6):340-347.
19. Marmor MF, Kellner U, Lai TY, et al; American Academy of Ophthalmology. Recommendations on screening for chloroquine and hydroxychloroquine retinopathy (2016 revision). *Ophthalmology.* 2016;123(6):1386-1394.
20. Fessler BJ, Alarcon GS, McGwin G Jr, et al; LUMINA Study Group. Systemic lupus erythematosus in three ethnic groups: XVI. Association of hydroxychloroquine use with reduced risk of damage accrual. *Arthritis Rheum.* 2005;52(5):1473-1480.
21. Parker BJ, Bruce IN. High dose methylprednisolone therapy for the treatment of severe systemic lupus erythematosus. *Lupus.* 2007; 16(6):387-393.

22. Fortin PR, Abrahamowicz M, Ferland D, et al; Canadian Network For Improved Outcomes in Systemic Lupus. Steroid-sparing effects of methotrexate in systemic lupus erythematosus: a double-blind, randomized, placebo-controlled trial. *Arthritis Rheum.* 2008;59(12):1796-1884.
23. FDA news release. *FDA Approves Benlysta to Treat Lupus.* www.fda.gov/NewsEvents/Newsroom/PressAnnouncements/ucm246489.htm. Accessed February 2012.
24. Erkan D, Lockshin MD. New treatments for antiphospholipid syndrome. *Rheum Dis Clin North Am.* 2006;32(1):129-148.
25. Eastham ABW, et al. Discoid lupus erythematosus treatment & management. *Medscape.* http://emedicine.medscape.com/article/1065529-treatment. Accessed January 2017.
26. Chasset F, Francès C, Barete S, et al. Influence of smoking on the efficacy of antimalarials in cutaneous lupus: a meta-analysis of the literature. *J Am Acad Dermatol.* 2015;72(4):634-639.

189 DERMATOMYOSITIS

Jordan E. Buckley, MD
Margaret L. Burks, MD
Anna Allred, MD
Richard P. Usatine, MD

PATIENT STORY

A 55-year-old Hispanic woman presents to her family physician with a diffuse rash and increasing muscle weakness. The initial rash (without weakness) 2 months prior was thought to be a photosensitivity reaction to her new hydrochlorothiazide (HCTZ) prescription. She stopped the HCTZ and the rash initially improved with some topical corticosteroids. At the time of her current presentation, she had trouble getting up from a chair, walking, and lifting her arms over her head. The rash was prominent in sun-exposed areas, but was also seen in a shawl-like distribution in non–sun-exposed areas (**Figure 189-1**). Aside from her hypertension and obesity, the patient did not have any previous chronic medical conditions. She was afebrile with no other pertinent findings on physical exam.

This is a classic presentation of dermatomyositis with the typical rash and proximal muscle weakness. Close attention to the rash around her eyes demonstrates the pathognomonic heliotrope rash of dermatomyositis (**Figures 189-2** and **189-3**). The patient also has Gottron papules on the fingers, seen best in this case over the proximal interphalangeal (PIP) joint of the third finger (**Figure 189-4**). There was periungual erythema and ragged cuticles. The scalp was red and scaly. Her neurologic exam was consistent with proximal myopathy. She also had some trouble swallowing bread; and dysphagia is not unusual in dermatomyositis. Laboratory tests showed mild elevations in muscle enzymes with the aspartate transaminase (AST) having the greatest elevation. In other cases, the creatine kinase (CK) can be very elevated.

The family physician started the patient on 60 mg of prednisone daily and topical steroids for the affected areas. The patient responded well to prednisone and 2 weeks later was feeling stronger and the rash was fading (**Figure 189-5**). After 4 weeks of 60 mg/day of prednisone she was started on 10 mg/wk of methotrexate in order to eventually taper her steroids. The patient has continued to do well, but the rash and muscle weakness tend to recur when her steroids are being tapered. The patient was sent for physical therapy and started on calcium and vitamin D supplementation to protect her from steroid-induced osteoporosis. She was also given 1 mg/day of folic acid to minimize the adverse effects of methotrexate. As dermatomyositis may be precipitated by an underlying malignancy, the physician screened the patient for internal cancers, especially ovarian cancer. Fortunately, the mammogram, Papanicolaou (Pap) smear, colonoscopy, transvaginal ultrasound for ovarian imaging, and abdominal/pelvic CT scans were all normal.

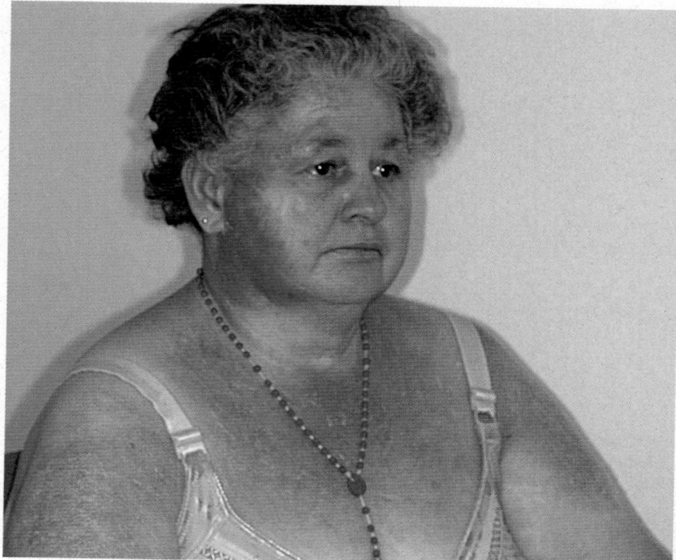

FIGURE 189-1 Initial presentation of dermatomyositis in a 55-year-old Hispanic woman. Prominent violaceous erythema with scale is visible on the chest, face, and arms. Deep-red erythema is especially visible on the side of the face. The scalp is red and scaling. (*Reproduced with permission from Richard P. Usatine, MD.*)

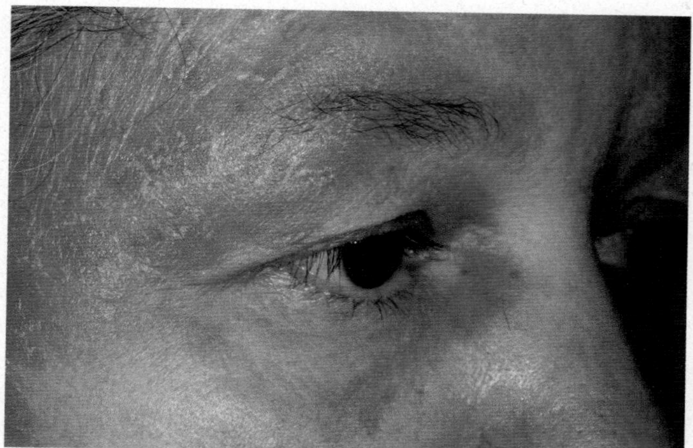

FIGURE 189-2 Close-up of the heliotrope (violaceous) rash around the eyes of the patient in **Figure 189-1**. (*Reproduced with permission from Richard P. Usatine, MD.*)

INTRODUCTION

Dermatomyositis is a rare, idiopathic inflammatory disease involving the striated muscles and the skin. The disease is characterized by progressive, symmetric, proximal muscle weakness. Dermatologic manifestations may occur with or without muscular disease and include the characteristic heliotrope rash (**Figures 189-2, 189-3, 189-5,** and **189-6**), "shawl sign," and Gottron papules of the PIP joints. Although primarily a disease of muscle and skin, dermatomyositis has a clear association with calcinosis, myocarditis, and interstitial lung disease, as well as an increased risk of underlying malignancy.

EPIDEMIOLOGY

- Annual incidence of 5 to 8.9 per 1 million population.[1]
- Seen more commonly in women.[1]
- Bimodal age distribution, most commonly affecting adults 45–64 years old and much less commonly children 5–14 years old; however, any age can be affected.[1]
- 35% to 40% of patients with dermatomyositis also have interstitial lung disease (ILD). It is the most common internal organ manifestation of the disease and greatly affects morbidity and mortality.[1,2]
- Has been linked to malignancy in up to 15% to 24% of adults.[3]
- Cancers most commonly associated are breast, ovarian, lung, GI tract, and hematologic.[4] The most common type of cancer is adenocarcinoma. Ovarian cancer is overrepresented in those patients with dermatomyositis and cancer. Cancer is not typically seen in children with dermatomyositis.
- Risk factors for malignancy include age over 45, male sex, and the presence of specific autoantibodies. TIF-1γ autoantibodies have been associated with increased risk, as well as anti-p155 autoantibodies, which have shown a 27-fold increase in odds.[5,6]
- Certain cutaneous manifestations have also been found to be risk factors for underlying malignancy. The finding of skin necrosis has the strongest association, with a twofold increase in odds. The presence of skin ulcerations has also been associated with increased risk.[7]
- Several protective factors have been identified. Younger age, TIF-1γ and p155 antibody–negative status, and concurrent ILD are associated with a lower risk of occult malignancy.[8]

ETIOLOGY AND PATHOPHYSIOLOGY

- Dermatomyositis is considered an autoimmune disease of unknown etiology. Environmental exposure and infectious agents may play a role in disease pathogenesis.
- Dermatomyositis has been shown to be a microangiopathy that affects the skin and muscle. The muscle weakness and skin manifestations may be a result of activation and deposition of complement, which cause lysis of endomysial capillaries and muscle ischemia.

DIAGNOSIS

- Diagnosis includes 5 criteria and may be categorized as: "definite" (skin findings plus any 3 of criteria 1 to 4), "probable" (skin

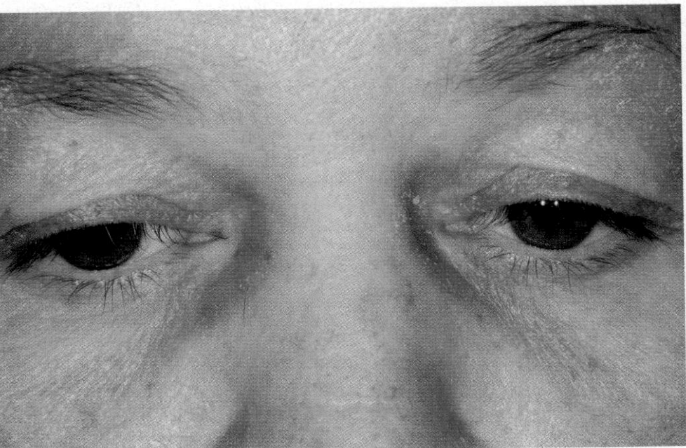

FIGURE 189-3 View showing the bilateral heliotrope rash of the patient in **Figure 189-1**. A pathognomonic sign of dermatomyositis. *(Reproduced with permission from Richard P. Usatine, MD.)*

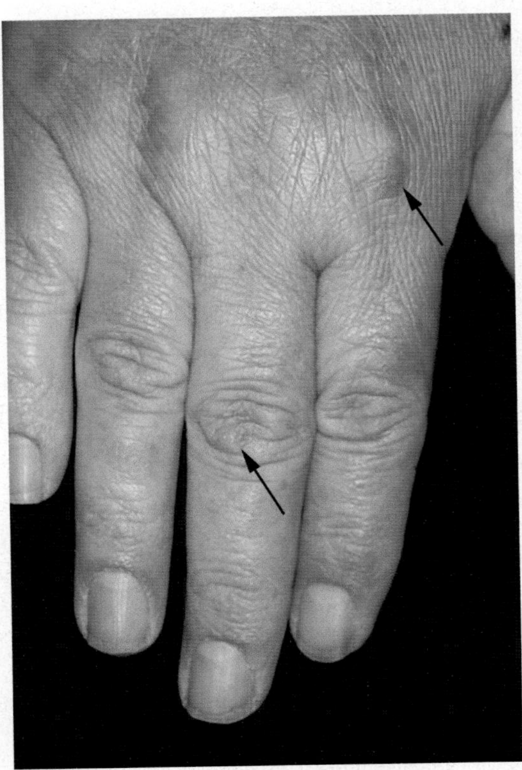

FIGURE 189-4 Hand involvement showing two Gottron papules over the knuckles (*arrows*) and erythematous nail folds (periungual erythema) in the patient in **Figure 189-1**. (*Reproduced with permission from Richard P. Usatine, MD.)*

findings plus 2 of any criteria 1 to 4), or "possible" (skin findings plus any 1 of criteria 1 to 4).[2,9,10]

- *Skin findings—The heliotrope rash and Gottron papules are considered pathognomonic (**Figures 189-2** to **189-8**). Nonpathognomonic manifestations include malar erythema and periungual and cuticular changes (**Figure 189-9**).*
    1. Proximal symmetric muscle weakness that progresses over weeks to months.
    2. Elevated serum levels of muscle enzymes (CK, AST, lactate dehydrogenase [LDH] and aldolase).
    3. Abnormal electromyogram (EMG).
    4. Abnormal muscle biopsy with muscle necrosis or inflammatory infiltrate.
- These criteria are still considered the "gold standard," although they are old (1975) and currently under critical review because of several limitations. Expanded criteria have been proposed that include MRI findings in the thigh muscles and specific autoantibodies.[2,8,11,12]

Recent studies indicate that the finding of dilated nail-fold capillary loops (**Figure 189-10**) often seen in patients with dermatomyositis may assist in earlier diagnosis and predicting patients with poor prognosis. Dilated nail-fold capillary loops have shown promise in juvenile dermatomyositis as a marker for both skin and muscle disease activity to guide treatment. Some authors propose adding this finding to criteria for diagnosis.[13,14]

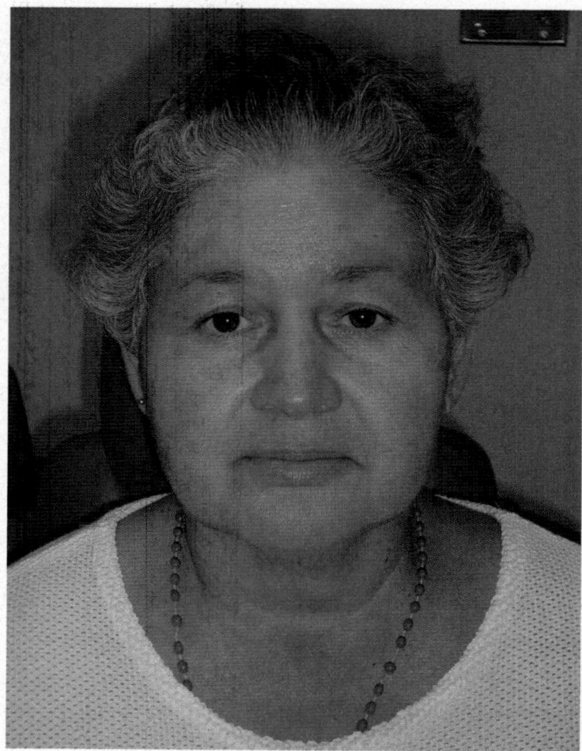

FIGURE 189-5 Patient improving after 2 weeks of oral prednisone. The heliotrope rash is still visible around the eyes and upper chest. The hairline erythema is from scalp involvement. (*Reproduced with permission from Richard P. Usatine, MD.*)

CLINICAL FEATURES

- Bilateral periorbital heliotrope erythema (pathognomonic) (see **Figures 189-2**, **189-3**, **189-5**, and **189-6**) and scaling violaceous papular dermatitis in a patient complaining of proximal muscle weakness points to dermatomyositis.
- The patient may classically complain of difficulty climbing stairs, rising from a seat, or combing their hair. Notably the skin manifestations may precede, follow, or present simultaneously with muscle involvement; a patient may even have skin manifestations for longer than a year prior to developing muscle weakness.
- Hand involvement includes abnormal nail folds and Gottron papules. "Moth-eaten" cuticles, also called the Samitz sign, are evidenced by periungual erythema and telangiectasias (see **Figures 189-7** to **189-9**).
- Gottron papules, smooth, purple-to-red papules and plaques, are classically located over the knuckles and on the sides of fingers (see **Figures 189-4**, **189-7**, and **189-8**). Plaques may be present over the knuckles instead of or in addition to papules. The papules are especially evident in juvenile-onset dermatomyositis (see **Figure 189-8**).
- Dysphagia can be present as a consequence of pharyngeal muscle involvement with risk of aspiration and pneumonia.
- Patients with concurrent interstitial lung disease may also present with fatigue, cough, dyspnea on exertion, and decreased exercise tolerance. Lung involvement usually appears following symptoms of myositis, although this is not always the case.[2]

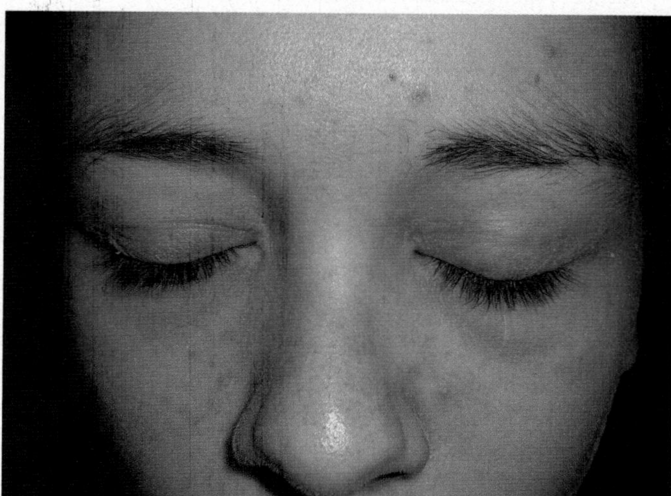

FIGURE 189-6 Classic heliotrope rash around the eyes of this 19-year-old woman newly diagnosed with dermatomyositis. The color "heliotrope" is a pink-purple tint named after the color of the heliotrope flower. As expected, her heliotrope rash is bilaterally symmetrical. This rash resolved on prednisone and hydroxychloroquine. (*Reproduced with permission from Goodall J, Usatine RP. Skin rash and muscle weakness, J Fam Pract. 2005;54(10):864-868. Frontline Medical Communications, Inc.*)

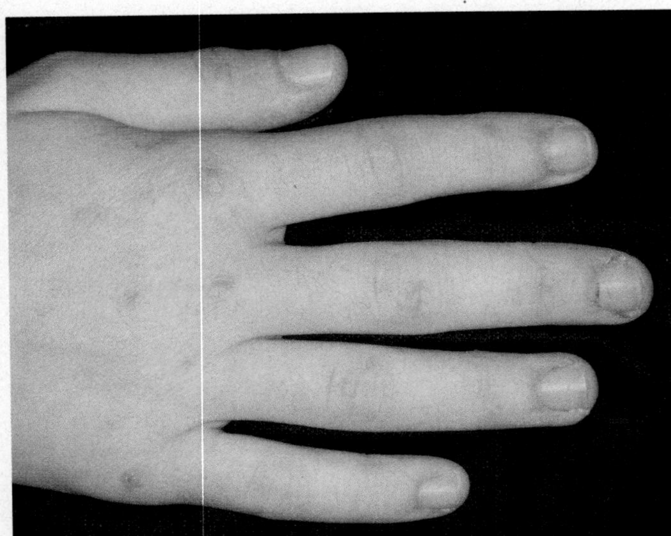

FIGURE 189-7 Hand involvement in the 19-year-old woman in **Figure 189-6** with Gottron papules over the finger joints. She has nail-fold erythema and ragged cuticles (Samitz sign). (*Reproduced with permission from Goodall J, Usatine RP. Skin rash and muscle weakness, J Fam Pract. 2005;54(10):864-868. Frontline Medical Communications, Inc.*)

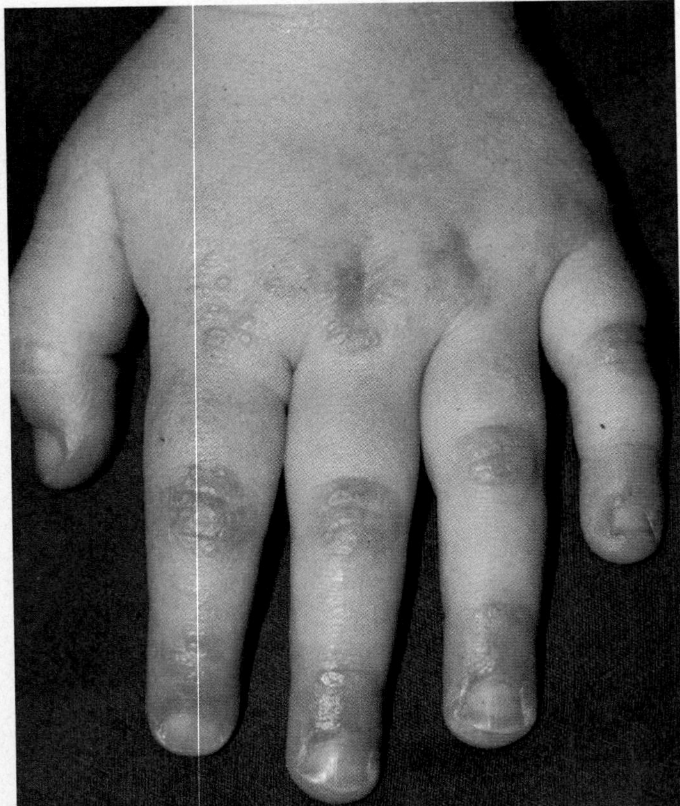

FIGURE 189-8 Juvenile dermatomyositis in a young boy. Note how the erythematous papules and plaques are most prominent over the finger joints and spare the space between joints. This is a good example of Gottron papules being very visible in juvenile dermatomyositis. (*Reproduced with permission from Goodall J, Usatine RP. Skin rash and muscle weakness, J Fam Pract. 2005;54(10):864-868. Frontline Medical Communications, Inc.*)

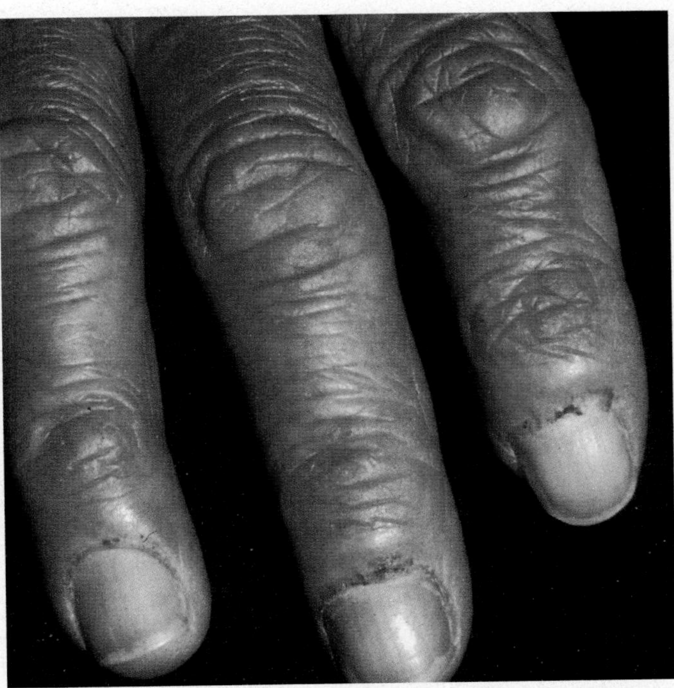

FIGURE 189-9 Dermatomyositis in a man showing cuticular changes that are thick, rough, and hyperkeratotic with telangiectasias. This moth-eaten appearance of the cuticles is called the Samitz sign. The hands also have the appearance of "mechanic's hands," another sign seen in dermatomyositis. (*Reproduced with permission from Richard P. Usatine, MD.*)

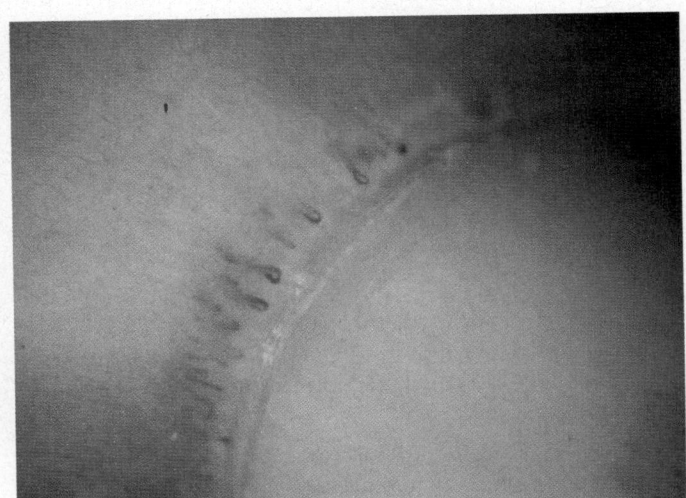

FIGURE 189-10 Dilated nail-fold capillary loops visible with dermoscopy in a young woman with newly diagnosed dermatomyositis. The nail-fold findings resolved with treatment. (*Reproduced with permission from Richard P. Usatine, MD.*)

TYPICAL DISTRIBUTION

- Face—The characteristic heliotrope rash occurs around the eyes. The color "heliotrope" is a pink-purple tint named after the color of the heliotrope flower. This color is best seen in **Figure 189-6**. The heliotrope rash can also be a dusky-red color as seen in **Figures 189-1** to **189-5**. This heliotrope rash is bilaterally symmetrical.
- Hands—There is usually hand involvement with Gottron papules (and plaques), visible nail-fold capillaries, and abnormal cuticles (see **Figures 189-4** and **189-7** to **189-9**).
- Neck and upper trunk—A red or poikiloderma-type rash can be seen in a V-neck (**Figure 189-11**) or shawl distribution (**Figure 189-12**). Poikiloderma refers to hyperpigmentation of the skin demonstrating a variety of shades with associated telangiectasias. The rash here can be scaling and look psoriasiform.
- Extremities may have erythematous plaques and papules with scale. If the erythema and scale is on the upper outer thigh, it is called the holster sign (**Figure 189-13**).
- Scalp is often involved with erythema, scale, and pruritus. This is similar to seborrhea or psoriasis.
- Sun-exposed areas are often involved and worsen with sun exposure. This is why so many of the skin findings are on the face and upper chest (**Figure 189-14**). However, patients rarely complain of sun sensitivity.

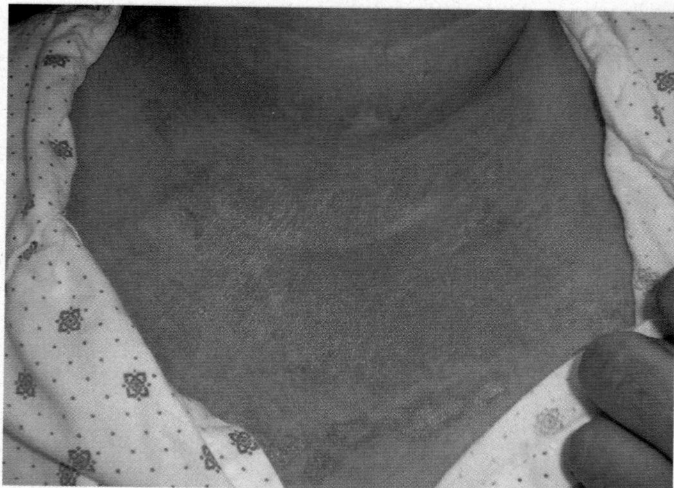

FIGURE 189-11 Poikiloderma (erythema and mottled hyperpigmentation) on the neck of a 35-year-old Hispanic woman with dermatomyositis. The V-neck distribution is related to sun exposure. (*Reproduced with permission from Goodall J, Usatine RP. Skin rash and muscle weakness, J Fam Pract. 2005;54(10):864-868. Frontline Medical Communications, Inc.*)

LABORATORY STUDIES AND DIAGNOSTIC TESTS

- Elevated muscle enzymes, evidence of inflammation on electromyography (EMG), and inflammatory infiltrates on muscle biopsy confirm the diagnosis of dermatomyositis. The following serum muscle enzymes can be drawn during the acute active phase and may be found to be elevated: CK, lactate dehydrogenase (LDH), alanine transaminase (ALT), AST, and aldolase. Of note, it is necessary to measure all of the aforementioned enzymes, as only one of them may be elevated.
- The diagnosis may be made with confidence in a patient with characteristic skin findings and elevated muscle enzymes. If the presentation is not straightforward, then EMG, MRI of the thigh muscle, and/or muscle biopsy should be performed.
- The diagnosis can be supported with positive antibodies such as antinuclear antibody (ANA), anti-Mi-2, and anti-Jo-1. It is not necessary to order these antibodies to make the diagnosis of dermatomyositis. In fact, these myositis-specific antibodies are positive in only 30% of patients with dermatomyositis. Patients with anti-Mi-2 generally have a better overall prognosis.
- Some experts recommend initial pulmonary function tests (PFTs), chest radiograph, and high-resolution CT to identify patients with interstitial lung disease early, regardless of the presence or absence of respiratory symptoms.[15]
- PFTs demonstrate a restrictive pattern and decreased diffusing capacity when interstitial lung disease is present. Abnormal results must be confirmed by CT scan, as PFT results may also reflect coexisting respiratory muscle weakness. Changes over time can be used to determine response to therapy, although intervals for testing are not clearly defined.[2]

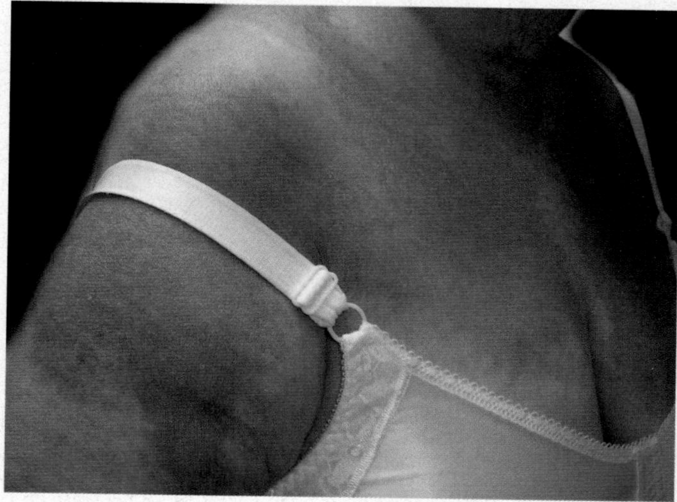

FIGURE 189-12 The shawl distribution of dermatomyositis. (*Reproduced with permission from Richard P. Usatine, MD.*)

DERMOSCOPY AND BIOPSY

- Dermoscopy of the proximal nail folds (cuticles) often shows dilated capillary loops with dropout of vessels between the loops (see **Figure 189-10**).
- Other papulosquamous diseases, such as lichen planus and psoriasis, may be differentiated from dermatomyositis with a 4-mm punch biopsy, but the histology of dermatomyositis is indistinguishable from cutaneous lupus erythematosus.
- Muscle biopsy of dermatomyositis will show inflammatory cells around intramuscular blood vessels. Atrophic muscle fibers are seen around the periphery of muscle fascicles ("perifascicular atrophy").[1]

DIFFERENTIAL DIAGNOSIS

- Polymyositis is another form of inflammatory myopathy. It is distinguished from dermatomyositis by its lack of cutaneous involvement. Dermatomyositis can also occur without muscle involvement. This is called *dermatomyositis sine myositis* or *amyopathic dermatomyositis*.
- Polymorphous light eruption or other photosensitivity reactions may be mistaken for the dermatologic findings of dermatomyositis. In the case of our patient, her cutaneous findings preceded her muscle weakness, and the cutaneous findings were only in light-exposed areas. Therefore, it is essential in the management and follow-up of patients with suspected photosensitivity reactions to inquire about muscle weakness and to look for other signs of dermatomyositis. Examination of the hands and tests for muscle enzyme elevations might help to distinguish dermatomyositis from photosensitivity reactions (see Chapter 208, Photosensitivity).
- Hypothyroidism can cause a proximal myopathy just like polymyositis and dermatomyositis. Although hypothyroidism can cause a dermopathy, it does not resemble the skin findings of dermatomyositis. All patients with proximal muscle weakness should have a screening thyroid-stimulating hormone (TSH) to rule out hypothyroidism regardless of their skin findings (see Chapter 235, Goitrous Hypothyroidism).
- Rosacea causes an erythematous rash on the face as is often seen in dermatomyositis. Of course rosacea does not cause muscle weakness and the erythema of rosacea is generally limited to the face (see Chapter 119, Rosacea).
- Steroid myopathy may develop as a side effect of systemic steroid therapy. The symptoms develop 4 to 6 weeks after starting oral steroids for dermatomyositis and other autoimmune diseases. Therefore, if muscle weakness recurs after initial improvement, it may be from the steroids, not the disease itself.
- Dermatomyositis-like reaction rarely may present with similar skin findings after initiation of the following medications and improve with their discontinuation: penicillamine, nonsteroidal anti-inflammatory drugs (NSAIDs), and carbamazepine.
- Overlap syndrome—The term *overlap* denotes that certain signs are seen in both dermatomyositis and other connective tissue diseases, such as scleroderma, rheumatoid arthritis, and lupus erythematosus. Scleroderma and dermatomyositis are the most commonly associated conditions and have been termed sclerodermatomyositis or

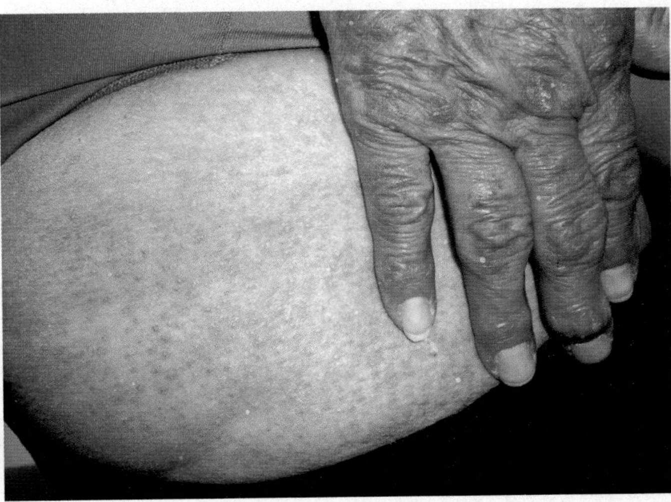

FIGURE 189-13 *Holster sign* showing erythema and scale on the lateral thigh. Note the Gottron papules on the fingers. (*Reproduced with permission from Richard P. Usatine, MD.*)

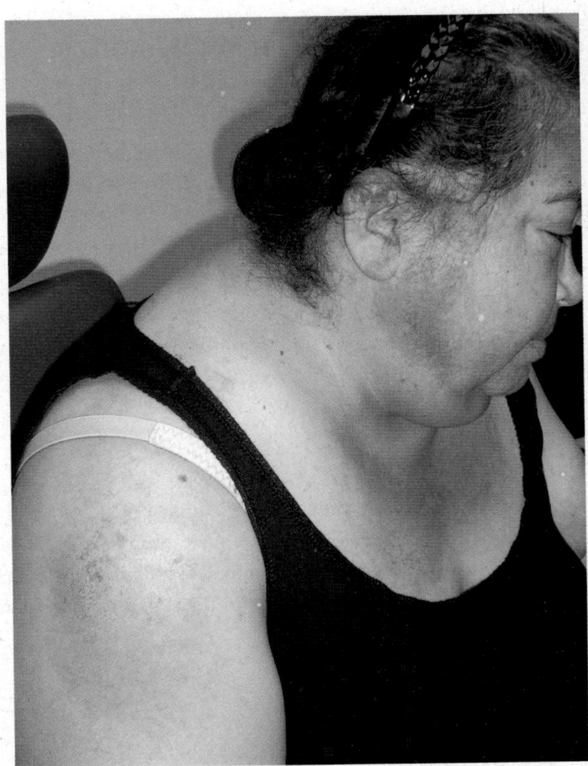

FIGURE 189-14 A flare of dermatomyositis in a patient previously under control on medications now showing erythema on the lateral face, upper chest, and proximal arm. (*Reproduced with permission from Richard P. Usatine, MD.*)

mixed connective disease. In mixed connective tissue disease, features of systemic lupus erythematosus (SLE), scleroderma, and polymyositis are evident, such as malar rash, alopecia, Raynaud phenomenon, waxy-appearing skin, and proximal muscle weakness.

MANAGEMENT

Given the autoimmune mechanism central to the disease process, treatment is geared toward the proximal muscle weakness and skin changes using immunosuppressive or immunomodulatory therapy. Treatment is nonspecific, as the target antigen remains elusive.[5] Cutaneous manifestations do not always parallel muscle disease in response to therapy. Clinical improvement should guide treatment, as serum CK level may falsely normalize during therapy and should not be used as a sole gauge of responsiveness to treatment. Effective therapies for the myopathy are oral corticosteroids, immunosuppressants, biologic agents, and/or intravenous immunoglobulin. Effective therapies for the skin disease are sun protection, topical corticosteroids, antimalarials, methotrexate, and/or immunoglobulin. Drug therapy for dermatomyositis continues to be based on empirical rather than evidence-based practice due to lack of controlled trials.[16]

FIRST LINE

NONPHARMACOLOGIC

- Physical and/or occupational therapy to regain strength is highly recommended. Physical therapy will preserve muscle function and help to prevent atrophy and contractures.[17]
- Aerobic exercise has been shown to improve muscle performance and the achievement of activities of daily living (ADLs), but regression to baseline performance was seen at follow-up, demonstrating the need for a sustained exercise regimen.[18]
- In combination with exercise, oral creatine supplement in juvenile dermatomyositis was shown to improve muscle endurance and functionality compared to placebo.[19] Although creatine supplementation was well tolerated in patients with juvenile dermatomyositis, it does not show therapeutic benefit in adult populations.[20]
- Patient education is crucial, emphasizing the photosensitive nature of the skin lesions and encouraging photoprotection consisting of broad-spectrum sunscreen, protective outerwear, and limiting sun exposure.[21-23] SOR Ⓑ

TOPICAL TREATMENT

- Therapy of the skin disease should include high-potency topical corticosteroids.[21,22,24] SOR Ⓑ Triamcinolone ointment may be used for less-severe areas or on the face at first. Consider a short course of a very high-potency steroid, such as clobetasol, for more severe involvement not on the face.[9]
- Topical tacrolimus 0.1% is a useful adjunct in the treatment of refractory skin manifestations.[17] SOR Ⓑ

ORAL TREATMENT

- If disease is limited to the skin, antimalarial agents in addition to topical corticosteroids are first-line therapy. Hydroxychloroquine is most commonly used at 200 mg to 400 mg daily in adults (maximum of 5 mg/kg of real body weight per day),[25] but patients with dermatomyositis are at increased risk of a drug eruption with this medication, and a morbilliform eruption may develop in 25% of patients. If this is the case, patients have been shown to tolerate chloroquine instead. These antimalarial agents have a rare side effect of retinopathy and require a baseline ophthalmologic exam before treatment is initiated, and yearly after 5 years during the duration of treatment.[25]
- First-line therapy for muscle disease is high-dose (1 mg/kg single daily dose) oral prednisone, with or without an immunosuppressive ("steroid-sparing") agent—methotrexate, cyclosporine, mycophenolate mofetil, or azathioprine.[3] The steroid-sparing immunosuppressive medication can be started after the patient is responding to the prednisone and be used to continue therapy while tapering down the dose of prednisone.
- Corticosteroids (either IV or oral) are also the first-line treatment for interstitial lung disease in patients with dermatomyositis. Approximately half of patients show response in respiratory symptoms. Refractory cases are treated with cyclosporine or cyclophosphamide, with or without corticosteroids. Methotrexate use is cautioned when there is coexisting lung disease, as it is a known cause of drug-induced interstitial lung disease.[2,26]
- To avoid the toxic effects of steroids, steroid taper (20% to 25% reduction monthly) should be initiated based on clinical responsiveness (increased muscle strength, energy) after 3 to 4 weeks on high-dose treatment.
- If no response by 3 months to oral high-dose steroids, another treatment approach should begin along with a reexamination of the diagnosis.[3,17] SOR Ⓑ
- Methotrexate is the most commonly used steroid-sparing agent in treating the muscular symptoms of childhood and adult refractory dermatomyositis. Methotrexate significantly improves skin lesions as well.[27] SOR Ⓑ
- Methotrexate dosing starts at 10 to 15 mg/wk. The dose is then increased 2.5 mg/wk until a total dose of 15 to 25 mg/wk is reached. The total dose of methotrexate is also determined by how well the patient can tolerate this medication. Improvement is typically noted after 4 to 8 weeks of therapy.[17,24]
- Using methotrexate safely requires a number of precautions. A purified protein derivative (PPD) should be placed or a QuantiFERON-TB Gold assay performed to make sure that latent tuberculosis will not be activated. Patients with active liver disease, including hepatitis C and alcoholic cirrhosis, should receive alternative forms of therapy, as methotrexate can be hepatotoxic. Women should avoid becoming pregnant during therapy, and men should also use contraception. Persons started on methotrexate should also be given 1 mg of folic acid daily to minimize the risk of side effects such as myelosuppression. The patient should be followed with regular laboratory testing, including complete blood counts and comprehensive metabolic profiles. Methotrexate should only be prescribed by doctors familiar with its risks and benefits.
- As the methotrexate dosage is increased, the dosage of prednisone should be tapered.
- Cyclosporine plus methotrexate has shown some benefit in the treatment of refractory juvenile and adult dermatomyositis.[17] SOR Ⓑ

Cyclosporine should be used cautiously, with monitoring of blood pressure, renal function, liver function, and hematologic parameters.

- New data show that methotrexate and cyclosporine both result in clinical improvement with no difference in efficacy or toxicity.[17]
- Azathioprine is commonly used in chronic inflammatory diseases as a steroid-sparing agent. It is usually administered up to 2 to 3 mg/kg per day. Azathioprine has been shown to have a slower clinical effect than methotrexate, but no difference was noted in efficacy of treatment of muscle disease.[17] Azathioprine is less effective for the treatment of cutaneous lesions. Like all the other immunosuppressive agents, azathioprine must be used cautiously and by physicians familiar with its risks.
- It is important to look at these medications' side-effect profile and monitor the patient accordingly during treatment. Patients must not get pregnant while on these medications, and various labs need to be followed. The role of liver biopsy in methotrexate use is debated and should be considered based on the most current guidelines and standards of care.

SECOND LINE

- Tacrolimus has effects similar to cyclosporine but has greater potency and is effective in refractory juvenile dermatomyositis.[17] In addition, tacrolimus has been shown to have great success in stabilizing or improving ILD and may be a good option for patients with comorbid interstitial lung disease.[28]
- Mycophenolate mofetil, an inhibitor of T- and B-cell proliferation, is a possible corticosteroid-sparing agent that has shown efficacy for both refractory cutaneous and muscular disease; however, concern regarding central nervous system (CNS) B-cell lymphoma and lack of controlled trials limits its use. It is also more costly than methotrexate or azathioprine.
- Hydroxychloroquine is one option for a steroid-sparing agent, especially for the rash of dermatomyositis, which may be considered for young women with mild disease. SOR C Quinacrine and isotretinoin have shown promise in rashes that are unresponsive to hydroxychloroquine.[17]
- Various combination therapies with two of the following agents have been studied but are still empirical: azathioprine, cyclosporine, intramuscular methotrexate, and oral methotrexate.[23,24,29] SOR C
- Biologics, including tumor necrosis factor (TNF)-α inhibitors, are currently being tested for use in juvenile and adult dermatomyositis. Conflicting and discouraging initial results prompt the need for further clinical trials. Interferon-β, monoclonal complement antibodies, and anti–T-cell signaling drugs are currently under investigation.
- Pulsed intravenous methylprednisolone has been advocated for severe disease (especially juvenile cases) and in refractory cases of myositis.[30] SOR C This treatment has also been recommended as first-line therapy for patients with associated interstitial lung disease.[1]
- In patients who are not responsive to traditional therapies, recent studies have found intravenous immunoglobulin (IVIG) to be an effective and relatively safe second-line therapy. Studies show improvement in muscle histology and cutaneous disease. Higher remission rates after 4 years are seen in patients receiving IVIG as part of therapy. IVIG is dosed 2 g/kg over 3 to 6 months with treatment for 2 to 5 consecutive days each month. As opposed to other agents that take months to show effect, IVIG may show clinical improvement within 15 days of the first infusion, and maximal efficacy is seen after the second or third infusion.[31] Recent studies reveal that there may be a survival benefit when IVIG is used as part of initial therapy.[31] High cost limits current use.[16,17] SOR C
- Rituximab, a chimeric antibody against CD20+ B cells, has shown mixed results in different studies. In some studies, it has shown efficacy in patents refractory to conventional therapy who have failed an average of 3 disease-modifying anti-rheumatic drugs (DMARDs).[32,33] However, the median time to measurable clinical improvement was 20 weeks.[33] Although rituximab is very expensive, these results are promising for patients who are unresponsive to prednisone, methotrexate, and other conventional therapies.[32]

MALIGNANCY WORK-UP

- All patients with dermatomyositis, regardless of age, should undergo an age- and gender-relevant malignancy work-up beginning at the time of diagnosis. Cancer may be diagnosed before or after the diagnosis of dermatomyositis, but malignancy risk is highest within 1 year of diagnosis. Some studies show an increased risk up to 5 years following diagnosis.[11,30]
- Cancer is rare in juvenile dermatomyositis, so these patients do not need an extensive malignancy evaluation.[6]
- For adults, evidence-based guidelines for cancer screening have not been defined, leading to ambiguity about how to approach the malignancy work-up. Screening should be performed with risks attributed to age, gender, ethnicity, and family history in mind.[6,11]
- Despite the lack of published guidelines, algorithms have been proposed that stratify adult patients based on the presence of anti-TIF-1γ. Individuals positive for the antibody are recommended to undergo the most aggressive evaluation for occult malignancy, which may consist of whole-body PET/CT at the time of diagnosis and annually for the next 3–5 years. For patients who are anti-TIF-1γ negative, a full-body PET/CT upon diagnosis may be sufficient.[6]
- Alternatively, if antibody testing is unavailable, women newly diagnosed should undergo a pelvic and transvaginal ultrasound, mammogram, and CT thorax and abdomen, or a full-body PET scan. Colonoscopy is recommended in patients older than age 50 years or with risk factors.[27]
- For men, a testicular and prostate exam should be performed at diagnosis with colonoscopy if age older than 50 years.[34]
- If primary screening is negative, some experts recommend that a patient should be screened again in 3 to 6 months and every 6 months up to 4 years following diagnosis. Risk factors for underlying malignancy should be kept in mind, such as male sex, age older than 45 years, and the presence of skin necrosis. The cumulative risk factors should be balanced against the risks of exposing the patient to repeated radiation with successive screening.[6,11,34]
- The value of surveillance of tumor markers such as CA-125 and CA-19-9 is debatable.[11,34]
- Given its suggestive high predictive value, some experts recommend more intensive and frequent screening for patients positive for the anti-p155 or anti-TIF-1γ antibodies.[5]
- In one study, conventional cancer screening (thoracoabdominal CT, mammography, gynecologic examination, ultrasound, and tumor

marker analysis) and fluorodeoxyglucose-positron emission tomography (FDG-PET)/CT total-body screening had equivalent overall predictive values for diagnosing malignancy in patients with myositis.[35]

PROGNOSIS

Recent reports indicate that approximately 20% to 40% of patients treated achieve remission, although 80% of treated patients remained disabled. One study found the mortality rate of patients with dermatomyositis to be threefold higher than the rest of the population. Cancer, lung, and cardiac complications are the most common cause of death. Poor prognostic indicators include older age, cardiac and lung involvement (ILD), and dysphagia. Certain antibodies have also been linked to higher mortality rates and greater risk of malignancy.[8]

FOLLOW-UP

Patients need very close and frequent follow-up to manage their medications and overall care, as well as continued surveillance for malignancy. High doses of steroids and steroid-sparing agents, such as methotrexate, have numerous potential side effects. Patients need to be closely followed with laboratory tests and careful titration of the toxic medicines used for treatment. Patients also need physical therapy, periodic eye exams for cataracts and glaucoma, and specific supplements including calcium, vitamin D, and folic acid to prevent some of the side effects of the strong medications being prescribed. Patients on long-term corticosteroids especially need efforts made to prevent and detect osteoporosis.

PATIENT EDUCATION

Discuss the importance of sun protection, as sun exposure makes the cutaneous manifestations worse. Counseling about the serious nature of the disease and prognosis is important, as many patients are left with residual weakness even after good disease control is obtained. Patients need to understand that the medications being used have many risks along with their benefits and need to report side effects to their physicians. Pregnancy prevention is needed for women of childbearing potential while on a number of the medications used to treat this disease.

PATIENT RESOURCES

- The Myositis Association. **www.myositis.org.**
- National Institute of Neurological Disorders and Stroke. *NINDS Dermatomyositis Information Page*—**www.ninds.nih.gov/Disorders/All-Disorders/Dermatomyositis-Information-Page.**

PROVIDER RESOURCES

- Medscape. *Dermatomyositis*—**http://emedicine.medscape.com/article/332783.**
- MedicineNet. *Polymyositis and Dermatomyositis*—**http://www.medicinenet.com/polymyositis/article.htm.**

REFERENCES

1. Robinson AB, Reed AM. Clinical features, pathogenesis and treatment of juvenile and adult dermatomyositis. *Nat Rev Rheumatol.* 2011;7(11):664-675.
2. Connors GR, Christopher-Stine L, Oddis CV, Danoff SK. Interstitial lung disease associated with the idiopathic inflammatory myopathies: what progress has been made in the past 35 years? *Chest.* 2010;138(6):1464-1474.
3. Dalakas MC. Immunotherapy of inflammatory myopathies: practical approach and future prospects. *Curr Treat Options Neurol.* 2011;13(3):311-323.
4. Olazagasti, JM, Baez PJ, Wetter DA, Erneste FC. Cancer risk in dermatomyositis: a meta-analysis of cohort studies. *Am J Clin Dermatol.* 2015;16(2):89-98.
5. Trallero-Araguás E, Rodrigo-Pendás J, Selva-O'Callaghan A, et al. Usefulness of anti-p155 autoantibody for diagnosing cancer-associated dermatomyositis. *Arthritis Rheum.* 2012;64(2):523-532.
6. Tiniakou E, Mammen AL. Idiopathic inflammatory myopathies and malignancy: a comprehensive review. *Clin Rev Allergy Immunol.* 2017;52(1):20-33.
7. Wang J, Guo G, Chen G, et al. Meta-analysis of the association of dermatomyositis and polymyositis with cancer. *Br J Dermatol.* 2013;169(4):838-847.
8. Marie I. Morbidity and mortality in adult polymyositis and dermatomyositis. *Curr Rheumatol Rep.* 2012;14(3):275-285.
9. Bohan A, Peter JB. Polymyositis and dermatomyositis (first of two parts). *N Engl J Med.* 1975;292(7):344-347.
10. Bohan A, Peter JB. Polymyositis and dermatomyositis (second of two parts). *N Engl J Med.* 1975;292(8):403-407.
11. Madan V, Chinoy H, Griffiths CE, Cooper RG. Defining cancer risk in dermatomyositis. Part I. *Clin Exp Dermatol.* 2009;34(4):451-455.
12. Sultan SM, Isenberg DA. Re-classifying myositis. *Rheumatology (Oxford).* 2010;49(5):831-833.
13. Schmeling H, Stevens S, Goia C, et al. Nailfold capillary density is importantly associated over time with muscle and skin disease activity in juvenile dermatomyositis. *Rheumatology.* 2011;50(5):885-893.
14. Selva-O'Callaghan A, Fonollosa-Pla V, Trallero-Araguás E, et al. Nailfold capillary microscopy in adults with inflammatory myopathy. *Semin Arthritis Rheum.* 2010;39(5):398-404.
15. Fathi M, Dastmalchi M, Rasmussen E, et al. Interstitial lung disease, a common manifestation of a newly diagnosed polymyositis and dermatomyositis. *Ann Rheum Dis.* 2004;63(3):297-301.
16. Wang DX, Shu XM, Tian XL, et al. Intravenous immunoglobulin therapy in adult patients with polymyositis/dermatomyositis: a systematic literature review. *Clin Rheumatol.* 2012;31(5):801-806.
17. Aggarwal R, Oddis CV. Therapeutic approaches in myositis. *Curr Rheumatol Rep.* 2011;13(3):182-191.
18. Alemo Munters L, Dastmalchi M, Andgren V, et al. Improvement in health and possible reduction in disease activity using endurance exercise in patients with established polymyositis and dermatomyositis: a multicenter randomized controlled trial with a 1-year open extension followup. *Arthritis Care Res (Hoboken).* 2013;65(12):1959-1968.

19. Chung Y, Alexanderson H, Pipitone N, et al. Creatine supplements in patients with idiopathic inflammatory myopathies who are clinically weak after conventional pharmacologic treatment: six-month, double-blind, randomized, placebo controlled trial. *Arthritis Rheum.* 2007;57(4):694-702.

20. Zieglschmid-Adams ME, Pandya AG, Cohen SB, Sontheimer RD. Treatment of dermatomyositis with methotrexate. *J Am Acad Dermatol.* 1995;32(5 Pt 1):754-757.

21. Callen JP. Dermatomyositis: diagnosis, evaluation and management. *Minerva Med.* 2002;93(3):157-167.

22. Callen JP, Wortmann RL. Dermatomyositis. *Clin Dermatol.* 2006; 24(5):363-373.

23. Choy EH, Isenberg DA. Treatment of dermatomyositis and polymyositis. *Rheumatology (Oxford).* 2002;41(1):7-13.

24. Habif T. *A Color Guide to Diagnosis and Therapy, Clinical Dermatology*, 4th ed. St. Louis, MO: Mosby; 2004.

25. Marmor MF, Kellner U, Lai TY, et al; American Academy of Ophthalmology. Recommendations on screening for chloroquine and hydroxychloroquine retinopathy (2016 revision). *Ophthalmology.* 2016;123(6):1386-1394.

26. Mimori T, Nakashima R, Hosono Y. Interstitial lung disease in myositis: clinical subsets, biomarkers, and treatment. *Curr Rheumatol Rep.* 2012;14(3):264-274.

27. Hornung T, Ko A, Tuting T, et al. Efficacy of low-dose methotrexate in the treatment of dermatomyositis skin lesions. *Clin Exp Dermatol.* 2011;37(2):139-142.

28. Ge Y, Zhou H, Shi J, et al. The efficacy of tacrolimus in patients with refractory dermatomyositis/polymyositis: a systematic review. *Clin Rheumatol.* 2015;34(12):2097-2103.

29. Choy EH, Hoogendijk JE, Lecky B, Winer JB. Immunosuppressant and immunomodulatory treatment for dermatomyositis and polymyositis. *Cochrane Database Syst Rev.* 2005;(3):CD003643.

30. Zahr ZA, Baer AN. Malignancy in myositis. *Curr Rheumatol Rep.* 2011;13(3):208-215.

31. Anh-Tu Hoa S, Hudson M. Critical review of the role of intravenous immunoglobulins in idiopathic inflammatory myopathies. *Semin Arthritis Rheum.* 2017;46(4):488-508.

32. Mahler EA, Blom M, Voermans NC, et al. Rituximab treatment in patients with refractory inflammatory myopathies. *Rheumatology.* 2011;50(12):2206-2213.

33. Oddis CV, Reed AM, Aggarwal R, et al. Rituximab in the treatment of refractory adult and juvenile dermatomyositis and adult polymyositis: a randomized, placebo-phase trial. *Arthritis Rheum.* 2013;65(2):314-324.

34. Titulaer MJ, Soffietti R, Dalmau J, et al; European Federation of Neurological Societies. Screening for tumors in paraneoplastic syndromes: report of an EFNS Task Force. *Eur J Neurol.* 2011; 18(1):19-27.

35. Selva-O'Callaghan A, Grau JM, Gámez-Cenzano C, et al. Conventional cancer screening versus PET/CT in dermatomyositis/polymyositis. *Am J Med.* 2010;123(6):558-562.

190 SCLERODERMA AND MORPHEA

E.J. Mayeaux, Jr., MD
Richard P. Usatine, MD

PATIENT STORY

A 49-year-old woman presents with skin changes on her face and hands and gastroesophageal reflux disease. Examination of her face shows multiple telangiectasias and tight skin over her nose and around her mouth (**Figure 190-1**). Examination of her hands shows tight skin over the fingers with some deformities due to the tightening of the skin (**Figure 190-2**). A closer look at an individual finger shows pitting of the skin and loss of the soft tissue of the distal phalanx (**Figure 190-3**). A "salt-and-pepper" appearance is noted on the forearms (**Figure 190-4**) and lower legs. Some firm nodules around the elbows are consistent with calcinosis. Her cardiopulmonary exam is normal. Further history reveals Raynaud's phenomenon. A diagnosis of CREST syndrome and scleroderma is made. The physician orders blood tests, chest X-ray (CXR), and pulmonary function tests (PFTs) to determine if this is limited cutaneous systemic sclerosis or diffuse systemic sclerosis.

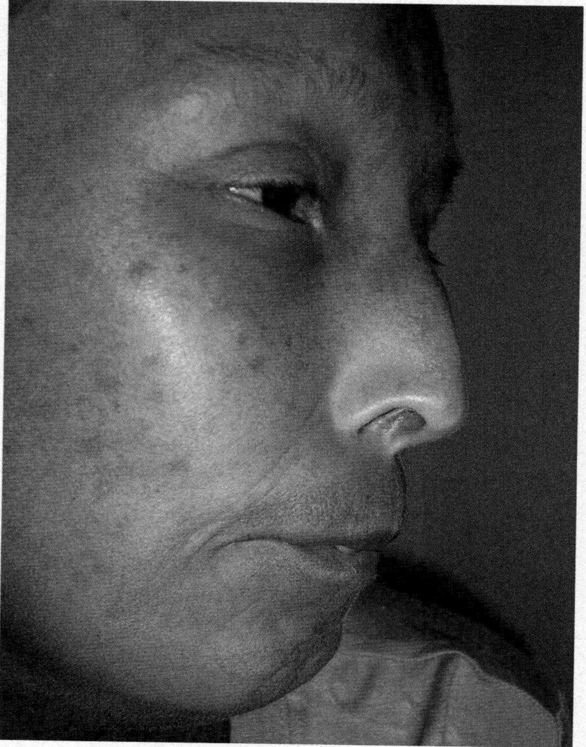

FIGURE 190-1 Scleroderma with CREST syndrome in a 49-year-old woman. Note the telangiectasias and tight skin around the mouth. The tight skin on the nose gives a "beak" appearance. (*Reproduced with permission from Richard P. Usatine, MD.*)

INTRODUCTION

Scleroderma (from the Greek *scleros*, to harden) is a term that describes the presence of thickened, hardened skin. It may affect only limited areas of the skin (morphea), most or all of the skin (scleroderma), or also involve internal organs (systemic sclerosis).

EPIDEMIOLOGY

- The prevalence rates of diseases that share scleroderma as a clinical feature are reported ranging from 4 to 253 cases per 1 million individuals.[1]
- Systemic sclerosis has an annual incidence of 1 to 2 per 100,000 individuals in the United States.[1] The peak onset is between the ages of 30 and 50 years.[1]
- In the United States, the incidence of morphea has been estimated at 25 cases per 1 million individuals per year.[1]
- Worldwide, there are higher rates in the United States and Australia than in Japan or Europe.[2]
- Pulmonary fibrosis and pulmonary arterial hypertension are the leading causes of death as a consequence of these diseases.[3]

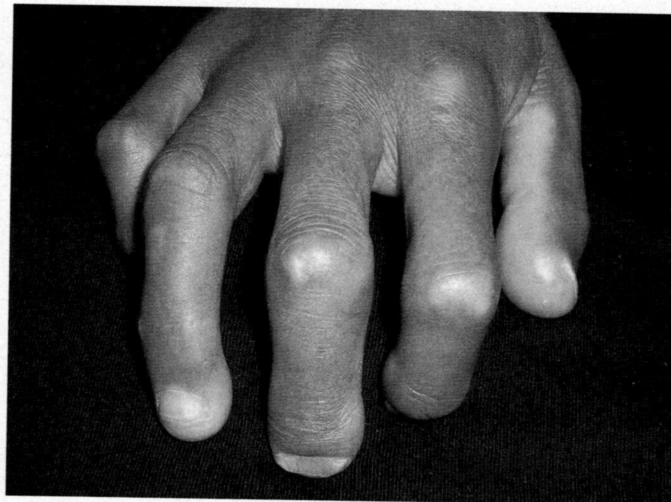

FIGURE 190-2 Sclerodactyly with tight skin over the fingers and some flexion deformities. (*Reproduced with permission from Richard P. Usatine, MD.*)

ETIOLOGY AND PATHOPHYSIOLOGY

- The scleroderma disorders can be subdivided into three groups: localized scleroderma (morphea; **Figures 190-5** and **190-6**),

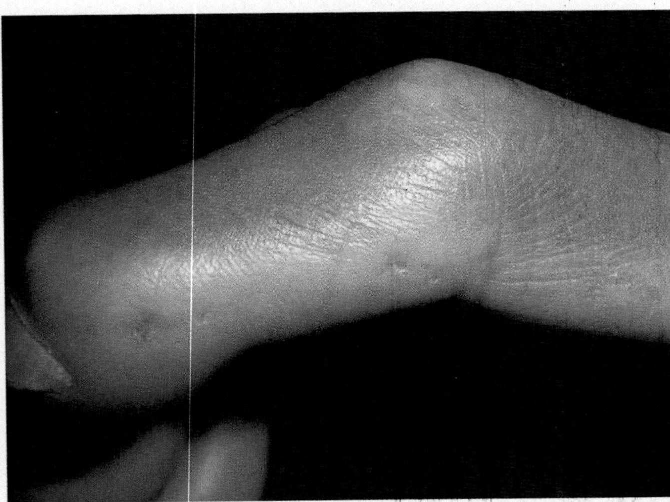

FIGURE 190-3 Sclerodactyly—close-up of a finger with pitting of skin and resorption of the distal phalanx. (*Reproduced with permission from Richard P. Usatine, MD.*)

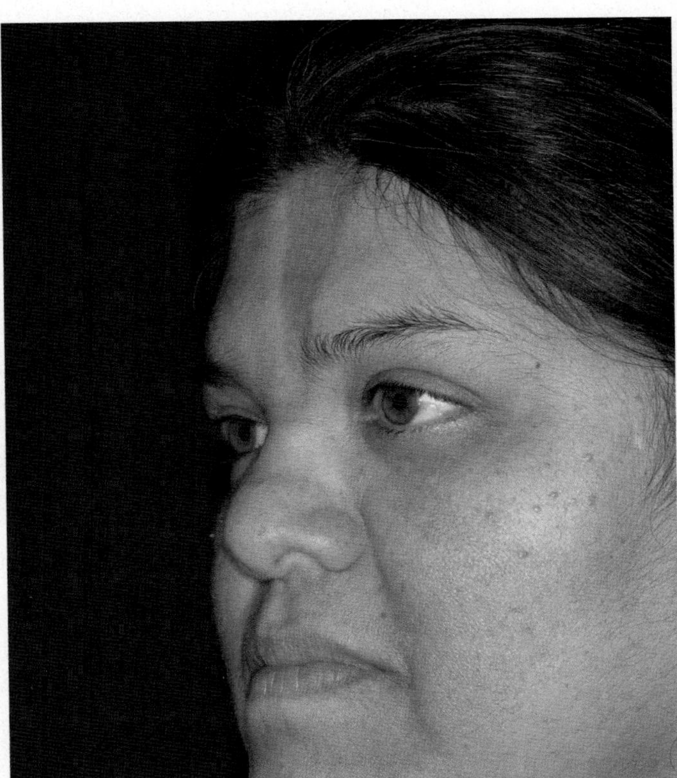

FIGURE 190-5 Linear morphea that started 3 years before on the forehead of a 41-year-old woman. An example of "en coup de sabre," meaning the blow of a sword. (*Reproduced with permission from Richard P. Usatine, MD.*)

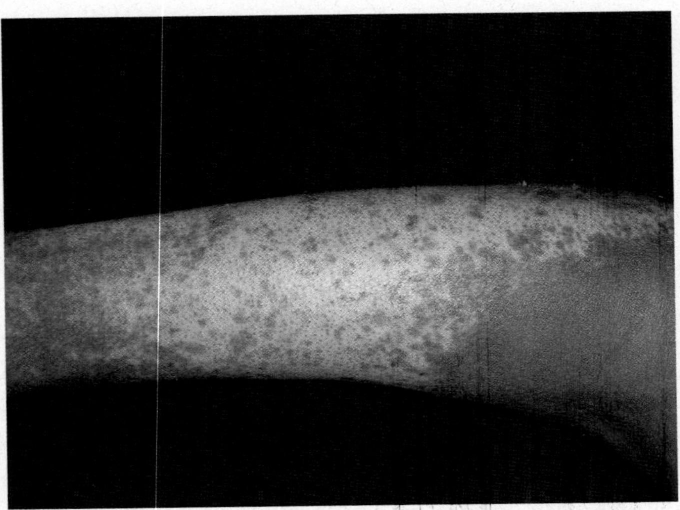

FIGURE 190-4 Scleroderma with salt-and-pepper appearance on the forearm of a 49-year-old woman with CREST syndrome. (*Reproduced with permission from Richard P. Usatine, MD.*)

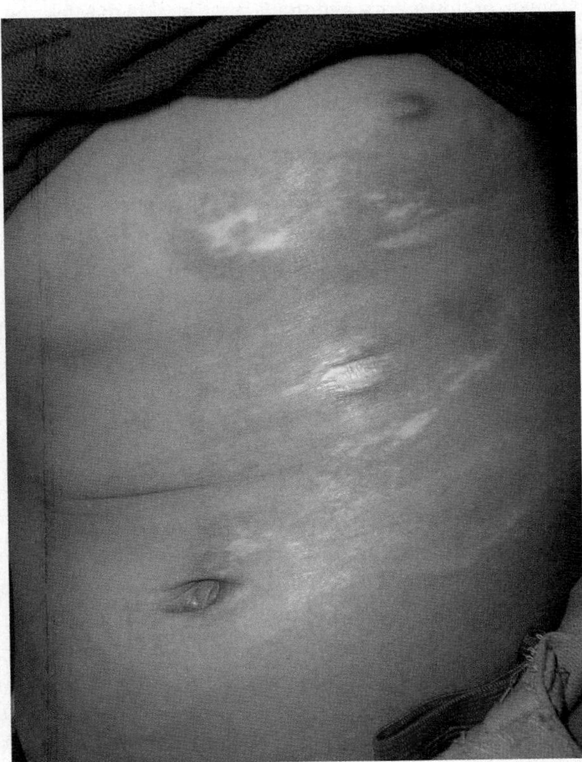

FIGURE 190-6 Morphea on the abdomen of this 5-year-old girl showing hypopigmentation. The skin is thickened and more firm on palpation. (*Reproduced with permission from Richard P. Usatine, MD.*)

systemic sclerosis (see **Figures 190-1** to **190-4**), and other scleroderma-like disorders that are marked by the presence of thickened, sclerotic skin lesions.

- The most common vascular dysfunction associated with scleroderma is Raynaud phenomenon (**Figure 190-7**). Raynaud phenomenon is produced by arterial constriction in the digits. The characteristic color changes progress from white pallor, to blue (acrocyanosis), to finally red (reperfusion hyperemia). Raynaud phenomenon generally precedes other disease manifestations, sometimes by years. Many patients develop progressive structural changes in their small blood vessels, which permanently impair blood flow and can result in digital ulceration or infarction. Other forms of vascular injury include pulmonary artery hypertension, renal crisis, and gastric antral vascular ectasia.
- Systemic sclerosis is used to describe a systemic disease characterized by skin induration and thickening accompanied by variable tissue fibrosis and inflammatory infiltration in numerous visceral organs. Systemic sclerosis can be diffuse (diffuse cutaneous systemic sclerosis [DcSSc]) or limited to the skin and adjacent tissues (limited cutaneous systemic sclerosis [LcSSc]).
- Patients with LcSSc usually have skin sclerosis restricted to the hands and, to a lesser extent, the face and neck. With time, some patients develop scleroderma of the distal forearm. They often display the CREST syndrome, which presents with Raynaud phenomenon (see **Figure 190-7**), esophageal dysmotility, sclerodactyly (**Figures 190-2** and **190-8**), telangiectasias (see **Figure 190-1**), and calcinosis cutis (**Figure 190-9**).
- Patients with DcSSc often present with sclerotic skin on the chest, abdomen, or upper arms and shoulders. The skin may take on a salt-and-pepper look (see **Figure 190-4**). They are more likely to develop internal organ damage caused by ischemic injury and fibrosis than those with LcSSc or morphea.
- Almost 90% of patients with systemic sclerosis have some GI involvement,[4] although half of these patients may be asymptomatic. Any part of the GI tract may be involved. Potential signs and symptoms include dysphagia, choking, heartburn, cough after swallowing, bloating, constipation and/or diarrhea, pseudo-obstruction, malabsorption, and fecal incontinence. Chronic gastroesophageal reflux and recurrent episodes of aspiration may contribute to the development of interstitial lung disease. Vascular ectasia in the stomach (often referred to as "watermelon stomach" on endoscopy) is common and may lead to GI bleeding and anemia.
- Pulmonary involvement is seen in more than 70% of patients, usually presenting as dyspnea on exertion and a nonproductive cough. Fine "Velcro" rales may be heard at the lung bases with lung auscultation. Pulmonary vascular disease occurs in 10% to 40% of patients with systemic sclerosis and is more common in patients with limited cutaneous disease. The risk of lung cancer is increased approximately fivefold in patients with scleroderma.
- Autopsy data suggest that 60% to 80% of patients with DcSSc have evidence of kidney damage.[5] Some degree of proteinuria, a mild elevation in the plasma creatinine concentration, and/or hypertension are observed in as many as 50% of patients.[6] Severe renal disease develops in 10% to 15% of patients, most commonly in patients with DcSSc.

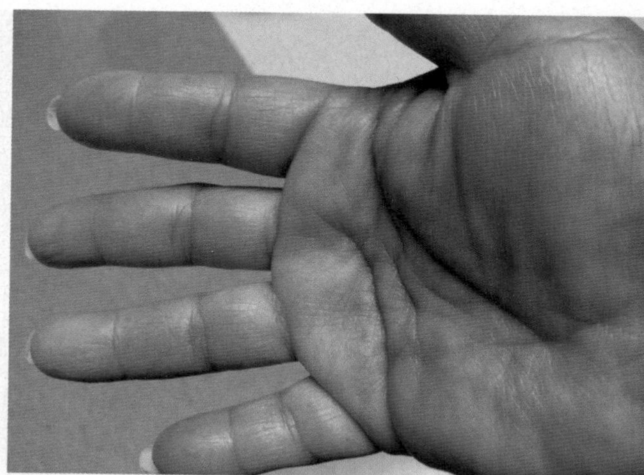

FIGURE 190-7 Raynaud's phenomenon with the fingers turning blue (purple) and pink after turning white. (*Reproduced with permission from Richard P. Usatine, MD.*)

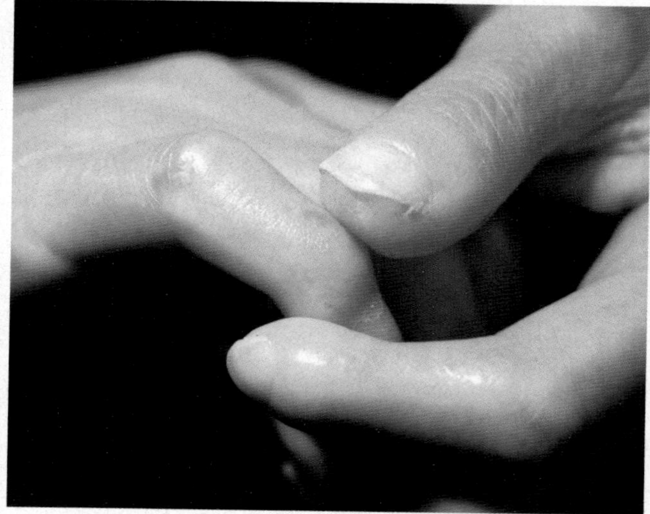

FIGURE 190-8 Scleroderma showing sclerodactyly with tight shiny skin over the fingers. (*Reproduced with permission from Everett Allen, MD.*)

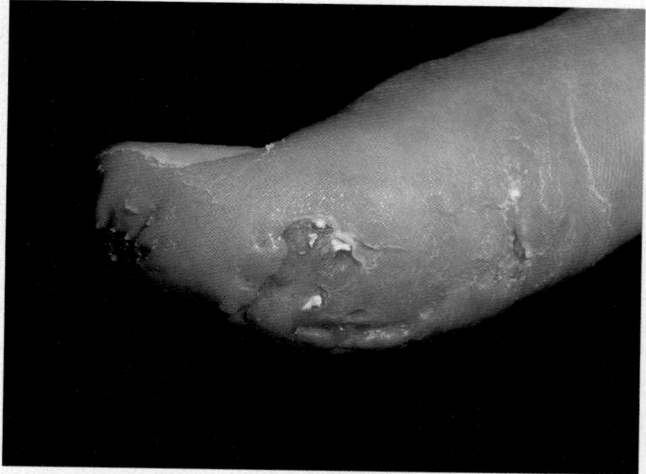

FIGURE 190-9 Calcinosis cutis on the thumb of a man with newly diagnosed scleroderma. All of his fingers were involved. The calcinosis resolved when the patient was treated with oral minocycline. (*Reproduced with permission from Richard P. Usatine, MD.*)

- Symptomatic pericarditis occurs in 7% to 20% of patients and has a 5-year mortality rate of 75%.[7] Primary cardiac involvement includes pericarditis, pericardial effusion, myocardial fibrosis, heart failure, myocarditis associated with myositis, conduction disturbances, and arrhythmias.[8] Patchy myocardial fibrosis is characteristic of systemic sclerosis and is thought to result from recurrent vasospasm of small vessels. Arrhythmias are common, and most are caused by fibrosis of the conduction system.
- Pulmonary vascular disease occurs in 10% to 40% of patients with scleroderma and is more common in patients with limited cutaneous disease. It may occur in the absence of significant interstitial lung disease, generally a late complication, and is usually progressive. Severe pulmonary arterial hypertension may develop, sometimes with pulmonale and right-sided heart failure or thrombosis of the pulmonary vessels.
- Joint pain, immobility, and contractures may develop, with contractures of the fingers being most common (**Figure 190-10**). Neuropathies and central nervous system involvement occur, including headache, seizures, stroke, vascular disease, radiculopathy, and myelopathy.
- Scleroderma produces sexual dysfunction in men and women. In men, it is very frequently associated with erectile dysfunction.

DIAGNOSIS

CLINICAL FEATURES

- The diagnosis of systemic sclerosis and related disorders is based primarily on the presence of characteristic clinical findings. Skin involvement is characterized by variable thickening and hardening of the skin. Skin pigmentary changes may occur, especially a salt-and-pepper appearance from spotty hypopigmentation (**Figure 190-11**). Other prominent skin manifestations include:
  - Pruritus and edema in the early stages.
  - Sclerodactyly (**Figure 190-12**).
  - Digital ulcers and pitting at the fingertips (**Figure 190-13**).
  - Telangiectasia (see **Figure 190-1**).
  - Calcinosis cutis (**Figure 190-14**).
- The diagnosis of localized scleroderma (morphea) is suggested by the presence of typical skin thickening and hardening confined to one area (see **Figures 190-5** and **190-6**). Generalized morphea typically spares the hands and face and is not associated with major vascular symptoms or with visceral disease. The diagnosis of systemic sclerosis is suggested by the presence of typical skin thickening and hardening (sclerosis) that is not confined to one area (i.e., not localized scleroderma) plus one or more of the typical systemic features. Variants of localized morphea include linear scleroderma, en coup de sabre (**Figure 190-15**), and guttate morphea.
- The American College of Rheumatology and the European League Against Rheumatism criteria[9] for the diagnosis of systemic sclerosis requires fibrosis of the skin and/or internal organs, production of specific autoantibodies, and evidence of vasculopathy.
  - Sclerodactyly—Skin thickening of the fingers extending proximal to the metacarpophalangeal joints is sufficient for the patient to be classified as having systemic sclerosis (SSc) (**Figure 190-16**).
  - If sclerodactyly is not present, seven additive items should be used: skin thickening of the fingers, fingertip lesions, telangiectasia,

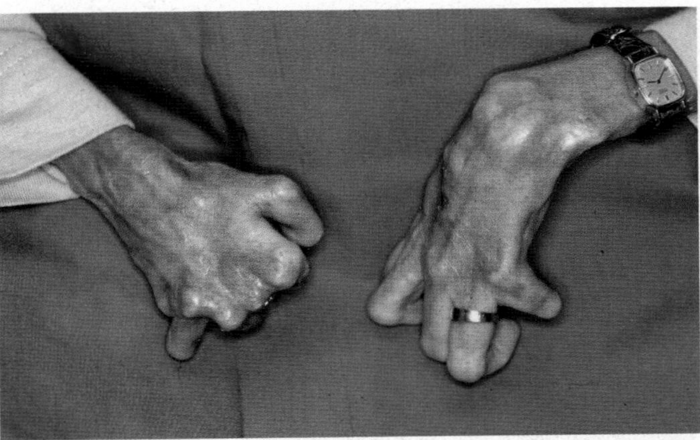

FIGURE 190-10 Severe scleroderma with deformity of hands as a result of sclerodactyly leading to severe flexion contractures. (*Reproduced with permission from Jeffrey Meffert, MD.*)

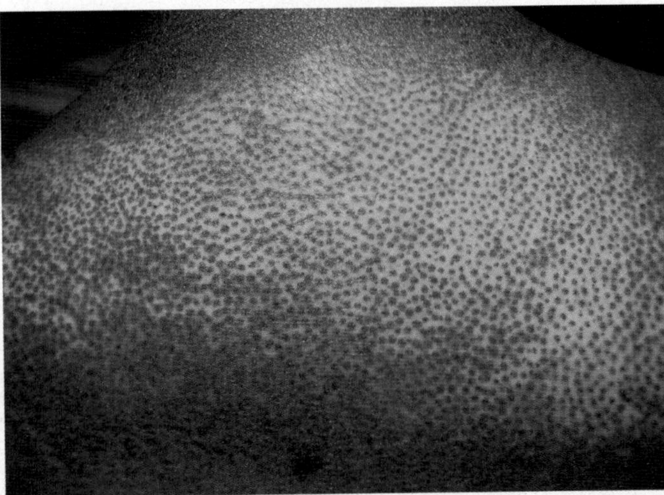

FIGURE 190-11 Scleroderma with mottled hypopigmentation. The skin may have a salt-and-pepper appearance as shown here. (*Reproduced with permission from Ricardo Zuniga-Montes, MD.*)

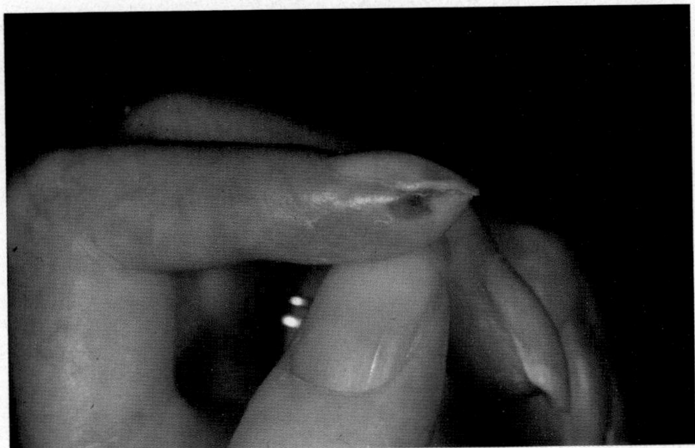

FIGURE 190-12 Sclerodactyly with tapering of the fingers and mottled hyperpigmentation. (*Reproduced with permission from Jeffrey Meffert, MD.*)

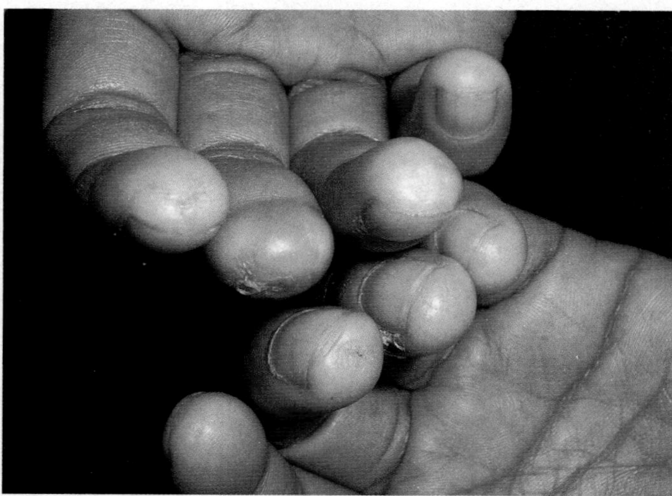

FIGURE 190-13 Digital pitting scars and loss of substance from finger pads in this 27-year-old woman with scleroderma and sclerodactyly. (*Reproduced with permission from Richard P. Usatine, MD.*)

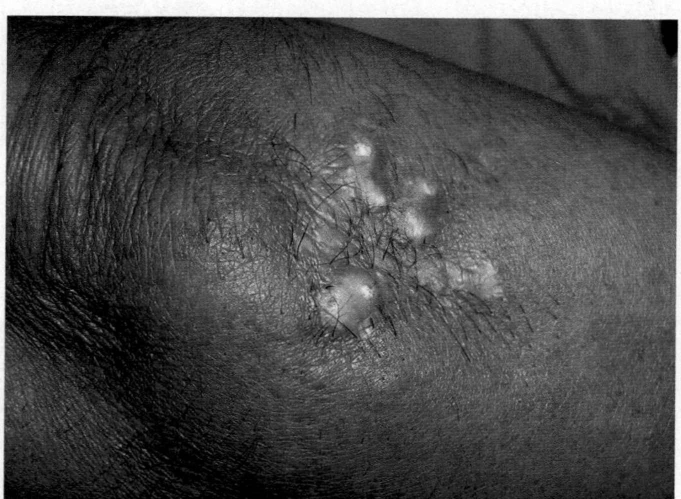

FIGURE 190-14 Calcinosis over the elbow in a patient with CREST syndrome. (*Reproduced with permission from Richard P. Usatine, MD.*)

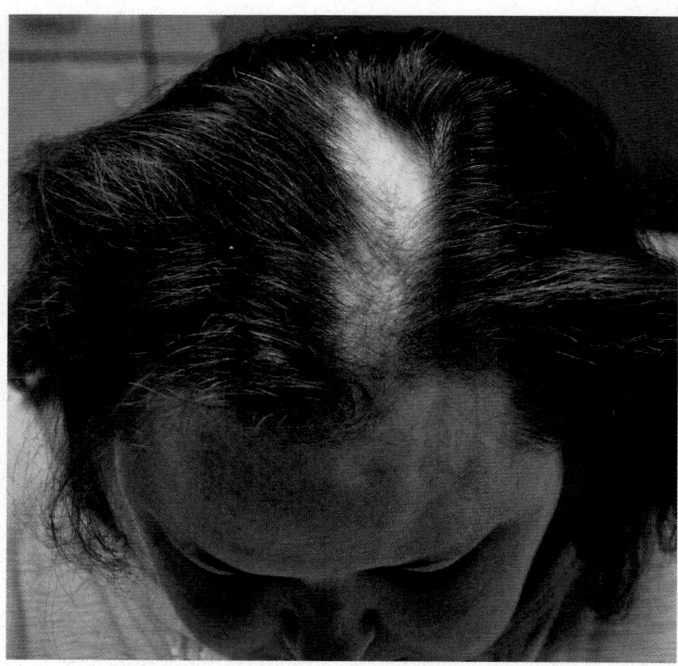

FIGURE 190-15 Linear morphea that cuts across the scalp and upper forehead like the blow of a sword known as "en coup de sabre." (*Reproduced with permission from Richard P. Usatine, MD.*)

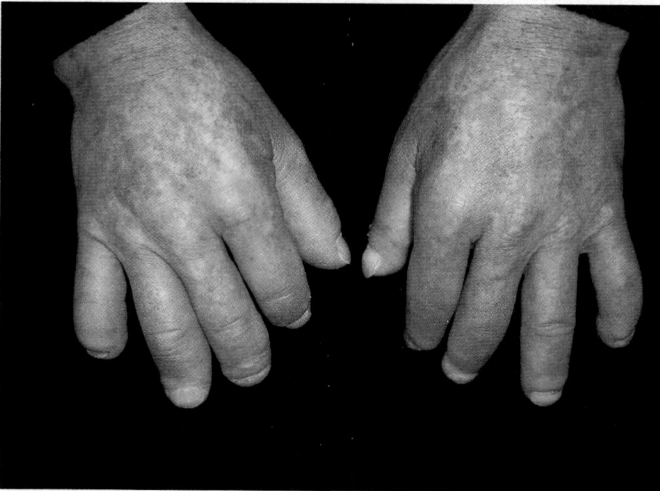

FIGURE 190-16 Sclerodactyly and sausage fingers in a 56-year-old woman with scleroderma and CREST syndrome. Note how the fingers are shortened secondary to digital tuft resorption and loss of substance from finger pads. There is also a salt-and-pepper appearance to the skin on the dorsum of the hands. (*Reproduced with permission from Richard P. Usatine, MD.*)

abnormal nail-fold capillaries, interstitial lung disease (ILD) or pulmonary arterial hypertension, Raynaud's phenomenon (RP), and SSc-related autoantibodies.

LABORATORY TESTING

- A positive antinuclear antibody (ANA) with a speckled, homogenous, or nucleolar staining pattern is common in scleroderma. Anticentromere antibodies are often associated with LcSSc. Anti-DNA topoisomerase I (Scl-70) antibodies are highly specific for both systemic sclerosis and related interstitial lung and renal disease.[10] Although not very sensitive, anti-RNA polymerases I and III antibodies are specific for systemic sclerosis. Other testing for specific organ dysfunction is routinely done, such as a serum creatinine.
- The presence of characteristic autoantibodies, such as anticentromere, antitopoisomerase I (Scl-70), anti-RNA polymerase, or U3-RNP antibodies, is supportive of the diagnosis of systemic sclerosis.

IMAGING

All patients with systemic sclerosis should have a CXR and PFTs screening for pulmonary involvement. The most common types of pulmonary involvement are interstitial lung disease and pulmonary hypertension.

The diffusing capacity (as part of PFTs) is the most sensitive test for pulmonary disease in systemic sclerosis. High-resolution CT may be indicated for further evaluation of active pulmonary disease.

BIOPSY

- A punch biopsy can be used to diagnose morphea and scleroderma when the clinical diagnosis is not clear. The biopsy specimen should be taken from an inflammatory or indurated border if present.

DIFFERENTIAL DIAGNOSIS

- Idiopathic occurrence of systemic sclerosis–associated diseases such as Raynaud phenomenon, renal failure, and gastroesophageal reflux disease.
- Systemic lupus erythematosus (SLE) presents with systemic symptoms and a typical rash that may be scarring. ANA testing may help to distinguish the diagnosis (see Chapter 188, Lupus: Systemic and Cutaneous).
- Discoid lupus erythematosus (DLE) presents as localized plaque lesion that eventually scar. Biopsy usually makes the diagnosis (see Chapter 188, Lupus: Systemic and Cutaneous).
- Myxedema is associated with hypothyroidism and is characterized by thickening and coarseness of the skin. Thyroid testing will make the diagnosis (see Chapter 235, Goitrous Hypothyroidism).
- Lichen sclerosus when it occurs away from the genital area can resemble morphea. Although it most commonly affects the genital and perianal area, it can occur on the upper trunk, breasts, and upper arms. The plaques appear atrophic, but a cigarette-paper crinkling appearance may help to differentiate it from morphea (**Figure 190-17**). A punch biopsy will lead to the correct diagnosis.
- Amyloidosis of the skin may result in localized thickening and stiffness of the skin (**Figure 190-18**). When it is a cutaneous condition

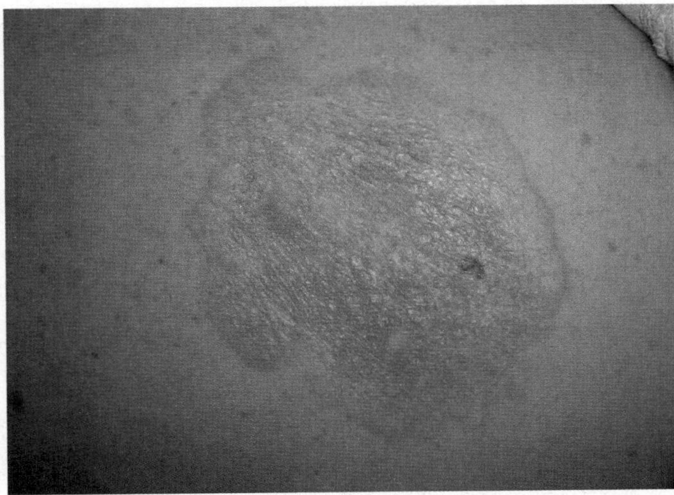

FIGURE 190-17 Extragenital lichen sclerosus on the back of a 44-year-old woman could be mistaken for morphea. Note that the crinkling (cigarette-paper appearance) of the skin helps to distinguish this from morphea. (*Reproduced with permission from Richard P. Usatine, MD.*)

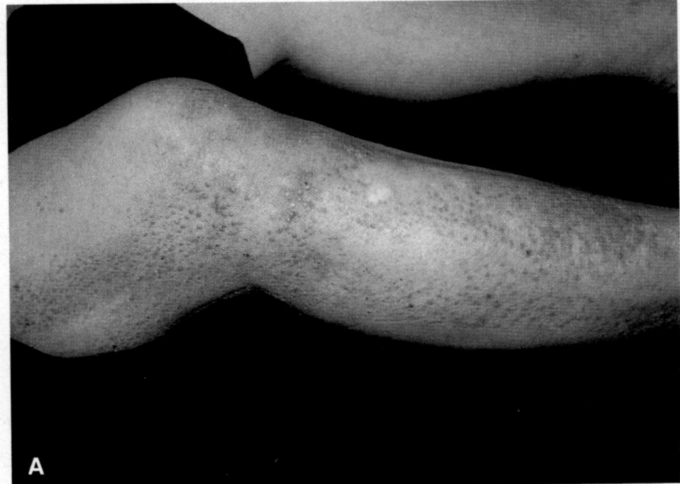

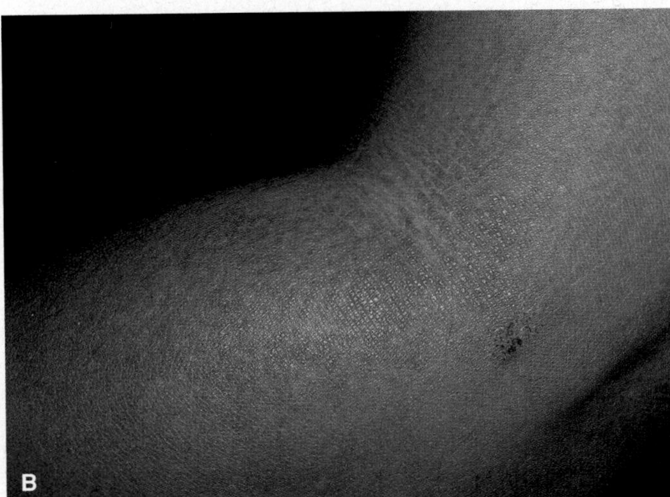

FIGURE 190-18 Cutaneous amyloidosis is caused by repeated scratching and rubbing of the skin and the thickened appearance may resemble morphea/scleroderma. **A.** Lichen amyloidosis. **B.** Macular amyloidosis. (*Reproduced with permission from Richard P. Usatine, MD.*)

rather than systemic amyloidosis, there is always a history of itching and scratching. Macular amyloidosis is flatter than lichen amyloidosis, but both are caused by repeated scratching or rubbing of the skin. Skin biopsy reveals amyloid infiltration.

- Mycosis fungoides presents with purplish macules and plaques throughout the body. Biopsy usually makes the diagnosis (see Chapter 180, Cutaneous T-Cell Lymphoma).

MANAGEMENT

NONPHARMACOLOGIC

- Localized scleroderma, including morphea, appears to soften with UVA light therapy.[11] SOR Ⓑ
- For symptomatic therapy, skin lubrication, histamine 1 (H_1) and histamine 2 (H_2) blockers, oral doxepin, and low-dose oral glucocorticoids may be used to treat pruritus. SOR Ⓒ
- Telangiectasias may be covered with foundation makeup or treated with laser therapy.

FIRST LINE

- Treatment options for morphea include high-potency topical steroids such as clobetasol and topical calcipotriol, topical calcipotriene 0.005%, topical tacrolimus 0.1%, and phototherapy (UVA or narrowband UVB).[12-14] SOR Ⓑ
- The combination of high-dose oral prednisone and low-dose oral methotrexate has been used successfully for generalized morphea and scleroderma.[15] SOR Ⓑ Methotrexate given orally or subcutaneously at a dose of 7.5 to 25 mg per week and titrated as needed. Taper the prednisone while using the oral methotrexate as a steroid-sparing agent.
- Calcium channel blockers, prazosin, prostaglandin derivatives, dipyridamole, aspirin, and topical nitrates may help symptoms of Raynaud phenomenon.[16,17] SOR Ⓑ Sildenafil (20 mg PO tid) has also been shown to be effective in patients with primary Raynaud phenomenon.[18] SOR Ⓑ Patients should be advised to avoid cold, nicotine, caffeine, and sympathomimetic decongestant medications. Acid-reducing agents may be used empirically for gastroesophageal reflux disease. Prokinetic agents, such as erythromycin, may be useful for patients with esophageal hypomotility. SOR Ⓒ
- Minocycline may be effective for calcinosis at a dose of 100 mg daily (see **Figure 190-9**).

SECOND LINE

- Unapproved therapies for skin disease include interferon-γ, mycophenolate mofetil (1 to 1.5 g PO bid), and cyclophosphamide (50 to 150 mg/day PO in a single a.m. dose). Extensive skin disease is being experimentally treated with d-penicillamine (250 to 1500 mg/day PO bid/tid on an empty stomach).[19] SOR Ⓑ Rituximab has also shown to be effective for skin fibrosis.[20]
- The mainstay of treatment of renal disease is control of blood pressure, with angiotensin-converting enzyme (ACE) inhibitors being the first-line agent. SOR Ⓒ Hemodialysis or peritoneal dialysis may be used as needed.
- Treatments of pulmonary hypertension associated with the systemic sclerosis being tested include the endothelin receptor antagonist bosentan (62.5 mg PO bid for 4 weeks, then increase to 125 mg PO bid), the phosphodiesterase-5 inhibitor sildenafil, and various prostacyclin analogs (e.g., epoprostenol, treprostinil, and iloprost). Pulmonary fibrosing alveolitis may be treated with cyclophosphamide.[21] SOR Ⓑ
- Myositis may be treated with oral prednisone, methotrexate, and azathioprine (50 to 150 mg daily). Doses of prednisone greater than 40 mg/day are associated with a higher incidence of sclerodermal renal crisis.[22] SOR Ⓑ Arthralgias can be treated with acetaminophen and nonsteroidal anti-inflammatory drugs (NSAIDs). SOR Ⓒ
- Arthritis is often treated with treatment with hydroxychloroquine 200 to 400 mg daily (maximum 6.5 mg/kg real body weight) and, if unresponsive, by adding methotrexate.[23]
- Any patient on long-term oral prednisone needs to be monitored for osteoporosis and diabetes. Osteoporosis prevention should include weight-bearing exercise, calcium, vitamin D supplements, and yearly dual-energy X-ray absorptiometry (DEXA) scanning to determine when and if additional medications are needed.

REFERRAL

Patients with systemic sclerosis should be referred to a rheumatologist, as this is a complicated disease that often requires the use of immunosuppressive medications. Depending on the complications, patients with scleroderma may also need referral to pulmonology, cardiology, and nephrology.

PROGNOSIS

- There is an increase in the risk of premature death with systemic sclerosis. Most deaths among these patients are a result of pulmonary fibrosis and/or pulmonary hypertension. Mortality also results from renal crisis, cardiac disease, infections, malignancies, and cardiovascular disease.[24]
- The prognosis for morphea is usually excellent, as it only affects the skin. Although the appearance may be disturbing to the patient, it is not life-threatening. If the morphea is extensive and over an extremity, it can affect function (**Figure 190-19**).

FOLLOW-UP

- The patient with systemic sclerosis needs to be evaluated at least every 3 months to monitor disease activity, medication side effects, and progression.

PATIENT EDUCATION

- Instruct the patient to avoid skin trauma (especially to the fingers), cold exposure, and smoking. Make patients aware of potential complications and have them watch for signs of systemic disease occurrence or progression.

PATIENT RESOURCES

- American College of Rheumatology. *Scleroderma (Also Known as Systemic Sclerosis)*—**http://www.rheumatology.org/I-Am-A/Patient-Caregiver/Diseases-Conditions/Scleroderma.**
- Scleroderma Foundation—**http://www.scleroderma.org.**
- International Scleroderma Network—**http://www.sclero.org.**

PROVIDER RESOURCES

- National Institute of Arthritis and Musculoskeletal and Skin Diseases. *Handout on Health: Scleroderma*—**http://www.niams.nih.gov/health-topics/scleroderma**.
- Medscape. *Scleroderma*—**http://emedicine.medscape.com/article/331864**.

REFERENCES

1. Lawrence RC, Helmick CG, Arnett FC, et al. Estimates of the prevalence of arthritis and selected musculoskeletal disorders in the United States. *Arthritis Rheum.* 1998;41(5):778-799.
2. Chifflot H, Fautrel B, Sordet C, et al. Incidence and prevalence of systemic sclerosis: a systematic literature review. *Semin Arthritis Rheum.* 2008;37(4):223-235.
3. Steen VD, Lucas M, Fertig N, Medsger TA Jr. Pulmonary arterial hypertension and severe pulmonary fibrosis in systemic sclerosis patients with a nucleolar antibody. *J Rheumatol.* 2007;34(11):2230-2235.
4. Akesson A, Wollheim FA. Organ manifestations in 100 patients with progressive systemic sclerosis: a comparison between the CREST syndrome and diffuse scleroderma. *Br J Rheumatol.* 1989;28(4):281-286.
5. Medsger TA Jr, Masi AT. Survival with scleroderma. II. A life-table analysis of clinical and demographic factors in 358 male U.S. veteran patients. *J Chronic Dis.* 1973;26(10):647-660.
6. Tuffanelli DL, Winkelmann RK. Systemic scleroderma, a clinical study of 727 cases. *Arch Dermatol.* 1961;84:359-371.
7. Janosik DL, Osborn TG, Moore TL, et al. Heart disease in systemic sclerosis. *Semin Arthritis Rheum.* 1989;19(3):191-200.
8. Byers RJ, Marshall DA, Freemont AJ. Pericardial involvement in systemic sclerosis. *Ann Rheum Dis.* 1997;56(6):393-394.
9. van den Hoogen F, Khanna D, Fransen J, et al. 2013 classification criteria for systemic sclerosis: an American college of rheumatology/European league against rheumatism collaborative initiative. *Ann Rheum Dis.* 2013;72:1747.
10. Reveille JD, Solomon DH. Evidence-based guidelines for the use of immunologic tests: Anticentromere, Scl-70, and nucleolar antibodies. *Arthritis Rheum.* 2003;49(3):399-412.
11. Kreuter A, Breuckmann F, Uhle A, et al. Low-dose UVA1 phototherapy in systemic sclerosis: effects on acrosclerosis. *J Am Acad Dermatol.* 2004;50(5):740-747.
12. Seyger MM, van den Hoogen FH, de Boo T, de Jong EM. Low-dose methotrexate in the treatment of widespread morphea. *J Am Acad Dermatol.* 1998;39(2 Pt 1):220-225.

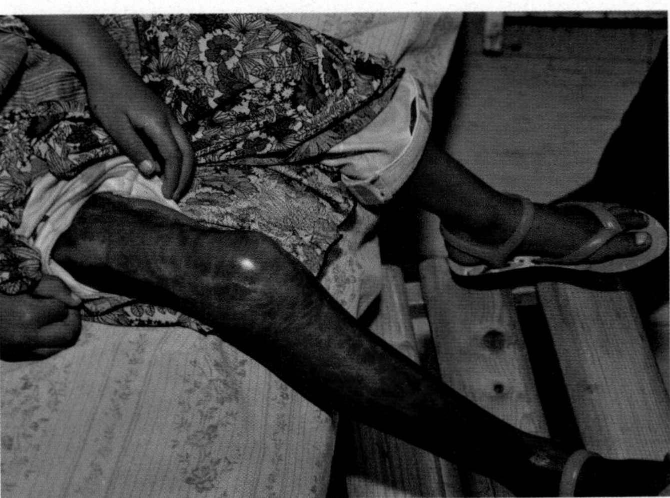

FIGURE 190-19 Localized morphea of the leg in this young girl. Although her disease is not systemic, the tightening of the skin around the knee does cause problems with knee movement and ambulation. *(Reproduced with permission from Richard P. Usatine, MD.)*

13. Zwischenberger BA, Jacobe HT. A systematic review of morphea treatments and therapeutic algorithm. *J Am Acad Dermatol.* 2011; 65:925.

14. Kreuter A, Hyun J, Stücker M, et al. A randomized controlled study of low-dose UVA1, medium-dose UVA1, and narrowband UVB phototherapy in the treatment of localized scleroderma. *J Am Acad Dermatol.* 2006;54:440.

15. Kreuter A, Gambichler T, Breuckmann F, et al. Pulsed high-dose corticosteroids combined with low-dose methotrexate in severe localized scleroderma. *Arch Dermatol.* 2005;141(7):847-852.

16. Thompson AE, Shea B, Welch V, et al. Calcium-channel blockers for Raynaud's phenomenon in systemic sclerosis. *Arthritis Rheum.* 2001;44(8):1841-1847.

17. Clifford PC, Martin MF, Sheddon EJ, et al. Treatment of vasospastic disease with prostaglandin E1. *Br Med J.* 1980;281(6247):1031-1034.

18. Fries R, Shariat K, von Wilmowsky H, Bohm M. Sildenafil in the treatment of Raynaud's phenomenon resistant to vasodilatory therapy. *Circulation.* 2005;112(19):2980-2985.

19. Falanga V, Medsger TA Jr. D-penicillamine in the treatment of localized scleroderma. *Arch Dermatol.* 1990;126(5):609-612.

20. Jordan S, Distler JH, Maurer B, et al. Effects and safety of rituximab in systemic sclerosis: an analysis from the European Scleroderma Trial and Research (EUSTAR) group. *Ann Rheum Dis.* 2015;74:1188.

21. Tashkin DP, Elashoff R, Clements PJ, et al. Cyclophosphamide versus placebo in scleroderma lung disease. *N Engl J Med.* 2006; 354(25):2655-2666.

22. Steen VD, Medsger TA Jr. Case-control study of corticosteroids and other drugs that either precipitate or protect from the development of scleroderma renal crisis. *Arthritis Rheum.* 1998;41(9): 1613-1619.

23. Avouac J, Clements PJ, Khanna D, et al. Articular involvement in systemic sclerosis. *Rheumatology (Oxford).* 2012;51:1347.

24. Tyndall AJ, Bannert B, Vonk M, et al. Causes and risk factors for death in systemic sclerosis: a study from the EULAR Scleroderma Trials and Research (EUSTAR) database. *Ann Rheum Dis.* 2010; 69(10):1809-1815.

SECTION Q BULLOUS DISEASE

191 OVERVIEW OF BULLOUS DISEASES

Richard P. Usatine, MD
Ana Treviño Sauceda, MD

PATIENT STORY

A 100-year-old black woman with diabetes was brought to the office by her family concerned about the large blister on her leg that started earlier that day (**Figure 191-1**). This large bulla appeared spontaneously without trauma, and there was no surrounding erythema. The bulla contained clear fluid, and there were no signs of infection. The bulla was drained with a sterile needle and no further bullae developed. The diagnosis is bullosis diabeticorum, a benign self-limited condition.

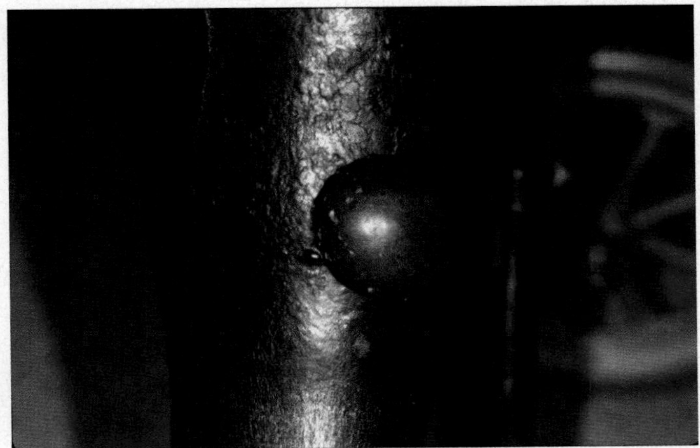

FIGURE 191-1 Bullosis diabeticorum on the lower leg of an older black woman with diabetes. This large bulla appeared spontaneously without trauma and there is no surrounding erythema. The bulla contained clear fluid and there was no infection. *(Reproduced with permission from Richard P. Usatine, MD.)*

INTRODUCTION

Bullae are fluid-filled lesions on the skin that are larger than 10 mm in diameter. Bullous diseases are defined by the presence of bullae and vesicles (less than 10 mm in diameter). Bullous diseases are caused by many factors, including infections, bites, drug reactions, inflammatory conditions, and genetic and autoimmune diseases.

APPROACH TO THE DIAGNOSIS

The approach to a patient with a blistering disorder begins with a complete history and physical examination. To make the final diagnosis, laboratory investigations or tissue biopsies may be needed.

DIAGNOSIS

HISTORY

- How did the eruption present?
- Has it changed in morphology or location?
- Has it responded to any therapies?
- Are there any associated symptoms or aggravating factors?
- How has it impacted the patient's life?
- Does the patient have any chronic medical conditions?
- Does the patient take any medications?
- Does the patient have any significant family history?

PHYSICAL EXAMINATION

- Note the location of the eruption.
- Are the bullae flaccid or tense (**Figure 191-2**)?

- Are there other lesions present (erosions, excoriations, papules, wheals)?
- Is Nikolsky sign positive or negative? (Does the skin shear off when lateral pressure is applied to unblistered skin?)
- Is Asboe-Hansen sign positive or negative (**Figure 191-3**)? (Do the bullae extend to surrounding skin when vertical pressure is applied?) Sometimes the Asboe-Hansen sign is also attributed to Nikolsky and called a Nikolsky sign, too.
- Is the Darier sign positive or negative? (Do wheals form with rubbing of the skin?)
- Note the skin background (sun-exposed skin, postinflammatory hyperpigmentation, lichenification, and scarring).
- Does the patient have lymphadenopathy or hepatosplenomegaly?

CLINICAL FEATURES

- Autoimmune:
  - In bullous pemphigoid, patients have large, tense bullae that primarily involve the trunk, groin, axilla, proximal extremities, and flexor surfaces (see **Figures 191-2A** and **191-3**; Chapter 192, Bullous Pemphigoid).[1]
  - Pemphigus vulgaris is characterized by erosions and flaccid bullae that frequently involve the mouth (**Figure 191-4**; Chapter 193, Pemphigus). In fact, mucosal membrane involvement may be the initial presentation. If the skin is involved, then Nikolsky and Asboe-Hansen signs are positive.[1]
  - Pemphigus foliaceus presents with cutaneous erosions and never involves the mucosal membranes (see **Figure 191-2B**; Chapter 193, Pemphigus). Nikolsky and Asboe-Hansen signs are positive.[1]
  - Pemphigoid gestationis is a condition during pregnancy or during the postpartum period that can have a bullous component. The patient usually presents with urticarial papules and plaques with bullae developing around the umbilicus and extremities. The eruption eventually generalizes and involves the palms and soles. There usually is sparing of the face, scalp, and oral mucosa (**Figure 191-5**).[1]
  - Cicatricial pemphigoid involves the oral mucosa in 90% of cases and the conjunctiva in 66% of cases (**Figures 192-3** to **192-5** in Chapter 192, Bullous Pemphigoid). Patients frequently present with a desquamative gingivitis. Cutaneous lesions are seen in 25% of patients.[1]
  - Epidermolysis bullosa acquisita presents with trauma-induced blistering and erosions usually on the distal extremities (**Figure 191-6**). The patient should have background scarring, milia, and nail dystrophy. This usually affects elderly persons.
  - Epidermolysis bullosa simplex also has trauma-induced blistering that can involve the trunk and extremities. This is the most common form of epidermolysis bullosa and usually starts at birth or early childhood. The bullae are intraepidermal (**Figure 191-7**).
  - Dermatitis herpetiformis classically is a symmetrical, pruritic eruption that involves the extensor surfaces, scalp, and buttocks. The patient presents with pruritic vesicles and crusted papules with overlying excoriations (see **Figures 194-11** and **194-12** in Chapter 194, Other Bullous Diseases).[1]
  - Linear immunoglobulin (Ig): A bullous dermatosis may produce a ringlike pattern of distribution and can occur in childhood (**Figure 191-8**). Patients may have mucous membrane involvement in up to 50% of cases.[1]

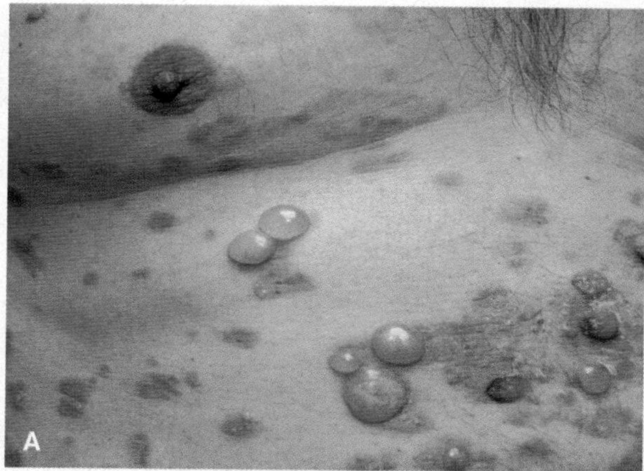

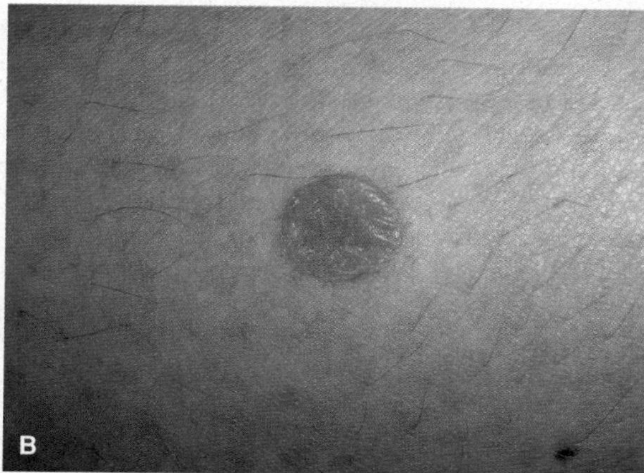

FIGURE 191-2 Comparison of the tense bullae seen in bullous pemphigoid and the more flaccid bullae seen in pemphigus. **A.** Tense bullae in bullous pemphigoid. **B.** Flaccid bulla on the leg of a patient with pemphigus foliaceus. *(Reproduced with permission from Richard P. Usatine, MD.)*

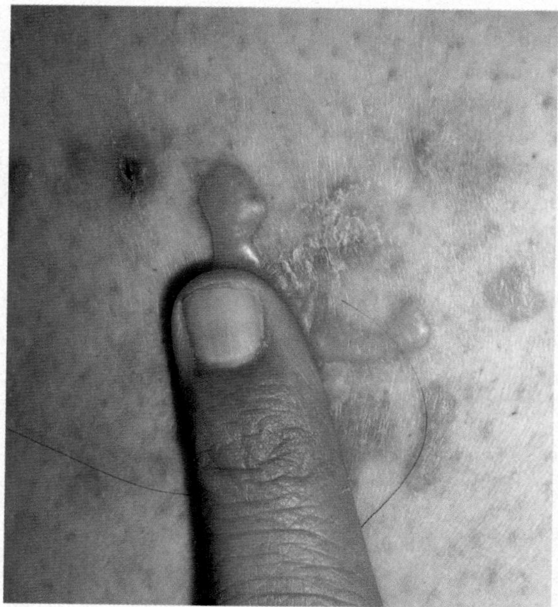

FIGURE 191-3 Testing for Asboe-Hansen sign on the back of a patient with bullous pemphigoid. The bulla did not extend with vertical pressure, so the sign was negative. *(Reproduced with permission from Richard P. Usatine, MD.)*

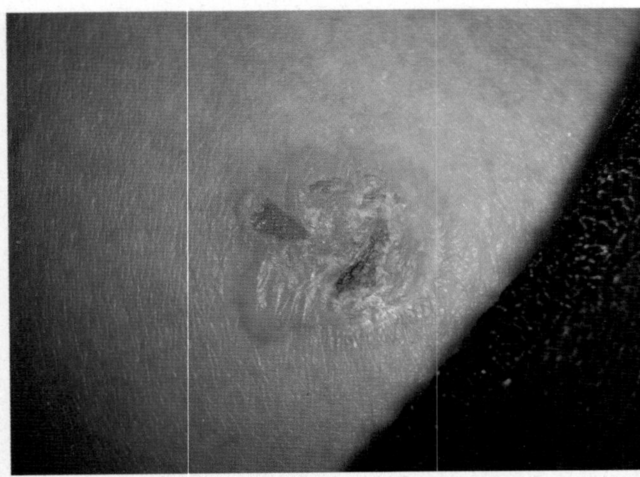

FIGURE 191-4 Flaccid and partially crusted bulla on the breast of a 51-year-old woman with pemphigus vulgaris. She also has severe oral involvement with large mucosal erosions. (*Reproduced with permission from Richard P. Usatine, MD.*)

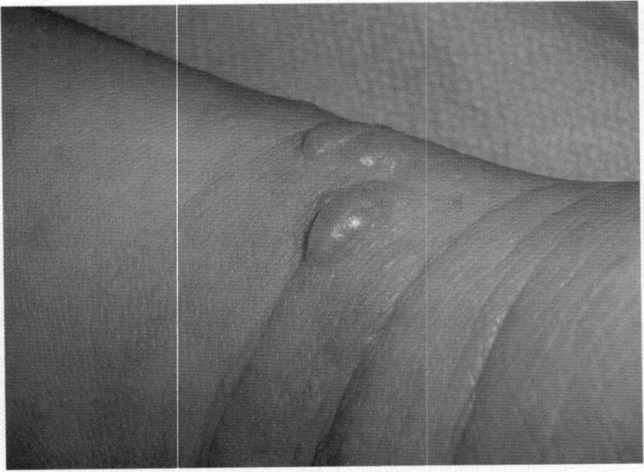

FIGURE 191-5 Pemphigoid gestationis with bullae on the wrist. (*Reproduced with permission from Richard P. Usatine, MD.*)

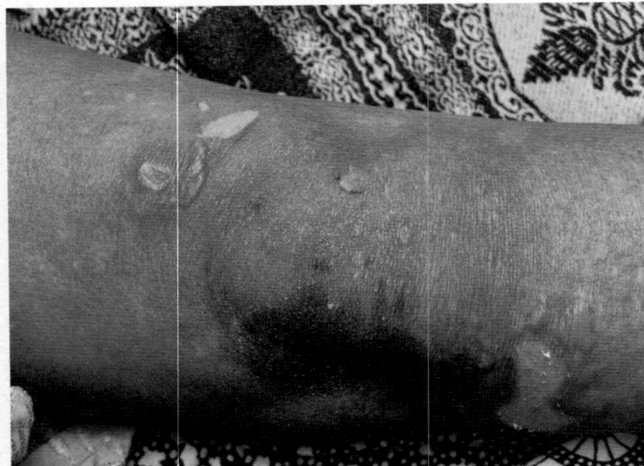

FIGURE 191-6 Epidermolysis bullosa acquisita in an elderly woman. Note the partially intact bulla over the knee along with other areas of erosions and hyperpigmentation. (*Reproduced with permission from Richard P. Usatine, MD.*)

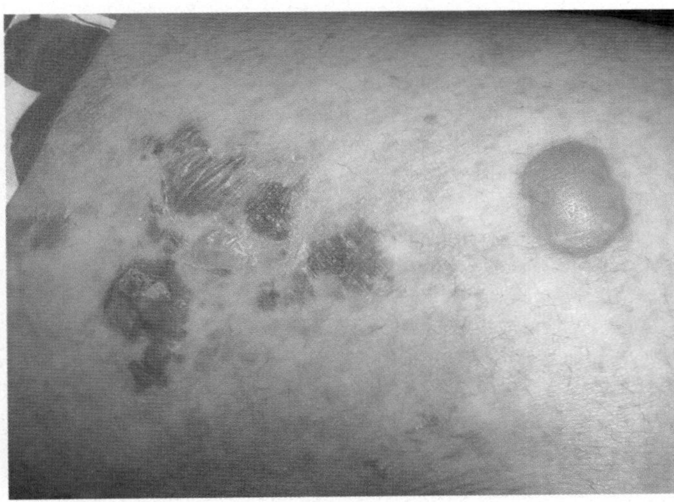

FIGURE 191-7 Large trauma-induced bulla on the leg of a 13-year-old girl with epidermolysis bullosa simplex. (*Reproduced with permission from Richard P. Usatine, MD.*)

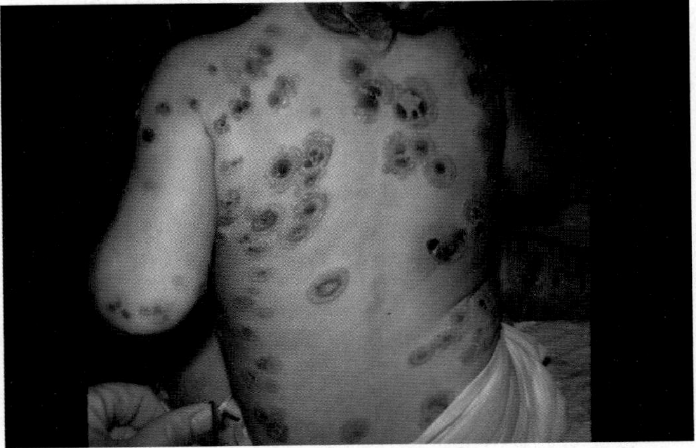

FIGURE 191-8 Bullae in a ringlike pattern in a young girl with IgA bullous dermatosis of childhood. (*Reproduced with permission from Jack Resneck, Sr., MD.*)

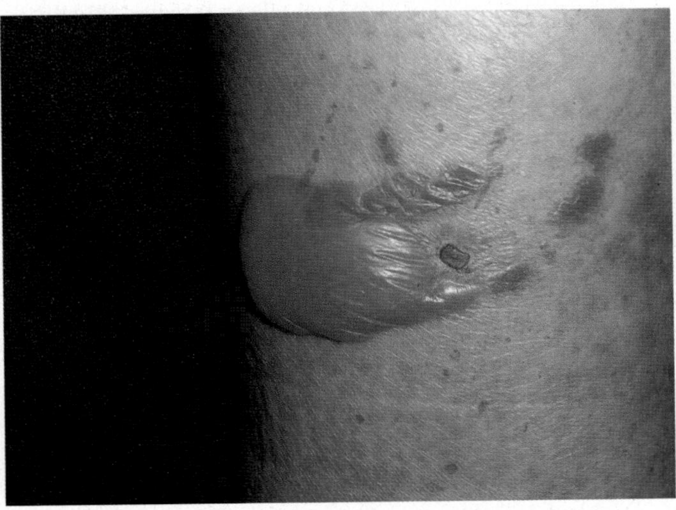

FIGURE 191-9 Large intact bulla on the lower leg of a woman with diabetes. This is bullosis diabeticorum, also known as a diabetic bulla. (*Reproduced with permission from Richard P. Usatine, MD.*)

- Traumatic/physical stress:
  - Friction blisters form at sites of pressure and friction, frequently on the distal lower extremities.[1]
  - Bullosis diabeticorum is trauma-induced, painless blistering, frequently in an acral distribution, in individuals with diabetes mellitus (**Figure 191-9**).[1]
  - Postburn blistering occurs in the hours after the insult, such as is seen in severe second-degree sunburns.[1] Blistering after cold injury can also occur rapidly (**Figure 191-10**).
  - Miliaria is caused by keratinous obstruction of the eccrine ducts in response to heat. Small superficial vesicles may involve the face, trunk, or extremities.[1]
- Metabolic:
  - Porphyria cutanea tarda (PCT) involves sun-exposed skin, particularly the dorsal hands, forearms, ears, and face. The patient will have associated milia, scarring, and background dyspigmentation. PCT has been associated with hepatitis C infection (see **Figure 191-11**).[1]
- Immunologic:
  - Pityriasis lichenoides et varioliformis acuta (PLEVA) usually presents as a papulonecrotic eruption but may have vesicles resembling varicella (see **Figure 191-12**). It usually involves the anterior trunk, flexor surfaces of the upper extremities, and the axilla. It is seen more frequently in young men and can go on to become chronic.
  - Allergic-contact and irritant-contact dermatitis, if severe, can cause blistering. Special attention should be given to the location and pattern of involvement. For example, linear vesicles and bullae would suggest a plant-induced dermatitis such as poison ivy, poison oak, or poison sumac (**Figure 191-13**). Blistering in the periumbilical area is consistent with nickel dermatitis from a belt buckle or pants snap. Involvement of the dorsal feet is frequently seen with footwear dermatitis due to chemicals in the leather (Chapter 152, Contact Dermatitis).[2]
- Drug:
  - Bullous drug eruptions may be localized to 2 mucosal surfaces with minimal cutaneous involvement or may be generalized, involving all mucosal surfaces and a majority of the skin surface area. Nikolsky and Asboe-Hansen signs are positive on affected skin. Even fixed-drug eruptions can be bullous (**Figure 191-14**).
- Infections and bites:
  - Bullous arthropod reaction can occur after an insect bite (**Figure 191-15**).[1]
  - Bacterial infections should be considered when evaluating a localized blistering eruption. Amongst these infections is bullous impetigo (**Figure 191-16**). When evaluating the extremities, vesiculation overlying cellulitis may be associated with the more severe staphylococcal and streptococcal infections, and a thorough evaluation should be conducted to rule out necrotizing fasciitis. As with most bacterial infections, the patient typically presents with fever and has an elevated white blood cell count.[2]
  - Herpes simplex viruses should always be considered when blistering of the mucosal surfaces is observed. Generalized blistering in the adult could be from disseminated herpes and should prompt an evaluation for immunosuppression. Blistering in a

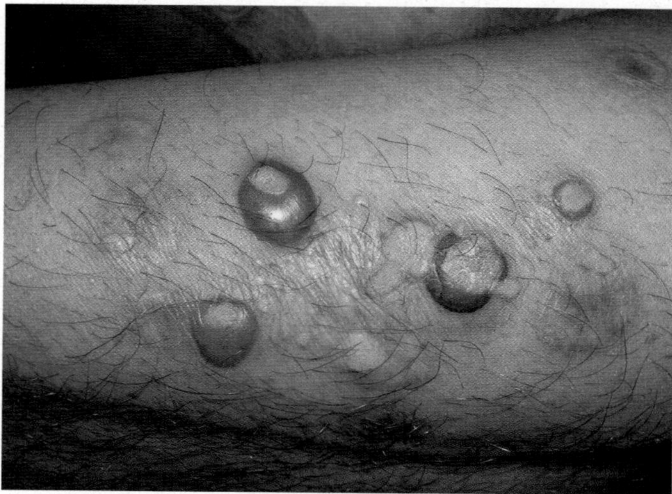

FIGURE 191-10 Bullae the day after cryotherapy for warts. (*Reproduced with permission from Richard P. Usatine, MD.*)

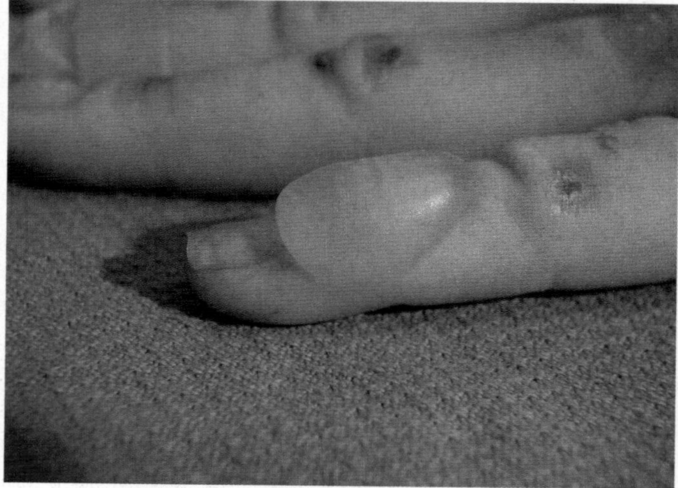

FIGURE 191-11 Porphyria cutanea tarda with a large bulla on the finger. (*Reproduced with permission from Lewis Rose, MD.*)

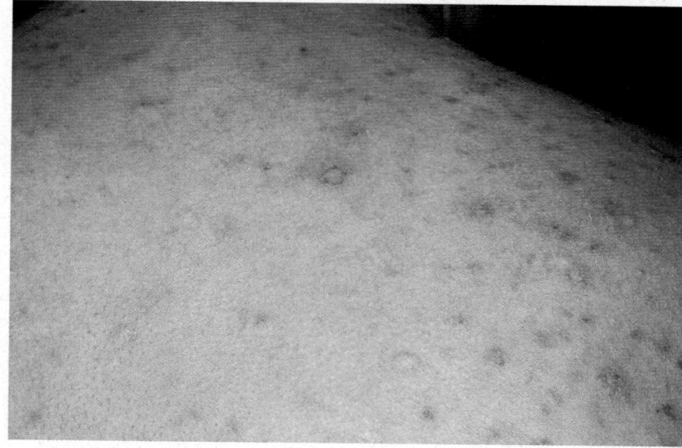

FIGURE 191-12 Pityriasis lichenoides et varioliformis acuta in a young man showing erosions where vesicles and bullae had been previously. (*Reproduced with permission from Richard P. Usatine, MD.*)

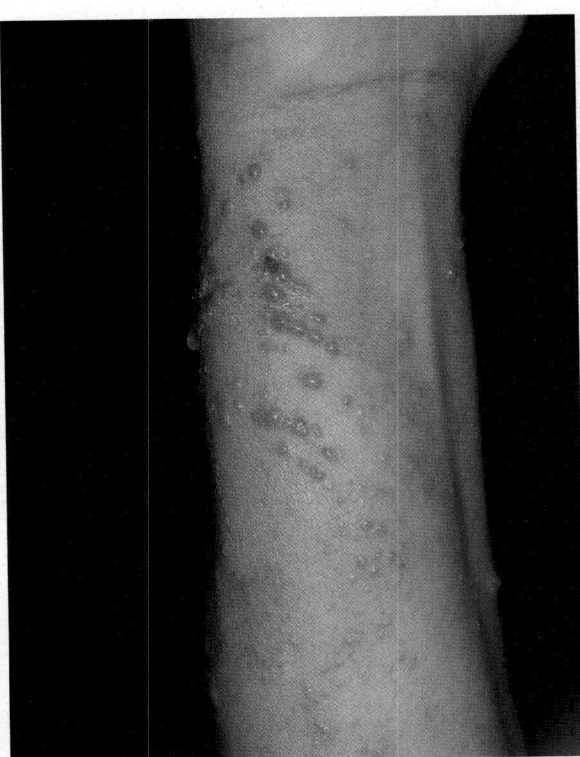

FIGURE 191-13 Bullae and vesicles on the extremity of a patient with poison ivy. Acute contact dermatitis can present with bullae and vesicles. (*Reproduced with permission from Richard P. Usatine, MD.*)

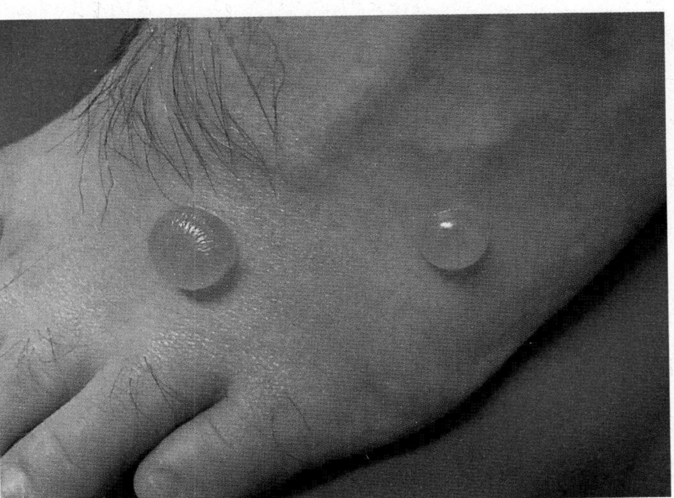

FIGURE 191-15 Bullous arthropod bites secondary to fire ants. (*Reproduced with permission from Lane K, Lumbang W. Pruritic blisters on legs and feet, J Fam Pract. 2008;57(3):177-180. Frontline Medical Communications. Inc.*)

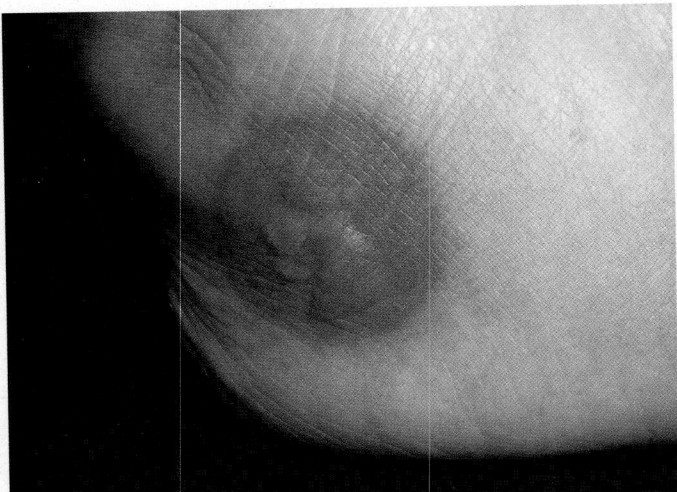

FIGURE 191-14 Bullous fixed-drug eruption on the ankle of a woman taking amoxicillin. She has had this reaction before in the same location while taking another penicillin antibiotic. Note the dusky color, annular erythema, and the central bullae. (*Reproduced with permission from Richard P. Usatine, MD.*)

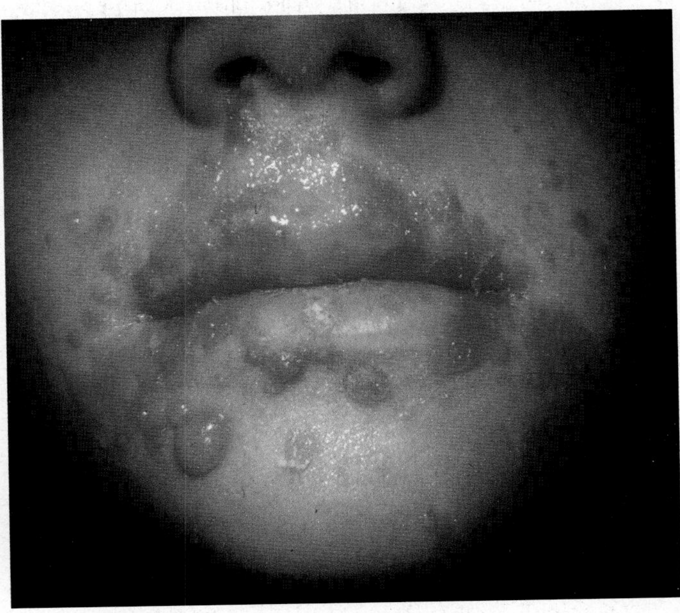

FIGURE 191-16 Bullous impetigo on the face of a child. Note the honey crusts, vesicles, and bullae. (*Reproduced with permission from Jack Resneck, Sr., MD.*)

dermatomal distribution is characteristic of herpes zoster (**Figures 191-17** and **191-18**).[2]
  - Scabies, tinea, and *Candida* can also have bullous or pustular presentations in the classic sites of involvement.[2]
- Hydrostatic.
  - Edema blisters form from the osmotic pressure experienced during the third-spacing of fluid. As such, patients usually have a diagnosis of heart failure, cirrhosis, or kidney failure.[1]
- Childhood.
  - Transient neonatal pustular melanosis (TNPM) involves pustules or vesicles without associated erythema located in clusters on the forehead, posterior ears, chin, neck, upper chest, back, buttocks, abdomen, and thighs, which spontaneously heal and leave behind pigmented macules. TNPM affects up to 4% of term infants and is more commonly seen in the African-American population (Chapter 116, Pustular Diseases of Childhood).[3]
  - Acropustulosis of infancy develops during the first few weeks to months of life and spontaneously remits at 2 to 3 years of age. In this condition, crops of vesicles and pustules involve palms and soles, causing pruritus (Chapter 116, Pustular Diseases of Childhood).[3]
  - Neonatal pemphigus occurs in neonates whose mothers have active pemphigus vulgaris. The patient is born with bullae that spontaneously resolve within 1 to 2 weeks.[3]
  - Epidermolysis bullosa simplex is a hereditary condition in which minimal friction or trauma causes vesicles, bullae, and erosions. The distal extremities are frequently involved.[4]
  - Congenital infections with herpes simplex virus usually present with vesicles. In addition, a vesicular eruption in the neonate could be caused by neonatal syphilis, which is the only form of syphilis with a vesicular presentation.[2]
  - Bullous mastocytosis is caused by mast cell accumulation in the skin. The bullous presentation is less common but may involve any area of the body (**Figure 191-19**). On examination, the Darier sign should be positive and dermatographism should be present. Work-up should be conducted to determine the presence of systemic involvement, which may include a mast cell leukemia. A good lymph node and abdominal examination is recommended to evaluate for lymphadenopathy and hepatosplenomegaly.[3]

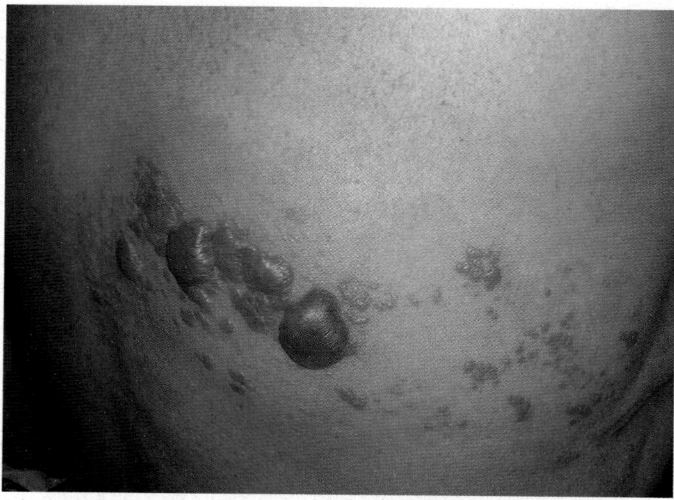

FIGURE 191-17 Herpes zoster with large bullae in a dermatomal pattern. (*Reproduced with permission from Rose Walczak, MD.*)

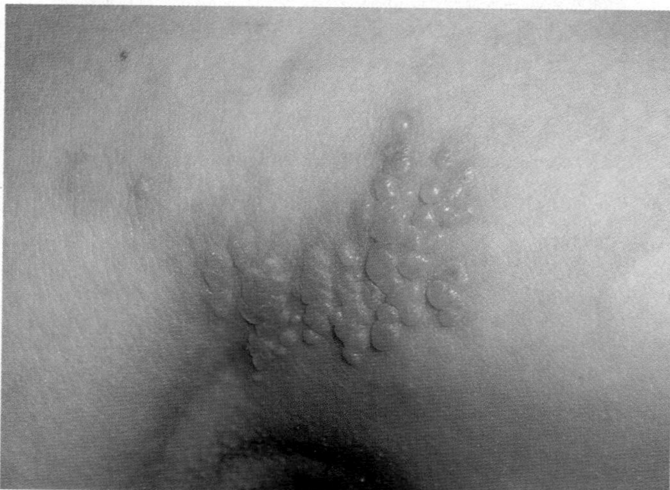

FIGURE 191-18 Cluster of intact bullae and vesicles on an erythematous base in a young woman with herpes zoster in the axilla. (*Reproduced with permission from Richard P. Usatine, MD.*)

LABORATORY STUDIES AND WORK-UP

If the clinical picture is not clear, various laboratory studies may assist the clinician in making the diagnosis. Some diagnoses should be confirmed by histology even if the diagnosis appears clear. For example, all cases of suspected pemphigus should be biopsied because the management will involve long-term use of potentially toxic medications and it is crucial to know the exact diagnosis. The information in Chapters 192, Bullous Pemphigoid, and 193, Pemphigus, will help one to decide which tests to use in some of the autoimmune blistering diseases. Consulting a dermatologist is very appropriate for many of the more rare and lethal conditions.

- Herpes simplex or varicella zoster virus testing can be done rapidly by polymerase chain reaction (PCR).
- Dermoscopy to see the scabies mites and burrows (Chapter 149, Scabies).

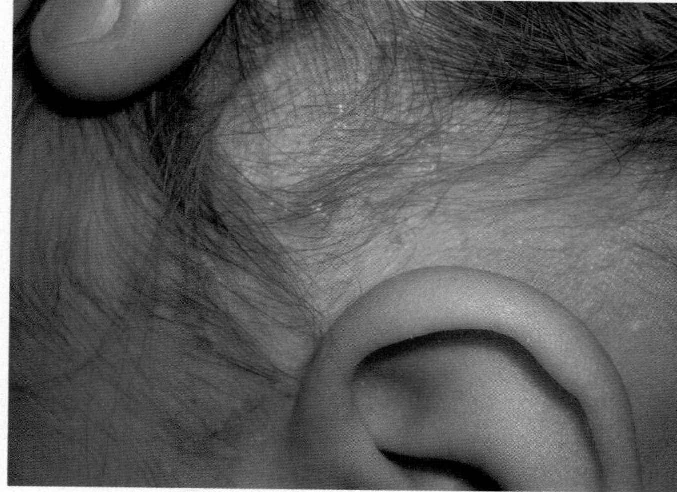

FIGURE 191-19 Bullous mastocytosis in a 9-month-old infant presenting with bullae on the scalp. (*Reproduced with permission from Richard P. Usatine, MD.*)

- KOH scraping for possible blistering tinea infections (such as bullous tinea pedis).
- Genetic studies for suspected genetic defects; consider referral to geneticist.

BIOPSY

- Four-millimeter punch biopsy for pathologic evaluation—Biopsy an established lesion including the edge of the blister. A shave biopsy is an alternative as long as the epidermis of the blister stays attached to the specimen.
- Biopsy for direct immunofluorescence (DIF)—Biopsy the perilesional skin and send the specimen in special Michel media or sterile saline and let the lab know to transfer it to Michel media when it arrives. The easiest way to do this is to take a shave biopsy that includes the bulla and the perilesional skin. Then cut the specimen in half and send the perilesional skin for DIF and the blister for standard pathology.
- Consider sending part of the biopsy for bacterial, fungal, and viral cultures and stains if infections are suspected and cultures and other less-invasive studies are not providing the diagnosis. Send the specimens in a sterile urine cup on top of a sterile gauze pad soaked with sterile saline.

FURTHER EVALUATIONS

Patients with cicatricial pemphigoid and toxic epidermal necrolysis need an ophthalmologic evaluation. Patients with several of the epidermolysis bullosa diseases and dermatitis herpetiformis need a gastroenterologic evaluation.

For possible paraneoplastic conditions, such as in epidermolysis bullosa acquisita and cicatricial pemphigoid, thorough cancer screening and studies targeting the patient's symptomatology are indicated.

REFERENCES

1. Bolognia JL, Jorizzo JL, Rapini RP. *Dermatology*. London, UK: Elsevier Health Sciences; 2003.
2. James WD, Berger TG, Elston DM. *Andrews' Diseases of the Skin: Clinical Dermatology*, 10th ed. Philadelphia, PA: Elsevier Health Sciences; 2005.
3. Schachner LA, Hansen RC. *Pediatric Dermatology*, 3rd ed. New York, NY: Mosby; 2003.
4. Spitz JL. *Genodermatoses: A Clinical Guide to Genetic Skin Disorders*. Philadelphia, PA: Lippincott Williams & Wilkins; 2004.

192 BULLOUS PEMPHIGOID

Richard P. Usatine, MD
Caitlin Morgan, MD

PATIENT STORY

A native of Panama was seen for extensive bullous disease that had a classic presentation for bullous pemphigoid (BP) (**Figure 192-1**). The classic presentation of BP is described as tense blisters that have an erythematous or urticarial base and are often pruritic. The presence of numerous intact bullae seen in this patient made pemphigus vulgaris very unlikely, as pemphigus has flaccid bullae. The Panama patient was treated with a systemic glucocorticoid (prednisone) and responded quickly. The patient eventually had a good outcome with the oral prednisone.

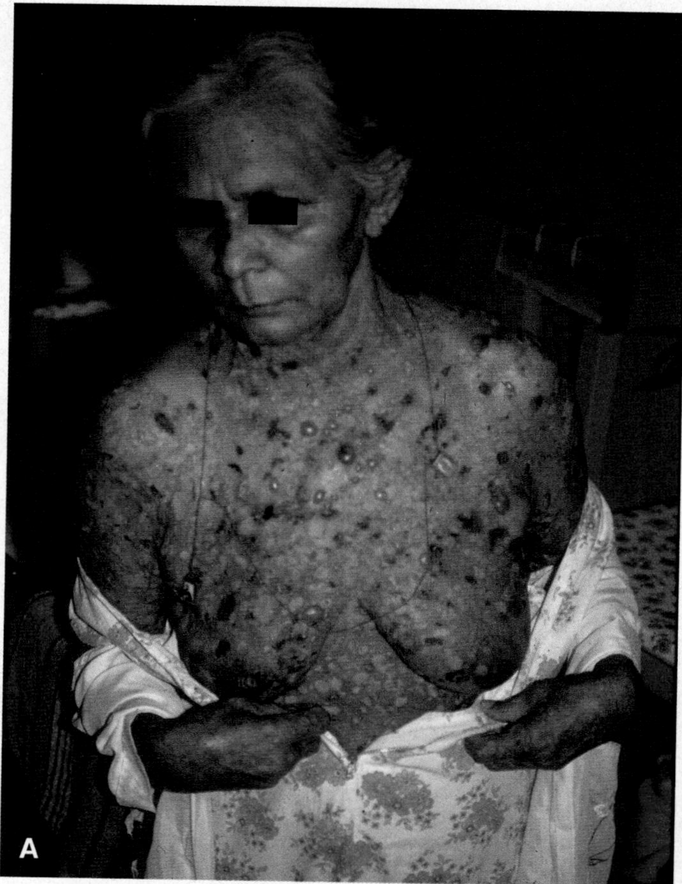

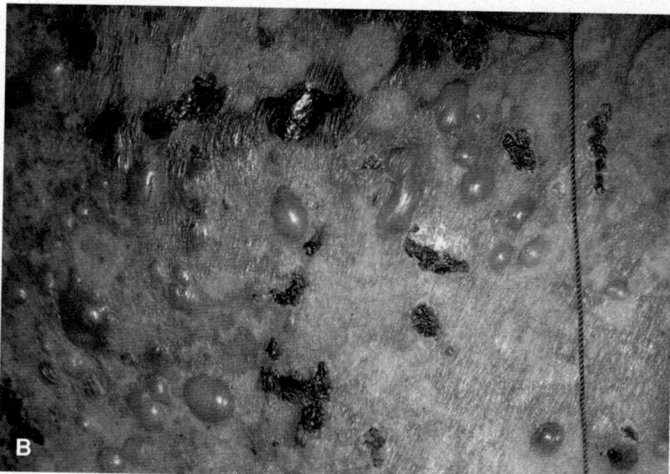

FIGURE 192-1 A. Extensive untreated bullous pemphigoid in a Panamanian woman. B. Close-up of intact bullae and dark crusts. *(Reproduced with permission from Eric Kraus, MD.)*

INTRODUCTION

BP is a chronic autoimmune blistering disease, more commonly of older adults, that may cause significant morbidity and poor quality of life. The term *pemphigoid* refers to its similarity to the blisters seen in pemphigus. However, BP is usually less severe than pemphigus vulgaris and is not considered a life-threatening condition.

EPIDEMIOLOGY

- BP is the most frequent autoimmune blistering disease of the skin and mucosa.
- It typically affects persons older than 65 years of age but can occur at any age.
- There is no racial or gender predilection (a recent British population study, however, suggested an increased prevalence in women).[1]
- Its incidence may be on the rise.[1]
- Although it is not considered life threatening, it has been associated with an increased risk of mortality (hazard ratio [HR] 2.3, 95% confidence interval [CI] 2 to 2.7).[1]

ETIOLOGY AND PATHOPHYSIOLOGY

- BP is a chronic autoimmune disorder of the skin.
- Immunoglobulin (Ig) G antibodies against BP180 antigen of the basement membrane protein are considered pathognomonic and can be found in up to 65% of patients.[2]
- Anti-BP230 antibodies are present in virtually all patients but are not considered pathognomonic.[3]
- Binding of antibodies to the basement membrane activates the complement system, leading to chemotaxis of inflammatory cells such as eosinophils and mast cells, which release proteases. The subsequent degradation of hemidesmosomal proteins leads to blister formation.

- There are several morphologically distinct clinical presentations:
  - Generalized bullous form is the most common (see **Figure 192-1**). Tense bullae occur on both erythematous and normal-appearing skin surfaces. The bullae usually heal without scarring.
  - Localized form of BP is less common and is limited to a small area of involvement (**Figure 192-2**).
  - Vesicular (also known as "eczematous") form is characterized by clusters of small tense blisters with an urticarial or erythematous base.
  - Other forms are less common and include vegetative (intertriginous vegetating plaques), urticarial (without any bullae), nodular (resembling prurigo nodularis), acral (bullae on palms, soles, and face in children associated with vaccination), and generalized erythroderma (exfoliative lesions with or without vesicles/bullae).
- Pemphigoid gestationis is a variant of BP that occurs during or after pregnancy. Lesions resolve after delivery but may recur with subsequent pregnancies, or in the nonpregnant state (Chapter 78, Pemphigoid Gestationis).[4]
- Drug-induced BP has been reported with drugs containing sulfhydryl groups, including penicillamine, furosemide, captopril, and sulfasalazine.

DIAGNOSIS

CLINICAL FEATURES

- Tense blisters that involve normal or inflamed skin or mucous membranes (see **Figures 192-1** and **192-2**).
- Development of bullae is typically preceded by a prodromal phase characterized by intense pruritus with or without excoriations and eczematous (or urticarial) lesions. This phase can last for months, making early diagnosis difficult.[5]
- Nikolsky sign, which is the wrinkling and sheetlike peeling of the skin when lateral pressure is applied to unblistered skin, is usually negative.[6]
- Asboe-Hansen sign, also termed indirect Nikolsky sign or Nikolsky II sign, will be negative as well. This sign describes bullae extending to surrounding skin when vertical pressure is applied (see **Figure 192-2B**).

TYPICAL DISTRIBUTION

- Flexural surfaces of the arms and legs.
- Lower abdomen and groin.
- Mucous membranes are involved in 10% to 25% of cases.

BIOPSY

Biopsy is required for establishing diagnosis and to differentiate BP from other conditions that can have a similar clinical presentation:

- A scoop shave or 4-mm punch biopsy from the edge of an early blister, including part of the normal-appearing skin for hematoxylin and eosin (H&E) staining, shows a subepidermal blister and an eosinophil-rich mixed dermal inflammatory infiltrate. If the scoop shave contains sufficient perilesional skin, cut this off and send it for direct immunofluorescence (DIF). DIF is considered the gold standard in the diagnosis of BP.
- The skin collected from around the lesion should be transported in Michel or Zeus medium for DIF. If these media are not available,

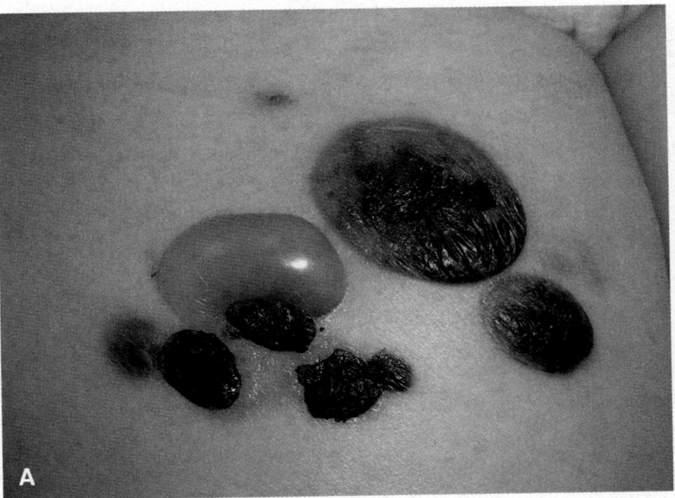

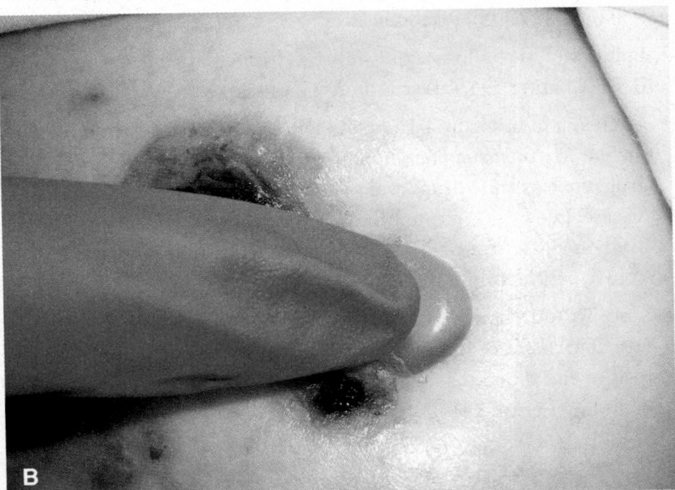

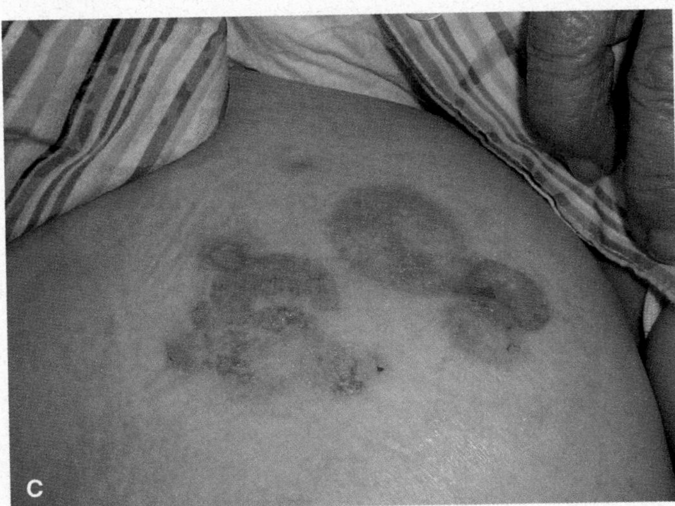

FIGURE 192-2 Localized bullous pemphigoid with large bullae on the thigh of a 91-year-old woman. Her biopsy for direct immunofluorescence demonstrated a linear band of IgG at the dermal–epidermal junction. **A.** Bullae on the thigh. **B.** New bulla 1 week later demonstrating a negative Asboe-Hansen sign. **C.** After being treated 1 week topically with clobetasol and orally with doxycycline and niacin. *(Reproduced with permission from Richard P. Usatine, MD.)*

send the specimen for DIF in sterile saline–soaked gauze and alert the laboratory to transfer the specimen into Michel medium as soon as possible. DIF demonstrates linear IgG and/or complement C3 deposits at the dermal–epidermal junction.

- Alternatively, an enzyme-linked immunosorbent assay (ELISA) blood test for BP180 antibodies can be performed for characterization of circulating antibodies.[7] If the ELISA blood test is negative for BP180 antibodies, then it can be performed for BP230 antibodies.

DIFFERENTIAL DIAGNOSIS

- Cicatricial pemphigoid (**Figures 192-3** to **192-5**)—Predominant mucosal involvement; lesions heal with prominent scarring; IgG localizes to blister floor on IDIF.
- Dermatitis herpetiformis—Grouped vesicles; extensor distribution (Chapter 194, Other Bullous Diseases).
- Epidermolysis bullosa acquisita—IgG localizes to blister floor on IDIF (Chapter 194, Other Bullous Diseases).
- Erythema multiforme—Targetoid lesions; associated with infections such as *Mycoplasma pneumoniae* and herpes simplex virus (HSV), drugs such as sulfa drugs and phenytoin, cancer, or autoimmune disease; linear IgG immunofluorescence is negative (Chapter 185, Erythema Multiforme, Stevens-Johnson Syndrome, and Toxic Epidermal Necrolysis).
- Linear IgA dermatosis—Usually drug-induced (e.g., vancomycin[8]); DIF demonstrates IgA deposits. Also called chronic bullous dermatosis of childhood (Chapter 191, Overview of Bullous Disease, including **Figure 191-4**).

MANAGEMENT

The objectives of therapy in BP are to decrease troublesome symptoms, resolve active lesions, and prevent recurrences associated with the blistering lesions.

FIRST LINE

High-potency topical corticosteroids are considered first-line treatment for moderate to severe generalized disease (e.g., clobetasol).[9] SOR Ⓐ Initial disease control and 1-year survival rates in extensive BP are better with the topical approach when compared with oral prednisolone.[10]

Oral corticosteroids.[9] SOR Ⓐ

- Prednisone 0.5 to 0.75 mg/kg per day.[11]
- Increase dose until new blisters cease to develop.
- Reduce dose approximately 10% every 2 to 3 weeks to reach dose of 15 to 20 mg/day.

Adjuvant antibiotic treatment should be considered for all patients:

- Tetracycline (1.5 to 2 g/day) with or without niacinamide (1.5 to 2 g/day).[12] SOR Ⓑ Both tetracycline and niacinamide come in 500-mg capsules and may be taken 3 to 4 times daily. Niacinamide contains niacin (vitamin B_3) and is available over the counter. Doxycycline 100 mg twice daily is an alternative.

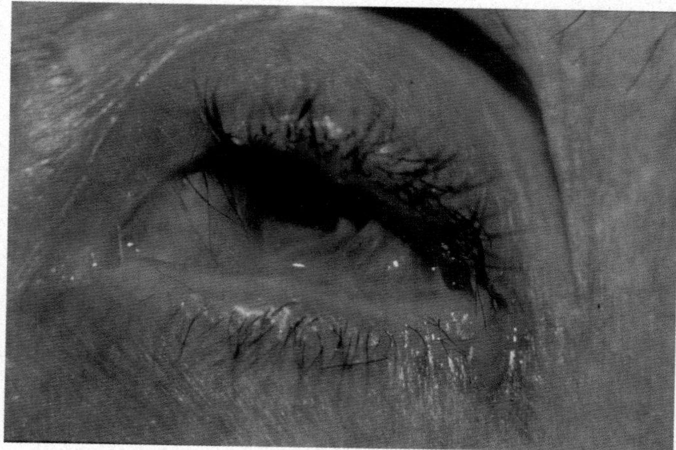

FIGURE 192-3 Cicatricial bullous pemphigoid of the eye, causing scarring and blindness. (*Reproduced with permission from Eric Kraus, MD.*)

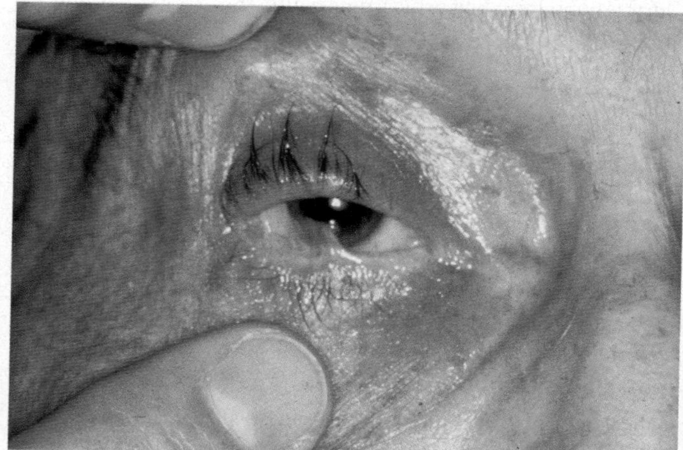

FIGURE 192-4 Cicatricial bullous pemphigoid with scarring connecting the lower lid to the cornea. (*Reproduced with permission from Eric Kraus, MD.*)

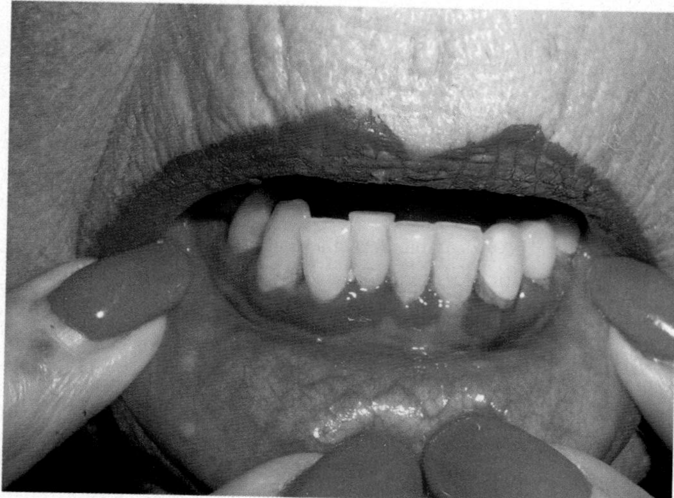

FIGURE 192-5 Cicatricial bullous pemphigoid of the mouth showing gingivitis. More than 50% of cases of BP have oral involvement. (*Reproduced with permission from Richard P. Usatine, MD.*)

SECOND LINE

Steroid-sparing drugs and adjuvant therapy for patients whose disease is not controlled with steroids and doxycycline. Before starting any of the following systemic medications, be aware of the laboratory tests needed to initiate and continue such therapy:

- Dapsone is an antineutrophilic antibiotic that is an alternative to tetracycline and doxycycline (**Figure 192-6**).[9] SOR B
- Azathioprine 50 to 200 mg divided bid or tid (first-line adjuvant).[9] SOR B
- Mycophenolate mofetil 0.5 to 2 g/day divided bid or tid (less hepatotoxic than azathioprine).[13] SOR C

Disease resistant to combination of corticosteroids and steroid-sparing agents:

- Intravenous immunoglobulin (IVIG) can produce a rapid and dramatic but very transient response; requires multiple cycles of IVIG. SOR C
- Plasmapheresis can be considered for patients with severe resistant disease requiring high doses of systemic steroids to improve symptoms and reduce steroid dose.[14] SOR C
- Case reports and small series of successful therapy of refractory BP with rituximab,[15] etanercept,[16,17] or omalizumab[18] have been published in the recent medical literature.
    - Rituximab has proved to offer promising results for recalcitrant bullous pemphigoid. In a retrospective study, the combination of rituximab and IVIG resulted in sustained remission for 83% of patients in the study with no side effects or complications.[19] SOR B
    - Etanercept has proven beneficial in patients with psoriasis coinciding with BP. Etanercept is a tumor necrosis factor (TNF) antagonist and can help to control symptoms of both BP and psoriasis which are mediated by TNF.[17] SOR B
    - Omalizumab has also been used as a treatment for select patients with BP. The exact mechanism for resolution of BP symptoms with omalizumab is not completely understood. One theory includes decreased numbers of IgE, eosinophils, and mast cells; another theory involves eosinophil apoptosis and decreased circulating cytokines.[20] SOR B

REFER

- Dermatology consultation for recommending therapy based on extent of disease and for changes in therapy when required. When second-line therapies are needed, referral to a dermatologist is especially important.
- Nutrition consultation if patient is having difficulty maintaining weight.

FOLLOW-UP

- Ask patient about recurrent lesions, pruritus, and side effects from treatment.
- Perform periodic skin examinations looking for new lesions to adjust dose of prednisone and to monitor for lymphadenopathy and skin cancer in patients using immunosuppressive medications.

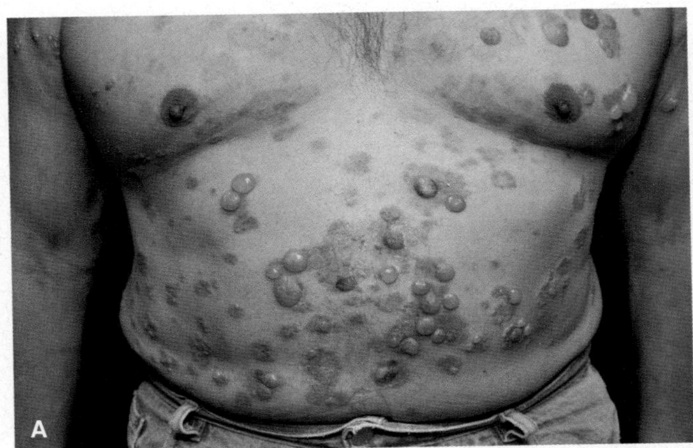

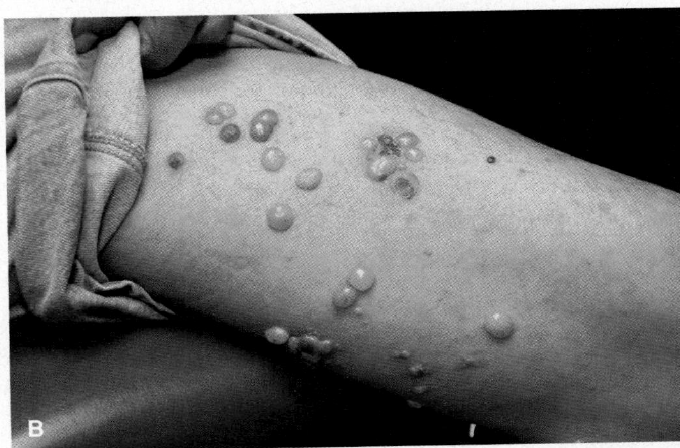

FIGURE 192-6 New-onset bullous pemphigoid in a 65-year-old man with previous psoriasis. His bullous pemphigoid is currently controlled with dapsone. **A.** Bullae on abdomen with some psoriatic plaques visible. **B.** Tense bullae on leg. (*Reproduced with permission from Richard P. Usatine, MD.*)

- Monitor for drug-specific laboratory abnormalities (e.g., glucose and triglycerides with steroid use; complete blood count [CBC], renal function, and liver function tests for azathioprine and other immunosuppressive medications).
- Make sure patients do not run out of their medications, because this can result in recurrent lesions (**Figure 192-7**).
- Adjust treatment if patient relapses by increasing steroid dose or adding an immunosuppressive agent.
- Taper steroids slowly after dissipation of disease flare.

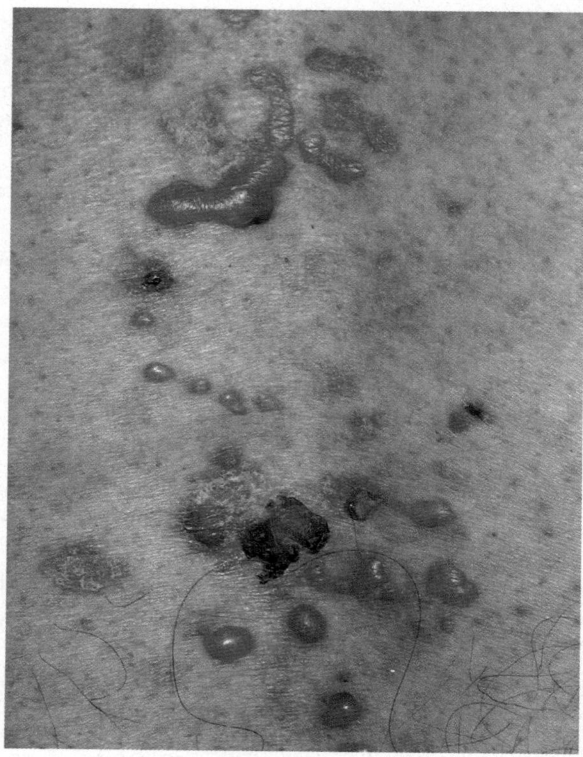

FIGURE 192-7 Recurrent bullous pemphigoid on the back of a 57-year-old man who ran out of his prednisone for a few days. *(Reproduced with permission from Richard P. Usatine, MD.)*

PATIENT EDUCATION

- Avoid mechanical irritation, direct sun exposure, dental prostheses, extremes of temperature.
- Recommend high-protein, low-carbohydrate, and low-fat diet; calcium and vitamin D supplementation for patients on corticosteroids.
- Provide information on wound care, stress reduction, appropriate exercise, and side effects of medications.

PATIENT RESOURCES

- **https://patient.info/health/bullous-pemphigoid-leaflet.**
- International Pemphigus & Pemphigoid Foundation—**http://www.pemphigus.org/patients-and-caregivers/.**

PROVIDER RESOURCES

- eMedicine—**http://emedicine.medscape.com/article/1062391.**

REFERENCES

1. Langan SM, Smeeth L, Hubbard R, et al. Bullous pemphigoid and pemphigus vulgaris—incidence and mortality in the UK: population based cohort study. *BMJ*. 2008;337:a180.
2. Zillikens D, Rose PA, Balding SD, et al. Tight clustering of extracellular BP180 epitopes recognized by bullous pemphigoid autoantibodies. *J Invest Dermatol*. 1997;109:573-579.
3. Yancey KB, Egan CA. Pemphigoid: clinical, histologic, immunopathologic, and therapeutic considerations. *JAMA*. 2000;284:350-356.
4. Kroumpouzos G, Cohen LM. Specific dermatoses of pregnancy: an evidence-based systematic review. *Am J Obstet Gynecol*. 2003;188(4):1083-1092.
5. Bingham EA, Burrows D, Sandford JC. Prolonged pruritus and bullous pemphigoid. *Clin Exp Dermatol*. 1984;9:564-570.
6. Habif TP. *Clinical Dermatology: A Color Guide to Diagnosis and Therapy*, 4th ed. St. Louis, MO: Mosby; 2004.
7. Schmidt E, Zillikens D. Modern diagnosis of auto-immune blistering skin diseases. *Autoimmun Rev*. 2010;10:84-89.
8. Kuechle MK, Stegemeir E, Maynard B, Gibson LE. Drug-induced linear IgA bullous dermatosis: report of six cases and review of the literature. *J Am Acad Dermatol*. 1994;30:187-192.

9. Khumalo N, Kirtschig G, Middleton P, et al. Interventions for bullous pemphigoid. *Cochrane Database Syst Rev.* 2003;(3):CD002292.
10. Joly P, Roujeau JC, Benichou J, et al. A comparison of oral and topical corticosteroids in patients with bullous pemphigoid. *N Engl J Med.* 2002;346:321-327.
11. Kirtschig G, Middleton P, Bennett C, et al. Interventions for bullous pemphigoid. *Cochrane Database Syst Rev.* 2010;(10):CD002292.
12. Fivenson DP, Breneman DL, Rosen GB, et al. Nicotinamide and tetracycline therapy of bullous pemphigoid. *Arch Dermatol.* 1994; 130(6):753-758.
13. Böhm M, Beissert S, Schwarz T, et al. Bullous pemphigoid treated with mycophenolate mofetil. *Lancet.* 1997;349(9051):541.
14. Mazzi G, Raineri A, Zanolli FA, et al. Plasmapheresis therapy in pemphigus vulgaris and bullous pemphigoid. *Transfus Apher Sci.* 2003;28(1):13-18.
15. Kasperkiewicz M, Shimanovich I, Ludwig RJ, et al. Rituximab for treatment-refractory pemphigus and pemphigoid: a case series of 17 patients. *J Am Acad Dermatol.* 2011;65(3):552-558.
16. Cusano F, Iannazzone SS, Riccio G, Piccirillo F. Coexisting bullous pemphigoid and psoriasis successfully treated with etanercept. *Eur J Dermatol.* 2010;20(4):520.
17. Yamauchi PS, Lowe NJ, Gindi V. Treatment of coexisting bullous pemphigoid and psoriasis with the tumor necrosis factor antagonist etanercept. *J Am Acad Dermatol.* 2006;54(3 Suppl 2):S121-S122. PubMed PMID: 16488323.
18. Fairley JA, Baum CL, Brandt DS, Messingham KA. Pathogenicity of IgE in autoimmunity: successful treatment of bullous pemphigoid with omalizumab. *J Allergy Clin Immunol.* 2009;123(3): 704-705.
19. Ahmed AR, Shetty S, Kaveri S, Spigelman ZS. Treatment of recalcitrant bullous pemphigoid (BP) with a novel protocol: a retrospective study with a 6-year follow-up. *J Am Acad Dermatol.* 2016; 74(4):700-708.e3.
20. Gönül MZ, Keseroglu HO, Ergin C, et al. Bullous pemphigoid successfully treated with omalizumab. *Indian J Dermatol Venereol Leprol.* 2016;82(5):577-579.

193 PEMPHIGUS

Richard P. Usatine, MD
Jenny Yeh, MD
Pavela G. Bambekova, BS

PATIENT STORY

A young man presented with painful blisters on his face and mouth (**Figure 193-1**). The patient was referred to dermatology. Suspecting pemphigus vulgaris (PV), the physician performed shave biopsies for histopathology and direct immunofluorescence of facial vesicles/bullae to confirm the presumed diagnosis. The patient was started on 60 mg of prednisone daily until the pathology confirmed PV. Steroid-sparing therapy was then discussed and started 2 weeks after initial presentation.

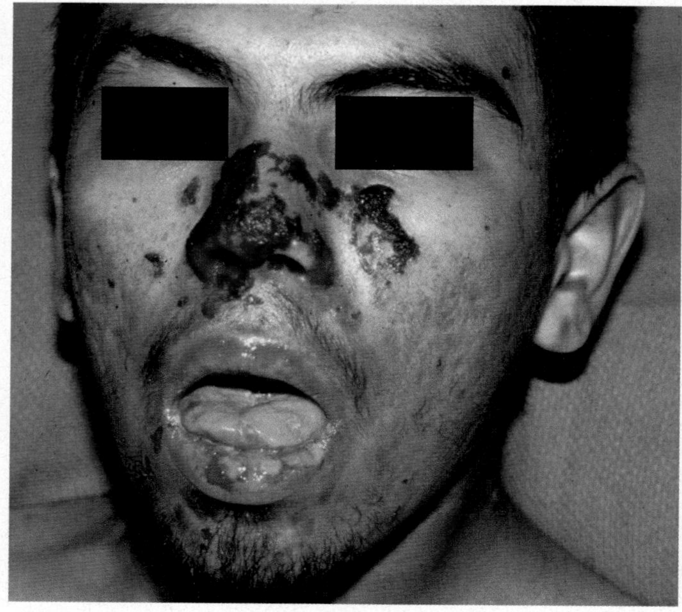

FIGURE 193-1 Pemphigus vulgaris with mouth involvement on the face of a young man. (*Reproduced with permission from Eric Kraus, MD.*)

INTRODUCTION

Pemphigus is a rare group of autoimmune bullous diseases of the skin and mucous membranes characterized by flaccid bullae and erosions. The word *pemphigus* is derived from the Greek word *pemphix,* which means bubble or blister. The three main types of pemphigus are PV, pemphigus foliaceus (PF), and paraneoplastic pemphigus (PNP). Pemphigus causes significant morbidity and mortality and can be fatal if left untreated. Although pemphigus is not curable, it can be controlled with systemic steroids and immunosuppressive medications. These medications can be lifesaving, but they also place pemphigus patients at risk for a number of complications.

EPIDEMIOLOGY

Epidemiology of the three major types of pemphigus:

- PV (**Figures 193-1** to **193-4**).
  - Most common form of pemphigus in the United States.
  - Annual incidence is 0.75 to 5 cases per 1 million.[1]
  - Usually occurs between 30 and 50 years of age.[2]
  - Increased incidence in people of Ashkenazi Jewish and Mediterranean origin.[2]
  - Pemphigus vegetans is an even rarer vegetative variant form of PV (**Figures 193-5** and **193-6**).
- Pemphigus foliaceus (**Figures 193-7** to **193-10**)—Superficial form of pemphigus.
  - More prevalent in Africa (**Figures 193-11** and **193-12**).[1]
  - Variant forms include pemphigus erythematosus (resembles the malar rash of lupus erythematosus) and fogo selvagem.
  - Fogo selvagem is an endemic form of PF seen in Brazil and affects teenagers and individuals in their twenties.[1]
- Paraneoplastic pemphigus.
  - Onset at age 60 years and older.
  - Associated with occult neoplasms, commonly lymphoreticular, (e.g., non-Hodgkin lymphoma and chronic lymphocytic leukemia).

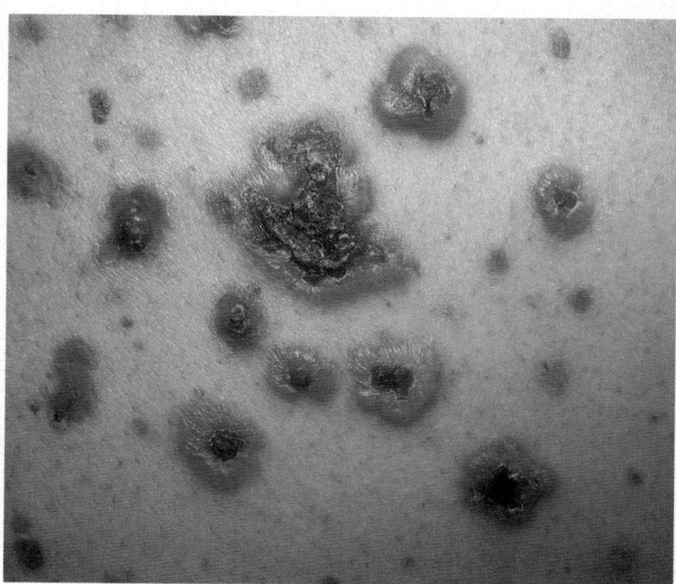

FIGURE 193-2 Pemphigus vulgaris seen on the back with crusted and intact bullae. Downward pressure on a bulla demonstrates a positive Asboe-Hansen sign with lateral spread of a fresh bulla. (*Reproduced with permission from Eric Kraus, MD.*)

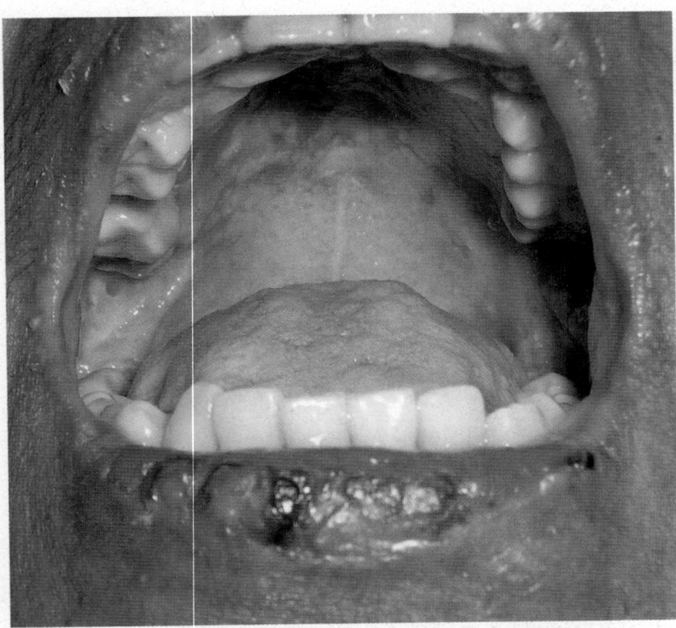

FIGURE 193-3 Pemphigus vulgaris involving the lips and palate of a 55-year-old woman. (*Reproduced with permission from Dan Shaked, MD.*)

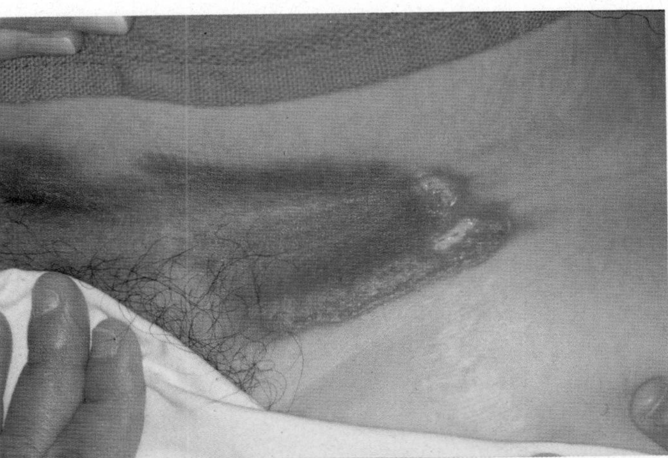

FIGURE 193-5 Pemphigus vegetans in the groin of a middle-aged woman. (*Reproduced with permission from Eric Kraus, MD.*)

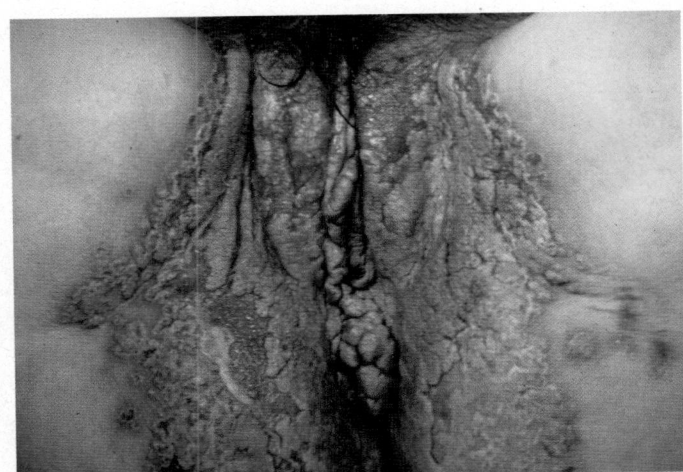

FIGURE 193-6 Pemphigus vegetans widespread over the external genitalia and buttocks. (*Reproduced with permission from Eric Kraus, MD.*)

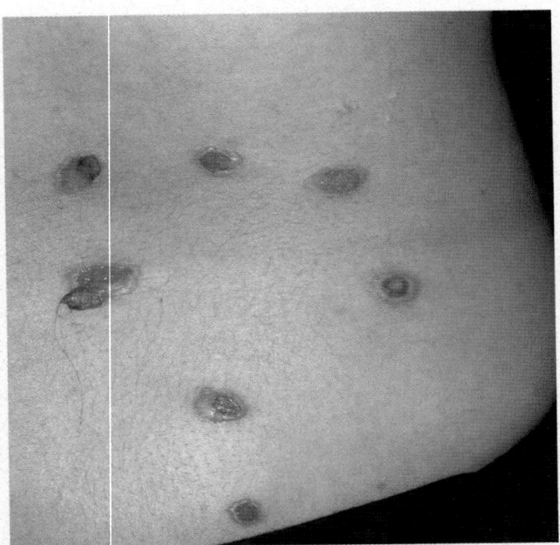

FIGURE 193-4 New onset pemphigus vulgaris on the trunk of a 29-year-old woman. She also has blisters and erosions on her scalp, groin, thighs and in her mouth and axillae. (*Reproduced with permission from Wolff K, Johnson RA. Fitzpatrick's Color Atlas & Synopsis of Clinical Dermatology, 6th ed. New York, NY: McGraw-Hill Education; 2009.*)

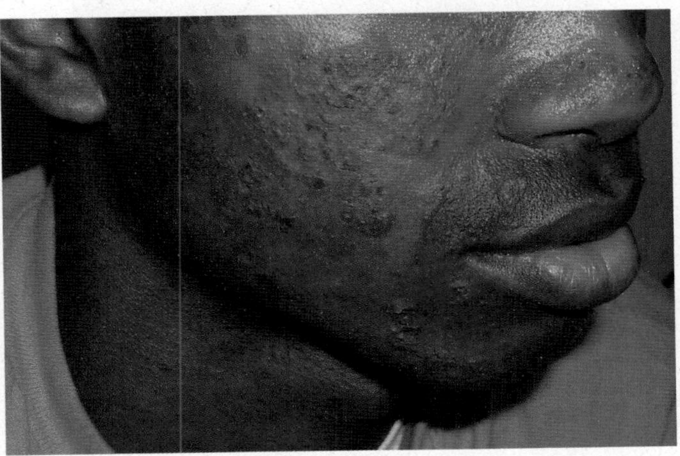

FIGURE 193-7 Pemphigus foliaceus on the face of a black man. (*Reproduced with permission from Jack Resneck, Sr., MD.*)

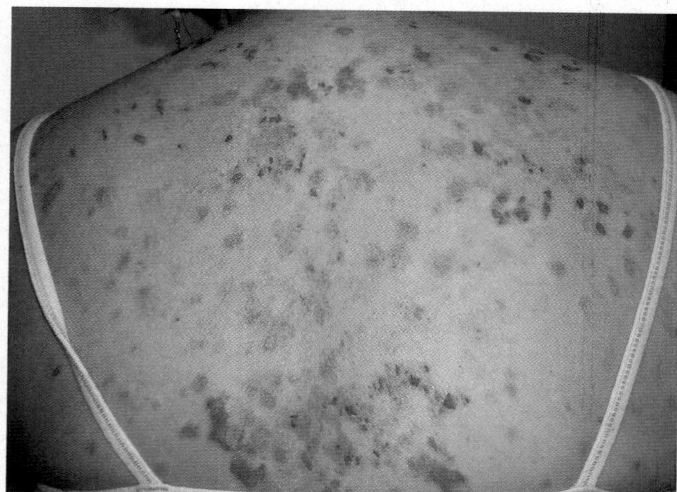

FIGURE 193-8 Pemphigus foliaceus on the back of a 55-year-old Hispanic woman. Note the absence of bullae and the cornflake crusting from the superficial erosions. (*Reproduced with permission from Richard P. Usatine, MD.*)

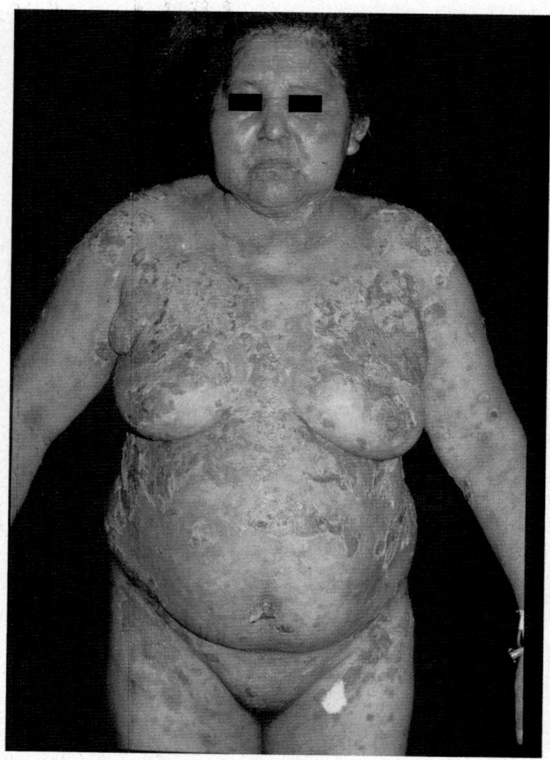

FIGURE 193-10 Widespread pemphigus foliaceus. (*Reproduced with permission from Eric Kraus, MD.*)

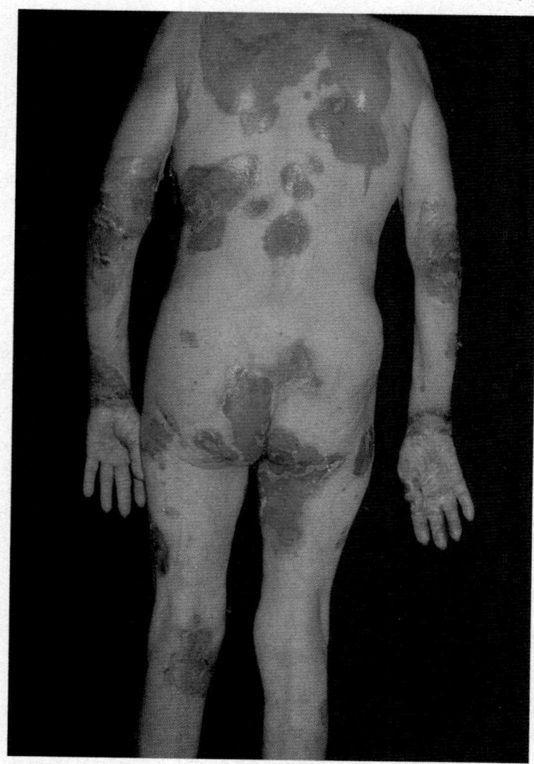

FIGURE 193-9 Pemphigus foliaceus with large erosions on the back and extremities of a patient. (*Reproduced with permission from Eric Kraus, MD.*)

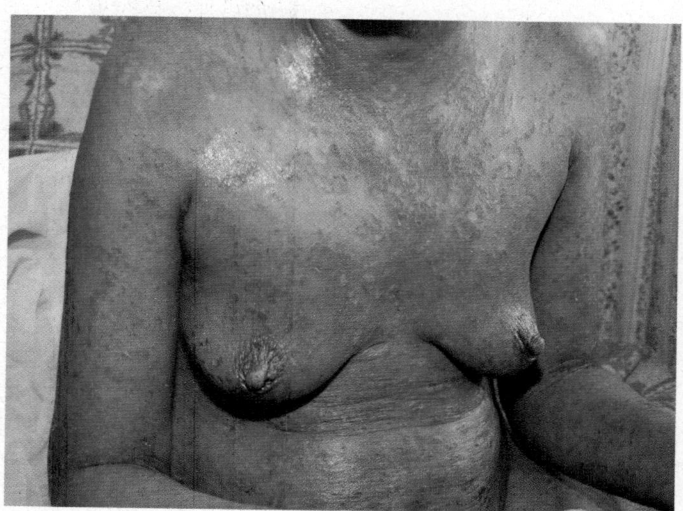

FIGURE 193-11 Pemphigus foliaceus on the trunk and arms of a woman in Africa. Some of the lesions appear annular, but they are all superficial erosions within the epidermis. (*Reproduced with permission from Richard P. Usatine, MD.*)

- Can also be associated with benign neoplasms, such as thymoma and Castleman disease (angiofollicular lymph node hyperplasia).[2]

ETIOLOGY AND PATHOPHYSIOLOGY

- The basic abnormality in all three types of pemphigus is acantholysis—a process in which keratinocytes separate from one another. This occurs as a result of autoantibody formation against desmoglein (the adhesive molecule that holds epidermal cells together). Separation of epidermal cells leads to formation of intraepidermal clefts, which enlarge to form bullae.[1]
- The mechanism that induces the production of these autoantibodies in most individuals is unknown. Yet PF may be triggered by drugs, most commonly thiol compounds such as penicillamine, captopril, piroxicam, and others like penicillin and imiquimod.[3] An environmental trigger in the presence of susceptible human leukocyte antigen (HLA) gene is suggested to induce autoantibodies in fogo selvagum.[1]
- The autoantibodies in pemphigus are usually directed against desmoglein 1 and 3 (Dsg1 and Dsg3). Dsg1 is present predominantly in the superficial layers of the epidermis, whereas Dsg3 is expressed in deeper epidermal layers and in mucous membranes. As a result, clinical presentation depends on the antibody profile. In PV, a limited mucosal disease occurs when only anti-Dsg3 antibody is present, but extensive mucosal and cutaneous disease occurs when both anti-Dsg1 and anti-Dsg3 antibodies are present. In PF, mucosal lesions are absent, and the cutaneous lesions are superficial because of isolated anti-Dsg1 antibody.
- Like PV, PNP demonstrate antibodies against desmogleins 1 and 3 but also against all the members of the plakin family. These autoantibodies form a reliable marker for this type of pemphigus.

DIAGNOSIS

CLINICAL FEATURES

- Pemphigus vulgaris (see **Figures 193-1** to **193-4**)—Classical lesions are flaccid bullae that rupture easily, creating erosions. Because bullae are short-lived, erosions are the more common presenting physical finding (**Figure 193-13**). Lesions are typically tender and heal with postinflammatory hyperpigmentation that resolves without scarring. A positive Asboe-Hansen or Nikolsky sign may be present, but neither of these signs is diagnostic. A positive Asboe-Hansen sign occurs when a bulla extends to surrounding skin while pressure is applied directly to the bulla. The Nikolsky sign is positive when skin shears off while lateral pressure is applied to unblistered skin during active disease.
- Pemphigus vegetans—A variant of PV commonly affecting intertriginous areas, where flaccid pustules and erosions heal with vegetating proliferation of the epidermis (see **Figures 193-5** and **193-6**).
- Pemphigus foliaceus—Characterized by the presence of multiple red, pruritic erosions with scale and crust described like "cornflakes." Intact blisters are rare as the disease is superficial, and mucosa is not involved. Lesions are distributed in seborrheic pattern (face, scalp, upper trunk) (see **Figures 193-7** to **193-12**).

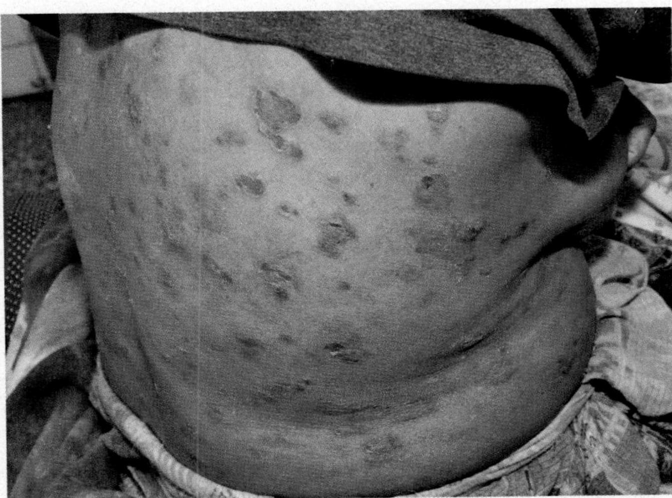

FIGURE 193-12 Another case of pemphigus foliaceus in Africa. Pemphigus foliaceus is more prevalent in Africa. Note the hyperpigmentation of the healing lesions after treatment has begun. *(Reproduced with permission from Richard P. Usatine, MD.)*

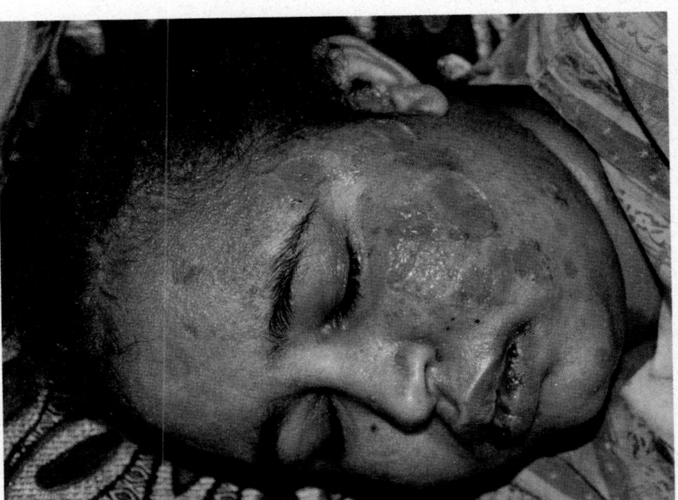

FIGURE 193-13 Pemphigus vulgaris involving the face and oral mucosa. The erosions are deeper than those seen in pemphigus foliaceus. The oral involvement points to pemphigus vulgaris. *(Reproduced with permission from Richard P. Usatine, MD.)*

- PNP (**Figure 193-14**)—Typically presents with severe and painful oral erosions. Skin lesions can be similar to PV, although lichen planus, morbilliform, or erythema multiforme–like lesions may also be seen in addition to blisters and erosions. Another distinctive feature is the presence of epithelial necrosis and lichenoid changes in the lesions as well as extensive and painful mucosal involvement. Pulmonary involvement secondary to acantholysis of bronchial mucosa is seen in 30% to 40% of cases of PNP.

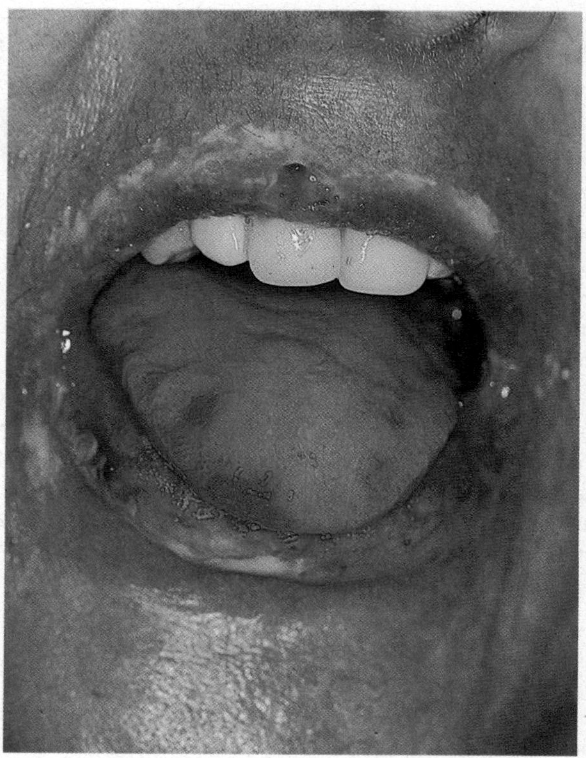

FIGURE 193-14 Paraneoplastic pemphigus with severe erosions covering almost the entire mucosa of the oral cavity with partial sparing of the dorsum of the tongue. Lesions are extremely painful, interfering with adequate food intake. This patient had non-Hodgkin lymphoma as the underlying malignancy. *(Reproduced with permission from Wolff K, Johnson RA. Fitzpatrick's Color Atlas & Synopsis of Clinical Dermatology, 6th ed. New York, NY: McGraw-Hill Education; 2009.)*

TYPICAL DISTRIBUTION

- PV—Common mucosal site is oral mucosa, although any stratified squamous epithelium may be involved. Skin lesions may follow mucosal lesions weeks to months after presentation of mucosal lesions. The skin lesions usually manifest on the scalp, face, and upper torso. PV should be suspected if an oral ulcer persists beyond one month (**Figures 193-1**, **193-3**, and **193-15**).
- Pemphigus vegetans—Usually seen in intertriginous areas such as the axilla, groin, and genital region (see **Figures 193-5** and **193-6**).
- PF—Initially affects face and scalp, though it may progress to involve the chest and back (see **Figures 193-7** to **193-12**). When the facial involvement in PF is in a lupus-like pattern, this is called pemphigus erythematosus (**Figure 193-16**).
- PNP—Common sites include oral mucosa and conjunctiva (see **Figure 193-14**). Columnar and transitional epithelia may also be involved in addition to stratified squamous epithelium.

LABORATORY STUDIES

- Circulating desmoglein antibody levels may be measured in the blood using indirect immunofluorescence. This is usually not necessary unless the diagnosis is suspected and further data is needed.
- A complete blood count and a comprehensive metabolic profile—including liver function tests, creatinine, and glucose—need to be provided with their baseline levels because systemic therapies have significant toxicities.
- Patients at risk for steroid-induced osteoporosis should have a dual-energy X-ray absorptiometry (DEXA) scan performed.

BIOPSY

- Skin biopsy is essential for accurate diagnosis. The depth of acantholysis and the site of deposition of antibody complexes help differentiate pemphigus from other bullous diseases. Two specimens should be sent. Perform a shave of the edge of the bulla to include the surrounding normal-appearing epidermis. This biopsy should be of the freshest lesion with an intact bulla, if possible. Cut the specimen in half, and send the portion with the bulla in formalin for routine histopathology. The second half should be perilesional adjacent normal skin. This is sent on a gauze pad soaked in normal saline or Michel solution for direct immunofluorescence (DIF). Routine histopathology demonstrates suprabasal acantholysis, and DIF shows antibody deposition in the intercellular spaces of the epidermis. The pattern of the DIF fluorescence is described as chicken wire (**Figure 193-17**).

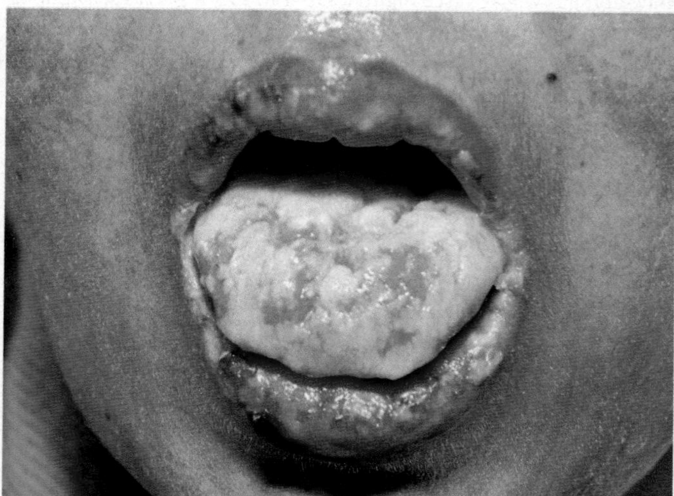

FIGURE 193-15 Pemphigus vulgaris involving the tongue and lips of a young woman. This is severely painful, making it difficult to eat or drink. *(Reproduced with permission from Richard P. Usatine, MD.)*

DIFFERENTIAL DIAGNOSIS

- Bullous pemphigus—Bullae are tense because they occur in the deeper subepidermal layer. Mucous membrane involvement is rare. Biopsy illustrates subepidermal acantholysis and immunoglobulin deposition along the basement membrane (Chapter 192, Bullous Pemphigoid).[3]
- Cicatricial pemphigoid—Also known as mucous membrane pemphigoid. Usually affects oral mucosa and conjunctiva. Lesions heal with scarring, which results in irreversible sequelae, such as blindness, subglottic stenosis, and esophageal strictures.[3] Histology demonstrates antibody complexes in the basement membrane with submucosal infiltrate and prominent fibroblast proliferation (Chapter 192, Bullous Pemphigoid).
- Dermatitis herpetiformis—Grouped vesicles and erosions resembling herpes commonly seen on extensor aspects of extremities and buttocks. It is associated with gluten-induced enteropathy. Biopsy reveals neutrophilic microabscesses at the tips of dermal papillae with deposition of immunoglobulin (Ig) A antibody complexes. Blood tests for antigliadin and antiendomysial antibodies can help diagnose the gluten-induced enteropathy (Chapter 194, Other Bullous Diseases).
- Linear IgA dermatosis—Typical lesions are described as "string of pearls," which is an urticarial plaque surrounded by vesicles. Histologically, IgA antibodies are deposited in a linear fashion along the basement membrane (Chapter 191, Overview of Bullous Diseases).[4]
- Porphyria cutanea tarda—Bullae seen on sun-exposed areas, especially on the dorsum of the hands. Serum iron, ferritin, transaminase, and 24-hour urine porphyrins levels are elevated. Elevations in urine porphyrins are diagnostic (Chapter 194, Other Bullous Diseases).
- Hailey-Hailey disease (benign familial pemphigus)—A genodermatosis with crusted erosions and flaccid vesicles distributed in the intertriginous areas (**Figure 193-18**). It most closely resembles pemphigus vegetans clinically, but its pathophysiology is completely different from that of true pemphigus. It is called benign because it is not life-threatening. A 4-mm punch biopsy is adequate to make this diagnosis, as the histology is different from pemphigus.

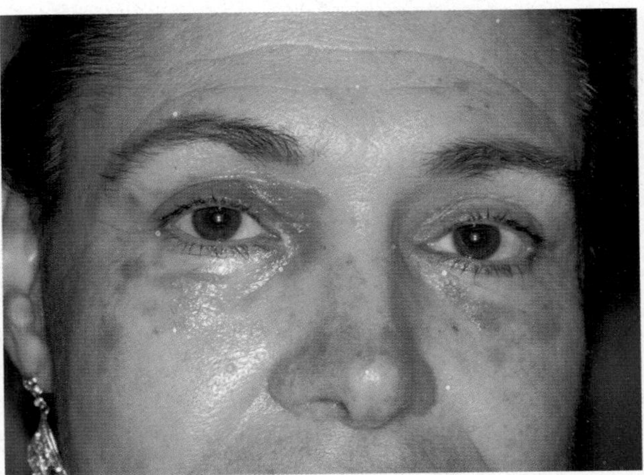

FIGURE 193-16 Pemphigus erythematosus creating a lupus-like pattern of facial involvement. Note how the pemphigus foliaceus lesions involve the malar areas bilaterally. *(Reproduced with permission from Richard P. Usatine, MD.)*

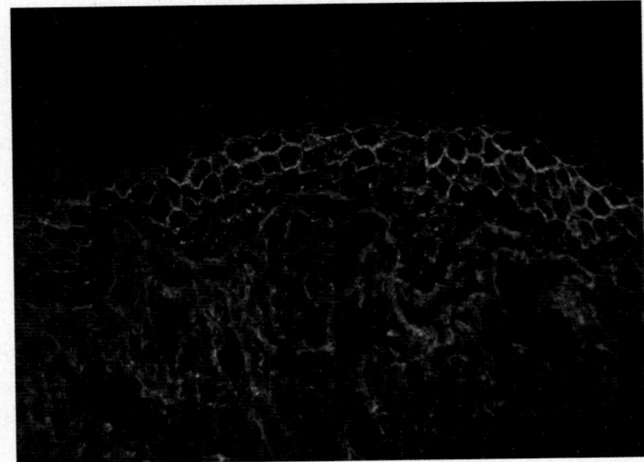

FIGURE 193-17 Direct immunofluorescence against immunoglobulin (Ig) G antibodies surrounding cells of the epidermis in a patient with pemphigus vulgaris. Note the chicken-wire appearance. *(Reproduced with permission from Martin Fernandez, MD, and Richard P. Usatine, MD.)*

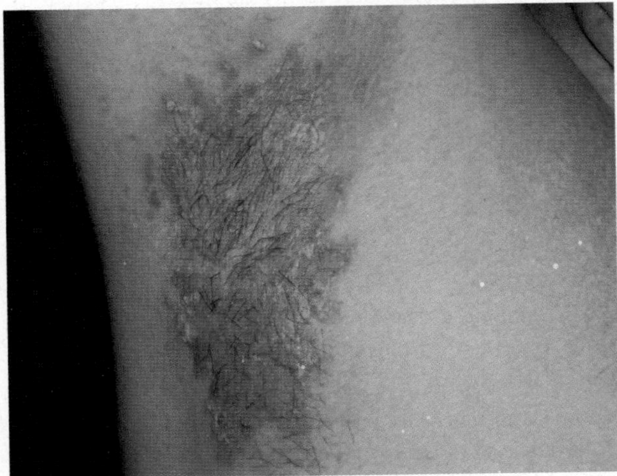

FIGURE 193-18 Hailey-Hailey disease (benign familial pemphigus) with erythema and pustules in the axilla. This is not true pemphigus but resembles pemphigus vegetans. *(Reproduced with permission from Jonathan B. Karnes, MD.)*

MANAGEMENT

Treatment of pemphigus should be undertaken in consultation with a dermatologist. Treatment is directed initially at disease control and remission followed by disease suppression. The goal is to eventually discontinue all medications and achieve complete remission. Unfortunately, this goal may be difficult to achieve.

SYSTEMIC THERAPY

▶ Corticosteroids

Systemic corticosteroids are considered first-line therapy in all types of pemphigus.[4-6] SOR Ⓑ

- Mild disease may be controlled with prednisone 40 mg/day, but for rapidly progressive and extensive disease, a higher dose of prednisone (60 to 80 mg/day) is initiated. SOR Ⓒ The dose may be increased by 50% every 1 to 2 weeks until disease activity is controlled. In most cases, a dose of approximately 60 mg of prednisone daily will need to be continued for at least 1 month. Once remission is induced, the dose is tapered by 25% every 1 to 2 weeks to the lowest dose needed to suppress recurrence of new lesions.[1]

- Pulse therapy with intravenous methylprednisolone 1 g/day for 5 days may be tried in severe cases in an attempt to decrease the cumulative dose of steroids, especially when high-dose oral steroids are ineffective.[7] SOR C
- High-dose and prolonged treatment with steroids can have serious side effects. Consequently, it is advisable to start adjuvant steroid-sparing therapy within 2 to 4 weeks of treatment. Adjuvant agents have a lag period of 4 to 6 weeks before they become effective, so starting them sooner allows for earlier steroid taper. They may be used alone to maintain remission after steroid withdrawal.

▶ Adjuvant agents

- Adjuvant therapies have improved the treatment of PV and help prevent chronic steroid use. Despite not achieving complete remission, adjuvant therapies lower the chance for PV relapse by 29%.[8]
- Adjuvant agents include azathioprine, cyclophosphamide, mycophenolate, dapsone, and intravenous immunoglobulin.[7-11] In addition, anti-CD20 biologics such as rituximab offer promising results for targeted therapy against autoreactive B cells. Steroid efficacy is enhanced when combined with a cytotoxic drug.[4]
- Azathioprine and mycophenolate mofetil (CellCept) are often the preferred adjuvants for PV.[7,8,10,12] SOR B
- Azathioprine was less effective than mycophenolate mofetil in achieving remission in one study with 40 participants (risk ratio 0.72; 95% confidence interval [CI] 0.52 to 0.99).[10,12] In 13 (72%) of 18 patients with pemphigus receiving oral methylprednisolone and azathioprine, complete remission was achieved after a mean of 74 (±127) days, compared with 20 (95%) of 21 patients receiving oral methylprednisolone and mycophenolate in whom complete remission occurred after a mean of 91 (±113) days. A greater percentage of patients treated with azathioprine suffered adverse effects compared with those on mycophenolate.
- In one open-label randomized controlled trial (RCT) of four treatment regimens for PV, the most efficacious cytotoxic drug that reduced the use of steroids was azathioprine, followed by cyclophosphamide (IV pulse therapy) and mycophenolate mofetil.[4] SOR B
- Standard dosing for azathioprine is 50 mg per day. Standard dosing for mycophenolate is 1000 mg to 1500 mg twice daily. Azathioprine is significantly less expensive, but patients may experience more side effects.[4,5,8,10-12] Monitoring while on azathioprine include frequent complete blood count and liver enzymes. Patients also need thiopurine methyltransferase (TPMT) levels checked before initiation of azathioprine. Deficiency of TPMT would render the patient unable to efficiently metabolize medication and may result in severe pancytopenia.
- Dapsone is an alternative adjuvant for pemphigus.[7] SOR C In one small study, 8 (73%) of 11 patients receiving dapsone versus 3 (30%) of 10 receiving placebo reached the primary outcome of a prednisone dosage of 7.5 mg per day or less. This was not statistically significant and only showed a trend to efficacy of dapsone as a steroid-sparing drug in maintenance-phase PV.[13]
- Intravenous immunoglobulin (IVIG) may be used as adjuvant therapy in refractory cases of pemphigus.[7,14-16] SOR B In one RCT, it was used as a 5-day cycle to treat pemphigus that was relatively resistant to systemic steroids. In this multicenter study of 61 patients with PV or foliaceus, there was a decrease in disease activity subsequent to the cycle of IVIG.[16] SOR B
- Rituximab is a chimeric monoclonal antibody against CD20 on B lymphocytes. It leads to depletion of pathogenic B cells for up to 12 months, resulting in a reduction of pathogenic autoantibodies. Rituximab is infused weekly for 4 consecutive weeks in addition to the standard immunosuppressive treatment. It has shown promise in several case reports and cohort studies in the treatment of PNP and refractory cases of PV and foliaceus.[6,17,18] SOR B Monoclonal antibody therapy with rituximab has shifted the treatment paradigm of PV from complete immune suppression to only targeting the pathologic B cells that eventually produce the disease-causing antibodies.
- In a recent, prospective, parallel-group, randomized trial of 25 hospitals in France, dual therapy of rituximab with short-term prednisone (tapered over 3–6 months) proved to be more effective and safer than using prednisone alone (tapered over 12–18 months) in newly diagnosed adult patients being treated for the first time. By 2 years, 89% of patients on the combined treatment achieved complete remission compared to only 34% of patients only on prednisone (95% CI 38.4-71.7; $p < 0.0001$).[19]
- Veltuzumab and ofatumumab are next-generation anti-CD20 biologics that offer promising effects for the treatment of PV. Studies show possible efficacy of veltuzumab in treating refractory PV and will have the added benefit of being administered subcutaneously. Ofatumumab is currently undergoing phase 3 clinical trials.[6]

▶ Treating and preventing complications of therapy

- Osteoporosis prevention—Long-term therapy with oral prednisone is a significant risk factor for osteoporosis. All patients should receive supplemental calcium and vitamin D based on their age, gender, and normal dietary intake. A DEXA scan early in the course of the disease can be a helpful baseline. One study showed that alendronate therapy given to patients with immunobullous disease on long-term steroids resulted in statistically significant increases in bone mineral density at the lumbar spine and femoral neck.[20]
- Thrush is a common complication of high-dose steroids in pemphigus (**Figure 193-19**). This should be treated with oral fluconazole or another antifungal to prevent *Candida* esophagitis. If the patient is complaining of pain or difficulty swallowing, consider the diagnosis of *Candida* esophagitis and treat accordingly.
- Steroid-induced diabetes may also occur. This can be treated with metformin and monitoring of blood sugars and hemoglobin A_{1c}.

LOCAL THERAPY

- Solitary lesions may be treated with topical high-potency steroids, such as clobetasol, or with intralesional steroid injections, for example, 20 mg/mL triamcinolone acetonide. Isolated oral lesions may be treated with steroid paste, sprays, or lozenges.
- Normal saline compresses or bacteriostatic solutions such as potassium permanganate are useful in keeping lesions clean. Oral

hygiene is crucial. Mouthwashes such as chlorhexidine 0.2% or 1:4 hydrogen peroxide may be used. Topical anesthetics may be used for pain.[7]

PROGNOSIS

Pemphigus is a chronic group of diseases that are potentially life-threatening. There is no cure, and the long-term use of steroids and immunosuppressive drugs puts patients at risk for a number of complications, including infections, sepsis, steroid-induced diabetes, and steroid-induced osteoporosis. Some patients can go into remission, while others will need systemic therapy for life. Complications of treatment have become the greatest source of morbidity and mortality in pemphigus.

FOLLOW-UP

Prolonged follow-up is needed for medication adjustment and to monitor disease activity and drug side effects.

PATIENT EDUCATION

- Educate patients regarding disease, complications, and side effects of medications.
- Advise patients on avoiding trauma to skin such as with contact sports. Similarly, oral lesions may be aggravated by nuts, spicy foods, chips, or dental appliances.
- Instruct patients on wound care to prevent infections and relieve local discomfort.
- Provide information on support groups such as the International Pemphigus Pemphigoid Foundation.

PATIENT RESOURCES

- MedlinePlus. *Pemphigus*—**http://www.nlm.nih.gov/medlineplus/pemphigus.html.**
- Mayo Clinic. *Pemphigus*—**http://www.mayoclinic.org/diseases-conditions/symptoms-causes/syc-20350404.**
- International Pemphigus Pemphigoid Foundation—**http://www.pemphigus.org.**

PROVIDER RESOURCES

- Medscape. *Pemphigus Vulgaris*—**http://emedicine.medscape.com/article/1064187.**
- Information on how to perform the appropriate biopsy can be found in Usatine R, Pfenninger J, Stulberg D, Small R. *Dermatologic and Cosmetic Procedures in Office Practice*. Philadelphia, PA: Elsevier; 2012. The text and the accompanying videos can also be purchased as an electronic application at: **http://www.usatinemedia.com.**

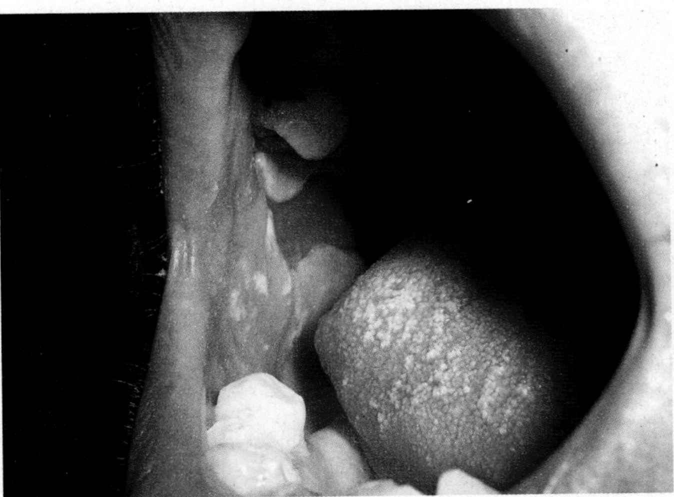

FIGURE 193-19 Thrush appearing in the mouth of a 50-year-old woman recently placed on oral prednisone for new-onset pemphigus vulgaris. Note the large erosion on the buccal mucosa and the adherent white *Candida* anterior as well as on the tongue. KOH was positive, and the patient was treated with fluconazole. (*Reproduced with permission from Richard P. Usatine, MD.*)

REFERENCES

1. Bystryn JC, Rudolph JL. Pemphigus. *Lancet.* 2005;366:61-73.
2. Ettlin DA. Pemphigus. *Dent Clin North Am.* 2005;49:107-125.
3. Bickle K, Roark TR, Hsu S. Autoimmune bullous dermatoses: a review. *Am Fam Physician.* 2002;65:1861-1870.
4. Chams-Davatchi C, Esmaili N, Daneshpazhooh M, et al. Randomized controlled open-label trial of four treatment regimens for pemphigus vulgaris. *J Am Acad Dermatol.* 2007;57:622-628.
5. Beissert S, Mimouni D, Kanwar AJ, et al. Treating pemphigus vulgaris with prednisone and mycophenolate mofetil: a multicenter, randomized, placebo-controlled trial. *J Invest Dermatol.* 2010;130: 2041-2048.
6. Huang A, Madan RK, Levitt J. Future therapies for pemphigus vulgaris: rituximab and beyond. *J Am Acad Dermatol.* 2016; 74(4):746-753.
7. Harman KE, Albert S, Black MM. Guidelines for the management of pemphigus vulgaris. *Br J Dermatol.* 2003;149:926-937.
8. Atzmony L, Hodak E, Leshem YA, et al. The role of adjuvant therapy in pemphigus: a systematic review and meta-analysis. *J Am Acad Dermatol.* 2015;73(2):264-271.
9. Frew JW, Martin LK, Murrell DF. Evidence-based treatments in pemphigus vulgaris and pemphigus foliaceus. *Dermatol Clin.* 2011;29:599-606.
10. Martin LK, Werth VP, Villaneuva EV, Murrell DF. A systematic review of randomized controlled trials for pemphigus vulgaris and pemphigus foliaceus. *J Am Acad Dermatol.* 2011;64:903-908.
11. Singh S. Evidence-based treatments for pemphigus vulgaris, pemphigus foliaceus, and bullous pemphigoid: a systematic review. *Indian J Dermatol Venereol Leprol.* 2011;77:456-469.
12. Beissert S, Werfel T, Frieling U, et al. A comparison of oral methylprednisolone plus azathioprine or mycophenolate mofetil for the treatment of pemphigus. *Arch Dermatol.* 2006;142:1447-1454.
13. Werth VP, Fivenson D, Pandya AG, et al. Multicenter randomized, double-blind, placebo-controlled, clinical trial of dapsone as a glucocorticoid-sparing agent in maintenance-phase pemphigus vulgaris. *Arch Dermatol.* 2008;144:25-32.
14. Sami N, Qureshi A, Ruocco E, Ahmed AR. Corticosteroid-sparing effect of intravenous immunoglobulin therapy in patients with pemphigus vulgaris. *Arch Dermatol.* 2002;138:1158-1162.
15. Gurcan HM, Jeph S, Ahmed AR. Intravenous immunoglobulin therapy in autoimmune mucocutaneous blistering diseases: a review of the evidence for its efficacy and safety. *Am J Clin Dermatol.* 2010;11:315-326.
16. Amagai M, Ikeda S, Shimizu H, et al. A randomized double-blind trial of intravenous immunoglobulin for pemphigus. *J Am Acad Dermatol.* 2009;60:595-603.
17. Hertl M, Zillikens D, Borradori L, et al. Recommendations for the use of rituximab (anti-CD20 antibody) in the treatment of autoimmune bullous skin diseases. *J Dtsch Dermatol Ges.* 2008;6: 366-373.
18. El Tal AK, Posner MR, Spigelman Z, Ahmed AR. Rituximab: a monoclonal antibody to CD20 used in the treatment of pemphigus vulgaris. *J Am Acad Dermatol.* 2006;55:449-459.
19. Joly P, Maho-Vaillant M, Prost-Squarcioni C, et al. First-line rituximab combined with short-term prednisone versus prednisone alone for the treatment of pemphigus (Ritux 3): a prospective, multicentre, parallel-group, open-label randomised trial. *Lancet.* 2017;389(10083):2031-2040.
20. Tee SI, Yosipovitch G, Chan YC, et al. Prevention of glucocorticoid-induced osteoporosis in immunobullous diseases with alendronate: a randomized, double-blind, placebo-controlled study. *Arch Dermatol.* 2012;148:307-314.

194 OTHER BULLOUS DISEASES

Lina M. Cardona, MD
Jimmy H. Hara, MD
Richard P. Usatine, MD

INTRODUCTION

There are a number of bullous diseases other than pemphigus and bullous pemphigoid that are important to recognize. Porphyria cutanea tarda is a disease that has no extracutaneous manifestations (**Figures 194-1** to **194-3**). Dystrophic epidermolysis bullosa belongs to a family of inherited diseases where blister formation can be caused by even minor skin trauma due to mechanical fragility. PLEVA (pityriasis lichenoides et varioliformis acuta) is a minor cutaneous lymphoid dyscrasia that can appear suddenly and persist for weeks to months. Dermatitis herpetiformis is a recurrent eruption that is usually associated with gluten-induced enteropathy.

PORPHYRIA CUTANEA TARDA

PATIENT STORY

A middle-aged woman presented with tense blisters on the dorsum of her hand (**Figure 194-1**). One bulla was intact, and the others had ruptured, showing erosions. Work-up showed elevated porphyrins in the urine (which fluoresced orange-red under a Wood lamp) and the patient was diagnosed with porphyria cutanea tarda.

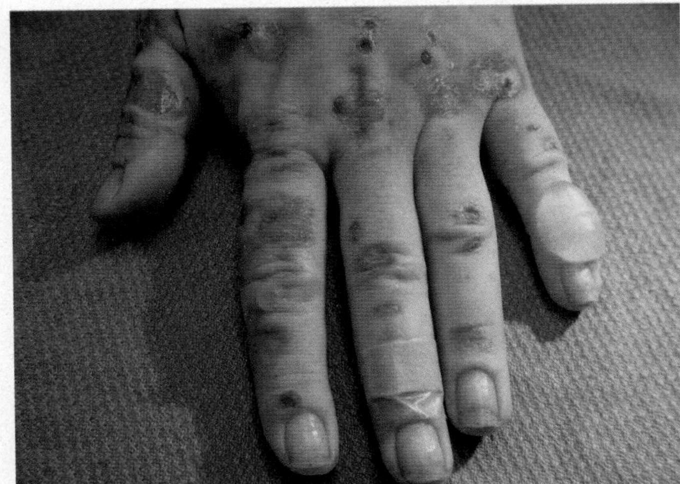

FIGURE 194-1 Porphyria cutanea tarda in a middle-aged woman. *(Reproduced with permission from Lewis Rose, MD.)*

EPIDEMIOLOGY

- Porphyria cutanea tarda (PCT) is the most common type of porphyria disorder.[1]
- PCT occurs mostly in middle-aged adults (typically 30 to 50 years of age) and is rare in children.
- It may occur in women on oral contraceptives and in men on estrogen therapy for prostate cancer.[2,3]
- Alcohol, pesticides, and chloroquine have been implicated as chemicals that induce PCT.[1,3]
- PCT is equally common in both genders.
- There is an increased incidence of PCT in persons with hepatitis C[4-6] and HIV[7] (see **Figure 194-2**).

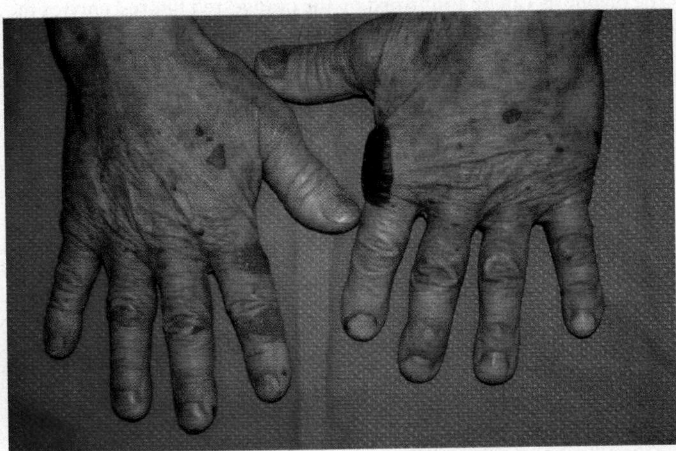

FIGURE 194-2 Porphyria cutanea tarda in a man with hepatitis C and alcohol abuse. *(Reproduced with permission from Richard P. Usatine, MD.)*

ETIOLOGY AND PATHOPHYSIOLOGY

- The porphyrias are a family of illnesses caused by various metabolic derangements in the metabolism of porphyrin, the chemical backbone of hemoglobin. Whereas the other porphyrias (acute intermittent porphyria and variegate porphyria) are associated with well-known systemic manifestations (abdominal pain, peripheral neuropathy, and pulmonary complications), PCT has no extracutaneous manifestations. Photosensitivity is seen (as with variegate porphyria). PCT is associated with a reduction in hepatic uroporphyrinogen decarboxylase (fifth enzyme in hemoglobin synthesis).

RISK FACTORS

- Hepatitis C.
- Alcohol-induced liver injury.
- Hemochromatosis[3] (iron overload)—50% of cases of PCT are associated with the same gene mutation for hemochromatosis.[3]
- Use of estrogens.
- Cigarette smoking.
- Patients on dialysis.
- Exposure to pesticides (halogenated hydrocarbons).
- HIV infection.[7]

DIAGNOSIS

CLINICAL FEATURES

The classic presentation is that of blistering (vesicles and tense bullae) on photosensitive "fragile skin" (similar to epidermolysis bullosa). Scleroderma-like heliotrope suffusion of the eyelids and face may be seen. As the blisters heal, the skin takes on an atrophic, scarlike appearance. Excoriations, erosions, and milia can be seen in sun exposure areas, mainly the dorsa of the hands. Hypertrichosis (especially on the cheeks and temples) (see **Figure 194-3**) may occur and even be the presenting feature.

TYPICAL DISTRIBUTION

Classically, the dorsa of the hands are affected (see **Figures 194-1** and **194-2**).

LABORATORY STUDIES

The diagnosis can be confirmed by the orange-red fluorescence of the urine when examined under a Wood lamp. Urine also can turn red to brown after exposure to sunlight for several hours. Increased plasma iron may be seen (associated with increased hepatic iron in the Kupffer cells). Diabetes is said to occur in 25% of individuals.

- Twenty-four-hour urine collection for porphyrins—These will be elevated in PCT.
- Skin biopsy may help confirm PCT if the other information is not clear.
- Once the diagnosis is made, secondary causes of PCT should be investigated:
  - Serum for ferritin, iron, and iron-binding capacity to look for hemochromatosis.
  - Order liver function tests, and if abnormal order tests for hepatitis B and C.
  - Consider α-fetoprotein and liver ultrasound if considering cirrhosis and/or hepatocellular carcinoma.
  - Order an HIV test.

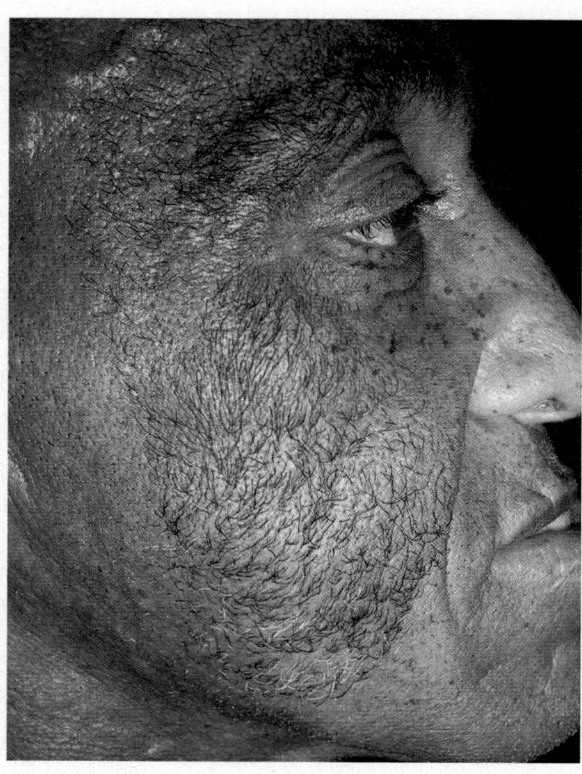

FIGURE 194-3 Hypertrichosis of the cheeks and temples secondary to porphyria cutanea tarda associated with his hepatitis C. This is sometimes referred to as the werewolf syndrome. (*Reproduced with permission from Richard P. Usatine, MD.*)

DIFFERENTIAL DIAGNOSIS

- The acral vesiculobullous lesions may suggest nummular or dyshidrotic eczema. In younger individuals, the acral blistering may suggest epidermolysis bullosa. The lesions may also suggest erythema multiforme bullosum. The heliotrope suffusion may suggest dermatomyositis, and the atrophic changes may suggest systemic sclerosis.
- Polymorphous light eruption; you also can see papules, plaques, vesicles in sun-exposed areas.
- Bullous drug eruptions; check for drug exposure.

MANAGEMENT

- If the onset is associated with alcohol ingestion, estrogen therapy, or exposure to pesticides, reducing exposure is warranted.[1,3]
- Phlebotomy of 450–500 mL of blood biweekly until the hemoglobin is decreased to 11 g or serum ferritin below 20 ng/mL is associated with biochemical and clinical remission within a year.[8]
- Low-dose hydroxychloroquine or chloroquine can help maintain remissions. Standard dose of hydroxychloroquine is 100–200 mg and chloroquine is 125 mg two times per week for at least 6–12 months,[9] whereas high-dose chloroquine can exacerbate the illness[2] due to hepatotoxicity.[10]
- Sun protection clothing, regular use of broad-spectrum sunscreens.
- Treatment of hepatitis C has shown resolution of PCT.[5,6]

FOLLOW-UP

- Periodic clinical follow-up until remission is achieved is necessary, along with constant education and reinforcement of the need to avoid precipitants.

PATIENT EDUCATION

- Avoidance of potential precipitants (alcohol, estrogens, pesticides, cigarette smoking) and avoidance of excess sunlight exposure (to avoid hypersensitivity) are important. Avoidance of trauma and careful wound care is also necessary.

EPIDERMOLYSIS BULLOSA

PATIENT STORY

A 34-year-old pregnant woman presents with active blistering in her axilla, and past history revealed that she lost her fingernails and toenails (**Figure 194-4A**) as a young child. She was diagnosed as a child with recessive dystrophic epidermolysis bullosa. None of her children had been affected because her husband was neither affected nor a carrier (**Figure 194-4B**). A topical steroid ointment helped relieve the pain and calm the blistering in her axilla.

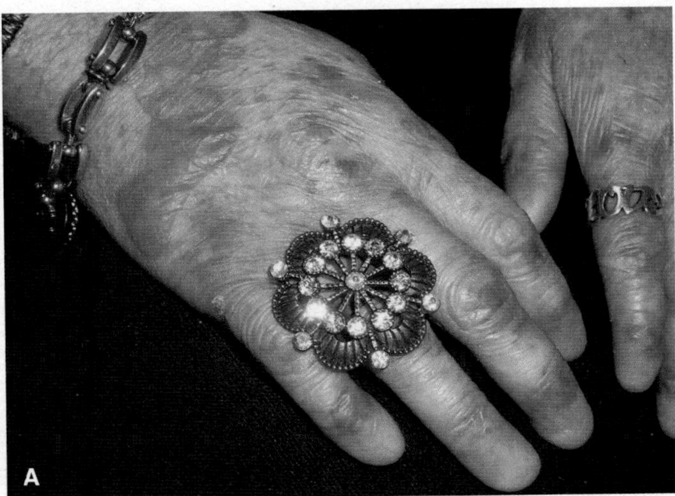

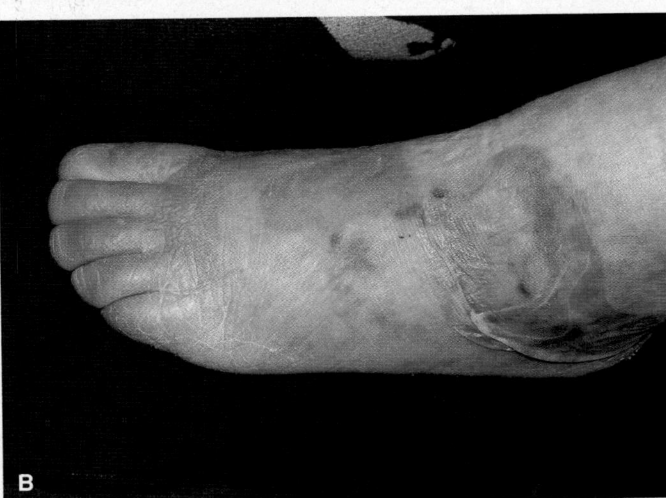

FIGURE 194-4 **A.** Recessive dystrophic epidermolysis bullosa showing a large blister on the dorsum of the hand with loss of fingernails. **B.** The same woman showing complete loss of her toenails and a large bulla that has broken over the ankle region. (*Reproduced with permission from Richard P. Usatine, MD.*)

EPIDEMIOLOGY

- Dystrophic epidermolysis bullosa belongs to a family of inherited diseases characterized by skin fragility and blister formation caused by minor skin trauma[11] due to mutations of the gene COL7A1, which encodes type VII collagen. The defect is located in the basal membrane zone (BMZ), altering the function, adhesion and integrity of the basal membrane of the skin and mucosa.[12] There are autosomal recessive, autosomal dominant, and sporadic types. The severity of this disease may vary widely, from mild skin blisters to gastrointestinal, cardiac, or ocular involvement, as well as scarring, milia, and deformities. Onset is in childhood, and in later years severe dystrophic deformities of hands and feet are characteristic, affecting quality of life[13] (**Figure 194-5**). Malignant degeneration, especially squamous cell carcinoma, is common in sun-exposed areas.[14]

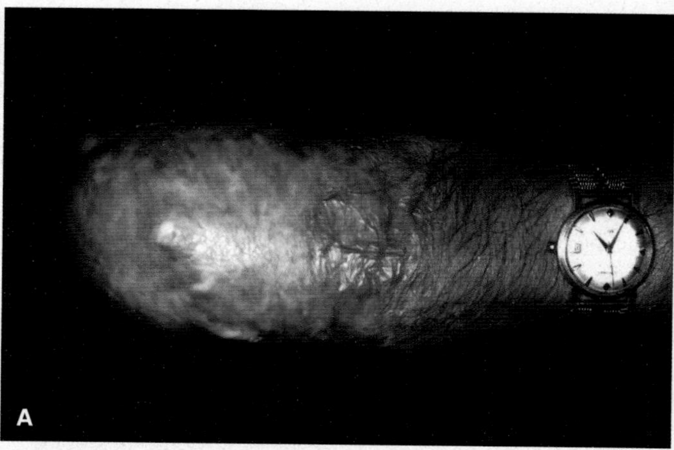

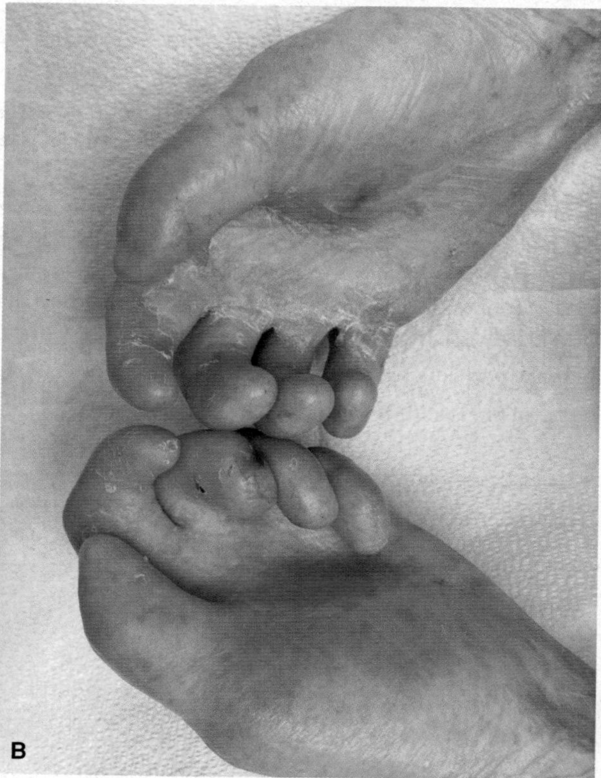

FIGURE 194-5 **A.** Severe recessive dystrophic epidermolysis bullosa in a 53-year-old Asian man. Complete loss of fingers from the disease on his hands. This is referred to as the mitten deformity. He has also had multiple squamous cell carcinomas excised from his hands. **B.** Less severe case of recessive dystrophic epidermolysis bullosa in which the fingers have not been fully lost yet. (*Reproduced with permission from Richard P. Usatine, MD.*)

ETIOLOGY AND PATHOPHYSIOLOGY

- Dystrophic epidermolysis bullosa has vesiculobullous skin separation occurring at the sub-basal lamina level, as opposed to junctional epidermolysis bullosa, which blisters at the intralamina lucida layer; epidermolysis bullosa simplex (**Figure 194-6**), which blisters at the intraepidermal layer; and Kindler syndrome, in which blisters are in multiple layers.[15]

DIAGNOSIS

CLINICAL FEATURES

Acral skin fragility and blistering are the hallmark in childhood. Minor trauma can induce severe blistering. As the disease progresses initially, painful and ultimately debilitating dystrophic deformities such as joint and tendon contractures, pseudosyndactyly, and dystrophic nails are typical. Repeated blistering of the hands can lead to fusion of the fingers and the "mitten" deformity (see **Figure 194-5**). Other clinical features include oral blisters, oral fibrosis, ankyloglossia (fusion of the tongue with mouth floor), esophageal erosions, and strictures.[16-18]

TYPICAL DISTRIBUTION

The typical distribution is acral (hands and feet), although blistering may extend proximally secondary to trauma. Other systems involved include gastrointestinal, commonly esophagus, small intestine; ocular with corneal abrasions; dilated cardiomyopathy; genitourinary stenosis; and osteoporosis.[16-19]

LABORATORY STUDIES AND BIOPSY

There are no laboratory tests to confirm the diagnosis. A punch biopsy can provide adequate tissue for the dermatopathologist to differentiate among the different forms of epidermolysis bullosa—simplex, junctional, dystrophic, and Kindler syndrome—via transmission electron microscopy (TEM), immunofluorescence antigen mapping (IFM), or genetic testing.[17]

DIFFERENTIAL DIAGNOSIS

- Erythema multiforme bullosum may have a similar appearance, but the distribution is less apt to be limited to the distal extremities.
- The appearance of an acral blistering on fragile skin is also characteristic of PCT, but the age of onset of PCT is typically in middle age and not in childhood.
- The first appearance of the condition may be confused, with staphylococcal scalded skin syndrome (see Chapter 122, Impetigo).[20]

MANAGEMENT

Management is primarily prevention of trauma, careful wound care, and treatment of complicating infections. Other supportive measures such as pain management, nutritional support, and electrolyte balance are often necessary with a multidisciplinary team.[21]

- Gentamicin (topical or intralesional) is a promising therapy in the treatment of recessive dystrophic epidermolysis bullosa that induces production of type VII collagen, accelerating wound healing and reducing blistering formation.[22]
- Occupational therapy may help with contractures. In some cases, surgical release of fingers/toes is necessary.[17]
- Screening the skin for squamous cell carcinoma is important in the dystrophic form.[17]
- Cyclosporine and mycophenolate mofetil have shown benefit as long-term therapy.[23]
- Bone marrow transplantation is currently under clinical investigation, and preliminary results are promising.[24]

FOLLOW-UP

Periodic skin examinations should be done to help manage symptoms and screen for malignancy.

PATIENT EDUCATION

Avoid trauma, and come in early if there are any signs of infection or malignancy.

PITYRIASIS LICHENOIDES ET VARIOLIFORMIS ACUTA (PLEVA)

PATIENT STORY

A 22-year-old man presented with a varicelliform eruption that he has had for 6 weeks (**Figure 194-7**). Initially, he was diagnosed with varicella and given a course of acyclovir. Then he was misdiagnosed with scabies and treated with permethrin. A correct diagnosis of PLEVA was made by clinical appearance and confirmed with biopsy. His skin lesions cleared with oral tetracycline.

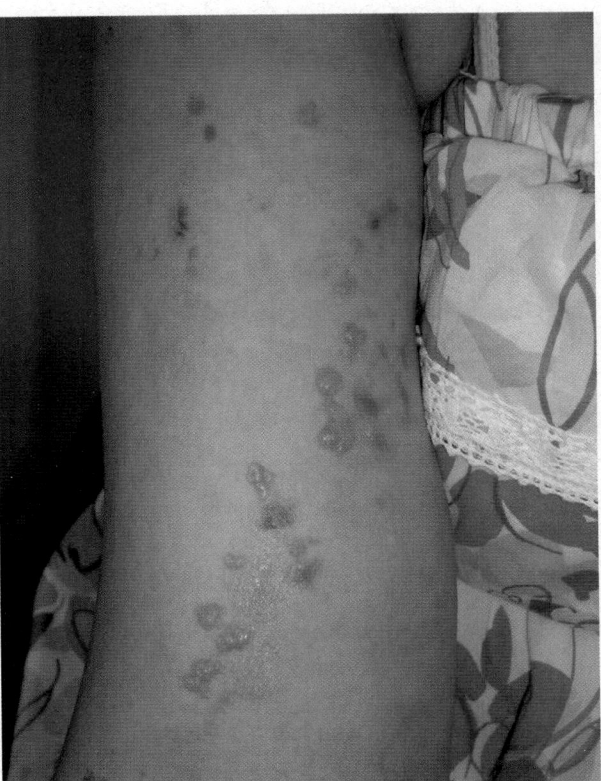

FIGURE 194-6 Epidermolysis bullosa simplex (Dowling-Meara type) in a teenage girl. She has extensive blistering over many areas of the body including, the trunk, extremities, and the hands. *(Reproduced with permission from Richard P. Usatine, MD.)*

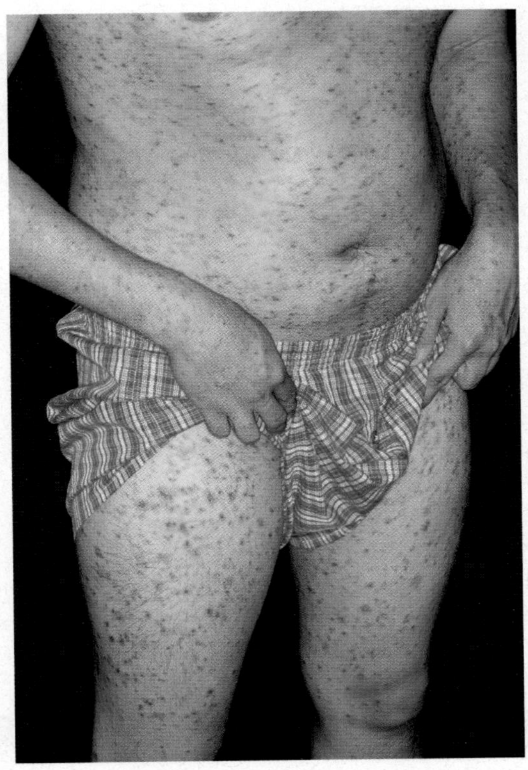

FIGURE 194-7 A 22-year-old man with pityriasis lichenoides et varioliformis acuta (PLEVA). His skin lesions cleared with oral tetracycline. *(Reproduced with permission from Richard P. Usatine, MD.)*

EPIDEMIOLOGY

- PLEVA or Mucha-Habermann disease and pityriasis lichenoides chronica are maculopapular erythematous eruptions that can occur in crops of vesicles that can become hemorrhagic over a course of weeks to months, leaving smallpox-like scars (**Figures 194-7** and **194-8**).[25]
- It occurs predominately in a pediatric population, median 8 years.[26]
- PLEVA occurs in preschool and preadolescent children as well.[27]
- There is a predilection for males in the second and third decades.

ETIOLOGY AND PATHOPHYSIOLOGY

- PLEVA has traditionally been classified as a benign papulosquamous disease. However, there is increasing evidence that suggests that PLEVA should be considered a form of cutaneous lymphoid dysregulation of T cells.[28] It may even evolve into an indolent form of mycosis fungoides (see Chapter 180, Cutaneous T-Cell Lymphoma).[29]
- Cases of PLEVA associated with human herpesvirus 7 (HHV-7) and human herpesvirus 8 (HHV-8), Epstein-Barr virus (EBV), and parvovirus B19 have been reported. This suggests that it could be an inflammatory condition due to dysregulation of T cells rather than a lymphoproliferative disorder.[30,31]

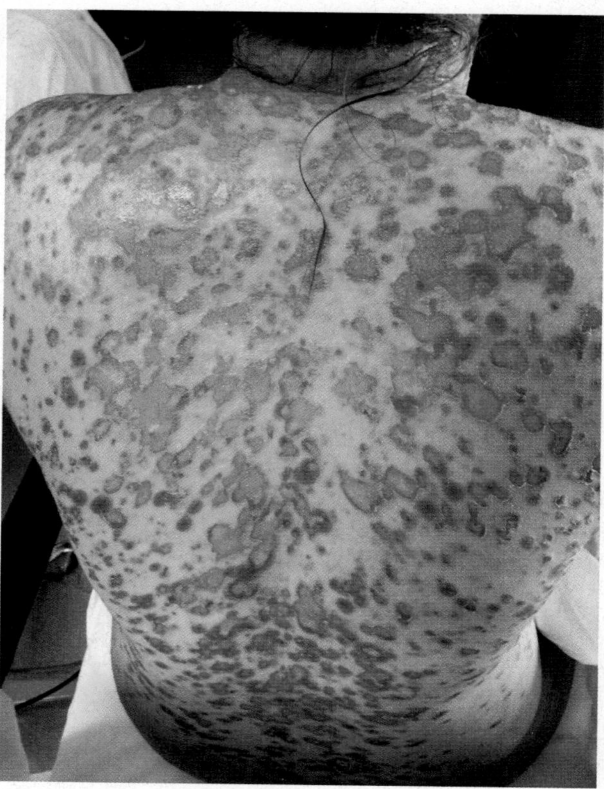

FIGURE 194-8 A young woman with severe ulceronecrotic pityriasis lichenoides et varioliformis acuta (PLEVA). (*Reproduced with permission from Luis Dehesa, MD.*)

DIAGNOSIS

CLINICAL FEATURES

PLEVA occurs with crops of maculopapular and papulosquamous lesions that can vesiculate and form hemorrhagic vesicles (see **Figures 194-7** and **194-8**). Although it resembles varicella, with multiple polymorphic lesions, new crops of lesions continue to appear over weeks and months. It can be thought of as "chickenpox that lasts for weeks to months."

TYPICAL DISTRIBUTION

Lesions typically occur over the anterior trunk and flexural aspects of the proximal extremities. The face is spared.

LABORATORY STUDIES

There are no specific laboratory tests for PLEVA except biopsy.

Dermoscopy findings have been described but do not replace biopsy for diagnosis.[32]

BIOPSY

A punch biopsy is helpful in making the diagnosis. It may be necessary to differentiate PLEVA from lymphomatoid papulosis (see "Differential Diagnosis" below).

DIFFERENTIAL DIAGNOSIS

- Varicella—A varicella direct fluorescent antibody test can confirm acute varicella. If no viral testing was done and what appeared to be varicella persists, PLEVA should be considered (Chapter 129, Chickenpox).

- Secondary syphilis—Direct fluoresce antibody, PCR and serology test help to establish the diagnosis (Chapter 225, Syphilis).
- Pityriasis lichenoides chronica is the chronic form of PLEVA and can be distinguished from PLEVA by length of time and biopsy (**Figure 194-9**). It has a more low-grade clinical course than PLEVA, and the lesions appear over a longer course of time with relapse and remission periods.
- Erythema multiforme (Chapter 185) is a hypersensitivity syndrome with abrupt onset in which symmetric target lesions are seen. The target lesions have epidermal disruption in the center with vesicles and/or erosions. Look for the target lesions to help differentiate this from PLEVA.
- Lymphomatoid papulosis presents in a manner similar to PLEVA with recurrent crops of pruritic papules at different stages of development that appear on the trunk and extremities. Usually it is chronic and self-limited. Although it has histologic features that suggest lymphoma, lymphomatoid papulosis (LP) alone is not fatal. It is important to differentiate LP from PLEVA, because patients with LP need to be worked up for coexisting malignancy. Patients with LP tend to be older, and a punch biopsy can make the diagnosis.
- Gianotti-Crosti syndrome (papular acrodermatitis of childhood) may resemble PLEVA, but the lesions are usually acral in distribution (**Figure 194-10**).[5] The erythematous papules and vesicles are found on the extremities and sometimes on the face. It is a benign syndrome associated with many childhood viruses that may last 2 to 8 weeks.
- Bullous arthropod reactions can be distinguished from PLEVA with a good clinical history and physical exam.

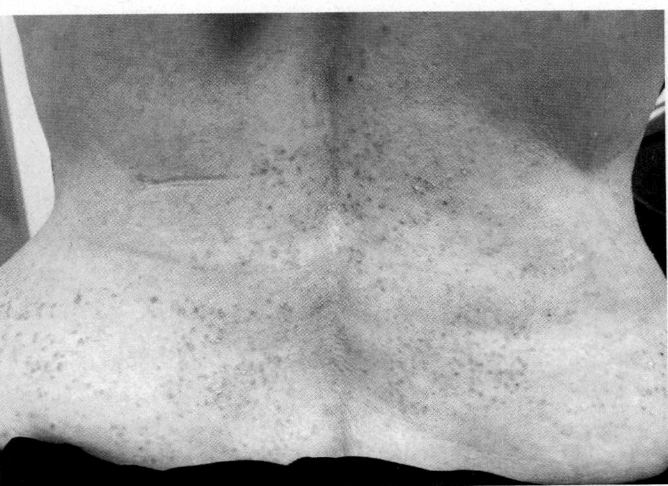

FIGURE 194-9 Pityriasis lichenoides chronica (PLC) is the chronic form of PLEVA that may persist for months to years. This woman has been suffering from PLC for years, and although this view shows the back involvement, she has PLC from her face down to her lower legs. *(Reproduced with permission from Richard P. Usatine, MD.)*

MANAGEMENT

FIRST LINE

- Oral macrolides are first-line treatment.[33] Oral erythromycin 30–50 mg /kg/day is given in divided dosing 3–4 times per day for 1–4 months.[34]
- Doxycycline 100 mg twice daily is an alternative. The efficacy of macrolides and tetracyclines is probably from their anti-inflammatory properties rather than their antibacterial effects.
- Narrowband UVB may be used 2–3 times per week.[33]
- Topical steroids such as triamcinolone 0.1% twice daily may decrease the itching.

SECOND LINE

- UVA1 phototherapy has been used with some success.[35]
- Recalcitrant cases or ulceronecrotic PLEVA can be treated with tumor necrosis factor (TNF)-α inhibitors, intravenous immunoglobulin, or methotrexate.[36,37]

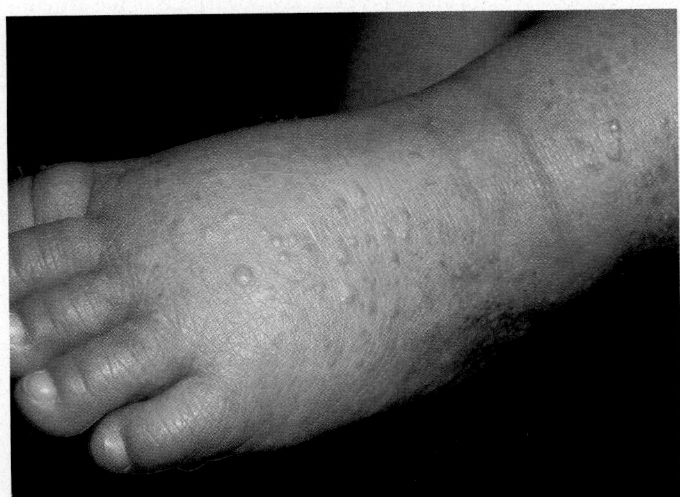

FIGURE 194-10 Gianotti-Crosti syndrome, "papular acrodermatitis of childhood," in a 7-month-old child. The acral eruption started just after a viral upper respiratory infection and involved the feet, lower legs, and buttocks. *(Reproduced with permission from Richard P. Usatine, MD.)*

FOLLOW-UP

Long term follow-up is recommended due to small risk of T-cell malignant transformation.[33]

PATIENT EDUCATION

PLEVA is usually a self-limited disease. There are treatments that can help the symptoms and may shorten the illness.

DERMATITIS HERPETIFORMIS

PATIENT STORY

A young man with a past history of diarrhea and malabsorption carries a past diagnosis of gluten-induced enteropathy. Despite a gluten-free diet, he continues to have a pruritic eruption on his elbows, knees, abdomen, and buttocks (**Figures 194-11** and **194-12**). Although the most likely diagnosis is dermatitis herpetiformis, a punch biopsy was performed to confirm this before starting the patient on oral dapsone.

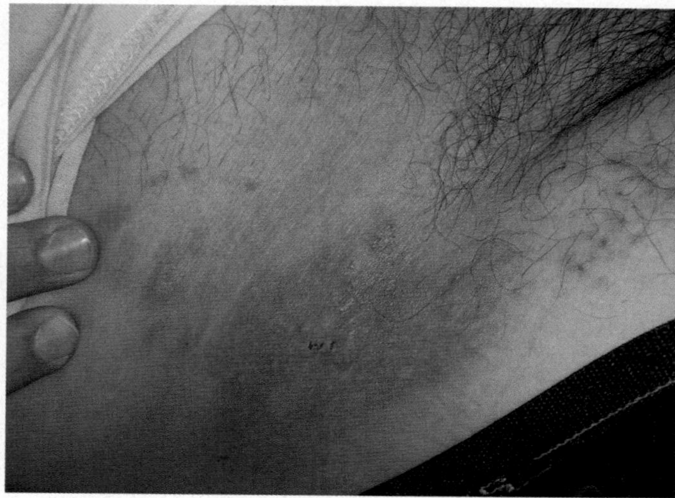

FIGURE 194-11 Vesicles and erosions on the abdomen of a young man with dermatitis herpetiformis and gluten-induced enteropathy. The vesicles that form are fragile and rapidly become small erosions. (*Reproduced with permission from Richard P. Usatine, MD.*)

EPIDEMIOLOGY

- Dermatitis herpetiformis is a chronic recurrent symmetric vesicular eruption that is usually associated with diet-related enteropathy, more specifically gluten hypersensitivity. It is a specific extraintestinal manifestation of gluten enteropathy.[38] It most commonly occurs in the 20- to 40-year-old age group. Men are affected more often than women. Usually more common in Caucasians. In 80% to 90% of cases there is a strong association with genotype HLA DQ2, HLA DQ8, and HLA DR3.[38,39]

ETIOLOGY AND PATHOPHYSIOLOGY

- The disease is related to gluten and other diet-related antigens that cause the development of circulating immune complexes and their subsequent deposition in the skin. The term *herpetiformis* refers to the grouped vesicles that appear on extensor aspects of the extremities and trunk; the disease is not a viral infection or related to the herpes viruses. It is characterized by the deposition of granular immunoglobulin (Ig) A along the tips of the dermal papillae. The majority of patients will also have blunting and flattening of jejunal villi, which leads to diarrhea even to the point of steatorrhea and malabsorption.

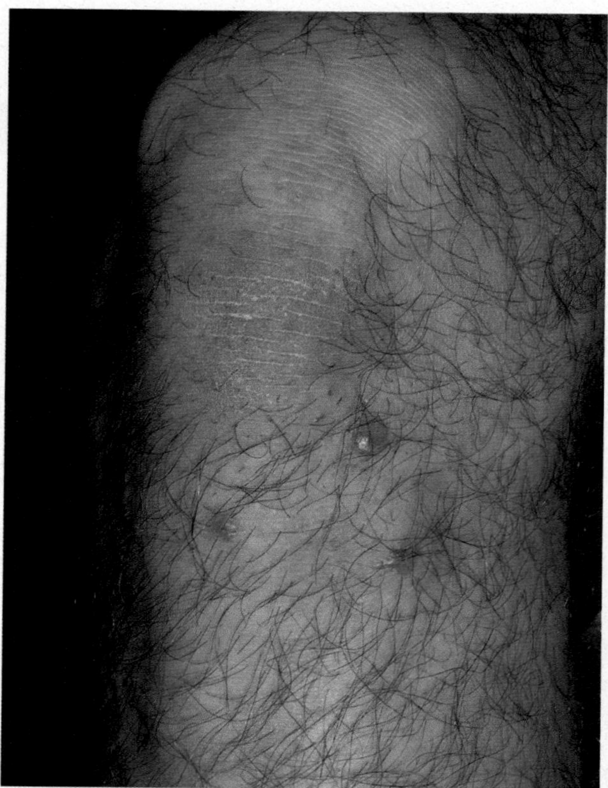

FIGURE 194-12 Dermatitis herpetiformis on the knees of a young man with gluten-induced enteropathy. He also has similar lesions on the elbows and abdomen. (*Reproduced with permission from Richard P. Usatine, MD.*)

DIAGNOSIS

CLINICAL FEATURES

The clinical eruption is characterized by severe itching, burning, or stinging in the characteristic extensor distribution (knees, elbows, back, buttocks, and the extensor aspect of the forearms). Herpetiform vesicles, papules, and urticarial plaques may be seen. Because of the intense pruritus, characteristic lesions may be excoriated beyond recognition (see **Figures 194-11** and **194-12**). The condition has relapses and remissions that are related to the gluten-restricted diet.

TYPICAL DISTRIBUTION

Classically, the lesions (or excoriations) are seen in the extensor aspects of the extremities, shoulders (see **Figure 194-11**), lower back, and buttocks (see **Figure 194-12**).

LABORATORY STUDIES

If the patient has gluten-induced enteropathy, antigliadin and antiendomysial antibodies may be present in 80% of the cases of dermatitis herpetiformis. A blood test for antigliadin antibody is a sensitive test for gluten-induced enteropathy.

BIOPSY

Diagnosis is confirmed by a punch biopsy. It is best to biopsy new crops of lesions or intact vesicles. A standard histologic examination will show microabscesses of neutrophils in the dermal papillae, subepidermal vesicles, perivascular lymphocytic infiltrate, and few eosinophils. Direct immunofluorescence reveals granular deposits of IgA and complement within the dermal papillae, with almost 100% specificity and sensitivity.[38]

DIFFERENTIAL DIAGNOSIS

- Scabies may have a similar appearance with pruritus, papules, and vesicles. If the lesions and distribution suggest scabies, it should be ruled out with skin scraping looking for the mite, feces, and eggs. If the scraping is negative, but the clinical appearance suggests scabies, empiric treatment with permethrin should be considered as well. If the lesions persist, consider a punch biopsy to look for dermatitis herpetiformis (Chapter 149, Scabies).
- Nummular and dyshidrotic eczema may also be diagnostic considerations, but response to steroids in eczema may be helpful in differentiation (Chapters 151, Atopic Dermatitis, and 153, Hand Eczema).
- The classic differential for PCT is pseudoporphyria (caused by nonsteroidal anti-inflammatory drugs [NSAIDs] such as naproxen), epidermolysis bullosa acquisita, and variegate porphyria.
- IgA bullous dermatosis: differs from dermatitis herpetiformis because in IgA bullous dermatosis the deposit of IgA is linear instead of the granular pattern seen in DH and often is caused by drugs.
- Bullous arthropod bites; patient may recall insect exposure.

MANAGEMENT

- With a gluten-free diet, 80% of patients will show improvement in the skin lesions (see **Figure 194-12**). The degree of benefit is dependent on the strictness of the diet.[38,39]
- A gluten-free diet may help the enteropathy and decrease the subsequent development of small bowel lymphoma.[38]
- Dapsone at an initial dose of 100–200 mg daily or 0.5–1 mg/kg/day with gradual reduction to a 25- to 50-mg maintenance level may be necessary indefinitely.[38] Monitor complete blood count (CBC), liver function test due to risk of hemolysis, methemoglobinemia. Some clinicians, recommend checking glucose-6-phosphate dehydrogenase (G6PD) activity prior to start of treatment.
- Rituximab has been used in recalcitrant cases with good outcome, serologic and immunologic remission.[40]

FOLLOW-UP

Follow-up is needed to control the disease and monitor nutritional status.

PATIENT EDUCATION

Nutritional counseling is important for all patients with gluten-induced enteropathy. Persons with dermatitis herpetiformis and gluten-induced, enteropathy should not eat wheat and barley but can eat rice, oats, and corn. Patients can get information, dietary guidelines, and educational materials online via support groups such as www.gluten.org and www.celiac.org.

PATIENT RESOURCES

- MedlinePlus. *Porphyria*—**https://medlineplus.gov/ency/article/001208.htm.**
- Genetics Home Reference. *Epidermolysis Bullosa Simplex*—**http://ghr.nlm.nih.gov/condition/epidermolysis-bullosa-simplex.**
- National Institute of Arthritis and Musculoskeletal and Skin Diseases. *Epidermolysis Bullosa*—**http://www.niams.nih.gov/health-topics/epidermolysis-bullosa.**
- **www.gluten.org** or **www.celiac.org.**

PROVIDER RESOURCES

- Medscape. *Porphyria Cutanea Tarda*—**http://emedicine.medscape.com/article/1103643.**
- Medscape. *Epidermolysis Bullosa*—**http://emedicine.medscape.com/article/1062939.**
- Medscape. *Dermatitis Herpetiformis*—**http://emedicine.medscape.com/article/1062640.**
- Medscape. *Pityriasis Lichenoides*—**http://emedicine.medscape.com/article/1099078.**

REFERENCES

1. Ramanujam VM, Anderson KE. Porphyria diagnostics—part 1: a brief overview of the porphyrias. *Curr Protoc Hum Genet.* 2015; 86:17.20.1-26.
2. Elder GH. Porphyria cutanea tarda and related disorders. In: Kadish K, Smith K, Guilard R, eds. *The Porphyrin Handbook.* Vol. 14. San Diego, CA: Elsevier Science; 2003:67ff.
3. Jalil S, Grady JJ, Lee C, Anderson KE. Associations among behavior-related susceptibility factors in porphyria cutanea tarda. *Clin Gastroenterol Hepatol.* 2010;8(3):297-302, 302e-1.
4. Sood S, Mingos N, Ross G. Porphyria. *N Engl J Med.* 2017;377(21): 2100.

5. Callen JP. Hepatitis C viral infection and porphyria cutanea tarda. *Am J Med Sci.* 2017;354(1):5-6.
6. Combalia A, To-Figueras J, Laguno M, et al. Direct-acting antivirals for hepatitis C virus induce a rapid clinical and biochemical remission of porphyria cutanea tarda. *Br J Dermatol.* 2017;177(5):e183-e184.
7. Guha SK, Bandyopadhyay D, Saha A, Lal NR. Human immunodeficiency virus associated sporadic nonfamilial porphyria cutanea tarda. *Indian J Dermatol.* 2016;61(3):318-320.
8. Assi TB, Baz E. Current applications of therapeutic phlebotomy. *Blood Transfus.* 2014;12 Suppl 1:s75-83.
9. Singal AK, Kormos-Hallberg C, Lee C, et al. Low-dose hydroxychloroquine is as effective as phlebotomy in treatment of patients with porphyria cutanea tarda. *Clin Gastroenterol Hepatol.* 2012;10(12):1402-1409.
10. Rossmann-Ringdahl I, Olsson R. Porphyria cutanea tarda: effects and risk factors for hepatotoxicity from high-dose chloroquine treatment. *Acta Derm Venereol.* 2007;87(5):401-405.
11. Horn HM, Tidman MJ. The clinical spectrum of epidermolysis bullosa. *Br J Dermatol.* 2002;146(2):267-274.
12. Uitto J, Richard G. Progress in epidermolysis bullosa: genetic classification and clinical implications. *Am J Med Genet C Semin Med Genet.* 2004;131C:61.
13. Horn HM, Tidman MJ. Quality of life in epidermolysis bullosa. *Clin Exp Dermatol.* 2002;27(8):707-710.
14. Fine JD, Johnson LB, Weiner M, et al. Epidermolysis bullosa and the risk of life-threatening cancers: the National EB Registry experience, 1986–2006. *J Am Acad Dermatol.* 2009;60(2):203-211.
15. Fine JD, Bruckner-Tuderman L, Eady RA, et al. Inherited epidermolysis bullosa: updated recommendations on diagnosis and classification. *J Am Acad Dermatol.* 2014;70(6):1103-1126.
16. Paller AS, Mancini AJ. Bullous diseases in children. In: Paller AS, Mancini AJ, eds. *Hurwitz's Clinical Pediatric Dermatology*, 5th ed. Philadelphia, PA: Elsevier; 2016:317-333.e5.
17. Pfendner EG, Lucky AW. Dystrophic epidermolysis bullosa. 2006 Aug 21 [updated 2015 Feb 26]. In: Adam MP, Ardinger HH, Pagon RA, editors. GeneReviews [Internet]. Seattle (WA): University of Washington; 1993-2018.
18. Kummer TR, Nagano HC, Tavares SS, et al. Oral manifestations and challenges in dental treatment of epidermolysis bullosa dystrophica. *J Dent Child (Chic).* 2013;80(2):97-100.
19. Tong L, Hodgkins PR, Denyer J, et al. The eye in epidermolysis bullosa. *Br J Ophthalmol.* 1999;83(3):323-326.
20. Patel GK, Finlay AY. Staphylococcal scalded skin syndrome: diagnosis and management. *Am J Clin Dermatol.* 2003;4(3):165-175.
21. Chiaverini C, Bourrat E, Mazereeuw-Hautier J, et al. [Hereditary epidermolysis bullosa: French national guidelines (PNDS) for diagnosis and treatment]. *Ann Dermatol Venereol.* 2017;144(1):6-35.
22. Woodley DT, Cogan J, Hou Y, et al. Gentamicin induces functional type VII collagen in recessive dystrophic epidermolysis bullosa patients. *J Clin Invest.* 2017;127(8):3028-3038.
23. El-Darouti MA, Fawzy MM, Amin IM, et al. Mycophenolate mofetil: a novel immunosuppressant in the treatment of dystrophic epidermolysis bullosa, a randomized controlled trial. *J Dermatolog Treat.* 2013;24(6):422-426.
24. Rashidghamat E, McGrath JA. Novel and emerging therapies in the treatment of recessive dystrophic epidermolysis bullosa. *Intractable Rare Dis Res.* 2017;6(1):6-20.
25. Bowers S, Warshaw EM. Pityriasis lichenoides and its subtypes. *J Am Acad Dermatol.* 2006;55(4):557-572.
26. Zang JB, Coates SJ, Huang J, et al. Pityriasis lichenoides: long-term follow-up study. *Pediatr Dermatol.* 2018;35(2):213-219.
27. Ersoy-Evans S, Greco MF, Mancini AJ, et al. Pityriasis lichenoides in childhood: a retrospective review of 124 patients. *J Am Acad Dermatol.* 2007;56(2):205-210.
28. Magro C, Crowson AN, Kovatich A, Burns F. Pityriasis lichenoides: a clonal T-cell lymphoproliferative disorder. *Hum Pathol.* 2002; 33(8):788-795.
29. Zaaroura H, Sahar D, Bick T, Bergman R. Relationship between pityriasis lichenoides and mycosis fungoides: a clinicopathological, immunohistochemical, and molecular study. *Am J Dermatopathol.* 2018;40(6):409-415.
30. Costa-Silva M, Calistru A, Sobrinho-Simões J, et al. Pityriasis lichenoides et varioliformis acuta associated with human herpesvirus 7. *Actas Dermosifiliogr.* 2017 Dec 5. pii: S0001-7310(17)30591-4. [Epub ahead of print]
31. Kim JE, Yun WJ, Mun SK, et al. Pityriasis lichenoides et varioliformis acuta and pityriasis lichenoides chronica: comparison of lesional T-cell subsets and investigation of viral associations. *J Cutan Pathol.* 2011;38(8):649-656.
32. Ankad BS, Beergouder SL. Pityriasis lichenoides et varioliformis acuta in skin of color: new observations by dermoscopy. *Dermatol Pract Concept.* 2017;7(1):27-34.
33. Geller L, Antonov NK, Lauren CT, et al. Pityriasis lichenoides in childhood: review of clinical presentation and treatment options. *Pediatr Dermatol.* 2015;32(5):579-592.
34. Hapa A, Ersoy-Evans S, Karaduman A. Childhood pityriasis lichenoides and oral erythromycin. *Pediatr Dermatol.* 2012;29(6):719-724.
35. Pinton PC, Capezzera R, Zane C, De Panfilis G. Medium-dose ultraviolet A1 therapy for pityriasis lichenoides et varioliformis acuta and pityriasis lichenoides chronica. *J Am Acad Dermatol.* 2002;47(3):410-414.
36. Meziane L, Caudron A, Dhaille F, et al. Febrile ulceronecrotic Mucha-Habermann disease: treatment with infliximab and intravenous immunoglobulins and review of the literature. *Dermatology.* 2012;225(4):344-348.
37. Lazaridou E, Fotiadou C, Tsorova C, et al. Resistant pityriasis lichenoides et varioliformis acuta in a 3-year-old boy: successful treatment with methotrexate. *Int J Dermatol.* 2010;49(2):215-217.
38. Antiga E, Caproni M. The diagnosis and treatment of dermatitis herpetiformis. *Clin Cosmet Investig Dermatol.* 2015;8:257-265.
39. Mendes FB, Hissa-Elian A, Abreu MA, Gonçalves VS. Review: dermatitis herpetiformis. *An Bras Dermatol.* 2013;88(4):594-599.
40. lbers LN, Zone JJ, Stoff BK, Feldman RJ. Rituximab treatment for recalcitrant dermatitis herpetiformis. *JAMA Dermatol.* 2017;153(3):315-318.

SECTION R HAIR AND NAIL CONDITIONS

195 ALOPECIA AREATA

Richard P. Usatine, MD

PATIENT STORY

A young woman presented to her physician with hair loss for 3 months. She is very worried that it will not grow back and that it might spread to other parts of her scalp. When she lifted her hair, one round area of hair loss was noted **(Figure 195-1)**. The scalp was smooth, and there were no signs of scale or inflammation. Some fine white hairs were also seen growing in the area of hair loss. A few "exclamation point" hairs were also seen. The physician readily diagnosed alopecia areata (AA) based on the clinical exam. He attempted to reassure the young woman that her hair is already growing back and would likely regrow fully in the coming months. He also explained that the new hairs may be white at first but will regain their natural dark color. He also offered her the option of intralesional steroid injection of the involved scalp. The physician did explain that the intralesional steroid is not a guarantee of 100% resolution but may increase the speed and likelihood of recovery. The young woman chose to have the steroid injection because she did not want to take any chances of not regaining her hair.

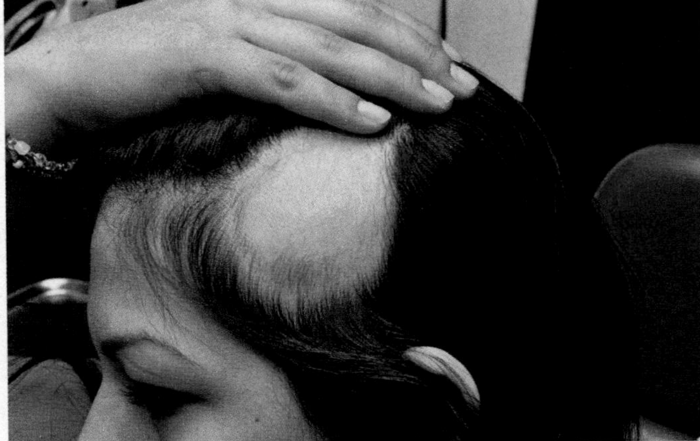

FIGURE 195-1 Alopecia areata in a young woman with a typical round area of alopecia. The scalp was smooth without scale or visible lesions. *(Reproduced with permission from Richard P. Usatine, MD.)*

INTRODUCTION

AA is a common disorder that causes patches of hair loss without scarring the hair follicle. This autoimmune process involves inflammation but does not damage the ability of the hair follicle to produce hairs again in the future. The areas of hair loss are often round, and the scalp is often very smooth at the site of hair loss.[1] AA can occur at any age, and the extent of the disease is variable. Alopecia totalis (AT) involves the whole scalp. Alopecia universalis (AU) involves loss of all hair including the whole scalp, eyebrows, eyelashes, and body (**Figure 195-2**).

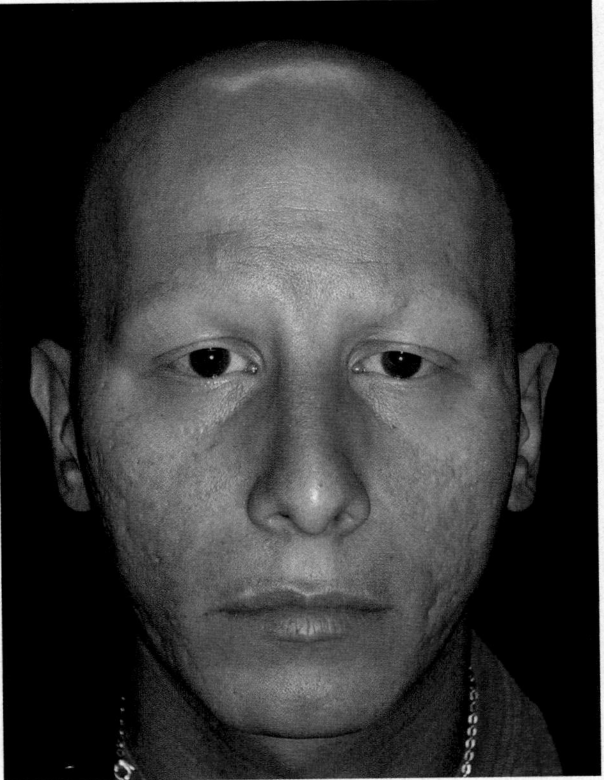

FIGURE 195-2 Alopecia universalis for more than 10 years in this man. Note that he has lost his eyebrows and eyelashes. *(Reproduced with permission from Richard P. Usatine, MD.)*

EPIDEMIOLOGY

Alopecia affects approximately 0.2% of the population at any given time with approximately 2.1% of the population experiencing an episode during their lifetime.[2,3]

- Men and women are equally affected.
- Most patients are younger than age 40 years at disease onset, with the average age being 25 to 27 years.[2,4] Children and teenagers are often affected.[5]

ETIOLOGY AND PATHOPHYSIOLOGY

- The preponderance of evidence supports that AA is an autoimmune condition in which autoreactive T cells infiltrate the hair follicle.[5] The inflammatory immune cells turn the growing anagen hair follicle into the resting telogen phase. This results in hair loss but not destruction of the stem cell compartment within the hair follicle.[5] This explains why hair growth can occur spontaneously or with treatment at any time after hair loss with AA.

- Janus kinase/signal transducers and activators of transcription pathway is upregulated in AA but not in normal hair follicles.[5] This is relevant to the use of Janus kinase inhibitors as treatment of AA.[5]

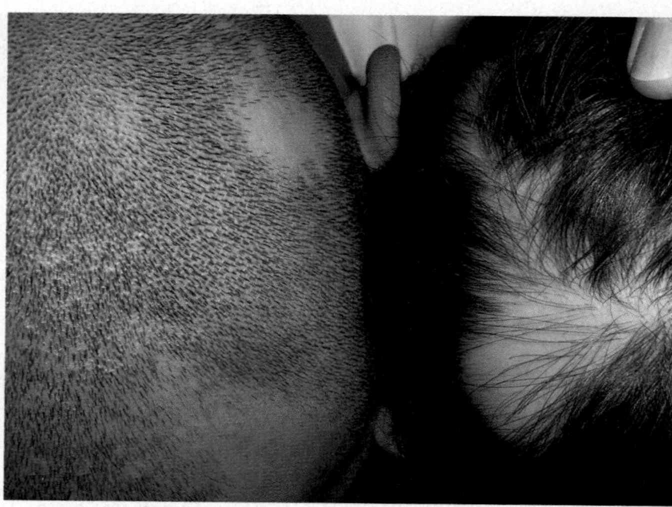

FIGURE 195-3 Alopecia areata in a father and daughter. AA in a parent is a risk factor for AA in the children. (*Reproduced with permission from Richard P. Usatine, MD.*)

RISK FACTORS

- Previous episode of AA.
- Family history of AA—In one study, the estimated lifetime risks were 7.1% in siblings, 7.8% in parents, and 5.7% in offspring of patients with AA (**Figure 195-3**).[6]
- Atopy (atopic dermatitis, asthma, and allergic rhinitis).[5,7]
- Other autoimmune conditions such as vitiligo, psoriasis, and thyroid disease.[5,7]
- Stress and psych problems.[5,7] This association is strong, but no causality is proven.

DIAGNOSIS

CLINICAL FEATURES

- Sudden onset of 1 or more 1- to 4-cm areas of hair loss on the scalp (**Figures 195-1** and **195-4**). This can occur in the beard, eyebrows, or other areas of hair (**Figure 195-5**).
- The affected skin is smooth and may have short stubble hair growth.
- "Exclamation point" hairs are often noted (**Figure 195-6**). These hairs are characterized by proximal thinning while the distal portion remains of normal caliber.
- When hair begins to regrow, it often comes in as fine white hair (**Figure 195-7**).

CLINICAL SUBTYPES

- Ophiasis (like a serpent)—This creates a bandlike alopecia resembling a serpent (**Figure 195-8**). This is often found at the occipital and temporal hairlines.
- Sisaipho (**Figure 195-9**)—This causes central hair loss that spares the hair at the margins of the scalp.
- Diffuse forms—Hair loss is diffuse and sudden.

TYPICAL DISTRIBUTION

- Scalp, beard, and eyebrows but can involve total-body hair loss.
- Nail changes can include pitting, longitudinal ridging, and trachyonychia (nails appear dull and rough) (**Figure 195-10**). Nail changes are more likely to be seen with severe disease and occur in approximately 10% to 20% of persons with AA.[5]

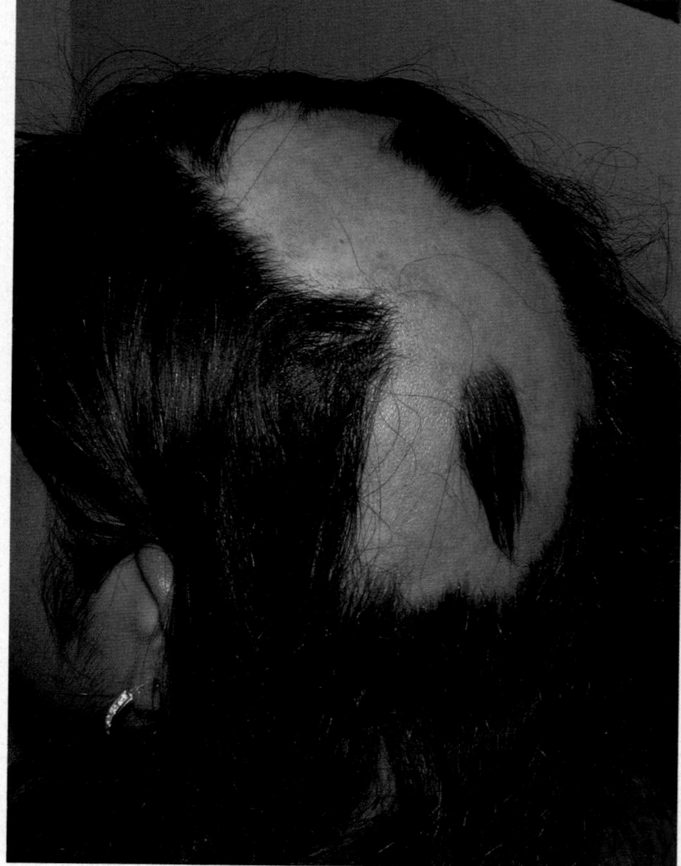

FIGURE 195-4 Extensive alopecia areata for more than 6 months in a woman. (*Reproduced with permission from Richard P. Usatine, MD.*)

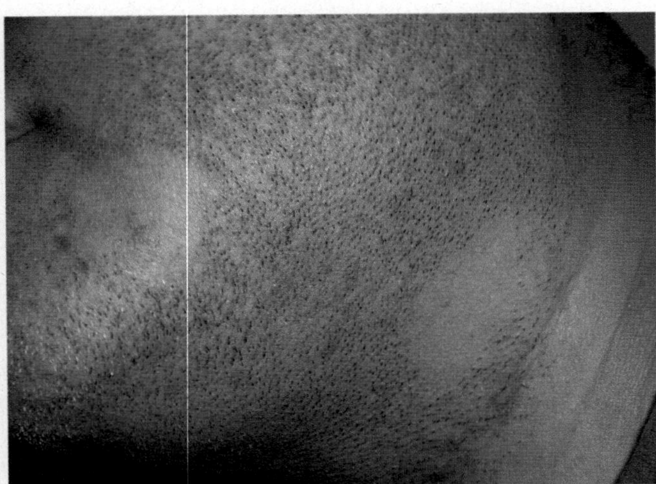

FIGURE 195-5 Alopecia areata can be seen in the beard in this young man. (*Reproduced with permission from Richard P. Usatine, MD.*)

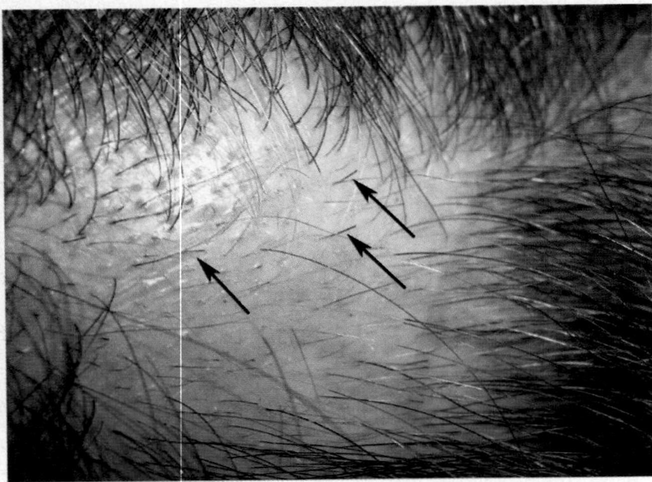

FIGURE 195-6 Exclamation point hairs (*arrows*) can be seen in this case of alopecia areata. The hair is narrow at the base, short and wide at the end. (*Reproduced with permission from Richard P. Usatine, MD.*)

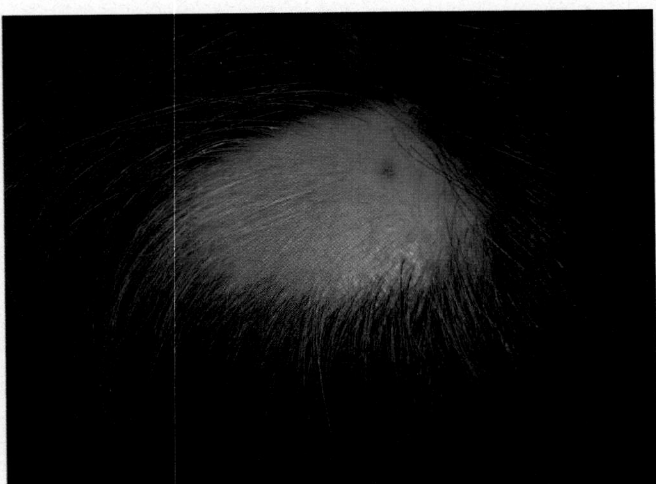

FIGURE 195-7 New growth of white hair after 7 months of alopecia areata in this middle-age woman. (*Reproduced with permission from Richard P. Usatine, MD.*)

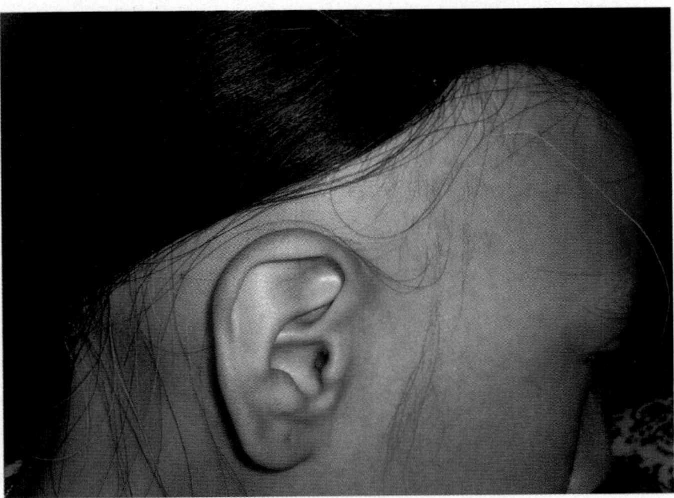

FIGURE 195-8 Ophiasis pattern of alopecia areata in a 12-year-old girl with atopic dermatitis. Ophiasis means "serpent-like." This is often found at the occipital and temporal hairline as seen here. The white hairs support the diagnosis of AA. (*Reproduced with permission from Richard P. Usatine, MD.*)

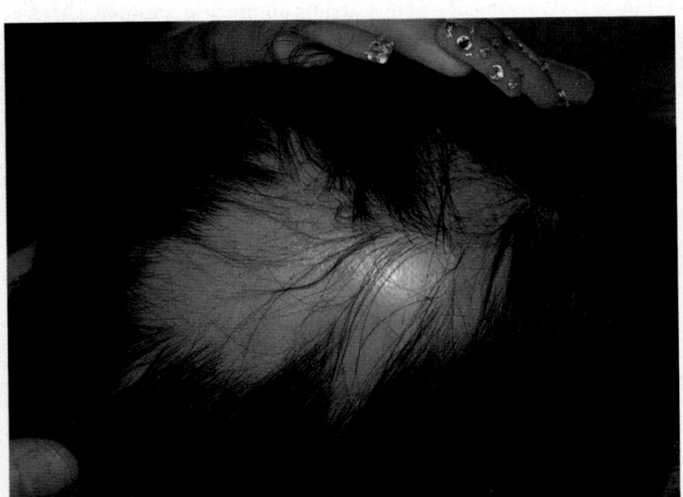

FIGURE 195-9 Sisaipho pattern of alopecia areata that causes central hair loss and spares the hair at the margins of the scalp. The hair loss began 1 year ago in this 3-year-old boy. (*Reproduced with permission from Richard P. Usatine, MD.*)

LABORATORY STUDIES

- Typically, the diagnosis can be made with history and physical examination alone.
- Thyroid abnormalities, vitiligo, and pernicious anemia often accompany AA. Consequently, screening laboratory tests (e.g., thyroid-stimulating hormone, complete blood count [CBC]) may be helpful to look for thyroid disorders and anemia (**Figure 195-11**).

DERMOSCOPY (TRICHOSCOPY)

The dermatoscope allows magnification of the scalp and remaining hairs. Exclamation point hairs (as described above) can be seen well and are pathognomonic of AA (**Figure 195-12**).

BIOPSY

Not needed unless the diagnosis is uncertain. Histology examination shows peribulbar lymphocytic infiltration in the acute stage. The findings vary according to the stages: acute, chronic, and recovery. When in doubt, the preferred biopsy is performed with a 4-mm punch and should include at least one hair or hair follicle in the affected area.

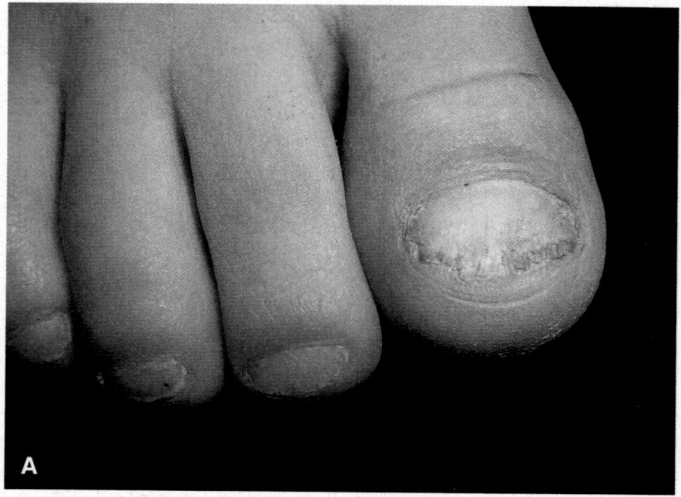

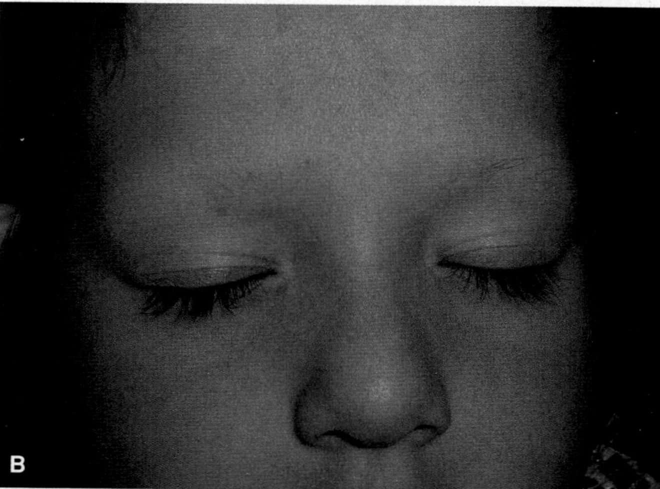

FIGURE 195-10 **A.** Nail changes in the 3-year-old boy with sisaipho alopecia areata. Note the longitudinal ridging and trachyonychia (nails appear dull and rough). **B.** Same boy showing the loss of his eyebrows. *(Reproduced with permission from Richard P. Usatine, MD.)*

DIFFERENTIAL DIAGNOSIS

- Trichotillomania—History of hair pulling; short, "broken" hairs are seen (see Chapter 196, Traction Alopecia and Trichotillomania).
- Telogen effluvium—Even distribution of hair loss; may be drug-induced (e.g., warfarin, β-blockers, lithium) or occur after pregnancy (see Chapter 76, Skin Findings in Pregnancy).
- Anagen effluvium—History of drug use (e.g., chemotherapeutic agents); even distribution of hair loss.
- Tinea capitis—Skin scaling and inflammation; KOH prep or fungal culture, if necessary (see Chapter 143, Tinea Capitis).
- Secondary syphilis—"Moth-eaten" appearance in scalp or beard; risk factors and rapid plasma reagin (RPR) will help distinguish (see Chapter 225, Syphilis).
- Lupus erythematosus—Skin scarring; antinuclear antibody (ANA) if clinical presentation compatible with this diagnosis (see Chapter 188, Lupus: Systemic and Cutaneous).
- Follicular mucinosis with or without mycosis fungoides can cause areas of hair loss similar to AA. These are rare diagnoses and require a punch biopsy if suspected.

MANAGEMENT

Consider extent of hair loss and age of patient to guide therapy.

FIRST LINE

- Intralesional steroids are first-line therapy in patients older than 10 years of age with less than 50% scalp involvement (**Figure 195-13**).[8] SOR B
  - In one large randomized controlled trial (RCT), adult patients with localized AA were randomized to receive either intralesional triamcinolone acetonide (10 mg/mL) or topical betamethasone cream 0.1% twice daily. Hair regrowth was seen in 84 (74.3%) of

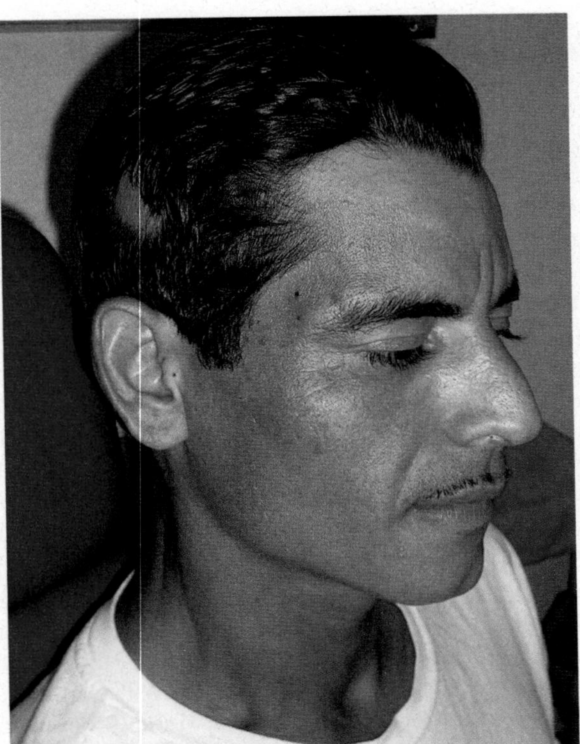

FIGURE 195-11 A patient with alopecia areata who was hyperthyroid. He had symptoms of hyperthyroidism and his thyroid-stimulating hormone was low. (*Reproduced with permission from Richard P. Usatine, MD.*)

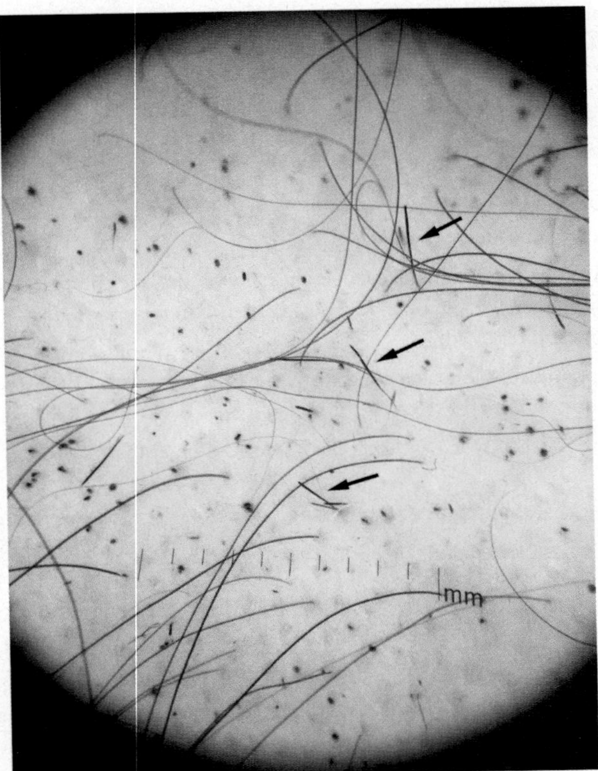

FIGURE 195-12 Trichoscopy (dermoscopy for hair) is a great tool to magnify the scalp to see such findings as exclamation point hairs. These are pathognomonic of AA. (*Reproduced with permission from Richard P. Usatine, MD.*)

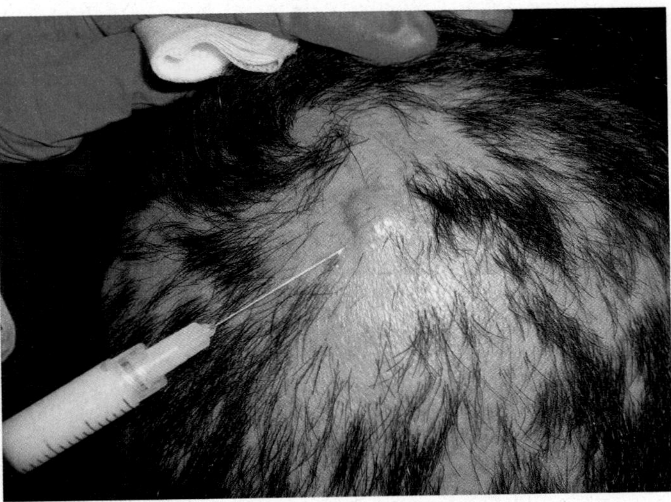

FIGURE 195-13 Injecting extensive patchy alopecia areata of the scalp with triamcinolone acetonide 5 mg/mL. The injections are intradermal to avoid scalp atrophy. This young woman had complete regrowth of her scalp hair after 3 monthly injections. (*Reproduced with permission from Richard P. Usatine, MD.*)

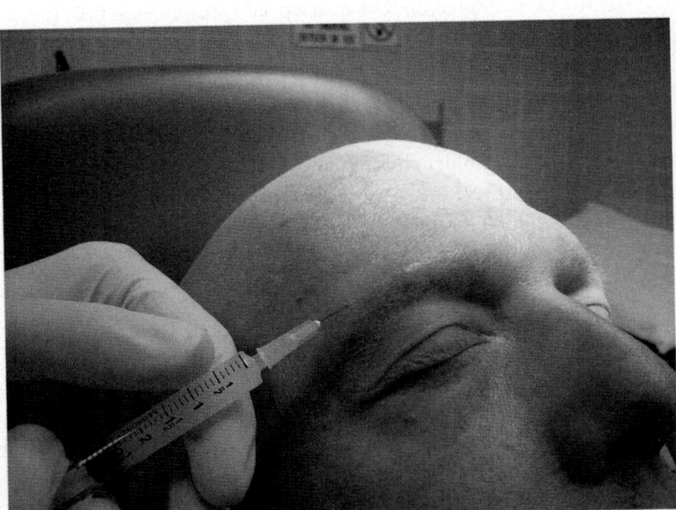

FIGURE 195-14 Injecting the eyebrows of a man with alopecia totalis using triamcinolone acetonide 2.5 mg/mL. This has worked in the past, but the patient has had new eyebrow hair loss and is coming in for another set of injections. (*Reproduced with permission from Richard P. Usatine, MD.*)

the intralesional steroid group and in 53 (46.9%) of the topical betamethasone group. The intralesional steroid was significantly better than the topical steroid.[9]

- In another RCT, intralesional triamcinolone acetonide (10 mg/mL every 3 weeks) was better than betamethasone valerate foam in management of localized AA.[10]
- In one small study, injection of 2.5 mg/mL triamcinolone acetonide was as beneficial as 5 or 10 mg/mL for limited, patchy alopecia areata.[11] The authors suggest that using the lowest effective concentration minimizes skin atrophy and allows for injection of a greater volume, increasing the maximal treatment area.[11] Using a 2.5 mg/mL concentration monthly allows for 8 mL of volume per treatment without exceeding 20 mg of triamcinolone per month. This is especially helpful to cover more extensive alopecia.
- Although 10 mg/mL triamcinolone is often used as treatment in practice and in research studies, we recommend using 2.5–5 mg/mL to avoid atrophy. Dilute triamcinolone acetonide (Kenalog) 10 mg/mL with sterile saline to 2.5 or 5 mg/mL for use on the scalp. Inject with a 27- or 30-gauge needle to minimize pain. Inject into the dermis of the involved areas of the scalp up to a total of 20 mg triamcinolone. Use 2.5 mg/mL for involved areas of the eyebrows or beard. Do not exceed 0.5 mL for each eyebrow (**Figure 195-14**). SOR C
- Do not reinject areas that show atrophy. In most cases, the atrophy will resolve spontaneously. SOR C
- Because spontaneous regrowth can occur, steroid injections should be discontinued after 6 months if there is no response.

- Topical steroids are first-line therapy in patients younger than 10 years of age with less than 50% scalp involvement.[8] SOR B This also applies to any older children or adults who are needle phobic and reject intralesional steroids.
  - Clobetasol 0.05% ointment under occlusion and clobetasol 0.05% foam have been studied in adults with AA, AT, and AU with good results in some patients.[12,13] The study in which half the scalp was treated showed that the effect is local and not from systemic absorption.[12] In the clobetasol foam study, greater hair regrowth was noted on 89% of scalp sites treated with the clobetasol versus 11% of sites treated with placebo after 12 weeks.[12] Although foam is a well-tolerated vehicle, the high pricing and prior authorization process may make it difficult to obtain. Cream and ointment vehicles of high-potency steroids are also worth trying in older children and adults who do not want intralesional therapy. It is easier to start without occlusion, but this could be added if no regrowth is noted. Experts in a recent review of AA recommended topical mometasone in children.[8] Triamcinolone 0.1% is a low-priced alternative.

SECOND LINE

- Other topical agents used to treat AA include 5% minoxidil and/or anthralin.[8] The combination of anthralin with topical steroids and/or minoxidil may be considered. SOR C
- For patients with more than 50% of scalp involvement, consider referral for topical immunotherapy with contact sensitizers. This treatment is very time consuming and challenging to administer. It involves weekly applications of irritating chemicals to the scalp for months at a time.
  - Topical diphenylcyclopropenone (DPCP) is a contact immunotherapy that has some proven benefit with extensive AA. In one study, 56 patients with chronic, extensive AA (duration ranging from 1 to 10 years, involving 30% to 100% of the scalp) were treated with progressively higher concentrations of DPCP in a randomized crossover trial. Twenty-five of 56 patients had total hair regrowth at 6 months, and no relapse occurred in 60% of patients.[14] SOR B Another contact sensitizer that has been used in a similar fashion is squaric acid.
  - These contact sensitizers have potential severe side effects, including mutagenesis, blistering, hyperpigmentation, and scarring.
- Other treatments being used by dermatology specialists for treatment resistant AA, AT, and AU span the spectrum of old affordable medications like oral methotrexate to the new highly expensive oral Janus kinase inhibitors.[8,15] Oral Janus kinase inhibitors, including tofacitinib and ruxolitinib, have been approved for rheumatoid arthritis and are off-label for AA. In the studies so far there is hair regrowth, but most patients experience recurrence of hair loss after discontinuation.[8,15] SOR B
- A Cochrane review in 2008 concluded that most trials have been reported poorly and are so small that any important clinical benefits are inconclusive.[9] They stated that considering the possibility of spontaneous remission (especially for those in the early stages of the disease), the options of not treating or wearing a wig are reasonable alternatives.[16]
- Hairpieces and camouflage techniques may be used for those patients with unresponsive, recalcitrant disease.
- One RCT showed aromatherapy with topical essential oils to be a safe and effective treatment for AA.[17] The active group massaged essential oils (thyme, rosemary, lavender, and cedarwood) in a mixture of carrier oils (jojoba and grapeseed) into their scalp daily. SOR B

PROGNOSIS AND PATIENT EDUCATION

- Discuss the patient's reaction to the hair loss and counsel and/or refer as needed.
- Although spontaneous recovery usually occurs, the course of AA is unpredictable and often characterized by recurrent periods of hair loss and regrowth.
- Spontaneous long-term regrowth in alopecia totalis and AU is poor.
- Prognosis is worse if the alopecia persists longer than 1 year.

FOLLOW-UP

- Spontaneous recovery usually occurs within 6 to 12 months, and the prognosis for total permanent regrowth with limited involvement (AA) is excellent.
- The regrown hair is usually of the same texture and color but may be fine and white at first (**Figure 195-5**).
- Ten percent of patients never regrow hair and advance to chronic disease. Clinicians should provide contact information to the National Alopecia Areata Foundation and offer follow-up in the office as necessary.

- Patients with a family history of AA, younger age at onset, coexisting immune disorders, nail dystrophy, atopy, and widespread hair loss have a poorer prognosis.[5]

PATIENT RESOURCES

- The National Alopecia Areata Foundation (**http://www.naaf.org**) publishes a newsletter and can provide information regarding these support groups as well as hairpiece information.

PROVIDER RESOURCES

- **http://emedicine.medscape.com/article/1069931-overview.**

REFERENCES

1. Usatine RP. Bald spots on a young girl. *J Fam Pract.* 2004;53:33-36.
2. Firooz A, Firoozabadi MR, Ghazisaidi B, Dowlati Y. Concepts of patients with alopecia areata about their disease. *BMC Dermatol.* 2005;5:1.
3. Mirzoyev SA, Schrum AG, Davis MDP, Torgerson RR. Lifetime incidence risk of alopecia areata estimated at 2.1 percent by Rochester Epidemiology Project, 1990–2009. *J Invest Dermatol.* 2014;134:1141.
4. Choi HJ, Ihm CW. Acute alopecia totalis. *Acta Dermatovenerol Alp Panonica Adriat.* 2006;15:27-34.
5. Strazzulla LC, Wang EHC, Avila L, et al. Alopecia areata: disease characteristics, clinical evaluation, and new perspectives on pathogenesis. *J Am Acad Dermatol.* 2018;78(1):1-12.
6. Blaumeiser B, van der Goot I, Fimmers R, et al. Familial aggregation of alopecia areata. *J Am Acad Dermatol.* 2006;54:627-632.
7. Huang KP, Mullangi S, Guo Y, Qureshi AA. Autoimmune, atopic, and mental health comorbid conditions associated with alopecia areata in the United States. *JAMA Dermatol.* 2013;149:789-794.
8. Strazzulla LC, Wang EHC, Avila L, et al. Alopecia areata: an appraisal of new treatment approaches and overview of current therapies. *J Am Acad Dermatol.* 2018;78(1):15-24.
9. Devi M, Rashid A, Ghafoor R. Intralesional triamcinolone acetonide versus topical betamethasone valerate in the management of localized alopecia areata. *J Coll Physicians Surg Pak.* 2015;25(12):860-862.
10. Kuldeep C, Singhal H, Khare AK, et al. Randomized comparison of topical betamethasone valerate foam, intralesional triamcinolone acetonide and tacrolimus ointment in management of localized alopecia areata. *Int J Trichol.* 2011;3:20-24.
11. Chu TW, AlJasser M, Alharbi A, et al. Benefit of different concentrations of intralesional triamcinolone acetonide in alopecia areata: an intrasubject pilot study. *J Am Acad Dermatol.* 2015;73(2):338-340.
12. Tosti A, Piraccini BM, Pazzaglia M, Vincenzi C. Clobetasol propionate 0.05% under occlusion in the treatment of alopecia totalis/universalis. *J Am Acad Dermatol.* 2003;49:96-98.
13. Tosti A, Iorizzo M, Botta GL, Milani M. Efficacy and safety of a new clobetasol propionate 0.05% foam in alopecia areata: a randomized, double-blind placebo-controlled trial. *J Eur Acad Dermatol Venereol.* 2006;20:1243-1247.
14. Cotellessa C, Peris K, Caracciolo E, et al. The use of topical diphenylcyclopropenone for the treatment of extensive alopecia areata. *J Am Acad Dermatol.* 2001;44:73-76.
15. Liu LY, Craiglow BG, Dai F, King BA. Tofacitinib for the treatment of severe alopecia areata and variants: a study of 90 patients. *J Am Acad Dermatol.* 2017;76:22-28.
16. Delamere FM, Sladden MM, Dobbins HM, Leonardi-Bee J. Interventions for alopecia areata. *Cochrane Database Syst Rev.* 2008;(2):CD004413.
17. Hay IC, Jamieson M, Ormerod AD. Randomized trial of aromatherapy. Successful treatment for alopecia areata. *Arch Dermatol.* 1998;134:1349-1352.

196 TRACTION ALOPECIA AND TRICHOTILLOMANIA

E.J. Mayeaux, Jr., MD
Jacqueline Bucher, MD

PATIENT STORY

A 38-year-old woman was found to have hair thinning on the anterior scalp. She had long, thick, heavy hair that she always styled in a bun on the top of her head. She was concerned about the slow, steady loss of hair that she was experiencing. **Figure 196-1** shows the appearance of the thinned hair as a result of chronic traction. A 4-mm punch biopsy was performed to confirm the clinical impression, and the histology was supportive of this diagnosis.

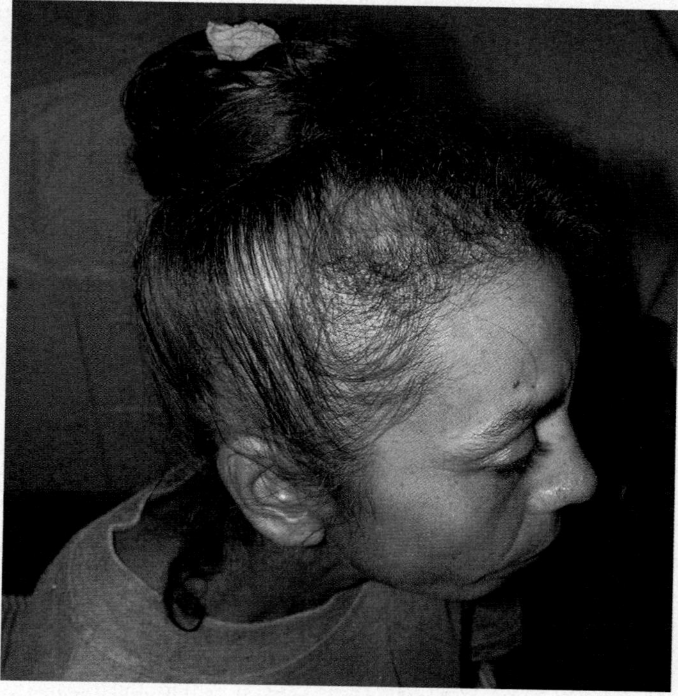

FIGURE 196-1 Traction alopecia from pulling the hair up in a tight bun. (*Reproduced with permission from Richard P. Usatine, MD.*)

INTRODUCTION

Traction alopecia is hair loss caused by damage to the dermal papilla and hair follicle by constant pulling or tension over a long period. It often occurs in persons who wear tight braids, especially "cornrows," that lead to high tension, pulling, and breakage of hair. Trichotillomania (Greek for "hair-pulling madness") is a traction alopecia related to a compulsive disorder caused when patients pull on and pluck hairs, often creating bizarre patterns of hair loss.

SYNONYMS

Traumatic alopecia, hair pulling.

EPIDEMIOLOGY

- Epidemiologic information on traction alopecia is limited (**Figures 196-1** and **196-2**) and varies by cultural hairstyle practices. It is most commonly seen in females and children of African descent.
- The prevalence of trichotillomania (**Figures 196-3** to **196-6**) is also difficult to determine but is estimated to be approximately 1.5% of males and 3.4% of females in the United States. The mean age of onset of trichotillomania is 8 years in boys and 12 years in girls, and it is the most common cause of childhood alopecia.[1]

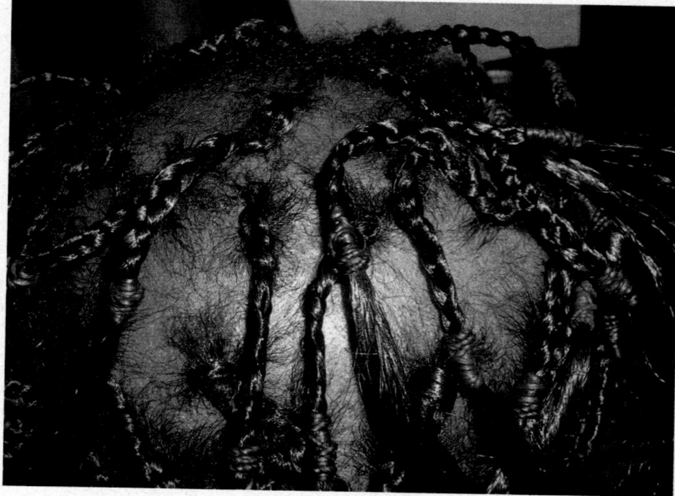

FIGURE 196-2 Traction alopecia in a young African-American girl whose mom braids her hair tightly. (*Reproduced with permission from Richard P. Usatine, MD.*)

ETIOLOGY AND PATHOPHYSIOLOGY

- Traction alopecia is seen in individuals who place chronic tension on the hair shafts with tight braids, heavy natural hair, use of hair prostheses, or chronic pulling (see **Figures 196-1** and **196-2**).[2] It also occurs commonly in female athletes who pull their hair into tight ponytails.
- Chronic tension on the hair shaft seems to create inflammation within the hair follicle that eventually leads to cessation of hair

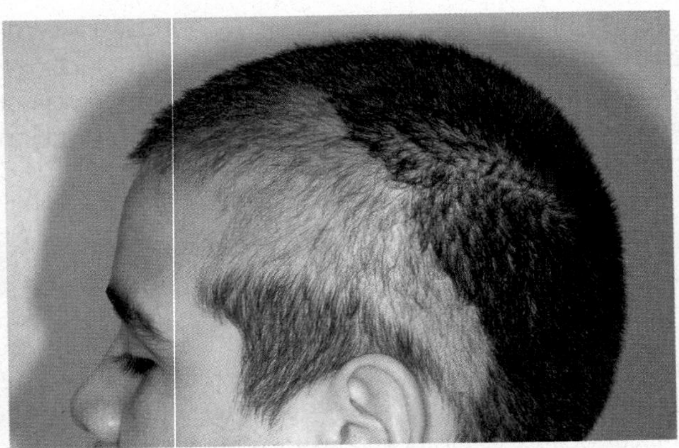

FIGURE 196-3 Trichotillomania in an 11-year-old boy. Note the incomplete hair loss and unusual geometric pattern. He was receiving help and the hair is now growing in. (*Reproduced with permission from Richard P. Usatine, MD.*)

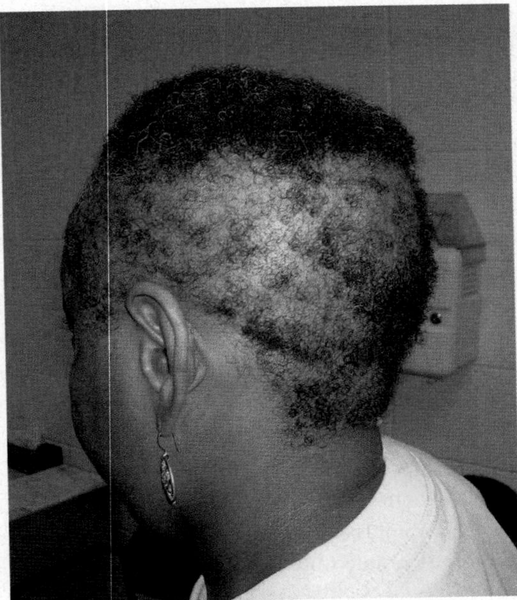

FIGURE 196-4 Chronic hair loss in a 39-year-old woman with trichotillomania. (*Reproduced with permission from E.J. Mayeaux, Jr., MD.*)

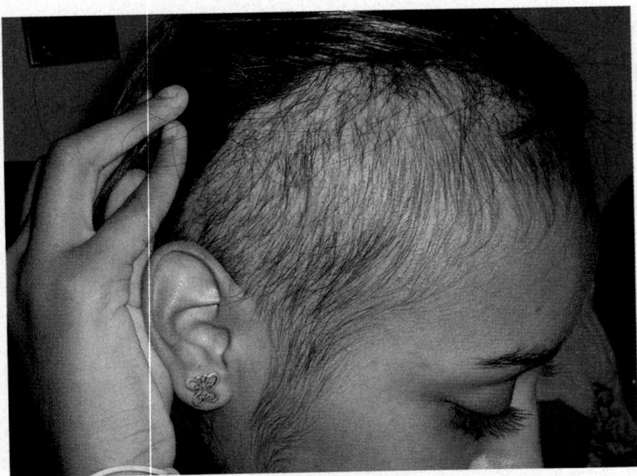

FIGURE 196-5 Trichotillomania in a 17-year-old honors student who is currently taking four Advanced Placement courses simultaneously. (*Reproduced with permission from Richard P. Usatine, MD.*)

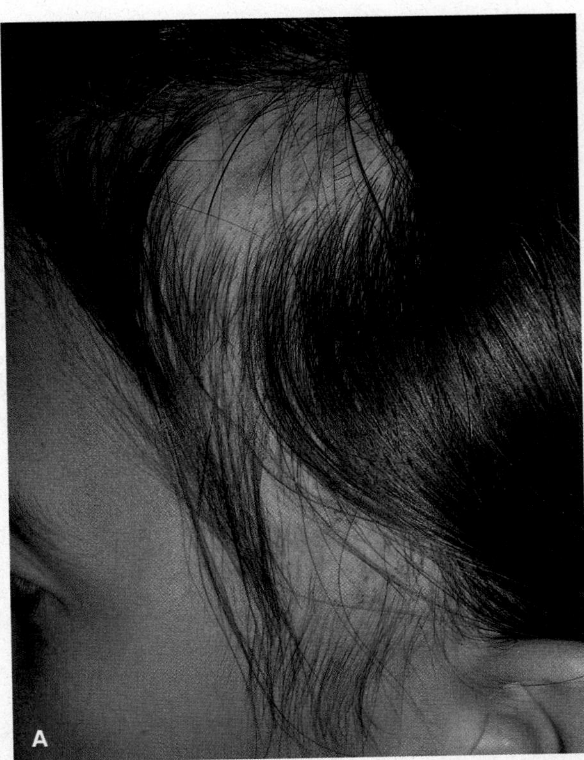

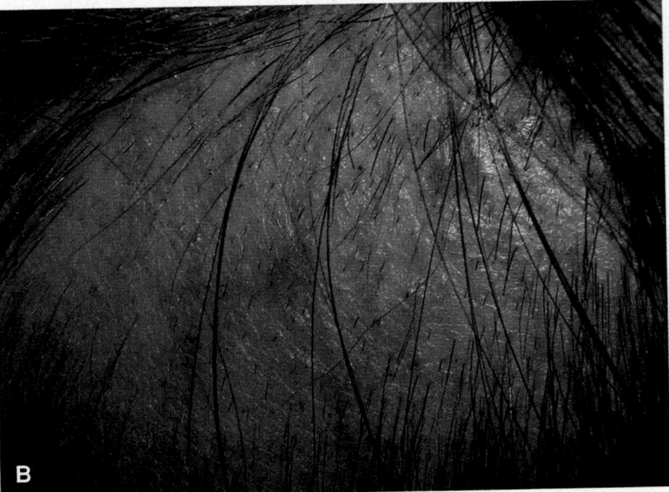

FIGURE 196-6 **A.** Trichotillomania in a 12-year-old girl undergoing significant stress because of conflict in her family. **B.** Close-up of trichotillomania showing broken hairs, black dots, and excoriations. (*Reproduced with permission from Richard P. Usatine, MD.*)

growth. Because hair loss from traction alopecia may become permanent and eventually lead to scarring, prevention and early treatment are important.

- It is seen most frequently in black women who tightly braid or pull the hair into a hairstyle during youth and on into adulthood. Traction alopecia may also be seen in individuals who wear hair prostheses or extensions for a prolonged period of time. It is also seen in Sikh men of India and Japanese women whose traditional hairstyles may pull and damage hair.
- Trichotillomania is a subtype of traction alopecia manifested by chronic hair pulling (see **Figures 196-3** to **196-6**) and sometimes hair eating (trichophagy), which can lead to a trichobezoar. It is classified as a psychiatric obsessive–compulsive-related disorder.[3]
- Trichotillomania may be a manifestation of the inability to cope with stress rather than more severe mental disorders.
- Children who exhibit trichotillomania may discontinue the hair pulling with parental support and maturity. Adults who exhibit trichotillomania, even though they are aware of the problem, may require psychiatric intervention to limit the behavior. The hair loss is initially reversible but may become permanent if the habits persist.

DIAGNOSIS

CLINICAL FEATURES

In patients with traction alopecia, there are decreased follicular ostia in the affected area coupled with decreased hair density. The hair loss usually occurs in the frontal and temporal areas but depends on the precipitating hairstyle (see **Figures 196-1** and **196-2**). There may be a lag time of a decade or more between the period the hair was in traction and the appearance of hair loss. No scalp inflammation or scaling is typically visible. No pain or other discomfort is associated with the condition. Patients with trichotillomania often demonstrate short, broken hairs (see **Figure 196-6**) without the presence of inflammation or skin scale early in the disease. The affected areas are not bald, but rather possess hairs of varying length. There may be telltale stubble of hairs too short to pull. The hair loss often follows bizarre patterns with incomplete areas of clearing. The scalp may appear normal or have areas of erythema and pustule formation. With chronic pulling, the hair loss becomes permanent (see **Figure 196-4**). Friends or family members may observe the patient pulling or twisting the hair.

TYPICAL DISTRIBUTION

Trichotillomania most commonly occurs on the scalp and can involve any area of the body that the patient can reach.[2] Traction alopecia can occur anywhere on the scalp but is most commonly seen at the anterior hairline. This is the site where the hair is pulled back from the face into braids or a bun.

LABORATORY STUDIES

Laboratory tests are not needed to make the diagnosis. A hand lens can be used to examine the affected scalp for decreased follicular ostia, if desired. A scalp biopsy (4-mm punch biopsy) may be necessary to make the diagnosis and rule out other etiologies, especially in trichotillomania, because patients may not acknowledge the habit.

Hypothyroidism or hyperthyroidism may be associated with telogen effluvium or alopecia areata. It may be worth ordering a thyroid-stimulating hormone (TSH) test if the history and physical exam are suggestive of thyroid dysfunction and are not completely convincing for self-induced hair loss.

DIFFERENTIAL DIAGNOSIS[1]

- Alopecia areata is characterized by the total absence of hair in an area and the presence of exclamation-point hairs. These hairs are thinner in diameter closer to the scalp and thicker in diameter away from the scalp, creating the appearance of an exclamation point. Hairs are often white when they start to regrow (see Chapter 195, Alopecia Areata).
- Tinea capitis exhibits hairs broken off at the skin surface and the presence of scale and/or inflammation. Some varieties fluoresce when examined with a Wood light (UV light). Microscopy of a KOH preparation may detect the dermatophyte. Sometimes it is necessary to culture some hairs and scale to make this diagnosis (see Chapter 143, Tinea Capitis).
- Scarring alopecia (lichen planopilaris, folliculitis decalvans) is observed as loss of the follicular ostia and the absence of hairs. The scalp may appear scarred with changes in pigmentation (see Chapter 197, Scarring Alopecia).
- Telogen effluvium (postpregnancy hair loss) is associated with hair loss during the postpartum period and can happen after other stressful events such as surgery or severe illness (see Chapter 76, Skin Findings in Pregnancy). The hair loss is evenly distributed across the head, and the hair is thinned all over rather than in patches as in traction alopecia.
- Androgenetic alopecia produces central thinning in women and temple and crown thinning in men. It should be considered in women with symptoms of hormonal abnormalities such as hirsutism, amenorrhea, or infertility.

MANAGEMENT

NONPHARMACOLOGIC

FIRST LINE

- Stop the hairstyling practices that led to the traction alopecia. No tight braiding or buns should be worn.[2] SOR C
  - Recommend lower-risk hair-styling practices including looser braids, leave braided hairstyles in for no longer than 2–3 months, opt for larger-diameter braids/dreadlocks, avoid bonding glues when applying weaves, decrease thermal straightening, and use lower heat settings on flat irons and blow dryers.[4] SOR C
  - When fibrosis and permanent hair loss has occurred, hair transplantation may be a therapeutic option. SOR C
- For trichotillomania, open discussions with the patient, and the family, if appropriate, are important to understand the reason for the behavior. Many times there are secondary social or emotional issues that must be resolved before the trichotillomania ceases.

- Cognitive behavioral treatment is the most effective treatment for trichotillomania.[2,5] SOR Ⓑ
- Cognitive behavioral therapy usually is successful if the patient is recalcitrant to simple education.[6] SOR Ⓒ

MEDICATIONS

SECOND LINE

- Topical or intralesional corticosteroids can be used to decrease scalp inflammation if erythema or itching is present. SOR Ⓒ
- Topical minoxidil 2% or 5% is sometimes used to speed hair regrowth in the area. SOR Ⓒ
- No medication class definitely demonstrates efficacy in the treatment of trichotillomania; treatment effects have been demonstrated with clomipramine, olanzapine, and *N*-acetylcysteine.[7] SOR Ⓑ

FOLLOW-UP

Specific follow-up is not required for traction alopecia, but psychiatric/behavioral counseling follow-up is indicated for trichotillomania.

PATIENT EDUCATION

Explain that in traction alopecia, current grooming practices are responsible for the hair loss, and a new hairstyle must be selected. It is important to tell the patient that some of the hair loss may be permanent and no guarantee can be given regarding the amount of expected hair regrowth. Similar hair grooming practices should be avoided in the patient's children to prevent traction alopecia from occurring. Prevention is definitely the best treatment.

Explain that trichotillomania is a self-induced disease that can often resolve if the hair pulling or twisting is discontinued. Patients may exhibit hair pulling or twisting unconsciously when stressed or use it as a calming activity when relaxing or going to sleep. The underlying reasons for the behavior should be explored and discussed. Sometimes trichotillomania can be substituted with another behavior, such as playing with beads or rubbing a stone.

PATIENT RESOURCES

- Trichotillomania Support and Therapy Site. *Emphasis on Growth*—**http://www.trichotillomania.co.uk.**
- WebMD. *Trichotillomania*—**http://www.webmd.com/anxiety-panic/guide/trichotillomania.**
- *Traction alopecia: Symptoms and prevention*—**https://www.medicalnewstoday.com/articles/320648.php**
- MedlinePlus. *Trichotillomania*—**http://medlineplus.gov/ency/article/001517.htm.**
- Mental Health America. *Trichotillomania*—**http://www.mentalhealthamerica.net/conditions/trichotillomania-hair-pulling.**

PROVIDER RESOURCES

- *Trichotillomania*—**http://emedicine.medscape.com/article/1071854-overview.**
- *Scarring Alopecia*—**https://emedicine.medscape.com/article/1073559-overview**

REFERENCES

1. Messinger ML, Cheng TL. Trichotillomania. *Pediatr Rev.* 1999;20:249-250.
2. Springer K, Brown M, Stulberg DL. Common hair loss disorders. *Am Fam Physician.* 2003;68:93-102, 107-108.
3. American Psychiatric Association. (2013). *Diagnostic and Statistical Manual of Mental Disorders: DSM-5.* Washington, DC: American Psychiatric Association.
4. Haskin A, Aguh C. All hairstyles are not created equal: what the dermatologist needs to know about black hairstyling practices and the risk of traction alopecia. *J Am Acad Dermatol.* 2016;75:606-611.
5. Bloch MH, Landeros-Weisenberger A, Dombrowski P, et al. Systematic review: pharmacological and behavioral treatment for trichotillomania. *Biol Psychiatry.* 2007;62(8):839-846.
6. Streichenwein SM, Thornby JI. A long-term, double-blind, placebo-controlled crossover trial of the efficacy of fluoxetine for trichotillomania. *Am J Psychiatry.* 1995;152:1192-1196.
7. Rothbart A, Amos T, Siegfried N. Pharmacotherapy for trichotillomania. *Cochrane Database Syst Rev.* 2013;(11):CD007662.

197 SCARRING ALOPECIA

Richard P. Usatine, MD
Amit Sharma, DO

PATIENT STORY

A 32-year-old man presents with hair loss along with chronic pustular eruptions of his scalp. Previous biopsy has shown folliculitis decalvans. He has had many courses of antibiotics, but the hair loss continues to progress. The active pustular lesions are cultured and grow out methicillin-resistant *Staphylococcus aureus*. The patient is treated with trimethoprim-sulfamethoxazole twice daily and mupirocin to the nasal mucosa, twice daily for 5 days. Two weeks later, the pustular lesions are less prominent, although the alopecia is permanent (**Figures 197-1** and **197-2**).

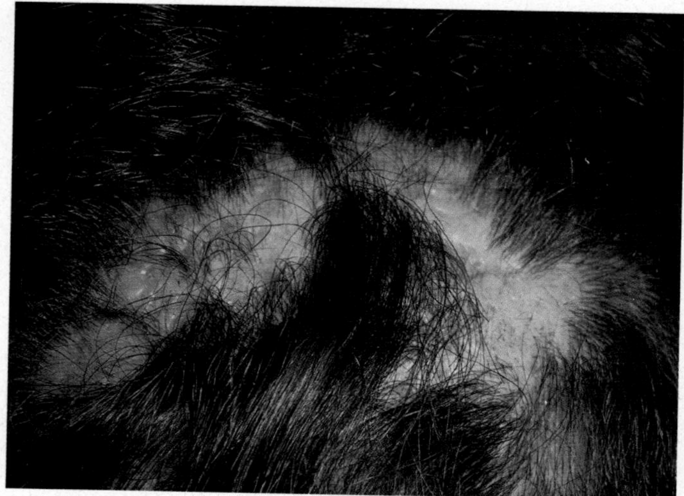

FIGURE 197-1 Folliculitis decalvans in a 32-year-old man. He has an active area of pustular lesions on the periphery with wide areas of scarring and hair loss. (*Reproduced with permission from Richard P. Usatine, MD.*)

INTRODUCTION

Scarring alopecia is a group of inflammatory disorders in which there is permanent destruction of the pilosebaceous unit. Although it is mostly seen on the scalp, it can involve other areas, such as the eyebrows.

In primary cicatricial alopecia, the hair follicle is the primary target of destruction by inflammation. In secondary cicatricial alopecia, the follicular destruction is incidental to a nonfollicular process such as infection, tumor, burn, radiation, or traction.

SYNONYM

Cicatricial alopecia.

EPIDEMIOLOGY

Primary cicatricial alopecias are rare.

The annual incidence rate of lichen planopilaris (LPP) in 4 hair loss centers in the United States varied from 1.15% to 7.59% as defined by new biopsy-proven LPP—all new patients with hair loss seen over a 1-year period.[1]

PATHOPHYSIOLOGY

Scarring alopecia occurs when there is inflammation and destruction of the hair follicles leading to fibrous tissue formation.[2]

Hair loss in scarring alopecia is irreversible because the inflammatory infiltrate results in destruction of the hair follicle stem cells and the sebaceous glands.[3]

The inflammatory infiltrates are either predominantly lymphocytic, neutrophilic, or mixed.[4] These differences are used to classify the scarring alopecias. See **Table 197-1**.

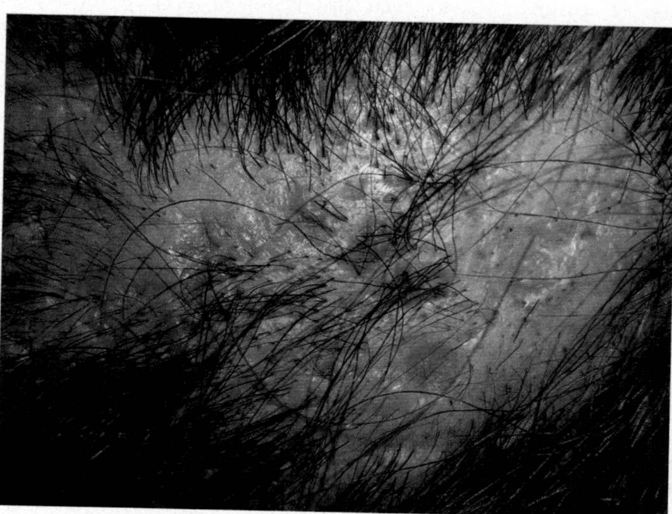

FIGURE 197-2 Same patient (**Figure 197-1**) showing permanent hair loss on the top of the head with some small active pustular lesions. (*Reproduced with permission from Richard P. Usatine, MD.*)

TABLE 197-1 Classification of Cicatricial Alopecia

Lymphocytic	Lichen planopilaris (LPP) Frontal fibrosing alopecia (FFA) Central centrifugal cicatricial alopecia (CCCA) Discoid lupus erythematosus (DLE)*
Neutrophilic	Folliculitis decalvans Tufted folliculitis
Mixed	Dissecting cellulitis* Acne keloidalis nuchae*
End-stage	Nonspecific

*Not a primary cicatricial alopecia.
Adapted with permission from Olsen EA, Bergfeld WF, Cotsarelis G, et al. Summary of North American Hair Research Society (NAHRS)-sponsored Workshop on Cicatricial Alopecia, Duke University Medical Center, February 10 and 11, 2001, J Am Acad Dermatol. 2003;48(1):103-10

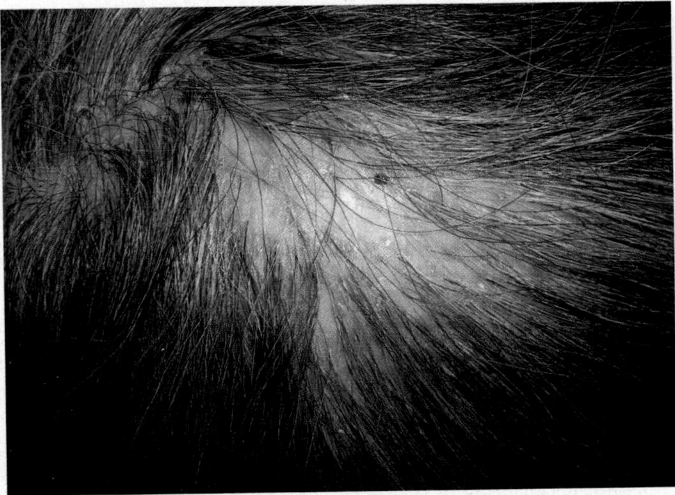

FIGURE 197-3 Lichen planopilaris in a 45-year-old woman causing hair loss with perifollicular scale. (*Reproduced with permission from Richard P. Usatine, MD.*)

DIAGNOSIS

Scarring alopecias can vary by distribution and appearance. Most patients will need a biopsy to confirm the clinical impression and determine the specific type of alopecia.

CLINICAL PRESENTATION

- Hair loss with itching, pain, and/or burning of the scalp. Some cases are asymptomatic.

PHYSICAL EXAM

The "pull test" is used to see how active the hair loss is in general and in specific areas of the scalp. Always ask the patient if you can pull on the hair as part of your diagnosis.

- With the thumb and forefinger grasp approximately 30 to 40 hairs close to the scalp.
- Gently, but firmly, slide the fingers away from the scalp at a 90-degree angle along the entire length of the hair swatch. Do not tug or jerk.

Interpreting the pull test results:

- Negative pull test = 1 to 4 telogen hairs (small bulbs at bottom).
- Positive pull test = 5 or more hairs (including anagen hairs that have longer follicle sheath at the bottom of the hair).[5]

Forms of primary cicatricial alopecia include:

- LPP most commonly affects middle-age women. It mostly occurs on the frontal and parietal scalp and causes follicular hyperkeratosis, pruritus, perifollicular erythema, violaceous color of scalp, and scalp pain (**Figure 197-3**).[2] It may also affect other hair-bearing sites such as the groin and axilla.[2] Most patients with LPP do not have lichen planus even though the names are very similar.
- Central centrifugal scarring alopecia (CCCA) is a slowly progressive alopecia that begins in the vertex and advances to surrounding areas. It may be related to chemicals used on the hair, heat from hot combs, or chronic tension on the hair.[2] It is seen more commonly in African-American women (**Figure 197-4**).

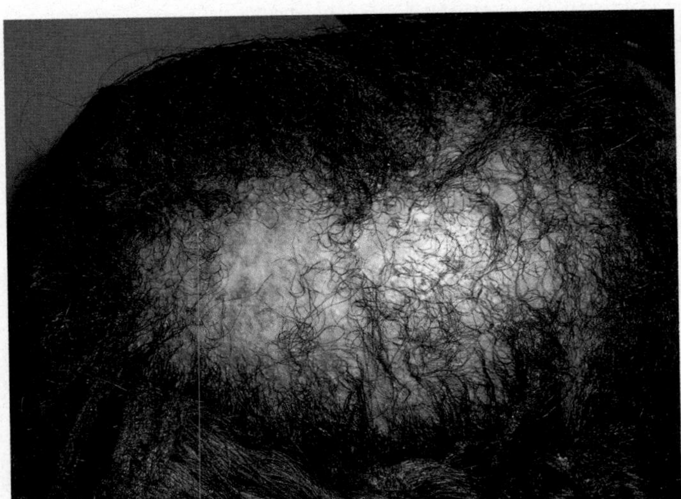

FIGURE 197-4 Central centrifugal scarring alopecia in a middle-age African-American woman. Note how the vertex is most affected. Patient has used many hair chemicals, hot combs, and braids over the years. (*Reproduced with permission from Richard P. Usatine, MD.*)

- Frontal fibrosing alopecia (FFA) presents with a progressive recession of the frontal hairline affecting particularly postmenopausal women. It is considered to be a variant of LPP on the basis of its clinical, histologic, and immunohistochemical features. The women typically lose their eyebrows and the temporal veins become prominent (**Figure 197-5**).[6]
- Folliculitis decalvans is a chronic painful neutrophilic bacterial folliculitis characterized by bogginess or induration of the scalp with pustules, erosions, crusts, and scale.[2] It is postulated that this results from an abnormal host response to *S. aureus*, which is often cultured from the lesions (see **Figures 197-1** and **197-2**). In one case series, the disease ran a protracted course with temporary improvement while on antibiotic and flare-up of disease when antibiotics were stopped.[7]
- Tufted folliculitis can be considered to be a milder version of folliculitis decalvans with less surface area of the scalp involved and a better prognosis (**Figure 197-6**). However, these hair tufts can be seen in other types of scarring alopecias.

Secondary forms of scarring alopecia:

- Dissecting cellulitis presents with deep inflammatory nodules, primarily over the occiput, that progress to coalescing regions of boggy scalp.[1] Sinus tracts may form, and *S. aureus* is frequently cultured from the inflamed lesions. When dissecting cellulitis occurs with acne conglobata and hidradenitis suppurativa, the syndrome is referred to as the follicular occlusion triad (**Figures 197-7** and **197-8**).
- Acne keloidalis nuchae (folliculitis keloidalis) presents with a chronic papular and pustular eruption at the nape of the neck. This can lead to scarring alopecia with large keloidal scarring. It is seen most commonly in men of color but also can be seen in women. It is often made worse by shaving the hair (see Chapter 120, Pseudofolliculitis and Acne Keloidalis Nuchae) (**Figure 197-9**).
- Discoid lupus erythematosus (DLE) presents with lesions that can be erythematous, atrophic, and/or hypopigmented. Scarring alopecia may be accompanied by follicular plugging on the scalp. Hypopigmentation may develop in the central area of the inflammatory lesions, and hyperpigmentation may develop at the active border. The external ear and ear canal are often involved (**Figure 197-10**) (see Chapter 188, Lupus: Systemic and Cutaneous).

LABORATORY STUDIES

If there is purulence, perform a bacterial culture. *S. aureus* and methicillin-resistant *S. aureus* are frequently seen in the neutrophilic alopecias. Consider obtaining various tests such as thyroid-stimulating hormone (TSH), serum iron level, complete blood count (CBC), and rapid plasma reagin (RPR) to rule out treatable causes of alopecia. Do a KOH smear and/or culture if tinea capitis is suspected.

DERMOSCOPY (TRICHOSCOPY)

Looking at the hair with dermoscopy is called trichoscopy. The dermoscope may be helpful in looking for the perifollicular scale that is found in LPP and FFA (**Figure 197-11**).

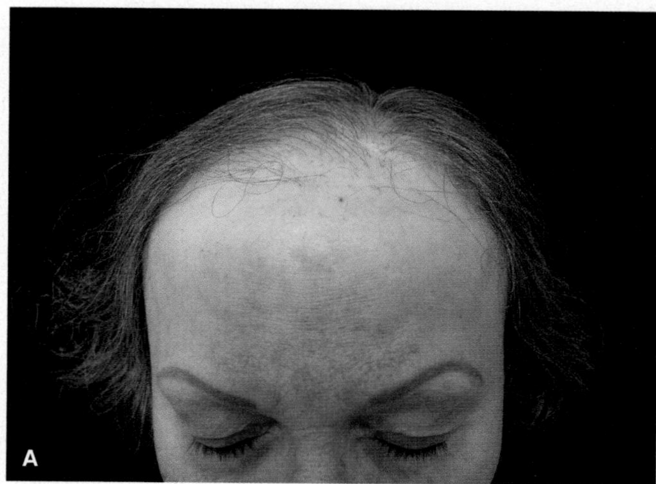

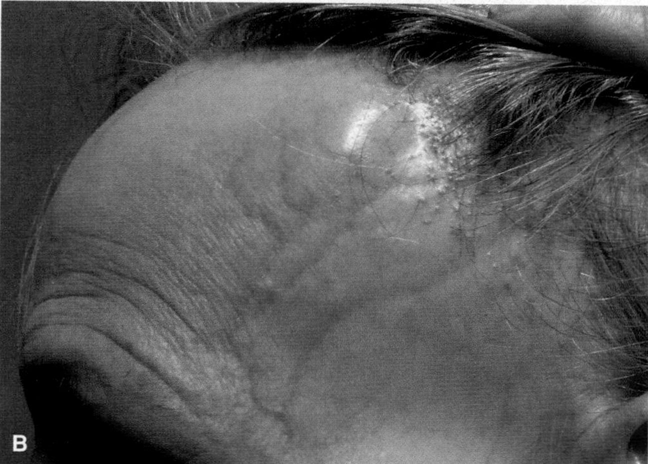

FIGURE 197-5 **A.** Frontal fibrosing alopecia (FFA) with progressive recession of the frontal hairline and loss of eyebrows. (*Reproduced with permission from Richard P. Usatine, MD.*) **B.** 66-year-old woman with FFA showing the receding frontal and parietal hairlines along with prominent temporal veins and erythematous papules at the active border of hair loss. (*Reproduced with permission from Power DV, Disse M, Hordinsky M. Progressive hair loss, J Fam Pract. 2017;66(8):521-523. Frontline Medical Communications. Inc.*)

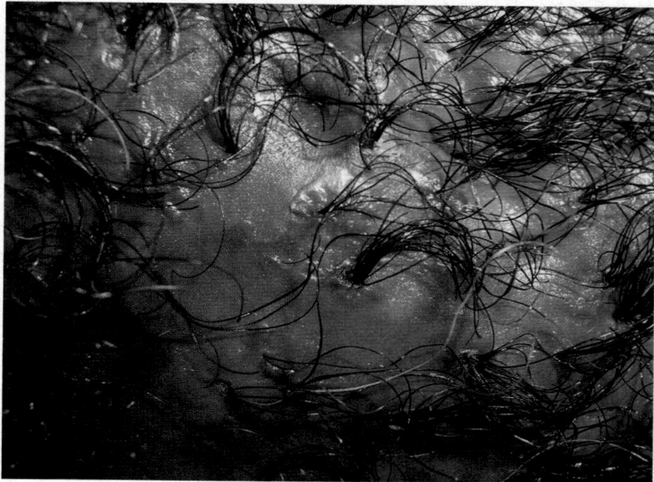

FIGURE 197-6 Tufted folliculitis showing multiple hairs growing from the same follicle along with purulence and hair loss. (*Reproduced with permission from Richard P. Usatine, MD.*)

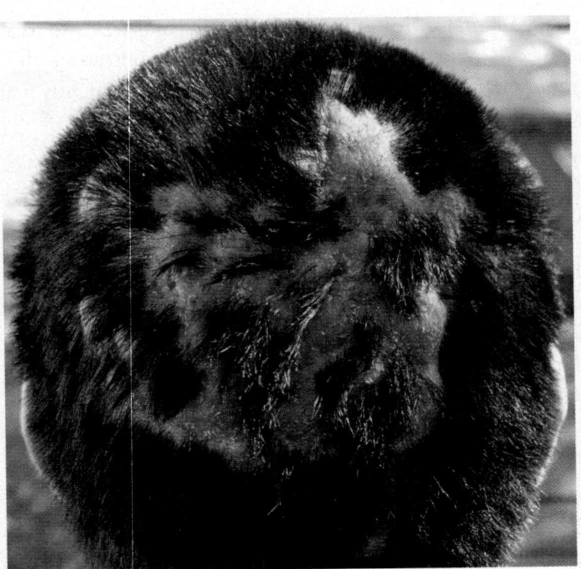

FIGURE 197-7 Dissecting cellulitis of the scalp in a young Hispanic man with many active sinus tracts and alopecia. (*Reproduced with permission from Richard P. Usatine, MD.*)

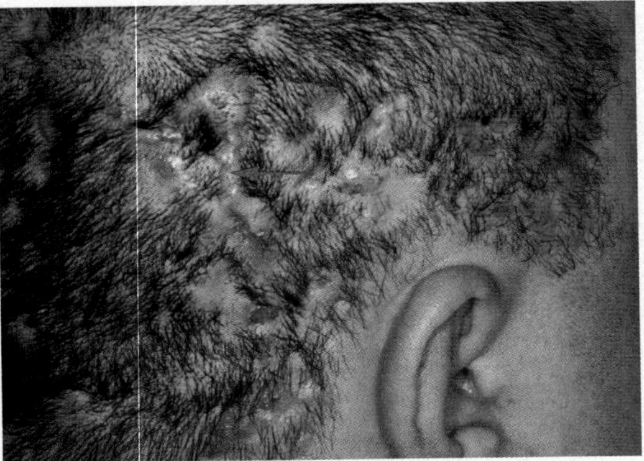

FIGURE 197-8 Dissecting cellulitis of the scalp causing painful purulent nodules and sinus tracts leading to scarring alopecia. The patient also has severe hidradenitis suppurativa and therefore has two of three elements of the follicular occlusion triad (he does not have acne conglobata). The *arrow* points to one sinus tract. (*Reproduced with permission from Richard P. Usatine, MD.*)

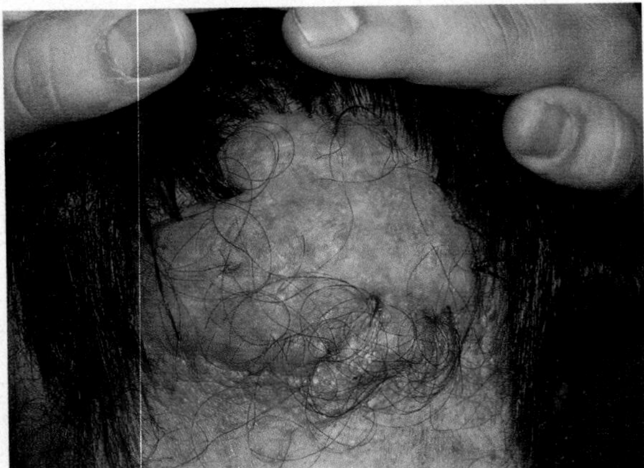

FIGURE 197-9 Acne keloidalis nuchae in a 32-year-old man with significant hair loss and a keloidal mass. Note that there are many hairs growing together in "tufts" as seen in tufted folliculitis. (*Reproduced with permission from Richard P. Usatine, MD.*)

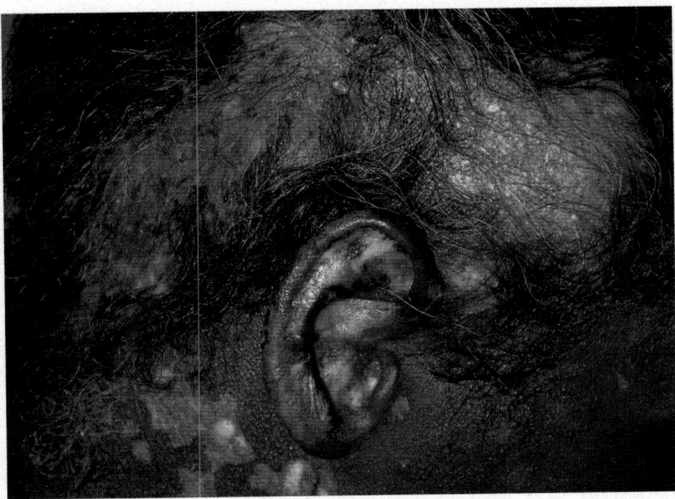

FIGURE 197-10 Chronic cutaneous lupus erythematosus showing scarring alopecia. Prominent hypopigmentation and skin atrophy are visible on the scalp and ear. (*Reproduced with permission from Richard P. Usatine, MD.*)

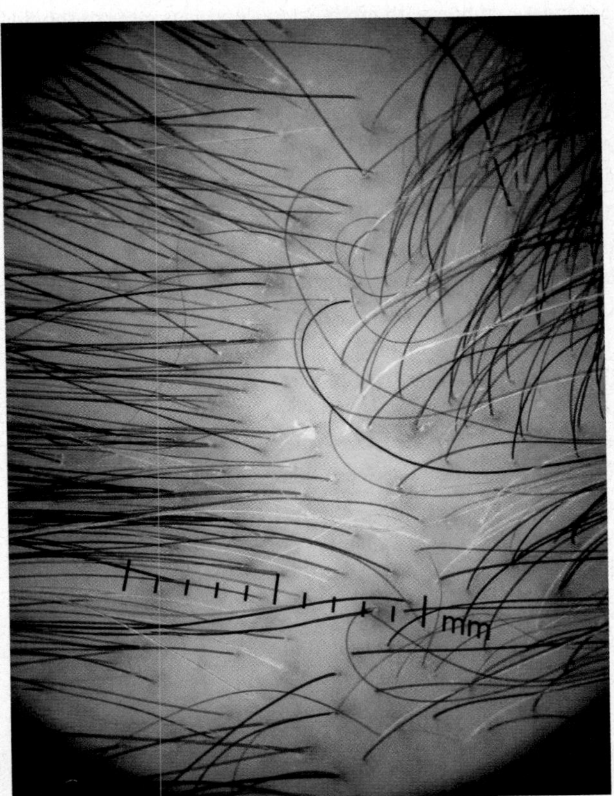

FIGURE 197-11 Dermoscopy (trichoscopy) demonstrating perifollicular scale in lichen planopilaris and frontal fibrosing alopecia. (*Reproduced with permission from Richard P. Usatine, MD.*)

BIOPSY

- Biopsy is almost always recommended to diagnose primary scarring alopecia.[5] Usually a single 4-mm punch biopsy for histology is adequate. Some dermatopathologists will prefer two 4-mm punch biopsies at the same time so that they may cut the specimens both tangentially and vertically for analysis. Discuss this with your dermatopathologist or pathologist. Make sure to biopsy at the margin of the active disease and include at least a few hair follicles in the specimen.

DIFFERENTIAL DIAGNOSIS

- Alopecia areata presents with hair loss and a very smooth scalp. The hair loss is usually in round punched-out patterns and the scalp otherwise appears normal (Chapter 195, Alopecia Areata).
- Androgenetic alopecia is the standard hair loss that males experience with aging. There are a number of male pattern types of hair loss. Women also get androgenetic alopecia, but the pattern tends to be more diffuse and frontal. Both are treatable with topical minoxidil and oral finasteride.
- Drug-induced alopecia is from chemotherapy and other toxic drugs.
- Sarcoidosis of the scalp can resemble DLE, but treatment will be different; hence the importance of a biopsy diagnosis (see Chapter 184, Sarcoidosis).[8]
- Seborrheic dermatitis may cause some hair loss. The presence of scale on the scalp with minimal to no hair loss helps to differentiate this from scarring alopecia (see Chapter 157, Seborrheic Dermatitis).
- Secondary syphilis with moth-eaten alopecia is rare but should be considered. A highly positive RPR can easily make this diagnosis (see Chapter 225, Syphilis).
- Telogen effluvium is a type of nonscarring alopecia that occurs after childbirth or other traumatic events. The skin on the scalp appears normal.
- Tinea capitis presents with scale and hair loss. It is diagnosed by a positive KOH and/or fungal culture. Do not miss this diagnosis because it is much easier to treat than any of the scarring alopecias (see Chapter 143, Tinea Capitis).
- Trichotillomania is defined as self-induced hair loss caused by pulling at the hairs. The pattern of hair loss may be distinctive, and the behavior may be discovered on history. The scalp appears normal and there is a distinctive pattern seen on biopsy (see Chapter 196, Traction Alopecia and Trichotillomania).
- Traction alopecia occurs when the hair is pulled too tight for braids or ponytails (see Chapter 196, Traction Alopecia and Trichotillomania).
- Various metabolic and nutritional problems can lead to alopecia. It is worth doing a CBC, ferritin, vitamin D 25-OH, and TSH to rule out iron deficiency, vitamin D deficiency, and hyper- or hypothyroidism.[5]

MANAGEMENT

- Scarring alopecias are such rare conditions that there are few randomized controlled trials available to guide therapy.
- One paradigm for treating primary scarring alopecia is to treat those containing predominantly lymphocytic infiltrates with immunomodulating agents and those with predominantly neutrophilic infiltrates with antimicrobial agents.[5,9] SOR Ⓒ

LYMPHOCYTIC INFILTRATE PREDOMINATES IN LPP, CCCA, AND FFA

FIRST LINE

- Start with one of the two oral agents combined with topical/intralesional medications:
  - Doxycycline 100 mg bid, or
  - Hydroxychloroquine 200 mg bid.
  - After 6 to 12 months, if symptoms and signs persist, move to second line.
- In a retrospective review of 40 patients with LPP and its variant FFA, the investigators found that those treated with hydroxychloroquine daily had a 69% reduction in symptoms and signs after 6 months, and 89% improved after 12 months.[10] SOR Ⓑ
- Topical/intralesional medications:
  - Intralesional triamcinolone acetonide 10 mg/mL to inflamed, symptomatic sites (inject margins where there are still hair follicles).
  - High-potency topical corticosteroids or topical tacrolimus or pimecrolimus.
  - Derma-Smoothe/FS scalp oil—Fluocinolone in peanut oil.

SECOND LINE

- Mycophenolate mofetil 0.5 g bid for 1 month, then 1 g bid for 5 months.
- Cyclosporine 3 to 5 mg/kg per day, or 100 mg tid.[11]
- Pioglitazone 15 mg daily.[12]
- In a retrospective review of 16 patients with LPP treated with at least 6 months of mycophenolate mofetil in an open-label, single-center study, 5 of 12 patients were complete responders, 5 of 12 patients were partial responders, and 2 of 12 patients were treatment failures. Four patients withdrew from the trial because of adverse events.[13]
- In FFA the loss of eyebrows is common. Intralesional injection of triamcinolone acetonide (5–10 mg/mL) showed regrowth response in 9 of 10 patients.[14]

NEUTROPHILIC INFILTRATE PREDOMINATES (FOLLICULITIS DECALVANS AND TUFTED FOLLICULITIS)

FIRST LINE

- Start by culturing pustules and using oral antibiotics based on the pathogens cultured.
- Powell et al. studied a treatment regimen for patients with folliculitis decalvans that combines oral rifampin 600 mg daily and oral clindamycin 300 mg bid together for 10 weeks.[15] SOR Ⓑ Ten of the 18 patients responded well with no evidence of recurrence 2 to 22 months after 1 course of treatment, and 15 of the 18 responded after 2 or 3 courses.[15] Patients need to be warned

about the risk of diarrhea and to stop the regimen if this occurs to avoid *C. difficile* enterocolitis.

- For methicillin-sensitive *S. aureus*, cephalexin 500 mg 4 times daily × 10 weeks with oral rifampin 600 mg daily × 10 days is an alternative treatment.
- For methicillin-resistant *S. aureus* (MRSA), treat with oral clindamycin 300 mg bid, or oral trimethoprim-sulfamethoxazole DS bid, or oral doxycycline 100 mg bid for 10 weeks combined with rifampin 600 mg daily × 10 days.[5]
- If the patient is a *S. aureus* carrier, add mupirocin ointment intranasally daily for 1 week, then monthly thereafter.[5] SOR Ⓒ

SECOND LINE

- Dapsone at 75 to 100 mg/day for 4 to 6 months was well tolerated and rapidly effective in treating 2 cases of folliculitis decalvans. Long-term low-dose (25 mg/day) maintenance treatment avoided disease relapses. Dapsone combines antimicrobial activity with anti-inflammatory action directed toward neutrophils.[16] SOR Ⓒ

MIXED INFILTRATES (DISSECTING CELLULITIS)

FIRST LINE

- Start by culturing any purulence and using oral antibiotics based on the pathogens cultured.
- For predominantly neutrophilic infiltrates, treat with oral clindamycin 300 mg bid, or oral trimethoprim-sulfamethoxazole DS bid, or oral doxycycline 100 mg bid for 10 weeks combined with rifampin 600 mg daily × 10 days.

SECOND LINE

- Isotretinoin may be effective in inducing a prolonged remission. Start with 20 mg daily, to avoid a flare, and then slowly increase to 1 mg/kg per day for at least 6 months.[5] SOR Ⓒ
- Other second-line therapies for dissecting cellulitis include prednisone, zinc sulfate, dapsone and cyclosporine.[17]

ALOPECIA SECONDARY TO DISCOID LUPUS

- Start with a high-potency topical steroid or injections of triamcinolone acetonide 5–10 mg/mL. SOR Ⓒ
- Imiquimod cream 5% was reported to cause regression of discoid lupus of the scalp and face in a single patient when applied to the lesions once a day 3 times a week. After 20 applications, Gul et al. reported that the lesions had regressed significantly.[18] SOR Ⓒ
- Milam et al. treated 3 patients with refractory DLE using 0.3% tacrolimus lotion. After 3 months patients demonstrated improvement in lesion severity and hair regrowth.[19] SOR Ⓒ

FOLLOW-UP

Follow-up is needed for patients who are prescribed oral agents. The timing and the monitoring for side effects is agent specific.

PATIENT EDUCATION

The following points are based on information from the Cicatricial Alopecia Research Foundation (http://www.carfintl.org).

- The goal of treatment is to control scalp inflammation and stop the progression of the disease. Hair regrowth is not possible.
- Scarring alopecias often reactivate after a quiet period of 1 or more years. Patients should be encouraged to self-monitor for recurrence and to seek care early to prevent hair loss.
- It is safe to wash the hair with gentle hair products, if desired, even daily.
- When severe hair loss occurs, hats, scarves, hairpieces, and wigs may be used safely for cosmetic purposes.

PATIENT RESOURCES

- Cicatricial Alopecia Research Foundation—**http://www.carfintl.org.**
- American Hair Loss Association—**http://www.americanhairloss.org.**

PROVIDER RESOURCES

- Scarring alopecia—**http://emedicine.medscape.com/article/1073559.**

REFERENCES

1. Ochoa BE, King LE Jr, Price VH. Lichen planopilaris: annual incidence in four hair referral centers in the United States. *J Am Acad Dermatol.* 2008;58:352-353.
2. Wolff K, Johnson RA, Suurmond D. *Fitzpatrick's Color Atlas & Synopsis of Clinical Dermatology*, 5th ed. New York, NY: McGraw-Hill; 2005.
3. Sperling LC, Cowper SE. The histopathology of primary cicatricial alopecia. *Semin Cutan Med Surg.* 2006;25:41-50.
4. Olsen EA, Bergfeld WF, Cotsarelis G, et al. Summary of North American Hair Research Society (NAHRS)-sponsored Workshop on Cicatricial Alopecia, Duke University Medical Center, February 10 and 11, 2001. *J Am Acad Dermatol.* 2003;48:103-110.
5. Price V, Mirmirani P. *Cicatricial Alopecia: An Approach to Diagnosis and Management.* New York, NY: Springer; 2011.
6. Moreno-Ramirez D, Camacho MF. Frontal fibrosing alopecia: a survey in 16 patients. *J Eur Acad Dermatol Venereol.* 2005;19:700-705.
7. Chandrawansa PH, Giam YC. Folliculitis decalvans—a retrospective study in a tertiary referred centre, over five years. *Singapore Med J.* 2003;44:84-87.
8. Henderson CL, Lafleur L, Sontheimer RD. Sarcoidal alopecia as a mimic of discoid lupus erythematosus. *J Am Acad Dermatol.* 2008;59:143-145.
9. Price VH. The medical treatment of cicatricial alopecia. *Semin Cutan Med Surg.* 2006;25:56-59.
10. Chiang C, Sah D, Cho BK, et al. Hydroxychloroquine and lichen planopilaris: efficacy and introduction of Lichen Planopilaris

Activity Index scoring system. *J Am Acad Dermatol.* 2010;62: 387-392.

11. Mirmirani P, Willey A, Price VH. Short course of oral cyclosporine in lichen planopilaris. *J Am Acad Dermatol.* 2003;49:667-671.
12. Mirmirani P, Karnik P. Lichen planopilaris treated with a peroxisome proliferator-activated receptor gamma agonist. *Arch Dermatol.* 2009;145:1363-1366.
13. Cho BK, Sah D, Chwalek J, et al. Efficacy and safety of mycophenolate mofetil for lichen planopilaris. *J Am Acad Dermatol.* 2010; 62:393-397.
14. Donovan JC, Samrao A, Ruben BS, Price VH. Eyebrow regrowth in patients with frontal fibrosing alopecia treated with intralesional triamcinolone acetonide. *Br J Dermatol.* 2010;163:1142-1144.
15. Powell JJ, Dawber RP, Gatter K. Folliculitis decalvans including tufted folliculitis: clinical, histological and therapeutic findings. *Br J Dermatol.* 1999;140:328-333.
16. Paquet P, Pierard GE. [Dapsone treatment of folliculitis decalvans] [in French]. *Ann Dermatol Venereol.* 2004;131:195-197.
17. Rossi A, Calvieri S. Treatment for alopecia. *G Ital Dermat Venereol.* 2014;149:103-106.
18. Gul U, Gonul M, Cakmak SK, et al. A case of generalized discoid lupus erythematosus: successful treatment with imiquimod cream 5%. *Adv Ther.* 2006;23:787-792.
19. Milam EC, Ramachandran S, Franks AG. Jr Treatment of scarring alopecia in discoid variant of chronic cutaneous lupus erythematosus with tacrolimus lotion, 0.3%. *JAMA Dermatol.* 2015;151(10): 113-116.

198 NORMAL NAIL VARIANTS

E.J. Mayeaux, Jr., MD

PATIENT STORY

A 28-year-old man is in the office for a work physical and asks about the white streaks on his fingernail (**Figure 198-1**). He has had them on and off all of his adult life, but recently developed more of them and was concerned that he might have a vitamin deficiency. He was reassured that this is a normal nail finding often associated with minor trauma.

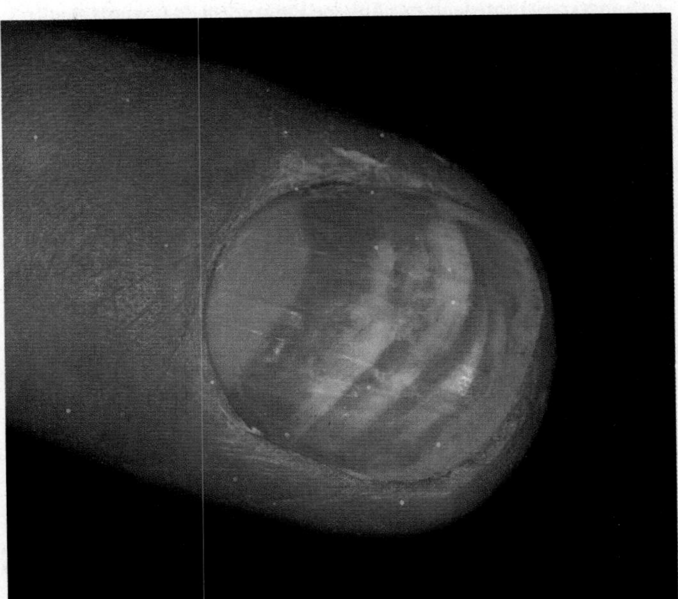

FIGURE 198-1 Transverse striate leukonychia (transverse white streaks) in a healthy patient. Note that the lines do not extend all of the way to the lateral folds, which indicates a probable benign process. *(Reproduced with permission from Richard P. Usatine, MD.)*

INTRODUCTION

The anatomy of the nail unit is shown in **Figure 198-2**. The nail unit includes the nail matrix, nail plate, nail bed, cuticle, proximal and lateral folds, and fibrocollagenous supportive tissues. The proximal matrix produces the superficial aspects of the plate, and the distal matrix the deeper portions. The nail plate is composed of hard and soft keratins and is formed via onychokeratinization, which is similar to hair sheath keratinization.[1] Most normal nail variants occur as a result of accentuation or disruption of normal nail formation.

SYNONYMS

- Leukonychia.
  - Transverse striate leukonychia.
  - Leukonychia punctata.
  - White nails.
- Longitudinal melanonychia (LM).
  - Ethnic melanonychia in patients with skin of color (see Chapter 199, Pigmented Nail Disorders).
- Nail hypertrophy and onychogryphosis (also known as onychogryphosis).
  - Ram's horn nail.
  - Oyster-like deformity.
  - Lateral nail hypertrophy.
  - Thickened toenail.

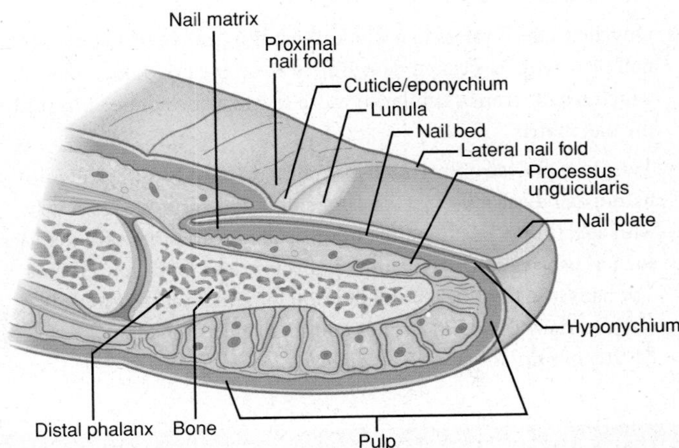

FIGURE 198-2 The anatomy of the nail unit. *(Reproduced with permission from Usatine R, Pfenninger J, Stulberg D, et al. Dermatologic and Cosmetic Procedures in Office Practice. Philadelphia, PA: Elsevier, Inc; 2012.)*

EPIDEMIOLOGY

Melanonychia often involves several nails and is a more common occurrence in patients with darker skin types. Among African Americans, benign melanonychia affects up to 77% of young adults and nearly 100% of those age 50 years or older. In the Japanese, LM affects 10% to 20% of adults.[1] The incidences of most other benign nail findings are not well established.

ETIOLOGY AND PATHOPHYSIOLOGY

- *Leukonychia* refers to benign, single or multiple white spots or lines in the nails. Patchy patterns of partial, transverse white streaks (transverse striate leukonychia, see **Figure 198-1**) or spots (leukonychia punctata, **Figure 198-3**) are the most common patterns of leukonychia.[2] Leukonychia is common in children and becomes less frequent with age. Parents may fear that it represents a dietary deficiency, in particular a lack of calcium, but this concern is almost always unfounded in industrialized countries.
- Most commonly, no specific cause for leukonychia can be found. It is usually the result of minor trauma to the nail cuticle or matrix and is the most commonly found nail condition in children.[3] When the lesions are caused by overly aggressive manicuring or nervous habit, behavior modification often is helpful. Leukonychia can also be an indirect manifestation of autoimmunity, including alopecia areata or thyroid disease. It results from defective keratinization from the distal matrix with persistence of parakeratotic cells in the ventral nail plate.
- *Nail hypertrophy and onychogryphosis* (ram's horn nail—lateral nail hypertrophy, **Figure 198-4**) is the development of opaque thickened nails with exaggerated upward or lateral growth. It may be associated with age, fungal infections, and trauma. It can cause pain with pressure.
- *Habit-tic deformity* (**Figures 198-5** and **198-6**) is caused by habitual picking of the proximal nail fold. The resulting inflammation induces the nail plate to be wavy and ridged, while its substance remains intact and hard.
- *Beau lines* are transverse linear depressions or grooves in the nail plate (**Figures 198-7** and **198-8**). They are thought to result from suppressed nail growth secondary to local trauma or severe illness.[4] They most commonly appear symmetrically in several or all nails and may have associated white lines. They usually grow out over several months. One may estimate the time since onset of systemic illness by measuring the distance from the Beau line to the proximal nail fold and applying the conversion factor of 6 to 10 days per millimeter of growth.[3]
- Onychomadesis refers to a whole-thickness groove or sulcus in the nail plate with associated detachment from the proximal nail fold, which results from a similar or more severe or prolonged insult to the nail matrix.
- Twenty-nail dystrophy (trachyonychia) (**Figure 198-9**) is an idiopathic nail dystrophy that starts in childhood and resolves slowly with age. It may be idiopathic or associated with other skin diseases such as psoriasis, lichen planus, alopecia areata, or atopic eczema.[5] The nails lose their luster and develop longitudinal striations. It often starts with the fingernails and then affects the toenails. All 20 nails do not have to be involved.

RISK FACTORS

- Leukonychia
  - Use of nail enamels, nail hardeners, or artificial nails as a result of trauma and allergic reactions.

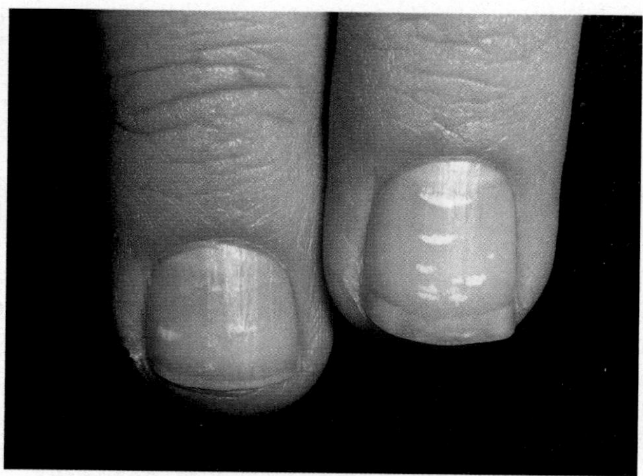

FIGURE 198-3 Leukonychia punctata showing distinct punctate white spots and lines on the fingernails. (*Reproduced with permission from Richard P. Usatine, MD.*)

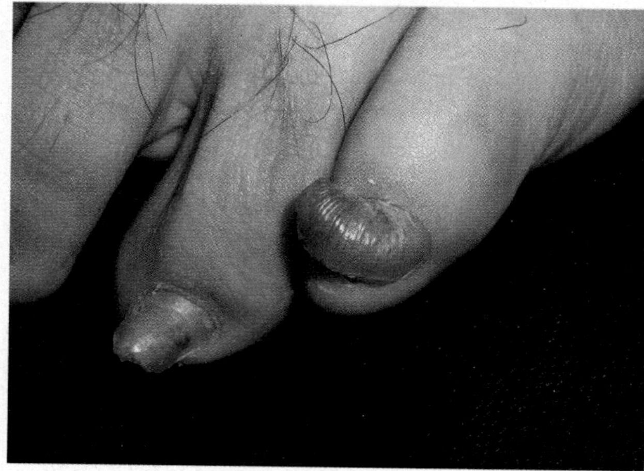

FIGURE 198-4 Onychogryphosis (ram's horn nail) is a type of lateral nail hypertrophy most frequently found in the toenails and often associated with onychomycosis. (*Reproduced with permission from Richard P. Usatine, MD.*)

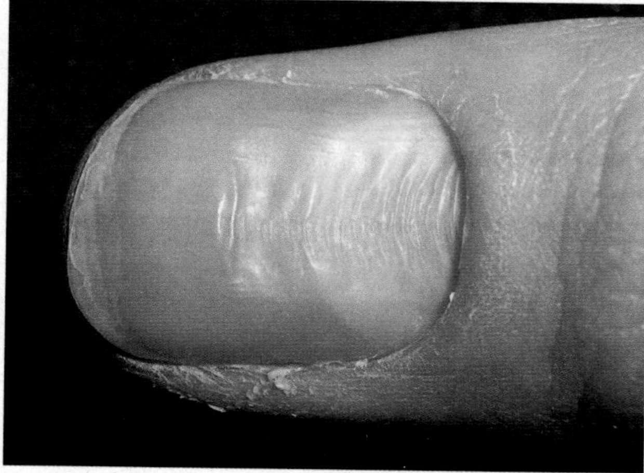

FIGURE 198-5 Habit-tic deformity of the thumbnail caused by a conscious or unconscious rubbing or picking of the proximal nails and nail folds. Horizontal grooves are formed proximally and move distally with fingernail growth. The thumbnails are most often affected. (*Reproduced with permission from Richard P. Usatine, MD.*)

- Repetitive trauma from work, sports, or leisure activities.
- Nail hypertrophy and onychogryphosis.
  - Age.
- Habit-tic deformity.
  - Psychological dysfunctions.
- Beau lines and onychomadesis.
  - Severe illness.
  - High fever.
  - Local trauma (e.g., manicure) and onychotillomania (habit tic deformity).
  - Local cutaneous disease (e.g., dermatitis, paronychia).
  - Drugs (e.g., retinoids, chemotherapy agents).[6]
  - Viral infections such as hand, foot, and mouth disease.[7]
  - Pemphigus.
  - Kawasaki disease.

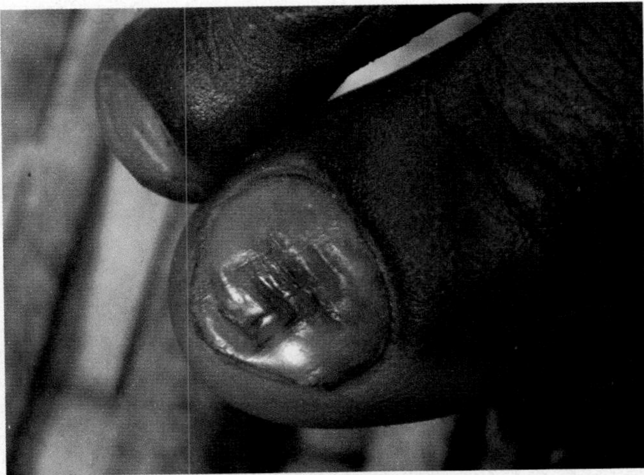

FIGURE 198-6 Habit-tic deformity of the large toenail in a man who walks barefoot often. He acknowledged that he picks at the nail and cuticle. *(Reproduced with permission from Richard P. Usatine, MD.)*

DIAGNOSIS

CLINICAL FEATURES

- All diagnoses of nail disorders should begin with a focused history and physical exam. It is especially important to ask about trauma and recent illnesses. All nails should be examined under adequate lighting with and without magnification. Natural sunlight is preferred over artificial light. Transillumination of the distal phalanx by using a penlight may help in localizing any abnormalities. To detect subtle changes of the nail plate surface, alcohol or acetone can be used to cleanse the surface. Digits should be relaxed and not pressed against a surface during the examination, since any alteration in the hemodynamics of the nail bed can change the nail appearance.

Dermoscopy is becoming the gold standard for examining hyperpigmentation of the nails (see Chapters 111, Dermoscopy and 199, Pigmented Nail Disorders). Ultrasound gel makes a great interface for dermoscopic examination.

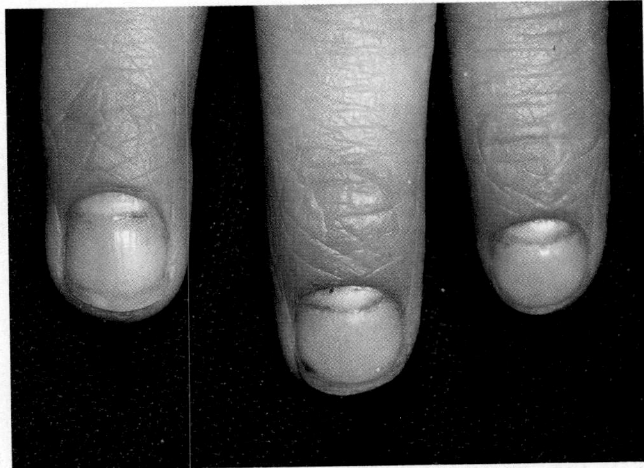

FIGURE 198-7 Beau lines in the fingernails of a young boy who had erythema multiforme and exfoliation approximately 2 months prior to this visit. *(Reproduced with permission from Richard P. Usatine, MD.)*

LABORATORY TESTING

- If renal disease is suspected, order a urinalysis and a serum creatinine.

DIFFERENTIAL DIAGNOSIS

- Hematoma may be confused with nail unit lesions, but the color grows out with the nail plate, exhibiting a proximal border that reproduces the shape of the lunula. A dermoscopic exam helps in visualizing how the blood is following the grooves in the underlying nail bed. (Figure 199-11).
- Mees and Muehrcke lines may be confused with leukonychia or Beau lines. Mees lines are multiple white transverse lines that begin in the nail matrix and extend completely across the nail plate (**Figure 198-10**). They are caused by heavy-metal poisoning or severe systemic insults. Muehrcke lines are white transverse lines that represent an abnormality of the nail vascular bed and may occur with chronic hypoalbuminemia or renal disease (**Figure 198-11**). In contrast to Beau lines, they are not grooved and they do not move with nail growth. **Table 198-1** lists the clinical signs that help

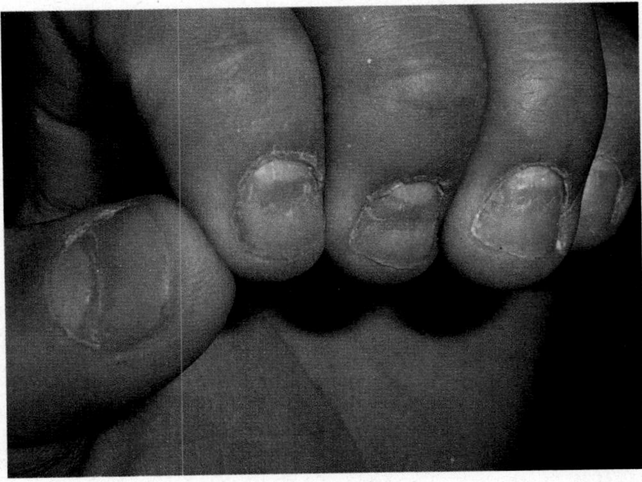

FIGURE 198-8 Beau lines in the fingernails of a young girl who was hospitalized with pneumonia 4 months prior to this visit. *(Reproduced with permission from Richard P. Usatine, MD.)*

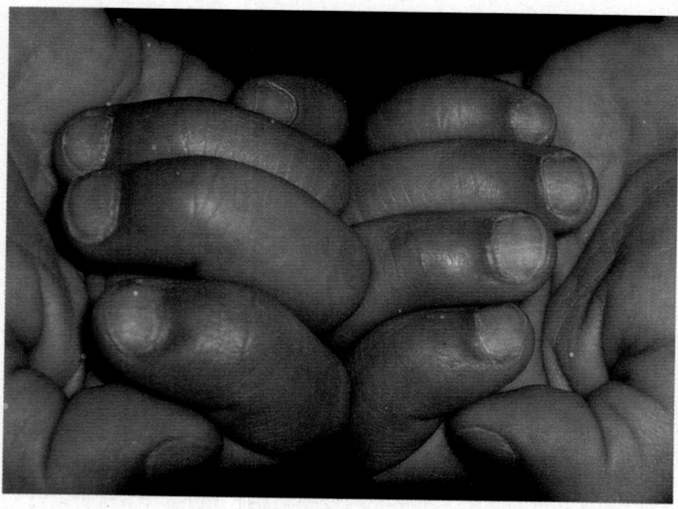

FIGURE 198-9 Twenty-nail dystrophy in a healthy 8-year-old girl. In this case all the fingernails are uniformly affected with longitudinal striations and loss of nail luster. Her skin is otherwise normal. (*Reproduced with permission from Richard P. Usatine, MD.*)

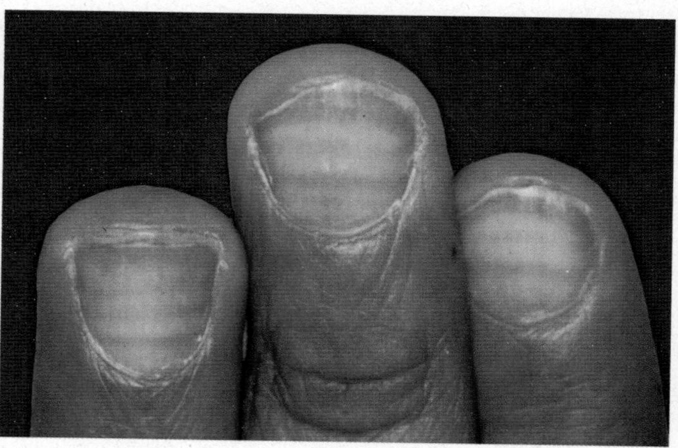

FIGURE 198-10 Mees lines that spread transversely across the entire breadth of the nail and are somewhat rounded with a contour similar to the distal lunula. (*Reproduced with permission from Jeffrey Meffert, MD.*)

TABLE 198-1 Signs That Help Differentiate Local Trauma-Induced Nail Changes from Those Associated with Systemic Disease

Characteristic	Mees Lines (Figure 198-10)	Muehrcke Lines (Figure 198-11)	Beau Lines (Figures 198-7 and 198-8)	Leukonychia (Figures 198-1 and 198-3)
Number of nails involved	Tend to be single but may occur on several nails at once	Tend to occur on several nails at once	Appear symmetrically in several or all nails	Usually on 1 or 2 nails
Nail coverage	Spread transversely across the entire breadth of the nail	Spread across the entire breadth of the nail bed or plate, often disappear with nail plate pressure	Spread transversely across the entire breadth of the nail	Often do not span the entire breadth of the nail plate
Line shape	Tend to have contour similar to the distal lunula, with a rounded distal edge	White transverse lines that have contour similar to the distal lunula, with a rounded distal edge	Tend to have contour similar to the distal lunula, with a rounded distal edge	More linear and resemble the contour of the proximal nail fold
Nail surface changes	Absent	Absent	Usually depressed	Absent
Etiology	Fragmented nail plate structure as a result of a compromised nail matrix	Abnormality of the nail vascular bed	Suppressed nail growth	Disruption of nail plate formation
Associated conditions	History of a systemic insult correlated with the onset of the lines such as chemotherapy, heart failure, or heavy-metal poisoning	Chronic hypoalbuminemia (hepatic and renal disease)	History of a physiologic stressor such as surgery or a severe illness	History of physical trauma (often not identified)

differentiate local trauma-induced lesions from those associated with systemic disease.
  - Leukonychia must also be differentiated from localized white onychomycosis; half-and-half nails, which are white proximal nails and pink or brown distal nails seen in renal failure (**Figure 198-12**); and Terry nails, which are white proximal nails and reddened distal nails that are seen in liver cirrhosis.
- The differential diagnosis of habit-tic deformity includes several nail dystrophies. In median nail, dystrophy produces a distinctive longitudinal split in the center of the nail plate with several cracks projecting laterally (**Figure 198-13**). Chronic paronychia is a *Candida*-induced inflammation of the proximal nail folds that may induce ripples that can mimic the habit-tic deformity. Chronic eczematous inflammation may produce similar changes. Onychomycosis, Beau lines, and psoriatic nail lesions may also appear similar to habit-tic deformity.[8]

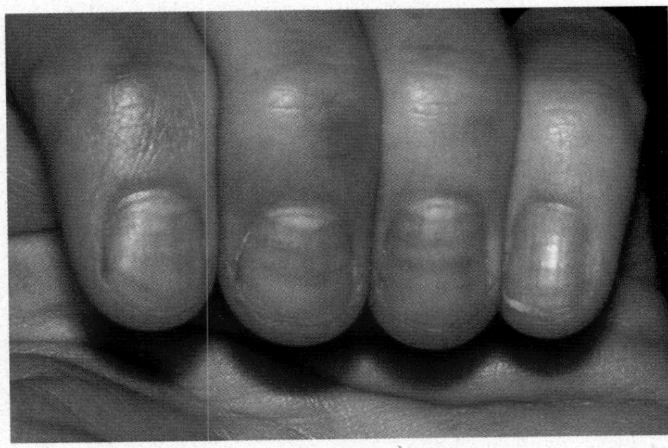

FIGURE 198-11 Muehrcke lines in a patient with chronic hypoalbuminemia from nephrotic syndrome. The white transverse lines extend across the full nail bed and represent an abnormality of the nail vascular bed. (*Reproduced with permission from Wikimedia Commons and Lyrl at http://commons.wikimedia.org/wiki/File:Muehrcke%27s_lines.JPG.*)

MANAGEMENT

NONPHARMACOLOGIC

- Grinding of the nail at regular intervals is useful for onychogryphosis.

MEDICATIONS

- Fluoxetine has been reported as being helpful in the treatment of habit-tic deformity.[9] SOR Ⓒ

SURGICAL

- Removal of the nail and ablation of the nail bed for onychogryphosis. SOR Ⓒ

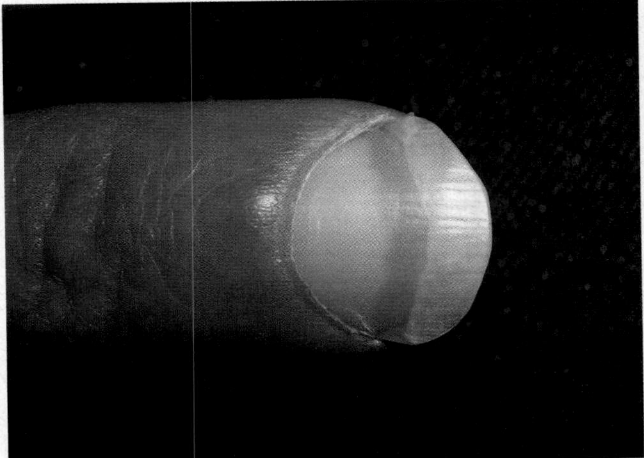

FIGURE 198-12 Half-and-half nail ("Lindsay nails") with the proximal portion of the nail being white and the distal portion pink. Note the sharp line of demarcation between the two halves. The patient has cirrhosis and HIV. (*Reproduced with permission from Richard P. Usatine, MD.*)

PATIENT RESOURCES

- University of Maryland Medical Center. *Nail Abnormalities*—**http://umm.edu/health/medical/ency/articles/nail-abnormalities.**
- Healthgrades Right Diagnosis. *Onychogryphosis*—**http://www.rightdiagnosis.com/o/onychogryphosis/intro.htm.**

PROVIDER RESOURCES

- eMedicine. *Nail Surgery*—**http://www.emedicine.com/derm/topic818.htm.**
- Color pictures at Dermatlas.org—**http://www.dermatlas.com/derm/** and select body site: *nails (all).*
- Medscape. *Melanonychia*—**http://emedicine.medscape.com/article/1375850-overview#showall.**
- Clinical Advisor. *Dystrophies of the Nail*—**http://www.clinicaladvisor.com/dermatologic-look-alikes/dystrophies-of-the-nail/article/180142/3/.**
- DermNet NZ. *Nail Diseases*—**http://dermnetnz.org/hair-nails-sweat/nails.html.**

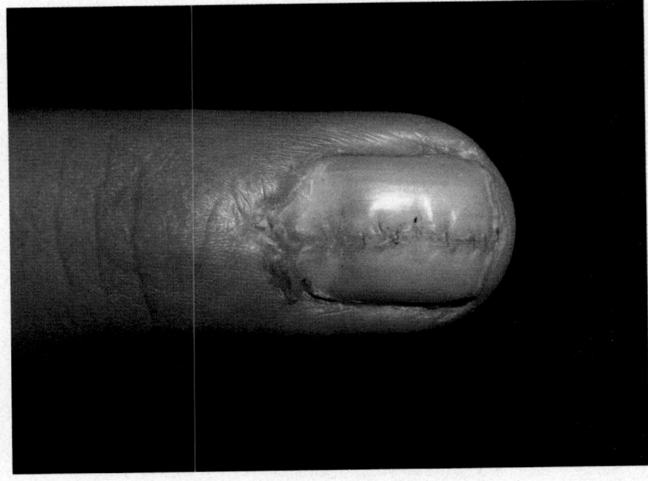

FIGURE 198-13 Median nail dystrophy that started with trauma in childhood. Note how it resembles a fir tree. (*Reproduced with permission from Richard P. Usatine, MD.*)

REFERENCES

1. Ruben B. Pigmented lesions of the nail unit: clinical and histopathologic features. *Semin Cutan Med Surg.* 2010;29:148-158.
2. Grossman M, Scher RK. Leukonychia. Review and classification. *Int J Dermatol.* 1990;29:535-541.
3. Baran R, Kechijian P. Diagnosis and management. *J Am Acad Dermatol.* 1989;21:1165-1175.
4. Daniel CR, Zaias N. Pigmentary abnormalities of the nails with emphasis on systemic diseases. *Dermatol Clin.* 1988;6:305-313.
5. Gordon KA, Vega JM, Tosti A. Trachyonychia: a comprehensive review. *Indian J Dermatol Venereol Leprol.* 2011;77:640.
6. Piraccini BM, Iorizzo M, Tosti A. Drug-induced nail abnormalities. *Am J Clin Dermatol.* 2003;4:31.
7. Wei SH, Huang YP, Liu MC, et al. An outbreak of coxsackievirus A6 hand, foot, and mouth disease associated with onychomadesis in Taiwan, 2010. *BMC Infect Dis.* 2011;11:346.
8. Farnell EA 4th. Bilateral thumbnail deformity. *J Fam Pract.* 2008; 57(11):743-745.
9. Vittorio CC, Phillips KA. Treatment of habit-tic deformity with fluoxetine. *Arch Dermatol.* 1997;133(10):1203-1204.

199 PIGMENTED NAIL DISORDERS

E.J. Mayeaux, Jr., MD

PATIENT STORY

An African-American medical student presented with a new dark band on her index finger for 1 year (**Figure 199-1**). The dark color and the lack of melanonychia in other fingers made this concerning. A biopsy of the nail matrix was performed, and the result showed a benign nevus.

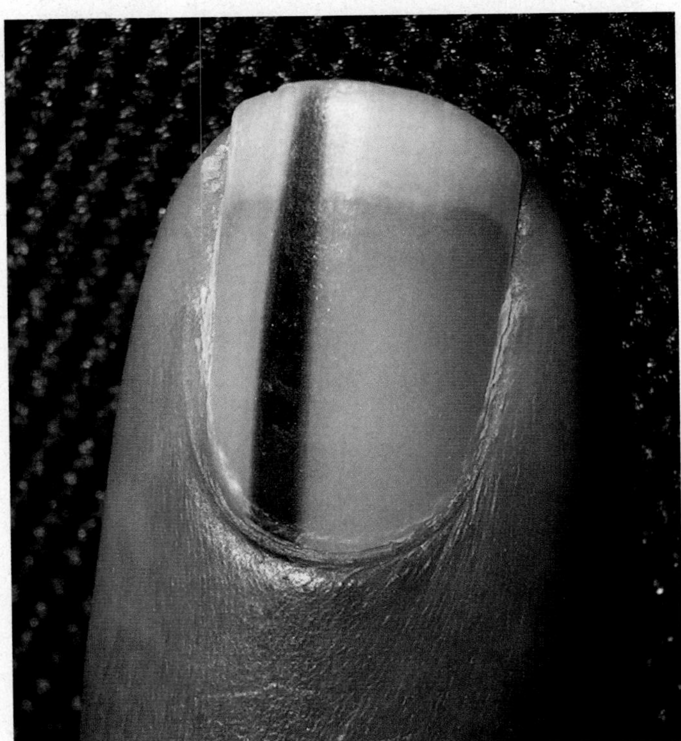

FIGURE 199-1 Longitudinal melanonychia—a single dark band of nail pigment appearing in the matrix region and extended to the tip of the nail. This is concerning for melanoma. The widening of the band in the proximal nail shows that the melanocytic lesion in the matrix is growing. This young woman had a biopsy that showed a benign nevus. *(Reproduced with permission from Richard P. Usatine, MD.)*

INTRODUCTION

Atypical pigmentation of the nail plate may result from many causes, such as melanin or hemosiderin within the nail plate, inflammatory changes, benign melanocytic hyperplasia, nevi, drugs, fungal infections, and endocrine disorders. It may also result from development of subungual melanoma. The challenge for the clinician is separating the malignant from the nonmalignant sources.

Longitudinal melanonychia (LM or melanonychia striata) is a pigmented band in the nail plate resulting from melanin deposition (**Figures 199-1** and **199-2**). This may result from activation or proliferation of nail matrix melanocytes. It may involve 1 or several digits, vary in color from light brown to black, vary in width (most range from 2 to 4 mm), and have sharp or blurred borders.

EPIDEMIOLOGY

- Benign LM is more common in more darkly pigmented persons. It occurs in 77% of African Americans older than age 20 years and in almost 100% of those older than age 50 years.[1,2] It also occurs in 10% to 20% of persons of Japanese descent. LM is common in Hispanic and other dark-skinned groups. LM is unusual in whites, occurring in only approximately 1% of the population.[1]
- Melanoma is the seventh most common cause of cancer in patients in the United States. Subungual melanoma is a relatively rare tumor with reported incidences between 0.7% and 3.5% of all melanoma cases in the general population.[3]
- Subungual melanoma arises on the hand in 45% to 60% of cases, and most of those occur in the thumb (**Figures 199-5** to **199-7**).[4] On the foot, subungual melanoma usually occurs in the great toe.[5] The median age at which subungual melanoma is usually diagnosed is in the sixth and seventh decades. It appears with equal frequency in males and females.[5] Amelanotic melanoma represents 25% to 30% of nail melanomas.[6]

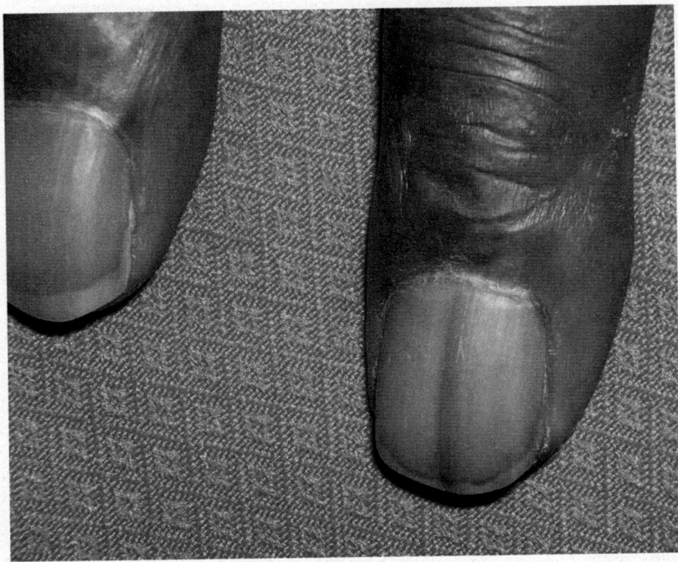

FIGURE 199-2 Close-up of longitudinal melanonychia in a single finger. Note that the color band is translucent with uniform color and width. *(Reproduced with permission from E.J. Mayeaux, Jr., MD.)*

ETIOLOGY AND PATHOPHYSIOLOGY

- LM originates in the nail matrix and results from increased deposition of melanin within the nail plate. Nail matrix melanocytes are

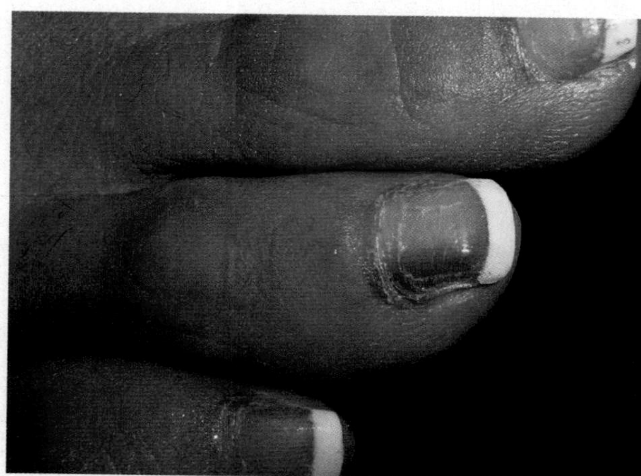

FIGURE 199-3 Longitudinal melanonychia in a single toe. Biopsy demonstrated changes consistent with melanocyte activation or lentigo, which is frequent in individuals with darkly pigmented skin. (*Reproduced with permission from Richard P. Usatine, MD.*)

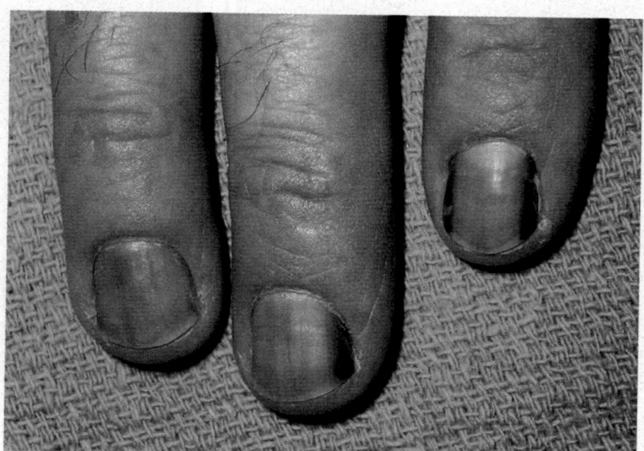

FIGURE 199-4 Melanonychia secondary to chemotherapy for metastatic penile cancer. (*Reproduced with permission from Richard P. Usatine, MD.*)

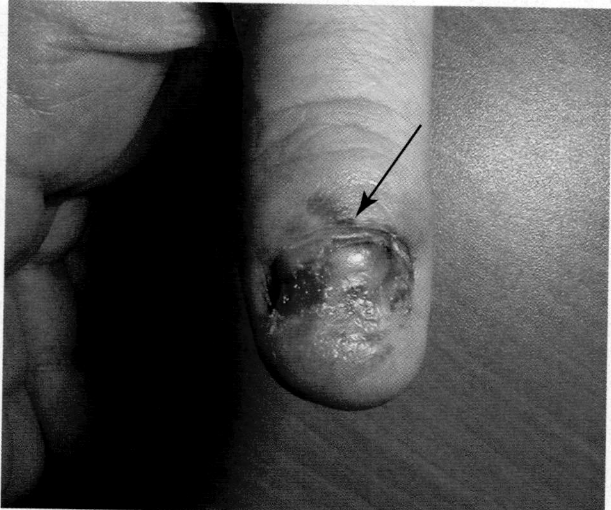

FIGURE 199-5 Advanced acral lentiginous melanoma of the thumb with destruction of the nail plate and ulceration. Note the hyperpigmentation of the proximal nail fold (Hutchinson sign), which is strongly indicative of melanoma. (*Reproduced with permission from Dr. Dubin at http://www.skinatlas.com.*)

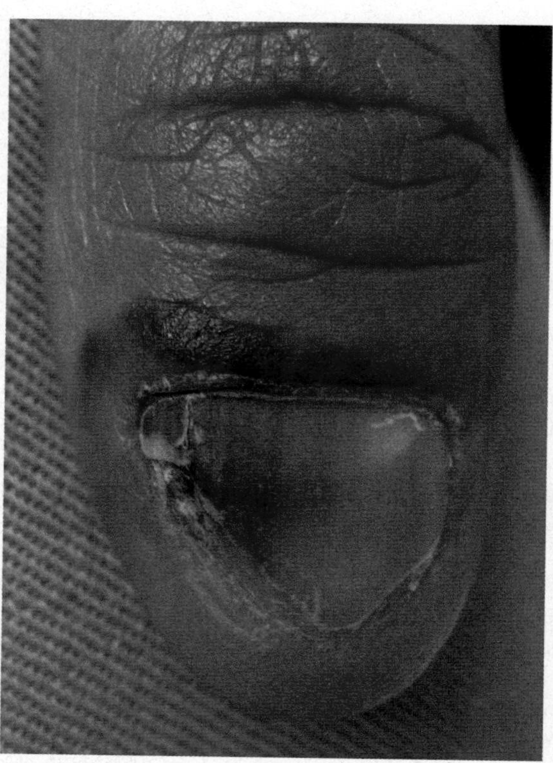

FIGURE 199-6 Acral lentiginous melanoma of the thumb with a very positive Hutchinson sign. Note how the pigmented band on the nail is greater than 3 mm in width. (*Reproduced with permission from Robert T. Gilson, MD.*)

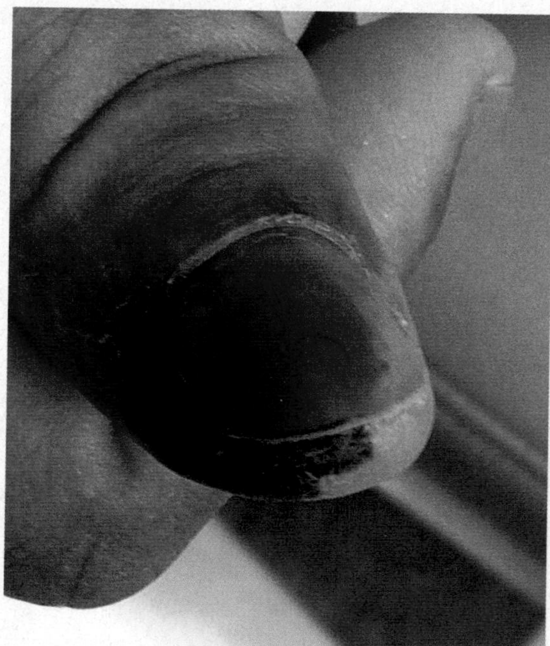

FIGURE 199-7 Acral lentiginous melanoma of the thumb with a very positive Hutchinson sign showing dark hyperpigmentation of the nail folds. Note how the light brown pigmented band on the nail is much greater than 3 mm in width. (*Reproduced with permission from Ryan O'Quinn, MD.*)

usually quiescent, frequently clustered, and not confined to the basal layer, and are more numerous in the distal matrix. Melanocytes of the proximal matrix are DOPA (3,4-dihydrooxyphenylalanine)-negative and cannot be activated, whereas melanocytes of the distal matrix are DOPA-positive and can be activated.[7] Distal matrix activation likely explains why most pigmented nail lesions are found in the ventral nail plate. Look at the distal edge of the nail in a cross-sectional view to see whether the pigment is dorsal or ventral (a dermatoscope may help).[8]

- Ethnic-type melanonychia is due to benign melanocyte activation that often involves several nails and is more common in skin of color.[9]
- Benign melanocytic hyperplasia (lentigo) is observed in 9% of the adult cases (see **Figure 199-3**) and 30% of the pediatric cases of single-biopsied LM.[4]
- Nevi represent 12% of LM in adults, but almost 50% of cases in children. A brown-black coloration is observed in two-thirds of cases and periungual pigmentation (benign pseudo-Hutchinson sign) in one-third.
- LM may also be caused by melanocytic activation from chronic trauma, especially in the great toes. It may occur in the fingernails of individuals who bite or traumatize the proximal nail fold and cuticle.
- Inflammatory changes accompanying skin diseases located in the nail unit, such as psoriasis, lichen planus, amyloidosis, and localized scleroderma, rarely may result in LM caused by melanocytic activation.[8]
- Drugs causing melanonychia include chemotherapy agents, antimalarials (mepacrine, amodiaquine, and chloroquine), and psoralens (see **Figure 199-4**). Drug-induced nail pigmentation typically causes longitudinal or transverse melanonychia and affects multiple nails.[10]
- Endocrine disorders, such as Addison disease, Cushing syndrome, hyperthyroidism, and acromegaly, can be responsible for LM.
- The diagnosis of subungual melanoma must always be considered in patients with LM (see **Figures 199-5** and **199-6**). Separating benign from malignant lesions is often difficult. Both arise most often in the thumb or index fingers, and both are more common in dark-skinned persons.[5] A biopsy should be performed in an adult if the cause of LM is uncertain. **Table 199-1** lists diagnostic clues for subungual melanomas.
- Hutchinson sign is the extension of pigmentation to the skin adjacent to the nail plate involving the nail folds or the fingertip. It is an important indicator for nail melanoma (see **Figures 199-5** to **199-7**).[11]
- Pseudo-Hutchinson sign is the presence of dark pigment around the proximal nail fold secondary to benign conditions such as ethnic melanosis and not melanoma (**Figure 199-8**). Another cause of pseudo-Hutchinson sign is a translucent cuticle below which the pigment of LM is visible. Trauma and drug-induced pigmentation can also produce a pseudo-Hutchinson sign.

RISK FACTORS

Table 199-1 lists diagnostic clues that indicate an increased risk for the presence of subungual melanoma.

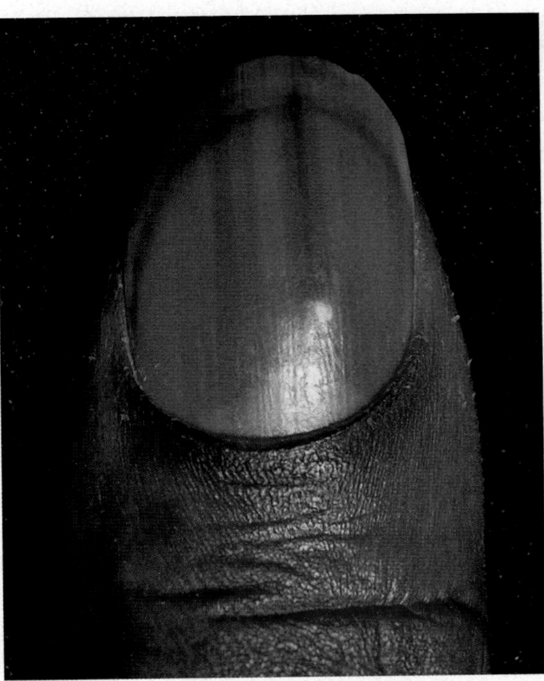

FIGURE 199-8 Benign longitudinal melanonychia in a black person demonstrating pseudo-Hutchinson sign (dark pigment around the proximal nail fold secondary to racial melanosis and not melanoma). *(Reproduced with permission from Richard P. Usatine, MD.)*

TABLE 199-1 Diagnostic Clues That Indicate Longitudinal Melanonychia (LM) Is Suspicious for Subungual Melanoma

Hutchinson sign (melanoma until proven otherwise)
In a single digit
Sixth decade of life or later
Develops abruptly in a previously normal nail plate
Suddenly darkens or widens (change in the LM morphology)
Occurs in the thumb, index finger, or great toe
History of digital trauma
Dark-skinned patient, particularly if the thumb or great toe is affected
Blurred, rather than sharp, lateral borders
Personal history of malignant melanoma
Increased risk for melanoma (e.g., familial atypical mole and melanoma [FAMM] syndrome)
Nail dystrophy, such as partial nail destruction or disappearance

DIAGNOSIS

CLINICAL FEATURES

There is an ABCDEF mnemonic system that applies to peri- or subungual melanoma:

- In this system "A" stands for age (peak incidence being between the fifth to seventh decades) and African Americans, Asians, and Native Americans in whom subungual melanoma accounts for one third of melanoma cases.
- "B" stands for "brown to black" and with "breadth" of 3 mm or more.
- "C" stands for change in the nail band coloration or lack of change after adequate treatment.
- "D" stands for the digit most commonly involved.
- "E" stands for extension of the pigment onto the proximal and/or lateral nail fold (Hutchinson sign and micro-Hutchinson sign).
- "F" stands for family or personal history of dysplastic nevus or melanoma.

TYPICAL DISTRIBUTION

The digits used for grasping (thumb, index finger, and middle finger) are the most commonly involved in LM and melanoma, but either may be found in any finger or toe.

DERMOSCOPY

Nail dermoscopy (onychoscopy) can greatly improve the diagnosis of nail pigmentation and help distinguish benign lesions from lesions that require biopsy or regular follow-up.[12] However, dermoscopy is not a substitute for pathology in the differential diagnosis of questionable cases of longitudinal melanonychia and should not prevent or delay biopsy. When evaluating nail pigmentation in an adult, determine if the pigment is melanin, and eliminate blood as the most important differential.

Determine if the lesion is more likely benign (e.g., lentigo, nevus) or malignant. Brown-black bands with a regular pattern showing individual lines that have similar shades of color, similar thickness, are regularly spaced, and are parallel are a sign of benign proliferation. Benign melanonychia may also exhibit a homogeneous gray background coloration with thin longitudinal gray lines.[12] A brown background is usually associated with melanocyte proliferation. When associated with regular parallel lines and regular spacing and with potential varying color and width, it suggests either a nevus or lentigo. There is usually homogeneity of color and width in each individual longitudinal line.[8]

Dermoscopic features of nail melanoma–related LM includes a brown to black background with or without longitudinal brown to black lines with irregular color, spacing, and thickness. Lines usually show loss of parallelism and may vary within single lines (**Figure 199-9**).[12] A brown background associated with longitudinal lines that are irregular in color, width, spacing, or parallelism may be benign *nevi* in children but is suggestive of malignant melanoma in adults.[12] Individual lines may show irregularity in color or width along their length, which is suspicious of melanoma, especially when associated with a diffuse dark background. Melanoma may also present as a dark background with barely visible lines.[8]

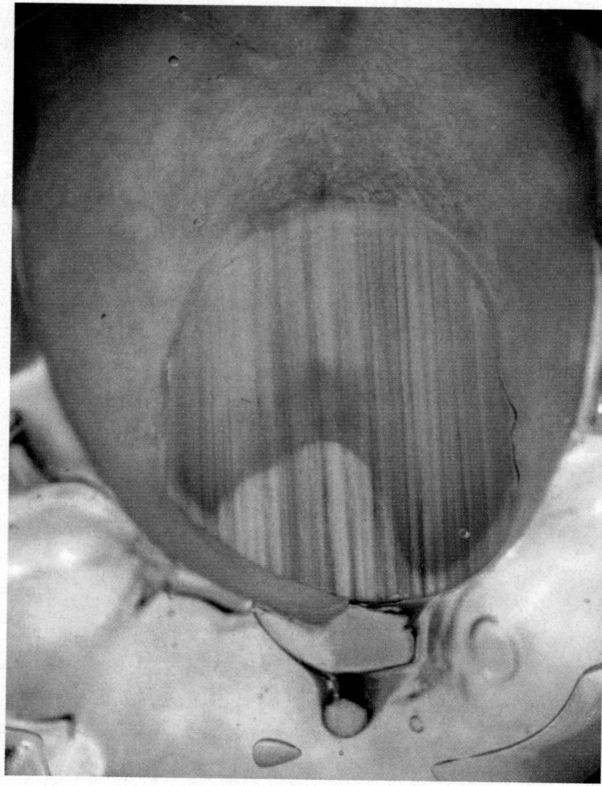

FIGURE 199-9 Dermoscopic view of a nail unit showing longitudinal melanonychia consistent with malignant melanoma. Note the brown background with longitudinal brown lines with irregular line color, spacing, and thickness. Micro-Hutchinson sign is present in the proximal nail fold. (*Reproduced with permission from Ashfaq A. Marghoob, MD.*)

Dermoscopic evaluation may reveal a micro-Hutchinson sign, which is pigmentation of the cuticle that is not visible to the naked eye. It is unusual but is very concerning for melanoma when found.[8,12] It has also been described in congenital nevi in children. Dark lesions may also be visible through the cuticle, and this is referred to as pseudo-Hutchinson sign. Pigmentation in the hyponychial skin is a true Hutchinson sign and is highly suggestive of melanoma. It may be associated with a parallel ridge pattern on dermoscopy.[2] Blood spots and micro-Hutchinson sign (see **Figure 199-9**) in the proximal nail fold may be found. In a retrospective observational study published in 2016, univariate and multivariable analyses determined that melanoma cases were significantly associated with a width of the pigmented band greater than two thirds of the nail plate, presence of gray and black colors, irregularly pigmented lines, Hutchinson and micro-Hutchinson signs, nail dystrophy, and granular pigmentation.[13]

BIOPSY

Definitive diagnosis of a nail discoloration may be made with a biopsy of the nail matrix. Patients with darker skin color and multiple digits with translucent LM often need only be observed. Single dark lines in whites should always be biopsied. As with melanomas in other parts of the body, excision is becoming preferred to biopsy because there are reports of false-negative incisional biopsies.[8] A 3-mm punch biopsy can be performed at the origin of the darkest part of a dark band within the nail matrix (**Figure 199-10**) of smaller lesions. Otherwise, a tangential matrix excision (shave biopsy of the matrix) is recommended.[8] Histologic diagnosis of atypical melanocytic hyperplasia necessitates the complete removal of the lesion.

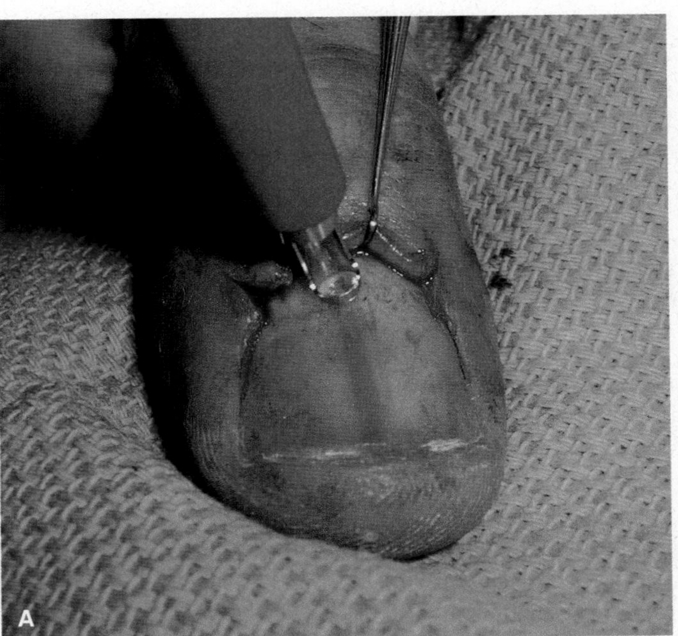

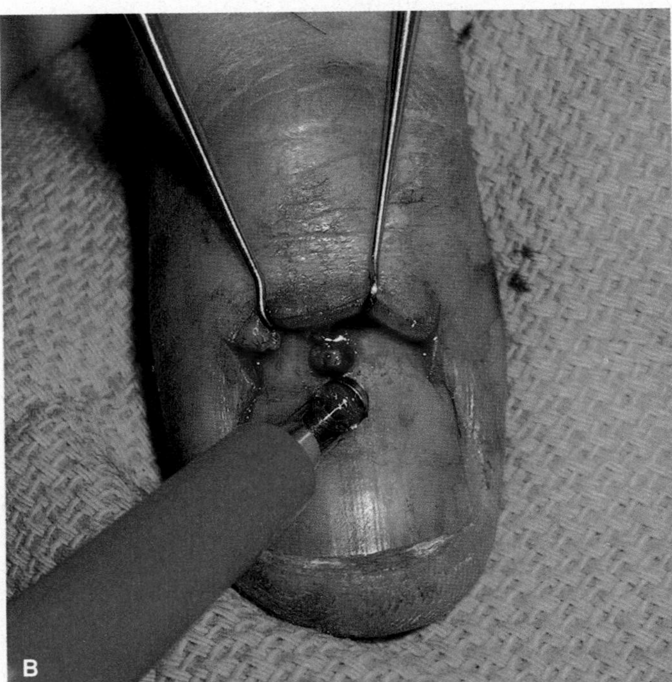

FIGURE 199-10 **A.** The proximal nail fold is reflected back to perform a nail matrix biopsy in a young man with new onset of longitudinal melanonychia. The 3-mm punch is placed over the origin of the dark band at the distal matrix. **B.** The 3-mm punch now contains the specimen for pathology. The longitudinal melanonychia was caused by melanocytic hyperplasia. (*Reproduced with permission from Richard P. Usatine, MD.*)

DIFFERENTIAL DIAGNOSIS

- Pigmented lesions in the nail bed usually do not cause LM and are viewed through the nail as a grayish to brown or black spot.[7]
- Subungual hematoma may be confused with LM, but the color grows out with the nail plate, exhibiting a proximal border that reproduces the shape of the lunula. Subungual hemorrhages have a distinct dermatoscopic pattern of globules, sometimes with distal streaks, with color ranging from red to brown to black (**Figure 199-11**). The dermoscopic diagnosis of subungual hematoma does not rule out a coincident nail tumor.[8,12] A hole punched in the nail plate allows for the visualization of the underlying nail bed and confirmation of a subungual hematoma (see Chapter 204, Subungual Hematoma).
- Some non-dermatophytic molds (particularly some *Neoscytalidium* and *Trichophyton* species) produce pigmented hyphae that cause nail pigmentation.

MANAGEMENT

NONPHARMACOLOGIC

No treatment is required for benign LM.

REFERRAL OR HOSPITALIZATION

Treatment of primary subungual melanomas includes amputation at the level of the interphalangeal joint for thumb lesions SOR Ⓑ, the distal interphalangeal joint for fingers SOR C, and the metatarsophalangeal joint for toes.[14] For melanoma in situ, it may be possible to remove the full nail apparatus and save the digit. Regional lymph node dissection can help with establishment of disease stage. Chemotherapy is recommended for nodal or visceral metastases.

PROGNOSIS

The 5-year survival is approximately 74% for patients with stage I and 40% for patients with stage II disease. Prognostic variables negatively affecting survival include stage at diagnosis, deeper Clark level of invasion, African-American race, and ulceration.[15]

FOLLOW-UP

Because LM may indicate an undiagnosed melanoma of the nail unit, regular monitoring is extremely important. Have the patient report any rapid changes in pigmentation of the nail plate or nail folds, and strongly consider biopsy in these individuals.

PATIENT RESOURCES

- Medscape. *Nail Diseases in Childhood*—**http://www.medscape.com/viewarticle/585158_8.**
- DermNet NZ. *Subungual Melanoma*—**http://dermnetnz.org/hair-nails-sweat/melanoma-nailunit.html.**

PROVIDER RESOURCES

- DermNet NZ. *Nail Disorders*—**https://www.dermnetnz.org/topics/nail-disorders/**
- DermNet NZ. *Dermatoscopy Dermoscopy of the Nail*—**http://www.dermnetnz.org/cme/dermoscopy-course/dermoscopy-of-the-nail/.**
- Di Chiacchio ND, Farias DC, Piraccini BM, et al. Consensus on melanonychia nail plate dermoscopy. *An Bras Dermatol.* 2013;88(2):309-313—**https://www.ncbi.nlm.nih.gov/pmc/articles/PMC3750907/.**
- eMedicine. *Nail Surgery*—**http://www.emedicine.com/derm/topic818.htm.**
- Braun RP, Baran R, Le Gal FA, et al. Diagnosis and management of nail pigmentation. *J Am Acad Dermatol.* 2007;56(5):835-847.
- Jellinek N. Nail matrix biopsy of longitudinal melanonychia: diagnostic algorithm including the matrix shave biopsy. *J Am Acad Dermatol.* 2007;56(5):803-810.
- Usatine R. Nail procedures. In: Usatine R, Pfenninger J, Stulberg D, Small R, eds. *Dermatologic and Cosmetic Procedures in Office Practice.* Philadelphia, PA: Elsevier; 2012:216-228. The whole procedure depicted in **Figure 199-8** is described in detail.

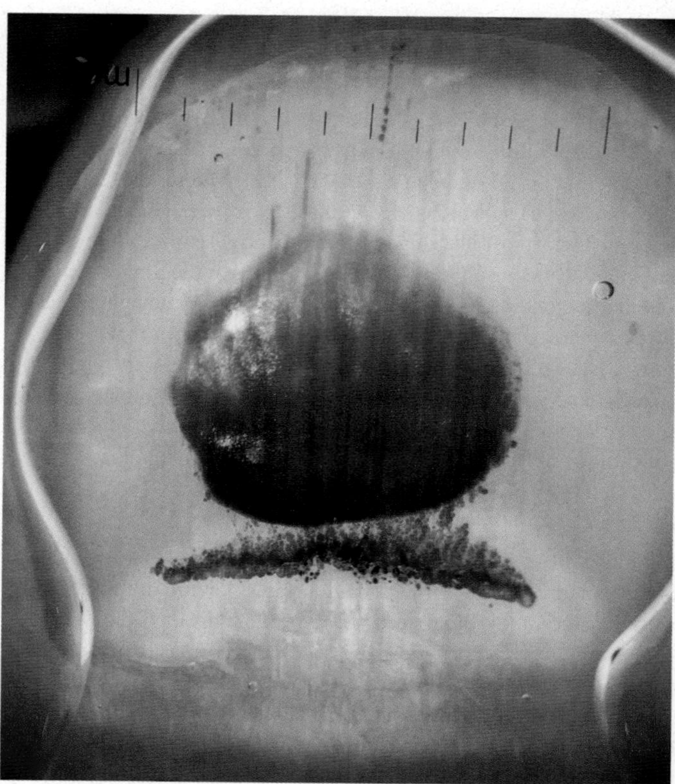

FIGURE 199-11 Dermoscopy of a subungual hemorrhage showing proximal globules and distal streaks. (*Reproduced with permission from Richard P. Usatine, MD.*)

REFERENCES

1. Baran R, Kechjijian P. Longitudinal melanonychia (melanonychia striata): diagnosis and management. *J Am Acad Dermatol.* 1989;21:1165-1175.
2. Ruben B. Pigmented lesions of the nail unit: clinical and histopathologic features. *Semin Cutan Med Surg.* 2010;29:148-158.
3. Finley RK, Driscoll DL, Blumenson LE, Karakousis CP. Subungual melanoma: an eighteen year review. *Surgery.* 1994;116:96-100.
4. Goettmann-Bonvallot S, André J, Belaich S. Longitudinal melanonychia in children: a clinical and histopathologic study of 40 cases. *J Am Acad Dermatol.* 1999;41:17-22.
5. Papachristou DN, Fortner JG. Melanoma arising under the nail. *J Surg Oncol.* 1982;21:219-222.
6. Tosti A, Piraccini BM, de Farias DC. Dealing with melanonychia. *Semin Cutan Med Surg.* 2009;28:49.
7. Perrin C, Michiels JF, Pisani A, Ortonne JP. Anatomic distribution of melanocytes in normal nail unit: an immunohistochemical investigation. *Am J Dermatopathol.* 1997;19:462.
8. Di Chiacchio ND, Farias DC, Piraccini BM, et al. Consensus on melanonychia nail plate dermoscopy. *An Bras Dermatol.* 2013;88(2):309-313.
9. Astur Mde M, Farkas CB, Junqueira JP, et al. Reassessing melanonychia striata in phototypes IV, V, and VI patients. *Dermatol Surg.* 2016;42:183.
10. Piraccini BM, Iorizzo M, Starace M, Tosti A. Drug-induced nail diseases. *Dermatol Clin.* 2006;24:387.
11. Mikhail GR. Hutchinson's sign. *J Dermatol Surg Oncol.* 1986;12:519-521.
12. Lencastre A, Lamas A, Sá D, Tosti A. Onychoscopy. *Clin Dermatol.* 2013;31:587.
13. Benati E, Ribero S, Longo C, et al. Clinical and dermoscopic clues to differentiate pigmented nail bands: an International Dermoscopy Society study. *J Eur Acad Dermatol Venereol.* 2017;31(4):732-736.
14. Moehrle M, Metzger S, Schippert W, et al. "Functional" surgery in subungual melanoma. *Dermatol Surg.* 2003;29(4):366-374.
15. O'Leary JA, Berend KR, Johnson JL, et al. Subungual melanoma: a review of 93 cases with identification of prognostic variables. *Clin Orthop Relat Res.* 2000;378:206-212.

200 INGROWN TOENAIL

E.J. Mayeaux, Jr., MD

PATIENT STORY

A 14-year-old boy presents with a history of multiple ingrown nails of both great toes. Today his right big toe is swollen and painful (**Figure 200-1**). He has a 2-week history of pain, redness, and swelling of the lateral nail fold of the right great toe. Soaking the toe in Epsom salts has not helped. A partial nail removal after a digital block was successful. The nail matrix was also ablated with phenol to prevent recurrence of the ingrown nail.

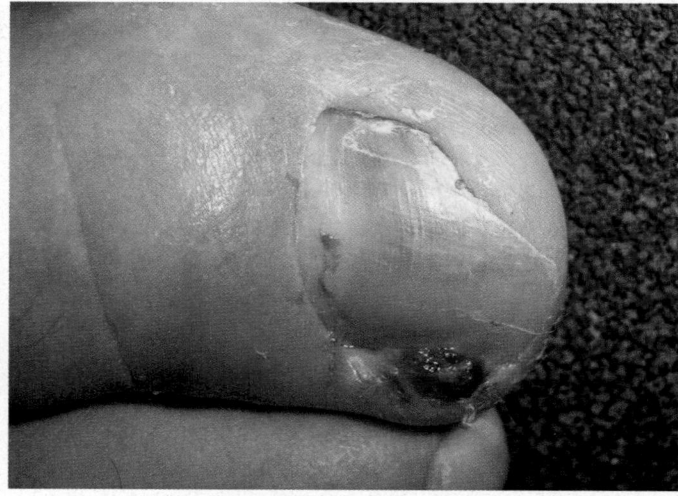

FIGURE 200-1 Ingrown toenail of the lateral aspect of the right great toe showing inflammation and granulation tissue. (*Reproduced with permission from Richard P. Usatine, MD.*)

INTRODUCTION

Onychocryptosis (ingrown toenails) is a common childhood and adult problem. Patients often seek treatment because of the significant levels of discomfort and disability associated with the condition.

SYNONYMS

Onychocryptosis, unguis incarnatus.

EPIDEMIOLOGY

The prevalence of onychocryptosis is unknown, as many patients do not seek medical care and it is not a reportable disease. The toenails, especially the great toenail, are most commonly affected. Ingrown toenails at birth and in early childhood do occur, but are very rare.

ETIOLOGY AND PATHOPHYSIOLOGY

Onychocryptosis occurs when the lateral nail plate damages the lateral nail fold. The lateral edge of the nail plate penetrates and perforates the adjacent nailfold skin. Perforation of the lateral fold skin results in painful inflammation that manifests clinically as mild edema, erythema, and pain. In advanced stages, drainage, infection, and ulceration may be present. Hypertrophy of the lateral nail wall occurs, and granulation tissue forms over the nail plate and the nailfold during healing of the ulcerated skin.[1] It is a common affliction that can result from a variety of conditions that cause improper fit of the nail plate in the lateral nail groove (see **Figure 200-1**).

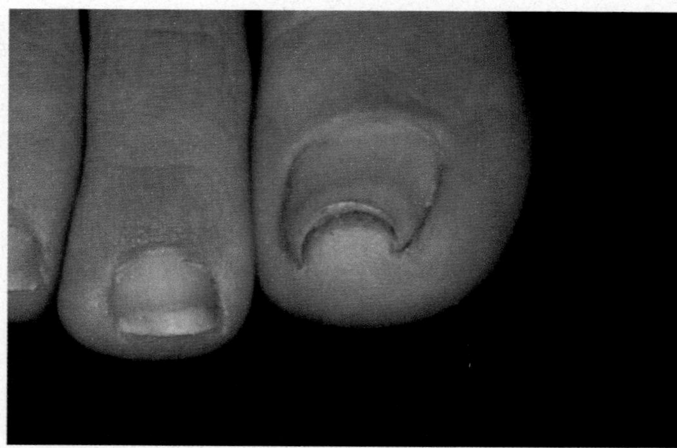

FIGURE 200-2 The curved infolding of the lateral edges of the nail plate indicates that this patient has a pincer nail, which predisposes to onychocryptosis. (*Reproduced with permission from Richard P. Usatine, MD.*)

RISK FACTORS[1]

- Genetic predisposition.
- Poor-fitting footwear.
- Excessive trimming of the lateral nail plate.
- Pincer nail deformity (**Figure 200-2**).

- Trauma.
- Sports in which kicking or running is important.
- Hyperhidrosis.
- Anatomic features such as nailfold width.
- Congenital malalignment of the digit.
- Overcurvature of the nail plate.
- Onychomycosis and other diseases that result in abnormal changes in the nail plate.

DIAGNOSIS

CLINICAL FEATURES: HISTORY AND PHYSICAL

The diagnosis is based on clinical appearance and rarely is difficult. Characteristic signs and symptoms include pain, edema, exudate, and granulation tissue (see **Figure 200-1**).

TYPICAL DISTRIBUTION

The great toe is most commonly affected; fingers are rarely involved except when nail biting is present.

DIFFERENTIAL DIAGNOSIS

- Cellulitis—Presents with redness, pain, and swelling beyond the nail fold (see Chapter 126, Cellulitis).
- Paronychia—Presents with redness and abscess formation (pus) in a nail fold (see Chapter 202, Paronychia).

MANAGEMENT

The treatment of ingrown toenails depends on the age of the patient and the severity of the lesion.

NONPHARMACOLOGIC

- Lesions characterized by minimal to moderate pain and no discharge can be treated conservatively with soaking the affected foot in warm water for 20 minutes, 3 times per day, and pushing the lateral nailfold away from the nail plate.[2] SOR Ⓒ
  - Other palliative measures include cotton wedging underneath the lateral nail plate and trimming the lateral part of the nail plate below the area of nailfold irritation.
- Gutter treatment (gutter removal or gutter splinting) involves placing a small vinyl or plastic tube that is slit from top to bottom over the side of the ingrowing plate and affixing it with tape or sutures. This separates the nail plate from the nail-fold wall, preventing it from growing further into the skin.[3,4] SOR Ⓑ
- Orthonyxia or brace treatment involves hooking a small metal brace around both edges of the nail plate after the painful part of the nail is removed. The metal brace has an omega shape that puts the brace under tension when it is attached to the nail plate with gel. This relieves nail pressure on the fold soft tissue. SOR Ⓑ Devices that have shown promise include shape memory alloys (SMAs), of either a Cu-Al-Mn base or a Ni-Ti base.[3-5]
- The tape or adhesive bandage method involves placing the adhesive band on the affected fold and pulling it under and the across the toe to reduce the pressure of the nail fold and the edge of the nail plate. SOR Ⓒ

MEDICATIONS

- Although many elect to treat apparent infections with oral antibiotics, studies show the use of antibiotics does not decrease healing time or postprocedure morbidity in otherwise normal patients.[6] SOR Ⓐ
- A medium- to high-potency topical corticosteroid can be applied after soaking to decrease inflammation but is often unnecessary.
- If nail avulsion and/or matrix ablation is used, pain relievers for mild to moderate pain may be necessary.
- When placing digital blocks for surgical procedures, the best evidence indicates that the use of lidocaine with epinephrine is equally safe and efficacious for anesthesia.[7]

SURGICAL

- Nonresponders to conservative therapy and patients with more severe lesions (substantial erythema, granulation tissue, and pus) need surgical therapy.[8,9] SOR Ⓒ Surgical interventions are more effective than nonsurgical interventions in preventing the recurrence of an ingrowing toenail.[10]
- Surgical intervention involves partial or full nail plate avulsion. Usually it is only necessary to remove the part of the nail that is placing pressure on the lateral nailfold (**Figure 200-3**). SOR Ⓒ
- Patients who develop recurrent ingrown toenails benefit from permanent nail ablation of the lateral nail matrix. This may be achieved with the combination of partial nail plate avulsion plus phenol matrixectomy, which can cut recurrence rates by 90% (**Figure 200-4**).[8-10] SOR Ⓐ
- Based on a Cochrane Systematic Review of surgical treatments for ingrowing toenails, nail avulsion with the use of phenol is more effective at preventing symptomatic recurrence than nail avulsion without the use of phenol.[10] They also found that postoperative treatments such as antibiotics, manuka honey, povidone-iodine with paraffin, hydrogel with paraffin, or paraffin gauze reduced the risk of postoperative infection or postoperative pain, or gave a shorter healing time.[10] SOR Ⓐ
- Chemical matrixectomy is performed mainly with phenol (full-strength 88%), but 10% sodium hydroxide is another alternative. In a comparison study of the use of chemical matrixectomy for the treatment of ingrown toenails, the overall success rates were 95% for both phenol and sodium hydroxide.[11] SOR Ⓐ
- One study found that partial nail avulsion with phenolization gave better results than partial avulsion with matrix excision.[12] Local antibiotics applied to the surgical site did not reduce signs of infection or recurrence. The use of phenol did not produce more signs of infection than matrix excision.[12] SOR Ⓑ
- Electrosurgical ablation can be performed with electrosurgery units on the fulguration setting or using a special matrixectomy electrode with a high-frequency electrosurgical unit (**Figure 200-5**). SOR Ⓒ

FOLLOW-UP

After surgical intervention, consider follow-up in 3 to 4 days to assess treatment and exclude cellulitis.

PATIENT EDUCATION

- Patients should be educated about proper nail trimming so as to minimize trauma to the lateral nailfold. The lateral nail plate should be allowed to grow well beyond the lateral nailfold before trimming horizontally.
- Patients should also be educated about the importance of avoiding shoes that are too tight over the toes to help minimize recurrences.

PATIENT RESOURCES

- Ingrown Toenails information at the familydoctor.org website—**https://familydoctor.org/condition/ingrown-toenails/.**
- eMedicineHealth. *Ingrown Toenails*—**http://www.emedicinehealth.com/ingrown_toenails/article_em.htm.**

PROVIDER RESOURCES

- Medscape eMedicine. *Ingrown Nails*—**http://emedicine.medscape.com/article/909807.**
- Usatine R, Pfenninger J, Stulberg D, Small R. *Dermatologic and Cosmetic Procedures in Office Practice.* Philadelphia: Elsevier; 2012 (with DVD). The "Nail Procedures" chapter provides details, photographs, and videos of how to perform ingrown toenail surgeries. Available as an electronic app as well—**http://usatinemedia.com.**
- **http://itunes.apple.com/us/app/dermatologic-cosmetic-procedures/id479310808?ls=1&mt=8.**

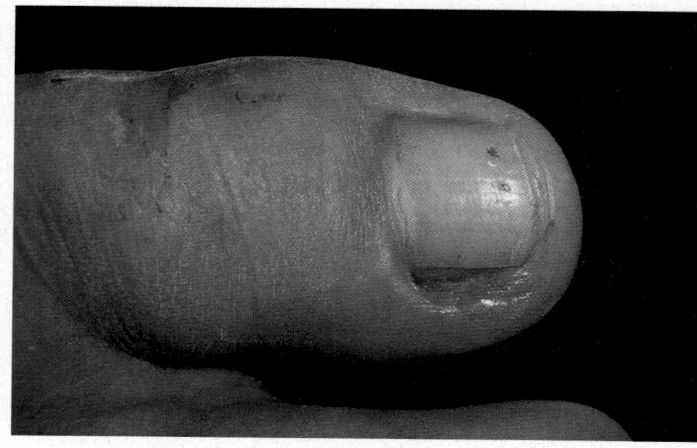

FIGURE 200-3 Status post partial nail avulsion procedure for an ingrown toenail. (*Reproduced with permission from Richard P. Usatine, MD.*)

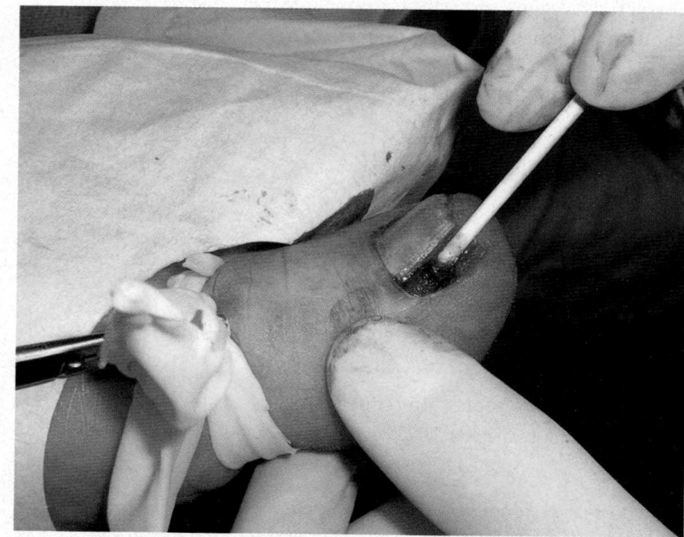

FIGURE 200-4 Phenol matrixectomy to destroy a portion of the nail matrix to prevent a recurrent ingrown toenail. Note the use of a tourniquet to decrease bleeding while applying the phenol with a twisting motion. (*Reproduced with permission from Richard P. Usatine, MD.*)

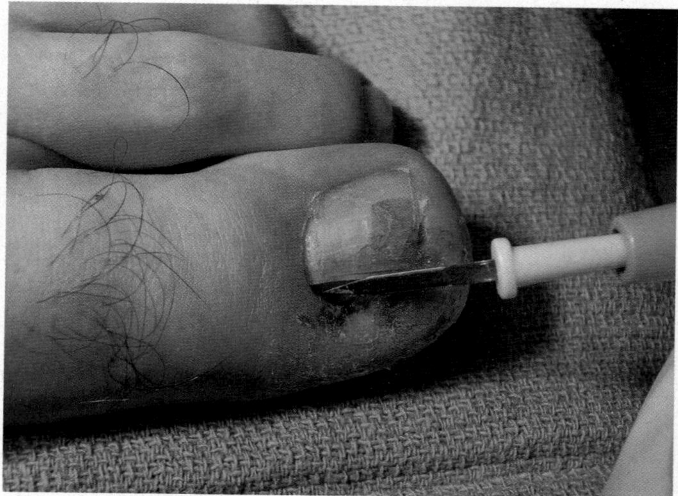

FIGURE 200-5 Use of electrosurgery to ablate the lateral nail matrix. This results in a narrower nail and a decreased likelihood of onychocryptosis recurrence. (*Reproduced with permission from Richard P. Usatine, MD.*)

REFERENCES

1. Siegle RJ, Swanson NA. Nail surgery: a review. *J Dermatol Surg Oncol.* 1982;8(8):659-666.
2. Connolly B, Fitzgerald RJ. Pledgets in ingrowing toenails. *Arch Dis Child.* 1988;63:71.
3. Nazari S. A simple and practical method in treatment of ingrown nails: splinting by flexible tube. *J Eur Acad Dermatol Venereol.* 2006;20(10):1302-1306.
4. Arai H. Formable acrylic treatment for ingrowing nail with gutter splint and sculptured nail. *Int J Dermatol.* 2004;43(10): 759-765.
5. Ishibashi M, Tabata N, Suetake T, et al. A simple method to treat an ingrowing toenail with a shape-memory alloy device. *J Dermatolog Treat.* 2008;19(5):291-292.
6. Reyzelman AM, Trombello KA, Vayser DJ, et al. Are antibiotics necessary in the treatment of locally infected ingrown toenails? *Arch Fam Med.* 2000;9:930.

7. Altinyazar HC, Demirel CB, Koca R, Hosnuter M. Digital block with and without epinephrine during chemical matricectomy with phenol. *Dermatol Surg.* 2010;36(10):1568-1571.
8. Grieg JD, Anderson JH, Ireland AJ, Anderson JR. The surgical treatment of ingrowing toenails. *J Bone Joint Surg Br.* 1991;73:131.
9. Vaccari S, Dika E, Balestri R, et al. Partial excision of matrix and phenolic ablation for the treatment of ingrowing toenail: a 36-month follow-up of 197 treated patients. *Dermatol Surg.* 2010;36(8):1288-1293.
10. Eekhof JAH, VanWijk B, Knuistingh Neven A, van der Wouden JC. Interventions for ingrowing toenails. *Cochrane Database Syst Rev.* 2012;(4):CD001541.
11. Bostanci S, Kocyigit P, Gurgey E. Comparison of phenol and sodium hydroxide chemical matricectomies for the treatment of ingrowing toenails. *Dermatol Surg.* 2007;33:680-685.
12. Bos AM, van Tilburg MW, van Sorge AA, Klinkenbijl JH. Randomized clinical trial of surgical technique and local antibiotics for ingrowing toenail. *Br J Surg.* 2007;94:292-296.

201 ONYCHOMYCOSIS

James O. Williams, Jr, MD
E.J. Mayeaux, Jr., MD

PATIENT STORY

A 29-year-old woman presents with thickened and discolored toenails for 1 year (**Figure 201-1**). She is embarrassed to wear sandals and wants treatment. The entire nail plates are involved and there is subungual keratosis. She did not realize that she had tinea pedis, but a fine scale was seen on the soles and sides of the feet indicative of tinea pedis in a moccasin distribution. A KOH scraping from the subungual debris was positive for hyphae. She has no history of liver disease or risk factors for liver disease. An oral antifungal was prescribed for 3 months.

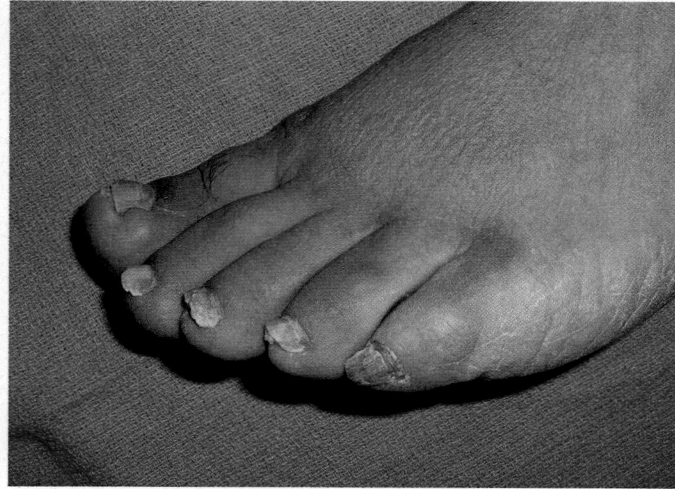

FIGURE 201-1 Onychomycosis in all toenails of this 29-year-old woman. Note the nail plate thickening and discoloration along with the subungual keratosis. She also has tinea pedis in a moccasin distribution. *(Reproduced with permission from Richard P. Usatine, MD.)*

INTRODUCTION

Onychomycosis is a term used to denote nail infections caused by any fungus, including dermatophytes, yeasts, and nondermatophyte molds, which are the predominant organism in patients with human immunodeficiency virus (HIV) infection.[1] One, some, and occasionally all of the toenails and/or fingernails may be involved. Although most toenail onychomycosis is caused by dermatophytes, many cases of fingernail onychomycosis are caused by yeast. Onychomycosis may involve the nail plate and other parts of the nail unit, including the nail matrix.

SYNONYMS

Toenail fungus, tinea unguium, dermatophytosis of nails.

EPIDEMIOLOGY

- The mean prevalence of onychomycosis in Europe and North America in population based studies is 4.3% (1.9% to 6.8%). In hospital-based studies the mean prevalence is 8.9% (4.3% to 13.6%).[2] Most patients (7.6%) have only toenail involvement, and only 0.15% have fingernail involvement alone.[3]
- The disease is very common in adults but may also occur in children.

ETIOLOGY AND PATHOPHYSIOLOGY

- Dermatophytes are responsible for most finger- and toenail infections.
- Nonpathogenic fungi and *Candida* (in the rare syndrome of chronic mucocutaneous candidiasis) also can infect the nail plate.

- Dermatophytic onychomycosis (tinea unguium) occurs in five distinct forms: distal lateral subungual (**Figure 201-2**), proximal white subungual (**Figure 201-3**), distal superficial white (**Figure 201-4**), endonyx, and total dystrophic (**Figure 201-5**).[4]
- The vast majority of distal and proximal subungual onychomycosis results from *Trichophyton rubrum* (**Figure 201-6**).
- Distal white superficial onychomycosis is usually caused by *Trichophyton mentagrophytes*, although cases caused by *T. rubrum* have also been reported[4] (**Figure 201-7**).
- Yeast onychomycosis is most common in the fingers and is caused by *Candida albicans*.

RISK FACTORS

- Tinea pedis.[5]
- Trauma predisposes to infection but can also cause a dysmorphic nail that can be confused for onychomycosis.[5]
- Older age.[5]
- Swimming.[5]
- Diabetes.[5]
- Living with family members who have onychomycosis.[5]
- Immunosuppression (**Figure 201**-8).[6]
- Microtrauma due to sports activity.[4]
- Psoriasis.[4]

DIAGNOSIS

CLINICAL FEATURES

- Distal subungual onychomycosis is the most common presentation.
- Distal subungual onychomycosis begins with a whitish, yellowish, or brownish discoloration of a distal corner of the nail, which gradually spreads to involve the entire width of the nail plate and extends slowly toward the cuticle. Keratin debris collecting between the nail plate and its bed is the cause of the discoloration (see **Figures 201-1** and **201-2**).
- Proximal subungual onychomycosis progresses in a manner similar to distal subungual onychomycosis but affects the nail in the vicinity of the cuticle first and extends distally. It usually occurs in individuals with a compromised immune system (see **Figure 201-3**).
- White superficial onychomycosis appears as dull white spots on the surface of the nail plate (see **Figure 201-4**). Eventually the whole nail plate may be involved. The white areas may be soft and can be lightly scraped to yield a chalky scale that may be examined or cultured.
- Endonyx onychomycosis presents as a diffuse milky-white discoloration of the nail without nail bed hyperkeratosis or onycholysis. The nail shows irregular wave patterns with pitting and lamellar splits. This pattern of onychomycosis is caused almost exclusively by *Trichophyton soudanense*.[4]

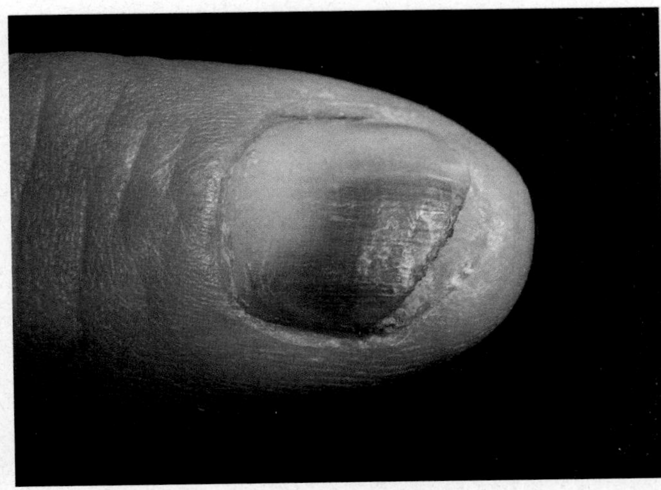

FIGURE 201-2 Distal lateral subungual onychomycosis. The dark color is created by the fungus and is not suspicious for melanoma, as the color does not begin in the matrix and the keratosis pattern is fungal. *(Reproduced with permission from Richard P. Usatine, MD.)*

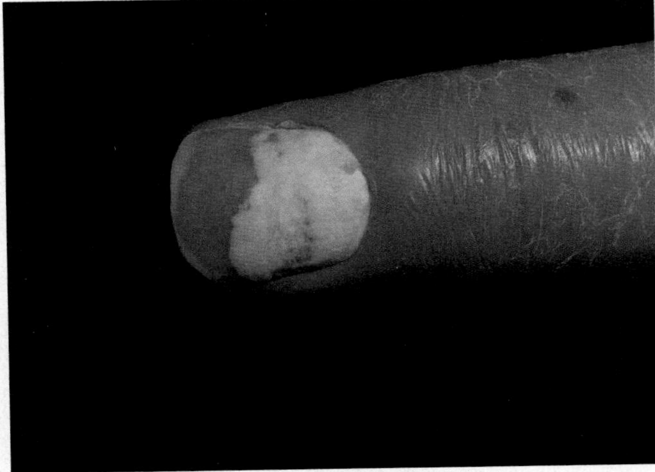

FIGURE 201-3 Proximal white subungual onychomycosis in an immunosuppressed man with scleroderma. The culture grew *Trichophyton rubrum*. *(Reproduced with permission from Richard P. Usatine, MD.)*

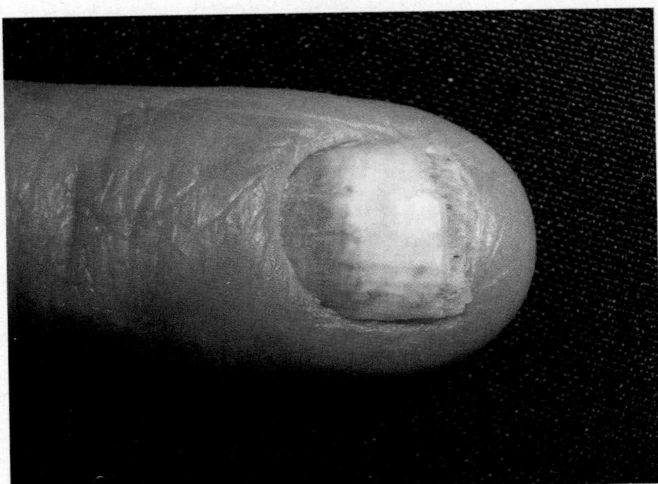

FIGURE 201-4 Distal white subungual onychomycosis. *(Reproduced with permission from Richard P. Usatine, MD.)*

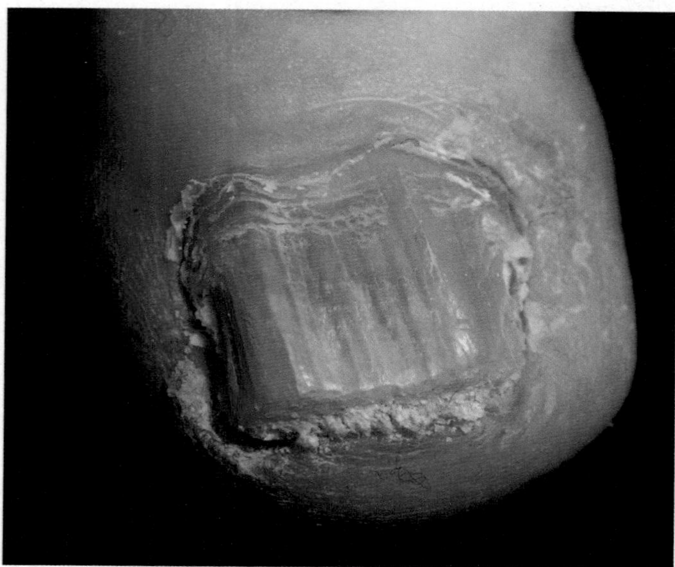

FIGURE 201-5 Total dystrophic onychomycosis. KOH was positive for branching hyphae. (*Reproduced with permission from Richard P. Usatine, MD.*)

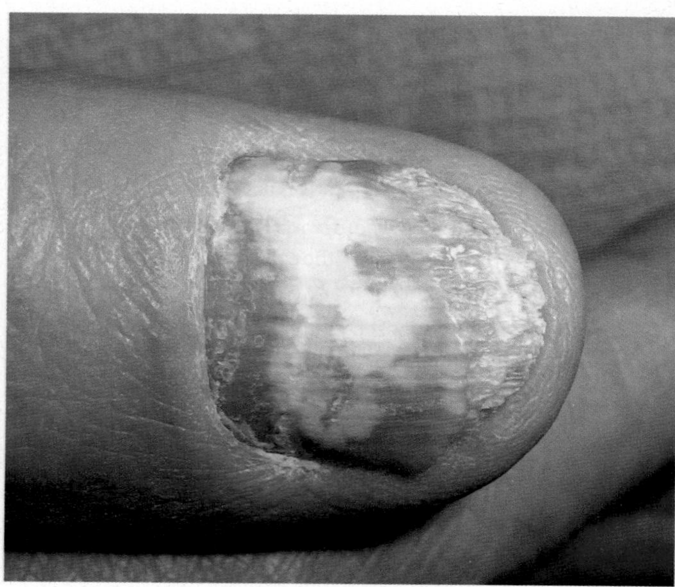

FIGURE 201-7 White superficial onychomycosis of the thumbnail. The culture was positive for *Trichophyton mentagrophytes*. (*Reproduced with permission from Richard P. Usatine, MD.*)

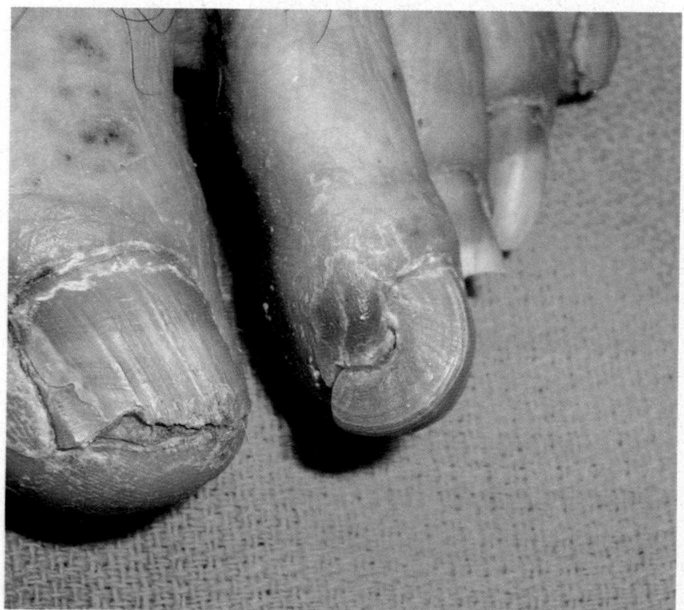

FIGURE 201-6 Severe toenail onychomycosis demonstrating subungual keratosis in the first nail and onychogryphosis (ram's horn nail) in the second nail because of the fungal infection. The culture grew *Trichophyton rubrum*. (*Reproduced with permission from Richard P. Usatine, MD.*)

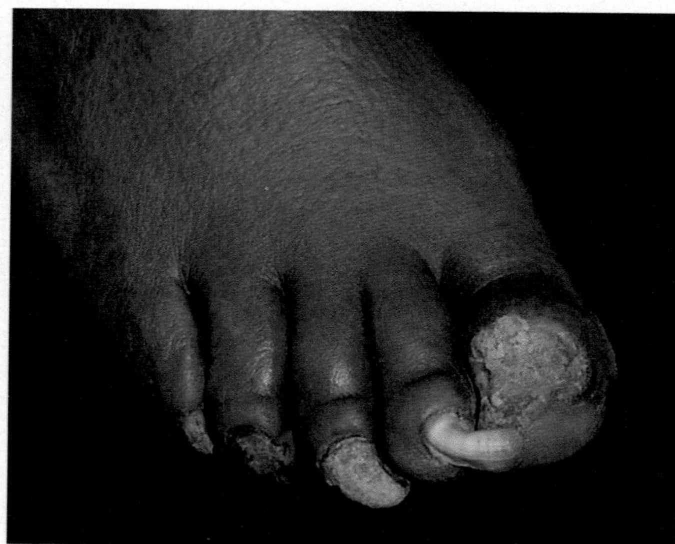

FIGURE 201-8 Extensive onychomycosis involving all toenails in an HIV-positive man. His second toenail shows onychogryphosis (ram's horn nail) secondary to the fungal infection. (*Reproduced with permission from Richard P. Usatine, MD.*)

TYPICAL DISTRIBUTION

- Nail infection may occur in a single digit but most often occurs simultaneously in multiple digits of the foot. Toenails and fingernails may be affected at the same time, especially in patients who are immunocompromised (see **Figures 201-5** and **201-6**).

LABORATORY TESTING

- KOH and culture—Clippings of nail plate and scrapings of subungual keratosis can be examined with KOH and microscopy and/or sent to the laboratory in a sterile container to be inoculated onto Sabouraud medium to culture.
- Dermatophyte test medium (DTM) culture is an alternative to Sabouraud medium culture and was once performed in the office before the current regulations changed this option.[6]
- Clippings—Nail clippings may be sent to pathology in formalin to be examined with periodic acid–Schiff (PAS) stain for fungal elements. This can be more sensitive than KOH and culture.
- Comparison of diagnostic methods:
    - In a 2003 study by Weinberg et al, the sensitivities for onychomycosis detection were KOH 80%, Bx/PAS 92%, and culture 59%. The specificities were KOH 72%, Bx/PAS 72%, and culture 82%. The positive predictive values were KOH 88%, Bx/PAS 89.7%, and culture 90%. The negative predictive values were KOH 58%, Bx/PAS 77%, and culture 43%.[7]
    - In a 2007 study of the diagnosis of onychomycosis by Hsiao et al, the sensitivities of KOH, PAS, and culture were 87%, 81%, and 67%, respectively, and the negative predictive values of KOH, PAS, and culture were 50%, 40%, and 28%, respectively. One reason that the KOH may have done so well is that the nail specimen was immersed in 20% KOH in a test tube for 30 minutes or longer before being examined under the microscope.[8]
    - KOH may be equivalent to PAS if done and read properly. It is less expensive and the results are available while the patient is in the office. PAS is a good second line if the KOH is negative and the suspicion for onychomycosis is still present.

DIFFERENTIAL DIAGNOSIS

- Nail trauma can cause a dysmorphic nail that is discolored and thickened. It is especially seen in the big toenail in runners. Ask about nail trauma before diagnosing onychomycosis. Although onychomycosis often starts in the big toenail, it usually spreads to other nails. Traumatic changes often present with only one nail involved.
- Psoriatic and lichen planus nail changes may easily be confused with onychomycosis, especially when the nail becomes thickened and discolored. Pitting of the nail plate surface, which is common in psoriasis, is not a feature of fungal infection. It is possible for a patient with psoriasis to get onychomycosis. Fungal studies can help determine if the changes are truly secondary to onychomycosis (see Chapter 203, Psoriatic Nails).
- Pseudomonal nail infection—Produces a blue-green tint to the nail plate (**Figure 201-9**).
- Leukonychia—White spots or bands that appear proximally and proceed out with the nail may be confused with white superficial onychomycosis (see Chapter 198, Normal Nail Variants).
- Habitual picking of the proximal nail fold—Induces the nail plate to be wavy and ridged, although its substance remains intact and hard (see Chapter 198, Normal Nail Variants).

MANAGEMENT

- Treating onychomycosis can be discouraging. Most topical creams and lotions do not penetrate the nail plate well and are of little value except in controlling inflammation at the nail folds.
- Surgical avulsion may be used to decrease pain caused by pressure on an elevated nail plate because of a dermatophytoma (a collection of dermatophytes and cellular debris under the nail plate). Recurrences are common in the absence of additional systemic or topical therapy with ciclopirox, as the infection typically involves the nail matrix and bed. SOR Ⓒ

MEDICATIONS

FIRST LINE

- Oral therapy (**Table 201-1**) is no longer expensive now that terbinafine is generic and on many discounted drug lists.
- Terbinafine dosing is 250 mg daily for 3 months for toenail onychomycosis and 2 months to treat fingernail involvement only.[9] SOR Ⓐ
- A Cochrane review found that the evidence suggests that terbinafine is more effective than griseofulvin and that terbinafine and itraconazole are more effective than no treatment.[10] SOR Ⓐ
- Another Cochrane review found two trials of nail infections that did not provide any evidence of benefit for topical treatments (ciclopirox not included) compared with placebo.[11] SOR Ⓐ
- Terbinafine has a preferable drug interaction profile and may have better long-term cure rates; daily dosing may be the most effective treatment.[9,11] SOR Ⓐ
- Itraconazole (Sporanox) has more drug interactions. Pulse dosing is as effective as daily dosing, but even with pulse dosing, therapy is more costly than terbinafine. Consider itraconazole if terbinafine does not effectively treat onychomycosis caused by fungus other than dermatophytes. SOR Ⓒ
- Fluconazole (Diflucan) is not currently approved by the U.S. Food and Drug Administration (FDA) for nail therapy and is not as effective as other oral therapies.[11,12] SOR Ⓑ

SECOND LINE

- Ciclopirox 8% nail lacquer (Penlac) used daily (with weekly nail cleaning and filing) is an FDA-approved topical treatment for mild to moderate onychomycosis. A meta-analysis of 2 randomized controlled trials showed a clinical cure rate of 8% versus 1% for vehicle alone.[13] Such a low cure rate is disappointing, but a larger group of patients had some improvement without cure. This is one option for persons able to afford this topical treatment but who are not able to take oral antifungals.

- Tavaborole (Kerydin) is a topical antifungal approved by the FDA in 2014. It exhibits activity against a broad range of dermatophytes. It is unique in that its low molecular weight allows for improved penetration through the nail plate. In clinical trials tavaborole was found to have a clinical cure rate of 6.5%–9.1%, a clear or almost clear nail rate of 26.1–27.5%, and a negative mycologic rate of 31.1%–35.9%. Dosing calls for covering the entire nail plate and under the distal edge of the nail once daily for 48 weeks. Exfoliation (2.7%), erythema (1.6%), and dermatitis (1.3%) were the most common adverse events.[14]
- Efinaconazole (Jublia) is another topical antifungal approved by the FDA in 2014 for the treatment of onychomycosis. Efinaconazole has a particularly low affinity for binding to keratin as compared to ciclopirox which significantly increases it penetration to the nail bed as compared to ciclopirox or amorolfine. The

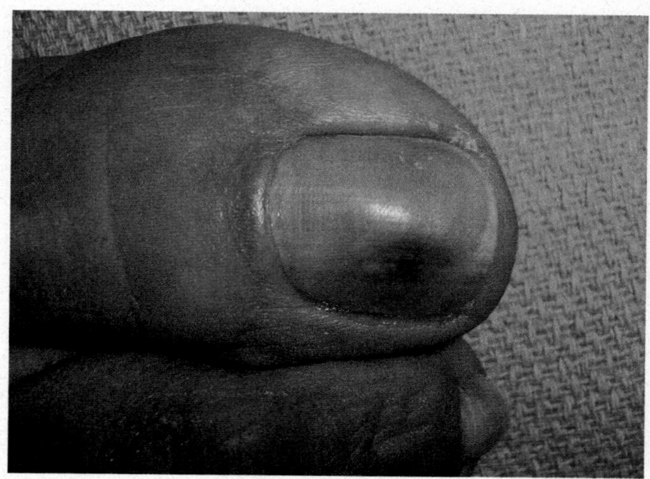

FIGURE 201-9 *Pseudomonas* of the nail showing a blue-green discoloration. (*Reproduced with permission from Richard P. Usatine, MD.*)

TABLE 201-1 Common Treatments for Onychomycosis

Drug	Pediatric Dose	Adult Dose	Course	Toenail Cure Rate
Griseofulvin (Grifulvin V)	Microsize 15 to 20 mg/kg per day	500 mg PO qd	4 to 9 months (f), 6 to 12 months (t)	60%–6%
Terbinafine (Lamisil)	10 to 20 kg: 62.5 mg/day 20 to 40 kg: 125 mg/day	250 mg PO qd	6 weeks (f), 12 weeks (t)	76%–3%
Terbinafine (Lamisil) pulse*	—	250 mg bid 1 wk/mo	2 months (f), 3 months (t)	NR
Itraconazole (Sporanox)	—	200 mg daily	6 weeks (f), 12 weeks (t)	59%–5%
Itraconazole (Sporanox) pulse	<20 kg: 5 mg/kg per day for 1 wk/mo 20 to 40 kg: 100 mg daily for 1 wk/mo	200 mg bid or 5 mg/kg per day capsules for 1 wk/mo	2 months (f), 3 months (t)	63%–7%
Fluconazole (Diflucan)	3 to 6 mg/kg once a wk	150 mg once a wk	12 to 16 weeks (f), 18 to 26 weeks (t)	48%–5%
Ciclopirox 8% nail lacquer (Penlac)	—	Apply daily to nail and surrounding 5 mm skin	Up to 48 weeks	Approximately 7%
Tavaborole (Kerydin)	—	Apply to the entire nail plate and under the distal edge of nail once daily	48 weeks	6.5%–9.1%
Efinaconazole (Jublia)	—	Apply to entire nail plate and under distal edge of nail once daily	48 weeks	15.2%–17.8%

Abbreviation: NR, not recorded.
*Not indicated for treating onychomycosis by the FDA.
Data from Harrell TK, Necomb WW, Replogle WH, et al. Onychomycosis: improved cure rates with itraconazole and terbinafine. *J Am Board Fam Pract.* 2000;13(4):268-273; Bell-Syer S, Porthouse J, Bigby M. Oral treatments for toenail onychomycosis. *Cochrane Database Syst Rev.* 2004;(2):CD004766; Crawford F, Hart R, Bell-Syer S, et al. Topical treatments for fungal infections of the skin and nails of the foot. *Cochrane Database Syst Rev.* 1999;(3):CD001434; Havu V, Heikkila H, Kuokkanen K, et al. A double-blind, randomized study to compare the efficacy and safety of terbinafine (Lamisil) with fluconazole (Diflucan) in the treatment of onychomycosis. *Br J Dermatol.* 2000;142(1):97-102; and Sanders J, Maki K, Koski R, Nybo SE. Tavaborole, efinaconazole, and luliconazole: three new antimycotic agents for the treatment of dermatophytic fungi. *J Pharm Pract.* 2017;30(6):621-630.

complete cure rate of efinaconazole in clinical trials was 15.2%–17.8%. The negative mycologic rate was 53.4%–55.2% and the treatment success rate ranged from 31.0% to 35.7%. Dosing is once daily for 48 weeks applied to the entire nail plate, nail folds, toenail bed, hyponychium, and undersurface of the nail. The most common adverse events were dermatitis at the application site (3.5%), application site vesicles (2.0%), and ingrown toenail (2.6%).[14]

- Amorolfine (Curanail, Loceryl, Locetar, Odenil) is a topical antifungal agent with activity against dermatophytes, yeasts, and fungi that is available over the counter in Australia, Russia, and the United Kingdom, but is not approved for use in the United States. Amorolfine 5% nail lacquer has been used as monotherapy for the treatment of onychomycosis. It is applied once weekly after the surface of the nail is filed with a disposable file and wiped with alcohol. Once-weekly application of amorolfine 5% nail lacquer for 6 months led to both clinical and mycologic cure in 38% and 46% of patients. It may also be used to increase cure rates when used in combination with oral antifungals.[15]
- Although these topical therapies can be effective, their use should still be considered second line to oral therapies terbinafine (preferred) and itraconazole because of the much lower efficacy rates of the topical therapies. Topical therapies should be considered only in those who have had an adverse reaction or contraindication to oral therapy.[14]

NONPHARMACOLOGIC

- Nine laser systems have been approved by the FDA to treat onychomycosis. The approval process is different for device-based therapy than for medical therapy, and the approval statement differs as well. The lasers are approved for a "temporary increase in clear nail in onychomycosis," and no reference is made to mycologic cure. Data from randomized controlled trials of efficacy are still lacking.[16]

COMPLEMENTARY AND ALTERNATIVE THERAPY

- There are numerous complementary and alternative medicine (CAM) therapies described on the Internet, most of which have minimal or no evidence of clinical efficacy.
- Mentholated chest rub—There is minimal data on the efficacy of a mentholated chest rub (Vicks VapoRub) in the treatment of onychomycosis. In a series of 18 patients who applied the medication to affected nails daily for 48 weeks, 4 patients (22%) achieved both clinical and mycologic cure.[17] Although these products are unlikely to be harmful, additional studies that support their efficacy in onychomycosis are necessary before widespread use can be recommended.

PREVENTION

Patients should be educated about the use of appropriate footwear, especially in high-exposure areas such as communal bathing facilities and health clubs.

PROGNOSIS

The condition may persist indefinitely if left untreated.

In patients with diabetes or other immunocompromised states, onychomycosis may increase the risk of secondary bacterial infections.[18]

FOLLOW-UP

Routine monitoring of liver function tests during therapy is probably not necessary in patients without underlying liver disease. However, because the manufacturer of terbinafine recommends checking pretreatment serum transaminases and monitoring for potential symptoms of hepatotoxicity during treatment, many clinicians routinely obtain pretreatment and mid-therapy values.

PATIENT EDUCATION

Patients should be advised that with treatment, nails may not appear normal for up to 1 year. The normal nail must grow out as treatment progresses. The appearance of normal-appearing nails at the proximal edge of the nail is an encouraging sign at the completion of therapy.

PATIENT RESOURCES

- eMedicineHealth. *Onychomycosis*—**http://www.emedicinehealth.com/onychomycosis/article_em.htm.**
- Familydoctor.org website. *Nail Fungal Infections*—**https://familydoctor.org/condition/nail-fungal-infections/.**
- MedicineNet. *Fungal Nails*—**http://www.medicinenet.com/fungal_nails/article.htm.**

PROVIDER RESOURCES

- Tosti A. *Onychomycosis*—**http://emedicine.medscape.com/article/1105828-overview.** Accessed January 2017.
- Westerberg DP, Voyack, MJ; American Family Physician. *Onychomycosis: Current Trends in Diagnosis and Treatment*—**http://www.aafp.org/afp/2013/1201/p762.html.** Accessed January 2017.
- Elewski BE. Onychomycosis: pathogenesis, diagnosis, and management. *Clin Microbiol Rev.* 1998;11(3):415-429—**http://www.ncbi.nlm.nih.gov/pmc/articles/PMC88888/.** Accessed January 2017.
- DermNet NZ. *Fungal Nail Infections*—**https://dermnetnz.org/topics/fungal-nail-infections/.** Accessed January 2017.

REFERENCES

1. Westerberg D, Voyac M. Onychomycosis: current trends in diagnosis and treatment. *Am Fam Physician.* 2013;88(11):762-770.
2. Sigurgeirsson B, Baran R. The prevalence of onychomycosis in the global population—a literature study. *J Eur Acad Dermatol Venereol.* 2014;28:1480-1491.

3. Gupta AK. Prevalence and epidemiology of onychomycosis in patients visiting physicians' offices: a multicenter Canadian survey of 15,000 patients. *J Am Acad Dermatol.* 2000;43:244.
4. Grover C, Khurana A. Onychomycosis: newer insights in pathogenesis and diagnosis. *Indian J Dermatol Venereol Leprol.* 2012; 78:263-269.
5. Sigurgeirsson B, Steingrímsson O. Risk factors associated with onychomycosis. *J Eur Acad Dermatol Venereol.* 2004;18:48.
6. Elewski BE, Leyden J, Rinaldi MG, Atillasoy E. Office practice-based confirmation of onychomycosis: a US nationwide prospective survey. *Arch Intern Med.* 2002;162:2133.
7. Weinberg JM, Koestenblatt EK, Tutrone WD, et al. Comparison of diagnostic methods in the evaluation of onychomycosis. *J Am Acad Dermatol.* 2003;49(2):193-197.
8. Hsiao YP, Lin HS, Wu TW, et al. A comparative study of KOH test, PAS staining and fungal culture in diagnosis of onychomycosis in Taiwan. *J Dermatol Sci.* 2007;45(2):138-140.
9. Bell-Syer S, Porthouse J, Bigby M. Oral treatments for toenail onychomycosis. *Cochrane Database Syst Rev. 2004;(2): CD004766.*
10. Crawford F, Hart R, Bell-Syer S, et al. Topical treatments for fungal infections of the skin and nails of the foot. *Cochrane Database Syst Rev.* 1999;(3):CD001434.
11. Harrell TK, Necomb WW, Replogle WH, et al. Onychomycosis: improved cure rates with itraconazole and terbinafine. *J Am Board Fam Pract.* 2000;13(4):268-273.
12. Havu V, Heikkila H, Kuokkanen K, et al. A double-blind, randomized study to compare the efficacy and safety of terbinafine (Lamisil) with fluconazole (Diflucan) in the treatment of onychomycosis. *Br J Dermatol.* 2000;142(1):97-102.
13. Gupta AK, Joseph WS. Ciclopirox 8% nail lacquer in the treatment of onychomycosis of the toenails in the United States. *J Am Podiatr Med Assoc.* 2000;90(10):495-501.
14. Sanders J, Maki K, Koski R, Nybo SE. Tavaborole, efinaconazole, and luliconazole:three new antimycotic agents for the treatment of dermatophytic fungi. *J Pharm Pract.* 2017;30(6):621-630.
15. Baran R, Kaoukhov A. Topical antifungal drugs for the treatment of onychomycosis: an overview of current strategies for monotherapy and combination therapy. *J Eur Acad Dermatol Venereol.* 2005;19:21.
16. Gupta AK, Paquet M, Simpson F. Therapies for the treatment of onychomycosis. *Clin Dermatol.* 2013;31:544-554.
17. Derby R, Rohal P, Jackson C, et al. Novel treatment of onychomycosis using over-the-counter mentholated ointment: a clinical case series. *J Am Board Fam Med.* 2011;24:69.
18. Bristow IR, Spruce MC. Fungal foot infection, cellulitis and diabetes: a review. *Diabet Med.* 2009;26:548.

202 PARONYCHIA

E.J. Mayeaux, Jr., MD

PATIENT STORY

A 41-year-old woman presented with a 3-day history of localized pain, redness, and tenderness of the lateral nail fold of the index finger. A small abscess had developed in the last 24 hours at the nail margin (**Figure 202-1**). After informed consent was given, a digital block was performed. This acute paronychia was treated with incision and drainage using a #11 scalpel (**Figure 202-2**). A significant amount of pus was drained. She soaked her finger four times daily as directed. Two days later the patient's finger was much better, and the culture grew out *Staphylococcus aureus*. Draining the abscess was sufficient treatment.

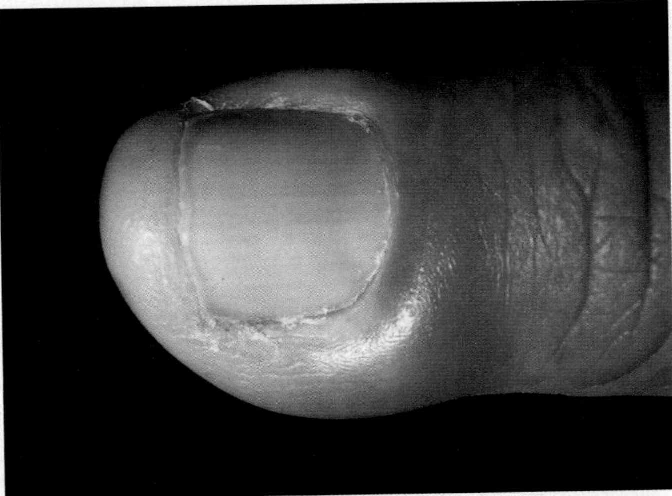

FIGURE 202-1 Painful acute paronychia around the fingernail of a 41-year-old woman. Note the swelling and erythema with a small white-yellow area suggesting underlying purulence. (*Reproduced with permission from Richard P. Usatine, MD.*)

INTRODUCTION

Paronychia is a localized, superficial infection or abscess of the nail folds. It is one of the most common infections of the hand. Paronychia can be acute or chronic. Acute paronychia usually presents as an acutely painful abscess in the nail fold. Chronic paronychia is defined as being present for longer than 6 weeks' duration. It is a generalized red, tender swelling of the proximal or lateral nail folds. It is usually nonsuppurative and is more difficult to treat.

EPIDEMIOLOGY

Paronychia is the most common infection of the hand, representing 35% of all hand infections in the United States.[1]

ETIOLOGY AND PATHOPHYSIOLOGY

- Paronychial infections develop when a disruption occurs between the seal of the nail fold and the nail plate or the skin of a nail fold is disrupted and allows a portal of entry for invading organisms.[2]
- Acute paronychia is most commonly caused by *S. aureus*, followed by streptococci and *Pseudomonas* (**Figures 202-1** to **202-5**).[1]
- In digits heavily exposed to oral flora, acute paronychia may be caused by oral flora including aerobic bacteria (streptococci and *Eikenella* species) and anaerobic bacteria (*Fusobacterium*, *Prevotella*, *Peptostreptococcus*, and *Porphyromonas* species).[3]
- Chronic paronychia is an irritant or allergic reaction, secondary to contact, allergic, or hypersensitivity, or irritative causes[4,5] (**Figures 202-6** and **202-7**). *Candida* or *Pseudomonas* infection is sometimes a secondary phenomenon, or it may be a sensitizing agent.[6]
- Untreated persistent chronic paronychia may cause horizontal ridging, undulations, and other changes to the nail plate (see **Figures 202-6** and **202-7**).

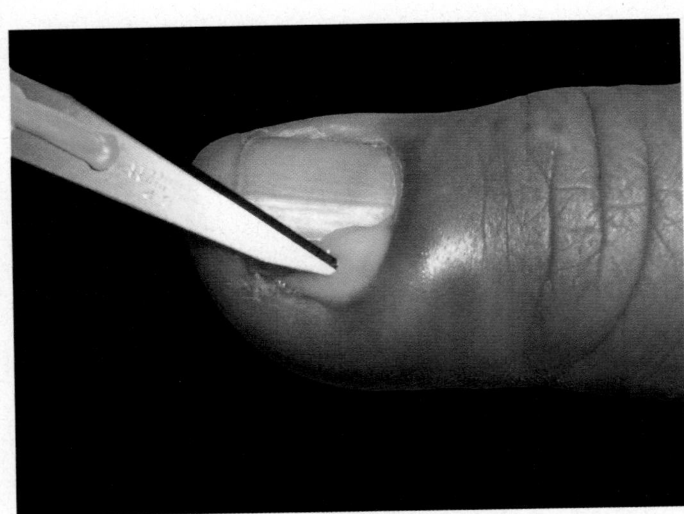

FIGURE 202-2 Incision and drainage of the acute paronychia in the previous figure with a #11 scalpel. Note the exuberant pus draining from the incision. (*Reproduced with permission from Richard P. Usatine, MD.*)

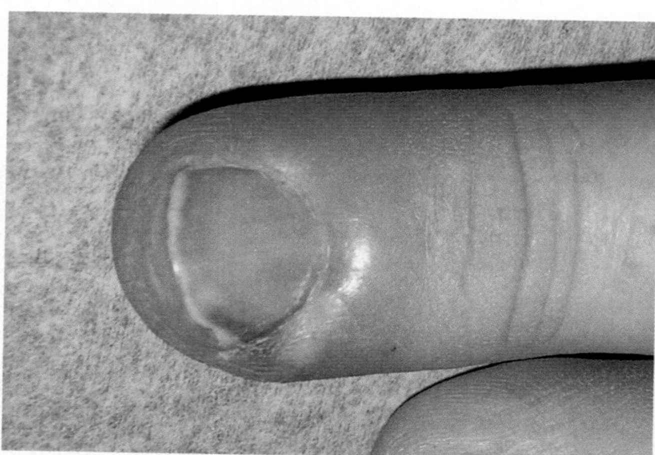

FIGURE 202-3 Acute paronychia from nail biting. Note abscess formation in the lateral nail fold that is extending into the proximal fold. (*Reproduced with permission from E.J. Mayeaux, Jr., MD.*)

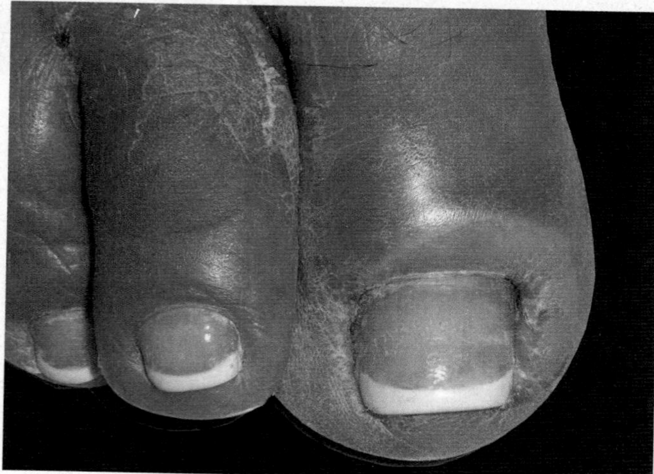

FIGURE 202-4 Acute paronychia of the great toe. Note extensive manicure of the nails, which may predispose to paronychia if the cuticle or nail folds are disrupted. (*Reproduced with permission from Jennifer P. Pierce, MD.*)

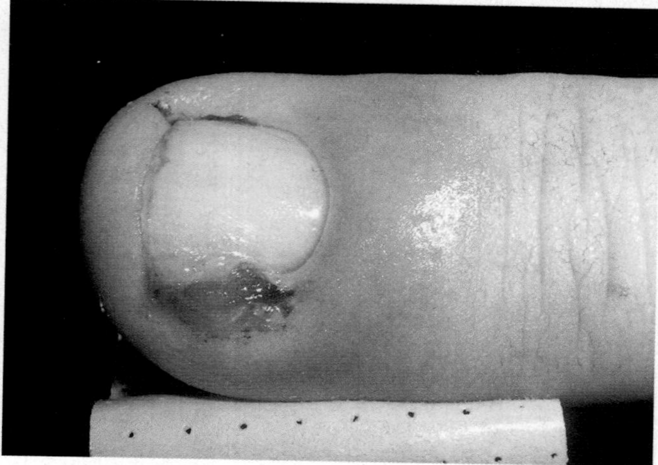

FIGURE 202-5 Acute paronychia with cellulitis of the skin of the fingertip and granulation tissue formation. This all started when the patient began manipulating a hangnail. (*Reproduced with permission from Richard P. Usatine, MD.*)

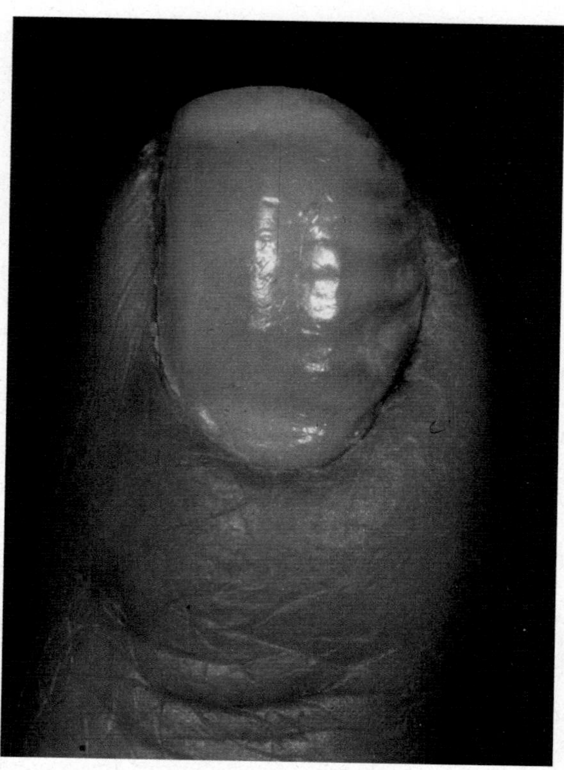

FIGURE 202-6 Chronic paronychia. Note horizontal ridges on one side of the nail plate as a result of chronic inflammation. (*Reproduced with permission from Richard P. Usatine, MD.*)

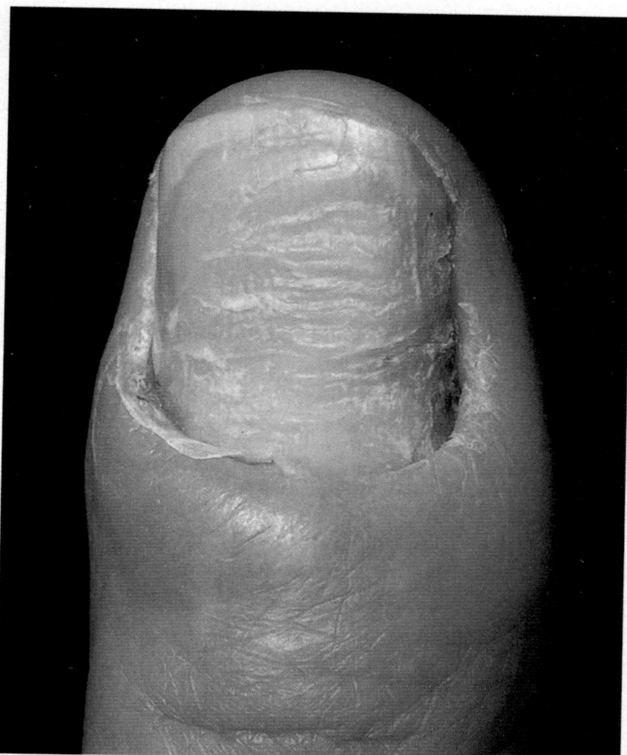

FIGURE 202-7 Chronic paronychia causing a dysmorphic fingernail with horizontal ridging. (*Reproduced with permission from Richard P. Usatine, MD.*)

RISK FACTORS

- Acute paronychia commonly results from nail biting (see **Figure 202-3**), finger sucking, aggressive manicuring (see **Figure 202-6**), hangnails (see **Figure 202-5**), trauma, excessive handwashing, obsessive nail biting or picking, aggressive cuticle removal, frequent contact with chemicals, and/or the application of artificial nails involving the use of chemicals that can result in damage to the cuticle.[2,5,7]
- Children are prone to acute paronychia through direct infection of fingers with mouth flora from finger sucking and nail biting.
- People at risk of developing chronic paronychia include those who are repeatedly exposed to liquid irritants or alkali, and those whose hands are chronically wet. People with occupations such as baker, bartender, housekeepers, and dishwashers are predisposed to developing chronic paronychia.[5]
- Patients with diabetes mellitus, compromised immune systems, or a history of oral steroid use are at increased risk for paronychia. Retroviral therapy use, especially indinavir and lamivudine, may be associated with an increased incidence of paronychia.[8]
- Other drugs associated with paronychia include oral retinoids, cephalexin, docetaxel, 5-fluorouracil, methotrexate, cyclophosphamide, vincristine, and intralesional injections of bleomycin.[5]
- Sculptured (artificial) nail placement is associated with the development of paronychia.[1]

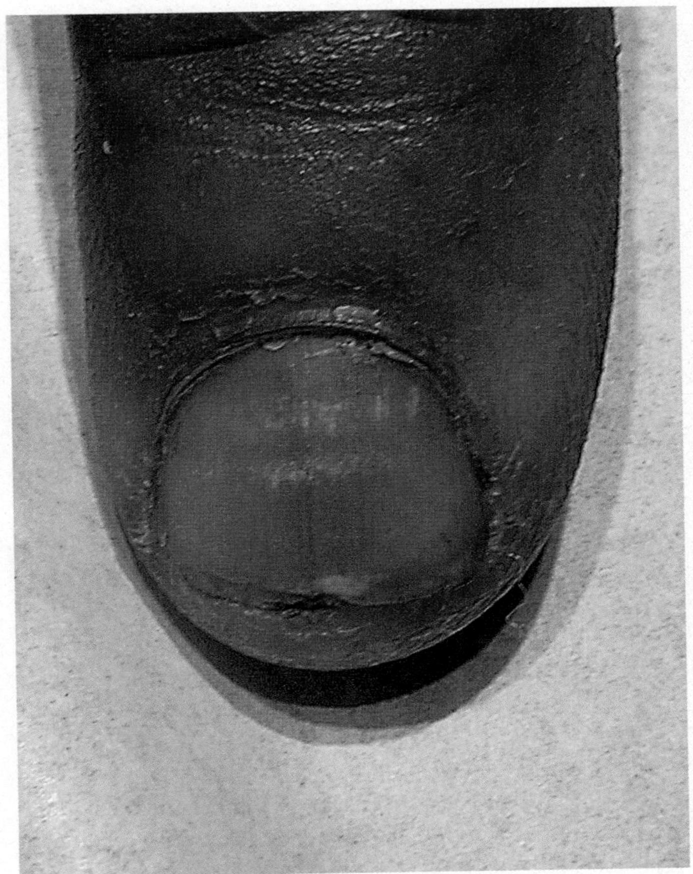

FIGURE 202-8 The proximal nail fold is tender to palpation but the erythema is less visible due to the dark skin type. (*Reproduced with permission from E.J. Mayeaux, Jr., MD.*)

DIAGNOSIS

CLINICAL FEATURES

- Acute paronychia presents with localized pain and tenderness. The nail fold appears erythematous and inflamed, and a collection of pus usually develops (see **Figures 202-1** to **202-5**). Granulation tissue may develop along the nail fold, and cellulitis may also develop (see **Figure 202-5**).
- Chronic paronychia is a red, tender, painful swelling of the proximal or lateral nail folds. A small collection of pus or abscess may form, but typically only redness and swelling are present. Eventually, the nail plates may become thickened and discolored, with pronounced horizontal ridges (see **Figures 202-6** and **202-7**) or transverse striate leukonychia **(Figure 202-8)**.[5,9]

DIFFERENTIAL DIAGNOSIS

- Mucus cyst—Presents as a painless swelling lateral and proximal to the nail plate (**Figure 202-9**); may be confused with paronychia. This can also cause changes in the nail morphology.
- Ingrown nail (onychocryptosis)—A condition in which the nail plate is too large for the nail bed. The pressure applied to the lateral nail fold causes a painful inflammation. Although this is sometimes called paronychia, it is different from the type of paronychia caused by an infection of the nail fold (see Chapter 200, Ingrown Toenail).

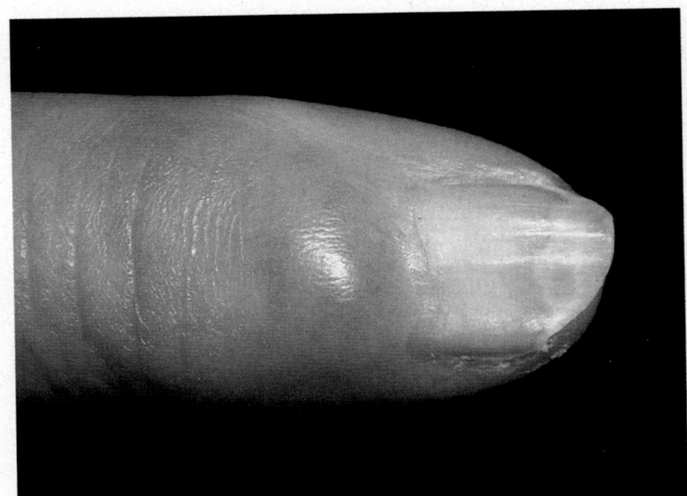

FIGURE 202-9 Digital mucus cyst presenting as a painless swelling of the nail fold in a young woman. Note the indented area of the nail caused by the pressure of the mucus cyst on the nail matrix. (*Reproduced with permission from Richard P. Usatine, MD.*)

- Glomus tumor—Presents with constant severe pain, nail plate elevation, bluish discoloration of the nail plate, and blurring of the lunula; may be confused with paronychia.
- Herpetic whitlow—Results from herpes simplex virus (HSV) infection. Presents with acute onset of vesicles or pustules, severe edema, erythema, and pain. Tzanck staining of vesicles will demonstrate multinucleated giant cells, and viral culture will grow HSV (see Chapter 135, Herpes Simplex).
- Felon—Paronychia must be distinguished from a felon, which is an infection of the digital pulp (**Figure 202-10**). It is characterized by severe pain, swelling, and erythema in the pad of the fingertip.
- Benign and malignant neoplasms, which may present early with redness and swelling, should always be ruled out when chronic paronychia does not respond to conventional treatment.

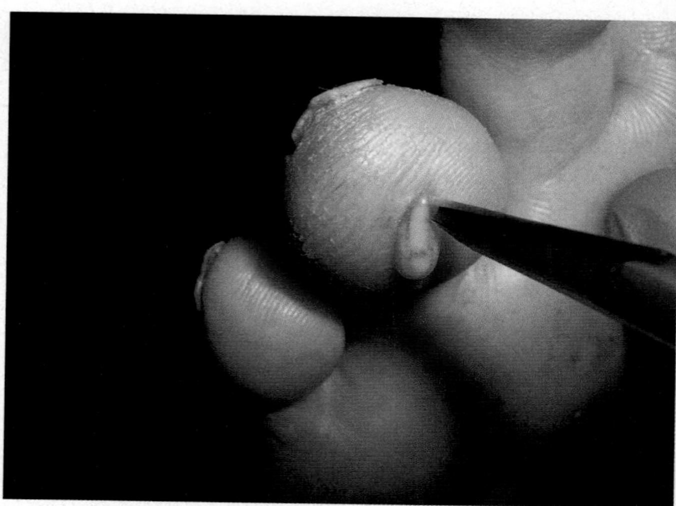

FIGURE 202-10 A felon being drained in a 45-year-old woman who presented with an extremely red, swollen, painful toe. The pus poured out and the pain subsided, even after the anesthesia wore off. *(Reproduced with permission from Richard P. Usatine, MD.)*

MANAGEMENT

NONPHARMACOLOGIC

- Milder cases of acute paronychia without abscess formation may be treated with warm soaks for 20 minutes 3 to 4 times a day with or without mupirocin.[2,10] SOR C
- When an abscess or fluctuance is present, drainage is necessary.[11] It is performed with digital block anesthesia. The affected nail fold is incised with a scalpel with the blade parallel to the edge of the nail plate and the pus expressed (see **Figure 202-2**). Warm soaks 3–4 times a day are initiated to keep the incision from sealing until all of the pus is gone.[12] Between soakings, an adhesive bandage can protect the nail fold. Antibiotic therapy is usually not necessary unless there is accompanying cellulitis. SOR C

MEDICATIONS

- Although antibiotics are not necessary for simple paronychia, addition of an oral antistaphylococcal agent (dicloxacillin 500 mg 3 times daily, cephalexin 500 mg 2 to 3 times daily for 7 to 10 days, erythromycin 333 to 500 mg 3 times daily, or azithromycin 500 mg on day 1 followed by 250 mg daily for 4 days) may be added for cases with coexisting cellulitis or that are unresponsive. SOR C
- Both children who suck their fingers and patients who bite their nails and who require antibiotics should be covered against anaerobes. Clindamycin and amoxicillin-clavulanate potassium are effective against most pathogens isolated from infections originating in the mouth.[13]
- Long-term treatment of chronic paronychia primarily involves avoiding predisposing factors such as prolonged exposure to water, nail trauma, and finger sucking.
- Treatment of chronic paronychia usually requires application of a mild-potency topical steroid (methylprednisolone aceponate 0.1% cream) at bedtime[14] or tacrolimus 0.1% ointment applied twice a day.[15] SOR B As methylprednisolone aceponate is not available in the United States, one generic alternative is triamcinolone 0.1% cream. Tacrolimus may require a prior authorization in the United States because of high pricing.

- Systemic steroids (methylprednisone 20 mg/kg/d) or triamcinolone acetonide 2.5 mg/mL into affected nail folds (monthly injections) may be used as an alternative in severe cases. SOR C Oral antifungal therapy is usually not necessary.[2,14] SOR B

PREVENTION

- Trim hangnails to a semilunar smooth edge with a clean, sharp nail plate trimmer. Trim toenails flush with the toe tip.
- Do not bite the nail plate or lateral nail folds.
- Avoid prolonged hand exposure to moisture. If handwashing must be frequent, use antibacterial soap, thoroughly dry hands with a clean towel, and apply an antibacterial moisturizer. Use cotton glove liners under waterproof gloves to keep hands dry from sweat and condensation.
- Wear rubber or latex-free gloves when there is potential exposure to pathogens.
- Control diabetes mellitus.
- Keep fingernails clean.
- Moisturize the skin; don't let it become chafed and cracked.

PROGNOSIS

Although the nail fold should improve with treatment, some chronic nail-plate changes may not resolve.

FOLLOW-UP

Patients can perform warm soaks 3 to 4 times per day and should have a follow-up examination several days after incision and drainage to ensure that the infection is resolving appropriately.

PATIENT EDUCATION

Educate patients on measures that may prevent or improve paronychia (above).

PATIENT RESOURCES

- eMedicineHealth. *Paronychia (Nail Infection)*—**http://www.emedicinehealth.com/paronychia_nail_infection/article_em.htm.**
- **Familydoctor.org.** Paronychia information—**http://familydoctor.org/condition/paronychia/.**

PROVIDER RESOURCES

- Rockwell PG. Acute and chronic paronychia. *Am Fam Physician.* 2001;63:1113-1116—**http://www.aafp.org/afp/20010315/1113.html.**
- Emedicine. *Paronychia*—**http://emedicine.medscape.com/article/1106062-overview.**

REFERENCES

1. Rockwell PG. Acute and chronic paronychia. *Am Fam Physician.* 2001;63(6):1113-1116.
2. Hochman LG. Paronychia: more than just an abscess. *Int J Dermatol.* 1995;34:385-386.
3. Brook I. Bacteriologic study of paronychia in children. *Am J Surg.* 1981;141:703.
4. Tosti A, Piraccini BM, Ghetti E, Colombo MD. Topical steroids versus systemic antifungals in the treatment of chronic paronychia: an open, randomized double-blind and double dummy study. *J Am Acad Dermatol.* 2002;47:73.
5. Chang P. Diagnosis using the proximal and lateral nail folds. *Dermatol Clin.* 2015;33(2):207-241.
6. Bahunuthula RK, Thappa DM, Kumari R, et al. Evaluation of role of *Candida* in patients with chronic paronychia. *Indian J Dermatol Venereol Leprol.* 2015;81:485-490.
7. Shemer A, Daniel CR 3rd. Common nail disorders. *Clin Dermatol.* 2013;31(5):578-586.
8. Tosti A, Piraccini BM, D'Antuono A, et al. Paronychia associated with antiretroviral therapy. *Br J Dermatol.* 1999;140(6):1165-1168.
9. Canales FL, Newmeyer WL 3d, Kilgore ES. The treatment of felons and paronychias. *Hand Clin.* 1989;5:515-523.
10. Wollina U. Acute paronychia: comparative treatment with topical antibiotic alone or in combination with corticosteroid. *J Eur Acad Dermatol Venereol.* 2001;15:82.
11. Keyser JJ, Littler JW, Eaton RG. Surgical treatment of infections and lesions of the perionychium. *Hand Clin.* 1990;6(1):137-153.
12. Mayeaux EJ Jr. Paronychia surgery. In: Mayeaux EJ Jr. *The Essential Guide to Primary Care Procedures*, 2nd ed. Philadelphia, PA: Lippincott Williams & Wilkins; 2015.
13. Brook I. Aerobic and anaerobic microbiology of paronychia. *Ann Emerg Med.* 1990;19:994-996.
14. Tosti A, Piraccini BM, Ghetti E, et al. Topical steroids versus systemic antifungals in the treatment of chronic paronychia: an open, randomized double-blind and double dummy study. *J Am Acad Dermatol.* 2002;47:73-76.
15. Rigopoulos D, Gregoriou S, Belyayeva E, et al. Efficacy and safety of tacrolimus ointment 0.1% vs. betamethasone 17-valerate 0.1% in the treatment of chronic paronychia: an unblinded randomized study. *Br J Dermatol.* 2009;160:858-860.

203 PSORIATIC NAILS

E.J. Mayeaux, Jr., MD

PATIENT STORY

A 19-year-old man with a 4-year history of plaque psoriasis presents with nail abnormalities in several fingers (**Figure 203-1**). He is particularly concerned about the recently acquired greenish discoloration of his fifth digit.

INTRODUCTION

Psoriasis is a hereditary disorder of skin with numerous clinical expressions. It affects millions of people throughout the world.[1] Nail involvement is common and can have a significant cosmetic impact.

EPIDEMIOLOGY

- Nails are involved in 30% to 66% of psoriasis patients at any given time, and 80% to 90% develop nail changes over their lifetime.[1,2] In most cases, nail involvement coexists with cutaneous psoriasis, although the skin surrounding the affected nails need not be involved. Psoriatic nail disease without overt cutaneous disease occurs in 1% to 5% of psoriasis cases.
- Patients with nail involvement are thought to have a higher incidence of associated arthritis.[2,3] Among patients with psoriatic arthritis, the prevalence of nail psoriasis is greater than 80%.[4] Psoriatic nail disease may be considered an indicator for patients at risk for future psoriatic joint damage.[5]
- The most common nail change seen with psoriasis is nail plate pitting (**Figures 203-1** and **203-2**).

ETIOLOGY AND PATHOPHYSIOLOGY

- In psoriasis, parakeratotic cells within the stratum corneum of the nail matrix alter normal keratinization.[4] The proximal nail matrix forms the superficial portion of the nail plate, so that involvement in this part of the matrix results in pitting of the nail plate (see **Figures 203-1** and **203-2**). The pits may range in size from pinpoint depressions to large punched-out lesions. People without psoriasis can have nail pitting.
- Longitudinal matrix involvement produces longitudinal nail ridging or splitting (see **Figure 203-2**). When transverse matrix involvement occurs, solitary or multiple "growth arrest" lines (Beau lines) may occur (see Chapter 198, Normal Nail Variants). Psoriatic involvement of the intermediate portion of the nail matrix leads to leukonychia and diminished nail plate integrity.
- Parakeratosis of the nail bed with thickening of the stratum corneum causes discoloration of the nail bed, producing the "salmon patch" or "oil drop" signs.[6]

FIGURE 203-1 Patient with nail psoriasis demonstrating the oil-drop sign (second digit), nail pitting (second and third digit), onycholysis (second, fourth and fifth digit), and secondary *Pseudomonas* infection (fifth digit). (*Reproduced with permission from E.J. Mayeaux, Jr., MD.*)

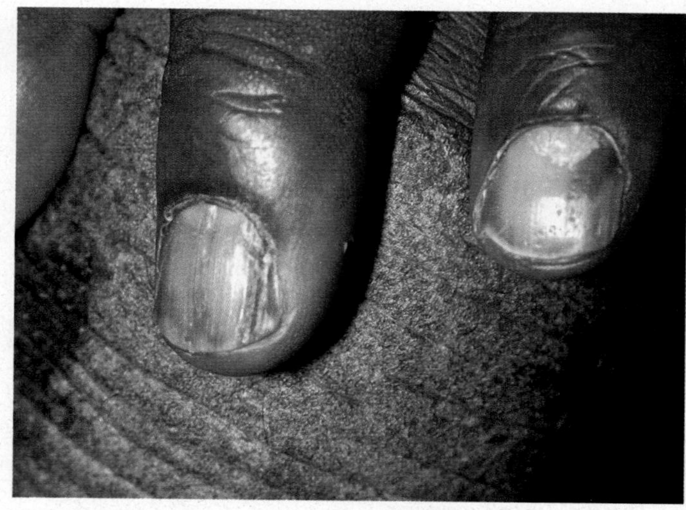

FIGURE 203-2 Nail psoriasis demonstrating nail pitting, onycholysis, oil-drop sign, and longitudinal ridging. Nails held over the silvery plaque on the knee. (*Reproduced with permission from Richard P. Usatine, MD.*)

- Desquamation of parakeratotic cells at the hyponychium leads to onycholysis, which may allow for bacterial and fungal infection.[7]

RISK FACTORS

- Psoriasis of the skin.
- Psoriatic arthritis.
- Nail unit trauma.
- Generalized psoriasis flare.

DIAGNOSIS

CLINICAL FEATURES

- The diagnosis of nail psoriasis is usually straightforward when characteristic nail findings coexist with cutaneous psoriasis. Nail pitting and onycholysis are the most common findings (**Figure 203-3**). Nail pitting is caused by intermittent psoriatic inflammation of the nail matrix.[4]
- Nail psoriasis and onychomycosis are often indistinguishable by clinical examination alone. Psoriasis at the hyponychium produces subungual hyperkeratosis and distal onycholysis (**Figures 203-4** and **203-5**). Trauma may accentuate this process. Secondary microbial colonization by *Candida* or *Pseudomonas* organisms may occur (see **Figures 203-1** and **203-5**).
- Nail-bed psoriasis produces localized onycholysis that often appears like a drop of oil on a piece of paper (oil-drop sign) (see **Figures 203-2, 203-4**, and **203-5**). This same condition is also called the salmon-patch sign.
- Extensive germinal matrix involvement may result in loss of nail integrity and transverse (horizontal) ridging (**Figure 203-6**).
- Psoriasis causes dermal vascular dilation and tortuosity, and in the nails it is associated with splinter hemorrhages of the nail bed caused by foci of capillary bleeding. Extravasated blood becomes trapped between the longitudinal troughs of the nail bed, and the overlying nail plate grows out distally along with the plate (**Figure 203-7**). The splinter hemorrhages of the psoriatic nail are analogous to the cutaneous Auspitz sign.

LABORATORY TESTING

- KOH preparation and fungal culture will usually provide an answer. However, it may be necessary to clip a portion of the nail plate and send it for fungal staining (periodic acid–Schiff [PAS] stain) if the first test results are not consistent with the clinical picture.[2] Psoriasis and onychomycosis can occur concomitantly.

IMAGING

- Dermoscopy can help visualize nail-bed changes such as oil-drop signs, salmon patches and splinter hemorrhages. In psoriasis, dermoscopy of the hyponychium demonstrate capillaries that are dilated, tortuous, and elongated, with irregular distribution. These changes correlate with disease severity and response to treatment. These capillary loops are seen as regular red with handheld

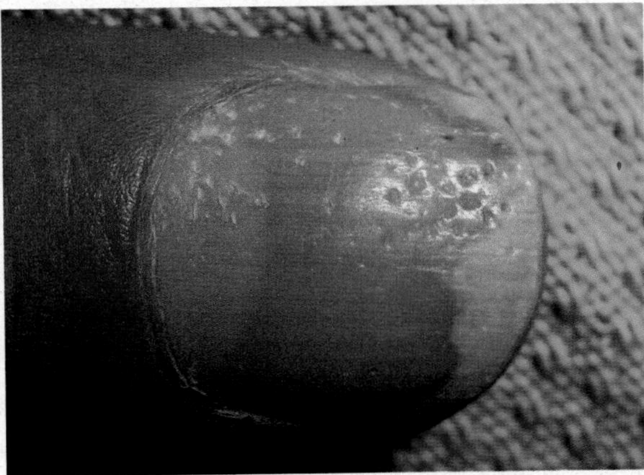

FIGURE 203-3 Nail pitting and onycholysis in a patient with psoriasis. *(Reproduced with permission from Richard P. Usatine, MD.)*

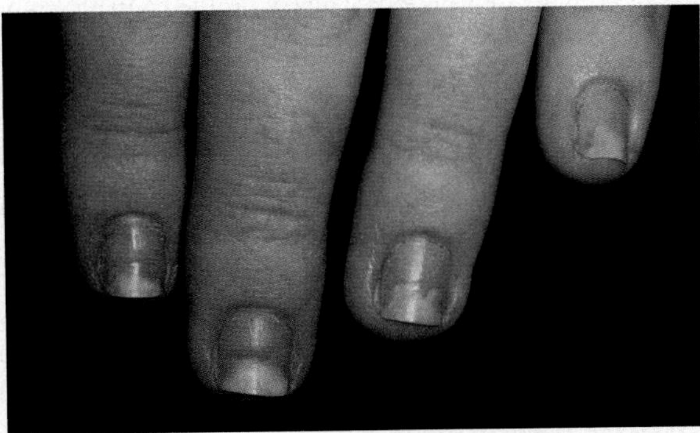

FIGURE 203-4 Nail psoriasis with onycholysis and oil-drop sign in a young woman. Note that the ends of the nail plates are no longer attached to the nail bed and there is a light brown discoloration where the nail loses its attachment. *(Reproduced with permission from Richard P. Usatine, MD.)*

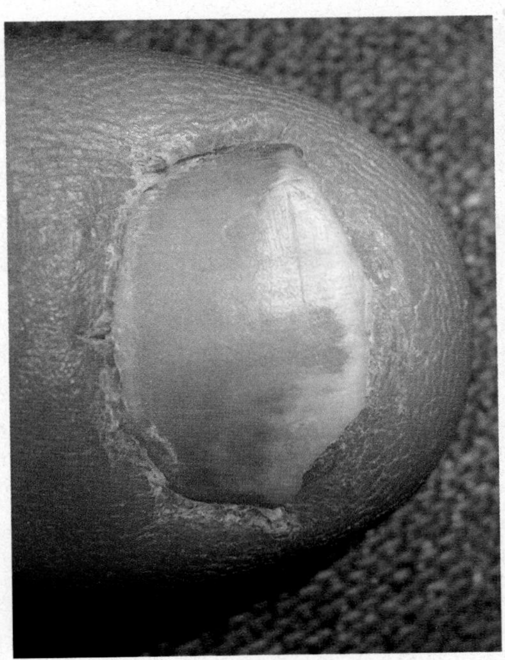

FIGURE 203-5 Nail psoriasis with the oil-drop sign proximal to the lighter onycholysis at the distal nail. *(Reproduced with permission from Richard P. Usatine, MD.)*

dermoscopy. The number and diameter of capillaries are decreased on the proximal nail folds of patients with nail psoriasis, which also improve with treatment.[8]

BIOPSY

- Biopsy of the nail unit is rarely necessary unless a malignancy is suspected.

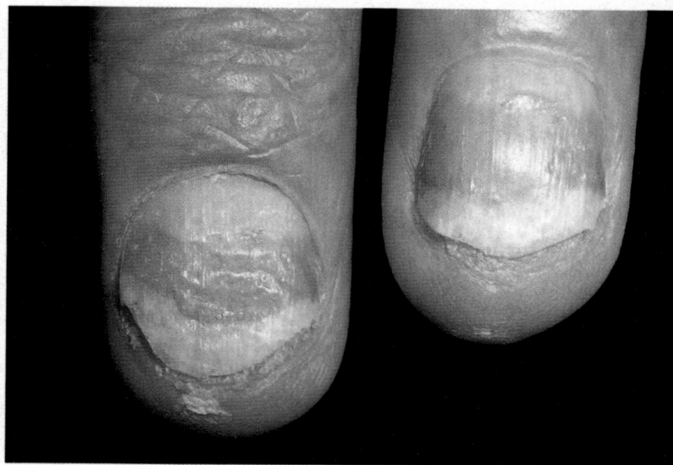

FIGURE 203-6 Nail psoriasis demonstrating onycholysis, pits, and transverse (horizontal) ridging. (*Reproduced with permission from Richard P. Usatine, MD.*)

DIFFERENTIAL DIAGNOSIS

- Onychomycosis produces distal onycholysis and hyperkeratosis that appear identical to psoriasis (see Chapter 201, Onychomycosis). Concomitant onychomycosis has a prevalence of 18.0% in psoriasis patients compared with a prevalence of 9.1% in control groups.[2]
- Lichen planus usually manifests in the nail as thin, grooved, or ridged nail plates and occasionally as scarring of the matrix to the ventral fold resulting in pterygium formation. The classic cutaneous manifestations of lichen planus are pruritic, violaceous, polygonal papules or plaques, especially on the wrists and mucosal erosions; reticular white plaques; or hyperkeratotic plaques (see Chapter 160, Lichen Planus.)
- Darier disease (keratosis follicularis) is an autosomal dominant disorder that results in abnormal keratinization and loss of adhesion between epidermal cells. It typically presents in the second decade of life with hyperkeratotic, yellow-brown, greasy-appearing papules that coalesce into verrucous plaques in a seborrheic distribution. Nails may demonstrate red/white longitudinal stripes, subungual hyperkeratosis, and notching of the distal nail margins (**Figure 203-8**). The course of the illness is chronic and persistent.
- Alopecia areata also can produce pitting of the nails. As a general rule, pitting in psoriasis is more irregular and broader based; pitting in alopecia areata is more regular, shallow, and geometric and produces fine pits (see Chapter 195, Alopecia Areata).
- Neoplastic and dysplastic diseases may produce psoriasiform nail changes in a single nail. Bowen disease, squamous cell carcinoma, and verruca vulgaris may appear as an isolated subungual or periungual plaque, possibly with accompanying nail plate destruction. A biopsy can establish a definitive diagnosis.

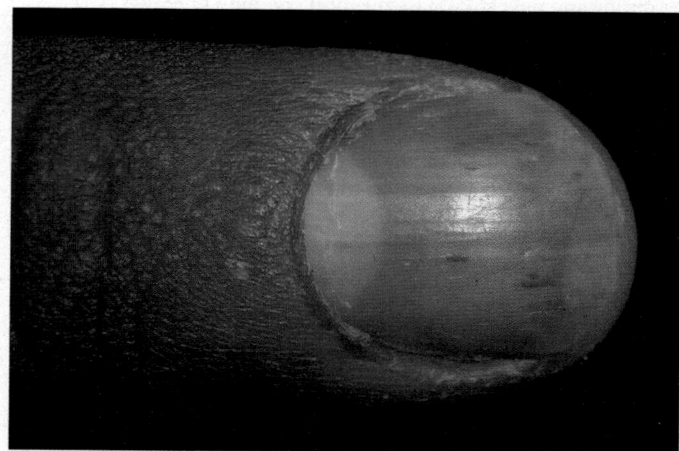

FIGURE 203-7 Prominent splinter hemorrhages in the nail of a person with psoriasis. (*Reproduced with permission from Richard P. Usatine, MD.*)

MANAGEMENT

NONPHARMACOLOGIC

- Psoriatic nail disease is often persistent and refractory to treatment. There is insufficient evidence to recommend a standard treatment.
- The nails should be kept short, to avoid traumatic exacerbation of onycholysis and to avoid the accumulation of exogenous material under the nail.[4] SOR Ⓒ
- Nail polish may be very helpful in concealing a range of nail unit changes.[9] SOR Ⓒ
- Nail plate buffing may diminish surface imperfections.[9] SOR Ⓒ

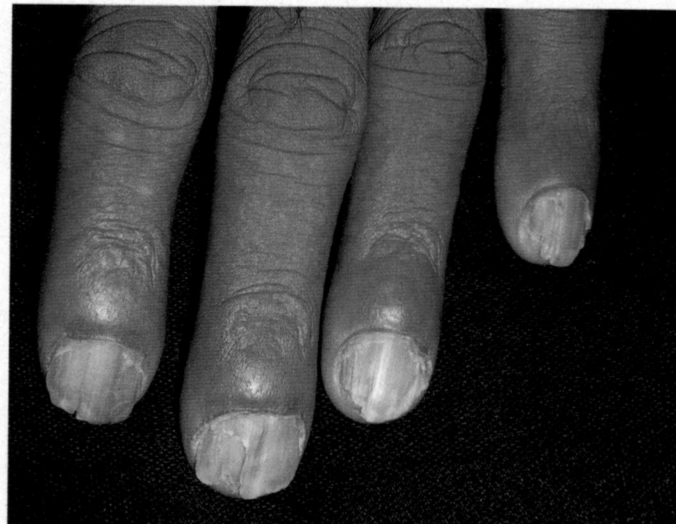

FIGURE 203-8 A woman with Darier disease (keratosis follicularis) demonstrating brittle nails with brown/white longitudinal stripes and notching of the distal nail plate. (*Reproduced with permission from Richard P. Usatine, MD.*)

MEDICATIONS

- The National Psoriasis Foundation recommends that treatment of nail psoriasis should balance consideration of the extent of skin disease, psoriatic arthritis, and severity of nail disease with concomitant impairment of quality of life.[10]

- For patients with local psoriasis limited to some nails, topical high-potency topical corticosteroids with or without calcipotriol are initial options, with intralesional corticosteroids also recommended.[10] In order to be effective, the medication must penetrate into the nail bed or nail matrix, in spite of the fact that the nail plate make it difficult for topical agents to penetrate. It is important to distinguish signs of nail matrix psoriasis from signs of nail bed psoriasis. When signs of nail matrix psoriasis are present, topical medications should be applied on the proximal nail fold above the nail matrix. If signs of nail bed psoriasis are present, the nail plate should be trimmed as much as possible during treatment and medication applied to the proximal and lateral folds and hyponychium.[4] Clinical improvement usually takes 4–6 months of treatment, and additional improvement can be seen during the first year.[4]
  - Betamethasone dipropionate ointment (64 mg/g) twice daily and clobetasol propionate 0.05% cream under occlusion once daily has been shown to be effective for subungual hyperkeratosis, salmon patches, pitting, and onycholysis after 12–20 weeks of use. Chronic topical therapy can lead to complications of atrophy and the "disappearing digit" with atrophy of the underlying phalanx.[4] SOR B
  - Calcipotriol ointment (50 mcg/g) twice daily has been shown to be effective in the treatment of nail bed psoriasis with severe fingernail and toenail hyperkeratosis.[4,11] SOR B
  - The combination of topical steroids (clobetasol propionate) two times per week with the vitamin D_3 analog calcipotriol (50 mcg/g) nightly five times per week is effective and is widely used.[4] SOR B
  - Intralesional injection of triamcinolone acetonide (0.1–0.2 mL, 10 mg/mL) into the nail bed and proximal and/or lateral folds following topical anesthetic or digital block, and then at 2-month intervals for 6–12 months.[4,10,12] SOR A Subungual hyperkeratosis, ridging, and thickening respond better than pitting and onycholysis, with benefit sustained for at least 9 months.[12] The steroid may be introduced into a digit by needle injection or high-pressure jet. Potential side effects include short-term paresthesia, focal pain, hematoma formation, depigmentation, loss of the nail plate, secondary infection, cyst formation, tendon rupture, and nail-fold atrophy.[4,10]
- For patients with significant skin and nail disease or for whom topical therapy has failed, treatment with adalimumab, etanercept, intralesional corticosteroids, ustekinumab, methotrexate sodium, acitretin, infliximab, apremilast, or golimumab is recommended.[10]
  - Adalimumab is a human anti-TNFa IgG1 monoclonal antibody. Studies have shown good improvement in psoriasis of the nail bed and the nail plate. Side effects are comparable with those of other biologics.[4] SOR A
  - Etanercept is approved by the U.S. Food and Drug Administration (FDA) for the treatment of skin and joint psoriasis and has shown excellent efficacy in nail psoriasis.[4] SOR A There is an increased risk of onychomycosis with etanercept.[4] SOR A
  - Ustekinumab self-administered as a subcutaneous injection is FDA approved for the treatment of skin and joint psoriasis. Patients weighing less than 100 kg are given 45 mg initially, again in 4 weeks, followed by 45 mg every 12 weeks. Patients weighing more than 100 kg are given 90 mg initially, again in 4 weeks, and then every 12 weeks thereafter. Patients using ustekinumab should be evaluated for tuberculosis infection and any active serious infection prior to administration. Ustekinumab may increase the risk of infections, reactivation of latent infections, and malignancy, especially nonmelanoma skin cancer.[4] SOR A
  - Oral or subcutaneously administered methotrexate 7.5 mg to 25 mg given once weekly is a commonly used systemic treatments for plaque psoriasis, psoriatic arthritis, and nail psoriasis. Potential side effects such as hepatotoxicity, ulcerative stomatitis, lymphopenia, nausea, low white blood cell count, and nausea limit its use. It has less efficacy than most modern biologics.[4] SOR A
  - Acitretin is a non-immunosuppressing antipsoriatic drug that can be used for years in patients. Side effects include cheilitis, dry mouth, and skin exfoliation. It is slow-acting with moderate efficacy for nail-bed signs of psoriasis. It can also be used as an adjuvant therapy to psoralen and UVA (PUVA) and UVB treatment.[4] SOR A
  - Infliximab is FDA approved for the treatment of skin and joint psoriasis. Infusion reactions can include chills, fever, headache, flushing and urticaria, myalgia and arthralgia, nausea, dyspnea, hypotension, anaphylactic reactions, and a serum sickness–like reaction. There is also an increased risk of onychomycosis.[4] SOR A
  - Oral apremilast is a phosphodiesterase inhibitor that is approved by the FDA and the European Medicines Agency (EMA) for treatment of psoriasis and psoriatic arthritis that has efficacy for nail psoriasis. It is administered in a dose titration schedule to minimize risk for drug-induced diarrhea. It is generally well tolerated and does not require labwork.[4] SOR A
  - Golimumab 50 mg every 4 weeks is FDA approved for the treatment of psoriatic arthritis. It has shown some efficacy for nail psoriasis.[4] SOR B
  - Systemic cyclosporine 3 and 5 mg/day shows reasonable efficacy in the treatment of both nail bed and nail matrix psoriasis but shows lack of efficacy in the often-coexisting psoriatic arthritis. Cyclosporine is comparable to biologics in treating nail psoriasis but has a relatively high rate of side effects, including reversible renal dysfunction, hypertension, fatigue, headache, paresthesia, hypertrichosis, gingival hyperplasia, and gastrointestinal disorders. After prolonged use, cyclosporine may play a role in the development of renal failure and several malignancies, so it is generally only used for 6 to 12 months.[4] SOR B
- Other treatments less commonly used or with less evidence[10]:
  - Topical tazarotene 0.1% cream applied nightly compared well with clobetasol propionate 0.05% cream under occlusion once daily for 12 weeks for improvement for pitting, onycholysis, hyperkeratosis, and salmon patches. Mild side effects occurred in 18.8% of the tazarotene-treated patients and included irritation, desquamation, and erythema of the nail-fold skin, periungual irritation, and paronychia.[4] SOR A
  - Topical tacrolimus 0.1% ointment applied once daily to the periungual skin has shown positive effects in one trial. It is usually well tolerated.[13] SOR B
  - Formulations with corticosteroids (8% clobetasol-17-propionate) in a nail lacquer have shown to improve onycholysis, pitting,

salmon patches, and subungual hyperkeratosis but are not yet commercially available in the United States. SOR Ⓐ

- One study found that topical 1% 5-fluorouracil solution or 5% cream applied twice daily to the matrix area for 6 months improved pitting and hyperkeratosis but worsened onycholysis.[4] SOR Ⓑ
- In a single-blinded study, Feliciani and colleagues found that combination therapy (oral cyclosporine and topical calcipotriol) was more effective than monotherapy (cyclosporine alone) on nail psoriasis.[4,14] SOR Ⓑ
- Anthralin ointment 0.4% to 2.0%, applied once daily and washed off after 30 minutes, is effective for onycholysis, subungual hyperkeratosis, and possibly pitting.[4] SOR Ⓑ
- Narrow-band UVB and PUVA phototherapy for 3 to 6 months is effective for cutaneous psoriasis, but its efficacy for nail psoriasis is poorly defined.[4] SOR Ⓑ
- A 595-nm pulsed dye laser is sometimes used to treat nail psoriasis. Pulsed dye laser treatments are typically given once monthly for 6 months. Side effects of pulsed dye laser therapy include petechiae, transient hyperpigmentation, moderate to severe pain, and burning sensations.[15] SOR Ⓑ
- Indigo naturalis is a dark-blue powder extracted from the leaves of indigo-bearing plants that is commonly used as a dye in the Western world. In China it has been used as a treatment for psoriasis but produces an intense and lasting blue color. The indigo naturalis oil extract has a slight purple–red color that is more cosmetically acceptable. Although not widely commercially available, this compound (0.1 and 0.2 mg/mL) has been found to improve nail psoriasis in three studies at 24 weeks after application of one drop onto the lateral nail folds, eponychium, and hyponychium. It showed better results than with topical calcipotriol solution for onycholysis and subungual hyperkeratosis. Irritation was the most common side effect of indigo naturalis.[4] SOR Ⓑ

PREVENTION[16]

- Wearing gloves during wet work and during exposure to harsh materials may minimize trauma to the skin and nail unit.
- It may help to trim the nail short to minimize leverage at the free edge and resulting trauma.
- If dry skin or scaling develop, application of emollients may be helpful.
- Cosmetic manipulations of the nail risk exacerbating the disease due to minor trauma. Discretion and care should be exercised when trimming the cuticle and clearing subungual debris.

PROGNOSIS

- Psoriatic nail changes may be reversible because scarring typically does not occur. An exception to this may develop in severe cases of generalized pustular psoriasis.
- If topical steroids are used frequently and for a prolonged period, telangiectasia and atrophy of the skin may occur.[4]

FOLLOW-UP

- Follow-up can be combined with regular follow-ups for cutaneous psoriasis.

PATIENT EDUCATION

- Nail psoriasis is mainly a cosmetic problem. Nail polish or artificial nails can be used in some patients to conceal psoriatic pitting and onycholysis. When subungual hyperkeratosis becomes uncomfortable because of pressure exerted by footwear, the nail can be pared down to relieve the pressure.
- Patients should be instructed to trim nails back to the point of firm attachment with the nail bed to minimize further nail-bed and nail-plate disassociation. Wearing gloves while working may minimize trauma to the nails. Tell patients to avoid vigorous cleaning and scraping under the nails, as this may break the skin where the nail is attached and lead to an infection.

PATIENT RESOURCES

- National Psoriasis Foundation. *Hands, Feet and Nails*—**https://www.psoriasis.org/about-psoriasis/specific-locations/hands-feet-nails.**
- National Psoriasis Foundation. *Managing Nail Psoriasis*—**https://www.psoriasis.org/about-psoriasis/specific-locations/hands-feet-nails/managing-nail-psoriasis.**
- eMedicineHealth. *Nail Psoriasis*—**http://www.emedicinehealth.com/nail_psoriasis/article_em.htm.**

PROVIDER RESOURCES

- Medscape. *Nail Psoriasis: Overview of Nail Psoriasis*—**https://emedicine.medscape.com/article/1107949-overview.**
- Schons KR, Knob CF, Murussi N, et al. Nail psoriasis: a review of the literature. *An Bras Dermatol.* 2014;89(2):312-317—**https://www.ncbi.nlm.nih.gov/pmc/articles/PMC4008063/.**
- DermNet NZ. *Nail Psoriasis*—**http://dermnetnz.org/topics/nail-psoriasis.html.**

REFERENCES

1. Jiaravuthisan MM, Sasseville D, Vender RB, et al. Psoriasis of the nail. Anatomy, pathology, clinical presentation, and a review of the literature on therapy. *J Am Acad Dermatol.* 2007;57(1):1-27.
2. Klaassen KM, van de Kerkhof PC, Pasch MC. Nail psoriasis: a questionnaire-based survey. *Br J Dermatol.* 2013;169(2):314-319.
3. Noronha PA, Zubkov B. Nails and nail disorders in children and adults. *Am Fam Physician.* 1997;55(6):2129-2140.
4. Pasch MC. Nail psoriasis: a review of treatment options. *Drugs.* 2016;76(6):675-705.
5. Langenbruch A, Radtke MA, Krensel M, et al. Nail involvement as a predictor of concomitant psoriatic arthritis in patients with psoriasis. *Br J Dermatol.* 2014;171(5):1123-1128.

6. Edwards F, de Berker D. Nail psoriasis: clinical presentation and best practice recommendations. *Drugs.* 2009;69(17):2351-2361.
7. Jiaravuthisan MM, Sasseville D, Vender RB, et al. Psoriasis of the nail: anatomy, pathology, clinical presentation, and a review of the literature on therapy. *J Am Acad Dermatol.* 2007;57(1):1-27.
8. Lencastre A, Lamas A, Sá D, Tosti A. Onychoscopy. *Clin Dermatol.* 2013;31(5):587-593.
9. de Berker D. Management of psoriatic nail disease. *Semin Cutan Med Surg.* 2009;28(1):39-43.
10. Crowley JJ, Weinberg JM, Wu JJ, et al; National Psoriasis Foundation. Treatment of nail psoriasis: best practice recommendations from the Medical Board of the National Psoriasis Foundation. *JAMA Dermatol.* 2015;151(1):87-94.
11. Tosti A, Piraccini BM, Cameli N, et al. Calcipotriol in nail psoriasis: a controlled double-blind comparison with betamethasone dipropionate and salicylic acid. *Br J Dermatol.* 1998;139(4):655-659.
12. de Berker DA, Lawrence CM. A simplified protocol of steroid injection for psoriatic nail dystrophy. *Br J Dermatol.* 1998;138(1):90-95.
13. De Simone C, Maiorino A, Tassone F, et al. Tacrolimus 0.1% ointment in nail psoriasis: a randomized controlled open-label study. *J Eur Acad Dermatol Venereol.* 2013;27:1003.
14. Feliciani C, Zampetti A, Forleo P, et al. Nail psoriasis: combined therapy with systemic cyclosporine and topical calcipotriol. *J Cutan Med Surg.* 2004;8(2):122-125.
15. Goldust M, Raghifar R. Clinical trial study in the treatment of nail psoriasis with pulsed dye laser. *J Cosmet Laser Ther 2013.* [Epub ahead of print]
16. André J. Artificial nails and psoriasis. *J Cosmet Dermatol.* 2005;4(2):103-106.

204 SUBUNGUAL HEMATOMA

E.J. Mayeaux, Jr., MD

PATIENT STORY

A 22-year-old woman dropped an iron on her toe the day before she visited our free clinic. Her toe was painful at rest and worse when walking (**Figure 204-1**). This subungual hematoma needed to be drained, and we did not have an electrocautery unit. A paperclip was bent open and held in a hemostat and heated with a torch. With some pressure it pierced the patient's nail plate and the blood spontaneously drained (**Figures 204-2** and **204-3**). This relieved the pressure and gave the patient immediate pain relief. The remaining old blood was drained with a little pressure on the proximal nail fold (**Figure 204-4**). Although we were concerned about a possible underlying fracture, the patient did not have health insurance and chose to postpone an X-ray. Her toe healed well and no radiographs were ever taken. (*Story by Richard P. Usatine, MD.*)

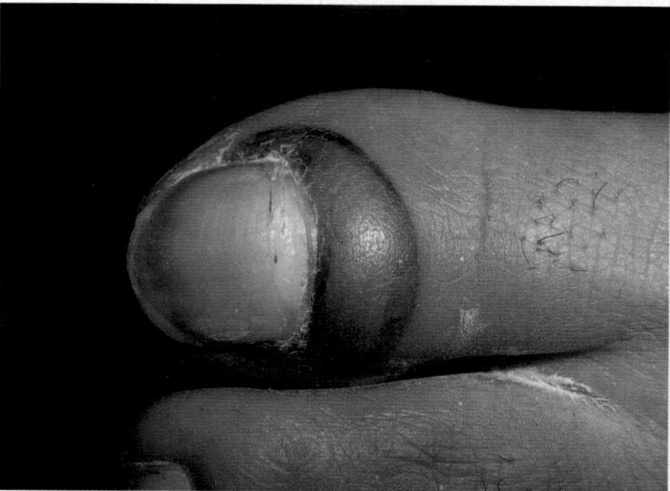

FIGURE 204-1 Acute subungual hematoma 1 day after dropping an iron on her toe. It was painful at rest and worse when walking. (*Reproduced with permission from Richard P. Usatine, MD.*)

INTRODUCTION

Subungual hematoma (blood under the fingernail or toenail) is a common injury. It is typically caused by a blow to the distal phalanx (e.g., smashing with a tool, crush in a door jamb, stubbing one's toe). The blow causes bleeding of the nail matrix or bed with resultant subungual hematoma formation. Patients usually present because of throbbing pain associated with blue-black discoloration under the nail plate. Subungual hematomas may be simple (i.e., the nail and nail fold are intact) or accompanied by significant injuries to the nail fold and digit.[1] The patient may not be aware of the precipitating trauma, because it may have been minor and/or chronic (e.g., rubbing in a tight shoe).

EPIDEMIOLOGY

Subungual hematoma is a common childhood and adult injury.

ETIOLOGY AND PATHOPHYSIOLOGY

- The injury causes bleeding of the nail matrix and nail bed, which results in subungual hematoma formation (**Figures 204-1** to **204-5**).
- In most cases it grows out with the nail plate, exhibiting a proximal border that reproduces the shape of the lunula. Occasionally, a hematoma does not migrate because of repeated daily trauma. An extended, nonmigrating hematoma should be considered suspicious. Nail plate punch biopsy will often reveal the dark streak to be a subungual hematoma as the color lifts off with nail plate (see **Figure 204-5**).
- Potential complications of subungual hematoma include onycholysis, nail deformity (usually splitting as in **Figure 204-6**), and

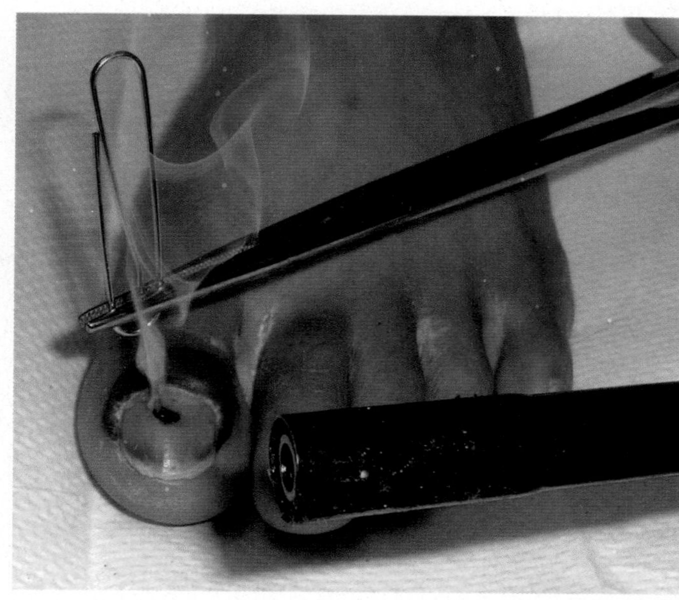

FIGURE 204-2 A paperclip was held in a hemostat and heated with a torch to pierce the patient's nail plate in order to relieve the subungual hematoma. (*Reproduced with permission from Richard P. Usatine, MD.*)

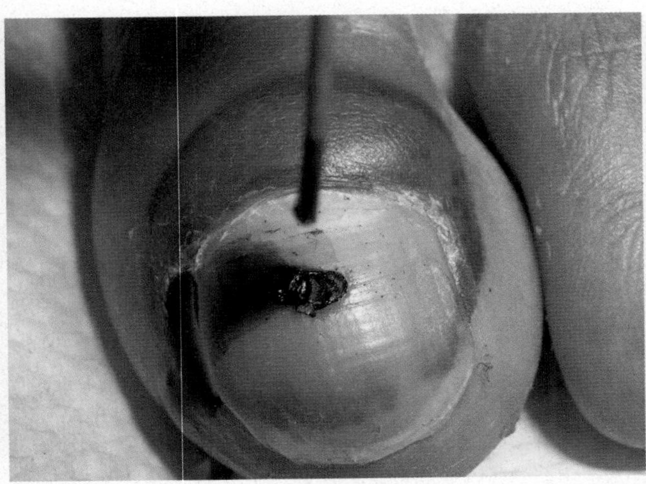

FIGURE 204-3 The hot paper clip formed a nice hole in the nail plate, and the blood drained out spontaneously. This relieved the pressure and gave the patient immediate pain relief. *(Reproduced with permission from Richard P. Usatine, MD.)*

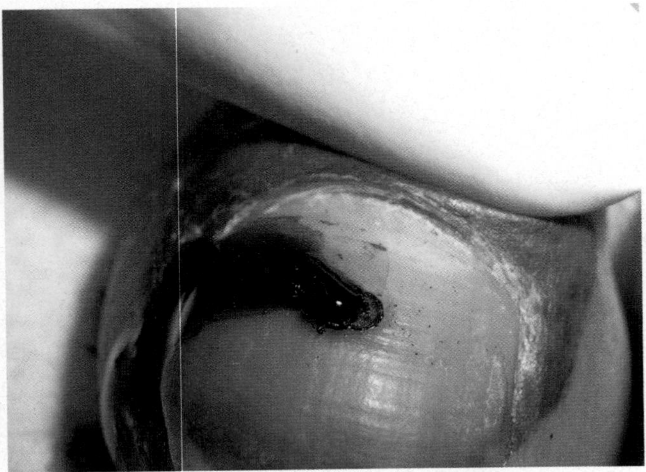

FIGURE 204-4 After the nail plate is pierced, the blood drains easily with a little pressure on the proximal nail fold. *(Reproduced with permission from Richard P. Usatine, MD.)*

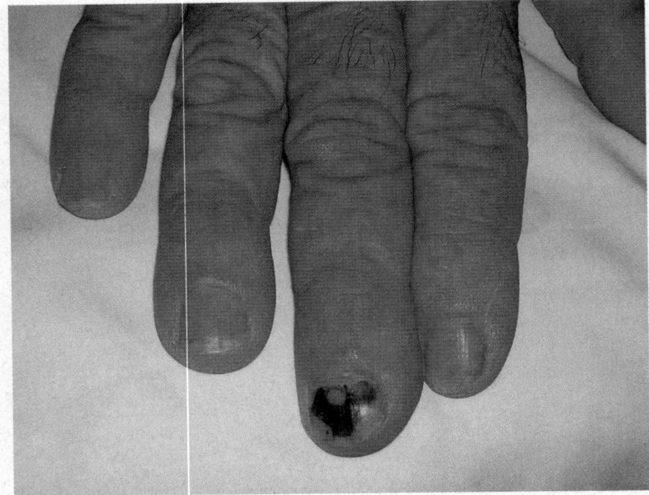

FIGURE 204-5 This persistent discoloration of the nail was found to be a subungual hematoma by nail plate biopsy using a punch biopsy instrument. *(Reproduced with permission from E.J. Mayeaux, Jr., MD.)*

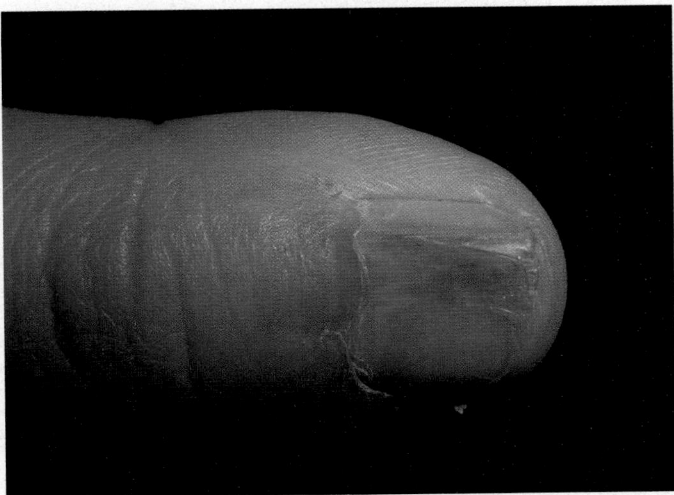

FIGURE 204-6 Split-nail deformity in a 6-year-old girl 1 year after her finger was closed in a car door and sutured in the emergency department. The matrix did not come together well, and the nail will remain split (onychoschizia). *(Reproduced with permission from Richard P. Usatine, MD.)*

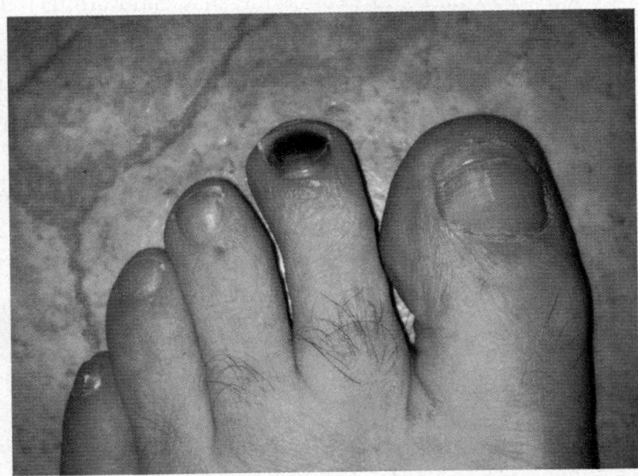

FIGURE 204-7 Patient with toenail onychomycosis and a subungual hematoma after very mild trauma. The infection can predispose to hematoma formation. *(Reproduced with permission from E.J. Mayeaux, Jr., MD.)*

infection (**Figure 204-7**). Complications are more likely to occur when presentation is delayed or there is an underlying fracture.[2]

DIAGNOSIS

CLINICAL FEATURES

- Patients complain of throbbing pain and blue-black discoloration under the nail as the hematoma progresses. Pain is relieved immediately in most patients with simple nail trephination (see **Figure 204-3**).

IMAGING

- If the mechanism of injury and clinical picture suggest a possible distal phalanx or distal interphalangeal (DIP) fracture, consider obtaining a radiograph. SOR Ⓒ
- With dermoscopy, the hematoma is characterized by a reddish to reddish-black pigmentation depending on the age of the bleed. There are usually black, purple, or reddish to brown peripheral globules or blood spots with a well defined, rounded, proximal edge and sometimes a streaked or filamentous distal end (**Figure 204-8**).[3,4] This pattern is highly characteristic of hematoma but is not sufficient to rule out melanoma.[5] SOR Ⓒ

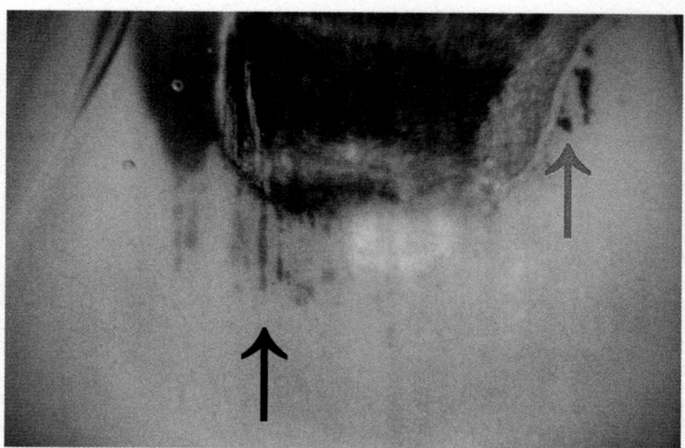

FIGURE 204-8 Dermoscopic image of a subungal hematoma demonstrating black peripheral globules or blood spots on the peripheral edge of the hematoma with well-defined, rounded edges (*red arrow*) and some with more streaked or filamentous distal ends (*black arrow*). (*Reproduced with permission from E.J. Mayeaux, Jr., MD.*)

DIFFERENTIAL DIAGNOSIS

- Nail bed nevus—Appears as a stable or slowly growing painless dark spot in the nail bed or matrix.
- Longitudinal melanonychia—Appears as painless pigmented bands that start in the matrix and extend the length of the nail (see Chapter 199, Pigmented Nail Disorders).
- Subungual melanoma—May start as a painless darkly pigmented band in the matrix and extend the length of the nail. It may be associated with pigment deposition in the proximal nail fold (Hutchinson sign) (see Chapter 199, Pigmented Nail Disorders).
- Splinter hemorrhages—Appear as reddish streaks in the nail bed and are seen in psoriasis more commonly than endocarditis (see Chapter 203, Psoriatic Nails).
- Subungual glomus tumor—A rare benign neoplasm mainly found in the nail unit or digit tip; appears as a red, purple, or blue lesion under the nail plate.
- The diagnosis of child abuse must be considered in cases of chronic or frequently recurrent subungual hematomas in children.[6]

MANAGEMENT

NONPHARMACOLOGIC

- Subungual hematomas are treated with nail trephination, which removes the extravasated blood and relieves the pressure and resulting pain. Beyond 48 hours, most subungual hematomas have clotted and pain has decreased, so trephination is ineffective (**Figure 204-9**). SOR Ⓒ

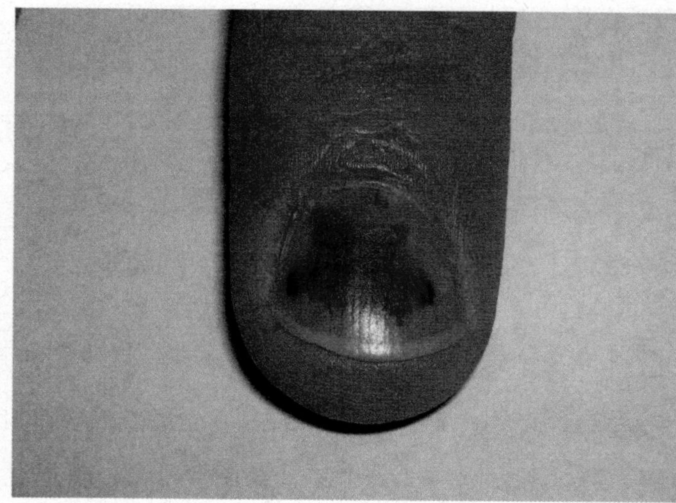

FIGURE 204-9 Finger hematoma 1 week after injury. It is now painless and starting to grow out distally. (*Reproduced with permission from E.J. Mayeaux, Jr., MD.*)

SURGERY

- Nail trephination is a painless procedure because there are no nerve endings in the nail plate that is perforated. The nail is perforated with a hot metal wire or steel paper clip (see **Figures 204-2** to **204-4**), an electrocautery device, or by spinning a large-bore needle against the nail plate like a mechanical spade bit. This allows the collected blood to drain out (see **Figures 204-3** and **204-4**). The hole must be large enough for continued drainage, which can continue for 24 to 36 hours. The puncture site should be kept covered with sterile gauze dressing while the wound drains, and the gauze should be changed daily.

MEDICATIONS

- The use of prophylactic antibiotics does not appear to improve outcomes in patients with subungual hematomas and intact nail folds.[7] SOR B
- Oral analgesia such as ibuprofen 10 mg/kg (maximum dose: 800 mg) every 6–8 hours may be used with more painful digits. SOR C

REFERRAL

- Some authors recommend removal of the nail with inspection instead of nail trephination when the hematoma involves more than 25% to 50% of the nail because of the increased likelihood of significant nail bed injury and fracture of the distal phalanx.[8,9] Other authors recommend trephination in most circumstances when the nail plate is adherent to the nail bed and is without laceration, unless the phalanx has a displaced fracture.[10,11] SOR C
- When deeper injuries are involved, nail plate removal after a digital block allows for nail bed repair.[12] SOR C

PROGNOSIS

The potential complications of a subungual hematoma include onycholysis (separation of the nail plate from the nail bed), nail deformity, nail loss, and infection. Complications are more likely to occur when care is delayed.

A retrospective analysis of 123 patients treated with simple trephination found that 85% of patients reported an excellent or very good outcome, 2% reported a poor outcome (nail splitting), and no correlation was found between outcome and size of the hematoma or the presence of fracture or infection.[2]

FOLLOW-UP

After trephination, instruct the patient to keep the affected digit clean and dry. There is no need to soak the affected digit because this may lead to additional bleeding and allow the introduction of bacteria.[13] Have the patient return with any signs of reaccumulation of blood or infection.

PATIENT EDUCATION

- Potential complications of subungual hematoma and nail trephination should be discussed with the patient and/or the patient's parents or guardian.
- Inform the patient that residual discoloration usually slowly grows out with the nail.

PATIENT RESOURCES

- eMedicineHealth. *Subungual Hematoma*—**http://www.emedicinehealth.com/subungual_hematoma_bleeding_under_nail/article_em.htm.**
- WebMD. *Subungual Hematoma*—**http://www.webmd.com/skin-problems-and-treatments/bleeding-under-nail#1.**
- Drugs.com. Subungual Hematoma—What You Need to Know—**https://www.drugs.com/cg/subungual-hematoma.html.**

PROVIDER RESOURCES

- American Family Physician. *Fingertip Injuries*—**https://www.aafp.org/afp/2001/0515/p1961.html.**
- American Osteopathic College of Dermatology. *Subungual Hematoma*—**https://www.aocd.org/page/SubungualHematoma.**
- Medscape. *Subungual Hematoma Drainage*—**http://emedicine.medscape.com/article/82926-overview.**
- Emergency Medicine News. *Evaluation and Treatment of Subungual Hematoma*—**http://journals.lww.com/em-news/Fulltext/2003/08000/Evaluation_and_Treatment_of_Subungual_Hematoma.12.aspx?trendmd-shared=0.**
- Dr ER. *Nail Trephination*—**https://www.youtube.com/watch?v=19XXTII8Zpk.**
- *Subungual Hematoma (Blood Under Nail) Relief*—**https://www.youtube.com/watch?v=T2s_b_Sr7eI.**

REFERENCES

1. Roser SE, Gellman H. Comparison of nail bed repair versus nail trephination for subungual hematomas in children. *J Hand Surg Am.* 1999;24:1166-1170.
2. Meek S, White M. Subungual haematomas: is simple trephining enough? *J Accid Emerg Med.* 1998;15:269-271.
3. Lencastre A, Lamas A, Sá D, Tosti A. Onychoscopy. *Clin Dermatol.* 2013;31(5):587-593.
4. Ronger S, Touzet S, Ligeron C, et al. Dermoscopic examination of nail pigmentation. *Arch Dermatol.* 2002;138:1327-1333.
5. Braun RP, Baran R, Le Gal FA, et al. Diagnosis and management of nail pigmentations. *J Am Acad Dermatol.* 2007;56(5):835-847.
6. Gavin LA, Lanz MJ, Leung DY, Roesler TA. Chronic subungual hematomas: a presumed immunologic puzzle resolved with a diagnosis of child abuse. *Arch Pediatr Adolesc Med.* 1997;151:103-105.
7. Seaberg DC, Angelos WJ, Paris PM. Treatment of subungual hematomas with nail trephination: a prospective study. *Am J Emerg Med.* 1991;9:209-210.

8. Zook EG, Guy RJ, Russell RC. A study of nail bed injuries: causes, treatment, and prognosis. *J Hand Surg Am.* 1984;9:247-252.
9. Zacher JB. Management of injuries of the distal phalanx. *Surg Clin North Am.* 1984;64:747-760.
10. Fehrenbacher V, Blackburn E. Nail bed injury. *J Hand Surg Am.* 2015;40(3):581-582.
11. Dean B, Becker G, Little C. The management of the acute traumatic subungual haematoma: a systematic review. *Hand Surg.* 2012;17(1):151-154.
12. Hart RG, Kleinert HE. Fingertip and nail bed injuries. *Emerg Med Clin North Am.* 1993;11:755-765.
13. Bonisteel PS. Practice tips. Trephining subungual hematomas. *Can Fam Physician.* 2008;54:693.

SECTION S PIGMENTARY AND LIGHT-RELATED CONDITIONS

205 MELASMA

E.J. Mayeaux, Jr., MD
Richard P. Usatine, MD

PATIENT STORY

A young Hispanic woman delivers a healthy baby boy. On the first postpartum day, she is sitting in the rocking chair after breastfeeding her son. Her doctor notes that she has melasma and asks her about it. She states that the hyperpigmented areas on her face have become darker during this pregnancy (**Figure 205-1**). She noted the dark spots started with her first pregnancy but they are worse this time. On physical examination, hyperpigmented patches are noted on the cheeks and upper lip (**Figure 205-2**). Although the patient hopes the pigment will fade, she does not want to treat the melasma at this time.

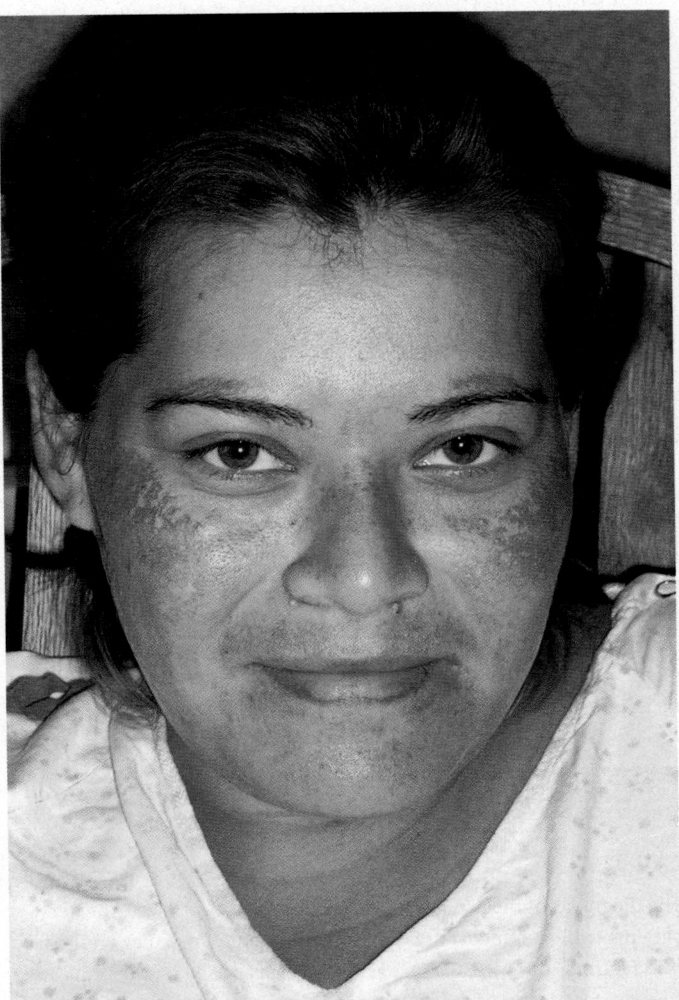

FIGURE 205-1 Melasma (chloasma) in the typical distribution in a woman who just gave birth to her second child. This is sometimes called the mask of pregnancy. (*Reproduced with permission from Richard P. Usatine, MD.*)

INTRODUCTION

Melasma is an acquired hyperpigmentary disorder characterized by symmetric light- to dark-brown macules and patches occurring in the sun-exposed areas of the face and neck. It is most commonly caused by pregnancy or the use of sex steroid hormones, such as oral contraceptive pills.

SYNONYMS

Chloasma, chloasma gravidarum, mask of pregnancy.

EPIDEMIOLOGY

- It is a relatively common disorder that affects sun-exposed areas of skin, most commonly the face. The prevalence within populations varies according to ethnic composition, dermal phototypes, and intensity of sun exposure. It is believed to affect 5% to 50% of women.[1]
- It affects predominantly women (**Figures 205-1** to **205-3**), with men accounting for only 10% of all cases (**Figure 205-4**.) It is particularly prevalent in women of Hispanic, East Asian, Indian, Pakistani, Middle Eastern, and Mediterranean-African origin (skin types IV to VI) and who live in areas of intense UV radiation exposure.[1]
- Melasma caused by pregnancy usually regresses within a year, but areas of hyperpigmentation never completely resolve in about 30% of patients.[1,2] There is a 6% rate of spontaneous remission. Melasma may increase, becoming more obvious with each subsequent pregnancy.
- There appears to be a genetic predisposition for the condition, because over 40% of patients reported having relatives affected with the disease.[1]

ETIOLOGY AND PATHOPHYSIOLOGY

The major etiologic factors include genetic influences, exposure to UV radiation, and sex hormones.

- The precise cause of melasma has not been determined. Multiple trigger factors have been implicated, including pregnancy, oral contraceptives, genetics, sun exposure, cosmetic use, thyroid dysfunction, antiepileptic medications, ovarian tumors, intestinal parasitoses, liver disease, photosensitizing drug use, inflammatory processes of the skin, and stressful events.[1,3,4]
- Women with melasma not related to pregnancy or oral contraceptive use may have hormonal alterations that are consistent with mild ovarian dysfunction.
- Melasma in men (see **Figure 205-4**) shares the same clinical features as in women, but it is not known if hormonal factors play a role.[5]

Other factors associated with melasma include certain cosmetic ingredients (oxidized linoleic acid, salicylate, citral, preservatives) and certain antiepileptic drugs. Some medications or topical preparations in combination with sun exposure worsen melasma.[1]

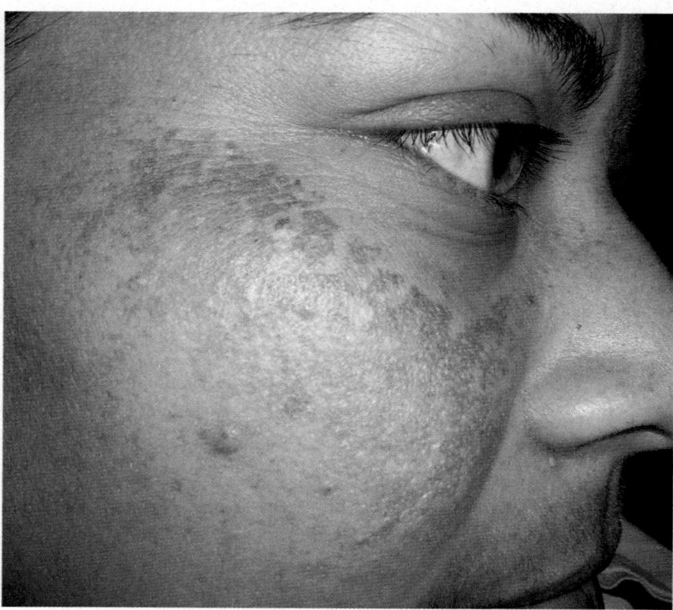

FIGURE 205-2 Close-up of the melasma showing the hyperpigmented patches on cheeks and upper lip. (*Reproduced with permission from Richard P. Usatine, MD.*)

RISK FACTORS

A recent global survey of 324 women with melasma demonstrated that a combination of the known triggers, including pregnancy, hormonal birth control, family history, and sun exposure, affects onset of melasma.[6]

Individuals with skin types I and VI rarely demonstrate melasma. In theory, individuals with skin type I are unable to produce the additional pigmentation and individuals with skin type VI always produce pigment maximally.[1]

DIAGNOSIS

CLINICAL FEATURES

The diagnosis of melasma is based on clinical appearance. Affected patients exhibit splotchy areas of hyperpigmented macules on the face (see **Figures 205-1** to **205-4**), neck, and occasionally on the arms and sternal area.[1] In natural light, epidermal melasma appears light to dark brown, and the dermal pattern is blue or gray.

Melasma is divided into four clinical types:

1. Epidermal type—The hyperpigmentation is usually light brown, and Wood light enhances the color contrast between hyperpigmented areas and normal skin. It is the most common type, and it best responds to the use of depigmenting agents.
2. Dermal type—The hyperpigmentation is ashen or bluish-gray and exhibits no accentuation of color contrast under Wood light. Depigmenting agents are generally not effective for this type.
3. Mixed type—The hyperpigmentation is usually dark brown, and Wood light enhances the color contrast in some areas but not in others.
4. Indeterminate type—Presents in patients with darker complexions (skin types V to VI) and cannot be categorized under Wood light.[1]

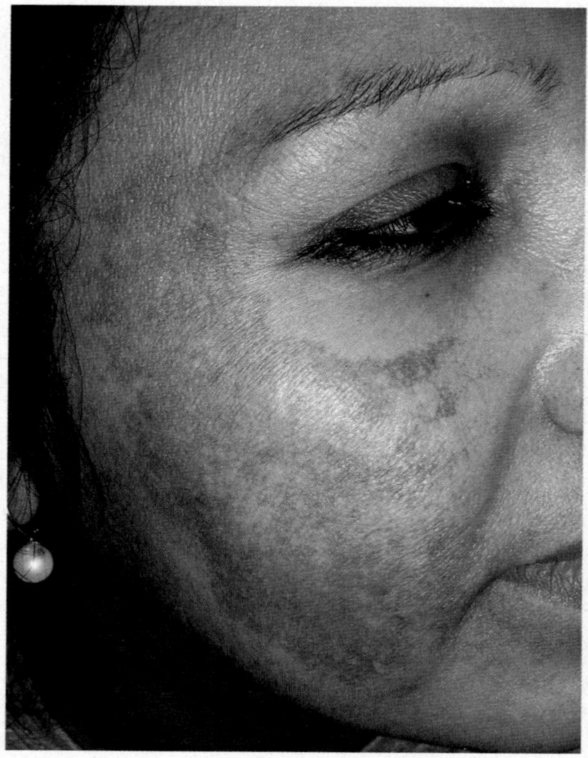

FIGURE 205-3 A 39-year-old Hispanic woman with melasma seeking treatment. She is disturbed by this dark color on her face. Note that the hyperpigmentation reaches the eyebrows but does not cover the upper lip. She has not been pregnant for years and is not taking hormonal contraceptives. (*Reproduced with permission from Richard P. Usatine, MD.*)

TYPICAL DISTRIBUTION

The lesion is found typically on sun-exposed areas. The three typical patterns of involvement are[1]:

1. Centrofacial, involving the cheeks, forehead, upper lip, nose, and chin.
2. Malar, involving the cheeks and nose.
3. Mandibular, involving the ramus of the mandible.
4. Peripheral, involving the frontotemporal, preauricular, and mandibular branch areas.

IMAGING

A Wood light may be used to determine the type of melasma.[1] This does not change the choices of standard topical therapies.

Dermoscopy of melasma shows very characteristic changes including more intense telangiectasis in the affected area. The melanin presents as a dark brown color and well defined network when located in the stratum corneum; shades of light brown color and irregularity of the network when located in the lower layers of the epidermis; and blue to bluish-gray color when located in the dermis.[1]

BIOPSY

Histologically, there is not an increased number of melanocytes, but they are hypertrophied and show a greater number of dendrites.[1]

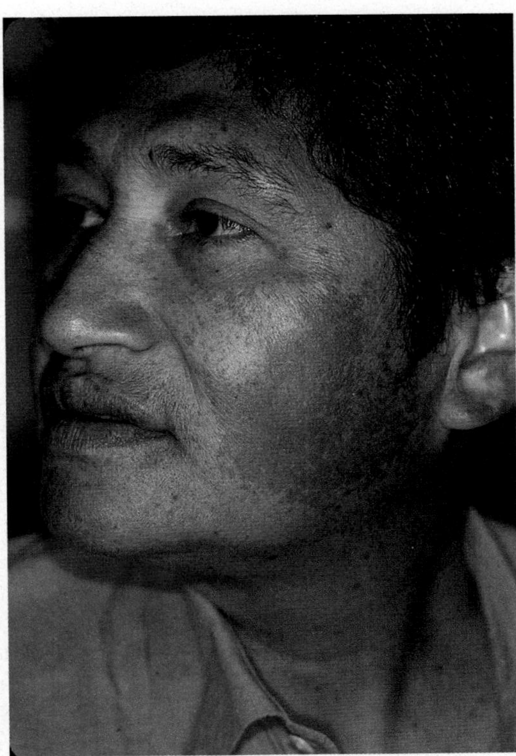

FIGURE 205-4 Melasma in a man. *(Reproduced with permission from Richard P. Usatine, MD.)*

DIFFERENTIAL DIAGNOSIS

- The facial rash of systemic lupus erythematosus (SLE) may be confused with melasma, as they both can have a butterfly pattern. Melasma is hyperpigmented, whereas the lupus facial rash is usually inflammatory. An antinuclear antibody (ANA) test should be positive in SLE and negative in melasma. False-positive antinuclear antibodies are usually low titer, and the patient does not have other criteria for lupus (see Chapter 188, Lupus: Systemic and Cutaneous).
- Discoid lupus or cutaneous lupus can occur across the face but is usually seen with scarring. In this condition, the ANA is often negative (see Chapter 188, Lupus: Systemic and Cutaneous).
- Contact dermatitis will be inflamed in the acute stage, but the postinflammatory hyperpigmentation could be confused with melasma (see Chapter 152, Contact Dermatitis).
- Benign chronic skin pigmented macules such as freckles, solar lentigo, and postinflammatory hyperpigmentation must be excluded.
- Poikiloderma of Civatte is a rare skin condition characterized by mottled pigmentation and telangiectasias on the lateral neck with sparing of the submental area due to chronic sun exposure.

MANAGEMENT

Melasma is challenging because of its chronic and relapsing nature, and treatment for melasma is generally unsatisfactory.[7] Numerous less-than-adequate treatment options exist, including topical agents and chemical peels. Melasma treatment is started only when the patient is disturbed by the hyperpigmentation. All patients can benefit from sun protection, and this is always a good place to start.

It is important to give the patient realistic treatment goals. The treatments that follow may lighten the hyperpigmentation but do not generally remove it completely. Side effects of all topical treatments include contact dermatitis, depigmentation of surrounding normal skin, and postinflammatory hyperpigmentation. Tretinoin should not be used during pregnancy. Discontinue oral contraceptives or other estrogen/progesterone agents, if possible.

FIRST LINE

MEDICATIONS

- Hydroquinone applied twice daily for up to 3 months with subsequent tapering to once daily is the main bleaching agent used to treat melasma.[7] SOR Ⓐ It is available over the counter in 2% or 3% formulations (some including sunscreens). The prescription strength is 4% and is available with or without a sunscreen. Generic 4% hydroquinone comes in many sizes and formulations, so write the prescription to be flexible to avoid hassles for you and the patient. Although hydroquinone with sunscreen may be somewhat better than hydroquinone alone, a combination product has not been shown to be better than using these two topical agents together as two separate products. SOR Ⓒ If the patient has not noticed a benefit by 3 months, the treatment should be stopped. SOR Ⓒ
    - Ochronosis—If the skin becomes darker with treatment, then the hydroquinone should be discontinued, as there is a known side effect of hydroquinone, called ochronosis, that causes hyperpigmentation. Ochronosis only occurs in the treated area, but the hyperpigmentation can be permanent.[8]
    - Hydroquinone can also cause a contact dermatitis, so it is a good idea for the patient to try it on a small area of skin before applying it to large areas of the face. Hydroquinone should be avoided on inflamed skin to avoid additional postinflammatory hyperpigmentation.
- Topical tretinoin 0.1% (Retin-A) cream is applied once daily at bedtime to lighten melasma. In two studies where tretinoin was compared to placebo, participants rated their melasma as significantly improved in one but not the other. In both studies, by other objective measures, tretinoin treatment significantly reduced the severity of melasma.[7] SOR Ⓐ
    - Combining tretinoin and hydroquinone is believed to potentiate their effects. SOR Ⓒ
    - There is a triple combination cream (Tri-Luma) containing 4% hydroquinone, retinoic acid, and fluocinolone (corticosteroid). It is used once daily before bed for a duration of 8 weeks. Studies show that it has efficacy superior to that of hydroquinone monotherapy for melasma.[9,10] SOR Ⓐ However, the side effect of skin irritation is very common, and it is not recommended for long-term use.[9,10] Triple-combination cream was significantly more effective at lightening melasma than hydroquinone alone (relative risk [RR] 1.58) or when compared to the dual combinations of tretinoin and hydroquinone (RR 2.75).[7] SOR Ⓐ Note that Tri-Luma is very expensive. Individual prescriptions for 4% hydroquinone, tretinoin cream, and a mild topical steroid cream can be given to keep the cost down. Desonide or 1% hydrocortisone are good options for the topical steroid. The steroid should not be used daily for longer than 8 weeks to avoid adverse effects.
- Mequinol is a phenolic agent that that is a competitive inhibitor of tyrosinase. It is sometimes used daily in a combination medication with tretinoin, although it has not been specifically studied in melasma treatment. Adverse effects may include erythema, stinging, desquamation, and pruritus. SOR Ⓒ
- Azelaic acid (20% cream or 15% gel) twice a day is significantly more effective than 2% hydroquinone at lightening melasma but not better than 4% hydroquinone.[7] SOR Ⓐ
- Kojic acid 2% applied twice daily blocks the conversion of tyrosine to melanin. It is usually applied with other agents. Kojic acid may cause local irritation and allergic contact dermatitis. SOR Ⓒ
- The adverse events most commonly reported with topical agents were mild and transient, such as skin irritation, itching, burning, and stinging.[7] SOR Ⓐ

SECOND LINE

SURGICAL PROCEDURES

- Chemical peels are one option for patients who have moderate to severe melasma that has not responded to bleaching agents and who are seeking further treatment. SOR Ⓒ
- Dermabrasion treatment is one aggressive option.[11] SOR Ⓒ
- Q-switched pigmentary lasers, intense pulsed light, and fractional laser treatments have some efficacy but can cause postinflammatory hyperpigmentation, and relapses may occur, so these options should be used only in refractory cases and are usually not recommended.[12] SOR Ⓑ

PREVENTION

Strict avoidance of sun exposure is important to prevent further hyperpigmentation. SOR Ⓒ Broad-spectrum, >30 sun protection-factor sunscreens (with UVB and UVA protection), such as titanium dioxide, micronized zinc oxide, Mexoryl, or avobenzone/Parsol, are essential.[13] Broad-spectrum sunscreens likely enhance the efficacy of skin-lightening agents.[14]

FOLLOW-UP

Follow-up is advisable when using bleaching agents. Long-term follow-up and reinforcement of limiting sun exposure can be accomplished during routine prevention visits.

PATIENT EDUCATION

- Provide the patient with realistic treatment goals.
- If the topical medications are irritating the skin, stop them and return for further evaluation.
- If after 3 months hydroquinone has not worked, stop it in favor of other or combination agents.
- If the skin is darkening rather than lightening, stop the medications and return for further evaluation.

- Bleaching agents are often not covered by insurance. The price of hydroquinone formulations can vary widely, so it helps to shop around when cost is a major concern.

PATIENT RESOURCES

- WebMD. *Skin Problems of Pregnancy*—**http://www.webmd.com/baby/skin-conditions-pregnancy#1.**
- American Pregnancy Association. *Skin Changes During Pregnancy*—**http://americanpregnancy.org/pregnancy-health/skin-changes-during-pregnancy/.**
- WebMD. *Cosmetic Procedures, Birthmarks, and Other Abnormal Skin Pigmentation*—**http://www.webmd.com/skin-problems-and-treatments/cosmetic-procedures-birthmarks#1.**
- American Academy of Dermatology. *Melasma*—**https://www.aad.org/public/diseases/color-problems/melasma.**

PROVIDER RESOURCES

- American Academy of Family Physicians. *Common Hyperpigmentation Disorders in Adults: Part II*—**https://www.aafp.org/afp/2003/1115/p1963.html**.
- Kang HY, Ortonne JP. What should be considered in treatment of melasma. *Ann Dermatol.* 2010;22(4):373-378—**http://pdf.medrang.co.kr/Aod/022/Aod022-04-01.pdf.**
- Handel AC, Miot LD, Miot HA. Melasma: a clinical and epidemiological review. *An Bras Dermatol.* 2014;89(5):771-782—**https://www.ncbi.nlm.nih.gov/pmc/articles/PMC4155956/.**

REFERENCES

1. Handel AC, Miot LD, Miot HA. Melasma: a clinical and epidemiological review. *An Bras Dermatol.* 2014;89(5):771-782.
2. Elling SV, Powell FC. Physiological changes in the skin during pregnancy. *Clin Dermatol.* 1997;15:35-43.
3. Grimes PE. Melasma. Etiologic and therapeutic considerations. *Arch Dermatol.* 1995;131:1453-1457.
4. Hassan I, Kaur I, Sialy R, Dash RJ. Hormonal milieu in the maintenance of melasma in fertile women. *J Dermatol.* 1998;25:510-512.
5. Vazquez M, Maldonado H, Benmaman C, Sanchez JL. Melasma in men. A clinical and histologic study. *Int J Dermatol.* 1988;27:25-27.
6. Ortonne JP, Arellano I, Berneburg M, et al. A global survey of the role of ultraviolet radiation and hormonal influences in the development of melasma. *J Eur Acad Dermatol Venereol.* 2009;23:1254-1262.
7. Rajaratnam R, Halpern J, Salim A, Emmett C. Interventions for melasma. *Cochrane Database Syst Rev.* 2010;(7):CD003583.
8. Ribas J, Schettini AP, Cavalcante Mde S. Exogenous ochronosis hydroquinone induced: a report of four cases. *An Bras Dermatol.* 2010;85(5):699-703.
9. Kang HY, Valerio L, Bahadoran P, Ortonne JP. The role of topical retinoids in the treatment of pigmentary disorders: an evidence-based review. *Am J Clin Dermatol.* 2009;10:251-260.
10. Taylor SC, Torok H, Jones T, et al. Efficacy and safety of a new triple-combination agent for the treatment of facial melasma. *Cutis.* 2003;72(1):67-72.
11. Kunachak S, Leelaudomlipi P, Wongwaisayawan S. Dermabrasion: a curative treatment for melasma. *Aesthetic Plast Surg.* 2001;25:114-117.
12. Kang HY, Ortonne J. What should be considered in treatment of melasma. *Ann Dermatol.* 2010;22:373-378.
13. Vazquez M, Sanchez JL. The efficacy of a broad-spectrum sunscreen in the treatment of chloasma. *Cutis.* 1983;32:92.
14. Lakhdar H, Zouhair K, Khadir K, et al. Evaluation of the effectiveness of a broad-spectrum sunscreen in the prevention of chloasma in pregnant women. *J Eur Acad Dermatol Venereol.* 2007; 21:738.

206 VITILIGO AND HYPOPIGMENTATION

Karen A. Hughes, MD
Richard P. Usatine, MD
Mindy A. Smith, MD, MS

PATIENT STORY

An 8-year-old Hispanic boy is brought in to the clinic by his mother, who is concerned about his pigment loss (**Figure 206-1**). He is starting to develop vitiligo around the eyes, and his mother wants him to be treated. The child was started on a topical steroid, and the use of narrow-band UVB was discussed if the steroid does not prove helpful. Realistic expectations of the treatments were provided to the mother and her son.

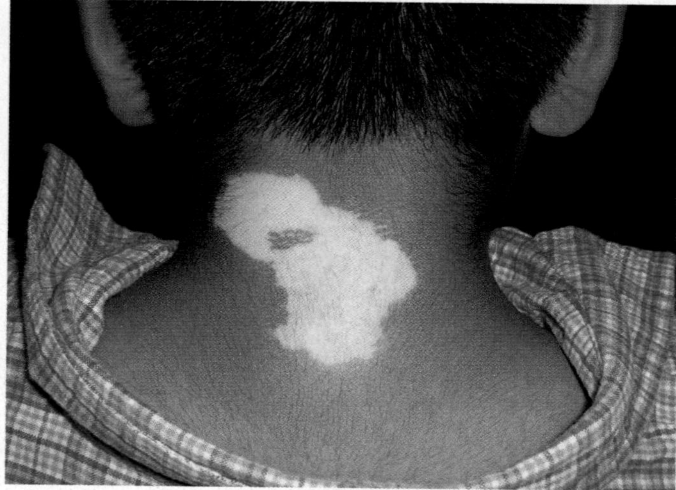

FIGURE 206-1 Vitiligo on the neck of an 8-year-old Hispanic boy. *(Reproduced with permission from Richard P. Usatine, MD.)*

INTRODUCTION

Vitiligo is an acquired, progressive loss of pigmentation of the epidermis. The Vitiligo European Task Force defines nonsegmental vitiligo, the most common form, as "an acquired chronic pigmentation disorder characterized by white patches, often symmetrical, which usually increase in size with time, corresponding to a substantial loss of functioning epidermal and sometimes hair follicle melanocytes."[1] Segmental vitiligo is defined similarly except for a unilateral distribution that may totally or partially match a dermatome; occasionally more than one segment is involved.[1]

SYNONYMS

Vitiligo vulgaris.

EPIDEMIOLOGY

- Vitiligo occurs in approximately 0.5% to 2% of the worldwide population.[2,3]
- Nonsegmental vitiligo can occur at any age but typically develops between the ages of 10 and 30 years; segmental vitiligo develops before age 30 years with 41.3% of cases occurring before age 10 years.[2]
- Vitiligo has equal rates in men and women.[2]
- It occurs in all races but has the highest incidence in India, followed by Mexico and Japan.[2]

ETIOLOGY AND PATHOPHYSIOLOGY

- Autoimmune or autoinflammatory disease with destruction of melanocytes. Evidence also points to melanocyte-intrinsic abnormalities that may induce an inflammatory cascade.[2]

- Genetic factors have been observed. Susceptibility loci have been identified including a gene encoding tyrosinase, a melanocyte enzyme that catalyzes the rate-limiting steps of melanin biosynthesis.[2] ApaI or the BsmI gene polymorphism are associated with risk of vitiligo in East Asian populations.[4]
- Environmental factors, as yet unknown, may play a role; in one study, vitiligo extent was associated with birthplace, and significant regional variation was noted.[5]
- Can trigger or worsen with illness, emotional stress, and/or skin trauma (Koebner phenomenon).

DIAGNOSIS

CLINICAL FEATURES

- Macules and patches of depigmentation with scalloped, well-defined borders (**Figures 206-1** and **206-2**).
- Depigmented areas often coalesce over time to form larger areas (**Figures 206-3** and **206-4**).
- Nonsegmental vitiligo has two identified phenotypes: early onset (before age 12 years), often associated with halo nevus (**Figures 206-5**) (see Chapter 168, Benign Nevi) and a familial history of premature hair greying, and late onset usually associated with an acrofacial pattern.[2]
- Segmental vitiligo is further subdivided into uni-, bi-, or plurisegmental (**Figure 206-6**).[2] Patients with small focal lesions not clearly falling into one of these two categories over 1–2 years are considered to have unclassifiable vitiligo.
- Minor vitiligo is a subgroup of nonsegmental vitiligo that appears limited to dark-skinned individuals with an incomplete defect in pigmentation showing as pale (vs. chalk-white) skin color compared with healthy skin.[2]
- Depigmented areas are more susceptible to sunburn. Tanning of the normal surrounding skin makes the depigmented areas more obvious.
- There is no standardized method for assessing vitiligo; strategies include subjective clinical assessment, semiobjective assessment (e.g., Vitiligo Area Scoring Index [VASI] and point-counting methods), macroscopic morphologic assessment (e.g., visual, photographic in natural or UV light, computerized image analysis), micromorphologic assessment (e.g., confocal laser microscopy), and objective assessment (e.g., software-based image analysis, tristimulus colorimetry, spectrophotometry).[6] Authors of a literature review concluded that the VASI, the rule of 9, and Wood lamp were the best techniques for assessing the degree of pigmentary lesions and measuring the extent and progression of vitiligo.[6]
- Active lesions were associated with hypomelanotic vs. amelanotic appearance with poorly defined borders and, histologically, by infiltration of CD8+ T lymphocytes in the epidermis and dermis, with a strong expression of E-cadherin on immunostaining in one study.[7]
- Associated autoimmune disorders include thyroid disease and the presence of thyroid antibodies, rheumatoid arthritis, psoriasis, alopecia areata,[8] Addison disease, and atopy.[2] Other conditions associated with vitiligo include halo nevi (see **Figure 206-5**)[1,2] and possibly primary open-angle glaucoma (57% of patients in one case series).[9]

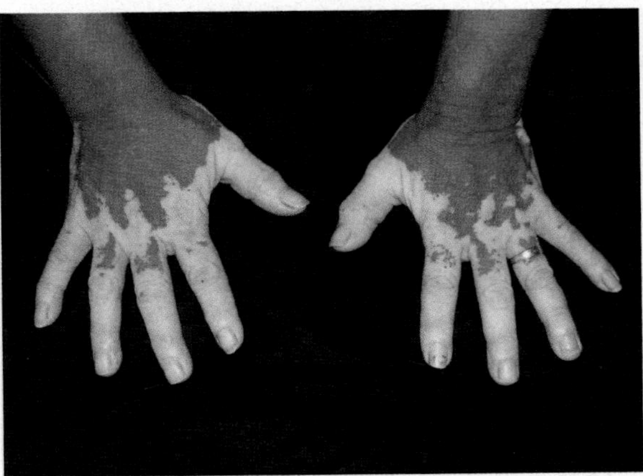

FIGURE 206-2 Vitiligo on the hands of a Hispanic man. (*Reproduced with permission from Richard P. Usatine, MD.*)

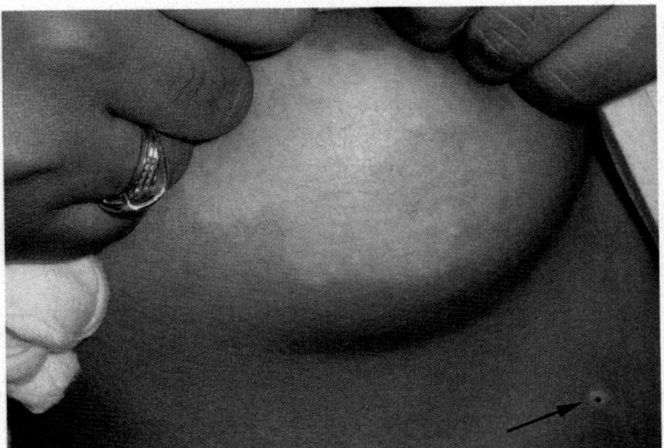

FIGURE 206-3 Vitiligo on the breast and a halo-nevus (arrow) below the breast in this 17-year-old adolescent. She has had multiple halo nevi and vitiligo for years. (*Reproduced with permission from Richard P. Usatine, MD.*)

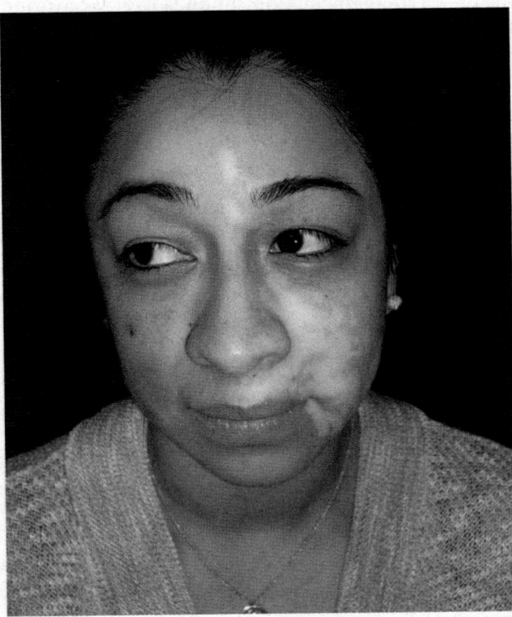

FIGURE 206-4 Segmental vitiligo on the left side of the face. Note how it stops in the midline. (*Reproduced with permission from Richard P. Usatine, MD.*)

TYPICAL DISTRIBUTION

- Widespread, but generally seen first on the face, hands, arms, and genitalia (**Figure 206-7**). Nonsegmental vitiligo has a predilection for extensor surfaces.[2]
- Depigmentation around body openings such as eyes, mouth, umbilicus, and anus is common (**Figure 206-8**). When the eyelashes are involved it is called *leukotrichia*.

LABORATORY AND IMAGING

- Evaluation for endocrine disorders such as hyper- or hypothyroidism (e.g., thyroid-stimulating hormone [TSH]) and diabetes mellitus (e.g., fasting blood sugar) is indicated, as vitiligo can be associated with these disorders.[2]
- Pernicious anemia and lupus erythematosus should be considered; obtain complete blood count (CBC) with indices and an antinuclear antibody (ANA).

BIOPSY

Not indicated unless the diagnosis is not clear, and then a 4-mm punch biopsy will suffice.

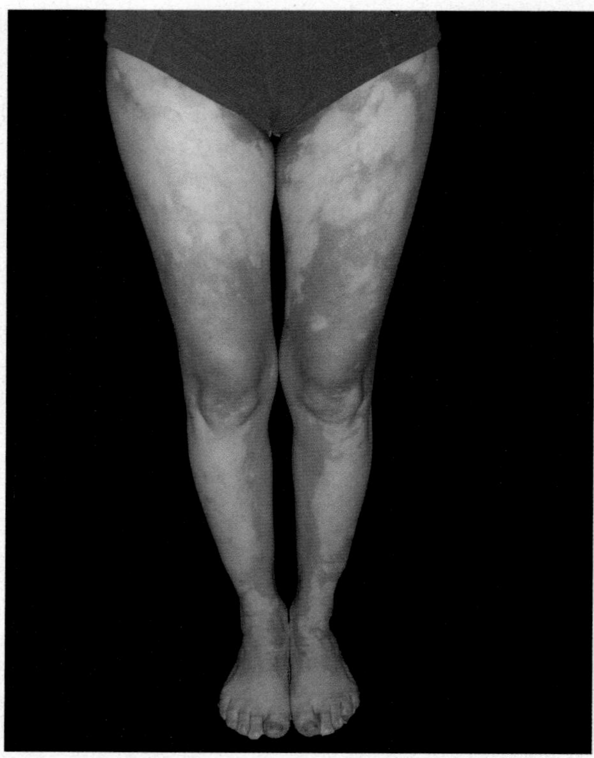

FIGURE 206-5 Vitiligo covering more than 50% of this young Hispanic woman's body. The patient is starting topical monobenzone to attempt to bleach the unaffected skin so that she has one matching skin color. *(Reproduced with permission from Richard P. Usatine, MD.)*

DIFFERENTIAL DIAGNOSIS

- Pityriasis alba—Areas of decreased pigmentation with scaling and mild itching. Seen in young children and usually associated with eczema and improves with age (see Chapter 151, Atopic Dermatitis).
- Ash leaf spots—Lance-shaped macules of hypopigmentation, which remain stable in size and shape over time (**Figure 206-9**). Often the earliest sign of tuberous sclerosis. More concerning if there are 3 or more present in one child.
- Halo nevus—Hypopigmentation confined to areas surrounding pigmented nevi that typically appear in adolescents and young adults (see Chapter 168, Benign Nevi).
- Idiopathic guttate hypomelanosis—Confetti-like 2- to 5-mm areas of depigmentation predominantly on sun-exposed areas (**Figure 206-10**).
- Nevus depigmentosus is usually present at birth or starts in early childhood. There are fewer melanosomes within a normal number of melanocytes. It typically has a serrated or jagged edge. Its presence at birth or early in childhood helps to differentiate it from vitiligo (**Figure 206-11**).
- Nevus anemicus—A congenital hypopigmented macule or patch that is stable in relative size and distribution. It occurs as a result of localized hypersensitivity to catecholamines and not a decrease in melanocytes. On diascopy (pressure with a glass slide) the skin is indistinguishable from the surrounding skin. Its presence from birth helps distinguish it from vitiligo (**Figure 206-12**).
- Hypomelanosis of Ito is a rare syndrome with hypopigmented whorls of skin present at birth along the Blaschko lines of development. This pattern may be accompanied by congenital abnormalities involving the eyes, or neurologic or renal systems. Its presence at birth helps distinguish it from vitiligo (**Figure 206-13**).

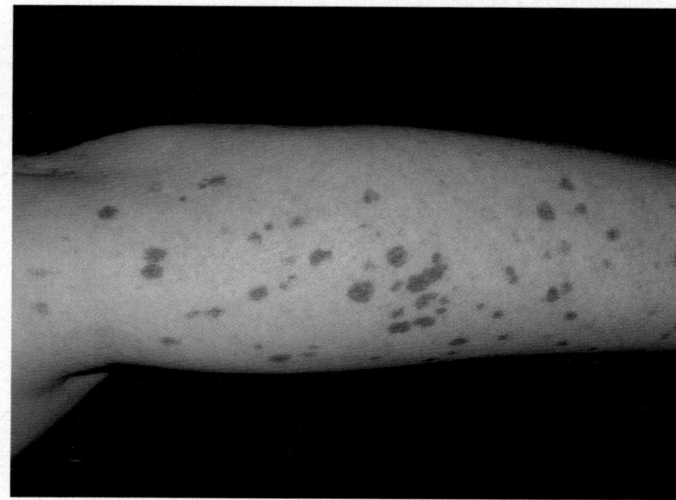

FIGURE 206-6 This previously dark-skinned woman has only a few spots of pigment remaining on her arm because of the extensive vitiligo. Her father has the same condition. *(Reproduced with permission from Richard P. Usatine, MD.)*

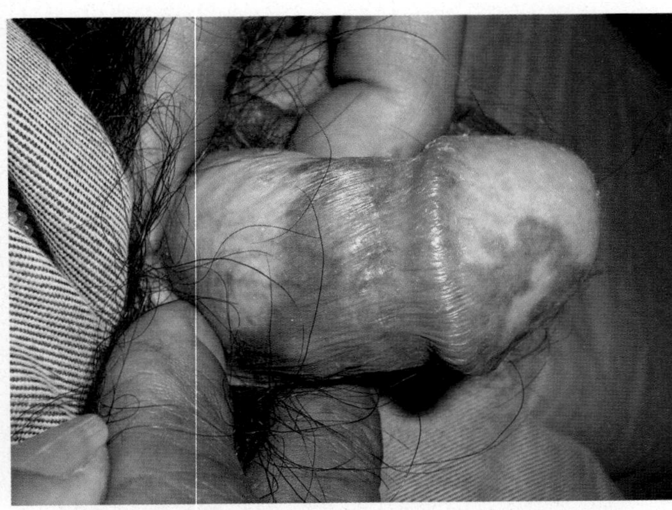

FIGURE 206-7 Vitiligo on the penis of a 72-year-old man. (*Reproduced with permission from Richard P. Usatine, MD.*)

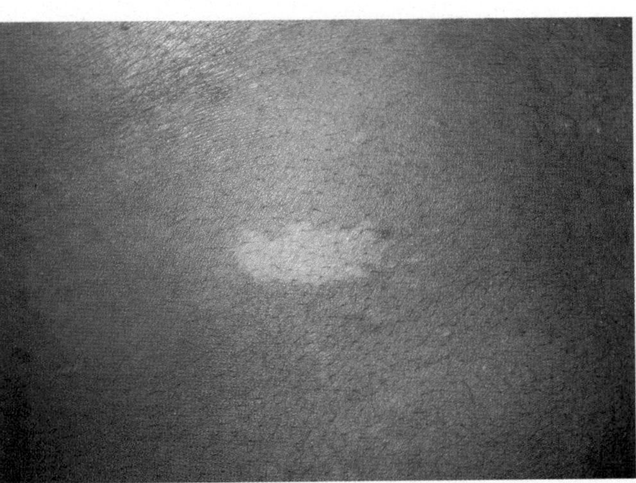

FIGURE 206-9 An ash leaf macule on a young man with tuberous sclerosus. He has angiofibromas on the face and collagenomas on the trunk as well. (*Reproduced with permission from Richard P. Usatine, MD.*)

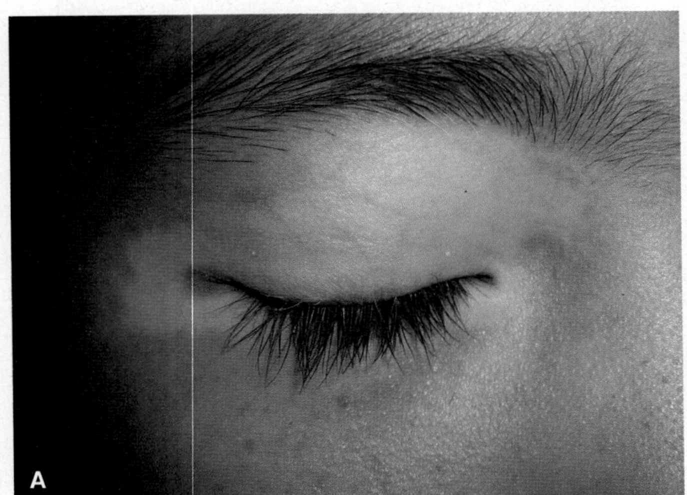

FIGURE 206-8 Vitiligo occurs commonly around the eye. **A.** Vitiligo with normal eyelashes. **B.** Vitiligo with leukotrichia. The loss of melanocytes has turned some of the eyelashes white. (*Reproduced with permission from Richard P. Usatine, MD.*)

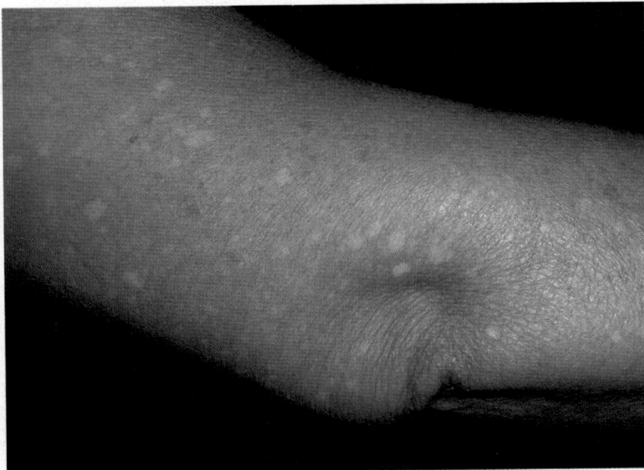

FIGURE 206-10 Idiopathic guttate hypomelanosis on the arm. This is usually seen in sun-exposed areas, especially of the arms and legs. (*Reproduced with permission from Richard P. Usatine, MD.*)

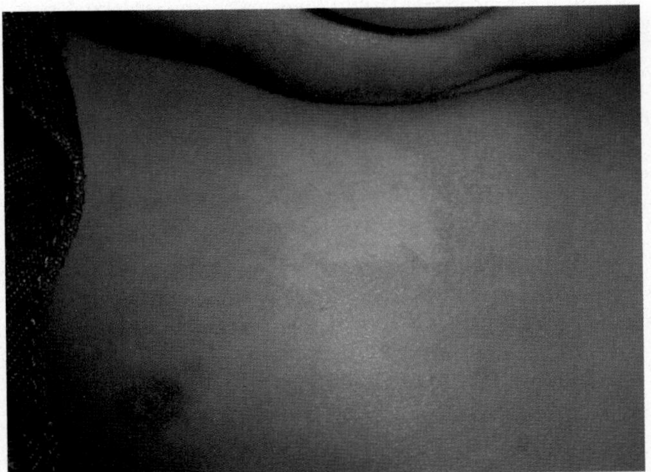

FIGURE 206-11 Nevus depigmentosus, present since birth, on the chest of this 4-month-old infant. Note the serrated or jagged edge. Vitiligo is not present at birth. (*Reproduced with permission from Richard P. Usatine, MD.*)

- Eruptive hypomelanosis, presenting as hypopigmented macules, has been reported associated with viral infections in children; lesions spontaneously resolve.[10]

MANAGEMENT

For assessing outcomes to treatment, the Vitiligo European Task Force suggests a system combining analysis of extent using percentage of body area involved (rule of 9), stage of disease based on cutaneous and hair pigmentation in vitiligo patches and staged 0 to 4 (with 0 representing normal pigment and 4 complete hair whitening) on the largest macule in each body region except hands and feet, and disease progression (spreading) assessed with Wood lamp examination of the same largest macule in each body area.[1] An evaluation sheet can be found in the citation.[1]

FIRST LINE

NONPHARMACOLOGIC

- Addressing the psychological distress that this disfiguring skin disorder causes should be a primary focus, as the clinical course is unpredictable, and in some cases little can be done to modify the condition itself.
- Management of inciting factors such as illness, stress, and skin trauma may be useful. SOR Ⓒ

MEDICATIONS

First-line topical treatments used for vitiligo include corticosteroids and calcineurin inhibitors,[2] with topical steroids having a higher rate of adverse events.[11] SOR Ⓑ Data on effectiveness (especially long-term), quality-of-life outcomes, and safety are limited. Ineffective topical agents include melagenina, topical phenylalanine, topical l-DOPA (levodopa), coal tar, anacarcin forte oil, and minoxidil.[12]

- Based on several reviews, topical corticosteroids (potent or very potent) are the preferred drugs for localized vitiligo (<20% of skin area)[11,12]; a less-than-2-month trial is recommended.[12] SOR Ⓑ A typical regimen would be 0.1% betamethasone valerate once daily in a discontinuous fashion (e.g., 15 days per month for 6 months) to avoid local side effects; adverse effects are rare but might include skin atrophy, telangiectasia, hypertrichosis, acneiform eruptions, and striae. Another option is topical 0.05% clobetasol cream daily—1 week on and 1 week off. For treatment of the face, 0.1% triamcinolone cream is a moderate potency steroid that is less likely to cause adverse effects and can be effective (**Figure 206-14**).
- In a retrospective study of 101 children with vitiligo treated with moderate- to high-potency topical corticosteroids, 64% (45/70) had repigmentation of the lesions, 24% (17/70) showed no change, and 11% (8/70) were worse than at the initial presentation.[13] Local steroid side effects were noted in 26% of patients at 81.7 ± 44 days of follow-up. Two children were given the diagnosis of steroid-induced adrenal suppression. Children with head and/or neck affected areas were eight times more likely to have an abnormal cortisol level compared with children who were affected in other body areas.[13]

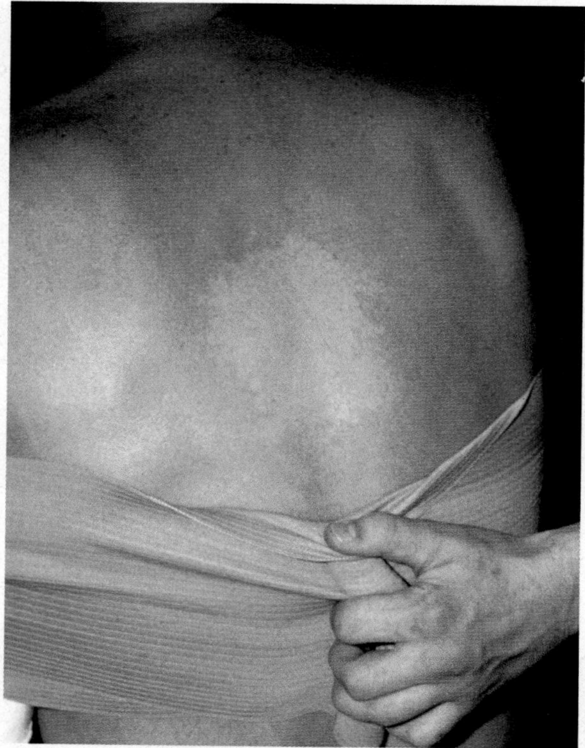

FIGURE 206-12 Nevus anemicus on the back of this woman, which has been there since birth. This is a congenital hypersensitivity to localized catecholamines. On diascopy the skin was indistinguishable from the surrounding skin. The irregular broken-up outline is seen in nevus anemicus and nevus depigmentosus. (*Reproduced with permission from Richard P. Usatine, MD.*)

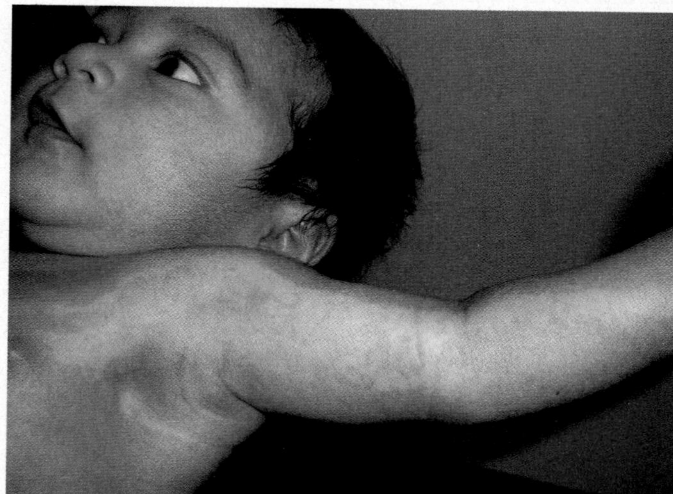

FIGURE 206-13 Hypomelanosis of Ito is a rare syndrome with hypopigmented whorls of skin present at birth along the Blaschko lines of development. It is typically unilateral and extends down an extremity such as an arm. Note the whorls on the chest and upper arm. (*Reproduced with permission from Richard P. Usatine, MD.*)

- Topical calcineurin inhibitors (tacrolimus, pimecrolimus) are an alternative for localized vitiligo, mainly head and neck.[2] SOR Ⓑ Authors of a review of 29 studies with 709 patients found that a treatment duration of at least 2 months was required to achieve 50% repigmentation of patches, with a peak at 6 months; best results were obtained using tacrolimus 0.1% ointment two times daily on lesions of the cephalic region.[14]
- Authors of a systematic review of vitiligo treatment in children found that the most commonly used drugs were tacrolimus alone (or combined with clobetasol), pimecrolimus, corticosteroids, and calcipotriol, but the authors were unable to determine the most effective treatment.[15]

SECOND LINE

MEDICATIONS

- Systemic steroids, such as oral minipulse of moderate doses of betamethasone or dexamethasone for 3–6 months, can be considered to stop progression in fast-spreading cases.[2]
- In a small case series (N = 6), various antitumor necrosis factor a agents (infliximab, etanercept, and adalimumab given according to treatment regimens used for psoriasis) were not effective for widespread nonsegmental vitiligo.[16] Authors of a case report found the Janus kinase inhibitor tofacitinib citrate effective for repigmentation.[17] These are all very expensive treatments that are not approved for vitiligo by the U.S. Food and Drug Administration (FDA).

COMPLEMENTARY AND ALTERNATIVE THERAPY

- Antioxidants may be useful adjunctive therapy.[11]
- Authors of a systematic review and meta-analysis of 5 randomized controlled trials found Chinese herbal medicine combined with phototherapy more effective than phototherapy alone for vitiligo.[18]

OTHER TREATMENT

- Use sunscreen to prevent burns to the depigmented areas and further trauma to unaffected skin, and to minimize contrast between these areas.[19] SOR Ⓐ
- Bleaching the unaffected skin in patients with widespread depigmentation (<50% of surface area) or disfiguring or highly visible recalcitrant facial or hand vitiligo to reduce contrast with depigmented areas can improve cosmetic appearance.[2,19] SOR Ⓑ Skin-bleaching methods include monobenzone ethyl ester or 4-methoxyphenol; laser treatment and cryotherapy can also be used. These skin areas are at higher risk for sunburn.

PROCEDURES

Phototherapy, narrow-band UVB, and psoralen and UVA (PUVA) are recommended as second-line therapy (**Figure 206-15**).[2,11] SOR Ⓑ

- Combination therapies including phototherapy are likely to be more effective than monotherapy. Authors of a Cochrane review found that majority of analyses showing statistically significant differences in treatment outcomes were from studies that assessed combination interventions including some form of light treatment.[20] In 3 of these studies, narrow-band UVB was associated with less nausea, and in 2 studies less erythema, than PUVA.

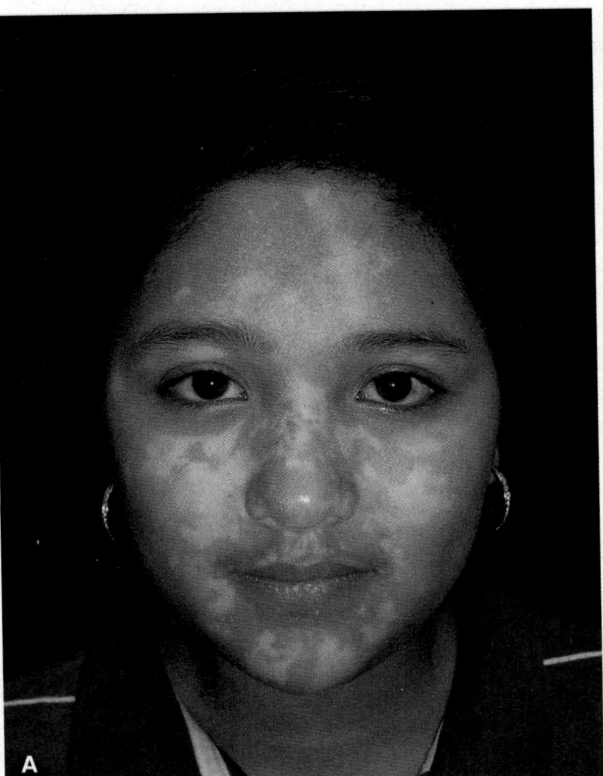

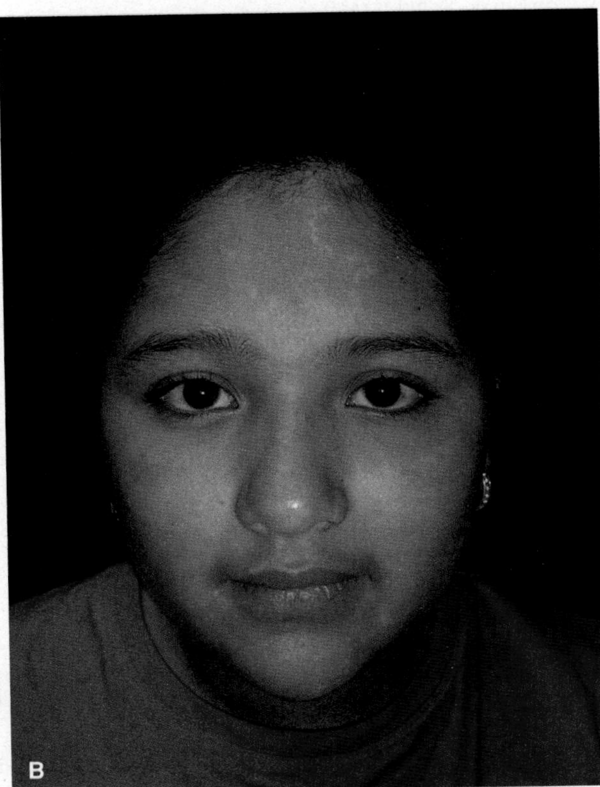

FIGURE 206-14 **A.** Vitiligo on the face of an 11-year-old girl. **B.** Significant resolution of the vitiligo 2 months later after using 0.1% triamcinolone cream once to twice daily. The patient and the mother were very happy with the results. There were no signs of skin atrophy or steroid side effects. (*Reproduced with permission from Richard P. Usatine, MD.*)

- Excimer laser is an alternative to UVB therapy, achieving good responses especially in localized vitiligo of the face, where the excimer laser may be superior to UVB therapy. By combining with topical immunomodulators, treatment response can be accelerated.[19] SOR Ⓑ In one prospective study of 14 patients, repigmentation rates for once-, twice-, and thrice-weekly treatment approached each other (60%, 79%, and 82%, respectively) at 12 weeks.[21] Although repigmentation occurred fastest with thrice-weekly treatment, the final repigmentation depends on the total number of treatments, not their frequency. SOR Ⓑ
- Surgical therapy can be considered in patients with segmental vitiligo or nonsegmental vitiligo who fail medical therapy and have stable disease for at least 1 year and absence of Koebner phenomenon.[2] Of surgical therapies, split-thickness skin grafts appear to have the highest repigmentation success.[22]
- No single therapy for vitiligo can be regarded as the most effective, as the success of each treatment modality depends on the type and location of vitiligo. SOR Ⓑ

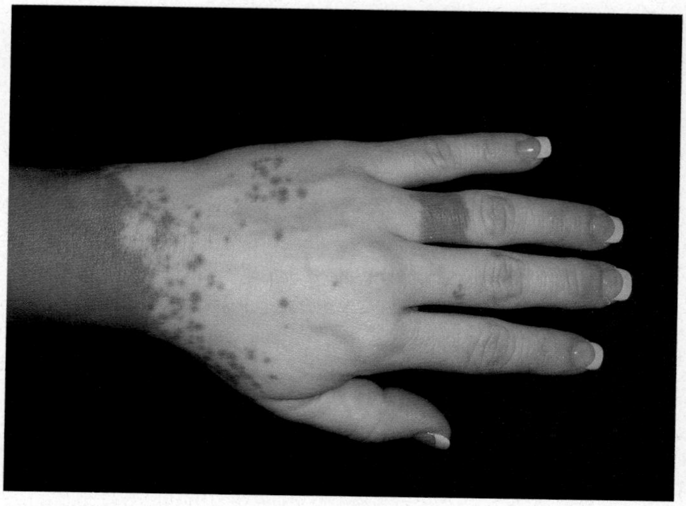

FIGURE 206-15 Vitiligo, which spared the area under a ring; the patient has spotty return of pigment on hand with narrow-band UVB treatment. (*Reproduced with permission from Richard P. Usatine, MD.*)

PROGNOSIS

The course of vitiligo varies but is usually progressive, with periods of activity interspersed with times of inactivity.[23] Spontaneous repigmentation can occur but is rare.

- The face and neck respond best to all therapeutic approaches, whereas the acral areas are least responsive.[19] SOR Ⓑ
- In a questionnaire-based study of 1541 adults with vitiligo, subjects reported reduced quality of life, especially those who had an affected body surface area (BSA) of >25% or more body parts affected.[24] Sexual dysfunction was reported by 18% of subjects, especially those with BSA >25% affected or if lesions were present in the genital area. Itching/skin burning was reported by 35%.
- Vitiligo does not appear to be associated with adverse outcomes in pregnancy.[25]

FOLLOW-UP

- Counseling and emotional support are a mainstay of follow-up treatment.
- Trials of various combination therapies may be needed.

PATIENT EDUCATION

- Offer reassurance that this is a benign condition while acknowledging associated symptoms and any psychological distress.
- Advise patients about the highly variable course of vitiligo with usually progressive periods of activity interspersed with times of inactivity.
- Inform patients about the multiple treatment options and possible need for prolonged or repeat treatment.

PATIENT RESOURCES

- National Institutes of Health. *Vitiligo*—**https://www.niams.nih.gov/health-topics/vitiligo.**
- National Organization for Albinism and Hypopigmentation—**https://healthfinder.gov/FindServices/Organizations/Organization.aspx?code=HR2242.**
- American Vitiligo Research Foundation—**http://www.avrf.org.**
- MedlinePlus. *Vitiligo*—**https://medlineplus.gov/ency/article/003224.htm.**

PROVIDER RESOURCES

- Medscape. *Vitiligo*—**http://emedicine.medscape.com/article/1068962-overview.**
- Vitiligo Support and Awareness Foundation. *A Handbook for Physicians*—**http://www.vitsaf.org/handbook-physicians.**

REFERENCES

1. Taïeb A, Picardo M; VETF Members. The definition and assessment of vitiligo: a consensus report of the Vitiligo European Task Force. *Pigment Cell Res.* 2007;20(1):27-35.
2. Ezzedine K, Eleftheriadou V, Whitton M, van Geel N. Vitiligo. *Lancet.* 2015;386(9988):74-84.
3. Krüger C, Schallreuter KU. A review of the worldwide prevalence of vitiligo in children/adolescents and adults. *Int J Dermatol.* 2012;51(10):1206-1212.
4. Li L, Wu Y, Li L, et al. Association of ApaI and BsmI polymorphisms with vitiligo risk: a meta-analysis. *Clin Exp Dermatol.* 2015;40(7):794-803.
5. Silverberg JI, Reja M, Silverberg NB. Regional variation of and association of US birthplace with vitiligo extent. *JAMA Dermatol.* 2014;150(12):1298-1305.
6. Alghamdi KM, Kumar A, Taïeb A, Ezzedine K. Assessment methods for the evaluation of vitiligo. *J Eur Acad Dermatol Venereol.* 2012;26(12):1463-1471.
7. Benzekri L, Gauthier Y. Clinical markers of vitiligo activity. *J Am Acad Dermatol.* 2017;76(5):856-862.
8. Mohan GC, Silverberg JI. Association of vitiligo and alopecia areata with atopic dermatitis: a systematic review and meta-analysis. *JAMA Dermatol.* 2015;151(5):522-528.
9. Rogosić V, Bojić L, Puizina-Ivić N, et al. Vitiligo and glaucoma—an association or a coincidence? A pilot study. *Acta Dermatovenerol Croat.* 2010;18(1):21-26.
10. Zawar V, Bharatia P, Chuh A. Eruptive hypomelanosis: a novel exanthem associated with viral symptoms in children. *JAMA Dermatol.* 2014;150(11):1197-201.
11. Bacigalupi RM, Postolova A, Davis RS. Evidence-based, non-surgical treatments for vitiligo: a review. *Am J Clin Dermatol.* 2012;13(4):217-237.
12. Hossani-Madani AR, Halder RM. Topical treatment and combination approaches for vitiligo: new insights, new developments. *G Ital Dermatol Venereol.* 2010;145(1):57-78.
13. Kwinter J, Pelletier J, Khambalia A, Pope E. High-potency steroid use in children with vitiligo: a retrospective study. *J Am Acad Dermatol.* 2007;56(2):236-241.
14. Sisti A, Sisti G, Oranges CM. Effectiveness and safety of topical tacrolimus monotherapy for repigmentation in vitiligo: a comprehensive literature review. *An Bras Dermatol.* 2016;91(2):187-195.
15. de Menezes AF, Oliveira de Carvalho F, Barreto RS, et al. Pharmacologic treatment of vitiligo in children and adolescents: a systematic review. *Pediatr Dermatol.* 2017;34(1):13-24.
16. Alghamdi KM, Khurrum H, Taieb A, Ezzedine K. Treatment of generalized vitiligo with anti-TNF-α agents. *J Drugs Dermatol.* 2012;11(4):534-539.
17. Craiglow BG, King BA. Tofacitinib citrate for the treatment of vitiligo: a pathogenesis-directed therapy. *JAMA Dermatol.* 2015;151(10):1110-1112.
18. Chen YJ, Chen YY, Wu CY, Chi CC. Oral Chinese herbal medicine in combination with phototherapy for vitiligo: a systematic review and meta-analysis of randomized controlled trials. *Complement Ther Med.* 2016 ;26:21-27.
19. Forschner T, Buchholtz S, Stockfleth E. Current state of vitiligo therapy—evidence-based analysis of the literature. *J Dtsch Dermatol Ges.* 2007;5(6):467-475.
20. Whitton ME, Pinart M, Batchelor J, et al. Interventions for vitiligo. *Cochrane Database Syst Rev.* 2015;(2):CD003263.
21. Hofer A, Hassan AS, Legat FJ, et al. Optimal weekly frequency of 308-nm excimer laser treatment in vitiligo patients. *Br J Dermatol.* 2005;152(5):981-985.
22. Mulekar SV, Isedeh P. Surgical interventions for vitiligo: an evidence-based review. *Br J Dermatol.* 2013;169(Suppl 3):57-66.
23. Viles J, Monte D, Gawkrodger DJ. Vitiligo. *BMJ.* 2010;341:c3780.
24. Silverberg JI, Silverberg NB. Association between vitiligo extent and distribution and quality-of-life impairment. *JAMA Dermatol.* 2013;149(2):159-164.
25. Horev A, Weintraub AY, Sergienko R, et al. Pregnancy outcome in women with vitiligo. *Int J Dermatol.* 2011;50(9):1083-1085.

207 POSTINFLAMMATORY HYPERPIGMENTATION

Sigrid M. Collier, MD, MPH
Jennifer Krejci-Manwaring, MD
Richard P. Usatine, MD

PATIENT STORY

A 7-year-old African American girl was brought to her family physician by her mom, who was worried that she was itching and that her skin was getting darker. The physician knew the girl well as a patient with asthma and allergic rhinitis. In fact the girl performed the allergic salute more than once in the office as she rubbed her itchy nose. Morgan-Dennie lines were seen under her eyes (**Figure 207-1A**). The mom undressed the girl to show the dark patches of skin around her knees (**Figure 207-1B**). Atopic dermatitis is common in the popliteal fossae, and this girl clearly demonstrated the atopic triad: atopic dermatitis, asthma, and allergic rhinitis. The darkening of the skin around the knees and also seen on the neck is related to the scratching and rubbing of the skin secondary to the pruritus of atopic dermatitis. The physician explained to the mom and child about the need to more aggressively treat the atopic dermatitis with emollients and topical steroids. No promises were made about the reversibility of the hyperpigmentation, as each patient will respond differently to treatment.

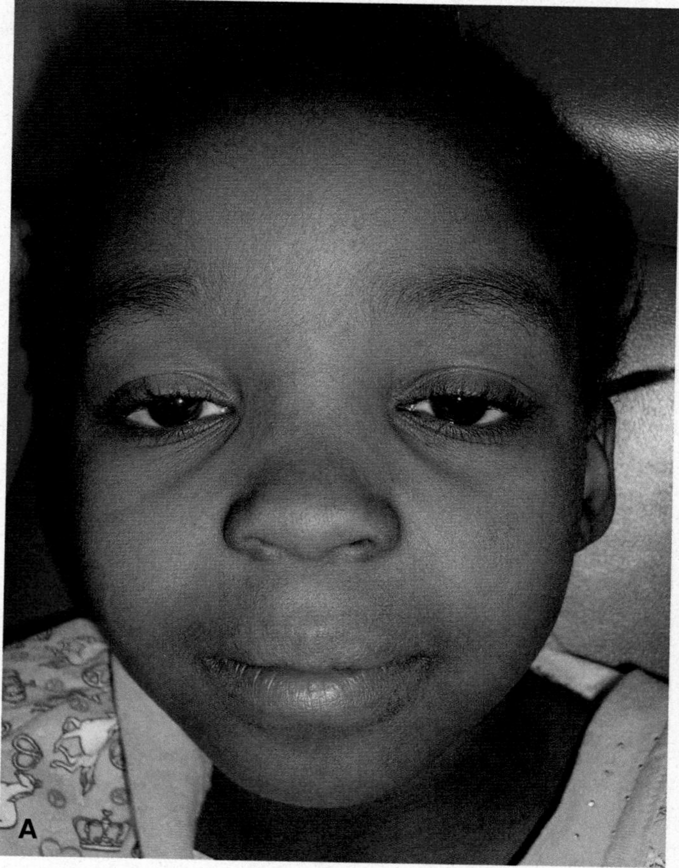

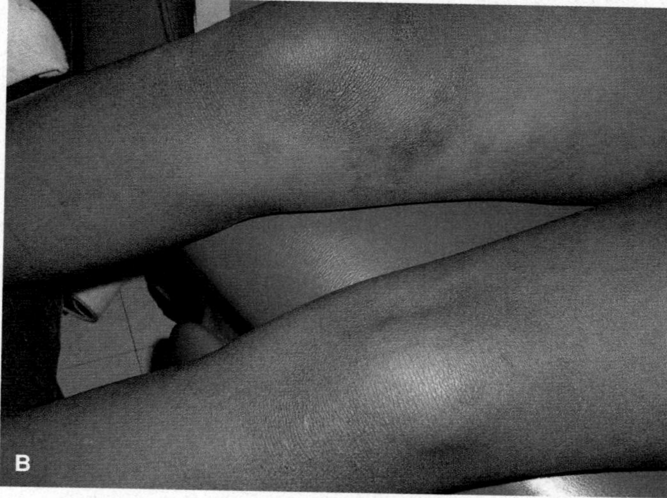

FIGURE 207-1 A. Atopic triad in a 7-year-old girl with Dennie-Morgan lines and a nasal crease. B. Postinflammatory hyperpigmentation around the knees in the same girl. *(Reproduced with permission from Richard P. Usatine, MD.)*

INTRODUCTION

Postinflammatory hyperpigmentation (PIH) is an accumulation of melanin in response to chronic inflammation that usually appears as brown, black, or gray macules or patches in the pattern of an underlying inflammatory condition. PIH can result from any kind of irritant to the skin, but is more common in conditions resulting in chronic irritation and inflammation and is more common in individuals with darker Fitzpatrick skin types IV, V, and VI. It is more severe and longer lasting if the underlying inflammatory condition goes untreated, though most PIH will fade within 6–12 months of treating the underlying inflammatory condition. For the girl in the case above, the PIH may resolve without treatment if her atopic dermatitis clears up, but if the atopic dermatitis persists, then the PIH will continue until the resolution of the underlying condition.

EPIDEMIOLOGY

- The prevalence of disorders of hyperpigmentation including PIH in the general population has been reported as low as 0.42% in Kuwait to as high as 55.9% in Michigan.[1]
- The prevalence in children in the United States is around 22% based on a sample of hospitalized children in Kentucky.[2]
- PIH is one of the most common types of cutaneous hyperpigmentation, and although there are no good estimates of its prevalence

in the children of the United States, studies in Nigeria estimate PIH to represent 49.5% of skin lesions present in hospitalized children.[3] In studies of adults, "dyschromia" is often used to combine disorders of hyperpigmentation, which would include melasma, lentigines, and PIH, so true prevalence is difficult to obtain. In one study dyschromia was the second most common diagnosis among African-American patients, but failed to make it into the top 10 for white patients.[4]

- The distribution of PIH is equal among males and females of all ages.[5]
- PIH is more common in dark-skinned individuals (Fitzpatrick skin types IV, V, and VI), and therefore is frequently found in individuals from Asia, Africa (**Figure 207-2**), and South America, and in Native Americans.[6]
- PIH, erythema ab igne, and confluent and reticulated papillomatosis (CARP) are more common in older children and young adults than in young children (**Figure 207-3**).[7]
- Other hyperpigmented lesions such as "linear and whorled hypermelanosis," nevus of Ota, and café-au-lait spots are linked to embryologic mosaicism or genetic abnormalities and may be seen at birth or within a few weeks after birth (**Figures 207-4** and **207-5**). Mongolian spots are nearly always present at birth (**Figure 207-6**).[7]
- Just as PIH is most common in darker-skinned individuals, nevus of Ota, Mongolian spot, café-au-lait macules, and CARP are more common in Asians and blacks.[7] Conversely, linear and whorled hypermelanosis shows no racial predilection.[8]

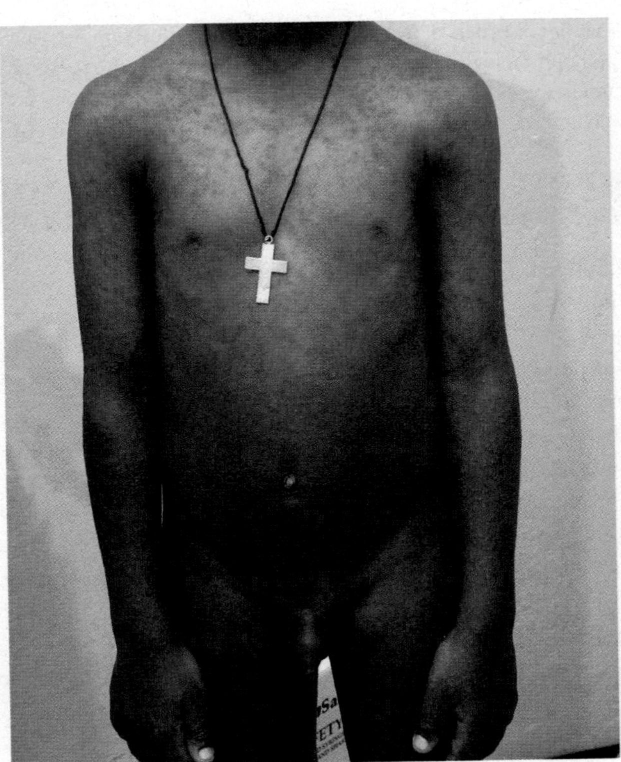

FIGURE 207-2 An African boy with a long history of atopic dermatitis and newly diagnosed scabies. Note how the postinflammatory hyperpigmentation is concentrated around the waist and forearms.

ETIOLOGY AND PATHOPHYSIOLOGY

- The most common causes of PIH are acne vulgaris, atopic dermatitis (see **Figure 207-1**), and impetigo, but any insult to the skin from bug bites and minor burns to drug reactions and other rashes can result in PIH.[1,5]
- PIH may be divided based on whether the pigment accumulates in the epidermis or in the dermis. This can be helpful in terms of understanding the pathophysiology, characteristic appearances, and treatment modalities associated with the two categories.
- Epidermal hyperpigmentation is thought to be in part caused by the release of inflammatory molecules such as prostanoids, cytokines, chemokines, and other products of arachidonic acid, which leads to increased melanocyte activity, increased melanin production and release, and accumulation of melanin in adjacent keratinocytes.[1,5,9,10]
- Dermal hyperpigmentation is thought to result from inflammatory mediated destruction of keratinocytes, which results in melanin release and its accumulation within macrophages in the upper dermis.[1] Histologically this is described as "pigment incontinence."
- The distinction between accumulation of pigment in the epidermis and accumulation of pigment in the dermis is reflected in the appearance of the lesion on the skin. Dermal lesions tend to be a blue-gray color with indistinct boundaries, and epidermal lesions tend to be tan, brown, or dark brown and with more sharply demarcated borders.[1,11]

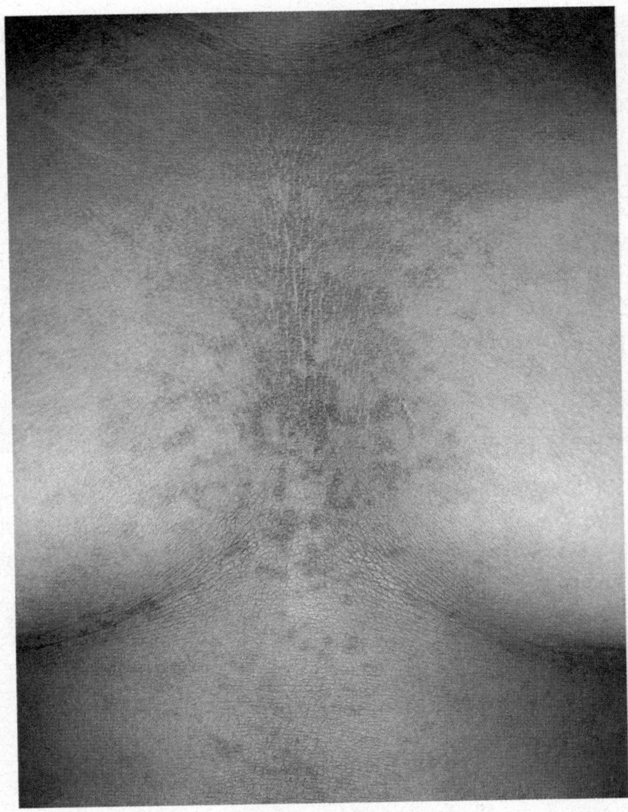

FIGURE 207-3 Confluent and reticulated papillomatosis (CARP) in an overweight 15-year-old boy with gynecomastia. *(Reproduced with permission from Richard P. Usatine, MD.)*

- In other disorders of hyperpigmentation the connection between the pathophysiology and the cutaneous appearance also exists; the color and shape of the pigment generally reflects both the location of melanin and the degree of melanocytic hyperplasia or release of melanin.[7]

DIAGNOSIS

CLINICAL FEATURES

- The degree of pigmentation is strongly correlated with the total duration of the inflammatory process, where chronic or relapsing inflammatory processes cause darker and longer-lasting hyperpigmentation.[1]
- Darker-skinned individuals have larger and more densely distributed melanin pigment in their skin. In turn, they tend to react to inflammation with more accumulation of pigment, and therefore PIH tends to present with darker lesions that last longer.[1,12]
- UV exposure is also associated with darkening and persistence of hyperpigmented lesions.[13]
- The location of the pigmentation in the skin also affects the persistence of PIH, and dermal hyperpigmentation tends to last longer since the dermis does not continuously turn over like the epidermis.[13]

TYPICAL DISTRIBUTION

- PIH typically follows the pattern of the initial inflammatory process and consists of macules or patches.[12]

LABORATORY AND IMAGING

- A Wood lamp examination can be used to distinguish between epidermal and dermal hyperpigmentation, where epidermal lesions will have distinct margins and a prominent border whereas dermal lesions will have fluffy, indistinct margins.[5]

BIOPSY

In general, skin biopsies are unnecessary, but if the etiology is uncertain, a 4-mm punch biopsy can help determine the underlying cause of PIH. The Fontana-Masson stain is used to identify melanin in the skin and is useful in distinguishing between epidermal and dermal hyperpigmentation.[5]

DIFFERENTIAL DIAGNOSIS

- Confluent and reticular papillomatosis (CARP) is characterized by hyperkeratotic or verrucous scaly brown papules that coalesce into plaques, with a peripheral reticular pattern with or without pruritus (**Figure 207-7**). It is generally first seen in the inframammary region or interscapular region, and it often spreads to the chest or abdomen (see **Figure 207-3**). It can be found on the face, neck, extremities, flanks, or gluteal cleft. The etiology is unknown, but potential causes include a keratinization disorder, a reaction to a fungal or bacterial infection, photosensitivity, amyloidosis, and genetic factors.[14,15]

CARP can be distinguished from PIH both clinically and by its unique histology. CARP is raised and keratotic papules and plaques on the torso while PIH is typically flat macules or patches where there

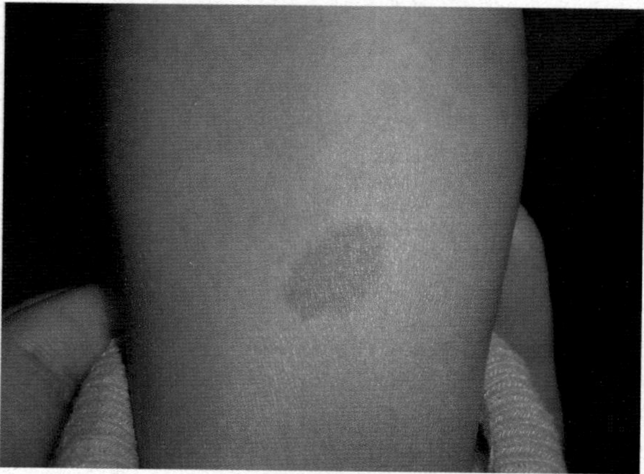

FIGURE 207-4 Café au lait macule in a girl found to have tuberous sclerosis. (*Reproduced with permission from Richard P. Usatine, MD.*)

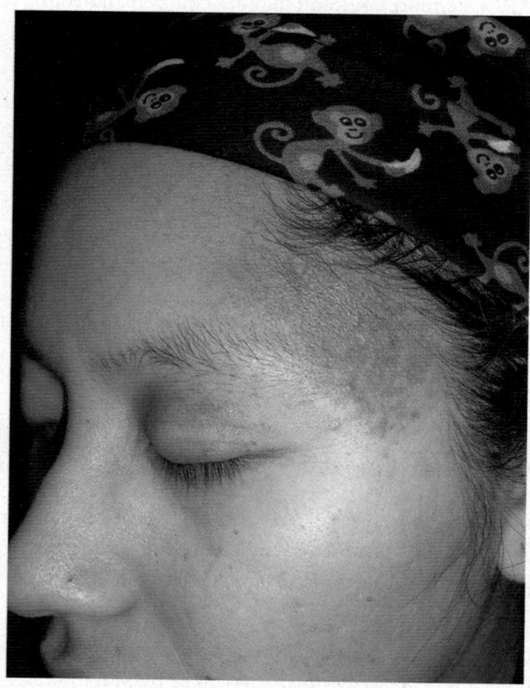

FIGURE 207-5 Nevus of Ota with a blue-gray coloration around the eye. (*Reproduced with permission from Richard P. Usatine, MD.*)

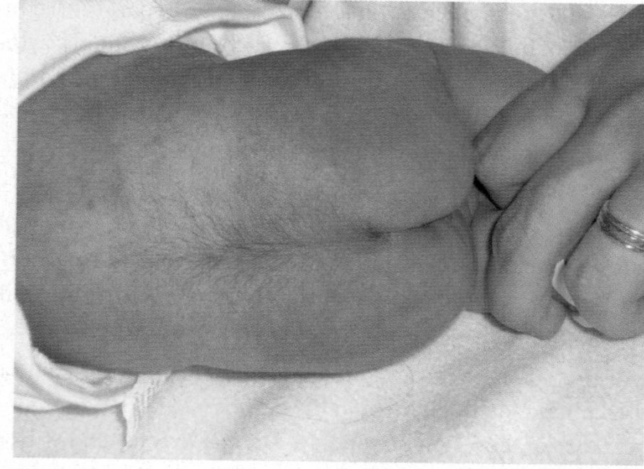

FIGURE 207-6 Dermal melanocytosis (Mongolian spot) over the buttocks of a newborn. (*Reproduced with permission from Richard P. Usatine, MD.*)

were previous lesions. Tinea versicolor occurs in a similar distribution to CARP (on the torso), but tinea versicolor is scaly patches and responds to oral or topical antifungal therapy (**Figure 207-8**).

CARP is a rare disorder, but it is most commonly seen in young adults (age 18–21) and people with skin of color. In the United States it is more common in females than in males, but the gender distribution varies in different parts of the world. Minocycline is considered the first-line treatment, but azithromycin, clarithromycin, fusidic acid, and retinoic acid have also been effective in case reports and case studies.[14]

- Linear and whorled hypermelanosis (LAWH) is characterized by linear and whorled patches that occur along the lines of Blaschko (lines of embryologic development).[16] The lesions can occur anywhere on the body, but typically spare the mucous membranes, palms, soles, and eyes.[16] LAWH appears within a few weeks of birth and will progressively expand and darken until the child is 1–2 years of age. The exact cause of LAWH is unknown, but it may be associated with underlying genetic mosaicism.[8] There have been a few cases where LAWH was associated with neurologic abnormalities, but the association is very rare.[16,17] In general, there is no need to do neurologic testing or brain imaging if the child seems normal and healthy.[8]
- Segmental hyperpigmentation presents at birth or in early childhood as a hyperpigmented patch on the trunk with a characteristic delineation at midline, usually ventral, giving them a dermatomal appearance (**Figure 207-9**). There are no known associated abnormalities, and segmental hyperpigmentation is thought to be due to a somatic mosaicism.[18]
- Erythema ab igne is a reticular tan-brown pigmented patch (see Chapter 209, Erythema Ab Igne). It is most commonly caused by prolonged exposure to heat or infrared.[19] It has been reported in persons who use laptop computers directly on their laps.[19] Other common causes include hot-water bottles, heating pads, and heated blankets. It is generally a self-limited condition, but prolonged exposure and recurrence of the lesions may predispose to squamous cell carcinoma or Merkel cell carcinoma.[19]
- Café-au-lait macules (CALMs) are evenly pigmented light brown macules or patches (see **Figure 207-4**). They are commonly solitary and present at birth, though they can appear any time in the first few years of life.[20] CALMs are also more common in blacks than whites. If CALMs continue to appear into adulthood or are multiple, this warrants further investigation, as these characteristics increase the likelihood of a coexisting condition such as neurofibromatosis, tuberous sclerosis, McCune-Albright, or Noonan syndrome (see Chapter 245, Neurofibromatosis).[20] There is no medical reason to treat CALMs. These lesions are caused by epidermal melanin, giant melanosomes, and increased melanocyte density. Skin lightening creams are not effective, but several lasers have been used with variable responses, including pulsed dye, erbium:YAG, Q-switched Nd:YAG, QS ruby, and QS alexandrite. The risks of laser surgery include hypo/hyperpigmentation, scarring, incomplete removal, and recurrence.[21]
- Dermal melanocytosis (Mongolian spot) is a blue-gray hyperpigmented patch that can vary in size, but is most commonly found on the gluteal region of newborns and infants (see **Figure 207-6**).[22] It is most prevalent in individuals of Asian and African ancestry, but

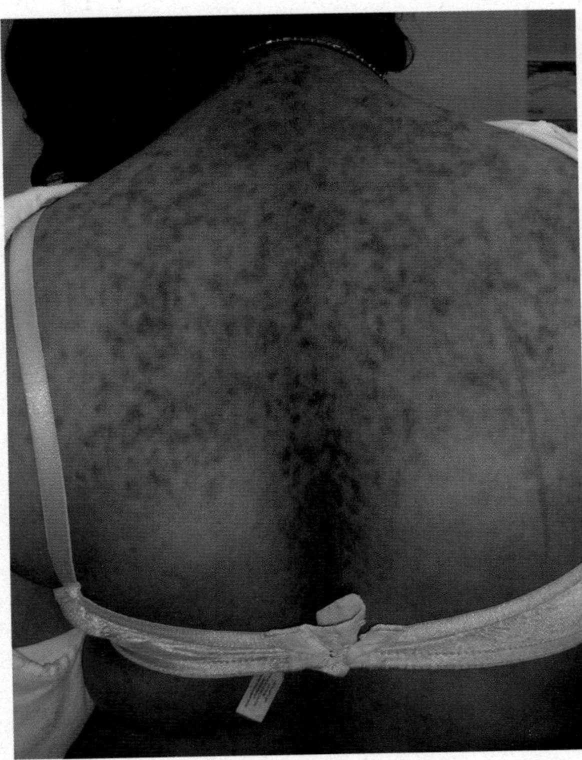

FIGURE 207-7 Confluent and reticulated papillomatosis (CARP) on the back of an African American girl. (*Reproduced with permission from Richard P. Usatine, MD.*)

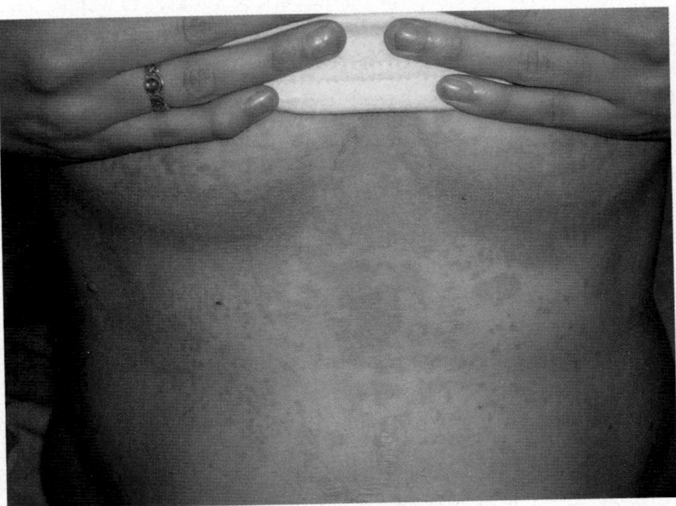

FIGURE 207-8 Tinea versicolor over the chest in a 22-year-old woman. Note how the *Malassezia* has caused a brown hyperpigmentation along with scale. (*Reproduced with permission from Richard P. Usatine, MD.*)

it can occur in individuals of any race. The lesion is benign, has no known association with other congenital abnormalities, and will disappear in most children by the age of 4 but sometimes persists.[22] Given the likelihood of spontaneous regression, there is no need for treatment.

- Ashy dermatosis (erythema dyschromicum perstans, EDP) is characterized by blue-gray macules that may have a raised erythematous border.[23] They are most often found on the trunk, extremities, and neck (**Figure 207-10**). These lesions of unknown etiology are chronic and may grow larger and multiply over time. The prevalence is highest among Latin Americans, though other races can be affected. EDP most commonly presents between the ages of 10 and 30, but can occur at any age.[23] The treatment of EDP is limited and lesions are often permanent. Many therapies have been attempted, but none are very effective.[24]
- Nevus of Ota (oculodermal melanocytosis) is a speckled blue-gray or brown macular lesion that follows a dermatomal distribution, usually unilaterally within the distribution of the ophthalmic and maxillary branches of the trigeminal nerve. In addition to skin, it may involve ocular and oral mucosal surfaces (see **Figures 207-5** and **16-8**).[25] These lesions represent a hamartoma of dermal melanocytes. Nevus of Ito is the same process on the body and is often found on the shoulder or back (**Figure 207-11**). These lesions are often present at birth and tend to darken and expand with age. It is more commonly seen in Asian children, but can occur in any race and shows no gender predilection. Malignant transformation in nevus of Ota/Ito is extremely rare, but there is up to 10% risk of glaucoma if the eye is involved. Nevus of Ota have also been associated with Sturge-Weber, Klippel-Trenaunay-Weber, and neurodevelopmental abnormalities.[25] These risks make close follow-up important in pediatric patients. This dermal pigmentation responds well to laser therapy with the Q-switched ruby, Q-switched alexandrite, or Q-switched Nd:YAG lasers for cosmesis, but they do not require treatment.[26-28]
- In children with pigmented lesions, it is especially important to consider and rule out child abuse as a possibly cause.[12] Bruising or PIH that is linear or geometric in nature should raise concern for abuse. Also, lesions of abuse on the back or buttocks in a child can mimic EDP or dermal melanocytosis; however, traumatic lesions will fade quickly compared to the latter.

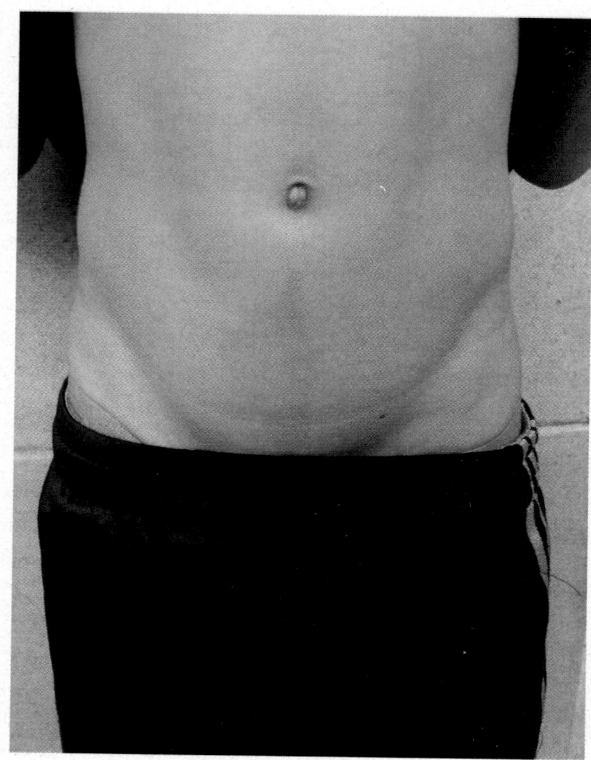

FIGURE 207-9 Segmental hyperpigmentation in a healthy 8-year-old boy. Lesion appeared shortly after birth as a faint patch and became more apparent in early childhood. (*Reproduced with permission from Jennifer Krejci-Mannwaring, MD.*)

MANAGEMENT

The first step in the management of PIH is to ascertain the underlying cause of cutaneous inflammation or trauma and rule out other causes of pigmented lesions.

The shape and distribution of the lesions should mirror the pattern of the underlying disorder, and most patients with PIH will have a history of chronic skin disease or trauma. When there is no history of a chronic skin condition, it is important to consider congenital diseases or other causes of hyperpigmentation; see Differential Diagnosis above.

If the underlying cause is a treatable condition, then prompt treatment is essential. Decreasing the development of additional PIH requires controlling the source of cutaneous inflammation.[12]

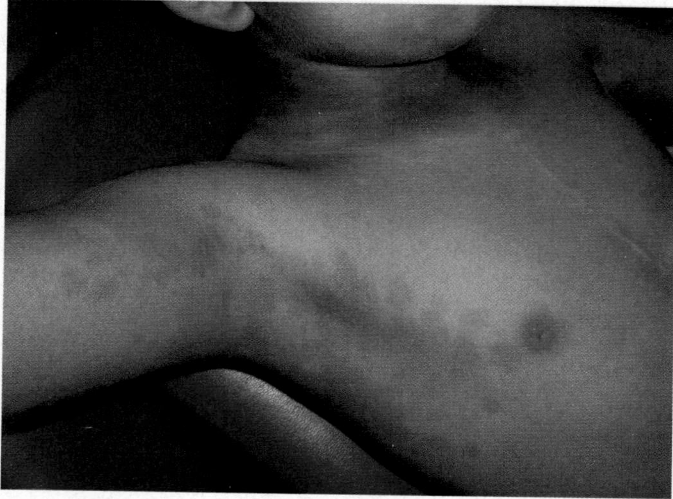

FIGURE 207-10 Ashy dermatosis (erythema dyschromicum perstans) in an 8-year-old boy that was confirmed by a punch biopsy. (*Reproduced with permission from Richard P. Usatine, MD.*)

NONPHARMACOLOGIC

- The first line of therapy for PIH is *daily* sunscreen use. Daily use of sunscreen with a sun protection factor (SPF) of 30 or greater has been shown to decrease the duration of PIH and to prevent darkening of existing lesions.[1] Any gains made with topical or other therapies can quickly be undone by short exposures to ultraviolet light. Behavior modification often requires additional patient/parent education. Although individuals with darker skin types are more prone to pigmentary disorder, they may not be familiar with sun protection behaviors, given that they have a lower propensity for sunburn. "Physical sunscreens" (ones that are zinc or titanium based) are preferred; however, on darkly pigmented skin they may leave a gray or violaceous hue when applied, and therefore finding an aesthetically acceptable product may be tricky. Sun protection should also include avoidance of peak sun hours (10 AM to 4 PM), the use of wide-brimmed hats, and long sleeves or pants depending on the body part affected.

TOPICAL TREATMENTS

Various topical skin-lightening agents have been used to treat PIH and other disorders of hyperpigmentation. The treatments include topical medication such as hydroquinone, retinoids, mequinol, azelaic acid, kojic acid, licorice extract, ascorbic acid, niacinamide, *N*-acetyl glucosamine, and soy.[1,12,29] In general, topical skin-lightening agents are most effective on epidermal pigmentation, and less effective for dermal hyperpigmentation.[12]

The first line in topical treatment for PIH is hydroquinone, which can be used at various concentrations, although there is no increase in efficacy at concentrations higher than 5%.[13,30] Controlled trials have shown a decrease in skin hyperpigmentation as compared to baseline by 4 weeks after beginning therapy.[31] The potential side effects include allergic dermatitis (most common), the development of a ring of hypopigmentation around the lesions, and, rarely, paradoxical darkening of the lesions (exogenous ochronosis).[32]

Combination therapies with hydroquinone show additional efficacy. Small trials of 4% hydroquinone and 0.15% retinol have shown significant improvement in the degree of pigmentation and the lesion size.[31] Triple therapies combining 4% hydroquinone, 0.1% tretinoin or 0.5% ascorbic acid, and topical steroids (dexamethasone or fluocinolone acetonide) resulted in higher rates of complete skin clearing of melasma than either hydroquinone monotherapy or dual therapy, but there is no such trial on the use of triple therapy in PIH.[33]

There is some evidence for the efficacy of tretinoin (retinoic acid) as monotherapy in the treatment of PIH. In one randomized controlled trial, 91% of the participants in the treatment group had significant lightening of their lesions compared to 57% in the control group based on clinical evaluation.[34]

- There is some limited clinical evidence for the efficacy of such compounds as kojic acid, arbutin, niacinamide, *N*-acetyl glucosamine, ascorbic acid, licorice extract, and soy in treating hyperpigmentation. Most of the evidence for the efficacy of these naturally occurring chemicals is from trials for the treatment of melasma.[29] Of the agents listed, topical soy extract is the only agent with significant evidence in PIH.[13] Many of these compounds are marketed in over-the-counter products and may also contain derivatives of retinoic acid such as retinol or retinyl.

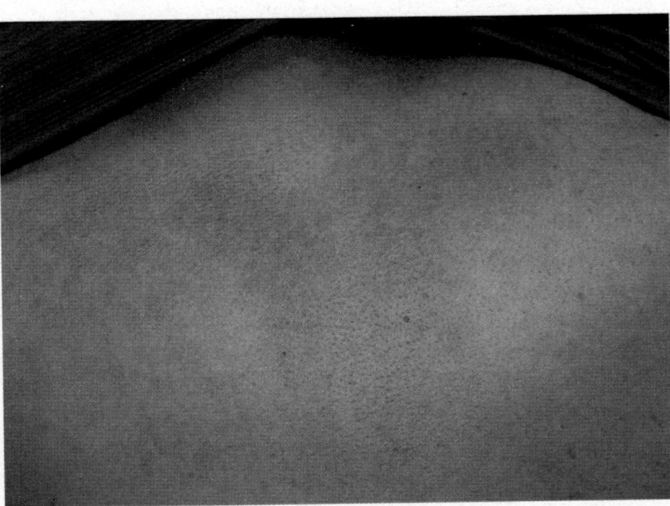

FIGURE 207-11 Nevus of Ito with blue-gray coloration on the back of a 57-year-old man. He has had this his whole life. (*Reproduced with permission from Richard P. Usatine, MD.*)

PROCEDURES

- The most common procedures used in the treatment of hyperpigmented lesions are chemical peels and laser therapy. Both have been shown to be efficacious in clinical trials.[21] They remain second-line treatments and are generally only indicated in combination with topical agents, or after treatment with topical agents has failed.[21]
- Chemical peels are used to treat hyperpigmentation.[13] The chemical agents used for these procedures include glycolic acid (GA), salicylic acid, and trichloroacetic acid.[35,36] In general, superficial peels are recommended for people with skin of color to decrease the risk of additional PIH. Side effects of chemical peels include erythema, burning/stinging, hypo/hyperpigmentation, ulceration, scarring, reactivation of herpes simplex virus (HSV), and superficial desquamation. Repeated peels (5 or more) are often needed to achieve results.

A few randomized controlled trials have indicated that the use of GA chemical peels in addition to hydroquinone therapy was as effective in PIH as hydroquinone therapy and tended to work more quickly with more dramatic results.[37] There are few data in the current literature assessing the safety of these therapies in children, though there are a few case reports of good outcomes in children with xeroderma pigmentosum and congenital melanocytic nevi.[38,39]

- Lasers are used in the treatment of hyperpigmentation. Q-switch alexandrite, Q-switch ruby, Q-switch Nd:YAG, and nonablative fractional proteolysis laser treatments have been effective in treatment of many hyperpigmented lesions including PIH, Mongolian spots, nevus of Ota, and café-au-lait macules.[21]

PROGNOSIS

- The course of PIH is strongly dependent on controlling the underlying inflammatory disease. Once the underlying disease is treated, most epidermal hyperpigmentation will resolve in 6–12 months, and with treatment the lesions may resolve as quickly as 4 weeks.[5,31] Dermal hyperpigmentation has a comparatively prolonged course, and lesions can persist for years or be permanent despite treatment.[5]

FOLLOW-UP

- The first step for children with PIH is to treat the underlying cause. Once the cause is treated, simple reassurance and regular follow-up may be sufficient. More aggressive treatment should be considered for lesions in aesthetically sensitive areas such as the face, or if the child experiences significant psychological distress.
- In children with congenital hyperpigmented lesions that may lead to psychological distress, consider initiating treatment early, but give parents realistic expectations. Most congenital or persistent lesions, if responsive, will do so to more invasive treatments such as laser therapy.

PATIENT EDUCATION

- PIH will generally resolve spontaneously over time, and the primary objective is to identify and eliminate the cause of inflammation in the skin.
- Strict sun protection may prevent worsening of PIH and can help it fade more quickly.
- If PIH persists, there are other treatment options, but they have variable effectiveness and side effects and should be reserved for cases that have not resolved with watchful waiting.

PATIENT RESOURCES

- **http://www.nlm.nih.gov/medlineplus/ency/article/003242.htm.**
- **http://www.skinsight.com/infant/cafeauLaitMacule.htm.**
- **http://www.dermnetnz.org/colour/pigmentation.html.**

PROVIDER RESOURCES

- **http://emedicine.medscape.com/article/1069191-overview.**

REFERENCES

1. Davis EC, Callender VD. Postinflammatory hyperpigmentation: a review of the epidemiology, clinical features, and treatment options in skin of color. *J Clin Aesthet Dermatol.* 2010;3(7):20-31.
2. Hubert JN, Callen JP, Kasteler JS. Prevalence of cutaneous findings in hospitalized pediatric patients. *Pediatr Dermatol.* 1997; 14(6):426-429.
3. Okafor OO, Akinbami FO, Orimadegun AE, et al. Prevalence of dermatological lesions in hospitalized children at the University College Hospital, Ibadan, Nigeria. *Niger J Clin Pract.* 2011;14(3): 287-292.
4. Alexis AF, Sergay AB, Taylor SC. Common dermatologic disorders in skin of color: a comparative practice survey. *Cutis.* 2007; 80(5):387-394.
5. Lacz NL, Vafaie J, Kihiczak NI, Schwartz RA. Postinflammatory hyperpigmentation: a common but troubling condition. *Int J Dermatol.* 2004;43(5):362-365.
6. Epstein JH. Postinflammatory hyperpigmentation. *Clin Dermatol.* 1989;7(2):55-65.
7. Taieb A, Boralevi F. Hypermelanoses of the newborn and of the infant. *Dermatol Clin.* 2007;25(3):327-336, viii.
8. Loomis CA. Linear hypopigmentation and hyperpigmentation, including mosaicism. *Semin Cutan Med Surg.* 1997;16(1):44-53.
9. Tomita Y, Maeda K, Tagami H. Melanocyte-stimulating properties of arachidonic acid metabolites: possible role in postinflammatory pigmentation. *Pigment Cell Res.* 1992;5(5 Pt 2):357-361.
10. Ortonne JP. Retinoic acid and pigment cells: a review of in-vitro and in-vivo studies. *Br J Dermatol.* 1992;127 Suppl 41:43-47.
11. Pandya AG, Guevara IL. Disorders of hyperpigmentation. *Dermatol Clin.* 2000;18(1):91-98, ix.
12. Ruiz-Maldonado R, Orozco-Covarrubias ML. Postinflammatory hypopigmentation and hyperpigmentation. *Semin Cutan Med Surg.* 1997;16(1):36-43.
13. Callender VD, St Surin-Lord S, Davis EC, Maclin M. Postinflammatory hyperpigmentation: etiologic and therapeutic considerations. *Am J Clin Dermatol.* 2011;12(2):87-99.

14. Jang HS, Oh CK, Cha JH, et al. Six cases of confluent and reticulated papillomatosis alleviated by various antibiotics. *J Am Acad Dermatol.* 2001;44(4):652-655.

15. Scheinfeld N. Confluent and reticulated papillomatosis: a review of the literature. *Am J Clin Dermatol.* 2006;7(5):305-313.

16. Di Lernia V. Linear and whorled hypermelanosis. *Pediatr Dermatol.* 2007;24(3):205-210.

17. Nehal KS, PeBenito R, Orlow SJ. Analysis of 54 cases of hypopigmentation and hyperpigmentation along the lines of Blaschko. *Arch Dermatol.* 1996;132(10):1167-1170.

18. Hogeling M, Frieden IJ. Segmental pigmentation disorder. *Br J Dermatol.* 2010;162(6):1337-1341.

19. Arnold AW, Itin PH. Laptop computer-induced erythema ab igne in a child and review of the literature. *Pediatrics.* 2010;126(5): e1227-1230.

20. Shah KN. The diagnostic and clinical significance of cafe-au-lait macules. *Pediatr Clin North Am.* 2010;57(5):1131-1153.

21. Polder KD, Landau JM, Vergilis-Kalner IJ, et al. Laser eradication of pigmented lesions: a review. *Dermatol Surg.* 2011;37(5):572-595.

22. Cordova A. The Mongolian spot: a study of ethnic differences and a literature review. *Clin Pediatr (Phila).* 1981;20(11):714-719.

23. Osswald SS, Proffer LH, Sartori CR. Erythema dyschromicum perstans: a case report and review. *Cutis.* 2001;68(1):25-28.

24. Torrelo A, Zaballos P, Colmenero I, et al. Erythema dyschromicum perstans in children: a report of 14 cases. *J Eur Acad Dermatol Venereol.* 2005;19(4):422-426.

25. Sinha S, Cohen PJ, Schwartz RA. Nevus of Ota in children. *Cutis.* 2008;82(1):25-29.

26. Chang CJ, Kou CS. Comparing the effectiveness of Q-switched ruby laser treatment with that of Q-switched Nd:YAG laser for oculodermal melanosis (nevus of Ota). *J Plast Reconstr Aesthet Surg.* 2011;64(3):339-345.

27. Liu J, Ma YP, Ma XG, et al. A retrospective study of q-switched alexandrite laser in treating nevus of Ota. *Dermatol Surg.* 2011; 37(10):1480-1485.

28. Fusade T, Lafaye S, Laubach HJ. Nevus of Ota in dark skin—an uncommon but treatable entity. *Lasers Surg Med.* 2011;43(10): 960-964.

29. Leyden JJ, Shergill B, Micali G, et al. Natural options for the management of hyperpigmentation. *J Eur Acad Dermatol Venereol.* 2011;25(10):1140-1145.

30. Perez-Bernal A, Munoz-Perez MA, Camacho F. Management of facial hyperpigmentation. *Am J Clin Dermatol.* 2000;1(5): 261-268.

31. Cook-Bolden FE, Hamilton SF. An open-label study of the efficacy and tolerability of microencapsulated hydroquinone 4% and retinol 0.15% with antioxidants for the treatment of hyperpigmentation. *Cutis.* 2008;81(4):365-371.

32. Lynde CB, Kraft JN, Lynde CW. Topical treatments for melasma and postinflammatory hyperpigmentation. *Skin Therapy Lett.* 2006;11(9):1-6.

33. Taylor SC, Torok H, Jones T, et al. Efficacy and safety of a new triple-combination agent for the treatment of facial melasma. *Cutis.* 2003;72(1):67-72.

34. Bulengo-Ransby SM, Griffiths CE, Kimbrough-Green CK, et al. Topical tretinoin (retinoic acid) therapy for hyperpigmented lesions caused by inflammation of the skin in black patients. *N Engl J Med.* 1993;328(20):1438-1443.

35. Grimes PE. The safety and efficacy of salicylic acid chemical peels in darker racial-ethnic groups. *Dermatol Surg.* 1999;25(1):18-22.

36. Grover C, Reddu BS. The therapeutic value of glycolic acid peels in dermatology. *Indian J Dermatol Venereol Leprol.* 2003;69(2):148-150.

37. Burns RL, Prevost-Blank PL, Lawry MA, et al. Glycolic acid peels for postinflammatory hyperpigmentation in black patients. A comparative study. *Dermatol Surg.* 1997;23(3):171-174; discussion 175.

38. Nelson BR, Fader DJ, Gillard M, et al. The role of dermabrasion and chemical peels in the treatment of patients with xeroderma pigmentosum. *J Am Acad Dermatol.* 1995;32(4):623-626.

39. O'Neill TB, Rawlins J, Rea S, Wood F. Treatment of a large congenital melanocytic nevus with dermabrasion and autologous cell suspension (ReCELL(R)): a case report. *J Plast Reconstr Aesthet Surg.* 2011;64(12):1672-1676.

208 PHOTOSENSITIVITY

E.J. Mayeaux, Jr., MD

PATIENT STORY

A 50-year-old woman presented to the clinic with an abrupt onset of an intensely pruritic rash that extended over the dorsal aspect of both arms (**Figure 208-1**). The patient noted no new medicines and no recent exposures to any new chemicals. She acknowledged recent time spent outside in the sun. The plaques were photodistributed, with sparing of her watch area. A clinical diagnosis of polymorphous light eruption (PMLE) was made, and the patient was started on oral antihistamines and topical steroids. It was recommended that she minimize her sun exposure.

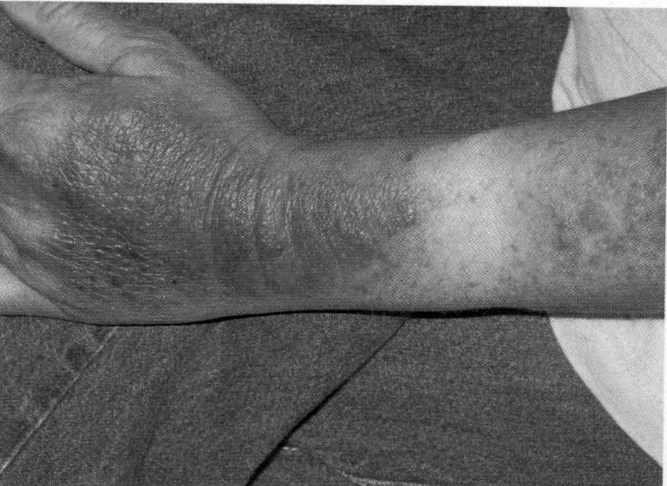

FIGURE 208-1 Polymorphous light eruption noted over dorsum of left forearm. Note absence of the lesion where the patient had been wearing her watch. *(Reproduced with permission from Wenner C, Lee A. A bright red pruritic rash on the forearms, J Fam Pract. 2007;56(8): 627-629. Frontline Medical Communications. Inc.)*

INTRODUCTION

Photosensitivity is an abnormal skin response to ultraviolet light that occurs on sun-exposed areas of the skin. There are three common types of photodermatitis:

- Polymorphous light eruption or PMLE (**Figures 208-1** and **208-2**).
- Phototoxic eruptions (**Figures 208-3** to **208-7**).
- Photoallergic eruptions (**Figure 208-8**). **Table 208-1** compares key characteristics of phototoxic and photoallergic reactions.

UV light radiating from the sun may be categorized into UVA (wavelength 320 to 400 nm), UVB (290 to 320 nm), and UVC (200 to 290 nm). UVC is completely absorbed by the earth's ozone layer and thus does not play a role in photosensitivity. Photosensitivity may be induced by UVA, UVB, or visible light (400 to 760 nm). Longer wavelength light penetrates deeper into the skin. UVA penetrates through to the dermis, but UVB mainly penetrates and affects the epidermis.

Ultraviolet light has multiple effects on the skin. Notably, it causes DNA damage and has immunosuppressive effects on skin inflammatory cells, increasing the risk of carcinogenesis. In patients with photosensitivity, it elicits an inflammatory response in the skin, leading to the development of a photodermatosis.

EPIDEMIOLOGY

- PMLE (see **Figures 208-1** and **208-2**) may affect up to 10% of the population, with a predilection for females.[1] The prevalence increases in northern latitudes. Onset typically occurs within the first three decades of life but may appear spontaneously at any age.[2] It typically occurs in the spring and early summer.
- The incidence of drug- and plant-induced phototoxic reactions in the United States is unknown. Photosensitivity incidence is low, and phototoxic reactions are much more common than photoallergic reactions. Data from photodermatology referral centers show 7% to 15% for phototoxic reactions and 4% to 8% for photoallergic reactions. Studies in the United States and Europe show the incidence of photoallergic contact dermatitis in patients who are photopatch-tested is between 1.4% and 12.0%.[3]

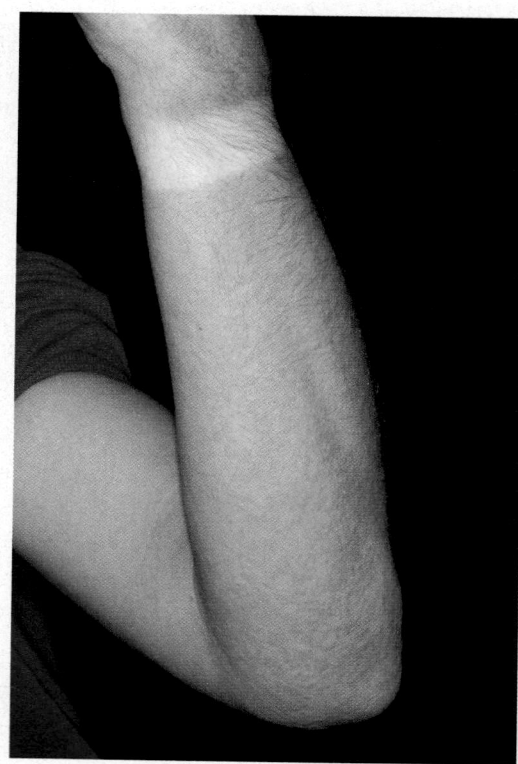

FIGURE 208-2 Polymorphous light eruption on the arm of a young man. Note the sparing of the skin under his watchband. *(Reproduced with permission from Richard P. Usatine, MD.)*

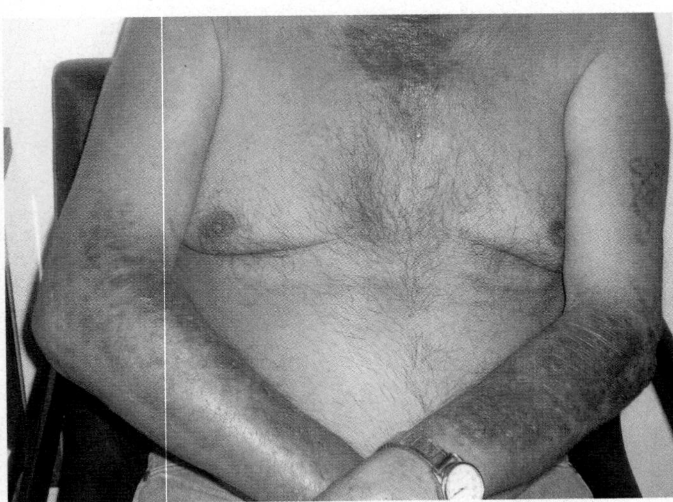

FIGURE 208-3 Severe phototoxic drug reaction secondary to hydrochlorothiazide use. (*Reproduced with permission from Richard P. Usatine, MD.*)

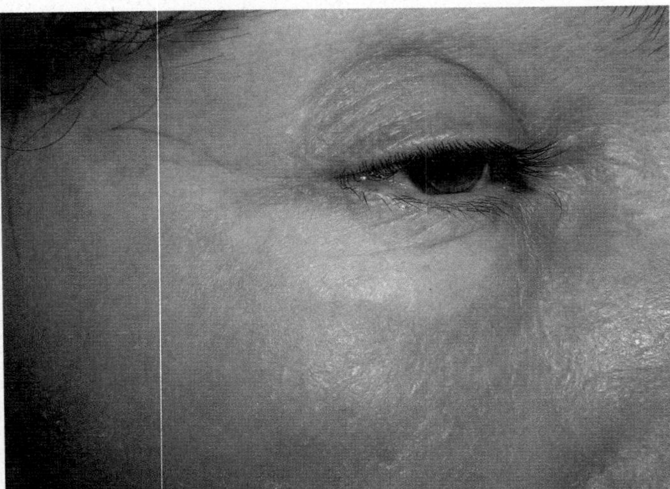

FIGURE 208-4 Phototoxic drug reaction secondary to ibuprofen. (*Reproduced with permission from Richard P. Usatine, MD.*)

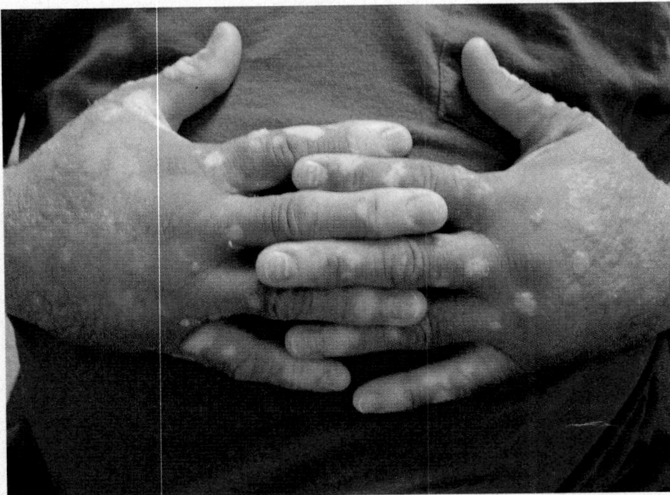

FIGURE 208-5 Phototoxic drug reaction secondary to treatment of vitiligo with oral psoralen and ultraviolet light (phytophotodermatitis). Note the bullae. (*Reproduced with permission from Richard P. Usatine, MD.*)

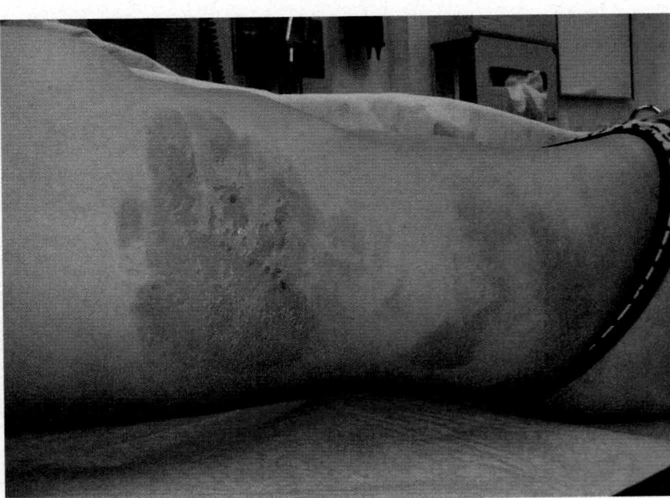

FIGURE 208-6 Phytophotodermatitis in a woman, caused by lime juice and sun exposure on the beach. Note the hand print of her fiancé who had been squeezing limes into their tropical drinks. This contact occurred when they posed for a photograph. (*Reproduced with permission from Darby-Stewart AL, Edwards FD, Perry KJ. Hyperpigmentation and vesicles after beach vacation. Phytophotodermatitis, J Fam Pract. 2006;55(12):1050-1053. Frontline Medical Communications. Inc.*)

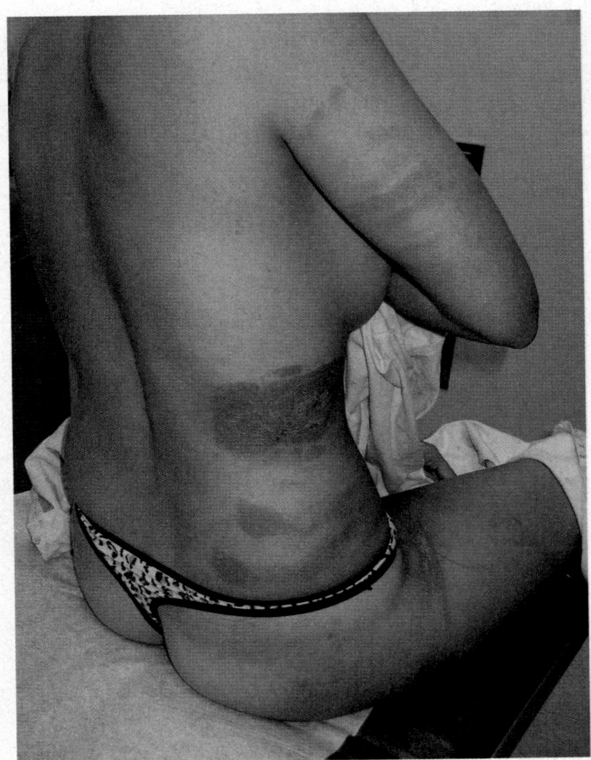

FIGURE 208-7 Phytophotodermatitis visible on the arm, trunk, and leg caused by lime juice and sun exposure on the beach. Note the hyperpigmentation that occurs in conjunction with the erythema. (*Reproduced with permission from Darby-Stewart AL, Edwards FD, Perry KJ. Hyperpigmentation and vesicles after beach vacation. Phytophotodermatitis, J Fam Pract. 2006;55(12):1050-1053. Frontline Medical Communications. Inc.*)

ETIOLOGY AND PATHOPHYSIOLOGY

PMLE (sun poisoning or sun allergy) is an idiopathic, delayed-type hypersensitivity reaction to UVA light and, to a lesser extent, UVB light (see **Figures 208-1** and **208-2**). PMLE is the most common photoeruption encountered in clinical practice. The reaction will remit spontaneously with time and absence of sun exposure, but occasionally it will last as long as sun exposure occurs. The rash develops within hours to days after exposure to sunlight and lasts for several days to a week.

There is a broad range of degrees of photosensitivity with PMLE. Extremely sensitive individuals can tolerate only minutes of exposure, whereas many people have a low sensitivity and require prolonged exposure to sunlight before developing a reaction. It is a recurrent condition that persists for many years in most patients.[4]

Phototoxic reactions are the most common drug-induced photoeruptions (see **Figures 208-3** to **208-7**). They are caused by absorption of ultraviolet rays by the causative drug, which releases energy and damages cell membranes, or, in the case of psoralens, DNA. The drugs that most frequently cause phototoxic reactions are nonsteroidal anti-inflammatory drugs (NSAIDs), quinolones, tetracyclines, amiodarone, and the phenothiazines[5] (**Table 208-2**). Most of these drugs have at least one resonating double bond or an aromatic ring that can absorb radiant energy. Most compounds are activated by wavelengths within the UVA (320 to 400 nm) range, although some compounds have a peak absorption within the UVB or visible range.

Phytophotodermatitis are phototoxic reactions to psoralens, which are plant compounds found in limes, celery, figs, and certain drugs. They can cause dramatic inflammation and bullae where the psoralen comes into contact with the skin (see **Figures 208-5** to **208-7**). The inflammation is frequently followed by hyperpigmentation.

Photoallergic eruptions are delayed-type hypersensitivity reactions. Photoactivation of a drug or agent results in the development of a metabolite that can bind to proteins in the skin to form a complete antigen. The subsequent pathogenesis and presentation of the reaction is identical to allergic contact dermatitis.[6] The antigen is presented to lymphocytes by Langerhans cells, causing an inflammatory response

TABLE 208-1 Characteristics of Phototoxic and Photoallergic Reactions

Feature	Phototoxic Reaction	Photoallergic Reaction
Incidence	High	Low
Amount of agent required for photosensitivity	Large	Small
Onset of reaction after exposure	Minutes to hours	24 to 72 hours
More than 1 exposure to agent required	No	Yes
Examination findings	Exaggerated sunburn	Dermatitis
Immunologically mediated	No	Yes

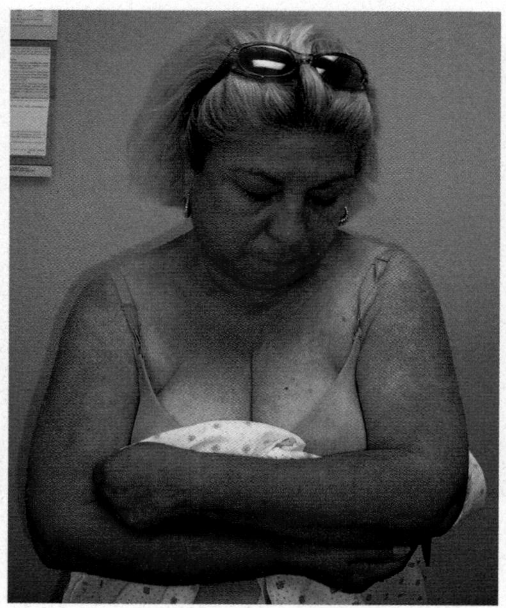

FIGURE 208-8 A photoallergic drug reaction characterized by widespread eczema in the photodistribution areas such as the face, upper chest, arms, and back of hands. A punch biopsy showed a spongiotic dermatitis. The exact photoallergen was not found. (*Reproduced with permission from Richard P. Usatine, MD.*)

TABLE 208-2 Common Medications That Cause Phototoxic Reactions

Class	Medication
Antibiotics	Tetracyclines Fluoroquinolones Sulfonamides Griseofulvin
NSAIDs	Ketoprofen Ibuprofen Naproxen Piroxicam
Diuretics	Furosemide Thiazides
Retinoids	Isotretinoin Acitretin
Photodynamic therapy prophotosensitizers	5-Aminolevulinic acid Methyl-5-aminolevulinic acid Verteporfin Photofrin
Neuroleptic drugs	Phenothiazines Thioxanthenes (chlorprothixene and thiothixene)
Other drugs	Itraconazole 5-Fluorouracil (5-FU) Amiodarone Diltiazem Quinidine Coal tar
Sunscreens	Paraaminobenzoic acid (PABA)

and spongiotic dermatitis (eczema). The eruption is characterized by widespread eczema in the photodistribution areas such as the face, upper chest, arms, and back of hands (see **Figure 208-8**). Most photoallergic reactions are caused by topical agents such as antibiotics and halogenated phenolic compounds added to soaps and fragrances (**Figure 208-9**).[6] Systemic photoallergens such as the phenothiazines, chlorpromazine, sulfa products, and NSAIDs can produce photoallergic reactions, although most of their photosensitive reactions are phototoxic (**Table 208-3**).

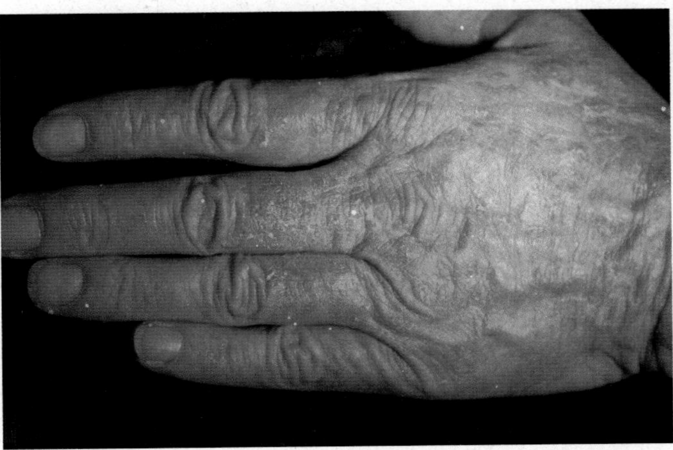

FIGURE 208-9 A photoallergic reaction to an ingredient in certain hand soaps characterized by eczema in the hands and lower arms. Note that the reaction only occurred with use of the offending agents and sun exposure. (*Reproduced with permission from E.J. Mayeaux, Jr., MD.*)

RISK FACTORS

Unprotected exposure to sunlight and the use of drugs associated with phototoxic and photoallergic eruptions are the main risk factors.

Patients with PMLE appear to have an as yet undefined genetic susceptibility with a probable dominant mode of inheritance with low penetrance.[7]

DIAGNOSIS

CLINICAL FEATURES

Most cases of photodermatitis can be diagnosed on the basis of the patient's history. Be sure to review the patient's medications for possible sources.

- The appearance of the PMLE varies from person to person but is consistent in a given patient. Erythematous pruritic papules, sometimes with vesicles, are most common (see **Figures 208-1** and **208-2**). Lesions may coalesce to form plaques. The rash typically involves the "V" of the neck and the arms, legs, or both. The face, which is exposed to sunlight in both summer and winter, tends to be spared. PMLE is most severe in the spring and early summer with early exposure to the sun, moderates as the summer progresses, and resolves in the autumn or winter, only to recur the next spring. The rash typically develops 1 to 4 days after sun exposure. In black and Asian patients, it may also present as pinpoint papules that sometimes involve the face and perioral areas.[8]
- Phototoxic reaction occurs 2 to 6 hours after exposure to sunlight. The eruption typically appears as an exaggerated sunburn, with mild cases causing slight erythema and severe cases causing vesicles or bullae (see **Figures 208-3** to **208-7**).
- Phytophotodermatitis reactions are asymmetric and localized to the area in which the plant psoralen was in contact with the skin. Accompanying hyperpigmentation is a good clue to a phytophotodermatitis reaction (see **Figures 208-5** to **208-7**). Ask the patient if he or she had any contact with limes, celery, or figs. Squeezing lime juice into drinks is a particularly common cause of this reaction.
- Photoonycholysis phototoxicity reactions (sun-induced separation of the nail plate from the nail bed) have been reported with the use of tetracycline, psoralen, chloramphenicol, fluoroquinolones, oral contraceptives, quinine, and mercaptopurine. Photoonycholysis may be the only manifestation of phototoxicity in individuals with heavily pigmented skin.

TABLE 208-3 Common Substances That Cause Photoallergic Reactions

5-Fluorouracil (5-FU)
6-Methylcoumarin
Fragrances (6-methylcoumarin, musk, sandalwood oil)
NSAIDs (e.g., ketoprofen, diclofenac, piroxicam, celecoxib)
Sunscreens (benzophenones, cinnamates, dibenzoylmethanes)
Hormonal contraceptives
Hydrochlorothiazide
Antimicrobial agents (bithionol, chlorhexidine, dapsone, hexachlorophene, fenticlor, griseofulvin, itraconazole, sulfonamides, quinolones)
Phenothiazines
Salicylates
Sulfonylureas (glipizide and glyburide)
Quinidine

Abbreviation: NSAID, nonsteroidal anti-inflammatory drug.

- Photoallergic eruptions are characterized by widespread eczema in the photodistribution areas such as the face, upper chest, arms, and backs of hands. They resemble allergic contact dermatitis, but the distribution is mostly limited to sun-exposed areas of the body (see **Figure 208-8**).

TYPICAL DISTRIBUTION

- All photodermatitis reactions occur in sun-exposed areas, such as the face, ears, dorsal forearms, and V-area of the neck and upper chest.

LABORATORY TESTING

- Laboratory studies that may be helpful include antinuclear antibody (ANA), anti-Ro (SSA), and anti-La (SSB) titers to rule out lupus, and porphyrin studies to exclude porphyria.
- Phototesting can be used to determine a patient's minimal erythema dose to light exposure and help to define the inciting spectrum of a photodermatosis (UVA versus UVB versus visible light). Phototesting involves irradiating the skin with varying doses of UVA, UVB, and visible light through an opaque screen with multiple openings.[9] Usually the test is performed on the back. The presence or absence of solar urticaria is recorded within the first hour and the minimal erythema dose is determined after 24 hours.
- Provocative phototesting involves irradiating normal-appearing previously affected skin with the suspected causative light, either by higher doses of UV light or by natural sunlight exposure.[9] Provocative phototesting is primarily used for suspected PMLE.
- Photopatch testing is useful when a topical photoallergen is suspected. It is performed by placing two identical sets of potential photoallergens on the patient's back and covering them. After 24 hours, one set is removed and that site is irradiated with UVA. The site is covered again. Twenty-four hours later, both the irradiated and control test sites are assessed for reactions. A reaction to a specific photoallergen in the irradiated site, but not the control site, indicates a photoallergy. A similar reaction in both sites suggests a contact dermatitis.[5]

BIOPSY

- Punch biopsy of PMLE demonstrates extensive spongiosis and edema of the dermis with a deep lymphohistiocytic infiltrate. In acute phototoxic reactions, necrotic keratinocytes are observed.
- Skin biopsy findings in phototoxic reactions are identical to those of ordinary sunburn.

DIFFERENTIAL DIAGNOSIS

- Systemic lupus erythematosus (SLE)—Sunlight can precipitate a lupus rash. Serum ANA is usually positive (see Chapter 188, Lupus: Systemic and Cutaneous).
- Porphyria cutanea tarda reactions can also be precipitated by sunlight. It tends to present with vesicles or bullae in sun-exposed areas such as the backs of the hands. The bullae generally do not have any surrounding erythema, and urine for porphyrins should be positive (see Chapter 194, Other Bullous Disease).
- Dermatomyositis may cause an erythematous or violaceous eruption in sun-exposed areas. If these cutaneous findings precede the muscle weakness, it can appear to be a photosensitivity reaction such as PMLE or a phototoxic drug reaction. Therefore, it is essential in the management and follow-up of patients with suspected PMLE or other photosensitivity to inquire about muscle weakness and to look for other signs of dermatomyositis on the hands and/or through laboratory tests for muscle enzyme elevations (see Chapter 189, Dermatomyositis). The dermatomyositis patient story in Chapter 189 is one in which the initial rash was thought to be a photosensitivity reaction to a new hydrochlorothiazide (HCTZ) prescription.
- Contact dermatitis appears the same as photoallergic dermatitis but is usually not limited to sun-exposed areas (see Chapter 152, Contact Dermatitis).
- Actinic prurigo is a photosensitive rash that occurs mainly in children and tends to persist through the summer and possibly into the winter months.

MANAGEMENT

NONPHARMACOLOGIC

- The management of PMLE is aimed mainly at prevention. Patients who have mild disease should adopt a program of sun avoidance (see "Prevention" below). Broad-spectrum (UVA and UVB blocking) sunscreen with a minimum sun protection factor (SPF) of 30 should be used whenever out of doors (**Table 208-4**).[10] However, the SPF value of a sunscreen describes its protection factor against sunburn, which is primarily caused by UVB. The SPF does not provide sufficient information on UVA protection.[11] SOR C Patients must use sunscreen liberally and frequently (reapply every 2 hours and after swimming), as an insufficiently thick application may reduce its effectiveness.[12] SOR B
- Patients with severe PMLE can be desensitized in the spring with the use of phototherapy and maintained in the nonreactive state with a weekly 1-hour unprotected exposure to sunlight. SOR C A course of psoralen and UVA radiation, or a course of narrow-band UVB, 3 times a week for 4 weeks, provides protection.[13] SOR B These treatments may induce a typical rash or erythema but otherwise have no major adverse effects.
- Avoid tobacco products because they may make PMLE worse.[14] SOR B

MEDICATIONS

Topical group 1 to 3 corticosteroids should provide symptomatic relief and decrease the inflammation. Topicals may be applied once or twice daily to the affected areas for 5 to 7 days. For more severe reactions, a course of prednisone 30 mg daily for 5 to 7 days may be used.[15,16] SOR B

- Oral antihistamines may be useful to control pruritus.
- Patients with acute drug-induced photodermatitis need to practice sun avoidance until well after the drug is discontinued. Topical and

TABLE 208-4 UV Blocking Characteristics of Sunscreens

Sunscreen	Blocks UVB	Blocks UVA
Aminobenzoic acid	X	
Avobenzone		X
Cinoxate	X	
Dioxybenzone	X	X
Ecamsule*		X
Ensulizole	X	
Homosalate	X	
Meradimate		X
Octocrylene	X	
Octinoxate	X	
Octisalate	X	
Oxybenzone	X	X
Padimate O	X	
Sulisobenzone	X	X
Titanium dioxide	X	X
Trolamine salicylate	X	
Zinc oxide	X	X
Drometrizole trisiloxane (Mexoryl XL)*	X	X
Methylene-bis-benzotriazolyl tetramethylbutylphenol (Tinosorb M)*	X	X
Bis-ethylhexyloxyphenol methoxyphenyl triazine (Tinosorb S)*		X

*Not available in the United States in 2012.

systemic corticosteroids may be used, especially with photoallergic reactions, but their efficacy is unproven. SOR C

- Nicotinamide was successful in 60% of 42 patients treated with 3 g/day orally for 2 weeks.[17] SOR B

PREVENTION

Sun protection is the primary preventative measure for patients with photosensitivity. Patients should avoid exposure to midday sun (between 10:00 a.m. and 3:00 p.m.). Protective clothing such as long-sleeved shirts and broad-brim hats should be worn while outdoors. Fabrics that are tightly woven, thick, and/or dark-colored are useful for protection.[18] Clothing treated with broad-spectrum UV absorbers is also helpful. Window film that blocks UV and some visible light can be applied to cars or homes.[19]

Sunscreen is important for daily use for patients with photosensitivity. Sunscreens are divided into chemical (organic) and physical (inorganic) products. Physical sunscreens block both UV and some visible light (see **Table 208-4**). Products containing avobenzone or ecamsule offer improved protection against UVA.

Physical blocker (inorganic) sunscreens, such as titanium dioxide and zinc oxide, work by reflecting and scattering UV and visible light. Older formulations were opaque, making them cosmetically less acceptable to patients. Newer nonopaque, micronized formulations of titanium and zinc oxide have been developed but are less capable of scattering visible light and the longer wavelengths of UVA. Chemical sunscreens may cause allergic contact dermatitis or photoallergic reactions in some patients. These patients should use titanium dioxide or zinc oxide sunscreens for protection.

Afamelanotide is a synthetic analog of alpha-melanocyte stimulating hormone that is used for the prevention of phototoxic reactions in patients with erythropoietic protoporphyria. It may be a potential prophylactic treatment for patients with PMLE and other photosensitizing diseases.[20]

PROGNOSIS

- Some patients with PMLE experience less-severe reactions with successive years, but they may also worsen over time without appropriate treatment.
- The prognosis is excellent with patients when the offending agent is removed. Complete resolution of the photosensitivity may take weeks to months. Patients with persistent light reactivity beyond this have a poorer prognosis.

FOLLOW-UP

- Follow-up is needed if the photosensitivity persists.

PATIENT EDUCATION

- Patients with any type of photodermatitis should apply strong broad-spectrum sunscreens daily and use protective clothing (hats and shirts that cover the arms and V-neck). The sunscreen should be water resistant and applied to exposed areas before sun exposure.[21] Sunscreens should be reapplied every 2 hours if there is continued sun exposure. Some of the most effective sunscreens contain stabilized avobenzone, Mexoryl, and/or titanium dioxide or zinc oxide to block UVA and UVB.
- Tell your patients that if they develop an allergy to one sunscreen, they should find another with different ingredients.
- It is important to avoid sunlight during the midday period whenever possible.
- Explain to patients that phototoxic reactions may cause hyperpigmentation, which can take weeks to months to resolve. There is no guarantee that all the hyperpigmentation will go away.
- Avoid repeated rubbing and scratching, which can lead to skin thickening and chronic lichenification. Use the topical medications prescribed to treat the itching and to avoid lichenification.

PATIENT RESOURCES

- DermNet NZ. *Photosensitivity (Sun Allergy)*—**http://www.dermnetnz.org/topics/photosensitivity/.**
- DermNet NZ. *Drug-Induced Photosensitivity*—**http://www.dermnetnz.org/topics/drug-induced-photosensitivity/.**
- The Skin Cancer Foundation. *Photosensitivity—photosensitivity report*—**http://www.skincancer.org/publications/photosensitivity-report/medications.**

PROVIDER RESOURCES

- American Academy of Family Physicians. *Common Hyperpigmentation Disorders in Adults: Part I*—**http://www.aafp.org/afp/2003/1115/p1955.html.**
- eMedicine. *Drug-Induced Photosensitivity*—**http://emedicine.medscape.com/article/1049648.**
- DermNet NZ. *Polymorphic Light Eruption*—**http://www.dermnetnz.org/topics/polymorphic-light-eruption/.**
- Darby-Stewart AL, Edwards FD, Perry KJ. Hyperpigmentation and vesicles after beach vacation. Phytophotodermatitis. *J Fam Pract.* 2006;55(12):1050-1053.
- Phytophotodermatitis case report and review—**https://www.mdedge.com/sites/default/files/Document/September-2017/021020099.pdf".**
- eMedicine. *Sunscreens and Photoprotection*—**https://emedicine.medscape.com/article/1119992-overview.**

REFERENCES

1. Morison WL, Stern RS. Polymorphous light eruption: a common reaction uncommonly recognized. *Acta Derm Venereol.* 1982;62:237-240.
2. Hönigsmann H. Polymorphous light eruption. *Photodermatol Photoimmunol Photomed.* 2008;24:155.
3. Kutlubay Z, Sevim A, Engin B, Tüzün Y. Photodermatoses, including phototoxic and photoallergic reactions (internal and external). *Clin Dermatol.* 2014;32:73-79.
4. Hasan T, Ranki A, Jansen CT, Karvonen J. Disease associations in polymorphous light eruption: a long-term follow-up study of 94 patients. *Arch Dermatol.* 1998;134:1081-1085.
5. Stern RS, Shear NH. Cutaneous reactions to drugs and biological modifiers. In: Arndt KA, LeBoit PE, Robinson JK, Wintroub BU, eds. *Cutaneous Medicine and Surgery*. Vol. 1. Philadelphia, PA: Saunders; 1996:412.
6. Gonzalez E, Gonzalez S. Drug photosensitivity, idiopathic photodermatoses, and sunscreens. *J Am Acad Dermatol.* 1996;35:871-875.
7. McGregor JM, Grabczynska S, Vaughan R, et al. Genetic modeling of abnormal photosensitivity in families with polymorphic light eruption and actinic prurigo. *J Invest Dermatol.* 2000;115:471.
8. Isedeh P, Lim HW. Polymorphous light eruption presenting as pinhead papular eruption on the face. *J Drugs Dermatol.* 2013;12:1285.
9. Yashar SS, Lim HW. Classification and evaluation of photodermatoses. *Dermatol Ther.* 2003;16(1):1-7.
10. Dawe RS, Ferguson J. Diagnosis and treatment of chronic actinic dermatitis. *Dermatol Ther.* 2003;16:45-51.
11. Fourtanier A, Moyal D, Seité S. Sunscreens containing the broad-spectrum UVA absorber, Mexoryl SX, prevent the cutaneous detrimental effects of UV exposure: a review of clinical study results. *Photodermatol Photoimmunol Photomed.* 2008;24:164-174.
12. Faurschou A, Wulf HC. The relation between sun protection factor and amount of sunscreen applied in vivo. *Br J Dermatol.* 2007;156:716-719.
13. Bilsland D, George SA, Gibbs NK, et al. A comparison of narrow band phototherapy (TL-01) and photochemotherapy (PUVA) in the management of polymorphic light eruption. *Br J Dermatol.* 1993;129:708-712.
14. Metelitsa AI, Lauzon GJ. Tobacco and the skin. *Clin Dermatol.* 2010;4:384-390.
15. Patel DC, Bellaney GJ, Seed PT, et al. Efficacy of short-course oral prednisolone in polymorphic light eruption: a randomized controlled trial. *Br J Dermatol.* 2000;143:828-831.
16. Gruber-Wackernagel A, Byrne SN, Wolf P. Polymorphous light eruption: clinic aspects and pathogenesis. *Dermatol Clin.* 2014;32:315.
17. Neumann R, Rappold E, Pohl-Markl H. Treatment of polymorphous light eruption with nicotinamide: a pilot study. *Br J Dermatol.* 1986;115(1):77-80.
18. Lautenschlager S, Wulf HC, Pittelkow MR. Photoprotection. *Lancet.* 2007;370:528-537.
19. Dawe R, Russell S, Ferguson J. Borrowing from museums and industry: two photoprotective devices. *Br J Dermatol.* 1996;135:1016-1017.
20. Biolcati G, Marchesini E, Sorge F, et al. Long-term observational study of afamelanotide in 115 patients with erythropoietic protoporphyria. *Br J Dermatol.* 2015;172:1601.
21. Morison WL. Photosensitivity. *N Engl J Med.* 2004;350:1111-1117.

209 ERYTHEMA AB IGNE

Edward Bae, MD
Amor Khachemoune, MD
Yoon-Soo Cindy Bae, MD
Khashayar Sarabi, MD

PATIENT STORY

A 50-year-old woman presented with bilateral erythematous lesions on the inner aspects of both of her lower extremities (**Figures 209-1** and **209-2**). The lesions had begun developing approximately 6 months ago. They became progressively more noticeable but remained localized in the inner aspects of the lower extremities. She mentioned using a hot-water bottle in the area to keep herself warm at night when sleeping in bed. Although our working clinical diagnosis was erythema ab igne, clinical entities such as livedo reticularis, poikiloderma atrophicans vasculare, and acanthosis nigricans were in the differential diagnosis. A skin biopsy confirmed the diagnosis of erythema ab igne. The patient was advised to discontinue use of the hot-water bottle on the skin. Over the course of 4 months, her skin lesions started to clear with no further intervention.

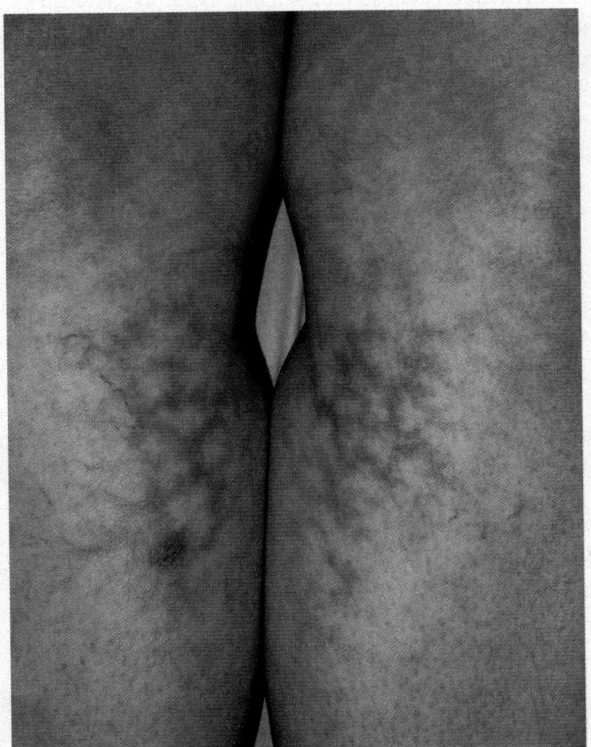

FIGURE 209-1 Mottled or meshlike pigmentary changes on the legs of a 50-year-old woman who slept with a hot-water bottle between her legs. *(Reproduced with permission from El-Ghandour A, Selim A, Khachemoune A. Bilateral lesions on the legs, J Fam Pract. 2007; 56(1):37-39. Frontline Medical Communications. Inc.)*

INTRODUCTION

Erythema ab igne (EAI) is a rare skin condition caused by chronic exposure to low-intensity heat that is insufficient to cause burns. Sources of this heat can include hot-water bottles, heating pads, electric blankets, car seat warmers, exposure to open fires, and laptops placed on the users' thighs or propped legs. EAI is typically characterized by pink, reticulated, and hyperpigmented mottled patches in the setting of prolonged exposure to heat. Patients may complain of associated pruritus or paresthesias, or they may be asymptomatic. Treatment is limited and patients are instructed to avoid triggers.

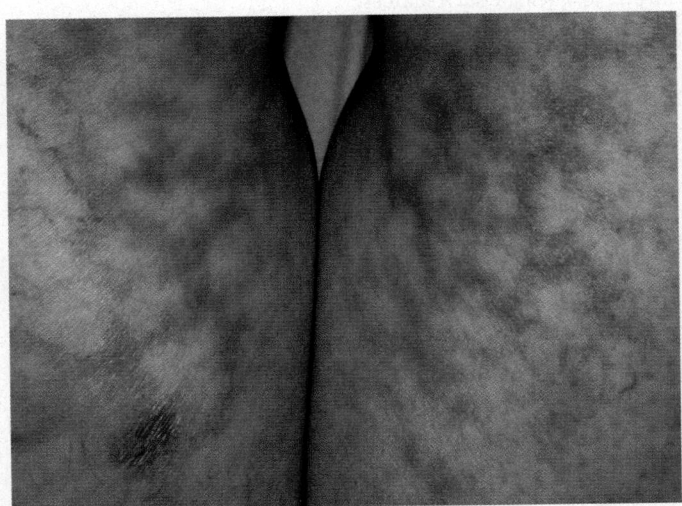

FIGURE 209-2 Close-up of legs in **Figure 209-1**. *(Reproduced with permission from El-Ghandour A, Selim A, Khachemoune A. Bilateral lesions on the legs, J Fam Pract. 2007;56(1):37-39. Frontline Medical Communications. Inc.)*

SYNONYMS

Chronic moderate heat dermatitis, chronic radiant heat dermatitis, toasted skin syndrome, fire stains, hot-water bottle rash, laptop thigh.

EPIDEMIOLOGY

- Rare disease.
- Women, in particular those who are overweight, are affected more often than men.

ETIOLOGY AND PATHOPHYSIOLOGY

- The skin findings form as a result of multiple exposures to low-intensity heat.

- EAI is thought to be caused by damage to superficial blood vessels from external heat, which leads to hemosiderin deposits in the superficial skin, usually in a reticulated pattern.[1]
- In the past, EAI was reported in women who were exposed to open fires, fireplaces, or furnaces to cook for extended periods of time.[2-5] As a result, most of the lesions would manifest on the medial side of the thigh and the lower legs.
- In modern times, newer sources of heat exposures have led to a wide variety of presentations of the disease manifesting in different parts of the body.
    - Hot packs, heating pads, ultrasound physiotherapy, and hot-water bottles used for chronic pain.
    - Seat warmers and other furniture with internal heating pads.
    - Laptop computers used on the legs without a barrier.
    - Occupational exposures such as chefs or cooks who stand in front of stoves and open fires; brick manufacturers exposed to hot bricks; exposure to infrared lamps.
    - Even domestic exposures such as microwave popcorn or taking frequent prolonged hot baths[6] have been implicated in causing EAI.

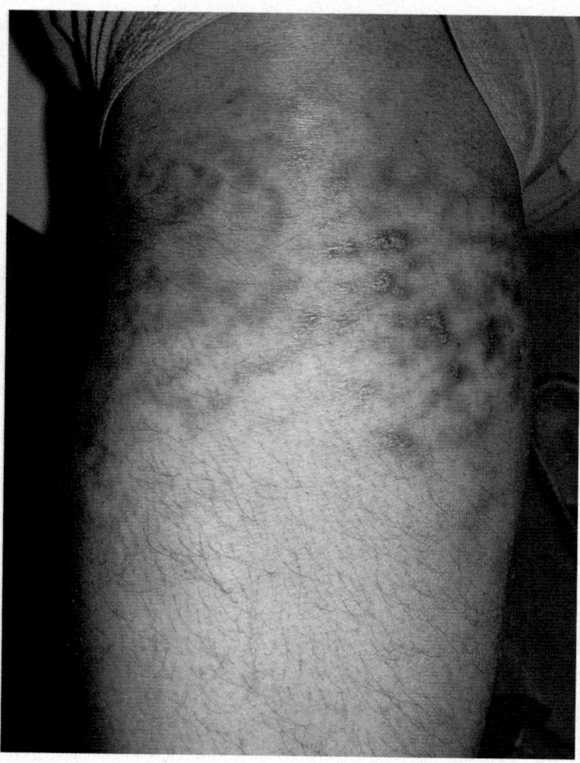

FIGURE 209-3 Mottled hyperpigmentation and hint of blistering and crusting on the anterior leg area in a 23-year-old woman who spent significant time close to a fireplace. (*Reproduced with permission from Amor Khachemoune, MD.*)

RISK FACTORS

- Persistent exposure to heat as described above.
- Occupations that involve chronic exposure to external heat sources (e.g., kitchen workers, silversmiths, jewelers, foundry workers).[7]

DIAGNOSIS

In most cases, EAI is diagnosed by taking a thorough history and physical exam with focus on exposing any potential sources of prolonged or repeated heat. Questions regarding management of chronic pain or exposures from occupational or domestic sources can be helpful to elucidate such sources.

CLINICAL FEATURES

- Some patients have mild pruritus or burning sensation, but the majority of patients are asymptomatic.
- Skin lesions may not appear immediately and may appear up to 1 month after exposure.
- Skin changes start as a reddish-brown pigmentation distributed as a mottled rash followed by skin atrophy (**Figures 209-1** to **209-3**).
- Telangiectasias with diffuse hyperpigmentation and subepidermal bullae may also develop.
- The rash appears meshlike or netlike in the area exposed to the heat. The heat can be from fireplaces, heating pads, laptop computers, open fires, place heaters, and hot-water bottles (**Figures 209-1** to **209-7**).
- Malignant melanoma and various sarcomas are reported to arise in burn scars; however, none arising in areas of erythema ab igne have been reported to date.

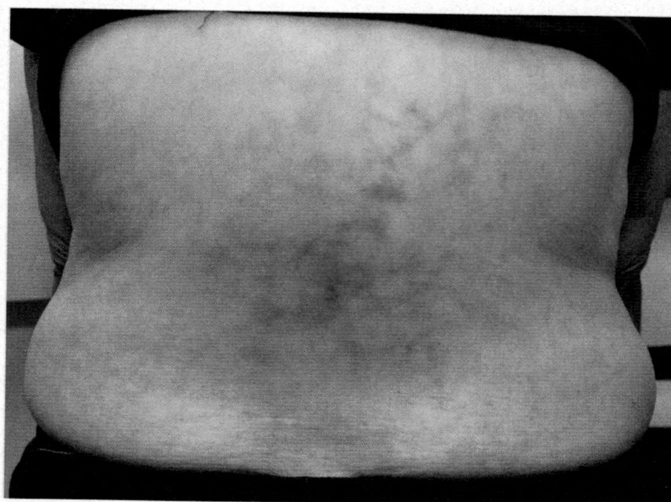

FIGURE 209-4 Erythema ab igne from the use of a heating pad in a woman with back pain. (*Reproduced with permission from Richard P. Usatine, MD.*)

- In some rare cases, actinic keratoses, squamous cell carcinomas, or Merkel cell carcinomas have developed in areas of erythema ab igne.[8-11]
- EAI may be a sign of internal malignancy. Several reports have detailed patients developing EAI on the lower back after using heat packs to alleviate pain caused by new-onset gastrointestinal or pancreatic cancers. A thorough evaluation for internal malignancy should be performed if there are troubling constitutional symptoms with EAI.[1]

TYPICAL DISTRIBUTION

Consistent with area of heat exposure, most often the legs or back (**Figure 209-4**).

LABORATORY STUDIES

None recommended.

SKIN BIOPSY

- Biopsy is warranted if there is suspicion of malignant transformation or if the history is unclear.

DIFFERENTIAL DIAGNOSIS

EAI should be differentiated from other diseases with skin changes that mimic its presentation.

LIVEDO RETICULARIS

- Reticular cyanotic cutaneous discoloration surrounding pale central areas caused by dilation of capillary blood vessels and stagnation of blood (**Figure 209-8**).
- Occurs mostly on the legs, arms, and trunk and appears to be a purplish mottling of the skin.
- More pronounced in cold weather.
- Idiopathic condition that may be associated with systemic diseases such as systemic lupus erythematosus (SLE).

POIKILODERMA ATROPHICANS VASCULARE

- A variant of mycosis fungoides (cutaneous T-cell lymphoma) (see 180, Cutaneous T Cell lymphoma). This is a diagnosis made by skin biopsy.
- Circumscribed violaceous erythema.
- Occurs mostly in posterior shoulders, back, buttocks, V-shaped area of anterior neck and chest.
- May be asymptomatic or mildly pruritic.

ACANTHOSIS NIGRICANS

- Velvety, light-brown-to-black patches usually on the neck, under the arms, or in the groin (see Chapter 229, Acanthosis Nigricans).
- Most often associated with being overweight and glucose intolerance.
- More common in people with darker skin pigmentation.
- May begin at any age and may be inherited as a primary condition or associated with various underlying syndromes.

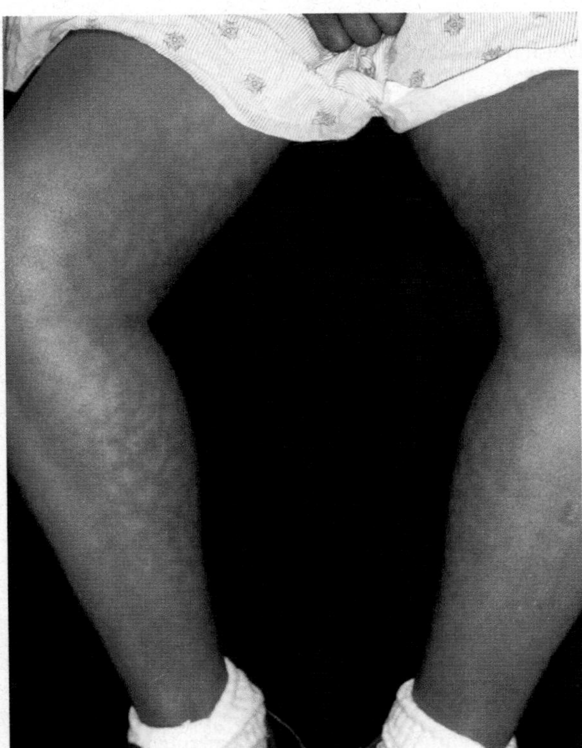

FIGURE 209-5 Erythema ab igne on the legs of a woman who was straddling a space heater to keep warm during the winter. (*Reproduced with permission from Richard P. Usatine, MD.*)

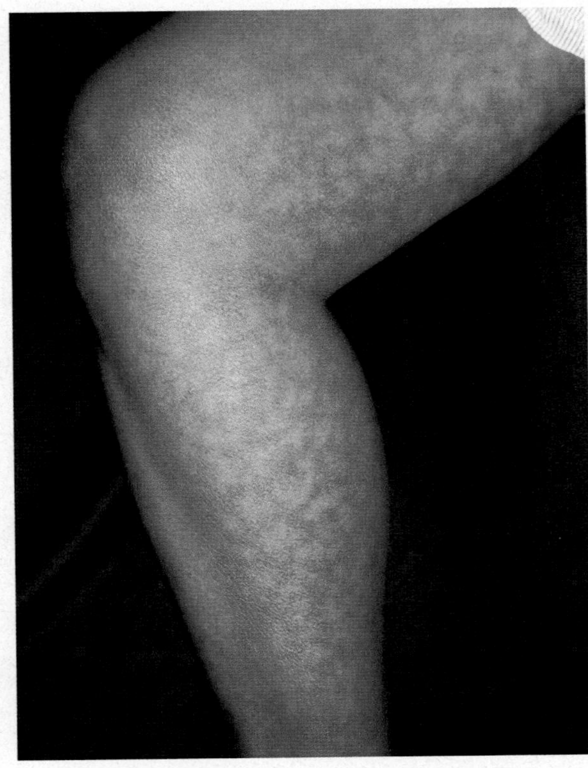

FIGURE 209-6 Close-up of leg in **Figure 209-5** showing the netlike pattern on the medial leg. (*Reproduced with permission from Richard P. Usatine, MD.*)

- The characteristic distribution of acanthosis nigricans helps to distinguish this condition from EAI.

MANAGEMENT

FIRST LINE

- The goal of treatment is to identify the source of heat radiation to avoid further exposure. For mild lesions, no intervention is needed after the heat source is removed, with a good probability of full resolution.

SECOND LINE

- Topical retinoids, vitamin A derivatives, hydroquinone, and 5-fluorouracil have been prescribed to treat the abnormal skin pigmentation.[12] Laser therapy has been used to even out the skin color.[5,13] SOR Ⓒ

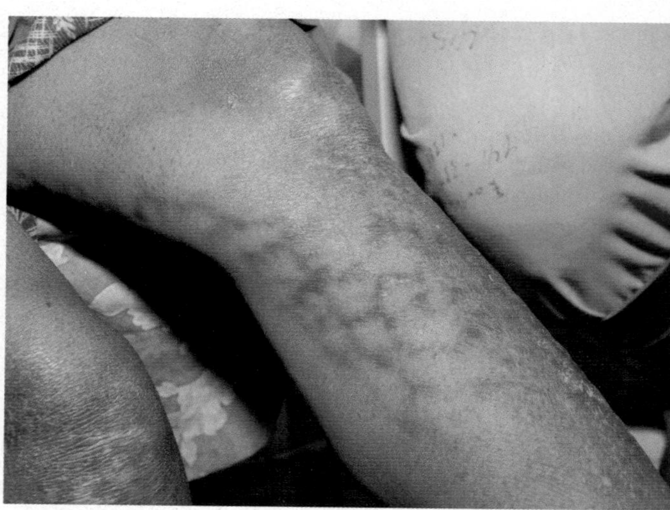

FIGURE 209-7 Erythema ab igne on the legs of an Ethiopian woman who cooks over an open fire. (*Reproduced with permission from Richard P. Usatine, MD.*)

PROGNOSIS

Prognosis is excellent for full resolution if the external heat source is removed or discontinued. However, the hyperpigmentation may remain, and various treatments may not succeed in returning the skin to its original pigmentation.

FOLLOW-UP

Follow-up visits are recommended if there are new changes to the skin after removing the source of heat. This may be a sign of malignant transformation.

PATIENT EDUCATION

Patients should avoid excessive and prolonged localized heat exposures. Personal protective equipment should also be used to shield the body from occupational heat sources when possible.

There are many ways to shield the thighs from the heat of a laptop computer, from the use of pillows and blankets to the purchase of special devices manufactured for this purpose.

PATIENT RESOURCES

- Wikipedia. *Erythema Ab Igne*—**http://en.wikipedia.org/wiki/Erythema_ab_igne.**

PROVIDER RESOURCES

- Medscape. *Erythema Ab Igne*—**http://emedicine.medscape.com/article/1087535.**
- DermNet NZ. *Erythema Ab Igne*—**http://dermnetnz.org/topics/erythema-ab-igne/**

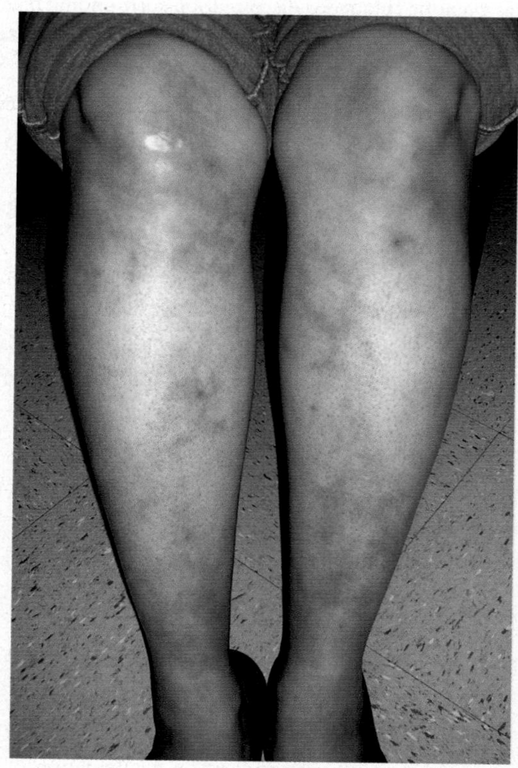

FIGURE 209-8 Livedo reticularis in a 27-year-old woman with lupus. The mottled purple color gets worse when she is exposed to colder temperatures. (*Reproduced with permission from Richard P. Usatine, MD.*)

REFERENCES

1. Bunick CG, Ibrahim O, King BA. When erythema ab igne warrants an evaluation for internal malignancy. *Int J Dermatol.* 2014;53(7): e353-e355.
2. Meffert JJ, Davis BM. Furniture-induced erythema ab igne. *J Am Acad Dermatol.* 1996;34(3):516-517.
3. Helm TN, Spigel GT, Helm KF. Erythema ab igne caused by a car heater. *Cutis.* 1997;59(2):81-82.
4. Bilic M, Adams BB. Erythema ab igne induced by a laptop computer. *J Am Acad Dermatol.* 2004;50(6):973-974.
5. El-Ghandour A, Selim A, Khachemoune A. Bilateral lesions on the legs. *J Fam Pract.* 2007;56(1):37-39.
6. Weber MB, Ponzio HA, Costa FB, Camini L. Erythema ab igne: a case report. *An Bras Dermatol.* 2005;80(2):187-188.
7. Runger TM. Disorders due to physical agents. In: Bolognia J, Jorizzo JL, Rapini RP, eds. *Dermatology.* Vol 2. London, UK: Mosby; 2003: 1385-1409.
8. Jones CS, Tyring SK, Lee PC, Fine JD. Development of neuroendocrine (Merkel cell) carcinoma mixed with squamous cell carcinoma in erythema ab igne. *Arch Dermatol.* 1988;124(1):110-113.
9. Arrington JH 3rd, Lockman DS. Thermal keratoses and squamous cell carcinoma in situ associated with erythema ab igne. *Arch Dermatol.* 1979;115(10):1226-1228.
10. Hewitt JB, Sherif A, Kerr KM, Stankler L. Merkel cell and squamous cell carcinomas arising in erythema ab igne. *Br J Dermatol.* 1993;128(5):591-592.
11. Miller K, Hunt R, Chu J, Meehan S, Stein J. Erythema ab igne. *Dermatol Online J.* 2011;17(10):28.
12. Sahl WJ Jr, Taira JW. Erythema ab igne: treatment with 5-fluorouracil cream. *J Am Acad Dermatol.* 1992;27(1):109-110.

SECTION T VASCULAR

210 ACQUIRED VASCULAR SKIN LESIONS

Nathan Hitzeman, MD
Richard P. Usatine, MD

PATIENT STORY

A 31-year-old woman presented with a new swelling on her lower lip. This was clinically recognized as a venous lake (**Figure 210-1**). The patient was bothered by its appearance and wanted it removed. She chose to have cryotherapy, which eradicated the venous lake.

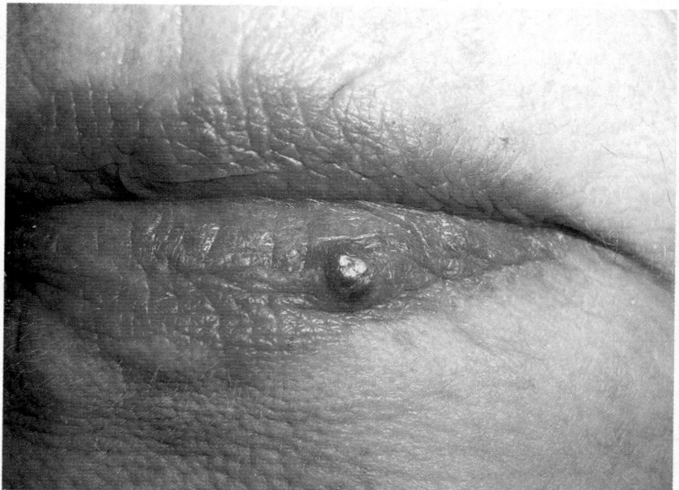

FIGURE 210-1 Venous lake on the lip of a young woman. This was eradicated with cryotherapy. (*Reproduced with permission from Richard P. Usatine, MD.*)

INTRODUCTION

Acquired vascular lesions are common skin findings. The most common one is the cherry angioma.

SYNONYMS

Cherry angiomas have been called senile angiomas, as they have a tendency to develop as adults become older.

EPIDEMIOLOGY

- Venous lakes are acquired vascular lesions of the face and ears.[1]
- Cherry angiomas are common vascular malformations that occur in many adults after the age of 30 years (**Figure 210-2**). Cherry angiomas sometimes proliferate during pregnancy.[1]
- Angiokeratomas, the most common form being angiokeratomas of the scrotum (Fordyce) or vulva, develop during adult years (**Figures 210-3** and **210-4**).[1]
- Glomangiomas, also known as glomuvenous malformations or glomus tumors, are a type of venous malformation (**Figure 210-5**). Most patients with glomangiomas are of Northern European descent and have a family history of similar lesions.[2]
- Cutaneous angiosarcomas are rare malignant vascular tumors most commonly found on the head and neck areas of elderly white men (**Figure 210-6**).[3]

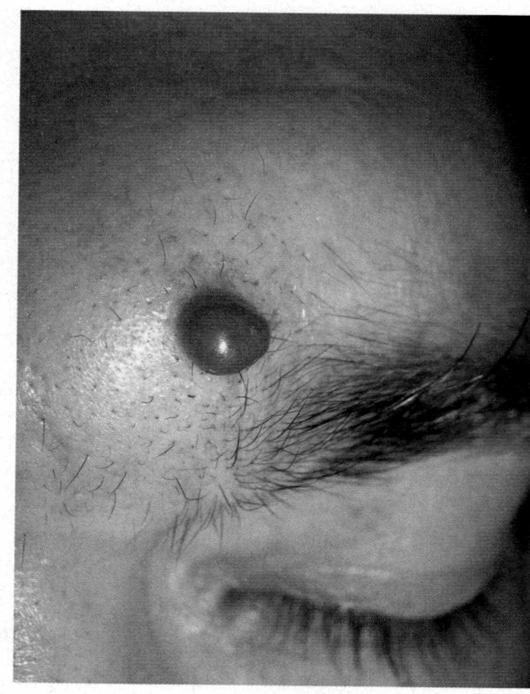

FIGURE 210-2 Large cherry angioma treated with shave excision and electrodesiccation of the base. (*Reproduced with permission from Richard P. Usatine, MD.*)

ETIOLOGY AND PATHOPHYSIOLOGY

- Venous lakes are benign dilated vascular channels (see **Figure 210-1**).
- Cherry angiomas are common benign vascular malformations (see **Figure 210-2**). They are most commonly part of normal aging of

the skin. Several case reports have cited increased cherry angiomas after exposure to toxins.[4]

- Angiokeratomas are dilated superficial blood vessels that may be associated with increased venous pressure (such as in pregnant patients and patients with hemorrhoids)[1] (see **Figures 210-3** and **210-4**).
- Glomangiomas are a distinct type of venous malformation caused by abnormal synthesis of the protein glomulin[2] (see **Figure 210-5**). Lesions may be acquired or congenital.
- Cutaneous angiosarcomas are rare malignant vascular tumors thought to arise from vascular endothelium. Most arise spontaneously, but risk factors include radiation, chronic lymphedema, toxins, and certain familial syndromes. Elevation of several growth factors and cytokines has been associated with this malignancy (**Figures 210-6** and **210-7**).[3]

DIAGNOSIS

CLINICAL FEATURES

- Venous lakes are dark blue or purple, slightly raised, and less than a centimeter in size. The lesions empty with firm compression. They may bleed with trauma.
- Cherry angiomas are deep red papules resembling the color of a cherry.
- Angiokeratomas are multiple red-to-purple papules with associated hyperkeratosis. They may bleed with trauma.
- Glomangiomas are typically tender, blue-purple, partially compressible nodules with a cobblestone appearance.
- Cutaneous angiosarcomas present as progressively enlarging erythematous plaques.

TYPICAL DISTRIBUTION

- Venous lakes are found on the face and ears, particularly the vermilion border of the lips (see **Figure 210-1**).
- Cherry angiomas favor the trunk but may occur on other parts of the body. The number of lesions on one person ranges from one to many.
- Angiokeratomas typically occur on the scrotum or vulva (see **Figures 210-3** and **210-4**).
- Glomangiomas tend to occur on the extremities (see **Figure 210-5**). Solitary glomangiomas (glomus tumor) may occur in the nail bed, especially in women. The number of lesions ranges from solitary to more than 100.[5]
- Cutaneous angiosarcomas often present on the head and neck areas (see **Figures 210-6** and **210-7**).

DERMOSCOPY AND BIOPSY

- Diagnosis of venous lakes, cherry angiomas, and angiokeratomas is usually by history and physical examination alone. If these are removed surgically, it is still best to send them to pathology for confirmation of diagnosis. If the diagnosis is not clear clinically, a biopsy is warranted to rule out malignancy.

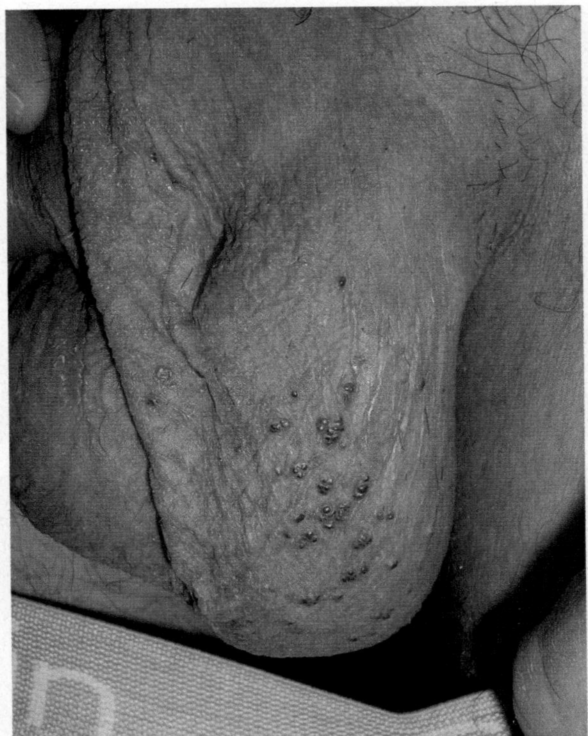

FIGURE 210-3 Angiokeratosis on the scrotum. Fordyce spots. *(Reproduced with permission from Lewis Rose, MD.)*

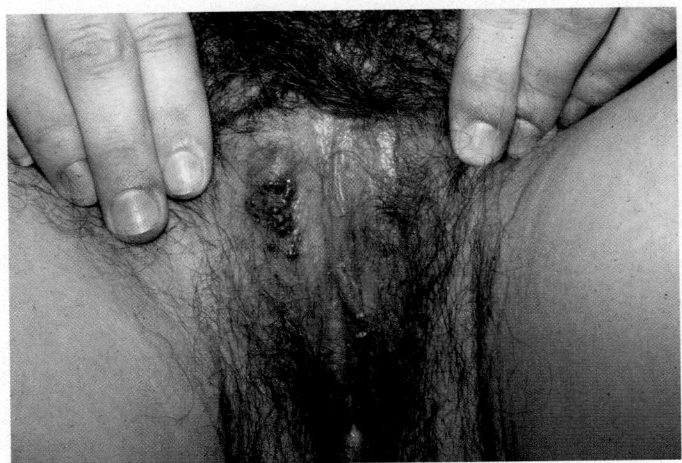

FIGURE 210-4 Angiokeratosis on the vulva. This might be mistaken for a melanoma. *(Reproduced with permission from Eric Kraus, MD.)*

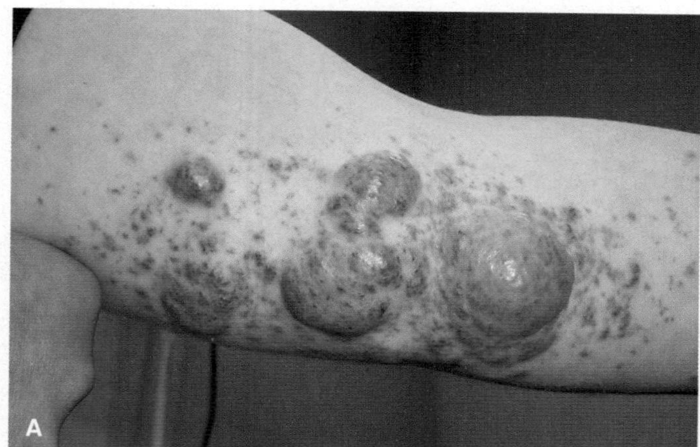

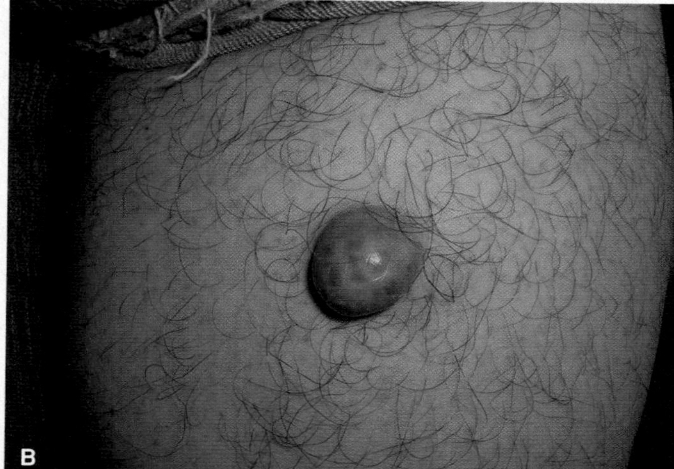

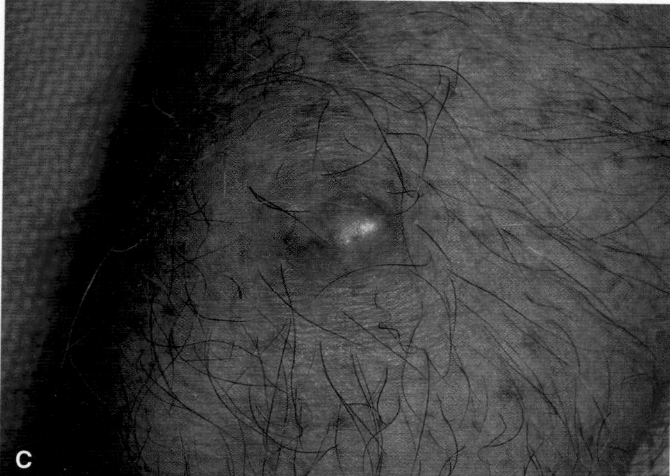

FIGURE 210-5 Glomangiomas can be multiple or solitary. **A.** Large glomangiomas of the arm. (*Reproduced with permission from Jack Resneck, Sr., MD.*) **B.** Solitary painful glomangioma on the leg of a young man. **C.** Small solitary painful glomangioma on the arm. These solitary glomangiomas were surgically resected. (*Reproduced with permission from Richard P. Usatine, MD.*)

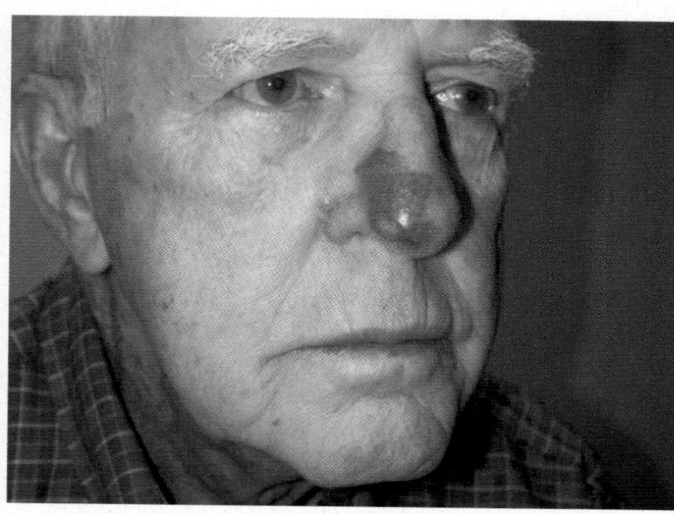

FIGURE 210-6 Angiosarcoma on the nose. A lesion like this requires an urgent biopsy. (*Reproduced with permission from Amor Khachemoune, MD.*)

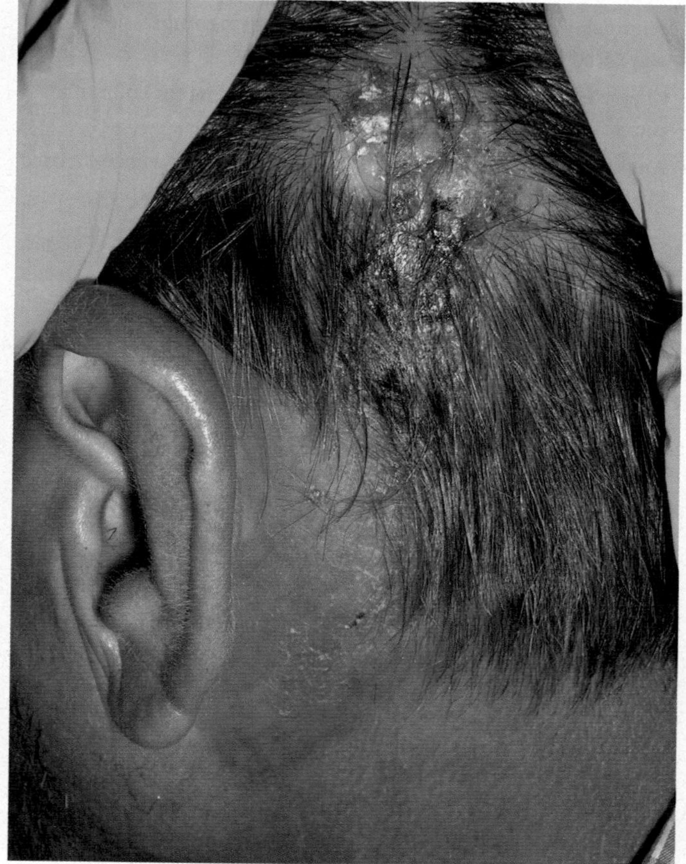

FIGURE 210-7 Angiosarcoma behind the ear and on the scalp of this 64-year-old man. (*Reproduced with permission from Richard P. Usatine, MD.*)

- Diascopy is a technique in which a microscope slide is used to compress a vascular lesion, allowing the clinician the ability to see the red or purple color of a vascular lesion blanch under pressure (**Figure 210-8**).
- Dermoscopy is a very useful method to aid in the diagnosis of all skin conditions including vascular lesions.[6] It combines excellent lighting with 10-fold magnification to improve imaging of all vascular lesions. Dermoscopy of hemangiomas and angiokeratomas is described in Chapter 111. Recognition of the classic pink-red lacunae (similar to a lake) with white septae between the lacunae can help to prevent an unnecessary biopsy of a benign hemangioma (**Figure 210-9**).
- Skin biopsy of glomangioma reveals distinct rows of glomus cells that surround distorted vascular channels.[2]
- Skin biopsy of cutaneous angiosarcoma reveals irregular vascular channels and atypical endothelial cells.[3]

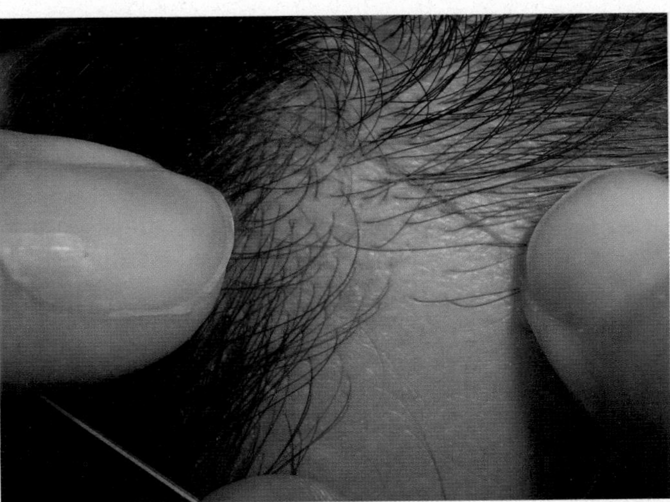

FIGURE 210-8 Diascopy in which a microscope slide is being used to compress a vascular lesion. The red color of this vascular hemangioma is blanching under pressure. *(Reproduced with permission from Richard P. Usatine, MD.)*

DIFFERENTIAL DIAGNOSIS

- Cutaneous angiosarcomas present as progressively enlarging erythematous plaques that may resemble bruising, cellulitis, rosacea, or erysipelas. The head-tilt maneuver has been described to aid in its detection.[5] Having a patient lower his or her head below the level of the heart for 5 to 10 seconds will make the lesion more engorged and violaceous, thus confirming its vascular nature.

MANAGEMENT

OBSERVATION

- Patients can be reassured that venous lakes and most other acquired vascular lesions (with the exception of angiosarcomas) are benign lesions that develop during adult years.

SURGICAL

- Venous lakes, cherry angiomas, and other acquired vascular lesions can be eradicated by cryotherapy, electrodesiccation, surgery, sclerotherapy, intralesional bleomycin, intense pulsed light, and other laser modalities.[1,7-11] SOR C Compared with intense pulsed light, the Nd:YAG (neodymium:yttrium-aluminum-garnet) laser system may yield superior results in the treatment of benign vascular lesions.[12] SOR B Hyperpigmentation is the most common complication of treatment.
- When using cryotherapy to treat vascular lesions, it can help to compress the lesion at the same time as it is frozen. This can be done with a cryogun that has a solid probe for compression. Liquid nitrogen spray is also an alternative. SOR C
- Small cherry angiomas can be treated with light electrodesiccation using an electrosurgical instrument on a low setting without anesthesia. The tip of the electrode is lightly applied to the lesion while the electrical current is engaged for one to a few bursts of electricity. A dull tip electrode is preferred over a sharp one. The desired endpoint is "charring" of the lesion with minimal surrounding tissue destruction. SOR C

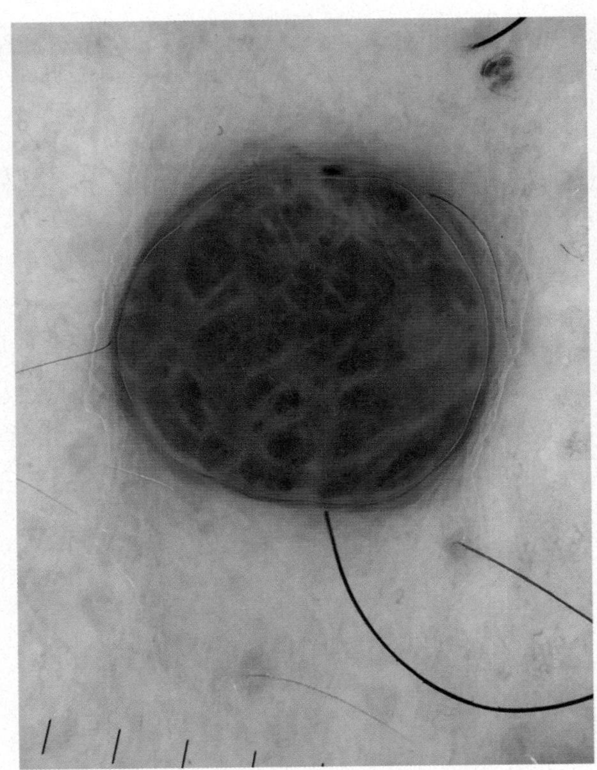

FIGURE 210-9 Dermoscopy of a cherry angioma in an adult showing the classic pink-red lacunae with whitish septae between them. *(Reproduced with permission from Richard P. Usatine, MD.)*

- Larger cherry angiomas can be removed with a shave excision after injecting with lidocaine and epinephrine. The base is then treated with electrodesiccation. SOR Ⓒ
- Isolated glomangiomas may be surgically excised. Sclerotherapy may be useful for multiple lesions or large segmental lesions.[13] SOR Ⓒ
- Cutaneous angiosarcoma is best treated with excision and wide surgical margins, as the primary tumor is often more extensive than appears on examination. Postoperative radiotherapy is then used at the primary site and regional lymphatics. If the tumor is inoperable, palliative chemotherapy may be considered.[3] SOR Ⓒ

PATIENT EDUCATION

- When discussing any new lesions in sun-exposed areas, the clinician should take the opportunity to counsel patients on sunscreen use, avoiding direct sun during peak hours, and performing periodic skin examination.
- Patients should be fully informed about the risk of pigmentary changes and chance of recurrence if they elect for cosmetic removal of benign lesions.

FOLLOW-UP

None typically needed for benign lesions unless lesions recur or the patient is concerned about growth or changes to the lesions.

PATIENT RESOURCES

- MedlinePlus. *Cherry Angioma*—**http://medlineplus.gov/ency/article/001441.htm.**

PROVIDER RESOURCES

- **http://emedicine.medscape.com/article/1082935.**

REFERENCES

1. Habif TP. Acquired vascular lesions. In: *Clinical Dermatology: A Color Guide to Diagnosis and Therapy*, 5th ed. Philadelphia, PA: Mosby; 2010:904-912. http:www.clinderm.com. Accessed March 2012.
2. Brauer JA, Anolik R, Tzu J, et al. Glomuvenous malformations (familial generalized multiple glomangiomas). *Dermatol Online J.* 2011;17(10):9. http://dermatology.cdlib.org/1710/2010-11/9_2010-11/article.html. Accessed March 2012.
3. Young RB, Brown NJ, Reed MW, et al. Angiosarcoma. *Lancet Oncol.* 2010;11(10):983-991. http://www.mdconsult.com/das/article/body/326552771-2/jorg=journal&source=&sp=23684736&sid=0/N/767926/s1470204510700231.pdf?issn=1470-2045. Accessed March 2012.
4. Hefazi M, Maleki M, Mahmoudi M, et al. Delayed complications of sulfur mustard poisoning in the skin and the immune system of Iranian veterans 16-20 years after exposure. *Int J Dermatol.* 2006;45(9):1025-1031.
5. Asgari MM, Cockerell CJ, Weitzul S. The head-tilt maneuver. *Arch Dermatol.* 2007;143:75-77.
6. Marghoob AA, Usatine RP, Jaimes N. Dermoscopy for the family physician. *Am Fam Physician.* 2013;88(7):441-450.
7. Suhonen R, Kuflik EG. Venous lakes treated by liquid nitrogen cryosurgery. *Br J Dermatol.* 1997;137:1018-1019.
8. Hong SK, Lee HJ, Seo JK, et al. Reactive vascular lesions treated using ethanolamine oleate sclerotherapy [21 patient study, 5 of whom had venous lakes; 95% of patients had complete remission]. *Dermatol Surg.* 2010;36(7):1148-1152.
9. Sainsbury DC, Kessell G, Fall AJ, et al. Intralesional bleomycin injection treatment for vascular birthmarks: a 5-year experience at a single United Kingdom unit [164-patient study]. *Plast Reconstr Surg.* 2011;127(5):2031-2044.
10. Bernstein EF. The pulsed-dye laser for treatment of cutaneous conditions. *G Ital Dermatol Venereol.* 2009;144(5):557-572.
11. Bekhor PS. Long-pulsed Nd:YAG laser treatment of venous lakes: report of a series of 34 cases. *Dermatol Surg.* 2006;32:1151-1154.
12. Fodor L, Ramon Y, Fodor A, et al. A side-by-side prospective study of intense pulsed light and Nd:YAG laser treatment for vascular lesions. *Ann Plastic Surg.* 2006;56:164-170.
13. Parsi K, Kossard S. Multiple hereditary glomangiomas: successful treatment with sclerotherapy. *Australas J Dermatol.* 2002;43:43.

211 HEREDITARY AND CONGENITAL VASCULAR LESIONS

Nathan Hitzeman, MD
Richard P. Usatine, MD

PATIENT STORY

A 56-year-old woman has had recurrent nosebleeds starting in childhood and has visible telangiectasias on her lips and tongue (**Figure 211-1**). In early adulthood, she was diagnosed with hereditary hemorrhagic telangiectasias (HHTs) (Osler-Weber-Rendu syndrome) and was found to have an arteriovenous malformation (AVM) in the lung requiring surgical resection. She has led a normal productive life and has two children who have not inherited this condition. Her mother had recurrent epistaxis, but never had an AVM.

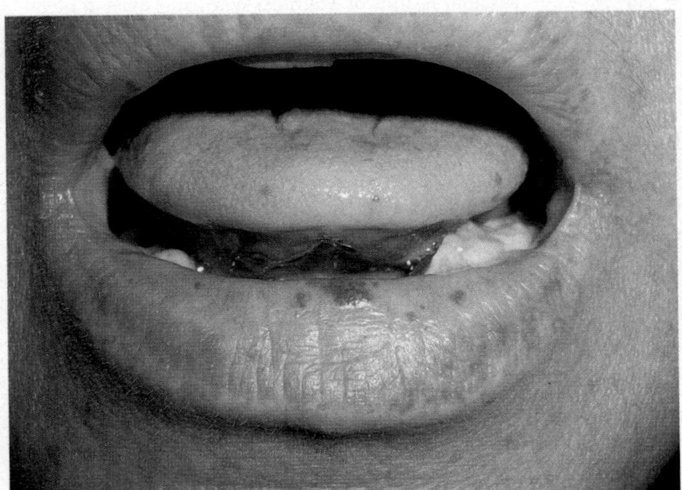

FIGURE 211-1 Hereditary hemorrhagic telangiectasias (Osler-Weber-Rendu syndrome) in a 56-year-old woman with recurrent nosebleeds and an arteriovenous malformation in the lung. (*Reproduced with permission from Richard P. Usatine, MD.*)

INTRODUCTION

Hereditary and congenital vascular lesions range from the very common and benign stork bite (a variation of nevus flammeus) to rare but serious neurocutaneous syndromes. Childhood hemangiomas are covered separately in Chapter 115, Childhood Hemangiomas.

EPIDEMIOLOGY

- Hereditary hemorrhagic telangiectasia (HHT) is an autosomal-dominant vascular disorder that affects one in several thousands of people (see **Figure 211-1**). Certain populations in Europe and the United States have a higher prevalence of this disease.[1]
- Nevus flammeus, or port-wine stains, are congenital vascular malformations that occur in 0.1% to 0.3% of infants as developmental anomalies. They persist into adulthood (**Figure 211-2**).[2] They may be associated with rare syndromes such as Klippel-Trenaunay and Sturge-Weber syndromes (**Figure 211-3**).
- Maffucci syndrome is a rare, nonhereditary condition characterized by hemangiomas and enchondromas involving the hands, feet, and long bones (**Figure 211-4**).[3]

ETIOLOGY AND PATHOPHYSIOLOGY

- HHT is associated with mutations in two genes: endoglin on chromosome 9 (HHT type 1) and activin receptor-like kinase-1 on chromosome 12 (HHT type 2). These genes are involved in vascular development and repair. With the mutations, arterioles become dilated and connect directly with venules without a capillary in between. Although manifestations are not present at birth, telangiectasias later develop on the skin, mucous membranes, and GI

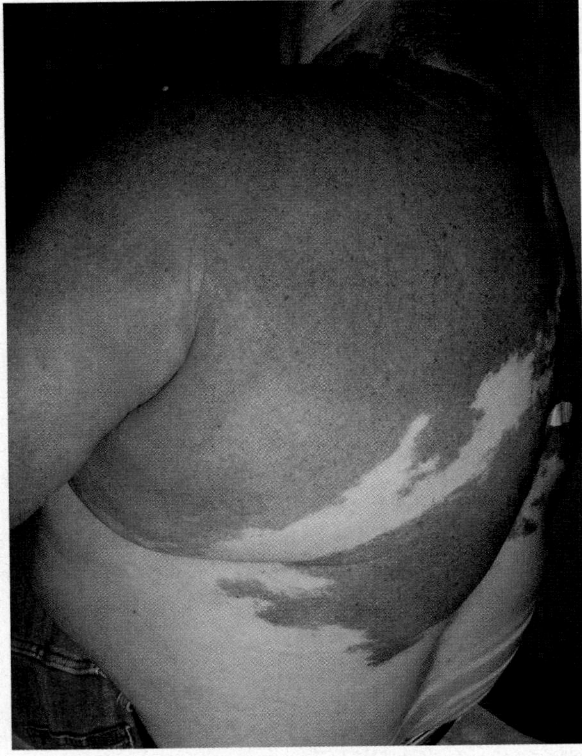

FIGURE 211-2 Large nevus flammeus or port-wine stain over the trunk of a 55-year-old man since birth. (*Reproduced with permission from Casey Pollard, MD.*)

tract. In addition, AVMs often develop in the hepatic (up to 70% of patients), pulmonary (5% to 300%), and cerebral circulations (10% to 15%). Any of these lesions may become fragile and prone to bleeding.[1]

- Port-wine stains are vascular ectasias or dilations thought to arise from a deficiency of sympathetic nervous innervation to the blood vessels. Dilated capillaries are present throughout the dermis layer of the skin.
- The bone and vascular lesions of Maffucci syndrome exist at birth or develop during childhood. Progression usually does not occur after completion of puberty.

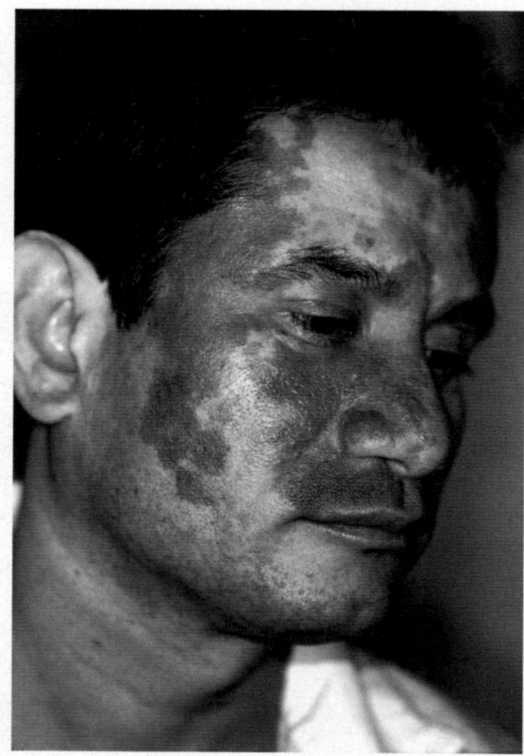

FIGURE 211-3 Port-wine stain, since birth, on the face of a man. Its distribution puts this patient at risk of Sturge-Weber syndrome. *(Reproduced with permission from Richard P. Usatine, MD.)*

DIAGNOSIS

CLINICAL FEATURES

- HHT is diagnosed if three of the following four Curaçao criteria are met (and suspected if two are present):
  1. Recurrent spontaneous nosebleeds (the presenting sign in more than 90% of patients, often during childhood);
  2. Mucocutaneous telangiectasia (typically develops in the third decade of life);
  3. Visceral involvement (lungs, brain, liver, and colon); and/or
  4. An affected first-degree relative.[4]
- Port-wine stains are irregular red-to-purple patches that start out smooth in infancy but may hypertrophy and develop a cobblestone texture with age. Nuchal port-wine stains are associated with alopecia areata.[5] Klippel-Trenaunay syndrome is characterized by vascular malformations, venous varicosities, and soft-tissue hyperplasia. Patients with Sturge-Weber syndrome often have mental retardation, epilepsy, and eye problems.[2]
- The cobblestone deformity of the hands and feet in Maffucci syndrome is striking (see **Figure 211-4**).

TYPICAL DISTRIBUTION

- HHT skin manifestations are few to numerous lesions on the tongue, lips, nasal mucosa, hands, and feet. However, any skin area or internal organ may be involved.
- Port-wine stains tend to affect the face and neck, although lesions may affect any body surface, including mucous membranes. Lesions of Klippel-Trenaunay syndrome tend to affect the lower extremities. A diagnosis of Sturge-Weber syndrome requires that a port-wine stain be present in the V1 trigeminal nerve distribution (aka ophthalmic branch). Patients with port-wine stains of the eyelids, bilateral trigeminal lesions (40% of patients with Sturge-Weber syndrome), and unilateral lesions involving all three divisions of the trigeminal nerve are particularly at risk of Sturge-Weber syndrome.[2]

LABORATORY STUDIES

- Check an annual complete blood count (CBC) and fecal occult blood in patients with HHT. They are at higher risk for iron-deficiency anemia because of recurrent nosebleeds and/or GI bleeding.

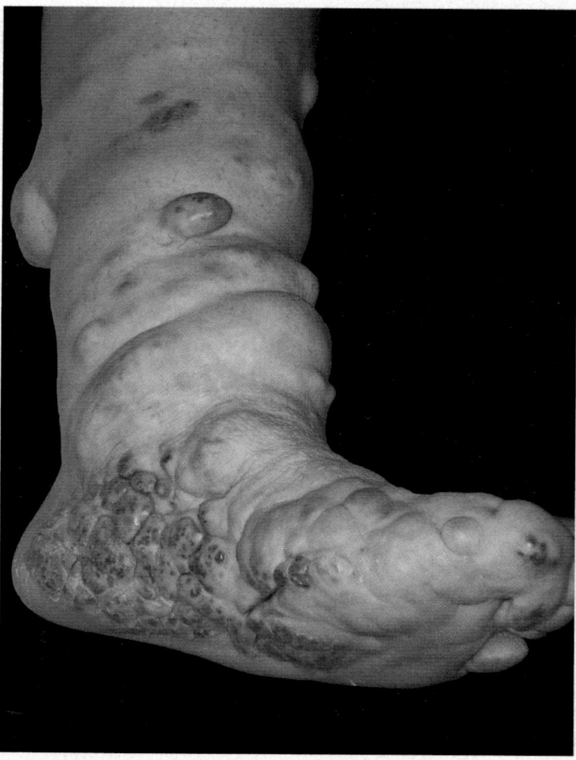

FIGURE 211-4 Hereditary hemangiomatosis, also called Maffucci syndrome. Note the cobblestone deformity of the foot. *(Reproduced with permission from Jeff Shellenberger, MD.)*

- Patients with benign-appearing port-wine stains, who lack other concerning symptoms, do not require laboratory testing (**Figure 211-5**).
- If Sturge-Weber syndrome is suspected, perform neuroimaging and glaucoma testing. Neuroimaging may reveal leptomeningeal malformations ipsilateral to the port-wine stain. An electroencephalogram may reveal epilepsy. Elevated ocular pressures or visual field deficits may indicate glaucoma.
- Investigate the musculoskeletal system in persons with Maffucci syndrome. It is associated with various benign and malignant tumors of the bone and cartilage.[3]

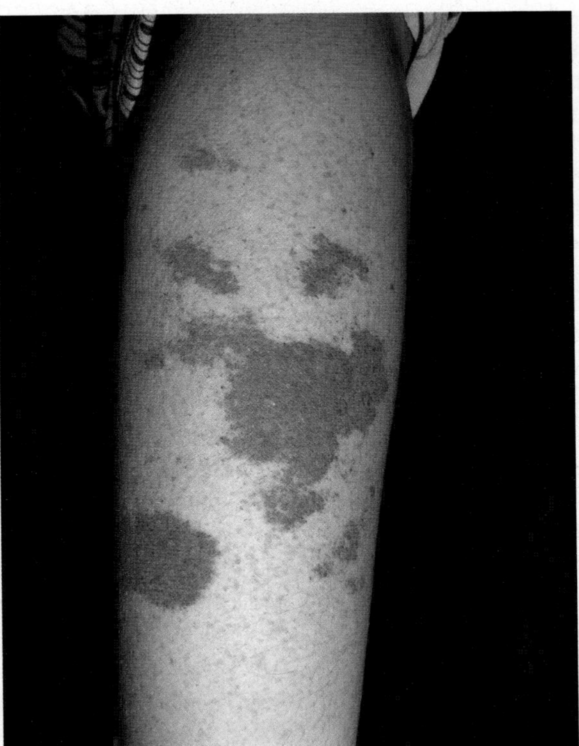

FIGURE 211-5 Nevus flammeus or port-wine stain, since birth, on the arm of a 34-year-old woman. She has had no problems with this benign capillary malformation. (*Reproduced with permission from Richard P. Usatine, MD.*)

DIFFERENTIAL DIAGNOSIS

- CREST (calcinosis, Raynaud phenomenon, esophageal involvement, sclerodactyly, and telangiectasia) syndrome and scleroderma usually have multiple telangiectasias as in HHT. Other clinical features and laboratory tests such as the antinuclear antibody (ANA) and skin biopsies can differentiate between these rheumatologic conditions and HHT (see Chapter 190, Scleroderma and Morphea).
- Port-wine stains are often isolated findings but may indicate underlying Klippel-Trenaunay or Sturge-Weber syndrome. Further investigations may be necessary when these syndromes are suspected.
- Glomangiomas are blue-purple, partially compressible nodules with a cobblestone appearance. These glomuvenous malformations may appear similar to Maffucci syndrome but lack the rheumatologic component (see Chapter 210, Acquired Vascular Skin Lesions).
- Salmon patches, also known as "stork bites" or "angel kisses" (present in 40% to 70% of newborns), are a type of nevus flammeus or port-wine stain. Salmon patches are pinker than purple but are true congenital vascular malformations, not hemangiomas. The angel kisses over the face tend to fade with time, but the stork bites on the nape of the neck often persist, as seen in **Figure 211-6** (see Chapter 115, Childhood Hemangiomas).[2]
- Lymphangioma circumscriptum is caused by cutaneous lymphatic malformations. It can be present at birth (**Figure 211-7**) or be acquired after trauma or surgery. Although it can have clear lymphatic fluid within the malformations, red blood cells are often also present. The red cells may layer out at the bottom in a manner that gives it a distinct appearance (**Figure 211-8**).

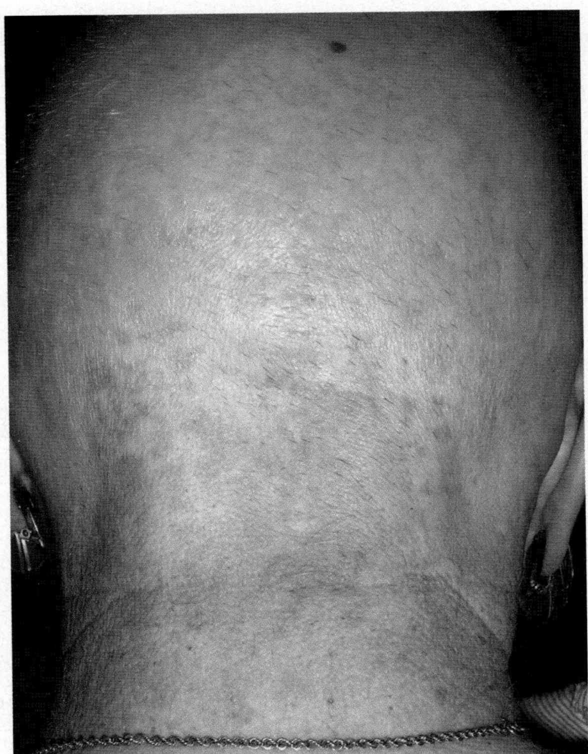

FIGURE 211-6 Stork bite (salmon patch) that has persisted since birth in this 72-year-old woman. This benign capillary malformation is more visible now because of the hair loss from chemotherapy. (*Reproduced with permission from Richard P. Usatine, MD.*)

MANAGEMENT

- HHT has no cure. Oral iron supplementation and transfusions are sometimes needed as a result of bleeding. Few randomized controlled trials exist regarding treatment of bleeding. Estrogen/progesterone supplementation for heavily transfusion-dependent patients decreases recurrent bleeding.[6] SOR Ⓑ Case reports and uncontrolled studies regarding epistaxis treatment show some benefit from laser treatment, surgery, embolization, and topical therapy. SOR Ⓒ Cauterization is not recommended because of complications from local tissue damage. Embolization procedures have been described for AVMs in the liver, lungs, and brain. Surgical resection of AVMs is sometimes done as a last resort when other measures fail.[1] In short, it is often best to do as little intervention as possible with HHT and, if any intervention is done, it is done with input from specialists experienced with this disease, as complications and recurrence are frequently encountered.

- The monoclonal antibody against vascular endothelial growth factor (VEGF), bevacizumab, is being used and studied in patients with HHT. In a review of 18 case reports, 14 reported improvements in epistaxis, and 11 reported hemoglobin improvement following intravenous bevacizumab.[7] SOR B
- Port-wine stains may be treated with makeup (see "Patient Resources" below). Pulsed-dye laser treatment is another option, albeit expensive. Laser treatments blanch most port-wine lesions to some degree, but complete resolution is difficult to achieve and the recurrence rate is high.[8] SOR C
- Patients with Maffucci syndrome often require multiple orthopedic surgeries for their enchondromatous deformities and for cosmetic purposes.[3,9]

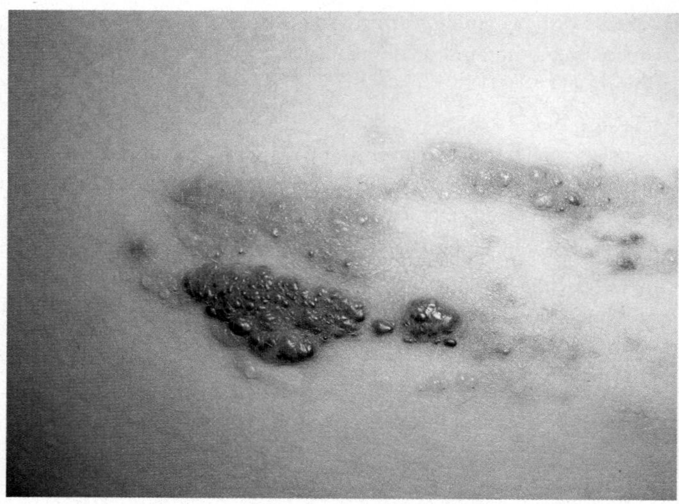

FIGURE 211-7 Close-up of lymphangioma circumscriptum present from birth on the trunk of this 7-year-old girl. Note the group of vesicles of different colors from pale yellow to pink and red. The red color is due to blood within the dilated lymphatic vessels. Note how this pattern resembles frogspawn. (*Reproduced with permission from Richard P. Usatine, MD.*)

PATIENT EDUCATION

- Whatever the vascular condition is, patients can benefit from reliable information about the current and future outlook for their condition.

FOLLOW-UP

- Patients with port-wine stains should have periodic skin checks, as other lesions may develop within the port-wine stains. Several case reports of basal cell cancers developing within port-wine stains have been described.[10]
- Patients with Sturge-Weber syndrome should have yearly eye examinations that include testing of intraocular pressures. SOR C
- Patients with Maffucci syndrome should be monitored closely for both skeletal and nonskeletal tumors, particularly of the brain and abdomen.[9] SOR C

PATIENT RESOURCES

- HHT Foundation International. Excellent patient information on HHT can be found at the Foundation's website—**http://www.curehht.org.**
- Covermark. Port-wine stains are often psychologically detrimental. Cosmetic makeup may be purchased through Covermark—**http://www.covermark.com.**
- Dermablend is another effective cosmetic product for port-wine stains—**http://www.dermablend.com.**

PROVIDER RESOURCES

- Medscape. *Vascular Malformations*—**http://emedicine.medscape.com/article/1018071.**

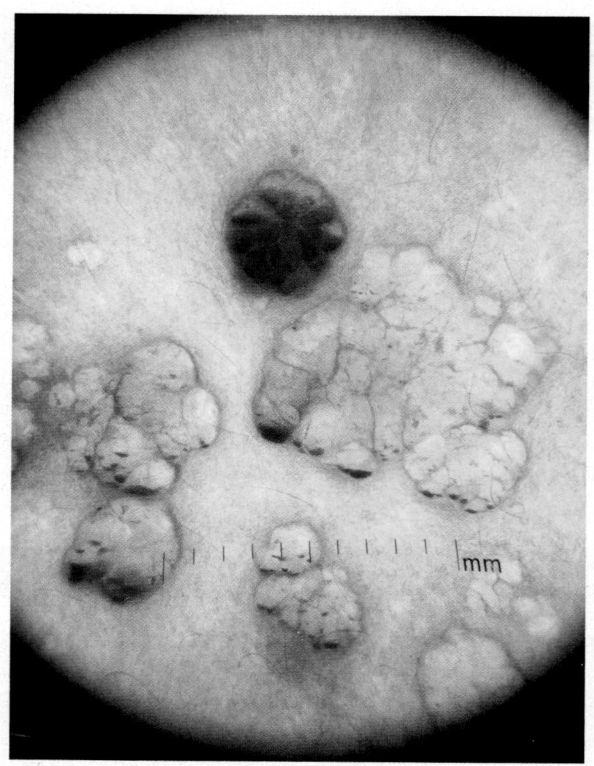

FIGURE 211-8 Dermoscopy of lymphangioma circumscriptum that started after trauma in a 35-year-old man. The red blood cells have settled out due to gravity and create a blood-lymph level within the dilated lymphatic vessels. (*Reproduced with permission from Richard P. Usatine, MD.*)

REFERENCES

1. Grand'Maison A. Hereditary hemorrhagic telangiectasia. *CMAJ.* 2009;180(8):833-835. http://www.ncbi.nlm.nih.gov/pmc/articles/PMC2665965/pdf/1800833.pdf. Accessed March 2012.
2. Habif TP. Vascular tumors and malformations. In: *Clinical Dermatology: A Color Guide to Diagnosis and Therapy*, 5th ed. Philadelphia, PA: Mosby, 2010:891-903.
3. Jermann M, Eid K, Pfammatter T, Stahel R. Maffucci's syndrome. *Circulation.* 2001;104:1693.
4. Shovlin CL, Guttmacher AE, Buscarini E, et al. Diagnostic criteria for hereditary haemorrhagic telangiectasia (Rendu-Osler-Weber syndrome). *Am J Med Genet.* 2000;91:66-67.
5. Akhyani M, Farnaghi F, Seirafi H, et al. The association between nuchal nevus flammeus and alopecia areata: a case-control study. *Dermatology.* 2005;211(4):334-337.
6. Van Cutsem E, Rutgeerts P, Vantrappen G. Treatment of bleeding GI vascular malformations with oestrogen-progesterone. *Lancet.* 1990;335:953-955.
7. Arizmendez NP, Rudmik L, Poetker DM. Intravenous bevacizumab for complications of hereditary hemorrhagic telangiectasia: a review of the literature. *Int Forum Allergy Rhinol.* 2015;5(11):1042-1047.
8. Lanigan SW, Taibjee SM. Recent advances in laser treatment of port-wine stains. *Br J Dermatol.* 2004;151(3):527-533.
9. Gupta N, Kabra M. Maffucci syndrome. *Indian Pediatr.* 2007;44(2):149-150.
10. Silapunt S, Goldberg LH, Thurber M, Friedman PM. Basal cell carcinoma arising in a port-wine stain. *Dermatol Surg.* 2004;30(9):1241-1245.

SECTION U OTHER SKIN DISORDERS

212 CUTANEOUS DRUG REACTIONS

Robert Christopher Gilson, MD
Anna Allred, MD
Mindy A. Smith, MD, MS
Richard P. Usatine, MD

PATIENT STORIES

A 20-year-old college student was seen for fatigue and an upper respiratory infection and started on amoxicillin for a sore throat. Six days later she broke out with a red rash all over her body (**Figure 212-1**). She went to see her family physician back home with the rash and lymphadenopathy. A monospot was drawn and found to be positive. This morbilliform rash (like measles) is typical of an amoxicillin drug eruption in a person with mononucleosis. Amoxicillin was stopped, and diphenhydramine was used for the itching.

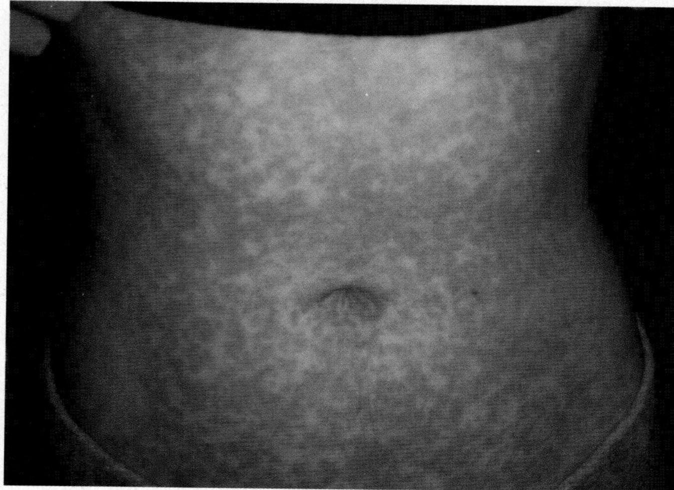

FIGURE 212-1 Amoxicillin rash in a young woman with mononucleosis. This is a morbilliform eruption. (*Reproduced with permission from Richard P. Usatine, MD.*)

INTRODUCTION

Cutaneous drug reactions are the visible skin manifestations of a drug hypersensitivity and can present in a wide myriad of dermatosis. This includes the most common manifestation as a morbilliform exanthem but also includes urticaria/angioedema, acneiform or pustular, fixed drug eruption, eruptions, and the Stevens-Johnson syndrome/toxic epidermal necrolysis (SJS/TEN) spectrum. The primary morphology often elucidates a typical time course for its occurrence which can help identify the culprit drug for discontinuation. One should also quickly identify the more serious life-threatening drug-induced conditions or severe cutaneous adverse reactions (SCARs).

Drug hypersensitivity may be defined as symptoms or signs initiated by a drug exposure at a dose normally tolerated by non-hypersensitive persons.[1] An adverse drug reaction (ADR) is defined by the World Health Organization as a noxious and unintended response to a drug at doses and indications normally used for treatment. They can be a predictable side effect of the pharmacologic action of the drug, type A (80%), or as an idiosyncratic reaction, which occurs only in susceptible patients, type B (10%–15%).[2] Cutaneous drug reactions range from mild skin eruptions (e.g., exanthem, urticaria, and angioedema) to SCARs, the latter category including acute generalized exanthematous pustulosis (AGEP); drug reaction with eosinophilia and systemic symptoms (DRESS), also known as drug-induced hypersensitivity syndrome (DIHS); SJS; and TEN.[3] Other serious adverse reactions include anticoagulant-induced skin necrosis, drug-induced vasculitis, and generalized fixed drug eruption. Features suggestive of a complicated or severe SCAR include fever, facial swelling, bullae or skin shedding, mucosal involvement, and systemic symptoms.[4]

SYNONYMS

Cutaneous adverse reactions, drug reactions, medication reactions, adverse effects to drugs, hypersensitivity reactions.

EPIDEMIOLOGY

- Cutaneous drug reactions are common complications of drug therapy occurring in 2% to 3% of hospitalized patients.[5]
- One study found that 4% to 5% of all adverse drug reactions were manifested in the skin.[5] Approximately 1 in 6 adverse drug reactions represents drug hypersensitivity and can be either allergic or non–immune-mediated (pseudoallergic) reactions.[2]
- Maculopapular eruptions, also known as exanthematous drug eruptions, are the most frequent of all cutaneous drug reactions, representing 95% of skin reactions.[6] They are often confused with viral exanthems. This occurs most commonly with aminopenicillins, sulfonamides, cephalosporins, anticonvulsants, and allopurinol (**Figures 212-1** and **212-2**).
- Urticarial drug reactions are the second most common skin eruptions, representing approximately 5% of cutaneous drug reactions.[6] This reaction can result from any drug but commonly occurs with aspirin, penicillin, sulfa, angiotensin-converting enzyme (ACE) inhibitors, aminoglycosides, and blood products. Urticaria results from immunoglobulin (Ig) E reactions within minutes to hours of drug administration (**Figures 212-3** and **212-4**).
- Drug-induced hyperpigmentation occurs with antiarrhythmics (amiodarone), antibiotics (minocycline), nonsteroidal anti-inflammatory drugs (NSAIDs), and chemotherapy agents (doxorubicin) (**Figure 212-5**).
- A lichenoid drug eruption can also lead to hyperpigmentation and requires drug identification and discontinuation for resolution (**Figure 212-6**).
- Warfarin-induced skin necrosis (WISN) is a rare but serious side effect predominantly seen in obese women and presents in the first few days of warfarin treatment. Skin lesions with purpura and necrosis usually occur in areas containing subcutaneous fat. WISN is more common in those with hypercoagulable abnormalities, given large loading doses (**Figure 212-7**).
- Heparin-induced skin necrosis can present similarly but occurs later, typically 5 to 10 days after starting unfractionated or even low-molecular-weight heparin products. The necrosis is frequently observed at the site of the heparin injections and often favors fat-rich areas such as the abdomen. It may be associated with a trend of falling platelet counts from heparin-induced thrombocytopenia (HIT) and can be confirmed when suspected by an enzyme-linked immunosorbent assay (ELISA) for anti-platelet factor 4 antibody detection.
- Fixed drug eruptions (FDEs) can occur with many medications, including phenolphthalein, doxycycline, ibuprofen, sulfonamide antibiotics, and barbiturates. FDEs are more commonly observed in men but occur in women as well (**Figures 212-8** to **212-14**).

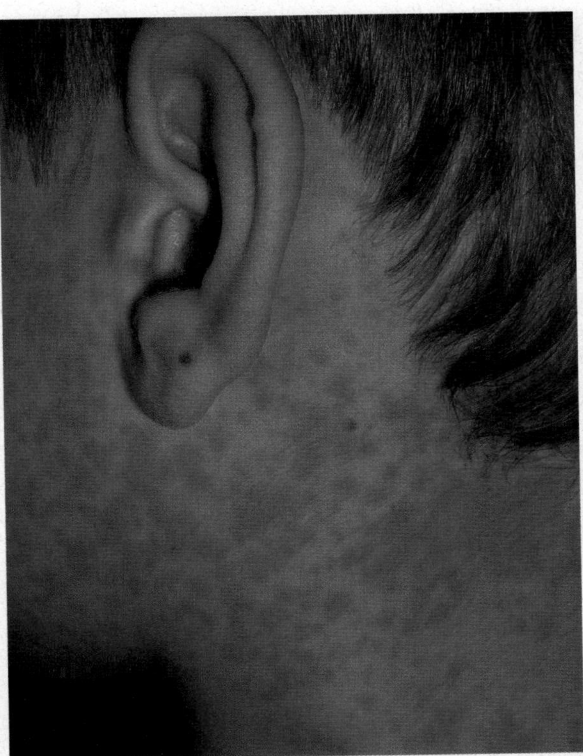

FIGURE 212-2 Maculopapular drug eruption in a 5-year-old boy with an upper respiratory infection started on amoxicillin for a questionable otitis media. Four days later he broke out with a red rash all over his face and body. This morbilliform rash (like measles) is typical of an amoxicillin drug eruption. (*Reproduced with permission from Robert Tunks, MD.*)

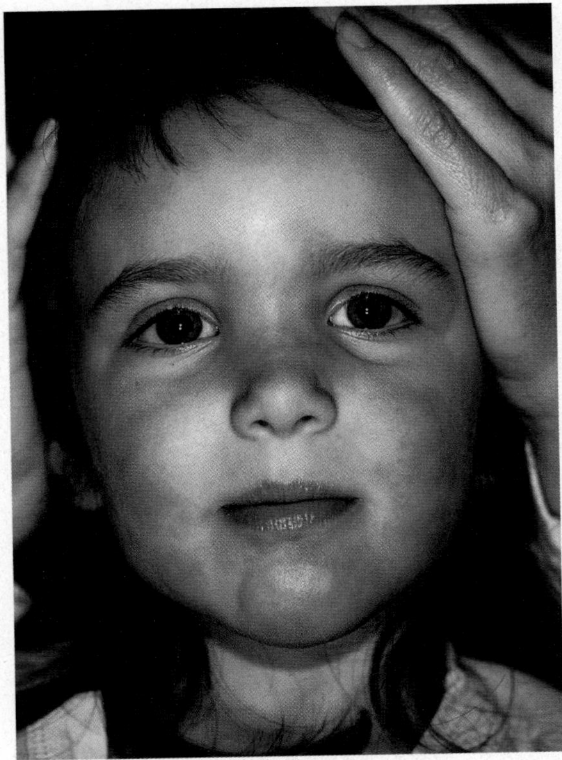

FIGURE 212-3 Urticarial drug eruption secondary to trimethoprim/sulfamethoxazole. This young girl had urticaria multiforme. (*Reproduced with permission from Richard P. Usatine, MD.*)

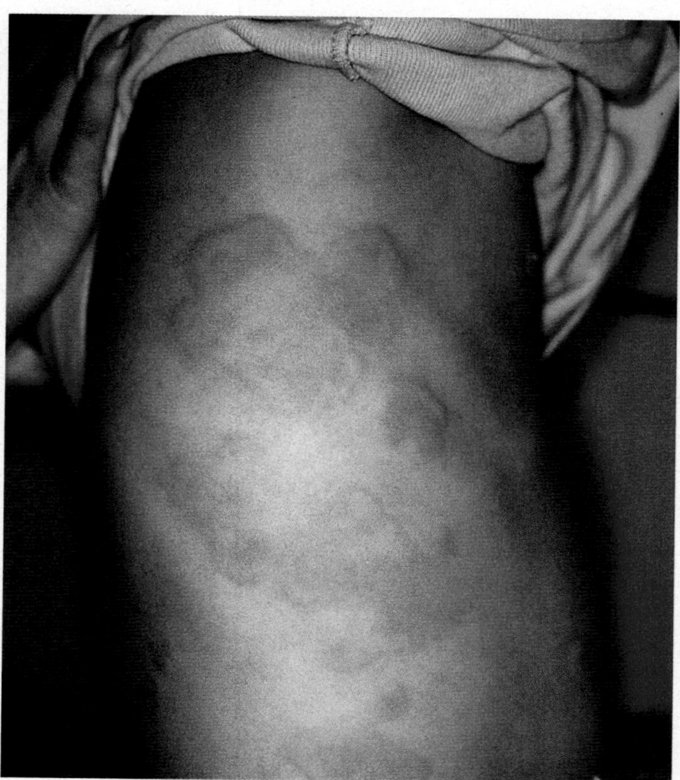

FIGURE 212-4 Giant urticarial eruption (urticaria multiforme) in the patient in **Figure 212-3** with drug reaction to sulfa. (*Reproduced with permission from Richard P. Usatine, MD.*)

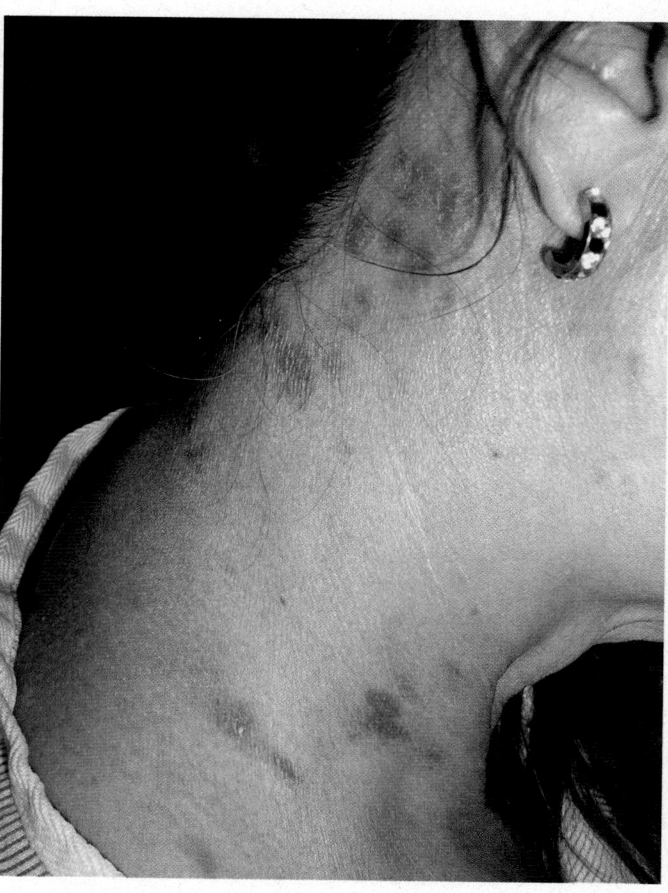

FIGURE 212-6 Hyperpigmented lesions from a biopsy-confirmed lichenoid drug eruption. This 61-year-old Hispanic woman developed these lichenoid lesions after starting medications for tuberculosis. (*Reproduced with permission from Richard P. Usatine, MD.*)

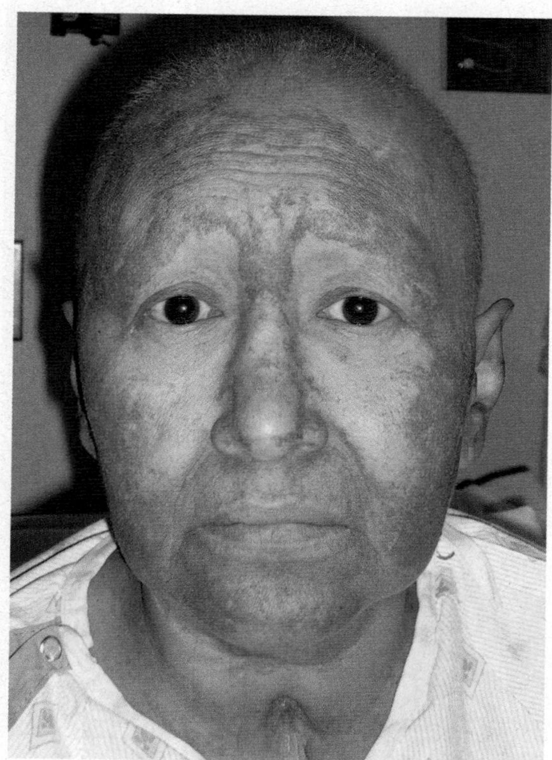

FIGURE 212-5 Facial hyperpigmentation secondary to doxorubicin. (*Reproduced with permission from Richard P. Usatine, MD.*)

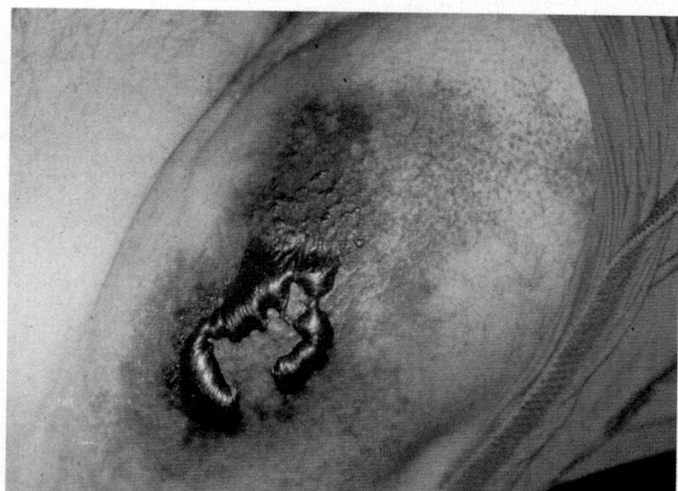

FIGURE 212-7 Warfarin (Coumadin) necrosis with dark bullae on the arm of a woman just started on Coumadin. (*Reproduced with permission from Eric Kraus, MD.*)

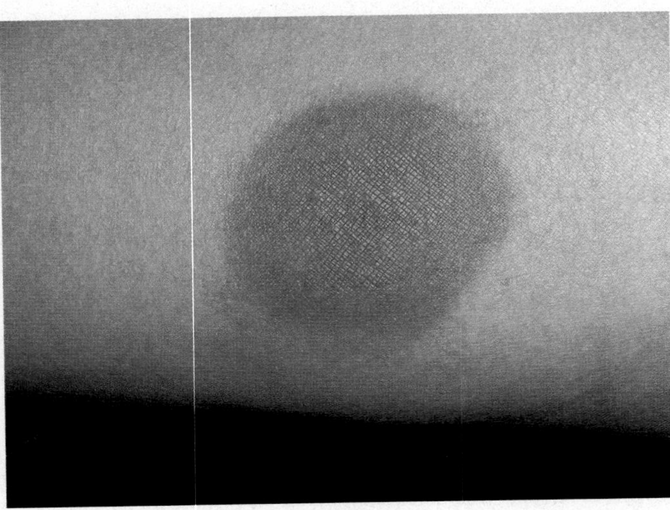

FIGURE 212-8 Annular-appearing fixed drug eruption with a dusky center on the leg. (*Reproduced with permission from Richard P. Usatine, MD.*)

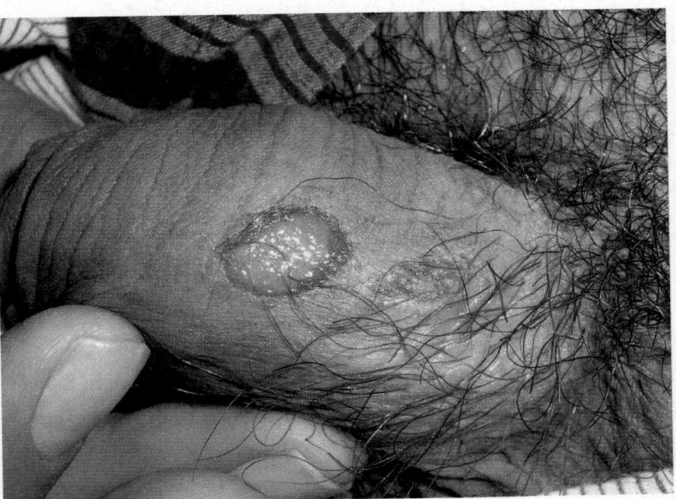

FIGURE 212-10 Fixed drug eruption to ibuprofen with violaceous and hyperpigmented macules and erosions on the penis. (*Reproduced with permission from Richard P. Usatine, MD.*)

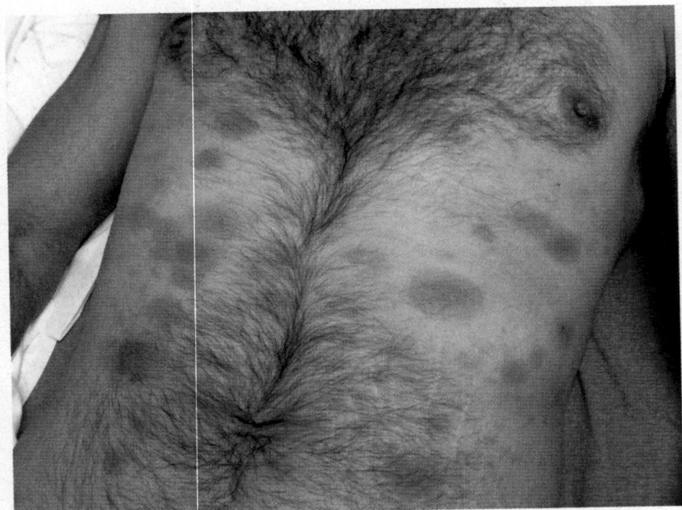

FIGURE 212-9 Disseminated (or generalized) fixed drug eruption in a 31-year-old man. He had similar-appearing lesions in the exact same initial locations of the chin and glans penis upon exposure to trimethoprim-sulfamethoxazole in the past. During this episode the lesions returned to the chin and penis and also involved the trunk and extremities. (*Reproduced with permission from Bucher J, Rahnama-Moghadam S, Osswald S. Generalized rash follows ankle ulceration. J Fam Pract. 2016 Jul;65(7):489-91. Frontline Medical Communications, Inc.*)

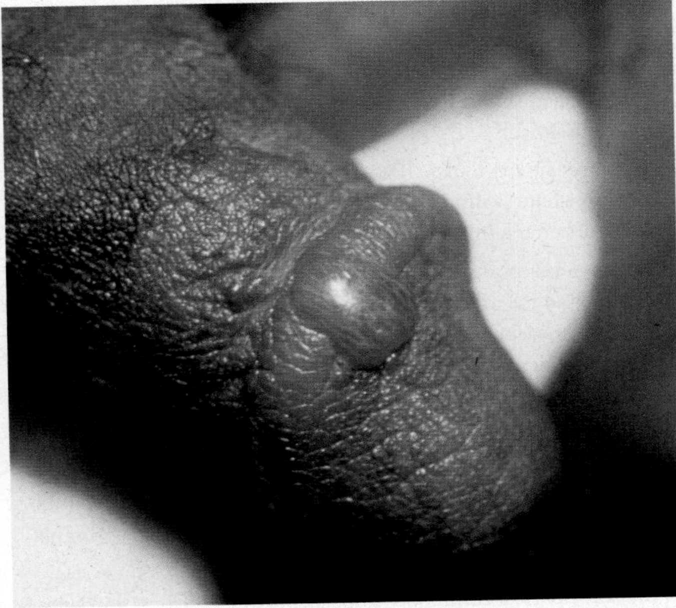

FIGURE 212-11 Bullous fixed drug eruptions. Bullous fixed drug eruption on the glans penis, a common location for these fixed drug eruptions. (*Reproduced with permission from Jeffrey Meffert, MD.*)

- Erythema multiforme (EM) is most often due to a preceding herpes simplex virus (HSV) or *Mycoplasma* infection (**Figure 212-15**).
- SJS is more often associated with medication reactions and drug-induced in its etiology (**Figure 212-16**). Incidence of SJS is estimated at 1.2 per 6 million people.[3]
- DRESS (**Figures 212-17** and **212-18**) is also a severe adverse drug-induced reaction characterized by eosinophilia and systemic symptoms, often with a rash, liver involvement, fever, and lymphadenopathy. In a case series (N = 172), 44 drugs were associated with DRESS.[7] The most common causes are aromatic anticonvulsants, especially phenytoin, carbamazepine, and phenobarbital, and sulfonamides like dapsone and sulfasalazine.[8] Also referred to as DIHS (drug-induced hypersensitivity syndrome), this syndrome is estimated to occur in 1 per 1000 to 1 per 10,000 exposures to antiepileptic drugs.[9]

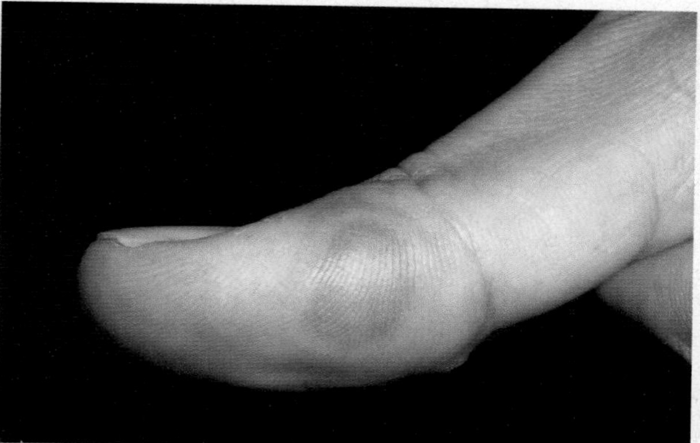

FIGURE 212-12 Third episode of fixed drug eruption to doxycycline. Note how the finger lesion is similar to a target lesion in erythema multiforme. However, there is no central epithelial disruption in this target lesion. The patient also had lesions on the palm, lips, and palate. *(Reproduced with permission from Richard P. Usatine, MD.)*

ETIOLOGY AND PATHOPHYSIOLOGY

- Two mechanisms are responsible for cutaneous drug reactions: immunologic, including all four types of hypersensitivity reactions, and, more commonly, nonimmunologic (pseudoallergic). Although the precise mechanism of immune stimulation is unknown, it may be triggered by drug-protein (hapten-carrier) complexes or through direct interaction with immune receptors (p-i concept).[2] The mechanism for pseudoallergic reactions is pathogenetically poorly defined.[2]
- Hypersensitivity to NSAIDs is a nonimmunologic reaction that can be immediate (within hours after exposure) or delayed (more than 24 hours after administration).[1]
- WISN develops during the hypercoagulable state as a result of a more rapid fall in concentration of protein C compared to the other vitamin-K–dependent procoagulant factors. Hypercoagulable abnormalities such as familial or acquired deficiency of protein C or S and factor V Leiden mutations have been implicated in WISN (see **Figure 212-7**).
- Specific mutations in genes that encode drug detoxification enzymes have been shown in those having a higher risk of DRESS (see **Figures 212-17 and 212-18**) and are felt to lead to accumulation of drug-reactive metabolites.[8]
- SJS/TEN is most commonly associated with penicillins and sulfonamide antibiotics but can also occur with anticonvulsants, NSAIDs, and allopurinol. It is hypothesized that a specific human leukocyte antigen (HLA)-B molecule may present the drug or its metabolites to naïve CD8 cells, resulting in clonal expansion of CD8 cytotoxic lymphocytes and induction of cytotoxic effector responses, resulting in apoptosis of keratinocytes.[10] This pathway is not likely to be specific to SJS.

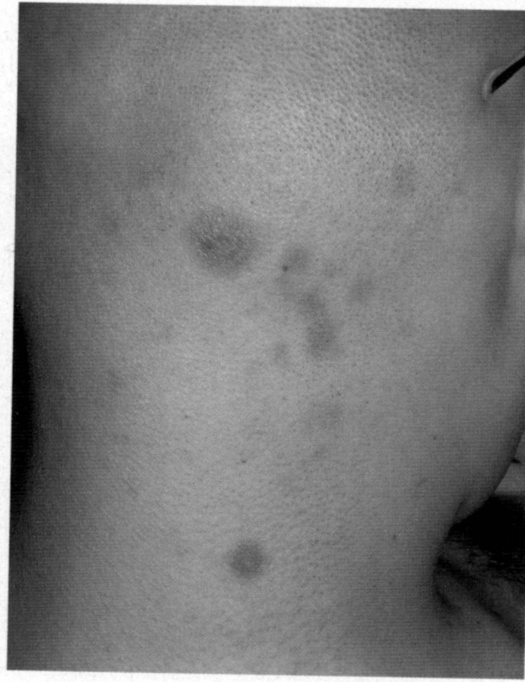

FIGURE 212-13 Fixed drug eruption to hydrocodone seen on the scalp and neck of this 22-year-old man. *(Reproduced with permission from Richard P. Usatine, MD.)*

RISK FACTORS

- Drug hypersensitivity reactions increase with the drug dose, duration, route of administration (topical < subcutaneous < intramuscular < oral < intravenous),[11] immune activation of the individual,

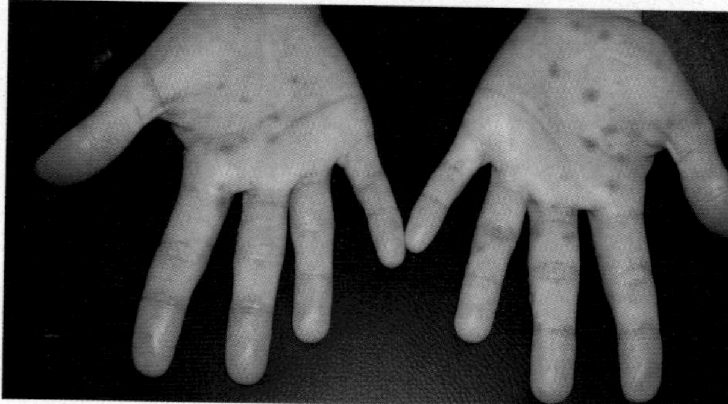

FIGURE 212-14 Erythema multiforme showing target lesions on the palms secondary to herpes simplex in a young woman. *(Reproduced with permission from Richard P. Usatine, MD.)*

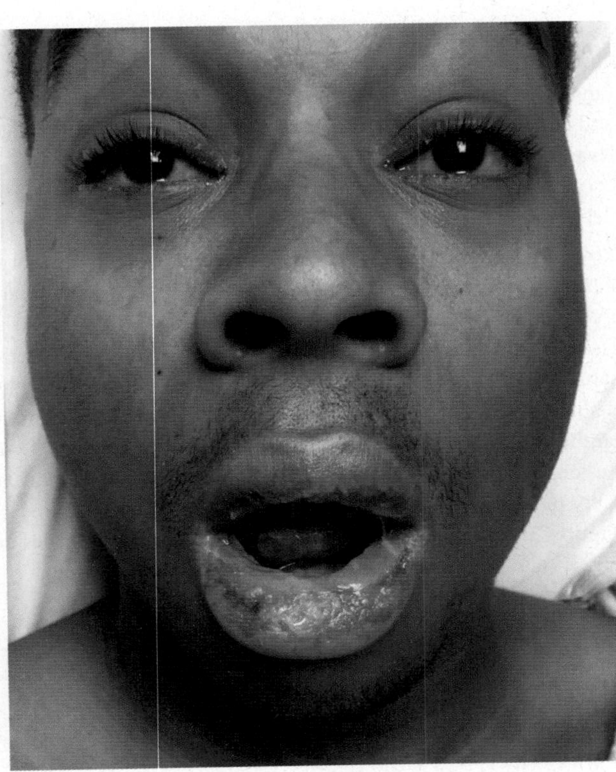

FIGURE 212-15 Erythema multiforme major with 2 mucus membranes involved secondary to mycoplasma. (*Reproduced with permission from Sahand Rahnama, MD.*)

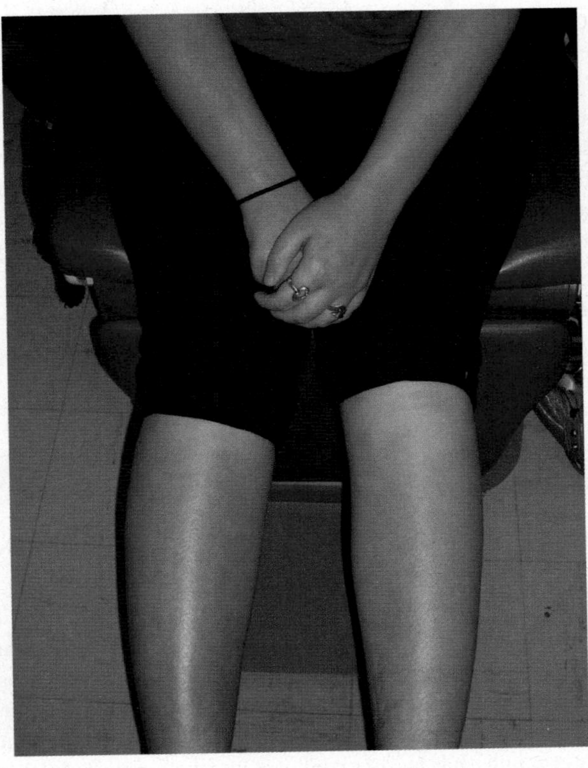

FIGURE 212-17 Drug reaction with eosinophilia and systemic symptoms (DRESS). Erythroderma has persisted, but the patient is feeling better after treatment and discharge from the hospital. (*Reproduced with permission from Richard P. Usatine, MD.*)

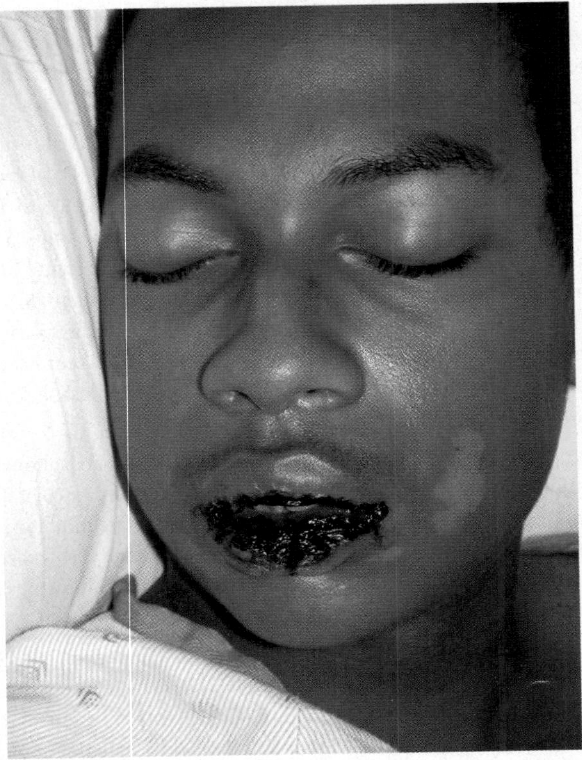

FIGURE 212-16 Stevens-Johnson syndrome secondary to a sulfa antibiotic. (*Reproduced with permission from Eric Kraus, MD.*)

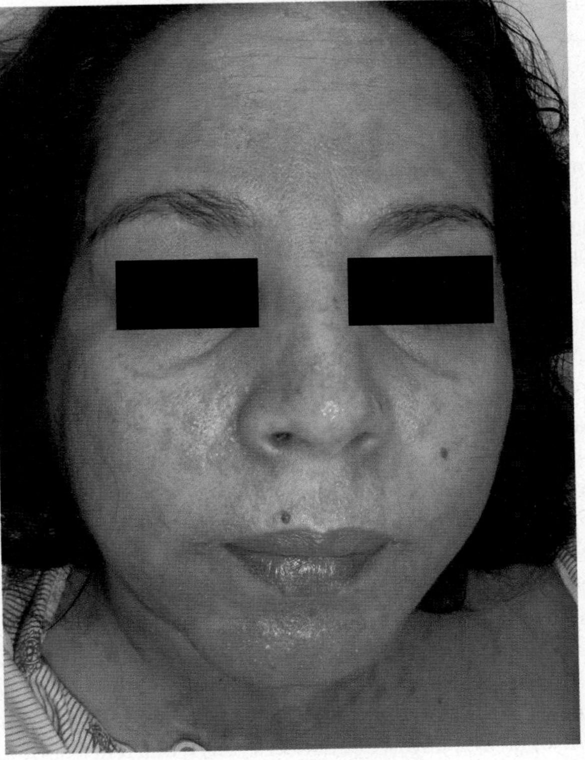

FIGURE 212-18 Drug reaction with eosinophilia and systemic symptoms (DRESS) on the face with facial swelling and erythema. This 40-year-old woman developed DRESS as a reaction to a new phenytoin prescription. (*Reproduced with permission from Robert T. Gilson, MD.*)

and immunogenetic predisposition; they are also more frequent in women.[2] Multiple drug therapy may also increase risk.[11]

- Patients with certain HLA types in certain ethnic groups can be at higher risk for cutaneous drug reactions: for example, HLA-B*5701 identifies a higher risk of hypersensitivity reactions to abacavir (an antiretroviral drug).[2,7] Other associations with specific medications have been further identified and can be screened for when the predictive value is deemed significant.
- Prior drug reaction may result in a faster recurrence on reexposure.[11]
- Concomitant illness, especially viral infections and autoimmune disorders.[11]

DIAGNOSIS

CLINICAL FEATURES AND TYPICAL DISTRIBUTION (THE MOST COMMON AND IMPORTANT DRUG ERUPTIONS)

- *Maculopapular*—These eruptions, red macules with papules, can occur any time after drug therapy is initiated (often 7 to 10 days) and last 1 to 2 weeks. The reaction usually starts on the upper trunk or head and neck then spreads symmetrically downward to limbs. The eruptions may become confluent in a symmetric, generalized distribution that often spares the face (see **Figure 212-1**). Mild desquamation is normal as the exanthematous eruption resolves.
- *Urticaria and angioedema*—Urticarial reactions present as circumscribed areas of blanching with raised erythema and edema of the superficial dermis (see **Figures 212-3** and **212-4**). They may occur on any skin area and are usually transient, migratory, and pruritic. Angioedema represents a deeper reaction, with swelling usually around the lips and eyes (see Chapter 156, Urticaria and Angioedema).
- *Hyperpigmentation*—Drug-induced hyperpigmentation presents in many ways. Amiodarone causes a dusky red coloration that turns blue-gray with time in photo-exposed areas. Minocycline can cause a blue-gray color in acne lesions, on the gingiva, and on the teeth. Phenytoin (Dilantin) and other hydantoins may cause melasma-like brown pigmentation on the face. Bleomycin can cause a streaking hyperpigmentation on the trunk and extremities. Doxorubicin (Adriamycin), as evident in the case above, can cause hyperpigmentation of the face and nails (see **Figure 212-5**).
- *NSAIDs*—The cutaneous reactions to NSAID-associated drug hypersensitivity are urticaria, angioedema, or anaphylaxis.[1] These reactions can be caused by a single NSAID or multiple NSAIDs. There is also an NSAID-exacerbated urticaria and angioedema that occurs in patients with chronic idiopathic urticaria.
- *Warfarin-induced skin necrosis*—WISN presents with sudden onset of a painful localized skin lesion that is initially erythematous and/or hemorrhagic and that becomes bullous, culminating in gangrenous necrosis (see **Figure 212-7**). It develops more often in obese women in their 50s in areas with high subcutaneous fat content such as breasts, thighs, and buttocks. This is different from a warfarin bleed secondary to too much anticoagulation (**Figure 212-19**).
- Cocaine-associated retiform purpura (**Figure 251-8** in Chapter 251, Cocaine). Nonprescription medications and substances should also be inquired into when suspecting a drug-induced rash. In particular, cocaine use is associated with a particularly unique retiform (angulated) purpura with necrosis, often affecting the ears, nose, and face. It has been determined to be induced by the contaminant levamisole now estimated to be in 70% of the U.S. supply of cocaine. ANCA antibodies and associated leukopenia are often detected.
- *Fixed drug eruption*—FDE presents with single or multiple sharply demarcated circular, violaceous or hyperpigmented plaques that may include central blisters (see **Figures 212-8** to **212-14**). The lesion(s) appear after drug exposure and reappear exactly at the same site and location each time the drug is taken, typically within 8 hours. As the site resolves, it leaves a round to oval area of macular dusky gray to reddish brown hyperpigmentation (**Figure 212-20**). Lesions can occur anywhere including the hands and feet, but also favor the lips and genitalia, commonly involving the penis (see **Figures 212-10** and **212-11**). Bullous FDEs occur when the lesion blisters and erodes, followed by desquamation and crusting (**Figures 212-11** and **212-21**).
- *Erythema multiforme*—EM presents with typical target (3 distinct zones) of raised edematous papules distributed acrally (see **Figures 212-14** and **212-15**; see Chapter 185, Erythema Multiforme, Stevens-Johnson Syndrome, and Toxic Epidermal Necrolysis). It is a more benign reaction, typically associated with HSV or less commonly *Mycoplasma pneumoniae* infections.
- *SJS*—It presents with erythematous or pruritic macules, widespread blisters on the trunk and face, and erosions of two or more mucous membranes, most commonly oral and conjunctival (see **Figure 212-16**). Prodromal symptoms may include fever, influenza-like symptoms, and painful skin. Burning or painful skin can be a sign of increased severity. Atypical 2-zoned macular target lesions or widespread erythema, particularly in the upper chest and back, are potential early signs of both SJS and TEN.[11] Epidermal detachment occurs and involves less than 10% of total body surface area.
- *Toxic epidermal necrolysis*—TEN is on the more severe side of the SJS/TEN spectrum. SJS is diagnosed when less than 10% of the body surface area is involved, SJS/TEN *overlap* when 10% to 30% is involved, and TEN when more than 30% is involved. A positive Nikolsky sign is present and induced by tangential pressure of the finger on the affected skin causing epidermal detachment. SJS and TEN are distinct from EM in that these are severe drug reactions with significant morbidity. Ocular involvement and complications can have long-term sequelae. Mortality ranges from less than 5% for SJS to more than 90% for those with severe TEN.
- Drugs most commonly known to cause SJS and TEN are sulfonamide antibiotics, aminopenicillins, allopurinol, NSAIDs, antiretroviral drugs (especially non-nucleoside reverse-transcriptase inhibitors [NNRTIs]), amine antiepileptic drugs (phenytoin and carbamazepine), and lamotrigine (see Chapter 185, Erythema Multiforme, Stevens-Johnson Syndrome, and Toxic Epidermal Necrolysis).[12]
- *Drug reaction with eosinophilia and systemic symptoms (DRESS) or drug-induced hypersensitivity syndrome (DIHS)*—Infiltrated, palpable lesions are potential heralds of this disorder.[11] Central facial edema and erythema (see **Figure 212-18**) and a maculopapular rash are seen along with high fever, generalized lymphadenopathy, and arthralgias. There may also be peripheral eosinophilia, atypical

lymphocytosis, and increased hepatic enzymes. The typical rash is morbilliform, and significant facial edema is often characteristic. DRESS can also cause an erythroderma (see **Figure 212-17**). There is usually a longer lag time between drug exposure and symptoms, typically 15 to 40 days. The most common drugs include anticonvulsants, β-lactam antibiotics, allopurinol, NSAIDs, antiretrovirals, and sulfonamide antibiotics.[4] It may be more common in certain populations with susceptible alleles or genetics. Certain screening can be done for at-risk populations and specific medications (carbamazepine, allopurinol, abacavir). There is often internal organ involvement, which includes hepatitis, nephritis, pneumonitis, myocarditis, and others. It has a significant mortality of up to 10%, and the symptoms can persist for weeks to several months.[13]

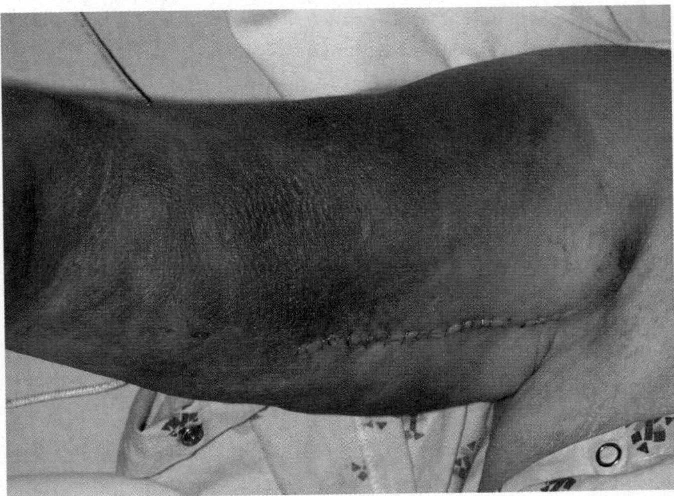

FIGURE 212-19 Large bleed in the arm secondary to overcoagulation with warfarin. The large hematoma was surgically evacuated to prevent neurovascular compromise to the arm. (*Reproduced with permission from Richard P. Usatine, MD.*)

LESS COMMON DRUG REACTIONS

- *Acute generalized exanthematous pustulosis (AGEP)*—A type of drug eruption occurring within 1–4 days of drug initiation. Antibiotics, specifically β-lactams, are among the most common culprits.[4] AGEP results in the sudden appearance of clusters of small pustules along with erythematous skin (**Figure 212-22**). The patients are often febrile, and the pustules are primarily nonfollicular and sterile on an erythematous base. Leukocytosis and eosinophilia are also typically present. Systemic treatment is not usually required, as it tends to resolve spontaneously following withdrawal of the offending medication, with mortality existing between 1% and 2%.[4]
- *Systemic drug-related intertriginous and flexural exanthema (SDRIFE)*—This is a type of drug eruption that causes erythema around the buttocks and genitalia along with intertriginous and flexural areas. If the pattern of erythema creates red buttocks, then it may also be called the baboon syndrome (**Figure 212-23**).

APPROACH TO A SUSPECTED CUTANEOUS DRUG REACTION

A drug-induced reaction should be considered in anyone taking medication who develops a sudden cutaneous eruption. In reviewing the history, obtain a full listing of all the patient's medications, including prescriptions and also over-the-counter medications or supplements, by any route—including topical, intermittent, or regular. Current and recent past medication history is important, as the reaction may be attributable to a medicine the patient stopped taking or took only intermittently. A historical timeline is critical in defining the interval between the time the drug was taken and the onset of the eruption, because many drug-related adverse reactions have a characteristic time interval. Fixed drug eruptions and AGEP occur often within days, whereas SJS/TEN occur within weeks, and DIHS and DRESS even longer after the offending medication was started.

The next step is the physical examination to define the morphology of the skin findings. There are a myriad presentations, and the exam findings will define the type of adverse drug reaction and subsequently help in determining the most likely offending medications known to cause that particular type of drug reaction. Once one has established the type of drug eruption, that pattern can help define the type of drugs most commonly associated or described to cause that type of eruption. The particular drug eruption pattern coupled with

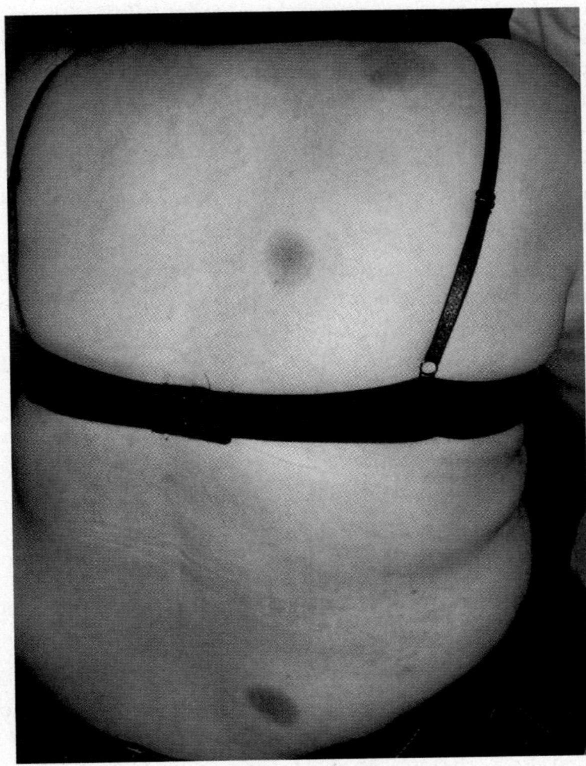

FIGURE 212-20 Fixed drug eruption with hyperpigmented patches in a Hispanic woman. Note how the patches are gray to brown with a velvet-like appearance. (*Reproduced with permission from Richard P. Usatine, MD.*)

its characteristic time course can then help define the likely offending medication in the drug history timeline (**Table 212-1**).

Examination should include a full cutaneous exam, including the groin and genitalia, mucosal surfaces of the eyes and oropharynx, and palpation for adenopathy. The clinician should specifically assess for the presence of facial edema or swelling, pustular or bullous lesions, and areas of denuded epithelium or skin at risk by evidence of a positive Nikolsky sign. This sign is induced by pushing a finger tangentially over involved skin and is positive if the epidermis detaches or sloughs with that frictional traction. The presence of any of the following are cause for concern for a more severe cutaneous adverse reaction: mucous membrane erosions, blisters or Nikolsky sign, confluent erythema, angioedema and tongue swelling, palpable purpura, skin necrosis, lymphadenopathy, fever, or hypotension.[14]

The ultimate goal is to identify and discontinue the offending medication if possible. Common causes of exanthematous morbilliform drug eruptions include antibiotics such as aminopenicillins, sulfonamides, and cephalosporins, although there are numerous culprits reported for this most common eruption. The most common attributable medications for the most severe drug eruptions such as SJS/TEN are sulfonamides, anticonvulsants, allopurinol, lamotrigine, and NSAIDs.

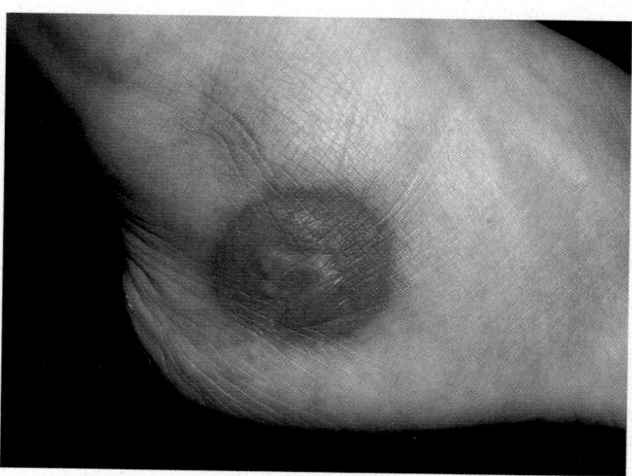

FIGURE 212-21 Bullous fixed drug eruption with a dusky color and an annular pink border on the ankle. (*Reproduced with permission from Richard P. Usatine, MD.*)

LABORATORY STUDIES

The diagnosis of drug eruptions is usually made based on history and physical examination, and with mild asymptomatic eruptions this is sufficient.

- Evaluation of suspected severe cutaneous drug reactions, however, should include a complete blood count (CBC) with differential (to assess for eosinophilia or atypical lymphocytes) and comprehensive serum chemistry panel to look for systemic involvement such as liver and kidney effects or other organs involved with DRESS. Urinalysis for protein or microscopic hematuria should also be included when vasculitis is suspected. Other serologies such as antinuclear antibodies (ANAs) can be considered with specific entities.
- Laboratory tests in patients with DRESS/DIHS may show atypical lymphocytes, eosinophilia, lymphocytopenia, and thrombocytopenia; and liver abnormalities are often seen. Eosinophilia may be seen with both AGEP and DRESS, but its absence does not exclude a drug-induced cause.[15]
- In more challenging cases or instances of SJS/TEN, a skin biopsy may be helpful to confirm the diagnosis. Immunofluorescence studies may be helpful for evaluation of bullous lesions.
- Intradermal skin testing may be hazardous to patients, and patch tests are not useful.
- Skin biopsies are usually not required for diagnosis of WISN, but may aid in the diagnosis.
- An FDE may be diagnosed by "provoking" the appearance of the lesion with an oral rechallenge with the suspected drug; however, this can be dangerous in bullous cases. Repeat drug challenge would also not be safe with angioedema, anaphylaxis, and suspected cases of SJS/TEN. Drug desensitization or induction of drug tolerance can be considered if no suitable alternative agent exists.[15]

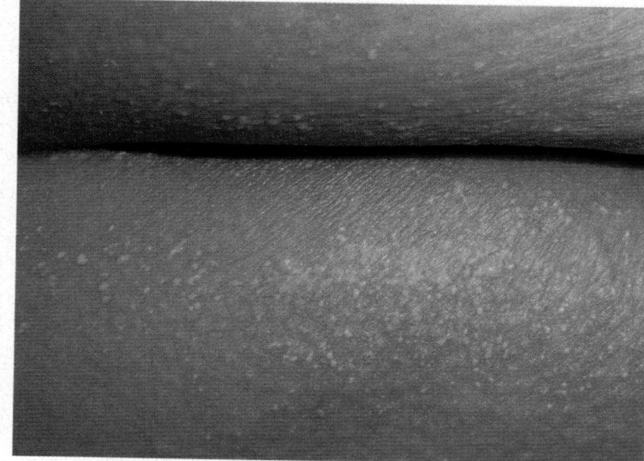

FIGURE 212-22 Acute generalized exanthematous pustulosis (AGEP) caused by a drug eruption. The clusters of small pustules with erythematous skin are seen on the buttocks. In this case the pustules and erythema covered major portions of the back and buttocks. (*Reproduced with permission from Robert T. Gilson, MD.*)

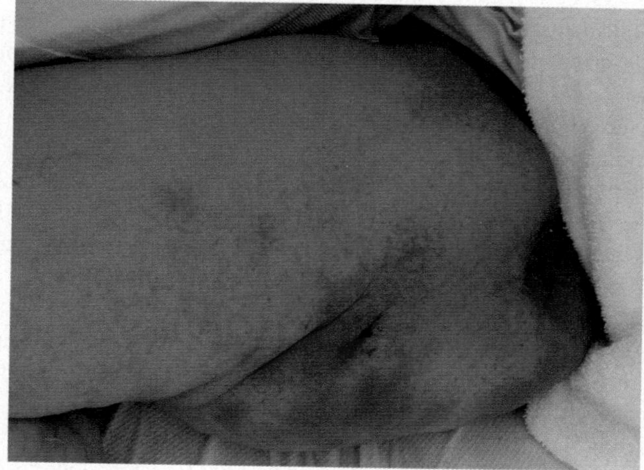

FIGURE 212-23 Systemic drug-related intertriginous and flexural exanthema. Because the pattern of erythema creates red buttocks, it may also be called the baboon syndrome. (*Reproduced with permission from Robert T. Gilson, MD.*)

TABLE 212-1 Types of Drug Eruptions*

Drug Eruption Type	Typical Time Interval	Commonly Responsible Drugs
Exanthematous eruption	4–14 days	Aminopenicillins Sulfonamides Cephalosporins Anticonvulsants Allopurinol Abacavir Nevirapine
Urticaria	Minutes to hours	Penicillins Cephalosporins NSAIDs Monoclonal antibodies X-ray contrast media
Fixed drug eruption	First exposure: 1–2 weeks Re-exposure: 1–2 days, usually within 24 hours	TMP-SMX NSAIDs Tetracyclines Pseudoephedrine
Acute generalized exanthematous pustulosis (AGEP)	<4 days	β-Lactam antibiotics Macrolides Calcium channel blockers
Stevens–Johnson syndrome/toxic epidermal necrolysis	7–21 days	Sulfonamides Anticonvulsants Lamotrigine Allopurinol NSAIDs NNRTIs Minocycline Nevirapine
Drug reaction with eosinophilia and systemic symptoms (DRESS)/ drug-induced hypersensitivity syndrome (DIHS)	15–40 days	Anticonvulsants Lamotrigine Sulfonamides Abacavir Allopurinol Dapsone

Abbreviations: NSAIDs, nonsteroidal anti-inflammatory drugs; TMP-SMX, trimethoprim-sulfamethoxazole; NNRTIs, non-nucleoside reverse-transcriptase inhibitors.
*Data from Bolognia JL, Schaffer JV, Cerroni L. Dermatology, 4th ed. Philadelphia, PA: Elsevier; 2018.

DIFFERENTIAL DIAGNOSIS

- Viral exanthems look just like generalized maculopapular drug eruptions. Sometimes when a patient is given an antibiotic for an upper respiratory infection, the rash that ensues may be the viral exanthem rather than a drug eruption. The best way to avoid this confusion is only to use antibiotics when the evidence for bacterial infection is sufficient to justify the risk of a drug reaction.
- Urticarial reactions present as transient migratory circumscribed areas of blanching-raised erythema and edema of the superficial dermis. Patients experience itching. Identifying urticaria is easy compared with finding the precipitating factors. If there is a temporal association with starting a new drug, it is best to stop the drug (in most cases) and see if the urticaria resolves. (See Chapter 156, Urticaria and Angioedema.)
- EM presents with sudden onset of rapidly progressive, symmetric, and cutaneous lesions with centripetal spread. The patient may have a burning sensation in affected areas but usually has no pruritus. EM is most often caused by a reaction to an infection such as HSV or *Mycoplasma pneumoniae* (see **Figures 212-14** and **212-15**) but may be caused by a drug reaction. Careful history and physical examination can help differentiate between the possible causes (see Chapter 185, Erythema Multiforme, Stevens-Johnson Syndrome, and Toxic Epidermal Necrolysis).
- SJS and TEN present with generalized cutaneous lesions with blisters, fever, malaise, arthralgias, headache, sore throat, nausea, vomiting, and diarrhea. The patient may also have difficulty in eating, drinking, or opening his or her mouth secondary to painful, often hemorrhagic crusted erosions of the oral mucous membranes (see **Figure 212-16**) and often have a mucopurulent conjunctivitis. Most cases of SJS or TEN are secondary to drug exposure, and it is

the job of the clinician to investigate this cause and stop any suspicious medications. SJS and TEN can be life-threatening (see Chapter 185, Erythema Multiforme, Stevens-Johnson Syndrome, and Toxic Epidermal Necrolysis).

- DRESS/DIHS (see **Figures 212-17** and **212-18**) can be distinguished by involvement of organs other than skin, including liver (hepatitis in 50% to 70%), kidney (nephritis in 10%), and, more rarely, pneumonitis, colitis, myocarditis, parotitis, meningitis, encephalitis, or pancreatitis; the pattern of organ involvement appears to depend on the drug trigger.[8,9] Some of the sequelae from DRESS/DHIS are strongly related to herpesvirus reactivation.[9] A recurrence of symptoms at the third week is common. Diagnostic criteria have been proposed to include all of the following: maculopapular rash developing more than 3 weeks after drug exposure, prolonged clinical symptoms after drug discontinuation, fever (>38°C [100.4°F]), liver abnormalities or other organ involvement, leukocyte abnormalities (atypical lymphocytosis, leukocytosis, eosinophilia), lymphadenopathy, and human herpesvirus-6 reactivation.[8]
- Pityriasis rosea (PR) is a mysterious eruption of unknown etiology that could easily mimic a maculopapular drug eruption. Look and ask for the herald patch to help make the diagnosis of PR. In PR, look for the collarette scale and observe whether the eruption follows the skin lines (causing a Christmas-tree pattern on the back). These clinical features should help positively identify PR, as there are no laboratory tests that are specific to PR or most drug eruptions (see Chapter 159, Pityriasis Rosea).
- Syphilis is the great imitator. Any generalized rash without a known etiology may be caused by secondary syphilis. A rapid plasma reagin (RPR) will always be positive in secondary syphilis and is easy to run (see Chapter 225, Syphilis).
- Bullous pemphigoid and pemphigus vulgaris can resemble a bullous drug eruption. Biopsies are the best way to diagnose these bullous diseases. Their clinical pictures are described in detail in Chapters 192, Bullous Pemphigoid, and 193, Pemphigus.
- Hematoma is a much more common complication of warfarin therapy and must be distinguished from WISN early to decrease permanent tissue damage; a high index of suspicion is needed, and a very elevated international normalized ratio (INR) will confirm that bleeding may be a result of overcoagulation (see **Figure 212-19**).

MANAGEMENT

NONPHARMACOLOGIC

- Discontinue the offending medication for all types of drug reactions whenever possible. Older patients with drug eruptions may be on multiple medications and may be very ill; however, efforts should be made to discontinue all nonessential medications.[6]
- Hyperpigmentation—Stop the drug if possible. In the case of doxorubicin-induced skin hyperpigmentation, the doxorubicin may be continued if it is the best chemotherapy for a life-threatening malignancy (see **Figure 212-5**).
- Local wound care, debridement, and skin grafting may need to be performed to repair resultant disfigurement from necrosis.

MEDICATIONS

- Treatment of the drug eruption depends on the specific type of reaction.
- Urticarial/angioedema-type drug reactions are treated with antihistamines. If the angioedema is causing airway compromise, epinephrine (10 mcg/kg intramuscular) and other treatments will be necessary. Usually an H_1-blocker is started. In some cases of urticaria/angioedema, an H_2-blocker is added on for broader antihistamine effects (see Chapter 156, Urticaria and Angioedema).
- Diphenhydramine (Benadryl)—Adult dosing is 25 to 50 mg orally every 4 to 6 hours (nonprescription). Hydroxyzine (Atarax)—Adults receive 25 mg orally every 6 hours. Pediatric dose is 0.5 to 1.0 mg/kg per day orally 4 times daily.
- Nonsedating nonprescription antihistamines such as cetirizine (Zyrtec), fexofenadine (Allegra), or loratadine (Claritin) may help reduce the sedation of earlier generation antihistamines. An H_2-blocker can be added if needed.
- Exanthematous or maculopapular eruptions are treated with topical steroids such as triamcinolone, which may be used for symptomatic relief of pruritus.
- FDEs are treated by discontinuing the drug and applying topical corticosteroids to the affected area.[5]
- Oral steroids are first line therapy in DRESS/DHIS, and the course is typically more prolonged.[16]

REFERRAL OR HOSPITALIZATION

Patients with WISN, SJS, TEN, and DRESS/DIHS, are usually hospitalized and those with SJS/TEN ideally referred and managed in a burn center familiar with the intensive skin care needs for this condition ("acute skin failure"). The prognosis for those with TEN is more guarded, with scarring, blindness, and death possible.

- WISN treatment is generally supportive, including discontinuing the warfarin, admission to the hospital, and administration of vitamin K and either protein C concentrate if available or fresh-frozen plasma.[17,18]
- Many clinicians recommend resuming heparin therapy if needed for the patient's underlying pathology that prompted the use of initial anticoagulation therapy.[17,18]
- SJS, TEN, DRESS/DIHS—Start with early diagnosis, rapid discontinuation of the culprit offending agent, admission to an intensive care unit (ICU) or burn unit, preferably where supportive therapy includes wound care, fluid and electrolyte management, nutritional support, temperature management, pain control, and monitoring or treatment of superinfections (see Chapter 185, Erythema Multiforme, Steven-Johnson Syndrome, and Toxic Epidermal Necrolysis).[5,6] Eye involvement merits an ophthalmologic consult, and severe disease may benefit from amniotic membrane transplantation. which, if performed early in the disease course (within 7–10 days), may prevent blindness and scarring. The first-line treatment is controversial but may include intravenous immunoglobulin (IVIG), short-term systemic steroids, cyclosporine, and now tumor necrosis factor (TNF)-α inhibitors.
- Patients are monitored for developing infection, but antibiotics are not used prophylactically and are started only when infection is suspected.[5]

- DRESS/DIH requires longer courses of steroids with slow tapering over months (often for liver or renal involvement), and complications of delayed hypothyroidism must be monitored for. Liver transplant has been used in patients with DRESS.[16]

PREVENTION

- Avoid reexposure to the drug.
- In the future, prevention may occur through screening for HLA associations and drug avoidance.[1]
- Screening for HLA-B*1502 is advised by the U.S. FDA and Health Canada for patients of southeastern Asian ethnicity before carbamazepine therapy.[1]

PROGNOSIS

- Most cutaneous drug reactions resolve with discontinuation of the causative agent.
- Mortality, however, is high at 5% for SJS and 30% to 50% for TEN.[6,19] In a case series of patients with possible or probable DRESS, the case fatality rate was 5% (9 of 172).[7]
- Studies show the occurrence of autoimmune diseases, including autoimmune thyroid disease, months to years after resolution of DIHS/DRESS, and thyroid function should be routinely screened for at least 2 years.[8]

FOLLOW-UP

- Follow-up is most important when the case is severe or the diagnosis is uncertain. Clear-cut mild drug reactions may not need scheduled follow-up.
- Continued surveillance for autoimmune disorders may be warranted in patients following DRESS/DHIS.

PATIENT EDUCATION

- Most patients with drug eruptions recover fully without any complications. The patient should be warned that even after the responsible medication is stopped, the eruptions may clear slowly or even worsen at first; the patient should be advised that the reaction may not resolve for 1 to 2 weeks.
- The patient should also be counseled that mild desquamation is normal as the exanthematous eruption resolves. Confirming the diagnosis of an FDE, especially for lesions presenting on the glans, may allay the patient's anxiety about the venereal origin of the disease.
- The family should be counseled as to the genetic predisposition of some drug-induced eruptions.
- If a severe ADR, the patient should be advised to enroll in a medical alert program and to wear a bracelet detailing the allergy.

PATIENT RESOURCES

- MedlinePlus. *Drug Reactions*—**https://medlineplus.gov/drugreactions.html.**
- Mayo Clinic. *Drug Allergy.* **https://www.mayoclinic.org/diseases-conditions/drug-allergy/symptoms-causes/syc-20371835.**

PROVIDER RESOURCES

- Medscape. *Drug Eruptions: Practice Essentials* (updated June 29, 2018)—**https://emedicine.medscape.com/article/1049474-overview.**
- DermNet New Zealand. *Drug Eruptions* (updated January 2016)—**https://www.dermnetnz.org/topics/drug-eruptions/.**
- Drug eruptions: Medical information about drug eruptions—**https://patient.info/doctor/drug-allergy-pro.**
- Litt's Drug Eruption and Reaction Database—**http://www.drugeruptiondata.com.** Electronic access subscription required, continually updated.
- If the skin eruption is rare, serious, or unexpected, the drug reaction should be reported to the manufacturer and to the FDA by telephone at 1-800-FDA-1088, or it can be done online.

REFERENCES

1. Sánchez-Borges M. NSAID hypersensitivity (respiratory, cutaneous, and generalized anaphylactic symptoms). *Med Clin North Am.* 2010;94(4):853-864.
2. Pichler WJ, Adam J, Daubner B, et al. Drug hypersensitivity reactions: pathomechanism and clinical symptoms. *Med Clin North Am.* 2010;94(4):645-664.
3. Phillips EJ, Chung WH, Mockenhaupt M, et al. Drug hypersensitivity: pharmacogenetics and clinical syndromes. *J Allergy Clin Immunol.* 2011;127(3 Suppl):S60-S66.
4. Swanson L, Colven RM. Approach to the patient with a suspected cutaneous adverse drug reaction. *Med Clin North Am.* 2015;99(6):1337-1348.
5. Nigen S, Knowles SR, Shear NH. Drug eruptions: approaching the diagnosis of drug-induced skin diseases. *J Drugs Dermatol.* 2003;2(3):278-299.
6. Bachot N, Roujeau JC. Differential diagnosis of severe cutaneous drug eruptions. *Am J Clin Dermatol.* 2003;4:561-572.
7. Cacoub P, Musette P, Descamps V, et al. The DRESS syndrome: a literature review. *Am J Med.* 2011;124(7):588-597.
8. Husain Z, Reddy BY, Schwartz RA. DRESS syndrome: part I. Clinical perspectives. *J Am Acad Dermatol.* 2013;68(5):693.e1-e14.
9. Kano Y, Ishida T, Kazuhisa K, Shiohara T. Visceral involvements and long-term sequelae in drug-induced hypersensitivity syndrome. *Med Clin North Am.* 2010;94(4):743-759.
10. Fernando SL, Broadfoot J. Prevention of severe cutaneous adverse drug reactions: the emerging value of pharmacogenetic screening. *CMAJ.* 2010;182(5):476-480.

11. Scherer K, Bircher AJ. Danger signs in drug hypersensitivity. *Med Clin North Am.* 2010;94(4):681-689.

12. Bolognia J, Jorizzo JL, Schaffer JV. *Dermatology,* 3rd ed. Philadelphia, PA: Elsevier Saunders; 2012:325-338.

13. Chung WH, Wang CW, Dao RL. Severe cutaneous adverse drug reactions. *J Dermatol.* 2016;43(7):758-766.

14. Drug eruptions. https://emedicine.medscape.com/article/1049474-overview. Accessed January 2018.

15. Khan DA, Solensky R. Drug allergy. *J Allergy Clin Immunol.* 2010; 125(2 Suppl 2):S126-S137.

16. Husain Z, Reddy BY, Schwartz RA. DRESS syndrome: Part II. Management and therapeutics. *J Am Acad Dermatol.* 2013;68(5):709.

17. Alves DW, Chen IA. Warfarin-induced skin necrosis. *Hosp Physician.* 2002;38(8):39-42.

18. Stewart AJ, Penman ID, Cook MK, Ludlam CA. Warfarin-induced skin necrosis. *Postgrad Med J.* 1999;75:233-235.

19. Mockenhaupt M, Norgauer J. Cutaneous adverse drug reactions: Stevens-Johnson syndrome and toxic epidermal necrolysis. *Allergy Clin Immunol Int.* 2002;14:143-150.

213 KELOIDS

E.J. Mayeaux, Jr., MD
Jacqueline Bucher, MD
Alexis Rae Tracy, MD
Richard P. Usatine, MD

PATIENT STORY

A 64-year-old black woman presents to the office with itching keloids on her chest (**Figure 213-1**). The horizontal keloid started during childhood when she was scratched by a branch of a tree. The vertical keloid is the result of bypass surgery 1 year ago. The lower portion of this area could be called a hypertrophic scar, as it does not advance beyond the borders of the original surgery. The patient was happy to receive intralesional steroids to decrease her symptoms. Intralesional triamcinolone did, in fact, decrease the itching and flatten the vertical keloid.

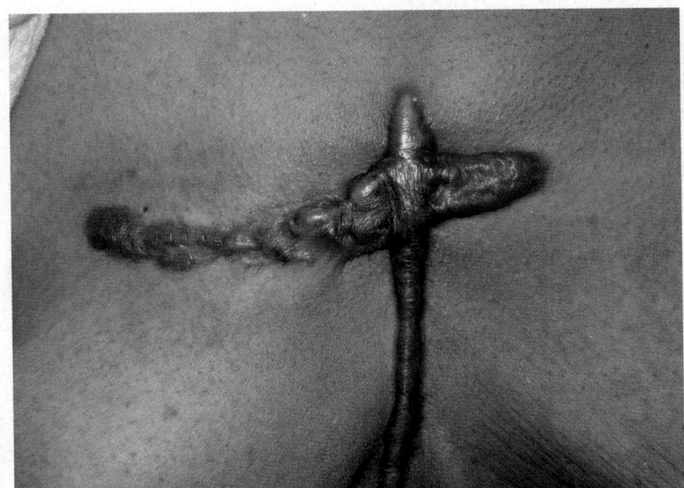

FIGURE 213-1 Two keloids that cross the chest of a 64-year-old black woman. The horizontal keloid came from a scratch during childhood, and the vertical keloid is a result of open-heart surgery. *(Reproduced with permission from Richard P. Usatine, MD.)*

INTRODUCTION

Keloids are benign dermal fibroproliferative tumors that form in scar secondary to altered wound healing. Keloids are characterized by their nature of extending beyond the original area of injury. They form as a result of overproduction of extracellular matrix and dermal fibroblasts that have a high mitotic rate.

EPIDEMIOLOGY

- Individuals with darker pigmentation are more likely to develop keloids. Sixteen percent of black persons reported having keloids in a random sampling.[1]
- Men and women are generally affected equally, except that keloids are more common in young adult women—probably secondary to a higher rate of piercing the ears (**Figure 213-2**).[2]
- There is evidence for a family tendency in developing keloids; studies thus far have suggested autosomal dominance with incomplete penetrance.[3]
- Rare in extremes of age; highest incidence is in individuals ages 10 to 20 years.[2,4]

ETIOLOGY AND PATHOPHYSIOLOGY

- Keloids are dermal fibrotic lesions that are a variation of the normal wound-healing process in the spectrum of fibroproliferative disorders.
- Keloids are more likely to develop in areas of the body that are subjected to high skin tension such as over the sternum (see **Figure 213-1**).
- May occur up to a year after the injury and will enlarge beyond the scar margin. Burns and other injuries can heal with a keloid in just one portion of the area injured (**Figure 213-3**).

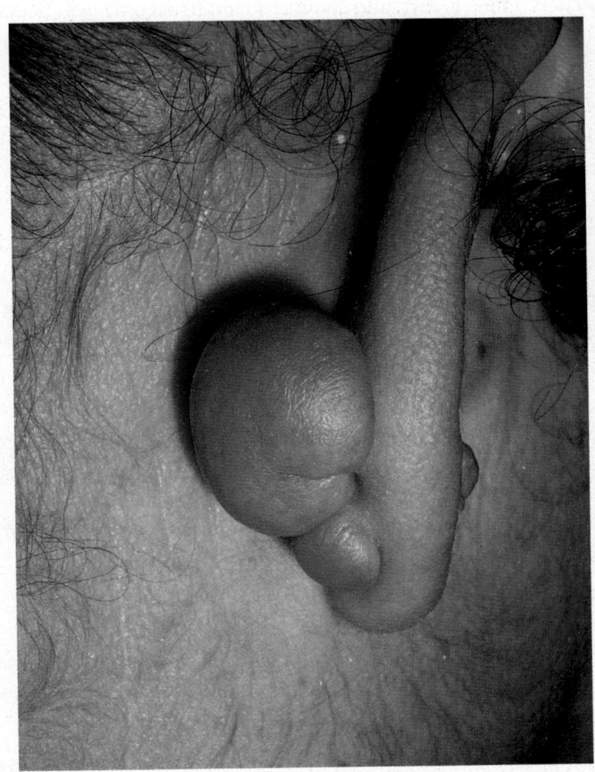

FIGURE 213-2 A keloid on the earlobe that started from piercing the ear. *(Reproduced with permission from Richard P. Usatine, MD.)*

- Wounds subjected to prolonged inflammation (acne cysts) are more likely to develop keloids.

RISK FACTORS[3]

- Darker skin pigmentation (African, Hispanic, or Asian ethnicity).
- A family history of keloids.
- Wound healing by secondary intention.
- Wounds subjected to prolonged inflammation.
- Sites of repeated trauma.
- Pregnancy.
- Body piercings (**Figure 213-4**).

DIAGNOSIS

CLINICAL FEATURES

- Some keloids present with pruritic pain or a burning sensation around the scar.
- Initially manifest as erythematous lesions devoid of hair follicles or other glandular tissue.
- Papules to nodules to large tuberous lesions (**Figure 213-5**).
- Range in consistency from soft and doughy to rubbery and hard. Most often, the lesions are the color of normal skin but can become brownish red or bluish and then pale as they age.[5]
- May extend in a clawlike fashion far beyond any slight injury.
- Lesions on neck, ears, and abdomen tend to become pedunculated.

TYPICAL DISTRIBUTION

- Most frequently found on anterior chest, shoulders, flexor surfaces of extremities, anterior neck, earlobes, and wounds that cross skin tension lines.

LABORATORY TESTING

- Biopsy is rarely needed to make a diagnosis because the clinical appearance is usually distinctive and clear. However, if the diagnosis is uncertain, a skin biopsy is beneficial in excluding potentially serious conditions that mimic keloids.

DIFFERENTIAL DIAGNOSIS

- Hypertrophic scars, unlike keloids, are confined to the site of original injury.
- Acne keloidalis nuchae is an inflammatory disorder around hair follicles of the posterior neck that results in keloidal scarring (**Figure 213-6**). Although the scarring is similar to keloids, the location and pathophysiology are unique. This process can also cause alopecia (Chapter 120, Pseudofolliculitis and Acne Keloidalis Nuchae).
- Dermatofibromas are common button-like dermal nodules usually found on the legs or arms. They may umbilicate when the surrounding skin is pinched. These often have a hyperpigmented halo

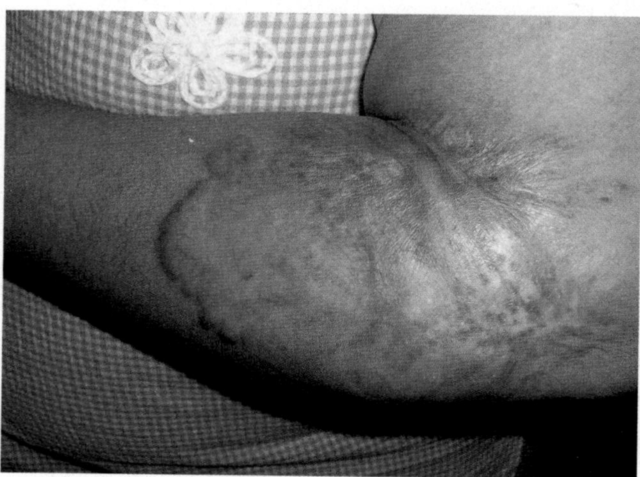

FIGURE 213-3 A keloid on the arm of a Hispanic woman burned accidentally by a hot iron at the age of 1 year. Most of the burn scar is not a keloid. The keloid is at the distal edge where the skin is raised nodular and pink. She has pruritus in that area. (*Reproduced with permission from Richard P. Usatine, MD.*)

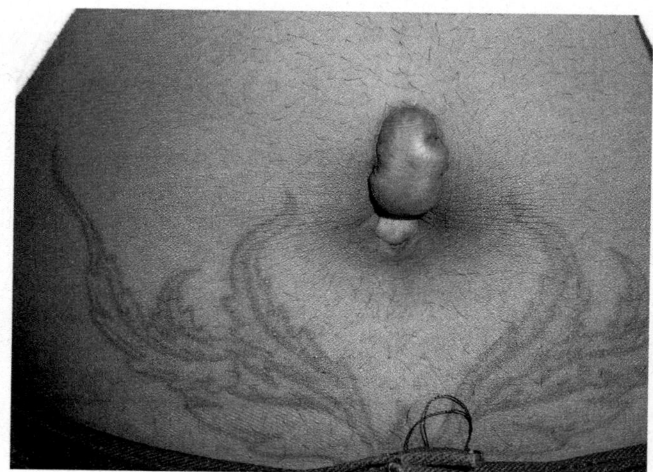

FIGURE 213-4 This keloid formed at the site of a belly button piercing in this young woman. (*Reproduced with permission from Richard P. Usatine, MD.*)

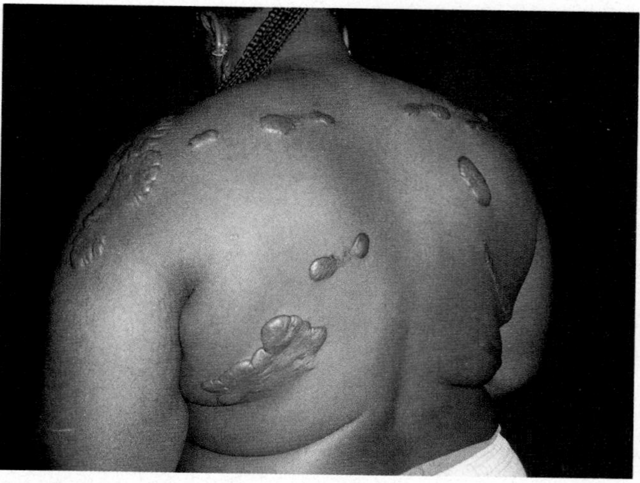

FIGURE 213-5 Many keloids in a woman who develops keloids with even the most minor skin injuries. (*Reproduced with permission from Richard P. Usatine, MD.*)

around them and are less elevated than keloids (Chapter 166, Dermatofibroma).

- Dermatofibrosarcoma protuberans is a rare, malignant version of the dermatofibroma. It usually presents as an atrophic, scarlike lesion developing into an enlarging firm and irregular nodular mass. If this is suspected, a biopsy is needed (Chapter 166, Dermatofibroma).
- Nodular scleroderma is a rare form of scleroderma, resulting in an excessive fibrosing reaction leading to formation of keloidal nodules.[6]

MANAGEMENT

- Numerous therapies are available; however, initially prevention and patient education is key.
- Management cannot be standardized because of variability in formation and presentation: location, age, type, ethnic/genetic predisposition. As no single modality is vastly superior or universally efficacious, combination therapies have led to the best success rates.[7]
- Patients frequently want keloids treated because of symptoms (i.e. pain, pruritus) and cosmetic appearance.
- A 2006 systematic review of 396 studies and an accompanying meta-analysis of 36 articles concluded that no optimal evidence-based therapy exists and recommended choosing treatment based on cost and adverse effect profile.[8]

FIRST LINE

- Intralesional corticosteroids, cryotherapy, intralesional 5-fluorouracil (5-FU).[7] SOR B
- Intralesional triamcinolone acetonide (10–40 mg/mL) significantly reduced the size and erythema of keloids compared to untreated controls. There was no statistically significant difference in pain or itch compared to controls. Treatment is typically repeated at 4- to 6-week intervals. There is no optimal number of treatments, and limited data on injection volume and keloid size (**Figure 213-7**). Intralesional triamcinolone was more effective in improving scar than silicone gel sheet, verapamil, or cryotherapy.[8] SOR A
- Intralesional triamcinolone acetonide in combination with 5-FU was more effective than intralesional triamcinolone acetonide 10 mg/mL alone. Combination treatment was not superior to intralesional triamcinolone acetonide alone when a higher concentration of 20 mg/mL was employed. To achieve keloid resolution, intralesional triamcinolone acetonide at high concentration (40 mg/mL) is recommended for monotherapy.[8] SOR B
- In a controlled study, 10 patients with 28 keloids were treated with cryotherapy alone, steroid injection alone, or cryotherapy combined with steroid injection. At 8-month follow-up, combination therapy had significantly better results with no keloid recurrence noted in this group.[9] SOR B The lesion is initially frozen with liquid nitrogen spray and allowed to thaw. Then it is injected with triamcinolone acetate (10 to 40 mg/mL). It is not necessary to freeze a margin of normal tissue.
- Cryotherapy alone was performed on 135 patients with a total of 166 keloids; 79.5% responded well with a volume reduction of 80% or more after three treatments.[10] SOR B

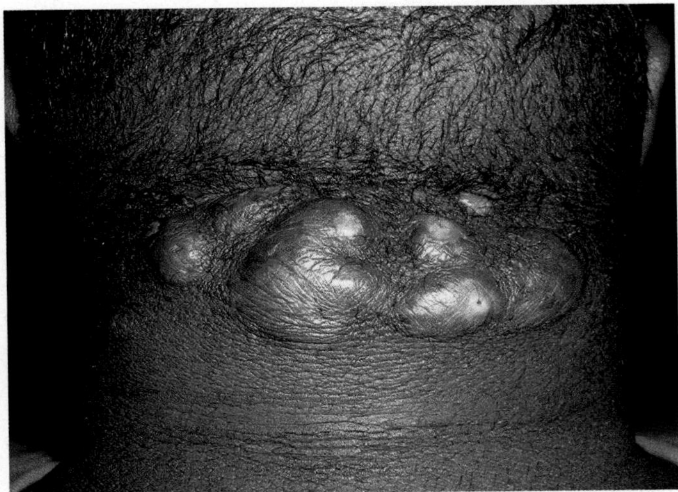

FIGURE 213-6 Acne keloidalis nuchae on the posterior neck of this young African-American man. (*Reproduced with permission from Richard P. Usatine, MD.*)

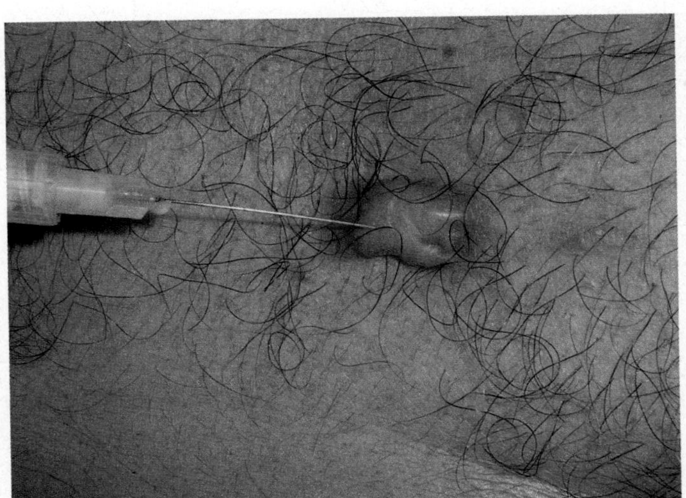

FIGURE 213-7 Triamcinolone injected into this symptomatic keloid on the chest. Note how the keloid is blanching white, demonstrating that the steroid is properly injected into the body of the keloid. A Luer-Lok syringe is used to avoid the needle popping off during the injection under pressure, and a 27-gauge needle is used to minimize patient discomfort. (*Reproduced with permission from Richard P. Usatine, MD.*)

SECOND LINE

- Intralesional interferon-α 2b (SOR Ⓑ), silicon gel sheeting (SOR Ⓑ), radiation (SOR Ⓑ), and laser therapy.[7]
- Intralesional verapamil 2.5 mg/mL, bleomycin 1.5 IU/mL, and interferon-α 2b injections 1.5 million IU twice daily for 4 days are less-studied alternatives to corticosteroid treatment.[4] SOR Ⓒ
- Superior results were seen in 19 patients treated with combined triamcinolone acetonide intralesional injection and interferon-α 2b therapy, with greater than 80% improvement in lesion depth and volume in most patients.[11] SOR Ⓑ
- Postoperative radiotherapy is an effective management for keloids; comparison revealed the lowest recurrence rate with brachytherapy (15%), versus X-ray and electron beam (23% and 23%, respectively).[12] SOR Ⓑ
- Silicone gel sheeting for treatment of hypertrophic and keloid scarring is supported by poor-quality trials susceptible to bias. There is only weak evidence of a benefit of silicone gel sheeting as prevention for abnormal scarring in high-risk individuals.[13] SOR Ⓑ
- Laser therapy with the 585/595-nm pulsed-dye laser and 532-nm laser may result in decreased size and erythema of hypertrophic scars; however, level of evidence for treatment of keloid scars is low.[14] SOR Ⓑ
- Laser and light-based treatment of keloids using CO_2, light-emitting diode (LED) phototherapy, or photodynamic therapy (PDT) may result in favorable patient outcomes; however, conclusions on efficacy cannot be made because of the scarcity of adequate studies.[15] SOR Ⓑ

COMPLEMENTARY AND ALTERNATIVE THERAPY

- There is limited clinical evidence to support efficacy of topical treatments including imiquimod, mitomycin C, and plant extracts such as onion extract, green tea, and aloe vera, as well as vitamins E and D, applied to healing wounds, mature scar tissue, or fibrotic scars following revision surgery, or in combination with other more established treatments such as steroid injections.[16] SOR Ⓑ

SURGICAL

- Earlobe keloids can be surgically excised with a shave or excisional technique and then injected with triamcinolone acetate (10 to 40 mg/mL) after hemostasis is obtained. The triamcinolone injection can be repeated in 1 month to decrease the chance of recurrence.[17] It is hard to get much volume of steroid into the base of these keloids, so 40 mg/mL triamcinolone is preferred as the concentration for injection after excision. SOR Ⓒ
- According to one article, simple excision of earlobe keloids can result in recurrence rates approaching 80%.[18] However, in clinical experience, keloids on the upper ear can be excised and the skin closed with sutures (**Figure 213-8**). SOR Ⓒ

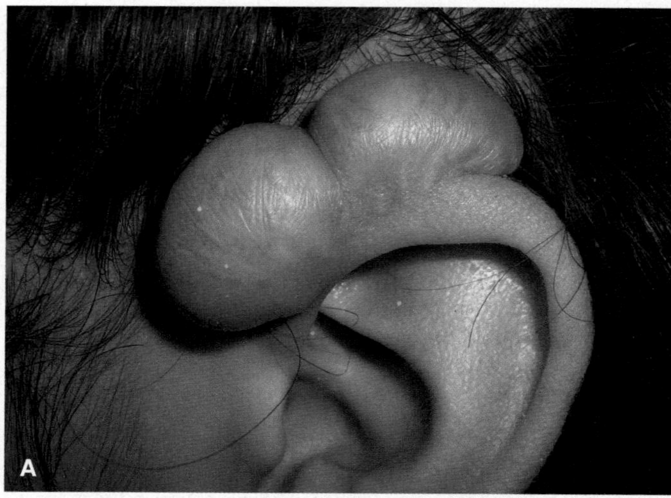

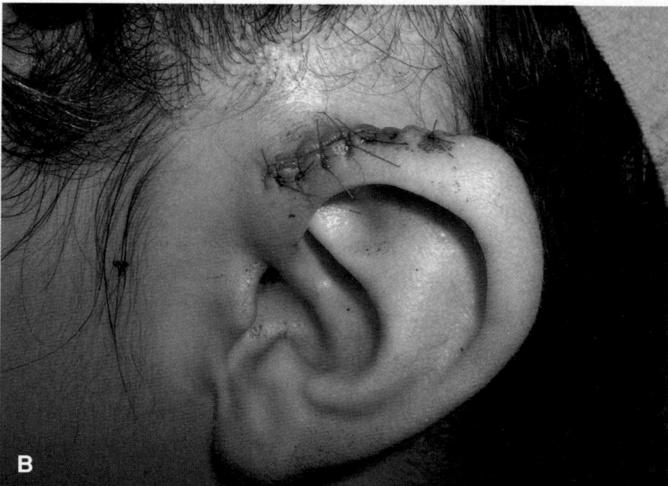

FIGURE 213-8 **A.** A large keloid has been present on the upper ear of this 14-year-old boy for more than 2 years, since he experienced trauma to this area. **B.** The keloid was excised in the office with local anesthetic and the defect sutured using 5-0 Prolene. The cosmetic result was excellent. (*Reproduced with permission from Richard P. Usatine, MD.*)

PREVENTION

- Persons prone to keloid formation should avoid piercings, tattoos, and cosmetic surgery.
- Treat skin problems, such as acne, aggressively in predisposed individuals to avoid keloid formation.

PROGNOSIS

- A 2006 systematic review of 396 studies and an accompanying meta-analysis of 36 articles concluded that any treatment gave patients an overall 70% (95% confidence interval, 49% to 91%) chance of improvement.[19]

FOLLOW-UP

- Follow-up is based on the chosen treatment. Follow-up for intralesional steroid injections is usually in 1 month.

PATIENT EDUCATION

- Advise patients to avoid local skin trauma, for example, ear piercing, body piercing, and tattoos, and to control inflammatory acne.

PATIENT RESOURCES

- MedlinePlus. *Keloids*—**https://medlineplus.gov/ency/article/000849.htm.**
- Skinsight. *Keloid Information for Adults*—**https://www.skinsight.com/skin-conditions/adult/keloid.**

PROVIDER RESOURCES

- Medscape. *Keloid and Hypertrophic Scar* (Dermatology)—**http://emedicine.medscape.com/article/1057599.**
- Medscape. *Keloids* Video on intralesional injections by Dr. Usatine—**https://www.youtube.com/watch?v=OKZCjptD_Eg.**
- Usatine R, Pfenninger J, Stulberg D, Small R. *Dermatologic and Cosmetic Procedures in Office Practice.* Philadelphia, PA: Elsevier; 2012. Available as a text with DVD or electronic application. Contains details, photographs, and videos on how to use cryosurgery and intralesional injections to treat keloids—**https://usatinemedia.com/app/dermatologic-and-cosmetic-procedures-in-office-practice/.**

REFERENCES

1. Chike-Obi CJ, Cole PD, Brissett AE. Keloids: pathogenesis, clinical features, and management. *Semin Plast Surg.* 2009;23:178-184.
2. Alhady SM, Sivanantharajah K. Keloids in various races. A review of 175 cases. *Plast Reconstr Surg.* 1969;44(6):564-566.
3. Brown JJ, Bayat A. Genetic susceptibility to raised dermal scarring. *Br J Dermatol.* 2009;161:8-18.
4. Juckett G, Hartman-Adams H. Management of keloids and hypertrophic scars. *Am Fam Physician.* 2009;80(3):253-260.
5. Urioste SS, Arndt KA, Dover JS. Keloids and hypertrophic scars: review and treatment strategies. *Semin Cutan Med Surg.* 1999;18:159-171.
6. Stadler B, Somacal APB, Weingraber A. Systemic sclerosis with keloidal nodules. *An Bras Dermatol.* 2013;88(6):75-77.
7. Lebwohl M, Heymann W, Berth-Jones J, Coulson I. *Treatment of Skin Disease. [Electronic Resource]: Comprehensive Therapeutic Strategies* [e-book]. Edinburgh, UK: Saunders; 2013.
8. Wong TS, Li JZ, Chen S. The efficacy of triamcinolone acetonide in keloid treatment: a systematic review and meta-analysis. *Front Med (Lausanne).* 2016;3:71.
9. Yosipovitch G, Widijanti MS, Goon A. A comparison of the combined effect of cryotherapy and corticosteroid injections versus corticosteroids and cryotherapy alone on keloids: a controlled study. *J Dermatol Treat.* 2001;12:87-90.
10. Rusciani L, Paradisi A, Alfano C. Cryotherapy in the treatment of keloids. *J Drugs Dermatol.* 2006;5:591-595.
11. Lee JH, Kim SE, Lee A-Y. Effects of interferon-α 2b on keloid treatment with triamcinolone acetonide intralesional injection. *Int J Dermatol.* 2008;47:183-186.
12. Mankowski P, Kanevsky J, Tomilson J. Optimizing radiotherapy for keloids: a meta-analysis systematic review comparing recurrence rates between different radiation modalities. *Ann Plast Surg.* 2017;78(4):403-411.
13. O'Brien L, Jones DJ. Silicone gel sheeting for preventing and treating hypertrophic and keloid scars. *Cochrane Database Syst Rev.* 2013;(9):CD003826.
14. Jin R, Huang X, Li H. Laser therapy for prevention and treatment of pathologic excessive scars. *Plast Reconstr Surg.* 2013;132(6):1747-1758.
15. Mamalis AD, Lev-Tov H, Nguyen DH. Laser and light-based treatment of keloids—a review. *J Eur Acad Dermatol Venereol.* 2014;28(6):689-699.
16. Sidgwick GP, McGeorge D, Bayat A. A comprehensive evidence-based review on the role of topicals and dressings in the management of skin scarring. *Arch Dermatol Res.* 2015;307(6):461-477.
17. Williams CC, De Groote S. Clinical inquiry: what treatment is best for hypertrophic scars and keloids? *J Fam Pract.* 2011;60(12):757-758.
18. Darougheh A, Asilian A, Shariati F. Intralesional triamcinolone alone or in combination with 5-fluorouracil for the treatment of keloid and hypertrophic scars. *Clin Exp Dermatol.* 2009;34:219-223.
19. Leventhal D, Furr M, Reiter D. Treatment of keloids and hypertrophic scars: a meta-analysis and review of the literature. *Arch Facial Plast Surg.* 2006;8:362-368.

214 GENODERMATOSES

Michael J. Babcock, MD
Richard P. Usatine, MD

PATIENT STORY

A 45-year-old black man presents with greasy scale over his face and large parts of his chest and back (**Figure 214-1**). A previous biopsy was diagnostic for Darier disease. His mother has the same condition. Other siblings are similarly affected (**Figure 214-2**). The patient has suffered with this condition for his entire life and believes that he has been ostracized from normal social life because of his appearance and body odor. He suffers from depression and has used various substances to treat his pain. Topical steroids provide some help for the itching and scaling, but the patient is looking for a more effective treatment. The cost of oral retinoids is currently prohibitive, but an application has been put in for patient assistance to receive acitretin.

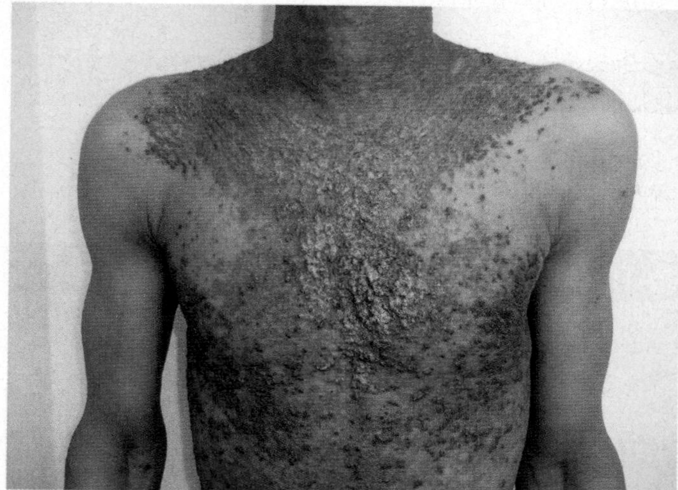

FIGURE 214-1 Darier disease with greasy scales and hyperkeratotic and hyperpigmented papules and plaques in a seborrheic distribution involving the neck and chest. He has similar lesions on the back and scalp and in the groin. Sunlight and heat make his disease worse. *(Reproduced with permission from Richard P. Usatine, MD.)*

INTRODUCTION

There are more than 100 genetic syndromes with cutaneous manifestations that are referred to as genodermatoses. For example, there are disorders of pigmentation (albinism), cornification (the ichthyoses and Darier disease), vascularization (Sturge-Weber syndrome), connective tissue (Ehlers-Danlos syndrome), porphyrin metabolism, other errors of metabolism (phenylketonuria), the immune system (Wiskott-Aldrich syndrome), and DNA repair (ataxia-telangiectasia and xeroderma pigmentosa), to name a few. Some textbooks are dedicated to the topic of genodermatoses alone.[1] This chapter introduces the topic and illustrates a couple of genodermatoses. We have chosen two disorders of cornification as an introduction to the genodermatoses: Darier disease and X-linked ichthyosis.

EPIDEMIOLOGY

- Darier disease (keratosis follicularis)—1:30,000 to 1:100,000. Males and females are equally affected. Clinically becomes apparent near puberty.
- X-linked ichthyosis—1:2000 to 1:6000 males. Clinical lesions present typically during the first 1 to 2 months of life.

ETIOLOGY AND PATHOPHYSIOLOGY

- Darier disease—An abnormal calcium pump in the sarco-/endoplasmic reticulum, SERCA2, results from a gene mutation in the ATP2A2 gene. It is inherited in an autosomal-dominant fashion and results in abnormal epidermal differentiation.
- X-linked ichthyosis—A deletion of the steroid sulfatase gene results in keratinocyte retention by inhibiting degradation of the desmosome. It is inherited in an X-linked recessive manner.

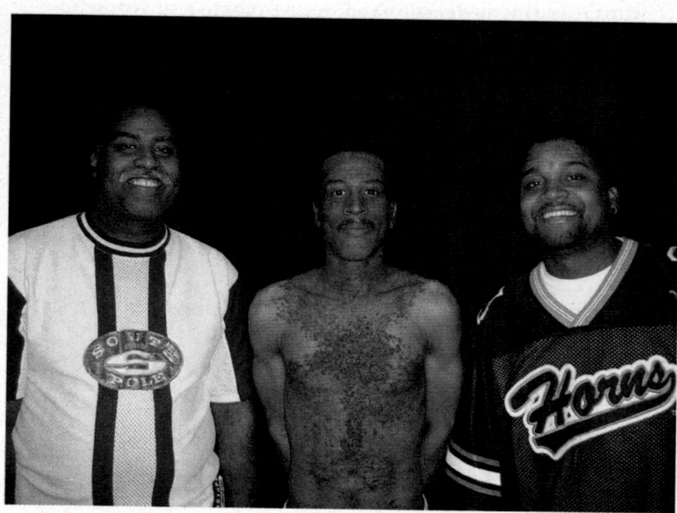

FIGURE 214-2 Darier disease present in three siblings. Their mother also has the disease. *(Reproduced with permission from Richard P. Usatine, MD.)*

DIAGNOSIS

DARIER DISEASE

- Clinical features—Greasy, hyperkeratotic, yellowish-brown papules in a seborrheic distribution (**Figures 214-1** to **214-3**). The feet can be covered with hyperkeratotic plaques. The palms may have pits or keratotic papules, and the nails can have V-shaped nicking and alternating longitudinal red and white bands (**Figure 214-4**). The keratotic papules can be malodorous such that it can interfere with normal social situations.
- Typical distribution—The clinical lesions involve skin in the seborrheic distribution (face, ears, scalp, upper chest, upper back, and groin) (**Figures 214-5** to **214-6**). The axillae and inframammary areas may be involved (**Figure 214-7**). In early, mild, or partially treated disease, only the skin behind the ears may be affected (**Figure 214-8**).[2] The nails are characteristically involved.
- Laboratories—Skin biopsy reveals the characteristic histopathology. A test for the ATP2A2 gene mutation can be performed.

X-LINKED ICHTHYOSIS

- Clinical features—Firm, adherent, fishlike brown scale noted early in the life of young affected boys whose mothers were carriers of the gene on one X chromosome (**Figures 214-9** and **214-10**). These boys have an increased incidence of cryptorchidism and are at an increased risk of testicular cancer, independent of the risk from cryptorchidism alone.[2,3] Often they are delivered by cesarean section because a placental sulfatase deficiency results in failure of labor progression. These patients can have corneal opacities on the Descemet membrane of the posterior capsule, which does not affect their vision.
- Typical distribution—The skin on most of the body is involved, except for the typical sparing of the flexures, face, palms, and soles. The antecubital fossae (see **Figure 214-10**) and popliteal fossae are notably spared (**Figure 214-11**). There is an accentuation noted on the neck, giving these patients a characteristic "dirty neck" appearance (**Figure 214-12**).
- Laboratories—Increased levels of serum cholesterol sulfate levels (steroid sulfatase hydrolyzes cholesterol sulfate). Steroid sulfatase activity can also be measured directly.

DIFFERENTIAL DIAGNOSIS

DARIER DISEASE[4]

- Hailey-Hailey disease (aka benign familial pemphigus)—Another genodermatosis with crusted erosions and flaccid vesicles distributed in the intertriginous areas as opposed to the greasy keratotic papules in the seborrheic distribution (**Figure 214-13**). A 4-mm punch biopsy is adequate to make this diagnosis.
- Grover disease—This presents sporadically as many small, pruritic, erythematous to reddish-brown hyperkeratotic papules on the trunks of older adults. These typically result from conditions that cause sweating or occlusion (such as lying in a hospital bed) (see Chapter 123, Folliculitis).
- Seborrheic dermatitis—Erythematous patches and thin plaques with yellow greasy scale on the scalp, central face, and chest. This is rarely as severe as Darier disease (see Chapter 157, Seborrheic Dermatitis).
- Pachyonychia congenita (**Figure 214-14**).

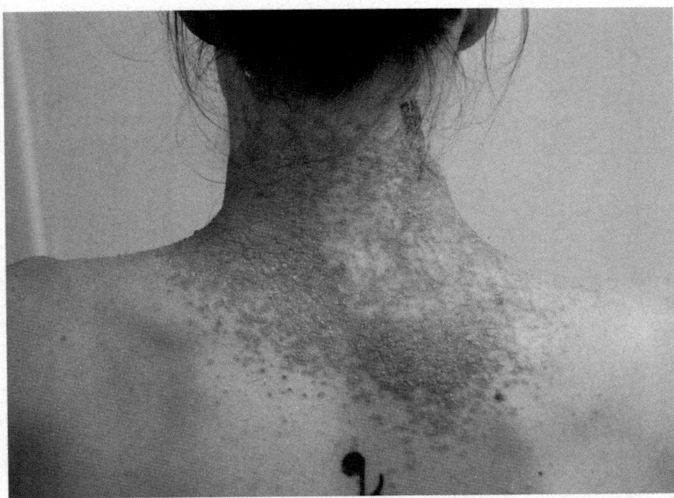

FIGURE 214-3 Darier disease flared up on the posterior neck and upper back. Note the erythema and greasy yellow hyperkeratotic scale in the seborrheic area. *(Reproduced with permission from Yoon Cohen, MD.)*

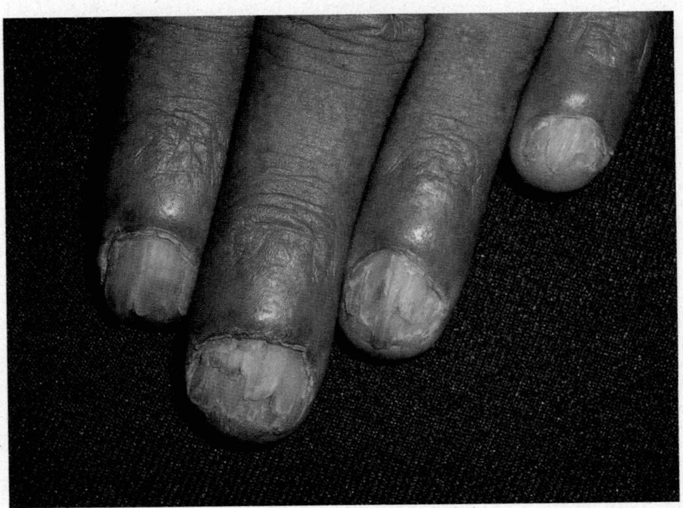

FIGURE 214-4 Typical nail findings in Darier disease showing longitudinal bands and longitudinal splitting. V-shaped nicks at the free margin of the fingernails are the most pathognomonic nail finding in Darier disease. *(Reproduced with permission from Richard P. Usatine, MD.)*

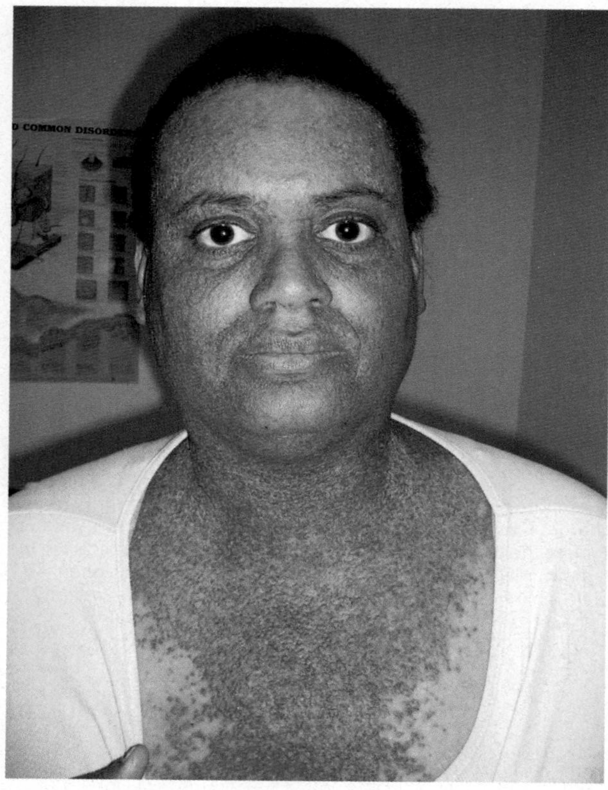

FIGURE 214-5 Darier disease with greasy, hyperkeratotic papules in a seborrheic distribution. She is the sister of the men in **Figure 214-2**. (*Reproduced with permission from Richard P. Usatine, MD.*)

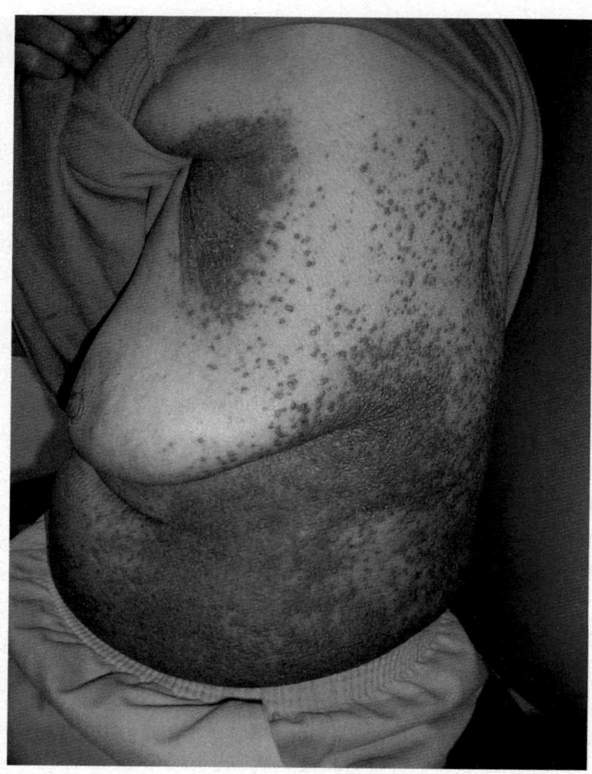

FIGURE 214-7 Darier disease with axillary and inframammary involvement in this 64-year-old woman. (*Reproduced with permission from Richard P. Usatine, MD.*)

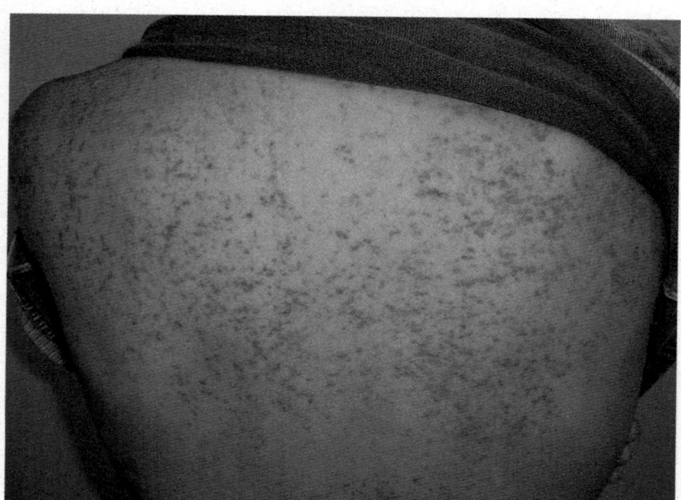

FIGURE 214-6 Darier disease with greasy, hyperkeratotic scaling papules in a seborrheic distribution on the back of a 33-year-old woman. Although this is a genodermatosis, she did not note skin changes until age 30. Her neck and arms are also involved. (*Reproduced with permission from Richard P. Usatine, MD.*)

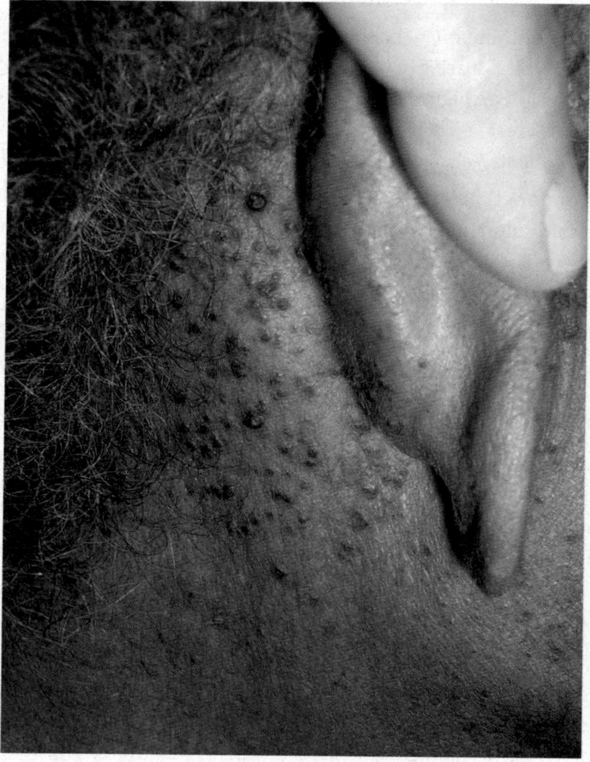

FIGURE 214-8 Darier disease with hyperkeratotic papules behind the ear of this 72-year-old woman. She has a mild case with skin changes only above the neck. (*Reproduced with permission from Richard P. Usatine, MD.*)

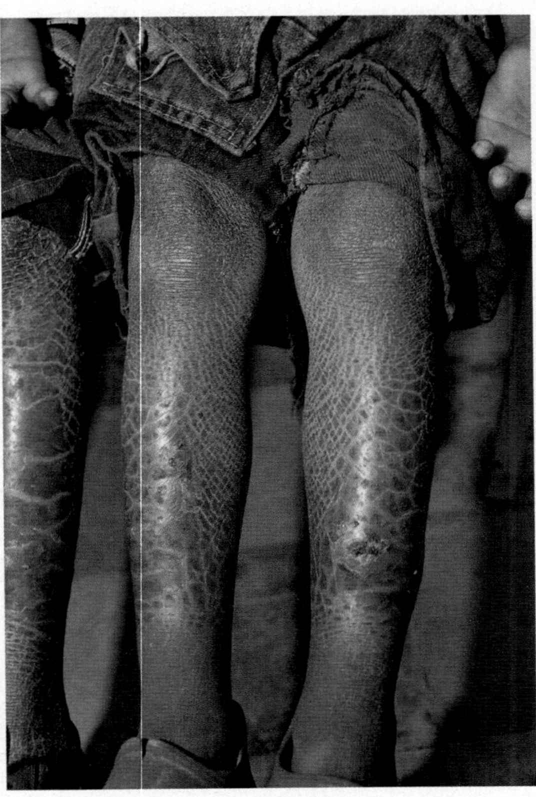

FIGURE 214-9 Heavy fish scale of X-linked ichthyosis on the legs of two affected brothers. (*Reproduced with permission from Richard P. Usatine, MD.*)

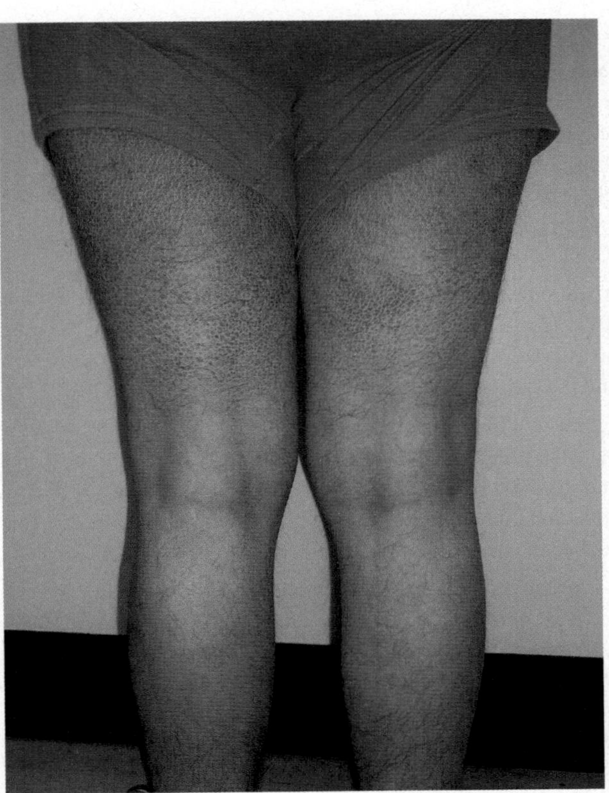

FIGURE 214-11 X-linked ichthyosis in a 17-year-old Hispanic young man showing sparing of the popliteal fossae. (*Reproduced with permission from Richard P. Usatine, MD.*)

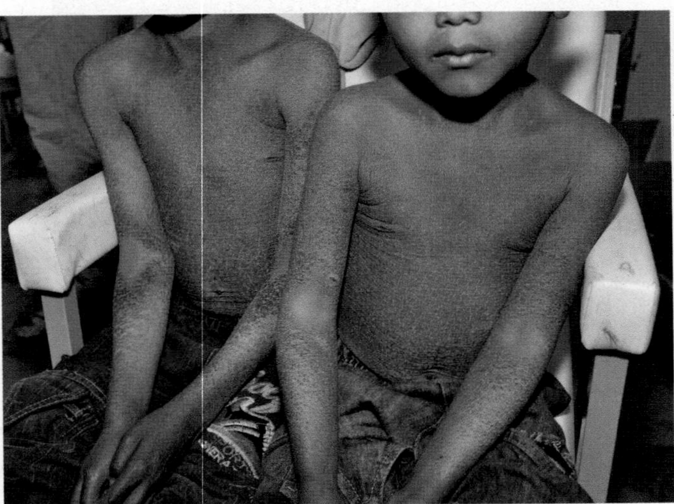

FIGURE 214-10 X-linked ichthyosis in two brothers showing sparing of the antecubital fossae of the arms amidst the heavy scales. (*Reproduced with permission from Richard P. Usatine, MD.*)

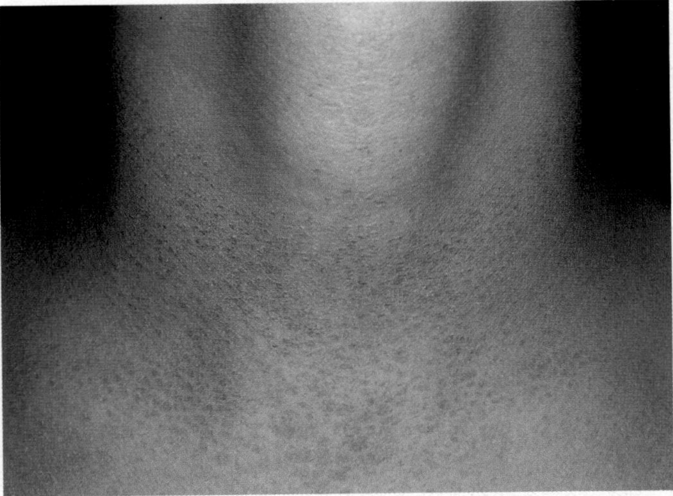

FIGURE 214-12 X-linked ichthyosis in a 13-year-old Hispanic boy showing the dirty-neck appearance. Of course his neck is not dirty—this is merely the hyperkeratosis. (*Reproduced with permission from Richard P. Usatine, MD.*)

X-LINKED ICHTHYOSIS

- Ichthyosis vulgaris—A relatively common condition that is inherited in an autosomal dominant manner (approximately 1 in 250 people affected). It presents in childhood with a fine adherent scale in a distribution similar to that of X-linked ichthyosis (**Figure 214-15**). These patients frequently have hyperlinear palms, keratosis pilaris, and atopic dermatitis, which are not commonly associated with X-linked ichthyosis.
- Acquired ichthyosis does not occur until adulthood. It is not inherited and may be associated with some systemic disease. The time of onset is the key to diagnosis. The legs are often are most involved, and the skin appears similar to fish scales (**Figure 214-16**).
- Lamellar ichthyosis—A more severe and rare disorder that has a platelike scale, which involves most of the body, including the face and flexures (**Figure 214-17**). These patients are typically born as a collodion baby (they have a thin translucent membrane that surrounds the baby at birth).
- Asteatotic eczema—Dry skin that has a "dried riverbed" or "cracked porcelain" appearance, which usually involves the lower extremities. There may be erythema and serous exudate associated with the cracks. It typically presents in the winter, improves during the rest of the year, and is also known as winter itch or eczema craquelé (see Chapter 151, Atopic Dermatitis).
- Xerosis—Dry scaly skin most notably on legs without significant inflammation. This is very common compared with any ichthyosis.

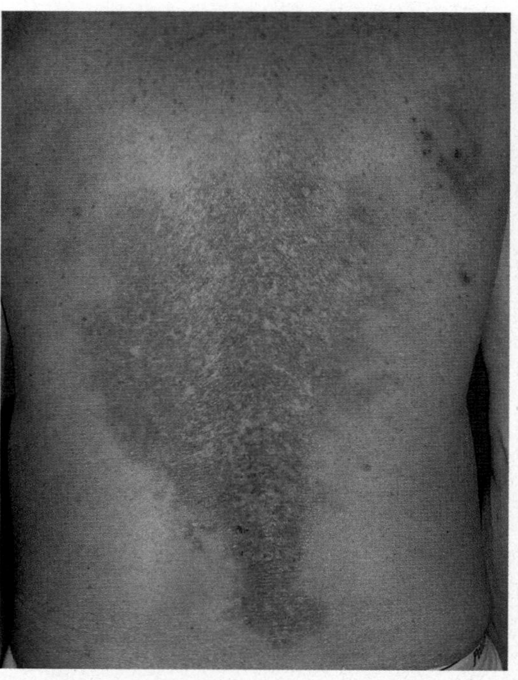

FIGURE 214-13 Hailey-Hailey disease, also known as benign familial pemphigus, on the back of a 54-year-old man. This genodermatosis has a similar appearance to Darier disease and also occurs in a seborrheic distribution. (*Reproduced with permission from Richard P. Usatine, MD.*)

MANAGEMENT

- Darier disease and X-linked ichthyosis are so rare that there are no randomized controlled trials to guide treatment.
- The odor that accompanies the disease, as well as the facial involvement, often adversely affects the patient's quality of life; thus, treatment is often warranted. Mild-to-moderate disease can be treated by avoiding exacerbating factors (sunlight, heat, and occlusion) and with topical medications, SOR Ⓒ but severe disease is best treated with oral retinoids. SOR Ⓒ
- Topical retinoids (adapalene, tretinoin, or tazarotene) are effective in some patients, but their main limitation is irritation. Adapalene gel may be effective in localized variants and is now available over the counter (OTC).[5] SOR Ⓒ All retinoids are contraindicated in pregnancy.
- Topical corticosteroids may be of some help. Lower-potency topical corticosteroids should be used on the face, groin, and axillae to minimize side effects in these areas. SOR Ⓒ
- Topical calcineurin inhibitors (pimecrolimus and tacrolimus) may also be helpful as noted in some case reports.[6,7] SOR Ⓒ These do not have a risk of skin atrophy like steroids, but are generally more expensive and have a controversial black box warning.
- Systemic retinoids (acitretin, alitretinoin, isotretinoin) are the most potent treatment.[8,9] SOR Ⓒ They should only be prescribed by physicians who have experience with these medications. Patients on systemic retinoids require close monitoring and careful selection, as these drugs are teratogenic (category X) and can cause hyperlipidemia, hypertriglyceridemia, mucous

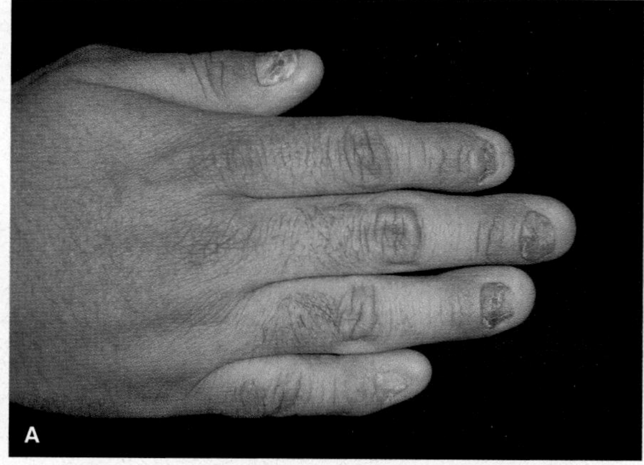

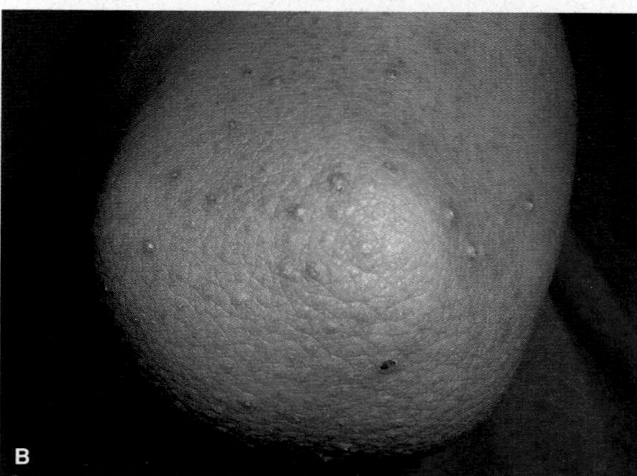

FIGURE 214-14 **A.** Pachyonychia congenita showing the hyperkeratotic nail dystrophy. **B.** He also has hyperkeratotic papules on the elbows, hands, and buttocks. (*Reproduced with permission from Richard P. Usatine, MD.*)

membrane dryness, alopecia, hepatotoxicity, and possible mood disturbances. Females must not get pregnant for at least 1 month after stopping isotretinoin and at least 3 years after stopping acitretin.

- Cyclosporine can be used for acute flares but should also only be prescribed by a physician who has experience with this medication. It should only be used temporarily and requires close follow-up for monitoring hypertension and nephrotoxicity. It is metabolized by the common cytochrome P450 3A4 system and has many medication interactions.
- In one case report, doxycycline 100 mg daily was effective in clearing the skin lesions within 2 weeks and the clearance was maintained for at least 3 months with ongoing daily therapy.[10] SOR Ⓒ
- Topical or oral antibiotics may be necessary for flares, as they often are secondarily infected with bacteria. SOR Ⓒ
- Laser, radiation, photodynamic, and gene therapy are newer treatment modalities that are being investigated.
- X-linked ichthyosis is rare and treatments are based on the clinical experience of experts and small studies.[11]
- In one systematic review of all congenital ichthyoses, topical treatments including 5% urea, 20% propylene glycol alone or in combination with 5% lactic acid, calcipotriol ointment showed therapeutic benefit.[11] SOR Ⓑ
- Frequent application of emollients, humectants, and keratinolytics is the mainstay of therapy. SOR Ⓑ There are many effective nonprescription and prescription products that contain propylene glycol, urea, or lactic acid. Ammonium lactate is affordable and easily available OTC as an emollient with keratolytic activity.
- Calcipotriol is a topical vitamin D preparation that is very expensive and is limited in use by the risk of vitamin D toxicity.[11]
- Topical retinoids can be used, but systemic retinoids are rarely used. SOR Ⓒ
- Refer to a urologist or ophthalmologist if testicular abnormality or corneal opacities are detected. SOR Ⓒ
- Gene therapy has also been studied but has not yet become a viable treatment option.

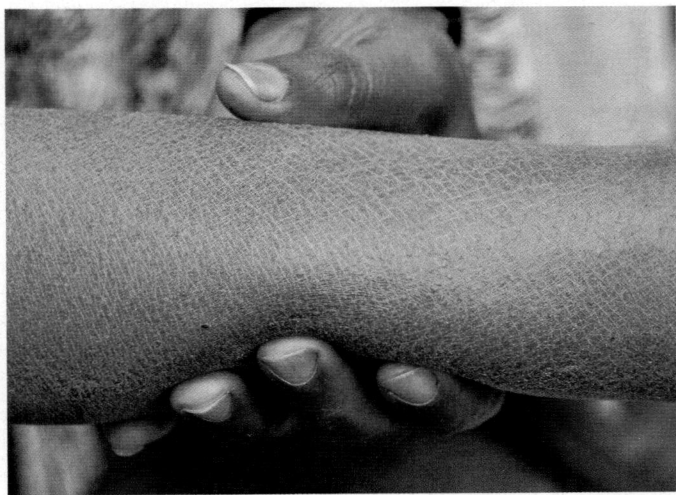

FIGURE 214-15 Ichthyosis vulgaris starts in childhood and has a fine scale. (*Reproduced with permission from Richard P. Usatine, MD.*)

FOLLOW-UP

- Darier disease—Follow-up is needed if patients are on oral retinoids to monitor patients' lipid panel and liver function tests approximately every 3 months. They should also be monitored for signs of secondary bacterial infection.
- X-linked ichthyosis—Monitoring for corneal opacities and for testicular cancer in men should be performed at follow-up visits.

PATIENT EDUCATION

DARIER DISEASE

- Avoid direct sunlight, heat, occlusion, and people acutely infected with herpes simplex virus (HSV) or varicella-zoster virus.
- Watch for signs of secondary cutaneous bacterial or viral infections.

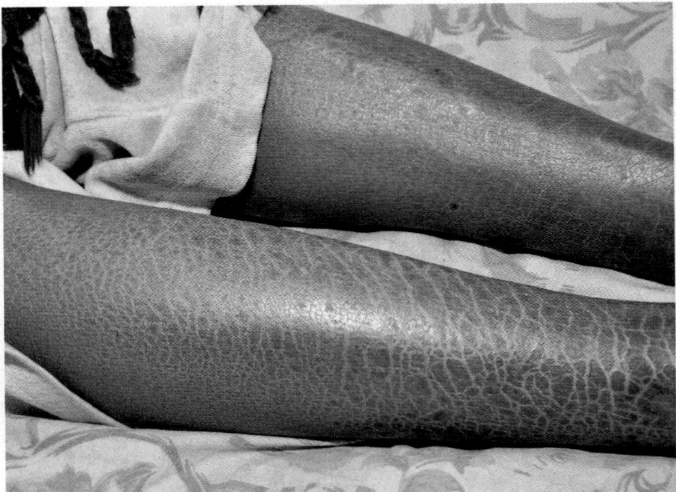

FIGURE 214-16 Acquired ichthyosis starts in adulthood and is especially prominent on the legs. (*Reproduced with permission from Richard P. Usatine, MD.*)

X-LINKED ICHTHYOSIS

- Use daily moisturizers, especially in dry climates and in the winter.

PATIENT RESOURCES

- There are patient advocacy groups for several genetic skin conditions. A quick search online can obtain their websites and contact information.
- The American Academy of Dermatology has a summer camp that is free of charge for children with skin conditions called Camp Discovery. Information can be found at **http://www.campdiscovery.org.**

PROVIDER RESOURCES

- A helpful free online resource for the genodermatoses, or any genetic disease for that matter, is the Online Mendelian Inheritance of Man website at **http://www.omim.org.**
- For information on laboratories that perform rare genetic tests and clinics that perform prenatal diagnostic testing for certain conditions, see **http://www.genetests.org.**
- Skin Advocate is a free application for mobile devices that is provided by the Society of Investigative Dermatology. It lists contact information for various patient advocacy groups.

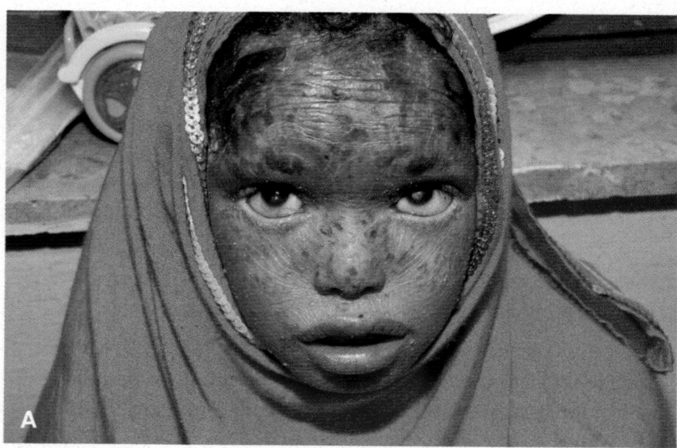

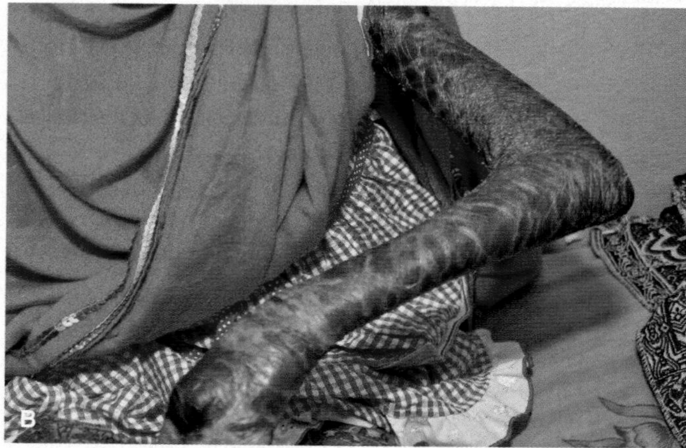

FIGURE 214-17 Lamellar ichthyosis is another genodermatosis that is more rare and severe than X-linked ichthyosis. **A.** Note the deep lines and severe dryness of the skin on the face of this girl with lamellar ichthyosis. **B.** Her arm is severely affected so that she cannot extend her elbow fully. *(Reproduced with permission from Richard P. Usatine, MD.)*

REFERENCES

1. Spitz J. *Genodermatoses: A Clinical Guide to Genetic Skin Disorders*, 2nd ed. Philadelphia, PA: Lippincott Williams & Wilkins; 2005.
2. James W, Berger T, Elston D. *Andrews' Diseases of the Skin: Clinical Dermatology*, 11th ed. Amsterdam, The Netherlands: Elsevier; 2011.
3. Hazan C, Orlow S, Schagger J. X-linked recessive ichthyosis. *Dermatol Online J*. 2005;11(4):12.
4. Khachemoune A, Lockshin B. Chronic papules on the back and extremities. *J Fam Pract*. 2004;53(5):361-363.
5. Casals M, Campoy A, Aspiolea F, et al. Successful treatment of linear Darier's disease with topical adapalene. *J Eur Acad Dermatol Venereol*. 2009;23(2):237-238.
6. Pérez-Carmona L, Fleta-Asín B, Moreno-García-Del-Real C, et al. Successful treatment of Darier's disease with topical pimecrolimus. *Eur J Dermatol*. 2011;21(2):301-302.
7. Rubegni P, Poggiali S, Sbano P, et al. A case of Darier's disease successfully treated with topical tacrolimus. *J Eur Acad Dermatol Venereol*. 2006;20(1):84-87.
8. Bolognia J, Jorizzo J, Rapini R. *Dermatology*. London, UK: Mosby; 2003.
9. Shreberk-Hassidim R, Sheffer S, Horev L, et al. Successful treatment of refractory Darier disease with alitretinoin with a follow up of over a year: a case report. *Dermatol Ther*. 2016;29(4):222-223.
10. Sfecci A, Orion C, Darrieux L, et al. Extensive Darier disease successfully treated with doxycycline monotherapy. *Case Rep Dermatol*. 2015;7(3):311-315.
11. Hernández-Martin A, Aranegui B, Martin-Santiago A, Garcia-Doval I. A systematic review of clinical trials of treatments for the congenital ichthyoses, excluding ichthyosis vulgaris. *J Am Acad Dermatol*. 2013;69(4):544-549.e8.

215 ERYTHEMA ANNULARE CENTRIFUGUM

Shehnaz Zaman Sarmast, MD
Richard P. Usatine, MD

PATIENT STORY

A 57-year-old farm worker presents with itchy red rings on his body that have come and gone for more than 13 years (**Figures 215-1** and **215-2**). The erythematous annular eruption was visible on his abdomen, legs, and arms. **Figure 215-2** shows the typical "trailing scale" of erythema annulare centrifugum (EAC). A KOH preparation was negative for fungal elements, and the patient was given the diagnosis of EAC. He recently began using paint thinner to "dry out the rash" and decrease the itching. Because topical steroids did not provide any relief for him in the past, we offered the option of using calcipotriol ointment. He chose to try the calcipotriol and stop using paint thinner.

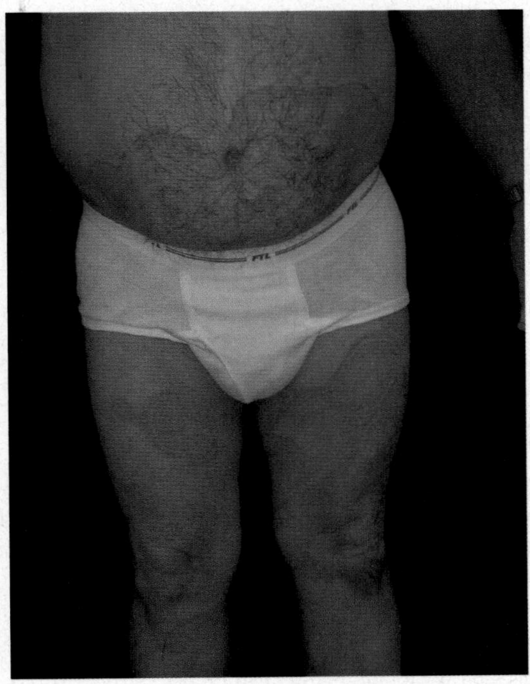

FIGURE 215-1 Erythema annulare centrifugum with large erythematous rings on the trunk and legs of a 57-year-old man. *(Reproduced with permission from Brand ME, Usatine RP. Persistent itchy pink rings, J Fam Pract. 2005;54(2):131-133. Frontline Medical Communications. Inc..)*

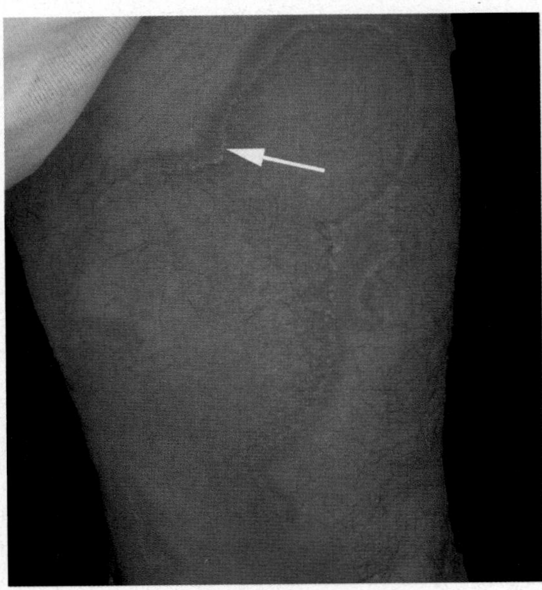

FIGURE 215-2 Erythema annulare centrifugum with conjoined rings on the thigh. *Arrow* pointing to "trailing scale," which appears as a white scaling line within the erythematous border. *(Reproduced with permission from Brand ME, Usatine RP. Persistent itchy pink rings, J Fam Pract. 2005;54(2):131-133. Frontline Medical Communications. Inc..)*

INTRODUCTION

EAC is an uncommon inflammatory skin disease characterized by slowly migrating annular or configurate erythematous lesions.

SYNONYMS

Erythema gyratum perstans, erythema exudativum perstans, erythema marginatum perstans, erythema perstans, erythema figuratum perstans, erythema microgyratum perstans, and erythema simplex gyratum.

EPIDEMIOLOGY

- It may begin at any age (mean age of onset: 39.7 years), with no predilection for either sex.[1]
- The mean duration of skin condition is 2.8 years but may last between 4 weeks and 34 years.[2]

ETIOLOGY AND PATHOPHYSIOLOGY

- Unknown etiology and pathogenesis, but EAC has been associated with other medical conditions, such as fungal infections (in 72% of cases),[1] malignancy, and other systemic illness. In one series of 66 patients, the most common underlying reported cause was tinea pedis.[1] A few case reports have reported the diagnosis of cancer 2 years after presentation of EAC.[2]
- Other infections identified as triggers for EAC include bacterial infections such as cystitis, appendicitis, and tuberculosis (TB); viral infections such as Epstein-Barr virus (EBV), molluscum contagiosum, and herpes zoster; and parasites, such as *Ascaris*.[2]

- Certain drugs, such as chloroquine, hydroxychloroquine, estrogen, cimetidine, penicillin, salicylates, piroxicam, hydrochlorothiazide, amitriptyline, lenalidomide, finasteride, and etizolam, can also trigger EAC.[2-6]
- Systemic diseases involving the liver, dysproteinemias, autoimmune disorders, HIV, and pregnancy are associated with EAC by various case reports.[2,7,8]
- Because injections of *Trichophyton*, *Candida*, tuberculin, and tumor extracts have been reported to induce EAC, a type IV hypersensitivity reaction is thought to be one possible mechanism for its development.[8]

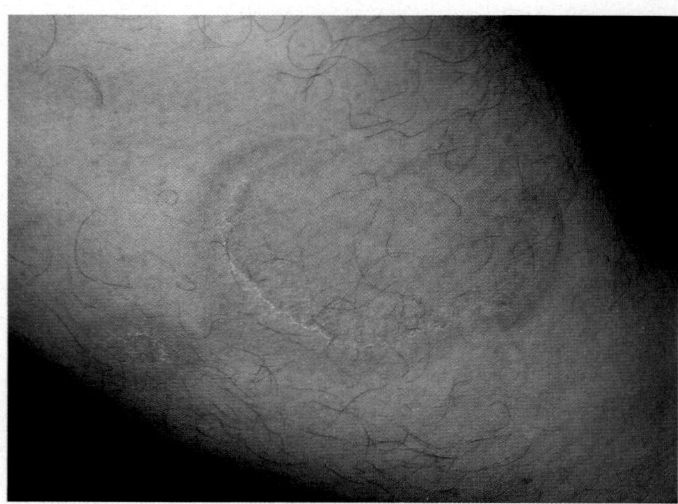

FIGURE 215-3 Erythema annulare centrifugum on the arm with trailing scale. Note the largest ring is not a complete circle. (*Reproduced with permission from Richard P. Usatine, MD.*)

DIAGNOSIS

CLINICAL FEATURES

- Large, scaly, erythematous plaques, which begin as papules and spread peripherally with a central clearing forming a "trailing" scale. The margins are indurated and may vary in width from 4 to 6 mm[1,2] (**Figures 215-1** to **215-4**).
- Pruritus is common but not always present.[2,9]
- Slowly progressing but may enlarge up to 2 to 5 mm/day.[2]
- Evaluation of a skin biopsy specimen by light microscopy reveals parakeratosis and spongiosis within the epidermis and a tightly cuffed lymphohistiocytic perivascular infiltrate with focal extravasation of erythrocytes in the papillary dermis.[10]

TYPICAL DISTRIBUTION

- Lesions typically found in lower extremities, particularly the thighs, but also can be found on trunk and face.[1,2]

LABORATORY STUDIES

- No specific laboratory tests are necessary to diagnose EAC, but laboratory tests may be obtained to rule out other common conditions. Consider a KOH prep to search for tinea corporis or cutaneous candidiasis. If the patient has been in an area with Lyme disease, consider *Borrelia* titers to rule out Lyme disease.[2,7]

BIOPSY

- If the diagnosis is uncertain, a punch biopsy can be performed to look for the typical histology of EAC, and a periodic acid–Schiff (PAS) stain can be performed on the specimen to look for fungal elements. Other diseases on the differential diagnosis, such as psoriasis, cutaneous lupus, and sarcoidosis, can be diagnosed with a punch biopsy.

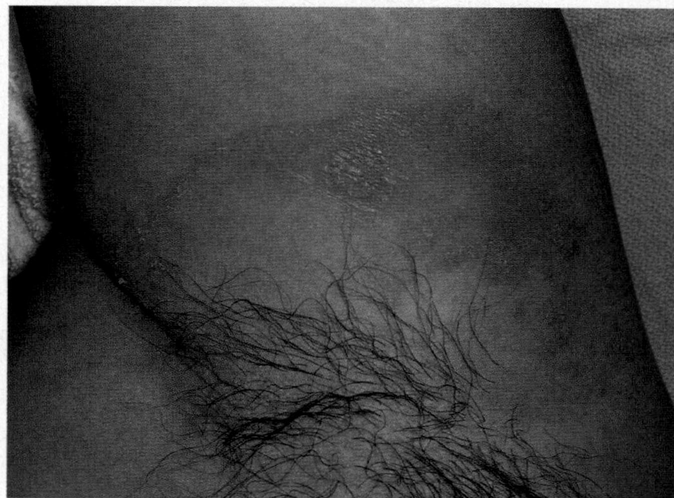

FIGURE 215-4 Erythema annular centrifugum in the axilla of a 28-year-old man, which had repeatedly been mistaken for tinea corporis. The trailing scale is visible and a punch biopsy confirmed the diagnosis of erythema annular centrifugum. (*Reproduced with permission from Richard P. Usatine, MD.*)

DIFFERENTIAL DIAGNOSIS

- Pityriasis rosea has erythematous patch distributed on trunk and lower extremities, but these patches have a distinctive collarette border and typically have a "herald patch" that appears first. Classically, the patches have a "Christmas tree" pattern in the back and, unlike EAC, last only 6 to 8 weeks[2] (see Chapter 159, Pityriasis Rosea).
- Tinea corporis (ringworm) presents with one or multiple areas of annular plaques caused by a dermatophyte fungal infection. Tinea

corporis often produces red scaling rings that resemble EAC. However, the scale in tinea corporis tends to lead with the erythema inside the ring and the scale on the outside (**Figure 215-5**). This is the opposite of the trailing scale seen with EAC (**Figure 215-6**). KOH prep shows branched hyphae with septae. Tinea corporis responds to antifungal treatment.[2] **Figure 215-4** shows a case of EAC that was mistaken for tinea corporis by a number of physicians (see Chapter 144, Tinea Corporis).

- Psoriatic plaques can be annular but do not have the trailing scale that is characteristic of EAC. Psoriasis will respond to steroid therapy[2] (see Chapter 158, Psoriasis).
- Erythema migrans seen in Lyme disease is a large annular rash with central clearing. The red ring in erythema migrans is usually smooth without the scale seen in EAC. Patients usually have other signs of infection, positive antibodies, and may have a history of tick bite (see Chapter 227, Lyme Disease).
- Erythema gyratum repens, which is typically seen in association with malignancies, has concentric rings but trailing scale is noted.
- Cutaneous lupus could present with annular or papulosquamous plaques, with or without scales, on sun-exposed areas. Patients with lupus generally have other systemic symptoms and positive antinuclear antibodies[9] (see Chapter 188, Lupus: Systemic and Cutaneous).
- Sarcoidosis may present with annular indurated papules and plaques, but they are more commonly found on the face. Patients may have other systemic manifestations of sarcoidosis. Sarcoidosis can effectively be treated with systemic corticosteroids[11] (see Chapter 184, Sarcoidosis).
- Mycosis fungoides, a type of cutaneous T-cell lymphoma, can mimic EAC (see Chapter 180, Cutaneous T-Cell Lymphoma).[12,13]

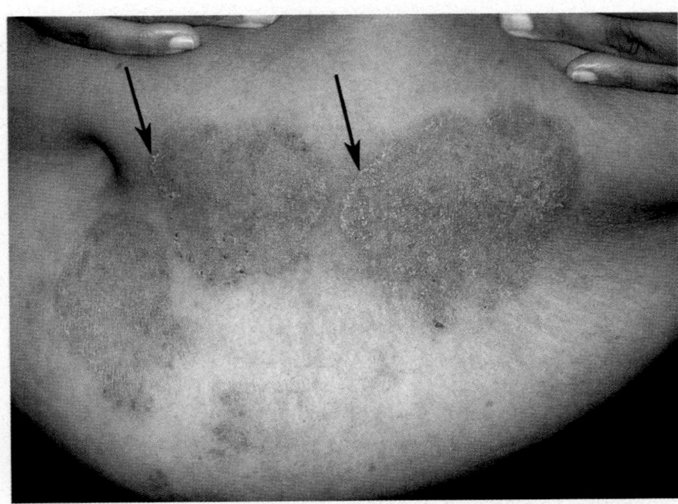

FIGURE 215-5 Tinea corporis with leading scale (*arrows*). The white scale is on the outside of the ring and the erythema is on the inside. KOH prep was positive. (*Reproduced with permission from Richard P. Usatine, MD.*)

MANAGEMENT

FIRST LINE

- There is no proven treatment for EAC. Identifying and treating underlying medical conditions may help resolve the skin condition. Because EAC is seen in association with certain drugs, discontinuing the offending medication may resolve the problem. SOR Ⓒ
- Erythromycin stearate tablet 1000 mg per day for 2 weeks was provided to 8 adults in a small series without a control group. The authors reported that all patients showed a rapid response with reduction in the size of the lesions and the erythema. Three patients with more extensive lesions had a recurrence, but another course of oral erythromycin was effective.[14] SOR Ⓒ
- Oral fluconazole was used to treat 5 children with EAC at a dose of 3–6 mg/kg/day (maximum dose of 200 mg per day) for a course of 2 to 14 weeks. Four of 5 also received a topical low to midpotency corticosteroid. This regimen was effective in all 5 children with EAC, although 2 needed a second course. There were many limitations to this study, but it is presented here due to lack of other studies of children with EAC. The authors postulated that there was an underlying fungal infection somewhere on the child and the EAC was a hypersensitivity reaction.[15] SOR Ⓒ

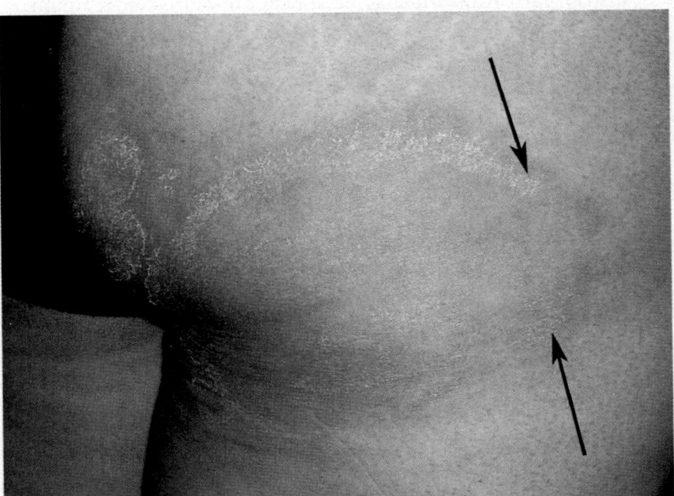

FIGURE 215-6 Erythema annulare centrifugum on the buttocks and upper thigh showing trailing scale (*arrows*) inside the ring of erythema. KOH prep was negative. (*Reproduced with permission from Richard P. Usatine, MD.*)

SECOND LINE

- Topical corticosteroids have been traditionally used, but there is little evidence to support their use. SOR C
- Case reports have reported benefits of using calcipotriol daily for EAC.[16] Another case report described a good outcome for a patient with EAC being treated with calcipotriol and narrow-band UVB phototherapy.[17] Case reports have also suggested that etanercept and metronidazole may be beneficial as well.[18,19]

PROGNOSIS

The prognosis is excellent if there is no underlying disease and may resolve in less than a year. It may resolve with effective treatment of an underlying disorder. If EAC is associated with pregnancy, it should resolve soon after delivery. If EAC is associated with a malignancy, the prognosis depends on that of the malignancy. Even if it resolves, EAC may recur repeatedly over many years.

FOLLOW-UP

Follow-up depends on the type of treatment provided and patient's preferences.

PATIENT EDUCATION

- EAC is not contagious or malignant.
- Although the treatment might not work and the condition may recur, it is not dangerous and is confined to the skin only.

PROVIDER RESOURCES

- Medscape. *Erythema Annulare Centrifugum*—**http://emedicine.medscape.com/article/1122701-overview.**
- **https://patient.info/doctor/erythema-annulare-centrifugum.**

REFERENCES

1. Kim KJ, Chang SE, Choi JH, et al. Clinicopathologic analysis of 66 cases of erythema annulare centrifugum. *J Dermatol.* 2002;29(2):61-67.
2. Brand ME, Usatine RP. Persistent itchy pink rings. *J Fam Pract.* 2005;54(2):131-133.
3. Garcia-Doval I, Pereiro C, Toribio J. Amitriptyline-induced erythema annulare centrifugum. *Cutis.* 1999;63(1):35-36.
4. Kuroda K, Yabunami H, Hisanaga Y. Etizolam-induced superficial erythema annulare centrifugum. *Clin Exp Dermatol.* 2002;27(1):34-36.
5. Tageja N, Giorgadze T, Zonder J. Dermatological complications following initiation of lenalidomide in a patient with chronic lymphocytic leukemia. *Intern Med J.* 2011;41(3):286-288.
6. Al Hammadi A, Asai Y, Patt M, Sasseville D. Erythema annulare centrifugum secondary to treatment with finasteride. *J Drugs Dermatol.* 2007;6(4):460-463.
7. Rosina P, Francesco S, Barba A. Erythema annulare centrifugum and pregnancy. *Int J Dermatol.* 2002;41(8):516-517.
8. Gonzalez-Vela MC, Gonzalez-Lopez MA, Val-Bernal JF, et al. Erythema annulare centrifugum in a HIV-positive patient. *Int J Dermatol.* 2006;45(12):1432-1435.
9. White JW. Gyrate erythema. *Dermatol Clin.* 1985;3:129-139.
10. Weyers W, Diaz-Cascajo C, Weyers I. Erythema annulare centrifugum: results of a clinicopathologic study of 73 patients. *Am J Dermatopathol.* 2003;25(6):451-462.
11. Hsu S, Le FH, Khoshevis MR. Differential diagnosis of annular lesions. *Am Fam Physician.* 2001;64(2):289-296.
12. Zackheim H, McCalmont T. Mycosis fungoides: the great imitator. *J Am Acad Dermatol.* 2002;47(6):914-918.
13. Ceyhan AM, Akkaya VB, Chen W, Bircan S. Erythema annulare centrifugum-like mycosis fungoides. *Australas J Dermatol.* 2011;52(4):e11-e13.
14. Kruse LL, Kenner-Bell BM, Mancini AJ. Pediatric erythema annulare centrifugum treated with oral fluconazole: a retrospective series. *Pediatr Dermatol.* 2016;33(5):501-506.
15. Chuang FC, Lin SH, Wu WM. Erythromycin as a safe and effective treatment option for erythema annulare centrifugum. *Indian J Dermatol.* 2015;60(5):519.
16. Gniadecki R. Case report: calcipotriol for erythema annulare centrifugum. British Association of Dermatologists. *Br J Dermatol.* 2002;146:317-319.
17. Reuter J, Braun-Falco M, Termeer C, Bruckner-Tuderman L. Erythema annulare centrifugum Darier: successful therapy with topical calcitriol and 311 nm-ultraviolet B narrow band phototherapy [in German]. *Hautarzt.* 2007;58(2):146-148.
18. Minni J, Sarro R. A novel therapeutic approach to erythema annulare centrifugum. *J Am Acad Dermatol.* 2006;54(3 Suppl 2):S134-S135.
19. De Aloe G, Rubegni P, Risulo M, et al. Erythema annulare centrifugum successfully treated with metronidazole. *Clin Exp Dermatol.* 2005;30(5):583-584.

PART XIV

PODIATRY

Strength of Recommendation (SOR)	Definition
A	Recommendation based on consistent and good-quality patient-oriented evidence.*
B	Recommendation based on inconsistent or limited-quality patient-oriented evidence.*
C	Recommendation based on consensus, usual practice, opinion, disease-oriented evidence, or case series for studies of diagnosis, treatment, prevention, or screening.*

*See Appendix A on pages 1603–1606 for further information.

216 CORN AND CALLUS

Naohiro Shibuya, DPM, MS
Javier La Fontaine, DPM, MS

PATIENT STORY

A 48-year-old woman with diabetes and mild sensory neuropathy presented with multiple calluses on the plantar feet (**Figure 216-1**). Most notably, the callus under the left hallux was hemorrhagic. Sharp debridement of the calluses was performed, and accommodating foot inserts to reduce pressure and friction on these calluses were dispensed. The patient walked out of the office with less pain and discomfort. She was instructed to watch out for hemorrhagic calluses, as they can have an underlying ulcer. One important goal, especially in a neuropathic patient, is to avoid such an ulcer (**Figure 216-2**), which occurred in another patient who did not get care for his callus in a timely manner.

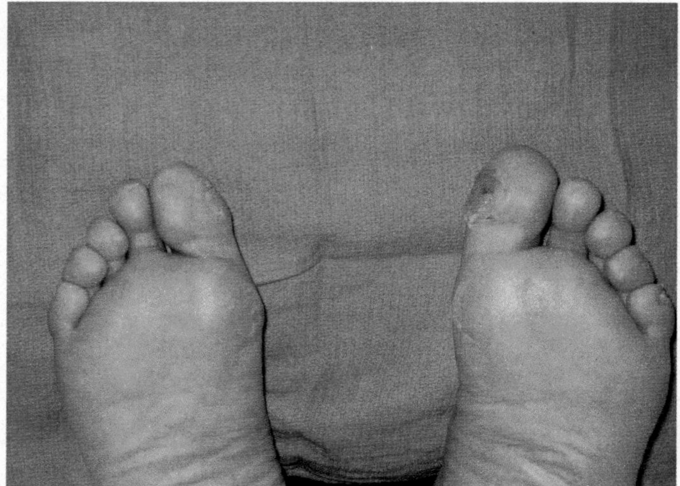

FIGURE 216-1 Multiple calluses are found on the plantar feet. The callus in the left hallux can represent an underlying ulcer. A physician should be alerted when a callus is hemorrhagic, especially in a diabetic, neuropathic patient. (*Reproduced with permission from Naohiro Shibuya, DPM.*)

INTRODUCTION

Corns and calluses are localized, thickened epidermis, resulting from mechanical pressure or shearing force applied repeatedly on the same area. A callus is located on the plantar surface and "grows in." A corn is located on the dorsal surface or between digits and often "grows out." An ulcer forms if the plantar or interdigital lesion penetrates the subcutaneous layer. Initial management includes removing the pressure by changing shoes or using pads followed by sharp debridement if needed.

SYNONYMS

Hyperkeratotic lesion, keratosis, heloma durum (hard corn) or heloma molle (soft corn), tyloma (callus), clavi (corns).

EPIDEMIOLOGY

In one population-based study, 20% of men and 40% of women reported corns or calluses.[1]

ETIOLOGY AND PATHOPHYSIOLOGY

Calluses and corns are caused by multiple factors:

- Mechanical pressure from abnormal biomechanics, underlying spur/exostosis, ill-fitting shoes, physiologic repetitive activities, and foot surgery or amputation that result in increased focal pressure at the distance site.
- Shearing force from ill-fitting shoes, foot deformities (e.g., hammer toe and bunion), and physiologic repetitive activities.
- A foreign body in the foot or shoe.

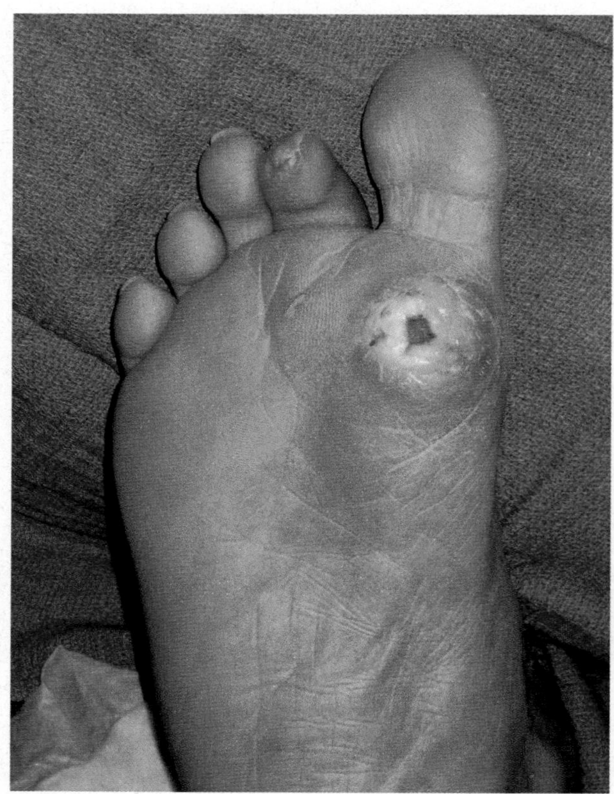

FIGURE 216-2 When neglected, an untreated hemorrhagic callus can turn into a full-thickness ulcer, which can result in infection in high-risk patients. (*Reproduced with permission from Naohiro Shibuya, DPM.*)

RISK FACTORS

- Bunion (**Figure 216-3**), hammer toe, flatfoot, high-arched (cavus) foot, Charcot arthropathy (**Figure 216-4**).
- Previous amputation in the foot (**Figure 216-5**).
- Older age, fat pad atrophy.
- Smoking.
- Female gender.
- Genodermatoses with abnormal keratin formation.

DIAGNOSIS

The diagnosis of callus or corn formation is made clinically. Radiographic examination is helpful in identifying underlying bony pathology.

CLINICAL FEATURES

- Pain at site, especially with pressure.
- Prominent underlying bony structure or deformity of the foot (high arch, flatfoot, or bunion).
- Hard, slightly hyperpigmented or skin colored, well demarcated.
- Hard or soft nucleus.

TYPICAL DISTRIBUTION

- Callus (weight-bearing surface)—Under the metatarsal heads, plantar-medial hallux interphalangeal joint, distal tip of the digits, plantar heel, fifth metatarsal base, dorsolateral fifth digit, and nail folds.
- Corns (non–weight-bearing surface)—Dorsal proximal interphalangeal joints in patients with hammer-toe deformity (see **Figure 216-3**), interdigital spaces, most commonly the fourth space.

IMAGING

- Dorsoplantar, lateral, and medial oblique weight-bearing plain radiographs with a metal marker on the lesion may detect an exostosis and/or spur. Underlying deformities can also be assessed with plain radiographs.

DIFFERENTIAL DIAGNOSIS

Other painful hyperkeratotic lesions in the foot can be caused by the following:

- Warts are common painful human papillomavirus (HPV) skin infections found in young or immunocompromised patients. Black dots (thrombosed capillaries) and disruption of skin lines differentiate these warts from callus or corns (**Figure 216-6**) (see Chapter 140, Planter Warts).
- Acrolentiginous melanoma can occur on the foot and become painful over time. These are usually pigmented with irregular borders and variations in color (**Figure 216-7**). If these are amelanotic, they may be harder to diagnose. Any unusual growth on the foot should be biopsied (see Chapter 179, Melanoma). If possible, examination by dermoscopy can increase diagnostic accuracy and help

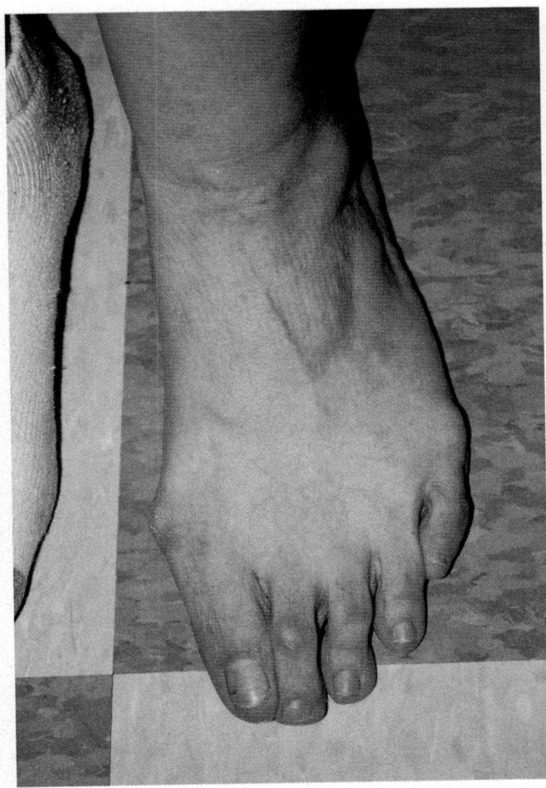

FIGURE 216-3 Bony prominences created by a bunion and hammertoe resulting in hyperkeratotic lesions (a corn on the second digit and a callus medial to the first metatarsophalangeal joint). (*Reproduced with permission from Naohiro Shibuya, DPM.*)

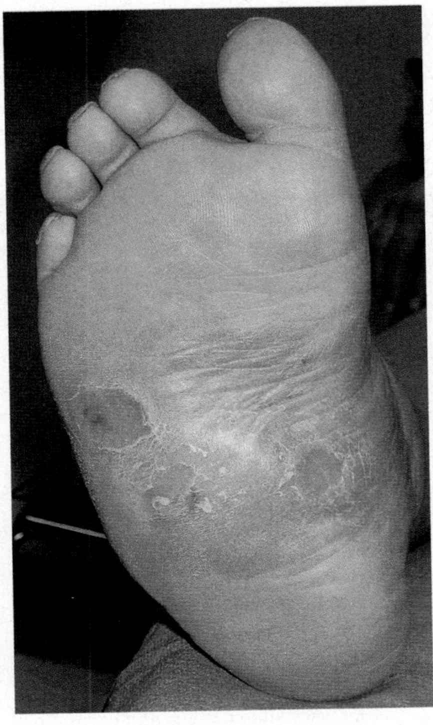

FIGURE 216-4 A mid-foot Charcot deformity results in a rocker-bottom foot and causes increased pressure points over the plantar midfoot. People with Charcot arthropathy have neuropathy, and their risk of developing plantar ulcers and infection is extremely high. (*Reproduced with permission from Naohiro Shibuya, DPM.*)

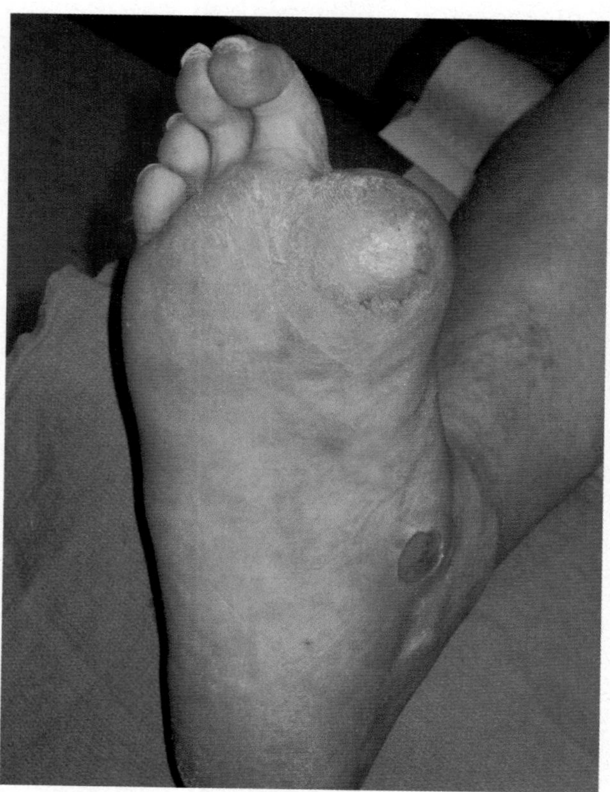

FIGURE 216-5 A previous amputation of part of a foot can alter biomechanics significantly and create pressure points that present with hyperkeratotic lesions. (*Reproduced with permission from Naohiro Shibuya, DPM.*)

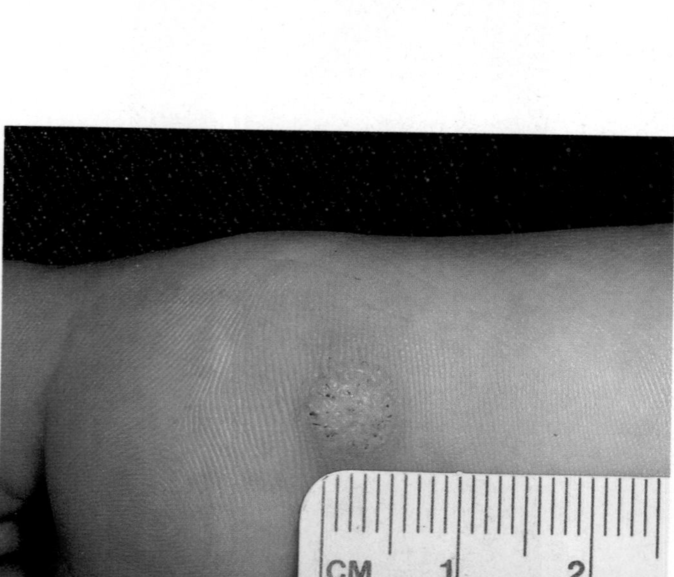

FIGURE 216-6 Plantar warts mimic callus and corns. They can be distinguished from a callus/corn by how they disrupt normal skin lines and have black dots from thrombosed capillaries. If this is not clear, superficial debridement with a scalpel will show pinpoint bleeding in a wart but not a callus/corn. (*Reproduced with permission from Richard P. Usatine, MD.*)

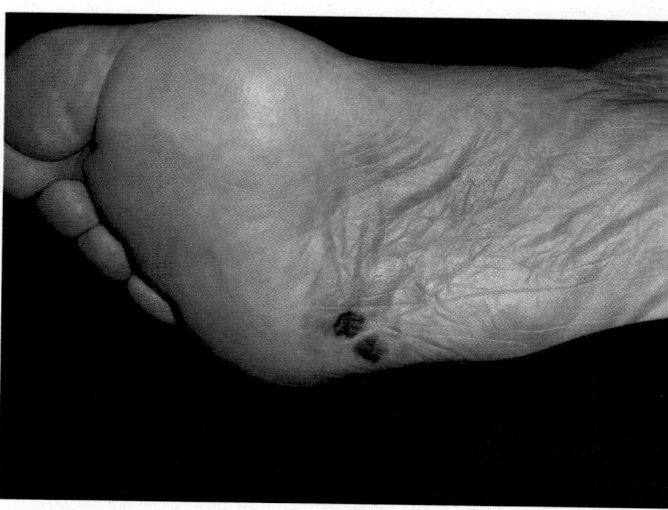

FIGURE 216-7 Acrolentiginous melanoma in situ. The variations in color and size of this lesion are red flags for melanoma. This requires immediate biopsy or direct referral to a clinician trained to do these biopsies. (*Reproduced with permission from Richard P. Usatine, MD.*)

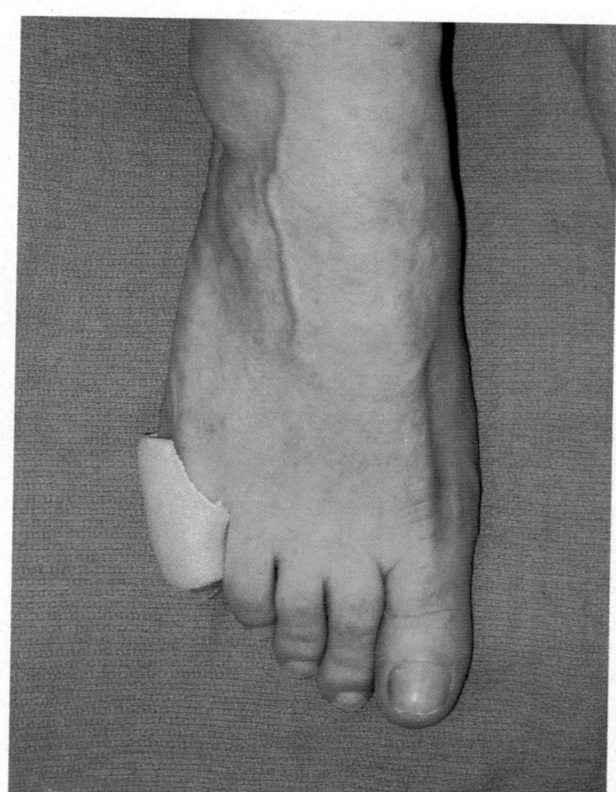

FIGURE 216-8 A padding can help protect a painful corn/callus; however, it can take up more space in a shoe and potentially increase pressure as well. A larger shoe may be needed to accommodate the padding. (*Reproduced with permission from Naohiro Shibuya, DPM.*)

determine whether a biopsy is needed (see Chapter 181, Advanced Dermoscopy of Skin Cancer).

- Nonmelanoma skin cancers rarely occur on the foot and are more likely to be on the dorsum of the foot where there is more sun exposure. These cancers are hyperkeratotic and may ulcerate. If suspicious, a shave biopsy should be adequate for diagnosis (see Chapters 177, Basal Cell Carcinoma, and 178, Squamous Cell Carcinoma).
- Porokeratosis is a deep, seeded callus that has been described as a "plugged sweat duct" and is not necessarily located in a weight-bearing area.
- Diseases with abnormal keratin production can cause painful and thick callus on the feet in the same areas, such as the heels and under the metatarsal heads.
- Surgical physiologic/hypertrophic scar can be easily identified by the surgical orientation of the incision and patient history.

MANAGEMENT

FIRST LINE

Conservative measures:

- Suggest that the patient change shoes to something that puts less pressure on the area involved.
- Pad the foot to limit shearing force from shoes (**Figure 216-8**).
- Use interdigital spacers to relieve pressure (**Figure 216-9**).
- Incorporate offloading devices or "cutoffs" in custom-made orthoses to realign an underlying deformity to minimize abnormal biomechanics.[2] SOR Ⓑ
- Suggest the patient reduce activity level on the feet.
- Encourage the patient to stop smoking and offer assistance.
- Intralesional bleomycin injection has been shown to be effective in short-term pain relief.[3] SOR Ⓑ
- Application of salicylic acid, often used in treatment of a verruca lesion, may have some benefit in treatment of a plantar callus.[4] SOR Ⓑ

SECOND LINE

If conservative measures fail to work, consider these surgical options:

- Sharp debridement of the lesion provides instant temporary relief from pain and discomfort, though it does not provide long-term solution.[5,6] SOR Ⓒ Infiltration of a local anesthetic may be necessary before debridement of an extremely painful lesion, but most calluses and corns can be debrided without anesthesia. Perform sharp debridement with a #10 or #15 surgical blade. Debride the lesion down to soft, nonkeratotic tissue and remove the hard nucleus.
- In a patient with recurring lesions, consider a surgical referral to a foot specialist to correct an underlying deformity, bony prominence, or spur.
- Exostectomy of the prominent underlying bone can be done with a minimal incision technique.
- Consider prophylactic correction of the deformity and/or removal of exostosis in a high-risk patient (e.g., patients with diabetes who are immunocompromised and neuropathic) to reduce the risk of future ulceration and infection.

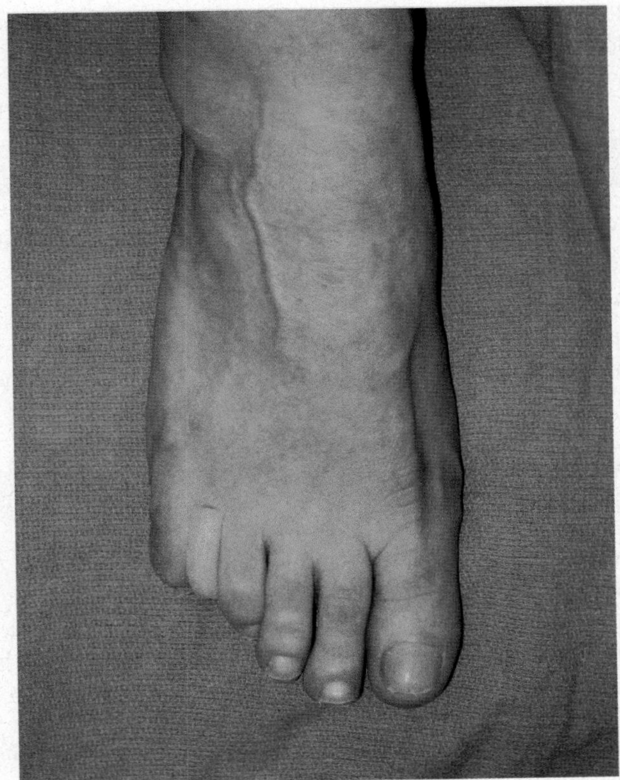

FIGURE 216-9 A toe spacer may be helpful for a corn found in a interdigital space. (*Reproduced with permission from Naohiro Shibuya, DPM.*)

- Plastic procedures (e.g., excisional biopsy with primary closure or local flap) may be necessary in patients with a chronic lesion of idiopathic origin.

PREVENTION

- Well-padded shoes and/or padded insoles can prevent hyperkeratotic lesion formation.
- Avoid activities when excessive pressure is felt in the feet.
- People with severe underlying deformity may benefit from foot orthoses and shoe management to relieve localized pressure in the foot.

PROGNOSIS

In healthy, younger patients, both conservative and surgical treatments have a good prognosis. Severe peripherally neuropathic patients neglect repetitive painful stimuli, and they are prone to ulceration from untreated hyperkeratotic lesions. Surgical management by changing the biomechanics of the foot is often successful, but it can cause a "transfer lesion"—a new lesion developing distant from the original lesion. Surgical excision of the skin lesion without addressing underlying pressure will likely result in recurrence.

FOLLOW-UP

- A healthy patient can be seen on an "as-needed" basis.
- A high-risk patient requires periodic follow-up and sharp debridement of the lesion to prevent development of a neurotrophic ulcer.
- If the patient develops an open lesion with infection, obtain plain radiographs to rule out osteomyelitis and gas gangrene. An irregular, hyperpigmented, fast-growing lesion must be biopsied.

PATIENT EDUCATION

Mild nonpainful lesions are physiologic. Conservative measures are effective in mild, painful lesions. If conservative measures fail, surgical management is indicated to correct the underlying cause of the problem. Surgical correction can result in a "transferred lesion" by shifting the pressure point away from the original site. Tell patients with neuropathy and/or their caregivers to examine the patient's feet daily for potential ulceration. An overlying hyperkeratotic lesion can mask an underlying ulcer. Drainage, maceration, and malodor are signs of underlying ulceration and infection.

PATIENT RESOURCES

- WebMD. *Calluses and Corns—Topic Overview*—**https://www.webmd.com/skin-problems-and-treatments/understanding-corns-calluses-basics.**

PROVIDER RESOURCES

- ePodiatry.com. *Foot Corns and Callus (Hyperkeratosis)*—**http://www.epodiatry.com/corns-callus.htm.**
- Classification system of diabetic foot ulcers—**http://www.medicalcriteria.com/criteria/dbt_foot.htm.**

REFERENCES

1. Garrow AP, Silman AJ, Macfarlane GJ. The Cheshire Foot Pain and Disability Survey: a population survey assessing prevalence and associations. *Pain.* 2004;110(1-2):378-384.
2. Colagiuri S, Marsden LL, Naidu V, Taylor L. The use of orthotic devices to correct plantar callus in people with diabetes. *Diabetes Res Clin Pract.* 1995;28(1):29-34.
3. Lee WJ, Lee SM, Won CH, et al. Efficacy of intralesional bleomycin for the treatment of plantar hard corns. *Int J Dermatol.* 2014;53(12):e572-577.
4. Akdemir O, Bilkay U, Tiftikcioglu YO, et al. New alternative in treatment of callus. *J Dermatol.* 2011;38(2):146-150.
5. Landorf KB, Morrow A, Spink MJ, et al. Effectiveness of scalpel debridement for painful plantar calluses in older people: a randomized trial. *Trials.* 2013;14:243.
6. Siddle HJ, Redmond AC, Waxman R, et al. Debridement of painful forefoot plantar callosities in rheumatoid arthritis: the CARROT randomised controlled trial. *Clin Rheumatol.* 2013;32(5):567-574.

217 BUNION DEFORMITY

Naohiro Shibuya, DPM, MS
Javier La Fontaine, DPM, MS

PATIENT STORY

A healthy 35-year-old woman has had "bunion pain" for more than 3 years. On examination, she has moderate lateral deviation of the hallux (**Figure 217-1**), a mildly contracted second digit, tenderness at the medial prominence, painless first metatarsophalangeal (MTP) range of motion, and a callus under the second metatarsal head. Radiographs (**Figure 217-2**) show medial angulation of the first metatarsal and lateral deviation of the hallux.

The patient was referred to podiatry for surgical correction of the bunion deformity. After surgery, she was placed in a post-op shoe for 4 weeks. She progressed to a regular shoe over the next month.

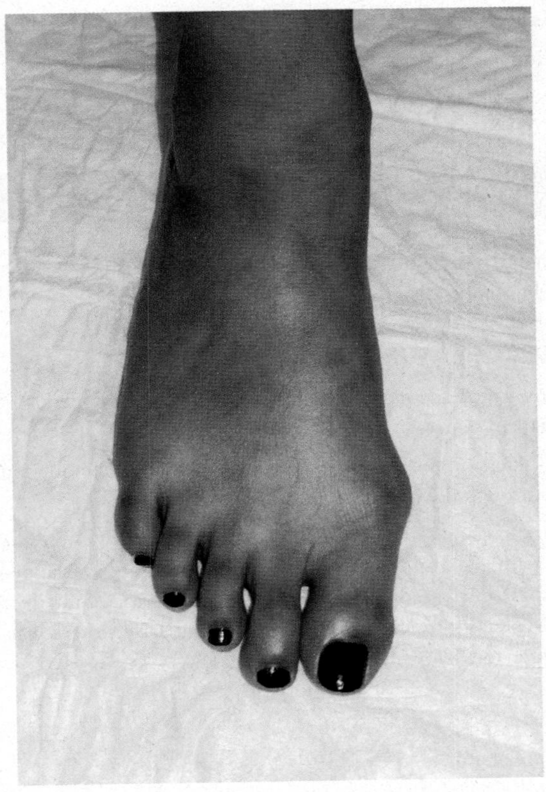

FIGURE 217-1 Laterally deviated hallux resulting in a bunion (hallux abducto valgus deformity). (*Reproduced with permission from Naohiro Shibuya, DPM.*)

INTRODUCTION

Bunion deformity is characterized by the presence of a medial prominence at the first MTP joint, caused by a laterally angulated hallux on a medially angulated first metatarsal. The deformity causes irritation in a tight shoe and/or pain in the MTP joint. Initial therapy can be conservative with correction of footwear and application of padding. Most of the surgical procedures correct the misalignment, rather than shave the medial prominence.

SYNONYMS

Hallux valgus, hallux abducto valgus, metatarsus adductovarus.

EPIDEMIOLOGY

- The prevalence of bunions ranges from 2% to 50%.
- It is far more common in women.[1]

ETIOLOGY AND PATHOPHYSIOLOGY

Bunion deformities are caused by multiple factors:

- Genetic and hereditary factors.
- Abnormal biomechanics (most common) such as limb length discrepancy, hypermobility/ligament laxity, flatfoot deformity, malaligned skeletal structures, and ankle equinus.
- Inflammatory arthritis such as rheumatoid arthritis (**Figure 217-3**).
- Neuromuscular diseases.
- Ill-fitting shoes.
- Trauma.
- Iatrogenic causes.
- Neoplasm.

RISK FACTORS

- Underlying flatfoot, metatarsus adductus (global medial angulation of the metatarsals) and equinus.
- Family history of bunion deformity.
- Ligamentous laxity.
- Having to wear dress shoes (narrowed toe shoes).
- Female gender.

DIAGNOSIS

The diagnosis of hallux abducto valgus deformity is made clinically and radiographically.

CLINICAL FEATURES

- Laterally deviated hallux with/out erythema and/or edema in the medial eminence.
- Tenderness on the medial eminence at the first MTP joint and/or pain through the first MTP joint range of motion.
- Associated signs—Hypermobility, flatfoot deformity, second MTP joint pain, pain under the second metatarsal head, overlapped second digit, decreased ankle dorsiflexion, concurrent gout, decreased first MTP joint range of motion, sesamoiditis, hyperkeratosis, and hammer-toe deformity.

TYPICAL DISTRIBUTION

- Often bilateral.
- A unilateral bunion deformity is often caused by a limb length discrepancy or trauma.

IMAGING

- Weight-bearing plain radiographs are obtained in dorsoplantar, lateral, sesamoid axial, and medial oblique views.
- Lateral deviation of the hallux and medial deviation of the first metatarsal bone are noted in the dorsoplantar view.
- The first MTP joint narrowing, osteophyte formation, subchondral cysts, and sclerosis are indicative of osteoarthritis (**Figure 217-4**).
- The lateral view is useful in assessing elevation of the first metatarsal, dorsal spur formation at the first MTP joint, and hammer-toe deformity.
- The sesamoid axial view may show incongruent metatarsal-sesamoid articulation and some arthritic changes.

BIOPSY

- Biopsy is not indicated unless a physician is suspicious about a neoplasm or infection causing inflammation or a medial prominence in the MTP joint in extremely rare cases.
- To rule out inflammatory arthritis, infection, gout, joint fluid can be aspirated from the first MTP joint. Because of its small size, it is difficult to collect the fluid from the MTP joint.

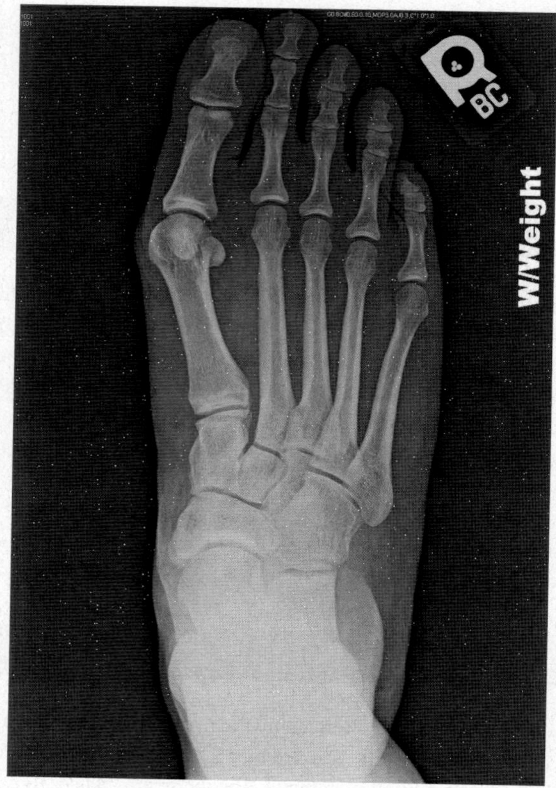

FIGURE 217-2 A weight-bearing dorsoplantar plain radiograph helps in assessing severity of the deformity and determining treatment plan. *(Reproduced with permission from Naohiro Shibuya, DPM.)*

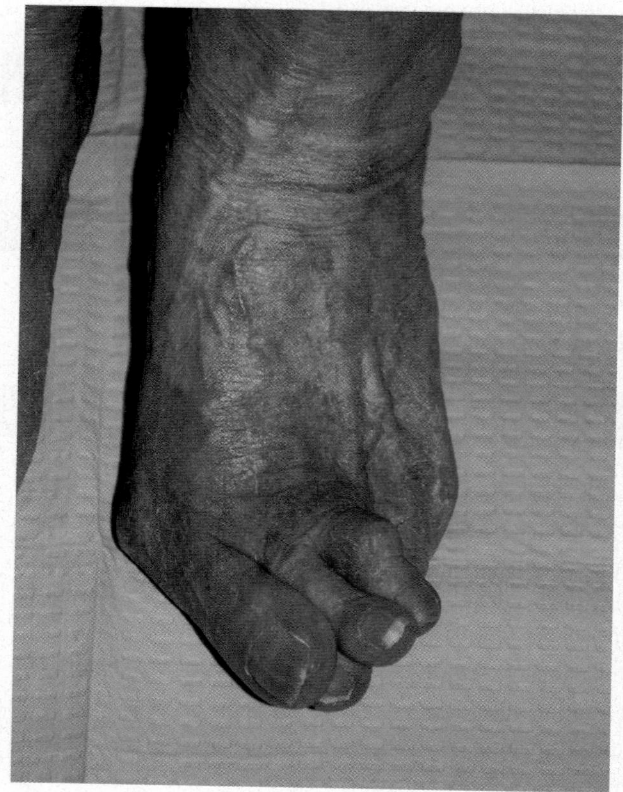

FIGURE 217-3 A bunion caused by rheumatoid arthritis. Note the lateral (fibular) deviation of all the lesser digits. *(Reproduced with permission from Naohiro Shibuya, DPM.)*

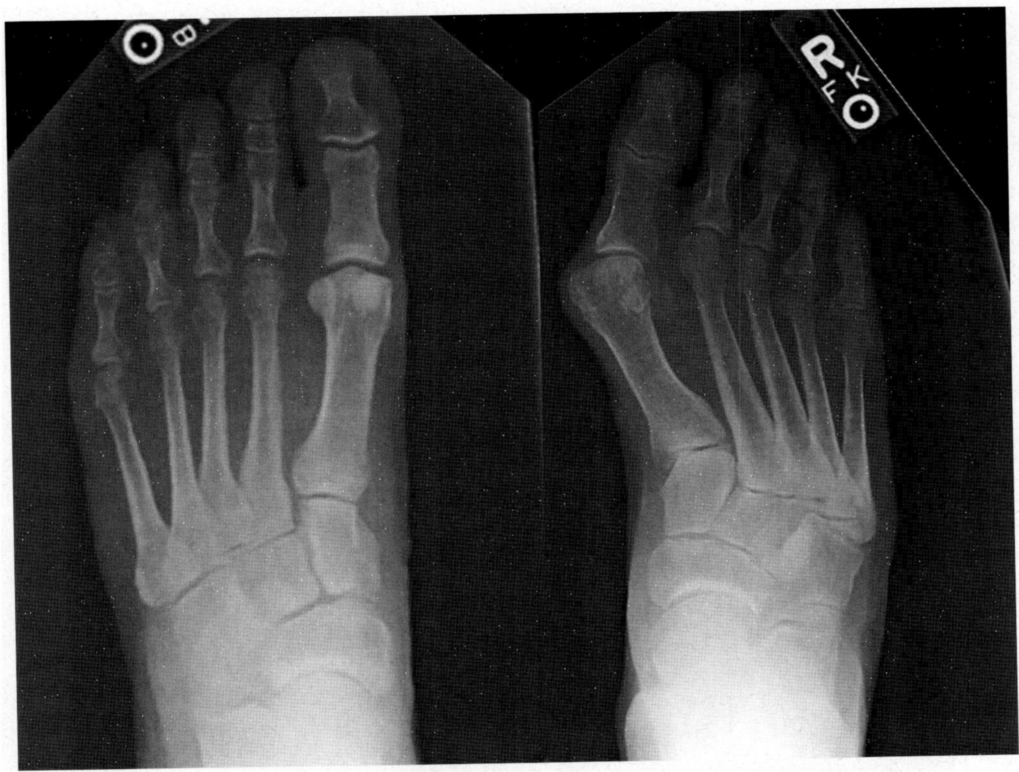

FIGURE 217-4 Compared with a normal foot (*left*), this bunion deformity (*right*) possesses a narrowed first metatarsophalangeal joint (MTPJ), indicative of concomitant osteoarthritis. (*Reproduced with permission from Naohiro Shibuya, DPM.*)

DIFFERENTIAL DIAGNOSIS

Pain and swelling around the first MTP joint may be caused by the following:

- Gout or pseudogout presents with acute pain with signs of inflammation and prior history of gout/pseudogout. Joint aspiration may be performed to rule out septic joint (see Chapter 102, Gout).
- Rheumatoid arthritis presents with pain, inflammation, and loss of range of motion and is often symmetrical. Radiographic evidence of other small pedal joint involvement is usually evident (see Chapter 99, Rheumatoid Arthritis). Rheumatoid arthritis often results in a bunion when the hallux starts to deviate laterally.
- Septic joint presents with acute pain, loss of range of motion, and systemic signs and symptoms of infectious process.
- Hallux limitus or rigidus is a condition where the first MTP joint range of motion is decreased. It is often presented with intra- and/or peri-articular arthritic changes that cause pain in the joint. It is also often presented with a prominence in the area. The prominence, however, is located more dorsally (**Figure 217-5**).

MANAGEMENT

FIRST LINE

Conservative measures:

- Change to shoes with a wider toe box.

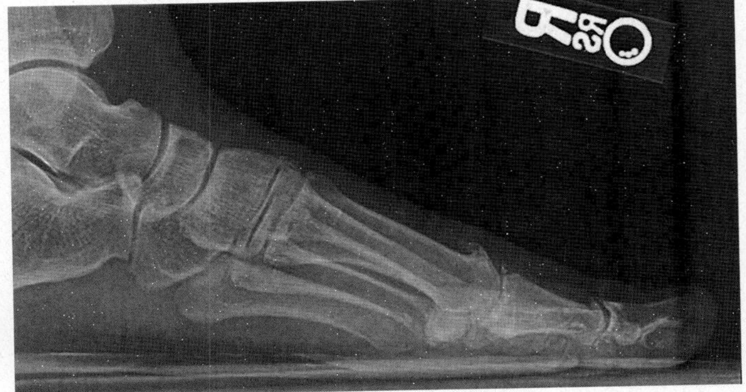

FIGURE 217-5 The dorsal spur in a patient with hallux limitus can cause pain and prominence in the first metatarsophalangeal (MTP) joint. (*Reproduced with permission from Naohiro Shibuya, DPM.*)

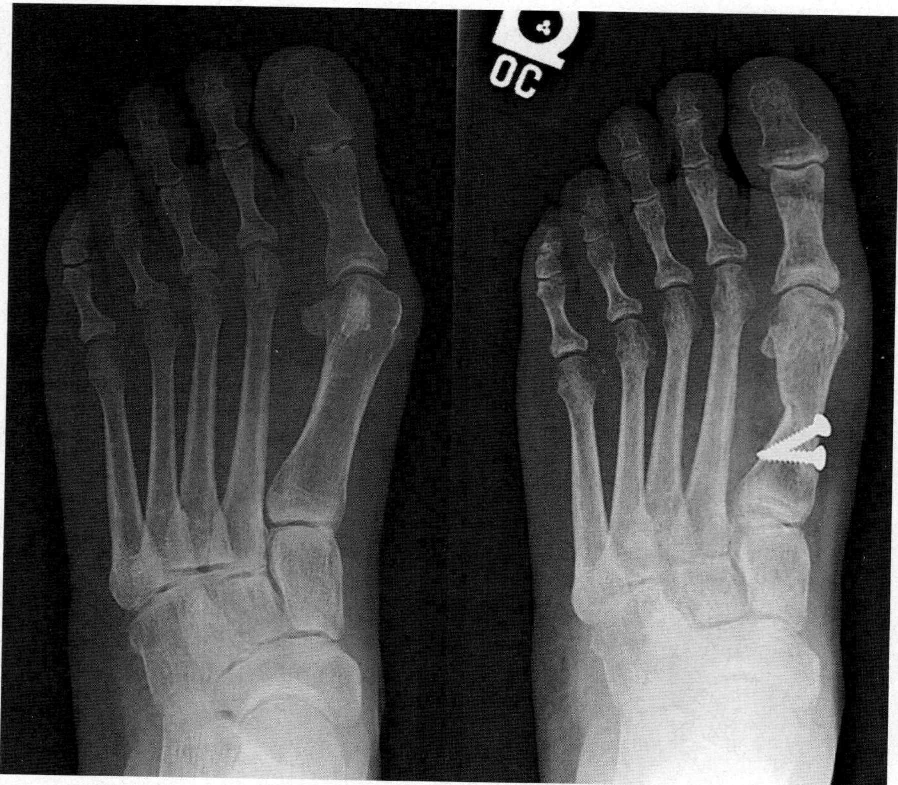

FIGURE 217-6 Surgical correction is indicated if conservative measures fail. (*Reproduced with permission from Naohiro Shibuya, DPM.*)

- Place a toe spacer in the first interdigital space to straighten the hallux and decrease the irritation caused by rubbing of the first and second digits.
- Pad the shoe to limit shearing force.
- Functional foot orthoses help reducing pain[2,3] SOR Ⓑ and slow progression of the deformity caused by biomechanical factors.
- Rest, nonsteroidal anti-inflammatory drugs (NSAIDs), and ice may help an inflamed joint and/or shoe irritation.
- Physical therapy may help improve joint range of motion, reduce edema, or decrease nerve pain.

SECOND LINE

Surgical treatment:

- Consider surgical referral to a foot specialist for correction of the deformity.
- The tendon and ligament balancing procedure is used for minor, flexible deformities.
- Exostectomy may help patients who have no joint pain, but complain about extraarticular "bump pain."
- Osteotomy to realign the bony structure is indicated for moderate to severe deformities (**Figure 217-6**).[4] SOR Ⓐ
- Arthrodesis of the first MTP or metatarsocuneiform joint is indicated in a severe deformity.
- Adjunctive procedures (e.g., correction of hammer-toe deformities, flatfoot deformity, ankle equinus, and resection of the sesamoid bone) may be required for a positive long-term outcome.

PREVENTION

- Treatment of underlying etiology, such as flatfoot, can prevent progression of bunion deformity.
- Avoid shoes that push the hallux laterally in patients who are starting to develop a bunion.

PROGNOSIS

- The prognosis worsens as the deformity progresses.[5]
- Function and quality of life can be affected in severe debilitating deformity. Surgical correction provides good prognosis in such patients.

FOLLOW-UP

The patient may be seen on an as-needed basis. Serial plain radiographs can be obtained to follow the progression of the deformity and arthritic changes in the first MTP joint.

PATIENT EDUCATION

Conservative measures may or may not provide temporary relief and prevent progression of the deformity. Surgical management is necessary to correct the deformity. Surgical treatment will typically require 2 to 6 weeks of non–weight-bearing status postoperatively, depending on the procedure performed. More severe deformities will require a more extensive surgical approach and longer recovery period.

PATIENT RESOURCES

- Foot Health Facts. *Bunions*—**https://www.foothealthfacts.org/conditions/bunions.**

PROVIDER RESOURCES

- Medscape. *Bunion*—**http://emedicine.medscape.com/article/1235796.**

REFERENCES

1. Shibuya N, Jupiter DC, Ciliberti LJ Jr, et al. Prevalence of podiatric medical problems in veterans versus nonveterans. *J Am Podiatr Med Assoc.* 2011;101:323-330.
2. Kripke C. Custom vs. prefabricated orthoses for foot pain. *Am Fam Physician.* 2009;79:758-759.
3. Hawke F, Burns J, Radford JA, du Toit V. Custom-made foot orthoses for the treatment of foot pain. *Cochrane Database Syst Rev.* 2008;(3):CD006801.
4. Torkki M, Malmivaara A, Seitsalo S, et al. Surgery vs orthosis vs watchful waiting for hallux valgus: a randomized controlled trial. *JAMA.* 2001;285:2474-2480.
5. Shibuya N, Thorud JC, Martin LR, et al. Evaluation of hallux valgus correction with versus without akin proximal phalanx osteotomy. *J Foot Ankle Surg.* 2016;55:910-914.

218 HAMMER TOE

Naohiro Shibuya, DPM, MS
Javier La Fontaine, DPM, MS

PATIENT HISTORY

A 44-year-old woman presented with pain in the ball of her left foot on weight-bearing. She works as a nurse and walks most of her 12-hour shift. Two months ago she noticed a new deformity of the second digit of her left foot (**Figure 218-1**). Her second digit was contracted with a nonreducible proximal interphalangeal (PIP) joint and reducible metatarsophalangeal (MTP) joint.

She was referred to a podiatrist who diagnosed an acute isolated hammer-toe deformity. At the time of surgery a plantar plate rupture at the MTP joint was found. The podiatrist fused her PIP joint and released her extensor tendon and dorsal capsule at the MTP joint to reduce the deformity. She began protective ambulation in a surgical shoe on postoperative day 3. An internal fixation wire, which was used to fixate the fusion site, was removed in 4 weeks. She returned to work and her regular activities within 6 weeks of the operation.

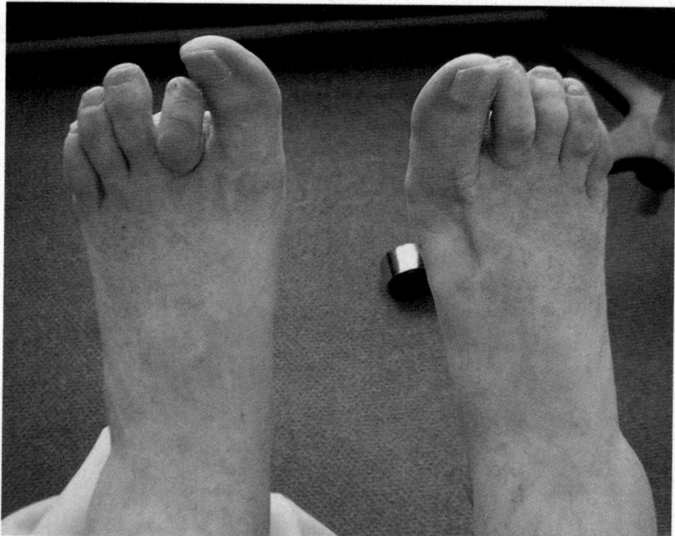

FIGURE 218-1 A plantar plate rupture at the metatarsophalangeal joint from overuse often causes an acute isolated hammer-toe deformity. (*Reproduced with permission from Naohiro Shibuya, DPM.*)

INTRODUCTION

Hammer-toe deformity is a flexion contracture in the PIP joint of a pedal digit, resulting in plantar flexion of the middle phalanx at the PIP joint with dorsal angulation of the proximal phalanx at the MTP joint. Hammer toes are associated with imbalance of soft-tissue structures around the joints in the digits and are often progressive. Surgical correction is required when deformity interferes with function.

SYNONYMS

- Hammer toe, claw toe, and mallet toe describe similar digital contractures.
- Claw toe refers to progression of hammer toe to include extension of the MTP joint along with flexion in the PIP joint.
- Mallet toe has a digital contracture at the distal interphalangeal (DIP) joint.

EPIDEMIOLOGY

Hammer-toe deformity is the most common digital deformity, and it can affect more women than men.[1,2]

ETIOLOGY AND PATHOPHYSIOLOGY

A hammer toe is caused by multiple factors:

- Genetic and hereditary factors.
- Abnormal biomechanics (cavus or high-arch foot, flatfoot deformity, loss of intrinsic muscle function, and hypermobile first ray) (**Figure 218-2**).

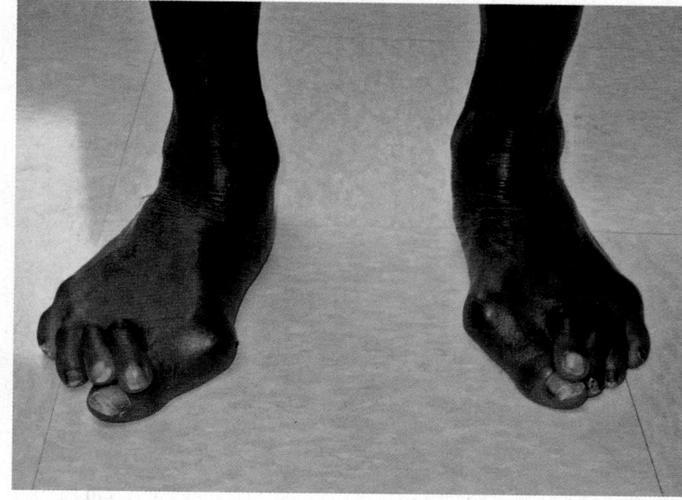

FIGURE 218-2 Biomechanically induced hammer toes. Underlying deformities, such as hallux valgus and pes planus, can cause contracture of the digits. (*Reproduced with permission from Naohiro Shibuya, DPM.*)

- Long metatarsal and/or digit.
- Systemic arthritides.
- Neuromuscular diseases such as Charcot-Marie-Tooth disease (**Figure 218-3**).
- Stroke.
- Ill-fitting shoes.
- Trauma.
- Iatrogenic causes.

RISK FACTORS

- High-arch foot type (cavus foot).
- Flatfeet.
- Bunion deformity.

DIAGNOSIS

The diagnosis of hammer-toe deformity is made clinically and radiographically.

CLINICAL FEATURES

- Pain and deformity in 1 or more of the lesser toes.
- Dorsiflexed proximal phalanx at the MTP joint and plantarflexed middle phalanx at the PIP joint of a lesser digit.
- Callus formation at the dorsal aspect of the PIP joint and/or distal aspect of the digit.
- Edema and tenderness on the plantar aspect of the lesser MTP joint(s).
- Associated signs—Cavus foot deformity, flatfoot deformity, bunion deformity, transverse deformity of the digits, decreased ankle dorsiflexion, and bowstringing of the extensor and/or flexor tendons.
- Evaluation of the digit in weight-bearing and non–weight-bearing conditions helps assess reducibility and rigidity of the deformity. In the case of predislocation syndrome (acute rupture or tear of the MTP joint capsule or plantar plate), the deformity may not be appreciated unless the foot is evaluated in the weight-bearing position.[3]

IMAGING

Obtain weight-bearing plain radiographs in dorsoplantar, lateral, and medial oblique views (**Figure 218-4**).

- Dorsal angulation and/or translation of the proximal phalanx on the metatarsal head with plantar angulation of the middle phalanx (lateral view).
- Degenerative changes in the digital joints and dislocation in the MTP joint.
- Transverse deformity and abnormal metatarsal length (dorsoplantar view).

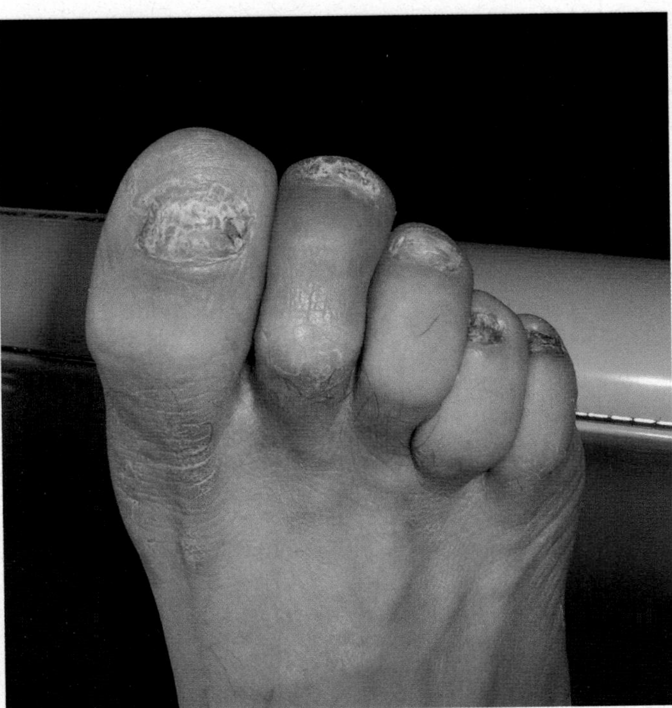

FIGURE 218-3 Severe hammer-toe deformity caused by Charcot-Marie-Tooth disease, an autosomal dominant neuromuscular disease. *(Reproduced with permission from Richard P. Usatine, MD.)*

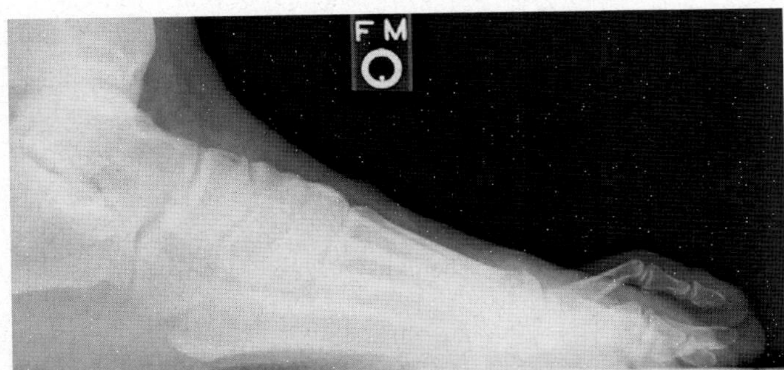

FIGURE 218-4 This lateral plain film shows dorsiflexion of the proximal phalanx at the metatarsophalangeal joint and plantarflexion of the middle phalanx at the proximal interphalangeal joint of the second digit. *(Reproduced with permission from Naohiro Shibuya, DPM.)*

DIFFERENTIAL DIAGNOSIS

Pain and swelling in the digit may be caused by the following:

- Gout or pseudogout presents with acute pain with signs of inflammation, and prior history of gout/pseudogout. Joint aspiration may be performed to rule out septic joint (see Chapter 102, Gout).
- Rheumatoid arthritis presents with pain, inflammation, and loss of range of motion and is often symmetrical. Radiographic evidence of other small foot joint involvement usually is evident (see Chapter 99, Rheumatoid Arthritis).
- Septic joint presents with acute pain, loss of range of motion, and systemic signs and symptoms of infectious process.
- Fractured toe caused by sudden trauma.
- Neuroma in the intermetatarsal space (Morton neuroma) with compression of the intermetatarsal nerves—Numbness and cramping of the innervated toes are the most common symptoms.

MANAGEMENT

Conservative measures and surgical treatment may be used to correct this condition. Note that a neglected hammer-toe deformity could result in ulceration in a patient with diabetes.

NONSURGICAL TREATMENT

Conservative measures:

- Change shoes.
- Pad shoes to limit shearing force. A crest pad can be used to prevent painful callus formation at the distal tip of the digit (**Figure 218-5**).
- Splinting can be used in an early flexible hammer toe.
- Custom-made orthoses may be helpful to slow down progression of the deformity if it is caused by biomechanical factors. SOR Ⓒ
- Rest, nonsteroidal anti-inflammatory drugs (NSAIDs), and ice help an inflamed joint and/or shoe irritation.

SURGICAL TREATMENT

- Consider surgical referral to a foot specialist to correct the deformity.
- Percutaneous tenotomy and/or capsulotomy are used for mild, flexible deformities.[4-6] SOR Ⓑ
- Resectional arthroplasty at the PIP joint may be beneficial for a more rigid deformity.[7] SOR Ⓑ
- Shortening osteotomy of the metatarsal is indicated in deformities resulting from the long metatarsal.
- Arthrodesis (fusion) of the PIP joint and/or flexor tendon transfer is indicated for a severe deformity (**Figure 218-6**).[8] SOR Ⓑ
- Adjunctive procedures (e.g., correction of bunion, cavus foot, flatfoot deformities, and ankle equinus) may be necessary for a good long-term outcome.

PREVENTION

- Proper shoes with an adequate toe box and heel counter prevent excessive contracture of the digits.

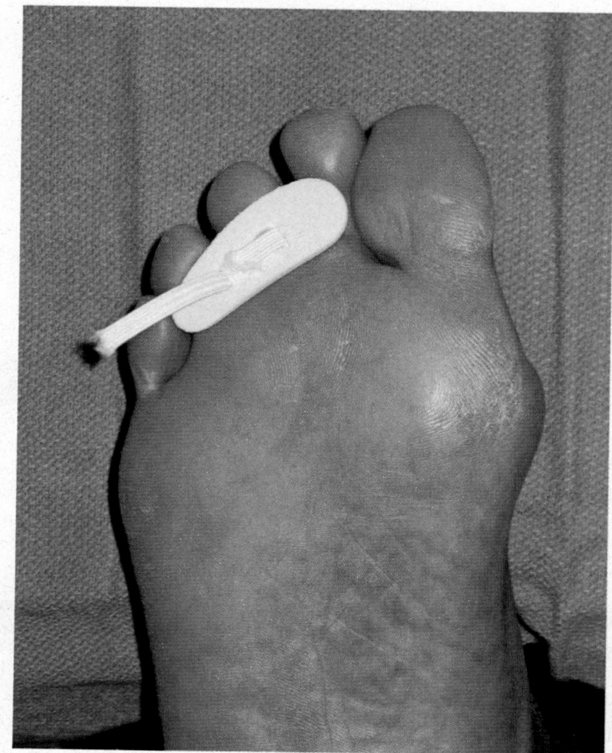

FIGURE 218-5 A crest pad prevents painful callus formation at the distal tip of the digit. (*Reproduced with permission from Naohiro Shibuya, DPM.*)

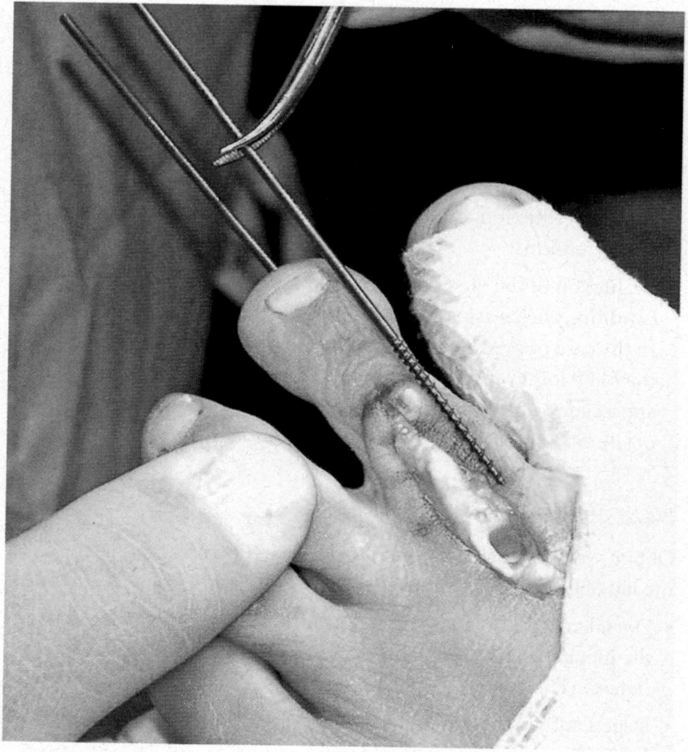

FIGURE 218-6 Proximal interphalangeal joint arthrodesis (fusion) is often used to correct hammer-toe deformity. (*Reproduced with permission from Naohiro Shibuya, DPM.*)

- Controlling associated deformities, such as bunion and flatfoot deformities, via orthotic management can prevent progression of hammer-toe deformity.

PROGNOSIS

- The prognosis worsens as the deformity progresses.
- Function and quality of life can be affected in severe debilitating deformity. Surgical correction provides good prognosis in such patients.

FOLLOW-UP

Periodic debridement of the calluses developed from the deformity may be sufficient in many patients if the deformity is not progressive. Serial plain radiographs can be obtained to follow the progression of the deformity and arthritic changes in the first MTP joint. In a high-risk, immunocompromised, neuropathic patient, prophylactic surgical correction of the deformity may be indicated.

PATIENT EDUCATION

Explain to patients that conservative measures may prevent progression of the deformity and provide temporary relief, but that surgical management is necessary to correct the deformity. Surgical treatment can require up to 2 to 4 weeks of non–weight-bearing status postoperatively in severe deformities. A less involved surgical approach to correct a mild deformity can allow a patient to walk on the same day as the surgery. In many cases, fixation with a pin, small screw, or implant is necessary to correct the deformity.

PATIENT RESOURCES

- American College of Foot and Ankle Surgeons. *Hammertoe*—**http://www.acfas.org/footankleinfo/hammertoes.htm.**

PROVIDER RESOURCES

- Medscape. *Hammertoe Deformity*—**http://emedicine.medscape.com/article/1235341.**

REFERENCES

1. Shibuya N, Jupiter DC, Ciliberti LJ Jr, et al. Prevalence of podiatric medical problems in veterans versus nonveterans. *J Am Podiatr Med Assoc.* 2011;101(4):323-330.
2. Nguyen US, Dufour AB, Positano RG, et al. The occurrence of ipsilateral or contralateral foot disorders and hand dominance: the Framingham foot study. *J Am Podiatr Med Assoc.* 2013;103(1):16-23.
3. Yu GV, Judge MS, Hudson JR, Seidelmann FE. Predislocation syndrome. Progressive subluxation/dislocation of the lesser metatarsophalangeal joint. *J Am Podiatr Med Assoc.* 2002;92(4):182-199.
4. Kearney TP, Hunt NA, Lavery LA. Safety and effectiveness of flexor tenotomies to heal toe ulcers in persons with diabetes. *Diabetes Res Clin Pract.* 2010;89(3):224-226.
5. Tamir E, Vigler M, Avisar E, Finestone AS. Percutaneous tenotomy for the treatment of diabetic toe ulcers. *Foot Ankle Int.* 2014;35(1):38-43.
6. Debarge R, Philippot R, Viola J, Besse JL. Clinical outcome after percutaneous flexor tenotomy in forefoot surgery. *Int Orthop.* 2009;33(5):1279-1282.
7. Sung W, Weil L Jr, Weil LS Sr. Retrospective comparative study of operative repair of hammertoe deformity. *Foot Ankle Spec.* 2014;7(3):185-192.
8. Lehman DE, Smith RW. Treatment of symptomatic hammertoe with a proximal interphalangeal joint arthrodesis. *Foot Ankle Int.* 1995;16(9):535-541.

219 ISCHEMIC ULCER

Javier La Fontaine, DPM, MS
Naohiro Shibuya, DPM, MS

PATIENT STORY

A 60-year-old woman with uncontrolled type 2 diabetes, hypercholesterolemia, and tobacco use presented with a 2-month history of a nonhealing ulceration on her left foot (**Figure 219-1**). She believes this started as a callus that peeled off. She presented with the ulcer, loss of protective sensation, and a nonpalpable posterior tibial pulse. She began treatment in a wound care center without any success. Noninvasive arterial studies showed severe vascular disease and thus, she underwent revascularization. While in the hospital, she quit smoking and gained control of her diabetes. Her ulcer healed, and she continues to take her diabetes medications and no longer smokes.

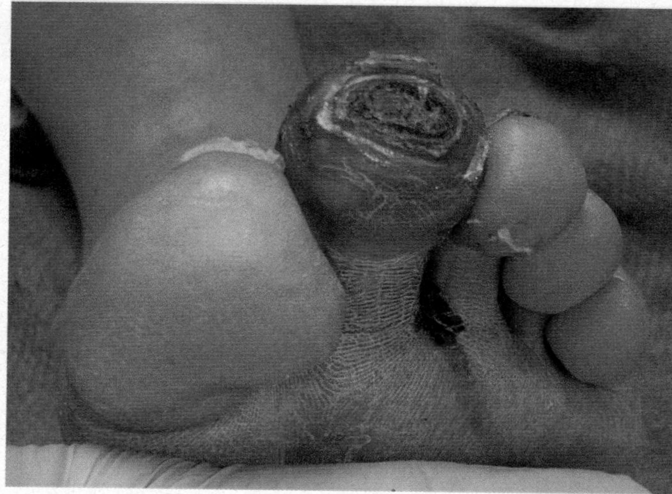

FIGURE 219-1 Ischemic ulcer on the second digit of the left foot. The base of the wound is black in color with callus surrounding wound margins. (*Reproduced with permission from Javier La Fontaine, DPM.*)

INTRODUCTION

Ulcerations occur from ongoing biomechanical forces or trauma in the insensate foot. Ulcers require adequate blood flow to heal. Nonhealing ulcers are often a result of peripheral ischemia seen in patients with diabetes and other vascular diseases. Treatment includes local wound care and improvement or correction of underlying factors causing ischemia. Untreated ischemic ulcers become infected and may require amputation.

SYNONYMS

Arterial ulcer.

EPIDEMIOLOGY

Of patients with diabetes, 15% to 25% will develop an ulcer at an annual incidence of 1% to 4%.[1]

ETIOLOGY AND PATHOPHYSIOLOGY

Microvascular dysfunction is an important component of the disease process that occurs in diabetic foot disease. The abnormalities observed in the endothelium in patients with diabetes are not well understood, and evidence suggests that endothelial dysfunction could be involved in the pathogenesis of diabetic macroangiopathy and microangiopathy.[2] Microangiopathy is a functional disease, in which neuropathy and autoregulation of capillaries lead to poor perfusion of the tissues, especially at the wound base. Also, an occlusion of the small vessels may occur.

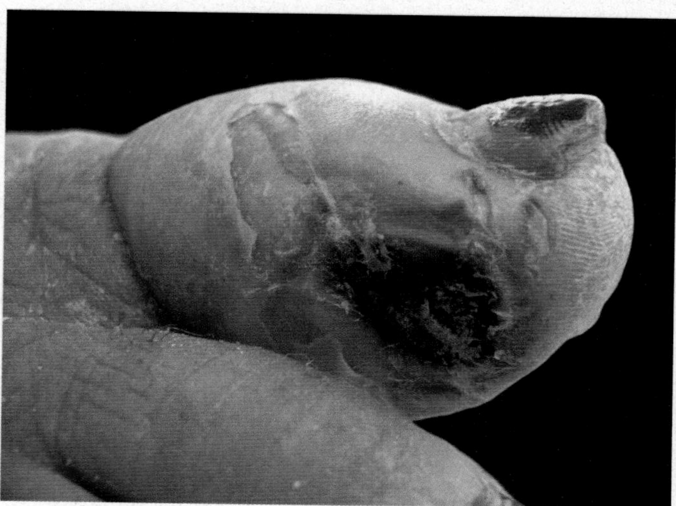

FIGURE 219-2 A 57-year-old man with diabetes for 25 years with an ischemic ulcer of the right great toe. A black base with surrounding gray/yellow rim is a common finding in this type of ulcer. (*Reproduced with permission from Javier La Fontaine, DPM.*)

RISK FACTORS

- Diabetes for more than 10 years, especially with poor glycemic control and the presence of other macro- or microvascular complications such as nephropathy and retinopathy.
- Peripheral vascular disease from any cause or other vascular risk factors, including dyslipidemia and tobacco use.
- Neuropathy caused by diabetes is a sign of microvascular disease, and an accompanying loss of protective sensation may delay detection.
- History of a previous ischemic ulcer.

DIAGNOSIS

CLINICAL FEATURES

- Pain.
- Gray/black fibrotic base (**Figures 219-1** and **219-2**).
- Undermined skin margins.
- Punched-out appearance.
- Nonpalpable pulses.
- Associated trophic skin changes (e.g., absent pedal hair and thin shiny skin).

TYPICAL DISTRIBUTION

- Distal aspect of the toes.

IMAGING

- Noninvasive studies (e.g., arterial Doppler and pulse volume recordings) are important for baseline assessment of the patient's blood flow.[3]
- Radiographs may be necessary to rule out osteomyelitis.

DIFFERENTIAL DIAGNOSIS

- Neuropathic ulcer usually presents with beefy red wound base and hyperkeratosis at the skin margins (see Chapter 220, Neuropathic Ulcer).
- Infected wounds present with localized redness, edema, drainage, and warmth in any of the diabetic-type wounds with lack of systemic symptoms of infection.
- Gangrene usually is well demarcated with black eschar in foot with vascular disease (see Chapter 222, Dry Gangrene).

MANAGEMENT

- A multidisciplinary approach is recommended for patients with ischemic ulcers.[4] SOR Ⓑ
    - Vascular surgery consultation to evaluate for revascularization.[4] SOR Ⓒ
    - Avoid aggressive debridement until optimization of blood flow occurs.
    - Change dressings twice daily to evaluate the wound and keep a low bacterial load. Many advanced therapies can be added to accomplish the same goals.
    - Offloading is important to prevent the wound from increasing in size.
- Carefully evaluate for a concomitant infection. Antibiotics are not indicated unless infection is present.[4] SOR Ⓒ
- Improve glycemic control.[4] SOR Ⓑ
- Assist with smoking cessation.[4] SOR Ⓑ

PREVENTION

- A yearly comprehensive foot examination should be performed in patients with diabetes.[4] SOR Ⓑ
- In patients with diabetes, adequate glycemic control is essential.[4] SOR Ⓑ
- Smoking cessation.[4] SOR Ⓑ

PROGNOSIS

Prognosis of an ischemic ulcer depends on the possibility of revascularization. Early recognition and treatment of underlying vascular disease is imperative for a successful outcome. Untreated or inadequately treated ulcers lead to infection and amputation.

FOLLOW-UP

- Schedule weekly to biweekly visits to monitor the ulcer.
- Obtain serial radiographs every 4 weeks to monitor for the development of osteomyelitis.
- Closely monitor the patient every 3 to 4 months once healing has occurred. Patients with a history of ulcerations are 36 times more likely to develop another ulcer.[5]

PATIENT EDUCATION

- Prevention measures, such as smoking cessation, are important to aid wound healing.[4]
- Promote successful treatment by encouraging adherence with use of offloading devices.
- Strive for normal glycemic control to optimize outcome for healing and surgical intervention.

PATIENT RESOURCES

- MedlinePlus. Patient information available in English and Spanish—**https://medlineplus.gov/ency/patientinstructions/000742.htm.**

PROVIDER RESOURCES

- ADA Standards of Medical Care in Diabetes—2016—**http://care.diabetesjournals.org/content/suppl/2015/12/21/39.Supplement_1.DC2/2016-Standards-of-Care.pdf.**

REFERENCES

1. Singh N, Armstrong DG, Lipsky BA. Preventing foot ulcers in patients with diabetes. *JAMA*. 2005;293:217-228.
2. La Fontaine J, Allen M, Davis C, et al. Current concepts in diabetic microvascular dysfunction. *J Am Podiatr Med Assoc.* 2006;96(3): 245-252.
3. Sykes MT, Godsey JB. Vascular evaluation of the problem diabetic foot. *Clin Podiatr Med Surg.* 1998;15(1):49-82.
4. American Diabetes Association Guidelines. Preventive foot care in people with diabetes. *Diabetes Care.* 2016;39(1):S72-S80.
5. Armstrong DG, Lavery LA, Harkless LB. Validation of a diabetic wound classification system. The contribution of depth, infection, and ischemia to risk of amputation. *Diabetes Care.* 1998;21(5): 855-859.

220 NEUROPATHIC ULCER

Javier La Fontaine, DPM, MS
Naohiro Shibuya, DPM, MS

PATIENT STORY

A 52-year-old man with type 2 diabetes, with a history of a third-toe amputation, presented with a new neuropathic ulceration to the right foot (**Figure 220-1**). The patient recalled having a callus for several months. He noticed blood on his sock a few days ago. He denied fever or chills, but noted that his glucose has been higher than normal. The patient demonstrated loss of protective sensation, but his vascular status was intact. He was referred to a podiatrist who immediately offloaded his foot with a total contact cast. His ulcer healed in 1 month, and he was subsequently fitted with extra-depth shoes.

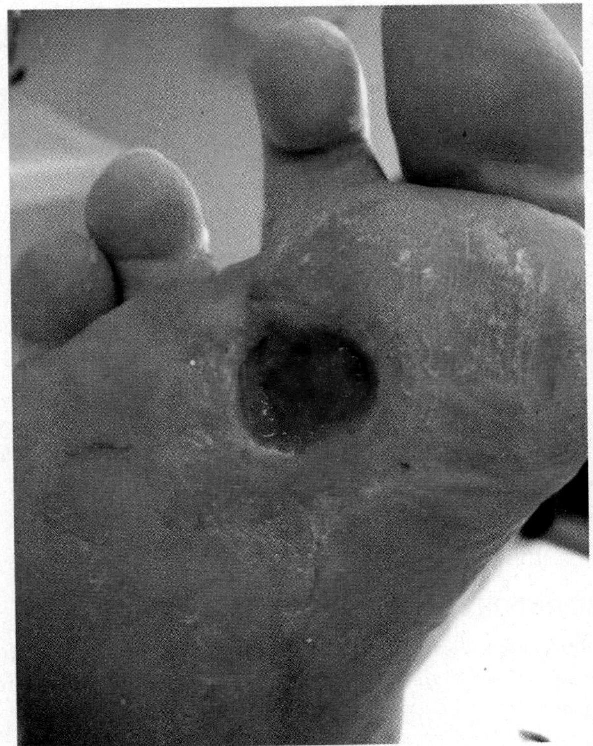

FIGURE 220-1 Neuropathic ulcer after the third metatarsal head of the right foot was resected in a patient with diabetes. Note the red base with a white rim of hyperkeratotic tissue, a classical finding of this type of ulcer. (*Reproduced with permission from Javier La Fontaine, DPM.*)

INTRODUCTION

Foot complications in patients with diabetes mellitus are common, costly, and affect quality of life. Neuropathic ulcers can lead to the most devastating outcome, which is an amputation. Eighty-five percent of all amputations related to diabetes are preceded by an ulcer. Prevention, early recognition, and treatment of foot ulcers are critical in avoiding infections and amputations.

EPIDEMIOLOGY

- Of people with diabetes, 15% will experience a foot ulcer during their lifetime, and 15% to 60% of these will develop osteomyelitis.[1]
- Neuropathy causes approximately 50% of diabetic foot ulcers.[2]
- The prevalence of neuropathic ulcer is 20% in patients with diabetic neuropathy.

ETIOLOGY AND PATHOPHYSIOLOGY

- Peripheral neuropathy is the most important factor in the development of a diabetic foot ulcer.
- Neuropathy causes loss of protective sensation. Also, autonomic neuropathy can lead to anhidrosis, which leads to skin fissuring.
- Moderate pressure with repetitive trauma occurs in a particular site, often from poorly fitting footwear, which then leads to ulceration.

RISK FACTORS

- Diabetic neuropathy increases the risk of developing a foot ulcer by 70%.[3]
- Patients with pedal deformity combined with diabetic neuropathy are 12 times more likely to develop a foot ulcer.[3]

- Patients who have a history of ulcerations are 36 times more likely to develop another ulcer.[3]
- Limited joint mobility, high level of activity, and poorly fitting footwear also increase the risk of the repetitive trauma that leads to ulceration.
- Puncture wounds may become neuropathic ulcers in the presence of neuropathy.

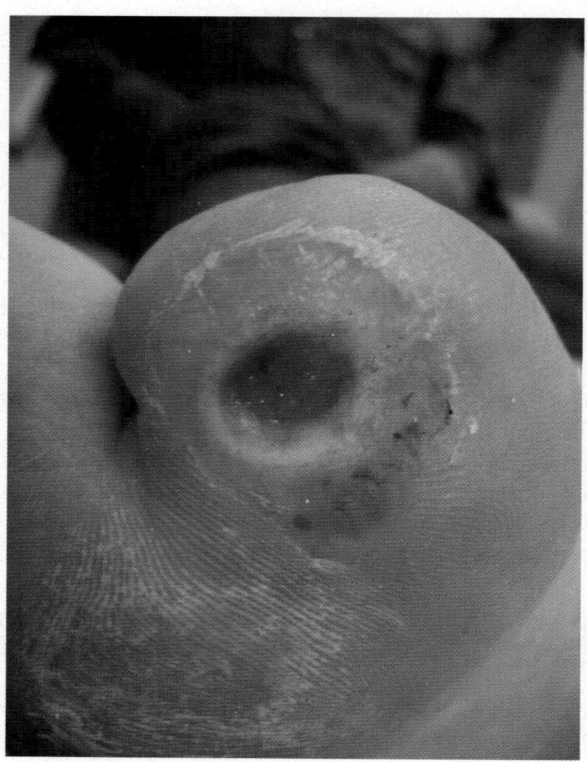

FIGURE 220-2 Neuropathic ulcers in the plantar aspect of a partially amputated great toe. The patient's amputation caused increased pressure in a different area of the foot, which, in combination with neuropathy, led to a new ulcer. (*Reproduced with permission from Javier La Fontaine, DPM.*)

DIAGNOSIS

The diagnosis of neuropathic ulceration is made clinically.

CLINICAL FEATURES

- A red, granular wound base (**Figures 220-1** and **220-2**).
- Surrounding hyperkeratosis with white, macerated margins (see **Figures 220-1** and **220-2**).

TYPICAL DISTRIBUTION

- Most common under the metatarsal heads, hallux, heel, or other weight-bearing areas.
- Can develop in any location of the foot such as the distal and dorsal aspects of the toes.

LABORATORY STUDIES

- Cultures are indicated only if infection is suspected. Swab cultures are not reliable. Curettage of the base of the wound may be more reliable.

IMAGING

- Radiographs may identify a foreign body or underlying osteomyelitis.

BIOPSY

- A biopsy may be necessary to rule out a suspected malignancy.

DIFFERENTIAL DIAGNOSIS

- Ischemic ulcer presents in the dysvascular foot, usually with pink to gray wound base, which may have black eschar (see Chapter 219, Ischemic Ulcer).
- Infected wounds present with localized redness, edema, drainage, and warmth in any of the diabetic-type wounds, and often lack systemic symptoms of infection.
- Gangrene is well demarcated with a black eschar and occurs in a foot with vascular disease (see Chapter 222, Dry Gangrene).

MANAGEMENT

NONPHARMACOLOGIC

- Offloading pressure from the foot is the standard of care and is best accomplished with a nonremovable device such as a total contact cast.[4] SOR Ⓐ

- Sharp tissue debridement removing callus tissue and exposing bleeding healthy tissue should be performed by a provider experienced in care of neuropathic foot ulcers.[4] SOR Ⓒ

MEDICATIONS

- Oral antibiotics are not indicated unless infection is suspected.
- If no improvement in 4 weeks with adherence to offloading, the ulcer should be considered a chronic wound, and adjunctive therapy such as topical growth factors and bioengineered skin products (i.e., Apligraf, Dermagraft, or Regranex) should be considered.

REFERRAL

- Consider early referral to a podiatrist, wound care center, or physician with experience treating neuropathic ulcers.

PREVENTION

- In patients with diabetes:
    - A yearly comprehensive foot examination should be performed.[5] SOR Ⓑ
    - Adequate glycemic control is essential.[5] SOR Ⓑ
    - General foot self-care education should be provided.[5,6] SOR Ⓑ

PROGNOSIS

Neuropathic ulcers should heal in approximately 4 to 6 weeks once aggressive offloading therapy has been implemented. Patient adherence to the treatment plan is essential to healing.

FOLLOW-UP

- Weekly to biweekly visits are needed to monitor and treat the ulcer.
- Serial radiographs every 4 weeks may be necessary to monitor for the development of osteomyelitis.
- Closely monitor the patient every 3 to 4 months once healing is accomplished.

PATIENT EDUCATION

- Tell patients that adherence with offloading devices is essential.
- Inform patients that control of blood sugar and blood pressure promotes healing.

PATIENT RESOURCES

- MedlinePlus. Patient information on diabetic foot ulcers in English and Spanish—**https://medlineplus.gov/ency/patientinstructions/000077.htm.**
- Information on total contact cast—**https://familydoctor.org/what-is-a-total-contact-cast/.**

PROVIDER RESOURCES

- Medscape. *Diabetic Ulcers*—**http://emedicine.medscape.com/article/460282-overview.**

REFERENCES

1. Levin ME. Pathogenesis and general management of foot lesions in the diabetic patient. In: Bowker JH, Pfeifer MA, eds. *Levin and O'Neal's The Diabetic Foot*, 6th ed. St. Louis, MO: CV Mosby; 2001:219-260.
2. Reiber GE, Smith DG, Wallace C, et al. Effect of therapeutic footwear on foot reulceration in patients with diabetes: a randomized controlled trial. *JAMA*. 2002;287:2552-2558.
3. Armstrong DG, Lavery LA, Harkless LB. Validation of a diabetic wound classification system. The contribution of depth, infection, and ischemia to risk of amputation. *Diabetes Care*. 1998;21(5):855-859.
4. Boulton AJM. The Diabetic Foot. In Endotext. Updated October 26, 2016. https://www.ncbi.nlm.nih.gov/books/NBK409609/. Accessed July 31, 2018.
6. American Diabetes Association Guidelines. Preventive foot care in people with diabetes. *Diabetes Care*. 2016;39(1):S72-S80.

221 CHARCOT ARTHROPATHY

Javier La Fontaine, DPM, MS
Naohiro Shibuya, DPM, MS

PATIENT STORY

A 48-year-old man with a 19-year history of diabetes mellitus, type 2, presents with a 2-week history of an erythematous, hot, swollen left foot (**Figure 221-1**). Three days ago, he noticed pain in his foot. The patient does not recall any trauma to his foot. He denies fever or chills. He takes multiple medications for diabetes, but he has been above his glycemic targets for many years. The radiograph of his foot (**Figure 221-2**) shows midfoot osteopenia, an early sign of acute Charcot arthropathy.

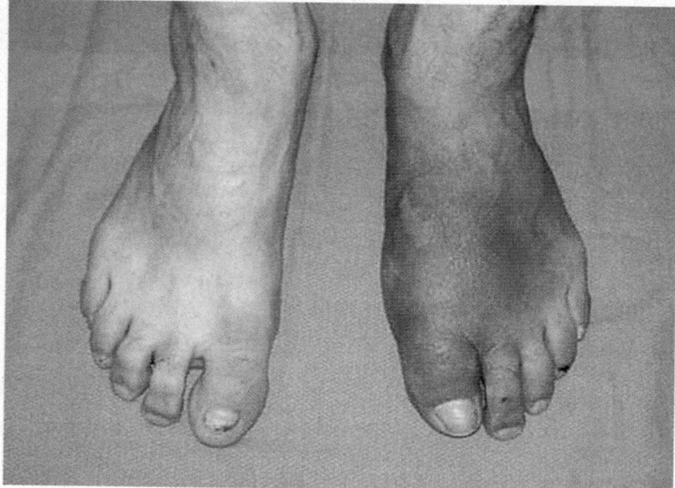

FIGURE 221-1 Charcot arthropathy in the right foot. Notice the swelling and discoloration compared to the contralateral side. *(Reproduced with permission from Javier La Fontaine, DPM.)*

INTRODUCTION

Charcot arthropathy is a rare but devastating complication in patients with neuropathy. Patients often present with pain, swelling, and erythema, similar to the presentation of a foot infection. Patients may have a rockerbottom foot deformity. Radiographs confirm the diagnosis.

SYNONYMS

Charcot foot, Charcot neuroarthropathy.

EPIDEMIOLOGY

The incidence of Charcot arthropathy in diabetes ranges from 0.1% to 5%.[1]

ETIOLOGY AND PATHOPHYSIOLOGY

Charcot arthropathy is a gradual destruction of the joint in patients with neurosensory loss, most commonly seen in patients with diabetic neuropathy.[2] The pathogenesis is unknown. Historical theories include:

- Neurotraumatic theory—Following sensory-motor neuropathy, the resulting sensory loss and muscle imbalance induces abnormal stress in the bones and joints of the affected limb, leading to bone destruction.
- Neurovascular theory—Following the development of autonomic neuropathy, there is an increased blood flow to the extremity, resulting in osteopenia from a mismatch in bone reabsorption and synthesis.
- Recently, it has been suggested that glycation of ligament, joint capsule, and bone abnormalities[3] along with a chronic prolonged inflammatory process may lead to joint destruction.
- Stretching of the ligaments because of joint effusion may lead to joint subluxation.

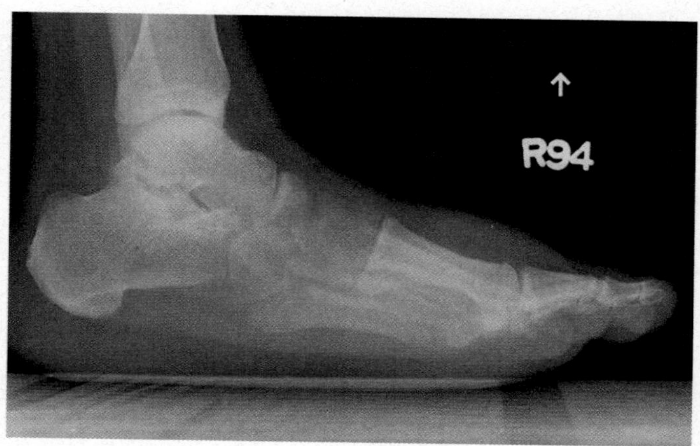

FIGURE 221-2 Lateral view of same foot demonstrating midfoot osteopenia, an early sign of acute Charcot arthropathy. *(Reproduced with permission from Javier La Fontaine, DPM.)*

RISK FACTORS

- Advanced peripheral neuropathy.
- Micro- or macrotrauma.
- Microangiopathy.
- Nephropathy.
- Genetic component might exist.

DIAGNOSIS

The diagnosis of Charcot arthropathy is suspected based on the presentation and confirmed with imaging.

CLINICAL FEATURES

- Red, hot, swollen foot (see **Figure 221-1**).
- Even with neurosensory loss, 71% of patients present with the chief complaint of pain.[4]
- Rockerbottom foot deformity is a classic finding of this entity (**Figure 221-3**).
- Patients may present with an open wound in the plantar aspect of the foot, which may complicate the distinction between Charcot arthropathy and infection.

IMAGING

Radiographs are imperative for diagnosis. Bone destruction and joint dislocation may be observed.

- Arch collapse within the joints of the midfoot (tarsometatarsal joints) (**Figure 221-4**).
- Erosions and cystic degeneration of the tarsometatarsal joints in Charcot arthropathy (**Figure 221-5**) may also be present.
- Bone scan and MRI may be ordered when infection is suspected, but are often inconclusive as cellulitis and osteomyelitis have similar findings.

CULTURE AND BIOPSY

- If osteomyelitis is suspected, bone cultures and bone biopsy are recommended. Cultures need to be taken during the bone biopsy so that the suspected infected bone can be visualized for accurate sampling. Send cultures for aerobic and anaerobic cultures as well as for acid-fast bacilli.

DIFFERENTIAL DIAGNOSIS

- Infections, including cellulitis and osteomyelitis, should be considered and treated if present (see Chapter 126, Cellulitis).
- Gouty arthropathy of the foot or ankle can resemble a Charcot foot (see Chapter 102, Gout).
- Acute trauma to the foot can cause swelling and erythema, but should be easy to distinguish from the history.
- Deep venous thrombosis in the leg will generally cause swelling that extends above the ankle.

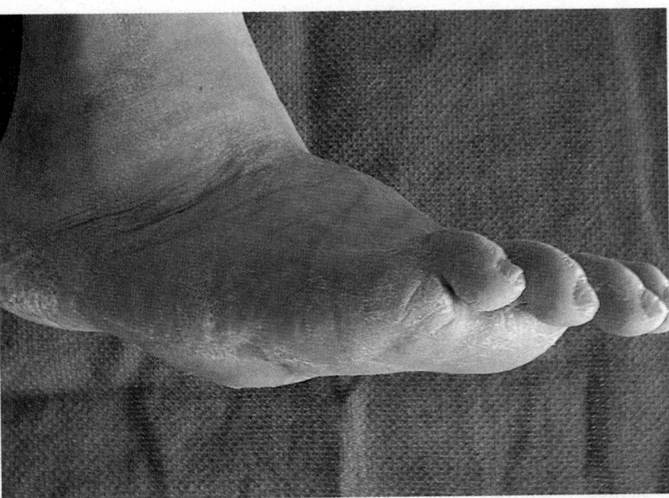

FIGURE 221-3 Lateral view of the right foot demonstrating the classic rockerbottom deformity. (*Reproduced with permission from Javier La Fontaine, DPM.*)

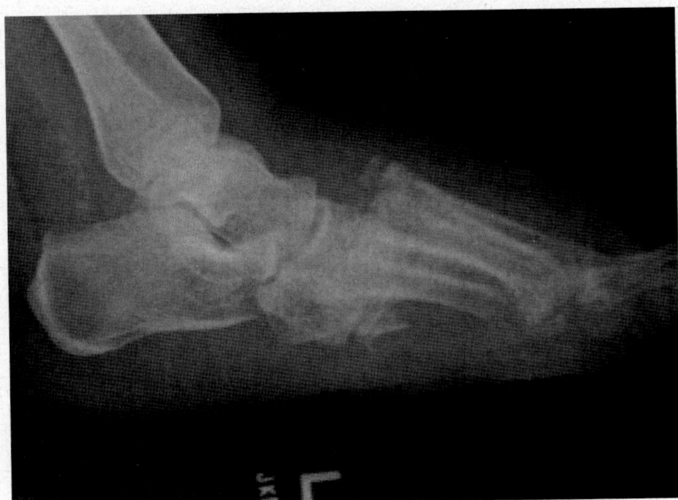

FIGURE 221-4 Lateral radiographic view of the left foot demonstrating the classic rockerbottom deformity in Charcot arthropathy with the arch collapsed at the tarsometatarsal joints. (*Reproduced with permission from Javier La Fontaine, DPM.*)

MANAGEMENT

- Immobilization and offloading of pressure from the foot is the standard of care.[2] SOR Ⓒ The total contact cast is commonly preferred. Other methods that are used include the removable cast boot, crutches, and wheelchair.
- Diabetic shoes should not be used as offloading devices for Charcot arthropathy.
- Skin temperature assessment with infrared thermometry has been demonstrated to be successful in monitoring improvement.[2] SOR Ⓒ
- Prevention of rockerbottom deformities, plantar ulcers, and amputations is the major goal of the treatment. Untreated Charcot foot may lead to a rockerbottom foot, which in turn leads to increased plantar pressure in the neuropathic foot. This cascade will lead to an ulceration (**Figure 221-6**) and possible amputation.[4]
- The bones will take approximately 4 to 5 months to heal in the presence of neuropathy.
- Oral antibiotics are not indicated unless infection is suspected.
- If deformity develops, custom-molded shoes and insoles must be ordered to prevent plantar ulcers that can lead to amputation.
- If the foot develops instability at the fracture sites, surgical reconstruction may be required.

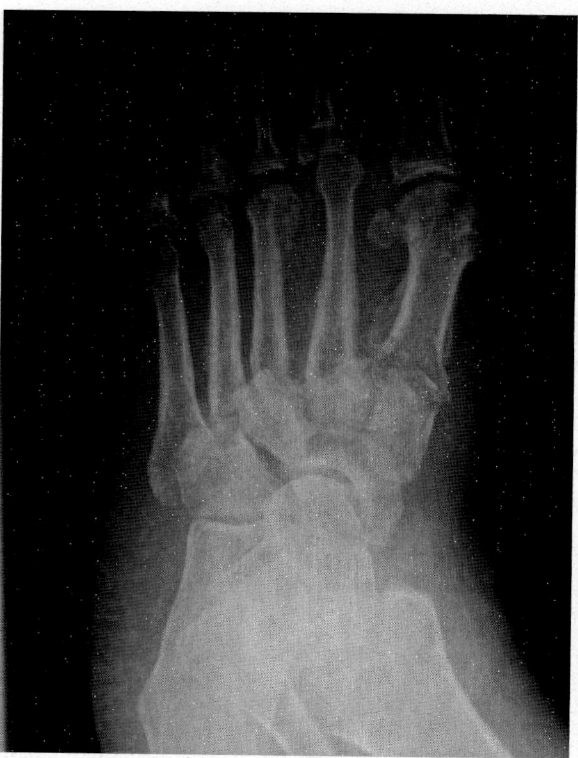

FIGURE 221-5 Anterior–posterior radiograph of the right foot demonstrating erosion and cystic degeneration at the tarsometatarsal joints in Charcot arthropathy. (*Reproduced with permission from Javier La Fontaine, DPM.*)

PREVENTION

- Control of blood glucose helps to prevent diabetic complications, including Charcot arthropathy.
- Appropriate footwear and foot care are essential to preventing many types of diabetic foot problems.

PROGNOSIS

Patients with history of Charcot arthropathy are at risk to develop further foot complications. The combination of severe foot deformity and neuropathy places them at risk for more ulceration and further amputation. Almost 50% of these patients will require complex foot surgery to fix the deformity.

FOLLOW-UP

- Weekly to biweekly visits to the podiatrist or other professional skilled in the management of Charcot arthropathy.
- Serial radiographs every 4 weeks to monitor bone healing and deformity.
- Once healing is accomplished, continue to monitor the patient every 3 to 4 months. Patients with a history of Charcot arthropathy are 36 times more likely to develop another ulcer and are at risk of amputation.[5]

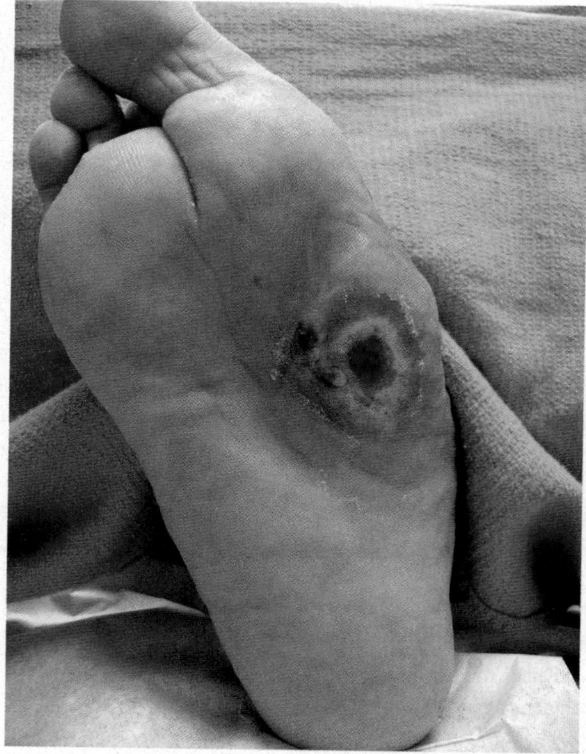

FIGURE 221-6 Foot ulcer as a result of diabetic neuropathy and a Charcot foot. Note the collapse of the arch. (*Reproduced with permission from Javier La Fontaine, DPM.*)

PATIENT EDUCATION

- Tell the patient that all efforts should be made to control blood sugar and blood pressure to promote healing.
- Educate the patient to recognize the clinical signs of Charcot arthropathy.
- Educate patient to wear shoe gear prescribed by physician.
- Ensure that patients with Charcot arthropathy understand that adherence with offloading devices is essential.

PATIENT RESOURCES

- ePodiatry.com. Information for patients—**http://www.epodiatry.com/charcot-foot.htm.**

PROVIDER RESOURCES

- Medscape. *Charcot Arthropathy*—**http://emedicine.medscape.com/article/1234293.**
- Sommer TC, Lee TH. Charcot foot: the diagnostic dilemma. *Am Fam Physician.* 2001;64:1591-1598—**https://www.aafp.org/afp/2001/1101/p1591.html.**

REFERENCES

1. Brodsky J, Rouse AM. Exostectomy for symptomatic bony prominences in diabetic Charcot feet. *Clin Orthop Relat Res.* 1993;296:21-26.
2. Fryksberg R, Zgonis T, Armstrong D, et al. Diabetic foot disorders: a clinical practice guideline (2006 revision). *J Foot Ankle Surg.* 2006;45(5 Suppl):S1-66.
3. La Fontaine J, Shibuya N, Sampson HW, Valderrama P. Trabecular quality and cellular characteristics of normal, diabetic, and Charcot bone. *J Foot Ankle Surg.* 2011;50(6):648-653.
4. Armstrong DG, Todd WF, Lavery LA, et al. The natural history of acute Charcot's arthropathy in a diabetic foot specialty clinic. *J Am Podiatr Med Assoc.* 1997;87(6):272-278.
5. Levin ME. Pathogenesis and general management of foot lesions in the diabetic patient. In: Bowker JH, Pfeifer MA, eds. *Levin and O'Neal's The Diabetic Foot*, 6th ed. St. Louis, MO: Mosby; 2001:219-260.

222 DRY GANGRENE

Javier La Fontaine, DPM, MS
Naohiro Shibuya, DPM, MS

PATIENT STORY

A 36-year-old woman with type 1 diabetes presented with a 4-week history of a dry, black great toe and third toe on the right foot (**Figure 222-1**). She said that she noticed severe maceration between the first and second interspace approximately 6 weeks ago. Subsequently, the toes changed color and became very painful. Two days ago, she noticed a foul odor from both toes. The patient reported smoking since she was 13 years old. On physical examination, there were no palpable pulses in the right foot. The patient was admitted for IV antibiotics and revascularization was performed. Subsequently, the toes were partially amputated and the wounds healed without any complications. Her physicians attempted to help her to quit smoking and she enrolled in a smoking cessation program.

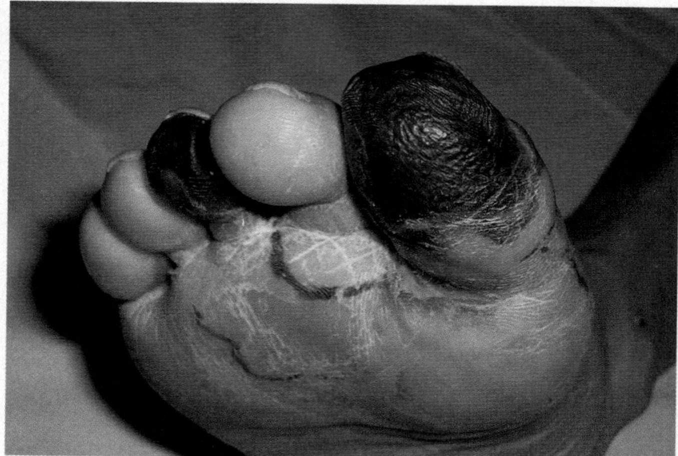

FIGURE 222-1 Dry gangrene of the first and third toes in a 36-year-old woman with poorly controlled diabetes demonstrating the typical demarcation of the necrotic eschar from the normal tissue. (*Reproduced with permission from Richard P. Usatine, MD.*)

INTRODUCTION

Dry gangrene develops following arterial obstruction and appears as dark brown/black dry tissue. Peripheral arterial disease is common in patients with diabetes, smoking history, and dyslipidemia. Dry gangrene is most commonly seen on the toes. The nonviable tissue becomes black in color from the iron sulfide released by the hemoglobin in the lysed red blood cells.

SYNONYMS

Mummification necrosis.

EPIDEMIOLOGY

- Peripheral arterial disease (PAD) is a common finding in patients with diabetes and is an important factor leading to lower-extremity amputation in patients with diabetes.[1]
- Thirty percent of diabetic patients with an absent pedal pulse will have some degree of coronary artery disease.[1]

ETIOLOGY AND PATHOPHYSIOLOGY

- PAD manifests in the lower extremity in two ways: macro- and microvascular diseases.
- The pattern of occlusion in the macrovascular tree is distal and multisegmental in the diabetic population.[2] In the nondiabetic population, the pattern of occlusion occurs proximal to the knee joint.
- In the diabetic population, multiple occlusions occur below the trifurcation of the popliteal artery into the anterior tibial artery, posterior tibial artery, and peroneal artery.

- Risk factors, such as hypercholesterolemia, hyperlipidemia, and hypertension, are often associated with patients with PAD.[3,4]

RISK FACTORS

- Diabetes.
- Dyslipidemia.
- Smoking.
- Neuropathy.

DIAGNOSIS

CLINICAL FEATURES

- Dry, black eschar, which most commonly begins distally at the extremities (**Figures 222-1** and **222-2**).
- There is a clear demarcation between healthy tissue and necrotic tissue (see **Figures 222-1** and **222-2**).
- Foul odor.
- Pain may be present.
- Trauma is the most common etiology.
- Nonpalpable pulses are common. Palpable pulses do not preclude the presence of limb-threatening ischemia. Also, the dorsalis pedis pulse is reported to be absent in 8% of healthy individuals, and the posterior tibial pulse is absent in 2% of the population.
- Associated trophic skin changes (e.g., absent pedal hair and thin shiny skin).
- Indicators of vascular insufficiency include pallor upon elevation of the limb and rubor upon dependency, along with prolonged digital capillary filling time.

TYPICAL DISTRIBUTION

- Distal extremities, especially the toes.

IMAGING

- Even in the presence of a palpable pulse, noninvasive studies (e.g., arterial Doppler and pulse volume recordings) are important for baseline assessment of the patient's blood flow.
- Angiogram is required to evaluate the possibility of revascularization.
- Radiographs may be necessary to rule out osteomyelitis.

DIFFERENTIAL DIAGNOSIS

- Wet gangrene is an acute, urgent problem that is a caused by a severe infection in the dysvascular foot (**Figure 222-3**). Wet gangrene usually presents with cyanosis, purulence, foul odor, and systemic signs and symptoms of infection.
- Embolization from a proximal vascular lesion needs to be ruled out as the source of the gangrenous process.
- Ischemic ulcer is an actual foot ulcer that usually presents with a pink to gray wound base (see Chapter 219, Ischemic Ulcer).

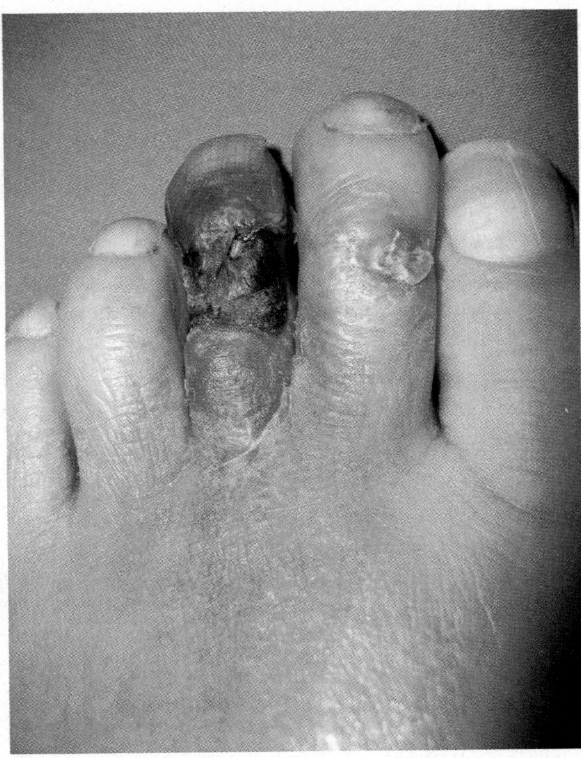

FIGURE 222-2 A 55-year-old man with type 2 diabetes presenting with dry gangrene of the third toe. Note a visible line of demarcation between the gangrene and normal tissue. The dry, black eschar is more distal than proximal. (*Reproduced with permission from Javier La Fontaine, DPM.*)

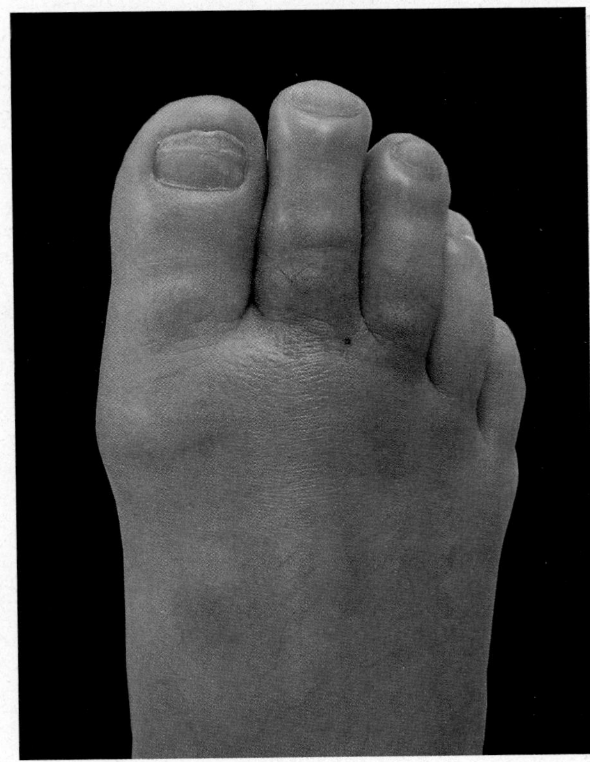

FIGURE 222-3 A 53-year-old diabetic man with wet gangrene of the second and third toes of the right foot. This diagnosis should always be considered when evaluating the ischemic limb. Wet gangrene is an emergency caused by an infectious process with severe ischemia. (*Reproduced with permission from Javier La Fontaine, DPM.*)

- Although diabetes is the most common cause of dry gangrene of the toes, severe frostbite and Buerger disease can also damage the microvasculature and lead to dry gangrene.

MANAGEMENT

- Consult vascular surgery.
- Rule out wet gangrene. Wet gangrene is an emergent infectious process in combination with severe ischemia. Consequently, immediate debridement of infected tissue is required with antibiotics.
- Avoid amputation or debridement until optimization of blood flow occurs. This may require an open revascularization and/or endovascular procedure.
- Antibiotics are not indicated for dry gangrene unless infection is suspected.

PREVENTION

- Smoking cessation.
- Diet and exercise to control blood sugar and lipids.
- Routine examination of the feet in patients with diabetes.
- Vascular examination at least on a yearly basis in patients with PAD.

PROGNOSIS

Once dry gangrene has been established, gangrenous tissue will need to be amputated. On occasion, the toes will autoamputate. Successful revascularization must occur for the patient to heal. If the problem is addressed early and aggressive wound care is provided, most amputations heal. Delaying revascularization increases the risk of infection. Early and aggressive management of vascular disease is imperative for a successful outcome.

FOLLOW-UP

Closely monitor the patient for new gangrene or ulcers every 3 to 4 months once healing has occurred.

PATIENT EDUCATION

- Avoid trauma to the amputated site.
- Advise and assist patients to stop smoking to help the wound heal and prolong the survival of the revascularization procedure.

PATIENT RESOURCES

- MedicineNet. *Gangrene*—**http://www.medicinenet.com/gangrene/article.htm.**
- eMedicineHealth. *Gangrene*—**http://www.emedicinehealth.com/gangrene/article_em.htm.**

PROVIDER RESOURCES

- Medscape. *Toe Amputation*—**http://emedicine.medscape.com/article/1829931.**
- Medscape. *Emergent Treatment of Gas Gangrene*—**http://emedicine.medscape.com/article/782709.**

REFERENCES

1. American Diabetes Association Guidelines. Preventive foot care in people with diabetes. *Diabetes Care.* 2016;39(Suppl 1):S72-S80.
2. Sykes MT, Godsey JB. Vascular evaluation of the problem diabetic foot. *Clin Podiatr Med Surg.* 1998;15(1):49-82.
3. La Fontaine J, Allen M, Davis C, et al. Current concepts in diabetic microvascular dysfunction. *J Am Podiatr Med Assoc.* 2006;96(3):245-252.
4. Tooke JE. A pathophysiological framework for the pathogenesis of diabetic microangiopathy. In: Tooke JE, ed. *Diabetic Angiopathy.* New York, NY: Oxford University Press; 1999:187.

PART XV

INFECTIOUS DISEASES

Strength of Recommendation (SOR)	Definition
A	Recommendation based on consistent and good-quality patient-oriented evidence.*
B	Recommendation based on inconsistent or limited-quality patient-oriented evidence.*
C	Recommendation based on consensus, usual practice, opinion, disease-oriented evidence, or case series for studies of diagnosis, treatment, prevention, or screening.*

*See Appendix A on pages 1603–1606 for further information.

223 INTESTINAL WORMS AND PARASITES

Heidi S. Chumley, MD, MBA

PATIENT STORY

A parent brings in a 4-year-old boy suffering with anal itching. On examination, the physician finds several excoriations around the anus and suspects pinworms. The physician then applies Scotch tape to the perianal area and places the tape on a glass slide. Review of the slide demonstrates adult worms and ova of *Enterobius vermicularis* (pinworms) (**Figure 223-1**). The boy is treated with a single dose of chewable mebendazole and his symptoms resolve. The parent is told to repeat the mebendazole dose in 2 weeks to increase the long-term cure rate. If the Scotch tape test were negative, the physician could choose to treat empirically or have the parent apply the Scotch tape to the boy's perianal area first thing in the morning and bring that back to the office (the yield is higher in the morning).

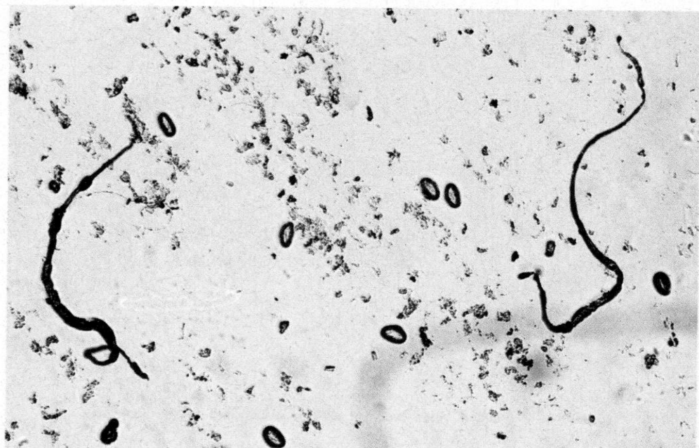

FIGURE 223-1 *Enterobius vermicularis* (pinworms and ova) seen under the microscope from a Scotch tape specimen taken of the perianal region of a 4-year-old boy with anal itching. (*Reproduced with permission from James L. Fishback, MD.*)

INTRODUCTION

Intestinal parasites are most common in places with warmer temperatures and high humidity, poor sanitation and unclean water, and a large number of individuals (especially children) living in close proximity. In general, the parasites are either asymptomatic or cause symptoms related to their presence in the GI tract. Several migrate through the lungs and can cause pulmonary symptoms during the migration. Diagnoses are made by history of worms being seen by the patient or parents or by laboratory examination for ova and parasites in the stool.

EPIDEMIOLOGY

- Nematoda is the phylum that contains pinworms, hookworms, *Ascaris*, *Strongyloides*, and whipworms.
  - *E. vermicularis* (pinworm) is the most prevalent nematode in the United States. Populations at risk include children under the age of 18, institutionalized persons, and household members of persons with pinworm infection[1] (see **Figure 223-1**).
  - *Necator americanus* (**Figures 223-2** and **223-3**) and *Ancylostoma duodenale* (hookworms) are found worldwide in areas with warm, moist climates. An estimated 576–740 million people in the world are infected with hookworms.[1]
  - *Ascaris lumbricoides*, uncommonly seen in the United States, is the largest and most common roundworm worldwide, affecting 1000 million people. It is found in tropical and subtropical areas where sanitation and hygiene are poor (**Figures 223-4** and **223-5**).[1]
  - *Strongyloides stercoralis* is seen mostly in tropical, subtropical, and temperate areas and affects 30–100 million people worldwide (**Figure 223-6**). It is more commonly found in immigrants, rural areas, institutional settings, and lower socioeconomic groups.[1]

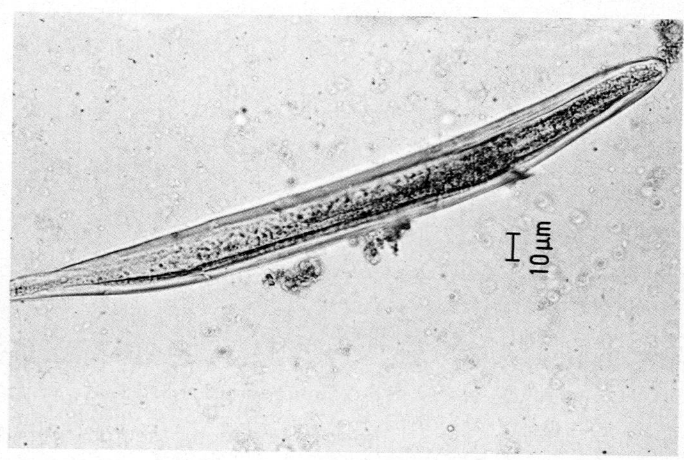

FIGURE 223-2 *Necator americanus* (hookworm) larvae can penetrate the skin and travel through veins to the heart, then the lungs. They then climb the bronchial tree to the pharynx, are swallowed, and attach to intestinal walls. (*Reproduced with permission from James L. Fishback, MD.*)

- *Trichuris trichiura* (whipworm) is the third most common roundworm, affecting 604–795 million people worldwide. Infections are more frequent in areas with tropical weather and poor sanitation practices, and among children (**Figure 223-7**). Trichuriasis occurs in the southern United States.[1]

- Cestodes (tapeworm) are a class in the phylum Platyhelminthes that contains *Taenia solium* (pork tapeworm), *T. saginata* (beef tapeworm), and *T. asiatica* (Asian pork tapeworm).
  - *T. solium* is found worldwide in underdeveloped communities with poor sanitation where pigs and humans live in close proximity.
  - *T. saginata* is rare in the United States, mostly found where cattle and humans live in close proximity in unsanitary conditions.
  - *T. asiatica* is limited to Asia where pigs and humans live in close proximity.
- Protozoa is the kingdom of one-celled organisms that includes *Giardia lamblia* and *Entamoeba histolytica.*
  - *G. lamblia (Giardia intestinalis)* is the most common intestinal parasite infection in the United States and affects 2% of adults and 6% to 8% of children worldwide (**Figure 223-8**).[1]
  - *E. histolytica* is seen worldwide, with higher incidence in developing countries. Risk groups include men who have sex with men, travelers, recent immigrants, and institutionalized populations.[1]

ETIOLOGY AND PATHOPHYSIOLOGY

- Nematodes (roundworms).
  - *E. vermicularis* (pinworm) (see **Figure 223-1**) is acquired through an oral route when hands that have contacted contaminated objects are placed in the mouth. Larvae hatch in the small intestine. Adults live in the cecum. The pregnant female goes to the perianal region at night to lay eggs.
  - *N. americanus* (hookworm) (see **Figure 223-2**) larvae penetrate the skin, travel through veins to the heart and then to the lungs, climb the bronchial tree to the pharynx, and then are swallowed and attach to intestine walls (see **Figure 223-3**).
  - When fertilized eggs of *A. lumbricoides* (see **Figure 223-4**) are ingested, they hatch and the larvae enter the circulation through intestinal mucosa, travel to the lungs, climb to the pharynx, then are swallowed, and finally the adult *Ascaris* worms live in the small intestine.
  - *S. stercoralis* have both a free-living and parasitic cycle. In the parasitic cycle, larvae penetrate the skin, travel through the circulation to the lungs, are swallowed, and travel to the small intestine (see **Figures 223-5** and **223-6**) to become adults. Adult females lay eggs, which become rhabditiform larvae, which either can become free living or can cause autoinfection by reentering the parasitic cycle or disseminating widely in the body.
  - *T. trichiura* (whipworm) (see **Figure 223-7**) eggs are ingested and hatch in the small intestine; worms live in the cecum or colon.
- Cestodes (tapeworms)—*T. solium* and *T. asiatica* are acquired by ingesting undercooked contaminated pork. *T. saginata* is acquired by ingesting undercooked beef.

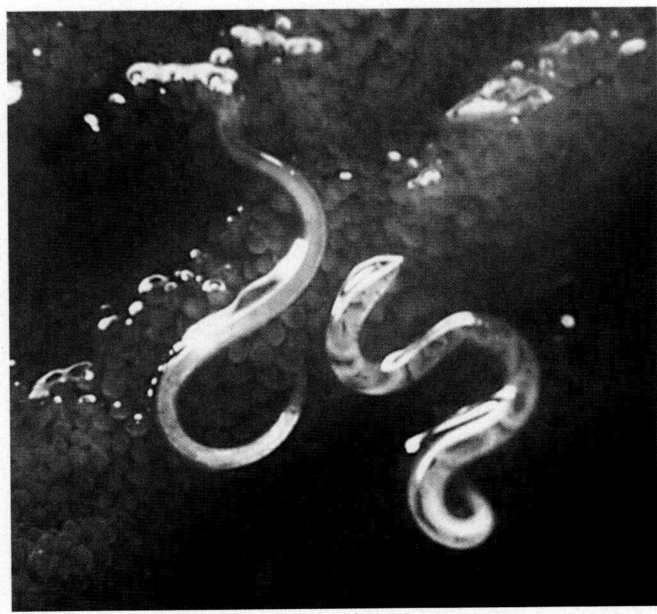

FIGURE 223-3 Adult hookworm attached to the intestinal wall. *(Reproduced with permission from Centers for Disease Control and Prevention.)*

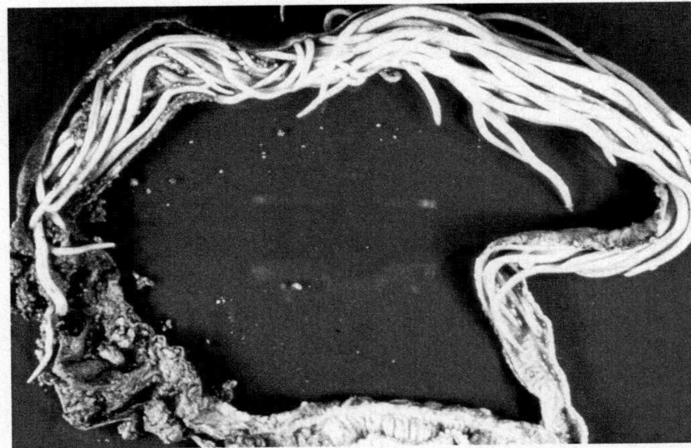

FIGURE 223-4 *Ascaris lumbricoides* in the resected bowel of a patient with bowel obstruction. *(Reproduced with permission from James L. Fishback, MD.)*

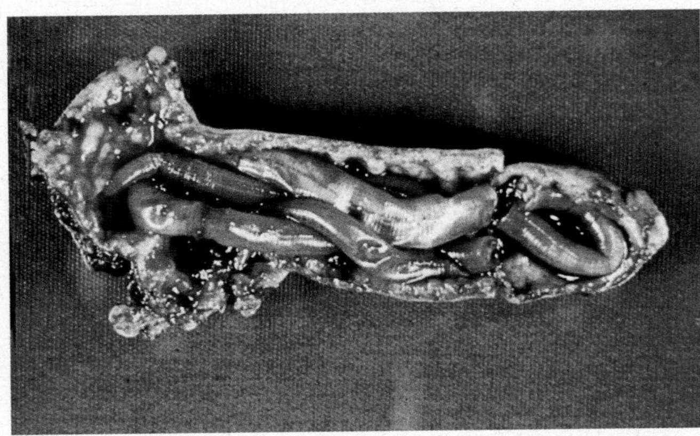

FIGURE 223-5 *Ascaris lumbricoides* in the appendix after being removed from a young adult with acute appendicitis. *(Reproduced with permission from James L. Fishback, MD.)*

- Protozoa.
  - *G. lamblia* cysts are ingested from contaminated water, food, or fomites and travel to the small intestine (**Figure 223-8**).
  - *E. histolytica* cysts or trophozoites are ingested from fecally contaminated food, water, or hands, or from fecal contact during sexual practices; these then travel to the large intestine, where they either remain or travel through the bloodstream to the brain, liver, or lungs.

RISK FACTORS

- Living in or immigrating from developing countries with limited access to clean water.
- Living in an environment conducive to parasites (warm, humid climate) and parasitic transfer (crowded conditions, contaminated water supply, poor hygiene).
- Residing in the same household or caring for persons with intestinal parasites.
- Children or others with poor hygiene are also at high risk.
- Immunocompromised patients, once infected, may have a more serious course.

DIAGNOSIS

CLINICAL FEATURES

- Nematodes.
  - *E. vermicularis* (pinworm)—Perianal pruritus is the most common; secondary bacterial infection from scratching may be present; female genital tract irritation also reported; rarely abdominal pain or appendicitis; infants show irritability, but can be asymptomatic.[1]
  - *N. americanus* (hookworm)—Most commonly presents with iron-deficiency anemia.[1]
  - *A. lumbricoides*—Frequently asymptomatic; high numbers of worms can cause abdominal pain or intestinal obstruction. When in the lungs, cough, dyspnea, hemoptysis, or eosinophilic pneumonitis may be present. Patients may cough up visible worms.
  - *S. stercoralis*—Frequently asymptomatic; eosinophilia; may cause abdominal complaints, diarrhea, cough, throat irritation, or rash at entry point or on thighs/buttocks; can disseminate in immunocompromised patients causing critical illness requiring hospitalization.
  - *T. trichiura* (whipworm)—Frequently asymptomatic; high number of worms can cause abdominal pain or intestinal obstruction, especially in children.
- Cestodes.
  - *T. solium*—Frequently asymptomatic; risk of developing cysticercosis with symptoms based on location of cysts in brain (e.g., seizures, focal neurologic signs, and death), eyes, heart, or spine.
  - *T. saginata*—More likely to cause abdominal symptoms because tapeworms are larger; not known to be associated with cysticercosis.
- Protozoa.
  - *G. lamblia*—Diarrhea, nausea, emesis, abdominal bloating may occur 1 to 14 days after ingestion for up to 3 weeks, or infection can be asymptomatic.

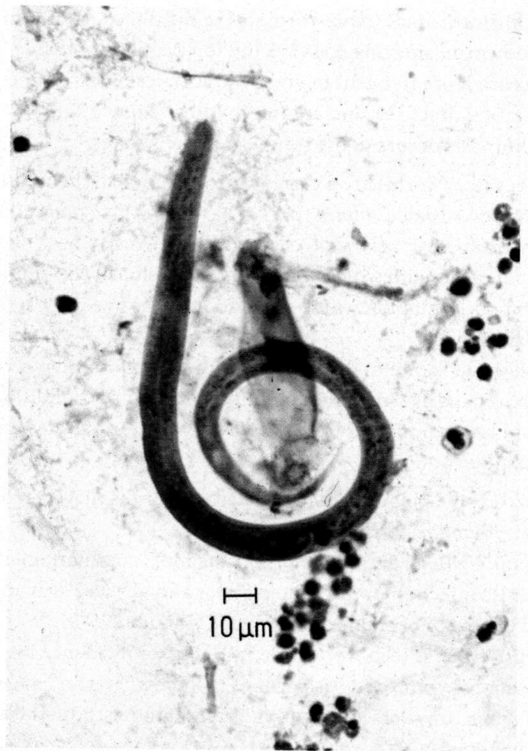

FIGURE 223-6 *Strongyloides stercoralis* ova and parasite in stool. (*Reproduced with permission from James L. Fishback, MD.*)

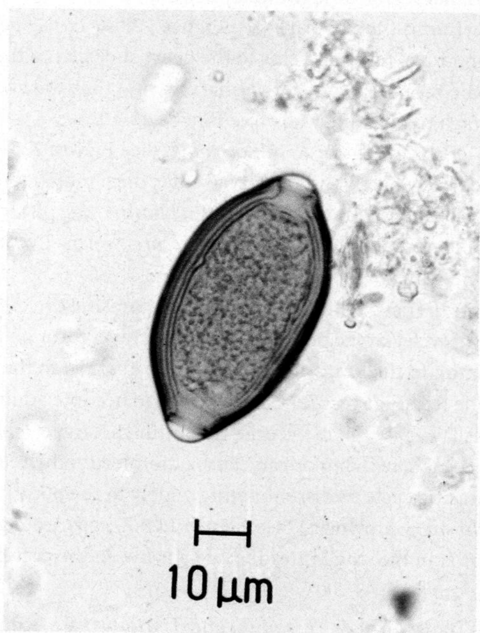

FIGURE 223-7 *Trichuris trichiura* (whipworm) egg in stool. (*Reproduced with permission from James L. Fishback, MD.*)

- *E. histolytica*—Asymptomatic, intestinal symptoms (e.g., colitis and appendicitis), or extraintestinal sign/symptoms (e.g., abscess in the liver or lungs, peritonitis, and skin or genital lesions).

LABORATORY TESTING

- Nematodes.
  - *E. vermicularis* (pinworm)—Microscopic identification of eggs (see **Figure 223-1**) collected from perianal area; apply transparent adhesive tape to the unwashed perianal area at the time of presentation or in the morning and then place tape on slide. Use the tape method on three consecutive mornings if needed.
  - *N. americanus* (hookworm)—Microscopic identification of eggs in the stool (see **Figure 223-2**).
  - *A. lumbricoides*—Microscopic identification of eggs in the stool.
  - *S. stercoralis*—Microscopic identification of larvae in stool (see **Figure 223-6**) or duodenal fluid; often requires several samples. Immunologic tests are highly sensitive and specificity continues to improve. Titers from newer tests change and may offer a method to test for cure.
  - *T. trichiura* (whipworm)—Microscopic identification of eggs in stool (see **Figure 223-7**).
- Cestodes.
  - *T. solium*—Microscopic identification of eggs or proglottids in stool indicates taeniasis, but does not differentiate among species; collect stool samples on three different days. Cysticercosis diagnosis may require serologic testing in addition to imaging.[1]
- Protozoa.
  - *G. lamblia*—Microscopic identification of cysts or trophozoites in stool or trophozoites in duodenal fluid or biopsy (see **Figure 223-8**). Antigen tests and immunofluorescence are available.
  - *E. histolytica*—Microscopic identification of cysts or trophozoites in stool (difficult to distinguish from nonpathogens); antibody detection for extraintestinal disease; antigen detection can distinguish pathogenic and nonpathogenic infections.[1]

IMAGING

- Cestodes.
  - *T. solium*—CT and MRI, often in combination, are used to identify brain cysts.

DIFFERENTIAL DIAGNOSIS

- Abdominal symptoms seen with several intestinal parasites can also be caused by the following:
  - Viral or bacterial infections—May present with acute onset of emesis and diarrhea often with fever.
  - Irritable bowel disease—Chronic symptoms of abdominal cramping with diarrhea or loose stools and/or constipation; usually no bloody stools, weight loss, or anemia.
  - Inflammatory bowel disease—Intermittent abdominal pain and bloody stools; diagnosis confirmed by colonoscopy with biopsy.
  - Iron-deficiency anemia seen with hookworms can be seen with blood loss from any site from one of many causes, and can be seen with a diet deficient in iron without having hookworms.
- GI blood loss can be seen with other infections or inflammation, polyps, or masses.

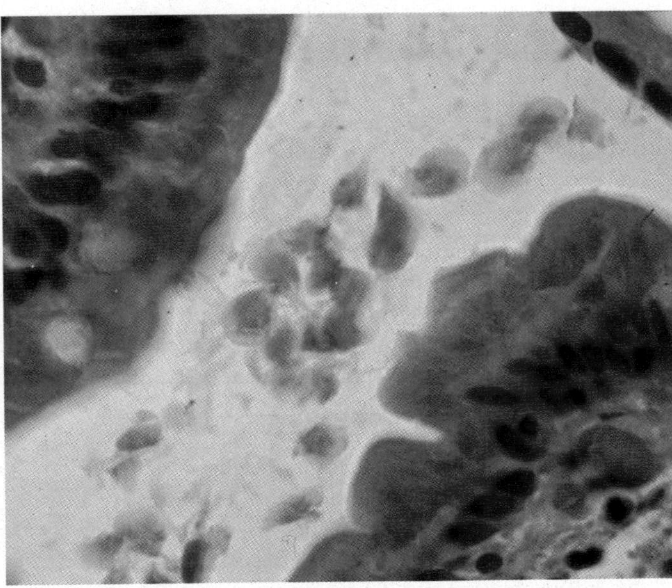

FIGURE 223-8 *Giardia lamblia* in a duodenal biopsy obtained by esophagogastroduodenoscopy in a patient with typical symptoms of chronic giardiasis (excessive flatulence and sulfurous belching) that failed to improve on metronidazole. (*Reproduced with permission from Tom Moore, MD.*)

MANAGEMENT

MEDICATIONS

All medication doses are from *The Medical Letter*[2] and apply to adults and children unless specified.

- Nematodes
  - *E. vermicularis* (pinworm)—Pyrantel pamoate 11 mg/kg once (maximum 1 g), repeat in 2 weeks; or mebendazole 100 mg once, repeat in 2 weeks; consider treating entire household.
  - *N. americanus* (hookworm)—Mebendazole 100 mg twice a day for 3 days or 500 mg once; or pyrantel pamoate 11 mg/kg (maximum 1 g) for 3 days.
  - *A. lumbricoides*—Mebendazole 500 mg once or 100 mg twice a day for 3 days; ivermectin 150 to 200 mcg/kg once.
  - *S. stercoralis*—Ivermectin 200 mcg/kg per day for 2 days; alternate therapy albendazole 400 mg bid for 7 days.
  - *T. trichiura* (whipworm)—Mebendazole 100 mg twice a day for 3 days; or ivermectin 200 mcg/kg per day for 3 days; alternate therapy albendazole 400 mg once a day for 3 days.
- Cestodes
  - *T. solium*—Praziquantel 5 to 10 mg/kg once for intestinal stage; cysticercosis requires longer therapy with albendazole 15 mg/kg per day divided into 2 doses (maximum 400 mg bid) for 8 to 30 days; patients with seizures or parenchymal inflammation require seizure prophylaxis and steroids; ophthalmologic examination for eye cysts is recommended.
- Protozoa
  - *G. lamblia*—Metronidazole 250 mg tid for 5 to 7 days (adults), 15 mg/kg per day divided tid for 5 to 7 days (children); or tinidazole 2 g once (adults), 50 mg/kg (maximum 2 g) once (children); or nitazoxanide 500 mg bid for 3 days (age >12 years), 200 mg PO bid for 3 days (age 4 to 11 years), 100 mg bid for 3 days (age 1 to 3 years)
  - *E. histolytica*—Two medications in sequence: Metronidazole 500 to 750 mg tid for 7 to 10 days (adults), 35 to 50 mg/kg per day divided in 3 doses for 7 to 10 days (children) or tinidazole 2 g once daily for 3 days (adults), 50 mg/kg per day in 3 doses up to 2 g for 3 days. Then iodoquinol 650 mg tid for 20 days (adults), 30 to 40 mg/kg per day up to 2 g in 3 doses for 20 days (children); or paromomycin 25 to 35 mg/kg per day in 3 doses for 7 days.

REFERRAL OR HOSPITALIZATION

Refer or hospitalize patients

- Who do not respond to initial therapy or have recurrent infections.
- Suspected of having cysticercosis; diagnosis must be confirmed; control of seizures, edema, intracranial hypertension, and hydrocephalus is critical; surgical removal of cysts may be necessary.[1]
- Experiencing severe abdominal symptoms suggesting obstruction or an acute abdomen.

PREVENTION

- Clean uncontaminated water for drinking and cooking—Use bottled water, chemically treated water, or boiled water in endemic areas.
- Good hygiene, especially handwashing.
- When traveling to endemic areas, drink bottled water when possible. Water can also be treated with chlorine, iodine, or boiled if bottled water is not available. Clean water should be used for brushing teeth. Avoid eating fresh salads washed in local water.
- Children in developing countries who are drinking contaminated water (and lack access to clean water) should be considered for deworming with albendazole every 3 to 6 months (see Chapter 7, Global Health).

PROGNOSIS

Prognosis is excellent for most infections if adequate therapy and clean water is available.

FOLLOW-UP

Follow-up at completion of therapy.

PATIENT EDUCATION

Most intestinal parasites are asymptomatic and easily treatable. Avoid infecting others by practicing good hygiene, including handwashing.

PATIENT RESOURCES

- The Centers for Disease Control and Prevention Division of Parasitic Diseases has information on many parasitic diseases—**http://www.cdc.gov/parasites.**

PROVIDER RESOURCES

- Centers for Disease Control and Prevention (CDC)—**http://www.cdc.gov/parasites.**
- Medical Letter. *Drugs for Parasitic Infections*—**www.medletter.com** for individual and institutional subscribers.

REFERENCES

1. Centers for Disease Control and Prevention. *Parasites*. http://www.cdc.gov/parasites. Accessed March 2017.
2. The Medical Letter. Drugs for parasitic infections. Treatment guidelines. Vol 11(Suppl), 2013. http://secure.medicalletter.org/system/files/private/parasitic.pdf. Accessed March 2017.

224 GONOCOCCAL AND CHLAMYDIA URETHRITIS

Heidi S. Chumley, MD, MBA
Richard P. Usatine, MD

PATIENT STORY

A 24-year-old man presents to a primary care clinic with 3 days of dysuria and heavy purulent penile discharge (**Figure 224-1**). He was diagnosed with gonococcal urethritis by clinical appearance, and a urine specimen was sent for testing to confirm the gonorrhea and test for *Chlamydia*. He was treated with ceftriaxone 250 mg IM for gonorrhea and 1 g of oral azithromycin. He was tested for other sexually transmitted infections. He was advised to inform his partners of the diagnosis and was counseled about safer sex. On his 1-week follow-up visit, his symptoms were gone and he had no further discharge. Nucleic acid amplification tests were positive for gonorrhea and *Chlamydia*. Rapid plasma reagin (RPR) and HIV tests were negative. His case was reported to the Health Department for contact tracing.

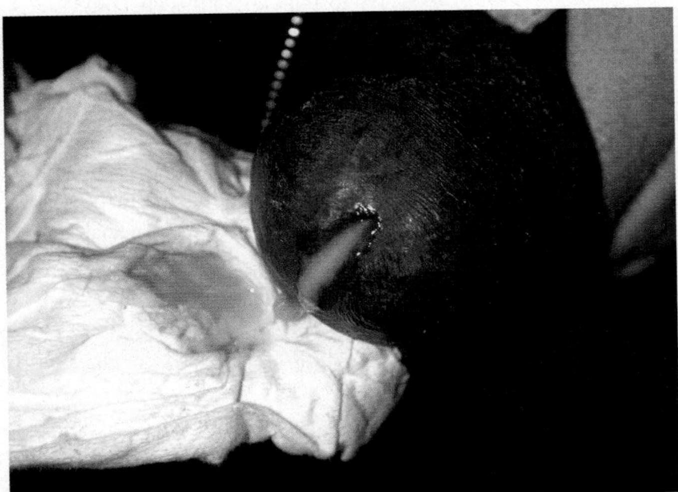

FIGURE 224-1 A 24-year-old man with gonococcal urethritis and a heavy purulent urethral discharge. (*Reproduced with permission from Richard P. Usatine, MD.*)

INTRODUCTION

Urethritis is urethral inflammation caused by infectious or noninfectious causes (i.e., trauma). Gonococcal and chlamydial infections in men occur most commonly between the ages of 20 and 24 years, and the prevalence is highest in black men. Diagnosis is suspected clinically, reinforced by an office urine test positive for leukocyte esterase, and confirmed by a urine nucleic acid amplification test. Treat for both gonorrhea and *Chlamydia* until one or both are ruled out by laboratory testing.

EPIDEMIOLOGY

- Worldwide, 151 million cases of gonococcal and nongonococcal urethritis are reported annually (**Figures 224-1** and **224-2**).[1]
- Urethritis of all types occurs in 4 million Americans each year.[1]
- The prevalence of gonorrhea in men was 140.9 per 100,000 population among men in the United States in 2015. The rate was highest among those men ages 20–24 years (539.1 per 100,000 population). Rates are 9.6 times higher among black men and women (424.9), compared to whites (44.2 per 100,000 population). The rate among Hispanics (80.5) was 1.8 times that of whites.[2]
- The prevalence of *Chlamydia* in men in the United States in 2015 was 305.2 cases per 100,000 males. The rate was highest among those men ages 20–24 years (1307.8 cases per 100,000 males). The rate of *Chlamydia* among black men and women was 5.9 times the rate among whites (1097.6 and 187.6 cases per 100,000 population, respectively). The rate among Hispanics was 2.0 times the rate among whites.[3]

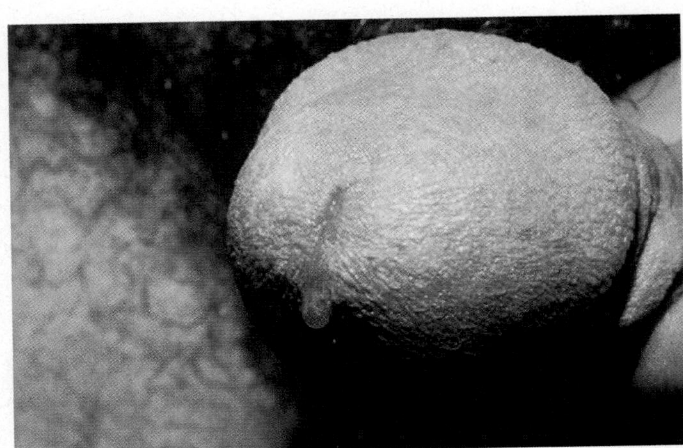

FIGURE 224-2 Nongonococcal urethritis caused by *Chlamydia*. Note that the discharge is clearer and less purulent than seen with gonorrhea. (*Reproduced with permission from Seattle STD/HIV Prevention Training Center, University of Washington.*)

ETIOLOGY AND PATHOPHYSIOLOGY

- Urethritis is urethral inflammation caused by infectious or noninfectious causes.
- *Neisseria gonorrhoeae* and *Chlamydia trachomatis* are the most important infectious causes. When transmitted, they can cause other illnesses and complications in men (epididymitis, prostatitis, and reactive arthritis) and women (pelvic inflammatory disease and infertility).
- Other infectious agents include *Mycoplasma genitalium*, *Ureaplasma urealyticum*, *Trichomonas vaginalis*, herpes simplex viruses 1 and 2, adenovirus, and enteric bacteria.
- Noninfectious causes include trauma, foreign bodies, granulomas or unusual tumors, allergic reactions, or voiding dysfunction (any abnormal holding or voiding pattern not caused by an anatomic or neurologic process).

DIAGNOSIS

CLINICAL FEATURES

Male patients with urethritis can be asymptomatic or present with urethral discharge, dysuria, or urethral pruritus.

Urethritis is diagnosed when one of the following is present[4]:

- Mucopurulent or purulent urethral discharge (see **Figures 224-1** and **224-2**).
- First-void urine positive leukocyte esterase test ≥10 white blood cells (WBCs) per high-power field. (This can also be seen with a urinary tract infection [UTI]; however, the incidence of UTI in men younger than 50 years of age is approximately 50 per 100,000 per year, much lower than the incidence of gonococcal or chlamydial urethritis in this age group.)

LABORATORY TESTING

- Nucleic acid amplification test (NAAT) is the recommended test for screening asymptomatic at-risk men and testing symptomatic men.[4] Urine is a better specimen than urethral swab and does not hurt.[4,5]
- Gram stain of urethral secretions with ≥5 WBC per oil immersion field. (If Gram-negative intracellular diplococci are seen, gonococcal urethritis is present.) Gram stain will identify most cases; ≥5 WBCs are seen in 82% of *Chlamydia* and 94% of gonococcal infections.[6] Government regulations concerning in-office laboratory testing have severely curtailed the use of Gram stains in the office.
- Consider culture when tests for gonorrhea and *Chlamydia* are negative, or symptoms persist despite adequate treatment in a patient who is unlikely to have been reinfected by an untreated partner.

DIFFERENTIAL DIAGNOSIS

Dysuria in men can be caused by the following[7]:

- Infections in other sites of the urogenital tract—Cystitis, prostatitis with perineal pain or prostate tenderness, or epididymitis with scrotal pain.
- Penile lesions—Vesicles of herpes simplex, ulcers of syphilis, chancroid, or lymphogranuloma venereum, and glans irritation from balanitis.
- Mechanical causes—Obstruction from benign prostatic hyperplasia (BPH) causing inflammation without infection, trauma including catheterization, urethral strictures, or genitourinary cancers.
- Inflammatory conditions—Spondyloarthropathies, drug reactions, or autoimmune diseases.

MANAGEMENT

Treat patients who meet criteria for urethritis. For patients with dysuria who do not meet criteria for urethritis, test for *N. gonorrhoeae* and *C. trachomatis* and treat if positive. Advise sex partners to be evaluated and treated.[8]

MEDICATIONS

- Gonococcal urethritis.
  - Ceftriaxone 250 mg IM with 1 g azithromycin is the standard of care.[8] SOR Ⓐ Dual therapy is recommended to lower the risk that antimicrobial resistance develops, and to empirically treat for *Chlamydia*.
  - Cefixime 400 mg orally (single dose) if ceftriaxone is unavailable[8] (with 1 g azithromycin).
  - Doxycyline 100 mg orally twice a day for 7 days is second-line therapy; use doxycycline (with ceftriaxone or cefixime) when azithromycin cannot be used (i.e., patient allergy).[8]
- *Chlamydia* urethritis.
  - Azithromycin 1 g orally in a single dose or doxycycline 100 mg orally twice a day for 7 days.[8] SOR Ⓐ
  - Acceptable alternative regimens include[8]:
    - Erythromycin base 500 mg 4 times a day for 7 days or erythromycin ethylsuccinate 800 mg 4 times a day for 7 days.
    - Ofloxacin 300 mg orally twice a day for 7 days or levofloxacin 500 mg orally once daily for 7 days.
- For persistent urethritis, consider *Trichomonas vaginalis* as a possible cause—Culture and treat with a single dose of metronidazole 2 g.
- Consider expedited partner therapy (EPT). EPT is the delivery of medications or prescriptions by persons infected with a sexually transmitted disease (STD) to their sex partners without clinical assessment of the partners. Legal status by state is available at http://www.cdc.gov/std/ept/legal/default.htm.

PREVENTION

- Educate patients on safer sex practices.
- Screening recommendations:
  - The U.S. Preventive Services Task Force concluded there was insufficient evidence to recommend screening for gonococcal or chlamydial infections in men.[9]
  - Centers for Disease Control and Prevention (CDC) guidelines suggest consideration of screening in settings with high

prevalence of *Chlamydia* (i.e., STD clinics or correctional facilities) or in populations with a high burden of infection (i.e., men who have sex with men).[8]

PROGNOSIS

Gonococcal and chlamydial urethritis respond well to appropriate antibiotic therapy. Partners must be treated to avoid reinfection.

FOLLOW-UP

- Reevaluate patients with persistent or recurrent symptoms after treatment. Reexamine for evidence of urethral inflammation and retest for gonorrhea and *Chlamydia*.
- Routine test-of-cure laboratory examination is not recommended by the CDC for gonorrhea or *Chlamydia* infections unless therapeutic compliance is in question, symptoms persist, or reinfection is suspected.[8]
- However, patients who have symptoms that persist after treatment of gonorrhea should be evaluated by culture for *N. gonorrhoeae*, and any gonococci isolated should be tested for antimicrobial susceptibility.[8]
- Consider chronic prostatitis if symptoms persist for more than 3 months.

PATIENT EDUCATION

The CDC recommends the following for patients diagnosed with gonorrhea or *Chlamydia*[8]:

- Return for evaluation if the symptoms persist or return after therapy is completed.
- Abstain from sexual intercourse until 7 days after starting therapy, symptoms have resolved, and sexual partners have been adequately treated.
- Undergo testing for other STDs, including HIV and syphilis.
- Advise sexual partners of the need for treatment and/or take medications directly to them using EPT.

PATIENT RESOURCES

- Centers for Disease Control and Prevention—**http://www.cdc.gov/std/Gonorrhea/STDFact-gonorrhea.htm.**
- Centers for Disease Control and Prevention—**http://www.cdc.gov/std/chlamydia/default.htm.**

PROVIDER RESOURCES

- The Centers for Disease Control and Prevention (CDC) website has the latest epidemiologic data and management recommendations—**http://www.cdc.gov/std/default.htm.**
- The newest CDC Treatment Guidelines are at **http://www.cdc.gov/std/treatment.**

REFERENCES

1. Terris MK. *Urethritis.* http://emedicine.medscape.com/article/438091. Updated September 8, 2016. Accessed March 2017.
2. U.S. Centers for Disease Control and Prevention. https://www.cdc.gov/std/stats15/gonorrhea.htm. Accessed March 2017.
3. U.S. Centers for Disease Control and Prevention. https://www.cdc.gov/std/stats15/chlamydia.htm. Accessed March 2017.
4. Brill JR. Diagnosis and treatment of urethritis in men. *Am Fam Physician.* 2010;81(7):873-878.
5. Sugunendran H, Birley HD, Mallinson H, et al. Comparison of urine, first and second endourethral swabs for PCR based detection of genital *Chlamydia trachomatis* infection in male patients. *Sex Transm Infect.* 2001;77(6):423-426.
6. Geisler WM, Yu S, Hook EW III. Chlamydial and gonococcal infection in men without polymorphonuclear leukocytes on Gram stain: implications for diagnostic approach and management. *Sex Transm Dis.* 2005;32(10):630-634.
7. Michels T, Sands J. Dysuria: Evaluation and differential diagnosis in adults. *Am Fam Physician.* 2015;92(9):778-788.
8. Centers for Disease Control and Prevention (CDC). *2015 Sexually Transmitted Diseases Treatment Guidelines.* https://www.cdc.gov/std/tg2015/default.htm. Accessed March 2017.
9. U.S. Preventive Services Task Force. Clinical Summary Chlamydia and Gonorrhea: Screening. Updated September 24, 2014. https://www.uspreventiveservicestaskforce.org.

225 SYPHILIS

Heidi S. Chumley, MD, MBA
Richard P. Usatine, MD

PATIENT STORY

A 39-year-old woman presents with a nonhealing ulcer over her upper lip for 1 week and a new-onset rash on her trunk (**Figures 225-1** and **225-2**). The ulcer on her upper lip was misdiagnosed as herpes simplex by another physician. Sexual history revealed that the patient had oral sex with a boyfriend who had a lesion on his penis and she suspected that he had been having sex with other women. The examining physician recognized the nonpainful ulcer and rash as a combination of primary and secondary (P&S) syphilis. An RPR (rapid plasma reagin) was drawn and the patient was treated immediately with IM benzathine penicillin. The RPR came back as 1:128 and the ulcer was healed within 1 week.

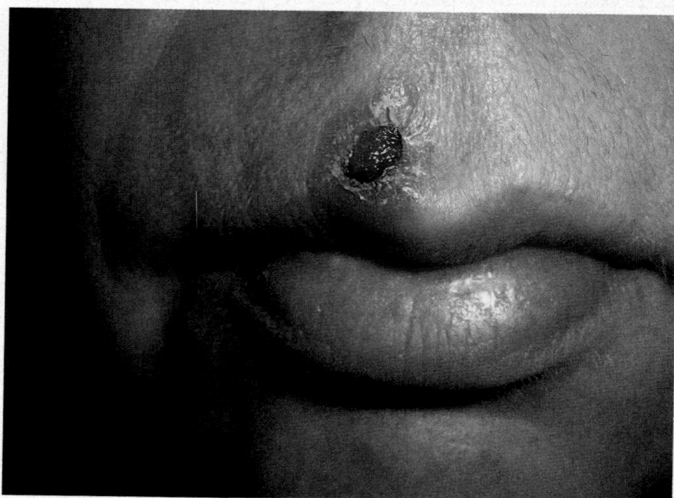

FIGURE 225-1 Primary syphilis with a chancre over the lip of a woman. *(Reproduced with permission from Richard P. Usatine, MD.)*

INTRODUCTION

Syphilis, caused by *Treponema pallidum*, is a systemic disease characterized by multiple overlapping stages: primary syphilis (ulcer), secondary syphilis (skin rash, mucocutaneous lesions, or lymphadenopathy), tertiary syphilis (cardiac or gummatous lesions), and early or late latent syphilis (positive serology without clinical manifestations). Neurosyphilis can occur at any stage. Diagnosis is made using treponemal and nontreponemal tests. Treatment is penicillin; the dose and duration depend on the stage.

SYNONYMS AND ACRONYMS

Lues is another word for syphilis.

Nontreponemal tests:

- VDRL—Venereal Disease Research Laboratory.
- RPR—Rapid plasma reagin.

Treponemal tests:

- EIA—Enzyme immunoassay.
- TP-PA—*T. pallidum* particle agglutination.
- FTA-ABS—Fluorescent treponemal antibody absorption.
- MHA-TP—Microhemagglutination assay for *T. pallidum*.

EPIDEMIOLOGY

- In 2015, 23,872 cases of primary and secondary (P&S) syphilis were reported to the Centers for Disease Control and Prevention (CDC), an increase of 19%, reaching a rate of 7.5 cases per 100,000 population.[1]
- During 2013–2015, the rate of P&S syphilis increased 18.1% among men (from 11.7 to 13.9 cases per 100,000 men) and 27.3% among women (from 1.1 to 1.4 cases per 100,000 women).[1]

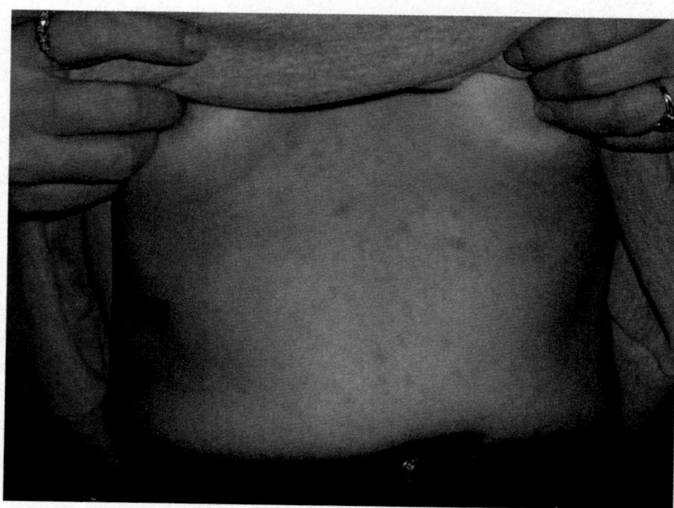

FIGURE 225-2 A nonpruritic rash of secondary syphilis on the abdomen of the patient shown in **Figure 225-1**. *(Reproduced with permission from Richard P. Usatine, MD.)*

- In 2015, the rate of P&S syphilis was highest among persons aged 20–24 years and 25–29 years (20.8 and 23.5 cases per 100,000 population, respectively).[1]
- Men who have sex with men (MSM) accounted for 59% of the syphilis cases reported in 2015.[1]
- Syphilis rates vary by races/ethnicities. In 2015, the rates among black, Hispanic, and white persons were 21.4, 9.1, and 4.1 cases per 100,000 persons, respectively.[1]
- HIV-infected patients were found to have syphilis rates of 62.3 per 1000 compared to 0.8 per 1000 in HIV uninfected patients in a population study in California.[2] In patients with syphilis, co-infection with HIV was found in 49.8% of MSM, 10.0% of men who have sex with women only, and 3.9% of women.[1]

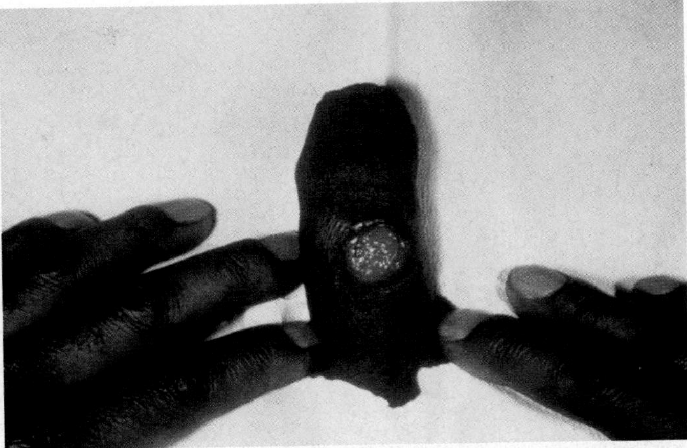

FIGURE 225-3 A painless chancre at the location of treponemal entry. *(Reproduced with permission from Public Health Image Library, Centers for Disease Control and Prevention.)*

ETIOLOGY AND PATHOPHYSIOLOGY

- Syphilis is caused by the spirochete *T. pallidum* and contracted through direct sexual contact with primary or secondary lesions. Congenital syphilis can be contracted across the placenta.

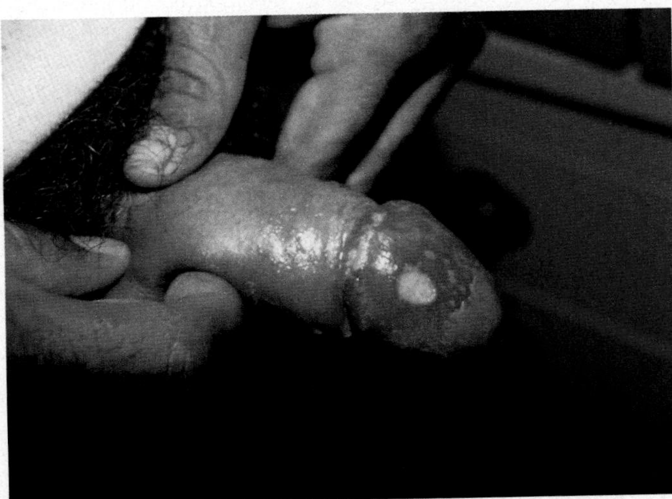

FIGURE 225-4 Primary syphilis with a large chancre on the glans of the penis. The multiple small surrounding ulcers are part of the syphilis and not a second disease. *(Reproduced with permission from Richard P. Usatine, MD.)*

RISK FACTORS

- Sexual contact, especially oral or anal, with a person with primary or secondary syphilis.
- MSM.
- Prostitution.
- Sex for drugs.
- HIV/AIDS.

DIAGNOSIS

CLINICAL FEATURES

- Primary syphilis is associated with a chancre, an ulcer that is usually not painful (**Figures 225-1, 225-3, and 225-4**). The presence of pain does not rule out syphilis, and the patient with a painful genital ulcer should be tested for both syphilis and herpes.
- Secondary syphilis occurs when the spirochetes become systemic and may present as a rash with protean morphologies, condyloma lata, and/or mucous patches (**Figures 225-2 and 225-5 to 225-11**).
- Tertiary syphilis may be visualized with gummas on the skin, but many of the manifestations are internal, such as the cardiac and neurologic diseases that occur (e.g., aortitis, tabes dorsalis, and iritis). **Figure 225-12** shows a gumma of the scrotum.
- Neurosyphilis can occur at any stage. Clinical symptoms include cognitive dysfunction, vision or hearing loss, uveitis or iritis, motor or sensory abnormalities, cranial nerve palsies, or symptoms of meningitis.

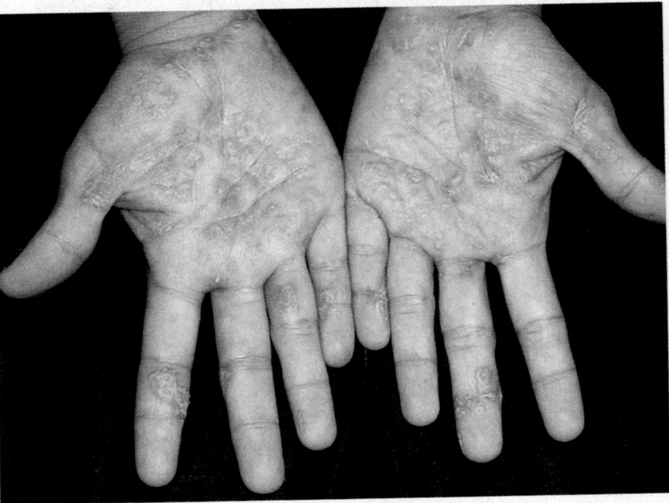

FIGURE 225-5 Papular squamous eruption on the hands of a woman with secondary syphilis. *(Reproduced with permission from Richard P. Usatine, MD.)*

TYPICAL DISTRIBUTION

- Primary syphilis is usually a single ulcer (chancre) that is not painful in the genital region (see **Figures 225-3 and 225-4**). A chancre can be seen on the lip (see **Figure 225-1**).

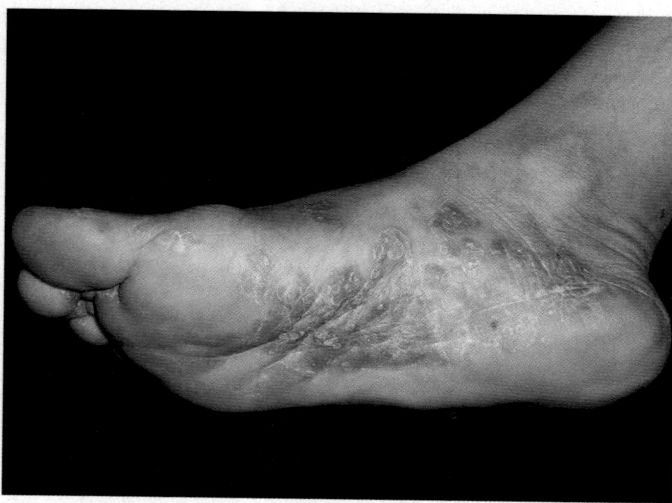

FIGURE 225-6 Papular squamous eruption on the foot of the woman in **Figure 225-5**, with secondary syphilis. (*Reproduced with permission from Richard P. Usatine, MD.*)

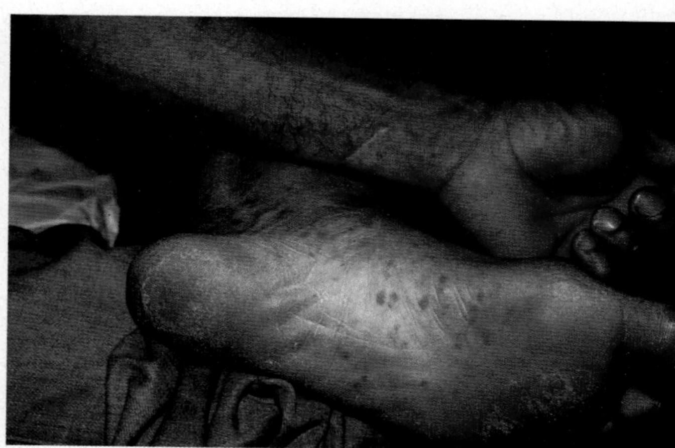

FIGURE 225-8 Pink macules on the feet and wrists of a man with secondary syphilis. (*Reproduced with permission from Richard P. Usatine, MD.*)

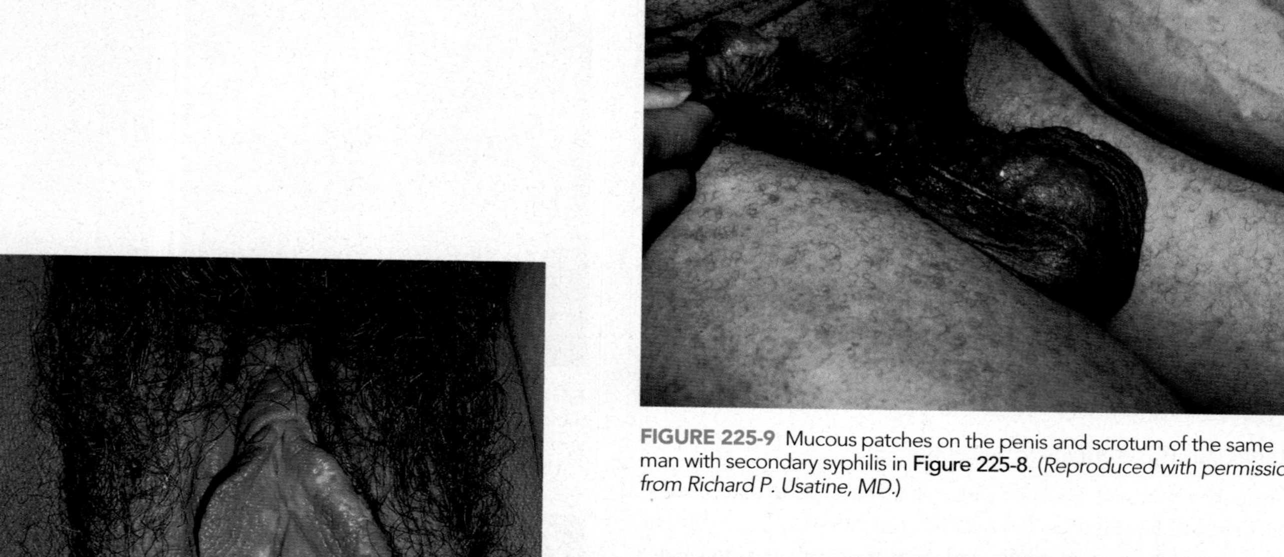

FIGURE 225-9 Mucous patches on the penis and scrotum of the same man with secondary syphilis in **Figure 225-8**. (*Reproduced with permission from Richard P. Usatine, MD.*)

FIGURE 225-7 Mucous patches on the labia of the woman in **Figure 225-5**, with secondary syphilis teeming with spirochetes. (*Reproduced with permission from Richard P. Usatine, MD.*)

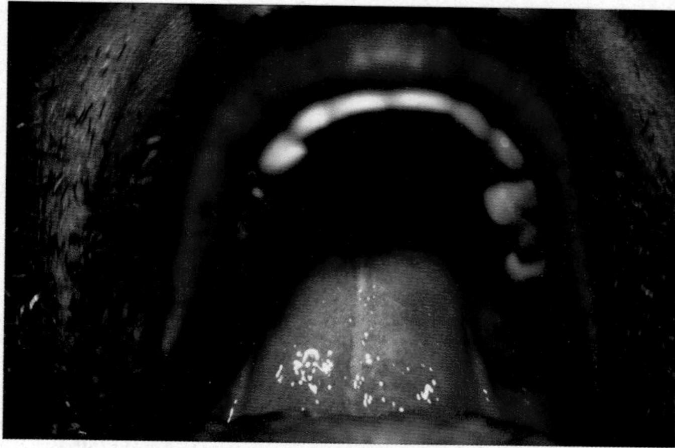

FIGURE 225-10 Oral lesion on the palate of the same man with secondary syphilis in **Figure 225-9**. (*Reproduced with permission from Richard P. Usatine, MD.*)

- Secondary syphilis may present with various eruptions on the trunk, palms, and soles (**Figures 225-2, 225-5, 225-6, 225-8, 225-13, 225-14, and 225-15**).
- Mucous patches are on the genitals or in the mouth (see **Figures 225-7, 225-9,** and **225-10**).

LABORATORY TESTING

- Serologic tests are either nontreponemal (RPR or VDRL), which measure anticardiolipin antibodies, or treponemal (EIA, TP-PA, FTA-ABS, or MHA-TP), which measure antibodies to *T. pallidum*.
- There are two algorithms for laboratory testing currently in use around the world:
    1. Start with a low-cost nontreponemal test and confirm a positive result with a treponemal test.
    2. Start with the EIA treponemal test, followed by a nontreponemal test for confirmation.
- Nontreponemal tests are reported qualitatively (reactive or nonreactive) and quantitatively (titer); a fourfold change in titer is considered significant. When testing sequentially, use the same test and same laboratory. Seventy-five percent to 85% of patients will remain reactive after successful treatment.[3]
- A positive treponemal test should be confirmed with a non-treponemal test. If the non-treponemal test is nonreactive, perform a second treponemal test. If the second treponemal test is positive and the patient was previously treated and not likely reinfected, no treatment is needed. If the patient was not previously treated, consider this a positive result and offer treatment.[3]
- Dark-field microscopy is useful in evaluating moist cutaneous lesions, such as chancre, mucous patches, and condyloma lata (**Figure 225-16**).
- Test all patients with syphilis for HIV.
- Patients with syphilis who have any signs or symptoms suggesting neurologic disease including vision or hearing need a cerebrospinal fluid (CSF) exam, a slit-lamp ophthalmologic examination, and an otologic examination to determine if neurosyphilis is present.

DIFFERENTIAL DIAGNOSIS

- Herpes simplex—Most common cause of genital ulcers in the United States. These ulcers are painful and often start as vesicles (see Chapter 135, Herpes Simplex).
- Chancroid—Painful beefy red ulcers on the penis or vulva, less common than syphilis. Chancroid is also known to cause large painful inguinal adenopathy (bubo) (**Figures 225-17** and **225-18**).
- Drug eruptions—Can be on the genital area such as seen in a fixed drug eruption. Also, whole-body drug eruptions can appear, similar to secondary syphilis (see Chapter 212, Cutaneous Drug Reactions).
- Erythema multiforme—Can look like the rash of secondary syphilis but may have target lesions (see Chapter 185, Erythema Multiforme, Stevens-Johnson Syndrome, and Toxic Epidermal Necrolysis).
- Pityriasis rosea—A self-limited cutaneous eruption that often begins with a herald patch and may have a Christmas-tree distribution on the back (see Chapter 159, Pityriasis Rosea).

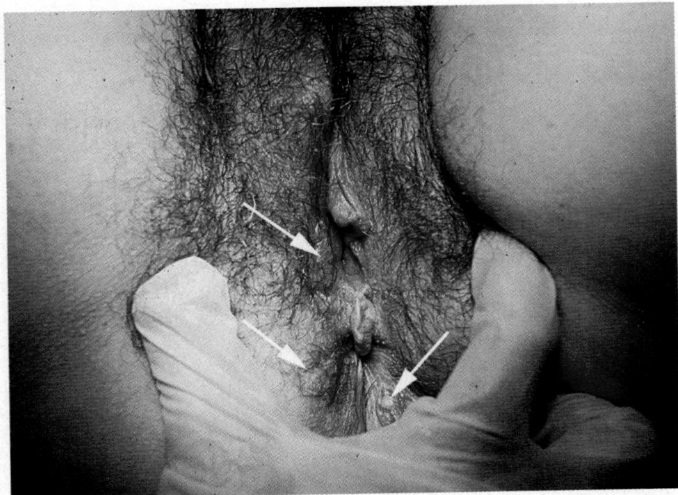

FIGURE 225-11 Condylomata lata (*arrows*) on the vulva of a woman with secondary syphilis. (*Reproduced with permission from Richard P. Usatine, MD.*)

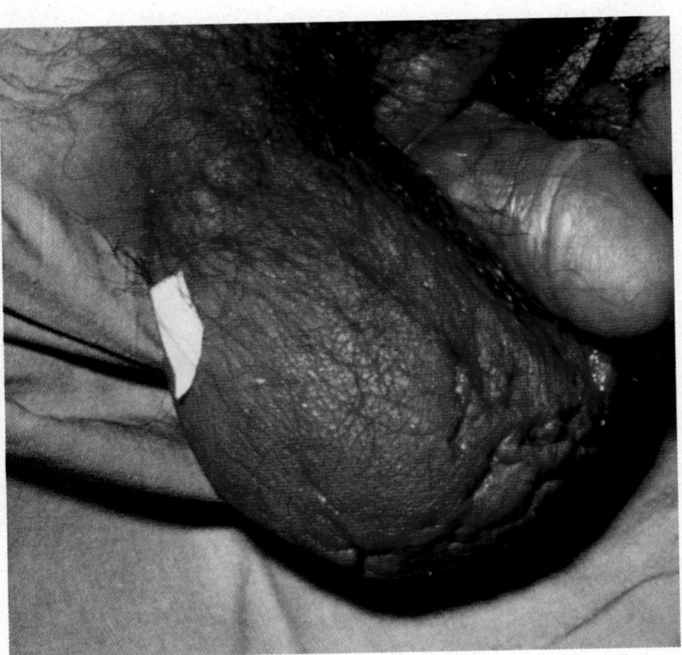

FIGURE 225-12 Tertiary syphilis presenting as a swollen scrotum, which was diagnosed as a syphilitic gumma of the testicle. (*Reproduced with permission from Public Health Image Library, Centers for Disease Control and Prevention.*)

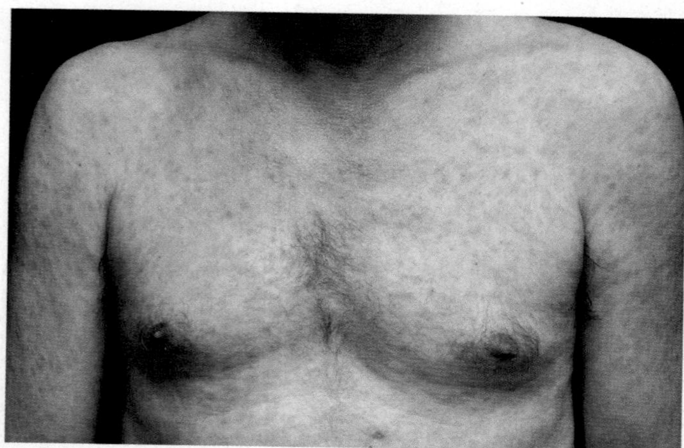

FIGURE 225-13 Middle-age married man with diffuse eruption of secondary syphilis from neck to feet. The eruption remained undiagnosed for months as the patient denied any risk factors. His RPR was 1:256. (*Reproduced with permission from Richard P. Usatine, MD.*)

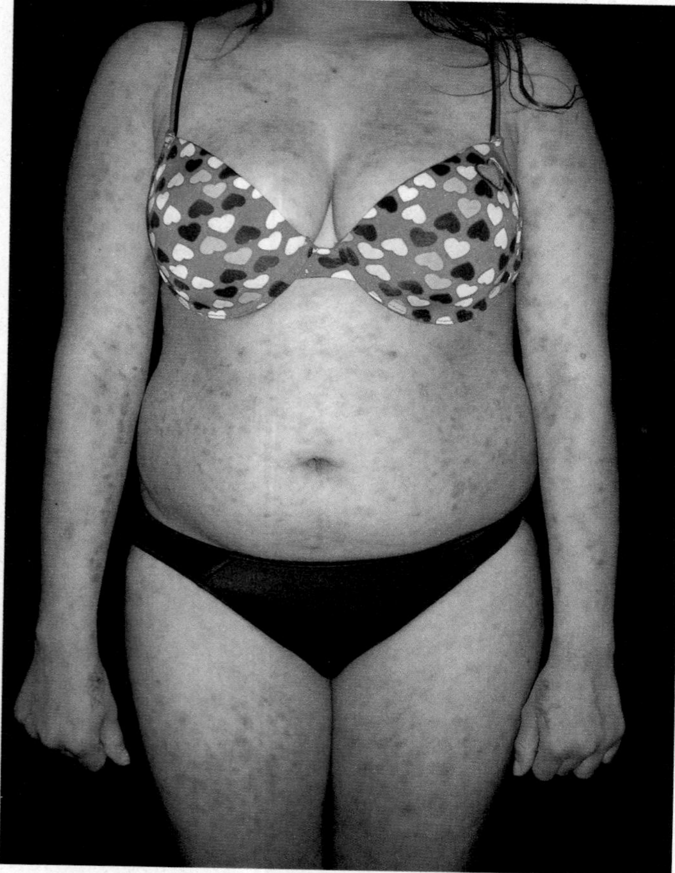

FIGURE 225-14 Secondary syphilis in a 20-year-old woman with a history of injection drug use and multiple sexual partners. Her HIV test was also positive. (*Reproduced with permission from Richard P. Usatine, MD.*)

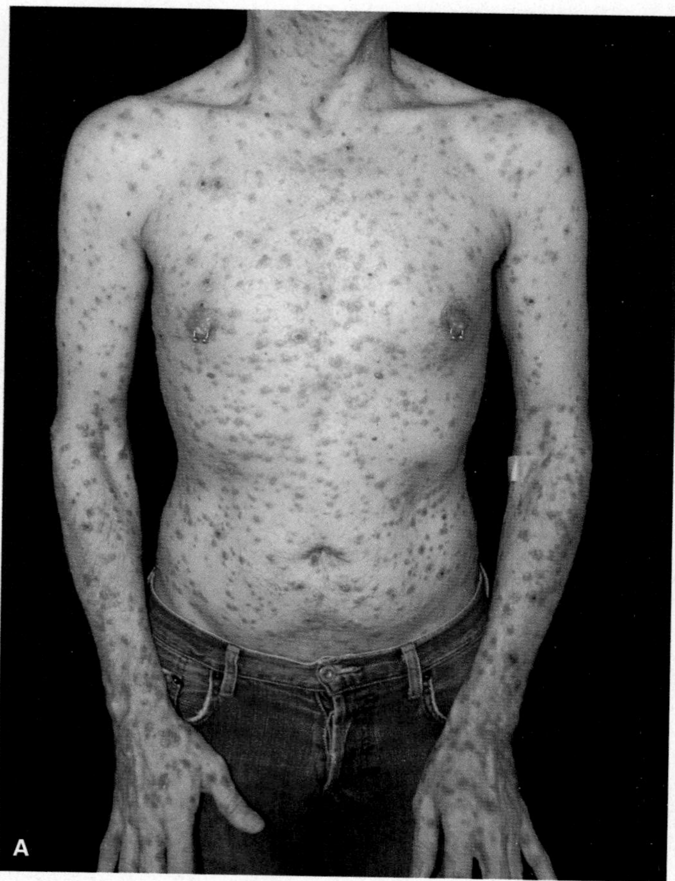

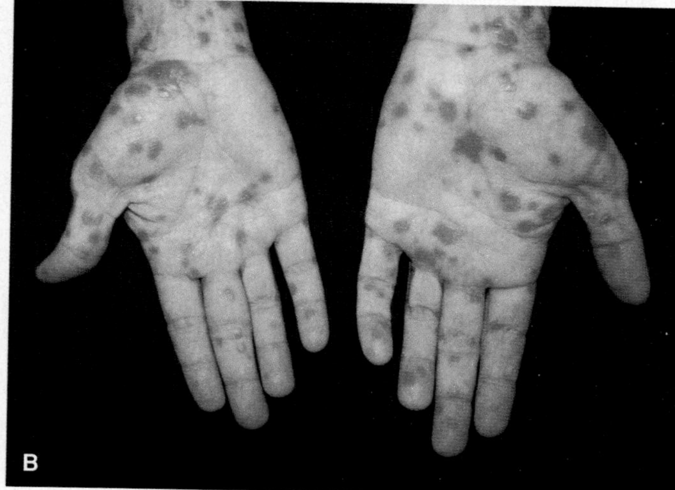

FIGURE 225-15 Secondary syphilis in a young man with known HIV/AIDS. **A.** Impressive red papulosquamous eruption from head to toe is present. **B.** Close-up showing the palmar patches and plaques. (*Reproduced with permission from Jonathan B. Karnes, MD.*)

MANAGEMENT

MEDICATIONS

Benzathine penicillin is the treatment of choice for all stages of syphilis. Dose and duration depend on stage.[3]

- Primary, secondary, and early latent (immunocompetent and nonpregnant):
  - Adults: Benzathine penicillin G 2.4 million U IM one time.
  - Children older than 1 month with acquired primary or secondary: 50,000 U/kg IM up to 2.4 million U one time.
- Penicillin allergy:
  - Doxycycline 100 mg twice daily × 14 days or tetracycline 500 mg four times a day for 14 days.
  - Ceftriaxone 1 g IM/IV daily × 10 to 14 days (limited studies) *or*
  - Azithromycin 2 g single oral dose; however, azithromycin resistance has been documented in several areas of the United States. Use only when penicillin or doxycycline cannot be used. Do not use in MSM, persons with HIV, or pregnant women.
  - Penicillin desensitization and subsequent treatment with benzathine penicillin.
- Late latent syphilis or syphilis of unknown duration:
  - Adults: Benzathine penicillin G 2.4 million U IM once a week for 3 weeks.
  - Children: 50,000 U/kg IM (up to 2.4 million U) once a week for 3 weeks.
- Penicillin allergy: Doxycycline 100 mg twice a day for 28 days (or tetracycline 500 mg 4 times a day for 28 days) are the only acceptable alternatives.
- For the management of congenital, tertiary, and neurosyphilis, see the *2015 Sexually Transmitted Diseases Treatment Guidelines* published by the CDC at: https://www.cdc.gov/std/tg2015/syphilis.htm.

REFERRAL OR HOSPITALIZATION

- Refer patients when the stage of syphilis is unclear. Consider referral to an infectious disease specialist in children younger than 1 month of age, pregnant women with a penicillin allergy, patients with tertiary or neurosyphilis, or patients who have failed treatment.

PREVENTION

Primary prevention: Safer sex practices—sexual transmission occurs when mucocutaneous syphilitic lesions are present.

Secondary prevention:

- Treat presumptively (regardless of serology) sexual partners who were exposed within 90 days of the partner's diagnosis of primary, secondary, or early latent syphilis.
- Consider presumptive treatment when exposure was more than 90 days before partner's diagnosis if serology is unavailable or follow-up is uncertain.[3]

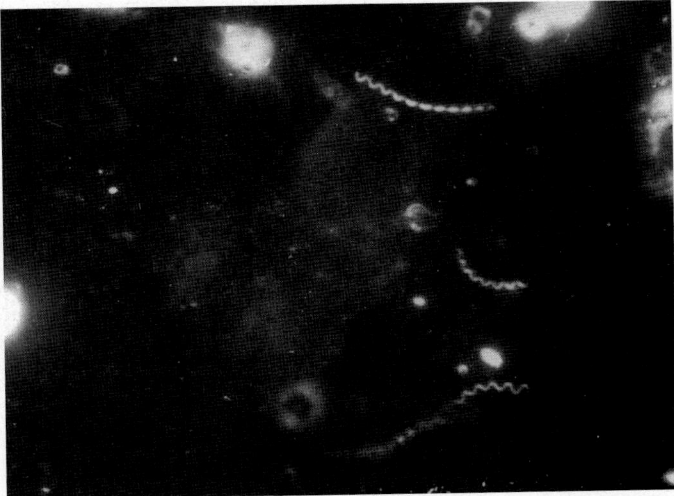

FIGURE 225-16 Live spirochetes of *T. pallidum* seen in a dark-field preparation. (*Reproduced with permission from Public Health Image Library, Centers for Disease Control and Prevention.*)

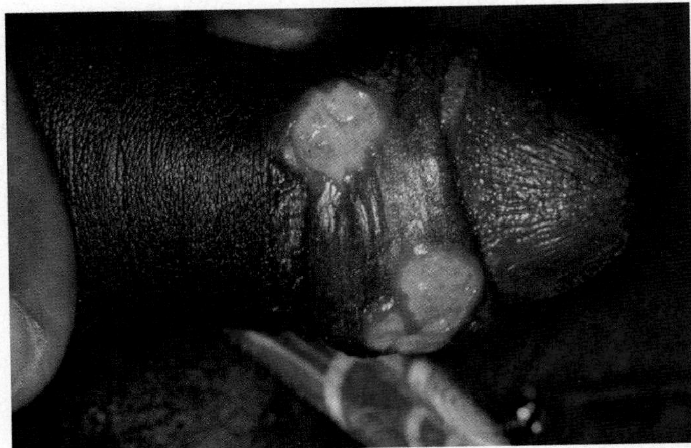

FIGURE 225-17 Culture-proven indurated beefy chancroidal ulcers in an HIV-positive man. (*Reproduced with permission from Richard P. Usatine, MD.*)

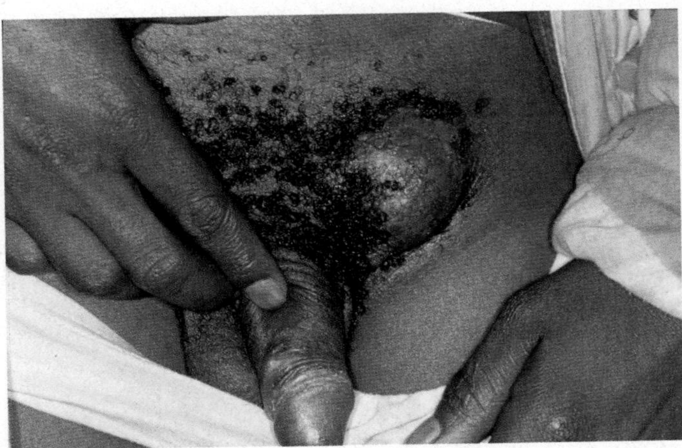

FIGURE 225-18 Left-side inguinal bubo in a patient with a culture-proven chancroidal ulcer. (*Reproduced with permission from Richard P. Usatine, MD.*)

PROGNOSIS

When syphilis is recognized and appropriately treated, the prognosis is excellent.

FOLLOW-UP

Reexamine clinically and attain a nontreponemal serologic test at 6, 12, and 24 months. Consider treatment failure if signs and/or symptoms persist or the nontreponemal test titer does not decline fourfold after 12 to 24 months of therapy.[3]

For treatment failures: Retest for HIV; perform a lumbar puncture for CSF analysis and treat for neurosyphilis if positive.[3]

PATIENT EDUCATION

Condoms can prevent the spread of syphilis. Patients should be advised to get HIV testing and need to know that syphilis is a risk factor for the spread of HIV. HIV/AIDS is also a risk factor for acquiring syphilis. Patients should be advised of the importance of completing treatment and follow-up to prevent complications.

PATIENT RESOURCES

- Centers for Disease Control and Prevention (CDC). *Sexually Transmitted Diseases (STDs): Syphilis—CDC Fact Sheet*—**http://www.cdc.gov/std/syphilis/stdfact-syphilis.htm.**

PROVIDER RESOURCES

- **http://emedicine.medscape.com/article/229461.**
- The Centers for Disease Control and Prevention. *2015 Sexually Transmitted Diseases Treatment Guidelines*—**https://www.cdc.gov/std/tg2015/default.htm.**

REFERENCES

1. Centers for Disease Control and Prevention (CDC). *2015 Sexually Transmitted Diseases Surveillance.* Syphilis. https://www.cdc.gov/std/stats15/syphilis.htm. Accessed March 2017.
2. Horberg MA, Ranatunga DK, Quesenberry CP, et al. Syphilis epidemiology and clinical outcomes in HIV-infected and HIV-uninfected patients in Kaiser Permanente Northern California. *Sex Transm Dis.* 2010;37(1):53-58.
3. Centers for Disease Control and Prevention (CDC). *2015 Sexually Transmitted Diseases Treatment Guidelines.* Syphilis. https://www.cdc.gov/std/tg2015/syphilis.htm. Accessed March 2017.

226 AIDS AND KAPOSI SARCOMA

Heidi S. Chumley, MD, MBA
Austin Baraki, MD

PATIENT STORY

A 35-year-old gay man presented with papular lesions on his elbow (**Figure 226-1**). Shave biopsy revealed Kaposi sarcoma (KS). He subsequently tested positive for HIV infection and began treatment with combination antiretroviral therapy. The KS lesions subsequently went into remission.

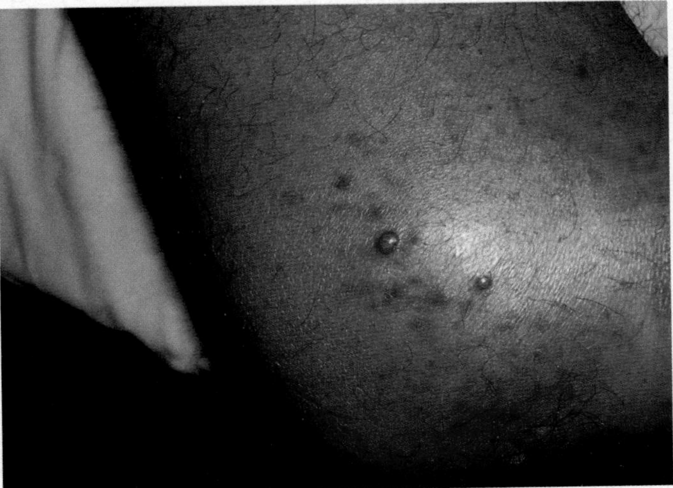

FIGURE 226-1 Several reddish-purple papular lesions of Kaposi sarcoma on the elbow of a man with human immunodeficiency virus/acquired immunodeficiency syndrome. (*Reproduced with permission from Heather Wickless, MD.*)

INTRODUCTION

In the United States, KS is most often seen in patients with AIDS and in organ transplant patients receiving immunosuppressive therapy. KS can also be classic-type (older Mediterranean men) or endemic-type (young men in sub-Saharan Africa). KS is caused by human herpesvirus 8 (HHV-8), also known as Kaposi sarcoma–associated herpesvirus (KSHV), which evades host immunity and promotes oncogenesis through multiple mechanisms. KS cannot be cured, but treatment can result in disease stabilization or remission. Current therapies aim to restore immune function or target KSHV directly. Therapies that directly target KSHV-mediated oncogenic signaling are being studied.

EPIDEMIOLOGY

- KS can be classic (older Mediterranean men), endemic (young men in sub-Saharan Africa), epidemic (AIDS patients), or organ transplant–associated.[1]
- In the United States, 81.6% of KS is seen in patients with AIDS[2] (see **Figure 226-1**).
- In HIV-positive patients, the prevalence is 7.2/1000 person years—451 times higher than general population.[3]
- In transplant patients, the prevalence is 1.4/1000 person years—128 times higher than general population.[3]
- The male-to-female ratio for epidemic KS in the United States is approximately 50:1 but is falling as the prevalence of AIDS increases among women.[4] The male-to-female ratio has been approximately 10:1 for classic and endemic KS.
- KS is the most common malignancy seen in AIDS patients, but incidence has been declining at a rate of approximately 6% to 8% per year in the highly active antiretroviral therapy (HAART) era since 2000–2005.

ETIOLOGY AND PATHOPHYSIOLOGY

- KS is caused by KSHV, also known as HHV-8. KSHV is a double-stranded DNA virus that infects numerous cell types throughout the body and expresses oncogenes that interfere with cell cycle regulation and host cell apoptosis.[5]

- KSHV contains a number of genes that allow it to evade host immunity by suppressing the interferon response, inhibiting autophagy, and blocking the natural killer (NK) cell–mediated response.[6]
- The specific mechanisms of viral transmission remain unknown; however, there is evidence implicating salivary shedding and sexual transmission in many cases.[7]
- KS is an angioproliferative neoplasm, demonstrating abnormal proliferation of endothelial cells, myofibroblasts, and monocytes.
- Lesions often begin as papules or patches and progress to plaques as proliferation continues. Some lesions ulcerate (nodular stage), and lymphedema can occur.

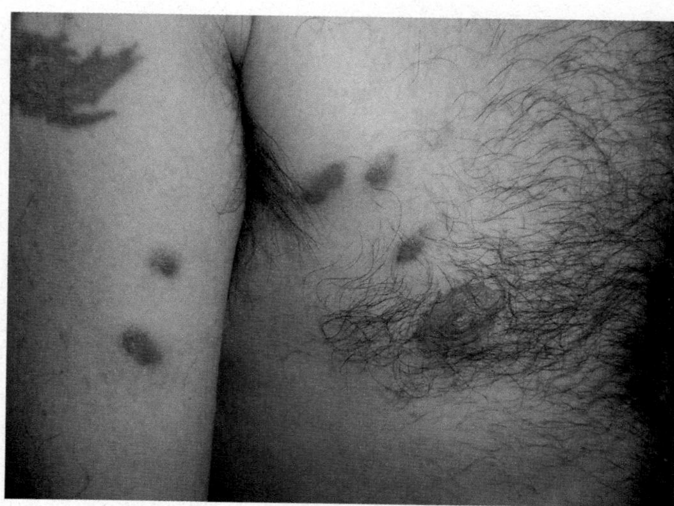

FIGURE 226-2 Kaposi sarcoma presenting as purplish-red papules on the chest and arm of an HIV-positive man. His KS was disseminated and was found in his colon. (*Reproduced with permission from Richard P. Usatine, MD.*)

RISK FACTORS

- HHV-8 infection.
- Immunodeficiency or immunosuppression (particularly T-cell immunity).
- Male gender, especially men who have sex with men (MSM).
- Cigarette smoking appears to provide a protective effect for KS but is otherwise terrible for one's health.[8]

DIAGNOSIS

A presumptive clinical diagnosis is often made in a patient who has AIDS and a typical presentation of KS. In atypical presentations, biopsy is required for diagnosis.

CLINICAL FEATURES

- Cutaneous lesions are usually multifocal, papular, and reddish-purple in color (**Figures 226-1** and **226-2**).
- Plaques or fungating lesions can be seen on the lower extremities, including the soles of the feet (**Figure 226-3**).
  - Vascular-appearing papules on the feet and lower legs are typical of classic KS without AIDS (**Figure 226-4**).
- Oral cavity lesions can be flat or nodular and are red to purple in color (**Figure 226-5**).
- Gastrointestinal lesions can be asymptomatic or can cause abdominal pain, nausea, vomiting, bleeding, diarrhea, obstruction, or weight loss.
- Pulmonary lesions can cause shortness of breath or may appear as infiltrates, nodules, or pleural effusions on chest radiograph.

TYPICAL DISTRIBUTION

AIDS-related KS[9]:

- Skin lesions are seen mainly on the lower extremities (**Figures 226-6** and **226-7**), face, and genitalia. Presence of skin lesions should prompt an oral examination, as oral involvement may change prognosis and management.
- Lesions in the oral cavity are common (33%), typically seen on the palate (see **Figure 226-5**) or gingiva (**Figure 226-8**).

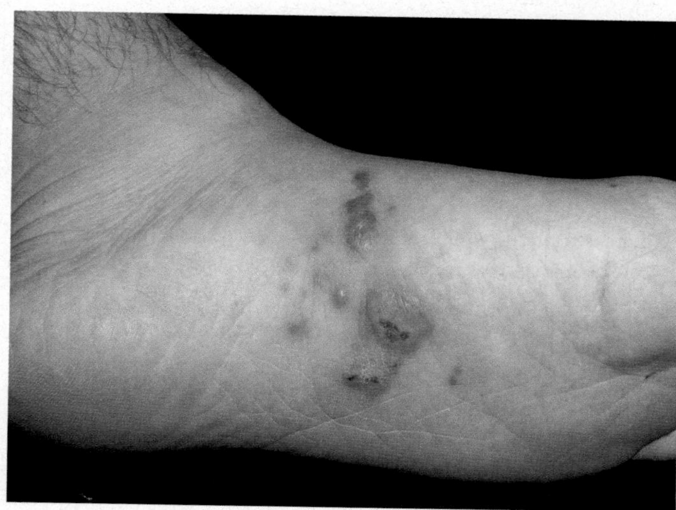

FIGURE 226-3 Kaposi sarcoma on the foot of a 28-year-old HIV-positive man. Note the purplish-red color. (*Reproduced with permission from Richard P. Usatine, MD.*)

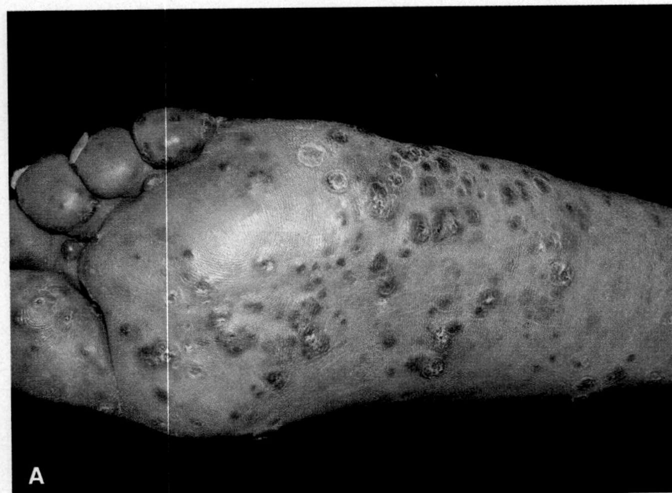

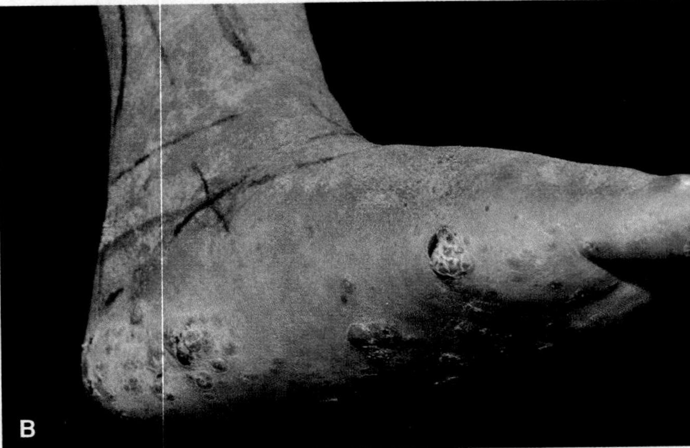

FIGURE 226-4 **A.** Classic Kaposi sarcoma on the foot of an 85-year-old Hispanic man from Mexico who is HIV negative. He initially declined radiation, and his lesions grew and multiplied over 3 years. **B.** He is receiving palliative radiation to improve his ability to walk. (*Reproduced with permission from Richard P. Usatine, MD.*)

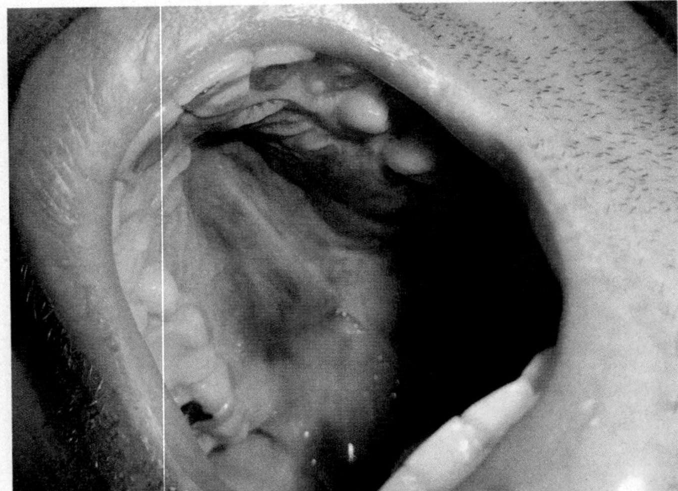

FIGURE 226-5 Kaposi sarcoma presenting with purplish-red color on the palate of the same man in **Figure 226-2.** Always look in the mouth when suspecting KS. (*Reproduced with permission from Richard P. Usatine, MD.*)

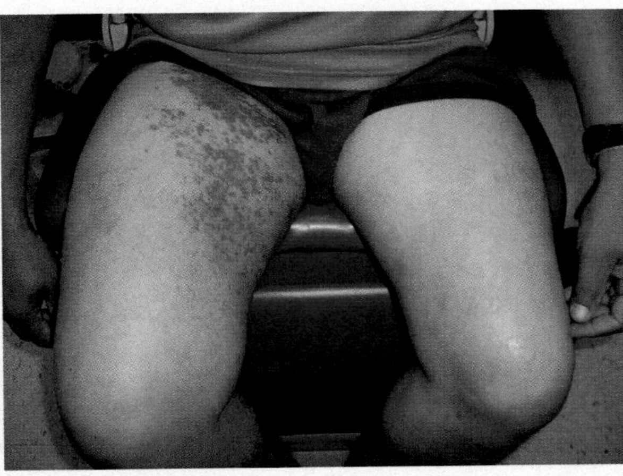

FIGURE 226-6 Kaposi sarcoma in a 43-year-old man with HIV/AIDS already on antiretroviral therapy. He presented with a diffuse rash and lymphedema in the right leg. The initial biopsy was negative, but a second biopsy demonstrated Kaposi sarcoma. The right leg is significantly larger than the left leg due to the lymphedema. (*Reproduced with permission from Richard P. Usatine, MD.*)

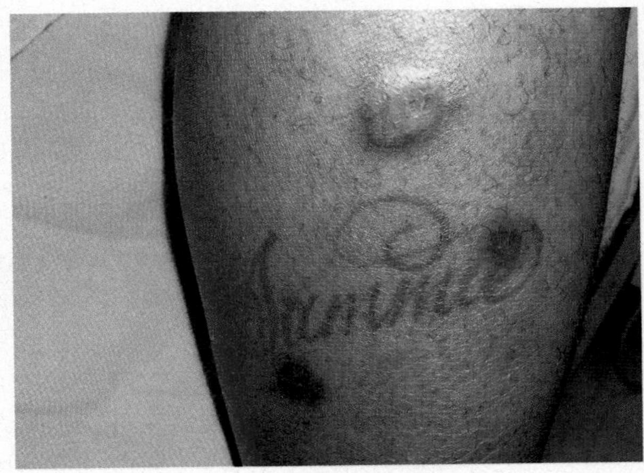

FIGURE 226-7 Kaposi sarcoma (KS) on the lower leg of a 23-year-old African-American man with HIV/AIDS. His lesions are dark brown to black rather than pink or purple. It is important to note that the classic colors described in white skin are often not found in dark skin. Any persistent skin nodule in an HIV-positive person should be suspect for KS, and a biopsy is the best method for a definitive diagnosis. (*Reproduced with permission from Richard P. Usatine, MD.*)

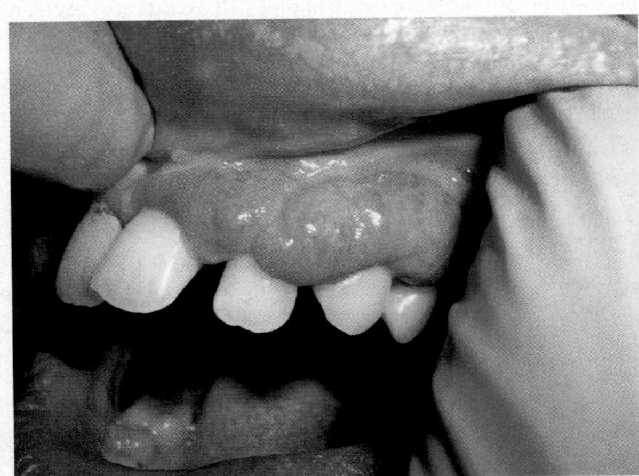

FIGURE 226-8 Kaposi sarcoma causing gingival hypertrophy. Always look in the mouth when suspecting KS. (*Reproduced with permission from Richard P. Usatine, MD.*)

- Gastrointestinal involvement is noted in 40% of newly diagnosed KS in HIV patients at diagnosis and up to 80% in autopsy studies. GI lesions can occur without skin lesions and may occur anywhere in the GI tract.
- Pulmonary involvement is common, and up to 15% may occur without skin lesions in patients with KS and AIDS. Pulmonary KS may involve the parenchyma, airways, lymph nodes, or pleura and may be seen on chest radiograph or CT.
- KS may occur in essentially all visceral organs.

LABORATORY TESTING

- Test for HIV infection in any patient with KS who is not already known to be infected.
- CD4+ T-lymphocyte count is an important prognostic indicator.
- Fecal occult blood testing may be used to screen for GI involvement.

IMAGING

Chest radiograph to evaluate for pulmonary involvement. Endoscopy may be performed if GI involvement is suspected based on symptoms or laboratory testing.

BIOPSY

Often required for definitive diagnosis. If the lesions are nodular, a simple shave biopsy should be sufficient (**Figure 226-9**). If the lesions are flat, a 4-mm punch biopsy should provide adequate tissue for diagnosis.

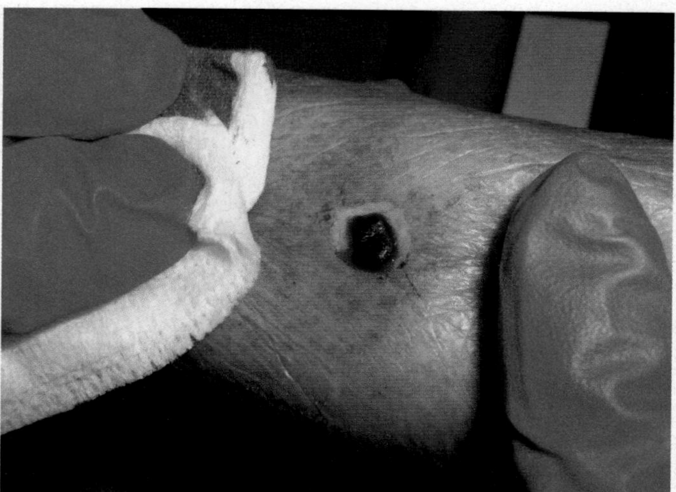

FIGURE 226-9 A shave biopsy of Kaposi sarcoma on the leg demonstrates the vascularity of these lesions. Curettage and electrodesiccation right after the shave biopsy can potentially remove this lesion. (*Reproduced with permission from Richard P. Usatine, MD.*)

DIFFERENTIAL DIAGNOSIS

The diagnosis of KS requires a biopsy, as several other lesions can mimic early KS.[9]

- Purpura—Bleeding under the skin caused by a variety of platelet, vascular, or coagulation disorders; usually not palpable and more widespread.
- Hematoma—Localized swelling, usually from a break in a blood vessel; often a history of trauma will be present and lesions may not be palpable.
- Hemangiomas or angiomas—Benign growths of small blood vessels that blanch with pressure (see Chapter 210, Acquired Vascular Skin Lesions).
- Dermatofibromas—Small, firm, red-to-brown nodules made up of histiocytes and collagen deposits in the mid-dermis, often seen on the legs; lesions are usually small (<6 mm) and dimple downward when compressed laterally (see Chapter 166, Dermatofibroma).
- Bacillary angiomatosis—A systemic infectious disease caused by *Bartonella* species. Cutaneous lesions appear as scattered papules and nodules or an abscess. Bacillary angiomatosis may occur when the CD4 count is below 200 cells/mm^3 and is treated with antibiotics (**Figure 226-10**).

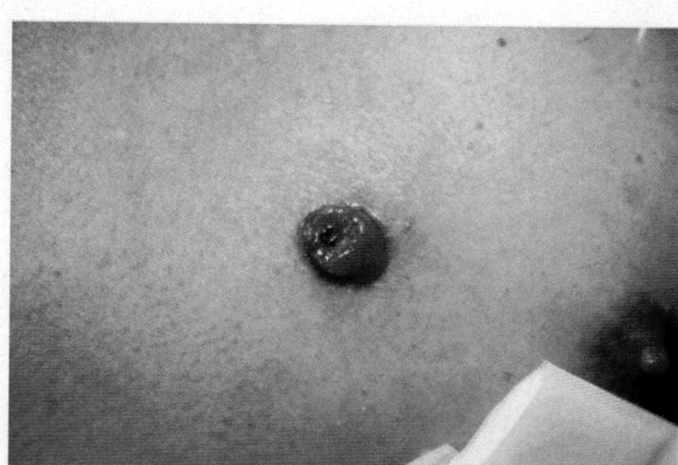

FIGURE 226-10 Cutaneous bacillary angiomatosis in a man with HIV/AIDS. (*Reproduced with permission from Usatine RP, Moy RL, Tobinick EL, et al. Skin Surgery: A Practical Guide. St. Louis, MO: Mosby; 1998.*)

MANAGEMENT

KS is not curable, but treatments can reduce disease burden and prevent progression (see **Figure 226-9**). Unfortunately, the U.S. Food and Drug Administration (FDA)-approved treatments for KS have not changed in 20 years.[10]

FIRST LINE

- In patients with HIV/AIDS, antiretroviral therapy (ART) is the first line of therapy. Treat with ART or refer to a physician with experience managing these medications. ART inhibits HIV replication and facilitates immune reconstitution. However, initiation of ART can trigger the immune reconstitution inflammatory syndrome (IRIS), which is associated with rapid progression of KS. SOR Ⓐ
- Consider KS-specific therapies:
  - Alitretinoin gel 0.1%—Patient applies gel to lesions 2 times a day, increasing to 3 to 4 times a day if tolerated, for 4 to 8 weeks (35% response rate).[11] SOR Ⓐ
  - Liposomal doxorubicin 20 mg/m^2 every 3 weeks or liposomal daunorubicin 40 mg/m^2 every 2 weeks (50% response rate).[12] SOR Ⓐ
  - Paclitaxel 100 mg/m^2 every 2 weeks or 135 mg/m^2 every 3 weeks; response rates 60% to 70% in patients who had failed a prior chemotherapy regiment.[13] SOR Ⓐ

  Premedication with dexamethasone is recommended.[13]
  - Interferon-α at 1 million U/day demonstrated the most benefit to patients with KS limited to the skin and CD4+ T-lymphocyte counts more than 200.[14]
  - Intralesional vinblastine (70% response rate)[15] or radiation therapy (80% response rate) are also effective for skin lesions.[16] SOR Ⓐ
- Removing immunosuppression or using radiation can treat transplant-related KS.

SECOND LINE

- In addition to the medications that target KSHV, experimental therapies are undergoing study that target KSHV-mediating signaling, including imatinib, imiquimod, thalidomide, *mTOR* inhibitors, and *VEGF* inhibitors, among others.[5]
- Topical timolol 0.1% and 0.5% has been used to successfully treat localized classic and HIV-related KS in a number of case reports.[18,19] Timolol 0.5% can be prescribed as ophthalmic timolol. Patients applied the timolol twice daily for 4–6 weeks without any side effects. Resolution was reported up to 10 months.
- Avoid high-dose corticosteroids, as they can severely aggravate KS, especially pulmonary KS.

RADIATION OR SURGERY

- Classic and endemic KS are often treated with radiation (see **Figure 226-4**) or surgery.
- Small numbers of skin lesions can be treated with electrodesiccation and curettage or cryosurgery. SOR Ⓒ

PROGNOSIS

- In severe disease requiring systemic therapy, 50% to 85% of patients will respond with either improvement or disease stability; however, the response lasts only 6 to 7 months before therapy has to be repeated. When therapy is repeated, the response times generally decrease.[5]
- Patients with AIDS-related KS have 5-year survival rates of greater than 80% when KS is the AIDS-defining illness and the CD4+ T-lymphocyte count is greater than 200. Survival rates fall to less than 10% when the patient is older than age 50 years and there is another AIDS-defining illness at the time of presentation.[17]

FOLLOW-UP

KS, particularly AIDS-related KS, is generally treated by physicians with advanced training in HIV/AIDS management and oncology. Follow-up is determined by disease progression and response to therapy.

PATIENT EDUCATION

- KS is not curable, but treatment can result in regression of lesions for a better cosmetic result.
- KS can affect most parts of the body, commonly the skin, oral cavity, GI tract, and lungs.
- During treatment, lesions typically flatten, shrink, and fade (see **Figure 226-8**).
- Rarely, starting ART may cause lesions to flare because of an inflammatory reaction as the immune system begins to recover (IRIS).

PATIENT RESOURCES

- The National Cancer Institute. *Kaposi Sarcoma Treatment*—**https://www.cancer.gov/types/soft-tissue-sarcoma/patient/kaposi-treatment-pdq.**

PROVIDER RESOURCES

- The National Cancer Institute has information for health professionals—**https://www.cancer.gov/types/soft-tissue-sarcoma/hp/kaposi-treatment-pdq.**

REFERENCES

1. Curtiss P, Strazzulla LC, Friedman-Kien AE. An update on Kaposi's sarcoma: epidemiology, pathogenesis and treatment. *Dermatol Ther (Heidelb)*. 2016;6(4):465-470.
2. Shiels MS, Pfeiffer RM, Hall HI, et al. Proportions of Kaposi sarcoma, selected non-Hodgkin lymphomas, and cervical cancer in the United States occurring in persons with AIDS, 1980–2007. *JAMA*. 2011;305(14):1450-1459.
3. Serraino D, Piselli P, Angeletti C, et al. Kaposi's sarcoma in transplant and HIV-infected patients: an epidemiologic study in Italy and France. *Transplantation*. 2005;80(12):1699-1704.
4. Onyango JF, Njiru A. Kaposi's sarcoma in a Nairobi hospital. *East Afr Med J*. 2004;81(3):120-123.
5. Dittmer DP, Damania B. Kaposi sarcoma-associated herpesvirus: immunobiology, oncogenesis, and therapy. *J Clin Invest*. 2016;126(9):3165-3175.
6. Jung J, Munz C. Immune control of oncogenic gamma-herpesviruses. *Curr Opin Virol*. 2015;14:79-86.

7. Koelle DM, Huang ML, Chandran B, et al. Frequent detection of Kaposi's sarcoma-associated herpesvirus (human herpesvirus 8) DNA in saliva of human immunodeficiency virus-infected men: clinical and immunologic correlates. *J Infect Dis.* 1997;176(1):94-102.
8. Goedert JJ, Vitale F, Lauria C, et al. Risk factors for classical Kaposi's sarcoma. *J Natl Cancer Inst.* 2002;94(22):1712-1718.
9. Cheung MC, Pantanowitz L, Dezube BJ. AIDS-related malignancies: emerging challenges in the era of highly active antiretroviral therapy. *Oncologist.* 2005;10(6):412-426.
10. Schneide JW, Dittmer DP. Diagnosis and treatment of Kaposi sarcoma. *Am J Clin Dermatol.* 2017;18:529.
11. Walmsley S, Northfelt DW, Melosky B, et al. Treatment of AIDS-related cutaneous Kaposi's sarcoma with topical alitretinoin (9-*cis*-retinoic acid) gel. Panretin Gel North American Study Group. *J Acquir Immune Defic Syndr.* 1999;22:235-246.
12. Cooley HD, Volberding P, Martin F, et al. Final results of a phase III randomized trial of pegylated liposomal doxorubicin versus liposomal daunorubicin in patients with AIDS-related Kaposi's sarcoma [abstract]. *Proc Am Soc Clin Oncol.* 2002;21:411a;1640.
13. Gill PS, Tulpule A, Espina BM, et al. Paclitaxel is safe and effective in the treatment of advanced AIDS related Kaposi's sarcoma. *J Clin Oncol.* 1999;17:1876-1883.
14. Krown SE, Li P, Von Roenn JH, et al. Efficacy of low-dose interferon with antiretroviral therapy in Kaposi's sarcoma: a randomized phase II AIDS Clinical Trials Group study. *J Interferon Cytokine Res.* 2002;22:295-303.
15. Boudreaux AA, Smith LL, Cosby CD, et al. Intralesional vinblastine for cutaneous Kaposi's sarcoma associated with acquired immunodeficiency syndrome. A clinical trial to evaluate efficacy and discomfort associated with infection. *J Am Acad Dermatol.* 1993;28:61-65.
16. Swift PS. The role of radiation therapy in the management of HIV-related Kaposi's sarcoma. *Hematol Oncol Clin North Am.* 1996;10:1069-1080.
17. Stebbing J, Sanitt A, Nelson M, et al. A prognostic index for AIDS-associated Kaposi's sarcoma in the era of highly active antiretroviral therapy. *Lancet.* 2006;367(9521):1495-1502.
18. Alcántara-Reifs CM, Salido-Vallejo R, Garnacho-Saucedo GM, Vélez García-Nieto A. Classic Kaposi's sarcoma treated with topical 0.5% timolol gel. *Dermatol Ther.* 2016;29(5):309-311.
19. Abdelmaksoud A, Filoni A, Giudice G, Vestita M. Classic and HIV-related Kaposi sarcoma treated with 0.1% topical timolol gel. *J Am Acad Dermatol.* 2017;76(1):153-155.

227 LYME DISEASE

Athena Andreadis, MD
Heidi S. Chumley, MD, MBA

PATIENT STORY

On a warm summer afternoon, a 32-year-old woman presents with a 5-day history of low-grade fever and a rash. On physical examination, the physician notes a large, erythematous, annular patch with central clearing on her back (**Figure 227-1**). The patient states that the rash has gotten progressively larger during the last 3 days and she has had a recent onset of intermittent joint pain. She does not recall being bitten by an insect. She denies taking medications within the past month and has no known allergies. When asked about recent travel, she admits to a camping trip in eastern Massachusetts, which she returned from 4 days ago. The patient was diagnosed with Lyme borreliosis and started on doxycycline 100 mg twice daily for 14 days. She responded quickly to the antibiotics and never developed the persistent stage of Lyme disease.

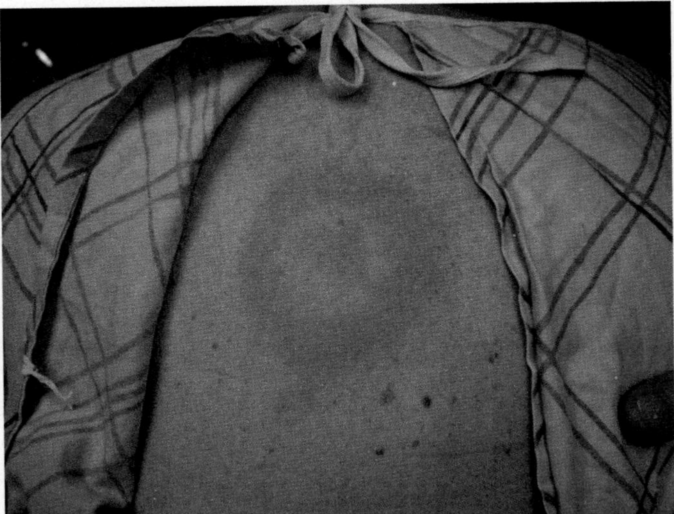

FIGURE 227-1 A 32-year-old woman with the typical eruption of erythema migrans on her upper back. Note the expanding annular lesion with a target-like morphology. (*Reproduced with permission from Thomas Corson, MD.*)

INTRODUCTION

Lyme disease is an infection caused by the spirochete *Borrelia burgdorferi*, transmitted via tick bite. Most cases of Lyme disease occur in the northeast United States between April and November. Patients experience flu-like symptoms and may develop the pathognomonic rash, erythema migrans. Lyme disease is prevented by avoiding exposure to the tick vector using insect repellant and protective clothing.

EPIDEMIOLOGY

- In 1977, clusters of patients in Old Lyme, Connecticut, began reporting symptoms originally thought to be juvenile rheumatoid arthritis.[1]
- In 1981, American entomologist Dr. Willy Burgdorfer isolated the infectious pathogen responsible for Lyme disease from the midgut of *Ixodes scapularis* (a.k.a., black-legged deer ticks) (**Figure 227-2**), which serve as the primary transmission vector in the United States.[1]
- The infectious agent was identified as a bacterial spirochete and named *B. burgdorferi* in honor of its discoverer.
- Based on Centers for Disease Control and Prevention (CDC) data reported in 2007, Lyme disease (or Lyme borreliosis) is the most common tick-borne illness in the United States, with an overall incidence of 7.9 per 100,000 persons.[2]
- In 2013, 95% of Lyme disease cases were reported from 14 states: Connecticut, Delaware, Maine, Maryland, Massachusetts, Minnesota, New Jersey, New Hampshire, New York, Pennsylvania, Rhode Island, Vermont, Virginia, and Wisconsin.[3]
- Patients living between Maryland and Maine accounted for 93% of all reported cases in the United States in 2005, with an overall incidence of 31.6 cases for every 100,000 persons.[2]
- More than 90% of cases report onset between April and November.[2]

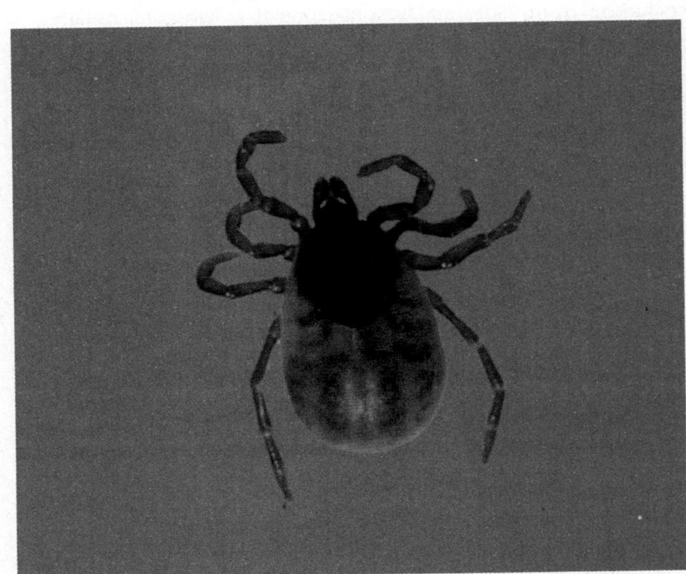

FIGURE 227-2 The deer tick transmits the *Borrelia* spirochete. This is an unengorged female black-legged deer tick. The tick is tiny and can be undetected in its unengorged state. (*Reproduced with permission from Thomas Corson, MD.*)

ETIOLOGY AND PATHOPHYSIOLOGY

- *B. burgdorferi* begins to multiply in the midgut of *I. scapularis* ticks upon attaching to humans.
- Migration from midgut to salivary glands of ticks requires 24 to 48 hours.
- Prior to this migration, host infection rarely occurs.
- Common hosts include field mice, white-tailed deer, and household pets.
- Ticks must feed on infested hosts in order to infect humans.
- Seventy percent to 75% of infected patients do not recall being bitten.[4]
- Once a human is infected, disease progression is categorized into three stages: localized, disseminated, and persistent.

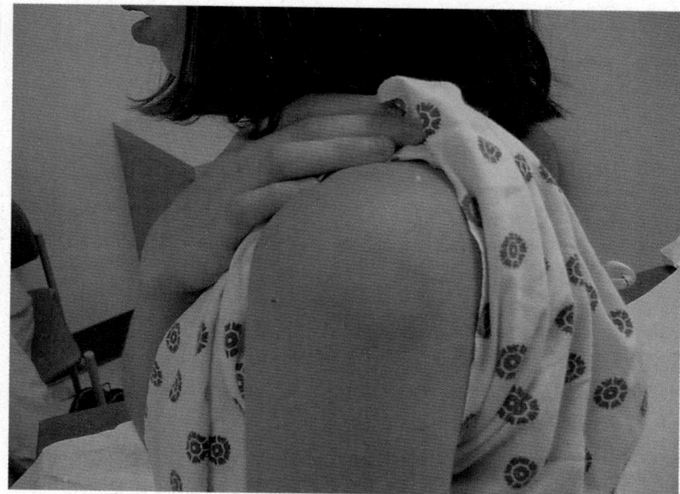

FIGURE 227-3 An 11-year-old girl with erythema migrans eruption on her shoulder. She is febrile and systemically ill. *(Reproduced with permission from Jeremy Golding, MD.)*

DIAGNOSIS

CLINICAL FEATURES

▶ Localized (days to weeks)

Erythema migrans (formerly known as erythema chronicum migrans)

This pathognomonic finding occurs in roughly 68% of Lyme disease cases.[4] Described as a "bull's-eye" eruption (**Figures 227-1** and **227-3** to **227-6**), this nonpruritic, maculopapular lesion typically occurs near the site of infection. The erythematous perimeter migrates outward over several days while the central area clears. Multiple lesions in different sites can develop in some individuals (see **Figures 227-3** and **227-4**). Erythema migrans can persist for 3 to 4 weeks if left untreated.

Flu-like symptoms

Roughly 67% of patients will develop flu-like symptoms that can include fever, myalgias, and lymphadenopathy. Symptoms usually subside within 7 to 10 days.

▶ Disseminated (days to months)

Inflammatory arthritis

Typical onset occurs around 3 to 6 months after localized infection. Patients will often present with polyarticular, migratory joint pain with or without erythema, and swelling, which is exacerbated with motion. After more than 24 to 48 hours, these symptoms localize to one joint (especially knee, ankle, or wrist) and last approximately 1 week. Recurrence is common and usually happens every few months, but typically resolves within 10 years even without treatment.

Cranial nerve palsy

Bell palsy (seventh cranial nerve) is the most common neurologic manifestation of Lyme disease. However, nearly every cranial nerve has been reported to be involved. Facial nerve palsy is a lower motor neuron lesion that results in weakness of both the lower face and the forehead. Lasting up to 8 weeks, the resolution of symptoms is gradual and begins shortly after initial onset (see Chapter 244, Bell Palsy).

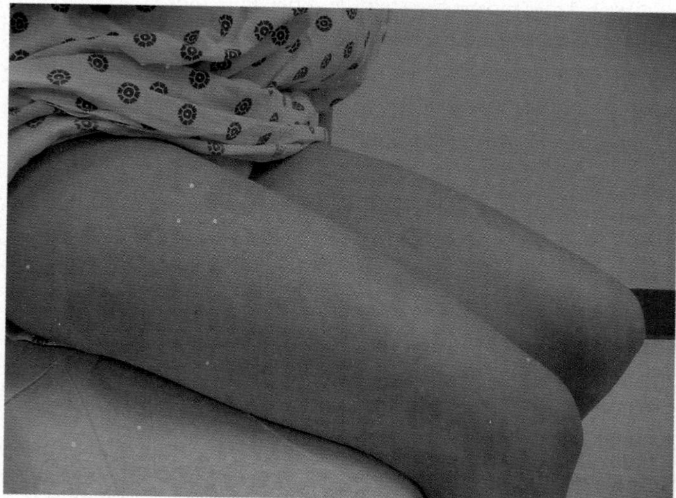

FIGURE 227-4 Same 11-year-old girl in **Figure 227-3** with multiple erythema migrans eruptions on her legs. *(Reproduced with permission from Jeremy Golding, MD.)*

Atrioventricular blockade

Present in only 1% of patients with Lyme disease, syncope, light-headedness, and dyspnea are classic symptoms consistent with atrioventricular (AV) dysfunction.[3] However, patients can be completely asymptomatic. The degree of Lyme-associated blockade varies so that symptoms are generally episodic. Most cases resolve spontaneously within 1 week.[4] Any patient with history and/or examination findings suspicious of Lyme disease should undergo ECG testing. Hospitalization and continuous monitoring are advisable for symptomatic patients and for patients with second- or third-degree AV block, as well as for those with first-degree heart block when the PR interval is prolonged to 30 or more milliseconds, because the degree of block may fluctuate and worsen very rapidly in such patients.[5]

Aseptic meningitis

Patients may present with complaints similar to bacterial meningitis (photophobia, nuchal rigidity, and headache), but symptoms are generally less severe in nature. This can also occur with or without concomitant cranial nerve palsy.[4]

Fatigue

A depressed level of activity as a result of fatigue is one of the most common complaints, affecting up to 80% of infected patients. Even after adequate treatment, symptoms consistent with chronic fatigue syndrome have developed in patients with known Lyme disease.

▶ Persistent (longer than 1 year)

Chronic arthritis

Generally occurs in the knee, although other sites such as the shoulder, ankle, elbow, or wrist are not uncommon. Approximately 10% of patients with intermittent arthritis will progress to this stage.[4]

Chronic fatigue

Commonly misdiagnosed as fibromyalgia or chronic fatigue syndrome, patients develop debilitating malaise and myalgias that can persist for months or years after infection.

Meningoencephalitis

Symptoms vary from mild (memory loss, mood lability, irritability, or panic attacks) to severe (manic or psychotic episodes, paranoia, and obsessive/compulsive symptoms).[5]

LABORATORY TESTING

Diagnosing Lyme disease is generally based on pertinent history findings and/or the presence of an erythema migrans lesion, especially in endemic areas. In cases where an erythema migrans lesion is absent, serologic testing may be warranted using the following tests:

- Enzyme-linked immunosorbent assay (ELISA) (sensitivity: 94%, specificity: 97%)[6]—Used as a *screening* test in patients lacking physical signs of erythema migrans. Up to 50% of patients with early infection can have a false-negative result. If strong suspicion remains, convalescent titers should be obtained in 6 weeks.[6] Prior infection does not indicate immunity. Lyme titers may be falsely positive in patients with mononucleosis, periodontal disease, connective tissue disease, and other less common conditions.[7]

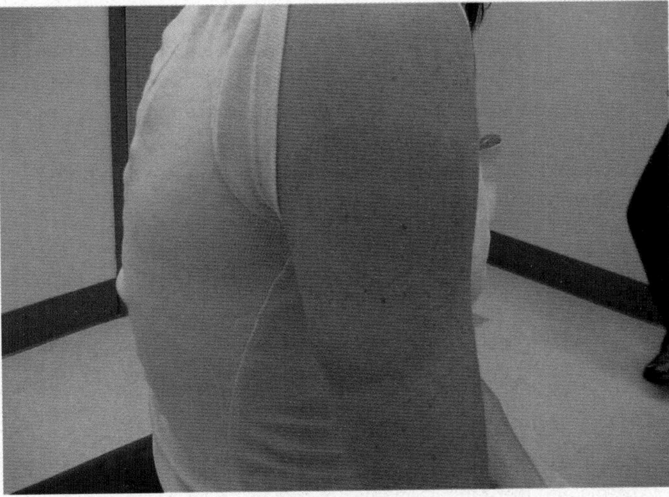

FIGURE 227-5 A 12-year-old girl with erythema migrans eruption on her right arm. The annular border is somewhat raised and there is central clearing. (*Reproduced with permission from Jeremy Golding, MD.*)

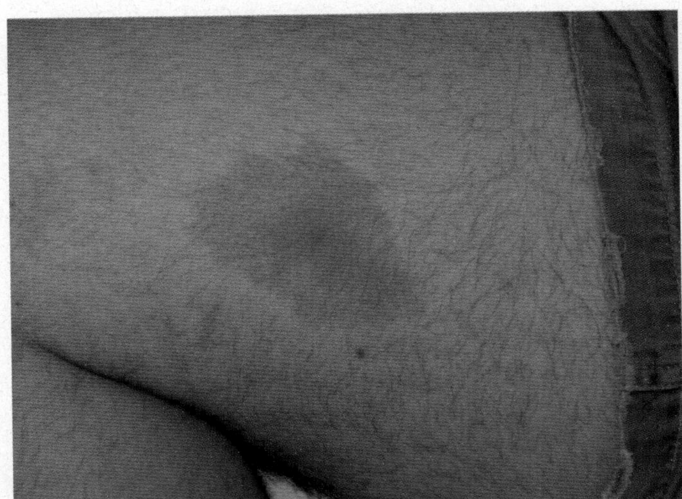

FIGURE 227-6 A 26-year-old man with erythema migrans eruption on his right medial thigh. The central papule is the site of the bite, and there has not been much central clearing yet. (*Reproduced with permission from Gil Shlamovitz, MD.*)

- Western blot (immunoglobulin [Ig] M and IgG for *B. burgdorferi*)—If ELISA test yields a positive result, Western blot test is used as a *confirmatory* test. IgM antibodies are detectable between 2 weeks and 6 months after inoculation. IgG may be present indefinitely after 6 weeks, despite appropriate antibiotic therapy. Once it is determined that a person is seropositive for Lyme disease, antibiotic therapy should be initiated promptly.

Empiric antibiotic therapy (no test necessary) should be considered in any of the following clinical presentations: presence of EM rash, flu-like symptoms (in absence of upper respiratory infection [URI] or GI symptoms) after known tick bite, Bell palsy in endemic areas, especially between June and September, and tick bites occurring during pregnancy.

▶ Characteristic laboratory findings

- Complete blood count (CBC)—Leukocytosis (11,000 to 18,000/μL). Anemia and thrombocytopenia are rare.
- Elevated erythrocyte sedimentation rate (ESR) (>20 mm/h).
- Elevated γ-glutamyl transpeptidase (GGT) and aspartate transaminase (AST).
- Cerebrospinal fluid—Pleocytosis and elevated protein levels if central nervous system (CNS) is involved. Spirochete antibodies may be detectable.
- Blood culture—Low yield; not recommended.
- Nerve conduction studies and electromyography (EMG)—Useful in patients with paresthesias or radicular pain.
- ECG should be performed in all patients with history and physical examination suspicious for Lyme disease to detect AV block and arrhythmias.

DIFFERENTIAL DIAGNOSIS[8]

- Cellulitis—Spreads more rapidly than Lyme disease. Induration and tenderness are more common. Negative Lyme serologies (see Chapter 126, Cellulitis).
- Urticaria—Can resemble erythema migrans (EM) when the urticarial lesions are annular. Urticaria is generally more widespread and the wheals come and go over time, whereas the lesion of EM is more fixed (see Chapter 156, Urticaria and Angioedema).
- Rocky Mountain spotted fever—Associated with *Dermacentor variabilis* (American dog) tick; rash is petechial and the spots are widely distributed over the body (see Chapter 187, Vasculitis, Figure 187-17). Patients often appear toxic.
- Cutaneous fungal infections—Usually pruritic and may be annular; associated with scaling, which is not characteristic of erythema migrans; and spread slowly if at all. The similarity is that the annular appearance of tinea corporis can mimic EM (see Chapter 144, Tinea Corporis).
- Local reaction to tick bites—Tick bites may cause a local reaction in skin and do not expand with time; generally less than 2 cm in diameter and are usually papular.
- Febrile viral illnesses (particularly enteroviruses during summer)—Rash, myalgias, arthralgias, and headache; GI symptoms; sore throat and/or cough. Perform Lyme serologic test in the absence of EM.
- Facial nerve palsy—May be bilateral in Lyme disease. This is uncommon in facial nerve palsy not associated with Lyme disease (see Chapter 244, Bell Palsy).
- Viral meningitis—Lymphocytic (aseptic) meningitis caused by viral infection generally results in transient illness that resolves within several days, usually after a monophasic course.
- Heart block—Idiopathic conduction system disease (sick sinus syndrome) can present with the same symptoms and signs as Lyme carditis. Use serologic testing and epidemiologic history to discriminate.
- Inflammatory arthritis (reactive arthritis, gout, pseudogout, and rheumatoid arthritis)—Acute, large joint monoarticular or oligoarticular arthritis from multiple causes; may be indistinguishable from acute arthritis associated with Lyme disease at the time of presentation; joint fluid examination, and culture and X-ray may help distinguish from Lyme arthritis (see Chapter 97, Arthritis Overview).
- Peripheral neuropathy is more often associated with diabetes mellitus, peripheral vascular disease, endocrinopathies, and nerve root impingement syndromes. If Lyme disease is the cause, the serologies should be positive.
- Radiculoneuropathy—Dermatomal pain, sensory loss, and/or weakness in a limb or the trunk. Check serologies if Lyme disease is suspected.
- Encephalomyelitis—Focal inflammation of the brain or spinal cord. Check serologies if Lyme disease is suspected.

MANAGEMENT

MEDICATIONS

Localized:

- Adults—Doxycycline 100 mg twice a day (nonpregnant patients only) or amoxicillin 500 mg 3 times a day or cefuroxime 500 mg twice a day for 14 days.[5] SOR Ⓐ
- Children—Amoxicillin 50 mg/kg divided 3 times a day up to 500 mg per dose or cefuroxime 30 mg/kg divided twice a day up to 500 mg per dose; older than 8 years of age—Doxycycline 4 mg/kg divided twice a day up to 100 mg/dose.[5] SOR Ⓐ

Meningitis or other neurologic manifestations:

- Adults—Ceftriaxone 2 g IV every day for 14 days; alternative therapy cefotaxime 2 g IV every 8 hours or penicillin G 18 to 24 million U every day divided into 6 daily doses for 14 days.[5] SOR Ⓑ
- Children—Ceftriaxone 50 to 75 mg/kg IV up to a maximum of 2 g/day for 14 days; alternative therapy cefotaxime 150 to 200 mg/kg per day up to a maximum of 6 g/day, divided into 3 to 4 doses per day.[5] SOR Ⓑ
- Doxycycline (oral) 100 to 200 mg twice a day for 10 to 28 days may be effective; consider for nonpregnant adults or children older than 8 years of age who are intolerant of β-lactam antibiotics.[5] SOR Ⓑ
- Lyme carditis—Oral or IV antibiotics as above with hospitalization and continuous cardiac monitoring in patients with symptoms including syncope, shortness of breath, or chest pain, or in patients with AV block.[5] SOR Ⓑ

Persistent Lyme disease:

- Arthritis without neurologic disease—Doxycycline, amoxicillin, or cefuroxime; amoxicillin, cefuroxime in children younger than 8 years of age; medications at doses shown under early disease with therapy extended to 28 days.[5] SOR Ⓑ If arthritis persists, treat for another 28 days with oral antibiotics or a 28-day regimen of IV antibiotics.
- Neurologic disease—IV therapy with ceftriaxone for 14 to 28 days.[5] SOR Ⓑ

REFERRAL OR HOSPITALIZATION

- Symptomatic patients with Lyme carditis should be hospitalized with continuous cardiac monitoring.
- Consider referring patients in whom the diagnosis is unclear or who do not respond to initial therapy.

PREVENTION

- Avoid exposure to ticks by using protective clothing and tick repellant. If hiking in tick-infested areas, check body daily for ticks and promptly remove any attached ticks.
- Prophylactic doxycycline (1 dose of 200 mg) is recommended only if the tick is identified as an adult or nymphal *I. scapularis* tick that has been attached for at least 36 hours; medication can be started within 72 hours of tick removal; local rate of infection of ticks with *B. burgdorferi* is at least 20%; and doxycycline is not contraindicated.[5]

PROGNOSIS

- Most patients respond to appropriate therapy with prompt resolution of symptoms within 4 weeks.
- Posttreatment Lyme disease syndrome (persistent or recurrent symptoms) occurs in 10% to 20% of patients despite appropriate treatment. Prolonged antibiotic treatment is not effective.[3] Most patients eventually feel completely well, but this can take months or years.
- True treatment failures are uncommon, and prolonged oral or parenteral antibiotic courses are emphatically discouraged. In patients who continue to present with residual subjective symptoms, providers should seek alternative diagnoses and/or referral to an appropriate specialist.

FOLLOW-UP

Follow patients during antibiotic therapy through recovery.

PATIENT EDUCATION

Prevention is accomplished by reducing exposure to ticks. If you live in an area that has Lyme disease, then use tick repellant, tick checks, and other simple measures to prevent tick bites. This is especially important during the high-risk months of April through November. Patients should know the early signs of Lyme disease so that they can get care early when it is most curable.

If a tick is found on the skin, remove it early using fine-tipped tweezers. See Patient Resources below.

PATIENT RESOURCES

- Centers for Disease Control and Prevention (CDC). *Lyme Disease*—**http://www.cdc.gov/lyme/.**
- Centers for Disease Control and Prevention (CDC). *Tick Removal*—**http://www.cdc.gov/lyme/removal/index.html.**

PROVIDER RESOURCES

- Centers for Disease Control and Prevention (CDC). *Lyme Disease*—**http://www.cdc.gov/lyme/.**

REFERENCES

1. Sternbach G, Dibble CL. Willy Burgdorfer: Lyme disease. *J Emerg Med.* 1996;14(5):631-634.
2. Centers for Disease Control and Prevention. Lyme disease—United States, 2003–2005. *MMWR Morb Mortal Wkly Rep.* 2007;56(23):573-576.
3. Centers for Disease Control and Prevention. *Lyme Disease.* http://www.cdc.gov/lyme/. Accessed March 2017.
4. Meyerhoff JO. *Lyme Disease.* http://emedicine.medscape.com/article/330178. Accessed March 2017.
5. Wormser GP, Dattwyler RJ, Shapiro ED, et al. The clinical assessment, treatment, and prevention of Lyme disease, human granulocytic anaplasmosis, and babesiosis: clinical practice guidelines by the Infectious Diseases Society of America. *Clin Infect Dis.* 2006;43(9):1089-1134.
6. *Lyme Disease Executive Summary.* http://www.harp.org/eng/kaiserslymesummary.htm. Accessed March 2017.
7. Columbia University Medical Center Lyme and Tick-Borne Diseases Research Center. http://www.columbia-lyme.org/index.html. Accessed March 2017.
8. American College of Physicians. *Differential Diagnosis of Lyme Disease.* http://www.acponline.org/journals/news/jun07/critters.pdf. Accessed March 2017.

PART XVI

ENDOCRINE

Strength of Recommendation (SOR)	Definition
A	Recommendation based on consistent and good-quality patient-oriented evidence.*
B	Recommendation based on inconsistent or limited-quality patient-oriented evidence.*
C	Recommendation based on consensus, usual practice, opinion, disease-oriented evidence, or case series for studies of diagnosis, treatment, prevention, or screening.*

*See Appendix A on pages 1603–1606 for further information.

228 DIABETES OVERVIEW

Mindy A. Smith, MD, MS

PATIENT STORY

A 66-year-old man with obesity and mild hypertension controlled with a diuretic presents with increasing nocturia and excessive thirst. He has no other urinary symptoms and denies any visual problems. His mother had diabetes and died at age 85 years from a heart attack. His only other concern is a recurrent fungal infection on his feet. His blood pressure in the office today is 135/85 mm Hg and his finger-stick blood sugar is 220 mg/dL. Physical exam findings confirm tinea pedis (**Figure 228-1**). A monofilament test demonstrates normal sensation in his feet.

You explain that based on his elevated blood sugar, he has diabetes mellitus. You order a fasting blood sugar, lipid profile, serum electrolytes, creatinine, and hemoglobin A_{1c}. You ask him to return next week for a more complete examination, review of his test results, and diabetes education. You encourage him and his wife to consider meeting with a nutritionist, and briefly review treatment options, including diet, exercise, and metformin, as well as a possible need to improve his blood pressure control or switch to another agent. You suggest a nonprescription antifungal cream and will see if he needs additional treatment for his feet at follow-up. The patient is referred to an ophthalmologist, who finds diabetic nonproliferative retinopathy (**Figure 228-2**).

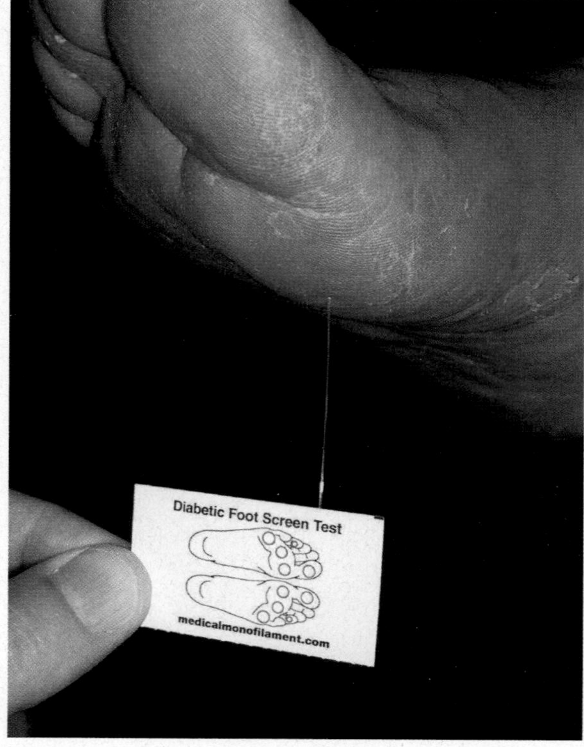

FIGURE 228-1 Patient with diabetes and tinea pedis being tested with a monofilament for sensation. (*Reproduced with permission from Richard P. Usatine, MD.*)

INTRODUCTION

Diabetes is a group of disorders caused by a complex interaction between genetic susceptibility, environmental factors, and personal lifestyle choices that share the phenotype of hyperglycemia. Type 2 diabetes mellitus (DM) is a heterogeneous group of chronic disorders caused by a progressive insulin secretory defect and increased glucose production in the setting of insulin resistance.

EPIDEMIOLOGY[1]

- Prevalence—In the United States, 29.1 million adults and children (9.3% of the population), including 21 million who have been diagnosed, have diabetes (2014). This includes about 1 in 400 children and adolescents and 25.9% of people age 65 years and older. Type 2 DM is the most common form, accounting for more than 90% of cases.
- Incidence—In the United States in 2012, there were 1.7 million new cases among individuals 20 years of age and older.
- Highest rates of diabetes, in decreasing order, are in American Indians/Alaska Natives (15.9%), non-Hispanic blacks (13.2%), Hispanics (12.8%), Asian Americans (9.0%), and non-Hispanic whites (7.6%).
- In 2012, total costs of diagnosed DM in the United States were \$245 billion (\$176 billion in direct medical costs).

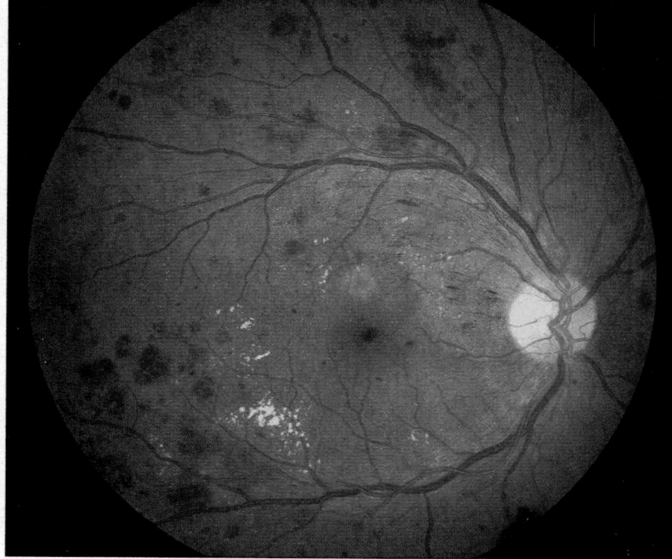

FIGURE 228-2 Nonproliferative diabetic retinopathy, with scattered intraretinal dot-blot and flame hemorrhages, along with macular exudates. Macular exudates can be related to diabetic macular edema, which accounts for a large portion of poor vision and disability secondary to diabetic retinopathy. (*Reproduced with permission from Andrew Sanchez, COA.*)

ETIOLOGY AND PATHOPHYSIOLOGY

- Insulin resistance is attributed to obesity, inactivity, and genetic factors (including defects in β-cell function and insulin action).
- Initially, the pancreatic β cells increase insulin production to overcome insulin resistance and maintain euglycemia. Eventually, β cells fail, resulting in hyperglycemia.
- Other contributing factors include diseases of the pancreas (e.g., pancreatitis, hemochromatosis), infection (e.g., cytomegalovirus), and other endocrinopathies (e.g., hyperthyroidism [see Chapter 236, Graves Disease and Goiter] and acromegaly [see Chapter 237, Acromegaly]).
- Microvascular and macrovascular diseases may result from hyperglycemia or other metabolic changes.

RISK FACTORS[1-4]

- Obesity (or overweight; body mass index >25 kg/m^2*).
- Red meat consumption (relative risk [RR] 1.51; 95% confidence interval [CI], 1.25, 1.83 for 50 g processed red meat/day).[5]
- Physical inactivity (also television viewing 2 h/day; odds ratio [OR] 1.20; 95% CI, 1.14–1.27).[6]*
- Nonwhite race.*
- First-degree relative with diabetes.*
- Prior gestational diabetes (or delivery of a baby weighing more than 4 kg*).
- Impaired glucose tolerance (hazard ratio [HR] 13.2, 95% CI, 10.8–16.2).[7]
- Elevated blood pressure (BP) (HR 1.58, 95% CI, 1.56–1.59 for a 20 mm Hg elevation over usual systolic BP and HR 1.52, 95% CI, 1.52–1.54 for a 10 mm Hg elevation over usual diastolic BP).[8]
- Polycystic ovarian syndrome, acanthosis nigricans, nonalcoholic fatty liver disease.*
- Coronary heart disease, hypertension, metabolic syndrome.*
- Acute pancreatitis (5-year relative risk 2.7, 95% CI, 1.9–3.8).[9]
- Smoking (OR [current smoker] 1.44; 95% CI, 1.31–1.58).
- Antipsychotic therapy for patients with schizophrenia or severe bipolar disease.*
- Prolonged use of oral corticosteroids.*
- Previously identified glucose intolerance; especially in patients with a sleep disorder.*
- HDL-C <35 mg/dL (0.90 mmol/L) and/or a triglyceride level >250 mg/dL (2.82 mmol/L).*

*Risk factors used by the American Association of Clinical Endocrinologists (AACE) in making decisions for screening patients for DM.[4]

Many risk models and scores have been developed to predict the development of DM.[10] One of these, the Framingham Offspring Study,[11] uses fasting plasma glucose levels, body mass index, high-density lipoprotein cholesterol and triglyceride levels, parental history of diabetes, and blood pressure to determine risk. Unfortunately, none of the models were developed on a cohort recruited prospectively, and no studies have demonstrated a reduction in incident DM using risk scoring and intervention.

DIAGNOSIS

The AACE guideline defines the diagnosis of diabetes as a fasting (8 or more hours of no caloric intake) glucose level 126 mg/dL or greater (≥7.0 mmol/L), *or* a 2-hour plasma glucose 200 mg/dL or greater (≥11.1 mmol/L) on a 75-g oral glucose tolerance test, *or* a random plasma glucose level of greater than 200 mg/dL with symptoms of diabetes, *or* a hemoglobin A_{1c} level of 6.5% or higher.[4] SOR Ⓐ The same test should be repeated on a different day to confirm the diagnosis unless the patient has a glucose level of greater than 200 mg/dL with diabetes symptoms. SOR Ⓒ

CLINICAL FEATURES

- Many patients with type 2 DM are asymptomatic.
- Patients may report polydipsia, polyuria, and blurred vision.
- Funduscopic examination may reveal signs of retinopathy (hard exudates, hemorrhages) (**Figure 228-2**; see Chapter 22, Diabetic Retinopathy).
- Patients with diabetic neuropathy may have abnormalities on monofilament, vibration, and superficial pain testing.
- Skin changes in patients with DM include diabetic dermopathy in 15% to 40% of patients (**Figure 228-3**; see Chapter 230, Diabetic Dermopathy),[12] acanthosis nigricans in approximately one-third of patients (**Figure 228-4**; see Chapter 229, Acanthosis Nigricans),[13] diabetic foot ulcers (**Figure 228-5**; see Chapter 219, Ischemic Ulcer), and, uncommonly, necrobiosis lipoidica (**Figure 228-6**; see Chapter 231, Necrobiosis Lipoidica).
- Hyperlipidemia may result in eruptive xanthomas (**Figure 228-7**) or xanthelasma.
- Patients with DM of prolonged duration may also have Charcot joints (**Figure 228-8**; see Chapter 221, Charcot Arthropathy).[14]

LABORATORY TESTS

- AACE prefers a fasting blood glucose or 2-hour result as the diagnostic test.[4] Other tests that can be used for diagnosis are listed above.

MANAGEMENT

AACE 2017 treatment goals are presented as algorithms for lifestyle optimization, atherosclerotic cardiovascular disease (ASCVD) risk factor modification, glycemic control, and insulin therapy.[15] Treatment goals emphasize lifestyle optimization for all and individualized targets for weight loss, hypertension management, lipids, and glucose.

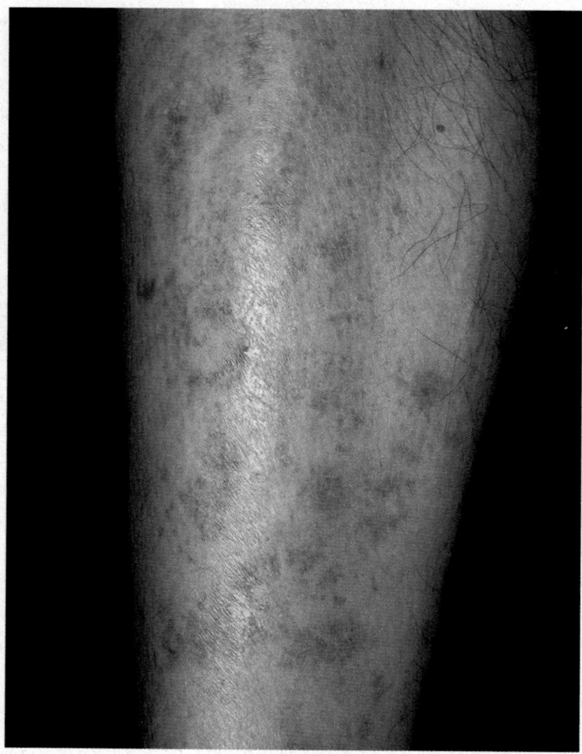

FIGURE 228-3 Diabetic dermopathy on the lower legs that is particularly prominent over the shins. (*Reproduced with permission from Richard P. Usatine, MD.*)

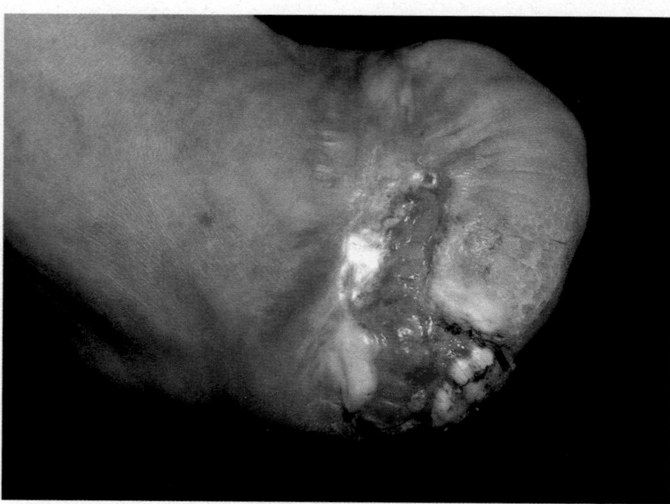

FIGURE 228-5 Diabetic foot ulcer that has occurred at the amputation site. (*Reproduced with permission from Richard P. Usatine, MD.*)

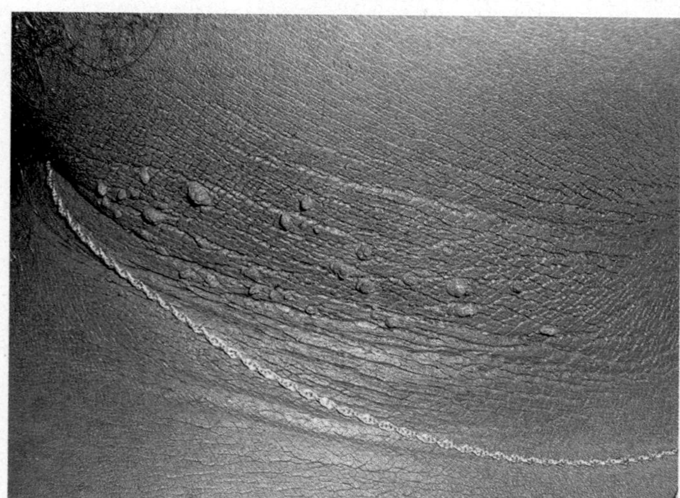

FIGURE 228-4 Acanthosis nigricans in a woman with type 2 diabetes and obesity. She is requesting that her skin tags be removed. (*Reproduced with permission from Richard P. Usatine, MD.*)

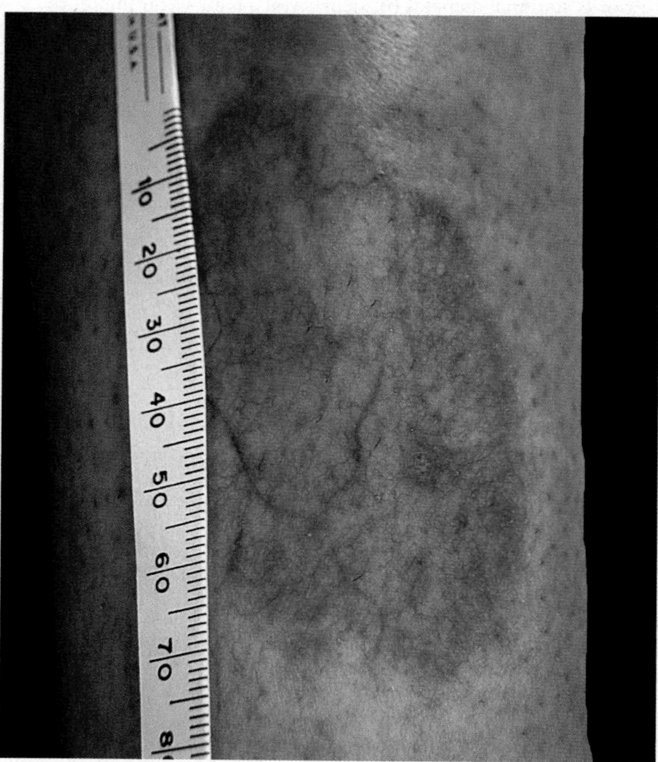

FIGURE 228-6 Necrobiosis lipoidica diabeticorum on the lower leg with typical findings of skin atrophy, yellow coloration, and prominent blood vessels. (*Reproduced with permission from Richard P. Usatine, MD.*)

The primary treatment goals for the patient with DM are to aggressively control blood pressure (<130/80 mm Hg) and lower lipids (low-density lipoprotein [LDL] goal is <100 mg/dL or <70 mg/dL in patients with DM and ASCVD or DM and 1 major ASCVD risk factor) to improve cardiovascular and all-cause mortality. Blood glucose control is usually undertaken with metformin, although combination therapy is often needed to achieve a target A_{1c} level; specific AACE recommendations are below.

This author believes that tight/strict control should no longer be stressed, especially in older patients, as it does not improve most outcomes and increases episodes of hypoglycemia. In the ADVANCE (Action in Diabetes and Vascular Disease: Preterax and Diamicron Modified-Release Controlled Evaluation) trial (N = 11,140), there were no differences seen in the rates of major macrovascular events or overall mortality between patients randomized to intense control (hemoglobin A_{1c} ≤6.5%) or standard control.[16] A meta-analysis of 14 trials also concluded that intensive control did not reduce all-cause mortality; data were insufficient to confirm a relative risk reduction for cardiovascular morbidity or mortality, composite microvascular complications, or retinopathy at a magnitude of 10%.[17] Intensive glycemic control increased the relative risk of severe hypoglycemia by 30%.[17]

In epidemiologic research, a hemoglobin A_{1c} level less than 7% is associated with the best outcomes, and the ADA uses a hemoglobin A_{1c} of less than 7% as the benchmark for adequate control. The AACE recommends a target A_{1c} of 6.5% or less in most nonpregnant adults if it can be achieved safely, as near-normal levels may prevent microvascular (e.g., retinopathy) complications.[4] SOR Ⓒ A less stringent A_{1c} of 7.0% to 8.0% is appropriate for patients with a history of severe hypoglycemia, limited life expectancy, advanced renal disease or macrovascular complications, extensive comorbid conditions, or long-standing DM in which the A_{1c} goal has been difficult to attain, so long as the patient remains hyperglycemia symptom free.[4]

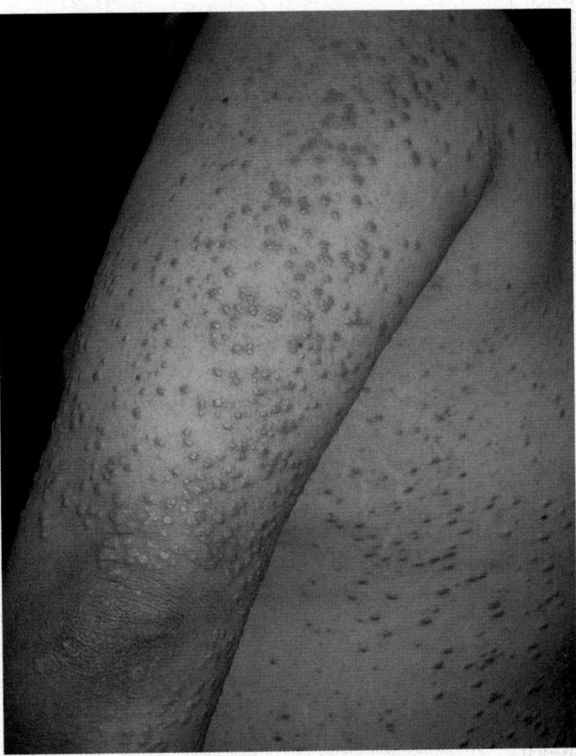

FIGURE 228-7 Eruptive xanthomas on the extremities and trunk of a young man with untreated type 2 diabetes and hyperlipidemia. *(Reproduced with permission from Richard P. Usatine, MD.)*

FIRST LINE

NONPHARMACOLOGIC

Lifestyle interventions:

- Diet—Nutrition advice may be best delivered by a registered dietician familiar with DM. AACE recommends a primarily plant-based diet high in polyunsaturated and monounsaturated fatty acids, limited intake of saturated fatty acids, and avoidance of *trans* fats.[4] SOR Ⓑ Patients should be instructed in portion control and consuming meals at regular times and in places where one can focus on the act of eating.[15] Caloric restriction is recommended for patients who are overweight with the goal of reducing body weight by at least 5% to 10%.[15]
    - At 5.5-year follow-up of 6213 individuals with type 2 diabetes without macroalbuminuria, those eating a healthy diet and moderate intake of alcohol (highest tertile based on modified Alternate Healthy Eating Index) had a lower risk of chronic kidney disease (adjusted OR 0.74; 95% CI, 0.64–0.84) and lower risk of mortality (OR, 0.61; 95% CI, 0.48–0.78) than those in the lowest tertile.[18]
    - A Cochrane review of 11 randomized controlled trials (RCTs) concluded that a low-glycemic-index diet improved glycemic control over a higher-glycemic-index diet with fewer hypoglycemic episodes in one trial and fewer hyperglycemic episodes in another trial.[19]

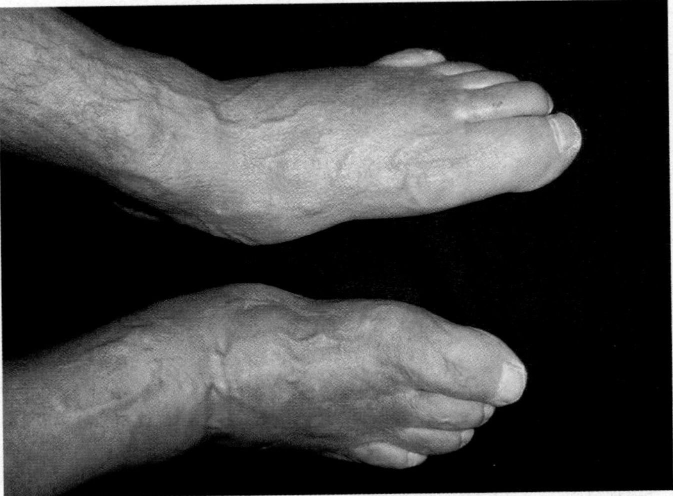

FIGURE 228-8 Charcot feet bilaterally in a person with poorly controlled diabetes. Note the pronation of the feet with the abnormal bulging of the medial foot. X-rays showed abnormal tarsal bones secondary to diabetic neuropathy. *(Reproduced with permission from Richard P. Usatine, MD.)*

  - Authors of a systematic review and meta-analysis of 20 RCTs found that the most effective diets for improving cardiovascular risk in people with DM were low-carbohydrate, low-GI, Mediterranean, and high-protein diets.[20] Long-term effects of intensive lifestyle interventions, however, have been disappointing. In the Look AHEAD RCT including 5145 overweight or obese patients with type 2 diabetes, an intensive lifestyle intervention focusing on weight loss did not reduce the rate of cardiovascular events at a median follow-up of 9.6 years.[21]
- Weight-loss strategies for those who are overweight include diet, physical activity, behavioral interventions, and surgery (recommended for those with a BMI ≥35; discussed below). Authors of a systematic review and meta-analysis fount that weight loss of at least 5% was required to confer benefit on A_{1c}, lipids and blood pressure.[22] The two studies that achieved this level of weight loss used regular physical activity and frequent contact with health professionals in addition to a Mediterranean-style diet in one study and an intensive lifestyle intervention in the other (Look AHEAD).
  - Even without weight loss, structured exercise (>150 min/wk of moderate exertion such as walking) significantly improves glycemic control in patients with type 2 DM.[23] SOR Ⓐ In this meta-analysis, a combination of dietary and exercise advice also lowered hemoglobin A_{1c}.[23]
- AACE also recommends adequate sleep (about 7 hours per night), behavioral support including assessment of mood, and assistance with smoking cessation.[4]

Education, self-management, and self-monitoring interventions:

- AACE recommends patient education and behavior modification such as self-monitoring of food intake and physical activity, and learning to cope with negative thoughts by means other than eating.[4] SOR Ⓐ Authors of a systematic review and meta-analysis found that most lifestyle and diabetes self-management education and support programs offering ≥11 contact hours led to clinically important improvements in A_{1c}, whereas most diabetes self-management education programs without added support provided little benefit.[24]
- Authors of a meta-analysis of 35 RCTs of various forms of telemedicine support (i.e., telephone call or a text message, videoconferencing and/or informational websites, and electronically transmitted clinician recommendations) found a small but statistically significant decrease in A_{1c} in the intervention compared to conventional treatment groups.[25]
- Authors of a Cochrane review of 12 trials on blood glucose self-monitoring in patients with type 2 DM not using insulin found a small effect of self-monitoring on glycemic control (reduced hemoglobin A_{1c}) that lasted up to 6 months after initiation but not at or beyond 12 months.[26] There was no evidence that self-monitoring affected patient satisfaction, general well-being, or general health-related quality of life.
  - In a small trial of 47 adults with newly diagnosed DM who were not on hypoglycemic medications, replacing high- with low-glycemic-load foods and increasing routine physical activities guided by systematic self-monitoring of blood glucose resulted in decreased A_{1c} from 8.4% to 7.4% compared with 8.3% to 8.3% among controls.[27]
  - Self-monitoring of glucose may be useful for assessing and preventing hypoglycemia and adjusting medications, medical nutrition therapy, and physical activity.
- Structured goal setting was shown in an RCT (N = 87) to improve glycemic control up to 1 year postintervention.[28]

MEDICATIONS

▶ Blood pressure

Agents that can be used for initial blood pressure control include diuretics, angiotensin-converting enzyme (ACE) inhibitors, and β blockers. AACE considers ACE inhibitors or angiotensin II receptor blockers (ARBs) the preferred choice in patients with DM.[15] SOR Ⓒ Combinations of medications may be needed. AACE recommends dual therapy for patients with an initial BP of >150/100 mm Hg with an ACE or ARB plus calcium channel blocker, beta-blocker, or thiazide.[15] The blood pressure target is less than 130/80 mm Hg.[4,15] SOR Ⓑ

- Authors of a systematic review and meta-analysis of 40 RCTs at low risk of bias confirmed the benefits of BP lowering in patients with DM.[29] For each 10-mm Hg lower systolic BP, there was an associated lower risk of cardiovascular events (absolute RR [ARR] 3.90; 95% CI, 1.57–6.06) and stroke (ARR 4.06; 95% CI, 2.53–5.40), and a lower relative risk of mortality (RR 0.87; 95% CI, 0.78–0.96).
- In patients with DM and chronic kidney disease, no specific blood pressure–lowering strategy was shown in one meta-analysis to prolong survival, but use of ACE inhibitors or ARBs lowered the risk of end-stage kidney disease.[30] The combination of an ACE inhibitor plus an ARB showed borderline increases in hyperkalemia and acute kidney injury
- In the ACCORD trial of intensive blood pressure control in 4733 patients with type 2 DM, there were no additional cardiovascular benefits to targeting a systolic blood pressure of 120 mm Hg versus 140 mm Hg. Patients treated with intensive blood pressure lowering were more likely to experience serious adverse effects (3.3% vs. 1.3%).[31] This finding was supported by a meta-analysis of 49 trials that showed a reduced risk of mortality and cardiovascular morbidity in people with DM who had a systolic BP >140 mm Hg, but an increased risk of cardiovascular death and no observed benefit if baseline systolic BP was <140 mm Hg.[32]

▶ Glycemic control

AACE recommends initiating therapy with metformin (biguanide that suppresses hepatic glucose production), a glucagon-like peptide 1 (GLP-1) receptor agonist (increases insulin release and slows glucose absorption), a dipeptidyl peptidase 4 (DPP-4) inhibitor (blocks enzyme destruction of incretin, increasing insulin production and decreasing glucagon), a sodium glucose cotransporter 2 (SGLT2) inhibitor (prevents glucose reabsorption through the kidney), or an α-glucosidase inhibitor (e.g., acarbose that decreases intestinal carbohydrate absorption) for patients with an entry A_{1c} <7.5%. For patients with entry A_{1c} levels >7.5%, AACE recommends initiating treatment with metformin (unless contraindicated) plus a second agent, with preference given to GLP-1 receptor agonists, SGLT2 inhibitors, or DPP-4 inhibitors agents due to their low potential for hypoglycemia and weight gain. SOR Ⓒ

Details on these and other hypoglycemic agents can be found in the AACE 2017 document cited.[15]

- Of the oral hypoglycemic agents, no significant differences in cardiovascular mortality or all-cause mortality were found between any drug class as monotherapy or dual or triple therapy.[33] Metformin as monotherapy, however, has the greatest effect on lowering A_{1c}[33] and, given its safety profile and beneficial effects on weight, is a good choice for initial therapy.[34] SOR Ⓐ Monotherapy, although initially effective for many patients, fails to sustain control in approximately half of patients at 3 years.[35]

▶ Lipid control

Lipid control in patients whose lipids are not controlled by diet and exercise is usually achieved with statin therapy.[4] Patients with DM and elevated lipids fall into one of the four benefit groups for treatment with a high-intensity statin—atorvastatin (80 mg) or rosuvastatin (20 mg) (see Chapter 232, Hyperlipidemia and Xanthomas); atorvastatin may be more renoprotective.[36] SOR Ⓐ

SECOND LINE

MEDICATIONS

▶ Glycemic control

- Addition of a second oral agent should be considered when monotherapy does not provide adequate control after 3 months; drugs recommended by AACE include GLP-1 receptor agonists, SGLT2 inhibitors, DPP-4 inhibitors with consideration of colesevelam (bile acid sequestrant), bromocriptine quick release (uncertain mechanism of action), or an α-glucosidase inhibitor.[15] SOR Ⓒ In the meta-analysis noted above, drugs added to metformin are associated with similar HbA_{1c} levels, although SGLT-2 inhibitors are associated with the lowest odds of hypoglycemia.[33]
- Triple therapy is considered if the patient is still not at goal on dual therapy using the same preferred drugs. Other agents including insulin can be used with caution. A meta-analysis of 18 trials did not find a clear difference in benefit between drug classes when adding a third agent for patients who were already on metformin and a sulfonylurea.[37]
- If triple therapy does not provide adequate control, add or intensify insulin.[15] In the United Kingdom Prospective Diabetes Study (UKPDS) trial, the use of insulin therapy for patients with type 2 DM was not associated with decreased cardiovascular (CV) or all-cause mortality despite reductions in blood sugar.[38] A Cochrane review of six trials also did not find evidence of major clinical benefit for use of long-acting insulin analogs for patients with type 2 DM.[39]
    - In addition, although intensified therapy with insulin increased survival by about 2 years in patients with DM following myocardial infarction in one study,[40] insulin therapy was associated with increased mortality in patients with DM undergoing coronary artery bypass grafting based on a meta-analysis of 11 studies.[41]
    - For patients with type 2 DM on monotherapy with insulin, adding oral hypoglycemic agents has positive effects on glycemic control and insulin requirements.[42]
    - Finally, if insulin is added, continuing metformin if possible is advised, as there is less weight gain associated with this combination.[42]
- Consultation with an endocrinologist is suggested if a third agent is needed, and the choice of agent should be made with consideration of the patient's age (decline in renal and cardiac function may preclude use of metformin or a thiazolidinedione), weight (e.g., metformin, acarbose, exenatide, sitagliptin, and human amylin are more often associated with weight loss or maintenance), and comorbidities.[15] SOR Ⓒ

▶ Lipid control

If the initial statin does not result in adequate control, AACE recommends addition of a bile acid sequestrant, niacin, and/or cholesterol absorption inhibitor.[4]

SURGERY

- Bariatric surgery plus intensive medical therapy is more effective than intensive medical therapy alone in decreasing, or sometimes resolving, hyperglycemia and for improving cardiovascular risk factors and quality of life in patients with DM who are overweight or obese.[43,44] Nutritional adverse effects and anemia occur following biliopancreatic diversion procedures.

COMPLEMENTARY AND ALTERNATIVE THERAPY

- Several Chinese herbal medicines (e.g., Xianzhen Pian, Qidan Tongmai) show hypoglycemic effects in patients with type 2 DM, but current evidence does not support widespread use.[45]
- In another Cochrane review of herbal mixtures, significant reductions in hemoglobin A_{1c}, fasting blood sugar or both were observed with Diabecon, Inolter, and Cogent db compared to placebo; however, small sample sizes precluded definite conclusions regarding efficacy.[46]
- Psyllium fiber appears useful for both prevention and adjunctive treatment of DM for glycemic control.[47]

REFERRAL OR HOSPITALIZATION

- Consider referral for bariatric surgery for patients with DM who have a body mass index (BMI) of 35 kg/m^2 or more, as this facilitates weight loss and improvement or reversal of hyperglycemia[4]; surgery has not yet been shown to decrease all-cause mortality, and long-term risk, beyond 5 years, is unknown. SOR Ⓐ
- Consultation with a foot specialist should be considered for patients with DM and foot deformity, infected lesions, foot ulcers, or deformed nails or thick calluses. SOR Ⓒ
- Refer patients with diabetic retinopathy to an ophthalmologist for evaluation and treatment. SOR Ⓑ
- Consider consultation with a vascular surgeon for patients with peripheral vascular disease. SOR Ⓒ
- Patients with type 2 DM may require hospitalization for hyperglycemic crises (e.g., hyperosmolar hyperglycemic state, ketoacidosis) or severe hypoglycemia.

PREVENTION AND SCREENING

Primary prevention is considered for patients who have prediabetes, defined by the AACE as the presence of impaired glucose tolerance (i.e., an oral glucose tolerance test glucose value of 140 to 199 mg/dL, 2 hours after ingesting 75 g of glucose and/or a fasting glucose value of 100 to 125 mg/dL).[4] Each year 3% to 10% of individuals with prediabetes will progress to type 2 DM.[48]

- Lifestyle changes that can prevent or at least delay type 2 DM in persons who have prediabetes include weight loss of 5% to 10% of body weight in overweight individuals and participation in moderate physical activity.[4,49] SOR Ⓐ
- Smoking cessation should be encouraged; tobacco smoking increases the risk of macrovascular complications approximately 4% to 400% in adults with type 2 DM (see Chapter 248, Smoking and Tobacco Addiction).
- Provide annual influenza immunization and pneumococcal vaccine as needed; repeat the pneumococcal vaccine at 5 years for patients with nephrotic syndrome, or chronic renal disease, or who are immunocompromised, or who are receiving the vaccine before age 65 years if 5 years has passed since the primary vaccine was given.[4]
- The AACE also suggests that metformin, acarbose, or thiazolidinediones be considered for those with prediabetes.[4]
- In a meta-analysis of lifestyle and pharmacologic interventions for the prevention or delay of DM in patients with impaired glucose tolerance, the number needed to treat to benefit was 6.4 for lifestyle (95% CI, 5.0–8.4), 10.8 for oral diabetes drugs (95% CI, 8.1–15.0), and 5.4 for orlistat (95% CI, 4.1–7.6).[50] SOR Ⓐ In a recent 15-year follow-up of 2776 (88%) of the surviving cohort initially enrolled in the 3-year Diabetes Prevention Program, cumulative incidences of diabetes were 55% in the lifestyle group, 56% in the metformin group, and 62% in the placebo group.[51]
- In a Swedish study of 1658 patients without DM who underwent bariatric surgery and 1771 obese matched controls, type 2 DM developed in 392 participants in the control group (incidence rate 28.4 cases per 1000 person years) and in 110 in the bariatric-surgery group (incidence rate 6.8 cases per 1000 person years).[52] Surgical complications included postoperative mortality in 0.2% and reoperation for complications in 2.8% of patients who underwent bariatric surgery.
- Low-dose aspirin is recommended for patients with DM who have risk factors for CV disease and are older than age 40 years.[4]

Secondary prevention for micro- and macrovascular disease:

- Use of an ACE inhibitor can prevent new-onset diabetic nephropathy and death in patients with diabetes and normoalbuminuria.[53] SOR Ⓐ
- Patients with DM should undergo a dilated comprehensive eye examination at diagnosis and annually.[4] SOR Ⓒ Panretinal scatter photocoagulation reduces the risk of severe visual loss by more than 50% in eyes with high-risk characteristics, and immediate focal laser photocoagulation reduces the risk of moderate visual loss by at least 50% in patients with clinically significant macular edema.[54]
- Patients with DM should also undergo screening for peripheral neuropathy at diagnosis or 5 years after diagnosis and then annually.[4] Testing may include inspection and assessment of pulses and sensation; use of a monofilament for sensory testing; vibration perception using a 128-Hz tuning fork; ankle reflexes; and touch, pinprick, and warm and cold thermal sensations.[4] Patients with peripheral vascular disease, foot ulcers, or diabetic foot deformity should be considered for referral (as above) to prevent limb loss.
- As discussed above, patients with well-controlled BP, lipids, and good glycemic control have a lower risk of macrovascular and microvascular disease and diabetic dermopathy.[4,10] For example, estimates for years of life saved with lipid lowering in patients with diabetes are 3 years to 3.4 years for men and 1.6 years to 2.4 years for women—greater increases than for patients without diabetes.[55]
- The U.S. Preventive Services Task Force (USPSTF) recommends screening for type 2 DM as part of cardiovascular risk assessment in adults aged 40 to 70 years who are overweight or obese.[56] SOR Ⓑ
- Screening for type 2 DM should be considered in the presence of risk factors for DM (see "Risk Factors" above) every 2 to 3 years.[4] SOR Ⓒ However, in a United Kingdom sample of 16,047 high-risk individuals, screening for DM was not associated with a reduction in all-cause, cardiovascular, or diabetes-related mortality within 10 years.[57]

▶ Pregnancy

- AACE and the American Diabetes Association recommend that pregnant women with DM risk factors should be screened at the first prenatal visit for undiagnosed DM, and all pregnant women should be screened for gestational diabetes mellitus (GDM) at 24 to 28 weeks' gestation, using a 75-g (glucose), 2-hour oral glucose tolerance test.[4] SOR Ⓑ There are limited supporting data on screening and a lack of consensus on optimal screening; the American College of Obstetricians and Gynecologists recommends selective (risk-based) screening at 24 to 28 weeks' gestation, with earlier screening recommended in women with a history of gestational diabetes, known impaired glucose metabolism, or obesity, and the USPSTF recommends universal screening for GDM in asymptomatic pregnant women after 24 weeks of gestation.

PROGNOSIS

- Sustained elevation in fasting blood glucose levels and 2-hour post-load glucose testing, even when below the threshold for a diabetes diagnosis, is significantly associated with future CV events and mortality.
- Poorly controlled diabetes before conception and during the first trimester of pregnancy can cause major birth defects in 3% to 10% of pregnancies and perinatal mortality rates of 31.7% to 32.3% of pregnancies.[58] These rates are much higher than those in the general population (2% and 8.5%, respectively).
- In 2010, diabetes was listed as the underlying cause on 69,071 death certificates and was listed as a contributing factor on an additional 234,051 death certificates.[1] Complications of diabetes contributing to death included heart disease (death rates 1.7 times higher than for adults without DM) and stroke (1.5 times higher than for adults without DM).
- Diabetes is the leading cause of new cases of blindness (4.4% have advanced diabetic retinopathy), kidney failure (49,677 people began treatment for end-stage renal disease in 2011), and nontraumatic lower-limb amputation (73,000 amputations in 2010).[1]

FOLLOW-UP

- Routine follow-up is recommended to continue to assist patients with risk factor reduction, adherence to treatment, and screening for diabetes complications (including depression), as well as to provide ongoing support and guidance. Visit frequency depends on the patient's needs, recent changes in management, and severity of complications.
- The AACE recommends development of a comprehensive care plan that includes modification of CVD risk factors.[4,15] Hypoglycemic therapy is evaluated frequently (e.g., every 3 months) until stable using multiple criteria (e.g., A_{1c}, self-monitoring [fasting and postprandial glucose], documented and suspected hypoglycemic events, lipid and BP values, adverse events [weight gain, fluid retention, hepatic or renal impairment, or CVD], comorbidities, other relevant laboratory data, concomitant drug administration, diabetic complications, and psychosocial factors affecting patient care). Less frequent monitoring is acceptable once targets are achieved.
    - Monitoring frequency for patients with kidney impairment is based on degree of albuminuria (mild to severe) and glomerular filtration rate, ranging from once to four or more times annually.
- A fasting lipid profile is recommended by AACE annually.
    - Remind the patient to schedule dilated ophthalmic exams with an optometrist or ophthalmologist.
    - Monitor foot exams annually or more frequently and educate the patient on appropriate recognition, prevention, and management of infections.

PATIENT EDUCATION

- Patient education includes information about DM (e.g., treatment options), primary and secondary prevention recommendations, and self-management.
- Recommended self-management activities include goal setting, incorporating nutrition management and physical activity into lifestyle, and prevention and early detection of complications (e.g., medication adherence, foot care).[4]

PATIENT RESOURCES

- American Diabetes Association. Provides information and support—**https://www.diabetes.org.**
- MedlinePlus. *Diabetes*—**https://medlineplus/diabetes.html.**

PROVIDER RESOURCES

- Handelsman Y, Bloomgarden ZT, Grunberger G, et al. American Association of Clinical Endocrinologists and American College of Endocrinology—clinical practice guidelines for developing a DM comprehensive care plan—2015. *Endocr Pract.* 2015; 21(Suppl 1):1-87.
- Garber AJ, Abrahamson MJ, Barzilay JI, et al. Consensus statement by the American Association of Clinical Endocrinologists and American College of Endocrinology on the comprehensive type 2 diabetes management algorithm—2017 Executive Summary. *Endocr Pract.* 2017;23(2):207-237.
- Centers for Disease Control and Prevention. *Diabetes Home*—**https://www.cdc.gov/diabetes/home/index.html.**
- National Institute of Diabetes and Digestive and Kidney Diseases. *Diabetes*—**https://www.niddk.nih.gov/health-information/diabetes.**

REFERENCES

1. Centers for Disease Control and Prevention. *2014 National Diabetes Statistics Report.* https://www.cdc.gov/diabetes/pubs/statsreport14/national-diabetes-report-web.pdf. Accessed June 2017.
2. Burchfiel CM, Hamman RF, Marshall JA, et al. Cardiovascular risk factors and impaired glucose tolerance: the San Luis Valley Diabetes Study. *Am J Epidemiol.* 1990;131(1):57-70.
3. Juonala M, Magnussen CG, Berenson GS, et al. Childhood adiposity, adult adiposity, and cardiovascular risk factors. *N Engl J Med.* 2011;365(20):1876-1885.
4. Handelsman Y, Bloomgarden ZT, Grunberger G, et al. American Association of Clinical Endocrinologists and American College of Endocrinology—clinical practice guidelines for developing a diabetes mellitus comprehensive care plan—2015. *Endocr Pract.* 2015;21(Suppl 1):1-87.
5. Pan A, Sun Q, Bernstein AM, et al. Red meat consumption and risk of type 2 diabetes: 3 cohorts of US adults and an updated meta-analysis. *Am J Clin Nutr.* 2011;94(4):1088-1096.
6. Grøntved A, Hu FB. Television viewing and risk of type 2 diabetes, cardiovascular disease, and all-cause mortality: a meta-analysis. *JAMA.* 2011;305(23):2448-2455.
7. Yeboah J, Bertoni AG, Herrington DM, et al. Impaired fasting glucose and the risk of incident diabetes mellitus and cardiovascular events in an adult population: MESA (Multi-Ethnic Study of Atherosclerosis). *J Am Coll Cardiol.* 2011;58(2): 140-146.
8. Emdin CA, Anderson SG, Woodward M, Rahimi K. Usual blood pressure and risk of new-onset diabetes: evidence from 4.1 million adults and a meta-analysis of prospective studies. *J Am Coll Cardiol.* 2015;66(14):1552-1562.
9. Das SL, Singh PP, Phillips AR, et al. Newly diagnosed diabetes mellitus after acute pancreatitis: a systematic review and meta-analysis. *Gut.* 2014;63(5):818-831.
10. Noble D, Mathur R, Dent T, et al. Risk models and scores for type 2 diabetes: systematic review. *BMJ.* 2011;343:d7163.
11. Wilson PW, Meigs JB, Sullivan L, et al. Prediction of incident diabetes mellitus in middle-aged adults: the Framingham Offspring Study. *Arch Intern Med.* 2007;167:1068-1074.
12. Sibbald RG, Landolt SJ, Toth D. Skin and diabetes. *Endocrinol Metab Clin North Am.* 1996;25(2):463-472.
13. Litonjua P, Pinero-Pilona A, Aviles-Santa L, et al. Prevalence of acanthosis nigricans in newly-diagnosed type 2 diabetes. *Endocr Pract.* 2004;10:101-106.

14. van der Ven A, Chapman CB, Bowker JH. Charcot neuroarthropathy of the foot and ankle. *J Am Acad Orthop Surg*. 2009;17(9):562-571.
15. Garber AJ, Abrahamson MJ, Barzilay JI, et al. Consensus statement by the American Association of Clinical Endocrinologists and American College of Endocrinology on the comprehensive type 2 diabetes management algorithm—2017 Executive Summary. *Endocr Pract*. 2017;23(2):207-237.
16. Patel A, MacMahon S, Chalmers J, et al. The Advance Collaborative Group. Intensive blood glucose control and vascular outcomes in patients with type 2 diabetes. *N Engl J Med*. 2008;358(24):2560-2572.
17. Hemmingsen B, Lund SS, Gluud C, et al. Intensive glycaemic control for patients with type 2 diabetes: systematic review with meta-analysis and trial sequential analysis of randomised clinical trials. *BMJ*. 2011;343:d6898.
18. Dunkler D, Dehghan M, Teo KK, et al; ONTARGET Investigators. Diet and kidney disease in high-risk individuals with type 2 diabetes mellitus. *JAMA Intern Med*. 2013;173(18):1682-1692.
19. Thomas D, Elliott EJ. Low glycaemic index, or low glycaemic load, diets for diabetes mellitus. *Cochrane Database Syst Rev*. 2009;(1):CD006296.
20. Ajala O, English P, Pinkney J. Systematic review and meta-analysis of different dietary approaches to the management of type 2 diabetes. *Am J Clin Nutr*. 2013;97(3):505-516.
21. Look AHEAD Research Group, Wing RR, Bolin P, Brancati FL, et al. Cardiovascular effects of intensive lifestyle intervention in type 2 diabetes. *N Engl J Med*. 2013;369(2):145-154.
22. Franz MJ, Boucher JL, Rutten-Ramos S, VanWormer JJ. Lifestyle weight-loss intervention outcomes in overweight and obese adults with type 2 diabetes: a systematic review and meta-analysis of randomized clinical trials. *J Acad Nutr Diet*. 2015;115(9):1447-1463.
23. Umpierre D, Ribeiro PA, Kramer CK, et al. Physical activity advice only or structured exercise training and association with HbA1c levels in type 2 diabetes: a systematic review and meta-analysis. *JAMA*. 2011;305(17):1790-1799.
24. Pillay J, Armstrong MJ, Butalia S, et al. Behavioral programs for type 2 diabetes mellitus: a systematic review and network meta-analysis. *Ann Intern Med*. 2015;163(11):848-860.
25. Zhai YK, Zhu WJ, Cai YL, et al. Clinical- and cost-effectiveness of telemedicine in type 2 diabetes mellitus: a systematic review and meta-analysis. *Medicine (Baltimore)*. 2014;93(28):e312.
26. Malanda UL, Welschen LM, Riphagen II, et al. Self-monitoring of blood glucose in patients with type 2 diabetes mellitus who are not using insulin. *Cochrane Database Syst Rev*. 2012;(1):CD005060.
27. Cox DJ, Taylor AG, Singh H, et al. Glycemic load, exercise, and monitoring blood glucose (GEM): a paradigm shift in the treatment of type 2 diabetes mellitus. *Diabetes Res Clin Pract*. 2016;111:28-35.
28. Naik AD, Palmer N, Petersen NJ, et al. Comparative effectiveness of goal setting in diabetes mellitus group clinics: randomized clinical trial. *Arch Intern Med*. 2011;171(5):453-459.
29. Emdin CA, Rahimi K, Neal B, et al. Blood pressure lowering in type 2 diabetes: a systematic review and meta-analysis. *JAMA*. 2015;313(6):603-615.
30. Palmer SC, Mavridis D, Navarese E, et al. Comparative efficacy and safety of blood pressure-lowering agents in adults with diabetes and kidney disease: a network meta-analysis. *Lancet*. 2015;385(9982):2047-2056.
31. ACCORD Study Group, Cushman WC, Evans GW, Byington RP. Effects of intensive blood-pressure control in type 2 diabetes mellitus. *N Engl J Med*. 2010;362(17):1575-1585.
32. Brunström M, Carlberg B. Effect of antihypertensive treatment at different blood pressure levels in patients with diabetes mellitus: systematic review and meta-analyses. *BMJ*. 2016;352:i717.
33. Palmer SC, Mavridis D, Nicolucci A, et al. Comparison of clinical outcomes and adverse events associated with glucose-lowering drugs in patients with type 2 diabetes: a meta-analysis. *JAMA*. 2016;316(3):313-324.
34. Maruthur NM, Tseng E, Hutfless S, et al. Diabetes medications as monotherapy or metformin-based combination therapy for type 2 diabetes: a systematic review and meta-analysis. *Ann Intern Med*. 2016;164(11):740-751.
35. Turner RC, Cull CA, Frighi V, et al. Glycemic control with diet, sulfonylurea, metformin, or insulin in patients with type 2 diabetes mellitus: progressive requirement for multiple therapies (UKPDS 49). *JAMA*. 1999;281:2005-2012.
36. de Zeeuw D, Anzalone DA, Cain VA, et al. Renal effects of atorvastatin and rosuvastatin in patients with diabetes who have progressive renal disease (PLANET I): a randomised clinical trial. *Lancet Diabetes Endocrinol*. 2015;3(3):181-190.
37. Gross JL, Kramer CK, Leitao CB, et al. Effect of antihyperglycemic agents added to metformin and a sulfonylurea on glycemic control and weight gain in type 2 diabetes: a network meta-analysis. *Ann Intern Med*. 2011;154(10):672-679.
38. Effect of intensive blood-glucose control with metformin on complications in overweight patients with type 2 diabetes (UKPDS 34). UK Prospective Diabetes Study (UKPDS) Group. *Lancet*. 1998;352(9131):854-865.
39. Horvath K, Jeitler K, Berghold A, et al. Long-acting insulin analogues versus NPH insulin (human isophane insulin) for type 2 diabetes mellitus. *Cochrane Database Syst Rev*. 2007;(2):CD005613.
40. Ritsinger V, Malmberg K, Mårtensson A, et al. Intensified insulin-based glycaemic control after myocardial infarction: mortality during 20 year follow-up of the randomised Diabetes Mellitus Insulin Glucose Infusion in Acute Myocardial Infarction (DIGAMI 1) trial. *Lancet Diabetes Endocrinol*. 2014;2(8):627-633.
41. Munnee K, Bundhun PK, Quan H, Tang Z. Comparing the clinical outcomes between insulin-treated and non-insulin-treated patients with type 2 diabetes mellitus after coronary artery bypass surgery: a systematic review and meta-analysis. *Medicine (Baltimore)*. 2016;95(10):e3006.
42. Vos RC, van Avendonk MJP, Jansen H, et al. Insulin monotherapy compared with the addition of oral glucose-lowering agents to insulin for people with type 2 diabetes already on insulin therapy

and inadequate glycaemic control. *Cochrane Database Syst Rev.* 2016;(9):CD006992.

43. Schauer PR, Bhatt DL, Kirwan JP, et al; STAMPEDE Investigators. Bariatric surgery versus intensive medical therapy for diabetes—5-year outcomes. *N Engl J Med.* 2017;376(7):641-651.
44. Yan Y, Sha Y, Yao G, et al. Roux-en-Y gastric bypass versus medical treatment for type 2 diabetes mellitus in obese patients: a systematic review and meta-analysis of randomized controlled trials. *Medicine (Baltimore).* 2016;95(17):e3462.
45. Liu JP, Zhang M, Wang W, Grimsgaard S. Chinese herbal medicines for type 2 diabetes mellitus. *Cochrane Database Syst Rev.* 2004;(3):CD003642.
46. Sridharan K, Mohan R, Ramaratnam S, Panneerselvam D. Ayurvedic treatments for diabetes mellitus. *Cochrane Database Syst Rev.* 2011;(12):CD008288.
47. Gibb RD, McRorie JW Jr, Russell DA, et al. Psyllium fiber improves glycemic control proportional to loss of glycemic control: a meta-analysis of data in euglycemic subjects, patients at risk of type 2 diabetes mellitus, and patients being treated for type 2 diabetes mellitus. *Am J Clin Nutr.* 2015;102(6):1604-1614.
48. Twigg SM, Kamp MC, Davis TM, et al. Prediabetes: a position statement from the Australian Diabetes Society and Australian Diabetes Educators Association. *Med J Aust.* 2007;186(9):461-465.
49. Lindström J, Ilanne-Parikka P, Peltonen M, et al, for the Finnish Diabetes Prevention Study Group. Sustained reduction in the incidence of type 2 diabetes by lifestyle intervention: follow-up of the Finnish Diabetes Prevention Study. *Lancet.* 2006;368(9548):1673-1679.
50. Gillies CL, Abrams KR, Lambert PC, et al. Pharmacological and lifestyle interventions to prevent or delay type 2 diabetes in people with impaired glucose tolerance: systematic review and meta-analysis. *BMJ.* 2007;334(7588):299.
51. Diabetes Prevention Program Research Group. Long-term effects of lifestyle intervention or metformin on diabetes development and microvascular complications over 15-year follow-up: the Diabetes Prevention Program Outcomes Study. *Lancet Diabetes Endocrinol.* 2015;3(11):866-875.
52. Carlsson LM, Peltonen M, Ahlin S, et al. Bariatric surgery and prevention of type 2 diabetes in Swedish obese subjects. *N Engl J Med.* 2012;367(8):695-704.
53. Lv J, Perkovic V, Foote CV, et al. Antihypertensive agents for preventing diabetic kidney disease. *Cochrane Database Syst Rev.* 2012;(12):CD004136.
54. Neubauer AS, Ulbig MW. Laser treatment in diabetic retinopathy. *Ophthalmologica.* 2007;221(2):95-102.
55. Grover SA, Coupal L, Zowall H, et al. Evaluating the benefits of treating dyslipidemia: the importance of diabetes as a risk factor. *Am J Med.* 2003;115(2):122-128.
56. U.S. Preventive Services Task Force. *Final Update Summary: Abnormal Blood Glucose and Type 2 Diabetes Mellitus: Screening.* September 2016. https://www.uspreventiveservicestaskforce.org/Page/Document/UpdateSummaryFinal/screening-for-abnormal-blood-glucose-and-type-2-diabetes?ds=1&s=diabetes. Accessed June 2017.
57. Simmons RK, Echouffo-Tcheugui JB, Sharp SJ, et al. Screening for type 2 diabetes and population mortality over 10 years (ADDITION-Cambridge): a cluster-randomised controlled trial. *Lancet.* 2012;380(9855):1741-1748.
58. Ali S, Dornhorst A. Diabetes in pregnancy: health risks and management. *Postgrad Med J.* 2011;87(1028):417-427.

229 ACANTHOSIS NIGRICANS

Mindy A. Smith, MD, MS
Sarah J. James, DO

PATIENT STORY

A 13-year-old Hispanic girl presents to her family physician with concerns about "dirty areas" under her arms and on her neck that "can't be cleaned" (**Figure 229-1**). Her periods have stopped and she is getting new hair growth on her face. She is overweight and has a family history of diabetes. The physician makes the diagnosis of acanthosis nigricans.

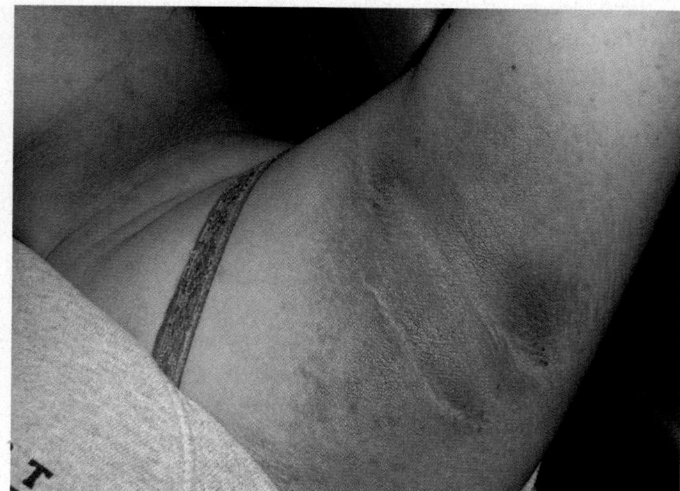

FIGURE 229-1 Acanthosis nigricans on the neck and in the axilla of an overweight 13-year-old Hispanic girl. She also has hirsutism, secondary amenorrhea, and a family history of diabetes. (*Reproduced with permission from Richard P. Usatine, MD.*)

INTRODUCTION

- Acanthosis nigricans (AN) is a localized form of hyperpigmentation that involves epidermal alteration. AN is usually associated with insulin resistance or hyperinsulinemia and is seen in patients with endocrine disorders (e.g., type 2 diabetes mellitus [DM], Cushing syndrome, acromegaly), obesity, and polycystic ovary syndrome.[1-3]

EPIDEMIOLOGY

- In a cross-sectional study of prevalence conducted in a nationwide underserved practice-based research network (N = 1730), AN was found in 18.2% of children and 19.5% of adults. Those with AN were twice as likely to have DM as those without AN (35.4% vs. 17.6%, $p < 0.001$).[4]
- Several studies have used AN as a predictor of metabolic syndrome[5,6]; AN observed on the knuckles of Latin American youth had been reported as an early clinical indicator.[7]
- AN is sometimes associated with malignancy, primarily adenocarcinoma (60%) of the stomach, gallbladder, colon, ovary, pancreas, rectum, and uterus.[2,8,9]
- Although most cases are idiopathic, there are also genetic causes of AN.[2,8]
- A condition of hyperandrogenism (HA), insulin resistance (IR), and AN called HAIR-AN syndrome occurs in approximately 1% to 3% of women with HA.[10] This syndrome may also be seen in patients with autoimmune disorders such as Hashimoto thyroiditis.
- AN can be an adverse effect from hormonal therapies.[11]

ETIOLOGY AND PATHOPHYSIOLOGY

- AN results from long-term exposure of keratinocytes to insulin.[2]
- Keratinocytes have insulin and insulin-like growth receptors on their surface. The pathogenesis of this condition is linked to insulin

binding to insulin-like growth receptors in the epidermis stimulating keratinocyte proliferation.[2]

- Fibroblast growth factor receptor 3 (FGFR3) gene mutations should be considered in patients with coexistent AN and skeletal dysplasia.[12]

DIAGNOSIS

The diagnosis of AN is made clinically, with histopathology only when confirmation is needed, and can be classified by severity on a scale of 0–4. Increased scores correlate with increased BMI and fasting insulin levels.[2]

CLINICAL FEATURES

- AN ranges in appearance from diffuse streaky thickened brown velvety lesions to leathery verrucous papillomatous lesions (**Figures 229-1** to **229-9**).
- Women with HAIR-AN syndrome have evidence of virilization (e.g., increased body hair in male distribution, enlarged clitoris) in addition to AN.[10]

TYPICAL DISTRIBUTION

- Commonly located on the neck (see **Figures 229-3** to **229-5**) or skin folds (i.e., axillae [see **Figures 229-1**, **229-2**, and **229-9**], inframammary folds, groin, and perineum).[2]
- Less often AN can be seen on the nipples or areolae, perineum, and extensor surfaces of the legs.[2,8]
- Verrucous AN may affect the eyelids, lips, and buccal mucosa.[8]
- In patients with malignancy, the onset of AN can be abrupt, and the distribution of lesions is more widespread and may include the palms and soles.[9]
- AN is a possible consequence of repetitively used insulin injection sites.[2,13]

LABORATORY TESTING

- Obtain blood test for blood glucose or insulin level, and consider lipid testing.[1,5-7,14]

BIOPSY

- May be needed in unusual cases.
- Histologic examination reveals hyperkeratosis and papillary hypertrophy, although the epidermis is only mildly thickened.[15]

DIFFERENTIAL DIAGNOSIS

Other hyperpigmented lesions that may be confused with AN include:

- Seborrheic keratosis (see Chapter 164, Seborrheic Keratosis)—Most commonly found on the trunk or the face; these lesions are more plaque-like with adherent, greasy scale and have a "stuck-on" appearance.
- Tinea versicolor around the neck could be confused with acanthosis nigricans when it is hyperpigmented in the neck region (see Chapter 147, Tinea Versicolor). However, most AN extends to the

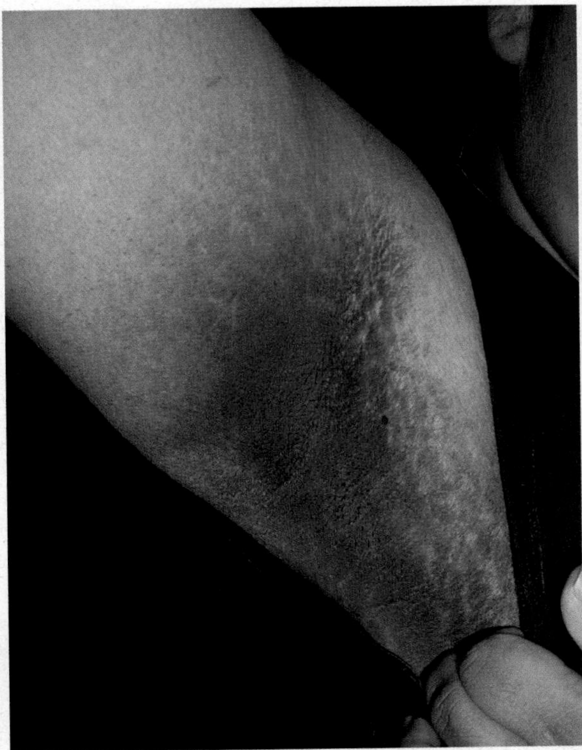

FIGURE 229-2 Acanthosis nigricans in the right axilla of a 25-year-old woman with type 2 diabetes. The skin appears velvety. *(Reproduced with permission from Richard P. Usatine, MD.)*

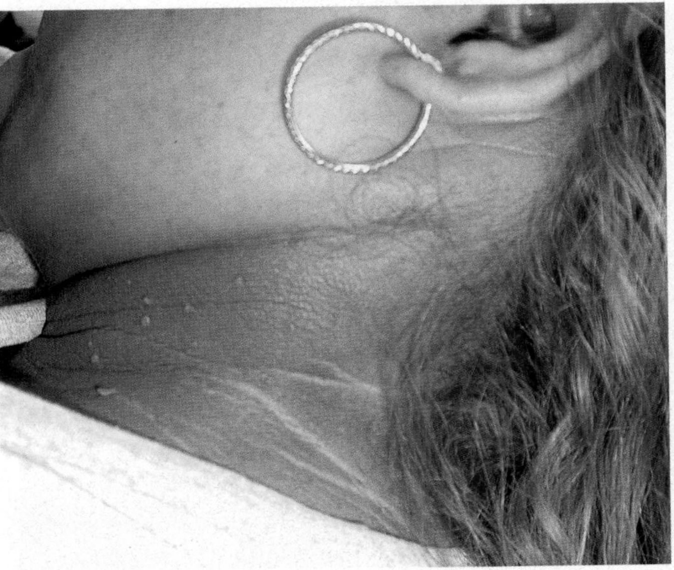

FIGURE 229-3 Acanthosis nigricans on the neck of an obese Hispanic woman with type 2 diabetes. Note that multiple skin tags are also present. *(Reproduced with permission from Richard P. Usatine, MD.)*

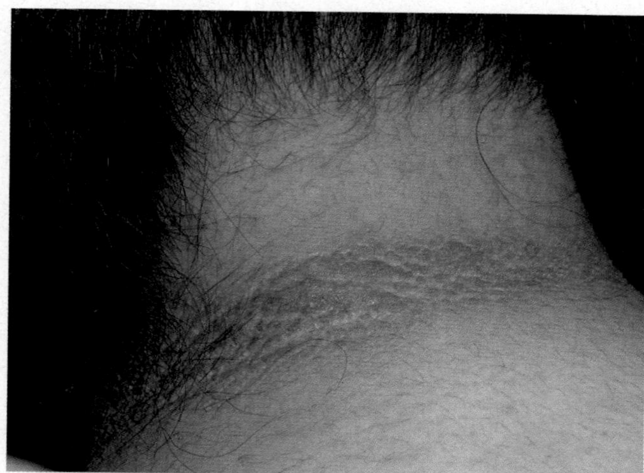

FIGURE 229-4 Acanthosis nigricans on the neck of an obese woman with type 2 diabetes. Note the hypertrophic thickening of the darker skin. (*Reproduced with permission from Richard P. Usatine, MD.*)

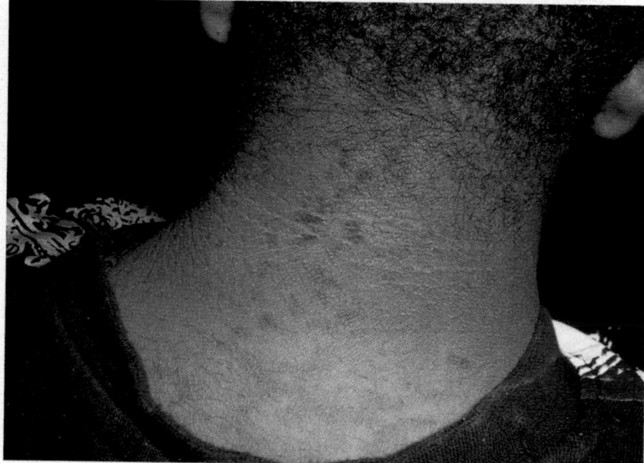

FIGURE 229-5 Acanthosis nigricans on the neck of a 15-year-old boy with no obesity or diabetes. His mother has very prominent acanthosis nigricans. (*Reproduced with permission from Richard P. Usatine, MD.*)

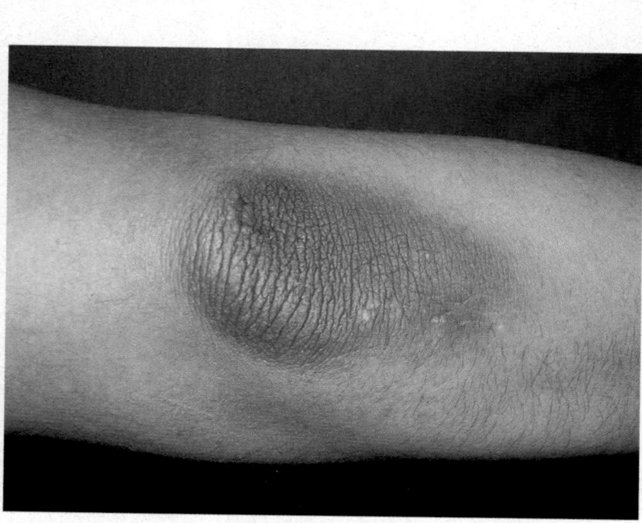

FIGURE 229-6 Acanthosis nigricans on the elbow of a young obese Hispanic woman. (*Reproduced with permission from Richard P. Usatine, MD.*)

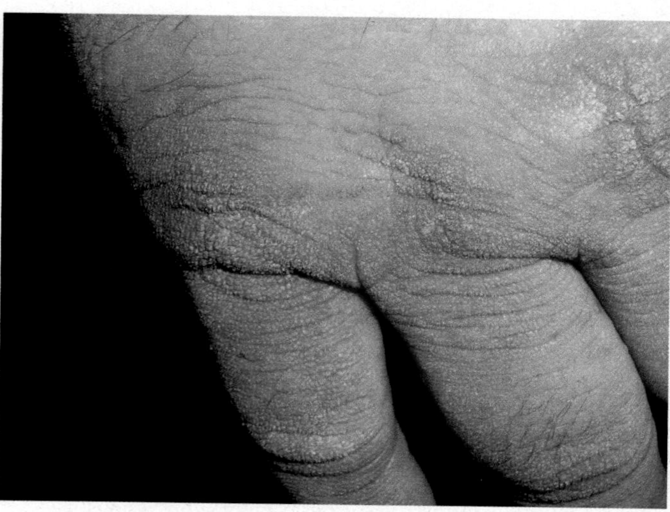

FIGURE 229-7 Acanthosis nigricans on the dorsum of the hand in a morbidly obese young man. Note the hyperpigmentation and tiny papules present. (*Reproduced with permission from Richard P. Usatine, MD.*)

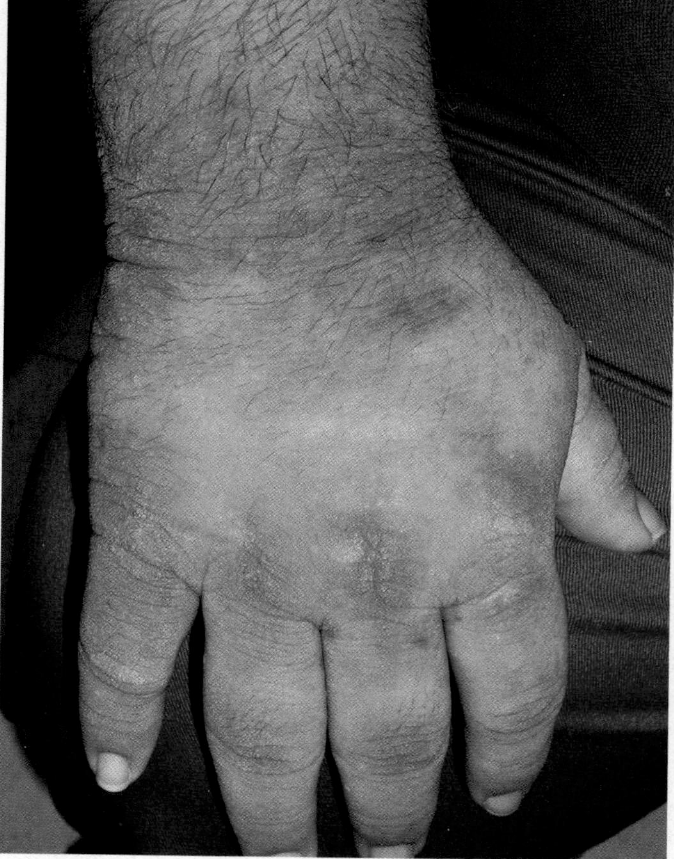

FIGURE 229-8 Acanthosis nigricans on the hand and wrist of a morbidly obese young man with widespread acanthosis. Note the texture of the skin along with the skin darkening. (*Reproduced with permission from Richard P. Usatine, MD.*)

trunk in a capelike distribution, is less raised, has more scale, and is not velvety by palpation.

MANAGEMENT

NONPHARMACOLOGIC

- Weight loss through diet and exercise helps reverse the process, probably by reducing both IR and compensatory hyperinsulinemia.

MEDICATIONS

- Keratolytic agents, such as salicylic, glycolic, or trichloroacetic acid, can improve the cosmetic appearance.[2,16] Other topical therapies, including 0.1% adapalene gel[17] or 0.1% tretinoin cream (to lighten the lesion), combination tretinoin cream with 12% ammonium lactate cream, or topical vitamin D ointments,[18] may be useful.[2,8] SOR Ⓒ Adapalene gel is now, so no prior authorizations are needed.
- Metformin and rosiglitazone have also been used to manage AN.[2] SOR Ⓒ

COMPLEMENTARY AND ALTERNATIVE THERAPY

- The use of omega-3-fatty acid and dietary fish oil supplementation has also been reported to improve AN.[2] SOR Ⓒ

PROCEDURES

- Long-pulsed alexandrite laser therapy[2] and dermabrasion are alternative treatments.[8]
- Some patients have many skin tags within the area of acanthosis and request them to be removed (**Figure 229-9**). (See Chapter 163, Skin Tag, for details on treatment.)

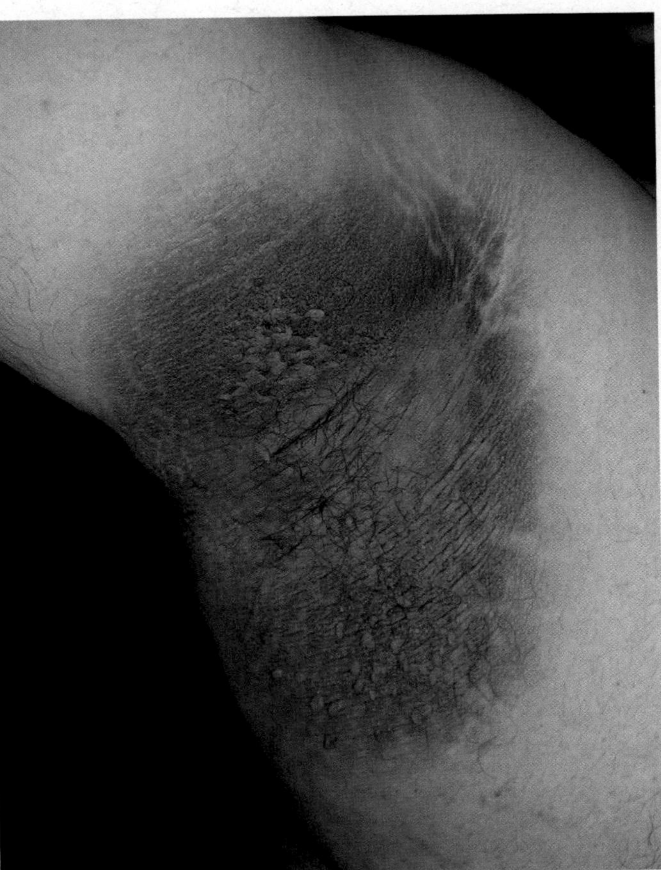

FIGURE 229-9 Acanthosis nigricans in the axilla of a man with type 2 diabetes. Note the many skin tags also present. (*Reproduced with permission from Richard P. Usatine, MD.*)

PROGNOSIS

- AN usually regresses when the underlying condition (e.g., diabetes, malignancy) is treated.[8]

PATIENT EDUCATION

- Patients who are overweight should be encouraged to lose weight through diet and exercise, because weight loss may cause AN to improve or resolve.

PATIENT RESOURCES

- **http://www.diabetes.org/living-with-diabetes/complications/skin-complications.html?loc=lwd-slabnav.**
- **http://www.nlm.nih.gov/medlineplus/ency/article/000852.htm.**

PROVIDER RESOURCES

- Centers for Disease Control and Prevention. *Diabetes Home*—**https://www.cdc.gov/diabetes/home/index.html.**

REFERENCES

1. Schilling WHK, Crook MA. Cutaneous stigmata associated with insulin resistance and increased cardiovascular risk. *Int J Dermatol.* 2014;53:1064-1065.
2. Phiske MM. An approach to acanthosis nigricans. *Indian Dermatol Online J.* 2014;5(3):239-249.
3. Huang L, Huang J, Dong Z. Associations of acanthosis nigricans with metabolic abnormalities in polycystic ovary syndrome women with normal body mass index. *J Dermatol.* 2013;40: 188-192.
4. Kong AS, Williams RL, Rhyne R, et al. Acanthosis nigricans: high prevalence and association with diabetes in practice-based research network consortium—a PRImary care Multi-Ethnic Network (PRIME Net) study. *J Am Board Fam Med.* 2010;23(4): 476-485.
5. Koh YK, Lee JH, Kim EY, et al. Acanthosis nigricans as a clinical predictor of insulin resistance in obese children. *Pediatr Gastroenterol Hepatol Nutr.* 2016;19(4):251-258.
6. Verma S, Vasani R, Joshi R, et al. A descriptive student of facial acanthosis nigricans and its association with body mass index, waist circumference and insulin resistance using HOMA2 IR. *Indian Dermatol Online J.* 2016;7(6):498-503.
7. Gomez-Flores M, Gonzalez-Saldivar G, Santos-Santos OR, et al. Implication of a clinically ignored site of acanthosis nigricans: the knuckles. *Exp Clin Endocrinol Diabetes.* 2015;123:27-33.
8. Kapoor S. Diagnosis and treatment of acanthosis nigricans. *Skinmed.* 2010;8(3):161-164.
9. Stulberg DL, Clark N. Common hyperpigmented disorders in adults: part II. *Am Fam Physician.* 2003;68:1963-1968.
10. Elmer KB, George RM. HAIR-AN syndrome: a multisystem challenge. *Am Fam Physician.* 2001;63:2385-2390.
11. Downs AM, Kennedy CT. Somatotrophin-induced acanthosis nigricans. *Br J Dermatol.* 1999;141:390-391.
12. Mir A, Wu T, Orlow S. Cutaneous features of Crouzon syndrome with acanthosis nigricans. *JAMA Dermatol.* 2013;149(6):737-741.
13. Brodell JD, Cannella JD, Helms SE. Acanthosis nigricans resulting from repetitive same-site insulin injections. *J Drugs Dermatol.* 2012;11(12):e85-e87.
14. Rafalson L, Pham T, Willi S, et al. The association between acanthosis nigricans and dysglycemia in an ethnically diverse group of eighth grade students. *Obesity.* 2013;21(3):E328-E333.
15. Sibbald RG, Landolt SJ, Toth D. Skin and diabetes. *Endocrinol Metab Clin North Am.* 1996;25(2):463-472.
16. Ichiyama S, Funasaka Y, Otsuka Y, et al. Effective treatment by glycolic acid peeling for cutaneous manifestation of familial generalized acanthosis nigricans caused by FGFR3 mutation. *J Eur Acad Dermatol Venereol.* 2016;30:442-445.
17. Treesirichod A, Chaithirayanon S, Wongjitrat N, et al. The efficacy of topical 0.1% adapalene gel for the use in the treatment of childhood acanthosis nigricans: a pilot study. *Indian J Dermatol.* 2015; 60(1):103.
18. Hermanns-Le T, Scheen A, Pierard GE. Acanthosis nigricans associated with insulin resistance: pathophysiology and management. *Am J Clin Dermatol.* 2004;5(3):199-203.

230 DIABETIC DERMOPATHY

Mindy A. Smith, MD, MS

PATIENT STORY

A 60-year-old woman with diabetes mellitus (DM) for the past 10 years noticed reddish-colored lesions on both anterior shins that turned brown over the past year (**Figure 230-1**). She reported no pain with the hyperpigmented areas but has neuropathic foot pain. The patient is diagnosed with diabetic dermopathy and begins working with her physician on achieving better control of her diabetes.

INTRODUCTION

Diabetic dermopathy is a constellation of well-demarcated, hyperpigmented, atrophic depressions, macules, or papules located on the anterior surface of the lower legs that is usually found in patients with DM. It is the most common cutaneous marker of DM.

EPIDEMIOLOGY

- Diabetic dermopathy is found in 12.5% to 40% of patients and most often in the elderly. It is less common in women.[1]
- In a case series of 100 consecutive inpatients or outpatients in India with DM and skin lesions, diabetic dermopathy was found in 36%.[2] The incidence was much lower in a second case series of 500 patients attending a diabetes clinic in India, with only 0.2% diagnosed with diabetic dermopathy; the authors concluded that because most patients were well controlled (fasting blood sugar <130 mg/mL in 60%), cutaneous signs of chronic hyperglycemia were decreased.[3] It is also possible that dermopathy is more difficult to see in dark-skinned individuals.
- Sometimes seen in persons without DM, especially patients with circulatory compromise.

ETIOLOGY AND PATHOPHYSIOLOGY

The cause of diabetic dermopathy is unknown.

- Diabetic dermopathy may be related to mechanical or thermal trauma, especially in patients with neuropathy.
- Lesions have been classified as vascular because histology sections demonstrate red blood cell extravasation and capillary basement membrane thickening. In one study, patients with type 1 DM and diabetic dermopathy had marked reduction in skin blood flow at normal-appearing skin areas on the pretibial surface of the legs compared with type 1 control and nondiabetic control patients.[4]
- Dermal changes include fibroblastic proliferation, thickening of collagen bundles and fragmentation or separation of the collagen fibers and edema.[5]
- There is an association between diabetic dermopathy and the presence of retinopathy, nephropathy, and neuropathy.[6,7] In a Turkish study, women with diabetic dermopathy appeared to have a more severe sensorial neuropathy (e.g., loss of deep tendon reflexes, superficial sensory loss, and the loss of vibration sense) than did patients without these skin lesions; a high prevalence of carpel tunnel syndrome (63.8%) was also found in these patients.[8]

DIAGNOSIS

CLINICAL FEATURES

The diagnosis is usually clinical. Lesions often begin as pink patches (0.5 to 1 cm), which become hyperpigmented with surface atrophy and fine scale (**Figures 230-1** to **230-4**).

TYPICAL DISTRIBUTION

Pretibial and lateral areas of the shin (see **Figures 230-1** to **230-4**) in a bilateral asymmetrical distribution; rarely lesions are seen on the arms, thighs, trunk, and abdomen.[5]

BIOPSY

Histology shows epidermal atrophy, thickened small superficial dermal blood vessels, increased epidermal melanin, and hemorrhage with hemosiderin deposits. These findings are not all present in biopsy specimens; in an autopsy series, only 4 of 14 skin biopsies of diabetic dermopathy lesions showed moderate to severe wall thickening of arterioles or medium-sized arteries, 11 of 14 showed mild basement membrane thickening, and 9 of 14 had markedly increased epidermal melanin.[9]

DIFFERENTIAL DIAGNOSIS

Consider the following when evaluating patients with similar skin conditions:

- Early lesions of necrobiosis lipoidica—Erythematous papules or plaques beginning in the pretibial area, but becoming larger and darker with irregular margins and raised erythematous borders. Telangiectasias, atrophy, and yellow discoloration may be seen. The lesion may be painful (see Chapter 231, Necrobiosis Lipoidica).
- Schamberg disease (pigmented purpuric dermatosis) is a capillaritis that produces brown hemosiderin deposits along with visible pink-to-red spots like cayenne pepper on the lower extremities. It is not more common in patients with diabetes but may resemble diabetic dermopathy. A biopsy could be used to distinguish between them (see Chapter 187, Vasculitis).

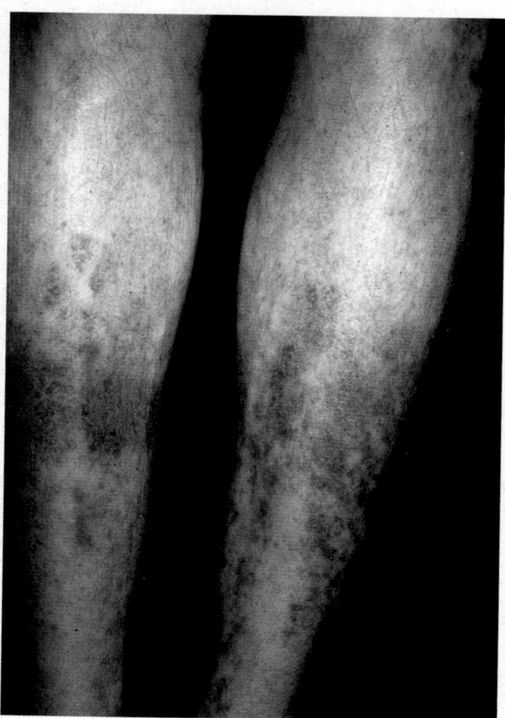

FIGURE 230-1 Lesions of diabetic dermopathy (also called pigmented pretibial papules) on both lower extremities of a 60-year-old woman with diabetes. The skin appears atrophic, and the lesions are flat and hyperpigmented. *(Reproduced with permission from Richard P. Usatine, MD.)*

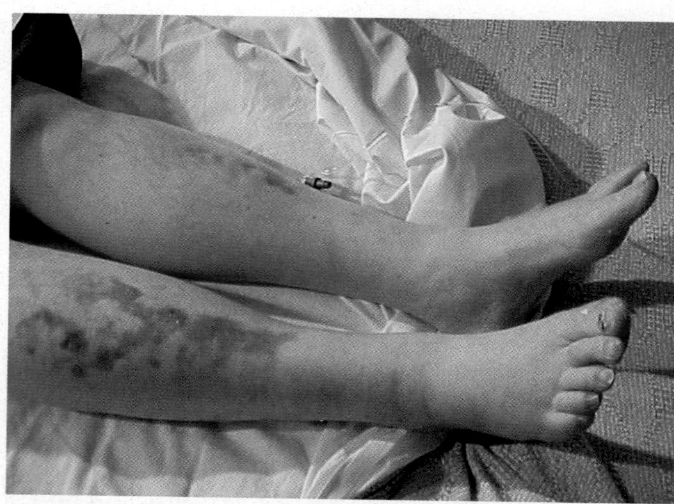

FIGURE 230-3 Diabetic dermopathy on both lower extremities of a middle-age man with diabetes. The sparse hair is secondary to his vasculopathy. *(Reproduced with permission from Dan Stulberg, MD.)*

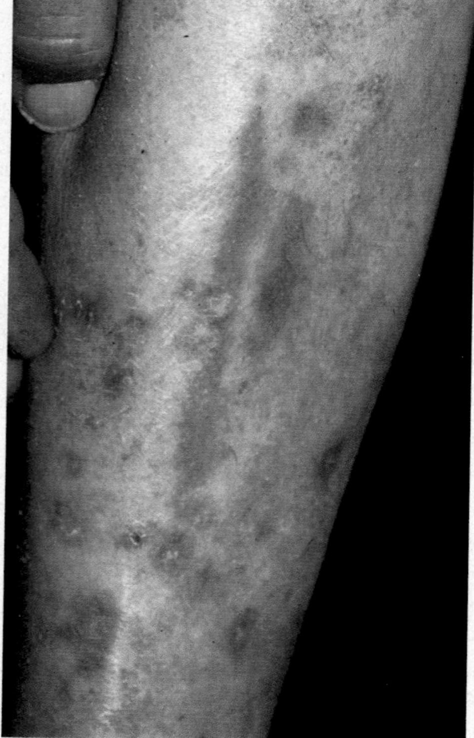

FIGURE 230-2 Diabetic dermopathy on the leg showing pretibial hyperpigmentation and healed ulcers with hypopigmentation. There are also signs of erythema and fine scale. *(Reproduced with permission from Richard P. Usatine, MD.)*

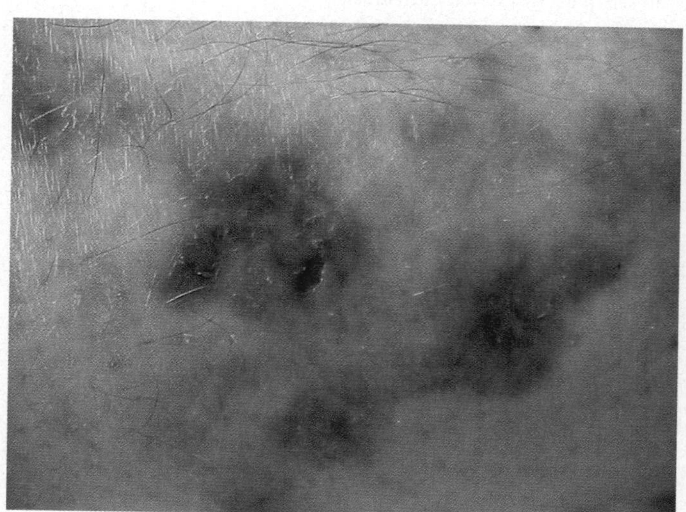

FIGURE 230-4 Close-up of diabetic dermopathy on the right leg showing atrophy, hyperpigmentation, a shallow ulcer, and fine scale. The hyperpigmentation is from hemosiderin deposition. *(Reproduced with permission from Dan Stulberg, MD.)*

- Stasis dermatitis—The typical site is the medial aspect of the ankle. Early lesions are erythematous, scaly, and sometimes pruritic, becoming progressively hyperpigmented (see Chapter 54, Venous Insufficiency).
- Traumatic scars—There is no scale, lesions are permanent, and edema is not usually present.

MANAGEMENT

- There is no effective treatment.
- It is not known whether the lesions improve with better control of diabetes.
- One informal case report stated that patients may benefit from 15 to 25 mg chelated zinc daily for several weeks.[10] SOR Ⓒ

PREVENTION

- It is possible that patients with well-controlled DM have a lower risk of diabetic dermopathy.

PROGNOSIS

- Lesions may resolve spontaneously.

PATIENT EDUCATION

- Reassure patients that the lesions are asymptomatic and may resolve spontaneously within 1 to 2 years, although new lesions may form.

PATIENT RESOURCES

- American Diabetes Association. *Skin Complications*—**http://www.diabetes.org/living-with-diabetes/complications/skin-complications.html?loc=DropDownLWD-skin.**

REFERENCES

1. Sibbald RG, Landolt SJ, Toth D. Skin and diabetes. *Endocrinol Metab Clin North Am.* 1996;25(2):463-472.
2. Goyal A, Raina S, Kaushal SS, et al. Pattern of cutaneous manifestations in diabetes mellitus. *Indian J Dermatol.* 2010;55(1):39-41.
3. Ragunatha S, Anitha B, Inamadar AC, et al. Cutaneous disorders in 500 diabetic patients attending diabetic clinic. *Indian J Dermatol.* 2011;56(2):160-164.
4. Brugler A, Thompson S, Turner S, et al. Skin blood flow abnormalities in diabetic dermopathy. *J Am Acad Dermatol.* 2011;65(3):559-563.
5. George SMC, Walton S. Diabetic dermopathy. *Brit J Diabetes Vasc Dis.* 2014;14(3):95-97.
6. Shemer A, Bergnan R, Linn S, et al. Diabetic dermopathy and internal complications in diabetes mellitus. *Int J Dermatol.* 1998;37(2):113-115.
7. Abdollahi A, Daneshpazhooh M, Amirchaghmaghi E, et al. Dermopathy and retinopathy in diabetes: is there an association? *Dermatology.* 2007;214(2):133-136.
8. Kiziltan ME, Benbir G. Clinical and nerve conduction studies in female patients with diabetic dermopathy. *Acta Diabetol.* 2008;45(2):97-105.
9. McCash S, Emanuel PO. Defining diabetic dermopathy. *J Dermatol.* 2011;38(10):988-992.
10. DiabetesNet.com. *Skin Complications: Necrobiosis Lipoidica.* http://www.diabetesnet.com/diabetes_complications/diabetes_skin_changes.php. Accessed August 2018.

231 NECROBIOSIS LIPOIDICA

Mindy A. Smith, MD, MS

PATIENT STORY

A 30-year-old woman presents with discoloration on both lower legs. She has no personal history of diabetes; however, type 2 diabetes runs in her family. Visible inspection of the lesions is highly suggestive of necrobiosis lipoidica (NL) (**Figure 231-1**). There is hyperpigmentation, yellow discoloration, atrophy, and telangiectasias. The patient is not overweight and had no symptoms of diabetes. Her blood sugar at this visit is 142 after eating lunch 1 hour prior to testing. The following day, the patient's fasting blood sugar is 121, with a glycosylated hemoglobin of 6.1. The patient is informed of her borderline diabetes, and diet and exercise are prescribed. She is disturbed by her skin appearance and chooses to try a moderate-strength topical corticosteroid for treatment.

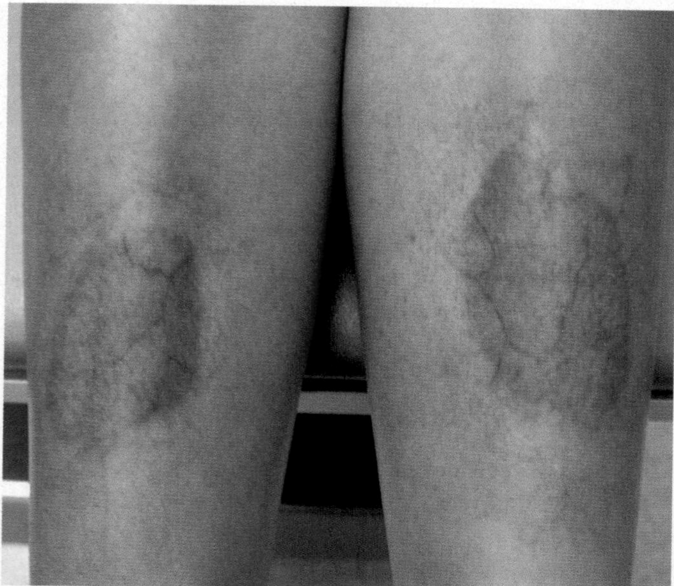

FIGURE 231-1 Necrobiosis lipoidica in a 30-year-old woman with impaired glucose tolerance (borderline diabetes). Note the brown pigmentation and prominent blood vessels. *(Reproduced with permission from Suraj Reddy, MD.)*

INTRODUCTION

- NL is a chronic granulomatous skin condition with degenerative connective-tissue changes most often seen in patients with diabetes mellitus (DM). It was previously called *necrobiosis lipoidica diabeticorum* before the recognition of the significant minority of patients with NL who do not have DM.

EPIDEMIOLOGY

- NL is a rare condition that occurs in approximately 1% (0.3% to 2.3%) of patients with DM.[1-4]
- NL primarily affects women (80%), particularly those with type 1 DM, but it can occur with type 2 DM.[1,2] Lesions, however, may be more prone to ulceration in men (58% vs. 15% in one study).[5] Approximately 75% of patients with NL have or will develop DM.[6]
- Average age of onset is 34 years.[1,2]
- In a study comparing 212 young patients with type 1 DM, ages 2 to 22 years, with sex- and age-matched control patients, most (68% vs. 26.5% of controls) had at least 1 cutaneous disorder, with 2.3% versus 0% of control patients having NL.[4]
- NL has also been reported in patients with Hashimoto thyroiditis.[3]
- Cases of familial NL not associated with DM have also been reported.[7]

ETIOLOGY AND PATHOPHYSIOLOGY

- The cause of NL remains unknown.
- Angiopathy leading to thrombosis and occlusion of the cutaneous vessels has been implicated in its etiology. However, microangiopathic changes are less common in lesions on areas other than the shins and, therefore, are not necessary for developing the lesions.[2]

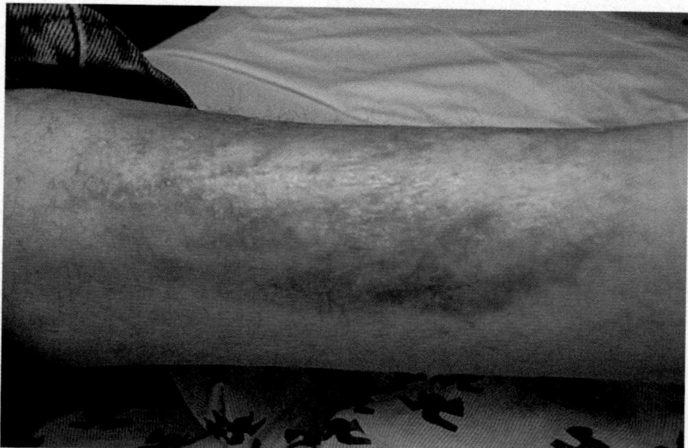

FIGURE 231-2 Necrobiosis lipoidica in a patient with type 1 diabetes. Note the pink area at the site of a healed superficial ulcer. *(Reproduced with permission from Amber Tully, MD.)*

- Antibodies and C3 have been found at the dermal–epidermal junction, suggesting vasculitis.
- The presence of fibrin in these lesions associated with palisading histiocytes may indicate a delayed hypersensitivity reaction.
- In a microscopy study, *Borrelia* was detected in 75% of NL lesions overall and 92.7% of inflammatory-rich (38 of 41) versus inflammatory-poor (4 of 15, 26.7%) cases.[8] The authors posit that these findings indicate a potential role for *Borrelia burgdorferi* or other similar strains in the development of or trigger for NL.

RISK FACTORS

- Among patients with type 1 DM, those with NL have poorer metabolic control (hemoglobin A_{1c} 8.7% vs. 8.3% in those without NL) and longer duration of DM (6.24 vs. 5.11 years).[9] There were no significant differences between groups in the frequency of microvascular complications.

DIAGNOSIS

CLINICAL FEATURES

- The lesions begin as erythematous papules or plaques in the pretibial area and become larger and darker with irregular margins and raised erythematous borders (**Figures 231-1** to **231-4**). The lesion's center atrophies and turns yellow in color, appearing waxy (**Figures 231-3**, **231-4**, and **231-5A**).
- There is often a prominent brown color or hyperpigmentation visible (see **Figures 231-1** to **231-4**).
- The lesions may ulcerate (occurs in approximately one third) and become painful (see **Figure 231-5B**).
- Telangiectasias and prominent blood vessels may be seen within the lesions (see **Figures 231-1** to **231-4**).
- The yellow color may be because of lipid deposits or beta-carotene.

TYPICAL DISTRIBUTION

- The lesions are usually located on the shins (90%) (see **Figures 231-1** to **231-4**).
- NL lesions have been reported on many skin areas, including the face, scalp, and penis.[10,11]

DERMOSCOPY/BIOPSY

- Dermoscopy of NL is characterized by sharply focused, elongated, and serpentine telangiectasias (see **Figure 231-5**).
- Biopsy is not always needed, as the clinical picture is often clear. The dangers of a biopsy include delayed healing and infection in a patient who often has diabetes. The shin region of the leg is notorious for delayed healing even in healthy persons, and so biopsy should be avoided in most cases.
- If the diagnosis is uncertain, a 4-mm punch biopsy will show a thin atrophic epidermis with dermal granulomatous inflammation and obliterative endarteritis. The dermal change shows increased necrobiosis or degeneration of collagen with absence of elastic tissue.

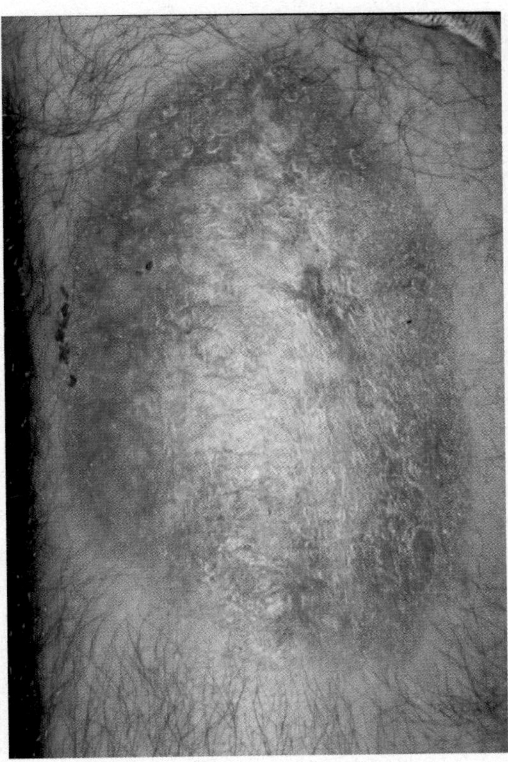

FIGURE 231-3 Necrobiosis lipoidica on the leg of a man with type 2 diabetes. Note the central atrophy and yellow discoloration with a well-demarcated brown border. (*Reproduced with permission from Richard P. Usatine, MD.*)

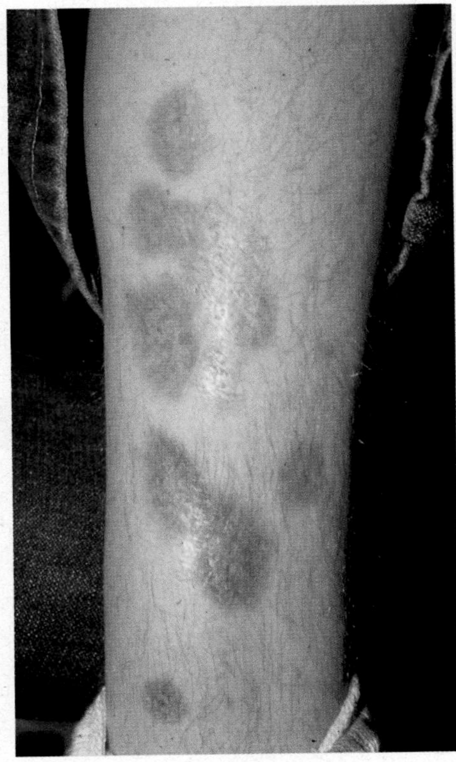

FIGURE 231-4 Multiple lesions of necrobiosis lipoidica in a young adult with type 1 diabetes. Note the central yellow discoloration and well-circumscribed brown borders. (*Reproduced with permission from Richard P. Usatine, MD.*)

DIFFERENTIAL DIAGNOSIS

NL may be confused with the following conditions:

- Erythema nodosum (EN) is an inflammatory panniculitis that occurs in the same areas as NL (especially shins). These nodules are pink in color and the skin is smooth above them. The color and lack of epidermal changes should differentiate EN from NL (see Chapter 186, Erythema Nodosum).
- Granuloma annulare—Appears as asymmetric annular red plaques on the dorsum of the hands, extensor surface of the extremities, or posterior neck. They lack the yellow discoloration of NL. These lesions are so visibly like red, raised rings that they appear different from NL.
  - If biopsy is needed, the presence of abundant mucin deposits helps to distinguish these lesions from NL (see Chapter 182, Granuloma Annulare).[2]
  - Dermoscopy appears useful in differentiating NL from granuloma annulare. In one study, NL was characterized by sharply focused, elongated, and serpentine telangiectasias, typically located over a whitish, structureless background, whereas granuloma annulare was typified by peripheral, structureless orange-reddish borders sometimes associated with isolated, unfocused small vessels.[12]
- Lichen simplex chronicus—A chronic pruritic eczematous lesion. The lesions are well-circumscribed plaques or papules with lichenified or thickened skin caused by chronic scratching or rubbing. Lesions are commonly located on the ankles, wrists, or posterior nuchal region. The prominent scale and lichenification should help differentiate these lesions from NL (see Chapter 151, Atopic Dermatitis).
- Sarcoidosis skin lesions—Including EN, maculopapular eruptions on the face, nose, back, and extremities; skin plaques that are often purple and raised; and broad macules with telangiectasias that are most commonly seen on the face or hands. Punch biopsy will distinguish between sarcoidosis and NL (see Chapter 184, Sarcoidosis).
- Stasis dermatitis—Occurs on the lower extremities secondary to venous incompetence and edema. Affected patients are usually older, and the typical site is the medial aspect of the ankle. Early lesions are erythematous, scaly, and sometimes pruritic that progressively become hyperpigmented. These lesions are rarely well circumscribed, as seen in NL (see Chapter 54, Venous Insufficiency).

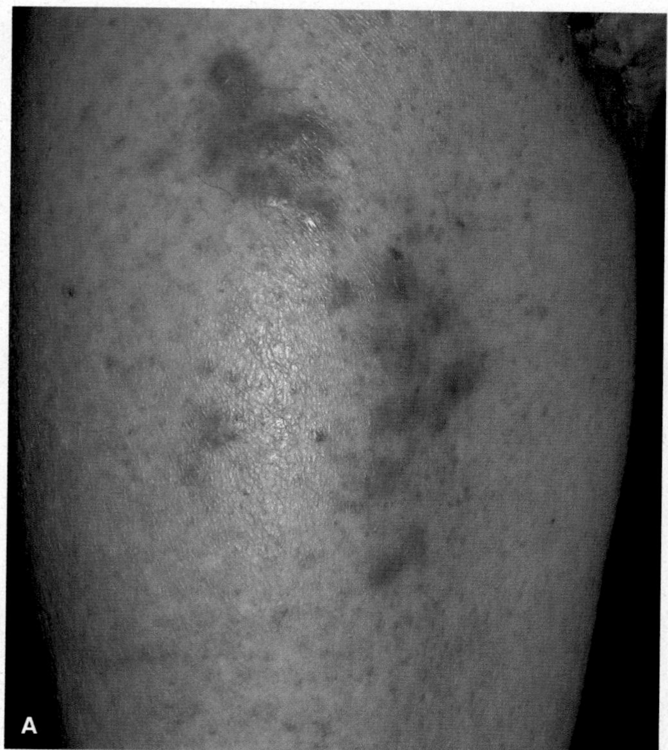

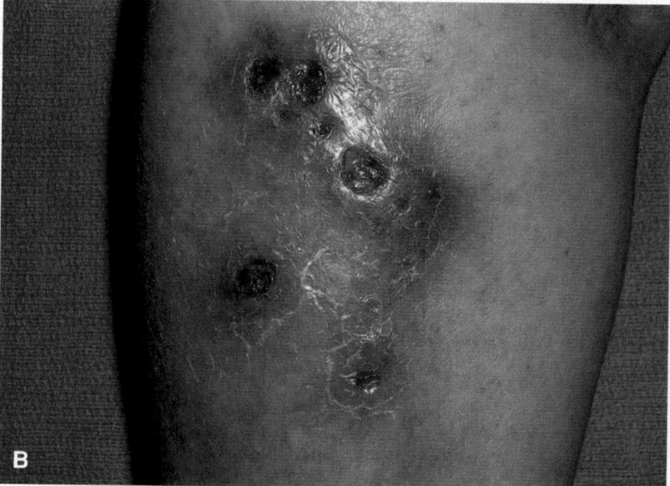

FIGURE 231-5 **A.** Necrobiosis lipoidica on the leg of a woman with no diabetes. It was biopsy proven and treated. **B.** Worsening and ulcerations of necrobiosis lipoidica despite treatment with topical steroids. *(Reproduced with permission from Richard P. Usatine, MD.)*

MANAGEMENT

Evaluate patients not previously diagnosed with DM for diabetes. Even though glycemic control does not correlate with progression of these lesions, DM should be treated to decrease the risk of macro- and microvascular complications.

MEDICATIONS

Data on successful treatment is largely based on case reports.

FIRST LINE

- Local application of potent steroids or intralesional injections of 2.5 mg/mL of triamcinolone.[2] SOR Ⓒ The major risk of these treatments includes increasing the existing atrophy, so patients should be informed of risks and benefits before initiating steroid treatments.

- Topical tacrolimus (0.1% ointment twice daily for 8 weeks followed by once daily for 8 weeks) was successful in several case reports.[5,13] SOR Ⓒ

SECOND LINE

- Pentoxifylline (400 mg 2 to 3 times daily), an agent that improves blood flow and decreases red cell and platelet aggregation, was shown in 2 case reports to completely resolve the lesions at 8 weeks in one[3] and at 6-month follow-up in the other.[4] The latter patient continued therapy and remained in remission at a 2-year follow-up. SOR Ⓒ
- Phototherapy and photodynamic therapy have been partially successful in some case reports.[5] Interestingly, in a review of therapies including topical psoralen and UVA (PUVA) therapy, photodynamic therapy, and systemic fumaric acid esters, authors found that as numbers treated increased, successful treatment decreased, which they interpreted as likely publication bias and lack of efficacy.[14]
- Ulcerative NL has been reported to respond to tetracycline,[15] antimalarial agents (e.g., hydroxychloroquine),[16] clofazimine,[17] colchicine,[18] systemic steroids,[19] antiplatelet therapy,[20] and biologic agents (e.g., infliximab infusion, subcutaneous etanercept).[21,22] SOR Ⓒ

REFERRAL

- Refer patients with intractable skin ulcers for consideration of skin grafting. In one study that included patients with NL, application of allogeneic cultured dermal substitute was successful in improving healing.[23]

PROGNOSIS

- Spontaneous resolution occurs in 10% to 20% of cases.
- In a study of 11 patients with DM undergoing pancreatic transplantation, all 5 patients with NL achieved resolution of NL following transplantation; 1 patient had recurrent NL associated with transplant rejection.[24] The single patient with NL who underwent kidney transplantation had persistent NL.
- Squamous cell carcinoma can arise within long-standing NL lesions.[5]

PATIENT EDUCATION

- Patients with NL without DM should be advised about the increased risk of developing the disease and counseled about symptoms and periodic surveillance.
- NL may resolve spontaneously and does respond to several treatments.

PATIENT RESOURCES

- American Diabetes Association—**http://www.diabetes.org.**
- American Diabetes Association. *Skin Complications*—**http://www.diabetes.org/living-with-diabetes/complications/skin-complications.html?loc=DropDownLWD-skin.**
- American Osteopathic College of Dermatology. *Necrobiosis Lipoidica Diabeticorum*—**http://www.aocd.org/?page=NLD.**

PROVIDER RESOURCES

- **http://emedicine.medscape.com/article/1103467-overview.**

REFERENCES

1. Noz KC, Korstanje MJ, Vermeer BJ. Cutaneous manifestations of endocrine disorders: a guide for dermatologists. *Am J Clin Dermatol.* 2003;4(5):315-331.
2. Sibbald RG, Landolt SJ, Toth D. Skin and diabetes. *Endocrinol Metab Clin North Am.* 1996;25(2):463-472.
3. Ahmed K, Muhammad Z, Qayum I. Prevalence of cutaneous manifestations of diabetes mellitus. *J Ayub Med Coll Abbottabad.* 2009;21(2):76-79.
4. Pavlović MD, Milenković T, Dinić M, et al. The prevalence of cutaneous manifestations in young patients with type 1 diabetes. *Diabetes Care.* 2007;30(8):1964-1967.
5. Erfurt-Berge C, Seitz AT, Rehse C, et al. Update on clinical and laboratory features in necrobiosis lipoidica: a retrospective multicentre study of 52 patients. *Eur J Dermatol.* 2012;22:770-775.
6. O'Reilly K, Chu J, Meehan S, et al. Necrobiosis lipoidica. *Dermatol Online J.* 2011;17(10):18.
7. Roche-Gamón E, Vilata-Corell JJ, Velasco-Pastor M. Familial necrobiosis lipoidica not associated with diabetes. *Dermatol Online J.* 2007;13(3):26.
8. Eisendle K, Baltaci M, Kutzner H, Zelger B. Detection of spirochaetal microorganisms by focus floating microscopy in necrobiosis lipoidica in patients from central Europe. *Histopathology.* 2008;52(7):877-884.
9. Hammer E, Lilienthal E, Hofer SE, et al; DPV Initiative and the German BMBF Competence Network for Diabetes Mellitus. Risk factors for necrobiosis lipoidica in Type 1 diabetes mellitus. *Diabet Med.* 2017;34(1):86-92.
10. Lynch M, Callagy G, Mahon S, Murphy LA. Arcuate plaques of the face and scalp. Atypical necrobiosis lipoidica (ANL) of the face and scalp. *Clin Exp Dermatol.* 2010;35(7):799-800.
11. Alonso ML, Riós JC, González-Beato MJ, Herranz P. Necrobiosis lipoidica of the glans penis. *Acta Derm Venereol.* 2011;91(1): 105-106.
12. Pellicano R, Caldarola G, Filabozzi P, Zalaudek I. Dermoscopy of necrobiosis lipoidica and granuloma annulare. *Dermatology.* 2013; 226(4):319-323.
13. Patsatsi A, Kyriakou A, Sotiriadis D. Necrobiosis lipoidica: early diagnosis and treatment with tacrolimus. *Case Rep Dermatol.* 2011;3(1):89-93.
14. Peckruhn M, Tittelbach J, Elsner P. Update: treatment of necrobiosis lipoidica. *J Dtsch Dermatol Ges.* 2017;15(2):151-157.
15. Mahé E, Zimmermann U. Significant improvement in ulcerative necrobiosis lipoidica with doxycycline. *Ann Dermatol Venereol.* 2011;138(10):686-688.

16. Durupt F, Dalle S, Debarbieux S, et al. Successful treatment of necrobiosis lipoidica with antimalarial agents. *Acta Derm Venereol.* 2009;89(6):651-652.
17. Benedix F, Geyer A, Lichte V, et al. Response of ulcerated necrobiosis lipoidica to clofazimine. *Acta Derm Venereol.* 2010;90(1):104-106.
18. Schofield C, Sladden MJ. Ulcerative necrobiosis responsive to colchicine. *Australas J Dermatol.* 2012;53(3):e54-57.
19. Tan E, Patel V, Berth-Jones J. Systemic corticosteroids for the outpatient treatment of necrobiosis lipoidica in a diabetic patient. *J Dermatolog Treat.* 2007;18(4):246-248.
20. Moore AF, Abourizk NN. Necrobiosis lipoidica: an important cutaneous manifestation of diabetes that may respond to antiplatelet therapy. *Endocr Pract.* 2008;14(7):947-948.
21. Hu SW, Bevona C, Winterfield L, et al. Treatment of refractory ulcerative necrobiosis lipoidica diabeticorum with infliximab: report of a case. *Arch Dermatol.* 2009;145(4):437-439.
22. Suárez-Amor O, Pérez-Bustillo A, Ruiz-González I, Rodríguez-Prieto MA. Necrobiosis lipoidica therapy with biologicals: an ulcerated case responding to etanercept and a review of the literature. *Dermatology.* 2010;221(2):117-121.
23. Taniguchi T, Amoh Y, Tanabe K, et al. Treatment of intractable skin ulcers caused by vascular insufficiency with allogeneic cultured dermal substitute: a report of eight cases. *J Artif Organs.* 2012;15(1):77-82.
24. Souza AD, El-Azhary RA, Gibson LE. Does pancreas transplant in diabetic patients affect the evolution of necrobiosis lipoidica? *Int J Dermatol.* 2009;48(9):964-970.

232 HYPERLIPIDEMIA AND XANTHOMAS

Mindy A. Smith, MD, MS

PATIENT STORY

A 27-year-old Hispanic man reported new painful nonpruritic bumps, which started 6 months ago, over his entire body. The patient had not seen a physician for 10 months and had run out of his oral medicines for type 2 diabetes mellitus. His grandmother had a milder version of bumps like this years ago. The firm yellowish papules were present all over his body from the neck down (**Figures 232-1** to **232-3**). Laboratory evaluation revealed a random blood sugar of 203, a fasting triglyceride level greater than 7000 mg/dL, and total cholesterol greater than 700 mg/dL. High-density lipoproteins were 32 mg/dL, and there were no chylomicrons present. The patient was diagnosed with xanthomas, poorly controlled diabetes mellitus, and hyperlipidemia, and was started on metformin, gemfibrozil, and a β-hydroxy-β-methylglutaryl-coenzyme A (HMG-CoA)-reductase inhibitor.

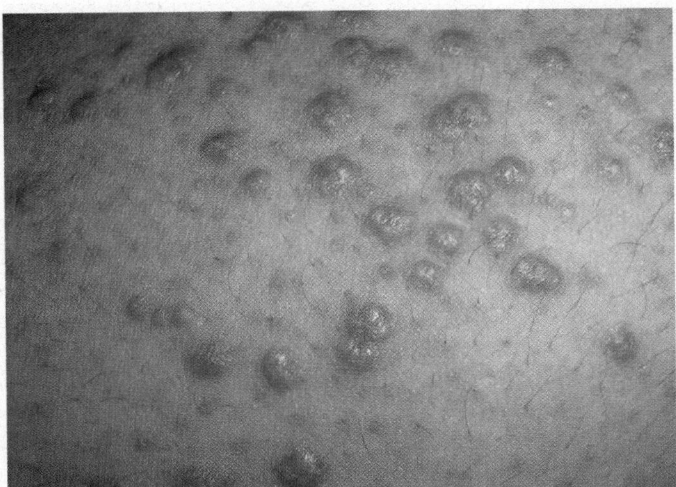

FIGURE 232-1 Close-up of eruptive xanthomas on the arm of a 27-year-old man with untreated hyperlipidemia and diabetes. *(Reproduced with permission from Richard P. Usatine, MD.)*

INTRODUCTION

Hyperlipidemia refers to an elevated concentration of one or more of the measured serum lipid components (total cholesterol [TC; ≥240 mg/dL], low-density lipoprotein [LDL; ≥160 mg/dL], and triglycerides [TGs; ≥200 mg/dL]), often accompanied by low high-density lipoprotein (HDL; ≤40 mg/dL). Most patients have a combination of genetic predisposition and an acquired component (see Etiology). Xanthomas are a skin manifestation of familial or severe secondary hyperlipidemia, although they can occur in patients with normal lipid levels. Hyperlipidemia is a major modifiable risk factor for cardiovascular disease.

SYNONYMS

Collectively referred to as dyslipidemias.

EPIDEMIOLOGY

- During 2011 to 2014, 27.8% of adults in the United States had a serum TC level ≥240 mg/dL or were taking cholesterol-lowering medications.[1]
- An estimated 31.7% of the adult population had high LDL-C in 2015 and less than half were receiving treatment to lower their levels.[2]
- Among young adults (ages 12 to 19 years), 20.3% had abnormal lipids; boys are more likely than girls to have at least 1 lipid abnormality (24.3% vs. 15.9%, respectively).[3]
- Patients with homozygous familial hypercholesterolemia (FH) (1 in 1 million persons worldwide) have mutations in both alleles of the LDL receptor and present in childhood with cutaneous xanthomas on the hands, wrists, elbows, knees, heels, or buttocks.[4,5]

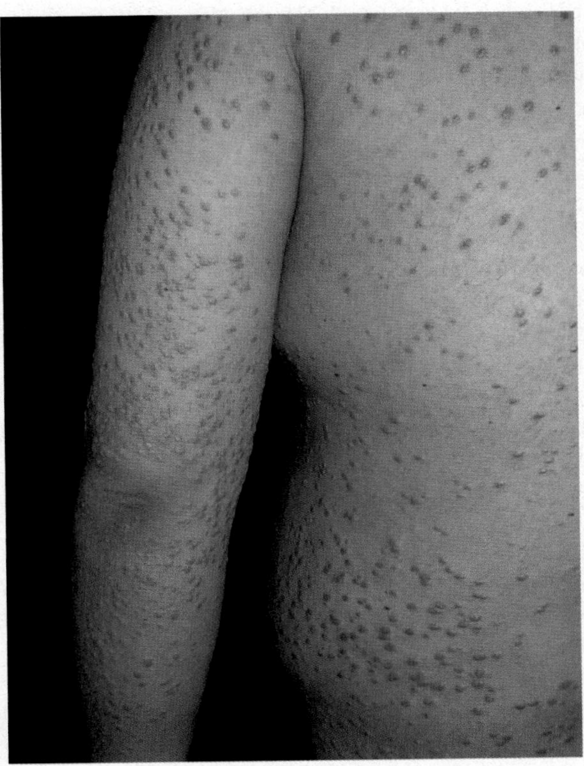

FIGURE 232-2 Eruptive xanthomas on the arm and trunk of the man in **Figure 232-1**. *(Reproduced with permission from Richard P. Usatine, MD.)*

- Patients with heterozygous FH (1 in 250 to 500 persons worldwide) can present as adults with tendon xanthomas.
- Patients with familial defective apolipoprotein B-100, another inherited autosomal dominant dyslipidemia, resemble those with heterozygous FH and may also develop tendon xanthomas.[4]

ETIOLOGY AND PATHOPHYSIOLOGY

- Lipoproteins are complexes of lipids and proteins essential for transporting cholesterol, TGs, and fat-soluble vitamins. Apolipoproteins are proteins associated with lipoproteins that are required for their assembly, structure, function, and metabolism.
- Elevated lipoprotein levels can result from genetically based derangement of lipid metabolism and/or transport (primary lipid disorder) or from secondary causes such as diet, medical disorders (e.g., type 2 diabetes mellitus [DM], hypothyroidism, chronic kidney disease, cholestatic liver disease), cigarette smoking, obesity, or drugs (e.g., corticosteroids, estrogens, retinoids, high-dose β-blockers). For a complete review of these disorders, see reference 4.
- Increased circulating LDL becomes incorporation into atherosclerotic plaques. These plaques can grow to block blood supply and oxygen delivery, resulting in ischemia to vital organs. In addition, if the plaque ruptures, it can precipitate a clot, causing, for example, myocardial infarction (MI).
- Elevated TG is an independent risk factor for coronary heart disease (CHD) and increases the risk of hepatomegaly, splenomegaly, hepatic steatosis, and pancreatitis. Contributing factors include obesity, physical inactivity, cigarette smoking, excess alcohol intake, medical diseases (e.g., type 2 DM, chronic renal failure, nephrotic syndrome), drugs (as above), and genetic disorders (e.g., familial combined hyperlipidemia).
- Xanthomas are deposits of lipid in the skin or subcutaneous tissue, usually occurring because of primary or secondary hyperlipidemia. Xanthomas can also be seen in association with monoclonal gammopathy.[6] There are five basic types of xanthomas:
  - Eruptive xanthomas (also called tuberoeruptive) are the most common form. These appear as crops of yellow or hyperpigmented papules with erythematous halos in white persons (**Figures 232-1** to **232-3**), appearing hyperpigmented in black persons (**Figures 232-4** and **232-5**).
  - Tendon xanthomas are frequently seen on the Achilles and extensor finger tendons.
  - Plane xanthomas are flat and commonly seen on the palmar creases, face, upper trunk, and on scars.
  - Tuberous xanthomas are found most frequently on the hand or over large joints.
  - Xanthelasma are yellow papules found on the eyelids (**Figure 232-6**). Fifty percent of individuals with xanthelasmas have normal lipid profiles.

RISK FACTORS

The 2013 American College of Cardiology (ACC)/American Heart Association (AHA) Guideline on Treatment of Blood Cholesterol to

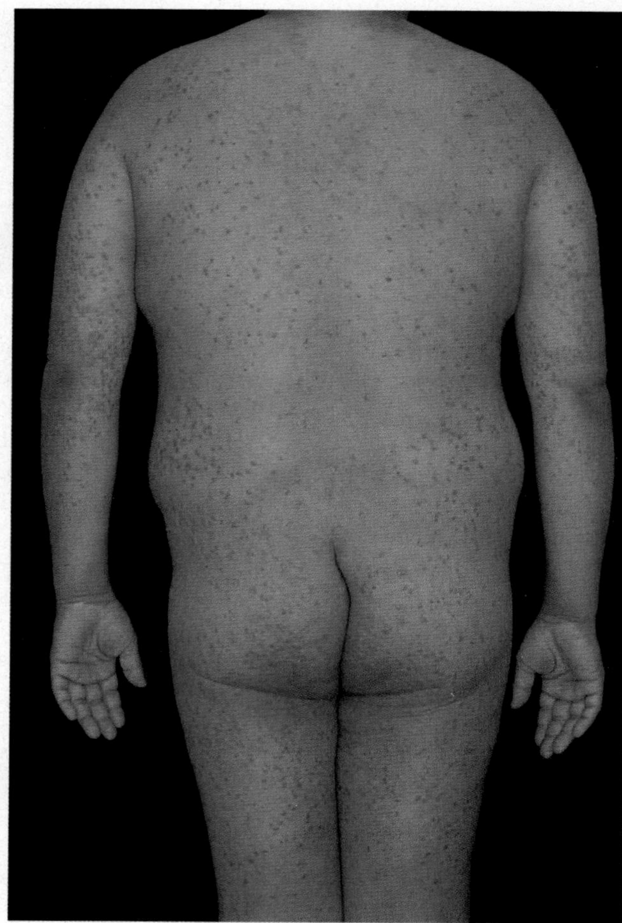

FIGURE 232-3 Eruptive xanthomas covering most of the body of the man in **Figure 232-1**. (*Reproduced with permission from Richard P. Usatine, MD.*)

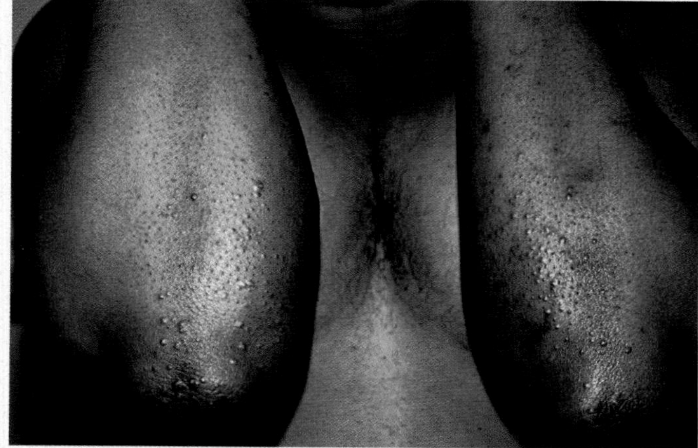

FIGURE 232-4 Eruptive xanthomas on the elbows of a hyperlipidemic black man with type 2 diabetes. His triglycerides and total cholesterol levels were high. (*Reproduced with permission from Richard P. Usatine, MD. Previously published in the Western Journal of Medicine.*)

Reduce Atherosclerotic Cardiovascular Risk in Adults focuses on atherosclerotic cardiovascular disease (ASCVD) risk reduction (primarily addressing DM, hypertension, obesity, sedentary lifestyle, and smoking) and the identification of 4 statin-benefit groups (**Table 232-1**).[7] Other risk factors considered by ACC/AHA for those not falling into the treatment benefit groups are:

- Genetic hyperlipidemia or elevated lifetime risk of ASCVD.
- Family history of premature ASCVD in a first-degree relative (onset in men <55 years and women <65 years).
- Abnormal laboratory tests: Primary LDL cholesterol ≥160 mg/dL or C-reactive protein elevation ≥2 mg/L.
- Other abnormal test results: Coronary artery calcium score ≥300 Agatston units or ≥75 percentile for age, sex, and ethnicity or ankle-brachial index <0.9.
- For those without known ASCVD and an LDL between 70 and 189 mg/dL, 10-year risk for ASCVD can be estimated using a risk calculator available at https://www.mdcalc.com/ascvd-atherosclerotic-cardiovascular-disease-2013-risk-calculator-aha-acc.
- Risk factors in children that track into adulthood include elevated blood pressure and cholesterol, DM, obesity, tobacco use, and poor physical fitness (to some degree).[8]

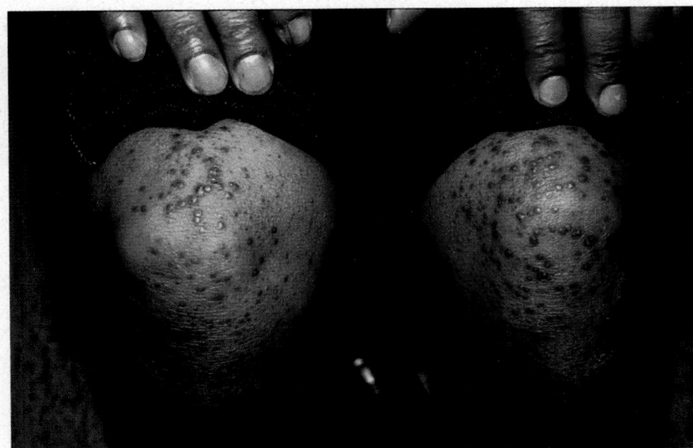

FIGURE 232-5 Eruptive xanthomas on the knees in the patient in Figure 232-4. *(Reproduced with permission from Richard P. Usatine, MD. Previously published in the Western Journal of Medicine.)*

DIAGNOSIS

CLINICAL FEATURES

- Most patients with hyperlipidemia are asymptomatic.
- A very high TC level (>2000 mg/dL) may result in eruptive xanthomas or lipemia retinalis (white appearance of the retina; also seen with isolated high TG). Very high LDL may lead to the formation of tendinous xanthomas.
- Xanthomas manifest clinically as yellowish papules, nodules, or tumors (**Figure 232-1**).
- Eruptive xanthomas (**Figures 232-2** to **232-5**) begin as clusters of small papules on the elbows, knees, and buttocks that can grow to the size of grapes.
- There is a case report of a patient with normolipidemic xanthomatosis with lesions involving the bones and mucous membranes in addition to skin.[9]

TYPICAL DISTRIBUTION

Xanthomas are most commonly found in superficial soft tissues, such as skin and subcutis, or on tendon sheaths.

LABORATORY TESTING

- The ACC/AHA guidelines recommend a fasting lipid profile (FLP) as the initial test[7]; alternatively patients may be tested initially with a random TC and HDL. If the nonfasted total cholesterol is ≥200 mg/dL or HDL <40 mg/dL, an FLP should be obtained.
- If a screening lipid profile shows elevated LDL cholesterol, low HDL cholesterol, or high TGs, obtain a second, fasting lipid profile before starting treatment to confirm elevation and establish an accurate baseline.

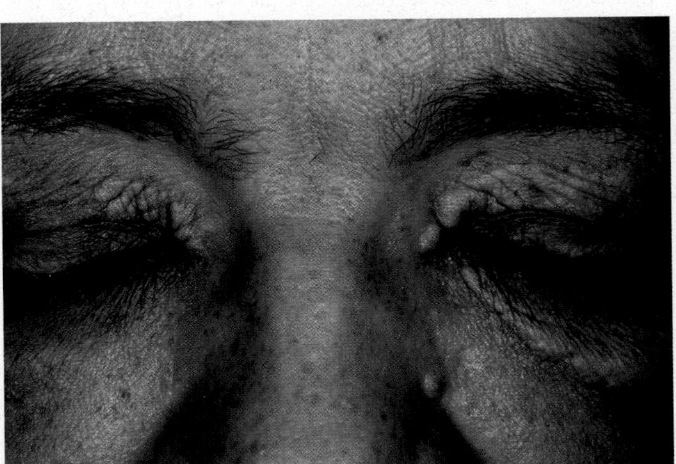

FIGURE 232-6 Xanthelasma around the eyes (xanthoma palpebrarum); most often seen on the medial aspect of the eyelids, with upper lids being more commonly involved than lower lids. *(Reproduced with permission from Richard P. Usatine, MD.)*

TABLE 232-1 Benefit Groups for Statin Therapy and Treatment Recommendations

Benefit Groups for Statin Therapy	High-Intensity Statin Therapy (daily dose lowers LDL by approximately 50% or more)*	Moderate-Intensity Statin Therapy (daily dose lowers LDL by 30% to 49%)
Patients with known ASCVD	Age ≤75 years (SOR Ⓐ)	Age >75 years or not a candidate for high-intensity therapy (SOR Ⓐ)
Patients with primary elevation of LDL ≥190 mg/dL	All candidates (SOR Ⓑ)	Not a candidate for high-intensity therapy (SOR Ⓑ)
Patients ages 40–75 years without ASCVD who have DM, and an LDL of 70–189 mg/dL	Estimated 10-year ASCVD risk ≥7.5%† (SOR Ⓒ)	All others with DM (SOR Ⓐ)
Other patients ages 40–75 years without ASCVD or DM with an estimated 10-year ASCVD risk ≥7.5%†	Clinical decision (SOR Ⓐ)	Clinical decision (SOR Ⓐ)

Abbreviations: LDL, low-density lipid; ASCVD, atherosclerotic cardiovascular disease; DM, diabetes mellitus.
*Percent LDL reduction can be used as a measure of treatment response and adherence but is not in itself a treatment goal.
†10-year risk of ASCVD, defined as nonfatal myocardial infarction, coronary heart disease death, and nonfatal and fatal stroke.
Reproduced with permission from Smith MA, Shimp LA: Lange Family Medicine: Ambulatory Care and Practice, 6th ed. New York, NY: McGraw-Hill Education; 2014.

- The predominant hyperlipidemic pattern in children is one associated with obesity, moderate to severe TG elevation, and reduced HDL (laboratory values used are similar to those for adults).[8]
- The Endocrine Society guideline recommends evaluation of abnormalities of glucose metabolism and liver dysfunction in patients with primary hypertriglyceridemia.[10]
- If thyroid dysfunction is suspected, obtain a thyroid-stimulating hormone level to determine whether thyroid dysfunction is contributing to the lipid abnormalities.
- Other secondary causes to consider include anorexia nervosa, Cushing syndrome, hepatitis, nephrotic syndrome, renal failure, and systemic lupus erythematosus.
- If a statin is under consideration, baseline measurement of alanine transaminase (ALT) levels should be obtained.[7] Measurement of baseline creatine phosphokinase (CPK) is considered for those at increased risk of adverse muscle events (e.g., personal or family history of statin intolerance or muscle disease, concomitant drug therapy that might increase the likelihood of myopathy).[7]

BIOPSY

Biopsy of xanthomas is rarely needed and shows collections of lipid-filled macrophages.

DIFFERENTIAL DIAGNOSIS

Other skin papules that can be mistaken for xanthomas include the following:

- Gouty tophi—Deposits of monosodium urate that are usually firm and occasionally discharge a chalky material (**Figure 232-7**; see Chapter 102, Gout).

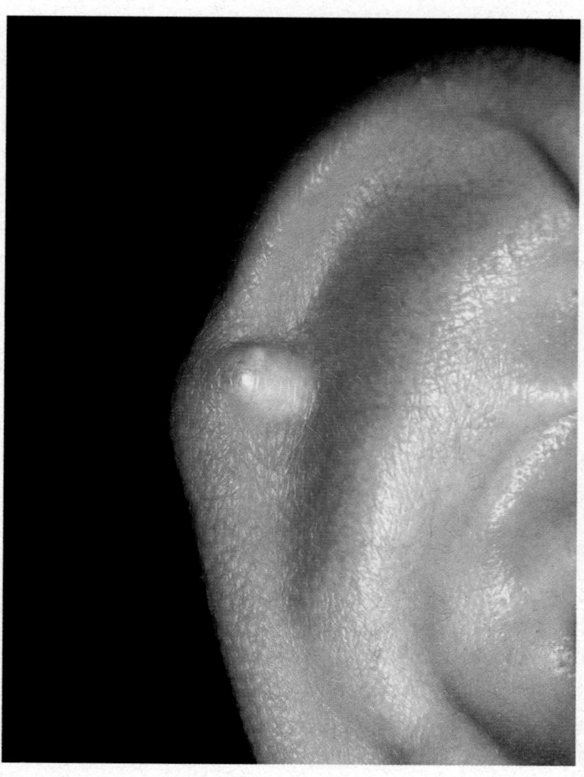

FIGURE 232-7 Ear gouty tophus in a young man with gout. (*Reproduced with permission from Richard P. Usatine, MD.*)

- Pseudoxanthoma elasticum—A disorder caused by abnormal deposits of calcium on the elastic fibers of the skin and eye.
- Molluscum contagiosum—Caused by a virus; lesions can be papular and widespread but generally have a central depression (see Chapter 136, Molluscum Contagiosum). The patient in **Figures 232-1** to **232-3** was originally misdiagnosed with molluscum.

MANAGEMENT

FIRST LINE

Management of patients with hyperlipidemia emphasizes reduction of cardiovascular risk factors (as noted above). Lifestyle approaches often improve lipids sufficiently. The ACC/AHA guidelines have moved away from categorizing lipid target levels in favor of benefit groups for medication that includes those with high LDL levels (see **Table 232-1**).[7] The use of lipid goals, however, is still a topic of debate.[11]

- For children with elevated lipids, diet is recommended as first-line treatment to achieve a TC of less than 215 mg/dL or an LDL of less than 155 mg/dL.[8] Referral to a pediatric endocrinologist or dietician may be beneficial.

NONPHARMACOLOGIC

- Smoking cessation should be encouraged and attempts actively supported; cessation lowers both cardiovascular risk and lipid levels. SOR Ⓐ
- Patients with hyperlipidemia should be encouraged to modify their risk factors through exercise and dietary changes. Running and walking exercise lowers risk of diabetes, hypertension, and CVD in patients with elevated TC.[12] High cholesterol can be lowered through dietary changes. SOR Ⓐ
- Patients who are overweight should be encouraged to reduce calories to achieve weight loss. SOR Ⓒ
- Features of a lipid-lowering diet for adults includes emphasizing intake of vegetables, fruits, and whole grains; including low-fat dairy products, poultry, fish, legumes, nontropical vegetable oils, and nuts in the diet; and limiting intake of sweets, sugar-sweetened beverages, and red meats.[13] SOR Ⓐ In addition, aim for a diet that achieves 5% to 6% of total calories as saturated fat. Recommended diets include the DASH dietary pattern, the USDA Food Pattern, or the AHA Diet adjusted for other medical conditions such as diabetes.
- Authors of a Cochrane review, however, found no trials on long-term (>6 months) effects of a low-fat diet in patients with hyperlipidemia.[14]
- Similarly, of 15 small trials of dietary intervention for familial hypercholesterolemia identified by authors of a Cochrane review, only short-term outcomes were reported.[15] There was some benefit of plant sterols over a low-cholesterol diet for lowering TC and LDL.[15] The addition of guar gum to bezafibrate also appeared to effectively reduce TC and LDL compared to the drug alone.
- For children, a diet with total fat at 25% to 30% of calories, saturated fat less than 10% of calories, and cholesterol intake less than 300 mg/d (the original NCEP Pediatric Panel diet) has been shown to be safe and effective in reducing TC LDL.[8] SOR Ⓐ A more stringent diet with saturated fat <7% of calories and dietary cholesterol limited to 200 mg/d is also safe and modestly effective for those with higher elevations of LDL.
    - In children with elevated TG, reduce simple carbohydrate intake, increase intake of complex carbohydrates, and reduce saturated fat intake. SOR Ⓑ
    - For children with obesity and TG elevation, strive to achieve weight loss through decreasing caloric intake and increasing activity levels. Behavioral approaches including a registered dietician are most effective.
- Reducing saturated fat through fat modification diets reduces the risk of cardiovascular events by 14% (relative risk [RR] 0.86, 95% confidence interval [CI] 0.77 to 0.96).[16] SOR Ⓐ This reduction in cardiovascular events was directly related to the degree of effect on serum total and LDL cholesterol and TGs. The strongest evidence was for trials of at least 2 years' duration and in studies of men (not of women). However, there were no clear effects of dietary fat changes on total mortality (RR 0.98, 95% CI 0.93 to 1.04) or cardiovascular mortality (RR 0.94, 95% CI 0.85 to 1.04).
- Initial treatment of xanthomas should target the underlying hyperlipidemia (when present).

MEDICATIONS

- The intensity of statin therapy is based on the patient's age and risk status (see **Table 232-1**).[7]

The use of combination therapy has not been supported by outcome-based studies.

- Statins (HMG-CoA reductase inhibitors; lovastatin [10–80 mg or 20–60 mg extended release], pravastatin [40–80 mg], simvastatin [5–40 mg], fluvastatin [20–40 mg or 80 mg XL], atorvastatin [10–80 mg], pitavastatin [2 mg], and rosuvastatin [5–40 mg]) are considered first-line for most patients. High intensity statins include atorvastatin [80 mg] and rosuvastatin [20 mg]. Safety has not been established for use of statins in children under 8–10 years of age.
    - Evidence supports use of statins in patients with risk factors for CHD (lowers all-cause mortality [odds ratio (OR) 0.88, 95% CI 0.81 to 0.96], major coronary events [OR 0.70, 95% CI 0.61 to 0.81], and major cerebrovascular events [OR 0.81, 95% CI 0.71 to 0.93]).[17] SOR Ⓐ In a systematic review of 19 randomized clinical trials of statin therapy, investigators found a decreased risk of all-cause mortality (absolute risk difference [ARD], −0.40%; 95% CI, −0.64% to −0.17% and number needed to treat [NNT] 250), stroke (ARD, −0.38%; 95% CI, −0.53% to −0.23% and NNT 263), and MI (ARD, −0.81%; 95% CI, −1.19 to −0.43% and NNT 123).[18]
    - For secondary prevention, authors of a meta-analysis found reduced rates of recurrent cardiovascular events for both men and women, but all-cause mortality and stroke benefit were only observed in men.[19]
- Statin side effects include myopathy and increased liver enzymes; statins are associated with a small increase in the risk of developing DM (number needed to harm = 255).[20] The major contraindication is liver disease.
- High-dose statins, however, appear to increase admission for acute kidney injury, especially within the first 120 days after initiation.[21]
- Fibrates (gemfibrozil [600 mg bid], fenofibrate [200 mg], clofibrate [1000 mg bid]) are recommended as primary therapy for patients with very high TG who are at risk for triglyceride-induced

pancreatitis.[10] Side effects include dyspepsia, gallstones, myopathy, and unexplained non-CHD deaths. Contraindications are severe renal or hepatic disease.

Hypolipidemic drug treatment often results in regression of xanthomas. SOR Ⓒ In patients with xanthomas associated with monoclonal gammopathy, hematologic remission following chemotherapy was associated with improvement in the xanthomas in several patients.[6]

SECOND LINE

NONPHARMACOLOGIC

- Addition of plant sterols/stanols up to 2 g/day may be considered to reduce LDL in addition to diet modification and exercise. SOR Ⓑ Plant sterol or stanol esters can be effective and safe in children with familial hyperlipidemia.[8] SOR Ⓐ However, long-term studies are needed.

MEDICATIONS

Secondary therapy includes statins, niacin, fibric acids, ezetimibe, and a bile acid sequestrant. The use of combination therapy or titration of single drug therapy to achieve a specific LDL level has not been supported by outcome-based studies, although combination therapy can further reduce lipid levels.[7]

- Niacin (immediate release [crystalline] nicotinic acid [1.5–3 g], extended-release nicotinic acid [Niaspan] [1–2 g], sustained release) can be used as a first-line agent for patients with very high TG. Start with low dose and titrate upward every few weeks. Evidence supports reduction in major CHD events with niacin. SOR Ⓐ Niacin is nonprescription.
  - Niacin side effects include GI distress, flushing (can be reduced by aspirin 325 mg dose 30 minutes prior to niacin), hyperuricemia, hyperglycemia in patients with DM, and hepatotoxicity. Contraindications are chronic liver disease and severe gout; use with caution in patients with DM, hyperuricemia, or peptic ulcer disease.
- Fibrates (gemfibrozil [600 mg twice daily], fenofibrate [200 mg], clofibrate [1000 mg twice daily]) have been shown to reduce major CHD events but not overall mortality.[22] SOR Ⓐ Fibrates can be used as primary therapy for very high TG. Side effects and contraindications are described above.
- Bile acid sequestrants (cholestyramine [4–16 g], colestipol [5–20 g], colesevelam [2.6–3.8 g]) can reduce CHD mortality.[16] SOR Ⓐ These drugs are considered first-line agents for children.[10] Side effects include GI distress, constipation, and decreased absorption of other drugs. Contraindications are dysbetalipoproteinemia or TG greater than 400 mg/dL.
- The newest lipid-lowering approach is use of monoclonal antibodies targeting proprotein convertase subtilisin/kexin type 9 (e.g., evolocumab, alirocumab). Based on a meta-analysis of 24 randomized controlled trials, authors found marked reductions in LDL (–47.49%; 95% CI, –69.64% to –25.35%) accompanied by reductions in all-cause mortality (odds ratio 0.45; 95% CI, 0.23 to 0.86).[23] SOR Ⓐ There were no serious adverse events.

COMPLEMENTARY AND ALTERNATIVE THERAPY

- Artichoke leaf extract, red yeast rice, and several Chinese herbal medicines (in particular Xuezhikang) lower cholesterol compared with placebo; data on patient-oriented outcomes are lacking.[24-26]
- It is not clear whether supplementing with omega-3 fatty acids reduces mortality when combined primary and secondary prevention data are analyzed. A 2006 meta-analysis failed to find a reduction in overall mortality or cardiovascular events.[27]
- Benefit is suggested for whole flaxseed and lignan, especially for women, but not for flaxseed oil.[28] Flaxseed supplementation increased TG and decreased HDL in a trial with children.[29]
- In a randomized crossover trial, consuming walnuts (42.5 g walnuts/10.1 mJ) and fatty fish (113 g salmon, twice a week) in a healthy diet significantly lowered serum cholesterol and triglyceride concentrations, respectively.[30] In a meta-analysis, nut consumption (67 g [1/4 cup is 50 g]) reduced lipid levels (TC by 10.9 mg/dL [5.1% change] and LDL by 10.2 mg/dL [7.4% change]).[31] In a more recent systematic review and meta-analysis of 61 trials, tree nut intake lowered TC, LDL, apolipoprotein B, and TG by less than half as much as the previous study and had no effect on patient-oriented outcomes.[32] The major determinant of cholesterol lowering was nut dose and not nut type.

SURGICAL PROCEDURES

- Xanthelasma lesions may be treated for cosmetic purposes. Methods of treatment include surgery, electrosurgery, cryotherapy, topical trichloroacetic acid 50% to 100%, and laser therapy (e.g., diode, argon, yttrium-aluminum-garnet [YAG]).[33] SOR Ⓒ

REFERRAL

- Referral for nutritional counseling should be considered, especially if initial attempts at dietary control fail. Dietary advice has been shown to result in modest improvements in cardiovascular risk factors, such as blood pressure and total and TC and LDL levels.[34] SOR Ⓐ

PREVENTION AND SCREENING

- The U.S. Preventive Services Task Force (USPSTF) recommends a low- to moderate-dose statin for prevention of cardiovascular disease (CVD) events and mortality in adults without symptomatic coronary artery disease or ischemic stroke who meet all the following criteria: (1) ages 40 to 75 years; (2) 1 or more CVD risk factors (i.e., dyslipidemia, diabetes, hypertension, or smoking); and (3) have a calculated 10-year risk of a cardiovascular event of 10% or greater.[35] SOR Ⓑ
- The USPSTF recommends universal screening for dyslipidemia in adults ages 40–75 years to identify those who require treatment; TC and HDL levels are needed to calculate 10-year CVD event risk (http://www.cvriskcalculator.com).[35] A Cochrane review confirmed reductions in all-cause mortality, major vascular events, and revascularizations with no cancer excess in 18 trials, 14 recruiting patients with risk factors.[36] SOR Ⓐ In one meta-analysis, NNT for primary prevention in patients (primarily men) with risk factors was 173 to prevent 1 premature death, 81 to prevent 1 CHD event, and 245 to prevent 1 stroke.[17]
- Secondary prevention trials show reductions in CHD mortality, CHD events, nonfatal MI, and revascularization for women that is similar to reductions seen for men and demonstrate decreased mortality for older men.[7] SOR Ⓐ
- Retest adults every 3 to 5 years based on CHD risk.

- The USPSTF found insufficient evidence to assess the balance of benefits and harms of screening for lipid disorders in children and adolescents 20 years or younger.[35] However, the Expert Panel recommended the following (SOR C)[8]:
    - Ages 2–8 years: No routine lipid screening. Measure fasting lipid profile twice for an average level if the family history is positive for elevated cardiovascular risk or the child has a high-level risk factor (e.g., hypertension requiring drug therapy, obesity, or smoker) or condition (e.g., diabetes mellitus, chronic kidney disease).
    - Ages 9–11 years: Universal screening with non-fasting lipid profile; calculate non-HDL and if ≥145 mg/dL and HDL <40 mg/dL, repeat fasting lipid profile twice to obtain an average level.
    - Ages 12–16 years: No routine screening. If new knowledge of positive family history, new risk factor, or new high-risk condition is identified, obtain fasting lipid panel twice to obtain an average level.
    - Ages 17–21 years: Universal screening once with a non-fasting lipid profile. Calculate non-HDL and if ≥145 mg/dL and HDL <40 mg/dL, obtain fasting lipid panel (average of two readings).

PROGNOSIS

- Based on observational data, each 30-mg/dL increase in LDL increases the relative risk of CHD by 30%.
- Use of strategies to lower elevated lipid levels will likely reduce CHD events and all-cause mortality, especially in patients with CHD or CVD risk factors.
- With medical (diet or drugs) treatment of hyperlipidemia, eruptive xanthomas usually resolve within a few weeks, and many xanthomas resolve over months; tendinous xanthomas may take years to resolve or may persist. With surgical treatment, recurrence is uncommon.[33]

FOLLOW-UP

- ACC/AHA guidelines recommend obtaining a fasting lipid panel to assess adherence, response to therapy, and adverse effects within 4–12 wk following statin initiation or change in therapy.[7] Anticipated therapeutic response is an approximately 50% reduction in LDL from baseline for high-intensity statin and 30% to <50% for moderate-intensity statin. Decreasing the statin dose may be considered when 2 consecutive LDL values are <40 mg/dL.
- If adequate lowering of lipids is not observed, evaluate the patient for secondary causes of hyperlipidemia, if indicated, and increase statin intensity or, if on maximally tolerated statin intensity, consider addition of nonstatin therapy in selected high-risk individuals.[7] SOR C
- There is no recommendation to monitor ALT level because no significant difference was shown in rates of ALT elevation between placebo and statin treatment groups in clinical trials.[7] It is reasonable to check ALT if symptoms occur suggesting hepatotoxicity (e.g., unusual fatigue or weakness, loss of appetite, abdominal pain, dark-colored urine, or yellowing of skin or sclera).[7]
- Similarly, it is reasonable to measure CPK in individuals with muscle symptoms such as pain, tenderness, stiffness, cramping, weakness, or generalized fatigue.[7] Statin therapy should be discontinued if the CPK is more than 10 times normal. For patients with myopathy and moderate or no CPK elevation, conduct weekly monitoring until symptoms improve, or halve the dose or discontinue statins if there is worsening or failure to resolve.[7]

PATIENT EDUCATION

- Patients should be counseled about benefits and risks of screening.
- Lifestyle changes should be stressed as primary prevention for patients with hyperlipidemia.
- Patients in the 4 benefit groups should be recommended for statin use (see **Table 232-1**).
- If persistent elevations in lipids continue despite lifestyle change for those outside of the 4 benefit groups, especially for those with risk factors listed above, consider medications.
- Patients with hyperlipidemia and/or DM should be encouraged to establish and maintain good control of these diseases, as this often results in regression of xanthomas.

PATIENT RESOURCES

- Centers for Disease Control and Prevention. *High Cholesterol Facts*. **https://www.cdc.gov/cholesterol/facts.htm.**
- MedlinePlus. *Cholesterol*—**https://medlineplus.gov/cholesterol.html.**

PROVIDER RESOURCES

- 2013 ACC/AHA Guideline on the treatment of blood cholesterol to reduce atherosclerotic cardiovascular risk in adults. *J Am Clin Cardiol*. 2014;63(25):2889-2934.
- Expert Panel on Integrated Guidelines for Cardiovascular Health and Risk Reduction in Children and Adolescents: Summary Report. **https://www.nhlbi.nih.gov/health-pro/guidelines/current/cardiovascular-health-pediatric-guidelines/summary.**
- 10-year risk calculator for ASCVD—**https://www.mdcalc.com/ascvd-atherosclerotic-cardiovascular-disease-2013-risk-calculator-aha-acc.**

REFERENCES

1. United States Department of Health and Human Services, Centers for Disease Control and Prevention, and National Center for Health Statistics. *Health, United States, 2015*. https://www.cdc.gov/nchs/data/hus/hus15.pdf#055. Accessed May 2017.
2. High Cholesterol Facts. Centers for Disease Control and Prevention. *High Cholesterol Facts*. https://www.cdc.gov/cholesterol/facts.htm. Accessed May 2017.
3. Prevalence of abnormal lipid levels among youths—United States, 1999–2006. *MMWR Morb Mortal Wkly Rep*. 2010;59(02):29-33. http://www.cdc.gov/mmwr/preview/mmwrhtml/mm5902a1.htm. Accessed January 2012.
4. Rader DJ, Hobbs HH. Disorders of lipoprotein metabolism. In: Kasper DL, Fauci AS, Hauser SL, et al, eds. *Harrison's Principles of Internal Medicine*, 19th ed. New York, NY: McGraw-Hill; 2014.

5. Cuchel M, Bruckert E, Ginsberg HN, et al; European Atherosclerosis Society Consensus Panel on Familial Hypercholesterolaemia. Homozygous familial hypercholesterolaemia: new insights and guidance for clinicians to improve detection and clinical management. A position paper from the Consensus Panel on Familial Hypercholesterolaemia of the European Atherosclerosis Society. *Eur Heart J*. 2014;35(32):2146-2157.
6. Szalat R, Arnulf B, Karlin L, et al. Pathogenesis and treatment of xanthomatosis associated with monoclonal gammopathy. *Blood*. 2011;118(14):3777-3784.
7. 2013 ACC/AHA Guideline on the treatment of blood cholesterol to reduce atherosclerotic cardiovascular risk in adults. *J Am Clin Cardiol*. 2014;63(25):2889-2934.
8. Expert Panel on Integrated Guidelines for Cardiovascular Health and Risk Reduction in Children and Adolescents. *Summary Report*. https://www.nhlbi.nih.gov/health-pro/guidelines/current/cardiovascular-health-pediatric-guidelines/summary. Accessed May 2017.
9. Akasaka E, Matsuzaki Y, Kimura K, et al. Normolipidaemic xanthomatosis with systemic involvement of the skin, bone and pharynx. *Clin Exp Dermatol*. 2012;37(3):305-307.
10. Berglund L, Brunzell JD, Goldberg AC, et al. Evaluation and treatment of hypertriglyceridemia: an Endocrine Society clinical practice guideline. *J Clin Endocrinol Metab*. 2012;97(9):2969-2989.
11. Martin SS, Abd TT, Jones SR, et al. 2013 ACC/AHA cholesterol treatment guideline: what was done well and what could be done better. *J Am Coll Cardiol*. 2014;63(24):2674-2678.
12. Williams PT, Franklin BA. Incident diabetes mellitus, hypertension, and cardiovascular disease risk in exercising hypercholesterolemic patients. *Am J Cardiol*. 2015;116(10):1516-1520.
13. Eckel RH, Jakicic JM, Ard JD, et al. 2013 ACC/AHA Guideline on the lifestyle management to reduce cardiovascular risk. *J Am Clin Cardiol*. 2014;63(25):2889-2934.
14. Smart NA, Marshall BJ, Daley M, et al. Low-fat diets for acquired hypercholesterolaemia. *Cochrane Database Syst Rev*. 2011;(2):CD007957.
15. Malhotra A, Shafiq N, Arora A, et al. Dietary interventions (plant sterols, stanols, omega-3 fatty acids, soy protein and dietary fibers) for familial hypercholesterolaemia. *Cochrane Database Syst Rev*. 2014;(6):CD001918.
16. Hooper L, Summerbell CD, Thompson R, et al. Reduced or modified dietary fat for preventing cardiovascular disease. *Cochrane Database Syst Rev*. 2012;(5):CD002137.
17. Brugts JJ, Yetgin T, Hoeks SE, et al. The benefits of statins in people without established cardiovascular disease but with cardiovascular risk factors: meta-analysis of randomised controlled trials. *BMJ*. 2009;338:b2376.
18. Chou R, Dana T, Blazina I, et al. Statins for prevention of cardiovascular disease in adults: evidence report and systematic review for the US Preventive Services Task Force. *JAMA*. 2016;316(19):2008-2024.
19. Gutierrez J, Ramirez G, Rundek T, Sacco RL. Statin therapy in the prevention of recurrent cardiovascular events: a sex-based meta-analysis. *Arch Intern Med*. 2012;172(12):909-919.
20. Sattar N, Preiss D, Murray HM, et al. Statins and risk of incident diabetes: a collaborative meta-analysis of randomised statin trials. *Lancet*. 2010;375:735-742.
21. Dormuth CR, Hemmelgarn BR, Paterson JM, et al. Use of high potency statins and rates of admission for acute kidney injury: multicenter, retrospective observational analysis of administrative databases. *BMJ*. 2013;346:f880.
22. Abourbih S, Filion KB, Joseph L, et al. Effect of fibrates on lipid profiles and cardiovascular outcomes: a systematic review. *Am J Med*. 2009;122:962.e1-8.
23. Navarese EP, Kolodziejczak M, Schulze V, et al. Effects of proprotein convertase subtilisin/kexin type 9 antibodies in adults with hypercholesterolemia: a systematic review and meta-analysis. *Ann Intern Med*. 2015;163(1):40-51.
24. Wider B, Pittler MH, Thompson-Coon J, Ernst E. Artichoke leaf extract for treating hypercholesterolaemia. *Cochrane Database Syst Rev*. 2009;(4):CD003335.
25. Becker DJ, Gordon RY, Halbert SC, et al. Red yeast rice for dyslipidemia in statin-intolerant patients: a randomized trial. *Ann Intern Med*. 2009;150(12):830-839.
26. Liu ZL, Liu JP, Zhang AL, et al. Chinese herbal medicines for hypercholesterolemia. *Cochrane Database Syst Rev*. 2011;(7):CD008305.
27. Hooper L, Thompson RL, Harrison RA, et al. Risks and benefits of omega 3 fats for mortality, cardiovascular disease, and cancer: systematic review. *BMJ*. 2006;332:752-760.
28. Pan A, Yu D, Demark-Wahnefried W, et al. Meta-analysis of the effects of flaxseed interventions on blood lipids. *Am J Clin Nutr*. 2009;90(2):288-297.
29. Wong H, Chahal N, Manlhiot C, et al. Flaxseed in pediatric hyperlipidemia: a placebo-controlled, blinded, randomized clinical trial of dietary flaxseed supplementation for children and adolescents with hypercholesterolemia. *JAMA Pediatr*. 2013;167(8):708-713.
30. Rajaram S, Haddad EH, Mejia A, Sabaté J. Walnuts and fatty fish influence different serum lipid fractions in normal to mildly hyperlipidemic individuals: a randomized controlled study. *Am J Clin Nutr*. 2009;89(5):1657S-1663S.
31. Sabaté J, Oda K, Ros E. Nut consumption and blood lipid levels: a pooled analysis of 25 intervention trials. *Arch Intern Med*. 2010;170(9):821-827.
32. Del Gobbo LC, Falk MC, Feldman R, et al. Effects of tree nuts on blood lipids, apolipoproteins, and blood pressure: systematic review, meta-analysis, and dose-response of 61 controlled intervention trials. *Am J Clin Nutr*. 2015;102(6):1347-1356.
33. Torres KMT. Xanthoma treatment and management. In: eMedicine. Medscape. http://emedicine.medscape.com/article/1103971-treatment#d9, updated March 25, 2018. Accessed May 2017.
34. Rees K, Dyakova M, Wilson N, et al. Dietary advice for reducing cardiovascular risk. *Cochrane Database Syst Rev*. 2013;(12):CD002128.
35. US Preventive Services Task Force. *https://www.uspreventiveservicestaskforce.org/BrowseRec/Search?s=lipids*. Accessed May 2017.
36. Taylor F, Huffman MD, Macedo AF, et al. Statins for the primary prevention of cardiovascular disease. *Cochrane Database Syst Rev*. 2013;(1):CD004816.

233 OBESITY

Mindy A. Smith, MD, MS

PATIENT STORY

Diane is a 35-year-old woman who has struggled with obesity for most of her life. Her current body mass index (BMI) is 36. She has tried "every kind of diet you can imagine" but has always gotten stuck after losing the first 10 pounds and gets discouraged. She is not currently exercising regularly. She is concerned about all the skin tags on her neck and wants them removed if possible. She and her husband are talking about having another baby and she would like to be in better shape before she attempts pregnancy. She wants to discuss risks of pregnancy considering her weight and asks for any advice that you can give her on how to successfully lose weight. You obtain a random blood sugar because of her acanthosis and obesity (**Figure 233-1**). The result is 150 mg/dL and you order a fasting blood sugar (FBS) before her next visit, at which time you will remove her skin tags. After discussing diet and exercise, you encourage her to pursue Weight Watchers or a similar program.

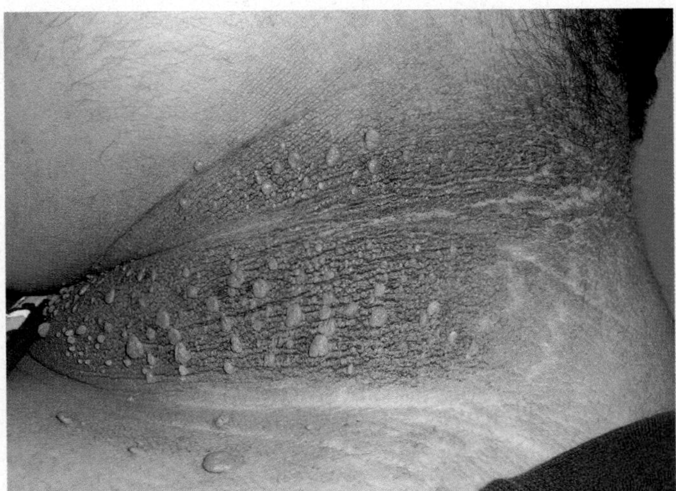

FIGURE 233-1 Neck circumference enlargement with acanthosis nigricans and many skin tags in a woman with obesity and impaired glucose tolerance. (*Reproduced with permission from Richard P. Usatine, MD.*)

INTRODUCTION

Obesity is defined as a BMI greater than or equal to 30. BMI is calculated as weight in kilograms divided by height in meters squared, rounded to 1 decimal place.[1] Obesity in children is defined as a BMI greater than or equal to the age- and sex-specific 95th percentiles of the 2000 Centers for Disease Control and Prevention (CDC) growth charts. Adults with a BMI greater than 40 have substantially more serious health consequences, including heart disease and diabetes, and a reduced life expectancy.

EPIDEMIOLOGY

- Based on the National Health and Nutrition Examination Surveys, more than one-third of U.S. adults (34.9%) and 16.9% of children and adolescents are obese (2012).[1] Slightly more women than men are obese (36.1% vs. 33.5%), although more men than women are classified as overweight or obese (BMI ≥25) (71.3% vs. 65.8%). The prevalence of obesity appears stable since 2003–2004.
- The medical care costs of obesity in the United States (2014 dollars) are approximately $149.4 billion, with medical spending attributable to an obese individual of $1901 annually ($1239–$2582).[2]

ETIOLOGY AND PATHOPHYSIOLOGY

Obesity is a complex problem involving genetics, health behaviors, environment, and sometimes medical diseases (see "Differential Diagnosis" below) or drugs (e.g., steroids, antidepressants). The simplest explanation of obesity is an imbalance between intake (calories eaten) and output (physical activity).

GENETICS

The genetic contribution to interindividual variation in common obesity has been estimated at 40% to 70%.[3] Despite this relatively high heritability, the search for obesity susceptibility genes has been difficult. At least five variants in four candidate genes are associated with obesity-related traits. Although genome-wide linkage studies have been unable to pinpoint genetic loci for common obesity, high-density genome-wide association studies have discovered at least 15 previously unanticipated genetic loci associated with BMI and extreme obesity risk.[3] Genetic influences, however, cannot explain the recent increased prevalence in the rate of weight gain by age; rather, significant changes in lifestyle factors are likely responsible.[4]

- Two GI "hormones" that appear to integrate into the brain may regulate appetite; these hormones—ghrelin (increases appetite) and obestatin (slows gastric emptying, blocking ghrelin action)—may also play a role in obesity. Authors of a meta-analysis concluded that obestatin and total and active ghrelin were significantly higher in normal-weight subjects than in those of obese groups.[5] Lower levels of ghrelin in obese subjects may be a response to hyperinsulinemia.

HEALTH BEHAVIORS

Lifestyle factors associated with obesity include physical activity level (low levels and associated behaviors such as television viewing), diet, and sleep.

- In the Nurses' Health Study, each 2-hour per day increment in TV watching was associated with a 23% (95% confidence interval [CI], 17% to 30%) and each 2-hour per day increment in sitting at work was associated with a 5% (95% CI, 0% to 10%) increase in obesity.[6]
- Based on second-wave interview data from the National Longitudinal Study of Adolescent Health (N = more than 14,000 adolescents), increasing levels of vigorous physical activities lowered the risk for obesity among all adolescents, while eating sufficient fruits and vegetables was inversely associated with adolescents' obesity.[4] As in the above study, sedentary lifestyle was associated with adolescents' obesity. However, in models based on race, low family socioeconomic status and being sedentary were associated with overweight and obesity among whites, and increased nighttime sleep hours was associated with obesity among African Americans.
- In one study, belief that obesity was inherited was associated with lower reported levels of physical activity and fruit and vegetable consumption, while the belief that obesity was caused by lifestyle behaviors was associated with greater reported physical activity but not diet.[7]
- In a study of Latino men and women, men who did not exercise, rarely trimmed fat from meat, and ate fried foods the previous day were 16 pounds heavier than men with healthier habits.[8] Women who had limited exercise (<2.5 hours per week), watched television regularly, ate chips and snacks, and ate no fruit the previous day were 45 pounds heavier than women with healthier habits.

ENVIRONMENT

Factors that have been discussed include location of grocery stores versus fast-food restaurants and safe places to exercise in relation to home proximity. Research studies suggest that neighborhood residents who have better access to supermarkets and limited access to convenience stores tend to have healthier diets and lower levels of obesity.[9] Poor neighborhoods are often characterized by just the opposite. In fact, in one study, having the opportunity to move from a poor neighborhood to one with a lower level of poverty through housing vouchers was associated with modest reductions (4.6%) in the prevalence of extreme obesity and diabetes.[10]

RISK FACTORS

- Family history of obesity.
- Diet—High calorie, low fruits and vegetables,[11] snack foods, and fast-food consumption (obesity prevalence 24% of those going to fast-food restaurants less than once a week to 33% of those going 3 or more times per week).[12]
- Low levels of physical activity.

DIAGNOSIS

The diagnosis of obesity is based on a BMI greater than 30.

CLINICAL FEATURES

- Although elevated weight alone is a risk factor for the development of hypertension, diabetes mellitus (DM), and heart disease, increased waist circumference confers additional mortality risk (**Figure 233-2**).[13]
- Neck circumference enlargement (**Figure 233-1)** along with increased BMI and waist circumference are significant risk factors for obstructive sleep apnea and metabolic syndrome.[14,15]
- There is a strong direct correlation between epicardial fat and abdominal visceral adiposity with evidence supporting a role for epicardial fat in the pathogenesis of coronary artery disease.[16]
- Nonalcoholic fatty liver disease (NAFLD) is present in 57% of overweight individuals attending outpatient clinics compared to 98% of nondiabetic obese patients and in contrast to 10% to 30% of adults in the general population (see Chapter 63, Liver Disease).[17]
- Obesity is also associated with an increased risk of varicose veins (odds ratio [OR] 3.28; 95% CI 1.25 to 8.63) (see Chapter 54, Venous Insufficiency) (**Figure 233-3**).
- Skin conditions associated with obesity include acanthosis nigricans (**Figures 233-1** and **233-4**), eruptive xanthomas (**Figure 233-5**), hidradenitis suppurativa (**Figure 233-6**), and psoriasis (see **Figure 233-2**) (see Chapters 121, Hidradenitis Suppurativa; 158, Psoriasis; 229, Acanthosis Nigricans; and 232, Hyperlipidemia and Xanthomas).

LABORATORY TESTING

Although no specific tests are suggested for patients with obesity, assessing a patient's cardiovascular risk status in addition to BMI, waist circumference, and a patient's motivation to lose weight may be helpful in planning treatment. Consider screening for DM and NAFLD.

DIFFERENTIAL DIAGNOSIS

Several classes of medications (e.g., antidepressants, antidiabetic agents, antipsychotic agents, antiseizure agents, and hormones) can

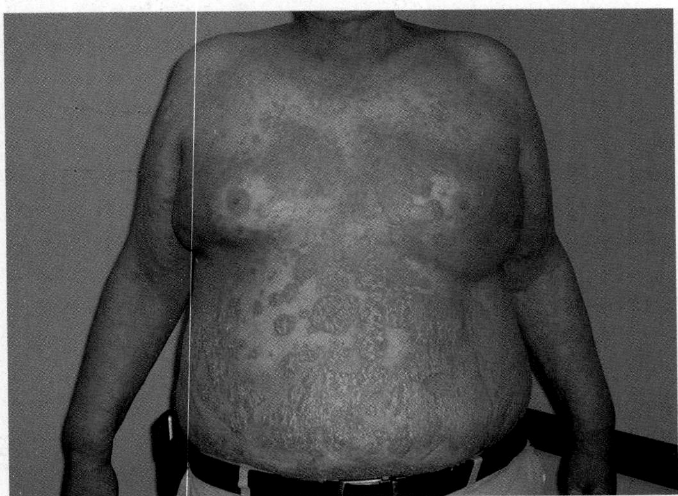

FIGURE 233-2 Central obesity in a man with extensive plaque psoriasis. *(Reproduced with permission from Richard P. Usatine, MD.)*

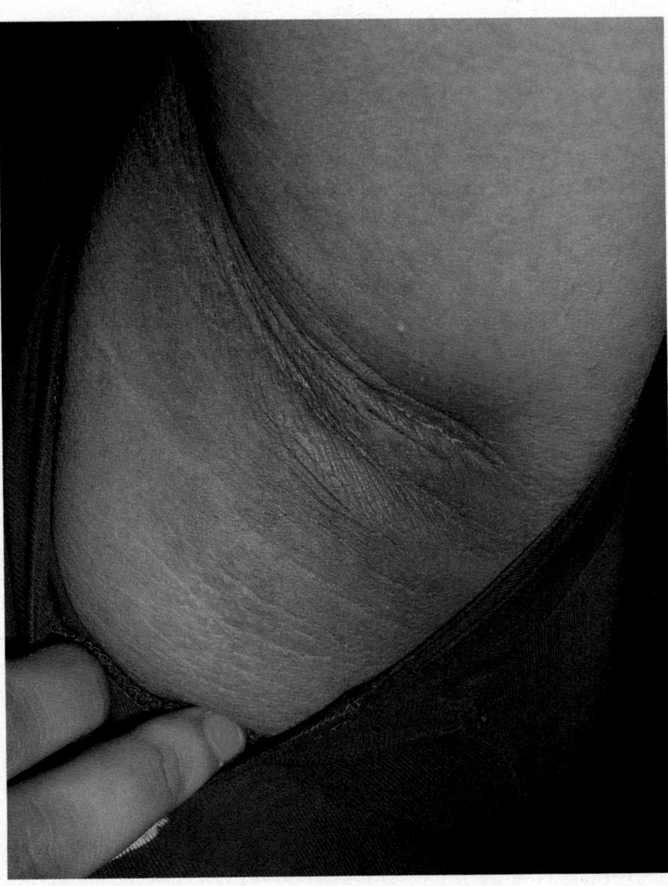

FIGURE 233-4 Acanthosis nigricans in a 14-year-old Hispanic girl with obesity, insulin resistance, and a strong family history of type 2 diabetes. *(Reproduced with permission from Richard P. Usatine, MD.)*

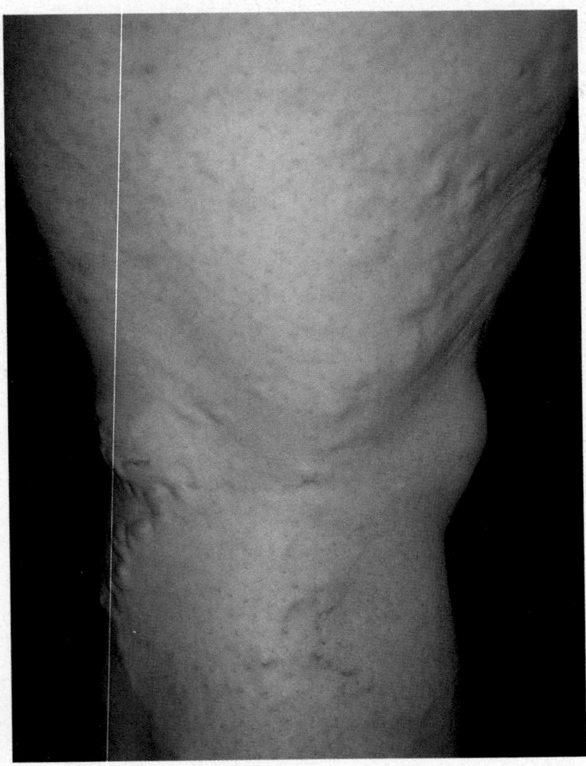

FIGURE 233-3 Serpiginous varicose veins in a woman with obesity. *(Reproduced with permission from Richard P. Usatine, MD.)*

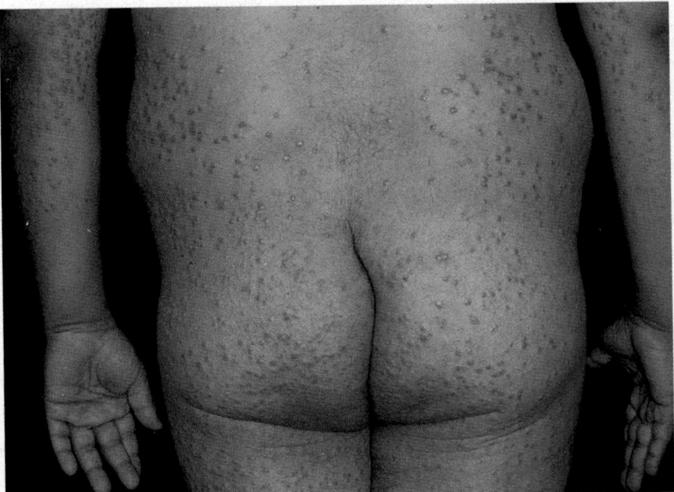

FIGURE 233-5 Eruptive xanthomas in a young man with untreated type 2 diabetes, hyperlipidemia, and obesity. *(Reproduced with permission from Richard P. Usatine, MD.)*

promote weight gain and should be considered for discontinuation or substitution, if able.[18] The differential diagnosis of a patient with obesity includes the following medical conditions:

- Cushing syndrome—Caused by prolonged exposure to endogenous or exogenous glucocorticoids; in addition to truncal obesity, clinical features include moon facies, supraclavicular fat pads, buffalo hump, purple striae, proximal muscle weakness, and hirsutism. Diagnosis is confirmed with inappropriately high serum or urine cortisol levels.
- Polycystic ovarian syndrome (PCOS)—Criteria include two of three of oligo-ovulation or anovulation, hyperandrogenism, and polycystic ovaries. Diagnosis is more strict for adolescent girls because of higher rates of anovulation and cystic ovaries. Diagnosis of PCOS in this age group includes oligomenorrhea for >2 years or primary amenorrhea after age 16 years, hyperandrogenemia (rather than just clinical signs of androgen excess), and presence of polycystic ovaries with ovarian size >10 cm^3.[19]
- Obesity is also a finding in many single-gene disorders such as Prader-Willi syndrome (abnormality of proximal arm of chromosome 15 with associated characteristics of obesity, hypotonia, mental retardation, short stature, hypogonadotropic hypogonadism, strabismus, and small hands and feet) and Bardet-Biedl syndrome (associated with truncal obesity, childhood-onset visual loss preceded by night blindness, and polydactyly).

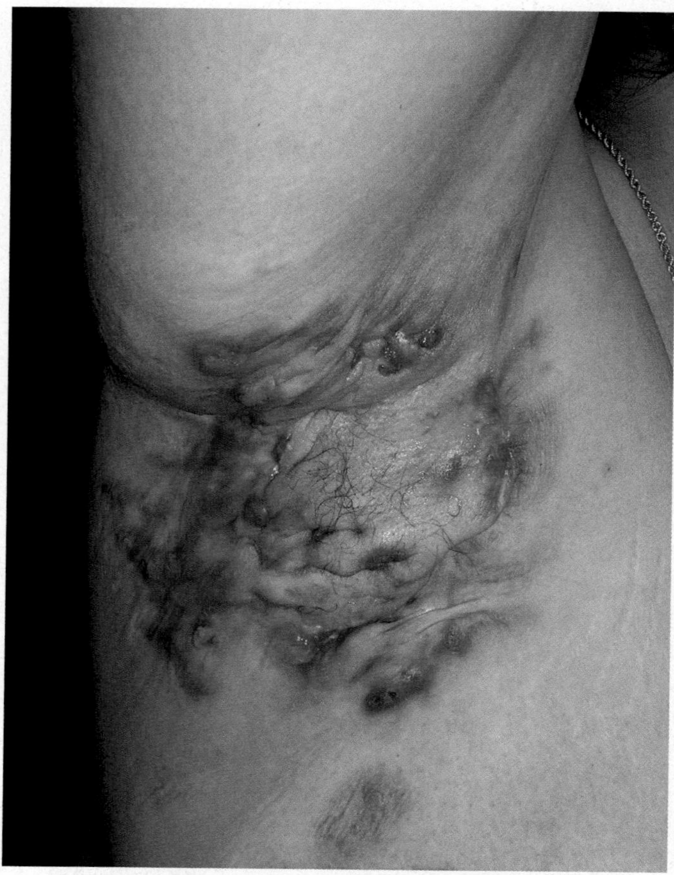

FIGURE 233-6 Hidradenitis suppurativa with significant scarring and sinus tract formation in an obese woman with a body mass index greater than 30. *(Reproduced with permission from Richard P. Usatine, MD.)*

MANAGEMENT

Patients with obesity should be screened for conditions associated with obesity and managed as appropriate. An initial weight loss goal is set to produce an average weight loss of about 1 pound/week for a clinically meaningful weight loss of 3% to 5%.[20] This level of weight loss results in clinically meaningful reductions in triglycerides, blood glucose, hemoglobin A_{1c}, and risk of developing type 2 diabetes. Additional weight loss can be attempted if this goal is achieved.

FIRST LINE

NONPHARMACOLOGIC

- Dietary changes may be useful. In a meta-analysis of long-term weight loss strategies in adults, however, dietary/lifestyle therapy provided less than 5 kg weight loss after 2 to 4 years.[21] SOR A
  - Patients should be prescribed a diet that creates a deficiency of about 500–750 kcal/d below what is needed to maintain weight. As there is no single diet that is better than any other,[22] choose based on patient preference and experience. Diet options include specific diets (e.g., Mediterranean, low-carbohydrate, low-fat), eliminating specific high-calorie foods, or substituting low-calorie drinks for meals.
  - Commercial weight management services appear to be more effective and cheaper than primary care–based services led by specially trained staff (range: 4.4 kg [Weight Watchers] to 1.4 kg [general practice]).[23] SOR A
- Exercise should be encouraged and can result in small weight losses and improvement in cardiovascular risk factors; greater intensity exercise results in additional small weight loss (weighted mean

difference [WMD] approximately −1.5 kg).[24] SOR Ⓐ The addition of diet to exercise also increases weight loss (WMD −1 kg).

- High-intensity (i.e., ≥14 sessions in 6 months) comprehensive (diet, exercise, and behavioral strategies) weight-loss interventions provided in individual or group sessions by a trained interventionist are effective and recommended when available.[20]
- Although data are limited, lifestyle interventions appear to reduce overweight in children,[25] and multicomponent interventions appear effective for infants and children up to age 6 years.[26] SOR Ⓑ
- Enhanced brief lifestyle counseling, including meal replacements, was more effective than usual care for initial weight loss and sustained weight loss at 2 years (1.7 ± 0.7 and 4.6 ± 0.7 kg, respectively) in one randomized controlled trial (RCT) of adults with obesity.[27] SOR Ⓑ

SECOND LINE

NONPHARMACOLOGIC

- The Cochrane library is currently reviewing behavioral and cognitive behavioral strategies that, in the past, have been minimally effective, especially when used in combination with diet and exercise.
  - Behavioral strategies found to be effective include various forms of support, motivational interviewing, and reducing TV screen time.
  - Both remote weight-loss support (study-specific website and email) and in-person support during group and individual sessions along with remote support resulted in greater sustained weight loss at 24 months than the control group (−4.6 kg, −5.1 kg, and −0.8 kg, respectively).[28]

MEDICATIONS

- The Endocrine Society *Clinical Practice Guideline* recommends offering pharmacologic therapy to patients with obesity (or with a BMI of 27 kg/m^2 or 30 kg/m^2 or more with concomitant obesity-related risk factors or diseases) who fail to achieve their weight loss goals through diet and exercise alone.[29] SOR Ⓑ
- Medication options that are FDA-approved as of 2017 include orlistat (both prescription and nonprescription), lorcaserin, phentermine/topiramate, naltrexone/bupropion, and liraglutide.[29] Phentermine and diethylpropion are approved for short-term use. Most weight loss occurs in the first 6 months of treatment.[30]
  - Average weight loss ranges from 2.9 to 8.6 kg over 6–12 months; detailed information is available in the Endocrine Society guideline.[29]
  - Side effects vary, based on mechanism of action, and include nausea and vomiting (liraglutide, naltrexone/bupropion), dry mouth and constipation (lorcaserin, phentermine/topiramate), and steatorrhea, flatulence, and oily spotting (orlistat).

COMPLEMENTARY AND ALTERNATIVE THERAPY

- A number of therapies have been proposed to assist in weight loss, including herbal and nonherbal food supplements, homeopathy, hypnotherapy, acupuncture, and acupressure.[31] Of these, only *Ephedra sinica* and other ephedrine-containing dietary supplements had convincing evidence of small reductions in body weight over placebo.
- A systematic review of food supplements (e.g., guar gum, chromium, chitosan) for weight reduction by some of the same authors also failed to find evidence of a clinically relevant weight loss (WMDs in the range of no benefit to −1.7 kg) using these preparations.[32]

DEVICES

Several devices are on the market to assist with weight loss, including two new gastric balloon devices (Obera and ReShape) that are FDA-approved for use up to 6 months for patients with a BMI of 30–40 who have failed to lose weight with a weight loss program and, for ReShape, who have at least one obesity-related comorbidity.[33] Weight loss ranges from 15 to 32 pounds over 6 months with a regain of up to one half of the weight lost at up to 5 years follow-up.[33,34] Success with these devices is likely in part due to the intensive counseling and support provided.

Other available devices in addition to space-occupying ones are aspiration, restrictive implants, and nonsurgical intestinal bypass (EndoBarrier).[35] There are limited data on adverse effects, which range from nausea, gastric ulceration, gastritis, and abdominal or oropharyngeal pain to obstruction and perforation; each has specific contraindications.

SURGERY

Weight loss surgery is an option for well-informed, carefully selected patients with clinically severe obesity (BMI ≥40 or ≥35 with comorbid conditions) when less-invasive methods of weight loss have failed and the patent is at high risk for obesity-associated morbidity or mortality.[20] SOR Ⓐ Bariatric surgery has been shown to reduce all-cause mortality as well as rates of diabetes, sleep apnea and symptoms of dyspnea and chest pain. Surgical therapy provides approximately 25 to 75 kg of weight loss after 2 to 4 years.[21] Potential long-term side effects include vitamin B_{12} deficiency, incisional hernia, possible need for reoperation, gastritis, gallbladder disease, and malabsorption; operative mortality is about 1% for gastric bypass and 0.4% for gastric banding, but appears lower when performed in high-volume centers.[20] There are no RCTs investigating longer-term effects of surgery compared to conventional treatment on weight loss, comorbidities, and health-related quality of life.[36]

Two types of surgical procedures (gastric banding and gastric bypass) are in current use; all induce substantial weight loss and serve to reduce weight-associated risk factors and comorbidities.

- In a Cochrane review, authors found that weight loss was greater from gastric bypass than from adjustable gastric banding, but similar to isolated sleeve gastrectomy and duodenojejunal bypass with sleeve gastrectomy.[36] Biliopancreatic diversion with duodenal switch is associated with a higher rate of adverse events than gastric bypass.
- Bariatric surgery was also found to be cost-effective compared to other treatments for obesity.[37] Authors identified several remaining questions to be answered, including the influence of surgery on quality of life, late complications leading to reoperation, duration of comorbidity remission, and resource use.
- Laparoscopic bariatric surgery may be safer than open surgery with respect to wound infection (relative risk [RR] 0.21; 95% CI, 0.07 to 0.65) and incisional hernia (RR 0.11; 95% CI, 0.03 to 0.35). Risks appear similar for reoperation, anastomotic leak, and all-cause mortality.[38]
- In one study, the rate of hospitalization in the year following gastric bypass surgery was more than double the rate in the preceding year

(19.3% vs. 7.9%).[39] The most common reasons for admission prior to surgery were obesity-related problems (e.g., osteoarthritis, lower extremity cellulitis) and elective operation (e.g., hysterectomy). The most common reasons for admission after gastric bypass surgery were complications thought to be procedure related, such as ventral hernia repair and gastric revision.[36]

- To prevent nutritional deficiencies after bariatric surgery, patients should take 1–2 adult multivitamins plus minerals containing iron, folic acid, and thiamine; 1200–1500 mg elemental calcium from dietary sources and/or supplements; 3000 IU of vitamin D (titrated to therapeutic 25-D levels >30 ng/mL); and vitamin B_{12}.[40]

REFERRAL

The American Association of Clinical Endocrinologists guideline provides detailed information about preoperative screening for patients considering bariatric surgery and early and late postoperative care for surgical patients. Care should be provided by a team including the surgeon and a nutritionist.

PREVENTION AND SCREENING

- For pregnant women, a behavioral intervention (face-to-face visit; weekly mailed materials promoting appropriate weight gain, healthy eating, and exercise; individual weight gain graphs; and telephone-based feedback) was effective in reducing the number of women with excessive weight gain in pregnancy by approximately 10%,[41] but authors of a systematic review found insufficient quality data from four earlier trials to provide evidence-based recommendations.[42]
- A behavioral approach of lifestyle counseling from nurse practitioners was not effective compared with usual care in preventing weight gain in overweight or obese adults, although approximately 60% of patients in both groups achieved weight maintenance after 3 years.[43]
- Authors of a Cochrane review of 37 studies found strong evidence supporting beneficial effects of child obesity prevention programs on BMI, particularly for programs targeting children ages 6–12 years.[44] However, the overall effect was small (−0.15 kg/m² [95% CI, −0.21 to −0.09]).
- The U.S. Preventive Services Task Force (USPSTF) recommends that clinicians screen children age 6 years and older for obesity and offer them or refer them to comprehensive, intensive behavioral interventions to promote improvement in weight status; these recommendations are under review.[45] SOR Ⓑ This recommendation is based in part on data showing that moderate- to high-intensity programs (>25 hours of contact with the child and/or the family over a 6-month period) improve weight status primarily in children with obesity.
- For adults, the USPSTF recommends that clinicians screen all adult patients for obesity and offer intensive counseling and behavioral interventions to promote sustained weight loss for obese adults.[46] SOR Ⓑ Evidence, however, was insufficient to recommend for or against the use of moderate- or low-intensity counseling together with behavioral interventions to promote sustained weight loss in obese adults or use of counseling of any intensity and behavioral interventions to promote sustained weight loss in overweight adults.

PROGNOSIS

Obesity increases the risk in adults for the following[47]:

- Chronic health diseases such as coronary heart disease, type 2 DM, stroke, osteoarthritis, and gallbladder disease.
- Cancers (i.e., endometrial, breast, colon, kidney, gallbladder and liver).
- Cardiovascular risk factors such as hypertension and dyslipidemia.
- Sleep apnea and respiratory problems.
- Gynecologic problems (e.g., abnormal menses, infertility).

Overweight adolescents are also more susceptible than their leaner peers to hypertension, type 2 DM, dyslipidemia, lung problems (e.g., asthma, obstructive sleep apnea), orthopedic problems (e.g., genu varum, slipped capital femoral epiphysis), and nonalcoholic steatohepatitis.[48] Obese adolescents may also suffer from depression and low self-esteem. In addition, children with obesity are more likely than their leaner counterparts to have obesity as adults.[48]

Among pregnant women, obesity increases the risk for prenatal complications (gestational diabetes and hypertensive disorders),[49] intrapartum complications (cesarean section, induced preterm birth),[50] and stillbirth (OR 2.8; 95% CI, 1.5 to 5.3) and neonatal death (OR 2.6; 95% CI, 1.2 to 5.8) compared with women of normal weight.[51] In addition, women whose gestational weight gain is above the recommendations retain an additional 3 kg after 3 years and 4.7 kg on average after 15 or more years postpartum.[52]

FOLLOW-UP

- Authors of the 2013 guideline encourage clinicians to provide support and encouragement to patients attempting to lose weight, to be prepared to assist patients with addressing small weight gains before they become larger ones, and to reinstitute weight management efforts as early as possible in the course of regain.[20] While visit frequency is not specified, the usual pattern of weight loss in patients undergoing a lifestyle intervention is that maximum weight loss is achieved at 6 months, followed by plateau and gradual regain over time. Referral to comprehensive programs is recommended.
    - For patients on medication for weight loss, if weight loss is <5% at 3 months or if there are safety or tolerability issues at any time, medication should be discontinued and alternative medications or referral for alternative treatment approaches should be considered.
    - Following bariatric surgery, follow-up intervals are based on type of surgery and provided in reference 42.
- For children, health providers should calculate and plot BMI (or weight percentile) at every healthcare visit and watch for excessive weight gain compared with linear growth, identify and track patients at risk of obesity based on risk factors, encourage and support breastfeeding, routinely promote healthy diets and levels of physical activity, and monitor changes in obesity-associated risk factors.[53]

PATIENT EDUCATION

- Advise patients to strive for a healthy lifestyle with a diet that is high in fruits and vegetables and to pursue daily physical activity. Maintaining normal weight and treating obstructive sleep apnea and diabetes may help prevent NAFLD.
- Weight loss can improve cardiovascular risk factors. Commercial weight-reduction programs may be most helpful.[23] The addition of cognitive behavioral strategies may enhance weight loss.
- For patients who are obese and fail to achieve their weight-loss goals through diet and exercise alone, pharmacologic therapy can be considered, but pharmacologic therapy adds cost, can be associated with adverse effects, and lacks long-term safety data; also, weight loss may be temporary.
- Surgery is also an option for carefully selected patients with clinically severe obesity (BMI ≥40 or ≥35 with comorbid conditions) when less-invasive methods of weight loss have failed and the patient is at high risk for obesity-associated morbidity or mortality.

RESOURCES

- MedlinePlus. *Obesity*—**https://medlineplus.gov/obesity.html.**

PROVIDER RESOURCES

- *2013 AHA/ACC/TOS Guideline for the Management of Overweight and Obesity in Adults*—**https://www.ncbi.nlm.nih.gov/pmc/articles/PMC5819889/.**
- Centers for Disease Control and Prevention. *Overweight & Obesity*—**http://www.cdc.gov/obesity/index.html.**

REFERENCES

1. Ogden CL, Carroll MD, Kit BK, Flegal KM. Prevalence of childhood and adult obesity in the United States, 2011–2012. *JAMA*. 2014;311(8):806-814.
2. Kim DD, Basu A. Estimating the medical care costs of obesity in the United States: systematic review, meta-analysis, and empirical analysis. *Value Health*. 2016;19(5):602-613.
3. Loos RJ. Recent progress in the genetics of common obesity. *Br J Clin Pharmacol*. 2009;68(6):811-829.
4. Dodor BA, Shelley MC, Hausafus CO. Adolescents' health behaviors and obesity: does race affect this epidemic? *Nutr Res Pract*. 2010;4(6):528-534.
5. Zhang N, Yuan C, Li Z, et al. Meta-analysis of the relationship between obestatin and ghrelin levels and the ghrelin/obestatin ratio with respect to obesity. *Am J Med Sci*. 2011;341(1):48-55.
6. Hu FB, Li TY, Colditz GA, et al. Television watching and other sedentary behaviors in relation to risk of obesity and type 2 diabetes mellitus in women. *JAMA*. 2003;289(14):1785-1791.
7. Wang C, Coups EJ. Causal beliefs about obesity and associated health behaviors: results from a population-based survey. *Int J Behav Nutr Phys Act*. 2010;7:19.
8. Hubert HB, Snider J, Winkleby MA. Health status, health behaviors, and acculturation factors associated with overweight and obesity in Latinos from a community and agricultural labor camp survey. *Prev Med*. 2005;50(6):642-651.
9. Larson NI, Story MT, Nelson MC. Neighborhood environments: disparities in access to healthy foods in the U.S. *Am J Prev Med*. 2009;36(1):74-81.
10. Ludwig J, Sanbonmastu L, Gennetian L, et al. Neighborhoods, obesity, and diabetes—a randomized social experiment. *N Engl J Med*. 2011;365(16):1509-1519.
11. Mozaffarian D, Hao T, Rimm EB, et al. Changes in diet and lifestyle and long-term weight gain in women and men. *N Engl J Med*. 2011;364(25):2392-2404.
12. Anderson B, Rafferty AP, Lyon-Callo S, et al. Fast-food consumption and obesity among Michigan adults. *Prev Chronic Dis*. 2011; Jul;8(4):A71.
13. Cerhan JR, Moore SC, Jacobs EJ, et al. A pooled analysis of waist circumference and mortality in 650,000 adults. *Mayo Clin Proc*. 2014;89(3):334-345.
14. Soylu AC, Levent E, Sariman N, et al. Obstructive sleep apnea syndrome and anthropometric obesity indexes. *Sleep Breath*. 2012; 16(4):1151-1158.
15. Onat A, Hergenc G, Yuksel H, et al. Neck circumference as a measure of central obesity: associations with metabolic syndrome and obstructive sleep apnea syndrome beyond waist circumference. *Clin Nutr*. 2009;28(1):46-51.
16. Rabkin SW. Epicardial fat: properties, function and relationship to obesity. *Obes Rev*. 2007;8(3):253-261.
17. Vernon G, Baranova A, Younossi ZM. Systematic review: the epidemiology and natural history of non-alcoholic fatty liver disease and non-alcoholic steatohepatitis in adults. *Aliment Pharmacol Ther*. 2011;34(3):274-285.
18. Domecq JP, Prutsky G, Leppin A, et al. Clinical review: drugs commonly associated with weight change: a systematic review and meta-analysis. *J Clin Endocrinol Metab*. 2015;100(2):363-370.
19. Fauser BC, Tarlatzis BC, Rebar RW, et al. Consensus on women's health aspects of polycystic ovary syndrome (PCOS): the Amsterdam ESHRE/ASRM-Sponsored 3rd PCOS Consensus Workshop Group. *Fertil Steril*. 2012;97(1):28-38.e25.
20. Jensen MD, Ryan DH, Apovian CM, et al. 2013 AHA/ACC/TOS Guideline for the Management of Overweight and Obesity in Adults. *Circulation*. https://www.guideline.gov/summaries/summary/48339/2013-ahaacctos-guideline-for-the-management-of-overweight-and-obesity-in-adults-a-report-of-the-american-college-of-cardiologyamerican-heart-association-task-force-on-practice-guidelines-and-the-obesity-society. Accessed April 2017.
21. Douketis JD, Macie C, Thabane L, Williamson DF. Systematic review of long-term weight loss studies in obese adults: clinical significance and applicability to clinical practice. *Int J Obes (Lond)*. 2005;29(10):1153-1167.
22. Johnston BC, Kanters S, Bandayrel K, et al. Comparison of weight loss among named diet programs in overweight and obese adults. A meta-analysis. *JAMA*. 2014;312(9):923-933.
23. Jolly K, Lewis A, Beach J, et al. Comparison of range of commercial or primary care led weight reduction programmes with minimal

intervention control for weight loss in obesity: Lighten Up randomised controlled trial. *BMJ.* 2011;343:d6500.

24. Thorogood A, Mottillo S, Shimony A, et al. Isolated aerobic exercise and weight loss: a systematic review and meta-analysis of randomized controlled trials. *Am J Med.* 2011;124(8):747-755.
25. Oude Luttikhuis H, Baur L, Jansen H, et al. Interventions for treating obesity in children. *Cochrane Database Syst Rev.* 2009;(1): CD001872.
26. Colquitt JL, Loveman E, O'Malley C, et al. Diet, physical activity, and behavioural interventions for the treatment of overweight or obesity in preschool children up to the age of 6 years. *Cochrane Database Syst Rev.* 2016;(3):CD012105.
27. Wadden TA, Volger S, Sarwer DB, et al. A two-year randomized trial of obesity treatment in primary care practice. *N Engl J Med.* 2011;365(21):1969-1979.
28. Appel LJ, Clark JM, Yeh HC, et al. Comparative effectiveness of weight-loss interventions in clinical practice. *N Engl J Med.* 2011;365(21):1959-1968.
29. Apovian CM, Aronne LJ, Bessesen DH, et al. Pharmacologic management of obesity: an Endocrine Society clinical practice guideline. *J Clin Endocrinol Metab.* 2015;100(2):342-362.
30. Greenway FL, Caruso MK. Safety of obesity drugs. *Expert Opin Drug Saf.* 2005;4(6):1083-1095.
31. Pitter MH, Ernst E. Complementary therapies for reducing body weight: a systematic review. *Int J Obes (Lond).* 2005;29(9):1030-1038.
32. Onakpoya IJ, Wider B, Pittler MH, Ernst E. Food supplements for body weight reduction: as systematic review of systematic reviews. *Obesity (Silver Spring).* 2011;19(2):239-244.
33. *ReShape* and *Orbera*—Two gastric balloon devices for weight loss. *Medical Lett.* 2015;57(1476):122-123.
34. Kotzampassi K, Grosomanidis V, Papakostas P, et al. 500 intragastric balloons: what happens 5 years thereafter? *Obes Surg.* 2012; 22:896-903.
35. Kumar N. Endoscopic therapy for weight loss: gastroplasty, duodenal sleeves, intragastric balloons, and aspiration. *World J Gastrointest Endosc.* 2015;7(9):847-859.
36. Colquitt JL, Pickett K, Loveman E, Frampton GK. Surgery for obesity. *Cochrane Database Syst Rev.* 2014:(8):CD003641.
37. Picot J, Jones J, Colquitt JL, et al. The clinical effectiveness and cost-effectiveness of bariatric (weight loss) surgery for obesity: a systematic review and economic evaluation. *Health Technol Assess.* 2009;13(41):1-190.
38. Reoch J, Mottillo S, Shimony A, et al. Safety of laparoscopic vs open bariatric surgery: a systematic review and meta-analysis. *Arch Surg.* 2011;146(11):1314-1322.
39. Zingmond DS, McGory ML, Ko CY. Hospitalization before and after gastric bypass surgery. *JAMA.* 2005;294(15):1918-1924.
40. Mechanick JI, Youdim A, Jones DB, et al. Clinical practice guidelines for the perioperative nutritional, metabolic, and nonsurgical support of the bariatric surgery patient—2013 update: cosponsored by American Association of Clinical Endocrinologists, The Obesity Society, and American Society for Metabolic & Bariatric Surgery. *Surg Obes Relat Dis.* 2013;9(2):159-191.
41. Phelan S, Phipps MG, Abrams B, et al. Randomized trial of a behavioral intervention to prevent excessive gestational weight gain: the Fit for Delivery Study. *Am J Clin Nutr.* 2011;93(4):772-779.
42. Ronnberg AK, Nilsson K. Interventions during pregnancy to reduce excessive gestational weight gain: a systematic review assessing current clinical evidence using the Grading of Recommendations, Assessment, Development and Evaluation (GRADE) system. *BJOG.* 2010;117(11):1327-1334.
43. ter Bogt NC, Bemelmans WJ, Beltman FW, et al. Preventing weight gain by lifestyle intervention in a general practice setting: three-year results of a randomized controlled trial. *Arch Intern Med.* 2011;171(4):306-313.
44. Waters E, de Silva-Sanigorski A, Hall BJ, et al. Interventions for preventing obesity in children. *Cochrane Database Syst Rev.* 2011 Dec 7;(12):CD001871
45. US Preventive Services Task Force, Barton M. Screening for obesity in children and adolescents: US Preventive Services Task Force recommendation statement. *Pediatrics.* 2010;125(2):361-367.
46. US Preventive Services Task Force. *Screening for Obesity in Adults.* http://www.uspreventiveservicestaskforce.org/uspstf/uspsobes.htm. Accessed April 2017.
47. Centers for Disease Control and Prevention. *Adult Obesity Causes and Consequences.* https://www.cdc.gov/obesity/adult/causes.html. Accessed April 2017.
48. Centers for Disease Control and Prevention. https://www.cdc.gov/obesity/childhood/causes.html. Accessed April 2017.
49. Arendas K, Qiu Q, Gruslin A. Obesity in pregnancy: pre-conceptional to postpartum consequences. *J Obstet Gynaecol Can.* 2008;30(6): 477-488.
50. McDonald SD, Han Z, Mulla S, et al. Obesity is associated with fatal coronary heart disease independently of traditional risk factors and deprivation. *BMJ.* 2010;341:c3428.
51. Kristensen J, Vestergaard M, Wisborg K, et al. Pre-pregnancy weight and the risk of stillbirth and neonatal death. *BJOG.* 2005; 112(4):403-408.
52. Nehring I, Schmoll S, Beverlein A, et al. Gestational weight gain and long-term postpartum weight retention: a meta-analysis. *Am J Clin Nutr.* 2011;94(5):1225-1231.
53. Daniels SR, Hassink SG; Committee on nutrition. The role of the pediatrician in primary prevention of obesity. *Pediatrics.* 2015; 136(1):e275-e292.

234 OSTEOPOROSIS AND OSTEOPENIA

Mindy A. Smith, MD, MS
Jeffrey H. Baker, MD

PATIENT STORY

An 83-year-old woman accompanied by her 56-year-old daughter presents to the office with severe upper back pain over the past 2 days. Her medical problems include hypothyroidism, for which she is on replacement medication, and mild hypertension, which is controlled with a diuretic. She has known osteopenia and was taking calcium and vitamin D but had not tolerated a bisphosphonate. Physical examination reveals moderate thoracic kyphosis and tenderness over several lower thoracic vertebrae. A plain radiograph demonstrates vertebral compression fractures (**Figure 234-1A**). The daughter asks about management options for pain and prevention of future fractures and also about screening for herself. As there was a suggestion of multiple compression fractures, a CT was ordered to better visualize the fractures (**Figure 234-1B**).

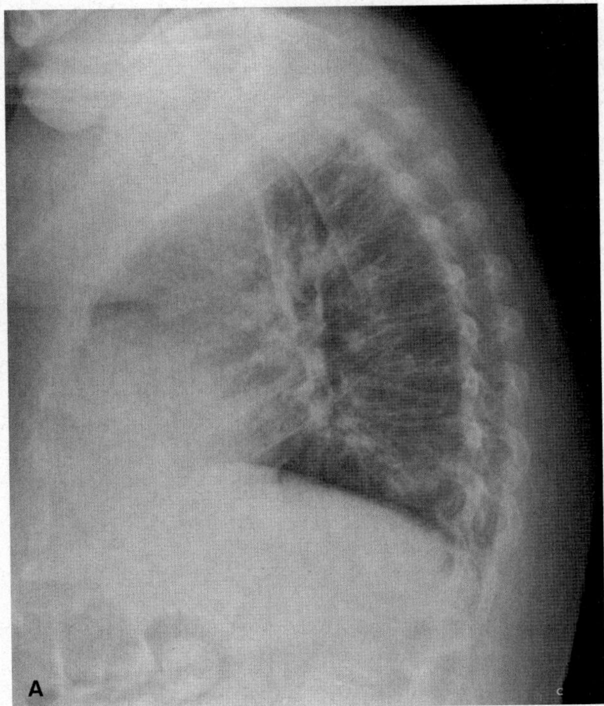

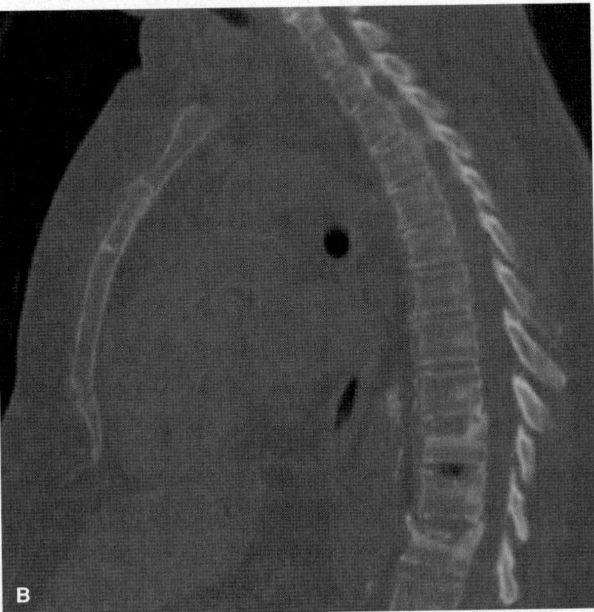

FIGURE 234-1 Osteoporosis-related thoracic vertebral compression fractures in an 83-year-old woman with kyphosis. **A.** Lower thoracic vertebral compression fractures seen on the lateral plain radiograph. **B.** Same fractures visualized more clearly on a lateral CT of the spine. (*Reproduced with permission from Rebecca Loredo-Hernandez, MD.*)

INTRODUCTION

- Osteoporosis is a skeletal disorder characterized by low bone mineral density (BMD) ≤2.5 standard deviations (SD) of the mean for a gender-matched young white adult and compromised bone strength predisposing a person to fracture from minimal trauma.
- Osteopenia is defined as a BMD measurement of between 1.0 and 2.5 SD below the gender-matched young white adult mean. The World Health Organization also defines osteoporosis as a history of fragility fractures and osteopenia.[1]
- The National Osteoporosis Foundation reported in 2014 that fewer than 25% of elderly women who had an osteoporotic fracture received a BMD study or medication to treat osteoporosis 6 months after the fracture, despite availability of cost-effective therapy.[2]

EPIDEMIOLOGY

- Approximately 12 million Americans older than age 50 years have osteopenia.[3]
- Half of all postmenopausal women will have an osteoporosis-related fracture in their lifetime; 25% will experience a vertebral deformity and 15% will suffer a hip fracture.[3]
- Low BMD at the femoral neck (T-score of −2.5 or below) is found in 21% of postmenopausal white women,16% of postmenopausal Mexican American women, and 10% of postmenopausal African-American women.
- About 1 in 5 older men are at risk of an osteoporosis-related fracture.[3]

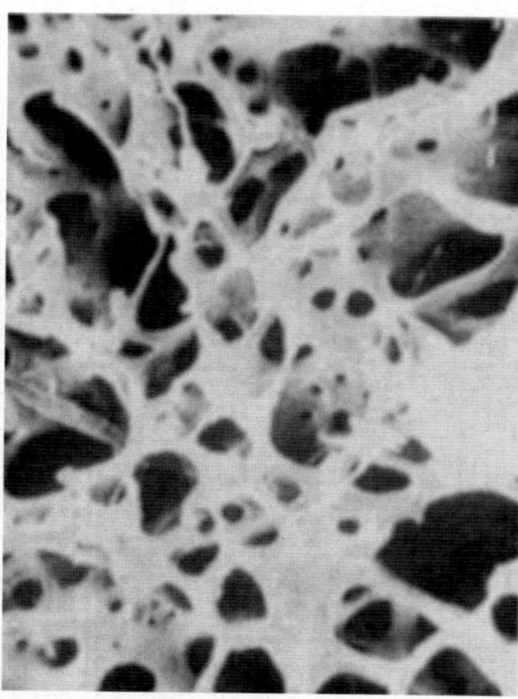

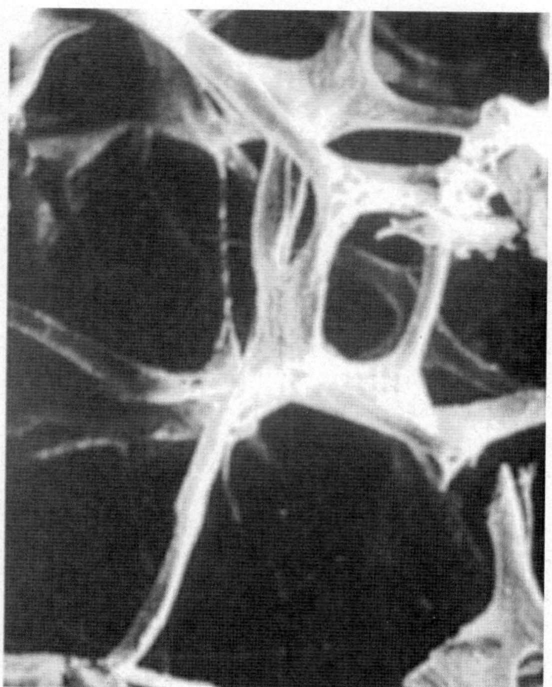

FIGURE 234-2 Normal trabecular bone (*left*) compared with trabecular bone in a patient with osteoporosis (*right*). The loss of mass in osteoporosis leaves these bones more susceptible to breakage. (*Reproduced with permission from Barrett KE, Barman SM, Boitano S, et al. Ganong's Review of Medical Physiology, 25th ed. New York, NY: McGraw-Hill Education; 2016.*)

- Vertebral fractures can cause severe pain and lead to 150,000 hospital admissions per year in the United States.
- Following a hip fracture, up to 20% of women die within 2 years and more than half are unable to return to independent living.[4]

ETIOLOGY AND PATHOPHYSIOLOGY

- Primary osteoporosis is a result of either aging changes or menopause.
  - Usually affects those older than age 70 years.
  - Proportionate loss of cortical and trabecular bone density (**Figure 234-2**). Bone mass peaks at approximately age 30 years and declines thereafter. This bone loss can lead to an increase in vertebral, hip, and radius fractures.
  - In the 15 years following menopause, there is a disproportionate loss of trabecular bone. This can lead to an increase in fractures of the vertebrae, distal forearm, and ankle.
- Secondary osteoporosis is a result of medical conditions or medications (**Table 234-1**). Long-term oral prednisone used to treat several autoimmune diseases is a major contributing cause of secondary osteoporosis (**Figure 234-3**).

RISK FACTORS

- See **Table 234-1**.
- Previous low-trauma fracture.[5] Other risk factors for an osteoporosis-related fracture include advanced age, low BMD, low body mass index (BMI), and starred items in **Table 234-1**.[4]
- An extensively validated online tool developed by the World Health Organization, the Fracture Risk Assessment (FRAX) (http://www.shef.ac.uk/FRAX/, Android and iPhone apps), can be used to estimate 10-year risk for fractures for women and men based on easily obtainable clinical information, such as age, BMI, parental fracture history, and tobacco and alcohol use.

DIAGNOSIS

CLINICAL FEATURES

- Height loss (>1 cm or >0.8 inch) can alert the clinician to osteoporosis.
- Kyphosis and cervical lordosis (dowager's hump).
- Acute pain is often the first symptom from a fracture, usually of the vertebrae (vertebral body collapse), hip, or forearm, especially occurring after minor trauma. Pain may also be elicited from palpation over spinous processes, and paraspinous muscle spasm may be noted.
- Osteoporosis may be identified on X-ray done for another purpose.

TYPICAL DISTRIBUTION

- Fractures caused by menopausal osteoporosis typically occur in thoracic vertebrae, distal forearm, and ankle; occasionally there is loss of teeth.
- Fractures caused by senile osteoporosis are in the vertebrae, hip, and radius.

TABLE 234-1 Factors Associated with Osteoporosis

Genetic factors
- White or Asian ethnicity
- Family history of osteoporosis*
- Low body weight (<127 pounds)*
- Late menarche or early menopause

Nutritional factors
- Low intake of calcium or vitamin D
- High animal protein intake
- Low protein intake

Medical disorders
- Endocrine disorders (e.g., hyperthyroidism, hyperparathyroidism, diabetes mellitus type 1, Cushing disease, hypogonadism)
- Hematologic disorders (e.g., multiple myeloma, anemia [hemolytic, pernicious], lymphoma, leukemia)
- GI disorders (e.g., malabsorption syndromes, chronic liver disease)
- Renal disorders (e.g., chronic renal failure)
- Rheumatologic disorders (e.g., rheumatoid arthritis, ankylosing spondylitis)
- Other disorders (e.g., anorexia, osteogenesis imperfecta)

Medications (commonly used)
- Systemic corticosteroids,* antiepileptic drugs, proton pump inhibitors, chemotherapy, diuretics producing calciuria, GnRH agonist or antagonist, Depo Provera, heparin, extended tetracycline use, SSRIs

Lifestyle factors
- Sedentary
- Excessive exercise
- Current smoking or alcohol use (≥3 drinks/day)*

Abbreviations: GnRH, Gonadotropin-releasing hormone; SSRI, selective serotonin reuptake inhibitors.
*Also risk factors for osteoporosis-related fractures.
Data from Kaplan-Machlis B, Bors KP, Brown SR. Osteoporosis. In: Smith MA, Shimp LA, eds. *Twenty Common Problems in Women's Health Care.* New York, NY: McGraw-Hill; 2000; Osteoporosis. In: Ebell MH, Ferenchik G, Smith MA, et al, eds. *Essential Evidence Plus.* Hoboken, NJ: John Wiley; 2009; Camacho PM, Petak SM, Binkley N, et al. American Association of Clinical Endocrinologists and American College of Endocrinology clinical practice guidelines for the diagnosis and treatment of postmenopausal osteoporosis—2016. *Endocr Pract.* 2016;22(Suppl 4):1-42.

LABORATORY TESTING

- Laboratory testing is recommended for women with osteoporosis to identify secondary causes including a complete blood cell count (for anemia or malignancy), serum chemistry (calcium, phosphorus, total protein, albumin, liver enzymes, alkaline phosphatase, creatinine, and electrolytes), 24-hour urine collection (calcium, sodium, and creatinine excretion to identify calcium malabsorption or hypercalciuria), and serum 25-hydroxyvitamin D.[4]
- Other laboratory tests may be indicated for patients with suspected secondary causes (e.g., serum thyrotropin, erythrocyte sedimentation rate, testosterone, acid–base studies).[4,5] The American Association of Clinical Endocrinologists (AACE) guidelines suggest consideration of bone turnover markers (e.g., serum C-terminal telopeptide and serum carboxy-terminal propeptide) in the initial evaluation and follow-up of patients with osteoporosis, as elevated levels can predict more rapid rates of bone loss and higher fracture risk, and these markers respond quickly to intervention.[4]
- Central dual-energy X-ray absorptiometry (DEXA) measurement of BMD is the accepted gold standard for diagnosis (T-score less than or equal to −2.5 in the spine, femoral neck or hip in the absence of fracture) (**Figures 234-4** and **234-5**).
- Additional imaging with X-ray can confirm osteoporosis-related fracture (**Figures 234-1** and **234-3**).
- The presence of a hip or vertebral fracture in the absence of other bone conditions can also be considered osteoporosis.[4] Two types of

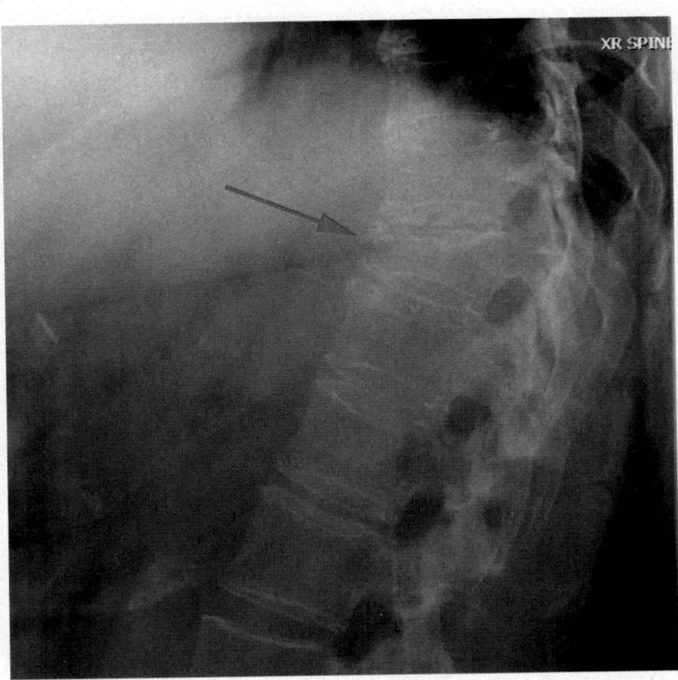

FIGURE 234-3 Wedge compression fracture of T11 vertebra in a postmenopausal woman on long-term prednisone for dermatomyositis. The patient presented with acute back pain. (*Reproduced with permission from Richard P. Usatine, MD.*)

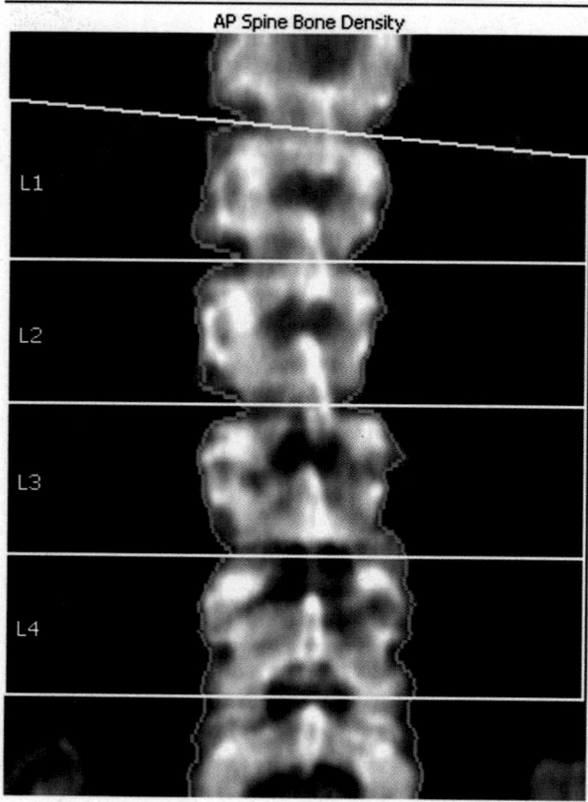

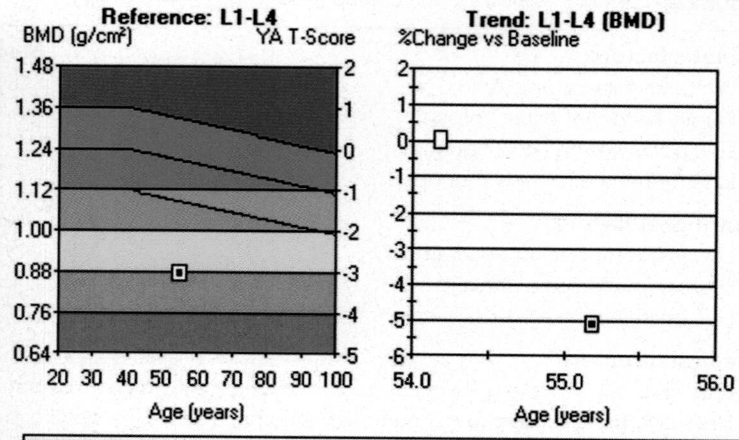

Region	BMD[1] (g/cm²)	Young-Adult[2] (%)	Young-Adult T-Score	Age-Matched[3] (%)	Age-Matched Z-Score
L1	0.871	75	-2.5	77	-2.2
L2	0.895	72	-2.9	73	-2.7
L3	0.867	70	-3.1	72	-2.9
L4	0.854	69	-3.2	71	-2.9
L1-L4	0.871	71	-2.9	73	-2.7

Trend: L1-L4

Measured Date	Age (years)	BMD[1] (g/cm²)	Change vs Previous (g/cm²)	Change vs Previous (%)
12/23/2011	55.1	0.871	-0.047	-5.1
12/21/2010	54.1	0.918	-	-

COMMENTS: PREVIOUS EXAM 2011, TAKING CALCIUM SUPPLEMENT, VITAMIN D, DECREASE IN HEIGHT BY A 1/2 INCH

FIGURE 234-4 Dual-energy X-ray absorptiometry bone density scan showing osteoporosis in the vertebral spine showing 5% loss of vertebral bone density in 1 year. (*Reproduced with permission from Richard P. Usatine, MD.*)

hip fractures related to osteoporosis are femoral neck fractures (**Figure 234-6**) and intertrochanteric fractures.

- Quantitative techniques are being developed to appraise additional characteristics of osteoporosis including three-dimensional bone architecture with quantitative computed tomography (QCT) and magnetic resonance imaging (MRI).[6]

DIFFERENTIAL DIAGNOSIS

Thoracic kyphosis of recent onset in adults can also be caused by:

- Degenerative arthritis of the spine—Pain and swelling in other joints, morning stiffness.
- Poor mobility in an older population.[7]
- Ankylosing spondylitis—Male gender, night pain, and limited motion in sacroiliac joints, uveitis.
- Tuberculosis (TB) and other infections of the spine—History of TB, positive cultures, X-ray showing joint destruction (see Chapter 56, Tuberculosis).
- Cancer—History of cancer, imaging distinguishes.

MANAGEMENT

FIRST LINE

NONPHARMACOLOGIC

- Identify and treat secondary causes (see **Table 234-1**).
- Dietary advice includes adequate calcium, vitamin D, and protein intake.[4] SOR B
- Recommend regular weight-bearing exercise.[4] The Institute for Clinical Systems Improvement (ICSI) notes that 3 components of an exercise program are needed for strong bone health: impact exercise (e.g., jogging, brisk walking, stair climbing), strengthening exercise with weights, and balance training such as tai chi or dancing.[5]
- Encourage smoking cessation and moderate alcohol use (<3 drinks per day).[4] SOR B
- Hip protectors may reduce hip fractures in the nursing home.[8] SOR B
- Address other risk factors for falling (e.g., home safety assessment, low vision, neurologic disorders, gait disturbance, use of sedatives, narcotics, and antihypertensives) and consider referral for physical or occupational therapy, if indicated.

DualFemur Bone Density

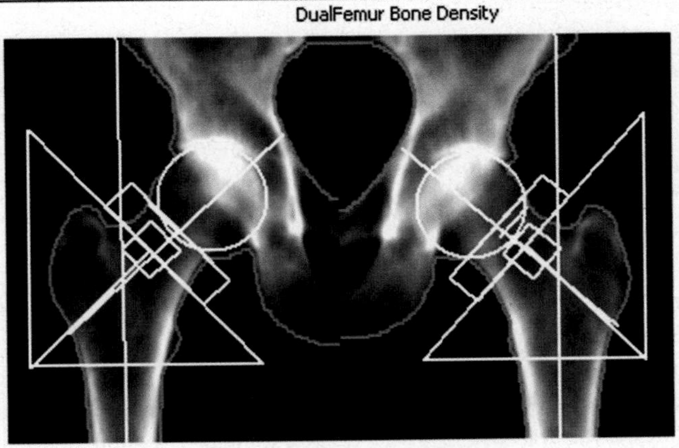

Image not for diagnosis

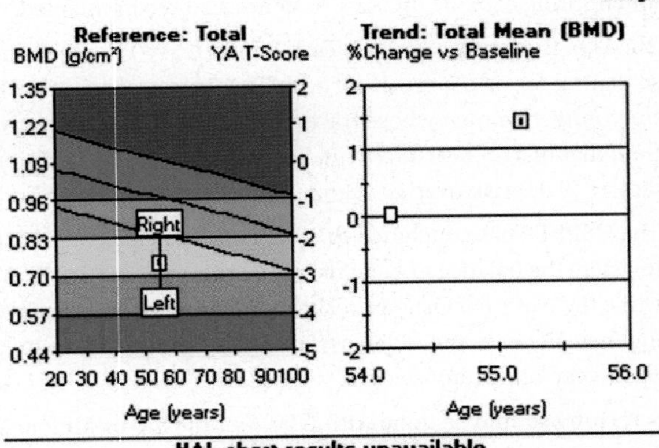

Region	BMD[1,6] (g/cm²)	Young-Adult[2,7] (%)	T-Score	Age-Matched[3] (%)	Z-Score
Neck					
Left	0.720	67	-2.7	78	-1.5
Right	0.712	67	-2.8	78	-1.6
Mean	0.716	67	-2.7	78	-1.6
Difference	0.008	1	0.1	1	0.1
Total					
Left	0.740	68	-2.7	76	-1.8
Right	0.741	68	-2.7	76	-1.8
Mean	0.740	68	-2.7	76	-1.8
Difference	0.001	0	0.0	0	0.0

Trend: Total Mean

Measured Date	Age (years)	BMD[1,6] (g/cm²)	Change vs Previous (g/cm²)	Change vs Previous (%)
12/23/2011	55.1	0.740	0.010	1.4
12/21/2010	54.1	0.730	-	-

COMMENTS: PREVIOUS EXAM 2011, TAKING CALCIUM SUPPLEMENT, VITAMIN D, DECREASE IN HEIGHT BY A 1/2 INCH

FIGURE 234-5 Dual-energy X-ray absorptiometry bone density scan showing osteoporosis of the hips with 2% gain of bone density in 1 year. *(Reproduced with permission from Richard P. Usatine, MD.)*

MEDICATIONS

- Calcium (1200 mg/day from diet plus supplement for women ≥50 years) and vitamin D (at least 800–1000 IU/day).[4,9] SOR Ⓐ A Cochrane review of 53 studies of vitamin D therapy without supplemental calcium found it unlikely to be effective in preventing hip fractures or any new fractures, while combining with calcium supplementation would result in a small reduction in hip fracture and a significant reduction in new non-vertebral fractures.[10] One study found that a single large dose of vitamin D (100,000 IU given orally every 4 months) over 5 years reduced fractures in elderly British women (number needed to treat [NNT] = 20).[11] AACE recommends measuring serum 25-hydroxyvitamin D in patients with osteoporosis and supplementing vitamin D to maintain a level ≥30 ng/mL.[4]
- Women with osteoporosis, osteopenia, or low bone mass and a previous hip or spine fragility fracture should receive medication therapy, beginning with a bisphosphonate.[4] Women should also be considered for medication if they have a T-score of between −1.0 and −2.5, if FRAX major osteoporotic fracture probability is ≥20%, or if hip fracture probability is ≥3%.[4]

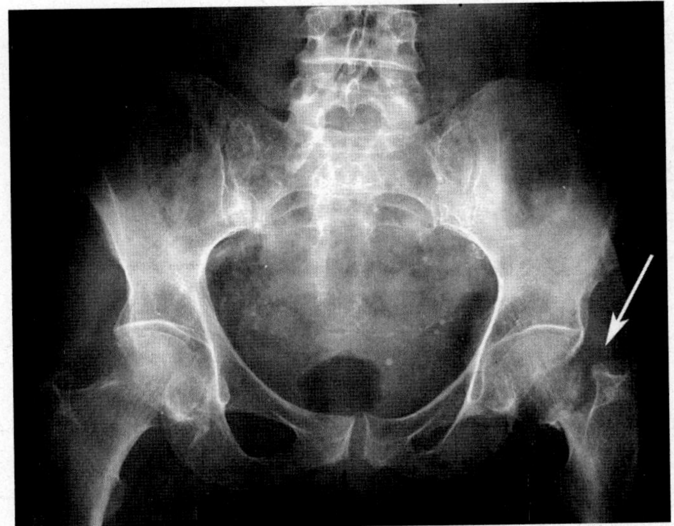

FIGURE 234-6 Femoral neck fracture *(arrow)* in an elderly woman with osteoporosis. The woman fell on her left hip when coming out of the shower. *(Reproduced with permission from Rebecca Loredo-Hernandez, MD.)*

- First-line agents include alendronate, risedronate, zoledronic acid, and denosumab.[4] SOR Ⓐ Based on a Cochrane review of 11 studies, use of alendronate prevented hip (absolute risk reduction [ARR] 1%), vertebral (ARR 6%), and nonvertebral fractures (ARR 2%).[12] Potential side effects of bisphosphonates include rare atypical femoral shaft fracture (0.13% in the subsequent year for women with at least 5 years of treatment)[13] and jaw osteonecrosis (0.7 per 100,000 patient-years with oral bisphosphonate therapy).[14]
- Other drug therapies approved by the U.S. Food and Drug Administration to reduce fractures include parathyroid hormone (PTH, teriparatide [e.g., Forteo]), raloxifene (a selective estrogen receptor modulator [SERM]), and estrogen (women only). AACE recommends PTH, denosumab, or zoledronic acid as first-line agents for patients with the highest fracture risk or those who are unable to use oral therapy. Ibandronate and raloxifene may be appropriate initial agents for patients requiring drugs with spine-specific efficacy.[4] AACE recommends against combination therapy. SOR Ⓑ
- The first-line agents listed above for treatment of osteoporosis have been approved for use in men as well as women; however, data are limited for men, especially for fracture reduction. In a randomized controlled trial of 265 men on glucocorticoid therapy, both risedronate and zoledronic acid prevented bone loss in the prevention population, while zoledronic acid increased BMD slightly more than risedronate (4.7% vs. 3.3% lumbar spine and 1.8% vs. 0.2% total hip, respectively) in the treatment group.[15]
- Denosumab is a human monoclonal antibody that inhibits osteoclast-mediated bone resorption; denosumab was shown to reduce new vertebral fractures in women with multiple and/or severe prevalent vertebral fractures (ARR 9.1%) and hip fractures in subjects age 75 years or older (ARR 1.4%). Both denosumab and zoledronic acid appear to reduce fracture risk in men with castration-resistant prostate cancer metastatic to bone, and denosumab and toremifene (a SERM) reduced osteoporotic fracture risk in men on androgen-deprivation treatment.[16] Denosumab has not been compared with bisphosphonates or other interventions. AACE considers this a first-line agent, but it is very expensive.[4] SOR Ⓐ Risks of treatment include endocarditis, cancer, and skin rash.

SECOND LINE

MEDICATIONS

- Nasal calcitonin (200 IU intranasally once daily, or 100 IU subcutaneously every other day) may preserve BMD and reduce new vertebral fractures; this drug also has an analgesic effect for some women with painful acute vertebral fractures.[17]

COMPLEMENTARY AND ALTERNATIVE THERAPY

- Limited data support use of phytoestrogens, synthetic isoflavones such as ipriflavone, or natural progesterone cream for prevention or treatment of osteoporosis. A 2-year multicenter, randomized trial of ipriflavone showed some effect on total body BMD but no significant effect on regional bone density at common fracture sites.[18]

REFERRAL

- AACE recommends referral of patients to a clinical endocrinologist if a patient with a normal BMD sustains a low-trauma fracture, has recurrent fractures or continued bone loss despite therapy, has a less common secondary condition (e.g., hyperparathyroidism), has unexpectedly severe osteoporosis or unusual features, or has a complicating condition (e.g., renal failure).[4] SOR Ⓒ

PREVENTION AND SCREENING

- The AACE guideline recommends adequate calcium and vitamin D intake to reduce bone loss.[4] SOR Ⓑ Maintaining an active lifestyle SOR Ⓑ, smoking cessation SOR Ⓑ, limiting alcohol intake SOR Ⓑ, and limiting caffeine intake SOR Ⓒ are also recommended.
- The U.S. Preventive Services Task Force (USPSTF) recommends screening for osteoporosis for women 65 years of age and older and for younger women whose fracture risk is the same as or greater than that of a 65-year-old white woman who has no additional risk factors (9.3% risk over 10 years).[3]
- The USPSTF has concluded that the current evidence is insufficient to assess the balance of benefits and harms of screening in men, while the National Osteoporosis Foundation recommends screening men 70 years and older, assuming this group has a similar risk as 65-year-old white women.[3]
- Screening should be done with DEXA of the hip or lumbar spine or quantitative ultrasonography of the calcaneus; appropriate cutoffs for diagnosis and treatment using ultrasound, however, have not been established.
- Bisphosphonate therapy should be considered for postmenopausal women and men age >50 years who are starting glucocorticoid therapy planned for over 3 months or on chronic glucocorticoid therapy; teriparatide is considered if the patient is at high risk of fracture.[19] For premenopausal women of nonchildbearing potential and younger men, a bisphosphonate is recommended for fracture prevention if 1–3 months of corticosteroid use is planned and a bisphosphonate or teriparatide is recommended and ≥3 months of use is planned; there are insufficient data to guide recommendations for women of childbearing age. Authors of a Cochrane review found bisphosphonates for steroid-induced osteoporosis reduced the risk of vertebral fractures and prevented steroid-induced bone loss.[20]

FOLLOW-UP

- Repeat DEXA (same machine if possible) every 1 to 2 years until findings are stable and then continue with follow-up DEXA every 1–2 years or less, depending on clinical circumstances (see **Figures 234-4** and **234-5**).[4] A 2012 Agency for Healthcare Research and Quality update noted that although the practice of follow-up DEXA remains popular, the rationale for it is unclear; treatment trial analyses showed that changes in BMD while on treatment only modestly predicted fracture reduction, while patients whose BMD declined still showed significant fracture risk reduction.[21]

- There is insufficient evidence to determine which bone turnover marker, if any, to use in routine clinical practice to monitor osteoporosis treatment response.[4,22]
- Consider discontinuation of a bisphosphonates after 5 years of stability or after 6–10 years of stability for high-risk patients.[4] Reinstitute treatment if BMD declines substantially, bone turnover markers increase, or a fracture occurs.
- Treatment with teriparatide should be limited to 2 years, and patients on intravenous zoledronic acid should be considered for a drug holiday after 3 annual doses in moderate-risk patients and after 6 annual doses in higher-risk patients.[4]

PATIENT EDUCATION

- Encourage home-based fall prevention by removing throw rugs, reducing clutter in high-traffic areas, increasing lighting, and using safety step stools and safety hand rails in the bathroom, and walking aids.
- Encourage healthy lifestyle and diet.

PATIENT RESOURCES

- MedlinePlus. *Osteoporosis*—**https://medlineplus.gov/osteoporosis.html.**
- MedlinePlus. *Kyphosis*—**https://medlineplus.gov/ency/article/001240.htm.**
- Osteoporosis Foundation—**https://www.nof.org.**

PROVIDER RESOURCES

- **https://www.bones.nih.gov.**
- **https://www.aace.com/files/final-appendix.pdf.**
- The FRAX tool has been developed by the World Health Organization (WHO) to evaluate fracture risk of patients. It can be very helpful in making treatment choices: **https://www.sheffield.ac.uk/FRAX/.** It is also available as a smartphone application at **www.itunes.apple.com and www.play.google.com.**

REFERENCES

1. The WHO Study Group. *Assessment of Fracture Risk and Its Application to Screening for Postmenopausal Osteoporosis*. Technical Report Series. No. 843. Geneva, Switzerland: World Health Organization; 1994.
2. National Osteoporosis Foundation. *Clinician's Guide to Prevention and Treatment of Osteoporosis*. Washington, DC: National Osteoporosis Foundation; 2014:2359-2381.
3. U.S. Preventive Services Task Force. Screening for osteoporosis: U.S. Preventive Services Task Force Recommendation Statement. *Ann Intern Med.* 2011;154(5):356-364.
4. Camacho PM, Petak SM, Binkley N, et al. American Association of Clinical Endocrinologists and American College of Endocrinology clinical practice guidelines for the diagnosis and treatment of postmenopausal osteoporosis—2016. *Endocr Pract.* 2016; 22(Suppl 4):1-42. https://www.aace.com/sites/default/files/OsteoGuidelines2010.pdf. Accessed October 2011.
5. National Guideline Clearinghouse (NGC). Guideline summary: Diagnosis and treatment of osteoporosis. In: National Guideline Clearinghouse (NGC) [website]. Rockville (MD): Agency for Healthcare Research and Quality (AHRQ); 2013 Jul 01. Accessed March 2017.
6. Oei L, Koromani F, Rivadeneira F, et al. Quantitative imaging methods in osteoporosis. *Quant Imaging Med Surg.* 2016;6(6): 680-698.
7. Eum R, Leveille SG, Kiely DK, et al. Is kyphosis related to mobility, balance and disability? *Am J Phys Med Rehabil.* 2013;90(11): 980-989.
8. Sawka AM, Boulos P, Beattie K, et al. Hip protectors decrease hip fracture risk in elderly nursing home residents: a bayesian meta-analysis. *J Clin Epidemiol.* 2007;60:336-344.
9. Bischoff-Ferrari HA, Willett WC, Wong JB, et al. Prevention of nonvertebral fractures with oral vitamin D dose dependency. A meta-analysis of randomized controlled trials. *Arch Intern Med.* 2009;169(6):551-561.
10. Avenell A, Mak JCS, O'Connell D. Vitamin D and vitamin D analogues for preventing fractures in post-menopausal women and older men. *Cochrane Database Syst Rev.* 2014;(4):CD000227.
11. Trivedi DP, Doll R, Khaw KT. Effect of four monthly oral vitamin D_3 (cholecalciferol) supplementation on fractures and mortality in men and women living in the community: randomised double blind controlled trial. *BMJ.* 2003;326:469-472.
12. Wells GA, Cranney A, Peterson J, et al. Alendronate for the primary and secondary prevention of osteoporotic fractures in postmenopausal women. *Cochrane Database Syst Rev.* 2008;(1): CD001155.
13. Park-Wyllie LY, Mamdani MM, Juurlink DN, et al. Bisphosphonate use and the risk of subtrochanteric or femoral shaft fractures in older women. *JAMA.* 2011;305:783-789.
14. Ruggiero SL, Dodson TB, Assael LA, et al. Association of Oral and Maxillofacial Surgeons. American Association of Oral and Maxillofacial Surgeons position paper on bisphosphonate-related osteonecrosis of the jaws. *J Oral Maxillofac Surg.* 2009; 67(5 Suppl):2-12.
15. Sambrook PN, Roux C, Devogelaer JP, et al. Bisphosphonate and glucocorticoid osteoporosis in men: results of a randomized controlled trial comparing zoledronic acid with risedronate. *Bone.* 2012;50(1):289-295.
16. Saylor PJ, Lee RJ, Smith MR. Emerging therapies to prevent skeletal morbidity in men with prostate cancer. *J Clin Oncol.* 2011; 29(27):3705-3714.
17. Chesnut CH, Silverman S, Andriano K, et al. A randomized trial of nasal spray salmon calcitonin in postmenopausal women with established osteoporosis: the Prevent Recurrence of Osteoporotic Fractures Study. *Am J Med.* 2000;109:267-276.

18. Wong WW, Lewis RD, Steinberg FM, et al. Soy isoflavone supplementation and bone mineral density in menopausal women: a 2-y multicenter clinical trial. *Am J Clin Nutr.* 2009;90(5):1433-1439.
19. American College of Rheumatology 2010 recommendations for the prevention and treatment of glucocorticoid-induced osteoporosis. *Arthritis Care Res.* 2010;62(11):1515-1526.
20. Allen CS, Yeung JHS, Vandermeer B, et al. Bisphosphonates for steroid-induced osteoporosis. *Cochrane Database Syst Rev.* 2016;(10):CD001347.
21. Crandall CJ, Newberry SJ, Gellad WG, et al. Treatment to prevent fractures in men and women with low bone density or osteoporosis: update of a 2007 report. Comparative Effectiveness Review No. 53. Rockville, MD: Agency for Healthcare Research and Quality; March 2012.
22. Burch J, Rice S, Yang H, et al. Systematic review of the use of bone turnover markers for monitoring the response to osteoporosis treatment: the secondary prevention of fractures, and primary prevention of fractures in high-risk groups. *Health Technol Assess.* 2014;18(11):1-180.

235 GOITROUS HYPOTHYROIDISM

Mindy A. Smith, MD, MS

PATIENT STORY

A 55-year-old woman presented with a several-month history of fatigue and weight gain. She reported that she felt puffy and swollen. She had difficulty buttoning the top button of her blouse because her neck was so large, but she reported no neck pain. Review of systems was positive for constipation, dry skin, and cold intolerance. On physical examination, a large goiter was found (**Figure 235-1**). Laboratory testing revealed an elevated thyroid-stimulating hormone (TSH) and a low free thyroxine (FT_4) level, confirming hypothyroidism. The patient was started on levothyroxine.

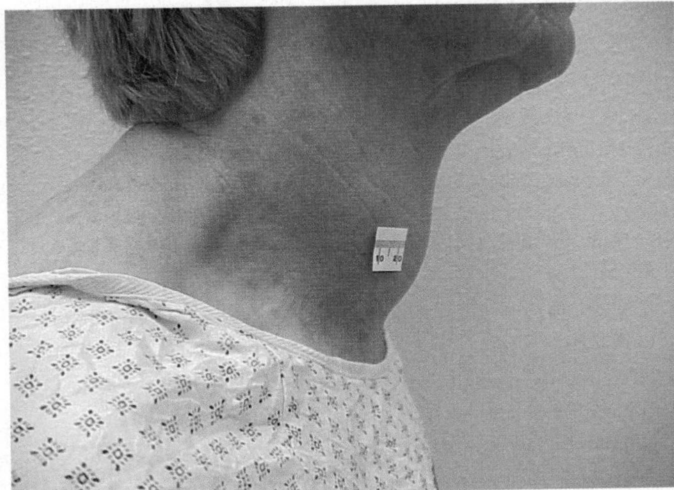

FIGURE 235-1 Goiter that extends approximately 2 cm forward when viewed from the patient's side. (*Reproduced with permission from Dan Stulberg, MD.*)

INTRODUCTION

- Goiter is a spectrum of changes in the thyroid gland ranging from diffuse enlargement to nodular enlargement depending on the cause. In the United States, the most common etiology of goiter with normal thyroid function or transient dysfunction is thyroiditis.
- Hypothyroidism is a condition caused by lack of thyroid hormone and usually develops because of thyroid failure from intrinsic thyroid disease. The most common cause of goitrous hypothyroidism is chronic lymphocytic (Hashimoto) thyroiditis.
- Subclinical thyroid disease refers to abnormal laboratory values (elevated TSH and thyroxine level within the normal range) in a patient with no or minimal thyroid-related symptoms.

EPIDEMIOLOGY

- Worldwide, goiter is the most common endocrine disorder, with rates of 4% to 15% in areas of adequate iodine intake and more than 90% where there is iodine deficiency.[1] Endemic goiter is defined as goiter that affects more than 5% of the population (**Figures 235-2** and **235-3**).
- Most goiters are not associated with thyroid dysfunction.
- The prevalence of goitrous hypothyroidism varies from 0.7% to 4% of the population.
- Subclinical hypothyroidism is present in 3% to 10% of population groups and in 10% to 18% of elderly persons.[2,3]
- The female-to-male ratio of goiter is 3:1, and 6:1 for goitrous hypothyroidism.
- The annual incidence of autoimmune hypothyroidism is 4 in 1000 women and 1 in 1000 men, with a mean age at diagnosis of 60 years.[4]

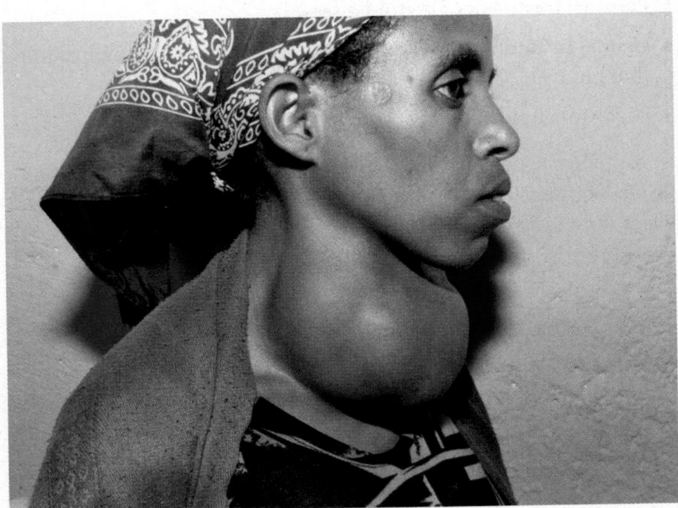

FIGURE 235-2 Massive goiter in an Ethiopian woman who lives in an endemic area for goiters. Many adults have large goiters in Ethiopia where there is little iodine in their diets. (*Reproduced with permission from Richard P. Usatine, MD.*)

ETIOLOGY AND PATHOPHYSIOLOGY

Contributing factors for goiter are:

- Iodine deficiency or excess (**Figures 235-2** and **235-3**).
- TSH stimulation.
- Drugs, including lithium, amiodarone, and α-interferon.
- Autoimmunity/heredity.

Hypothyroidism may be caused by disease of the thyroid gland itself (e.g., Hashimoto thyroiditis), radioiodine thyroid ablation, thyroidectomy, high-dose head and neck radiation therapy, and medications (as above), or, rarely, by pituitary or hypothalamic disorders (e.g., tumors, inflammatory conditions, infiltrative diseases, infections, pituitary surgery, pituitary radiation therapy, and head trauma).[2]

- Hashimoto thyroiditis is caused by thyroid peroxidase antibodies (TPOAbs).
- Human leukocyte antigen-D related (HLA-DR) and cytotoxic T-lymphocyte antigen 4 (CTLA-4) are the best-documented genetic risk factors for this disorder.[4]
- There is marked lymphocytic infiltration of the thyroid in Hashimoto thyroiditis; the infiltrate is composed of activated CD4+ and CD8+ T cells, as well as B cells.
- Thyroid destruction in Hashimoto thyroiditis is believed to be primarily mediated by CD8+ cytotoxic T cells.

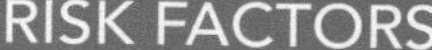

RISK FACTORS

Risk factors for hypothyroidism include[2]:

- Symptoms of thyroid hormone deficiency.
- Goiter.
- Personal or family history of thyroid disease.
- Personal treatment of thyroid disease.
- History of autoimmune disease, especially type 1 diabetes mellitus (but not type 2 diabetes).[5]
- High-dose head and neck radiation therapy.

Myxedema coma usually occurs in elderly patients with untreated or inadequately treated hypothyroidism who develop a precipitating event, such as myocardial infarction, stroke, sepsis, or prolonged cold exposure.[2]

DIAGNOSIS

CLINICAL FEATURES

The history can be the key to the diagnosis:

- A painful neck mass is usually a form of thyroiditis.
- Large goiters are easily visible before palpating the neck (**Figures 235-1** to **235-5**).
- Asymmetric goiters can shift the trachea away from the midline (**Figure 235-6**).

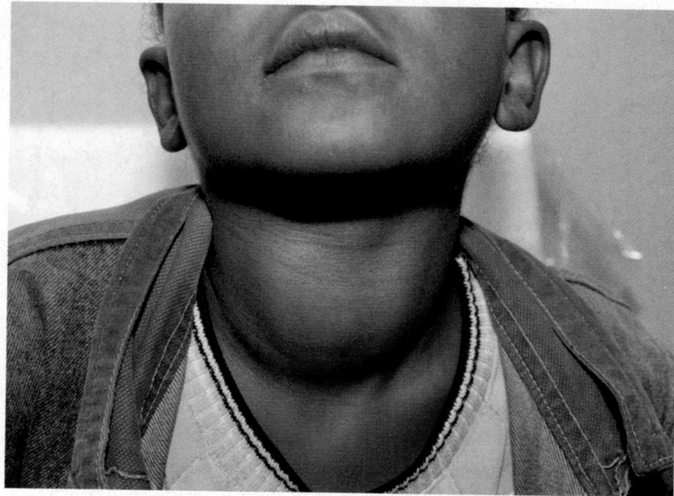

FIGURE 235-3 Goiter developing in a 12-year-old girl in an endemic area for goiters. (*Reproduced with permission from Richard P. Usatine, MD.*)

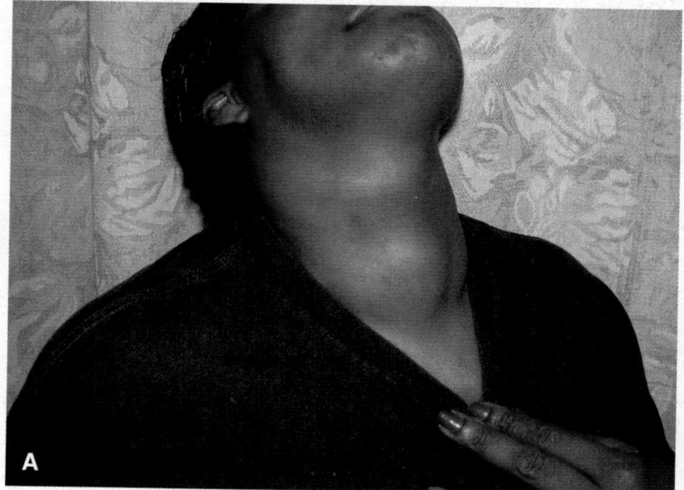

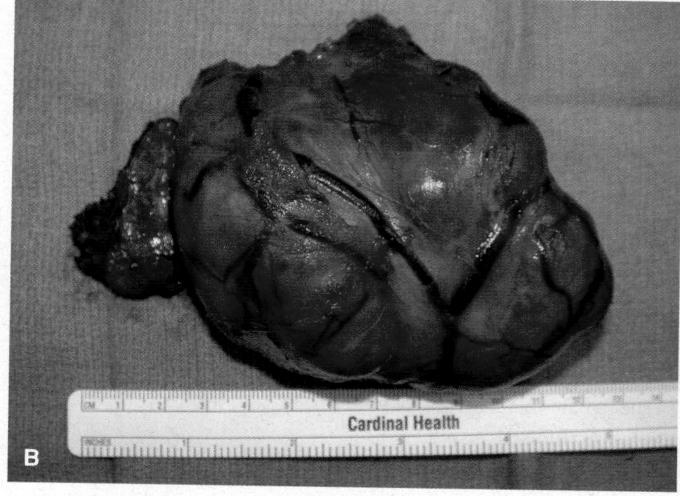

FIGURE 235-4 **A.** A 36-year-old woman with large goiter. **B.** The resected goitrous thyroid gland. (*Reproduced with permission from Frank Miller, MD.*)

Common signs and symptoms of hypothyroidism are:

- Fatigue and/or weakness.
- Dry and cool skin.
- Diffuse hair loss or thinning of the lateral eyebrows.
- Difficulty concentrating.
- Puffy face/hands/feet from myxedema (**Figure 235-7**).
- Bradycardia.
- Delayed deep tendon reflex relaxation.
- Weight gain despite poor appetite.
- Constipation.
- The most useful signs for diagnosing hypothyroidism are puffiness (likelihood ratio positive [LR+] 16.2) and delayed ankle reflex relaxation (LR+ 11.8).[6]

Clues to a central cause of hypothyroidism include a history of pituitary/hypothalamic surgery or radiation, headache, visual field defects, or ophthalmoplegia.[2]

Physical examination maneuvers that help detect goiter are[7]:

- Neck extension.
- Observation from the side.
- Palpation by locating the isthmus first.
- Having the patient swallow.
- Myxedema coma.

LABORATORY STUDIES

Laboratory tests include an erythrocyte sedimentation rate (ESR) if thyroiditis is suspected, and TSH (elevated in hypothyroidism and subclinical disease) and FT_4 levels (low in hypothyroidism).

- In acute granulomatous thyroiditis, ESR is greater than 50 (LR+ 95) and the TSH and FT_4 are usually normal.
- In primary hypothyroidism, the TSH is greater than 10 mU/L (LR+ 16) and FT_4 is less than 8 (LR+ 11).
  - An upper limit of normal TSH of 4.12 mU/L should be considered if an age-based upper limit of normal for a third-generation TSH assay is not available in an iodine-sufficient area.[8]
  - For pregnant women, recommended normal reference ranges are: first trimester, 2.5 mIU/L; second trimester, 3.0 mIU/L; third trimester, 3.5 mIU/L in absence of trimester-specific ranges for that laboratory.[8]
- The presence of antibodies to TPO and thyroglobulin helps establish the diagnosis of Hashimoto thyroiditis but is unnecessary for treatment. TPOAb will be positive in 90% to 95% of patients.[4]
  - Measuring TPOAb should be considered in the following patients: women with recurrent miscarriage, with or without infertility (SOR Ⓐ); those with subclinical hypothyroidism (SOR Ⓑ); and those with nodular thyroid disease suspected to be due to autoimmune thyroid disease.[8]
- In pituitary causes of hypothyroidism (central hypothyroidism), the TSH may be normal or elevated, but FT_4 will be low.[2]
- In the future, reference limits may need to change as TSH distribution and reference limits shift to higher concentrations with age and are unique for different racial/ethnic groups.[9]

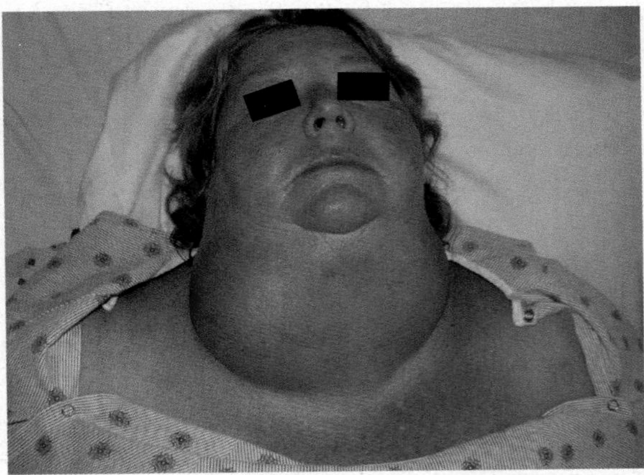

FIGURE 235-5 Massive multinodular goiter before surgery. (*Reproduced with permission from Frank Miller, MD.*)

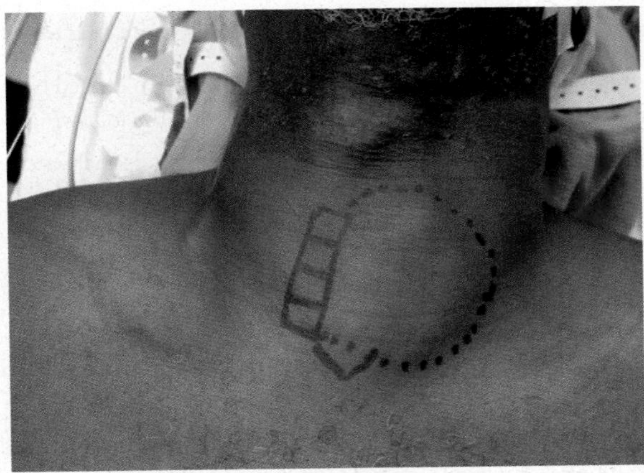

FIGURE 235-6 Asymmetric multinodular goiter causing trachea to deviate from the midline prior to resection. (*Reproduced with permission from Frank Miller, MD.*)

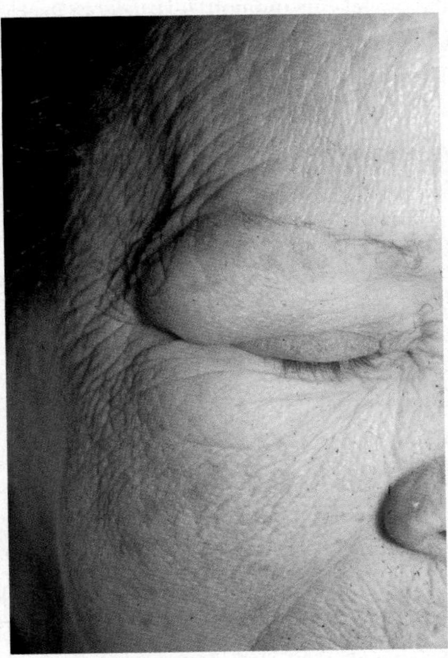

FIGURE 235-7 Myxedema of the face with puffiness around the eye. (*Reproduced with permission from Richard P. Usatine, MD.*)

DIFFERENTIAL DIAGNOSIS

Goiter presenting as a painful neck mass is most commonly caused by subacute granulomatous (de Quervain) thyroiditis (likely viral) or hemorrhage into a thyroid cyst or adenoma. Other causes include the following:

- Painful Hashimoto thyroiditis—Hypothyroidism with the presence of antibodies helps to confirm this diagnosis.
- Infected thyroglossal duct or branchial cleft cyst—Mass palpates as cystic and may be fluctuant; focal (e.g., erythema and warmth) and systemic symptoms of infection (e.g., fever) may be present. Even a noninfected thyroglossal duct cyst can be confused for an enlarged thyroid (**Figure 235-8**).
- Acute suppurative thyroiditis (microbial)—Focal (e.g., erythema and warmth) and systemic symptoms of infection (e.g., fever) are usually present.
- Thyroid carcinoma—Hard mass within thyroid gland (**Figure 235-9**).

Painless goiter and hypothyroidism are most often caused by Hashimoto thyroiditis, but may also be caused by the following:

- Environmental goitrogens (e.g., excess iodine, foods such as cassava, cabbage, and soybeans).
- Iodine deficiency.
- Pharmacologic inhibition (rare)—Drugs include lithium, amiodarone, and interferon-α.

Painless goiter and hyperthyroidism may be caused by the following:

- Graves disease (common, 0.5% to 2.5% of the population)—Symptoms of nervousness, fatigue, weight loss, heat intolerance, palpitations, and exophthalmos (see Chapter 236, Graves Disease and Goiter).
- Postpartum thyroiditis (2% to 16% within 3 to 6 months of delivery)—Recent delivery.
- Toxic nodular goiter (uncommon)—Usually in the elderly; thyroid gland feels nodular (see **Figure 235-4**) and thyroid scan shows multiple foci of increased uptake.

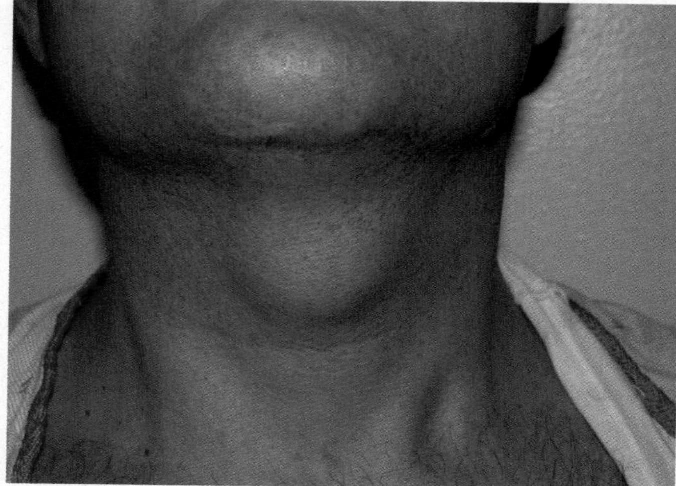

FIGURE 235-8 Thyroglossal duct cyst in the midline superior to the thyroid. (*Reproduced with permission from Frank Miller, MD.*)

MANAGEMENT

NONPHARMACOLOGIC

- For nonendemic goiter, identify and remove goitrogens.

MEDICATIONS

Patients with endemic goiter should be provided with iodine.

For nonendemic goiter, also consider the following:

- TSH suppression with levothyroxine (1 to 2.2 mg/kg per day) (variable but limited effect on goiter size and can cause hyperthyroidism, so monitoring of TSH is needed during therapy).[10] SOR Ⓑ
- Radioactive iodine treatment if enough functioning tissue is present. SOR Ⓒ

Treat patients with acute microbial thyroiditis with antibiotics against the most common pathogens (i.e., *Staphylococcus aureus,*

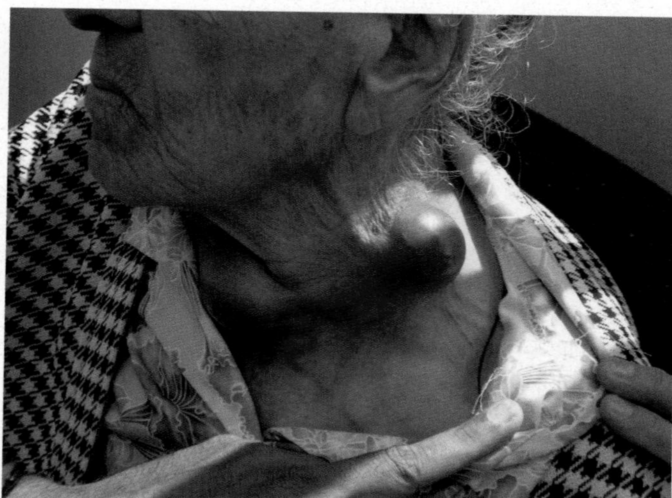

FIGURE 235-9 A 93-year-old woman with thyroid cancer that went untreated for 3 years. Two large, firm masses are visible in the neck. (*Reproduced with permission from Dustin Williams, MD.*)

Streptococcus pyogenes, and *Streptococcus pneumoniae*). Therapeutic agents, used for 7 to 10 days, include: SOR C

- Amoxicillin/clavulanate (500 mg/125 mg 3 times daily),
- A first- or second-generation cephalosporin (e.g., cephalexin 500 mg 4 times daily), and
- Penicillinase-resistant penicillin (e.g., dicloxacillin 500 mg 4 times daily).

In patients with subacute thyroiditis:

- Oral corticosteroids can reduce pain and swelling. SOR C
- Symptoms of hyperthyroidism can be treated with β-blockers or calcium channel blockers (see Chapter 236, Graves Disease and Goiter). SOR B
- Symptoms of hypothyroidism can be treated with levothyroxine.[10] SOR B

Nonpregnant patients should be considered for treatment with levothyroxine if they have a TSH level >10 mU/L OR TSH between the upper limit of the normal laboratory reference range and 10 mU/L AND symptoms suggestive of hypothyroidism, positive TPOAb, or evidence of atherosclerotic cardiovascular disease, heart failure, or associated risk factors for these diseases.[8] SOR B

- For those with subclinical hypothyroidism, treatment should be considered if they are pregnant or considering pregnancy AND have TPOAb, especially if they have a history of overt hypothyroidism or recurrent miscarriage.[8]

Patients are treated with levothyroxine as follows:

- Start with 50 to 100 mcg/day increasing by 25 to 50 mcg/day at 6- to 8-week intervals until the TSH is normal (approximately 1.6 mcg/kg per day of levothyroxine).[2] SOR B
  - Young, healthy adults with overt hypothyroidism can be started on the full replacement dose.[8]
  - Older patients who have overt hypothyroidism and no cardiac disease can begin with 50 mcg/day.[8] Otherwise, begin with 25 mcg/day and increase by 12.5 to 25 mcg/day every 6 to 8 weeks to normalize the TSH (approximately 1 mcg/kg per day of levothyroxine). SOR C
- Dosing in the evening appears to normalize the laboratory values more effectively, but may not influence symptoms or quality of life.[2,11]

Authors of a Cochrane review of 12 small randomized controlled trials (RCTs) determined that treatment of subclinical hypothyroidism did not improve survival or decrease cardiovascular morbidity.[12] In a more recent evidence review, treatment of subclinical hypothyroidism was associated with decreased risk for coronary heart disease events but not improved quality of life, cognitive function, blood pressure, or body mass index compared to no treatment.[13]

- Levothyroxine treatment of pregnant euthyroid women with TPOAb appears to reduce rates of preterm delivery.[14] Treatment does not influence cognitive development in children born to women with subclinical hypothyroidism versus euthyroid women.[15]
- A daily dose of 25 to 75 mcg/day is usually sufficient for those with subclinical hypothyroidism.[8] SOR C

REFERRAL

- Large goiters that impinge on the trachea or do not respond to medications may be treated with surgery (see **Figure 235-4**).
- Subtotal thyroidectomy can be considered for nodular goiters, but recurrence rates can be high.[16] SOR A About 1 in 5 patients undergoing hemithyroidectomy become hypothyroid.[17]
- Consultation with an endocrinologist may be helpful if the diagnosis is uncertain and for patients with central hypothyroidism, severe hypothyroidism (i.e., myxedema coma), or coexisting cardiovascular disease.[2]
- The American Association of Clinical Endocrinologists (AACE)/American Thyroid Association (ATA) guidelines recommend consultation or shared care with an endocrinologist for patients who are: children and infants; difficult to render and maintain in a euthyroid state; pregnant or planning conception; have cardiac disease; have a goiter, nodule, or other structural change in the thyroid gland; have other endocrine disease such as adrenal and pituitary disorders; have an unusual constellation of thyroid function test results; or have unusual causes of hypothyroidism (e.g., medications that interfere with absorption of L-thyroxine).[8]
- Patients with myxedema coma should be hospitalized in an intensive care unit; without treatment, mortality approaches 100%.

PREVENTION AND SCREENING

- There is insufficient evidence to support screening for hypothyroidism in pregnant and nonpregnant patients[18]; however, pregnant women with overt hyper- and hypothyroidism are more likely to have preterm delivery (odds ratio [OR] 1.19; 95% confidence index [CI], 1.12–1.26),[19] and subclinical hypothyroidism is associated with miscarriage (OR 1.45 and 2.47 if accompanied by thyroid autoimmunity).[20] The AACE/ATA suggest "aggressive case finding" rather than universal screening for women who are planning pregnancy, and consideration of screening for patients over age 60 years.[8]
- One expert panel recommended TSH testing in women with symptoms of thyroid dysfunction, personal or family history of thyroid disease, an abnormal thyroid gland on palpation, or type 1 diabetes mellitus or other autoimmune disorders.[21] In support of this approach, a clinical trial of universal screening versus case finding did not demonstrate a difference in adverse outcomes; however, treatment of women with thyroid dysfunction identified by screening a low-risk group was associated with a lower rate of adverse outcomes.[22]

PROGNOSIS

- In the most extensive community survey on goiter (Whickham, England), goiter was present in 15.5% of the population.[1] At the 20-year follow-up, 20% of women and 5% of men no longer had goiter and 4% of women and no men had acquired a goiter.
- Suppression of TSH with levothyroxine effectively reduces the goiter of Hashimoto thyroiditis and should be continued indefinitely. In one study, withdrawal of medication after 1 year resulted in only 11.4% remaining euthyroid.[23]

- Large goiter, TSH greater than 10 mU/L, and a family history of thyroid disease are associated with failure to recover normal thyroid function and treatment should continue indefinitely.
- In patients with subclinical hypothyroidism, progression to clinically overt hypothyroidism is 2.6% each year if TPOAbs are absent, and 4.3% each year if they are present.[24]
- Patients with hypothyroidism have an increased risk of heart failure, and those with both hypothyroidism and heart failure have an increased risk of mortality.[25]

FOLLOW-UP

- TSH should be rechecked approximately 4 to 8 weeks after initiation of levothyroxine therapy and again in 6 months if normal, and annually thereafter unless otherwise clinically indicated.[8] SOR Ⓑ
- Although the need for thyroid replacement is lifelong, dose requirements may change over time. Thyroxine dose may need to be increased during pregnancy (20%–40%), with use of estrogens, or in situations of weight gain, malabsorption, *Helicobacter pylori*–related gastritis and atrophic gastritis, and with use of some medications. Requirements may decrease with increased age, androgen use, reactivation of Graves disease, or the development of autonomous thyroid nodules.[2]
- There is some evidence that use of ultrasound can help predict progression to overt hypothyroidism in patients with subclinical hypothyroidism[26]; in one study, patients with TPOAb and/or ultrasound abnormalities had a greater progression to overt disease than those without either finding (31.2% vs. 9.5% at 3 years).[27]
- The frequency of other autoimmune disease is increased in patients with Hashimoto thyroiditis (14.3% in one study), including rheumatoid arthritis, pernicious anemia, systemic lupus erythematosus, Addison disease, celiac disease, and vitiligo, and increased monitoring should be considered.[28]

PATIENT EDUCATION

- Most goiters are not associated with thyroid hormone changes but are a risk factor for hypothyroidism.
- Goiters may be treated with thyroid hormone, radioactive iodine, or surgery.
- Risk factors for hypothyroidism include a personal or family history of thyroid disease, neck irradiation, or a history of autoimmune disease.
- Symptoms of hypothyroidism include puffy face/hands/feet, fatigue, and diffuse hair loss.
- Patients with hypothyroidism are treated with thyroid hormone replacement.
- Treatment is considered for those with subclinical hypothyroidism if there are suggestive symptoms, a positive TPO antibody or heart disease, or if they are pregnant or considering pregnancy and have a positive TPO antibody.

PATIENT RESOURCES

- Booklet from the American Thyroid Association—**https://www.thyroid.org/hypothyroidism/.**
- Web-based resources—**http://www.nlm.nih.gov/medlineplus/thyroiddiseases.html.**

PROVIDER RESOURCES

- Clinical practice guidelines for hypothyroidism in adults: cosponsored by the American Association of Clinical Endocrinologists and the American Thyroid Association—**https://www.liebertpub.com/doi/full/10.1089/thy.2012.0205.**

REFERENCES

1. Wang C, Crapo LM. The epidemiology of thyroid disease and implications for screening. *Endocrinol Metab Clin North Am.* 1997;26(1):189-218.
2. McDermott MT. In the clinic. Hypothyroidism. *Ann Intern Med.* 2009;151(11):ITC61.
3. Fatourechi V. Subclinical hypothyroidism: an update for primary care physicians. *Mayo Clin Proc.* 2009;84(1):65-71.
4. Jameson JL, Weetman AP. Disorders of the thyroid gland. In: Kasper DL, Braunwald E, Fauci AS, et al, eds. *Harrison's Principles of Internal Medicine*, 16th ed. New York, NY: McGraw-Hill; 2005: 2109-2113.
5. Fleiner HF, Bjøro T, Midthjell K, et al. Prevalence of thyroid dysfunction in autoimmune and type 2 diabetes: the population-based HUNT study in Norway. *J Clin Endocrinol Metab.* 2016; 101(2):669-677.
6. Zulewski H, Müller B, Exer P, et al. Estimation of tissue hypothyroidism by a new clinical score: evaluation of patients with various grades of hypothyroidism and controls. *J Clin Endocrinol Metab.* 1997;82:771-776.
7. Siminoski K. Does this patient have a goiter? *JAMA.* 1995;273(10): 813-819.
8. National Guideline Clearinghouse (NGC). Guideline summary: Clinical practice guidelines for hypothyroidism in adults: cosponsored by the American Association of Clinical Endocrinologists and the American Thyroid Association. In: National Guideline Clearinghouse (NGC) [website]. Rockville (MD): Agency for Healthcare Research and Quality (AHRQ); 2012 Nov 01. [cited 2017 May 22]. Available: https://www.liebertpub.com/doi/full/10.1089/thy.2012.0205.
9. Surks MI, Boucai L. Age- and race-based serum thyrotropin reference limits. *J Clin Endocrinol Metab.* 2010;95(2):496-502.
10. Zelmanovitz F, Genro S, Gross JL. Suppressive therapy with levothyroxine for solitary thyroid nodules: a double-blind controlled clinical study and cumulative meta-analyses. *J Clin Endocrinol Metab.* 1998;3:3881-3885.
11. Bolk N, Visser TJ, Nijman J, et al. Effects of evening vs morning levothyroxine intake: a randomized double-blind crossover trial. *Ann Intern Med.* 2010;170(22):1996-2003.

12. Villar HCCE, Saconato H, Valente O, Atallah ÁN. Thyroid hormone replacement for subclinical hypothyroidism. *Cochrane Database Syst Rev*. 2007;(3):CD003419.
13. Rugge JB, Bougatsos C, Chou R. Screening and treatment of thyroid dysfunction: an evidence review for the U.S. Preventive Services Task Force. *Ann Intern Med*. 2015;162(1):35-45.
14. Reid SM, Middleton P, Cossich MC, et al. Interventions for clinical and subclinical hypothyroidism pre-pregnancy and during pregnancy. *Cochrane Database Syst Rev*. 2013;(5):CD007752.
15. Casey BM, Thom EA, Peaceman AM, et al. Treatment of subclinical hypothyroidism or hypothyroxinemia in pregnancy. *N Engl J Med*. 2017;376(9):815-825.
16. Rojdmark J, Jarhult J. High long term recurrence rate after subtotal thyroidectomy for nodular goitre. *Eur J Surg*. 1995;161:725-727.
17. Verloop H, Louwerens M, Schoones JW, et al. Risk of hypothyroidism following hemithyroidectomy: systematic review and meta-analysis of prognostic studies. *J Clin Endocrinol Metab*. 2012;97(7):2243-2255.
18. U.S. Preventive Services Task Force. *Screening for Thyroid Disease*. https://www.uspreventiveservicestaskforce.org/Page/Document/UpdateSummaryFinal/thyroid-disease-screening. Accessed May 2017.
19. Sheehan PM, Nankervis A, Araujo Júnior E, Da Silva Costa F. Maternal thyroid disease and preterm birth: systematic review and meta-analysis. *J Clin Endocrinol Metab*. 2015;100(11):4325-4331.
20. Zhang Y, Wang H, Pan X, et al. Patients with subclinical hypothyroidism before 20 weeks of pregnancy have a higher risk of miscarriage: a systematic review and meta-analysis. *PLoS One*. 2017;12(4):e0175708.
21. Surks MI, Ortiz E, Daniels GH, et al. Subclinical thyroid disease: scientific review and guidelines for diagnosis and management. *JAMA*. 2004;291:228-238.
22. Negro R, Schwartz A, Gismondi R, et al. Universal screening versus case finding for detection and treatment of thyroid hormonal dysfunction during pregnancy. *J Clin Endocrinol Metab*. 2010;95(4):1699-1707.
23. Comtois R, Faucher L, Lafleche L. Outcome of hypothyroidism cause by Hashimoto's thyroiditis. *Arch Intern Med*. 1995;155(13):1404-1408.
24. Vanderpump MP, Tunbridge WM, French JM, et al. The incidence of thyroid disorders in the community: a twenty-year follow-up of the Whickham Survey. *Clin Endocrinol (Oxf)*. 1995;43(1):55-68.
25. Ning N, Gao D, Triggiani V, et al. Prognostic role of hypothyroidism in heart failure: a meta-analysis. *Medicine (Baltimore)*. 2015;94(30):e1159.
26. Shin DY, Kim EK, Lee EJ. Role of ultrasonography in outcome prediction in subclinical hypothyroid patients treated with levothyroxine. *Endocr J*. 2010;57(1):15-22.
27. Rosário PW, Bessa B, Valadão MM, Purisch S. Natural history of mild subclinical hypothyroidism: prognostic value of ultrasound. *Thyroid*. 2009;19(1):9-12.
28. Boelaert K, Newby PR, Simmonds MJ, et al. Prevalence and relative risk of other autoimmune diseases in subjects with autoimmune thyroid disease. *Am J Med*. 2010;123(2):183.e1-e9.

236 GRAVES DISEASE AND GOITER

Mindy A. Smith, MD, MS

PATIENT STORY

A 32-year-old woman presents with fatigue and "eye strain" (**Figure 236-1**). She had been working as a secretary and noticed difficulty focusing her eyes. She said she was anxious and was having difficulty writing. She reported that her sister was taking medication for "thyroid trouble." A low thyroid-stimulating hormone (TSH) and an elevated free thyroxine (T_4) level were found on laboratory testing, and the patient was diagnosed with Graves disease (GD). Her thyroid scan showed an enlarged thyroid with increased uptake (**Figure 236-2**). The patient chose radioactive iodine (RAI) as her treatment and her symptoms resolved. One year later she required levothyroxine treatment.

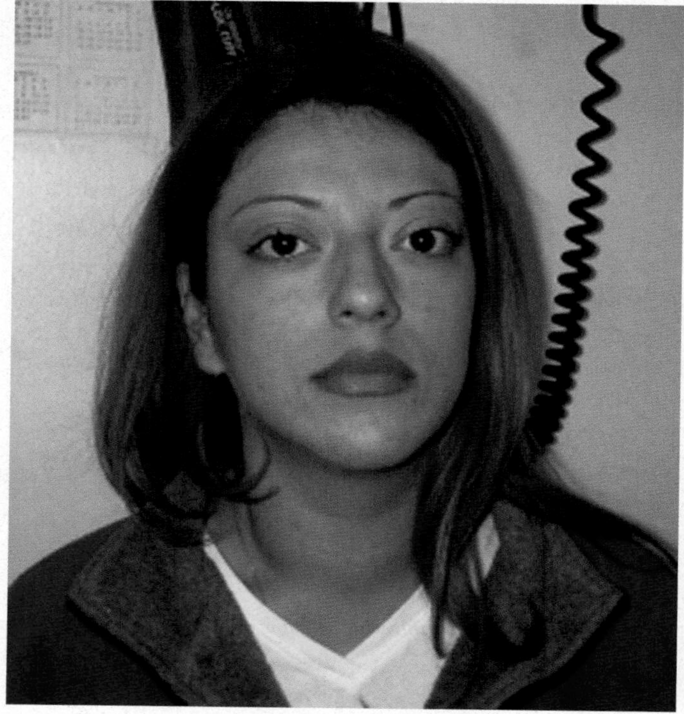

FIGURE 236-1 This patient displays the following common findings of Graves disease: lid retraction and mild proptosis (exophthalmos), particularly evident on the left eye, and goiter. (*Reproduced with permission from Dan Stulberg, MD.*)

INTRODUCTION

GD is an autoimmune thyroid disorder characterized by circulating antibodies that stimulate the TSH receptor, resulting in hyperthyroidism.[1] GD is caused by a combination of environmental and genetic factors. Risk factors include stress, smoking, and sudden increases in iodine uptake.[1] Goiter is an enlargement of the thyroid gland.

SYNONYMS

Thyrotoxicosis (clinical state resulting from inappropriately high thyroid hormone levels), hyperthyroidism (thyrotoxicosis caused by elevated synthesis and secretion of thyroid hormone).

EPIDEMIOLOGY

- GD is a common disorder affecting about 2% to 3% of women and 0.5% of men in their lifetime.[1,2] Peak onset is between ages 20 and 50 years.[1]
- The annual incidence of GD is 20 to 50 cases per 100,000 persons.[3]
- Among patients with hyperthyroidism (1.2% of the U.S. population), 60% to 80% have GD; younger patients (younger than age 64 years) with hyperthyroidism are more likely to have GD than are older patients with hyperthyroidism.[1]
- Graves ophthalmopathy (GO; see "Clinical Features" below) occurs in about 75% of patients within 1 year before or after diagnosis of GD.[1]
- Goiter is typically present; the thyroid gland is diffusely enlarged to two to three times its normal size with a firm consistency.[1]
- Untreated hyperthyroidism can lead to osteoporosis, atrial fibrillation, cardiomyopathy, and congestive heart failure; mortality rate prior to satisfactory treatment was 10% to 30%.[1]

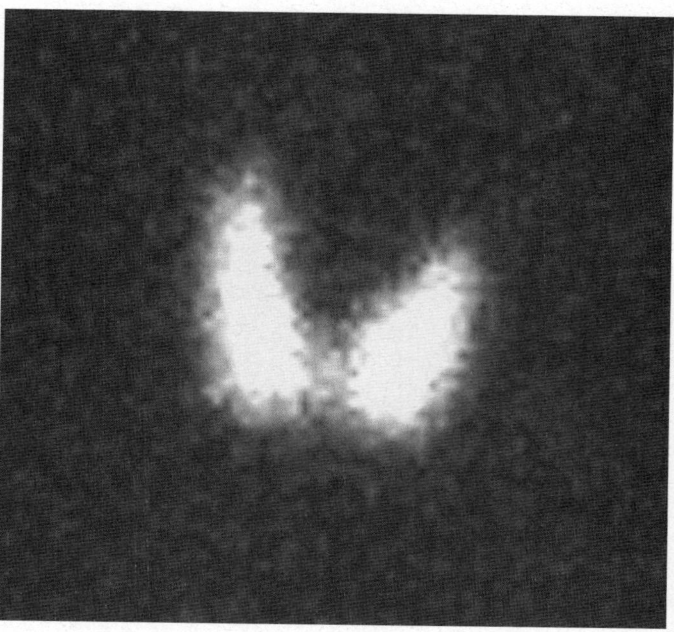

FIGURE 236-2 Nuclear scan of the thyroid in Graves disease showing increased uptake (61%). (*Reproduced with permission from Michael Freckleton, MD.*)

ETIOLOGY AND PATHOPHYSIOLOGY

- The hyperthyroidism of GD results from circulating immunoglobulin (Ig) G antibodies directed against the thyrotropin receptor that mimic the action of thyrotropin and stimulate thyroid hormone production.[3] These antibodies are synthesized in the thyroid gland, bone marrow, and lymph nodes. In addition to thyrotropin-receptor antibodies, antibodies directed at thyroglobulin and thyroperoxidase are frequently found in patients with GD; these antibodies have no known pathologic role.[3]
- Activation of the TSH receptor stimulates follicular hypertrophy and hyperplasia causing thyroid enlargement (goiter) and an increase in thyroid hormone production.
- Both T and B cells are involved in the pathogenesis of GD, resulting in production of thyroid-stimulating antibodies and cytokines (e.g., interleukins, CD40, tumor necrosis factor alpha), the latter creating thyroid cell inflammation and altered behavior.[3] In addition, insulin-like growth factor-1 receptor (IGF-1R)-bearing fibroblasts and B-cells exhibiting the IGF-1R(+) phenotype are involved in the connective tissue manifestations.[3] Siblings have higher incidence of both GD and Hashimoto thyroiditis (see Chapter 235, Goitrous Hypothyroidism). The concordance for GD in monozygotic twins is 20% to 30% but <5% in dizygotic twins.[1]
- The ophthalmopathy is believed to result from an autoimmune response directed toward an antigen shared by the thyroid and the eye's orbit. There is infiltration of orbital tissues with lymphocytes. Similar to the pathogenesis of GD hyperthyroidism, interactions between T cells and fibroblasts, mediated by cytokines, result in tissue activation, inflammation, and remodeling.[3] Activated fibroblasts increase the synthesis of glycosaminoglycans that trap water, causing orbital muscle swelling; later in the disease, irreversible muscle fibrosis occurs and leads to diplopia.[1]

RISK FACTORS

- Family history of thyroid disease, especially in maternal relatives.
- Smoking (a strong risk factor for GO).
- Physical or emotional stress.[2]
- GD may occur during the postpartum period, after sudden increases in iodine intake, or during immune reconstitution after highly active antiretroviral therapy (HAART) or alemtuzumab treatment.[1]

DIAGNOSIS

CLINICAL FEATURES

Symptoms depend on the severity of thyrotoxicosis, duration of disease, and age (findings are more subtle in the elderly). More than half of patients diagnosed with GD have these common symptoms:

- Nervousness.
- Fatigue.
- Weight loss.
- Heat intolerance.
- Palpitations.

Signs of disease include:

- Tachycardia (atrial fibrillation is more common in patients >50 years of age).[1]
- Goiter—Listening over the goiter with a stethoscope may reveal a thyroid bruit (**Figure 236-3**).
- Resting tremor.
- Hyperreflexia.
- Flushing and temporal wasting (**Figure 236-4**).
- Fine hair texture, with diffuse alopecia in 40%.[1]
- Skin and nail changes include:
  - Warm, erythematous, moist skin (from increased peripheral circulation).
  - Palmar erythema.
  - Pretibial myxedema—Occurring in a small percentage of patients (0.5% to 4%), it consists of nonpitting scaly thickening and induration of the skin, usually on the anterior shin and dorsa of the feet (**Figures 236-5** and **236-6**).[4] It can also appear as a few well-demarcated pink, flesh-colored, or purple-brown papules or nodules.
  - Nails are soft and shiny and may develop onycholysis (distal separation of the nail plate from the underlying nail bed).
- Eye involvement begins with mild discomfort (a gritty sensation with increased tearing is the earliest manifestation). Ophthalmopathy typically worsens over 3–6 months then plateaus over the next 12–18 months, with spontaneous improvement in the soft tissue changes.[1] The eye findings in GD[1] are:
  - Lid retraction (drawing back of the eyelid allowing more sclera to be visible) (**Figures 236-1** and **236-7**).
  - Frank proptosis (displacement of the eye in the anterior direction); occurs in one-third (**Figures 236-1** and **236-7**).
  - Unilateral eye involvement in up to 10% with GO (**Figure 236-8**).
  - Extraocular muscle dysfunction (e.g., diplopia).
  - Corneal exposure keratitis or ulcer.
  - Periorbital edema, chemosis, and scleral injection (5% to 10%).
  - Most severe manifestation is optic nerve compression leading to papilledema and possibly permanent visual loss.

LABORATORY TESTING AND IMAGING

- With typical symptoms, you can confirm the diagnosis of GD with a low or undetectable sensitive assay for TSH and an elevated free T_4 level. In 2% to 5% of cases, only triiodothyronine (T_3) is elevated (measured as total T_3).[1]
- The presence of thyroid receptor antibodies (TRAbs, present in 70% to 100% of patients at diagnosis) has a positive and negative likelihood ratio of 247 and 0.01, respectively.[5] These antibodies are not usually required for diagnosis.
- If the clinical picture is uncertain or there is thyroid nodularity, obtain an RAI scan and uptake.[6] Elevated uptake (>30%) and a homogeneous pattern on scan are diagnostic (see **Figure 236-2**).

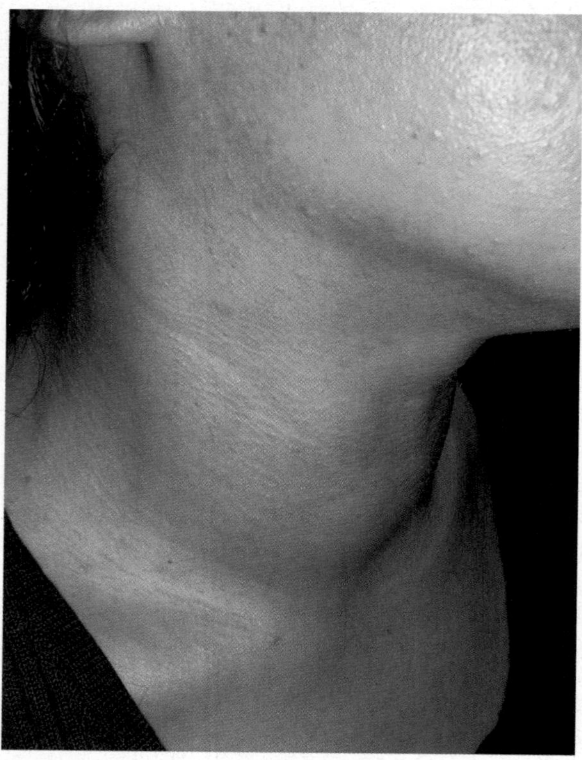

FIGURE 236-3 This 37-year-old woman has Graves disease and a loud bruit over her enlarged hyperactive thyroid gland. She was thyrotoxic at this time. (*Reproduced with permission from Richard P. Usatine, MD.*)

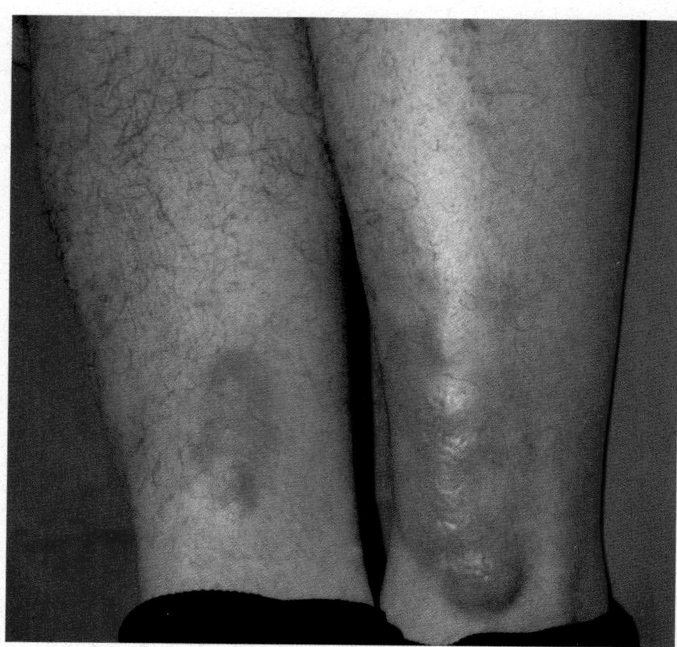

FIGURE 236-5 Early bilateral pretibial myxedema in a patient with Graves eye disease. These asymmetrical erythematous plaques and nodules are firm and nonpitting. (*Reproduced with permission from Richard P. Usatine, MD.*)

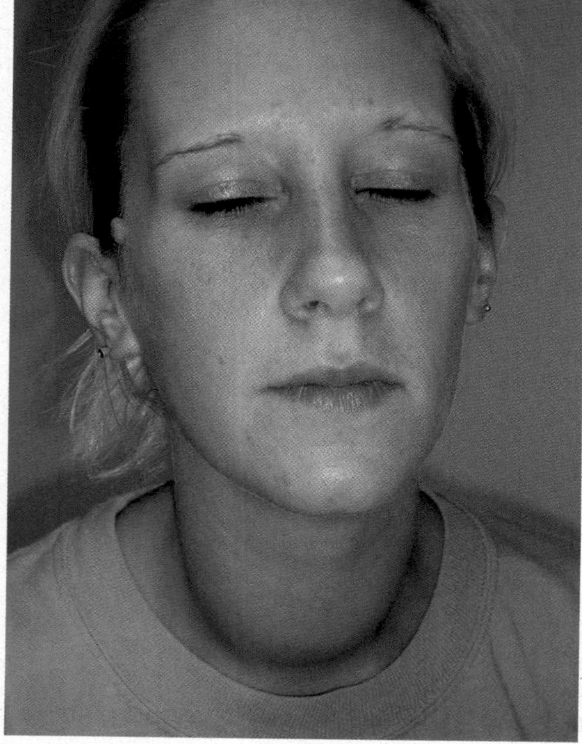

FIGURE 236-4 Enlarged thyroid, visible flushed skin and temporal wasting in this thyrotoxic woman with new-onset Graves disease. (*Reproduced with permission from Richard P. Usatine, MD.*)

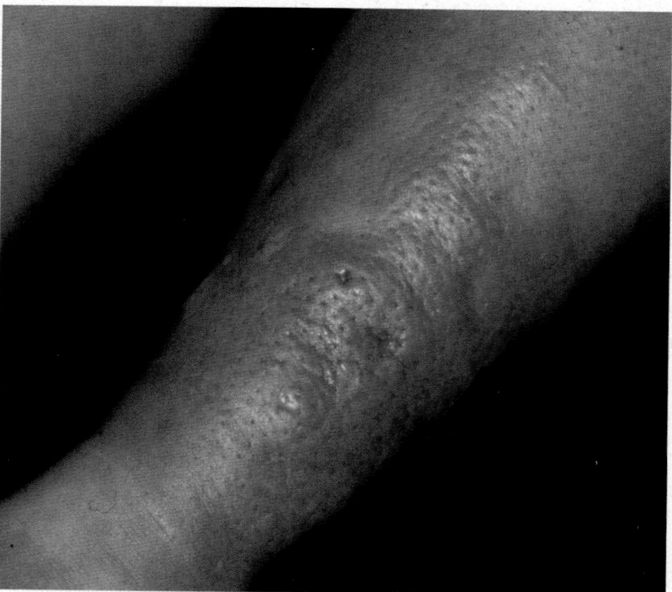

FIGURE 236-6 Pretibial myxedema in a patient with Graves ophthalmopathy. Hair follicles are prominent, giving a peau d'orange appearance. (*Reproduced with permission from Richard P. Usatine, MD.*)

DIFFERENTIAL DIAGNOSIS

Other causes of hyperthyroidism:

- Autonomous functioning nodule—This is an uncommon cause of thyrotoxicosis (present in 1.6% to 9% of patients with hyperthyroidism),[7] and most nodules do not cause hyperthyroidism. These present as a discrete swelling in an otherwise normal thyroid gland, and thyroid scan would show a discrete nodule.
- Toxic multinodular goiter—More common cause of hyperthyroidism in the elderly; thyroid scan shows multiple foci of increased uptake.
- Thyrotropin-secreting pituitary adenoma (rare)—Adenomas may cause visual disturbance (in the absence of exophthalmos), and other hormonal stimulation may occur (e.g., elevated serum prolactin). These can be confirmed on computed tomography or magnetic resonance scan.
- Thyroiditis—May be painless or painful, short duration, low update on RAI scan.
- Exogenous thyroid hormone ingestion—History of overdosage of prescribed or acquired thyroid medication.

The differential diagnoses for the eye findings include the following:

- Metastatic disease to the extraocular muscles.
- Pseudotumor—This condition's rapid onset and pain differentiate it from GO.

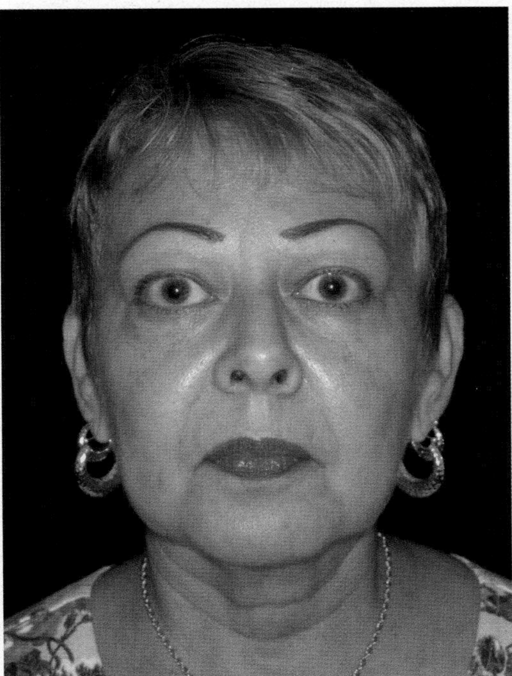

FIGURE 236-7 Bilateral exophthalmos that has been present for 5 years since patient was diagnosed with Graves disease. Although the radioactive iodine returned her thyroid function to normal, the exophthalmos continues to bother the patient. *(Reproduced with permission from Richard P. Usatine, MD.)*

MANAGEMENT

- Three options are available to treat the hyperthyroidism: antithyroid drugs, RAI therapy, and surgery, as discussed below.[1,2,6] SOR Ⓐ These three options are considered equivalent for patients with Graves hyperthyroidism and no or mild active ophthalmopathy and no risk factors for eye disease.[6] Specific guidance is offered for GD in pregnant women and children in the American Thyroid Association (ATA) guidelines.[6]

FIRST LINE

NONPHARMACOLOGIC

- Supportive measures for eye symptoms include dark glasses, artificial tears, propping up the head, and taping the eyelids closed at night.

MEDICATIONS

- Symptoms of hyperthyroidism can be controlled with β-adrenergic blockers (e.g., propranolol, 10 to 40 mg 3–4 times daily) or calcium channel blockers (e.g., diltiazem, 30 to 90 mg twice daily) if unable to tolerate or not candidates for beta-blockers. SOR Ⓑ Authors of the recent ATA guidelines recommend β-adrenergic blockage in elderly patients with symptomatic disease, those who are thyrotoxic with cardiovascular disease or a resting heart rate greater than 90 beats/min, and prior to RAI treatment in patients with GD at risk for complications of extreme hyperthyroidism (e.g., elderly, comorbidities).[6]

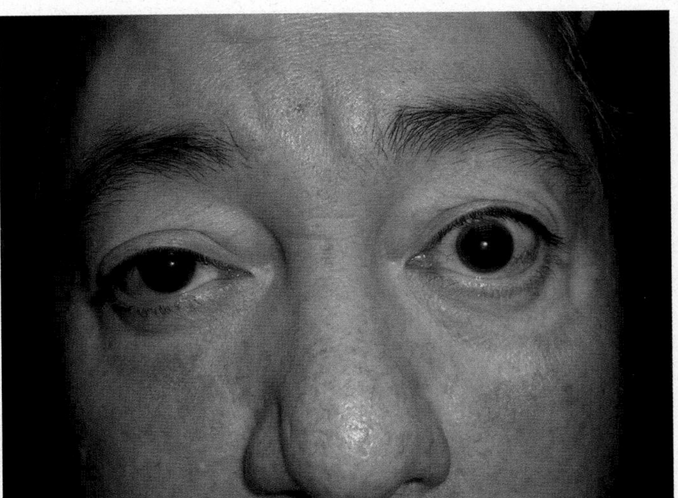

FIGURE 236-8 Woman with unilateral Graves ophthalmopathy and vitiligo. There is a strong association between autoimmune thyroid diseases and vitiligo. *(Reproduced with permission from Richard P. Usatine, MD.)*

- Antithyroid drugs (ATDs): methimazole (MMI) is used for virtually all patients. The initial once-daily dose is based on elevation of free T_4: 5–10 mg if free T_4 is 1–1.5 times the upper limit of normal, 10–20 mg for free T_4 1.5–2 times the upper limit of normal, and 30–40 mg for free T_4 2–3 times the upper limit of normal.[6] Propylthiouracil (PTU) is recommended during the first trimester of pregnancy, for those being treated for thyroid storm, and for those who have reactions to MMI (initial dose 100 to 150 mg 3 times daily depending on severity).[6] MMI is associated with higher rates of congenital anomalies when used in the first trimester; in one study the rate of major anomalies was 4% compared to control groups or PTU (2% and 1.9%, respectively).[8]
  - Baseline complete blood cell count and liver profile is suggested by ATA prior to ATDs.[6]
  - Potential side effects of these medications occur in about 13% to 28% and include rash, joint pain, hepatotoxicity (cholestatic for MMI and hepatocellular injury for PTU), and, rarely, agranulocytosis or vasculitis.[2,6] Liver enzymes should be assessed in patients taking ATDs who experience pruritic rash, jaundice, light-colored stool or dark urine, joint pain, abdominal pain or bloating, anorexia, nausea, or fatigue. Patients should be counseled to watch for and report these symptoms. A white blood cell count and differential is recommended during febrile illness or at onset of pharyngitis for those taking ATDs.[6]
  - ATDs are favored by the ATA during pregnancy, in patients with high likelihood of remission (mild disease, small goiter, and lower antibody levels), elderly patients or those with comorbidities, patients with previously operated or irradiated necks, patients with lack of access to high-volume thyroid surgeons, patients with moderate to severe active Graves ophthalmopathy, and patients who need more rapid biochemical disease control.[6] Patients who value avoidance of lifelong thyroid hormone treatment, surgery, or exposure to radioactivity may elect to use ATDs.
  - Prior adverse drug reaction is a contraindication to ATDs.[6]
  - Pretreatment with MMI prior to RAI is suggested for patients with GD who are at high risk for complications of extreme hyperthyroidism.[6]

The optimal duration of titrated antithyroid drug therapy is 12 to 18 months to minimize relapse.[6] SOR Ⓐ Medications can be discontinued if the TSH and TRAb are normal.

- Patients with severe (and possibly moderate) GO are usually treated with a 12-week course of high-dose intravenous (IV) glucocorticoid pulses (total <8 g of methylprednisolone); approximately 80% of patients respond to this regimen.[9]
  - In one randomized controlled trial (RCT) of three cumulative doses of IV methylprednisolone tested in 159 patients with moderate to severe GO, initial improvement was more common in the high-dose (7.49 g) group (52% vs. 35% and 28% for intermediate and low-dose), but relapse at 12 weeks among responders was similar (33%, 21%, and 40%, respectively).[10]
  - Response rate was higher using a weekly IV glucocorticoid protocol than daily medication in another RCT (77% vs. 41% by week 12).[11]
  - Potential side effects of high-dose steroids include sleep and mood disturbance, gastric upset, and elevated blood sugar. Liver failure and cardiovascular and cerebrovascular complications are serious but rare side effects that can be fatal.[12]

RADIOTHERAPY

- RAI—It is the most commonly prescribed treatment in the United States, but is contraindicated in pregnancy or with breastfeeding and should be used with caution in patients with cardiovascular disease. ATA recommends obtaining a pregnancy test within 48 hours of administering RAI to women of childbearing age. They also recommend optimizing medical therapy for patients with comorbid conditions prior to RAI initiation.[6]
  - RAI may also be used after initial treatment with antithyroid drugs; these drugs should be discontinued for 3 to 7 days before treatment.[6]
  - RAI is given in a single dose (typically 10–15 mCi) sufficient to render a patient hypothyroid.[6]
  - The half-life of iodine-131 is about 1 week; however, it is recommended that women not attempt pregnancy for 6 to 12 months after RAI treatment. Agents with shorter half-lives are available.
  - RAI may cause painful thyroid inflammation for a few weeks in approximately 1% of patients; this condition can be treated with nonsteroidal antiinflammatory agents, β-blockers, and possibly steroids.[6]
  - ATA favors use of RAI in women planning pregnancy after 6 months, individuals with comorbidities increasing surgical risk, patients with previously operated or externally irradiated necks, those who lack access to a high-volume thyroid surgeon, patients with contraindications to ATD use or failure to achieve euthyroidism during ATD treatment, or patients with right heart failure, pulmonary hypertension, or congestive heart failure.[6] Patients who value definitive control of hyperthyroidism or avoidance of surgery or potential ATD side effects may elect to use RAI.
  - Contraindications to RAI include pregnancy, lactation, coexisting or suspected thyroid cancer, and inability of the individual to comply with radiation safety guidelines. RAI is used with informed caution in women planning a pregnancy within 4–6 months.[6]
- Radiation-induced thyroiditis can aggravate ophthalmopathy. This side effect can be minimized by early levothyroxine replacement and prednisone prophylaxis (0.4–0.5 mg/kg per day or at least 30 mg, started 1–3 days after RAI administration, continued for 1 month, and then tapered over 2 months).[6] ATA recommends oral prednisone following RAI for patients with mild ophthalmopathy, especially if risk factors are present.[6]

SURGICAL TREATMENT

- Near-total to total thyroidectomy by a high-volume thyroid surgeon is recommended for patients with GD.[6]
  - Indications for surgery are very large goiters or large nodules, presence of suspicious nodules or suspected thyroid malignancy, pregnant women requiring high doses of antithyroid drugs or planning pregnancy within 6 months, relatively low uptake of RAI, coexisting hyperparathyroidism requiring surgery, and failure of other therapies.[6] Patients who value prompt and definitive control of hyperthyroidism and avoidance of exposure to radioactivity or potential ATD side effects may elect surgery. Contraindications to surgery include substantial comorbidity (e.g., cardiopulmonary disease, end-stage cancer) or lack of access to a high-volume thyroid surgeon. Pregnancy is a relative contraindication.[6]

- Authors of a Cochrane review of 5 RCTs of thyroid surgeries with 886 participants with GD found that total thyroidectomy was more effective than subtotal thyroidectomy at preventing recurrent hyperthyroidism but conferred a greater risk of permanent hypocalcemia/hypoparathyroidism. GO and permanent recurrent laryngeal nerve palsy were unrelated to type of surgery.[13]
- In most cases for patients with GD, pretreatment with MMI until euthyroid is recommended followed by potassium iodide (3 drops SSKI orally three times daily), prior to surgery and levothyroxine is started following surgery.[1,6]
- Complications following surgery are uncommon and include bleeding, laryngeal edema, hypoparathyroidism, and recurrent laryngeal nerve damage; recurrence rates are <2%.[1]

- With respect to the eye findings, most symptoms except for proptosis improve with control of the hyperthyroidism. Thyroidectomy, alone or in combination with medical therapy, is associated with a decreased risk of ophthalmopathy compared to RAI.[14]

SECOND LINE

MEDICATIONS

- In an RCT of 159 patients with mild GO who were given selenium (100 mcg twice daily), pentoxifylline (600 mg twice daily), or placebo (twice daily) orally for 6 months, selenium significantly improved quality of life, reduced ocular involvement, and slowed progression of the disease compared to the other treatments.[15]
- Trials of rituximab, an anti-CD20 monoclonal antibody, in patients with active moderate to severe GO have shown mixed results, with one trial showing no difference versus placebo and another demonstrating more benefit than intravenous methylprednisolone with respect to eye motility outcome, visual functioning, and reduced number of surgical procedures at 1 year.[16,17]

PROCEDURES

- Treatment options for the persistent severe GO include high-dose systemic steroids (40 to 80 mg/day), orbital radiotherapy, and orbital decompression surgery.[6,18] SOR B

REFERRAL

- Patients with significant eye symptoms or clinical findings should be referred to an ophthalmologist.

PREVENTION OF OPHTHALMOPATHY

- Prevention of GO includes smoking cessation, maintenance of euthyroidism after GD treatment, and glucocorticoids for patients with mild active GO who are treated with RAI.[6]

PROGNOSIS

- With use of antithyroid medications, symptoms improve in 3 to 4 weeks. Remission rates following ATDs vary based on a number of factors, but early U.S. studies show lasting remission after 12–18 months of 20% to 30%.[6]
- Following RAI for GD, most patients become euthyroid after 4 to 8 weeks, but eventually become hypothyroid.
- Authors of a systematic review and meta-analysis of 8 studies comparing GD treatments found higher relapse rates among patients who received ATDs (52.7%) versus patients following RAI (15%) and surgery (20%).[19]

FOLLOW-UP

- The goals of therapy are to resolve hyperthyroid symptoms and to restore the euthyroid state. Close follow-up is needed in the initial treatment period; medications for symptoms of hyperthyroidism may be withdrawn slowly following treatment.
- Obtain thyroid function tests and monitor clinical manifestations 4–6 weeks after starting an ATD.[1] ATD dosages may be reduced after the patient is euthyroid (typically PTU 50 mg 2–3 times daily or methimazole 2.5 to 10 mg/day), but drugs should be continued for 12 to 18 months to minimize relapse.[6] SOR A Medication can be discontinued after 12–18 months in patients with a normal TRAb and TSH. Patients with persistently high TRAb could continue ATD therapy or elect more definitive treatment.
- Following treatment with RAI, most patients become hypothyroid (>80% by 16 weeks) and so periodic monitoring of thyroid function is important. Follow-up within the first 1 to 2 months (TSH, free T_4, and total T_3) is recommended and then every 4 to 6 weeks for 6 months or until the patient becomes hypothyroid and is on stable thyroid replacement; consider retreatment with RAI if GD persists after 6 months.[6]
- Following surgery, patients may become hypothyroid or have a recurrence of hyperthyroidism, depending on the size of the remnant; patients should be monitored with periodic blood tests and for symptoms. For those with GD following surgery and levothyroxine, a TSH level is recommended at 6 to 8 weeks postsurgery.[6]
- Patients with GD are at high risk for development of other autoimmune disease; in one cross-sectional study in the United Kingdom of patients attending a thyroid clinic, the frequency of another autoimmune disorder (e.g., rheumatoid arthritis [3.15%], pernicious anemia, systemic lupus erythematosus, Addison disease, celiac disease, and vitiligo) was 9.67% in patients with GD.[20]

PATIENT EDUCATION

- Patients should be told that the goals of therapy are to resolve the symptoms of thyroid excess and to restore the thyroid function to normal, often with thyroid replacement medication.
- The treatment choices should be discussed, as each has advantages and disadvantages; treatment should be individualized.
- Regardless of the therapy chosen, long-term follow-up is needed to monitor thyroid status; there is a high risk of becoming hypothyroid in the future or of relapsing into hyperthyroidism. Patients should be made aware of symptoms to watch for and advised to report any recurrent symptoms.

- Following RAI, patients should avoid close and prolonged contact with children and pregnant women for 5–7 days.[1] Detailed instructions for patients for reducing radiation exposure to others after RAI can be found at the ATA website (https://www.thyroid.org/radioactive-iodine/).
- Ophthalmopathy usually runs its own course independent of the thyroid function; most patients improve or stabilize. Additional treatment may be needed in consultation with an ophthalmologist.
- Smoking cessation may have a beneficial effect on the course of ophthalmopathy.
- Siblings and children should be made aware of their increased risk of developing thyroid disease or associated disorders and should monitor themselves for symptoms.

PATIENT RESOURCES

- Booklets from the American Thyroid Association—**https://www.thyroid.org/thyroid-information/.**
- National Library of Medicine. *Thyroid Diseases*—**https://www.nlm.nih.gov/medlineplus/thyroiddiseases.html.**
- Graves' Disease and Thyroid Foundation—**https://www.gdatf.org.**

PROVIDER RESOURCES

- Ross DS, Burch HB, Cooper DS, et al. 2016 American Thyroid Association guidelines for diagnosis and management of hyperthyroidism and other causes of thyrotoxicosis. *Thyroid*. 2016; 26(10):1343-1421.
- Alexander EK, Pearce EN, Brent GA, et al. 2017 Guidelines of the American Thyroid Association for the diagnosis and management of thyroid disease during pregnancy and the postpartum. *Thyroid*. 2017;27(3):315-389.

REFERENCES

1. Jameson JL, Mandel SJ, Weetman AP. Disorders of the thyroid gland. In: Kasper DL, Fauci AS, Hauser SL, et al, eds. *Harrison's Principles of Internal Medicine*, 19th ed. New York, NY: McGraw-Hill; 2015.
2. Burch HB, Cooper DS. Management of Graves disease: a review. *JAMA*. 2015;314(23):2544-2554.
3. Smith TJ, Hegedüs L. Graves' disease. *N Engl J Med*. 2016;375(16):1552-1565.
4. Jabbour SA. Cutaneous manifestations of endocrine disorders. *Am J Clin Dermatol*. 2003;4(5):315-331.
5. Costagliola S, Marganthaler NG, Hoermann R, et al. Second generation assay for thyrotropin receptor antibodies has superior diagnostic sensitivity for Graves' disease. *J Clin Endocrinol Metab*. 1999;84:90-97.
6. Ross DS, Burch HB, Cooper DS, et al. 2016 American Thyroid Association guidelines for diagnosis and management of hyperthyroidism and other causes of thyrotoxicosis. *Thyroid*. 2016; 26(10):1343-1421.
7. Siegel RD, Lee SL. Toxic nodular goiter—toxic adenoma and toxic multinodular goiter. *Endocrinol Metab Clin North Am*. 1998;27(1):151-166.
8. Yoshihara A, Noh J, Yamaguchi T, et al. Treatment of Graves' disease with antithyroid drugs in the first trimester of pregnancy and the prevalence of congenital malformation. *J Clin Endocrinol Metab*. 2012;97(7):2396-2403.
9. Zang S, Ponto KA, Kahaly GJ. Clinical review: Intravenous glucocorticoids for Graves' orbitopathy: efficacy and morbidity. *J Clin Endocrinol Metab*. 2011;96(2):320-332.
10. Bartalena L, Krassas GE, Wiersinga W, et al; European Group on Graves' Orbitopathy. Efficacy and safety of three different cumulative doses of intravenous methylprednisolone for moderate to severe and active Graves' orbitopathy. *J Clin Endocrinol Metab*. 2012;97(12):4454-4463.
11. Zhu W, Ye L, Shen L, et al. A prospective, randomized trial of intravenous glucocorticoids therapy with different protocols for patients with Graves' ophthalmopathy. *J Clin Endocrinol Metab*. 2014;99(6):1999-2007.
12. Marcocci C, Watt T, Altea MA, et al. Fatal and non-fatal adverse events of glucocorticoid therapy for Graves' orbitopathy: a questionnaire survey among members of the European Thyroid Association. *Eur J Endocrinol*. 2012;166(2):247-253.
13. Liu ZW, Masterson L, Fish B, et al. Thyroid surgery for Graves' disease and Graves' ophthalmopathy. *Cochrane Database Sys Rev*. 2015;25;(11):CD010576.
14. Stein JD, Childers D, Gupta S, et al. Risk factors for developing thyroid-associated ophthalmopathy among individuals with Graves disease. *JAMA Ophthalmol*. 2015;133(3):290-296.
15. Marcocci C, Kahaly GJ, Krassas GE, et al. Selenium and the course of mild Graves' orbitopathy. *N Engl J Med*. 2011;364(20):1920-1931.
16. Stan MN, Garrity JA, Carranza Leon BG, et al. Randomized controlled trial of rituximab in patients with Graves' orbitopathy. *J Clin Endocrinol Metab*. 2015;100(2):432-441.
17. Salvi M, Vannucchi G, Currò N, et al. Efficacy of B-cell targeted therapy with rituximab in patients with active moderate to severe Graves' orbitopathy: a randomized controlled study. *J Clin Endocrinol Metab*. 2015;100(2):422-431.
18. Tanda ML, Bartalena L. Efficacy and safety of orbital radiotherapy for Graves' orbitopathy. *J Clin Endocrinol Metab*. 2012;97(11):3857-3865.
19. Sundaresh V, Brito JP, Wang Z, et al. Comparative effectiveness of therapies for Graves' hyperthyroidism: a systematic review and network meta-analysis. *J Clin Endocrinol Metab*. 2013;98(9):3671-3677.
20. Boelaert K, Newby PR, Simmonds MJ, et al. Prevalence and relative risk of other autoimmune diseases in subjects with autoimmune thyroid disease. *Am J Med*. 2010;123(2):183.e1-e9.

237 ACROMEGALY

Mindy A. Smith, MD, MS

PATIENT STORY

A 60-year-old man presents to his family physician with severe headache and weakness (**Figure 237-1**). He also noted enlargement of his hands (**Figure 237-2**), which made him remove his wedding ring when it became too tight, and feet (his shoe size had increased). He said his voice seemed to be deeper and his hands feel doughy and sweaty. Laboratory testing reveals an elevated insulin-like growth factor (IGF)-1, and there is a failure of growth hormone (GH) suppression following an oral glucose load confirming the diagnosis of acromegaly. Computed tomography (CT) scan of the head demonstrates a pituitary adenoma.

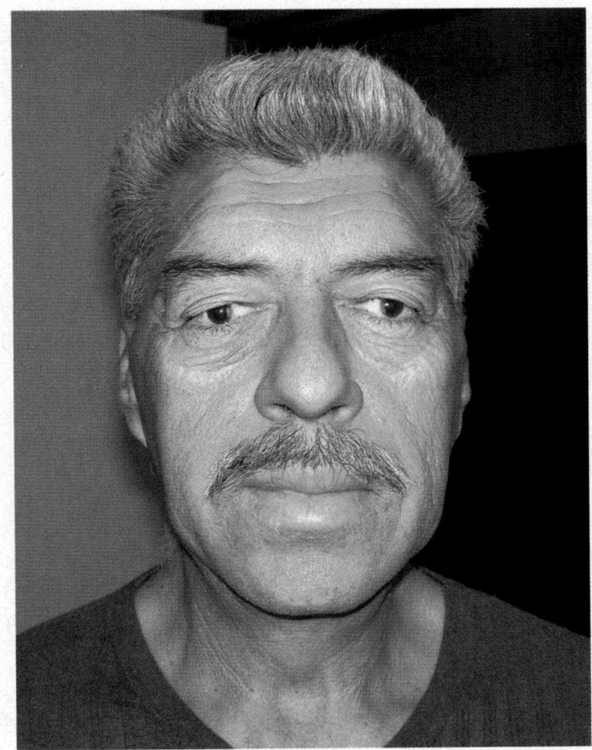

FIGURE 237-1 A 60-year-old man with acromegaly. Note the coarse facial features and moderate prognathism (Protrusion of the lower jaw). *(Reproduced with permission from Richard P. Usatine, MD.)*

INTRODUCTION

Acromegaly is a condition of excessive linear and organ growth usually caused by autonomous GH hypersecretion from a pituitary tumor.

EPIDEMIOLOGY

- Rare (5/1,000,000 adults).[1]
- Most typically caused by a pituitary somatotroph macroadenoma. It may also be caused by growth hormone–releasing hormone (GHRH) excess from lesions of the pancreas, lung, or ovaries, or from a chest or abdominal carcinoid tumor.
- The disorder is usually sporadic, but may be familial (<5%) and has been associated with other endocrine tumors (e.g., multiple endocrine neoplasia type I).[1]
- In a Spanish multicenter epidemiologic study, the reported mean age at diagnosis was 45 years.[2]
- The occurrence of GH hypersecretion in children and adolescents, prior to epiphyseal closure, causes gigantism. In one study, early-onset gigantism was caused by an Xq26.3 genomic duplication.[3]

ETIOLOGY AND PATHOPHYSIOLOGY

- The clinical signs and symptoms of acromegaly result from GH excess that stimulates linear and organ growth (through IGF-1), soft-tissue swelling, and chondrocyte action.
- Acromegaly is also associated with insulin resistance and an increased risk of cardiovascular disease; the latter appears to be a result of pressure-related arterial and left ventricular stiffening rather than atherosclerotic disease.[4] There may be gender-specific metabolic profiles in patients with acromegaly, with women having greater insulin resistance and features of metabolic syndrome compared to men.[5]
- An increased risk for several cancers among these patients may be a result of the proliferative and antiapoptotic activity associated with increased circulating levels of IGF-1.

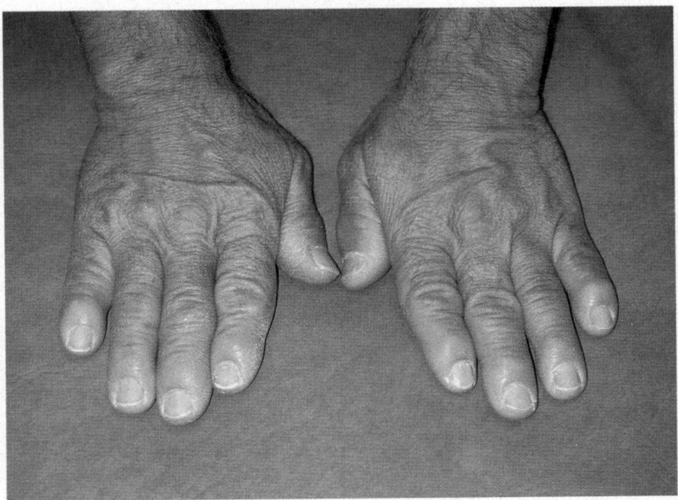

FIGURE 237-2 The man in **Figure 237-1** with acromegaly producing hands that are large and doughy with widened fingers. *(Reproduced with permission from Richard P. Usatine, MD.)*

DIAGNOSIS

The diagnosis of acromegaly is established by documenting autonomous GH hypersecretion and by pituitary imaging.

CLINICAL FEATURES

The clinical manifestations of acromegaly are often subtle and may not be noticed for many years. Gigantism occurs if excessive GH exposure occurs *before* closure of the epiphyses; acromegaly develops *after* closure of the epiphyses. Clinical features of acromegaly include[1]:

- Soft-tissue swelling resulting in hand and foot enlargement (see **Figure 237-2**).
- Kyphoscoliosis and skeletal hyperostosis.
- Coarse facial features and a large fleshy nose (**Figures 237-1** and **237-3**).
- Frontal bossing.
- Jaw malocclusion and overbite.
- Hyperhidrosis and oily skin.
- Other common features are deep voice (soft-tissue swelling of vocal cords), arthropathy, carpal tunnel syndrome, kyphosis, proximal muscle weakness, and fatigue; patients may complain of headache and visual field defects (expanding tumor), paresthesias, and sexual dysfunction.[1]
- Associated medical conditions include sleep apnea (60%), coronary heart disease (20% to 90% depending on duration and associated hypertension), and diabetes mellitus (25%). There also appears to be an increase in intracranial aneurysms.[6]
- In one study, approximately two-thirds of 55 women had anovulatory cycles, some believed related to elevated hormone levels.[7]

LABORATORY AND IMAGING

- An elevated total serum IGF-1 concentration (age and gender matched) is extremely useful in the diagnosis of acromegaly.[8,9] SOR Ⓐ Lack of standardization and normative data, however, has hampered diagnosis and monitoring.
- Failure of GH suppression to less than 1 mcg/L within 1 to 2 hours of an oral glucose load (75 g) can confirm the diagnosis, although 20% of patients exhibit a paradoxical increase in GH. SOR Ⓐ Failure to suppress GH levels may also be seen in patients with diabetes, renal or hepatic failure, and obesity, in those receiving estrogen replacement, and in pregnant women.[1]
- A single measure of GH is not helpful because of its pulsatile secretion.
- Another associated laboratory abnormality is elevated prolactin (30% of patients).
- Following biochemical confirmation of acromegaly, the Endocrine Society guidelines recommend magnetic resonance imaging (MRI) to assess tumor size and appearance, as well as parasellar extent.[9] SOR Ⓑ
  - If MRI is contraindicated or unavailable, use computed tomography.
  - If a tumor is found that abuts the optic chiasm, perform formal visual field testing.[9]

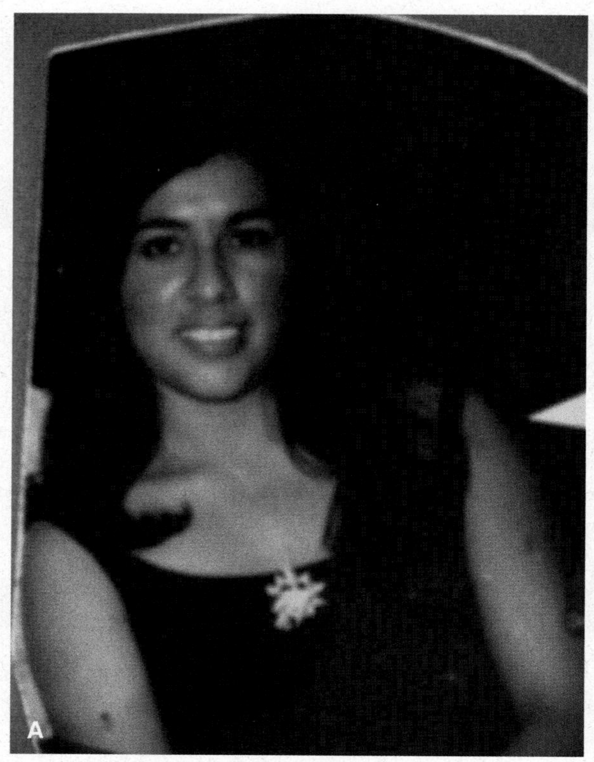

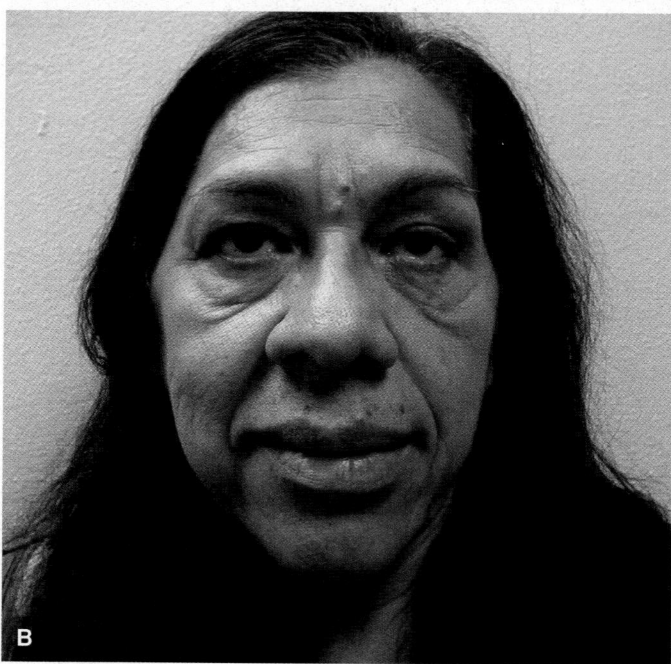

FIGURE 237-3 **A.** A 26-year-old attractive woman prior to acromegaly changes. **B.** Facial changes 20 years later in the same woman. Note the coarse facial features with large nose, lips, and chin. Protrusion of the lower jaw is visible. (*Reproduced with permission from Vernon Burke, DMD.*)

MANAGEMENT

The Endocrine Society recommends a multidisciplinary team approach.[9] This might include an experienced surgeon, an endocrinologist with pituitary expertise, and a physician with radiotherapy experience. Treatment is usually surgical followed by medication (usually a somatostatin receptor ligand [SRL]) if the disease is not controlled.

- Patients should be evaluated and monitored for associated comorbidities, including hypertension, diabetes mellitus, cardiovascular disease, osteoarthritis, and sleep apnea.[9] SOR B
  - Screening colonoscopy should be considered.
  - If thyroid nodularity is identified, obtain a thyroid ultrasound.
  - Assess for hypopituitarism and replace hormones as needed.

FIRST LINE

MEDICATIONS

There are 3 types of medications used in the treatment of patients with acromegaly: SRLs, a GH receptor antagonist, and a dopamine agonist. Although GH reduction may alleviate symptoms, attempts to normalize levels of both GH and its target growth factor (i.e., IGF-1) should be made because persistent secretion of either poses significant long-term health risks.

- The Endocrine Society recommends against presurgical medical therapy except for patients with severe pharyngeal thickness and sleep apnea, or high-output heart failure who may benefit from presurgical treatment with SRLs.[9]
- Somatostatin analogs (for most patients) or pegvisomant are first-line therapies for those with significant disease and non–surgically resectable tumors; after surgery; or during radiation treatment until control is achieved by that therapy (which can take several years).
  - Long-acting somatostatin depot formulations, octreotide LAR and lanreotide Autogel, are available and appear equivalent. Patients should be treated with the same dose for 3 months before reassessment and dose titration if needed.[9] An oral octreotide as well as an octreotide implant are undergoing testing and appear promising.[9,10] Pasireotide, a novel SRL that has enhanced binding to more somatostatin receptor subtypes, was shown in one RCT to be more effective than octreotide in achieving normal IGF-1 (38.6% and 23.6%) with similar rates of GH <2.5 μg/L (48.3% and 51.6%).[11] There were more hyperglycemic adverse effects with pasireotide.
    - Side effects are injection pain, sinus bradycardia, and symptoms related to suppression of GI motility and secretion (nausea, abdominal pain, diarrhea, and flatulence); gallstones or sludge occur in 30%, but few develop cholecystitis.[1]
  - Subcutaneous pegvisomant, a GH receptor antagonist, can also be used as initial adjuvant medical therapy for acromegaly. Pegvisomant may be particularly useful in patients with comorbid diabetes.[9]
    - Side effects include injection site pain and lipohypertrophy. Elevated liver enzymes are seen in approximately 5% to 25% of patients (usually transient) and should be monitored.
- In patients with only modest elevations of serum IGF-1 and mild signs and symptoms of GH excess, the Endocrine Society guidelines suggest a trial of a dopamine agonist, usually cabergoline, as the initial adjuvant medical therapy.[9] Response appears to decrease over time.
  - Common side effects are GI (nausea, constipation), psychiatric and central nervous system (sleep disturbance, vertigo, depression), and cardiovascular (hypertension, peripheral edema); cardiac valve abnormalities have been reported in patients with Parkinson disease (who usually use high doses).

PROCEDURES

- Surgical resection (adenomectomy via transsphenoidal approach) is the cornerstone of treatment for intrasellar microadenomas, noninvasive macroadenomas, and when the tumor is causing compression symptoms.
  - The Endocrine Society recommends transsphenoidal surgery as primary therapy because it results in immediate lowering of GH levels and provides tissue for pathology.[9] SOR A Repeat surgery is considered in patients with residual intrasellar disease.[9] SOR B
    - Surgical complications include bleeding, spinal fluid leak, meningitis, sodium and water imbalance, and hypopituitarism.
  - Debulking surgery should be considered in patients with parasellar disease when total surgical resection is unlikely to improve response to medication.[9]

SECOND LINE

- If initial medical treatment (following dose titration) fails to normalize GH and IGF-1, patients with tumor mass on MRI may consider radiation therapy while those without a mass effect may be tried on combination medical therapy.[9]

MEDICATIONS

- In patients who have an inadequate response to SRLs, the Endocrine Society guidelines suggest the addition of pegvisomant or cabergoline.
- In a case series of 16 men with acromegaly who remained uncontrolled after surgery, radiotherapy, and/or medical treatment, the addition of clomiphene citrate 50 mg/d resulted in 7 patients achieving normal IGF-1 levels.[12]

RADIATION THERAPY

- Radiation therapy, conventional and stereotactic procedures (the latter is preferred), is also effective in decreasing GH levels, but takes 10 to 15 years to work and carries a risk of hypopituitarism (>50%). It is recommended by the Endocrine Society guidelines for residual tumor mass following surgery or in cases where medical therapy is unavailable or unsuccessful.[9] Radiation has been used in an attempt to discontinue medical therapy.
  - Five-year remission rates from gamma knife radiotherapy (after surgical debulking) are between 29% and 60%.[9]
  - Conventional radiotherapy has potential risks of second tumors (approximately 1% intracranial) and cerebrovascular events, but long-term data are lacking.[9]

PROGNOSIS

- After surgical resection, 70% to 95% of patients with microadenomas and 40% to 68% of patients with macroadenomas have

normalization of IGF-1.[8,9] Five-year disease recurrence ranges between 2% and 8%.[9]
  - Irradiation of adenomas results in attenuation of IGF-1 secretion in more than 60% of subjects after 10 to 15 years.[9]
  - Less than half of patients (44%) receiving somatostatin analogs achieve normal IGF-1 levels, and a third achieve normal GH levels.[9]
- In the past, patients with acromegaly had a 10-year reduction in life span because of cardiac (heart failure, arrhythmia), cerebrovascular, metabolic (diabetes, osteoporosis), and respiratory (airway obstruction from macroglossia and hypertrophied mucosal tissues, sleep apnea) disease; radiotherapy may also increase the mortality rate.[1] Both IGF-1 and GH levels correlate with mortality, and normalizing these levels (IGF-1 to age/sex standards and GH <2.5 ng/mL) appears to normalize the life span.[9]
- Successful pregnancy can occur in women with acromegaly,[7] although one case series found cases of gestational diabetes and gestational hypertension in women with uncontrolled disease; symptomatic (e.g., visual field defect, headache) enlargement of GH-secreting pituitary macroadenomas occurred in a few women.[13]

FOLLOW-UP

- Continued monitoring and treatment of comorbidities should be pursued.[9]
- The Acromegaly Consensus Group and Endocrine Society define optimal disease control (i.e., posttreatment remission of acromegaly) as IGF-1 level (determined by a reliable standardized assay) in the age-adjusted normal range, and a GH level less than 1 g/L from a random GH measurement, using an ultrasensitive assay.[8,9] In patients who are controlled, monitor levels every 6 months and use the same GH and IGF-1 assay in the same patient throughout management.[9]
- Based on a cohort study of patients hospitalized for acromegaly (Denmark 1977–1993; Sweden 1965–1993) linked to tumor registry data for up to 28 years of follow-up, individuals with acromegaly have higher rates of small intestine, colon, rectal, kidney, and bone cancer.[14] The researchers also found that these patients had elevated rates for cancers of the brain and thyroid that may be related to pituitary irradiation.
- A higher rate of vertebral fractures has been reported for patients with acromegaly, especially those with active acromegaly compared to controls.[15]
- In patients receiving pegvisomant, the Endocrine Society guidelines suggest serial imaging with MRI scan to evaluate tumor size and monitoring liver function tests monthly for the first 6 months and then every 6 months with consideration of discontinuation of pegvisomant if the transaminases are greater than 3-fold elevated.[9]
- Monitoring treatment success postoperatively or following radiation therapy includes:
  - Measurement of GH and IGF-1 levels 12 weeks or later following surgery and annually following medication withdrawal after radiation therapy.[9]
  - Postoperative MRI 12 weeks postsurgery and 3 to 6 months following medical therapy, and yearly for those who remain uncontrolled. There is no consensus on frequency of continued MRI once remission is achieved.[9]
  - Full pituitary function should be measured 3 months after surgery and annually for those receiving radiotherapy.[9]

PATIENT EDUCATION

- Patients should be advised that untreated, one's life span is decreased by an average of 10 years. Survival improves greatly if GH and IGF-1 can be normalized.
- Patients should consider increased surveillance for colorectal cancer and encouraged to actively manage comorbid conditions.

PATIENT RESOURCES

- National Institute of Diabetes and Digestive and Kidney Diseases. *Acromegaly*—**https://www.niddk.nih.gov/health-information/endocrine-diseases/acromegaly.**

PROVIDER RESOURCES

- Medscape. *Acromegaly*—**https://emedicine.medscape.com/article/925446-overview.**

REFERENCES

1. Melmed S. Acromegaly pathogenesis and treatment. *J Clin Invest.* 2009;119(11):3189-3202.
2. Mestron A, Webb SM, Astorga R, et al. Epidemiology, clinical characteristics, outcome, morbidity and mortality in acromegaly based on the Spanish Acromegaly Registry (Registro Espanol de Acromegalia, REA). *Eur J Endocrinol.* 2004;151(4):439-446.
3. Trivellin G, Daly AF, Faucz FR, et al. Gigantism and acromegaly due to Xq26 microduplications and GPR101 mutation. *N Engl J Med.* 2014;371(25):2363-2374.
4. Paisley AN, Banerjee M, Rezai M, et al. Changes in arterial stiffness but not carotid intimal thickness in acromegaly. *J Clin Endocrinol Metab.* 2011;96(5):1486-1492.
5. Ciresi A, Amato MC, Pivonello R, et al. The metabolic profile in active acromegaly is gender-specific. *J Clin Endocrinol Metab.* 2013 Jan;98(1):E51-E59.
6. Manara R, Maffei P, Citton V, et al. Increased rate of intracranial saccular aneurysms in acromegaly: an MR angiography study and review of the literature. *J Clin Endocrinol Metab.* 2011;96(5):1292-1300.
7. Grynberg M, Salenave S, Young J, Chanson P. Female gonadal function before and after treatment of acromegaly. *J Clin Endocrinol Metab.* 2010;95(10):4518-4525.
8. Giustina A, Chanson P, Bronstein MD, et al. Acromegaly Consensus Group. A consensus on criteria for cure of acromegaly. *J Clin Endocrinol Metab.* 2010;95(7):3141-3148.

9. Katznelson L, Laws ER, Melmed S, et al. Acromegaly: an Endocrine Society clinical practice guideline. *J Clin Endocrinol Metab.* 2014; 99:3933-3951.

10. Chieffo C, Cook D, Xiang Q, Frohman LA. Efficacy and safety of an octreotide implant in the treatment of patients with acromegaly. *J Clin Endocrinol Metab.* 2013;98(10):4047-4054.

11. Colao A, Bronstein MD, Freda P, et al. Pasireotide versus octreotide in acromegaly: a head-to-head superiority study. *J Clin Endocrinol Metab.* 2014;99(3):791-799.

12. Duarte FH, Jallad RS, Bronstein MD. Clomiphene citrate for treatment of acromegaly not controlled by conventional therapies. *J Clin Endocrinol Metab.* 2015;100(5):1863-1869.

13. Caron P, Broussaud S, Bertherat J, et al. Acromegaly and pregnancy: a retrospective multicenter study of 59 pregnancies in 46 women. *J Clin Endocrinol Metab.* 2010;95(10):4680-4687.

14. Baris D, Gridley G, Ron E, et al. Acromegaly and cancer risk: a cohort study in Sweden and Denmark. *Cancer Causes Control.* 2002;13(5):395-400.

15. Mazziotti G, Bianchi A, Maffezzoni F, et al. Bone turnover, bone mineral density, and fracture risk in acromegaly: a meta-analysis. *J Clin Endocrinol Metab.* 2015;100(2):384-394.

PART XVII

THE BRAIN AND NERVOUS SYSTEM

Strength of Recommendation (SOR)	Definition
A	Recommendation based on consistent and good-quality patient-oriented evidence.*
B	Recommendation based on inconsistent or limited-quality patient-oriented evidence.*
C	Recommendation based on consensus, usual practice, opinion, disease-oriented evidence, or case series for studies of diagnosis, treatment, prevention, or screening.*

*See Appendix A on pages 1603–1606 for further information.

238 MENTAL HEALTH

Mindy A. Smith, MD, MS
Richard P. Usatine, MD

PATIENT STORY

A 21-year-old woman is seen by a family physician in a student-run free clinic within a residential chemical dependency program for women. She has just finished withdrawing from intravenous heroin. She is experiencing anxiety and insomnia and is asking for medications to help her sleep at night and function during the day. The young woman has a 10-month-old baby. She had been on a methadone program during her pregnancy. The patient states that her mother is bipolar and often uses various drugs including heroin. Her brother sells heroin but claims to not use it anymore. He does sell heroin to her and her mother at a discount. The patient admits to having been sexually abused as a child and states that the heroin numbs some of the pain from her childhood. Unfortunately, she has bad nightmares (related to posttraumatic stress disorder [PTSD]) that make sleeping difficult. She did return to injecting heroin after the baby was born and lost custody of her child. She is motivated to maintain sobriety so she can be with her baby again. The family physician listens with compassion and empathy and prescribes some non-addicting medications to help her with the anxiety, insomnia, and nightmares. A follow-up appointment is set for the following week, as it is clear that this young woman needs a lot of support in addition to close management of pharmacologic therapy.

INTRODUCTION

Over half of mental health treatment in the United States occurs within primary care, and about 25% of all primary care patients have diagnosable mental health disorders (most commonly, depression and anxiety).[1] Frequent mental distress, defined in one study as 14 or more days of poor mental health in the past month, was reported by 9.4% of U.S. adults for the combined periods 1993–2001 and 2003–2006.[2]

Access to mental health services is difficult in many areas of the country. In a study based on National Health Interview Survey data, unmet need for mental healthcare increased from 4.3 million in 1997 to 7.2 million in 2010.[3] Unmet need was higher among children (ages 2–17 years); working-age adults (ages 18–64 years); women; uninsured persons; and persons with low incomes, those in fair or poor health, and those with chronic conditions. This makes it vital that primary care clinicians be well versed in the identification and care of these conditions.

Mental health disorders include anxiety disorders, mood disorders, schizophrenia and other psychotic disorders, dementia, and eating disorders. This chapter covers the first three of these categories; information on dementia can be found in Chapter 243, Dementia.

- Anxiety disorders are the most common class of mental disorders in the general population and include PTSD, generalized anxiety disorder (GAD), panic disorder, social anxiety disorder, phobias, and separation anxiety disorder.[4]
- The most common mood disorders are major depressive disorder (MDD) (**Figure 238-1**), dysthymic disorder, mood disorders due to a general medical condition (or substance), and bipolar disorder types I and II. MDD is also a common comorbidity of many chronic diseases such as stroke, diabetes, heart disease, and chronic obstructive pulmonary disease. Bipolar disorder is defined by episodes of depression and episodes of mania or hypomania.
- Psychotic disorders are characterized by dysregulation of thought. Schizophrenia is the most common disorder in which psychosis is observed; patients with schizophrenia may report symptoms of delusions (false beliefs) and visual and auditory hallucinations. Psychosis, however, can be present in other mental and substance use disorders.

EPIDEMIOLOGY

- **Anxiety:** Estimated lifetime prevalence of any anxiety disorder is approximately 16%; 12-month prevalence is approximately 11%.[4]
  - More prevalent in women than men (1.7:1, lifetime), except for social anxiety; women have greater illness burden.[5]
  - Specific anxiety disorders in primary care include PTSD (8.6%), GAD (7.6%), panic disorder with or without agoraphobia (6.8%), and social anxiety disorder (6.2%).[6] In this study, 19.5% (95% confidence index [CI], 17.0%–22.1%) of the 965 patients had at least 1 anxiety disorder and 41% reported no current treatment.
  - Annual associated cost in the United States was estimated at $42.3 billion (1990s).[7]
- **Major Depression** (see **Figure 238-1**): Lifetime rates of MDD are reported by approximately12% globally; 12-month prevalence is approximately 6%.[4]
  - Like anxiety, overall rates of MDD are higher among women (1.7:1)[4]; global annual prevalence in women and men was 5.5% and 3.2%, respectively.[8]
  - Based on 2009–2012 data from the National Health and Nutrition Examination Survey, 7.6% of persons aged 12 years and over reported depression in any 2-week period and 3% had severe depression.[9]
  - Nearly 90% of those with severe depression report difficulty with home, work, and social activities. However, only about one-third (35.3%) of them have seen a mental health professional in the past year.[10]
- **Bipolar Disorder:** Lifetime prevalence is 4.4% for diagnosed bipolar disorder.[11] The condition is likely underdiagnosed.
  - Incidence rates for bipolar disorder in a study in the Netherlands were 0.70/10,000 person years (PY) (95% CI: 0.57–0.83) overall, 0.43/10,000 PY for bipolar I disorder and 0.19/10,000 PY for bipolar II disorder.[12] For bipolar I there were two peaks in age of onset: 15–24 years and a larger peak in later life (45–54 years; 1.2/10,000 PY). In bipolar II disorder, age of onset was 45–54 years.

- Based on a multinational study using household surveys of adults, lifetime prevalence of bipolar I disorder was 0.6%, bipolar II was 0.4%, subthreshold bipolar disorder was 1.4%, and bipolar spectrum was 2.4%.[13] Symptom severity was greater for depressive versus manic episodes, and 75% of respondents with depression and 50% of respondents with mania reported severe role impairment. Of those with bipolar spectrum disorder, 75% met criteria for at least one other disorder; anxiety disorders, particularly panic attacks, were the most common comorbid condition.
- Bipolar disorder is more common in women than men (ratio 3:2). The median age of onset is 25 years, with men having an earlier age of onset than women.[10]
- Bipolar disorder is associated with a high medical burden, in part due to the high rate of medical comorbidity of 60%.[14] Comorbid conditions include obesity, hyperlipidemia, hypertension, asthma, thyroid disease, migraine headaches, and osteoarthritis.[14]
- Comorbid psychiatric conditions were reported in 57% of patients with bipolar disorder in one study, and 30% had more than one diagnosis.[15] The inpatient hospitalization rate of patients with bipolar disorder is greater than that of all other patients with behavioral health diagnoses (39.1% vs. 4.5%, respectively).[10]

- **Schizophrenia:** Lifetime prevalence, based on estimates from 46 countries, is 4 per 1000 persons (10% to 90% quartiles, 1.6–12.1).[16] Symptom onset is between late adolescence and mid-30s[16]; by age 30 years, 9 of 10 men, but only 2 of 10 women, will manifest the illness.[17,18]
  - There is no gender difference in rates of schizophrenia; however, there appears to be a higher rate in blacks than in non-Hispanic whites.[19]
  - In Canada, direct healthcare and non-healthcare costs of schizophrenia were estimated at 2.02 billion Canadian dollars (2004).[20]

ETIOLOGY AND PATHOPHYSIOLOGY

- **Anxiety** is likely caused by biopsychosocial factors in a genetically susceptible individual that interact with situations, stress, or trauma to produce clinically significant syndromes.[21] Serotonergic, noradrenergic, glutamatergic, and gamma-aminobutyric acid (GABA) systems are implicated.[22]
  - It is not known why some people experience PTSD following a traumatic event, but it is likely a combination of genetic, neurobiology, risk factors (see below), and lack of positive coping strategies.[23]
  - Patients with panic disorder have a heightened sensitivity to internal autonomic cues (e.g., tachycardia). Panic episodes can be triggered by many factors including injury, illness, interpersonal conflict, and substance use (e.g., cannabis, caffeine).[22]
  - Social phobia can be initiated by a traumatic social experience or by social-skill deficits that produce recurring negative experiences; genetics likely play a role.[22]

- **Depression** is likely caused by a combination of genetic, biologic, environmental, and psychological factors. Depression can be triggered by stressful life events, adverse childhood experiences, dysfunctional attitudes such as low self-esteem, and personality traits that inhibit satisfactory social functioning, such as pessimism.[24]
  - Pathophysiologic features include defects of serotonin and postsynaptic serotonin receptors; brain morphology and cellular deficits (e.g., reduced neural connections and cerebral blood flow,

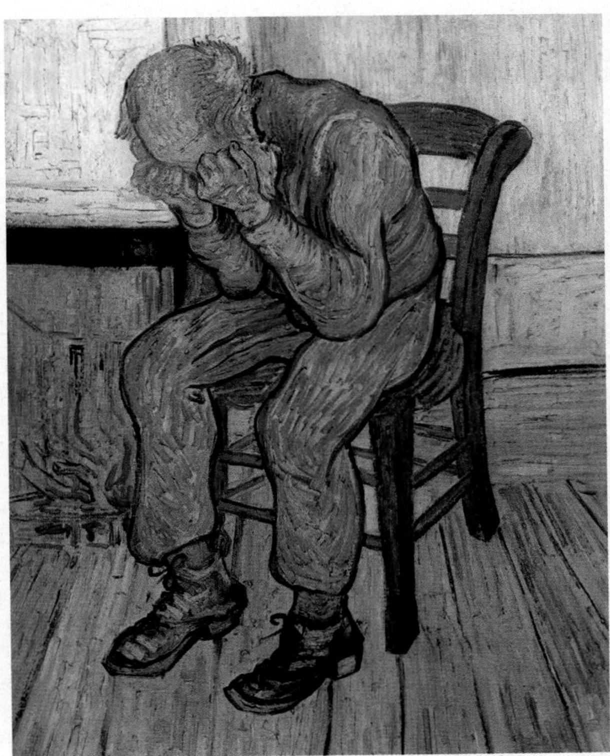

FIGURE 238-1 Van Gogh's *Old Man in Sorrow* is a depiction of depression by an artist who suffered from depression himself.

TABLE 238-1 Risk Factors for Selected Mental Health Conditions

Anxiety	Depression	Bipolar Disorder (BD)	Schizophrenia
• Intolerance for uncertainty • High neuroticism • Family history of GAD • Increased stress • History of physical or emotional trauma	• Prior depression • Family history MDD • Single/divorced/widowed • Female sex • Younger age • Chronic minor or recent major stress • Chronic medical illness • Systemic use of glucocorticoids • Low social support	• Family history of BD • Early-onset panic attacks and disorder • Separation anxiety • Presence of GAD, conduct symptoms and disorder, ADHD, impulsivity, and criminal behavior	• Lower IQ • Polygenic risk score • Socioeconomic status • Family history of schizophrenia or psychoses • CNS infection in early childhood • Born and raised in urban area

Abbreviations: GAD, generalized anxiety disorder; MDD, major depressive disorder; ADHD, attention-deficit/hyperactivity disorder; IQ, intelligence quotient.

Data from Shearer SL. Generalized anxiety disorder. http://www.essentialevidenceplus.com.proxy1.cl.msu.edu/content/eee/623. Updated November 24, 2016. Accessed January 2018; Faedda GL, Serra G, Marangoni C, et al. Clinical risk factors for bipolar disorders: a systematic review of prospective studies. *J Affect Disord.* 2014;168:314-321; Kendler KS, Ohlsson H, Sundquist J, Sundquist K. IQ and schizophrenia in a Swedish national sample: their causal relationship and the interaction of IQ with genetic risk. *Am J Psychiatry.* 2015;172(3):259-265; Agerbo E, Sullivan PF, Vilhjálmsson BJ, et al. Polygenic risk score, parental socioeconomic status, family history of psychiatric disorders, and the risk for schizophrenia: a Danish population-based study and meta-analysis. *JAMA Psychiatry.* 2015;72(7):635-641; Holder SD, Wayhs A. Schizophrenia. *Am Fam Physician.* 2014;90(11):775-782.

blunted amygdala hemodynamic activity to positive stimuli); and increased corticotropin-releasing hormone, vasopressin, and pro-inflammatory cytokine (e.g., interleukin-6 [IL-6]) secretion.[24]
  - Among women, evidence supports a hormonal influence; there is an increased incidence of depression at puberty, postpartum, and at menopause (for at-risk women), and depressive symptoms are linked to the luteal phase of the menstrual cycle.[25]

- **Bipolar disorder** is likely caused by a complex interplay of neurologic, genetic, and environmental factors. Neuroimaging studies show abnormalities in neural circuits that support emotion processing and regulation as well as reward processing.[26] Genetic factors, including several common polymorphisms, contribute to bipolar disorder, and there is overlap of susceptibility between bipolar disorder and schizophrenia for several individual risk alleles.[27] Environmental factors among adolescents include early cannabis use, brain maturation, and genetic risk.[28]
- **Schizophrenia** also has neurobiologic, genetic, and environmental components. There are many abnormalities observed in the brain, including decrements in both gray and white matter, *N*-methyl-D-aspartate (NMDA)-receptor hypofunction, low-grade brain inflammation, and increased striatal dopamine synthesis.[29] Although most patients with schizophrenia do not have a family history of psychosis, relatives of patients with schizophrenia have a higher risk of many psychiatric disorders, including schizoaffective disorder, schizotypal personality disorder, bipolar disorder, depression, and autism spectrum disorder.[17]

RISK FACTORS

- Authors of a meta-analysis of 293 predominantly U.S. studies published between 1983 and 2013 found that being subjected to racism was associated with poorer mental, physical, and general health.[30]
- Risk factors for anxiety, depression, bipolar disorder, and schizophrenia are shown in **Table 238-1**.

DIAGNOSIS

The *Diagnostic and Statistical Manual of Mental Disorders, Fifth Edition* (DSM-5),[31] is a critical tool in the diagnosis of mental health disorders to be used in conjunction with a detailed history and good clinical judgment.

CLINICAL FEATURES

- **Anxiety disorders** have in common feelings of worry, nervousness, unease, or excessive fear and related behavioral disturbances. Symptoms vary depending on the disorder; GAD diagnostic criteria are shown in **Table 238-2**. Other common symptoms include restlessness or feeling on edge, being easily fatigued, having difficulty concentrating, irritability, muscle tension, and sleep disturbance.
  - Individuals with PTSD experience hyperarousal and worry about safety following a traumatic event (**Figure 238-2**).
  - Panic disorder includes experiencing recurrent panic attacks—abrupt periods of intense fear/terror or discomfort accompanied by 4 or more of 13 systemic symptoms including physical symptoms (palpitations, sweating, shortness of breath, trembling) or fears (fear of losing control, of dying).[31] Patients have one or more attacks followed by at least 1 month of fear of another panic attack or significant maladaptive behavior related to the attacks.[21]
  - Patients with social phobia worry about embarrassment or inferior performance in social situations (e.g., public speaking).
- **MDD** is characterized by depressed mood and/or diminished pleasure lasting at least 2 weeks (see **Table 238-2**). The illness causes significant distress and/or occupational, social, or other

TABLE 238-2 Diagnostic Criteria for Major Depressive Disorder and Generalized Anxiety Disorder

Major Depressive Disorder	Generalized Anxiety Disorder
A person must experience five or more symptoms below for a continuous period of at least 2 weeks. Most symptoms must be present every day or nearly every day and must cause significant distress or problems in daily life functioning and not be attributable to another disorder.	A person must experience excessive anxiety and worry associated with three (or more) of the following six symptoms (or one or more for children). Symptoms occur on more days than not for at least 6 months and about a number of events or activities. The symptoms must cause clinically significant distress or impairment in social, occupational, or other important areas of functioning and not be attributable to another disorder.
• Feelings of sadness, hopelessness, depressed mood • Loss of interest or pleasure in activities that used to be enjoyable • Change in weight or appetite (either increase or decrease) • Change in activity: psychomotor agitation (being more active than usual) or psychomotor retardation (being less active than usual) • Insomnia (difficulty sleeping) or sleeping too much • Feeling tired or not having any energy • Feelings of guilt or worthlessness • Difficulties concentrating and paying attention • Thoughts of death or suicide	• Restlessness, feeling keyed up or on edge • Being easily fatigued • Difficulty concentrating or mind going blank • Irritability • Muscle tension • Sleep disturbance (difficulty falling or staying asleep, or restless, unsatisfying sleep)

impairment that is a change from previous functioning. Psychic pain can be every bit as devastating as chronic physical pain (**Figure 283-3**). DSM-5 no longer excludes individuals from receiving a diagnosis of MDD within 2 months of a significant death.

- **Bipolar disorder** with *mania* requires episodic abnormally and persistently elevated, expansive, or irritable mood lasting at least 7 consecutive days, or nearly every day, in association with 3 (or 4 if irritable mood) of the following symptoms: inflated self-esteem or grandiosity, sleeplessness, being more talkative than usual, flight of ideas or racing thoughts, distractibility, increased goal-directed activity, and/or excessive risk-taking activities.[31] Symptoms must cause marked functional impairment, and psychotic symptoms are present.[31,32] Symptom severity can be assessed using the Young Mania Rating Scale and the Montgomery-Ashbery Depression Rating Scale.[33] Bipolar disorder with *hypomanic episodes* requires symptoms lasting 4 consecutive days or nearly every day that do not cause marked functional impairment or associated psychosis.

- There are four types of bipolar disorder[34]:
    - **Bipolar I Disorder**—Defined by manic episodes lasting at least 7 days or by manic symptoms so severe that immediate hospital care is needed. Usually, depressive episodes occur as well, typically lasting at least 2 weeks. Episodes of depression with mixed features (three manic symptoms concurrently) and episodes of mania with mixed features (three depressive symptoms concurrently) are also possible.[14]
    - **Bipolar II Disorder**—Defined by a pattern of depressive episodes and hypomanic episodes, but not the full-blown manic episodes.

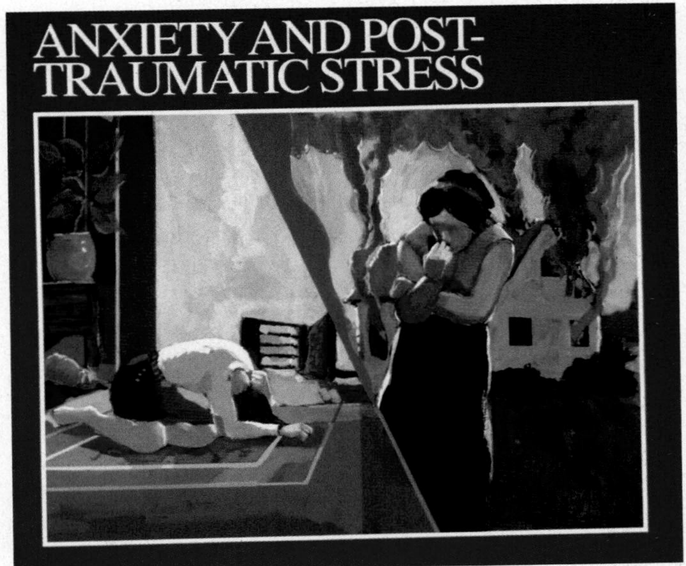

FIGURE 238-2 This image has two components that depict both anxiety and posttraumatic stress disorder (PTSD). The right side displays a young woman suffering from anxiety and PTSD as she recalls her house burning down, and on the left side she is doing yoga to relieve her anxiety and PTSD. This image was used in a poster for an Office of Research on Women's Health Seminar Series on anxiety and posttraumatic stress.

- **Cyclothymic Disorder**—Defined by numerous periods of hypomanic symptoms as well numerous periods of depressive symptoms lasting for at least 2 years (1 year in children and adolescents). However, the symptoms do not meet the diagnostic requirements for a hypomanic episode and a depressive episode.
- **Other Specified and Unspecified Bipolar and Related Disorders**—Defined by bipolar disorder symptoms that do not match the three categories listed above.

- **Schizophrenia** is characterized by positive (delusions, hallucinations, disorganized speech, grossly disorganized or catatonic behavior) and negative (diminished emotional expression, or avolition) symptoms for a significant portion of time during a 1-month period (see DSM-5 for full criteria).[31] During this active phase, at least one of delusions, hallucinations, or disorganized speech must be present.
  - As with other disorders, level of function must be compromised, and the disturbance cannot be attributable to use of a substance or another medical illness.
  - Continuous signs of the disturbance must persist intermittently for at least 6 months and must include at least 1 month of active-phase symptoms (or less if successfully treated).
  - There may be a prodromal phase during which there is social withdrawal, loss of interest in school or work, lack of attention to personal hygiene, angry outbursts, or unusual behavior.[17]

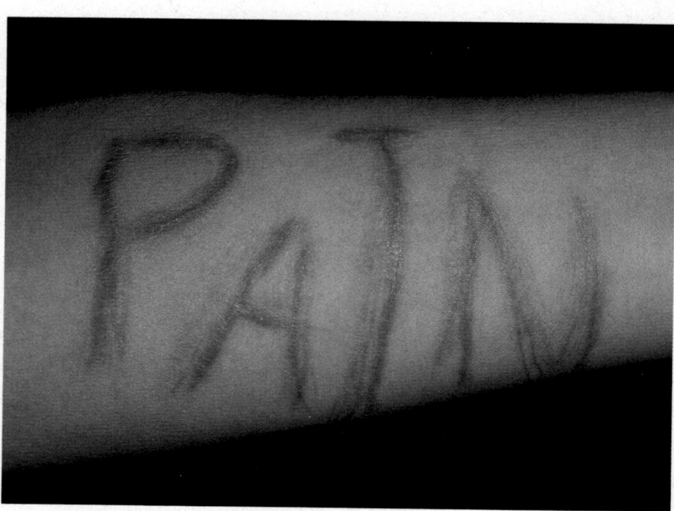

FIGURE 238-3 This middle-aged woman was seen in a homeless shelter free clinic. She had a significant history of mental illness including depression and showed her arm to the attending physician. One day, in the midst of despair and psychic pain, she had taken a knife and cut the word *pain* into her arm. The physical pain seemed to numb some of the psychic pain. The cuts healed and the scars have remained. *(Reproduced with permission from Richard P. Usatine, MD.)*

LABORATORY TESTS

- For patients presenting with **anxiety**, consider tests for substance use and hyperthyroidism, if clinically suspected (thyroid-stimulating hormone [TSH] and free thyroxine [T_4] level; see Chapter 236, Graves Disease and Goiter).
- For patients presenting with **depressed mood**, consider obtaining a complete blood count (CBC) (anemia) and TSH level (hypothyroidism; see Chapter 235, Goitrous Hypothyroidism).
- Because of the frequency of comorbid conditions, patients with **bipolar disorder** should be screened for hypertension, smoking, and substance use; recommended laboratory tests include lipids and fasting blood sugar or hemoglobin A_{1c}.[14]
- For patients with suspected **schizophrenia**, consider testing for substance abuse (elevated alcohol level, drug screen) or medical disorders (e.g., thyroid disorder, electrolyte disturbance, systemic or brain infection), based on history (see Differential Diagnosis).

DIFFERENTIAL DIAGNOSIS

- **Anxiety disorders** should be differentiated based on presenting symptoms. Other considerations include:
  - Medications—Medication review, particularly use of stimulants.
  - Substance abuse—Alcoholism/delirium tremens, cocaine, amphetamines, caffeine; these can also exacerbate anxiety disorders.
  - Hyperthyroidism—In addition to nervousness and fatigue, may report weight loss, heat intolerance, and palpitations or experience resting tremor, goiter, and exophthalmos; low TSH and elevated T_4.
- **Depression**
  - Minor depression—Requires only 2 to 4 major depressive episode symptoms, minimum symptom duration 2 weeks or more.

- Persistent depressive disorder (previously called dysthymia)—Requires only 3 to 4 depression symptoms, minimum symptom duration at least 2 years; core symptom is depressed mood.
- Premenstrual Dysphoric Disorder—Specific cyclic symptoms associated with the luteal and menstrual phases of the menstrual cycle and evidence of dysfunction.
- Hypothyroidism—Elevated TSH, dry skin, constipation, goiter, puffiness, weight gain.
- Anemia—Low hemoglobin/hematocrit, pallor, fatigue, dyspnea with exertion or at rest, and palpitations.

- **Bipolar Disorder**
  - Unipolar depression—Because patients with bipolar disorder report more depressive than manic or hypomanic symptoms (3 times more for bipolar I disorder and 39 times more for bipolar II disorder) and may already have a diagnosis of MDD, care must be taken to ask about manic behaviors/episodes.[32] In addition to the presence of manic behaviors, features that may help to distinguish bipolar disorder from unipolar depression include ability to function with few hours of sleep, early onset of depressive symptoms (e.g., adolescence), family history of bipolar disorder or unpredictable behavior (e.g., multiple relocations, marriages, bankruptcies), risky behaviors, paradoxic response to antidepressants, or treatment-resistant depression.[32]
  - Anxiety disorder—Frequent comorbidity with bipolar disorder (see **Table 238-2**).
- **Schizophrenia**
  - Other psychiatric conditions associated with psychosis: MDD, bipolar disorder, PTSD, brief psychotic disorder (duration less than 1 month), and delusional disorder (nonbizarre delusions and absence of hallucinations, disorganized speech, and negative symptoms).[17]
    - Obsessive–compulsive disorder and body dysmorphic disorder—Prominent obsessions, compulsions, and preoccupations with appearance or body odor, hoarding, or body-focused repetitive behaviors.
    - Autism spectrum disorder—Although encompassing a wide range of symptoms, skills, and levels of disability, often includes deficits in social interaction and repetitive behaviors.
    - Schizoaffective disorder—Mood episode concurrent for a substantial portion of active-phase symptoms; delusions present for 2 weeks without prominent mood symptoms.
    - Schizophreniform disorder—Duration of symptoms at least 1 month but less than 6 months.
  - Medical conditions (AFP)—Hypo- or hyperthyroidism, dementia, vitamin B_{12} deficiency, systemic lupus erythematosus, Cushing syndrome, brain tumor, temporal lobe epilepsy, Wilson disease, porphyria.[17]

MANAGEMENT

INTEGRATED CARE

Although a challenge in today's healthcare system, primary care practices should strive to employ an interdisciplinary team that delivers integrated healthcare services, including mental healthcare. The transition of our offices to patient-centered medical homes offers an opportunity to explore more effective ways of providing this care. Integrating behavioral healthcare providers into primary care settings can result in improved patient functioning and cost savings.[35-37]

Collaborative care has been shown to result in significant improvement in depression and anxiety outcomes compared with usual care based on a Cochrane review of 79 randomized controlled trials (RCTs) involving 24,308 participants.[38] Collaborative services can be provided through a traditional consultation service, by use of telemedicine,[39] or by incorporating co-located or fully integrated behavioral healthcare providers. Newer models of care include the Primary Mental Health Care model and the Integrated Behavioral Healthcare Model (IBHM).[40,41] In the former, a behavioral healthcare provider offers brief, time-limited contacts with patients (e.g., several sessions of 15–30 minutes' duration) and works closely with primary care providers to effect behavior change. In the latter, a behavioral healthcare provider, often a psychiatrist who is usually co-located in the practice, reviews the treatment of patients with mental health conditions and is available to provide direct care; a care manager is assigned to this group of patients to provide regular patient contact and follow-up.

FIRST LINE: ANXIETY

NONPHARMACOLOGIC

- Supportive counseling, education, and cognitive behavioral therapy (CBT) can be considered first-line treatment for anxiety disorders for adults and children.[42] SOR Ⓐ
  - Authors of a Cochrane review found that therapist-supported Internet CBT was more effective than a wait list, attention, information, or online discussion group–only controls.[43] It was not clear if unguided CBT was equally effective, or if therapist-supported Internet CBT was equivalent to therapist-delivered CBT.
  - For patients with PTSD, effective psychological therapies include trauma-focused CBT and eye movement desensitization and reprocessing.[44]

MEDICATION

- Selective serotonin reuptake inhibitors (SSRIs) are well tolerated. SOR Ⓐ Authors of a systematic review and meta-analysis found fluoxetine to be most likely to induce remission; sertraline was best tolerated.[45] Reducing the starting dose and increasing slowly may help reduce initial side effects (e.g., insomnia, jitteriness, gastrointestinal, sexual dysfunction). Use caution if suspecting an underlying bipolar disorder, as SSRIs can unmask or potentiate mania.
- For patients with panic disorder, authors of a meta-analysis found that tricyclic antidepressants (TCAs) were as effective as SSRIs.[46] SOR Ⓐ
- For patients with social anxiety, beta blockers can be considered.[47] SOR Ⓑ

FIRST LINE: DEPRESSION

NONPHARMACOLOGIC

- Psychotherapy is as effective as antidepressant medications after the first 3 months of treatment, and combination treatment with an antidepressant is more effective than either modality alone (number needed to treat [NNT] 4).[24] SOR Ⓐ The 2016 Institute for Clinical Systems Improvement guideline recommends consideration of

combined psychological interventions and pharmacologic interventions for adults with MDD.[48]
  - About one-quarter to one-half of patients respond to some form of psychotherapy.[24]
  - Types of therapy that have proven to be effective include CBT and interpersonal therapy.[24,49] In an RCT of 440 patients with depression, behavioral activation was non-inferior to CBT for depression symptoms score and more cost effective; serious depression-related adverse events occurred in 3 versus 12 cases, respectively.[50] Long-term CBT can prevent recurrence like antidepressants.[51]
- For those who do not respond to initial therapy or who present with more severe depression, the National Institute for Health and Care Excellence (NICE) suggests use of medication, high-intensity psychological therapy, or both and referral to a behavioral health provider for further assessment.[52] Those with severe or complex depression or who are at risk of suicide should be considered for crisis referral, inpatient care, and/or electroconvulsive therapy (ECT).
- Care management programs can decrease depression severity better than usual care,[53] although the degree of integration does not appear to be related to depression outcomes.[54]

MEDICATION

- About one-third to one-half of patients respond to the first medication tried, regardless of class selected. SOR B
- Both TCAs and SSRIs are effective, compared to placebo, for depression treated in primary care settings.[55] For TCAs, the NNT ranges from 7 to 16 and for SSRIs from 7 to 8. The number needed to treat to harm (NNTH for withdrawal due to side effects) ranges from 4 to 30 for TCAs and from 20 to 90 for SSRIs. Data are insufficient to determine the relative effectiveness of antidepressant medication, psychological interventions, or combination interventions in children and adolescents.[56]
- Most commonly used antidepressants have similar reported efficacy and safety; side effects vary and should be considered during shared decision-making with patients. There are also reported differences in efficacy and acceptability within and between classes of medications; for example, authors of one Cochrane review found citalopram to be more effective than paroxetine and reboxetine, more acceptable than TCAs, reboxetine, and venlafaxine, but less effective than escitalopram.[57] Findings for most comparison studies, however, are of limited trustworthiness because of possible treatment overestimation from sponsorship and publication bias.
- Antidepressants such as TCAs, SSRIs, and monoamine oxidase inhibitors are effective in the treatment of dysthymia compared to placebo, with an NNT of about 5.[58] Cochrane authors found no differences between and within drug classes.

FIRST LINE: BIPOLAR DISORDER

Bipolar disorder can be conceptualized as a chronic disease.[33] Treatment goals include stabilizing the mood disturbance (depression or mania), preventing relapse, maximizing function, and identifying and treating comorbidities.

NONPHARMACOLOGIC

- As cognitive impairment and risky behavioral patterns are often present in patients with bipolar disorder, psychological therapies may be needed. Psychological therapies that may be effective in improving symptoms and reducing relapse in patients with bipolar disorder include CBT, patient education, and family-focused therapy.[33] NICE recommends offering patients a psychological intervention designed specifically for bipolar disorder and conducted by psychological therapists trained to care for patients with bipolar disorder.[59] Exercise can also be of benefit.

MEDICATION

- Medication options for bipolar disorder include mood stabilizers and anticonvulsants (**Table 238-3**).[33] NICE recommends that a patient who develops mania or hypomania and who is not currently taking an antipsychotic or mood stabilizer should be offered haloperidol, olanzapine, quetiapine, or risperidone, taking into account the person's preference and clinical context.[59] In primary care settings, NICE recommends starting lithium only for people who have taken lithium before, except under shared care arrangements; NICE recommends against starting valproate in primary care.[59]
  - Monotherapy for mania is associated with fewer side effects and less discontinuation than combination therapy.[60] The three atypical antipsychotics approved by the U.S. Food and Drug Administration (FDA) for bipolar disorder are olanzapine/fluoxetine, quetiapine, and lurasidone; weight gain is associated with all three.
  - For relapse prevention, lithium monotherapy is more effective than divalproex monotherapy.[33] In addition, authors of a systematic review and meta-analysis found lithium effective for reducing risk of suicide (odds ratio [OR] 0.13; 95% CI 0.03–0.66) and death from any cause (OR 0.38; 95% CI 0.15–0.95) compared to placebo.[61]
- Patients with mixed features do not respond as well to pharmacotherapy as those presenting with either depression or mania.[33] Consider use of atypical antipsychotics or divalproex.

FIRST LINE: SCHIZOPHRENIA

For patients presenting with psychosis, first determine whether the condition requires hospitalization for evaluation and treatment of a medical, substance use, or psychiatric condition that poses danger to themselves or others. An urgent psychiatric referral may be helpful in this regard. NICE recommends that primary care clinicians only initiate treatment with medication in consultation with a psychiatrist.[62]

The treatment goal is for remission, defined as a period of 6 months with no symptoms or mild symptoms that do not interfere with a person's behavior.[17]

NONPHARMACOLOGIC

- CBT, family intervention, or social skills training should be offered to patients with schizophrenia.[16,57,63] Authors of a Cochrane review did not find differences in most outcomes, including relapse or rehospitalization, between CBT and other psychosocial therapies.[64] Combination psychosocial treatment plus medication was found in one randomized trial to improve treatment adherence and quality of life, and it decreased hospital admissions in early-stage schizophrenia.[65]

TABLE 238-3 Matching Pharmacotherapeutic Agents to Bipolar States

Medication	Type I Maintenance	Type II Maintenance	Acute Mania	Acute Depression
Aripiprazole	++	++	++	–
Carbamazepine	+++	+++	++	–
Lamotrigine	+++	+++	–	+
Lithium	+++	+++	+++	+ (+++ suicidal thoughts)
Lurasidone	–	–	+	+++
Olanzapine	++	+	+++	++
Olanzapine/Fluoxetine	–	–	–	+++
Oxcarbazepine	+++	+++	+	–
Quetiapine	+	+	+++	+++
Risperidone	++	+	+++	–
Valproic Acid	+++	+++	+++	–
Ziprasidone	++	+	+++	–

(–) No evidence to support; (+) weak evidence; (++) moderate evidence; (+++) strong evidence.
Reproduced with permission from Wells MJ, Kodner CM: Bipolar disorder: Making the Dx, selecting the right Rx, J Fam Pract. 2017 Jun;66(6):375-379. Frontline Medical Communications, Inc.

MEDICATION

- Treatment is initiated with a single antipsychotic (monotherapy); the choice is based on cost, side-effect profile, dosing regimen, and patient preference. Authors of an overview of meta-analyses concluded that although some combination strategies had medium to large effect sizes for symptom control, no pharmacologic combination treatment was supported by sufficiently high-quality or consistent efficacy to recommend them over antipsychotic monotherapy.[66]
  - First-generation antipsychotics include chlorpromazine (300–100 mg daily), haloperidol (5–20 mg daily), perphenazine (16–64 mg daily), or thiothixene (15–60 mg daily).[17] Common side effects include drowsiness, dry mouth, and extrapyramidal symptoms; the most serious complications are neuroleptic malignant syndrome and tardive dyskinesia.
  - Second-generation antipsychotics include aripiprazole (10–30 mg daily), clozapine (150–600 mg daily), lurasidone (40–160 mg daily), olanzapine (10–30 mg daily), paliperidone (3–12 mg daily), quetiapine (300–800 mg daily), risperidone (2–8 mg daily), or ziprasidone (120–200 mg daily). Side effects vary but, for most, include akathisia, hypotension, and weight gain; agranulocytosis, neuroleptic malignant syndrome, and tardive dyskinesia are the most serious complications.[17]
  - There do not appear to be differences in effectiveness of first- or second-generation antipsychotics.[17] However, authors of a multiple treatment meta-analysis were able to develop hierarchies of the comparative efficacy of antipsychotic drugs and of major side effects.[67] Widely accepted guidelines for interpreting the following standardized mean differences (SMDs) are 0.2 as small effect, 0.5 as medium effect, and 0.8 as large effect. All drugs were more effective than placebo, and SMDs were: clozapine 0.88, amisulpride 0.66, olanzapine 0.59, risperidone 0.56, paliperidone 0.50, zotepine 0.49, haloperidol 0.45, quetiapine 0.44, aripiprazole 0.43, sertindole 0.39, ziprasidone 0.39, chlorpromazine 0.38, asenapine 0.38, lurasidone 0.33, and iloperidone 0.33. Odds of discontinuation versus placebo ranged from 0.43 for amisulpride to 0.80 for haloperidol. Odds ratio for extrapyramidal side effects versus placebo ranged from 0.30 for clozapine to 4.76 for haloperidol.
  - Response to medication at 2 to 4 weeks is predictive of long-term response, but it may take several months for maximal effect.[68]

SECOND LINE

ANXIETY

- Other medications to consider are serotonergic norepinephrine reuptake inhibitors (side effects include nausea, insomnia, and headaches) and pregabalin (side effects include dizziness, dry mouth, loss of balance, tremors, and weight gain); the latter can be useful for GAD, and onset of efficacy is often within the first few days of treatment.[22]
- Benzodiazepines can be useful adjuncts to SSRIs in the initiation phase of treatment. While useful for anxiety symptoms, side effects include sedation, dizziness, and prolonged reaction time with negative effects on cognitive function and driving skills. Risks include dependency, and a history of alcoholism or substance dependence is a contraindication; use of longer-acting agents can help reduce risk of dependency.
- Azapirones such as buspirone are also an option for patients suffering from GAD. Authors of a Cochrane review found that azapirones appear to be superior to placebo in the short term (4–9 weeks) but may not be superior to benzodiazepines or as acceptable to patients as benzodiazapines.[69]
- With respect to second-generation antipsychotics, authors of a Cochrane review found data supporting use of quetiapine for symptoms of GAD; however, side effects limited tolerability.[70]

- Alternative therapies with supporting evidence of efficacy include massage, exercise, and relaxation.[22]

DEPRESSION

- Aerobic exercise is effective and recommended for patients without contraindications (NNT = 5 for high-intensity aerobic exercise), but medication therapy works faster with less treatment discontinuation.[24] In a Cochrane review of exercise for depression treatment, however, the effect size was small.[71]
- Other medications that can useful in patients with depression include vilazodone, a selective serotonin 1a receptor partial agonist and reuptake inhibitor, and anti-glucocorticoids (e.g., mifepristone, metyrapone, and DHEA).[24] Use caution if prescribing mirtazapine (Remeron) and venlafaxine (Effexor), as these drugs have been associated with higher rates of completed suicide in primary care patients compared to other antidepressants (1-year absolute suicide risk ranged from 0.02% for amitriptyline to 0.19% for mirtazapine).[72] For patients with treatment-resistant depression, antidepressant agents can be augmented with thyroid hormone or benzodiazepines (the latter for patients with prominent anxiety symptoms).[24]
- Complementary and alternative therapies that may be helpful for patients with depression include St. John's wort, saffron stigma and petal, lavender (as an adjunct), Rhodiola, tryptophan, and 5-hydroxytryptophan.[73,74]

BIPOLAR DISORDER

- For patients who fail the initial mediation, whether due to lack of efficacy or unacceptable side effects, NICE recommends selecting an alternative antipsychotic, taking into account any the person's preference and clinical context.[59] If the second medication fails to control symptoms, consider the addition of lithium.
- Antidepressants can be used as adjunctive therapy, but not monotherapy; combination fluoxetine and olanzapine has been approved, but authors of a meta-analysis found that such augmentation did not improve remission or relapse rates over mood stabilizers alone.[75]
- In an RCT of 73 inpatients with treatment-resistant bipolar disorder, ECT was significantly more effective than algorithm-based pharmacologic treatment at 6 weeks for response rate (73.9% vs. 35.0%), but the remission rate did not differ between the groups (34.8% vs. 30.0%).[76]

SCHIZOPHRENIA

- Antidepressants and anxiolytics can be helpful as adjunctive therapy for treating comorbid psychiatric disorders.[17] Adjunctive treatment with valproate also appears to be more effective than antipsychotic monotherapy.[77] It is not known which antipsychotic is more effective for patients with treatment-resistant schizophrenia.
- Extrapyramidal symptoms can be treated with propranolol, lorazepam, amantadine, benztropine, or diphenhydramine; tardive dyskinesia is usually irreversible, but medication discontinuation may lessen symptoms.[17]
- ECT was shown to be effective in a small crossover trial of clozapine-resistant schizophrenia.[78]

SCREENING

- Screening for anxiety, bipolar disorder, or schizophrenia is not recommended in the general population. In fact, the NICE guideline on bipolar disorder recommends against using questionnaires for case finding.[59] Of note, authors of one study found that children of patients with MDD and bipolar disorder had much higher rates of mood and anxiety disorders (MDD probands: 25.5% any mood and 44.6% any anxiety disorder; bipolar disorder probands: 34.5% any mood and 42.5% any anxiety disorder; controls: 12.6% any mood and 22.8% any anxiety disorder), which might justify screening.[79]
- Depression screening is recommended by the U.S. Preventive Service Task Force in the general adult population, including pregnant and postpartum women, and for MDD in adolescents ages 12–18 years, provided there are adequate systems in place to ensure accurate diagnosis, effective treatment, and appropriate follow-up (2016). SOR Ⓑ

PROGNOSIS

- All-cause mortality is significantly higher among patients with mental disorders compared to the general population or controls (relative risk 2.22; 95% CI 2.12–2.33); most deaths (67%) are due to natural causes, and the median years of potential life lost is 10 years.[80] This is likely due to multiple factors including behavioral and lifestyle factors (e.g., tobacco use), access to and quality of healthcare, and social determinants of health such as poverty and social connectedness.[80]
- **Anxiety:** Remission rates following treatment are about 30% to 40%. Discontinuing antidepressant treatment for patients with anxiety disorders results in relapse in almost one-third, and 1 in 6 patients previously treated successfully will relapse despite continued treatment.[81]

Patients with GAD often have prolonged symptoms that wax and wane over time.[22] In one 40-year follow-up study, GAD remitted by age 50 years, but many patients had continued difficulty with undifferentiated somatic disorders.[82] Treatment response is poorer in patients with concomitant depression.[22]

- **Depression:** Patients with untreated recurrent major depressive episodes experience remission within 3–6 months.[83] Two-thirds of patients with one prior episode of MDD will experience recurrence during the next 10 years; risk of recurrence increases with each subsequent episode.[24]
- **Bipolar disorder:** In one study of inpatients diagnosed with bipolar I or II and treated with a variety of mood stabilizers, time to remission in months was significantly longer in those with depressive mixed-state and subthreshold mixed-state than in the pure depressive state group.[84] Those with bipolar disorder have a reduced life expectancy of up to 9 years compared to the general population, likely due to unrecognize comorbid conditions and lack of access to care.[32]
- **Schizophrenia:** The clinical course is varied, with about 20% expected to have a positive outcome and the remainder having remissions and exacerbations or a more chronic course.[17] Authors of a meta-analysis found that after a first psychotic episode, over half (57.9%) achieved symptomatic and/or functional improvement

with an average follow-up of 5.5 years. Remission rates were higher among patients with affective psychosis (84.6%).[85]

- Persons with schizophrenia pose a high risk for suicide; lifetime risk is about 5%.[17] Patients with auditory hallucinations, delusions, substance abuse, and history of prior suicide attempts are at higher risk.
- The overall mortality rate for patients with schizophrenia is 2 to 3 times higher than that for the general public, attributed primarily to cardiovascular disease, stroke, thromboembolic events, respiratory disease, and cancer.[86] The high prevalence of smoking contributes to many of these conditions.

FOLLOW-UP

- For patients with **depression**, monitor for suicidality, symptom severity, functional status, mania, and new psychiatric symptoms. If on medication, assess side effects and adherence.
  - Reevaluate patients every 1 to 4 weeks in the acute phase and at least monthly until symptom remission. NICE guidelines recommend follow-up for patients treated only with antidepressants at least every 2–4 weeks for at least the first 3 months of treatment.[52] If symptoms have not remitted after 4–8 weeks on a given regimen, adjust treatment. All antidepressant classes are equally effective at inducing remission following treatment failure with another class.[24]
  - For maintenance, follow patients every 2–3 months. All antidepressant classes prevent relapse and recurrence during continuation and maintenance phases. NICE recommends continuing antidepressants for those who benefit from treatment for at least 6 months after remission, extending to at least 2 years for people at risk of relapse.[52]
  - Discontinuation of SSRIs has been associated with a withdrawal reaction (i.e., antidepressant treatment discontinuation syndrome) that includes sensory, gastrointestinal-related, somatic, and psychiatric symptoms.[87] SSRIs should be tapered off slowly if possible to minimize the withdrawal reactions.
- Patients with **bipolar disorder** should undergo comprehensive health screening annually with attention focused on early detection of metabolic syndrome, cardiovascular disease, diabetes, respiratory disease, and comorbid psychiatric illness. NICE recommends development of a risk management plan with the person and their caregiver, if possible, to address personal, social, occupational, or environmental triggers and early warning signs and symptoms of relapse.[59]
- For patients on long-term lithium therapy, the NICE guidelines recommend obtaining yearly renal and thyroid function, and calcium levels.[59] For patients with bipolar disorder who are under the care of their primary care provider, consider referral to secondary care for any one of the following[59]:
  - Poor or partial response to treatment
  - Functioning declines significantly
  - Treatment adherence is poor
  - The person develops intolerable or medically important side effects from medication
  - Comorbid alcohol or drug misuse is suspected
  - The person is considering stopping medication after a period of relatively stable mood
  - A woman with bipolar disorder is pregnant or planning a pregnancy
- For patients with schizophrenia on antipsychotics, follow-up is recommended as needed or every 6 weeks to monitor adherence and response to treatment, medication side effects, blood pressure, weight, and fasting glucose and lipid levels—the latter two if second-generation antipsychotics are prescribed.[17]

PATIENT EDUCATION

- Patients and their caregivers and families should be educated about their diagnosis, treatment options, and prognosis.
- For most patients, combining some form of psychosocial therapy with medication may be optimal. Recurrence is common, and maintaining vigilance for symptoms and a relationship with a primary care provider should be encouraged.

PATIENT RESOURCES

- National Institute of Mental Health. *Mental Health Information*—**https://www.nimh.nih.gov/health/topics/index.shtml.**
- Anxiety and Depression Association of America. *Understanding the Facts* (includes information on support groups)—**https://adaa.org/understanding-anxiety#.**
- MedlinePlus. *Anxiety* (also depression, bipolar disorder, and schizophrenia topics)—**https://medlineplus.gov/anxiety.html.**

PROVIDER RESOURCES

- American Psychiatric Association. *Diagnostic and Statistical Manual of Mental Disorders (DSM-5).* 5th ed. Washington, DC: American Psychiatric Publishing; 2013.
- Centers for Disease Control and Prevention. *Mental Health Basics*—**https://www.cdc.gov/mentalhealth/learn/index.htm.**
- National Institute of Mental Health. *Health Topics: Mental Disorders and Related Topics*—**https://www.nimh.nih.gov/health/topics/index.shtml.**

REFERENCES

1. World Health Organization. *The Global Burden of Disease: 2004 Update*. Geneva, Switzerland: WHO Press; 2008.
2. Moriarty DG, Zack MM, Holt JB, et al. Geographic patterns of frequent mental distress: U.S. adults, 1993–2001 and 2003–2006. *Am J Prev Med.* 2009;46:497-505.
3. Roll JM, Kennedy J, Tran M, Howell D. Disparities in unmet need for mental health services in the United States, 1997–2010. *Psychiatr Serv*. 2013;64(1):80-82.
4. Kessler RC, Aguilar-Gaxiola S, Alonso J, et al. The global burden of mental disorders: an update from the WHO World Mental Health (WMH) surveys. *Epidemiol Psichiatr Soc.* 2009;18(1):23-33.
5. McLean CP, Asnaani A, Litz BT, Hofmann SG. Gender differences in anxiety disorders: Prevalence, course of illness, comorbidity and burden of illness. *J Psychiatr Res.* 2011;45(8):1027-1035.
6. Kroenke K, Spitzer RL, Williams J, et al. Anxiety disorders in primary care: prevalence, impairment, comorbidity, and detection. *Ann Intern Med.* 2007;146(5):317-325.

7. Greenberg PE, Sisitsky T, Kessler RC, et al. The economic burden of anxiety disorders in the 1990s. *J Clin Psychiatry.* 1999;60(7): 427-435.
8. Albert PR. Why is depression more common in women? *J Psychiatry Neurosci.* 2015;40(4):219-221.
9. National Center for Health Statistics. *Depression in the U.S. Household Population, 2009–2012.* https://www.cdc.gov/nchs/data/databriefs/db172.htm. Accessed January 2, 2018.
10. Centers for Disease Control and Prevention. *Burden of Mental Illness.* https://www.cdc.gov/mentalhealth/basics/burden.htm. Accessed January 2018.
11. Kessler RC, Berglund P, Demler O, et al. Lifetime prevalence and age-of-onset distributions of DSM-IV disorders in the National Comorbidity Survey Replication. *Arch Gen Psychiatry.* 2006; 62(6):593-602.
12. Kroon JS, Wohlfarth TD, Dieleman J, et al. Incidence rates and risk factors of bipolar disorder in the general population: a population-based cohort study. *Bipolar Disord.* 2013;15(3): 306-313.
13. Merikangas KR, Jin R, He JP, et al. Prevalence and correlates of bipolar spectrum disorder in the World Mental Health Survey Initiative. *Arch Gen Psychiatry.* 2011;68(3):241-251.
14. Manning JS. Bipolar disorder, bipolar depression and comorbid illness. *J Fam Pract.* 2015;64(6 Suppl):S10-15.
15. Bauer MS, Aktsheuler L, Evans DR, et al. Prevalence and distinct correlates of anxiety, substance, and combined comorbidity in a multisite public sector sample with bipolar disorder. *J Affect Disord.* 2005;85(3):301-315.
16. Saha S, Chant D, Welham J, McGrath J. A systematic review of the prevalence of schizophrenia. *PLoS Med.* 2005 May;2(5):e141.
17. Holder SD, Wayhs A. Schizophrenia. *Am Fam Physician.* 2014; 90(11):775-782.
18. Andreasen NC, Black DW. *Introductory Textbook of Psychiatry.* 4th ed. Washington, DC: American Psychiatric Publishing; 2006.
19. Gara MA, Vega WA, Arndt S, et al. Influence of patient race and ethnicity on clinical assessment in patients with affective disorders. *Arch Gen Psychiatry.* 2012;69(6):593-600.
20. Goeree R, Farahati F, Burke N, et al. The economic burden of schizophrenia in Canada in 2004. *Curr Med Res Opin.* 2005;21: 2017-2028.
21. Bhatt, NV. *Anxiety Disorders.* https://emedicine.medscape.com/article/286227-overview. Updated Jun 09, 2017. Accessed January 2018.
22. Shearer SL. *Generalized Anxiety Disorder.* http://www.essentialevidenceplus.com.proxy1.cl.msu.edu/content/eee/623. Updated November 24, 2016. Accessed January 2018.
23. National Institutes of Mental Health. *Post-Traumatic Stress Disorder.* https://www.nimh.nih.gov/health/topics/post-traumatic-stress-disorder-ptsd/index.shtml. Accessed January 2018.
24. Rubin SR. *Depression.* http://www.essentialevidenceplus.com.proxy1.cl.msu.edu/content/eee/624. Updated December 28, 2017. Accessed January 2018.
25. Bromberger JT, Kravitz HM, Chang YF, et al. Major depression during and after the menopausal transition: Study of Women's Health Across the Nation (SWAN). *Psychol Med.* 2011;41(9): 1879-1888.
26. Phillips ML, Swartz HA. A critical appraisal of neuroimaging studies of bipolar disorder: toward a new conceptualization of underlying neural circuitry and a road map for future research. *Am J Psychiatry.* 2014;171(8):829-843.
27. Craddock N, Sklar P. Genetics of bipolar disorder. *Lancet.* 2013; 381(9878):1654-1662.
28. French L, Gray C, Leonard G, et al. Early cannabis use, polygenic risk score for schizophrenia and brain maturation in adolescence. *JAMA Psychiatry.* 2015;72(10):1002-1011.
29. Kahn RS, Sommer IE. The neurobiology and treatment of first-episode schizophrenia. *Mol Psychiatry.* 2015;20(1):84-97.
30. Paradies Y, Ben J, Denson N, et al. Racism as a determinant of health: a systematic review and meta-analysis. *PLoS One.* 2015; 10(9):e0138511.
31. American Psychiatric Association. *Diagnostic and Statistical Manual of Mental Disorders (DSM-5).* 5th ed. Washington, DC: American Psychiatric Publishing; 2013.
32. Culpepper L. Pathways to the diagnosis of bipolar disorder. *J Fam Pract.* 2015;64(6):S4-S9.
33. McIntyre RS. Evidence-based treatment of bipolar disorder, bipolar depression and mixed features. *J Fam Pract.* 2015;64(6):S16-S23.
34. National Institute of Mental Health. *Bipolar Disorder.* https://www.nimh.nih.gov/health/topics/bipolar-disorder/index.shtml. Accessed January 2018.
35. Bryan CJ, Morrow C, Appolonio KK. Impact of behavioral health consultant interventions on patient symptoms and functioning in an integrated family medicine clinic. *J Clin Psychol.* 2009;65(3): 281-293.
36. Ray-Sannerud BN, Dolan DC, Morrow CE, et al. Longitudinal outcomes after brief behavioral intervention in an integrated primary care clinic. *Fam Syst Health.* 2012;30(1):60-71.
37. Katon WJ, Roy-Byrne P, Russo J, Cowley D. Cost-effectives and cost offset of a collaborative care intervention for primary care patients with panic order. *Arch Gen Psychiatry.* 2002;59:1098-1104.
38. Archer J, Bower P, Gilbody S, et al. Collaborative care for depression and anxiety problems. *Cochrane Database Syst Rev.* 2012; (10):CD006525.
39. Hilty DM, Ferrer DC, Parish MB, et al. The effectiveness of telemental health: a 2013 review. *Telemed J E Health.* 2013;19(6): 444-454.
40. Strosahl K. Integrating behavioral health and primary care services: The primary mental health care model. In: Blount A (ed.): *Integrated Primary Care: The Future of Medical and Mental Health Collaboration.* New York, NY: WW Norton; 1998: 139-166.
41. Agency for Healthcare Research and Quality. *What Is Integrated Behavioral Health Care?* https://integrationacademy.ahrq.gov/resources/ibhc-measures-atlas/what-integrated-behavioral-health-care-ibhc. Accessed January 2018.

42. James AC, James G, Cowdrey FA, et al. Cognitive behavioural therapy for anxiety disorders in children and adolescents. *Cochrane Database Syst Rev*. 2015;(2):CD004690.
43. Olthuis JV, Watt MC, Bailey K, et al. Therapist-supported Internet cognitive behavioural therapy for anxiety disorders in adults. *Cochrane Database Syst Rev*. 2016;(3):CD011565.
44. Greenberg N, Brooks S, Dunn R. Latest developments in post-traumatic stress disorder: diagnosis and treatment. *Br Med Bull*. 2015;114(1):147-155.
45. Baldwin D, Woods R, Lawson R, Taylor D. Efficacy of drug treatments for generalised anxiety disorder: systematic review and meta-analysis. *BMJ*. 2011;342:d1199.
46. Otto MW, Tuby KS, Gould RA, et al. An effect-size analysis of the relative efficacy and tolerability of serotonin selective reuptake inhibitors for panic disorder. *Am J Psychiatry*. 2001;158:1989-1992.
47. Steenen SA, Wijk AJ, van der Heijden G, et al. Propranolol for the treatment of anxiety disorders: systematic review and meta-analysis. *J Psychopharmacol*. 2016;30(2):128-139.
48. National Guideline Clearinghouse (NGC). *Guideline Summary: Adult Depression in Primary Care*. National Guideline Clearinghouse (NGC) [website]. Rockville (MD): Agency for Healthcare Research and Quality (AHRQ). Accessed March 2016.
49. Twomey C, O'Reilly G, Byrne M. Effectiveness of cognitive behavioural therapy for anxiety and depression in primary care: a meta-analysis. *Fam Pract*. 2015;32:3-15.
50. Richards DA, Ekers D, McMillan D, et al. Cost and outcome of behavioural activation versus cognitive behavioural therapy for depression (COBRA): a randomised, controlled, non-inferiority trial. *Lancet*. 2016;388(10047):871-880.
51. Kuyken W, Hayes R, Barrett B, et al. Effectiveness and cost-effectiveness of mindfulness-based cognitive therapy compared with maintenance antidepressant treatment in the prevention of depressive relapse or recurrence (PREVENT): a randomised controlled trial. *Lancet*. 2015;386(9988):63-73.
52. National Institute for Health and Care Excellence. *Depression in Adults*. March 2011. https://www.nice.org.uk/guidance/qs8/chapter/List-of-statements. Accessed January 2018.
53. Neumeyer-Gromen A, Lampert T, Stark K, Kallischnigg G. Disease management programs for depression: a systematic review and meta-analysis of randomized controlled trials. *Med Care*. 2004;42:1211-1221.
54. Butler M, Kane RL, McAlpine D, et al. Does integrated care improve treatment for depression? A systematic review. *J Ambul Care Manage*. 2011;34:113-125.
55. Arroll B, Elley CR, Fishman T, et al. Antidepressants versus placebo for depression in primary care. *Cochrane Database Syst Rev*. 2009;(3):CD007954.
56. Cox GR, Callahan P, Churchill R, et al. Psychological therapies versus antidepressant medication, alone and in combination for depression in children and adolescents. *Cochrane Database Syst Rev*. 2014;(11):CD008324.
57. Cipriani A, Purgato M, Furukawa TA, et al. Citalopram versus other anti-depressive agents for depression. *Cochrane Database Syst Rev*. 2012;(7):CD006534.
58. Silva de Lima M, Moncrieff J, Soares BG. Drugs versus placebo for dysthymia. *Cochrane Database Syst Rev*. 2015;(6):CD001130.
59. National Institute for Health and Care Excellence. *Assessment and Management of Bipolar Disorder: Summary of Updated NICE Guidance*. https://www.nice.org.uk/guidance/cg185. Accessed January 2018.
60. Geoffroy PA, Etain B, Henry C, Bellivier F. Combination therapy for manic phases: a critical review of common practice. *CNS Neurosci Ther*. 2012;18(12):957-964.
61. Cipriani A, Hawton K, Stockton S, Geddes JR. Lithium in the prevention of suicide in mood disorders: updated systematic review and meta-analysis. *BMJ*. 2013;346:f3646.
62. National Institute for Health and Care Excellence. NICE Guidelines for Schizophrenia. http://www.nice.org.uk/Guidenace/CG178. Accessed January 2018.
63. Morrison AP, Turkington D, Pyle M, et al. Cognitive therapy for people with schizophrenia spectrum disorders not taking antipsychotic drugs: a single-blind randomised controlled trial. *Lancet*. 2014;383(9926):1395-1403.
64. Jones C, Hacker D, Cormac I, et al. Cognitive behaviour therapy versus other psychosocial treatments for schizophrenia. *Cochrane Database Syst Rev*. 2012;(4):CD008712.
65. Guo X, Zhai J, Liu Z, et al. Effect of antipsychotic medication alone vs combined with psychosocial intervention on outcomes of early-stage schizophrenia: a randomized 1-year study. *Arch Gen Psychiatry*. 2010;67(9):895-904.
66. Correll CU, Rubio JM, Inczedy-Farkas G, et al. Efficacy of 42 pharmacologic cotreatment strategies added to antipsychotic monotherapy in schizophrenia: systematic overview and quality appraisal of the meta-analytic evidence. *JAMA Psychiatry*. 2017;74(7):675-684.
67. Leeucht S, Cipriani A, Spineli L, et al. Comparative efficacy and tolerability of 15 antipsychotic drugs in schizophrenia: a multiple-treatments meta-analysis. *Lancet*. 2013;382(9896):951-962.
68. Lieberman JA, Stroup TS, McEvoy JP, et al. Effectiveness of antipsychotic drugs in patients with chronic schizophrenia. *N Engl J Med*. 2005;353(12):1209-1223.
69. Chessick CA, Allen MH, Thase M, et al. Azapirones for generalized anxiety disorder. *Cochrane Database Syst Rev*. 2006;(3):CD006115.
70. Depping AM, Komossa K, Kissling W, Leucht S. Second-generation antipsychotics for anxiety disorders. *Cochrane Database Syst Rev*. 2010;(12):CD008120.
71. Cooney GM, Dwan K, Greig CA, et al. Exercise for depression. *Cochrane Database Syst Rev*. 2013;(9):CD004366.
72. Coupland C, Hill T, Morriss R, et al. Antidepressant use and risk of suicide and attempted suicide or self harm in people aged 20 to 64: cohort study using a primary care database. *BMJ*. 2015;350:h517.
73. Carpenter DJ. St. John's wort and *S*-adenosyl methionine as "natural" alternatives to conventional antidepressants in the era of the suicidality boxed warning: what is the evidence for clinically relevant benefit? *Altern Med Rev*. 2011;16(1):17-39.

74. Shaw K, Turner J, Del Mar C. Tryptophan and 5-hydroxytryptophan for depression. *Cochrane Database Syst Rev*. 2002;(1):CD003198.

75. Sidor MM, MacQueen GM. Antidepressants for the acute treatment of bipolar depression: a systematic review and meta-analysis. *J Clin Psychiatry*. 2011;72(2):156-167.

76. Schoeyen HK, Kessler U, Andreassen OA, et al. Treatment-resistant bipolar depression: a randomized controlled trial of electroconvulsive therapy versus algorithm-based pharmacological treatment. *Am J Psychiatry*. 2015;172(1):41-51.

77. Tseng PT, Chen YW, Chung W, et al. Significant effect of valproate augmentation therapy in patients with schizophrenia: a meta-analysis study. *Medicine (Baltimore)*. 2016;95(4):e2475.

78. Petrides G, Malur C, Braga RJ, et al. Electroconvulsive therapy augmentation in clozapine-resistant schizophrenia: a prospective, randomized study. *JAMA Psychiatry*. 2015;172(1):52-58.

79. Vandeleur C, Rothen S, Gholam-Rezaee M, et al. Mental disorders in offspring of parents with bipolar and major depressive disorders. *Bipolar Disord*. 2012;14(6):641-653.

80. Walker ER, McGee RE, Druss BG. Mortality in mental disorders and global disease burden implications: a systematic review and meta-analysis. *JAMA Psychiatry*. 2015;72(4):334-341.

81. Batelaan NM, Bosman RC, Muntingh A, et al. Risk of relapse after antidepressant discontinuation in anxiety disorders, obsessive-compulsive disorder, and post-traumatic stress disorder: systematic review and meta-analysis of relapse prevention trials. *BMJ*. 2017;358:j3927.

82. Rubio G, Lopez-Ibor JJ. Generalized anxiety disorder: a 40-year follow-up study. *Acta Psychiatr Scand*. 2007;115:372-379.

83. Posternak MA, Solomon DA, Leon AC, et al. The naturalistic course of unipolar major depression in the absence of somatic therapy. *J Nerv Ment Dis*. 2006;194:324-329.

84. Shim IH, Woo YS, Jun TY, Bahk WM. Mixed-state bipolar I and II depression: time to remission and clinical characteristics. *J Affect Disord*. 2014;152-154:340-346.

85. Lally J, Ajnakina O, Stubbs B, et al. Remission and recovery from first-episode psychosis in adults: systematic review and meta-analysis of long-term outcome studies. *Br J Psychiatry*. 2017;211(6):350-358.

86. Lwin AM, Symeon C, Jan F, Sule A. Morbidity and mortality in schizophrenia. *Br J Hosp Med*. 2011;72(11):628-630.

87. Renoir T. Selective serotonin reuptake inhibitor antidepressant treatment discontinuation syndrome: a review of the clinical evidence and the possible mechanisms involved. *Front Pharmacol*. 2013;4:45.

239 HEADACHE

Heidi S. Chumley, MD, MBA

PATIENT STORY

A 35-year-old woman presented to the office to discuss her migraines. She has episodic unilateral throbbing headaches accompanied by nausea, photophobia, and phonophobia. She used to have a migraine about every 3 months, but is now having one almost every 2 weeks. As this frequency interferes with her life, prophylactic therapy is discussed. She accepts, and her migraine frequency decreases dramatically.

INTRODUCTION

More than 77% of adults experience headaches during their lifetime. Headaches are either primary (migraine, tension-type, trigeminal autonomic cephalgias, or other primary) or secondary (headaches attributed to another cause, including headache medication overuse). The presence or absence of red flags is useful to distinguish dangerous causes of secondary headaches. The most common primary headaches are tension-type and migraine; cluster headache is the most common trigeminal autonomic cephalgia. Medication overuse can complicate headache therapy. Treatment and prognosis depend on type of headache.

EPIDEMIOLOGY

- Lifetime prevalence estimated to be greater than 77% in adults.[1]
- Fifty-three percent of adults (61% of women and 45% of men), and 53% of children have had a headache in the past year.[1] Elderly adults have a lower rate of headaches, with 36% reporting a headache in the past year.
- Episodic tension-type headache (TTH) prevalence is 62.6% in adults and 15.9% in children.[1]
- Chronic (>15 days per month) TTH has a prevalence of 3.3% in adults and 0.9% in children.[1]
- Migraine has a prevalence of 14.7% in adults (8% in men, 17.6% in women) and 9.2% in children.[1]
- Medication overuse contributes to daily headache in approximately 1% of adults in the general population.[1]
- Cluster headache has a lifetime prevalence of 0.2% to 0.3%.[1]

ETIOLOGY AND PATHOPHYSIOLOGY

- TTH etiology is uncertain, but likely caused by activation of peripheral afferent neurons in head and neck muscles.[2]
- Migraine headache is thought to be caused by genetically influenced neuronal hypersensitivity and anatomic alterations that contribute to extreme sensitivity to changes in homeostasis, which is experienced as recurrent headaches.[3] Nociceptive input from the meningeal vessels is abnormally modulated in the dorsal raphe nucleus, locus coeruleus, and nucleus raphe magnus. This activation can be seen on positron emission tomography (PET) scan during an acute attack (**Figure 239-1**).
- Trigeminal autonomic cephalgias (TACs), which include cluster headaches, are caused by trigeminal activation with hypothalamic involvement, but the inciting mechanism is unknown.[4]

RISK FACTORS

- For migraines—Family history.
- For TACs—Family history.[5]
- For medication overuse headache—Regular use of any medication used to treat acute headaches, most commonly simple analgesics and triptans.

DIAGNOSIS

CLINICAL FEATURES

- Red flags for dangerous secondary cause—Sudden onset; worsening pattern; history of cancer, HIV, or systemic illness (fever, rash, etc.); focal neurologic signs or seizures; vision changes; papilledema; headache worsened by Valsalva or position changes; new headache during pregnancy or postpartum; new headache after age 50 years.[6,7]
- Tension-type headache—At least two of the following: bilateral location, mild to moderate intensity, pressure (nonpulsating) type pain, and not aggravated by physical activity, and without nausea or vomiting, or photophobia and phonophobia. Classified as infrequent episodic, frequent episodic, or chronic based on headache pattern.[8]
- Migraine headache—At least 5 episodes with at least two of the following: unilateral location, pulsating, moderate-to-severe headache, and aggravated by physical activity; and accompanied by nausea or emesis or photophobia and phonophobia. Classified as without aura, with aura, or chronic based on presence or absence of aura and frequency.[8]
- Trigeminal autonomic cephalgias (TAC)—Cluster headache is the most common TAC: severe unilateral orbital, suborbital, or temporal pain with either ipsilateral autonomic feature (i.e., conjunctival injection, lacrimation, nasal congestion, ptosis, etc.) or agitation/restlessness (as opposed to migraine sufferers, who are quiet and still).[5] Classified as episodic or chronic[8] (**Figure 239-2**).
- Medication overuse headache—Secondary headache that accompanies a preexisting headache disorder; frequency ≥15 days per month, with regular overuse of acute medications, such as triptans or opiates, for more than 3 months.[8]

TYPICAL DISTRIBUTION

- Tension headaches are typically bilateral (**Figure 239-3**).
- Migraine and cluster headaches are typically unilateral.

LABORATORY TESTING

- Generally not indicated.
- May be used when a secondary cause such as infection is suspected.

IMAGING

- Generally not indicated.
- MRI when red flags are present.

DIFFERENTIAL DIAGNOSIS

- Common primary headaches include infrequent and episodic TTH and migraine.
- Secondary causes of headache, other than medication overuse headache, are less common and include systemic illnesses/infections, brain masses, subarachnoid hemorrhage (**Figure 239-4**), or increased intracranial pressure.
- Medication overuse headache is predominantly seen with a primary headache, but may also accompany a secondary headache.

MANAGEMENT

Tension-type headache:

- Acute therapy.
  - Aspirin 1000 mg, ibuprofen 400 mg, or naproxen 500 mg; acetaminophen 1000 mg when nonsteroidal anti-inflammatory drugs (NSAIDs) cannot be used.[9]
  - Avoid opiates.
  - Limit acute medications to less than 3 times a week to reduce the risk of medication overuse headache.
- Consider preventive therapy if headaches occur once a week.
  - First line: Amitriptyline or nortriptyline—Begin at 10 mg a day and titrate up to 100 mg a day using the lowest effective dose.[9]
  - Second line: Mirtazapine 30 mg a day or venlafaxine 150 mg a day.[9]
  - Acupuncture may be helpful.[10]

Migraine headache:

- Use a stepped approach to treat acute migraine episodes.
  - Start with aspirin 1000 mg, ibuprofen 400 mg, naproxen 500 mg, or acetaminophen 1000 mg.[9]
  - Second line: triptan (i.e., sumatriptan 100 mg oral or 6 mg subcutaneously if vomiting); add an antiemetic if needed.[9]
  - Third line: naproxen 500 mg with a triptan.[9]
  - Fourth line: combinational analgesic (with opioid if needed); do not use routinely.[9]
- Consider prophylaxis for patients whose migraines have a negative impact on their lives, or to decrease risk of developing medication overuse headache when frequency requires use of simple analgesics more than 15 days a month or use of opioids, triptans, or combination analgesics more than 10 days a month.

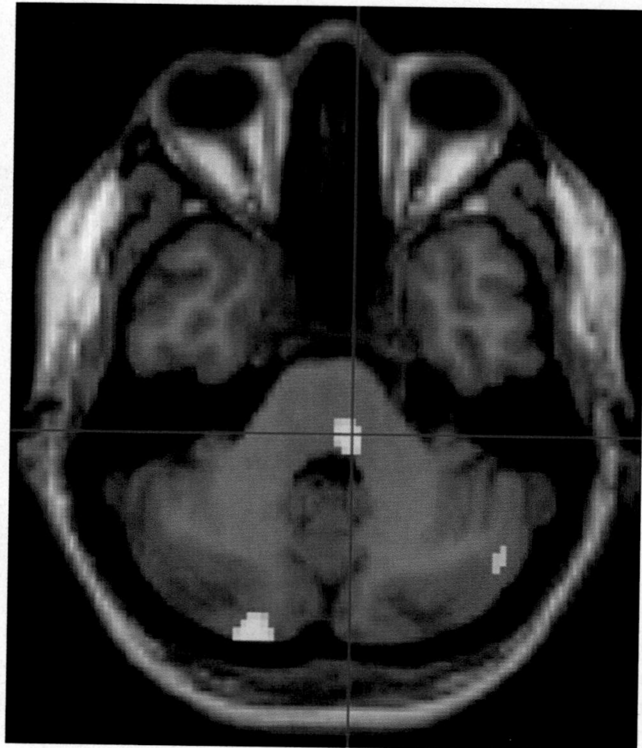

FIGURE 239-1 Imaging has helped clarify the etiology of migraine disorder. This positron emission tomography image shows activation in the dorsolateral pons, which includes the noradrenergic locus coeruleus, an area that modulates nociceptive input from the meningeal vessels. (*Reproduced with permission from Longo D, Fauci A, Kasper D, et al: Harrison's Principles of Internal Medicine, 18th ed. New York, NY: McGraw-Hill Education; 2011.*)

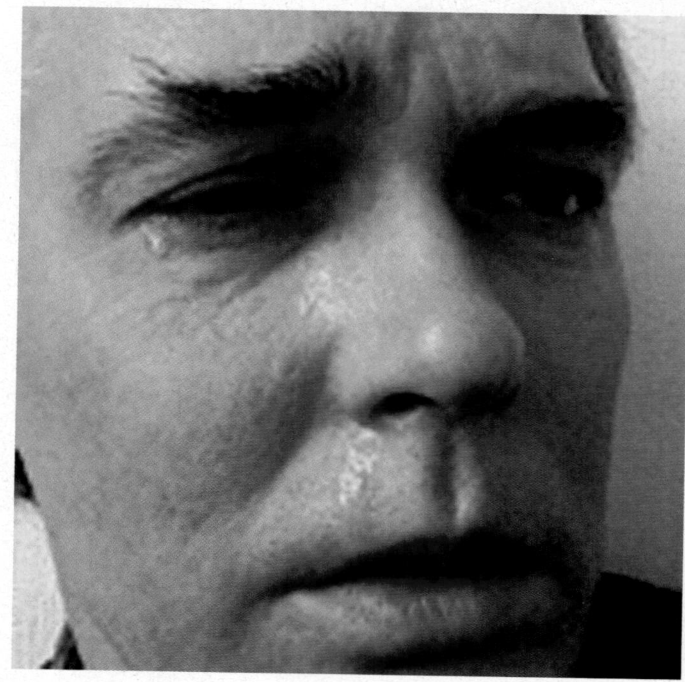

FIGURE 239-2 Lacrimation, ptosis, and lid edema seen in cluster headache. (*Reproduced with permission from The International Headache Society, http://ihs-classification.org/en/. Copyright www.ihs-classification.org; Copyright (2012) Prof. Hartmut Göbel, Germany, www.schmerzklinik.de.*)

- Amitriptyline (before bedtime starting with 10 or 25 mg and titrate up as needed and tolerated), divalproex sodium 500 to 1500 mg daily, topiramate 100 mg daily, venlafaxine 150 mg daily, and multiple β-blockers have each demonstrated 50% reduction in migraine frequency.[11]
- Riboflavin 400 mg daily, coenzyme Q10 300 mg daily, butterbur 50 mg twice daily have each demonstrated 50% reduction in migraine frequency.[11]
- Magnesium citrate 600 mg daily also reduces migraine frequency and has an A rating in pregnancy.[11]

- Cognitive behavioral therapy, biofeedback, stress management, and lifestyle modification may also be useful.[12]
- Acupuncture may provide additional benefit.[13]

Cluster headache:

- Acute episode:
  - Inhaled high-flow oxygen 10 to 15 L per minute.[5]
  - Sumatriptan 6 mg subcutaneously[5]; contraindicated in pregnancy, lactation, coronary artery disease, stroke, peripheral artery disease.
- Several agents may be effective for prophylactic therapy including verapamil or topiramate.[5]
- Refer refractory patients for evaluations for other medical or surgical therapies.

Medication overuse headaches:

- Educate patients that chronic medication use is contributing to their daily headaches.[14]
- Abruptly stop (when safe) or taper the overused medication.[14]
- Inpatient withdrawal is recommended for patients overusing opiates, benzodiazepines, or barbiturates.[14]
- Start prophylactic therapy with topiramate 100 to 200 mg daily prior to initiating withdrawal or as soon as possible after withdrawal has been initiated.[14]

REFERRAL

- Refer patients when the diagnosis is unclear or response to therapy is inadequate.
- Consider referral for medication overuse headaches, as these are difficult to treat.

PREVENTION

- Closely monitor use of medications for acute episodes. Advise patients to limit simple analgesics to less than 15 days per month and triptans, opiates, and combination medications to less than 10 days per month.
- Appropriately prescribe preventive therapies to reduce frequency of headaches and avoid development of chronic headaches.

PROGNOSIS

- Prospective studies lasting up to 8 years found that 45% of teenagers or young adults with tension-type or migraine headaches showed improvement and 25% to 33% became headache-free.

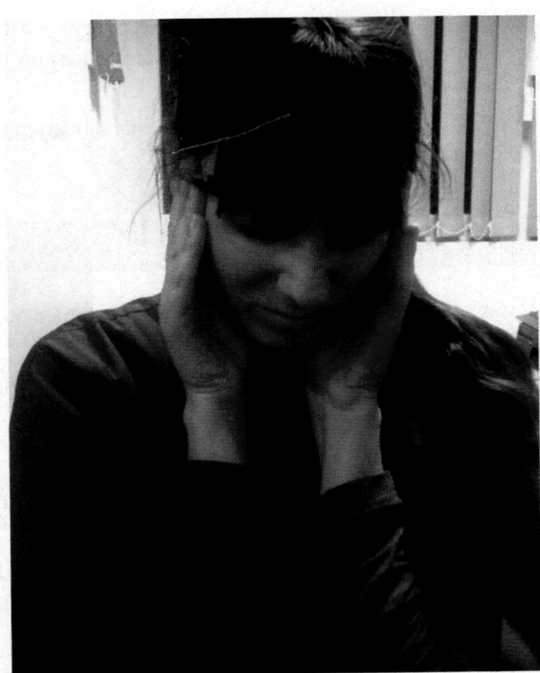

FIGURE 239-3 Woman with daily tension-type headache. This is a primary headache. (*Source: Wikimedia Commons and Shanghai killer whale at http://commons.wikimedia.org/wiki/File:Tension-headache.jpg.*)

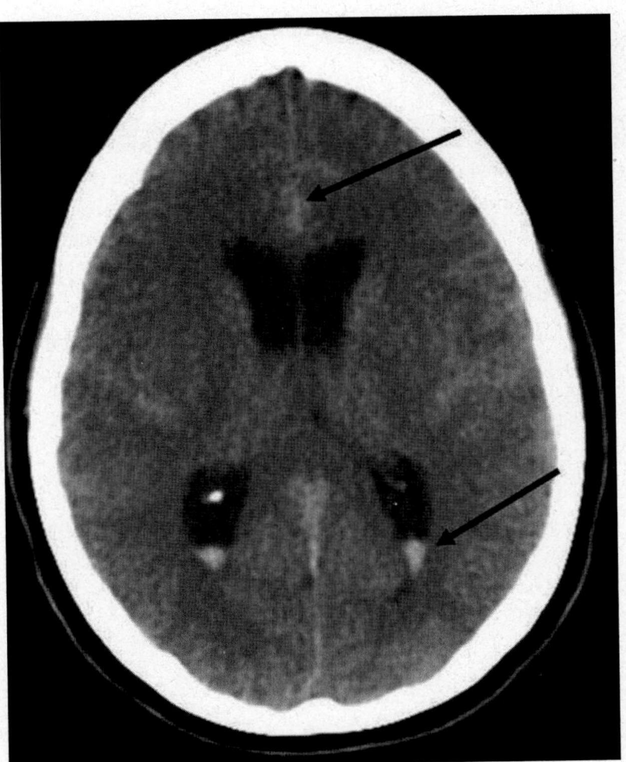

FIGURE 239-4 Sudden onset of a thunderclap headache prompted imaging that showed diffuse subarachnoid hemorrhage with associated ventricular hemorrhage. Top arrow indicates blood in interhemispheric fissure. Bottom arrow indicates blood in lateral ventricle. (*Reproduced with permission from James Anderson, MD, Department of Radiology, Oregon Health & Science University.*)

More than one-third had a change in type of primary headache from tension-type to migraine or from migraine to tension-type during the study.[15]

- Cluster headaches—Unknown; ranges from total remission to chronic form.[15]

FOLLOW-UP

- Dangerous causes of secondary headaches require immediate evaluation and management.
- Frequency of follow-up for primary headaches is determined by type and severity of headache and response to therapy.

PATIENT EDUCATION

Advise patients to limit frequency of acute medications to less than 2 to 3 times a week to reduce the risk of medication overuse headache.

PATIENT RESOURCES

National Headache Foundation has information for patients on many topics including:

- *Migraine*—**https://headaches.org/2012/10/25/migraine/.**
- *Tension-Type Headache*—**https://headaches.org/2007/10/25/tension-type-headache/.**
- *Cluster Headache*—**https://headaches.org/2013/10/25/cluster-headaches/.**

PROVIDER RESOURCES

- The Institute for Clinical Systems Improvement has a comprehensive guideline on the diagnosis and treatment of headache—**https://www.icsi.org/guidelines__more/catalog_guidelines_and_more/catalog_guidelines/catalog_neurological_guidelines/headache/.**
- The International Headache Society has a searchable website to assist with headache classification using ICHD-3 criteria—**https://www.ichd-3.org/_klassifikation/.**

REFERENCES

1. Stovner LJ, Andree C. Prevalence of headache in Europe: a review for the Eurolight project. *J Headache Pain.* 2010;11(4):289-299.
2. Loder E, Rizzoli P. Tension-type headache. *BMJ.* 2008:336(7635):88-92.
3. Burstein R, Noseda R, Borsook D. Migraine: multiple processes, complex pathophysiology. *J Neurosci.* 2015;35(17):6619-6629.
4. Costa A, Antonaci F, Ramusino MC, Nappi G. The neuropharmacology of cluster headache and other trigeminal autonomic cephalalgias. *Curr Neuropharmacol.* 2015;13(3):304-323.
5. Benoliel R. Trigeminal autonomic cephalgias. *Br J Pain.* 2012;6(3):106-123.
6. Hainer BL, Matheson EM. Approach to acute headache in adults. *Am Fam Physician.* 2013;87(10):682-687.
7. Beran RG. Management of chronic headache. *Aust Fam Phys.* 2014:43(3):106-110.
8. International Headache Society Headache Classification Committee. ICHD-3 Beta. The Primary Headaches. https://www.ichd-3.org. Accessed December 2017.
9. Becker WJ, Findlay T, Moga C, et al. Guideline for primary care management of headache in adults. *Can Fam Physician.* 2015;61(8):670-679.
10. Linde K, Allais G, Brinkhaus B, et al. Acupuncture for the prevention of tension-type headache. *Cochrane Database Syst Rev.* 2016;(4):CD007587.
11. Pringsheim T, Davenport WJ, Becker WJ. Prophylaxis of migraine headache. *CMAJ.* 2010;182(7):E269-E276.
12. Buse DC, Rupnow MFT, Lipton RB. Assessing and managing all aspects of migraine: migraine attacks, migraine-related functional impairment, common comorbidities, and quality of life. *Mayo Clin Proc.* 2009;84(5):422-435.
13. Linde K, Allais G, Brinkhaus B, et al. Acupuncture for preventing migraine attacks. *Cochrane Database Syst Rev.* 2016;(6):CD001218.
14. Evers S, Jensen R. Treatment of medication overuse headache—guideline of the EFNS headache panel. *Eur J Neurol.* 2011;18(9):1115-1121.
15. Antonaci F, Voiticovschi-Iosob C, Di Stefano AL, et al. The evolution of headache from childhood to adulthood: a review of the literature. *J Headache Pain.* 2014;15(1):15.

240 SPORTS-RELATED HEAD INJURY

Heidi S. Chumley, MD, MBA

PATIENT STORY

A professional soccer player bumped heads with another player while heading a ball in a game (**Figure 240-1**). She fell, sat up slowly, and then lay down on the field. She was noted to have a vacant stare and confused responses when evaluated on the field by a certified trainer. She was removed from the field, underwent a complete evaluation, and was diagnosed with a concussion. She complied with her cognitive and physical rest and her gradual return to activities. Her recovery was without incident, and she was released to return to play after 10 days.

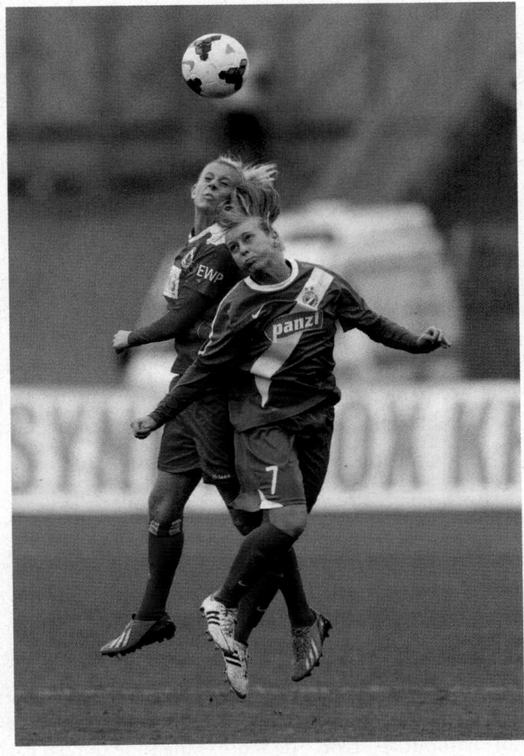

FIGURE 240-1 Young women soccer players hit heads while heading a soccer ball. This is a common mechanism by which concussion occurs in soccer players. (*Laszlo Szirtesi/licensed from Shutterstock.*)

INTRODUCTION

Sports-related concussions occur in athletes of all ages and skill levels engaged in many different sports (**Figures 240-1** and **240-2**). After a head impact, athletes are evaluated immediately and removed from play if there is any concern for a concussion. A full evaluation, performed shortly after, is needed to make the clinical diagnosis. The mainstay of therapy is cognitive and physical rest, with a gradual return to activities. Most adults recover within 10 days, whereas children may require up to 4 weeks for a normal recovery. Returning to play requires a release by a certified health practitioner.

EPIDEMIOLOGY

- Sports-related concussion (SRC) occurs in more than 10,000 U.S. college athletes each year, at a concussion rate of 4.47 per 10,000 athlete exposures.[1] SRC is more common in competition (12.81 per 10,000) than in practice (2.57 per 10,000).[1]
- Men's football, women's soccer, and women's basketball have the most reported SRCs among college sports; the highest concussive rates occur in men's wrestling (10.92 per 10,000), men's ice hockey (7.91 per 10,000), and women's ice hockey (7.5 per 10,000).[1]
- SRC occurred at an incidence rate of 26.1 per 100,000 athlete-exposures in high school athletes playing football (men), or soccer, lacrosse, or hockey (men and women).[2]
- High school athletes in the above sports have a 1.3% to 2.6% chance of concussion in a season.[2]
- Nine percent of sports-related concussions are recurrent[1]; a concussion in the previous 24 months increases the risk of a second concussion by more than five times.[2]
- Chronic traumatic encephalopathy has been described in athletes, particularly American football players and boxers, with repetitive concussive and sub-concussive head blows; however, the prevalence is unknown.[3]

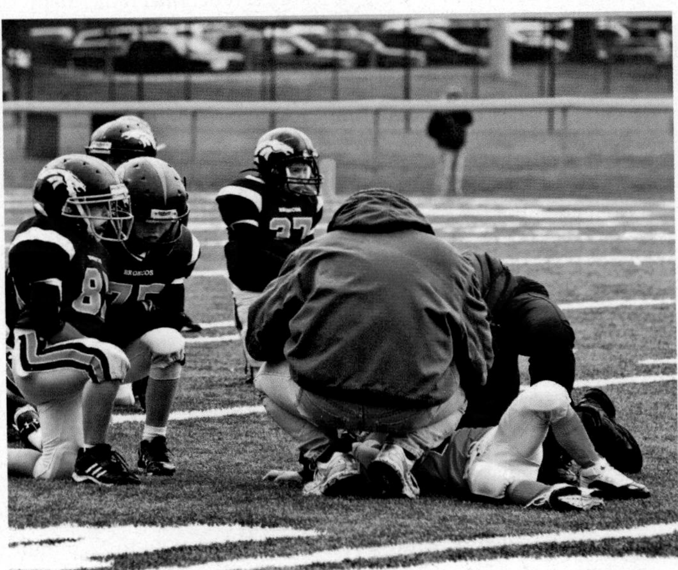

FIGURE 240-2 Young football players take a knee while a coach and parent attend to a player who sustained a head impact while tackling another player. Both the coach and parent completed concussion education prior to the season. (*Licensed from Shutterstock.*)

ETIOLOGY AND PATHOPHYSIOLOGY

The force of direct or indirect head trauma increases neuronal glucose requirements beyond availability, resulting in common symptoms. Trauma injures neuronal cell walls, increasing ion exchange. The increased movement of potassium outside the cell triggers the release of excitatory amino acids (i.e., glutamate) and depolarizes the cell wall, suppressing neuronal activity. The cell activates the sodium-potassium pump to restore ion balance, which increases metabolism and requires more glucose. Increased blood flow would bring more glucose, but the injury has decreased blood flow. This mismatch lasts for 1 to 10 days, during which symptoms may continue and susceptibility to future injury is increased.[4]

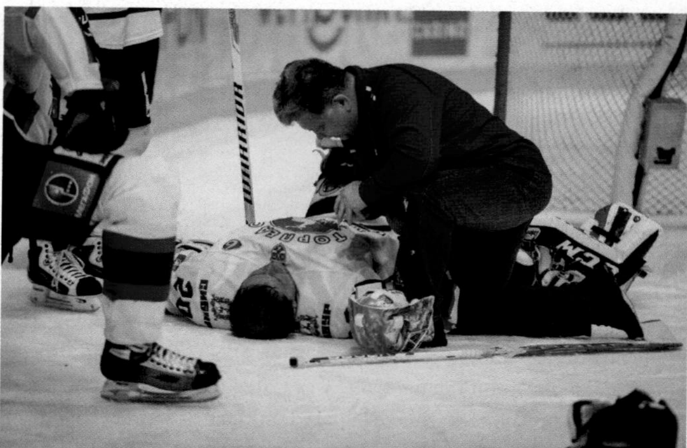

FIGURE 240-3 An international professional hockey player is attended to on the ice after a shoulder-to-head collision resulting in loss of consciousness. (*Licensed from Shutterstock.*)

DIAGNOSIS

SRC is a clinical diagnosis requiring a forceful impact directly or indirectly transmitted to the head that is associated with symptoms reported by the athlete, visible signs, and clinical suspicion from the medical staff.[5]

- Assessment tools, such as the Sport Concussion Assessment Tool 5 (SCAT5),[6] provide a structured approach to collecting pertinent information to make the diagnosis.
- Neurocognitive assessments are commonly used. In a review of the most common assessments[7]:
  - ImPACT computerized test had the highest sensitivity (81.9%–91.4%) and specificity (69.1%–89.4%).[7] A pediatric version is available.
  - King-Devick test is a card reading test that is easily performed on the sideline. The athlete reads single-digits numbers as quickly as possible without an error. The score is the time to read each card without an error.

CLINICAL FEATURES

Rapid onset of transient neurologic features, functional rather than structural, resolve spontaneously.

Symptoms:

- Physical (i.e., headache, neck pain, nausea/vomiting, dizziness, blurry vision, difficulty with balance, sensitivity to light or sound, fatigue).
- Cognitive (i.e., feeling "not right" or in a fog, difficulty concentrating or remembering, confusion).
- Emotional/sleep (i.e., more emotional, sad, nervous or anxious, trouble falling asleep).

Physical signs:

- Immediate: lying motionless on playing surface or loss of consciousness (**Figure 240-3**), balance disturbance or motor incoordination, disorientation or inappropriate (confused) responses, vacant stare.
- Off-field examination: disturbances of orientation, poor performance on memory or concentration testing, finger to nose, gait/balance.
- Computerized neurocognitive testing: ImPACT, a 20- to 25-minute computer-based assessment tool, produces scores for verbal memory, reaction time, visual-motor speed, and visual-memory composites. Abnormalities are seen within the first few days and resolve over time.[7]

LABORATORY TESTING

- Generally not indicated when signs and symptoms consistent with concussion follow a sports-related head injury.
- Newly approved biomarkers to aid in evaluation of concussion, ubiquitin carboxy-terminal hydrolase-L1 and glial fibrillary acidic protein, may be helpful in identifying patients who do not need CT scanning after a head injury. Not tested in children or adolescents.

IMAGING

- Structural imaging (non-contrast CT or MRI) is generally not indicated and routinely normal, as SRC is a functional, not a structural, issue.
- Consider CT or MRI if symptoms/signs are worsening, resolution is not occurring as expected, or loss of consciousness exceeded 1 minute.[4]
- Functional imaging is being developed as a diagnostic tool for concussion; for example, MRI with CO_2 stress demonstrated higher cerebrovascular responsiveness; not yet used clinically.[8]

DIFFERENTIAL DIAGNOSIS

- Concussion can be accompanied by a cervical spine injury or a concurrent intracranial injury, both of which require urgent consultation and management.
- With prolonged symptoms, consider post-concussive syndrome, migraine headaches, depression, or anxiety.
- If unknown if head trauma occurred, migraine headaches or hypoglycemia may cause similar symptoms.

MANAGEMENT

- Perform emergency care (i.e., assess airway, breathing, circulation) or first aid (i.e., stop bleeding) if needed.
- Perform an on-site assessment using an instrument such as the SCAT5. Assess for red flags (i.e., loss of consciousness) and observable signs. Evaluate memory with Maddock's questions. Perform the Glasgow Coma Scale and a cervical spine assessment.
- Immediately remove an athlete suspected of having a concussion from play. Athletes with red flags should be evaluated immediately by a physician.
- When the athlete can be safely moved to an office setting, perform a standardized concussion evaluation including relevant history, symptom evaluation, cognitive screen, and neurologic screen. Arrange for neurocognitive testing.

NONPHARMACOLOGIC

- Advise physical and cognitive rest for 1–2 days. Use a graded approach to return to cognitive, then physical activities.[5] SOR Ⓒ
- Increase mental activity (i.e., reading, screen time) for time periods that do not exacerbate symptoms. Begin with 5–15 minutes.[6] SOR Ⓒ
- As symptoms allow, restart schoolwork outside of the classroom, return to school part-time, then return to school full-time.[5,6] SOR Ⓒ
- Add back physical activity as follows: light aerobic exercise, sports-specific exercises without contact (i.e., skating), non-contact training drills, full-contact practice, regular game play. Spend 24 hours at each step before advancing to the next one.[5,6] SOR Ⓒ

MEDICATIONS

- In general, medications are only used if needed for pain relief within the first 1–2 days or for prolonged symptoms (more than 10 days).[5] SOR Ⓒ
- Medications are not typically needed. Acetaminophen may be used sparingly in some cases. A common cause of prolonged headache, especially in pediatric patients, is chronic medication use following concussion.[9]
- Medications to treat prolonged sleep disturbances or anxiety can be considered after 10 days in adults and 4 weeks in children.[5]
- Medication use interferes with assessing when to increase cognitive and physical activity by masking symptoms. In general, athletes should be off medications started after a concussion before returning to play.[5]

REFERRAL OR HOSPITALIZATION

If you do not routinely manage sports-related concussions, refer patients:

- With an unclear diagnosis or an unusual symptom complex.
- With red flags: neck pain/tenderness, weakness/tingling/burning in arms or legs, severe or worsening headache, double vision, seizure, loss of consciousness or deteriorating consciousness, emesis, restless or agitated behavior.[6]
- Whose condition deteriorates after the initial evaluation.
- With symptoms lasting longer than 10 days in adults and 4 weeks in children.[5] SOR Ⓒ

PREVENTION

- Rule changes in some sports have decreased the incidence of sports-related concussion (i.e., head tackling in American football, heading in soccer, and body-checking in hockey).[10]
- Protective equipment (e.g., helmets in football) reduces the severity of injuries, but not the incidence of concussion. Ongoing improvements in helmet technology may result in decreases in concussion in the near future.[10]
- Laws and public policy requiring education of athletes, coaches, and trainers and evaluation by a certified health professional prior to return to play have not yet resulted in decreased incidence of concussion[10] (see **Figure 240-2**).
- Prevention of a second concussion is best accomplished by ensuring a full recovery from the first concussion. After multiple concussions, prevention may be best achieved by removal from sports.[10]

PROGNOSIS

- With appropriate cognitive and physical rest, 85% of patients have complete resolution of symptoms within 10 days. Normal recovery time may be longer (up to 4 weeks) for children and adolescents.[5]

- Predictors of slow recovery include severe symptoms, pre-injury mental health problems, and perhaps being a high school girl. Attention-deficit/hyperactivity disorder (ADHD) or learning disabilities are not associated with slower recovery.[11]

FOLLOW-UP

Patients should be seen if their recovery stalls. Consider reevaluating at any time during the recovery period if patients are unable to advance cognitive or physical symptoms after 24–48 hours at the previous stage. Reevaluate all athletes before allowing them to return to play.

PATIENT EDUCATION

Advise patients and caregivers of the following[6]:

- Cognitive and physical rest is critical to recovery.
- Avoid alcohol and medications, including sleeping tablets, aspirin, nonsteroidal anti-inflammatory drugs (NSAIDs), or narcotics.
- Do not drive until cleared by a physician.
- You must be cleared to return to play.

PATIENT RESOURCES

- HEADS UP to Youth Sports has information for athletes, coaches, trainers, and parents—**https://www.cdc.gov/headsup/youthsports/index.html.**
- Safe Kids Worldwide has a discussion guide for parents in English or Spanish—**https://www.safekids.org.**

PROVIDER RESOURCES

- Consensus Statement on Concussion in Sport—**http://bjsm.bmj.com/content/51/11/838.**
- Sport Concussion Assessment Tool, 5th edition (SCAT 5) is available free online—**http://bjsm.bmj.com/content/bjsports/early/2017/04/26/bjsports-2017-097506SCAT5.full.pdf.**
- ImPACT application site—**https://impacttest.com.**

REFERENCES

1. Zuckerman SL, Kerr ZY, Yengo-Kahn A, et al. epidemiology of sports-related concussion in NCAA athletes from 2009-2010 to 2013-2014: incidence, recurrence, and mechanisms. *Am J Sports Med.* 2015;43(11):2654-2662.
2. Marshall SW, Guskiewicz KM, Shankar V, et al. Epidemiology of sports-related concussion in seven US high school and collegiate sports. *Inj Epidemiol.* 2015;2(1):13.
3. Meehan W, Mannix R, Zafonte R, Pascual-Leone A. Chronic traumatic encephalopathy and athletes. *Neurology.* 2015;85(17):1504-1511.
4. Patel DR, Parachuri V, Shettigar A. Evaluation and management of sport-related concussions in adolescent athletes. *Translational Pediatrics.* 2017;6(3):121-128.
5. McCrory P, Meeuwisse W, Dvorak J, et al. Consensus statement on concussion in sport—the 5th International Conference on Concussion in Sport held in Berlin, October 2016. *Br J Sports Med.* 2017;51:838-847.
6. Echemendia RJ, Meeuwisse W, McCrory P, et al. The Sport Concussion Assessment Tool, 5th Edition (SCAT5): background and rationale. *Br J Sports Med.* 2017:51(11):848-850.
7. Dessy AM, Yuk FJ, Maniya AY, et al. Review of assessment scales for diagnosing and monitoring sports-related concussion. *Cureus.* 2017;9(12):e1922.
8. Mutch WAC, Ellis MJ, Ryner LN, et al. Patient-specific alterations in CO_2 cerebrovascular responsiveness in acute and sub-acute sports-related concussion. *Front Neurol.* 2018;9:23.
9. Halstead ME. Pharmacologic therapies for pediatric concussions. *Sports Health.* 2016;8(1):50-52.
10. Patel DR, Fidrocki D, Parachuri V. Sport-related concussions in adolescent athletes: a critical public health problem for which prevention remains an elusive goal. *Transl Pediatr.* 2017;6(3):114-120.
11. Iverson GL, Gardner AJ, Terry DP, et al. Predictors of clinical recovery from concussion: a systematic review. *Br J Sports Med.* 2017;51(12):941-948.

241 CEREBRAL VASCULAR ACCIDENT

J. William Hayden, Jr, MD, EdD
Heidi S. Chumley, MD, MBA

PATIENT STORY

A 65-year-old hypertensive black man presented to the emergency department with onset of right face, arm, and hand paralysis, and difficulty communicating. Rapid diagnostic testing using MRI revealed an ischemic infarct in the left middle cerebral artery (**Figure 241-1**). He was evaluated by a stroke response team and was found to be a candidate for tissue plasminogen activator (TPA). After the stroke, he was treated with aspirin, antihypertensives, and cholesterol-lowering medication. He recovered 80% of his neurologic deficit over the next 3 months. **Figure 241-2** is a noncontrast CT image of this patient 2 weeks later.

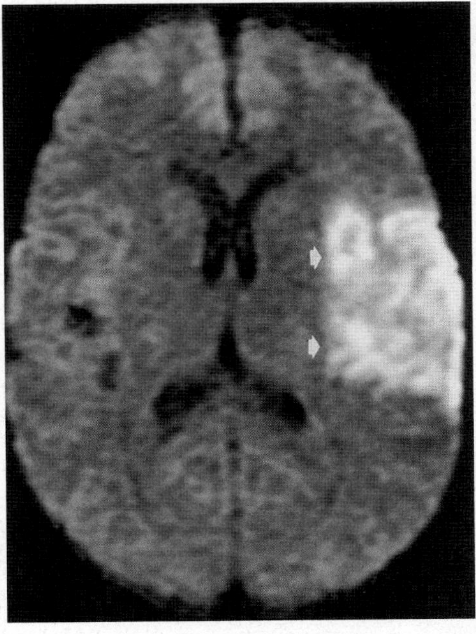

FIGURE 241-1 Acute left middle cerebral artery infarct on MRI of a 65-year-old hypertensive man. The MRI demonstrates increased signal intensity (*arrows*). Abnormalities in MRI occur before those seen on CT during ischemic strokes. (*Reproduced with permission from Chen MYM, Pope TL, Ott DJ. Basic Radiology. New York, NY: McGraw-Hill Education; 2004.*)

INTRODUCTION

Cerebral vascular accidents or strokes are common, especially in older populations. Most strokes are ischemic or hemorrhagic. Risk factors include hypertension, smoking, diabetes mellitus, and atrial fibrillation. Thirty-day mortality for a first stroke is greater than 20%.

SYNONYMS

Stroke.

EPIDEMIOLOGY

- Cerebral vascular accidents (CVAs) affect approximately 795,000 people per year in the United States, most being older than age 65 years, although strokes can and do occur at any age.[1]
- As many as 46% to 51% of strokes are cryptogenic or have an undetermined cause.[2] Other known causes account for 2% to 4% of strokes. Of the remaining, approximately 80% are caused by ischemic infarction, while 20% result from intracerebral or subarachnoid hemorrhage, each accounting for 10%.[3]
- Among ages 18 and older, stroke prevalence rates for ethnic groups in the United States are as follows: Asian/Pacific Islanders, 1.8%, Hispanics of any race, 2.4%, Non-Hispanic whites, 2.5%, Non-Hispanic blacks, 4.5%, American Indian/Alaska natives, 5.4%.[3]
- Black patients at ages 45 and 65 are 2.9 and 1.66 times more likely to have a stroke compared to white patients.[4]
- Mortality is higher in blacks than in whites: 95.8 versus 73.7 per 100,000 for black and white men, respectively.[1]
- Hispanics have witnessed an increase in death rates due to stroke since 2013.[2]

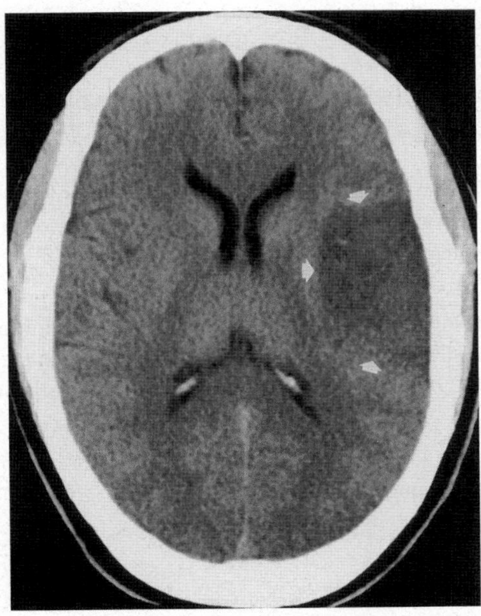

FIGURE 241-2 Noncontrast CT image of a subacute left middle cerebral artery infarct (*arrows*). This was done 2 weeks after the stroke in the same patient as previous figure. CT findings occur later than MRI findings in ischemic strokes. (*Reproduced with permission from Chen MYM, Pope TL, Ott DJ. Basic Radiology. New York, NY: McGraw-Hill Education; 2004.*)

- Each year in the United States, an estimated $34 billion for health-care services, medications, and missed days of work are due to stroke.[5]

ETIOLOGY AND PATHOPHYSIOLOGY

- CVAs are classified into two categories: brain ischemia and brain hemorrhage. Brain ischemia may result from cardioaortic emboli (15% to 22%), atherothrombotic emboli from both large vessels (10% to 12%) and small vessels (15% to 18%), and hypoperfusion.
- Thrombotic brain ischemia occurs when atherosclerosis progresses to a plaque, which ruptures acutely, initiating an ischemic cascade. Ischemic cascade leads to cellular hypoxia, depletion of ATP, and loss of ion gradients. Cytotoxic edema develops with release of free radicals, vasogenic edema, and eventual brain swelling.[6]
- Each step of this process is mediated by inflammation.[7]
- An estimated 5% of uncomplicated ischemic strokes may experience hemorrhagic transformation usually within the first week with or without neurologic decline.[6]
- Intracerebral hemorrhage occurs when vessels bleed into the brain. The most common causes are elevated blood pressure, trauma, bleeding diatheses, amyloid angiopathy, illicit drug use (mostly amphetamines and cocaine), and vascular malformations.[3]
- Arterial aneurysmal rupture is the major cause of subarachnoid hemorrhage.[3]
- Other known causes of CVAs include inflammatory disorders (giant cell arteritis, systemic lupus erythematosus [SLE], polyarteritis nodosa, granulomatous angiitis, syphilis, and AIDS), fibromuscular dysplasia, hematologic disorders (thrombocytopenia, polycythemia, and sickle cell), and hypercoagulable states.

RISK FACTORS

Nonmodifiable risk factors include age, race, sex, ethnicity, history of migraines, fibromuscular dysplasia, and family history of stroke or transient ischemic attack (TIA).[6]

Modifiable risk factors include:

- Hypertension (HTN)—The predominant risk factor for more than 50% of all strokes. Prehypertension (blood pressure in the range of 130 to 139/85 to 89) carries a hazard ratio of 2.5 for women and 1.6 for men.[8]
- Cigarette smoking carries a hazard ratio of 1.62 for ischemic stroke and 2.56 for hemorrhagic stroke.[9]
- Type 2 diabetes mellitus (DM) increases the risk of having a stroke six-fold.[8]
- Atrial fibrillation increases the risk of stroke. The CHADS2 (congestive heart failure [CHF], HTN, age >75, DM, stroke) scoring system (see below) separates patients into low risk (stroke rate 1% to 1.5% per year), moderate risk (2.5%), high risk (4%), and very high risk (7%).[8]
- Body mass index (BMI) greater than 30 carries a hazard ratio of 1.45 for ischemic stroke but does not increase the risk of hemorrhagic stroke.[9]

DIAGNOSIS

Diagnosis of CVA must be made expediently to minimize mortality and morbidity. Critical in patient management is early triage to CT scan or MRI to rule out intracerebral or subarachnoid bleed. If either is present, the use of thrombolytics is contraindicated.

- If there is strong suspicion for subarachnoid bleed, a lumbar puncture is mandatory despite a normal head CT.[10]

CLINICAL FEATURES

- Obtain focused history. For older patients, include age, HTN, cigarette smoking, type 2 DM, high cholesterol, coronary artery disease, arrhythmias, or previous TIA or stroke.
- In younger patients, history should include any recent trauma; coagulopathies; illicit drug use, especially cocaine; migraines; and oral contraceptive use.
- Document acute onset of neurologic signs and symptoms based on the site of the CVA (see "Typical Distribution" below).

TYPICAL DISTRIBUTION

TIA or stroke can occur in any area of the brain; common areas with typical constellation of symptoms include the following:

- Middle cerebral artery is the most common ischemic site (**Figure 241-3**):
    - Superior branch occlusion causes contralateral hemiparesis and sensory deficit in face, hand, and arm, and an expressive aphasia if the lesion is in the dominant hemisphere.
    - Inferior branch occlusion causes a homonymous hemianopia, impairment of contralateral graphesthesia and stereognosis, anosognosia and neglect of the contralateral side, and a receptive aphasia if the lesion is in the dominant hemisphere.
- Internal carotid artery (approximately 20% of ischemic strokes) occlusion causes contralateral hemiplegia, hemisensory deficit, and homonymous hemianopia; aphasia is also present with dominant hemisphere involvement.
- Posterior cerebral artery occlusion causes a homonymous hemianopia affecting the contralateral visual field.

LABORATORY EVALUATION

These tests may be helpful in the context of an acute stroke, particularly when the cause of the stroke is not immediately evident:

- Complete blood count (CBC) for thrombocytosis or polycythemia.
- Coagulation profile including prothrombin time, partial thromboplastin time (PTT), international normalized ratio (INR), thrombin time and/or ecarin clotting time if patient is known to be taking a direct thrombin or factor Xa inhibitor such as hirudin or rivaroxaban.[5]
- Lipid panel including HDL, LDL, cholesterol and triglycerides.[5]
- Erythrocyte sedimentation rate (ESR) for diseases such as giant cell arteritis or SLE.

- Testing for syphilis using a treponemal enzyme immunoassay (EIA), with positive results confirmed by a nontreponemal test (Venereal Disease Research Laboratory [VDRL]).
- Serum glucose to eliminate hypoglycemia as the cause of the neurologic symptoms.
- A pregnancy test in all women of childbearing age presenting with stroke symptoms, as rt-PA thrombolytic therapy has not been studied in pregnancy—must weigh risk versus benefits. U.S. Food and Drug Administration (FDA) pregnancy category C.[4]
- Electrocardiogram.[7] SOR Ⓑ

IMAGING

CT or MRI can distinguish ischemic from hemorrhagic and localize the lesion (**Figure 241-4**).

Brain imaging should be completed with interpretation within 45 minutes of patient arrival in the emergency department by a physician competent to read CT and MRI studies.[7] SOR Ⓒ, Class I

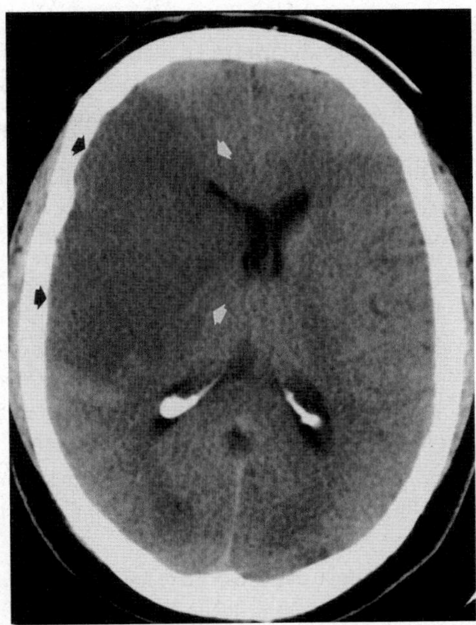

FIGURE 241-3 CT image of right middle cerebral artery infarct; the hypodense (darker) area (*arrows*) indicates the infarct. The midline structures are shifted to the left. (*Reproduced with permission from Chen MYM, Pope TL, Ott DJ. Basic Radiology. New York, NY: McGraw-Hill Education; 2004.*)

DIFFERENTIAL DIAGNOSIS

Other causes of acute neurologic dysfunction include the following:

- TIA—This precursor to a CVA can appear identical; however, no lesion is seen on imaging, and symptoms resolve within 48 hours.
- Multiple sclerosis—Multiple anatomically distinct neurologic signs and symptoms that occur over time and resolve; vision is often affected. MRI findings should help to distinguish multiple sclerosis from CVA.
- Brain mass—More common presentation is headache or seizure; however, may present with focal neurologic signs based on location. CT or MRI will help to diagnose a brain mass and differentiate this from stroke.
- Migraines—Throbbing, unilateral headache with photophobia and nausea; hemiparesis or aphasia may be part of the aura.
- Vertigo from benign positional vertigo or acute labyrinthitis—Can mimic a CVA in the posterior circulation; however, symptoms such as dysarthria, dysphagia, and diplopia are typically absent.
- Hypoglycemia—Confused state is similar to large stroke syndromes but is easily differentiated by a blood glucose measurement.
- Wernicke encephalopathy—Triad of ophthalmoplegia, ataxia, and confusion due to depletion of B vitamin reserves, especially thiamine.

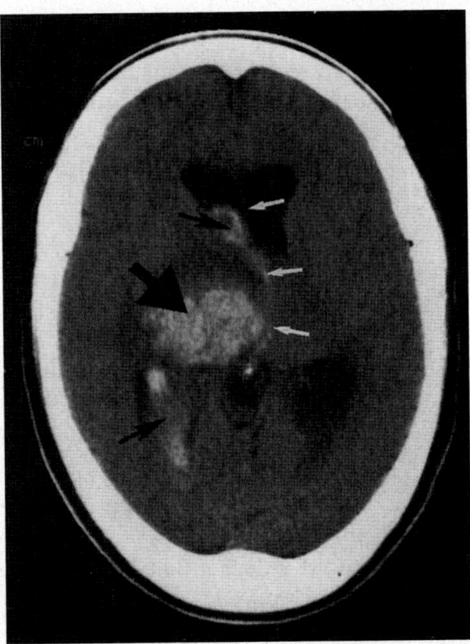

FIGURE 241-4 Hemorrhagic stroke. CT image demonstrates bleeding in the right basal ganglia (*large black arrow*) and into the ventricles (*small black arrows*). Blood appears white on the CT scan. The *white arrows* illustrate midline shift. (*Reproduced with permission from Chen MYM, Pope TL, Ott DJ. Basic Radiology. New York, NY: McGraw-Hill Education; 2004.*)

MANAGEMENT

ACUTE STROKE (WITHIN THE FIRST 3 HOURS)

- Initial assessment and management priorities are airway, breathing, and circulation (blood pressure). If patient has decreased level of consciousness and poor airway protection, intubation may be necessary to protect airway and prevent hypoventilation, hypercarbia, and further elevation of intracranial pressure.[5]
- An acute elevation of blood pressure may represent an appropriate physiologic response to maintain cerebral perfusion. Blood pressure management requires a balance between permissive HTN

versus lowering blood pressure with risk for further neurologic impairment. For acute ischemic stroke eligible for thrombolytic therapy, antihypertensive treatment is recommended to maintain systolic blood pressure ≤185 mm Hg and diastolic blood pressure ≤110 mm Hg.[6] SOR C
  - For patients who are **not** treated with thrombolytic therapy, cautious lowering of blood pressure by approximately 15% during the first 24 hours after stroke onset is recommended.[6] SOR C
- Fever may occur with stroke and worsen brain ischemia. Normothermia should be maintained.[5]
- Rapidly evaluate or consult specialists to identify candidates for TPA. Odds for a favorable 3-month outcome for TPA compared to no TPA are 2.8 (95% confidence interval [CI], 1.8–4.5) for 0 to 90 minutes, 1.6 (95% CI, 1.1–2.2) for 91 to 180 minutes.[7] SOR A
- In this context, stroke care units with specially trained nursing staff and allied healthcare personnel have clearly been demonstrated to improve outcomes.[4]
- Favorable outcomes at 90 days poststroke have also been demonstrated when TPA is given up to 4.5 hours after the onset of symptoms.[8] SOR B
- Currently, only 3% of patients who meet the criteria receive TPA.[4]
- Preliminary studies cautioned about using TPA in community settings; recent studies, however, indicate several options to improve outcomes, including telephone consultation with a regional stroke center.[9]
- In all patients with suspected embolic stroke, cardiac emboli may account for up to 20% of acute strokes.[4] An echocardiogram and cardiac monitoring to identify occult atrial fibrillation or other arrhythmias should be performed for a minimum of 24 hours.[5]
- Vascular studies should include duplex ultrasound of the neck and transcranial Doppler of intracranial arteries, as these may be sources for brain embolism.[5]

After stabilization, management of ischemic stroke includes antithrombotics, antihypertensives, statins, and lifestyle changes as secondary measures to prevent stroke re-occurrence.[4]

- Prescribe 81-mg or 325-mg aspirin for secondary stroke prevention in patients with prior ischemic stroke or TIA (relative risk [RR] reduction 28%; number needed to treat [NNT] to prevent 1 stroke per year = 77).[4] SOR A
- Lower blood pressure (RR reduction 28%; NNT to prevent 1 stroke per year = 51).[4] Current data demonstrate that thiazide-type diuretic and angiotensin-converting enzyme inhibitor (ACEI) (or angiotensin receptor blocker [ARB]) may provide additional risk reduction beyond blood pressure (BP) control and should be used first. ACEI and ARB may not be as effective as monotherapy in black populations.[4] SOR A
- Lower low-density lipoprotein (LDL) cholesterol to less than 100 mg/dL for patients with a prior stroke or who are at high risk of stroke using a statin (RR reduction 25%; NNT to prevent 1 stroke per year = 57).[4] SOR A
- Assist patients to stop smoking (RR reduction 33%; NNT to prevent 1 stroke per year = 43).[4] SOR A
- Advise patients to adopt a healthy lifestyle by eating more fruits and vegetables, losing weight, and maintaining a physical exercise program. SOR B

Consider the following to further decrease morbidity and mortality:

- Avoid indwelling urinary catheters to reduce the risk of urinary tract infection.
- Encourage early ambulation to reduce the risk of a deep venous thrombosis.
- Use antiembolism stockings to reduce the risk of a deep venous thrombosis.
- Consider a swallowing study to identify patients at risk of aspiration, as dysphagia is common after stroke and a major risk factor for developing aspiration pneumonia.

SPECIAL SITUATIONS

- Hemorrhagic stroke:
  - Acutely—Do not aggressively lower BP. Some authorities recommend lowering BP only when mean arterial pressure (MAP) is more than 130 mm Hg (MAP = [(2 × diastolic BP) + systolic BP]/3).
  - After the hemorrhagic stroke is over, treat BP aggressively; modest decreases (12/5 mm Hg) from one of many classes of hypertensive drugs lower recurrent stroke risk by 50% to 75%.[4]
- Nonvalvular atrial fibrillation (AF)—Use the CHADS2 scoring system to identify patients with AF who can be managed with aspirin or should be anticoagulated with coumadin.[4]
- The CHADS/CHADS2 scoring table is shown below[2]:

C: Congestive heart failure	= 1 point
H: HTN (or treated HTN)	= 1 point
A: Age >75 years	= 1 point
D: Diabetes	= 1 point
S: Prior TIA or stroke	= 2 points

  - For 0 to 1 point, use aspirin; 2 points, weigh risk of bleeding, adequacy of follow-up versus benefit; 3 or greater, use warfarin if at all possible.
- Seizure activity occurs in 4% to 28% of patients with hemorrhagic stroke. Patients with clinical seizure activity or electroencephalographic (EEG) evidence of seizure activity accompanied by a change in mental status should receive a benzodiazepine such as lorazepam or diazepam.[8]
- To control intracranial pressure (ICP), elevate the head of the bed to 30 degrees to improve venous jugular outflow. More aggressive measures such as IV mannitol and barbiturate anesthesia require continuous intracranial blood pressure and systemic blood pressure monitoring. Hyperventilation is not recommended because its effect is transient and may result in rebound ICP.[8]
- Initiation of inpatient statin use and maintenance may improve outcomes in hemorrhagic stroke.[8]
- Patients with symptomatic carotid stenosis: Refer for carotid endarterectomy patients with 70% to 99% carotid stenosis (without near-occlusion) with ipsilateral focal neurologic signs (absolute risk reduction [ARR] 16.0%).[10] Consider referring symptomatic patients with moderate stenosis of 50% to 69% (ARR 4.6%).[10] SOR A
- Patients with asymptomatic carotid artery stenosis greater than 60%. Consider referral for carotid endarterectomy in patients younger than the age of 75 years (NNT = 20 to prevent 1 stroke in 5 years).[4]

PREVENTION

- Address modifiable risk factors: control HTN, high cholesterol, and DM; stop smoking; and maintain a healthy body weight.
- The U.S. Preventive Services Task Force (USPSTF) recommends the use of aspirin for stroke prevention in adults ages 50–59 years with a ≥10% 10-year cardiovascular disease risk, who are not at risk for bleeding, and have a life expectancy of at least 10 years.[11] SOR Ⓑ
- In adults ages 60–69 years, the decision to use low-dose aspirin for stroke prevention should be made on an individual basis.[11]
- In adults younger than 50 or older than 70 years of age, current evidence is insufficient to make any recommendation regarding low-dose aspirin and stroke prevention.[11]

PROGNOSIS

CVA prognosis varies based on size and location of ischemia or hemorrhage, time to TPA administration (for ischemic stroke), and availability of aggressive poststroke rehabilitation.

- The 30-day mortality rate after a first or second stroke is 22% and 41%, respectively.[4]
- Five-year observed survival is 40% to 68% for stroke.[12]

FOLLOW-UP

- Patients with symptoms of an acute stroke should be hospitalized, evaluated immediately for appropriateness of TPA and treatment of reversible causes, and managed, if possible, in a stroke unit or using the "best practices" associated with these units.
- After a stroke and rehabilitation, patients should be followed at regular intervals to evaluate risk reduction strategies.

PATIENT EDUCATION

Educate patients who have had a stroke about the high risk of having a second stroke, the high morbidity and mortality associated with a recurrent stroke, and the need for lifestyle modifications and medications to reduce this risk.

PATIENT RESOURCES

- The National Stroke Association has patient information including signs of a stroke and resources for recovery—**http://www.stroke.org.**
- The Internet Stroke Center has a section for patients and families with patient education about signs of a stroke and living after a stroke—**http://www.strokecenter.org.**
- The National Institute of Neurologic Diseases and Stroke has written and auditory patient information in English and Spanish—**http://www.ninds.nih.gov.**

PROVIDER RESOURCES

- The Internet Stroke Center has a large collection of stroke scales and clinical assessment tools, a neurology image library, listings of professional resources, and evidence-based diagnosis and management strategies—**http://www.strokecenter.org.**
- Guidelines for early management of adults with ischemic stroke from the American Heart Association and other partners—**https://www.ahajournals.org/doi/full/10.1161/strokeaha.107.181486.**

REFERENCES

1. Stansbury JP, Jia H, Williams LS, et al. Ethnic disparities in stroke: epidemiology, acute care, and postacute outcomes [see comment] [review] [91 refs]. *Stroke.* 2005;36(2):374-386.
2. Schneider AT, Kissela B, Woo D, et al. Ischemic stroke subtypes: a population-based study of incidence rates among blacks and whites. *Stroke.* 2004;35(7):1552-1556.
3. Elkind MS. Inflammation, atherosclerosis, and stroke [review] [72 refs]. *Neurologist.* 2006;12(3):140-148.
4. Sanossian N, Ovbiagele B. Multimodality stroke prevention [review] [179 refs]. *Neurologist.* 2006;12(1):14-31.
5. Zhang Y, Tuomilehto J, Jousilahti P, et al. Lifestyle factors on the risks of ischemic and hemorrhagic stroke. *Arch Intern Med.* 2011;171(20):1811-1818.
6. Howard G, Cushman M, Kissela BM, et al; REasons for Geographic And Racial Differences in Stroke (REGARDS) Investigators. Traditional risk factors as the underlying cause of racial disparities in stroke: lessons from the half-full (empty?) glass. *Stroke.* 2011;42(12):3369-3375.
7. Tonarelli SB, Hart RG. What's new in stroke? The top 10 for 2004/05 [review] [25 refs]. *J Am Geriatr Soc.* 2006;54(4):674-679.
8. Maiser SJ, Georgiadis AL, Suri MF, et al. Intravenous recombinant tissue plasminogen activator administered after 3 h following onset of ischaemic stroke: a metaanalysis. *Int J Stroke.* 2011;6(1):25-32.
9. Frey JL, Jahnke HK, Goslar PW, et al. TPA by telephone: extending the benefits of a comprehensive stroke center. *Neurology.* 2005;64(1):154-156.
10. Orrapin S, Rerkasem K. Carotid endarterectomy for symptomatic carotid stenosis. *Cochrane Database Syst Rev.* 2017;(6):CD001081.
11. U.S. Preventive Services Task Force, *Aspirin for the Prevention of Cardiovascular Disease and Colorectal Cancer: Preventive Medicine.* https://www.uspreventiveservicestaskforce.org/Page/Document/UpdateSummaryFinal/aspirin-to-prevent-cardiovascular-disease-and-cancer?ds=1&s=aspirin. Updated April 2016.
12. Askoxylakis V, Thieke C, Pleger ST, et al. Long-term survival of cancer patients compared to heart failure and stroke: a systematic review. *BMC Cancer.* 2010;10:105.

242 SUBDURAL HEMATOMA

J. William Hayden, Jr, MD, EdD
Heidi S. Chumley, MD, MBA

PATIENT STORY

A 34-year-old driver was hit from behind at approximately 25 mph. He hit his head, but did not lose consciousness and did not seek care. Approximately 12 hours later, he developed a headache and confusion and was taken to the emergency department by a family member. He was found to have an acute subdural hematoma (**Figure 242-1**). He was hospitalized, and a neurosurgeon was consulted for surgical management.

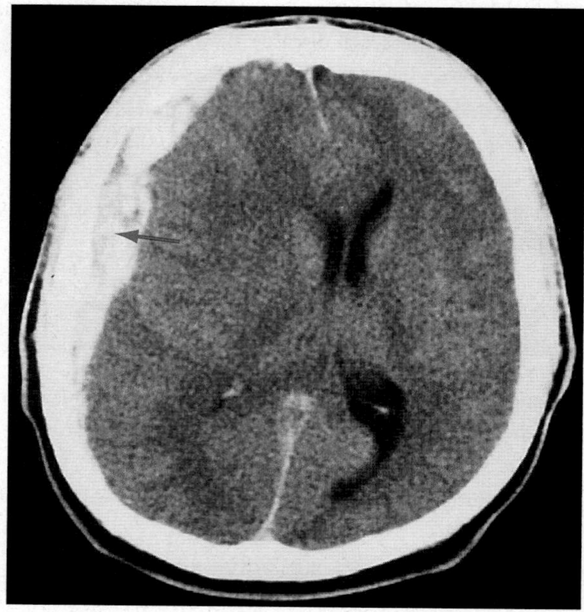

FIGURE 242-1 CT scan of an acute subdural hematoma (*arrow*) seen as a hyperdense clot with an irregular border. There is a midline shift from the mass effect of the accumulated blood. (*Reproduced with permission from Kasper DL, Braunwald E, Fauci AS, et a: Harrison's Principles of Internal Medicine, 16th ed. New York, NY: McGraw-Hill Education; 2005.*)

INTRODUCTION

Subdural hematoma (SH) is a collection of blood between the dura and arachnoid membranes, but external to the brain. SH may be acute or chronic. While most SHs are caused by trauma, they can occur at any age, most commonly in infants (abusive or unintentional head injury) and older adults due to cerebral atrophy with traction and rupture of bridging veins. Rarely, SH may occur spontaneously, associated with a ruptured aneurysm, bleeding from intracranial tumors, or malignancy-induced coagulopathy.[1] Presentation varies widely in acute SH. While many patients are initially comatose, lucid intervals are reported in up to 38% of cases.[1] Often, symptoms may be nonspecific, such as irritability or poor feeding in infants and confusion or headaches in adults. Treatment is prompt consultation with a neurosurgeon.

EPIDEMIOLOGY

- SHs occur at all ages. In adults, SHs are more common in men than in women with a male-to-female ratio of 3:1.[1,2]
- In a study of 111 asymptomatic newborns, 8% were found to have an SH; all resolved by 4 weeks without intervention.[3]
- Incidence of SH in infants ages 0 to 1 year in the United Kingdom was found to be 24 of 100,000.[4]
- Fewer than 1 in 100,000 adults per year have a traumatic SH.[2]
- SH accounts for 42 of every 100,000 adult hospitalizations.[5]
- Incidence of chronic SH is highest in the fifth through seventh decades of life.[1]
- Cost is $1.6 billion per year in 2007 dollars.[5]
- Mortality rates in treated older adults are approximately 8% for patients younger than age 65 years and 33% for patients older than age 65 years.[6]
- Estimated overall mortality rate in patients with acute SH requiring surgery is 40% to 60%.[7]

ETIOLOGY AND PATHOPHYSIOLOGY

- Most SHs are caused by trauma, either accidental or intentional, from a direct injury to the head or shaking injury in an infant (shaken baby syndrome).[1]
- The most common causes of traumatic SH are falls/assaults (72%) and vehicular trauma (24%).[1,2]
- SHs have even been attributed to trivial trauma such as chronic jarring from rapid walking in older patients.
- SH may occur in up to 8% of term deliveries, particularly with vacuum extraction and forceps deliveries.[3]
- Motion of the brain within the skull causes a shearing force to the cortical surface and interhemispheric bridging veins.[4]
- This force tears the weakest bridging veins as they cross the subdural space, resulting in an acute SH as seen in **Figure 242-1**.[4]
- Three days to 3 weeks after the injury, the body breaks down the blood in an SH; water is drawn into the collection, causing hemodilution, which appears less white, that is, less dense, and more gray on noncontrast CT.[4]
- If the hematoma fails to resolve, the collection has an even higher content of water and appears darker on a noncontrast CT, referred to as a hygroma; it may have fresh bleeding or may calcify (chronic SH; **Figure 242-2**).[4] This is often of the same density as brain parenchyma on noncontrast CT.
- Nontraumatic causes reported in the literature include spontaneous bleeding because of bleeding disorders or anticoagulation, meningitis, and complications of neurologic procedures, including lumbar puncture and spinal anesthesia.[7]

RISK FACTORS

Increased mortality associated with acute SHs ranges from 36% to 79%,[1] especially in patients:

- Older than 80 years of age.[5]
- With lower income.[5]
- With acquired clotting abnormalities.[5,7]
- Who experienced trauma.[5]
- With a higher APACHE (Acute physiology, Age, and Chronic Health Evaluation) III score on presentation.[7]

Comorbidity risk factors for chronic SH include[1]:

- Chronic alcoholism.
- Epilepsy.
- Cardiovascular disease, such as hypertension or arteriosclerosis.
- Thrombocytopenia.
- Diabetes mellitus.
- Anticoagulant therapy, including aspirin.
- Arachnoid cysts.

DIAGNOSIS

In the absence of known trauma, clinical features are often nonspecific, making the diagnosis difficult. With chronic SH, 25% to 50% of patients have no history of head trauma.[1] In 8.7% to 32%, chronic SHs have been reported to be bilateral.[1]

- Infants may present with drowsiness, irritability, poor tone, poor feeding, or new seizures.[4]
- Older adults may present with headaches, confusion, subtle changes in mental status, personality change, gait disturbances, hemiparesis, or other focal neurologic signs.[1,8]

With traumatic injuries, physical findings may include signs of a basilar skull fracture:

- Bilateral periorbital ecchymoses (raccoon eyes).
- Retroauricular ecchymoses (Battle sign).
- Cerebrospinal rhinorrhea or otorrhea.

TYPICAL DISTRIBUTION

SHs by definition occur in the subdural space, most commonly seen in the parietal region.

With children, an SH found in the interhemispheric space or posterior fossa highly suggests physical abuse, as do hematomas in multiple sites.[9]

IMAGING

Acute SHs are seen easily on a noncontrast CT scan (see **Figure 242-1**). Subacute and chronic SHs (see **Figure 242-2**) can be similar in color—that is, density—to the brain parenchyma and may be easier to see on a contrast CT or an MRI. Although MRI is superior in delineating the size of an acute SH and its effect on the brain, CT remains the primary diagnostic imaging study for immediate management decisions, as images can be produced quickly and are highly sensitive to acute blood.[1] Moreover, MRI cannot be used in the presence of metallic objects often needed in resuscitating trauma victims, such as ventilators and oxygen tanks.

- The initial CT scan may underestimate the size of parenchymal contusions. Clinical deterioration should prompt repeat imaging in salvageable patients.[1]
- In traumatic head injuries, cervical spine series are critical to evaluate possible concomitant cervical spine fractures.[1]

DIFFERENTIAL DIAGNOSIS

Prior to CT availability, 72% of chronic SHs were misdiagnosed because of their variable clinical presentation and frequently absent history of head trauma.[1]

In conjunction with CT neuroimaging, SH can be more accurately differentiated from the following conditions:

- Infections such as sepsis or meningitis—Fever, elevated white blood cells, positive blood cultures, and cerebrospinal fluid consistent with meningitis.
- Hemorrhagic (**Figure 242-3**) or ischemic stroke or transient ischemic attacks—Consider risk factors for stroke such as hypertension, diabetes, atrial fibrillation, and smoking (see Chapter 241, Cerebral Vascular Accident).
- Dementia or depression—Less acute onset, advanced age, and other symptoms consistent with depression.

- Primary or metastatic brain neoplasms—History of cancer and risk factors for cancer.
- Epidural hematoma (**Figure 242-4**)—Well-defined biconvex bright white density that resembles the shape of the lens of the eye.
- Subarachnoid hemorrhage (**Figure 242-5**)—Bright white blood outlines cerebral sulci.
- Hemorrhage in brain parenchyma—Bright white lesion apart from dura.

MANAGEMENT

Most SHs are managed surgically. While there is little evidence for conservative management other than limited observational data, expert panel guidelines published in 2006 recommended nonoperative management in an intensive care unit with intracranial pressure monitoring for patients meeting the following criteria: they are neurologically stable, have clot thickness <10 mm, midline shift <5 mm, no pupillary abnormalities, and no intracranial hypertension.[7] SOR Ⓒ

- Observational studies in patients with SH suggest that surgery performed within 2 to 4 hours after the onset of neurological deterioration have mortality rates between 30% and 47%, as opposed to 80%°90% percent mortality with surgery delayed beyond 4 hours.[7]
- Determine the Glasgow Coma Scale in patients with serious head trauma and consider airway protection in patients with a score less than 12.
- Obtain an urgent noncontrast CT scan on any patient suspected of having an SH.
- Blood studies should include[1]:
  - Complete blood count
  - Coagulation profile (important for patients on anticoagulants and with history of alcohol abuse)
  - Basic metabolic profile for electrolyte abnormalities
  - Type and screen/cross-match
- If the noncontrast CT scan is nonrevealing, obtain a contrast CT or MRI, if available and no contraindications, particularly if the traumatic event occurred 2 to 3 days prior.
- Emergently refer patients with an SH and deteriorating neurologic status or evidence of brain edema or midline shift to a hospital with neurosurgeons.
- Consult a neurosurgeon expediently in patients with an SH and stable focal neurologic signs.
- Avoid hypotension and hypoxia, as they are independent predictors of poor outcomes.[1]
- Maintain pCO_2 between 30 and 35 mm Hg with continuous mainstream or sidestream capnometry monitoring.
- Medications may include[1]:
  - Anticonvulsants to prevent seizure-induced ischemia and surges in intracranial pressure.
  - Short-acting sedatives and paralytics only when necessary to facilitate ventilation or with elevated intracranial pressure.

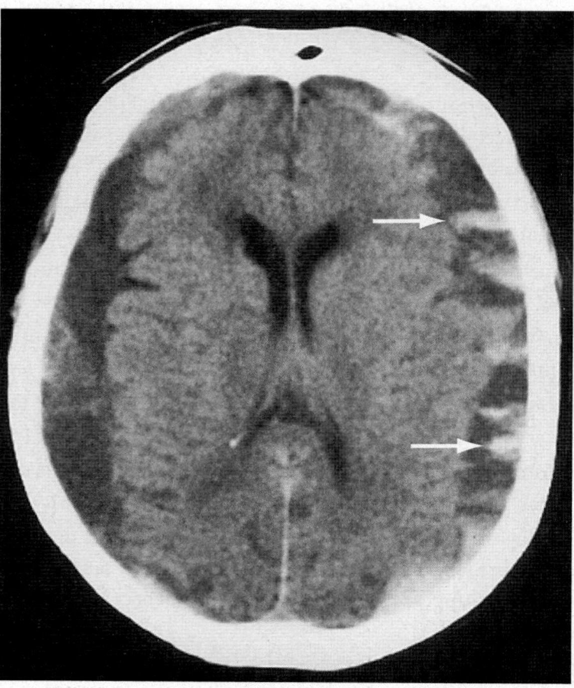

FIGURE 242-2 CT scan of chronic bilateral subdural hematomas. As subdural hematomas age, these become isodense gray and then hypodense (darker gray to black) compared to the brain. Some resolving blood is still visible on the left (*arrows*). (*Reproduced with permission from Kasper DL, Braunwald E, Fauci AS, et a: Harrison's Principles of Internal Medicine, 16th ed. New York, NY: McGraw-Hill Education; 2005.*)

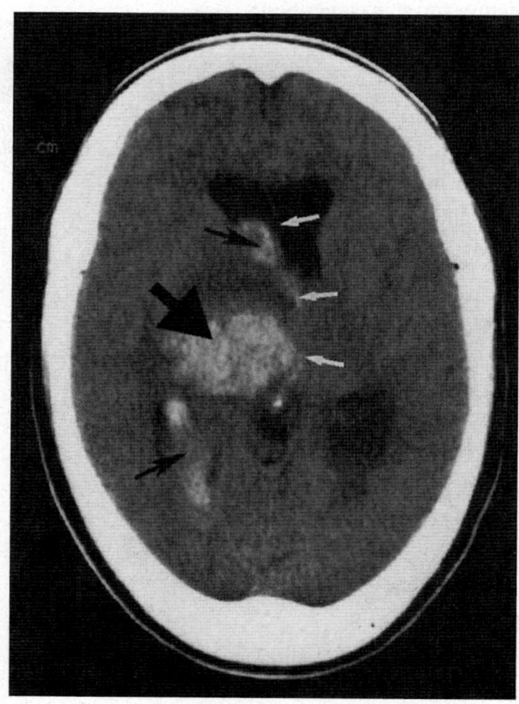

FIGURE 242-3 Hemorrhagic stroke seen on CT. The CT image demonstrates bleeding in the right basal ganglia (*large black arrow*) into the ventricles (*small black arrows*) with midline shift (*white arrows*). (*Reproduced with permission from Chen MYM, Pope TL, Ott DJ. Basic Radiology. New York, NY: McGraw-Hill Education; 2004.*)

- Prothrombin complex concentrate, fresh frozen plasma, and/or platelets in patients with coagulopathies or receiving anticoagulant medications. Maintain prothrombin time within reference range and platelets above 100,000.
- With herniation syndrome, administer mannitol 1 g/kg rapidly via IV push.
- Avoid steroids, as they have been found ineffective in head-injury patients.

- With traumatic injury, serial follow-up CT scans should be obtained during the first 36 hours following injury because of the high incidence of clot expansion during this period. Perform the first repeat scan within 6 to 8 hours of admission.[7]
- Consider neurosurgical consultation in asymptomatic patients or those with only a headache and a small acute SH without brain edema or midline shift. These patients may be followed by serial CT scans without surgical treatment, but this should be done in consultation with experts in CT interpretation and management of SHs.[7] SOR C
- Evaluate any infant with an SH for child abuse or neglect.[3] SOR C

PREVENTION

- Follow safety measures that reduce motor vehicle accidents, and falls in the elderly.
- Use recommended protective gear for sports and recreational activities and follow evidence-based guidelines for return to play after a head injury. (See Chapter 240, Sports-related Head Injury)
- Carefully evaluate the risks and benefits of chronic use of antiplatelet and anticoagulation medications.

PROGNOSIS

- In-hospital mortality for acute SH is 12%.[5,6]
- In-hospital mortality for traumatic SH is 26%.[2]
- Best predictor of in-hospital mortality is neurologic status on admission.[8]
- Younger patients have more favorable outcomes: age <40 years—20% mortality rate; age 40–80 years—65% mortality rate; age >80 years—88% mortality rate.[9]
- In patients older than age 65 years, the mortality rate for chronic SH remains elevated until 1 year after diagnosis, independent of treatment.[10]

FOLLOW-UP

- Follow-up is determined by severity of SH and type of treatment.
- Ideally, follow-up is conducted jointly between the neurosurgeon and primary care physician to ensure resolution of the SH and maximal return of function, especially in elderly patients.

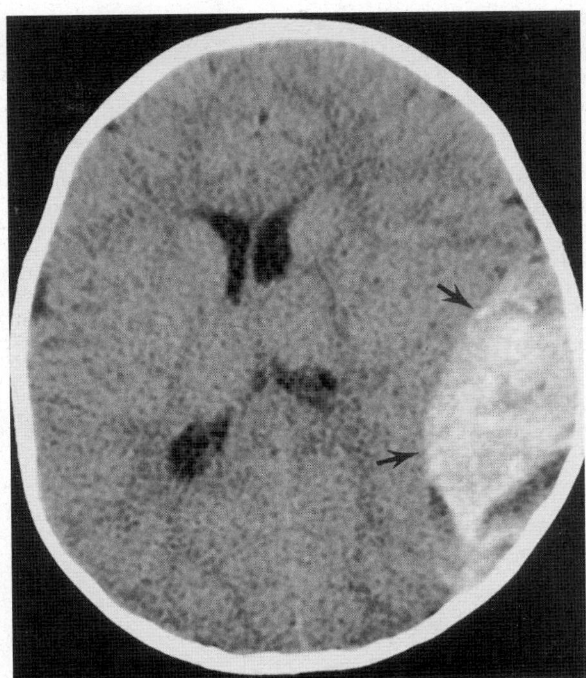

FIGURE 242-4 This head CT demonstrates an epidural hematoma, with the typical biconvex appearance (*arrows*). Note how the biconvex appearance resembles the lens of an eye. (*Reproduced with permission from Chen MYM, Pope TL, Ott DJ. Basic Radiology. New York, NY: McGraw-Hill Education; 2004.*)

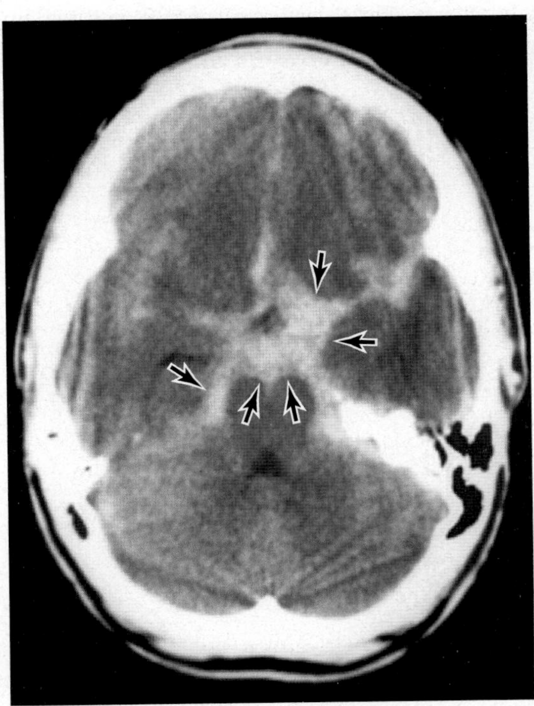

FIGURE 242-5 A subarachnoid hemorrhage appears as areas of high density (more white like bone rather than the darker gray of brain tissue) in the subarachnoid space (*arrows*). (*Reproduced with permission from Aminoff MJ, Greenberg DA, Simon RP. Clinical Neurology, 6th ed. New York, NY: McGraw-Hill Education; 2005.*)

PATIENT EDUCATION

- Advise patients to seek medical care immediately for head trauma, which can cause several emergencies including an SH.
- Discuss with parents or guardians the need for a thorough evaluation for child abuse and neglect in infants with an SH.

PATIENT RESOURCES

- MedlinePlus. *Subdural Hematoma*—**https://medlineplus.gov/ency/article/000713.htm.**

PROVIDER RESOURCES

- *Head injury: assessment and early management*—**https://www.nice.org.uk/guidance/cg176**.
- *Pediatric Glasgow Coma Scale*—**https://www.mdcalc.com/pediatric-glasgow-coma-scale-pgcs**.
- *Glasgow Coma Scale Calculator*—**https://www.mdcalc.com/glasgow-coma-scale-score-gcs**.

REFERENCES

1. Meagher RJ, Lutsep HL, et al. Subdural hematoma. http://emedicine.medscape.com/article/1137207-clinical. Updated August 4, 2016. Accessed April 2017.
2. Tallon JM, Ackroyd-Stolarz S, Karim SA, Clarke DB. The epidemiology of surgically treated acute subdural and epidural hematomas in patients with head injuries: a population-based study. *Can J Surg.* 2008;51(5):339-345.
3. Whitby EH, Griffiths PD, Rutter S, et al. Frequency and natural history of subdural haemorrhages in babies and relation to obstetric factors [see comment]. *Lancet.* 2004;363(9412):846-851.
4. Minns RA. Subdural haemorrhages, haematomas, and effusions in infancy [comment] [review] [9 refs]. *Arch Dis Child.* 2005;90(9):883-884.
5. Frontera JA, Egorova N, Moskowitz AJ. National trend in prevalence, cost, and discharge disposition after subdural hematoma from 1998-2007. *Crit Care Med.* 2011;39(7):119-125.
6. Munro PT, Smith RD, Parke TR. Effect of patients' age on management of acute intracranial haematoma: prospective national study. *BMJ.* 2002;325(7371):1001.
7. McBride W. Subdural hematoma in adults: prognosis and management. https://uptodate.com/contents/subdural-hematoma-in-adults-prognosis-and-management. Updated March 25, 2014. Accessed April 2017.
8. Bershad EM, Farhadi S, Suri MF, et al. Coagulopathy and in hospital deaths in patients with acute subdural hematoma. *J Neurosurg.* 2008;109(4):664-669.
9. Proctor MR. Intracranial subdural hematoma in children: epidemiology, anatomy, and pathophysiology. https://uptodate.com/contents/intracranial-subdural-hematoma-in-children-epidemiology-anatomy-and-physiology. UpToDate March 2, 2016. Accessed April 2017.
10. Miranda LB, Braxton E, Hobbs J, Quigley MR. Chronic subdural hematoma in the elderly: not a benign disease. *J Neurosurg.* 2011;114(1):72-76.

243 DEMENTIA

Heidi S. Chumley, MD, MBA

PATIENT STORY

A 70-year-old woman is brought to the physician by her daughter, who is concerned that she is becoming forgetful. She has hypertension but is otherwise healthy and lives independently. A neurologic examination is normal, with the exception of mild cognitive decline on an objective assessment. You recommend testing to evaluate for reversible causes of cognitive decline, including an MRI.

INTRODUCTION

Dementia is present in approximately 6% of adults over the age of 60 and increases with age. Dementia is now called minor or major neurocognitive disorder based on severity and can be due to many different disease processes. Alzheimer disease, vascular dementia, frontotemporal dementia, and dementia with Lewy bodies are the most common types of dementia. Dementia is a clinical diagnosis, although biomarkers can now assist with differentiating types of dementia. Treatments may slow decline, but the course is progressive.

EPIDEMIOLOGY

- In most areas of the world, 5% to 7% of adults over 60 years of age have dementia. The prevalence is slightly higher in Latin America (8.5%) and lower in sub-Saharan Africa (2%–4%).[1]
- In 2010, approximately 36 million people were living with dementia, a number that is expected to double every 20 years.[1]
- The pooled prevalence of dementia increases with age. Almost 45% of adults age 95 or older have dementia.[2]
- In 2010, Alzheimer disease (AD) was the 6th leading cause of death in the United States and the leading cause of death in people over the age of 65.[3]
- In the United States, health care for people age 65 and older with dementia costs an estimated $214 billion each year; unpaid caregivers provide a contribution estimated to be an additional $220 billion.[3]

ETIOLOGY AND PATHOPHYSIOLOGY

Dementia can be due to a number of different disease processes.

- AD, 50% to 70% of dementia cases—Progressive loss of neurons, buildup of amyloid plaques and neurofibrillary tangles, and decline in presynaptic cholinergic function.
- Vascular dementia, 20% of dementia cases—Cerebrovascular disease in large or small vessels.
- Frontotemporal dementia (FTD), 5% of dementia cases—Atrophy of frontal and temporal lobes, tau or protein TDP-43 accumulation; Pick disease is a subtype with intracellular tau (Pick bodies).
- DLB, 5% of dementia cases—Progressive loss of neurons due to alpha-synuclein misfolding and aggregation within Lewy bodies.
- Less common causes of dementia are Parkinson disease (although dementia is common in patients with Parkinson disease), Huntington disease, prion disease, HIV/AIDS, or multiple sclerosis.

DIAGNOSIS

Criteria for major neurocognitive disorder (dementia) from the *Diagnostic and Statistical Manual of Mental Disorders, Fifth Edition* (DSM-5):

- Significant cognitive decline (observed by a clinician or reliable informant or documented on an objective cognitive assessment).
- Substantial loss of independence in everyday activities.
- Not present only during delirium or better explained by another diagnosis.

DSM-5 criteria for mild neurocognitive disorder (dementia):

- Mild cognitive decline (observed by a clinician or reliable informant or documented on an objective cognitive assessment).
- Maintains independence in everyday activities, although they may take longer or require a compensatory strategy.
- Not present only during delirium or better explained by another diagnosis.

Objective cognitive assessments routinely used in the ambulatory setting include the Mini-Mental Status Exam, Montreal Cognitive Assessment, St. Louis University Mental Status Examination, and the Mini-Cog.[4]

CLINICAL FEATURES

Different causes of dementia have different patterns of cognitive decline. Cognitive domains affected include complex attention, executive function (i.e., planning or multitasking), learning and memory, language, perceptual-motor/visuospatial (i.e., getting lost), and social cognition (i.e., inappropriate behavior).[5]

- Alzheimer disease—Gradual onset and progressive impairments, memory deficits early, language and social deficits later; late stage may also include psychosis, agitation, and wandering. Depressive symptoms or apathy may be present throughout the course.
- Vascular dementia—History of stroke or transient ischemic attack preceding cognitive decline, course may be stepwise or gradual, complex attention and executive function deficits are common,

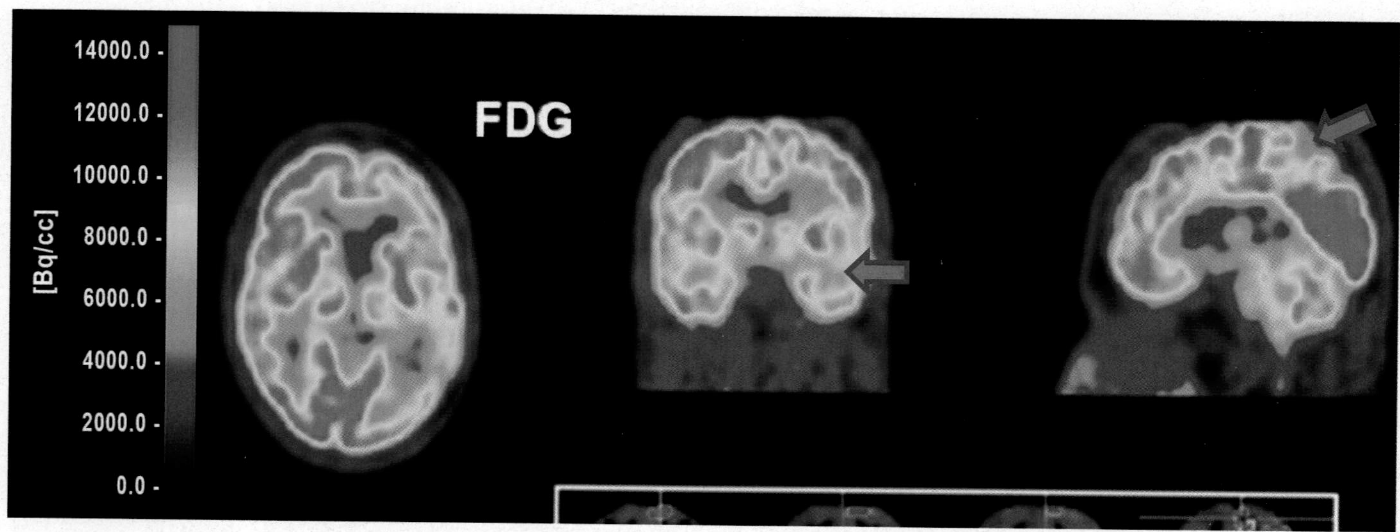

FIGURE 243-1 Positron emission tomography (PET) brain imaging of a patient with Alzheimer disease. *Red arrows* point to the decreased metabolic activity (*green color*) in the temporoparietal lobes and posterior cingulate gyri. (*Reproduced with permission from Bundhit Tantiwongkosi, MD.*)

other neurologic findings depending on location of vascular insults, may coexist with Alzheimer disease.

- FTD—Gradual onset and progressive impairments, 75% of patients experience symptoms before age 65,[5] two variants are described with deficits in behavior or language.
- Dementia with Lewy bodies—Gradual onset and progressive impairments; deficits in complex attention, visuospatial, and executive function are common; parkinsonian features that occur after the cognitive decline.

LABORATORY TESTING

- Screen for potential contributors to cognitive decline with a complete blood count, comprehensive metabolic panel, thyroid function tests, and vitamin B_{12}; consider HIV and syphilis testing in at-risk patients.
- Alzheimer disease:
  - Biomarkers associated with AD include CSF T-tau, P-tau, Aβ42, and NFL, and plasma T-tau; however, they are not routinely used in diagnosis or monitoring.[6]
  - Consider genetics testing (or referral for genetic testing/counseling) for patients with onset of dementia before age 65 and a positive family history. Genes associated with early-onset AD include PSEN1, APP, and PSEN2.[7]

IMAGING

- Structural imaging (non-contrast CT or MRI) is indicated in many patients presenting with cognitive decline to their primary care physician.
  - Patients with rapid progression, atypical course, focal neurologic signs, or head trauma.
  - Patients with a history or physical examination that suggests tumors, subdural hematoma, normal-pressure hydrocephalus, or stroke (vascular dementia).
  - Patients for whom the "unsuspected presence of cerebrovascular disease would alter management."[8]
- Functional imaging may be helpful in differentiating AD from DLB[9] (**Figures 243-1** and **243-2**).
  - MRI—AD shows atrophy in temporal lobes, which is preserved in DLB.
  - FP-CIT SPECT—AD shows generous uptake in the caudate and putamen; DLB uptake is minimal and restricted to the caudate.
- Frontotemporal dementia has atrophy in the frontal and temporal lobes that can be seen on MRI (**Figure 243-3**).

DIFFERENTIAL DIAGNOSIS

- Delirium—Often has a more acute onset, a trigger such as an infection or recent hospitalization, and a predominance of attention and orientation deficits.
- Depression—More commonly presents with somatic complaints and insomnia, but often coexists with dementias.
- Parkinson disease with dementia—Motor features precede cognitive deficits.
- Schizophrenia or bipolar spectrum disorders—Typically occur at a younger age and have a predominance of psychotic or mood symptoms; most likely confused with FTD.
- Tumors—May have presence of constitutional symptoms and are seen on structural imaging.
- Stroke—Risk factor for or history of vascular disease, seen on structural imaging.
- Subdural hematoma—History of fall or head trauma, visible on structural imaging.

MANAGEMENT

- The goals of treatment are to prevent further cognitive decline, maintain function and independence, and address quality-of-life issues.

- Manage comorbidities, especially depression and those contributing to vascular disease.
- Review medications, including over-the-counter, and consider replacing those that can worsen cognition.

NONPHARMACOLOGIC

- Exercise may be of benefit in slowing cognitive decline[4] and preserving function SOR B and is an important component of a healthy lifestyle.
- Cognitive training may also be of benefit.[4] SOR C
- Caregiver training and support may also be of benefit.[4] SOR C

MEDICATIONS

- Alzheimer disease:
  - Cholinesterase inhibitors (i.e., rivastigmine or donepezil) may improve cognition and function or slow deterioration.[10] SOR A
  - *N*-Methyl-D-aspartate (NMDA) receptor antagonist (memantine) may have a small beneficial effect on cognition, can be taken with a cholinesterase inhibitor, and is generally well tolerated.[5] SOR B
- Vascular dementia—Pharmacologic treatment is aimed at preventing further vascular incidences.
- FTD—No disease-modifying agents; treat behavioral symptoms as needed using selective serotonin reuptake inhibitor (SSRI) or trazadone; neuroleptics may help with aggression or psychosis but have more side effects.
- DLB—Cholinesterase inhibitors (i.e., rivastigmine or donepezil) improve cognition and function and slow deterioration.[11] SOR A

REFERRAL OR HOSPITALIZATION

- Dementia diagnosis is evolving rapidly; refer patients when the diagnosis is in question.
- Refer patients with difficult-to-control symptoms to a physician skilled in the management of dementias.

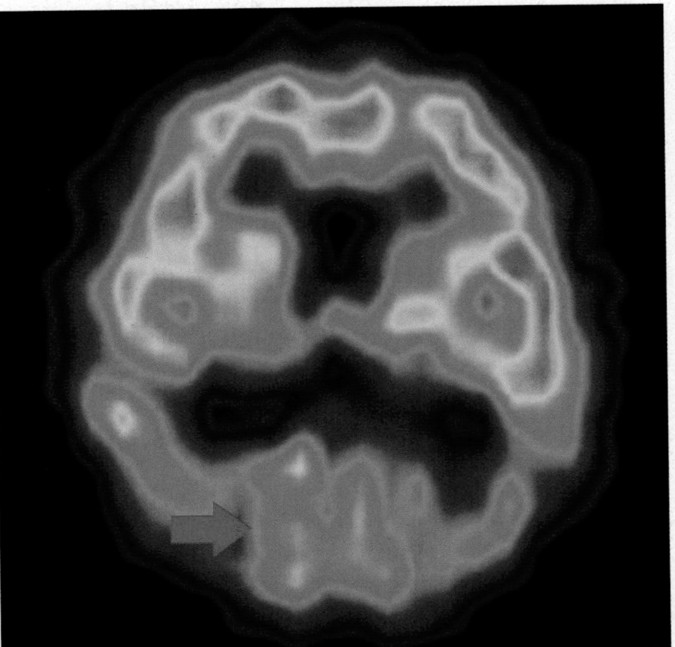

FIGURE 243-2 Dementia with Lewy bodies (DLB) has hypometabolism (*green color*) throughout the entire cerebral cortex, including occipital lobe involvement (*red arrow*), which helps to differentiate DLB from Alzheimer disease. (*Reproduced with permission from Bundhit Tantiwongkosi, MD.*)

PROGNOSIS

At present, dementia is a progressive disease. Prognosis depends on the type of dementia as well as the stage of cognitive impairment.

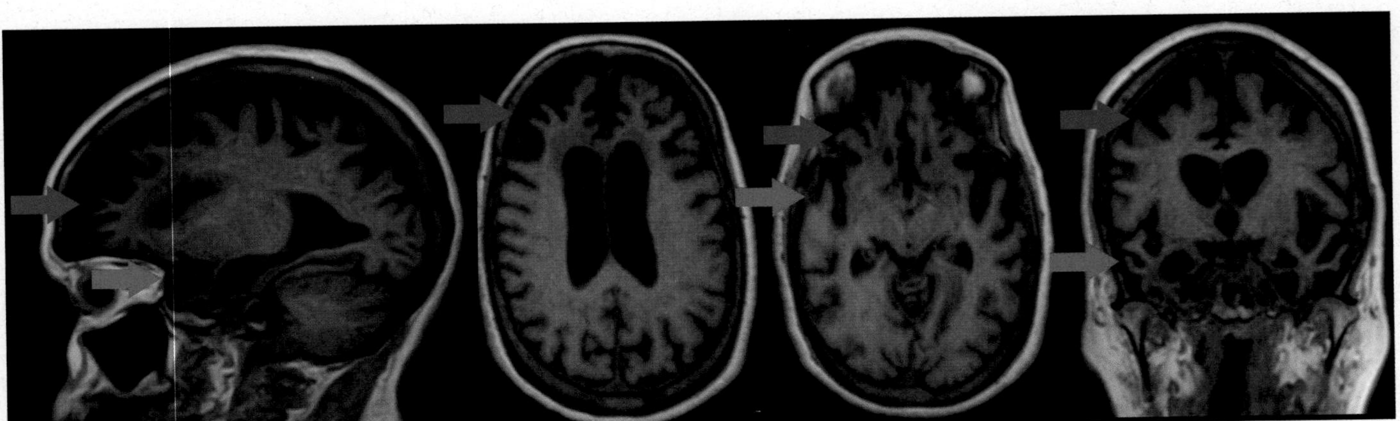

FIGURE 243-3 Frontotemporal dementia has atrophy of the bilateral frontal (*blue arrows*) and temporal (*red arrows*) lobes that can be seen with these T1-weighted MRI images. (*Reproduced with permission from Bundhit Tantiwongkosi, MD.*)

- AD patients progress from mild to moderate to severe, spending 3–5 years in each stage.[12]
- Vascular dementia patients seem to progress more quickly, with a life expectancy of 3–5 years.[12]

FOLLOW-UP

Patients with dementia should be seen regularly by their managing physician to monitor and adjust medications when used, follow the course and assist with life planning, and attend to caregiver needs.

PATIENT EDUCATION

Advise patients and caregivers of the progressive nature of dementia and the need for ongoing evaluation of function. When possible, establish patient wishes and power of attorney in the early stages. Advise on issues such as driving and financial management.

PATIENT RESOURCES

- Alzheimer's Association has information for patients and caregivers—**https://www.alz.org.**
- Family Caregiver Alliance National Center on Caregiving has the Caregiver's Guide to Understanding Dementia Behaviors—**https://www.caregiver.org**.

PROVIDER RESOURCES

- NIH National Institute on Aging has an Alzheimer's and Dementia Resources for Professionals with links to assessment tools, curricula, patient care guidelines, and research trials—**https://www.nia.nih.gov.**
- Alzheimer's Association has patient and informant assessment tools available in multiple languages—**https://www.alz.org.**

REFERENCES

1. Prince M, Bryce R, Albanese E, et al. The global prevalence of dementia: a systematic review and metaanalysis. *Alzheimers Dement.* 2013;9(1):63-75.e2.
2. Alexander M, Perera G, Ford L, et al. Age-stratified prevalence of mild cognitive impairment and dementia in European populations: a systematic review. *J Alzheimers Dis.* 2015;48(2):355-359.
3. Alzheimer's Association. 2014 Alzheimer's disease facts and figures. *Alzheimers Dement.* 2014:10(2):e47-e92.
4. Hildreth KL, Church S. Evaluation and management of the elderly patient presenting with cognitive complaints. *Medical Clin North Am.* 2015;99(2):311-335.
5. Hugo J, Ganguli M. Dementia and cognitive impairment: epidemiology, diagnosis, and treatment. *Clin Geriatr Med.* 2014;30(3): 421-442.
6. Olsson B, Lautner R, Andreasson U, et al. CSF and blood biomarkers for the diagnosis of Alzheimer's disease: a systematic review and meta-analysis. *Lancet Neurol.* 2016;15(7):673-684.
7. Zou Z, Liu C, Che C, Huang H. Clinical genetics of Alzheimer's disease. *BioMed Res Int.* 2014;2014:291862.
8. Moore A, Patterson C, Lee L, et al. Fourth Canadian Consensus Conference on the Diagnosis and Treatment of Dementia Recommendations for family physicians. *Can Fam Physician.* 2014;60:433-438.
9. McKeith IG, Boeve BF, Dickson DW, et al. Diagnosis and management of dementia with Lewy bodies: fourth consensus report of the DLB Consortium. *Neurology.* 2017;89(1):88-100.
10. Birks J. Cholinesterase inhibitors for Alzheimer's disease. *Cochrane Database Syst Rev.* 2006;(1):CD005593.
11. Stinton C, McKeith I, Taylor JP, et al. Pharmacological management of Lewy body dementia: a systematic review and meta-analysis. *Am J Psychiatry.* 2015;172:731-742.
12. Kua EH, Ho E, Tan HH, et al. The natural history of dementia. *Psychogeriatrics.* 2014:14(3)196-201.

244 BELL PALSY

J. William Hayden, Jr, MD, EdD
Heidi S. Chumley, MD, MBA

PATIENT STORY

Five years ago, a young woman awoke with the inability to move the left side of her face and presented to her family physician. She was pregnant at that time. On examination, she had absent brow furrowing, weak eye closure, and dropping of her mouth angle (**Figure 244-1**). She was diagnosed with Bell palsy and was provided eye lubricants and guidance on keeping her left eye moist. Her physician discussed the available evidence about treatment with steroids. She chose not to take the steroids because of her pregnancy.

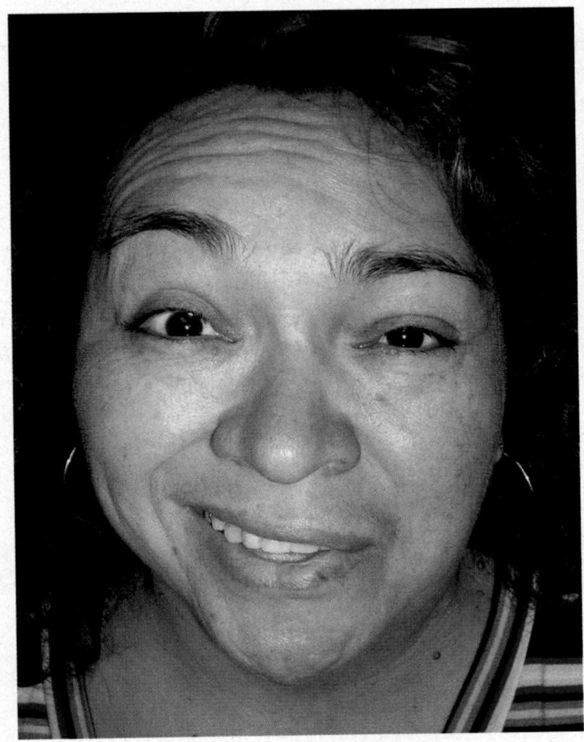

FIGURE 244-1 Bell palsy with loss of brow furrowing and dropped angle of the mouth on the affected left side of her face demonstrated during a request to smile and raise her eyebrows. The Bell palsy has been present for 5 years and the patient is being evaluated by ear, nose, and throat (ENT) for surgery to restore facial movement. *(Reproduced with permission from Richard P. Usatine, MD.)*

INTRODUCTION

Bell palsy is an acute paralysis of the facial nerve of unproven etiology resulting in loss of brow furrowing, weak eye closure, and dropped angle of mouth. Treatment is oral steroids as soon after the onset of symptoms as possible. Most patients have a full recovery within 6 months.

SYNONYMS

Bell palsy is a diagnosis of exclusion. Although Bell palsy has been synonymous with idiopathic facial paralysis, peripheral facial nerve palsy is a clinical syndrome with many causes. In most cases of Bell palsy, herpes simplex or other suspected viral etiology is likely the causative agent. If some degree of facial nerve function fails to return within 4 months, a diagnosis of Bell palsy is questionable and a more extensive evaluation is warranted.[1]

The syndrome is named after Sir Charles Bell, a 19th-century Scottish anatomist who described the facial nerve and its possible association to this condition.[2]

EPIDEMIOLOGY

- In a Canadian study, incidence was 13.1 to 15.2 per 100,000 adults.[3]
- In the United States, Bell palsy affects approximately 40,000 Americans annually.[2]
- In a study of U.S. military members, the incidence was 42.77 per 100,000, with higher incidence in females, blacks, and Hispanics; arid climate and cold months were independent predictors of risk with adjusted relative risk ratios of 1.34 and 1.31, respectively.[4]
- Women who develop Bell palsy in pregnancy have a 5-fold increased risk of preeclampsia or gestational hypertension.[5]
- Seventy percent of cases of acute peripheral facial nerve palsy are idiopathic (Bell palsy); 30% have known etiologic factors such as trauma, diabetes mellitus, polyneuritis, tumors, or infections such as herpes zoster, leprosy (**Figure 244-2**), or *Borrelia*.[6]

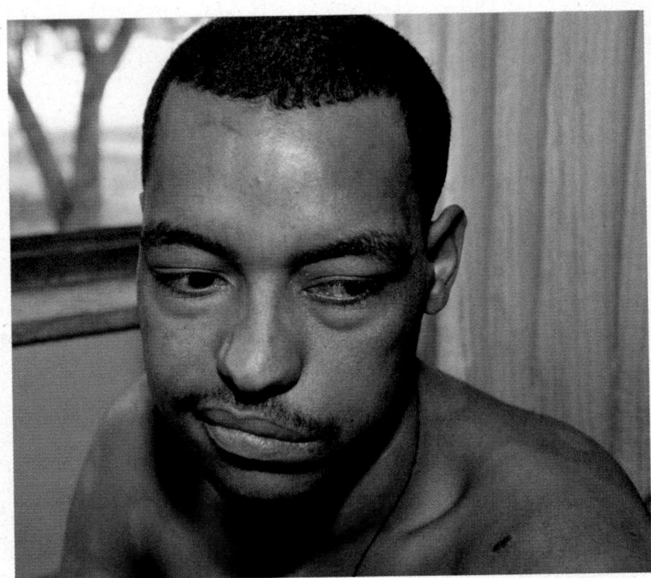

FIGURE 244-2 Bell palsy secondary to leprosy. The hypopigmented patches on his back are further signs of the leprosy. *(Reproduced with permission from Richard P. Usatine, MD.)*

- Seven percent to 15% of patients with Bell palsy may experience recurrent attacks. Mean time to recurrence is approximately 10 years.[7]

ETIOLOGY AND PATHOPHYSIOLOGY

- Etiology of Bell palsy is currently unknown and under debate; the prevailing theory suggests a herpes virus reactivation—herpes simplex I or herpes zoster.
- The facial nerve becomes inflamed, resulting in nerve compression, often in the setting of a flu-type illness.
- Compression of the facial nerve compromises muscles of facial expression, taste fibers to the anterior tongue, pain fibers, and secretory fibers to the salivary and lacrimal glands.
- This is a lower motor neuron lesion; the upper and lower portions of the face are affected (see **Figure 244-1**). In upper motor neuron lesions (e.g., cortical stroke), the upper third of the face is spared, while the lower two thirds are affected as a result of the bilateral innervation of the orbicularis, frontalis, and corrugator muscles, which allows sparing of upper face movement.

DIAGNOSIS

CLINICAL FEATURES

- A diagnosis of Bell palsy is made on the basis of the initial clinical presentation, as there is no specific laboratory test to confirm the diagnosis. A careful history and physical examination are essential to exclude identifiable causes of facial nerve paresis or paralysis.
- Weakness of all facial muscles on the affected side—Loss of brow furrowing, weak eye closure, and dropped angle of mouth.
- Postauricular pain.
- Dry eyes.
- Involuntary tearing.
- Hyperacusis.
- Altered tastes.
- The House-Brackmann grading system may be useful for guiding therapy and prognosis.[8]
  - Grade I: normal facial function
  - Grade II: mild dysfunction (i.e., slight weakness noticeable on close inspection, complete eye closure with minimal effort)
  - Grade III: moderate dysfunction (i.e., obvious but not disfiguring asymmetry, eye closure with moderate effort)
  - Grade IV: moderately severe dysfunction (i.e., disfiguring asymmetry, incomplete eye closure)
  - Grade V: severe dysfunction (i.e., barely perceptible motion with asymmetry at rest)
  - Grade VI: total paralysis

LABORATORY TESTING

Laboratory testing is not usually indicated but may be useful in selected patients:

- In endemic areas of Lyme disease, facial paralysis may be present in up to 25% of cases.[9]
- Blood glucose or hemoglobin A_{1c} for diabetes mellitus in patients with risk factors.
- Herpes virus titers are not usually helpful due to the ubiquitous nature of herpes simplex virus.

IMAGING

- The American Academy of Otolaryngology—Head and Neck Surgery advises against routine imaging in patients with new-onset Bell palsy.[10]
- For presentations of facial nerve paralysis inconsistent with Bell palsy, consider MRI to look for space-occupying lesions. Should MRI be contraindicated or unavailable, contrast-enhanced CT may be an alternative.

DIFFERENTIAL DIAGNOSIS

- Upper motor neuron diseases including stroke—Normal brow furrowing, eye closure, and blinking.
- Space-occupying lesion—Symptoms are dependent on the location of the mass; consider with an isolated facial nerve palsy that does not affect all three branches of the facial nerve.
- A slow, progressive paralysis of the facial nerve beyond 3 weeks should be evaluated for neoplasm.[11]
- Cerebellopontine tumors may affect the 5th, 7th, and 8th cranial nerves simultaneously.[11]
- Lyme disease—Occurs in endemic area with skin rash, joint inflammation, and flu-like symptoms. Bell palsy is the most common neurologic manifestation of Lyme disease (see Chapter 227, Lyme Disease).
- Suppurative ear disease (otitis media)—Ear pain, abnormal tympanic membrane, and more common in children.
- Ramsay Hunt syndrome (herpes zoster)—Sudden hearing loss with severe pain and onset of facial paralysis. An erythematous vesicular rash involving the ear canal, auricle, and/or oropharynx may be present.
- Guillain-Barré syndrome—Consider in patients with facial weakness and progressive, mostly symmetric muscle weakness with absent or depressed deep tendon reflexes.
- Facial nerve damage from microvascular disease—Most commonly in diabetes mellitus.
- Facial nerve damage from trauma—History of trauma differentiates this from Bell palsy that is idiopathic or from an infectious etiology.
- Isolated third nerve palsy—Manifestations include diplopia and drooping of the upper eyelid (ptosis) (**Figure 244-3**). The affected eye may deviate out and down in straight-ahead gaze; adduction is slow and cannot proceed past the midline. Upward gaze is impaired. When downward gaze is attempted, the superior oblique muscle causes the eye to adduct. The pupil may be normal or dilated; its response to direct or consensual light may be sluggish or absent (efferent defect). Pupil dilation (mydriasis) may be an early sign.

MANAGEMENT

NONPHARMACOLOGIC

- Provide eye protection with artificial tears, lubricants, or closing of the eyelid. SOR Ⓒ

MEDICATIONS

- A Cochrane systematic review supports treating patients with systemic corticosteroids. Steroids significantly decrease a patient's risk for incomplete recovery from 28% to 17%, risk ratio 0.63 (confidence index [CI] 0.50–0.80).[12] SOR Ⓐ
    - Dosing of steroids in the studies included in the Cochrane review varied from oral methylprednisolone 1 mg/kg daily for 10 days, and then gradually withdrawn for another 3 to 5 days, to prednisone given as a single dose of 60 mg daily for 5 days, followed by a dose reduced by 10 mg per day, with a total treatment of 10 days. One trial used high-dose prednisolone given intravenously.
- A Cochrane systematic review does not support using antiviral medications. There is no significant benefit from acyclovir or valacyclovir when compared to placebo. Antivirals are less likely than steroids to produce complete recovery.[13] SOR Ⓐ
- The addition of antiviral therapy in combination with oral steroids may be of benefit, especially for a subgroup of patients with severe or complete facial palsy, House-Brackmann grade V or VI (relative risk [RR] 0.64, 95% CI 0.41–0.99).[13] SOR Ⓑ

COMPLEMENTARY AND ALTERNATIVE THERAPY

Acupuncture and physical therapy have been studied; the data, however, are inadequate to determine their efficacy.[14,15]

REFERRAL

- In long-standing facial paralysis, consider referral to an ear, nose, and throat (ENT) surgeon or plastic surgeon with experience in treating Bell palsy with surgery. It is possible to restore some facial movement with specialized surgical procedures including regional muscle transfer and microvascular free tissue transfer.[16] SOR Ⓒ Because only two small randomized trials have compared surgery and nonsurgical control groups, no recommendation can be made regarding surgical decompression, and this should be decided on a case-by-case basis.

PROGNOSIS

Seventy-seven percent of patients treated with systemic steroids have complete recovery of facial motor function in 6 months.

A simple rule to recall is that clinically incomplete lesions tend to recover. In the House-Brackmann grading system, groups I and II have the best outcomes.[7]

FOLLOW-UP

Consider seeing patients in 2 to 3 weeks to evaluate recovery and to reconsider diagnosis if there has been no recovery, particularly in children.

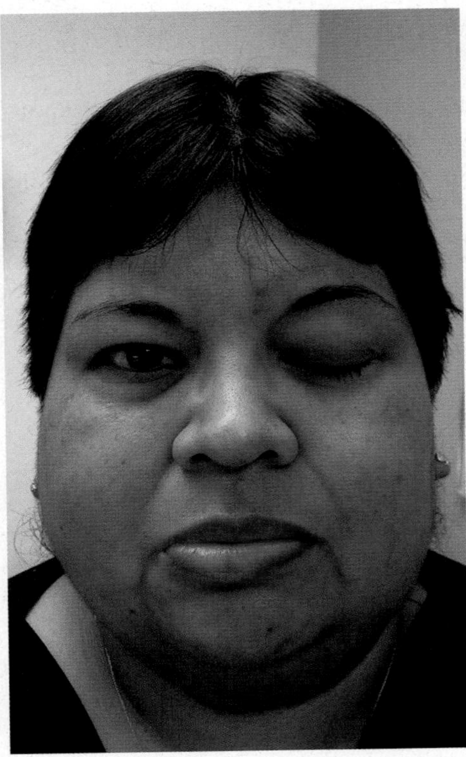

FIGURE 244-3 Ptosis from an isolated third nerve palsy in a patient with diabetes. Note the symmetry of the facial creases, which would be absent in Bell palsy. This patient would also have abnormal eye movements. The eye would deviate down and out, adduction would not pass the midline, and upward gaze would be impaired. (*Reproduced with permission from Richard P. Usatine, MD.*)

PATIENT EDUCATION

- Most patients recover spontaneously. Steroid treatment improves a patient's chance of complete recovery.
- Ninety-five percent of children recover; 70% recover within 3 weeks.

PATIENT RESOURCES

- The American Academy of Family Physicians has written and auditory information in English and in Spanish—**https://www.familydoctor.org.**
- **FamilyDoctor.org.** *Bell's Palsy Overview*—**https://familydoctor.org/condition/bells-palsy.**

PROVIDER RESOURCES

- The Cochrane Collaborative contains updated systematic reviews of steroid and/or antiviral treatment of Bell palsy—**http://www.cochranelibrary.com/cochrane-database-of-systematic-reviews/.**
- House-Brackmann classification calculator—**https://www.thecalculator.co/health/House-Brackmann-Scale-For-Facial-Paralysis-Calculator-1019.html.**

REFERENCES

1. Ronthal, M. Bell's palsy: pathogenesis, clinical features, and diagnosis in adults. December 1, 2016, http://www.uptodate. Accessed November 2017.
2. National Institute of Neurological Disorders and Stroke. *Bell's Palsy Fact Sheet.* https://www.ninds.nih.gov/Disorders/Patient-Caregiver-Educ ation/Fact-Sheets/Bells-Palsy-Fact-Sheet. Accessed December 2017.
3. Morris AM, Deeks SL, Hill MD, et al. Annualized incidence and spectrum of illness from an outbreak investigation of Bell's palsy. *Neuroepidemiology.* 2002;(5):255-261.
4. Campbell KE, Brundage JF. Effects of climate, latitude, and season on the incidence of Bell's palsy in the U.S. Armed Forces, October 1997 to September 1999. *Am J Epidemiol.* 2002;156(1):32-39.
5. Shmorgun D, Chan WS, Ray JG. Association between Bell's palsy in pregnancy and pre-eclampsia. *QJM.* 2002;95(6):359-362.
6. Berg T, Jonsson L, Engstrom M. Agreement between the Sunnybrook, House-Brackmann, and Yanagihara facial nerve grading systems in Bell's palsy. *Otol Neurotol.* 2004;25(6):1020-1026.
7. Ronthal, M. Bell's palsy: treatment and prognosis in adults. April 27, 2017, http://www.uptodate. Accessed December 2017.
8. Facial Paralysis Institute. *House-Brackmann Grading System.* https://www.facialparalysisinstitute.com/conditions/house-brackmann-grading-system/. Accessed January 2018.
9. Centers for Disease Control and Prevention. *Lyme Disease: Two-Step Laboratory Testing Process.* https://www.cdc.gov/lyme/diagnosistesting/labtest/twostep/index.html. Accessed December 2017.
10. Baugh R, Ishil L, Drumheller C, et al. Clinical practice guideline. *Am Acad Otolaryngol Head Neck Surg.* 2013. http://journals.sagepub.com/doi/pdf/10.1177/0194599813505967. Accessed December 2017.
11. Taylor, D. Bell palsy clinical presentation. July 12, 2017. https://emedicine.medscape.com/article/1146903-clinical. Accessed November 2017.
12. Madhok VB, Gagyor I, Daly F, et al. Corticosteroids for Bell's palsy (idiopathic facial paralysis). *Cochrane Database Syst Rev.* 2016;(7):CD001942.
13. Gagyor I, Madhok VB, Daly F, et al. Antiviral treatment for Bell's palsy (idiopathic facial paralysis). *Cochrane Database Syst Rev.* 2015;(11):CD001869.
14. Chen N, Zhou M, He L, et al. Acupuncture for Bell's palsy. *Cochrane Database Syst Rev.* 2010;(8):CD002914.
15. Teixeira LJ, Valbuza JS, Prado GF. Physical therapy for Bell's palsy (idiopathic facial paralysis). *Cochrane Database Syst Rev.* 2011;(12):CD006283.
16. Chuang DC. Free tissue transfer for the treatment of facial paralysis. *Facial Plast Surg.* 2008;24(2):194-203.

245 NEUROFIBROMATOSIS

Naira Chobanyan, MD, PhD
Heidi S. Chumley, MD, MBA

PATIENT STORY

A 44-year-old Hispanic man has neurofibromatosis type 1 (NF-1). He has typical features of NF-1, including eight café-au-lait spots, axillary freckling, and neurofibromas all over his body (**Figures 245-1** to **245-4**). He states that he is used to having the neurofibromas and they do not currently affect his work or life. He is happily married but never had children. No intervention is necessary at this time other than recommending yearly visits to his family physician and ophthalmologist.

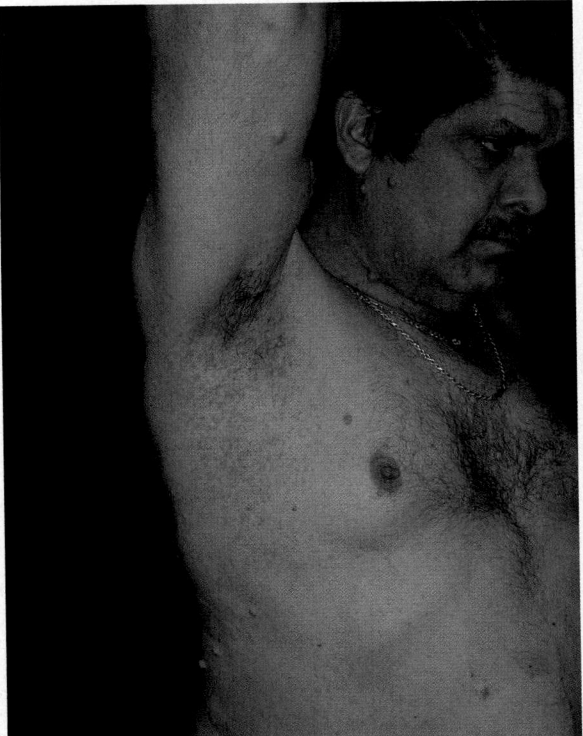

FIGURE 245-1 A 44-year-old Hispanic man with neurofibromatosis type 1 showing all the typical findings including neurofibromas, café-au-lait spots, and axillary freckling. (*Reproduced with permission from Richard P. Usatine, MD.*)

INTRODUCTION

NF-1, formerly known as von Recklinghausen disease, is a common autosomal dominant disorder that predisposes to tumor formation. Café-au-lait macules are often the first clinical sign. Other clinical signs include neurofibromas, axillary or inguinal freckling, optic gliomas, Lisch nodules (iris hamartomas), and sphenoid bone dysplasia. Treatment is early recognition and monitoring for complications such as cognitive dysfunction, scoliosis or other orthopedic problems, tumor pressure on vital structures, or malignant transformation.

EPIDEMIOLOGY

- NF-1 is relatively common—Birth incidence is 1 in 3000 and prevalence in the general population is 1 in 5000.[1]
- Autosomal-dominant inheritance; however, up to 50% of cases are sporadic[1]; likelihood of sporadic cases increases with advanced paternal age.
- Diagnosis is typically made during childhood.
- Segmental NF-1, a condition in which lesions are limited to part of the body, is less common, with an incidence of 1 in 36,000 to 40,000.[2]

ETIOLOGY AND PATHOPHYSIOLOGY

- Mutations in the *NF1* gene (on the long arm of chromosome 17) result in loss of function of neurofibromin, which helps keep protooncogene ras (which increases tumorigenesis) in an inactive form.
- Loss of neurofibromin results in increased protooncogene ras activity in neurocutaneous tissues, leading to tumorigenesis.[1]
- Segmental NF-1 is caused by somatic mosaicism due to a postzygotic mutation in the *NF1* gene.[2]

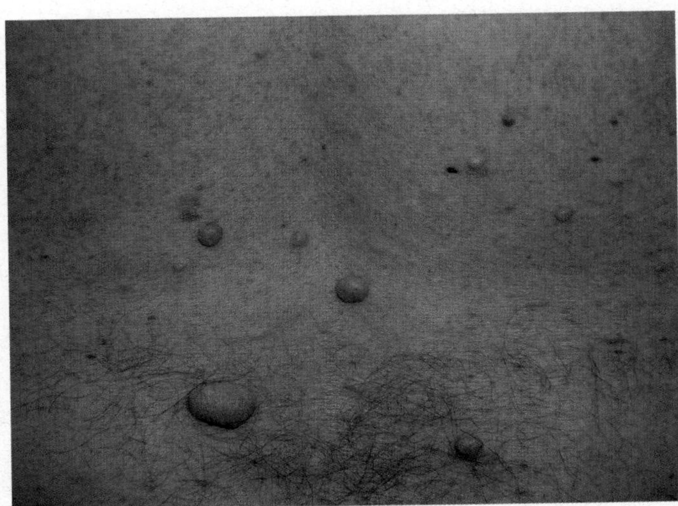

FIGURE 245-2 Close-up of neurofibromas on the back of the man in **Figure 234-1**. These are soft and round. (*Reproduced with permission from Richard P. Usatine, MD.*)

RISK FACTORS

A first-degree relative with NF-1.

DIAGNOSIS

For a diagnosis of NF-1, patients need to have at least 2 of the following[3]:

1. Two or more neurofibromas (**Figures 245-1** to **245-6**) or at least one plexiform neurofibroma (**Figure 245-7**).
2. Six or more café-au-lait spots, 0.5 cm or larger before puberty and 1.5 cm or larger after puberty (see **Figures 245-3** and **245-4**).
3. Axillary or inguinal freckling (see **Figures 245-1** and **245-4**).
4. Optic glioma.
5. Two or more Lisch nodules (melanotic iris hamartomas) (**Figure 245-8**).
6. Dysplasia of the sphenoid bone or dysplasia/thinning of long bone cortex.
7. A first-degree relative with NF-1.

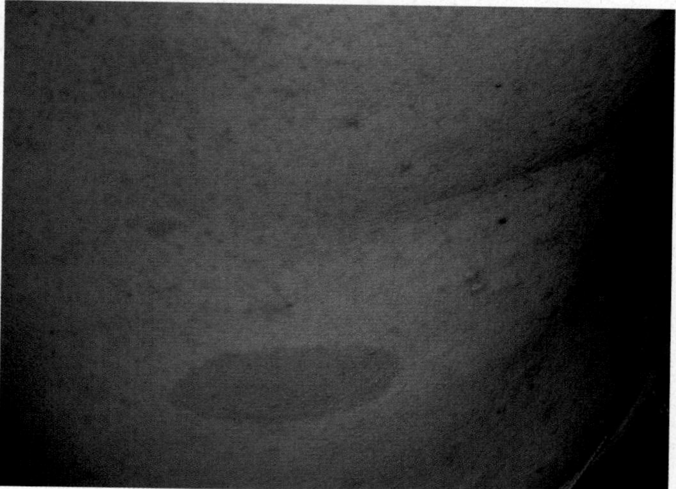

FIGURE 245-3 Large café-au-lait spot on the back of the man in **Figure 234-1**. Café-au-lait spots are ovoid hyperpigmented macules, 10 to 40 mm in diameter, with smooth borders. (*Reproduced with permission from Richard P. Usatine, MD.*)

CLINICAL FEATURES

History and physical:

- Ninety-five percent have café-au-lait macules, mostly before the age of 1 year.
- Ninety percent have axillary or inguinal freckling (see **Figures 245-1** and **245-4**).
- Eighty-one percent have cognitive dysfunction manifest as learning disorder, attention-deficit/hyperactivity disorder, or mild cognitive impairment.[4]
- Nerve sheath, intracranial, or spinal tumors.
- Cutaneous or subcutaneous neurofibromas (see **Figures 245-1** to **245-6**).
- Soft tissue sarcomas, including rhabdomyosarcoma (RMS), and gastrointestinal stromal tumors (GISTs).
- **Glomus tumors that** arise in the tips of the fingers and toes under the nail bed and present with pain, tenderness, and sensitivity to cold.
- Bony pathology, including dysplasia of the sphenoid or long bones, scoliosis, osteoporosis, or short stature.
- Eye abnormalities, including Lisch nodules or early glaucoma (see **Figure 245-7**).
- Other manifestations: **macrocephaly**, **seizures**, **hypertension.**
- Segmental NF—cutaneous neurofibromas limited to specific dermatome(s).

LABORATORY TESTING

- Genetic testing for couples considering having children.

IMAGING

- Not typically used for diagnosis, but imaging is helpful if tumor compression of vital structures is suspected.
- Neuroimaging abnormalities include NF-associated bright spots (focal areas of increased T2-weighted signal intensity on MRI of child's brain) and increased brain volume.[5]

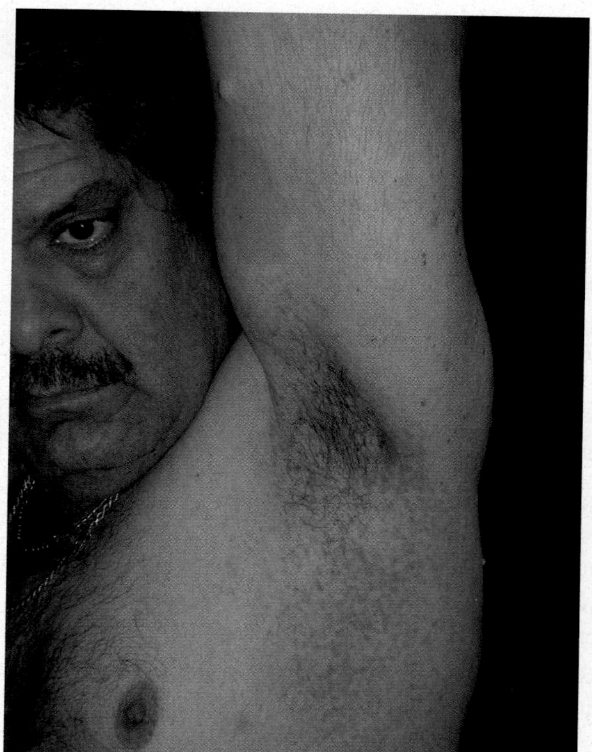

FIGURE 245-4 Close-up of axillary freckling (Crow sign) with large café-au-lait spot on arm. (*Reproduced with permission from Richard P. Usatine, MD.*)

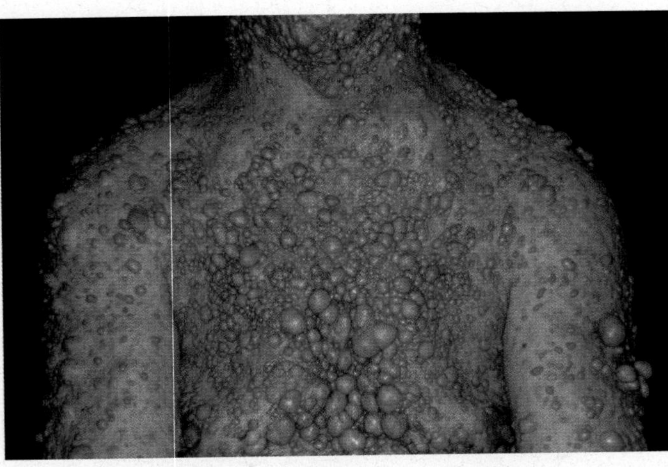

FIGURE 245-5 A man with neurofibromatosis covered with neurofibromas. (*Reproduced with permission from Jack Resneck, Sr., MD.*)

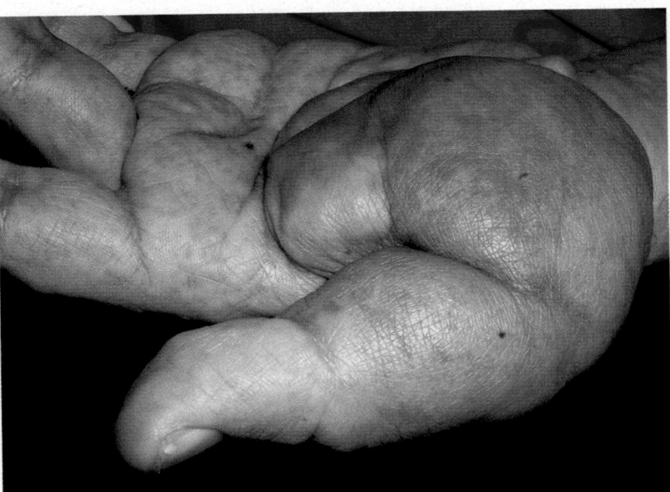

FIGURE 245-7 Plexiform neurofibroma on the thenar eminence feels like a bag of worms in this man with neurofibromatosis. It is a benign tumor of the peripheral nerve sheath and is most often asymptomatic. (*Reproduced with permission from Richard P. Usatine, MD.*)

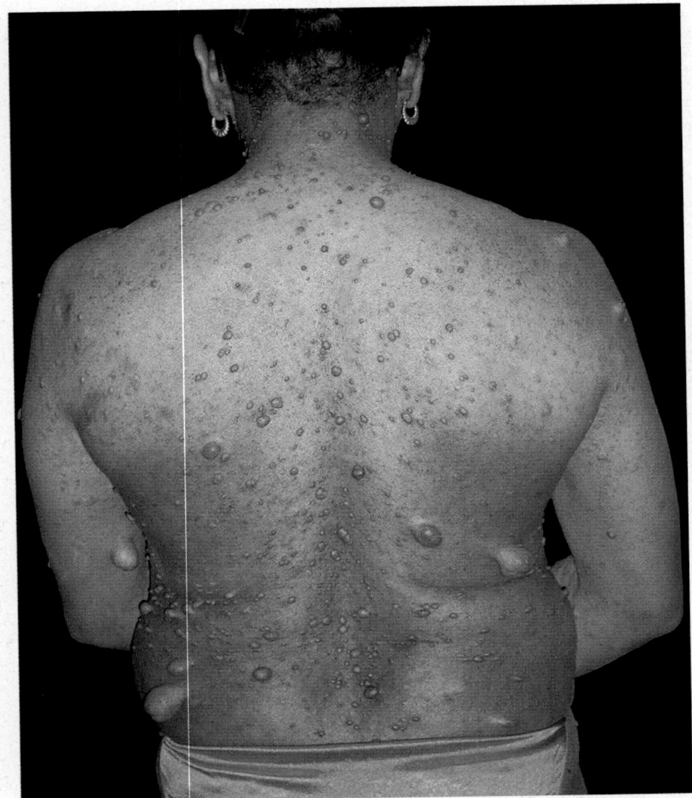

FIGURE 245-6 Neurofibromatosis in a 62-year-old black woman. Note how large some the neurofibromas can become. (*Reproduced with permission from Richard P. Usatine, MD.*)

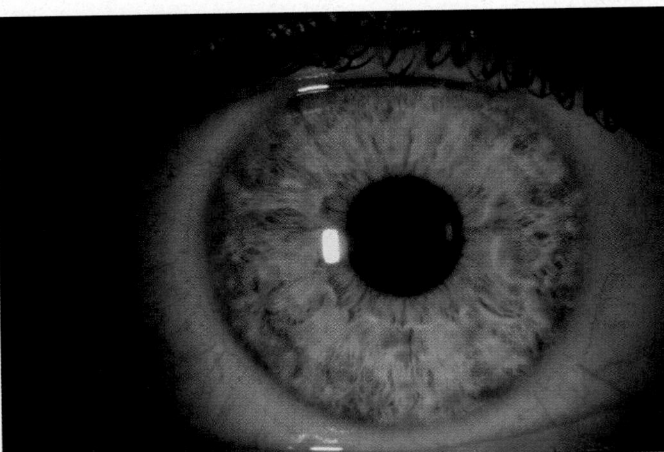

FIGURE 245-8 Lisch nodules (melanotic hamartomas of the iris) are clear yellow-to-brown, dome-shaped elevations that project from the surface of this blue iris. These hamartomas are the most common type of ocular involvement in neurofibromatosis type 1 and do not affect vision. (*Reproduced with permission from Paul Comeau.*)

DIFFERENTIAL DIAGNOSIS

NF-1 is the predominant cause of café-au-lait macules, which can also be seen in the following conditions:

- Normal childhood—13% to 27% of children younger than 10 years of age have at least one macule.
- Neurofibromatosis type 2 (NF-2)—Vestibular schwannomas, family history of NF-2, meningioma, glioma, schwannoma, juvenile posterior subcapsular lenticular opacities, or juvenile cortical cataracts.
- Tuberous sclerosis—Angiofibromas (skin-colored telangiectatic papules most commonly in the nasolabial folds, cheek, or chin; **Figure 245-9**) and hypopigmented ovoid or ash leaf–shaped macules.
- McCune-Albright syndrome—Fibrous dysplasia of bone and endocrine gland hyperactivity.
- Fanconi anemia—Decreased production of all blood cells, short stature, upper limb anomalies, genital changes, skeletal anomalies, eye/eyelid anomalies, kidney malformations, ear anomalies/deafness, and GI/cardiopulmonary malformations.
- Segmental NF—Cutaneous neurofibromas limited to specific dermatome(s); very rare.
- Bloom syndrome—Growth delay and short stature, increased risk of cancer, telangiectatic erythema on the face, cheilitis, narrow face, prominent nose, large ears, and long limbs.
- Ataxia telangiectasia—Progressive neurologic impairment, cerebellar ataxia, immunodeficiency, impaired organ maturation, ocular and cutaneous telangiectasia, and a predisposition to malignancy.
- Proteus syndrome—Very rare condition with hamartomatous and multisystem involvement. Joseph Merrick (also known as "the elephant man") is now, in retrospect, thought by clinical experts to have had Proteus syndrome and not NF.
- Legius syndrome—an autosomal dominant NF-1–like disorder with multiple café-au-lait macules, axillary freckling, and macrocephaly, but importantly lack of neurofibromas and central nervous system tumors.
- Constitutional mismatch repair-deficiency syndrome—CMMR-D syndrome is a rare autosomal recessive disorder with hematologic malignancies that typically develop in infancy to early childhood, brain tumors (primarily glioblastoma) in mid-childhood, and colorectal cancer in adolescence to young adulthood.
- Noonan syndrome—Short stature, webbed neck, characteristic facial features, and pulmonic stenosis.

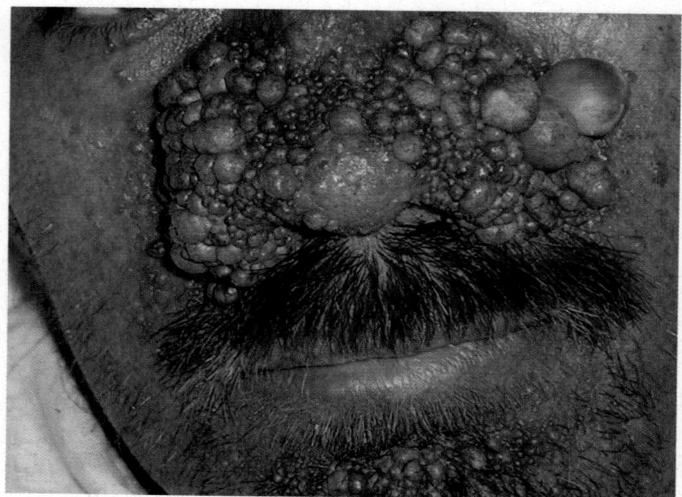

FIGURE 245-9 Angiofibromas (previously called adenoma sebaceum) on the face of a patient with tuberous sclerosis. The patient was originally thought to have neurofibromatosis. He also has epilepsy and cognitive impairment, which accompanies tuberous sclerosis. (*Reproduced with permission from Natalie Norman, MD.*)

MANAGEMENT

Management focuses on early recognition and treatment of manifestations.

- Evaluate children twice a year and adults annually. SOR Ⓒ
- Screen for cognitive impairment and refer early for intervention. SOR Ⓒ
- Screen for scoliosis and treat accordingly.

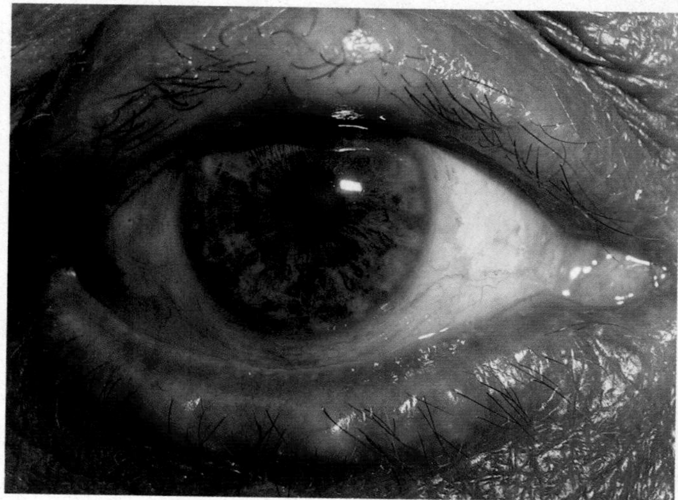

FIGURE 245-10 Neurofibromas on the lower lid with Lisch nodules (dark brown spots) on the iris of this 64-year-old man with neurofibromatosis type 1. (*Reproduced with permission from Richard P. Usatine, MD.*)

- Refer patients annually for ophthalmologic evaluation.
- Consider treatment or referral for treatment of café-au-lait spots if desired by the patient.
  - Topical vitamin D_3 analogs (calcipotriene [Dovonex]) and laser therapy independently may improve the appearance of café-au-lait spots.[6,7] SOR Ⓑ
  - One small study suggests that intense pulsed light–radio frequency (IPL-RF) in combination with topical application of vitamin D_3 ointment may lighten small pigmented lesions in patients with NF-1.[8] SOR Ⓑ
  - Although calcipotriene is approved for use in psoriasis, it can be prescribed off-label to patients disturbed by their hyperpigmented macules.[6,8] SOR Ⓑ
- Examine other undiagnosed first-degree relatives. SOR Ⓒ
- Surgical excision of tumors is required for tumors pressing on vital structures (i.e., spinal cord impingement) or when characteristics such as rapid enlargement are worrisome for malignant transformation.

PROGNOSIS

- Clinical manifestations are variable leading to difficulty in prognosis.
- There is a 10% lifetime risk of developing a malignant peripheral nerve sheath tumor.

FOLLOW-UP

- Primary care evaluation biannually for children; annually for adults, including monitoring of blood pressure.
- Ophthalmologic examination annually for children and adults for early detection of optic gliomas and glaucoma. Neurofibromas and plexiform neuromas can occur on the eyelids. Neurofibromas on the eyelids usually are not a problem (**Figure 245-10**), but a plexiform neuroma can present with ptosis and need surgical intervention.
- Genetic counseling for patients with NF-1 considering having children.

PROVIDER RESOURCES

- Neurofibromatosis Network has a variety of resources including NF specialists by location—**https://nfnetwork.org.**

PATIENT RESOURCES

- Neurofibromatosis, Inc. has a variety of patient education materials, information about local support groups, ongoing clinical trials, and Camp New Friends for children with NF—**https://nfnetwork.org.**
- The National Institute of Neurological Diseases and Stroke has patient information at its *Neurofibromatosis Information Page*—**https://www.ninds.nih.gov/disorders/NF/NF.htm.**

REFERENCES

1. Yohay K. Neurofibromatosis types 1 and 2 [review] [65 refs]. *Neurologist*. 2006;12(2):86-93.
2. Ruggieri M, Huson SM. The clinical and diagnostic implications of mosaicism in the neurofibromatoses. *Neurology*. 2001;56:1433.
3. Hirsch NP, Murphy A, Radcliffe JJ. Neurofibromatosis: clinical presentations and anaesthetic implications [review] [114 refs]. *Br J Anaesth*. 2001;86(4):555-564.
4. Hyman SL, Shores A, North KN. The nature and frequency of cognitive deficits in children with neurofibromatosis type 1. *Neurology*. 2005;65(7):1037-1044.
5. Payne JM, Moharir MD, Webster R, North KN. Brain structure and function in neurofibromatosis type 1: current concepts and future directions. *J Neurol Neurosurg Psychiatry*. 2010;81:304.
6. Nakayama J, Kiryu H, Urabe K, et al. Vitamin D3 analogues improve café au lait spots in patients with von Recklinghausen's disease: experimental and clinical studies. *Eur J Dermatol*. 1999;9(3):202-206.
7. Shimbashi T, Kamide R, Hashimoto T. Long-term follow-up in treatment of solar lentigo and café-au-lait macules with Q-switched ruby laser. *Aesthetic Plast Surg*. 1997;21(6):445-448.
8. Yoshida Y, Sato N, Furumura M, Nakayama J. Treatment of pigmented lesions of neurofibromatosis 1 with intense pulsed-radio frequency in combination with topical application of vitamin D_3 ointment. *J Dermatol*. 2007;34(4):227-230.

PART XVIII

SUBSTANCE ABUSE

Strength of Recommendation (SOR)	Definition
A	Recommendation based on consistent and good-quality patient-oriented evidence.*
B	Recommendation based on inconsistent or limited-quality patient-oriented evidence.*
C	Recommendation based on consensus, usual practice, opinion, disease-oriented evidence, or case series for studies of diagnosis, treatment, prevention, or screening.*

*See Appendix A on pages 1603–1606 for further information.

246 SUBSTANCE ABUSE DISORDER

Richard P. Usatine, MD
Heidi S. Chumley, MD, MBA
Kelli H. Foulkrod, MS, LPC, LPA
Stacy L. Speedlin, PhD

PATIENT STORY

A 21-year-old mother and her 4 children are being seen in a free clinic within a homeless shelter for various health reasons (**Figure 246-1**). The woman is currently clean and sober, but has a long history of cocaine use and addiction (**Figure 246-2**). Her children span the ages of 3 months to 5 years. She was recently living with her mother after the birth of her youngest child, but was kicked out of her mother's home when she went out to use cocaine once again. The patient gave written consent to the photograph, and when she was shown the image on the digital camera, she noted how depressed she looked. She asked for us to tell the viewers of this photograph that these can be the consequences of drug abuse—being depressed, homeless, and a single mom.

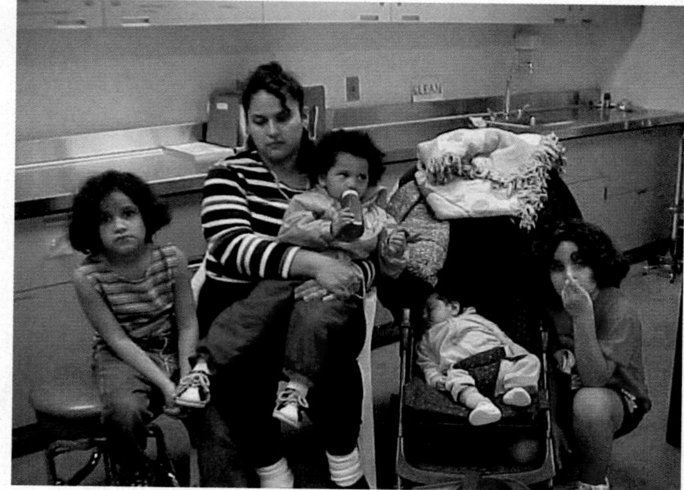

FIGURE 246-1 A cocaine-addicted mother with her children in a homeless shelter. Her drug addiction resulted in their homelessness. *(Reproduced with permission from Richard P. Usatine, MD.)*

INTRODUCTION

Addiction occurs when substance use has altered brain function to an extent that an individual loses a degree of control over his or her behaviors. Addiction is an epigenetic phenomenon. Many genes influence the brain functions that affect behavior and genetic variants. These genes differ in their susceptibility to environmental conditions, which trigger the changes in brain circuitry and contribute to the development of addiction. Addiction must be recognized and treated as a chronic illness with an interprofessional team and social support. While opioid addiction has received an enormous amount of press lately for good reasons, there are many substances that, when used by some persons, lead to addictions. This chapter provides an overview of the disease of addiction. Some of the most addictive substances dealt with here and in the substance abuse section are tobacco, alcohol, marijuana, cocaine, methamphetamine, hallucinogens, and opioids.

EPIDEMIOLOGY

- An estimated 66.9 million Americans age 12 years or older were current users of a tobacco product in 2014. This represents 25.2% of the population in that age range. In addition, 55.2 million persons (20.8% of the population) were current cigarette smokers, 12.0 million (4.5%) smoked cigars, 8.7 million (3.3%) used smokeless tobacco, and 2.2 million (0.8%) smoked tobacco in pipes.[1]
- An estimated 27.0 million Americans age 12 years or older were current illicit drug users in 2014. This represents 10.2% of the population in that age range.[1]

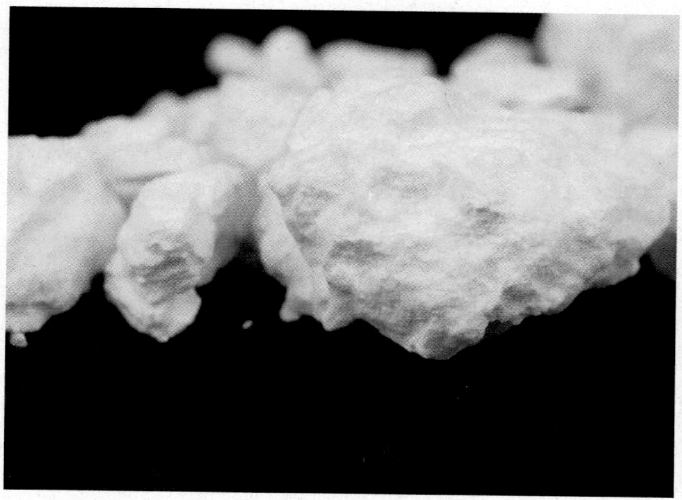

FIGURE 246-2 Purified cocaine. *(Reproduced with permission from U.S. Drug Enforcement Administration.)*

- Marijuana was the most commonly used illicit drug (22.2 million users) (**Figures 246-3** and **246-4**). Marijuana is still the most widely used illicit drug, according to the 2014 National Survey of Drug Use and Health.[1]
- There were 1.5 million persons who were current cocaine users in 2014.[1]
- There were 569,000 persons who were current methamphetamine users in 2014 (**Figure 246-5**).[1]
- In 2014, 1.2 million people (0.4%) had used hallucinogens in the past month, including 609,000 (0.2%) who had used Ecstasy (**Figure 246-6**) and 287,000 (0.1%) who had used LSD.[1]
- In 2014, 914,000 persons had used heroin in the past year (**Figure 246-7**).[1]
- There were 6.5 million people age 12 years or older (2.5%) who were current users of illicit drugs other than marijuana in 2014. Most used psychotherapeutic drugs (including prescription drugs) nonmedically. Of these, 5.1 million used pain relievers, 1.9 million used tranquilizers, 1.6 million used stimulants, and 0.3 million used sedatives.[1]
- Among persons who had used pain relievers nonmedically in the past 12 months, 55% reported that the drug was obtained from a friend or relative for free. Another 17.3% reported that they got the drug from a physician. Only 4.4% obtained the pain relievers from a drug dealer or other stranger, and only 0.4% reported buying the drug on the Internet.[2]

ASSOCIATION WITH CIGARETTE AND ALCOHOL USE

- In 2010, the rate of current illicit drug use was 8.5 times higher among youths ages 12 to 17 years who had smoked cigarettes in the past month (52.9%) than it was among youths who had not smoked cigarettes in the past month (6.2%).[2]
- Past-month illicit drug use was also associated with the level of past-month alcohol use. Among youths age 12 to 17 years in 2010 who were heavy drinkers (i.e., drank 5 or more drinks on the same occasion [i.e., at the same time or within a couple of hours] on each of 5 or more days in the past 30 days), 70.6% were also current illicit drug users, which was higher than among nondrinkers (5.1%).[2]

ETIOLOGY AND PATHOPHYSIOLOGY

- "Drug addiction is a brain disease. Although initial drug use might be voluntary, drugs of abuse have been shown to alter gene expression and brain circuitry, which in turn affect human behavior. Once addiction develops, these brain changes interfere with an individual's ability to make voluntary decisions, leading to compulsive drug craving, seeking and use."[3]
- Addiction is a polygenic disorder. Many genes have direct or indirect influences on neurotransmitters, drug metabolic pathways, and behavioral patterns. For example, variants of receptors for dopamine or opiates influence perceived reward.[4]
- Epigenetic mechanisms, external influences that trigger changes in gene expression, are believed to play a role through

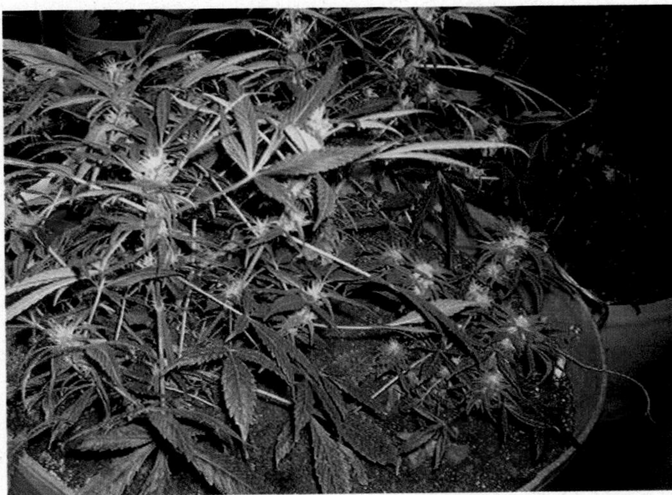

FIGURE 246-3 Home-grown marijuana plant. *(Reproduced with permission from U.S. Drug Enforcement Administration.)*

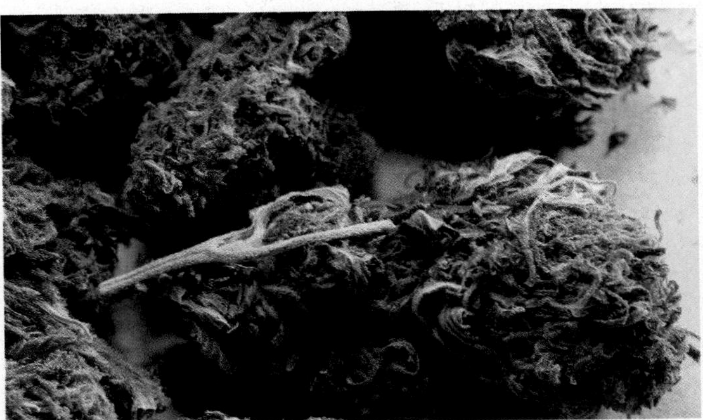

FIGURE 246-4 Marijuana ready to be smoked. *(Reproduced with permission from U.S. Drug Enforcement Administration.)*

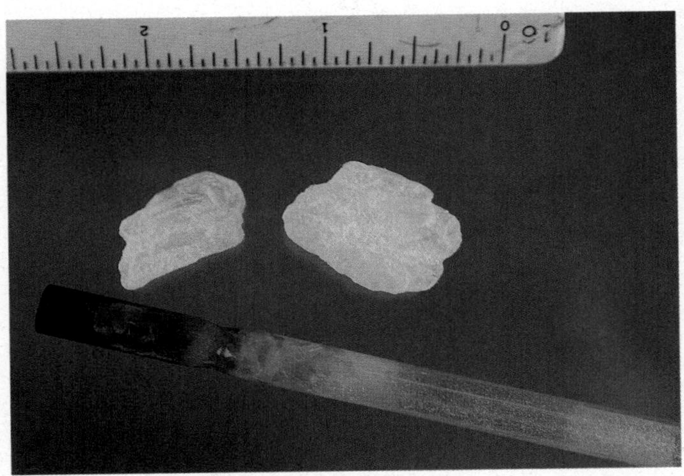

FIGURE 246-5 Methamphetamine ice with pipe. *(Reproduced with permission from U.S. Drug Enforcement Administration.)*

modulation of reward and emotion.[4] As such, both genetics and environment/learned behaviors can increase a person's risk for substance abuse.

- Family, twin, and adoption studies convincingly demonstrate that genes play an important role in the development of alcohol dependence, with heritability estimates in the range of 50% to 60% for both men and women. Important genes include those involved in alcohol metabolism, and those involved in γ-aminobutyric acid (GABA), endogenous opioid, dopaminergic, cholinergic, and serotonergic transmission.[5]
- Several drinking behaviors, including alcohol dependence, history of blackouts, age at first drunkenness, and level of response to alcohol, are associated with single-nucleotide polymorphisms (SNPs) within 1 of 4 GABA receptor genes on chromosome 5q.[5]
- Comorbid mental health issues and chronic pain disorders are highly prevalent among persons with substance abuse disorders. Commonly, a person begins using drugs to self-treat feelings of depression and symptoms of pain.
- The medical consequences of addiction are far reaching and very costly to society. Cardiovascular disease, stroke, cancer, HIV/AIDS, hepatitis, and lung disease can all be increased by drug abuse. Some of these effects occur when drugs are used at high doses or after prolonged use. Some consequences occur after just one use.[3]
- Classes of substances that are frequently abused and involved in addiction include:
  - Depressants—Alcohol, sedatives, hypnotics, opioids, and anxiolytics.
  - Stimulants—Cocaine, amphetamines, and nicotine.
  - Hallucinogens—Cannabis, phencyclidine (PCP), and lysergic acid diethylamide (LSD).
  - Toxic inhalants—Including glue and compressed air dusters (**Figure 246-8**).
- The onset of drug effects is approximately:
  - Seven to 10 seconds for inhaling or smoking.
  - Fifteen to 30 seconds for intravenous injection.
  - Three to 5 minutes for intramuscular or subcutaneous injection.
  - Three to 5 minutes for intranasal use (snorting).

DISEASE MODEL OF ADDICTION

- In 2011, the American Society of Addiction Medicine established a practical and working definition for the identification and treatment of the addicted patient:
  - Addiction is a neurological disorder affecting brain chemistry homeostasis that affects primary brain function including autonomic, regulatory mechanisms as well as global depletion of neuro-chemicals associated with co-morbid mood disorders.[7] It is a disease that is chronic and progressive and may lead to disability or premature death if not treated.[8]
- There are several manifestations of the addicted brain, all of which must be treated for long-term recovery: (1) biologic/physiologic/medical, (2) psychological/emotional (which include all mood disorders that may be acute or chronic complications in the addicted patient), (3) social/cultural, and (4) spiritual.[8]

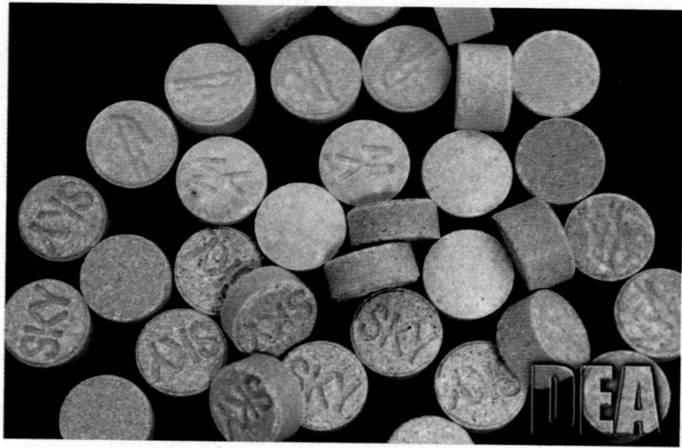

FIGURE 246-6 Ecstasy tablets used at raves where people dance all night long and some collapse in dehydration. (*SReproduced with permission from U.S. Drug Enforcement Administration.*)

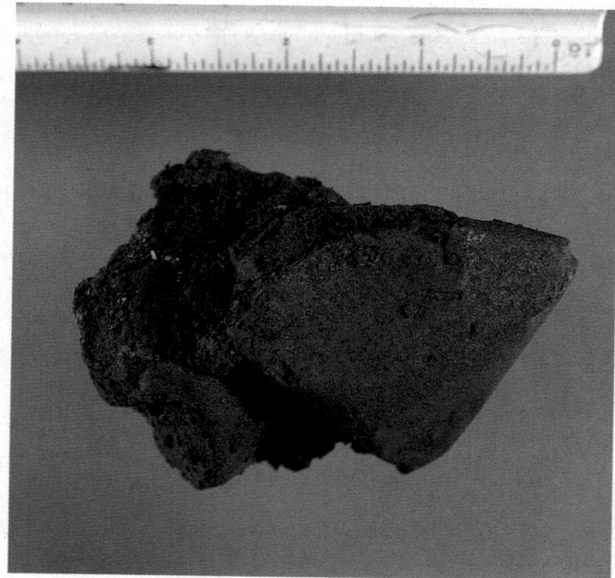

FIGURE 246-7 Black tar heroin for injection. (*Reproduced with permission from U.S. Drug Enforcement Administration.*)

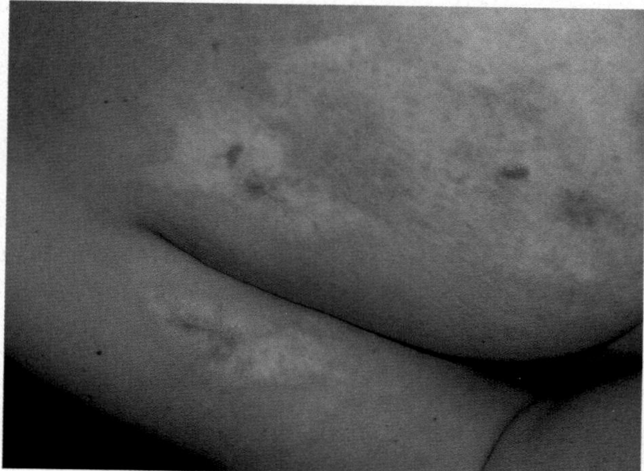

FIGURE 246-8 Freeze-induced burn scars on the chest of a woman using a compressed air duster to get high. She would use four or five canisters until she passed out. Then the cold cans would lie on her skin and cause second-degree burns. (*Reproduced with permission from Richard P. Usatine, MD.*)

RISK FACTORS

- Family history.
- Personal history of prior addiction.

DIAGNOSIS

The diagnosis of a substance use disorder is based on a pathologic pattern of behaviors related to use of the substance. The *Diagnostic and Statistical Manual of Mental Disorders, Fifth Edition* (DSM-5) uses 11 criteria to make this diagnosis.[9] One example of these criteria is the following 11 symptoms for alcohol abuse disorder. If one substitutes other substances such as cannabis or cocaine, the same criteria still apply.

A problematic pattern of alcohol use leading to clinically significant impairment or distress, as manifested by at least two of the following, occurring within a 12-month period[8]:

1. Alcohol is often taken in larger amounts or over a longer period than was intended.
2. There is a persistent desire or unsuccessful efforts to cut down or control alcohol use.
3. A great deal of time is spent in activities necessary to obtain alcohol, use alcohol, or recover from its effects.
4. Craving, or a strong desire or urge to use alcohol.
5. Recurrent alcohol use resulting in a failure to fulfill major role obligations at work, school, or home.
6. Continued alcohol use despite having persistent or recurrent social or interpersonal problems caused or exacerbated by the effects of alcohol.
7. Important social, occupational, or recreational activities are given up or reduced because of alcohol use.
8. Recurrent alcohol use in situations in which it is physically hazardous.
9. Alcohol use is continued despite knowledge of having a persistent or recurrent physical or psychological problem that is likely to have been caused or exacerbated by alcohol.
10. Tolerance, as defined by either of the following:
    - A need for markedly increased amounts of alcohol to achieve intoxication or desired effect.
    - A markedly diminished effect with continued use of the same amount of alcohol.
11. Withdrawal, as manifested by either of the following:
    - The characteristic withdrawal syndrome for alcohol (refer to Criteria A and B of the criteria set for alcohol withdrawal).
    - Alcohol (or a closely related substance, such as a benzodiazepine) is taken to relieve or avoid withdrawal symptoms.

Severity is graded based on the number of symptoms present:

- Mild: Presence of 2–3 symptoms.
- Moderate: Presence of 4–5 symptoms.
- Severe: Presence of 6 or more symptoms.[9]

CLINICAL FEATURES VISIBLE WITH SUBSTANCE ABUSE

- With intoxication, the following signs may be visible:
    - Via stimulants—Dilated pupils and increase in blood pressure, respiratory rate, pulse, and body temperature.
    - Via depressants—Decrease in blood pressure, respiratory rate, pulse, and body temperature. Opioids produce pinpoint pupils. Alcohol intoxication produces dilated pupils.
    - Withdrawal develops with decline of substance in the central nervous system (CNS). Withdrawal reactions vary by the substance used. Alcohol withdrawal is one of the most deadly and dangerous types of withdrawal.

LABORATORY TESTING

- All injection-drug users and persons engaged in high-risk sexual activities should be screened for HIV (with consent), hepatitis B and hepatitis C, and syphilis (rapid plasma reagin [RPR]).
- Women should have Papanicolaou (Pap) smears performed and be screened for chlamydia and gonorrhea based on age, risk factors, and previous history of screening.
- Men or women who have multiple sex partners or use sex to obtain drugs are at high risk for sexually transmitted diseases (STDs) and should be tested.
- Homeless, HIV-positive, and previously incarcerated patients should be screened for tuberculosis using a purified protein derivative (PPD) test or QuantiFERON TB Gold.
- ECG is warranted if there are any cardiac symptoms or if the physical examination reveals signs of cardiac disease.
- Urine screen for common drugs of abuse may reveal other drugs not admitted to in the history. Substances have different physiologic half-lives in the body and show up for varying amounts of time in the urine. Marijuana has a long excretion half-life and may be detectable for 1 month after its use. Other substances may last for only days.

DIFFERENTIAL DIAGNOSIS

Substance abuse disorders coexist with and complicate the course and treatment of numerous psychiatric conditions.

- Mood/anxiety disorders—Especially depression, bipolar affective disorder, panic disorder, and generalized anxiety disorder. Persons with addictions can develop the symptoms of these disorders from the drugs of abuse. However, mood and anxiety disorders can predate the use of drugs, and some of the motivation for drug use can stem from the desire to self-treat these psychological conditions. It is best to evaluate persons for coexisting psychiatric problems when they are off the drugs whenever possible.
- Schizophrenia—Although drugs can cause temporary psychosis and paranoia, if these symptoms persist after the drugs have been stopped for some time, consider schizophrenia and other causes of psychosis.
- Personality disorders—These are a complicated set of disorders that can coexist and be confused with substance abuse disorder. An addict may appear to have an antisocial personality disorder when

committing crimes to get money for expensive drugs. It is best not to use this diagnosis unless the behaviors continue when the person is off the drugs.

MANAGEMENT

- Recognize and diagnose addiction. One simple mnemonic device is the "three C's of addiction":
  - Compulsion to use.
  - Lack of Control.
  - Continued use despite adverse consequences.
- Use the "5 *As*"—Ask, Advise, Assess, Assist, and Arrange—to help smokers who are willing to quit (see Chapter 248, Smoking and Tobacco Addiction). This model can be applied to any substance of abuse.[10]
- Offer counseling and pharmacotherapy to aid your patients to become free of addiction.
- Take a good alcohol history rather than relying on the CAGE[11] questionnaire:
  - Cut down (Have you ever felt you should *cut* down on your drinking?).
  - Annoyed (Have people *annoyed* you by criticizing your drinking?).
  - Guilty (Have you ever felt bad or *guilty* about your drinking?).
  - Eye opener (Have you ever had a drink first thing in the morning to steady your nerves or get rid of a hangover [eye-opener[?).

It is more important to inquire about quantity and frequency of drinking in order to identify at-risk drinkers and patients with functional alcohol dependence (see Chapter 249, Alcohol Use Disorder).

- Refer to addiction specialists and pain specialists as needed.
- Refer to substance abuse programs. Such programs include hospital- and community-based programs. Some programs include detoxification, and others require the patient to have gone through detoxification before starting the program. There are residential treatment units, outpatient programs, and ongoing self-help programs. Learn about the programs in your community and work with them.
- When prescribing opioid analgesics for chronic pain consider the outcomes in 4 domains, or the "4 *As*." Is the patient:
  - Receiving adequate Analgesia?
  - Experiencing improvements in Activities of daily life?
  - Experiencing any Adverse effects?
  - Demonstrating Aberrant medication-taking behaviors that may be linked to addiction?[1]
- When patients are exhibiting aberrant drug-taking behaviors, consider the following:
  - They may have an addiction.
  - They may not be getting adequate pain relief taking the drug as prescribed.
  - They may have a comorbid mental illness.
  - They may be distributing (diverting) pain medications illegally.[7]
- Use state drug monitoring programs to check if patients are receiving multiple psychoactive substances from multiple doctors and pharmacies.
- Use urine screening to check for drug abuse and to find out if patients who are receiving opioid medications are truly using these medications rather than diverting them for sale.
- Help your patients acknowledge that they have a problem and offer them help in a nonjudgmental manner.
- Enlist family members to help whenever the patient gives your permission to do so.
- Demonstrate genuine concern and care; suspend judgment and you will have a higher chance of successfully helping your patients overcome addiction.
- Recommend the 12-step programs to your patients with addiction. These have been very effective for millions of people worldwide.
- Discuss overdose prevention and consider writing a prescription for or recommending naloxone to be purchased and kept available to prevent opioid overdose (see Chapter 252, Injection-Drug Use).
- Advanced brain imaging and genetic tests are helping us to understand the physiologic basis of addiction and will ultimately provide us with better treatments for the medical disease of addiction.

PHARMACOGENETIC TESTING

- Pharmacogenetic testing (PGT) is a new field of pharmacology and genomics used to develop patient specific pharmacotherapy.[12] This tool is now used in several disciplines of medicine, including addiction medicine.[12]
- PGT can be used to predict relative risk for substance abuse and for genetic counseling for patients with substance use disorders.[12]

PREVENTION/HARM REDUCTION

- See Chapter 252, Injection-Drug Use, for information on naloxone use, needle/syringe exchange programs, and supervised injection facilities. While the goal is complete abstinence from injection drug use, these programs can save lives and prevent complications of drug use.

PERSONS IN RECOVERY

- Be careful how you prescribe medications to persons in recovery. A "simple" prescription for hydrocodone postoperatively can start a recovered person down the road of active addiction.
- Avoid giving opioids and benzodiazepines whenever there are good alternatives. Use nonsteroidal anti-inflammatory drugs (NSAIDs) for pain if possible. Use selective serotonin reuptake inhibitors (SSRIs), other antidepressants, or buspirone for anxiety if a medication is needed.
- If an opioid is needed, work with the patient to monitor the amount and manner of use. Involving a third person or sponsor to help meter out the dose may prevent relapse.
- Be upfront and honest about a shared goal to avoid relapse.

FOLLOW-UP

- Follow-up is critical to the treatment of all types of substance abuse. Substance abuse is a chronic condition (similar to hypertension or diabetes mellitus) and requires ongoing intervention to maintain sobriety.
- The frequency and intensity of follow-up depends on the substance, the addiction, and the patient.
- Do not give up on patients who relapse, because it often takes more than one attempt before long-term cessation can be achieved.

PATIENT EDUCATION

Explain to patients that addiction is a disease and not a failing of their moral character. Inform patients about the existing treatment programs in their community and offer them names and phone numbers so that they may get help. If your patient is not ready for help today, give the numbers and names for tomorrow. Speak about the value of 12-step programs because these are effective, and everyone can afford a 12-step program (they are free). There are 12-step programs in the community for everyone, including nonsmokers and agnostics.

PATIENT RESOURCES

- Alcoholics Anonymous (AA). Meetings and the Big Book are free. The Big Book is online for free in three languages—**https://www.aa.org.**
- Narcotics Anonymous (NA). Meetings are free. The "Basic Text" costs $10; it is similar to the AA Big Book, but the language is more up to date and readable—**https://www.na.org.**
- Cocaine Anonymous (CA). Meetings are free. Their first book, *Hope, Faith and Courage: Stories from the Fellowship of Cocaine Anonymous*, was published in 1994 and sells for $10—**https://ca.org.**
- Crystal Meth Anonymous (12-step meetings)—**https://crystalmeth.org.**

PROVIDER RESOURCES

- American Society of Addiction Medicine—**https://www.asam.org/resources/guidelines-and-consensus-documents.**
- Collected resources for physicians on prescription drug abuse—**http://www.universityhealthsystem.com/services/pharmacy/prescription-drug-abuse/provider-resources.**
- The National Institute on Drug Abuse (NIDA). *Medical Consequences of Drug Abuse*—**https://www.drugabuse.gov/related-topics/health-consequences-drug-misuse.**
- Substance Abuse and Mental Health Services Administration—**https://www.samhsa.gov.**
- Drug Enforcement Administration. *Multi-Media Library* (includes many images of illegal drugs)—**https://www.dea.gov/media.shtml.**

REFERENCES

1. Passik SD, Kirsh KL, Whitcomb L, et al. A new tool to assess and document pain outcomes in chronic pain patients receiving opioid therapy. *Clin Ther.* 2004;26(4):552-561.
2. Substance Abuse and Mental Health Services Administration, *Results from the 2010 National Survey on Drug Use and Health: Summary of National Findings*, NSDUH Series H-41, HHS Publication No. (SMA) 11-4658. Rockville, MD: Substance Abuse and Mental Health Services Administration; 2011. http://www.samhsa.gov/data/NSDUH/2k10NSDUH/2k10Results.pdf. Accessed April 2018.
3. The National Institute on Drug Abuse (NIDA). *Medical Consequences of Drug Abuse.* http://www.nida.nih.gov/consequences/. Accessed April 2018.
4. Baler RD, Volkow ND. Addiction as a systems failure: focus on adolescence and smoking. *J Am Acad Child Adolesc Psychiatry.* 2011;50(4):329-339.
5. Dick DM, Bierut LJ. The genetics of alcohol dependence. *Curr Psychiatry Rep.* 2006;8:151-157.
6. Dick DM, Plunkett J, Wetherill LF, et al. Association between GABRA1 and drinking behaviors in the collaborative study on the genetics of alcoholism sample. *Alcohol Clin Exp Res.* 2006; 30(7):1101-1110.
7. Substance Abuse and Mental Health Services Administration. *Behavioral Health Trends in the United States: Results from the 2014 National Survey on Drug Use and Health.* (HHS Publication No. SMA 15-4927, NSDUH Series H-50). 2015.
8. American Society of Addiction Medicine. *Public Policy Statement: Definition of Addiction.* August 2011. www.asam.org.
9. The American Psychiatric Association. *Diagnostic and Statistical Manual of Mental Disorders, Fifth Edition* (DSM-5). Washington, DC: American Psychiatric Association; 2013.
10. Fiore MC, Bailey WC, Cohen SJ, et al. *Treating Tobacco Use and Dependence. Quick Reference Guide for Clinicians.* Rockville, MD: U.S. Department of Health and Human Services, Public Health Service; 2000.
11. Ewing JA. Detecting alcoholism: the CAGE questionnaire. *JAMA.* 1984;252(14):1905-1907.
12. Mayo Clinic, Center for Individualized Medicine. *Drug-Gene Testing: PGT in Clinical Practice.* www.mayoclinic.org.

247 THE OPIOID CRISIS AND THE WAR ON DRUGS

Leo Lopez III, MD

The opioid crisis lies at the intersection of two public health challenges: reducing the burden of suffering from pain, and the rising toll of harms related to opioid use.
—National Academies of Sciences, Engineering, and Medicine, 2018.

THE OPIOID CRISIS

Opioid addiction and related deaths increased at an alarming and unprecedented rate over the past 15 years in the United States. In fact, opioid overdoses have quadrupled since 1999.[1] Pain medications such as methadone, oxycodone, and hydrocodone, and illicit opioids such as fentanyl, account for 1 in 6 drug overdose deaths in the United States.[1] In 2016, nearly 43,000 people died from opioid-related deaths.[2] Without strategic action and intervention, this number is projected to rise to nearly 100,000 per year by 2027.[3] At the current rate, the crisis may result in more than 500,000 deaths over the next decade,[3] largely due to the accessibility of synthetic variants such as fentanyl, and delays in addiction treatment. In addition to opioid overdose, misuse, addictions, and use disorders pose significant public health challenges, to say nothing of the suffering affecting families and communities nationwide.

PRESCRIPTION OPIOIDS

At the forefront of the crisis is the supply of prescription opioids, in addition to the ready availability of heroin and fentanyl on the streets. In 2015 alone, more than 20,000 people died from overdoses involving prescription opioids.[4] Sales of prescription opioids in the United States more than tripled from 1999 to 2014.[5] Between 2007 and 2012, the rate of prescribing opioids increased among surgeons, pain management and emergency room physicians, and other specialists who manage pain regularly. Primary care providers accounted for nearly 50% of opioid pain medications prescribed.[5]

Fortunately, the rate began to decline in 2012 and hit a 10-year low in 2016.[6] This decrease may be attributed to strong messaging doctors received about decreasing opioid prescriptions and added barriers to prescribing hydrocodone products. This occurred after the Drug Enforcement Administration (DEA) moved hydrocodone combination products from Schedule III to Schedule II in October 2014. Even so, the rate of prescribing opioids varies greatly by region in the United States. In 2016, the average rate of opioid prescriptions in U.S. counties was 66 per 1000 people. In areas most affected by the opioid crisis, such as Ohio, West Virginia, and Kentucky, the rate was up to seven times the average.[6]

HEROIN

In addition to prescription opioids, the crisis is fueled by illicit drugs such as heroin (**Figure 247-1**). From 2002 to 2013, heroin use and addiction increased among young people, which was attributed to heroin being cheaper and more accessible than prescription opioids.[7] Heroin-related deaths more than doubled between 2010 and 2015, with more than 12,000 heroin-related deaths in 2015.[8] Data suggest that 3 in 4 heroin users in the United States started their opioid use with prescription opioids.[8] Patients who are addicted to prescription opioids are 40 times more likely to be addicted to heroin,[9] suggesting that the transition from prescription opioids to heroin is linked in addiction. Note that between 2012 and 2016, when there was a decrease in prescribed opioids, there was an increase in heroin-related deaths. It is clear that the complex issues of drug abuse and addiction cannot be dealt with by changes in the supply of prescription opioids alone. We need solutions that target the root of addiction. For example, in cases where patients are opioid-naïve, even a modest miscalculation in heroin dosing leads to fatal outcomes.

SYNTHETIC OPIOID USE

In 2016, nearly 20,000 people died from overdoses involving fentanyl and other synthetic opioids (excluding methadone).[10] Scientific data regarding fentanyl use have proven difficult to collect, but law enforcement confiscation and seizure data indicate that much of the synthetic opioid overdose increase may be due to fentanyl. These forensic data show a sharp, 7-fold increase in fentanyl seizures from 2012 to 2014, suggesting increased access to illicitly acquired fentanyl.[10]

THE WAR ON DRUGS

HISTORICAL AND SOCIETAL PERSPECTIVE

To understand the current opioid epidemic, physicians, policy makers, and the public should understand the cultural shifts, innovations, milestones, special interests, and scientific advancements that evolved over time. In the early 20th century, post–Civil War veterans struggled with chronic pain, and concerns grew regarding the increasing use of morphine to treat their conditions. Bayer began producing heroin, commercially, as an analgesic for minor pain. In 1914, the Harrison Act was passed, in the nation's first attempt to regulate heroin; however, the act allowed physicians to manage addiction with "compassion." Years later heroin became illegal, obstructing physicians from using opioids to treat pain and addiction. However, in 1925, the Supreme Court ruled in favor of physicians' ability to prescribe opioids for withdrawal and addiction under the Harrison Act.

The next decade saw the installation of Harry Anslinger as the head of the Federal Bureau of Narcotics, under the U.S. Treasury Department. Anslinger used his position to garner public support for his hard-line stance on criminalizing drug use (**Figure 247-2**). Anslinger is criticized for his racist, fear-mongering tactics used in public media and in swaying Congressional funding for his department's initiatives. He created and propagated narratives of African Americans and

Mexican and Chinese immigrants as sexual deviants forming the majority of known drug addicts and posing a threat to the American way of life. His rhetoric engendered fear within federal bureaucracies and in the public at large. Anslinger targeted racial minorities with impunity. His office led the prosecution of Latinos and African Americans, and raided the homes and business of Chinese-Americans, exacerbating racial tension in communities across the US. As Anslinger took action on criminalizing substance use, physicians such as Dr. Edward Williams opened free medical clinics aimed at treating opioid addiction. Anslinger perceived Dr. Williams' work as a threat to the public. In 1931, in defiance of the 1925 Supreme Court Harrison Act ruling, and under Anslinger's leadership, Dr. Williams and more than 15,000 other physicians were arrested for treating their patients' addictions with opioids. More than 90% of these physicians were convicted.[11] Addiction clinics from Los Angeles to Portland were closed. This set a notable precedent in physicians' approach to treating substance use disorder as the paradigm of compassionate addiction treatment shifted to criminalization.

The 1940s saw a new wave of suffering, as wounded World War II veterans flooded physician offices. Pain treatment clinics developed in the United States in response. Harry Anslinger stepped down from the Federal Bureau of Narcotics in the early 1960s, a decade in which the social stigma surrounding drug use softened. In 1970, President Nixon funded Dr. Robert DuPont's novel methadone treatment initiative, based in Washington, DC. The following year, the Nixon administration declared a "war on drugs," making drug use public enemy number one (**Figure 247-3**). Nixon launched the Drug Enforcement Administration. Later, President Gerald Ford created a federal task force to study substance abuse. While societal and cultural concerns regarding marijuana use mounted in this era, this task force instructed federal law enforcement agencies to shift their focus and resources to heroin users. In the 1970s, acetaminophen/oxycodone (Percocet) and acetaminophen/hydrocodone (Vicodin) became available to treat pain. Physicians began to increasingly prescribe opioids to treat terminally ill patients, as patients rightly asked not to be forced to die in pain because of fears of addiction at the end of life.

The Reagan administration reaffirmed the war on drugs. Nancy Reagan's famous admonition, "Just say no," framed the conversation on substance use and addiction as a moral dilemma, not a public health issue. In 1986, the Reagan administration passed the Anti-Drug Abuse Act as part of a wave of political mantras calling on public officials to be "tough on crime." This legislation instituted harsh, mandatory minimum sentences; allocated hundreds of millions of dollars toward prisons, education, and treatment; and called for the death penalty for some drug-related crimes. Of note, during this period substance use was already declining nationwide. Yet incarceration climbed to unprecedented rates. This was partly due to the ethos entrenched in society at the time, depicting addicts as moral failures and criminals, as opposed to patients in need of treatment. President George H. W. Bush continued the "tough on crime" approach. Many drug arrests were for possession of marijuana. Continuing with criminalization of substance use, the Clinton Administration supported the "three strikes and you're out" mandatory life sentences for felony offenses. Clinton also endorsed the lifetime ban on the receipt of welfare benefits for felony drug offenses. As in Harry Anslinger's time, U.S. drug policies of the 1980s and 1990 disproportionately devastated African-American and Latino families and communities.

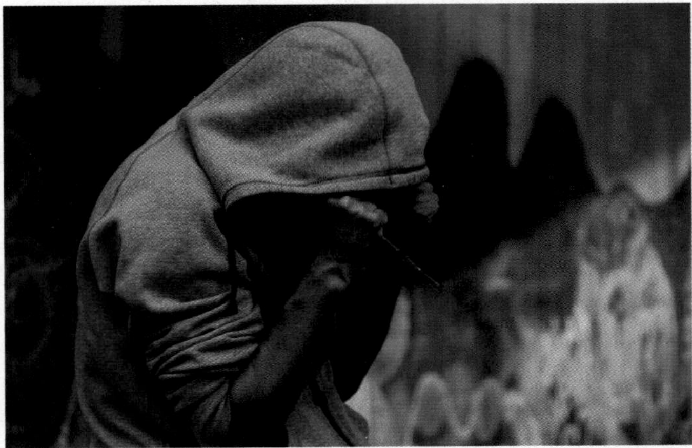

FIGURE 247-1 A young man in anguish about to inject himself with heroin.

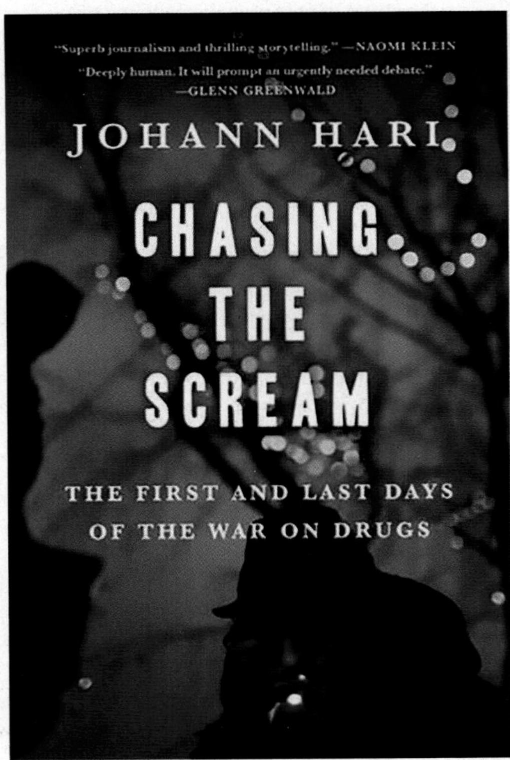

FIGURE 247-2 *Chasing the Scream: The First and Last Days of the War on Drugs*. Cover of this powerful book by journalist Johann Hari.

PRESENT-DAY REALITIES

In the 1980s, physicians' fears and overall restrictions around the use of opioids resulted in many patients being inadequately treated for pain. Then in 1996, pure extended-release oxycodone (OxyContin from Purdue Pharma) hit U.S. markets. Shortly thereafter, the number of opioid prescriptions written for pain increased by more than 7 million.[12] In the late 1990s, the Purdue Pharma OxyContin marketing campaign swept the nation. The number of opioid prescriptions for pain increased by an additional 10 million.[12] The turn of the century was marred by controversy as Purdue Pharma and executives were charged by the U.S. government for misbranding OxyContin, as well as suppressing its possible link to addiction. Purdue Pharma Executives pled guilty and settled the case for more than $500 million.

In 2001, the nonprofit accreditation body currently known as The Joint Commission (then the Joint Commission on Accreditation of Healthcare Organizations, or JCAHO) made patient pain assessments an institutional standard because of concerns that pain was often undertreated. This policy led to the labeling of pain as the fifth vital sign. The power of JCAHO should not be underestimated, and this emphasis on pain affected hospital culture, physician assessment, and prescribing patterns. Under scrutiny from the commission and a culture that attempted to promote compassionate care, physicians increasingly evaluated and treated patient pain—often with opioids.

The Joint Commission now faces criticism for fueling the opioid crisis with concerns over inadequate pain control for hospitalized patients. They released a public statement with the intent to debunk "misconceptions" regarding their role in the opioid crisis.[13] As part of a national effort to address the opioid crisis and increase the quality and safety of patients, The Joint Commission revised its pain assessment and management standards in 2016. The R3 Report, released in 2017, addresses the issues of pain management at a time of opioid crisis.[14] When pendulums of clinical practice swing between "inadequate pain control" and "overuse of opioids," looking for blame is not unusual. Analyzing and addressing these problems with science and understanding allows for more objective assessments and solutions and minimizes blame placement.

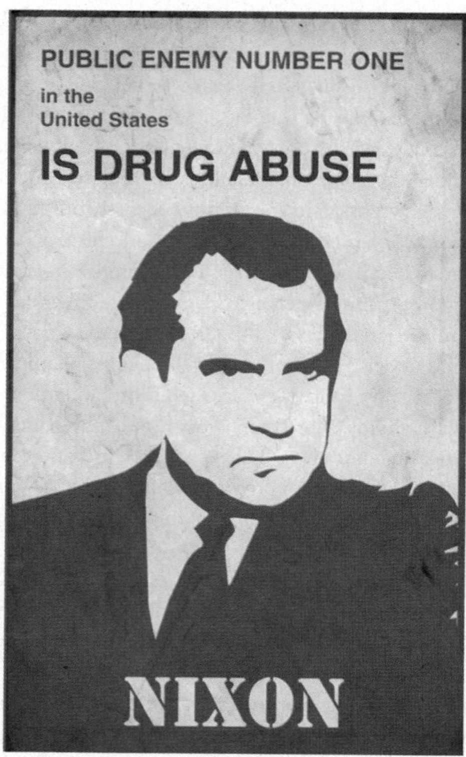

FIGURE 247-3 Nixon declares war on drugs in 1971.

HEALTH DISPARITIES AND OPIOID ADDICTION

Although all people are susceptible to suffering from substance-use disorders and addictions, disparities in disease prevalence, mortality, and morbidity exist across specific subsets of the population.

GEOGRAPHY

States most affected by the opioid epidemic in 2016 included Kentucky, Pennsylvania, New Hampshire, Ohio, and West Virginia. These states posted the highest rates of opioid-overdose deaths in the nation. Rural America has been most affected by the epidemic, young people in particular. Rural Americans tend to have less access to healthcare, are more likely to be of lower socioeconomic status, and are generally less healthy. There are higher rates of unemployment with greater risks for despair and depression, making these Americans more vulnerable to opioid use and substance-use disorder.

WOMEN

Tens of thousands of women have died from opioid prescription overdoses since 1999. Differences in physiology and substance metabolism, as well as a higher ratio of body fat to water, account for the more rapid progression from substance use to dependency in women compared to men. Women also suffer more severe states of withdrawal and have a higher risk of opioid overdose. Further, women have a higher likelihood of suffering co-occurring disorders, with higher rates of anxiety and depression (see Chapter 238, Mental Health).

Healthcare workers tend to overlook signs of addiction in women, particular in the young and the elderly, and among pregnant women. The epidemic has carried over to neonatal intensive care units nationwide. Between 2000 and 2012, there was a fivefold increase in infants born with symptoms of opioid withdrawal.[15]

RACE

Opioid use disorder and overdose affect patients across class, gender, and race. However, 82% of deaths from opioid overdoses in 2015 were in people who identify as white.[16] People identifying as black accounted for 8% of U.S. deaths due to opioid overdose during this period.[16] Data available suggest the state with the lowest mortality rate for opioid overdose in people identifying as black was posted in Arizona at 3%, and the highest in Maryland at 27%. People identifying as Hispanic accounted for 8% of U.S. opioid overdose deaths in 2015; the highest rates occurred in Texas at 22%, and the lowest in Virginia, Georgia, Maryland, Tennessee, Ohio, and North Carolina, all posting 2%.[16]

VETERANS

Veterans are twice as likely as the general population to suffer death from opioid overdose.[17] Veterans suffer chronic pain nearly twice as much as non-veterans and, for much of the past decade, this pain was often managed with prescription opioids. Veterans with mental health disorders such as posttraumatic stress disorder (PTSD) are at higher risk. Veterans with PTSD receive opioid prescriptions at higher doses and are more likely to receive a concurrent benzodiazepine prescription.[18]

SOCIAL DETERMINISM

Enrollment in Medicaid, like living in a rural area and having low income, serves as a high-risk indicator for opioid abuse and overdose.[19] While pathophysiology describes addiction, in part, as a disorder of the reward mechanism of the brain, one's environment, including the availability of health insurance, access to healthcare, neighborhood, and poverty, play a crucial role in developing addiction. Experts suggest that patients insured through Medicaid tend to be sicker, and poorer in general, increasing biopsychosocial anguish and vulnerability and requiring higher dosages of opioids for pain control. Further, many patients on Medicaid suffer from dually diagnosed mental health disorders and tend to lack adequate, timely access to mental health services. Coupled with economic instability, these stressors exacerbate comorbid mental health conditions, drive social isolation, and worsen addiction.

PHYSICIANS

Physicians have been blamed and criticized for their role in the opioid epidemic. Some physicians have run "pill-mills," but most doctors thought to be overprescribing have not had malicious intent. Physician opioid-prescribing behavior slowed in recent years as the "opioid epidemic" received daily press and regulations clamped down on opioid prescriptions.

Ironically, long-acting opioid maintenance therapy with buprenorphine and methadone is currently promoted as the standard of care to treat opioid use disorder. Some say that this therapy is underused because it is significantly restricted and regulated. Approximately 2.3 million U.S. patients would benefit from treatment of their opioid-use disorder, but only about 20% of patients access treatment.[20]

To prescribe buprenorphine, primary care physicians must obtain a waiver from the Substance Abuse and Mental Health Services Administration. Even if physicians choose to obtain this waiver, they are capped at treating 30 patients in their first year, and 275 per year thereafter. In addition, over 50% of rural counties lack physicians with waivers. Even so, data from 2012 showed that even if all waivered U.S. physicians maximized their buprenorphine prescription ability, more than 50% of patients in need of treatment would still lack access to this type of therapy.[8]

Buprenorphine and methadone are not panaceas for addiction treatment. Both have been diverted by patients and sold on the street for illicit use. These medications are most beneficial when used in conjunction with other programs that address mental health, chronic pain, homelessness, and joblessness.

CLINICAL RECOMMENDATIONS

The Centers for Disease Control and Prevention (CDC) outlined a three-pronged approach to curbing the epidemic.[22] The proposed steps include improving opioid prescribing behavior, increasing access to and use of addiction treatment methods, and eliminating access to illicit forms of opioids. The CDC published clinical guidelines aimed at empowering clinicians in managing chronic pain, while working to prevent misuse and addiction. Of note, these clinical recommendations are intended for use in adult patients who are older than 18 years of age, have had pain for longer than 3 months, and are not currently at end of life, receiving palliative care, or receiving active management for cancer.

The CDC recommendations for prescribing opioids for chronic pain are grouped into three areas[22]:

1. Determining when to initiate or continue opioids for chronic pain.
2. Opioid selection, dosage, duration, follow-up, and discontinuation.
3. Assessing risk and addressing harms of opioid use.

Opioids should not serve as first-line treatment for chronic pain. First-line options include nonsteroidal anti-inflammatory drugs (NSAIDs), physical therapy, and analgesic injections, among others. One should manage expectations and create tangible goals for quality of life, daily activities, and overall function. Clinicians should discuss risks and benefits before initiating opioids, and periodically thereafter.

With respect to opioid selection, clinicians are encouraged to choose a medication that is immediate release (as opposed to extended release) when initiating treatment; begin with the lowest effective dose; and for acute pain, use the shortest duration possible.

Reassess patients with chronic pain for risks, harms, and benefits at 1- to 4-week intervals after initiating opioid treatment and at least every 12 weeks thereafter. Managing risks and harms includes considering prescribing naloxone should a patient require higher dose opioids, have a history of overdose, or a history of a use disorder. Clinicians should routinely check their state's prescription drug monitoring program to ensure that each patient on opioids is not at increased risk for overdose by obtaining excessive dosages or other medications such as a benzodiazepine. Co-prescribing benzodiazepines and opioids should be avoided. Clinicians should perform urine drug screening at least annually. Clinicians are encouraged to facilitate treatment for substance use disorders with medication-assisted treatment.

These guidelines have faced criticism. Implementation may be particularly challenging when caring for patients who have been taking prescription opioids continuously for chronic pain. In addition, the new guideline may have deleterious effects on patient well-being by shifting prescribing patterns to rapid tapers or restricting access. Other organizations, such as the American Medical Association, warn that the CDC language regarding managing opioid medication dosages greater than "fifty morphine milligram equivalents" per day will have downstream effects on access, insurance coverage, and pharmacy restrictions, and will worsen stigma on patients with high dosing requirements.[23]

CONCLUSION

Many complicated public health, medical, societal, economic, and law-enforcement issues surround the use and abuse of opioids worldwide, creating short- and long-term challenges. For clinicians searching for solutions in treating their patients, the clinical effectiveness of opioids in the treatment of acute pain creates a real-time conundrum. Opioids provide one effective option for pain control, but carry risks of overdose and addiction. Unless other pain modalities are made more accessible, it is likely that pain will continue to be undertreated. (See Appendix B, Chronic Non-Cancer Pain, for other options in pain management.)

Clinicians should also consider that the opioid crisis is not occurring in a vacuum. A simple solution will not address chronic pain, addiction, mental health, personal suffering, poverty, unemployment, homelessness, and law enforcement, and ultimately end the current opioid crisis. Ending today's crisis requires inter-institutional cooperation, funding scientific efforts, and endorsing sound public policies. The following chapters in this section address specific addictions and drug use, including tobacco, alcohol, methamphetamine, cocaine, and injection drug use.

PATIENT RESOURCES

- SAMHSA's Treatment Locator and National Helpline. A confidential and anonymous source of information for persons seeking treatment facilities in the United States or U.S. Territories for substance abuse/addiction and/or mental health problems—**https://findtreatment.samhsa.gov.**
- Centers for Disease Control and Prevention. Alternative approaches to chronic pain—**https://www.samhsa.gov/sites/default/files/programs_campaigns/wellness_initiative/paw-opioid-prevention-fact-sheet.pdf.**

PHYSICIAN RESOURCES

- Centers for Disease Control and Prevention. *CDC Guideline for Prescribing Opioids for Chronic Pain*—**https://www.cdc.gov/drugoverdose/prescribing/guideline.html.**
- Centers for Disease Control and Prevention. *Applying CDC's Guideline for Prescribing Opioids*—**https://www.cdc.gov/drugoverdose/training/overview/index.html.**
- American Medical Association. *Reversing the Opioid Epidemic*—**https://www.ama-assn.org/delivering-care/reversing-opioid-epidemic.**
- American Medical Association. *End the Epidemic*—**https://www.end-opioid-epidemic.org.**
- Dineen K, DuBois JM. *Between a Rock and a Hard Place: Can Physicians Prescribe Opioids to Treat Pain Adequately While Avoiding Legal Sanction?*—**https://www.ncbi.nlm.nih.gov/pmc/articles/PMC5494184/.**
- From the author of *Chasing the Scream*, Johann Hari. Links on how to get involved as an advocate to end the "War on Drugs" and create good public health policies for drug use and addiction—**http://chasingthescream.com/getinvolved/.**

REFERENCES

1. Centers for Disease Control and Prevention. *Opioid Overdose—Understanding the Epidemic.* https://www.cdc.gov/drugoverdose/epidemic/index.html. Accessed April 2018.
2. Centers for Disease Control and Prevention. *Opioid Overdose—Drug Overdose Death Data.* https://www.cdc.gov/drugoverdose/data/statedeaths.html. Accessed April 2018.
3. Blau, Max. *Opioids Could Kill Nearly 500,000 Americans Next Decade.* STAT News, June 27, 2017. https://www.statnews.com/2017/06/27/opioid-deaths-forecast/. Accessed April 2018.
4. Centers for Disease Control and Prevention. *Opioid Overdose—Opioid Data Analysis.* https://www.cdc.gov/drugoverdose/data/analysis.html. Accessed April 2018.
5. Centers for Disease Control and Prevention. *Opioid Overdose—Prescribing Data.* https://www.cdc.gov/drugoverdose/data/prescribing.html. Accessed April 2018.
6. Centers for Disease Control and Prevention. *Opioid Overdose—U.S. Prescribing Rate Maps.* https://www.cdc.gov/drugoverdose/maps/rxrate-maps.html. Accessed April 2018.
7. Centers for Disease Control and Prevention. *Opioid Overdose—Heroin Overdose Data.* https://www.cdc.gov/drugoverdose/data/heroin.html. Accessed April 2018.
8. Lopez, German. *The Opioid Epidemic Explained.* Vox. https://www.vox.com/science-and-health/2017/8/3/16079772/opioid-epidemic-drug-overdoses. Accessed April 2018.
9. Jones CM, Logan J, Gladden RM, Bohm MK. Vital signs: demographic and substance use trends among heroin users—United States, 2002–2013. *MMWR Morb Mortal Wkly Rep.* 64(26): 719-725. https://www.cdc.gov/mmwr/preview/mmwrhtml/mm6426a3.htm. Accessed April 2018.

10. Centers for Disease Control and Prevention. *Opioid Overdose—Fentanyl.* https://www.cdc.gov/drugoverdose/opioids/fentanyl.html. Accessed April 2018.
11. Hari J. *Chasing the Scream: the First and Last Days of the War on Drugs.* New York, NY: Bloomsbury Publishing; 2016.
12. Moghe S. *Opioid History—From Wonder Drug to Abuse Epidemic.* CNN. http://www.cnn.com/2016/05/12/health/opioid-addiction-history/index.html. Accessed April 2018.
13. Baker DW. Joint Commission statement on pain management. April 18, 2016. The Joint Commission. https://www.jointcommission.org/joint_commission_statement_on_pain_management/. Accessed April 2018.
14. The Joint Commission. Pain assessment and management standards for hospitals. *Requirement, Rationale, Reference.* https://www.jointcommission.org/assets/1/18/R3_Report_Issue_11_Pain_Assessment_8_25_17_FINAL.pdf. Accessed April 2018.
15. Sagynbekov K. The terrible toll of the opioid crisis is even worse for women. *Los Angeles Times*, December 18, 2017. http://www.latimes.com/opinion/op-ed/la-oe-sagynbekov-opioids-and-women-20171218-story.html. Accessed April 2018.
16. Kaiser Family Foundation. *Opioid Overdose Deaths by Race/Ethnicity.* https://www.kff.org/other/state-indicator/opioid-overdose-deaths-by-raceethnicity/?dataView=1¤tTimeframe=1&sortModel=%7B%22colId%22:%22Location%22,%22sort%22:%22asc%22%. Accessed April 2018.
17. Childress S. *Veterans Face Greater Risks Amid Opioid Crisis.* PBS. https://www.pbs.org/wgbh/frontline/article/veterans-face-greater-risks-amid-opioid-crisis/. Accessed April 2018.
18. Seal KH, Shi Y, Cohen G, et al. Association of mental health disorders with prescription opioids and high-risk opioid use in US veterans of Iraq and Afghanistan. *JAMA.* 2012;307(9):940-947.
19. Centers for Disease Control and Prevention. *Opioid Overdose—Prescription Opioids.* https://www.cdc.gov/drugoverdose/opioids/prescribed.html. Accessed April 2018.
20. O'Reilly KB. Critical treatment gap seen in effort to stem opioid epidemic [Editorial]. April 25, 2017. *AMA Wire.* https://wire.ama-assn.org/practice-management/critical-treatment-gap-seen-effort-stem-opioid-epidemic. Accessed April 2018.
21. Crawford C. *Overcoming Barriers to Opioid Treatment Takes Centers Stage.* American Academy of Family Physicians. https://www.aafp.org/news/health-of-the-public/20170811opioidsstudy.html. Accessed April 2018.
22. Centers for Disease Control and Prevention. *Opioid Overdose—CDC Guideline for Prescribing Opioids for Chronic Pain.* https://www.cdc.gov/drugoverdose/prescribing/guideline.html. Accessed April 2018.
23. Gordon AL, Connolly SL. Treating pain in an established patient: sifting through the guidelines. *R I Med J.* 2017;100(10):41-44. http://rimed.org/rimedicaljournal/2017/10/2017-10-41-cont-gordon.pdf

248 SMOKING AND TOBACCO ADDICTION

Nehman Moses Andry, MD
Carlos Roberto Jaén, MD, PhD

PATIENT STORY

A 55-year-old woman presents for follow-up of hypertension. She has been smoking 1.5 packs of cigarettes per day since her late teens and reports that she is now ready to stop smoking. She realizes that smoking is bad for her health and does not like how smoking causes more wrinkles on her face (**Figure 248-1**). She has tried unsuccessfully to stop smoking on multiple occasions. Her efforts have included stopping "cold turkey"; using nicotine replacement therapy (patches and gum); 12 weeks of bupropion; and most recently, trying electronic cigarettes (though this was not recommended by her physician). She has no history of psychiatric disorders and does not have unstable cardiovascular disease. She would like to try stopping smoking with varenicline and is interested in setting a quit date. She is also willing to return for 4 follow-up sessions at weekly intervals. She agrees to call a stop smoking telephone helpline (1-800-QUIT-NOW) for counseling help. The patient tolerates the varenicline well and is able to stop successfully without any adverse effects. Two years after treatment she continues to be abstinent and very glad of this outcome. The clinician used elements of the "5 A's" model for treating tobacco use and dependence to successfully help this patient quit smoking (**Table 248-1**).

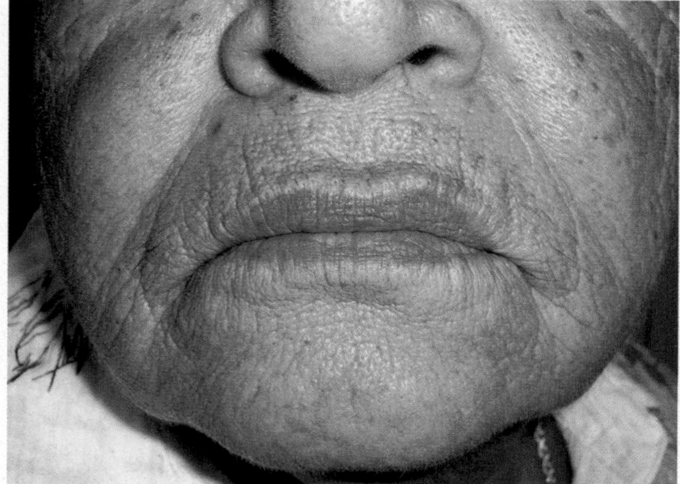

FIGURE 248-1 55-year-old woman with premature wrinkling from years of heavy smoking. Note the numerous lines around her mouth and lips. (*Reproduced with permission from Richard P. Usatine, MD.*)

TABLE 248-1 The "5 A's" Model for Treating Tobacco Use and Dependence

Ask about tobacco use.	Identify and document tobacco use status for every patient at every visit.
Advise to quit.	In a clear, strong, and personalized manner, urge every tobacco user to quit.
Assess willingness to make a quit attempt.	Is the tobacco user willing to make a quit attempt at this time?
Assist in quit attempt.	For the patient willing to make a quit attempt, offer medication and provide or refer for counseling or additional treatment to help the patient quit. For patients unwilling to quit at the time, provide interventions designed to increase future quit attempts.
Arrange follow-up.	For the patient willing to make a quit attempt, arrange for follow-up contacts, beginning within the first week after the quit date. For patients unwilling to make a quit attempt at the time, address tobacco dependence and willingness to quit at next clinic visit.

Reproduced with permission from *Treating Tobacco Use and Dependence*: 2008 Update. US Department of Health and Human Services; 2008. http://www.ahrq.gov/clinic/tobacco/treating_tobacco_use08.pdf

INTRODUCTION

Tobacco use is the leading cause of preventable death across the world.[1] In the United States, cigarette smoking causes nearly 500,000 deaths per year, including those resulting from secondhand smoke exposure.[2] Tobacco addiction is a chronic disease, often developed during adolescence and early adulthood, that requires ongoing assessment and repeated intervention. Effective treatments do exist and can significantly increase rates of long-term abstinence. There are also effective interventions that can prevent the initiation of tobacco use and reduce its prevalence among youth.

SYNONYMS

Tobacco use and dependence, tobacco use disorder, nicotine addiction, nicotine dependence.

EPIDEMIOLOGY

- Nearly 9 of 10 adult smokers in the United States begin before age 18, and nearly all (99%) of adult smokers start before age 26.[3,4]
- The rate of adults in the United States who smoke every day or on some days declined to 15.1% in 2015.[3]

TABLE 248-2 Fast Facts About E-Cigarettes

- E-cigarettes, e-pens, e-hookah, e-pipes, and e-cigars are collectively known as electronic nicotine delivery systems (ENDS)
- 900 percent increase in use among high school students from 2011 to 2015
- Nearly 500 brands and 7700 flavors are on the market
- Flavors are one of the main reasons for popularity among youth
- Aerosol from ENDS is not safe
- Expose users to nicotine and several potentially harmful chemicals
- Use is strongly associated with use of other tobacco products
- In May 2016, the Food and Drug Administration (FDA) extended its authority to include ENDS
- Not approved as safe or effective for smoking cessation
- Long-term safety not established and FDA evaluation in progress

- Smoking rates remain highest among the following groups[3]:
  - Men
  - Young adults
  - Non-Hispanic American Indians/Alaska Natives
  - Persons with low levels of education
  - Persons of low socioeconomic status
  - Lesbian/gay/bisexual adults
  - Persons with a disability/limitation
  - Persons with mental illness and/or substance abuse
  - Persons living in the midwestern and southern United States
- Smoking rates have also declined among U.S. youth in recent years, but the use of electronic cigarettes, hookahs, and smokeless tobacco products has all increased (**Tables 248-2** and **248-3**).[5]
- Electronic cigarettes are currently the most commonly used tobacco product among U.S. youth.[5]
- Patterns of tobacco use among youth also differ by gender (**Table 248-4**).
- Secondhand smoke exposure is higher in African-American children and adults, persons with low socioeconomic status, and persons with low levels of education.[6,7]

ETIOLOGY AND PATHOPHYSIOLOGY

- The evidence on the mechanisms by which smoking causes disease indicates that there is no risk-free level of exposure to tobacco smoke.[8]
- Inhaling the complex chemical mixture of combustion compounds in tobacco smoke causes adverse health outcomes, particularly cancer and cardiovascular and pulmonary diseases, through mechanisms that include DNA damage, inflammation, and oxidative stress.[8]
- There is sufficient evidence to infer that a causal relationship exists between active smoking and (a) impaired lung growth during childhood and adolescence; (b) early onset of decline in lung function during late adolescence and early adulthood; (c) respiratory signs and symptoms in children and adolescents, including coughing, phlegm, wheezing, and dyspnea; and (d) asthma-related symptoms (e.g., wheezing) in childhood and adolescence.[9]
- The evidence is suggestive but not sufficient to conclude that smoking by adolescents and young adults is *not* associated with significant weight loss, contrary to young people's belief.[9]

Through multiple defined mechanisms, the risk and severity of many adverse health outcomes caused by smoking are directly related to the duration and level of exposure to tobacco smoke.[8]

TABLE 248-3 Prevalence of Tobacco Products Used by Youth in Last 30 Days

Type of Tobacco	High School Students	Middle School Students
Any product	25.3%	7.4%
Use of 2 or more products	13.0%	3.3%
Electronic cigarettes	16.0%	5.3%
Cigars	8.6%	1.6%
Cigarettes	9.3%	2.3%
Smokeless tobacco	6.0%	1.8%
Hookahs	7.2%	2.0%
Pipes	1.0%	0.4%
Bidis*	0.6%	0.2%

*Small hand-rolled cigarettes that have been infused with sweet flavors to attract young smokers.
Reproduced with permission from Singh T, Arrazola RA, Corey CG, et al. Tobacco use among middle and high school students—United States, 2011–2015. *Morb Mortal Wkly Rep.* 2016;65(14):361–367. https://www.cdc.gov/mmwr/volumes/65/wr/mm6514a1.htm. Accessed February 2017.

TABLE 248-4 Patterns of Tobacco Use in High School Males and Females Who Used Tobacco in Last 30 Days

Type of Tobacco	Males	Females
Electronic cigarettes	19%	12.8%
Cigars	11.5%	5.6%
Cigarettes	10.7%	7.7%
Smokeless tobacco	10.0%	1.8%
Hookahs	7.4%	6.9%
Pipes	1.4%	0.7%
Bidis*	0.9%	0.4%

*Small hand-rolled cigarettes that have been infused with sweet flavors to attract young smokers.
Reproduced with permission from Singh T, Arrazola RA, Corey CG, et al. Tobacco use among middle and high school students—United States, 2011–2015. *Morb Mortal Wkly* R3ep. 2016;65(14):361–367. https://www.cdc.gov/mmwr/volumes/65/wr/mm6514a1.htm. Accessed February 2017.

- Sustained use and long-term exposures to tobacco smoke are caused by the powerfully addicting effects of tobacco products, which are mediated by diverse actions of nicotine and perhaps other compounds, at multiple types of nicotinic receptors in the brain.[8]
- Nicotine stimulates the release of multiple neurotransmitters, including dopamine, norepinephrine, acetylcholine, glutamate, serotonin, b-endorphin, and g-aminobutyric acid.[10]
- Nicotine exposure during pregnancy harms the developing fetus and causes lasting consequences for the developing brain and lung function in newborns. Nicotine exposure during pregnancy can also result in low birth weight, preterm delivery, stillbirth, and sudden infant death syndrome.[5]
- Nicotine also has a negative impact on adolescent brain development and has been associated with lasting cognitive and behavioral impairments, including effects on attention and working memory.[2]
- Low levels of exposure, including exposures to secondhand tobacco smoke, lead to a rapid and sharp increase in endothelial dysfunction and inflammation, which are implicated in acute cardiovascular events and thrombosis.[8]
- There is insufficient evidence that product modification strategies to lower emissions of specific toxicants in tobacco smoke reduce risk for the major adverse health outcomes.[8]

RISK FACTORS

Given their developmental stage, adolescents and young adults are uniquely susceptible to social and environmental influences to use tobacco.

- Socioeconomic factors and educational attainment influence the development of youth smoking behavior. The adolescents most likely to begin to use tobacco and progress to regular use are those who have lower academic achievement.[9]
- The evidence is sufficient to conclude that there is a causal relationship between peer group social influences and the initiation and maintenance of smoking behaviors during adolescence.[9]
- Adolescents whose parents are tobacco dependent are at greater risk of developing more intense smoking patterns, and those who have a longer duration of exposure to parental tobacco use are at an even higher risk.[11]
- Affective processes play an important role in youth smoking behavior, with a strong association between youth smoking and negative affect.[9]
- The evidence is suggestive that tobacco use is a heritable trait, more so for regular use than for onset. The expression of genetic risk for smoking among young people may be moderated by small-group and larger social–environmental factors.[9]

DIAGNOSIS

CLINICAL FEATURES

- History—Most tobacco users express a desire to stop using tobacco but report repeated failures in their attempts. All patients should be asked if they use tobacco and should have their tobacco use status documented on a regular basis. Evidence shows that clinic screening systems, such as expanding the vital signs to include tobacco use status, or the use of other reminder systems, such as chart stickers or computer prompts, significantly increase rates of clinician intervention.[12] SOR Ⓐ
- Physical—Individuals with tobacco addiction may easily be detected by:
  - Distinctive odor of tobacco smoke.
  - Smoker's cough.
  - Raspy or hoarse voice (see Chapter 38, The Larynx [Hoarseness])
  - Pack of cigarettes in the front pocket of the shirt.
  - Wrinkles in excess of what would be expected for their age (**Figure 248-2**).
- *Smoker's face* is described as:
  - "Lines or wrinkles on the face, typically radiating at right angles from the upper and lower lips or corners of the eyes, deep lines on the cheeks, or numerous shallow lines on the cheeks and lower jaw" (see **Figure 248-2**).
  - "A subtle gauntness of the facial features with prominence of the underlying bony contours."[13]
- The oral cavity of smokers often shows signs of prolonged exposure to tobacco in the form:
  - Yellow and brown teeth (**Figures 248-3** to **248-5**).
  - Angular cheilitis (see **Figure 248-3**) (see Chapter 34, Angular Cheilitis).
  - Gingivitis and periodontitis (see **Figure 248-4**) (see Chapter 41, Gingivitis and Periodontal Disease).
- There may be other serious conditions within the oral cavity such as:
  - Leukoplakia—A pre-malignant condition (see **Figure 248-5**) (see Chapter 44, Leukoplakia).
  - Nicotine stomatitis (**Figure 248-6**).
  - Squamous cell carcinoma (**Figures 248-7** and **248-8**) (see Chapter 45, Oropharyngeal Cancer).
- Withdrawal symptoms—Symptoms associated with tobacco addiction withdrawal include a dysphoric or depressed mood, insomnia, irritability, frustration or anger, anxiety, difficulty concentrating, restlessness, decreased heart rate, and increased appetite or weight gain.[14] None of the withdrawal symptoms are life-threatening, as they can be with other drugs such as alcohol and opiates. Their intensity peaks during the first week, and most last no more than 2 to 4 weeks following abstinence.[15]
- Complications—Continuing use of tobacco causes multiple cancers and the development and/or exacerbation of multiple chronic diseases, as summarized in **Figure 248-9**.
- Emphysema may significantly impair lung function and lead to death (see Chapter 58, Chronic Obstructive Pulmonary Disease). Centrilobular emphysema occurs with carbon deposits in the destroyed lung tissue.

LABORATORY TESTING

- Some specialized assessments of individual and environmental attributes provide information for tailoring treatment and may predict quitting success. Specialized assessments refer to the use of formal instruments (e.g., questionnaires, clinical interviews, or physiologic indices such as carbon monoxide, serum nicotine/cotinine levels,

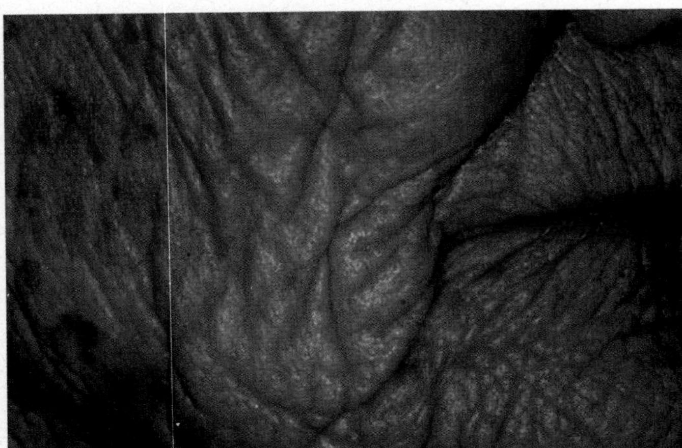

FIGURE 248-2 **Smoker's face** described as "one or more of the following: (a) lines or wrinkles on the face, typically radiating at right angles from the upper and lower lips or corners of the eyes, deep lines on the cheeks, or numerous shallow lines on the cheeks and lower jaw. (b) A subtle gauntness of the facial features with prominence of the underlying bony contours."[6] *(Reproduced with permission from Usatine R, Moy R, Tobinick E, et al: Skin Surgery: A Practical Guide. St. Louis, MO: Mosby; 1998.)*

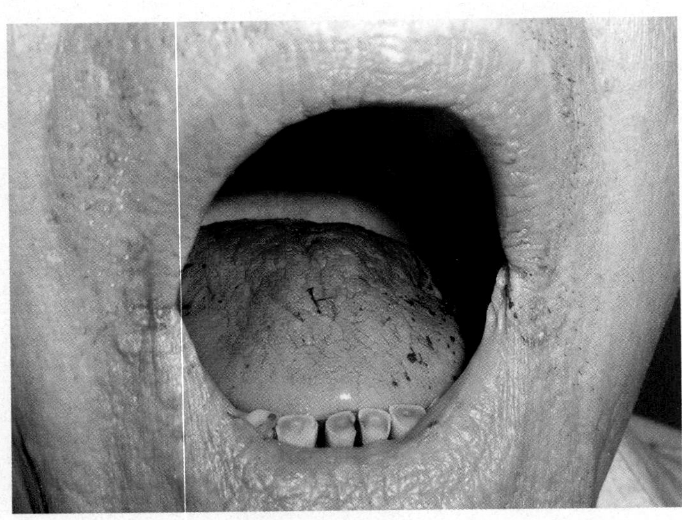

FIGURE 248-3 Angular cheilitis and tobacco staining of the tongue from chewing tobacco. (*Reproduced with permission from Richard P. Usatine, MD.*)

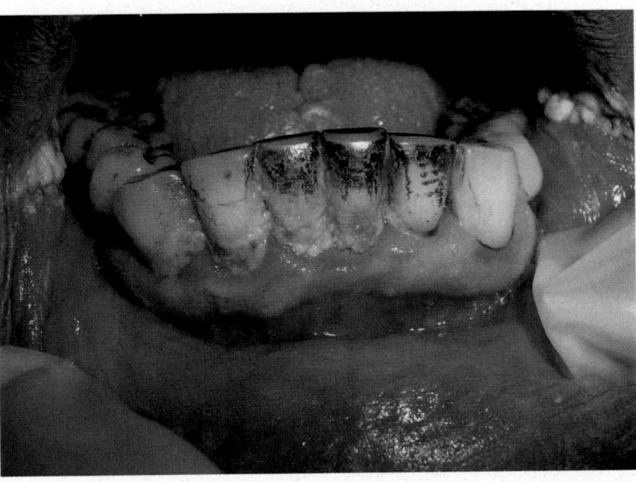

FIGURE 248-4 Tobacco stained teeth and periodontitis from smoking tobacco. (*Reproduced with permission from Richard P. Usatine, MD.*)

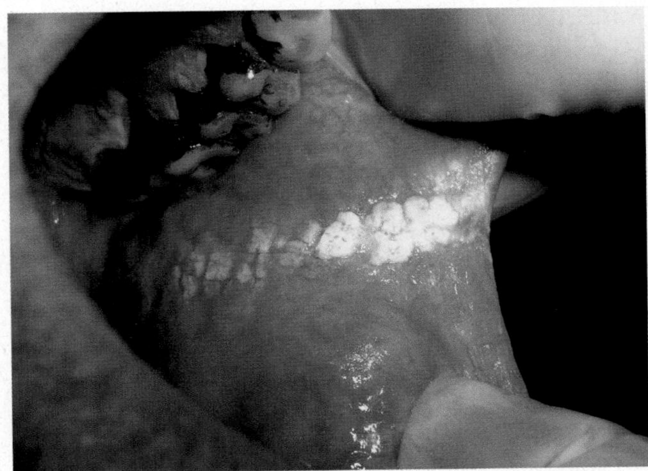

FIGURE 248-5 Leukoplakia on the buccal mucosa and gingiva in a tobacco smoker. Although much of the leukoplakia is on the bite line, the risk of squamous cell carcinoma of the oral cavity must be assessed with appropriate biopsies. (*Reproduced with permission from Richard P. Usatine, MD.*)

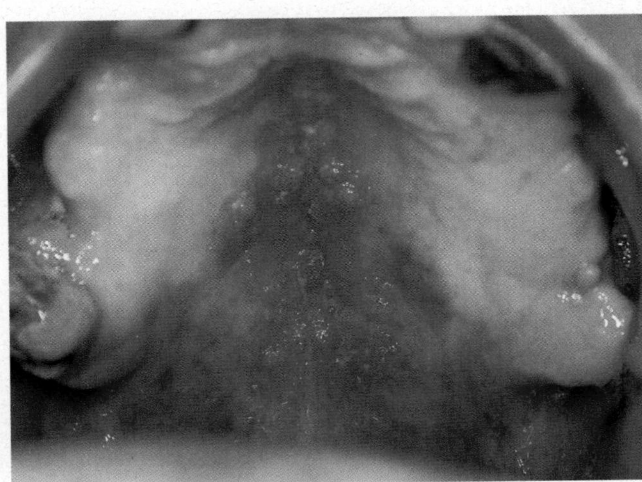

FIGURE 248-6 Nicotine stomatitis over the hard palate from smoking tobacco. (*Reproduced with permission from Rizzolo D, Chiodo TA. Lesion on the hard palate. J Fam Pract, 2008;57(1):33-35. Frontline Medical Communications.*)

and/or pulmonary function) that may be associated with cessation outcome. In addition, clinicians may find other assessments relevant to medication use and specific populations when selecting treatment. The use of biochemical confirmation (use of biologic samples, such as expired air, saliva, urine, or blood, to measure tobacco-related compounds, such as nicotine, cotinine, and carboxyhemoglobin) is particularly useful to verify abstinence during pregnancy treatment where reports of deception have been documented.[12] Variables targeted by specialized assessments that predict treatment success include:
  - High motivation.
  - Readiness to change in the next month.
  - Moderate to high self-efficacy (confidence in his or her ability to stop using tobacco successfully).
  - Supportive social network.
- Variables associated with lower abstinence rates include:
  - High nicotine dependence.
  - Psychiatric comorbidity and substance use (particularly elevated depressive symptoms, schizophrenia, and current alcohol abuse).
  - High stress level.
  - Exposure to other smokers.[12]

IMAGING

While there are currently no practical clinical applications for imaging studies that are helpful when treating individuals with tobacco addiction, imaging can be used to help diagnose complications related to tobacco addiction.

The U.S. Preventive Services Task Force (USPSTF) recommends:

- One-time abdominal aortic aneurysm (AAA) screening with ultrasonography in men between ages 65 and 75 years who have ever smoked.[16] SOR B
- Annual lung cancer screening using low-dose chest computed tomography (LDCT) in adults between ages 55 to 80 years who have a 30 pack-year smoking history and currently smoke or have stopped within the past 15 years. Screening should be stopped once a person has not smoked for 15 years or develops a life-limiting health condition that would prevent curative lung surgery.[17] SOR B

FIGURE 248-7 Squamous cell carcinoma of buccal mucosa in a man who used chewing tobacco along with smoking. (*Reproduced with permission from Richard P. Usatine, MD.*)

MANAGEMENT

Management of smoking and tobacco addiction involves measures to promote cessation and prevent disease complications.

- The Advisory Committee on Immunization Practice recommends vaccinating adult smokers ages 19–64 with one dose of pneumococcal polysaccharide vaccine (PPSV23) to prevent pneumococcal disease in this "at risk" group.[18]
- Behavioral counseling is the mainstay of treatment for all tobacco users.[12]
- FDA-approved pharmacotherapy should be offered to all adult nonpregnant smokers who smoke at least 10 cigarettes daily and lack specific medication contraindications.[12] SOR A
- The combination of counseling and medication is more effective for smoking cessation than either medication or counseling alone. Therefore, whenever feasible and appropriate, both counseling and medication should be offered and provided to patients trying to stop smoking.[12] SOR A

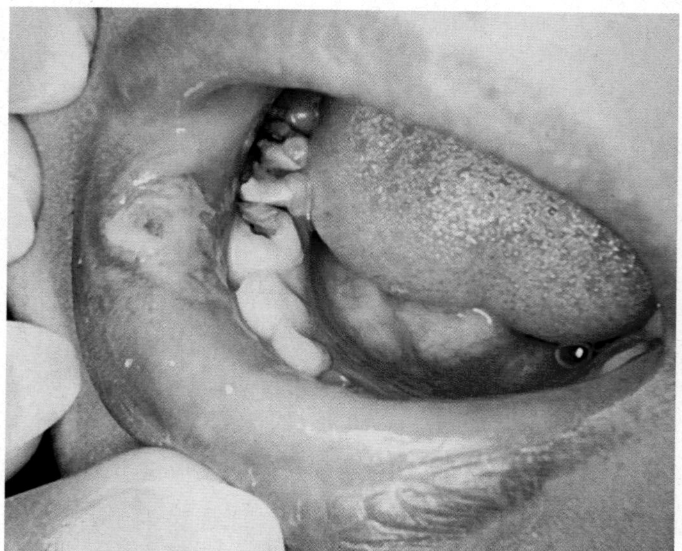

FIGURE 248-8 Squamous cell carcinoma of the inner lip in a cigar smoker. (*Reproduced with permission from Gerald Ferritti, DDS.*)

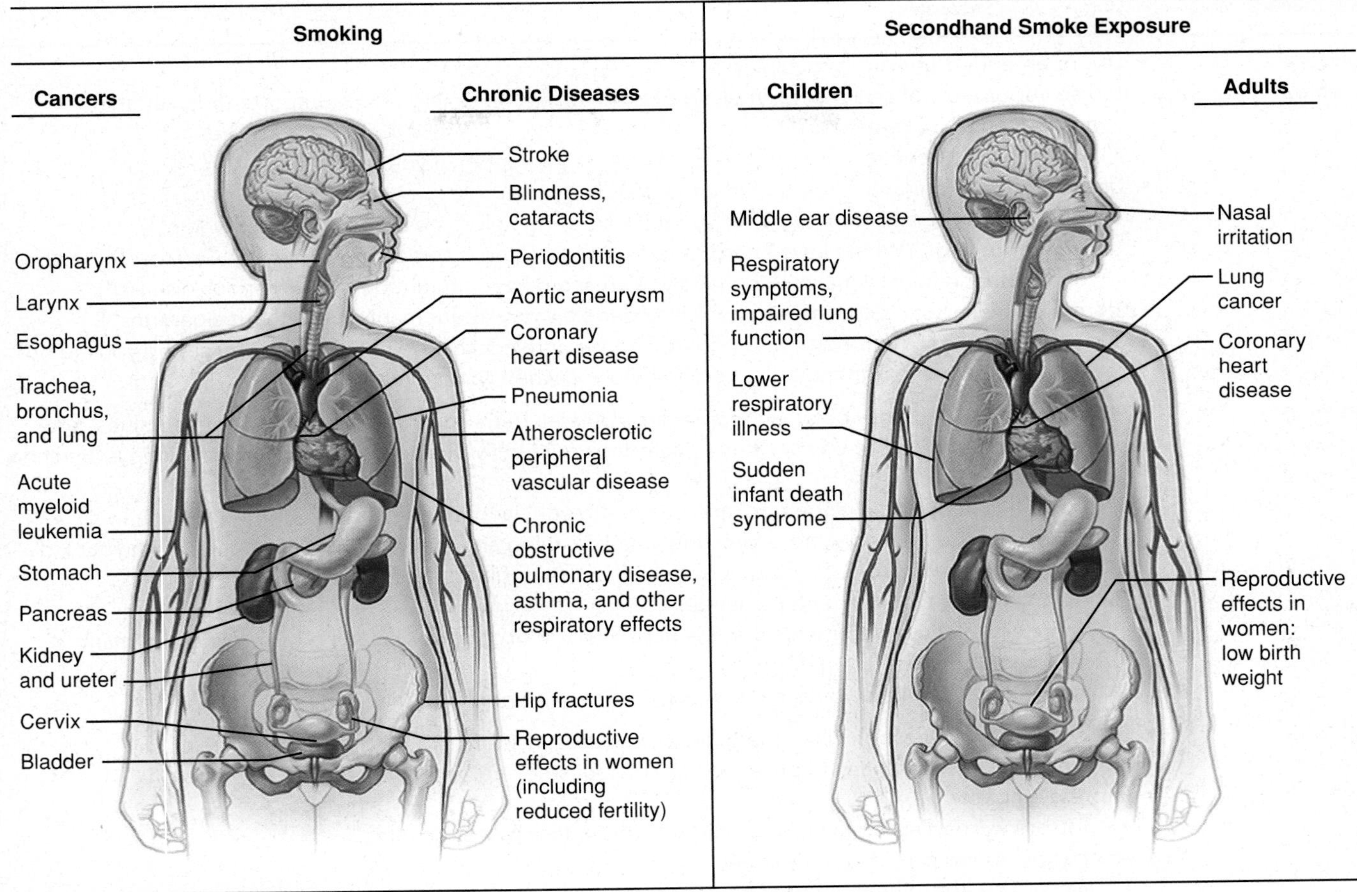

FIGURE 248-9 Health consequences causally linked to smoking and secondhand smoking. (*Reproduced with permission from U.S. Department of Health and Human Services. How Tobacco Smoke Causes Disease: The Biology and Behavioral Basis for Smoking-Attributable Disease: A Report of the Surgeon General. Atlanta, GA: U.S. Department of Health and Human Services, Centers for Disease Control and Prevention, National Center for Chronic Disease Prevention and Health Promotion, Office on Smoking and Health; 2010.*)

FIRST LINE

NONPHARMACOLOGIC (COUNSELING INTERVENTIONS)

- Minimal interventions lasting less than 3 minutes increase overall tobacco abstinence rates. Every tobacco user should be offered at least a minimal intervention, whether or not he or she is referred to an intensive intervention.[12] SOR Ⓐ
- Two types of counseling and behavioral therapies result in higher abstinence rates: (1) providing smokers with practical counseling (problem-solving skills/skills training), and (2) providing support and encouragement as part of treatment. These types of counseling elements should be included in smoking cessation interventions.[12] SOR Ⓑ
- There is a strong dose–response relationship between the session length of person-to-person contact and successful treatment outcomes. Intensive interventions are more effective than less-intensive interventions and should be used whenever possible.[12] SOR Ⓐ
- Proactive telephone counseling, group counseling, and individual counseling formats are effective and should be used in smoking cessation interventions.[12] SOR Ⓐ
- Person-to-person treatment delivered for 4 or more sessions appears especially effective in increasing abstinence rates. Therefore, if feasible, clinicians should strive to meet 4 or more times with individuals quitting tobacco use.[12] SOR Ⓐ
- Motivational interviewing for smokers not willing to make an attempt to stop tobacco use:
  - Motivational intervention techniques appear to be effective in increasing a patient's likelihood of making a future quit attempt. Therefore, clinicians should use motivational techniques to encourage smokers who are not currently willing to quit to consider making a quit attempt in the future.[12] SOR Ⓑ
  - The four general principles that underlie motivational intervention are: (a) *express empathy,* (b) *develop discrepancy,* (c) *roll with resistance,* and (d) *support self-efficacy* (**Table 248-5**). Motivational intervention researchers have found that having patients use their own words to commit to change is more effective than clinician exhortations, lectures, or arguments for quitting, which tend to increase rather than lessen patient resistance to change.[12]

MEDICATIONS

Clinicians should encourage all patients attempting to quit to use effective medications for tobacco dependence treatment, except where contraindicated or for specific populations for which there is

TABLE 248-5 Motivational Interviewing Strategies

Express empathy.	• Use open-ended questions to explore: ◦ The importance of addressing smoking or other tobacco use (e.g., "How important do you think it is for you to quit smoking?") ◦ Concerns and benefits of quitting (e.g., "What might happen if you quit?") • Use reflective listening to seek shared understanding: ◦ Reflect words or meaning (e.g., "So you think smoking helps you to maintain your weight"). ◦ Summarize (e.g., "What I have heard so far is that smoking is something you enjoy. On the other hand, your boyfriend hates your smoking, and you are worried you might develop a serious disease"). • Normalize feelings and concerns (e.g., "Many people worry about managing without cigarettes"). • Support the patient's autonomy and right to choose or reject change (e.g., "I hear you saying you are not ready to quit smoking right now. I'm here to help you when you are ready").
Develop discrepancy.	• Highlight the discrepancy between the patient's present behavior and expressed priorities, values, and goals (e.g., "It sounds like you are very devoted to your family. How do you think your smoking is affecting your children?"). • Reinforce and support "change talk" and "commitment" language: ◦ "So, you realize how smoking is affecting your breathing and making it hard to keep up with your kids." ◦ "It's great that you are going to quit when you get through this busy time at work." • Build and deepen commitment to change: ◦ "There are effective treatments that will ease the pain of quitting, including counseling and many medication options." ◦ "We would like to help you avoid a stroke like the one your father had."
Roll with resistance.	• Back off and use reflection when the patient expresses resistance: ◦ "Sounds like you are feeling pressured about your smoking." • Express empathy: ◦ "You are worried about how you would manage withdrawal symptoms." • Ask permission to provide information: ◦ "Would you like to hear about some strategies that can help you address that concern when you quit?"
Support self-efficacy.	• Help the patient to identify and build on past successes: ◦ "So you were fairly successful the last time you tried to quit." • Offer options for achievable small steps toward change: ◦ Call the quitline (1-800-QUIT-NOW) for advice and information. ◦ Read about quitting benefits and strategies. ◦ Change smoking patterns (e.g., no smoking in the home). ◦ Ask the patient to share his or her ideas about quitting strategies.

Reproduced with permission from *Treating Tobacco Use and Dependence*: 2008 Update. U.S. Department of Health and Human Services; 2008. http://www.ahrq.gov/clinic/tobacco/treating_tobacco_use08.pdf

insufficient evidence of effectiveness (e.g., pregnant women, smokeless tobacco users, light smokers, and adolescents).[12] SOR Ⓐ

- In the United States, there are 7 FDA-approved medications for treating tobacco use, and these first-line medications should be recommended: bupropion SR (Zyban), nicotine gum, nicotine inhaler, nicotine lozenge, nicotine nasal spray, nicotine patch, and varenicline (Chantix). Dosing guidelines for these 7 meds are found in **Table 248-6**.
- 2 mg/day varenicline or the combination of long-term nicotine patch use + ad libitum nicotine replacement therapy (NRT) are first-line options shown to be more effective than the nicotine patch alone.[12]
- Certain combinations of first-line medications have been shown to be effective smoking cessation treatments. Therefore, clinicians should consider using these combinations of medications with their patients who are willing to quit. Effective combination medications are:
    - Long-term (>14 weeks) nicotine patch + other NRT (gum and spray).
    - The nicotine patch + the nicotine inhaler.
    - The nicotine patch + bupropion SR.[12] SOR Ⓐ
- There is a strong relationship between the number of sessions of counseling combined with medication and the likelihood of successful smoking cessation. Therefore, to the extent possible, clinicians should provide multiple counseling sessions, in addition to medication, to their patients who are trying to quit smoking.[12] SOR Ⓐ

SECOND LINE

- Second-line medications include clonidine and nortriptyline.[12] These agents should be considered for persons unable to use first-line medications because of contraindications or intolerable side effects or in persons whom first-line medications were not

TABLE 248-6 Pharmacologic Product Guide: FDA-Approved Medications for Smoking Cessation

	Nicotine Replacement Therapy (NRT) Formulations						
	Gum	Lozenge	Transdermal Patch	Nasal Spray	Oral Inhaler	Bupropion SR	Varenicline
Product	**Nicorette,**[1] **Generic** **OTC** 2 mg, 4 mg original, cinnamon, fruit, mint, orange $14.00/40 pieces	**Nicorette Lozenge,**[1] **Nicorette Mini Lozenge,**[1] **Generic** OTC 2 mg, 4 mg cherry, mint $39.00/81 pieces (2 mg)	**NicoDerm CQ,**[1] **Generic** OTC (NicoDerm CQ, generic) Rx (generic) 7 mg, 14 mg, 21 mg (24-hour release) $101.00/28 days	**Nicotrol NS**[2] Rx Metered spray 0.5 mg nicotine in 50 mcL aqueous nicotine solution $471.00/nasal spray	**Nicotrol Inhaler**[2] Rx10 mg cartridge delivers 4 mg inhaled nicotine vapor $471.00/inhaler	**Zyban,**[1] **Generic** Rx150 mg sustained-release tablet $49.00/month	**Chantix**[2] Rx 0.5 mg, 1 mg tablet $434.00 for starting month
Precautions	• Recent (≤2 weeks) myocardial infarction • Serious underlying arrhythmias • Serious or worsening angina pectoris • Temporomandibular joint disease • Pregnancy[3] and breastfeeding • Adolescents (<18 years)	• Recent (≤2 weeks) myocardial infarction • Serious underlying arrhythmias • Serious or worsening angina pectoris • Pregnancy[3] and breastfeeding • Adolescents (<18 years)	• Recent (≤2 weeks) myocardial infarction • Serious underlying arrhythmias • Serious or worsening angina pectoris • Pregnancy[3] (Rx formulations, category D) and breastfeeding • Adolescents (<18 years)	• Recent (≤2 weeks) myocardial infarction • Serious underlying arrhythmias • Serious or worsening angina pectoris • Underlying chronic nasal disorders (rhinitis, nasal polyps, sinusitis) • Severe reactive airway disease • Pregnancy[3] (category D) and breastfeeding • Adolescents (<18 years)	• Recent ≤2 weeks) myocardial infarction • Serious underlying arrhythmias • Serious or worsening angina pectoris • Bronchospastic disease • Pregnancy[3] (category D) and breastfeeding • Adolescents (<18 years)	• Concomitant therapy with medications or medical conditions known to lower the seizure threshold • Severe hepatic cirrhosis • Pregnancy[3] (category C) and breastfeeding • Adolescents (<18 years) **Warning:** • Black-box warning for neuropsychiatric symptoms[4] **Contraindications:** • Seizure disorder • Concomitant bupropion (e.g., Wellbutrin) therapy • Current or prior diagnosis of bulimia or anorexia nervosa • Simultaneous abrupt discontinuation of alcohol or sedatives/benzodiazepines • MAO inhibitor therapy in previous 14 days	• Severe renal impairment (dosage adjustment is necessary) • Pregnancy[3] (category C) and breastfeeding • Adolescents (<18 years) **Warnings:** • Black-box warning for neuropsychiatric symptoms[4] • Cardiovascular adverse events in patients with existing cardiovascular disease

(continued)

TABLE 248-6 Pharmacologic Product Guide: FDA-Approved Medications for Smoking Cessation (*Continued*)

	Nicotine Replacement Therapy (NRT) Formulations						
	Gum	Lozenge	Transdermal Patch	Nasal Spray	Oral Inhaler	Bupropion SR	Varenicline
Dosing	*≥25 cigarettes/day:* 4 mg *<25 cigarettes/day:* 2 mg Weeks 1–6: 1 piece q 1–2 hours Weeks 7–9: 1 piece q 2–4 hours Weeks 10–12: 1 piece q 4–8 hours • Maximum, 24 pieces/day • Chew each piece slowly • Park between cheek and gum when peppery or tingling sensation appears (~15–30 chews) • Resume chewing when tingle fades • Repeat chew/park steps until most of the nicotine is gone (tingle does not return: generally 30 min) • Park in different areas of mouth • No food or beverages 15 minutes before or during use • Duration: up to 12 weeks	*1st cigarette ≤30 minutes after waking:* 4 mg *1st cigarette >30 minutes after waking:* 2 mg Weeks 1–6:1 lozenge q 1–2 hours Weeks 7–9: 1 lozenge q 2–4 hours Weeks 10–12:1 lozenge q 4–8 hours • Maximum, 20 lozenges/day • Allow to dissolve slowly (20–30 minutes for standard: 10 minutes for mini) • Nicotine release may cause a warm, tingling sensation • Do not chew or swallow • Occasionally rotate to different areas of the mouth • No food or beverages 15 minutes before or during use • Duration: up to 12 weeks	*>10 cigarettes/day:* 21 mg/day × 4 weeks (generic) 6 weeks (NicoDerm CQ) 14 mg/day × 2 weeks 7 mg/day × 2 weeks *≤10 cigarettes/day:* 14 mg/day × 6 weeks 7 mg/day × 2 weeks • May wear patch for 16 hours if patient experiences sleep disturbances (remove at bedtime) • Duration: 8–10 weeks	1–2 doses/hour (8–40 doses/day) One dose = 2 sprays (one in **each** nostril): each spray delivers 0.5 mg of nicotine to the nasal mucosa • Maximum – 5 doses/hour or – 40 doses/day • For best results, initially use at least 8 doses/day • Do not sniff, swallow, or inhale through the nose as the spray is being administered • Duration: 3–6 months	6–16 cartridges/day Individualize dosing: initially use 1 cartridge q 1–2 hours • Best effects with continuous puffing for 20 minutes • Initially use at least 6 cartridges/day • Nicotine in cartridge is depleted after 20 minutes of active puffing • Inhale into back of throat or puff in short breaths • Do NOT inhale into the lungs (like a cigarette) but "puff" as if lighting a pipe • Open cartridge retains potency for 24 hours • No food or beverages 15 minutes before or during use • Duration: 3–6 months	150 mg po q AM × 3 days, then 150 mg po bid • Do not exceed 300 mg/day • Begin therapy 1–2 weeks **prior** to quit date • Allow at least 8 hours between doses • Avoid bedtime dosing to minimize insomnia • Dose tapering is not necessary • Can be used safely with NRT • Duration: 7–12 weeks, with maintenance up to 6 months in selected patients	Days 1–3:0.5 mg po q AM Days 4–7: 0.5 mg po bid Weeks 2–12:1 mg po bid • Begin therapy 1 week **prior** to quit date • Take dose after eating and with a full glass of water • Dose tapering is not necessary • Duration: 12 weeks: an additional 12-week course may be used in selected patients
Adverse Effects	• Mouth/jaw soreness • Hiccups • Dyspepsia • Hypersalivation • Effects associated with incorrect chewing technique: – Lightheadedness – Nausea/vomiting – Throat and mouth irritation	• Nausea • Hiccups • Cough • Heartburn • Headache • Flatulence • Insomnia	• Local skin reactions (erythema, pruritus, burning) • Headache • Sleep disturbances (insomnia, abnormal/vivid dreams); associated with nocturnal nicotine absorption	• Nasal and/or throat irritation (hot, peppery, or burning sensation) • Rhinitis • Tearing • Sneezing • Cough • Headache	• Mouth and/or throat irritation • Cough • Headache • Rhinitis • Dyspepsia • Hiccups	• Insomnia • Dry mouth • Nervousness/difficulty concentrating • Rash • Constipation • Seizures (risk is 0.1%) • Neuropsychiatric symptoms (rare; see PRECAUTIONS)	• Nausea • Sleep disturbances (insomnia, abnormal/vivid dreams) • Constipation • Flatulence • Vomiting • Neuropsychiatric symptoms (rare; see PRECAUTIONS)

Advantages	• Might satisfy oral cravings • Might delay weight gain • Patients can titrate therapy to manage withdrawal symptoms • Variety of flavors are available	• Might satisfy oral cravings • Might delay weight gain • Easy to use and conceal • Patients can titrate therapy to manage withdrawal symptoms • Variety of flavors are available	• Provides consistent nicotine levels over 24 hours • Easy to use and conceal • Once-daily dosing associated with fewer compliance problems	• Patients can titrate therapy to rapidly manage withdrawal symptoms	• Patients can titrate therapy to manage withdrawal symptoms • Mimics hand-to-mouth ritual of smoking (could also be perceived as a disadvantage)	• Easy to use; oral formulation might be associated with fewer compliance problems • Might delay weight gain • Can be used with NRT • Might be beneficial in patients with depression	• Easy to use; oral formulation might be associated with fewer compliance problems • Offers a new mechanism of action for patients who have failed other agents
Disadvantages	• Need for frequent dosing can compromise compliance • Might be problematic for patients with significant dental work • Patients must use proper chewing technique to minimize adverse effects • Gum chewing may not be socially acceptable	• Need for frequent dosing can compromise compliance • Gastrointestinal side effects (nausea, hiccups, heartburn) might be bothersome	• Patients cannot titrate the dose to acutely manage withdrawal symptoms • Allergic reactions to adhesive might occur • Patients with dermatologic conditions should not use the patch	• Need for frequent dosing can compromise compliance • Nasal/throat irritation may be bothersome • Patients must wait 5 minutes before driving or operating heavy machinery • Patients with chronic nasal disorders or severe reactive airway disease should not use the spray	• Need for frequent dosing can compromise compliance • Initial throat or mouth irritation can be bothersome • Cartridges should not be stored in very warm conditions or used in very cold conditions • Patients with underlying bronchospastic disease must use with caution	• Seizure risk is increased • Several contraindications and precautions preclude use in some patients (see PRECAUTIONS) • Patients should be monitored for potential neuropsychiatric symptoms[4] (see PRECAUTIONS)	• May induce nausea in up to one third of patients • Patients should be monitored for potential neuropsychiatric symptoms[4] (see PRECAUTIONS)

[1]Marketed by GlaxoSmithKline.
[2]Marketed by Pfizer.
[3]The U.S. Clinical Practice Guideline states that pregnant smokers should be encouraged to quit without medication based on insufficient evidence of effectiveness and theoretical concerns with safety. Pregnant smokers should be offered behavioral counseling interventions that exceed minimal advice to quit.
[4]In July 2009, the FDA mandated that the prescribing information for all bupropion- and varenicline-containing products include a black-box warning highlighting the risk of serious neuropsychiatric symptoms, including changes in behavior, hostility, agitation, depressed mood, suicidal thoughts and behavior, and attempted suicide. Clinicians should advise patients to stop taking varenicline or bupropion SR and contact a healthcare provider immediately if they experience agitation, depressed mood, and any changes in behavior that are not typical of nicotine withdrawal, or if they experience suicidal thoughts or behavior. If treatment is stopped due to neuropsychiatric symptoms, patients should be monitored until the symptoms resolve.
Abbreviations: MAO, monoamine oxidase; NRT, nicotine replacement therapy; OTC, over-the-counter (non-prescription product); Rx, prescription product.
For complete prescribing information, please refer to the manufacturers' package inserts.

helpful.[12] Use of clonidine and nortriptyline may be limited by contraindications and side effects as well.

COMPLEMENTARY AND ALTERNATIVE THERAPY

- Acupuncture—A meta-analysis of 5 studies did not show effectiveness of acupuncture as a tobacco use treatment. There is also lack of scientific evidence for the effectiveness of electrostimulation or laser acupuncture for the treatment of tobacco addiction.[12]
- Hypnotherapy—There is insufficient evidence to recommend hypnotherapy as an effective treatment for tobacco addiction.[12]
- Novel tobacco products—There is insufficient evidence to determine whether novel tobacco products reduce individual and population health risks. The evidence indicates that changing cigarette designs over the past 5 decades, including filtered, low-tar, and "light" variations, have not reduced overall disease risk among smokers and may have hindered prevention and cessation efforts. The overall health of the public could be harmed if the introduction of novel tobacco products encourages tobacco use among people who would otherwise be unlikely to use a tobacco product or delays cessation among persons who would otherwise quit using tobacco altogether.[8]

REFERRAL

For patients who are unsuccessful with therapies available in primary care, it is reasonable to refer them to a tobacco-cessation specialist. These specialists typically provide intensive tobacco interventions. Specialists are not defined by their professional affiliation or by the field in which they trained. Rather, specialists view tobacco dependence treatment as a primary professional role. Specialists possess the skills, knowledge, and training to provide effective interventions across a range of intensities and often are affiliated with programs offering intensive treatment interventions or services.

PREVENTION

Nearly all adults who smoke every day started smoking when they were age 26 years or younger, so youth prevention is the key to stopping the tobacco epidemic.

The USPSTF recommends that primary care clinicians provide interventions, including patient education or brief counseling, to prevent initiation of tobacco use among children and adolescents.[19] SOR Ⓐ

Advertising and promotional activities by tobacco companies have been shown to cause the onset and continuation of smoking among adolescents and young adults.[9] The tobacco industry spends almost $10 billion a year to market its products, half of all movies for children younger than age 13 years contain scenes of tobacco use, and images and messages normalize tobacco use in magazines, on the Internet, and at retail stores frequented by youth.[9] Tobacco use is also prevalent in video games played by youth.[20]

- The evidence is sufficient to conclude that there is a causal relationship between depictions of smoking in the movies and the initiation of smoking among young people.[9]
- Additionally, tobacco companies use flavorings to make products more appealing to youth.[4] In 2014, 73% of high school students and 56% of middle school students who used tobacco in the past 30 days reported using a flavored product.[4]
- The evidence is sufficient to conclude that mass media campaigns, comprehensive community programs, and comprehensive statewide tobacco control programs can prevent the initiation of tobacco use and reduce its prevalence among youth.[9]
- The evidence is sufficient to conclude that increases in cigarette prices reduce the initiation, prevalence, and intensity of smoking among youth and young adults.[9]
- The evidence is sufficient to conclude that school-based programs with evidence of effectiveness, containing specific components, can produce at least short-term effects and reduce the prevalence of tobacco use among school-age youth.[9] One tobacco-free education program for kids from the American Academy of Family Physicians (AAFP) is *Tar Wars*: http://www.tarwars.org/online/tarwars/home.html.

PROGNOSIS

- Each day in the United States, more than 3200 youths younger than age 18 years start smoking, and an additional 2100 youth and young adults become daily cigarette smokers.[9] If smoking continues at the current rate among youth in this country, 5.6 million of today's Americans younger than age 18 will die early from a smoking-related illness.[2] Most of these young people never considered the long-term health consequences associated with tobacco use when they started smoking; and nicotine, a highly addictive drug, causes many to continue smoking well into adulthood, often with deadly consequences.[9]
- Those with serious mental illnesses die, on average, 25 years earlier than the general population, with most deaths related to tobacco-related diseases such as heart disease, diabetes, and chronic lung disease.[21]

FOLLOW-UP

- All patients who receive a tobacco dependence intervention should be assessed for abstinence at the completion of treatment and during subsequent contacts.[9] Abstinent patients should have their quitting success acknowledged, and the clinician should offer to assist the patient with problems associated with quitting.[21] Patients who have relapsed should be assessed to determine whether they are willing to make another quit attempt. SOR Ⓒ

PATIENT RESOURCES

- **1-800-QUIT-NOW**—This free telephone quit line service refers callers to their own state's quit line via this national routing number. In some counties free nicotine patches are available to callers.
- The American Legacy Foundation's Became an EX Program—**https://www.becomeanex.org.** The EX Plan is a free quit smoking program that helps you relearn life without cigarettes. Before you actually stop smoking, they'll show you how to deal

with the very things that trip up so many people when they try to stop. So you'll be more prepared to stop and stay off tobacco.

- Office on Smoking and Health at the Centers for Disease Control and Prevention. *Smoking & Tobacco Use*—**http://www.cdc.gov/tobacco.** The Smoking and Tobacco Use website of the Centers for Disease Control and Prevention (CDC) provides tobacco use data and statistics; information about the health effects of smoking, smokeless tobacco products, and secondhand smoke; resources for tobacco cessation and youth smoking prevention; and products and materials that can help motivate behavior change. Visitors to the CDC website can find links to clinician and patient resources, such as a quit guideline.

PROVIDER RESOURCES

- American Academy of Family Physicians' Tobacco Cessation Program—**https://www.aafp.org/patient-care/public-health/tomacco-nicotine/ask-act.html.** The American Academy of Family Physicians' (AAFP) tobacco cessation program, "Ask and Act," encourages family physicians to ASK their patients about tobacco use, then ACT to help them quit. Through the Ask and Act program, AAFP members have access to a variety of free resources to help patients quit using tobacco, such as a quit smoking prescription pad and a wallet card with quitline information.
- American Academy of Family Physicians. *Pharmacologic Product Guide: FDA-Approved Medications*—**https://www.aafp.org/dam/AAFP/documents/patient_care/tobacco/pharmacologic-guide.pdf.** This is an excellent guide to pharmacologic intervention that summarizes precautions, dosing, adverse effects, advantages, disadvantages, and costs for the 7 FDA-approved medications for treatment of tobacco addiction.
- Smoking Cessation Leadership Center—**https://smokingcessationleadership.ucsf.edu.** The Smoking Cessation Leadership Center aims to increase smoking cessation rates and increase the number of health professionals who help smokers quit. The site not only provides tobacco cessation resources for providers to pass on to patients, it also offers a variety of tools, materials, and training courses aimed toward improving the delivery of tobacco cessation intervention in clinical settings. 1-800-QUIT-NOW cards can be ordered online at this website, which provides telephone cessation resources for all 50 states in the United States.
- Nicotine and Tobacco Dependence Website—**http://www.nicotineandtobaccodependence.com.** A companion to the book *Nicotine and Tobacco Dependence* (Peterson, Vander Werg, and Jaén, 2011), it provides book owners with easy-to-print forms, including a Nicotine and Tobacco Dependence Intake Form; Minnesota Nicotine Withdrawal Scale-Revised (MSW-R); Decisional Balance Exercise; Tobacco Use Diary; Physical, Behavioral, and Psychologic Strategies to Quit Tobacco; and a Sample Treatment Manual for 8 sessions for intensive tobacco treatment.
- American Academy of Family Physicians. *Tar Wars*—**https://www.aafp.org/patient-care/public-health/obacco-nicotine/tar-wars.html.** This is a tobacco-free education program for kids from the AAFP involving classroom presentations and poster contests.

REFERENCES

1. World Health Organization. *WHO Report on the Global Tobacco Epidemic, 2013.* Geneva: World Health Organization, 2013. http://www.who.int/tobacco/global_report/2013/en/. Accessed February 2017.
2. U.S. Department of Health and Human Services. *The Health Consequences of Smoking—50 Years of Progress: A Report of the Surgeon General.* Atlanta, GA: U.S. Department of Health and Human Services, Centers for Disease Control and Prevention, National Center for Chronic Disease Prevention and Health Promotion, Office on Smoking and Health, 2014. https://www.surgeongeneral.gov/library/reports/50-years-of-progress/index.html. Accessed February 2017.
3. Jamal A, King BA, Neff LJ, et al. Cigarette smoking among adults—United States, 2005–2015. *Morb Mortal Wkly Rep.* 2016;65(44):1205-1211. https://www.cdc.gov/mmwr/volumes/65/wr/mm6544a2.htm. Accessed February 2017.
4. Singh T, Arrazola RA, Corey CG, et al. Tobacco use among middle and high school students—United States, 2011–2015. *Morb Mortal Wkly Rep.* 2016;65(14):361-367. https://www.cdc.gov/mmwr/volumes/65/wr/mm6514a1.htm. Accessed February 2017.
5. U.S. Department of Health and Human Services. *E-Cigarette Use Among Youth and Young Adults: A Report of the Surgeon General—Executive Summary.* Atlanta, GA: U.S. Department of Health and Human Services, Centers for Disease Control and Prevention, National Center for Chronic Disease Prevention and Health Promotion, Office on Smoking and Health, 2016. https://e-cigarettes.surgeongeneral.gov/documents/2016_SGR_Exec_Summ_508.pdf. Accessed February 2017.
6. Centers for Disease Control and Prevention. Vital signs: disparities in nonsmokers' exposure to secondhand smoke—United States 1999–2012. *Morb Mortal Wkly Rep.* 2015;64 (Early Release):1-7. https://www.cdc.gov/tobacco/data_statistics/mmwrs/byyear/2015/mm64e0203a1/intro.htm. Accessed February 2017.
7. Centers for Disease Control and Prevention. Vital signs: disparities in nonsmokers' exposure to secondhand smoke—United States 1999–2012. *Morb Mortal Wkly Rep.* 2015;64(04):103-108. https://www.cdc.gov/mmwr/preview/mmwrhtml/mm6404a7.htm?s_cid=mm6404a7_w. Accessed February 2017.
8. U.S. Department of Health and Human Services. *How Tobacco Smoke Causes Disease: The Biology and Behavioral Basis for Smoking-Attributable Disease: A Report of the Surgeon General.* Atlanta, GA: U.S. Department of Health and Human Services, Centers for Disease Control and Prevention, National Center for Chronic Disease Prevention and Health Promotion, Office on Smoking and Health; 2010. https://www.ncbi.nlm.nih.gov/books/NBK53017/. Accessed February 2017.
9. U.S. Department of Health and Human Services. *Preventing Tobacco Use Among Youth and Young Adults: A Report of the Surgeon General.* Atlanta, GA: U.S. Department of Health and Human Services, Centers for Disease Control and Prevention, National Center for Chronic Disease Prevention and Health Promotion, Office on Smoking and Health; 2012. https://www.surgeongeneral.gov/library/reports/preventing-youth-tobacco-use/index.html. Accessed February 2017.

10. Benowitz NL. Clinical pharmacology of nicotine: implications for understanding, preventing, and treating tobacco addiction. *Clin Pharmacol Ther*. 2008;83(4):531-541.
11. Mays D, Gilman SE, Rende R, et al. Parental smoking exposure and adolescent smoking trajectories. *Pediatrics*. 2014;133(6): 983-991.
12. Fiore MC, Jaén CR, Baker TB, et al. *Treating Tobacco Use and Dependence: 2008 Update. Clinical Practice Guideline*. Rockville, MD: U.S. Department of Health and Human Services, Public Health Service; 2008.
13. Model D. Smoker's face. An underrated clinical sign? *Br Med J (Clin Res Ed)*. 1985;291(6511):1760-1762.
14. American Psychiatric Association. *Diagnostic and Statistical Manual of Mental Disorders, Fourth Edition, Text Revision (DSM-IV-TR)*. Arlington, VA: American Psychiatric Publishing; 2000.
15. Peterson AL, Vander Weg MW, Jaén CR. *Advances in Psychotherapy—Evidence-Based Practice. Vol. 21. Nicotine and Tobacco Dependence*. Cambridge, MA: Hogrefe; 2011.
16. U.S. Preventive Services Task Force. *Final Update Summary: Abdominal Aortic Aneurysm: Screening. September 2016*. https://www.uspreventiveservicestaskforce.org/Page/Document/UpdateSummaryFinal/abdominal-aortic-aneurysm-screening?ds=1&s=aaa. Accessed February 2017.
17. U.S. Preventive Services Task Force. *Final Update Summary: Lung Cancer: Screening*. July 2015. https://www.uspreventiveservicestaskforce.org/Page/Document/UpdateSummaryFinal/lung-cancer-screening?ds=1&s=lung cancer. Accessed February 2017.
18. Centers for Disease Control and Prevention. Use of 13-valent pneumococcal conjugate vaccine and 23-valent pneumococcal polysaccharide vaccine for adults with immunocompromising conditions: recommendations of the Advisory Committee on Immunization Practices (ACIP). *Morb Mortal Wkly Rep*. 2012;61(40):816-819. https://www.cdc.gov/mmwr/pdf/wk/mm6140.pdf. Accessed February 2017.
19. U.S. Preventive Services Task Force. *Final Update Summary: Tobacco Use in Children and Adolescents: Primary Care Interventions*. September 2016. https://www.uspreventiveservicestaskforce.org/Page/Document/UpdateSummaryFinal/tobacco-use-in-children-and-adolescents-primary-care-interventions?ds=1&s=tobacco. Accessed February 2017.
20. Barrientos-Gutierrez T, Barrientos-Gutierrez I, Lazcano-Ponce E, Thrasher JF. Tobacco content in video games: 1994–2011. *Lancet Oncol*. 2012;13(3):237-238.
21. Schroeder SA. A 51-year-old woman with bipolar disorder who wants to quit smoking. *JAMA*. 2009;301(5):522-531.

249 ALCOHOL USE DISORDER

Mark L. Willenbring, MD
Stacy L. Speedlin, PhD
Donald L. Hilton Jr, MD

PATIENT STORY

Theresa is a 39-year-old, white, single woman who presents with insomnia and depression. After exploring the presenting symptoms, her physician reviews some screening questions about potentially related problems. In response to a question about heavy drinking in the past year, Theresa responds that she is drinking about 2 bottles (10 drinks) of wine nightly. She acknowledges going over limits repeatedly and a persistent desire to quit or cut down, as well as continuing to drink in spite of hangovers and nausea in the morning. She denies withdrawal symptoms, driving while intoxicated, job or serious relationship problems, but admits that her social activities have decreased over the past year because she spends her evenings drinking alone. No one else knows she is struggling with drinking. Her depression and insomnia started after her drinking increased about 2 years ago.

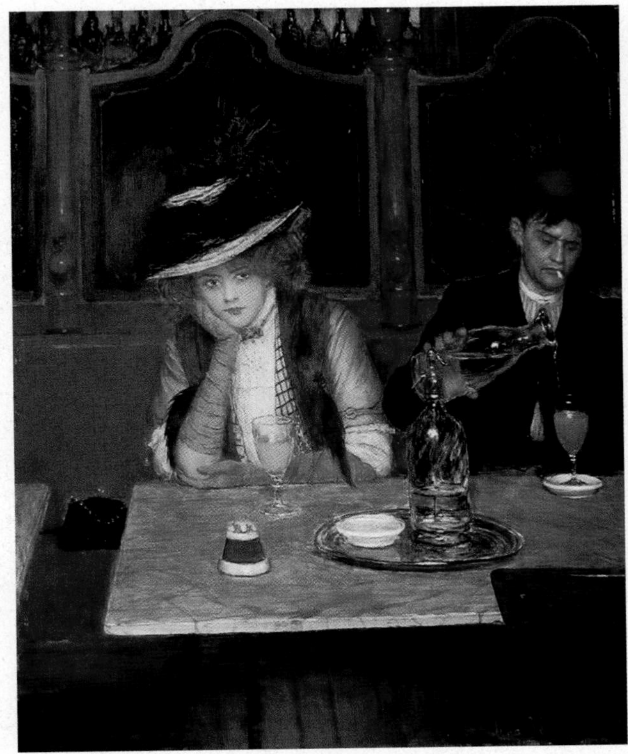

FIGURE 249-1 *The Drinkers* by Jean Béraud depicting a disheveled man pouring another drink of alcohol as a cigarette dangles from his mouth. The woman looks directly at us as she appears ready to leave with her handbag on the seat. She is dressed for a night out and appears to have expected more than sitting in a booth as her male partner drinks himself into oblivion. Painted in France in 1908 but touches us even today, as alcoholism is a worldwide and universal human issue.

INTRODUCTION

Excessive drinking of alcohol (**Figure 249-1**) is a common behavior encountered in primary care, yet few clinicians feel prepared to address it. Most clinicians are unclear about the best way to screen for heavy drinking and lack confidence in how to address it. Physicians often lack the knowledge and skill to screen and evaluate excessive drinking, let alone address it other than suggesting a referral to an addiction counselor or treatment program. Regrettably, few patients accept referral to a counselor or program. Fortunately, research over the past 20 years has provided evidence-based, efficient ways to screen, evaluate, and treat heavy drinking in primary care.

SYNONYMS (TERMINOLOGY)

Heavy drinking refers to drinking in excess of low-risk guidelines (see below).

Alcohol dependence (alcoholism) is a disorder of compulsive drinking associated with impaired control over intake, such as repeatedly exceeding self-defined limits, a persistent desire to quit or cut down and difficulty doing so, and continued use despite adverse consequences.

The terms *alcohol use disorder, alcohol dependence*, and *alcoholism* can be used interchangeably.

EPIDEMIOLOGY

- In any given year, approximately 30% of U.S. adults 18 years of age and older exceed the National Institute on Alcohol Abuse and Alcoholism (NIAAA) low-risk drinking guidelines at least once.[1]

BOX 249-1 Common Presentations of 3 Categories of Excessive Drinkers*

	Diagnosis of Alcohol Use Disorder
Category	**Common Presentation**
At-risk drinkers	None or driving while drinking only (no DWI)
Functional alcohol use disorder	• "Internal symptoms" of impaired control – Going over limits repeatedly – Desire to cut down/quit without success – Use despite "internal" problems associated with drinking (e.g., hangover, nausea) – Drinking and driving (no DWI) • Usually 2 to 4 criteria positive (out of 11)* • No legal, job, or serious interpersonal problems • Maximum drinks about 5 to 8 per drinking day • Single episode lasting 3 to 4 years on average, no recurrence
Severe recurrent alcohol use disorder	• "Internal" symptoms of impaired control (above) plus – Spending a lot of time drinking – Giving up non-drinking activities – Physical withdrawal and morning drinking – Serious medical complications (e.g. liver disease) • Usually >5 criteria positive • "External" symptoms of dysfunction – Social and family disruption – Problems with job, school, parenting – Legal problems (e.g., DWI) • Maximum drinks about 10 to 24 per drinking day • Recurrent episodes over years to decades (average of 5)

*The approach of DSM-5 diagnosis.[14]

The low-risk drinking limits for healthy adult women is defined as drinking no more than 3 drinks in any day and 7 drinks in any week, and for men, no more than 4 drinks in any day and 14 drinks in any week.

- A drink refers to 12 oz of beer, 5 oz of wine, or 1.5 oz of spirits, each of which contains about 14 g of absolute ethanol.[1] Within that group, the frequency varies from occasional to daily or near daily, and the amount of drinking varies from 5 to more than 20 drinks daily. Most excessive drinkers who exceed the limits (72%) do not meet diagnostic criteria for an alcohol use disorder and are considered at-risk drinkers.[1]
- At-risk drinkers are analogous to asymptomatic patients with hyperlipidemia or hypertension: they do not currently have a disorder (other than the risk factor) but are at elevated risk for developing one if the risk factor is not decreased. Reduction in excessive drinking significantly reduces risk of developing an alcohol use disorder, liver disease, or social problems.[2]
- In 2014, 139.7 million Americans (age 12 and older) reported current alcohol use, with 60.9 million reporting binge alcohol use within the past month[3]; 16.3 million Americans identified heavy drinking behavior in the past month.[3] Many individuals worldwide meet criteria for functional alcohol dependence, which is characterized by a predominance of "internal symptoms" of impaired control such as going over limits and persistent desire to quit or cut down and a limited course. People with functional alcohol dependence have a single episode, lasting on average 3 to 4 years, usually with resolution of the episode and no recurrence. A quarter of those with dependence, 1% of the general population in any year, have recurrent alcohol dependence, demonstrating an average of 5 episodes over a period of years to decades.[4]
- Thus, there are 3 categories of heavy drinkers the primary care provider is apt to encounter (**Box 249-1**):
  - At-risk drinkers (the predominant group);
  - Functional alcohol dependence; and
  - Recurrent, more severe alcohol dependence.
- Based on DSM-5 criteria, alcohol use disorder is generally treated according to the level of severity (mild, moderate, and severe).[5]

ETIOLOGY AND PATHOPHYSIOLOGY

Alcohol use disorder is a heritable disease: Approximately 50% of the risk is genetic, while environmental factors account for the remainder, the most clearly established factor being early childhood abuse or neglect.[6,7] Multigenerational alcohol dependence often appears in the early to mid-teens, but functional alcohol dependence can begin at any age.[8]

RISK FACTORS

The most important risk factors are:

- Family history of alcohol dependence,[9] and
- Early life stress in the form of early childhood abuse or neglect.[10]

Other risk factors include:

- An early history of externalizing personality factors, such as:
  - Extroversion
  - Attention-deficit disorder
  - Oppositional defiant disorder
  - Conduct disorder
- Antisocial and borderline personality disorders among adults[11]

Onset of drinking before the age of 14 years markedly increases risk for later development of alcohol dependence, especially for adolescents with a positive family history.[12]

DIAGNOSIS

CLINICAL FEATURES

- Contrary to common belief, heavy drinkers are very likely to answer questions about their drinking honestly, provided the questions are skillful. Asking about quantity and frequency ("On any single occasion during the past 3 months, have you had more than 5 drinks containing alcohol?") is most likely to elicit an informative answer, whereas any question that suggests even the possibility of moral judgment (e.g., "How much do you drink?") is less likely to yield helpful answers. See **Box 249-2** for the specific screening question recommended by the NIAAA.
- Most heavy drinkers are not symptomatic. Thus, they do not have alcohol-related symptoms. They can only be detected through screening for quantity and frequency of drinking. Screening focused on symptoms of alcohol use disorder, such as the well-known CAGE ("Have you ever tried to cut down on your drinking? Have you ever felt annoyed by criticism of your drinking? Have you ever felt guilty about your drinking? Have you ever had a morning eye-opener?"), will not detect asymptomatic at-risk drinkers, and it performs poorly compared to almost all other methods.[13] It is important to inquire about quantity and frequency of drinking in order to identify at-risk drinkers and patients with functional alcohol dependence. The AUDIT (Alcohol Use Disorders Identification Test) (**Figure 249-2**) is the gold standard for a written questionnaire; it only takes about 3 minutes to complete and is easy to score. A score of 8 or more for men or 4 or more for women suggests excessive drinking.[1]
- Current diagnostic criteria for alcohol use disorder are based on the DSM-5.[14] The presence of any 2 of the following 11 symptoms is enough to establish a diagnosis, where the number of symptoms met is highly correlated with severity of the disorder:

"1. Alcohol is often taken in larger amounts or over a longer period than was intended.
2. There is a persistent desire or unsuccessful efforts to cut down or control alcohol use.
3. A great deal of time is spent in activities necessary to obtain alcohol, use alcohol, or recover from its effects.
4. Craving, or a strong desire or urge to use alcohol.
5. Recurrent alcohol use resulting in a failure to fulfill major role obligations at work, school, or home.

BOX 249-2 Screening Question Recommended by the National Institute on Alcohol Abuse and Alcoholism (NIAAA)

How many times in the past year have you had...

- 5 or more drinks in a day? (for men)
- 4 or more drinks in a day? (for women)

One standard drink is equivalent to 12 oz of beer, 5 oz of wine, or 1.5 oz of 80-proof spirits.

Reproduced with permission from http://www.niaaa.nih.gov/guide.

6. Continued alcohol use despite having persistent or recurrent social or interpersonal problems caused or exacerbated by the effects of alcohol.
7. Important social, occupational, or recreational activities are given up or reduced because of alcohol use.
8. Recurrent alcohol use in situations in which it is physically hazardous.
9. Alcohol use is continued despite knowledge of having a persistent or recurrent physical or psychological problem that is likely to have been caused or exacerbated by alcohol.
10. Tolerance, as defined by either of the following:
    - A need for markedly increased amounts of alcohol to achieve intoxication or desired effect.
    - A markedly diminished effect with continued use of the same amount of alcohol.
11. Withdrawal, as manifested by either of the following:
    - The characteristic withdrawal syndrome for alcohol (refer to Criteria A and B of the criteria set for alcohol withdrawal).
    - Alcohol (or a closely related substance, such as a benzodiazepine) is taken to relieve or avoid withdrawal symptoms."[14]

- According to NIAAA, healthy adult men should not drink in excess of 4 standard U.S. drinks in any day, or 14 in any week, and adult women should not exceed 3 drinks in any day and 7 in any week.[1] Low-risk drinking limits may be less for certain groups, such as adults older than age 65 years, or in the presence of medical illnesses, such as liver disease. Women who are pregnant or are trying to become pregnant should be advised to abstain completely.
- A recent meta-analysis concluded that light drinking increases the risk of cancer of the oral cavity and pharynx, esophagus, and female breast.[15] This data and other studies prompted the American Society of Clinical Oncology to release a statement in 2018 that a proactive stance to "minimize excessive exposure to alcohol has important implications for cancer prevention."[16]
- Drinking in excess of the limits above is surely unhealthy, placing heavy drinkers at elevated risk for developing an alcohol use disorder (AUD) and associated complications such as liver disease.[16] Approximately 30% of U.S. adults age 18 years and older drink in excess of low-risk limits at least once in any year. About 4 of 5 of them do not meet diagnostic criteria for a disorder and are considered to be "at risk" for developing one.[1] In other words, this group has an asymptomatic risk factor similar to

AUDIT

PATIENT: Because alcohol use can affect your health and can interfere with certain medications and treatments, it is important that we ask some questions about your use of alcohol. Your answers will remain confidential, so please be honest.

For each question in the chart below, place an X in one box that best describes your answer.

NOTE: In the U.S., a single drink serving contains about 14 grams of ethanol or "pure" alcohol. Although the drinks below are different sizes, each one contains the same amount of pure alcohol and counts as a single drink:

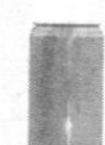
12 oz. of beer (about 5% alcohol) =

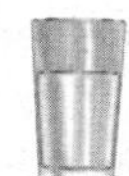
8-9 oz. of malt liquor (about 7% alcohol) =

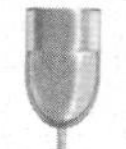
5 oz. of wine (about 12% alcohol) =

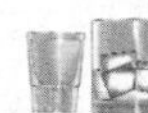
1.5 oz. of hard liquor (about 40% alcohol)

Questions	0	1	2	3	4	
1. How often do you have a drink containing alcohol?	Never	Monthly or less	2 to 4 times a month	2 to 3 times a week	4 or more times a week	
2. How many drinks containing alcohol do you have on a typical day when you are drinking?	1 or 2	3 or 4	5 or 6	7 to 9	10 or more	
3. How often do you have 5 or more drinks on one occasion?	Never	Less than monthly	Monthly	Weekly	Daily or almost daily	
4. How often during the last year have you found that you were not able to stop drinking once you had started?	Never	Less than monthly	Monthly	Weekly	Daily or almost daily	
5. How often during the last year have you failed to do what was normally expected of you because of drinking?	Never	Less than monthly	Monthly	Weekly	Daily or almost daily	
6. How often during the last year have you needed a first drink in the morning to get yourself going after a heavy drinking session?	Never	Less than monthly	Monthly	Weekly	Daily or almost daily	
7. How often during the last year have you had a feeling of guilt or remorse after drinking?	Never	Less than monthly	Monthly	Weekly	Daily or almost daily	
8. How often during the last year have you been unable to remember what happened the night before because of your drinking?	Never	Less than monthly	Monthly	Weekly	Daily or almost daily	
9. Have you or someone else been injured because of your drinking?	No		Yes, but not in the last year		Yes, during the last year	
10. Has a relative, friend, doctor, or other health care worker been concerned about your drinking or suggested you cut down?	No		Yes, but not in the last year		Yes, during the last year	
					Total	

Note: This questionnaire (the AUDIT) is reprinted with permission from the World Health Organization. To reflect drink serving sizes in the United States (14g of pure alcohol), the number of drinks in question 3 was changed from 6 to 5. A free AUDIT manual with guidelines for use in primary care settings is available online at *www.who.org*.

FIGURE 249-2 The AUDIT questionnaire. Scores are added to determine the total. Positive screens are indicated by total scores ≥8 in men and ≥4 in women. Higher scores indicate more severe alcohol involvement. Scores >16 suggest the possibility of alcohol dependence. (*Reproduced with permission from World Health Organization, available online at www.who.org. NIH Publication No. 07-3769 National Institute on Alcohol and Alcoholism www.niaaa.nih.gov/guide.*)

hypertension or hyperlipidemia. At-risk drinkers are typically unaware that their drinking constitutes a health risk. This does not reflect "denial" but rather the lack of information available to the public about what constitutes high-risk drinking or how to measure consumption. For example, how many standard U.S. drinks are in a 7 oz. martini? (Depending on the specific way it is mixed, the answer is about 4.) It is much easier to obtain dietary information about food than information about alcohol content in a beverage.

- Patients with functional alcohol dependence are aware of struggling with their alcohol consumption, but lack serious life consequences at this time. Most are open to changing their drinking, but they may need to be identified through screening, rather than presenting with this problem.
- Patients with more severe, recurrent alcohol dependence often present with intoxication, withdrawal, or medical complications of heavy drinking, such as liver disease or pancreatitis. If these disorders are present, they demonstrate the expected physical manifestations. Like other patients with chronic, treatment-refractory illness, they have a chronic course, with periodic relapses or even with ongoing chronic illness.

TYPICAL DISTRIBUTION

- In a given year, 30% of the adult U.S. population engages in unhealthy drinking at least once. In an average primary care practice, approximately 10% to 15% of outpatients are heavy drinkers.

LABORATORY TESTING

- The most sensitive way to detect heavy drinking is to ask about the frequency of heavy drinking. Use of a written questionnaire such as the AUDIT can be helpful (see **Figure 249-2**).[17]
- The most sensitive but least specific laboratory test is γ-glutamyl transferase (GGT). Carbohydrate-deficient transferrin provides similar sensitivity but better specificity, but this test is not widely available.[18]
- Other transaminases such as aspartate transaminase (AST) and alanine transaminase (ALT) are less sensitive and require hepatic cell destruction before they are elevated. Thus, they are not very sensitive for detecting heavy drinking, but they may be helpful in following patients who have elevated values at baseline.

IMAGING

- There are no imaging tests that detect heavy drinking itself. Abdominal ultrasound is often helpful in evaluating alcoholic liver disease.

DIFFERENTIAL DIAGNOSIS

- It is important to distinguish between AUD and asymptomatic at-risk drinking. AUD is characterized by preoccupation with and impaired control over drinking.

MANAGEMENT

Box 249-3: Clinical Prevention and Treatment of Alcohol Use Disorder.

NONPHARMACOLOGIC

- Brief counseling and advice to reduce drinking is effective for at-risk drinking, resulting in 15% to 20% reduction in drinking for at least 1 year.[2]
- Alcohol use disorder requires either more intensive counseling and/or anti-relapse medications. The relationship between intensity and setting (inpatient, residential, or outpatient) is complex. Most studies show no difference in 1-year outcomes based on intensity or setting.[19] For example, in a highly controlled, well-done study, 174 persons with alcoholism were randomly assigned to partial hospital treatment or extended inpatient rehabilitation after inpatient evaluation and/or detoxification. The outpatient group attended daily Monday through Friday therapy alongside the group that was assigned to 6 months of psychiatric inpatient hospitalization. The study found no additional benefit to extended hospitalization.[20]
- However, there are circumstances that make providing structured sober housing important: among people who are homeless, those

BOX 249-3 Clinical Prevention and Treatment of Alcohol Use Disorder

Category	Management
At-risk drinkers Goal: risk reduction	• Brief counseling to quit or cut down • Hand patients *Rethinking Drinking* booklet • Repeated counseling increases effectiveness
Functional alcohol use disorder Goal: long-term abstinence or low-risk drinking (e.g., recovery)	• Anti-relapse medications – Naltrexone (oral, injection) – Topiramate (Topamax) – Disulfiram (Antabuse) • Brief behavioral support (medication management) • Recommend Alcoholics Anonymous • Offer referral to addiction specialist, especially if fails to respond to primary care treatment
Severe recurrent alcohol use disorder Goals: • Reduce frequency, severity, and length of relapses • Treat complications • Slow the rate of deterioration • Aim for full recovery, but recognize it may not be achieved	• Offer referral to addiction specialist • Recommend Alcoholics Anonymous • Medications – Treat withdrawal if needed – Anti-relapse medications • Care coordination • Integrate medical, psychiatric, addiction treatment • Treatment for as long as needed; usually years to decades

who cannot stop drinking while living independently, and people with significant coexisting psychiatric illness.[19] The degree of housing structure required, however, is relatively independent of the intensity or type of treatment given. Some patients require a great deal of housing structure but very few treatment services, whereas others are stably housed but require intensive and prolonged treatment. Thus, it makes sense to uncouple housing structure from treatment decisions, as there is no apparent benefit to having patients stay in a facility overnight while they are receiving treatment services.

- Increasingly, treatment for recurrent AUD (dependence) is being conceptualized as management of a chronic illness.[21] A recent study found that continued care that included primary care management as well as continued access to specialty addiction care resulted in improved outcomes and reduced costs.[22]
- Long-term regular medical follow-up that simply attends to drinking and encourages abstinence is effective for reducing drinking among patients with medical complications such as liver cirrhosis or pancreatitis.[23]

MEDICATIONS

- Several anti-relapse medications are available for alcohol use disorder. Their average efficacy is similar to that for selective serotonin reuptake inhibitor (SSRI) antidepressants in treating depression.[24,25]
- Naltrexone 50 mg daily or as needed for each drinking occasion reduces relapse rates and quantity of drinking per occasion. It reduces craving for alcohol and the reward or "kick" an individual experiences when first beginning a drinking episode. This reduces the compulsive quality of drinking, making it easier to stop before a full relapse occurs. Its effectiveness is determined by genetic factors; it is most effective among northern Europeans and least likely to be effective among African Americans. In the author's experience, naltrexone 25 to 50 mg as needed per drinking occasion may help at-risk drinkers reduce excessive alcohol use, especially in social situations. Approximately 10% of patients will experience nausea. Patients should be warned that usual doses of oral opioids such as hydrocodone will not work because of the opioid blockade, so naltrexone should be stopped at least 3 days prior to elective procedures. In emergencies the blockade can be overridden, but the therapeutic index is reduced. Although initially quite concerning, in practice this has not proved to be a significant problem. Naltrexone also is available in a long-acting injectable formulation that only requires monthly administration.
- Disulfiram 250 mg daily acts by blocking the breakdown of ethanol, resulting in increased levels of acetaldehyde, which causes an adverse flushing reaction. The disulfiram-ethanol reaction is thus dose related; a small amount of alcohol such as might exist in wine vinegar, for example, might cause mild facial flushing, whereas drinking several glasses of wine or beer, or several ounces of distilled spirits, will cause a more severe reaction. Disulfiram-ethanol reactions may be very unpleasant but are unlikely to be harmful in the absence of preexisting ischemic heart disease. Reactions can occur up to several days after discontinuation, so patients should be warned. Some patients will not develop a disulfiram-ethanol reaction at the standard dose and require 500 mg daily. Disulfiram therapy is the most effective for maintaining abstinence, because any significant alcohol use will cause a reaction. It works best when administration is monitored by a family member, roommate, or friend. The most common side effect is a metallic taste. Less common are peripheral neuropathy, optical neuritis, and delirium or psychosis. A rare but serious idiosyncratic risk is that of fulminant hepatitis, often leading to liver failure and death.
- Topiramate and gabapentin can reduce alcohol ingestion.[25] These meds are thought to work by normalizing the γ-aminobutyric acid (GABA)-glutamate imbalance that occurs with severe alcohol use disorder. They can reduce the desire to drink and the reward that occurs with drinking. Because of side effects, it is important to start at a low dose of topiramate, for example, 25 mg before bedtime, and ramp up slowly over 4 to 8 weeks to a target dose of 200 to 800 mg daily. The most distressing side effect is cognitive dysfunction, best described as difficulty with word finding. Perioral paresthesias are common but reversible. Topiramate increases the excretion of calcium, thus increasing the risk for renal calculi, especially in patients with a previous history.
- Antidepressants can also decrease alcohol ingestion for patients with mood disorders. Equally, these drugs are typically not effective with patients without mood disorders.[26]
- Acamprosate is licensed for alcohol use disorder by the FDA, but the last 3 large multisite trials demonstrated no effectiveness.[27-29] It is expensive and must be taken 3 times a day. If it is effective at all, it would be in very severe dependence with a history of physical withdrawal.
- Ondansetron may reduce the use of alcohol in patients with AUD, particularly those of select subpopulations.[26]

COMPLEMENTARY AND ALTERNATIVE THERAPY

- No complementary/alternative therapies have proven efficacy in alcohol use disorder.
- Unfortunately, some treatment programs continue to offer "nutritional therapy," treatment guided by single-photon emission computed tomography (SPECT) scans, acupuncture, and other unproven therapies, but there is no evidence of their effectiveness.
- 12-Step community support groups such as Alcoholics Anonymous (AA) help some patients with severe alcohol dependence. People who affiliate and stay with AA have better outcomes than those who do not.

REFER OR HOSPITALIZE

- Alcohol withdrawal is best managed in the hospital for patients with histories of alcohol withdrawal seizures or delirium, or who have medical conditions that might destabilize during withdrawal, such as ischemic heart disease or fragile diabetes.
- Alcohol withdrawal delirium requires hospitalization, usually in an intensive care unit.
- Consider a referral to an addiction medical specialist.
- Inpatient psychiatric hospitalization conferred no added benefit compared with outpatient treatment, but inpatient treatment might be useful for patients who are unable to abstain for the 4 to 8 weeks necessary for outpatient treatment.[30] Sober housing coupled with an outpatient treatment program can also be beneficial for some.

- Anti-relapse medication along with medical management is as effective as high-quality addiction counseling for more functional patients with alcohol dependence.[31]
- Patients with severe recurrent alcohol dependence with medical comorbidities fare best with long-term regular medical management, which includes discussion of alcohol consumption and its relationship to medical conditions, as well as encouragement to abstain. When sustained over 1 to 2 years, such medical management results in a substantial proportion of patients who are abstinent.[32]
- The presence of severe psychiatric conditions such as psychosis, mania, or severe depression with suicidal ideation requires referral to a psychiatrist or hospital. Long-term comanagement by primary care physicians and psychiatrists is likely to be necessary.

PREVENTION

- Most heavy drinkers are asymptomatic but are drinking at a rate that puts them at increased risk for developing mild alcohol use disorder and associated medical and social complications. These "at-risk" drinkers respond well to brief counseling by physicians, resulting in significant reductions in heavy drinking. This finding is based on extensive research, such that the U.S. Preventive Services Task Force has rated screening and brief counseling to be a "B" recommendation (both have also been determined to be cost-effective).[33] Because the prevalence of at-risk drinking is so high (26% of U.S. adults in any given year), the potential public health impact of broad implementation of screening and brief counseling is large.
- The NIAAA has published a guide to help physicians with screening, assessment, and brief counseling techniques. There is also an online continuing medical education (CME) activity available. This online training uses 4 video case series, along with advanced interactive educational techniques, to improve physicians' skills and knowledge (available at http://www.niaaa.nih.gov/publications/clinical-guides-and-manuals/niaaa-clinicians-guide-online-training). CME credit is available and it has been approved by the American Academy of Family Physicians.
- *Rethinking Drinking*, available as a booklet and online, is an educational tool for at-risk drinkers (available at https://pubs.niaaa.nih.gov/publications/RethinkingDrinking/Rethinking_Drinking.pdf). This publication takes the drinker through a process of increasing awareness of drinking, deciding whether to change and what the drinking goal is, and developing a plan to implement change. Using this publication substantially enhances the value while decreasing the time it takes to counsel a patient to reduce or stop drinking.

PROGNOSIS

- Most at-risk drinkers eventually reduce their drinking or abstain, and do not develop an AUD or other complications of heavy drinking.
- Nearly three-fourths of people who have an episode where they meet criteria for an AUD experience remission of the disorder (either through abstaining or reducing drinking to low-risk levels) after a few years. Once remitted, the AUD generally does not recur, and 20 years after onset, fewer than 10% still meet full diagnostic criteria for a disorder.[4]
- Those with recurrent or chronic dependence have an average of 5 episodes over a period of decades. However, many eventually do remit. Almost all patients who enter rehab programs have severe recurrent dependence.[8] Rehab outcomes are very similar across different programs.[34] In the first year following an episode of rehab, roughly one-third of patients will be in stable recovery (approximately 25% will abstain and 10% will be in non-abstinent recovery, defined as engaging in no high-risk drinking and having no alcohol-related problems), a third will not respond and will remain in stable non-recovery, and the remainder will show variability.
- Patients with moderate-severe, recurrent dependence usually must make multiple quit attempts over several years before long-term abstinence is established.[35]
- Recent research suggests that heavy drinking in mid-life tends to persist over time and may be resistant to available treatment approaches.[36] Consequently, repeated and ongoing efforts to support change are often required. It is helpful under these circumstances to think in terms of "quit attempts," much as for smoking cessation.
- A minority of patients have chronic dependence or periodic relapses for many years, and as is true with all chronic illnesses, some will die of the disease and its medical complications, in spite of availability of all available current treatments and motivated effort by the patient. The science of behavior change is in its infancy, so much of what we do is nonspecific and modestly effective.

FOLLOW-UP

- *At-risk drinkers:* Although a single brief counseling session has significant efficacy, the effect may be magnified by repeated counseling. For this reason, it is best to inquire about drinking quantity and frequency at each follow-up visit and to reinforce advice about low-risk drinking limits.
- *Patients with alcohol dependence:* Approach this group of patients with the same attitude you adopt for smoking cessation. Most people require multiple quit attempts before achieving lasting remission, so it is important to anticipate the possibility of recurrence, and to plan for it if it occurs. Let the patient know that you won't be angry or disappointed with them if recurrence occurs. In fact, if they have a relapse to heavy drinking, that is exactly when they should seek care; a relapse is similar to an asthma attack or an increase in chest pain from ischemic heart disease. Exacerbations or recurrences of chronic illnesses are common and can be managed. The goal is to seek care quickly if a recurrence occurs, as well as to keep relapses infrequent and short and to reduce their severity. If withdrawal is a concern, it can generally be managed on an outpatient basis.[37] Reevaluate pharmacotherapy and behavioral approaches. Support learning from the recurrence: How did it happen? What could prevent the next one? Address guilt and shame and encourage patients to minimize time spent on this relapse and to look to the future and get right back on track.
- For patients with functional alcohol dependence, consider referral to an addiction medicine or psychiatry specialist.

- For patients with complex chronic addiction, treat complications, recruit social and environmental resources (family, community, etc.) as indicated, and provide support.

PATIENT EDUCATION

- A patient handbook is available from the NIAAA. Titled *Rethinking Drinking*, it takes patients through a scientifically based process of education, evaluation of their drinking, and decision making regarding whether to change it. Free copies of the printed version are available from the Institute and it is also available on the Internet—https://pubs.niaaa.nih.gov/publications/RethinkingDrinking/Rethinking_Drinking.pdf.
- General principles in approaching patients:
  - Heavy drinking and AUDs are similar to other common complex diseases such as diabetes: they have about a 50:50 combination of genetic and environmental etiologies.
  - Alcohol dependence occurs when the brain changes after exposure to large doses of alcohol, causing an impairment of control over intake. In all but mild cases, this is irreversible and good control over drinking will always be problematic. Thus, abstinence is the best and easiest approach for most people.
  - Acknowledge that friends and family may take a long time to trust an individual in early recovery, as most have been disappointed numerous times in the past.
  - Emphasize that slips and relapses are common and encourage patients to keep trying in spite of them.

PATIENT RESOURCES

- The National Institute on Alcohol Abuse and Alcoholism—**https://www.niaaa.nih.gov.**
- *Rethinking Drinking*, a booklet for people who wish to consume alcohol—**https://pubs.niaaa.nih.gov/publications/RethinkingDrinking/Rethinking_Drinking.pdf.**
- Faces and Voices of Recovery—**https://facesandvoicesofrecovery.org.**
- Alcoholics Anonymous—**https://www.aa.org.**

PROVIDER RESOURCES

- *Helping Patients Who Drink Too Much: A Clinician's Guide*—**http://www.niaaa.nih.gov/publications/clinical-guides-and-manuals/helping-patients-who-drink-too-much-clinicians-guide.**

REFERENCES

1. *Helping Patients Who Drink Too Much: A Clinician's Guide.* Bethesda, MD: National Institutes of Health; 2007.
2. Whitlock EP, Polen MR, Green CA, et al. Behavioral counseling interventions in primary care to reduce risky/harmful alcohol use by adults: a summary of the evidence for the U.S. Preventive Services Task Force. *Ann Intern Med.* 2004;140(7):557-568, I564.
3. Substance Abuse and Mental Health Services Administration. *Behavioral Health Trends in the United States: Results from the 2014 National Survey on Drug Use and Health.* (HHS Publication No. SMA 15-4927, NSDUH Series H-50). 2015.
4. Hasin DS, Stinson FS, Ogburn E, Grant BF. Prevalence, correlates, disability, and comorbidity of DSM-IV alcohol abuse and dependence in the United States: results from the national epidemiologic survey on alcohol and related conditions. *Arch Gen Psychiatry.* 2007;64(7):830-842.
5. Grant BF, Goldstein RB, Saha TD, et al. Epidemiology of DSM-5 alcohol use disorder: results From the National Epidemiology Survey on Alcohol and Related Conditions III. *JAMA Psychiatry.* 2015;72:757.
6. Dick DM, Bierut LJ. The genetics of alcohol dependence. *Curr Psychiatry Rep.* 2006;8(2):151-157.
7. Enoch M-A. The influence of gene-environment interactions on the development of alcoholism and drug dependence. *Curr Psychiatry Rep.* 2012;14(2):150-158.
8. Moss HB, Chen CM, Yi Hy. Subtypes of alcohol dependence in a nationally representative sample. *Drug Alcohol Depend.* 2007;91(2-3):149-158.
9. Lynskey MT, Agrawal A, Heath AC. Genetically informative research on adolescent substance use: methods, findings, and challenges. *J Am Acad Child Adolesc Psychiatry.* 2010;49(12):1202-1214.
10. Enoch M-A. The role of early life stress as a predictor for alcohol and drug dependence. *Psychopharmacology (Berl).* 2011;214(1):17-31.
11. Chartier KG, Hesselbrock MN, Hesselbrock VM. Development and vulnerability factors in adolescent alcohol use. *Child Adolesc Psychiatr Clin N Am.* 2010;19(3):493-504.
12. Hingson RW, Heeren T, Winter MR. Age of alcohol-dependence onset: associations with severity of dependence and seeking treatment. *Pediatrics.* 2006;118(3):e755-e763.
13. Rubinsky AD, Kivlahan DR, Volk RJ, et al. Estimating risk of alcohol dependence using alcohol screening scores. *Drug Alcohol Depend.* 2010;108(1-2):29-36.
14. American Psychiatric Association. *Diagnostic and Statistical Manual of Psychiatric Disorders, Fifth Edition.* Washington, DC: American Psychiatric Publishing; 2013.
15. Bagnardi V, Rota M, Botteri E, et al. Light alcohol drinking and cancer: a meta-analysis. *Ann Oncol.* 2013;24:301-308.
16. LoConte NK, Brewster AM, Kaur JS, et al. Alcohol and cancer: A statement of the American Society of Clinical Oncology. *J Clin Oncol.* 2018;36(1):83-93.
17. Boschloo L, Vogelzangs N, Smit JH, et al. The performance of the Alcohol Use Disorder Identification Test (AUDIT) in detecting alcohol abuse and dependence in a population of depressed or anxious persons. *J Affect Disord.* 2010;126(3):441-446.
18. Hock B, Schwarz M, Limmer C, et al. Validity of carbohydrate-deficient transferrin (%CDT), gamma-glutamyltransferase (gamma-GT) and mean corpuscular erythrocyte volume (MCV) as biomarkers for chronic alcohol abuse: a study in patients with alcohol dependence and liver disorders of non-alcoholic and alcoholic origin. *Addiction.* 2005;100(10):1477-1486.

19. Finney JW, Hahn AC, Moos RH. The effectiveness of inpatient and outpatient treatment for alcohol abuse: the need to focus on mediators and moderators of setting effects. *Addiction.* 1996; 91(12):1773-1796.

20. Longabaugh R, McCrady B, Fink E, et al. Cost effectiveness of alcoholism treatment in partial vs inpatient settings. Six-month outcomes. *J Stud Alcohol.* 1983;44(6):1049-1071.

21. McLellan AT, Lewis DC, O'Brien CP, Kleber HD. Drug dependence, a chronic medical illness: implications for treatment, insurance, and outcomes evaluation. *JAMA.* 2000;284(13): 1689-1695.

22. Parthasarathy S, Chi FW, Mertens JR, Weisner C. The role of continuing care in 9-year cost trajectories of patients with intakes into an outpatient alcohol and drug treatment program. *Med Care.* 2012;50(6):540-546.

23. Willenbring ML, Olson DH. A randomized trial of integrated outpatient treatment for medically ill alcoholic men. *Arch Intern Med.* 1999;159(16):1946-1952.

24. Bouza C, Angeles M, Munoz A, Amate JM. Efficacy and safety of naltrexone and acamprosate in the treatment of alcohol dependence: a systematic review. *Addiction.* 2004;99(7):811-828.

25. Johnson BA, Rosenthal N, Capece J, et al. Topiramate for the treatment of alcohol dependence: results from a multi-site trial. *Alcohol Clin Exp Res.* 2007;31(s2):261A-261A.

26 Winslow BT, Onysko M, Hebert M. Medications for alcohol use disorder. *Am Fam Physician.* 2016;93(6):457-465.

27. Anton RF, O'Malley SS, Ciraulo DA, et al. Combined pharmacotherapies and behavioral interventions for alcohol dependence: the COMBINE study: a randomized controlled trial. *JAMA.* 2006;295(17):2003-2017.

28. Mason BJ, Goodman AM, Chabac S, Lehert P. Effect of oral acamprosate on abstinence in patients with alcohol dependence in a double-blind, placebo-controlled trial: the role of patient motivation. *J Psychiatr Res.* 2006;40(5):383-393.

29. Mann KF, Lemenager KF, Smolka M; the Project PREDICT Research Group. Craving subtypes as predictors for treatment response: results from the PREDICT Study. *Alcohol Clin Exp Res.* 2008;32(Suppl 1a):281A.

30. Fink EB, Longabaugh R, McCrady BM, et al. Effectiveness of alcoholism treatment in partial versus inpatient settings: twenty-four month outcomes. *Addict Behav.* 1985;10(3):235-248.

31. O'Malley SS, Rounsaville BJ, Farren C, et al. Initial and maintenance naltrexone treatment for alcohol dependence using primary care vs specialty care: a nested sequence of 3 randomized trials. *Arch Intern Med.* 2003;163(14):1695-1704.

32. Willenbring ML, Olson DH, Bielinski J. Integrated outpatient treatment for medically ill alcoholic men: results from a quasi-experimental study. *J Stud Alcohol.* 1995;56(3):337-343.

33. Solberg LI, Maciosek MV, Edwards NM. Primary care intervention to reduce alcohol misuse. ranking its health impact and cost effectiveness. *Am J Prev Med.* 2008;34(2).

34. Miller WR, Walters ST, Bennett ME. How effective is alcoholism treatment in the United States? *J Stud Alcohol.* 2001;62(2):211-220.

35. Dawson DA, Grant BF, Stinson FS, et al. Recovery from DSM-IV alcohol dependence: United States, 2001-2002. *Addiction.* 2005; 100(3):281-292.

36. Delucchi KL, Kline Simon AH, Weisner C. Remission from alcohol and other drug problem use in public and private treatment samples over seven years. *Drug Alcohol Depend.* 2012;124(1-2): 57-62.

37. Hayashida M, Alterman AI, McLellan AT, et al. Comparative effectiveness and costs of inpatient and outpatient detoxification of patients with mild-to-moderate alcohol withdrawal syndrome. *N Engl J Med.* 1989;320(6):358-365.

250 METHAMPHETAMINE

Andrew D. Schechtman, MD
Stacy L. Speedlin, PhD
Donald L. Hilton Jr, MD
Lina M. Cardona, MD

PATIENT STORY

A 40-year-old woman with diabetes comes to the clinic with blood sugars in the 400s because she ran out of insulin a few weeks ago. She appears poorly groomed and has nicotine stains on her fingertips. Excoriated lesions (**Figure 250-1**) are noted on her forearms and face. She reports no itching at this moment, but when asked confirms that she regularly smokes methamphetamine. The diagnosis of her skin condition is meth mites. She acknowledges that she picks at her skin when she is high on meth. The physician asks her if she wants help to get off the meth so she can care for her health and well-being. She breaks down in tears and says that her craving for meth is very strong, but she is willing to try something because she knows the meth is ruining her body and life.

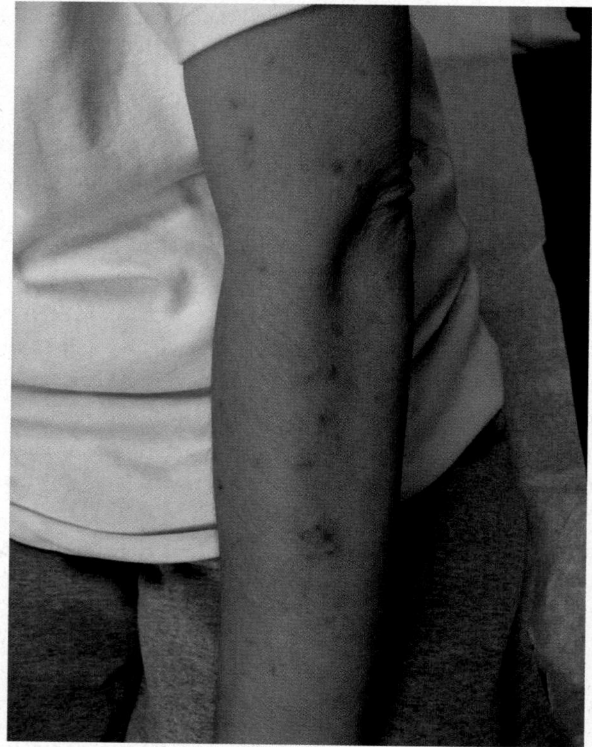

FIGURE 250-1 A 40-year-old woman with sores on her arm caused by picking at her skin while using methamphetamine. Also called meth mites, although there are no mites. (*Reproduced with permission from Andrew Schechtman, MD.*)

INTRODUCTION

Methamphetamine is a powerfully addictive stimulant that can be smoked, snorted, or injected. This drug can be produced using common household products and pseudoephedrine. Methamphetamine is similar chemically to other stimulants, contains many adulterants, and is manufactured illegally.[1] There is a worldwide epidemic of methamphetamine abuse and addiction.

SYNONYMS

Meth, crank (powder), ice (crystal meth), croak (with cocaine), shabu (with cocaine), twisters (with crack), speed kills, crystal, and yaba (oral tablets).[2]

EPIDEMIOLOGY

- Worldwide, compared to other drugs of abuse, only marijuana is used more often than amphetamine/methamphetamine.[1-3]
- According to the 2015 report of the United Nations Office on Drugs and Crime, between 14 and 55 million people worldwide are estimated to use amphetamines/methamphetamines, and ages varies between 15 and 64.[2]
- The lifetime prevalence ("ever-used") rate for methamphetamine was 1.2%, 0.7%, 0.6% for 12th, 10th, and 8th graders respectively, in the 2016 Monitoring the Future study, which surveys 45,500 students in 8th, 10th, and 12th grades in 372 schools nationwide annually.[3] In 2014, an estimated 569,000 people age 12 and older were

meth users. These statistics were similar to previous trends for most years in between 2002 and 2014.[4]

- Stimulants (methamphetamine and amphetamine) accounted for 12.8% of nationwide emergency department visits involving use of illicit drugs in 2011, with the highest incidence in those from 18 to 44 years old.[5] The number of emergency room visits increased 71% from 2009 to 2011.[5] Net numbers of emergency room visits involving methamphetamines were 67,954 in 2007 and 102,961 in 2011, with congruent patterns for males and females.[6]
- Methamphetamine use is associated with white, Native American, Hispanic, and Asian race; residence in the west or south, in rural areas; having an ever-incarcerated father; marijuana, cocaine, and intravenous drug use; men who have sex with men (MSM); traumatic childhood events; and history of mood disorders.[1,7]
- Methamphetamine is the most common substance abused by vulnerable women (homeless, sex workers, those with psychiatric disorders, and survivors of intimate partner violence). During pregnancy it leads to pre-eclampsia, preterm birth, and low birth weight.[8]
- An analysis of methamphetamine found in workforce drug testing, done nationwide by Quest Diagnostics and released in 2011, showed the highest rates of use in western, midwestern, and southern states, with relative sparing of eastern states. Highest prevalence (more than twice the national average) was found in Hawaii, Arkansas, Oklahoma, Nevada, California, Wyoming, Utah, Arizona, and Kansas.[9]
- Methamphetamine is a Schedule II stimulant with legitimate medical uses, including the treatment of narcolepsy and attention-deficit/hyperactivity disorder.
- Methamphetamine is known on the street as meth, crank, ice (**Figure 250-2**), and crystal. The drug is abused by smoking, injecting, snorting, or oral ingestion. Smoking or injecting the drug gives an intense, short-lived "flash" or rush. Snorting or oral ingestion creates euphoria but no rush. Methamphetamine is also available in the form of tablets (called yaba), that can be swallowed whole or chewed.[2]
- Methamphetamine can be manufactured from inexpensive, readily available chemicals using recipes easily found on the Internet and in books (**Figure 250-3**).
- Common household and industrial chemicals used to make methamphetamine include pseudoephedrine and ephedrine (cold tablets), red phosphorus (matches/road flares), iodine (teat dip or flakes/crystal), methanol (gasoline additives), muriatic acid (used in swimming pools), anhydrous ammonia (farm fertilizer), sodium hydroxide (lye), sulfuric acid (drain cleaner), toluene (brake cleaner), ether (engine starter), and acetone (paint thinner).[10]
- The "meth laboratory," the site of small-scale methamphetamine production (**Figure 250-4**), brings with it many hazards, including exposure to toxic chemicals for the meth cooks themselves, their children, and law enforcement, medical, and fire personnel entering the laboratory in the course of their duties. Explosions and fires at meth laboratories are common. Improper disposal of the toxic chemicals used in the laboratories frequently leads to environmental contamination.[10,11]
- Effects of methamphetamine, such as euphoria, increased libido, and impaired judgment, may lead to increased high-risk sexual behaviors, such as unprotected sexual intercourse and contact with multiple

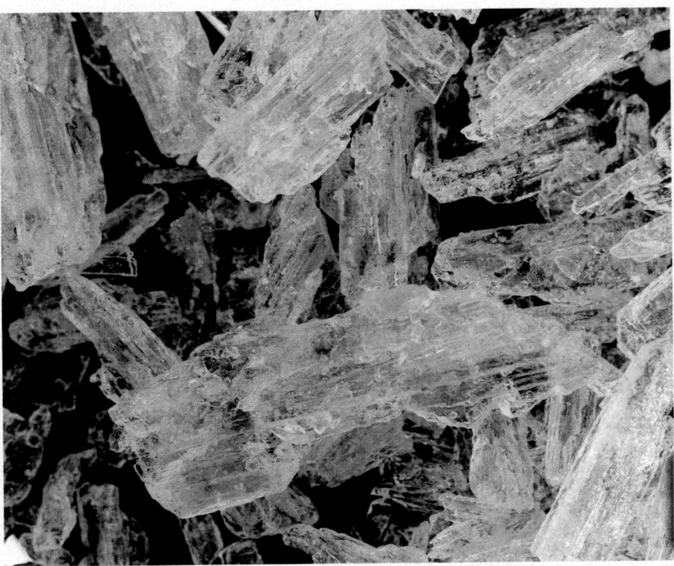

FIGURE 250-2 Methamphetamine in its ice format. (*Reproduced with permission from DEA.*)

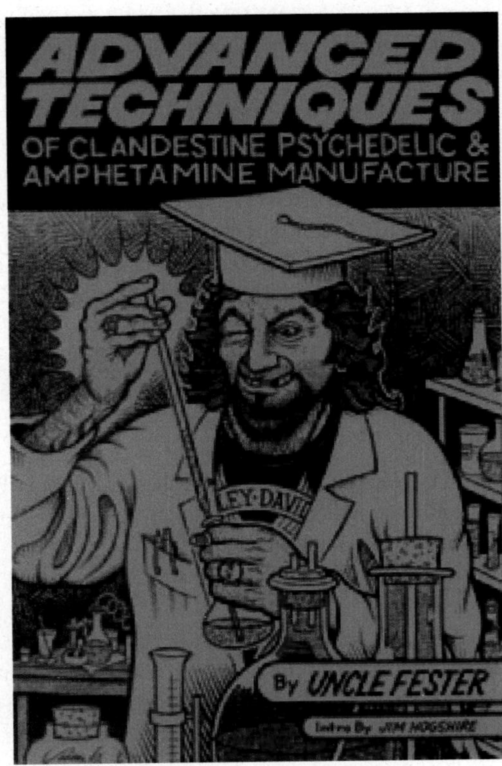

FIGURE 250-3 One of many books by Uncle Fester that can be purchased on the Internet. The information to manufacture methamphetamine is readily available. (*Reproduced with permission from Uncle Fester, www.unclefesterbooks.com.*)

sexual partners. As a result, methamphetamine users are at increased risk of contracting sexually transmitted infections, including HIV.

ETIOLOGY AND PATHOPHYSIOLOGY

- Methamphetamine acts as a central nervous system stimulant by blocking presynaptic reuptake of dopamine, norepinephrine, and serotonin.
- Compared to amphetamines, methamphetamine has an increased ability to cross the blood-brain barrier and has a prolonged half-life (10 to 12 hours). This leads to faster onset and more intense and longer-lasting effects when compared to amphetamine.
- Intended effects of methamphetamine use include euphoria, increased energy, a heightened sense of alertness, and increased libido.
- Unintended effects include increased heart rate, blood pressure, and body temperature; headaches; nausea; anxiety; aggression; paranoia; visual and auditory hallucinations; insomnia; tremors; cardiac arrhythmias; and strokes.
- With chronic abuse, neurologic manifestations include confusion, poor concentration, cognitive impairment,[12] depression, paranoia, and psychosis. Weight loss and dental decay can occur. The face and body become atrophic and gaunt, making the chronic methamphetamine user appear older than their stated age.
- Methamphetamine users may experience formication, the hallucination that bugs are crawling under the skin. The skin excoriations resulting from picking at the imagined bugs are known as "meth mites" (**Figures 250-1**, **250-5**, and **250-6**).
- Dental caries and gingivitis commonly seen in methamphetamine users is known as "meth mouth" (**Figures 250-7** and **250-8**). The causes of meth mouth are multiple. Vasoconstriction leads to decreased saliva production and lower pH, which leads to dry mouth and more dental caries. Meth users are more likely to consume large amounts of sugar-containing beverages and neglect their oral hygiene when preoccupied with obtaining and using the drug. These factors also worsen caries and gingivitis. Methamphetamine-induced bruxism damages the teeth. Neglect of early symptoms and lack of access to or failure to seek dental care often lead to unsalvageable teeth that can only be extracted.[13-15]

DIAGNOSIS

ACUTE INTOXICATION

This can lead to tachycardia, hypertension, chest pain, hyperthermia, diaphoresis, mydriasis, agitation, irritability, hypervigilance, paranoia, hallucinations, and tremor.

CHRONIC USE

Chronic use of methamphetamine can cause violent behavior, anxiety, depression, confusion, insomnia, cognitive impairment and psychotic symptoms (paranoia, auditory hallucinations, delusions, and formication).[16,17]

WITHDRAWAL SYMPTOMS

Withdrawal symptoms include drug cravings, depressed mood, disturbed sleep patterns, increased appetite, fatigue, and cognitive disorders.

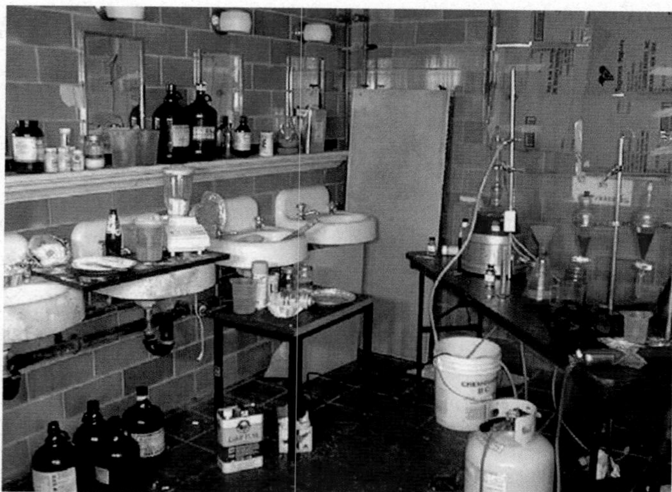

FIGURE 250-4 A methamphetamine laboratory with visible toxic and flammable substances.

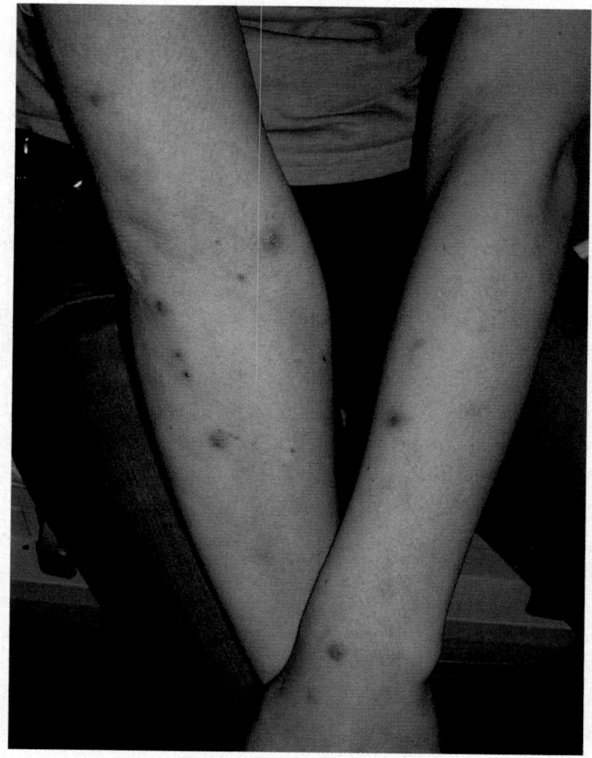

FIGURE 250-5 A 19-year-old woman with sores on her arms from picking at her skin while using methamphetamine. Also called meth mites. *(Reproduced with permission from Richard P. Usatine, MD.)*

COMPLICATIONS

- Neurologic: seizures; primary psychosis[1]; stroke caused by intracerebral hemorrhage or vasospasm, especially in users 45 years old or younger; associated with poor outcomes.[18]
- Cardiovascular: cardiac arrhythmias, myocardial ischemia or infarction, dilated cardiomyopathy, pulmonary hypertension, valvular disorders, and infective endocarditis.[19]
- Hyperthermia (potentially fatal) and rhabdomyolysis.
- Consequences of injection drug abuse (skin infections and abscesses).
- Dental: "meth mouth," xerostomia, dental cavities, bruxism.
- High-risk sexual behavior, increasing risks of contracting sexually transmitted infections including hepatitis B, hepatitis C, and HIV.

LABORATORY STUDIES

- Urine drug screening is commonly done with immunoassays. These tests are highly cross-reactive and may give false-positive results for methamphetamine or amphetamine caused by the presence of other sympathomimetic amines such as pseudoephedrine or ephedrine. Unexpected positive results on a screening test can be confirmed with more specific tests such as gas chromatography/mass spectrometry (GC/MS) and stereospecific chromatography.[20] One limitation of urine drug testing for methamphetamine is that the drug may only be detectable for up to 3 days after use. Hair testing is available and remains positive for weeks or months; the validity of this test is debatable.[20]
- Methamphetamine users are at increased risk of sexually transmitted diseases and diseases transmitted through the use of shared needles. Consider screening for HIV, syphilis, hepatitis C, chlamydia, and gonorrhea, especially now that the prevalence of STDs is on the rise.[21]
- For patients with signs and symptoms of acute intoxication, consider excluding complications of methamphetamine abuse by ordering creatinine phosphokinase (CK), complete blood count (CBC), chemistry panel, and toxicology test.
- Based on recent studies, electrocardiogram abnormalities are very common in this population and include tachyarrhythmias, QT prolongation, left ventricular dysfunction and hypertrophy, and right axis deviation. An electrocardiogram (ECG) should be considered in all active methamphetamine users.[19]

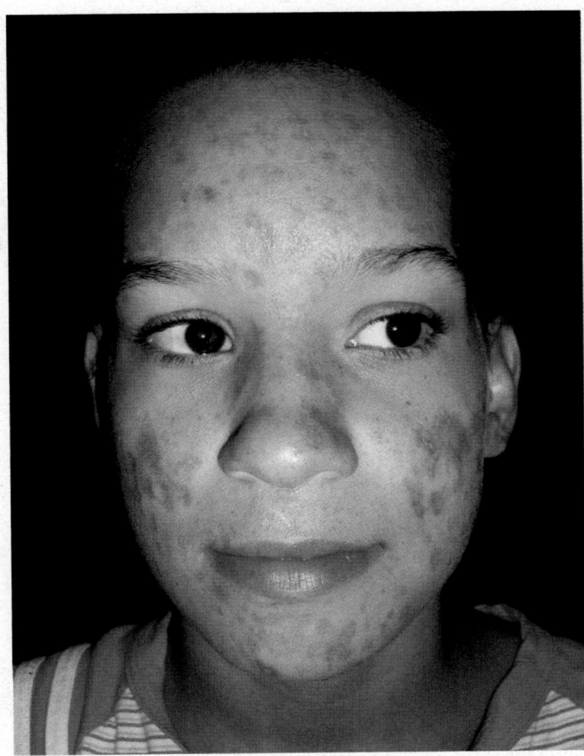

FIGURE 250-6 Postinflammatory hyperpigmentation in a young woman who has picked at her skin while addicted to methamphetamine. *(Reproduced with permission from Richard P. Usatine, MD.)*

DIFFERENTIAL DIAGNOSIS

ACUTE METHAMPHETAMINE INTOXICATION

- Intoxication with other substances causing sympathetic stimulation and/or altered mental status (cocaine, ecstasy, phencyclidine [PCP], theophylline, aspirin, monoamine oxidase inhibitors, serotonin syndrome).
- Psychiatric disorders (bipolar disorder, panic attack, and schizophrenia).
- Hyperthyroidism and thyroid storm (see Chapter 236, Graves Disease and Goiter).

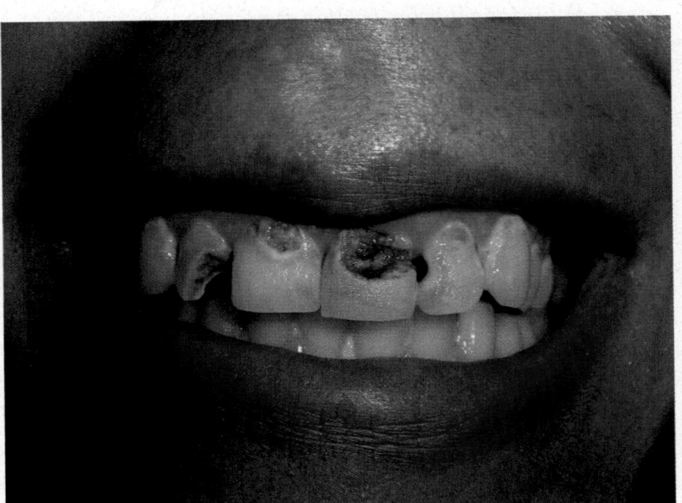

FIGURE 250-7 Methamphetamine mouth (meth mouth) in a young woman with 1 year of methamphetamine use. The meth use has led to visible caries in her teeth. *(Reproduced with permission from Richard P. Usatine, MD.)*

METHAMPHETAMINE-INDUCED SKIN LESIONS (METH MITES)

- Scabies—Burrows may be present; located on wrists, fingers, or genital region, but spares face; very pruritic. Family members may be infected as well (see Chapter 149, Scabies).
- Atopic dermatitis—Persistent pruritus (pruritus from meth stops after acute intoxication clears). In most cases there is a long history of the dermatitis before the meth use had begun (see Chapter 151, Atopic Dermatitis).
- Contact dermatitis is pruritic but is generally localized to the area in which the contact allergen has touched the skin. A good history should allow this to be differentiated from meth mites (see Chapter 152, Contact Dermatitis).
- Neurodermatitis and prurigo nodularis—Persistent complaints of severe pruritus. In many ways, these are similar to meth mites in that the stimulus to scratch is from the brain, not just the skin. Absence of meth use should be present in these self-inflicted dermatoses to distinguish them from meth mites (see Chapter 155, Psychocutaneous Disorders).

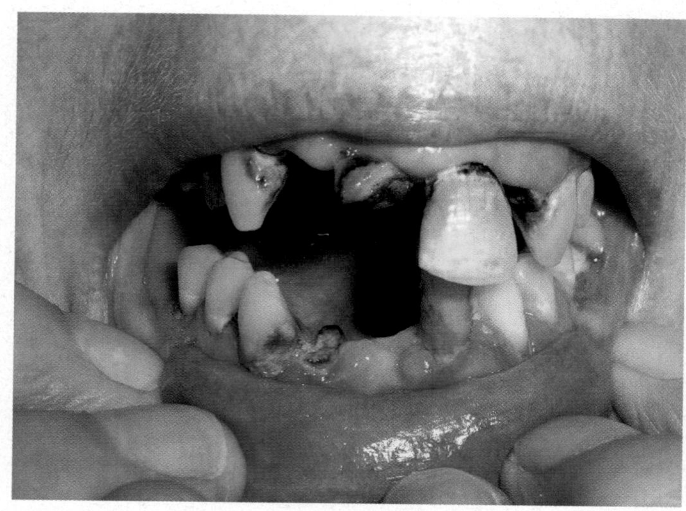

FIGURE 250-8 Meth mouth in a young woman using methamphetamine. Note how destructive the caries has been to her teeth. *(Reproduced with permission from Richard P. Usatine, MD.)*

MANAGEMENT

- Acute methamphetamine intoxication is treated with supportive measures. Sedation with haloperidol, droperidol, olanzapine, risperidone, or benzodiazepines (diazepam, lorazepam, or midazolam) can be used for agitated patients. Methamphetamine-induced cardiac ischemia is treated with oxygen, nitrates, and β blockers. Seizures and rhabdomyolysis are treated in the standard fashion.[22] SOR Ⓑ
- There are no medications with proven efficacy for treatment of methamphetamine withdrawal. Mirtazapine and modafinil have shown some benefit in preliminary studies.[23] SOR Ⓒ
- Treatment of methamphetamine dependence and addiction is challenging. In clinical trials, pharmacologic treatments have not demonstrated strong benefits for methamphetamine abstinence.[24,25] Inpatient detoxification may be required initially, followed by a long-term program of behavioral interventions. SOR Ⓒ
- Evidence-based behavioral approaches have moderate impact in reducing the use of methamphetamines.[17]
- Refer patients to 12-step programs, which are valuable and free. Crystal Meth Anonymous is a 12-step program modeled on the 12 steps of Alcoholics Anonymous and the White Book of Narcotics Anonymous. If Crystal Meth Anonymous meetings are not available, any 12-step program can be of help in recovery and maintaining sobriety.[26] The use of a sponsor is helpful to maintain abstinence from methamphetamine.[27] SOR Ⓑ
- The Matrix model, a behavioral treatment method initially developed for treatment of cocaine addiction, has been used successfully to treat methamphetamine addiction. It consists of a 16-week program, including group and individual therapy, relapse prevention, family involvement, participation in a 12-step program or other spiritual group, and weekly drug testing.[28] SOR Ⓒ

- In the context of outpatient behavioral treatment programs, providing small incentives for drug-free urine samples can help promote abstinence. One study found that 19% of incentivized patients achieved 12 weeks of continuous abstinence, whereas only 5% of non-incentivized patients did so (number needed to treat [NNT] = 7.1) at a cost of only $2.42 per day per participant.[29] However, further analysis of the same data showed that this method did not have any impact on retention rates in both groups (<50%). It also demonstrated that who entered into the program with negative urine tests had better success with abstinence.[30] SOR Ⓑ
- Recent meta-analysis reinforced that the initial period of abstinence prior to entering into the 12-step program correlated with a positive impact on continued abstinence.[31]
- Although no medications to help treat methamphetamine dependence are currently approved by the U.S. Food and Drug Administration (FDA), several medications under study have shown favorable early results, including modafinil, bupropion, and naltrexone. SOR Ⓑ "Replacement" therapy using low-dose stimulants, similar to the way methadone and nicotine are used for opioid and nicotine dependence, respectively, has also shown some benefit.[32]
- In a pilot study, tai chi (traditional Chinese exercise) had favorable benefits for improving quality of life in persons with meth addiction.[33]
- Methamphetamine-related skin excoriation should heal without treatment if the picking behavior stops. However, postinflammatory hyperpigmentation may never resolve (see Figure 250-6). Antibiotic treatment with an antistaphylococcal agent, such as cephalexin or dicloxacillin, is indicated if the excoriations become infected. If methicillin-resistant *Staphylococcus aureus* (MRSA) is suspected, choose an antibiotic that covers MRSA (see Chapter 122, Impetigo).
- Referral for dental care is indicated for patients with gingivitis and dental caries caused by chronic methamphetamine use. Recommend daily use of a soft-bristled toothbrush and dental floss for treatment and prevention of oral pathology. SOR Ⓐ Rinsing with a chlorhexidine-containing mouthwash may be a reasonable alternative for patients who find it too painful to floss SOR Ⓒ (see Chapters 41, Gingivitis and Periodontal Disease, and 47, Adult Dental Caries).

FOLLOW-UP

- Methamphetamine users who have recently quit are at high risk of relapse. Close follow-up is indicated to identify relapses and to reinitiate treatment.
- Maintenance of abstinence can be aided by participation in an outpatient treatment program and 12-step programs with sponsorship.
- Methamphetamine-induced skin lesions should heal when the picking behavior ceases. Resolution is unlikely if methamphetamine abuse continues.

PATIENT EDUCATION

- Encourage patients to stop using methamphetamine. Offer referral to a treatment program in the community.
- Inform patients that methamphetamine use carries risks of heart attack, stroke, and death that can result from a single dose. There is no safe level of methamphetamine use.
- Counsel patients who have sex while using methamphetamine that this combination increases the likelihood of unsafe sexual practices and their risk of getting a sexually transmitted infection.
- Advise users who inject methamphetamine to use clean needles and to avoid sharing needles to decrease their risk of contracting hepatitis B, hepatitis C, and HIV.
- Counsel patients to engage in physical activity, such as tai chi, which has shown to improve the quality of life in methamphetamine users.[33]

PATIENT RESOURCES

- Crystal Meth Anonymous (12-step meetings)—**https://crystalmeth.org.**
- Substance Abuse & Mental Health Services Administration (SAMHSA). *Substance Abuse Treatment Facility Locator*—**https://www.findtreatment.samhsa.gov.**
- ADA Division of Communications; Journal of the American Dental Association; ADA Division of Scientific Affairs. For the dental patient . . . methamphetamine use and oral health. *J Am Dent Assoc.* 2005;136(10):1491—**https://www.ada.org/~/media/ADA/Publications/Files/patient_55.pdf?la=en.**
- PBS. *Frontline: the Meth Epidemic: How Meth Destroys the Body*—**http://www.pbs.org/wgbh/pages/frontline/meth/body/.**

PROVIDER RESOURCES

- National Institute on Drug Abuse—**https://www.drugabuse.gov/drugs-abuse/methamphetamine.html.**
- American Society of Addiction Medicine. *Research & Treatment*—**https://elearning.asam.org/products/the-asam-review-course-in-addiction-medicine-2017.**

REFERENCES

1. Mullen JM, Crawford AT. *Amphetamine Related Psychiatric Disorders.* Jan 23, 2018. Treasure Island, FL: StatPearls Publishing. http://www.ncbi.nlm.nih.gov/books/NBK482368/.
2. United Nations Office of Drugs and Crime (UNODC). *2015 World Drug Report*. Vienna, Austria: UNODC; 2015. https://www.unodc.org/documents/wdr2015/World_Drug_Report_2015.pdf. Accessed April 2018.
3. Monitoring the future. National survey results on drug use 1975-2016. 2016 Overview. Key Findings on Adolescent Drug Use. http://www.monitoringthefuture.org/pubs/monographs/mtf-overview2016.pdf. Accessed April 2018.
4. Substance Abuse and Mental Health Services Administration. Behavioral health trends in the United States: Results from the 2014 National Survey on Drug Use and Health.(HHS Publication No. SMA 15-4927, NSDUH Series H-50). 2015.
5. Substance Abuse and Mental Health Services Administration, Drug Abuse Warning Network. *2009: National Estimates of Drug-Related Emergency Department Visits.* HHS Publication No.

(SMA) 11-4659, DAWN Series D-35. Rockville, MD: Substance Abuse and Mental Health Services Administration; 2011.

6. Mattson ME. *Emergency Department Visits Involving Methamphetamine: 2007 to 2011.* Jun 19, 2014. In: The CBHSQ Report. Rockville (MD): Substance Abuse and Mental Health Services Administration (US); 2013..
7. Iritani BJ, Hallfors DD, Bauer DJ. Crystal methamphetamine use among young adults in the USA. *Addiction.* 2007;102:1102-1113.
8. Kittirattanapaiboon P, Srikosai S, Wittayanookulluk A. Methamphetamine use and dependence in vulnerable female populations. *Curr Opin Psychiatry.* 2017;30(4):247-252.
9. Quest Diagnostics. Press Release: "Hawaii, Arkansas and Oklahoma lead the nation for methamphetamine use in the workforce, reveals Quest Diagnostics Drug Testing Index(TM): five-year data suggest methamphetamine's national decline has halted and that the drug's stronghold may be moving eastward." Madison, NJ: PRNewswire; September 2, 2011. https://www.questdiagnostics.com/dms/Documents/DTI-Reports/2011-09-02_DTI.pdf. Accessed April 2018.
10. United States Department of Justice. Achieve. Meth awareness. https://www.justice.gov/archive/olp/methawareness/. Accessed April 2018.
11. Lineberry TW, Bostwick JM. Methamphetamine abuse: a perfect storm of complications. *Mayo Clin Proc.* 2006;81(1):77-84.
12. Potvin S, Pelletier J, Grot S, et al. Cognitive deficits in individuals with methamphetamine use disorder: a meta-analysis. *Addict Behav.* 2018;80:154-160.
13. American Dental Association. *Methamphetamine.* https://www.ada.org/en/member-center/oral-health-topics/methamphetamine. Accessed April 2018.
14. Hamamoto D, Rhodus N. Methamphetamine abuse and dentistry. *Oral Dis.* 2009;15:27-37.
15. Rommel N, Rohleder NH, Koerdt S, et al. Sympathomimetic effects of chronic methamphetamine abuse on oral health: a cross-sectional study. *BMC Oral Health.* 2016;16(1):59.
16. Rawson RA, Condon TP. Why do we need an *Addiction* supplement focused on methamphetamine? *Addiction.* 2007;102(Suppl 1):1-4.
17. Courtney KE, Ray LA. Methamphetamine: an update on epidemiology, pharmacology, clinical phenomenology, and treatment literature. *Drug Alcohol Depend.* 2014;143:11-21.
18. Lappin JM, Darke S, Farrell M. Stroke and methamphetamine use in young adults: a review. *J Neurol Neurosurg Psychiatry.* 2017;88(12):1079-1091.
19. Paratz ED, Zhao J, Sherwen AK, et al. Is an abnormal ECG just the tip of the ICE-berg? Examining the utility of electrocardiography in detecting methamphetamine-induced cardiac pathology. *Heart Lung Circ.* 2017;26(7):684-689.
20. Gourlay DL, Heit HA, Caplan YH. Urine drug testing in clinical practice. Edition 6, 2015. https://www.remitigate.com/wp-content/uploads/2015/11/Urine-Drug-Testing-in-Clinical-Practice-Ed6_2015-08.pdf. Accessed April 2018.
21. CDC Newsroom. STDs at record high, indicating urgent need for prevention. September 26, 2017. https://www.cdc.gov/media/releases/2017/p0926-std-prevention.html. Accessed April 2018.
22. Richard J. *Methamphetamine Toxicity.* https://emedicine.medscape.com/article/820918-overview. Accessed April 2018.
23. Pennay AE, Lee NK. Putting the call out for more research: the poor evidence base for treating methamphetamine withdrawal. *Drug Alcohol Rev.* 2011;30:216-222.
24. Morley KC, Cornish JL, Faingold A, et al. Pharmacotherapeutic agents in the treatment of methamphetamine dependence. *Expert Opin Investig Drugs.* 2017;26(5):563-578.
25. Karila L, Weinstein W, Aubin HJ, et al. Pharmacological approaches to methamphetamine dependence: a focused review. *Br J Clin Pharmacol.* 2010;69(6):578-592.
26. Hatch-Maillette M, Wells EA, Doyle SR, et al. Predictors of 12-Step attendance and participation for individuals with stimulant use disorders. *J Subst Abuse Treat.* 2016;68:74-82.
27. Wendt DC, Hallgren KA, Daley DC, Donovan DM. Predictors and outcomes of twelve-step sponsorship of stimulant users: secondary analyses of a multisite randomized clinical trial. *J Stud Alcohol Drugs.* 2017;78(2):287-295.
28. Rawson RA, Marinelli-Casey P, Anglin MD, et al. A multisite comparison of psychosocial approaches for the treatment of methamphetamine dependence. *Addiction.* 2004;99:708-717.
29. Petry NM, Peirce JM, Stitzer ML, et al. Effect of prize-based incentives on outcomes in stimulant abusers in outpatient psychosocial treatment programs: A National Drug Abuse Treatment Clinical Trials Network Study. *Arch Gen Psychiatry.* 2005;62(10):1148-1156.
30. Stitzer ML, Petry N, Peirce J, et al. Effectiveness of abstinence-based incentives: interaction with intake stimulant test results. *J Consult Clin Psychol.* 2007;75(5):805-811.
31. Cook R, Quinn B, Heinzerling K, Shoptaw S. Dropout in clinical trials of pharmacological treatment for methamphetamine dependence: the role of initial abstinence. *Addiction.* 2017;112(6):1077-1085.
32. Ling W, Chang L, Hillhouse M, et al. Sustained-release methylphenidate in a randomized trial of treatment of methamphetamine use disorder: methylphenidate for methamphetamine use. *Addiction.* 2014;109:1489-1500.
33. Zhu D, Xu D, Dai G, et al. Beneficial effects of Tai Chi for amphetamine-type stimulant dependence: a pilot study. *Am J Drug Alcohol Abuse.* 2016;42(4):469-478.

251 COCAINE

Heidi S. Chumley, MD, MBA
Mindy A. Smith, MD, MS
Enrique R. Perez-Rodriguez, MD
Stacy L. Speedlin, PhD

PATIENT STORY

A 26-year-old man in status epilepticus is brought into the emergency department by his "friends," who promptly flee the scene. His seizures spontaneously cease, and he is noted to have an altered mental status. IV access is obtained and he is stabilized. A urine toxicology screen is positive for cocaine and his creatine phosphokinase is markedly elevated. He is admitted for cocaine-induced seizures and rhabdomyolysis. He survives the hospitalization and consents to a photograph of his eyes before discharge. **Figure 251-1** shows the bilateral subconjunctival hemorrhages that occurred during his seizures. The patient states that he understands the gravity of the situation and will enter a drug rehabilitation program when he leaves the hospital.

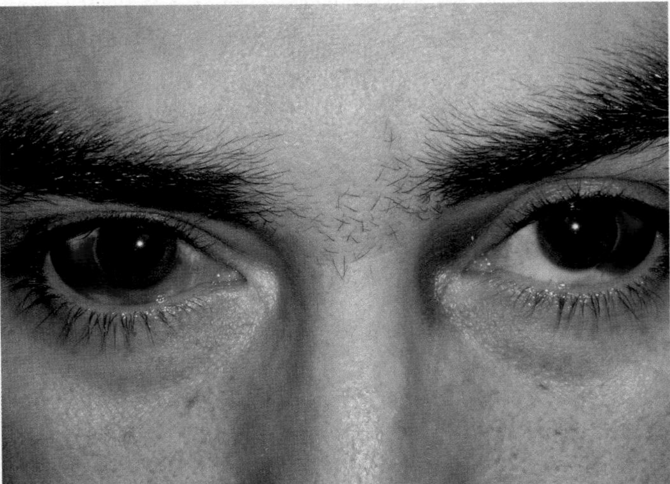

FIGURE 251-1 Bilateral subconjunctival hemorrhages after severe cocaine-induced seizures in a young man. This patient also developed rhabdomyolysis and was hospitalized. *(Reproduced with permission from Beau Willison, MD.)*

INTRODUCTION

Cocaine is a natural alkaloid and is extracted from the Andean shrub known as *Erythroxylum coca*. Cocaine remains the primary nonalcoholic drug of abuse globally. It is available as a free base in cocaine hydrochloride salt. The water solubility of cocaine lends itself to various routes of administration. Cocaine use is common, and 5% to 6% of users develop dependence within the first year of use. Acutely intoxicated patients have increased heart rates, blood pressures, temperatures, and, initially, respiratory rates; mood changes, involuntary movements; and dilated pupils. Chronic addiction can be treated with a comprehensive program, although only one-third of patients will become and remain abstinent.

SYNONYMS

Cocaine is also called blow, C, coke, crack, flake, snow, bump, rock, toot, nose candy, and line.

EPIDEMIOLOGY

- Based on the National Comorbidity Survey Replication (NCS-R) using interviews with a nationally representative sample of 9282 English-speaking respondents ages 18 years and older (conducted in 2001 to 2003), the cumulative incidence of cocaine use was 16%.[1]
- Similar numbers were reported from the National Survey on Drug Use and Health in 2005[2]:
  - Of Americans ages 12 years and older, 13.8% reported lifetime cocaine use in 2005.[2]

- A total of 33.7 million Americans ages 12 years and older reported lifetime use of cocaine, and 7.9 million reported using crack cocaine.[2]
- An estimated 2.4 million Americans reported current use of cocaine (682,000 of whom reported using crack).[2]
- Of the estimated 860,000 new users of cocaine in 2005, most were age 18 years or older, with the average age of first use being 20 years.[2]
- The percentage of youth ages 12 to 17 years reporting lifetime use of cocaine was 2.3%, and among young adults ages 18 to 25 years the rate was 15.1%.[2]

- For both male and female cocaine users, the estimated risk for developing cocaine dependence, based on data from the NCS-R, was 5% to 6% within the first year after first use.[3] Thereafter, the estimated risk decreased from the peak value, with a somewhat faster decline for females in the next 3 years after first use.
- Females may be more susceptible to crack/cocaine dependence; in a study of 152 individuals (37% female) in a residential substance-use treatment program, females evidenced greater use of crack/cocaine (current and lifetime heaviest) and were significantly more likely to show crack/cocaine dependence than males.[4]
- In one study, siblings of cocaine-dependent individuals had an elevated risk of developing cocaine dependence (relative risk [RR] = 1.71).[5]
- The highest rate of cocaine use is among persons 18–24 years of age.[6]

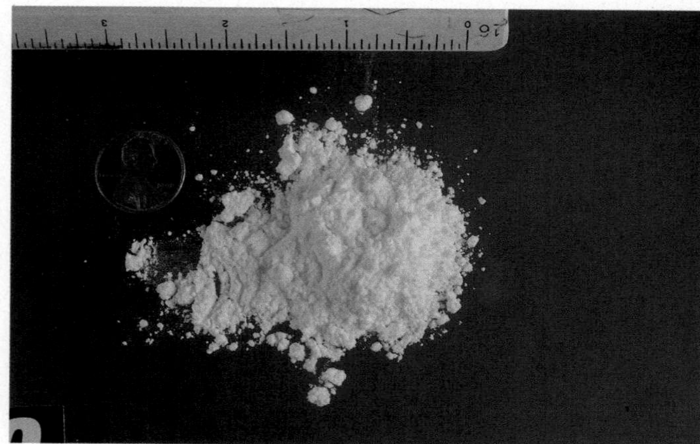

FIGURE 251-2 Cocaine in a powder form used for snorting and injecting. (*Reproduced with permission from U.S. Drug Enforcement Agency.*)

ETIOLOGY AND PATHOPHYSIOLOGY

- Cocaine is a potent stimulant that affects the both the central nervous system and peripheral nervous system. Cocaine's effects on the cardiovascular system are widespread, and because it is a global vasoconstrictor, it compromises oxygen consumption in all vital organs. This contributes to multiple comorbid conditions in individuals with chronic cocaine use.[7-9]
- It produces stimulant effects by causing increased synaptic concentration of neurotransmitters, most notably dopamine and serotonin, but eventually leads to subphysiologic depletion of these chemicals. This ultimately contributes to the mood disorders that are associated with cocaine use.
- It produces its stimulant effects by causing increasing synaptic concentration of monoamine neurotransmitters (i.e., dopamine, norepinephrine, and serotonin).[10]
- Similar to other local anesthetics, cocaine blocks the generation and conduction of electrical impulses in excitable tissues (e.g., neurons and cardiac muscle), blocking the voltage-gated fast sodium channels in the cell membrane and abolishing the ability of the tissue to generate an action potential.[11]
- Effects are seen following oral, intranasal (as a powder [**Figure 251-2**]), IV, and inhalation administration (as crack cocaine [**Figure 251-3**], coca paste, and free-base).

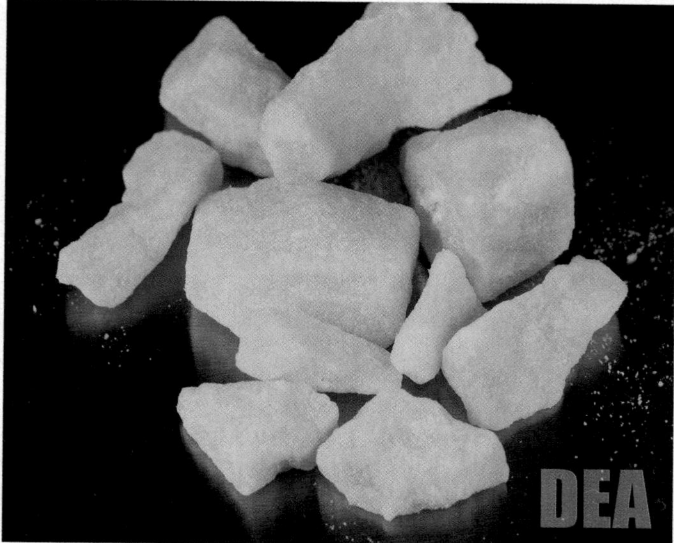

FIGURE 251-3 Crack cocaine used for smoking. (*Reproduced with permission from U.S. Drug Enforcement Agency.*)

RISK FACTORS

- Family history/genetic predisposition.
- In a study of inner-city incarcerated male adolescents (23% of whom had used cocaine or crack in the month before arrest and

32% of whom had used cocaine at least once), current cocaine/crack users were more likely to have the following characteristics[12]:
  - Alcohol, marijuana, and intranasal heroin use.
  - Multiple previous arrests.
  - To be out of school.
  - To be psychologically distressed.
  - To have been sexually molested as a child.
  - To have substance-abusing parents.
  - To have frequent sex with girls, to be gay or bisexual, and to engage in anal intercourse.
- Among those who died from an accidental drug overdose in New York City, those dying from cocaine-only versus opiates were more likely to be male, black or Hispanic, have alcohol detected at autopsy, and to be of older age.[13]

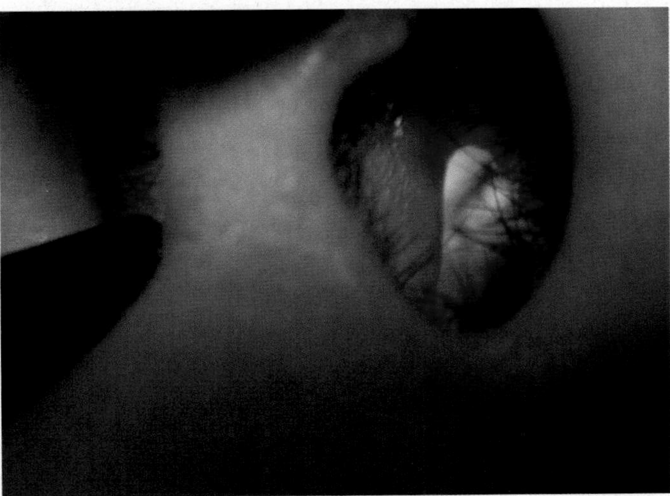

FIGURE 251-4 Shining a light through a hole in the nasal septum caused by 10 years of snorting cocaine. *(Reproduced with permission from Richard P. Usatine, MD.)*

DIAGNOSIS

CLINICAL FEATURES

- Acute effects occur within 3 to 5 minutes with intranasal administration (8 to 10 seconds with free base) and last approximately 1 hour, after which there is an abrupt disappearance of the effects.[10] When used IV or smoked as crack cocaine, the onset of action is immediate and the peak effect occurs 3 to 5 minutes later, lasting for 20 to 30 minutes.[11]
- Cocaine use is more frequently associated with acute rather than chronic sympathetic toxicity. However, prolonged cocaine use causes global neurochemical depletion and general hypoxemia of vital organs, which contribute to chronic comorbidities. In clinical practice, cocaine users presenting to a primary care facility or emergency department have a spectrum of complaints and subjective symptoms, particularly chest pain.[7-9] In such patients, diagnostic evaluation and treatment should target acute cardiovascular, neurologic, or metabolic syndromes.[8] When a patient on cocaine presents with chest pain and/or tachycardia, consider myocardial infarction, malignant arrhythmias, and aortic dissection.
- Findings on physical examination during cocaine use may include:
  - Elevated heart rate, blood pressure, and temperature.
  - Increased respiratory rate and/or dyspnea followed by decreased respiratory rate.
  - Mood changes including enhanced mood/euphoria, hyperactivity, irritability and anxiety, excessive talking, and long periods without eating or sleeping.
  - Involuntary movements (e.g., tremors, chorea, and dystonic reactions).
  - Dilated pupils, nystagmus, and/or retinal hemorrhages.
  - Nasal septum perforation (**Figure 251-4**), epistaxis, and/or cerebrospinal fluid (CSF) rhinorrhea.
  - Wheezing, rales, and/or pneumothorax.
  - Absent bowel sounds (mesenteric ischemia) and/or right upper quadrant tenderness (hepatic necrosis).
  - Skin tracks from intravenous use (**Figure 251-5**).
  - Multiple areas of atrophic skin scars are from skin popping—injecting cocaine directly into the skin without finding a vein for intravenous injections (**Figure 251-6**).

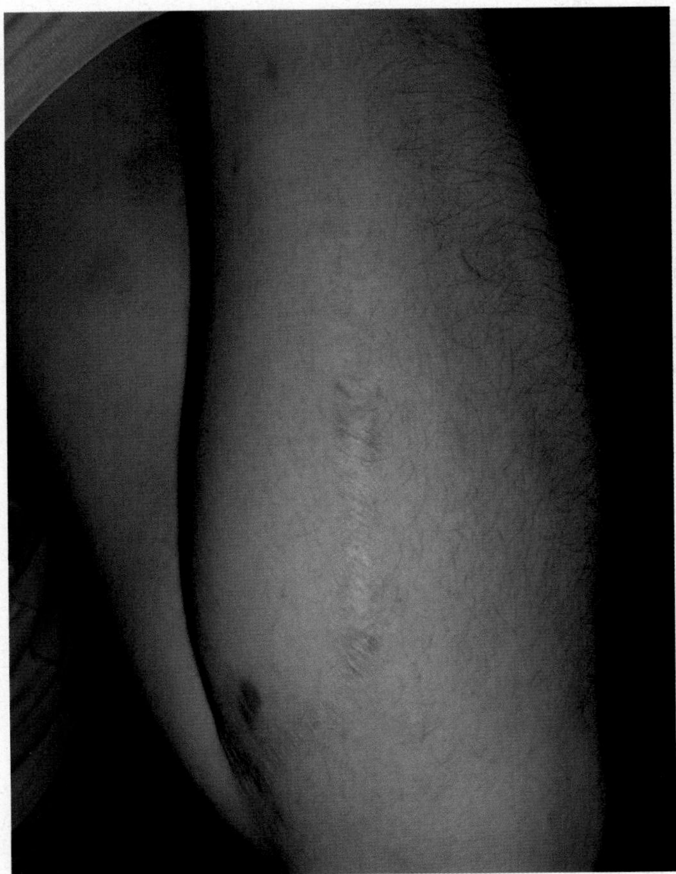

FIGURE 251-5 An injection track along the vein of a young woman in recovery from IV cocaine use and addiction. *(Reproduced with permission from Richard P. Usatine, MD.)*

- Acute effects may be altered by concomitant use of other drugs or alcohol.
- Adverse effects of cocaine use can include[10]:
  - Respiratory depression that may result in death.
  - Cardiac arrhythmias, chest pain, and myocardial infarction (MI).
  - Neurologic symptoms, including headache, tonic-clonic seizures, ischemic or hemorrhagic stroke, and subarachnoid hemorrhage.
  - Myalgias and rhabdomyolysis.
  - Severe pulmonary disease (e.g., alveolar hemorrhage and pulmonary edema) and hepatic necrosis caused by crack cocaine.
  - Exacerbation of existing hypertension, cardiac, and cerebrovascular disease.
  - Recurrent diabetic ketoacidosis.[14]
- Cocaine is being laced with levamisole around the world because it boosts the profits of the seller and it potentiates the psychoactive effects of the cocaine. Cutaneous vasculitis secondary to levamisole-adulterated cocaine has been reported many times in the literature.[15-17] Levamisole is an antihelminthic drug approved only for veterinary purposes. It had been previously used as an immune modulator in autoimmune disorders but is considered no longer safe for human use, as it can cause agranulocytosis. Levamisole-associated vasculitis presents with ear purpura (**Figure 251-7**), retiform (like a net) purpura (**Figure 251-8**) of the trunk or extremities, neutropenia, and positive tests for perinuclear antineutrophil cytoplasmic antibody (pANCA).[17] This cutaneous vasculitis may also present on the nose or face (**Figure 251-9**). Now, there are reports of cocaine/levamisole-associated autoimmune syndrome (CLAAS) involving agranulocytosis and cutaneous vasculitis and affecting other organ systems.[18]
- Chronic cardiovascular complications include thrombus formation via platelet activation and potentiation of prothrombotic proteins (thromboxane) that contribute to atherosclerotic heart disease.
- Neurologic complications—Cocaine blocks the initiation and conduction of electrical impulses within nerve cells (anesthetic effect), as well as being a potent stimulant to the CNS; it causes alteration of uptake and metabolism of neurotransmitters such as norepinephrine, dopamine, and serotonin. The resultant hyperstimulation of the central and autonomic nervous system produces an array of multi-organ effects such as mydriasis, hyperglycemia, and hyperthermia. Neuro psychiatric effect of dopamine flooding with eventual depletion is involved in production of acute euphoria and chronic mood disorders in the addicted patient.
- Chronic cocaine use is associated with decreased libido and impaired reproductive function.
  - In men, cocaine can cause impotence and gynecomastia.
  - In women, cocaine can cause galactorrhea, amenorrhea, and infertility.
  - In pregnant women, crack cocaine is associated with an increase in placental abruption, miscarriage, and congenital malformation.
- Protracted use can cause paranoid ideation and visual and auditory hallucinations. Severe depression can follow recovery from cocaine intoxication (called "crashing").
- Withdrawal from chronic cocaine use can cause depression, insomnia, and anorexia.

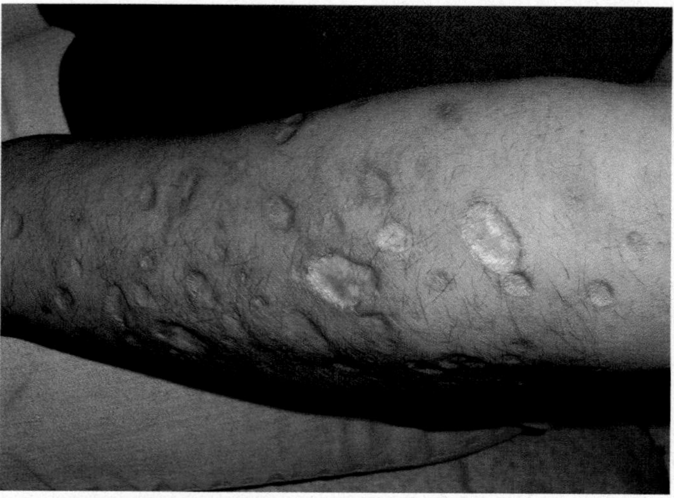

FIGURE 251-6 Multiple areas of atrophic skin scarring from skin popping cocaine. Note how the scars are depressed and relatively round. Some cocaine addicts inject the cocaine directly into the skin rather than look for a vein for intravenous injections. (*Reproduced with permission from Richard P. Usatine, MD.*)

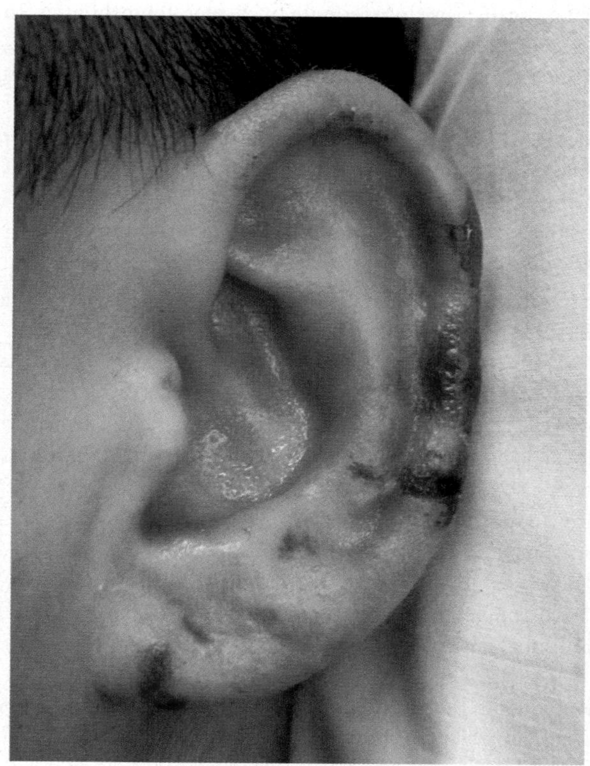

FIGURE 251-7 Cutaneous vasculitis of the ear caused by levamisole-adulterated cocaine. (*Reproduced with permission from Robert T. Gilson, MD.*)

LABORATORY STUDIES

- Urine toxicology screen (using immunoassays) for commonly abused drugs (e.g., cocaine, marijuana, and opiates) is the gold standard.
  - Cocaine may be detected in the urine for 24 hours after use and the metabolite of cocaine, benzoylecgonine, may be detected as long as 60 hours after a single use.
  - In chronic cocaine users, benzoylecgonine may be detected for up to 22 days.
- All injection-drug users should be screened for human immunodeficiency virus (HIV) and hepatitis C.
- If there is a history of multiple sexual partners, unsafe sex, and/or sex for drugs, cocaine users should be screened for sexually transmitted diseases (STDs). This might include *Chlamydia*, gonorrhea, hepatitis C, HIV, and syphilis (**Figure 251-10**). Because the prevalence of syphilis and other STDs is increasing in the United States, syphilis screening is particularly important.[19]
- In an unconscious patient and in patients denying cocaine use, the following laboratory tests can be considered to rule out other diseases with similar symptoms:
  - Serum glucose, magnesium, and phosphorus.
  - Serum electrolytes.
- Laboratory tests that can be completed to detect or monitor acute complications of cocaine overdose include[11]:
  - Arterial blood gas (respiratory acidosis or alkalosis).
  - Blood urea nitrogen (BUN) and/or creatinine (renal infarction).
  - Creatine kinase (CK) (rhabdomyolysis) and isoenzyme of creatine kinase (CK-MB) (MI).
  - Liver function tests (liver necrosis).
  - Urine dipstick (rhabdomyolysis).

IMAGING AND OTHER TESTS

- Plain films of the abdomen (supine and upright) can be useful in the diagnosis of body packing or stuffing of cocaine (swallowing or inserting packets of cocaine into a body orifice), but false-negative results may occur.
- A chest X-ray and head CT can be considered for respiratory and neurologic symptoms, respectively.

DIFFERENTIAL DIAGNOSIS

- Delirium—Defined as a state of confusion accompanied by agitation, hallucinations, tremor, and illusions, delirium can be caused by drug toxicity or withdrawal, seizure, head injury, systemic infections, metabolic disorders, or a chronic dementing condition. The history, physical examination, and laboratory tests (many noted earlier) can help to identify the etiology.
- Hypoglycemia—Low blood sugar, most commonly caused by taking insulin or oral drugs used to treat diabetes mellitus. Symptoms include confusion, fatigue, seizures, and loss of consciousness. Autonomic responses to hypoglycemia include palpitations, sweating, tremor, and anxiety. Laboratory testing for serum glucose will document the condition, and symptoms resolve with administration of oral or IV glucose.

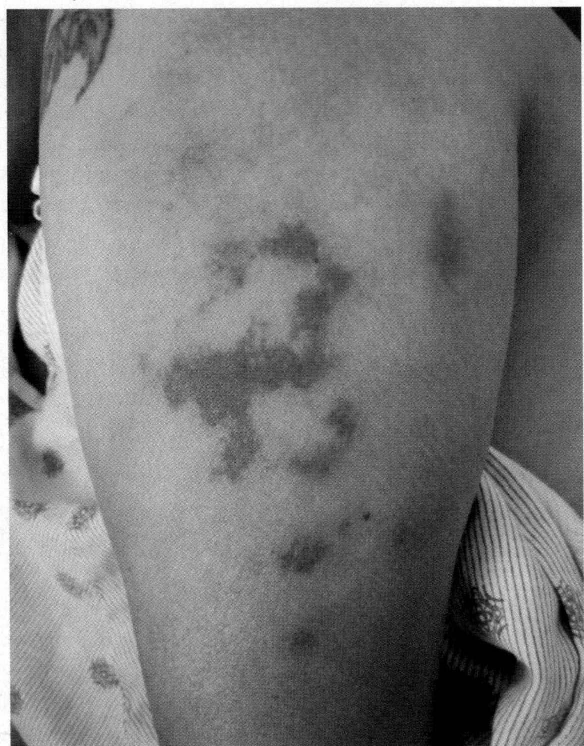

FIGURE 251-8 Cutaneous vasculitis in a retiform (netlike) pattern caused by the use of levamisole-adulterated cocaine. This is also called retiform purpura. (*Reproduced with permission from Richard P. Usatine, MD.*)

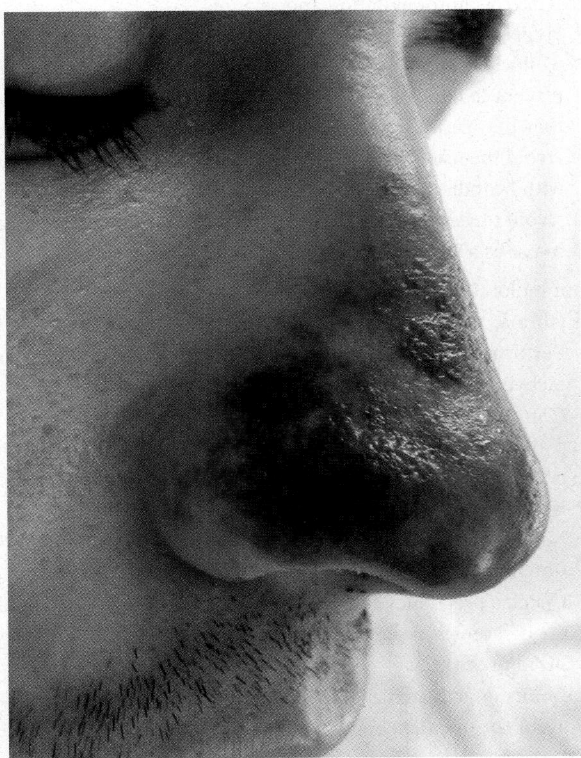

FIGURE 251-9 Cutaneous vasculitis of the nose secondary to the use of levamisole-adulterated cocaine. (*Reproduced with permission from Robert T. Gilson, MD.*)

- Meningitis—Acute infection within the subarachnoid space presenting within hours or days with fever, headache, and stiff neck (more than 90% of patients); additional potential signs are change in mental status (e.g., confusion and decreased consciousness), seizures, increased intracranial pressure, and stroke. The appearance of a rash/petechiae can aid in the diagnosis (meningococcemia). Diagnosis is made with examination of the CSF following lumbar puncture (LP).
- Encephalitis—Acute infection of the central nervous system that involves the brain parenchyma; usually caused by viruses. The clinical features include fever, altered level of consciousness, and focal (e.g., aphasia, ataxia, hemiparesis, and involuntary movements) or diffuse (e.g., agitation, hallucinations, and personality change) symptoms. Diagnosis is established with examination of the CSF following LP.

MANAGEMENT

MANAGEMENT OF ACUTE OVERDOSE

- Acute overdose is a medical emergency best managed in the intensive care unit because of the hyperadrenergic state and seizures.
  - Hyperthermia and severe psychomotor agitation are the most immediately life-threatening complications of cocaine poisoning.[11] Temperatures as high as 45.6°C (114°F) have been recorded. Rapid physical cooling with sponging, fans, ice baths, and cooling blankets can be used, and gastric or peritoneal lavage with iced saline is considered if persistent.
  - IV diazepam up to 0.5 mg/kg given over 8 hours is used to control psychomotor agitation and seizures.[11]
    - Hypertension may also respond to benzodiazepines. β-Blockers should not be used in the setting of cocaine toxicity (except to control ventricular arrhythmia, as below) because they may result in unopposed alpha effects of cocaine.
    - Avoid the use of neuroleptic agents because they can interfere with heat dissipation and, perhaps, lower the seizure threshold.
    - Avoid physical restraints if possible. Benzodiazepines are safe to use as a pharmacologic restraint.
- Propranolol (0.5 to 1 mg IV) can be used to control ventricular arrhythmia.[11]
    - Perform defibrillation in all patients with pulseless ventricular tachycardia.
    - Consider electrical cardioversion in all unstable patients.
    - β-Blockers should not be used in cocaine-induced cardiac ischemia. Nitroglycerin may be used for cocaine-induced cardiac ischemia or infarct.
    - Monitor for rhabdomyolysis and provide rapid fluid resuscitation as needed.
    - Check a pregnancy test on women of childbearing potential, as 6% of women in the emergency room may have an unrecognized pregnancy.
  - Administer activated charcoal to alert patients with oral ingestions of cocaine (i.e., body stuffers and body packers) to reduce absorption. Whole-bowel irrigation may be used to reduce transit time in these patients.[11]
  - Medical providers should be prepared to manage multiple drug effects, especially heroin.

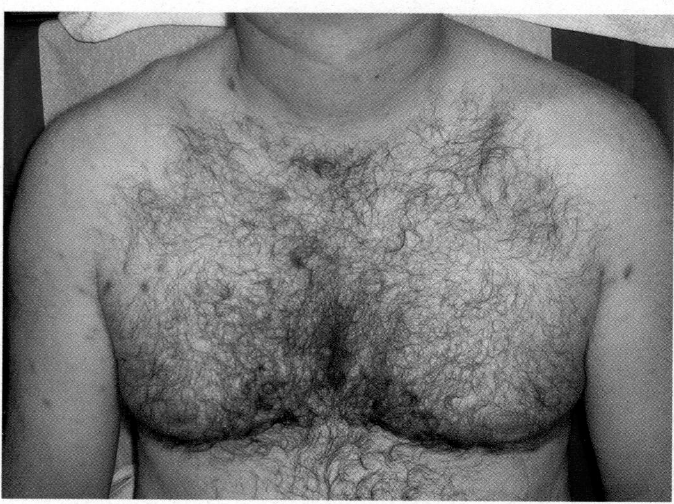

FIGURE 251-10 Secondary syphilis in a man who was involved in unsafe sex while addicted to cocaine. The papulonodular eruption is an unusual presentation of secondary syphilis that was diagnosed with a skin biopsy and confirmed with a rapid plasma reagin (RPR) titer of 1:512. The specific treponemal blood test was also positive. (*Reproduced with permission from Richard P. Usatine, MD.*)

MANAGEMENT OF CHRONIC ADDICTION

- Cognitive behavioral therapy is effective in the treatment of cocaine-dependent outpatients.[20]
- There is no current evidence supporting the clinical use of carbamazepine, antidepressants, dopamine agonists, disulfiram, mazindol, phenytoin, nimodipine, lithium, or NeuRecover-SA in the treatment of cocaine dependence.[21]
- Antidepressant medication exerts a modest beneficial effect for patients with combined depressive and substance-use disorders but should be used as part of a program to directly target the addiction.[22]

REFERRAL

- Referral to specialists may be needed to assist patients with upper respiratory tract (e.g., CSF rhinorrhea and nasal septum perforation) or ophthalmologic complications (e.g., central retinal artery occlusion).
- Following withdrawal from chronic cocaine use, patients may benefit from individual, group, and/or family therapy and peer assistance.

PROGNOSIS

- Cocaine addiction is difficult to treat.
- Of patients enrolled in cocaine addiction programs, 42% do not complete treatment.[23]
- One-third of patients treated for cocaine addiction remain abstinent.[23] Some comprehensive therapy programs have demonstrated abstinence rates at 1 year of up to 58%.[24]
    - Of 131 persons addicted to crack cocaine, 107 were able to be followed for 12 years: 43 (33%) were crack-free for at least 12 months, 22 (17%) continued to use, 13 (10%) were imprisoned, 2 (1.5%) were lost to follow-up, and 27 (20.5%) were deceased.[25]

FOLLOW-UP

- Patients and their families may need ongoing support, home healthcare, and physical and occupational therapy to address long-term neurologic and cardiovascular complications of cocaine, including anoxic encephalopathy, stroke, intracerebral hemorrhage, congestive heart failure, and cardiomyopathy.
- Physicians should closely monitor and assist patients in managing depression, insomnia, and anorexia that may follow cessation of chronic cocaine use.
- Among individuals leaving residential detoxification, chronic pain is a common problem and is associated independently with long-term substance use after detoxification; management of pain may improve long-term outcomes.[26]

PATIENT EDUCATION

- Encourage patients to quit cocaine use and offer assistance.
- Recommend 12-step programs including Cocaine Anonymous.
- Patients should be made aware of the potential complications associated with use of cocaine, including its powerful psychologically addictive properties.
- Instruct IV drug users who continue to use not to reuse or share needles or syringes; cleaning the skin before injection can also decrease risk of infection. Harm reduction programs exist that help addicts obtain and maintain clean needles and syringes.

PATIENT RESOURCES

- eMedicineHealth. *Cocaine Abuse*—**https://www.emedicinehealth.com/cocaine_abuse/article_em.htm.**
- The Substance Abuse and Mental Health Services Administration (SAMHSA) provides an online resource for locating drug and alcohol abuse treatment programs—**https://findtreatment.samhsa.gov/**.
- The SAMHSA referral helpline in English and Spanish is: **1-800-662-HELP.**
- Cocaine Anonymous (CA). Meetings are free. "Hope, Faith and Courage: Stories from the Fellowship of Cocaine Anonymous" now has a new second volume to go with the first volume—both can be ordered online—**https://.ca.org.**
- MedlinePlus. *Cocaine*—**https://www.nlm.nih.gov/medlineplus/cocaine.html.**

PROVIDER RESOURCES

- National Institute on Drug Abuse. *Cocaine*—**http://medlineplus.gov/cocaine.html.**
- U.S. Drug Enforcement Administration. *Cocaine*—**https://www.dea.gov/pr/multimedia-library/image-gallery/images_cocaine.shtml.**

REFERENCES

1. Degenhardt L, Chiu WT, Sampson N, et al. Epidemiological patterns of extra-medical drug use in the United States: evidence from the National Comorbidity Survey Replication, 2001–2003. *Drug Alcohol Depend.* 2007;90(2-3):210-223.
2. Substance Abuse and Mental Health Services Administration. *National Survey on Drug Use and Health.* http://www.samhsa.gov. Accessed May 2012.
3. Wagner FA, Anthony JC. Male–female differences in the risk of progression from first use to dependence upon cannabis, cocaine, and alcohol. *Drug Alcohol Depend.* 2007;86(2-3):191-198.
4. Lejuez CW, Bornovalova MA, Reynolds EK, et al. Risk factors in the relationship between gender and crack/cocaine. *Exp Clin Psychopharmacol.* 2007;15(2):165-175.
5. Bierut LJ, Dinwiddie SH, Begleiter H, et al. Familial transmission of substance dependence: alcohol, marijuana, cocaine, and habitual smoking: a report from the Collaborative Study on the Genetics of Alcoholism. *Arch Gen Psychiatry.* 1998;55(11):982-988.
6. Substance Abuse and Mental Health Services Administration. Behavioral health trends in the United States: Results from the 2014 National Survey on Drug Use and Health. (HHS Publication No. SMA 15-4927, NSDUH Series H-50). 2015.

7. Lange RA, Hills LD. Cardiovascular complications of cocaine use. *N Engl J Med.* 2001;345:351.
8. Maraj S, Figueredo VM, Lynn Morris D. Cocaine and the heart. *Clin Cardiol.* 2010; 33:264.
9. McCord J, Jneid H, Hollaner JE, et al. Management of cocaine-associated chest pain and myocardial infarction: a scientific statement from the American Heart Association Acute Cardiac Care Committee of the Council on Clinical Cardiology. *Circulation.* 2008;117:1897.
10. Mendelson JH, Mello NK. Cocaine and other commonly abused drugs. In: Kasper DL, Braunwald E, Fauci AS, et al, eds. *Harrison's Principles of Internal Medicine*, 16th ed. New York, NY: McGraw-Hill; 2005:2570-2573.
11. Burnett LB. *Cocaine Toxicity in Emergency Medicine Treatment and Management.* http://emedicine.medscape.com/article/813959, updated 2016. Accessed April 2018.
12. Kang SY, Magura S, Shapiro JL. Correlates of cocaine/crack use among inner-city incarcerated adolescents. *Am J Drug Alcohol Abuse.* 1994;20(4):413-429.
13. Bernstein KT, Bucciarelli A, Piper TM, et al. Cocaine- and opiate-related fatal overdose in New York City, 1990–2000. *BMC Public Health.* 2007;7:31.
14. Nyenwe EA, Loganathan RS, Blum S, et al. Active use of cocaine: an independent risk factor for recurrent diabetic ketoacidosis in a city hospital. *Endocr Pract.* 2007;13(1):22-29.
15. Chung C, Tumeh PC, Birnbaum R, et al. Characteristic purpura of the ears, vasculitis, and neutropenia—a potential public health epidemic associated with levamisole-adulterated cocaine. *J Am Acad Dermatol.* 2011;65:722-725.
16. Gross RL, Brucker J, Bahce-Altuntas A, et al. A novel cutaneous vasculitis syndrome induced by levamisole-contaminated cocaine. *Clin Rheumatol.* 2011;30:1385-1392.
17. Jenkins J, Babu K, Hsu-Hung E, et al. ANCA-positive necrotizing vasculitis and thrombotic vasculopathy induced by levamisole-adulterated cocaine: a distinctive clinicopathologic presentation. *J Am Acad Dermatol.* 2011;65:e14-e16.
18. Cascio MJ, Jen KY. Cocaine/levamisole-associated autoimmune syndrome: a disease of neutrophil-mediated autoimmunity. *Curr Opin Hematol.* 2018;25(1):29-36.
19. CDC Newsroom. STDs at record high, indicating urgent need for prevention. September 26, 2017. https://www.cdc.gov/media/releases/2017/p0926-std-prevention.html. Accessed April 2018.
20. Carroll KM, Onken LS. Behavioral therapies for drug abuse. *Am J Psychiatry.* 2005;162(8):1452-1460.
21. de Lima MS, de Oliveira Soares BG, Reisser AA, Farrell M. Pharmacological treatment of cocaine dependence: a systematic review. *Addiction.* 2002;97(8):931-949.
22. Nunes EX, Levin FR. Treatment of depression in patients with alcohol or other drug dependence: a meta-analysis. *JAMA.* 2004;291(15):1887-1896.
23. Dutra L, Stathopoulou G, Basden SL, et al. A meta-analytic review of psychosocial interventions for substance use disorders. *Am J Psychiatry.* 2008;165:179-187.
24. Secades-Villa R, García-Rodríguez O, García-Fernández G, et al. Community reinforcement approach plus vouchers among cocaine-dependent outpatients: twelve-month outcomes. *Psychol Addict Behav.* 2011;25(1):174-179.
25. Dias AC, Araujo MR, Laranjeira R. Evolution of drug use in a cohort of treated crack cocaine users. *Rev Saude Publica.* 2011;45(5):938-948.
26. Larson MJ, Paasche-Orlow M, Cheng DM, et al. Persistent pain is associated with substance use after detoxification: a prospective cohort analysis. *Addiction.* 2007;102(5):752-760.

252 INJECTION-DRUG USE

Richard P. Usatine, MD
Heidi S. Chumley, MD, MBA
Stacy L. Speedlin, PhD
Charles L. Roeth, MD
J. Michael Blair, MD

PATIENT STORY

A 23-year-old woman is seen for her intake physical in a residential treatment program for women recovering from substance abuse. She has not injected heroin for 2 days now, but her tracks are still visible (**Figure 252-1**). Her parents were both addicted to heroin, and she admits to having been born addicted to heroin herself. She began using heroin on her own in her early teens and has been on and off heroin since that time. She acknowledges a history of physical and sexual abuse as a child. She has had many suicide attempts and has cut herself with a knife across her arm many times. She has traded sex for money to buy heroin. Her 2 children are in foster care after having been removed by Child Protective Services. She is a young woman looking for help and is thankful to have been admitted to this program. She does not know whether she has acquired hepatitis B, hepatitis C, or HIV, but wants to be tested.

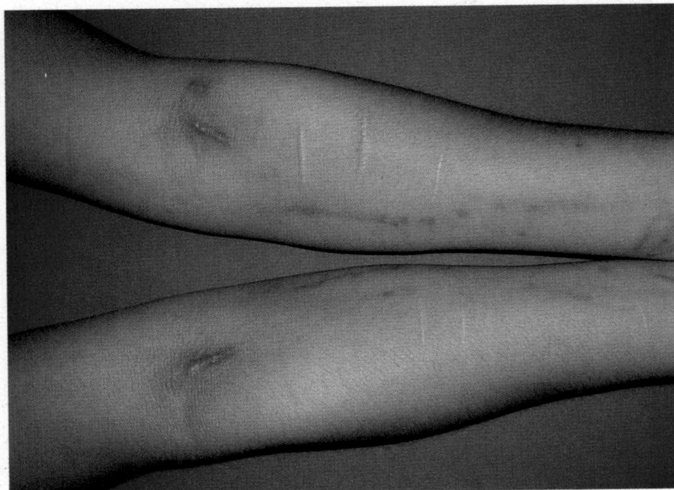

FIGURE 252-1 A 23-year-old woman with visible tracks on her arms from intravenous heroin use. She also has visible scars from self-mutilation with a knife. *(Reproduced with permission from Richard P. Usatine, MD.)*

INTRODUCTION

Injection-drug use of psychoactive drugs affects millions of people across the world. Combinations of genetic, environmental, and behavioral factors influence risk of drug use and addiction. People who inject drugs often have other medical and psychiatric diagnoses, as well as social, legal, and vocational problems. Comprehensive management includes acute treatment and continuing care. Relapse is common, but involvement in a treatment program improves outcomes. While the injection use of heroin has been on the rise for years, the rise in illicitly manufactured fentanyl (IMF) injection use has fueled the overdose problem in the United States.[1]

EPIDEMIOLOGY

- An estimated 16 million people inject drugs worldwide, based on data from 148 countries. The largest numbers of injection drug users are in China, the United States, and Russia.[2]
- In the United States in 2016, there were 63,632 drug overdose deaths (many from injection drug use). From 2015 to 2016, deaths increased across all drug categories examined. The largest overall rate increases occurred among deaths involving cocaine (52.4%) and synthetic opioids (100%), likely driven by IMF.[1]
- Synthetic opioid–involved deaths in 2016 accounted for 30.5% of all drug overdose deaths and 45.9% of all opioid-involved deaths. As of 2017, an average of 115 Americans die every day from opioid overdose.[3] Synthetic opioids propelled increases with 19,413 deaths (more than any drug examined) fueled by the contribution of

fentanyl. In addition, IMF is now being mixed into counterfeit opioid and benzodiazepine pills, heroin, and cocaine, likely contributing to increases in overdose death rates involving other substances.[1,4]

- A kilogram of heroin costs about $65,000; the same amount of fentanyl costs $6500.[4] People who inject drugs such as heroin are unaware of the increased prevalence of synthetic opioids including IMF, which may be referred to as China White (this term also describes high-purity heroin).[4,5] The adulterant is often not discovered until a series of emergency room presentations of overdose.[5]
- In 2011, an estimated 2.6% of the U.S. population over the age of 13 had injected drugs during their lifetime,[6] and 0.30% of the U.S. population had injected drugs in the past year.[5] The prevalence of injection-drug use (IDU) among adolescents and young adults ages 15–29 years, which was estimated at 0.97% in 1997 and 1.15% in 2002, is increasing.[7] An estimated 2.0% of the U.S. population ages 18–24 years had injected drugs during their lifetime as of 2011.
- In 2011, an estimated 3.4% of the U.S. population over the age of 18 were identified as persons who inject drugs during their lifetime. Among men in the United States, the estimated proportions of persons who inject drugs were 3.4% of African Americans, 3.8% of whites, and 2.3% of Hispanics. For women surveyed, the estimated proportions of persons who inject drugs were 1.5% of African Americans, 1.6% of whites, and 0.7% of Hispanics.[6]
- In 2002, the mean age of injection-drug users (IDUs) was 36 years compared to 21 years in 1979.[8] In 2011, the highest proportion of U.S. adults who had ever injected drugs were ages 35–49 years with an estimated prevalence of 3.0%; stratified by gender, the prevalence of IDU was 4.1% for men and 2.0% for women.[6]
- Needle sharing is common. In the previous 3 months, 46% of IDUs had lent a person a used syringe[9] and 54% had injected with a used syringe.[10]
- There were 278,371 substance-abuse treatment admissions for injection-drug use (14.2% of all admissions reported to Substance Abuse and Mental Health Services Administration's [SAMHSA] *Treatment Episode Data Set for 2009*).[11]
- The most commonly injected drug is heroin. Amphetamines, buprenorphine, benzodiazepines, cocaine, and barbiturates are also injected.[12] The 2013 National Survey on Drug Use and Health reported 1.9 million persons in the United States met criteria for opioid use disorder through the misuse of prescription opioids.[13]
- 4.5 million persons were current nonmedical users of prescription opioids in the past month.[13] Comparably, less than one million (289,000) people were users of heroin within the past month.[13]
- IDU is the highest-risk behavior for acquiring infectious diseases, such as hepatitis C virus (HCV), hepatitis B, and HIV. In 2010, 17,000 new cases of HCV surfaced; more than half (53%) were the result of IDU. Hepatitis B infection rates were also 20% higher for IDUs.[14] HIV prevalence among IDUs is estimated to be 20% to 40%.[2]
- The 2009 Monitoring the Future Survey showed that 2.5% of 12th-grade boys in the United States were using anabolic steroids (**Figure 252-2**).[15]
- Anabolic steroid abuse among athletes may range between 1% and 6%.[15]
- Some adolescents abuse steroids as part of a pattern of high-risk behaviors. These adolescents also take risks such as drinking and

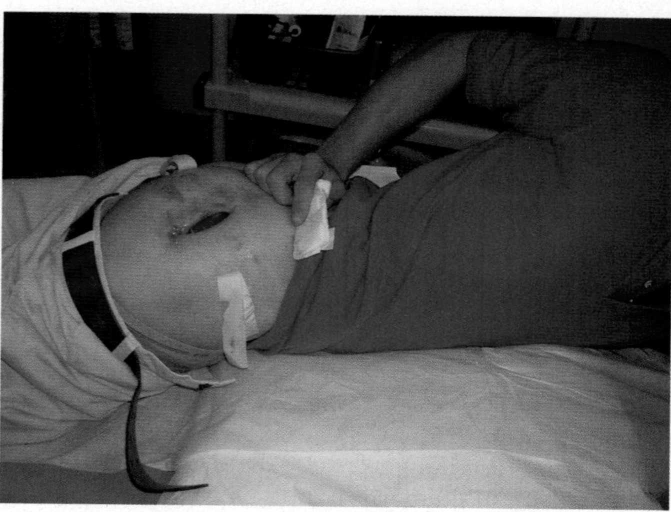

FIGURE 252-2 A high school athlete used injectable anabolic steroids for muscle building and developed a large abscess in his buttocks. This photograph was taken 2 months after the original abscess was drained, and the wound is healing by secondary intention. (*Reproduced with permission from William Rodney, MD.*)

driving, carrying a gun, driving a motorcycle without a helmet, and abusing other illicit drugs.[15]

ETIOLOGY AND PATHOPHYSIOLOGY

- Drug use disorders are thought to be a result of combinations of multiple factors, including genetic, environmental, and individual risk-conferring behaviors.[16]
- Drug use alters the brain's structure and function. These changes persist after drug use stops.[17]
- Most injection-drug users inject drugs intravenously, but subcutaneous injection (skin-popping) is also common.[12]
- Injected, snorted, or smoked heroin causes an almost immediate "rush" or brief period of euphoria that wears off very quickly, terminating in a "crash." The user then experiences an intense craving to use more heroin to stop the crash and bring back the euphoria. The cycle of euphoria, crash, and craving—repeated several times a day—leads to a cycle of addiction.
- Drug overdose surpasses HIV/AIDS and hepatitis C as the leading cause of death for IDUs.[18] The availability of synthetic fentanyl for IDU has increased the risk of overdose, as this drug is 50 to 100 times more potent than morphine, and the strength can be unpredictable.[4,5]
- A heroin overdose can lead to death from respiratory depression, coma, and pulmonary edema. Death from the direct effects of cocaine is usually associated with cardiac dysrhythmias and conduction disturbances, leading to myocardial infarction and stroke.[12]
- Anabolic steroids can lead to early heart attacks, strokes, liver tumors, kidney failure, and serious psychiatric problems. In addition, because steroids are often injected, users who share needles or use nonsterile techniques when they inject steroids are at risk of contracting dangerous infections, such as HIV/AIDS, hepatitis B, and hepatitis C (see **Figure 252-2**).[15]

RISK FACTORS

- Family history.

DIAGNOSIS

CLINICAL FEATURES

Heroin use produces the following clinical appearances:

- Pinpoint pupils and no response of pupils to light.
- A rush of pleasurable feelings.
- Cessation of physical pain.
- Lethargy and drowsiness.
- Slurred speech.
- Shallow breathing.
- Sweating.
- Vomiting.
- A drop in body temperature.
- Sleepiness.
- Loss of appetite.

Cocaine (by injection) can produce the following signs, symptoms, and adverse effects:

- Dilated pupils.
- Hyperactivity.
- Euphoria.
- Irritability and anxiety.
- Excessive talking.
- Depression or excessive sleeping.
- Long periods without eating or sleeping.
- Weight loss.
- Dry mouth and nose.
- Paranoia.
- Cardiac—arrhythmias, chest pain, myocardial infarction (MI), and congestive heart failure (CHF).
- Strokes and seizures.
- Respiratory failure.

COMPLICATIONS OF INJECTING DRUG USE

- Local problems—Abscess (**Figures 252-2** and **252-3**; see Chapter 127, Abscess), cellulitis, septic thrombophlebitis, local induration, necrotizing fasciitis, gas gangrene, pyomyositis, mycotic aneurysm, compartmental syndromes, and foreign bodies (e.g., broken needle parts) in local areas.[2]
  - IDUs are at higher risk of getting methicillin-resistant *Staphylococcus aureus* (MRSA) skin infections that the patient may think are spider bites (**Figure 252-4**).
  - Some IDUs give up trying to inject into their veins and put the cocaine directly into the skin. This causes local skin necrosis that produces round atrophic scars (**Figure 252-5**).
- IDUs are at risk for contracting systemic infections, including HIV and hepatitis B or hepatitis C.
  - Injecting drug users are at risk of endocarditis, osteomyelitis (**Figures 252-6** and **252-7**), and an abscess of the epidural region. These infections can lead to long hospitalizations for intravenous antibiotics. The endocarditis that occurs in IDUs involves the right-sided heart valves (see Chapter 52, Bacterial Endocarditis).[2] They are also at risk of septic emboli to the lungs, group A β-hemolytic streptococcal septicemia, septic arthritis, and candidal and other fungal infections.

LABORATORY TESTING

- All IDUs should be screened for HIV (with consent), hepatitis B, and hepatitis C.
- If there is a history of high-risk sexual behavior, screen for syphilis (rapid plasma reagin [RPR]), *Chlamydia*, and gonorrhea.
- QuantiFERON-TB Gold or purified protein derivative (PPD) test to screen for tuberculosis (especially if the patient is experiencing homelessness or living with HIV).

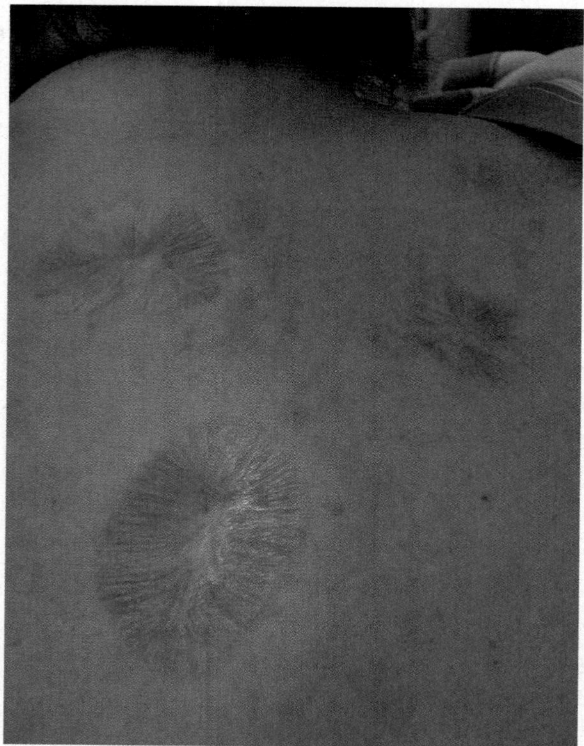

FIGURE 252-3 A 32-year-old woman with type 1 diabetes developed large abscesses all over her body secondary to injection of cocaine and heroin. Her back shows the large scars remaining after the healing of these abscesses. (*Reproduced with permission from Richard P. Usatine, MD.*)

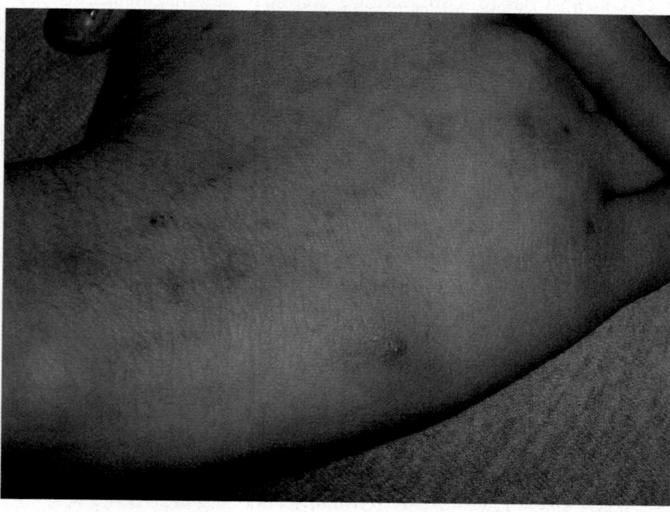

FIGURE 252-4 A young woman with methicillin-resistant *Staphylococcus aureus* infection from injection-drug use. Track marks are barely visible on her hand and wrist. Note one pustule from methicillin-resistant *S. aureus*. (*Reproduced with permission from Richard P. Usatine, MD.*)

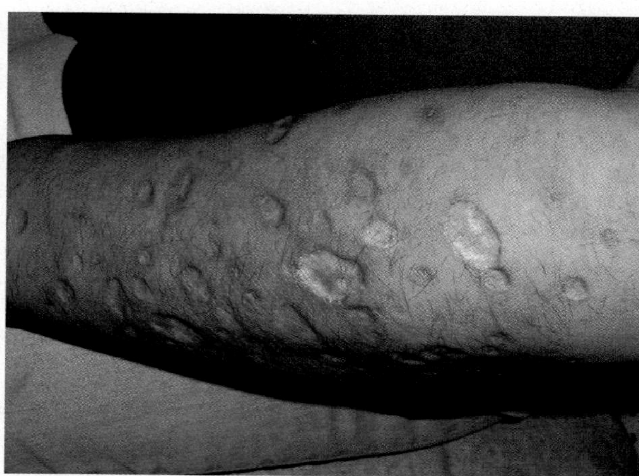

FIGURE 252-5 A young woman in a residential treatment program with multiple scars from skin-popping cocaine. She gave up trying to inject into her veins and put the cocaine directly into the skin. Note how the local skin necrosis caused round atrophic scars. (*Reproduced with permission from Richard P. Usatine, MD.*)

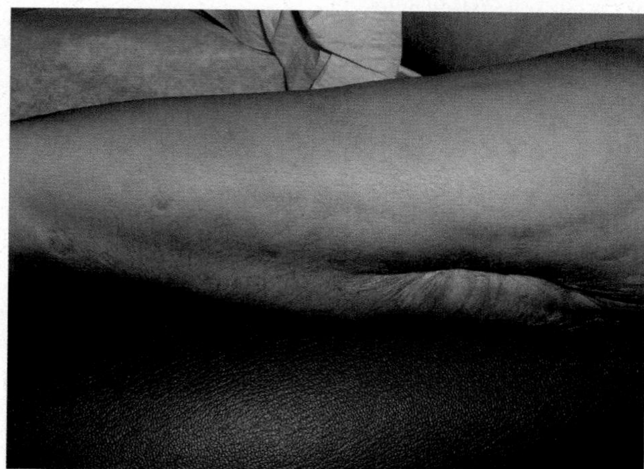

FIGURE 252-6 A 24-year-old woman with an 8-year history of injection-drug use. She has a large deep linear scar from osteomyelitis of the ulnar bone and smaller round scars from skin popping. A track is also visible above the deep scar. (*Reproduced with permission from Richard P. Usatine, MD.*)

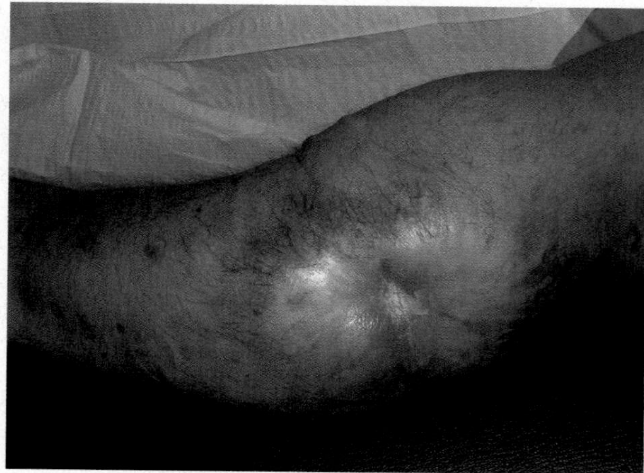

FIGURE 252-7 The other arm of the woman in **Figure 252-6** with deep scar from osteomyelitis secondary to injecting drugs that destroyed the bones in her left forearm. Her arm is deformed and poorly functional. (*Reproduced with permission from Richard P. Usatine, MD.*)

- Urine screen for common drugs of abuse may reveal other drugs not admitted to in the history.
- Women of childbearing age should be tested for pregnancy when indicated. This is especially important when prescribing medications to treat withdrawal.[14] Additionally, contraceptive counseling should be a routine part of substance use disorder treatment to prevent unplanned pregnancy.
- ECG is warranted if there are any cardiac symptoms or if the physical examination reveals signs of cardiac disease.

DIFFERENTIAL DIAGNOSIS

- Injection-drug use and dependence may be hidden problems. The differential diagnosis will differ based on the presenting complaints.

MANAGEMENT

- Drug-abuse therapy is cost-effective. For example, 1 year of methadone maintenance therapy is approximately $4700 compared to 1 year of imprisonment, which costs $18,400.[17,19]
- Every $1 invested in addiction treatment saves $12 in health, legal, and theft costs.[17]

NONPHARMACOLOGIC

- Recognize addiction as a chronic illness that requires a comprehensive approach during the treatment phase (e.g., residential/outpatient treatment) and continuing care (e.g., drug-abuse monitoring, booster sessions, and reevaluation of treatment needs).[17]
- Identify and address associated medical and psychiatric diagnoses, as well as social, legal, and work-related problems. Coexisting psychiatric illnesses are common.[17]
- Fifty-six percent to 90% of IDUs have been incarcerated in their lifetime.[14] For criminal justice–involved drug abusers and addicts, use this opportunity to engage individuals in treatment. Research supports the efficacy of combining criminal justice sanctions and drug-abuse treatment.[17]
- Test IDUs for HIV/AIDS, hepatitis B, and hepatitis C. Consider testing for tuberculosis and other infectious diseases as indicated.[17]
- Consider medically assisted detoxification to minimize withdrawal symptoms.
- Recommend an appropriate length of time for treatment. Most patients need at least 3 months to stop using drugs.[17]
- Encourage patients to engage in individual or group behavioral therapies and assist patients in finding programs that meet their individual needs.[17]
- Advise patients to join a self-help group, such as Narcotics Anonymous (NA) or Cocaine Anonymous (CA), which are based on the 12-step model. Most drug-addiction treatment programs encourage patients to participate in a self-help group during and after formal treatment.[11]

MEDICATIONS

- For opioid addiction, consider a methadone maintenance program.
  - Opioid replacement therapy reduces IDU and thus reduces the mortality and morbidity associated with IDU, including the transmission of HIV and hepatitis C virus (HCV).[12]
  - Opioid replacement combined with counseling, medical and psychiatric care, employment assistance, and family services is superior to opioid replacement alone.[17]
- Buprenorphine, a partial opioid agonist, is also used for opioid detoxification and for opioid replacement therapy.[12,17] Buprenorphine should be used cautiously in combination with HIV antiretroviral medications—particularly those that can inhibit or be metabolized by the P450 3A4 enzyme system, such as efavirenz (a component of Atripla).[19] In the United States, physicians who wish to prescribe buprenorphine must take a certification course.
- Naltrexone, a long-acting synthetic opioid antagonist, blocks opioid receptors, thereby preventing the effects of opioids. Treatment is initiated after patients have been opioid-free for several days to prevent a severe withdrawal.[17]
- Naloxone, a short-acting opioid antagonist, can be administered as an injection or nasal spray in the event of opioid overdose.[14] Because of elevated statistics on opioid-related deaths, more first responders are seeking training to administer naloxone as an auto-injector.[14] Naloxone can safely be administered to pregnant women experiencing an overdose.[14] In April 2018, the U.S. Surgeon General released a rare public health advisory urging Americans to be familiar and equipped with naloxone in the midst of the worsening opioid epidemic.[20] See Prevention/Harm Reduction below.
- Treating criminal justice–involved drug abusers and addicts—Drug abusers may come into contact with the criminal justice system earlier than with other health or social systems. Thus, the period of involvement with the criminal justice system may offer an opportunity to engage individuals in a treatment that can shorten a pattern of drug abuse and related crime. Research supports the efficacy of combining criminal justice sanctions and drug-abuse treatment.[21]
- Drug-abuse treatment is less expensive than alternatives, such as not treating addicts or incarcerating them. The average cost for 1 full year of methadone maintenance treatment is approximately $4700 per patient, whereas 1 full year of imprisonment costs approximately $18,400 per person. According to several conservative estimates, every $1 invested in addiction treatment programs yields up to $7 in savings, much of which results from reduced drug-related crime and criminal justice costs.[21] Although methadone maintenance is not as desirable as full abstinence, the comparative costs are in favor of drug treatment over incarceration.
- Recovery from drug addiction has two key components: treatment and continuing care. The clinical practices that make up the treatment phase (e.g., residential/outpatient treatment) must be followed up by management of the disorder over time (e.g., drug-abuse monitoring, booster sessions, and reevaluation of treatment needs).[21]
- Research shows that treatment must last, on average, at least 3 months to produce stable behavior change.[21] This accounts for the existence of 90-day residential treatment programs.

- A comprehensive assessment is the first step in the treatment process and includes identifying individual strengths to facilitate treatment and recovery. In addition, drug abuse cannot be treated in isolation from related issues and potential threats, such as criminal behavior, mental health status, physical health, family functioning, employment status, homelessness, and HIV/AIDS.[21]
- Treatments that use cognitive behavioral therapies, residential treatment, contingency management, and medications have demonstrated effectiveness in reducing drug abuse and criminal behavior.[21]
- Medications are a key treatment component for drug abusers and can stabilize the brain and help return it to normal functioning. Methadone and buprenorphine are effective in helping individuals addicted to heroin or other opiates reduce their drug abuse. Naltrexone is also an effective medication for some opiate-addicted patients and those with concurrent alcohol use disorder.[21]
- Family and friends can play critical roles in motivating individuals with drug problems to enter and stay in treatment. Family therapy is important, especially for adolescents. Involvement of a family member in an individual's treatment program can strengthen and extend the benefits of the program.[21]
- Buprenorphine (Subutex or, in combination with naloxone, Suboxone) is demonstrated to be a safe and acceptable addiction treatment. Congress passed the Drug Addiction Treatment Act (DATA 2000), permitting qualified physicians to prescribe narcotic medications (Schedules III to V) for the treatment of opioid addiction. This legislation created a major paradigm shift by allowing access to opiate treatment in a medical setting rather than limiting it to specialized drug treatment clinics. Approximately 10,000 physicians have taken the training needed to prescribe these 2 medications, and nearly 7000 have registered as potential providers.
- Methadone and levo-α-acetyl methadol (LAAM) have more gradual onsets of action and longer half-lives than heroin. Patients stabilized on these medications do not experience the heroin rush. Both medications wear off much more slowly than heroin, so there is no sudden crash, and the brain and body are not exposed to the marked fluctuations seen with heroin use. Maintenance treatment with methadone or LAAM markedly reduces the desire for heroin.
- If an individual maintained on adequate, regular doses of methadone (once a day) or LAAM (several times per week) tries to take heroin, the euphoric effects of heroin will be significantly blocked. According to research, patients undergoing maintenance treatment do not suffer the medical abnormalities and behavioral destabilization that rapid fluctuations in drug levels cause in heroin addicts.

PREVENTION/HARM REDUCTION

- Needle/syringe exchange programs can help patients injecting drugs from getting or giving others hepatitis C and HIV. In fact, many pharmacies will sell large boxes of insulin syringes with needles attached to anyone without a prescription and without proven diabetes. While the goal is complete abstinence from injection drug use, clean needles/syringes do prevent the transmission of hepatitis and HIV. This information can prevent disease, save health care dollars, and save lives. As physicians we can advocate for patient and community access to clean needles/syringes as prevention of costly infectious diseases to the patient and our society.
- Safe injection sites (supervised injection facilities) can prevent fatal overdoses, HIV, and hepatitis, as well as abscesses and skin necrosis. Although these are not legal in the United States, there are other countries that are successfully using this harm reduction method. Again, while the goal is complete abstinence from injection drug use, these programs can save lives and be the front door into treatment.
- Naloxone is a non-addictive, lifesaving drug that can reverse effects of an opioid overdose (**Figure 252-8**) when administered in time. Naloxone is now available at many local pharmacies without a prescription, and the U.S. Surgeon General encourages more adults to be familiar and equipped with naloxone in the midst of the current opioid epidemic. Providing patients with a prescription for naloxone may allow for purchase at a reduced cost. Naloxone comes as an easy-to-administer nasal spray under the brand name Narcan (**Figure 252-9**). By following the directions on the box, Narcan can be given to an unconscious person by anyone without the need for medical training.

PREVENTION AND SCREENING

- The U.S. Preventive Services Task Force concluded that there is insufficient evidence to screen for illicit drug use in adolescents, adults, or pregnant women, but advises clinicians to be alert for sign and symptoms of drug use.[22]
- Accurate and reliable office screening instruments include CRAFFT (adolescent drug use/misuse), and the ASSIST, CAGE-AID, and DAST (adults with drug misuse).[22]
- An empirically validated scale to measure withdrawal symptoms can guide physicians with appropriate, timely administration of methadone and buprenorphine. Scales such as the Objective Opioid Withdrawal Scale (OOWS), the Subjective Opioid Scale (SOWS), and the Clinical Opioid Withdrawal Scale (COWS) can identify moderate to severe withdrawal in patients.[14]

PROGNOSIS

- Most patients who enter and remain in treatment stop injecting drugs and see improvements in their work, relationships, and psychological functioning.[17]
- Forty percent to 60% of patients relapse.[17] Patients should be counseled on the possibility of relapse and encouraged to take measures to maintain abstinence from substance use.
- Patients with co-occurring psychiatric disorders will show higher levels of difficulty engaging and participating in treatment programs.[19] Furthermore, these patients have higher attrition rates and poorer prognosis rates compared to patients with opioid IDUs alone.[19]
- Drug injectors who do not enter treatment are up to 6 times more likely to become infected with HIV than are injectors who enter and remain in treatment. Drug users who enter and continue in treatment reduce activities that can spread disease, such as sharing injection equipment and engaging in unprotected sexual activity. Participation in treatment also presents opportunities for screening, counseling, and referral for additional services. The best drug-abuse treatment programs provide HIV counseling and offer HIV testing to their patients.[17]

FOLLOW-UP

- Follow-up is important for the treatment of IDUs. Addiction is a chronic (and relapsing) condition and requires long-term follow-up. Your intervention and caring attitude can help the patient to overcome addiction and to live a sober and drug-free life. Do not give up on patients who relapse, because it often takes more than one attempt before long-term cessation can be achieved. The frequency and intensity of follow-up depend on the substance, the addiction, and the patients and their complications.

PATIENT EDUCATION

- For patients who are not ready to stop their IDU, harm reduction and counseling programs can be helpful. Encourage patients to use clean and sterile needle/syringes and not to share these with anyone. Bleach can be used to clean and sterilize needles/syringes and prevent the spread of HIV and hepatitis.
- Encourage patients to get help to become drug-free and abstinent. There is no safe level of injection-drug use.
- Explain to patients that addiction is a disease and not a failure of their moral character.
- Inform patients about the existing treatment programs in their community and offer them names and phone numbers so that they may get help.
- If your patient is not ready for help today, give the numbers and names for tomorrow.
- Speak about the value of 12-step programs including NA and CA, because everyone can afford a 12-step program. There are 12-step programs in the community for everyone, including nonsmokers and agnostics.

PATIENT RESOURCES

- Narcotics Anonymous. Provides information about meetings and literature in more than 40 different languages—**https://www.na.org.**
- Nar-Anon Family Groups. Provides support for friends and family of people addicted to narcotics—**https://www.nar-anon.org.**
- Cocaine Anonymous. Provides information about meetings and other resources—**https://www.ca.org.**

PROVIDER RESOURCES

- The Center for Adolescent Substance Abuse Research. *The CRAFFT Screening Tool*—**http://www.ceasar-boston.org/clinicians/crafft.php.**
- The National Institute on Drug Abuse. *Medical Consequences of Drug Abuse*—**https://www.drugabuse.gov/related-topics/health-consequences-drug-misuse.**
- Substance Abuse and Mental Health Services Administration. *Substance Abuse Treatment Facility Locator* (information on treatment programs in the United States)—**https://www.findtreatment.samhsa.gov.**

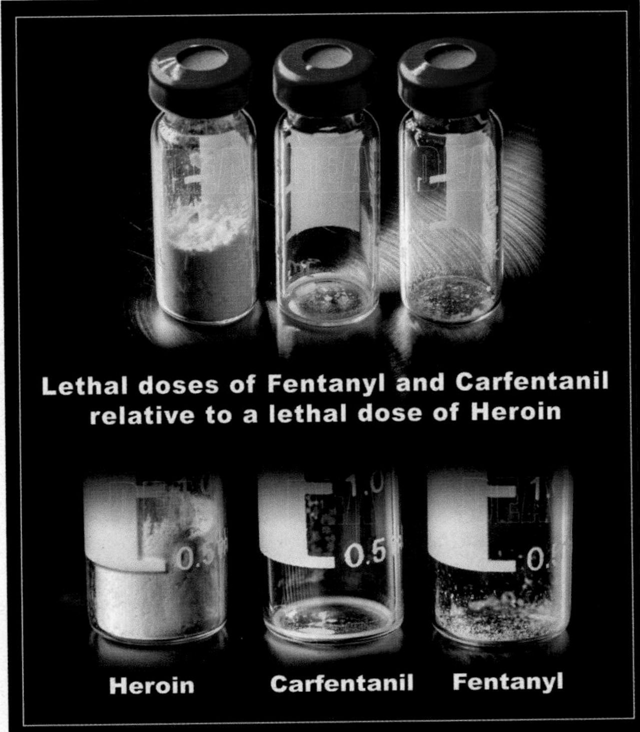

FIGURE 252-8 Lethal doses of heroin, fentanyl, and carfentanil are displayed by the U.S. Drug Enforcement Administration.

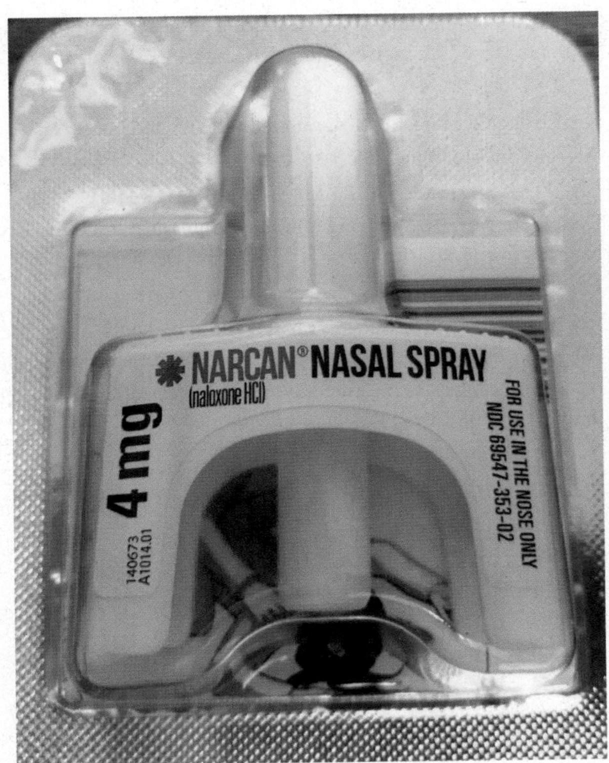

FIGURE 252-9 Naloxone comes as an easy-to-administer nasal spray under the brand name Narcan.

- Substance Abuse and Mental Health Services Administration. *Providers Clinical Support System* (evidence-based prevention and treatment of opioid use disorders and treatment of chronic pain)—**https://pcssnow.org.**

REFERENCES

1. Seth P, Scholl L, Rudd RA, Bacon S. Overdose deaths involving opioids, cocaine, and psychostimulants—United States, 2015-2016. *MMWR Morb Mortal Wkly Rep.* 2018;67(12):349-358.
2. Mathers BM, Degenhardt L, Phillips B, et al. Global epidemiology of injecting drug use and HIV among people who inject drugs: a systematic review. *Lancet.* 2008;372(9651):1733-1745.
3. CDC. *Understanding the Epidemic.* Updated August 30, 2017. https://www.cdc.gov/drugoverdose/epidemic/index.html. Accessed April 2018.
4. Pergolizzi JV, LeQuang JA, Taylor R., et al; NEMA Research Group. Going beyond prescription pain relievers to understand the opioid epidemic: the role of illicit fentanyl, new psychoactive substances, and street heroin. *Postgrad Med.* 2017;130:1-8.
5. Miller JM, Stogner JM, Miller BL, Blough S. Exploring synthetic heroin: accounts of acetyl fentanyl use from sample of dually diagnosed drug offenders. *Drug Alcohol Rev.* 2018;37:121-127.
6. Lansky A, Finlayson T, Johnson C, et al. Estimating the number of persons who inject drugs in the united states by meta-analysis to calculate national rates of HIV and hepatitis C virus infections. *PLoS One.* 2014;9(5):e97596. https://doi.org/10.1371/journal.pone.0097596.
7. Chatterjee A, Tempalski B, Pouget ER, et al. Changes in the prevalence of injection drug use among adolescents and young adults in large U.S. metropolitan areas. *AIDS Behav.* 2011;15(7):1570-1578.
8. Armstrong GL. Injection drug users in the United States, 1979–2002: an aging population. *Arch Intern Med.* 2007;167(2):166-173.
9. Golub ET, Strathdee SA, Bailey SL, et al; DUIT Study Team. Distributive syringe sharing among young adult injection drug users in five U.S. cities. *Drug Alcohol Depend.* 2007;91 Suppl 1:S30-S38.
10. Bailey SL, Ouellet LJ, Mackesy-Amiti ME, et al. DUIT Study Team. Perceived risk, peer influences, and injection partner type predict receptive syringe sharing among young adult injection drug users in five U.S. cities. *Drug Alcohol Depend.* 2007;91 Suppl 1:S18-S29.
11. Substance Abuse and Mental Health Services Administration. *Treatment Episode Data Set (TEDS). 1999–2009.* (National Admission to Substance Abuse Treatment Services, DASIS Series: S-56, HHS Publication No. 9SMA 11-4646.) Rockville, MD: Substance Abuse and Mental Health Services Administration; 2011.
12. Baciewicz GJ. *Injecting Drug Use.* Updated March 2016. https://emedicine.medscape.com/article/286976. Accessed April 2018.
13. Substance Abuse and Mental Health Services Administration. *Results from the 2012 National Survey on Drug Use and Health: Mental Health Findings,* NSDUH Series H-47, HHS Publication No. (SMA) 13-4805. 2013.
14. Kampman K, Jarvis M. American Society of Addiction Medicine (ASAM) National Practice Guideline for the use of medications in the treatment of addiction involving opioid use. *J Addict Med.* 2015;9(5):358-367.
15. Johnston LD, O'Malley PM, Bachman JG, Schulenberg JE. *Monitoring the Future: National Results on Adolescent Drug Use: Overview of Key Findings, 2009.* (NIH Publication No. 10-7583). Bethesda, MD: National Institute on Drug Abuse.
16. Schulden JD, Thomas YF, Compton W. Substance abuse in the United States: findings from recent epidemiologic studies. *Curr Psychiatry Rep.* 2009;11(5):353-359.
17. National Institute on Drug Abuse. *Principles of Drug Addiction Treatment: A Research Based Guide,* 2nd ed. (NIH Publication No. 09-4180, revised April 2009.) Bethesda, MD: National Institutes of Health and U.S. Department of Health and Human Services; 2009.
18. Martinez AN, D'Amico EJ, Kral AH, Bluthenthal RN. Nonmedical prescription drug use among injection drug users. *J Drug Iss.* 2012;42(3):216-225.
19. Kraus ML, Alford DP, Kotz MM, et al. Statement of the American Society of Addiction Medicine Consensus Panel on the use of buprenorphine in office-based treatment of opioid addiction. *J Addict Med.* 2011;5(4):254-263.
20. Adams JM. Increasing naloxone awareness and use: the role of health care practitioners. *JAMA.* 2018;319(20):2073-2074.
21. *Principles of Drug Abuse Treatment for Criminal Justice Populations—A Research-Based Guide.* http://www.drugabuse.gov/drugpages/cj.html. Accessed May 2012.
22. U.S. Preventive Services Task Force. *Screening for Illicit Drug Use.* http://www.uspreventiveservicestaskforce.org. Accessed April 2012.

APPENDIX

Strength of Recommendation (SOR)	Definition
A	Recommendation based on consistent and good-quality patient-oriented evidence.*
B	Recommendation based on inconsistent or limited-quality patient-oriented evidence.*
C	Recommendation based on consensus, usual practice, opinion, disease-oriented evidence, or case series for studies of diagnosis, treatment, prevention, or screening.*

*See Appendix A on pages 1603–1606 for further information.

APPENDIX A INTERPRETING EVIDENCE-BASED MEDICINE

Mindy A. Smith, MD, MS

"Evidence-based medicine—is this something new?" asked my father, incredulously. "What were you practicing before?"

Like my father, our patients assume that we provide recommendations to them based on scientific evidence. The idea that there might not be relevant evidence or that we might not have access to that evidence has not even occurred to most of them. This is certainly not to imply that such evidence is the be-all and end-all of medical practice, or that our patients would follow such recommendations blindly—rather, for me, it is a starting point from which to begin rational testing or outline a possible therapeutic plan. In fact, one definition of evidence-based medicine is "the conscientious, explicit, and judicious development and use of current best evidence in making decisions about the care of individual patients."[1]

The first time that I recall the term *evidence-based medicine* (EBM) being discussed was in the early 1990s.[2,3] It seemed that we would need to develop skills in evaluating the published literature and determining its quality, validity, and relevance to the care of our patients. As a teacher and researcher, I was intrigued by the challenges of critically appraising articles and teaching this newfound skill to others. As a clinician, however, I was most interested in answering clinical questions and doing so in a compressed time frame. I needed rapid access to tools or sources that provided summary answers to those questions tagged to information about the quantity and quality of the evidence and the consistency of information across studies.

There are many systems for rating literature, but few that met the needs of the busy practitioner trying to make sense of individual clinical trials and the hundreds of both evidence-based and consensus-based guidelines that seemed to spring up overnight. In 2004, the editors of the U.S. family medicine and primary care journals and the Family Practice Inquiries Network published a paper on a unified taxonomy called *Strength of Recommendation* (SOR) Taxonomy that seemed to fit the bill (**Figure A-1**).[4] This taxonomy made use of existing systems for judging study quality while incorporating the concept of patient-oriented (e.g., mortality, morbidity, symptom improvement) rather than disease-oriented (e.g., change in blood pressure, blood chemistry) outcomes as most relevant. A SOR Ⓐ recommendation is one based on consistent, good-quality patient-oriented evidence; SOR Ⓑ is a recommendation based on inconsistent or limited-quality patient-oriented evidence; and SOR Ⓒ is a recommendation based on consensus, usual practice, opinion, disease-oriented evidence, or case series (**Figures A-1** and **A-2**).

In this book, we made a commitment to search for patient-oriented evidence to support the diagnostic and therapeutic information that we provide in each of the chapters, and to provide a SOR rating for that evidence whenever possible. The bulleted format within the chapter divisions allows the practitioner to quickly find answers to their clinical questions while providing some direction about how confident we are that a recommendation had high-quality patient-oriented evidence to support it. Although textbooks, like this one, do not always contain the most current information, we believe that they are highly relevant for providing essential background information (who, what, why, when, where, how) and to guide the approach to patients—particularly in the case of this *Color Atlas*, in which visual findings are present. For those foreground questions (specific information to guide clinical decisions), we encourage the reader to also check online, regularly updated secondary data sources (e.g., Essential Evidence Plus, DynaMed, Cochrane Database) and guidelines (e.g., U.S. Preventive Services Task Force).

Several other concepts are used throughout the book that can assist practitioners in using evidence-based information and explaining that information to patients. Risk reductions from medical treatments are often presented in relative terms—the *relative risk reduction* (RRR) or the difference in the percentage of adverse outcomes between the intervention group and the control group divided by the percentage of adverse outcomes in the control group. These numbers are often large, and using them not only causes us to overestimate the importance of a treatment but misses its clinical relevance. A more meaningful term is the *absolute risk reduction* (ARR)—the risk difference between the two groups. This number can then be used to obtain a *number needed to treat* (NNT)—the number of patients who would need to be treated (over the same time period as used in the treatment trial) to prevent 1 bad outcome or produce 1 good outcome. This is calculated as 100% divided by the ARR. NNT is more easily understood by us and our patients. See the NNT example in **Box A-1**.

Most absolute risk reductions, and therefor NNT, are small. For example, the NNT to prevent one death for treatment of high blood pressure over 5 years is 125. This must be balanced against potential harm. Adverse effects from treatments are often downplayed or sometimes absent from these discussions. In the case of treating hypertension, 1 in 10 patients stop medication, often due to side effects. Information, including these figures, on NNT and number needed to harm, can be found online at http://www.thennt.com.

Another term that is used in this book is the *likelihood ratio* (LR). This number, based on the sensitivity and specificity of a diagnostic test, is used to determine the probability of a patient with a positive test (LR+) having the disease or the probability of a patient with a

BOX A-1 NNT Example

If a new drug was released for the treatment of postherpetic neuralgia and a randomized controlled trial found that 70% of the treated group reported significant pain control (based on a defined endpoint) and 20% of the placebo group reported significant pain control, this would produce an absolute risk reduction (ARR) of 50%. In this case the NNT would be 100%/50% = 2. On average, only 2 patients would need to be treated for 1 patient to receive the defined pain control benefit. If the ARR was only 10% (30% of the intervention group and 20% of the control group benefitted), then the NNT = 10 or 10 patients would need treatment on average for 1 to receive benefit.

Figure A-1

How recommendations are graded for strength, and underlying individual studies are rated for quality

In general, only key recommendations for readers require a grade of the "Strength of Recommendation." Recommendations should be based on the highest quality evidence available. For example, vitamin E was found in some cohort studies (level 2 study quality) to have a benefit for cardiovascular protection, but good-quality randomized trials (level 1) have not confirmed this effect. Therefore, it is preferable to base clinical recommendations in a manuscript on the level 1 studies.

Strength of recommendation	Definition
A	Recommendation based on consistent and good-quality patient-oriented evidence.*
B	Recommendation based on inconsistent or limited-quality patient-oriented evidence.*
C	Recommendation based on consensus, usual practice, opinion, disease-oriented evidence,* or case series for studies of diagnosis, treatment, prevention, or screening

Use the following scheme to determine whether a study measuring patient-oriented outcomes is of good or limited quality, and whether the results are consistent or inconsistent between studies.

	Type of Study		
Study quality	**Diagnosis**	**Treatment/prevention/ screening**	**Prognosis**
Level 1—good-quality patient-oriented evidence	Validated clinical decision rule SR/meta-analysis of high-quality studies High-quality diagnostic cohort study†	SR/meta-analysis of RCTs with consistent findings High-quality individual RCT‡ All-or-none study§	SR/meta-analysis of good-quality cohort studies Prospective cohort study with good follow-up
Level 2—limited-quality patient-oriented evidence	Unvalidated clinical decision rule SR/meta-analysis of lower-quality studies or studies with inconsistent findings Lower-quality diagnostic cohort study or diagnostic case-control study§	SR/meta-analysis lower-quality clinical trials or of studies with inconsistent findings Lower-quality clinical trial‡ or prospective cohort study Cohort study Case-control study	SR/meta-analysis of lower-quality cohort studies or with inconsistent results Retrospective cohort study with poor follow-up Case-control study Case series
Level 3—other evidence	Consensus guidelines, extrapolations from bench research, usual practice, opinion, other evidence disease-oriented evidence (intermediate or physiologic outcomes only), or case series for studies of diagnosis, treatment, prevention, or screening		

Consistency across studies	
Consistent	Most studies found similar or at least coherent conclusions (coherence means that differences are explainable); ***or*** If high-quality and up-to-date systematic reviews or meta-analyses exist, they support the recommendation
Inconsistent	Considerable variation among study findings and lack of coherence; ***or*** If high-quality and up-to-date systematic reviews or meta-analyses exist, they do not find consistent evidence in favor of the recommendation

*Patient-oriented evidence measures outcomes that matter to patients: morbidity, mortality, symptom improvement, cost reduction, and quality of life. Disease-oriented evidence measures intermediate, physiologic, or surrogate end points that may or may not reflect improvements in patient outcomes (ie, blood pressure, blood chemistry, physiologic function, and pathologic findings).

† High-quality diagnostic cohort study: cohort design, adequate size, adequate spectrum of patients, blinding, and a consistent, well-defined reference standard.

‡ High-quality RCT: allocation concealed, blinding if possible, intention-to-treat analysis, adequate statistical power, adequate follow-up (greater than 80 percent).

§ In an all-or-none study, the treatment causes a dramatic change in outcomes, such as antibiotics for meningitis or surgery for appendicitis, which precludes study in a controlled trial.

SR, systematic review; RCT, randomized controlled trial

FIGURE A-1 *(Reproduced with permission from Ebell MH, Siwek J, Weiss BD, et al. Simplifying the language of evidence to improve patient care: Strength of recommendation taxonomy (SORT), J Fam Pract. 2004 Feb;53(2):111–120. Frontline Medical Communications. Inc.)*

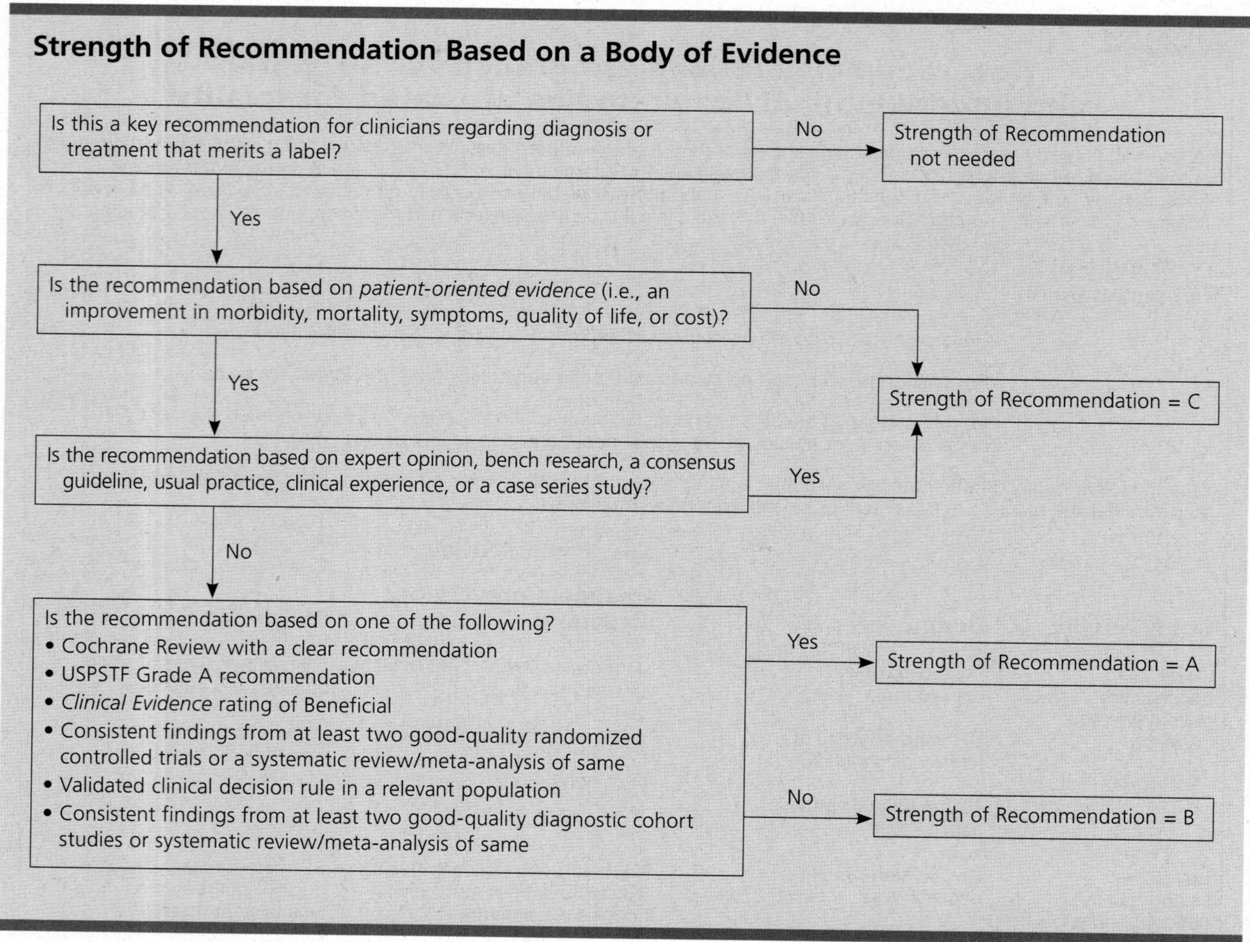

FIGURE A-2 Assigning a Strength-of-Recommendation grade based on a body of evidence. (USPSTF = U.S. Preventive Services Task Force.) *(Reproduced with permission from Ebell MH, Siwek J, Weiss BD, et al. Simplifying the language of evidence to improve patient care: Strength of recommendation taxonomy (SORT), J Fam Pract. 2004 Feb;53(2):111–120. Frontline Medical Communications. Inc.)*

negative test (LR−) not having the disease in question. The LR is defined as the likelihood that a given test result would be expected in a patient with the target disorder compared to the likelihood that the same result would be expected in a patient without the target disorder. The number obtained for the LR+ [Sensitivity/(100 − Specificity)] or the LR− [(100 − Sensitivity)/Specificity] can be multiplied by the pretest probability of disease to determine the posttest probability of disease. An LR+ over 10 is considered strong evidence to rule in disease, while an LR− of less than 0.1 is strong evidence to rule out disease. YouTube videos explaining LRs available, like this one: https://www.youtube.com/watch?v=lnZTOoGc_F0.

We both are privileged and cursed with practicing medicine in an information-rich environment. We have designed our *Color Atlas* to link evidence to clinical recommendations so that we can provide our patients the best science available. When the evidence is lacking, we make that clear and encourage you to engage in frank and honest discussions that lead to the shared responsibility for decisions. Our patients are justified in expecting science along with humanism—can we give them anything less?

REFERENCES

1. Center for Evidence-Based Medicine. http://www.cebm.net/evidence-based-medicine-whats-in-a-name/. Accessed June 2017.
2. Evidence-Based Medicine Working Group. Evidence-based medicine. A new approach to teaching the practice of medicine. *JAMA*. 1992;268:2420-2425.
3. Shaughnessy AF, Slawson DC, Bennett JH. Becoming an information master: a guidebook to the medical information jungle. *J Fam Pract.* 1994;39:489-499.
4. Ebell MA, Siwek J, Weiss BD, et al. Strength of Recommendation Taxonomy (SORT): a patient-centered approach to grading evidence in the medical literature. *J Fam Pract.* 2004;53(2):111-120.

APPENDIX B CHRONIC PAIN

Alan Remde, MD

INTRODUCTION

This appendix focuses on one of the most common scenarios in primary care—chronic non-cancer pain that does not have an easily identifiable physical source, and therefore is difficult to "fix" with simple interventions. Of course, as needed, arrange treatment for any clearly identifiable source that is not resolving with conservative measures. Examples of these include interventional treatments of severe persistent back pain due to verified disc herniation with clinically consistent exam findings, documented nerve impingements amenable to surgical release, or severe joint disease amenable to surgical repair or joint replacement.

But how should the practitioner approach the more common scenario, where their patient has chronic pain with no clearly identifiable lesion to fix, or their pain seems more widespread, out of proportion, or otherwise not correlating with or lasting longer than expected for any "nociceptive generator lesions" found? This scenario of chronic pain is common and increasing in prevalence, places an enormous burden on healthcare resources, is responsible for major loss of work productivity, causes untold misery to the patient, increases risk of many other chronic diseases, disrupts family and social life, and is a major driver of the opioid epidemic.

SCOPE

This appendix does not address specific issues in some important pain syndromes such as sickle cell anemia and chronic pancreatitis, nor does it specifically address palliative and end-of-life care issues (see Chapter 5, End of Life). While many of the principles reviewed here can be generalized to other chronic pain situations, the reader is encouraged to review standard resources for specific aspects of treating entities not addressed here.

KEY PRINCIPLES

Chronic pain is defined as pain persisting beyond the period of healing of the damaged tissues (sometimes arbitrarily set as >3 months). Much of nonspecific chronic pain is caused by alterations in the "psycho-neuro pain processing system" rather than solely or mainly due to persistent nociceptive input from a peripheral lesion. This type of chronic pain is believed to be a maladaptive psychophysiologic response. The pain processing neural networks get into a vicious cycle of danger-alarm triggering and facilitation leading to pain generation and hypersensitivity.[1,2] It is possible and common for the CNS pain processing neural networks to "learn" to manufacture pain with no actual nociceptive input from peripheral tissues, or to magnify any such nociceptive input to worsen pain. This pain is just as "real" as tissue injury–related pain. The patient's experience of pain produced by this subconscious psychophysiologic mechanism appears to be indistinguishable from pain due to a peripheral lesion; thus, misattribution of the source of pain is common, and it is critical to assess to effectively treat it. It is likely that much of the chronic pain syndromes seen in primary care are primarily due to this "psychophysiologic disorder" (PPD), also known by many other names such as mind/body and tension myositis syndrome.[1] These include the majority of chronic headache, neck, back, pelvic, abdominal pains, fibromyalgia, and related syndromes such as irritable bowel syndrome (IBS) and interstitial cystitis.[1,2] Fortunately, these pain-manufacturing neural networks can also be unlearned.[1-5] In addition, chronic inflammation, either in peripheral tissues or in the pain neurologic circuits themselves, may worsen pain hypersensitivity.[6,7] Chronic pain is not just longer-duration acute pain; therefore, its treatment is different from acute pain.

Figure B-1 displays possible risk and healing factors for chronic pain. Level of evidence varies widely for these, and proof of causality is sparse. For example, there is significant circumstantial evidence that poor diet increases inflammation and chronic pain, but outcomes research directly testing the effects of healthy nutrition on chronic pain is scant.

POTENTIAL RISK FACTORS FOR DERANGEMENT OF PAIN PROCESSING AND CHRONIC PAIN

- **Deficiencies/imbalances in the biochemical substrates** required for proper pain processing tend to increase chronic pain. Examples include vitamin D, magnesium, omega-3 fatty acid, and antioxidant deficiencies.
- **Any cause of excess inflammation**, especially increased inflammation of the central nervous system (CNS), tends to increase chronic pain. Common causes are poor nutrition, poor sleep, high stress, chronic inflammatory diseases, and some medications (possibly including opioids in some instances).[6-8]
- **Neuromuscular deconditioning and imbalances** lead to myofascial and joint dysfunction and pain. Musculoskeletal sources of chronic pain require a careful evaluation and specific treatment as appropriate, including related trigger points (which are common but often ignored pain generators) and their deactivation via myofascial release techniques.
- **Emotional pain** that persists from any source is intricately related to and overlaps with CNS processing of physical pain and tends to increase chronic pain. Unresolved or excess stress, fear, anger, and their many variations such as anxiety, worry, panic, complicated grief and loss, resentment, cynicism, and negativity disturb the mind/body axis and manifest as or amplify chronic pain. Patients who have an over-conscientious, perfectionistic, or unassertive personality style or who are entangled in dysfunctional family, workplace, or community dynamics may be especially susceptible to this subconscious process, and these patients benefit greatly from guidance and support in processing and expressing unresolved emotions in a healthy manner. Chronic pain itself is a source of stress

and may be highly emotionally charged. This can lead to a vicious cycle of increasing pain, stress, and defensive emotions, which further amplifies pain. Escaping this cycle is a central goal of psychological and mindfulness-based therapies.[1,2]

- Those suffering from the stress and indignities of **socioeconomic inequalities and injustices** tend to have more chronic pain.
- Reducing the above risk factors (red side of **Figure B-1**) and supporting healing factors (green side) are foundational in treating patients with chronic pain.

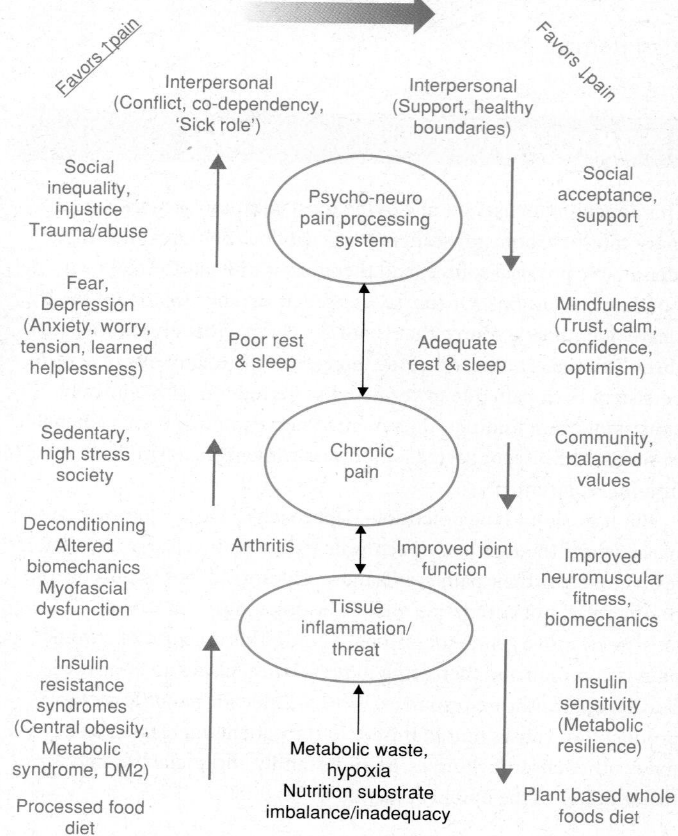

FIGURE B-1 Risk and healing factors for chronic pain.

FOUNDATIONS OF TREATMENT OF CHRONIC PAIN

- **Therapeutic alliance:** Chronic pain is complex—patients need a trusted ally to guide them. Schedule regular, longer visits (e.g., 30–45 minutes every month), use nonjudgmental empathic listening and support, and assemble a team to support the patient, including family/social/spiritual community. Prudently consult specialists, avoiding medical cascades of overtesting and overtreatments (see **Table B-1**). Physical and behavioral therapy is often key.
- **Education**: Accurate information empowers patients. Help patients understand that nonspecific chronic pain (i.e., after tissue healing is complete) is largely a disorder of the pain processing system, not just longer-lasting acute pain. Many patients are misinformed on the nature of their chronic pain, so this *reframing* may take some patience and repetition. Introduce one key element at a time to teach patients the following during their rehabilitation:
  - ***Patience:*** In initial stages of recovery even light movement or exercise can be painful, and misunderstood by the patient as harmful. To that extent, the patient's sensitized nervous system sets pain thresholds very low and does not accurately sense actual threats to tissue damage.
  - ***Pain spread is a false signal:*** There are no segregated parts of the nervous system, so more and more of the network may begin to participate in a persistent pain experience. As a result, the patient may feel as if the pain is spreading to other body parts. Knowing that pain spread is not caused by further tissue damage is very helpful in reducing fear, catastrophizing, and hypervigilance. Patients may need to challenge psychophysiologic pain triggers (such as a negative attitude toward a life disappointment) to overcome them, at the same time avoiding nociceptive triggers (such as overuse of an arthritic joint).
  - ***Pain may worsen but the patient is still safe:*** A sensitized nervous system may increase its warning in a misguided effort to stay safe. It is often helpful to teach a patient to "talk to" his or her nervous system, saying things like "thanks for the warning, but I'm okay." This is a primary form of reframing pain signals. At the same time, pacing so as to not overload a sensitized neuromuscular system is important.
  - ***Accept pain unpredictability***—Because of the myriad ways in which thoughts, emotions, and activities sum to create pain experiences, teach your patient to practice self-awareness of their emotional triggers, at the same time not dwelling on why their pain flared on any given day. Encourage maintaining reasonable activity. Teach patients to allow pain to arise and pass without strong emotion. Rather than feeling compelled to figure it out or

TABLE B-1 Mind/Body Therapies with Evidence of Efficacy

Finding a Qualified Practitioner/Credible Certification	Comments and Resources[a]
Cognitive Behavioral Therapy (CBT) and Variants	
Doctorate in psychology or Masters in Social Work	Well-studied. Good choice if there are psychological issues related to pain, such as distorted thoughts or "somatic symptom disorder." Requires professional intervention. Cochrane review: small benefit on treating chronic pain based on 40 studies.
Hypnosis/Guided Imagery	
American Society of Clinical Hypnosis	Well-studied. Requires ability to focus and imagine. Guided imagery is especially suited for creative patients. Often combined with other modalities such as music, progressive muscle relaxation. Effective as adjunct for cancer pain, low back pain, arthritis, temporal mandibular joint syndrome, and fibromyalgia. Gut-focused hypnotherapy is effective for irritable bowel syndrome-related pain. A useful resource for buying hypnosis materials is https://store.cdbaby.com/all/stevengurgevich.
Relaxation (e.g., progressive relaxation, autogenics, breath work)	
Doctorate in psychology or master's in social work and others	Simple, many self-help downloads. Providers can teach Yogic breathing and other simple relaxation techniques to patients in the office. See resources at www.integrativemedsource.com.
Biofeedback (skin conductance, thermal, heart rate variability, electromyogram QEEG, others)	
Biofeedback Certification Institute of America and others	Well-studied with wide applications. Especially effective for headaches and chronic myofascial neck and back pain. Can be a helpful "bridge" to mind/body connection.
Meditation/Mindfulness–Based Stress Reduction (MBSR) and variants	
MBSR and similar certifications	**MBSR** well studied in many chronic pain situations. Especially helpful in fibromyalgia spectrum and to enhance quality of life. Many schools of meditation, such as transcendental meditation, Zen. **Mindfulness-Oriented Recovery Enhancement** (MORE) Combines cognitive behavioral therapy, mindfulness, and positive psychology. Demonstrates moderate reductions in pain severity, functional interference.
Touch Therapies including therapeutic touch, Reiki, Shiatsu, and polarity therapy	
Choose experienced practitioner with good reputation	Level of experience of Reiki practitioners correlates with efficacy. Most of these are well suited to elderly patients. There are many schools and certifications that are not well standardized for most.
Mind/Body Integration Modalities (Hakomi, somatics, Feldenkrais, Alexander technique, Trager, among others)	
Hakomi therapy hakomiinstitute.com Hanna Somatics: www.hannasomatics.com Feldenkrais Institute www.feldenkrais.com/fgna U.S. Trager Association www.tragerus.org Am. Center for Alexander tech. https://www.amsatonline.org	Hakomi Mindfulness-Centered Somatic Psychotherapy is a relatively new form of therapy that accesses body (somatic) experience as part of the therapeutic process. Feldenkrais, Somatics, Alexander technique, and Trager are mind/body integrative modalities. Preliminary studies on these mind/body therapies suggest benefit. These gentle, safe modalities may be especially useful in cases of habitual and problematic muscular tension, posture or movement patterns. Requires ability to focus and maintain attention, though Trager less so.
Music Therapy	
Certification Board for Music Therapists	Preliminary studies. Effective in reducing discomfort in end-of-life care, ICU ventilated patients. Generally used combined with other modalities.
Meditative Movement Therapies (Yoga, Tai Chi, Chi Kung)	
Many schools. Choose experienced teacher with good reputation	Well studied. Gentler forms more appropriate for frail, elderly (e.g., gentle yoga, tai chi). Tai chi also has strong evidence for reducing fall risk in elderly.

[a]See references 11–15 for more details and supportive evidence.
*An inexpensive approach is daily use of app such as *Headspace or Calm. Headspace* (https://www.headspace.com) has a 30-session chronic pain packet that this author found useful for patients with chronic pain. Affective Self-Awareness program (https://www.unlearnyourpain.com) can be especially helpful for patients with fibromyalgia and other psycho-physiologic disorders.

heal it in the moment, learn to manage reactions to it. Dwelling on pain worsens it; developing and attending to larger fields of meaningful experience reduces it.
- ***Movement is healing*** (see below).
- ***Emphasize mindful use of language*** by both patient and clinician—use positive language such as "can", "will" rather than negative or unsure language such as "try". Language has powerful influence in clinical outcomes.
- ***Set therapeutic, verifiable goals focusing on improving psychosocial, physical, work function.*** Examples: increase walking distance from 10 to 11 blocks over the next 2 weeks, as evidenced by pedometer reading.

SUPPORT "PILLARS OF HEALTH"

- **Optimize nutrition:** Imbalance malnutrition leads to altered GI microbiome and function, chronic inflammation, and associated visceral or central obesity with metabolic syndrome or type 2 diabetes and possibly worsened pain hypersensitivity, all of which can increase chronic pain. Plant-based whole-foods diet, cultured foods (e.g., yoghurt, kefir) and weight loss may improve these issues and thus indirectly help healthier pain processing. Gastrointestinal disrupting factors to address include poor diet; medications such as proton pump inhibitors and opioids (alter digestive function and gut microbiome), antibiotics (alter gut microbiome), corticosteroids, infections and parasites, food intolerances and allergies.[9,10]
  - Nutrition can be optimized through a nutritionist referral (at least 6 visits are often needed) or managed within the office team. A simple aid to nutrition management is using "My Healthy Plate," shown in **Figure B-2** (1/2 plate of mostly vegetables/some whole fruit [eat "rainbow of colors"]; 1/4 healthy protein such as soy, beans, fish, lean poultry; 1/4 healthy carbohydrates such as whole grains [as opposed to flour products like bread]). This proportioning during main meals will solve many nutritional issues. For details and different ethnic variations, go to: https://www.institute.org/health-care/services/diabetes-care/healthyplates/. Supplements can be added if needed to ensure adequate intake of vitamins and minerals.
- **Encourage stress management to improve coping skills and mind/body integration:** Stress and mood disturbances increase pain. Relaxation and coping improve pain.[8] Assess the patient for significant comorbid emotional/mood disorders and, if meeting the diagnostic criteria, consider psychotherapy or medication. For all patients with chronic pain, facilitate psychosocial support.
- Motivational interviewing is also a useful tool. Match stress management/mind-body program to the needs of the patient, given logistics and local resources (**Table B-1**). Mind/body therapies help many chronic pain syndromes, especially fibromyalgia spectrum and similar disorders. Daily practice is likely as important as the method chosen.
- **Encourage safe and graded movement and fitness:** Conditioning improves fitness, healthy neuroplasticity, builds "neuromuscular resilience" to pain, and improves mood, confidence, and morale.[11-16] There are many options including physical therapy (PT), home rehabilitation, and meditative movement therapies (see **Table B-1**). Reconditioning requires thoughtful planning and consistent, skillful execution.
- **Correct anatomic malalignment** (which as a result of altered biomechanics from trauma, compensation, overuse or deconditioning may, over time, lead to physiologic dysfunction, including edema and inflammation). This somatic dysfunction may be treated using both exercise and manipulation. Sports medicine, Physical Medicine and Rehabilitation, or an orthopedic physician or physical therapist can assist in this.
- **Functional fitness evaluation & goal setting:** Assess level of fitness, hobbies, and leisure activities that are meaningful and fun for the patient. The best exercise is the one the patient will do consistently. Progress slowly if there is a high degree of irritability—increase duration first, then reps, and finally intensity. Generally a chronic pain/rheumatologic patient can find a balance among these three variables that allows for 30 minutes of exercise per day, 3 to 5 times per week. Such a program should help with pain reduction while increasing their tissue fitness. A major goal is to reverse the downward spiral of pain → fear of movement → deconditioning → pain & disturbed mood. Ideally includes aerobics, strengthening, neuromuscular control, stretching, mind/body integration, though may have to start very modestly. Have the patient set realistic functional goals to meet for next visit .
- **Promote adequate rest and sleep:** Insomnia can worsen pain, and adequate rest can reduce chronic pain. Assess the patient for obstructive sleep apnea and other sleep disorders and educate in good sleep hygiene. The best evidence for improving sleep in patients with insomnia is through use of cognitive behavioral therapy (CBT), stimulus control therapy, relaxation training, and sleep restriction (see resources at www.IntegrativeMedSource.com).

Figure B-3 displays an overview of how to incorporate these approaches into the practical clinical care of a patient with chronic pain. **Figure B-4** summarizes common "vicious cycles" that can exacerbate chronic pain and how to help patients escape them.

PHARMACEUTICALS FOR CHRONIC PAIN

Often as a treatment program begins, immediate pain control is needed to ease suffering and to allow the patient enough relief and free sufficient psychic (emotional) energy to devote him/herself to the usually more labor-intensive integrative approaches. Sometimes, integrative approaches cannot resolve chronic pain completely, so medication may be needed long-term.

1. **Acetaminophen** use has shown only limited efficacy in most chronic pain scenarios. Use caution to avoid exceeding maximum from all sources (1 g as a single dose or 4 g daily).
2. **NSAIDs**
   - Topical NSAIDs are best tried first when used for chronic musculoskeletal pain because of fewer gastrointestinal and other systemic side effects, although their efficacy is also limited.
   - Avoid systemic NSAIDs as first-line chronic treatment whenever possible, because of their potential GI, renal, and cardiovascular toxicities. However, they are useful for short-term treatment of pain flares. If one does not work well, try switching NSAID classes.

3. **Tramadol**
   - Weak activity at mu (opioid) receptors and some inhibition of serotonin and norepinephrine uptake. Similar side-effect profile to mild opioids; moderate efficacy in neuropathic and fibromyalgia pain.
   - Has multiple drug interactions. Decreases the seizure threshold, especially when used with neuroleptics and antidepressants. Potential for substance abuse, so use sparingly for flares rather than chronically for most patients.
4. **Opioids**
   - Very effective for acute, severe pain; however, there is little evidence of efficacy in most non-cancer chronic pain.[17-20] Chronic pain is not satisfactorily managed with opioids because opioids do not treat the peripheral and central sensitization or psychophysiologic disorder found in many chronic pain situations. Opioids can worsen neuroinflammation via glial activation, which may worsen chronic pain.[6,7] In fact, long-term opioid

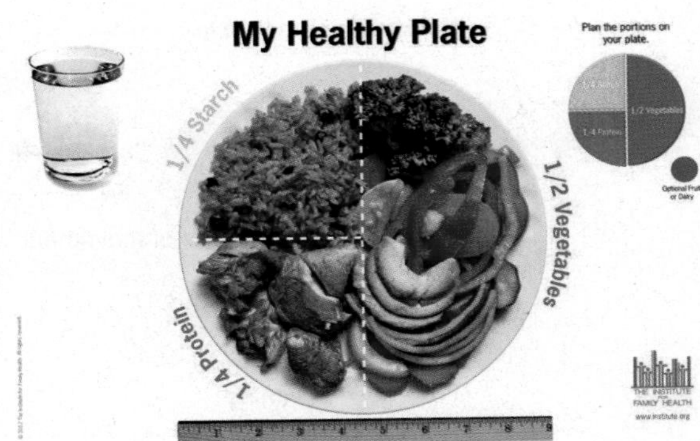

FIGURE B-2 My Plate healthy eating diagram. (*Reproduced with permission from The Institute for Family Health™. Copyright 2010–2018. All rights reserved.*)

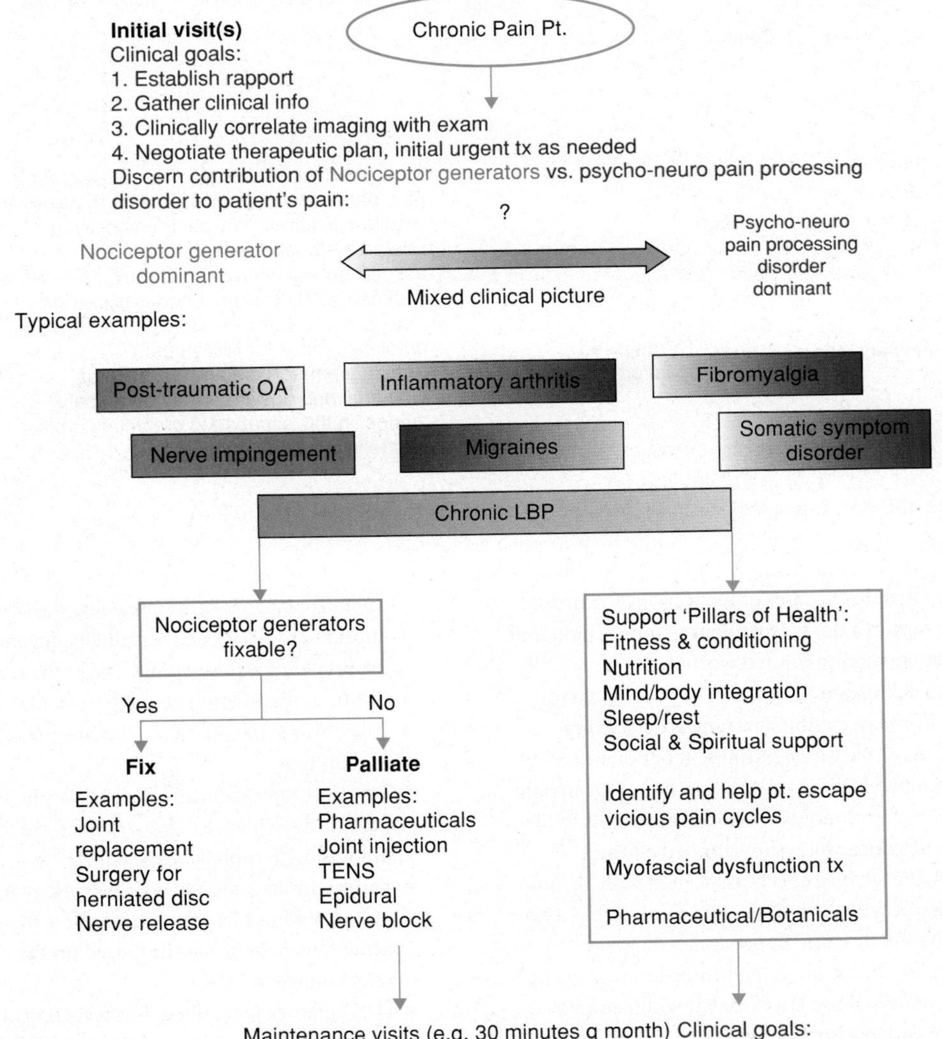

FIGURE B-3 Chronic pain evaluation and treatment algorithm.

Neuromuscular cycle

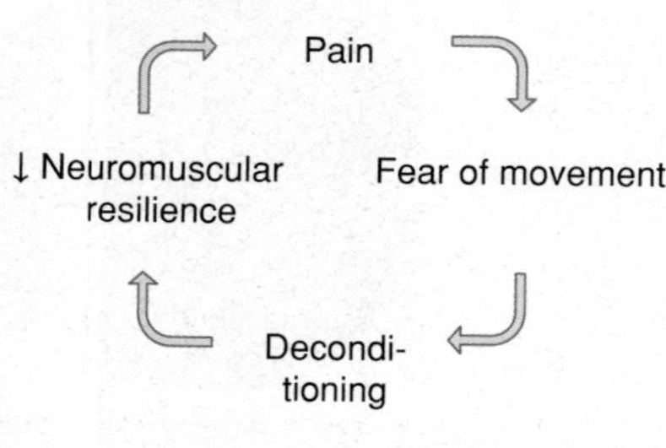

Encourage movement starting at a comfortable level and slowly build. If movement hurts too much, limiting progress, try improving other spheres first such as sleep, nutrition, and mood, which will allow the patient to exercise more

Emotional cycle

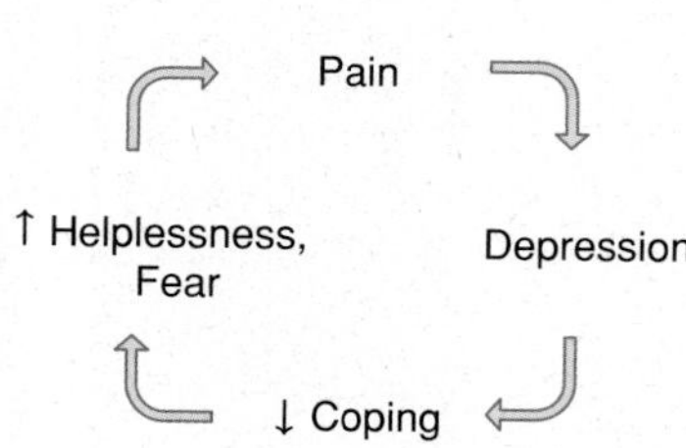

Evaluate for past trauma causing subconscious pain triggers and assist patient to overcome these (a good website is https://www.unlearnyourpain.com). Treat depression. Medications such as duloxetine also help pain. S- adenosylmethionine may help both depression and arthritis. Gradual but consistent increases in movement and activities of daily living can improve morale

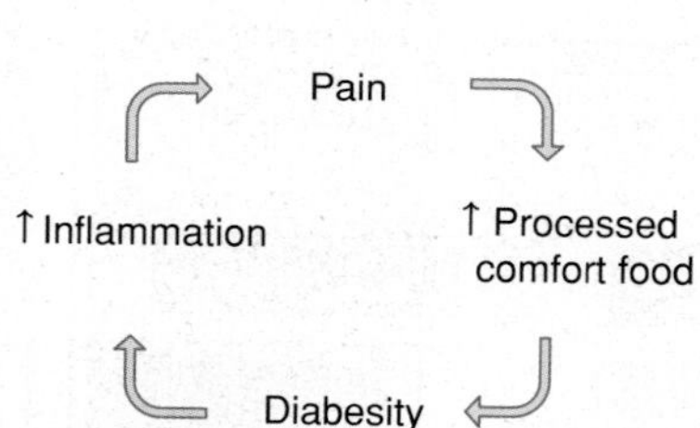

Processed foods are tempting to the chronic pain patient who is seeking comfort, however resultant inflammatory central obesity and related metabolic derangements are associated with increased chronic pain. While avoiding perfectionism, encourage healthy regular meals (see 'My Healthy Plate' in nutrition section for first steps). Anti-inflammatory botanicals, such as curcumin and boswellia may be a useful 'bridge' in this situation to break this cycle and relieve pain

FIGURE B-4 Examples of vicious cycles and solutions in chronic pain.

therapy is associated with lower rates of recovery from chronic pain and return to work in a dose-dependent manner compared to non-opioid treatment among injured workers.[21]

- Studies suggest that a significant proportion of patients taking prescription opioids for pain exhibit aberrant drug-seeking behavior/addiction. In primary care settings, about one-third of patients will likely exhibit aberrant use, and perhaps 5% outright addiction. Unfortunately, commonly used screening tools to identify those at risk for substance abuse show limited efficacy.[18,19]
- There are several notable adverse effects associated with chronic opioid use. Opiate use of >50 morphine equivalent dose is associated with double the fracture rate in patients >60 years.[22] Hypogonadism is especially common in chronic long-acting opioid use. In addition, maternal use is associated with neonatal abstinence syndrome and low birth weight.
- Avoid opioids in the following situations:
  - When under emotional/situational/time pressure to prescribe them, including "inheriting" a patient on opioids for unclear or dubious reasons. Rather, reassess the situation first. If a patient appears physically or emotionally dependent or is taking inappropriate high-dose opioids, refer them to specialists for detoxification or addiction recovery services.
  - Any chronic pain patient who likely has PPD as a main driver of their pain[1,2]
  - For most typical chronic low-back, hip, or knee osteoarthritis pain (little evidence of better effectiveness compared to non-opioids, with more adverse effects[20])
  - During initial visits with a new patient with chronic pain, opioids should not be prescribed unless there is genuine, verifiable acute, severe pain superimposed on the chronic pain (e.g., new crush injury to foot).
  - If opioids are prescribed, the best clinical practice is to be sure that the patient is showing clear, robust, and broad benefit (i.e., better pain, mood, and physical and social function) from an initial opioid trial before proceeding to long-term opioid therapy. Use state monitoring sites and CDC guidelines[17]

(https://www.cdc.gov/drugoverdose/prescribing/guideline.html).

5. **Antiepileptics** are mainly used for neuropathic pain. Monitor for fatigue, dizziness, and depression. Examples include gabapentin, pregabalin, and carbamazepine.
6. **Antidepressants** have some efficacy in treating neuropathic and fibromyalgia-related pain.
   - Tricyclic antidepressants such as amitriptyline (start at 10 mg nightly and slowly titrate as needed) can be used for patients with insomnia, especially in fibromyalgia and various neuropathic syndromes.
   - SNRIs (selective serotonin norepinephrine reuptake inhibitors)—Helpful for neuropathic pain, depression/anxiety, fibromyalgia, and chronic musculoskeletal pain. Examples with approval for pain syndromes include duloxetine (e.g., titrated to 60 mg daily) and milnacipran (titrated to 50 mg 2×/day; approved for fibromyalgia by the U.S. Food and Drug Administration [FDA]).
   - Other agents such as selective serotonin reuptake inhibitors (SSRIs) less studied for chronic pain but may occasionally be useful.
7. **Muscle relaxants** tend to have a narrow therapeutic window and modest benefit. May be most useful for sleep, although these agents may disturb sleep architecture. Examples include baclofen and cyclobenzaprine.

Topicals can be used in various musculoskeletal pain syndromes. Agents include lidocaine patches, capsaicin, NSAID topicals such as diclofenac gel, or as compounded mixtures (e.g., gabapentin, ketoprofen, ketamine, amitriptyline).

SELECT NATURAL MEDICINES USEFUL IN TREATING CHRONIC PAIN

1. **Overview**—Brief highlights of some commonly used natural medicines are listed here (refer to standard references for full details such as National Center for Complementary and Integrative Health, Natural Medicines database, and ConsumerLabs.com). Just like pharmaceuticals, avoid in pregnancy, lactation, infants/young children, and severe liver/kidney disease unless clear evidence of safety and benefit. Because of less FDA monitoring, the quality of supplements is variable; therefore, guide patients on specific reputable brands (can use ConsumerLabs.com) and focus on natural medicines supported by clinical trials.
2. **Glucosamine sulfate (GS)/chondroitin sulfate (CS)**—Efficacy is controversial; likely modest at best for osteoarthritis, but may be worth a 3-month trial. Unclear if sulfate form is better than HCl salt. Generally well tolerated.
   a. **Dose GS/CS**: 1500/1200 mg daily
3. **Curcumin**—Potent anti-inflammatory and antioxidant derived from the spice turmeric. Use only highly bioavailable curcumin for systemic indications, because little is absorbed otherwise. Multiple small randomized controlled trials (RCTs) (mid-level evidence) support efficacy in knee osteoarthritis. Preliminary evidence that curcumin benefits a multitude of other inflammatory conditions.[23]
   a. **Dose**—Generally follow serving size of individual brand products. Typical dose for plain curcumin for arthritis is 500 mg 3×/day with healthy fat and black pepper. Generally is well tolerated.
   b. **Cautions/avoid if**—On blood thinners, history of biliary colic or calcium oxalate kidney stones, on hypoglycemic meds (may further lower blood sugar), on critical drugs metabolized by the P450 3A system such as tacrolimus. Monitor iron levels in those deficient or with marginal stores and take curcumin at a different time than iron supplements. Bioperine theoretically could alter some drug levels, so if part of the curcumin complex, may be best to take at a different time than other meds.
4. ***Boswellia serrata*** (frankincense)—Ayurvedic botanical used for millennia to reduce inflammation. Preliminary RCTs suggest benefit for OA and rheumatoid arthritis (mixed results), as well as several other inflammatory conditions. Often combined with other botanicals to enhance efficacy.
   a. **Dose**—300–1200 mg three times daily of *Boswellia* extract standardized to contain 37.5%–65% boswellic acid. Start with lower dose and titrate upward. Take *Boswellia* with a fatty meal to enhance absorption.
   b. **Adverse effects**—Generally well tolerated. GI upset occasionally.
   c. **Contraindications/cautions**—Avoid in pregnancy (lack of studies).
   d. **Interactions**—No major interactions known.
5. **S-Adenosylmethionine (SAMe):** Many chronic pain patients also suffer from depression. SAMe is a natural substance that is synthesized in and supports the liver, supports neurotransmitter metabolism, with antidepressant (preliminary evidence) as well as analgesic, anti-inflammatory properties equivalent to NSAIDs in some RCTs. May stimulate cartilage growth helpful for joint support (preliminary evidence), with studies showing benefit for OA (moderate evidence) of knee, hip, hand, and spine and fibromyalgia (preliminary evidence).[24] It is expensive and sensitive to heat, moisture and stomach acid, so only use enteric-coated in blister packs. Uses folate, B_{12}, B_6 as cofactors—consider supplementing these if marginal nutritional status.
   a. **Doses** shown to be effective in clinical trials (these are all for the actual active SAMe component taken orally and are higher than what is often listed on the bottle) for OA: 800 to 1200 mg/day divided 2–3×/day.[4] For depression: 400–1600 mg/day in divided doses. For fibromyalgia: 800 mg/day. It can take a few weeks for SAMe to reach its full effect.
   b. **Adverse effects** of SAMe are generally minimal, but at higher doses can get GI upset, headache, agitation. Avoid taking in evening if insomnia is an issue. Does not cause weight gain or sex dysfunction.
   c. **Contraindications**—Bipolar (because it could trigger a manic phase)
   d. **Interactions** with SAMe appear to be few. Levodopa (L-dopa) used in Parkinson disease treatment may deplete brain SAMe levels, thus supplementation may improve depression. SAMe might decrease L-dopa effectiveness.

See www.integrativemedsource.com for further resources.

CLINICAL TREATMENT SUMMARIES FOR COMMON NON-CANCER CHRONIC PAIN SYNDROMES

Most patients with chronic pain will benefit from the foundational approaches listed above, wisely chosen based on individual clinical context and need. For specific syndromes, **Table B-2** highlights treatment approaches and modalities that may be helpful (assuming typical presentations with no alarm findings on clinical evaluation). For any musculoskeletal disorder, such as chronic low back, neck, or shoulder pain and OA, always correlate clinical exam findings with imaging, because severity of imaging findings generally has poor correlation with severity of chronic pain.

SUMMARY

Reductionistic solutions work for reductionistic problems, such as hip replacement for severe hip OA. However, the majority of chronic pain patients have a complex web of factors that resist simple solutions, often leading to disordered pain processing on multiple levels. Therefore, the main focus in treating chronic pain, in addition to fixing or palliating any identifiable nociceptive generators, is healing the causes of pain hypersensitivity on multiple levels—community/interpersonal, emotional/energetic, nutritional/metabolic, central and peripheral nervous system hypersensitivity, myofascial—all these levels ultimately may need treatment for an optimal outcome. Many chronic pain patients have at least an element of PPD and benefit from "unlearning" their pain-producing or pain-amplifying neural networks. Treating chronic pain as if it is a simple peripheral nociceptive phenomenon—that is, only with pain pills—is usually ineffective and often creates more problems than it solves. This integrative treatment process must be done with great compassion, tact, and patience, starting by meeting the patient where they are and celebrating small steps of success. It requires a keen, often intuitive sense of what factors are the highest priorities to address in an individual patient—what is within their ability to accomplish, and most likely to yield benefit—using as a "map" the plan presented in this appendix. It often requires months of work, with the patient leading the way under the guidance and coaching of their physician and team. Set expectations accordingly. Even if pain is not completely resolved, this approach may be more economical and effective than pharmaceutical-centered approaches[25] and can be deeply rewarding—a liberation of the patient from the shackles of debilitating chronic pain.

TABLE B-2 Treatment Approaches for Chronic Pain

First-Line Treatments	Second-/Third-Line Treatments	Comments and Resources
Chronic Low Back Pain (CLBP)		
Education on self-care including staying active as tolerated, safe exercise, posture, ergonomics, limit sitting to 30 minutes at a time. Somatics and other mind/body treatments If suffers from psychophysiologic disorder (PPD), then individualized treatment program** **Psychotherapies,** such as CBT or Emotional Awareness & Expression Training (EAET), others **Non-opioid analgesics** such as NSAIDs, curcumin **Manual therapies:** massage (short-term benefits) or manipulation (modest short-term benefits) **Acupuncture** (moderate benefits <3 months)	**SNRI** such as duloxetine (modest benefit) **Tramadol** to treat flares if not responsive to first-line treatments **Gabapentinoids** (gabapentin or pregabalin) not shown effective for *nonspecific* CLBP. Improvements for radicular symptoms are small **Non-benzodiazepine muscle relaxants** (e.g., cyclobenzaprine) for flares. Avoid long-term use because of narrow therapeutic window and side effects **Spine interventional modalities** in carefully selected patients (e.g., epidural glucocorticoids in persistent radiculopathy); no evidence supporting epidural steroid injections in nonspecific CLBP or acute lumbosacral radiculopathy or spinal stenosis **Surgery** if lumbar disc prolapse radiculopathy with severe or progressive neurologic deficits or other serious lesions.	**Differentiate subtypes of CLBP to ensure proper treatment.*** Avoid diagnosis and treatment of CLBP solely by imaging Sparse evidence of efficacy for most modalities overall, therefore use most benign modalities first. Emphasize activity as tolerated, modalities such as yoga, tai chi; mindfulness-based stress reduction, other relaxation techniques **Avoid benzodiazepines** in almost all cases of CLBP, due to their strong addictive potential and side effects **Avoid chronic opioids** in most cases of CLBP, as there is little evidence of efficacy and much potential harm. **Refer intractable severe CLBP** cases to a multi-disciplinary pain center
Chronic Neck Pain		
Individualized treatment program if PPD.** Posture, ergonomics, neck pillow; limit sitting to 30 minutes at a time; gentle exercise; qigong/tai chi; PT; gentle neck mobilization; NSAIDs or botanical analgesics	If symptoms persist, trials of trigger point injections, acupuncture, TENS If severe facet joint symptoms, trial of cervical medial branch blocks or percutaneous radiofrequency neurotomy Surgery if alarm or significant neurological symptoms	Conservative treatment is adequate in majority of cases Avoid prolonged use of cervical collars

TABLE B-2 Treatment Approaches for Chronic Pain (*Continued*)

First-Line Treatments	Second-/Third-Line Treatments	Comments and Resources
Osteoarthritis		
Exercise: aerobic and strengthening (strong evidence of benefit) **Non-opioid analgesics:** start with topical NSAIDs, capsaicin or oral botanicals such as curcumin **Acupuncture:** moderate benefits (conflicting evidence) **Walking and other aids** **Psychological support/therapy**	**Oral NSAIDs**, especially for flares **Supplements:** Glucosamine/ chondroitin sulfate (not HCl form), avocado soybean unsaponifiables (ASU), SAMe (*S*-adeno-syl-methionine; also may help mood) may be worth a 3-month trial **Surgical options if severe:** Joint replacement effective No evidence of benefit for arthroscopic knee surgery	**Treat related regional myofascial dysfunction** with myofascial release or dry needling techniques **Limit steroid injections**, perhaps maximum of 4 injections per joint per lifetime (overuse associated with cartilage thinning) Intra-articular hyaluronic acid may have small benefit (controversial)
Shoulder Pain (e.g., impingement, rotator cuff pathology, frozen shoulder)		
PT tailored to problem or home rehabilitation Individualized treatment program if PPD.**	**Steroid injections** if severe pain may be of short-term benefit and help patients succeed at PT **Surgery** may be indicated in rotator cuff severe tears or recalcitrant frozen shoulder	PT guided by diagnosis is key and will help resolve majority of shoulder pain syndromes Consider addressing "pain body memories" with mind/body therapies such as somatics and psychotherapies
Myofascial Dysfunction		
Individualized treatment program if PPD.** Emphasize self-management programs including self-help guides for de-activation of trigger points	Practitioner-dependent myofascial release techniques (e.g., strain-counterstrain, muscle energy, dry needling, manipulation)	Research is sparse. Individualize modalities to needs of patient. Adequate sleep, exercise, posture and mental health are key Treat underlying cause if possible
Fibromyalgia		
Individualized treatment program for PPD.** **Education, "Pillars of Health"** (see above)—key aspects include reducing stress, improving mood and sleep hygiene, creative outlets and adequate self-care. Empathic listening and affirmation through regular visits **CBT, EAET, other psychotherapies** **Graded exercise** (especially water based) **Mind/body:** Yoga, tai chi, biofeedback, daily meditation **Optimize nutrition**: Vitamin D; avoid excitotoxins like MSG, aspartame	**Medications** have only modest benefit, often used in combination (e.g., SNRIs, amitriptyline, and/or pregabalin) **Acupuncture** may be helpful (limited evidence) Less researched options include low-dose naltrexone, memantine, cannabinoids, and anti-inflammatory botanicals such as turmeric, ginger (weak evidence) Treat comorbidities such as depression	**Foundational and multidisciplinary approaches** are key NSAIDs generally are not helpful in fibromyalgia Opioids should be avoided. Tramadol can be used for severe flares (avoid chronic use) For difficult cases, consultation with fibromyalgia expert/multidisciplinary team. Pain clinics that focus on interventions without a well-rounded psychological/mind/body approach are generally not very helpful
Headache (e.g., chronic migraine, tension, chronic daily headache)		
Individualized treatment program if PPD.** **Behavioral self-management** including stress reduction, relaxation, biofeedback, posture, ergonomics **Focus on preventive measures and medication while minimizing acute medications** (can lead to chronic daily headache)	**Migraine preventive therapies:** **Natural agents:** *Petasites hybridus* (butterbur; Petadolex is a good brand), magnesium, riboflavin, CoQ10 **Pharmaceuticals:** beta blockers (e.g., metoprolol, propranolol), calcium blockers (e.g., verapamil), amitriptyline, topiramate, botulinum toxin type A injections **Acupuncture, myofascial release** (limited evidence)	**Focus on Pillars of Health and search for and treat common comorbidities** (depression, anxiety, insomnia, IBS) Many patients with chronic headache are medication sensitive—**start low, titrate up slowly** **Avoid opioids and barbiturates** in most chronic headache syndromes

(*continued*)

TABLE B-2 Treatment Approaches for Chronic Pain (*Continued*)

First-Line Treatments	Second-/Third-Line Treatments	Comments and Resources
Trial avoiding common diet triggers (e.g., caffeine, chocolate, cheese, citrus, red wine) **Trial of oligoantigenic diet** may reduce migraine frequency	**Calcitonin Gene Related Peptide monoclonal Ab** may improve migraine frequency and severity, sometimes with prolonged remission (see Schulte, 2015 doi: 10.1016/S1474-4422(14)70295-9).	
TMJ Syndrome		
Individualized treatment program if PPD.** **Stress reduction**, relaxation **Occlusal splint**, exercises if bruxism	**NSAIDs, muscle relaxants** for flares Consider surgery in severe, recalcitrant cases	Rule out serious dental causes
Irritable Bowel Syndrome (IBS)		
Psychosocial support, gut-focused hypnotherapy (www.healingwithhypnosis.com) **Nutritionist referral for trial of low FODMAP, traditional IBS or elimination diet**. Non-celiac gluten sensitivity may be a fructans sensitivity, avoidance of which improves symptoms	In constipation predominant (**IBS-C**): psyllium or polyethylene glycol (PEG) or other osmotic laxatives, other agents if refractory **Enteric-coated peppermint** or antispasmodics for bowel cramps **IBS-D**: Antidiarrheals, tricyclics	**Doctor–patient relationship is key** Consider **screening for SIBO** with a carbohydrate breath test in patients with prominent bloating, gas and watery diarrhea **Avoid benzodiazepines** Severe IBS with bloating/loose stool—consider trial of **rifaximin** if suspecting gut dysbiosis, then replace with healthy gut bacteria via healthy diet, cultured foods/pre and probiotics
Chronic Neuropathic Pain		
First-line neuropathic pain medication: TCAs, gabapentin, pregabalin, SNRIs, topical lidocaine **For diabetes-related neuropathic pain: prevention** with anti-inflammatory low glycemic load diet and glycemic control **For post-herpetic neuralgia**: TCAs, gabapentin, pregabalin, SNRIs; if local, lidocaine patches, capsaicin **For trigeminal neuralgia**: carbamazepine or oxcarbazepine	**Prevention/early treatment:** alpha lipoic acid (conflicting evidence), gamma linolenic acid (e.g., evening primrose oil)	Combination of medications are often needed Low-dose opioids often added for severe neuropathic chronic pain

*A useful resource for differentiating types of chronic low back pain is *A System of Orthopaedic Medicine* by Ludwig Ombregt.
**A good website to support relearning pain producing/amplifying neural networks is https://www.unlearnyourpain.com + https://www.feldenkraisresources.com.
Abbreviations: CBT, cognitive behavioral therapy; EAET, Emotional Awareness and Expression Therapy; FODMAP, fermentable oligo-, di-, and monosaccharides and polyols; IBS, irritable bowel syndrome; NSAID, nonsteroidal anti-inflammatory drug; PPD, psychophysiologic disorder; PT, physical therapy; SIBO, small intestinal bowl overgrowth; SNRI, selective serotonin norepinephrine reuptake inhibitor; TCA, tricyclic antidepressant; TENS, transcutaneous electrical nerve stimulation.

REFERENCES

1. Sarno JE, Leonard-Segal A, Rashbaum I, et al. *The Divided Mind: The Epidemic of Mindbody Disorders.* New York, NY: Harper Perennial; 2006
2. Schubiner H. Emotional awareness of pain. In: Rakel D, ed. *Integrative Medicine*, 4th Ed. Philadelphia, PA: Elsevier Health Sciences; 2017.
3. Williams A, Eccleston C, Morley S. Psychological therapies for the management of chronic pain (excluding headache) in adults. *Cochrane Database Syst Rev.* 2012;(11):CD007407.
4. Nicholson RA, Buse DC, Andrasik F, Lipton RB. Nonpharmacologic treatments for migraine and tension-type headache: how to choose and when to use. *Curr Treat Options Neurol.* 2011;13(1): 28-40.
5. Dhanani NM, Caruso TJ, Carinci AJ. Complementary and alternative medicine for pain: an evidence-based review. *Curr Pain Headache Rep.* 2011;15(1):39-46.
6. Giron SE, Griffis CA, Burkard JF. Chronic pain and decreased opioid efficacy: an inflammatory link. *Pain Manag Nurs.* 2015; 16(5):819-831.
7. Ji RR, Berta T, Nedergaard T. Glia and pain: is chronic pain a gliopathy? *Pain.* 2013;154:S10-S28.
8. Boakye PA, Olechowski C, Rashiq S, et al. A critical review of neurobiological factors involved in the interactions between chronic pain, depression, and sleep disruption. *Clin J Pain.* 2016; 32:327-336.
9. Tick H. Nutrition and pain. *Phys Med Rehabil Clin N Am.* 2015; 26:309-320.
10. Narouze S, Souzdalnitski D. Obesity and chronic pain—systematic review of prevalence and implications for pain practice. *Reg Anesth Pain Med.* 2015;40(2):91-111.
11. Hall AM, Mather CG, Lam P, et al. Tai chi exercise for treatment of pain and disability in people with persistent low back pain: a randomized controlled trial. *Arthritis Care Res (Hoboken).* 2011; 63(11):1576-1583.
12. Wieland LS, Skoetz N, Pilkington K, et al. Yoga treatment for chronic non-specific low back pain. *Cochrane Database Syst Rev.* 2017(1):CD010671.
13. Elkins G, Jensen MP, Patterson DR. Hypnotherapy for the management of chronic pain. *Int J Clin Exp Hypnosis.* 2007;55(3): 275-287.
14. Posadzki P, Lewandowski W, Terry R, et al. Guided imagery for non-musculoskeletal pain: a systematic review of randomized clinical trials. *J Pain Symptom Manage.* 2012;44(1):95-104.
15. Posadzki P, Ernst E. Guided imagery for musculoskeletal pain: a systematic review. *Clin J Pain.* 2011;27(7):648-653.
16. Qaseem A, Wilt TJ, McLean RM; Clinical Guidelines Committee of the American College of Physicians. Noninvasive treatments for acute, subacute, and chronic low back pain: a clinical practice guideline from the American College of Physicians. *Ann Intern Med.* 2017;166:514-530.
17. Centers for Disease Control and Prevention. *CDC Guideline for Prescribing Opioids for Chronic Pain.* https://www.cdc.gov/drugoverdose/prescribing/guideline.html. Accessed September 2018.
18. Franklin GM. Opioids for chronic non-cancer pain. A position paper of the American Academy of Neurology. *Neurology.* 2014; 83:1277-1284.
19. Sullivan MD, Howe CQ. Opioid therapy for chronic pain in the United States: promises and perils. *Pain.* 2013;154:S94-S100.
20. Krebs EE, Gravely A, Nugent S, et al. Effect of opioid vs. non-opioid medications on pain-related function in patients with chronic back pain or hip or knee osteoarthritis pain. The SPACE Randomized Clinical Trial. *JAMA.* 2018;319(9):872-882.
21. Volinn E, Fargo JD, Fine PG. Opioid therapy for nonspecific low back pain and the outcome of chronic work loss. *Pain.* 2009; 142(3):194-201.
22. Saunders KW, Dunn KM, Merrill JO, et al. Relationship of opioid use and dosage levels to fractures in older chronic pain patients. *J Gen Intern Med.* 2010;25:310-315.
23. Perkins K, Sahy W, Beckett RD. Efficacy of curcuma for treatment of osteoarthritis. J *Evid Based Complementary Altern Med.* 2017; 22(1):156-165.
24. Natural Medicines Database, *Curcumin, Boswellia, S-Adenosyl-L-methionine.* https://naturalmedicines.therapeuticresearch.com/Login.aspx. Accessed September 2018.
25. Sundberg T, Petzold M, Kohls N, Falkenberg T. Opposite drug prescription and cost trajectories following integrative and conventional care for pain—a case-control study. *PLoS One.* 2014; 9(5):e96717.

Note: Tables, figures, and boxes are indicated by t, f, and b, respectively, following the page number.

A

Abacavir, cutaneous reactions, 1346–1357, 1355t
ABCDE (advance directives), 31, 32
ABCDE guidelines, melanoma, 1044, 1049, 1113–1114, 1113f, 1114f, 1117, 1118f
ABCD rule, melanoma, 1117, 1119
Abdominal circumference, fetal, on second trimester ultrasound, 488, 489f, 490
Abortion
  first trimester ultrasound, 484–486
  medical, 22
  patient education, 24
  surgical, 22
Abruptio placentae, ultrasound
  second trimester, 489
  third trimester, 493
Abscess, 771–775
  breast, 562–565
  peritonsillar, pharyngitis, 228
Absolute risk reduction, 1604
Abstinence, periodic sexual, 14, 15t
Abuse
  intimate partner, 102–106
  sexual, adult, 108–113
  substance abuse disorder, 1546–1551 (*See also specific drugs*)
Abuse, child
  physical, 90–94
  sexual, 96–100
Acantholysis, in pemphigus, 1229, 1230
Acanthosis nigricans, 1442–1445
  diabetes, 1433, 1434f
  obesity, 1442, 1443f, 1463, 1463f, 1464, 1465f
  skin tags, 1010, 1010f
Access, healthcare
  disabilities, 42–43, 42f
  improved, 41–43, 41f, 42f
  racism, 40
Acetaminophen, for chronic pain, 1610
Acetowhite changes, on colposcopy
  high-grade lesions, 550–551, 550f, 552f
  low-grade disease, 545–548
Acne, cystic, intralesional triamcinolone acetonide for, 685, 686f, 686t, 722, 723f
Acne, neonatal, 717, 718f
  benign cephalic pustolosis, 694–699, 694f
  true, 694, 696
Acne conglobata, 719, 719f–720f
Acne fulminans, 719, 720f
Acne inversa, 738–743
Acne keloidalis nuchae, 719, 721, 733–737, 733f–734f, 750, 751f, 752
  scarring alopecia, 1257t, 1258, 1259f
Acne rosacea, 725–731
Acne vulgaris, 717–724
Acquired immunodeficiency syndrome (AIDS), 28, 1419–1423. *See also* HIV/AIDS
Acquired vascular lesions, 1336–1340
Acral, 644
Acral lentiginous melanoma, 1114, 1116f, 1120, 1270–1274, 1270f
Acral nevi, benign, 1134, 1138f, 1139f
Acral skin, 1137f
Acrochordon, 1010–1013
  diabetes mellitus, 1010, 1010f, 1011, 1434f, 1443f, 1445, 1445f
  obesity, 1462, 1462f, 1577f
  preauricular, 205–208
  pregnancy, 473, 475
Acrodermatitis enteropathica, 714, 714f
  zinc deficiency, 59–60, 60f
Acrolentiginous melanoma. *See also* Melanoma
  dermoscopy, 1134, 1138f–1140f, 1140
Acromegaly, 1493–1496
Acromioclavicular separation, 614, 614f, 614t
Acropustulosis, 708–710
  of infancy, 1218
Actinic cheilitis, 1072–1077, 1072f
Actinic comedones, 721, 721f
Actinic elastosis, 1064–1069
Actinic keratosis, 656, 661t, 662t, 1072–1077
  squamous cell carcinoma from, 1005f, 1103, 1103f, 1106f
Actinic superficial folliculitis, 753
Actinobacillus bacterial endocarditis, 299
Acute angle-closure glaucoma, 157–159
Acute generalized exanthematous pustulosis, 1346, 1353, 1354f, 1355t
Acute necrotizing ulcerative gingivitis, 250–252
Acute otitis media, 188–195
Addiction, 1546, 1548. *See also specific types*
  substance abuse disorder, 1546–1551
Adenocarcinoma
  cervical, 556–560, 558f
  gastric cancer, 381–385
  lung, 366–373
  mouth, 268, 269f
Adenomatous polyp, 401–405
Adenomatous polyposis coli *(APC)* gene mutation, 402, 408
Adenovirus
  conjunctivitis, 145
  urethritis, in men, 1410
Adoption, LGBTQ, 119
Adriamycin, cutaneous reactions, 1346–1357, 1348f
Adult education, peer-to-peer, 53
Advance care planning, 32
Adverse drug reaction, 1346–1357, 1351f
Affordable Care Act, 42, 43
Age-related macular degeneration, 172–175
Age spots, 1014–1020
Air pollution, 44
Alcohol consumption, mortality, 28
Alcoholic hepatitis, 386–393
Alcoholism (alcohol dependence, alcohol use disorder), 1571–1578
  liver disease, 386–393
  substance abuse disorders, 1546–1551
Allergic contact dermatitis, 919–927
  blistering, 1216, 1217f
Allergic triad, 338, 339f
Allopurinol, cutaneous reactions, 1346–1357, 1355t

Alopecia
- acne keloidalis nuchae, 1257t, 1258, 1259f
- androgenetic, pregnancy, 474
- central centrifugal scarring, 1257, 1257f, 1257t, 1260
- cicatricial, 1256–1261
- postpartum, 474
- scarring, 1256–1261
- traction, 1252–1255, 1252f
- traumatic, 1252–1255
- tufted folliculitis, 752, 752f, 1257t, 1258, 1258f, 1260–1261

Alopecia areata, 1245–1251
- intralesional triamcinolone acetonide for, 685, 686f, 686t

Alopecia totalis, 1245, 1249f, 1250
Alopecia universalis, 1245, 1245f, 1250
α_1-Antitrypsin deficiency, COPD from, 349, 350, 352f, 353f, 355
Alzheimer disease, dementia, 1531–1534, 1532f
Amelanotic melanoma, 1034, 1035f, 1117, 1117f–1118f
Aminoglycosides, cutaneous reactions, 1346–1357
Aminopenicillins, cutaneous reactions, 1346–1357, 1355t
Amiodarone, cutaneous reactions, 1346–1357
Amoxicillin, cutaneous reactions, 1217f, 1346–1357, 1346f, 1347f
Anabolic steroid abuse, injection, 1595–1601, 1596f
Anaerobic vaginosis, 508–512
Anal tumor, 407–413
Ancylostoma braziliense, cutaneous larva migrans, 906–908
Ancylostoma caninum, cutaneous larva migrans, 906–908
Ancylostoma duodenale, 1404–1408
Androgenetic alopecia, pregnancy, 474
Anemia, iron deficiency, 60
Anesthesia, for biopsy, 688–689
Aneuploidy, first trimester ultrasound, 485, 485f
"Angel's kisses," 702, 702f
Angioedema, 949–956
- drug-related, 1347–1357
- hereditary, 950, 951f

Angiokeratoma, 1336–1340, 1337f
Angioma, 700–706
- cherry, 1336–1340, 1336f
- spider, pregnancy, 472–475

Angioma/angiokeratoma, dermoscopy algorithms, 660, 667f, 668t
- red/blue/black lacunae, 660, 667f, 668t
- red lacunae, 660, 667f, 668t

Angiosarcoma, 1336–1340, 1338f
- cutaneous, 1336–1340

Angiotensin-converting enzyme (ACE) inhibitors, cutaneous reactions, 1346–1357
- angioedema, 949–956, 950f

Angiotensin receptor blocker, angioedema from, 949–956, 954f
Angle-closure glaucoma, 157–159
Angular cheilitis, 218–220, 856–860, 857f
- smoking, 1560, 1561f

Angular cheilosis, 218–220
Angular stomatitis, 218–220
Ankylosing spondylitis, 583t, 595–598
- uveitis, 153–156

Annular, 644, 647f
Anogenital warts, 837–843
Anorexia, end-of-life care, 34
Ant, 203f
Anterior cruciate ligament tear, 628–633, 628f
Anterior drawer test, 630
Anterior uveitis, 153–156
Antiarrhythmics, hyperpigmentation from, 1346–1357
Antibiotics, cutaneous reactions, 1346–1357, 1355t
Anticonvulsants, cutaneous reactions, 1346–1357, 1355t
Antidepressants, for chronic pain, 1613
Antiepileptics, for chronic pain, 1613
Antifungals. *See also specific types and disorders*
- triazoles, 10–11

Anxiety (disorder), 1500–1509
- after sexual assault, 112
- end-of-life care, 35

Aphthous stomatitis, 258–261
Aphthous ulcer, 258–261
Apophysis, 623
Arterial spiders, pregnancy, 473
Arterial ulcer (foot), 1390–1391
Arteriogram, coronary, 280
Arthritis, 578–584
- gouty, 604–608
- inflammatory, Lyme disease, 1426
- osteoarthritis, 585–589
- psoriatic, 578–581, 578f, 580f, 583, 583t, 965, 967f, 973, 973f
- reactive, 999–1003
  - *Chlamydia,* 525
  - with conjunctivitis, 999, 1000, 1001f
- rheumatoid, 590–594

Arthritis mutilans, 581, 581t
Arthropod reaction, bullous, 1216, 1217f
Asboe-Hansen sign
- bullous drug eruptions, 1216
- pemphigus foliaceus, 1214
- pemphigus vulgaris, 1214, 1229
- testing, 1214, 1214f

Ascaris, global health, 56–57, 56f
Ascaris lumbricoides, 1404–1408, 1405f
Asexuality, 116t
Aspergillus niger, otitis externa, 197–201
Aspirin, cutaneous reactions, 1346–1357
Assisted reproduction, LGBTQ, 119
Asteatotic eczema, 1368
Asthma, 336–345
- atelectasis, 339, 341f
- atopic dermatitis, 338, 339f, 340f
- pityriasis alba, 338, 340f
- pneumonia, 317, 318
- pulmonary function tests, 336, 337f, 338, 339, 340f
- pulsus paradoxus, 339
- status asthmaticus, 338

Atelectasis, in asthma, 339, 341f
Atherosclerotic disease, 280–282
Athlete's foot, 850–855, 880–886. *See also* Tinea pedis
- diabetes, 1432, 1432f

Atopic dermatitis, 909–917
- asthma with, 338, 339f, 340f
- hand (*See* Eczema, hand)
- *Malassezia,* 887
- steroids for, topical, 685

Atopic eczema, 909–917
Atopic eruption of pregnancy, 472–475
Atopic hand dermatitis, 928–934
Atopic triad, 338, 339f, 910, 915f, 916
Atrial fibrillation, cerebral vascular accident with, 1522
Atrioventricular blockage, Lyme disease, 1427

At-risk drinkers, 1572, 1572b, 1573, 1575, 1575b, 1577
Atrophic cervical epithelium, 541, 542, 543f, 544
colposcopy and diagnosis, 542
Atrophic gastritis, gastric cancer, 382
Atrophic vaginal epithelium, 541, 542, 543f, 544
Atrophic vaginitis, 501–506
Atrophy, 640, 644f
Atypical moles, 1057–1062
Atypical nevus, 1057–1062
AUDIT questionnaire, 1573, 1574f, 1575
Auspitz sign, 968
Autoimmune hepatitis, 390, 390t, 392
Autosomal-dominant polycystic kidney disease, 445–448
Autosomal-recessive polycystic kidney disease, 446
Avulsion fracture, metatarsal, 621–623, 621f
Axillary freckling, neurofibromatosis, 1539, 1539f, 1540f

B

Baboon syndrome, 1353, 1354f
Baby bottle caries, 271–274
Back pain, 599–602
low back, 599–602
low back, chronic, 1614t
Bacterial endocarditis, 297–305
Bacterial folliculitis, 750, 750f, 752, 753f, 754
Bacterial infections. *See also specific types*
blistering eruption, 1216, 1217f
Bacterial vaginosis, 497–499, 499t, 508–512
after sexual assault, 110
Bacteriuria, with urinary tract infection, 431
Bacteroides
necrotizing fasciitis, 776–779
otitis externa, 197–201
Bad news, delivering, 30–31
Balanitis, *Candida,* 856–860, 856f
Balanitis circinata, reactive arthritis, 999–1003, 1000f
Balsam of Peru, contact dermatitis, 919, 925f
Barbiturates
abuse (*See* Injection-drug use; Substance abuse disorder)
drug reactions, 1346–1357
Bardet-Biedl syndrome, obesity in, 1466
Barton fracture, 616–620, 618f
Basal cell carcinoma, 1093–1101
dermoscopy, 658t–659t, 1132, 1132f–1133f
dermoscopy algorithms, 656, 657f, 658t–659t
arborizing vessels, 656, 657f, 658t, 1132, 1133f
blue-gray ovoid nests, globules, and dots, 656, 657f, 659t, 1132, 1133f
concentric structures, and spoke-wheel areas, 657f, 658t, 1132
erosions, 659t
leaf-like areas, 656, 657f, 658t, 1132
shiny white structures, 656, 659t, 1132, 1132f–1133f
spoke wheel-like structures, 656, 657f, 658t, 1132
ulcerations, 656, 657f, 659t, 1132, 1133f
infiltrative, 1132, 1133f
of mouth (*See* Oropharyngeal cancer)
nodular, 1093–1101, 1093f–1094f, 1099f, 1132, 1133f
sclerosing (morpheaform), 1093–1101, 1093f, 1095f, 1098f, 1132, 1133f
superficial, 1093–1101, 1094f, 1101f, 1132, 1132f–1133f
Basal cell nevus syndrome, 1093, 1096f
BATHE method, 8
Bathing trunk nevus, 1046–1049
Beach sand, 203f
Bead, 202, 202f
Beau lines, 1264, 1265, 1265f, 1266t
psoriatic nails, 1292
Becker nevus, 1041, 1042f
Beck's triad, 293
Bed bugs, 903, 903f
Bell palsy, 1535–1538
Lyme disease, 1426, 1427
Benign cephalic pustulosis, 694–699, 694f
Benign fibrous histiocytoma, 1026–1030
Benign intracranial hypertension, papilledema, 168–170
Benign juvenile melanoma, 1039–1041, 1040f, 1041f, 1057–1062
Benign migratory glossitis, 246–249
Benign nevus, 1038–1044
Bereavement, 37
β-Human chorionic gonadotropin, 20
β-Lactams, cutaneous reactions, 1346–1357, 1355t
Bias, implicit, 40
Biliary cirrhosis, 386, 386f, 387, 388, 390, 390t, 392
Biofeedback, for chronic pain, 1609t
Biometric measurements, fetal, ultrasound
first trimester, 484–486
second trimester, 488–492
Biophysical profile, on third trimester ultrasound, 495–496
Biopsy principles and techniques, 688–693
anesthesia, 688–689
elliptical excisional, 692
punch biopsy, 690–692, 691f–692f
shave biopsy, 689–690, 689f–690f
skin cancers, 689f, 692–693
synonyms, 688
Biparietal diameter, on ultrasound
first trimester, 486, 486f
second trimester, 488, 488f, 490
third trimester, 494f
Bipolar disorder, 1500–1509, 1507t
Birthing, 23–24
Bisexual health issues, 115–119
Bisexuality, 116t
Bismuth subsalicylate, black tongue, 243
Black hairy tongue, 242–245
Blackheads, 718, 719f
Bladder cancer, 433, 456–460
Bleomycin, cutaneous reactions, 1352
Blepharitis, red eye, 180–185, 183f, 184f
Blindness
Chlamydia trachomatis, 66–67, 67f
diabetic retinopathy, 161–163, 1432, 1432f, 1433, 1435, 1438
glaucoma, 157–159
Blisters. *See also* Bullous diseases
after cryotherapy, 1216, 1216f
allergic contact dermatitis, 1216, 1217f
bacterial infections, 1216, 1217f
edema, 1218
friction, 1216
herpes simplex virus, 1216
herpes zoster, 1216–1218, 1218f
irritant contact dermatitis, 1216, 1217f
postburn, 1216, 1216f
trauma-induced, 1214, 1215f
Blood products, cutaneous reactions, 1346–1357
Bloody show, 20

Blue nevus, 1039, 1040f
Body dysmorphic disorder, 120
Bone mineral density
  osteopenia, 1471–1477
  osteoporosis, 1471–1477
Borrelia burgdorferi, 1425–1429, 1425f
Boswellia serrata, 1613
Bouchard nodes, 579f, 585, 585f, 586, 594f
Bourne toxemic rash of pregnancy, 477–479
Bowen disease, 662t, 663t, 1072–1077, 1132, 1133f–1134f
BRCA mutation, 568
Breakbone fever (dengue), 80–82, 81f
Breast abscess, 562–565
Breast cancer, 566–571
Breastfeeding, 23, 24f
Breathiness, 234–238
British Thoracic Society (BTS) rule, 320
Bronchoalveolar carcinoma, 366–373
Bronchopneumonia, 318f, 319, 320f, 321f
Bruises, child abuse, 90–94, 90f–91f, 93f
Buerger disease, dry gangrene, 1402
Bulla, 640, 642f
Bullosis diabeticorum, 1213, 1213f, 1215f, 1216
Bullous arthropod reaction, 1216, 1217f
Bullous diseases, 1213–1219. *See also specific diseases*
  autoimmune, 1213f–1214f, 1214
  childhood, 1218, 1218f
  drug eruptions, 1216, 1217f
  hydrostatic (edema blisters), 1218
  immunologic, 1215f, 1216, 1217f
  infections and bites, 1216, 1217f
  metabolic (porphyria cutanea tarda), 1216, 1216f, 1235–1237, 1235f–1236f
  traumatic/physical stress, 1216, 1216f
Bullous drug eruptions, 1216, 1217f
  fixed, 1346–1357, 1349f–1350f, 1354f
Bullous impetigo, 1216, 1217f
Bullous mastocytosis, 1218, 1218f
Bullous pemphigoid, 1214, 1214f, 1220–1224
Bunion, callus from, 1376–1377, 1377f
Bunion deformity, 1381–1385
Buprenorphine
  injection abuse, 1596
  for opioid addiction, 1555, 1599, 1600
Burns, child abuse, 90, 92f
Bursitis, olecranon, 609–611

C
Cachexia, end-of-life care, 34
Café-au-lait spots, neurofibromatosis, 1539, 1539f, 1540, 1540f, 1543
CAGE questionnaire, 1550, 1573, 1600
Calcinosis cutis, 1206, 1206f, 1207, 1208f, 1210
Calcium oxalate kidney stones, 435–439
Calcium phosphate kidney stones, 435–439
Calcium pyrophosphate dihydrate disease, 579, 581, 583
Calluses, 1376–1380
Cancer. *See also specific types*
  mortality, 28–29
Candida albicans, 856–860
  angular cheilitis, 218–220, 218f
  paronychia, 1287–1291
Candida diaper dermatitis, 712–715, 712f, 714f
Candida infection (candidiasis), dermal, 850–855, 851f
  bullous presentation, 1218
  hand dermatitis, 930, 930f
  microscopic appearance, 857, 858f
  onychomycosis, 1280–1281
Candida vulvovaginitis, 497–498, 499t, 513–517
  cutaneous, 497–499, 499t
Candidiasis, 513–517, 856–860
Candidiasis, mucocutaneous (thrush), 850–860, 851f, 856f, 857f
  angular cheilitis, 218–220, 218f
Canker sores, 258–261
Cardiobacterium bacterial endocarditis, 299
Cardiomegaly
  heart failure, 288–291
  pericardial effusion, 292f
Career Support Needs Assessment Tool, 35
Caries, 271
  adult, 275–278
  early childhood, 271–274
Caring, 8
Casts, urinary, 430–433. *See also* Urinary sediment
Cavernous hemangiomas, 700–706
Cavitated lesions, 275–278
Cavities, dental. *See* Caries
Cellulitis, 765–770
  breast, 562–564, 562f
  dissecting, scarring alopecia, 1257t, 1258, 1259f
Center for Disease Control and Prevention Healthy Places Site, 44–45
Center for Medical Humanities Ethics, 48
Central centrifugal scarring alopecia, 1257, 1257f, 1257t, 1260
Cephalic index, on second trimester ultrasound, 490
Cephalosporins, cutaneous reactions, 1346–1357, 1355t
Cerebral vascular accident, 1521–1525
Cervical cancer, 556–560
Cervical dysplasia, colposcopy, 545–548
Cervical epithelial atrophy, 541, 542, 543f, 544
Cervical erosion (ectropion), 540, 540f, 542, 543f, 544
Cervical intraepithelial neoplasia I (CIN I)
  CIN II/III and, 550–554
  colposcopy, 545–548
  human papillomavirus, 545
Cervical intraepithelial neoplasia II/III (CIN II/III), 550–554
Cervical length, on second trimester ultrasound, 488f, 489, 492f
Cervical os
  second trimester ultrasound, 489
  third trimester ultrasound, 494f
Cervical polyp, 542, 543f, 544
Cervical transformation zone, 540, 541f
Cervicitis, 542, 544
Cestodes, 1404–1408
CHADS/CHADS2 scoring table, 1522
Chadwick sign, 20
Chalazion, 132–134
Charcot arthropathy, 1396–1399
  callus, 1377, 1377f
  diabetes mellitus, 1433, 1435f, 1550–1553
Charcot foot, 1396–1399
Charcot-Marie-Tooth disease, hammer toe, 1387, 1387f

Charcot neuroarthropathy, 1396–1399
Chauffeur's fracture, 616–620, 618f
Cheilitis
  actinic, 1072–1077, 1072f
  angular, 218–220, 856–860, 857f
    smoking, 1560, 1561f
  with atopic dermatitis, 910
Cherry angioma, 1336–1340, 1336f, 1339f
Chickenpox, 780–784
Chikungunya, 82–84, 83f
Child abuse
  physical, 90–94
  sexual, 96–100
Childhood hemangioma, 700–706
Child mortality, global, 53
Child Protective Services, 90
Children's health, migrants and immigrants, 43
Chlamydia cervicitis, 524–528
Chlamydial pelvic inflammatory disease, with reactive arthritis, 999–1003, 1001f, 1002f
Chlamydial urethritis, 1409
Chlamydia trachomatis, 524–528
  blindness, 66–67, 67f
  conjunctivitis, 144–147
  sexual assault, 110, 111
  urethritis, in men, 1409–1411
Chloasma (gravidarum), 20, 20f, 1303–1307
Cholera, 55–56, 56f
Cholestatic disease, 386–393
Cholesterol stones, 396, 397
Chondrodermatitis nodularis (chronica) helicis, 205–208, 206f–207f
Chorioretinitis, 153–156
Choroiditis, 153–156
Chromophobic tumors, renal cell, 451
Chronic actinic damage of skin, 1064–1069
Chronic low back pain, 1614t
Chronic moderate heat dermatitis, 1331–1334
Chronic neck pain, 1614t
Chronic neuropathic pain, 1616t
Chronic obstructive pulmonary disease, 348–356
  α_1-antitrypsin deficiency, 349, 350, 352f, 353f, 355
  clubbing, 307–309
Chronic pain, 1607–1616
Chronic radiant heat dermatitis, 1331–1334
Chronic tension-type headache, 1513–1516
Chronic traumatic encephalopathy, 1517
Cicatricial alopecia, 1256–1261
Cicatricial pemphigoid, 1214, 1215f, 1219
Cirrhosis, 386–393
Citizens for a Clean Columbia, 45, 45f
Clark nevus, 1057–1062
Clavi (corns), 1376–1380
Clavicular fracture, 613–615
Claw toe, 1386–1389
Clear cell acanthoma, dermoscopy algorithms, 660, 669f
Clear cell carcinoma, renal cell, 451
Climate change, 44
Closed-angle glaucoma, 157–159
Clubbing, 307–309
Cluster headache, 1513–1516
Cocaine abuse, 1546f, 1587–1593
  injection, 1595–1601
  levamisole-adulterated, 1590, 1590f, 1591f
  skin popping, 1589, 1590f, 1597, 1598f
  substance use disorders, 1546–1551
Coccidiomycosis, erythema nodosum, 1170
Cognitive behavioral therapy, for chronic pain, 1609t
Coining, 94, 94f
Colitis
  NSAID-induced, 419
  ulcerative, 415–422
Collateral ligament injuries, 628–633
Colles fracture, 616–620, 616f
Colon cancer, 407–413
Colon polyps, 401–405
Color terminology, skin disorders, 640, 644, 645f
Colposcope, 540, 540f
Colposcopy, 540, 540f
  cervical cancer, 556–560
  high-grade lesions, 550–554
  low-grade lesions, 545–548
  normal and noncancerous findings, 540–544
Columnar epithelium, cervical, 540f, 541–542, 541f
Combination contraceptive patch, 13, 14f
Combined hormonal contraceptive, 13
Comedonal acne, 717–724, 718f, 719f, 721f
Comedonal nevus, 1041, 1043f
Coming out, 118
Commissural cheilitis, 218–220
Common River, 51, 51f–52f
Common warts, 826–831
Communication skills, 8
Community-acquired pneumonia, 316–323
Complexion-associated melanosis, 135–137
Compound nevi, benign, 1039, 1039f, 1043
Concussion, sports-related, 1517–1520
Condoms
  female, 11f, 12t, 14
  male, 11, 11f, 12t, 14
Condylar split fracture, lateral, 631, 631f
Condyloma lata, syphilis, 1413, 1414, 1415f
Condylomata acuminata, 837–843
Congenital dermal melanocytosis, 694–699, 695f
Congenital heart disease, clubbing, 307–309
Congenital melanocytic nevi, 1038, 1046–1049
Congenital nevus, 1038, 1046–1049
Congenital vascular lesions, 1341–1344
Congestive heart failure, 288–291
Conjunctival foreign body irritation, red eye, 182f
Conjunctival melanoma, 135–137
Conjunctival pigmentation, 135–137
Conjunctivitis, 144–147
  with reactive arthritis, 999, 1000, 1001f
  red eye, 180–185, 180f, 181t, 182f
  giant papillary, 145–146, 182f
Constipation, end-of-life care, 34
Contact dermatitis, 1035–1043, 1216, 1217f
  allergic, 919–927
  hand, 928–934, 928f
  irritant, 919–927
  occupational, 919

Contact lens
  conjunctivitis, 144–147
  corneal abrasions, 139–143
  giant papillary conjunctivitis, 145–146, 182f
  keratitis, 140
Contraception, 10–17
  effectiveness
    highly effective, 10f, 11–12, 11t, 12t, 13f, 14f
    less effective, 11t, 14, 15t
    moderately effective, 11t, 12t, 13–14, 14f
  emergency, 15, 21–22
  epidemiology, 10–11
  examinations and tests, 14, 16t
  follow-up, 15
  patient education, 15
  patient story, 10
  reversibility, 11t
  starting and switching methods, 14–15, 16t, 17t
Contraceptive patch, combination, 13, 14f
Copper-containing intrauterine device, 12
Corneal epithelial defect, 139–143
Corneal foreign body/abrasion, 139–143
Corneal ulceration, red eye, 180–185, 183f
Corns, 1376–1380
Coronary artery disease, 280–282
Coronary heart disease, 280–282
Corynebacterium, pitted keratolysis, 756–758
Corynebacterium minutissimum, erythrasma, 759–763
Corynebacterium vaginale vaginosis/vaginitis, 508–512
Coumadin (warfarin), warfarin-induced skin necrosis, 1346–1357, 1348f
Cowden's disease, gingival overgrowth, 254
Coxsackievirus, hand, foot, and mouth disease, 806–810
Crabs, 892–896, 893f, 894f
Cradle cap, 957–962, 959f, 960f
Cranial nerve palsy. *See also* Bell palsy
  Lyme disease, 1426, 1427
Crank, 1580–1585
Creeping eruption, 906–908
CREST syndrome, 1204, 1204f–1206f, 1206
Crohn disease, 415–422
  colon mucosa, 1147f
  pyoderma gangrenosum with, 1147–1151, 1147f–1148f
Crotch rot, 875–879
Crown-to-rump length, 21, 21f
  on first trimester ultrasound, 485–486, 486f
Crow sign, neurofibromatosis, 1539, 1539f, 1540f
Crust, 640, 642f
Crusted scabies, 898–905
Cryotherapy, blistering after, 1216, 1216f
Crystal meth, 1580–1585
Cucurmin, 1613
Culex quinquefasciatus, 79, 79f
Cup-to-disc ratio, glaucoma, 157–159
Cutaneous angiokeratomas, 1336–1340, 1338f
Cutaneous drug reactions, 1346–1357
Cutaneous horn, 1089–1092
Cutaneous larva migrans, 906–908
Cutaneous lupus erythematosus, chronic, 1183–1192
Cutaneous T-cell lymphoma, 1042–1048, 1124–1130
Cutaneous vasculitis, 1174–1181
Cutis marmorata, 698, 698f
Cutis rhomboidalis nuchae, 1065, 1066f
Cystic acne, intralesional triamcinolone acetonide for, 685, 686f, 686t, 722, 723f
Cystine kidney stones, 435–439
Cystitis
  hematuria, 431
  management, 433
  urinary sediment, 430–433
  white blood cell casts, 433

D

Dactylitis, 1000f
Dancer fracture, 621–623
Dandruff, 957–962
Darier disease, 1364–1370, 1364f–1366f
Darier-Roussy disease, 1153–1159, 1156f
Darier sign, 1218
  urticaria pigmentosa, 951f, 952, 952f
Dating scan, 484–486
DaVinci robot, for prostate cancer surgery, 467, 467f
Death. *See also* End of life
  epidemiology, 27
Decay, dental, 275–278
Decision-making, shared, 8
Deep hemangiomas of infancy, 700–706
Deep venous thrombosis
  pulmonary embolus, 358, 360, 362
  venous insufficiency, 310, 311
Delirium, end-of-life care, 35
Dementia, 1531–1534
  mortality, 29
Dementia with Lewy bodies, 1531–1534, 1533f
Demodex folliculitis, 752
Dengue (hemorrhagic) fever, 80–82, 81f
Dennie-Morgan lines, with atopic dermatitis, 910, 912f
Dental caries, 271
  adult, 275–278
  early childhood, 271–274
Dental cavities, 275–278
Dental decay, 275–278
Depigmentation, 644, 645f
Depo-Provera, 11f, 11t, 12t, 14
Depression, 1500–1509, 1503t
  end-of-life care, 34–35
  intimate partner violence, 103, 105
  sexual assault, 108, 109, 111, 112–113
de Quervain thyroiditis, 1482
Dermal melanocytosis, 694–699, 695f
Dermal nevi, 656, 656f, 1039, 1039f, 1040f, 1043
Dermatitis. *See also specific types*
  nummular, 936–939
  perioral, 730, 730f
Dermatitis herpetiformis, 1214, 1219, 1242–1243, 1242f
Dermatitis syphiloides posterosiva, 714
Dermatofibroma, 1026–1030
  dermoscopy algorithms, 656, 656f–657f
    network, with central white blotch, 656, 656f
    network, with ring-like globules, shiny white streaks, and pink hue, 656, 656f
  pregnancy, 473
Dermatographism, urticaria, 950, 950f
Dermatohelosis, 1064–1069

Dermatomyositis, 1194–1202
Dermatophilus congolensis, pitted keratolysis, 756–758
Dermatophytes, 850–855. *See also* Fungal infections, cutaneous; *specific types*
  tinea corporis, 868–873
Dermatophytic onychomycosis, 1280–1285, 1281f
Dermatophytid reaction, tinea pedis, 881, 882*f*
Dermatophytosis, 868–873
  nails, 1280–1285
Dermatoses, self-inflicted, 941–947
Dermatosis papulosa nigra, 1015, 1017f
Dermoscopes (dermatoscope), 649, 649f
  choosing, 677–678, 677t
Dermoscopy, 649–679
  applications and goals, 649
  non-polarized, 649, 650f, 677–678, 677t
  polarized, 649–650, 651f
  structures, 650, 651f
Dermoscopy, skin cancer, advanced, 1132–1140
  acrolentiginous melanoma, 1134, 1137f–1140f, 1140
  basal cell carcinoma, subtypes, 658t–659t, 1132, 1132f–1133f
  melanoma, face and scalp, 672t–675t, 1134, 1135t–1136t, 1136f–1137f
  squamous cell carcinoma, subtypes, 661t–663t, 1132–1134, 1133f–1134f
Dermoscopy algorithms, 650–677
  final step, melanoma, 671, 672f, 672t–675t, 675f
    angulated lines, 672f, 672t, 676
    atypical blotch, 672f, 675t, 677
    atypical/irregular globules, 672f, 673t, 676
    atypical/irregular pigment network, 671, 672f, 672t
    blue-whitish veil, 672f, 674t, 676, 676f
    negative pigment network, 672f, 673t, 676
    polymorphous vessels, 672f, 675t, 677
    regression structures, 672f, 674t, 676
    shiny white lines/streaks, 672f, 675t, 677
    streaks, 672f, 673t, 676
    tan structureless peripheral areas, 672f, 674t, 676
  step 1, level 1a, flat and slightly raised nevi, 652–656, 652f, 653t–655t
    diffuse globules, 654f
    diffuse network, 653f
    globular, 652, 652f
    globular, cobblestone pattern, 652, 652f, 654f
    homogenous blue, 652, 652f, 655f, 656
    homogenous brown, 652f, 655f, 656
    network or reticular pattern, 652, 652f
    patchy network/reticular pattern, 652, 652f, 653f
    peripheral network, with central brown globules, 652, 654f
    peripheral network, with central globules, 652, 652f, 654f
    peripheral network, with central hyperpigmentation, 652, 652f, 654f
    peripheral network, with central hypopigmentation, 652, 652f, 653f
    reticular pattern, with peripheral rim of globules, 652, 652f, 655f
  step 1, level 1b, sessile to dome shaped to pedunculated nevi; intradermal nevi, 656, 656f
  step 1, level 2, dermatofibromas, 656, 656f–657f
    network, with central white blotch, 656, 656f
    network, with ring-like globules, shiny white streaks, and pink hue, 656, 656f
  step 1, level 3, basal cell carcinoma, 656, 657f, 658t–659t
    arborizing vessels, 656, 657f, 658t, 1132, 1133f
    blue-gray ovoid nests, globules, and dots, 656, 657f, 659t, 1132, 1133f
    concentric structures, and spoke-wheel areas, 657f, 658t, 1132
    erosions, 659t
    leaf-like areas, 656, 657f, 658t, 1132
    shiny white structures, 656, 659t, 1132, 1132f–1133f
    spoke wheel-like structures, 656, 657f, 658t, 1132
    ulcerations, 656, 657f, 659t, 1132, 1133f
  step 1, level 4, squamous cell carcinoma
    arborizing vessels, 656, 660f, 661t–663t
    brown circles, 656, 660f
    brown dots radially arranged, 656, 660f
    glomerular vessels, 656, 660f
    hairpin vessels with halo, 656, 660f
    rosettes, 656, 660f
    strawberry pattern, 656, 660f
    white circles, 656, 660f
    yellow scale, 656, 660f
  step 1, level 5, seborrheic keratosis and lentigo, 660, 664f, 665t–667t
    comedo-like openings, 660, 664f, 665t
    fingerprint-like structures, 660, 664f, 666t
    fissures/sulci, ridges, 660, 664f, 665t
    gyri/ridges and sulci/fissures, 660, 664f, 667t
    hairpin vessels with whitish halo, 660, 664f, 667t
    milia-like cysts, 660, 664f, 665t
    moth-eaten border, 660, 664f, 666t
    sharp demarcation, 660, 664f, 666t
  step 1, level 6, angioma/angiokeratoma, 660, 667f, 668t
    red/blue/black lacunae, 660, 667f, 668t
    red lacunae, 660, 667f, 668t
  step 1, level 7, sebaceous hyperplasia and clear cell acanthoma, 660, 669f
  step 2, nevi requiring special attention, 667–671, 669f, 670t–671t
    multi-component pattern, symmetric, 667, 669f, 670t
    peripheral globules/tiered globules, Spitz/Reed, 667, 669f, 671, 671t
    starburst pattern, Spitz/Reed, 669f, 671, 671t
    structureless tan/pink nevi, 667, 669f, 670t
    two-component pattern, kissing nevus, 667, 669f, 670t
  triage amalgamated dermoscopy algorithm, 676f, 677
  two-step, 650–677
Diabetes mellitus, 1432–1439
  acanthosis nigricans, 1433, 1434f, 1442–1445
  cerebral vascular accident, 1522
  Charcot arthropathy, 1433, 1435f, 1550–1553
  diabetic dermopathy, 1433, 1434f, 1438, 1447–1449
  dry gangrene, 1400–1402
  foot ulcers, 1433, 1434f, 1437, 1438
    ischemic, 1390–1391
    neuropathic, 1393–1395
  insulin resistance, 1433
  necrobiosis lipoidica, 1433, 1434f, 1450–1453
  peripheral arterial disease, 1400
  psoriasis, 978
  skin tag, 1010, 1010f, 1011, 1434f, 1443f, 1445, 1445f
  tinea pedis, 1432, 1432f
  xanthoma and xanthelasma, 1455–1461
  xanthomas, eruptive, 1433, 1435f
Diabetic dermopathy, 1433, 1434f, 1438, 1447–1449
Diabetic retinopathy, 161–163
  nonproliferative, 161, 1432, 1432f, 1433, 1435, 1438

Diagnosis. *See also specific disorders*
  dermoscopy (*See* Dermoscopy)
  image banks, 3–4, 4t
  images, using, 2–4, 4t
  senses, 2
Diaper dermatitis, 712–715
Diaper rash, 712–715
Diaphragm with spermicide, 11f, 12t
Diarrheal diseases. *See also specific types*
  water and sanitation, 53–54, 53f–54f, 56, 56f
Diet
  for chronic pain, 1610, 1611f
  poor, mortality, 28
DIHS. *See* DRESS/DIHS
"Dinner fork" deformity, 616–620, 616f
Disabilities, healthcare access, 42–43, 42f
Discoid eczema, 936–939
Discoid hand dermatitis, 928, 929f
Discoid lupus erythematosus, 1183–1192
  scarring alopecia, 1187f, 1188f, 1189, 1189f, 1257t, 1258, 1259f
Dissecting cellulitis, scarring alopecia, 1257t, 1258, 1259f
Distal radius fracture, 616–620
Distribution terminology, skin disorders, 644, 647f
Doctor–patient relationship, 6–8
Domestic violence, 102–106
Double decidual sign, 21
Dowager's hump, 1471–1477, 1471f
Dowling-Meara epidermolysis bullosa simplex, 1237–1239, 1239f
Doxorubicin, cutaneous reactions, 1346–1357, 1348f
Doxycycline, cutaneous reactions, 1346–1357, 1350f
DRESS/DIHS, 1346–1357, 1351f
Drinking, heavy, 1571–1578
Drospirenone, 13–14
Drug-induced bullous pemphigoid, 1220–1224
Drug-induced gingival overgrowth, 254–256
Drug-induced hypersensitivity syndrome, 1346–1357, 1351f
Drug-induced liver disease, 387, 391. *See also* Liver disease
Drug-induced photosensitivity, 1324–1329, 1325f
Drug reactions, cutaneous, 1346–1357. *See also specific drugs*
  bullous drug eruptions, 1346–1357, 1349f, 1354f
  erythroderma, 1004–1009
  pityriasis rosea, 985
Drumstick fingers, 307–309
Drusen, age-related macular degeneration, 172–175
Dry gangrene, 1400–1402
Dry mouth, dental caries, 277, 278
Dupuytren disease (contracture), 635–637
Dust mites, 342f
  control, 338, 342–343
Dyshidrotic eczema, 928–934, 929f
Dyslipidemias, 1455–1461
Dysphonia, 234–238
Dysplastic nevus, 1057–1062
Dyspnea, end-of-life care, 34
Dystrophic epidermolysis bullosa, 1237–1239, 1238f

E

Ear foreign body, 202–204
Early childhood caries, 271–274
Ebola virus disease, 84–85, 85f
Ecchymosis, 644
Ecstasy, 1546–1551, 1548f
Ectopic pregnancy, 22
  first trimester ultrasound, 484–486
  IUD use, 12
Ectropion, 540, 540f, 542, 543f, 544
Eczema, 909–917
  asteatotic, 1368
  discoid, 936–939
  dyshidrotic, 928–934
  microbial, 936–939
  nummular, 936–939
  nummular, hand, 928, 929f
  orbicular, 936–939
  photoallergic drug reaction, 1324–1329, 1326f
  pregnancy, 472–475
  seborrheic, 957–962
Eczema, hand, 928–934
  atopic, 928, 929f
  chronic vesicular, 928, 930f
  contact, 928, 928f
  dyshidrotic (pompholyx), 928–934, 929f
  endogenous, 930
  exogenous, 930
  frictional, 928, 929f
  hyperkeratotic, 928, 929f
  infectious, 930, 930f
  nummular, 928, 929f
  rubber allergens, 930
Eczema herpeticum, with atopic dermatitis, 910, 910f
Eczema vaccinatum, with atopic dermatitis, 910, 911f
Edema blisters, 1218
Education
  family, end of life, 35–36
  patient (*See also specific disorders*)
    pregnancy and birthing, 24, 24f
Effusion
  otitis media with, 188–195
  pericardial, 292–295
Eikenella bacterial endocarditis, 299
Elliptical excisional biopsy, 692
Embolus, pulmonary, 358, 360, 362
Embryo, on first trimester ultrasound, 484–486
Embryonic disc, on first trimester ultrasound, 486, 486f
Emergency contraceptives, 15, 21–22
Emerging infections, 76–86. *See also* Infections, emerging
Emotional pain, 1607
Emphysema, 348–356
Encephalomyelitis, postinfectious, 798
"En coup de sabre," linear morphea, 1205f, 1207, 1208f
Endocarditis, bacterial, 297–305
Endocervical polyp, 541, 543f, 544
End of life, 26–37
  management, 30–35
Endometrial polyp, 541, 543f
End-stage liver disease, mortality, 30
End-stage renal disease, mortality, 29
  in diabetes, 1436, 1438
Entamoeba histolytica, 1404–1408
Enterobacter folliculitis, 752
Enterobacteriaceae necrotizing fasciitis, 776
Enterobius vermicularis, 1404–1408, 1404f

Enterococcus bacterial endocarditis, 299
Entropion, red eye, 182
Environmental protection and social justice, 44–46
Environmental Protection Agency, 44
Eosinophilic folliculitis, 750, 751f, 753, 754–755
Epidermal inclusion cyst, 772, 773f
Epidermal nevi, 1041, 1051–1055
Epidermolysis bullosa, 1237–1239, 1237f–1239f
Epidermolysis bullosa acquisita, 1214, 1215f, 1219
Epidermolysis bullosa simplex, 1214, 1215f
  children, 1218
Epidermophyton, 850–855
  tinea corporis, 868–873
Epidermophyton floccosum
  tinea cruris, 875–879
  tinea pedis, 880–886
Episcleritis, 149–152
  red eye, 180–185, 181t, 183f
Epithelial cyst, 540, 541, 541f, 542, 542f, 544
Epithelial keratitis, zoster ophthalmicus, 792f, 794
Epithelium, cervical, 541, 541f
  atrophic, 541, 542, 543f, 544
Epitheloid cell nevus, 1039–1041, 1040f, 1041f, 1057–1062
Erosio interdigitalis blastomycetica, 930f
Erosion, 640, 643f
Eruptive xanthomas, 1455f–1457f, 1456, 1457, 1461
Erysipelas, 765, 767f
Erythema ab igne, 1331–1334
Erythema annulare centrifugum, 1371–1374
Erythema exudativum perstans, 1371–1374
Erythema figuratum perstans, 1371–1374
Erythema gyratum perstans, 1371–1374
Erythema infectiosum, 802–805
Erythema marginatum perstans, 1371–1374
Erythema microgyratum perstans, 1371–1374
Erythema migrans, 1425, 1425f–1427f, 1426, 1427
Erythema multiforme, 1161–1167, 1162f, 1165f
  drug-induced, 1346–1357, 1350f
Erythema nodosum, 1169–1173
  sarcoidosis-related, 1153–1154
Erythema nodosum leprosum, 1171, 1172f
Erythema perstans (annulare), 1371–1374
Erythema simplex gyratum, 1371–1374
Erythematotelangiectatic rosacea, 726f, 727, 727f
Erythematous, 640, 644, 645f
Erythema toxicum neonatorum, 694–699, 695f
Erythrasma, 759–763
Erythroderma, 1004–1009
Erythrodermic psoriasis, 965, 967f, 970, 972f, 980, 1004–1009
Erythroleukoplakia, 263–266
  oropharyngeal cancer, 267, 268
Erythroplakia, 263–266
Erythroplasia, 263–266
Erythroplasia of Queyrat, 1072–1077, 1073f, 1104, 1104f–1105f
Erythroxylum coca, 1587
Escherichia coli
  folliculitis, 752
  mastitis, 562
  pneumonia, 317
Essure tubal occlusion device, 13, 13f, 14f
Estimated date of delivery, 20, 484, 495
Estimated fetal weight, 488, 490f
Estimated gestational age, ultrasound
  first trimester, 484–486
  second trimester, 488–492
  third trimester, 493–496, 493f, 494f
Estrogen-containing contraceptives, smoking with, 11
Estrogen deficiency, postmenopause, 501–504
Etonogestrel implant, 11t, 12t, 13, 13f
Evidence-based medicine, interpreting, 1604–1606
Exanthematous drug eruptions, 1346–1357, 1347f
Excisional biopsy, elliptical (fusiform), 692
Excoriation, 640, 643f
Excoriation disorder, 941–947
Exophthalmos, Graves, 1486–1492
Extramammary Paget disease, 530–533
Eyelid ecchymosis, 177
Eye trauma (hyphema), 176–178

F

Facial nerve palsy, peripheral, 1535–1538
Failure to thrive, child abuse, 90–94
False vocal cords, 234
Falx cerebri, on second trimester ultrasound, 489f, 492f
Familial atypical mole and melanoma syndrome, 1058
Familial hypercholesterolemia, 1455–1456, 1459, 1460
Family physicians, pregnancy care delivery and outcomes, 19, 19f
Family planning
  contraception, 10–17
  LGBTQ, 119
Fatigue, end-of-life care, 34
Favre-Racouchot disease, 1065, 1066f
Female sterilization, 11, 11f, 11t, 12t, 13, 13f
Feminizing treatment, transgender, 120–121
Femoral neck fracture, 624–626, 624f, 625f
Femur length, on second trimester ultrasound, 488, 490, 490f
Fentanyl addiction, 1552–1556
Fertility, 19
Fertility awareness, 14, 15t
Fetal biometric measurements, ultrasound
  first trimester, 484–486
  second trimester, 488–492
Fetal pole, 21, 486, 486f
Fever, end-of-life care, 35
Fibroepithelial polyps, 1010–1013
Fibromyalgia, 1615t
Fibrous histiocytoma, benign, 1026–1030
Fifth cranial nerve, sensory distribution, 794, 794f
Fifth disease, 802–805
Fifth metatarsal tuberosity fracture, 621–623, 621f
Fingernail clubbing, 307–309
Fire ants, bullous bites from, 1216, 1217f
Fire stains, 1331–1334
First cranial nerve, sensory distribution, 794, 794f
First trimester obstetrical ultrasound, 484–486
Fissure, 640, 643f
Fixed drug eruptions, 1346–1357, 1349f–1350f, 1354f
Flat warts, 832–835
Flesh-eating bacteria, 776–779
Flint, Michigan water crisis, 45
Fluid–air interface, liver disease, 388, 389f
Fluoride, early childhood caries, 271–274
Folic acid supplements, pregnancy, 23

Folliculitis, 750–755
acne keloidalis nuchae, 750, 751f, 752
actinic superficial, 753
bacterial, 750–752, 750f–751f, 754
eosinophilic, 750, 751f, 753, 754–755
folliculitis decalvans, 752, 752f
fungal, 750, 752, 753, 753f, 754
Gram-negative, 752
herpetic, 752–753
Malassezia, 752, 753f, 754, 887, 890f
molluscum contagiosum, 752–753
MRSA, 750, 751f
noninfectious, 750
parasitic *(Demodex),* 752
pseudofolliculitis barbae, 750, 751f, 752, 755
Pseudomonas ("hot tub"), 750, 750f, 752, 753f, 754
staphylococcus, 750–752, 750f–751f, 754
tufted, 752, 752f, 1257t, 1258, 1258f, 1260–1261
viral, 750, 752–753, 754
Folliculitis decalvans, 752, 752f, 1256f, 1257t, 1258, 1260–1261
Folliculitis keloidalis, 1257t, 1258, 1259f
Foot dermatitis, with atopic dermatitis, 910
Foot ulcers, diabetes mellitus, 1433, 1434f, 1437, 1438
Forchheimer spots, 224
Foreign body, ear, 202–204
Foreign body, eye
conjunctival irritation, 182f
conjunctivitis, 146, 147
corneal, 139–143
Foster parenting, LGBTQ, 119
Fourchette, posterior, child sexual abuse, 98
Fournier gangrene, 776–779
Fractures. *See also specific types*
child abuse, 90–94, 90f, 92f
Fragrances, contact dermatitis, 919, 920, 921f, 928, 928f
Frankincense, 1613
Friction blisters, 1216
Frontal fibrosing alopecia, 1257t, 1258, 1258f
Frontotemporal dementia, 1531–1534, 1533f
Frostbite, dry gangrene, 1402
Functional alcohol use disorder, 1572, 1572b
Fungal folliculitis, 750, 752, 753, 753f, 754
Fungal infections, cutaneous, 850–855. *See also specific types*
Fusiform excision biopsy, 692
Future of Family Medicine initiative, physician–patient relationship, 6–7

G

Gallbladder sludge, 395, 396
Gallstones, 395–399
intrahepatic cholestasis of pregnancy, 472, 475
Gangrene
dry, 1400–1402
necrotizing fasciitis with, 776–779, 778f
wet, 1401, 1401f
Gardnerella vaginalis vaginitis, 497–499, 498f
Gardnerella vaginalis vaginosis, 508–512
Garment trunk nevus, 1046–1049
Gastric cancer, 381–385
Gastric ulcers, 376–379
Gay health issues, 115–119
Gender, on second trimester ultrasound, 490, 491f, 492f
Gender dysphoria, 115–119
Gender-expansive, 115–119
Gender nonconformity, 119–122
Genital herpes, 812–818, 812f–814f, 816f
Genital warts, 837–843
Genodermatoses, 1364–1370
callus, 1377
Darier disease, 1364–1370, 1364f–1366f
X-linked ichthyosis, 1364–1370, 1367f
Geographic stomatitis, 246–249
Geographic tongue, 246–249
Gestational age, on ultrasound
first trimester, 484–486
second trimester, 488–492
third trimester, 493–496
Gestational sac, 21
on first trimester ultrasound, 485–486
Ghon complex, 326, 326f, 328
Ghrelin, 1464
Giant hairy nevus, 1046–1049
Giant papillary conjunctivitis, 145–146, 182f
Giant pigmented nevus, 1046–1049
Giant urticaria, 952f
Giardia lamblia, 1404–1408, 1407f
Gigantism, 1493–1496
Gingival fibromatosis, hereditary, 254–256
Gingival hyperplasia, 254–256
Gingival overgrowth, 254–256
Gingivitis, 250–252
acute necrotizing ulcerative, 250–252
smoking, 1560
Gingivostomatitis, herpes, 812–818, 813f, 818f
Glaucoma, 157–159
red eye, 180–185, 181t
Gleason grade and score, prostate cancer, 462, 464, 464f
Global health, 51–73
child mortality, 53
cholera, 55–56, 56f
Common River community, 51, 51f–52f
definition, 51
ethical dilemmas, 51–52
eye diseases, trachoma, 66–67, 66f–67f
infectious skin diseases, 67–69, 70–72, 71f
intestinal parasites, 56–57, 56f
kwashiorkor, 57–58, 57f–58f
malnutrition, 57–58, 57f–58f
marasmus, 57–58, 57f
peer-to-peer adult education in, 53
trust, local health providers, 53, 53f
typhoid fever, 54–55
water and sanitation, 53–54, 53f–54f
Global health, *Mycobacterium*
leprosy, 69–71, 70f–71f
tuberculosis, 71–73, 73f
tuberculosis, HIV and, 72–73, 72f
Global health, vector-borne diseases, 61–66
leishmaniasis, 64–66, 64f–66f
malaria, 61–63, 62f–63f
prevention, 66
prognosis, 66
Global Health and Disparities Path of Excellence, 43
Globe injury, red eye, 180–185, 184f
Glomangiomas, 1336–1340, 1338f

Glomerulocystic kidney, 446
Glucosamine sulfate (GS)/chondroitin sulfate (CS), 1613
Glue ear, 189
Gluten-induced enteropathy, dermatitis herpetiformis with, 1242–1243, 1242f
Goiter, 1486–1492
  iodine deficiency, 60–61, 62f
Goitrous hypothyroidism, 1479–1484
Goldenhar syndrome, 205
Gonococcal arthritis, 579, 581, 583
Gonococcal conjunctivitis, 144–147
Gonococcal urethritis, in men, 1409–1411
Gonorrhea (*Neisseria gonorrhoeae*)
  conjunctivitis, 144–147
  sexual assault, 110, 111
  urethritis, in men, 1409–1411
Google image search, 3–4, 4t
Gorlin syndrome, 1093, 1096f
Gottron's papules, dermatomyositis, 1194, 1195, 1195f, 1196, 1197f, 1198, 1199f
Gout, 583, 604–608
  arthritis, 578, 581, 581f
  tophaceous, 582f
Gouty arthritis, 604–608
Gram-negative folliculitis, 752
Granular casts, 430–433
Granuloma, pyogenic, 1032–1036
  pregnancy, 474, 474f, 475
Granuloma annulare, 1141–1146
Granuloma gluteale infantum, 714
Granuloma gravidarum, 474, 474f, 475
Granulomatous thyroiditis, subacute, 1482
Graves disease, 1486–1492
  with amenorrhea, 21
Graves ophthalmopathy, 1486, 1486f, 1487, 1489f
Grief, 37
Group A β-hemolytic *Streptococcus* (GABHS)
  cellulitis, 765
  erythema nodosum, 1169, 1169f, 1170
  impetigo, 745–749 (*See also* Impetigo)
  perianal dermatitis, 712–715, 712f, 713f
  pharyngitis, 227–232
  scarlet fever and strawberry tongue, 223–226
Guided imagery, for chronic pain, 1609t
Guttate psoriasis, 965, 966f, 968, 970, 970f, 971f, 980

H

Habit-tic deformity, 1264, 1264f, 1265, 1265f
Haemophilus
  bacterial endocarditis, 299
  conjunctivitis, 145
Haemophilus influenzae
  acute otitis media, 189
  pneumonia, 317
  sinusitis, 212–217
Haemophilus vaginalis vaginitis, 508–512
Hair. *See also specific disorders*
  pregnancy, 472–475
HAIR-AN syndrome, 1442
Hair pulling, 1252–1255, 1253f
Half-and-half nail, 1267, 1267f
Hallucinogens, 1546–1551, 1548f
Hallux valgus, 1381–1385
Halo nevus, 1038f, 1039
Hammer toe, 1386–1389
  callus from, 1376–1377
Hand, foot, and mouth disease, 806–810
Hand dermatitis, 928–934
  with atopic dermatitis, 910
Hand eczema, 928–934
Hands, on second trimester ultrasound, 490, 491f
Hansen disease, 69–71, 70f–71f
Hart line, 536
Haven for Hope Transformational Campus, 47–48
Head, on second trimester ultrasound, 488, 488f
Headache, 1513–1516. *See also specific types*
  pain management, 1615t–1616t
Head circumference, fetal, 488, 488f, 490
Head injury, sports-related, 1517–1520
Head lice, 892–896, 893f–894f
HEADSS, 96
Healthcare, universal, 41–43, 41f, 42f
Healthcare-associated pneumonia, 316–323
Heart disease. *See also specific types*
  coronary, 280–282
  mortality, 29, 29f
Heart failure, 288–291
  pericardial effusion, 292–295
Heat rash (miliaria), 697, 697f
Heavy drinking, 1571–1578, 1572b
Heberden nodes, 579, 579f, 585, 585f, 586, 587f
Hegar sign, 20
Helicobacter pylori
  colon polyps, 402
  gastric cancer, 382
  peptic ulcer disease, 376–379
Heloma durum, hard corn, 1376–1380
Heloma molle, soft corn, 1376–1380
Hemangioma, 668t
  childhood, 700–706
  vascular, 1339, 1339f
Hematoma
  subdural, 1526–1530
  subungual, 1298–1301
Hematuria, 430–433
  bladder cancer, 456–460
  polycystic kidney disease, 445–448
  renal cell carcinoma, 450–454
Hemochromatosis, liver disease, 387, 388, 390, 390t, 392
Hemorrhagic fevers, dengue, 80–82, 81f
Hemorrhoidal varicosities, pregnancy, 472–475
Hemorrhoids, 424–428
Hemosiderin deposition, lipodermatosclerosis with, 310, 311f
Henoch-Schönlein purpura, 1174–1181, 1174f, 1175f
Heparin-induced skin necrosis, 1346–1357
Hepatic artery, 387
Hepatic dysfunction, 386–393
Hepatic failure, 386–393
Hepatitis, 386–393
  alcoholic, 386–393
  autoimmune, 390, 390t, 392
  viral, 386–393
Hepatitis A, 387, 391
Hepatitis B, 387, 391, 393

Hepatitis B vaccination, after sexual assault, 111
Hepatitis C, 387, 391–392
Hepatocellular disease, 386–393
Hepatocytes, 387
Herald patch, pityriasis rosea, 984, 985, 985f, 986f
Hereditary angioedema, 950, 951f
Hereditary gingival fibromatosis, 254–256
Hereditary hemangiomatosis, 1341–1344, 1342f
Hereditary hemorrhagic telangiectasias, 1341–1344, 1341f
Hereditary nonpolyposis colorectal cancer, 382
Hereditary vascular lesions, 1341–1344
Heroin, 1546–1551, 1548f
  injection abuse, 1595–1601, 1595f, 1598f
  opioid crisis, 1552–1556
Herpes gestationis, 480–482
Herpes gingivostomatitis, 812–818, 813f, 818f
Herpes labialis, 812–819, 817t
Herpes simplex virus (HSV), 812–818
  blistering, 1216
  child sexual abuse, 97, 99f
  congenital, 1218
  urethritis, in men, 1410
Herpes zoster, 786–790
  blistering, 1216–1218, 1218f
  zoster ophthalmicus, 792–796
Herpes zoster oticus, 787, 787f
Herpetic folliculitis, 752–753
Herpetic whitlow, 812–818, 814f, 815f
Heterotopic pregnancies, 22
Hidradenitis suppurativa, 738–743
  obesity, 1464, 1466f
  pregnancy, 473
High-density lipoproteins, hyperlipidemia, 1455, 1456
High-grade squamous intraepithelial lesions, 550–554
Hip
  artificial, 625f
  fracture, 624–626
Hippocratic nails (fingers), 307–309
Hirsutism, pregnancy, 474
Histiocytoma, benign fibrous, 1026–1030
HIV/AIDS, 1419–1423
  angular cheilitis, 218–220, 220f
  child sexual abuse, 98, 100
  dementia, 1531–1534
  Kaposi sarcoma, 1419–1423
  molluscum contagiosum, 820–824
  mortality, 28, 29
  postexposure prophylaxis, sexual assault, 111
  seborrheic dermatitis, 957–962, 960f, 961f
  skin viral infections, 69
  tuberculosis co-infection, 72–73, 72f
Hives, 949–956
HLA-B27 positive, uveitis and iritis, 153–156
Hoarseness, 234–238
Homeless
  LGBTQ, 119
  medical care, 46–48, 47f
Home pregnancy kits, 20, 24
Homogenous leukoplakia, 263–266
Hookworms, 1404–1408, 1404f, 1405f
  cutaneous larva migrans, 906–908
  global health, 56–57
Hordeolum, 132–134
Hormonal vaginal ring, 10, 10f, 14
Horn, cutaneous, 1089–1092
Hospice care and services, 32–33
Hospital gangrene, 776–779
Hot flashes, premature menopause, 22
"Hot tub" folliculitis, 750, 750f, 752, 753f, 754
Hot-water bottle rash, 1331–1334
Human papillomavirus (HPV), 826
  cervical cancer, 556, 557
  cervical intraepithelial neoplasia, 545
  maternal, and juvenile onset recurrent respiratory papillomatosis, 235
  oropharyngeal cancer, 268
  with squamous intraepithelial lesions
    high-grade, 551, 552
    low-grade, 545–548
  vaccination, 548, 550
    after sexual assault, 111
  warts
    common, 826–831
    flat, 832–835
    genital, 837–843
    plantar, 844–849
Humerus, third trimester ultrasound, 493f
Huntington disease, dementia, 1531–1534
Hutchinson fracture, 616–620, 618f
Hutchinson melanotic freckle, 1084–1088
Hutchinson sign, 1270f, 1271
  acral lentiginous melanoma, 1114, 1116f, 1270f, 1271
  pseudo-, 1271, 1271f
  zoster ophthalmicus, 793f, 794, 794f
Hyaline casts, 430–433
Hydrocodone, cutaneous reactions, 1346–1357, 1350f
Hydrogen peroxide–producing *Lactobacillus*, vaginal, 509
Hydronephrosis, 440–443
Hydrops fetalis, on third trimester ultrasound, 493, 494f
Hydroureter, 440f, 441
Hygroma, 1527
Hymen, normal, 96, 96f
Hyperhidrosis, pregnancy, 473
Hyperkeratosis of the tongue, 242–245
Hyperkeratotic lesions, 1376–1380
Hyperlipidemia, 1455–1461
Hyperpigmentation, 644, 645f
  central, peripheral network with, 652, 652f, 654f
  drug-induced, 1346–1357, 1348f, 1349f, 1353f
  postinflammatory, 1316–1322
Hyperplastic polyp, 401–405
Hypersensitivity syndromes, 1161–1167
Hypersensitivity vasculitis, 1174–1181
Hypertension, 284–286
  cerebral vascular accident, 1522
  idiopathic (benign) intracranial, papilledema, 168–170
  pulmonary
    chronic obstructive pulmonary disease, 349, 350, 354, 355, 356
    pulmonary embolus, 361f, 363
Hypertensive retinopathy, 165–167
Hyperthyroidism, 154, 1486–1492
Hypertriglyceridemia, 1458
Hypertrophic scars, intralesional triamcinolone acetonide for, 685, 686f, 686t

Hypertrophy, 640, 644f
Hyperuricemia
  gout, 605
  medications, 605, 608
Hyphema, 176–178
  red eye, 180–185, 184f
Hypnosis, for chronic pain, 1609t
Hypopigmentation, 644, 645f, 1308–1314
Hypopyon, red eye, 182, 184f
Hypothyroidism
  definition, 1479
  goitrous, 1479–1484
Hysteroscopic tubal occlusion, 13, 13f, 14f

I

Ibuprofen, cutaneous reactions, 1346–1357, 1349f, 1355t
Ichthyosis
  acquired, 1368, 1369f
  with atopic dermatitis, 910, 913f
  lamellar, 1368, 1370f
  X-linked, 1364–1370
Ichthyosis vulgaris, 1368, 1369f
Idiopathic guttate hypomelanosis, 1065, 1066f
Idiopathic intracranial hypertension, papilledema, 168–170
ID reaction, tinea pedis, 881, 882*f*
IgA bullous dermatosis, 1214, 1215f
IgA vasculitis, 1174–1181, 1174f, 1175f
Images. *See also specific disorders*
  diagnosis, 2–4, 2f–3f, 4t
  internet sources, 3–4, 4t
  patient–physician relationship, 4
  taking your own, 4
Immigrant health, 43–44
Impetiginization, 747, 748f
Impetigo, 745–749
  with atopic dermatitis, 910
  with chickenpox, 780f
  global health, 68, 69f
Implant, etonogestrel, 11t, 12t, 13, 13f
Implantation, fertilized egg, 19
Implicit bias, 40
Inactivity, physical, on mortality, 28
Infantile hemangiomas, 700–706
Infant mortality rate, 27
Infections, emerging, 76–86
  chikungunya, 82–84, 83f
  dengue fever, 80–82, 81f
  Ebola virus disease, 84–85, 85f
  Middle East respiratory syndrome, 85–86, 85f
  patient story, 76
  severe acute respiratory syndrome, 85–86
  travel, 76
  West Nile virus, 79–80, 79f
  Zika, 76–78, 77f–78f
Infectious skin diseases, 70–72, 71f. *See also specific types*
  fungal, 69, 69f
  global health, 67–69
  impetigo and bacterial, 68, 69f
  lice, 68
  scabies, 68, 68f–70f
Inflammatory acne, 717–724, 718f
Inflammatory arthritis, Lyme disease, 1426
Inflammatory bowel disease, 415–422
Inflammatory breast cancer, 566–571
Inflammatory linear verrucous epidermal nevus, 1051–1055, 1052f
Influenza virus, sinusitis, 212–217
Ingrown toenail, 1276–1278
Inhalants, toxic, 1546–1551
Injection-drug use, 1595–1601
Injury. *See also specific types*
  child abuse, 90–94
  eye
    globe, red eye, 180–185, 184f
    retinal pigment epithelial, 172–173
  intimate partner violence, 102–106
  knee, 628–633
  Lisfranc, 621, 622, 623
  mortality, 28
  sexual abuse
    adult, 108–113
    child, 96–100
Insulin resistance, diabetes mellitus, 1433
International health, 51
Internet, images, 3–4, 4t
Interstitial pneumonia, 319, 321f
Intertriginous, 644, 647f
Intertriginous vegetating plaques, 1221
Intertrochanteric fracture, 624–626, 626f
Interview
  motivational, 8, 1562, 1563t
  patient-centered, 8
Intestinal worms and parasites, 1404–1408
  global health, 56–57, 56f
Intimate partner violence, 102–106
Intracranial pressure, increased, 169, 170
  papilledema, 168–170
Intradermal melanocytic nevus, 1039, 1039f, 1040f
Intradermal nevi (dermal nevi), 656, 656f, 1039, 1039f, 1040f, 1043
  melanocytic, 1039, 1039f, 1040f
Intrahepatic cholestasis of pregnancy, 472–475
Intraocular pressure, elevated, glaucoma, 157–159
Intrauterine device (IUD), 10, 10f, 11–12, 11f, 12t
  copper-containing, 12, 12t
  levonorgestrel, 10f, 11–12, 12t
Invasive squamous cell cancer, cervix, 556–560
Inverse psoriasis, 2, 2f, 3f, 859f, 877f, 964f, 965, 966f, 970, 971f, 980
Iodine
  deficiency, 60–61, 62f
  Lugol's, 546, 547f
Iridocyclitis, 153
Iris hamartomas, neurofibromatosis, 1539, 1540, 1541f, 1542f
Iritis, 153–156
  red eye, 180–185, 181t, 184f
  zoster ophthalmicus, 792–796, 792f
Iron deficiency, 60
Iron-deficiency anemia, from hookworms, 1406
Iron supplements, pregnancy, 23
Irritable bowel syndrome, 1616t
Irritant contact dermatitis, 919–927
  blistering, 1216, 1217f
Irritant diaper dermatitis, 712–715, 713f
Ischemic ulcer, foot, 1390–1391
Isothiazolinone, contact dermatitis, 919, 920, 922f–923f

J

Jaccoud arthropathy, 580f
Jacquemier sign, 474
Janeway lesions, 299, 299f
Jock itch, 875–879
Jones fracture, acute, 621–623, 622f
Junctional nevi, 1039, 1039f, 1043
Juvenile polyp, 401–405
Juvenile transformation zone, persistent, 540, 540f, 542, 543f, 544

K

Kala-azar, 64–66, 64f–66f
Kaposi sarcoma, 1419–1423
Karnofsky Performance Scale, 30
Kayser-Fleischer ring, 388, 389f
Keloids, 1359–1363
  intralesional triamcinolone acetonide for, 685, 686f, 686t
  pregnancy, 473
Keratinocyte carcinoma, 1064–1069
Keratitis
  red eye, 180–185, 181t, 183f
  zoster ophthalmicus, 792–796, 792f
Keratoacanthoma, 663t, 667t, 1079–1083, 1134, 1134f
Keratoconus, with atopic dermatitis, 914, 914f
Keratoderma blenorrhagicum, reactive arthritis, 999, 999f, 1000, 1001f
Keratosis, 1376–1380
  seborrheic, 1014–1020
    dermoscopy algorithms, 660, 664f, 665t–667t
Keratosis pilaris, with atopic dermatitis, 910, 913f
Kidney stones, 435–439
  polycystic kidneys, 446
Kingella bacterial endocarditis, 299
"Kissing warts," 826, 827f
Klebsiella folliculitis, 752
Klippel-Trenaunay, port-wine stains, 1341, 1342
Knee anatomy, 629f
Knee fracture, patellar, 630, 631f
Knee injury, 628–633
Knuckle pads, 932, 932f
Koebner phenomenon, 968, 970f
  lichen planus, 991f, 992
Koilocytosis, 550–551
Koplik spots, 798, 798f, 799
Kwashiorkor, 57–58, 57f–58f
Kyphosis, thoracic, 1471–1477, 1471f
Kytococcus sedentarius, pitted keratolysis, 756–758

L

Labial adhesion, child, 99, 100f
Labor, 20, 23–24
Lachman test, 628, 630
Lactobacillus, hydrogen peroxide–producing, vaginal, 509
Lane, Melanie, 47f
Laptop thigh, 1331–1334
Laryngeal cancer, hoarseness, 234–238
Laryngeal papillomatosis, 234–238
Laryngeal polyp, 234–238
Laryngitis, 234–238
Laryngopharyngeal reflux, 234–238
Larynx, 234–238
Latent tuberculosis infection, 72
Lateral collateral injury, 628–633
Lateral condylar split fracture, 631, 631f
Latrines, pit, in Ethiopia, 53, 53f–54f
Ledderhose disease, 635–637
Left portal vein, on third trimester ultrasound, 493f
Legionella pneumonia, 317
Leiomyoma
  pregnancy, 473
  uterine, 21
Leishmaniasis, 64–66, 64f–66f
Lentiginous nevus. *See* Nevus, benign
Lentigo, dermoscopy algorithms, 660, 664f, 665t–667t
  comedo-like openings, 660, 664f, 665t
  fingerprint-like structures, 660, 664f, 666t
  fissures/sulci, ridges, 660, 664f, 665t
  gyri/ridges and sulci/fissures, 660, 664f, 667t
  hairpin vessels with whitish halo, 660, 664f, 667t
  milia-like cysts, 660, 664f, 665t
  moth-eaten border, 660, 664f, 666t
  sharp demarcation, 660, 664f, 666t
Lentigo maligna, 1084–1088
Lentigo maligna melanoma, 1084–1088, 1085f, 1114, 1115f, 1119
  dermoscopic features and definitions, 1135t–1136t
  face and scalp, 672t–675t, 1134, 1136f–1137f
Leprosy, 69–71, 70f–71f
Lesbian gay bisexual transgender (LGBT) health issues, 115–119
Leukocytoclastic vasculitis, 1174–1181, 1176f, 1178f
Leukonychia, 1263–1267, 1263f, 1264f, 1266t
  transverse striate, 1263, 1263f, 1264, 1289f
Leukonychia punctata, 1263–1267, 1264f, 1266t
Leukoplakia, 263–266
  of cervix on colposcopy, 551, 551f
  oropharyngeal cancer and, 267, 268
  from smoking, 1560, 1561f
Levamisole-adulterated cocaine, 1590, 1590f, 1591f
Levonorgestrel
  EE pills, 14
  intrauterine device, 10, 10f, 11–12, 11f, 12t
Levo-α-acetyl methadol, 1600
Lice, 68, 892–896
  body lice, 892–896, 892f–894f
Lichenification, 640, 643f
Lichen nuchae, 942, 943f, 944f
Lichenoid drug eruption, 1346–1357, 1348f
Lichen planopilaris, 1256, 1257f, 1257t, 1259f, 1260
Lichen planus, 991–997
Lichen sclerosus, genitals, high-potency steroids for, 681–683, 683f
Lichen sclerosus et atrophicus, vulvar
  child sexual abuse, 99, 100f
  vulvar intraepithelial neoplasia, 535, 537, 537f
Lichen simplex chronicus, 941–947, 943f–944f
Lidocaine with epinephrine, for biopsy, 688–689
Life expectancy, at birth, 27
Life-sustaining treatment, withdrawal, 36–37
Likelihood ratio, 1604–1606
Lindsay nails, 1267, 1267f
Linea alba, pregnancy, 473, 473f, 478f
Linea nigra, 30, 473, 473f
Linear immunoglobulin A (IgA) dermatosis, bullous, 1214, 1215f
Linear immunoglobulin M (IgM) dermatosis, of pregnancy, 477–479
Lingua villosa nigra, 242–245

Lip cancer, 267–270
Lip licking, perlèche from, 218–220
Lipodermatosclerosis, with hemosiderin deposition, 310, 311f
Lipoproteins, 1455, 1456
Lisch nodules, neurofibromatosis, 1539, 1540, 1541f, 1542f
Liver disease, 386–393
Liver fibrosis, 386–393
Lobar pneumonia, 316f, 318f–319f, 319
Lobullary capillary hemangioma, 1032–1036
Locally advanced breast cancer, 566–571, 567f, 568f
Löfgren syndrome, 1153–1159
  erythema nodosum, 1169–1173
Longitudinal melanonychia, 1263, 1269–1274, 1269f–1270f, 1271t, 1273f
Lordosis, cervical, 1471–1477, 1471f
Low back pain, 599–602
  chronic, 1614t
Low-density lipoproteins, hyperlipidemia, 1456
Low-grade squamous intraepithelial lesion, 545–548
Lues, 1412–1418
Lugol's iodine, 546, 547f
Lung cancer, 366–373
Lung transplantation, for COPD, 355
Lung volume reduction surgery, for COPD, 355
Lupus
  discoid, 1183–1192
    scarring alopecia, 1187f, 1188f, 1189, 1189f, 1257t, 1258, 1259f
  lupus erythematosus, 1183–1192
  neonatal, 698, 698f, 1185, 1185f
  systemic lupus erythematosus, 1183–1192
    mother with, neonatal lupus from, 698f
    vasculitis, 1175, 1175f, 1176f
Lupus panniculitis, 1183, 1184f, 1190f
Lupus pernio, 1153–1159, 1153f–1155f, 1158f–1159f
Lupus profundus, 1183, 1184f, 1190f
Lyme disease, 1425–1429
Lymphadenitis, tuberculous, 72, 73f
Lymphangioma circumscriptum, 1343, 1344f

M

Macrolides, cutaneous reactions, 1346–1357, 1355t
Macular degeneration, age-related, 172–175
Macular-type blue nevi, 694–699, 695f
Macule, 640, 641f
Maculopapular eruptions, drug-related, 1346–1357, 1347f
Maffucci syndrome, 1341–1344, 1342f
Majocchi granuloma, 869, 870f, 873, 878–879, 878f
Major depressive disorders, 1500–1509, 1503t
Major neurocognitive disorder, 1531–1534
Malassezia (Pityrosporum), 850–855, 890f
  atopic dermatitis, 887
  folliculitis, 752, 753f, 754, 887, 890f
  seborrhea, 850, 863, 887, 958
  tinea versicolor, 850, 887–890
Malassezia furfur, 890f
  tinea versicolor, 887–890
Malassezia globosa, tinea versicolor, 887–890
Male sterilization, 11f, 11t, 12t
Mallet toe, 1386–1389
Malnutrition, 90–94
  childhood, global, 57–58, 57f–58f
Mammary candidiasis, 856–860, 856f, 858f
Mammogram, screening
  breast cancer, 566, 566f, 567f, 568, 569, 570
  Paget disease of breast, 573, 574
Marasmus, 57–58, 57f
Marijuana, 1546–1551, 1547f
Marjolin ulcer, 1104, 1104f
Masculinizing treatment, transgender, 121
Mask of pregnancy, 1303–1307
Mastitis, 562–565
Mastocytosis, bullous, 1218, 1218f
Matrix metalloproteinases, 1065
MCA-PSV, 493
McMurray test, 628, 630
Measles, 797–800
Medial collateral injury, 628–633
Medicare Hospice Benefit, 32–33
Medication overuse headache, 1513–1516
Meditation, for chronic pain, 1609t
Meditative movement therapies, for chronic pain, 1609t
Mee lines, 1265, 1266f, 1266t
Megaureter, children, 441, 442
Meibomian gland, blockage or infection, 132
Melanocytic atypia, 1057–1062
Melanocytic nevus, 1038–1044
  intradermal, 1039, 1039f, 1040f
Melanocytosis, oculodermal, 137
Melanoma, 1064–1065, 1112–1122
Melanoma in situ, 1112, 1112f, 1114, 1115f, 1119, 1120
  acquired nevus, 1048f
  conjunctival, 135–137
  face and scalp, dermoscopy, 672t–675t, 1134, 1135t–1136t, 1136f–1137f
  mouth, 268
  subungual, 1270–1274, 1270f, 1271t, 1272f
Melanoma, dermoscopy algorithms, 671, 672f, 672t–675t, 675f
  angulated lines, 672f, 672t, 676
  atypical blotch, 672f, 675t, 677
  atypical/irregular globules, 672f, 673t, 676
  atypical/irregular pigment network, 671, 672f, 672t
  blue-whitish veil, 672f, 674t, 676, 676f
  negative pigment network, 672f, 673t, 676
  polymorphous vessels, 672f, 675t, 677
  regression structures, 672f, 674t, 676
  shiny white lines/streaks, 672f, 675t, 677
  streaks, 672f, 673t, 676
  tan structureless peripheral areas, 672f, 674t, 676
Melanonychia striata, 1269–1274, 1269f–1270f, 1273f
Melanotic hamartomas of iris, neurofibromatosis, 1539, 1540, 1541f, 1542f
Melasma, 20, 20f, 1303–1307
Meningitis, aseptic, Lyme disease, 1427
Meningoencephalitis, Lyme disease, 1427
Meniscal tear, 628–633, 630f
Menopause, 501
  atrophic vaginitis, 501–506
  definition, 22
  premature, 22
Mental health, 1500–1509
Menzies method, 1117, 1119
Metal, contact dermatitis, 919, 920, 920f, 921f
Metatarsal fracture, 621–623
Metatarsus adductovarus, 1381–1385

Methadone, 1600
  addiction to, 1552–1553
  for opioid addiction, 1555, 1599, 1600
Methamphetamine (meth), 1580–1585
  substance abuse, 1546–1551, 1547f
Methicillin-resistant *Staphylococcus aureus* (MRSA)
  abscess, 771–775, 771f, 772f
  cellulitis, 766
  folliculitis, 750, 751f
  impetigo, 745–749
  necrotizing fasciitis, 776–779
  pneumonia, 322
Meth lab (oratory), 1581, 1581f, 1582f
Meth mites, 1580, 1580f, 1582, 1582f, 1583f, 1584
Meth mouth, 1582, 1583f, 1584f
Methylisothiazolinone, contact dermatitis, 919, 920
Microaneurysms, eye
  diabetic retinopathy, 161–162
  hypertensive retinopathy, 165, 166
Microbial agents. *See also specific agents and disorders*
  mortality, 28
Microbial eczema, 936–939
Micronutrient deficiencies, global, 57, 59–61
  iodine, 60–61, 61f
  iron, 60
  vitamin A, 59, 59f
  zinc, 59–60, 60f
Microsporum, 850–855. *See also* Fungal infections, cutaneous; Tinea
  tinea capitis, 861–866, 864f
  tinea corporis, 868–873
Microsporum canis, 864f
  tinea capitis, 861–866
Middle cerebral artery, third trimester, 496
Middle-ear effusion, acute otitis media, 189–195
Middle East respiratory syndrome (MERS), 85–86, 85f
Migraine headache, 1513–1516
Migrant health, 43–44
Migratory glossitis, benign, 246–249
Milia, 1024f
Milia, newborn, 694–699, 694f
Miliaria, 697, 697f, 1216
  neonatal, 697, 697f
  pregnancy, 473
Miliary pneumonia, 319
Milk spots, 694–699, 694f
Mind/body integration modalities, for chronic pain, 1609t
Mindfulness-Based Stress Reduction (MBSR), for chronic pain, 1609t
Minocycline
  black tongue, 243
  drug reactions, 1346–1357
Minority stress model, 118
Minor neurocognitive disorder, 1531–1534
Mirena intrauterine device, 10, 10f, 11–12, 11f, 12t
Miscarriage, after intimate partner violence, 105
Mites, folliculitis, 752
Moderate heat dermatitis, chronic, 1331–1334
Mohs surgery, 1109–1110, 1110t
Moles, 1038–1044
  atypical, 1057–1062
Molluscum contagiosum, 820–824
  folliculitis, 752–753
Mongolian (blue) spots, 694–699, 695f
Moniliasis, 513–517
Monoarticular inflammatory arthritis, 578, 579
Monoarticular noninflammatory arthritis, 578, 579
Monosodium urate crystal deposition, 581, 604, 604f
Montgomery tubercles, 473, 473f
Moraxella catarrhalis
  acute otitis media, 189
  sinusitis, 212–217
Morbillivirus, 798. *See also* Measles
Morbus Dupuytren, 635–637
Morphea, 122f, 1204–1210, 1205f
Morphology terminology, skin disorders, 640, 641f–644f
Mortality. *See also specific disorders*
  alcohol consumption, 28
  cancer, 28–29
  child, global, 53
  dementia, 29
  diet on, poor, 28
  heart disease, 29, 29f
  HIV/AIDS, 28, 29
  inactivity on, physical, 28
  infant rate, 27
  injury, 28
  liver disease, end-stage, 30
  maternal, pregnancy and birth, 18–19
  microbial agents, 28
  neurologic disease, 29
  pregnancy-related, 18–19
  pulmonary disease, 29
  renal disease, end-stage, 29
  sexually transmitted infections, 28
  stroke, 30
  substance abuse disorder, 28
  tobacco addiction, 27–28
  toxic agents, 28
Motivational interviewing, 8
  for smoking cessation, 1563, 1563t
Mouth cancer, 267–270
MRSA. *See* Methicillin-resistant *Staphylococcus aureus* (MRSA)
Mucha-Habermann disease, 1350f, 1351, 1374–1377, 1374f–1375f
Mucinous retention cyst, 540, 541, 541f, 542, 542f, 544
Mucopyocele, 214f, 215f
Mucormycosis sinusitis, 212–215, 213f
Muehrcke lines, 1265, 1266t, 1267
Multidrug-resistant pathogens, pneumonia, 316–323
Multiple sclerosis, dementia, 1531–1534
Mummification necrosis, 1400–1402
Muscle relaxants, for chronic pain, 1613
Music thanatology, 26, 26f
Music therapy, for chronic pain, 1609t
Mycobacterium infection, global health
  leprosy, 69–71, 70f–71f
  tuberculosis with HIV, 72–73, 72f
Mycobacterium tuberculosis
  pneumonia, 317
  tuberculosis, 325, 325f, 326f
Mycoplasma genitalium urethritis, in men, 1410
Mycosis fungoides
  cutaneous T-cell lymphoma, 1124–1130
  erythroderma with, 1004–1009, 1007f

My Healthy Plate, 1610, 1611f
Myofascial dysfunction, 1615t
Myoma, uterine, 21
Myrmecia, 844–849
Myxedema
  coma, hypothyroidism, 1480, 1481, 1481f, 1484
  pretibial, Graves disease, 1487, 1488f

N

Nabothian cyst, 540, 542f
  colposcopy and diagnosis, 541, 541f, 542, 542f
Naegele's rule, 20
Nail disorders, pigmented, 1269–1274
Nail hypertrophy, 1263, 1264f, 1265
Nail plate pitting, psoriatic nails, 1292, 1292f
Nail psoriasis, 965, 967f, 973
Nail splitting, 1298, 1299f
Nail trauma, subungual hematoma, 1298–1301
Nail trephination, 1298, 1298f–1299f, 1301
Nail unit, 1263, 1263f
Nail variants, normal, 1263–1267. *See also specific types*
  Beau lines, 1264, 1265, 1265f, 1266t
  habit-tic deformity, 1264, 1264f, 1265, 1265f
  half-and-half nail, 1267, 1267f
  leukonychia, 1263–1267, 1263f, 1264f, 1266t
  leukonychia punctata, 1263–1267, 1264f, 1266t
  longitudinal melanonychia, 1263
  Mee lines, 1265, 1266f, 1266t
  Muehrcke lines, 1265, 1266t, 1267
  onychogryphosis, 1263, 1264f, 1265
  onychomadesis, 1264, 1265
  transverse striate leukonychia, 1263, 1263f, 1264, 1289f
  twenty-nail dystrophy, 1264, 1266f
Naloxone (Narcan), 1599, 1600, 1601f
Naltrexone, 1599
Napkin dermatitis, 712–715
Nasal crease, horizontal, with atopic dermatitis, 914, 915f
Nasal polyps, 209–211
Natural family planning, 14, 15t
Nausea and vomiting, end-of-life care, 34
Necator americanus, 1404–1408, 1404f, 1405f
Neck pain, chronic, 1614t
Necrobiosis lipoidica, 1433, 1434f, 1450–1453
Necrotizing erysipelas, 776–779
Necrotizing fasciitis, 776–779
Necrotizing soft-tissue infection, 776–779
Neisseria gonorrhoeae infection
  conjunctivitis, 144–147
  sexual assault, 110, 111
  urethritis, in men, 1409–1411
Nematodes, 1404–1408, 1404f–1406f
Neomycin contact dermatitis, 919, 920, 921f
Neonatal acne, 715–721, 718f
  benign cephalic pustulosis, 694–699, 694f
  true, 694, 696
Neonatal lupus, 698, 698f, 1185, 1185f
Neonatal pemphigus, 1218
Neonatal pustular melanosis, 697
Neonatal syphilis, 1218
Nephrolithiasis, 435–439
Neurodermatitis, 941–947
Neurodermatitis circumscripta, 941–947
Neurofibroma
  with neurofibromatosis, 1541f
  pregnancy, 473
Neurofibromatosis type 1, 1539–1543
  with neurofibromas, 1541f
Neurologic disease. *See also specific types*
  mortality, 29
Neuropathic pain, 34
  chronic, 1616t
Neuropathic ulcer of foot, 1393–1395
Neurosyphilis, 1412–1418
Neurotic excoriation, 941–947, 941f–943f
Nevirapine, cutaneous reactions, 1346–1357, 1355t
Nevus. *See also specific types*
  with architectural disorder, 1057–1062
  atypical, 1057–1062
  benign, 1038–1044 (*See also specific types*)
    eye, conjunctival, 135–137
    eye, scleral, 135–137
  Clark, 1057–1062
  congenital melanocytic, 1038, 1046–1049
  dysplastic, 1057–1062
  epidermal, 1041, 1051–1055
  melanocytic, 1038–1044
    intradermal, 1039, 1039f, 1040f
  Spitz, 1039–1041, 1040f, 1041f, 1057–1062
Nevus, dermoscopy algorithms
  flat and slightly raised, 652–656, 652f, 653t–655t
    diffuse globules, 654f
    diffuse network, 653f
    globular, 652, 652f
    globular, cobblestone pattern, 652, 652f, 654f
    homogenous blue, 652, 652f, 655f, 656
    homogenous brown, 652f, 655f, 656
    network or reticular pattern, 652, 652f
    patchy network/reticular pattern, 652, 652f, 653f
    peripheral network, with central brown globules, 652, 654f
    peripheral network, with central globules, 652, 652f, 654f
    peripheral network, with central hyperpigmentation, 652, 652f, 654f
    peripheral network, with central hypopigmentation, 652, 652f, 653f
    reticular pattern, with peripheral rim of globules, 652, 652f, 655f
  sessile to dome shaped to pedunculated nevi; intradermal, 656, 656f
  special attention, requiring, 667–671, 669f, 670t–671t
    multi-component pattern, symmetric, 667, 669f, 670t
    peripheral globules/tiered globules, Spitz/Reed, 667, 669f, 671, 671t
    starburst pattern, Spitz/Reed, 669f, 671, 671t
    structureless tan/pink nevi, 667, 669f, 670t
    two-component pattern, kissing nevus, 667, 669f, 670t
Nevus anemicus, 1041, 1042f
Nevus comedonicus, 1041, 1043f
Nevus depigmentosus, 1041, 1042f
Nevus flammeus, 1341–1344, 1341f–1343f
Nevus of Ota, 137, 1041, 1041f
Nevus pigmentosus, 1046–1049
Nevus pigmentosus of pilus, 1046–1049
Nevus sebaceous, 1051–1055
Nevus spilus, 1039, 1040, 1040f, 1047f, 1048
Nexplanon, 13, 13f
Nickel contact dermatitis, 919, 920, 920f, 921f

Nicotine addiction, 1558–1569
Nicotine stomatitis, 1560, 1561f
Nikolsky sign
  bullous drug eruptions, 1216
  bullous pemphigoid, 1214, 1216, 1221, 1229, 1352, 1354
  cutaneous drug reactions, 1352, 1354
  pemphigus foliaceus, 1214
  pemphigus vulgaris, 1214
  toxic epidermal necrolysis, 1352
Nipple candidiasis, 856–860, 856f
Nits, 68, 892–896
Nodular elastosis, 1065, 1066f
Nodular leukoplakia, 263–266
Nodular melanoma, 1112, 1112f, 1114, 1115f, 1116f, 1117, 1120f, 1122f
  masking blue nevus, 1039
Nodule, 640, 642f
  Lisch, 1539, 1540, 1541f, 1542f
  palmar, 636–637
  rheumatoid arthritis, 579, 580f, 591, 592f
  thyroid, autonomous functioning, 1489
  vocal cord, 234–238
Nodulocystic acne, 717–724, 717f–718f
Nonalcoholic fatty liver disease, 386–388, 390–391, 391
  with obesity, 1464
Noncontact sexual abuse, 108
Nonhomogenous leukoplakia, 263–266
Nonimmune hydrops, on third trimester ultrasound, 493
Nonneoplastic hamartoma, 401–405
Non-polarized dermoscopy, 649, 650f, 677–678, 677t
Nonspecific vaginitis, 508–512
Nonsteroidal antiinflammatory drugs (NSAIDs)
  for ankylosing spondylitis, 595, 596, 597, 598
  for arthritis, 578
  for back pain, 599, 601, 602
  for chronic pain, 1610
  for colitis, 419
  cutaneous reactions, 1346–1357, 1349f, 1355t
  GI events from, risk factors, 604
  for gout, 604, 607
  for olecranon bursitis, 609, 611
  for osteoarthritis, 588–589, 588t
  in peptic ulcer disease, 376–379
  for rheumatoid arthritis, 593
Norwegian scabies, 898–905
Number needed to harm, 1604
Number needed to treat, 1604, 1605f
Nummular, 644, 646f
Nummular dermatitis, 936–939
Nummular eczema, 936–939
Nummular hand dermatitis, 928, 929f
NURSE, 32
Nurse's late-onset prurigo, 477–479
Nursing bottle caries, 271–274
Nutrition, for chronic pain, 1610, 1611f
NuvaRing, 10, 10f, 11–12, 11f, 12t, 14

O

Obesity, 1463–1469
  acanthosis nigricans, 1442, 1443f, 1463, 1463f, 1464, 1465f
  hidradenitis suppurativa, 1464, 1466f
  nonalcoholic fatty liver disease, 1464
  psoriasis, 1464, 1465f
  skin tag (acrochordon), 1462, 1462f, 1577f
  varicose veins, 1464, 1465f
  waist circumference, 1464, 1465f
  xanthomas, 1455–1461, 1464, 1464f
Obestatin, 1464
Obstructive acne, 717–724, 718f, 721f
Occupational contact dermatitis, 919–926, 919f, 921f, 926f
Ocular herpes zoster, 792–796
Ocular rosacea, 728, 729f, 731
  red eye, 180–185, 181t, 183f
Oculodermal melanocytosis, 137
Oil drop sign, psoriatic nails, 1292, 1292f, 1293f
Oil seed, 694–699, 694f
Olecranon bursitis, 609–611
  gout, 581, 582f
Onychocryptosis, 1276–1278
Onychogryphosis, 1263, 1264f, 1265, 1282f
Onychomadesis, 1264, 1265
Onychomycosis, 850–855, 1280–1285
  with tinea pedis, 880, 881, 885
Onychoschizia, 1298, 1299f
Open-angle glaucoma, 157–159
Open relationship, 116t
Ophthalmic nerve, sensory distribution, 794, 794f
Opioid crisis, 1552–1556
Opioids, for chronic pain, 1611–1613
Optic disc cupping, glaucoma, 157–159
Optic nerve atrophy, glaucoma, 158
Oral cancer, 267–270
Oral contraceptive pills, 11, 12t, 13–14, 14f
Oral squamous cell carcinoma, 267–270
Orbicular eczema, 936–939
Orolabial herpes, 812–818, 813f
Oropharyngeal cancer, 267–270
Ortho Evra, 13, 14f
Osler nodes, 299, 299f, 300
Osler-Weber-Rendu syndrome, 1341–1344, 1341f
Osteoarthritis, 585–589
  overview, 578, 579, 579f, 581, 583f, 583t
  pain management, 1615t
Osteoporosis and osteopenia, 1471–1477
Otitis externa, 197–201
Otitis media, acute, 188–195
Otitis media with effusion, 188–195
Ottawa ankle rules, 621, 621f, 623
Overlap syndrome, 1199
Oxycodone (OxyContin) addiction, 1554–1556

P

Paget disease of breast, 573–576
Paget disease of external genitalia, 530–533
Paget disease of the scrotum, 530–533
Paget disease of the vulva, 530–533
Pain
  chronic, 1607–1616
  emotional, 1607
  management (*see also specific disorders*)
    end-of-life care, 33–34
  neuropathic, 34
  shoulder, 1615t
Pain reliever addiction, 1546–1551

Palliative care, 33–35
Palliative Performance Scale, 30
Palmar erythema, pregnancy, 473
Palmar fibromatosis, 635–637
Palmar hyperlinearity, with atopic dermatitis, 910
Palmar nodule, 636–637
Palmar-plantar (palmoplantar) psoriasis, 965, 966f, 970, 971f, 972f, 974f, 980
Palmoplantar eczema, vesicular, 928–934
Palmoplantar warts, 844–849
Panniculitis, erythema nodosum, 1169–1173
Panretinal photocoagulation, for diabetic retinopathy, 161–163
Pansexuality, 116t
Pansusceptible *Mycobacterium tuberculosis*, 325
Panuveitis, 154
Papanicolaou (Pap) smear, 540, 541f
Papanicolaou (Pap) smear abnormalities
  colposcopy
    high-grade lesions, 550–554
    low-grade lesions, 545–548
  epidemiology, 545
Papillary carcinoma, renal cell, 451
Papilledema, 168–170
Papillomatosis
  laryngeal, 234–238
  recurrent respiratory, 234–238
Papule, 640, 641f
Papulopustular rosacea, 725f–726f, 728, 728f, 730–731
Parainfluenza virus sinusitis, 212–217
Parakeratosis, psoriatic nails, 1292
Paramyxoviridae, 798
Paraneoplastic pemphigus, 1226–1233, 1230f
Parapsoriasis variegata, 1125f
Parasitic folliculitis, 752
Parkinson disease, dementia, 1531–1534
Paronychia, 1287–1291
Parvovirus B19, fifth disease, 802–805
Pasteurella multocida cellulitis, 766
Pastia's lines, 223f, 224
Patch, 640, 641f
  combination contraceptive, 13, 14f
  contraceptive, 12t
Patch testing, contact dermatitis, 923–924, 924f
Patellar dislocation, 629
Patellar fracture, 630, 631f
Patellar subluxation/dislocation, 628–633
Pathergy, 1147, 1147f
Patient
  learning from, 7
  what physicians want from and for, 6
Patient-centered interview, 8
Patient–physician relationship, trust-building images, 4
Pautrier microabscess, 1129
Pearly, 644, 646f
Pediculosis, 892–896
Pediculus humanus capitis, 892–896, 893f–894f
Pediculus humanus corporis, 892–896, 892f–894f
Peer-to-peer adult education, 53
Pelvic inflammatory disease, after *Chlamydia* infection, 525
Pemphigoid gestationis, 480–482, 1214, 1215f, 1221
Pemphigus, 1226–1233
Pemphigus erythematosus, 1230, 1231f
Pemphigus foliaceous, 1214, 1214f, 1226–1233, 1228f–1229f
Pemphigus vegetans, 1226–1233, 1227f
Pemphigus vulgaris, 1214, 1215f, 1226–1233, 1226f–1227f, 1229f, 1230f
  black tongue, 243f
  neonatal, 1218
Penicillins, cutaneous reactions, 1346–1357, 1355t
Penile pyoderma gangrenosum, 1148
Penis, on second trimester ultrasound, 490, 490f
Peptic ulcer disease, 376–379
Peptostreptococcus
  necrotizing fasciitis, 776–779
  otitis externa, 197–201
Perfume, contact dermatitis, 928, 928f
Perianal dermatitis, childhood, 712–715
Perianal Paget disease, 530–533
Perianal pseudoverrucous papules, 714
Pericardial effusion, 292–295
Perinuclear cytoplasmic vacuolization, 550–551
Periodontal anatomy, healthy, 250
Periodontal disease (periodontitis), 250–252
  smoking, 156f, 1560
Perioral dermatitis, without rosacea symptoms, 730, 730f
Peripheral arterial disease, with diabetes and dry gangrene, 1400
Peristomal pyoderma gangrenosum, 1148
Perlèche, 218–220, 856–860, 857f
Persistent juvenile transformation zone, 540, 540f, 542, 543f, 544
Pesticide exposure, 46
Petechiae, 644, 645f
Petroleum products, contact dermatitis, 926f
PHACE syndrome, large segmental hemangioma, 703, 704f, 705f
Pharyngitis, 227–232
Phenolphthalein, cutaneous reactions, 1346–1357
Phenytoin, cutaneous reactions, 1346–1357, 1351f
Photoaging, 1064–1069
Photoallergic eruptions (drug reactions), 1324–1329, 1326f, 1326t, 1327f
  eczema as, 1324–1329, 1326f
Photocoagulation, panretinal, for diabetic retinopathy, 161–163
Photodermatitis, 1324–1329
Photo-distributed, 644
Photography, 4
Photoonycholysis phototoxicity reactions, 1327
Photosensitivity, 1324–1329
Phototoxic (drug) reactions, 1324–1329, 1325f, 1326f, 1326t
Phthirus pubis, 892–896, 893f, 894f
Phymatous rosacea, 726f, 728
Physical abuse
  child, 90–94
  intimate partner, 102–106
Physical inactivity, mortality, 28
Physician orders for life-sustaining treatment (POLST), 32
Physicians
  family, pregnancy care delivery and outcomes, 19, 19f
  physician–patient relationships, 4, 6–7
  what patients want from, 6
Physicians for a National Health Plan, 42
Phytophotodermatitis, 1324–1329, 1325f
Picker's nodules, 941–947, 944f–945f
Pigmentation terminology, skin disorders, 640, 644, 645f
Pigmented hairy nevus, 1046–1049

Pigmented nail disorders, 1269–1274
acral lentiginous melanoma, 1270–1274, 1270f
Hutchinson sign, 1270f, 1271
longitudinal melanonychia, 1269–1274, 1269f–1270f, 1271t, 1273f
pseudo-Hutchinson sign, 1271, 1271f
subungual melanoma, 1270–1274, 1270f, 1271t, 1272f
Pigmented pretibial papules, 1447–1449, 1448f
Pigmented stones, 396, 397
Piles, 424–428
Pillars of health, 1610
Pilonidal cyst, 773, 774f
Pincer nail, 1276, 1276f
Pink eye, 144–147
Pinworm infestation, 1404–1408, 1404f
Pit latrines, in Ethiopia, 53, 53f–54f
Pitted keratolysis, 756–758
Pituitary adenoma, somatotrope, acromegaly from, 1493–1496
Pityriasis alba
with asthma, 338, 340f
with atopic dermatitis, 910, 913f
Pityriasis lichenoides chronica, 1216, 1239–1242, 1239f–1240f, 1241, 1241f
Pityriasis lichenoides et varioliformis acuta (PLEVA), 1216, 1216f, 1239–1242, 1239f–1240f
Pityriasis rosea, 984–989
Pityriasis versicolor, 850–855, 851f, 887–890
Pityrosporum. See Malassezia
Pivot shift test, 630
Placenta, on ultrasound
second trimester, 488–492
third trimester, 493–495
Placenta previa, ultrasound
second trimester, 489, 492
third trimester, 493, 494f, 496
Plane warts, 832–835
Plane xanthomas, 1456
Plantar hyperlinearity, with atopic dermatitis, 910
Plantar warts, 844–849
Plaque, 640, 641f
Plaque psoriasis, 964f, 965, 965f, 968, 968f–970f, 976t, 979f, 980
Plasmodium falciparum, 61–63, 62f–63f
Plasmodium malariae, 61–63, 62f–63f
Plasmodium ovale, 61–63, 62f–63f
Plasmodium vivax, 61–63, 62f–63f
Plumber's itch, 906–908
Pneumococcal polysaccharide vaccination, 322
Pneumonia, 316–323
asthma, 317, 318
bronchopneumonia, 318f, 319, 320f, 321f
community-acquired, 316–323
healthcare-associated, 316–323
interstitial, 319, 321f
lobar, 316f, 318f–319f, 319
miliary, 319 (*See also* Tuberculosis)
vaccination, 322
Podagra, 606f, 607. *See also* Gout
Poikiloderma
cutaneous T-cell lymphoma, 1127
dermatomyositis, 1198, 1198f
Poikiloderma of Civatte, 1065, 1066f
Poison ivy/oak, contact dermatitis, 1035, 1036, 1037f, 1039, 1039f, 1216, 1217f
Polarized dermoscopy, 649–650, 651f, 677–678, 677t. *See also* Dermoscopy
POLST, 32
Polyamory, 116t
Polyarticular inflammatory arthritis, 579
Polyarticular noninflammatory arthritis, 579
Polycystic kidney disease, 445–448
Polymorphic eruption of pregnancy, 477–479
Polymorphous light eruption, 1324–1329, 1324f
Polyp
colon, 401–405
laryngeal, 234–238
nasal, 209–211
Pompholyx, 928–934. *See also* Eczema, hand
Pork tapeworm, 1404–1408
Porphyria cutanea tarda, 1216, 1216f, 1235–1237, 1235f–1236f
Portal vein, 387
on third trimester ultrasound, 493f
Port-wine stains, 1341–1344, 1341f–1343f
Klippel-Trenaunay syndrome, 1341, 1342
Sturge-Weber syndrome, 1341, 1342, 1342f
Postburn blistering, 1216, 1216f
Postcholecystectomy syndrome, 399
Postherpetic neuralgia, 786–790
Postinfectious encephalomyelitis, 798
Postinflammatory hyperpigmentation, 1316–1322
Postscabies syndrome, 708
Posttraumatic stress disorder (PTSD)
after intimate partner violence, 103, 105
after sexual assault, 110, 111, 112–113
Pott disease, from tuberculosis, 327, 327f
Prader-Willi syndrome, obesity in, 1466
Preauricular tags, 205–208, 207f
Primary biliary cirrhosis, 386, 386f, 387, 388, 390, 390t, 392
Pregnancy and birth, 18–24
acrochordon, 473, 475
after sexual assault, 111, 112
atopic eruption of, 472–475
definition, 19–20
diagnosis, 20–21, 20f, 21f
differential diagnosis, 21–22
ectopic, 22
epidemiology, 18–19
etiology and pathophysiology, 19–20
home pregnancy kits, 20, 24
intimate partner violence, 103–105
intrahepatic cholestasis of, 472–475
labor and birthing, 23–24
management, 22–24
mask of, 1303–1307 (*See also* Melasma)
maternal mortality, 18–19
patient education, 24, 24f
patient story, 18, 18f
planned, 18
planning, 24
prevention, 24
prurigo of, 472–475
ruling out, 15, 16t, 17t
skin findings, 472–475
tubal, 525
unplanned (unintended), 18
Pregnancy epulis, 474, 474f, 475

Pregnancy-related mortality, 18–19
Pregnancy tests, 20
Pregnancy tumor, 474, 474f, 475
Premature menopause, 22
Prenatal care, 22–23
Presbyphonia, 234–238
Preservatives, contact dermatitis, 919, 920
Prickly heat (miliaria), 697, 697f
  neonatal, 697, 697f
  pregnancy, 473
Primary acquired melanosis, 135–137
Prion disease, dementia, 1531–1534
Progestin-only injectable contraceptive, 11f, 11t, 12t, 14
Progestin-only oral contraceptive pills, 12t
Proliferative verrucous leukoplakia, 263–266
Prostate cancer, 462–468
Prostate zones, 464, 464f
Prosthetic valve endocarditis, 297–305
Protein–calorie malnutrition, 57–58, 57f–58f
Proteus folliculitis, 752
Protozoa, 1404–1408, 1407f
Prurigo nodularis, 941–947, 944f–945f
Prurigo of pregnancy, 472–475
Pruritic folliculitis of pregnancy, 472–475
Pruritic urticarial papules and plaques of pregnancy, 477–479
Pruritus gravidarum, 472–475
PSA screening, 462, 465, 466t
Pseudofolliculitis, 733–737
Pseudofolliculitis barbae, 733–737, 733f–734f, 750, 751f, 752, 755
Pseudofolliculitis pubis, 733–737
Pseudo-Hutchinson sign, 1271, 1271f
Pseudo-Jones fracture, 621–623
Pseudomonas aeruginosa
  folliculitis, 750, 750f, 752, 753f, 754
  otitis externa, 197–201
Pseudomonas paronychia, 1287–1291, 1287f, 1288f
Pseudopregnancy, 22
Pseudotumor cerebri, 168–170
Pseudoverrucous papules, perianal, 714
Psoriasis, 3, 3f, 964–981, 1292
  with diabetes mellitus, 978
  erythrodermic, 965, 967f, 970, 972f, 980, 1004–1009
  inverse, 2, 2f, 3f, 859f, 877f, 964f, 965, 966f, 970, 971f, 980
  obesity, 1464, 1465f
  steroids for, topical, 685
Psoriatic arthritis, 578–581, 578f, 580f, 583, 583t, 965, 967f, 973, 973f
  arthritis mutilans, 581, 581t
  swan-neck deformities, 580f, 597f
Psoriatic arthritis mutilans, 581, 581f
Psoriatic nails, 581, 1292–1296
P-SPIKES approach, 31
Psychocutaneous disorders, 941–947
Psychogenic dermatoses, 941–947
Psychophysiologic disorder, 1607, 1612
Psychotherapeutic drug abuse, 1546–1551
Psychotic disorders, 1500–1509
Pterygium, 128–130
  red eye, 182, 184f
Pubic lice, 892–896, 893f, 894f
Pulmonary disease. *See also specific types*
  mortality, 29
Pulmonary embolus, 358–364
Pulmonary function tests
  abbreviations, 336t
  asthma, 336, 337f, 338, 339, 340f
Pulmonary hypertension
  chronic obstructive pulmonary disease, 349, 350, 354, 355, 356
  pulmonary embolus, 361f, 363
Pulmonary thromboembolism, 358–364
Punch biopsy, 690–692, 691f–692f
  skin cancers, 692
Puncture wound, neuropathic ulcer from, 1394
Purpura, 644, 646f
Pustular diseases of childhood, 708–710
Pustular psoriasis, 965, 967f, 970, 972f, 973, 980–981
Pustule, 640, 642f
Pyelonephritis, 432–433
Pyloric ulcers, 376–379
Pyoderma faciale, 729f, 730
Pyoderma gangrenosum, 1147–1151
Pyogenic granuloma, 1032–1036
  pregnancy, 474, 474f, 475
Pyonephrosis, 440–443
Pyostomatitis vegetans, 1148
Pyuria, 430–433

Q

Queer, 116t
Queer health issues, 115–119

R

Racial melanosis, eye, 135–137
Racism, 40–41
Radiant heat dermatitis, chronic, 1331–1334
Radicular syndrome, 600
Radius fracture
  distal, 616–620
  Universal Classification, 618, 619t
Ramsay Hunt syndrome, 787
Ram's horn nail, 1263, 1264f, 1265, 1282f
Rash, newborn, 694
Raspiness, 234–238
Raynaud phenomenon, 1204, 1206, 1206f, 1210
Reactive arthritis, 999–1003
  Chlamydia, 525
  with conjunctivitis, 999, 1000, 1001f
Reactive oxygen species, 1065
Rectal bleeding. *See also specific disorders*
  colon cancer, 407, 408
  hemorrhoids, 424–428
  inflammatory bowel disease, 415–422
Recurrent aphthous ulcer, 258–261
Recurrent respiratory papillomatosis, 234–238
Red blood cell casts, 430–433
Red dye, contact dermatitis, 925f
Red eye, 180–185, 181t
Reed nevus, 1058
Relapsing polychondritis, vasculitis, 1175
Relative risk reduction, 1604
Relaxation, for chronic pain, 1609t
Renal artery stenosis, hypertension, 285–286, 285f
Renal calculus, 435–439
Renal cell carcinoma, 450–454
Renal stone, 435–439

Reticular, 644, 647f
Retinal necrosis, from zoster ophthalmicus, 794
Retinal pigment epithelial injury, 172–173
Retinopathy
  diabetic, 161–163
  hypertensive, 165–167
Reverse Colles fracture, 616–620, 617f
Rheumatoid arthritis, 590–594
  vasculitis, 1175
Rheumatoid nodules, 579, 580f
Rhinocerebral mucormycosis sinusitis, 212–217, 213f
Rhinophyma, 726f, 728, 731
Rhinophymatous rosacea, 726f, 728
Rhinosinusitis, 212–217
Rhus dermatitis, 1035, 1036, 1037f, 1039, 1039f, 1216, 1217f
Ring, vaginal, 14
  hormonal, 10, 10f, 11–12, 11f, 12t, 14
Ringworm of the scalp, 861–866, 868–873
Rockerbottom foot deformity, 1396–1399
Rosacea, 725–731
  ocular, red eye, 180–185, 181t, 183f
Rosacea fulminans, 729f, 730
Roth spots, 297, 297f, 298f, 299, 300
Roundworm, 1404–1408, 1405f
Rubber allergens, in hand eczema, 930

S

S-adenosylmethionine (SAMe), 1613
SAFE Kit, 110
Safety plan, intimate partner violence, 103
Salivary gland tumors, 268, 269
Salmonella typhi, 54–55
Salmon patch, 836, 836f, 837f, 1343f
Salmon spot, psoriatic nails, 1292, 1292f, 1293f
Samitz sign, 1196, 1197f
Sandpaper rash, 223–226
Sanitation, global health, 53–54, 53f–54f
Saphenous varicosities, pregnancy, 473–475
Sarcoidosis, 1153–1159
  annular (circinate), 1153f, 1155
  erythema nodosum, 1169–1173, 1169f
  granulomas, 1155, 1156f
  lupus pernio, 1153f–1155f
  maculopapular, 1154, 1154f
  plaque, 1155, 1155f
  systemic, advanced, 1155, 1156f
Sarcoptes scabiei, 899, 899f
Saucerization (deep shave biopsy), 689–690, 689f–690f
  skin cancers, 692–693
Scabies, 898–905
  bullous presentation, 1218
  global health, 68, 68f–69f
Scale, 640, 642f
Scalp edema, on third trimester ultrasound, 494f
Scalp hair, pregnancy, 473–474, 474f
Scalp psoriasis, 965, 965f, 968, 980
Scar, hypertrophic, 1359–1363
Scarlatiniform rash, 223–226
Scarlet fever, 223–226
Scarring alopecia, 1256–1261
Schamroth sign, 308, 308f
Schiller test, 546, 547f
Schistosomiasis, 56–57
Schizophrenia, 1500–1509
Scleral nevus, 135–137
Scleral pigmentation, 135–137
Scleritis, 149–152
  red eye, 180–185, 181t, 183f
Sclerodactyly, 1204f, 1205f–1208f, 1206, 1207
Scleroderma, 1204–1210
Sclerodermatomyositis, 1199
Screening mammogram
  breast cancer, 566, 566f, 567f, 568, 569, 570
  Paget disease of breast, 573, 574
Scrofula, 72, 72f
Scrofuloderma, from tuberculosis, 327f, 328, 329f
Scrotum
  angiokeratosis of, 1336–1340, 1337f
  Paget disease of, 530–533
Sebaceous hyperplasia, 1021–1024
  dermoscopy, 660, 669f
Seborrhea (seborrheic dermatitis)
  Malassezia, 850, 863, 887, 958
  scalp (dandruff), 957–962
Seborrheic eczema, 957–962
Seborrheic keratosis, 1014–1020
  dermoscopy algorithms, 660, 664f, 665t–667t
    comedo-like openings, 660, 664f, 665t
    fingerprint-like structures, 660, 664f, 666t
    fissures/sulci, ridges, 660, 664f, 665t
    gyri/ridges and sulci/fissures, 660, 664f, 667t
    hairpin vessels with whitish halo, 660, 664f, 667t
    milia-like cysts, 660, 664f, 665t
    moth-eaten border, 660, 664f, 666t
    sharp demarcation, 660, 664f, 666t
Second hand smoke, 1558–1560, 1563f
Second trimester obstetrical ultrasound, 488–492
Sedative abuse, 1546–1551
Sediment, urinary, 430–433
Self-healing squamous cell carcinoma, 663t, 667t, 1079–1083
Self-inflicted dermatoses, 941–947
Senile angioma, 1336–1340, 1336f, 1339f
Senile keratosis, 1014–1020
Senile vaginitis, 501–506
Senses, diagnosis, 2
Sentinel tumor lymph node biopsy, skin cancers, 692
Septic arthritis, 579, 581, 582f, 584, 631, 632f
Serpiginous, 644, 646f
Seven-year itch, 898–905
Severe acute respiratory syndrome (SARS), 85–86
Severe recurrent alcohol use disorder, 1572, 1572b
Sex, on second trimester ultrasound, 490, 491f, 492f
Sexual abstinence, periodic, 14, 15t
Sexual abuse
  child, 96–100
  intimate partner, 102
  noncontact, 108
Sexual assault/violence
  adult, 108–113
  child, 96–100
  intimate partner, 102
Sexually transmitted infections
  child abuse, 98, 100
  LGBTQ, 116–117, 117t
  mortality, 28
  sexual assault, 109, 110–111

Sexual minority, 115
Sézary syndrome, cutaneous T-cell lymphoma, 1124–1130
Shaken baby syndrome, subdural hematoma, 1527
Shapes terminology, skin disorders, 644, 646f–647f
Shared decision-making, 8
Shave biopsy, 689–690, 689f–690f
deep, skin cancers, 692–693
Sheehan syndrome, 21–22
Shingles, 786–790
Shoes, contact dermatitis, 920, 921f, 922f
Shoulder pain, 1615t
Single rod implant, 13, 13f
Sinusitis, 212–217
Skin
infant care, routine, 715
pediatric, normal changes, 694–699
pregnancy, 472–475
Skin cancers, 1064–1065. *See also* Melanoma; *specific types*
biopsy, 689f, 692–693
diagnosis (*See* Dermoscopy)
prevention, 1064–1069
screening, 1068
Skin-picking disorder, 941–947
Skin popping, 1589, 1590f, 1597, 1598f
Skin tag (acrochordon), 1010–1013
diabetes mellitus, 1010, 1010f, 1011, 1434f, 1443f, 1445, 1445f
obesity, 1462, 1462f, 1577f
preauricular, 205–208
pregnancy, 473, 475
Skin tape, contact dermatitis, 920
Slapped cheek syndrome, 802–805
Slate grey patches, 694–699, 695f
Sleep disorders in obesity, 1464, 1468
after intimate partner violence, 103
after sexual assault, 112
Slit lamp examination
corneal foreign body/abrasion, 139, 140, 141
scleritis, 149
uveitis, acute anterior, 154
uveitis, nontraumatic, 155
Small-vessel vasculitis, 1174–1181
Smith fracture, 616–620, 617f
Smoker's face, 1560, 1561f
Smoking, 1558–1569. *See also* Tobacco addiction
Smoking cessation, 1562–1564, 1564t
pregnancy, 22
Smooth, 644, 646f
Social justice, 40–48
air pollution and climate change, 44
environmental protection, 44–46
homelessness, 46–48, 47f
migrant and immigrant health, 43–44
patient stories, 40
pesticide exposure, 46
racism, 40–41
universal healthcare and improved access to care, 41–43, 41f, 42f
water pollution, 44–46, 45f
Social needs, end of life, 35
Solar elastosis, 1064–1069
Solar keratosis, 1072–1077
Solar lentigines (solar lentigo), 666t, 1065, 1066f
Solar purpura, 1065, 1067f
Solomon syndrome, 1051–1055
Specked nevus, 1039, 1040f
Speckled congenital nevus, 1039, 1040, 1040f, 1047f, 1048
Speckled leukoplakia, 263–266
Spermicide, 11f, 11t, 12t, 14
Sperm viability, 19
Spider angiomas, pregnancy, 473
Spider nevi, pregnancy, 473
Spider telangiectasias, pregnancy, 472–475
Spindle-cell nevus, 1039–1041, 1040f, 1041f, 1057–1062
Spine. *See also specific disorders*
on third trimester ultrasound, 493f
Spiritual distress, end-of-life care, 34
Spiritual needs, end of life, 35
Spitz nevus (tumor), 1039–1041, 1040f, 1041f, 1057–1062
Spondylitis, 581
Spontaneous venous pulsations, 169
Sports-related head injury, 1517–1520
Squamocolumnar junction, cervical, 541, 543f
Squamous cell carcinoma, 1103–1111
dermoscopy, 661t–663t, 1132–1134, 1133f–1134f
dermoscopy algorithms
arborizing vessels, 656, 660f, 661t–663t
brown circles, 656, 660f
brown dots radially arranged, 656, 660f
glomerular vessels, 656, 660f
hairpin vessels with halo, 656, 660f
rosettes, 656, 660f
strawberry pattern, 656, 660f
white circles, 656, 660f
yellow scale, 656, 660f
laryngeal cancer, 234–238
lung, 366–373
oral, 267–270
self-healing, 663t, 667t, 1079–1083
of skin, in situ, 1072–1077
smoking, 1560, 1561f, 1562f
Squamous epithelium, cervical, 540f, 541, 541f
Squamous intraepithelial lesion, low-grade, 545–548
Staghorn calculi, 436, 437
Standard Sexual Assault Forensic Evidence (AFE) Kit, 110
Staphylococcus aureus. See also specific diseases
acute otitis media, 189
atopic dermatitis, 909–910
bacterial endocarditis, 298, 299
cellulitis, 765–766
hand dermatitis, 930
hordeolum, 132
impetigo, 745–749
mastitis, 562
necrotizing fasciitis, 776–779
otitis externa, 197–201
paronychia, 1287–1291, 1287f, 1288f
pneumonia, 317
sinusitis, 212–217
Staphylococcus epidermis bacterial endocarditis, 298
Staphylococcus folliculitis, 750, 750f, 752, 753f, 754
Status asthmaticus, 338
Sterilization
female, 11, 11f, 11t, 12t, 13, 13f
male, 11f, 11t, 12t
Steroid abuse, anabolic, 1595–1601, 1596f
Steroid-induced acneiform eruption, 730, 730f

Steroids, intralesional, 681–686
concentrations, 686t
for cystic acne, 685, 686f, 686t
side effects, 681, 681t
Steroids, topical, 681–686
application frequency, 684
for lichen sclerosus, genital, 681–683, 683f
for long-term use, 685
potency, 681–683, 682t–683t
prescribing amounts, 684–685, 684t
price issues, 683–684
side effects, 681, 681t
vehicles, 684
Stevens-Johnson syndrome, 1161–1167, 1161f–1162f, 1164f, 1346–1357, 1351f
Stimulant abuse, 1546–1551
S-to-D ratio, 495
Stomach, on third trimester ultrasound, 493f
Stomach cancer. *See* Gastric cancer
Stomatitis. *See also specific types*
angular, 218–220
aphthous, 258–261
geographic, 246–249
nicotine, 1560, 1561f
Stones
gallbladder, 395–399
kidney, 435–439
Stork bite, 836, 836f, 837f, 1343f
Strawberry cervix, 519–522, 542, 542f
Strawberry hemangioma, 700–706, 700f, 703f, 704f
Strawberry tongue, 223–226
Strength of Recommendation (SOR) Taxonomy, 1603, 1604, 1605f, 1606f
Streptococcus
mastitis, 562
paronychia, 1287–1291, 1287f, 1288f
Streptococcus gallolyticus bacterial endocarditis, 298, 299
Streptococcus mutans dental caries
adult, 275–278
early childhood, 271–274
Streptococcus pneumoniae
pneumonia, 317
sinusitis, 212–217
Streptococcus pyogenes
cellulitis, 765
necrotizing fasciitis, 776–779
pneumonia, 317
scarlet fever and strawberry tongue, 223–226
Stress, sexual minorities, 118–119
Stress fracture, diaphyseal metatarsal, 621–623
Stretch marks, pregnancy, 472–475
Striae distensae, 472–475
Striae gravidarum, 472–475
Stroke, 1521–1525
mortality, 30
Stromal keratitis, from zoster ophthalmicus, 794
Strongyloides stercoralis, 1404–1408, 1406f
global health, 56–57
Struvite kidney stones, 435–439
Stucco keratosis, 1015, 1017f
Sturge-Weber syndrome, port-wine stains, 1341, 1342, 1342f
Stye, 132–134
Subacute granulomatous thyroiditis, 1482
Subacute sclerosing panencephalitis, 799
Subclinical thyroid disease, 1478
Subconjunctival hemorrhage, 142, 177
red eye, 180, 181t, 182, 183f
Subdural hematoma, 1526–1530
Substance abuse disorder, 1546–1551. *See also specific substances*
addiction, 1546, 1548
injection-drug use, 1595–1601
mortality, 28
Subtrochanteric fracture, 624–626
Subungual hematoma, 1298–1301
Subungual melanoma, 1270–1274, 1270f, 1271t, 1272f
Suicide attempt
intimate partner violence, 105
LGBTQ, 119
sexual assault, 110, 112
Sulfa antibiotics, drug reactions, 1239f, 1346–1357, 1347f, 1348f, 1351f, 1355t
Sulfonamides, cutaneous reactions, 1346–1357, 1355t
Sunburn, blistering after, 1216
Sun damage, 1064–1069
Sun exposure, skin cancer and, 1064–1069
Superficial capillary malformations, 702, 702f, 703f
Superficial hemangiomas of infancy, 700–706, 700f, 703f, 704f
Superficial spreading (malignant) melanoma, 1113, 1114, 1114f, 1118f, 1120f
Suppurative fasciitis, 776–779
Surface characteristics terminology, skin disorders, 644, 646f
Swab test, 526, 526f
Swan-neck deformities
lupus erythematosus, 580f
psoriatic arthritis, 580f, 597f
Swimmer's ear, 197–201
Swinging, 116t
Syndesmophytes, 595, 595f, 597, 600
Syphilis, 1412–1418
neonatal, 1218
Syphilis, secondary, 1412–1418
Syringocystadenoma papilliferum, 1054f, 1055
Syringoma, 1024f
Systemic drug-related intertriginous and flexural exanthema (SDRIFE), 1353, 1354f
Systemic lupus erythematosus, 1183–1192
mother with, neonatal lupus from, 698f
vasculitis, 1175, 1175f, 1176f
Systemic sclerosis, 1204–1210, 1204f–1205f

T

Taenia asiatica, 1404–1408
Taenia saginata, 1404–1408
Taenia solium, 1404–1408
Tai chi, for chronic pain, 1609t
Tape, skin, contact dermatitis, 920
Tapeworm, 1404–1408
Tardive congenital nevus, 1046
Tattoo dyes, contact dermatitis, 925f
T-cell lymphoma
cutaneous, 1042–1048
erythroderma with, 1005–1007, 1007f

Telangiectasias, 644, 646f
sun exposure, 1065
Telogen effluvium, postpartum, 474, 474f
Temporomandibular joint disease, 1616t
Tendon xanthomas, 1456
Tension-type headache, 1513–1516
Terminology, skin disorders, 640–647. *See also specific terms*
color and pigmentation, 640, 644, 645f
distribution, 644, 647f
morphology, 640, 641f–644f
shapes, 644, 646f–647f
surface characteristics, 644, 646f
vascular, 644, 645f–646f
Tetracycline, cutaneous reactions, 1346–1357, 1355t
Third nerve palsy, 1535–1538
Third trimester obstetrical ultrasound, 493–496
Thoracic back pain, 599–602
Thoracic kyphosis, osteoporosis, 1471–1477, 1471f
Thrush (oral candidiasis), 850–855, 851f, 856–860, 856f, 857f
angular cheilitis, 218–220, 218f
Thyroid disease. *See also specific types*
subclinical, 1478
Thyrotoxicosis, 1486–1492
Tierfell nevus, 1046–1049
Tinea. *See also specific types*
bullous presentation, 1218
hand dermatitis, 930
Tinea capitis, 850–855, 851f, 861–866
folliculitis, 752
global health, 69, 69f
Tinea corporis, 850–855, 850f, 851f, 858f, 868–873
Tinea cruris, 850–855, 851f, 875–879
Tinea faciei, 850–855, 850f, 868–873, 871f
Tinea incognito, 882, 883f
Tinea manus, 850–855
Tinea pedis, 850–855, 880–886
diabetes, 1432, 1432f
Tinea unguium, 1280–1285, 1281f
Tinea versicolor, 850–855, 851f, 887–890
Toasted skin syndrome, 1331–1334
Tobacco addiction, 1558–1569
chronic obstructive pulmonary disease, 348–356
estrogen-containing contraceptives with, 11
lung cancer, 366–373
mortality, 27–28
substance abuse overview, 1546–1551
Toenail fungus, 1280–1285
Tongue cancer, 267–270
Tooth (teeth) decay
adult, 275–278
early childhood, 271–274
Tophaceous gout, 582f, 604–608, 606f
Torus palatinus, 221–222
Toxic agents. *See also specific agents*
mortality, 28
Toxic epidermal necrolysis, 1161–1167, 1165f–1166f, 1346–1357, 1351f
Toxic erythema of pregnancy, 477–479
Toxic erythema of the newborn, 694–699, 695f
Toxicodendron (Rhus) dermatitis, 919, 920, 921f, 923, 923f, 926, 1216, 1217f
Trabecular bone
normal, 1472f
osteoporotic, 1472, 1472f
Trachoma, 66–67, 66f–67f
Trachyonychia, 1264, 1266f
Traction alopecia, 1252–1255, 1252f
Tramadol, for chronic pain, 1611
Tranquilizer abuse, 1546–1551
Transformation zone, 541, 541f
atypical, 546
persistent juvenile, 540, 540f, 542, 543f, 544
Transgender health issues, 119–122
Transient neonatal pustular melanosis, 824–826, 1218
Transitional cell carcinoma, of bladder, 456–460
Transplantation, lung, for COPD, 355
Transrectal ultrasound, 466
Transvaginal ultrasound, 21, 21f
Transverse striate leukonychia, 1263, 1263f, 1264, 1289f
Trauma-induced blistering, 1214, 1215f
Traumatic alopecia, 1252–1255
Trench mouth, 250–252
Treponema pallidum infection, 1412–1418, 1417f
Triage amalgamated dermoscopy algorithm, 676f, 677
Triamcinolone acetonide, intralesional, 685, 686t
for alopecia areata, 685, 686f, 686t
for cystic acne, 685, 686f, 686t, 722, 723f
for keloids and hypertrophic scars, 685, 686f, 686t
Triazoles, 10–11
Trichomonas cervicitis, colposcopy of, 542, 542f
Trichomonas vaginalis
urethritis, male, 1410
vaginitis, 497–499, 498f, 499t, 519–522
Trichomoniasis (trich, tricky monkeys), 519–522
sexual assault, 110, 111
Trichophagy, 1254
Trichophyton, 850–855. *See also* Tinea
tinea capitis, 861–866, 861f, 864f
tinea corporis, 868–873
Trichophyton mentagrophytes
onychomycosis, 1281, 1282f
tinea cruris, 875–879
tinea pedis, 880–886
Trichophyton rubrum, 850–855, 853f
onychomycosis, 1281, 1281f
tinea capitis, 861–866, 865f
tinea cruris, 875–879, 877f
tinea pedis, 880–886
Trichophyton soudanense, onychomycosis, 1281
Trichophyton tonsurans, tinea capitis, 861–866, 861f, 864f
Trichophyton verrucosum, tinea cruris, 875–879
Trichotillomania, 1252–1255, 1253f
Trichuris trichiura, 1404–1408, 1406f
Tricyclic antidepressants, for chronic pain, 1613
Trigeminal autonomic cephalgias, 1513–1516
Trigeminal nerve
sensory distribution, 794, 794f
zoster ophthalmicus, 792–796
Triglycerides, high, hyperlipidemia, 1456
Trimethoprim/sulfamethoxazole
cutaneous reactions, 1346–1357, 1347f, 1349f
urticaria, 949–956, 949f
T.R.U.E. Test, 923–924, 924f, 924t

Tubal occlusion, hysteroscopic, 13, 13f, 14f
Tubal pregnancy, 525
Tuberculosis, 71–73, 73f, 325–334
  erythema nodosum in, 1170
  HIV with, 72–73, 72f
Tuberculous lymphadenitis, 72, 73f
Tuberoeruptive xanthomas, 1455f–1457f, 1456, 1457, 1461
Tuberous xanthomas, 1456
Tuboovarian abscesses, 21
Tufted folliculitis, 752, 752f, 1257t, 1258, 1258f, 1260–1261
Tumor, 640, 642f
Twenty-nail dystrophy, 1264, 1266f
Twin pregnancy, third trimester ultrasound, 495
Two-foot, one-hand syndrome, 851f, 852, 932, 932f
Tyloma, 1376–1380. *See also* Calluses
Tympanic membrane
  acute otitis media, 188, 188f–190f
  bullous myringitis, 193f
  normal, 191f
  otitis media with effusion, 188, 188f
Tympanosclerosis, 189f, 194, 195f
Tympanostomy tubes, 194
Tyndall effect, 1039, 1040f
Typhoid fever, 54–55

U

Ulcer, 640, 643f
  aphthous, 258–261 (*See also specific ulcers*)
  corneal, red eye, 180–185, 181t, 183f
  foot
    ischemic, 1390–1391
    neuropathic, 1393–1395
  gastric/peptic, 376–379
  Marjolin, 1104, 1104f
  pyloric, 376–379
  venous stasis, 310–313, 312f
Ulcerative colitis, 415–422
Ulipristal acetate, 22
Ultrasound, obstetrical
  first trimester, 484–486
  second trimester, 488–492
  third trimester, 493–495
  transvaginal, 21, 21f
Ultraviolet radiation, 1065
Umbilical artery, third trimester, 496
Umbilicated, 644, 647f
Uncinaria stenocephala, cutaneous larva migrans, 906–908
Unguis incarnatus, 1276–1278, 1276f
Unintended (unplanned) pregnancy, 18
Universal healthcare, 41–43, 41f, 42f
Ureaplasma urealyticum urethritis, in men, 1410
Ureterolithiasis, 435–439
Urethritis, gonococcal, 1409–1411
Uric acid kidney stones, 435–439
Urinary casts, 430–433
Urinary sediment, 430–433
Urinary tract infection
  bacteriuria, 431
  pyuria, 431
Urinary tract stone, 435–439
Urogenital atrophy, 501–506
Urolithiasis, 435–439
Urothelial carcinoma, 456–460
Urticaria, 949–956
  giant, 952f
Urticarial drug reactions, 1346–1357, 1347f, 1348f
Urticaria multiforme, 952f
  drug reaction, 1346–1357, 1348f
Urticaria pigmentosa, 949–956, 951f, 952f
  Darier sign, 951f, 952, 952f
Uterine cervix, invasive cancer, 556–560. *See also* Colposcopy, high-grade lesions
  pregnancy, 556
Uterine leiomyomas, 21
Uteroplacental insufficiency, third trimester ultrasound, 495
Uveitis, 153–156
  ankylosing spondylitis, 596
  red eye, 180–185, 181t, 184f
  zoster ophthalmicus, 792–796, 792f
UV light, 1324

V

Vaccination
  hepatitis B, sexual assault, 111
  human papillomavirus, 548, 550
    sexual assault, 111
  pneumococcal polysaccharide, 322
  pneumonia, 322
Vaginal atrophy, 501–506
Vaginal bacteriosis, 508–512
Vaginal bleeding, ultrasound
  first trimester, 484–486
  second trimester, 489
  third trimester, 493, 494f, 496
Vaginal discharge, 497–499, 499t
Vaginal dryness, 501
Vaginal epithelium, atrophic, 541, 542, 543f, 544
Vaginal ring, 14
  hormonal, 10, 10f, 11–12, 11f, 12t, 14
Vaginitis, 497–499, 499t
  atrophic, 501–506
  Candida, 497–499, 499t, 513–517
  nonspecific, 508–512
  Trichomonas, 497–499, 498f, 499t, 519–522
  yeast, 497–499, 499t, 513–517
Vaginocervicitis, 544
Valgus stress test, 630
Varicella-zoster virus
  chickenpox, 780–784
  herpes zoster, 786–790
  zoster ophthalmicus, 792–796
Varicose veins, 310–313
  obesity, 1464, 1465f
Varicosities, pregnancy, 473–475
Varus stress test, 630
Vascular dementia, 1531–1534
Vascular lesions
  acquired, 1336–1340
  hereditary and congenital, 1341–1344
Vascular malformations, childhood, 700–706
Vascular terminology, skin disorders, 644, 645f–646f
Vasculitis, 1174–1181. *See also specific types*
  Henoch-Schönlein purpura, 1174–1181, 1174f, 1175f

Vector-borne diseases, 61–66. *See also specific diseases*
  leishmaniasis, 64–66, 64f–66f
  malaria, 61–63, 62f–63f
  prevention, 66
  prognosis, 66
Venice Family Clinic, 47
Venous insufficiency, 310–313
Venous insufficiency (stasis) ulcer, 310–313, 312f, 1151f
Venous lake, 1336–1340, 1336f
Venous pulsations, spontaneous, 169
Verrucae, 826–831
Verruca plana, 832–835
Verruca plana juvenilis, 832–835
Verruca plantaris, 844–849
Verruca vulgaris, 826–831
Verrucous, 644, 646f
Verrucous leukoplakia, 263–266
Vesicle, 640, 641f
Vesicular palmoplantar eczema, 928–934
Vibrio cholerae, 55–56, 56f
Vibrio vulnificus
  cellulitis, 765, 767f
  necrotizing fasciitis, 776–779
Villous adenomas, 401–405
Vincent disease, 250–252
Violence
  intimate partner, 102–106
  prevention–intervention programs, 112
  sexual assault
    adult, 108–113
    child, 96–100
    intimate partner, 102
Viral hepatitis, 386–393
Viridans streptococcus pneumonia, 317
Vision loss, age-related macular degeneration, 172–175
Vision loss, blindness
  Chlamydia trachomatis, 66–67, 67f
  diabetic retinopathy, 161–163, 1432, 1432f, 1433, 1435, 1438
  glaucoma, 157–159
Vitamin A deficiency, 59, 59f
Vitamin B deficiency, angular cheilitis, 218–220
Vitiligo, 1308–1314
Vocal cords
  false, 234–238
  nodules, 234–238
  paresis or paralysis, 234–238
Vulva, Paget disease of, 530–533
Vulvar angiokeratosis, 1336–1340, 1337f
Vulvar cancer, 534–535. *See also specific types*
Vulvar intraepithelial neoplasia, 534–538
Vulvar pyoderma gangrenosum, 1148
Vulvar varicosities, pregnancy, 473–475
Vulvovaginal atrophy, 501–506
Vulvovaginal candidiasis, 513–517
Vulvovaginitis, *Candida,* 497–499, 499t, 513–517

W

Waist circumference, obesity, 1464, 1465f
Warfarin, drug reactions, 1346–1357, 1348f
Warfarin-induced skin necrosis, 1346–1357, 1348f
War on drugs, 1552–1553, 1554f
Warts
  common, 826–831
  flat, 832–835
  genital (condylomata acuminata), 837–843
  plantar, 844–849
Water
  global health, 53–54, 53f–54f
  pollution, 44–46, 45f
West Nile virus, 79–80, 79f
Wet gangrene, 1401, 1401f
Wet wipes, contact dermatitis, 920, 922f–923f
Wheal, 640, 641f
  urticaria, 949, 950, 950f, 951f
"Whiff" test, 499, 499t
Whipworm, 1404–1408, 1406f
White blood cell casts, 430–433
White coat hypertension, 286
Whiteheads, 719, 719f
Wickham striae (lines), 992, 992f, 996f
Wife-battering, 102–106
Wilson disease, liver disease, 387, 388, 389f, 390, 390t, 392
Withdrawal, birth control, 12t
Wood chip, in cornea, 139
Woodard, Laurie, 42f, 43
World health, 51–73. *See also* Global health
Worms, intestinal, 1404–1408

X

Xanthelasma, 1456, 1457f, 1460
Xanthomas, 1455–1461
  eruptive, diabetes mellitus, 1433, 1435f
  obesity, 1455–1461, 1464, 1464f
Xerophthalmia, vitamin A deficiency, 59, 59f
Xerosis, with atopic dermatitis, 914, 914f
Xerostomia, dental caries with, 277, 278
X-linked ichthyosis, 1364–1370, 1367f

Y

Yeast infection, 513–517
  Candida vulvovaginitis, 497–499, 499t, 513–517
Yeast onychomycosis, 1280–1285
Yeast vaginitis, 497–499, 499t, 513–517
Yolk sac, on first trimester ultrasound, 485–486

Z

Zika virus, 76–78, 77f–78f
Zinc deficiency, 59–60, 60f
  acrodermatitis enteropathica, 714, 714f
Zoster, 786–790
Zoster ophthalmicus, 792–796